D0840391

GERIATRIC DOSAGE HANDBOOK

Including Clinical Recommendations and Monitoring Guidelines

Senior Editors:
Todd P. Semla, MS, PharmD, BCPS, FCCP, AGSF
Judith L. Beizer, PharmD, CGP, FASCP
Martin D. Higbee, PharmD

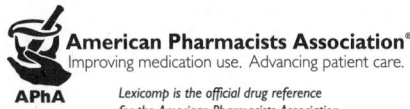

American Pharmacists Association®
Improving medication use. Advancing patient care.

APhA   *Lexicomp is the official drug reference
for the American Pharmacists Association*

17th Edition

GERIATRIC DOSAGE HANDBOOK

Including Clinical Recommendations and Monitoring Guidelines

Todd P. Semla, MS, PharmD, BCPS, FCCP, AGSF
Senior Editor
Clinical Pharmacy Specialist
Department of Veterans Affairs
Pharmacy Benefits Management Services
Associate Professor, Clinical
Departments of Medicine and Psychiatry and Behavioral Health
Feinberg School of Medicine
Northwestern University
Chicago, Illinois

Judith L. Beizer, PharmD, CGP, FASCP
Senior Editor
Clinical Professor
Department of Clinical Pharmacy Practice
St John's University College of Pharmacy and Allied Health Professions
Jamaica, New York

Martin D. Higbee, PharmD
Senior Editor
Adjunct Professor
Department of Pharmacy Practice and Science
The University of Arizona
Tucson, Arizona

NOTICE

This data is intended to serve the user as a handy reference and not as a complete drug information resource. It does not include information on every therapeutic agent available. The publication covers 980 commonly used drugs and is specifically designed to present important aspects of drug data in a more concise format than is typically found in medical literature or product material supplied by manufacturers.

The nature of drug information is that it is constantly evolving because of ongoing research and clinical experience and is often subject to interpretation. While great care has been taken to ensure the accuracy of the information and recommendations presented, the reader is advised that the authors, editors, reviewers, contributors, and publishers cannot be responsible for the continued currency of the information or for any errors, omissions, or the application of this information, or for any consequences arising therefrom. Therefore, the author(s) and/or the publisher shall have no liability to any person or entity with regard to claims, loss, or damage caused, or alleged to be caused, directly or indirectly, by the use of information contained herein. Because of the dynamic nature of drug information, readers are advised that decisions regarding drug therapy must be based on the independent judgment of the clinician, changing information about a drug (eg, as reflected in the literature and manufacturer's most current product information), and changing medical practices. Therefore, this data is designed to be used in conjunction with other necessary information and is not designed to be solely relied upon by any user. The user of this data hereby and forever releases the authors and publishers of this data from any and all liability of any kind that might arise out of the use of this data. The editors are not responsible for any inaccuracy of quotation or for any false or misleading implication that may arise due to the text or formulas as used or due to the quotation of revisions no longer official.

Certain of the authors, editors, and contributors have written this book in their private capacities. No official support or endorsement by any federal or state agency or pharmaceutical company is intended or inferred.

The publishers have made every effort to trace any third party copyright holders, if any, for borrowed material. If they have inadvertently overlooked any, they will be pleased to make the necessary arrangements at the first opportunity.

If you have any suggestions or questions regarding any information presented in this data, please contact our drug information pharmacists at (330) 650-6506. Book revisions are available at our website at http://www.lexi.com/home/revisions/.

Copyright © 2012 by Lexi-Comp Inc. All rights reserved.

Copyright © 1993-2011, 1st-16th Editions.

Printed in the United States. No part of this publication may be reproduced, stored in a retrieval system, used as a source of information for transcription into a hospital information system or electronic health or medical record, or transmitted in any form or by any means, electronic, mechanical, photocopying, recording or otherwise, without the prior written permission of the publisher. Should you or your institution have a need for this information in a format we protect, we have solutions for you. Please contact our office at the number below.

This manual was produced using Lexi-Comp's Information Management System™ (LIMS) — A complete publishing service of Lexi-Comp Inc.

1100 Terex Road • Hudson, Ohio 44236
(330) 650-6506

ISBN 978-1-59195-302-9

TABLE OF CONTENTS

ABOUT THE EDITORS

Todd P. Semla, MS, PharmD, BCPS, FCCP, AGSF

Dr Semla received his Bachelor of Science in Pharmacy, his Master of Science in Clinical Pharmacy, and his Doctor of Pharmacy degrees from the University of Iowa. After earning his doctorate, Dr Semla was awarded the American Society of Health-System Pharmacists Fellowship in Geriatric Pharmacotherapy which he completed at the University of Iowa.

Dr Semla has more than 30 years experience in geriatric pharmacotherapy in a variety of clinical settings including ambulatory care, acute care and rehabilitation, and the nursing home. He is a Clinical Pharmacy Specialist in the Department of Veterans Affairs Pharmacy Benefits Management Service and an Associate Professor of Medicine and Clinical Psychiatry at the Feinberg School of Medicine, Northwestern University.

Dr Semla is the Editor for the section "Drugs and Pharmacology," for the *Journal of the American Geriatrics Society* and Chair of the Panel on Alzheimer's Disease for *The Annals of Pharmacotherapy*. He is an active member of several professional organizations, including the American College of Clinical Pharmacy (ACCP). He is a past President and Chair of the Board of Directors of the American Geriatrics Society.

Judith L. Beizer, PharmD, CGP, FASCP

Dr Beizer received her Bachelor of Science in Pharmacy from the St Louis College of Pharmacy and then earned a Doctor of Pharmacy degree from the University of Tennessee. After pursuing a residency in clinical pharmacy at the Hospital of the University of Pennsylvania, she completed a fellowship in geriatric pharmacy at Montefiore Medical Center, Bronx, NY. During her fellowship, Dr Beizer was involved in a National Institute on Aging (NIA) grant concerning medication use and pharmacist intervention in community-dwelling elderly.

Dr Beizer is a Clinical Professor in the Department of Clinical Pharmacy Practice at St John's University College of Pharmacy and Allied Health Professions. As part of her teaching responsibilities, she serves as the Clinical Pharmacist at the Center for Extended Care and Rehabilitation, a long-term care facility in Manhasset, NY. At this facility, Dr Beizer has expanded clinical pharmacy services and precepts pharmacy students. Dr Beizer speaks regularly on the topic of medication use in the elderly and has published articles and abstracts on various issues in geriatric pharmacotherapy.

Dr Beizer is a member of a number of professional organizations, including the American Society of Health-System Pharmacists (ASHP), American Society of Consultant Pharmacists (ASCP), American College of Clinical Pharmacy (ACCP), American Pharmacists Association (APhA), and the American Geriatrics Society (AGS). She is a past president of ASCP. She previously served on the Board of Commissioners for the Commission for Certification in Geriatric Pharmacy. She is a past chairperson of the ASHP Special Interest Group on Geriatric Pharmacy Practice. Dr Beizer is on the Editorial Advisory Board of *The Consultant Pharmacist*.

Martin D. Higbee, PharmD

Dr Higbee received his Bachelor of Science in Pharmacy from The University of Utah in 1973. After a year of pharmacy practice and clinical pharmacy experience at The University of Utah, he entered the Doctor of Pharmacy degree program at The University of Texas at San Antonio. After graduation in 1977, he joined the University of Utah College of Pharmacy faculty. He became involved in development of the Salt Lake Veteran Administration Medical Center's Geriatric Treatment and Evaluation Unit, and after the establishment of this unit, Dr Higbee created an ASHP accredited post-doctoral Geriatric Residency through the Veteran's Administration Medical Center and The University of Utah College of Pharmacy. Dr Higbee was also on the editorial staff for the Eli Lily - AACP Geriatric Curriculum for Pharmacists project which created a geriatric textbook and curriculum for educators.

Dr Higbee joined the faculty at The University of Arizona in 1987. As part of his teaching responsibilities, he was a Clinical Pharmacist Consultant for the Hospital-Based Primary Care Team (division of Geriatric Care Center) at the Veterans Administration Medical Center in Tucson, Arizona, where he is preceptor for doctor of pharmacy students. Currently, he serves as an adjunct professor for the university. Dr Higbee has joined a nursing home consulting group, Donohue and Associates, a long-term care and assisted living consulting group based in Arizona. In addition, Dr Higbee frequently is called upon as an expert witness in legal proceedings.

Dr Higbee regularly speaks locally and nationally on geriatric drug therapy topics and has published articles, chapters, and abstracts on various geriatric research and pharmacotherapy topics. He is a member of numerous professional organizations. He is a past chairman of the ASHP Special Interest Group on Geriatric Pharmacy Practice and past member of the AACP Task Force on Aging.

Irene H. Chenowith, MD, FACP
Senior Medical Staff
Department of Internal Medicine
Summa Health Systems
Akron, Ohio
Medical Consultant
Lexi-Comp, Inc
Hudson, Ohio
Associate Professor of Internal Medicine
Northeast Ohio Medical University (NEOMED)
Rootstown, Ohio

M. Petrea Cober, PharmD, BCNSP
Clinical Pharmacy Coordinator
Neonatal Intensive Care Unit
Children's Hospital of Akron
Akron, Ohio
Assistant Professor, Pharmacy Practice
Northeastern Ohio Medical University
Rootstown, Ohio

Amanda H. Corbett, PharmD, BCPS, FCCP, AAHIVE
Clinical Assistant Professor
University of North Carolina
Eshelman School of Pharmacy
Chapel Hill, North Carolina

Harold L. Crossley, DDS, PhD
Associate Professor of Pharmacology
Baltimore College of Dental Surgery
Dental School
University of Maryland Baltimore
Baltimore, Maryland

Melanie W. Cucchi, BS, PharmD, RPh
Pharmacotherapy Contributor
Lexi-Comp, Inc
Hudson, Ohio

Laura Cummings, PharmD, BCPS
Clinical Pharmacy Specialist, Pediatrics
The Children's Hospital at MetroHealth
Cleveland, Ohio

William J. Dana, PharmD, FASHP
Pharmacy Quality Assurance
Harris County Hospital District
Houston, Texas

Beth Deen, PharmD, BDNSP
Senior Pediatric Clinical Pharmacy Specialist
Cook Children's Medical Center
Fort Worth, Texas

Julie A. Dopheide, PharmD, BCPP
*Associate Professor of Clinical Pharmacy,
Psychiatry and the Behavioral Sciences*
University of Southern California
Schools of Pharmacy and Medicine
Los Angeles, California

Teri Dunsworth, PharmD, FCCP, BCPS
Pharmacotherapy Specialist
Lexi-Comp, Inc
Hudson, Ohio

Eve Echt, MD
Medical Staff
Department of Radiology
Akron General Medical Center
Akron, Ohio

Michael S. Edwards, PharmD, MBA, BCOP
*Chief, Oncology Pharmacy
Director, Oncology Pharmacy
Residency Program*
Walter Reed Army Medical Center
Washington, D.C.

Vicki L. Ellingrod, PharmD, BCPP
*Head, Clinical Pharmacogenomics Laboratory
Associate Professor*
College of Pharmacy
Associate Professor
College of Medicine
Department of Psychiatry
University of Michigan
Ann Arbor, Michigan

Kelley K. Engle, BSPharm
Medical Science Pharmacist
Lexi-Comp, Inc
Hudson, Ohio

Christopher Ensor, PharmD, BCPS (AQ-CV)
Clinical Specialist
Cardiothoracic Transplantation and
Mechanical Circulatory Support
The Johns Hopkins Hospital
Baltimore, Maryland

Erin Fabian, PharmD, RPh
Pharmacotherapy Specialist
Lexi-Comp, Inc
Hudson, Ohio

Elizabeth A. Farrington, PharmD, FCCP, FCCM, FPPAG, BCPS
Pharmacist III - Pediatrics
New Hanover Regional Medical Center
Wilmington, North Carolina

Margaret A. Fitzgerald, MS, APRN, BC, NP-C, FAANP
President
Fitzgerald Health Education Associates, Inc.
North Andover, Massachusetts
Family Nurse Practitioner
Greater Lawrence Family Health Center
Lawrence, Massachusetts

Lawrence A. Frazee, PharmD, BCPS
*Pharmacotherapy Specialist in
Internal Medicine*
Akron General Medical Center
Akron, Ohio

Michael Klepser, PharmD, FCCP
Professor of Pharmacy
Department of Pharmacy Practice
Ferris State University
Kalamazoo, Michigan

Daren Knoell, PharmD
Associate Professor of Pharmacy Practice and Internal Medicine
Davis Heart and Lung Research Institute
The Ohio State University
Columbus, Ohio

David Knoppert, MScPhm, FCCP, MSc, FCSHP
Clinical Leader - Paediatrics
Pharmacy Services
London Health Sciences Centre
Children's Health Research Institute
London, Ontario, Canada

Sandra Knowles, RPh, BScPhm
Drug Safety Pharmacist
Sunnybrook and Women's College HSC
Toronto, Ontario

Jill M. Kolesar, PharmD, FCCP, BCPS
Associate Professor
School of Pharmacy
Associate Professor
University of Wisconsin Paul P. Carbone
Comprehensive Cancer Center
University of Wisconsin
Madison, Wisconsin

Susannah E. Koontz, PharmD, BCOP
Principal and Consultant
Pediatric Hematology/Oncology and Stem Cell
Transplantation/Cellular Therapy
Koontz Oncology Consulting, LLC
Houston, Texas

Donna M. Kraus, PharmD, FAPhA, FPPAG
Associate Professor of Pharmacy Practice
Departments of Pharmacy Practice
and Pediatrics
Pediatric Clinical Pharmacist
University of Illinois
Chicago, Illinois

Daniel L. Krinsky, RPh, MS
Manager, MTM Services
Giant Eagle Pharmacy
Ravenna, Ohio
Assistant Professor
Department of Pharmacy Practice
Northeast Ohio Medical University (NEOMED)
Rootstown, Ohio

Kay Kyllonen, PharmD
Clinical Specialist
The Cleveland Clinic Children's Hospital
Cleveland, Ohio

Charles Lacy, MS, PharmD, FCSHP
Vice President for Executive Affairs
Professor, Pharmacy Practice
Professor, Business Leadership
University of Southern Nevada
Las Vegas, Nevada

Brenda R. Lance, RN, MSN
Program Development Director
Northcoast HealthCare
Management Company
Northcoast Infusion Network
Beachwood, Ohio

Leonard L. Lance, RPh, BSPharm
Pharmacist
Lexi-Comp, Inc
Hudson, Ohio

Tim T.Y. Lau, PharmD, ACPR, FCSHP
Pharmacotherapeutic Specialist in Infectious Diseases
Pharmaceutical Sciences
Vancouver General Hospital
Clinical Associate Professor
Faculty of Pharmaceutical Sciences
Associate Member
Division of Infectious Diseases
Faculty of Medicine
University of British Columbia
Vancouver, British Columbia, Canada

Mandy C. Leonard, PharmD, BCPS
Assistant Professor
Cleveland Clinic Lerner College of Medicine of
Case Western University
Assistant Director, Drug Information Services
Cleveland Clinic
Cleveland, Ohio

John J. Lewin III, PharmD, BCPS
Clinical Specialist, Neurosciences
Critical Care
The Johns Hopkins Hospital
Baltimore, Maryland

Jeffrey D. Lewis, PharmD, MACM
Assistant Dean and
Associate Professor of Pharmacy Practice
Cedarville University School of Pharmacy
Cedarville, Ohio

John Lindsley, PharmD, BCPS
Cardiology Clinical Pharmacy Specialist
The Johns Hopkins Hospital
Baltimore, Maryland

Jennifer Fisher Lowe, PharmD, BCOP
Pharmacotherapy Contributor
Lexi-Comp, Inc
Hudson, Ohio

Curtis M. Rimmermann, MD, MBA, FACC
Gus P. Karos Chair
Clinical Cardiovascular Medicine
Department of Cardiovascular Medicine
Cleveland Clinic Foundation
Cleveland, Ohio

P. David Rogers, PharmD, PhD, FCCP
Professor and Associate Dean for Translational Research
University of Tennessee College of Pharmacy
Memphis, Tennessee

Amy Rybarczyk, PharmD, BCPS
Pharmacotherapy Specialist, Internal Medicine
Akron General Medical Center
Akron, Ohio

Jennifer K. Sekeres, PharmD, BCPS
Infectious Diseases Clinical Specialist
The Cleveland Clinic Foundation
Cleveland, Ohio

Todd P. Semla, MS, PharmD, BCPS, FCCP, AGSF
Clinical Pharmacy Specialist
Department of Veterans Affairs
Pharmacy Benefits Management Services
Associate Professor, Clinical
Department of Medicine and Psychiatry and Behavioral Health
Feinberg School of Medicine
Northwestern University
Chicago, Illinois

Chasity M. Shelton, PharmD, BCPS, BCNSP
Assistant Professor of Clinical Pharmacy
Department of Clinical Pharmacy
Neonatal Clinical Pharmacy Specialist
University of Tennessee
Health Science Center
Memphis, Tennessee

Joseph Snoke, RPh, BCPS
Manager
Core Pharmacology Group
Lexi-Comp, Inc
Hudson, Ohio

Joni Lombardi Stahura, BS, PharmD, RPh
Pharmacotherapy Specialist
Lexi-Comp, Inc
Hudson, Ohio

Stephen Marc Stout, PharmD, MS, BCPS
Pharmacotherapy Specialist
Lexi-Comp, Inc
Hudson, Ohio

Dan Streetman, PharmD, RPh
Pharmacotherapy Specialist
Lexi-Comp, Inc
Hudson, Ohio

Darcie-Ann Streetman, PharmD, RPh
Clinical Pharmacist
University of Michigan Health System
Ann Arbor, Michigan

Carol K. Taketomo, PharmD
Director of Pharmacy and Nutrition Services
Children's Hospital Los Angeles
Los Angeles, California

Mary Temple-Cooper, PharmD
Pediatric Clinical Research Specialist
Hillcrest Hospital
Mayfield Heights, Ohio

Elizabeth A. Tomsik, PharmD, BCPS
Manager
Adverse Drug Reactions Group
Lexi-Comp, Inc
Hudson, Ohio

Dana Travis, RPh
Pharmacotherapy Specialist
Lexi-Comp, Inc
Hudson, Ohio

Jennifer Trofe-Clark, PharmD
Clinical Transplant Pharmacist
Hospital of The University of Pennsylvania
Philadelphia, Pennsylvania

Beatrice B. Turkoski, RN, PhD
Associate Professor, Graduate Faculty,
Pharmacology for Advanced Practice Nurses
College of Nursing
Kent State University
Kent, Ohio

John N. van den Anker, MD, PhD, FCP, FAAP
Vice Chair of Pediatrics for Experimental Therapeutics
Evan and Cindy Jones Professor of Pediatric Clinical Pharmacology
Chief, Division of Pediatric Clinical Pharmacology
Children's National Medical Center
Professor of Pediatrics, Pharmacology & Physiology
George Washington University School of Medicine and Health Sciences
Washington, D.C.

Heather L. VandenBussche, PharmD
Professor of Pharmacy, Pediatrics
Pharmacy Practice
Ferris State University College of Pharmacy
Kalamazoo, Michigan

9

DESCRIPTION OF SECTIONS AND FIELDS

The *Geriatric Dosage Handbook* is organized into four sections: Introductory information, drug information section, appendix, and pharmacologic category index.

Alphabetical Listing of Drugs

The drug information section of the handbook, wherein all drug monographs are arranged alphabetically by generic name, details information pertinent to geriatric use for each drug. U.S. brand names and index terms are cross-referenced between monographs and marked with diamonds ♦ for easy visibility.

Individual monographs contain most or all of the following fields of information:

Generic Name	U.S. adopted name
Pronunciation	Phonetic pronunciation guide
Related Information	Cross-reference to other pertinent information found elsewhere in this handbook
Medication Safety Issues	In an effort to promote the safe use of medications, this field is intended to highlight possible sources of medication errors such as look-alike/sound-alike drugs or highly concentrated formulations which require vigilance on the part of healthcare professionals. In addition, medications which have been associated with severe consequences in the event of a medication error are also identified in this field.
Brand Names: U.S.	Trade names (manufacturer-specific) found in the United States. The symbol [DSC] appears after trade names that have been recently discontinued.
Brand Names: Canada	Trade name(s) found in Canada
Index Terms	Includes names or accepted abbreviations of the generic drug; may include common brand names no longer available; this field is used to create cross-references to monographs
Generic Availability (U.S.)	Indicates availability of generic products in the United States
Pharmacologic Category	Unique systematic classification of medications
Use	Information pertaining to appropriate FDA-approved indications of the drug.
Unlabeled/Investigational Use	Information pertaining to non-FDA-approved and investigational indications of the drug
Prescribing and Access Restrictions	Provides information on any special requirements regarding the prescribing, obtaining or dispensing of drugs, including access restrictions pertaining to drugs with REMS elements and those drugs whose access restrictions are not REMS-related.
Medication Guide Available	Identifies drugs that have an FDA-approved Medication Guide.
Contraindications	Information pertaining to inappropriate use of the drug as dictated by approved labeling.
Warnings/Precautions	Precautionary considerations, hazardous conditions related to use of the drug, and disease states or patient populations in which the drug should be cautiously used. Boxed warnings, when present, are clearly identified and are adapted from the FDA approved labeling. Consult the product labeling for the exact black box warning through the manufacturer's or the FDA website.
Adverse Reactions	Side effects are grouped by percentage of incidence (if known) and/or body system; <1% effects are not listed, please consult manufacturer's product labeling regarding rare serious or life threatening events; **percentages are reflective of the adult population in general, not specific for older adults**

DESCRIPTION OF SECTIONS AND FIELDS

Drug Interactions

Metabolism/Transport Effects

If a drug has demonstrated involvement with cytochrome P450 enzymes, or other metabolism or transport proteins, this field will identify the drug as an inhibitor, inducer, or substrate of the specific enzyme(s) (eg, CYP1A2 or UGT1A1). CYP450 isoenzymes are identified as substrates (minor or major), inhibitors (weak, moderate, or strong), and inducers (weak or strong).

Avoid Concomitant Use

Designates drug combinations which should not be used concomitantly, due to an unacceptable risk:benefit assessment. Frequently, the concurrent use of the agents is explicitly prohibited or contraindicated by the product labeling.

Increased Effect/Toxicity

Drug combinations that result in an increased or toxic therapeutic effect between the drug listed in the monograph and other drugs or drug classes.

Decreased Effect

Drug combinations that result in a decreased therapeutic effect between the drug listed in the monograph and other drugs or drug classes.

Ethanol/Nutrition/Herb Interactions

Presents a description of the interaction between the drug listed in the monograph and ethanol, food, or herb/nutraceuticals.

Stability

Information regarding storage of product or steps for reconstitution. Provides the time and conditions for which a solution or mixture will maintain full potency. For example, some solutions may require refrigeration after reconstitution while stored at room temperature prior to preparation. Also includes compatibility information. **Note:** Professional judgment of the individual pharmacist in application of this information is imperative. While drug products may exhibit stability over longer durations of time, it may not be appropriate to utilize the drug product due to concerns in sterility.

Mechanism of Action

How drugs work in the body to elicit a response

Pharmacodynamics/Kinetics

The magnitude of a drug's effect depends on the drug concentration at the site of action. The pharmacodynamics are expressed in terms of onset of action and duration of action. Pharmacokinetics are expressed in terms of absorption, distribution (including appearance in breast milk and crossing of the placenta), protein binding, metabolism, bioavailability, half-life, time to peak serum concentration, and elimination.

Dosage

The amount of drug to be typically given or taken during therapy; may include the following:

Geriatric

Suggested amount of drug to be given to geriatric patients; for the purpose of this publication, the terms *elderly*, *geriatric*, or *older adult* include patients ≥65 years of age unless otherwise specified; may include adjustments from adult dosing; lack of this information in the monograph may imply that the drug is not used in the elderly patient or that no specific adjustments could be identified

Geriatric & Adult

This combined field is only used to indicate that no specific adjustments for elderly patients were identified. However, other issues should be considered (ie, renal or hepatic impairment). Also refer to Special Geriatric Considerations for additional information related to the elderly.

Adult

The recommended amount of drug to be given to adult patients

Renal Impairment

Suggested dosage adjustments or comments based on compromised renal function; may include dosing instructions for patients on dialysis

Hepatic Impairment

Suggested dosage adjustments or comments based on compromised liver function

Administration

Information regarding the recommended final concentrations, rates of administration for parenteral drugs, or other guidelines when giving the medication

Monitoring Parameters

Laboratory tests and patient physical parameters that should be monitored for safety and efficacy of drug therapy

Reference Range

Therapeutic and toxic serum concentrations listed including peak and trough levels

Test Interactions	Listing of assay interference when relevant
Pharmacotherapy Pearls	Information about sodium content and/or pertinent information about specific brands
Special Geriatric Considerations	Pertinent information specific to older adults
Product Availability	Provides availability information on products that have been approved by the FDA, but not yet available for use. Estimates for when a product may be available are included, when this information is known. May also provide any unique or critical drug availability issues.
Controlled Substance	Contains controlled substance schedule information as assigned by the United States Drug Enforcement Administration (DEA) or Canadian Controlled Substance Act (CDSA). CDSA information is only provided for drugs available in Canada and not available in the U.S.
Dosage Forms	Information with regard to form, strength, and availability of the drug in the United States. **Note:** Additional formulation information (eg, excipients, preservatives) is included when available. Please consult product labeling for further information.
Dosage Forms: Canada	Information with regard to form, strength, and availability of products that are uniquely available in Canada, but currently not available in the United States.
Extemporaneously Prepared	Directions for preparing liquid formulations from solid drug products. May include stability information and references.
Selected References	Bibliographic information referring to specific geriatric literature findings

Appendix

The appendix offers a compilation of tables, guidelines, and conversion information which can often be helpful when considering patient care.

Pharmacologic Category Index

This index provides a useful listing of drugs by their pharmacologic classification.

PREVENTING PRESCRIBING ERRORS

Prescribing errors account for the majority of reported medication errors and have prompted healthcare professionals to focus on the development of steps to make the prescribing process safer. Prescription legibility has been attributed to a portion of these errors and legislation has been enacted in several states to address prescription legibility. However, eliminating handwritten prescriptions and ordering medications through the use of technology [eg, computerized prescriber order entry (CPOE)] has been the primary recommendation. Whether a prescription is electronic, typed, or hand-printed, additional safe practices should be considered for implementation to maximize the safety of the prescribing process. Listed below are suggestions for safer prescribing:

- Ensure correct patient by using at least 2 patient identifiers on the prescription (eg, full name, birth date, or address). Review prescription with the patient or patient's caregiver.

- If pediatric patient, document patient's birth date or age and most recent weight. If geriatric patient, document patient's birth date or age.

- Prevent drug name confusion:

  - Use TALLman lettering (eg, buPROPion, busPIRone, predniSONE, predniso-LONE). For more information see: http://www.fda.gov/Drugs/DrugSafety/Medica-tionErrors/ucm164587.htm.

  - Avoid abbreviated drug names (eg, MSO_4, $MgSO_4$, MS, HCT, 6MP, MTX), as they may be misinterpreted and cause error.

  - Avoid investigational names for drugs with FDA approval (eg, FK-506, CBDCA).

  - Avoid chemical names such as 6-mercaptopurine or 6-thioguanine, as sixfold overdoses have been given when these were not recognized as chemical names. The proper names of these drugs are mercaptopurine or thioguanine.

  - Use care when prescribing drugs that look or sound similar (eg, look- alike, sound-alike drugs). Common examples include: Celebrex® vs Celexa®, hydroxyzine vs hydralazine, Zyprexa® vs Zyrtec®.

- Avoid dangerous, error-prone abbreviations (eg, regardless of letter-case: U, IU, QD, QOD, µg, cc, @). Do not use apothecary system or symbols. Additionally, text messaging abbreviations (eg, "2Day") should never be used.

  - For more information see: http://www.ismp.org/Tools/errorproneabbreviations.pdf

- Always use a leading zero for numbers less than 1 (0.5 mg is correct and .5 mg is **incorrect**) and never use a trailing zero for whole numbers (2 mg is correct and 2.0 mg is **incorrect**).

- Always use a space between a number and its units as it is easier to read. There should be no periods after the abbreviations mg or mL (10 mg is correct and 10mg is **incorrect**).

- For doses that are greater than 1,000 dosing units, use properly placed commas to prevent 10-fold errors (100,000 units is correct and 100000 units is **incorrect**).

- Do not prescribe drug dosage by the type of container in which the drug is available (eg, do not prescribe "1 amp", "2 vials", etc).

- Do not write vague or ambiguous orders which have the potential for misinterpretation by other healthcare providers. Examples of vague orders to avoid: "resume pre-op medi-cations," "give drug per protocol," or "continue home medications."

- Review each prescription with patient (or patient's caregiver) including the medication name, indication, and directions for use.

- Take extra precautions when prescribing *high alert drugs* (drugs that can cause significant patient harm when prescribed in error). Common examples of these drugs include: Anticoagulants, chemotherapy, insulins, opiates, and sedatives.

  - For more information see: http://www.ismp.org/Tools/highalertmedications.pdf

To Err is Human: Building a Safer Health System, Kohn LT, Corrigan JM, and Donaldson MS, eds, Washington, D.C.: National Academy Press, 2000.

A Complete Outpatient Prescription[1]

A complete outpatient prescription can prevent the prescriber, the pharmacist, and/or the patient from making a mistake and can eliminate the need for further clarification. The complete outpatient prescription should contain:

- Patient's full name

- Medication indication

- Allergies

- Prescriber name and telephone or pager number

- For pediatric patients: Their birth date or age and current weight

- For geriatric patients: Their birth date or age

- Drug name, dosage form and strength

- For pediatric patients: Intended daily weight-based dose so that calculations can be checked by the pharmacist (ie, mg/kg/day or units/kg/day)

- Number or amount to be dispensed

- Complete instructions for the patient or caregiver, including the purpose of the medication, directions for use (including dose), dosing frequency, route of administration, duration of therapy, and number of refills.

- Dose should be expressed in convenient units of measure.

- When there are recognized contraindications for a prescribed drug, the prescriber should indicate knowledge of this fact to the pharmacist (ie, when prescribing a potassium salt for a patient receiving an ACE inhibitor, the prescriber should write "K serum leveling being monitored").

Upon dispensing of the final product, the pharmacist should ensure that the patient or caregiver can effectively demonstrate the appropriate administration technique. An appropriate measuring device should be provided or recommended. Household teaspoons and tablespoons should not be used to measure liquid medications due to their variability and inaccuracies in measurement; oral medication syringes are recommended.

For additional information see: http://www.ppag.org/attachments/files/111/Guidelines_Peds.pdf
[1]Levine SR, Cohen MR, Blanchard NR, et al, "Guidelines for Preventing Medication Errors in Pediatrics," *J Pediatr Pharmacol Ther*, 2001, 6:426-42.

FDA NAME DIFFERENTIATION PROJECT: THE USE OF TALL-MAN LETTERS

Confusion between similar drug names is an important cause of medication errors. For years, The Institute For Safe Medication Practices (ISMP), has urged generic manufacturers to use a combination of large and small letters as well as bolding (ie, chlorpro**MAZINE** and chlorpro**PA-MIDE**) to help distinguish drugs with look-alike names, especially when they share similar strengths. Recently the FDA's Division of Generic Drugs began to issue recommendation letters to manufacturers suggesting this novel way to label their products to help reduce this drug name confusion. Although this project has had marginal success, the method has successfully eliminated problems with products such as diphenhydr**AMINE** and dimenhy**DRINATE**. Hospitals should also follow suit by making similar changes in their own labels, preprinted order forms, computer screens and printouts, and drug storage location labels.

Lexi-Comp, Inc. Medical Publishing will use "Tall-Man" letters for the drugs suggested by the FDA or recommended by ISMP.

The following is a list of generic and brand name product names and recommended revisions.

Drug Product	Recommended Revision
acetazolamide	aceta**ZOLAMIDE**
alprazolam	**ALPRAZ**olam
amiloride	a**MIL**oride
amlodipine	am**LODIP**ine
aripiprazole	**ARIP**iprazole
Avinza	**AVIN**za
azacitidine	aza**CITID**ine
azathioprine	aza**THIO**prine
bupropion	bu**PROP**ion
buspirone	bus**PIR**one
carbamazepine	car**BAM**azepine
carboplatin	**CARBO**platin
cefazolin	ce**FAZ**olin
cefotetan	cefo**TE**tan
cefoxitin	cef**OX**itin
ceftazidime	cef**TAZ**idime
ceftriaxone	cef**TRIAX**one
Celebrex	Cele**BREX**
Celexa	Cele**XA**
chlordiazepoxide	chlordiaze**POXIDE**
chlorpromazine	chlorpro**MAZINE**
chlorpropamide	chlorpro**PAMIDE**
cisplatin	**CIS**platin
clomiphene	clomi**PHENE**
clomipramine	clomi**PRAMINE**
clonazepam	clonaze**PAM**
clonidine	clo**NID**ine
clozapine	clo**ZAP**ine
cycloserine	cyclo**SERINE**
cyclosporine	cyclo**SPORINE**
dactinomycin	**DACTIN**omycin
daptomycin	**DAPTO**mycin

Drug Product	Recommended Revision
daunorubicin	**DAUNO**rubicin
dimenhydrinate	dimenhy**DRINATE**
diphenhydramine	diphenhydr**AMINE**
dobutamine	**DOBUT**amine
docetaxel	**DOCE**taxel
dopamine	**DOP**amine
doxorubicin	**DOXO**rubicin
duloxetine	**DUL**oxetine
ephedrine	e**PHED**rine
epinephrine	**EPINEPH**rine
fentanyl	fenta**NYL**
flavoxate	flavox**ATE**
fluoxetine	**FLU**oxetine
fluphenazine	flu**PHENAZ**ine
fluvoxamine	fluvoxa**MINE**
glipizide	glipi**ZIDE**
glyburide	gly**BURIDE**
guaifenesin	guai**FEN**esin
guanfacine	guan**FACINE**
Humalog	Huma**LOG**
Humulin	Humu**LIN**
hydralazine	hydr**ALAZINE**
hydrocodone	**HYDRO**codone
hydromorphone	**HYDRO**morphone
hydroxyzine	hydr**OXY**zine
idarubicin	**IDA**rubicin
infliximab	in**FLIX**imab
Invanz	**INV**anz
isotretinoin	**ISO**tretinoin
Klonopin	Klono**PIN**
Lamictal	La**MIC**tal
Lamisil	Lam**ISIL**
lamivudine	lami**VUD**ine
lamotrigine	lamo**TRI**gine
levetiracetam	Lev**ETIRA**cetam
levocarnitine	lev**OCARN**itine
lorazepam	**LOR**azepam
medroxyprogesterone	medroxy**PROGESTER**one
metformin	met**FORMIN**
methylprednisolone	methyl**PREDNIS**olone
methyltestosterone	methyl**TESTOSTER**one
metronidazole	metro**NIDAZOLE**
mitomycin	mito**MY**cin
mitoxantrone	Mito**XAN**trone
Nexavar	Nex**AVAR**
Nexium	Nex**IUM**
nicardipine	ni**CAR**dipine
nifedipine	**NIFE**dipine
nimodipine	ni**MOD**ipine
Novolin	Novo**LIN**

Drug Product	Recommended Revision
Novolog	NovoLOG
olanzapine	OLANZapine
oxcarbazepine	OXcarbazepine
oxycodone	oxyCODONE
Oxycontin	OxyCONTIN
paclitaxel	PACLitaxel
paroxetine	PARoxetine
pemetrexed	PEMEtrexed
pentobarbital	PENTobarbital
phenobarbital	PHENobarbital
pralatrexate	PRALAtrexate
prednisolone	prednisoLONE
prednisone	predniSONE
Prilosec	PriLOSEC
Prozac	PROzac
quetiapine	QUEtiapine
quinidine	quiNIDine
quinine	quiNINE
rabeprazole	RABEprazole
Risperdal	RisperDAL
risperidone	risperiDONE
rituximab	riTUXimab
romidepsin	romiDEPsin
romiplostim	romiPLOStim
ropinirole	rOPINIRole
Sandimmune	sandIMMUNE
Sandostatin	SandoSTATIN
Seroquel	SEROquel
Sinequan	SINEquan
sitagliptin	sitaGLIPtin
Solu-Cortef	Solu-CORTEF
Solu-Medrol	Solu-MEDROL
sorafenib	SORAfenib
sufentanil	SUFentanil
sulfadiazine	sulfADIAZINE
sulfasalazine	sulfaSALAzine
sumatriptan	SUMAtriptan
sunitinib	SUNItinib
Tegretol	TEGretol
tiagabine	tiaGABine
tizanidine	tiZANidine
tolazamide	TOLAZamide
tolbutamide	TOLBUTamide
tramadol	traMADol
trazodone	traZODone
Trental	TRENtal
valacyclovir	valACYclovir
valganciclovir	valGANciclovir
vinblastine	vinBLAStine
vincristine	vinCRIStine

Drug Product	Recommended Revision
zolmitriptan	**ZOLM**itriptan
Zyprexa	Zy**PREXA**
Zyrtec	Zyr**TEC**

"FDA and ISMP Lists of Look-Alike Drug Names with Recommended Tall Man Letter." Available at http://www.ismp.org/tools/tallmanletters.pdf. Last accessed January 6, 2011.

"Name Differentiation Project." Available at http://www.fda.gov/Drugs/DrugSafety/MedicationErrors/ucm164587.htm. Last accessed January 6, 2011.

U.S. Pharmacopeia, "USP Quality Review: Use Caution-Avoid Confusion," March 2001, No. 76. Available at http://www.usp.org

♦ **A200® Lice [OTC]** *see* Permethrin *on page 1429*

Abatacept (ab a TA sept)

Medication Safety Issues
Sound-alike/look-alike issues:
Orencia® may be confused with Oracea®
Brand Names: U.S. Orencia®
Brand Names: Canada Orencia®
Index Terms BMS-188667; CTLA-4lg
Generic Availability (U.S.) No
Pharmacologic Category Antirheumatic, Disease Modifying; Selective T-Cell Costimulation Blocker
Use
Treatment of moderately- to severely-active adult rheumatoid arthritis (RA); may be used as monotherapy or in combination with other DMARDs
Treatment of moderately- to severely-active juvenile idiopathic arthritis (JIA); may be used as monotherapy or in combination with methotrexate
Note: Abatacept should **not** be used in combination with anakinra or TNF-blocking agents
Contraindications There are no contraindications listed within the FDA-approved labeling.
Warnings/Precautions Caution should be exercised when considering the use of abatacept in patients with a history of recurrent infections, with conditions that predispose them to infections, or with chronic, latent, or localized infections. Patients who develop a new infection while undergoing treatment should be monitored closely. If a patient develops a serious infection, abatacept should be discontinued. Screen patients for latent tuberculosis infection prior to initiating abatacept; safety in tuberculosis-positive patients has not been established. Treat patients testing positive according to standard therapy prior to initiating abatacept. Adult patients receiving abatacept in combination with TNF-blocking agents had higher rates of infections (including serious infections) than patients on TNF-blocking agents alone. The manufacturer does not recommend concurrent use with anakinra or TNF-blocking agents. Monitor for signs and symptoms of infection when transitioning from TNF-blocking agents to abatacept. Due to the affect of T-cell inhibition on host defenses, abatacept may affect immune responses against infections and malignancies; impact on the development and course of malignancies is not fully defined.

Use caution with chronic obstructive pulmonary disease (COPD), higher incidences of adverse effects (COPD exacerbation, cough, rhonchi, dyspnea) have been observed; monitor closely. Rare cases of hypersensitivity, anaphylaxis, or anaphylactoid reactions have been reported; medications for the treatment of hypersensitivity reactions should be available for immediate use. Patients should be screened for viral hepatitis prior to use; antirheumatic therapy may cause reactivation of hepatitis B. Patients should be brought up to date with all immunizations before initiating therapy. Live vaccines should not be given concurrently or within 3 months of discontinuation of therapy; there is no data available concerning secondary transmission of live vaccines in patients receiving therapy. May contain maltose, which may result in falsely-elevated serum glucose readings on the day of infusion. Higher incidences of infection and malignancy were observed in the elderly; use with caution.
Adverse Reactions (Reflective of adult population; not specific for elderly) Note: Percentages not always reported; COPD patients experienced a higher frequency of COPD-related adverse reactions (COPD exacerbation, cough, dyspnea, pneumonia, rhonchi)

>10%:
Central nervous system: Headache (≤18%)
Gastrointestinal: Nausea
Respiratory: Nasopharyngitis (12%), upper respiratory tract infection
Miscellaneous: Infection (54%), antibody formation (2% to 41%)
1% to 10%:
Cardiovascular: Hypertension (7%)
Central nervous system: Dizziness (9%), fever
Dermatologic: Rash (4%)
Gastrointestinal: Dyspepsia (6%), abdominal pain, diarrhea
Genitourinary: Urinary tract infection (6%)
Neuromuscular & skeletal: Back pain (7%), limb pain (3%)
Respiratory: Cough (8%), bronchitis, pneumonia, rhinitis, sinusitis
Miscellaneous: Infusion-related reactions (2% to 9%), herpes simplex, influenza

Drug Interactions

Avoid Concomitant Use

Avoid concomitant use of Abatacept with any of the following: Anti-TNF Agents; BCG; Belimumab; Natalizumab; Pimecrolimus; Tacrolimus (Topical); Vaccines (Live)

Increased Effect/Toxicity

Abatacept may increase the levels/effects of: Belimumab; Leflunomide; Natalizumab; Vaccines (Live)

The levels/effects of Abatacept may be increased by: Anti-TNF Agents; Denosumab; Pimecrolimus; Roflumilast; Tacrolimus (Topical); Trastuzumab

Decreased Effect

Abatacept may decrease the levels/effects of: BCG; Sipuleucel-T; Vaccines (Inactivated); Vaccines (Live)

The levels/effects of Abatacept may be decreased by: Echinacea

Ethanol/Nutrition/Herb Interactions Herb/Nutraceutical: Avoid echinacea (has immunostimulant properties; consider therapy modifications).

Stability Prior to reconstitution, store at 2°C to 8°C (36°F to 46°F). Protect from light. Reconstitute each vial with 10 mL SWFI using the provided silicone-free disposable syringe (discard solutions accidentally reconstituted with siliconized syringe as they may develop translucent particles). Inject SWFI down the side of the vial to avoid foaming. The reconstituted solution contains 25 mg/mL abatacept. Further dilute (using a silicone-free syringe) in 100 mL NS to a final concentration of ≤10 mg/mL. Prior to adding abatacept to the 100 mL bag, the manufacturer recommends withdrawing a volume of NS equal to the abatacept volume required, resulting in a final volume of 100 mL. Mix gently; do not shake.

After dilution, may be stored for up to 24 hours at room temperature or refrigerated at 2°C to 8°C (36°F to 46°F). Must be used within 24 hours of reconstitution.

Mechanism of Action Selective costimulation modulator; inhibits T-cell (T-lymphocyte) activation by binding to CD80 and CD86 on antigen presenting cells (APC), thus blocking the required CD28 interaction between APCs and T cells. Activated T lymphocytes are found in the synovium of rheumatoid arthritis patients.

Pharmacodynamics/Kinetics

Distribution: V_{ss}: 0.02-0.13 L/kg

Half-life elimination: 8-25 days

Dosage

Geriatric Refer to adult dosing. Due to potential for higher rates of infections and malignancies, use caution.

Adult Rheumatoid arthritis: I.V.: Dosing is according to body weight. Repeat dose at 2 weeks and 4 weeks after initial dose, and every 4 weeks thereafter:

<60 kg: 500 mg

60-100 kg: 750 mg

>100 kg: 1000 mg

Administration Infuse over 30 minutes. Administer through a 0.2-1.2 micron low protein-binding. filter

Monitoring Parameters Signs and symptoms of infection, signs and symptoms of infusion reaction; hepatitis and TB screening prior to therapy initiation

Test Interactions Contains maltose; may result in falsely elevated blood glucose levels with dehydrogenase pyrroloquinolinequinone or glucose-dye-oxidoreductase testing methods on the day of infusion. Glucose monitoring methods which utilize glucose dehydrogenase nicotine adenine dinucleotide (GDH-NAD), glucose oxidase, or glucose hexokinase are recommended.

Special Geriatric Considerations The number of elderly (≥65 years of age) were insufficient to draw significant clinical conclusions. The studies to date have not demonstrated any differences in safety and efficacy between young adults and elderly. However, the frequency of infections and malignancy was higher in those >65 years of age than those <65 years. Since elderly experience a higher incidence of infections and malignancies, use abatacept with caution in this population.

Product Availability

Orencia® 125 mg/mL prefilled syringe: FDA approved August 2011; availability expected in September 2011

Orencia® 125 mg/mL prefilled syringe is a subcutaneously administered once-weekly formulation approved for the treatment of adult rheumatoid arthritis.

Dosage Forms Excipient information presented when available (limited, particularly for generics); consult specific product labeling.

Injection, powder for reconstitution [preservative free]:

Orencia®: 250 mg [contains maltose]

◄ **Selected References**
Doan T and Massarotti E, "Rheumatoid Arthritis: An Overview of New and Emerging Therapies," *J Clin Pharmacol*, 2005, 45(7):751-62.

Furst DE, Breedveld FC, Kalden JR, et al, "Updated Consensus Statement on Biological Agents for the Treatment of Rheumatic Diseases, 2007," *Ann Rheum Dis*, 2007, 66(Suppl 3):2-22.

Genovese MC, Becker JC, Schiff M, et al, "Abatacept for Rheumatoid Arthritis Refractory to Tumor Necrosis Factor Alpha Inhibition," *N Engl J Med*, 2005, 353(11):1114-23.

Kremer JM, Dougados M, Emery P, et al, "Treatment of Rheumatoid Arthritis With the Selective Costimulation Modulator Abatacept: Twelve-Month Results of a Phase IIb, Double-Blind, Randomized, Placebo-Controlled Trial," *Arthritis Rheum*, 2005, 52(8):2263-71.

Kremer JM, Genant HK, Moreland LW, et al, "Effects of Abatacept in Patients With Methotrexate-Resistant Active Rheumatoid Arthritis: A Randomized Trial," *Ann Intern Med*, 2006, 144(12):865-76.

Kremer JM, Westhovens R, Leon M, et al, "Treatment of Rheumatoid Arthritis by Selective Inhibition of T-Cell Activation With Fusion Protein CTLA4Ig," *N Engl J Med*, 2003, 349(20):1907-15.

Tay L, Leon F, Vratsanos G, et al, "Vaccination Response to Tetanus Toxoid and 23-Valent Pneumococcal Vaccines Following Administration of a Single Dose of Abatacept: A Randomized, Open-Label, Parrallel Group Study in Healthy Subjects," *Arthritis Res Ther*, 2007, 9(2): R38.

Weinblatt M, Combe B, Covucci A, et al, "Safety of the Selective Costimulation Modulator Abatacept in Rheumatoid Arthritis Patients Receiving Background Biologic and Nonbiologic Disease-Modifying Antirheumatic Drugs: A One-Year Randomized, Placebo-Controlled Study," *Arthritis Rheum*, 2006, 54(9):2807-16.

◆ **Abbott-43818** *see* Leuprolide *on page 1039*
◆ **ABCD** *see* Amphotericin B Cholesteryl Sulfate Complex *on page 120*
◆ **Abelcet®** *see* Amphotericin B (Lipid Complex) *on page 125*
◆ **Abilify®** *see* ARIPiprazole *on page 143*
◆ **Abilify Discmelt®** *see* ARIPiprazole *on page 143*

Abiraterone Acetate (a bir A ter one AS e tate)

Brand Names: U.S. Zytiga™
Brand Names: Canada Zytiga™
Index Terms CB7630
Generic Availability (U.S.) No
Pharmacologic Category Antiandrogen
Use Treatment of metastatic, castration-resistant prostate cancer (in combination with prednisone) in patients previously treated with docetaxel
Warnings/Precautions Hazardous agent; use appropriate precautions for handling and disposal. Significant increases in liver enzymes have been reported; may require dosage reduction or discontinuation. ALT, AST, and bilirubin should be monitored prior to treatment, every 2 weeks for 3 months and monthly thereafter; patients with hepatic impairment, elevations in liver function tests, or experiencing hepatotoxicity require more frequent monitoring (see Dosage: Hepatic Impairment and Monitoring Parameters). Evaluate liver function promptly with signs or symptoms of hepatotoxicity. The safety of retreatment after significant elevations (ALT or AST >20 times the upper limit of normal [ULN] or total bilirubin >10 times ULN) has not been evaluated. Avoid use in patients with pre-existing severe hepatic impairment; dosage reduction is recommended in patients with baseline moderate impairment. Canadian labeling (not in U.S. labeling) also recommends avoiding use in patients with pre-existing moderate hepatic impairment.

Concurrent infection, stress, or interruption of daily corticosteroids is associated with reports of adrenocortical insufficiency. Monitor closely for signs and symptoms of adrenocorticoid insufficiency, which could be masked by adverse events associated with mineralocorticoid excess. Diagnostic testing for insufficiency may be clinically indicated. Increased corticosteroid doses may be required before, during, and after stress. May cause increased mineralocorticoid levels, which may result in hypertension, hypokalemia and fluid retention. Concomitant administration with corticosteroids reduces the incidence and severity of these adverse events. Due to potential for hypertension, hypokalemia, or fluid retention, use with caution in patients with cardiovascular disease (particularly heart failure, recent MI, or ventricular arrhythmia); patients with left ventricular ejection fraction (LVEF) <50% or NYHA class III or IV heart failure were excluded from clinical trials. Monitor at least monthly for hypertension, hypokalemia, and fluid retention.

Must be administered on an empty stomach (administer at least 1 hour before and 2 hours after any food). Avoid (or use caution) with concomitant CYP3A4 strong inhibitors and inducers. Avoid concurrent administration with CYP2D6 substrates with a narrow therapeutic index (eg, thioridazine); if concurrent administration cannot be avoided, consider a dose reduction of the CYP2D6 substrate.
Adverse Reactions (Reflective of adult population; not specific for elderly) Note:
Adverse reactions reported for use in combination with prednisone.
>10%:
Cardiovascular: Edema (27%)

Endocrine & metabolic: Triglycerides increased (63%), hypokalemia (28%; grades 3/4: 5%), hypophosphatemia (24%; grades 3/4: 7%), hot flush (19%)

Gastrointestinal: Diarrhea (18%)

Genitourinary: Urinary tract infection (12%)

Hepatic: AST increased (31%; grades 3/4: 2%), ALT increased (11%; grades 3/4: 1%)

Neuromuscular & skeletal: Joint swelling/discomfort (30%), muscle discomfort (26%)

Respiratory: Cough (11%)

1% to 10%:

Cardiovascular: Hypertension (9%; grades 3/4: 1%), arrhythmia (7%), chest pain/discomfort (4%), heart failure (2%)

Gastrointestinal: Dyspepsia (6%)

Genitourinary: Polyuria (7%), nocturia (6%)

Hepatic: Bilirubin increased (7%; grades 3/4: <1%)

Respiratory: Upper respiratory infection (5%)

Drug Interactions

Avoid Concomitant Use

Avoid concomitant use of Abiraterone Acetate with any of the following: Clopidogrel; Conivaptan; Silodosin; Tamoxifen; Thioridazine; Topotecan

Increased Effect/Toxicity

Abiraterone Acetate may increase the levels/effects of: Atomoxetine; Bendamustine; Carvedilol; Colchicine; CYP1A2 Substrates; CYP2C19 Substrates; CYP2C9 Substrates (High risk); CYP2D6 Substrates; Dabigatran Etexilate; Everolimus; Fesoterodine; Iloperidone; Nebivolol; P-Glycoprotein Substrates; Rivaroxaban; Silodosin; Tamoxifen; Tetrabenazine; Thioridazine; Topotecan

The levels/effects of Abiraterone Acetate may be increased by: Conivaptan; CYP3A4 Inhibitors (Moderate); CYP3A4 Inhibitors (Strong); Dasatinib

Decreased Effect

Abiraterone Acetate may decrease the levels/effects of: Clopidogrel; Codeine; Iloperidone; TraMADol

The levels/effects of Abiraterone Acetate may be decreased by: CYP3A4 Inducers (Strong); Deferasirox; Herbs (CYP3A4 Inducers); Tocilizumab

Ethanol/Nutrition/Herb Interactions Food: Do not administer with food (will increase systemic exposure).

Stability Store at 20°C to 25°C (68°F to 77°F); excursions permitted to 15°C to 30°C (59°F to 86°F).

Mechanism of Action Selectively and irreversibly inhibits CYP17 (17 alpha-hydroxylase/C17,20-lyase), an enzyme required for androgen biosynthesis which is expressed in testicular, adrenal, and prostatic tumor tissues. Inhibits the formation of the testosterone precursors dehydroepiandrosterone (DHEA) and androstenedione.

Pharmacodynamics/Kinetics

Distribution: V_{dss}: 19,669 ± 13,358 L

Protein binding: >99%; to albumin and alpha$_1$-acid glycoprotein

Metabolism: Abiraterone acetate is hydrolyzed to the active metabolite abiraterone; further metabolized to inactive metabolites abiraterone sulphate and N-oxide abiraterone sulphate via CYP3A4 and SULT2A1

Bioavailability: Systemic exposure is increased by food

Half-life elimination: 12 ± 5 hours

Time to peak: 2 hours

Excretion: Feces (~88%); urine (~5%)

Dosage

Geriatric & Adult Prostate cancer, metastatic, castration-resistant: Oral: 1000 mg once daily (in combination with prednisone 5 mg twice daily)

Renal Impairment No adjustment required.

Hepatic Impairment

Hepatic impairment *prior to* treatment initiation:

Mild (Child-Pugh class A): No adjustment required

Moderate (Child-Pugh class B): 250 mg once daily (**Note:** Canadian labeling does not recommend use). Permanently discontinue treatment if ALT and/or AST >5 times the upper limit of normal (ULN) or total bilirubin >3 times ULN.

Severe (Child-Pugh class C): Avoid use

Hepatotoxicity *during* treatment:

U.S. labeling:

ALT and/or AST >5 times ULN or total bilirubin >3 times ULN: Withhold treatment until liver function tests return to baseline or ALT and AST ≤2.5 times ULN and total bilirubin ≤1.5 times ULN, then reinitiate at 750 mg once daily.

Recurrent hepatotoxicity on 750 mg/day: Withhold treatment until liver function tests return to baseline or ALT and AST ≤2.5 times ULN and total bilirubin ≤1.5 times ULN, then reinitiate at 500 mg once daily.

Recurrent hepatotoxicity on 500 mg/day: Discontinue treatment

Canadian labeling:

ALT and/or AST >5 times ULN or total bilirubin >3 times ULN:

Withhold treatment until liver function tests return to baseline, then reinitiate at 500 mg once daily

Recurrent hepatotoxicity on 500 mg/day: Discontinue treatment

ALT >20 times ULN (any time during treatment): Discontinue permanently.

Administration Administer orally on an empty stomach, at least 1 hour before and 2 hours after food. Swallow tablets whole with water.

Monitoring Parameters ALT, AST, and bilirubin prior to treatment, every 2 weeks for 3 months and monthly thereafter; if baseline moderate hepatic impairment (Child-Pugh class B), monitor ALT, AST, and bilirubin prior to treatment, weekly for the first month, every 2 weeks for 2 months then monthly thereafter. If hepatotoxicity develops during treatment (and only after therapy is interrupted and liver function tests have returned to safe levels), monitor ALT, AST, and bilirubin every 2 weeks for 3 months and monthly thereafter. Monitoring of testosterone levels is not necessary.

Monitor for signs and symptoms of adrenocorticoid insufficiency; monthly for hypertension, hypokalemia, and fluid retention.

Special Geriatric Considerations According to the manufacturer, 71% of men in clinical trials were ≥65 years; 28% were ≥75 years. No difference in efficacy or safety was noted between younger and older men.

Dosage Forms Excipient information presented when available (limited, particularly for generics); consult specific product labeling.

Tablet, oral:

Zytiga™: 250 mg

Selected References

Attard G, Reid AH, A'Hern R, et al, "Selective Inhibition of CYP17 With Abiraterone Acetate is Highly Active in the Treatment of Castration-Resistant Prostate Cancer," *J Clin Oncol*, 2009, 27(23):3742-8.

Danila DC, Morris MJ, de Bono JS, et al, "Phase II Multicenter Study of Abiraterone Acetate Plus Prednisone Therapy in Patients With Docetaxel-Treated Castration-Resistant Prostate Cancer," *J Clin Oncol*, 2010, 28(9):1496-501.

de Bono JS, Logothetis CJ, Fizazi K, et al, "Aberiterone Acetate (AA) Plus Low Dose Prednisone (P) Improves Overall Survival in Patients (PTS) With Metastatic Castration-Resistant Prostate Cancer (MCRPC) Who Have Progressed After Docetaxel-Based Chemotherapy (CHEMO): Results of COU-AA-301, a Randomized Double-Blind Placebo-Controlled Phase III Study," *Ann Oncol*, 2010, 21(8s):LBA5 [abstract LBA5 from 2010 ESMO Annual Meeting].

de Bono JS, Logothetis CJ, Molina A, et al, "Abiraterone and Increased Survival in Metastatic Prostate Cancer," *New Engl J Med*, 2011, 364(21):1995-2005.

Reid AH, Attard G, Danila DC, et al, "Significant and Sustained Antitumor Activity in Post-Docetaxel, Castration-Resistant Prostate Cancer With the CYP17 Inhibitor Abiraterone Acetate," *J Clin Oncol*, 2010, 28(9):1489-95.

Ryan CJ, Smith MR, Fong L, et al, "Phase I Clinical Trial of the CYP17 Inhibitor Abiraterone Acetate Demonstrating Clinical Activity in Patients With Castration-Resistant Prostate Cancer Who Received Prior Ketoconazole Therapy," *J Clin Oncol*, 2010, 28(9):1481-8.

◆ **ABLC** *see* Amphotericin B (Lipid Complex) *on page 125*

AbobotulinumtoxinA (aye bo BOT yoo lin num TOKS in aye)

Medication Safety Issues

Administration issues:

Botulinum products are not interchangeable; potency differences may exist between the products.

Brand Names: U.S. Dysport™

Index Terms Botulinum Toxin Type A

Generic Availability (U.S.) No

Pharmacologic Category Neuromuscular Blocker Agent, Toxin

Use Treatment of cervical dystonia in both toxin-naive and previously treated patients; temporary improvement in the appearance of moderate-severe glabellar lines associated with procerus and corrugator muscle activity

Medication Guide Available Yes

Dosage

Geriatric

Cervical dystonia: Refer to adult dosing. No specific adjustment recommended.

Glabellar lines: Not recommended in patients ≥65 years of age.

Adult

Cervical dystonia: I.M.: Initial: 500 units divided among affected muscles in toxin-naïve or toxin-experienced patients. May re-treat at intervals of ≥12 weeks

Dosage adjustments: Adjust dosage in 250-unit increments; do not administer at intervals <12 weeks; dosage range used in studies: 250-1000 units

Glabellar lines: Adults <65 years: I.M.: Inject 10 units (0.05 mL or 0.08 mL) into each of 5 sites (2 injections in each corrugator muscle and 1 injection in the procerus muscle) for a total dose of 50 units; do not administer at intervals <3 months; efficacy has been demonstrated up to 4 repeated administrations

Renal Impairment No adjustment necessary.

Hepatic Impairment No adjustment necessary.

Special Geriatric Considerations No specific dosage adjustment recommended.

Dosage Forms Excipient information presented when available (limited, particularly for generics); consult specific product labeling.

Injection, powder for reconstitution:

Dysport™: 500 units [contains albumin (human), lactose 2.5 mg]

♦ **Abstral®** *see* FentaNYL *on page* 709
♦ **ABT-335** *see* Fenofibric Acid *on page* 704
♦ **AC 2993** *see* Exenatide *on page* 687

Acamprosate (a kam PROE sate)

Brand Names: U.S. Campral®
Brand Names: Canada Campral®
Index Terms Acamprosate Calcium; Calcium Acetylhomotaurinate
Generic Availability (U.S.) No
Pharmacologic Category GABA Agonist/Glutamate Antagonist
Use Maintenance of alcohol abstinence
Contraindications Hypersensitivity to acamprosate or any component of the formulation; severe renal impairment (Cl_{cr} <30 mL/minute)
Warnings/Precautions Should be used as part of a comprehensive program to treat alcohol dependence. Treatment should be initiated as soon as possible following the period of alcohol withdrawal, when the patient has achieved abstinence. Acamprosate does not eliminate or diminish the symptoms of alcohol withdrawal. Use caution in moderate renal impairment (Cl_{cr} 30-50 mL/minute). Suicidal ideation, attempted and completed suicides have occurred in acamprosate-treated patients; monitor for depression and/or suicidal thinking. Traces of sulfites may be present in the formulation.
Adverse Reactions (Reflective of adult population; not specific for elderly) Note: Many adverse effects associated with treatment may be related to alcohol abstinence; reported frequency range may overlap with placebo.

>10%: Gastrointestinal: Diarrhea (10% to 17%)
1% to 10%:
  Cardiovascular: Syncope, palpitation, edema (peripheral)
  Central nervous system: Insomnia (6% to 9%), anxiety (5% to 8%), depression (4% to 8%), dizziness (3% to 4%), pain (2% to 4%), paresthesia (2% to 3%), headache, somnolence, amnesia, tremor, chills
  Dermatologic: Pruritus (3% to 4%), rash
  Endocrine & metabolic: Weight gain, libido decreased
  Gastrointestinal: Anorexia (2% to 5%), flatulence (1% to 3%), nausea (3% to 4%), abdominal pain, dry mouth (1% to 3%), vomiting, dyspepsia, constipation, appetite increased, taste perversion
  Genitourinary: Impotence
  Neuromuscular & skeletal: Weakness (5% to 7%), back pain, myalgia, arthralgia
  Ocular: Abnormal vision
  Respiratory: Rhinitis, dyspnea, pharyngitis, bronchitis
  Miscellaneous: Diaphoresis (2% to 3%), suicide attempt
Drug Interactions
  Avoid Concomitant Use There are no known interactions where it is recommended to avoid concomitant use.
  Increased Effect/Toxicity There are no known significant interactions involving an increase in effect.
  Decreased Effect There are no known significant interactions involving a decrease in effect.
Ethanol/Nutrition/Herb Interactions
  Ethanol: Abstinence is required during treatment. Ethanol does not affect the pharmacokinetics of acamprosate; however, the continued use of ethanol will decrease desired efficacy of acamprosate.
  Food: Food decreases absorption of acamprosate (not clinically significant).
Stability Store at 25°C (77°F); excursions permitted to 15°C to 30°C (59°F to 86°F).

◀ **Mechanism of Action** Mechanism not fully defined. Structurally similar to gamma-amino butyric acid (GABA), acamprosate appears to increase the activity of the GABA-ergic system, and decreases activity of glutamate within the CNS, including a decrease in activity at N-methyl D-aspartate (NMDA) receptors; may also affect CNS calcium channels. Restores balance to GABA and glutamate activities which appear to be disrupted in alcohol dependence. During therapeutic use, reduces alcohol intake, but does not cause a disulfiram-like reaction following alcohol ingestion.

Pharmacodynamics/Kinetics
Distribution: V_d: 1 L/kg
Protein binding: Negligible
Metabolism: Not metabolized
Bioavailability: 11%
Half-life elimination: 20-33 hours
Excretion: Urine (as unchanged drug)

Dosage
Geriatric & Adult Alcohol abstinence: Oral: 666 mg 3 times/day (a lower dose may be effective in some patients).
Adjustment in patients with low body weight (unlabeled): A lower dose (4 tablets/day) may be considered in patients with low body weight (eg, <60 kg).
Note: Treatment should be initiated as soon as possible following the period of alcohol withdrawal, when the patient has achieved abstinence.

Renal Impairment
Cl_{cr} 30-50 mL/minute: Initial dose should be reduced to 333 mg 3 times/day.
Cl_{cr} <30 mL/minute: Contraindicated in severe renal impairment.

Administration May be administered without regard to meals.

Special Geriatric Considerations Initial studies did not include sufficient geriatric patients to be able to derive sufficient data to compare elderly to younger adults. Only 41 out of 4234 patients in clinical trials were ≥65 years of age with none ≥75 years. However, since this medication is cleared renally exclusively, caution should be used since many elderly have Cl_{cr} 30-50 mL/minute where dosage reduction is required (see Dosage).

Dosage Forms Excipient information presented when available (limited, particularly for generics); consult specific product labeling.
Tablet, delayed release, enteric coated, oral, as calcium:
Campral®: 333 mg [contains calcium 33 mg/tablet, sulfites]

Selected References
Brasser SM, McCaul ME, and Houtsmuller EJ, "Alcohol Effects During Acamprosate Treatment: A Dose-Response Study in Humans," Alcohol Clin Exp Res, 2004, 28(7):1074-83.
Graham R, Wodak AD, and Whelan G, "New Pharmacotherapies for Alcohol Dependence," Med J Aust, 2002, 177 (2):103-7.
Overman GP, Teter CJ, and Guthrie SK, "Acamprosate For the Adjunctive Treatment of Alcohol Dependence," Ann Pharmacother, 2003, 37(7-8):1090-9.

◆ **Acamprosate Calcium** see Acamprosate on page 27

Acarbose (AY car bose)

Related Information
Diabetes Mellitus Management, Adults on page 2073
Medication Safety Issues
Sound-alike/look-alike issues:
Precose® may be confused with PreCare®
International issues:
Precose® [U.S., Malaysia] may be confused with Precosa brand name for *Saccharomyces boulardii* [Finland, Sweden]
Brand Names: U.S. Precose®
Brand Names: Canada Glucobay™
Generic Availability (U.S.) Yes
Pharmacologic Category Antidiabetic Agent, Alpha-Glucosidase Inhibitor
Use Adjunct to diet and exercise to lower blood glucose in patients with type 2 diabetes mellitus (noninsulin dependent, NIDDM)
Contraindications Hypersensitivity to acarbose or any component of the formulation; patients with diabetic ketoacidosis or cirrhosis; patients with inflammatory bowel disease, colonic ulceration, partial intestinal obstruction, or in patients predisposed to intestinal obstruction; patients who have chronic intestinal diseases associated with marked disorders of digestion or absorption, and in patients who have conditions that may deteriorate as a result of increased gas formation in the intestine

Warnings/Precautions Acarbose given in combination with a sulfonylurea or insulin will cause a further lowering of blood glucose and may increase the hypoglycemic potential of the sulfonylurea or insulin. Treatment-emergent elevations of serum transaminases (AST and/or ALT) occurred in up to 14% of acarbose-treated patients in long-term studies. These serum transaminase elevations appear to be dose related and were asymptomatic, reversible, more common in females, and, in general, were not associated with other evidence of liver dysfunction. Fulminant hepatitis has been reported rarely. It may be necessary to discontinue acarbose and administer insulin if the patient is exposed to stress (ie, fever, trauma, infection, surgery). Use not recommended in patients with significant impairment (S_{cr} >2 mg/dL); use with caution in other patients with renal impairment.

Adverse Reactions (Reflective of adult population; not specific for elderly) >10%:
Gastrointestinal: Diarrhea (31%) and abdominal pain (19%) tend to return to pretreatment levels over time; frequency and intensity of flatulence (74%) tend to abate with time
Hepatic: Transaminases increased (≤4%)

Drug Interactions
Avoid Concomitant Use There are no known interactions where it is recommended to avoid concomitant use.
Increased Effect/Toxicity
Acarbose may increase the levels/effects of: Hypoglycemic Agents

The levels/effects of Acarbose may be increased by: Herbs (Hypoglycemic Properties); Neomycin; Pegvisomant
Decreased Effect
Acarbose may decrease the levels/effects of: Digoxin

The levels/effects of Acarbose may be decreased by: Corticosteroids (Orally Inhaled); Corticosteroids (Systemic); Luteinizing Hormone-Releasing Hormone Analogs; Somatropin; Thiazide Diuretics
Ethanol/Nutrition/Herb Interactions Ethanol: Limit ethanol.
Stability Store at <25°C (77°F). Protect from moisture.
Mechanism of Action Competitive inhibitor of pancreatic α-amylase and intestinal brush border α-glucosidases, resulting in delayed hydrolysis of ingested complex carbohydrates and disaccharides and absorption of glucose; dose-dependent reduction in postprandial serum insulin and glucose peaks; inhibits the metabolism of sucrose to glucose and fructose
Pharmacodynamics/Kinetics
Absorption: <2% as active drug; ~35% as metabolites
Metabolism: Exclusively via GI tract, principally by intestinal bacteria and digestive enzymes; 13 metabolites identified (major metabolites are sulfate, methyl, and glucuronide conjugates)
Bioavailability: Low systemic bioavailability of parent compound; acts locally in GI tract
Half-life elimination: ~2 hours
Time to peak: Active drug: ~1 hour
Excretion: Urine (~34% as inactive metabolites, <2% parent drug and active metabolite); feces (~51% as unabsorbed drug)
Dosage
Geriatric & Adult Type 2 diabetes: Oral:
Initial: 25 mg 3 times/day with the first bite of each main meal; to reduce GI effects, some patients may benefit from initiating at 25 mg once daily with gradual titration to 25 mg 3 times/day as tolerated
Maintenance dose: Should be adjusted at 4- to 8-week intervals based on 1-hour post-prandial glucose levels and tolerance until maintenance dose is reached; maintenance dose: 50-100 mg 3 times/day. Dosage must be individualized on the basis of effectiveness and tolerance while not exceeding the maximum recommended dose.
Maximum:
≤60 kg: 50 mg 3 times/day
>60 kg: 100 mg 3 times/day
Patients receiving sulfonylureas or insulin: Acarbose given in combination with a sulfonylurea or insulin will cause a further lowering of blood glucose and may increase the hypoglycemic potential of the sulfonylurea or insulin. If hypoglycemia occurs, appropriate adjustments in the dosage of these agents should be made.
Renal Impairment
Cl_{cr} <25 mL/minute: Peak plasma concentrations were 5 times higher and AUCs were 6 times larger than in volunteers with normal renal function.
Significant renal dysfunction (S_{cr} >2 mg/dL): Use is not recommended.
Administration Should be administered with the first bite of each main meal.
Monitoring Parameters Postprandial glucose, glycosylated hemoglobin levels, serum transaminase levels should be checked every 3 months during the first year of treatment and periodically thereafter, renal function (serum creatinine); blood pressure

◀ **Reference Range**
Recommendations for glycemic control in adults with diabetes:
Hb A_{1c}: <7%
Preprandial capillary plasma glucose: 70-130 mg/dL
Peak postprandial capillary blood glucose: <180 mg/dL
Blood pressure: <130/80 mm Hg
Recommendations for glycemic control in older adults with diabetes:
Relatively healthy, cognitively intact, and with a ≥5-year life expectancy: See Adults
Frail, life expectancy <5 years or those for whom the risks of intensive glucose control outweigh the benefits:
Hb A_{1c}: <8% to 9%
Blood pressure: <140/80 mm Hg or <130/80 mm Hg if tolerated

Special Geriatric Considerations Intensive glucose control (HbA$_{1c}$ <6.5%) has been linked to increased all-cause and cardiovascular mortality, hypoglycemia requiring assistance, and weight gain in adult type 2 diabetes. How "tightly" to control a geriatric patient's blood glucose needs to be individualized. Such a decision should be based on several factors, including the patient's functional and cognitive status, how well he/she recognizes hypoglycemic or hyperglycemic symptoms, and how to respond to them and other disease states. An HbA$_{1c}$ <7.5% is an acceptable endpoint for a healthy older adult, while <8% is acceptable for frail elderly patients, those with a duration of illness >10 years, or those with comorbid conditions and requiring combination diabetes medications. Patients who are unable to accurately draw up their dose will need assistance, such as prefilled syringes. Initial doses may require considerations for renal function in the elderly with dosing adjusted subsequently based on blood glucose monitoring. For elderly patients with diabetes who are relatively healthy, attaining target goals for aspirin use, blood pressure, lipids, smoking cessation, and diet and exercise may be more important than normalized glycemic control.

Dosage Forms Excipient information presented when available (limited, particularly for generics); consult specific product labeling.
Tablet, oral: 25 mg, 50 mg, 100 mg
Precose®: 25 mg, 50 mg, 100 mg

Selected References

Action to Control Cardiovascular Risk in Diabetes Study Group, Gerstein HC, Miller ME, et al, "Effects of Intensive Glucose Lowering in Type 2 Diabetes," *N Engl J Med*, 2008, 358(24):2545-59.
ADVANCE Collaborative Group, Patel A, MacMahon S, et al, "Intensive Blood Glucose Control and Vascular Outcomes in Patients With Type 2 Diabetes," *N Engl J Med*, 2008, 358(24):2560-72.
American Diabetes Association, "Standards of Medical Care in Diabetes – 2011," *Diabetes Care*, 2011, 34(Suppl 1):11-61.
Brown AF, Mangione CM, Saliba D, et al, "Guidelines for Improving the Care of the Older Person With Diabetes Mellitus," *J Am Geriatr Soc*, 2003, 51(5 Suppl Guidelines):265-80.
"VA/DoD Clinical Practice Guideline for the Management of Diabetes Mellitus," 2010. Available at http://www.healthquality.va.gov/Diabetes_Mellitus.asp

◆ **Accolate®** *see* Zafirlukast *on page* 1937
◆ **AccuNeb®** *see* Albuterol *on page* 50
◆ **Accupril®** *see* Quinapril *on page* 1561
◆ **Accuretic®** *see* Quinapril and Hydrochlorothiazide *on page* 1564
◆ **ACE** *see* Captopril *on page* 264

Acebutolol (a se BYOO toe lole)

Related Information
Beta-Blockers *on page* 2001
Medication Safety Issues
Sound-alike/look-alike issues:
Sectral® may be confused with Seconal®, Septra®
Brand Names: U.S. Sectral®
Brand Names: Canada Apo-Acebutolol®; Mylan-Acebutolol; Mylan-Acebutolol (Type S); Novo-Acebutolol; Nu-Acebutolol; Rhotral; Sandoz-Acebutolol; Sectral®; Teva-Acebutolol
Index Terms Acebutolol Hydrochloride
Generic Availability (U.S.) Yes
Pharmacologic Category Antiarrhythmic Agent, Class II; Beta Blocker With Intrinsic Sympathomimetic Activity
Use Treatment of hypertension; management of ventricular arrhythmias
Unlabeled/Investigational Use Treatment of chronic stable angina
Contraindications Overt cardiac failure; cardiogenic shock; persistently-severe bradycardia or second- and third-degree heart block (except in patients with a functioning artificial pacemaker)

Warnings/Precautions Consider pre-existing conditions such as sick sinus syndrome before initiating. Beta-blocker therapy should not be withdrawn abruptly (particularly in patients with CAD), but gradually tapered to avoid acute tachycardia, hypertension, and/or ischemia. Chronic beta-blocker therapy should not be routinely withdrawn prior to major surgery. Use with caution in diabetic patients. Beta-blockers may impair glucose tolerance, potentiate hypoglycemia, and/or mask symptoms of hypoglycemia in a diabetic patient. Use with caution in bronchospastic lung disease, hepatic impairment, myasthenia gravis, psychiatric disease (may cause CNS depression), or renal dysfunction. May precipitate or aggravate symptoms of arterial insufficiency in patients with PVD and Raynaud's disease; use with caution and monitor for progression of arterial obstruction. Use reduced doses in the elderly since metabolism and elimination are reduced. Beta-blockers with intrinsic sympathomimetic activity (eg, acebutolol) are likely to worsen survival in HF and should be avoided. Adequate alpha$_1$-receptor blockade is required prior to use of any beta-blocker for patients with untreated pheochromocytoma. May mask signs of hyperthyroidism (eg, tachycardia); use caution if hyperthyroidism is suspected, abrupt withdrawal may precipitate thyroid storm. Alterations in thyroid function tests may be observed. May induce or exacerbate psoriasis. Use caution with history of severe anaphylaxis to allergens; patients taking beta-blockers may become more sensitive to repeated challenges. Treatment of anaphylaxis (eg, epinephrine) in patients taking beta-blockers may be ineffective or promote undesirable effects. Use with caution in patients on concurrent digoxin, verapamil, or diltiazem; bradycardia or heart block can occur. Use with caution in patients receiving inhaled anesthetic agents known to depress myocardial contractility.

Adverse Reactions (Reflective of adult population; not specific for elderly)
>10%: Central nervous system: Fatigue (11%)
1% to 10%:
  Cardiovascular: Chest pain (2%), edema (2%), bradycardia, hypotension, CHF
  Central nervous system: Headache (6%), dizziness (6%), insomnia (3%), depression (2%), abnormal dreams (2%), anxiety, hyper-/hypoesthesia
  Dermatologic: Rash (2%), pruritus
  Gastrointestinal: Constipation (4%), diarrhea (4%), dyspepsia (4%), nausea (4%), flatulence (3%), abdominal pain, vomiting
  Genitourinary: Micturition frequency (3%), dysuria, impotence, nocturia
  Neuromuscular & skeletal: Myalgia (2%), back pain, joint pain
  Ocular: Abnormal vision (2%), conjunctivitis, dry eyes, eye pain
  Respiratory: Dyspnea (4%), rhinitis (2%), cough (1%), pharyngitis, wheezing

Potential adverse effects (based on experience with other beta-blocking agents) include agranulocytosis, allergic reactions, alopecia, catatonia, claudication, depression (reversible), disorientation, emotional lability, erythematous rash, ischemic colitis, laryngospasm, mesenteric artery thrombosis, Peyronie's disease, purpura, respiratory distress, short-term memory loss, slightly clouded sensorium, thrombocytopenia

Drug Interactions
  Metabolism/Transport Effects Inhibits CYP2D6 (weak)
  Avoid Concomitant Use
    Avoid concomitant use of Acebutolol with any of the following: Floctafenine; Methacholine
  Increased Effect/Toxicity
    Acebutolol may increase the levels/effects of: Alpha-/Beta-Agonists (Direct-Acting); Alpha1-Blockers; Alpha2-Agonists; Amifostine; Antihypertensives; Antipsychotic Agents (Phenothiazines); Bupivacaine; Cardiac Glycosides; Fingolimod; Hypotensive Agents; Insulin; Lidocaine; Lidocaine (Systemic); Lidocaine (Topical); Mepivacaine; Methacholine; Midodrine; RiTUXimab; Sulfonylureas

    The levels/effects of Acebutolol may be increased by: Acetylcholinesterase Inhibitors; Aminoquinolines (Antimalarial); Amiodarone; Anilidopiperidine Opioids; Antipsychotic Agents (Phenothiazines); Calcium Channel Blockers (Dihydropyridine); Calcium Channel Blockers (Nondihydropyridine); Diazoxide; Dipyridamole; Disopyramide; Dronedarone; Floctafenine; Herbs (Hypotensive Properties); MAO Inhibitors; Pentoxifylline; Phosphodiesterase 5 Inhibitors; Propafenone; Propoxyphene; Prostacyclin Analogues; QuiNIDine; Reserpine

  Decreased Effect
    Acebutolol may decrease the levels/effects of: Beta2-Agonists; Theophylline Derivatives

    The levels/effects of Acebutolol may be decreased by: Barbiturates; Herbs (Hypertensive Properties); Methylphenidate; Nonsteroidal Anti-Inflammatory Agents; Rifamycin Derivatives; Yohimbine

◀ **Ethanol/Nutrition/Herb Interactions**
Food: Peak serum acebutolol levels may be slightly decreased if taken with food.
Herb/Nutraceutical: Avoid dong quai if using for hypertension (has estrogenic activity). Avoid yohimbe, ginseng (may worsen hypertension).

Stability Store at controlled room temperature of 20°C to 25°C (68°F to 77°F). Protect from light and dispense in a light-resistant, tight container.

Mechanism of Action Competitively blocks beta$_1$-adrenergic receptors with little or no effect on beta$_2$-receptors except at high doses; exhibits membrane stabilizing and intrinsic sympathomimetic activity

Pharmacodynamics/Kinetics
Onset of action: 1-2 hours
Duration: 12-24 hours
Absorption: Oral: 40%
Distribution: V_d: 1.2 L/kg
Protein binding: ~26%
Metabolism: Extensive first-pass effect to equipotent and cardioselective diacetolol metabolite
Bioavailability: Acebutolol: 40%
Half-life elimination: Parent drug: 3-4 hours; Metabolite: 8-13 hours
Time to peak: 2-4 hours
Excretion: Feces (50% to 60%); urine (30% to 40%); diacetolol eliminated primarily in the urine

Dosage
Geriatric Refer to adult dosing. Consider dose reduction due to age-related increase in bioavailability; do not exceed 800 mg/day. In the management of hypertension, consider lower initial dose (eg, 200-400 mg/day) and titrate to response (Aronow, 2011).
Adult
Angina, ventricular arrhythmia: Oral: 400 mg/day in divided doses; maintenance: 600-1200 mg/day in divided doses; maximum: 1200 mg/day
Hypertension: Oral: 400-800 mg/day (larger doses may be divided); maximum: 1200 mg/day; usual dose range (JNC 7): 200-800 mg/day in 2 divided doses
Chronic stable angina (unlabeled use): 400 mg/day in divided doses; maintenance: 600-1200 mg/day in divided doses; maximum: 1200 mg/day

Renal Impairment
Cl_{cr} 25-49 mL/minute: Reduce dose by 50%.
Cl_{cr} <25 mL/minute: Reduce dose by 75%.

Hepatic Impairment Use with caution.

Administration To discontinue therapy, taper dose gradually. May be administered without regard to meals.

Monitoring Parameters Blood glucose; blood pressure, orthostatic hypotension, heart rate, CNS effects, ECG

Test Interactions Increased AST, ALT, alkaline phosphatase, bilirubin, cholesterol, glucose, LDH, potassium, thyroxine, triglycerides, uric acid; decreased HDL

Special Geriatric Considerations Since bioavailability increased in elderly about twofold, geriatric patients may require lower maintenance doses, therefore, as serum and tissue concentrations increase beta$_1$ selectivity diminishes; due to alterations in the beta-adrenergic autonomic nervous system, beta-adrenergic blockade may result in less hemodynamic response than seen in younger adults. Studies indicate that despite decreased sensitivity to the chronotropic effects of beta-blockade with age, there appears to be an increased myocardial sensitivity to the negative inotropic effect during stress (ie, exercise). Controlled trials have shown the overall response rate for propranolol to be only 20% to 50% in elderly populations. Therefore, all beta-adrenergic blocking drugs may result in a decreased response as compared to younger adults. Adjust dose for renal function.

Dosage Forms Excipient information presented when available (limited, particularly for generics); consult specific product labeling.
Capsule, oral, as hydrochloride: 200 mg, 400 mg
Sectral®: 200 mg, 400 mg

Selected References
Chobanian AV, Bakris GL, Black HR, et al, "The Seventh Report of the Joint National Committee on Prevention, Detection, Evaluation, and Treatment of High Blood Pressure: The JNC 7 Report," *JAMA*, 2003, 289(19):2560-71.
Kligman EW and Higbee MD, "Drug Therapy for Hypertension in the Elderly," *J Fam Pract*, 1989, 28(1):81-7.
Vestal RE, Wood AJ, and Shand DG, "Reduced Beta-Adrenoceptor Sensitivity in the Elderly," *Clin Pharmacol Ther*, 1979, 26(2):181-6.
Yin FC, Raizes GS, Guarnieri T, et al, "Age-Associated Decrease in Ventricular Response to Haemodynamic Stress During Beta-Adrenergic Blockade," *Br Heart J*, 1978, 40(12):1349-55.

◆ **Acebutolol Hydrochloride** *see* Acebutolol *on page 30*
◆ **Aceon®** *see* Perindopril Erbumine *on page 1426*
◆ **Acephen™ [OTC]** *see* Acetaminophen *on page 33*
◆ **Acerola [OTC]** *see* Ascorbic Acid *on page 149*

Acetaminophen (a seet a MIN oh fen)

Medication Safety Issues

Sound-alike/look-alike issues:

Acephen® may be confused with AcipHex®

FeverALL® may be confused with Fiberall®

Triaminic™ Children's Fever Reducer Pain Reliever may be confused with Triaminic® cough and cold products

Tylenol® may be confused with atenolol, timolol, Tylenol® PM, Tylox®

Other safety concerns:

Duplicate therapy issues: This product contains acetaminophen, which may be a component of combination products. Do not exceed the maximum recommended daily dose of acetaminophen.

International issues:

Depon [Greece] may be confused with Depen brand name for penicillamine [U.S.]; Depin brand name for nifedipine [India]; Dipen brand name for dilitazem [Greece]

Duorol [Spain] may be confused with Diuril brand name for chlorothiazide [U.S., Canada]

Paralen [Czech Republic] may be confused with Aralen brand name for chloroquine [U.S., Mexico]

Brand Names: U.S. Acephen™ [OTC]; APAP 500 [OTC]; Aspirin Free Anacin® Extra Strength [OTC]; Cetafen® Extra [OTC]; Cetafen® [OTC]; Excedrin® Tension Headache [OTC]; Feverall® [OTC]; Infantaire [OTC]; Little Fevers™ [OTC]; Mapap® Arthritis Pain [OTC]; Mapap® Children's [OTC]; Mapap® Extra Strength [OTC]; Mapap® Infant's [OTC]; Mapap® Junior Rapid Tabs [OTC]; Mapap® [OTC]; Nortemp Children's [OTC]; Ofirmev™; Pain & Fever Children's [OTC]; Pain Eze [OTC]; Silapap Children's [OTC]; Silapap Infant's [OTC]; Triaminic™ Children's Fever Reducer Pain Reliever [OTC]; Tylenol® 8 Hour [OTC]; Tylenol® Arthritis Pain Extended Relief [OTC]; Tylenol® Children's Meltaways [OTC]; Tylenol® Children's [OTC]; Tylenol® Extra Strength [OTC]; Tylenol® Infant's Concentrated [OTC]; Tylenol® Jr. Meltaways [OTC]; Tylenol® [OTC]; Valorin Extra [OTC]; Valorin [OTC]

Brand Names: Canada Abenol®; Apo-Acetaminophen®; Atasol®; Novo-Gesic; Pediatrix; Tempra®; Tylenol®

Index Terms APAP; N-Acetyl-P-Aminophenol; Paracetamol

Generic Availability (U.S.) Yes: Excludes extended release products; injectable formulation

Pharmacologic Category Analgesic, Miscellaneous

Use Treatment of mild-to-moderate pain and fever (analgesic/antipyretic)

I.V.: Additional indication: Management of moderate-to-severe pain when combined with opioid analgesia

Contraindications Hypersensitivity to acetaminophen or any component of the formulation; severe hepatic impairment or severe active liver disease (Ofirmev™)

Warnings/Precautions Limit dose to <4 g/day. May cause severe hepatotoxicity on acute overdose; in addition, chronic daily dosing in adults has resulted in liver damage in some patients. Use with caution in patients with alcoholic liver disease; consuming ≥3 alcoholic drinks/day may increase the risk of liver damage. Use caution in patients with hepatic impairment or active liver disease. Use of intravenous formulation is contraindicated in patients with severe hepatic impairment or severe active liver disease. Use caution in patients with known G6PD deficiency; rare reports of hemolysis have occurred. Use caution in patients with chronic malnutrition and hypovolemia (intravenous formulation). Use caution in patients with severe renal impairment; consider dosing adjustments. Hypersensitivity and anaphylactic reactions have been reported; discontinue immediately if symptoms of allergic or hypersensitivity reactions occur.

OTC labeling: When used for self-medication, patients should be instructed to contact healthcare provider if used for fever lasting >3 days or for pain lasting >10 days in adults.

Adverse Reactions (Reflective of adult population; not specific for elderly) Oral, Rectal: Frequency not defined:

Dermatologic: Rash

Endocrine & metabolic: May increase chloride, uric acid, glucose; may decrease sodium, bicarbonate, calcium

Hematologic: Anemia; blood dyscrasias (neutropenia, pancytopenia, leukopenia)

Hepatic: Bilirubin increased, alkaline phosphatase increased

Renal: Ammonia increased, nephrotoxicity with chronic overdose, analgesic nephropathy

Miscellaneous: Hypersensitivity reactions (rare)

I.V.:

>10%: Gastrointestinal: Nausea (adults 34%; children ≥5%), vomiting (adults 15%; children ≥5%)

1% to 10%:

Cardiovascular: Edema (peripheral), hypervolemia, hypo/hypertension, tachycardia

Central nervous system: Headache (adults 10%; children ≥1%), insomnia (adults 7%; children ≥1%), agitation (children ≥5%), anxiety, fatigue

Dermatologic: Pruritus (children ≥5%), rash

Endocrine & metabolic: Hypoalbuminemia, hypokalemia, hypomagnesemia, hypophosphatemia

Gastrointestinal: Constipation (children ≥5%), abdominal pain, diarrhea

Hematologic: Anemia

Hepatic: Transaminases increased

Local: Infusion site pain

Neuromuscular & skeletal: Muscle spasms, pain in extremity, trismus

Ocular: Periorbital edema

Renal: Oliguria (children ≥1%)

Respiratory: Atelectasis (children ≥5%), breath sounds abnormal, dyspnea, hypoxia, pleural effusion, pulmonary edema, stridor, wheezing

Drug Interactions

Metabolism/Transport Effects Substrate (minor) of CYP1A2, 2A6, 2C9, 2D6, 2E1, 3A4; **Inhibits** CYP3A4 (weak)

Avoid Concomitant Use There are no known interactions where it is recommended to avoid concomitant use.

Increased Effect/Toxicity

Acetaminophen may increase the levels/effects of: Dasatinib; Imatinib; SORAfenib; Vitamin K Antagonists

The levels/effects of Acetaminophen may be increased by: Conivaptan; Dasatinib; Imatinib; Isoniazid; Metyrapone; Probenecid; SORAfenib

Decreased Effect

The levels/effects of Acetaminophen may be decreased by: Anticonvulsants (Hydantoin); Barbiturates; CarBAMazepine; Cholestyramine Resin; Cyproterone; Peginterferon Alfa-2b; Tocilizumab

Ethanol/Nutrition/Herb Interactions

Ethanol: Excessive intake of ethanol may increase the risk of acetaminophen-induced hepatotoxicity. Avoid ethanol or limit to <3 drinks/day.

Food: Rate of absorption may be decreased when given with food.

Herb/Nutraceutical: St John's wort may decrease acetaminophen levels.

Stability

Injection: Store intact vials at room temperature of 20°C to 25°C (68°F to 77°F); do not refrigerate or freeze. Injectable solution may be administered directly from the vial without further dilution. For doses <1000 mg, withdraw the appropriate volume and transfer to a separate sterile container (eg, glass bottle, plastic I.V. container, syringe) for administration. Use within 6 hours of opening vial or transferring to another container. Discard any unused portion; single use vials only.

Oral formulations: Store at controlled room temperature.

Suppositories: Store at <27°C (80°F); do not freeze.

Mechanism of Action Although not fully elucidated, believed to inhibit the synthesis of prostaglandins in the central nervous system and work peripherally to block pain impulse generation; produces antipyresis from inhibition of hypothalamic heat-regulating center

Pharmacodynamics/Kinetics

Onset of action:

Oral: <1 hour

I.V.: Analgesia: 5-10 minutes; Antipyretic: Within 30 minutes

Peak effect: I.V.: Analgesic: 1 hour

Duration:

I.V., Oral: Analgesia: 4-6 hours

I.V.: Antipyretic: ≥6 hours

Absorption: Primarily absorbed in small intestine (rate of absorption dependent upon gastric emptying); minimal absorption from stomach; varies by dosage form

Distribution: ~1 L/kg at therapeutic doses

Protein binding: 10% to 25% at therapeutic concentrations; 8% to 43% at toxic concentrations

Metabolism: At normal therapeutic dosages, primarily hepatic metabolism to sulfate and glucuronide conjugates, while a small amount is metabolized by CYP2E1 to a highly reactive intermediate, N-acetyl-p-benzoquinone imine (NAPQI), which is conjugated rapidly with glutathione and inactivated to nontoxic cysteine and mercapturic acid conjugates. At toxic doses (as little as 4 g daily) glutathione conjugation becomes insufficient to meet the metabolic demand causing an increase in NAPQI concentrations, which may cause hepatic cell necrosis. Oral administration is subject to first pass metabolism.

Half-life elimination: Prolonged following toxic doses; ~2 hours (range: 2-3 hours); may be slightly prolonged in severe renal insufficiency (Cl_{cr}<30 mL/minute): 2-5.3 hours

Time to peak, serum: Oral: Immediate release: 10-60 minutes (may be delayed in acute overdoses); I.V.: 15 minutes

Excretion: Urine (<5% unchanged; 60% to 80% as glucuronide metabolites; 20% to 30% as sulphate metabolites; ~8% cysteine and mercapturic acid metabolites)

Dosage

Geriatric & Adult Note: No dose adjustment required if converting between different acetaminophen formulations.

Pain or fever:

Oral, rectal: 325-650 mg every 4-6 hours or 1000 mg 3-4 times/day; do **not** exceed 4 g/day

I.V.:

<50 kg: 15 mg/kg every 6 hours or 12.5 mg/kg every 4 hours; maximum single dose: 750 mg/dose; maximum daily dose: 75 mg/kg/day (≤3.75 g/day)

≥50 kg: 650 mg every 4 hours or 1000 mg every 6 hours; maximum single dose: 1000 mg/dose; maximum daily dose: 4 g/day

Renal Impairment

Oral (Aronoff, 2007):

Adults:

Cl_{cr} 10-50 mL/minute: Administer every 6 hours.

Cl_{cr} <10 mL/minute: Administer every 8 hours.

Intermittent hemodialysis or peritoneal dialysis: No adjustment necessary.

CRRT: Administer every 8 hours.

I.V.: Cl_{cr} ≤30 mL/minute: Use with caution; consider decreasing daily dose and extending dosing interval.

Hepatic Impairment Use with caution. Limited, low-dose therapy is usually well tolerated in hepatic disease/cirrhosis. However, cases of hepatotoxicity at daily acetaminophen dosages <4 g/day have been reported. Avoid chronic use in hepatic impairment.

Administration

Suspension, oral: Shake well before pouring a dose.

Injection: For I.V. infusion only. May administer undiluted over 15 minutes.

Doses <1000 mg (<50 kg): Withdraw appropriate dose from vial and place into separate empty, sterile container prior to administration. Small volume pediatric doses (up to 60 mL) may be placed in a syringe and infused over 15 minutes via syringe pump.

Doses of 1000 mg (≥50 kg): Insert vented I.V. set through vial stopper.

Monitoring Parameters Relief of pain or fever

Dosage Forms Excipient information presented when available (limited, particularly for generics); consult specific product labeling. [DSC] = Discontinued product

Caplet, oral: 500 mg

Cetafen® Extra: 500 mg

Mapap® Extra Strength: 500 mg

Mapap® Extra Strength: 500 mg [scored]

Pain Eze: 650 mg

Tylenol®: 325 mg

Tylenol® Extra Strength: 500 mg

Caplet, extended release, oral:

Mapap® Arthritis Pain: 650 mg

Tylenol® 8 Hour: 650 mg

Tylenol® Arthritis Pain Extended Relief: 650 mg

Capsule, oral:

Mapap® Extra Strength: 500 mg

Captab, oral: 500 mg

Elixir, oral:

Mapap® Children's: 160 mg/5 mL (118 mL, 480 mL) [ethanol free; contains benzoic acid, propylene glycol, sodium benzoate; cherry flavor]

Gelcap, oral:

Mapap®: 500 mg

Gelcap, rapid release, oral:

Tylenol® Extra Strength: 500 mg

Geltab, oral:

Excedrin® Tension Headache: 500 mg [contains caffeine 65 mg/geltab]

Injection, solution [preservative free]:

Ofirmev™: 10 mg/mL (100 mL)

Liquid, oral:
APAP 500: 500 mg/5 mL (237 mL) [ethanol free, sugar free; cherry flavor]
Silapap Children's: 160 mg/5 mL (118 mL, 237 mL, 473 mL) [ethanol free, sugar free; contains propylene glycol, sodium benzoate; cherry flavor]
Tylenol® Extra Strength: 500 mg/15 mL (240 mL) [ethanol free; contains propylene glycol, sodium benzoate; cherry flavor]
Solution, oral: 160 mg/5 mL (5 mL, 10 mL, 20 mL)
Pain & Fever Children's: 160 mg/5 mL (118 mL, 473 mL) [ethanol free; contains benzoic acid, propylene glycol, sodium benzoate; cherry flavor]
Solution, oral [drops]: 80 mg/0.8 mL (15 mL)
Infantaire: 80 mg/0.8 mL (15 mL, 30 mL)
Little Fevers™: 80 mg/mL (30 mL) [dye free, ethanol free, gluten free; contains propylene glycol, sodium benzoate; berry flavor]
Mapap®: 80 mg/0.8 mL (15 mL) [fruit flavor]
Silapap Infant's: 80 mg/0.8 mL (15 mL, 30 mL) [ethanol free; contains propylene glycol, sodium benzoate; cherry flavor]
Suppository, rectal: 120 mg (12s); 325 mg (12s); 650 mg (12s)
Acephen™: 120 mg (12s, 50s, 100s); 325 mg (6s, 12s, 50s, 100s); 650 mg (12s, 50s, 100s, 500s [DSC])
Feverall®: 80 mg (6s, 50s); 120 mg (6s, 50s); 325 mg (6s, 50s); 650 mg (50s)
Suspension, oral: 160 mg/5 mL (5 mL, 10 mL, 10.15 mL, 20 mL, 20.3 mL)
Mapap® Children's: 160 mg/5 mL (118 mL) [ethanol free; contains propylene glycol, sodium benzoate; cherry flavor]
Nortemp Children's: 160 mg/5 mL (118 mL) [ethanol free; contains propylene glycol, sodium benzoate; cotton candy flavor]
Tylenol® Children's: 160 mg/5 mL (120 mL) [dye free, ethanol free; contains propylene glycol, sodium benzoate; cherry flavor]
Tylenol® Children's: 160 mg/5 mL (120 mL) [ethanol free; contains propylene glycol, sodium 2 mg/5 mL, sodium benzoate; bubblegum flavor]
Tylenol® Children's: 160 mg/5 mL (60 mL, 120 mL) [ethanol free; contains propylene glycol, sodium 2 mg/5 mL, sodium benzoate; cherry flavor]
Tylenol® Children's: 160 mg/5 mL (120 mL) [ethanol free; contains propylene glycol, sodium 2 mg/5 mL, sodium benzoate; grape flavor]
Tylenol® Children's: 160 mg/5 mL (120 mL) [ethanol free; contains propylene glycol, sodium 2 mg/5 mL, sodium benzoate; strawberry flavor]
Suspension, oral [drops]:
Mapap® Infant's: 80 mg/0.8 mL (15 mL, 30 mL) [ethanol free; contains propylene glycol, sodium benzoate; cherry flavor]
Tylenol® Infant's Concentrated: 80 mg/0.8 mL (30 mL) [dye free; contains propylene glycol; cherry flavor]
Tylenol® Infant's Concentrated: 80 mg/0.8 mL (15 mL, 30 mL) [ethanol free; contains sodium benzoate; cherry flavor]
Tylenol® Infant's Concentrated: 80 mg/0.8 mL (15 mL, 30 mL) [ethanol free; contains sodium benzoate; grape flavor]
Syrup, oral:
Triaminic™ Children's Fever Reducer Pain Reliever: 160 mg/5 mL (118 mL) [contains benzoic acid, sodium 6 mg/5 mL; bubblegum flavor]
Triaminic™ Children's Fever Reducer Pain Reliever: 160 mg/5 mL (118 mL) [contains sodium 5 mg/5 mL, sodium benzoate; grape flavor]
Tablet, oral: 325 mg, 500 mg
Aspirin Free Anacin® Extra Strength: 500 mg
Cetafen®: 325 mg
Mapap®: 325 mg
Tylenol®: 325 mg
Valorin: 325 mg [sugar free]
Valorin Extra: 500 mg [sugar free]
Tablet, chewable, oral: 80 mg
Mapap® Children's: 80 mg [fruit flavor]
Tablet, orally disintegrating, oral:
Mapap® Children's: 80 mg [bubblegum flavor]
Mapap® Children's: 80 mg [grape flavor]
Mapap® Junior Rapid Tabs: 160 mg [bubblegum flavor]
Tylenol® Children's Meltaways: 80 mg [scored; bubblegum flavor]
Tylenol® Children's Meltaways: 80 mg [scored; grape flavor]
Tylenol® Jr. Meltaways: 160 mg [bubblegum flavor]
Tylenol® Jr. Meltaways: 160 mg [grape flavor]

Selected References

American Geriatrics Society Panel on Pharmacological Management of Persistent Pain in Older Persons, "Pharmacological Management of Persistent Pain in Older Persons," *J Am Geriatr Soc,* 2009, 57(8):1331-46.

"Recommendations for the Medical Management of Osteoarthritis of the Hip and Knee: 2000 Update. American College of Rheumatology Subcommittee on Osteoarthritis Guidelines," *Arthritis Rheum,* 2000, 43(9):1905-15.

Acetaminophen and Codeine (a seet a MIN oh fen & KOE deen)

Related Information

Acetaminophen *on page 33*

Codeine *on page 407*

Medication Safety Issues

Sound-alike/look-alike issues:

Tylenol® may be confused with atenolol, timolol, Tylox®

High alert medication:

The Institute for Safe Medication Practices (ISMP) includes this medication among its list of drug classes which have a heightened risk of causing significant patient harm when used in error.

Other safety concerns:

Duplicate therapy issues: This product contains acetaminophen, which may be a component of other combination products. Do not exceed the maximum recommended daily dose of acetaminophen.

T3 is an error-prone abbreviation (mistaken as liothyronine)

International issues:

Codex: Brand name for acetaminophen/codeine [Brazil], but also the brand name for *saccharomyces boulardii* [Italy]

Codex [Brazil] may be confused with Cedax brand name for ceftibuten [U.S. and multiple international markets]

Brand Names: U.S. Capital® and Codeine; Tylenol® with Codeine No. 3; Tylenol® with Codeine No. 4

Brand Names: Canada ratio-Emtec; ratio-Lenoltec; Triatec-30; Triatec-8; Triatec-8 Strong; Tylenol Elixir with Codeine; Tylenol No. 1; Tylenol No. 1 Forte; Tylenol No. 2 with Codeine; Tylenol No. 3 with Codeine; Tylenol No. 4 with Codeine

Index Terms Codeine and Acetaminophen; Tylenol #2; Tylenol #3; Tylenol Codeine

Generic Availability (U.S.) Yes

Pharmacologic Category Analgesic, Opioid

Use Relief of mild-to-moderate pain

Dosage

Geriatric Doses should be titrated to appropriate analgesic effect.

One Tylenol® No. 3 tablet every 4 hours; do **not** exceed 4 g/day acetaminophen.

Adult Doses should be adjusted according to severity of pain and response of the patient. Adult doses ≥60 mg codeine fail to give commensurate relief of pain but merely prolong analgesia and are associated with an appreciably increased incidence of side effects.

Cough (Antitussive): Oral: Based on codeine (15-30 mg/dose) every 4-6 hours (maximum: 360 mg/24 hours based on codeine component)

Pain (Analgesic): Oral: Based on codeine (30-60 mg/dose) every 4-6 hours (maximum: 4000 mg/24 hours based on acetaminophen component)

1-2 tablets every 4 hours to a maximum of 12 tablets/24 hours

Renal Impairment See individual agents.

Hepatic Impairment Use with caution. Limited, low-dose therapy is usually well tolerated in hepatic disease/cirrhosis; however, cases of hepatotoxicity at daily acetaminophen dosages <4 g/day have been reported. Avoid chronic use in hepatic impairment.

Controlled Substance C-III; C-V

Dosage Forms Excipient information presented when available (limited, particularly for generics); consult specific product labeling.

Solution, oral [C-V]: Acetaminophen 120 mg and codeine phosphate 12 mg per 5 mL (5 mL, 10 mL, 12.5 mL, 15 mL, 120 mL, 480 mL) [contains alcohol 7%]

Suspension, oral [C-V] (Capital® and Codeine): Acetaminophen 120 mg and codeine phosphate 12 mg per 5 mL (480 mL) [alcohol free; contains propylene glycol, sodium benzoate; fruit punch flavor]

Tablet [C-III]: Acetaminophen 300 mg and codeine phosphate 15 mg; acetaminophen 300 mg and codeine phosphate 30 mg; acetaminophen 300 mg and codeine phosphate 60 mg

Tylenol® with Codeine No. 3: Acetaminophen 300 mg and codeine phosphate 30 mg [contains sodium metabisulfite]

Tylenol® with Codeine No. 4: Acetaminophen 300 mg and codeine phosphate 60 mg [contains sodium metabisulfite]

Dosage Forms: Canada Excipient information presented when available (limited, particularly for generics); consult specific product labeling. **Note:** In countries outside of the U.S., some formulations of Tylenol® with Codeine include caffeine.

Caplet:

ratio-Lenoltec No. 1, Tylenol No. 1: Acetaminophen 300 mg, codeine phosphate 8 mg, and caffeine 15 mg

Tylenol No. 1 Forte: Acetaminophen 500 mg, codeine phosphate 8 mg, and caffeine 15 mg

Solution, oral:

Tylenol Elixir with Codeine: Acetaminophen 160 mg and codeine phosphate 8 mg per 5 mL (500 mL) [contains alcohol 7%, sucrose 31%; cherry flavor]

Tablet:

ratio-Emtec, Triatec-30: Acetaminophen 300 mg and codeine phosphate 30 mg

ratio-Lenoltec No. 1: Acetaminophen 300 mg, codeine phosphate 8 mg, and caffeine 15 mg

ratio-Lenoltec No. 2, Tylenol No. 2 with Codeine: Acetaminophen 300 mg, codeine phosphate 15 mg, and caffeine 15 mg

ratio-Lenoltec No. 3, Tylenol No. 3 with Codeine: Acetaminophen 300 mg, codeine phosphate 30 mg, and caffeine 15 mg

ratio-Lenoltec No. 4, Tylenol No. 4 with Codeine: Acetaminophen 300 mg and codeine phosphate 60 mg

Triatec-8: Acetaminophen 325 mg, codeine phosphate 8 mg, and caffeine 30 mg

Triatec-8 Strong: Acetaminophen 500 mg, codeine phosphate 8 mg, and caffeine 30 mg

◆ **Acetaminophen and Hydrocodone** see Hydrocodone and Acetaminophen on page 880
◆ **Acetaminophen and Oxycodone** see Oxycodone and Acetaminophen on page 1371

Acetaminophen and Phenylephrine (a seet a MIN oh fen & fen il EF rin)

Related Information
Acetaminophen on page 33
Medication Safety Issues
Other safety concerns:
Duplicate therapy issues: This product contains acetaminophen, which may be a component of combination products. Do not exceed the maximum recommended daily dose of acetaminophen.
Brand Names: U.S. Alka-Seltzer Plus® Sinus Formula [OTC]; Cetafen Cold® [OTC]; Contac® Cold + Flu Maximum Strength Non-Drowsy [OTC]; Excedrin® Sinus Headache [OTC]; Mapap® Sinus Congestion and Pain Daytime [OTC]; Sinus Pain & Pressure [OTC]; Sinutab® Sinus [OTC]; Sudafed PE® Pressure + Pain [OTC]; Tylenol® Sinus Congestion & Pain Daytime [OTC]; Vicks® DayQuil® Sinus [OTC]
Index Terms Phenylephrine Hydrochloride and Acetaminophen
Generic Availability (U.S.) Yes: Caplet
Pharmacologic Category Analgesic, Miscellaneous; Decongestant
Use Temporary relief of sinus/nasal congestion and pressure, headache, and minor aches and pains
Dosage
Geriatric & Adult Sinus pain/pressure: Oral: General dosing guidelines, refer to specific product labeling: Acetaminophen 325 mg and phenylephrine 5 mg/caplet: Take 2 caplets every 4 hours as needed; maximum: 12 caplets/24 hours
Special Geriatric Considerations Elderly are more predisposed to the adverse effects of sympathomimetics since they frequently have cardiovascular disease and diabetes mellitus, and are on multiple medications. Since oral and topical phenylephrine can be obtained OTC, elderly patients should be counseled about their proper use and in what disease states they should be avoided.
Dosage Forms Excipient information presented when available (limited, particularly for generics); consult specific product labeling.
Caplet, oral:
Contac® Cold + Flu Maximum Strength Non Drowsy: Acetaminophen 500 mg and phenylephrine hydrochloride 5 mg
Excedrin® Sinus Headache: Acetaminophen 325 mg and phenylephrine hydrochloride 5 mg
Mapap® Sinus Congestion and Pain Daytime, Sinutab® Sinus, Sudafed PE® Pressure + Pain: Acetaminophen 325 mg and phenylephrine hydrochloride 5 mg
Tylenol® Sinus Congestion & Pain Daytime: Acetaminophen 325 mg and phenylephrine hydrochloride 5 mg [Cool Burst™ flavor]
Capsule, liquicap, oral:
Vicks® DayQuil® Sinus: Acetaminophen 325 mg and phenylephrine hydrochloride 5 mg [ethanol free]

Gelcap, oral:
Tylenol® Sinus Congestion & Pain Daytime: Acetaminophen 325 mg and phenylephrine hydrochloride 5 mg
Gelcap, rapid release, oral:
Tylenol® Sinus Congestion & Pain Datyime: Acetaminophen 325 mg and phenylephrine hydrochloride 5 mg
Tablet for solution, oral [effervescent]:
Alka-Seltzer Plus® Sinus Formula: Acetaminophen 250 mg and phenylephrine hydrochloride 5 mg [contains sodium 477 mg/tablet and phenylalanine 4.2 mg/tablet; lemon zest flavor]
Tablet, oral:
Cetafen Cold®: Acetaminophen 500 mg and phenylephrine hydrochloride 5 mg
Sinus Pain & Pressure: Acetaminophen 500 mg and phenylephrine hydrochloride 5 mg

AcetaZOLAMIDE (a set a ZOLE a mide)

Related Information
Glaucoma Drug Therapy *on page 2008*
Medication Safety Issues
International issues:
Diamox [Canada and multiple international markets] may be confused with Diabinese brand name for chlorpropamide [Multiple international markets]; Dobutrex brand name for dobutamine [Multiple international markets]; Trimox brand name for amoxicillin [Brazil]; Zimox brand name for amoxicillin [Italy] and carbidopa/levodopa [Greece]
Brand Names: U.S. Diamox® Sequels®
Brand Names: Canada Apo-Acetazolamide®; Diamox®
Generic Availability (U.S.) Yes
Pharmacologic Category Anticonvulsant, Miscellaneous; Carbonic Anhydrase Inhibitor; Diuretic, Carbonic Anhydrase Inhibitor; Ophthalmic Agent, Antiglaucoma
Use Treatment of glaucoma (chronic simple open-angle, secondary glaucoma, preoperatively in acute angle-closure); drug-induced edema or edema due to congestive heart failure (adjunctive therapy); centrencephalic epilepsies (immediate release dosage form); prevention or amelioration of symptoms associated with acute mountain sickness
Unlabeled/Investigational Use Metabolic alkalosis; respiratory stimulant in COPD; urine alkalinization
Contraindications Hypersensitivity to acetazolamide, sulfonamides, or any component of the formulation; hepatic disease or insufficiency; decreased sodium and/or potassium levels; adrenocortical insufficiency, cirrhosis; hyperchloremic acidosis, severe renal disease or dysfunction; severe pulmonary obstruction; long-term use in noncongestive angle-closure glaucoma
Warnings/Precautions Use with caution in patients with hepatic dysfunction; in cirrhosis, avoid electrolyte and acid/base imbalances that might lead to hepatic encephalopathy. Use with caution in patients with respiratory acidosis and diabetes mellitus (may change glucose control). Use with caution in the elderly; may be more sensitive to side effects. Impairment of mental alertness and/or physical coordination may occur. Chemical similarities are present among sulfonamides, sulfonylureas, carbonic anhydrase inhibitors, thiazides, and loop diuretics (except ethacrynic acid). Use in patients with sulfonamide allergy is specifically contraindicated in product labeling, however, a risk of cross-reaction exists in patients with allergy to any of these compounds; avoid use when previous reaction has been severe. Discontinue if signs of hypersensitivity are noted.

I.M. administration is painful because of the alkaline pH of the drug; use by this route is not recommended.
Adverse Reactions (Reflective of adult population; not specific for elderly) Frequency not defined.
Cardiovascular: Flushing
Central nervous system: Ataxia, confusion, convulsions, depression, dizziness, drowsiness, excitement, fatigue, fever, headache, malaise
Dermatologic: Allergic skin reactions, photosensitivity, Stevens-Johnson syndrome, toxic epidermal necrolysis, urticaria
Endocrine & metabolic: Electrolyte imbalance, hyperglycemia, hypoglycemia, hypokalemia, hyponatremia, metabolic acidosis
Gastrointestinal: Appetite decreased, diarrhea, melena, nausea, taste alteration, vomiting
Genitourinary: Crystalluria, glycosuria, hematuria, polyuria, renal failure
Hematologic: Agranulocytosis, aplastic anemia, leukopenia, thrombocytopenia, thrombocytopenic purpura

◀ Hepatic: Cholestatic jaundice, fulminant hepatic necrosis, hepatic insufficiency, liver function tests abnormal
Local: Pain at injection site
Neuromuscular & skeletal: Flaccid paralysis, paresthesia
Ocular: Myopia
Otic: Hearing disturbance, tinnitus
Miscellaneous: Anaphylaxis

Drug Interactions

Metabolism/Transport Effects Inhibits CYP3A4 (weak)

Avoid Concomitant Use

Avoid concomitant use of AcetaZOLAMIDE with any of the following: Carbonic Anhydrase Inhibitors

Increased Effect/Toxicity

AcetaZOLAMIDE may increase the levels/effects of: Alcohol (Ethyl); Alpha-/Beta-Agonists; Amifostine; Amphetamines; Anticonvulsants (Barbiturate); Anticonvulsants (Hydantoin); Antihypertensives; CarBAMazepine; Carbonic Anhydrase Inhibitors; CNS Depressants; Flecainide; Hypotensive Agents; Memantine; Methotrimeprazine; Primidone; QuiNIDine; RiTUXimab; Selective Serotonin Reuptake Inhibitors; Sodium Phosphates

The levels/effects of AcetaZOLAMIDE may be increased by: Alfuzosin; Diazoxide; Droperidol; Herbs (Hypotensive Properties); HydrOXYzine; MAO Inhibitors; Methotrimeprazine; Pentoxifylline; Phosphodiesterase 5 Inhibitors; Prostacyclin Analogues; Salicylates

Decreased Effect

AcetaZOLAMIDE may decrease the levels/effects of: Lithium; Methenamine; Primidone; Trientine

The levels/effects of AcetaZOLAMIDE may be decreased by: Herbs (Hypertensive Properties); Ketorolac; Ketorolac (Nasal); Ketorolac (Systemic); Mefloquine; Methylphenidate; Yohimbine

Stability

Capsules, tablets: Store at controlled room temperature.
Injection: Store vial for injection (prior to reconstitution) at controlled room temperature. Reconstitute with at least 5 mL sterile water to provide a solution containing not more than 100 mg/mL. Reconstituted solution may be refrigerated (2°C to 8°C) for 1 week, however, use within 12 hours is recommended. Further dilute in D_5W or NS for I.V. infusion. Stability of IVPB solution is 5 days at room temperature (25°C) and 44 days at refrigeration (5°C).

Mechanism of Action Reversible inhibition of the enzyme carbonic anhydrase resulting in reduction of hydrogen ion secretion at renal tubule and an increased renal excretion of sodium, potassium, bicarbonate, and water to decrease production of aqueous humor; also inhibits carbonic anhydrase in central nervous system to retard abnormal and excessive discharge from CNS neurons

Pharmacodynamics/Kinetics

Onset of action: Capsule, extended release: 2 hours; I.V.: 2 minutes
Peak effect: Capsule, extended release: 8-12 hours; I.V.: 15 minutes; Tablet: 2-4 hours
Duration: Inhibition of aqueous humor secretion: Capsule, extended release: 18-24 hours; I.V.: 4-5 hours; Tablet: 8-12 hours
Distribution: Erythrocytes, kidneys; blood-brain barrier
Excretion: Urine (70% to 100% as unchanged drug)

Dosage

Geriatric Oral: Initial: 250 mg once or twice daily; use lowest effective dose possible.
Adult Note: I.M. administration is not recommended.

Glaucoma:
Chronic simple (open-angle): Oral: 250 mg 1-4 times/day or 500 mg extended release capsule twice daily
Secondary, acute (closed-angle): I.V.: 250-500 mg, may repeat in 2-4 hours to a maximum of 1 g/day

Edema: Oral, I.V.: 250-375 mg once daily

Epilepsy: Oral: 8-30 mg/kg/day in 1-4 divided doses, not to exceed 1 g/day. **Note:** Extended release capsule is not recommended for treatment of epilepsy.

Metabolic alkalosis (unlabeled use): I.V. 250 mg every 6 hours for 4 doses or 500 mg single dose; reassess need based upon acid-base status

Mountain sickness: Oral: Manufacturer's labeling: 500-1000 mg daily, in divided doses every 8-12 hours (immediate release tablets) or divided every 12-24 hours (extended release capsules). Alternative recommendations suggest use of lower doses to reduce side effects: 125-250 mg twice daily for prevention or treatment of mild sickness, and 250 mg twice daily for treatment of moderate sickness (Hackett, 2001). Therapy should begin 24-48 hours before and continue during ascent and for at least 48 hours after arrival at the high altitude.

Note: In situations of rapid ascent (such as rescue or military operations), 1000 mg/day is recommended (manufacturer's labeling).

Urine alkalinization (unlabeled use): Oral: 5 mg/kg/dose repeated 2-3 times over 24 hours

Respiratory stimulant in COPD (unlabeled use): Oral, I.V.: 250 mg twice daily

Renal Impairment

Cl_{cr} 10-50 mL/minute: Administer every 12 hours.

Cl_{cr} <10 mL/minute: Avoid use (ineffective).

Moderately dialyzable (20% to 50%)

Administration

Oral: May be administered with food. May cause an alteration in taste, especially carbonated beverages. Short-acting tablets may be crushed and suspended in cherry or chocolate syrup to disguise the bitter taste of the drug; do not use fruit juices. Alternatively, submerge tablet in 10 mL of hot water and add 10 mL honey or syrup.

I.M.: I.M. administration is painful because of the alkaline pH of the drug; use by this route is not recommended.

I.V.: No specific guidance given by manufacturer, but I.V. push at a rate of up to 500 mg over 3 minutes has been reported in a clinical trial (Mazur, 1999); a study to assess cerebrovascular reserve has used rapid I.V. push of up to 1 g over ≤1 minute (Piepgras, 1990)

Monitoring Parameters Intraocular pressure, potassium, serum bicarbonate; serum electrolytes, periodic CBC with differential

Test Interactions May cause false-positive results for urinary protein with Albustix®, Labstix®, Albutest®, Bumintest®; interferes with HPLC theophylline assay and serum uric acid levels

Pharmacotherapy Pearls Drug may cause substantial increase in blood glucose in some diabetic patients; sustained release capsule is not recommended for treatment of epilepsy; the use of analgesic doses of salicylates should be avoided in patients treated with acetazolamide, especially older adults

Special Geriatric Considerations Oral carbonic anhydrase inhibitors are useful for patients who have difficulty administering ophthalmic drugs, who do not achieve sufficient lowering of intraocular pressure, or who cannot tolerate other agents. Malaise and complaints of tiredness and myalgia are signs of excessive dosing and acidosis in older adults. Orthostatic hypotension may occur; assess blood pressure. Note renal impairment recommendations; many elderly have Cl_{cr} <50 mL/minute.

Dosage Forms Excipient information presented when available (limited, particularly for generics); consult specific product labeling.

Capsule, extended release, oral: 500 mg

Capsule, sustained release, oral:

Diamox® Sequels®: 500 mg

Injection, powder for reconstitution: 500 mg

Tablet, oral: 125 mg, 250 mg

Selected References

Chapron DJ, Gomolin IH, and Sweeney KR, "Acetazolamide Blood Concentrations are Excessive in the Elderly: Propensity for Acidosis and Relationship to Renal Function," *J Clin Pharmacol*, 1989, 29(4):348-53.

Chapron DJ, Sweeney KR, Feig PU, et al, "Influence of Advanced Age on the Disposition of Acetazolamide," *Br J Clin Pharmacol*, 1985, 19(3):363-71.

Rousseau P and Fuentevilla-Clifton A, "Acetazolamide and Salicylate Interaction in the Elderly: A Case Report," *J Am Geriatr Soc*, 1993, 41(8):868-9.

◆ **Acetoxymethylprogesterone** see MedroxyPROGESTERone *on page 1122*

Acetylcholine (a se teel KOE leen)

Medication Safety Issues

Sound-alike/look-alike issues:

Acetylcholine may be confused with acetylcysteine

Brand Names: U.S. Miochol®-E

Brand Names: Canada Miochol®-E

Index Terms Acetylcholine Chloride

Generic Availability (U.S.) No

Pharmacologic Category Cholinergic Agonist; Ophthalmic Agent, Miotic

Use Produces complete miosis in cataract surgery, keratoplasty, iridectomy, and other anterior segment surgery where rapid miosis is required

Contraindications Hypersensitivity to acetylcholine chloride or any component of the formulation; acute iritis and acute inflammatory disease of the anterior chamber

Warnings/Precautions During cataract surgery, use only after lens is in place. Systemic effects rarely occur but can cause problems for patients with acute cardiac failure, bronchial asthma, peptic ulcer, hyperthyroidism, GI spasm, urinary tract obstruction, and Parkinson's disease; open under aseptic conditions only.

◀ **Adverse Reactions (Reflective of adult population; not specific for elderly)** Frequency not defined.
Cardiovascular: Bradycardia, flushing, hypotension
Central nervous system: Headache
Ocular: Clouding, corneal edema, decompensation
Respiratory: Dyspnea
Miscellaneous: Diaphoresis

Drug Interactions

Avoid Concomitant Use There are no known interactions where it is recommended to avoid concomitant use.

Increased Effect/Toxicity
The levels/effects of Acetylcholine may be increased by: Acetylcholinesterase Inhibitors

Decreased Effect There are no known significant interactions involving a decrease in effect.

Stability Store unopened vial at 4°C to 25°C (39°F to 77°F); prevent from freezing. Prepare solution immediately before use and discard unused portion. Acetylcholine solutions are unstable; reconstitute immediately before use.

Mechanism of Action Causes contraction of the sphincter muscles of the iris, resulting in miosis and contraction of the ciliary muscle, leading to accommodation spasm

Pharmacodynamics/Kinetics
Onset of action: Rapid
Duration: ~10 minutes

Dosage

Geriatric & Adult To produce miosis: Intraocular: 0.5-2 mL of 1% injection (5-20 mg) instilled into anterior chamber before or after securing one or more sutures

Administration Discard any solution that is not used; open under aseptic conditions only

Dosage Forms Excipient information presented when available (limited, particularly for generics); consult specific product labeling.
Powder for solution, intraocular, as chloride:
Miochol®-E: 20 mg (2 mL) [supplied with diluent; reconstitution results in 1:100 solution]

◆ **Acetylcholine Chloride** *see* Acetylcholine *on page 41*
◆ **Acetylcysteine, Methylcobalamin, and Methylfolate** *see* Methylfolate, Methylcobalamin, and Acetylcysteine *on page 1178*
◆ **Acetylcysteine, Methylfolate, and Methylcobalamin** *see* Methylfolate, Methylcobalamin, and Acetylcysteine *on page 1178*
◆ **Acetylsalicylic Acid** *see* Aspirin *on page 153*
◆ **Achromycin** *see* Tetracycline *on page 1772*
◆ **Aciclovir** *see* Acyclovir (Systemic) *on page 43*
◆ **Aciclovir** *see* Acyclovir (Topical) *on page 46*
◆ **Acid Gone [OTC]** *see* Aluminum Hydroxide and Magnesium Carbonate *on page 80*
◆ **Acid Gone Extra Strength [OTC]** *see* Aluminum Hydroxide and Magnesium Carbonate *on page 80*
◆ **Acidulated Phosphate Fluoride** *see* Fluoride *on page 751*
◆ **AcipHex®** *see* RABEprazole *on page 1571*
◆ **Aclovate®** *see* Alclometasone *on page 53*
◆ **Act® [OTC]** *see* Fluoride *on page 751*
◆ **Actemra®** *see* Tocilizumab *on page 1816*
◆ **Acticin® [DSC]** *see* Permethrin *on page 1429*
◆ **Actigall®** *see* Ursodiol *on page 1882*
◆ **Actiq®** *see* FentaNYL *on page 709*
◆ **Activase®** *see* Alteplase *on page 75*
◆ **Activated Dimethicone** *see* Simethicone *on page 1679*
◆ **Activated Ergosterol** *see* Ergocalciferol *on page 618*
◆ **Activated Methylpolysiloxane** *see* Simethicone *on page 1679*
◆ **Act® Kids [OTC]** *see* Fluoride *on page 751*
◆ **Actonel®** *see* Risedronate *on page 1619*
◆ **Actonel® and Calcium** *see* Risedronate and Calcium *on page 1621*
◆ **Actoplus Met®** *see* Pioglitazone and Metformin *on page 1461*
◆ **Actoplus Met® XR** *see* Pioglitazone and Metformin *on page 1461*
◆ **Actos®** *see* Pioglitazone *on page 1458*
◆ **Act® Restoring™ [OTC]** *see* Fluoride *on page 751*
◆ **Act® Total Care™ [OTC]** *see* Fluoride *on page 751*
◆ **Acular®** *see* Ketorolac (Ophthalmic) *on page 1012*
◆ **Acular LS®** *see* Ketorolac (Ophthalmic) *on page 1012*
◆ **Acuvail®** *see* Ketorolac (Ophthalmic) *on page 1012*
◆ **ACV** *see* Acyclovir (Systemic) *on page 43*
◆ **ACV** *see* Acyclovir (Topical) *on page 46*
◆ **Acycloguanosine** *see* Acyclovir (Systemic) *on page 43*

♦ **Acycloguanosine** *see* Acyclovir (Topical) *on page 46*

Acyclovir (Systemic) (ay SYE kloe veer)

Medication Safety Issues
Sound-alike/look-alike issues:
Acyclovir may be confused with ganciclovir, Retrovir®, valacyclovir
Zovirax® may be confused with Doribax®, Valtrex®, Zithromax®, Zostrix®, Zyloprim®, Zyvox®
Brand Names: U.S. Zovirax®
Brand Names: Canada Apo-Acyclovir®; Gen-Acyclovir; Mylan-Acyclovir; Novo-Acyclovir; Nu-Acyclovir; ratio-Acyclovir; Teva-Acyclovir; Zovirax®
Index Terms Aciclovir; ACV; Acycloguanosine
Generic Availability (U.S.) Yes
Pharmacologic Category Antiviral Agent
Use Treatment of genital herpes simplex virus (HSV) and HSV encephalitis
Unlabeled/Investigational Use Prevention of HSV reactivation in HIV-positive patients; prevention of HSV reactivation in hematopoietic stem cell transplant (HSCT); prevention of HSV reactivation during periods of neutropenia in patients with cancer; prevention of varicella zoster virus (VZV) reactivation in allogenic HSCT; prevention of CMV reactivation in low-risk allogeneic HSCT; treatment of disseminated HSV or VZV in immunocompromised patients with cancer; empiric treatment of suspected encephalitis in immunocompromised patients with cancer; treatment of initial and prophylaxis of recurrent mucosal and cutaneous herpes simplex (HSV-1 and HSV-2) infections in immunocompromised patients
Contraindications Hypersensitivity to acyclovir, valacyclovir, or any component of the formulation
Warnings/Precautions Use with caution in immunocompromised patients; thrombocytopenic purpura/hemolytic uremic syndrome (TTP/HUS) has been reported. Use caution in the elderly, pre-existing renal disease (may require dosage modification), or in those receiving other nephrotoxic drugs. Renal failure (sometimes fatal) has been reported. Maintain adequate hydration during oral or intravenous therapy. Use I.V. preparation with caution in patients with underlying neurologic abnormalities, serious hepatic or electrolyte abnormalities, or substantial hypoxia.

Varicella-zoster: Treatment should begin within 24 hours of appearance of rash; oral route not recommended for routine use in otherwise healthy children with varicella, but may be effective in patients at increased risk of moderate-to-severe infection (>12 years of age, chronic cutaneous or pulmonary disorders, long-term salicylate therapy, corticosteroid therapy).

Adverse Reactions (Reflective of adult population; not specific for elderly)
Oral:
>10%: Central nervous system: Malaise (≤12%)
1% to 10%:
Central nervous system: Headache (≤2%)
Gastrointestinal: Nausea (2% to 5%), vomiting (≤3%), diarrhea (2% to 3%)
Parenteral:
1% to 10%:
Dermatologic: Hives (2%), itching (2%), rash (2%)
Gastrointestinal: Nausea/vomiting (7%)
Hepatic: Liver function tests increased (1% to 2%)
Local: Inflammation at injection site or phlebitis (9%)
Renal: BUN increased (5% to 10%), creatinine increased (5% to 10%), acute renal failure
Drug Interactions
Avoid Concomitant Use
Avoid concomitant use of Acyclovir (Systemic) with any of the following: Zoster Vaccine
Increased Effect/Toxicity
Acyclovir (Systemic) may increase the levels/effects of: Mycophenolate; Tenofovir; Zidovudine

The levels/effects of Acyclovir (Systemic) may be increased by: Mycophenolate
Decreased Effect
Acyclovir (Systemic) may decrease the levels/effects of: Zoster Vaccine
Ethanol/Nutrition/Herb Interactions Food: Does not affect absorption of oral acyclovir.
Stability
Capsule, tablet: Store at controlled room temperature of 15°C to 25°C (59°F to 77°F); protect from moisture.
Injection: Store powder at controlled room temperature of 15°C to 25°C (59°F to 77°F). Reconstitute acyclovir 500 mg powder with SWFI 10 mL; do not use bacteriostatic water

containing benzyl alcohol or parabens. For intravenous infusion, dilute in D_5W, D_5NS, $D_5\frac{1}{4}NS$, $D_5\frac{1}{2}NS$, LR, or NS to a final concentration ≤7 mg/mL. Concentrations >10 mg/mL increase the risk of phlebitis. Reconstituted solutions remain stable for 12 hours at room temperature. Do not refrigerate reconstituted solutions or solutions diluted for infusion as they may precipitate. Once diluted for infusion, use within 24 hours.

Mechanism of Action Acyclovir is converted to acyclovir monophosphate by virus-specific thymidine kinase then further converted to acyclovir triphosphate by other cellular enzymes. Acyclovir triphosphate inhibits DNA synthesis and viral replication by competing with deoxyguanosine triphosphate for viral DNA polymerase and being incorporated into viral DNA.

Pharmacodynamics/Kinetics

Absorption: Oral: 15% to 30%

Distribution: V_d: 0.8 L/kg (63.6 L): Widely (eg, brain, kidney, lungs, liver, spleen, muscle, uterus, vagina, CSF)

Protein binding: 9% to 33%

Metabolism: Converted by viral enzymes to acyclovir monophosphate, and further converted to diphosphate then triphosphate (active form) by cellular enzymes

Bioavailability: Oral: 10% to 20% with normal renal function (bioavailability decreases with increased dose)

Half-life elimination: Terminal: Adults: 3 hours

Time to peak, serum: Oral: Within 1.5-2 hours

Excretion: Urine (62% to 90% as unchanged drug and metabolite)

Dosage

Geriatric & Adult Note: Obese patients should be dosed using ideal body weight

Genital herpes simplex virus (HSV) infection:

I.V.: Immunocompetent: Initial episode, severe: 5 mg/kg/dose every 8 hours for 5-7 days **or** 5-10 mg/kg/dose every 8 hours for 2-7 days, follow with oral therapy to complete at least 10 days of therapy (CDC, 2010)

Oral:

Initial episode: 200 mg every 4 hours while awake (5 times/day) for 10 days **or** 400 mg 3 times/day for 7-10 days (CDC, 2010)

Recurrence: 200 mg every 4 hours while awake (5 times/day) for 5 days (per manufacturer's labeling; begin at earliest signs of disease)

Alternatively, the following regimens are also recommended by the CDC: 400 mg 3 times/day for 5 days; 800 mg twice daily for 5 days; 800 mg 3 times/day for 2 days (CDC, 2010)

Chronic suppression: 400 mg twice daily or 200 mg 3-5 times/day, for up to 12 months followed by re-evaluation (per manufacturer's labeling)

Herpes zoster (shingles):

Oral: Immunocompetent: 800 mg every 4 hours (5 times/day) for 7-10 days

I.V.: Immunocompromised: 10 mg/kg/dose or 500 mg/m²/dose every 8 hours for 7 days

HSV encephalitis: I.V.: 10 mg/kg/dose every 8 hours for 10 days (per manufacturer's labeling); 10-15 mg/kg/dose every 8 hours for 14-21 days also reported

Mucocutaneous HSV:

I.V.: Immunocompromised: Treatment: 5 mg/kg/dose every 8 hours for 7 days (Leflore, 2000); dosing for up to 14 days also reported

Oral (unlabeled use): Immunocompromised: 400 mg 5 times/day for 7 days (Leflore, 2000)

Orolabial HSV (unlabeled use): Oral (immunocompetent):

Treatment: 200-400 mg 5 times/day for 5 days (Cernik, 2008; Leflore, 2000; Spruance, 1990) for episodic/recurrent treatment; for initial treatment, limited data are available, 200 mg 5 times/day or 400 mg 3 times/day for 7-10 days has been recommended by some clinicians.

Chronic suppression: 400 mg 2 times/day (has been clinically evaluated for up to 1 year) (Cernik, 2008; Rooney, 1993)

Varicella-zoster (chickenpox): Begin treatment within the first 24 hours of rash onset:

Oral: >40 kg (immunocompetent): 800 mg/dose 4 times a day for 5 days

I.V.:

Manufacturer's labeling (immunocompromised): 10 mg/kg/dose every 8 hours for 7 days

CDC HIV guidelines (immunocompromised): 10-15 mg/kg/dose every 8 hours for 7-10 days

Prevention of HSV reactivation in HIV-positive patients (unlabeled use): Oral: 400-800 mg 2-3 times/day (CDC, 2010)

Prevention of HSV reactivation in HSCT (unlabeled use): CDC recommendation: **Note:** Start at the beginning of conditioning therapy and continue until engraftment or until mucositis resolves (~30 days)

Oral: 200 mg 3 times/day

I.V.: 250 mg/m²/dose every 12 hours

Prevention of VZV reactivation in allogeneic HSCT (unlabeled use): *NCCN guidelines:* Oral: 800 mg twice a day

Prevention of CMV reactivation in low-risk allogeneic HSCT (unlabeled use): *NCCN guidelines:* **Note:** Requires close monitoring (due to weak activity); not for use in patients at high risk for CMV disease: Oral: 800 mg 4 times/day

Treatment of disseminated HSV or VZV or empiric treatment of suspected encephalitis in immunocompromised patients with cancer: (unlabeled use): *NCCN guidelines:* I.V.: 10-12 mg/kg/dose every 8 hours

Treatment of episodic HSV infection in HIV-positive patient (unlabeled use): Oral: 400 mg 3 times/day for 5-10 days (CDC, 2010)

Renal Impairment

Oral:

Cl_{cr} 10-25 mL/minute/1.73 m^2: Normal dosing regimen 800 mg every 4 hours: Administer 800 mg every 8 hours

Cl_{cr} <10 mL/minute/1.73 m^2:

Normal dosing regimen 200 mg every 4 hours or 400 mg every 12 hours: Administer 200 mg every 12 hours

Normal dosing regimen 800 mg every 4 hours: Administer 800 mg every 12 hours

I.V.:

Cl_{cr} 25-50 mL/minute/1.73 m^2: Administer recommended dose every 12 hours

Cl_{cr} 10-25 mL/minute/1.73 m^2: Administer recommended dose every 24 hours

Cl_{cr} <10 mL/minute/1.73 m^2: Administer 50% of recommended dose every 24 hours

Intermittent hemodialysis (IHD) (administer after hemodialysis on dialysis days): Dialyzable (60% reduction following a 6-hour session): I.V.: 2.5-5 mg/kg every 24 hours (Heintz, 2009). **Note:** Dosing dependent on the assumption of 3 times/week, complete IHD sessions.

Peritoneal dialysis (PD): Administer 50% of normal dose once daily; no supplemental dose needed

Continuous renal replacement therapy (CRRT) (Heintz, 2009; Trotman, 2005): Drug clearance is highly dependent on the method of renal replacement, filter type, and flow rate. Appropriate dosing requires close monitoring of pharmacologic response, signs of adverse reactions due to drug accumulation, as well as drug concentrations in relation to target trough (if appropriate). The following are general recommendations only (based on dialysate flow/ultrafiltration rates of 1-2 L/hour and minimal residual renal function) and should not supersede clinical judgment:

CVVH: I.V.: 5-10 mg/kg every 24 hours

CVVHD/CVVHDF: I.V.: 5-10 mg/kg every 12-24 hours

Note: The higher end of dosage range (eg, 10 mg/kg every 12 hours for CVVHDF) is recommended for viral meningoencephalitis and varicella-zoster virus infections.

Administration

Oral: May be administered with or without food.

I.V.: Avoid rapid infusion; infuse over 1 hour to prevent renal damage; maintain adequate hydration of patient; check for phlebitis and rotate infusion sites. Avoid I.M. or SubQ administration.

Monitoring Parameters Urinalysis, BUN, serum creatinine, liver enzymes, CBC

Special Geriatric Considerations For herpes zoster, acyclovir should be started within 72 hours of the appearance of the rash to be effective. Dose adjustment may be necessary depending on creatinine clearance.

Dosage Forms Excipient information presented when available (limited, particularly for generics); consult specific product labeling.

Capsule, oral: 200 mg

Zovirax®: 200 mg

Injection, powder for reconstitution, as sodium [strength expressed as base]: 500 mg, 1000 mg

Injection, solution, as sodium [strength expressed as base, preservative free]: 50 mg/mL (10 mL, 20 mL)

Suspension, oral: 200 mg/5 mL (473 mL)

Zovirax®: 200 mg/5 mL (473 mL) [banana flavor]

Tablet, oral: 400 mg, 800 mg

Zovirax®: 400 mg

Zovirax®: 800 mg [scored]

Acyclovir (Topical) (ay SYE kloe veer)

Medication Safety Issues
  Sound-alike/look-alike issues:
  Acyclovir may be confused with ganciclovir, Retrovir®, valacyclovir
  Zovirax® may be confused with Doribax®, Valtrex®, Zithromax®, Zostrix®, Zyloprim®, Zyvox®
  International issues:
  Opthavir [Mexico] may be confused with Optivar brand name for azelastine [U.S.]
Brand Names: U.S. Zovirax®
Brand Names: Canada Zovirax®
Index Terms Aciclovir; ACV; Acycloguanosine
Generic Availability (U.S.) No
Pharmacologic Category Antiviral Agent, Topical
Use Treatment of herpes labialis (cold sores), mucocutaneous HSV in immunocompromised patients
Dosage
  Geriatric & Adult
  Genital HSV: Topical: Immunocompromised: Ointment: Initial episode: 1/2" ribbon of ointment for a 4" square surface area every 3 hours (6 times/day) for 7 days
  Herpes labialis (cold sores): Topical: Apply 5 times/day for 4 days
  Mucocutaneous HSV: Topical: Ointment: Non-life-threatening, immunocompromised: 1/2" ribbon of ointment for a 4" square surface area every 3 hours (6 times/day) for 7 days
Dosage Forms Excipient information presented when available (limited, particularly for generics); consult specific product labeling.
  Cream, topical:
    Zovirax®: 5% (2 g, 5 g)
  Ointment, topical:
    Zovirax®: 5% (15 g, 30 g)

◆ **Adacel®** see Diphtheria and Tetanus Toxoids, and Acellular Pertussis Vaccine on page 531
◆ **Adalat® CC** see NIFEdipine on page 1300

Adalimumab (a da LIM yoo mab)

Medication Safety Issues
  Sound-alike/look-alike issues:
  Humira® may be confused with Humulin®, Humalog®
  Humira® Pen may be confused with HumaPen® Memoir®
Brand Names: U.S. Humira®; Humira® Pen
Brand Names: Canada Humira®
Index Terms Antitumor Necrosis Factor Alpha (Human); D2E7; Human Antitumor Necrosis Factor Alpha
Generic Availability (U.S.) No
Pharmacologic Category Antirheumatic, Disease Modifying; Gastrointestinal Agent, Miscellaneous; Monoclonal Antibody; Tumor Necrosis Factor (TNF) Blocking Agent
Use
  Treatment of active rheumatoid arthritis (moderate-to-severe) and active psoriatic arthritis; may be used alone or in combination with disease-modifying antirheumatic drugs (DMARDs); treatment of ankylosing spondylitis
  Treatment of moderately- to severely-active Crohn's disease in patients with inadequate response to conventional treatment, or patients who have lost response to or are intolerant of infliximab
  Treatment of moderate-to-severe plaque psoriasis
Medication Guide Available Yes
Contraindications There are no contraindications listed within the FDA-approved labeling.

  Canadian labeling: Additional contraindications (not in U.S. labeling): Hypersensitivity to adalimumab or any component of the formulation; severe infection (eg, sepsis, tuberculosis, opportunistic infection)
Warnings/Precautions [U.S. Boxed Warnings]: Patients should be evaluated for latent tuberculosis infection with a tuberculin skin test prior to therapy. Treatment of latent tuberculosis should be initiated before adalimumab is used. Tuberculosis (disseminated or extrapulmonary) has been reactivated while on adalimumab. Most cases have been reported within the first 8 months of treatment. Doses higher than recommended are associated with an increased risk for tuberculosis reactivation. **Patients with initial negative**

tuberculin skin tests should receive continued monitoring for tuberculosis throughout treatment; active tuberculosis has developed in this population during treatment. Rare reactivation of hepatitis B virus (HBV) has occurred in chronic virus carriers; evaluate prior to initiation, during, and for several months after treatment. Evaluate patients at risk for HBV infection prior to therapy to determine HBV status. Adalimumab may affect defenses against infections and malignancies.

[U.S. Boxed Warning]: Serious and potential fatal infections (including invasive fungal and other opportunistic infections) have been reported in patients receiving TNF-blocking agents, including adalimumab. Cases of unrecognized invasive fungal infections (eg, histoplasmosis, blastomycosis, coccidioidomycosis) have also been reported with anti-TNF agent use. Use caution with chronic infection, history of recurrent infection, or predis-position to infection (eg, diabetes or residence/travel from areas of endemic mycoses). Do not give to patients with an active chronic or localized infection. Many of the serious infections have occurred in patients on concomitant immunosuppressive therapy. Other opportunistic infections included *Aspergillus* and *Nocardia*. Use caution in patients who have resided in regions where histoplasmosis and tuberculosis are endemic. Patients who develop a new infection while undergoing treatment with adalimumab should be monitored closely. If a patient develops a serious infection or sepsis, adalimumab should be discontinued. Serious infections were reported when abatacept or anakinra was used with TNF-blocking agents; therefore, concurrent use of adalimumab and abatacept or anakinra is not recommended. [U.S. Boxed Warning]: Lymphoma and other malignancies have been reported in children and adolescent patients receiving other TNF-blocking agents. Half the cases are lymphomas (Hodgkin's and non-Hodgkin's) and the other cases are varied, but include malignancies not typically observed in this population. Most patients were receiving concomitant immunosup-pressants. [U.S. Boxed Warning]: Hepatosplenic T-cell lymphoma (HSTCL), a rare T-cell lymphoma, has also been reported primarily in patients with Crohn's disease or ulcerative colitis treated with adalimumab and who received concomitant azathioprine or mercaptopurine; reports occurred predominantly in adolescent and young adult males. Rare cases of lymphoma have also been reported in association with adalimumab. A higher incidence of nonmelanoma skin cancers was noted in adalimumab treated patients, when compared to the control group. Impact on the development and course of malignancies is not fully defined. May exacerbate pre-existing or recent-onset central or peripheral nervous system demyelinating disorders. Consider discontinuing use in patients who develop periph-eral or central nervous system demyelinating disorders during treatment.

May exacerbate pre-existing or recent-onset demyelinating CNS disorders. Worsening and new-onset heart failure (HF) has been reported; use caution in patients with decreased left ventricular function. Use caution in patients with HF. Patients should be brought up to date with all immunizations before initiating therapy. No data are available concerning the effects of adalimumab on vaccination. Live vaccines should not be given concurrently. No data are available concerning secondary transmission of live vaccines in patients receiving adalimu-mab. Rare cases of pancytopenia (including aplastic anemia) have been reported with TNF-blocking agents; with significant hematologic abnormalities, consider discontinuing therapy. Positive antinuclear antibody titers have been detected in patients (with negative baselines) treated with adalimumab. Rare cases of autoimmune disorder, including lupus-like syndrome, have been reported; monitor and discontinue adalimumab if symptoms develop. May cause hypersensitivity reactions, including anaphylaxis; monitor. Infection and malignancy has been reported at a higher incidence in elderly patients compared to younger adults; use caution in elderly patients. The packaging (needle cover of prefilled syringe) may contain latex. Product may contain polysorbate 80.

Adverse Reactions (Reflective of adult population; not specific for elderly)
>10%:
  Central nervous system: Headache (12%)
  Dermatologic: Rash (6% to 12%)
  Local: Injection site reaction (12% to 20%; includes erythema, itching, hemorrhage, pain, swelling)
  Neuromuscular & skeletal: CPK increased (15%)
  Respiratory: Upper respiratory tract infection (17%), sinusitis (11%)
  Miscellaneous: Antibodies to adalimumab (3% to 26%; significance unknown), positive ANA (12%)
5% to 10%:
  Cardiovascular: Hypertension (5%)
  Endocrine & metabolic: Hyperlipidemia (7%), hypercholesterolemia (6%)
  Gastrointestinal: Nausea (9%), abdominal pain (7%)
  Genitourinary: Urinary tract infection (8%)
  Hepatic: Alkaline phosphatase increased (5%)
  Local: Injection site reaction (8%; other than erythema, itching, hemorrhage, pain, swelling)

Neuromuscular & skeletal: Back pain (6%)

Renal: Hematuria (5%)

Miscellaneous: Accidental injury (10%), flu-like syndrome (7%)

<5%:

Cardiovascular: Arrhythmia, atrial fibrillation, chest pain, CHF, coronary artery disorder, heart arrest, MI, palpitation, pericardial effusion, pericarditis, peripheral edema, syncope, tachycardia, thrombosis (leg), vascular disorder

Central nervous system: Confusion, fever, hypertensive encephalopathy, multiple sclerosis, subdural hematoma

Dermatologic: Cellulitis, erysipelas

Endocrine & metabolic: Dehydration, menstrual disorder, parathyroid disorder

Gastrointestinal: Diverticulitis, esophagitis, gastroenteritis, gastrointestinal hemorrhage, vomiting

Genitourinary: Cystitis, pelvic pain

Hematologic: Agranulocytosis, granulocytopenia, leukopenia, pancytopenia, paraproteinemia, polycythemia

Hepatic: Cholecystitis, cholelithiasis, hepatic necrosis

Neuromuscular & skeletal: Arthralgia, arthritis, bone fracture, bone necrosis, joint disorder, muscle cramps, myasthenia, pain in extremity, paresthesia, pyogenic arthritis, synovitis, tendon disorder, tremor

Ocular: Cataract

Renal: Kidney calculus, pyelonephritis

Respiratory: Asthma, bronchospasm, dyspnea, lung function decreased, pleural effusion, pneumonia

Miscellaneous: Adenoma, allergic reactions (1%), carcinoma (including breast, gastrointestinal, skin, urogenital), healing abnormality, herpes zoster, ketosis, lupus erythematosus syndrome, lymphoma, melanoma, postsurgical infection, sepsis, tuberculosis (reactivation of latent infection; miliary, lymphatic, peritoneal and pulmonary)

Drug Interactions

Avoid Concomitant Use

Avoid concomitant use of Adalimumab with any of the following: Abatacept; Anakinra; BCG; Belimumab; Canakinumab; Certolizumab Pegol; Natalizumab; Pimecrolimus; Rilonacept; Tacrolimus (Topical); Vaccines (Live)

Increased Effect/Toxicity

Adalimumab may increase the levels/effects of: Abatacept; Anakinra; Belimumab; Canakinumab; Certolizumab Pegol; Leflunomide; Natalizumab; Rilonacept; Vaccines (Live)

The levels/effects of Adalimumab may be increased by: Abciximab; Denosumab; Pimecrolimus; Roflumilast; Tacrolimus (Topical); Trastuzumab

Decreased Effect

Adalimumab may decrease the levels/effects of: BCG; Sipuleucel-T; Vaccines (Inactivated); Vaccines (Live)

The levels/effects of Adalimumab may be decreased by: Echinacea

Ethanol/Nutrition/Herb Interactions Herb/nutraceutical: Echinacea may decrease the therapeutic effects of adalimumab; avoid concurrent use.

Stability Store under refrigeration at 2°C to 8°C (36°F to 46°F); do not freeze. Protect from light.

Mechanism of Action Adalimumab is a recombinant monoclonal antibody that binds to human tumor necrosis factor alpha (TNF-alpha), thereby interfering with binding to TNFα receptor sites and subsequent cytokine-driven inflammatory processes. Elevated TNF levels in the synovial fluid are involved in the pathologic pain and joint destruction in immune-mediated arthritis. Adalimumab decreases signs and symptoms of psoriatic arthritis, rheumatoid arthritis, and ankylosing spondylitis. It inhibits progression of structural damage of rheumatoid and psoriatic arthritis. Reduces signs and symptoms and maintains clinical remission in Crohn's disease; reduces epidermal thickness and inflammatory cell infiltration in plaque psoriasis.

Pharmacodynamics/Kinetics

Distribution: V_d: 4.7-6 L; Synovial fluid concentrations: 31% to 96% of serum

Bioavailability: Absolute: 64%

Half-life elimination: Terminal: ~2 weeks (range: 10-20 days)

Time to peak, serum: SubQ: 131 ± 56 hours

Excretion: Clearance increased in the presence of anti-adalimumab antibodies; decreased in patients ≥40 years of age

Dosage

Geriatric & Adult

Rheumatoid arthritis: SubQ: 40 mg every other week; may be administered with other DMARDs; patients not taking methotrexate may increase dose to 40 mg every week

Ankylosing spondylitis, psoriatic arthritis: SubQ: 40 mg every other week

Crohn's disease: SubQ: Initial: 160 mg (given as 4 injections on day 1 or as 2 injections/day over 2 consecutive days), then 80 mg 2 weeks later (day 15); Maintenance: 40 mg every other week beginning day 29. **Note:** Some patients may require 40 mg every week as maintenance therapy (Lichtenstein, 2009).

Plaque psoriasis: SubQ: Initial: 80 mg as a single dose; maintenance: 40 mg every other week beginning 1 week after initial dose

Administration For SubQ injection; rotate injection sites. Do not use if solution is discolored. Do not administer to skin which is red, tender, bruised, or hard. Needle cap of the prefilled syringe may contain latex.

Monitoring Parameters Place and read PPD before initiation. Monitor improvement of symptoms and physical function assessments; CBC; signs of infection, bleeding, or bruising; signs of HBV reactivation in patients who are carriers (during therapy and several months following discontinuation)

Special Geriatric Considerations In studies, the elderly have an increased incidence of infection and malignancy compared to younger adults <65 years of age. Given the higher incidence of infections and malignancies in the elderly population, caution and close monitoring are recommended when using adalimumab in this population. Additionally, elderly patients with a history of HF may be at risk for HF exacerbation.

Dosage Forms Excipient information presented when available (limited, particularly for generics); consult specific product labeling.

Injection, solution [preservative free]:
  Humira®: 40 mg/0.8 mL (0.8 mL) [contains natural rubber/natural latex in packaging, polysorbate 80; prefilled syringe]
  Humira® Pen: 40 mg/0.8 mL (0.8 mL) [contains natural rubber/natural latex in packaging, polysorbate 80]

Injection, solution [pediatric, preservative free]:
  Humira®: 20 mg/0.4 mL (0.4 mL) [contains natural rubber/natural latex in packaging, polysorbate 80; prefilled syringe]

Selected References

Kwon HJ, Coté TR, Cuffe MS, et al, "Case Reports of Heart Failure After Therapy With a Tumor Necrosis Factor Antagonist," *Ann Intern Med*, 2003, 138(10):807-11.

- **Akwa Tears® [OTC]** *see* Artificial Tears *on page 148*
- **ALA** *see* Aminolevulinic Acid *on page 93*
- **5-ALA** *see* Aminolevulinic Acid *on page 93*
- **Ala-Cort** *see* Hydrocortisone (Topical) *on page 886*
- **Alamag [OTC]** *see* Aluminum Hydroxide and Magnesium Hydroxide *on page 81*
- **Alamag Plus [OTC]** *see* Aluminum Hydroxide, Magnesium Hydroxide, and Simethicone *on page 84*
- **Ala-Scalp** *see* Hydrocortisone (Topical) *on page 886*
- **Alavert® Allergy 24 Hour [OTC]** *see* Loratadine *on page 1087*
- **Alavert® Children's Allergy [OTC]** *see* Loratadine *on page 1087*
- **Alaway™ [OTC]** *see* Ketotifen *on page 1013*

Albuterol (al BYOO ter ole)

Related Information
Inhalant Agents *on page 2010*

Medication Safety Issues
Sound-alike/look-alike issues:
Albuterol may be confused with Albutein®, atenolol
Proventil® may be confused with Bentyl®, PriLOSEC®, Prinivil®
Salbutamol may be confused with salmeterol
Ventolin® may be confused with phentolamine, Benylin®, Vantin

Brand Names: U.S. AccuNeb®; ProAir® HFA; Proventil® HFA; Ventolin® HFA; VoSpire ER®

Brand Names: Canada Airomir; Apo-Salvent®; Apo-Salvent® AEM; Apo-Salvent® CFC Free; Apo-Salvent® Sterules; Dom-Salbutamol; Med-Salbutamol; Mylan-Salbutamol Respirator Solution; Mylan-Salbutamol Sterinebs P.F.; Novo-Salbutamol HFA; Nu-Salbutamol; PHL-Salbutamol; PMS-Salbutamol; ratio-Ipra-Sal; ratio-Salbutamol; Sandoz-Salbutamol; Ventolin®; Ventolin® Diskus; Ventolin® HFA; Ventolin® I.V. Infusion; Ventolin® Nebules P.F.

Index Terms Albuterol Sulfate; Salbutamol; Salbutamol Sulphate

Generic Availability (U.S.) Yes

Pharmacologic Category Beta$_2$-Adrenergic Agonist

Use Treatment or prevention of bronchospasm in patients with reversible obstructive airway disease; prevention of exercise-induced bronchospasm

Contraindications Hypersensitivity to albuterol, adrenergic amines, or any component of the formulation

Injection formulation (not available in U.S.): Patients with tachyarrhythmias

Warnings/Precautions Optimize anti-inflammatory treatment before initiating maintenance treatment with albuterol. Do not use as a component of chronic therapy without an anti-inflammatory agent. Only the mildest forms of asthma (Step 1 and/or exercise-induced) would not require concurrent use based upon asthma guidelines. Patient must be instructed to seek medical attention in cases where acute symptoms are not relieved or a previous level of response is diminished. The need to increase frequency of use may indicate deterioration of asthma, and treatment must not be delayed.

Use caution in patients with cardiovascular disease (arrhythmia or hypertension or HF), convulsive disorders, diabetes, glaucoma, hyperthyroidism, or hypokalemia. Beta-agonists may cause elevation in blood pressure, heart rate, and result in CNS stimulation/excitation. Beta$_2$-agonists may increase risk of arrhythmia, increase serum glucose, or decrease serum potassium.

Immediate hypersensitivity reactions (urticaria, angioedema, rash, bronchospasm) have been reported. Do not exceed recommended dose; serious adverse events, including fatalities, have been associated with excessive use of inhaled sympathomimetics. Rarely, paradoxical bronchospasm may occur with use of inhaled bronchodilating agents; this should be distinguished from inadequate response. All patients should utilize a spacer device or valved holding chamber when using a metered-dose inhaler.

Patient response may vary between inhalers that contain chlorofluorocarbons and those which are chlorofluorocarbon-free.

Adverse Reactions (Reflective of adult population; not specific for elderly) Incidence of adverse effects is dependent upon age of patient, dose, and route of administration.

Cardiovascular: Angina, atrial fibrillation, arrhythmias, chest discomfort, chest pain, extrasystoles, flushing, hyper-/hypotension, palpitation, supraventricular tachycardia, tachycardia
Central nervous system: CNS stimulation, dizziness, drowsiness, headache, insomnia, irritability, lightheadedness, migraine, nervousness, nightmares, restlessness, seizure
Dermatologic: Angioedema, rash, urticaria
Endocrine & metabolic: Hyperglycemia, hypokalemia, lactic acidosis

Gastrointestinal: Diarrhea, dry mouth, dyspepsia, gastroenteritis, nausea, unusual taste, vomiting

Genitourinary: Micturition difficulty

Local: Injection: Pain, stinging

Neuromuscular & skeletal: Muscle cramps, musculoskeletal pain, tremor, weakness

Otic: Otitis media, vertigo

Respiratory: Asthma exacerbation, bronchospasm, cough, epistaxis, laryngitis, oropharyngeal drying/irritation, oropharyngeal edema, pharyngitis, rhinitis, upper respiratory inflammation, viral respiratory infection

Miscellaneous: Allergic reaction, anaphylaxis, diaphoresis, lymphadenopathy

Drug Interactions

Avoid Concomitant Use

Avoid concomitant use of Albuterol with any of the following: Iobenguane I 123

Increased Effect/Toxicity

Albuterol may increase the levels/effects of: Loop Diuretics; Sympathomimetics

The levels/effects of Albuterol may be increased by: Atomoxetine; Cannabinoids; MAO Inhibitors; Tricyclic Antidepressants

Decreased Effect

Albuterol may decrease the levels/effects of: Iobenguane I 123

The levels/effects of Albuterol may be decreased by: Alpha-/Beta-Blockers; Beta-Blockers (Beta1 Selective); Beta-Blockers (Nonselective); Betahistine

Ethanol/Nutrition/Herb Interactions

Food: Avoid or limit caffeine (may cause CNS stimulation).

Herb/Nutraceutical: Avoid ephedra, yohimbe (may cause CNS stimulation). Avoid St John's wort (may decrease the levels/effects of albuterol).

Stability

HFA aerosols: Store at 15°C to 25°C (59°F to 77°F).

Ventolin® HFA: Discard when counter reads 000 or 12 months after removal from protective pouch, whichever comes first. Store with mouthpiece down.

Infusion solution (Canadian labeling; product not available in U.S.): Ventolin® I.V.: Store at 15°C to 30°C (59°F to 86°F). Protect from light. After dilution, discard unused portion after 24 hours.

Inhalation solution: Solution for nebulization (0.5%): Store at 2°C to 25°C (36°F to 77°F). To prepare a 2.5 mg dose, dilute 0.5 mL of solution to a total of 3 mL with normal saline; also compatible with cromolyn or ipratropium nebulizer solutions.

AccuNeb®: Store at 2°C to 25°C (36°F to 77°F). Do not use if solution changes color or becomes cloudy. Use within 1 week of opening foil pouch.

Syrup: Store at 20°C to 25°C (68°F to 77°F).

Tablet: Store at 20°C to 25°C (68°F to 77°F).

Tablet, extended release: Store at 20°C to 25°C (68°F to 77°F)

Mechanism of Action
Relaxes bronchial smooth muscle by action on beta$_2$-receptors with little effect on heart rate

Pharmacodynamics/Kinetics

Onset of action: Peak effect:

Nebulization/oral inhalation: 0.5-2 hours

CFC-propelled albuterol: 10 minutes

Ventolin® HFA: 25 minutes

Oral: 2-3 hours

Duration: Nebulization/oral inhalation: 3-4 hours; Oral: 4-6 hours

Metabolism: Hepatic to an inactive sulfate

Half-life elimination: Inhalation: 3.8 hours; Oral: 3.7-5 hours

Excretion: Urine (30% as unchanged drug)

Dosage

Geriatric

Inhalation: Refer to adult dosing.

Bronchospasm (treatment): Oral: 2 mg 3-4 times/day; maximum: 8 mg 4 times/day

Adult

Bronchospasm:

Metered-dose inhaler: 2 puffs every 4-6 hours as needed (NIH Guidelines, 2007):

Solution for nebulization: 2.5 mg 3-4 times daily as needed; Quick relief: 1.25-5 mg every 4 to 8 hours as needed (NIH Guidelines, 2007)

Oral: 2-4 mg/dose 3-4 times/day; maximum dose not to exceed 32 mg/day (divided doses)

Extended release: 8 mg every 12 hours; maximum dose not to exceed 32 mg/day (divided doses). A 4 mg dose every 12 hours may be sufficient in some patients, such as adults of low body weight.

I.V. continuous infusion (Canadian labeling; product not available in U.S.]): Severe bronchospasm and status asthmaticus: Initial: 5 mcg/minute; may increase up to 10-20 mcg/minute at 15- to 30-minute intervals if needed

Exacerbation of asthma (acute, severe) (NIH Guidelines, 2007):

Metered-dose inhaler: 4-8 puffs every 20 minutes for up to 4 hours, then every 1-4 hours as needed

Solution for nebulization: 2.5-5 mg every 20 minutes for 3 doses, then 2.5-10 mg every 1-4 hours as needed, **or** 10-15 mg/hour by continuous nebulization

Exercise-induced bronchospasm (prevention): *Metered-dose inhaler:* 2 puffs 5-30 minutes prior to exercise

Renal Impairment Use with caution in patients with renal impairment. No dosage adjustment required (including patients on hemodialysis, peritoneal dialysis, or CRRT; Aronoff, 2007).

Administration

Metered-dose inhaler: Shake well before use; prime prior to first use, and whenever inhaler has not been used for >2 weeks or when it has been dropped, by releasing 3-4 test sprays into the air (away from face). HFA inhalers should be cleaned with warm water at least once per week; allow to air dry completely prior to use. A spacer device or valved holding chamber is recommended for use with metered-dose inhalers.

Solution for nebulization: Concentrated solution should be diluted prior to use. Blow-by administration is not recommended, use a mask device if patient unable to hold mouthpiece in mouth for administration.

Infusion solution (Canadian labeling; product not available in U.S.): Do not inject undiluted. Reduce concentration by at least 50% before infusing. Administer as a continuous infusion via infusion pump.

Oral: Do not crush or chew extended release tablets.

Monitoring Parameters FEV_1, peak flow, and/or other pulmonary function tests; blood pressure, heart rate; CNS stimulation; serum glucose, serum potassium; asthma symptoms; arterial or capillary blood gases (if patients condition warrants)

Test Interactions Increased renin (S), increased aldosterone (S)

Pharmacotherapy Pearls The 2007 National Heart, Lung, and Blood Institute Guidelines for the Diagnosis and Management of Asthma do not recommend the use of oral systemic albuterol as a quick-relief medication and do not recommend regularly scheduled daily, chronic use of inhaled beta-agonists for long-term control of asthma.

Special Geriatric Considerations Because of its minimal effect on $beta_1$-receptors and its relatively long duration of action, albuterol is a rational choice in elderly when a beta-agonist is indicated. Elderly patients may find it beneficial to utilize a spacer device when using a metered dose inhaler. Oral use should be avoided due to adverse effects.

Dosage Forms Excipient information presented when available (limited, particularly for generics); consult specific product labeling.

Aerosol, for oral inhalation:

ProAir® HFA: 90 mcg/inhalation (8.5 g) [chlorofluorocarbon free; 200 metered actuations]

Proventil® HFA: 90 mcg/inhalation (6.7 g) [chlorofluorocarbon free; 200 metered actuations]

Ventolin® HFA: 90 mcg/inhalation (18 g) [chlorofluorocarbon free; 200 metered actuations]

Ventolin® HFA: 90 mcg/inhalation (8 g) [chlorofluorocarbon free; 60 metered actuations]

Solution, for nebulization: 0.083% [2.5 mg/3 mL] (25s, 30s, 60s); 0.5% [100 mg/20 mL] (1s)

Solution, for nebulization [preservative free]: 0.021% [0.63 mg/3 mL] (25s); 0.042% [1.25 mg/3 mL] (25s, 30s); 0.083% [2.5 mg/3 mL] (25s, 30s, 60s); 0.5% [2.5 mg/0.5 mL] (30s)

AccuNeb®: 0.021% [0.63 mg/3 mL] (25s); 0.042% [1.25 mg/3 mL] (25s)

Syrup, oral: 2 mg/5 mL (473 mL)

Tablet, oral: 2 mg, 4 mg

Tablet, extended release, oral: 4 mg, 8 mg

VoSpire ER®: 4 mg, 8 mg

Dosage Forms: Canada Excipient information presented when available (limited, particularly for generics); consult specific product labeling.

Injection, solution, as sulphate:

Ventolin® I.V.: 1 mg/1mL (5 mL)

Selected References

National Asthma Education and Prevention Program, "Expert Panel Report 3 (EPR-3): Guidelines for the Diagnosis and Management of Asthma-Summary Report 2007," *J Allergy Clin Immunol*, 2007, 120(5 Suppl):94-138.

◆ **Albuterol and Ipratropium** *see* Ipratropium and Albuterol *on page 975*

◆ **Albuterol Sulfate** *see* Albuterol *on page 50*

Alcaftadine (al KAF ta deen)

Brand Names: U.S. Lastacaft™

Generic Availability (U.S.) No

Pharmacologic Category Histamine H$_1$ Antagonist; Histamine H$_1$ Antagonist, Second Generation; Mast Cell Stabilizer
Use Prevention of itching associated with allergic conjunctivitis
Dosage
  Geriatric & Adult Allergic conjunctivitis: Ophthalmic: Instill 1 drop into each eye once daily.
  Dosage Forms Excipient information presented when available (limited, particularly for generics); consult specific product labeling.
  Solution, ophthalmic [drops]:
    Lastacaft™: 0.25% (3 mL) [contains benzalkonium chloride]

Alclometasone (al kloe MET a sone)

Related Information
  Corticosteroids *on page 2005*
Medication Safety Issues
  Sound-alike/look-alike issues:
    Aclovate® may be confused with Accolate®
  International issues:
    Cloderm: Brand name for alclometasone [Indonesia], but also brand name for clobetasol [China, India, Malaysia, Singapore, Thailand]; clocortolone [U.S., Canada]; clotrimazole [Germany]
Brand Names: U.S. Aclovate®
Index Terms Alclometasone Dipropionate
Generic Availability (U.S.) Yes
Pharmacologic Category Corticosteroid, Topical
Use Treatment of inflammation of corticosteroid-responsive dermatosis (low to medium potency topical corticosteroid)
Dosage
  Geriatric & Adult Steroid-responsive dermatoses: Topical: Apply a thin film to the affected area 2-3 times/day. **Note:** Therapy should be discontinued when control is achieved; if no improvement is seen within 2 weeks, reassessment of diagnosis may be necessary.
  Special Geriatric Considerations Due to age-related changes in skin, limit use of topical corticosteroids.
  Dosage Forms Excipient information presented when available (limited, particularly for generics); consult specific product labeling.
  Cream, topical, as dipropionate: 0.05% (15 g, 45 g, 60 g)
    Aclovate®: 0.05% (15 g, 60 g)
  Ointment, topical, as dipropionate: 0.05% (15 g, 45 g, 60 g)
    Aclovate®: 0.05% (15 g, 60 g)

♦ **Alclometasone Dipropionate** *see* Alclometasone *on page 53*
♦ **Aldactazide®** *see* Hydrochlorothiazide and Spironolactone *on page 878*
♦ **Aldactone®** *see* Spironolactone *on page 1707*
♦ **Aldomet** *see* Methyldopa *on page 1176*
♦ **Aldroxicon I [OTC]** *see* Aluminum Hydroxide, Magnesium Hydroxide, and Simethicone *on page 84*
♦ **Aldroxicon II [OTC]** *see* Aluminum Hydroxide, Magnesium Hydroxide, and Simethicone *on page 84*

Alendronate (a LEN droe nate)

Related Information
  Osteoporosis Management *on page 2027*
Medication Safety Issues
  Sound-alike/look-alike issues:
    Alendronate may be confused with risedronate
    Fosamax® may be confused with Flomax®, Fosamax Plus D®, fosinopril, Zithromax®
  International issues:
    Fosamax [U.S., Canada, and multiple international markets] may be confused with Fisamox brand name for amoxicillin [Australia]
Brand Names: U.S. Fosamax®
Brand Names: Canada Alendronate-FC; Apo-Alendronate®; CO Alendronate; Dom-Alendronate; Fosamax®; Mylan-Alendronate; Novo-Alendronate; PHL-Alendronate; PMS-Alendronate; PMS-Alendronate-FC; ratio-Alendronate; Riva-Alendronate; Sandoz-Alendronate; Teva-Alendronate

◄ **Index Terms** Alendronate Sodium; Alendronic Acid Monosodium Salt Trihydrate; MK-217

Generic Availability (U.S.) Yes: Tablet

Pharmacologic Category Bisphosphonate Derivative

Use Treatment and prevention of osteoporosis in postmenopausal females; treatment of osteoporosis in males; Paget's disease of the bone in patients who are symptomatic, at risk for future complications, or with alkaline phosphatase ≥2 times the upper limit of normal; treatment of glucocorticoid-induced osteoporosis in males and females with low bone mineral density who are receiving a daily dosage ≥7.5 mg of prednisone (or equivalent)

Medication Guide Available Yes

Contraindications Hypersensitivity to alendronate, other bisphosphonates, or any component of the formulation; hypocalcemia; abnormalities of the esophagus which delay esophageal emptying such as stricture or achalasia; inability to stand or sit upright for at least 30 minutes; oral solution should not be used in patients at risk of aspiration

Warnings/Precautions Use caution in patients with renal impairment (not recommended for use in patients with Cl$_{cr}$ <35 mL/minute); hypocalcemia must be corrected before therapy initiation; ensure adequate calcium and vitamin D intake. May cause irritation to upper gastrointestinal mucosa. Esophagitis, dysphagia, esophageal ulcers, esophageal erosions, and esophageal stricture (rare) have been reported; risk increases in patients unable to comply with dosing instructions. Use with caution in patients with dysphagia, esophageal disease, gastritis, duodenitis, or ulcers (may worsen underlying condition). Discontinue use if new or worsening symptoms develop.

Osteonecrosis of the jaw (ONJ) has been reported in patients receiving bisphosphonates. Risk factors include invasive dental procedures (eg, tooth extraction, dental implants, boney surgery); a diagnosis of cancer, with concomitant chemotherapy or corticosteroids; poor oral hygiene, ill-fitting dentures; and comorbid disorders (anemia, coagulopathy, infection, pre-existing dental disease). Most reported cases occur after I.V. bisphosphonate therapy; however, cases have been reported following oral therapy. A dental exam and preventative dentistry should be performed prior to placing patients with risk factors on chronic bisphosphonate therapy. The manufacturer's labeling states that discontinuing bisphosphonates in patients requiring invasive dental procedures may reduce the risk of ONJ. However, other experts suggest that there is no evidence that discontinuing therapy reduces the risk of developing ONJ (Assael, 2009). The benefit/risk must be assessed by the treating physician and/or dentist/surgeon prior to any invasive dental procedure. Patients developing ONJ while on bisphosphonates should receive care by an oral surgeon.

Atypical femur fractures have been reported in patients receiving bisphosphonates for treatment/prevention of osteoporosis. The fractures include subtrochanteric femur (bone just below the hip joint) and diaphyseal femur (long segment of the thigh bone). Some patients experience prodromal pain weeks or months before the fracture occurs. It is unclear if bisphosphonate therapy is the cause for these fractures, although the majority have been reported in patients taking bisphosphonates. Patients receiving long-term (>3-5 years) therapy may be at an increased risk. Discontinue bisphosphonate therapy in patients who develop a femoral shaft fracture.

Severe (and occasionally debilitating) bone, joint, and/or muscle pain have been reported during bisphosphonate treatment. The onset of pain ranged from a single day to several months. Consider discontinuing therapy in patients who experience severe symptoms; symptoms usually resolve upon discontinuation. Some patients experienced recurrence when rechallenged with same drug or another bisphosphonate; avoid use in patients with a history of these symptoms in association with bisphosphonate therapy.

Adverse Reactions (Reflective of adult population; not specific for elderly) Note: Incidence of adverse effects (mostly GI) increases significantly in patients treated for Paget's disease at 40 mg/day.

>10%: Endocrine & metabolic: Hypocalcemia (transient, mild, 18%); hypophosphatemia (transient, mild, 10%)

1% to 10%:
Central nervous system: Headache (up to 3%)
Gastrointestinal: Abdominal pain (1% to 7%), acid reflux (1% to 4%), dyspepsia (1% to 4%), nausea (1% to 4%), flatulence (up to 4%), diarrhea (1% to 3%), gastroesophageal reflux disease (1% to 3%), constipation (up to 3%), esophageal ulcer (up to 2%), abdominal distension (up to 1%), gastritis (up to 1%), vomiting (up to 1%), dysphagia (up to 1%), gastric ulcer (1%), melena (1%)
Neuromuscular & skeletal: Musculoskeletal pain (up to 6%), muscle cramps (up to 1%)

Drug Interactions

Avoid Concomitant Use There are no known interactions where it is recommended to avoid concomitant use.

Increased Effect/Toxicity

  Alendronate may increase the levels/effects of: Deferasirox; Phosphate Supplements

  The levels/effects of Alendronate may be increased by: Aminoglycosides; Aspirin; Non-steroidal Anti-Inflammatory Agents

Decreased Effect

  The levels/effects of Alendronate may be decreased by: Antacids; Calcium Salts; Iron Salts; Magnesium Salts; Proton Pump Inhibitors

Ethanol/Nutrition/Herb Interactions

  Ethanol: Avoid ethanol (may increase risk of osteoporosis and gastric irritation).

  Food: All food and beverages interfere with absorption. Coadministration with caffeine may reduce alendronate efficacy. Coadministration with dairy products may decrease alendronate absorption. Beverages (especially orange juice and coffee) and food may reduce the absorption of alendronate as much as 60%.

Stability Store tablets and oral solution at room temperature of 15°C to 30°C (59°F to 86°F). Keep in well-closed container.

Mechanism of Action A bisphosphonate which inhibits bone resorption via actions on osteoclasts or on osteoclast precursors; decreases the rate of bone resorption, leading to an indirect increase in bone mineral density. In Paget's disease, characterized by disordered resorption and formation of bone, inhibition of resorption leads to an indirect decrease in bone formation; but the newly-formed bone has a more normal architecture.

Pharmacodynamics/Kinetics

  Distribution: 28 L (exclusive of bone)

  Protein binding: ~78%

  Metabolism: None

  Bioavailability: Fasting: 0.6%; reduced up to 60% with food or drink

  Half-life elimination: Exceeds 10 years

  Excretion: Urine; feces (as unabsorbed drug)

Dosage

  Geriatric & Adult Note: Patients should receive supplemental calcium and vitamin D if dietary intake is inadequate.

  Osteoporosis in postmenopausal females: Oral:

    Prophylaxis: 5 mg once daily **or** 35 mg once weekly

    Treatment: 10 mg once daily **or** 70 mg once weekly

  Osteoporosis in males: Oral: 10 mg once daily **or** 70 mg once weekly

  Osteoporosis secondary to glucocorticoids in males and females: Oral: Treatment: 5 mg once daily; a dose of 10 mg once daily should be used in postmenopausal females who are not receiving estrogen

  Paget's disease of bone in males and females: Oral: 40 mg once daily for 6 months

    Retreatment: Relapses during the 12 months following therapy occurred in 9% of patients who responded to treatment. Specific retreatment data are not available. Following a 6-month post-treatment evaluation period, treatment with alendronate may be considered in patients who have relapsed based on increases in serum alkaline phosphatase, which should be measured periodically. Retreatment may also be considered in those who failed to normalize their serum alkaline phosphatase.

Renal Impairment

  Cl_{cr} 35-60 mL/minute: None necessary.

  Cl_{cr} <35 mL/minute: Alendronate is not recommended due to lack of experience.

Hepatic Impairment No adjustment necessary.

Administration Alendronate must be taken with plain water (tablets 6-8 oz; oral solution follow with 2 oz) first thing in the morning and ≥30 minutes before the first food, beverage, or other medication of the day. Do not take with mineral water or with other beverages. Patients should be instructed to stay upright (not to lie down) for at least 30 minutes **and** until after first food of the day (to reduce esophageal irritation).

Monitoring Parameters

  Osteoporosis: Bone mineral density as measured by central dual-energy x-ray absorptiometry (DXA) of the hip or spine (prior to initiation of therapy and at least every 2 years; after 6-12 months of combined glucocorticoid and alendronate treatment); annual measurements of height and weight, assessment of chronic back pain; serum calcium and 25(OH)D; may consider monitoring biochemical markers of bone turnover

  Paget's disease: Alkaline phosphatase; pain; serum calcium and 25(OH)D

Reference Range Calcium (total): Adults: 9.0-11.0 mg/dL (2.05-2.54 mmol/L), may slightly decrease with aging; phosphorus: 2.5-4.5 mg/dL (0.81-1.45 mmol/L)

Test Interactions Bisphosphonates may interfere with diagnostic imaging agents such as technetium-99m-diphosphonate in bone scans.

◀ **Pharmacotherapy Pearls** Esophageal irritation and gastric pain have been reported frequently. Proper administration may prevent or decrease this common adverse effect. Patients need to take supplemental calcium while treated with alendronate appropriate for age and hormonal status; vitamin D supplements suggested if patient is deficient in this vitamin. Patients treated with 10 mg of alendronate daily had significant increases in bone mineral density. Increases were absorbed as early as 3 months and continued throughout the 3 years of study. Mean bone mineral density increases at 3 years were: spine, trochanter 8%; femoral neck 6%; total body bone mineral density 2.5%.

Special Geriatric Considerations The elderly are frequently treated long-term for osteoporosis. Elderly patients should be advised to report any lower extremity, jaw (osteonecrosis), or muscle pain that cannot be explained or lasts longer than 2 weeks. Additionally, elderly often receive concomitant diuretic therapy and therefore their electrolyte status (eg, calcium, phosphate) should be periodically evaluated.

Dosage Forms Excipient information presented when available (limited, particularly for generics); consult specific product labeling. [DSC] = Discontinued product
Solution, oral:
Fosamax®: 70 mg/75 mL (75 mL [DSC]) [raspberry flavor]
Tablet, oral: 5 mg, 10 mg, 35 mg, 40 mg, 70 mg
Fosamax®: 5 mg [DSC], 10 mg, 35 mg [DSC], 40 mg [DSC], 70 mg

Selected References
Assael LA, "Oral Bisphosphonates as a Cause of Bisphosphonate-Related Osteonecrosis of the Jaws: Clinical Findings, Assessment of Risks, and Preventive Strategies," *J Oral Maxillofac Surg*, 2009, 67(5 Suppl):35-43.
Chesnut CH 3rd, McClung MR, Ensrud KE, et al, "Alendronate Treatment of the Postmenopausal Osteoporotic Woman: Effect of Multiple Dosages on Bone Mass and Bone Remodeling," *Am J Med*, 1995, 99(2):144-52.
Hillner BE, Ingle JN, Chlebowski RT, et al, "American Society of Clinical Oncology 2003 Update on the Role of Bisphosphonates and Bone Health Issues in Women With Breast Cancer," *J Clin Oncol*, 2003, 21(21):4042-57.
"Management of Osteoporosis in Postmenopausal Women: 2010 Position Statement of The North American Menopause Society," *Menopause*, 2010, 17(1):25-54.
National Osteoporosis Foundation, "Clinician's Guide to Prevention and Treatment of Osteoporosis," Washington, DC, 2010. Available at http://www.nof.org
Watts NB, "Treatment of Osteoporosis With Bisphosphonates," *Rheum Dis Clin North Am*, 1994, 20(3):717-34.
Whyte MP, "Clinical Practice. Paget's Disease of Bone," *N Engl J Med*, 2006, 355(6):593-600.

Alendronate and Cholecalciferol (a LEN droe nate & kole e kal SI fer ole)

Related Information
Alendronate *on page 53*
Cholecalciferol *on page 346*
Medication Safety Issues
Sound-alike/look-alike issues:
Fosamax Plus D® may be confused with Fosamax®
Brand Names: U.S. Fosamax Plus D®
Brand Names: Canada Fosavance
Index Terms Alendronate Sodium and Cholecalciferol; Cholecalciferol and Alendronate; Vitamin D_3 and Alendronate
Generic Availability (U.S.) No
Pharmacologic Category Bisphosphonate Derivative; Vitamin D Analog
Use Treatment of osteoporosis in postmenopausal females; increase bone mass in males with osteoporosis
Medication Guide Available Yes
Dosage
Geriatric & Adult Osteoporosis: Oral: One tablet (alendronate 70 mg/cholecalciferol 2800 int. units **or** alendronate 70 mg/cholecalciferol 5600 int. units) once weekly. Appropriate dose in most osteoporotic women or men: Alendronate 70 mg/cholecalciferol 5600 int. units once weekly. Supplemental calcium and vitamin D may be necessary if dietary intake is inadequate.

Renal Impairment
Cl_{cr} 35-60 mL/minute: No adjustment needed.
Cl_{cr} <35 mL/minute: Not recommended.

Hepatic Impairment Alendronate: None necessary. Cholecalciferol: May not be adequately absorbed in patients who have malabsorption due to inadequate bile production.

Special Geriatric Considerations The elderly are frequently treated long-term for osteoporosis. Elderly patients should be advised to report any lower extremity, jaw (osteonecrosis), or muscle pain that cannot be explained or lasts longer than 2 weeks. Additionally, elderly often receive concomitant diuretic therapy and therefore their electrolyte status (eg, calcium, phosphate) should be periodically evaluated.

Dosage Forms Excipient information presented when available (limited, particularly for generics); consult specific product labeling.
Tablet:
  Fosamax Plus D® 70/2800: Alendronate 70 mg and cholecalciferol 2800 int. units
  Fosamax Plus D® 70/5600: Alendronate 70 mg and cholecalciferol 5600 int. units

- ◆ **Alendronate Sodium** *see* Alendronate *on page 53*
- ◆ **Alendronate Sodium and Cholecalciferol** *see* Alendronate and Cholecalciferol *on page 56*
- ◆ **Alendronic Acid Monosodium Salt Trihydrate** *see* Alendronate *on page 53*
- ◆ **Aler-Cap [OTC]** *see* DiphenhydrAMINE (Systemic) *on page 520*
- ◆ **Aler-Dryl [OTC]** *see* DiphenhydrAMINE (Systemic) *on page 520*
- ◆ **Aler-Tab [OTC]** *see* DiphenhydrAMINE (Systemic) *on page 520*
- ◆ **Aleve® [OTC]** *see* Naproxen *on page 1263*

Alfuzosin (al FYOO zoe sin)

Related Information
  Pharmacotherapy of Urinary Incontinence *on page 2032*
Brand Names: U.S. Uroxatral®
Brand Names: Canada Apo-Alfuzosin®; Sandoz-Alfuzosin; Teva-Alfuzosin PR; Xatral
Index Terms Alfuzosin Hydrochloride
Generic Availability (U.S.) Yes
Pharmacologic Category Alpha$_1$ Blocker
Use Treatment of the functional symptoms of benign prostatic hyperplasia (BPH)
Unlabeled/Investigational Use Facilitation of expulsion of ureteral stones
Contraindications Hypersensitivity to alfuzosin or any component of the formulation; moderate or severe hepatic insufficiency (Child-Pugh class B and C); concurrent use with potent CYP3A4 inhibitors (eg, itraconazole, ketoconazole, ritonavir) or other alpha$_1$-blocking agents
Warnings/Precautions Not intended for use as an antihypertensive drug. May cause significant orthostatic hypotension and syncope, especially with first dose; anticipate a similar effect if therapy is interrupted for a few days, if dosage is rapidly increased, or used with antihypertensives (particularly vasodilators), PDE-5 inhibitors, nitrates or other medications which may result in hypotension. Discontinue if symptoms of angina occur or worsen. Alfuzosin has been shown to prolong the QT interval alone (minimal) and with other drugs with comparable effects on the QT interval (additive); use with caution in patients with known QT prolongation (congenital or acquired). Patients should be cautioned about performing hazardous tasks when starting new therapy or adjusting dosage upward. Discontinue if symptoms of angina occur or worsen. Rule out prostatic carcinoma before beginning therapy. Use caution with severe renal or mild hepatic impairment; contraindicated in moderate-to-severe hepatic impairment. Intraoperative floppy iris syndrome has been observed in cataract surgery patients who were on or were previously treated with alpha$_1$-blockers. Causality has not been established and there appears to be no benefit in discontinuing alpha-blocker therapy prior to surgery. May cause priapism. Contraindicated in patients taking strong CYP3A4 inhibitors or other alpha$_1$-blockers.
Adverse Reactions (Reflective of adult population; not specific for elderly) 1% to 10%:
  Central nervous system: Dizziness (6%), fatigue (3%), headache (3%), pain (1% to 2%)
  Gastrointestinal: Abdominal pain (1% to 2%), constipation (1% to 2%), dyspepsia (1% to 2%), nausea (1% to 2%)
  Genitourinary: Impotence (1% to 2%)
  Respiratory: Upper respiratory tract infection (3%), bronchitis (1% to 2%), pharyngitis (1% to 2%), sinusitis (1% to 2%)
Drug Interactions
  Metabolism/Transport Effects Substrate of CYP3A4 (major)
  Avoid Concomitant Use
    Avoid concomitant use of Alfuzosin with any of the following: Alpha1-Blockers; CYP3A4 Inhibitors (Strong); Protease Inhibitors; Telaprevir
  Increased Effect/Toxicity
    Alfuzosin may increase the levels/effects of: Alpha1-Blockers; Antihypertensives; Calcium Channel Blockers; Nitroglycerin; QTc-Prolonging Agents

    The levels/effects of Alfuzosin may be increased by: Beta-Blockers; CYP3A4 Inhibitors (Moderate); CYP3A4 Inhibitors (Strong); MAO Inhibitors; Phosphodiesterase 5 Inhibitors; Protease Inhibitors; Telaprevir
  Decreased Effect
    The levels/effects of Alfuzosin may be decreased by: CYP3A4 Inducers (Strong); Deferasirox; Herbs (CYP3A4 Inducers); Tocilizumab

Ethanol/Nutrition/Herb Interactions
Food: Food increases the extent of absorption.
Herb/Nutraceutical: Avoid St John's wort (may decrease alfuzosin levels).

Stability Store at room temperature of 25°C (77°F); excursions permitted to 15°C to 30°C (59°F to 86°F). Protect from light and moisture.

Mechanism of Action An antagonist of alpha$_1$-adrenoreceptors in the lower urinary tract. Smooth muscle tone is mediated by the sympathetic nervous stimulation of alpha$_1$-adrenoreceptors, which are abundant in the prostate, prostatic capsule, prostatic urethra, and bladder neck. Blockade of these adrenoreceptors can cause smooth muscles in the bladder neck and prostate to relax, resulting in an improvement in urine flow rate and a reduction in BPH symptoms.

Pharmacodynamics/Kinetics
Absorption: Decreased 50% under fasting conditions
Distribution: V_d: 3.2 L/kg
Protein binding: 82% to 90%
Metabolism: Hepatic, primarily via CYP3A4; metabolism includes oxidation, O-demethylation, and N-dealkylation; forms metabolites (inactive)
Bioavailability: 49% following a meal
Half-life elimination: 10 hours
Time to peak, plasma: 8 hours following a meal
Excretion: Feces (69%); urine (24%; 11% as unchanged drug)

Dosage
Geriatric & Adult
Benign prostatic hyperplasia (BPH): Oral: 10 mg once daily
Ureteral stones, expulsion (unlabeled use): Oral: 10 mg once daily, discontinue after successful expulsion (average time to expulsion 1-2 weeks) (Gurbuz, 2011; Ahmed, 2010; Agrawal, 2009). **Note:** Patients with stones >10 mm were excluded from studies.
Renal Impairment Bioavailability and maximum serum concentrations are increased by ~50% with mild (Cl$_{cr}$ 60-80 mL/minute), moderate (Cl$_{cr}$ 30-59 mL/minute), or severe (Cl$_{cr}$ <30 mL/minute) renal impairment.
Note: Safety data is limited in patients with severe renal impairment (Cl$_{cr}$ <30 mL/minute). Use with caution.
Hepatic Impairment
Mild hepatic impairment: Use has not been studied; use caution.
Moderate or severe hepatic impairment (Child-Pugh class B and C): Clearance is decreased $1/3$ to $1/4$ and serum concentration is increased three- to fourfold; use is contraindicated.

Administration Tablet should be swallowed whole; do not crush or chew. Administer once daily (immediately following a meal); should be taken at the same time each day.

Monitoring Parameters Urine flow, blood pressure, PSA

Special Geriatric Considerations Alfuzosin is a functionally uroselective alpha-blocker, therefore, having minimal effects on the cardiovascular system. Alfuzosin has been available in Europe for many years and appears to be well tolerated in elderly. In one study, orthostatic changes were minimal and not influenced by age.

Dosage Forms Excipient information presented when available (limited, particularly for generics); consult specific product labeling.
Tablet, extended release, oral, as hydrochloride: 10 mg
Uroxatral®: 10 mg

Selected References
Lee, M, "Alfuzosin Hydrochloride for the Treatment of Benign Prostatic Hyperplasia," *Am J Health Syst Pharm*, 2003, 60(14):1426-39.
van Kerrebroeck P, Jardin A, van Cangh P, et al, "Long-term Safety and Efficacy of a Once-daily Formulation of Alfuzosin 10 mg in Patients With Symptomatic Benign Prostatic Hyperplasia: Open-label Extension Study," *Eur Urol*, 2002, 41(1):54-61.

♦ **Alfuzosin Hydrochloride** see Alfuzosin on page 57
♦ **Aliclen™** see Salicylic Acid on page 1648

Aliskiren (a lis KYE ren)

Related Information
Angiotensin Agents on page 1985
Medication Safety Issues
Sound-alike/look-alike issues:
Tekturna® may be confused with Valturna®
Brand Names: U.S. Tekturna®
Brand Names: Canada Rasilez®
Index Terms Aliskiren Hemifumarate; SPP100

Generic Availability (U.S.) No

Pharmacologic Category Renin Inhibitor

Use Treatment of hypertension, alone or in combination with other antihypertensive agents

Unlabeled/Investigational Use Treatment of persistent proteinuria in patients with type 2 diabetes mellitus, hypertension, and nephropathy despite administration of optimized recommended renoprotective therapy (eg, angiotensin II receptor blocker)

Contraindications

U.S. labeling: There are no contraindications listed in manufacturer's labeling.

Canada labeling: Hypersensitivity to aliskiren or any component of the formulation

Warnings/Precautions Since the effect of aliskiren on bradykinin levels is unknown, the risk of kinin-mediated etiologies of angioedema occurring is also unknown. Use with caution in any patient with a history of angioedema (of any etiology) as angioedema, some cases necessitating hospitalization and intubation, has been observed (rarely) with aliskiren use. Discontinue immediately following any signs and symptoms of angioedema; do not readminister. Prolonged frequent monitoring may be required especially if tongue, glottis, or larynx are involved as they are associated with airway obstruction. Patients with a history of airway surgery may have a higher risk of airway obstruction. Early, aggressive, and appropriate management is critical. Hyperkalemia may occur (rarely) during monotherapy; risk may increase in patients with predisposing factors (eg, renal dysfunction, diabetes mellitus or concomitant use with ACE inhibitors, potassium-sparing diuretics, potassium supplements, and/or potassium-containing salts). Symptomatic hypotension may occur (rarely) during the initiation of therapy, particularly in patients with an activated renin-angiotensin system (ie, volume or salt-depleted patients). Use with caution in patients with severe renal impairment; not studied in patients with severe renal impairment (eGFR <30 mL/minute and/or S_{cr} ≥1.7 mg/dL [women]; S_{cr} ≥2 mg/dL [men]), history of dialysis, nephrotic syndrome, or renovascular hypertension. Use with caution or avoid in patients with deteriorating renal function or renal artery stenosis (bilateral or unilateral). Avoid concurrent use with strong inhibitors of P-glycoprotein (eg, cyclosporine, itraconazole).

Adverse Reactions (Reflective of adult population; not specific for elderly)

1% to 10%:

Dermatologic: Rash (1%)

Endocrine & metabolic: Hyperkalemia (monotherapy ≤1%; concurrent with ACE inhibitor in patients with diabetes 6%)

Gastrointestinal: Diarrhea (2%)

Hematologic: Creatine kinase increased (>300%: 1%)

Renal: BUN increased (≤7%), serum creatinine increased (≤7%)

Respiratory: Cough (1%)

Drug Interactions

Metabolism/Transport Effects Substrate of CYP3A4 (minor), P-glycoprotein

Avoid Concomitant Use

Avoid concomitant use of Aliskiren with any of the following: CycloSPORINE; Cyclo-SPORINE (Systemic); Itraconazole

Increased Effect/Toxicity

Aliskiren may increase the levels/effects of: Amifostine; Antihypertensives; Hypotensive Agents; RiTUXimab

The levels/effects of Aliskiren may be increased by: Alfuzosin; Atorvastatin; Conivaptan; CycloSPORINE; CycloSPORINE (Systemic); Diazoxide; Herbs (Hypotensive Properties); Itraconazole; Ketoconazole; Ketoconazole (Systemic); MAO Inhibitors; Pentoxifylline; P-Glycoprotein Inhibitors; Phosphodiesterase 5 Inhibitors; Prostacyclin Analogues; Verapamil

Decreased Effect

Aliskiren may decrease the levels/effects of: Furosemide

The levels/effects of Aliskiren may be decreased by: Grapefruit Juice; Herbs (Hypertensive Properties); Methylphenidate; P-Glycoprotein Inducers; Tocilizumab; Yohimbine

Ethanol/Nutrition/Herb Interactions

Food: High-fat meals decrease absorption.

Herb/Nutraceutical: Avoid herbs with *hypertensive* properties (bayberry, blue cohosh, cayenne, ephedra, ginger, ginseng [American], kola, licorice). Avoid herbs with *hypotensive* properties (black cohosh, California poppy, coleus, garlic, goldenseal, hawthorn, mistletoe, periwinkle, quinine, shepherd's purse).

Stability Store at 25°C (77°F); excursions permitted to 15°C to 30°C (59°F to 86°F). Protect from moisture.

Mechanism of Action Aliskerin is a direct renin inhibitor, resulting in blockade of the conversion of angiotensinogen to angiotensin I. Angiotensin I suppression decreases the formation of angiotensin II (Ang II), a potent blood pressure-elevating peptide (via direct vasoconstriction, aldosterone release, and sodium retention). Ang II also functions within the Renin-Angiotensin-Aldosterone System (RAAS) as a negative inhibitory feedback mediator

◀ within the renal parenchyma to suppress the further release of renin. Thus, reductions in Ang II levels suppress this feedback loop, leading to further increased plasma renin concentrations (PRC) and subsequent activity (PRA). This disinhibition effect can be potentially problematic for ACE inhibitor and ARB therapy, as increased PRA could partially overcome the pharmacologic inhibition of the RAAS. As aliskiren is a direct inhibitor of renin activity, blunting of PRA despite the increased PRC (from loss of the negative feedback) may be clinically advantageous. The effect of aliskiren on bradykinin levels is unknown.

Pharmacodynamics/Kinetics
Onset of action: Maximum antihypertensive effect: Within 2 weeks
Absorption: Poor; absorption decreased by high-fat meal. Aliskiren is a substrate of P-glycoprotein; concurrent use of P-glycoprotein inhibitors may increase absorption.
Metabolism: Extent of metabolism unknown; *in vitro* studies indicate metabolism via CYP3A4
Bioavailability: ~3%
Half-life elimination: ~24 hours (range: 16-32 hours)
Time to peak, plasma: 1-3 hours
Excretion: Urine (~25% of absorbed dose excreted unchanged in urine); feces (unchanged via biliary excretion)

Dosage
Geriatric Refer to adult dosing. No initial dosage adjustment required.
Adult Hypertension: Initial: 150 mg once daily; may increase to 300 mg once daily (maximum: 300 mg/day). **Note:** Prior to initiation, correct hypovolemia and/or closely monitor volume status in patients on concurrent diuretics during treatment initiation.
Renal Impairment
Mild-to-moderate impairment (eGFR ≥30 mL/minute and/or S_{cr} <1.7 mg/dL [women]; S_{cr} <2 mg/dL [men]): No dose adjustment required
Severe impairment (eGFR <30 mL/minute and/or S_{cr} ≥1.7 mg/dL [women]; S_{cr} ≥2 mg/dL [men]): Use caution; not studied in severe renal impairment
Hepatic Impairment No dosage adjustment required.

Administration Administer at the same time daily; may take with or without a meal, but consistent administration with regards to meals is recommended. Avoid taking with high-fat meals.

Monitoring Parameters Blood pressure; serum potassium, BUN, serum creatinine

Special Geriatric Considerations The pharmacokinetic studies in elderly (≥65 years of age) demonstrated an increased AUC; however, adjustments in starting dose are not necessary. Blood pressure response and adverse effects were similar to younger adults in studies where 19% of patients were >65 years of age.

Dosage Forms Excipient information presented when available (limited, particularly for generics); consult specific product labeling.
Tablet, oral:
Tekturna®: 150 mg, 300 mg

Selected References
Straessen JA, Li Y, and Richart T, "Oral Renin Inhibitors," *Lancet*, 2006, 368(9545):1449-56.
Vaidyanathan S, Warren V, Yeh C, et al, "Pharmacokinetics, Safety, and Tolerability of the Oral Renin Inhibitor Aliskiren in Patients With Hepatic Impairment," *J Clin Pharmacol*, 2007, 47(2):192-200.

Aliskiren, Amlodipine, and Hydrochlorothiazide
(a lis KYE ren, am LOE di peen, & hye droe klor oh THYE a zide)

Related Information
Aliskiren *on page 58*
AmLODIPine *on page 106*
Hydrochlorothiazide *on page 876*
Medication Safety Issues
Sound-alike/look-alike issues:
Amturnide™ may be confused with AMILoride
Brand Names: U.S. Amturnide™
Index Terms Aliskiren, Hydrochlorothiazide, and Amlodipine; Amlodipine Besylate, Aliskiren Hemifumarate, and Hydrochlorothiazide; Amlodipine, Aliskiren, and Hydrochlorothiazide; Amlodipine, Hydrochlorothiazide, and Aliskiren; Hydrochlorothiazide, Aliskiren, and Amlodipine; Hydrochlorothiazide, Amlodipine, and Aliskiren
Generic Availability (U.S.) No
Pharmacologic Category Calcium Channel Blocker; Calcium Channel Blocker, Dihydropyridine; Diuretic, Thiazide; Renin Inhibitor
Use Treatment of hypertension (not for initial therapy)
Contraindications Hypersensitivity to sulfonamide-derived drugs; anuria
Warnings/Precautions See individual agents.

Adverse Reactions (Reflective of adult population; not specific for elderly) Also see individual agents.

1% to 10%:

Cardiovascular: Peripheral edema (7%)

Central nervous system: Dizziness (4%), headache (4%)

Respiratory: Nasopharyngitis (3%)

Drug Interactions

Avoid Concomitant Use

Avoid concomitant use of Aliskiren, Amlodipine, and Hydrochlorothiazide with any of the following: Conivaptan; CycloSPORINE; CycloSPORINE (Systemic); Dofetilide; Itraconazole

Increased Effect/Toxicity

Aliskiren, Amlodipine, and Hydrochlorothiazide may increase the levels/effects of: ACE Inhibitors; Allopurinol; Amifostine; Antihypertensives; Beta-Blockers; Calcium Channel Blockers (Nondihydropyridine); Calcium Salts; CarBAMazepine; CYP1A2 Substrates; Dofetilide; Fosphenytoin; Hypotensive Agents; Lithium; Magnesium Salts; Neuromuscular-Blocking Agents (Nondepolarizing); Nitroprusside; OXcarbazepine; Phenytoin; Porfimer; QuiNIDine; RiTUXimab; Simvastatin; Sodium Phosphates; Tacrolimus; Tacrolimus (Systemic); Topiramate; Toremifene; Vitamin D Analogs

The levels/effects of Aliskiren, Amlodipine, and Hydrochlorothiazide may be increased by: Alcohol (Ethyl); Alpha1-Blockers; Analgesics (Opioid); Antifungal Agents (Azole Derivatives, Systemic); Atorvastatin; Barbiturates; Calcium Channel Blockers (Nondihydropyridine); Conivaptan; Corticosteroids (Orally Inhaled); Corticosteroids (Systemic); CycloSPORINE; CycloSPORINE (Systemic); CYP3A4 Inhibitors (Moderate); CYP3A4 Inhibitors (Strong); Dasatinib; Fluconazole; Grapefruit Juice; Herbs (Hypotensive Properties); Itraconazole; Ketoconazole; Ketoconazole (Systemic); Licorice; Macrolide Antibiotics; Magnesium Salts; MAO Inhibitors; Pentoxifylline; P-Glycoprotein Inhibitors; Phosphodiesterase 5 Inhibitors; Prostacyclin Analogues; Protease Inhibitors; QuiNIDine; Verapamil

Decreased Effect

Aliskiren, Amlodipine, and Hydrochlorothiazide may decrease the levels/effects of: Antidiabetic Agents; Clopidogrel; Furosemide; QuiNIDine

The levels/effects of Aliskiren, Amlodipine, and Hydrochlorothiazide may be decreased by: Barbiturates; Bile Acid Sequestrants; Calcium Salts; CarBAMazepine; CYP3A4 Inducers (Strong); Deferasirox; Grapefruit Juice; Herbs (CYP3A4 Inducers); Herbs (Hypertensive Properties); Methylphenidate; Nafcillin; Nonsteroidal Anti-Inflammatory Agents; P-Glycoprotein Inducers; Rifamycin Derivatives; Tocilizumab; Yohimbine

Ethanol/Nutrition/Herb Interactions

Food: High-fat meals decrease aliskiren absorption. Grapefruit juice may modestly increase amlodipine levels. Hydrochlorothiazide may deplete potassium, sodium, and magnesium.

Herb/Nutraceutical: St John's wort may decrease amlodipine levels. Avoid herbs with *hypertensive* properties (bayberry, blue cohosh, cayenne, ephedra, ginger, ginseng [American], kola, licorice). Avoid herbs with *hypotensive* properties (black cohosh, California poppy, coleus, garlic, goldenseal, hawthorn, mistletoe, periwinkle, quinine, shepherd's purse).

Stability Store at 25°C (77°F); excursions permitted between 15°C to 30°C (59°F to 86°F) in original container; protect from heat. Protect from moisture.

Mechanism of Action

Aliskiren: Direct renin inhibitor, resulting in blockade of the conversion of angiotensinogen to angiotensin I. Angiotensin I suppression decreases the formation of angiotensin II (Ang II), a potent blood pressure-elevating peptide (via direct vasoconstriction, aldosterone release, and sodium retention). Ang II also functions within the Renin-Angiotensin-Aldosterone System (RAAS) as a negative inhibitory feedback mediator within the renal parenchyma to suppress the further release of renin. Thus, reductions in Ang II levels suppress this feedback loop, leading to further increased plasma renin concentrations (PRC) and subsequent activity (PRA). This disinhibition effect can be potentially problematic for ACE inhibitor and ARB therapy, as increased PRA could partially overcome the pharmacologic inhibition of the RAAS. As aliskiren is a direct inhibitor of renin activity, blunting of PRA despite the increased PRC (from loss of the negative feedback) may be clinically advantageous. The effect of aliskiren on bradykinin levels is unknown.

Amlodipine: Inhibits calcium ion from entering the "slow channels" or select voltage-sensitive areas of vascular smooth muscle and myocardium during depolarization, producing a relaxation of coronary vascular smooth muscle and coronary vasodilation; increases myocardial oxygen delivery in patients with vasospastic angina. Amlodipine directly acts on vascular smooth muscle to produce peripheral arterial vasodilation reducing peripheral vascular resistance and blood pressure.

Hydrochlorothiazide: Inhibits sodium reabsorption in the distal tubules causing increased excretion of sodium and water as well as potassium and hydrogen ions.

◀ **Pharmacodynamics/Kinetics** See individual agents.
Dosage
Geriatric Hypertension: Oral:
Patients ≥65 and <75 years: Refer to adult dosing.
Patients ≥75 years: Initial: Amlodipine 2.5 mg (strength not available in combination product)
Adult Note: Not for initial therapy. Dose is individualized; combination product may be substituted for individual components in patients currently maintained on all three agents separately, used to switch a patient on any dual combination of the components who is experiencing dose-limiting adverse reactions from an individual component (to a lower dose of that component), or used as add-on therapy in patients not adequately controlled with any two of the following: Aliskiren, dihydropyridine calcium channel blockers, and thiazide diuretics.

Hypertension: Oral: *Add-on/switch therapy/replacement therapy:* Aliskiren 150-300 mg and amlodipine 5-10 mg and hydrochlorothiazide 12.5-25 mg once daily; dose may be titrated after 2 weeks of therapy. Maximum recommended daily dose: Aliskiren 300 mg; amlodipine 10 mg; hydrochlorothiazide 25 mg
Renal Impairment Cl$_{cr}$ ≤30 mL/minute: Use of combination product is not recommended.
Hepatic Impairment Severe hepatic impairment: Initial: Amlodipine 2.5 mg daily (strength not available in combination product).
Administration Administer at the same time daily. May take with or without a meal, but consistent administration with regard to meals is recommended.
Monitoring Parameters Heart rate, blood pressure; serum electrolytes, BUN, serum creatinine; assess weight, I & O reports daily to determine fluid loss; peripheral edema
Special Geriatric Considerations No overall differences in safety or efficacy were observed in older adults compared to younger adults receiving aliskiren, amlodipine, and hydrochlorothiazide (Amturnide™) during short-term clinical trials involving 19% of patients ≥65 years of age. Also see individual agents.
Dosage Forms Excipient information presented when available (limited, particularly for generics); consult specific product labeling.
Tablet, oral:
Amturnide™: Aliskiren 150 mg, amlodipine 5 mg, and hydrochlorothiazide 12.5 mg
Amturnide™: Aliskiren 300 mg, amlodipine 5 mg, and hydrochlorothiazide 12.5 mg
Amturnide™: Aliskiren 300 mg, amlodipine 5 mg, and hydrochlorothiazide 25 mg
Amturnide™: Aliskiren 300 mg, amlodipine 10 mg, and hydrochlorothiazide 12.5 mg
Amturnide™: Aliskiren 300 mg, amlodipine 10 mg, and hydrochlorothiazide 25 mg

---

Aliskiren and Amlodipine (a lis KYE ren & am LOE di peen)

Related Information
Aliskiren *on page 58*
AmLODIPine *on page 106*
Brand Names: U.S. Tekamlo™
Index Terms Aliskiren Hemifumarate and Amlodipine Besylate; Amlodipine and Aliskiren
Generic Availability (U.S.) No
Pharmacologic Category Calcium Channel Blocker; Calcium Channel Blocker, Dihydropyridine; Renin Inhibitor
Use Treatment of hypertension, alone or in combination with other antihypertensive agents, including use as initial therapy in patients likely to need multiple antihypertensives for adequate control
Contraindications There are no contraindications listed in manufacturer's labeling.
Warnings/Precautions See individual agents.
Adverse Reactions (Reflective of adult population; not specific for elderly) Frequencies reported with combination product. See individual monographs for additional adverse effects reported with each agent.
1% to 10%: Cardiovascular: Peripheral edema (6% to 9%)
Drug Interactions
Avoid Concomitant Use
Avoid concomitant use of Aliskiren and Amlodipine with any of the following: Conivaptan; CycloSPORINE; CycloSPORINE (Systemic); Itraconazole
Increased Effect/Toxicity
Aliskiren and Amlodipine may increase the levels/effects of: Amifostine; Antihypertensives; Beta-Blockers; Calcium Channel Blockers (Nondihydropyridine); CYP1A2 Substrates; Fosphenytoin; Hypotensive Agents; Magnesium Salts; Neuromuscular-Blocking Agents (Nondepolarizing); Nitroprusside; Phenytoin; QuiNIDine; RiTUXimab; Simvastatin; Tacrolimus; Tacrolimus (Systemic)

The levels/effects of Aliskiren and Amlodipine may be increased by: Alpha1-Blockers; Antifungal Agents (Azole Derivatives, Systemic); Atorvastatin; Calcium Channel Blockers (Nondihydropyridine); Conivaptan; CycloSPORINE; CycloSPORINE (Systemic); CYP3A4 Inhibitors (Moderate); CYP3A4 Inhibitors (Strong); Dasatinib; Diazoxide; Fluconazole; Grapefruit Juice; Herbs (Hypotensive Properties); Itraconazole; Ketoconazole; Ketoconazole (Systemic); Macrolide Antibiotics; Magnesium Salts; MAO Inhibitors; Pentoxifylline; P-Glycoprotein Inhibitors; Phosphodiesterase 5 Inhibitors; Prostacyclin Analogues; Protease Inhibitors; QuiNIDine; Verapamil

Decreased Effect

Aliskiren and Amlodipine may decrease the levels/effects of: Clopidogrel; Furosemide; QuiNIDine

The levels/effects of Aliskiren and Amlodipine may be decreased by: Barbiturates; Calcium Salts; CarBAMazepine; CYP3A4 Inducers (Strong); Deferasirox; Grapefruit Juice; Herbs (CYP3A4 Inducers); Herbs (Hypertensive Properties); Methylphenidate; Nafcillin; P-Glycoprotein Inducers; Rifamycin Derivatives; Tocilizumab; Yohimbine

Ethanol/Nutrition/Herb Interactions Food: High-fat meals decrease absorption.

Herb/Nutraceutical: Avoid herbs with *hypertensive* properties (bayberry, blue cohosh, cayenne, ephedra, ginger, ginseng [American], kola, licorice). Avoid herbs with *hypotensive* properties (black cohosh, California poppy, coleus, garlic, goldenseal, hawthorn, mistletoe, periwinkle, quinine, shepherd's purse).

Stability Store at 25°C (77°F); excursions permitted to 15°C to 30°C (59°F to 86°F). Protect from moisture.

Mechanism of Action

Aliskiren: Direct renin inhibitor, resulting in blockade of the conversion of angiotensinogen to angiotensin I. Angiotensin I suppression decreases the formation of angiotensin II (Ang II), a potent blood pressure-elevating peptide (via direct vasoconstriction, aldosterone release, and sodium retention). Ang II also functions within the Renin-Angiotensin-Aldosterone System (RAAS) as a negative inhibitory feedback mediator within the renal parenchyma to suppress the further release of renin. Thus, reductions in Ang II levels suppress this feedback loop, leading to further increased plasma renin concentrations (PRC) and subsequent activity (PRA). This disinhibition effect can be potentially problematic for ACE inhibitor and ARB therapy, as increased PRA could partially overcome the pharmacologic inhibition of the RAAS. As aliskiren is a direct inhibitor of renin activity, blunting of PRA despite the increased PRC (from loss of the negative feedback) may be clinically advantageous. The effect of aliskiren on bradykinin levels is unknown.

Amlodipine: Inhibits calcium ion from entering the "slow channels" or select voltage-sensitive areas of vascular smooth muscle and myocardium during depolarization, producing a relaxation of coronary vascular smooth muscle and coronary vasodilation; increases myocardial oxygen delivery in patients with vasospastic angina. Amlodipine directly acts on vascular smooth muscle to produce peripheral arterial vasodilation reducing peripheral vascular resistance and blood pressure.

Pharmacodynamics/Kinetics See individual agents.

Dosage

Geriatric Refer to adult dosing. No initial dosage adjustment required.

Adult

Hypertension: Oral: Dosage must be individualized. Combination product may be used as initial therapy or substituted for individual components in patients currently maintained on both agents separately or in patients not adequately controlled with monotherapy (using one of the agents or an agent within same antihypertensive class).

Initial therapy: Aliskiren 150 mg and amlodipine 5 mg once daily; dose may be titrated at 2- to 4-week intervals; maximum recommended daily doses: Aliskiren 300 mg; amlodipine 10 mg

Add-on therapy: Initiate by adding the lowest available dose of the alternative component (aliskiren 150 mg or amlodipine 5 mg); dose may be titrated at 2- to 4-week intervals; maximum recommended daily doses: Aliskiren 300 mg; amlodipine 10 mg

Replacement therapy: Substitute for the individually titrated components

Note: Prior to initiation, correct hypovolemia and/or closely monitor volume status in patients on concurrent diuretics during treatment initiation.

Renal Impairment

Mild-to-moderate impairment (eGFR ≥30 mL/minute and/or S_{cr} <1.7 mg/dL [women]; S_{cr} <2 mg/dL [men]): No dose adjustment required

Severe impairment (eGFR <30 mL/minute and/or S_{cr} ≥1.7 mg/dL [women]; S_{cr} ≥2 mg/dL [men]): Use caution; not studied in severe renal impairment

Hepatic Impairment Use caution; no dosage adjustment required; titrate slowly.

Administration Administer at the same time daily. May take with or without a meal, but consistent administration with regards to meals is recommended.

Monitoring Parameters Blood pressure; serum potassium, BUN, serum creatinine

Special Geriatric Considerations No overall differences in safety or efficacy were observed in older adults compared to younger adults receiving aliskiren and amlodipine (Tekamlo™) during short-term clinical trials involving 17% of patients ≥65 years of age. Also see individual agents.

Dosage Forms Excipient information presented when available (limited, particularly for generics); consult specific product labeling.

Tablet, oral:

Tekamlo™ 150/5: Aliskiren 150 mg and amlodipine 5 mg
Tekamlo™ 150/10: Aliskiren 150 mg and amlodipine 10 mg
Tekamlo™ 300/5: Aliskiren 300 mg and amlodipine 5 mg
Tekamlo™ 300/10: Aliskiren 300 mg and amlodipine 10 mg

Selected References

Littlejohn TW 3rd, Trenkwalder P, Hollanders G, et al, "Long-Term Safety, Tolerability and Efficacy of Combination Therapy With Aliskiren and Amlodipine in Patients With Hypertension," *Curr Med Res Opin*, 2009, 25(4):951-9.

Aliskiren and Valsartan (a lis KYE ren & val SAR tan)

Related Information

Aliskiren *on page 58*
Valsartan *on page 1892*

Medication Safety Issues

Sound-alike/look-alike issues:

Valturna® may be confused with Tekturna®, valsartan

Brand Names: U.S. Valturna®

Index Terms Aliskiren Hemifumarate and Valsartan; Valsartan and Aliskiren

Generic Availability (U.S.) No

Pharmacologic Category Angiotensin II Receptor Blocker; Renin Inhibitor

Use Treatment of hypertension, including use as initial therapy in patients likely to need multiple antihypertensives for adequate control

Dosage

Geriatric & Adult Hypertension: Oral: Dose is individualized; combination product may be used as initial therapy or substituted for individual components in patients currently maintained on both agents separately or in patients not adequately controlled with mono-therapy (using one of the agents or an agent within same antihypertensive class). Titrate at 2- to 4-week intervals as necessary.

Initial therapy: Aliskiren 150 mg and valsartan 160 mg once daily; titrate to effect (max-imum daily aliskiren dose: 300 mg; maximum daily valsartan dose: 320 mg)

Patients not controlled with single-agent therapy: Aliskiren 150 mg and valsartan 160 mg once daily; titrate to effect (maximum daily aliskiren dose: 300 mg; maximum daily valsartan dose: 320 mg)

Renal Impairment

Mild-to-moderate impairment (Cl_{cr} ≥30 mL/minute): No dose adjustment required.

Severe impairment (Cl_{cr} <30 mL/minute): Use caution; not studied in severe renal impairment.

Hepatic Impairment In mild-to-moderate liver disease no adjustment is needed. Use caution in patients with severe hepatic impairment; clinical experience is limited.

Special Geriatric Considerations See individual agents.

Dosage Forms Excipient information presented when available (limited, particularly for generics); consult specific product labeling.

Tablet:

Valturna®:

150/160: Aliskiren 150 mg and valsartan 160 mg
300/320: Aliskiren 300 mg and valsartan 320 mg

◆ **Aliskiren Hemifumarate** *see* Aliskiren *on page 58*
◆ **Aliskiren Hemifumarate and Amlodipine Besylate** *see* Aliskiren and Amlodipine *on page 62*
◆ **Aliskiren Hemifumarate and Valsartan** *see* Aliskiren and Valsartan *on page 64*
◆ **Aliskiren, Hydrochlorothiazide, and Amlodipine** *see* Aliskiren, Amlodipine, and Hydro-chlorothiazide *on page 60*
◆ **Alka-Mints® [OTC]** *see* Calcium Salts (Oral) *on page 256*
◆ **Alka-Seltzer Plus® Sinus Formula [OTC]** *see* Acetaminophen and Phenylephrine *on page 38*
◆ **Alkeran®** *see* Melphalan *on page 1131*
◆ **All Day Allergy [OTC]** *see* Cetirizine *on page 327*
◆ **Allegra®** *see* Fexofenadine *on page 730*

♦ **Allegra® Allergy 12 Hour [OTC]** *see* Fexofenadine *on page 730*
♦ **Allegra® Allergy 24 Hour [OTC]** *see* Fexofenadine *on page 730*
♦ **Allegra® Children's Allergy [OTC]** *see* Fexofenadine *on page 730*
♦ **Allegra® Children's Allergy ODT [OTC]** *see* Fexofenadine *on page 730*
♦ **Allegra® ODT [DSC]** *see* Fexofenadine *on page 730*
♦ **Aller-Chlor® [OTC]** *see* Chlorpheniramine *on page 337*
♦ **Allerfrim [OTC]** *see* Triprolidine and Pseudoephedrine *on page 1872*
♦ **AllerMax® [OTC]** *see* DiphenhydrAMINE (Systemic) *on page 520*
♦ **Allfen [OTC]** *see* GuaiFENesin *on page 846*
♦ **Allfen CD** *see* Guaifenesin and Codeine *on page 848*
♦ **Allfen CDX** *see* Guaifenesin and Codeine *on page 848*
♦ **Allfen DM [OTC] [DSC]** *see* Guaifenesin and Dextromethorphan *on page 848*
♦ **Alli® [OTC]** *see* Orlistat *on page 1351*

Allopurinol (al oh PURE i nole)

Medication Safety Issues
Sound-alike/look-alike issues:
Allopurinol may be confused with Apresoline
Zyloprim® may be confused with ZORprin®, Zovirax®
Brand Names: U.S. Aloprim®; Zyloprim®
Brand Names: Canada Alloprin®; Apo-Allopurinol®; Novo-Purol; Zyloprim®
Index Terms Allopurinol Sodium
Generic Availability (U.S.) Yes
Pharmacologic Category Antigout Agent; Xanthine Oxidase Inhibitor
Use
Oral: Management of primary or secondary gout (acute attack, tophi, joint destruction, uric acid lithiasis, and/or nephropathy); management of hyperuricemia associated with cancer treatment for leukemia, lymphoma, or solid tumor malignancies; management of recurrent calcium oxalate calculi (with uric acid excretion >800 mg/day in men and >750 mg/day in women)
I.V.: Management of hyperuricemia associated with cancer treatment for leukemia, lymphoma, or solid tumor malignancies
Contraindications Hypersensitivity to allopurinol or any component of the formulation
Warnings/Precautions Do not use to treat asymptomatic hyperuricemia. Has been associated with a number of hypersensitivity reactions, including severe reactions (vasculitis and Stevens-Johnson syndrome); discontinue at first sign of rash. Reversible hepatotoxicity has been reported; use with caution in patients with pre-existing hepatic impairment. Bone marrow suppression has been reported; use caution with other drugs causing myelosuppression. Caution in renal impairment, dosage adjustments needed. Use with caution in patients taking diuretics concurrently. Risk of skin rash may be increased in patients receiving amoxicillin or ampicillin. The risk of hypersensitivity may be increased in patients receiving thiazides, and possibly ACE inhibitors. Use caution with mercaptopurine or azathioprine; dosage adjustment necessary. Full effect on serum uric acid levels in chronic gout may take several weeks to become evident; gradual titration is recommended.
Adverse Reactions (Reflective of adult population; not specific for elderly)
Dermatologic: Rash
Endocrine & metabolic: Gout (acute)
Gastrointestinal: Diarrhea, nausea
Hepatic: Alkaline phosphatase increased, liver enzymes increased
Drug Interactions
Avoid Concomitant Use
Avoid concomitant use of Allopurinol with any of the following: Didanosine
Increased Effect/Toxicity
Allopurinol may increase the levels/effects of: Amoxicillin; Ampicillin; Anticonvulsants (Hydantoin); AzaTHIOprine; CarBAMazepine; ChlorproPAMIDE; Cyclophosphamide; Didanosine; Mercaptopurine; Theophylline Derivatives; Vitamin K Antagonists

The levels/effects of Allopurinol may be increased by: ACE Inhibitors; Loop Diuretics; Thiazide Diuretics
Decreased Effect
The levels/effects of Allopurinol may be decreased by: Antacids
Ethanol/Nutrition/Herb Interactions
Ethanol: May decrease effectiveness.
Iron supplements: Hepatic iron uptake may be increased.
Vitamin C: Large amounts of vitamin C may acidify urine and increase kidney stone formation.

Stability

Powder for injection: Store at controlled room temperature of 20°C to 25°C (68°F to 77°F). Reconstitute powder for injection with SWFI. Further dilution with NS or D_5W (50-100 mL) to ≤6 mg/mL is recommended. Following preparation, intravenous solutions should be stored at 20°C to 25°C (68°F to 77°F). Do not refrigerate reconstituted and/or diluted product. Must be administered within 10 hours of solution preparation.

Tablet: Store at controlled room temperature of 20°C to 25°C (68°F to 77°F). Protect from moisture and light.

Mechanism of Action

Allopurinol inhibits xanthine oxidase, the enzyme responsible for the conversion of hypoxanthine to xanthine to uric acid. Allopurinol is metabolized to oxypurinol which is also an inhibitor of xanthine oxidase; allopurinol acts on purine catabolism, reducing the production of uric acid without disrupting the biosynthesis of vital purines.

Pharmacodynamics/Kinetics

Onset of action: Peak effect: 1-2 weeks

Absorption: Oral: ~80%; Rectal: Poor and erratic

Distribution: V_d: ~1.6 L/kg; V_{ss}: 0.84-0.87 L/kg; enters breast milk

Protein binding: <1%

Metabolism: ~75% to active metabolites, chiefly oxypurinol

Bioavailability: 49% to 53%

Half-life elimination:

Normal renal function: Parent drug: 1-3 hours; Oxypurinol: 18-30 hours

End-stage renal disease: Prolonged

Time to peak, plasma: Oral: 30-120 minutes

Excretion: Urine (76% as oxypurinol, 12% as unchanged drug)

Allopurinol and oxypurinol are dialyzable

Dosage

Geriatric & Adult Note: Oral doses >300 mg should be given in divided doses.

Gout (chronic): Oral:

Manufacturer's labeling: Mild: 200-300 mg/day; Severe: 400-600 mg/day; to reduce the possibility of acute gouty attacks, initiate dose at 100 mg/day and increase weekly to recommended dosage, also consider using low-dose colchicine or an NSAID to reduce the risk of a gouty attack. Maximum daily dose: 800 mg/day.

Alternative recommendations (unlabeled dosing): Initial: 100 mg/day, increasing the dose gradually every 4 weeks, while monitoring plasma uric acid levels to achieve a goal of <6 mg/dL; dosages of 600 mg/day and rarely, 900 mg/day may be required (McGill, 2010) **or** Initial: 100 mg/day, increasing the dose by 100 mg/day at 2-4 weeks intervals as required to achieve desired uric acid level of ≤6 mg/dL (EULAR gout guidelines; Zhang, 2006).

Management of hyperuricemia associated with chemotherapy:

Oral:

Manufacturer's labeling: 600-800 mg/day in 2-3 divided doses

Alternative recommendations (unlabeled dosing; intermediate-risk for tumor lysis syndrome): Intermediate-risk for tumor lysis syndrome: 10 mg/kg/day (maximum dose/day: 800 mg) in 3 divided doses **or** 50-100 mg/m² every 8 hours (maximum dose: 300 mg/m²/day), begin 1-2 days before initiation of induction chemotherapy; may continue for 3-7 days after chemotherapy (Coiffier, 2008)

I.V.:

Manufacturer's labeling: 200-400 mg/m²/day (maximum: 600 mg/day) beginning 1-2 days before chemotherapy

Alternative recommendations (unlabeled dosing; intermediate-risk for tumor lysis syndrome): 200-400 mg/m²/day (maximum dose/day: 600 mg) in 1-3 divided doses beginning 1-2 days before the start of induction chemotherapy; may continue for 3-7 days after chemotherapy (Coiffier, 2008)

Note: Intravenous daily dose can be given as a single infusion or in equally divided doses at 6-, 8-, or 12-hour intervals. A fluid intake sufficient to yield a daily urinary output of at least 2 L in adults is desirable.

Recurrent calcium oxalate stones: Oral: 200-300 mg/day in single or divided doses

Renal Impairment

Manufacturer's labeling: Oral, I.V.: Lower doses are required in renal impairment due to potential for accumulation of allopurinol and metabolites.

Cl_{cr} 10-20 mL/minute: 200 mg/day

Cl_{cr} 3-10 mL/minute: ≤100 mg/day

Cl_{cr} <3 mL/minute: 100 mg/dose at extended intervals

Alternative recommendations (unlabeled dosing):

Management of hyperuricemia associated with chemotherapy: Dosage reduction of 50% is recommended in renal impairment (Coiffier, 2008)

Gout: Oral:

Initiate therapy with 50-100 mg daily, and gradually increase to a maintenance dose to achieve a serum uric acid level of ≤6 mg/dL (with close monitoring of serum uric acid levels and for hypersensitivity) (Dalbeth, 2007).

Maintenance: The following maintenance dose recommendations (see table) have been proposed to reduce the risk of allopurinol hypersensitivity syndrome (AHS) (Hande, 1984). However, the utility of these recommendations has been questioned in recent literature due to observations that AHS risk is not altered and the reduced dosing may not adequately reduce serum uric acid levels to control hyperuricemia effectively (Dalbeth, 2007).

Hemodialysis: Initial: 100 mg alternate days given postdialysis, increase cautiously to 300 mg based on response. If dialysis is on a daily basis, an additional 50% of the dose may be required postdialysis (Dalbeth, 2007)

Adult Maintenance Doses of Allopurinol[1]

Creatinine Clearance (mL/min)	Maintenance Dose of Allopurinol (mg)
140	400 daily
120	350 daily
100	300 daily
80	250 daily
60	200 daily
40	150 daily
20	100 daily
10	100 every 2 days
0	100 every 3 days

[1]This table is based on a standard maintenance dose of 300 mg of allopurinol per day for a patient with a creatinine clearance of 100 mL/min.

I.V.:

Cl_{cr} 10-20 mL/minute: Administer 200 mg/day.

Cl_{cr} 3-10 mL/minute: Administer 100 mg/day.

Cl_{cr} <3 mL/minute: Administer 100 mg/day at extended intervals.

Administration

Oral: Should administer oral forms after meals with plenty of fluid.

I.V.: The rate of infusion depends on the volume of the infusion. Whenever possible, therapy should be initiated at 24-48 hours before the start of chemotherapy known to cause tumor lysis (including adrenocorticosteroids). I.V. daily dose can be administered as a single infusion or in equally divided doses at 6-, 8-, or 12-hour interval.

Monitoring Parameters CBC, serum uric acid levels, I & O, hepatic and renal function, especially at start of therapy; signs and symptoms of hypersensitivity

Reference Range Uric acid, serum: An increase occurs during childhood

Adults:

Male: 3.4-7 mg/dL or slightly more

Female: 2.4-6 mg/dL or slightly more

Target: ≤6 mg/dL

Values >7 mg/dL are sometimes arbitrarily regarded as hyperuricemia, but there is no sharp line between normals on the one hand, and the serum uric acid of those with clinical gout. Normal ranges cannot be adjusted for purine ingestion, but high purine diet increases uric acid. Uric acid may be increased with body size, exercise, and stress.

Special Geriatric Considerations Adjust dose based on renal function.

Dosage Forms Excipient information presented when available (limited, particularly for generics); consult specific product labeling.

Injection, powder for reconstitution, as sodium: 500 mg (base)

Aloprim®: 500 mg (base)

Tablet, oral: 100 mg, 300 mg

Zyloprim®: 100 mg, 300 mg [scored]

◆ **Allopurinol Sodium** see Allopurinol on page 65

◆ **Almacone® [OTC]** see Aluminum Hydroxide, Magnesium Hydroxide, and Simethicone on page 84

◆ **Almacone Double Strength® [OTC]** see Aluminum Hydroxide, Magnesium Hydroxide, and Simethicone on page 84

◆ **Almora® [OTC]** *see* Magnesium Salts (Various Salts) *on page 1114*

Almotriptan (al moh TRIP tan)

Medication Safety Issues
Sound-alike/look-alike issues:
Axert® may be confused with Antivert®
Brand Names: U.S. Axert®
Brand Names: Canada Axert®
Index Terms Almotriptan Malate
Generic Availability (U.S.) No
Pharmacologic Category Antimigraine Agent; Serotonin 5-HT$_{1B, 1D}$ Receptor Agonist
Use Acute treatment of migraine with or without aura in adults (with a history of migraine)
Contraindications Hypersensitivity to almotriptan or any component of the formulation; hemiplegic or basilar migraine; known or suspected ischemic heart disease (eg, angina pectoris, MI, documented silent ischemia, coronary artery vasospasm, Prinzmetal's variant angina); cerebrovascular syndromes (eg, stroke, transient ischemic attacks); peripheral vascular disease (eg, ischemic bowel disease); uncontrolled hypertension; use within 24 hours of another 5-HT$_1$ agonist; use within 24 hours of ergotamine derivatives and/or ergotamine-containing medications (eg, dihydroergotamine, ergotamine)
Warnings/Precautions Almotriptan is only indicated for the treatment of acute migraine headache; not indicated for migraine prophylaxis, or the treatment of cluster headaches, hemiplegic migraine, or basilar migraine. If a patient does not respond to the first dose, the diagnosis of acute migraine should be reconsidered.

Almotriptan should not be given to patients with documented ischemic or vasospastic CAD. Patients with risk factors for CAD (eg, hypertension, hypercholesterolemia, smoker, obesity, diabetes, strong family history of CAD, menopause, male >40 years of age) should undergo adequate cardiac evaluation prior to administration; if the cardiac evaluation is "satisfactory," the first dose of almotriptan should be given in the healthcare provider's office (consider ECG monitoring). All patients should undergo periodic evaluation of cardiovascular status during treatment. Cardiac events (coronary artery vasospasm, transient ischemia, myocardial infarction, ventricular tachycardia/fibrillation, cardiac arrest, and death), cerebral/subarachnoid hemorrhage, stroke, peripheral vascular ischemia, and colonic ischemia have been reported with 5-HT$_1$ agonist administration. Patients who experience sensations of chest pain/pressure/tightness or symptoms suggestive of angina following dosing should be evaluated for coronary artery disease or Prinzmetal's angina before receiving additional doses; if dosing is resumed and similar symptoms recur, monitor with ECG. Significant elevation in blood pressure, including hypertensive crisis, has also been reported on rare occasions following 5-HT$_1$ agonist administration in patients with and without a history of hypertension.

Transient and permanent blindness and partial vision loss have been reported (rare) with 5-HT$_1$ agonist administration. Almotriptan contains a sulfonyl group which is structurally different from a sulfonamide. Cross-reactivity in patients with sulfonamide allergy has not been evaluated; however, the manufacturer recommends that caution be exercised in this patient population. Use with caution in liver or renal dysfunction. Symptoms of agitation, confusion, hallucinations, hyper-reflexia, myoclonus, shivering, and tachycardia (serotonin syndrome) may occur with concomitant proserotonergic drugs (ie, SSRIs/SNRIs or triptans) or agents that reduce almotriptan's metabolism. Concurrent use of serotonin precursors (eg, tryptophan) is not recommended. If concomitant administration with SSRIs is warranted, monitor closely, especially at initiation and with dose increases. Efficacy has not been demonstrated in improvement of migraine-associated symptoms (eg, phonophobia, nausea, photophobia) in patients aged 12-17 years (Linder, 2008).
Adverse Reactions (Reflective of adult population; not specific for elderly)
1% to 10%:
Central nervous system: Somnolence (≤5%), dizziness (≤4%), headache (≤2%)
Gastrointestinal: Nausea (1% to 3%), vomiting (≤2%), xerostomia (1%)
Neuromuscular & skeletal: Paresthesia (≤1%)
Drug Interactions
Metabolism/Transport Effects Substrate (minor) of CYP2D6, 3A4
Avoid Concomitant Use
Avoid concomitant use of Almotriptan with any of the following: Ergot Derivatives; MAO Inhibitors; Sibutramine
Increased Effect/Toxicity
Almotriptan may increase the levels/effects of: Ergot Derivatives; Serotonin Modulators

The levels/effects of Almotriptan may be increased by: CYP3A4 Inhibitors (Strong); Ergot Derivatives; MAO Inhibitors; Sibutramine

Decreased Effect

The levels/effects of Almotriptan may be decreased by: Peginterferon Alfa-2b; Tocilizumab

Stability Store at 25°C (77°F); excursions permitted to 15°C to 30°C (59°F to 86°F).

Mechanism of Action Selective agonist for serotonin (5-HT$_{1B}$ and 5-HT$_{1D}$ receptors) in cranial arteries; causes vasoconstriction and reduces sterile inflammation associated with antidromic neuronal transmission correlating with relief of migraine

Pharmacodynamics/Kinetics Geriatrics: Pharmacokinetic disposition is similar to that in young adults.

Absorption: Well absorbed

Distribution: V$_d$: 180-200 L

Protein binding: ~35%

Metabolism: MAO type A oxidative deamination (~27% of dose)

Bioavailability: 12.5 mg dose - 80%; 25 mg dose - 70%

Half-life: 3-4 hours

Time to peak: 1-3 hours

Elimination: Urine (40% as unchanged drug); feces (13% unchanged and metabolized)

Dosage

Geriatric & Adult Migraine: Oral: Initial: 6.25-12.5 mg in a single dose; if the headache returns, repeat the dose after 2 hours; no more than 2 doses (maximum daily dose: 25 mg)
Note: The safety of treating more than 4 migraines/month has not been established.

Dosage adjustment with concomitant use of an enzyme inhibitor:

Patients receiving a potent CYP3A4 inhibitor: Initial: 6.25 mg in a single dose; maximum daily dose: 12.5 mg

Patients with renal impairment and concomitant use of a potent CYP3A4 inhibitor: Avoid use

Patients with hepatic impairment and concomitant use of a potent CYP3A4 inhibitor: Avoid use

Renal Impairment Severe renal impairment (Cl$_{cr}$ ≤30 mL/minute): Initial: 6.25 mg in a single dose; maximum daily dose: 12.5 mg

Hepatic Impairment Initial: 6.25 mg in a single dose; maximum daily dose: 12.5 mg

Administration Administer without regard to meals.

Special Geriatric Considerations Use cautiously in elderly, particularly since many have cardiovascular disease, which would put them at risk for cardiovascular adverse effects. Safety and efficacy in elderly patients >65 years of age have not been established.

Dosage Forms Excipient information presented when available (limited, particularly for generics); consult specific product labeling.

Tablet, oral, as maleate:

Axert®: 6.25 mg, 12.5 mg

◆ **Almotriptan Malate** *see Almotriptan on page 68*
◆ **Alocril®** *see Nedocromil on page 1275*
◆ **Alodox™** *see Doxycycline on page 570*
◆ **Aloe Vesta® Antifungal [OTC]** *see Miconazole on page 1206*
◆ **Alomide®** *see Lodoxamide on page 1085*
◆ **Alophen® [OTC]** *see Bisacodyl on page 205*
◆ **Aloprim®** *see Allopurinol on page 65*
◆ **Alora®** *see Estradiol (Systemic) on page 641*

Alpha-Galactosidase (AL fa ga lak TOE si days)

Medication Safety Issues

Sound-alike/look-alike issues:

beano® may be confused with B&O (belladonna and opium)

Brand Names: U.S. beano® [OTC]

Index Terms *Aspergillus niger*

Generic Availability (U.S.) No

Pharmacologic Category Enzyme

Use Prevention of flatulence and bloating attributed to a variety of grains, cereals, nuts, and vegetables containing the sugars raffinose, stachyose, and/or verbascose

Dosage

Geriatric & Adult Flatulence and bloating: Oral:

Drops: Take 5 drops per serving of problem food; adjust according to number of problem foods per meal; usual dose/meal: 10-15 drops

Tablet: One tablet per serving of problem food; adjust according to number of problem foods per meal; usual dose/meal: 2-3 tablets

ALPHA-GALACTOSIDASE

◀ **Dosage Forms** Excipient information presented when available (limited, particularly for generics); consult specific product labeling.
Liquid, oral [drops]:
beano®: 150 Galactosidase units/5 drops (15 mL) [contains sodium 5 mg/5 drops]
Tablet, oral:
beano®: 150 Galactosidase units [scored]

◆ **Alphagan® P** see Brimonidine on page 211
◆ **1α-Hydroxyergocalciferol** see Doxercalciferol on page 567
◆ **Alph-E [OTC]** see Vitamin E on page 1921
◆ **Alph-E-Mixed [OTC]** see Vitamin E on page 1921

ALPRAZolam (al PRAY zoe lam)

Related Information
Anxiolytic, Sedative / Hypnotic, and Miscellaneous Benzodiazepines on page 2000
Beers Criteria – Potentially Inappropriate Medications for Geriatrics on page 2089
Medication Safety Issues
Sound-alike/look-alike issues:
ALPRAZolam may be confused with alprostadil, LORazepam, triazolam
Xanax® may be confused with Fanapt®, Lanoxin®, Tenex®, Tylox®, Xopenex®, Zantac®, ZyrTEC®
BEERS Criteria medication:
This drug may be inappropriate for use in geriatric patients (high severity risk).
Brand Names: U.S. Alprazolam Intensol™; Niravam™; Xanax XR®; Xanax®
Brand Names: Canada Apo-Alpraz®; Apo-Alpraz® TS; Mylan-Alprazolam; Novo-Alprazol; Nu-Alpraz; Teva-Alprazolam; Xanax TS™; Xanax®
Generic Availability (U.S.) Yes: Excludes oral solution
Pharmacologic Category Benzodiazepine
Use Treatment of anxiety disorder (GAD); panic disorder, with or without agoraphobia; anxiety associated with depression
Contraindications Hypersensitivity to alprazolam or any component of the formulation (cross-sensitivity with other benzodiazepines may exist); narrow-angle glaucoma; concurrent use with ketoconazole or itraconazole
Warnings/Precautions Rebound or withdrawal symptoms, including seizures, may occur 18 hours to 3 days following abrupt discontinuation or large decreases in dose (more common in patients receiving >4 mg/day or prolonged treatment). Breakthrough anxiety may occur at the end of dosing interval. Use with caution in patients receiving concurrent CYP3A4 inhibitors. Use with caution in renal impairment or predisposition to urate nephropathy. Use with caution in elderly or debilitated patients, patients with hepatic disease (including alcoholics), renal impairment, or obese patients.

Causes CNS depression (dose related) which may impair physical and mental capabilities. Patients must be cautioned about performing tasks that require mental alertness (eg, operating machinery or driving). Effects with other sedative drugs or ethanol may be potentiated. Benzodiazepines have been associated with falls and traumatic injury and should be used with extreme caution in patients who are at risk of these events. Due to increased sensitivity in the elderly, smaller doses of benzodiazepines may be safer and as effective. Avoid using doses >2 mg daily of alprazolam (Beers Criteria). Use with caution in patients with respiratory disease or impaired gag reflex.

Use caution in patients with depression, particularly if suicidal risk may be present. Episodes of mania or hypomania have occurred in depressed patients treated with alprazolam. May cause physical or psychological dependence. Acute withdrawal may be precipitated in patients after administration of flumazenil.

Benzodiazepines have been associated with anterograde amnesia. Paradoxical reactions have been reported with benzodiazepines, particularly in adolescent/pediatric or psychiatric patients. Does not have analgesic, antidepressant, or antipsychotic properties.
Adverse Reactions (Reflective of adult population; not specific for elderly)
>10%:
Central nervous system: Abnormal coordination, cognitive disorder, depression, drowsiness, fatigue, irritability, lightheadedness, memory impairment, sedation, somnolence
Gastrointestinal: Appetite increased/decreased, constipation, salivation decreased, weight gain/loss, xerostomia
Genitourinary: Micturition difficulty
Neuromuscular & skeletal: Dysarthria

1% to 10%:
Cardiovascular: Hypotension
Central nervous system: Agitation, attention disturbance, confusion, depersonalization, derealization, disorientation, disinhibition, dizziness, dream abnormalities, fear, hallucinations, hypersomnia, nightmares, seizure, talkativeness
Dermatologic: Dermatitis, pruritus, rash
Endocrine & metabolic: Libido decreased/increased, menstrual disorders
Gastrointestinal: Salivation increased
Genitourinary: Incontinence
Hepatic: Bilirubin increased, jaundice, liver enzymes increased
Neuromuscular & skeletal: Arthralgia, ataxia, myalgia, paresthesia
Ocular: Diplopia
Respiratory: Allergic rhinitis, dyspnea

Drug Interactions

Metabolism/Transport Effects Substrate of CYP3A4 (major)

Avoid Concomitant Use

Avoid concomitant use of ALPRAZolam with any of the following: Conivaptan; Indinavir; OLANZapine

Increased Effect/Toxicity

ALPRAZolam may increase the levels/effects of: Alcohol (Ethyl); CloZAPine; CNS Depressants; Methotrimeprazine; Selective Serotonin Reuptake Inhibitors

The levels/effects of ALPRAZolam may be increased by: Antifungal Agents (Azole Derivatives, Systemic); Aprepitant; Boceprevir; Calcium Channel Blockers (Nondihydropyridine); Cimetidine; Conivaptan; Contraceptives (Estrogens); Contraceptives (Progestins); CYP3A4 Inhibitors (Moderate); CYP3A4 Inhibitors (Strong); Dasatinib; Droperidol; Fluconazole; Fosaprepitant; Grapefruit Juice; HydrOXYzine; Indinavir; Isoniazid; Macrolide Antibiotics; Methotrimeprazine; Nefazodone; OLANZapine; Protease Inhibitors; Proton Pump Inhibitors; Selective Serotonin Reuptake Inhibitors; Telaprevir

Decreased Effect

The levels/effects of ALPRAZolam may be decreased by: CarBAMazepine; CYP3A4 Inducers (Strong); Deferasirox; Rifamycin Derivatives; St Johns Wort; Theophylline Derivatives; Tocilizumab; Yohimbine

Ethanol/Nutrition/Herb Interactions

Cigarette smoking: May decrease alprazolam concentrations up to 50%.
Ethanol: May increase CNS depression; monitor for increased effects with coadministration. Caution patients about effects.
Food: Alprazolam serum concentration is unlikely to be increased by grapefruit juice because of alprazolam's high oral bioavailability. The C_{max} of the extended release formulation is increased by 25% when a high-fat meal is given 2 hours before dosing. T_{max} is decreased 30% when food is given immediately prior to dose. T_{max} is increased by 30% when food is given ≥1 hour after dose.
Herb/Nutraceutical: St John's wort may decrease alprazolam levels. Avoid valerian, St John's wort, kava kava, gotu kola (may increase CNS depression).

Stability Orally-disintegrating tablet: Store at room temperature of 20°C to 25°C (68°F to 77°F). Protect from moisture. Seal bottle tightly and discard any cotton packaged inside bottle.

Mechanism of Action Binds to stereospecific benzodiazepine receptors on the postsynaptic GABA neuron at several sites within the central nervous system, including the limbic system, reticular formation. Enhancement of the inhibitory effect of GABA on neuronal excitability results in increased neuronal membrane permeability to chloride ions. This shift in chloride ions results in hyperpolarization (a less excitable state) and stabilization.

Pharmacodynamics/Kinetics

Onset of action: Immediate release and extended release formulations: 1 hour
Duration: Immediate release: 5.1 ± 1.7 hours; Extended release: 11.3 ± 4.2 hours
Absorption: Extended release: Slower relative to immediate release formulation resulting in a concentration that is maintained 5-11 hours after dosing
Distribution: V_d: 0.9-1.2 L/kg
Protein binding: 80%; primarily to albumin
Metabolism: Hepatic via CYP3A4; forms two active metabolites (4-hydroxyalprazolam and α-hydroxyalprazolam)
Bioavailability: 90%
Half-life elimination:
Adults: 11.2 hours (immediate release range: 6.3-26.9 hours; extended release range: 10.7-15.8 hours)
Elderly: 16.3 hours (range: 9-26.9 hours)
Alcoholic liver disease: 19.7 hours (range: 5.8-65.3 hours)
Obesity: 21.8 hours (range: 9.9-40.4 hours)

◄

Time to peak, serum: Immediate release: 1-2 hours; Extended release: ~9 hours; decreased by 1 hour following bedtime dosing compared to morning dosing

Excretion: Urine (as unchanged drug and metabolites)

Dosage

Geriatric Initial: 0.125-0.25 mg twice daily; increase by 0.125 mg/day as needed. The smallest effective dose should be used.

Immediate release: Initial: 0.25 mg 2-3 times/day

Extended release: Initial: 0.5 mg once daily

Adult Note: Treatment >4 months should be re-evaluated to determine the patient's continued need for the drug

Anxiety: Oral: *Immediate release:* Effective doses are 0.5-4 mg/day in divided doses; the manufacturer recommends starting at 0.25-0.5 mg 3 times/day; titrate dose upward; usual maximum: 4 mg/day. Patients requiring doses >4 mg/day should be increased cautiously. Periodic reassessment and consideration of dosage reduction is recommended.

Anxiety associated with depression: Oral: *Immediate release:* Average dose required: 2.5-3 mg/day in divided doses

Ethanol withdrawal (unlabeled use): Oral: *Immediate release:* Usual dose: 2-2.5 mg/day in divided doses

Panic disorder: Oral:

Immediate release: Initial: 0.5 mg 3 times/day; dose may be increased every 3-4 days in increments ≤1 mg/day. Mean effective dosage: 5-6 mg/day; many patients obtain relief at 2 mg/day, as much as 10 mg/day may be required

Extended release: 0.5-1 mg once daily; may increase dose every 3-4 days in increments ≤1 mg/day (range: 3-6 mg/day)

Switching from immediate to extended release: Patients may be switched to extended release tablets by taking the total daily dose of the immediate release tablets and giving it once daily using the extended release preparation.

Preoperative sedation: Oral: 0.5 mg in evening at bedtime and 0.5 mg 1 hour before procedure

Dose reduction: Abrupt discontinuation should be avoided. Daily dose may be decreased by 0.5 mg every 3 days, however, some patients may require a slower reduction. If withdrawal symptoms occur, resume previous dose and discontinue on a less rapid schedule.

Renal Impairment No guidelines for adjustment; use caution.

Hepatic Impairment Oral: Reduce dose by 50% to 60% or avoid in cirrhosis.

Administration

Immediate release preparations: Can be administered sublingually with comparable onset and completeness of absorption.

Extended release tablet: Should be taken once daily in the morning; do not crush, break, or chew.

Orally-disintegrating tablets: Using dry hands, place tablet on top of tongue. If using one-half of tablet, immediately discard remaining half (may not remain stable). Administration with water is not necessary.

Monitoring Parameters Respiratory and cardiovascular status

Pharmacotherapy Pearls Not intended for management of anxieties and minor distresses associated with everyday life. Treatment longer than 4 months should be re-evaluated to determine the patient's need for the drug. Patients who become physically dependent on alprazolam tend to have a difficult time discontinuing it; withdrawal symptoms may be severe. To minimize withdrawal symptoms, taper dosage slowly; do not discontinue abruptly. Abrupt discontinuation after sustained use (generally >10 days) may cause withdrawal symptoms.

Special Geriatric Considerations This medication is considered to be potentially inappropriate in this patient population (Beers Criteria severity: High).

Controlled Substance C-IV

Dosage Forms Excipient information presented when available (limited, particularly for generics); consult specific product labeling.

Solution, oral [concentrate]:

Alprazolam Intensol™: 1 mg/mL (30 mL) [dye free, ethanol free, sugar free; contains propylene glycol]

Tablet, oral: 0.25 mg, 0.5 mg, 1 mg, 2 mg

Xanax®: 0.25 mg, 0.5 mg, 1 mg, 2 mg [scored]

Tablet, extended release, oral: 0.5 mg, 1 mg, 2 mg, 3 mg

Xanax XR®: 0.5 mg, 1 mg, 2 mg, 3 mg

Tablet, orally disintegrating, oral: 0.25 mg, 0.5 mg, 1 mg, 2 mg

Niravam™: 0.25 mg, 0.5 mg, 1 mg, 2 mg [scored; orange flavor]

Selected References
Greenblatt DJ, Divoll M, Abernethy DR, et al, "Alprazolam Kinetics in the Elderly: Relation to Antipyrine Disposition," *Arch Gen Psychiatry*, 1983, 40(3):287-90.

Reidenberg MM, Levy M, Warner H, et al, "Relationship Between Diazepam Dose, Plasma Level, Age, and Central Nervous System Depression," *Clin Pharmacol Ther*, 1978, 23(4):371-4.

◆ **Alprazolam Intensol™** *see* ALPRAZolam *on page 70*

Alprostadil (al PROS ta dill)

Medication Safety Issues
Sound-alike/look-alike issues:
Alprostadil may be confused with alPRAZolam
Brand Names: U.S. Caverject Impulse®; Caverject®; Edex®; Muse®
Brand Names: Canada Caverject®; Muse® Pellet
Index Terms PGE$_1$; Prostaglandin E$_1$
Generic Availability (U.S.) Yes: Solution for injection
Pharmacologic Category Prostaglandin; Vasodilator
Use
Caverject®: Treatment of erectile dysfunction of vasculogenic, psychogenic, or neurogenic etiology; adjunct in the diagnosis of erectile dysfunction
Edex®, Muse®: Treatment of erectile dysfunction of vasculogenic, psychogenic, or neurogenic etiology
Contraindications Hypersensitivity to alprostadil or any component of the formulation; conditions predisposing patients to priapism (sickle cell anemia, multiple myeloma, leukemia); patients with anatomical deformation of the penis, penile implants; use in men for whom sexual activity is inadvisable or contraindicated
Warnings/Precautions Use cautiously in neonates with bleeding tendencies. **[U.S. Boxed Warning]: Apnea may occur in 10% to 12% of neonates with congenital heart defects, especially in those weighing <2 kg at birth.** Apnea usually appears during the first hour of drug infusion. When used for patency of ductus arteriosus infuse for the shortest time at the lowest dose consistent with good patient care. Use for >120 hours has been associated with antral hyperplasia and gastric outlet obstruction.

When used in erectile dysfunction, priapism may occur; treat prolonged priapism (erection persisting for >4 hours) immediately to avoid penile tissue damage and permanent loss of potency; discontinue therapy if signs of penile fibrosis develop (penile angulation, cavernosal fibrosis, or Peyronie's disease). When used in erectile dysfunction (Muse®), syncope occurring within 1 hour of administration has been reported. The potential for drug-drug interactions may occur when Muse® is prescribed concomitantly with antihypertensives.

Adverse Reactions (Reflective of adult population; not specific for elderly)
Intraurethral:
>10%: Genitourinary: Penile pain, urethral burning
2% to 10%:
Central nervous system: Headache, dizziness, pain
Genitourinary: Vaginal itching (female partner), testicular pain, urethral bleeding (minor)
Intracavernosal injection:
>10%: Genitourinary: Penile pain
1% to 10%:
Cardiovascular: Hypertension
Central nervous system: Headache, dizziness
Genitourinary: Prolonged erection (>4 hours, 4%), penile fibrosis, penis disorder, penile rash, penile edema
Local: Injection site hematoma and/or bruising
Drug Interactions
Avoid Concomitant Use There are no known interactions where it is recommended to avoid concomitant use.
Increased Effect/Toxicity There are no known significant interactions involving an increase in effect.
Decreased Effect There are no known significant interactions involving a decrease in effect.
Ethanol/Nutrition/Herb Interactions Ethanol: Avoid concurrent use (vasodilating effect).
Stability
Caverject® Impulse™: Store at controlled room temperature of 15°C to 30°C (59°F to 86°F). Provided as a dual-chamber syringe with diluent in one chamber. To mix, hold syringe with needle pointing upward and turn plunger clockwise; turn upside down several times to mix. Device can be set to deliver specified dose, each device can be set at various increments. Following reconstitution, use within 24 hours and discard any unused solution.

ALPROSTADIL

Caverject® powder: The 5 mcg, 10 mcg, and 20 mcg vials should be stored at or below 25°C (77°F). The 40 mcg vial should be stored at 2°C to 8°C until dispensed. After dispensing, stable for up to 3 months at or below 25°C. Use only the supplied diluent for reconstitution (ie, bacteriostatic/sterile water with benzyl alcohol 0.945%). Following reconstitution, all strengths should be stored at or below 25°C (77°F); do not refrigerate or freeze; use within 24 hours.

Caverject® solution: Prior to dispensing, store frozen at -20°C to -10°C (-4°F to -14°F); once dispensed, may be stored frozen for up to 3 months, or under refrigeration at 2°C to 8°C (36°F to 46°F) for up to 7 days. Do not refreeze. Once removed from foil wrap, solution may be allowed to warm to room temperature prior to use. If not used immediately, solution should be discarded. Shake well prior to use.

Edex®: Store at controlled room temperature of 15°C to 30°C (59°F to 86°F); following reconstitution with NS, use immediately and discard any unused solution.

Muse®: Refrigerate at 2°C to 8°C (36°F to 46°F); may be stored at room temperature for up to 14 days.

Mechanism of Action Causes vasodilation by means of direct effect on vascular and ductus arteriosus smooth muscle; relaxes trabecular smooth muscle by dilation of cavernosal arteries when injected along the penile shaft, allowing blood flow to and entrapment in the lacunar spaces of the penis (ie, corporeal veno-occlusive mechanism)

Pharmacodynamics/Kinetics

Onset of action: Rapid

Duration: <1 hour

Distribution: Insignificant following penile injection

Protein binding, plasma: 81% to albumin

Metabolism: ~75% by oxidation in one pass via lungs

Half-life elimination: 5-10 minutes

Excretion: Urine (90% as metabolites) within 24 hours

Dosage

Geriatric Elderly patients may have a greater frequency of renal dysfunction; lowest effective dose should be used. In clinical studies with Edex®, higher minimally effective doses and a higher rate of lack of effect were noted.

Adult

Erectile dysfunction:

Intracavernous (Caverject®, Edex®): Individualize dose by careful titration; doses >40 mcg (Edex®) or >60 mcg (Caverject®) are not recommended: Initial dose must be titrated in physician's office. Patient must stay in the physician's office until complete detumescence occurs; if there is no response, then the next higher dose may be given within 1 hour; if there is still no response, a 1-day interval before giving the next dose is recommended; increasing the dose or concentration in the treatment of impotence results in increasing pain and discomfort.

Vasculogenic, psychogenic, or mixed etiology: Initiate dosage titration at 2.5 mcg, increasing by 2.5 mcg to a dose of 5 mcg and then in increments of 5-10 mcg depending on the erectile response until the dose produces an erection suitable for intercourse, not lasting >1 hour; if there is absolutely no response to initial 2.5 mcg dose, the second dose may be increased to 7.5 mcg, followed by increments of 5-10 mcg

Neurogenic etiology (eg, spinal cord injury): Initiate dosage titration at 1.25 mcg, increasing to a dose of 2.5 mcg and then 5 mcg; increase further in increments 5 mcg until the dose is reached that produces an erection suitable for intercourse, not lasting >1 hour

Maintenance: Once appropriate dose has been determined, patient may self-administer injections at a frequency of no more than 3 times/week with at least 24 hours between doses

Intraurethral (Muse® Pellet):

Initial: 125-250 mcg

Maintenance: Administer as needed to achieve an erection; duration of action is about 30-60 minutes; use only two systems per 24-hour period

Administration Erectile dysfunction: Use a ½", 27- to 30-gauge needle; inject into the dorsolateral aspect of the proximal third of the penis, avoiding visible veins; alternate side of the penis for injections

Monitoring Parameters Arterial pressure, respiratory rate, heart rate, temperature, degree of penile pain, length of erection, signs of infection

Special Geriatric Considerations Elderly may have concomitant diseases which would contraindicate the use of alprostadil. Other forms of attaining penile tumescence are recommended.

Dosage Forms Excipient information presented when available (limited, particularly for generics); consult specific product labeling. [DSC] = Discontinued product
Injection, powder for reconstitution:
  Caverject®: 20 mcg, 40 mcg [contains lactose; diluent contains benzyl alcohol]
  Caverject Impulse®: 10 mcg, 20 mcg [prefilled injection system; contains lactose; diluent contains benzyl alcohol]
  Edex®: 10 mcg, 20 mcg, 40 mcg [contains lactose; packaged in kits containing diluent, syringe, and alcohol swab]
Pellet, urethral:
  Muse®: 125 mcg (6s) [DSC], 250 mcg (6s), 500 mcg (6s), 1000 mcg (6s)

◆ **Alrex®** *see* Loteprednol *on page 1096*
◆ **Alsuma™** *see* SUMAtriptan *on page 1723*
◆ **Altabax™** *see* Retapamulin *on page 1600*
◆ **Altace®** *see* Ramipril *on page 1581*
◆ **Altachlore [OTC]** *see* Sodium Chloride *on page 1690*
◆ **Altafrin** *see* Phenylephrine (Ophthalmic) *on page 1443*
◆ **Altamist [OTC]** *see* Sodium Chloride *on page 1690*
◆ **Altaryl [OTC]** *see* DiphenhydrAMINE (Systemic) *on page 520*

Alteplase (AL te plase)

Medication Safety Issues
Sound-alike/look-alike issues:
Activase® may be confused with Cathflo® Activase®, TNKase®
Alteplase may be confused with Altace®
"tPA" abbreviation should not be used when writing orders for this medication; has been misread as TNKase (tenecteplase)
High alert medication:
The Institute for Safe Medication Practices (ISMP) includes this medication (I.V.) among its list of drugs which have a heightened risk of causing significant patient harm when used in error.
Brand Names: U.S. Activase®; Cathflo® Activase®
Brand Names: Canada Activase® rt-PA; Cathflo® Activase®
Index Terms Alteplase, Recombinant; Alteplase, Tissue Plasminogen Activator, Recombinant; tPA
Generic Availability (U.S.) No
Pharmacologic Category Thrombolytic Agent
Use Management of ST-elevation myocardial infarction (STEMI) for the lysis of thrombi in coronary arteries; management of acute ischemic stroke (AIS); management of acute pulmonary embolism (PE)
Recommended criteria for treatment:
STEMI: Chest pain ≥20 minutes duration, onset of chest pain within 12 hours of treatment (or within prior 12-24 hours in patients with continuing ischemic symptoms), and ST-segment elevation >0.1 mV in at least two contiguous precordial leads or two adjacent limb leads on ECG or new or presumably new left bundle branch block (LBBB)
AIS: Onset of stroke symptoms within 3 hours of treatment
Acute pulmonary embolism: Age ≤75 years: Documented massive PE (defined as acute PE with sustained hypotension [SBP <90 mm Hg for ≤15 minutes or requiring inotropic support], persistent profound bradycardia [HR <40 bpm with signs or symptoms of shock], or pulselessness); alteplase may be considered for submassive PE with clinical evidence of adverse prognosis (eg, new hemodynamic instability, worsening respiratory insufficiency, severe RV dysfunction, or major myocardial necrosis) and low risk of bleeding complications. **Note:** Not recommended for patients with low-risk PE (eg, normotensive, no RV dysfunction, normal biomarkers) or submassive acute PE with minor RV dysfunction, minor myocardial necrosis, and no clinical worsening (Jaff, 2011).
Cathflo® Activase®: Restoration of central venous catheter function
Unlabeled/Investigational Use Treatment of peripheral arterial thrombotic obstruction
Contraindications Hypersensitivity to alteplase or any component of the formulation

Treatment of STEMI or PE: Active internal bleeding; history of CVA; recent intracranial or intraspinal surgery or trauma; intracranial neoplasm; arteriovenous malformation or aneurysm; known bleeding diathesis; severe uncontrolled hypertension

Treatment of acute ischemic stroke: Evidence of intracranial hemorrhage or suspicion of subarachnoid hemorrhage on pretreatment evaluation; recent (within 3 months) intracranial or intraspinal surgery; prolonged external cardiac massage; suspected aortic dissection; serious head trauma or previous stroke; history of intracranial hemorrhage; uncontrolled hypertension at time of treatment (eg, >185 mm Hg systolic or >110 mm Hg diastolic); seizure at the onset of stroke; active internal bleeding; intracranial neoplasm; arteriovenous malformation or aneurysm; known bleeding diathesis including but not limited to: current use of anticoagulants or an INR >1.7, administration of heparin within 48 hours preceding the onset of stroke and an elevated aPTT at presentation, platelet count <100,000/mm^3.

Other exclusion criteria (NINDS recombinant tPA study): Stroke or serious head injury within 3 months, major surgery or serious trauma within 2 weeks, GI or urinary tract hemorrhage within 3 weeks, aggressive treatment required to lower blood pressure, glucose level <50 mg/dL or >400 mg/dL, arterial puncture at a noncompressible site or lumbar puncture within 1 week, clinical presentation suggesting post-MI pericarditis.

Warnings/Precautions Concurrent heparin anticoagulation may contribute to bleeding. In the treatment of acute ischemic stroke, concurrent use of anticoagulants was not permitted during the initial 24 hours of the <3 hour window trial (NINDS, 1995). Initiation of SubQ heparin (≤10,000 units) or equivalent doses of low molecular weight heparin for prevention of DVT during the first 24 hours of the 3-4.5 hour window trial was permitted and did not increase the incidence of intracerebral hemorrhage (Hacke, 2008). For acute PE, withhold heparin during the 2-hour infusion period. Monitor all potential bleeding sites. Do not use doses >150 mg; associated with increased risk of intracranial hemorrhage. Intramuscular injections and nonessential handling of the patient should be avoided. Venipunctures should be performed carefully and only when necessary. If arterial puncture is necessary, use an upper extremity vessel that can be manually compressed. If serious bleeding occurs, the infusion of alteplase and heparin should be stopped. Avoid aspirin for 24 hours following administration of alteplase; administration within 24 hours increases the risk of hemorrhagic transformation.

For the following conditions, the risk of bleeding is higher with use of thrombolytics and should be weighed against the benefits of therapy: Recent major surgery (eg, CABG, obstetrical delivery, organ biopsy, previous puncture of noncompressible vessels), prolonged CPR with evidence of thoracic trauma, lumbar puncture within 1 week, cerebrovascular disease, recent gastrointestinal or genitourinary bleeding, recent trauma, hypertension (systolic BP >175 mm Hg and/or diastolic BP >110 mm Hg), high likelihood of left heart thrombus (eg, mitral stenosis with atrial fibrillation), acute pericarditis, subacute bacterial endocarditis, hemostatic defects including ones caused by severe renal or hepatic dysfunction, significant hepatic dysfunction, diabetic hemorrhagic retinopathy or other hemorrhagic ophthalmic conditions, septic thrombophlebitis or occluded AV cannula at seriously infected site, advanced age (eg, >75 years), any other condition in which bleeding constitutes a significant hazard or would be particularly difficult to manage because of location. When treating acute MI or pulmonary embolism, use with caution in patients receiving oral anticoagulants. In the treatment of acute ischemic stroke within 3 hours of stroke symptom onset, the current use of oral anticoagulants producing an INR >1.7 is contraindicated.

Coronary thrombolysis may result in reperfusion arrhythmias. Patients who present **within 3 hours** of stroke symptom onset should be treated with alteplase unless contraindications exist. A longer time window (**3-4.5 hours** after symptom onset) has now been formally evaluated and shown to be safe and efficacious for select individuals (del Zoppo, 2009; Hacke, 2008). Treatment of patients with minor neurological deficit or with rapidly improving symptoms is not recommended. Follow standard management for STEMI while infusing alteplase.

Cathflo® Activase®: When used to restore catheter function, use Cathflo® cautiously in those patients with known or suspected catheter infections. Evaluate catheter for other causes of dysfunction before use. Avoid excessive pressure when instilling into catheter.

Adverse Reactions (Reflective of adult population; not specific for elderly) As with all drugs which may affect hemostasis, bleeding is the major adverse effect associated with alteplase. Hemorrhage may occur at virtually any site. Risk is dependent on multiple variables, including the dosage administered, concurrent use of multiple agents which alter hemostasis, and patient predisposition. Rapid lysis of coronary artery thrombi by thrombolytic agents may be associated with reperfusion-related atrial and/or ventricular arrhythmia. **Note:** Lowest rate of bleeding complications expected with dose used to restore catheter function.

1% to 10%:
  Cardiovascular: Hypotension
  Central nervous system: Fever
  Dermatologic: Bruising (1%)
  Gastrointestinal: GI hemorrhage (5%), nausea, vomiting
  Genitourinary: GU hemorrhage (4%)
  Hematologic: Bleeding (0.5% major, 7% minor: GUSTO trial)
  Local: Bleeding at catheter puncture site (15.3%, accelerated administration)

Additional cardiovascular events associated **with use in STEMI:** AV block, cardiogenic shock, heart failure, cardiac arrest, recurrent ischemia/infarction, myocardial rupture, electromechanical dissociation, pericardial effusion, pericarditis, mitral regurgitation, cardiac tamponade, thromboembolism, pulmonary edema, asystole, ventricular tachycardia, bradycardia, ruptured intracranial AV malformation, seizure, hemorrhagic bursitis, cholesterol crystal embolization

Additional events associated **with use in pulmonary embolism:** Pulmonary re-embolization, pulmonary edema, pleural effusion, thromboembolism

Additional events associated **with use in stroke:** Cerebral edema, cerebral herniation, seizure, new ischemic stroke

Drug Interactions

Avoid Concomitant Use There are no known interactions where it is recommended to avoid concomitant use.

Increased Effect/Toxicity

Alteplase may increase the levels/effects of: Anticoagulants; Drotrecogin Alfa

The levels/effects of Alteplase may be increased by: Antiplatelet Agents; Herbs (Anticoagulant/Antiplatelet Properties); Nonsteroidal Anti-Inflammatory Agents; Salicylates

Decreased Effect

The levels/effects of Alteplase may be decreased by: Aprotinin; Nitroglycerin

Ethanol/Nutrition/Herb Interactions Herb/Nutraceutical: Avoid cat's claw, dong quai, evening primrose, feverfew, red clover, horse chestnut, garlic, green tea, ginseng, ginkgo (all have additional antiplatelet activity).

Stability

Activase®: The lyophilized product may be stored at room temperature (not to exceed 30°C/86°F), or under refrigeration. Once reconstituted, it should be used within 8 hours. Reconstitution:

50 mg vial: Use accompanying diluent; mix by gentle swirling or slow inversion; do not shake. Vacuum is present in 50 mg vial. Final concentration: 1 mg/mL.

100 mg vial: Use transfer set with accompanying diluent (100 mL vial of sterile water for injection). No vacuum is present in 100 mg vial. Final concentration: 1 mg/mL.

Cathflo® Activase®: Store lyophilized product under refrigeration. The following stability information has also been reported: Intact vials may be stored at room temperature for up to 4 months (Cohen, 2007).

To reconstitute, add 2.2 mL SWFI to vial; do not shake. Final concentration: 1 mg/mL. Once reconstituted, store at 2°C to 30°C (36°F to 86°F) and use within 8 hours. Do not mix other medications into infusion solution.

Mechanism of Action Initiates local fibrinolysis by binding to fibrin in a thrombus (clot) and converts entrapped plasminogen to plasmin

Pharmacodynamics/Kinetics

Duration: >50% present in plasma cleared ~5 minutes after infusion terminated, ~80% cleared within 10 minutes

Excretion: Clearance: Rapidly from circulating plasma (550-650 mL/minute), primarily hepatic; >50% present in plasma is cleared within 5 minutes after the infusion is terminated, ~80% cleared within 10 minutes

Dosage

Geriatric & Adult

ST-elevation myocardial infarction (STEMI): I.V. (Activase®): Front loading dose (weight-based):

Patients >67 kg: Total dose: 100 mg over 1.5 hours; infuse 15 mg over 1-2 minutes. Infuse 50 mg over 30 minutes. Infuse remaining 35 mg of alteplase over the next hour. See **"Note."**

Patients ≤67 kg: Infuse 15 mg I.V. bolus over 1-2 minutes, then infuse 0.75 mg/kg (not to exceed 50 mg) over next 30 minutes, followed by 0.5 mg/kg over next 60 minutes (not to exceed 35 mg). See **"Note."**

Note: All patients should receive 162-325 mg of chewable nonenteric coated aspirin as soon as possible and then daily. Administer concurrently with heparin 60 units/kg bolus (maximum: 4000 units) followed by continuous infusion of 12 units/kg/hour (maximum: 1000 units/hour) and adjust to aPTT target of 50-70 seconds (or 1.5-2 times the upper limit of control).

Acute massive or submassive pulmonary embolism (PE): I.V. (Activase®): 100 mg over 2 hours; may be administered as a 10 mg bolus followed by 90 mg over 2 hours as was done in patients with submassive PE (Konstantinides, 2002). **Note:** Not recommended for submassive PE with minor RV dysfunction, minor myocardial necrosis, and no clinical worsening or low-risk PE (ie, normotensive, no RV dysfunction, normal biomarkers) (Jaff, 2011).

◄ **Acute ischemic stroke:** I.V. (Activase®): Within 3 hours of the onset of symptom onset (labeled use) **or** within 3-4.5 hours of symptom onset (unlabeled use; del Zoppo, 2009; Hacke, 2008): **Note:** Initiation of anticoagulants (eg, heparin) or antiplatelet agents (eg, aspirin) within 24 hours after starting alteplase is not recommended; however, initiation of aspirin between 24-48 hours after stroke onset is recommended (Adams, 2007). Initiation of SubQ heparin (≤10,000 units) or equivalent doses of low molecular weight heparin for prevention of DVT during the first 24 hours of the 3-4.5 hour window trial did not increase incidence of intracerebral hemorrhage (Hacke, 2008).

Recommended total dose: 0.9 mg/kg (maximum total dose: 90 mg)

Patients ≤100 kg: Load with 0.09 mg/kg (10% of 0.9 mg/kg dose) as an I.V. bolus over 1 minute, followed by 0.81 mg/kg (90% of 0.9 mg/kg dose) as a continuous infusion over 60 minutes.

Patients >100 kg: Load with 9 mg (10% of 90 mg) as an I.V. bolus over 1 minute, followed by 81 mg (90% of 90 mg) as a continuous infusion over 60 minutes.

Central venous catheter clearance: Intracatheter (Cathflo® Activase® 1 mg/mL):

Patients <30 kg: 110% of the internal lumen volume of the catheter, not to exceed 2 mg/2 mL; retain in catheter for 0.5-2 hours; may instill a second dose if catheter remains occluded

Patients ≥30 kg: 2 mg (2 mL); retain in catheter for 0.5-2 hours; may instill a second dose if catheter remains occluded

Acute peripheral arterial occlusive disease (unlabeled use): Intra-arterial: 0.02-0.1 mg/kg/hour for up to 36 hours

Advisory Panel to the Society for Cardiovascular and Interventional Radiology on Thrombolytic Therapy recommendation: ≤2 mg/hour and subtherapeutic heparin (aPTT <1.5 times baseline)

Administration

Activase®: ST-elevation MI: Accelerated infusion: Bolus dose may be prepared by one of three methods:

1) Removal of 15 mL reconstituted (1 mg/mL) solution from vial
2) Removal of 15 mL from a port on the infusion line after priming
3) Programming an infusion pump to deliver a 15 mL bolus at the initiation of infusion

Activase®: Acute ischemic stroke: Bolus dose (10% of total dose) may be prepared by one of three methods:

1) Removal of the appropriate volume from reconstituted solution (1 mg/mL)
2) Removal of the appropriate volume from a port on the infusion line after priming
3) Programming an infusion pump to deliver the appropriate volume at the initiation of infusion

Note: Remaining dose for STEMI, AIS, or total dose for acute pulmonary embolism may be administered as follows: Any quantity of drug not to be administered to the patient must be removed from vial(s) prior to administration of remaining dose.

50 mg vial: Either PVC bag or glass vial and infusion set

100 mg vial: Insert spike end of the infusion set through the same puncture site created by transfer device and infuse from vial

If further dilution is desired, may be diluted in equal volume of 0.9% sodium chloride or D_5W to yield a final concentration of 0.5 mg/mL.

Cathflo® Activase®: Intracatheter: Instill dose into occluded catheter. Do not force solution into catheter. After a 30-minute dwell time, assess catheter function by attempting to aspirate blood. If catheter is functional, aspirate 4-5 mL of blood in patients ≥10 kg or 3 mL in patients <10 kg to remove Cathflo® Activase® and residual clots. Gently irrigate the catheter with NS. If catheter remains nonfunctional, let Cathflo® Activase® dwell for another 90 minutes (total dwell time: 120 minutes) and reassess function. If catheter function is not restored, a second dose may be instilled.

Monitoring Parameters

Acute ischemic stroke: In addition to monitoring for bleeding complications, the 2007 AHA/ASA Guidelines for the early management of acute ischemic stroke recommends the following:

Perform neurological assessments every 15 minutes during infusion and every 30 minutes thereafter for the next 6 hours, then hourly until 24 hours after treatment.

If severe headache, acute hypertension, nausea, or vomiting occurs, discontinue the infusion and obtain emergency CT scan.

Measure BP every 15 minutes for the first 2 hours then every 30 minutes for the next 6 hours, then hourly until 24 hours after initiation of alteplase. Increase frequency if a systolic BP is ≥180 mm Hg or if a diastolic BP is ≥105 mm Hg; administer antihypertensive medications to maintain BP at or below these levels.

Obtain a follow-up CT scan at 24 hours before starting anticoagulants or antiplatelet agents.

Central venous catheter clearance: Assess catheter function by attempting to aspirate blood.

ST-elevation MI: Assess for evidence of cardiac reperfusion through resolution of chest pain, resolution of baseline ECG changes, preserved left ventricular function, cardiac enzyme washout phenomenon, and/or the appearance of reperfusion arrhythmias; assess for bleeding potential through clinical evidence of GI bleeding, hematuria, gingival bleeding, fibrinogen levels, fibrinogen degradation products, prothrombin times, and partial thromboplastin times.

Reference Range Not routinely measured; literature supports therapeutic levels of 0.52-1.8 mcg/mL

Fibrinogen: 200-400 mg/dL

Activated partial thromboplastin time (aPTT): 22.5-38.7 seconds

Prothrombin time (PT): 10.9-12.2 seconds

Test Interactions Altered results of coagulation and fibrinolytic agents

Special Geriatric Considerations No specific changes in use in elderly patients are necessary.

Dosage Forms Excipient information presented when available (limited, particularly for generics); consult specific product labeling.

Injection, powder for reconstitution [recombinant]:

Activase®: 50 mg [29 million int. units], 100 mg [58 million int. units] [contains polysorbate 80; derived from or manufactured using Chinese hamster ovary cells; supplied with diluent]

Cathflo® Activase®: 2 mg [contains polysorbate 80; derived from or manufactured using Chinese hamster ovary cells]

Selected References

Ansell J, Hirsh J, Hylek E, et al, "Pharmacology and Management of the Vitamin K Antagonists: American College of Chest Physicians Evidence-Based Clinical Practice Guidelines (8th Edition)," Chest, 2008, 133:160-98.

◆ **Alteplase, Recombinant** see Alteplase on page 75
◆ **Alteplase, Tissue Plasminogen Activator, Recombinant** see Alteplase on page 75
◆ **ALternaGel® [OTC]** see Aluminum Hydroxide on page 79
◆ **Altoprev®** see Lovastatin on page 1097

Aluminum Hydroxide (a LOO mi num hye DROKS ide)

Brand Names: U.S. ALternaGel® [OTC]; Dermagran® [OTC]

Brand Names: Canada Amphojel®; Basaljel®

Generic Availability (U.S.) Yes: Suspension

Pharmacologic Category Antacid; Antidote; Protectant, Topical

Use Treatment of hyperacidity; hyperphosphatemia; temporary protection of minor cuts, scrapes, and burns

Contraindications Hypersensitivity to aluminum salts or any component of the formulation

Warnings/Precautions Oral: Hypophosphatemia may occur with prolonged administration or large doses; aluminum intoxication and osteomalacia may occur in patients with uremia. Use with caution in patients with HF, renal failure, edema, cirrhosis, and low sodium diets, and patients who have recently suffered gastrointestinal hemorrhage; uremic patients not receiving dialysis may develop osteomalacia and osteoporosis due to phosphate depletion.

Elderly may be predisposed to constipation and fecal impaction. Careful evaluation of possible drug interactions must be done. When used as an antacid in ulcer treatment, consider buffer capacity (mEq/mL) to calculate dose.

Topical: Not for application over deep wounds, puncture wounds, infected areas, or lacerations. When used for self medication (OTC use), consult with healthcare provider if needed for >7 days.

Adverse Reactions (Reflective of adult population; not specific for elderly) Frequency not defined.

Gastrointestinal: Constipation, discoloration of feces (white speckles), fecal impaction, nausea, stomach cramps, vomiting

Endocrine & metabolic: Hypomagnesemia, hypophosphatemia

Drug Interactions

Avoid Concomitant Use

Avoid concomitant use of Aluminum Hydroxide with any of the following: Deferasirox; QuiNINE; Vitamin D Analogs

Increased Effect/Toxicity

Aluminum Hydroxide may increase the levels/effects of: Amphetamines; Calcium Polystyrene Sulfonate; Dexmethylphenidate; Methylphenidate; Sodium Polystyrene Sulfonate

The levels/effects of Aluminum Hydroxide may be increased by: Ascorbic Acid; Calcium Polystyrene Sulfonate; Citric Acid Derivatives; Sodium Polystyrene Sulfonate; Vitamin D Analogs

ALUMINUM HYDROXIDE

◄ **Decreased Effect**
Aluminum Hydroxide may decrease the levels/effects of: ACE Inhibitors; Allopurinol; Anticonvulsants (Hydantoin); Antipsychotic Agents (Phenothiazines); Atazanavir; Bisacodyl; Bisphosphonate Derivatives; Cefditoren; Cefpodoxime; Cefuroxime; Chenodiol; Chloroquine; Corticosteroids (Oral); Dabigatran Etexilate; Dasatinib; Deferasirox; Delavirdine; Eltrombopag; Erlotinib; Ethambutol; Fexofenadine; Gabapentin; HMG-CoA Reductase Inhibitors; Iron Salts; Isoniazid; Itraconazole; Ketoconazole; Ketoconazole (Systemic); Levothyroxine; Mesalamine; Methenamine; Mycophenolate; Penicillamine; Phosphate Supplements; Protease Inhibitors; QuiNINE; Quinolone Antibiotics; Rilpivirine; Tetracycline Derivatives; Trientine; Ursodiol

Mechanism of Action Neutralizes hydrochloride in stomach to form Al $(Cl)_3$ salt + H_2O

Dosage
Geriatric & Adult
Hyperphosphatemia: Oral: Initial: 300-600 mg 3 times/day with meals
Hyperacidity: Oral: 600-1200 mg between meals and at bedtime
Skin protectant: Topical: Apply to affected area as needed; reapply at least every 12 hours
Renal Impairment Aluminum may accumulate in renal impairment.

Administration
Oral: Dose should be followed with water.
Topical: Apply as needed to affected area; reapply at least every 12 hours

Monitoring Parameters Monitor phosphorus levels periodically when patient is on chronic therapy.

Test Interactions Decreased phosphorus, inorganic (S)

Pharmacotherapy Pearls When used primarily as a phosphate binder, dose should be followed with water; when used for peptic ulcer treatment, deliver 144 mEq neutralizing capacity 1 and 3 hours after meals as needed to control symptoms; often alternated with aluminum and magnesium combinations to decrease diarrhea

Special Geriatric Considerations Elderly, due to disease and/or drug therapy, may be predisposed to constipation and fecal impaction. Careful evaluation of possible drug interactions must be done. When used as an antacid in ulcer treatment, consider buffer capacity (mEq/mL) to calculate dose. Consider renal insufficiency (<30 mL/minute) as predisposition to aluminum toxicity.

Dosage Forms Excipient information presented when available (limited, particularly for generics); consult specific product labeling. [DSC] = Discontinued product
Ointment, topical:
Dermagran®: 0.275% (113 g)
Suspension, oral: 320 mg/5 mL (30 mL, 355 mL [DSC], 473 mL); 600 mg/5 mL (355 mL)
ALternaGel®: 600 mg/5 mL (360 mL) [sugar free]

Aluminum Hydroxide and Magnesium Carbonate
(a LOO mi num hye DROKS ide & mag NEE zhum KAR bun nate)

Related Information
Aluminum Hydroxide *on page 79*

Medication Safety Issues
International issues:
Remegel [Netherlands] may be confused with Renagel brand name for sevelamer [U.S., Canada, and multiple international markets]
Remegel: Brand name for aluminum hydroxide and magnesium carbonate [Netherlands], but also the brand name for calcium carbonate [Great Britain, Hungary, and Ireland]

Brand Names: U.S. Acid Gone Extra Strength [OTC]; Acid Gone [OTC]; Gaviscon® Extra Strength [OTC]; Gaviscon® Liquid [OTC]; Genaton™ [OTC]

Index Terms Magnesium Carbonate and Aluminum Hydroxide

Generic Availability (U.S.) Yes

Pharmacologic Category Antacid

Use Temporary relief of symptoms associated with gastric acidity

Adverse Reactions (Reflective of adult population; not specific for elderly)
1% to 10%:
Endocrine & metabolic: Hypermagnesemia, aluminum intoxication (prolonged use and concomitant renal failure), hypophosphatemia
Gastrointestinal: Constipation, diarrhea
Neuromuscular & skeletal: Osteomalacia

Drug Interactions
Avoid Concomitant Use
Avoid concomitant use of Aluminum Hydroxide and Magnesium Carbonate with any of the following: Deferasirox; QuiNINE; Vitamin D Analogs

Increased Effect/Toxicity
Aluminum Hydroxide and Magnesium Carbonate may increase the levels/effects of: Alpha-/ Beta-Agonists; Amphetamines; Calcium Polystyrene Sulfonate; Dexmethylphenidate; Methylphenidate; Misoprostol; QuiNIDine; Sodium Polystyrene Sulfonate

The levels/effects of Aluminum Hydroxide and Magnesium Carbonate may be increased by: Ascorbic Acid; Calcium Polystyrene Sulfonate; Citric Acid Derivatives; Sodium Polystyrene Sulfonate; Vitamin D Analogs

Decreased Effect
Aluminum Hydroxide and Magnesium Carbonate may decrease the levels/effects of: ACE Inhibitors; Allopurinol; Anticonvulsants (Hydantoin); Antipsychotic Agents (Phenothiazines); Atazanavir; Bisacodyl; Bisphosphonate Derivatives; Cefditoren; Cefpodoxime; Cefuroxime; Chenodiol; Chloroquine; Corticosteroids (Oral); Dabigatran Etexilate; Dasatinib; Deferasirox; Delavirdine; Eltrombopag; Erlotinib; Ethambutol; Fexofenadine; Gabapentin; HMG-CoA Reductase Inhibitors; Iron Salts; Isoniazid; Itraconazole; Ketoconazole; Ketoconazole (Systemic); Levothyroxine; Mesalamine; Methenamine; Mycophenolate; Penicillamine; Phosphate Supplements; Protease Inhibitors; QuiNINE; Quinolone Antibiotics; Rilpivirine; Tetracycline Derivatives; Trientine; Ursodiol

Dosage
Geriatric & Adult Dyspepsia, gastric acidity: Oral:
Liquid:
 Gaviscon® Regular Strength: 15-30 mL 4 times/day after meals and at bedtime
 Gaviscon® Extra Strength: 15-30 mL 4 times/day after meals
Tablet (Gaviscon® Extra Strength): Chew 2-4 tablets 4 times/day
Renal Impairment Aluminum and/or magnesium may accumulate in renal impairment.

Administration Administer 1-3 hours after meals with water, milk or juice.

Special Geriatric Considerations Elderly, due to disease or drug therapy, may be predisposed to diarrhea or constipation. Diarrhea may result in electrolyte imbalance. Decreased renal function (Cl$_{cr}$ <30 mL/minute) may result in toxicity of aluminum or magnesium. Drug interactions must be considered. If possible, administer antacid 1-2 hours apart from other drugs. When treating ulcers, consider buffer capacity (mEq/mL) to calculate dose of antacid.

Dosage Forms Excipient information presented when available (limited, particularly for generics); consult specific product labeling. [DSC] = Discontinued product
Liquid:
 Acid Gone: Aluminum hydroxide 31.7 mg and magnesium carbonate 119.3 mg per 5 mL (360 mL)
 Gaviscon®: Aluminum hydroxide 31.7 mg and magnesium carbonate 119.3 mg per 5 mL (355 mL) [contains sodium 0.57 mEq/5 mL and benzyl alcohol; cool mint flavor]
 Gaviscon® Extra Strength: Aluminum hydroxide 84.6 mg and magnesium carbonate 79.1 mg per 5 mL (355 mL) [contains sodium 0.9 mEq/5 mL and benzyl alcohol; cool mint flavor]
 Genaton™: Aluminum hydroxide 31.7 mg and magnesium carbonate 119.3 mg per 5 mL (360 mL)
Tablet, chewable:
 Acid Gone Extra Strength: Aluminum hydroxide 160 mg and magnesium carbonate 105 mg
 Gaviscon® Extra Strength: Aluminum hydroxide 160 mg and magnesium carbonate 105 mg [contains sodium 19 mg/tablet (1.3 mEq/tablet); cherry and original flavors]

Aluminum Hydroxide and Magnesium Hydroxide
(a LOO mi num hye DROKS ide & mag NEE zhum hye DROK side)

Related Information
Aluminum Hydroxide *on page 79*
Magnesium Hydroxide *on page 1109*
Brand Names: U.S. Alamag [OTC]; Mag-Al Ultimate [OTC]; Mag-Al [OTC]
Brand Names: Canada Diovol®; Diovol® Ex; Gelusil® Extra Strength; Mylanta™
Index Terms Magnesium Hydroxide and Aluminum Hydroxide
Generic Availability (U.S.) Yes: Suspension
Pharmacologic Category Antacid
Use Antacid for symptoms related to hyperacidity associated with heartburn, hiatal hernia, upset stomach, peptic ulcer, peptic esophagitis, or gastritis
Warnings/Precautions Prolonged antacid therapy may result in hypophosphatemia; aluminum in antacid may form insoluble complexes with phosphate leading to decreased phosphate absorption in the GI tract. Rarely, severe hypophosphatemia can lead to anorexia, muscle weakness, malaise, and osteomalacia. Use with caution in patients with renal impairment; avoid use in severe renal impairment; hypermagnesemia or aluminum

intoxication may occur in severe renal impairment, particularly with prolonged use. Aluminum intoxication may lead to osteomalacia or dialysis encephalopathy. Use with caution in the elderly; the population group may be predisposed to diarrhea or constipation. Some products may contain phenylalanine.

Self-medication (OTC use): Patients with renal disease or on a magnesium-restricted diet should consult a healthcare provider prior to use. Unless directed by a physician, do not use for >2 weeks or exceed the recommended daily dose.

Adverse Reactions (Reflective of adult population; not specific for elderly) Frequency not defined.

Gastrointestinal: Constipation, chalky taste, cramping, fecal discoloration (white speckles), fecal impaction, nausea, vomiting

Endocrine & metabolic: Hypophosphatemia (rare), hypermagnesemia (rare)

Drug Interactions

Avoid Concomitant Use

Avoid concomitant use of Aluminum Hydroxide and Magnesium Hydroxide with any of the following: Calcium Polystyrene Sulfonate; Deferasirox; QuiNINE; Sodium Polystyrene Sulfonate; Vitamin D Analogs

Increased Effect/Toxicity

Aluminum Hydroxide and Magnesium Hydroxide may increase the levels/effects of: Alpha-/Beta-Agonists; Amphetamines; Calcium Channel Blockers; Calcium Polystyrene Sulfonate; Dexmethylphenidate; Methylphenidate; Misoprostol; Neuromuscular-Blocking Agents; QuiNIDine; Sodium Polystyrene Sulfonate

The levels/effects of Aluminum Hydroxide and Magnesium Hydroxide may be increased by: Alfacalcidol; Ascorbic Acid; Calcitriol; Calcium Channel Blockers; Calcium Polystyrene Sulfonate; Citric Acid Derivatives; Sodium Polystyrene Sulfonate; Vitamin D Analogs

Decreased Effect

Aluminum Hydroxide and Magnesium Hydroxide may decrease the levels/effects of: ACE Inhibitors; Allopurinol; Anticonvulsants (Hydantoin); Antipsychotic Agents (Phenothiazines); Atazanavir; Bisacodyl; Bisphosphonate Derivatives; Cefditoren; Cefpodoxime; Cefuroxime; Chenodiol; Chloroquine; Corticosteroids (Oral); Dabigatran Etexilate; Dasatinib; Deferasirox; Delavirdine; Eltrombopag; Erlotinib; Ethambutol; Fexofenadine; Gabapentin; HMG-CoA Reductase Inhibitors; Iron Salts; Isoniazid; Itraconazole; Ketoconazole; Ketoconazole (Systemic); Levothyroxine; Mesalamine; Methenamine; Mycophenolate; Penicillamine; Phosphate Supplements; Protease Inhibitors; QuiNINE; Quinolone Antibiotics; Rilpivirine; Tetracycline Derivatives; Trientine; Ursodiol

The levels/effects of Aluminum Hydroxide and Magnesium Hydroxide may be decreased by: Trientine

Dosage

Geriatric & Adult Hyperacidity: Oral: OTC labeling:

Liquid (aluminum hydroxide 200 mg and magnesium hydroxide 200 mg per 5 mL): 10-20 mL 4 times/day (maximum:80 mL/day)

Suspension (aluminum hydroxide 500 mg and magnesium hydroxide 500 mg per 5 mL): 10-20 mL 4 times/day, between meals and at bedtime (maximum: 45 mL/day)

Tablet (aluminum hydroxide 300 mg and magnesium hydroxide 150 mg): 1-2 tablets after meals or at bedtime, or as needed (maximum: 16 tablets/day)

Renal Impairment Aluminum and/or magnesium may accumulate in severe renal impairment.

Administration

Liquid, suspension: Shake well before use; administer 1-3 hours after meals when stomach acidity is highest

Tablet: Chew tablet thoroughly before swallowing or allow tablets to dissolve slowly in mouth. Follow with a full glass of water.

Pharmacotherapy Pearls Sodium content varies with product; check for each product if important for patient

Special Geriatric Considerations Elderly, due to disease or drug therapy, may be predisposed to diarrhea or constipation. Diarrhea may result in electrolyte imbalance. Decreased renal function (Cl_{cr} <30 mL/minute) may result in toxicity of aluminum or magnesium. Drug interactions must be considered. If possible, administer antacid 1-2 hours apart from other drugs. When treating ulcers, consider buffer capacity (mEq/mL) to calculate dose of antacid.

Dosage Forms Excipient information presented when available (limited, particularly for generics); consult specific product labeling. [DSC] = Discontinued product

Liquid, oral:

Mag-Al: Aluminum hydroxide 200 mg and magnesium hydroxide 200 mg per 5 mL (30 mL) [contains propylene glycol, sodium 4 mg/5 mL; peppermint flavor]

Suspension, oral: Aluminum hydroxide 225 mg and magnesium hydroxide 200 mg per 5 mL (360 mL)

Alamag: Aluminum hydroxide 225 mg and magnesium hydroxide 200 mg per 5 mL (360 mL) [DSC]

Mag-Al Ultimate: Aluminum hydroxide 500 mg and magnesium hydroxide 500 mg per 5 mL (20 mL) [contains propylene glycol, sodium 4 mg/5 mL; peppermint flavor]

Tablet, chewable:

Alamag: Aluminum hydroxide 300 mg and magnesium hydroxide 150 mg [contains phenylalanine 2.63 mg; wild cherry flavor]

Aluminum Hydroxide and Magnesium Trisilicate
(a LOO mi num hye DROKS ide & mag NEE zhum trye SIL i kate)

Related Information
Aluminum Hydroxide *on page 79*
Brand Names: U.S. Gaviscon® Tablet [OTC]
Index Terms Magnesium Trisilicate and Aluminum Hydroxide
Generic Availability (U.S.) Yes
Pharmacologic Category Antacid
Use Temporary relief of hyperacidity
Drug Interactions

Avoid Concomitant Use

Avoid concomitant use of Aluminum Hydroxide and Magnesium Trisilicate with any of the following: Deferasirox; Nitrofurantoin; QuiNINE; Vitamin D Analogs

Increased Effect/Toxicity

Aluminum Hydroxide and Magnesium Trisilicate may increase the levels/effects of: Alpha-/Beta-Agonists; Amphetamines; Calcium Polystyrene Sulfonate; Dexmethylphenidate; Methylphenidate; Misoprostol; QuiNIDine; Sodium Polystyrene Sulfonate

The levels/effects of Aluminum Hydroxide and Magnesium Trisilicate may be increased by: Ascorbic Acid; Calcium Polystyrene Sulfonate; Citric Acid Derivatives; Sodium Polystyrene Sulfonate; Vitamin D Analogs

Decreased Effect

Aluminum Hydroxide and Magnesium Trisilicate may decrease the levels/effects of: ACE Inhibitors; Allopurinol; Anticonvulsants (Hydantoin); Antipsychotic Agents (Phenothiazines); Atazanavir; Bisacodyl; Bisphosphonate Derivatives; Cefditoren; Cefpodoxime; Cefuroxime; Chenodiol; Chloroquine; Corticosteroids (Oral); Dabigatran Etexilate; Dasatinib; Deferasirox; Delavirdine; Eltrombopag; Erlotinib; Ethambutol; Fexofenadine; Gabapentin; HMG-CoA Reductase Inhibitors; Iron Salts; Isoniazid; Itraconazole; Ketoconazole; Ketoconazole (Systemic); Levothyroxine; Mesalamine; Methenamine; Mycophenolate; Nitrofurantoin; Penicillamine; Phosphate Supplements; Protease Inhibitors; QuiNINE; Quinolone Antibiotics; Rilpivirine; Tetracycline Derivatives; Trientine; Ursodiol

Dosage

Geriatric & Adult Dyspepsia, gastric acidity: Oral: Chew 2-4 tablets 4 times/day or as directed by healthcare provider

Renal Impairment Aluminum and/or magnesium may accumulate in renal impairment.

Administration Tablets should be chewed and not swallowed whole.

Special Geriatric Considerations Elderly, due to disease or drug therapy, may be predisposed to diarrhea or constipation. Diarrhea may result in electrolyte imbalance. Decreased renal function (Cl_{cr} <30 mL/minute) may result in toxicity of aluminum or magnesium. Drug interactions must be considered. If possible, administer antacid 1-2 hours apart from other drugs. When treating ulcers, consider buffer capacity (mEq/mL) to calculate dose of antacid.

Dosage Forms Excipient information presented when available (limited, particularly for generics); consult specific product labeling. [DSC] = Discontinued product

Tablet, chewable: Aluminum hydroxide 80 mg and magnesium trisilicate 20 mg

Gaviscon®: Aluminum hydroxide 80 mg and magnesium trisilicate 20 mg [contains sodium 0.8 mEq/tablet; butterscotch flavor]

Aluminum Hydroxide, Magnesium Hydroxide, and Simethicone
(a LOO mi num hye DROKS ide, mag NEE zhum hye DROKS ide, & sye METH i kone)

Related Information
Aluminum Hydroxide *on page 79*
Magnesium Hydroxide *on page 1109*
Simethicone *on page 1679*
Medication Safety Issues
Sound-alike/look-alike issues:
Maalox® may be confused with Maox®, Monodox®
Mylanta® may be confused with Mynatal®
Other safety concerns:
Liquid Maalox® products contain a different formulation than Maalox® Total Relief® which contains bismuth subsalicylate.
Brand Names: U.S. Alamag Plus [OTC]; Aldroxicon I [OTC]; Aldroxicon II [OTC]; Almacone Double Strength® [OTC]; Almacone® [OTC]; Gelusil® [OTC]; Maalox® Advanced Maximum Strength [OTC]; Maalox® Advanced Regular Strength [OTC]; Mi-Acid Maximum Strength [OTC] [DSC]; Mi-Acid [OTC]; Mintox Plus [OTC]; Mylanta® Classic Maximum Strength Liquid [OTC]; Mylanta® Classic Regular Strength Liquid [OTC]; Rulox [OTC]
Brand Names: Canada Diovol Plus®; Gelusil®; Mylanta® Double Strength; Mylanta® Extra Strength; Mylanta® Regular Strength
Index Terms Magnesium Hydroxide, Aluminum Hydroxide, and Simethicone; Simethicone, Aluminum Hydroxide, and Magnesium Hydroxide
Generic Availability (U.S.) Yes
Pharmacologic Category Antacid; Antiflatulent
Use Temporary relief of hyperacidity associated with gas; may also be used for indications associated with other antacids
Adverse Reactions (Reflective of adult population; not specific for elderly)
>10%: Gastrointestinal: Chalky taste, stomach cramps, constipation, bowel motility decreased, fecal impaction, hemorrhoids
1% to 10%: Gastrointestinal: Nausea, vomiting, discoloration of feces (white speckles)
Drug Interactions
Avoid Concomitant Use
Avoid concomitant use of Aluminum Hydroxide, Magnesium Hydroxide, and Simethicone with any of the following: Calcium Polystyrene Sulfonate; Deferasirox; QuiNINE; Sodium Polystyrene Sulfonate; Vitamin D Analogs
Increased Effect/Toxicity
Aluminum Hydroxide, Magnesium Hydroxide, and Simethicone may increase the levels/ effects of: Alpha-/Beta-Agonists; Amphetamines; Calcium Channel Blockers; Calcium Polystyrene Sulfonate; Dexmethylphenidate; Methylphenidate; Misoprostol; Neuromuscular-Blocking Agents; QuiNIDine; Sodium Polystyrene Sulfonate*

The levels/effects of Aluminum Hydroxide, Magnesium Hydroxide, and Simethicone may be increased by: Alfacalcidol; Ascorbic Acid; Calcitriol; Calcium Channel Blockers; Calcium Polystyrene Sulfonate; Citric Acid Derivatives; Sodium Polystyrene Sulfonate; Vitamin D Analogs*
Decreased Effect
Aluminum Hydroxide, Magnesium Hydroxide, and Simethicone may decrease the levels/ effects of: ACE Inhibitors; Allopurinol; Anticonvulsants (Hydantoin); Antipsychotic Agents (Phenothiazines); Atazanavir; Bisacodyl; Bisphosphonate Derivatives; Cefditoren; Cefpodoxime; Cefuroxime; Chenodiol; Chloroquine; Corticosteroids (Oral); Dabigatran Etexilate; Dasatinib; Deferasirox; Delavirdine; Eltrombopag; Erlotinib; Ethambutol; Fexofenadine; Gabapentin; HMG-CoA Reductase Inhibitors; Iron Salts; Isoniazid; Itraconazole; Ketoconazole; Ketoconazole (Systemic); Levothyroxine; Mesalamine; Methenamine; Mycophenolate; Penicillamine; Phosphate Supplements; Protease Inhibitors; QuiNINE; Quinolone Antibiotics; Rilpivirine; Tetracycline Derivatives; Trientine; Ursodiol*

The levels/effects of Aluminum Hydroxide, Magnesium Hydroxide, and Simethicone may be decreased by: Trientine*
Dosage
Geriatric & Adult Dyspepsia, abdominal bloating: Oral: 10-20 mL or 2-4 tablets 4-6 times/ day between meals and at bedtime; may be used every hour for severe symptoms
Renal Impairment Aluminum and/or magnesium may accumulate in renal impairment.
Administration Administer 1-2 hours apart from oral drugs; administer 1-3 hours after meals.

Dosage Forms Excipient information presented when available (limited, particularly for generics); consult specific product labeling. [DSC] = Discontinued product

Liquid, oral: Aluminum hydroxide 200 mg, magnesium hydroxide 200 mg, and simethicone 20 mg per 5 mL (360 mL); aluminum hydroxide 400 mg, magnesium hydroxide 400 mg, and simethicone 40 mg per 5 mL (360 mL)

Aldroxicon I: Aluminum hydroxide 200 mg, magnesium hydroxide 200 mg, and simethicone 20 mg per 5 mL (30 mL)

Aldroxicon II: Aluminum hydroxide 400 mg, magnesium hydroxide 400 mg, and simethicone 40 mg per 5 mL (30 mL)

Almacone®: Aluminum hydroxide 200 mg, magnesium hydroxide 200 mg, and simethicone 20 mg per 5 mL (360 mL)

Almacone Double Strength®: Aluminum hydroxide 400 mg, magnesium hydroxide 400 mg, and simethicone 40 mg per 5 mL (360 mL)

Maalox® Advanced Maximum Strength: Aluminum hydroxide 400 mg, magnesium hydroxide 400 mg, and simethicone 40 mg per 5 mL (355 mL, 769 mL) [contains magnesium 167 mg/5 mL; cherry flavor]

Maalox® Advanced Maximum Strength: Aluminum hydroxide 400 mg, magnesium hydroxide 400 mg, and simethicone 40 mg per 5 mL (355 mL, 769 mL) [contains magnesium 167 mg/5 mL; lemon flavor]

Maalox® Advanced Maximum Strength: Aluminum hydroxide 400 mg, magnesium hydroxide 400 mg, and simethicone 40 mg per 5 mL (355 mL) [contains magnesium 167 mg/5 mL; mint flavor]

Maalox® Advanced Maximum Strength: Aluminum hydroxide 400 mg, magnesium hydroxide 400 mg, and simethicone 40 mg per 5 mL (355 mL) [contains magnesium 167 mg/5 mL; vanilla crème flavor]

Maalox® Advanced Regular Strength: Aluminum hydroxide 200 mg, magnesium hydroxide 200 mg, and simethicone 20 mg per 5 mL (360 mL, 780 mL) [contains magnesium 75 mg/5 mL, potassium 5 mg/5 mL, propylene glycol; mint flavor]

Mi-Acid: Aluminum hydroxide 200 mg, magnesium hydroxide 200 mg, and simethicone 20 mg per 5 mL (360 mL)

Mi-Acid Maximum Strength: Aluminum hydroxide 400 mg, magnesium hydroxide 400 mg, and simethicone 40 mg per 5 mL (360 mL)

Mylanta® Classic Maximum Strength: Aluminum hydroxide 400 mg, magnesium hydroxide 400 mg, and simethicone 40 mg per 5 mL (360 mL, 720 mL) [original, cherry, orange creme, and mint flavors]

Mylanta® Classic Regular Strength: Aluminum hydroxide 200 mg, magnesium hydroxide 200 mg, and simethicone 20 mg per 5 mL (360 mL) [original and mint flavors]

Suspension, oral: Aluminum hydroxide 225 mg, magnesium hydroxide 200 mg, and simethicone 25 mg per 5 mL (360 mL)

Alamag Plus: Aluminum hydroxide 225 mg, magnesium hydroxide 200 mg, and simethicone 25 mg per 5 mL (360 mL) [DSC]

Rulox: Aluminum hydroxide 200 mg, magnesium hydroxide 200 mg, and simethicone 25 mg per 5 mL (355 mL) [contains magnesium 85 mg/5 mL; mint flavor]

Tablet, chewable: Aluminum hydroxide 200 mg, magnesium hydroxide 200 mg, and simethicone 25 mg

Alamag Plus: Aluminum hydroxide 200 mg, magnesium hydroxide 200 mg, and simethicone 25 mg [contains magnesium 83 mg/tablet, phenylalanine 2.6 mg/tablet; cherry flavor]

Almacone®: Aluminum hydroxide 200 mg, magnesium hydroxide 200 mg, and simethicone 20 mg [dye free; contains magnesium 82 mg/tablet; peppermint flavor]

Gelusil®: Aluminum hydroxide 200 mg, magnesium hydroxide 200 mg, and simethicone 25 mg [peppermint flavor]

Mintox Plus: Aluminum hydroxide 200 mg, magnesium hydroxide 200 mg, and simethicone 25 mg [lemon crème flavor]

◆ **Aluminum Sucrose Sulfate, Basic** *see* Sucralfate *on page 1711*

Aluminum Sulfate and Calcium Acetate
(a LOO mi num SUL fate & KAL see um AS e tate)

Related Information
Calcium Acetate *on page 247*
Brand Names: U.S. Domeboro® [OTC]; Gordon Boro-Packs [OTC]; Pedi-Boro® [OTC]
Index Terms Calcium Acetate and Aluminum Sulfate
Generic Availability (U.S.) No
Pharmacologic Category Topical Skin Product
Use Astringent wet dressing for relief of inflammatory conditions of the skin; reduce weeping that may occur in dermatitis

ALUMINUM SULFATE AND CALCIUM ACETATE

◀ **Dosage**
  Geriatric & Adult Dermal inflammation, dermatitis: Topical: Soak affected area in the
  solution 2-4 times/day for 15-30 minutes or apply wet dressing soaked in the solution for
  more extended periods; rewet dressing with solution 2-4 times/day every 15-30 minutes
  Special Geriatric Considerations No special considerations necessary
  Dosage Forms Excipient information presented when available (limited, particularly for
  generics); consult specific product labeling.
    Powder, for topical solution:
      Domeboro®: Aluminum sulfate 1191 mg and calcium acetate 839 mg per packet (12s, 100s)
      Gordon Boro-Packs: Aluminum sulfate 49% and calcium acetate 51% per packet (100s)
      Pedi-Boro®: Aluminum sulfate 1191 mg and calcium acetate 839 mg per packet (12s, 100s)

◆ **Alupent** see Metaproterenol on page 1153
◆ **Alvesco®** see Ciclesonide (Oral Inhalation) on page 351

Amantadine (a MAN ta deen)

Related Information
  Antiparkinsonian Agents on page 1995
Medication Safety Issues
  Sound-alike/look-alike issues:
    Amantadine may be confused with ranitidine, rimantadine
    Symmetrel may be confused with Synthroid®
Brand Names: Canada Endantadine®; Mylan-Amantadine; PMS-Amantadine; Symmetrel®
Index Terms Adamantanamine Hydrochloride; Amantadine Hydrochloride; Symmetrel
Generic Availability (U.S.) Yes
Pharmacologic Category Anti-Parkinson's Agent, Dopamine Agonist; Antiviral Agent;
  Antiviral Agent, Adamantane
Use Prophylaxis and treatment of influenza A viral infection (per manufacturer labeling; also
  refer to current ACIP guidelines for recommendations during current flu season); treatment of
  parkinsonism; treatment of drug-induced extrapyramidal symptoms
Contraindications Hypersensitivity to amantadine or any component of the formulation
Warnings/Precautions May cause CNS depression, which may impair physical or mental
  abilities; patients must be cautioned about performing tasks which require mental alertness
  (eg, operating machinery or driving). There have been reports of suicidal ideation/attempt in
  patients with and without a history of psychiatric illness. Use with caution in patients with liver
  disease, a history of recurrent and eczematoid dermatitis, uncontrolled psychosis or severe
  psychoneurosis, seizures and in those receiving CNS stimulant drugs; reduce dose in renal
  disease; when treating Parkinson's disease, do not discontinue abruptly. In many patients, the
  therapeutic benefits of amantadine are limited to a few months. Abrupt discontinuation may
  cause agitation, anxiety, delirium, delusions, depression, hallucinations, paranoia, parkinsonian crisis, slurred speech, or stupor. Upon discontinuation of amantadine therapy, gradually
  taper dose. Elderly patients may be more susceptible to the CNS effects (using 2 divided daily
  doses may minimize this effect); may require dosage reductions based on renal function. Use
  with caution in patients with HF, peripheral edema, or orthostatic hypotension; dosage
  reduction may be required. Avoid in untreated angle closure glaucoma.

  Dopamine agonists have been associated with compulsive behaviors and/or loss of impulse
  control, which has manifested as pathological gambling, libido increases (hypersexuality),
  and/or binge eating. Causality has not been established, and controversy exists as to whether
  this phenomenon is related to the underlying disease, prior behaviors/addictions, and/or drug
  therapy. Dose reduction or discontinuation of therapy has been reported to reverse these
  behaviors in some, but not all cases. Risk for melanoma development is increased in
  Parkinson's disease patients; drug causation or factors contributing to risk have not been
  established. Patients should be monitored closely and periodic skin examinations should be
  performed.

  Due to increased resistance, the ACIP has recommended that rimantadine and amantadine
  no longer be used for the treatment or prophylaxis of influenza A in the United States until
  susceptibility has been re-established; consult current guidelines.
Adverse Reactions (Reflective of adult population; not specific for elderly)
  1% to 10%:
  Cardiovascular: Orthostatic hypotension, peripheral edema
  Central nervous system: Agitation, anxiety, ataxia, confusion, delirium, depression, dizziness,
    dream abnormality, fatigue, hallucinations, headache, insomnia, irritability, lightheadedness,
    nervousness, somnolence
  Dermatologic: Livedo reticularis

Gastrointestinal: Anorexia, constipation, diarrhea, nausea, xerostomia
Respiratory: Dry nose

Drug Interactions

Avoid Concomitant Use There are no known interactions where it is recommended to avoid concomitant use.

Increased Effect/Toxicity

Amantadine may increase the levels/effects of: Glycopyrrolate; Trimethoprim

The levels/effects of Amantadine may be increased by: Antipsychotics (Typical); MAO Inhibitors; Methylphenidate; Trimethoprim

Decreased Effect

Amantadine may decrease the levels/effects of: Antipsychotics (Typical); Influenza Virus Vaccine (Live/Attenuated)

The levels/effects of Amantadine may be decreased by: Antipsychotics (Atypical); Metoclopramide

Ethanol/Nutrition/Herb Interactions Ethanol: Avoid ethanol (may increase CNS adverse effects).

Stability Store at 25°C (77°F); excursions permitted to 15°C to 30°C (59°F to 86°F).

Mechanism of Action As an antiviral, blocks the uncoating of influenza A virus preventing penetration of virus into host; antiparkinsonian activity may be due to its blocking the reuptake of dopamine into presynaptic neurons or by increasing dopamine release from presynaptic fibers

Pharmacodynamics/Kinetics

Onset of action: Antidyskinetic: Within 48 hours

Absorption: Well absorbed

Distribution: V_d: Normal: 1.5-6.1 L/kg; Renal failure: 5.1 ± 0.2 L/kg; in saliva, tear film, and nasal secretions; in animals, tissue (especially lung) concentrations higher than serum concentrations; crosses blood-brain barrier

Protein binding: Normal renal function: ~67%; Hemodialysis: ~59%

Metabolism: Not appreciable; small amounts of an acetyl metabolite identified

Bioavailability: 86% to 90%

Half-life elimination: Normal renal function: 16 ± 6 hours (9-31 hours); Healthy, older (≥60 years) males: 29 hours (range: 20-41 hours); End-stage renal disease: 7-10 days

Time to peak, plasma: 2-4 hours

Excretion: Urine (80% to 90% unchanged) by glomerular filtration and tubular secretion

Dosage

Geriatric Patients ≥65 years: Adjust dose based on renal function; some patients tolerate the drug better when it is given in 2 divided daily doses (to avoid adverse neurologic reactions). Influenza A treatment/prophylaxis: 100 mg once daily

Adult

Influenza A treatment/prophylaxis: Note: Due to issues of resistance, amantadine is no longer recommended for the treatment or prophylaxis of influenza A. Please refer to the current ACIP recommendations. The following is based on the manufacturer's labeling:

Influenza A treatment: Oral: 200 mg once daily **or** 100 mg twice daily (may be preferred to reduce CNS effects); **Note:** Initiate within 24-48 hours after onset of symptoms; continue for 24-48 hours after symptom resolution (duration of therapy is generally 3-5 days).

Influenza A prophylaxis: Oral: 200 mg once daily **or** 100 mg twice daily (may be preferred to reduce CNS effects). **Note:** Continue prophylaxis throughout the peak influenza activity in the community or throughout the entire influenza season in patients who cannot be vaccinated. Development of immunity following vaccination takes ~2 weeks; amantadine therapy should be considered for high-risk patients from the time of vaccination until immunity has developed.

Drug-induced extrapyramidal symptoms: Oral: 100 mg twice daily; may increase to 300 mg/day in divided doses, if needed

Parkinson's disease: Oral: Usual dose: 100 mg twice daily as monotherapy; may increase to 400 mg/day in divided doses, if needed, with close monitoring. **Note:** Patients with a serious concomitant illness or those receiving high doses of other anti-parkinson drugs should be started at 100 mg/day; may increase to 100 mg twice daily, if needed, after one to several weeks.

Renal Impairment

Cl_{cr} 30-50 mL/minute: Administer 200 mg on day 1, then 100 mg/day

Cl_{cr} 15-29 mL/minute: Administer 200 mg on day 1, then 100 mg on alternate days

Cl_{cr} <15 mL/minute: Administer 200 mg every 7 days

Hemodialysis: Administer 200 mg every 7 days

Peritoneal dialysis: No supplemental dose is needed

Continuous arteriovenous or venous-venous hemofiltration: No supplemental dose is needed

Monitoring Parameters Renal function, Parkinson's symptoms, mental status, influenza symptoms, blood pressure

Test Interactions May interfere with urine detection of amphetamines/methamphetamines (false-positive).

Pharmacotherapy Pearls Patients with intolerable CNS side effects often do better with rimantadine.

Special Geriatric Considerations Amantadine is no longer recommended for the treatment or chemoprophylaxis of influenza A infection. Elderly patients may be more susceptible to the CNS effects of amantadine. Adjust dose based on renal function. Liquid forms may be used to administer doses <100 mg.

Dosage Forms Excipient information presented when available (limited, particularly for generics); consult specific product labeling.

Capsule, oral, as hydrochloride: 100 mg

Capsule, softgel, oral, as hydrochloride: 100 mg

Solution, oral, as hydrochloride: 50 mg/5 mL (473 mL)

Syrup, oral, as hydrochloride: 50 mg/5 mL (10 mL, 473 mL, 480 mL)

Tablet, oral, as hydrochloride: 100 mg

Selected References

Aoki FY and Sitar DS, "Amantadine Kinetics in Healthy Elderly Men: Implications for Influenza Prevention," *Clin Pharmacol Ther*, 1985, 37(2):137-44.

Aoki FY and Sitar DS, "Clinical Pharmacokinetics of Amantadine Hydrochloride," *Clin Pharmacokinet*, 1988, 14 (1):35-51.

Factor SA, "Current Status of Symptomatic Medical Therapy in Parkinson's Disease," *Neurotherapeutics*, 2008, 5 (2):164-80.

Fiore AE, Uyeki TM, Broder K, et al, "Prevention and Control of Influenza With Vaccines: Recommendations of the Advisory Committee on Immunization Practices (ACIP), 2010," *MMWR Recomm Rep*, 2010, 59(RR-8):1-62.

Olanow CW, Watts RL, and Koller WC, "An Algorithm (Decision Tree) for the Management of Parkinson's Disease (2001): Treatment Guidelines," *Neurology*, 2001, 56(11 Suppl 5):S1-S88.

Somani SK, Degelau J, Cooper SL, et al, "Comparison of Pharmacokinetic and Safety Profiles of Amantadine 50- and 100-mg Daily Doses in Elderly Nursing Home Residents," *Pharmacotherapy*, 1991, 11(6):460-6.

Weintraub D, Siderowf AD, Potenza MN, et al, "Association of Dopamine Agonist Use With Impulse Control Disorders in Parkinson Disease," *Arch Neurol*, 2006, 63(7):969-73.

◆ **Amantadine Hydrochloride** *see* Amantadine *on page 86*

◆ **Amaryl®** *see* Glimepiride *on page 820*

◆ **Ambien®** *see* Zolpidem *on page 1960*

◆ **Ambien CR®** *see* Zolpidem *on page 1960*

Amcinonide (am SIN oh nide)

Related Information

Corticosteroids *on page 2005*

Brand Names: Canada Amcort®; Cyclocort®; ratio-Amcinonide; Taro-Amcinonide

Generic Availability (U.S.) Yes

Pharmacologic Category Corticosteroid, Topical

Use Relief of the inflammatory and pruritic manifestations of corticosteroid-responsive dermatoses (high potency corticosteroid)

Dosage

Geriatric & Adult Steroid-responsive dermatoses: Topical: Apply in a thin film 2-3 times/day. Therapy should be discontinued when control is achieved; if no improvement is seen, reassessment of diagnosis may be necessary.

Special Geriatric Considerations Due to age-related changes in skin, limit use of topical corticosteroids.

Dosage Forms Excipient information presented when available (limited, particularly for generics); consult specific product labeling. [DSC] = Discontinued product

Cream, topical: 0.1% (15 g, 30 g, 60 g)

Lotion, topical: 0.1% (60 mL)

Ointment, topical: 0.1% (30 g [DSC], 60 g)

◆ **Amerge®** *see* Naratriptan *on page 1268*

◆ **A-Methapred** *see* MethylPREDNISolone *on page 1183*

◆ **A-Methapred®** *see* MethylPREDNISolone *on page 1183*

◆ **Amethopterin** *see* Methotrexate *on page 1168*

◆ **AMG-162** *see* Denosumab *on page 468*

Amikacin (am i KAY sin)

Related Information
Aminoglycoside Dosing and Monitoring *on page 2050*

Medication Safety Issues
Sound-alike/look-alike issues:
Amikacin may be confused with Amicar®, anakinra
Amikin® may be confused with Amicar®, Kineret®

Brand Names: Canada Amikacin Sulfate Injection, USP; Amikin®

Index Terms Amikacin Sulfate

Generic Availability (U.S.) Yes

Pharmacologic Category Antibiotic, Aminoglycoside

Use Treatment of serious infections (bone infections, respiratory tract infections, endocarditis, and septicemia) due to organisms resistant to gentamicin and tobramycin, including *Pseudomonas*, *Proteus*, *Serratia*, and other gram-negative bacilli; documented infection of mycobacterial organisms susceptible to amikacin

Unlabeled/Investigational Use Bacterial endophthalmitis

Contraindications Hypersensitivity to amikacin sulfate or any component of the formulation; cross-sensitivity may exist with other aminoglycosides

Warnings/Precautions [U.S. Boxed Warning]: Amikacin may cause neurotoxicity, nephrotoxicity, and/or neuromuscular blockade and respiratory paralysis; usual risk factors include pre-existing renal impairment, concomitant neuro-/nephrotoxic medications, advanced age and dehydration. Dose and/or frequency of administration must be monitored and modified in patients with renal impairment. Drug should be discontinued if signs of ototoxicity, nephrotoxicity, or hypersensitivity occur. Ototoxicity is proportional to the amount of drug given and the duration of treatment. Tinnitus or vertigo may be indications of vestibular injury and impending bilateral irreversible damage. Renal damage is usually reversible. Use with caution in patients with neuromuscular disorders, hearing loss and hypocalcemia. Prolonged use may result in fungal or bacterial superinfection, including *C. difficile*-associated diarrhea (CDAD) and pseudomembranous colitis; CDAD has been observed >2 months postantibiotic treatment. Solution contains sodium metabisulfate; use caution in patients with sulfite allergy.

Adverse Reactions (Reflective of adult population; not specific for elderly)
1% to 10%:
Central nervous system: Neurotoxicity
Otic: Ototoxicity (auditory), ototoxicity (vestibular)
Renal: Nephrotoxicity

Drug Interactions
Avoid Concomitant Use
Avoid concomitant use of Amikacin with any of the following: BCG; Gallium Nitrate
Increased Effect/Toxicity
Amikacin may increase the levels/effects of: AbobotulinumtoxinA; Bisphosphonate Derivatives; CARBOplatin; Colistimethate; CycloSPORINE; CycloSPORINE (Systemic); Gallium Nitrate; Neuromuscular-Blocking Agents; OnabotulinumtoxinA; RimabotulinumtoxinB

The levels/effects of Amikacin may be increased by: Amphotericin B; Capreomycin; CISplatin; Loop Diuretics; Nonsteroidal Anti-Inflammatory Agents; Vancomycin
Decreased Effect
Amikacin may decrease the levels/effects of: BCG; Typhoid Vaccine

The levels/effects of Amikacin may be decreased by: Penicillins

Stability Store at controlled room temperature. Following admixture at concentrations of 0.25-5 mg/mL, amikacin is stable for 24 hours at room temperature and 2 days at refrigeration when mixed in D_5W, NS, and LR.

Mechanism of Action Inhibits protein synthesis in susceptible bacteria by binding to 30S ribosomal subunits

Pharmacodynamics/Kinetics
Absorption: I.M.: Aminoglycosides may be delayed in the bedridden patient
Half-life:
Adults: 2-3 hours
Anuria: 28-86 hours
Half-life and clearance are dependent on renal function primarily distributed into extracellular fluid (highly hydrophilic); penetrates the blood-brain barrier when meninges are inflamed
Time to peak serum concentration:
I.M.: Within 45-120 minutes
I.V.: Within 30 minutes

Elimination: 94% to 98% excreted unchanged in urine via glomerular filtration within 24 hours

Clearance (renal) may be reduced and half-life prolonged in geriatric patients

The pharmacokinetics of the aminoglycosides are heterogeneous in older adults; it is best to assume that clearance is reduced and half-life prolonged in older adults, while volume of distribution is usually unchanged. The establishment of each patient's pharmacokinetic parameters is important for proper dosing in order to achieve optimal therapeutic benefit and minimize the risk of toxicity.

Dosage

Geriatric & Adult Individualization is critical because of the low therapeutic index

Note: Use of ideal body weight (IBW) for determining the mg/kg/dose appears to be more accurate than dosing on the basis of total body weight (TBW)

In morbid obesity, dosage requirement may best be estimated using a dosing weight of IBW + 0.4 (TBW - IBW)

Initial and periodic peak and trough plasma drug levels should be determined, particularly in critically-ill patients with serious infections or in disease states known to significantly alter aminoglycoside pharmacokinetics (eg, cystic fibrosis, burns, or major surgery). Manufacturer recommends a maximum daily dose of 15 mg/kg/day (or 1.5 g/day in heavier patients). Higher doses may be warranted based on therapeutic drug monitoring or susceptibility information.

Usual dosage range:

I.M., I.V.: 5-7.5 mg/kg/dose every 8 hours; **Note:** Some clinicians suggest a daily dose of 15-20 mg/kg for all patients with normal renal function. This dose is at least as efficacious with similar, if not less, toxicity than conventional dosing.

Intrathecal/intraventricular (unlabeled route): Meningitis (susceptible gram-negative organisms): 5-50 mg/day

Indication-specific dosing:

Endophthalmitis, bacterial (unlabeled use): Intravitreal: 0.4 mg/0.1 mL NS in combination with vancomycin

Hospital-acquired pneumonia (HAP): I.V.: 20 mg/kg/day with antipseudomonal beta-lactam or carbapenem (American Thoracic Society/ATS guidelines)

Meningitis (susceptible gram-negative organisms):

I.V.: 5 mg/kg every 8 hours (administered with another biocidal drug)

Intrathecal/intraventricular (unlabeled route): Usual dose: 30 mg/day (IDSA, 2004); Range: 5-50 mg/day (with concurrent systemic antimicrobial therapy) (Gilbert, 1986; Guardado, 2008; IDSA, 2004; Kasiakou, 2005)

Mycobacterium fortuitum, M. chelonae, or M. abscessus: I.V.: 10-15 mg/kg daily for at least 2 weeks with high dose cefoxitin

Renal Impairment Some patients may require larger or more frequent doses if serum levels document the need (ie, cystic fibrosis or febrile granulocytopenic patients).

Cl_{cr} ≥60 mL/minute: Administer every 8 hours

Cl_{cr} 40-60 mL/minute: Administer every 12 hours

Cl_{cr} 20-40 mL/minute: Administer every 24 hours

Cl_{cr} <20 mL/minute: Loading dose, then monitor levels

Intermittent hemodialysis (IHD) (administer after hemodialysis on dialysis days): Dialyzable (20%; variable; dependent on filter, duration, and type of HD): 5-7.5 mg/kg every 48-72 hours. Follow levels. Redose when pre-HD concentration <10 mg/L; redose when post-HD concentration <6-8 mg/L (Heintz, 2009). **Note:** Dosing dependent on the assumption of 3 times/week, complete IHD sessions.

Peritoneal dialysis (PD): Dose as Cl_{cr} <20 mL/minute: Follow levels.

Continuous renal replacement therapy (CRRT) (Heintz, 2009; Trotman, 2005): Drug clearance is highly dependent on the method of renal replacement, filter type, and flow rate. Appropriate dosing requires close monitoring of pharmacologic response, signs of adverse reactions due to drug accumulation, as well as drug concentrations in relation to target trough (if appropriate). The following are general recommendations only (based on dialysate flow/ultrafiltration rates of 1-2 L/hour and minimal residual renal function) and should not supersede clinical judgment:

CVVH/CVVHD/CVVHDF: Loading dose of 10 mg/kg followed by maintenance dose of 7.5 mg/kg every 24-48 hours

Note: For severe gram-negative rod infections, target peak concentration of 15-30 mg/L; redose when concentration <10 mg/L (Heintz, 2009).

Administration Administer I.M. injection in large muscle mass

Monitoring Parameters Urinalysis, BUN, serum creatinine, appropriately timed peak and trough concentrations, vital signs, temperature, weight, I & O, hearing parameters

Some penicillin derivatives may accelerate the degradation of aminoglycosides *in vitro*. This may be clinically-significant for certain penicillin (ticarcillin, piperacillin, carbenicillin) and aminoglycoside (gentamicin, tobramycin) combination therapy in patients with significant renal impairment. Close monitoring of aminoglycoside levels is warranted.

Reference Range
Sample size: 0.5-2 mL blood (red top tube) or 0.1-1 mL serum (separated)
Therapeutic levels:
Peak:
Life-threatening infections: 25-40 mcg/mL
Serious infections: 20-25 mcg/mL
Urinary tract infections: 15-20 mcg/mL
Trough: <8 mcg/mL
The American Thoracic Society (ATS) recommends trough levels of <4-5 mcg/mL for patients with hospital-acquired pneumonia.
Toxic concentration: Peak: >40 mcg/mL; Trough: >10 mcg/mL
Timing of serum samples: Draw peak 30 minutes after completion of 30-minute infusion or at 1 hour following initiation of infusion or I.M. injection; draw trough within 30 minutes prior to next dose

Test Interactions Some penicillin derivatives may accelerate the degradation of aminoglycosides *in vitro*, leading to a potential underestimation of aminoglycoside serum concentration.

Pharmacotherapy Pearls Drug should be discontinued if signs of ototoxicity, nephrotoxicity, or hypersensitivity occurs; hearing should be tested before, during, and after treatment, when indicated; sodium content of 1 g: 29.9 mg (1.3 mEq). Aminoglycoside serum concentrations measured from blood taken from silastic central catheters can sometimes give falsely high readings.

Special Geriatric Considerations The aminoglycosides are important therapeutic interventions for infections due to susceptible organisms and as empiric therapy in seriously ill patients. Their use is not without risk of toxicity, however, these risks can be minimized if initial dosing is adjusted for estimated renal function and appropriate monitoring performed. High dose, once daily aminoglycosides have been advocated as an alternative to traditional dosing regimens. Once daily or extended interval dosing is as effective and may be safer than traditional dosing. Interval must be adjusted for renal function.

Dosage Forms Excipient information presented when available (limited, particularly for generics); consult specific product labeling. [DSC] = Discontinued product
Injection, solution, as sulfate: 50 mg/mL (2 mL [DSC]); 250 mg/mL (2 mL, 4 mL)

Selected References
Bauer LA and Blouin RA, "Influence of Age on Amikacin Pharmacokinetics in Patients Without Renal Disease. Comparison With Gentamicin and Tobramycin," *Eur J Clin Pharmacol*, 1983, 24(5):639-42.
Yasuhara H, Kobayashi S, Sakamoto K, et al, "Pharmacokinetics of Amikacin and Cephalothin in Bedridden Elderly Patients," *J Clin Pharmacol*, 1982, 22(8-9):403-9.

◆ **Amikacin Sulfate** *see* Amikacin *on page* 89

AMILoride (a MIL oh ride)

Medication Safety Issues
Sound-alike/look-alike issues:
AMILoride may be confused with amiodarone, amLODIPine, inamrinone
Brand Names: Canada Apo-Amiloride®; Midamor
Index Terms Amiloride Hydrochloride
Generic Availability (U.S.) Yes
Pharmacologic Category Diuretic, Potassium-Sparing
Use Counteracts potassium loss induced by other diuretics in the treatment of hypertension or edematous conditions including CHF, hepatic cirrhosis, and hypoaldosteronism; usually used in conjunction with more potent diuretics such as thiazides or loop diuretics
Unlabeled/Investigational Use Investigational: Cystic fibrosis; reduction of lithium-induced polyuria
Contraindications Hypersensitivity to amiloride or any component of the formulation; presence of elevated serum potassium levels (>5.5 mEq/L); if patient is receiving other potassium-conserving agents (eg, spironolactone, triamterene) or potassium supplementation (medicine, potassium-containing salt substitutes, potassium-rich diet); anuria; acute or chronic renal insufficiency; evidence of diabetic nephropathy. Patients with evidence of renal impairment or diabetes mellitus should not receive this medicine without close, frequent monitoring of serum electrolytes and renal function.
Warnings/Precautions [U.S. Boxed Warning]: Hyperkalemia can occur; patients at risk include those with renal impairment, diabetes, the elderly, and the severely ill. Serum potassium levels must be monitored at frequent intervals especially when dosages are changed or with any illness that may cause renal dysfunction. Excess amounts can lead to profound diuresis with fluid and electrolyte loss; close medical supervision and dose evaluation are required. Watch for and correct electrolyte disturbances; adjust dose to avoid dehydration. In cirrhosis, avoid electrolyte and acid/base imbalances that might lead to hepatic encephalopathy. Use with extreme caution in patients with diabetes mellitus; monitor ▶

closely. Discontinue amiloride 3 days prior to glucose tolerance testing. Use with caution in patients who are at risk for metabolic or respiratory acidosis (eg, cardiopulmonary disease, uncontrolled diabetes).

Adverse Reactions (Reflective of adult population; not specific for elderly)
1% to 10%:

Central nervous system: Headache, fatigue, dizziness

Endocrine & metabolic: Hyperkalemia (up to 10%; risk reduced in patients receiving kaliuretic diuretics), hyperchloremic metabolic acidosis, dehydration, hyponatremia, gynecomastia

Gastrointestinal: Nausea, diarrhea, vomiting, abdominal pain, gas pain, appetite changes, constipation

Genitourinary: Impotence

Neuromuscular & skeletal: Muscle cramps, weakness

Respiratory: Cough, dyspnea

Drug Interactions

Avoid Concomitant Use

Avoid concomitant use of AMILoride with any of the following: Tacrolimus

Increased Effect/Toxicity

AMILoride may increase the levels/effects of: ACE Inhibitors; Amifostine; Ammonium Chloride; Antihypertensives; Cardiac Glycosides; Dofetilide; Hypotensive Agents; RiTUXimab; Sodium Phosphates; Tacrolimus

The levels/effects of AMILoride may be increased by: Alfuzosin; Angiotensin II Receptor Blockers; Diazoxide; Drospirenone; Eplerenone; Herbs (Hypotensive Properties); MAO Inhibitors; Nonsteroidal Anti-Inflammatory Agents; Pentoxifylline; Phosphodiesterase 5 Inhibitors; Potassium Salts; Prostacyclin Analogues; Tolvaptan

Decreased Effect

AMILoride may decrease the levels/effects of: Cardiac Glycosides; QuiNIDine

The levels/effects of AMILoride may be decreased by: Herbs (Hypertensive Properties); Methylphenidate; Nonsteroidal Anti-Inflammatory Agents; Yohimbine

Ethanol/Nutrition/Herb Interactions Food: Hyperkalemia may result if amiloride is taken with potassium-containing foods.

Mechanism of Action Blocks epithelial sodium channels in the late distal convoluted tubule (DCT), and collecting duct which inhibits sodium reabsorption from the lumen. This effectively reduces intracellular sodium, decreasing the function of Na+/K+ATPase, leading to potassium retention and decreased calcium, magnesium, and hydrogen excretion. As sodium uptake capacity in the DCT/collecting duct is limited, the natriuretic, diuretic, and antihypertensive effects are generally considered weak.

Pharmacodynamics/Kinetics

Onset of action: 2 hours

Duration: 24 hours

Absorption: ~15% to 25%

Distribution: V_d: 350-380 L

Protein binding: 23%

Metabolism: No active metabolites

Half-life elimination: Normal renal function: 6-9 hours; End-stage renal disease: 8-144 hours

Time to peak, serum: 6-10 hours

Excretion: Urine and feces (equal amounts as unchanged drug)

Dosage

Geriatric Oral: Initial: 5 mg once daily or every other day

Adult Hypertension, edema (to limit potassium loss): Oral: Initial: 5-10 mg/day (up to 20 mg)

Hypertension (JNC 7): 5-10 mg/day in 1-2 divided doses

Renal Impairment Oral:

Cl_{cr} 10-50 mL/minute: Administer 50% of normal dose.

Cl_{cr} <10 mL/minute: Avoid use.

Administration Administer with food or meals to avoid GI upset.

Monitoring Parameters I & O, daily weights, blood pressure, serum electrolytes, renal function

Test Interactions May falsely elevate serum digoxin levels done by radioimmunoassay

Pharmacotherapy Pearls Medication should be discontinued if potassium level exceeds 6.5 mEq/L. Combined with hydrochlorothiazide as Moduretic®. Amiloride is considered an alternative to triamterene or spironolactone.

Special Geriatric Considerations Use lower initial dose, and adjust dose for renal impairment. Potassium excretion may be decreased in the elderly, increasing the risk of hyperkalemia, which may occur with potassium-sparing diuretics such as amiloride.

Dosage Forms Excipient information presented when available (limited, particularly for generics); consult specific product labeling.
Tablet, oral, as hydrochloride: 5 mg

Amiloride and Hydrochlorothiazide
(a MIL oh ride & hye droe klor oh THYE a zide)

Related Information
AMILoride *on page 91*
Hydrochlorothiazide *on page 876*
Brand Names: Canada Ami-Hydro; Apo-Amilzide®; Gen-Amilazide; Moduret; Novamilor; Nu-Amilzide
Index Terms Hydrochlorothiazide and Amiloride
Generic Availability (U.S.) Yes
Pharmacologic Category Diuretic, Combination
Use Potassium-sparing diuretic; antihypertensive
Dosage
Geriatric Oral: Initial: 1/2 to 1 tablet/day
Adult Hypertension, edema: Oral: Initial: 1 tablet/day; may be increased to 2 tablets/day if needed; usually given in a single dose
Renal Impairment See individual agents.
Special Geriatric Considerations Hydrochlorothiazide is not effective in patients with a Cl_{cr} <30 mL/minute; therefore, it may not be a useful agent in many elderly patients. Potassium excretion may be decreased in the elderly, increasing the risk of hyperkalemia with potassium-sparing diuretics such as amiloride.
Dosage Forms Excipient information presented when available (limited, particularly for generics); consult specific product labeling.
Tablet: 5/50: Amiloride hydrochloride 5 mg and hydrochlorothiazide 50 mg

◆ **Amiloride Hydrochloride** *see* AMILoride *on page 91*
◆ **2-Amino-6-Trifluoromethoxy-benzothiazole** *see* Riluzole *on page 1615*
◆ **Aminobenzylpenicillin** *see* Ampicillin *on page 127*

Aminolevulinic Acid (a MEE noh lev yoo lin ik AS id)

Medication Safety Issues
Sound-alike/look-alike issues:
Aminolevulinic acid may be confused with methyl aminolevulinate
Brand Names: U.S. Levulan® Kerastick®
Brand Names: Canada Levulan® Kerastick®
Index Terms 5-ALA; 5-Aminolevulinic Acid; ALA; Amino Levulinic Acid; Aminolevulinic Acid Hydrochloride
Generic Availability (U.S.) No
Pharmacologic Category Photosensitizing Agent, Topical; Topical Skin Product
Use Treatment of minimally to moderately thick actinic keratoses (grade 1 or 2) of the face or scalp; to be used in conjunction with blue light illumination
Unlabeled/Investigational Use Photodynamic treatment of low-risk superficial basal cell skin cancer and low-risk squamous cell skin cancer *in situ* (Bowen's disease)
Dosage
Geriatric & Adult Actinic keratoses: Topical: Apply to actinic keratoses (**not** perilesional skin) followed 14-18 hours later by blue light illumination. Application/treatment may be repeated at a treatment site (once) after 8 weeks.
Special Geriatric Considerations Complaints by elderly with skin lesions increase with age. Common skin lesions are actinic keratoses, squamous cell carcinoma, and basal cell carcinoma. Although other agents for treatment are commonly used for these diseases, this agent is an alternative agent.
Dosage Forms Excipient information presented when available (limited, particularly for generics); consult specific product labeling.
Powder for solution, topical, as hydrochloride:
Levulan® Kerastick®: 20% (6s) [contains ethanol 48% (in diluent); supplied with diluent]

◆ **Amino Levulinic Acid** *see* Aminolevulinic Acid *on page 93*
◆ **5-Aminolevulinic Acid** *see* Aminolevulinic Acid *on page 93*
◆ **Aminolevulinic Acid Hydrochloride** *see* Aminolevulinic Acid *on page 93*

Aminophylline (am in OFF i lin)

Medication Safety Issues
Sound-alike/look-alike issues:
Aminophylline may be confused with amitriptyline, ampicillin
Brand Names: Canada Phyllocontin®; Phyllocontin®-350
Index Terms Theophylline Ethylenediamine
Generic Availability (U.S.) Yes
Pharmacologic Category Theophylline Derivative
Use Treatment of symptoms and reversible airway obstruction due to asthma or other chronic lung diseases (eg, emphysema, chronic bronchitis)

Note: The National Heart, Lung, and Blood Institute Guidelines (2007) do not recommend aminophylline I.V. for the treatment of asthma exacerbations.
Unlabeled/Investigational Use Reversal of adenosine-, dipyridamole-, or regadenoson-induced adverse reactions (eg, angina, hypotension) during nuclear cardiac stress testing
Contraindications Hypersensitivity to theophylline, ethylenediamine, or any component of the formulation

Canadian labeling: Additional contraindications (not in U.S. labeling): Coronary artery disease where cardiac stimulation might prove harmful; patients with peptic ulcer disease
Warnings/Precautions If a patient develops signs and symptoms of theophylline toxicity, a serum level should be measured and subsequent doses held. Theophylline clearance may be decreased in patients with acute pulmonary edema, congestive heart failure, cor pulmonale, fever, hepatic disease, acute hepatitis, cirrhosis, hypothyroidism, sepsis with multiorgan failure, and shock; clearance may also be decreased in the elderly >60 years of age and patients following cessation of smoking. Due to potential saturation of theophylline clearance at serum levels within (or in some patients less than) the therapeutic range, dosage adjustment should be made in small increments (maximum: 25% dose increase). Due to wide interpatient variability, theophylline serum level measurements must be used to optimize therapy and prevent serious toxicity. Use caution with peptic ulcer (use is contraindicated in the Canadian labeling), hyperthyroidism, seizure disorder, hypertension, or tachyarrhythmias.
Adverse Reactions (Reflective of adult population; not specific for elderly) Frequency not defined. Adverse events observed at therapeutic serum levels:
Cardiovascular: Flutter, tachycardia
Central nervous system: Behavior alterations (children), headache, insomnia, irritability, restlessness, seizures
Dermatologic: Allergic skin reactions, exfoliative dermatitis
Gastrointestinal: Diarrhea, nausea, vomiting
Neuromuscular & skeletal: Tremor
Renal: Diuresis (transient)
Drug Interactions
Metabolism/Transport Effects Substrate of CYP1A2 (major), 2E1 (minor), 3A4 (minor)
Avoid Concomitant Use
Avoid concomitant use of Aminophylline with any of the following: Iobenguane I 123
Increased Effect/Toxicity
Aminophylline may increase the levels/effects of: Formoterol; Pancuronium; Sympathomimetics

The levels/effects of Aminophylline may be increased by: Abiraterone Acetate; Allopurinol; Atomoxetine; Cannabinoids; Cimetidine; Contraceptives (Estrogens); CYP1A2 Inhibitors (Moderate); CYP1A2 Inhibitors (Strong); Deferasirox; Disulfiram; Febuxostat; FluvoxaMINE; Interferons; Isoniazid; Macrolide Antibiotics; Methotrexate; Mexiletine; Pentoxifylline; Propafenone; QuiNINE; Quinolone Antibiotics; Thiabendazole; Ticlopidine; Zafirlukast
Decreased Effect
Aminophylline may decrease the levels/effects of: Adenosine; Benzodiazepines; CarBAMazepine; Fosphenytoin; Iobenguane I 123; Lithium; Pancuronium; Phenytoin; Regadenoson; Zafirlukast

The levels/effects of Aminophylline may be decreased by: Aminoglutethimide; Barbiturates; Beta-Blockers (Beta1 Selective); Beta-Blockers (Nonselective); CarBAMazepine; CYP1A2 Inducers (Strong); Cyproterone; Fosphenytoin; Isoproterenol; Phenytoin; Protease Inhibitors; Thyroid Products
Ethanol/Nutrition/Herb Interactions Food: Food does not appreciably affect absorption. Avoid extremes of dietary protein and carbohydrate intake. Changes in diet may affect the elimination of theophylline; charcoal-broiled foods may increase elimination, reducing half-life by 50%. Ethanol may decrease theophylline clearance.

Stability

Solution: Vials should be stored at room temperature of 20°C to 25°C (68°F to 77°F). Protect from light. Do not use solutions if discolored or if crystals are present.

Tablets, immediate release: Store at room temperature of 20°C to 25°C (68°F to 77°F). Protect from light and moisture.

Tablets, sustained release (Canadian labeling, not available in the U.S.): Store at <30°C (<86°F).

Mechanism of Action

Causes bronchodilatation, diuresis, CNS and cardiac stimulation, and gastric acid secretion by blocking phosphodiesterase which increases tissue concentrations of cyclic adenine monophosphate (cAMP) which in turn promote catecholamine stimulation of lipolysis, glycogenolysis, and gluconeogenesis and induce release of epinephrine from adrenal medulla cells

Pharmacodynamics/Kinetics

Theophylline:

Absorption: Oral: Immediate release tablet: Rapid and complete

Distribution: 0.45 L/kg based on ideal body weight

Protein binding: 40%, primarily to albumin

Metabolism: Adults: Hepatic; involves CYP1A2, 2E1, and 3A4; forms active metabolites (caffeine and 3-methylxanthine)

Half-life elimination: Highly variable and dependent upon age, liver function, cardiac function, lung disease, and smoking history

Adults 16-60 years with asthma, nonsmoking, otherwise healthy: 8.7 hours (range: 6.1-12.8 hours)

Time to peak, serum:

Oral: Immediate release tablet: 1-2 hours; Sustained release tablet (Canadian labeling; not available in U.S.): 4-5 hours

I.V.: Within 30 minutes

Excretion: Adults: Urine (10% as unchanged drug)

Dosage

Geriatric Adults >60 years: Refer to adult dosing. Do not exceed a dose of aminophylline 507 mg/day (equivalent to theophylline 400 mg/day)

Adult Note: Doses should be individualized based on peak serum concentrations and should be based on ideal body weight. Theophylline dose is 80% of aminophylline dose.

Acute symptoms: Loading dose: Oral, I.V.:

Patients **not currently receiving** aminophylline or theophylline: Aminophylline 5.7 mg/kg (equivalent to theophylline 4.6 mg/kg) administered I.V. or theophylline 5 mg/kg administered orally.

Patients **currently receiving** aminophylline or theophylline: A loading dose is not recommended without first obtaining a serum theophylline concentration in patients who have received aminophylline or theophylline within the past 24 hours. The loading dose should be calculated as follows:

Dose = (desired serum theophylline concentration - measured serum theophylline concentration) (V_d)

Acute symptoms: Maintenance dose: I.V.: **Note:** To achieve a target theophylline concentration of 10 mcg/mL unless otherwise noted. Lower initial doses may be required in patients with reduced theophylline clearance. Dosage should be adjusted according to serum level measurements during the first 12- to 24-hour period.

Adults 16-60 years (otherwise healthy, nonsmokers): 0.51 mg/kg/hour (equivalent to theophylline 0.4 mg/kg/hour); maximum: 900 mg/day unless serum levels indicate need for larger dose

Adults >60 years: 0.38 mg/kg/hour (equivalent to theophylline 0.3 mg/kg/hour); maximum: 400 mg/day unless serum levels indicate need for larger dose

Dosage adjustment for cardiac decompensation, cor pulmonale, hepatic dysfunction, sepsis with multiorgan failure, shock: 0.25 mg/kg hour (equivalent to theophylline 0.2 mg/kg/hour); maximum: 400 mg/day unless serum levels indicate need for larger dose

Dosage adjustment after serum theophylline measurement:

Within normal limits: Asthma: 5-15 mcg/mL: Maintain dosage if tolerated. Recheck serum theophylline concentration at 24-hour intervals (for acute I.V. dosing) or at 6- to 12-month intervals (for oral dosing). Finer adjustments in dosage may be needed for some patients. If levels ≥15 mcg/mL, consider 10% dose reduction to improve safety margin.

AMINOPHYLLINE

Too high:

20-24.9 mcg/mL: Decrease dose by ~25%. Recheck serum theophylline concentrations (see "**Note**").

25-30 mcg/mL: Skip next dose (oral) or stop infusion for 24 hours and decrease subsequent doses by ~25%. Recheck serum theophylline concentrations (see "**Note**").

>30 mcg/mL: Stop dosing and treat overdose; if resumed, decrease subsequent doses by 50%. Recheck serum theophylline concentrations (see "**Note**").

Too low: <9.9 mcg/mL: If tolerated, but symptoms remain, increase dose by ~25%. Recheck serum theophylline concentrations (see "**Note**").

Note: Recheck serum theophylline levels after 3 days when using oral dosing, or after 24 hours when dosing intravenously. Patients maintained with oral therapy may be reassessed at 6- to 12-month intervals.

Chronic conditions: Oral:

Immediate release tablets: **Note:** Increase dose only if tolerated. Consider lowering dose or using a slower titration if caffeine-like adverse events occur. Smaller doses given more frequently may be used in patients with a more rapid metabolism to prevent breakthrough symptoms which could occur due to low trough concentration prior to the next dose.

Adults 16-60 years **without** risk factors for impaired theophylline clearance:

Aminophylline 380 mg/day (equivalent to theophylline 300 mg/day) in divided doses every 6-8 hours for 3 days;

Then increase to 507 mg/day (equivalent to theophylline 400 mg/day) in divided doses every 6-8 hours for 3 days

Maintenance dose: 760 mg/day (equivalent to theophylline 600 mg/day) in divided doses every 6-8 hours

Dose adjustment in patients **with** risk factors for impaired theophylline clearance and patients in whom monitoring serum theophylline levels is not feasible: Do not exceed a dose of aminophylline 507 mg/day (equivalent to theophylline 400 mg/day)

Sustained release tablets: Canadian labeling: Initial: 1 tablet (225-350 mg) every 12 hours (equivalent to theophylline 182.25-283.5 mg every 12 hours); may increase dose by $1/2$ tablet per dose at 3- to 4-day intervals; maximum dose: 1125 mg/day (equivalent to theophylline 900 mg/day); do not exceed maximum dose without monitoring theophylline concentrations.

Reversal of adenosine-, dipyridamole-, or regadenoson-induced adverse reactions (eg, angina, hypotension) during nuclear cardiac stress testing (unlabeled use): I.V.: 50-250 mg administered over 30-60 seconds, repeat as necessary. **Note:** Since adenosine-induced side effects are short lived after discontinuation of the infusion, aminophylline administration is only very rarely required.

Administration

I.M.: Not recommended

I.V.: Loading doses should be administered I.V. over 30 minutes. Infusion rate should not exceed 21 mg/hour (equivalent to theophylline 17 mg/hour) in patients with cor pulmonale, cardiac decompensation, liver dysfunction, patients >60 years of age, or patients taking medications which reduce theophylline clearance.

For reversal of adenosine-, dipyridamole-, or regadenoson-induced adverse events during nuclear cardiac stress testing, administer I.V. undiluted over 30-60 seconds, repeat as necessary. Since adenosine-induced side effects are short lived after discontinuation of the infusion, aminophylline administration is only very rarely required.

Tablet, immediate release: If dose is missed, administer the next dose at the scheduled time (do not make up missed dose).

Tablet, sustained release (Canadian labeling, not available in the U.S.): Administer every 12 hours with a full glass of water. Patient should be in the standing or sitting position. Tablets may be halved, however do not crush, chew or dissolve. Evening dose should be administered with or shortly following the evening meal. May administer a missed dose if within 4 hours of scheduled dosing time.

Monitoring Parameters Monitor heart rate; CNS effects (insomnia, irritability); respiratory rate (COPD patients often have resting controlled respiratory rates in low 20s); arterial or capillary blood gases (if applicable)

Theophylline levels: Serum theophylline levels should be monitored prior to making dose increases; in the presence of signs or symptoms of toxicity; or when a new illness, worsening of a present illness, or medication changes occur that may change theophylline clearance

I.V. loading dose: Measure serum concentrations 30 minutes after the end of an I.V. loading dose

I.V. infusion: Measure serum concentrations one half-life after starting a continuous infusion, then every 12-24 hours

Reference Range
Therapeutic levels: Asthma: 5-15 mcg/mL (peak level)
Toxic concentration: >20 mcg/mL

Test Interactions Plasma glucose, uric acid, free fatty acids, total cholesterol, HDL, HDL/LDL ratio, and urinary free cortisol excretion may be increased by theophylline. Theophylline may decrease triiodothyronine.

Pharmacotherapy Pearls 100 mg aminophylline = 79 mg theophylline
Older adults, the acutely ill, and patients with severe respiratory problems, pulmonary edema, or liver dysfunction are at greater risk of toxicity because of reduced drug clearance.

Special Geriatric Considerations Although there is a great intersubject variability for half-lives of methylxanthines (2-10 hours), elderly, as a group, have slower hepatic clearance. Therefore, use lower initial doses and monitor closely for response and adverse reactions. Additionally, elderly patients are at greater risk for toxicity due to concomitant disease (eg, congestive heart failure, arrhythmias), and drug use (eg, cimetidine, ciprofloxacin, etc).

Dosage Forms Excipient information presented when available (limited, particularly for generics); consult specific product labeling.
Injection, solution, as dihydrate: 25 mg/mL (10 mL, 20 mL)
Injection, solution, as dihydrate [preservative free]: 25 mg/mL (10 mL, 20 mL)
Tablet, oral, as dihydrate: 100 mg, 200 mg

Dosage Forms: Canada Excipient information presented when available (limited, particularly for generics); consult specific product labeling.
Tablet, oral, sustained release as dihydrate
Phyllocontin® 225 mg
Phyllocontin®-350: 350 mg

◆ **4-aminopyridine** *see* Dalfampridine *on page 444*
◆ **Aminosalicylate Sodium** *see* Aminosalicylic Acid *on page 97*

Aminosalicylic Acid (a mee noe sal i SIL ik AS id)

Brand Names: U.S. Paser®

Index Terms 4-Aminosalicylic Acid; Aminosalicylate Sodium; Para-Aminosalicylate Sodium; PAS; Sodium PAS

Generic Availability (U.S.) No

Pharmacologic Category Salicylate

Use Adjunctive treatment of tuberculosis used in combination with other antitubercular agents

Unlabeled/Investigational Use Treatment of Crohn's disease

Dosage
Geriatric & Adult
Tuberculosis: Oral: 150 mg/kg/day in 2-3 equally divided doses
Crohn's disease (unlabeled use): 1.5 g/day
Renal Impairment
Cl_{cr} 10-50 mL/minute: Administer 50% to 75% of dose.
Cl_{cr} <10 mL/minute: Administer 50% of dose.
Administer after hemodialysis: Administer 50% of dose.
Continuous arteriovenous hemofiltration: Dose for Cl_{cr} <10 mL/minute
Hepatic Impairment Use with caution

Special Geriatric Considerations The elderly may require a lower recommended dose due to age-related changes in renal function.

Dosage Forms Excipient information presented when available (limited, particularly for generics); consult specific product labeling.
Granules, delayed release, oral:
Paser®: 4 g/packet (30s) [sugar free]

◆ **4-Aminosalicylic Acid** *see* Aminosalicylic Acid *on page 97*
◆ **5-Aminosalicylic Acid** *see* Mesalamine *on page 1150*
◆ **Aminoxin® [OTC]** *see* Pyridoxine *on page 1552*

Amiodarone (a MEE oh da rone)

Related Information
Beers Criteria − Potentially Inappropriate Medications for Geriatrics *on page 2089*

◄ **Medication Safety Issues**
    Sound-alike/look-alike issues:
      Amiodarone may be confused with aMILoride, inamrinone
      Cordarone® may be confused with Cardura®, Cordran®
    High alert medication:
      The Institute for Safe Medication Practices (ISMP) includes this medication among its list of
        drugs which have a heightened risk of causing significant patient harm when used in error.
    BEERS Criteria medication:
      This drug may be inappropriate for use in geriatric patients (high severity risk).

Brand Names: U.S. Cordarone®; Nexterone®; Pacerone®

Brand Names: Canada Apo-Amiodarone®; Cordarone®; Dom-Amiodarone; Mylan-Amiodarone; Novo-Amiodarone; PHL-Amiodarone; PMS-Amiodarone; PRO-Amiodarone; ratio-Amiodarone; ratio-Amiodarone I.V.; Riva-Amiodarone; Sandoz-Amiodarone; Teva-Amiodarone

Index Terms Amiodarone Hydrochloride

Generic Availability (U.S.) Yes

Pharmacologic Category Antiarrhythmic Agent, Class III

Use Management of life-threatening recurrent ventricular fibrillation (VF) or hemodynamically-unstable ventricular tachycardia (VT) refractory to other antiarrhythmic agents or in patients intolerant of other agents used for these conditions

Unlabeled/Investigational Use
    Cardiac arrest with persistent ventricular tachycardia (VT) or ventricular fibrillation (VF) if defibrillation, CPR, and vasopressor administration have failed (ACLS/PALS guidelines)
    Control of hemodynamically-stable monomorphic VT, polymorphic VT with a normal baseline QT interval, or wide-complex tachycardia of uncertain origin (ACLS/PALS guidelines)
    Control of rapid ventricular rate due to accessory pathway conduction in pre-excited atrial arrhythmias (ACLS guidelines)
    Control of stable narrow-complex tachycardia (ACLS guidelines)
    Heart rate control in patients with atrial fibrillation and heart failure [no accessory pathway] (ACC/AHA/ESC Practice Guidelines)
    Paroxysmal supraventricular tachycardia (SVT) (not initial drug of choice)
    Prevention of postoperative atrial fibrillation associated with cardiothoracic surgery
    Pharmacologic adjunct to ICD therapy to suppress symptomatic ventricular tachyarrhythmias in otherwise optimally-treated patients with heart failure (ACC/AHA/ESC Practice Guidelines)
    Pharmacologic conversion of atrial fibrillation to normal sinus rhythm; maintenance of normal sinus rhythm

Medication Guide Available Yes

Contraindications Hypersensitivity to amiodarone, iodine, or any component of the formulation; severe sinus-node dysfunction; second- and third-degree heart block (except in patients with a functioning artificial pacemaker); bradycardia causing syncope (except in patients with a functioning artificial pacemaker); cardiogenic shock

Warnings/Precautions [U.S. Boxed Warning]: Only indicated for patients with life-threatening arrhythmias because of risk of toxicity. Alternative therapies should be tried first before using amiodarone. Patients should be hospitalized when amiodarone is initiated. Currently, the 2005 ACLS guidelines recommend I.V. amiodarone as the preferred antiarrhythmic for the treatment of pulseless VT/VF, both life-threatening arrhythmias. In patients with non-life-threatening arrhythmias (eg, atrial fibrillation), amiodarone should be used only if the use of other antiarrhythmics has proven ineffective or are contraindicated.

[U.S. Boxed Warning]: Lung damage (abnormal diffusion capacity) may occur without symptoms. Monitor for pulmonary toxicity. Evaluate new respiratory symptoms; pre-existing pulmonary disease does not increase risk of developing pulmonary toxicity, but if pulmonary toxicity develops then the prognosis is worse. The lowest effective dose should be used as appropriate for the acuity/severity of the arrhythmia being treated. **[U.S. Boxed Warning]: Liver toxicity is common, but usually mild with evidence of increased liver enzymes. Severe liver toxicity can occur and has been fatal in a few cases.**

[U.S. Boxed Warning]: Amiodarone can exacerbate arrhythmias, by making them more difficult to tolerate or reverse; other types of arrhythmias have occurred, including significant heart block, sinus bradycardia new ventricular fibrillation, incessant ventricular tachycardia, increased resistance to cardioversion, and polymorphic ventricular tachycardia associated with QT_c prolongation (torsade de pointes [TdP]). Risk may be increased with concomitant use of other antiarrhythmic agents or drugs that prolong the QT_c interval. Proarrhythmic effects may be prolonged.

Monitor pacing or defibrillation thresholds in patients with implantable cardiac devices (eg, pacemakers, defibrillators). Use very cautiously and with close monitoring in patients with thyroid or liver disease. May cause hyper- or hypothyroidism. Hyperthyroidism may result in thyrotoxicosis and may aggravate or cause breakthrough arrhythmias. If any new signs of arrhythmia appear, hyperthyroidism should be considered. Thyroid function should be monitored prior to treatment and periodically thereafter.

May cause optic neuropathy and/or optic neuritis, usually resulting in visual impairment. Corneal microdeposits occur in a majority of patients, and may cause visual disturbances in some patients (blurred vision, halos); these are not generally considered a reason to discontinue treatment. Corneal refractive laser surgery is generally contraindicated in amiodarone users. Avoid excessive exposure to sunlight; may cause photosensitivity.

Amiodarone is a potent inhibitor of CYP enzymes and transport proteins (including p-glycoprotein), which may lead to increased serum concentrations/toxicity of a number of medications. Particular caution must be used when a drug with QT_c-prolonging potential relies on metabolism via these enzymes, since the effect of elevated concentrations may be additive with the effect of amiodarone. Carefully assess risk:benefit of coadministration of other drugs which may prolong QT_c interval. Patients may still be at risk for amiodarone–related drug interactions after the drug has been discontinued. The pharmacokinetics are complex (due to prolonged duration of action and half-life) and difficult to predict. Correct electrolyte disturbances, especially hypokalemia or hypomagnesemia, prior to use and throughout therapy.

May cause hypotension and bradycardia (infusion-rate related). Caution in surgical patients; may enhance hemodynamic effect of anesthetics; associated with increased risk of adult respiratory distress syndrome (ARDS) postoperatively. May be inappropriate in the elderly due to a risk of QT_c-interval prolongation, torsade de pointes, and lack of efficacy in the elderly (Beers Criteria). Injection contains benzyl alcohol.

Adverse Reactions (Reflective of adult population; not specific for elderly) In a recent meta-analysis, patients taking lower doses of amiodarone (152-330 mg daily for at least 12 months) were more likely to develop thyroid, neurologic, skin, ocular, and bradycardic abnormalities than those taking placebo (Vorperian, 1997). Pulmonary toxicity was similar in both the low dose amiodarone group and in the placebo group but there was a trend towards increased toxicity in the amiodarone group. Gastrointestinal and hepatic events were seen to a similar extent in both the low dose amiodarone group and placebo group. As the frequency of adverse events varies considerably across studies as a function of route and dose, a consolidation of adverse event rates is provided by Goldschlager, 2000.

>10%:
  Cardiovascular: Hypotension (I.V. 16%, refractory in rare cases)
  Central nervous system (3% to 40%): Abnormal gait/ataxia, dizziness, fatigue, headache, malaise, impaired memory, involuntary movement, insomnia, poor coordination, peripheral neuropathy, sleep disturbances, tremor
  Dermatologic: Photosensitivity (10% to 75%)
  Endocrine & Metabolic: Hypothyroidism (1% to 22%)
  Gastrointestinal: Nausea, vomiting, anorexia, and constipation (10% to 33%)
  Hepatic: AST or ALT level >2x normal (15% to 50%)
  Ocular: Corneal microdeposits (>90%; causes visual disturbance in <10%)
1% to 10%:
  Cardiovascular: CHF (3%), bradycardia (3% to 5%), AV block (5%), conduction abnormalities, SA node dysfunction (1% to 3%), cardiac arrhythmia, flushing, edema. Additional effects associated with I.V. administration include asystole, atrial fibrillation, cardiac arrest, electromechanical dissociation, pulseless electrical activity (PEA), ventricular tachycardia, and cardiogenic shock.
  Dermatologic: Slate blue skin discoloration (<10%)
  Endocrine & metabolic: Hyperthyroidism (3% to 10%; more common in iodine-deficient regions of the world), libido decreased
  Gastrointestinal: Abdominal pain, abnormal salivation, abnormal taste (oral), diarrhea, nausea (I.V.)
  Hematologic: Coagulation abnormalities
  Hepatic: Hepatitis and cirrhosis (<3%)
  Local: Phlebitis (I.V., with concentrations >3 mg/mL)
  Ocular: Visual disturbances (2% to 9%), halo vision (<5% occurring especially at night), optic neuritis (1%)
  Respiratory: Pulmonary toxicity has been estimated to occur at a frequency between 2% and 7% of patients (some reports indicate a frequency as high as 17%). Toxicity may present as hypersensitivity pneumonitis; pulmonary fibrosis (cough, fever, malaise); pulmonary inflammation; interstitial pneumonitis; or alveolar pneumonitis. ARDS has been reported in up to 2% of patients receiving amiodarone, and postoperatively in patients receiving oral amiodarone.
  Miscellaneous: Abnormal smell (oral)

◀ **Drug Interactions**

Metabolism/Transport Effects Substrate of CYP1A2 (minor), CYP2C8 (major at low concentration), CYP2C19 (minor), CYP2D6 (minor), CYP3A4 (major), P-glycoprotein; **Inhibits** CYP1A2 (weak), CYP2A6 (moderate), CYP2B6 (weak), CYP2C9 (moderate), CYP2C19 (weak), CYP2D6 (moderate), CYP3A4 (moderate), P-glycoprotein

Avoid Concomitant Use

Avoid concomitant use of Amiodarone with any of the following: Agalsidase Alfa; Agalsidase Beta; Artemether; Conivaptan; Dronedarone; Grapefruit Juice; Lumefantrine; Nilotinib; Pimozide; Protease Inhibitors; QUEtiapine; QuiNINE; Silodosin; Tetrabenazine; Thioridazine; Tolvaptan; Topotecan; Toremifene; Vandetanib; Vemurafenib; Ziprasidone

Increased Effect/Toxicity

Amiodarone may increase the levels/effects of: Antiarrhythmic Agents (Class Ia); Beta-Blockers; Budesonide (Systemic, Oral Inhalation); Cardiac Glycosides; Colchicine; Cyclo-SPORINE; CycloSPORINE (Systemic); CYP2A6 Substrates; CYP2C9 Substrates (High risk); CYP2D6 Substrates; CYP3A4 Substrates; Dabigatran Etexilate; Dronedarone; Eplerenone; Everolimus; FentaNYL; Fesoterodine; Flecainide; Fosphenytoin; HMG-CoA Reductase Inhibitors; Lidocaine; Lidocaine (Systemic); Lidocaine (Topical); Loratadine; Lurasidone; P-Glycoprotein Substrates; Phenytoin; Pimecrolimus; Pimozide; Porfimer; QTc-Prolonging Agents; QuiNINE; Rivaroxaban; Salmeterol; Saxagliptin; Silodosin; Tamoxifen; Tetrabenazine; Thioridazine; Tolvaptan; Topotecan; Toremifene; Vandetanib; Vemurafenib; Vilazodone; Vitamin K Antagonists; Ziprasidone

The levels/effects of Amiodarone may be increased by: Alfuzosin; Artemether; Azithromycin; Azithromycin (Systemic); Boceprevir; Calcium Channel Blockers (Nondihydropyridine); Chloroquine; Cimetidine; Ciprofloxacin; Ciprofloxacin (Systemic); Conivaptan; CYP2C8 Inhibitors (Moderate); CYP2C8 Inhibitors (Strong); CYP3A4 Inhibitors (Moderate); CYP3A4 Inhibitors (Strong); Deferasirox; Eribulin; Fingolimod; Gadobutrol; Grapefruit Juice; Lumefantrine; Nilotinib; P-Glycoprotein Inhibitors; Protease Inhibitors; QUEtiapine; QuiNINE; Telaprevir

Decreased Effect

Amiodarone may decrease the levels/effects of: Agalsidase Alfa; Agalsidase Beta; Clopidogrel; Codeine; Sodium Iodide I131; TraMADol

The levels/effects of Amiodarone may be decreased by: Bile Acid Sequestrants; CYP2C8 Inducers (Highly Effective); CYP3A4 Inducers (Strong); Cyproterone; Deferasirox; Etravirine; Fosphenytoin; Grapefruit Juice; Herbs (CYP3A4 Inducers); Orlistat; Peginterferon Alfa-2b; P-Glycoprotein Inducers; Phenytoin; Rifamycin Derivatives; Tocilizumab

Ethanol/Nutrition/Herb Interactions

Food: Increases the rate and extent of absorption of amiodarone. Grapefruit juice increases bioavailability of oral amiodarone by 50% and decreases the conversion of amiodarone to N-DEA (active metabolite); altered effects are possible; use should be avoided during therapy.

Herb/Nutraceutical: St John's wort may decrease amiodarone levels or enhance photosensitization. Avoid ephedra (may worsen arrhythmia). Avoid dong quai.

Stability Store undiluted vials and premixed solutions at 20°C to 25°C (68°F to 77°F). Protect from light.

Vials for injection: When admixed in D_5W to a final concentration of 1-6 mg/mL, the solution is stable at room temperature for 24 hours in polyolefin or glass, or for 2 hours in PVC. Infusions >2 hours must be administered in a non-PVC container (eg, glass or polyolefin). Do not use evacuated glass containers; buffer may cause precipitation.

Mechanism of Action Class III antiarrhythmic agent which inhibits adrenergic stimulation (alpha- and beta-blocking properties), affects sodium, potassium, and calcium channels, prolongs the action potential and refractory period in myocardial tissue; decreases AV conduction and sinus node function

Pharmacodynamics/Kinetics

Absorption: Slow and variable

Onset of action: Oral: 2 days to 3 weeks; I.V.: May be more rapid

Peak effect: 1 week to 5 months

Duration after discontinuing therapy: 7-50 days

Distribution: V_d: 66 L/kg (range: 18-148 L/kg)

Protein binding: 96%

Metabolism: Hepatic via CYP2C8 and 3A4 to active N-desethylamiodarone metabolite; possible enterohepatic recirculation

Bioavailability: Oral: 35% to 65%

Half-life elimination: Terminal: 40-55 days (range: 26-107 days)

Time to peak, serum: 3-7 hours

Excretion: Feces; urine (<1% as unchanged drug)

Dosage

Geriatric Refer to adult dosing. No specific guidelines available. Dose selection should be cautious, at low end of dosage range, and titration should be slower to evaluate response. Although not supported by clinical evidence, a maintenance dose of 100 mg/day is commonly used especially for the elderly or patients with low body mass (Fuster, 2006; Zimetbaum, 2007).

Adult Note: Lower loading and maintenance doses are preferable in women and all patients with low body weight.

Atrial fibrillation pharmacologic cardioversion (ACC/AHA/ESC Practice Guidelines) (unlabeled use):

Oral: *Inpatient:* 1.2-1.8 g/day in divided doses until 10 g total, then 200-400 mg/day maintenance. *Outpatient:* 600-800 mg/day in divided doses until 10 g total, then 200-400 mg/day maintenance; although not supported by clinical evidence, a maintenance dose of 100 mg/day is commonly used especially for the elderly or patients with low body mass (Fuster, 2006; Zimetbaum, 2007). **Note:** Other regimens have been described and may be used clinically:

400 mg 3 times/day for 5-7 days, then 400 mg/day for 1 month, then 200 mg/day

or

10 mg/kg/day for 14 days, followed by 300 mg/day for 4 weeks, followed by maintenance dosage of 200 mg/day (Roy, 2000)

I.V.: 5-7 mg/kg over 30-60 minutes, then 1.2-1.8 g/day continuous infusion or in divided oral doses until 10 g total. Maintenance: See oral dosing.

Atrial fibrillation prophylaxis following open heart surgery (unlabeled use): Note: A variety of regimens have been used in clinical trials, including oral and intravenous regimens:

Oral: Starting in postop recovery, 400 mg twice daily for up to 7 days. Alternative regimen of amiodarone: 600 mg/day for 7 days prior to surgery, followed by 200 mg/day until hospital discharge, has also been shown to decrease the risk of postoperative atrial fibrillation.

I.V.: Starting at postop recovery, 1000 mg infused over 24 hours for 2 days has been shown to reduce the risk of postoperative atrial fibrillation.

Recurrent atrial fibrillation (unlabeled use): No standard regimen defined; examples of regimens include: Oral: Initial: 10 mg/kg/day for 14 days; followed by 300 mg/day for 4 weeks, followed by maintenance dosage of 200 mg/day (Roy, 2000). Other regimen have been described and are used clinically (ie, 400 mg 3 times/day for 5-7 days, then 400 mg/day for 1 month, then 200 mg/day).

Ventricular arrhythmias: Oral: 800-1600 mg/day in 1-2 doses for 1-3 weeks, then when adequate arrhythmia control is achieved, decrease to 600-800 mg/day in 1-2 doses for 1 month; maintenance: 400 mg/day; lower doses are recommended for supraventricular arrhythmias.

Pulseless VT or VF (ACLS, 2010): I.V. push, I.O.: Initial: 300 mg; if pulseless VT or VF continues after subsequent defibrillation attempt or recurs, administer supplemental dose of 150 mg. **Note:** In this setting, administering **undiluted** is preferred (Dager, 2006; Skrifvars, 2004). *The Handbook of Emergency Cardiovascular Care* (Hazinski, 2010) and the 2010 ACLS guidelines, do not make any specific recommendations regarding dilution of amiodarone in this setting. Experience limited with I.O. administration of amiodarone (ACLS, 2010).

Upon return of spontaneous circulation, follow with an infusion of 1 mg/minute for 6 hours, then 0.5 mg/minute for 18 hours (mean daily doses >2.1 g/day have been associated with hypotension).

Stable VT or SVT (unlabeled use): First 24 hours: 1050 mg according to following regimen

Step 1: 150 mg (100 mL) over first 10 minutes (mix 3 mL in 100 mL D_5W)

Step 2: 360 mg (200 mL) over next 6 hours (mix 18 mL in 500 mL D_5W): 1 mg/minute

Step 3: 540 mg (300 mL) over next 18 hours: 0.5 mg/minute

Note: After the first 24 hours: 0.5 mg/minute utilizing concentration of 1-6 mg/mL

Breakthrough stable VT or SVT: 150 mg supplemental doses in 100 mL D_5W or NS over 10 minutes (mean daily doses >2.1 g/day have been associated with hypotension)

I.V. to oral therapy conversion: Use the following as a guide:

<1 week I.V. infusion: 800-1600 mg/day

1- to 3-week I.V. infusion: 600-800 mg/day

>3 week I.V. infusion: 400 mg/day

Note: Conversion from I.V. to oral therapy has not been formally evaluated. Some experts recommend a 1-2 day overlap when converting from I.V. to oral therapy especially when treating ventricular arrhythmias.

◄ **Recommendations for conversion to intravenous amiodarone after oral administration:** During long-term amiodarone therapy (ie, ≥4 months), the mean plasma-elimination half-life of the active metabolite of amiodarone is 61 days. Replacement therapy may not be necessary in such patients if oral therapy is discontinued for a period <2 weeks, since any changes in serum amiodarone concentrations during this period may **not** be clinically significant.

Renal Impairment No dosage adjustment necessary.

Hemodialysis: Not dialyzable (0% to 5%); supplemental dose is not necessary

Peritoneal dialysis: Not dialyzable (0% to 5%); supplemental dose is not necessary

Hepatic Impairment Dosage adjustment is probably necessary in substantial hepatic impairment. No specific guidelines available. If hepatic enzymes exceed 3 times normal or double in a patient with an elevated baseline, consider decreasing the dose or discontinuing amiodarone.

Administration

Oral: Administer consistently with regard to meals. Take in divided doses with meals if GI upset occurs or if taking large daily dose. If GI intolerance occurs with single-dose therapy, use twice daily dosing.

I.V.: For infusions >1 hour, use concentrations ≤2 mg/mL unless a central venous catheter is used; commercially-prepared premixed solutions in concentrations of 1.5 mg/mL and 1.8 mg/mL are available. Use only volumetric infusion pump; use of drop counting may lead to underdosage. Administer through an I.V. line located as centrally as possible. During pulseless VT/VF, administering **undiluted** is preferred (Dager, 2006; Skrifvars, 2004). *The Handbook of Emergency Cardiovascular Care* (Hazinski, 2010) and the 2010 ACLS guidelines do not make any specific recommendations regarding dilution of amiodarone in this setting.

Adjust administration rate to urgency (give more slowly when perfusing arrhythmia present). Slow the infusion rate if hypotension or bradycardia develops. Infusions >2 hours must be administered in a non-PVC container (eg, glass or polyolefin). PVC tubing is recommended for administration regardless of infusion duration. **Note:** I.V. administration at lower flow rates (potentially associated with use in pediatrics) and higher concentrations than recommended may result in leaching of plasticizers (DEHP) from intravenous tubing. DEHP may adversely affect male reproductive tract development. Alternative means of dosing and administration (1 mg/kg aliquots) may need to be considered.

Monitoring Parameters Blood pressure, heart rate (ECG) and rhythm throughout therapy; assess patient for signs of lethargy, edema of the hands or feet, weight loss, and pulmonary toxicity (baseline pulmonary function tests and chest X-ray; continue monitoring chest X-ray annually during therapy); liver function tests (semiannually); monitor serum electrolytes, especially potassium and magnesium. Assess thyroid function tests before initiation of treatment and then periodically thereafter (some experts suggest every 3-6 months). If signs or symptoms of thyroid disease or arrhythmia breakthrough/exacerbation occur then immediate re-evaluation is necessary. Amiodarone partially inhibits the peripheral conversion of thyroxine (T_4) to triiodothyronine (T_3); serum T_4 and reverse triiodothyronine (rT_3) concentrations may be increased and serum T_3 may be decreased; most patients remain clinically euthyroid, however, clinical hypothyroidism or hyperthyroidism may occur.

Perform regular ophthalmic exams.

Patients with implantable cardiac devices: Monitor pacing or defibrillation thresholds with initiation of amiodarone and during treatment.

Reference Range Therapeutic: 0.5-2.5 mg/L (SI: 1-4 μmol/L) (parent); desethyl metabolite is active and is present in equal concentration to parent drug

Pharmacotherapy Pearls Hospitalization required for initiation of therapy; CNS symptoms normally develop within 7 days, muscle weakness may present a great hazard for ambulation.

Special Geriatric Considerations Information describing the clinical use and pharmacokinetics in the elderly is lacking; however, the elderly may be predisposed to toxicity. Half-life may be prolonged due to decreased clearance; monitor closely. It is recommended to start dosing at the lower end of the dosing range. Elderly patients may be predisposed to toxicity due to reduced renal, hepatic, or cardiac function.

This medication is considered to be potentially inappropriate in this patient population (Beers Criteria severity: High).

Dosage Forms Excipient information presented when available (limited, particularly for generics); consult specific product labeling.

Infusion, premixed iso-osmotic dextrose solution, as hydrochloride:

Nexterone®: 150 mg (100 mL); 360 mg (200 mL) [contains cyclodextrin]

Injection, solution, as hydrochloride: 50 mg/mL (3 mL, 9 mL, 18 mL)

Tablet, oral, as hydrochloride: 200 mg, 400 mg
  Cordarone®: 200 mg [scored]
  Pacerone®: 100 mg
  Pacerone®: 200 mg, 400 mg [scored]

Selected References
"2005 American Heart Association Guidelines for Cardiopulmonary Resuscitation and Emergency Cardiovascular Care," *Circulation*, 2005, 112(24 Suppl):1-211.

Martino E, Bartalena L, Bogazzi, et al, "The Effects of Amiodarone on the Thyroid," *Endocr Rev*, 2001, 22(2):240-54.

◆ **Amiodarone Hydrochloride** *see* Amiodarone *on page 97*
◆ **Amitiza®** *see* Lubiprostone *on page 1102*
◆ **Amitone® [OTC]** *see* Calcium Salts (Oral) *on page 256*

Amitriptyline (a mee TRIP ti leen)

Related Information
Antidepressant Agents *on page 1991*
Beers Criteria – Potentially Inappropriate Medications for Geriatrics *on page 2089*

Medication Safety Issues
Sound-alike/look-alike issues:
Amitriptyline may be confused with aminophylline, imipramine, nortriptyline
Elavil® may be confused with Aldoril®, Eldepryl®, enalapril, Equanil®, Plavix®

BEERS Criteria medication:
This drug may be inappropriate for use in geriatric patients (high severity risk).

Brand Names: Canada Apo-Amitriptyline®; Bio-Amitriptyline; Dom-Amitriptyline; Elavil; Levate®; Novo-Triptyn; PMS-Amitriptyline

Index Terms Amitriptyline Hydrochloride; Elavil

Generic Availability (U.S.) Yes

Pharmacologic Category Antidepressant, Tricyclic (Tertiary Amine)

Use Relief of symptoms of depression

Unlabeled/Investigational Use Analgesic for certain chronic and neuropathic pain; prophylaxis against migraine headaches

Medication Guide Available Yes

Contraindications Hypersensitivity to amitriptyline or any component of the formulation (cross-sensitivity with other tricyclics may occur); use of MAO inhibitors within past 14 days; acute recovery phase following myocardial infarction; concurrent use of cisapride

Warnings/Precautions [U.S. Boxed Warning]: Antidepressants increase the risk of suicidal thinking and behavior in children, adolescents, and young adults (18-24 years of age) with major depressive disorder (MDD) and other psychiatric disorders; consider risk prior to prescribing. Short-term studies did not show an increased risk in patients >24 years of age and showed a decreased risk in patients ≥65 years. Closely monitor for clinical worsening, suicidality, or unusual changes in behavior; the patient's family or caregiver should be instructed to closely observe the patient and communicate condition with healthcare provider. Such observation would generally include at least weekly face-to-face contact with patients or their family members or caregivers during the first 4 weeks of treatment, then every other week visits for the next 4 weeks, then at 12 weeks, and as clinically indicated beyond 12 weeks. Additional contact by telephone may be appropriate between face-to-face visits. Adults treated with antidepressants should be observed similarly for clinical worsening and suicidality, especially during the initial few months of a course of drug therapy, or at times of dose changes, either increases or decreases. A medication guide should be dispensed with each prescription. **Amitriptyline is not FDA-approved for use in children <12 years of age.**

The possibility of a suicide attempt is inherent in major depression and may persist until remission occurs. Monitor for worsening of depression or suicidality, especially during initiation of therapy (generally first 1-2 months) or with dose increases or decreases. Worsening depression and severe abrupt suicidality that are not part of the presenting symptoms may require discontinuation or modification of drug therapy. The patient's family or caregiver should be alerted to monitor patients for the emergence of suicidality and associated behaviors (such as agitation, irritability, hostility, impulsivity, and hypomania) and notify healthcare provider.

May worsen psychosis in some patients or precipitate a shift to mania or hypomania in patients with bipolar disorder. Patients presenting with depressive symptoms should be screened for bipolar disorder. Monotherapy in patients with bipolar disorder should be avoided. **Amitriptyline is not FDA approved for bipolar depression.**

The degree of sedation, anticholinergic effects, orthostasis, and conduction abnormalities are high relative to other antidepressants. Amitriptyline often causes drowsiness/sedation, resulting in impaired performance of tasks requiring alertness (eg, operating machinery or driving). Sedative effects may be additive with other CNS depressants and/or ethanol. Use with caution in patients with a history of cardiovascular disease (including previous MI, stroke, tachycardia, or conduction abnormalities). Use with caution in patients with urinary retention, benign prostatic hyperplasia, narrow-angle glaucoma, xerostomia, visual problems, constipation, or a history of bowel obstruction.

TCAs may rarely cause bone marrow suppression; monitor for any signs of infection and obtain CBC if symptoms (eg, fever, sore throat) evident. May alter glucose control - use with caution in patients with diabetes. Consider discontinuing, when possible, prior to elective surgery. Therapy should not be abruptly discontinued in patients receiving high doses for prolonged periods. May lower seizure threshold - use caution in patients with a previous seizure disorder or condition predisposing to seizures such as brain damage, alcoholism, or concurrent therapy with other drugs which lower the seizure threshold. Hyperpyrexia has been observed with TCAs in combination with anticholinergics and/or neuroleptics, particularly during hot weather. May increase the risks associated with electroconvulsive therapy. Use with caution in hyperthyroid patients or those receiving thyroid supplementation. Use with caution in patients with hepatic or renal dysfunction. Use with caution in the elderly; may be inappropriate in this age group due to its potent anticholinergic and sedative properties (Beers Criteria).

Adverse Reactions (Reflective of adult population; not specific for elderly) Anticholinergic effects may be pronounced; moderate to marked sedation can occur (tolerance to these effects usually occurs).

Frequency not defined.

Cardiovascular: Orthostatic hypotension, tachycardia, ECG changes (nonspecific), AV conduction changes, cardiomyopathy (rare), MI, stroke, heart block, arrhythmia, syncope, hypertension, palpitation

Central nervous system: Restlessness, dizziness, insomnia, sedation, fatigue, anxiety, cognitive function (impaired), seizure, extrapyramidal symptoms, coma, hallucinations, confusion, disorientation, coordination impaired, ataxia, headache, nightmares, hyperpyrexia

Dermatologic: Allergic rash, urticaria, photosensitivity, alopecia

Endocrine & metabolic: Syndrome of inappropriate ADH secretion

Gastrointestinal: Weight gain, xerostomia, constipation, paralytic ileus, nausea, vomiting, anorexia, stomatitis, peculiar taste, diarrhea, black tongue

Genitourinary: Urinary retention

Hematologic: Bone marrow depression, purpura, eosinophilia

Neuromuscular & skeletal: Numbness, paresthesia, peripheral neuropathy, tremor, weakness

Ocular: Blurred vision, mydriasis, ocular pressure increased

Otic: Tinnitus

Miscellaneous: Diaphoresis, withdrawal reactions (nausea, headache, malaise)

Drug Interactions

Metabolism/Transport Effects Substrate of CYP1A2 (minor), 2B6 (minor), 2C9 (minor), 2C19 (minor), 2D6 (major), 3A4 (minor); **Inhibits** CYP1A2 (weak), 2C9 (weak), 2C19 (weak), 2D6 (weak), 2E1 (weak)

Avoid Concomitant Use

Avoid concomitant use of Amitriptyline with any of the following: Artemether; Cisapride; Dronedarone; Iobenguane I 123; Lumefantrine; MAO Inhibitors; Methylene Blue; Nilotinib; Pimozide; QUEtiapine; QuiNINE; Sibutramine; Tetrabenazine; Thioridazine; Toremifene; Vandetanib; Vemurafenib; Ziprasidone

Increased Effect/Toxicity

Amitriptyline may increase the levels/effects of: Alpha-/Beta-Agonists (Direct-Acting); Alpha1-Agonists; Amphetamines; Anticholinergics; Aspirin; Beta2-Agonists; Cisapride; Desmopressin; Dronedarone; Methylene Blue; NSAID (COX-2 Inhibitor); NSAID (Nonselective); Pimozide; QTc-Prolonging Agents; QuiNIDine; QuiNINE; Serotonin Modulators; Sodium Phosphates; Sulfonylureas; Tetrabenazine; Thioridazine; Toremifene; TraMADol; Vandetanib; Vemurafenib; Vitamin K Antagonists; Yohimbine; Ziprasidone

The levels/effects of Amitriptyline may be increased by: Abiraterone Acetate; Alfuzosin; Altretamine; Artemether; BuPROPion; Chloroquine; Cimetidine; Cinacalcet; Ciprofloxacin; Ciprofloxacin (Systemic); Conivaptan; CYP2D6 Inhibitors (Moderate); CYP2D6 Inhibitors (Strong); Dexmethylphenidate; Divalproex; DULoxetine; Gadobutrol; Lithium; Lumefantrine; MAO Inhibitors; Methylphenidate; Metoclopramide; Nilotinib; Pramlintide; Propoxyphene; Protease Inhibitors; QUEtiapine; QuiNIDine; QuiNINE; Selective Serotonin Reuptake Inhibitors; Sibutramine; Terbinafine; Terbinafine (Systemic); Valproic Acid

Decreased Effect

Amitriptyline may decrease the levels/effects of: Acetylcholinesterase Inhibitors (Central); Alpha2-Agonists; Iobenguane I 123

The levels/effects of Amitriptyline may be decreased by: Acetylcholinesterase Inhibitors (Central); Barbiturates; CarBAMazepine; Cyproterone; Peginterferon Alfa-2b; St Johns Wort; Tocilizumab

Ethanol/Nutrition/Herb Interactions

Ethanol: May increase CNS depression; monitor for increased effects with coadministration. Caution patients about effects.

Food: Grapefruit juice may inhibit the metabolism of some TCAs and clinical toxicity may result.

Herb/Nutraceutical: St John's wort may decrease amitriptyline levels. Avoid valerian, St John's wort, kava kava, gotu kola (may increase CNS depression).

Mechanism of Action Increases the synaptic concentration of serotonin and/or norepinephrine in the central nervous system by inhibition of their reuptake by the presynaptic neuronal membrane

Pharmacodynamics/Kinetics

Geriatrics: Plasma concentrations increase with age and steady-state plasma concentrations are significantly increased in older patients compared to younger patients after equal doses. Plasma concentrations do not always correlate with clinical effectiveness.

Metabolism: In the liver to nortriptyline (active), hydroxy derivatives and conjugated derivatives

Half-life: Adults: 9-25 hours (15-hour average); half-life prolonged (mean: 21.7 hours)

Time to peak serum concentration: Within 4 hours

Elimination: Renal excretion of 18% as unchanged drug; small amounts eliminated in feces by bile

Dosage

Geriatric Depression: Oral: Initial: 10-25 mg at bedtime; dose should be increased in 10-25 mg increments every week if tolerated; dose range: 25-150 mg/day. See Dosage: Renal Impairment and Dosage: Hepatic Impairment.

Adult

Depression: Oral: 50-150 mg/day single dose at bedtime or in divided doses; dose may be gradually increased up to 300 mg/day.

Chronic pain management (unlabeled use): Oral: Initial: 25 mg at bedtime; may increase as tolerated to 100 mg/day.

Diabetic neuropathy (unlabeled use): Oral: 25-100 mg/day (Bril, 2011)

Migraine prophylaxis (unlabeled use): Oral: Initial: 10-25 mg at bedtime; usual dose: 150 mg; reported dosing ranges: 10-400 mg/day

Post-traumatic stress disorder (PTSD) (unlabeled use): Oral: 75-200 mg/day

Renal Impairment Nondialyzable

Hepatic Impairment Use with caution and monitor plasma levels and patient response.

Monitoring Parameters Monitor blood pressure and pulse rate prior to and during initial therapy; evaluate mental status, suicidal ideation (especially at the beginning of therapy or when doses are increased or decreased); monitor weight; ECG in older adults and patients with cardiac disease

Reference Range Therapeutic: Amitriptyline and nortriptyline 100-250 ng/mL (SI: 360-900 nmol/L); nortriptyline 50-150 ng/mL (SI: 190-570 nmol/L); Toxic: >0.5 mcg/mL; plasma levels do not always correlate with clinical effectiveness

Test Interactions May cause false-positive reaction to EMIT immunoassay for imipramine

Special Geriatric Considerations Not a drug of choice for the elderly. The most anticholinergic and sedating of the antidepressants; pronounced effects on the cardiovascular system (hypotension).

This medication is considered to be potentially inappropriate in this patient population (Beers Criteria severity: High).

Dosage Forms Excipient information presented when available (limited, particularly for generics); consult specific product labeling.

Tablet, oral, as hydrochloride: 10 mg, 25 mg, 50 mg, 75 mg, 100 mg, 150 mg

Selected References

Nies A, Robinson DS, Friedman MJ, et al, "Relationship Between Age and Tricyclic Antidepressant Plasma Levels," *Am J Psychiatry*, 1977, 134:790-3.

Schulz P, Turner-Tamiyasu K, Smith G, et al, "Amitriptyline Disposition in Young and Elderly Normal Men," *Clin Pharmacol Ther*, 1983, 33(3):360-6.

◆ **Amitriptyline Hydrochloride** see Amitriptyline on page 103

AmLODIPine (am LOE di peen)

Related Information
Calcium Channel Blockers *on page 2003*

Medication Safety Issues
Sound-alike/look-alike issues:
AmLODIPine may be confused with aMILoride
Norvasc® may be confused with Navane®, Norvir®, Vascor®
International issues:
Norvasc [U.S., Canada, and multiple international markets] may be confused with Vascor brand name for imidapril [Philippines] and simvastatin [Malaysia, Singapore, and Thailand]

Brand Names: U.S. Norvasc®

Brand Names: Canada Accel-Amlodipine; Apo-Amlodipine®; CO Amlodipine; Dom-Amlodipine; GD-Amlodipine; JAMP-Amlodipine; Mint-Amlodipine; Mylan-Amlodipine; Norvasc®; PHL-Amlodipine; PMS-Amlodipine; RAN™-Amlodipine; ratio-Amlodipine; Riva-Amlodipine; Sandoz Amlodipine; Septa-Amlodipine; Teva-Amlodipine; ZYM-Amlodipine

Index Terms Amlodipine Besylate

Generic Availability (U.S.) Yes

Pharmacologic Category Calcium Channel Blocker; Calcium Channel Blocker, Dihydropyridine

Use Treatment of hypertension; treatment of symptomatic chronic stable angina, vasospastic (Prinzmetal's) angina (confirmed or suspected); prevention of hospitalization due to angina with documented CAD (limited to patients without heart failure or ejection fraction <40%)

Contraindications Hypersensitivity to amlodipine or any component of the formulation

Warnings/Precautions Increased angina and/or MI has occurred with initiation or dosage titration of calcium channel blockers. Symptomatic hypotension with or without syncope can rarely occur; blood pressure must be lowered at a rate appropriate for the patient's clinical condition. Use caution in severe aortic stenosis and/or hypertrophic cardiomyopathy with outflow tract obstruction. Use caution in patients with hepatic impairment; may require lower starting dose; titrate slowly with severe hepatic impairment. The most common side effect is peripheral edema; occurs within 2-3 weeks of starting therapy. Reflex tachycardia may occur with use. Peak antihypertensive effect is delayed; dosage titration should occur after 7-14 days on a given dose. Initiate at a lower dose in the elderly.

Adverse Reactions (Reflective of adult population; not specific for elderly)
>10%: Cardiovascular: Peripheral edema (2% to 15% dose related; HF patients: 27% [Packer, 1996])
1% to 10%:
Cardiovascular: Flushing (1% to 5% dose related), palpitation (1% to 5% dose related)
Central nervous system: Dizziness (1% to 3% dose related), fatigue (5%), somnolence (1% to 2%)
Dermatologic: Rash (1% to 2%), pruritus (1% to 2%)
Endocrine & metabolic: Male sexual dysfunction (1% to 2%)
Gastrointestinal: Nausea (3%), abdominal pain (1% to 2%), dyspepsia (1% to 2%)
Neuromuscular & skeletal: Muscle cramps (1% to 2%), weakness (1% to 2%)
Respiratory: Dyspnea (1% to 2%), pulmonary edema (HF patients: 27% [Packer, 1996])

Drug Interactions
Metabolism/Transport Effects Substrate of CYP3A4 (major); **Inhibits** CYP1A2 (moderate), 2A6 (weak), 2B6 (weak), 2C8 (weak), 2C9 (weak), 2D6 (weak), 3A4 (weak)

Avoid Concomitant Use
Avoid concomitant use of AmLODIPine with any of the following: Conivaptan

Increased Effect/Toxicity
AmLODIPine may increase the levels/effects of: Amifostine; Antihypertensives; Beta-Blockers; Calcium Channel Blockers (Nondihydropyridine); CYP1A2 Substrates; Fosphenytoin; Hypotensive Agents; Magnesium Salts; Neuromuscular-Blocking Agents (Nondepolarizing); Nitroprusside; Phenytoin; QuiNIDine; RiTUXimab; Simvastatin; Tacrolimus; Tacrolimus (Systemic)

The levels/effects of AmLODIPine may be increased by: Alpha1-Blockers; Antifungal Agents (Azole Derivatives, Systemic); Calcium Channel Blockers (Nondihydropyridine); Conivaptan; CycloSPORINE; CycloSPORINE (Systemic); CYP3A4 Inhibitors (Moderate); CYP3A4 Inhibitors (Strong); Dasatinib; Diazoxide; Fluconazole; Grapefruit Juice; Herbs (Hypotensive Properties); Macrolide Antibiotics; Magnesium Salts; MAO Inhibitors; Pentoxifylline; Phosphodiesterase 5 Inhibitors; Prostacyclin Analogues; Protease Inhibitors; QuiNIDine

Decreased Effect

AmLODIPine may decrease the levels/effects of: Clopidogrel; QuiNIDine

The levels/effects of AmLODIPine may be decreased by: Barbiturates; Calcium Salts; CarBAMazepine; CYP3A4 Inducers (Strong); Deferasirox; Herbs (CYP3A4 Inducers); Herbs (Hypertensive Properties); Methylphenidate; Nafcillin; Rifamycin Derivatives; Tocilizumab; Yohimbine

Ethanol/Nutrition/Herb Interactions

Food: Grapefruit juice may modestly increase amlodipine levels.

Herb/Nutraceutical: St John's wort may decrease amlodipine levels. Avoid herbs with *hypertensive* properties (bayberry, blue cohosh, cayenne, ephedra, ginger, ginseng [American], kola, licorice). Avoid herbs with *hypotensive* properties (black cohosh, California poppy, coleus, garlic, goldenseal, hawthorn, mistletoe, periwinkle, quinine, shepherd's purse).

Stability Store at room temperature of 15°C to 30°C (59°F to 86°F).

Mechanism of Action Inhibits calcium ion from entering the "slow channels" or select voltage-sensitive areas of vascular smooth muscle and myocardium during depolarization, producing a relaxation of coronary vascular smooth muscle and coronary vasodilation; increases myocardial oxygen delivery in patients with vasospastic angina. Amlodipine directly acts on vascular smooth muscle to produce peripheral arterial vasodilation reducing peripheral vascular resistance and blood pressure.

Pharmacodynamics/Kinetics

Duration of antihypertensive effect: 24 hours

Absorption: Oral: Well absorbed

Distribution: V_d: 21 L/kg

Protein binding: 93% to 98%

Metabolism: Hepatic (>90%) to inactive metabolites

Bioavailability: 64% to 90%

Half-life elimination: Terminal: 30-50 hours; increased with hepatic dysfunction

Time to peak, plasma: 6-12 hours

Excretion: Urine (10% of total dose as unchanged drug, 60% of total dose as metabolites)

Dosage

Geriatric Dosing should start at the lower end of dosing range and titrated to response due to possible increased incidence of hepatic, renal, or cardiac impairment. Elderly patients also show decreased clearance of amlodipine.

Hypertension: Oral: 2.5 mg once daily

Angina: Oral: 5 mg once daily

Adult

Hypertension: Oral: Initial dose: 5 mg once daily; maximum dose: 10 mg once daily. In general, titrate in 2.5 mg increments over 7-14 days. Usual dosage range (JNC 7): 2.5-10 mg once daily.

Angina: Oral: Usual dose: 5-10 mg; most patients require 10 mg for adequate effect.

Renal Impairment Dialysis: Hemodialysis and peritoneal dialysis do not enhance elimination. Supplemental dose is not necessary.

Hepatic Impairment

Hypertension: Administer 2.5 mg once daily

Angina: Administer 5 mg once daily

Administration May be administered without regard to meals.

Monitoring Parameters Heart rate, blood pressure, peripheral edema

Special Geriatric Considerations Elderly may experience a greater hypotensive response. Constipation may be more of a problem in elderly. Calcium channel blockers are no more effective in elderly than other therapies, however, they do not cause significant CNS effects which is an advantage over some antihypertensive agents.

Dosage Forms Excipient information presented when available (limited, particularly for generics); consult specific product labeling.

Tablet, oral: 2.5 mg, 5 mg, 10 mg

Norvasc®: 2.5 mg, 5 mg, 10 mg

Selected References

Chobanian AV, Bakris GL, Black HR, et al, "The Seventh Report of the Joint National Committee on Prevention, Detection, Evaluation, and Treatment of High Blood Pressure: The JNC 7 Report," *JAMA*, 2003, 289(19):2560-71.

◆ **Amlodipine, Aliskiren, and Hydrochlorothiazide** *see* Aliskiren, Amlodipine, and Hydrochlorothiazide *on page 60*

◆ **Amlodipine and Aliskiren** *see* Aliskiren and Amlodipine *on page 62*

Amlodipine and Benazepril (am LOE di peen & ben AY ze pril)

Related Information
AmLODIPine *on page 106*
Benazepril *on page 188*
Brand Names: U.S. Lotrel®
Index Terms Benazepril Hydrochloride and Amlodipine Besylate
Generic Availability (U.S.) Yes
Pharmacologic Category Angiotensin-Converting Enzyme (ACE) Inhibitor; Calcium Channel Blocker; Calcium Channel Blocker, Dihydropyridine
Use Treatment of hypertension
Dosage
  Geriatric Initial dose: 2.5 mg (based on amlodipine component). Refer to adult dosing.
  Adult Note: Dose is individualized; combination product may be substituted for individual components in patients currently maintained on both agents separately or in patients not adequately controlled with monotherapy (using one of the agents or an agent within same antihypertensive class).
    Hypertension: Oral: 2.5-10 mg (amlodipine) and 10-40 mg (benazepril) once daily; maximum: Amlodipine: 10 mg/day; benazepril: 80 mg/day
  Renal Impairment Cl_{cr} ≤30 mL/minute: Use of combination product is not recommended.
  Hepatic Impairment Initial dose: 2.5 mg based on amlodipine component.
Special Geriatric Considerations See individual agents. Combination products are not recommended as first-line treatment. Use only if doses of individual agents correspond to the combination available.
Dosage Forms Excipient information presented when available (limited, particularly for generics); consult specific product labeling.
  Capsule:
    2.5/10: Amlodipine 2.5 mg and benazepril hydrochloride 10 mg
    5/10: Amlodipine 5 mg and benazepril hydrochloride 10 mg
    5/20: Amlodipine 5 mg and benazepril hydrochloride 20 mg
    5/40: Amlodipine 5 mg and benazepril hydrochloride 40 mg
    10/20: Amlodipine 10 mg and benazepril hydrochloride 20 mg
    10/40: Amlodipine 10 mg and benazepril hydrochloride 40 mg
      Lotrel® 2.5/10: Amlodipine 2.5 mg and benazepril hydrochloride 10 mg
      Lotrel® 5/10: Amlodipine 5 mg and benazepril hydrochloride 10 mg
      Lotrel® 5/20: Amlodipine 5 mg and benazepril hydrochloride 20 mg
      Lotrel® 5/40: Amlodipine 5 mg and benazepril hydrochloride 40 mg
      Lotrel® 10/20: Amlodipine 10 mg and benazepril hydrochloride 20 mg
      Lotrel® 10/40: Amlodipine 10 mg and benazepril hydrochloride 40 mg

Amlodipine and Olmesartan (am LOE di peen & olme SAR tan)

Related Information
AmLODIPine *on page 106*
Olmesartan *on page 1333*
Brand Names: U.S. Azor™
Index Terms Amlodipine Besylate and Olmesartan Medoxomil; Olmesartan and Amlodipine
Generic Availability (U.S.) No
Pharmacologic Category Angiotensin II Receptor Blocker; Calcium Channel Blocker; Calcium Channel Blocker, Dihydropyridine
Use Treatment of hypertension, including initial treatment in patients who will require multiple antihypertensives for adequate control
Dosage
  Geriatric Initial therapy is not recommended in patients ≥75 years of age.
  Adult Dose is individualized; combination product may be substituted for individual components in patients currently maintained on both agents separately or in patients not adequately controlled with monotherapy (using one of the agents or an agent within the same antihypertensive class). May also be used as initial therapy in patients who are likely to need >1 antihypertensive to control blood pressure.
    Hypertension: Oral:
      Initial therapy (antihypertensive naive): Amlodipine 5 mg/olmesartan 20 mg once daily; dose may be increased after 1-2 weeks of therapy. Maximum recommended dose: Amlodipine 10 mg/day; olmesartan 40 mg/day.

Add-on/replacement therapy: Amlodipine 5-10 mg and olmesartan 20-40 mg once daily depending upon previous doses, current control, and goals of therapy; dose may be titrated after 2 weeks of therapy. Maximum recommended dose: Amlodipine 10 mg/day; olmesartan 40 mg/day.

Renal Impairment No specific guidelines for dosage adjustment.

Hepatic Impairment Initial therapy is not recommended.

Special Geriatric Considerations See individual agents. Combination products are not recommended as first-line treatment. Use only if doses of individual agents correspond to the combination available.

Dosage Forms Excipient information presented when available (limited, particularly for generics); consult specific product labeling.

Tablet:

Azor™ 5/20: Amlodipine 5 mg and olmesartan medoxomil 20 mg

Azor™ 5/40: Amlodipine 5 mg and olmesartan medoxomil 40 mg

Azor™ 10/20: Amlodipine 10 mg and olmesartan medoxomil 20 mg

Azor™ 10/40: Amlodipine 10 mg and olmesartan medoxomil 40 mg

◆ **Amlodipine and Telmisartan** *see* Telmisartan and Amlodipine *on page 1749*

Amlodipine and Valsartan (am LOE di peen & val SAR tan)

Related Information

AmLODIPine *on page 106*

Valsartan *on page 1892*

Brand Names: U.S. Exforge®

Index Terms Amlodipine Besylate and Valsartan; Valsartan and Amlodipine

Generic Availability (U.S.) No

Pharmacologic Category Angiotensin II Receptor Blocker; Calcium Channel Blocker; Calcium Channel Blocker, Dihydropyridine

Use Treatment of hypertension

Dosage

Geriatric Refer to adult dosing. Initiate amlodipine at 2.5 mg/day; due to decreased clearance.

Adult Note: Dose is individualized; combination product may be used as initial therapy or substituted for individual components in patients currently maintained on both agents separately or in patients not adequately controlled with monotherapy (using one of the agents or an agent within same antihypertensive class).

Hypertension: Oral:

Initial therapy: Amlodipine 5 mg and valsartan 160 mg once daily, dose may be titrated after 1-2 weeks of therapy. Maximum recommended doses: Amlodipine 10 mg/day; valsartan 320 mg/day

Add-on/replacement therapy: Amlodipine 5-10 mg and valsartan 160-320 mg once daily; dose may be titrated after 3-4 weeks of therapy. Maximum recommended doses: Amlodipine 10 mg/day; valsartan 320 mg/day

Renal Impairment

Cl_{cr} >10 mL/minute: No dosage adjustment necessary.

Cl_{cr} ≤10 mL/minute: Use caution; titrate slowly.

Hepatic Impairment Mild-to-moderate hepatic impairment: No initial dosage adjustment required, titrate slowly. Amlodipine and valsartan exposure increased in presence of hepatic impairment.

Amlodipine: Use caution in severe hepatic impairment; lower initial doses may be required.

Valsartan: Mild-to-moderate hepatic impairment: No dosage adjustment required; however, patients with mild-to-moderate chronic disease have twice the exposure as healthy volunteers.

Special Geriatric Considerations See individual agents. Combination products are not recommended as first-line treatment. Use only if doses of individual agents correspond to the combination available.

Dosage Forms Excipient information presented when available (limited, particularly for generics); consult specific product labeling.

Tablet:

Exforge®:

5/160: Amlodipine 5 mg and valsartan 160 mg

5/320 mg: Amlodipine 5 mg and valsartan 320 mg

10/160: Amlodipine 10 mg and valsartan 160 mg

10/320: Amlodipine 10 mg and valsartan 320 mg

◆ **Amlodipine Besylate** *see* AmLODIPine *on page 106*

- ◆ **Amlodipine Besylate, Aliskiren Hemifumarate, and Hydrochlorothiazide** *see* Aliskiren, Amlodipine, and Hydrochlorothiazide *on page 60*
- ◆ **Amlodipine Besylate and Olmesartan Medoxomil** *see* Amlodipine and Olmesartan *on page 108*
- ◆ **Amlodipine Besylate and Telmisartan** *see* Telmisartan and Amlodipine *on page 1749*
- ◆ **Amlodipine Besylate and Valsartan** *see* Amlodipine and Valsartan *on page 109*
- ◆ **Amlodipine Besylate, Olmesartan Medoxomil, and Hydrochlorothiazide** *see* Olmesartan, Amlodipine, and Hydrochlorothiazide *on page 1335*
- ◆ **Amlodipine Besylate, Valsartan, and Hydrochlorothiazide** *see* Amlodipine, Valsartan, and Hydrochlorothiazide *on page 110*
- ◆ **Amlodipine, Hydrochlorothiazide, and Aliskiren** *see* Aliskiren, Amlodipine, and Hydrochlorothiazide *on page 60*
- ◆ **Amlodipine, Hydrochlorothiazide, and Olmesartan** *see* Olmesartan, Amlodipine, and Hydrochlorothiazide *on page 1335*
- ◆ **Amlodipine, Hydrochlorothiazide, and Valsartan** *see* Amlodipine, Valsartan, and Hydrochlorothiazide *on page 110*

Amlodipine, Valsartan, and Hydrochlorothiazide
(am LOE di peen, val SAR tan, & hye droe klor oh THYE a zide)

Related Information
AmLODIPine *on page 106*
Hydrochlorothiazide *on page 876*
Valsartan *on page 1892*
Brand Names: U.S. Exforge HCT®
Index Terms Amlodipine Besylate, Valsartan, and Hydrochlorothiazide; Amlodipine, Hydrochlorothiazide, and Valsartan; Hydrochlorothiazide, Amlodipine, and Valsartan; Valsartan, Hydrochlorothiazide, and Amlodipine
Generic Availability (U.S.) No
Pharmacologic Category Angiotensin II Receptor Blocker; Calcium Channel Blocker; Calcium Channel Blocker, Dihydropyridine; Diuretic, Thiazide
Use Treatment of hypertension (not for initial therapy)
Dosage

 Geriatric & Adult Note: Not for initial therapy. Dose is individualized; combination product may be substituted for individual components in patients currently maintained on all three agents separately or in patients not adequately controlled with any two of the following antihypertensive classes: Calcium channel blockers, angiotensin II receptor blockers, and diuretics.

 Hypertension: Oral: Add-on/switch/replacement therapy: Amlodipine 5-10 mg and valsartan 160-320 mg and hydrochlorothiazide 12.5-25 mg once daily; dose may be titrated after 2 weeks of therapy. Maximum recommended daily dose: Amlodipine 10 mg/valsartan 320 mg/hydrochlorothiazide 25 mg

 Renal Impairment
 Cl$_{cr}$ >30 mL/minute: No adjustment needed.
 Cl$_{cr}$ ≤30 mL/minute: Use of combination not recommended; contraindicated in patients with anuria.

 Hepatic Impairment Use of combination is not recommended in severe hepatic impairment. Use with caution in mild-to-moderate hepatic impairment; monitor for worsening of hepatic or renal function and adverse reactions.

 Special Geriatric Considerations In controlled trials, no overall differences in efficacy or safety were noted between elderly and younger adults. See individual agents. Combination products are not recommended as first-line treatment. Use only if doses of individual agents correspond to the combination available.

 Dosage Forms Excipient information presented when available (limited, particularly for generics); consult specific product labeling.
 Tablet, oral:
  Exforge HCT®:
   Amlodipine 5 mg, valsartan 160 mg, and hydrochlorothiazide 12.5 mg
   Amlodipine 5 mg, valsartan 160 mg, and hydrochlorothiazide 25 mg
   Amlodipine 10 mg, valsartan 160 mg, and hydrochlorothiazide 12.5 mg
   Amlodipine 10 mg, valsartan 160 mg, and hydrochlorothiazide 25 mg
   Amlodipine 10 mg, valsartan 320 mg, and hydrochlorothiazide 25 mg

Ammonium Chloride (a MOE nee um KLOR ide)

Generic Availability (U.S.) Yes

Pharmacologic Category Electrolyte Supplement, Parenteral

Use Treatment of hypochloremic states or metabolic alkalosis

Contraindications Severe hepatic or renal dysfunction

Warnings/Precautions Monitor closely for signs and symptoms of ammonia toxicity, including diaphoresis, altered breathing, bradycardia, arrhythmias, retching, twitching, and coma. Use caution in patients with primary respiratory acidosis or pulmonary insufficiency.

Adverse Reactions (Reflective of adult population; not specific for elderly) Frequency not defined.

Central nervous system: Coma, drowsiness, EEG abnormalities, headache, mental confusion, seizure

Dermatologic: Rash

Endocrine & metabolic: Calcium-deficient tetany, hyperchloremia, hypokalemia, metabolic acidosis, potassium may be decreased, sodium may be decreased

Gastrointestinal: Abdominal pain, gastric irritation, nausea, vomiting

Hepatic: Ammonia may be increased

Local: Pain at site of injection

Neuromuscular & skeletal: Twitching

Respiratory: Hyperventilation

Drug Interactions

Avoid Concomitant Use There are no known interactions where it is recommended to avoid concomitant use.

Increased Effect/Toxicity

The levels/effects of Ammonium Chloride may be increased by: Potassium-Sparing Diuretics

Decreased Effect

Ammonium Chloride may decrease the levels/effects of: Amphetamines; Analgesics (Opioid)

Stability Prior to use, vials should be stored at controlled room temperature of 15°C to 30°C (59°F to 86°F). Solution may crystallize if exposed to low temperatures. If crystals are observed, warm vial to room temperature in a water bath prior to use. Dilute prior to use; final concentration should not exceed 1% to 2% ammonium chloride. Suggested dilution: Mix contents of 1-2 vials (100-200 mEq) in 500-1000 mL NS.

Mechanism of Action Increases acidity by increasing free hydrogen ion concentration

Pharmacodynamics/Kinetics

Metabolism: Hepatic; forms urea and hydrochloric acid

Excretion: Urine

Dosage

Geriatric & Adult Metabolic alkalosis: The following equations represent different methods of correction utilizing either the serum HCO_3^-, the serum chloride, or the base excess

Dosing of mEq NH_4 Cl via the chloride-deficit method (hypochloremia):

Dose of mEq NH_4Cl = [0.2 L/kg x body weight (kg)] x [103 - observed serum chloride]; administer 50% of dose over 12 hours, then re-evaluate

Note: 0.2 L/kg is the estimated chloride volume of distribution and 103 is the average normal serum chloride concentration (mEq/L)

Dosing of mEq NH_4 Cl via the bicarbonate-excess method (refractory hypochloremic metabolic alkalosis):

Dose of NH_4Cl = [0.5 L/kg x body weight (kg)] x (observed serum HCO_3^- - 24); administer 50% of dose over 12 hours, then re-evaluate

Note: 0.5 L/kg is the estimated bicarbonate volume of distribution and 24 is the average normal serum bicarbonate concentration (mEq/L)

These equations will yield different requirements of ammonium chloride

Administration Administer by slow intravenous infusion to avoid local irritation and adverse effects. Rate of infusion should not exceed 5 mL/minute in an adult.

Monitoring Parameters Serum bicarbonate; signs and symptoms of ammonia toxicity

Pharmacotherapy Pearls Do not exceed a 1% to 2% concentration of ammonium chloride or an administration rate of more than 5 mL/minute; administer over approximately 3 hours for I.V. infusion

Special Geriatric Considerations No specific data available for elderly; monitor closely with hepatic disease for signs of toxicity.

◀ **Dosage Forms** Excipient information presented when available (limited, particularly for generics); consult specific product labeling.

Injection, solution: Ammonium 5 mEq/mL and chloride 5 mEq/mL (20 mL) [equivalent to ammonium chloride 267.5 mg/mL]

◆ **Amoclan** *see* Amoxicillin and Clavulanate Potassium *on page 116*

Amoxapine (a MOKS a peen)

Related Information
Antidepressant Agents *on page 1991*

Medication Safety Issues
Sound-alike/look-alike issues:
Amoxapine may be confused with amoxicillin, Amoxil
Asendin may be confused with aspirin

Index Terms Asendin [DSC]

Generic Availability (U.S.) Yes

Pharmacologic Category Antidepressant, Tricyclic (Secondary Amine)

Use Treatment of depression, psychotic depression, depression accompanied by anxiety or agitation

Medication Guide Available Yes

Contraindications Hypersensitivity to amoxapine or any component of the formulation; use of MAO inhibitors within past 14 days; acute recovery phase following myocardial infarction

Warnings/Precautions [U.S. Boxed Warning]: Antidepressants increase the risk of suicidal thinking and behavior in children, adolescents, and young adults (18-24 years of age) with major depressive disorder (MDD) and other psychiatric disorders; consider risk prior to prescribing. Short-term studies did not show an increased risk in patients >24 years of age and showed a decreased risk in patients ≥65 years. Closely monitor for clinical worsening, suicidality, or unusual changes in behavior; the patient's family or caregiver should be instructed to closely observe the patient and communicate condition with healthcare provider. A medication guide should be dispensed with each prescription. **Amoxapine is not FDA approved for use in patients <16 years of age.**

The possibility of a suicide attempt is inherent in major depression and may persist until remission occurs. Monitor for worsening of depression or suicidality, especially during initiation of therapy (generally first 1-2 months) or with dose increases or decreases. Use caution in high-risk patients. Worsening depression and severe abrupt suicidality that are not part of the presenting symptoms may require discontinuation or modification of drug therapy. The patient's family or caregiver should be alerted to monitor patients for the emergence of suicidality and associated behaviors (such as agitation, irritability, hostility, impulsivity, and hypomania) and notify the healthcare provider.

May worsen psychosis in some patients or precipitate a shift to mania or hypomania in patients with bipolar disorder. Patients presenting with depressive symptoms should be screened for bipolar disorder. Monotherapy in patients with bipolar disorder should be avoided. **Amoxapine is not FDA approved for bipolar depression.** May cause extrapyramidal symptoms, including pseudoparkinsonism, acute dystonic reactions, akathisia, and tardive dyskinesia (risk of these reactions is low). May be associated with neuroleptic malignant syndrome.

The degree of sedation, anticholinergic effects, orthostasis, and conduction abnormalities are moderate relative to other antidepressants. May cause drowsiness/sedation, resulting in impaired performance of tasks requiring alertness (eg, operating machinery or driving). Sedative effects may be additive with other CNS depressants and/or ethanol. Use with caution in patients with a history of cardiovascular disease (including previous MI, stroke, tachycardia, or conduction abnormalities). Use with caution in patients with urinary retention, benign prostatic hyperplasia, narrow-angle glaucoma, xerostomia, visual problems, constipation, or a history of bowel obstruction.

Consider discontinuing, when possible, prior to elective surgery. Therapy should not be abruptly discontinued in patients receiving high doses for prolonged periods. May lower seizure threshold - use caution in patients with a previous seizure disorder or condition predisposing to seizures such as brain damage, alcoholism, or concurrent therapy with other drugs which lower the seizure threshold. May increase the risks associated with electroconvulsive therapy. Use with caution in hyperthyroid patients or those receiving thyroid supplementation. Use with caution in patients with hepatic or renal dysfunction and in elderly patients.

Adverse Reactions (Reflective of adult population; not specific for elderly)

>10%:
Central nervous system: Drowsiness
Gastrointestinal: Xerostomia, constipation

1% to 10%:
Central nervous system: Anxiety, ataxia, confusion, dizziness, excitement, headache, insomnia, nervousness, restlessness
Dermatologic: Edema, skin rash
Endocrine: Prolactin levels increased
Gastrointestinal: Nausea
Neuromuscular & skeletal: Tremor, weakness
Ocular: Blurred vision
Miscellaneous: Diaphoresis

Drug Interactions

Metabolism/Transport Effects Substrate of CYP2D6 (major)

Avoid Concomitant Use

Avoid concomitant use of Amoxapine with any of the following: Artemether; Dronedarone; Iobenguane I 123; Lumefantrine; MAO Inhibitors; Methylene Blue; Nilotinib; Pimozide; QUEtiapine; QuiNINE; Sibutramine; Tetrabenazine; Thioridazine; Toremifene; Vandetanib; Vemurafenib; Ziprasidone

Increased Effect/Toxicity

Amoxapine may increase the levels/effects of: Alpha-/Beta-Agonists (Direct-Acting); Alpha1-Agonists; Amphetamines; Anticholinergics; Beta2-Agonists; Desmopressin; Dronedarone; Methylene Blue; Pimozide; QTc-Prolonging Agents; QuiNIDine; QuiNINE; Serotonin Modulators; Sodium Phosphates; Sulfonylureas; Tetrabenazine; Thioridazine; Toremifene; TraMADol; Vandetanib; Vemurafenib; Vitamin K Antagonists; Yohimbine; Ziprasidone

The levels/effects of Amoxapine may be increased by: Abiraterone Acetate; Alfuzosin; Altretamine; Artemether; Chloroquine; Cimetidine; Cinacalcet; Ciprofloxacin; Ciprofloxacin (Systemic); CYP2D6 Inhibitors (Moderate); CYP2D6 Inhibitors (Strong); Dexmethylphenidate; Divalproex; DULoxetine; Gadobutrol; Lithium; Lumefantrine; MAO Inhibitors; Methylphenidate; Metoclopramide; Nilotinib; Pramlintide; Propoxyphene; Protease Inhibitors; QUEtiapine; QuiNIDine; QuiNINE; Selective Serotonin Reuptake Inhibitors; Sibutramine; Terbinafine; Terbinafine (Systemic); Valproic Acid

Decreased Effect

Amoxapine may decrease the levels/effects of: Acetylcholinesterase Inhibitors (Central); Alpha2-Agonists; Iobenguane I 123

The levels/effects of Amoxapine may be decreased by: Acetylcholinesterase Inhibitors (Central); Barbiturates; CarBAMazepine; Peginterferon Alfa-2b; St Johns Wort

Ethanol/Nutrition/Herb Interactions

Ethanol: May increase CNS depression; monitor for increased effects with coadministration. Caution patients about effects.
Food: Grapefruit juice may inhibit the metabolism of some TCAs and clinical toxicity may result.
Herb/Nutraceutical: Avoid valerian, St John's wort, SAMe, kava kava.

Mechanism of Action Reduces the reuptake of serotonin and norepinephrine. The metabolite, 7-OH-amoxapine has significant dopamine receptor blocking activity similar to haloperidol.

Pharmacodynamics/Kinetics

Onset of antidepressant effect: Usually occurs after 1-2 weeks, but may require 4-6 weeks
Absorption: Rapid and well absorbed
Distribution: V_d: 0.9-1.2 L/kg
Protein binding: 80%
Metabolism: Primarily hepatic
Half-life elimination: Parent drug: 11-16 hours; Active metabolite (8-hydroxy): Adults: 30 hours
Time to peak, serum: 1-2 hours
Excretion: Urine (as unchanged drug and metabolites)

Dosage

Geriatric Oral: Initial: 25 mg at bedtime increased by 25 mg weekly for outpatients and every 3 days for inpatients if tolerated; usual dose: 50-150 mg/day, but doses up to 300 mg may be necessary. **Note:** Once symptoms are controlled, decrease gradually to lowest effective dose.

Adult Once symptoms are controlled, decrease gradually to lowest effective dose. Maintenance dose is usually given at bedtime to reduce daytime sedation.

Depression: Oral: Initial: 25 mg 2-3 times/day. If tolerated, dosage may be increased to 100 mg 2-3 times/day. May be given in a single bedtime dose when dosage <300 mg/day. Maximum daily dose: 600 mg (inpatients); 400 mg (outpatients)

◀ **Administration** May be administered with food to decrease GI distress.

Monitoring Parameters Monitor blood pressure and pulse rate prior to and during initial therapy evaluate mental status, suicide ideation (especially at the beginning of therapy or when doses are increased or decreased); monitor weight; ECG in older adults

Reference Range Therapeutic: Amoxapine: 20-100 ng/mL (SI: 64-319 nmol/L); 8-OH amoxapine: 150-400 ng/mL (SI: 478-1275 nmol/L); both: 200-500 ng/mL (SI: 637-1594 nmol/L)

Test Interactions Increased glucose, liver function tests; decreased WBC

Pharmacotherapy Pearls May take up to 2 weeks for full therapeutic effects to be apparent; maintenance dose is usually given at bedtime to reduce daytime sedation; tolerance develops in 1-3 months in some patients, close medical follow-up is essential

Special Geriatric Considerations Amoxapine is not the drug of choice in the elderly. Significant anticholinergic and orthostatic effects can occur and there is a risk for tardive dyskinesia and neuroleptic malignant syndrome.

Dosage Forms Excipient information presented when available (limited, particularly for generics); consult specific product labeling.
Tablet, oral: 25 mg, 50 mg, 100 mg, 150 mg

Amoxicillin (a moks i SIL in)

Related Information
Community-Acquired Pneumonia in Adults *on page 2059*
Helicobacter pylori Treatment in Adult Patients *on page 2009*
Prevention of Infective Endocarditis *on page 2064*

Medication Safety Issues
Sound-alike/look-alike issues:
Amoxicillin may be confused with amoxapine, Augmentin®
Amoxil may be confused with amoxapine
International issues:
Fisamox [Australia] may be confused with Fosamax brand name for alendronate [U.S., Canada, and multiple international markets] and Vigamox brand name for moxifloxacin [U.S., Canada, and multiple international markets]
Limoxin [Mexico] may be confused with Lanoxin brand name for digoxin [U.S., Canada, and multiple international markets]; Lincocin brand name for lincomycin [U.S., Canada, and multiple international markets]
Zimox: Brand name for amoxicillin [Italy], but also the brand name for carbidopa/levodopa [Greece]
Zimox [Italy] may be confused with Diamox which is the brand name for acetazolamide [Canada and multiple international markets]

Brand Names: U.S. Moxatag™

Brand Names: Canada Apo-Amoxi®; Gen-Amoxicillin; Lin-Amox; Mylan-Amoxicillin; Nova-moxin®; Nu-Amoxi; PHL-Amoxicillin; PMS-Amoxicillin

Index Terms *p*-Hydroxyampicillin; Amoxicillin Trihydrate; Amoxil; Amoxycillin

Generic Availability (U.S.) Yes: Excludes extended-release formulation

Pharmacologic Category Antibiotic, Penicillin

Use Treatment of otitis media, sinusitis, and infections caused by susceptible organisms involving the upper and lower respiratory tract, skin, and urinary tract; prophylaxis of infective endocarditis in patients undergoing surgical or dental procedures; as part of a multidrug regimen for *H. pylori* eradication

Unlabeled/Investigational Use Postexposure prophylaxis for anthrax exposure with documented susceptible organisms

Contraindications Hypersensitivity to amoxicillin, penicillin, other beta-lactams, or any component of the formulation

Warnings/Precautions In patients with renal impairment, doses and/or frequency of administration should be modified in response to the degree of renal impairment; in addition, use of certain dosage forms (eg, extended release 775 mg tablet and immediate release 875 mg tablet) should be avoided in patients with Cl_{cr} <30 mL/minute or patients requiring hemodialysis. A high percentage of patients with infectious mononucleosis have developed rash during therapy with amoxicillin; ampicillin-class antibiotics not recommended in these patients. Serious and occasionally severe or fatal hypersensitivity (anaphylactoid) reactions have been reported in patients on penicillin therapy, especially with a history of beta-lactam hypersensitivity, history of sensitivity to multiple allergens, or previous IgE-mediated reactions (eg, anaphylaxis, angioedema, urticaria). Use with caution in asthmatic patients. Prolonged use may result in fungal or bacterial superinfection, including *C. difficile*-associated diarrhea (CDAD) and pseudomembranous colitis; CDAD has been observed >2 months postantibiotic treatment. Chewable tablets contain phenylalanine.

Adverse Reactions (Reflective of adult population; not specific for elderly) Frequency not defined.

Central nervous system: Agitation, anxiety, behavioral changes, confusion, dizziness, headache, hyperactivity (reversible), insomnia, seizure

Dermatologic: Acute exanthematous pustulosis, erythematous maculopapular rash, erythema multiforme, exfoliative dermatitis, hypersensitivity vasculitis, mucocutaneous candidiasis, Stevens-Johnson syndrome, toxic epidermal necrolysis, urticaria

Gastrointestinal: Black hairy tongue, diarrhea, hemorrhagic colitis, nausea, pseudomembranous colitis, tooth discoloration (brown, yellow, or gray; rare), vomiting

Hematologic: Agranulocytosis, anemia, eosinophilia, hemolytic anemia, leukopenia, thrombocytopenia, thrombocytopenia purpura

Hepatic: Acute cytolytic hepatitis, ALT increased, AST increased, cholestatic jaundice, hepatic cholestasis

Renal: Crystalluria

Miscellaneous: Anaphylaxis, serum sickness-like reaction

Drug Interactions

Avoid Concomitant Use

Avoid concomitant use of Amoxicillin with any of the following: BCG

Increased Effect/Toxicity

Amoxicillin may increase the levels/effects of: Methotrexate

The levels/effects of Amoxicillin may be increased by: Allopurinol; Probenecid

Decreased Effect

Amoxicillin may decrease the levels/effects of: BCG; Mycophenolate; Typhoid Vaccine

The levels/effects of Amoxicillin may be decreased by: Fusidic Acid; Tetracycline Derivatives

Stability

Amoxil®: Oral suspension remains stable for 14 days at room temperature or if refrigerated (refrigeration preferred). Unit-dose antibiotic oral syringes are stable at room temperature for at least 72 hours (Tu, 1988).

Moxatag™: Store at 25°C (77°F); excursions permitted to 15°C to 30°C (59°F to 86°F).

Mechanism of Action Inhibits bacterial cell wall synthesis by binding to one or more of the penicillin-binding proteins (PBPs) which in turn inhibits the final transpeptidation step of peptidoglycan synthesis in bacterial cell walls, thus inhibiting cell wall biosynthesis. Bacteria eventually lyse due to ongoing activity of cell wall autolytic enzymes (autolysins and murein hydrolases) while cell wall assembly is arrested.

Pharmacodynamics/Kinetics

Absorption: Oral: Rapid and nearly complete; food does not interfere

Extended-release tablet: Rate of absorption is slower compared to immediate-release formulations; food decreases the rate but not extent of absorption

Distribution: Widely to most body fluids and bone; poor penetration into cells, eyes, and across normal meninges

Pleural fluids, lungs, and peritoneal fluid; high urine concentrations are attained; also into synovial fluid, liver, prostate, muscle, and gallbladder; penetrates into middle ear effusions, maxillary sinus secretions, tonsils, sputum, and bronchial secretions

CSF:blood level ratio: Normal meninges: <1%; Inflamed meninges: 8% to 90%

Protein binding: 17% to 20%

Metabolism: Partially hepatic

Half-life elimination: Normal renal function: 0.7-1.4 hours

Cl_{cr} <10 mL/minute: 7-21 hours

Time to peak: Capsule: 2 hours; Extended-release tablet: 3.1 hours; Suspension: 1 hour

Excretion: Urine (60% as unchanged drug)

Note: Extended-release tablets: In healthy volunteers, serum drug concentrations were below 0.25 mcg/mL and undetectable at 16 hours following dosing.

Dosage

Geriatric & Adult

Usual dosage range: Oral: 250-500 mg every 8 hours or 500-875 mg twice daily **or** extended-release tablet 775 mg once daily

Anthrax exposure (CDC guidelines): Oral: **Note:** Postexposure prophylaxis in pregnant or nursing women only with documented susceptible organisms: 500 mg every 8 hours

Ear, nose, throat, genitourinary tract, or skin/skin structure infections:

Mild-to-moderate: Oral: 500 mg every 12 hours **or** 250 mg every 8 hours

Severe: Oral: 875 mg every 12 hours **or** 500 mg every 8 hours

Tonsillitis and/or pharyngitis: Oral: Extended release tablet: 775 mg once daily

Helicobacter pylori **eradication:** Oral: 1000 mg twice daily; requires combination therapy with at least one other antibiotic and an acid-suppressing agent (proton pump inhibitor or H_2 blocker)

Lower respiratory tract infections: Oral: 875 mg every 12 hours **or** 500 mg every 8 hours

Lyme disease: Oral: 500 mg every 6-8 hours (depending on size of patient) for 21-30 days

Prophylaxis against infective endocarditis: Oral: 2 g 30-60 minutes before procedure.

Note: American Heart Association (AHA) guidelines now recommend prophylaxis only in patients undergoing invasive procedures and in whom underlying cardiac conditions may predispose to a higher risk of adverse outcomes should infection occur. As of April 2007, routine prophylaxis for GI/GU procedures is no longer recommended by the AHA.

Prophylaxis in total joint replacement patients undergoing dental procedures which produce bacteremia: 2 g 1 hour prior to procedure

Renal Impairment

Use of certain dosage forms (eg, extended-release 775 mg tablet and immediate-release 875 mg tablet) should be avoided in patients with Cl_{cr} <30 mL/minute or patients requiring hemodialysis

Cl_{cr} 10-30 mL/minute: 250-500 mg every 12 hours

Cl_{cr} <10 mL/minute: 250-500 mg every 24 hours

Moderately dialyzable (20% to 50%) by hemodialysis or peritoneal dialysis; approximately 50 mg of amoxicillin per liter of filtrate is removed by continuous arteriovenous or venovenous hemofiltration. Dose as per Cl_{cr} <10 mL/minute guidelines.

Administration Administer around-the-clock to promote less variation in peak and trough serum levels. The appropriate amount of suspension may be mixed with formula, milk, fruit juice, water, ginger ale or cold drinks; administer dose immediately after mixing.

DisperMox™: Dissolve 1 tablet in ~10 mL of water immediately before administration. Rinse container with additional water and drink entire contents to ensure that complete dose is taken. Do not chew or swallow tablet whole.

Monitoring Parameters With prolonged therapy, monitor renal, hepatic, and hematologic function periodically; assess patient at beginning and throughout therapy for infection; monitor for signs of anaphylaxis during first dose

Test Interactions May interfere with urinary glucose tests using cupric sulfate (Benedict's solution, Clinitest®)

Some penicillin derivatives may accelerate the degradation of aminoglycosides *in vitro*, leading to a potential underestimation of aminoglycoside serum concentration.

Pharmacotherapy Pearls Food does not interfere with absorption; urticarial rash that appears after a few days of therapy may indicate hypersensitivity

Special Geriatric Considerations Resistance to amoxicillin has been a problem in patients on frequent antibiotics or in nursing homes. Alternative antibiotics may be necessary in these populations. Consider renal function.

Dosage Forms Excipient information presented when available (limited, particularly for generics); consult specific product labeling.

Capsule, oral: 250 mg, 500 mg

Powder for suspension, oral: 125 mg/5 mL (80 mL, 100 mL, 150 mL); 200 mg/5 mL (50 mL, 75 mL, 100 mL); 250 mg/5 mL (80 mL, 100 mL, 150 mL); 400 mg/5 mL (50 mL, 75 mL, 100 mL)

Tablet, oral: 500 mg, 875 mg

Tablet, chewable, oral: 125 mg, 200 mg, 250 mg, 400 mg

Tablet, extended release, oral:

Moxatag™: 775 mg

Selected References

Mandell LA, Wunderink RG, Anzueto A, et al, "Infectious Diseases Society of America/American Thoracic Society Consensus Guidelines on the Management of Community-Acquired Pneumonia in Adults," *Clin Infect Dis*, 2007, 44 Suppl 2:S27-72.

Amoxicillin and Clavulanate Potassium

(a moks i SIL in & klav yoo LAN ate poe TASS ee um)

Related Information

Amoxicillin *on page 114*

Community-Acquired Pneumonia in Adults *on page 2059*

Medication Safety Issues

Sound-alike/look-alike issues:

Augmentin® may be confused with amoxicillin, Azulfidine®

Brand Names: U.S. Amoclan; Augmentin ES-600® [DSC]; Augmentin XR®; Augmentin®

Brand Names: Canada Amoxi-Clav; Apo-Amoxi-Clav®; Clavulin®; Novo-Clavamoxin; ratio-Aclavulanate

Index Terms Amoxicillin and Clavulanic Acid; Clavulanic Acid and Amoxicillin

Generic Availability (U.S.) Yes

Pharmacologic Category Antibiotic, Penicillin

Use Treatment of otitis media, sinusitis, and infections caused by susceptible organisms involving the lower respiratory tract, skin and skin structure, and urinary tract; spectrum same as amoxicillin with additional coverage of beta-lactamase producing *B. catarrhalis*, *H. influenzae*, *N. gonorrhoeae*, and *S. aureus* (not MRSA). The expanded coverage of this combination makes it a useful alternative when amoxicillin resistance is present and patients cannot tolerate alternative treatments.

Contraindications Hypersensitivity to amoxicillin, clavulanic acid, penicillin, or any component of the formulation; history of cholestatic jaundice or hepatic dysfunction with amoxicillin/clavulanate potassium therapy; Augmentin XR™: severe renal impairment (Cl_{cr} <30 mL/minute) and hemodialysis patients

Warnings/Precautions Hypersensitivity reactions, including anaphylaxis (some fatal), have been reported. Prolonged use may result in fungal or bacterial superinfection, including *C. difficile*-associated diarrhea (CDAD) and pseudomembranous colitis; CDAD has been observed >2 months postantibiotic treatment. In patients with renal impairment, doses and/or frequency of administration should be modified in response to the degree of renal impairment. High percentage of patients with infectious mononucleosis have developed rash during therapy; ampicillin-class antibiotics not recommended in these patients. Incidence of diarrhea is higher than with amoxicillin alone. Due to differing content of clavulanic acid, not all formulations are interchangeable. Low incidence of cross-allergy with cephalosporins exists. Some products contain phenylalanine.

Adverse Reactions (Reflective of adult population; not specific for elderly)

>10%: Gastrointestinal: Diarrhea (3% to 34%; incidence varies upon dose and regimen used)

1% to 10%:

Dermatologic: Diaper rash, skin rash, urticaria

Gastrointestinal: Abdominal discomfort, loose stools, nausea, vomiting

Genitourinary: Vaginitis, vaginal mycosis

Miscellaneous: Moniliasis

Additional adverse reactions seen with **ampicillin-class antibiotics:** Agitation, agranulocytosis, alkaline phosphatase increased, anemia, angioedema, anxiety, behavioral changes, bilirubin increased, black "hairy" tongue, confusion, convulsions, crystalluria, dizziness, enterocolitis, eosinophilia, erythema multiforme, exanthematous pustulosis, exfoliative dermatitis, gastritis, glossitis, hematuria, hemolytic anemia, hemorrhagic colitis, indigestion, insomnia, hyperactivity, interstitial nephritis, leukopenia, mucocutaneous candidiasis, pruritus, pseudomembranous colitis, serum sickness-like reaction, Stevens-Johnson syndrome, stomatitis, transaminases increased, thrombocytopenia, thrombocytopenic purpura, tooth discoloration, toxic epidermal necrolysis

Drug Interactions

Avoid Concomitant Use

Avoid concomitant use of Amoxicillin and Clavulanate Potassium with any of the following: BCG

Increased Effect/Toxicity

Amoxicillin and Clavulanate Potassium may increase the levels/effects of: Methotrexate

The levels/effects of Amoxicillin and Clavulanate Potassium may be increased by: Allopurinol; Probenecid

Decreased Effect

Amoxicillin and Clavulanate Potassium may decrease the levels/effects of: BCG; Mycophenolate; Typhoid Vaccine

The levels/effects of Amoxicillin and Clavulanate Potassium may be decreased by: Fusidic Acid; Tetracycline Derivatives

Stability

Powder for oral suspension: Store dry powder at room temperature of 25°C (77°F). Reconstitute powder for oral suspension with appropriate amount of water as specified on the bottle. Shake vigorously until suspended. Reconstituted oral suspension should be kept in refrigerator. Discard unused suspension after 10 days. Unit-dose antibiotic oral syringes are stable under refrigeration for 24 hours (Tu, 1988).

Tablet: Store at room temperature of 25°C (77°F).

Mechanism of Action Clavulanic acid binds and inhibits beta-lactamases that inactivate amoxicillin resulting in amoxicillin having an expanded spectrum of activity. Amoxicillin inhibits bacterial cell wall synthesis by binding to one or more of the penicillin-binding proteins (PBPs) which in turn inhibits the final transpeptidation step of peptidoglycan synthesis in bacterial cell walls, thus inhibiting cell wall biosynthesis. Bacteria eventually lyse due to ongoing activity of cell wall autolytic enzymes (autolysins and murein hydrolases) while cell wall assembly is arrested.

Pharmacodynamics/Kinetics Amoxicillin pharmacokinetics are not affected by clavulanic acid.

Amoxicillin: See Amoxicillin monograph.

◄ **Clavulanic acid:**
Protein binding: ~25%
Metabolism: Hepatic
Half-life elimination: 1 hour
Time to peak: 1 hour
Excretion: Urine (30% to 40% as unchanged drug)

Dosage
Geriatric & Adult Note: Dose is based on the amoxicillin component; see "Augmentin® Product-Specific Considerations" table.
Susceptible infections: Oral: 250-500 mg every 8 hours or 875 mg every 12 hours

Augmentin® Product-Specific Considerations

Strength	Form	Consideration
125 mg	CT, S	q8h dosing
	S	For adults having difficulty swallowing tablets, 125 mg/5 mL suspension may be substituted for 500 mg tablet.
200 mg	CT, S	q12h dosing
	CT	Contains phenylalanine
	S	For adults having difficulty swallowing tablets, 200 mg/5 mL suspension may be substituted for 875 mg tablet.
250 mg	CT, S, T	q8h dosing
	CT	Contains phenylalanine
	T	Not for use in patients <40 kg
	CT, T	Tablet and chewable tablet are not interchangeable due to differences in clavulanic acid.
	S	For adults having difficulty swallowing tablets, 250 mg/5 mL suspension may be substituted for 500 mg tablet.
400 mg	CT, S	q12h dosing
	CT	Contains phenylalanine
	S	For adults having difficulty swallowing tablets, 400 mg/5 mL suspension may be substituted for 875 mg tablet.
500 mg	T	q8h or q12h dosing
600 mg	S	q12h dosing
		Contains phenylalanine
		Not for use in adults ≥40 kg
		600 mg/5 mL suspension is not equivalent to or interchangeable with 200 mg/5 mL or 400 mg/5 mL due to differences in clavulanic acid.
875 mg	T	q12h dosing; not for use in Cl_{cr} <30 mL/minute
1000 mg	XR	q12h dosing
		Not interchangeable with two 500 mg tablets
		Not for use if Cl_{cr} <30 mL/minute or hemodialysis

Legend: CT = chewable tablet, S = suspension, T = tablet, XR = extended release.

Acute bacterial sinusitis: Oral: Extended release tablet: Two 1000 mg tablets every 12 hours for 10 days
Bite wounds (animal/human): Oral: 875 mg every 12 hours **or** 500 mg every 8 hours
Chronic obstructive pulmonary disease: Oral: 875 mg every 12 hours **or** 500 mg every 8 hours
Diabetic foot: Oral: Extended release tablet: Two 1000 mg tablets every 12 hours for 7-14 days
Diverticulitis, perirectal abscess: Oral: Extended release tablet: Two 1000 mg tablets every 12 hours for 7-10 days
Erysipelas: Oral: 875 mg every 12 hours **or** 500 mg every 8 hours
Febrile neutropenia: Oral: 875 mg every 12 hours
Pneumonia:
Aspiration: Oral: 875 mg every 12 hours
Community-acquired: Oral: Extended release tablet: Two 1000 mg tablets every 12 hours for 7-10 days
Pyelonephritis (acute, uncomplicated): Oral: 875 mg every 12 hours **or** 500 mg every 8 hours
Skin abscess: Oral: 875 mg every 12 hours

Renal Impairment

Cl_{cr} <30 mL/minute: Do not use 875 mg tablet or extended release tablets.
Cl_{cr} 10-30 mL/minute: 250-500 mg every 12 hours
Cl_{cr} <10 mL/minute: 250-500 every 24 hours
Hemodialysis: Moderately dialyzable (20% to 50%)
  250-500 mg every 24 hours; administer dose during and after dialysis. Do not use extended release tablets.
Peritoneal dialysis: Moderately dialyzable (20% to 50%)
  Amoxicillin: Administer 250 mg every 12 hours
  Clavulanic acid: Dose for Cl_{cr} <10 mL/minute
Continuous arteriovenous or venovenous hemofiltration effects:
  Amoxicillin: ~50 mg of amoxicillin/L of filtrate is removed
  Clavulanic acid: Dose for Cl_{cr} <10 mL/minute

Administration Administer around-the-clock to promote less variation in peak and trough serum levels. Administer with food to increase absorption and decrease stomach upset; shake suspension well before use. Extended release tablets should be administered with food.

Some penicillins (eg, carbenicillin, ticarcillin, and piperacillin) have been shown to inactivate aminoglycosides in vitro. This has been observed to a greater extent with tobramycin and gentamicin, while amikacin has shown greater stability against inactivation. Concurrent use of these agents may pose a risk of reduced antibacterial efficacy in vivo, particularly in the setting of profound renal impairment. However, definitive clinical evidence is lacking. If combination penicillin/aminoglycoside therapy is desired in a patient with renal dysfunction, separation of doses (if feasible), and routine monitoring of aminoglycoside levels, CBC, and clinical response should be considered.

Monitoring Parameters Assess patient at beginning and throughout therapy for infection; with prolonged therapy, monitor renal, hepatic, and hematologic function periodically; monitor for signs of anaphylaxis during first dose

Test Interactions May interfere with urinary glucose tests using cupric sulfate (Benedict's solution, Clinitest®, Fehling's solution); may inactivate aminoglycosides in vitro.
Some penicillin derivatives may accelerate the degradation of aminoglycosides in vitro, leading to a potential underestimation of aminoglycoside serum concentration.

Pharmacotherapy Pearls Both "250" and "500" tablets contain the same amount of clavulanic acid, thus two "250" tablets are not equivalent to one "500" tablet. Clavulanic acid inhibits beta-lactamase destruction of amoxicillin.

Special Geriatric Considerations Expanded coverage of this combination makes it a useful alternative when amoxicillin resistance is present and patients cannot tolerate alternative treatments; consider renal function. Considered one of the drugs of choice in the outpatient treatment of community-acquired pneumonia in elderly.

Dosage Forms Excipient information presented when available (limited, particularly for generics); consult specific product labeling. [DSC] = Discontinued product
Powder for suspension, oral: 200: Amoxicillin 200 mg and clavulanate potassium 28.5 mg per 5 mL (50 mL, 75 mL, 100 mL) [contains phenylalanine]; 250: Amoxicillin 250 mg and clavulanate potassium 62.5 mg per 5 mL (75 mL, 100 mL, 150 mL) [contains phenylalanine]; 400: Amoxicillin 400 mg and clavulanate potassium 57 mg per 5 mL (50 mL, 75 mL, 100 mL) [contains phenylalanine]; 600: Amoxicillin 600 mg and clavulanate potassium 42.9 mg per 5 mL (75 mL, 125 mL, 200 mL)
Amoclan:
  200: Amoxicillin 200 mg and clavulanate potassium 28.5 mg per 5 mL (50 mL, 75 mL, 100 mL) [contains phenylalanine 7 mg/5 mL and potassium 0.14 mEq/5 mL; fruit flavor]
  400: Amoxicillin 400 mg and clavulanate potassium 57 mg per 5 mL (50 mL, 75 mL, 100 mL) [contains phenylalanine 7 mg/5 mL and potassium 0.29 mEq/5 mL; fruit flavor]
  600: Amoxicillin 600 mg and clavulanate potassium 42.9 mg per 5 mL (75 mL, 125 mL) [contains phenylalanine 7 mg/5 mL, potassium 0.248 mEq/5 mL; orange flavor]
Augmentin®:
  125: Amoxicillin 125 mg and clavulanate potassium 31.25 mg per 5 mL (75 mL, 100 mL, 150 mL) [contains potassium 0.16 mEq/5 mL; banana flavor]
  200: Amoxicillin 200 mg and clavulanate potassium 28.5 mg per 5 mL (50 mL, 75 mL, 100 mL) [contains phenylalanine 7 mg/5 mL and potassium 0.14 mEq/5 mL; orange flavor] [DSC]
  250: Amoxicillin 250 mg and clavulanate potassium 62.5 mg per 5 mL (75 mL, 100 mL, 150 mL) [contains potassium 0.32 mEq/5 mL; orange flavor]
  400: Amoxicillin 400 mg and clavulanate potassium 57 mg per 5 mL (50 mL, 75 mL, 100 mL) [contains phenylalanine 7 mg/5 mL and potassium 0.29 mEq/5 mL; orange flavor] [DSC]
Augmentin ES-600®: Amoxicillin 600 mg and clavulanate potassium 42.9 mg per 5 mL (75 mL, 125 mL, 200 mL) [contains phenylalanine 7 mg/5 mL and potassium 0.23 mEq/5 mL; strawberry cream flavor] [DSC]

Tablet: 250: Amoxicillin 250 mg and clavulanate potassium 125 mg; 500: Amoxicillin 500 mg and clavulanate potassium 125 mg; 875: Amoxicillin 875 mg and clavulanate potassium 125 mg

Augmentin®:

250: Amoxicillin 250 mg and clavulanate potassium 125 mg [contains potassium 0.63 mEq/tablet] [DSC]

500: Amoxicillin 500 mg and clavulanate potassium 125 mg [contains potassium 0.63 mEq/tablet]

875: Amoxicillin 875 mg and clavulanate potassium 125 mg [contains potassium 0.63 mEq/tablet]

Tablet, chewable: 200: Amoxicillin 200 mg and clavulanate potassium 28.5 mg [contains phenylalanine]; 400: Amoxicillin 400 mg and clavulanate potassium 57 mg [contains phenyl-alanine]

Tablet, extended release: Amoxicillin 1000 mg and clavulanate acid 62.5 mg

Augmentin XR®: 1000: Amoxicillin 1000 mg and clavulanate acid 62.5 mg [contains potassium 12.6 mg (0.32 mEq) and sodium 29.3 mg (1.27 mEq) per tablet; packaged in either a 7-day or 10-day package]

Selected References

Ancill RJ, Ballard JH, and Capewell MA, "Urinary Tract Infections in Geriatric Inpatients: A Comparative Study of Amoxicillin-Clavulanic Acid and Co-trimoxazole," *Curr Ther Res*, 1987, 41(4):444-8.

Mandell LA, Bartlett JG, Dowell SF, et al, "Update of Practice Guidelines for the Management of Community-Acquired Pneumonia in Immunocompetent Adults," *Clin Infect Dis*, 2003, 37(11):1405-33.

◆ **Amoxicillin and Clavulanic Acid** *see* Amoxicillin and Clavulanate Potassium *on page 116*
◆ **Amoxicillin Trihydrate** *see* Amoxicillin *on page 114*
◆ **Amoxil** *see* Amoxicillin *on page 114*
◆ **Amoxycillin** *see* Amoxicillin *on page 114*
◆ **Amphadase™** *see* Hyaluronidase *on page 873*
◆ **Amphotec®** *see* Amphotericin B Cholesteryl Sulfate Complex *on page 120*

Amphotericin B Cholesteryl Sulfate Complex
(am foe TER i sin bee kole LES te ril SUL fate KOM plecks)

Medication Safety Issues
High alert medication:
The Institute for Safe Medication Practices (ISMP) includes this medication among its list of drugs which have a heightened risk of causing significant patient harm when used in error.
Other safety concerns:
Lipid-based amphotericin formulations (Amphotec®) may be confused with conventional formulations (Amphocin®, Fungizone®)
Large overdoses have occurred when conventional formulations were dispensed inadvertently for lipid-based products. Single daily doses of conventional amphotericin formulation never exceed 1.5 mg/kg.

Brand Names: U.S. Amphotec®
Brand Names: Canada Amphotec®
Index Terms ABCD; Amphotericin B Colloidal Dispersion
Generic Availability (U.S.) No
Pharmacologic Category Antifungal Agent, Parenteral
Use Treatment of invasive aspergillosis in patients who have failed amphotericin B deoxy-cholate treatment, or who have renal impairment or experience unacceptable toxicity which precludes treatment with amphotericin B deoxycholate in effective doses.
Unlabeled/Investigational Use Effective in patients with serious *Candida* species infections
Contraindications Hypersensitivity to amphotericin B or any component of the formulation
Warnings/Precautions Anaphylaxis has been reported with amphotericin B-containing drugs. If severe respiratory distress occurs, the infusion should be immediately discontinued. During the initial dosing, the drug should be administered under close clinical observation. Infusion reactions, sometimes severe, usually subside with continued therapy - manage with decreased rate of infusion and pretreatment with antihistamines/corticosteroids.
Adverse Reactions (Reflective of adult population; not specific for elderly)
>10%: Central nervous system: Chills, fever
1% to 10%:
  Cardiovascular: Hypotension, tachycardia
  Central nervous system: Headache
  Dermatologic: Rash
  Endocrine & metabolic: Hypokalemia, hypomagnesemia
  Gastrointestinal: Nausea, diarrhea, abdominal pain
  Hematologic: Thrombocytopenia
  Hepatic: LFT change

Neuromuscular & skeletal: Rigors

Renal: Creatinine increased

Respiratory: Dyspnea

Note: Amphotericin B colloidal dispersion has an improved therapeutic index compared to conventional amphotericin B, and has been used safely in patients with amphotericin B-related nephrotoxicity; however, continued decline of renal function has occurred in some patients.

Drug Interactions

Avoid Concomitant Use

Avoid concomitant use of Amphotericin B Cholesteryl Sulfate Complex with any of the following: Gallium Nitrate

Increased Effect/Toxicity

Amphotericin B Cholesteryl Sulfate Complex may increase the levels/effects of: Aminoglycosides; Colistimethate; CycloSPORINE; CycloSPORINE (Systemic); Flucytosine; Gallium Nitrate

The levels/effects of Amphotericin B Cholesteryl Sulfate Complex may be increased by: Corticosteroids (Orally Inhaled); Corticosteroids (Systemic)

Decreased Effect

Amphotericin B Cholesteryl Sulfate Complex may decrease the levels/effects of: Saccharomyces boulardii

The levels/effects of Amphotericin B Cholesteryl Sulfate Complex may be decreased by: Antifungal Agents (Azole Derivatives, Systemic)

Stability Store intact vials under refrigeration. Reconstitute 50 mg and 100 mg vials with 10 mL and 20 mL of SWI, respectively. The reconstituted vials contain 5 mg/mL of amphotericin B. Shake the vial gently by hand until all solid particles have dissolved. After reconstitution, the solution should be refrigerated at 2°C to 8°C (36°F to 46°F) and used within 24 hours. Further dilute amphotericin B colloidal dispersion with D_5W. Concentrations of 0.1-2 mg/mL in D_5W are stable for 14 days at 4°C and 23°C if protected from light, however, due to the occasional formation of subvisual particles, solutions should be used within 48 hours.

Mechanism of Action Binds to ergosterol altering cell membrane permeability in susceptible fungi and causing leakage of cell components with subsequent cell death. Proposed mechanism suggests that amphotericin causes an oxidation-dependent stimulation of macrophages (Lyman, 1992).

Pharmacodynamics/Kinetics

Distribution: V_d: Total volume increases with higher doses, reflects increasing uptake by tissues (with 4 mg/kg/day = 4 L/kg); predominantly distributed in the liver; concentrations in kidneys and other tissues are lower than observed with conventional amphotericin B

Half-life elimination: 28-29 hours; prolonged with higher doses

Dosage

Geriatric & Adult

Note: Premedication: For patients who experience chills, fever, hypotension, nausea, or other nonanaphylactic infusion-related immediate reactions, premedicate with the following drugs 30-60 minutes prior to drug administration: A nonsteroidal (eg, ibuprofen, choline magnesium trisalicylate) with or without diphenhydramine **or** acetaminophen with diphenhydramine **or** hydrocortisone 50-100 mg. If the patient experiences rigors during the infusion, meperidine may be administered.

Usual dosage: I.V.: 3-4 mg/kg/day (infusion of 1 mg/kg/hour); maximum: 7.5 mg/kg/day

A regimen of 6 mg/kg/day has been used for treatment of life-threatening invasive mold infections in immunocompromised patients; maximum: 7.5 mg/kg/day

Initially infuse at 1 mg/kg/hour. Rate of infusion may be increased with subsequent doses to 3 mg/kg/hour as patient tolerance allows. Treatment should continue as patient tolerance allows, until complete resolution of microbiologic and clinical evidence of fungal disease.

Administration Avoid injection faster than 1 mg/kg/hour. For a patient who experiences chills, fever, hypotension, nausea, or other nonanaphylactic infusion-related reactions, premedicate with the following drugs 30-60 minutes prior to drug administration: A nonsteroidal (eg, ibuprofen, choline magnesium trisalicylate) with or without diphenhydramine **or** acetaminophen with diphenhydramine **or** hydrocortisone 50-100 mg. If the patient experiences rigors during the infusion, meperidine may be administered. If severe respiratory distress occurs, the infusion should be immediately discontinued.

Monitoring Parameters Liver function tests, electrolytes, BUN, Cr, temperature, CBC, I/O, signs of hypokalemia (muscle weakness, cramping, drowsiness, ECG changes)

Pharmacotherapy Pearls Controlled trials which compare the original formulation of amphotericin B to the newer liposomal formulations (ie, Amphotec®) are lacking. Thus, comparative data discussing differences among the formulations should be interpreted cautiously. Although the risk of nephrotoxicity and infusion-related adverse effects may be less with Amphotec®, the efficacy profiles of Amphotec® and the original amphotericin formulation are comparable. Consequently, Amphotec® should be restricted to those patients who cannot tolerate or fail a standard amphotericin B formulation.

Special Geriatric Considerations The pharmacokinetics and dosing of amphotericin have not been studied in the elderly. It appears that use is similar to young adults. Caution should be exercised and renal function and desired effect monitored closely.

Dosage Forms Excipient information presented when available (limited, particularly for generics); consult specific product labeling.

Injection, powder for reconstitution:
Amphotec®: 50 mg [contains edetate disodium, lactose 950 mg]
Amphotec®: 100 mg [contains edetate disodium, lactose 1900 mg]

♦ **Amphotericin B Colloidal Dispersion** see Amphotericin B Cholesteryl Sulfate Complex on page 120

Amphotericin B (Conventional) (am foe TER i sin bee con VEN sha nal)

Medication Safety Issues

High alert medication:
The Institute for Safe Medication Practices (ISMP) includes this medication (intrathecal administration) among its list of drugs which have a heightened risk of causing significant patient harm when used in error.

Other safety concerns:
Conventional amphotericin formulations (Amphocin®, Fungizone®) may be confused with lipid-based formulations (AmBisome®, Abelcet®, Amphotec®).

Large overdoses have occurred when conventional formulations were dispensed inadvertently for lipid-based products. Single daily doses of conventional amphotericin formulation never exceed 1.5 mg/kg.

Brand Names: Canada Fungizone®

Index Terms Amphotericin B Deoxycholate; Amphotericin B Desoxycholate

Generic Availability (U.S.) Yes

Pharmacologic Category Antifungal Agent, Parenteral

Use Treatment of severe systemic and central nervous system infections caused by susceptible fungi such as *Candida* species, *Histoplasma capsulatum*, *Cryptococcus neoformans*, *Aspergillus* species, *Blastomyces dermatitidis*, *Torulopsis glabrata*, and *Coccidioides immitis*; fungal peritonitis; irrigant for bladder fungal infections; used in fungal infection in patients with bone marrow transplantation, amebic meningoencephalitis, ocular aspergillosis (intraocular injection), candidal cystitis (bladder irrigation), chemoprophylaxis (low-dose I.V.), immunocompromised patients at risk of aspergillosis (intranasal/nebulized), refractory meningitis (intrathecal), coccidioidal arthritis (intra-articular/I.M.).

Low-dose amphotericin B has been administered after bone marrow transplantation to reduce the risk of invasive fungal disease.

Contraindications Hypersensitivity to amphotericin or any component of the formulation

Warnings/Precautions Anaphylaxis has been reported with amphotericin B-containing drugs. During the initial dosing, the drug should be administered under close clinical observation. May cause nephrotoxicity; usual risk factors include underlying renal disease, concomitant nephrotoxic medications and daily and/or cumulative dose of amphotericin. Avoid use with other nephrotoxic drugs; drug-induced renal toxicity usually improves with interrupting therapy, decreasing dosage, or increasing dosing interval. However permanent impairment may occur, especially in patients receiving large cumulative dose (eg, >5 g) and in those also receiving other nephrotoxic drugs. Hydration and sodium repletion prior to administration may reduce the risk of developing nephrotoxicity. Frequent monitoring of renal function is recommended. Acute reactions (eg, fever, shaking chills, hypotension, anorexia, nausea, vomiting, headache, tachypnea) are most common 1-3 hours after starting the infusion and diminish with continued therapy. Avoid rapid infusion to prevent hypotension, hypokalemia, arrhythmias, and shock. If therapy is stopped for >7 days, restart at the lowest dose recommended and increase gradually. Leukoencephalopathy has been reported following administration of amphotericin. Total body irradiation has been reported to be a possible predisposition.

[U.S. Boxed Warning]: Should be used primarily for treatment of progressive, potentially life-threatening fungal infections, not noninvasive forms of infection. [U.S. Boxed warning]: Verify the product name and dosage if dose exceeds 1.5 mg/kg.

Adverse Reactions (Reflective of adult population; not specific for elderly)
>10%:
Central nervous system: Fever, chills, headache, malaise, generalized pain
Endocrine & metabolic: Hypokalemia, hypomagnesemia
Gastrointestinal: Anorexia
Hematologic: Anemia
Renal: Nephrotoxicity
1% to 10%:
Cardiovascular: Hypotension, hypertension, flushing
Central nervous system: Delirium, arachnoiditis, pain along lumbar nerves
Gastrointestinal: Nausea, vomiting
Genitourinary: Urinary retention
Hematologic: Leukocytosis
Local: Thrombophlebitis
Neuromuscular & skeletal: Paresthesia (especially with I.T. therapy)
Renal: Renal tubular acidosis, renal failure

Drug Interactions

Avoid Concomitant Use
Avoid concomitant use of Amphotericin B (Conventional) with any of the following: Gallium Nitrate

Increased Effect/Toxicity
Amphotericin B (Conventional) may increase the levels/effects of: Aminoglycosides; Colistimethate; CycloSPORINE; CycloSPORINE (Systemic); Flucytosine; Gallium Nitrate

The levels/effects of Amphotericin B (Conventional) may be increased by: Corticosteroids (Orally Inhaled); Corticosteroids (Systemic)

Decreased Effect
Amphotericin B (Conventional) may decrease the levels/effects of: Saccharomyces boulardii

The levels/effects of Amphotericin B (Conventional) may be decreased by: Antifungal Agents (Azole Derivatives, Systemic)

Stability Store intact vials under refrigeration. Protect from light. Add 10 mL of SWFI (without a bacteriostatic agent) to each vial of amphotericin B. Further dilute with 250-500 mL D_5W; final concentration should not exceed 0.1 mg/mL (peripheral infusion) or 0.25 mg/mL (central infusion).

Reconstituted vials are stable, protected from light, for 24 hours at room temperature and 1 week when refrigerated. Parenteral admixtures are stable, protected from light, for 24 hours at room temperature and 2 days under refrigeration. Short-term exposure (<24 hours) to light during I.V. infusion does **not** appreciably affect potency.

Mechanism of Action Binds to ergosterol altering cell membrane permeability in susceptible fungi and causing leakage of cell components with subsequent cell death. Proposed mechanism suggests that amphotericin causes an oxidation-dependent stimulation of macrophages (Lyman, 1992).

Pharmacodynamics/Kinetics
Distribution: Minimal amounts enter the aqueous humor, bile, CSF (inflamed or noninflamed meninges), amniotic fluid, pericardial fluid, pleural fluid, and synovial fluid
Protein binding, plasma: 90%
Half-life elimination: Biphasic: Initial: 15-48 hours; Terminal: 15 days
Time to peak: Within 1 hour following a 4- to 6-hour dose
Excretion: Urine (2% to 5% as biologically active form); ~40% eliminated over a 7-day period and may be detected in urine for at least 7 weeks after discontinued use

Dosage
Geriatric & Adult Note: Premedication: For patients who experience infusion-related immediate reactions, premedicate with the following drugs 30-60 minutes prior to drug administration: NSAID (with or without diphenhydramine) **or** acetaminophen with diphenhydramine **or** hydrocortisone 50-100 mg. If the patient experiences rigors during the infusion, meperidine may be administered.
Test dose: I.V.: 1 mg infused over 20-30 minutes. Many clinicians believe a test dose is unnecessary.
Susceptible fungal infections: I.V.: Adults: 0.3-1.5 mg/kg/day; 1-1.5 mg/kg over 4-6 hours every other day may be given once therapy is established; aspergillosis, rhinocerebral mucormycosis, often require 1-1.5 mg/kg/day; do not exceed 1.5 mg/kg/day
Aspergillosis, disseminated: I.V.: 0.6-0.7 mg/kg/day for 3-6 months
Bone marrow transplantation (prophylaxis): I.V.: Low-dose amphotericin B 0.1-0.25 mg/kg/day has been administered after bone marrow transplantation to reduce the risk of invasive fungal disease.

Candidemia (neutropenic or non-neutropenic): I.V.: 0.5-1 mg/kg/day until 14 days after first negative blood culture and resolution of signs and symptoms (Pappas, 2009)

Candidiasis, chronic, disseminated: I.V.: 0.5-0.7 mg/kg/day for 3-6 months and resolution of radiologic lesions (Pappas, 2009)

Dematiaceous fungi: I.V.: 0.7 mg/kg/day in combination with an azole

Endocarditis: I.V.: 0.6-1 mg/kg/day (with or without flucytosine) for 6 weeks after valve replacement; **Note:** If isolates susceptible and/or clearance demonstrated, guidelines recommend step-down to fluconazole; also for long-term suppression therapy if valve replacement is not possible (Pappas, 2009)

Endophthalmitis, fungal:
Intravitreal (unlabeled use): 10 mcg in 0.1 mL (in conjunction with systemic therapy)
I.V.: 0.7-1 mg/kg/day (with or without flucytosine) for at least 4-6 weeks (Pappas, 2009)

Esophageal candidiasis: I.V.: 0.3-0.7 mg/kg/day for 14-21 days after clinical improvement (Pappas, 2009)

Histoplasmosis: Chronic, severe pulmonary or disseminated: I.V.: 0.5-1 mg/kg/day for 7 days, then 0.8 mg/kg every other day (or 3 times/week) until total dose of 10-15 mg/kg; may continue itraconazole as suppressive therapy (lifelong for immunocompromised patients)

Meningitis:
Candidal: I.V.: 0.7-1 mg/kg/day (with or without flucytosine) for at least 4 weeks; **Note:** Liposomal amphotericin favored by IDSA guidelines based on decreased risk of nephrotoxicity and potentially better CNS penetration (Pappas, 2009)

Cryptococcal or Coccidioides: I.T.: Initial: 0.01-0.05 mg as single daily dose; may increase daily in increments of 0.025-0.1 mg as tolerated (maximum: 1.5 mg/day; most patients will tolerate a maximum dose of ~0.5 mg/treatment). Once titration to a maximum tolerated dose is achieved, that dose is administered daily. Once CSF improvement noted, may decrease frequency on a weekly basis (eg, 5 times/week, then 3 times/week, then 2 times/week, then once weekly, then once every other week, then once every 2 weeks, etc) until administration occurs once every 6 weeks. Typically, concurrent oral azole therapy is maintained (Stevens, 2001). **Note:** IDSA notes that the use of I.T. amphotericin for cryptococcal meningitis is generally discouraged and rarely necessary (Perfect, 2010).

Histoplasma: I.V.: 0.5-1 mg/kg/day for 7 days, then 0.8 mg/kg every other day (or 3 times/week) for 3 months total duration; follow with fluconazole suppressive therapy for up to 12 months

Meningoencephalitis, cryptococcal (Perfect, 2010): I.V.:
HIV positive: Induction: 0.7-1 mg/kg/day (plus flucytosine 100 mg/kg/day) for 2 weeks, then change to oral fluconazole for at least 8 weeks; alternatively, amphotericin (0.7-1 mg/kg/day) may be continued uninterrupted for 4-6 weeks; maintenance: amphotericin 1 mg/kg/week for ≥1 year may be considered, but inferior to use of azoles

HIV negative: Induction: 0.7-1 mg/kg/day (plus flucytosine 100 mg/kg/day) for 2 weeks (low-risk patients), ≥4 weeks (non-low-risk, but without neurologic complication, immunosuppression, underlying disease, and negative CSF culture at 2 weeks), >6 weeks (neurologic complication or patients intolerant of flucytosine) Follow with azole consolidation/maintenance treatment.

Oropharyngeal candidiasis: I.V.: 0.3 mg/kg/day for 7-14 days (Pappas, 2009)

Osteoarticular candidiasis: I.V.: 0.5-1 mg/kg/day for several weeks, followed by fluconazole for 6-12 months (osteomyelitis) or 6 weeks (septic arthritis) (Pappas, 2009)

Penicillium marneffei: I.V.: 0.6 mg/kg/day for 2 weeks

Pneumonia: Cryptococcal (mild-to-moderate): I.V.:
HIV positive: 0.5-1 mg/kg/day
HIV negative: 0.5-0.7 mg/kg/day (plus flucytosine) for 2 weeks

Sporotrichosis: Pulmonary, meningeal, osteoarticular or disseminated: I.V.: Total dose of 1-2 g, then change to oral itraconazole or fluconazole for suppressive therapy

Urinary tract candidiasis (Pappas, 2009):
Fungus balls: I.V.: 0.5-0.7 mg/kg/day with or without flucytosine 25 mg/kg 4 times daily
Pyelonephritis: I.V.: 0.5-0.7 mg/kg/day with or without flucytosine 25 mg/kg 4 times daily for 2 weeks
Symptomatic cystitis: I.V.: 0.3-0.6 mg/kg/day for 1-7 days
Bladder irrigation: Irrigate with 50 mcg/mL solution instilled periodically or continuously for 5-10 days or until cultures are clear for fluconazole-resistant *Candida*

Renal Impairment
If renal dysfunction is due to the drug, the daily total can be decreased by 50% or the dose can be given every other day. I.V. therapy may take several months.
Renal replacement therapy: Poorly dialyzed; no supplemental dose or dosage adjustment necessary, including patients on intermittent hemodialysis or CRRT.

Peritoneal dialysis (PD): Administration in dialysate: 1-2 mg/L of peritoneal dialysis fluid either with or without low-dose I.V. amphotericin B (a total dose of 2-10 mg/kg given over 7-14 days). Precipitate may form in ionic dialysate solutions.

Administration May be infused over 4-6 hours. For a patient who experiences chills, fever, hypotension, nausea, or other nonanaphylactic infusion-related reactions, premedicate with the following drugs 30-60 minutes prior to drug administration: A nonsteroidal (eg, ibuprofen, choline magnesium trisalicylate) with or without diphenhydramine **or** acetaminophen with diphenhydramine **or** hydrocortisone 50-100 mg. If the patient experiences rigors during the infusion, meperidine may be administered. Bolus infusion of normal saline immediately preceding, or immediately preceding and following amphotericin B may reduce drug-induced nephrotoxicity. Risk of nephrotoxicity increases with amphotericin B doses >1 mg/kg/day. Infusion of admixtures more concentrated than 0.25 mg/mL should be limited to patients absolutely requiring volume contraction.

Monitoring Parameters Renal function (monitor frequently during therapy), electrolytes (especially potassium and magnesium), liver function tests, temperature, PT/PTT, CBC; monitor input and output; monitor for signs of hypokalemia (muscle weakness, cramping, drowsiness, ECG changes, etc)

Reference Range Therapeutic: 1-2 mcg/mL (SI: 1-2.2 µmol/L)

Test Interactions Increased BUN (S), serum creatinine, alkaline phosphate, bilirubin; decreased magnesium, potassium (S)

Pharmacotherapy Pearls Premedication with diphenhydramine and acetaminophen may reduce the severity of acute infusion-related reactions. Meperidine reduces the duration of amphotericin B-induced rigors and chilling. Hydrocortisone may be used in patients with severe or refractory infusion-related reactions. Bolus infusion of normal saline immediately preceding, or immediately preceding and following amphotericin B may reduce drug-induced nephrotoxicity. Risk of nephrotoxicity increases with amphotericin B doses >1 mg/kg/day. Infusion of admixtures more concentrated than 0.25 mg/mL should be limited to patients absolutely requiring volume restriction. Amphotericin B does not have a bacteriostatic constituent, subsequently admixture expiration is determined by sterility more than chemical stability.

Special Geriatric Considerations The pharmacokinetics and dosing of amphotericin have not been studied in elderly. It appears that use is similar to young adults; caution should be exercised and renal function and desired effect monitored closely.

Dosage Forms Excipient information presented when available (limited, particularly for generics); consult specific product labeling.

Injection, powder for reconstitution, as desoxycholate: 50 mg

♦ **Amphotericin B Deoxycholate** *see* Amphotericin B (Conventional) *on page 122*
♦ **Amphotericin B Desoxycholate** *see* Amphotericin B (Conventional) *on page 122*

Amphotericin B (Lipid Complex) (am foe TER i sin bee LIP id KOM pleks)

Medication Safety Issues
  High alert medication:
    The Institute for Safe Medication Practices (ISMP) includes this medication among its list of drugs which have a heightened risk of causing significant patient harm when used in error.
  Other safety concerns:
    Lipid-based amphotericin formulations (Abelcet®) may be confused with conventional formulations (Amphocin®, Fungizone®)
    Large overdoses have occurred when conventional formulations were dispensed inadvertently for lipid-based products. Single daily doses of conventional amphotericin formulation never exceed 1.5 mg/kg.

Brand Names: U.S. Abelcet®
Brand Names: Canada Abelcet®
Index Terms ABLC
Generic Availability (U.S.) No
Pharmacologic Category Antifungal Agent, Parenteral
Use Treatment of aspergillosis or any type of progressive fungal infection in patients who are refractory to or intolerant of conventional amphotericin B therapy
Unlabeled/Investigational Use Effective in patients with serious *Candida* species infections
Contraindications Hypersensitivity to amphotericin or any component of the formulation
Warnings/Precautions Anaphylaxis has been reported with amphotericin B-containing drugs. If severe respiratory distress occurs, the infusion should be immediately discontinued. During the initial dosing, the drug should be administered under close clinical observation. Acute reactions (including fever and chills) may occur 1-2 hours after starting an intravenous infusion. These reactions are usually more common with the first few doses and generally diminish with subsequent doses.

◄ **Adverse Reactions (Reflective of adult population; not specific for elderly)** Nephrotoxicity and infusion-related hyperpyrexia, rigor, and chilling are reduced relative to amphotericin deoxycholate.

>10%:
  Central nervous system: Chills, fever
  Renal: Serum creatinine increased
  Miscellaneous: Multiple organ failure
1% to 10%:
  Cardiovascular: Hypotension, cardiac arrest
  Central nervous system: Headache, pain
  Dermatologic: Rash
  Endocrine & metabolic: Bilirubinemia, hypokalemia, acidosis
  Gastrointestinal: Nausea, vomiting, diarrhea, gastrointestinal hemorrhage, abdominal pain
  Renal: Renal failure
  Respiratory: Respiratory failure, dyspnea, pneumonia

Drug Interactions
  Avoid Concomitant Use
    Avoid concomitant use of Amphotericin B (Lipid Complex) with any of the following: Gallium Nitrate
  Increased Effect/Toxicity
    Amphotericin B (Lipid Complex) may increase the levels/effects of: Aminoglycosides; Colistimethate; CycloSPORINE; CycloSPORINE (Systemic); Flucytosine; Gallium Nitrate

    The levels/effects of Amphotericin B (Lipid Complex) may be increased by: Corticosteroids (Orally Inhaled); Corticosteroids (Systemic)
  Decreased Effect
    Amphotericin B (Lipid Complex) may decrease the levels/effects of: Saccharomyces boulardii

    The levels/effects of Amphotericin B (Lipid Complex) may be decreased by: Antifungal Agents (Azole Derivatives, Systemic)

Stability Intact vials should be stored at 2°C to 8°C (35°F to 46°F); do not freeze. Protect intact vials from exposure to light. Solutions for infusion are stable for 48 hours under refrigeration and for 6 hours at room temperature. Shake the vial gently until there is no evidence of any yellow sediment at the bottom. Dilute with D_5W to 1-2 mg/mL. Protect from light.
  Do not dilute with saline solutions or mix with other drugs or electrolytes - compatibility has not been established
  Do not use an in-line filter during administration.

Mechanism of Action Binds to ergosterol altering cell membrane permeability in susceptible fungi and causing leakage of cell components with subsequent cell death. Proposed mechanism suggests that amphotericin causes an oxidation-dependent stimulation of macrophages.

Pharmacodynamics/Kinetics
  Distribution: V_d: Increases with higher doses; reflects increased uptake by tissues (131 L/kg with 5 mg/kg/day)
  Half-life elimination: ~24 hours
  Excretion: Clearance: Increases with higher doses (5 mg/kg/day): 400 mL/hour/kg

Dosage
  Geriatric & Adult Note: Premedication: For patients who experience infusion-related immediate reactions, premedicate with the following drugs 30-60 minutes prior to drug administration: A nonsteroidal anti-inflammatory agent ± diphenhydramine **or** acetaminophen with diphenhydramine **or** hydrocortisone 50-100 mg. If the patient experiences rigors during the infusion, meperidine may be administered.

    Usual dosage range: I.V.: 2.5-5 mg/kg/day as a single infusion
  Renal Impairment The effects of renal impairment on drug pharmacokinetics or pharmacodynamics are currently unknown. The dose of amphotericin B lipid complex may be adjusted or drug administration may have to be interrupted in patients with acute kidney dysfunction to reduce the magnitude of renal impairment.

    Hemodialysis: Supplemental dose is not necessary.
    Peritoneal dialysis: Supplemental dose is not necessary.
    Continuous renal replacement therapy (CRRT): No supplemental dosage necessary
  Administration For patients who experience nonanaphylactic infusion-related reactions, premedicate 30-60 minutes prior to drug administration with a nonsteroidal anti-inflammatory agent ± diphenhydramine **or** acetaminophen with diphenhydramine **or** hydrocortisone 50-100 mg. If the patient experiences rigors during the infusion, meperidine may be administered.

Administer at an infusion rate of 2.5 mg/kg/hour (over 2 hours). Invert infusion container several times prior to administration and every 2 hours during infusion if it exceeds 2 hours.

Monitoring Parameters Renal function (monitor frequently during therapy), electrolytes (especially potassium and magnesium), liver function tests, temperature, PT/PTT, CBC; monitor input and output; monitor for signs of hypokalemia (muscle weakness, cramping, drowsiness, ECG changes, etc)

Test Interactions Increased BUN (S), serum creatinine, alkaline phosphate, bilirubin; decreased magnesium, potassium (S)

Pharmacotherapy Pearls As a modification of dimyristoyl phosphatidylcholine:dimyristoyl phosphatidylglycerol 7:3 (DMPC:DMPG) liposome, amphotericin B lipid-complex has a higher drug to lipid ratio and the concentration of amphotericin B is 33 M. ABLC is a ribbon-like structure, not a liposome.

Controlled trials which compare the original formulation of amphotericin B to the newer liposomal formulations (ie, Abelcet®) are lacking. Thus, comparative data discussing differences among the formulations should be interpreted cautiously. Although the risk of nephrotoxicity and infusion-related adverse effects may be less with Abelcet®, the efficacy profiles of Abelcet® and the original amphotericin formulation are comparable. Consequently, Abelcet® should be restricted to those patients who cannot tolerate or fail a standard amphotericin B formulation.

Special Geriatric Considerations The pharmacokinetics and dosing of amphotericin have not been studied in elderly. It appears that use is similar to young adults; caution should be exercised and renal function and desired effect monitored closely.

Dosage Forms Excipient information presented when available (limited, particularly for generics); consult specific product labeling.
Injection, suspension [preservative free]:
Abelcet®: 5 mg/mL (20 mL)

Ampicillin (am pi SIL in)

Related Information
Antibiotic Treatment of Adults With Infective Endocarditis *on page 2053*
Prevention of Infective Endocarditis *on page 2064*
Medication Safety Issues
Sound-alike/look-alike issues:
Ampicillin may be confused with aminophylline
Brand Names: Canada Apo-Ampi®; Novo-Ampicillin; Nu-Ampi
Index Terms Aminobenzylpenicillin; Ampicillin Sodium; Ampicillin Trihydrate
Generic Availability (U.S.) Yes
Pharmacologic Category Antibiotic, Penicillin

Use Treatment of susceptible bacterial infections (nonbeta-lactamase-producing organisms); treatment or prophylaxis of infective endocarditis; susceptible bacterial infections caused by streptococci, pneumococci, nonpenicillinase-producing staphylococci, *Listeria*, meningococci; some strains of *H. influenzae*, *Salmonella*, *Shigella*, *E. coli*, *Enterobacter*, and *Klebsiella*

Contraindications Hypersensitivity to ampicillin, any component of the formulation, or other penicillins

Warnings/Precautions Dosage adjustment may be necessary in patients with renal impairment. Serious and occasionally severe or fatal hypersensitivity (anaphylactoid) reactions have been reported in patients on penicillin therapy, especially with a history of beta-lactam hypersensitivity, history of sensitivity to multiple allergens, or previous IgE-mediated reactions (eg, anaphylaxis, angioedema, urticaria). Use with caution in asthmatic patients. High percentage of patients with infectious mononucleosis have developed rash during therapy with ampicillin; ampicillin-class antibiotics not recommended in these patients. Appearance of a rash should be carefully evaluated to differentiate a nonallergic ampicillin rash from a hypersensitivity reaction. Ampicillin rash occurs in 5% to 10% of children receiving ampicillin and is a generalized dull red, maculopapular rash, generally appearing 3-14 days after the start of therapy. It normally begins on the trunk and spreads over most of the body. It may be most intense at pressure areas, elbows, and knees. Prolonged use may result in fungal or bacterial superinfection, including *C. difficile*-associated diarrhea (CDAD) and pseudomembranous colitis; CDAD has been observed >2 months postantibiotic treatment.

Adverse Reactions (Reflective of adult population; not specific for elderly) Frequency not defined.
Central nervous system: Fever, penicillin encephalopathy, seizure
Dermatologic: Erythema multiforme, exfoliative dermatitis, rash, urticaria
Note: Appearance of a rash should be carefully evaluated to differentiate (if possible) nonallergic ampicillin rash from hypersensitivity reaction. Incidence is higher in patients ▶

with viral infection, *Salmonella* infection, lymphocytic leukemia, or patients that have hyperuricemia.

Gastrointestinal: Black hairy tongue, diarrhea, enterocolitis, glossitis, nausea, oral candidiasis, pseudomembranous colitis, sore mouth or tongue, stomatitis, vomiting

Hematologic: Agranulocytosis, anemia, hemolytic anemia, eosinophilia, leukopenia, thrombocytopenia purpura

Hepatic: AST increased

Renal: Interstitial nephritis (rare)

Respiratory: Laryngeal stridor

Miscellaneous: Anaphylaxis, serum sickness-like reaction

Drug Interactions

Avoid Concomitant Use

Avoid concomitant use of Ampicillin with any of the following: BCG

Increased Effect/Toxicity

Ampicillin may increase the levels/effects of: Methotrexate

The levels/effects of Ampicillin may be increased by: Allopurinol; Probenecid

Decreased Effect

Ampicillin may decrease the levels/effects of: Atenolol; BCG; Mycophenolate; Typhoid Vaccine

The levels/effects of Ampicillin may be decreased by: Chloroquine; Fusidic Acid; Lanthanum; Tetracycline Derivatives

Ethanol/Nutrition/Herb Interactions Food: Food decreases ampicillin absorption rate; may decrease ampicillin serum concentration.

Stability

Oral: Oral suspension is stable for 7 days at room temperature or for 14 days under refrigeration.

I.V.:

I.V. minimum volume: Concentration should not exceed 30 mg/mL due to concentration-dependent stability restrictions. Solutions for I.M. or direct I.V. should be used within 1 hour. Solutions for I.V. infusion will be inactivated by dextrose at room temperature. If dextrose-containing solutions are to be used, the resultant solution will only be stable for 2 hours versus 8 hours in the 0.9% sodium chloride injection. D_5W has limited stability.

Stability of parenteral admixture in NS at room temperature (25°C) is 8 hours.

Stability of parenteral admixture in NS at refrigeration temperature (4°C) is 2 days.

Standard diluent: 500 mg/50 mL NS; 1 g/50 mL NS; 2 g/100 mL NS

Mechanism of Action Inhibits bacterial cell wall synthesis by binding to one or more of the penicillin-binding proteins (PBPs) which in turn inhibits the final transpeptidation step of peptidoglycan synthesis in bacterial cell walls, thus inhibiting cell wall biosynthesis. Bacteria eventually lyse due to ongoing activity of cell wall autolytic enzymes (autolysins and murein hydrolases) while cell wall assembly is arrested.

Pharmacodynamics/Kinetics

Absorption: Oral: 50%

Distribution: Bile, blister, and tissue fluids; penetration into CSF occurs with inflamed meninges only, good only with inflammation (exceeds usual MICs)

Normal meninges: Nil; Inflamed meninges: 5% to 10%

Protein binding: 15% to 25%

Half-life elimination:

Adults: 1-1.8 hours

Anuria/end-stage renal disease: 7-20 hours

Time to peak: Oral: Within 1-2 hours

Excretion: Urine (~90% as unchanged drug) within 24 hours

Dosage

Geriatric Administer usual adult dose unless renal function is markedly reduced.

Adult

Usual dosage range:

Oral: 250-500 mg every 6 hours

I.M., I.V.: 250-500 mg every 6 hours

Actinomycosis: I.V.: 50 mg/kg/day for 4-6 weeks then oral amoxicillin

Cholangitis (acute): I.V.: 2 g every 4 hours with gentamicin

Diverticulitis: I.M., I.V.: 2 g every 6 hours with metronidazole

Endocarditis:

Infective: I.V.: 12 g/day via continuous infusion or divided every 4 hours

Prophylaxis: Dental, oral, or respiratory tract procedures: I.M., I.V.: 2 g within 30-60 minutes prior to procedure in patients not allergic to penicillin and unable to take oral amoxicillin. Intramuscular injections should be avoided in patients who are receiving anticoagulant therapy. In these circumstances, orally administered regimens should be given whenever possible. Intravenously administered antibiotics should be used for patients who are unable to tolerate or absorb oral medications. **Note:** American Heart Association (AHA) guidelines now recommend prophylaxis only in patients undergoing invasive procedures and in whom underlying cardiac conditions may predispose to a higher risk of adverse outcomes should infection occur.

Prophylaxis in total joint replacement patient: I.M., I.V.: 2 g 1 hour prior to the procedure

Genitourinary and gastrointestinal tract procedures: I.M., I.V.:

High-risk patients: 2 g within 30 minutes prior to procedure, followed by ampicillin 1 g (or amoxicillin 1 g orally) 6 hours later; must be used in combination with gentamicin. **Note:** As of April 2007, routine prophylaxis for GI/GU procedures is no longer recommended by the AHA.

Moderate-risk patients: 2 g within 30 minutes prior to procedure

Group B strep prophylaxis (intrapartum): I.V.: 2 g initial dose, then 1 g every 4 hours until delivery

Listeria **infections:** I.V.: 2 g every 4 hours (consider addition of aminoglycoside)

Sepsis/meningitis: I.M., I.V.: 150-250 mg/kg/day divided every 3-4 hours (range: 6-12 g/day)

Urinary tract infections (*Enterococcus* suspected): I.V.: 1-2 g every 6 hours with gentamicin

Renal Impairment

Cl_{cr} >50 mL/minute: Administer every 6 hours

Cl_{cr} 10-50 mL/minute: Administer every 6-12 hours

Cl_{cr} <10 mL/minute: Administer every 12-24 hours

Intermittent hemodialysis (IHD) (administer after hemodialysis on dialysis days): Dialyzable (20% to 50%): I.V.: 1-2 g every 12-24 hours (Heintz, 2009). **Note:** Dosing dependent on the assumption of 3 times/week, complete IHD sessions.

Peritoneal dialysis (PD): 250 mg every 12 hours

Continuous renal replacement therapy (CRRT) (Heintz, 2009): Drug clearance is highly dependent on the method of renal replacement, filter type, and flow rate. Appropriate dosing requires close monitoring of pharmacologic response, signs of adverse reactions due to drug accumulation, as well as drug concentrations in relation to target trough (if appropriate). The following are general recommendations only (based on dialysate flow/ultrafiltration rates of 1-2 L/hour and minimal residual renal function) and should not supersede clinical judgment:

CVVH: Loading dose of 2 g followed by 1-2 g every 8-12 hours

CVVHD: Loading dose of 2 g followed by 1-2 g every 8 hours

CVVHDF: Loading dose of 2 g followed by 1-2 g every 6-8 hours

Administration Administer around-the-clock to promote less variation in peak and trough serum levels.

Oral: Administer on an empty stomach (ie, 1 hour prior to, or 2 hours after meals) to increase total absorption.

I.V.: Administer over 3-5 minutes (125-500 mg) or over 10-15 minutes (1-2 g). More rapid infusion may cause seizures. Ampicillin and gentamicin should not be mixed in the same I.V. tubing.

Some penicillins (eg, carbenicillin, ticarcillin, and piperacillin) have been shown to inactivate aminoglycosides *in vitro*. This has been observed to a greater extent with tobramycin and gentamicin, while amikacin has shown greater stability against inactivation. Concurrent use of these agents may pose a risk of reduced antibacterial efficacy *in vivo*, particularly in the setting of profound renal impairment. However, definitive clinical evidence is lacking. If combination penicillin/aminoglycoside therapy is desired in a patient with renal dysfunction, separation of doses (if feasible), and routine monitoring of aminoglycoside levels, CBC, and clinical response should be considered.

Monitoring Parameters With prolonged therapy, monitor renal, hepatic, and hematologic function periodically; observe signs and symptoms of anaphylaxis during first dose

Test Interactions May interfere with urinary glucose tests using cupric sulfate (Benedict's solution, Clinitest®)

Some penicillin derivatives may accelerate the degradation of aminoglycosides *in vitro*, leading to a potential underestimation of aminoglycoside serum concentration.

Pharmacotherapy Pearls Appearance of a rash should be carefully evaluated to differentiate a nonallergic ampicillin rash from a hypersensitivity reaction; ampicillin rash is dull red, macular or maculopapular, and only mildly pruritic; normally appears on pressure areas like knees, elbows, palms, or soles, and may spread in symmetric pattern over most of the body; incidence of ampicillin rash is higher in patients with viral infections, *Salmonella* infections, lymphocytic leukemia, or patients that have hyperuricemia.

Special Geriatric Considerations Adjust dose for renal function.

◀ **Dosage Forms** Excipient information presented when available (limited, particularly for generics); consult specific product labeling.

Capsule, oral: 250 mg, 500 mg

Injection, powder for reconstitution, as sodium [strength expressed as base]: 125 mg, 250 mg, 500 mg, 1 g, 2 g, 10 g

Powder for suspension, oral: 125 mg/5 mL (100 mL, 200 mL); 250 mg/5 mL (100 mL, 200 mL)

Selected References

Triggs EJ, Johnson JM, and Learoyd B, "Absorption and Disposition of Ampicillin in the Elderly," *Eur J Clin Pharmacol*, 1980, 18(2):195-8.

Ampicillin and Sulbactam (am pi SIL in & SUL bak tam)

Related Information

Ampicillin *on page 127*

Community-Acquired Pneumonia in Adults *on page 2059*

Brand Names: U.S. Unasyn®

Brand Names: Canada Unasyn®

Index Terms Sulbactam and Ampicillin

Generic Availability (U.S.) Yes

Pharmacologic Category Antibiotic, Penicillin

Use Treatment of susceptible bacterial infections involved with skin and skin structure, intra-abdominal infections, gynecological infections; spectrum is that of ampicillin plus organisms producing beta-lactamases such as *S. aureus*, *H. influenzae*, *E. coli*, *Klebsiella*, *Acinetobacter*, *Enterobacter*, and anaerobes

Contraindications Hypersensitivity to ampicillin, sulbactam, penicillins, or any component of the formulations

Warnings/Precautions Dosage adjustment may be necessary in patients with renal impairment. Serious and occasionally severe or fatal hypersensitivity (anaphylactoid) reactions have been reported in patients on penicillin therapy, especially with a history of beta-lactam hypersensitivity, history of sensitivity to multiple allergens, or previous IgE-mediated reactions (eg, anaphylaxis, angioedema, urticaria). Use with caution in asthmatic patients. High percentage of patients with infectious mononucleosis have developed rash during therapy with ampicillin; ampicillin-class antibiotics not recommended in these patients. Appearance of a rash should be carefully evaluated to differentiate a nonallergic ampicillin rash from a hypersensitivity reaction. Prolonged use may result in fungal or bacterial superinfection, including *C. difficile*-associated diarrhea (CDAD) and pseudomembranous colitis; CDAD has been observed >2 months postantibiotic treatment.

Adverse Reactions (Reflective of adult population; not specific for elderly) Also see Ampicillin.

>10%: Local: Pain at injection site (I.M.)

1% to 10%:

Dermatologic: Rash

Gastrointestinal: Diarrhea

Local: Pain at injection site (I.V.), thrombophlebitis

Miscellaneous: Allergic reaction (may include serum sickness, urticaria, bronchospasm, hypotension, etc)

Drug Interactions

Avoid Concomitant Use

Avoid concomitant use of Ampicillin and Sulbactam with any of the following: BCG

Increased Effect/Toxicity

Ampicillin and Sulbactam may increase the levels/effects of: Methotrexate

The levels/effects of Ampicillin and Sulbactam may be increased by: Allopurinol; Probenecid

Decreased Effect

Ampicillin and Sulbactam may decrease the levels/effects of: Atenolol; BCG; Mycophenolate; Typhoid Vaccine

The levels/effects of Ampicillin and Sulbactam may be decreased by: Chloroquine; Fusidic Acid; Lanthanum; Tetracycline Derivatives

Stability Prior to reconstitution, store at ≤30°C (86°F).

I.M. and direct I.V. administration: Use within 1 hour after preparation. Reconstitute with sterile water for injection or 0.5% or 2% lidocaine hydrochloride injection (I.M.). Sodium chloride 0.9% (NS) is the diluent of choice for I.V. piggyback use. Solutions made in NS are stable up to 72 hours when refrigerated whereas dextrose solutions (same concentration) are stable for only 4 hours.

Mechanism of Action The addition of sulbactam, a beta-lactamase inhibitor, to ampicillin extends the spectrum of ampicillin to include some beta-lactamase-producing organisms; inhibits bacterial cell wall synthesis by binding to one or more of the penicillin-binding proteins (PBPs) which in turn inhibits the final transpeptidation step of peptidoglycan synthesis in bacterial cell walls, thus inhibiting cell wall biosynthesis. Bacteria eventually lyse due to ongoing activity of cell wall autolytic enzymes (autolysins and murein hydrolases) while cell wall assembly is arrested.

Pharmacodynamics/Kinetics

Ampicillin: See Ampicillin.

Sulbactam:

Distribution: Bile, blister, and tissue fluids

Protein binding: 38%

Half-life elimination: Normal renal function: 1-1.3 hours

Excretion: Urine (~75% to 85% as unchanged drug) within 8 hours

Dosage

Geriatric & Adult Doses expressed as ampicillin/sulbactam combination.

Susceptible infections: I.M., I.V.: 1.5-3 g every 6 hours (maximum: Unasyn® 12 g)

Amnionitis, cholangitis, diverticulitis, endometritis, endophthalmitis, epididymitis/ orchitis, liver abscess, osteomyelitis (diabetic foot), peritonitis: I.V.: 3 g every 6 hours; **Note:** Due to high rates of *E. coli* resistance, not recommended for the treatment of community-acquired intra-abdominal infections (Solomkin, 2010)

Endocarditis: I.V.: 3 g every 6 hours with gentamicin or vancomycin for 4-6 weeks

Orbital cellulitis: I.V.: 1.5 g every 6 hours

Parapharyngeal space infections: I.V.: 3 g every 6 hours

***Pasteurella multocida* (human, canine/feline bites):** I.V.: 1.5-3 g every 6 hours

Pelvic inflammatory disease: I.V.: 3 g every 6 hours with doxycycline

Peritonitis (CAPD): Intraperitoneal:

Anuric, intermittent: 3 g every 12 hours

Anuric, continuous: Loading dose: 1.5 g; maintenance dose: 150 mg

Pneumonia:

Aspiration, community-acquired: I.V.: 1.5-3 g every 6 hours

Hospital-acquired: I.V.: 3 g every 6 hours

Urinary tract infections, pyelonephritis: I.V.: 3 g every 6 hours for 14 days

Renal Impairment Note: Estimation of renal function for the purpose of drug dosing should be done using the Cockcroft-Gault formula.

Cl_{cr} 15-29 mL/minute/1.73 m^2: 1.5-3 g every 12 hours

Cl_{cr} 5-14 mL/minute/1.73 m^2: 1.5-3 g every 24 hours

Intermittent hemodialysis (IHD) (administer after hemodialysis on dialysis days): 1.5-3 g every 12-24 hours (Heintz, 2009). **Note:** Dosing dependent on the assumption of 3 times/ week, complete IHD sessions.

Peritoneal dialysis (PD): 3 g every 24 hours

Continuous renal replacement therapy (CRRT): Drug clearance is highly dependent on the method of renal replacement, filter type, and flow rate. Appropriate dosing requires close monitoring of pharmacologic response, signs of adverse reactions due to drug accumulation, as well as drug levels in relation to target trough (if appropriate). The following are general recommendations only (based on dialysate flow/ultrafiltration rates of 1-2 L/hour and minimal residual renal function) and should not supersede clinical judgment (Heintz, 2009; Trotman, 2005):

CVVH: Initial: 3 g; maintenance: 1.5-3 g every 8-12 hours

CVVHD: Initial: 3 g; maintenance: 1.5-3 g every 8 hours

CVVHDF: Initial: 3 g; maintenance: 1.5-3 g every 6-8 hours

Administration Administer around-the-clock to promote less variation in peak and trough serum levels. Administer by slow injection over 10-15 minutes or I.V. over 15-30 minutes. Ampicillin and gentamicin should not be mixed in the same I.V. tubing.

Some penicillins (eg, carbenicillin, ticarcillin, and piperacillin) have been shown to inactivate aminoglycosides *in vitro*. This has been observed to a greater extent with tobramycin and gentamicin, while amikacin has shown greater stability against inactivation. Concurrent use of these agents may pose a risk of reduced antibacterial efficacy *in vivo*, particularly in the setting of profound renal impairment. However, definitive clinical evidence is lacking. If combination penicillin/aminoglycoside therapy is desired in a patient with renal dysfunction, separation of doses (if feasible), and routine monitoring of aminoglycoside levels, CBC, and clinical response should be considered.

Monitoring Parameters With prolonged therapy, monitor hematologic, renal, and hepatic function; monitor for signs of anaphylaxis during first dose

◀ **Test Interactions** May interfere with urinary glucose tests using cupric sulfate (Benedict's solution, Clinitest®).

Some penicillin derivatives may accelerate the degradation of aminoglycosides *in vitro*, leading to a potential underestimation of aminoglycoside serum concentration.

Special Geriatric Considerations Adjust dose for renal function.

Dosage Forms Excipient information presented when available (limited, particularly for generics); consult specific product labeling.

Injection, powder for reconstitution: 1.5 g: Ampicillin 1 g and sulbactam 0.5 g; 3 g: Ampicillin 2 g and sulbactam 1 g; 15 g: Ampicillin 10 g and sulbactam 5 g

Unasyn®:

1.5 g: Ampicillin 1 g and sulbactam 0.5 g [contains sodium 115 mg (5 mEq)/1.5 g)]

3 g: Ampicillin 2 g and sulbactam 1 g [contains sodium 115 mg (5 mEq)/1.5 g)]

15 g: Ampicillin 10 g and sulbactam 5 g [bulk package; contains sodium 115 mg (5 mEq)/1.5 g)]

Selected References

Mandell LA, Wunderink RG, Anzueto A, et al, "Infectious Diseases Society of America/American Thoracic Society Consensus Guidelines on the Management of Community-Acquired Pneumonia in Adults," *Clin Infect Dis*, 2007, 44 Suppl 2:S27-72.

Meyers BR, Wilkinson P, Mendelson MH, et al, "Pharmacokinetics of Ampicillin-Sulbactam in Healthy Elderly and Young Volunteers," *Antimicrob Agents Chemother*, 1991, 35(10):2098-101.

Rho SP, Jones A, Woo M, et al, "Single Dose Pharmacokinetics of Intravenous Ampicillin plus Sulbactam in Healthy Elderly and Young Subjects," *J Antimicrob Chemother*, 1989, 24(4):573-80.

◆ **Ampicillin Sodium** *see* Ampicillin *on page* 127
◆ **Ampicillin Trihydrate** *see* Ampicillin *on page* 127
◆ **Ampyra™** *see* Dalfampridine *on page* 444
◆ **Amrinone Lactate** *see* Inamrinone *on page* 928
◆ **Amrix®** *see* Cyclobenzaprine *on page* 426
◆ **Amturnide™** *see* Aliskiren, Amlodipine, and Hydrochlorothiazide *on page* 60
◆ **Amylase, Lipase, and Protease** *see* Pancrelipase *on page* 1387
◆ **Anafranil®** *see* ClomiPRAMINE *on page* 383

Anakinra (an a KIN ra)

Medication Safety Issues
  Sound-alike/look-alike issues:
    Anakinra may be confused with amikacin, Ampyra™
    Kineret® may be confused with Amikin®
Brand Names: U.S. Kineret®
Brand Names: Canada Kineret®
Index Terms IL-1Ra; Interleukin-1 Receptor Antagonist
Generic Availability (U.S.) No
Pharmacologic Category Antirheumatic, Disease Modifying; Interleukin-1 Receptor Antagonist
Use Treatment of moderately- to severely-active rheumatoid arthritis in adult patients who have failed one or more disease-modifying antirheumatic drugs (DMARDs); may be used alone or in combination with DMARDs (other than tumor necrosis factor-blocking agents)
Contraindications Hypersensitivity to *E. coli*-derived proteins, anakinra, or any component of the formulation; patients with active infections (including chronic or local infection)
Warnings/Precautions Anakinra may affect defenses against infections and malignancies. Safety and efficacy in patients with immunosuppression or chronic infections have not been evaluated. Discontinue administration if patient develops a serious infection. Do not start drug administration in patients with an active infection. Patients with asthma may be at an increased risk of serious infections. Should not be used in combination with tumor necrosis factor antagonists, unless no satisfactory alternatives exist, and then only with extreme caution. Impact on the development and course of malignancies is not fully defined. As compared to the general population, an increased risk of lymphoma has been noted in clinical trials; however, rheumatoid arthritis has been previously associated with an increased rate of lymphoma.

Use caution in patients with a history of significant hematologic abnormalities; has been associated with uncommon, but significant decreases in hematologic parameters (particularly neutrophil counts). Patients must be advised to seek medical attention if they develop signs and symptoms suggestive of blood dyscrasias. Discontinue if significant hematologic abnormalities are confirmed.

Patients should be brought up to date with all immunizations before initiating therapy. Live vaccines should not be given concurrently. Patients with a significant exposure to varicella virus should temporarily discontinue anakinra. Hypersensitivity reactions may occur. Impact on the development and course of malignancies is not fully defined. Use caution in patients with renal impairment; consider increased dosing intervals for severe renal dysfunction (Cl_{cr} <30 mL/minute). Use caution in the elderly due to the potential for higher risk of infections. The packaging (needle cover) contains latex.

Adverse Reactions (Reflective of adult population; not specific for elderly)

>10%:

Central nervous system: Headache (12%)

Local: Injection site reaction (majority mild, typically lasting 14-28 days, characterized by erythema, ecchymosis, inflammation, and pain; up to 71%)

Miscellaneous: Infection (39% versus 37% in placebo; serious infection 2% to 3%)

1% to 10%:

Gastrointestinal: Nausea (8%), diarrhea (7%), abdominal pain (5%)

Hematologic: Neutropenia (8%; grades 3/4: 0.4%)

Respiratory: Sinusitis (7%)

Miscellaneous: Flu-like syndrome (6%)

Drug Interactions

Avoid Concomitant Use

Avoid concomitant use of Anakinra with any of the following: Anti-TNF Agents; BCG; Canakinumab; Natalizumab; Pimecrolimus; Tacrolimus (Topical); Vaccines (Live)

Increased Effect/Toxicity

Anakinra may increase the levels/effects of: Canakinumab; Leflunomide; Natalizumab; Vaccines (Live)

The levels/effects of Anakinra may be increased by: Anti-TNF Agents; Denosumab; Pimecrolimus; Roflumilast; Tacrolimus (Topical); Trastuzumab

Decreased Effect

Anakinra may decrease the levels/effects of: BCG; Sipuleucel-T; Vaccines (Inactivated); Vaccines (Live)

The levels/effects of Anakinra may be decreased by: Echinacea

Stability Store in refrigerator at 2°C to 8°C (36°F to 46°F); do not freeze. Do not shake. Protect from light.

Mechanism of Action Antagonist of the interleukin-1 (IL-1) receptor. Endogenous IL-1 is induced by inflammatory stimuli and mediates a variety of immunological responses, including degradation of cartilage (loss of proteoglycans) and stimulation of bone resorption.

Pharmacodynamics/Kinetics

Bioavailability: SubQ: 95%

Half-life elimination: Terminal: 4-6 hours

Time to peak: SubQ: 3-7 hours

Dosage

Geriatric & Adult Rheumatoid arthritis: SubQ: 100 mg once daily (administer at approximately the same time each day)

Renal Impairment Cl_{cr} <30 mL/minute and/or end-stage renal disease: 100 mg every other day

Administration Rotate injection sites (thigh, abdomen, upper arm); injection should be given at least 1 inch away from previous injection site. Do not shake. Provided in single-use, preservative free syringes with 27 gauge needles; discard any unused portion.

Monitoring Parameters CBC with differential (baseline, then monthly for 3 months, then every 3 months); serum creatinine

Pharmacotherapy Pearls Anakinra is produced by recombinant DNA/*E. coli* technology.

Special Geriatric Considerations Clinical trials with older adults (65% to 75%) demonstrated no clinical differences between elderly patients and younger adults in safety and efficacy. Since elderly may be more liable to infections in general, use with caution. Also, since many elderly patients may have Cl_{cr} <30 mL/minute, close monitoring should be followed with calculation of creatinine clearance prior to initiating therapy with anakinra.

Dosage Forms Excipient information presented when available (limited, particularly for generics); consult specific product labeling.

Injection, solution [preservative free]:

Kineret®: 100 mg/0.67 mL (0.67 mL) [contains edetate disodium, natural rubber/natural latex in packaging, polysorbate 80]

Selected References

Cohen S, Hurd E, Cush J, et al, "Treatment of Rheumatoid Arthritis With Anakinra, a Recombinant Human Interleukin-1 Receptor Antagonist, in Combination With Methotrexate: Results of a Twenty-Four-Week, Multicenter, Randomized, Double-Blind, Placebo-Controlled Trial," *Arthritis Rheum*, 2002, 46(3):614-24.

Fleischmann RM, Schechtman J, Bennett R, et al, "Anakinra, a Recombinant Human Interleukin-1 Receptor Antagonist (r-metHuIL-1ra), in Patients With Rheumatoid Arthritis: A Large, International, Multicenter, Placebo-Controlled Trial," *Arthritis Rheum*, 2003, 48(4):927-34.

Fleischmann RM, Tesser J, Schiff MH, et al, Safety of Extended Treatment With Anakinra in Patients With Rheumatoid Arthritis, *Ann Rheum Dis*, 2006, 65(8):1006-12.

◀   Genovese MC, Cohen S, Moreland L, et al, "Combination Therapy With Etanercept and Anakinra in the Treatment of Patients With Rheumatoid Arthritis Who Have Been Treated Unsuccessfully With Methotrexate," *Arthritis Rheum*, 2004, 50(5):1412-9.

◆ **Anaprox®** *see* Naproxen *on page 1263*
◆ **Anaprox® DS** *see* Naproxen *on page 1263*
◆ **Anaspaz®** *see* Hyoscyamine *on page 902*

Anastrozole (an AS troe zole)

Medication Safety Issues
Sound-alike/look-alike issues:
Anastrozole may be confused with anagrelide, letrozole
Arimidex® may be confused with Aromasin®
Brand Names: U.S. Arimidex®
Brand Names: Canada Arimidex®
Index Terms ICI-D1033; ZD1033
Generic Availability (U.S.) Yes
Pharmacologic Category Antineoplastic Agent, Aromatase Inhibitor
Use First-line treatment of locally-advanced or metastatic breast cancer (hormone receptor-positive or unknown) in postmenopausal women; treatment of advanced breast cancer in postmenopausal women with disease progression following tamoxifen therapy; adjuvant treatment of early hormone receptor-positive breast cancer in postmenopausal women
Unlabeled/Investigational Use Treatment of recurrent or metastatic endometrial or uterine cancers, treatment of recurrent ovarian cancer
Contraindications Hypersensitivity to anastrozole or any component of the formulation
Warnings/Precautions Hazardous agent - use appropriate precautions for handling and disposal. Anastrozole offers no clinical benefit in premenopausal women with breast cancer. Patients with pre-existing ischemic cardiac disease have an increased risk for ischemic cardiovascular events.

Due to decreased circulating estrogen levels, anastrozole is associated with a reduction in bone mineral density (BMD); decreases (from baseline) in total hip and lumbar spine BMD have been reported. Patients with pre-existing osteopenia are at higher risk for developing osteoporosis (Eastell, 2008). When initiating anastrozole treatment, follow available guidelines for bone mineral density management in postmenopausal women with similar fracture risk; concurrent use of bisphosphonates may be useful in patients at risk for fractures.

Elevated total cholesterol levels (contributed to by LDL cholesterol increases) have been reported in patients receiving anastrozole; use with caution in patients with hyperlipidemias; cholesterol levels should be monitored/managed in accordance with current guidelines for patients with LDL elevations. Plasma concentrations in patients with stable hepatic cirrhosis were within the range of concentrations seen in normal subjects across all clinical trials; use has not been studied in patients with severe hepatic impairment.

Adverse Reactions (Reflective of adult population; not specific for elderly)
>10%:
  Cardiovascular: Vasodilatation (25% to 36%), ischemic cardiovascular disease (4%; 17% in patients with pre-existing ischemic heart disease), hypertension (2% to 13%), angina (2%; 12% in patients with pre-existing ischemic heart disease)
  Central nervous system: Mood disturbance (19%), fatigue (19%), pain (11% to 17%), headache (9% to 13%), depression (5% to 13%)
  Dermatologic: Rash (6% to 11%)
  Endocrine & metabolic: Hot flashes (12% to 36%)
  Gastrointestinal: Nausea (11% to 19%), vomiting (8% to 13%)
  Neuromuscular & skeletal: Weakness (16% to 19%), arthritis (17%), arthralgia (2% to 15%), back pain (10% to 12%), bone pain (6% to 11%), osteoporosis (11%)
  Respiratory: Pharyngitis (6% to 14%), cough increased (8% to 11%)
1% to 10%:
  Cardiovascular: Peripheral edema (5% to 10%), chest pain (5% to 7%), edema (7%), venous thromboembolic events (2% to 4%), ischemic cerebrovascular events (2%), MI (1%)
  Central nervous system: Insomnia (2% to 10%), dizziness (6% to 8%), anxiety (2% to 6%), fever (2% to 5%), malaise (2% to 5%), confusion (2% to 5%), nervousness (2% to 5%), somnolence (2% to 5%), lethargy (1%)
  Dermatologic: Alopecia (2% to 5%), pruritus (2% to 5%)
  Endocrine & metabolic: Hypercholesterolemia (9%), breast pain (2% to 8%)
  Gastrointestinal: Diarrhea (8% to 9%), constipation (7% to 9%), abdominal pain (7% to 9%), weight gain (2% to 9%), anorexia (5% to 7%), xerostomia (6%), dyspepsia (7%), weight loss (2% to 5%)

Genitourinary: Urinary tract infection (2% to 8%), vulvovaginitis (6%), pelvic pain (5%), vaginal bleeding (1% to 5%), vaginitis (4%), vaginal discharge (4%), vaginal hemorrhage (2% to 4%), leukorrhea (2% to 3%), vaginal dryness (2% to 5%)

Hematologic: Anemia (2% to 5%), leukopenia (2% to 5%)

Hepatic: Liver function tests increased (1% to 10%), alkaline phosphatase increased (1% to 10%), gamma GT increased (≤5%)

Local: Thrombophlebitis (2% to 5%)

Neuromuscular & skeletal: Fracture (1% to 10%), arthrosis (7%), paresthesia (5% to 7%), joint disorder (6%), myalgia (2% to 6%), neck pain (2% to 5%), carpal tunnel syndrome (3%), hypertonia (3%)

Ocular: Cataracts (6%)

Respiratory: Dyspnea (8% to 10%), sinusitis (2% to 6%), bronchitis (2% to 5%), rhinitis (2% to 5%)

Miscellaneous: Lymphedema (10%), infection (2% to 9%), flu-like syndrome (2% to 7%), diaphoresis (2% to 5%), cyst (5%), neoplasm (5%), tumor flare (3%)

Drug Interactions

Metabolism/Transport Effects Inhibits CYP1A2 (weak), 2C8 (weak), 2C9 (weak), 3A4 (weak)

Avoid Concomitant Use

Avoid concomitant use of Anastrozole with any of the following: Estrogen Derivatives

Increased Effect/Toxicity There are no known significant interactions involving an increase in effect.

Decreased Effect

The levels/effects of Anastrozole may be decreased by: Estrogen Derivatives; Tamoxifen

Stability Store at 20°C to 25°C (68°F to 77°F).

Mechanism of Action Potent and selective nonsteroidal aromatase inhibitor. By inhibiting aromatase, the conversion of androstenedione to estrone, and testosterone to estradiol, is prevented, thereby decreasing tumor mass or delaying progression in patients with tumors responsive to hormones. Anastrozole causes an 85% decrease in estrone sulfate levels.

Pharmacodynamics/Kinetics

Onset of estradiol reduction: 70% reduction after 24 hours; 80% after 2 weeks therapy

Duration of estradiol reduction: 6 days

Absorption: Well absorbed; extent of absorption not affected by food

Protein binding, plasma: 40%

Metabolism: Extensively hepatic (~85%) via N-dealkylation, hydroxylation, and glucuronidation; primary metabolite (triazole) inactive

Half-life elimination: ~50 hours

Time to peak, plasma: ~2 hours without food; 5 hours with food

Excretion: Feces; urine (urinary excretion accounts for ~10% of total elimination, mostly as metabolites)

Dosage

Geriatric & Adult Females: Postmenopausal:

Breast cancer, advanced: Oral: 1 mg once daily; continue until tumor progression

Breast cancer, early (adjuvant treatment): Oral: 1 mg once daily; optimal duration unknown, duration in clinical trial is 5 years

Renal Impairment Dosage adjustment is not necessary.

Hepatic Impairment

Mild-to-moderate impairment or stable hepatic cirrhosis: Dosage adjustment is not required.

Severe hepatic impairment: Has not been studied in this population.

Administration May be administered with or without food.

Monitoring Parameters Bone mineral density; total cholesterol and LDL

Pharmacotherapy Pearls Oncology Comment: The American Society of Clinical Oncology (ASCO) guidelines for adjuvant endocrine therapy in postmenopausal women with HR-positive breast cancer (Burstein, 2010) recommend considering aromatase inhibitor (AI) therapy at some point in the treatment course (primary, sequentially, or extended). Optimal duration at this time is not known; however, treatment with an AI should not exceed 5 years in primary and extended therapies, and 2-3 years if followed by tamoxifen in sequential therapy (total of 5 years). If initial therapy with AI has been discontinued before the 5 years, consideration should be taken to receive tamoxifen for a total of 5 years. The optimal time to switch to an AI is also not known, but data supports switching after 2-3 years of tamoxifen (sequential) or after 5 years of tamoxifen (extended). If patient becomes intolerant or has poor adherence, consideration should be made to switch to another AI or initiate tamoxifen.

Special Geriatric Considerations No age-related changes in pharmacokinetics were noted in clinical trials.

◀ **Dosage Forms** Excipient information presented when available (limited, particularly for generics); consult specific product labeling.

Tablet, oral: 1 mg
Arimidex®: 1 mg

Selected References

National Comprehensive Cancer Network® (NCCN), "Clinical Practice Guidelines in Oncology™: Breast Cancer," Version 1.2009. Available at http://www.nccn.org/professionals/physician_gls/PDF/breast.pdf.

National Comprehensive Cancer Network® (NCCN), "Clinical Practice Guidelines in Oncology™: Breast Cancer Risk Reduction, Version 1.2009." Accessible at http://www.nccn.org/professionals/physician_gls/PDF/breast_risk.pdf

Visvanathan K, Chlebowski RT, Hurley P, et al, "American Society of Clinical Oncology Clinical Practice Guideline Update on the Use of Pharmacologic Interventions Including Tamoxifen, Raloxifene, and Aromatase Inhibition for Breast Cancer Risk Reduction," *J Clin Oncol*, 2009, 27(19):3235-58.

♦ **Ancef** see CeFAZolin *on page 290*
♦ **Ancobon®** see Flucytosine *on page 744*
♦ **Androderm®** see Testosterone *on page 1761*
♦ **AndroGel®** see Testosterone *on page 1761*
♦ **Android®** see MethylTESTOSTERone *on page 1188*
♦ **AneCream™ [OTC]** see Lidocaine (Topical) *on page 1064*
♦ **Anestafoam™ [OTC]** see Lidocaine (Topical) *on page 1064*
♦ **Aneurine Hydrochloride** see Thiamine *on page 1779*
♦ **Angeliq®** see Drospirenone and Estradiol *on page 579*
♦ **Ansamycin** see Rifabutin *on page 1607*
♦ **Antara®** see Fenofibrate *on page 701*
♦ **Anti-Diarrheal [OTC]** see Loperamide *on page 1085*
♦ **Antidiuretic Hormone** see Vasopressin *on page 1904*
♦ **Anti-Fungal™ [OTC]** see Clotrimazole (Topical) *on page 399*
♦ **Anti-Hist [OTC]** see DiphenhydrAMINE (Systemic) *on page 520*
♦ **Antitumor Necrosis Factor Alpha (Human)** see Adalimumab *on page 46*
♦ **Antivert®** see Meclizine *on page 1118*
♦ **Anucort-HC™** see Hydrocortisone (Topical) *on page 886*
♦ **Anu-Med [OTC]** see Phenylephrine (Topical) *on page 1443*
♦ **Anu-med HC** see Hydrocortisone (Topical) *on page 886*
♦ **Anusol-HC®** see Hydrocortisone (Topical) *on page 886*
♦ **Anzemet®** see Dolasetron *on page 552*
♦ **4-AP** see Dalfampridine *on page 444*
♦ **APAP** see Acetaminophen *on page 33*
♦ **APAP 500 [OTC]** see Acetaminophen *on page 33*
♦ **APC8015** see Sipuleucel-T *on page 1684*
♦ **Apidra®** see Insulin Glulisine *on page 952*
♦ **Apidra® SoloStar®** see Insulin Glulisine *on page 952*
♦ **Aplenzin™** see BuPROPion *on page 229*
♦ **Aplisol®** see Tuberculin Tests *on page 1877*
♦ **Aplonidine** see Apraclonidine *on page 138*
♦ **Apokyn®** see Apomorphine *on page 136*

Apomorphine (a poe MOR feen)

Related Information
Antiparkinsonian Agents *on page 1995*

Brand Names: U.S. Apokyn®

Index Terms Apomorphine Hydrochloride; Apomorphine Hydrochloride Hemihydrate

Generic Availability (U.S.) No

Pharmacologic Category Anti-Parkinson's Agent, Dopamine Agonist

Use Treatment of hypomobility, "off" episodes with Parkinson's disease

Unlabeled/Investigational Use Treatment of erectile dysfunction

Prescribing and Access Restrictions Apokyn® is only available through a select group of specialty pharmacies and cannot be obtained through a retail pharmacy. Apokyn® may be obtained from the following specialty pharmacies: Accredo Nova Factor or PharmaCare. To obtain the medication, contact the APOKYN Call Center at 1-877-7APOKYN (1-877-727-6596).

Contraindications Hypersensitivity to apomorphine or any component of the formulation; concomitant use with 5HT₃ antagonists; intravenous administration

Warnings/Precautions May cause orthostatic hypotension, especially during dosage escalation; use extreme caution, especially in patients on antihypertensives and/or vasodilators. If patient develops clinically-significant orthostatic hypotension with test dose then apomorphine should not be used. Ergot-derived dopamine agonists have also been associated with fibrotic complications (eg, retroperitoneal fibrosis, pleural thickening, and pulmonary infiltrates).

Pretreatment with antiemetic is necessary. Monitor patients for drowsiness. May cause hallucinations/psychosis. Use caution in patients with risk factors for torsade de pointes. Use caution in cardiovascular and cerebrovascular disease. Use caution in patients with hepatic or renal dysfunction. Use with caution in patients with pre-existing dyskinesias; may be exacerbated.

Dopamine agonists have been associated with compulsive behaviors and/or loss of impulse control, which has manifested as pathological gambling, libido increases (hypersexuality), and/or binge eating. Causality has not been established, and controversy exists as to whether this phenomenon is related to the underlying disease, prior behaviors/addictions and/or drug therapy. Dose reduction or discontinuation of therapy has been reported to reverse these behaviors in some, but not all cases. Dopaminergic agents have been associated with a syndrome resembling neuroleptic malignant syndrome on abrupt withdrawal or significant dosage reduction after long-term use. Retinal degeneration has been observed in animal studies when using dopamine agonists for prolonged periods. Rare cases of abuse have been reported. Risk for melanoma development is increased in Parkinson's disease patients; drug causation or factors contributing to risk have not been established. Patients should be monitored closely and periodic skin examinations should be performed. Contains metabisulfite. Do not give intravenously; thrombus formation or pulmonary embolism may occur.

Adverse Reactions (Reflective of adult population; not specific for elderly)
>10%:
  Cardiovascular: Chest pain/pressure or angina (15%)
  Central nervous system: Drowsiness or somnolence (35%), dizziness or orthostatic hypotension (20%)
  Gastrointestinal: Nausea and/or vomiting (30%)
  Neuromuscular & skeletal: Falls (30%), dyskinesias (24% to 35%)
  Respiratory: Yawning (40%), rhinorrhea (20%)
1% to 10%:
  Cardiovascular: Edema (10%), vasodilation (3%), hypotension (2%), syncope (2%), CHF
  Central nervous system: Hallucinations or confusion (10%), anxiety, depression, fatigue, headache, insomnia, pain
  Dermatologic: Bruising
  Endocrine & metabolic: Dehydration
  Gastrointestinal: Constipation, diarrhea
  Local: Injection site reactions
  Neuromuscular & skeletal: Arthralgias, weakness
  Miscellaneous: Diaphoresis increased

Drug Interactions
  Metabolism/Transport Effects Substrate (minor) of CYP1A2, 3A4, 2C19; **Inhibits** CYP1A2 (weak), 3A4 (weak), 2C19 (weak)
  Avoid Concomitant Use
    Avoid concomitant use of Apomorphine with any of the following: Antiemetics (5HT3 Antagonists); Artemether; Dronedarone; Lumefantrine; Nilotinib; Pimozide; QUEtiapine; QuiNINE; Tetrabenazine; Thioridazine; Toremifene; Vandetanib; Vemurafenib; Ziprasidone
  Increased Effect/Toxicity
    Apomorphine may increase the levels/effects of: Dronedarone; Pimozide; QTc-Prolonging Agents; QuiNINE; Tetrabenazine; Thioridazine; Toremifene; Vandetanib; Vemurafenib; Ziprasidone

    The levels/effects of Apomorphine may be increased by: Alfuzosin; Antiemetics (5HT3 Antagonists); Antipsychotics (Typical); Artemether; Chloroquine; Ciprofloxacin; Ciprofloxacin (Systemic); COMT Inhibitors; Conivaptan; Gadobutrol; Lumefantrine; MAO Inhibitors; Methylphenidate; Nilotinib; QUEtiapine; QuiNINE
  Decreased Effect
    Apomorphine may decrease the levels/effects of: Antipsychotics (Typical)

    The levels/effects of Apomorphine may be decreased by: Antipsychotics (Atypical); Cyproterone; Metoclopramide; Tocilizumab

Ethanol/Nutrition/Herb Interactions Ethanol: Caution with ethanol consumption; may increase risk of hypotension.
Stability Store at 15°C to 30°C (59°F to 86°F).
Mechanism of Action Stimulates postsynaptic D2-type receptors within the caudate putamen in the brain.
Pharmacodynamics/Kinetics
  Onset of action: SubQ: Rapid
  Distribution: V_d: Mean: 218 L

Metabolism: Not established; potential routes of metabolism include sulfation, N-demethylation, glucuronidation, and oxidation; catechol-O methyltransferase and nonenzymatic oxidation. CYP isoenzymes do not appear to play a significant role.

Half-life elimination: Terminal: 40 minutes

Time to peak, plasma: Improved motor scores: 20 minutes

Excretion: Urine 93% (as metabolites); feces 16%

Dosage

Geriatric & Adult Begin antiemetic therapy 3 days prior to initiation and continue for 2 months before reassessing need.

Parkinson's disease, "off" episode: SubQ: Initial test dose 2 mg, **medical supervision required; see "Note"**. Subsequent dosing is based on both tolerance and response to initial test dose.

If patient tolerates test dose and responds: Starting dose: 2 mg as needed; may increase dose in 1 mg increments every few days; maximum dose: 6 mg

If patient tolerates but does not respond to 2 mg test dose: Second test dose: 4 mg

If patient tolerates and responds to 4 mg test dose: Starting dose: 3 mg, as needed for "off" episodes; may increase dose in 1 mg increments every few days; maximum dose 6 mg

If patient does not tolerate 4 mg test dose: Third test dose: 3 mg

If patient tolerates 3 mg test dose: Starting dose: 2 mg as needed for "off" episodes; may increase dose in 1 mg increments to a maximum of 3 mg

If therapy is interrupted for >1 week, restart at 2 mg and gradually titrate dose.

Note: Medical supervision is required for all test doses with standing and supine blood pressure monitoring predose and 20-, 40-, and 60 minutes postdose. If subsequent test doses are required, wait >2 hours before another test dose is given; next test dose should be timed with another "off" episode. If a single dose is ineffective for a particular "off" episode, then a second dose should not be given. The average dosing frequency was 3 times/day in the development program with limited experience in dosing >5 times/day and with total daily doses >20 mg. Apomorphine is intended to treat the "off" episodes associated with levodopa therapy of Parkinson's disease and has not been studied in levodopa-naive Parkinson's patients.

Renal Impairment

Mild-to-moderate impairment: Reduce test dose and starting dose: 1 mg

Severe impairment: Has not been studied

Hepatic Impairment

Mild-to-moderate impairment: Use caution

Severe impairment: Has not been studied

Administration SubQ: Initiate antiemetic 3 days before test dose of apomorphine and continue for 2 months (if patient to be treated) before reassessment. Administer in abdomen, upper arm, or upper leg; change site with each injection. 3 mL cartridges are used with a manual, reusable, multidose injector pen. Injector pen can deliver doses up to 1 mL in 0.02 mL increments. Do not give intravenously; thrombus formation or pulmonary embolism may occur.

Monitoring Parameters Each test dose: Supine and standing blood pressure predose and 20, 40, and 60 minutes postdose; drowsiness

Dosage Forms Excipient information presented when available (limited, particularly for generics); consult specific product labeling.

Injection, solution, as hydrochloride:

Apokyn®: 10 mg/mL (3 mL) [contains benzyl alcohol, sodium metabisulfite]

Selected References

Factor SA, "Current Status of Symptomatic Medical Therapy in Parkinson's Disease," *Neurotherapeutics*, 2008, 5 (2):164-80.

Olanow CW, Watts RL, and Koller WC, "An Algorithm (Decision Tree) for the Management of Parkinson's Disease (2001): Treatment Guidelines," *Neurology*, 2001, 56(11 Suppl 5):S1-S88.

Weintraub D, Siderowf AD, Potenza MN, et al, "Association of Dopamine Agonist Use With Impulse Control Disorders in Parkinson Disease," *Arch Neurol*, 2006, 63(7):969-73.

◆ **Apomorphine Hydrochloride** *see* Apomorphine *on page* 136

◆ **Apomorphine Hydrochloride Hemihydrate** *see* Apomorphine *on page* 136

◆ **APPG** *see* Penicillin G Procaine *on page* 1420

Apraclonidine (a pra KLOE ni deen)

Related Information

Glaucoma Drug Therapy *on page* 2008

Medication Safety Issues

Sound-alike/look-alike issues:

Iopidine® may be confused with indapamide, iodine, Lodine®

Brand Names: U.S. Iopidine®

Brand Names: Canada Iopidine®

Index Terms Aplonidine; Apraclonidine Hydrochloride; p-Aminoclonidine
Generic Availability (U.S.) Yes
Pharmacologic Category Alpha$_2$ Agonist, Ophthalmic
Use Prevention and treatment of postsurgical intraocular pressure (IOP) elevation; short-term, adjunctive therapy in patients who require additional reduction of IOP
Dosage
Geriatric & Adult Postsurgical intraocular pressure elevation (prevention/treatment): Ophthalmic:
0.5%: Instill 1-2 drops in the affected eye(s) 3 times/day
1%: Instill 1 drop in operative eye 1 hour prior to anterior segment laser surgery, second drop in eye immediately upon completion of procedure
Renal Impairment Although the topical use of apraclonidine has not been studied in renal failure patients, structurally-related clonidine undergoes a significant increase in half-life in patients with severe renal impairment. Close monitoring of cardiovascular parameters in patients with impaired renal function is advised.
Hepatic Impairment Close monitoring of cardiovascular parameters in patients with impaired liver function is advised because the systemic dosage form of clonidine is partially metabolized in the liver.
Special Geriatric Considerations Evaluate the patient's or caregiver's ability to safely administer the correct dose of ophthalmic medication.
Dosage Forms Excipient information presented when available (limited, particularly for generics); consult specific product labeling.
Solution, ophthalmic [drops]: 0.5% (5 mL, 10 mL)
Iopidine®: 0.5% (5 mL, 10 mL); 1% (0.1 mL) [contains benzalkonium chloride]

♦ **Apraclonidine Hydrochloride** see Apraclonidine on page 138

Aprepitant (ap RE pi tant)

Medication Safety Issues
Sound-alike/look-alike issues:
Aprepitant may be confused with fosaprepitant
Emend® (aprepitant) oral capsule formulation may be confused with Emend® for injection (fosaprepitant).
Brand Names: U.S. Emend®
Brand Names: Canada Emend®
Index Terms L 754030; MK 869
Generic Availability (U.S.) No
Pharmacologic Category Antiemetic; Substance P/Neurokinin 1 Receptor Antagonist
Use Prevention of acute and delayed nausea and vomiting associated with moderately- and highly-emetogenic chemotherapy (in combination with other antiemetics); prevention of postoperative nausea and vomiting (PONV)
Contraindications Hypersensitivity to aprepitant or any component of the formulation; concurrent use with cisapride or pimozide
Warnings/Precautions Use caution with agents primarily metabolized via CYP3A4; aprepitant is a 3A4 inhibitor. Effect on orally administered 3A4 substrates is greater than those administered intravenously. Chronic continuous use is not recommended; however, a single 40 mg aprepitant oral dose is not likely to alter plasma concentrations of CYP3A4 substrates. Use caution with severe hepatic impairment; has not been studied in patients with severe hepatic impairment (Child-Pugh class C). Not studied for treatment of existing nausea and vomiting. Chronic continuous administration is not recommended.
Adverse Reactions (Reflective of adult population; not specific for elderly) Note: Adverse reactions reported as part of a combination chemotherapy regimen or with general anesthesia.

>10%:
Central nervous system: Fatigue (≤18%)
Gastrointestinal: Nausea (6% to 13%), constipation (9% to 10%)
Neuromuscular & skeletal: Weakness (≤18%)
Miscellaneous: Hiccups (11%)
1% to 10%:
Cardiovascular: Hypotension (≤6%), bradycardia (≤4%)
Central nervous system: Dizziness (≤7%)
Endocrine & metabolic: Dehydration (≤6%)
Gastrointestinal: Diarrhea (≤10%), dyspepsia (≤6%), abdominal pain (≤5%), epigastric discomfort (4%), gastritis (4%), stomatitis (3%)

Hepatic: ALT increased (≤6%), AST increased (3%)

Renal: Proteinuria (7%), BUN increased (5%)

Drug Interactions

Metabolism/Transport Effects Substrate of CYP1A2 (minor), 2C19 (minor), 3A4 (major); **Inhibits** CYP2C9 (weak), 2C19 (weak), 3A4 (moderate); **Induces** CYP2C9 (weak), 3A4 (weak)

Avoid Concomitant Use

Avoid concomitant use of Aprepitant with any of the following: Cisapride; Conivaptan; Pimozide; Tolvaptan

Increased Effect/Toxicity

Aprepitant may increase the levels/effects of: Benzodiazepines (metabolized by oxidation); Budesonide (Systemic, Oral Inhalation); Cisapride; Colchicine; Corticosteroids (Systemic); CYP3A4 Substrates; Diltiazem; Eplerenone; Everolimus; FentaNYL; Halofantrine; Lurasidone; Pimecrolimus; Pimozide; Ranolazine; Salmeterol; Saxagliptin; Tolvaptan; Vilazodone

The levels/effects of Aprepitant may be increased by: Antifungal Agents (Azole Derivatives, Systemic); Conivaptan; CYP3A4 Inhibitors (Moderate); CYP3A4 Inhibitors (Strong); Dasatinib; Diltiazem

Decreased Effect

Aprepitant may decrease the levels/effects of: Contraceptives (Estrogens); Contraceptives (Progestins); CYP2C9 Substrates (High risk); Diclofenac; PARoxetine; Saxagliptin; TOLBUTamide; Warfarin

The levels/effects of Aprepitant may be decreased by: CYP3A4 Inducers (Strong); Cyproterone; Deferasirox; Herbs (CYP3A4 Inducers); PARoxetine; Rifamycin Derivatives; Tocilizumab

Ethanol/Nutrition/Herb Interactions

Food: Aprepitant serum concentration may be increased when taken with grapefruit juice; avoid concurrent use.

Herb/Nutraceutical: Avoid St John's wort (may decrease aprepitant levels).

Stability Store at room temperature of 20°C to 25°C (68°F to 77°F).

Mechanism of Action Prevents acute and delayed vomiting by inhibiting the substance P/ neurokinin 1 (NK$_1$) receptor; augments the antiemetic activity of 5-HT$_3$ receptor antagonists and corticosteroids to inhibit acute and delayed phases of chemotherapy-induced emesis.

Pharmacodynamics/Kinetics

Distribution: V$_d$: ~70 L; crosses the blood brain barrier

Protein binding: >95%

Metabolism: Extensively hepatic via CYP3A4 (major); CYP1A2 and CYP2C19 (minor); forms 7 metabolites (weakly active)

Bioavailability: ~60% to 65%

Half-life elimination: Terminal: ~9-13 hours

Time to peak, plasma: ~3-4 hours

Dosage

Geriatric & Adult

Prevention of chemotherapy-induced nausea/vomiting: Oral: 125 mg 1 hour prior to chemotherapy on day 1, followed by 80 mg once daily on days 2 and 3 (in combination with a corticosteroid and 5-HT$_3$ antagonist antiemetic)

Prevention of PONV: Oral: 40 mg within 3 hours prior to induction

Renal Impairment No dose adjustment necessary in patients with renal disease or end-stage renal disease maintained on hemodialysis.

Hepatic Impairment

Mild-to-moderate impairment (Child-Pugh classes A and B): No adjustment necessary.

Severe impairment (Child-Pugh class C): Use caution; no data available.

Administration Administer with or without food.

Chemotherapy induced nausea/vomiting: First dose should be given 1 hour prior to antineoplastic therapy; subsequent doses should be given in the morning.

PONV: Administer within 3 hours prior to induction

Pharmacotherapy Pearls Oncology Comment: Aprepitant is recommended in the American Society of Clinical Oncology (ASCO) oncology antiemetic guidelines for use in combination with a serotonin receptor antagonist and dexamethasone for chemotherapy with high emetic risk and for chemotherapy regimens of moderate emetic risk which contain an anthracycline and cyclophosphamide (Kris, 2006). The National Comprehensive Cancer Network (NCCN) Clinical Practice Guidelines in Oncology for Antiemesis (version 2.2009) recommend the same use of aprepitant as is in the ASCO recommendation. In addition to the moderately emetogenic chemotherapy listed above, the NCCN guidelines suggest that aprepitant may also be used for select moderately emetogenic regimens containing carboplatin, cisplatin, doxorubicin, epirubicin, ifosfamide, irinotecan and methotrexate. Either fosaprepitant 115 mg or aprepitant (125 mg orally) are administered on day 1; for day 2 and 3, patients should receive aprepitant 80 mg orally.

Special Geriatric Considerations In two studies by the manufacturer, with a total of 544 patients, 31% were >65 years of age, while 5% were >75 years. No differences in safety and efficacy were noted between elderly subjects and younger adults. No dosing adjustment is necessary.

Dosage Forms Excipient information presented when available (limited, particularly for generics); consult specific product labeling.

Capsule, oral:
 Emend®: 40 mg, 80 mg, 125 mg
 Combination package, oral [each package contains]:
 Emend®: Capsule: 80 mg (2s) and Capsule: 125 mg (1s)

Selected References

Kris MG, Hesketh PJ, Somerfield MR, et al, "American Society of Clinical Oncology Guideline for Antiemetics in Oncology: Update 2006," *J Clin Oncol*, 2006, 24(18):2932-47.

National Comprehensive Cancer Network (NCCN), "Clinical Practice Guidelines in Oncology™: Antiemesis," Version 1, 2008. Available at http://www.nccn.org/professionals/physician_gls/PDF/antiemesis.pdf.

◆ **Aprepitant Injection** *see* Fosaprepitant *on page 788*
◆ **Apresoline [DSC]** *see* HydrALAZINE *on page 874*
◆ **Apriso™** *see* Mesalamine *on page 1150*
◆ **Aprodine [OTC]** *see* Triprolidine and Pseudoephedrine *on page 1872*
◆ **Aqua Gem-E™ [OTC]** *see* Vitamin E *on page 1921*
◆ **Aquanil HC® [OTC]** *see* Hydrocortisone (Topical) *on page 886*
◆ **Aquasol E® [OTC]** *see* Vitamin E *on page 1921*
◆ **Aqueous Procaine Penicillin G** *see* Penicillin G Procaine *on page 1420*
◆ **Aquoral™** *see* Saliva Substitute *on page 1652*
◆ **Aranesp®** *see* Darbepoetin Alfa *on page 456*
◆ **Aranesp® SingleJect®** *see* Darbepoetin Alfa *on page 456*
◆ **Arava®** *see* Leflunomide *on page 1034*
◆ **Aredia®** *see* Pamidronate *on page 1383*

Arformoterol (ar for MOE ter ol)

Related Information
 Inhalant Agents *on page 2010*
Brand Names: U.S. Brovana®
Index Terms (R,R)-Formoterol L-Tartrate; Arformoterol Tartrate
Generic Availability (U.S.) No
Pharmacologic Category Beta$_2$-Adrenergic Agonist; Beta$_2$-Adrenergic Agonist, Long-Acting
Use Long-term maintenance treatment of bronchoconstriction in chronic obstructive pulmonary disease (COPD), including chronic bronchitis and emphysema
Medication Guide Available Yes
Contraindications Hypersensitivity to arformoterol, racemic formoterol, or any component of the formulation

Additional contraindication for all long-acting beta$_2$-agonists: Use in patients with asthma (without concomitant use of a long-term asthma control medication)

Warnings/Precautions [U.S. Boxed Warning]: Long-acting beta$_2$-agonists (LABAs) increase the risk of asthma-related deaths. Monotherapy with an LABA is contraindicated in the treatment of asthma. In a large, randomized, placebo-controlled U.S. clinical trial (SMART, 2006), salmeterol was associated with an increase in asthma-related deaths (when added to usual asthma therapy); risk is considered a class effect among all LABAs. LABAs should not be used for acute bronchospasm. **Safety and efficacy of arformoterol in patients with asthma have not been established.** Do not exceed recommended dose; serious adverse events, including fatalities, have been associated with excessive use of inhaled sympathomimetics.

Use with caution in patients with cardiovascular disease (eg, arrhythmia, hypertension, HF); beta-agonists may cause elevation in blood pressure, heart rate and result in CNS stimulation/ excitation. Beta$_2$-agonists may also increase risk of arrhythmias and prolong QT$_c$ interval. Do **not** use for acute episodes of COPD. Do not initiate in patients with significantly worsening or acutely deteriorating COPD. Data are not available to determine if LABA use increases the risk of death in patients with COPD. Use with caution in patients with diabetes mellitus; beta$_2$-agonists may increase serum glucose. Use caution in hepatic impairment; systemic clearance prolonged in hepatic dysfunction. Use with caution in hyperthyroidism; may stimulate thyroid activity. Use with caution in patients with hypokalemia; beta$_2$-agonists may decrease serum potassium. Use with caution in patients with seizure disorders; beta$_2$-agonists may result in CNS stimulation/excitation.

Tolerance/tachyphylaxis to the bronchodilator effect, measured by FEV_1, has been observed in studies. Patients using inhaled, short-acting beta$_2$-agonists (eg, albuterol) should be instructed to discontinue routine use of these medications prior to beginning treatment; short-acting agents should be reserved for symptomatic relief of acute symptoms. Patients must be instructed to seek medical attention in cases where acute symptoms are not relieved or a previous level of response is diminished. The need to increase frequency of use may indicate deterioration of COPD, and treatment must not be delayed. Arformoterol is approved for COPD.

Adverse Reactions (Reflective of adult population; not specific for elderly)
2% to 10%:
Cardiovascular: Chest pain (7%), peripheral edema (3%)
Central nervous system: Pain (8%)
Dermatologic: Rash (4%)
Gastrointestinal: Diarrhea (6%)
Neuromuscular & skeletal: Back pain (6%), leg cramps (4%)
Respiratory: Dyspnea (4%), sinusitis (5%), congestive conditions (2%)
Miscellaneous: Flu-like syndrome (3%)

Drug Interactions
Metabolism/Transport Effects Substrate of CY2D6 (minor) and CYP2C19 (minor)
Avoid Concomitant Use
Avoid concomitant use of Arformoterol with any of the following: Iobenguane I 123
Increased Effect/Toxicity
Arformoterol may increase the levels/effects of: Loop Diuretics; Sympathomimetics

The levels/effects of Arformoterol may be increased by: Atomoxetine; Cannabinoids; MAO Inhibitors; Tricyclic Antidepressants
Decreased Effect
Arformoterol may decrease the levels/effects of: Iobenguane I 123

The levels/effects of Arformoterol may be decreased by: Alpha-/Beta-Blockers; Beta-Blockers (Beta1 Selective); Beta-Blockers (Nonselective); Betahistine
Stability Prior to dispensing, store in protective foil pouch under refrigeration at 2°C to 8°C (36°F to 46°F). Protect from light and excessive heat. After dispensing, unopened foil pouches may be stored at room temperature at 20°C to 25°C (68°F to 77°F) for up to 6 weeks. Only remove vial from foil pouch immediately before use.
Mechanism of Action Arformoterol, the (R,R)-enantiomer of the racemic formoterol, is a long-acting beta$_2$-agonist that relaxes bronchial smooth muscle by selective action on beta$_2$-receptors with little effect on cardiovascular system.

Pharmacodynamics/Kinetics
Onset of action: 7-20 minutes
Peak effect: 1-3 hours
Absorption: A portion of inhaled dose is absorbed into systemic circulation
Protein binding: 52% to 65%
Metabolism: Hepatic via direct glucuronidation and secondarily via O-demethylation; CYP2D6 and CYP2C19 (to a lesser extent) involved in O-demethylation
Half-life elimination: 26 hours
Time to peak: 0.5-3 hours

Dosage
Geriatric & Adult COPD: Nebulization: 15 mcg twice daily; maximum: 30 mcg/day
Renal Impairment No adjustment required.
Hepatic Impairment No dosage adjustment required, but use caution; systemic drug exposure prolonged (1.3- to 2.4-fold).
Administration Nebulization: Remove each vial from individually sealed foil pouch immediately before use. Use with standard jet nebulizer connected to an air compressor, administer with mouthpiece or face mask. Administer vial undiluted and do not mix with other medications in nebulizer.
Monitoring Parameters FEV_1, peak flow, and/or other pulmonary function tests; blood pressure, heart rate; CNS stimulation; serum glucose, serum potassium. Monitor for increased use of short-acting beta$_2$-agonist inhalers; may be marker of a deteriorating COPD condition.
Special Geriatric Considerations In clinical trials, no significant difference was seen in the AUC and C_{max} between younger and older subjects. In addition, no significant difference in clinical response was noted.
Dosage Forms Excipient information presented when available (limited, particularly for generics); consult specific product labeling.
Solution, for nebulization:
Brovana®: 15 mcg/2 mL (30s, 60s)

◆ **Arformoterol Tartrate** *see* Arformoterol *on page 141*

♦ **8-Arginine Vasopressin** see Vasopressin on page 1904
♦ **Aricept®** see Donepezil on page 554
♦ **Aricept® ODT** see Donepezil on page 554
♦ **Arimidex®** see Anastrozole on page 134

ARIPiprazole (ay ri PIP ray zole)

Related Information
Antipsychotic Agents on page 1997
Atypical Antipsychotics on page 1999
Liquid Compatibility of Antidepressants, Antipsychotics, and Mood Stabilizers on page 2111
Medication Safety Issues
Sound-alike/look-alike issues:
Abilify® may be confused with Ambien®
ARIPiprazole may be confused with proton pump inhibitors (dexlansoprazole, esomeprazole, lansoprazole, omeprazole, pantoprazole, RABEprazole)
Brand Names: U.S. Abilify Discmelt®; Abilify®
Brand Names: Canada Abilify®
Index Terms BMS 337039; OPC-14597
Generic Availability (U.S.) No
Pharmacologic Category Antipsychotic Agent, Atypical
Use
Oral: Acute and maintenance treatment of schizophrenia; acute (manic and mixed episodes) and maintenance treatment of bipolar I disorder as monotherapy or as an adjunct to lithium or valproic acid; adjunctive treatment of major depressive disorder; treatment of irritability associated with autistic disorder
Injection: Agitation associated with schizophrenia or bipolar I disorder
Unlabeled/Investigational Use Depression with psychotic features; psychosis/agitation related to Alzheimer's dementia
Medication Guide Available Yes
Contraindications Hypersensitivity to aripiprazole or any component of the formulation
Warnings/Precautions [U.S. Boxed Warning]: Elderly patients with dementia-related psychosis treated with antipsychotics are at an increased risk of death compared to placebo. Most deaths appeared to be either cardiovascular (eg, heart failure, sudden death) or infectious (eg, pneumonia) in nature. In addition, an increased incidence of cerebrovascular effects (eg, transient ischemic attack, cerebrovascular accidents) has been reported in studies of placebo-controlled trials of aripiprazole in elderly patients with dementia-related psychosis. Aripiprazole is not approved for the treatment of dementia-related psychosis.

[U.S. Boxed Warning]: Antidepressants increase the risk of suicidal thinking and behavior in children, adolescents, and young adults (18-24 years of age) with major depressive disorder (MDD) and other psychiatric disorders; consider risk prior to prescribing. The possibility of a suicide attempt is inherent in major depression and may persist until remission occurs. Patients treated with antidepressants should be observed for clinical worsening and suicidality, especially during the initial few months of a course of drug therapy, or at times of dose changes, either increases or decreases. Prescriptions should be written for the smallest quantity consistent with good patient care. The patient's family or caregiver should be alerted to monitor patients for the emergence of suicidality and associated behaviors; patients should be instructed to notify their healthcare provider if any of these symptoms or worsening depression or psychosis occur.

Leukopenia, neutropenia, and agranulocytosis (sometimes fatal) have been reported in clinical trials and postmarketing reports with antipsychotic use; presence of risk factors (eg, pre-existing low WBC or history of drug-induced leuko-/neutropenia) should prompt periodic blood count assessment. Discontinue therapy at first signs of blood dyscrasias or if absolute neutrophil count <1000/mm^3.

A medication guide concerning the use of antidepressants should be dispensed with each prescription.

May cause extrapyramidal symptoms (EPS), including pseudoparkinsonism, acute dystonic reactions, akathisia, and tardive dyskinesia (risk of these reactions is very low relative to typical/conventional antipsychotics, frequencies reported are similar to placebo). Risk of dystonia (and probably other EPS) may be greater with increased doses, use of conventional antipsychotics, males, and younger patients. May be associated with neuroleptic malignant syndrome (NMS).

May be sedating, use with caution in disorders where CNS depression is a feature. May cause orthostatic hypotension (although reported rates are similar to placebo); use caution in patients at risk of this effect or those who would not tolerate transient hypotensive episodes (cerebrovascular disease, cardiovascular disease, or other medications which may predispose).

Use caution in patients with Parkinson's disease; predisposition to seizures; and severe cardiac disease. May alter cardiac conduction; life-threatening arrhythmias have occurred with therapeutic doses of antipsychotics. Esophageal dysmotility and aspiration have been associated with antipsychotic use; use caution in patients at risk of pneumonia (eg, Alzheimer's disease). May alter temperature regulation. Significant weight gain has been observed with antipsychotic therapy; incidence varies with product. Monitor waist circumference and BMI.

Atypical antipsychotics have been associated with development of hyperglycemia; in some cases, may be extreme and associated with ketoacidosis, hyperosmolar coma, or death. Reports of hyperglycemia with aripiprazole therapy have been few and specific risk associated with this agent is not known. Use caution in patients with diabetes or other disorders of glucose regulation; monitor for worsening of glucose control.

Abilify Discmelt®: Use caution in phenylketonuria; contains phenylalanine.

Adverse Reactions (Reflective of adult population; not specific for elderly) Unless otherwise noted, frequency of adverse reactions is shown as reported for adult patients receiving oral administration. Spectrum and incidence of adverse effects similar in children; exceptions noted when incidence much higher in children.

>10%:

Central nervous system: Headache (27%; injection 12%), agitation (19%), insomnia (18%), anxiety (17%), EPS (dose related; 5% to 16%; children 6% to 26%), akathisia (dose related; 8% to 13%; injection 2%), sedation (dose related; 5% to 11%; children 8% to 24%; injection 3% to 9%)

Gastrointestinal: Weight gain (2% to 30%; highest frequency in patients with baseline BMI <23 and prolonged use), nausea (15%; injection 9%), constipation (11%), vomiting (11%; children 9% to 14%; injection 3%), dyspepsia (9%)

1% to 10%:

Cardiovascular: Orthostatic hypotension (1% to 4%; injection 1% to 3%), tachycardia (injection 2%), chest pain, hypertension, peripheral edema

Central nervous system: Dizziness (10%; injection 8%), pyrexia (children 5% to 9%), restlessness (5% to 6%), fatigue (dose related; 6%; children 8% to 17%; injection 2%), lethargy (children 2% to 5%), lightheadedness (4%), pain (3%), dystonia (children 1%), hypersomnia (1%), irritability (children 1%), coordination impaired, suicidal ideation

Dermatologic: Rash (children 2%), hyperhidrosis

Endocrine & metabolic: Dysmenorrhea (children 2%)

Gastrointestinal: Salivation increased (dose related; children 4% to 9%), appetite decreased (children 4% to 7%), appetite increased (children 7%), xerostomia (5%), toothache (4%), abdominal discomfort (3%), diarrhea (children 5%), weight loss

Local: Injection site reaction (injection)

Neuromuscular & skeletal: Tremor (dose related; 5% to 6%; children 6% to 10%), extremity pain (4%), stiffness (4%), myalgia (2%), spasm (2%), arthralgia (children 1%), dyskinesia (children 1%), CPK increased, weakness

Ocular: Blurred vision (3%; children 3% to 8%)

Respiratory: Nasopharyngitis (children 6%), pharyngolaryngeal pain (3%), cough (3%), rhinorrhea (children 2%), aspiration pneumonia, dyspnea, nasal congestion

Miscellaneous: Thirst (children 1%)

Drug Interactions

Metabolism/Transport Effects Substrate (major) of CYP2D6, 3A4

Avoid Concomitant Use

Avoid concomitant use of ARIPiprazole with any of the following: Conivaptan; Metoclopramide

Increased Effect/Toxicity

ARIPiprazole may increase the levels/effects of: Alcohol (Ethyl); CNS Depressants; Methotrimeprazine; Methylphenidate; Selective Serotonin Reuptake Inhibitors

The levels/effects of ARIPiprazole may be increased by: Abiraterone Acetate; Acetylcholinesterase Inhibitors (Central); Conivaptan; CYP2D6 Inhibitors (Moderate); CYP2D6 Inhibitors (Strong); CYP3A4 Inhibitors (Moderate); CYP3A4 Inhibitors (Strong); Darunavir; Dasatinib; Droperidol; HydrOXYzine; Lithium formulations; Methotrimeprazine; Methylphenidate; Metoclopramide; Tetrabenazine

Decreased Effect

ARIPiprazole may decrease the levels/effects of: Amphetamines; Anti-Parkinson's Agents (Dopamine Agonist); Quinagolide

The levels/effects of ARIPiprazole may be decreased by: CarBAMazepine; CYP3A4 Inducers (Strong); Deferasirox; Herbs (CYP3A4 Inducers); Lithium formulations; Peginterferon Alfa-2b; Tocilizumab

Ethanol/Nutrition/Herb Interactions

Ethanol: May increase CNS depression; monitor for increased effects with coadministration. Caution patients about effects.

Food: Ingestion with a high-fat meal delays time to peak plasma level.

Herb/Nutraceutical: St John's wort may decrease aripiprazole levels. Avoid kava kava, gotu kola, valerian, St John's wort (may increase CNS depression).

Stability

Injection solution: Store at controlled room temperature of 25°C (77°F); excursions permitted to 15°C to 30°C (59°F to 86°F). Protect from light.

Oral solution: Store at controlled room temperature of 25°C (77°F); excursions permitted to 15°C to 30°C (59°F to 86°F). Use within 6 months after opening.

Tablet: Store at controlled room temperature of 25°C (77°F); excursions permitted to 15°C to 30°C (59°F to 86°F).

Mechanism of Action

Aripiprazole is a quinolinone antipsychotic which exhibits high affinity for D_2, D_3, 5-HT$_{1A}$, and 5-HT$_{2A}$ receptors; moderate affinity for D_4, 5-HT$_{2C}$, 5-HT$_7$, alpha$_1$ adrenergic, and H$_1$ receptors. It also possesses moderate affinity for the serotonin reuptake transporter; has no affinity for muscarinic (cholinergic) receptors. Aripiprazole functions as a partial agonist at the D_2 and 5-HT$_{1A}$ receptors, and as an antagonist at the 5-HT$_{2A}$ receptor.

Pharmacodynamics/Kinetics

Onset of action: Initial: 1-3 weeks

Absorption: Well absorbed

Distribution: V_d: 4.9 L/kg

Protein binding: ≥99%, primarily to albumin

Metabolism: Hepatic, via CYP2D6, CYP3A4 (dehydro-aripiprazole metabolite has affinity for D_2 receptors similar to the parent drug and represents 40% of the parent drug exposure in plasma)

Bioavailability: I.M.: 100%; Tablet: 87%

Half-life elimination: Aripiprazole: 75 hours; dehydro-aripiprazole: 94 hours

CYP2D6 poor metabolizers: Aripiprazole: 146 hours

Time to peak, plasma: I.M.: 1-3 hours; Tablet: 3-5 hours

With high-fat meal: Aripiprazole: Delayed by 3 hours; dehydro-aripiprazole: Delayed by 12 hours

Excretion: Feces (55%, ~18% of the total dose as unchanged drug); urine (25%, <1% of the total dose as unchanged drug)

Dosage

Geriatric & Adult Note: Oral solution may be substituted for the oral tablet on a mg-per-mg basis, up to 25 mg. Patients receiving 30 mg tablets should be given 25 mg oral solution. Orally disintegrating tablets (Abilify Discmelt®) are bioequivalent to the immediate release tablets (Abilify®).

Acute agitation (schizophrenia/bipolar mania): I.M.: 9.75 mg as a single dose (range: 5.25-15 mg); repeated doses may be given at ≥2-hour intervals to a maximum of 30 mg/day. **Note:** If ongoing therapy with aripiprazole is necessary, transition to oral therapy as soon as possible.

Bipolar I disorder (acute manic or mixed episodes): Oral:

Stabilization:

Monotherapy: Initial: 15 mg once daily. May increase to 30 mg once daily if clinically indicated; safety of doses >30 mg/day has not been evaluated

Adjunct to lithium or valproic acid: Initial: 10-15 mg once daily. May increase to 30 mg once daily if clinically indicated; safety of doses >30 mg/day has not been evaluated.

Maintenance: Continue stabilization dose for up to 6 weeks; efficacy of continued treatment >6 weeks has not been established.

Depression (adjunctive with antidepressants): Oral: Initial: 2-5 mg/day (range: 2-15 mg/day); dose adjustments of up to 5 mg/day may be made in intervals of ≥1 week. **Note:** Dosing based on patients already receiving antidepressant therapy.

Schizophrenia: Oral: 10-15 mg once daily; may be increased to a maximum of 30 mg once daily (efficacy at dosages above 10-15 mg has not been shown to be increased). Dosage titration should not be more frequent than every 2 weeks.

◄ **Dosage adjustment with concurrent CYP450 inducer or inhibitor therapy:** Oral:
CYP3A4 inducers (eg, carbamazepine): Aripiprazole dose should be doubled (20-30 mg/day); dose should be subsequently reduced (10-15 mg/day) if concurrent inducer agent discontinued.
CYP3A4 inhibitors (eg, ketoconazole): Aripiprazole dose should be reduced to $1/2$ of the usual dose, and proportionally increased upon discontinuation of the inhibitor agent.
CYP2D6 inhibitors (eg, fluoxetine, paroxetine): Aripiprazole dose should be reduced to $1/2$ of the usual dose, and proportionally increased upon discontinuation of the inhibitor agent.

Renal Impairment No dosage adjustment required.

Hepatic Impairment No dosage adjustment required.

Administration

Injection: For I.M. use only; do not administer SubQ or I.V.; inject slowly into deep muscle mass

Oral: May be administered with or without food. Tablet and oral solution may be interchanged on a mg-per-mg basis, up to 25 mg. Doses using 30 mg tablets should be exchanged for 25 mg oral solution. Orally disintegrating tablets (Abilify Discmelt®) are bioequivalent to the immediate release tablets (Abilify®).

Orally-disintegrating tablet: Remove from foil blister by peeling back (do not push tablet through the foil). Place tablet in mouth immediately upon removal. Tablet dissolves rapidly in saliva and may be swallowed without liquid. If needed, can be taken with liquid. Do not split tablet.

Monitoring Parameters Vital signs; fasting lipid profile and fasting blood glucose/Hb A_{1c} (prior to treatment, at 3 months, then annually); CBC frequently during first few months of therapy in patients with pre-existing low WBC or a history of drug-induced leukopenia/neutropenia; BMI, personal/family history of diabetes, waist circumference, blood pressure, mental status, abnormal involuntary movement scale (AIMS), extrapyramidal symptoms (EPS). Weight should be assessed prior to treatment, at 4 weeks, 8 weeks, 12 weeks, and then at quarterly intervals. Consider titrating to a different antipsychotic agent for a weight gain ≥5% of the initial weight.

Special Geriatric Considerations Elderly patients have an increased risk of adverse response to side effects or adverse reactions to antipsychotics. Aripiprazole has been studied in elderly patients with psychosis associated with Alzheimer's disease. The package insert does not provide the outcomes of this study other than somnolence was more frequent with aripiprazole (8%) than placebo (1%). Clinical data have shown an increased incidence of serious cerebrovascular events in the elderly, some fatal. In light of significant risks and adverse effects in the elderly population (compared with limited data demonstrating efficacy in the treatment of dementia-related psychosis, aggression, and agitation), an extensive risk: benefit analysis should be performed prior to use. Aripiprazole's delayed onset of action and long half-life may limit its role in treating older persons with psychosis. Not approved for the treatment of patients with dementia-related psychosis.

Dosage Forms Excipient information presented when available (limited, particularly for generics); consult specific product labeling.

Injection, solution:
Abilify®: 7.5 mg/mL (1.3 mL)
Solution, oral:
Abilify®: 1 mg/mL (150 mL) [contains fructose 200 mg/mL, propylene glycol, sucrose 400 mg/mL; orange cream flavor]
Tablet, oral:
Abilify®: 2 mg, 5 mg, 10 mg, 15 mg, 20 mg, 30 mg
Tablet, orally disintegrating, oral:
Abilify Discmelt®: 10 mg [contains phenylalanine 1.12 mg/tablet; creme de vanilla flavor]
Abilify Discmelt®: 15 mg [contains phenylalanine 1.68 mg/tablet; creme de vanilla flavor]

Selected References

Rabins PV, Blacker D, Rovner BW, et al, "Practice Guidelines for the Treatment of Patients With Alzheimer's Disease and Other Dementias," *Am J Psychiatry*, 2007, 164(12 Suppl):5-56. Available at http://www.psych.org/psych_pract/treatg/pg/prac_guide.cfm.
Schneider LS, Tariot PN, Dagerman KS, et al, "Effectiveness of Atypical Antipsychotic Drugs in Patients With Alzheimer's Disease," *N Engl J Med*, 2006, 355(15):1525-38.

◆ **Aristospan®** see Triamcinolone (Systemic) on page 1853
◆ **Arixtra®** see Fondaparinux on page 782

Armodafinil (ar moe DAF i nil)

Brand Names: U.S. Nuvigil®
Index Terms R-modafinil
Generic Availability (U.S.) No

Pharmacologic Category Stimulant

Use Improve wakefulness in patients with excessive daytime sleepiness associated with narcolepsy and shift work sleep disorder (SWSD); adjunctive therapy for obstructive sleep apnea/hypopnea syndrome (OSAHS)

Medication Guide Available Yes

Contraindications Hypersensitivity to armodafinil, modafinil, or any component of the formulation

Warnings/Precautions For use following complete evaluation of sleepiness and in conjunction with other standard treatments (eg, CPAP). The degree of sleepiness should be reassessed frequently; some patients may not return to a normal level of wakefulness. Use is not recommended with a history of angina, cardiac ischemia, recent history of myocardial infarction, left ventricular hypertrophy, or patients with mitral valve prolapse who have developed mitral valve prolapse syndrome with previous CNS stimulant use. Blood pressure monitoring may be required in patients on armodafinil. New or additional antihypertensive therapy may be needed.

Serious and life-threatening rashes including Stevens-Johnson syndrome, toxic epidermal necrolysis, and drug rash with eosinophilia and systemic symptoms have been reported with modafinil, the racemate of armodafinil. In clinical trials of modafinil, these rashes were more likely to occur in children; however, in the postmarketing period, serious reactions have occurred in both adults and children. Most cases have been reported within the first 5 weeks of initiating therapy; however, rare cases have occurred after prolonged therapy.

Caution should be exercised when modafinil is given to patients with a history of psychosis; may impair the ability to engage in potentially hazardous activities. Stimulants may unmask tics in individuals with coexisting Tourette's syndrome. Use caution with renal or hepatic impairment (dosage adjustment in hepatic dysfunction is recommended). Use reduced doses in elderly patients.

Adverse Reactions (Reflective of adult population; not specific for elderly)
>10%: Central nervous system: Headache (14% to 23%; dose-related)
1% to 10%:
  Cardiovascular: Palpitation (2%), increased heart rate (1%)
  Central nervous system: Dizziness (5%), insomnia (4% to 6%; dose related), anxiety (4%), depression (1% to 3%; dose related), fatigue (2%), agitation (1%), attention disturbance (1%), depressed mood (1%), migraine (1%), nervousness (1%), pain (1%), pyrexia (1%), tremor (1%)
  Dermatologic: Rash (1% to 4%; dose related), contact dermatitis (1%), hyperhidrosis (1%)
  Gastrointestinal: Nausea (6% to 9%; dose related), xerostomia (2% to 7%; dose related), diarrhea (4%), abdominal pain (2%), dyspepsia (2%), anorexia (1%), appetite decreased (1%), constipation (1%), loose stools (1%), vomiting (1%)
  Genitourinary: Polyuria (1%)
  Hepatic: GGT increased (1%)
  Neuromuscular & skeletal: Paresthesia (1%)
  Respiratory: Dyspnea (1%)
  Miscellaneous: Flu-like syndrome (1%), thirst (1%)

Drug Interactions
  Metabolism/Transport Effects
    Substrate of CYP3A4 (major); **Inhibits** CYP2C19 (moderate); **Induces** CYP1A2 (weak), 3A4 (moderate)
  Avoid Concomitant Use
    Avoid concomitant use of Armodafinil with any of the following: Clopidogrel; Conivaptan; Iobenguane I 123
  Increased Effect/Toxicity
    Armodafinil may increase the levels/effects of: CYP2C19 Substrates; Sympathomimetics

    The levels/effects of Armodafinil may be increased by: Atomoxetine; Cannabinoids; Conivaptan; CYP3A4 Inhibitors (Moderate); CYP3A4 Inhibitors (Strong); Dasatinib
  Decreased Effect
    Armodafinil may decrease the levels/effects of: Clopidogrel; Contraceptives (Estrogens); CycloSPORINE; CycloSPORINE (Systemic); Iobenguane I 123; Saxagliptin

    The levels/effects of Armodafinil may be decreased by: CYP3A4 Inducers (Strong); Deferasirox; Herbs (CYP3A4 Inducers); Tocilizumab
  Ethanol/Nutrition/Herb Interactions
    Ethanol: Avoid or limit ethanol.
    Food: Delays absorption, but minimal effects on bioavailability. Food may affect the onset and time course of armodafinil.

Stability Store at 20°C to 25°C (68°F to 77°F).

◀ **Mechanism of Action** The exact mechanism of action of armodafinil is unknown. It is the R-enantiomer of modafinil. Armodafinil binds to the dopamine transporter and inhibits dopamine reuptake, which may result in increased extracellular dopamine levels in the brain. However, it does not appear to be a dopamine receptor agonist and also does not appear to bind to or inhibit the most common receptors or enzymes that are relevant for sleep/wake regulation.

Pharmacodynamics/Kinetics
Absorption: Readily absorbed
Distribution: V_d: 42 L
Protein binding: ~60% (based on modafinil; primarily albumin)
Metabolism: Hepatic, multiple pathways, including CYP3A4/5; metabolites include R-modafinil acid and modafinil sulfone
Clearance: 33 mL/minute, mainly via hepatic metabolism
Half-life elimination: 15 hours; Steady state: ~7 days
Time to peak, plasma: 2 hours (fasted)
Excretion: Urine (80% predominantly as metabolites; <10% as unchanged drug)

Dosage
Geriatric Refer to adult dosing. Consider lower initial dosage. Concentrations were almost doubled in clinical trials (based on modafinil).
Adult
Narcolepsy: Oral: 150-250 mg once daily in the morning
Obstructive sleep apnea/hypopnea syndrome (OSAHS): Oral: 150-250 mg once daily in the morning; 250 mg was not shown to have any increased benefit over 150 mg
Shift work sleep disorder (SWSD): Oral: 150 mg given once daily ~1 hour prior to work shift
Renal Impairment Inadequate data to determine safety and efficacy in severe renal impairment.
Hepatic Impairment Severe hepatic impairment (Child-Pugh classes B and C): Based on modafinil, dose should be reduced by half.
Administration May be administered without regard to food.
Monitoring Parameters Signs of hypersensitivity, rash, psychiatric symptoms, levels of sleepiness, blood pressure, and drug abuse
Special Geriatric Considerations There are no specific pharmacokinetic data for armodafinil, but the clearance of modafinil may be reduced in the elderly. Safety and effectiveness in persons >65 years of age have not been established.
Controlled Substance C-IV
Dosage Forms Excipient information presented when available (limited, particularly for generics); consult specific product labeling.
Tablet, oral:
Nuvigil®: 50 mg, 150 mg, 250 mg

◆ **Armour® Thyroid** see Thyroid, Desiccated on page 1786
◆ **Aromasin®** see Exemestane on page 685
◆ **Artane** see Trihexyphenidyl on page 1865
◆ **Arthropan®** see Salicylates (Various Salts) on page 1647
◆ **Arthrotec®** see Diclofenac and Misoprostol on page 501
◆ **Artificial Saliva** see Saliva Substitute on page 1652

Artificial Tears (ar ti FISH il tears)

Medication Safety Issues
Sound-alike/look-alike issues:
Isopto® Tears may be confused with Isoptin®
Brand Names: U.S. Akwa Tears® [OTC]; Bion® Tears [OTC]; HypoTears PF [OTC]; HypoTears [OTC]; Liquifilm® Tears [OTC]; Moisture® Eyes PM [OTC]; Moisture® Eyes [OTC]; Murine Tears® [OTC]; Murocel® [OTC]; Nature's Tears® [OTC]; Nu-Tears® II [OTC]; Nu-Tears® [OTC]; Refresh Plus® [OTC]; Refresh Tears® [OTC]; Refresh® [OTC]; Soothe® [OTC]; Systane® Free [OTC]; Systane® [OTC]; Teargen® II [OTC]; Teargen® [OTC]; Tearisol® [OTC]; Tears Again® [OTC]; Tears Naturale® Free [OTC]; Tears Naturale® II [OTC]; Tears Naturale® [OTC]; Tears Plus® [OTC]; Tears Renewed® [OTC]; Ultra Tears® [OTC]; Viva-Drops® [OTC]
Brand Names: Canada Teardrops®
Index Terms Hydroxyethylcellulose; Polyvinyl Alcohol
Generic Availability (U.S.) Yes
Pharmacologic Category Ophthalmic Agent, Miscellaneous
Use Ophthalmic lubricant; for relief of dry eyes and eye irritation
Dosage
Geriatric & Adult Ocular dryness/irritation: Ophthalmic: Use as needed to relieve symptoms, 1-2 drops into eye(s) 3-4 times/day

Special Geriatric Considerations Evaluate the patient's or caregiver's ability to safely administer the correct dose of ophthalmic medication.

Dosage Forms Excipient information presented when available (limited, particularly for generics); consult specific product labeling.

Solution, ophthalmic: 15 mL and 30 mL dropper bottles

Ascorbic Acid (a SKOR bik AS id)

Medication Safety Issues

International issues:

Rubex [Ireland] may be confused with Brivex brand name for brivudine [Switzerland]

Rubex: Brand name for ascorbic acid [Ireland], but also the brand name for doxorubicin [Brazil]

Brand Names: U.S. Acerola [OTC]; Asco-Caps-1000 [OTC]; Asco-Caps-500 [OTC]; Asco-Tabs-1000 [OTC]; Ascocid® [OTC]; Ascocid®-500 [OTC]; Ascor L 500®; Ascor L NC®; C-Gel [OTC]; C-Gram [OTC]; C-Time [OTC]; Cemill 1000 [OTC]; Cemill 500 [OTC]; Chew-C [OTC]; Dull-C® [OTC]; Mild-C® [OTC]; One Gram C [OTC]; Time-C® [OTC]; Vicks® Vitamin C [OTC]; Vita-C® [OTC]

Brand Names: Canada Proflavanol C™; Revitalose C-1000®

Index Terms Vitamin C

Generic Availability (U.S.) Yes

Pharmacologic Category Vitamin, Water Soluble

Use Prevention and treatment of scurvy; acidify the urine

Unlabeled/Investigational Use Investigational: In large doses to decrease the severity of "colds"; dietary supplementation; a 20-year study was recently completed involving 730 individuals which indicates a possible decreased risk of death by stroke when ascorbic acid at doses ≥45 mg/day was administered

Warnings/Precautions Patients with diabetes and patients prone to recurrent renal calculi (eg, dialysis patients) should not take excessive doses for extended periods of time. Some parenteral products contain aluminum; use caution in patients with impaired renal function.

Adverse Reactions (Reflective of adult population; not specific for elderly)

1% to 10%: Renal: Hyperoxaluria with large doses

Drug Interactions

Avoid Concomitant Use There are no known interactions where it is recommended to avoid concomitant use.

Increased Effect/Toxicity

Ascorbic Acid may increase the levels/effects of: Aluminum Hydroxide; Deferoxamine; Estrogen Derivatives

Decreased Effect

Ascorbic Acid may decrease the levels/effects of: Amphetamines; Bortezomib; Cyclo-SPORINE; CycloSPORINE (Systemic)

The levels/effects of Ascorbic Acid may be decreased by: Copper

Stability Injectable form should be stored under refrigeration (2°C to 8°C). Protect oral dosage forms from light. Rapidly oxidized when in solution in air and alkaline media.

Mechanism of Action Not fully understood; necessary for collagen formation and tissue repair; involved in some oxidation-reduction reactions as well as other metabolic pathways, such as synthesis of carnitine, steroids, and catecholamines and conversion of folic acid to folinic acid

Pharmacodynamics/Kinetics

Absorption: Oral: Readily absorbed; an active process thought to be dose dependent

Distribution: Large

Metabolism: Hepatic via oxidation and sulfation

Excretion: Urine (with high blood levels)

◄ **Dosage**
  Geriatric & Adult
    Recommended daily allowance (RDA): Upper limit of intake should not exceed 2000 mg/day
      Male: 90 mg
      Female: 75 mg;
      Adult smoker: Add an additional 35 mg/day
    Scurvy: Oral, I.M., I.V., SubQ: 100-250 mg 1-2 times/day for at least 2 weeks
    Urinary acidification: Oral, I.V.: 4-12 g/day in 3-4 divided doses
    Prevention and treatment of colds: Oral: 1-3 g/day
    Dietary supplement: Oral: 50-200 mg/day
  Administration Avoid rapid I.V. injection
  Monitoring Parameters Monitor pH of urine when using as an acidifying agent
  Test Interactions False-positive urinary glucose with cupric sulfate reagent, false-negative urinary glucose with glucose oxidase method; false-negative stool occult blood 48-72 hours after ascorbic acid ingestion
  Pharmacotherapy Pearls Sodium content of 1 g of sodium ascorbate: ~5 mEq
  Special Geriatric Considerations Minimum RDA for elderly is not established. Vitamin C is provided mainly in citrus fruits and tomatoes. The elderly, however, avoid citrus fruits due to cost and difficulty preparing (peeling). Daily replacement through a single multiple vitamin is recommended. Use of natural vitamin C or rose hips offers no advantages. Acidity may produce GI complaints.
  Dosage Forms Excipient information presented when available (limited, particularly for generics); consult specific product labeling.
  Caplet, oral: 1000 mg
  Caplet, timed release, oral: 500 mg, 1000 mg
  Capsule, oral:
    Mild-C®: 500 mg
  Capsule, softgel, oral:
    C-Gel: 1000 mg
  Capsule, sustained release, oral:
    C-Time: 500 mg
  Capsule, timed release, oral: 500 mg
    Asco-Caps-500: 500 mg
    Asco-Caps-1000: 1000 mg [sugar free]
    Time-C®: 500 mg
  Crystals for solution, oral: (170 g, 1000 g)
    Mild-C®: (170 g, 1000 g)
    Vita-C®: (113 g, 454 g) [dye free, gluten free, sugar free]
  Injection, solution: 500 mg/mL (50 mL)
    Ascor L 500®: 500 mg/mL (50 mL) [contains edetate disodium]
  Injection, solution [preservative free]: 500 mg/mL (50 mL)
    Ascor L NC®: 500 mg/mL (50 mL) [contains edetate disodium]
  Liquid, oral: 500 mg/5 mL (118 mL, 473 mL)
  Lozenge, oral:
    Vicks® Vitamin C: 25 mg (20s) [contains sodium 5 mg/lozenge; orange flavor]
  Powder for solution, oral:
    Ascocid®: (227 g, 454 g)
    Dull-C®: (113 g, 454 g) [dye free, gluten free, sugar free]
  Tablet, oral: 100 mg, 250 mg, 500 mg, 1000 mg
    Asco-Tabs-1000: 1000 mg [sugar free]
    Ascocid®-500: 500 mg [sugar free]
    C-Gram: 1000 mg [dye free, gluten free, sugar free]
    One Gram C: 1000 mg
  Tablet, chewable, oral: 250 mg, 500 mg
    Acerola: 500 mg [cherry flavor]
    Mild-C®: 250 mg [orange-tangerine flavor]
  Tablet, chewable, oral [buffered]:
    Chew-C: 500 mg [orange flavor]
  Tablet, timed release, oral: 500 mg, 1000 mg
    Cemill 500: 500 mg
    Cemill 1000: 1000 mg
    Mild-C®: 1000 mg

◆ **Asco-Tabs-1000 [OTC]** *see* Ascorbic Acid *on page* 149
◆ **Ascriptin® Maximum Strength [OTC]** *see* Aspirin *on page* 153
◆ **Ascriptin® Regular Strength [OTC]** *see* Aspirin *on page* 153

Asenapine (a SEN a peen)

Related Information

Antipsychotic Agents *on page 1997*
Atypical Antipsychotics *on page 1999*

Brand Names: U.S. Saphris®

Pharmacologic Category Antimanic Agent; Antipsychotic Agent, Atypical

Use Acute and maintenance treatment of schizophrenia; treatment of acute mania or mixed episodes associated with bipolar I disorder (as monotherapy or in combination with lithium or valproate)

Contraindications Hypersensitivity to asenapine or any component of the formulation

Warnings/Precautions [U.S. Boxed Warning]: Elderly patients with dementia-related psychosis treated with atypical antipsychotics are at an increased risk of death compared to placebo. Most deaths appeared to be either cardiovascular (eg, heart failure, sudden death) or infectious (eg, pneumonia) in nature. In addition, an increased incidence of cerebrovascular effects (eg, transient ischemic attack, cerebrovascular accidents) has been reported in studies of placebo-controlled trials of antipsychotics in elderly patients with dementia-related psychosis. Asenapine is not approved for the treatment of dementia-related psychosis.

Leukopenia, neutropenia, and agranulocytosis (sometimes fatal) have been reported in clinical trials and postmarketing reports with antipsychotic use; presence of risk factors (eg, pre-existing low WBC or history of drug-induced leuko/neutropenia) should prompt periodic blood count assessment. Discontinue therapy at first signs of blood dyscrasias or if absolute neutrophil count <1000/mm^3.

May be sedating; use with caution in disorders where CNS depression is a feature. Use with caution in Parkinson's disease. Use with caution in patients at risk of seizures, including those with a history of seizures, head trauma, brain damage, alcoholism, or concurrent therapy with medications which may lower seizure threshold. Use is not recommended in severe hepatic impairment; increased drug concentrations may occur. Esophageal dysmotility and aspiration have been associated with antipsychotic use; use with caution in patients at risk of aspiration pneumonia (ie, Alzheimer's disease). Elevates prolactin levels; use with caution in breast cancer or other prolactin-dependent tumors. May alter temperature regulation.

Use with caution in patients with cardiovascular diseases (eg, heart failure, history of myocardial infarction or ischemia, cerebrovascular disease, conduction abnormalities). May cause orthostatic hypotension; use with caution in patients at risk of this effect (eg, concurrent medication use which may predispose to hypotension/bradycardia or presence of hypovolemia) or in those who would not tolerate transient hypotensive episodes. May result in QT$_c$ prolongation. Risk may be increased by conditions or concomitant medications which cause bradycardia, hypokalemia, and/or hypomagnesemia. Avoid use in combination with QT$_c$-prolonging drugs and in patients with congenital long QT syndrome or patients with history of cardiac arrhythmia.

May cause extrapyramidal symptoms (EPS), including pseudoparkinsonism, acute dystonic reactions, akathisia, and tardive dyskinesia. Risk of dystonia (and probably other EPS) may be greater with increased doses, use of conventional antipsychotics, males, and younger patients. Risk of neuroleptic malignant syndrome (NMS) may be increased in patients with Parkinson's disease or Lewy body dementia. May cause hyperglycemia; in some cases may be extreme and associated with ketoacidosis, hyperosmolar coma, or death. Use with caution in patients with diabetes or other disorders of glucose regulation; monitor for worsening of glucose control. Significant weight gain has been observed with antipsychotic therapy; incidence varies with product. Monitor waist circumference and BMI. May cause anaphylaxis or hypersensitivity reactions.

The possibility of a suicide attempt is inherent in psychotic illness or bipolar disorder; use caution in high-risk patients during initiation of therapy. Prescriptions should be written for the smallest quantity consistent with good patient care. Use caution in elderly patients.

Adverse Reactions (Reflective of adult population; not specific for elderly) Actual frequency may be dependent upon dose and/or indication.

>10%:
  Central nervous system: Somnolence (13% to 24%), insomnia (6% to 16%), extrapyramidal symptoms (6% to 12%), headache (12%), akathisia (4% to 11%; dose related), dizziness (3% to 11%)
  Endocrine & metabolic: Hypertriglyceridemia (13% to 15%)
1% to 10%:
  Cardiovascular: Peripheral edema (3%), hypertension (2% to 3%)

◄ Central nervous system: Hypoesthesia (4% to 7%), fatigue (3% to 4%), anxiety (4%), depression (2%), irritability (1% to 2%)

Endocrine & metabolic: Cholesterol increased (8% to 9%), glucose increased (5% to 7%), hyperprolactinemia (2% to 3%)

Gastrointestinal: Constipation (4% to 7%), vomiting (4% to 7%), weight gain (2% to 5%), dyspepsia (3% to 4%), appetite increased (≤4%), salivation increased (≤4%), abnormal taste (3%), toothache (3%), abdominal discomfort (≤3%), xerostomia (1% to 3%)

Hematologic: Creatine kinase increased (6%)

Hepatic: Transaminases increased (<1% to 3%)

Neuromuscular & skeletal: Arthralgia (3%), extremity pain (2%)

Drug Interactions

Avoid Concomitant Use

Avoid concomitant use of Asenapine with any of the following: Artemether; Dronedarone; Lumefantrine; Metoclopramide; Nilotinib; Pimozide; QUENINE; Tetrabenazine; Thioridazine; Toremifene; Vandetanib; Vemurafenib; Ziprasidone

Increased Effect/Toxicity

Asenapine may increase the levels/effects of: Alcohol (Ethyl); CNS Depressants; Dronedarone; Methylphenidate; PARoxetine; Pimozide; QTc-Prolonging Agents; QuiNINE; Selective Serotonin Reuptake Inhibitors; Tetrabenazine; Thioridazine; Toremifene; Vandetanib; Vemurafenib; Ziprasidone

The levels/effects of Asenapine may be increased by: Abiraterone Acetate; Acetylcholinesterase Inhibitors (Central); Alfuzosin; Artemether; Chloroquine; Ciprofloxacin; Ciprofloxacin (Systemic); Conivaptan; CYP1A2 Inhibitors (Moderate); CYP1A2 Inhibitors (Strong); Deferasirox; FluvoxaMINE; Gadobutrol; HydrOXYzine; Lithium formulations; Lumefantrine; MAO Inhibitors; Methylphenidate; Metoclopramide; Nilotinib; QUEtiapine; QuiNINE; Tetrabenazine

Decreased Effect

Asenapine may decrease the levels/effects of: Amphetamines; Anti-Parkinson's Agents (Dopamine Agonist); Quinagolide

The levels/effects of Asenapine may be decreased by: CYP1A2 Inducers (Strong); Cyproterone; Lithium formulations; Peginterferon Alfa-2b; Tocilizumab

Ethanol/Nutrition/Herb Interactions Ethanol: May increase CNS depression; monitor for increased effects with coadministration. Caution patients about effects.

Stability Store at 15°C to 30°C (59°F to 86°F).

Mechanism of Action Asenapine is a dibenzo-oxepino pyrrole atypical antipsychotic with mixed serotonin-dopamine antagonist activity. It exhibits high affinity for 5-HT$_{1A}$, 5-HT$_{1B}$, 5-HT$_{2A}$, 5-HT$_{2B}$, 5-HT$_{2C}$, 5-HT$_{5-7}$, D$_{1-4}$, H$_1$ and, alpha$_1$- and alpha$_2$-adrenergic receptors; moderate affinity for H$_2$ receptors. Asenapine has no significant affinity for muscarinic receptors. The binding affinity to the D$_2$ receptor is 19 times lower than the 5-HT$_{2A}$ affinity (Weber, 2009). The addition of serotonin antagonism to dopamine antagonism (classic neuroleptic mechanism) is thought to improve negative symptoms of psychoses and reduce the incidence of extrapyramidal side effects as compared to typical antipsychotics.

Pharmacodynamics/Kinetics

Absorption: Rapid

Distribution: V$_d$: ~20-25 L/kg

Protein binding: 95% (including albumin and α$_1$-acid glycoprotein)

Metabolism: Hepatic via CYP1A2 oxidation and UGT1A4 glucuronidation

Bioavailability: Sublingual: 35%; decreased if swallowed (<2%); decreased if administered with food or liquid

Half-life elimination: Terminal: ~24 hours

Time to peak, plasma: 0.5-1.5 hours

Excretion: Urine (~50%); feces (~40%)

Dosage

Geriatric & Adult Note: Safety of doses >20 mg/day has not been evaluated:

Schizophrenia: Sublingual:

Acute treatment: Initial: 5 mg twice daily. Daily doses >20 mg/day in clinical trials did not appear to offer any additional benefits and increased risk of adverse effects.

Maintenance treatment: Initial: 5 mg twice daily; may increase to 10 mg twice daily after 1 week based on tolerability

Bipolar disorder: Sublingual:

Monotherapy: Initial: 10 mg twice daily; decrease to 5 mg twice daily if dose not tolerated

Combination therapy (with lithium or valproate): 5 mg twice daily; may increase to 10 mg twice daily based on tolerability

Renal Impairment No dosage adjustment is necessary.

Hepatic Impairment

Mild-to-moderate hepatic impairment (Child-Pugh class A or B): No dosage adjustment is necessary

Severe hepatic impairment (Child-Pugh class C): Use is not recommended

Administration Sublingual tablets should be placed under the tongue and allowed to disintegrate. Do not crush, chew, or swallow. Avoid eating or drinking for at least 10 minutes after administration.

Monitoring Parameters Vital signs; fasting lipid profile and fasting blood glucose/Hgb A_{1c} (baseline and periodically); CBC frequently during first few months of therapy in patients with pre-existing low WBC or a history of drug-induced leukopenia/neutropenia; BMI, personal/ family history of obesity, waist circumference; blood pressure; mental status, abnormal involuntary movement scale (AIMS), extrapyramidal symptoms; orthostatic blood pressure changes for 3-5 days after starting or increasing dose. Weight should be assessed prior to treatment and regularly throughout therapy. Consider titrating to a different antipsychotic agent for a weight gain ≥5% of the initial weight.

Special Geriatric Considerations Studies to date have not had sufficient numbers of patients to determine if elderly respond differently than younger adults. Given the high percentages of CNS adverse effects, patients should be monitored closely for somnolence, insomnia, EPS, akathisia, and dizziness. Elderly (with dementia-related psychosis) were determined, in initial studies with antipsychotics, to have an increased risk of death (1.6-1.7 times that seen in placebo groups). Asenapine is not approved for the treatment of dementia-related psychosis.

Dosage Forms Excipient information presented when available (limited, particularly for generics); consult specific product labeling.

Tablet, sublingual:

Saphris®: 5 mg [unflavored]

Saphris®: 5 mg [black cherry flavor]

Saphris®: 10 mg [unflavored]

Saphris®: 10 mg [black cherry flavor]

Selected References

Potkin SG, Cohen M, and Panagides J. "Efficacy and Tolerability of Asenapine in Acute Schizophrenia: A Placebo- and Risperidone-Controlled Trial," *J Clin Psychiatry*, 2007, 68(10):1492-1500.

Weber J and McCormack PL, "Asenapine," *CNS Drugs*, 2009, 23(9):781-92.

◆ **Asendin [DSC]** see Amoxapine on page 112
◆ **Asmanex® Twisthaler®** see Mometasone (Oral Inhalation) on page 1231
◆ **Aspart Insulin** see Insulin Aspart on page 943
◆ **Aspercin [OTC]** see Aspirin on page 153
◆ *Aspergillus niger* see Alpha-Galactosidase on page 69
◆ **Aspergum® [OTC]** see Aspirin on page 153

Aspirin (AS pir in)

Related Information

Beers Criteria – Potentially Inappropriate Medications for Geriatrics on page 2089

Medication Safety Issues

Sound-alike/look-alike issues:

Aspirin may be confused with Afrin®

Ascriptin® may be confused with Aricept®

Ecotrin® may be confused with Edecrin®, Epogen®

Halfprin® may be confused with Haltran®

ZORprin® may be confused with Zyloprim®

International issues:

Cartia [multiple international markets] may be confused with Cartia XT brand name for diltiazem [U.S.]

Brand Names: U.S. Ascriptin® Maximum Strength [OTC]; Ascriptin® Regular Strength [OTC]; Aspercin [OTC]; Aspergum® [OTC]; Aspir-low [OTC]; Aspirtab [OTC]; Bayer® Aspirin Extra Strength [OTC]; Bayer® Aspirin Regimen Adult Low Strength [OTC]; Bayer® Aspirin Regimen Children's [OTC]; Bayer® Aspirin Regimen Regular Strength [OTC]; Bayer® Genuine Aspirin [OTC]; Bayer® Plus Extra Strength [OTC]; Bayer® Women's Low Dose Aspirin [OTC]; Buffasal [OTC]; Bufferin® Extra Strength [OTC]; Bufferin® [OTC]; Buffinol [OTC]; Ecotrin® Arthritis Strength [OTC]; Ecotrin® Low Strength [OTC]; Ecotrin® [OTC]; Halfprin® [OTC]; St Joseph® Adult Aspirin [OTC]; Tri-Buffered Aspirin [OTC]

Brand Names: Canada Asaphen; Asaphen E.C.; Entrophen®; Novasen; Praxis ASA EC 81 Mg Daily Dose

Index Terms Acetylsalicylic Acid; ASA; Baby Aspirin

Generic Availability (U.S.) Yes: Excludes gum

Pharmacologic Category Antiplatelet Agent; Salicylate

Use Treatment of mild-to-moderate pain, inflammation, and fever; prevention and treatment of myocardial infarction (MI), acute ischemic stroke, and transient ischemic episodes; management of rheumatoid arthritis, rheumatic fever, osteoarthritis; adjunctive therapy in revascularization procedures (coronary artery bypass graft [CABG], percutaneous transluminal coronary angioplasty [PTCA], carotid endarterectomy), stent implantation

Unlabeled/Investigational Use Low doses have been used in complications associated with autoimmune disorders such as lupus or antiphospholipid syndrome; alternative therapy for prevention of thromboembolism associated with atrial fibrillation in patients not candidates for warfarin; pericarditis associated with MI; prosthetic valve thromboprophylaxis

Contraindications Hypersensitivity to salicylates, other NSAIDs, or any component of the formulation; asthma; rhinitis; nasal polyps; inherited or acquired bleeding disorders (including factor VII and factor IX deficiency)

Warnings/Precautions Use with caution in patients with platelet and bleeding disorders, renal dysfunction, dehydration, erosive gastritis, or peptic ulcer disease. Heavy ethanol use (>3 drinks/day) can increase bleeding risks. Avoid use in severe renal failure or in severe hepatic failure. Low-dose aspirin for cardioprotective effects is associated with a two- to fourfold increase in UGI events (eg, symptomatic or complicated ulcers); risks of these events increase with increasing aspirin dose; during the chronic phase of aspirin dosing, doses >81 mg are not recommended unless indicated (Bhatt, 2008).

Discontinue use if tinnitus or impaired hearing occurs. Caution in mild-to-moderate renal failure (only at high dosages). Patients with sensitivity to tartrazine dyes, nasal polyps, and asthma may have an increased risk of salicylate sensitivity. In the treatment of acute ischemic stroke, avoid aspirin for 24 hours following administration of alteplase; administration within 24 hours increases the risk of hemorrhagic transformation. Surgical patients should avoid ASA if possible, for 1-2 weeks prior to surgery, to reduce the risk of excessive bleeding (except in patients with cardiac stents that have not completed their full course of dual antiplatelet therapy [aspirin, clopidogrel]; patient-specific situations need to be discussed with cardiologist; AHA/ACC/SCAI/ACS/ADA Science Advisory provides recommendations). When used concomitantly with ≤325 mg of aspirin, NSAIDs (including selective COX-2 inhibitors) substantially increase the risk of gastrointestinal complications (eg, ulcer); concomitant gastroprotective therapy (eg, proton pump inhibitors) is recommended (Bhatt, 2008).

When used for self-medication (OTC labeling): Changes in behavior (along with nausea and vomiting) may be an early sign of Reye's syndrome; patients should be instructed to contact their healthcare provider if these occur.

Adverse Reactions (Reflective of adult population; not specific for elderly) As with all drugs which may affect hemostasis, bleeding is associated with aspirin. Hemorrhage may occur at virtually any site. Risk is dependent on multiple variables including dosage, concurrent use of multiple agents which alter hemostasis, and patient susceptibility. Many adverse effects of aspirin are dose related, and are rare at low dosages. Other serious reactions are idiosyncratic, related to allergy or individual sensitivity. Accurate estimation of frequencies is not possible. The reactions listed below have been reported for aspirin (frequency not defined).

Cardiovascular: Hypotension, tachycardia, dysrhythmias, edema

Central nervous system: Fatigue, insomnia, nervousness, agitation, confusion, dizziness, headache, lethargy, cerebral edema, hyperthermia, coma

Dermatologic: Rash, angioedema, urticaria

Endocrine & metabolic: Acidosis, hyperkalemia, dehydration, hypoglycemia (children), hyperglycemia, hypernatremia (buffered forms)

Gastrointestinal: Nausea, vomiting, dyspepsia, epigastric discomfort, heartburn, stomach pain, gastrointestinal ulceration (6% to 31%), gastric erosions, gastric erythema, duodenal ulcers

Hematologic: Anemia, disseminated intravascular coagulation (DIC), prothrombin times prolonged, coagulopathy, thrombocytopenia, hemolytic anemia, bleeding, iron deficiency anemia

Hepatic: Hepatotoxicity, transaminases increased, hepatitis (reversible)

Neuromuscular & skeletal: Rhabdomyolysis, weakness, acetabular bone destruction (OA)

Otic: Hearing loss, tinnitus

Renal: Interstitial nephritis, papillary necrosis, proteinuria, renal impairment, renal failure (including cases caused by rhabdomyolysis), BUN increased, serum creatinine increased

Respiratory: Asthma, bronchospasm, dyspnea, laryngeal edema, hyperpnea, tachypnea, respiratory alkalosis, noncardiogenic pulmonary edema

Miscellaneous: Anaphylaxis, prolonged pregnancy and labor, stillbirths, low birth weight, peripartum bleeding, Reye's syndrome

Drug Interactions

Metabolism/Transport Effects Substrate of CYP2C9 (minor)

Avoid Concomitant Use

Avoid concomitant use of Aspirin with any of the following: Floctafenine; Influenza Virus Vaccine (Live/Attenuated); Ketorolac; Ketorolac (Nasal); Ketorolac (Systemic)

Increased Effect/Toxicity

Aspirin may increase the levels/effects of: Alendronate; Anticoagulants; Carbonic Anhydrase Inhibitors; Collagenase (Systemic); Corticosteroids (Systemic); Divalproex; Drotrecogin Alfa; Heparin; Ibritumomab; Methotrexate; PRALAtrexate; Rivaroxaban; Salicylates; Sulfonylureas; Thrombolytic Agents; Ticagrelor; Tositumomab and Iodine I 131 Tositumomab; Valproic Acid; Varicella Virus-Containing Vaccines; Vitamin K Antagonists

The levels/effects of Aspirin may be increased by: Antidepressants (Tricyclic, Tertiary Amine); Antiplatelet Agents; Calcium Channel Blockers (Nondihydropyridine); Dasatinib; Floctafenine; Ginkgo Biloba; Glucosamine; Herbs (Anticoagulant/Antiplatelet Properties); Influenza Virus Vaccine (Live/Attenuated); Ketorolac; Ketorolac (Nasal); Ketorolac (Systemic); Loop Diuretics; Nonsteroidal Anti-Inflammatory Agents; NSAID (Nonselective); Omega-3-Acid Ethyl Esters; Pentosan Polysulfate Sodium; Pentoxifylline; Prostacyclin Analogues; Selective Serotonin Reuptake Inhibitors; Serotonin/Norepinephrine Reuptake Inhibitors; Treprostinil; Vitamin E

Decreased Effect

Aspirin may decrease the levels/effects of: ACE Inhibitors; Loop Diuretics; NSAID (Nonselective); Probenecid; Ticagrelor; Tiludronate

The levels/effects of Aspirin may be decreased by: Corticosteroids (Systemic); Nonsteroidal Anti-Inflammatory Agents; NSAID (Nonselective)

Ethanol/Nutrition/Herb Interactions

Ethanol: Avoid ethanol (may enhance gastric mucosal damage).

Food: Food may decrease the rate but not the extent of oral absorption.

Folic acid: Hyperexcretion of folate; folic acid deficiency may result, leading to macrocytic anemia.

Iron: With chronic aspirin use and at doses of 3-4 g/day, iron-deficiency anemia may result.

Sodium: Hypernatremia resulting from buffered aspirin solutions or sodium salicylate containing high sodium content. Avoid or use with caution in CHF or any condition where hypernatremia would be detrimental.

Benedictine liqueur, prunes, raisins, tea, and gherkins: Potential salicylate accumulation.

Fresh fruits containing vitamin C: Displace drug from binding sites, resulting in increased urinary excretion of aspirin.

Herb/Nutraceutical: Avoid cat's claw, dong quai, evening primrose, feverfew, garlic, ginger, ginkgo, red clover, horse chestnut, green tea, ginseng (all have additional antiplatelet activity). Limit curry powder, paprika, licorice; may cause salicylate accumulation. These foods contain 6 mg salicylate/100 g. An ordinary American diet contains 10-200 mg/day of salicylate.

Stability Keep suppositories in refrigerator; do not freeze. Hydrolysis of aspirin occurs upon exposure to water or moist air, resulting in salicylate and acetate, which possess a vinegar-like odor. Do not use if a strong odor is present.

Mechanism of Action Irreversibly inhibits cyclooxygenase-1 and 2 (COX-1 and 2) enzymes, via acetylation, which results in decreased formation of prostaglandin precursors; irreversibly inhibits formation of prostaglandin derivative, thromboxane A_2, via acetylation of platelet cyclooxygenase, thus inhibiting platelet aggregation; has antipyretic, analgesic, and anti-inflammatory properties

Pharmacodynamics/Kinetics

Duration: 4-6 hours

Absorption: Rapid

Distribution: V_d: 10 L; readily into most body fluids and tissues

◄ Metabolism: Hydrolyzed to salicylate (active) by esterases in GI mucosa, red blood cells, synovial fluid, and blood; metabolism of salicylate occurs primarily by hepatic conjugation; metabolic pathways are saturable

Bioavailability: 50% to 75% reaches systemic circulation

Half-life elimination: Parent drug: 15-20 minutes; Salicylates (dose dependent): 3 hours at lower doses (300-600 mg), 5-6 hours (after 1 g), 10 hours with higher doses

Time to peak, serum: ~1-2 hours

Excretion: Urine (75% as salicyluric acid, 10% as salicylic acid)

Dosage

Geriatric & Adult

Acute ischemic stroke: Oral: 150-325 mg once daily, initiated within 48 hours (in patients who are not candidates for alteplase and not receiving systemic anticoagulation)

Analgesic and antipyretic:

Oral: 325-650 mg every 4-6 hours up to 4 g/day

Rectal: 300-600 mg every 4-6 hours up to 4 g/day

Anti-inflammatory: Oral: Initial: 2.4-3.6 g/day in divided doses; usual maintenance: 3.6-5.4 g/day; monitor serum concentrations

Atrial fibrillation (in patients not candidates for warfarin or at low risk of ischemic stroke): Oral: 75-325 mg once daily

Bioprosthetic aortic valve: Oral: 50-100 mg once daily; usual dose: 81 mg once daily

Bioprosthetic mitral valve (following 3 months of anticoagulation): Oral: 50-100 mg once daily; usual dose: 81 mg once daily

CABG: Oral: 75-100 mg once daily (usual dose: 81 mg) initiated 6 hours following surgery; if bleeding prevents administration at 6 hours after CABG, initiate as soon as possible

CABG (internal mammary bypass graft): Oral: 75-162 mg once daily

Carotid artery stenting: Oral: 81-325 mg once daily beginning at least 24 hours (preferably 4 days) prior to procedure with concomitant clopidogrel

Carotid endarterectomy: Oral: 50-100 mg once daily preoperatively and daily thereafter; usual dose: 81 mg once daily

Infrainguinal arterial reconstruction/bypass: Oral: 75-100 mg once daily (begin preoperatively); usual dose: 81 mg once daily

Mechanical heart valve (with additional risk factors for thromboembolism): Oral: 50-100 mg once daily (in addition to warfarin); usual dose: 81 mg once daily

Mitral annular calcification (with documented stroke, TIA, or systemic embolism): Oral: 50-100 mg once daily; usual dose: 81 mg once daily

Mitral valve prolapse (with documented stroke or TIA): Oral: 50-100 mg once daily; usual dose: 81 mg once daily

Myocardial infarction (primary prevention): Oral: 75-162 mg once daily (Antman, 2004) or 75-100 mg (usual dose: 81 mg) once daily (Hirsh, 2008)

Non-ST-segment elevation myocardial infarction (NSTEMI): Oral: Initial: 162-325 mg; Maintenance: 75-100 mg once daily indefinitely; usual maintenance dose: 81 mg once daily

PCI: Oral: Initial: 75-325 mg (300-325 mg in aspirin naive patients) starting at least 2 hours (preferably 24 hours) before procedure; post procedure: 162-325 mg once daily (dose and duration varies with type of stent implanted); **Note:** Dose may be reduced to 75-162 mg once daily after appropriate duration based on stent-type is complete

Pericarditis associated with myocardial infarction: Oral: 162-325 mg once daily; doses as high as 650 mg every 4-6 hours may be required

Peripheral arterial disease: 75-100 mg once daily; usual dose: 81 mg once daily

ST-segment elevation myocardial infarction (STEMI): Initial: 162-325 mg given on presentation (patient should chew nonenteric-coated aspirin especially if not taking before presentation); for patients unable to take oral, may use rectal suppository (300 mg). Maintenance (secondary prevention): 75-162 mg once daily indefinitely

Stroke (cardioembolic; anticoagulation contraindicated): Oral: 75-325 mg once daily

Stroke/TIA (noncardioembolic; secondary prevention): Oral: 50-325 mg once daily (Adams, 2008) or 50-100 mg once daily; usual dose: 81 mg once daily (Hirsh, 2008)

Renal Impairment

Cl_{cr} <10 mL/minute: Avoid use.

Dialyzable (50% to 100%)

Hepatic Impairment Avoid use in severe liver disease.

Administration Do not crush enteric coated tablet. Administer with food or a full glass of water to minimize GI distress. For acute myocardial infarction, have patient chew tablet.

Reference Range Timing of serum samples: Peak levels usually occur 2 hours after ingestion. Salicylate serum concentrations correlate with the pharmacological actions and adverse effects observed. The serum salicylate concentration (mcg/mL) and the corresponding clinical correlations are as follows: See table on next page.

Serum Salicylate: Clinical Correlations

Serum Salicylate Concentration (mcg/mL)	Desired Effects	Adverse Effects / Intoxication
~100	Antiplatelet Antipyresis Analgesia	GI intolerance and bleeding, hypersensitivity, hemostatic defects
150-300	Anti-inflammatory	Mild salicylism
250-400	Treatment of rheumatic fever	Nausea/vomiting, hyperventilation, salicylism, flushing, sweating, thirst, headache, diarrhea, and tachycardia
>400-500		Respiratory alkalosis, hemorrhage, excitement, confusion, asterixis, pulmonary edema, convulsions, tetany, metabolic acidosis, fever, coma, cardiovascular collapse, renal and respiratory failure

Test Interactions False-negative results for glucose oxidase urinary glucose tests (Clinistix®); false-positives using the cupric sulfate method (Clinitest®); also, interferes with Gerhardt test, VMA determination; 5-HIAA, xylose tolerance test and T_3 and T_4

Special Geriatric Considerations Elderly are a high-risk population for adverse effects from nonsteroidal anti-inflammatory agents. As much as 60% of elderly with GI complications to NSAIDs can develop peptic ulceration and/or hemorrhage asymptomatically. The concomitant use of H_2 blockers and sucralfate is not effective as prophylaxis with the exception of NSAID-induced duodenal ulcers which may be prevented by the use of ranitidine. Misoprostol and proton pump inhibitors are the only prophylactic agents proven to help prevent the development of NSAID-induced ulcers. Also, concomitant disease and drug use contribute to the risk for GI adverse effects. Use lowest effective dose for shortest period possible. Consider renal function decline with age. Use of NSAIDs can compromise existing renal function especially when Cl_{cr} is ≤30 mL/minute. Tinnitus may be a difficult and unreliable indication of toxicity due to age-related hearing loss or eighth cranial nerve damage. CNS adverse effects such as confusion, agitation, and hallucination are generally seen in overdose or high dose situations, but elderly may demonstrate these adverse effects at lower doses than younger adults.

Dosage Forms Excipient information presented when available (limited, particularly for generics); consult specific product labeling.

Caplet, oral:
  Bayer® Aspirin Extra Strength: 500 mg
  Bayer® Genuine Aspirin: 325 mg
  Bayer® Women's Low Dose Aspirin: 81 mg [contains elemental calcium 300 mg]
Caplet, oral [buffered]:
  Ascriptin® Maximum Strength: 500 mg [contains aluminum hydroxide, calcium carbonate, magnesium hydroxide]
  Bayer® Plus Extra Strength: 500 mg [contains calcium carbonate]
Caplet, enteric coated, oral:
  Bayer® Aspirin Regimen Regular Strength: 325 mg
Gum, chewing, oral:
  Aspergum®: 227 mg (12s) [cherry flavor]
  Aspergum®: 227 mg (12s) [orange flavor]
Suppository, rectal: 300 mg (12s); 600 mg (12s)
Tablet, oral: 325 mg
  Aspercin: 325 mg
  Aspirtab: 325 mg
  Bayer® Genuine Aspirin: 325 mg
Tablet, oral [buffered]: 325 mg
  Ascriptin® Regular Strength: 325 mg [contains aluminum hydroxide, calcium carbonate, magnesium hydroxide]
  Buffasal: 325 mg [contains magnesium oxide]
  Bufferin®: 325 mg [contains calcium carbonate, magnesium carbonate, magnesium oxide]
  Bufferin® Extra Strength: 500 mg [contains calcium carbonate, magnesium carbonate, magnesium oxide]
  Buffinol: 324 mg [sugar free; contains magnesium oxide]
  Tri-Buffered Aspirin: 325 mg [contains calcium carbonate, magnesium carbonate, magnesium hydroxide]
  Tri-Buffered Aspirin: 325 mg [contains calcium carbonate, magnesium oxide]

◀ Tablet, chewable, oral: 81 mg
    Bayer® Aspirin Regimen Children's: 81 mg [cherry flavor]
    Bayer® Aspirin Regimen Children's: 81 mg [orange flavor]
    St Joseph® Adult Aspirin: 81 mg
Tablet, enteric coated, oral: 81 mg, 325 mg, 650 mg
    Aspir-low: 81 mg
    Bayer® Aspirin Regimen Adult Low Strength: 81 mg
    Ecotrin®: 325 mg
    Ecotrin® Arthritis Strength: 500 mg
    Ecotrin® Low Strength: 81 mg
    Halfprin®: 81 mg, 162 mg
    St Joseph® Adult Aspirin: 81 mg

Aspirin and Dipyridamole (AS pir in & dye peer ID a mole)

Related Information
Aspirin *on page 153*
Dipyridamole *on page 537*
Medication Safety Issues
  Sound-alike/look-alike issues:
    Aggrenox® may be confused with Aggrastat®
Brand Names: U.S. Aggrenox®
Brand Names: Canada Aggrenox®
Index Terms Aspirin and Extended-Release Dipyridamole; Dipyridamole and Aspirin
Generic Availability (U.S.) No
Pharmacologic Category Antiplatelet Agent
Use Reduction in the risk of stroke in patients who have had transient ischemia of the brain or ischemic stroke due to thrombosis
Unlabeled/Investigational Use Hemodialysis graft patency
Contraindications Hypersensitivity to dipyridamole, aspirin, or any component of the formulation; allergy to NSAIDs; patients with asthma, rhinitis, and nasal polyps; bleeding disorders (factor VII or IX deficiencies)
Warnings/Precautions Patients who consume ≥3 alcoholic drinks per day may be at risk of bleeding. Use cautiously use in patients with inherited or acquired bleeding disorders, renal impairment, hypotension, unstable angina, recent MI or hepatic dysfunction. Avoid use in patients with a history of active peptic ulcer disease, severe hepatic failure, or severe renal impairment (Cl_{cr} <10 mL/minute). Monitor for signs and symptoms of GI ulcers and bleeding. Discontinue use if dizziness, tinnitus, or impaired hearing occurs. Discontinue use 24 hours prior to pharmacologic (I.V. dipyridamole) stress testing. Discontinue 1-2 weeks before elective surgical procedures to reduce the risk of bleeding. Use caution in the elderly who are at high risk for adverse events. Dose of aspirin in this combination may not be adequate to prevent for cardiac indications (eg, MI prophylaxis). Formulation may contain lactose and/or sucrose. Use in patients with fructose and/or galactose intolerance is contraindicated in the Canadian labeling.
Adverse Reactions (Reflective of adult population; not specific for elderly)
>10%:
  Central nervous system: Headache (39%; tolerance usually develops)
  Gastrointestinal: Abdominal pain (18%), dyspepsia (18%), nausea (16%), diarrhea (13%)
1% to 10%:
  Cardiovascular: Cardiac failure (2%), syncope (1%)
  Central nervous system: Fatigue (6%), pain (6%), amnesia (2%), malaise (2%), seizure (2%), confusion (1%), somnolence (1%)
  Dermatologic: Purpura (1%)
  Gastrointestinal: Vomiting (8%), GI bleeding (4%), melena (2%), rectal bleeding (2%), hemorrhoids (1%), GI hemorrhage (1%), anorexia (1%)
  Hematologic: Hemorrhage (3%), anemia (2%)
  Neuromuscular & skeletal: Arthralgia (6%), back pain (5%), weakness (2%), arthritis (2%), arthrosis (1%), myalgia (1%)
  Respiratory: Cough (2%), epistaxis (2%), upper respiratory tract infection (1%)
Drug Interactions
  Metabolism/Transport Effects
    Aspirin: **Substrate** of CYP2C9 (minor)
    Dipyridamole: **Inhibits** ABCG2, P-glycoprotein

Avoid Concomitant Use

Avoid concomitant use of Aspirin and Dipyridamole with any of the following: Floctafenine; Influenza Virus Vaccine (Live/Attenuated); Ketorolac; Ketorolac (Nasal); Ketorolac (Systemic); Silodosin

Increased Effect/Toxicity

Aspirin and Dipyridamole may increase the levels/effects of: Adenosine; Alendronate; Anticoagulants; Beta-Blockers; Carbonic Anhydrase Inhibitors; Colchicine; Collagenase (Systemic); Corticosteroids (Systemic); Dabigatran Etexilate; Divalproex; Drotrecogin Alfa; Everolimus; Heparin; Hypotensive Agents; Ibritumomab; Methotrexate; P-Glycoprotein Substrates; PRALAtrexate; Regadenoson; Rivaroxaban; Salicylates; Silodosin; Sulfonylureas; Thrombolytic Agents; Ticagrelor; Topotecan; Tositumomab and Iodine I 131 Tositumomab; Valproic Acid; Varicella Virus-Containing Vaccines; Vitamin K Antagonists

The levels/effects of Aspirin and Dipyridamole may be increased by: Antidepressants (Tricyclic, Tertiary Amine); Antiplatelet Agents; Calcium Channel Blockers (Nondihydropyridine); Dasatinib; Floctafenine; Ginkgo Biloba; Glucosamine; Herbs (Anticoagulant/Antiplatelet Properties); Influenza Virus Vaccine (Live/Attenuated); Ketorolac; Ketorolac (Nasal); Ketorolac (Systemic); Loop Diuretics; Nonsteroidal Anti-Inflammatory Agents; NSAID (Nonselective); Omega-3-Acid Ethyl Esters; Pentosan Polysulfate Sodium; Pentoxifylline; Prostacyclin Analogues; Selective Serotonin Reuptake Inhibitors; Serotonin/Norepinephrine Reuptake Inhibitors; Treprostinil; Vitamin E

Decreased Effect

Aspirin and Dipyridamole may decrease the levels/effects of: ACE Inhibitors; Loop Diuretics; NSAID (Nonselective); Probenecid; Ticagrelor; Tiludronate

The levels/effects of Aspirin and Dipyridamole may be decreased by: Corticosteroids (Systemic); Nonsteroidal Anti-Inflammatory Agents; NSAID (Nonselective)

Ethanol/Nutrition/Herb Interactions Ethanol: Avoid ethanol (due to GI irritation).

Stability Store at 25°C (77°F); excursions permitted to 15°C to 30°C (59°F to 86°F). Protect from excessive moisture.

Mechanism of Action The antithrombotic action results from additive antiplatelet effects. Dipyridamole inhibits the uptake of adenosine into platelets, endothelial cells, and erythrocytes. Aspirin inhibits platelet aggregation by irreversible inhibition of platelet cyclooxygenase and thus inhibits the generation of thromboxane A_2.

Pharmacodynamics/Kinetics See individual agents.

Dosage

Geriatric & Adult

Stroke prevention: Oral: One capsule (dipyridamole 200 mg, aspirin 25 mg) twice daily
  Alternative regimen for patients with intolerable headache: Oral: One capsule at bedtime and low-dose aspirin in the morning. Return to usual dose (1 capsule twice daily) as soon as tolerance to headache develops (usually within a week).
  Hemodialysis graft patency (unlabeled use): Oral: One capsule (dipyridamole 200 mg, aspirin 25 mg) twice daily

Renal Impairment Avoid use in patients with severe renal dysfunction (Cl_{cr} <10 mL/minute).

Hepatic Impairment Avoid use in patients with severe hepatic impairment.

Administration Capsule should be swallowed whole; do not crush or chew. May be given with or without food.

Monitoring Parameters Hemoglobin, hematocrit, signs or symptoms of bleeding, signs or symptoms of stroke or transient ischemic attack

Special Geriatric Considerations Plasma concentrations were 40% higher, but specific dosage adjustments have not been recommended. Some evidence suggests that the doses of dipyridamole commonly used are ineffective for prevention of platelet aggregation, however, the addition of aspirin will add substantial efficacy. The dose of aspirin is effective for platelet inhibition, but low enough to offer a low adverse drug reaction rate.

Dosage Forms Excipient information presented when available (limited, particularly for generics); consult specific product labeling.
  Capsule, variable release:
    Aggrenox®: Aspirin 25 mg [immediate release] and dipyridamole 200 mg [extended release] [contains lactose, sucrose]

◆ **Aspirin and Extended-Release Dipyridamole** see Aspirin and Dipyridamole *on page 158*
◆ **Aspirin and Oxycodone** see Oxycodone and Aspirin *on page 1373*
◆ **Aspirin Free Anacin® Extra Strength [OTC]** see Acetaminophen *on page 33*
◆ **Aspir-low [OTC]** see Aspirin *on page 153*
◆ **Aspirtab [OTC]** see Aspirin *on page 153*
◆ **Asproject®** see Salicylates (Various Salts) *on page 1647*
◆ **Astelin®** see Azelastine (Nasal) *on page 172*
◆ **Astepro®** see Azelastine (Nasal) *on page 172*

◆ **Astramorph®/PF** *see* Morphine (Systemic) *on page 1238*
◆ **Atacand®** *see* Candesartan *on page 257*
◆ **Atacand HCT®** *see* Candesartan and Hydrochlorothiazide *on page 259*
◆ **Atelvia™** *see* Risedronate *on page 1619*

Atenolol (a TEN oh lole)

Related Information
  Beta-Blockers *on page 2001*
Medication Safety Issues
  Sound-alike/look-alike issues:
    Atenolol may be confused with albuterol, Altenol®, timolol, Tylenol®
    Tenormin® may be confused with Imuran®, Norpramin®, thiamine, Trovan®
Brand Names: U.S. Tenormin®
Brand Names: Canada Apo-Atenol®; CO Atenolol; Dom-Atenolol; JAMP-Atenolol; Mint-Atenolol; Mylan-Atenolol; Nu-Atenol; PHL-Atenolol; PMS-Atenolol; RAN™-Atenolol; ratio-Atenolol; Riva-Atenolol; Sandoz-Atenolol; Septa-Atenolol; Tenormin®; Teva-Atenolol
Generic Availability (U.S.) Yes
Pharmacologic Category Beta Blocker, Beta-1 Selective
Use Treatment of hypertension, alone or in combination with other agents; management of angina pectoris; secondary prevention postmyocardial infarction
Unlabeled/Investigational Use Treatment of acute ethanol withdrawal, supraventricular and ventricular arrhythmias; migraine headache prophylaxis
Contraindications Hypersensitivity to atenolol or any component of the formulation; sinus bradycardia; sinus node dysfunction; heart block greater than first-degree (except in patients with a functioning artificial pacemaker); cardiogenic shock; uncompensated cardiac failure; pulmonary edema
Warnings/Precautions Consider pre-existing conditions such as sick sinus syndrome before initiating. Administer cautiously in compensated heart failure and monitor for a worsening of the condition (efficacy of atenolol in heart failure has not been established). **[U.S. Boxed Warning]: Beta-blocker therapy should not be withdrawn abruptly (particularly in patients with CAD), but gradually tapered to avoid acute tachycardia, hypertension, and/or ischemia.** Chronic beta-blocker therapy should not be routinely withdrawn prior to major surgery. Beta-blockers should be avoided in patients with bronchospastic disease (asthma). Atenolol, with B_1 selectivity, has been used cautiously in bronchospastic disease with close monitoring. May precipitate or aggravate symptoms of arterial insufficiency in patients with PVD and Raynaud's disease; use with caution and monitor for progression of arterial obstruction. Use cautiously in patients with diabetes - may mask hypoglycemic symptoms. May mask signs of hyperthyroidism (eg, tachycardia); use caution if hyperthyroidism is suspected, abrupt withdrawal may precipitate thyroid storm. Alterations in thyroid function tests may be observed. Use cautiously in the renally impaired (dosage adjustment required). Caution in myasthenia gravis or psychiatric disease (may cause CNS depression). Bradycardia may be observed more frequently in elderly patients (>65 years of age); dosage reductions may be necessary. Adequate alpha-blockade is required prior to use of any beta-blocker for patients with untreated pheochromocytoma. May induce or exacerbate psoriasis. Use caution with history of severe anaphylaxis to allergens; patients taking beta-blockers may become more sensitive to repeated challenges. Treatment of anaphylaxis (eg, epinephrine) in patients taking beta-blockers may be ineffective or promote undesirable effects. Use with caution in patients on concurrent digoxin, verapamil, or diltiazem; bradycardia or heart block can occur. Use with caution in patients receiving inhaled anesthetic agents known to depress myocardial contractility.
Adverse Reactions (Reflective of adult population; not specific for elderly)
  1% to 10%:
    Cardiovascular: Persistent bradycardia, hypotension, chest pain, edema, heart failure, second- or third-degree AV block, Raynaud's phenomenon
    Central nervous system: Dizziness, fatigue, insomnia, lethargy, confusion, mental impairment, depression, headache, nightmares
    Gastrointestinal: Constipation, diarrhea, nausea
    Genitourinary: Impotence
    Miscellaneous: Cold extremities
Drug Interactions
  Avoid Concomitant Use
    Avoid concomitant use of Atenolol with any of the following: Floctafenine; Methacholine

Increased Effect/Toxicity

Atenolol may increase the levels/effects of: Alpha-/Beta-Agonists (Direct-Acting); Alpha1-Blockers; Alpha2-Agonists; Amifostine; Antihypertensives; Bupivacaine; Cardiac Glycosides; Fingolimod; Hypotensive Agents; Insulin; Lidocaine; Lidocaine (Systemic); Lidocaine (Topical); Mepivacaine; Methacholine; Midodrine; RiTUXimab; Sulfonylureas

The levels/effects of Atenolol may be increased by: Acetylcholinesterase Inhibitors; Amiodarone; Anilidopiperidine Opioids; Calcium Channel Blockers (Dihydropyridine); Calcium Channel Blockers (Nondihydropyridine); Diazoxide; Dipyridamole; Disopyramide; Dronedarone; Floctafenine; Glycopyrrolate; Herbs (Hypotensive Properties); MAO Inhibitors; Pentoxifylline; Phosphodiesterase 5 Inhibitors; Prostacyclin Analogues; Reserpine

Decreased Effect

Atenolol may decrease the levels/effects of: Beta2-Agonists; Theophylline Derivatives

The levels/effects of Atenolol may be decreased by: Ampicillin; Herbs (Hypertensive Properties); Methylphenidate; Nonsteroidal Anti-Inflammatory Agents; Yohimbine

Ethanol/Nutrition/Herb Interactions

Food: Atenolol serum concentrations may be decreased if taken with food.

Herb/Nutraceutical: Avoid dong quai if using for hypertension (has estrogenic activity). Avoid ephedra, yohimbe, ginseng (may worsen hypertension). Avoid garlic (may have increased antihypertensive effect).

Stability Protect from light.

Mechanism of Action Competitively blocks response to beta-adrenergic stimulation, selectively blocks beta$_1$-receptors with little or no effect on beta$_2$-receptors except at high doses

Pharmacodynamics/Kinetics

Onset of action: Peak effect: Oral: 2-4 hours

Duration: Normal renal function: 12-24 hours

Absorption: Oral: Rapid, incomplete (~50%)

Distribution: Low lipophilicity; does not cross blood-brain barrier

Protein binding: 6% to 16%

Metabolism: Limited hepatic

Half-life elimination: Beta: Normal renal function: 6-7 hours, prolonged with renal impairment; End-stage renal disease: 15-35 hours

Time to peak, plasma: Oral: 2-4 hours

Excretion: Feces (50%); urine (40% as unchanged drug)

Dosage

Geriatric Refer to adult dosing. In the management of hypertension, consider lower initial doses and titrate to response (Aronow, 2011).

Adult

Hypertension: Oral: 25-50 mg once daily, may increase to 100 mg/day. Doses >100 mg are unlikely to produce any further benefit.

Angina pectoris: Oral: 50 mg once daily; may increase to 100 mg/day. Some patients may require 200 mg/day.

Postmyocardial infarction: Oral: 100 mg/day or 50 mg twice daily for 6-9 days postmyocardial infarction.

Renal Impairment

Cl$_{cr}$ 15-35 mL/minute: Administer 50 mg/day maximum.

Cl$_{cr}$ <15 mL/minute: Administer 50 mg every other day maximum.

Hemodialysis effects: Moderately dialyzable (20% to 50%) via hemodialysis. Administer dose postdialysis or administer 25-50 mg supplemental dose. Elimination is not enhanced with peritoneal dialysis. Supplemental dose is not necessary.

Administration Administer I.V. at 1 mg/minute; intravenous administration requires a cardiac monitor and blood pressure monitor

Monitoring Parameters Blood pressure, orthostatic hypotension, heart rate, CNS effects, ECG

Test Interactions Increased glucose; decreased HDL

Pharmacotherapy Pearls May potentiate hypoglycemia in a diabetic patient and mask signs and symptoms; patients who receive hemodialysis should receive 50 mg oral dose after each dialysis

Special Geriatric Considerations Due to alterations in the beta-adrenergic autonomic nervous system, beta-adrenergic blockade may result in less hemodynamic response than seen in younger adults. Studies indicate that despite decreased sensitivity to the chronotropic effects of beta-blockade with age, there appears to be an increased myocardial sensitivity to the negative inotropic effect during stress (ie, exercise). Controlled trials have shown the overall response rate for propranolol to be only 20% to 50% in the elderly. Therefore, all beta-adrenergic blocking drugs may result in a decreased response as compared to younger adults. Since many elderly have Cl$_{cr}$ <35 mL/minute, creatinine clearance should be estimated or measured such that appropriate dose adjustment can be made.

Dosage Forms Excipient information presented when available (limited, particularly for generics); consult specific product labeling.
Tablet, oral: 25 mg, 50 mg, 100 mg
Tenormin®: 25 mg
Tenormin®: 50 mg [scored]
Tenormin®: 100 mg

Selected References
Fleisher LA, Beckman JA, Brown KA, et al, "ACC/AHA 2006 Guideline Update on Perioperative Cardiovascular Evaluation for Noncardiac Surgery: Focused Update on Perioperative Beta-Blocker Therapy. A Report of the American College of Cardiology/American Heart Association Task Force on Practice Guidelines (Writing Committee to Update the 2002 Guidelines on Perioperative Cardiovascular Evaluation for Noncardiac Surgery) Developed in Collaboration With the American Society of Echocardiography, American Society of Nuclear Cardiology, Heart Rhythm Society, Society of Cardiovascular Anesthesiologists, Society for Cardiovascular Angiography and Interventions, and Society for Vascular Medicine and Biology," *J Am Coll Cardiol*, 2006, 47(11):2343-55.
Juul AB, Wetterslev J, Gluud C, et al, "Effect of Perioperative Beta Blockade in Patients With Diabetes Undergoing Major Non-Cardiac Surgery: Randomized Placebo Controlled, Blinded Multicentre Trial. DIPOM Trial Group," *BMJ*, 2006, 332(7556):1482.

◆ **Ativan®** *see* LORazepam *on page 1089*
◆ **Atlizumab** *see* Tocilizumab *on page 1816*

Atorvastatin (a TORE va sta tin)

Related Information
Hyperlipidemia Management *on page 2021*
Medication Safety Issues
Sound-alike/look-alike issues:
Atorvastatin may be confused with atomoxetine, lovastatin, nystatin, pitavastatin, pravastatin, rosuvastatin, simvastatin
Lipitor® may be confused with labetalol, Levatol®, lisinopril, Loniten®, Lopid®, Mevacor®, Zocor®, ZyrTEC®
Brand Names: U.S. Lipitor®
Brand Names: Canada Apo-Atorvastatin®; CO Atorvastatin; GD-Atorvastatin; Lipitor®; Novo-Atorvastatin; PMS-Atorvastatin; RAN™-Atorvastatin; ratio-Atorvastatin; Sandoz-Atorvastatin
Index Terms Atorvastatin Calcium
Generic Availability (U.S.) No
Pharmacologic Category Antilipemic Agent, HMG-CoA Reductase Inhibitor
Use Treatment of dyslipidemias or primary prevention of cardiovascular disease (atherosclerotic) as detailed below:

Primary prevention of cardiovascular disease (high-risk for CVD): To reduce the risk of MI or stroke in patients without evidence of heart disease who have multiple CVD risk factors or type 2 diabetes. Treatment reduces the risk for angina or revascularization procedures in patients with multiple risk factors.
Secondary prevention of cardiovascular disease: To reduce the risk of nonfatal MI, nonfatal stroke, revascularization procedures, hospitalization for heart failure, and angina in patients with evidence of coronary heart disease.
Treatment of dyslipidemias: To reduce elevations in total cholesterol (C), LDL-C, apolipoprotein B, and triglycerides in patients with elevations of one or more components, and/or to increase low HDL-C as present in Fredrickson type IIa, IIb, III, and IV hyperlipidemias, heterozygous familial and nonfamilial hypercholesterolemia, and homozygous familial hypercholesterolemia
Treatment of heterozygous familial hypercholesterolemia (HeFH) in adolescent patients (10-17 years of age, females >1 year postmenarche) having LDL-C ≥190 mg/dL or LDL-C ≥160 mg/dL with positive family history of premature cardiovascular disease (CVD) or with two or more CVD risk factors.
Unlabeled/Investigational Use Secondary prevention in patients who have experienced a noncardioembolic stroke/TIA or following an ACS event regardless of baseline LDL-C using intensive lipid-lowering therapy
Contraindications Hypersensitivity to atorvastatin or any component of the formulation; active liver disease; unexplained persistent elevations of serum transaminases
Warnings/Precautions Secondary causes of hyperlipidemia should be ruled out prior to therapy. Atorvastatin has not been studied when the primary lipid abnormality is chylomicron elevation (Fredrickson types I and V). Liver function must be monitored by periodic laboratory assessment. May cause hepatic dysfunction. Use with caution in patients who consume large amounts of ethanol or have a history of liver disease; use is contraindicated in patients with active liver disease or unexplained persistent elevations of serum transaminases. Monitoring

is recommended. Patients with a history of hemorrhagic stroke may be at increased risk for another hemorrhagic stroke with use.

Rhabdomyolysis with acute renal failure has occurred. Risk is dose related and is increased with concurrent use of lipid-lowering agents which may cause rhabdomyolysis (fibric acid derivatives or niacin at doses ≥1 g/day) or during concurrent use with potent CYP3A4 inhibitors (including amiodarone, clarithromycin, cyclosporine, erythromycin, itraconazole, ketoconazole, nefazodone, grapefruit juice in large quantities, verapamil, or protease inhibitors such as indinavir, nelfinavir, or ritonavir). Ensure patient is on the lowest effective atorvastatin dose. If concurrent use of clarithromycin or combination protease inhibitors (eg, lopinavir/ritonavir or ritonavir/saquinavir) is warranted consider dose adjustment of atorvastatin. Monitor closely if used with other drugs associated with myopathy. Weigh the risk versus benefit when combining any of these drugs with atorvastatin. The manufacturer recommends temporary discontinuation for elective major surgery, acute medical or surgical conditions, or in any patient experiencing an acute or serious condition predisposing to renal failure (eg, sepsis, hypotension, trauma, uncontrolled seizures). However, based upon current evidence, HMG-CoA reductase inhibitor therapy should be continued in the perioperative period unless risk outweighs cardioprotective benefit. Use with caution in patients with advanced age, these patients are predisposed to myopathy. Safety and efficacy have not been established in patients <10 years of age or in premenarchal girls.

Adverse Reactions (Reflective of adult population; not specific for elderly)
>10%:
  Gastrointestinal: Diarrhea (5% to 14%)
  Neuromuscular & skeletal: Arthralgia (4% to 12%)
  Respiratory: Nasopharyngitis (4% to 13%)
2% to 10%:
  Central nervous system: Insomnia (1% to 5%)
  Gastrointestinal: Nausea (4% to 7%), dyspepsia (3% to 6%)
  Genitourinary: Urinary tract infection (4% to 8%)
  Hepatic: Transaminases increased (2% to 3% with 80 mg/day dosing)
  Neuromuscular & skeletal: Limb pain (3% to 9%), myalgia (3% to 8%), muscle spasms (2% to 5%), musculoskeletal pain (2% to 5%)
  Respiratory: Pharyngolaryngeal pain (1% to 4%)
Additional class-related events or case reports (not necessarily reported with atorvastatin therapy): Cataracts, cirrhosis, dermatomyositis, eosinophilia, erectile dysfunction, extraocular muscle movement impaired, fulminant hepatic necrosis, gynecomastia, hemolytic anemia, interstitial lung disease, ophthalmoplegia, peripheral nerve palsy, polymyalgia rheumatica, positive ANA, renal failure (secondary to rhabdomyolysis), systemic lupus erythematosus-like syndrome, thyroid dysfunction, tremor, vasculitis, vertigo

Drug Interactions
  Metabolism/Transport Effects Substrate of CYP3A4 (major), P-glycoprotein; **Inhibits** CYP3A4 (weak), P-glycoprotein
  Avoid Concomitant Use
    Avoid concomitant use of Atorvastatin with any of the following: Conivaptan; Red Yeast Rice; Silodosin; Telaprevir; Topotecan
  Increased Effect/Toxicity
    Atorvastatin may increase the levels/effects of: Aliskiren; DAPTOmycin; Digoxin; Diltiazem; Everolimus; Midazolam; P-Glycoprotein Substrates; Rivaroxaban; Silodosin; Topotecan; Trabectedin; Verapamil

    The levels/effects of Atorvastatin may be increased by: Amiodarone; Antifungal Agents (Azole Derivatives, Systemic); Boceprevir; Colchicine; Conivaptan; CycloSPORINE; Cyclo-SPORINE (Systemic); CYP3A4 Inhibitors (Moderate); CYP3A4 Inhibitors (Strong); Cyproterone; Danazol; Dasatinib; Diltiazem; Dronedarone; Eltrombopag; Fenofibrate; Fenofibric Acid; Fluconazole; Fusidic Acid; Gemfibrozil; Grapefruit Juice; Macrolide Antibiotics; Niacin; Niacinamide; P-Glycoprotein Inhibitors; Protease Inhibitors; QuiNINE; Red Yeast Rice; Rifamycin Derivatives; Sildenafil; Telaprevir; Verapamil
  Decreased Effect
    Atorvastatin may decrease the levels/effects of: Dabigatran Etexilate; Lanthanum

    The levels/effects of Atorvastatin may be decreased by: Antacids; Bexarotene; Bexarotene (Systemic); Bosentan; CYP3A4 Inducers (Strong); Deferasirox; Efavirenz; Etravirine; Fosphenytoin; P-Glycoprotein Inducers; Phenytoin; Rifamycin Derivatives; St Johns Wort; Tocilizumab

◀ **Ethanol/Nutrition/Herb Interactions**
Ethanol: Avoid excessive ethanol consumption (due to potential hepatic effects).
Food: Atorvastatin serum concentrations may be increased by grapefruit juice; avoid concurrent intake of large quantities (>1 quart/day). Red yeast rice contains an estimated 2.4 mg lovastatin per 600 mg rice.
Herb/Nutraceutical: St John's wort may decrease atorvastatin levels.

Stability Store at controlled room temperature of 20°C to 25°C (68°F to 77°F).

Mechanism of Action Inhibitor of 3-hydroxy-3-methylglutaryl coenzyme A (HMG-CoA) reductase, the rate-limiting enzyme in cholesterol synthesis (reduces the production of mevalonic acid from HMG-CoA); this then results in a compensatory increase in the expression of LDL receptors on hepatocyte membranes and a stimulation of LDL catabolism

Pharmacodynamics/Kinetics
Onset of action: Initial changes: 3-5 days; Maximal reduction in plasma cholesterol and triglycerides: 2 weeks
Absorption: Rapid
Distribution: V_d: ~381 L
Protein binding: ≥98%
Metabolism: Hepatic; forms active ortho- and parahydroxylated derivates and an inactive beta-oxidation product
Bioavailability: ~14% (parent drug); ~30% (parent drug and equipotent metabolites)
Half-life elimination: Parent drug: 14 hours; Equipotent metabolites: 20-30 hours
Time to peak, serum: 1-2 hours
Excretion: Bile; urine (<2% as unchanged drug)

Dosage
Geriatric & Adult
Primary prevention: **Note:** Doses should be individualized according to the baseline LDL-cholesterol concentrations, the recommended goal of therapy, and patient response; adjustments should be made at intervals of 2-4 weeks
Hypercholesterolemia (heterozygous familial and nonfamilial) and mixed hyperlipidemia (Fredrickson types IIa and IIb): Oral: Initial: 10-20 mg once daily; patients requiring >45% reduction in LDL-C may be started at 40 mg once daily; range: 10-80 mg once daily
Homozygous familial hypercholesterolemia: Oral: 10-80 mg once daily
Secondary prevention:
Clinically-evident coronary heart disease: Oral: Initial: 80 mg once daily; adjust based on patient tolerability and recommended goal LDL-C (LaRosa, 2005)
Intensive lipid-lowering after an ACS event regardless of baseline LDL (unlabeled use): Oral: Initial: 80 mg once daily; adjust based on patient tolerability and recommended goal LDL-C (Cannon, 2004; Pederson, 2005; Schwartz, 2001). **Note:** Currently, the ACC/AHA guidelines for UA/NSTEMI do not specify which statin to use (Anderson, 2007).
Noncardioembolic stroke/TIA (unlabeled use): Oral: Initial: 80 mg once daily; adjust based on patient tolerability and recommended goal LDL-C (Adams, 2008; Amarenco, 2006)

Dosage adjustment for atorvastatin with concomitant medications:
Cyclosporine: Atorvastatin dose should not exceed 10 mg/day
Clarithromycin, itraconazole, ritonavir plus saquinavir, or lopinavir plus ritonavir when atorvastatin dose >20 mg: Ensure that the lowest dose necessary of atorvastatin is used.
Renal Impairment No adjustment is necessary.
Hepatic Impairment Contraindicated in active liver disease or in patients with unexplained persistent elevations of serum transaminases.
Administration May take with food if desired; may take without regard to time of day.
Monitoring Parameters Lipid levels after 2-4 weeks; LFTs; baseline CPK (recheck CPK in any patient with symptoms suggestive of myopathy)

It is recommended that liver function tests (LFTs) be performed prior to and at 12 weeks following both the initiation of therapy and any elevation in dose, and periodically (eg, semiannually) thereafter. Monitor LDL-C at intervals no less than 4 weeks.

Special Geriatric Considerations Effective and well tolerated in the elderly. The definition of and, therefore, when to treat hyperlipidemia in the elderly is a controversial issue. The National Cholesterol Education Program recommends that all adults maintain a plasma cholesterol <160 mg/dL. For elderly patients with one additional risk factor, goal LDL would be <130 mg/dL. It is the authors' belief that pharmacologic treatment be reserved for those who are unable to obtain a desirable plasma cholesterol concentration by diet alone and for whom the benefits of treatment are believed to outweigh the potential adverse effects, drug interactions, and cost of treatment. Age ≥65 years is a risk factor for myopathy.

Dosage Forms Excipient information presented when available (limited, particularly for generics); consult specific product labeling.

Tablet, oral:

Lipitor®: 10 mg, 20 mg, 40 mg, 80 mg

Selected References

Gibson DM, Bron NJ, Richens A, et al, "Effect of Age and Gender on Pharmacokinetics of Atorvastatin in Humans," *J Clin Pharmacol*, 1996, 36(3):242-6.

Grundy SM, Cleeman JI, Merz CN, et al, "Implications of Recent Clinical Trials for the National Cholesterol Education Program Adult Treatment Panel III Guidelines," *J Am Coll Cardiol*, 2004, 44(3):720-32.

National Cholesterol Education Program (NCEP) Expert Panel on Detection, Evaluation, and Treatment of High Blood Cholesterol in Adults (Adult Treatment Panel III), "Third Report of the National Cholesterol Education Program (NCEP) Expert Panel on Detection, Evaluation, and Treatment of High Blood Cholesterol in Adults (Adult Treatment Panel III) Final Report," *Circulation*, 2002, 106(25):3143-421.

◆ **Atorvastatin Calcium** *see* Atorvastatin *on page 162*
◆ **AtroPen®** *see* Atropine *on page 165*

Atropine (A troe peen)

Brand Names: U.S. AtroPen®; Atropine Care™; Isopto® Atropine; Sal-Tropine™ [DSC]
Brand Names: Canada Dioptic's Atropine Solution; Isopto® Atropine
Index Terms Atropine Sulfate
Generic Availability (U.S.) Yes: Excludes tablet
Pharmacologic Category Anticholinergic Agent; Anticholinergic Agent, Ophthalmic; Antidote; Antispasmodic Agent, Gastrointestinal; Ophthalmic Agent, Mydriatic
Use

Injection: Preoperative medication to inhibit salivation and secretions; treatment of symptomatic sinus bradycardia, AV block (nodal level); antidote for acetylcholinesterase inhibitor poisoning (carbamate insecticides, nerve agents, organophosphate insecticides); adjuvant use with anticholinesterases (eg, edrophonium, neostigmine) to decrease their side effects during reversal of neuromuscular blockade

Note: Use is no longer recommended in the management of asystole or pulseless electrical activity (PEA) (ACLS, 2010).

Ophthalmic: Produce mydriasis and cycloplegia for examination of the retina and optic disc and accurate measurement of refractive errors; uveitis

Oral: Inhibit salivation and secretions

Prescribing and Access Restrictions The AtroPen® formulation is available for use primarily by the Department of Defense.

Contraindications Hypersensitivity to atropine or any component of the formulation; narrow-angle glaucoma; adhesions between the iris and lens; tachycardia; obstructive GI disease; paralytic ileus; intestinal atony of the elderly or debilitated patient; severe ulcerative colitis; toxic megacolon complicating ulcerative colitis; hepatic disease; obstructive uropathy; renal disease; myasthenia gravis (unless used to treat side effects of acetylcholinesterase inhibitor); asthma; thyrotoxicosis; Mobitz type II block

Warnings/Precautions Use with caution in elderly patients. Low doses cause a paradoxical decrease in heart rates. Some commercial products contain sodium metabisulfite, which can cause allergic-type reactions. May accumulate with multiple inhalational administration, particularly in the elderly. Heat prostration may occur in hot weather. Use with caution in patients with autonomic neuropathy, prostatic hyperplasia, hyperthyroidism, HF, cardiac arrhythmias, chronic lung disease, biliary tract disease; anticholinergic agents are generally not well tolerated in the elderly and their use should be avoided when possible. Atropine is rarely used except as a preoperative agent or in the acute treatment of bradyarrhythmias. In heart transplant recipients, atropine will likely be ineffective in treatment of asystole or bradycardia due to lack of vagal innervation of the transplanted heart; cholinergic reinnervation may occur over time (years), so atropine may be used cautiously (ACLS, 2005).

AtroPen®: There are no absolute contraindications for the use of atropine in severe organophosphate poisonings, however in mild poisonings, use caution in those patients where the use of atropine would be otherwise contraindicated. Formulation for use by trained personnel only.

Adverse Reactions (Reflective of adult population; not specific for elderly) Severity and frequency of adverse reactions are dose related and vary greatly; listed reactions are limited to significant and/or life-threatening.

Cardiovascular: Arrhythmia, flushing, hypotension, palpitation, tachycardia
Central nervous system: Ataxia, coma, delirium, disorientation, dizziness, drowsiness, excitement, fever, hallucinations, headache, insomnia, nervousness
Dermatologic: Anhidrosis, urticaria, rash, scarlatiniform rash

Gastrointestinal: Bloating, constipation, delayed gastric emptying, loss of taste, nausea, paralytic ileus, vomiting, xerostomia, dry throat, nasal dryness

Genitourinary: Urinary hesitancy, urinary retention

Neuromuscular & skeletal: Weakness

Ocular: Angle-closure glaucoma, blurred vision, cycloplegia, dry eyes, mydriasis, ocular tension increased

Respiratory: Dyspnea, laryngospasm, pulmonary edema

Miscellaneous: Anaphylaxis

Drug Interactions

Avoid Concomitant Use There are no known interactions where it is recommended to avoid concomitant use.

Increased Effect/Toxicity

Atropine may increase the levels/effects of: AbobotulinumtoxinA; Anticholinergics; Cannabinoids; OnabotulinumtoxinA; Potassium Chloride; RimabotulinumtoxinB

The levels/effects of Atropine may be increased by: Pramlintide

Decreased Effect

Atropine may decrease the levels/effects of: Acetylcholinesterase Inhibitors (Central); Secretin

The levels/effects of Atropine may be decreased by: Acetylcholinesterase Inhibitors (Central)

Stability Store injection at controlled room temperature of 15°C to 30°C (59°F to 86°F); avoid freezing. In addition, AtroPen® should be protected from light.

Mechanism of Action Blocks the action of acetylcholine at parasympathetic sites in smooth muscle, secretory glands, and the CNS; increases cardiac output, dries secretions. Atropine reverses the muscarinic effects of cholinergic poisoning. The primary goal in cholinergic poisonings is reversal of bronchorrhea and bronchoconstriction. Atropine has no effect on the nicotinic receptors responsible for muscle weakness, fasciculations, and paralysis.

Pharmacodynamics/Kinetics

Onset of action: I.V.: Rapid

Absorption: Complete

Distribution: Widely throughout the body; crosses placenta; trace amounts enter breast milk; crosses blood-brain barrier

Metabolism: Hepatic

Half-life elimination: 2-3 hours

Excretion: Urine (30% to 50% as unchanged drug and metabolites)

Dosage

Geriatric Refer to adult dosing.

Nerve agent toxicity management: See Note. I.M.: Elderly and frail patients:

Prehospital ("in the field"): Mild-to-moderate symptoms: 1 mg; severe symptoms: 2-4 mg

Hospital/emergency department: Mild-to-moderate symptoms: 1 mg; severe symptoms: 2 mg

Note: Pralidoxime is a component of the management of nerve agent toxicity.

Prehospital ("in the field") management: Repeat atropine I.M. (2 mg) at 5-10 minute intervals until secretions have diminished and breathing is comfortable or airway resistance has returned to near normal.

Hospital management: Repeat atropine I.M. (2 mg) at 5-10 minute intervals until secretions have diminished and breathing is comfortable or airway resistance has returned to near normal.

Adult Doses <0.5 mg have been associated with paradoxical bradycardia.

Inhibit salivation and secretions (preanesthesia):

I.M., I.V., SubQ: 0.4-0.6 mg 30-60 minutes preop and repeat every 4-6 hours as needed.

Oral: 0.4 mg; may repeat in 4 hours if necessary; 0.4 mg initial dose may be exceeded in certain cases and may repeat in 4 hours if necessary

Bradycardia (Note: Atropine may be ineffective in heart transplant recipients): *I.V.:* 0.5 mg every 3-5 minutes, not to exceed a total of 3 mg or 0.04 mg/kg (ACLS, 2010)

Neuromuscular blockade reversal: *I.V.:* 25-30 mcg/kg 30-60 seconds before neostigmine or 7-10 mcg/kg 30-60 seconds before edrophonium

Organophosphate or carbamate poisoning: Note: The dose of atropine required varies considerably with the severity of poisoning. Total amount of atropine used in carbamate poisoning is usually less. Severely poisoned patients may exhibit significant tolerance to atropine; ≥2 times the suggested doses may be needed. Titrate to pulmonary status (decreased bronchial secretions). Once patient is stable for a period of time, the dose/dosing frequency may be decreased. If atropinization occurs after 1-2 mg of atropine then re-evaluate working diagnosis.

I.V.: Initial: 1-5 mg; doses should be doubled every 5 minutes until signs of muscarinic excess abate (clearing of bronchial secretions, bronchospasm, and adequate oxygenation). Overly aggressive dosing may cause anticholinergic toxicity (eg, delirium, hyperthermia, and muscle twitching).

I.V. Infusion: 0.5-1 mg/hour or 10% to 20% of loading dose/hour

I.M.: AtroPen®: Mild symptoms: Administer 2 mg as soon as exposure is known or suspected. If severe symptoms develop after first dose, 2 additional doses should be repeated in 10 minutes; do not administer more than 3 doses. Severe symptoms: Immediately administer three 2 mg doses.

Nerve agent toxicity management: *I.M.:* See **Note**. Prehospital ("in the field") or hospital/emergency department: Mild-to-moderate symptoms: 2-4 mg; severe symptoms: 6 mg

Note: Pralidoxime is a component of the management of nerve agent toxicity; consult Pralidoxime for specific route and dose.

Prehospital ("in the field") management: Repeat atropine I.M. (2 mg) at 5-10 minute intervals until secretions have diminished and breathing is comfortable or airway resistance has returned to near normal.

Hospital management: Repeat atropine I.M. (2 mg) at 5-10 minute intervals until secretions have diminished and breathing is comfortable or airway resistance has returned to near normal.

Mydriasis, cycloplegia (preprocedure): *Ophthalmic* (1% solution): Instill 1-2 drops 1 hour before the procedure.

Uveitis: *Ophthalmic:*
1% solution: Instill 1-2 drops 4 times/day.
Ointment: Apply a small amount in the conjunctival sac up to 3 times/day. Compress the lacrimal sac by digital pressure for 1-3 minutes after instillation.

Administration

I.M.: AtroPen®: Administer to outer thigh. May be given through clothing as long as pockets at the injection site are empty. Hold autoinjector in place for 10 seconds following injection; massage the injection site.

I.V.: Administer undiluted by rapid I.V. injection; slow injection may result in paradoxical bradycardia. In bradycardia, atropine administration should not delay treatment with external pacing.

Intratracheal: Dilute in NS or sterile water (absorption may be greater with sterile water). Spray drug quickly down tube. Follow immediately with several quick insufflations.

Monitoring Parameters Heart rate, blood pressure, pulse, mental status; intravenous administration requires a cardiac monitor

Pharmacotherapy Pearls Because of its bothersome and potentially dangerous side effects, atropine is rarely used except as a preoperative agent or in the acute treatment of bradyarrhythmias

Special Geriatric Considerations Anticholinergic agents are generally not well tolerated in the elderly and their use should be avoided when possible. In elderly, anticholinergic agents should not be used as prophylaxis against extrapyramidal symptoms.

Dosage Forms Excipient information presented when available (limited, particularly for generics); consult specific product labeling. [DSC] = Discontinued product

Injection, solution, as sulfate: 0.05 mg/mL (5 mL); 0.1 mg/mL (5 mL, 10 mL); 0.4 mg/mL (1 mL [DSC], 20 mL [DSC]); 1 mg/mL (1 mL [DSC])

AtroPen®: 0.25 mg/0.3 mL (0.3 mL); 0.5 mg/0.7 mL (0.7 mL); 1 mg/0.7 mL (0.7 mL); 2 mg/0.7 mL (0.7 mL)

Injection, solution, as sulfate [preservative free]: 0.4 mg/0.5 mL (0.5 mL); 0.4 mg/mL (1 mL); 1 mg/mL (1 mL)

Ointment, ophthalmic, as sulfate: 1% (3.5 g)

Solution, ophthalmic, as sulfate [drops]: 1% (2 mL, 5 mL, 15 mL)

Atropine Care™: 1% (2 mL, 5 mL, 15 mL) [contains benzalkonium chloride]

Isopto® Atropine: 1% (5 mL, 15 mL) [contains benzalkonium chloride]

Tablet, oral, as sulfate:

Sal-Tropine™: 0.4 mg [DSC]

Selected References

Feinberg M, "The Problems of Anticholinergic Adverse Effects in Older Patients," *Drugs Aging*, 1993, 3(4):335-48.

◆ **Augmentin XR®** *see* Amoxicillin and Clavulanate Potassium *on page 116*

Auranofin (au RANE oh fin)

Medication Safety Issues
Sound-alike/look-alike issues:
Ridaura® may be confused with Cardura®
Brand Names: U.S. Ridaura®
Brand Names: Canada Ridaura®
Generic Availability (U.S.) No
Pharmacologic Category Gold Compound
Use Management of active stage of classic or definite rheumatoid arthritis in patients who do not respond to or tolerate other agents; psoriatic arthritis; adjunctive or alternative therapy for pemphigus
Contraindications Hypersensitivity to auranofin or any component of the formulation; renal disease, history of blood dyscrasias, congestive heart failure, exfoliative dermatitis, necrotizing enterocolitis, history of anaphylactic reactions
Warnings/Precautions [U.S. Boxed Warning]: May cause significant toxicity involving dermatologic, gastrointestinal, hematologic, pulmonary, renal and hepatic systems; patient education is required. Dermatitis and lesions of the mucous membranes are common and may be serious; pruritus may precede the early development of a skin reaction. Signs of toxicity include hematologic depression (depressed hemoglobin, leukocytes, granulocytes, or platelets); stomatitis, persistent diarrhea, enterocolitis, cholestatic jaundice; proteinuria (nephritic syndrome), and interstitial pulmonary fibrosis. Avoid use in patients with prior inflammatory bowel disease.

Concurrent use with ACE inhibitors may increase the risk of nitritoid reactions. Laboratory monitoring should be completed prior to each new prescription. Frequent monitoring of patients for signs and symptoms of toxicity will prevent serious adverse reactions.
Adverse Reactions (Reflective of adult population; not specific for elderly)
>10%:
Dermatologic: Rash (24%), pruritus (17%)
Gastrointestinal: Diarrhea/loose stools (47%), abdominal pain (14%), stomatitis (13%)
Ocular: Conjunctivitis
Renal: Proteinuria
1% to 10%:
Dermatologic: Alopecia, urticaria
Gastrointestinal: Anorexia, constipation, dyspepsia, dysgeusia, flatulence, glossitis
Hematologic: Anemia, eosinophilia, leukopenia, thrombocytopenia
Hepatic: Transaminases increased
Renal: Hematuria, proteinuria
Drug Interactions
Avoid Concomitant Use There are no known interactions where it is recommended to avoid concomitant use.
Increased Effect/Toxicity There are no known significant interactions involving an increase in effect.
Decreased Effect There are no known significant interactions involving a decrease in effect.
Stability Store in tight, light-resistant containers at 15°C to 30°C.
Mechanism of Action The exact mechanism of action of gold is unknown; gold is taken up by macrophages which results in inhibition of phagocytosis and lysosomal membrane stabilization; other actions observed are decreased serum rheumatoid factor and alterations in immunoglobulins. Additionally, complement activation is decreased, prostaglandin synthesis is inhibited, and lysosomal enzyme activity is decreased.
Pharmacodynamics/Kinetics
Onset of action: Delayed; therapeutic response may require as long as 3-4 months
Duration: Prolonged
Absorption: Oral: ~20% gold in dose is absorbed
Protein binding: 60%
Half-life elimination (single or multiple dose dependent): 21-31 days
Time to peak, serum: ~2 hours
Excretion: Urine (60% of absorbed gold); remainder in feces
Dosage
Geriatric & Adult Rheumatoid arthritis, psoriatic arthritis, pemphigus: Oral: Initial: 6 mg/day in 1-2 divided doses; after 3 months may be increased to 9 mg/day in 3 divided doses; if still no response after 3 months at 9 mg/day, discontinue drug

Renal Impairment
Cl$_{cr}$ 50-80 mL/minute: Administer 50% of dose.
Cl$_{cr}$ <50 mL/minute: Avoid use.

Monitoring Parameters Patients should have a CBC with differential, platelet count, hemoglobin determination and urinalysis for protein, white cells, red cells and casts; at baseline and periodically during therapy (at least monthly). Skin and oral mucosa should be inspected for skin rash, bruising or oral ulceration/stomatitis. Specific questioning for symptoms such as pruritus, rash, stomatitis or metallic taste should be included. Dosing should be withheld in patients with significant gastrointestinal, renal, dermatologic, or hematologic effects (platelet count falls to <100,000/mm^3, WBC <4000, granulocytes <1500/mm^3

Reference Range Gold: Normal: 0-0.1 mcg/mL (SI: 0-0.0064 μmol/L); Therapeutic: 1-3 mcg/mL (SI: 0.06-0.18 μmol/L); Urine: <0.1 mcg/24 hours

Test Interactions May enhance the response to a tuberculin skin test

Pharmacotherapy Pearls Metallic taste may indicate stomatitis

Special Geriatric Considerations Tolerance to gold decreases with advanced age; use cautiously only after traditional therapy and other disease modifying antirheumatic drugs (DMARDs) have been attempted.

Dosage Forms Excipient information presented when available (limited, particularly for generics); consult specific product labeling.
Capsule, oral:
Ridaura®: 3 mg [gold 29%]

AzaTHIOprine (ay za THYE oh preen)

Medication Safety Issues
Sound-alike/look-alike issues:
AzaTHIOprine may be confused with azaCITIDine, azidothymidine, azithromycin, Azulfidine®
Imuran® may be confused with Elmiron®, Enduron®, Imdur®, Inderal®, Tenormin®
Other safety concerns:
Azathioprine is metabolized to mercaptopurine; concurrent use of these commercially-available products has resulted in profound myelosuppression.

Brand Names: U.S. Azasan®; Imuran®

Brand Names: Canada Apo-Azathioprine®; Imuran®; Mylan-Azathioprine; Teva-Azathioprine

Index Terms Azathioprine Sodium

Generic Availability (U.S.) Yes

◀ **Pharmacologic Category** Immunosuppressant Agent

Use Adjunctive therapy in prevention of rejection of kidney transplants; management of active rheumatoid arthritis (RA)

Unlabeled/Investigational Use Adjunct in prevention of rejection of solid organ (nonrenal) transplants; steroid-sparing agent for corticosteroid-dependent Crohn's disease (CD) and ulcerative colitis (UC); maintenance of remission in CD; fistulizing CD; dermatomyositis/ polymyositis; erythema multiforme; pemphigus vulgaris

Contraindications Hypersensitivity to azathioprine or any component of the formulation; patients with rheumatoid arthritis and a history of treatment with alkylating agents (eg, cyclophosphamide, chlorambucil, melphalan) may have a prohibitive risk of neoplasia with azathioprine treatment

Warnings/Precautions [U.S. Boxed Warning]: Chronic immunosuppression increases the risk of neoplasia and serious infections. Azathioprine has mutagenic potential to both men and women. Dose-related, delayed hematologic toxicities (leukopenia, thrombocytopenia, macrocytic anemia, pancytopenia) may occur; may be more severe with renal transplants undergoing rejection; dosage modification for hematologic toxicity may be necessary. Use with caution in patients with liver disease or renal impairment; monitor hematologic function closely. Azathioprine is metabolized to mercaptopurine; concomitant use may result in profound myelosuppression and should be avoided. Patients with genetic deficiency of thiopurine methyltransferase (TPMT) or concurrent therapy with drugs which may inhibit TPMT may be sensitive to myelosuppressive effects. Patients with intermediate TPMT activity may be at risk for increased myelosuppression; those with low or absent TPMT activity are at risk for developing severe myelotoxicity. TPMT genotyping or phenotyping may assist in identifying patients at risk for developing toxicity. TPMT testing does not substitute for CBC monitoring. Xanthine oxidase inhibitors may increase risk for hematologic toxicity; reduce azathioprine dose when used concurrently with allopurinol; patients with low or absent TPMT activity may require further dose reductions or discontinuation.

Hepatotoxicity (transaminase, bilirubin, and alkaline phosphatase elevations) may occur, usually in renal transplant patients and generally within 6 months of transplant; normally reversible with discontinuation; monitor liver function periodically. Rarely, hepatic sinusoidal obstruction syndrome (SOS; formerly called veno-occlusive disease) has been reported; discontinue if hepatic SOS is suspected. Gastrointestinal toxicity may occur within the first several weeks of therapy and is reversible. Symptoms may include severe nausea, vomiting, diarrhea, rash, fever, malaise, myalgia, hypotension, and liver enzyme abnormalities. **[U.S. Boxed Warning]: Should be prescribed by physicians familiar with the risks, including hematologic toxicities and mutagenic potential.** Immune response to vaccines may be diminished. Hazardous agent - use appropriate precautions for handling and disposal.

Adverse Reactions (Reflective of adult population; not specific for elderly) Frequency not always defined; dependent upon dose, duration, indication, and concomitant therapy.

Central nervous system: Fever, malaise

Gastrointestinal: Nausea/vomiting (RA: 12%), diarrhea

Hematologic: Leukopenia (renal transplant: >50%; RA: 28%), thrombocytopenia

Hepatic: Alkaline phosphatase increased, bilirubin increased, hepatotoxicity, transaminases increased

Neuromuscular & skeletal: Myalgia

Miscellaneous: Infection (renal transplant: 20%; RA: <1%; includes bacterial, fungal, protozoal, viral); neoplasia (other than lymphoma: 3%)

Drug Interactions

Avoid Concomitant Use

Avoid concomitant use of AzaTHIOprine with any of the following: BCG; Febuxostat; Mercaptopurine; Natalizumab; Pimecrolimus; Tacrolimus (Topical)

Increased Effect/Toxicity

AzaTHIOprine may increase the levels/effects of: Leflunomide; Mercaptopurine; Natalizumab; Vaccines (Live)

The levels/effects of AzaTHIOprine may be increased by: 5-ASA Derivatives; ACE Inhibitors; Allopurinol; Denosumab; Febuxostat; Pimecrolimus; Ribavirin; Roflumilast; Sulfamethoxazole; Tacrolimus (Topical); Trastuzumab; Trimethoprim

Decreased Effect

AzaTHIOprine may decrease the levels/effects of: BCG; Sipuleucel-T; Vaccines (Inactivated); Vitamin K Antagonists

The levels/effects of AzaTHIOprine may be decreased by: Echinacea

Ethanol/Nutrition/Herb Interactions Herb/Nutraceutical: Avoid cat's claw, echinacea (have immunostimulant properties).

Stability
Tablet: Store at room temperature of 15°C to 25°C (59°F to 77°F); protect from light.

Powder for injection: Store intact vials at room temperature of 15°C to 25°C (59°F to 77°F). Protect from light. Reconstitute each vial with 10 mL sterile water for injection; may further dilute for infusion (in D$_5$W, ^{1}/$_2$NS, or NS). Reconstituted solution is stable for up to 2 weeks at room temperature or up to 4 days refrigerated; solutions diluted in D$_5$W, ^{1}/$_2$NS, or NS for infusion are stable at room temperature or refrigerated for up to 16 days; however, the manufacturer recommends use within 24 hours of reconstitution. Use appropriate precautions for handling and disposal.

Mechanism of Action Azathioprine is an imidazolyl derivative of mercaptopurine; antagonizes purine metabolism and may inhibit synthesis of DNA, RNA, and proteins; may also interfere with cellular metabolism and inhibit mitosis. The 6-thioguanine nucleotides appear to mediate the majority of azathioprine's immunosuppressive and toxic effects.

Pharmacodynamics/Kinetics
Absorption: Oral: Well absorbed

Protein binding: ~30%

Metabolism: Hepatic, to 6-mercaptopurine (6-MP), possibly by glutathione S-transferase (GST). Further metabolism of 6-MP (in the liver and GI tract), via three major pathways: Hypoxanthine guanine phosphoribosyltransferase (to 6-thioguanine-nucleotides, or 6-TGN), xanthine oxidase (to 6-thiouric acid), and thiopurine methyltransferase (TPMT), which forms 6-methylmercaptopurine (6-MMP).

Half-life elimination: Parent drug: 12 minutes; mercaptopurine: 0.7-3 hours; End-stage renal disease: Slightly prolonged

Time to peak, plasma: 1-2 hours (including metabolites)

Excretion: Urine (primarily as metabolites)

Dosage
Geriatric & Adult Note: Patients with intermediate TPMT activity may be at risk for increased myelosuppression; those with low or absent TPMT activity receiving conventional azathioprine doses are at risk for developing severe, life-threatening myelotoxicity. Dosage reductions are recommended for patients with reduced TPMT activity.

I.V. dose is equivalent to oral dose (dosing should be transitioned from I.V. to oral as soon as tolerated):

Renal transplantation (treatment usually started the day of transplant, however, has been initiated [rarely] 1-3 days prior to transplant): Oral, I.V.: Initial: 3-5 mg/kg/day usually given as a single daily dose, then 1-3 mg/kg/day maintenance

Rheumatoid arthritis: Oral:

Initial: 1 mg/kg/day given once daily or divided twice daily, for 6-8 weeks; increase by 0.5 mg/kg every 4 weeks until response or up to 2.5 mg/kg/day; an adequate trial should be a minimum of 12 weeks

Maintenance dose: Reduce dose by 0.5 mg/kg every 4 weeks until lowest effective dose is reached; optimum duration of therapy not specified; may be discontinued abruptly

Adjunctive management of severe recurrent aphthous stomatitis (unlabeled use): Oral: 50 mg once daily in conjunction with prednisone

Adjunctive management of dermatomyositis/polymyositis (unlabeled use): Oral: 50 mg/day in conjunction with prednisone; increase by 50 mg/week to total dose of 2-3 mg/kg/day (Briemberg, 2003); **Note:** Onset of beneficial effects may take 3-6 months; however, may be preferred over methotrexate in patients with pulmonary or hepatic toxicity.

Reduction of steroid use in CD or UC, maintenance of remission in CD or fistulizing disease (unlabeled uses): Oral: Initial: 50 mg once daily; may increase by 25 mg/day every 1-2 weeks as tolerated to target dose of 2-3 mg/kg/day

Dosage adjustment for concomitant use with allopurinol: Reduce azathioprine dose to one-third or one-fourth the usual dose when used concurrently with allopurinol. Patients with low or absent TPMT activity may require further dose reductions or discontinuation.

Renal Impairment Although dosage reductions are recommended, specific guidelines are not available in the FDA-approved labeling; the following guidelines have been used by some clinicians (Aronoff, 2007):

Cl$_{cr}$ >50 mL/minute: No adjustment recommended.

Cl$_{cr}$ 10-50 mL/minute: Administer 75% of normal dose.

Cl$_{cr}$ <10 mL/minute: Administer 50% of normal dose.

Hemodialysis (dialyzable; ~45% removed in 8 hours): Supplement: 0.25 mg/kg

CAPD: Unknown

CRRT: Administer 75% of normal dose

Administration
I.V.: Azathioprine can be administered IVP over 5 minutes at a concentration not to exceed 10 mg/mL **or** azathioprine can be further diluted with normal saline or D$_5$W and administered by intermittent infusion usually over 30-60 minutes; may be extended up to 8 hours.

Oral: Administering tablets after meals or in divided doses may decrease adverse GI events.

◀ **Monitoring Parameters** CBC with differential and platelets (weekly during first month, twice monthly for months 2 and 3, then monthly; monitor more frequently with dosage modifications), total bilirubin, liver function tests, TPMT genotyping or phenotyping

For use as immunomodulatory therapy in CD or UC, monitor CBC with differential weekly for 1 month, then biweekly for 1 month, followed by monitoring every 1-2 months throughout the course of therapy. LFTs should be assessed every 3 months.

Test Interactions TPMT phenotyping results will not be accurate following recent blood transfusions.

Special Geriatric Considerations Toxicity to immunosuppressives is increased in elderly. Start with lowest recommended adult doses. Signs of infection, such as fever and WBC rise, may not occur. Lethargy and confusion may be more prominent signs of infection. In the elderly, adjust dose to creatinine clearance.

Dosage Forms Excipient information presented when available (limited, particularly for generics); consult specific product labeling.

Injection, powder for reconstitution: 100 mg

Tablet, oral: 50 mg

    Azasan®: 75 mg, 100 mg [scored]

    Imuran®: 50 mg [scored]

Selected References

Aronoff GR, Bennett WM, Berns JS, et al, *Drug Prescribing in Renal Failure: Dosing Guidelines for Adults and Children*, 5th ed. Philadelphia, PA: American College of Physicians; 2007, p 97, 177.

Brookes MJ and Green JR, "Maintenance of Remission in Crohn's Disease: Current and Emerging Therapeutic Options," *Drugs*, 2004, 64(10):1069-89.

Hodgins C, Mosley M, and Pola-Strowd M, "Recommendations for the Diagnosis and Management of Recurrent Aphthous Stomatitis," University of Texas at Austin, School of Nursing, Family Nurse Practitioner Program, Austin; May 2003.

Lichtenstein GR, Abreu MT, Cohen R, et al, "American Gastroenterological Association Institute Medical Position Statement on Corticosteroids, Immunomodulators, and Infliximab in Inflammatory Bowel Disease," *Gastroenterology*, 2006, 130(3):935-9.

Simon L, Lipman AG, Jacox A, et al, "Guideline for the Management of Osteoarthritis, Rheumatoid Arthritis and Juvenile Chronic Arthritis Pain," 2nd ed, Glenview IL, American Pain Society, 2002.

◆ **Azathioprine Sodium** *see* AzaTHIOprine *on page 169*

Azelastine (Nasal) (a ZEL as teen)

Medication Safety Issues

  Sound-alike/look-alike issues:

    Astelin® may be confused with Astepro®

Brand Names: U.S. Astelin®; Astepro®

Brand Names: Canada Astelin®

Index Terms Azelastine Hydrochloride

Generic Availability (U.S.) Yes

Pharmacologic Category Histamine H_1 Antagonist; Histamine H_1 Antagonist, Second Generation

Use Treatment of the symptoms of seasonal allergic rhinitis such as rhinorrhea, sneezing, and nasal pruritus; treatment of the symptoms of vasomotor rhinitis

Dosage

  Geriatric & Adult

    Seasonal allergic rhinitis (Astelin®, Astepro®): Intranasal: 1-2 sprays each nostril twice daily.

    Vasomotor rhinitis (Astelin®): Intranasal: 2 sprays each nostril twice daily.

Special Geriatric Considerations Only a small number of older subjects were included in premarketing trials. In those patients, side effects were no different than in younger patients.

Dosage Forms Excipient information presented when available (limited, particularly for generics); consult specific product labeling.

Solution, intranasal, as hydrochloride [spray]: 0.1% [137 mcg/spray] (30 mL)

    Astelin®: 0.1% [137 mcg/spray] (30 mL) [contains benzalkonium chloride; 200 metered sprays]

    Astepro®: 0.15% [205.5 mcg/spray] (30 mL) [contains benzalkonium chloride; 200 metered sprays]

Azelastine (Ophthalmic) (a ZEL as teen)

Medication Safety Issues

  Sound-alike/look-alike issues:

    Optivar® may be confused with Optiray®, Optive™

  International issues:

    Optivar [U.S.] may be confused with Opthavir brand name for acyclovir [Mexico]

Brand Names: U.S. Optivar®
Index Terms Azelastine Hydrochloride
Generic Availability (U.S.) Yes
Pharmacologic Category Histamine H$_1$ Antagonist; Histamine H$_1$ Antagonist, Second Generation
Use Treatment of itching of the eye associated with seasonal allergic conjunctivitis
Dosage
  Geriatric & Adult Seasonal allergic conjunctivitis: Ophthalmic: Instill 1 drop into affected eye(s) twice daily.
Dosage Forms Excipient information presented when available (limited, particularly for generics); consult specific product labeling.
  Solution, ophthalmic, as hydrochloride [drops]: 0.05% (6 mL)
  Optivar®: 0.05% (6 mL) [contains benzalkonium chloride]

◆ **Azelastine Hydrochloride** see Azelastine (Nasal) on page 172
◆ **Azelastine Hydrochloride** see Azelastine (Ophthalmic) on page 172
◆ **Azilect®** see Rasagiline on page 1591

Azilsartan (ay zil SAR tan)

Related Information
  Angiotensin Agents on page 1985
Brand Names: U.S. Edarbi™
Index Terms Azilsartan Medoxomil; AZL-M
Generic Availability (U.S.) No
Pharmacologic Category Angiotensin II Receptor Blocker
Use Treatment of hypertension; may be used alone or in combination with other antihypertensives
Contraindications There are no contraindications listed in manufacturer's labeling.
Warnings/Precautions Angiotensin II receptor blockers may cause hyperkalemia; avoid potassium supplementation unless specifically required by healthcare provider. Avoid use or use a smaller dose in patients who are volume depleted; correct depletion first. May be associated with deterioration of renal function and/or increases in serum creatinine, particularly in patients with low renal blood flow (eg, renal artery stenosis, heart failure, volume depletion) whose glomerular filtration rate (GFR) is dependent on efferent arteriolar vasoconstriction by angiotensin II. Use with caution in unstented unilateral/bilateral renal artery stenosis. When unstented bilateral renal artery stenosis is present, use is generally avoided due to the elevated risk of deterioration in renal function unless possible benefits outweigh risks. Use with caution in pre-existing renal insufficiency; significant aortic/mitral stenosis. Concurrent use with ACE inhibitors may increase the risk of clinically-significant adverse events (eg, renal dysfunction, hyperkalemia).
Adverse Reactions (Reflective of adult population; not specific for elderly)
  Cardiovascular: Hypotension, orthostatic hypotension
  Central nervous system: Dizziness, fatigue
  Gastrointestinal: Diarrhea (2%), nausea
  Hematologic: Hemoglobin decreased, hematocrit decreased, RBC decreased
  Neuromuscular & skeletal: Muscle spasm, weakness
  Renal: Serum creatinine increased
  Respiratory: Cough
Drug Interactions
  Metabolism/Transport Effects Substrate of CYP2C9 (minor)
  Avoid Concomitant Use There are no known interactions where it is recommended to avoid concomitant use.
  Increased Effect/Toxicity
    Azilsartan may increase the levels/effects of: ACE Inhibitors; Amifostine; Antihypertensives; Hypotensive Agents; Lithium; Nonsteroidal Anti-Inflammatory Agents; Potassium-Sparing Diuretics; RiTUXimab; Sodium Phosphates

    The levels/effects of Azilsartan may be increased by: Alfuzosin; Diazoxide; Eplerenone; Herbs (Hypotensive Properties); MAO Inhibitors; Pentoxifylline; Phosphodiesterase 5 Inhibitors; Potassium Salts; Prostacyclin Analogues; Tolvaptan; Trimethoprim
  Decreased Effect
    The levels/effects of Azilsartan may be decreased by: Herbs (Hypertensive Properties); Methylphenidate; Nonsteroidal Anti-Inflammatory Agents; Rifamycin Derivatives; Yohimbine
  Ethanol/Nutrition/Herb Interactions Herb/Nutraceutical: Avoid ephedra, yohimbe, ginseng (may worsen hypertension). Avoid garlic (may have increased antihypertensive effect).

◀ **Stability** Store at 25°C (77°F); excursions permitted to 15°C to 30°C (59°F to 86°F). Protect from moisture and light.

Mechanism of Action Angiotensin II (which is formed by enzymatic conversion from angiotensin I) is the primary pressor agent of the renin-angiotensin system. Effects of angiotensin II include vasoconstriction, stimulation of aldosterone synthesis/release, cardiac stimulation, and renal sodium reabsorption. Azilsartan inhibits angiotensin II's vasoconstrictor and aldosterone-secreting effects by selectively blocking the binding of angiotensin II to the AT_1 receptor in vascular smooth muscle and adrenal gland tissues (azilsartan has a stronger affinity for the AT_1 receptor than the AT_2 receptor). The action is independent of the angiotensin II synthesis pathways. Azilsartan does not inhibit ACE (kininase II), therefore it does not affect the response to bradykinin (the clinical relevance of this is unknown) and does not bind to or inhibit other receptors or ion channels of importance in cardiovascular regulation.

Pharmacodynamics/Kinetics

Distribution: V_d: ~16 L

Protein binding: >99%; primarily to serum albumin

Metabolism: Gut: prodrug hydrolyzed to active metabolite; Hepatic: primarily via CYP2C9 to inactive metabolites

Bioavailability: ~60%

Half-life elimination: ~11 hours

Time to peak, serum: 1.5-3 hours

Excretion: Feces (~55%); urine (~42%, 15% as unchanged drug)

Clearance: 2.3 mL/minute

Dosage

Geriatric Refer to adult dosing.

Adult Hypertension: Oral: 80 mg once daily; consider initial dose of 40 mg once daily in patients with volume depletion (eg, patients receiving high-dose diuretics)

Renal Impairment No starting dosage adjustment is necessary; however, carefully monitor the patient.

Hepatic Impairment No starting dosage adjustment is necessary in patients with mild-to-moderate impairment; however, carefully monitor the patient. Not studied in patients with severe impairment.

Administration Administer without regard to food.

Monitoring Parameters Electrolytes, serum creatinine, BUN; blood pressure

Special Geriatric Considerations No dosage adjustment based on age is necessary with azilsartan. In clinical studies with this drug, 26% of the patients were elderly (≥65 years of age), with 5% of these being ≥75 years. Significant increases in serum creatinine was seen more often in those ≥75 years. No other differences in safety and efficacy were noted between elderly and younger adults. Recommend monitoring serum creatinine when employing this agent in the geriatric population.

Dosage Forms Excipient information presented when available (limited, particularly for generics); consult specific product labeling.

Tablet, oral, as medoxomil:

Edarbi™: 40 mg, 80 mg

Selected References

American Diabetes Association, "Standards of Medical Care in Diabetes Mellitus – 2011," *Diabetes Care*, 2011, 34 (Suppl 1):11-61.

Anderson JL, Adams CD, Antman EM, et al, "ACC/AHA 2007 Guidelines for the Management of Patients With Unstable Angina/Non-ST-Elevation Myocardial Infarction: A Report of the American College of Cardiology/American Heart Association Task Force on Practice Guidelines (Writing Committee to Revise the 2002 Guidelines for the Management of Patients With Unstable Angina/Non-ST-Elevation Myocardial Infarction) Developed in Collaboration With the American College of Emergency Physicians, the Society for Cardiovascular Angiography and Interventions, and the Society of Thoracic Surgeons Endorsed by the American Association of Cardiovascular and Pulmonary Rehabilitation and the Society for Academic Emergency Medicine," *J Am Coll Cardiol*, 2007, 50(7):e1-e157.

Antman EM, Hand M, Armstrong PW, et al, "2007 Focused Update of the ACC/AHA 2004 Guidelines for the Management of Patients With ST-Elevation Myocardial Infarction. A Report of the American College of Cardiology/American Heart Association Task Force on Practice Guidelines," *J Am Coll Cardiol*, 2008, 51(2):210-49.

Chobanian AV, Bakris GL, Black HR, et al, "The Seventh Report of the Joint National Committee on Prevention, Detection, Evaluation, and Treatment of High Blood Pressure: The JNC 7 Report," *JAMA*, 2003, 289(19):2560-71.

Epstein BJ and Gums JG, "Angiotensin Receptor Blockers Versus ACE Inhibitors: Prevention of Death and Myocardial Infarction in High-Risk Populations," *Ann Pharmacother*, 2005, 39(3):470-80.

"K/DOQI Clinical Practice Guidelines for Chronic Kidney Disease: Evaluation, Classification, and Stratification. Kidney Disease Outcome Quality Initiative," *Am J Kidney Dis*, 2002, 39(2 Suppl 2):1-246. Available at http://www.kidney.org/professionals/KDOQI/guidelines_ckd/toc.htm

Sipahi I, Debanne SM, Rowland DY, et al, "Angiotensin-Receptor Blockade and Risk of Cancer: Meta-Analysis of Randomised Controlled Trials," *Lancet Oncol*, 2010, 11(7):627-36.

White WB, Weber MA, Sica D, et al, "Effects of the Angiotensin Receptor Blocker Azilsartan Medoxomil Versus Olmesartan and Valsartan on Ambulatory and Clinic Blood Pressure in Patients With Stages 1 and 2 Hypertension," *Hypertension*, 2011, 57(3):413-20.

◆ **Azilsartan Medoxomil** see Azilsartan on page 173

Azithromycin (Systemic) (az ith roe MYE sin)

Related Information
Community-Acquired Pneumonia in Adults *on page 2059*
Prevention of Infective Endocarditis *on page 2064*
Medication Safety Issues
Sound-alike/look-alike issues:
Azithromycin may be confused with azathioprine, erythromycin
Zithromax® may be confused with Fosamax®, Zinacef®, Zovirax®
Brand Names: U.S. Zithromax®; Zithromax® TRI-PAK™; Zithromax® Z-PAK®; Zmax®
Brand Names: Canada Apo-Azithromycin®; CO Azithromycin; Dom-Azithromycin; Mylan-Azithromycin; Novo-Azithromycin; PHL-Azithromycin; PMS-Azithromycin; PRO-Azithromycin; ratio-Azithromycin; Riva-Azithromycin; Sandoz-Azithromycin; Zithromax®
Index Terms Azithromycin Dihydrate; Azithromycin Hydrogencitrate; Azithromycin Monohydrate; Z-Pak; Zithromax TRI-PAK™; Zithromax Z-PAK®
Generic Availability (U.S.) Yes: Excludes extended release microspheres
Pharmacologic Category Antibiotic, Macrolide
Use Oral, I.V.: Treatment of acute otitis media due to *H. influenzae, M. catarrhalis,* or *S. pneumoniae*; pharyngitis/tonsillitis due to *S. pyogenes*; treatment of mild-to-moderate upper and lower respiratory tract infections, infections of the skin and skin structure, community-acquired pneumonia, pelvic inflammatory disease (PID), sexually-transmitted diseases (urethritis/cervicitis), and genital ulcer disease (chancroid) due to susceptible strains of *Chlamydophila pneumoniae, C. trachomatis, M. catarrhalis, H. influenzae, S. aureus, S. pneumoniae, Mycoplasma genitalium, Mycoplasma pneumoniae,* and *C. psittaci*; acute bacterial exacerbations of chronic obstructive pulmonary disease (COPD) due to *H. influenzae, M. catarrhalis,* or *S. pneumoniae*; acute bacterial sinusitis; prevention, alone or in combination with rifabutin, of MAC in patients with advanced HIV infection; treatment, in combination with ethambutol, of disseminated MAC in patients with advanced HIV infection
Unlabeled/Investigational Use Prophylaxis of infective endocarditis in patients who are allergic to penicillin and undergoing surgical or dental procedures; pertussis
Contraindications Hypersensitivity to azithromycin, other macrolide (eg, azalide or ketolide) antibiotics, or any component of the formulation; history of cholestatic jaundice/hepatic dysfunction associated with prior azithromycin use
Warnings/Precautions Use with caution in patients with pre-existing liver disease; hepatic impairment, including hepatocellular and/or cholestatic hepatitis, with or without jaundice, has been observed. Discontinue if symptoms of malaise, nausea, vomiting, abdominal colic, and fever. Allergic reactions have been reported (rare); reappearance of allergic reaction may occur without further azithromycin exposure. May mask or delay symptoms of incubating gonorrhea or syphilis, so appropriate culture and susceptibility tests should be performed prior to initiating azithromycin. Prolonged use may result in fungal or bacterial superinfection, including *C. difficile*-associated diarrhea (CDAD) and pseudomembranous colitis; CDAD has been observed >2 months postantibiotic treatment. Use caution with renal dysfunction. Prolongation of the QT$_c$ interval has been reported with macrolide antibiotics; use caution in patients at risk of prolonged cardiac repolarization. Use with caution in patients with myasthenia gravis.

Oral suspensions (immediate release and extended release) are not interchangeable.
Adverse Reactions (Reflective of adult population; not specific for elderly)
>10%: Gastrointestinal: Diarrhea (4% to 9%; high single-dose regimens 12% to 14%), nausea (≤7%; high single-dose regimens 18%)
2% to 10%:
Dermatologic: Pruritus, rash
Gastrointestinal: Abdominal pain, anorexia, cramping, vomiting (especially with high single-dose regimens)
Genitourinary: Vaginitis
Local: (with I.V. administration): Injection site pain, inflammation
Drug Interactions
Metabolism/Transport Effects Substrate of CYP3A4 (minor); **Inhibits** CYP3A4 (weak)
Avoid Concomitant Use
Avoid concomitant use of Azithromycin (Systemic) with any of the following: Artemether; BCG; Dronedarone; Lumefantrine; Nilotinib; Pimozide; QUEtiapine; QuiNINE; Terfenadine; Tetrabenazine; Thioridazine; Toremifene; Vandetanib; Vemurafenib; Ziprasidone

Increased Effect/Toxicity

Azithromycin (Systemic) may increase the levels/effects of: Amiodarone; Cardiac Glycosides; CycloSPORINE; CycloSPORINE (Systemic); Dronedarone; Pimozide; QTc-Prolonging Agents; QuiNINE; Tacrolimus; Tacrolimus (Systemic); Tacrolimus (Topical); Terfenadine; Tetrabenazine; Thioridazine; Toremifene; Vandetanib; Vemurafenib; Vitamin K Antagonists; Ziprasidone

The levels/effects of Azithromycin (Systemic) may be increased by: Alfuzosin; Artemether; Chloroquine; Ciprofloxacin; Ciprofloxacin (Systemic); Conivaptan; Gadobutrol; Lumefantrine; Nelfinavir; Nilotinib; QUEtiapine; QuiNINE

Decreased Effect

Azithromycin (Systemic) may decrease the levels/effects of: BCG; Typhoid Vaccine

The levels/effects of Azithromycin (Systemic) may be decreased by: Tocilizumab

Ethanol/Nutrition/Herb Interactions Food: Rate and extent of GI absorption may be altered depending upon the formulation. Azithromycin suspension, not tablet form, has significantly increased absorption (46%) with food.

Stability

Injection (Zithromax®): Store intact vials of injection at room temperature. Reconstitute the 500 mg vial with 4.8 mL of sterile water for injection and shake until all of the drug is dissolved. Each mL contains 100 mg azithromycin. Reconstituted solution is stable for 24 hours when stored below 30°C (86°F). Use of a standard syringe is recommended due to the vacuum in the vial (which may draw additional solution through an automated syringe).

The initial solution should be further diluted to a concentration of 1 mg/mL (500 mL) to 2 mg/mL (250 mL) in 0.9% sodium chloride, 5% dextrose in water, or lactated Ringer's. The diluted solution is stable for 24 hours at or below room temperature (30°C or 86°F) and for 7 days if stored under refrigeration (5°C or 41°F).

Suspension, immediate release (Zithromax®): Store dry powder below 30°C (86°F). Following reconstitution, store at 5°C to 30°C (41°F to 86°F).

Suspension, extended release (Zmax®): Store dry powder ≤30°C (86°F). Following reconstitution, store at 25°C (77°F); excursions permitted to 15°C to 30°C (59°F to 86°F); do not refrigerate or freeze. Should be consumed within 12 hours following reconstitution.

Tablet (Zithromax®): Store between 15°C to 30°C (59°F to 86°F).

Mechanism of Action Inhibits RNA-dependent protein synthesis at the chain elongation step; binds to the 50S ribosomal subunit resulting in blockage of transpeptidation

Pharmacodynamics/Kinetics

Absorption: Oral: Rapid

Distribution: Extensive tissue; distributes well into skin, lungs, sputum, tonsils, and cervix; penetration into CSF is poor; I.V.: 33.3 L/kg; Oral: 31.1 L/kg

Protein binding (concentration dependent): Oral, I.V.: 7% to 51%

Metabolism: Hepatic

Bioavailability: Oral: 38%, decreased by 17% with extended release suspension; variable effect with food (increased with immediate or delayed release oral suspension, unchanged with tablet)

Half-life elimination: Oral, I.V.: Terminal: Immediate release: 68-72 hours; Extended release: 59 hours

Time to peak, serum: Oral: Immediate release: 2-3 hours; Extended release: 5 hours

Excretion: Oral, I.V.: Biliary (major route); urine (6%)

Dosage

Geriatric & Adult Note: Extended release suspension (Zmax®) is not interchangeable with immediate release formulations. Use should be limited to approved indications. All doses are expressed as immediate release azithromycin unless otherwise specified.

Bacterial sinusitis: Oral: 500 mg/day for a total of 3 days
Extended release suspension (Zmax®): 2 g as a single dose

Cat scratch disease (unlabeled use): Oral: >45.5 kg: 500 mg as a single dose, then 250 mg once daily for 4 days

Chancroid due to *H. ducreyi*: Oral: 1 g as a single dose (CDC, 2010)

Community-acquired pneumonia:
Oral: Extended release suspension (Zmax®): 2 g as a single dose
I.V.: 500 mg as a single dose for at least 2 days, follow I.V. therapy by the oral route with a single daily dose of 500 mg to complete a 7- to 10-day course of therapy.

Disseminated *M. avium* complex disease in patients with advanced HIV infection: Oral:
Treatment: 600 mg/day in combination with ethambutol
Primary prophylaxis: 1200 mg once weekly (preferred), with or without rifabutin **or** alternatively, 600 mg twice weekly (CDC, 2009)
Secondary prophylaxis: 500-600 mg/day in combination with ethambutol (CDC, 2009)

Gonococcal infection, uncomplicated (cervix, pharynx, rectum, urethra): Oral: 1 g as a single dose (in combination with a cephalosporin) (CDC, 2010)

Note: Monotherapy with azithromycin (1 g and 2 g) have been associated with resistance and/or treatment failure; use in combination with a cephalosporin (CDC, 2010). However, a single 2 g azithromycin dose is still an FDA-approved dose for gonococcal urethritis and cervicitis and also may be appropriate for treatment of a gonococcal infection in pregnant women who cannot tolerate a cephalosporin (CDC, 2010).

Granuloma inguinale (donovanosis): Oral: 1 g once a week for at least 3 weeks (and until lesions have healed) (CDC, 2010)

Mild-to-moderate respiratory tract, skin, and soft tissue infections: Oral: 500 mg in a single loading dose on day 1 followed by 250 mg/day as a single dose on days 2-5

Alternative regimen: Bacterial exacerbation of COPD: 500 mg/day for a total of 3 days

Pelvic inflammatory disease (PID): I.V.: 500 mg as a single dose for 1-2 days, follow I.V. therapy by the oral route with a single daily dose of 250 mg to complete a 7-day course of therapy.

Pertussis (CDC, 2005): Oral: 500 mg on day 1 followed by 250 mg/day on days 2-5 (maximum: 500 mg/day)

Prophylaxis against infective endocarditis (unlabeled use): Oral: 500 mg 30-60 minutes prior to the procedure. **Note:** American Heart Association (AHA) guidelines now recommend prophylaxis only in patients undergoing invasive procedures and in whom underlying cardiac conditions may predispose to a higher risk of adverse outcomes should infection occur. As of April 2007, routine prophylaxis for GI/GU procedures is no longer recommended by the AHA.

Prophylaxis against sexually-transmitted diseases following sexual assault: Oral: 1 g as a single dose (in combination with a cephalosporin and metronidazole) (CDC, 2010)

Urethritis/cervicitis: Oral: *Due to C. trachomatis or M. genitalium:* 1 g as a single dose

Renal Impairment Use caution in patients with GFR <10 mL/minute.

Poorly dialyzed; no supplemental dose or dosage adjustment necessary, including patients on intermittent hemodialysis, peritoneal dialysis, or continuous renal replacement therapy (eg, CVVHD).

Hepatic Impairment Use with caution due to potential for hepatotoxicity (rare). Specific guidelines for dosing in hepatic impairment have not been established.

Administration

I.V.: Infusate concentration and rate of infusion for azithromycin for injection should be either 1 mg/mL over 3 hours or 2 mg/mL over 1 hour. Other medications should not be infused simultaneously through the same I.V. line.

Oral: Immediate release suspension and tablet may be taken without regard to food; extended release suspension should be taken on an empty stomach (at least 1 hour before or 2 hours following a meal), within 12 hours of reconstitution.

Monitoring Parameters Liver function tests, CBC with differential

Pharmacotherapy Pearls Zithromax® tablets and immediate release suspension may be interchanged (eg, two Zithromax® 250 mg tablets may be substituted for one Zithromax® 500 mg tablet or the tablets may be substituted with the immediate release suspension); however, the extended release suspension (Zmax®) is not bioequivalent with Zithromax® and therefore should not be interchanged.

Special Geriatric Considerations Dosage adjustment does not appear to be necessary in the elderly. Considered to be one of the drugs of choice in the outpatient treatment of community-acquired pneumonia in elderly.

Dosage Forms Excipient information presented when available (limited, particularly for generics); consult specific product labeling. [DSC] = Discontinued product

Injection, powder for reconstitution, as dihydrate [strength expressed as base]: 500 mg

Zithromax®: 500 mg [contains sodium 114 mg (4.96 mEq)/vial]

Injection, powder for reconstitution, as hydrogencitrate [strength expressed as base]: 500 mg [DSC], 2.5 g [DSC]

Injection, powder for reconstitution, as monohydrate [strength expressed as base]: 500 mg

Microspheres for suspension, extended release, oral, as dihydrate [strength expressed as base]:

Zmax®: 2 g/bottle (60 mL) [contains sodium 148 mg/bottle, sucrose 19 g/bottle; cherry-banana flavor; product contains azithromycin 27 mg/mL after constitution]

Powder for suspension, oral, as dihydrate [strength expressed as base]: 100 mg/5 mL (15 mL); 200 mg/5 mL (15 mL, 22.5 mL, 30 mL); 1 g/packet (3s)

Zithromax®: 100 mg/5 mL (15 mL) [contains sodium 3.7 mg/5 mL; cherry-crème de vanilla-banana flavor]

Zithromax®: 200 mg/5 mL (15 mL, 22.5 mL, 30 mL) [contains sodium 7.4 mg/5 mL; cherry-crème de vanilla-banana flavor]

Zithromax®: 1 g/packet (3s, 10s) [contains sodium 37 mg/packet; banana-cherry flavor]

Powder for suspension, oral, as monohydrate: 200 mg/5 mL (15 mL, 22.5 mL)
Powder for suspension, oral, as monohydrate [strength expressed as base]: 100 mg/5 mL (15 mL); 200 mg/5 mL (15 mL, 22.5 mL [DSC], 30 mL)
Tablet, oral, as anhydrous: 250 mg, 500 mg, 600 mg
Tablet, oral, as dihydrate [strength expressed as base]: 250 mg, 500 mg, 600 mg
Zithromax®: 250 mg [contains sodium 0.9 mg/tablet]
Zithromax®: 500 mg [contains sodium 1.8 mg/tablet]
Zithromax®: 600 mg [contains sodium 2.1 mg/tablet]
Zithromax® TRI-PAK™: 500 mg [contains sodium 1.8 mg/tablet]
Zithromax® Z-PAK®: 250 mg [contains sodium 0.9 mg/tablet]
Tablet, oral, as monohydrate [strength expressed as base]: 250 mg, 500 mg, 600 mg

Selected References

Coates P, Daniel R, Houston AC, et al, "An Open Study to Compare the Pharmacokinetics, Safety, and Tolerability of a Multiple-Dose Regimen of Azithromycin in Young and Elderly Volunteers," *Eur J Clin Microbiol Infect Dis*, 1991, 10 (10):850-2.
Mandell LA, Wunderink RG, Anzueto A, et al, "Infectious Diseases Society of America/American Thoracic Society Consensus Guidelines on the Management of Community-Acquired Pneumonia in Adults," *Clin Infect Dis*, 2007, 44 Suppl 2:S27-72.

Azithromycin (Ophthalmic) (az ith roe MYE sin)

Medication Safety Issues
Sound-alike/look-alike issues:
Azithromycin may be confused with azathioprine, erythromycin
Brand Names: U.S. AzaSite®
Generic Availability (U.S.) No
Pharmacologic Category Antibiotic, Macrolide; Antibiotic, Ophthalmic
Use Bacterial conjunctivitis
Dosage
Geriatric & Adult Bacterial conjunctivitis: Ophthalmic: Instill 1 drop into affected eye(s) twice daily (8-12 hours apart) for 2 days, then 1 drop once daily for 5 days
Special Geriatric Considerations Evaluate the patient's or caregiver's ability to safely administer the correct dose of ophthalmic medication.
Dosage Forms Excipient information presented when available (limited, particularly for generics); consult specific product labeling.
Solution, ophthalmic [drops]:
AzaSite®: 1% (2.5 mL) [contains benzalkonium chloride]

♦ **Azithromycin Dihydrate** *see* Azithromycin (Systemic) *on page 175*
♦ **Azithromycin Hydrogencitrate** *see* Azithromycin (Systemic) *on page 175*
♦ **Azithromycin Monohydrate** *see* Azithromycin (Systemic) *on page 175*
♦ **AZL-M** *see* Azilsartan *on page 173*
♦ **Azo-Gesic™ [OTC]** *see* Phenazopyridine *on page 1433*
♦ **Azopt®** *see* Brinzolamide *on page 212*
♦ **Azor™** *see* Amlodipine and Olmesartan *on page 108*
♦ **AZO Standard® [OTC]** *see* Phenazopyridine *on page 1433*
♦ **AZO Standard® Maximum Strength [OTC]** *see* Phenazopyridine *on page 1433*
♦ **Azthreonam** *see* Aztreonam *on page 178*

Aztreonam (AZ tree oh nam)

Related Information
Community-Acquired Pneumonia in Adults *on page 2059*
Medication Safety Issues
Sound-alike/look-alike issues:
Aztreonam may be confused with azidothymidine
Brand Names: U.S. Azactam®; Cayston®
Index Terms Azthreonam
Generic Availability (U.S.) Yes: Injection (powder for reconstitution)
Pharmacologic Category Antibiotic, Miscellaneous
Use
Injection: Treatment of patients with urinary tract infections, lower respiratory tract infections, septicemia, skin/skin structure infections, intra-abdominal infections, and gynecological infections caused by susceptible gram-negative bacilli
Inhalation: Improve respiratory symptoms in cystic fibrosis (CF) patients with *Pseudomonas aeruginosa*

Prescribing and Access Restrictions Cayston® (aztreonam inhalation solution) is only available through a select group of specialty pharmacies and cannot be obtained through a retail pharmacy. Because Cayston® may only be used with the Altera® Nebulizer System, it can only be obtained from the following specialty pharmacies: Cystic Fibrosis Services, Inc; IV Solutions; Foundation Care; and Pharmaceutical Specialties, Inc. This network of specialty pharmacies ensures proper access to both the drug and device. To obtain the medication and proper nebulizer, contact the Cayston Access Program at 1-877-7CAYSTON (1-877-722-9786) or at www.cayston.com.

Contraindications Hypersensitivity to aztreonam or any component of the formulation

Warnings/Precautions Rare cross-allergenicity to penicillins and cephalosporins has been reported. Use caution in renal impairment; dosing adjustment required for the injectable formulation. Prolonged use may result in fungal or bacterial superinfection, including *C. difficile*-associated diarrhea (CDAD) and pseudomembranous colitis; CDAD has been observed >2 months postantibiotic treatment. Patients colonized with *Burkholderia cepacia* have not been studied. Safety and efficacy has not been established in patients with FEV_1 <25% or >75% predicted. To reduce the development of resistant bacteria and maintain efficacy reserve use for CF patients with known *Pseudomonas aeruginosa*. Bronchospasm may occur occur following nebulization; administer a bronchodilator prior to treatment.

Adverse Reactions (Reflective of adult population; not specific for elderly)
Injection: Adults: 1% to 10%:
Dermatologic: Rash
Gastrointestinal: Diarrhea, nausea, vomiting
Local: Thrombophlebitis, pain at injection site

Inhalation:
>10%:
   Central nervous system: Pyrexia (13%; more often observed in children)
   Respiratory: Cough (54%), nasal congestion (16%), pharyngeal pain (12%), wheezing (16%)
1% to 10%:
   Cardiovascular: Chest discomfort (8%)
   Dermatologic: Rash (2%)
   Gastrointestinal: Abdominal pain (7%), vomiting (6%)
   Respiratory: Bronchospasm (3%)

Drug Interactions
Avoid Concomitant Use
Avoid concomitant use of Aztreonam with any of the following: BCG
Increased Effect/Toxicity There are no known significant interactions involving an increase in effect.
Decreased Effect
Aztreonam may decrease the levels/effects of: BCG; Typhoid Vaccine

Stability
Inhalation: Prior to reconstitution, store at 2°C to 8°C (36°F to 46°F). Once removed from refrigeration, aztreonam and the diluent may be stored at room temperature (up to 25°C/77°F) for ≤28 days. Protect from light. Reconstitute immediately prior to use. Squeeze diluent into opened glass vial. Replace rubber stopper and gently swirl vial until contents have completely dissolved. Use immediately after reconstitution.
Injection: Prior to reconstitution, store at room temperature; avoid excessive heat. Reconstituted solutions are colorless to light yellow straw and may turn pink upon standing without affecting potency. Use reconstituted solutions and I.V. solutions (in NS and D_5W) within 48 hours if kept at room temperature (25°C) or 7 days under refrigeration (4°C).
I.M.: Reconstitute with at least 3 mL SWFI, sterile bacteriostatic water for injection, NS, or bacteriostatic sodium chloride.
I.V.:
   Bolus injection: Reconstitute with 6-10 mL SWFI.
   Infusion: Reconstitute to a final concentration ≤2%; the final concentration should not exceed 20 mg/mL. Solution for infusion may be frozen at less than -2°C (less than -4°F) for up to 3 months. Thawed solution should be used within 24 hours if thawed at room temperature or within 72 hours if thawed under refrigeration. **Do not refreeze.**

Mechanism of Action Inhibits bacterial cell wall synthesis by binding to one or more of the penicillin-binding proteins (PBPs) which in turn inhibits the final transpeptidation step of peptidoglycan synthesis in bacterial cell walls, thus inhibiting cell wall biosynthesis. Bacteria eventually lyse due to ongoing activity of cell wall autolytic enzymes (autolysins and murein hydrolases) while cell wall assembly is arrested. Monobactam structure makes cross-allergenicity with beta-lactams unlikely.

Pharmacodynamics/Kinetics
Absorption: I.M.: Well absorbed
Distribution: V_d (adults): 0.2 L/kg

Protein binding: 56%

Half-life: 1.3-2.2 hours (half-life prolonged in renal failure)

Time to peak serum concentration: Within 60 minutes following a dose

Elimination: 60% to 70% excreted unchanged in urine and partially excreted in feces

In healthy older adults with normal renal function (mean Cl_{cr}: 99 mL/minute), there were no significant changes in pharmacokinetic parameters. However, in older adults with impaired renal function (mean Cl_{cr}: 24 mL/minute) serum concentrations were inversely related to Cl_{cr}

Dosage

Geriatric & Adult

Urinary tract infection: I.M., I.V.: 500 mg to 1 g every 8-12 hours

Moderately severe systemic infections:

I.M.: 1 g every 8-12 hours

I.V.: 1-2 g every 8-12 hours

Severe systemic or life-threatening infections (especially caused by *Pseudomonas aeruginosa*): I.V.: 2 g every 6-8 hours; maximum: 8 g/day

Meningitis (gram-negative): I.V.: 2 g every 6-8 hours

***Pseudomonas aeruginosa* infection in cystic fibrosis:** Inhalation (nebulizer): 75 mg 3 times daily (at least 4 hours apart) for 28 days. Do not repeat for 28 days after completion.

Renal Impairment

Oral inhalation: Dosage adjustment not required for mild, moderate or severe renal impairment.

I.M., I.V.: Adults: Following initial dose, maintenance doses should be given as follows:

Cl_{cr} 10-30 mL/minute: 50% of usual dose at the usual interval

Cl_{cr} <10 mL/minute: 25% of usual dosage at the usual interval

Intermittent hemodialysis (IHD): Dialyzable (20% to 50%): Loading dose of 500 mg, 1 g, or 2 g, followed by 25% of initial dose at usual interval; for serious/life-threatening infections, administer one-eighth ($1/8$) of initial dose after each hemodialysis session (given in addition to the maintenance doses). Alternatively, may administer 500 mg every 12 hours (Heintz, 2009). **Note:** Dosing dependent on the assumption of 3 times/week, complete IHD sessions.

Peritoneal dialysis (PD): Administer as for Cl_{cr} <10 mL/minute

Continuous renal replacement therapy (CRRT) (Heintz, 2009; Trotman, 2005): Drug clearance is highly dependent on the method of renal replacement, filter type, and flow rate. Appropriate dosing requires close monitoring of pharmacologic response, signs of adverse reactions due to drug accumulation, as well as drug concentrations in relation to target trough (if appropriate). The following are general recommendations only (based on dialysate flow/ultrafiltration rates of 1-2 L/hour and minimal residual renal function) and should not supersede clinical judgment:

CVVH: Loading dose of 2 g followed by 1-2 g every 12 hours

CVVHD/CVVHDF: Loading dose of 2 g followed by either 1 g every 8 hours **or** 2 g every 12 hours (Heintz, 2009)

Administration

Inhalation: Administer using only an Altera® nebulizer system; **administer alone; do not mix with other nebulizer medications**. Administer a bronchodilator before administration of aztreonam (short-acting: 15 minutes to 4 hours before; long-acting: 30 minutes to 12 hours before). For patients on multiple inhaled therapies, administer bronchodilator first, then mucolytic, and lastly, aztreonam.

To administer Cayston®, pour reconstituted solution into the handset of the nebulizer system, turn unit on. Place the mouthpiece in the patient's mouth and encourage to breath normally through the mouth. Administration time is usually 2-3 minutes. Administer doses ≥4 hours apart.

Injection: Doses >1 g should be administered I.V.

I.M.: Administer by deep injection into large muscle mass, such as upper outer quadrant of gluteus maximus or the lateral part of the thigh

I.V.: Administer by slow I.V. push over 3-5 minutes or by intermittent infusion over 20-60 minutes.

Monitoring Parameters

Injection: Periodic liver function test; monitor for signs of anaphylaxis during first dose

Inhalation: Consider measuring FEV_1 prior to initiation of therapy

Test Interactions May interfere with urine glucose tests containing cupric sulfate (Benedict's solution, Clinitest®); positive Coombs' test

Pharmacotherapy Pearls Normally used with other antibiotics in life-threatening situations; member of new class of antibiotics called monobactams, with excellent gram-negative bacteria effectiveness, without ototoxicity or nephrotoxicity

Special Geriatric Considerations Injection: Adjust dose relative to renal function.

Dosage Forms Excipient information presented when available (limited, particularly for generics); consult specific product labeling.

Infusion, premixed iso-osmotic solution:

Azactam®: 1 g (50 mL); 2 g (50 mL)

Injection, powder for reconstitution: 1 g, 2 g

Azactam®: 1 g, 2 g

Powder for reconstitution, for oral inhalation [preservative free]:

Cayston®: 75 mg [supplied with diluent]

Selected References

Creasey WA, Platt TB, Frantz M, et al, "Pharmacokinetics of Aztreonam in Elderly Male Volunteers," *Br J Clin Pharmacol*, 1985, 19(2):233-7.

Mandell LA, Wunderink RG, Anzueto A, et al, "Infectious Diseases Society of America/American Thoracic Society Consensus Guidelines on the Management of Community-Acquired Pneumonia in Adults," *Clin Infect Dis*, 2007, 44 Suppl 2:S27-72.

Sattler FR, Schramm M, Swabb EA, "Safety of Aztreonam and SQ 26,992 in Elderly Patients With Renal Insufficiency," *Rev Infect Dis*, 1985, (Suppl 4):5622.

♦ **Azulfidine®** *see* SulfaSALAzine *on page 1719*
♦ **Azulfidine EN-tabs®** *see* SulfaSALAzine *on page 1719*
♦ **B6** *see* Pyridoxine *on page 1552*
♦ **Baby Aspirin** *see* Aspirin *on page 153*
♦ **Bacid® [OTC]** *see* Lactobacillus *on page 1020*

Baclofen (BAK loe fen)

Medication Safety Issues
Sound-alike/look-alike issues:
Baclofen may be confused with Bactroban®
Lioresal® may be confused with lisinopril, Lotensin®
High alert medication:
The Institute for Safe Medication Practices (ISMP) includes this medication (intrathecal administration) among its list of drugs which have a heightened risk of causing significant patient harm when used in error.

Brand Names: U.S. Gablofen®; Lioresal®

Brand Names: Canada Apo-Baclofen®; Dom-Baclofen; Lioresal®; Liotec; Med-Baclofen; Mylan-Baclofen; Novo-Baclofen; Nu-Baclo; PHL-Baclofen; PMS-Baclofen; ratio-Baclofen; Riva-Baclofen

Generic Availability (U.S.) Yes: Tablets

Pharmacologic Category Skeletal Muscle Relaxant

Use Treatment of reversible spasticity associated with multiple sclerosis or spinal cord lesions
Orphan drug: Intrathecal: Treatment of intractable spasticity caused by spinal cord injury, multiple sclerosis, and other spinal disease (spinal ischemia or tumor, transverse myelitis, cervical spondylosis, degenerative myelopathy)

Unlabeled/Investigational Use Treatment of intractable hiccups, intractable pain relief, bladder spasticity, trigeminal neuralgia, cerebral palsy, Huntington's chorea

Contraindications Hypersensitivity to baclofen or any component of the formulation

Warnings/Precautions Use with caution in patients with seizure disorder or impaired renal function. **[U.S. Boxed Warning]: Avoid abrupt withdrawal of the drug; abrupt withdrawal of intrathecal baclofen has resulted in severe sequelae (hyperpyrexia, obtundation, rebound/exaggerated spasticity, muscle rigidity, and rhabdomyolysis), leading to organ failure and some fatalities.** Risk may be higher in patients with injuries at T-6 or above, history of baclofen withdrawal, or limited ability to communicate. May cause CNS depression, which may impair physical or mental abilities; patients must be cautioned about performing tasks which require mental alertness (eg, operating machinery or driving). Elderly are more sensitive to the effects of baclofen and are more likely to experience adverse CNS effects at higher doses.

Cases (most from pharmacy compounded preparations) of intrathecal mass formation at the implanted catheter tip have been reported; may lead to loss of clinical response, pain or new/ worsening neurological effects. Neurosurgical evaluation and/or an appropriate imaging study should be considered if a mass is suspected.

Adverse Reactions (Reflective of adult population; not specific for elderly)
>10%:
Central nervous system: Drowsiness, vertigo, psychiatric disturbances, insomnia, slurred speech, ataxia, hypotonia
Neuromuscular & skeletal: Weakness
1% to 10%:
Cardiovascular: Hypotension
Central nervous system: Fatigue, confusion, headache

Dermatologic: Rash
Gastrointestinal: Nausea, constipation
Genitourinary: Polyuria

Drug Interactions

Avoid Concomitant Use There are no known interactions where it is recommended to avoid concomitant use.

Increased Effect/Toxicity

Baclofen may increase the levels/effects of: Alcohol (Ethyl); CNS Depressants; Methotrimeprazine; Selective Serotonin Reuptake Inhibitors

The levels/effects of Baclofen may be increased by: Droperidol; HydrOXYzine; Methotrimeprazine

Decreased Effect There are no known significant interactions involving a decrease in effect.

Ethanol/Nutrition/Herb Interactions

Ethanol: May increase CNS depression; monitor for increased effects with coadministration. Caution patients about effects.

Herb/Nutraceutical: Avoid valerian, St John's wort, kava kava, gotu kola.

Mechanism of Action Inhibits the transmission of both monosynaptic and polysynaptic reflexes at the spinal cord level, possibly by hyperpolarization of primary afferent fiber terminals, with resultant relief of muscle spasticity

Pharmacodynamics/Kinetics

Onset of action: 3-4 days
Peak effect: 5-10 days
Absorption (dose dependent): Oral: Rapid
Protein binding: 30%
Metabolism: Hepatic (15% of dose)
Half-life elimination: 3.5 hours
Time to peak, serum: Oral: Within 2-3 hours
Excretion: Urine and feces (85% as unchanged drug)

Dosage

Geriatric Oral (the lowest effective dose is recommended): Initial: 5 mg 2-3 times/day, increasing gradually as needed; if benefits are not seen withdraw the drug slowly.

Adult

Spasticity:

Oral: 5 mg 3 times/day, may increase 5 mg/dose every 3 days to a maximum of 80 mg/day
Intrathecal:
  Test dose: 50-100 mcg, doses >50 mcg should be given in 25 mcg increments, separated by 24 hours. A screening dose of 25 mcg may be considered in very small patients. Patients not responding to screening dose of 100 mcg should not be considered for chronic infusion/implanted pump.
  Maintenance: After positive response to test dose, a maintenance intrathecal infusion can be administered via an implanted intrathecal pump. Initial dose via pump: Infusion at a 24-hourly rate dosed at twice the test dose. Avoid abrupt discontinuation.

Hiccups (unlabeled use): Oral: 10-20 mg 2-3 times/day

Renal Impairment May be necessary to reduce dosage; no specific guidelines have been established

Hemodialysis: Poor water solubility allows for accumulation during chronic hemodialysis. Low-dose therapy is recommended. There have been several case reports of accumulation of baclofen resulting in toxicity symptoms (organic brain syndrome, myoclonia, deceleration and steep potentials in EEG) in patients with renal failure who have received normal doses of baclofen.

Administration Intrathecal: For screening dosages, dilute with preservative-free sodium chloride to a final concentration of 50 mcg/mL for bolus injection into the subarachnoid space. For maintenance infusions, concentrations of 500-2000 mcg/mL may be used.

Test Interactions Increased alkaline phosphatase, AST, glucose, ammonia (B); decreased bilirubin (S)

Pharmacotherapy Pearls Not indicated for muscle spasm associated with rheumatic disorders; not recommended in Parkinson's disease or stroke since the efficacy has not been established

Special Geriatric Considerations The elderly are more sensitive to the effects of baclofen and are more likely to experience adverse CNS effects at higher doses.

Dosage Forms Excipient information presented when available (limited, particularly for generics); consult specific product labeling.

Injection, solution, intrathecal [preservative free]:
  Gablofen®: 50 mcg/mL (1 mL); 500 mcg/mL (20 mL); 2000 mcg/mL (20 mL)
  Lioresal®: 500 mcg/mL (20 mL); 2000 mcg/mL (5 mL, 20 mL)

Injection, solution, intrathecal [for screening, preservative free]:
  Lioresal®: 50 mcg/mL (1 mL)
Tablet, oral: 10 mg, 20 mg

◆ **Bactrim™** see Sulfamethoxazole and Trimethoprim on page 1714
◆ **Bactrim™ DS** see Sulfamethoxazole and Trimethoprim on page 1714
◆ **Bactroban®** see Mupirocin on page 1250
◆ **Bactroban Cream®** see Mupirocin on page 1250
◆ **Bactroban Nasal®** see Mupirocin on page 1250
◆ **Baking Soda** see Sodium Bicarbonate on page 1688
◆ **Balsam Peru, Castor Oil, and Trypsin** see Trypsin, Balsam Peru, and Castor Oil on page 1876
◆ **Band-Aid® Hurt Free™ Antiseptic Wash [OTC]** see Lidocaine (Topical) on page 1064
◆ **Banophen™ [OTC]** see DiphenhydrAMINE (Systemic) on page 520
◆ **Banophen™ Anti-Itch [OTC]** see DiphenhydrAMINE (Topical) on page 523
◆ **Banzel®** see Rufinamide on page 1644
◆ **Baridium [OTC]** see Phenazopyridine on page 1433
◆ **Baycadron™** see Dexamethasone (Systemic) on page 483
◆ **Bayer® Aspirin Extra Strength [OTC]** see Aspirin on page 153
◆ **Bayer® Aspirin Regimen Adult Low Strength [OTC]** see Aspirin on page 153
◆ **Bayer® Aspirin Regimen Children's [OTC]** see Aspirin on page 153
◆ **Bayer® Aspirin Regimen Regular Strength [OTC]** see Aspirin on page 153
◆ **Bayer® Genuine Aspirin [OTC]** see Aspirin on page 153
◆ **Bayer® Plus Extra Strength [OTC]** see Aspirin on page 153
◆ **Bayer® Women's Low Dose Aspirin [OTC]** see Aspirin on page 153
◆ **Baza® Antifungal [OTC]** see Miconazole on page 1206
◆ **beano® [OTC]** see Alpha-Galactosidase on page 69

Becaplermin (be KAP ler min)

Medication Safety Issues
  Sound-alike/look-alike issues:
    Regranex® may be confused with Granulex®, Repronex®
Brand Names: U.S. Regranex®
Brand Names: Canada Regranex®
Index Terms Recombinant Human Platelet-Derived Growth Factor B; rPDGF-BB
Generic Availability (U.S.) No
Pharmacologic Category Growth Factor, Platelet-Derived; Topical Skin Product
Use Adjunctive treatment of diabetic neuropathic ulcers occurring on the lower limbs and feet that extend into subcutaneous tissue (or beyond) and have adequate blood supply
Contraindications Hypersensitivity to becaplermin or any component of the formulation; known neoplasm(s) at the site(s) of application
Warnings/Precautions For external use only; do not use in wounds that close by primary intention. Use with caution in ulcer wounds related to arterial or venous insufficiency when there are thermal, electrical, or radiation burns at wound site. **[U.S. Boxed Warning]: In a retrospective study, an increase in mortality secondary to malignancy has been observed in patients treated with ≥3 tubes of becaplermin.** Malignancies of varying types have been reported; all were remote from the becaplermin treatment site; use with caution in patients with known malignancy. Effects on exposed joints, tendons, ligaments and bone have not been established.
Adverse Reactions (Reflective of adult population; not specific for elderly)
  1% to 10%: Dermatologic: Erythematous rash (2%)
Drug Interactions
  Avoid Concomitant Use There are no known interactions where it is recommended to avoid concomitant use.
  Increased Effect/Toxicity There are no known significant interactions involving an increase in effect.
  Decreased Effect There are no known significant interactions involving a decrease in effect.
Stability Refrigerate at 2°C to 8°C (36°F to 46°F); do not freeze. The following stability information has also been reported: May be stored at room temperature for up to 6 days (Cohen, 2007).
Mechanism of Action Recombinant B-isoform homodimer of human platelet-derived growth factor (rPDGF-BB) which enhances formation of new granulation tissue, induces fibroblast proliferation and differentiation to promote wound healing; also promotes angiogenesis.

Pharmacodynamics/Kinetics
Onset of action: Complete healing: 15% of patients within 8 weeks, 25% at 10 weeks
Absorption: Minimal
Distribution: Binds to PDGF beta-receptors in normal skin and granulation tissue

Dosage
Geriatric & Adult Diabetic ulcers (lower extremity): Topical: Apply appropriate amount of gel once daily with a cotton swab or similar tool, as a coating over the ulcer. The amount of becaplermin to be applied will vary depending on the size of the ulcer area.
Note: If the ulcer does not decrease in size by ~30% after 10 weeks of treatment or complete healing has not occurred in 20 weeks, continued treatment with becaplermin gel should be reassessed.
Estimation of gel requirement: To calculate the length of gel applied to the ulcer, measure the greatest length of the ulcer by the greatest width of the ulcer. Tube size and unit of measure will determine the formula used in the calculation. Recalculate amount of gel needed every 1-2 weeks, depending on the rate of change in ulcer area.
Centimeters:
15 g tube: [ulcer length (cm) x width (cm)] divided by 4 = length of gel (cm)
2 g tube: [ulcer length (cm) x width (cm)] divided by 2 = length of gel (cm)
Inches:
15 g tube: [length (in) x width (in)] x 0.6 = length of gel (in)
2 g tube: [length (in) x width (in)] x 1.3 = length of gel (in)

Administration For external use only. Squeeze appropriate amount of gel onto clean measuring surface (eg, wax paper), spread onto entire ulcer area in a thin, continuous layer ~1/16 inch thick. Cover with saline moistened dressing; leave dressing in place ~12 hours. After 12 hours, remove dressing, rinse with saline or water to remove residual becaplermin gel and cover with saline moistened dressing (without becaplermin gel) for remainder of the day. Continue use once daily until ulcer is completely healed.

Monitoring Parameters Ulcer volume (pressure ulcers); wound area; evidence of closure; drainage (diabetic ulcers); signs/symptoms of toxicity (erythema, local infections)

Special Geriatric Considerations No specific information for use in elderly.

Dosage Forms Excipient information presented when available (limited, particularly for generics); consult specific product labeling. [DSC] = Discontinued product
Gel, topical:
Regranex®: 0.01% (2 g [DSC], 15 g)

Beclomethasone (Oral Inhalation) (be kloe METH a sone)

Related Information
Asthma *on page 2016*
Inhalant Agents *on page 2010*
Medication Safety Issues
Sound-alike/look-alike issues:
Vanceril® may be confused with Vancenase
Brand Names: U.S. QVAR®
Brand Names: Canada QVAR®; Vanceril® AEM
Index Terms Vancenase
Generic Availability (U.S.) No
Pharmacologic Category Corticosteroid, Inhalant (Oral)
Use Oral inhalation: Maintenance and prophylactic treatment of asthma; includes those who require corticosteroids and those who may benefit from a dose reduction/elimination of systemically-administered corticosteroids. Not for relief of acute bronchospasm.
Contraindications Hypersensitivity to beclomethasone or any component of the formulation; status asthmaticus
Warnings/Precautions May cause hypercorticism or suppression of hypothalamic-pituitary-adrenal (HPA) axis, particularly in patients receiving high doses for prolonged periods. HPA axis suppression may lead to adrenal crisis. Withdrawal and discontinuation of a corticosteroid should be done slowly and carefully. Particular care is required when patients are transferred from systemic corticosteroids to inhaled products due to possible adrenal insufficiency or withdrawal from steroids, including an increase in allergic symptoms. Patients receiving >20 mg per day of prednisone (or equivalent) may be most susceptible. Fatalities have occurred due to adrenal insufficiency in asthmatic patients during and after transfer from systemic corticosteroids to aerosol steroids; aerosol steroids do **not** provide the systemic steroid needed to treat patients having trauma, surgery, or infections.

Bronchospasm may occur with wheezing after inhalation; if this occurs, stop steroid and treat with a fast-acting bronchodilator. Supplemental steroids (oral or parenteral) may be needed during stress or severe asthma attacks. Not to be used in status asthmaticus or for the relief of acute bronchospasm. Corticosteroid use may cause psychiatric disturbances, including depression, euphoria, insomnia, mood swings, and personality changes. Pre-existing psychiatric conditions may be exacerbated by corticosteroid use. Prolonged use of corticosteroids may also increase the incidence of secondary infection, mask acute infection (including fungal infections), prolong or exacerbate viral infections, or limit response to vaccines. Exposure to chickenpox should be avoided; corticosteroids should not be used to treat ocular herpes simplex. Corticosteroids should not be used for cerebral malaria. Close observation is required in patients with latent tuberculosis and/or TB reactivity; restrict use in active TB (only in conjunction with antituberculosis treatment). Prolonged treatment with corticosteroids has been associated with the development of Kaposi's sarcoma (case reports); if noted, discontinuation of therapy should be considered.

Use with caution in patients with thyroid disease, hepatic impairment, renal impairment, cardiovascular disease, diabetes, glaucoma, cataracts, myasthenia gravis, patients at risk for osteoporosis, patients at risk for seizures, or GI diseases (diverticulitis, peptic ulcer, ulcerative colitis) due to perforation risk. Use caution following acute MI (corticosteroids have been associated with myocardial rupture). Because of the risk of adverse effects, systemic corticosteroids should be used cautiously in the elderly in the smallest possible effective dose for the shortest duration.

Adverse Reactions (Reflective of adult population; not specific for elderly) Frequency not defined.

Central nervous system: Agitation, depression, dizziness, dysphonia, headache, lightheadedness, mental disturbances

Dermatologic: Acneiform lesions, angioedema, atrophy, bruising, pruritus, purpura, striae, rash, urticaria

Endocrine & metabolic: Cushingoid features, growth velocity reduction in children and adolescents, HPA function suppression, weight gain

Gastrointestinal: Dry/irritated nose, throat and mouth, hoarseness, localized *Candida* or *Aspergillus* infection, loss of smell, loss of taste, nausea, unpleasant smell, unpleasant taste, vomiting

Ocular: Cataracts, glaucoma, intraocular pressure increased

Respiratory: Cough, paradoxical bronchospasm, pharyngitis, sinusitis, wheezing

Miscellaneous: Anaphylactic/anaphylactoid reactions, death (due to adrenal insufficiency, reported during and after transfer from systemic corticosteroids to aerosol in asthmatic patients), immediate and delayed hypersensitivity reactions

Drug Interactions

Avoid Concomitant Use

Avoid concomitant use of Beclomethasone (Oral Inhalation) with any of the following: Aldesleukin; BCG; Natalizumab; Pimecrolimus; Tacrolimus (Topical)

Increased Effect/Toxicity

Beclomethasone (Oral Inhalation) may increase the levels/effects of: Amphotericin B; Deferasirox; Leflunomide; Loop Diuretics; Natalizumab; Thiazide Diuretics

The levels/effects of Beclomethasone (Oral Inhalation) may be increased by: Denosumab; Pimecrolimus; Tacrolimus (Topical); Telaprevir; Trastuzumab

Decreased Effect

Beclomethasone (Oral Inhalation) may decrease the levels/effects of: Aldesleukin; Antidiabetic Agents; BCG; Corticorelin; Sipuleucel-T; Telaprevir; Vaccines (Inactivated)

The levels/effects of Beclomethasone (Oral Inhalation) may be decreased by: Echinacea

Stability Do not store near heat or open flame. Do not puncture canisters. Store at 25°C (77°F); excursions permitted between 15°C to 30°C (59°F to 86°F). Rest QVAR® on concave end of canister with actuator on top.

Mechanism of Action Controls the rate of protein synthesis; depresses the migration of polymorphonuclear leukocytes, fibroblasts; reverses capillary permeability and lysosomal stabilization at the cellular level to prevent or control inflammation

Pharmacodynamics/Kinetics

Onset of action: Therapeutic effect: 1-4 weeks

Absorption: Readily; quickly hydrolyzed by pulmonary esterases to active metabolite (beclomethasone-17-monoproprionate [17-BMP]) prior to absorption

Distribution: Beclomethasone dipropionate (BDP): 20 L; 17-BMP: 424 L

Protein binding: 17-BMP: 94% to 96%

Metabolism: Pro-drug; undergoes rapid conversion to 17-BMP during absorption; followed by additional metabolism via CYP3A4 to other, less active metabolites (beclomethasone-21-monopropionate [21-BMP] and beclomethasone [BOH])

Half-life elimination: BDP: 0.5 hours; 17-BMP: 3 hours

Time to peak, plasma: Oral inhalation: BDP: 0.5 hours; 17-BMP: 0.7 hours

Excretion: Feces (60%); urine (<10% to 12%)

BECLOMETHASONE (ORAL INHALATION)

◄ **Dosage**

Geriatric & Adult Nasal inhalation and oral inhalation dosage forms are not to be used interchangeably.

Asthma: Inhalation, oral (doses should be titrated to the lowest effective dose once asthma is controlled) (QVAR®):

Patients previously on bronchodilators only: Initial dose 40-80 mcg twice daily; maximum dose 320 mcg twice daily

Patients previously on inhaled corticosteroids: Initial dose 40-160 mcg twice daily; maximum dose 320 mcg twice daily

NIH Asthma Guidelines (NIH, 2007): HFA formulation (eg, QVAR®): Administer in divided doses:

"Low" dose: 80-240 mcg/day
"Medium" dose: >240-480 mcg/day
"High" dose: >480 mcg/day

Administration QVAR®: Rinse mouth and throat after use to prevent *Candida* infection. Do not wash or put inhaler in water; mouth piece may be cleaned with a dry tissue or cloth. Prime canister before using.

Pharmacotherapy Pearls Not used in status asthmaticus; shake thoroughly before using; oral inhalation and nasal inhalation dosage forms are **not** to be used interchangeably

Special Geriatric Considerations Elderly patients may have difficulty with oral metered dose inhalers and may benefit from the use of a spacer or chamber device.

Dosage Forms Excipient information presented when available (limited, particularly for generics); consult specific product labeling. [DSC] = Discontinued product

Aerosol, for oral inhalation, as dipropionate:

QVAR®: 40 mcg/inhalation (7.3 g [DSC]) [chlorofluorocarbon free; contains ethanol; 100 metered actuations]

QVAR®: 40 mcg/inhalation (8.7 g) [chlorofluorocarbon free; contains ethanol; 120 metered actuations]

QVAR®: 80 mcg/inhalation (7.3 g [DSC]) [chlorofluorocarbon free; contains ethanol; 100 metered actuations]

QVAR®: 80 mcg/inhalation (8.7 g) [chlorofluorocarbon free; contains ethanol; 120 metered actuations]

Beclomethasone (Nasal) (be kloe METH a sone)

Brand Names: U.S. Beconase AQ®
Brand Names: Canada Apo-Beclomethasone®; Gen-Beclo; Nu-Beclomethasone; Rivanase AQ
Index Terms Beclomethasone Dipropionate
Generic Availability (U.S.) No
Pharmacologic Category Corticosteroid, Nasal
Use Symptomatic treatment of seasonal or perennial rhinitis; prevent recurrence of nasal polyps following surgery.
Dosage

Geriatric & Adult Nasal inhalation and oral inhalation dosage forms are not to be used interchangeably.

Rhinitis, nasal polyps: Inhalation, nasal (Beconase® AQ): 1-2 inhalations each nostril twice daily; total dose 168-336 mcg/day

Dosage Forms Excipient information presented when available (limited, particularly for generics); consult specific product labeling.

Suspension, intranasal, as dipropionate [spray]:

Beconase AQ®: 42 mcg/inhalation (25 g) [contains benzalkonium chloride, ethanol 0.25%; 180 metered actuations]

◆ **Beclomethasone Dipropionate** *see* Beclomethasone (Nasal) *on page 186*
◆ **Beconase AQ®** *see* Beclomethasone (Nasal) *on page 186*

Belimumab (be LIM yoo mab)

Brand Names: U.S. Benlysta®
Pharmacologic Category Monoclonal Antibody
Use Treatment of autoantibody-positive (antinuclear antibody [ANA] and/or anti-double-stranded DNA [anti-ds-DNA]) systemic lupus erythematosus (SLE) in addition to standard therapy
Medication Guide Available Yes
Contraindications Hypersensitivity to belimumab or any component of the formulation

Warnings/Precautions Hazardous agent - use appropriate precautions for handling and disposal. Deaths due to infection, cardiovascular disease, and suicide were higher in belimumab patients compared to placebo during clinical trials. Use is not recommended if severe active infection is present; consider discontinuing in patients who develop infections and initiate appropriate anti-infective treatment. Hypersensitivity and infusion reactions have been associated with use; discontinue for severe reactions (anaphylaxis, angioedema); infusion may be slowed or temporarily interrupted for minor reactions (headache, nausea, skin reactions). May increase risk of malignancy. May cause psychiatric adverse effects, including anxiety, insomnia, or new/worsening depression. Combined use with other immune modifying therapy or intravenous cyclophosphamide is not recommended. Live vaccines should not be given within 30 days or concurrently with belimumab. African-American patients may have a lower response rate. Has not been studied in patients with severe active lupus nephritis or CNS lupus; use not recommended.

Adverse Reactions (Reflective of adult population; not specific for elderly)
>10%: Gastrointestinal: Nausea (15%), diarrhea (12%)
≥3% to 10%:
  Central nervous system: Fever (10%), insomnia (7%), migraine (5%), depression (5%), anxiety (4%)
  Gastrointestinal: Viral gastroenteritis (3%)
  Genitourinary: Cystitis (4%)
  Hematologic: Leukopenia (4%)
  Neuromuscular & skeletal: Pain in extremity (6%)
  Respiratory: Bronchitis (9%), nasopharyngitis (9%), pharyngitis (5%)

Drug Interactions
  Avoid Concomitant Use
  Avoid concomitant use of Belimumab with any of the following: Abatacept; Alefacept; BCG; Belatacept; Cyclophosphamide; Denileukin Diftitox; Etanercept; Monoclonal Antibodies; Natalizumab; Pimecrolimus; Tacrolimus (Topical); Vaccines (Live)

  Increased Effect/Toxicity
  Belimumab may increase the levels/effects of: Cyclophosphamide; Leflunomide; Natalizumab; Vaccines (Live)

  The levels/effects of Belimumab may be increased by: Abatacept; Abciximab; Alefacept; Belatacept; Denileukin Diftitox; Denosumab; Etanercept; Monoclonal Antibodies; Pimecrolimus; Roflumilast; Tacrolimus (Topical); Trastuzumab

  Decreased Effect
  Belimumab may decrease the levels/effects of: BCG; Sipuleucel-T; Vaccines (Inactivated); Vaccines (Live)

  The levels/effects of Belimumab may be decreased by: Echinacea

Stability Prior to reconstitution, store unused vials between 2°C to 8°C (36°F to 46°F); do not freeze. Protect from light. To reconstitute, allow vial to reach room temperature. Reconstitute 120 mg vial with 1.5 mL of SWFI. Reconstitute 400 mg vial with 4.8 mL of SWFI. Gently swirl for 60 seconds every 5 minutes until powder has dissolved (usual reconstitution time is 10-15 minutes, but may take up to 30 minutes); do not shake. Further dilute reconstituted solution in 250 mL of 0.9% sodium chloride by first removing and discarding the volume equivalent to the volume of the reconstituted solution to be added to prepare the appropriate dose; add the appropriate volume of the reconstituted solution to the infusion container and invert to mix solution. Protect from light. Solution may be stored refrigerated or at room temperature. Storage time, including infusion to the patient, must be completed within 8 hours of reconstitution.

Mechanism of Action Belimumab is an IgG1λ monoclonal antibody that prevents the survival of B lymphocytes by blocking the binding of soluble human B lymphocyte stimulator protein (BLyS) to receptors on B lymphocytes. This reduces the activity of B-cell mediated immunity and the autoimmune response.

Pharmacodynamics/Kinetics
Onset of action: B cells: 8 weeks; Clinical improvement (SLE Responder Index and flare reduction): 16 weeks (Navarra, 2011)
Distribution: V_d: 5.29 L
Half-life elimination: 19.4 days

Dosage
  Geriatric & Adult SLE: I.V.: Initial: 10 mg/kg every 2 weeks for 3 doses; Maintenance: 10 mg/kg every 4 weeks
  Renal Impairment No dosage adjustment necessary for Cl_{cr} ≥15 mL/minute; has not been studied in Cl_{cr} <15 mL/minute
  Hepatic Impairment Has not been studied.

◀ **Administration** Administer intravenously over 1 hour through a dedicated I.V. line. Do not give as an I.V. push or bolus. Discontinue infusion for severe hypersensitivity reaction (eg, anaphylaxis, angioedema). The infusion may be slowed or temporarily interrupted for minor reactions. Consider premedicating for prophylaxis against infusion reactions.

Monitoring Parameters Monitor for infusion reactions; worsening of depression, mood changes, or suicidal thoughts

Special Geriatric Considerations Clinical studies did not include sufficient numbers of elderly subjects to note differences in efficacy or toxicity; therefore, use with caution in the elderly.

Dosage Forms Excipient information presented when available (limited, particularly for generics); consult specific product labeling.

Injection, powder for reconstitution:

Benlysta®: 120 mg, 400 mg [contains polysorbate 80, sucrose 80 mg/mL]

Selected References

Navarra SV, Guzmán RM, Gallacher AE, et al, "Efficacy and Safety of Belimumab in Patients With Active Systemic Lupus Erythematosus: A Randomised, Placebo-Controlled, Phase 3 Trial," *Lancet*, 2011, 26(377):721-31.

Wallace DJ, Stohl W, Furie RA, et al, "A Phase II, Randomized, Double-Blind, Placebo-Controlled, Dose-Ranging Study of Belimumab in Patients With Active Systemic Lupus Erythematosus," *Arthritis Rheum*, 2009, 61(9):1168-78.

◆ **Belladonna Alkaloids With Phenobarbital** *see* Hyoscyamine, Atropine, Scopolamine, and Phenobarbital *on page 905*
◆ **Benadryl® Allergy [OTC]** *see* DiphenhydrAMINE (Systemic) *on page 520*
◆ **Benadryl® Allergy Quick Dissolve [OTC]** *see* DiphenhydrAMINE (Systemic) *on page 520*
◆ **Benadryl® Children's Allergy [OTC]** *see* DiphenhydrAMINE (Systemic) *on page 520*
◆ **Benadryl® Children's Allergy FastMelt® [OTC]** *see* DiphenhydrAMINE (Systemic) *on page 520*
◆ **Benadryl® Children's Allergy Perfect Measure™ [OTC]** *see* DiphenhydrAMINE (Systemic) *on page 520*
◆ **Benadryl® Children's Dye Free Allergy [OTC]** *see* DiphenhydrAMINE (Systemic) *on page 520*
◆ **Benadryl® Dye-Free Allergy [OTC]** *see* DiphenhydrAMINE (Systemic) *on page 520*
◆ **Benadryl® Extra Strength Itch Stopping [OTC]** *see* DiphenhydrAMINE (Topical) *on page 523*
◆ **Benadryl® Itch Relief Extra Strength [OTC]** *see* DiphenhydrAMINE (Topical) *on page 523*
◆ **Benadryl® Itch Stopping [OTC]** *see* DiphenhydrAMINE (Topical) *on page 523*
◆ **Benadryl® Itch Stopping Extra Strength [OTC]** *see* DiphenhydrAMINE (Topical) *on page 523*

Benazepril (ben AY ze pril)

Related Information

Angiotensin Agents *on page 1985*

Medication Safety Issues

Sound-alike/look-alike issues:

Benazepril may be confused with Benadryl®

Lotensin® may be confused with Lioresal®, lovastatin

Brand Names: U.S. Lotensin®

Brand Names: Canada Lotensin®

Index Terms Benazepril Hydrochloride

Generic Availability (U.S.) Yes

Pharmacologic Category Angiotensin-Converting Enzyme (ACE) Inhibitor

Use Treatment of hypertension, either alone or in combination with other antihypertensive agents

Unlabeled/Investigational Use Treatment of left ventricular dysfunction after myocardial infarction

Contraindications Hypersensitivity to benazepril or any component of the formulation; patients with a history of angioedema (with or without prior ACE inhibitor therapy)

Warnings/Precautions Anaphylactic reactions may occur rarely with ACE inhibitors. At any time during treatment (especially following first dose) angioedema may occur rarely with ACE inhibitors. It may involve the head and neck (potentially compromising airway) or the intestine (presenting with abdominal pain). African-Americans and patients with idiopathic or hereditary angioedema may be at an increased risk. Prolonged frequent monitoring may be required especially if tongue, glottis, or larynx are involved as they are associated with airway obstruction. Patients with a history of airway surgery may have a higher risk of airway obstruction. Aggressive early and appropriate management is critical. Contraindicated in patients with history of angioedema with or without prior ACE inhibitor therapy. Hypersensitivity reactions may be seen during hemodialysis (eg, CVVHD) with high-flux dialysis membranes (eg, AN69), and rarely, during low density lipoprotein apheresis with dextran sulfate cellulose. Rare cases of anaphylactoid reactions have been reported in patients undergoing sensitization treatment with hymenoptera (bee, wasp) venom while receiving ACE inhibitors.

Symptomatic hypotension with or without syncope can occur with ACE inhibitors (usually with the first several doses); effects are most often observed in volume depleted patients; close monitoring of patient is required especially with initial dosing and dosing increases; blood pressure must be lowered at a rate appropriate for the patient's clinical condition. Initiation of therapy in patients with ischemic heart disease or cerebrovascular disease warrants close observation due to the potential consequences posed by falling blood pressure (eg, MI, stroke). Use with caution in hypertrophic cardiomyopathy with outflow tract obstruction, severe aortic stenosis, or before, during, or immediately after major surgery.

Hyperkalemia may occur with ACE inhibitors; risk factors include renal dysfunction, diabetes mellitus, concomitant use of potassium-sparing diuretics, potassium supplements and/or potassium containing salts. Use cautiously, if at all, with these agents and monitor potassium closely. Cough may occur with ACE inhibitors. Other causes of cough should be considered (eg, pulmonary congestion in patients with heart failure) and excluded prior to discontinuation. Use with caution in patients with diabetes receiving insulin or oral antidiabetic agents; may be at increased risk for episodes of hypoglycemia.

May be associated with deterioration of renal function and/or increases in serum creatinine, particularly in patients with low renal blood flow (eg, renal artery stenosis, heart failure) whose glomerular filtration rate (GFR) is dependent on efferent arteriolar vasoconstriction by angiotensin II; deterioration may result in oliguria, acute renal failure, and progressive azotemia. Small increases in serum creatinine may occur following initiation; consider discontinuation only in patients with progressive and/or significant deterioration in renal function. Use with caution in patients with unstented unilateral/bilateral renal artery stenosis. When unstented bilateral renal artery stenosis is present, use is generally avoided due to the elevated risk of deterioration in renal function unless possible benefits outweigh risks. Concurrent use of angiotensin receptor blockers may increase the risk of clinically-significant adverse events (eg, renal dysfunction, hyperkalemia).

Rare toxicities associated with ACE inhibitors include cholestatic jaundice (which may progress to fulminant hepatic necrosis), agranulocytosis, neutropenia, or leukopenia with myeloid hypoplasia. Patients with collagen vascular diseases (especially with concomitant renal impairment) or renal impairment alone may be at increased risk for hematologic toxicity; periodically monitor CBC with differential in these patients.

Adverse Reactions (Reflective of adult population; not specific for elderly)
1% to 10%:
Cardiovascular: Postural dizziness (2%)
Central nervous system: Headache (6%), dizziness (4%), somnolence (2%)
Renal: Serum creatinine increased (2%), worsening of renal function may occur in patients with bilateral renal artery stenosis or hypovolemia
Respiratory: Cough (1% to 10%)
Eosinophilic pneumonitis, anaphylaxis, renal insufficiency, and renal failure have been reported with other ACE inhibitors. In addition, a syndrome including fever, myalgia, arthralgia, interstitial nephritis, vasculitis, rash, eosinophilia, and elevated ESR has been reported to be associated with ACE inhibitors.

Drug Interactions

Avoid Concomitant Use There are no known interactions where it is recommended to avoid concomitant use.

Increased Effect/Toxicity
Benazepril may increase the levels/effects of: Allopurinol; Amifostine; Antihypertensives; AzaTHIOprine; CycloSPORINE; CycloSPORINE (Systemic); Ferric Gluconate; Gold Sodium Thiomalate; Hypotensive Agents; Iron Dextran Complex; Lithium; Nonsteroidal Anti-Inflammatory Agents; RiTUXimab; Sodium Phosphates

The levels/effects of Benazepril may be increased by: Alfuzosin; Angiotensin II Receptor Blockers; Diazoxide; DPP-IV Inhibitors; Eplerenone; Everolimus; Herbs (Hypotensive Properties); Loop Diuretics; MAO Inhibitors; Pentoxifylline; Phosphodiesterase 5 Inhibitors; Potassium Salts; Potassium-Sparing Diuretics; Prostacyclin Analogues; Sirolimus; Temsirolimus; Thiazide Diuretics; TiZANidine; Tolvaptan; Trimethoprim

Decreased Effect
The levels/effects of Benazepril may be decreased by: Antacids; Aprotinin; Herbs (Hypertensive Properties); Icatibant; Lanthanum; Methylphenidate; Nonsteroidal Anti-Inflammatory Agents; Salicylates; Yohimbine

◀ **Ethanol/Nutrition/Herb Interactions** Herb/Nutraceutical: Avoid bayberry, blue cohosh, cayenne, ephedra, ginger, ginseng (American), kola, licorice (may worsen hypertension). Avoid black cohosh, California poppy, coleus, golden seal, hawthorn, mistletoe, periwinkle, quinine, shepherd's purse (may have increased antihypertensive effect).

Stability Store at ≤30°C (86°F). Protect from moisture.

Mechanism of Action Competitive inhibition of angiotensin I being converted to angiotensin II, a potent vasoconstrictor, through the angiotensin I-converting enzyme (ACE) activity, with resultant lower levels of angiotensin II which causes an increase in plasma renin activity and a reduction in aldosterone secretion

Pharmacodynamics/Kinetics

Reduction in plasma angiotensin-converting enzyme (ACE) activity:
  Onset of action: Peak effect: 1-2 hours after 2-20 mg dose
  Duration: >90% inhibition for 24 hours after 5-20 mg dose
Reduction in blood pressure:
  Peak effect: Single dose: 2-4 hours; Continuous therapy: 2 weeks
Absorption: Rapid (37%); food does not alter significantly; metabolite (benazeprilat) itself unsuitable for oral administration due to poor absorption
Distribution: V_d: ~8.7 L
Protein binding:
  Benazepril: ~97%
  Benazeprilat: ~95%
Metabolism: Rapidly and extensively hepatic to its active metabolite, benazeprilat, via enzymatic hydrolysis; extensive first-pass effect
Half-life elimination: Benazeprilat: Effective: 10-11 hours; Terminal: Adults: 22 hours
Time to peak: Parent drug: 0.5-1 hour
Excretion:
  Urine (trace amounts as benazepril; 20% as benazeprilat; 12% as other metabolites)
  Clearance: Nonrenal clearance (ie, biliary, metabolic) appears to contribute to the elimination of benazeprilat (11% to 12%), particularly patients with severe renal impairment; hepatic clearance is the main elimination route of unchanged benazepril
  Dialysis: ~6% of metabolite removed within 4 hours of dialysis following 10 mg of benazepril administered 2 hours prior to procedure; parent compound not found in dialysate

Dosage

Geriatric Oral: Initial: 5-10 mg/day in single or divided doses; usual range: 20-40 mg/day; adjust for renal function. Also see "Note" in adult dosing.

Adult Hypertension: Oral: Initial: 10 mg/day in patients not receiving a diuretic; 20-80 mg/day as a single dose or 2 divided doses; the need for twice-daily dosing should be assessed by monitoring peak (2-6 hours after dosing) and trough responses.

Note: Patients taking diuretics should have them discontinued 2-3 days prior to starting benazepril. If they cannot be discontinued, then initial dose should be 5 mg; restart after blood pressure is stabilized if needed.

Renal Impairment

Cl_{cr} <30 mL/minute: Administer 5 mg/day initially; maximum daily dose: 40 mg.
Hemodialysis: Moderately dialyzable (20% to 50%); administer dose postdialysis or administer 25% to 35% supplemental dose.
Peritoneal dialysis: Supplemental dose is not necessary.

Monitoring Parameters Blood pressure; serum creatinine and potassium; if patient has collagen vascular disease and/or renal impairment, periodically monitor CBC with differential

Pharmacotherapy Pearls Watch for hypotensive effect within 1-3 hours of first dose or new higher dose.

Special Geriatric Considerations Due to frequent decreases in glomerular filtration (also Cl_{cr}) with aging, elderly patients may have exaggerated responses to ACE inhibitors; differences in clinical response due to hepatic changes are not observed. ACE inhibitors may be preferred agents in elderly patients with congestive heart failure and diabetes mellitus. Diabetic proteinuria is reduced and insulin sensitivity is enhanced. In general, the side effect profile is favorable in elderly and causes little or no CNS confusion; use lowest dose recommendations initially. Many elderly may be volume depleted due to diuretic use and/or blunted thirst reflex resulting in inadequate fluid intake.

Benazepril and benazeprilat are substantially excreted by the kidney. Because elderly are more likely to have decreased renal function, care should be taken in dose selection, and it may be useful to monitor renal function.

Dosage Forms Excipient information presented when available (limited, particularly for generics); consult specific product labeling. [DSC] = Discontinued product
Tablet, oral, as hydrochloride: 5 mg, 10 mg, 20 mg, 40 mg
  Lotensin®: 5 mg [DSC], 10 mg, 20 mg, 40 mg

Extemporaneously Prepared To prepare a 2 mg/mL suspension, mix 15 benazepril 20 mg tablets in a bottle with Ora-Plus® 75 mL. Shake for 2 minutes, allow suspension to stand for ≥1 hour, then shake again for at least 1 additional minute. Add Ora-Sweet® 75 mL to suspension and shake to disperse. Will make 150 mL of a 2 mg/mL suspension. Store under refrigeration at 2°C to 8°C (36°F to 46°F) for up to 30 days. Shake prior to each use.

Selected References

American Diabetes Association, "Standards of Medical Care in Diabetes Mellitus – 2009," *Diabetes Care*, 2009, 32 (Suppl 1):13-61.

Miller DR, Oliveria SA, Berlowitz DR, et al, "Angioedema Incidence in US Veterens Initiating Angiotensin-Converting Enzyme Inhibitors," *Hypertension*, 2008, 51(6):1-7.

Benazepril and Hydrochlorothiazide
(ben AY ze pril & hye droe klor oh THYE a zide)

Related Information
Benazepril *on page 188*
Hydrochlorothiazide *on page 876*

Brand Names: U.S. Lotensin HCT®

Index Terms Benazepril Hydrochloride and Hydrochlorothiazide; Hydrochlorothiazide and Benazepril

Generic Availability (U.S.) Yes

Pharmacologic Category Angiotensin-Converting Enzyme (ACE) Inhibitor; Diuretic, Thiazide

Use Treatment of hypertension

Dosage

Geriatric Dose is individualized.

Adult Note: Not for initial therapy; dose should be individualized.

Hypertension: Oral: Range: Benazepril: 5-20 mg; Hydrochlorothiazide: 6.25-25 mg/day
Add-on therapy:
Patients not adequately controlled on benazepril monotherapy: Initiate benazepril 10-20 mg/hydrochlorothiazide 12.5 mg; titrate to effect at 2- to 3-week intervals
Patients controlled on hydrochlorothiazide 25 mg/day but experience significant potassium loss with this regimen: Initiate benazepril 5 mg/hydrochlorothiazide 6.25 mg
Replacement therapy: Substitute for the individually titrated components

Renal Impairment Cl_{cr} ≤30 mL/minute: Not recommended; loop diuretics are preferred.

Special Geriatric Considerations Hydrochlorothiazide is not effective in patients with a Cl_{cr} <30 mL/minute; therefore, it may not be a useful agent in many elderly patients.

Dosage Forms Excipient information presented when available (limited, particularly for generics); consult specific product labeling.
Tablet: 5/6.25: Benazepril hydrochloride 5 mg and hydrochlorothiazide 6.25 mg; 10/12.5: Benazepril hydrochloride 10 mg and hydrochlorothiazide 12.5 mg; 20/12.5: Benazepril hydrochloride 20 mg and hydrochlorothiazide 12.5 mg; 20/25: Benazepril hydrochloride 20 mg and hydrochlorothiazide 25 mg
Lotensin HCT® 10/12.5: Benazepril hydrochloride 10 mg and hydrochlorothiazide 12.5 mg
Lotensin HCT® 20/12.5: Benazepril hydrochloride 20 mg and hydrochlorothiazide 12.5 mg
Lotensin HCT® 20/25: Benazepril hydrochloride 20 mg and hydrochlorothiazide 25 mg

♦ **Benazepril Hydrochloride** *see Benazepril on page 188*
♦ **Benazepril Hydrochloride and Amlodipine Besylate** *see Amlodipine and Benazepril on page 108*
♦ **Benazepril Hydrochloride and Hydrochlorothiazide** *see Benazepril and Hydrochlorothiazide on page 191*
♦ **Benefiber® [OTC]** *see Wheat Dextrin on page 1933*
♦ **Benefiber® Plus Calcium [OTC]** *see Wheat Dextrin on page 1933*
♦ **Benemid [DSC]** *see Probenecid on page 1519*
♦ **Benicar®** *see Olmesartan on page 1333*
♦ **Benicar HCT®** *see Olmesartan and Hydrochlorothiazide on page 1336*
♦ **Benlysta®** *see Belimumab on page 186*
♦ **Bentyl®** *see Dicyclomine on page 504*
♦ **Benzathine Benzylpenicillin** *see Penicillin G Benzathine on page 1414*
♦ **Benzathine Penicillin G** *see Penicillin G Benzathine on page 1414*
♦ **Benzene Hexachloride** *see Lindane on page 1068*
♦ **Benzhexol Hydrochloride** *see Trihexyphenidyl on page 1865*

Benzonatate (ben ZOE na tate)

Brand Names: U.S. Tessalon®; Zonatuss™

◀ **Index Terms** Tessalon Perles
Generic Availability (U.S.) Yes: Capsule (softgel)
Pharmacologic Category Antitussive
Use Symptomatic relief of nonproductive cough
Contraindications Hypersensitivity to benzonatate, related compounds (such as tetracaine), or any component of the formulation
Warnings/Precautions Severe reactions, including bronchospasm, cardiovascular collapse and laryngospasm have been reported. May be related to localized anesthetic effects due to sucking or chewing the capsule. Isolated cases of abnormal behavior including mental confusion and visual hallucinations have been reported; may be related to prior sensitivity to related agents (eg, tetracaine, procaine) or interaction with concurrent medications. Signs and symptoms of overdose (restlessness, tremors, convulsion, coma, cardiac arrest) may occur within 15-20 minutes after ingestion. Death has been reported within 1 hour.
Adverse Reactions (Reflective of adult population; not specific for elderly) Frequency not defined.
Central nervous system: Confusion, dizziness, hallucinations, headache, sedation
Dermatologic: Pruritus, skin eruptions
Gastrointestinal: Constipation, GI upset, nausea
Neuromuscular & skeletal: Chest numbness
Ocular: Burning sensation in eyes
Respiratory: Nasal congestion
Miscellaneous: Chill sensation, hypersensitivity reactions (bronchospasm, laryngospasm, cardiovascular collapse)
Drug Interactions
  Avoid Concomitant Use There are no known interactions where it is recommended to avoid concomitant use.
  Increased Effect/Toxicity There are no known significant interactions involving an increase in effect.
  Decreased Effect There are no known significant interactions involving a decrease in effect.
Stability Store at room temperature of 25°C (77°F); excursions permitted to 15°C to 30°C (59°F to 86°F).
Mechanism of Action Tetracaine congener with antitussive properties; suppresses cough by topical anesthetic action on the respiratory stretch receptors
Pharmacodynamics/Kinetics
Onset of action: Therapeutic: 15-20 minutes
Duration: 3-8 hours
Dosage
  Geriatric & Adult Cough: Oral: 100-200 mg 3 times/day as needed; maximum dose: 600 mg/day
Administration Swallow capsule whole (do not break. chew, dissolve, cut, or crush).
Monitoring Parameters Monitor patient's chest sounds and respiratory pattern
Special Geriatric Considerations No specific geriatric information is available about benzonatate. Avoid use in patients with impaired gag reflex or who cannot swallow the capsule whole.
Dosage Forms Excipient information presented when available (limited, particularly for generics); consult specific product labeling.
Capsule, oral:
  Zonatuss™: 150 mg
Capsule, softgel, oral: 100 mg, 200 mg
  Tessalon®: 100 mg, 200 mg

Benztropine (BENZ troe peen)

Related Information
Antiparkinsonian Agents *on page 1995*
Medication Safety Issues
  Sound-alike/look-alike issues:
  Benztropine may be confused with bromocriptine
Brand Names: U.S. Cogentin®
Brand Names: Canada Apo-Benztropine®
Index Terms Benztropine Mesylate
Generic Availability (U.S.) Yes
Pharmacologic Category Anti-Parkinson's Agent, Anticholinergic; Anticholinergic Agent
Use Adjunctive treatment of Parkinson's disease; treatment of drug-induced extrapyramidal symptoms (except tardive dyskinesia)

Contraindications Hypersensitivity to benztropine or any component of the formulation; pyloric or duodenal obstruction, stenosing peptic ulcers; bladder neck obstructions; achalasia; myasthenia gravis

Warnings/Precautions Use with caution in hot weather or during exercise. May cause anhydrosis and hyperthermia, which may be severe. The risk is increased in hot environments, particularly in the elderly, alcoholics, patients with CNS disease, and those with prolonged outdoor exposure.

Elderly patients frequently develop increased sensitivity and require strict dosage regulation - side effects may be more severe in elderly patients with atherosclerotic changes. Use with caution in patients with tachycardia, cardiac arrhythmias, hypertension, hypotension, glaucoma, prostatic hyperplasia (especially in the elderly), any tendency toward urinary retention, liver or kidney disorders, and obstructive disease of the GI or GU tract. When given in large doses or to susceptible patients, may cause weakness and inability to move particular muscle groups.

May be associated with confusion or hallucinations (generally at higher dosages). Intensification of symptoms or toxic psychosis may occur in patients with mental disorders. May cause CNS depression, which may impair physical or mental abilities; patients must be cautioned about performing tasks which require mental alertness (eg, operating machinery or driving). Benztropine does not relieve symptoms of tardive dyskinesia.

Adverse Reactions (Reflective of adult population; not specific for elderly) Frequency not defined.
Cardiovascular: Tachycardia
Central nervous system: Confusion, disorientation, memory impairment, toxic psychosis, visual hallucinations
Dermatologic: Rash
Endocrine & metabolic: Heat stroke, hyperthermia
Gastrointestinal: Constipation, dry throat, ileus, nasal dryness, nausea, vomiting, xerostomia
Genitourinary: Urinary retention, dysuria
Ocular: Blurred vision, mydriasis
Miscellaneous: Fever

Drug Interactions
  Metabolism/Transport Effects Substrate of CYP2D6 (minor)
  Avoid Concomitant Use There are no known interactions where it is recommended to avoid concomitant use.
  Increased Effect/Toxicity
  Benztropine may increase the levels/effects of: AbobotulinumtoxinA; Anticholinergics; Cannabinoids; OnabotulinumtoxinA; Potassium Chloride; RimabotulinumtoxinB

  The levels/effects of Benztropine may be increased by: Pramlintide
  Decreased Effect
  Benztropine may decrease the levels/effects of: Acetylcholinesterase Inhibitors (Central); Secretin

  The levels/effects of Benztropine may be decreased by: Acetylcholinesterase Inhibitors (Central); Peginterferon Alfa-2b

Ethanol/Nutrition/Herb Interactions Ethanol: Avoid ethanol (may increase CNS depression).

Mechanism of Action Possesses both anticholinergic and antihistaminic effects. *In vitro* anticholinergic activity approximates that of atropine; *in vivo* it is only about half as active as atropine. Animal data suggest its antihistaminic activity and duration of action approach that of pyrilamine maleate. May also inhibit the reuptake and storage of dopamine, thereby prolonging the action of dopamine.

Pharmacodynamics/Kinetics
Onset of action: Oral: Within 1 hour; Parenteral: Within 15 minutes
Duration: 6-48 hours
Metabolism: Hepatic (N-oxidation, N-dealkylation, and ring hydroxylation)
Bioavailability: 29%

Dosage
  Geriatric Oral: Initial: 0.5 mg once or twice daily; titrate dose in 0.5 mg increments at every 5-6 days; maximum: 4 mg/day.
  Adult
    Drug-induced extrapyramidal symptom: Oral, I.M., I.V.: 1-4 mg/dose 1-2 times/day
    Acute dystonia: I.M., I.V.: 1-2 mg
    Parkinsonism: Oral: 0.5-6 mg/day in 1-2 divided doses; if one dose is greater, give at bedtime. Titrate dose in 0.5 mg increments at 5- to 6-day intervals.

BENZTROPINE

◄ **Monitoring Parameters** Symptoms of EPS or Parkinson's, pulse, anticholinergic effects (ie, CNS, bowel, and bladder function)

Pharmacotherapy Pearls No significant difference in onset of I.M. or I.V. injection, therefore, there is usually no need to use the I.V. route. Improvement is sometimes noticeable a few minutes after injection. Do not discontinue drug abruptly.

Special Geriatric Considerations Anticholinergic agents are generally not well tolerated in the elderly (often results in bowel, bladder, and CNS adverse effects) and their use should be avoided when possible. In the elderly, anticholinergic agents should not be used as prophylaxis against extrapyramidal symptoms.

Dosage Forms Excipient information presented when available (limited, particularly for generics); consult specific product labeling.
Injection, solution, as mesylate: 1 mg/mL
   Cogentin®: 1 mg/mL
Tablet, oral, as mesylate: 0.5 mg, 1 mg, 2 mg

Selected References
Feinberg M, "The Problems of Anticholinergic Adverse Effects in Older Patients," *Drugs Aging*, 1993, 3(4):335-48.
Olanow CW, Watts RL, and Koller WC, "An Algorithm (Decision Tree) for the Management of Parkinson's Disease (2001): Treatment Guidelines," *Neurology*, 2001, 56(11 Suppl 5):S1-S88.

♦ **Benztropine Mesylate** *see* Benztropine *on page 192*
♦ **Benzylpenicillin Benzathine** *see* Penicillin G Benzathine *on page 1414*
♦ **Benzylpenicillin Potassium** *see* Penicillin G (Parenteral/Aqueous) *on page 1417*
♦ **Benzylpenicillin Sodium** *see* Penicillin G (Parenteral/Aqueous) *on page 1417*

Bepotastine (be poe TAS teen)

Brand Names: U.S. Bepreve®
Index Terms Bepotastine Besilate
Generic Availability (U.S.) No
Pharmacologic Category Histamine H_1 Antagonist; Histamine H_1 Antagonist, Second Generation; Mast Cell Stabilizer
Use Treatment of itching associated with allergic conjunctivitis
Dosage
   Geriatric & Adult Allergic conjunctivitis: Ophthalmic: Instill 1 drop into the affected eye(s) twice daily
Dosage Forms Excipient information presented when available (limited, particularly for generics); consult specific product labeling.
Solution, ophthalmic, as besilate [drops]:
   Bepreve®: 1.5% (5 mL, 10 mL) [contains benzalkonium chloride]

♦ **Bepotastine Besilate** *see* Bepotastine *on page 194*
♦ **Bepreve®** *see* Bepotastine *on page 194*

Besifloxacin (be si FLOX a sin)

Brand Names: U.S. Besivance™
Index Terms Besifloxacin Hydrochloride; BOL-303224-A; SS734
Generic Availability (U.S.) No
Pharmacologic Category Antibiotic, Ophthalmic; Antibiotic, Quinolone
Use Treatment of bacterial conjunctivitis
Dosage
   Geriatric & Adult Bacterial conjunctivitis: Ophthalmic: Instill 1 drop into affected eye(s) 3 times/day (4-12 hours apart) for 7 days
Special Geriatric Considerations Evaluate the patient's or caregiver's ability to safely administer the correct dose of ophthalmic medication.
Dosage Forms Excipient information presented when available (limited, particularly for generics); consult specific product labeling.
Suspension, ophthalmic [drops]:
   Besivance™: 0.6% (5 mL) [contains benzalkonium chloride]

♦ **Besifloxacin Hydrochloride** *see* Besifloxacin *on page 194*
♦ **Besivance™** *see* Besifloxacin *on page 194*
♦ **β,β-Dimethylcysteine** *see* Penicillamine *on page 1412*
♦ **Betagan®** *see* Levobunolol *on page 1048*
♦ **Beta-HC® [OTC]** *see* Hydrocortisone (Topical) *on page 886*

Betamethasone (bay ta METH a sone)

Related Information
Corticosteroids *on page 2005*

Medication Safety Issues
Sound-alike/look-alike issues:
Luxiq® may be confused with Lasix®

International issues:
Beta-Val [U.S.] may be confused with Betanol brand name for metipranolol [Monaco]

Brand Names: U.S. Beta-Val® [DSC]; Celestone®; Celestone® Soluspan®; Diprolene®; Diprolene® AF; Luxiq®

Brand Names: Canada Betaderm; Betaject™; Betnesol®; Betnovate®; Celestone® Soluspan®; Diprolene®; Diprolene® Glycol; Diprosone®; Ectosone; Prevex® B; ratio-Ectosone; ratio-Topilene; ratio-Topisone; Rivasone; Rolene; Rosone; Taro-Sone®; Topilene®; Topisone®; Valisone® Scalp Lotion

Index Terms Betamethasone Dipropionate; Betamethasone Dipropionate, Augmented; Betamethasone Sodium Phosphate; Betamethasone Valerate; Flubenisolone

Generic Availability (U.S.) Yes: Excludes aerosol, solution

Pharmacologic Category Corticosteroid, Systemic; Corticosteroid, Topical

Use Inflammatory dermatoses such as seborrheic or atopic dermatitis, neurodermatitis, anogenital pruritus, psoriasis, inflammatory phase of xerosis

Unlabeled/Investigational Use Accelerate fetal lung maturation in patients with preterm labor

Contraindications Hypersensitivity to betamethasone, other corticosteroids, or any component of the formulation; systemic fungal infections; I.M. administration contraindicated in idiopathic thrombocytopenia purpura

Warnings/Precautions Very high potency topical products are not for treatment of rosacea, perioral dermatitis; not for use on face, groin, or axillae; not for use in a diapered area. Avoid concurrent use of other corticosteroids.

May cause hypercorticism or suppression of hypothalamic-pituitary-adrenal (HPA) axis, particularly in patients receiving high doses for prolonged periods. HPA axis suppression may lead to adrenal crisis. Withdrawal and discontinuation of a corticosteroid should be done slowly and carefully. Particular care is required when patients are transferred from systemic corticosteroids to inhaled products due to possible adrenal insufficiency or withdrawal from steroids, including an increase in allergic symptoms. Patients receiving >20 mg per day of prednisone (or equivalent) may be most susceptible. Fatalities have occurred due to adrenal insufficiency in asthmatic patients during and after transfer from systemic corticosteroids to aerosol steroids; aerosol steroids do not provide the systemic steroid needed to treat patients having trauma, surgery, or infections. In stressful situations, HPA axis-suppressed patients should receive adequate supplementation with natural glucocorticoids (hydrocortisone or cortisone) rather than betamethasone (due to lack of mineralocorticoid activity).

Acute myopathy has been reported with high dose corticosteroids, usually in patients with neuromuscular transmission disorders; may involve ocular and/or respiratory muscles; monitor creatine kinase; recovery may be delayed. Corticosteroid use may cause psychiatric disturbances, including depression, euphoria, insomnia, mood swings, and personality changes. Pre-existing psychiatric conditions may be exacerbated by corticosteroid use. Prolonged use of corticosteroids may also increase the incidence of secondary infection, mask acute infection (including fungal infections), prolong or exacerbate viral infections, or limit response to vaccines. Exposure to chickenpox should be avoided; corticosteroids should not be used to treat ocular herpes simplex. Corticosteroids should not be used for cerebral malaria or viral hepatitis. Close observation is required in patients with latent tuberculosis and/or TB reactivity; restrict use in active TB (only in conjunction with antituberculosis treatment). Prolonged treatment with corticosteroids has been associated with the development of Kaposi's sarcoma (case reports); if noted, discontinuation of therapy should be considered. High-dose corticosteroids should not be used to manage acute head injury.

Use with caution in patients with thyroid disease, hepatic impairment, renal impairment, cardiovascular disease, diabetes, glaucoma, cataracts, myasthenia gravis, patients at risk for osteoporosis, patients at risk for seizures, or GI diseases (diverticulitis, peptic ulcer, ulcerative colitis) due to perforation risk. Use caution following acute MI (corticosteroids have been associated with myocardial rupture). Because of the risk of adverse effects, systemic corticosteroids should be used cautiously in the elderly in the smallest possible effective dose for the shortest duration. Do not use occlusive dressings on weeping or exudative lesions and general caution with occlusive dressings should be observed; adverse effects may be

◀ increased. Discontinue if skin irritation or contact dermatitis should occur; do not use in patients with decreased skin circulation. Withdraw therapy with gradual tapering of dose.

Adverse Reactions (Reflective of adult population; not specific for elderly)

Systemic:

Cardiovascular: Congestive heart failure, edema, hyper-/hypotension

Central nervous system: Dizziness, headache, insomnia, intracranial pressure increased, lightheadedness, nervousness, pseudotumor cerebri, seizure, vertigo

Dermatologic: Ecchymoses, facial erythema, fragile skin, hirsutism, hyper-/hypopigmentation, perioral dermatitis (oral), petechiae, striae, wound healing impaired

Endocrine & metabolic: Amenorrhea, Cushing's syndrome, diabetes mellitus, growth suppression, hyperglycemia, hypokalemia, menstrual irregularities, pituitary-adrenal axis suppression, protein catabolism, sodium retention, water retention

Local: Injection site reactions (intra-articular use), sterile abscess

Neuromuscular & skeletal: Arthralgia, muscle atrophy, fractures, muscle weakness, myopathy, osteoporosis, necrosis (femoral and humeral heads)

Ocular: Cataracts, glaucoma, intraocular pressure increased

Miscellaneous: Anaphylactoid reaction, diaphoresis, hypersensitivity, secondary infection

Topical:

Dermatologic: Acneiform eruptions, allergic dermatitis, burning, dry skin, erythema, folliculitis, hypertrichosis, irritation, miliaria, pruritus, skin atrophy, striae, vesiculation

Endocrine and metabolic effects have occasionally been reported with topical use.

Drug Interactions

Metabolism/Transport Effects Inhibits CYP3A4 (weak)

Avoid Concomitant Use

Avoid concomitant use of Betamethasone with any of the following: Aldesleukin; BCG; Natalizumab; Pimecrolimus; Tacrolimus (Topical)

Increased Effect/Toxicity

Betamethasone may increase the levels/effects of: Acetylcholinesterase Inhibitors; Amphotericin B; Deferasirox; Leflunomide; Loop Diuretics; Natalizumab; NSAID (COX-2 Inhibitor); NSAID (Nonselective); Thiazide Diuretics; Vaccines (Live); Warfarin

The levels/effects of Betamethasone may be increased by: Antifungal Agents (Azole Derivatives, Systemic); Aprepitant; Calcium Channel Blockers (Nondihydropyridine); Denosumab; Estrogen Derivatives; Fluconazole; Fosaprepitant; Macrolide Antibiotics; Neuromuscular-Blocking Agents (Nondepolarizing); Pimecrolimus; Quinolone Antibiotics; Roflumilast; Salicylates; Tacrolimus (Topical); Telaprevir; Trastuzumab

Decreased Effect

Betamethasone may decrease the levels/effects of: Aldesleukin; Antidiabetic Agents; BCG; Calcitriol; Corticorelin; Isoniazid; Salicylates; Sipuleucel-T; Telaprevir; Vaccines (Inactivated)

The levels/effects of Betamethasone may be decreased by: Aminoglutethimide; Antacids; Barbiturates; Bile Acid Sequestrants; Echinacea; Mitotane; Primidone; Rifamycin Derivatives

Ethanol/Nutrition/Herb Interactions

Ethanol: Avoid ethanol (may enhance gastric mucosal irritation).

Food: Betamethasone interferes with calcium absorption.

Herb/Nutraceutical: Avoid cat's claw, echinacea (have immunostimulant properties).

Mechanism of Action Controls the rate of protein synthesis; depresses the migration of polymorphonuclear leukocytes, fibroblasts; reverses capillary permeability and lysosomal stabilization at the cellular level to prevent or control inflammation

Pharmacodynamics/Kinetics

Protein binding: 64%

Metabolism: Hepatic

Half-life elimination: 6.5 hours

Time to peak, serum: I.V.: 10-36 minutes

Excretion: Urine (<5% as unchanged drug)

Dosage

Geriatric Refer to adult dosing. Use the lowest effective dose.

Adult Base dosage on severity of disease and patient response

Inflammatory conditions:

Oral: 2.4-4.8 mg/day in 2-4 doses; range: 0.6-7.2 mg/day

I.M.: Betamethasone sodium phosphate and betamethasone acetate: 0.6-9 mg/day (generally, $\frac{1}{3}$ to $\frac{1}{2}$ of oral dose) divided every 12-24 hours

Psoriasis (scalp): Topical (foam): Apply to the scalp twice daily, once in the morning and once at night.

Rheumatoid arthritis/osteoarthritis:
Intrabursal, intra-articular, intradermal: 0.25-2 mL
Intralesional:
Very large joints: 1-2 mL
Large joints: 1 mL
Medium joints: 0.5-1 mL
Small joints: 0.25-0.5 mL

Steroid-responsive dermatoses: Therapy should be discontinued when control is achieved; if no improvement is seen, reassessment of diagnosis may be necessary.
Gel, augmented formulation: Apply once or twice daily; rub in gently. **Note:** Do not exceed 2 weeks of treatment or 50 g/week.
Lotion: Apply a few drops twice daily
Augmented formulation: Apply a few drops once or twice daily; rub in gently. **Note:** Do not exceed 2 weeks of treatment or 50 mL/week.
Cream/ointment: Apply once or twice daily
Augmented formulation: Apply once or twice daily. **Note:** Do not exceed 2 weeks of treatment or 45 g/week.

Hepatic Impairment Adjustments may be necessary in patients with liver failure because betamethasone is extensively metabolized in the liver

Administration
Oral: Not for alternate day therapy; once daily doses should be given in the morning.
I.M.: Do **not** give injectable sodium phosphate/acetate suspension I.V.
Topical: Apply topical sparingly to areas. Not for use on broken skin or in areas of infection. Do not apply to wet skin unless directed; do not cover with occlusive dressing. Do not apply very high potency agents to face, groin, axillae, or perianal area.
Foam: Invert can and dispense a small amount onto a saucer or other cool surface. Do not dispense directly into hands. Pick up small amounts of foam and gently massage into affected areas until foam disappears. Repeat until entire affected scalp area is treated.

Monitoring Parameters Blood pressure, blood glucose, electrolytes

Test Interactions May suppress the wheal and flare reactions to skin test antigens

Pharmacotherapy Pearls
Very High Potency: Augmented betamethasone dipropionate ointment, lotion
High Potency: Augmented betamethasone dipropionate cream, betamethasone dipropionate cream and ointment
Intermediate Potency: Betamethasone dipropionate lotion, betamethasone valerate cream

Special Geriatric Considerations Because of the risk of adverse effects, systemic corticosteroids should be used cautiously in the elderly, in the smallest possible dose, and for the shortest possible time.

Dosage Forms Excipient information presented when available (limited, particularly for generics); consult specific product labeling. [DSC] = Discontinued product
Aerosol, topical, as valerate [foam]:
Luxiq®: 0.12% (50 g, 100 g) [contains ethanol 60.4%]
Cream, topical, as dipropionate [strength expressed as base]: 0.05% (15 g, 45 g, 50 g)
Cream, topical, as dipropionate [strength expressed as base, augmented]: 0.05% (15 g, 50 g)
Diprolene® AF: 0.05% (15 g, 50 g)
Cream, topical, as valerate [strength expressed as base]: 0.1% (15 g, 45 g)
Beta-Val®: 0.1% (15 g [DSC], 45 g [DSC])
Gel, topical, as dipropionate [strength expressed as base, augmented]: 0.05% (15 g, 50 g)
Injection, suspension: Betamethasone sodium phosphate 3 mg and betamethasone acetate 3 mg per 1 mL (5 mL)
Celestone® Soluspan®: Betamethasone sodium phosphate 3 mg and betamethasone acetate 3 mg per 1 mL (5 mL) [contains benzalkonium chloride, edetate disodium; total of 6 mg/mL]
Lotion, topical, as dipropionate [strength expressed as base]: 0.05% (60 mL)
Lotion, topical, as dipropionate [strength expressed as base, augmented]: 0.05% (30 mL, 60 mL)
Diprolene®: 0.05% (30 mL, 60 mL) [contains isopropyl alcohol 30%]
Lotion, topical, as valerate [strength expressed as base]: 0.1% (60 mL)
Beta-Val®: 0.1% (60 mL [DSC]) [contains isopropyl alcohol]
Ointment, topical, as dipropionate [strength expressed as base]: 0.05% (15 g, 45 g)
Ointment, topical, as dipropionate [strength expressed as base, augmented]: 0.05% (15 g, 45 g, 50 g [DSC])
Diprolene®: 0.05% (15 g, 50 g)
Ointment, topical, as valerate [strength expressed as base]: 0.1% (15 g, 45 g)
Solution, oral, as base:
Celestone®: 0.6 mg/5 mL (118 mL) [contains ethanol <1%, propylene glycol, sodium benzoate]

◆ **Betamethasone Dipropionate** *see* Betamethasone *on page 195*
◆ **Betamethasone Dipropionate, Augmented** *see* Betamethasone *on page 195*
◆ **Betamethasone Sodium Phosphate** *see* Betamethasone *on page 195*
◆ **Betamethasone Valerate** *see* Betamethasone *on page 195*
◆ **Betapace®** *see* Sotalol *on page 1702*
◆ **Betapace AF®** *see* Sotalol *on page 1702*
◆ **Beta Sal® [OTC]** *see* Salicylic Acid *on page 1648*
◆ **Betaseron®** *see* Interferon Beta-1b *on page 970*
◆ **Beta-Val® [DSC]** *see* Betamethasone *on page 195*

Betaxolol (Systemic) (be TAKS oh lol)

Related Information
Beta-Blockers *on page 2001*
Medication Safety Issues
Sound-alike/look-alike issues:
Betaxolol may be confused with bethanechol, labetalol
Brand Names: U.S. Kerlone®
Brand Names: Canada Sandoz-Betaxolol
Index Terms Betaxolol Hydrochloride
Generic Availability (U.S.) Yes
Pharmacologic Category Beta Blocker, Beta-1 Selective
Use Management of hypertension
Unlabeled/Investigational Use Treatment of coronary artery disease

Contraindications Hypersensitivity to betaxolol or any component of the formulation; sinus bradycardia; heart block greater than first-degree (except in patients with a functioning artificial pacemaker); cardiogenic shock; uncompensated cardiac failure

Warnings/Precautions Consider pre-existing conditions (such as sick sinus syndrome) before initiating. Administer cautiously in compensated heart failure and monitor for a worsening of the condition. Beta-blocker therapy should not be withdrawn abruptly (particularly in patients with CAD), but gradually tapered to avoid acute tachycardia, hypertension, and/or ischemia. Use caution with concurrent use of beta-blockers, either verapamil or diltiazem, or digoxin; bradycardia or heart block can occur. Bradycardia may be observed more frequently in elderly patients (>65 years of age); dosage reductions may be necessary.

May precipitate or aggravate symptoms of arterial insufficiency in patients with peripheral vascular disease (PVD) and Raynaud's disease; use with caution; monitor for progression of arterial obstruction. In general, beta-blockers should be avoided in patients with bronchospastic disease. Betaxolol, with beta$_1$ selectivity, may be used cautiously in bronchospastic disease with the lowest possible dose (eg, 5-10 mg/day), availability of a bronchodilator, and close monitoring; if dosage increase is indicated, administer in divided doses. Use cautiously in patients with diabetes because it may potentiate and/or mask prominent hypoglycemic symptoms. May mask signs of hyperthyroidism (eg, tachycardia); use caution if hyperthyroidism is suspected, abrupt withdrawal may precipitate thyroid storm. May induce or exacerbate psoriasis. Use with caution in patients with cerebrovascular insufficiency; hypotension and decreased heart rate may reduce cerebral blood flow. Dosage adjustment required in severe renal impairment and in patients on dialysis. Use care with anesthetic agents which decrease myocardial function. Use with caution in patients with myasthenia gravis (may potentiate myasthenia-related muscle weakness, including diplopia and ptosis) or psychiatric disease (may cause CNS depression). Adequate alpha-blockade is required prior to use of any beta-blocker for patients with untreated pheochromocytoma. Use caution with history of severe anaphylaxis to allergens; patients taking beta-blockers may become more sensitive to repeated challenges. Treatment of anaphylaxis (eg, epinephrine) in patients taking beta-blockers may be ineffective or promote undesirable effects.

Adverse Reactions (Reflective of adult population; not specific for elderly)
2% to 10%:
Cardiovascular: Bradycardia (6% to 8%; symptomatic bradycardia: <1% to 2%; dose-dependent), chest pain (2% to 7%), palpitation (2%), edema (≤2%; similar to placebo)
Central nervous system: Fatigue (3% to 10%), insomnia (1% to 5%), lethargy (3%)
Gastrointestinal: Nausea (2% to 6%), dyspepsia (4% to 5%), diarrhea (2%)
Neuromuscular & skeletal: Arthralgia (3% to 5%), paresthesia (2%)
Respiratory: Dyspnea (2%), pharyngitis (2%)
Miscellaneous: Antinuclear antibody positive (5%), cold extremities (2%)
Drug Interactions
Metabolism/Transport Effects Substrate (major) of CYP1A2, 2D6; **Inhibits** CYP2D6 (weak)

Avoid Concomitant Use

Avoid concomitant use of Betaxolol (Systemic) with any of the following: Floctafenine; Methacholine

Increased Effect/Toxicity

Betaxolol (Systemic) may increase the levels/effects of: Alpha-/Beta-Agonists (Direct-Acting); Alpha1-Blockers; Alpha2-Agonists; Amifostine; Antihypertensives; Antipsychotic Agents (Phenothiazines); Bupivacaine; Cardiac Glycosides; Fingolimod; Hypotensive Agents; Insulin; Lidocaine; Lidocaine (Systemic); Lidocaine (Topical); Mepivacaine; Methacholine; Midodrine; RiTUXimab; Sulfonylureas

The levels/effects of Betaxolol (Systemic) may be increased by: Abiraterone Acetate; Acetylcholinesterase Inhibitors; Aminoquinolines (Antimalarial); Amiodarone; Anilidopiperidine Opioids; Antipsychotic Agents (Phenothiazines); Calcium Channel Blockers (Dihydropyridine); Calcium Channel Blockers (Nondihydropyridine); CYP1A2 Inhibitors (Moderate); CYP1A2 Inhibitors (Strong); Deferasirox; Diazoxide; Dipyridamole; Disopyramide; Dronedarone; Floctafenine; Herbs (Hypotensive Properties); MAO Inhibitors; Pentoxifylline; Phosphodiesterase 5 Inhibitors; Propafenone; Propoxyphene; Prostacyclin Analogues; QuiNIDine; Reserpine

Decreased Effect

Betaxolol (Systemic) may decrease the levels/effects of: Beta2-Agonists; Theophylline Derivatives

The levels/effects of Betaxolol (Systemic) may be decreased by: Barbiturates; CYP1A2 Inducers (Strong); Cyproterone; Herbs (Hypertensive Properties); Methylphenidate; Nonsteroidal Anti-Inflammatory Agents; Peginterferon Alfa-2b; Rifamycin Derivatives; Yohimbine

Ethanol/Nutrition/Herb Interactions Herb/Nutraceutical: Avoid bayberry; blue cohosh, cayenne, ephedra, ginger, ginseng (American), gotu kola, and licorice (may worsen hypertension). Avoid black cohosh, California poppy, coleus, golden seal, hawthorn, mistletoe, periwinkle, quinine, shepherd's purse (may have increased antihypertensive effects).

Stability Avoid freezing. Store tablets at room temperature of 15°C to 25°C (59°F to 77°F).

Mechanism of Action Competitively blocks beta$_1$-receptors, with little or no effect on beta$_2$-receptors

Pharmacodynamics/Kinetics

Onset of action: 1-1.5 hours
Absorption: ~100%
Metabolism: Hepatic to multiple metabolites
Protein binding: ~50%
Bioavailability: 89%
Half-life elimination: 14-22 hours; prolonged in hepatic disease and/or chronic renal failure
Time to peak: 1.5-6 hours
Excretion: Urine (>80%, as unchanged drug [15%] and inactive metabolites)

Dosage

Geriatric Hypertension: Oral: Refer to adult dosing. Initial: 5 mg/day.

Adult Hypertension (labeled use), coronary artery disease (unlabeled use): Oral: 5-10 mg/day; may increase dose to 20 mg/day after 7-14 days if desired response is not achieved

Renal Impairment

Severe impairment: Initial dose: 5 mg/day; may increase every 2 weeks up to a maximum of 20 mg/day.

Hemodialysis: Initial dose: 5 mg/day; may increase every 2 weeks up to a maximum of 20 mg/day. Supplemental dose not required.

Administration Absorption is not affected by food.

Monitoring Parameters Blood pressure; pulse; baseline renal function

Test Interactions Oral betaxolol may interfere with glaucoma screening tests.

Pharmacotherapy Pearls Because of betaxolol's low lipid solubility, it is less likely to enter the CNS, decreasing the likelihood of CNS side effects.

Special Geriatric Considerations Due to alterations in the beta-adrenergic autonomic nervous system, beta-adrenergic blockade may result in less hemodynamic response than seen in younger adults. Studies indicate that despite decreased sensitivity to the chronotropic effects of beta-blockade with age, there appears to be an increased myocardial sensitivity to the negative inotropic effect during stress (ie, exercise). Controlled trials have shown the overall response rate for propranolol to be only 20% to 50% in elderly populations. Therefore, all beta-adrenergic blocking drugs may result in a decreased response as compared to younger adults.

◄ **Dosage Forms** Excipient information presented when available (limited, particularly for generics); consult specific product labeling.
Tablet, oral, as hydrochloride: 10 mg, 20 mg
Kerlone®: 10 mg [scored]
Kerlone®: 20 mg

Selected References

Brauchli YB, Jick SS, Curtin F, et al, "Association Between Beta-Blockers, Other Antihypertensive Drugs and Psoriasis: Population-Based Case-Control Study," *Br J Dermatol*, 2008, 158(6):1299-307.

Fleisher LA, Beckman JA, Brown KA, et al, "ACC/AHA 2006 Guideline Update on Perioperative Cardiovascular Evaluation for Noncardiac Surgery: Focused Update on Perioperative Beta-Blocker Therapy. A Report of the American College of Cardiology/American Heart Association Task Force on Practice Guidelines (Writing Committee to Update the 2002 Guidelines on Perioperative Cardiovascular Evaluation for Noncardiac Surgery) Developed in Collaboration With the American Society of Echocardiography, American Society of Nuclear Cardiology, Heart Rhythm Society, Society of Cardiovascular Anesthesiologists, Society for Cardiovascular Angiography and Interventions, and Society for Vascular Medicine and Biology," *J Am Coll Cardiol*, 2006, 47(11):2343-55.

Juul AB, Wetterslev J, Gluud C, et al, "Effect of Perioperative Beta Blockade in Patients With Diabetes Undergoing Major Non-Cardiac Surgery: Randomized Placebo Controlled, Blinded Multicentre Trial. DIPOM Trial Group," *BMJ*, 2006, 332(7556):1482.

Schön MP and Boehncke WH, "Psoriasis," *N Eng J Med*, 2005, 352(18):1899-1912.

Betaxolol (Ophthalmic) (be TAKS oh lol)

Related Information
Glaucoma Drug Therapy *on page 2008*

Medication Safety Issues
Sound-alike/look-alike issues:
Betoptic® S may be confused with Betagan®, Timoptic®

Brand Names: U.S. Betoptic S®

Brand Names: Canada Betoptic® S

Index Terms Betaxolol Hydrochloride

Generic Availability (U.S.) Yes: Solution

Pharmacologic Category Ophthalmic Agent, Antiglaucoma

Use Treatment of chronic open-angle glaucoma or ocular hypertension

Dosage
Geriatric & Adult
Glaucoma: Ophthalmic:
Solution: Instill 1-2 drops into affected eye(s) twice daily.
Suspension (Betoptic® S): Instill 1 drop into affected eye(s) twice daily.

Dosage Forms Excipient information presented when available (limited, particularly for generics); consult specific product labeling.
Solution, ophthalmic [drops]: 0.5% (5 mL, 10 mL, 15 mL) [contains benzalkonium chloride]
Suspension, ophthalmic [drops]:
Betoptic S®: 0.25% (10 mL, 15 mL) [contains benzalkonium chloride]

♦ **Betaxolol Hydrochloride** *see* Betaxolol (Ophthalmic) *on page 200*
♦ **Betaxolol Hydrochloride** *see* Betaxolol (Systemic) *on page 198*

Bethanechol (be THAN e kole)

Medication Safety Issues
Sound-alike/look-alike issues:
Bethanechol may be confused with betaxolol

Brand Names: U.S. Urecholine®

Brand Names: Canada Duvoid®; PMS-Bethanechol

Index Terms Bethanechol Chloride

Generic Availability (U.S.) Yes

Pharmacologic Category Cholinergic Agonist

Use Treatment of acute postoperative and postpartum nonobstructive (functional) urinary retention; treatment of neurogenic atony of the urinary bladder with retention

Unlabeled/Investigational Use Gastroesophageal reflux

Contraindications Hypersensitivity to bethanechol or any component of the formulation; mechanical obstruction of the GI or GU tract or when the strength or integrity of the GI or bladder wall is in question; hyperthyroidism, peptic ulcer disease, epilepsy, asthma, bradycardia, vasomotor instability, coronary artery disease, hypotension, or parkinsonism

Warnings/Precautions Potential for reflux infection if the sphincter fails to relax as bethanechol contracts the bladder.

Adverse Reactions (Reflective of adult population; not specific for elderly) Frequency not defined.

Cardiovascular: Hypotension, tachycardia, flushed skin

Central nervous system: Headache, malaise, seizure

Gastrointestinal: Abdominal cramps, belching, borborygmi, colicky pain, diarrhea, nausea, vomiting, salivation

Genitourinary: Urinary urgency

Ocular: Lacrimation, miosis

Respiratory: Asthmatic attacks, bronchial constriction

Miscellaneous: Diaphoresis

Drug Interactions

Avoid Concomitant Use There are no known interactions where it is recommended to avoid concomitant use.

Increased Effect/Toxicity

The levels/effects of Bethanechol may be increased by: Acetylcholinesterase Inhibitors

Decreased Effect There are no known significant interactions involving a decrease in effect.

Stability Store at room temperature of 15°C to 30°C (59°F to 86°F).

Mechanism of Action Due to stimulation of the parasympathetic nervous system, bethanechol increases bladder muscle tone causing contractions which initiate urination. Bethanechol also stimulates gastric motility, increases gastric tone and may restore peristalsis.

Pharmacodynamics/Kinetics

Onset of action: 30-90 minutes

Duration: Up to 6 hours

Absorption: Variable

Dosage

Geriatric Refer to adult dosing. Use the lowest effective dose.

Adult

Urinary retention, neurogenic bladder: Oral: Initial: 10-50 mg 3-4 times/day (some patients may require dosages of 50-100 mg 4 times/day). To determine effective dose, may initiate at a dose of 5-10 mg, with additional doses of 5-10 mg hourly until an effective cumulative dose is reached. Cholinergic effects at higher oral dosages may be cumulative.

Gastroesophageal reflux (unlabeled): Oral: 25 mg 4 times/day

Administration Should be administered 1 hour before meals or 2 hours after meals.

Monitoring Parameters Urinary output, blood pressure, pulse

Test Interactions Increased lipase, amylase (S), bilirubin, aminotransferase [ALT/AST] (S)

Special Geriatric Considerations Urinary incontinence in elderly patients should be investigated. Bethanechol may be used for overflow incontinence (ie, dribbling) caused by an atonic or hypotonic bladder, but clinical efficacy is variable.

Dosage Forms Excipient information presented when available (limited, particularly for generics); consult specific product labeling.

Tablet, oral, as chloride: 5 mg, 10 mg, 25 mg, 50 mg

Urecholine®: 5 mg, 10 mg, 25 mg, 50 mg [scored]

Dosage Forms: Canada Excipient information presented when available (limited, particularly for generics); consult specific product labeling.

Tablet, as chloride:

Duvoid®: 10 mg, 25 mg, 50 mg

◆ **Bethanechol Chloride** *see* Bethanechol *on page 200*

◆ **Betimol®** *see* Timolol (Ophthalmic) *on page 1799*

◆ **Betoptic S®** *see* Betaxolol (Ophthalmic) *on page 200*

◆ **BI-1356** *see* Linagliptin *on page 1066*

◆ **Biaxin®** *see* Clarithromycin *on page 369*

◆ **Biaxin® XL** *see* Clarithromycin *on page 369*

Bicalutamide (bye ka LOO ta mide)

Medication Safety Issues

Sound-alike/look-alike issues:

Casodex® may be confused with Kapidex [DSC]

International issues:

Casodex [U.S., Canada, and multiple international markets] may be confused with Capadex brand name for propoxyphene/acetaminophen [Australia, New Zealand]

Brand Names: U.S. Casodex®

Brand Names: Canada Apo-Bicalutamide®; Casodex®; CO Bicalutamide; Dom-Bicalutamide; JAMP-Bicalutamide; Mylan-Bicalutamide; Novo-Bicalutamide; PHL-Bicalutamide; PMS-Bicalutamide; PRO-Bicalutamide; ratio-Bicalutamide; Sandoz-Bicalutamide

Index Terms CDX; ICI-176334

BICALUTAMIDE

Generic Availability (U.S.) Yes

Pharmacologic Category Antineoplastic Agent, Antiandrogen

Use Treatment of metastatic prostate cancer (in combination with an LHRH agonist)

Unlabeled/Investigational Use Monotherapy for locally-advanced prostate cancer

Contraindications Hypersensitivity to bicalutamide or any component of the formulation; use in women

Warnings/Precautions Hazardous agent - use appropriate precautions for handling and disposal. Rare cases of death or hospitalization due to hepatitis have been reported postmarketing. Use with caution in moderate-to-severe hepatic dysfunction. Hepatotoxicity generally occurs within the first 3-4 months of use; patients should be monitored for signs and symptoms of liver dysfunction. Bicalutamide should be discontinued if patients have jaundice or ALT is >2 times the upper limit of normal. Androgen-deprivation therapy may increase the risk for cardiovascular disease (Levine, 2010). May cause gynecomastia, breast pain, or lead to spermatogenesis inhibition. When used in combination with LHRH agonists, a loss of glycemic control and decrease in glucose tolerance has been reported in patients with diabetes; monitor. May cause gynecomastia or breast pain (at higher, unlabeled doses), or lead to spermatogenesis inhibition.

Adverse Reactions (Reflective of adult population; not specific for elderly) Adverse reaction percentages reported as part of combination regimen with an LHRH analogue unless otherwise noted.

>10%:
  Cardiovascular: Peripheral edema (13%)
  Central nervous system: Pain (35%)
  Endocrine & metabolic: Hot flashes (53%), breast pain (6%; monotherapy [150 mg]: 39% to 85%), gynecomastia (9%; monotherapy [150 mg]: 38% to 73%)
  Gastrointestinal: Constipation (22%), nausea (15%), diarrhea (12%), abdominal pain (11%)
  Genitourinary: Pelvic pain (21%), hematuria (12%), nocturia (12%)
  Hematologic: Anemia (11%)
  Neuromuscular & skeletal: Back pain (25%), weakness (22%)
  Respiratory: Dyspnea (13%)
  Miscellaneous: Infection (18%)

≥2% to 10%:
  Cardiovascular: Chest pain (8%), hypertension (8%), angina pectoris (2% to <5%), cardiac arrest (2% to <5%), CHF (2% to <5%), edema (2% to <5%), MI (2% to <5%), coronary artery disorder (2% to <5%), syncope (2% to <5%)
  Central nervous system: Dizziness (10%), headache (7%), insomnia (7%), anxiety (5%), depression (4%), chills (2% to <5%), confusion (2% to <5%), fever (2% to <5%), nervousness (2% to <5%), somnolence (2% to <5%)
  Dermatologic: Rash (9%), alopecia (2% to <5%), dry skin (2% to <5%), pruritus (2% to <5%), skin carcinoma (2% to <5%)
  Endocrine & metabolic: Hyperglycemia (6%), dehydration (2% to <5%), gout (2% to <5%), hypercholesterolemia (2% to <5%), libido decreased (2% to <5%)
  Gastrointestinal: Dyspepsia (7%), weight loss (7%), anorexia (6%), flatulence (6%), vomiting (6%), weight gain (5%), dysphagia (2% to <5%), gastrointestinal carcinoma (2% to <5%), melena (2% to <5%), periodontal abscess (2% to <5%), rectal hemorrhage (2% to <5%), xerostomia (2% to <5%)
  Genitourinary: Urinary tract infection (9%), impotence (7%), polyuria (6%), urinary retention (5%), urinary impairment (5%), urinary incontinence (4%), dysuria (2% to <5%), urinary urgency (2% to <5%)
  Hepatic: LFTs increased (7%), alkaline phosphatase increased (5%)
  Neuromuscular & skeletal: Bone pain (9%), paresthesia (8%), myasthenia (7%), arthritis (5%), pathological fracture (4%), hypertonia (2% to <5%), leg cramps (2% to <5%), myalgia (2% to <5%), neck pain (2% to <5%), neuropathy (2% to <5%)
  Ocular: Cataract (2% to <5%)
  Renal: BUN increased (2% to <5%), creatinine increased (2% to <5%), hydronephrosis (2% to <5%)
  Respiratory: Cough (8%), pharyngitis (8%), bronchitis (6%), pneumonia (4%), rhinitis (4%), asthma (2% to <5%), epistaxis (2% to <5%), sinusitis (2% to <5%)
  Miscellaneous: Flu-like syndrome (7%), diaphoresis (6%), cyst (2% to <5%), hernia (2% to <5%), herpes zoster (2% to <5%), sepsis (2% to <5%)

Drug Interactions

Avoid Concomitant Use

  Avoid concomitant use of Bicalutamide with any of the following: Tolvaptan

Increased Effect/Toxicity

Bicalutamide may increase the levels/effects of: Budesonide (Systemic, Oral Inhalation); Colchicine; CYP3A4 Substrates; Eplerenone; Everolimus; FentaNYL; Halofantrine; Lurasidone; Pimecrolimus; Ranolazine; Salmeterol; Saxagliptin; Tolvaptan; Vilazodone; Vitamin K Antagonists

Decreased Effect There are no known significant interactions involving a decrease in effect.

Stability Store at room temperature of 20°C to 25°C (68°F to 77°F).

Mechanism of Action Androgen receptor inhibitor; pure nonsteroidal antiandrogen that binds to androgen receptors; specifically a competitive inhibitor for the binding of dihydrotestosterone and testosterone; prevents testosterone stimulation of cell growth in prostate cancer

Pharmacodynamics/Kinetics

Absorption: Rapid and complete; unaffected by food

Protein binding: 96%

Metabolism: Extensively hepatic; glucuronidation and oxidation of the R (active) enantiomer to inactive metabolites; the S enantiomer is inactive

Half-life elimination: Active enantiomer: ~6 days, ~10 days in severe liver disease

Time to peak, plasma: Active enantiomer: ~31 hours

Excretion: Urine (36%, as inactive metabolites); feces (42%, as unchanged drug and inactive metabolites)

Dosage

Geriatric & Adult

Prostate cancer, metastatic: Oral: 50 mg once daily (in combination with an LHRH analogue)

Prostate cancer, locally-advanced (unlabeled use): Oral: 150 mg once daily (as monotherapy) (McLeod, 2006)

Renal Impairment No adjustment required

Hepatic Impairment No adjustment required for mild, moderate, or severe hepatic impairment; use caution with moderate-to-severe impairment. Discontinue if ALT >2 times ULN or patient develops jaundice.

Administration Dose should be taken at the same time each day with or without food. Treatment for metastatic cancer should be started concomitantly with an LHRH analogue.

Monitoring Parameters Periodically monitor CBC, ECG, echocardiograms, serum testosterone, luteinizing hormone, and prostate specific antigen (PSA). Liver function tests should be obtained at baseline and repeated regularly during the first 4 months of treatment, and periodically thereafter; monitor for signs and symptoms of liver dysfunction (discontinue if jaundice is noted or ALT is >2 times the upper limit of normal). Monitor blood glucose in patients with diabetes. If initiating bicalutamide in patients who are on warfarin, closely monitor prothrombin time.

Pharmacotherapy Pearls Oncology Comment: According to the 2007 update of the American Society of Clinical Oncology (ASCO) guidelines for initial hormonal management of androgen-sensitive advanced prostate cancer, the standard of care is initial treatment with a luteinizing hormone-releasing hormone (LHRH) agonist, however, bicalutamide should be considered in combination with an LHRH agonist for combined androgen blockade (CAB) treatment. Although the incidence of adverse effects is increased, the addition of a nonsteroidal antiandrogen (NSAA) such a s bicalutamide, increases overall survival (OS) (Loblaw, 2007).

The National Comprehensive Cancer Network (NCCN) Guidelines for Prostate Cancer (v.2.2009) also recommend an LHRH agonist as medical castration, which may be given alone or in combination with an NSAA. Certain patients (with evidence of metastases) receiving LHRH agonists are at risk for tumor flare, a condition in which an initial transient increase in testosterone levels induced by an LHRH agonist, results in worsening symptoms. These patients, according to the NCCN guidelines, should receive an antiandrogen with the LHRH agonist for at least 7 days, which may begin with or just prior to the LHRH agonist. The NCCN guidelines also address monotherapy with bicalutamide (150 mg orally daily) and while, to date, no OS advantage has been demonstrated in early, localized, or locally advanced prostate cancer, an improvement in progression-free survival has been demonstrated in locally advanced prostate cancer.

Special Geriatric Considerations Renal impairment has no clinically-significant changes in elimination of the parent compound or active metabolite; therefore, no dosage adjustment is needed in the elderly. In dosage studies, no difference was found between young adults and elderly with regard to steady-state serum concentrations for bicalutamide and its active R-enantiomer metabolite.

Dosage Forms Excipient information presented when available (limited, particularly for generics); consult specific product labeling.

Tablet, oral: 50 mg

Casodex®: 50 mg

◀ **Selected References**
National Comprehensive Cancer Network® (NCCN), "Clinical Practice Guidelines in Oncology™: Prostate Carci-noma," Version 2, 2009. Available at http://www.nccn.org/professionals/physician_gls/PDF/prostate.pdf

◆ **Bicillin® L-A** *see* Penicillin G Benzathine *on page* 1414
◆ **Bicillin® C-R** *see* Penicillin G Benzathine and Penicillin G Procaine *on page* 1416
◆ **Bicillin® C-R 900/300** *see* Penicillin G Benzathine and Penicillin G Procaine *on page* 1416
◆ **Bicitra** *see* Sodium Citrate and Citric Acid *on page* 1693
◆ **Bidex®-400 [OTC]** *see* GuaiFENesin *on page* 846
◆ **BiDil®** *see* Isosorbide Dinitrate and Hydralazine *on page* 990

Bimatoprost (bi MAT oh prost)

Related Information
Glaucoma Drug Therapy *on page* 2008
Brand Names: U.S. Latisse®; Lumigan®
Brand Names: Canada Lumigan®; Lumigan® RC
Generic Availability (U.S.) No
Pharmacologic Category Ophthalmic Agent, Antiglaucoma; Ophthalmic Agent, Miscella-neous; Prostaglandin, Ophthalmic
Use Reduction of intraocular pressure (IOP) in patients with open-angle glaucoma or ocular hypertension; hypotrichosis treatment of the eyelashes
Contraindications
Latisse®: Hypersensitivity to bimatoprost or any component of the formulation
Lumigan®: There are no contraindications listed in the manufacturer's prescribing information.
Warnings/Precautions May cause permanent changes in eye color (increases the amount of brown pigment in the iris), the eyelid skin, and eyelashes. In addition, may increase the length and/or number of eyelashes (may vary between eyes). Use caution in patients with intraocular inflammation, aphakic patients, pseudophakic patients with a torn posterior lens capsule, or patients with risk factors for macular edema. Contains benzalkonium chloride (may be adsorbed by contact lenses). Safety and efficacy have not been determined for use in patients with angle-closure, inflammatory, or neovascular glaucoma.

Latisse®: Additional warnings: Patients receiving medications to reduce intraocular pressure should consult their healthcare provider prior to using; may interfere with desired reduction of intraocular pressure. Unintentional hair growth may occur on skin that has repeated contact with solution; apply to upper eyelid only, blot away excess.
Adverse Reactions (Reflective of adult population; not specific for elderly) Adverse reactions and percentages are for Lumigan® unless noted:

>10%: Ocular: Conjunctival hyperemia (25% to 45%; Latisse®: <4%), growth of eyelashes, ocular pruritus (Latisse®: <4%)
1% to 10%:
Central nervous system: Headache (1% to 5%)
Dermatologic: Skin hyperpigmentation (Latisse®: <4%), abnormal hair growth
Hepatic: Liver function tests abnormal (1% to 5%)
Neuromuscular & skeletal: Weakness (1% to 5%)
Ocular: Dryness (Latisse®: <4%), erythema of the eyelid (Latisse®: <4%), irritation (Lat-isse®: <4%), allergic conjunctivitis, asthenopia, blepharitis, burning, cataract, conjunctival edema, conjunctival hemorrhage, discharge, eyelash darkening, foreign body sensation, iris pigmentation increased (may be delayed), pain, photophobia, pigmentation of peri-ocular skin, superficial punctate keratitis, tearing, visual disturbance
Miscellaneous: Infections (10%; primarily colds and upper respiratory tract infections)
Drug Interactions
Avoid Concomitant Use There are no known interactions where it is recommended to avoid concomitant use.
Increased Effect/Toxicity
The levels/effects of Bimatoprost may be increased by: Latanoprost
Decreased Effect There are no known significant interactions involving a decrease in effect.
Stability Store between 2°C to 25°C (36°F to 77°F).
Mechanism of Action As a synthetic analog of prostaglandin with ocular hypotensive activity, bimatoprost decreases intraocular pressure by increasing the outflow of aqueous humor. Bimatoprost may increase the percent and duration of hairs in the growth phase, resulting in eyelash growth.
Pharmacodynamics/Kinetics
Onset of action: Reduction of IOP: ~4 hours
Peak effect: Maximum reduction of IOP: ~8-12 hours
Distribution: V_d: 0.67 L/kg

Protein binding: ~88%

Metabolism: Undergoes oxidation, N-deethylation, and glucuronidation after reaching systemic circulation; forms metabolites

Half-life elimination: I.V.: ~45 minutes

Time to peak: ≤10 minutes

Excretion: Urine (≤67%); feces (25%)

Dosage

Geriatric & Adult

Open-angle glaucoma or ocular hypertension: Ophthalmic: Instill 1 drop into affected eye(s) once daily in the evening; do not exceed once-daily dosing (may decrease IOP-lowering effect). If used with other topical ophthalmic agents, separate administration by at least 5 minutes.

Hypotrichosis of the eyelashes: Ophthalmic, topical: Place one drop on applicator and apply evenly along the skin of the upper eyelid at base of eyelashes once daily at bedtime; repeat procedure for second eye (use a clean applicator).

Administration

Latisse®: Remove make-up and contact lenses prior to application; ensure face is clean. Apply with the sterile applicator provided only; do not use other brushes or applicators. Use a tissue or cloth to blot any excess solution on the outside of the upper eyelid margin; do not apply to lower eyelash line. Do not reuse applicators; use new applicator for second eye. Applying more than once nightly will not increase eyelash growth; eyelash growth is expected to return to baseline when therapy is discontinued. May reinsert contacts 15 minutes after application.

Lumigan®: May be used with other eye drops to lower intraocular pressure. If using more than one ophthalmic product, wait at least 5 minutes in between application of each medication. Remove contact lenses prior to administration and wait 15 minutes before reinserting.

Pharmacotherapy Pearls The IOP-lowering effect was shown to be 7-8 mm Hg in clinical studies.

Special Geriatric Considerations Evaluate the patient's or caregiver's ability to safely administer the correct dose of ophthalmic medication.

Dosage Forms Excipient information presented when available (limited, particularly for generics); consult specific product labeling.

Solution, ophthalmic [drops]:

Latisse®: 0.03% (3 mL) [contains benzalkonium chloride]

Lumigan®: 0.01% (2.5 mL, 5 mL, 7.5 mL); 0.03% (2.5 mL, 5 mL, 7.5 mL) [contains benzalkonium chloride]

- ◆ **Bio-D-Mulsion® [OTC]** *see* Cholecalciferol *on page 346*
- ◆ **Bio-D-Mulsion Forte® [OTC]** *see* Cholecalciferol *on page 346*
- ◆ **Bion® Tears [OTC]** *see* Artificial Tears *on page 148*
- ◆ **Bird Flu Vaccine** *see* Influenza Virus Vaccine (H5N1) *on page 936*
- ◆ **Bisac-Evac™ [OTC]** *see* Bisacodyl *on page 205*

Bisacodyl (bis a KOE dil)

Related Information

Beers Criteria − Potentially Inappropriate Medications for Geriatrics *on page 2089*

Laxatives, Classification and Properties *on page 2012*

Treatment Options for Constipation *on page 2035*

Medication Safety Issues

Sound-alike/look-alike issues:

Doxidan® may be confused with doxepin

Dulcolax® (bisacodyl) may be confused with Dulcolax® (docusate)

BEERS Criteria medication:

This drug may be inappropriate for use in geriatric patients (high severity risk).

Brand Names: U.S. Alophen® [OTC]; Bisac-Evac™ [OTC]; Biscolax™ [OTC]; Correctol® Tablets [OTC]; Dacodyl™ [OTC]; Doxidan® [OTC]; Dulcolax® [OTC]; ex-lax® Ultra [OTC]; Femilax™ [OTC]; Fleet® Bisacodyl [OTC]; Fleet® Stimulant Laxative [OTC]; Veracolate® [OTC]

Brand Names: Canada Apo-Bisacodyl®; Carter's Little Pills®; Dulcolax®; Gentlax®

Generic Availability (U.S.) Yes: Excludes enema

Pharmacologic Category Laxative, Stimulant

Use Treatment of constipation; colonic evacuation prior to procedures or examination

Contraindications Hypersensitivity to bisacodyl or any component of the formulation; abdominal pain or obstruction, nausea, or vomiting

Warnings/Precautions In the elderly, long-term use may exacerbate bowel dysfunction, except in the setting of chronic pain requiring opioid use (Beers Criteria).

◄ **Drug Interactions**

Avoid Concomitant Use There are no known interactions where it is recommended to avoid concomitant use.

Increased Effect/Toxicity There are no known significant interactions involving an increase in effect.

Decreased Effect

The levels/effects of Bisacodyl may be decreased by: Antacids

Ethanol/Nutrition/Herb Interactions Food: Milk or dairy products may disrupt enteric coating, increasing stomach irritation.

Mechanism of Action Stimulates peristalsis by directly irritating the smooth muscle of the intestine, possibly the colonic intramural plexus; alters water and electrolyte secretion producing net intestinal fluid accumulation and laxation

Pharmacodynamics/Kinetics

Onset of action: Oral: 6-10 hours; Rectal: 0.25-1 hour

Absorption: Oral, rectal: Systemic, <5%

Dosage

Geriatric & Adult

Relief of constipation:

Oral: 5-15 mg as single dose (up to 30 mg when complete evacuation of bowel is required)

Rectal: Suppository: 10 mg as single dose

Administration Administered with glass of water on empty stomach for rapid effect. Do not administer within 1 hour of milk, any dairy products, or taking an antacid, to protect the coating.

Monitoring Parameters Monitor stools daily or weekly; fluid/electrolyte status

Special Geriatric Considerations The chronic use of stimulant cathartics is inappropriate and should be avoided; although constipation is a common complaint from elderly, such complaints require evaluation; elderly are often predisposed to constipation due to disease, drugs, immobility, and a decreased fluid intake, partially because they have a blunted "thirst reflex" with aging; short-term use of stimulants is best; if prophylaxis is desired, this can be accomplished with bulk agents (psyllium), stool softeners, and hyperosmotic agents (sorbitol 70%); stool softeners are unnecessary if stools are well hydrated, soft, or "mushy".

This medication is considered to be potentially inappropriate in this patient population (Beers Criteria severity: High).

Dosage Forms Excipient information presented when available (limited, particularly for generics); consult specific product labeling.

Solution, rectal [enema]:

Fleet® Bisacodyl: 10 mg/30 mL (37 mL)

Suppository, rectal: 10 mg (12s, 50s, 100s)

Bisac-Evac™: 10 mg (8s, 12s, 50s, 100s, 500s, 1000s)

Biscolax™: 10 mg (12s, 100s)

Dulcolax®: 10 mg (4s, 8s, 16s, 28s, 50s)

Tablet, delayed release, oral: 5 mg

Doxidan®: 5 mg

Fleet® Stimulant Laxative: 5 mg

Tablet, enteric coated, oral: 5 mg

Alophen®: 5 mg

Bisac-Evac™: 5 mg

Correctol® Tablets: 5 mg

Dacodyl™: 5 mg

Dulcolax®: 5 mg

ex-lax® Ultra: 5 mg [contains sodium 0.1 mg/tablet]

Femilax™: 5 mg

Veracolate®: 5 mg

◆ **Bisacodyl and Polyethylene Glycol-Electrolyte Solution** *see* Polyethylene Glycol-Electrolyte Solution and Bisacodyl *on page 1481*

◆ **Biscolax™ [OTC]** *see* Bisacodyl *on page 205*

◆ **Bismatrol** *see* Bismuth *on page 207*

◆ **Bismatrol [OTC]** *see* Bismuth *on page 207*

◆ **Bismatrol Maximum Strength [OTC]** *see* Bismuth *on page 207*

Bismuth (BIZ muth)

Related Information
Helicobacter pylori Treatment in Adult Patients *on page* 2009

Medication Safety Issues
Sound-alike/look-alike issues:
Kaopectate® may be confused with Kayexalate®
Other safety concerns:
Maalox® Total Relief® is a different formulation than other Maalox® liquid antacid products which contain aluminum hydroxide, magnesium hydroxide, and simethicone.
Canadian formulation of Kaopectate® does not contain bismuth, the active ingredient in the Canadian formulation is attapulgite.

Brand Names: U.S. Bismatrol Maximum Strength [OTC]; Bismatrol [OTC]; Diotame [OTC]; Kao-Tin [OTC]; Kaopectate® Extra Strength [OTC]; Kaopectate® [OTC]; Maalox® Total Relief® [OTC] [DSC]; Peptic Relief [OTC]; Pepto Relief [OTC]; Pepto-Bismol® Maximum Strength [OTC]; Pepto-Bismol® [OTC]

Index Terms Bismatrol; Bismuth Subsalicylate; Pink Bismuth

Generic Availability (U.S.) Yes

Pharmacologic Category Antidiarrheal

Use Subsalicylate formulation: Symptomatic treatment of mild, nonspecific diarrhea; control of traveler's diarrhea (enterotoxigenic *Escherichia coli*); as part of a multidrug regimen for *H. pylori* eradication to reduce the risk of duodenal ulcer recurrence

Contraindications Hypersensitivity to bismuth or any component of the formulation

Subsalicylate formulation: Do not use subsalicylate in patients with influenza or chickenpox because of risk of Reye's syndrome; hypersensitivity to salicylates or any component of the formulation; history of severe GI bleeding; history of coagulopathy

Warnings/Precautions Bismuth subsalicylate should be used with caution if patient is taking aspirin. Bismuth products may be neurotoxic with very large doses.

When used for self-medication (OTC labeling): Changes in behavior (along with nausea and vomiting) may be an early sign of Reye's syndrome; patients should be instructed to contact their healthcare provider if these occur. Patients should be instructed to contact healthcare provider for diarrhea lasting >2 days, hearing loss, or ringing in the ears.

Adverse Reactions (Reflective of adult population; not specific for elderly) Frequency not defined; subsalicylate formulation:
Central nervous system: Anxiety, confusion, headache, mental depression, slurred speech
Gastrointestinal: Discoloration of the tongue (darkening), grayish black stools, impaction may occur in infants and debilitated patients
Neuromuscular & skeletal: Muscle spasms, weakness
Otic: Hearing loss, tinnitus

Drug Interactions
Avoid Concomitant Use There are no known interactions where it is recommended to avoid concomitant use.
Increased Effect/Toxicity There are no known significant interactions involving an increase in effect.
Decreased Effect
Bismuth may decrease the levels/effects of: Tetracycline Derivatives

Mechanism of Action Bismuth subsalicylate exhibits both antisecretory and antimicrobial action. This agent may provide some anti-inflammatory action as well. The salicylate moiety provides antisecretory effect and the bismuth exhibits antimicrobial directly against bacterial and viral gastrointestinal pathogens.

Pharmacodynamics/Kinetics
Absorption: Bismuth: <1%; Subsalicylate: >90%
Metabolism: Bismuth subsalicylate is converted to salicylic acid and insoluble bismuth salts in the GI tract.
Half-life elimination: Terminal: Bismuth: Highly variable
Excretion: Bismuth: Urine and feces; Salicylate: Urine

Dosage
Geriatric & Adult
Treatment of nonspecific diarrhea, control/relieve traveler's diarrhea: Subsalicylate: Oral: 524 mg every 30 minutes to 1 hour as needed up to 8 doses/24 hours
Helicobacter pylori **eradication:** Oral: Subsalicylate: 524 mg 4 times/day with meals and at bedtime; requires combination therapy
Renal Impairment Bismuth has been associated with nephrotoxicity in overdose (Leussnik, 2002); although there are no specific recommendations by the manufacturer, consider using with caution in patients with renal impairment.

◄ **Administration** Liquids must be shaken prior to use. Chewable tablets should be chewed thoroughly. Nonchewable caplets should be swallowed whole with a full glass of water.

Monitoring Parameters Signs/symptoms of nausea, diarrhea, tinnitus, CNS toxic effects, GI bleeding

Test Interactions Increased uric acid, increased AST; bismuth absorbs x-rays and may interfere with diagnostic procedures of GI tract

Pharmacotherapy Pearls Pepto-Bismol® contains bismuth 58% and salicylate 42%; do not exceed 4.2 g/day dosage; bismuth is radiopaque; 2 tablets yield 204 mg salicylate; 30 mL of suspension yields 258 mg

Special Geriatric Considerations Tinnitus and CNS side effects (confusion, dizziness, high tone deafness, delirium, psychosis) may be difficult to assess in some elderly patients. Limit use of this agent in elderly.

Dosage Forms Excipient information presented when available (limited, particularly for generics); consult specific product labeling. [DSC] = Discontinued product

Caplet, oral, as subsalicylate:
Pepto-Bismol®: 262 mg [sugar free; contains sodium 2 mg/caplet]
Liquid, oral, as subsalicylate: 262 mg/15 mL (240 mL)
Bismatrol: 262 mg/15 mL (240 mL)
Bismatrol Maximum Strength: 525 mg/15 mL (240 mL)
Diotame: 262 mg/15 mL (30 mL) [sugar free]
Kao-Tin: 262 mg/15 mL (240 mL, 473 mL) [contains sodium benzoate]
Kaopectate®: 262 mg/15 mL (236 mL) [contains potassium 5 mg/15 mL, sodium 5 mg/15 mL; peppermint flavor]
Kaopectate®: 262 mg/15 mL (177 mL) [contains sodium 4 mg/15 mL; cherry flavor]
Kaopectate®: 262 mg/15 mL (236 mL, 354 mL) [contains sodium 4 mg/15 mL; vanilla flavor]
Kaopectate® Extra Strength: 525 mg/15 mL (236 mL) [contains potassium 5 mg/15 mL, sodium 5 mg/15 mL; peppermint flavor]
Maalox® Total Relief®: 525 mg/15 mL (360 mL [DSC]) [contains sodium 3.3 mg/15 mL; peppermint flavor]
Maalox® Total Relief®: 525 mg/15 mL (360 mL [DSC]) [contains sodium 3.3 mg/15 mL; strawberry flavor]
Peptic Relief: 262 mg/15 mL (237 mL) [sugar free; mint flavor]
Pepto-Bismol®: 262 mg/15 mL (240 mL, 360 mL, 480 mL) [sugar free; contains benzoic acid, sodium 6 mg/15 mL; cherry flavor]
Pepto-Bismol®: 262 mg/15 mL (120 mL, 240 mL, 360 mL, 480 mL) [sugar free; contains benzoic acid, sodium 6 mg/15 mL; wintergreen flavor]
Pepto-Bismol® Maximum Strength: 525 mg/15 mL (120 mL, 240 mL, 360 mL) [sugar free; contains benzoic acid, sodium 6 mg/15 mL; wintergreen flavor]
Suspension, oral, as subsalicylate: 262 mg/15 mL (30 mL)
Tablet, chewable, oral, as subsalicylate: 262 mg [DSC]
Bismatrol: 262 mg
Diotame: 262 mg [sugar free]
Peptic Relief: 262 mg
Pepto Relief: 262 mg
Pepto-Bismol®: 262 mg [sugar free; contains sodium <1 mg/tablet; cherry flavor]
Pepto-Bismol®: 262 mg [sugar free; contains sodium <1 mg/tablet; wintergreen flavor]

◆ **Bismuth Subsalicylate** see Bismuth on page 207

Bisoprolol (bis OH proe lol)

Related Information
Beta-Blockers on page 2001
Medication Safety Issues
Sound-alike/look-alike issues:
Zebeta® may be confused with DiaBeta®, Zetia®
Brand Names: U.S. Zebeta®
Brand Names: Canada Apo-Bisoprolol®; Novo-Bisoprolol; PHL-Bisoprolol; PMS-Bisoprolol; PRO-Bisoprolol; Sandoz-Bisoprolol; ZYM-Bisoprolol
Index Terms Bisoprolol Fumarate
Generic Availability (U.S.) Yes
Pharmacologic Category Beta Blocker, Beta-1 Selective
Use Treatment of hypertension, alone or in combination with other agents
Unlabeled/Investigational Use Treatment of angina pectoris, supraventricular arrhythmias, PVCs
Contraindications Cardiogenic shock; overt cardiac failure; marked sinus bradycardia; heart block greater than first-degree (except in patients with a functioning artificial pacemaker)

Warnings/Precautions Consider pre-existing conditions such as sick sinus syndrome before initiating. Use caution in patients with heart failure; use gradual and careful titration; monitor for symptoms of congestive heart failure. Use with caution in patients with myasthenia gravis, psychiatric disease (may cause CNS depression), bronchospastic disease, undergoing anesthesia; and in those with impaired hepatic function. Bradycardia may be observed more frequently in elderly patients (>65 years of age); dosage reductions may be necessary. Beta-blocker therapy should not be withdrawn abruptly (particularly in patients with CAD), but gradually tapered to avoid acute tachycardia, hypertension, and/or ischemia. Chronic beta-blocker therapy should not be routinely withdrawn prior to major surgery. Can precipitate or aggravate symptoms of arterial insufficiency in patients with PVD and Raynaud's disease; use with caution and monitor for progression of arterial obstruction. Use caution with concurrent use of digoxin, verapamil, or diltiazem; bradycardia or heart block may occur. Use with caution in patients receiving inhaled anesthetic agents known to depress myocardial contractility. Bisoprolol, with beta$_1$-selectivity, may be used cautiously in bronchospastic disease with close monitoring. Use cautiously in patients with diabetes because it can mask prominent hypoglycemic symptoms. May mask signs of hyperthyroidism (eg, tachycardia); use caution if hyperthyroidism is suspected, abrupt withdrawal may precipitate thyroid storm. Dosage adjustment is required in patients with significant hepatic or renal dysfunction. Adequate alpha-blockade is required prior to use of any beta-blocker for patients with untreated pheochromocytoma. May induce or exacerbate psoriasis. Use caution with history of severe anaphylaxis to allergens; patients taking beta-blockers may become more sensitive to repeated challenges. Treatment of anaphylaxis (eg, epinephrine) in patients taking beta-blockers may be ineffective or promote undesirable effects.

Adverse Reactions (Reflective of adult population; not specific for elderly)
1% to 10%:
Cardiovascular: Chest pain (1% to 2%)
Central nervous system: Fatigue (dose related; 6% to 8%), insomnia (2% to 3%), hypoesthesia (1% to 2%)
Gastrointestinal: Diarrhea (dose related; 3% to 4%), nausea (2%), vomiting (1% to 2%)
Neuromuscular & skeletal: Arthralgia, asthenia (dose related; ≤2%)
Respiratory: Upper respiratory infection (5%), rhinitis (3% to 4%), sinusitis (dose related; 2%), dyspnea (1% to 2%)

Drug Interactions
Metabolism/Transport Effects Substrate of CYP2D6 (minor), 3A4 (major)
Avoid Concomitant Use
Avoid concomitant use of Bisoprolol with any of the following: Conivaptan; Floctafenine; Methacholine

Increased Effect/Toxicity
Bisoprolol may increase the levels/effects of: Alpha-/Beta-Agonists (Direct-Acting); Alpha1-Blockers; Alpha2-Agonists; Amifostine; Antihypertensives; Antipsychotic Agents (Phenothiazines); Bupivacaine; Cardiac Glycosides; Fingolimod; Hypotensive Agents; Insulin; Lidocaine; Lidocaine (Systemic); Lidocaine (Topical); Mepivacaine; Methacholine; Midodrine; RiTUXimab; Sulfonylureas

The levels/effects of Bisoprolol may be increased by: Acetylcholinesterase Inhibitors; Aminoquinolines (Antimalarial); Amiodarone; Anilidopiperidine Opioids; Antipsychotic Agents (Phenothiazines); Calcium Channel Blockers (Dihydropyridine); Calcium Channel Blockers (Nondihydropyridine); Conivaptan; CYP3A4 Inhibitors (Moderate); CYP3A4 Inhibitors (Strong); Dasatinib; Diazoxide; Dipyridamole; Disopyramide; Dronedarone; Floctafenine; Herbs (Hypotensive Properties); MAO Inhibitors; Pentoxifylline; Phosphodiesterase 5 Inhibitors; Propafenone; Propoxyphene; Prostacyclin Analogues; QuiNIDine; Reserpine

Decreased Effect
Bisoprolol may decrease the levels/effects of: Beta2-Agonists; Theophylline Derivatives

The levels/effects of Bisoprolol may be decreased by: Barbiturates; CYP3A4 Inducers (Strong); Deferasirox; Herbs (CYP3A4 Inducers); Herbs (Hypertensive Properties); Methylphenidate; Nonsteroidal Anti-Inflammatory Agents; Peginterferon Alfa-2b; Rifamycin Derivatives; Tocilizumab; Yohimbine

Ethanol/Nutrition/Herb Interactions Herb/Nutraceutical: Avoid dong quai if using for hypertension (has estrogenic activity). Avoid ephedra, yohimbe, ginseng (may worsen hypertension). Avoid garlic (may have increased antihypertensive effect).

Mechanism of Action Selective inhibitor of beta$_1$-adrenergic receptors; competitively blocks beta$_1$-receptors, with little or no effect on beta$_2$-receptors at doses ≤20 mg

Pharmacodynamics/Kinetics
Onset of action: 1-2 hours
Absorption: Rapid and almost complete
Distribution: Widely; highest concentrations in heart, liver, lungs, and saliva; crosses blood-brain barrier

◄ Protein binding: ~30%

Metabolism: Extensively hepatic; significant first-pass effect (~20%)

Bioavailability: ~80%

Half-life elimination: Normal renal function: 9-12 hours; Cl_{cr} <40 mL/minute: 27-36 hours; Hepatic cirrhosis: 8-22 hours

Time to peak: 2-4 hours

Excretion: Urine (50% as unchanged drug, remainder as inactive metabolites); feces (<2%)

Dosage

  Geriatric Oral: Initial: 2.5 mg/day; may be increased by 2.5-5 mg/day; maximum recommended dose: 20 mg/day

  Adult

    Hypertension: Oral: 2.5-5 mg once daily; may be increased to 10 mg and then up to 20 mg once daily, if necessary; usual dose range (JNC 7): 2.5-10 mg once daily

    HF (unlabeled use): Initial: 1.25 mg once daily; maximum recommended dose: 10 mg once daily. **Note:** Increase dose gradually and monitor for signs and symptoms of CHF.

  Renal Impairment

    Cl_{cr} <40 mL/minute: Oral: Initial: 2.5 mg/day; increase cautiously

    Not dialyzable

Administration May be administered without regard to meals.

Monitoring Parameters Blood pressure, ECG, orthostatic hypotension, heart rate, CNS effects

Pharmacotherapy Pearls May potentiate hypoglycemia in a diabetic patient and mask signs and symptoms

Special Geriatric Considerations Due to alterations in the beta-adrenergic autonomic nervous system, beta-adrenergic blockade may result in less hemodynamic response than seen in younger adults. Studies indicate that despite decreased sensitivity to the chronotropic effects of beta-blockade with age, there appears to be an increased myocardial sensitivity to the negative inotropic effect during stress (ie, exercise). Controlled trials have shown the overall response rate for propranolol to be only 20% to 50% in elderly populations. Therefore, all beta-adrenergic blocking drugs may result in a decreased response as compared to younger adults.

Dosage Forms Excipient information presented when available (limited, particularly for generics); consult specific product labeling.

Tablet, oral, as fumarate: 5 mg, 10 mg

  Zebeta®: 5 mg [scored]

  Zebeta®: 10 mg

Selected References

Chobanian AV, Bakris GL, Black HR, et al, "The Seventh Report of the Joint National Committee on Prevention, Detection, Evaluation, and Treatment of High Blood Pressure: The JNC 7 Report," *JAMA*, 2003, 289(19):2560-71.

Brimonidine (bri MOE ni deen)

Related Information
Glaucoma Drug Therapy *on page 2008*

Medication Safety Issues
Sound-alike/look-alike issues:
Brimonidine may be confused with bromocriptine

Brand Names: U.S. Alphagan® P

Brand Names: Canada Alphagan®; Apo-Brimonidine P®; Apo-Brimonidine®; PMS-Brimonidine Tartrate; ratio-Brimonidine; Sandoz-Brimonidine

Index Terms Brimonidine Tartrate

Generic Availability (U.S.) Yes

Pharmacologic Category Alpha$_2$ Agonist, Ophthalmic; Ophthalmic Agent, Antiglaucoma

Use Lowering of intraocular pressure (IOP) in patients with open-angle glaucoma or ocular hypertension

Contraindications Hypersensitivity to brimonidine tartrate or any component of the formulation; during or within 14 days of MAO inhibitor therapy

Warnings/Precautions Exercise caution in treating patients with severe cardiovascular disease. Use with caution in patients with depression, cerebral or coronary insufficiency, Raynaud's phenomenon, orthostatic hypotension, or thromboangiitis obliterans. Use with caution in patients with hepatic or renal impairment. Systemic absorption has been reported; children are at higher risk of systemic adverse events (Levy, 2004). May cause CNS depression, which may impair physical or mental abilities; patients must be cautioned about performing tasks which require mental alertness (eg, operating machinery or driving).

Some formulations may contain benzalkonium chloride which may be absorbed by soft contact lenses; remove contacts prior to administration and wait 15 minutes before reinserting. The IOP-lowering efficacy observed with brimonidine tartrate during the first of month of therapy may not always reflect the long-term level of IOP reduction. Routinely monitor IOP.

Adverse Reactions (Reflective of adult population; not specific for elderly) Actual frequency of adverse reactions may be formulation dependent; percentages reported with Alphagan® P:

>10%:
Central nervous system: Somnolence (adults 1% to 4%; children 25% to 83%)
Ocular: Allergic conjunctivitis, conjunctival hyperemia, eye pruritus
1% to 10% (unless otherwise noted 1% to 4%):
Cardiovascular: Hypertension (5% to 9%), hypotension
Central nervous system: Alertness decreased (children), dizziness, fatigue, headache, insomnia
Dermatologic: Rash
Endocrine & metabolic: Hypercholesterolemia
Gastrointestinal: Xerostomia (5% to 9%), dyspepsia
Neuromuscular & skeletal: Weakness
Ocular: Burning sensation (5% to 9%), conjunctival folliculosis (5% to 9%), ocular allergic reaction (5% to 9%), visual disturbance (5% to 9%), blepharitis, blepharoconjunctivitis, blurred vision, cataract, conjunctival edema, conjunctival hemorrhage, conjunctivitis, dry eye, epiphora, eye discharge, eyelid disorder, eyelid edema, eyelid erythema, follicular conjunctivitis, foreign body sensation, irritation, keratitis, pain, photophobia, stinging, superficial punctate keratopathy, visual acuity worsened, visual field defect, vitreous detachment, vitreous floaters, watery eyes
Respiratory: Bronchitis, cough, dyspnea, pharyngitis, rhinitis, sinus infection, sinusitis
Miscellaneous: Allergic reaction, flu-like syndrome, infection

Drug Interactions
Avoid Concomitant Use
Avoid concomitant use of Brimonidine with any of the following: MAO Inhibitors

Increased Effect/Toxicity
Brimonidine may increase the levels/effects of: Alcohol (Ethyl); CNS Depressants; Hypotensive Agents; Methotrimeprazine; Selective Serotonin Reuptake Inhibitors

The levels/effects of Brimonidine may be increased by: Droperidol; HydrOXYzine; MAO Inhibitors; Methotrimeprazine

Decreased Effect There are no known significant interactions involving a decrease in effect. ▶

◀ **Ethanol/Nutrition/Herb Interactions** Herb/Nutraceutical: Avoid herbs with **hypertensive** properties (bayberry, blue cohosh, cayenne, ephedra, ginger, ginseng, gotu kola, licorice); may diminish antihypertensive effect. Avoid herbs with **hypotensive** properties (black cohosh, California poppy, coleus, golden seal, hawthorn, mistletoe, periwinkle, quinine, shepherd's purse); may enhance hypotensive effect.

Stability Store between 15°C to 25°C (59°F to 77°F).

Mechanism of Action Selective agonism for alpha₂-receptors; causes reduction of aqueous humor formation and increased uveoscleral outflow

Pharmacodynamics/Kinetics
Onset of action: Peak effect: 2 hours
Metabolism: Hepatic
Half-life elimination: ~2 hours
Time to peak, plasma: 0.5-2.5 hours
Excretion: Urine (74%)

Dosage
 Geriatric & Adult Glaucoma, ocular hypertension: Ophthalmic: Instill 1 drop in affected eye(s) 3 times/day (approximately every 8 hours)

Administration Remove contact lenses prior to administration; wait 15 minutes before reinserting if using products containing benzalkonium chloride. Separate administration of other ophthalmic agents by 5 minutes.

Monitoring Parameters Closely monitor patients who develop fatigue or drowsiness; IOP

Pharmacotherapy Pearls The use of Purite® as a preservative in Alphagan® P has lead to a reduced incidence of certain adverse effects associated with products using benzalkonium chloride as a preservative. The 0.1% and 0.15% solutions are comparable to the 0.2% solution in lowering intraocular pressure.

Special Geriatric Considerations Evaluate the patient's or caregiver's ability to safely administer the correct dose of ophthalmic medication.

Dosage Forms Excipient information presented when available (limited, particularly for generics); consult specific product labeling.
Solution, ophthalmic, as tartrate [drops]: 0.15% (5 mL, 10 mL, 15 mL); 0.2% (5 mL, 10 mL, 15 mL)
 Alphagan® P: 0.1% (5 mL, 10 mL, 15 mL); 0.15% (5 mL, 10 mL, 15 mL) [contains Purite®]

Selected References
Byles DB, Frith P, and Salmon JF, "Anterior Uveitis as a Side Effect of Topical Brimonidine," *Am J Ophthalmol*, 2000, 130(3):287-91.

◆ **Brimonidine Tartrate** *see* Brimonidine *on page 211*

Brinzolamide (brin ZOH la mide)

Related Information
Glaucoma Drug Therapy *on page 2008*
Brand Names: U.S. Azopt®
Brand Names: Canada Azopt®
Generic Availability (U.S.) No
Pharmacologic Category Carbonic Anhydrase Inhibitor; Ophthalmic Agent, Antiglaucoma
Use Lowers intraocular pressure in patients with ocular hypertension or open-angle glaucoma
Contraindications Hypersensitivity to brinzolamide, sulfonamides, or any component of the formulation
Warnings/Precautions Although administered topically, systemic absorption occurs. Similar adverse reactions attributed to sulfonamides may occur with topical administration. Effects of prolonged use on corneal epithelial cells have not been evaluated; has not been studied in acute angle-closure glaucoma. Use caution with renal impairment (parent and metabolite may accumulate). Systemic absorption may cause serious hypersensitivity reactions to recur. Chemical similarities are present among sulfonamides, sulfonylureas, carbonic anhydrase inhibitors, thiazides, and loop diuretics (except ethacrynic acid). In patients with allergy to one of these compounds, a risk of cross-reaction exists; avoid use when previous reaction has been severe. Safety and efficacy have not been established with hepatic impairment.

Adverse Reactions (Reflective of adult population; not specific for elderly)
1% to 10%:
Dermatologic: Dermatitis (1% to 5%)
Gastrointestinal: Taste disturbances (5% to 10%)
Ocular: Blurred vision (5% to 10%), blepharitis (1% to 5%), dry eye (1% to 5%), foreign body sensation (1% to 5%), eye discharge (1% to 5%), eye pain (1% to 5%), itching of eye (1% to 5%)
Respiratory: Rhinitis (1% to 5%)

Drug Interactions
Metabolism/Transport Effects Substrate of CYP3A4 (minor)
Avoid Concomitant Use
Avoid concomitant use of Brinzolamide with any of the following: Carbonic Anhydrase Inhibitors
Increased Effect/Toxicity
Brinzolamide may increase the levels/effects of: Carbonic Anhydrase Inhibitors

The levels/effects of Brinzolamide may be increased by: CYP3A4 Inhibitors (Strong)
Decreased Effect
The levels/effects of Brinzolamide may be decreased by: Tocilizumab
Stability Store at 4°C to 30°C (39°F to 86°F). Shake well before use.
Mechanism of Action Brinzolamide inhibits carbonic anhydrase, leading to decreased aqueous humor secretion. This results in a reduction of intraocular pressure.
Pharmacodynamics/Kinetics
Onset of action: Peak effect: 2 hours
Duration: 8-12 hours
Absorption: Topical: Into systemic circulation
Distribution: Accumulates in red blood cells, binding to carbonic anhydrase (brinzolamide and metabolite)
Metabolism: To N-desmethyl brinzolamide
Excretion: Urine (as unchanged drug and metabolites)
Dosage
Geriatric & Adult Glaucoma: Ophthalmic: Instill 1 drop in affected eye(s) 3 times/day

Administration Shake well; may be used concomitantly with other topical ophthalmic drug products to lower intraocular pressure. If more than one topical ophthalmic drug is being used, administer drugs at least 10 minutes apart.
Monitoring Parameters Intraocular pressure
Special Geriatric Considerations The oral carbonic anhydrase inhibitors are useful for patients who have difficulty administering ophthalmic drugs, who do not achieve sufficient lowering of intraocular pressure, or who cannot tolerate other agents. Brinzolamide is a useful agent apart from those who need a carbonic anhydrase inhibitor and can administer ophthalmic drops.
Dosage Forms Excipient information presented when available (limited, particularly for generics); consult specific product labeling.
Suspension, ophthalmic [drops]:
Azopt®: 1% (10 mL, 15 mL) [contains benzalkonium chloride]

♦ **Brioschi® [OTC]** *see* Sodium Bicarbonate *on page 1688*
♦ **BRL 43694** *see* Granisetron *on page 842*
♦ **Bromax** *see* Brompheniramine *on page 217*
♦ **Bromday™** *see* Bromfenac *on page 213*

Bromfenac (BROME fen ak)

Brand Names: U.S. Bromday™; Xibrom® [DSC]
Index Terms Bromfenac Sodium
Generic Availability (U.S.) No
Pharmacologic Category Nonsteroidal Anti-inflammatory Drug (NSAID), Ophthalmic
Use Treatment of postoperative inflammation and reduction in ocular pain following cataract removal
Contraindications
Bromday™: There are no contraindications listed in the manufacturer's prescribing information.
Xibrom®: Hypersensitivity to bromfenac or any components of the formulation
Warnings/Precautions Use with caution in patients with previous sensitivity to acetylsalicylic acid and phenylacetic acid derivatives, including patients who experience bronchospasm, asthma, rhinitis, or urticaria following NSAID or aspirin therapy. May slow/delay healing or prolong bleeding time following surgery. Use caution in patients with a predisposition to bleeding (bleeding tendencies or medications which interfere with coagulation).

May cause keratitis; continued use of bromfenac in a patient with keratitis may cause severe corneal adverse reactions, potentially resulting in loss of vision. Immediately discontinue use in patients with evidence of corneal epithelial damage.

Use caution in patients with complicated ocular surgeries, corneal denervation, corneal epithelial defects, diabetes mellitus, ocular surface disease, rheumatoid arthritis, or repeat ocular surgeries (within a short timeframe); may be at risk of corneal adverse events, potentially resulting in loss of vision. Patients using ophthalmic drops should not wear contact lenses during administration. Use for more than 1 day prior to surgery or for 14 days beyond surgery may increase risk and severity of corneal adverse events.

Contains sulfites, which may cause allergic reactions.

Adverse Reactions (Reflective of adult population; not specific for elderly)
2% to 7%:
Central nervous system: Headache
Ocular: Abnormal sensation, conjunctival hyperemia, iritis, irritation (burning/stinging), pain, pruritus, redness

Drug Interactions
Avoid Concomitant Use There are no known interactions where it is recommended to avoid concomitant use.
Increased Effect/Toxicity There are no known significant interactions involving an increase in effect.
Decreased Effect
Bromfenac may decrease the levels/effects of: Latanoprost

Stability Store at 15°C to 25°C (59°F to 77°F).

Mechanism of Action Inhibits prostaglandin synthesis by decreasing the activity of the enzyme, cyclooxygenase, which results in decreased formation of prostaglandin precursors.

Pharmacodynamics/Kinetics
Absorption: Theoretically, systemic absorption may occur following ophthalmic use (not characterized); anticipated levels are below the limits of assay detection
Metabolism: Hepatic
Half-life elimination: 0.5-4 hours (following oral administration)

Dosage
Geriatric & Adult
Bromday™: Ophthalmic: Instill 1 drop into affected eye(s) once daily beginning 1 day prior to surgery and continuing on the day of surgery and for 2 weeks postoperatively
Xibrom®: Ophthalmic: Instill 1 drop into affected eye(s) twice daily beginning 24 hours after surgery and continuing for 2 weeks postoperatively

Administration Remove contact lenses prior to administration and wait 15 minutes before reinserting.
Bromday™: May be used with other eye drops. If using more than 1 ophthalmic product, wait at least 5 minutes between application of each medication.

Pharmacotherapy Pearls An oral formulation of bromfenac was previously available and was withdrawn from the market following reports of idiosyncratic hepatotoxicity.

Special Geriatric Considerations No differences in safety and efficacy noted between elderly and younger adults. No dosage adjustment necessary. Elderly may be taking other medications that will increase bleeding.

Dosage Forms Excipient information presented when available (limited, particularly for generics); consult specific product labeling. [DSC] = Discontinued product
Solution, ophthalmic [drops]: 0.09% (2.5 mL)
Bromday™: 0.09% (1.7 mL) [contains benzalkonium chloride, sodium sulfite]
Xibrom®: 0.09% (2.5 mL [DSC], 5 mL [DSC]) [contains benzalkonium chloride, sodium sulfite]

Selected References
Fontana RJ, McCashland TM, Benner KG, et al, "Acute Liver Failure Associated With Prolonged Use of Bromfenac Leading to Liver Transplantation. The Acute Liver Failure Study Group," *Liver Transpl Surg*, 1999, 5(6):480-4.
Kashiwagi K and Tsukahara S, "Effect of Non-Steroidal Anti-Inflammatory Ophthalmic Solution on Intraocular Pressure Reduction by Latanoprost," *Br J Ophthalmol*, 2003, 87(3):297-301.
Miyake-Kashima M, Takano Y, Tanaka M, et al, "Comparison of 0.1% Bromfenac Sodium and 0.1% Pemirolast Potassium for the Treatment of Allergic Conjunctivitis," *Jpn J Ophthalmol*, 2004, 48(6):587-90.
Rabkin JM, Smith MJ, Orloff SL, et al, "Fatal Fulminant Hepatitis Associated With Bromfenac Use," *Ann Pharmacother*, 1999, 33(9):945-7.
Skjodt NM and Davies NM, "Clinical Pharmacokinetics and Pharmacodynamics of Bromfenac," *Clin Pharmacokinet*, 1999, 36(6):399-408.

♦ **Bromfenac Sodium** *see* Bromfenac *on page 213*

Bromocriptine (broe moe KRIP teen)

Related Information
Antiparkinsonian Agents *on page 1995*
Diabetes Mellitus Management, Adults *on page 2073*
Medication Safety Issues
Sound-alike/look-alike issues:
Bromocriptine may be confused with benztropine, brimonidine
Cycloset® may be confused with Glyset®

Parlodel® may be confused with pindolol, Provera®

Brand Names: U.S. Cycloset®; Parlodel®; Parlodel® SnapTabs®

Brand Names: Canada Apo-Bromocriptine®; Dom-Bromocriptine; PMS-Bromocriptine

Index Terms Bromocriptine Mesylate; Cycloset®

Generic Availability (U.S.) Yes: Excludes Cycloset®

Pharmacologic Category Anti-Parkinson's Agent, Dopamine Agonist; Antidiabetic Agent, Dopamine Agonist; Ergot Derivative

Use Treatment of hyperprolactinemia associated with amenorrhea with or without galactorrhea, infertility, or hypogonadism; treatment of prolactin-secreting adenomas; treatment of acromegaly; treatment of Parkinson's disease

Cycloset®: Management of type 2 diabetes mellitus (noninsulin dependent, NIDDM) as an adjunct to diet and exercise

Unlabeled/Investigational Use Treatment of neuroleptic malignant syndrome

Contraindications Hypersensitivity to bromocriptine, ergot alkaloids, or any component of the formulation; ergot alkaloids are contraindicated with potent inhibitors of CYP3A4 (includes protease inhibitors, azole antifungals, and some macrolide antibiotics); uncontrolled hypertension; severe ischemic heart disease or peripheral vascular disorders

Warnings/Precautions Complete evaluation of pituitary function should be completed prior to initiation of treatment of any hyperprolactinemia-associated dysfunction. Use caution in patients with a history of peptic ulcer disease, dementia, or cardiovascular disease (myocardial infarction, arrhythmia). Use with extreme caution or avoid in patients with psychosis. Symptomatic hypotension may occur in a significant number of patients. In addition, hypertension, seizures, MI, and stroke have been rarely associated with bromocriptine therapy. Severe headache or visual changes may precede events. The onset of reactions may be immediate or delayed (often may occur in the second week of therapy). Sudden sleep onset and somnolence have been reported with use, primarily in patients with Parkinson's disease. Patients must be cautioned about performing tasks which require mental alertness.

Use with caution in patients taking strong CYP3A4 inhibitors and/or major CYP3A4 substrates (includes protease inhibitors, azole antifungals, and some macrolide antibiotics); consider alternative agents that avoid or lessen the potential for CYP-mediated interactions. Concurrent antihypertensives or drugs which may alter blood pressure should be used with caution. Concurrent use with levodopa has been associated with an increased risk of hallucinations. Consider dosage reduction and/or discontinuation in patients with hallucinations. Hallucinations may require weeks to months before resolution.

Dopamine agonists have been associated with compulsive behaviors and/or loss of impulse control, which has manifested as pathological gambling, libido increases (hypersexuality), and/or binge eating. Causality has not been established, and controversy exists as to whether this phenomenon is related to the underlying disease, prior behaviors/addictions and/or drug therapy. Dose reduction or discontinuation of therapy has been reported to reverse these behaviors in some, but not all cases. Risk for melanoma development is increased in Parkinson's disease patients; drug causation or factors contributing to risk have not been established. Patients should be monitored closely and periodic skin examinations should be performed.

In the treatment of acromegaly, discontinuation is recommended if tumor expansion occurs during therapy. Digital vasospasm (cold sensitive) may occur in some patients with acromegaly; may require dosage reduction. Use of bromocriptine in patients with uncontrolled hypertension is not recommended.

Monitoring and careful evaluation of visual changes during the treatment of hyperprolactinemia is recommended to differentiate between tumor shrinkage and traction on the optic chiasm; rapidly progressing visual field loss requires neurosurgical consultation. Discontinuation of bromocriptine in patients with macroadenomas has been associated with rapid regrowth of tumor and increased prolactin serum levels. Pleural and retroperitoneal fibrosis have been reported with prolonged daily use. Cardiac valvular fibrosis has also been associated with ergot alkaloids.

In the management of type 2 diabetes mellitus, Cycloset® ('quick-release' tablet) should not be interchanged with any other bromocriptine product due to formulation differences and resulting pharmacokinetics. Therapy is not appropriate in patients with diabetic ketoacidosis (DKA) or type 1 diabetes mellitus due to lack of efficacy in these patient populations. There is limited efficacy of use in combination with thiazolidinediones or in combination with insulin. Combination therapy with other hypoglycemic agents may increase risk for hypoglycemic events; dose reduction of concomitant hypoglycemics may be warranted.

Safety and efficacy have not been established in patients with hepatic or renal dysfunction.

◀ **Adverse Reactions (Reflective of adult population; not specific for elderly) Note:**
Frequency of adverse effects may vary by dose and/or indication.

>10%:
  Central nervous system: Dizziness, fatigue, headache
  Gastrointestinal: Constipation, nausea
  Neuromuscular & skeletal: Weakness
  Respiratory: Rhinitis

1% to 10%:
  Cardiovascular: Hypotension (including postural/orthostatic), Raynaud's syndrome exacer-
    bation, syncope
  Central nervous system: Drowsiness, fatigue, lightheadedness, somnolence
  Endocrine & metabolic: Hypoglycemia (4%; in combination with sulfonylureas or other
    antidiabetic agents: 7% to 9%)
  Gastrointestinal: Abdominal cramps, anorexia, diarrhea, dyspepsia, GI bleeding, vomiting,
    xerostomia
  Neuromuscular & skeletal: Digital vasospasm
  Ocular: Amblyopia
  Respiratory: Nasal congestion, sinusitis
  Miscellaneous: Infection, flu-like syndrome

Drug Interactions
  Metabolism/Transport Effects Substrate of CYP3A4 (major); **Inhibits** CYP1A2 (weak),
  3A4 (weak)

Avoid Concomitant Use
  Avoid concomitant use of Bromocriptine with any of the following: Conivaptan; Efavirenz;
  Itraconazole; Nitroglycerin; Posaconazole; Protease Inhibitors; Serotonin 5-HT1D Receptor
  Agonists; Sibutramine; Voriconazole

Increased Effect/Toxicity
  Bromocriptine may increase the levels/effects of: CycloSPORINE; CycloSPORINE (Systemic); Serotonin 5-HT1D Receptor Agonists; Serotonin Modulators

  The levels/effects of Bromocriptine may be increased by: Alpha-/Beta-Agonists; Antipsy-
  chotics (Typical); Conivaptan; CYP3A4 Inhibitors (Moderate); CYP3A4 Inhibitors (Strong);
  Dasatinib; Efavirenz; Itraconazole; Macrolide Antibiotics; MAO Inhibitors; Methylphenidate;
  Nitroglycerin; Posaconazole; Protease Inhibitors; Serotonin 5-HT1D Receptor Agonists;
  Sibutramine; Voriconazole

Decreased Effect
  Bromocriptine may decrease the levels/effects of: Antipsychotics (Typical); Nitroglycerin

  The levels/effects of Bromocriptine may be decreased by: Antipsychotics (Atypical);
  Metoclopramide; Tocilizumab

Ethanol/Nutrition/Herb Interactions
  Ethanol: Avoid ethanol (may increase GI side effects or ethanol intolerance).
  Herb/Nutraceutical: St John's wort may decrease bromocriptine levels.

Stability Store at or below 25°C (77°F).

Mechanism of Action Semisynthetic ergot alkaloid derivative and a dopamine receptor
agonist which activates postsynaptic dopamine receptors in the tuberoinfundibular (inhibiting
pituitary prolactin secretion) and nigrostriatal pathways (enhancing coordinated motor control).

In the treatment of type 2 diabetes mellitus, the mechanism of action is unknown; however,
bromocriptine is believed to affect circadian rhythms which are mediated, in part, by
dopaminergic activity, and are believed to play a role in obesity and insulin resistance. It is
postulated that bromocriptine (when administered during the morning and released into the
systemic circulation in a rapid, 'pulse-like' dose) may reset hypothalamic circadian activities
which have been altered by obesity, thereby resulting in the reversal of insulin resistance and
decreases in glucose production, without increasing serum insulin concentrations.

Pharmacodynamics/Kinetics
  Onset of action: Parlodel®: Prolactin decreasing effect: 1-2 hours
  Distribution: V_d: ~61L
  Protein binding: 90% to 96% (primarily albumin)
  Metabolism: Primarily hepatic via CYP3A; extensive first-pass biotransformation (Cyclo-
    set®: ~93%)
  Bioavailability: Parlodel®: 28%; Cycloset®: 65% to 95%
  Half-life elimination: Cycloset®: ~6 hours; Parlodel®: Biphasic: Terminal: 15 hours (range: 8-20
    hours)
  Time to peak, serum: Parlodel®: 1-3 hours; Cycloset®: 53 minutes
  Excretion: Feces; urine (2% to 6% as unchanged drug and metabolites)

Dosage
  Geriatric & Adult
    Acromegaly: Oral: Initial: 1.25-2.5 mg daily increasing by 1.25-2.5 mg daily as necessary every 3-7 days; usual dose: 20-30 mg/day (maximum: 100 mg/day)
    Hyperprolactinemia: Oral: Initial: 1.25-2.5 mg/day; may be increased by 2.5 mg/day as tolerated every 2-7 days until optimal response (range: 2.5-15 mg/day)
    Parkinsonism: Oral: 1.25 mg twice daily, increased by 2.5 mg/day in 2- to 4-week intervals as needed (maximum: 100 mg/day)
    Type 2 diabetes (Cycloset®): Oral: Initial: 0.8 mg once daily; may increase at weekly intervals in 0.8 mg increments as tolerated; usual dose: 1.6-4.8 mg/day (maximum: 4.8 mg/day)
    Neuroleptic malignant syndrome (unlabeled use): Oral: 2.5 mg (orally or via gastric tube) every 8-12 hours, increased to a maximum of 45 mg/day, if needed; continue therapy until NMS is controlled, then taper slowly (Gortney, 2009; Strawn, 2007)
    Hepatic Impairment No guidelines are available; however, adjustment may be necessary due to extensive hepatic metabolism.
Administration Administer with food to decrease GI distress.
  Cycloset®: Administer within 2 hours of waking in the morning.
Monitoring Parameters Monitor blood pressure closely as well as hepatic, hematopoietic, and cardiovascular function
Reference Range Recommendations for glycemic control in adults with diabetes:
  Hb A_{1c}: <7%
  Preprandial capillary plasma glucose: 70-130 mg/dL
  Peak postprandial capillary blood glucose: <180 mg/dL
Pharmacotherapy Pearls Usually used with levodopa or levodopa/carbidopa to treat Parkinson's disease. When adding bromocriptine, the dose of levodopa/carbidopa can usually be decreased.
Special Geriatric Considerations No special considerations are recommended since drug is dosed to response; however, elderly patients may have concomitant diseases or drug therapy which may complicate therapy. Because newer, more specific dopamine agonists have fewer side effects, bromocriptine is rarely the drug of choice in Parkinson's disease.
Dosage Forms Excipient information presented when available (limited, particularly for generics); consult specific product labeling.
  Capsule, oral: 5 mg
    Parlodel®: 5 mg
  Tablet, oral: 2.5 mg
    Cycloset®: 0.8 mg
    Parlodel® SnapTabs®: 2.5 mg [scored]
Selected References
Factor SA, "Current Status of Symptomatic Medical Therapy in Parkinson's Disease," *Neurotherapeutics*, 2008, 5 (2):164-80.
Olanow CW, Watts RL, and Koller WC, "An Algorithm (Decision Tree) for the Management of Parkinson's Disease (2001): Treatment Guidelines," *Neurology*, 2001, 56(11 Suppl 5):S1-S88.
Weintraub D, Siderowf AD, Potenza MN, et al, "Association of Dopamine Agonist Use With Impulse Control Disorders in Parkinson Disease," *Arch Neurol*, 2006, 63(7):969-73.

◆ **Bromocriptine Mesylate** *see* Bromocriptine *on page 214*

Brompheniramine (brome fen IR a meen)

Brand Names: U.S. Bromax; Lodrane® 24 [DSC]; LoHist-12; Respa®-BR [DSC]; TanaCof-XR [DSC]
Index Terms Brompheniramine Maleate; Brompheniramine Tannate
Generic Availability (U.S.) Yes: Chewable tablet
Pharmacologic Category Alkylamine Derivative; Histamine H_1 Antagonist; Histamine H_1 Antagonist, First Generation
Use Symptomatic relief of perennial and seasonal allergic rhinitis, vasomotor rhinitis, and other respiratory allergies
Contraindications Hypersensitivity to brompheniramine or any component of the formulation; use with or within 14 days of MAO inhibitor therapy; narrow-angle glaucoma; urinary retention; peptic ulcer disease; during acute asthmatic attacks
Warnings/Precautions Causes sedation; caution must be used in performing tasks which require alertness (eg, operating machinery or driving). Sedative effects of CNS depressants or ethanol are potentiated. Use with caution in patients with hyperthyroidism, increased intra-ocular pressure, prostatic hyperplasia, history of asthma, and cardiovascular disease (including hypertension and ischemic heart disease). Use with caution in the elderly; may be more sensitive to adverse effects. Some products may contain tartrazine or phenylalanine.

Adverse Reactions (Reflective of adult population; not specific for elderly) Frequency not defined.

Cardiovascular: Angina, blood pressure increased, chest tightness, circulatory collapse, extrasystoles, hypotension, palpitation, tachycardia

Central nervous system: Anxiety, chills, confusion, coordination impaired, dizziness, drowsiness, euphoria, excitation, fatigue, headache, hysteria, insomnia, irritability, nervousness, neuritis, restlessness, sedation, seizure, stimulation, tension, vertigo

Dermatologic: Photosensitivity, rash, urticaria

Endocrine & metabolic: Early menses

Gastrointestinal: Abdominal cramps, anorexia, constipation, diarrhea, dry throat, epigastric distress, heartburn, nausea, vomiting, xerostomia

Genitourinary: Dysuria, polyuria, urinary retention

Hematologic: Agranulocytosis, hemolytic anemia, hypoplastic anemia, thrombocytopenia

Neuromuscular & skeletal: Paresthesia, tremor, weakness

Ocular: Blurred vision, diplopia, mydriasis

Otic: Labyrinthitis (acute), tinnitus

Respiratory: Dry nose, nasal congestion, thickening of bronchial secretions, wheezing

Miscellaneous: Anaphylactic shock, diaphoresis

Drug Interactions

Avoid Concomitant Use There are no known interactions where it is recommended to avoid concomitant use.

Increased Effect/Toxicity

Brompheniramine may increase the levels/effects of: Alcohol (Ethyl); Anticholinergics; CNS Depressants; Selective Serotonin Reuptake Inhibitors

The levels/effects of Brompheniramine may be increased by: Droperidol; HydrOXYzine; Pramlintide

Decreased Effect

Brompheniramine may decrease the levels/effects of: Acetylcholinesterase Inhibitors (Central); Benzylpenicilloyl Polylysine; Betahistine

The levels/effects of Brompheniramine may be decreased by: Acetylcholinesterase Inhibitors (Central); Amphetamines

Ethanol/Nutrition/Herb Interactions Ethanol: May increase CNS depression; monitor for increased effects with coadministration. Caution patients about effect.

Stability Store between 15°C to 30°C (59°F to 86°F). Protect from light.

Mechanism of Action Competes with histamine for H_1-receptor sites on effector cells

Pharmacodynamics/Kinetics

Metabolism: Hepatic

Excretion: Urine

Dosage

Adult Allergic rhinitis, allergic symptoms, vasomotor rhinitis: Oral:

Bromax, Respa®-BR: One tablet twice daily

Lodrane® 24: 1-2 capsules once daily

LoHist-12: 1-2 tablets every 12 hours (maximum: 4 tablets/day)

Administration Extended release tablets are to be swallowed whole; do not crush or chew. Shake suspensions well before use.

Test Interactions May interfere with urine detection of amphetamine/methamphetamine (false-positive). May interfere with skin tests using allergen extracts.

Special Geriatric Considerations Anticholinergic action may cause significant confusional symptoms, constipation, or problems voiding urine. If an antihistamine is indicated, a second generation nonsedating antihistamine would be a more appropriate choice.

Dosage Forms Excipient information presented when available (limited, particularly for generics); consult specific product labeling. [DSC] = Discontinued product

Capsule, extended release, oral, as maleate:

Lodrane® 24: 12 mg [DSC] [dye free]

Suspension, oral, as tannate:

TanaCof-XR: 8 mg/5 mL (480 mL [DSC]) [ethanol free, sugar free; contains phenylalanine; strawberry cream flavor]

Tablet, chewable, oral, as tannate: 12 mg [DSC]

Tablet, extended release, oral, as maleate:

Bromax: 11 mg [dye free]

LoHist-12: 6 mg [scored; dye free]

Tablet, prolonged release, oral, as maleate:

Respa®-BR: 11 mg [DSC] [dye free]

Tablet, timed release, oral, as maleate: 6 mg [DSC]

◆ **Brompheniramine Maleate** *see* Brompheniramine *on page 217*

- ◆ **Brompheniramine Tannate** *see* Brompheniramine *on page* 217
- ◆ **Brovana®** *see* Arformoterol *on page* 141
- ◆ **BTX-A** *see* OnabotulinumtoxinA *on page* 1345
- ◆ **B-type Natriuretic Peptide (Human)** *see* Nesiritide *on page* 1285
- ◆ **Budeprion XL®** *see* BuPROPion *on page* 229
- ◆ **Budeprion SR®** *see* BuPROPion *on page* 229

Budesonide (Systemic, Oral Inhalation) (byoo DES oh nide)

Related Information
Asthma *on page* 2016
Inhalant Agents *on page* 2010
Brand Names: U.S. Entocort® EC; Pulmicort Flexhaler®; Pulmicort Respules®
Brand Names: Canada Entocort®; Pulmicort®
Generic Availability (U.S.) Yes: Capsule; suspension for nebulization
Pharmacologic Category Corticosteroid, Inhalant (Oral); Corticosteroid, Systemic
Use
Nebulization: Maintenance and prophylactic treatment of asthma
Oral capsule: Treatment of active Crohn's disease (mild-to-moderate) involving the ileum and/ or ascending colon; maintenance of remission (for up to 3 months) of Crohn's disease (mild-to-moderate) involving the ileum and/or ascending colon
Oral inhalation: Maintenance and prophylactic treatment of asthma; includes patients who require oral corticosteroids and those who may benefit from systemic dose reduction/ elimination
Contraindications Hypersensitivity to budesonide or any component of the formulation; primary treatment of status asthmaticus, acute episodes of asthma; not for relief of acute bronchospasm
Canadian labeling: Additional contraindications (not in U.S. labeling): Moderate-to-severe bronchiectasis, pulmonary tuberculosis (active or quiescent), untreated respiratory infection (bacterial, fungal, or viral)
Warnings/Precautions May cause hypercorticism or suppression of hypothalamic-pituitary-adrenal (HPA) axis, particularly in patients receiving high doses for prolonged periods. HPA axis suppression may lead to adrenal crisis. Withdrawal and discontinuation of a corticosteroid should be done slowly and carefully. Particular care is required when patients are transferred from systemic corticosteroids to inhaled products due to possible adrenal insufficiency or withdrawal from steroids, including an increase in allergic symptoms. Patients receiving >20 mg per day of prednisone (or equivalent) may be most susceptible. Fatalities have occurred due to adrenal insufficiency in asthmatic patients during and after transfer from systemic corticosteroids to aerosol steroids; aerosol steroids do not provide the systemic steroid needed to treat patients having trauma, surgery, or infections. Do not use this product to transfer patients directly from oral corticosteroid therapy.

Bronchospasm may occur with wheezing after inhalation; if this occurs stop steroid and treat with a fast-acting bronchodilator (eg, albuterol). Supplemental steroids (oral or parenteral) may be needed during stress or severe asthma attacks. Not to be used in status asthmaticus or for the relief of acute bronchospasm. Acute myopathy has been reported with high-dose corticosteroids, usually in patients with neuromuscular transmission disorders; may involve ocular and/or respiratory muscles; monitor creatine kinase; recovery may be delayed. Corticosteroid use may cause psychiatric disturbances, including depression, euphoria, insomnia, mood swings, and personality changes. Pre-existing psychiatric conditions may be exacerbated by corticosteroid use. Prolonged use of corticosteroids may also increase the incidence of secondary infection, mask acute infection (including fungal infections), prolong or exacerbate viral infections, or limit response to vaccines. Exposure to chickenpox should be avoided; corticosteroids should not be used to treat ocular herpes simplex. Corticosteroids should not be used for cerebral malaria or viral hepatitis. Close observation is required in patients with latent tuberculosis and/or TB reactivity; restrict use in active TB (only in conjunction with antituberculosis treatment). *Candida albicans* infections may occur in the mouth and pharynx; rinsing (and spitting) with water after inhaler use may decrease risk. Prolonged treatment with corticosteroids has been associated with the development of Kaposi's sarcoma (case reports); if noted, discontinuation of therapy should be considered.

Use with caution in patients with thyroid disease, hepatic impairment, renal impairment, cardiovascular disease, diabetes, glaucoma, cataracts, myasthenia gravis, patients at risk for osteoporosis, patients at risk for seizures, or GI diseases (diverticulitis, peptic ulcer, ulcerative colitis) due to perforation risk. Use caution following acute MI (corticosteroids have been associated with myocardial rupture). Because of the risk of adverse effects, systemic ▶

◀ corticosteroids should be used cautiously in the elderly in the smallest possible effective dose for the shortest duration.

Pulmicort Flexhaler™ contains lactose; very rare anaphylactic reactions have been reported in patients with severe milk protein allergy.

Adverse Reactions (Reflective of adult population; not specific for elderly) Reaction severity varies by dose and duration; not all adverse reactions have been reported with each dosage form.

>10%:
  Central nervous system: Headache (≤21%)
  Gastrointestinal: Nausea (≤11%)
  Respiratory: Respiratory infection, rhinitis
  Miscellaneous: Symptoms of HPA axis suppression and/or hypercorticism may occur in >10% of patients following administration of dosage forms which result in higher systemic exposure (ie, oral capsule), but may be less frequent than rates observed with comparator drugs (prednisolone). These symptoms may be rare (<1%) following administration via methods which result in lower exposures (topical).

1% to 10%:
  Cardiovascular: Chest pain, edema, flushing, hypertension, palpitation, syncope, tachycardia
  Central nervous system: Amnesia, dizziness, dysphonia, emotional lability, fatigue, fever, insomnia, malaise, migraine, nervousness, pain, sleep disorder, somnolence, vertigo
  Dermatologic: Acne, alopecia, bruising, contact dermatitis, eczema, hirsutism, pruritus, pustular rash, rash, striae
  Endocrine & metabolic: Adrenal insufficiency, hypokalemia, menstrual disorder
  Gastrointestinal: Abdominal pain, anorexia, diarrhea, dyspepsia, flatulence, gastroenteritis (including viral), glossitis, intestinal obstruction, oral candidiasis, taste perversion, tongue edema, vomiting, weight gain, xerostomia
  Genitourinary: Dysuria, hematuria, nocturia, pyuria
  Hematologic: Cervical lymphadenopathy, leukocytosis, purpura
  Hepatic: Alkaline phosphatase increased
  Neuromuscular & skeletal: Arthralgia, back pain, fracture, hyperkinesis, hypertonia, myalgia, neck pain, paresthesia, weakness
  Ocular: Conjunctivitis, eye infection
  Otic: Earache, ear infection, external ear infection
  Respiratory: Bronchitis, bronchospasm, cough, epistaxis, hoarseness, nasal congestion, nasal irritation, pharyngitis, sinusitis, stridor, throat irritation
  Miscellaneous: Abscess, allergic reaction, C-reactive protein increased, erythrocyte sedimentation rate increased, fat distribution (moon face, buffalo hump); flu-like syndrome, herpes simplex, infection, moniliasis, viral infection, voice alteration

Drug Interactions
  Metabolism/Transport Effects Substrate of CYP3A4 (major)
  Avoid Concomitant Use
    Avoid concomitant use of Budesonide (Systemic, Oral Inhalation) with any of the following: Aldesleukin; BCG; Grapefruit Juice; Natalizumab; Pimecrolimus; Tacrolimus (Topical)
  Increased Effect/Toxicity
    Budesonide (Systemic, Oral Inhalation) may increase the levels/effects of: Amphotericin B; Deferasirox; Leflunomide; Loop Diuretics; Natalizumab; Thiazide Diuretics

    The levels/effects of Budesonide (Systemic, Oral Inhalation) may be increased by: CYP3A4 Inhibitors (Moderate); CYP3A4 Inhibitors (Strong); Dasatinib; Denosumab; Grapefruit Juice; Pimecrolimus; Tacrolimus (Topical); Telaprevir; Trastuzumab
  Decreased Effect
    Budesonide (Systemic, Oral Inhalation) may decrease the levels/effects of: Aldesleukin; Antidiabetic Agents; BCG; Corticorelin; Sipuleucel-T; Telaprevir; Vaccines (Inactivated)

    The levels/effects of Budesonide (Systemic, Oral Inhalation) may be decreased by: Antacids; Bile Acid Sequestrants; Echinacea; Tocilizumab
  Ethanol/Nutrition/Herb Interactions Food: Grapefruit juice may double systemic exposure of orally-administered budesonide. Administration of capsules with a high-fat meal delays peak concentration, but does not alter the extent of absorption.

Stability
  Suspension for nebulization: Store upright at 20°C to 25°C (68°F to 77°F). Protect from light. Do not refrigerate or freeze. Once aluminum package is opened, solution should be used within 2 weeks. Continue to protect from light.
  Oral inhaler (Pulmicort Flexhaler™): Store at controlled room temperature of 20°C to 25°C (68°F to 77°F). Protect from moisture.

Mechanism of Action Controls the rate of protein synthesis; depresses the migration of polymorphonuclear leukocytes, fibroblasts; reverses capillary permeability and lysosomal stabilization at the cellular level to prevent or control inflammation. Has potent glucocorticoid activity and weak mineralocorticoid activity.

Pharmacodynamics/Kinetics

Onset of action: Pulmicort Respules®: 2-8 days; Inhalation: 24 hours
  Peak effect: Pulmicort Respules®: 4-6 weeks; Inhalation: 1-2 weeks
Distribution: 2.2-3.9 L/kg
Protein binding: 85% to 90%
Metabolism: Hepatic via CYP3A4 to two metabolites: 16 alpha-hydroxyprednisolone and 6 beta-hydroxybudesonide; minor activity
Bioavailability: Limited by high first-pass effect; Capsule: 9% to 21%; Pulmicort Respules®: 6%; Inhalation: 6% to 13%
Half-life elimination: 2-3.6 hours
Time to peak: Capsule: 0.5-10 hours (variable in Crohn's disease); Pulmicort Respules®: 10-30 minutes; Inhalation: 1-2 hours
Excretion: Urine (60%) and feces as metabolites

Dosage

Geriatric & Adult

Asthma: *Oral inhalation:*

Pulmicort Flexhaler™: Initial: 360 mcg twice daily (selected patients may be initiated at 180 mcg twice daily); maximum: 720 mcg twice daily
  NIH Asthma Guidelines (NIH, 2007) (administer in divided doses twice daily):
  "Low" dose: 180-600 mcg/day
  "Medium" dose: >600-1200 mcg/day
  "High" dose: >1200 mcg/day

Pulmicort® Turbuhaler®: [CAN, not available in the U.S.]: Initial (during periods of severe asthma or when switching from oral corticosteroid therapy): 400-2400 mcg daily in 2-4 divided doses; Maintenance: 200-400 mcg twice daily (higher doses may be needed for short periods of time). **Note:** Patients taking 400 mcg/day may take as a single daily dose

Crohn's disease (active): *Oral:* 9 mg once daily in the morning for up to 8 weeks; recurring episodes may be treated with a repeat 8-week course of treatment. **Note:** Patients receiving CYP3A4 inhibitors should be monitored closely for signs and symptoms of hypercorticism; dosage reduction may be required. If switching from oral prednisolone, prednisolone dosage should be tapered while budesonide (Entocort™ EC) treatment is initiated.

Maintenance of remission: Following treatment of active disease (control of symptoms with CDAI <150), treatment may be continued at a dosage of 6 mg once daily for up to 3 months. If symptom control is maintained for 3 months, tapering of the dosage to complete cessation is recommended. Continued dosing beyond 3 months has not been demonstrated to result in substantial benefit.

Hepatic Impairment Monitor closely for signs and symptoms of hypercorticism; dosage reduction may be required.

Administration

Oral capsule: Capsule should be swallowed whole; do not crush or chew.
Powder for inhalation:
Pulmicort Flexhaler™: Hold inhaler in upright position (mouthpiece up) to load dose. Do not shake prior to use. Unit should be primed prior to first use only. It will not need primed again, even if not used for a long time. Place mouthpiece between lips and inhale forcefully and deeply. Do not exhale through inhaler; do not use a spacer. Dose indicator does not move with every dose, usually only after 5 doses. Discard when dose indicator reads "0". Rinse mouth with water after each use to reduce incidence of candidiasis.
Pulmicort Turbuhaler® [CAN, not available in the U.S.]: Hold inhaler in upright position (mouthpiece up) to load dose. Do not shake inhaler after dose is loaded. Unit should be primed prior to first use. Place mouthpiece between lips and inhale forcefully and deeply; mouthpiece should face up. Do not exhale through inhaler; do not use a spacer. When a red mark appears in the dose indicator window, 20 doses are left. When the red mark reaches the bottom of the window, the inhaler should be discarded. Rinse mouth with water after use to reduce incidence of candidiasis.
Suspension for nebulization: Shake well before using. Use Pulmicort Respules® with jet nebulizer connected to an air compressor; administer with mouthpiece or facemask. Do not use ultrasonic nebulizer. Do not mix with other medications in nebulizer. Rinse mouth following treatments to decrease risk of oral candidiasis (wash face if using face mask).

Monitoring Parameters Monitor blood pressure, serum glucose, weight with high-dose or long-term oral use
Asthma: FEV_1, peak flow, and/or other pulmonary function tests

Pharmacotherapy Pearls No geriatric-specific information.

◀ **Special Geriatric Considerations** Ensure that patients can correctly use inhaler.
Dosage Forms Excipient information presented when available (limited, particularly for generics); consult specific product labeling.
Capsule, enteric coated, oral: 3 mg
  Entocort® EC: 3 mg
Powder, for oral inhalation:
  Pulmicort Flexhaler®: 90 mcg/inhalation (165 mg) [contains lactose; delivers ~80 mcg/inhalation; 60 actuations]
  Pulmicort Flexhaler®: 180 mcg/inhalation (225 mg) [contains lactose; delivers ~160 mcg/inhalation; 120 actuations]
Suspension, for nebulization: 0.25 mg/2 mL (30s); 0.5 mg/2 mL (30s)
  Pulmicort Respules®: 0.25 mg/2 mL (30s); 0.5 mg/2 mL (30s); 1 mg/2 mL (30s)
Dosage Forms: Canada Excipient information presented when available (limited, particularly for generics); consult specific product labeling.
Powder for oral inhalation:
  Pulmicort Turbuhaler®: 100 mcg/inhalation [delivers 200 metered actuations]; 200 mcg/inhalation [delivers 200 metered actuations]; 400 mcg/inhalation [delivers 200 metered actuations]
Selected References
National Asthma Education and Prevention Program, "Expert Panel Report 3 (EPR-3): Guidelines for the Diagnosis and Management of Asthma-Summary Report 2007," *J Allergy Clin Immunol*, 2007, 120(5 Suppl):94-138.

Budesonide (Nasal) (byoo DES oh nide)

Brand Names: U.S. Rhinocort Aqua®
Brand Names: Canada Gen-Budesonide AQ; Mylan-Budesonide AQ; Rhinocort® Aqua™; Rhinocort® Turbuhaler®
Generic Availability (U.S.) No
Pharmacologic Category Corticosteroid, Nasal
Use Management of symptoms of seasonal or perennial rhinitis

Canadian labeling: Additional use (not in U.S. labeling): Prevention and treatment of nasal polyps
Dosage
Geriatric & Adult
Nasal polyps: *Nasal inhalation:*
  Canadian labeling:
    Rhinocort® Aqua®: 256 mcg/day administered as a single 64 mcg spray in each nostril twice daily; maximum dose: 256 mcg/day
    Rhinocort® Turbuhaler®: 100 mcg into each nostril twice daily; maximum: 400 mcg/day

Rhinitis: *Nasal inhalation:*
  U.S. labeling (Rhinocort® Aqua®): 64 mcg/day as a single 32 mcg spray in each nostril. Some patients who do not achieve adequate control may benefit from increased dosage. A reduced dosage may be effective after initial control is achieved (maximum dose: 256 mcg/day)
  Canadian labeling:
    Rhinocort® Aqua®: Initial: 256 mcg/day administered as two 64 mcg sprays in each nostril once daily or a single 64 mcg spray in each nostril twice daily; Maintenance: Individualize, lowest effective dose (maximum dose: 256 mcg/day)
    Rhinocort® Turbuhaler®: Initial: 200 mcg into each nostril once daily; Maintenance: Individualize, lowest effective dose (maximum: 400 mcg/day)
Hepatic Impairment Monitor closely for signs and symptoms of hypercorticism; dosage reduction may be required.
Special Geriatric Considerations Ensure that patients can correctly use nasal inhaler.
Dosage Forms Excipient information presented when available (limited, particularly for generics); consult specific product labeling.
Suspension, intranasal [spray]:
  Rhinocort Aqua®: 32 mcg/inhalation (8.6 g) [120 metered actuations]
Dosage Forms: Canada Excipient information presented when available (limited, particularly for generics); consult specific product labeling.
Powder for nasal inhalation:
  Rhinocort® Turbuhaler®: 100 mcg/inhalation [delivers 200 metered actuations]
Suspension, intranasal [spray]:
  Rhinocort® Aqua®: 64 mcg/inhalation [120 metered actuations]

◆ **Buffasal [OTC]** *see Aspirin on page 153*
◆ **Bufferin® [OTC]** *see Aspirin on page 153*

◆ **Bufferin® Extra Strength [OTC]** *see* Aspirin *on page* 153
◆ **Buffinol [OTC]** *see* Aspirin *on page* 153
◆ **Bulk-K [OTC]** *see* Psyllium *on page* 1547

Bumetanide (byoo MET a nide)

Medication Safety Issues
Sound-alike/look-alike issues:
Bumetanide may be confused with Buminate®
Bumex® may be confused with Brevibloc®, Buprenex®
International issues:
Bumex [U.S.] may be confused with Permax brand name for pergolide [multiple international markets]
Brand Names: Canada Burinex®
Index Terms Bumex
Generic Availability (U.S.) Yes
Pharmacologic Category Diuretic, Loop
Use Management of edema secondary to heart failure or hepatic or renal disease (including nephrotic syndrome)
Unlabeled/Investigational Use Treatment of hypertension
Contraindications Hypersensitivity to bumetanide or any component of the formulation; anuria; patients with hepatic coma or in states of severe electrolyte depletion until the condition improves or is corrected
Warnings/Precautions [U.S. Boxed Warning]: Excessive amounts can lead to profound diuresis with fluid and electrolyte loss; close medical supervision and dose evaluation are required. Potassium supplementation and/or use of potassium-sparing diuretics may be necessary to prevent hypokalemia. In cirrhosis, initiate bumetanide therapy with conservative dosing and close monitoring of electrolytes; avoid sudden changes in fluid and electrolyte balance and acid/base status which may lead to hepatic encephalopathy. *In vitro* studies using pooled sera from critically-ill neonates have shown bumetanide to be a potent displacer of bilirubin; avoid use in neonates at risk for kernicterus. Coadministration of antihypertensives may increase the risk of hypotension.

Monitor fluid status and renal function in an attempt to prevent oliguria, azotemia, and reversible increases in BUN and creatinine; close medical supervision of aggressive diuresis required. Bumetanide-induced ototoxicity (usually transient) may occur with rapid I.V. administration, renal impairment, excessive doses, and concurrent use of other ototoxins (eg, aminoglycosides). Asymptomatic hyperuricemia has been reported with use.

Chemical similarities are present among sulfonamides, sulfonylureas, carbonic anhydrase inhibitors, thiazides, and loop diuretics (except ethacrynic acid); the manufacturer's labeling states that bumetanide may be used in patients allergic to furosemide. Use in patients with sulfonylurea allergy is not specifically contraindicated in product labeling; however, a risk of cross-reaction exists in patients with allergy to any of these compounds; avoid use when previous reaction has been severe. Discontinue if signs of hypersensitivity are noted.
Adverse Reactions (Reflective of adult population; not specific for elderly)
>10%:
Endocrine & metabolic: Hyperuricemia (18%), hypochloremia (15%), hypokalemia (15%)
Renal: Azotemia (11%)
1% to 10%:
Central nervous system: Dizziness (1%)
Endocrine & metabolic: Hyponatremia (9%), hyperglycemia (7%), phosphorus altered (5%), CO_2 content altered (4%), bicarbonate altered (3%), calcium altered (2%)
Neuromuscular & skeletal: Muscle cramps (1%)
Renal: Serum creatinine increased (7%)
Miscellaneous: LDH altered (1%)
Drug Interactions
Avoid Concomitant Use There are no known interactions where it is recommended to avoid concomitant use.
Increased Effect/Toxicity
Bumetanide may increase the levels/effects of: ACE Inhibitors; Allopurinol; Amifostine; Aminoglycosides; Antihypertensives; Cardiac Glycosides; CISplatin; Dofetilide; Hypotensive Agents; Lithium; Methotrexate; Neuromuscular-Blocking Agents; RisperiDONE; RiTUXimab; Salicylates; Sodium Phosphates

◀

The levels/effects of Bumetanide may be increased by: Alfuzosin; Beta2-Agonists; Corticosteroids (Orally Inhaled); Corticosteroids (Systemic); CycloSPORINE (Systemic); Diazoxide; Herbs (Hypotensive Properties); Licorice; MAO Inhibitors; Methotrexate; Pentoxifylline; Phosphodiesterase 5 Inhibitors; Probenecid; Prostacyclin Analogues

Decreased Effect

Bumetanide may decrease the levels/effects of: Lithium; Neuromuscular-Blocking Agents

The levels/effects of Bumetanide may be decreased by: Bile Acid Sequestrants; Fosphenytoin; Herbs (Hypertensive Properties); Methotrexate; Methylphenidate; Phenytoin; Probenecid; Salicylates; Yohimbine

Ethanol/Nutrition/Herb Interactions

Food: Bumetanide serum levels may be decreased if taken with food. It has been recommended that bumetanide be administered without food (Bard, 2004).

Herb/Nutraceutical: Avoid ephedra, yohimbe, ginseng (may worsen hypertension). Avoid dong quai if using for hypertension (has estrogenic activity). Avoid garlic (may have increased antihypertensive effect).

Stability

I.V.: Store vials at 15°C to 30°C (59°F to 86°F). Infusion solutions should be used within 24 hours after preparation. Light sensitive; discoloration may occur when exposed to light.

Tablet: Store at 15°C to 30°C (59°F to 86°F).

Mechanism of Action Inhibits reabsorption of sodium and chloride in the ascending loop of Henle and proximal renal tubule, interfering with the chloride-binding cotransport system, thus causing increased excretion of water, sodium, chloride, magnesium, phosphate, and calcium; it does not appear to act on the distal tubule

Pharmacodynamics/Kinetics

Onset of action: Oral, I.M.: 0.5-1 hour; I.V.: 2-3 minutes

Peak effect: Oral: 1-2 hours; I.V.: 15-30 minutes

Duration: 4-6 hours

Distribution: V_d: Adults: 9-25 L

Protein binding: 94% to 96%

Metabolism: Partially hepatic

Bioavailability: 59% to 89% (median: 80%)

Half-life elimination: Adults: 1-1.5 hours

Excretion: Urine (81% of total dose; 45% of which is unchanged drug); feces (2% of total dose)

Dosage

Geriatric & Adult

Edema:

Oral: 0.5-2 mg/dose 1-2 times/day; if diuretic response to initial dose is not adequate, may repeat in 4-5 hours for up to 2 doses (maximum dose: 10 mg/day)

I.M., I.V.: 0.5-1 mg/dose; if diuretic response to initial dose is not adequate, may repeat in 2-3 hours for up to 2 doses (maximum dose: 10 mg/day)

Continuous I.V. infusion (unlabeled dose): Initial: 1 mg I.V. load then 0.5-2 mg/hour (Hunt, 2009)

Hypertension (unlabeled use): Oral: 0.5 mg daily (maximum dose: 5 mg/day); usual dosage range (JNC 7): 0.5-2 mg/day in 2 divided doses (Chobanian, 2003)

Administration

I.V.: Administer slowly, over 1-2 minutes.

Oral: An alternate-day schedule or a 3-4 daily dosing regimen with rest periods of 1-2 days in between may be the most tolerable and effective regimen for the continued control of edema.

Monitoring Parameters Blood pressure; serum electrolytes, renal function; fluid status (weight and I & O), blood pressure

Pharmacotherapy Pearls Can be used in furosemide-allergic patients; 1 mg = 40 mg furosemide. Administer I.V. slowly, over 1-2 minutes.

Special Geriatric Considerations Loop diuretics are potent diuretics; excess amounts can lead to profound diuresis with fluid and electrolyte loss; close medical supervision and dose evaluation is required, particularly in the elderly. Severe loss of sodium and/or increases in BUN can cause confusion; for any change in mental status in patients on bumetanide, monitor electrolytes and renal function.

Dosage Forms Excipient information presented when available (limited, particularly for generics); consult specific product labeling.

Injection, solution: 0.25 mg/mL (2 mL, 4 mL, 10 mL)

Tablet, oral: 0.5 mg, 1 mg, 2 mg

◆ **Bumex** see Bumetanide on page 223

◆ **Buprenex®** see Buprenorphine on page 225

Buprenorphine (byoo pre NOR feen)

Related Information
Opioid Analgesics on page 2013

Medication Safety Issues
Sound-alike/look-alike issues:
Buprenex® may be confused with Brevibloc®, Bumex®

High alert medication:
The Institute for Safe Medication Practices (ISMP) includes this medication among its list of drug classes which have a heightened risk of causing significant patient harm when used in error.

Brand Names: U.S. Buprenex®; Butrans™; Subutex®

Brand Names: Canada Buprenex®; Subutex®

Index Terms Buprenorphine Hydrochloride

Generic Availability (U.S.) Yes; Excludes patch

Pharmacologic Category Analgesic, Opioid; Analgesic, Opioid Partial Agonist

Use
Injection: Management of moderate-to-severe pain
Sublingual tablet: Treatment of opioid dependence
Transdermal patch: Management of moderate-to-severe chronic pain in patients requiring an around-the-clock opioid analgesic for an extended period of time

Unlabeled/Investigational Use Injection: Management of opioid withdrawal in heroin-dependent hospitalized patients

Prescribing and Access Restrictions Prescribing of tablets for opioid dependence is limited to physicians who have met the qualification criteria and have received a DEA number specific to prescribing this product. Tablets will be available through pharmacies and wholesalers which normally provide controlled substances.

Medication Guide Available Yes

Contraindications Hypersensitivity to buprenorphine or any component of the formulation

Transdermal patch: Additional contraindications: Significant respiratory depression; severe asthma; known or suspected paralytic ileus; management of mild, acute, or intermittent pain; management of pain requiring short-term opioid analgesia; management of postoperative pain

Warnings/Precautions An opioid-containing analgesic regimen should be tailored to each patient's needs and based upon the type of pain being treated (acute versus chronic), the route of administration, degree of tolerance for opioids (naive versus chronic user), age, weight, and medical condition. The optimal analgesic dose varies widely among patients. Doses should be titrated to pain relief/prevention.

May cause CNS depression, which may impair physical or mental abilities. Effects with other sedative drugs or ethanol may be potentiated. Elderly may be more sensitive to CNS depressant and constipating effects. May cause respiratory depression - use caution in patients with respiratory disease or pre-existing respiratory depression. Hypersensitivity reactions, including bronchospasm, angioneurotic edema, and anaphylactic shock, have also been reported. Potential for drug dependency exists, abrupt cessation may precipitate withdrawal. Use caution in elderly, debilitated, depression or suicidal tendencies. Tolerance, psychological and physical dependence may occur with prolonged use. Partial antagonist activity may precipitate acute narcotic withdrawal in opioid-dependent individuals.

Hepatitis has been reported with buprenorphine use; hepatic events ranged from transient, asymptomatic transaminase elevations to hepatic failure; in many cases, patients had preexisting hepatic dysfunction. Monitor liver function tests in patients at increased risk for hepatotoxicity (eg, history of alcohol abuse, pre-existing hepatic dysfunction, I.V. drug abusers) prior to and during therapy. Use with caution in patients with hepatic impairment; dosage adjustments are recommended in hepatic impairment.

Use with caution in patients with pulmonary or renal function impairment. Also use caution in patients with head injury or increased ICP, biliary tract dysfunction, patients with history of hyperthyroidism, morbid obesity, adrenal insufficiency, prostatic hyperplasia, urinary stricture, CNS depression, toxic psychosis, pancreatitis, alcoholism, delirium tremens, or kyphoscoliosis. May cause hypotension; use with caution in patients with hypovolemia, cardiovascular disease (including acute MI), or drugs which may exaggerate hypotensive effects (including phenothiazines or general anesthetics). May obscure diagnosis or clinical course of patients with acute abdominal conditions. Opioid therapy may lower seizure threshold; use caution in patients with a history of seizure disorders.

Transdermal patch: **[U.S. Boxed Warning]: Do not exceed one 20 mcg/hour transdermal patch due to the risk of QT$_c$-interval prolongation.** Avoid using in patients with history of long QT syndrome or in patients with predisposing factors increasing the risk of QT abnormalities (eg, concurrent medications such as antiarrhythmics, hypokalemia, unstable heart failure, unstable atrial fibrillation). **[U.S. Boxed Warning]: Healthcare provider should be alert to problems of abuse, misuse, and diversion.**

Sublingual tablets, which are used for induction treatment of opioid dependence, should not be started until effects of withdrawal are evident.

Adverse Reactions (Reflective of adult population; not specific for elderly)

Injection:
>10%: Central nervous system: Sedation
1% to 10%:
    Cardiovascular: Hypotension
    Central nervous system: Respiratory depression, dizziness, headache
    Gastrointestinal: Vomiting, nausea
    Ocular: Miosis
    Otic: Vertigo
    Miscellaneous: Diaphoresis

Tablet:
>10%:
    Central nervous system: Headache (30%), pain (24%), insomnia (21% to 25%), anxiety (12%), depression (11%)
    Gastrointestinal: Nausea (10% to 14%), abdominal pain (12%), constipation (8% to 11%)
    Neuromuscular & skeletal: Back pain (14%), weakness (14%)
    Respiratory: Rhinitis (11%)
    Miscellaneous: Withdrawal syndrome (19%; placebo 37%), infection (12% to 20%), diaphoresis (12% to 13%)
1% to 10%:
    Central nervous system: Chills (6%), nervousness (6%), somnolence (5%), dizziness (4%), fever (3%)
    Gastrointestinal: Vomiting (5% to 8%), diarrhea (5%), dyspepsia (3%)
    Ocular: Lacrimation (5%)
    Respiratory: Cough (4%), pharyngitis (4%)
    Miscellaneous: Flu-like syndrome (6%)

Transdermal patch:
>10%:
    Central nervous system: Headache (16%), dizziness (16%), somnolence (14%),
    Gastrointestinal: Nausea (23%), constipation (14%), vomiting (11%)
    Local: Application site pruritus (15%)
1% to 10%:
    Cardiovascular: Peripheral edema (7%), chest pain, hypertension
    Central nervous system: Fatigue (5%), insomnia (3%), hypoesthesia (2%), anxiety, depression, fever, migraine
    Dermatologic: Pruritus (4%), rash (2%)
    Gastrointestinal: Xerostomia (7%), diarrhea (3%), abdominal discomfort (2%), anorexia (2%), upper abdominal pain
    Genitourinary: Urinary tract infection (3%)
    Local: Application site erythema (7%); application site rash (6%), application site irritation
    Neuromuscular & skeletal: Pain in extremity (3%), back pain (3%), joint swelling (3%), paresthesia (2%), tremor (2%), muscles spasms, musculoskeletal pain, myalgia, neck pain, weakness
    Respiratory: Dyspnea (3%), bronchitis, cough, nasopharyngitis, pharyngolaryngeal pain, sinusitis, upper respiratory tract infection
    Miscellaneous: Hyperhidrosis (4%), fall (4%), flu-like syndrome

Drug Interactions

Metabolism/Transport Effects Substrate of CYP3A4 (major); **Inhibits** CYP1A2 (weak), 2A6 (weak), 2C19 (weak), 2D6 (weak)

Avoid Concomitant Use
Avoid concomitant use of Buprenorphine with any of the following: Atazanavir; Conivaptan; MAO Inhibitors

Increased Effect/Toxicity
Buprenorphine may increase the levels/effects of: Alcohol (Ethyl); Alvimopan; CNS Depressants; Desmopressin; MAO Inhibitors; Selective Serotonin Reuptake Inhibitors; Thiazide Diuretics

The levels/effects of Buprenorphine may be increased by: Amphetamines; Antipsychotic Agents (Phenothiazines); Atazanavir; Boceprevir; Conivaptan; CYP3A4 Inhibitors (Moderate); CYP3A4 Inhibitors (Strong); Dasatinib; Droperidol; HydrOXYzine; Succinylcholine

Decreased Effect

Buprenorphine may decrease the levels/effects of: Analgesics (Opioid); Atazanavir; Pegvisomant

The levels/effects of Buprenorphine may be decreased by: Ammonium Chloride; Boceprevir; CYP3A4 Inducers (Strong); Deferasirox; Efavirenz; Herbs (CYP3A4 Inducers); Mixed Agonist / Antagonist Opioids; Tocilizumab

Ethanol/Nutrition/Herb Interactions

Ethanol: May increase CNS depression; monitor for increased effects with coadministration. Caution patients about effect.

Herb/Nutraceutical: Avoid valerian, St John's wort, kava kava, gotu kola (may increase CNS depression).

Stability

Injection: Protect from excessive heat >40°C (>104°F). Protect from light.

Patch, tablet: Store at room temperature of 25°C (77°F).

Mechanism of Action Buprenorphine exerts its analgesic effect via high affinity binding to μ opiate receptors in the CNS; displays partial mu agonist and weak kappa antagonist activity

Pharmacodynamics/Kinetics

Onset of action: Analgesic: I.M: Within 15 minutes

Peak effect: I.M.: ~1 hour; Transdermal patch: Steady state achieved by day 3

Duration: I.M.: ≥6 hours

Absorption: I.M., SubQ: 30% to 40%

Distribution: V_d: 97-187 L/kg

Protein binding: High (~96%, primarily to alpha- and beta globulin)

Metabolism: Primarily hepatic via N-dealkylation by CYP3A4 to norbuprenorphine (active metabolite), and to a lesser extent via glucuronidation by UGT1A1 and 2B7 to buprenorphine 3-O-glucuronide; the major metabolite, norbuprenorphine, also undergoes glucuronidation via UGT1A3; extensive first-pass effect

Bioavailability (relative to I.V. administration): I.M.: 70%; Sublingual tablet: 29%; Transdermal patch: ~15%

Half-life elimination: I.V.: 2.2-3 hours; Apparent terminal half-life: Sublingual tablet: ~37 hours; Transdermal patch: ~26 hours. **Note:** Extended elimination half-life for sublingual administration may be due to depot effect (Kuhlman, 1996).

Time to peak, plasma: Sublingual: 30 minutes to 1 hour (Kuhlman, 1996)

Excretion: Feces (~70%); urine (27% to 30%)

Dosage

Geriatric

Acute pain (moderate-to-severe): I.M., slow I.V.: 0.15 mg every 6 hours; elderly patients are more likely to suffer from confusion and drowsiness compared to younger patients. **Long-term use is not recommended.**

Chronic pain (moderate-to-severe): Transdermal patch: No specific dosage adjustments required; use caution due to potential for increased risk of adverse events.

Adult

Acute pain (moderate-to-severe): Note: Long-term use is not recommended. The following recommendations are guidelines and do not represent the maximum doses that may be required in all patients. Doses should be titrated to pain relief/prevention. In high-risk patients (eg, elderly, debilitated, presence of respiratory disease) and/or concurrent CNS depressant use, reduce dose by one-half. Buprenorphine has an analgesic ceiling.

I.M.: Initial: Opiate-naive: 0.3 mg every 6-8 hours as needed; initial dose (up to 0.3 mg) may be repeated once in 30-60 minutes after the initial dose if needed; usual dosage range: 0.15-0.6 mg every 4-8 hours as needed

Slow I.V.: Initial: Opiate-naive: 0.3 mg every 6-8 hours as needed; initial dose (up to 0.3 mg) may be repeated once in 30-60 minutes after the initial dose if needed

Chronic pain (moderate-to-severe): Transdermal patch:

Opioid-naive patients: Initial: 5 mcg/hour applied once every 7 days

Opioid-experienced patients (conversion from other opioids to buprenorphine): Taper the current around-the-clock opioid for up to 7 days to ≤30 mg/day of oral morphine or equivalent before initiating therapy. Short-acting analgesics as needed may be continued until analgesia with transdermal buprenorphine is attained. There is a potential for buprenorphine to precipitate withdrawal in patients already receiving opioids.

Patients who were receiving daily dose of <30 mg of oral morphine equivalents: Initial: 5 mcg/hour applied once every 7 days

Patients who were receiving daily dose of 30-80 mg of oral morphine equivalents: Initial: 10 mcg/hour applied once every 7 days

Dose titration (opioid-naive or opioid-experienced patients): May increase dose, based on patient's supplemental short-acting analgesic requirements, with a minimum titration interval of 72 hours (maximum dose: 20 mcg/hour applied once every 7 days; risk for QT_c prolongation increases with doses ≥20 mcg/hour patch).

◀

Discontinuation of therapy: Taper dose gradually to prevent withdrawal; consider initiating immediate-release opioids, if needed.

Opiate withdrawal in heroin-dependent hospitalized patients (unlabeled use): I.V. infusion: 0.3-0.9 mg (diluted in 50-100 mL of NS) over 20-30 minutes every 6-12 hours (Welsh, 2002)

Opioid dependence: Sublingual tablet: **Note:** The combination product, buprenorphine and naloxone, is preferred therapy over buprenorphine monotherapy for induction treatment (and stabilization/maintenance treatment) for short-acting opioid dependence (U.S. Department of Health and Human Services, 2005).

Manufacturer's labeling:

Induction: Day 1: 8 mg; Day 2 and subsequent induction days: 16 mg; usual induction dosage range: 12-16 mg/day (induction usually accomplished over 3-4 days). Treatment should begin at least 4 hours after last use of heroin or other short-acting opioids, preferably when first signs of withdrawal appear. Titrating dose to clinical effectiveness should be done as rapidly as possible to prevent undue withdrawal symptoms and patient drop-out during the induction period. There is little controlled experience with induction in patients on methadone or other long-acting opioids; consult expert physician experienced with this procedure.

Maintenance: Target dose: 16 mg/day; in some patients 12 mg/day may be effective; patients should be switched to the buprenorphine/naloxone combination product for maintenance and unsupervised therapy

Hepatic Impairment

Injection, sublingual tablet: Use caution due to extensive hepatic metabolism; dosage adjustments recommended although no specific recommendations are provided by the manufacturer.

Transdermal patch:

Mild-to-moderate impairment: Initial: 5 mcg/hour applied once every 7 days.

Severe impairment: Not studied; consider alternative therapy with more flexibility for dosing adjustments.

Administration

I.M.: Administer via deep I.M. injection

I.V.: Administer slowly, over at least 2 minutes. Administration over 20-30 minutes preferred when managing opioid withdrawal in heroin-dependent hospitalized patients (Welsh, 2002).

Oral: Sublingual tablet: Tablet should be placed under the tongue until dissolved; should not be swallowed. If two or more tablets are needed per dose, all may be placed under the tongue at once, or two at a time. To ensure consistent bioavailability, subsequent doses should always be taken the same way.

Transdermal patch: Apply to patch to intact, nonirritated skin only. Apply to a hairless or nearly hairless skin site. If hairless site is not available, do not shave skin; hair at application site should be clipped. Prior to application, if the site must be cleaned, clean with clear water and allow to dry completely; do not use soaps, alcohol, lotions or abrasives due to potential for increased skin absorption. Do not use any patch that has been damaged, cut or manipulated in any way. Remove patch from protective pouch immediately before application. Remove the protective backing, and apply the sticky side of the patch to one of eight possible application sites (upper outer arm, upper chest, upper back or the side of the chest [on either side of the body]). Firmly press patch in place and hold for ~15 seconds. Change patch every 7 days. Rotate patch application sites; wait ≥21 days before reapplying another patch to the same skin site. Avoid exposing application site to external heat sources (eg, heating pad, electric blanket, heat lamp, hot tub). If there is difficulty with patch adhesion, the edges of the system may be taped in place with first-aid tape. If the patch falls off during the 7-day dosing interval, dispose of the patch and apply a new patch to a different skin site.

Monitoring Parameters Pain relief, respiratory and mental status, CNS depression, blood pressure; LFTs (prior to initiation and during therapy); symptoms of withdrawal; application site reactions (transdermal patch)

Special Geriatric Considerations One postmarketing study found that elderly patients were more likely to suffer from confusion and drowsiness after buprenorphine as compared to younger patients. Use transdermal system with caution in the elderly. Respiratory depression occurs more frequently in the elderly. In clinical trials, the incidence of adverse events was higher in older subjects.

Controlled Substance C-III

Dosage Forms Excipient information presented when available (limited, particularly for generics); consult specific product labeling.

Injection, solution: 0.3 mg/mL (1 mL)

Buprenex®: 0.3 mg/mL (1 mL)

Patch, transdermal:
Butrans™: 5 mcg/hr (4s) [total buprenorphine 5 mg]
Butrans™: 10 mcg/hr (4s) [total buprenorphine 10 mg]
Butrans™: 20 mcg/hr (4s) [total buprenorphine 25 mg]
Tablet, sublingual: 2 mg, 8 mg
Subutex®: 2 mg, 8 mg

Selected References

American Geriatrics Society Panel on Pharmacological Management of Persistent Pain in Older Persons, "Pharmaco-logical Management of Persistent Pain in Older Persons," *J Am Geriatr Soc*, 2009, 57(8):1331-46.

Harcus AH, Ward AE, and Smith DW, "Buprenorphine: Experience in an Elderly Population of 975 Patients During a Year's Monitored Release," *Br J Clin Pract*, 1980, 34(5):144-6.

◆ **Buprenorphine Hydrochloride** *see* Buprenorphine *on page 225*
◆ **Buproban®** *see* BuPROPion *on page 229*

BuPROPion (byoo PROE pee on)

Related Information

Antidepressant Agents *on page 1991*
Beers Criteria – Potentially Inappropriate Medications for Geriatrics *on page 2089*

Medication Safety Issues

Sound-alike/look-alike issues:
Aplenzin™ may be confused with Albenza®, Relenza®
BuPROPion may be confused with busPIRone
Wellbutrin SR® may be confused with Wellbutrin XL®
Wellbutrin XL® may be confused with Wellbutrin SR®
Zyban® may be confused with Zagam®, Diovan®

Brand Names: U.S. Aplenzin™; Budeprion SR®; Budeprion XL®; Buproban®; Wellbutrin SR®; Wellbutrin XL®; Wellbutrin®; Zyban®

Brand Names: Canada Bupropion SR®; Novo-Bupropion SR; PMS-Bupropion SR; ratio-Bupropion SR; Sandoz-Bupropion SR; Wellbutrin® SR; Wellbutrin® XL; Zyban®

Index Terms Bupropion Hydrobromide; Bupropion Hydrochloride

Generic Availability (U.S.) Yes: Excludes bupropion hydrobromide tablet, sustained release hydrochloride tablet

Pharmacologic Category Antidepressant, Dopamine-Reuptake Inhibitor; Smoking Cessation Aid

Use Treatment of major depressive disorder, including seasonal affective disorder (SAD); adjunct in smoking cessation

Unlabeled/Investigational Use Attention-deficit/hyperactivity disorder (ADHD); depression associated with bipolar disorder

Medication Guide Available Yes

Contraindications Hypersensitivity to bupropion or any component of the formulation; seizure disorder; history of anorexia/bulimia; use of MAO inhibitors within 14 days; patients undergoing abrupt discontinuation of ethanol or sedatives (including benzodiazepines); patients receiving other dosage forms of bupropion

Warnings/Precautions [U.S. Boxed Warning]: Use in treating psychiatric disorders: Antidepressants increase the risk of suicidal thinking and behavior in children, adolescents, and young adults (18-24 years of age) with major depressive disorder (MDD) and other psychiatric disorders; consider risk prior to prescribing. Short-term studies did not show an increased risk in patients >24 years of age and showed a decreased risk in patients ≥65 years. All patients must be closely monitored for clinical worsening, suicidality, or unusual changes in behavior, especially during the initiation of therapy (generally first 1-2 months) or following an increase or decrease in dosage. The patient's family or caregiver should be instructed to closely observe the patient and communicate condition with healthcare provider. A medication guide should be dispensed with each prescription. **Bupropion is not FDA approved for use in children.**

[U.S. Boxed Warning]: Use in smoking cessation: Serious neuropsychiatric events, including depression, suicidal thoughts, and suicide, have been reported with use; some cases may have been complicated by symptoms of nicotine withdrawal following smoking cessation. Smoking cessation (with or without treatment) is associated with nicotine withdrawal symptoms and the exacerbation of underlying psychiatric illness; however, some of the behavioral disturbances were reported in treated patients who continued to smoke. These neuropsychiatric symptoms (eg, mood disturbances, psychosis, hostility) have occurred in patients with and without pre-existing psychiatric disease; many cases resolved following therapy discontinuation although in some cases, symptoms persisted. Monitor all patients for behavioral changes and psychiatric symptoms (eg, agitation, depression, suicidal behavior, suicidal ideation); inform patients to discontinue treatment and contact their health-care provider immediately if they experience any behavioral and/or mood changes.

The possibility of a suicide attempt is inherent in major depression and may persist until remission occurs. Use caution in high-risk patients. Worsening depression and severe abrupt suicidality that are not part of the presenting symptoms may require discontinuation or modification of drug therapy. The patient's family or caregiver should be alerted to monitor patients for the emergence of suicidality and associated behaviors (such as agitation, irritability, hostility, impulsivity, and hypomania) and notify the healthcare provider.

May worsen psychosis in some patients or precipitate a shift to mania or hypomania in patients with bipolar disorder. Patients presenting with depressive symptoms should be screened for bipolar disorder. Monotherapy in patients with bipolar disorder should be avoided. **Bupropion is not FDA approved for bipolar depression.**

The risk of seizures is dose-dependent and increased in patients with a history of seizures, anorexia/bulimia, head trauma, CNS tumor, severe hepatic cirrhosis, abrupt discontinuation of sedative-hypnotics or ethanol, medications which lower seizure threshold (antipsychotics, antidepressants, theophyllines, systemic steroids), stimulants, or hypoglycemic agents. Risk of seizures may also be increased by chewing, crushing, or dividing long-acting products. Risk may be reduced by limiting the daily dose to bupropion hydrochloride ≤450 mg or bupropion hydrobromide 522 mg. Gradually increase dose incrementally to reduce risk. Discontinue and do not restart in patients experiencing a seizure.

May cause CNS stimulation (restlessness, anxiety, insomnia) or anorexia. May increase the risks associated with electroconvulsive therapy. Consider discontinuing, when possible, prior to elective surgery. May cause weight loss; use caution in patients where weight loss is not desirable. The incidence of sexual dysfunction with bupropion is generally lower than with SSRIs.

Use caution in patients with cardiovascular disease, history of hypertension, or coronary artery disease; treatment-emergent hypertension (including some severe cases) has been reported, both with bupropion alone and in combination with nicotine transdermal systems. Use with caution in patients with hepatic or renal dysfunction and in elderly patients; reduced dose and/or frequency may be recommended. Elderly patients may be at greater risk of accumulation during chronic dosing. May cause motor or cognitive impairment in some patients; use with caution if tasks requiring alertness such as operating machinery or driving are undertaken. Arthralgia, myalgia, and fever with rash and other symptoms suggestive of delayed hypersensitivity resembling serum sickness have been reported.

Extended release tablet: Insoluble tablet shell may remain intact and be visible in the stool.
Adverse Reactions (Reflective of adult population; not specific for elderly) Frequencies, when reported, reflect highest incidence reported with sustained release product.

>10%:
Cardiovascular: Tachycardia (11%)
Central nervous system: Headache (25% to 34%), insomnia (11% to 20%), dizziness (6% to 11%)
Gastrointestinal: Xerostomia (17% to 26%), weight loss (14% to 23%), nausea (1% to 18%)
Respiratory: Pharyngitis (3% to 13%)
1% to 10%:
Cardiovascular: Palpitation (2% to 6%), arrhythmias (5%), chest pain (3% to 4%), hypertension (2% to 4%; may be severe), flushing (1% to 4%), hypotension (3%)
Central nervous system: Agitation (2% to 9%), confusion (8%), anxiety (5% to 7%), hostility (6%), nervousness (3% to 5%), sleep disturbance (4%), sensory disturbance (4%), migraine (1% to 4%), abnormal dreams (4%), irritability (2% to 3%), somnolence (2% to 3%), pain (2% to 3%), memory decreased (≤3%), fever (1% to 2%), CNS stimulation (1% to 2%), depression
Dermatologic: Rash (1% to 5%), pruritus (2% to 4%), urticaria (1% to 2%)
Endocrine & metabolic: Menstrual complaints (2% to 5%), hot flashes (1% to 3%), libido decreased (3%)
Gastrointestinal: Constipation (5% to 10%), abdominal pain (2% to 9%), diarrhea (5% to 7%), flatulence (6%), anorexia (3% to 5%), appetite increased (4%), taste perversion (2% to 4%), vomiting (2% to 4%), dyspepsia (3%), dysphagia (≤2%)
Genitourinary: Polyuria (2% to 5%), urinary urgency (≤2%), vaginal hemorrhage (≤2%), UTI (≤1%)
Neuromuscular & skeletal: Tremor (3% to 6%), myalgia (2% to 6%), weakness (2% to 4%), arthralgia (1% to 4%), arthritis (2%), akathisia (≤2%), paresthesia (1% to 2%), twitching (1% to 2%), neck pain
Ocular: Blurred vision (2% to 3%), amblyopia (2%)
Otic: Tinnitus (3% to 6%), auditory disturbance (5%)

Respiratory: Upper respiratory infection (9%), cough increased (1% to 4%), sinusitis (1% to 5%)

Miscellaneous: Infection (8% to 9%), diaphoresis (5% to 6%), allergic reaction (including anaphylaxis, pruritus, urticaria)

Drug Interactions

Metabolism/Transport Effects Substrate of CYP1A2 (minor), 2A6 (minor), 2B6 (major), 2C9 (minor), 2D6 (minor), 2E1 (minor), 3A4 (minor); **Inhibits** CYP2D6 (strong)

Avoid Concomitant Use

Avoid concomitant use of BuPROPion with any of the following: MAO Inhibitors; Methylene Blue; Tamoxifen; Thioridazine

Increased Effect/Toxicity

BuPROPion may increase the levels/effects of: Alcohol (Ethyl); Atomoxetine; CYP2D6 Substrates; Fesoterodine; Iloperidone; Methylene Blue; Nebivolol; Tamoxifen; Tetrabenazine; Thioridazine; Tricyclic Antidepressants

The levels/effects of BuPROPion may be increased by: Alcohol (Ethyl); Conivaptan; CYP2B6 Inhibitors (Moderate); CYP2B6 Inhibitors (Strong); MAO Inhibitors; Quazepam

Decreased Effect

BuPROPion may decrease the levels/effects of: Codeine; Iloperidone; TraMADol

The levels/effects of BuPROPion may be decreased by: CYP2B6 Inducers (Strong); Cyproterone; Efavirenz; Lopinavir; Peginterferon Alfa-2b; Ritonavir; Tocilizumab

Ethanol/Nutrition/Herb Interactions

Ethanol: May increase CNS depression; monitor for increased effects with coadministration. Caution about effects.

Herb/Nutraceutical: Avoid valerian, St John's wort, SAMe, gotu kola, kava kava (may increase CNS depression).

Stability Store at controlled room temperature of 20°C to 25°C (68°F to 77°F).

Aplenzin™, Wellbutrin XL®: Store at 15°C to 30°C (59°F to 86°F).

Mechanism of Action Aminoketone antidepressant structurally different from all other marketed antidepressants; like other antidepressants the mechanism of bupropion's activity is not fully understood. Bupropion is a relatively weak inhibitor of the neuronal uptake of norepinephrine and dopamine, and does not inhibit monoamine oxidase or the reuptake of serotonin. Metabolite inhibits the reuptake of norepinephrine. The primary mechanism of action is thought to be dopaminergic and/or noradrenergic.

Pharmacodynamics/Kinetics

Absorption: Rapid

Distribution: V_d: ~20-47 L/kg (Laizure, 1985)

Protein binding: 84%

Metabolism: Extensively hepatic via CYP2B6 to hydroxybupropion; non-CYP-mediated metabolism to erythrohydrobupropion and threohydrobupropion. Metabolite activity ranges from 20% to 50% potency of bupropion.

Half-life:

Distribution: 3-4 hours

Elimination: 21 ± 9 hours; Metabolites: Hydroxybupropion: 20 ± 5 hours; Erythrohydrobupropion: 33 ± 10 hours; Threohydrobupropion: 37 ± 13 hours

Extended release (Aplenzin™): 21 ± 7 hours; Metabolites: Hydroxybupropion: 24 ± 5 hours; Erythrohydrobupropion: 31 ± 8 hours; Threohydrobupropion: 51 ± 9 hours

Time to peak, serum:

Bupropion: Immediate release: Within 2 hours; Sustained release: Within 3 hours; Extended release: ~5 hours

Metabolite: Hydroxybupropion: Immediate release: ~3 hours; Extended release, sustained release: ~6-7 hours

Excretion: Urine (87%, primarily as metabolites); feces (10%, primarily as metabolites)

Dosage

Geriatric

Depression: Oral (hydrochloride salt): Initial: 37.5 mg of immediate release tablets twice daily or 100 mg/day of sustained release tablets; increase by 37.5-100 mg every 3-4 days as tolerated. There is evidence that the elderly respond at 150 mg/day in divided doses, but some may require a higher dose. **Note:** Patients with Alzheimer's dementia-related depression may require a lower starting dosage of 37.5 mg once or twice daily (100 mg/day sustained release), increased as needed up to 300 mg/day in divided doses (300 mg/day for sustained release)

Smoking cessation: Refer to adult dosing.

Adult

Depression: Oral:

Immediate release hydrochloride salt: 100 mg 3 times/day; begin at 100 mg twice daily; may increase to a maximum dose of 450 mg/day

Sustained release hydrochloride salt: Initial: 150 mg/day in the morning; may increase to 150 mg twice daily by day 4 if tolerated; target dose: 300 mg/day given as 150 mg twice daily; maximum dose: 400 mg/day given as 200 mg twice daily

Extended release:

Hydrochloride salt: Initial: 150 mg/day in the morning; may increase as early as day 4 of dosing to 300 mg/day; maximum dose: 450 mg/day

Hydrobromide salt (Aplenzin™): Target dose: 348 mg/day in the morning. Patients not previously on bupropion: Initial: 174 mg/day in the morning; may increase as early as day 4 of dosing to 348 mg/day; maximum dose: 522 mg/day. **Note:** 174 mg strength not currently available; 348 mg tablet cannot be split.

Switching from hydrochloride salt formulation (eg, Wellbutrin® immediate release, SR®, XL®) to hydrobromide salt formulation (Aplenzin™): **Note:** Patients being treated twice daily with bupropion hydrochloride would be switched to the equivalent once daily dose of bupropion hydrobromide.

Bupropion hydrochloride 150 mg is equivalent to bupropion hydrobromide 174 mg

Bupropion hydrochloride 300 mg is equivalent to bupropion hydrobromide 348 mg

Bupropion hydrochloride 450 mg is equivalent to bupropion hydrobromide 522 mg

SAD (Wellbutrin XL®): Oral: Initial: 150 mg/day in the morning; if tolerated, may increase after 1 week to 300 mg/day

Note: Prophylactic treatment should be reserved for those patients with frequent depressive episodes and/or significant impairment. Initiate treatment in the Autumn prior to symptom onset, and discontinue in early Spring with dose tapering to 150 mg/day for 2 weeks

Smoking cessation (Zyban®): Oral: Initiate with 150 mg once daily for 3 days; increase to 150 mg twice daily; treatment should continue for 7-12 weeks

Note: Therapy should begin at least 1 week before target quit date. Target quit dates are generally in the second week of treatment. If patient successfully quits smoking after 7-12 weeks, may consider ongoing maintenance therapy based on individual patient risk: benefit. Efficacy of maintenance therapy (300 mg/day) has been demonstrated for up to 6 months. Conversely, if significant progress has not been made by the seventh week of therapy, success is unlikely and treatment discontinuation should be considered.

Dosing conversion between hydrochloride salt (eg, Wellbutrin®) immediate, sustained, and extended release products: Convert using same total daily dose (up to the maximum recommended dose for a given dosage form), but adjust frequency as indicated for sustained (twice daily) or extended (once daily) release products.

Renal Impairment Use with caution and consider a reduction in dosing frequency; limited pharmacokinetic information suggests elimination of bupropion and/or the active metabolites may be reduced.

Moderate-to-severe renal impairment: Bupropion exposure was approximately twofold higher compared to normal subjects following a 150 mg single dose administration.

End-stage renal failure: Per the manufacturer, the elimination of hydroxybupropion and threohydrobupropion are reduced in patients with end-stage renal failure.

Hepatic Impairment

Mild-to-moderate hepatic impairment: Use with caution and/or reduced dose/frequency

Severe hepatic cirrhosis: Use with extreme caution; maximum dose:

Aplenzin™: 174 mg every other day

Wellbutrin®: 75 mg/day;

Wellbutrin SR®: 100 mg/day or 150 mg every other day

Wellbutrin XL®: 150 mg every other day

Zyban®: 150 mg every other day

Note: The mean AUC increased by ~1.5-fold for hydroxybupropion and ~2.5-fold for erythro/threohydrobupropion; median T_{max} was observed 19 hours later for hydroxybupropion, 31 hours later for erythro/threohydrobupropion; mean half-life for hydroxybupropion increased fivefold, and increased twofold for erythro/threohydrobupropion in patients with severe hepatic cirrhosis compared to healthy volunteers.

Administration May be taken without regard to meals. Zyban® and extended release tablets (hydrochloride and hydrobromide salt formulations) should be swallowed whole; do not crush, chew, or divide. The insoluble shell of the extended-release tablet may remain intact during GI transit and is eliminated in the feces. Data from the manufacturer states that dividing Wellbutrin SR® tablets resulted in an increased rate of release at 15 minutes: "However, the divided tablet retained its sustained-release characteristics with similar increases of released bupropion at each sampling point beyond 15 minutes when compared to the intact Wellbutrin SR® tablet..." Bupropion is hygroscopic and therefore should be stored in a dry place. Splitting of large quantities in advance of administration is not advised since loss of potency may result. If necessary, splitting should be done cleanly without crushing.

Monitoring Parameters Body weight; mental status for depression, suicidal ideation (especially at the beginning of therapy or when doses are increased or decreased), anxiety, social functioning, mania, panic attacks

Reference Range Therapeutic levels (trough, 12 hours after last dose): 50-100 ng/mL

Test Interactions May interfere with urine detection of amphetamine/methamphetamine (false-positive). Decreased prolactin levels.

Pharmacotherapy Pearls Risk of seizures: When using bupropion hydrochloride immediate release tablets, seizure risk is increased at total daily dosage >450 mg, individual dosages >150 mg, or by sudden, large increments in dose. Data for the immediate-release formulation of bupropion revealed a seizure incidence of 0.4% in patients treated at doses in the 300-450 mg/day range. The estimated seizure incidence increases almost 10-fold between 450 mg and 600 mg per day. Data for the sustained release dosage form revealed a seizure incidence of 0.1% in patients treated at a dosage range of 100-300 mg/day, and increases to ~0.4% at the maximum recommended dose of 400 mg/day.

Special Geriatric Considerations Studies have found bupropion effective as an antidepressant for older persons with major depressive disorder and as effective as paroxetine and imipramine. Its side effect profile (minimal anticholinergic and blood pressure effects) is favorable and makes it an alternative to other first-line antidepressants. A single- and multiple-dose pharmacokinetic study suggested that accumulation of bupropion and its metabolites may occur in the elderly.

Dosage Forms Excipient information presented when available (limited, particularly for generics); consult specific product labeling.
Tablet, oral, as hydrochloride: 75 mg [generic for Wellbutrin®], 100 mg [generic for Wellbutrin®]
    Wellbutrin®: 75 mg, 100 mg
Tablet, extended release, oral, as hydrobromide:
    Aplenzin™: 174 mg, 348 mg, 522 mg
Tablet, extended release, oral, as hydrochloride: 100 mg [generic for Wellbutrin SR®], 150 mg [generic for Wellbutrin SR®], 150 mg [generic for Wellbutrin XL®], 150 mg [generic for Zyban®], 200 mg [generic for Wellbutrin SR®], 300 mg [generic for Wellbutrin XL®]
    Budeprion SR®: 100 mg [contains tartrazine; generic for Wellbutrin SR®]
    Budeprion SR®: 150 mg [generic for Wellbutrin SR®]
    Budeprion XL®: 150 mg [generic for Wellbutrin XL®]
    Budeprion XL®: 300 mg [contains tartrazine; generic for Wellbutrin XL®]
    Buproban®: 150 mg [generic for Zyban®]
    Wellbutrin XL®: 150 mg, 300 mg
Tablet, sustained release, oral, as hydrochloride:
    Wellbutrin SR®: 100 mg, 150 mg, 200 mg
    Zyban®: 150 mg

Selected References

Branconnier RJ, Cole JO, Ghazvinian S, et al, "Clinical Pharmacology of Bupropion and Imipramine in Elderly Depressives," *J Clin Psychiatry*, 1983, 44(5 Pt 2):130-3.
Fiore M, Jaen CR, Baker TB, et al, "A Clinical Practice Guideline for Treating Tobacco Use and Dependence: 2008 Update. A U.S. Public Health Service Report," *Am J Prev Med*, 2008, 35(2):158-76.
Weihs KL, Settle EC Jr, Batey SR, et al, "Bupropion Sustained Release Versus Paroxetine for the Treatment of Depression in the Elderly," *J Clin Psychiatry*, 2000, 61(3):196-202.

◆ **Bupropion Hydrobromide** *see* BuPROPion *on page 229*
◆ **Bupropion Hydrochloride** *see* BuPROPion *on page 229*
◆ **Burn Jel® [OTC]** *see* Lidocaine (Topical) *on page 1064*
◆ **Burn Jel Plus [OTC]** *see* Lidocaine (Topical) *on page 1064*
◆ **BuSpar** *see* BusPIRone *on page 233*

BusPIRone (byoo SPYE rone)

Medication Safety Issues
    Sound-alike/look-alike issues:
        BusPIRone may be confused with buPROPion

Brand Names: Canada Apo-Buspirone®; BuSpar®; Buspirex; Bustab®; CO Buspirone; Dom-Buspirone; Gen-Buspirone; Lin-Buspirone; Mylan-Buspirone; Novo-Buspirone; Nu-Buspirone; PMS-Buspirone; ratio-Buspirone; Riva-Buspirone

Index Terms BuSpar; Buspirone Hydrochloride

Generic Availability (U.S.) Yes

Pharmacologic Category Antianxiety Agent, Miscellaneous

Use Management of generalized anxiety disorder (GAD)

Unlabeled/Investigational Use Management of aggression in mental retardation and secondary mental disorders, major depression; potential augmenting agent for antidepressants

◀ **Contraindications** Hypersensitivity to buspirone or any component of the formulation

Warnings/Precautions Use in severe hepatic or renal impairment is not recommended; does not prevent or treat withdrawal from benzodiazepines. Low potential for cognitive or motor impairment. Use with MAO inhibitors may result in hypertensive reactions. Restlessness syndrome has been reported in small number of patients; monitor for signs of any dopamine-related movement disorders. Buspirone does not exhibit cross-tolerance with benzodiazepines or other sedative/hypnotic agents. If substituting buspirone for any of these agents, gradually withdraw the drug(s) prior to initiating buspirone.

Adverse Reactions (Reflective of adult population; not specific for elderly)

>10%: Central nervous system: Dizziness (12%)

1% to 10%:

Cardiovascular: Chest pain (≥1%)

Central nervous system: Drowsiness (10%), headache (6%), nervousness (5%), light-headedness (3%), anger/hostility (2%), confusion (2%), excitement (2%), dream disturbance (≥1%)

Dermatologic: Rash (1%)

Gastrointestinal: Nausea (8%), diarrhea (2%)

Neuromuscular & skeletal: Numbness (2%), weakness (2%), musculoskeletal pain (1%), paresthesia (1%), incoordination (1%), tremor (1%)

Ocular: Blurred vision (2%)

Otic: Tinnitus (≥1%)

Respiratory: Nasal congestion (≥1%), sore throat (≥1%)

Miscellaneous: Diaphoresis (1%)

Drug Interactions

Metabolism/Transport Effects Substrate of CYP2D6 (minor), 3A4 (major)

Avoid Concomitant Use

Avoid concomitant use of BusPIRone with any of the following: Conivaptan; MAO Inhibitors; Methylene Blue; Sibutramine

Increased Effect/Toxicity

BusPIRone may increase the levels/effects of: Alcohol (Ethyl); Antidepressants (Serotonin Reuptake Inhibitor/Antagonist); CNS Depressants; MAO Inhibitors; Methotrimeprazine; Methylene Blue; Selective Serotonin Reuptake Inhibitors; Serotonin Modulators

The levels/effects of BusPIRone may be increased by: Antifungal Agents (Azole Derivatives, Systemic); Calcium Channel Blockers (Nondihydropyridine); Conivaptan; CYP3A4 Inhibitors (Moderate); CYP3A4 Inhibitors (Strong); Dasatinib; Droperidol; Grapefruit Juice; HydrOX-Yzine; Macrolide Antibiotics; Methotrimeprazine; Selective Serotonin Reuptake Inhibitors; Sibutramine

Decreased Effect

The levels/effects of BusPIRone may be decreased by: CYP3A4 Inducers (Strong); Deferasirox; Peginterferon Alfa-2b; Rifamycin Derivatives; Tocilizumab; Yohimbine

Ethanol/Nutrition/Herb Interactions

Ethanol: May increase CNS depression; monitor for increased effects with coadministration. Caution patients about effects.

Food: Food may decrease the absorption of buspirone, but it may also decrease the first-pass metabolism, thereby increasing the bioavailability of buspirone. Grapefruit juice may cause increased buspirone concentrations; avoid intake of large quantities of grapefruit juice.

Herb/Nutraceutical: St John's wort may decrease buspirone levels or increase CNS depression. Avoid valerian, gotu kola, kava kava (may increase CNS depression).

Stability Store at USP controlled room temperature of 25°C (77°F). Protect from light.

Mechanism of Action The mechanism of action of buspirone is unknown. Buspirone has a high affinity for serotonin 5-HT$_{1A}$ and 5-HT$_2$ receptors, without affecting benzodiazepine-GABA receptors. Buspirone has moderate affinity for dopamine D$_2$ receptors.

Pharmacodynamics/Kinetics

Absorption: Rapid

Distribution: V$_d$: 5.3 L/kg

Protein binding: 86% to 95%

Metabolism: Hepatic oxidation, primarily via CYP3A4; extensive first-pass effect

Bioavailability: ~4%

Half-life elimination: 2-3 hours

Time to peak, serum: 40-90 minutes

Excretion: Urine: 29% to 63% (<0.1% dose excreted unchanged); feces: 18% to 38%

Dosage

Geriatric Oral: Initial: 5 mg twice daily, increase by 5 mg/day every 2-3 days as needed up to 20-30 mg/day; maximum daily dose: 60 mg/day

Adult Anxiety disorders (GAD): Oral: 15 mg/day (7.5 mg twice daily); may increase in increments of 5 mg/day every 2-3 days to a maximum of 60 mg/day. Target dose for most people is 20-30 mg/day (10-15 mg twice daily).

Renal Impairment Patients with impaired renal function demonstrated increased plasma levels and a prolonged half-life of buspirone. Use in patients with severe renal impairment not recommended.

Hepatic Impairment Patients with impaired hepatic function demonstrated increased plasma levels and a prolonged half-life of buspirone. Use in patients with severe hepatic impairment not recommended.

Monitoring Parameters Mental status, symptoms of anxiety

Pharmacotherapy Pearls Has shown little potential for abuse; not effective when used prn; maximal effect may not be achieved until 3-4 weeks after adequate dose is achieved. Some response may be seen in 1-2 weeks after initiation of therapy. Buspirone, in the treatment of agitation, has been shown to be effective in older adults at an average daily dose of 30-35 mg; slow titration, as described in Dosage, is necessary to avoid side effects and achieve maximum tolerable doses for individual patients.

Special Geriatric Considerations Because buspirone is less sedating than other anxiolytics, it may be a useful agent in geriatric patients when an anxiolytic is indicated.

Dosage Forms Excipient information presented when available (limited, particularly for generics); consult specific product labeling.

Tablet, oral, as hydrochloride: 5 mg, 7.5 mg, 10 mg, 15 mg, 30 mg

Selected References

Gammans RE, Westrick ML, Shea JP, et al, "Pharmacokinetics of Buspirone in Elderly Subjects," *J Clin Pharmacol*, 1989, 29(1):72-8.

♦ **Buspirone Hydrochloride** see BusPIRone on page 233
♦ **Bussulfam** see Busulfan on page 235

Busulfan (byoo SUL fan)

Medication Safety Issues

Sound-alike/look-alike issues:

Busulfan may be confused with Butalan®

Myleran® may be confused with Alkeran®, Leukeran®, melphalan, Mylicon®

High alert medication:

This medication is in a class the Institute for Safe Medication Practices (ISMP) includes among its list of drug classes which have a heightened risk of causing significant patient harm when used in error.

Brand Names: U.S. Busulfex®; Myleran®

Brand Names: Canada Busulfex®; Myleran®

Index Terms Bussulfam; Busulfanum; Busulphan

Generic Availability (U.S.) No

Pharmacologic Category Antineoplastic Agent, Alkylating Agent

Use

Oral: Chronic myelogenous leukemia (CML); conditioning regimens for bone marrow transplantation

I.V.: Combination therapy with cyclophosphamide as a conditioning regimen prior to allogeneic hematopoietic progenitor cell transplantation for chronic myelogenous leukemia

Unlabeled/Investigational Use Oral: Bone marrow disorders, such as polycythemia vera and myeloid metaplasia; thrombocytosis

Contraindications Hypersensitivity to busulfan or any component of the formulation; oral busulfan is contraindicated in patients without a definitive diagnosis of CML

Warnings/Precautions Hazardous agent - use appropriate precautions for handling and disposal. **[U.S. Boxed Warning]: May induce severe bone marrow suppression.** May result in severe neutropenia, thrombocytopenia and/or anemia. Seizures have been reported with use; use caution in patients predisposed to seizures; initiate prophylactic anticonvulsant therapy (eg, phenytoin) prior to treatment; use caution with history of seizures or head trauma. May cause delayed pulmonary toxicity (known as "busulfan lung" - bronchopulmonary dysplasia with pulmonary fibrosis); the average onset is 4 years (range: 4 months to 10 years). Busulfan has been causally related to the development of secondary malignancies (tumors and acute leukemias). Busulfan has been associated with ovarian failure (including failure to achieve puberty).

High busulfan area under the concentration versus time curve (AUC) values (>1500 µM/minute) are associated with increased risk of hepatic veno-occlusive disease during conditioning for allogenic BMT; patients with of history of radiation therapy, prior chemotherapy (≥3 cycles) and prior stem cell transplantation are at increased risk. Oral busulfan doses above 16 mg/kg (based on IBW) and concurrent use with alkylating agents may also increase ▶

◄ the risk for hepatic VOD. The solvent in I.V. busulfan, DMA, may impair fertility. DMA may also be associated with hepatotoxicity, hallucinations, somnolence, lethargy, and confusion. **[U.S. Boxed Warning]: Should be administered under the supervision of an experienced cancer chemotherapy physician.**

Adverse Reactions (Reflective of adult population; not specific for elderly)

I.V.:

>10%:

Cardiovascular: Tachycardia (44%), hypertension (36%; grades 3/4: 7%), edema (28% to 79%), thrombosis (33%), chest pain (26%), vasodilation (25%), hypotension (11%; grades 3/4: 3%)

Central nervous system: Insomnia (84%), fever (80%), anxiety (72% to 75%), headache (69%), chills (46%), pain (44%), dizziness (30%), depression (23%), confusion (11%)

Dermatologic: Rash (57%), pruritus (28%), alopecia (2% to 15%)

Endocrine & metabolic: Hypomagnesemia (77%), hyperglycemia (66%; grades 3/4: 15%), hypokalemia (64%), hypocalcemia (49%), hypophosphatemia (17%)

Gastrointestinal: Nausea (98%), mucositis/stomatitis (97%; grades 3/4: 26%), vomiting (43% to 95%), anorexia (85%), diarrhea (84%; grades 3/4: 5%), abdominal pain (72%), dyspepsia (44%), constipation (38%), xerostomia (26%), rectal disorder (25%), abdominal fullness (23%)

Hematologic: Myelosuppression (≤100%), neutropenia (100%; median recovery: 13 days), thrombocytopenia (98%; median onset: 5-6 days), lymphopenia (children: 79%), anemia (69%)

Hepatic: Hyperbilirubinemia (49%; grades 3/4: 30%), ALT increased (31%; grades 3/4: 7%), hepatic sinusoidal obstruction syndrome (SOS; veno-occlusive disease) (adults: 8% to 12%; children: 21%), jaundice (12%)

Local: Injection site inflammation (25%), injection site pain (15%)

Neuromuscular & skeletal: Weakness (51%), back pain (23%), myalgia (16%), arthralgia (13%)

Renal: Creatinine increased (21%), oliguria (15%)

Respiratory: Rhinitis (44%), lung disorder (34%), cough (28%), epistaxis (25%), dyspnea (25%), pneumonia (children: 21%), hiccup (18%), pharyngitis (18%)

Miscellaneous: Infection (51%), allergic reaction (26%)

1% to 10%:

Cardiovascular: Arrhythmia (5%), cardiomegaly (5%), atrial fibrillation (2%), ECG abnormal (2%), heart block (2%), heart failure (grade 3/4: 2%), pericardial effusion (2%), tamponade (children with thalassemia: 2%), ventricular extrasystoles (2%), hypervolemia

Central nervous system: Lethargy (7%), hallucination (5%), agitation (2%), delirium (2%), encephalopathy (2%), seizure (2%), somnolence (2%), cerebral hemorrhage (1%)

Dermatologic: Vesicular rash (10%), vesiculobullous rash (10%), skin discoloration (8%), maculopapular rash (8%), acne (7%), exfoliative dermatitis (5%), erythema nodosum (2%)

Endocrine & metabolic: Hyponatremia (2%)

Gastrointestinal: Ileus (8%), weight gain (8%), hematemesis (2%), pancreatitis (2%)

Hematologic: Prothrombin time increased (2%)

Hepatic: Hepatomegaly (6%)

Renal: Hematuria (8%), dysuria (7%), hemorrhagic cystitis (grade 3/4: 7%), BUN increased (3%)

Respiratory: Asthma (8%), alveolar hemorrhage (5%), hyperventilation (5%), hemoptysis (3%), pleural effusion (3%), sinusitis (3%), atelectasis (2%), hypoxia (2%)

Oral: Frequency not defined:

Central nervous system: Seizure

Dermatologic: Hyperpigmentation of skin (busulfan tan 5% to 10%), alopecia, rash, urticaria

Endocrine & metabolic: Amenorrhea, ovarian suppression

Hematologic: Myelosuppression (anemia, leukopenia, thrombocytopenia), pancytopenia

Drug Interactions

Metabolism/Transport Effects Substrate of CYP3A4 (major)

Avoid Concomitant Use

Avoid concomitant use of Busulfan with any of the following: BCG; Conivaptan; Natalizumab; Pimecrolimus; Tacrolimus (Topical); Vaccines (Live)

Increased Effect/Toxicity

Busulfan may increase the levels/effects of: Leflunomide; Natalizumab; Vaccines (Live); Vitamin K Antagonists

The levels/effects of Busulfan may be increased by: Antifungal Agents (Azole Derivatives, Systemic); Conivaptan; CYP3A4 Inhibitors (Moderate); CYP3A4 Inhibitors (Strong); Dasatinib; Denosumab; MetroNIDAZOLE; MetroNIDAZOLE (Systemic); Pimecrolimus; Roflumilast; Tacrolimus (Topical); Trastuzumab

Decreased Effect

Busulfan may decrease the levels/effects of: BCG; Sipuleucel-T; Vaccines (Inactivated); Vaccines (Live); Vitamin K Antagonists

The levels/effects of Busulfan may be decreased by: CYP3A4 Inducers (Strong); Deferasirox; Echinacea; Herbs (CYP3A4 Inducers); Tocilizumab

Ethanol/Nutrition/Herb Interactions

Ethanol: Avoid ethanol due to GI irritation.

Food: No clear or firm data on the effect of food on busulfan bioavailability.

Herb/Nutraceutical: Avoid St John's wort (may decrease busulfan levels).

Stability

Injection: Store unopened ampuls and vials under refrigeration at 2°C to 8°C (36°F to 46°F). Dilute (using manufacturer provided 5-micron filters for ampuls) in 0.9% sodium chloride injection or dextrose 5% in water. The dilution volume should be ten times the volume of busulfan injection, ensuring that the final concentration of busulfan is 0.5 mg/mL. This solution is stable for up to 8 hours at room temperature (25°C); the infusion must also be completed within that 8-hour timeframe. Dilution of busulfan injection in 0.9% sodium chloride is stable for up to 12 hours at refrigeration (2°C to 8°C); the infusion must be completed within that 12-hour timeframe.

Tablet: Store at room temperature at 15°C to 30°C (59°F to 86°F).

Mechanism of Action Busulfan is an alkylating agent which reacts with the N-7 position of guanosine and interferes with DNA replication and transcription of RNA. Busulfan has a marked effect on myeloid cells than on lymphoid cells and is also very toxic to hematopoietic stem cells. Busulfan exhibits little immunosuppressive activity. Interferes with the normal function of DNA by alkylation and cross-linking the strands of DNA.

Pharmacodynamics/Kinetics

Duration: 28 days

Absorption: Rapid and complete

Distribution: V_d: ~1 L/kg; into CSF and saliva with levels similar to plasma

Protein binding: 32% to plasma proteins and 47% to red blood cells

Metabolism: Extensively hepatic (may increase with multiple doses); glutathione conjugation followed by oxidation

Half-life elimination: After first dose: 3.4 hours; After last dose: 2.3 hours

Time to peak, serum: Oral: Within 4 hours; I.V.: Within 5 minutes

Excretion: Urine (10% to 50% as metabolites) within 24 hours (<2% as unchanged drug)

Dosage

Geriatric Oral (refer to individual protocols): Start with lowest recommended doses for adults.

Adult Note: Premedicate with prophylactic anticonvulsant therapy (eg, phenytoin) prior to high-dose busulfan treatment.

CML remission induction: Oral: 60 mcg/kg/day or 1.8 mg/m^2/day; usual range: 4-8 mg/day (may be as high as 12 mg/day); Maintenance doses: 1-4 mg/day to 2 mg/week to maintain WBC 10,000-20,000 cells/mm^3

BMT marrow-ablative conditioning regimen:

Oral: 1 mg/kg/dose (ideal body weight) every 6 hours for 16 doses

I.V.: 0.8 mg/kg (ideal body weight or actual body weight, whichever is lower); for obese or severely-obese patients adjusted ideal body weight is recommended) every 6 hours for 4 days (a total of 16 doses)

Polycythemia vera (unlabeled use): Oral: 2-6 mg/day

Thrombocytosis (unlabeled use): Oral: 4-6 mg/day

Renal Impairment I.V.: Has not been studied in patients with renal impairment per the FDA-approved labeling. Some clinicians suggest adjustment is not necessary (Aronoff, 2007).

Hepatic Impairment I.V.: Has not been administered in clinical studies in patients with hepatic impairment per the FDA-approved labeling. Busulfan has extensive hepatic metabolism and risk of hepatic veno-occlusive disease with high doses; dosage adjustment may be needed.

Administration Intravenous busulfan should be administered as a 2-hour via central line.

BMT only: To facilitate ingestion of high oral doses, insert multiple tablets into gelatin capsules.

Monitoring Parameters CBC with differential and platelet count, liver function tests (evaluate transaminases, alkaline phosphatase, and bilirubin daily for at least 28 days post transplant)

Pharmacotherapy Pearls Oncology Comment: Low-dose monotherapy with oral busulfan for the palliative treatment of CML is no longer common. Treatment with imatinib or hematopoietic stem cell transplant (HSCT) are considered the primary treatments for CML (NCCN v1.2008).

◀ **Special Geriatric Considerations** Toxicity to immunosuppressives is increased in the elderly. Start with lowest recommended adult doses. Signs of infection, such as fever and rise in WBCs, may not occur. Lethargy and confusion may be more prominent signs of infection.

Dosage Forms Excipient information presented when available (limited, particularly for generics); consult specific product labeling.

Injection, solution:

Busulfex®: 6 mg/mL (10 mL) [contains N,N-dimethylacetamide (DMA)]

Tablet, oral:

Myleran®: 2 mg [scored]

Selected References

NCCN (National Comprehensive Cancer Network) "Practice Guidelines in Oncology: Antiemesis Version 1.2007." Available at http://www.nccn.org/professionals/physician_gls/PDF/antiemesis.pdf

NCCN (National Comprehensive Cancer Network) "Practice Guidelines in Oncology: Chronic Myelogenous Leukemia Version 1.2008." Available at http://www.nccn.org/professionals/physician_gls/PDF/cml.pdf

Tosti A, Piraccini BM, Vincenzi C, et al, "Permanent Alopecia After Busulfan Chemotherapy," Br J Dermatol, 2005, 152 (5):1056-8.

◆ **Busulfanum** see Busulfan on page 235
◆ **Busulfex®** see Busulfan on page 235
◆ **Busulphan** see Busulfan on page 235

Butorphanol (byoo TOR fa nole)

Related Information

Opioid Analgesics on page 2013

Medication Safety Issues

Sound-alike/look-alike issues:

Stadol may be confused with Haldol®, sotalol

High alert medication:

The Institute for Safe Medication Practices (ISMP) includes this medication among its list of drug classes which have a heightened risk of causing significant patient harm when used in error.

Brand Names: Canada Apo-Butorphanol®; PMS-Butorphanol

Index Terms Butorphanol Tartrate; Stadol

Generic Availability (U.S.) Yes

Pharmacologic Category Analgesic, Opioid; Analgesic, Opioid Partial Agonist

Use

Parenteral: Management of moderate-to-severe pain; preoperative medication; supplement to balanced anesthesia; management of pain during labor

Nasal spray: Management of moderate-to-severe pain, including migraine headache pain

Contraindications Hypersensitivity to butorphanol or any component of the formulation; avoid use in opiate-dependent patients who have not been detoxified, may precipitate opiate withdrawal

Warnings/Precautions An opioid-containing analgesic regimen should be tailored to each patient's needs and based upon the type of pain being treated (acute versus chronic), the route of administration, degree of tolerance for opioids (naive versus chronic user), age, weight, and medical condition. The optimal analgesic dose varies widely among patients. Doses should be titrated to pain relief/prevention. May cause CNS depression; use with caution in patients with head trauma, morbid obesity, thyroid dysfunction, hepatic/renal dysfunction, adrenal insufficiency, prostatic hyperplasia and/or urinary stricture, may elevate CSF pressure, may increase cardiac workload; tolerance of drug dependence may result from extended use. Use with caution in patients with biliary tract dysfunction; acute pancreatitis may cause constriction of sphincter of Oddi.

Partial antagonist activity may precipitate acute narcotic withdrawal in opioid-dependent individuals. Use with caution in patients with pre-existing respiratory compromise (hypoxia and/or hypercapnia), COPD or other obstructive pulmonary disease; critical respiratory depression may occur, even at therapeutic dosages. May cause hypotension; use with caution in patients with hypovolemia, cardiovascular disease (including acute MI), or drugs which may exaggerate hypotensive effects (including phenothiazines or general anesthetics). May obscure diagnosis or clinical course of patients with acute abdominal conditions.

Concurrent use of sumatriptan nasal spray and butorphanol nasal spray may increase risk of transient high blood pressure. Healthcare provider should be alert to problems of abuse, misuse, and diversion. Use with caution in the elderly and debilitated patients; may be more sensitive to adverse effects.

Adverse Reactions (Reflective of adult population; not specific for elderly)

>10%:

Central nervous system: Somnolence (43%), dizziness (19%), insomnia (nasal spray 11%)

Gastrointestinal: Nausea/vomiting (13%)

Respiratory: Nasal congestion (nasal spray 13%)

1% to 10%:

Cardiovascular: Palpitation, vasodilation

Central nervous system: Anxiety, confusion, headache, lethargy, lightheadedness

Dermatologic: Pruritus

Gastrointestinal: Anorexia, constipation, stomach pain, unpleasant aftertaste, xerostomia

Neuromuscular & skeletal: Tremor, paresthesia, weakness

Ocular: Blurred vision

Otic: Ear pain, tinnitus

Respiratory: Bronchitis, cough, dyspnea, epistaxis, nasal irritation, pharyngitis, rhinitis, sinus congestion, sinusitis, upper respiratory infection

Miscellaneous: Diaphoresis increased

Drug Interactions

Avoid Concomitant Use There are no known interactions where it is recommended to avoid concomitant use.

Increased Effect/Toxicity

Butorphanol may increase the levels/effects of: Alcohol (Ethyl); Alvimopan; CNS Depressants; Desmopressin; Selective Serotonin Reuptake Inhibitors; Thiazide Diuretics

The levels/effects of Butorphanol may be increased by: Amphetamines; Antipsychotic Agents (Phenothiazines); Droperidol; HydrOXYzine; Succinylcholine

Decreased Effect

Butorphanol may decrease the levels/effects of: Analgesics (Opioid); Pegvisomant

The levels/effects of Butorphanol may be decreased by: Ammonium Chloride; Mixed Agonist/ Antagonist Opioids

Ethanol/Nutrition/Herb Interactions

Ethanol: May increase CNS depression; monitor for increased effects with coadministration. Caution patients about effects.

Herb/Nutraceutical: Avoid valerian, St John's wort, kava kava, gotu kola (may increase CNS depression).

Stability Store at room temperature; protect from freezing.

Mechanism of Action Agonist of kappa opiate receptors and partial agonist of mu opiate receptors in the CNS, causing inhibition of ascending pain pathways, altering the perception of and response to pain; produces analgesia, respiratory depression, and sedation similar to opioids

Pharmacodynamics/Kinetics

Onset of action: I.M.: 5-10 minutes; I.V.: <10 minutes; Nasal: Within 15 minutes

Peak effect: I.M.: 0.5-1 hour; I.V.: 4-5 minutes

Duration: I.M., I.V.: 3-4 hours; Nasal: 4-5 hours

Absorption: Rapid and well absorbed

Protein binding: 80%

Metabolism: Hepatic

Bioavailability: Nasal: 60% to 70%

Half-life elimination:

Geriatrics: 5.5 hours

Adults: 2.5-4 hours

Excretion: Primarily urine

Dosage

Geriatric

I.M., I.V.: Initial dosage should generally be ¹/₂ of the recommended dose; repeated dosing must be based on initial response rather than fixed intervals, but generally should be at least 6 hours apart

Nasal spray: Initial dose should not exceed 1 mg; a second dose may be given after 90-120 minutes

Adult Note: These are guidelines and do not represent the maximum doses that may be required in all patients. Doses should be titrated to pain relief/prevention. Butorphanol has an analgesic ceiling.

Acute pain (moderate-to-severe):

I.M.: Initial: 2 mg, may repeat every 3-4 hours as needed; usual range: 1-4 mg every 3-4 hours as needed

I.V.: Initial: 1 mg, may repeat every 3-4 hours as needed; usual range: 0.5-2 mg every 3-4 hours as needed

◄ *Intranasal (spray)* (includes use for migraine headache pain): Initial: 1 spray (~1 mg per spray) in 1 nostril; if adequate pain relief is not achieved within 60-90 minutes, an additional 1 spray in 1 nostril may be given; may repeat initial dose sequence in 3-4 hours after the last dose as needed

Alternatively, an initial dose of 2 mg (1 spray in each nostril) may be used in patients who will be able to remain recumbent (in the event drowsiness or dizziness occurs); additional 2 mg doses should not be given for 3-4 hours

Note: In some clinical trials, an initial dose of 2 mg (as 2 doses 1 hour apart or 2 mg initially - 1 spray in each nostril) has been used, followed by 1 mg in 1 hour; side effects were greater at these dosages

Migraine: *Nasal spray:* Refer to "moderate-to-severe pain" indication

Preoperative medication: *I.M.:* 2 mg 60-90 minutes before surgery

Supplement to balanced anesthesia: *I.V.:* 2 mg shortly before induction and/or an incremental dose of 0.5-1 mg (up to 0.06 mg/kg), depending on previously administered sedative, analgesic, and hypnotic medications

Renal Impairment

I.M., I.V.: Initial dosage should generally be ½ of the recommended dose; repeated dosing must be based on initial response rather than fixed intervals, but generally should be at least 6 hours apart

Nasal spray: Initial dose should not exceed 1 mg; a second dose may be given after 90-120 minutes

Hepatic Impairment

I.M., I.V.: Initial dosage should generally be ½ of the recommended dose; repeated dosing must be based on initial response rather than fixed intervals, but generally should be at least 6 hours apart

Nasal spray: Initial dose should not exceed 1 mg; a second dose may be given after 90-120 minutes

Administration Intranasal: Consider avoiding simultaneous intranasal migraine sprays; may want to separate by at least 30 minutes

Monitoring Parameters Pain relief, respiratory and mental status, blood pressure

Reference Range 0.7-1.5 ng/mL

Special Geriatric Considerations Adjust dose for renal function in the elderly.

Controlled Substance C-IV

Dosage Forms Excipient information presented when available (limited, particularly for generics); consult specific product labeling.

Injection, solution, as tartrate: 1 mg/mL (1 mL); 2 mg/mL (1 mL, 2 mL, 10 mL)

Injection, solution, as tartrate [preservative free]: 1 mg/mL (1 mL); 2 mg/mL (1 mL, 2 mL)

Solution, intranasal, as tartrate [spray]: 10 mg/mL (2.5 mL)

Selected References

American Geriatrics Society Panel on Pharmacological Management of Persistent Pain in Older Persons, "Pharmacological Management of Persistent Pain in Older Persons," *J Am Geriatr Soc,* 2009, 57(8):1331-46.

Ramsey R, Higbee M, Maesner J, et al, "Influence of Age on the Pharmacokinetics of Butorphanol," *Acute Care,* 1986, 12(Suppl 1):8-16.

◆ **Butorphanol Tartrate** *see* Butorphanol *on page* 238
◆ **Butrans™** *see* Buprenorphine *on page* 225
◆ **BW-430C** *see* LamoTRIgine *on page* 1024
◆ **Byetta®** *see* Exenatide *on page* 687
◆ **Bystolic®** *see* Nebivolol *on page* 1273
◆ **311C90** *see* ZOLMitriptan *on page* 1958
◆ **Cafergot®** *see* Ergotamine and Caffeine *on page* 623
◆ **Caffeine and Ergotamine** *see* Ergotamine and Caffeine *on page* 623
◆ **Cal-C-Caps [OTC]** *see* Calcium Citrate *on page* 252
◆ **Calan®** *see* Verapamil *on page* 1909
◆ **Calan® SR** *see* Verapamil *on page* 1909
◆ **Cal Carb-HD® [OTC]** *see* Calcium Salts (Oral) *on page* 256
◆ **Cal-Cee [OTC]** *see* Calcium Citrate *on page* 252
◆ **Calci-Chew™ [OTC]** *see* Calcium Salts (Oral) *on page* 256
◆ **Calciday-667® [OTC]** *see* Calcium Salts (Oral) *on page* 256
◆ **Calciferol™ [OTC]** *see* Ergocalciferol *on page* 618
◆ **Calcijex®** *see* Calcitriol *on page* 243
◆ **Calci-Mix™ [OTC]** *see* Calcium Salts (Oral) *on page* 256

Calcipotriene (kal si POE try een)

Brand Names: U.S. Calcitrene™; Dovonex®
Brand Names: Canada Dovonex®
Generic Availability (U.S.) Yes: Excludes cream

Pharmacologic Category Topical Skin Product; Vitamin D Analog

Use Treatment of plaque psoriasis; chronic, moderate-to-severe psoriasis of the scalp

Unlabeled/Investigational Use Vitiligo

Contraindications Hypersensitivity to calcipotriene or any component of the formulation; patients with demonstrated hypercalcemia or evidence of vitamin D toxicity; use on the face; patients with acute psoriatic eruptions (scalp solution)

Warnings/Precautions Discontinue use if irritation occurs. May cause transient increases in serum calcium (reversible); if hypercalcemia occurs, discontinue treatment until levels return to normal. For external use only; not for ophthalmic, oral, or intravaginal use. Avoid or limit excessive exposure to natural or artificial sunlight, or phototherapy. Use with caution in elderly patients; severity of skin related adverse reactions may be increased compared to younger adults.

Adverse Reactions (Reflective of adult population; not specific for elderly) Frequency may vary with site of application.

>10%: Dermatologic: Burning, itching, rash, skin irritation, stinging, tingling

1% to 10%: Dermatologic: Dermatitis, dry skin, erythema, peeling, pruritus, worsening of psoriasis

Drug Interactions

Avoid Concomitant Use

Avoid concomitant use of Calcipotriene with any of the following: Aluminum Hydroxide; Sucralfate; Vitamin D Analogs

Increased Effect/Toxicity

Calcipotriene may increase the levels/effects of: Aluminum Hydroxide; Cardiac Glycosides; Sucralfate; Vitamin D Analogs

The levels/effects of Calcipotriene may be increased by: Calcium Salts; Thiazide Diuretics

Decreased Effect

The levels/effects of Calcipotriene may be decreased by: Orlistat

Stability Store at controlled room temperature of 15°C to 25°C (59°F to 77°F); do not freeze. Solution should be kept away from open flame; avoid sunlight.

Mechanism of Action Synthetic vitamin D_3 analog which regulates skin cell production and proliferation

Pharmacodynamics/Kinetics

Onset of action: Improvement begins after 2 weeks; marked improvement seen after 8 weeks

Absorption: When applied to psoriasis plaques: Cream, ointment: ~6%; Solution: <1%

Metabolism: Converted in the skin to inactive metabolites

Dosage

Geriatric & Adult Psoriasis: Topical:

Cream: Apply a thin film to the affected skin twice daily for up to 8 weeks

Ointment: Apply a thin film to the affected skin once or twice daily

Solution: Apply to the affected scalp twice daily for up to 8 weeks

Administration For external use only.

Cream, ointment: Apply to affected skin; rub in gently and completely. Wash hands thoroughly before and after use.

Solution: Prior to using scalp solution, comb hair to remove debris; apply only to lesions. Rub in gently and completely. Avoid solution spreading or dripping onto forehead. Avoid contact with eyes. Wash hands thoroughly before and after use.

Monitoring Parameters Serum calcium

Dosage Forms Excipient information presented when available (limited, particularly for generics); consult specific product labeling.

Cream, topical:

Dovonex®: 0.005% (60 g, 120 g)

Ointment, topical:

Calcitrene™: 0.005% (60 g)

Solution, topical: 0.005% (60 mL)

Dovonex®: 0.005% (60 mL) [contains isopropyl alcohol 51% v/v]

Calcitonin (kal si TOE nin)

Related Information

Osteoporosis Management *on page 2027*

Medication Safety Issues

Sound-alike/look-alike issues:

Calcitonin may be confused with calcitriol

◄   Miacalcin® may be confused with Micatin®

Administration issues:

Calcitonin nasal spray is administered as a single spray into **one** nostril daily, using alternate nostrils each day.

Brand Names: U.S. Fortical®; Miacalcin®

Brand Names: Canada Apo-Calcitonin®; Calcimar®; Caltine®; Miacalcin® NS; PRO-Calcitonin; Sandoz-Calcitonin

Index Terms Calcitonin (Salmon)

Generic Availability (U.S.) Yes: Intranasal solution

Pharmacologic Category Antidote; Hormone

Use Treatment of Paget's disease of bone (osteitis deformans); adjunctive therapy for hypercalcemia; treatment of osteoporosis in women >5 years postmenopause

Contraindications Hypersensitivity to calcitonin salmon or any component of the formulation

Warnings/Precautions A skin test should be performed prior to initiating therapy of calcitonin salmon in patients with suspected sensitivity; have epinephrine immediately available for a possible hypersensitivity reaction. A detailed skin testing protocol is available from the manufacturers. Temporarily withdraw use of nasal spray if ulceration of nasal mucosa occurs. Discontinue for ulcerations >1.5 mm or those that penetrate below the mucosa. Patients >65 years of age may experience a higher incidence of nasal adverse events with calcitonin nasal spray.

Adverse Reactions (Reflective of adult population; not specific for elderly) Unless otherwise noted, frequencies reported are with nasal spray.

>10%: Respiratory: Rhinitis (≤12%, including ulcerative)

1% to 10%:

Cardiovascular: Flushing (nasal spray: <1%; injection: 2% to 5%), angina (1% to 3%), hypertension (1% to 3%)

Central nervous system: Depression (1% to 3%), dizziness (1% to 3%), fatigue (1% to 3%)

Dermatologic: Erythematous rash (1% to 3%)

Gastrointestinal: Nausea (injection: 10%; nasal spray: 2%), abdominal pain (1% to 3%), constipation (1% to 3%), diarrhea (1% to 3%), dyspepsia (1% to 3%)

Genitourinary: Cystitis (1% to 3%)

Local: Injection site reactions (injection: 10%)

Neuromuscular & skeletal: Back pain (5%), arthrosis (1% to 3%), myalgia (1% to 3%), paresthesia (1% to 3%)

Ocular: Conjunctivitis (1% to 3%), lacrimation abnormality (1% to 3%)

Respiratory: Nasal ulcerations (3%), bronchospasm (1% to 3%), sinusitis (1% to 3%), upper respiratory tract infection (1% to 3%)

Miscellaneous: Flu-like syndrome (1% to 3%), infection (1% to 3%), lymphadenopathy (1% to 3%)

Drug Interactions

Avoid Concomitant Use There are no known interactions where it is recommended to avoid concomitant use.

Increased Effect/Toxicity There are no known significant interactions involving an increase in effect.

Decreased Effect

Calcitonin may decrease the levels/effects of: Lithium

Ethanol/Nutrition/Herb Interactions Ethanol: Avoid ethanol (may increase risk of osteoporosis).

Stability

Injection: Store under refrigeration at 2°C to 8°C (36°F to 46°F); protect from freezing. NS has been recommended for the dilution to prepare a skin test in patients with suspected sensitivity. The following stability information has also been reported: May be stored at room temperature for up to 14 days (Cohen, 2007).

Nasal: Store unopened bottle under refrigeration at 2°C to 8°C (36°F to 46°F); do not freeze.

Fortical®: After opening, store for up to 30 days at 20°C to 25°C (68°F to 77°F); excursions permitted to 15°C to 30°C (59°F to 86°F). Store in upright position.

Miacalcin®: After opening, store for up to 35 days at room temperature of 15°C to 30°C (59°F to 86°F). Store in upright position.

Mechanism of Action Peptide sequence similar to human calcitonin; functionally antagonizes the effects of parathyroid hormone. Directly inhibits osteoclastic bone resorption; promotes the renal excretion of calcium, phosphate, sodium, magnesium, and potassium by decreasing tubular reabsorption; increases the jejunal secretion of water, sodium, potassium, and chloride

Pharmacodynamics/Kinetics

Onset of action:

Hypercalcemia: I.M., SubQ: ~2 hours

Paget's disease: Within a few months; may take up to 1 year for neurologic symptom improvement

Duration: Hypercalcemia: I.M., SubQ: 6-8 hours

Distribution: V_d: 0.15-0.3 L/kg

Metabolism: Metabolized in kidneys, blood and peripheral tissue

Bioavailability: I.M.: 66%; SubQ: 71%; Nasal: ~3% to 5% (relative to I.M.)

Half-life elimination (terminal): I.M. 58 minutes; SubQ 59-64 minutes; Nasal: ~18 minutes

Time to peak, plasma: SubQ ~23 minutes; Nasal: ~13 minutes

Excretion: Urine (as inactive metabolites)

Dosage

Geriatric & Adult

Paget's disease *(Miacalcin®)*: I.M., SubQ: Initial: 100 units/day; maintenance: 50 units/day or 50-100 units every 1-3 days

Hypercalcemia *(Miacalcin®)*: Initial: I.M., SubQ: 4 units/kg every 12 hours; may increase up to 8 units/kg every 12 hours; if the response remains unsatisfactory, a further increase up to a maximum of 8 units/kg every 6 hours may be considered

Postmenopausal osteoporosis:
Miacalcin®: I.M., SubQ: 100 units/every other day
Fortical®, Miacalcin®: Intranasal: 200 units (1 spray) in one nostril daily

Administration

Injection solution: May be administered I.M. or SubQ. I.M route is preferred if the injection volume is >2 mL. SubQ route is preferred for outpatient self-administration unless the injection volume is >2 mL.

Nasal spray: Before first use, allow bottle to reach room temperature, then prime pump by releasing at least 5 sprays until full spray is produced. To administer, place nozzle into nostril with head in upright position. Alternate nostrils daily. Do not prime pump before each daily use. Discard after 30 doses.

Monitoring Parameters Serum electrolytes and calcium; alkaline phosphatase and 24-hour urine collection for hydroxyproline excretion (Paget's disease), urinalysis (urine sediment); bone mineral density

Nasal formulation: Visualization of nasal mucosa, turbinate, septum, and mucosal blood vessels (at baseline and with nasal complaints)

Special Geriatric Considerations Studies have shown calcitonin's effects on bone density and fracture rates are positive, but less than other treatments. Calcium and vitamin D supplements should also be given. Calcitonin may also be effective in steroid-induced osteoporosis and other states associated with high bone turnover. Nasal spray may provide faster onset of analgesic effects than I.M.

Dosage Forms Excipient information presented when available (limited, particularly for generics); consult specific product labeling.

Injection, solution [calcitonin-salmon]:
Miacalcin®: 200 int. units/mL (2 mL)

Solution, intranasal [calcitonin-salmon/rDNA origin/spray]:
Fortical®: 200 int. units/actuation (3.7 mL) [contains benzyl alcohol; delivers 30 doses]

Solution, intranasal [calcitonin-salmon/spray]: 200 int. units/actuation (3.7 mL)
Miacalcin®: 200 int. units/actuation (3.7 mL) [contains benzalkonium chloride; delivers 30 doses]

Selected References

Lyritis GP, Tsakalakos N, Magiasis B, et al, "Analgesic Effect of Salmon Calcitonin in Osteoporotic Vertebral Fractures: A Double-Blind, Placebo-Controlled Clinical Study," *Calcif Tissue Int*, 1991, 49(6):369-72.

Pontiroli AE, Pajetta E, Scaglia L, et al, "Analgesic Effect of Intranasal and Intramuscular Salmon Calcitonin in Postmenopausal Osteoporosis: A Double-Blind, Double-Placebo Study," *Aging (Milane)*, 1994, 6(6):459-63.

◆ **Calcitonin (Salmon)** see Calcitonin on page 241
◆ **Calcitrate [OTC]** see Calcium Citrate on page 252
◆ **Cal-Citrate™ 225 [OTC]** see Calcium Citrate on page 252
◆ **Calcitrene™** see Calcipotriene on page 240

Calcitriol (kal si TRYE ole)

Medication Safety Issues

Sound-alike/look-alike issues:

Calcitriol may be confused with alfacalcidol, calcifediol, Calciferol®, calcitonin, calcium carbonate, captopril, colestipol, paricalcitol, ropinirole

Administration issues:

Dosage is expressed in mcg (micrograms), **not** mg (milligrams); rare cases of acute overdose have been reported

Brand Names: U.S. Calcijex®; Rocaltrol®; Vectical™

Brand Names: Canada Calcijex®; Rocaltrol®

Index Terms 1,25 Dihydroxycholecalciferol
Generic Availability (U.S.) Yes: Excludes ointment
Pharmacologic Category Vitamin D Analog
Use

Oral, injection: Management of hypocalcemia in patients on chronic renal dialysis; management of secondary hyperparathyroidism in patients with chronic kidney disease (CKD); management of hypocalcemia in hypoparathyroidism and pseudohypoparathyroidism

Topical: Management of mild-to-moderate plaque psoriasis
Unlabeled/Investigational Use Reduction in severity of psoriatic lesions in psoriatic vulgaris; treatment of vitamin D-resistant rickets
Contraindications Hypersensitivity to calcitriol or any component of the formulation; hypercalcemia, vitamin D toxicity

Topical: There are no contraindications listed in the manufacturer's labeling.
Warnings/Precautions

Oral, injection: Adequate dietary (supplemental) calcium is necessary for clinical response to vitamin D. Excessive vitamin D may cause severe hypercalcemia, hypercalciuria, and hyperphosphatemia; calcium-phosphate product (serum calcium times phosphorus) must not exceed 70 mg^2/dL^2. Other forms of vitamin D should be withheld during therapy. Immobilization may increase risk of hypercalcemia and/or hypercalciuria. Maintain adequate hydration. Use caution in patients with malabsorption syndromes (efficacy may be limited and/or response may be unpredictable). Use of calcitriol for the treatment of secondary hyperparathyroidism associated with CKD is not recommended in patients with rapidly worsening kidney function or in noncompliant patients. Increased serum phosphate levels in patients with renal failure may lead to calcification; the use of an aluminum-containing phosphate binder is recommended along with a low phosphate diet in these patients. Use with caution in patients taking cardiac glycosides; digitalis toxicity is potentiated by hypocalcemia. Products may contain coconut (capsule) or palm seed oil (oral solution). Some products may contain tartrazine.

Topical: May cause hypercalcemia; if alterations in calcium occur, discontinue treatment until levels return to normal. For external use only; not for ophthalmic, oral, or intravaginal use. Do not apply to facial skin, eyes, or lips. Absorption may be increased with occlusive dressings. Avoid or limit excessive exposure to natural or artificial sunlight, or phototherapy. The safety and effectiveness has not been evaluated in patients with erythrodermic, exfoliative, or pustular psoriasis.
Adverse Reactions (Reflective of adult population; not specific for elderly)
Oral, I.V.: Frequency not defined.

Cardiovascular: Cardiac arrhythmia, hypertension

Central nervous system: Apathy, headache, hypothermia, psychosis, sensory disturbances, somnolence

Dermatologic: Erythema multiforme, pruritus

Endocrine & metabolic: Dehydration, growth suppression, hypercalcemia, hypercholesterolemia, hypermagnesemia, hyperphosphatemia, libido decreased, polydipsia

Gastrointestinal: Abdominal pain, anorexia, constipation, metallic taste, nausea, pancreatitis, stomach ache, vomiting, weight loss, xerostomia

Genitourinary: Nocturia, urinary tract infection

Hepatic: ALT increased, AST increased

Local: Injection site pain (mild)

Neuromuscular & skeletal: Bone pain, myalgia, dystrophy, soft tissue calcification, weakness

Ocular: Conjunctivitis, photophobia

Renal: Albuminuria, BUN increased, creatinine increased, hypercalciuria, nephrocalcinosis, polyuria

Respiratory: Rhinorrhea

Miscellaneous: Allergic reaction

Topical:

>10%: Endocrine: Hypercalcemia (≤24%)

1% to 10%:

Dermatologic: Skin discomfort (3%), pruritus (1% to 3%)

Genitourinary: Urine abnormality (4%)

Renal: Hypercalciuria (3%)
Drug Interactions

Metabolism/Transport Effects Substrate of CYP3A4 (major); **Induces** CYP3A4 (weak)
Avoid Concomitant Use

Avoid concomitant use of Calcitriol with any of the following: Aluminum Hydroxide; Conivaptan; Sucralfate; Vitamin D Analogs

Increased Effect/Toxicity

Calcitriol may increase the levels/effects of: Aluminum Hydroxide; Cardiac Glycosides; Magnesium Salts; Sucralfate; Vitamin D Analogs

The levels/effects of Calcitriol may be increased by: Calcium Salts; Conivaptan; CYP3A4 Inhibitors (Moderate); CYP3A4 Inhibitors (Strong); Dasatinib; Thiazide Diuretics

Decreased Effect

Calcitriol may decrease the levels/effects of: Saxagliptin

The levels/effects of Calcitriol may be decreased by: Bile Acid Sequestrants; Corticosteroids (Systemic); CYP3A4 Inducers (Strong); Deferasirox; Herbs (CYP3A4 Inducers); Mineral Oil; Orlistat; Sevelamer; Tocilizumab

Stability

Injection: Store at room temperature of 15°C to 30°C (59°F to 86°F). Protect from light.

Oral capsule, solution: Store at room temperature of 20°C to 25°C (68°F to 77°F). Protect from light.

Topical: Store at room temperature of 25°C (77°F); excursions permitted to 15°C to 30°C (59°F to 86°F); do not refrigerate; do not freeze.

Mechanism of Action Calcitriol is a potent active metabolite of vitamin D. Vitamin D promotes absorption of calcium in the intestines and retention at the kidneys thereby increasing calcium levels in the serum; decreases excessive serum phosphatase levels, parathyroid hormone levels, and decreases bone resorption; increases renal tubule phosphate resorption

The mechanism by which calcitriol is beneficial in the treatment of psoriasis has not been established.

Pharmacodynamics/Kinetics

Onset of action: Oral: ~2-6 hours

Duration: Oral, I.V.: 3-5 days

Absorption: Oral: Rapid

Protein binding: 99.9%

Metabolism: Primarily to 1,24,25-trihydroxycholecalciferol and 1,24,25-trihydroxy ergocalciferol

Half-life elimination: Normal adults: 5-8 hours; Hemodialysis: 16-22 hours

Time to peak, serum: Oral: 3-6 hours; Hemodialysis: 8-12 hours

Excretion: Primarily feces; urine

Dosage

Geriatric Refer to adult dosing. No dosage recommendations, but start at the lower end of the dosage range.

Adult

Hypocalcemia in patients on chronic renal dialysis (manufacturer labeling):

Oral: 0.25 mcg/day or every other day (may require 0.5-1 mcg/day); increases should be made at 4- to 8-week intervals

I.V.: Initial: 1-2 mcg 3 times/week (0.02 mcg/kg) approximately every other day. Adjust dose at 2-4 week intervals; dosing range: 0.5-4 mcg 3 times/week

Hypocalcemia in hypoparathyroidism/pseudohypoparathyroidism (manufacturers labeling): Oral (evaluate dosage at 2- to 4-week intervals): Initial: 0.25 mcg/day, range: 0.5-2 mcg once daily

Secondary hyperparathyroidism associated with moderate-to-severe CKD in patients not on dialysis (manufacturer labeling): Oral: 0.25 mcg/day; may increase to 0.5 mcg/day

K/DOQI guidelines for vitamin D therapy in CKD:

CKD stage 3: Oral: 0.25 mcg/day. Treatment should only be started with serum 25(OH) D >30 ng/mL, serum iPTH >70 pg/mL, serum calcium <9.5 mg/dL and serum phosphorus <4.6 mg/dL

CKD stage 4: Oral: 0.25 mcg/day. Treatment should only be started with serum 25(OH) D >30 ng/mL, serum iPTH >110 pg/mL, serum calcium <9.5 mg/dL and serum phosphorus <4.6 mg/dL

CKD stage 5:

Peritoneal dialysis: Oral: Initial: 0.5-1 mcg 2-3 times/week or 0.25 mcg/day

Hemodialysis: **Note:** The following initial doses are based on plasma PTH and serum calcium levels for patients with serum phosphorus <5.5 mg/dL and Ca-P product <55. Adjust dose based on serum phosphate, calcium, and PTH levels. Intermittent I.V. administration may be more effective than daily oral dosing.

Plasma PTH 300-600 pg/mL and serum Ca <9.5 mg/dL: Oral, I.V.: 0.5-1.5 mcg

Plasma PTH 600-1000 pg/mL and serum Ca <9.5 mg/dL:

Oral: 1-4 mcg

I.V.: 1-3 mcg

Plasma PTH >1000 pg/mL and serum Ca <10 mg/dL:
Oral: 3-7 mcg
I.V.: 3-5 mcg
Psoriasis: Topical: Apply twice daily to affected areas (maximum: 200 g/week)
Vitamin D-dependent rickets (unlabeled use): Oral: 1 mcg once daily

Administration

I.V.: May be administered as a bolus dose I.V. through the catheter at the end of hemodialysis.
Oral: May be administered without regard to food. Administer with meals to reduce GI problems.
Topical: Apply externally; not for ophthalmic, oral, or intravaginal use. Do not apply to eyes, lips, or facial skins. Rub in gently so that no medication remains visible. Limit application to only the areas of skin affected by psoriasis.

Monitoring Parameters

Serum calcium and phosphorus: Frequency of measurement may be dependent upon the presence and magnitude of abnormalities, the rate of progression of CKD, and the use of treatments for CKD-mineral and bone disorders (KDIGO, 2009):
CKD stage 3: Every 6-12 months
CKD stage 4: Every 3-6 months
CKD stage 5 and 5D: Every 1-3 months
Periodic 24-hour urinary calcium and phosphorus; magnesium; alkaline phosphatase every 12 months or more frequently in the presence of elevated PTH; creatinine, BUN, albumin; intact parathyroid hormone (iPTH) every 3-12 months depending on CKD severity

Reference Range

CKD K/DOQI guidelines definition of stages; chronic disease is kidney damage or GFR <60 mL/minute/1.73 m^2 for ≥3 months:
Stage 2: GFR 60-89 mL/minute/1.73 m^2 (kidney damage with mild decrease GFR)
Stage 3: GFR 30-59 mL/minute/1.73 m^2 (moderate decrease GFR)
Stage 4: GFR 15-29 mL/minute/1.73 m^2 (severe decrease GFR)
Stage 5: GFR <15 mL/minute/1.73 m^2 or dialysis (kidney failure)
Target range for iPTH:
Stage 3 CKD: 35-70 pg/mL
Stage 4 CKD: 70-110 pg/mL
Stage 5 CKD: 150-300 pg/mL
Serum phosphorus:
Stage 3 and 4 CKD: ≥2.7 to <4.6 mg/dL
Stage 5 CKD: 3.5-5.5 mg/dL
Serum calcium-phosphorus product:
Stage 3-5 CKD: <55 mg^2/dL^2

Pharmacotherapy Pearls Calcitriol degrades upon prolonged exposure to light; not used as a daily supplement due to dosage forms, strengths, and cost

Special Geriatric Considerations Vitamin D, folate, and B_{12} (cyanocobalamin) have decreased absorption with age (clinical significance unknown); studies in ill geriatrics demonstrated that low serum concentrations of vitamin D result in greater bone loss. Calorie requirements decrease with age and therefore, nutrient density must be increased to ensure adequate nutrient intake, including vitamins and minerals. The use of a daily supplement with a multiple vitamin with minerals is recommended because elderly consume less vitamin D, absorption may be decreased, and many have decreased sun exposure. This is a recommendation of particular need to those with high risk for osteoporosis.

Vitamin D supplementation has been shown to increase muscle function and strength, as well as improve balance. Patients at risk for falls should have vitamin D serum concentrations measured and be evaluated for supplementation.

Dosage Forms Excipient information presented when available (limited, particularly for generics); consult specific product labeling.
Capsule, softgel, oral: 0.25 mcg, 0.5 mcg
Rocaltrol®: 0.25 mcg, 0.5 mcg [contains coconut oil]
Injection, solution: 1 mcg/mL (1 mL)
Calcijex®: 1 mcg/mL (1 mL) [contains aluminum]
Ointment, topical:
Vectical™: 3 mcg/g (100 g)
Solution, oral: 1 mcg/mL (15 mL)
Rocaltrol®: 1 mcg/mL (15 mL) [contains palm oil]

Selected References

Letsou AP and Price LS, "Health Aging and Nutrition: An Overview," *Clin Geriatr Med*, 1987, 3(2):253-60.
Myrianthopoulos M, "Dietary Treatment of Hyperlipidemia in the Elderly," *Clin Geriatr Med*, 1987, 3(2):343-59.
Riggs BL and Melton LJ, "The Prevention and Treatment of Osteoporosis," *N Engl J Med*, 1992, 327(9):620-7.

Calcium Acetate (KAL see um AS e tate)

Medication Safety Issues
  Sound-alike/look-alike issues:
    PhosLo® may be confused with Phos-Flur®, ProSom™
Brand Names: U.S. Eliphos™; PhosLo®; Phoslyra™
Brand Names: Canada PhosLo®
Generic Availability (U.S.) Yes: Gelcap
Pharmacologic Category Antidote; Calcium Salt; Phosphate Binder
Use Control of hyperphosphatemia in end-stage renal failure; does not promote aluminum absorption
Contraindications Hypersensitivity to any component of the formulation; hypercalcemia, renal calculi
Warnings/Precautions Constipation, bloating, and gas are common with calcium supplements. Hypercalcemia and hypercalciuria are most likely to occur in hypoparathyroid patients receiving high doses of vitamin D. Use with caution in patients who may be at risk of cardiac arrhythmias. Use with caution in digitalized patients; hypercalcemia may precipitate cardiac arrhythmias. Calcium administration interferes with absorption of some minerals and drugs; use with caution. Oral solution may contain maltitol (a sugar substitute) which may cause a laxative effect.
Adverse Reactions (Reflective of adult population; not specific for elderly)
  >10%:
    Endocrine & metabolic: Hypercalcemia
    Gastrointestinal: Diarrhea (oral solution)
  1% to 10%: Gastrointestinal: Nausea, vomiting
Drug Interactions
  Avoid Concomitant Use
    Avoid concomitant use of Calcium Acetate with any of the following: Calcium Salts
  Increased Effect/Toxicity
    Calcium Acetate may increase the levels/effects of: CefTRIAXone; Vitamin D Analogs

    The levels/effects of Calcium Acetate may be increased by: Calcium Salts; Thiazide Diuretics
  Decreased Effect
    Calcium Acetate may decrease the levels/effects of: Bisphosphonate Derivatives; Calcium Channel Blockers; DOBUTamine; Eltrombopag; Estramustine; Phosphate Supplements; Quinolone Antibiotics; Tetracycline Derivatives; Thyroid Products; Trientine

    The levels/effects of Calcium Acetate may be decreased by: Trientine
Ethanol/Nutrition/Herb Interactions
  Ethanol: Ethanol may decrease calcium absorption.
  Food: Caffeine may decrease calcium absorption and increase calcium excretion. Foods that contain maltitol may have an additive laxative effect with the oral solution formulation (contains maltitol).
Mechanism of Action Combines with dietary phosphate to form insoluble calcium phosphate which is excreted in feces
Pharmacodynamics/Kinetics
  Absorption: Requires vitamin D; minimal unless chronic, high doses are given; calcium is absorbed in soluble, ionized form; solubility of calcium is increased in an acid environment
  Excretion: Primarily feces (as unabsorbed calcium); urine (20%)
Dosage
  Geriatric Control of hyperphosphatemia (ESRD, on dialysis): Refer to adult dosing.
  Adult Control of hyperphosphatemia (ESRD, on dialysis): Oral: Initial: 1334 mg with each meal, can be increased gradually (ie, every 2-3 weeks) to bring the serum phosphate value <6 mg/dL as long as hypercalcemia does not develop (usual dose: 2001-2668 mg calcium acetate with each meal); do not give additional calcium supplements
Administration Administer with meals.
Monitoring Parameters Serum calcium (twice weekly during initial dose adjustments), serum phosphorus; serum calcium-phosphorus product; intact parathyroid hormone (iPTH)
Reference Range
  Corrected total serum calcium (K/DOQI, 2003): CKD stages 3 and 4: 8.4-10.2 mg/dL (2.1-2.6 mmol/L); CKD stage 5: 8.4-9.5 mg/dL (2.1-2.37 mmol/L); KDIGO guidelines recommend maintaining normal ranges for all stages of CKD (3-5D) (KDIGO, 2009)

◄ Phosphorus (K/DOQI, 2003):
CKD stages 3 and 4: 2.7-4.6 mg/dL (0.87-1.48mmol/L) (adults); maintain within age-appropriate limits (children)
CKD stage 5 (including those treated with dialysis): 3.5-5.5 mg/dL (1.13-1.78 mmol/L) (children >12 years and adults); 4-6 mg/dL (1.29-1.94 mmol/L) (children 1-12 years)
KDIGO guidelines recommend maintaining normal ranges for CKD stages 3-5 and lowering elevated phosphorus levels toward the normal range for CKD stage 5D (KDIGO, 2009)
Serum calcium-phosphorus product (K/DOQI, 2003): CKD stage 3-5: <55 mg^2/dL^2 (children >12 years and adults); <65 mg^2/dL^2 (children ≤12 years)
PTH: Whole molecule, immunochemiluminometric assay (ICMA): 1.0-5.2 pmol/L; whole molecule, radioimmunoassay (RIA): 10.0-65.0 pg/mL; whole molecule, immunoradiometric, double antibody (IRMA): 1.0-6.0 pmol/L
Target ranges by stage of chronic kidney disease (KDIGO, 2009): CKD stage 3-5: Optimal iPTH is unknown; maintain normal range (assay-dependent); CKD stage 5D: Maintain iPTH within 2-9 times the upper limit of normal for the assay used

Pharmacotherapy Pearls Calcium acetate binds to phosphorus in the GI tract better than other calcium salts due to its lower solubility and subsequent reduced absorption and increased formation of calcium phosphate.

12.7 mEq calcium/g; 250 mg/g elemental calcium (25% elemental calcium)

Special Geriatric Considerations Constipation and gas can be significant in the elderly, but are usually mild.

Dosage Forms Excipient information presented when available (limited, particularly for generics); consult specific product labeling.
Gelcap, oral: 667 mg [equivalent to elemental calcium 169 mg (8.45 mEq)]
    PhosLo®: 667 mg [equivalent to elemental calcium 169 mg (8.45 mEq)]
Solution, oral:
    Phoslyra™: 667 mg/5 mL (473 mL) [contains maltitol 1 g/5 mL, propylene glycol; black-cherry-menthol flavor; equivalent to elemental calcium 169 mg (8.45 mEq)/5 mL]
Tablet, oral:
    Eliphos™: 667 mg [equivalent to elemental calcium 169 mg (8.45 mEq)]

◆ **Calcium Acetate and Aluminum Sulfate** see Aluminum Sulfate and Calcium Acetate on page 85
◆ **Calcium Acetylhomotaurinate** see Acamprosate on page 27
◆ **Calcium and Risedronate** see Risedronate and Calcium on page 1621

Calcium and Vitamin D (KAL see um & VYE ta min dee)

Medication Safety Issues
Sound-alike/look-alike issues:
Os-Cal® may be confused with Asacol®
Brand Names: U.S. Cal-CYUM [OTC]; Caltrate® 600+D [OTC]; Caltrate® 600+Soy™ [OTC]; Caltrate® ColonHealth™ [OTC]; Chew-Cal [OTC]; Citracal® Maximum [OTC]; Citracal® Petites [OTC]; Citracal® Regular [OTC]; Liqua-Cal [OTC]; Os-Cal® 500+D [OTC]; Oysco 500+D [OTC]; Oysco D [OTC]; Oyst-Cal-D 500 [OTC]; Oyst-Cal-D [OTC]
Index Terms Vitamin D and Calcium Carbonate
Generic Availability (U.S.) Yes
Pharmacologic Category Calcium Salt; Electrolyte Supplement, Oral; Vitamin, Fat Soluble
Use Dietary supplement, antacid
Contraindications Hypersensitivity to any component of the formulation; hypophosphatemia, hypercalcemia, evidence of vitamin D toxicity; history of kidney stones
Warnings/Precautions Constipation, bloating, and gas are common with calcium supplements. Use with caution patients with respiratory failure, renal impairment or respiratory acidosis. Use with caution in patients with renal failure to avoid hypercalcemia; frequent monitoring of serum calcium and phosphorus is necessary. Use caution when administering calcium supplements to patients with a history of kidney stones. Hypercalcemia and hypercalciuria are most likely to occur in hypoparathyroid patients receiving high doses of vitamin D. Calcium absorption is impaired in achlorhydria; common in elderly, use an alternate salt (eg, citrate) and administer with food. Calcium administration interferes with absorption of some minerals and drugs; use with caution. Taking calcium (≤500 mg) with food improves absorption.

Some products may contain soy, tartrazine, or phenylalanine, or may be derived from shellfish.

Adverse Reactions (Reflective of adult population; not specific for elderly) Frequency not defined; also see individual agents
Central nervous system: Headache

Endocrine & metabolic: Hypercalcemia, hypercalciuria
Gastrointestinal: Gastrointestinal discomfort

Drug Interactions

Avoid Concomitant Use

Avoid concomitant use of Calcium Carbonate and Vitamin D with any of the following: Calcium Acetate

Increased Effect/Toxicity

Calcium Carbonate and Vitamin D may increase the levels/effects of: Alpha-/Beta-Agonists; Amphetamines; Calcium Acetate; Calcium Polystyrene Sulfonate; Dexmethylphenidate; Methylphenidate; QuiNIDine; Sodium Polystyrene Sulfonate; Vitamin D Analogs

The levels/effects of Calcium Carbonate and Vitamin D may be increased by: Thiazide Diuretics

Decreased Effect

Calcium Carbonate and Vitamin D may decrease the levels/effects of: ACE Inhibitors; Allopurinol; Anticonvulsants (Hydantoin); Antipsychotic Agents (Phenothiazines); Atazanavir; Bisacodyl; Bisphosphonate Derivatives; Calcium Channel Blockers; Cefditoren; Cefpodoxime; Cefuroxime; Chloroquine; Corticosteroids (Oral); Dabigatran Etexilate; Dasatinib; Delavirdine; DOBUTamine; Eltrombopag; Erlotinib; Estramustine; Gabapentin; HMG-CoA Reductase Inhibitors; Iron Salts; Isoniazid; Itraconazole; Ketoconazole; Ketoconazole (Systemic); Mesalamine; Methenamine; Mycophenolate; Penicillamine; Phosphate Supplements; Protease Inhibitors; Quinolone Antibiotics; Rilpivirine; Tetracycline Derivatives; Thyroid Products; Trientine

The levels/effects of Calcium Carbonate and Vitamin D may be decreased by: Trientine

Ethanol/Nutrition/Herb Interactions

Ethanol: Avoid ethanol (may increase risk of osteoporosis).
Food: Food may increase calcium absorption. Calcium may decrease iron absorption. Bran, foods high in oxalates, or whole grain cereals may decrease calcium absorption.

Dosage

Geriatric & Adult Calcium supplement, hyperphosphatemia: Oral: Refer to individual monographs for dietary reference intake.

Renal Impairment Use caution in severe renal impairment.

Administration Administer, preferably with food, 2 hours before or after other medications.

Monitoring Parameters Monitor serum calcium (particularly if used in patients with severe renal impairment)

Dosage Forms Excipient information presented when available (limited, particularly for generics); consult specific product labeling.

Caplet, oral:
Citracal® Maximum: Calcium 315 mg and vitamin D 250 int. units [gluten free]
Capsule, softgel, oral: Calcium 500 mg and vitamin D 500 int. units; calcium 600 mg and vitamin D 100 int. units; calcium 600 mg and vitamin D 200 int. units
Liqua-Cal: Calcium 600 mg and vitamin D 200 int. units [contains beeswax, lecithin, and soybean oil]
Tablet, oral: Calcium 250 mg and vitamin D 125 int. units; calcium 500 mg and vitamin D 125 int. units; calcium 500 mg and vitamin D 200 int. units; calcium 600 mg and vitamin D 125 int. units; calcium 600 mg and vitamin D 200 int. units
Caltrate® 600+D: Calcium 600 mg and vitamin D 200 int. units [contains soybean oil]
Caltrate® 600+Soy™: Calcium 600 mg and vitamin D 200 int. units [contains soy isoflavones 25 mg]
Caltrate® ColonHealth™: Calcium 600 mg and vitamin D 200 int. units [contains soybean oil]
Citracal® Petites: Calcium 200 mg and vitamin D 250 int. units [gluten free]
Citracal® Regular: Calcium 250 mg and vitamin D 200 int. units [gluten free]
Oysco D: Calcium 250 mg and vitamin D 125 int. units
Oysco 500+D: Calcium 500 mg and vitamin D 200 int. units [contains tartrazine]
Oyst-Cal-D: Calcium 250 mg and vitamin D 125 int. units [sodium free, sugar free; contains tartrazine]
Oyst-Cal-D 500: Calcium 500 mg and vitamin D 200 int. units [sodium free, sugar free; contains tartrazine]
Tablet, chewable: Calcium 500 mg and vitamin D 100 int. units; Calcium 600 mg and vitamin D 400 int. units
Os-Cal® 500+D: Calcium 500 mg and vitamin D 400 int. units [sugar free; contains phenylalanine; light lemon flavor]
Wafer, chewable:
Cal-CYUM: Calcium 519 mg and vitamin D 150 int. units (50s) [dye free; vanilla flavor]
Chew-Cal: Calcium 333 mg and vitamin D 40 int. units (100s, 250s)

◆ **Calcium Carbonate, Magnesium Hydroxide, and Famotidine** *see* Famotidine, Calcium Carbonate, and Magnesium Hydroxide *on page 696*

Calcium Chloride (KAL see um KLOR ide)

Medication Safety Issues
Sound-alike/look-alike issues:
Calcium chloride may be confused with calcium gluconate
Administration issues:
Calcium chloride may be confused with calcium gluconate.
Confusion with the different intravenous salt forms of calcium has occurred. There is a threefold difference in the primary cation concentration between calcium chloride (in which 1g = 13.6 mEq [270 mg] of elemental Ca++) and calcium gluconate (in which 1g = 4.65 mEq [90 mg] of elemental Ca++).
Prescribers should specify which salt form is desired. Dosages should be expressed either as mEq, mg, or grams of the salt form.

Generic Availability (U.S.) Yes

Pharmacologic Category Calcium Salt; Electrolyte Supplement, Parenteral

Use Treatment of acute symptomatic hypocalcemia; cardiac disturbances of hyperkalemia or hypocalcemia; emergent treatment of hypocalcemic tetany; treatment of severe hypermagnesemia

Unlabeled/Investigational Use Calcium channel blocker overdose; severe hyperkalemia (K+ >7 mEq/L with toxic ECG changes) [ACLS guidelines]; malignant arrhythmias associated with hypermagnesemia [ACLS guidelines]

Contraindications Hypercalcemia, known or suspected digoxin toxicity; not recommended as routine treatment in cardiac arrest (includes asystole, ventricular fibrillation, pulseless ventricular tachycardia, or pulseless electrical activity)

Warnings/Precautions For I.V. use only; do not inject SubQ or I.M.; avoid rapid I.V. administration (<100 mg/minute) unless being given emergently. Avoid extravasation. Use with caution in patients with hyperphosphatemia, respiratory acidosis, renal impairment, or respiratory failure; acidifying effect of calcium chloride may potentiate acidosis. Use with caution in patients with chronic renal failure to avoid hypercalcemia; frequent monitoring of serum calcium and phosphorus is necessary. Use with caution in hypokalemic or digitalized patients since acute rises in serum calcium levels may precipitate cardiac arrhythmias. Solutions may contain aluminum; toxic levels may occur following prolonged administration in patients with renal impairment. Avoid metabolic acidosis (ie, administer only 2-3 days then change to another calcium salt).

Adverse Reactions (Reflective of adult population; not specific for elderly) Frequency not defined. I.V.:
Cardiovascular: Arrhythmia, bradycardia, cardiac arrest, hypotension, syncope, vasodilation
Endocrine & metabolic: Hypercalcemia
Gastrointestinal: Irritation, chalky taste
Hepatic: Serum amylase increased
Neuromuscular & skeletal: Tingling sensation
Renal: Renal calculi
Miscellaneous: Hot flashes
Postmarketing and/or case reports: Calcinosis cutis

Drug Interactions
Avoid Concomitant Use
Avoid concomitant use of Calcium Chloride with any of the following: Calcium Acetate
Increased Effect/Toxicity
Calcium Chloride may increase the levels/effects of: Calcium Acetate; CefTRIAXone; Vitamin D Analogs

The levels/effects of Calcium Chloride may be increased by: Thiazide Diuretics
Decreased Effect
Calcium Chloride may decrease the levels/effects of: Bisphosphonate Derivatives; Calcium Channel Blockers; DOBUTamine; Eltrombopag; Phosphate Supplements; Tetracycline Derivatives; Thyroid Products; Trientine

The levels/effects of Calcium Chloride may be decreased by: Trientine

Stability Do not refrigerate solutions; IVPB solutions/I.V. infusion solutions are stable for 24 hours at room temperature.
Although calcium chloride is not routinely used in the preparation of parenteral nutrition, it is important to note that phosphate salts may precipitate when mixed with calcium salts. Solubility is improved in amino acid parenteral nutrition solutions. Check with a pharmacist to determine compatibility.

Mechanism of Action Moderates nerve and muscle performance via action potential excitation threshold regulation

Pharmacodynamics/Kinetics

Absorption: I.V. calcium salts are absorbed directly into the circulation

Excretion: Primarily feces (80% as insoluble calcium); urine (20%)

Dosage

Geriatric & Adult Note: One gram of calcium chloride is equal to 270 mg of elemental calcium.

Dosages are expressed in terms of the calcium chloride salt based on a solution concentration of 100 mg/mL (10%) containing 1.4 mEq (27.3 mg)/mL elemental calcium.

Acute, symptomatic ionized hypocalcemia, hyperkalemia, or magnesium toxicity: **Note:** Routine use in cardiac arrest is not recommended due to the lack of improved survival (ACLS, 2010): I.V.: 500-1000 mg, may repeat as necessary

Beta-blocker overdose, refractory to glucagon and high-dose vasopressors (unlabeled use): I.V.: 1000 mg bolus via central line reported to quickly increase blood pressure (O'Grady, 2001)

Calcium channel blocker overdose (unlabeled use):

I.V.: 1000 mg every 10-20 minutes (total of 4 doses) **or** 1000 mg every 2-3 minutes until clinical effect is achieved; if favorable response obtained, consider I.V. infusion

I.V. infusion: 20-50 mg/kg/hour

Hypocalcemia secondary to citrated blood transfusion: I.V.: 200-500 mg per 500 mL of citrated blood (infused into another vein)

Note: Routine administration of calcium, in the absence of signs/symptoms of hypocalcemia, is generally not recommended. A number of recommendations have been published seeking to address potential hypocalcemia during massive transfusion of citrated blood; however, many practitioners recommend replacement only as guided by clinical evidence of hypocalcemia and/or serial monitoring of ionized calcium. In adults, clinically-significant hypocalcemia usually dose not occur until >5 units of packed red blood cells have been administered.

Hypocalcemic tetany: I.V.: 1000 mg over 10-30 minutes; may repeat after 6 hours

Renal Impairment Cl_{cr} <25 mL/minute: Dosage adjustments may be necessary depending on the serum calcium concentration.

Administration For I.V. administration only; avoid extravasation. Avoid rapid administration (do not exceed 100 mg/minute). May be given over 2-5 minutes if rapid increase in serum calcium concentration is required. For I.V. infusion, dilute to a maximum concentration of 20 mg/mL and infuse over 1 hour or no greater than 45-90 mg/kg/hour (0.6-1.2 mEq/kg/hour); administration via a central or deep vein is preferred; do not use scalp, small hand or foot veins for I.V. administration since severe necrosis and sloughing may occur. Monitor ECG if calcium is infused faster than 2.5 mEq/minute; **stop the infusion if the patient complains of pain or discomfort.** Warm to body temperature. **Do not infuse calcium chloride in the same I.V. line as phosphate-containing solutions.**

Monitoring Parameters Monitor infusion site, ECG when appropriate; serum calcium and ionized calcium (normal: 8.5-10.2 mg/dL [total]; 4.5-5.0 mg/dL [ionized]), albumin, serum phosphate

Calcium channel blocker overdose, beta-blocker overdose: Hemodynamic response, serum ionized calcium levels

Reference Range

Serum total calcium: 8.4-10.2 mg/dL. **Note:** Due to a poor correlation between the serum ionized calcium (free) and total serum calcium, particularly in states of low albumin or acid/base imbalances, direct measurement of ionized calcium is recommended.

In low albumin states, the corrected **total** serum calcium may be estimated by the following equation (assuming a normal albumin of 4 g/dL).

Corrected total calcium = total serum calcium + 0.8 (4.0 - measured serum albumin)

or

Corrected calcium = measured calcium - measured albumin + 4.0

Serum/plasma chloride: 95-108 mEq/L

Test Interactions Increased calcium

Pharmacotherapy Pearls 14 mEq/g/10 mL; 270 mg elemental calcium/g (27% elemental calcium)

Special Geriatric Considerations When using in the elderly, check albumin status and make appropriate decisions concerning reference serum concentrations. Elderly, especially the ill, often have low albumin due to malnutrition.

CALCIUM CHLORIDE

◀ **Dosage Forms** Excipient information presented when available (limited, particularly for generics); consult specific product labeling.

Injection, solution: 10% (10 mL) [equivalent to elemental calcium 27.2 mg (1.36 mEq)/mL]

Injection, solution [preservative free]: 10% (10 mL) [equivalent to elemental calcium 27.2 mg (1.36 mEq)/mL]

Selected References

Ariyan CE and Sosa JA, "Assessment and Management of Patients With Abnormal Calcium," *Crit Care Med*, 2004, 32 (4 Suppl):146-54.

Chin RL, Garmel GM, and Harter PM, "Development of Ventricular Fibrillation After Intravenous Calcium Chloride Administration in a Patient With Supraventricular Tachycardia," *Ann Emerg Med*, 1995, 25(3):416-9.

DeRoos F, "Calcium Channel Blockers," Goldfrank LG, et al, ed, *Goldfrank's Toxicologic Emergencies*, 7th ed, New York, (NY):McGraw-Hill Medical Publishing, 2002, 762-74.

Dickerson RN, "Treatment of Hypocalcemia in Critical Illness - Part 1," *Nutrition*, 2007, 23(4):358-61.

Dickerson RN, "Treatment of Hypocalcemia in Critical Illness - Part 2," *Nutrition*, 2007, 23(5):436-37.

ECC Committee, Subcommittees and Task Forces of the American Heart Association,"2005 American Heart Association Guidelines for Cardiopulmonary Resuscitation and Emergency Cardiovascular Care," *Circulation*, 2005, 112(24 Suppl):IV1-203.

Isbister GK, "Delayed Asystolic Cardiac Arrest After Diltiazem Overdose: Resuscitation With High Dose Intravenous Calcium", *Emerg Med J*, 2002, 19(4):355-7.

Lam YM, Tse HF, and Lau CP, "Continuous Calcium Chloride Infusion for Massive Nifedipine Overdose,"*Chest*, 2001, 119(4):1280-2.

Mokhlesi B, Leikin JB, Murray P, et al, "Adult Toxicology in Critical Care: Part II: Specific Poisonings," *Chest*, 2003, 123 (3):897-922.

Salhanick SD and Shannon MW, "Management of Calcium Channel Antagonist Overdose," *Drug Saf*, 2003, 26 (2):65-79.

Shepherd G, "Treatment of Poisoning Caused by β-adrenergic and Calcium-Channel Blockers," *Am J Health-Syst Pharm*, 2006, 63(19):1828-35.

Calcium Citrate (KAL see um SIT rate)

Medication Safety Issues

Sound-alike/look-alike issues:

Citracal® may be confused with Citrucel®

Brand Names: U.S. Cal-C-Caps [OTC]; Cal-Cee [OTC]; Cal-Citrate™ 225 [OTC]; Calcitrate [OTC]

Brand Names: Canada Osteocit®

Generic Availability (U.S.) Yes

Pharmacologic Category Calcium Salt

Use Antacid; treatment and prevention of calcium deficiency or hyperphosphatemia (eg, osteoporosis, osteomalacia, mild/moderate renal insufficiency, hypoparathyroidism, postmenopausal osteoporosis, rickets)

Contraindications Hypersensitivity to any component of the formulation; hypercalcemia, renal calculi, ventricular fibrillation

Warnings/Precautions Constipation, bloating, and gas are common with calcium supplements. Use with caution in patients with renal failure to avoid hypercalcemia; frequent monitoring of serum calcium and phosphorus is necessary. Use caution when administering calcium supplements to patients with a history of kidney stones. Hypercalcemia and hypercalciuria are most likely to occur in hypoparathyroid patients receiving high doses of vitamin D. Calcium absorption is impaired in achlorhydria; common in elderly. Citrate may be preferred because better absorbed. Calcium administration interferes with absorption of some minerals and drugs; use with caution. It is recommended to concomitantly administer vitamin D for optimal calcium absorption. Taking calcium (≤500 mg) with food improves absorption.

Adverse Reactions (Reflective of adult population; not specific for elderly) Frequency not defined:

Mild hypercalcemia (calcium: >10.5 mg/dL) may be asymptomatic or manifest itself as constipation, anorexia, nausea, and vomiting

More severe hypercalcemia (calcium: >12 mg/dL) is associated with confusion, delirium, stupor, and coma

Central nervous system: Headache

Endocrine & metabolic: Hypophosphatemia, hypercalcemia

Gastrointestinal: Nausea, anorexia, vomiting, abdominal pain, constipation

Miscellaneous: Thirst

Drug Interactions

Avoid Concomitant Use

Avoid concomitant use of Calcium Citrate with any of the following: Calcium Acetate

Increased Effect/Toxicity

Calcium Citrate may increase the levels/effects of: Aluminum Hydroxide; Calcium Acetate; Vitamin D Analogs

The levels/effects of Calcium Citrate may be increased by: Thiazide Diuretics

Decreased Effect
Calcium Citrate may decrease the levels/effects of: Bisphosphonate Derivatives; Calcium Channel Blockers; DOBUTamine; Eltrombopag; Estramustine; Phosphate Supplements; Quinolone Antibiotics; Tetracycline Derivatives; Thyroid Products; Trientine

The levels/effects of Calcium Citrate may be decreased by: Trientine

Ethanol/Nutrition/Herb Interactions Ethanol: Avoid ethanol (may increase risk of osteoporosis).

Mechanism of Action Moderates nerve and muscle performance via action potential excitation threshold regulation

Pharmacodynamics/Kinetics Absorption: Requires vitamin D

Dosage
Geriatric
Dietary Reference Intake for Calcium: RDA:
Females: Refer to adult dosing.
Males ≤70 years: Refer to adult dosing.
Males >70 years: 1200 mg/day
Dietary supplement: Refer to adult dosing.
Adult Oral: Dosage is in terms of **elemental** calcium
Dietary Reference Intake for Calcium:
Adults, Female/Male: RDA:
19-50 years: 1000 mg/day
≥51 years, females: 1200 mg/day
51-70 years, males: 1000 mg/day
Dietary supplement: Oral: Usual dose: 500-2000 mg divided 2-4 times/day

Reference Range
Serum calcium: 8.5-10.5 mg/dL. Monitor plasma calcium levels if using calcium salts as electrolyte supplements for deficiency.

Due to a poor correlation between the serum ionized calcium (free) and total serum calcium, particularly in states of low albumin or acid/base imbalances, direct measurement of ionized calcium is recommended

In low albumin states, the corrected **total** serum calcium may be estimated by:
Corrected total calcium = total serum calcium + 0.8 (4.0 - measured serum albumin)

Dosage Forms
Excipient information presented when available (limited, particularly for generics); consult specific product labeling. [DSC] = Discontinued product
Capsule, oral:
Cal-C-Caps: Elemental calcium 180 mg
Cal-Citrate™ 225: Elemental calcium 225 mg
Granules, oral: (480 g)
Tablet, oral: Elemental calcium 200 mg [DSC], Elemental calcium 250 mg
Cal-Cee: Elemental calcium 250 mg
Calcitrate: Elemental calcium 200 mg

Selected References
"Dietary Reference Intakes for Calcium, Phosphorus, Magnesium, Vitamin D, and Fluoride. Standing Committee on the Scientific Evaluation of Dietary Reference Intakes, Food and Nutrition Board, Institute of Medicine," National Academy of Sciences, Washington, DC: National Academy Press, 1997. Available at: http://www.nap.edu.

Calcium Gluconate (KAL see um GLOO koe nate)

Medication Safety Issues
Sound-alike/look-alike issues:
Calcium gluconate may be confused with calcium glubionate

Brand Names: U.S. Cal-G [OTC]; Cal-GLU™ [OTC]

Generic Availability (U.S.) Yes

Pharmacologic Category Calcium Salt; Electrolyte Supplement, Oral; Electrolyte Supplement, Parenteral

Use Treatment and prevention of hypocalcemia; treatment of tetany, cardiac disturbances of hyperkalemia, cardiac resuscitation when epinephrine fails to improve myocardial contractions, hypocalcemia; calcium supplementation; hydrofluoric acid (HF) burns

Unlabeled/Investigational Use Hydrofluoric acid (HF) burns; calcium channel blocker overdose

Contraindications Hypersensitivity to calcium gluconate or any component of the formulation; ventricular fibrillation during cardiac resuscitation; digitalis toxicity or suspected digoxin toxicity; hypercalcemia

Warnings/Precautions Injection solution is for I.V. use only; do not inject SubQ or I.M. Avoid too rapid I.V. administration and avoid extravasation. Use with caution in digitalized patients, severe hyperphosphatemia, respiratory failure, or acidosis. May produce cardiac arrest.

Hypercalcemia may occur in patients with renal failure; frequent determination of serum calcium is necessary. Use caution with renal disease. Use caution when administering calcium supplements to patients with a history of kidney stones. Solutions may contain aluminum; toxic levels may occur following prolonged administration in patients with renal dysfunction. Oral: Constipation, bloating, and gas are common with oral calcium supplements (especially carbonate salt). Taking calcium (≤500 mg) with food improves absorption. Calcium administration interferes with absorption of some minerals and drugs; use with caution. It is recommended to concomitantly administer vitamin D for optimal calcium absorption.

Adverse Reactions (Reflective of adult population; not specific for elderly) Frequency not defined.

I.V.:
Cardiovascular: Arrhythmia, bradycardia, cardiac arrest, hypotension, vasodilation, and syncope may occur following rapid I.V. injection
Central nervous system: Sense of oppression
Gastrointestinal: Chalky taste
Local: Abscess and necrosis following I.M. administration
Neuromuscular & skeletal: Tingling sensation
Miscellaneous: Heat waves
Oral: Gastrointestinal: Constipation

Drug Interactions

Avoid Concomitant Use

Avoid concomitant use of Calcium Gluconate with any of the following: Calcium Acetate

Increased Effect/Toxicity

Calcium Gluconate may increase the levels/effects of: Calcium Acetate; CefTRIAXone; Vitamin D Analogs

The levels/effects of Calcium Gluconate may be increased by: Thiazide Diuretics

Decreased Effect

Calcium Gluconate may decrease the levels/effects of: Bisphosphonate Derivatives; Calcium Channel Blockers; DOBUTamine; Eltrombopag; Estramustine; Phosphate Supplements; Quinolone Antibiotics; Tetracycline Derivatives; Thyroid Products; Trientine

The levels/effects of Calcium Gluconate may be decreased by: Trientine

Stability

Do not refrigerate solutions. IVPB solutions/I.V. infusion solutions are stable for 24 hours at room temperature.

Standard diluent: 1 g/100 mL D_5W or NS; 2 g/100 mL D_5W or NS.

Maximum concentration in parenteral nutrition solutions is variable depending upon concentration and solubility (consult detailed reference).

Mechanism of Action As dietary supplement, used to prevent or treat negative calcium balance; in osteoporosis, it helps to prevent or decrease the rate of bone loss. The calcium in calcium salts moderates nerve and muscle performance and allows normal cardiac function.

Pharmacodynamics/Kinetics

Absorption: Requires vitamin D; calcium is absorbed in soluble, ionized form; solubility of calcium is increased in an acid environment
Distribution: Primarily in bones and teeth; crosses placenta; enters breast milk
Protein binding: Primarily albumin
Excretion: Primarily feces (as unabsorbed calcium); urine (20%)

Dosage

Geriatric

Dietary Reference Intake for Calcium: RDA:
Females: Refer to adult dosing.
Males ≤70 years: Refer to adult dosing.
Males >70 years: 1200 mg/day
All other indications: Refer to adult dosing.

Adult

Dietary Reference Intake for Calcium:
Adults, Female/Male: RDA:
19-50 years: 1000 mg/day
≥51 years, females: 1200 mg/day
51-70 years, males: 1000 mg/day

Dosage note: Calcium chloride has 3 times more elemental calcium than calcium gluconate. Calcium chloride is 27% elemental calcium; calcium gluconate is 9% elemental calcium. One gram of calcium chloride is equal to 270 mg of elemental calcium; 1 gram of calcium gluconate is equal to 90 mg of elemental calcium. The following dosages are expressed in terms of the calcium gluconate salt based on a solution concentration of 100 mg/mL (10%) containing 0.465 mEq (9.3 mg)/mL elemental calcium:

Hypocalcemia:

I.V.: 2-15 g/24 hours as a continuous infusion or in divided doses

Oral: 500 mg to 2 g 2-4 times/day

Hypocalcemia secondary to citrated blood infusion: I.V.: 500 mg to 1 g per 500 mL of citrated blood (infused into another vein). Single doses up to 2 g have also been recommended.

Note: Routine administration of calcium, in the absence of signs/symptoms of hypocalcemia, is generally not recommended. A number of recommendations have been published seeking to address potential hypocalcemia during massive transfusion of citrated blood; however, many practitioners recommend replacement only as guided by clinical evidence of hypocalcemia and/or serial monitoring of ionized calcium.

Hypocalcemic tetany: I.V.: 1-3 g/dose may be administered until therapeutic response occurs

Magnesium intoxication or cardiac arrest in the presence of hyperkalemia or hypocalcemia: I.V.: 500-800 mg/dose (maximum: 3 g/dose)

Maintenance electrolyte requirements for TPN: I.V.: Daily requirements: 1.7-3.4 g/1000 kcal/24 hours

Calcium channel blocker overdose (unlabeled use): I.V. infusion: 10% solution: 0.6-1.2 mL/kg/hour or I.V. 0.2-0.5 ml/kg every 15-20 minutes for 4 doses (maximum: 2-3 g/dose). In life-threatening situations, 1 g has been given every 1-10 minutes until clinical effect is achieved (case reports of resistant hypotension reported use of 12-18 g total).

Renal Impairment Cl_{cr} <25 mL/minute: Dosage adjustments may be necessary depending on the serum calcium levels.

Administration Not for I.M. or SubQ administration. For I.V. administration only; administer slowly (~1.5 mL calcium gluconate 10% per minute) through a small needle into a large vein in order to avoid too rapid increased in serum calcium and extravasation.

Extravasation treatment example: Hyaluronidase: Add 1 mL NS to 150 unit vial to make 150 units/mL of concentration; mix 0.1 mL of above with 0.9 mL NS in 1 mL syringe to make final concentration = 15 units/mL

Monitoring Parameters ECG, plasma and urine calcium concentrations

Reference Range

Serum calcium: 8.5-10.5 mg/dL. Monitor plasma calcium levels if using calcium salts as electrolyte supplements for deficiency.

Due to a poor correlation between the serum ionized calcium (free) and total serum calcium, particularly in states of low albumin or acid/base imbalances, direct measurement of ionized calcium is recommended

In low albumin states, the corrected **total** serum calcium may be estimated by:

Corrected total calcium = total serum calcium + 0.8 (4.0 - measured serum albumin)

Test Interactions Increased calcium (S); decreased magnesium

Pharmacotherapy Pearls A topical 2.5% to 5% calcium gel for the treatment of hydrofluoric acid (HF) burns can be prepared by adding calcium gluconate to a surgical lubricant (water soluble such as K-Y® Jelly). Calcium chloride should not be used for this purpose. Use of injectable calcium gluconate (I.V., SubQ) has also been reported in the literature for the treatment of HF burns not amenable to topical treatment.

Special Geriatric Considerations Constipation and gas can be significant in elderly, but are usually mild.

Dosage Forms Excipient information presented when available (limited, particularly for generics); consult specific product labeling. [DSC] = Discontinued product

Capsule, oral:

Cal-G: 700 mg [gluten free; equivalent to elemental calcium 65 mg]

Cal-GLU™: 515 mg [dye free, sugar free; equivalent to elemental calcium 50 mg]

Injection, solution [preservative free]: 10% (10 mL, 50 mL, 100 mL) [equivalent to elemental calcium 9.3 mg (0.465 mEq)/mL]

Powder, oral: (480 g)

Tablet, oral: 500 mg [equivalent to elemental calcium 45 mg], 648 mg [equivalent to elemental calcium 60 mg], 972 mg [DSC] [equivalent to elemental calcium 90 mg]

Selected References

DeRoos F, "Calcium Channel Blockers," Goldfrank LG, et al, ed, *Goldfrank's Toxicologic Emergencies*, 7th ed, New York, (NY):McGraw-Hill Medical Publishing, 2002, 762-74.

Isbister GK, "Continuous Calcium Chloride Infusion for Massive Nifedipine Overdose," *Emerg Med J*, 2002, 19 (4):355-7.

CALCIUM GLUCONATE

Lam YM, Tse HF, and Lau CP, "Delayed Asystolic Cardiac Arrest After Diltiazem Overdose: Resuscitation With High Dose Intravenous Calcium," *Chest*, 2001, 119(4):1280-2.

Millard TP, Harris AJ, and MacDonald DM, "Calcinosis Cutis Following Intravenous Infusion of Calcium Gluconate," *Br J Dermatol*, 1999, Jan;140(1):184-6.

Mokhlesi B, Leikin JB, Murray P, et al, "Adult Toxicology in Critical Care: Part II: Specific Poisonings," *Chest*, 2003, 123 (3):897-922.

Salhanick SD and Shannon MW, "Management of Calcium Channel Antagonist Overdose," *Drug Saf*, 2003, 26 (2):65-79.

Calcium Salts (Oral) (KAL see um salts OR al)

Brand Names: U.S. Alka-Mints® [OTC]; Amitone® [OTC]; Cal Carb-HD® [OTC]; Cal-Plus® [OTC]; Calci-Chew™ [OTC]; Calci-Mix™ [OTC]; Calciday-667® [OTC]; Caltrate® 600 [OTC]; Chooz® [OTC]; Citracal® [OTC]; Dicarbosil® [OTC]; Equilet® [OTC]; Florical® [OTC]; Gencalc® 600 [OTC]; Mallamint® [OTC]; Mylanta® Soothing Antacids [OTC]; Neo-Calglucon® [OTC]; Nephro-Calci® [OTC]; Os-Cal® 500 [OTC]; Oyst-Cal 500 [OTC]; Oystercal® 500; Posture® [OTC]; Rolaids® Calcium Rich [OTC]; Titralac® Plus Liquid [OTC]; Tums® E-X Extra Strength Tablet [OTC]; Tums® Extra Strength Liquid [OTC]; Tums® Ultra [OTC]; Tums® [OTC]

Generic Availability (U.S.) Yes

Stability Admixture incompatibilities: carbonates, phosphates, sulfates, tartrates

Mechanism of Action Moderates nerve and muscle performance via action potential excitation threshold regulation; may prevent negative calcium balance when used as dietary supplement as treatment or for osteoporosis; calcium carbonate is used as an antacid for acute dyspepsia

Pharmacodynamics/Kinetics Calcium is absorbed in soluble, ionized form; solubility of calcium is increased in an acid environment (except calcium lactate); therefore, administer with meals to maximize acidity and solubility to enhance absorption

Monitoring Parameters Plasma and urine calcium concentrations; ECG if hypercalcemic

Test Interactions Increased calcium (S); decreased magnesium; decreased phosphorus

Pharmacotherapy Pearls Doses for calcium supplementation are given in elemental calcium; calcium salts vary in their amount of elemental calcium

Calcium glubionate (6.5% elemental calcium)
Calcium carbonate (40% elemental calcium)
Calcium gluconate (9% elemental calcium)
Calcium lactate (13% elemental calcium)
Calcium citrate (21% elemental calcium)
Dibasic calcium phosphate (23% elemental calcium)
Calcium acetate (25% elemental calcium)
Tricalcium phosphate (39% elemental calcium)

All calcium preparations should be administered in divided doses to maximize calcium absorption; no more than 300-350 mg of elemental calcium should be given at a time. Women receiving estrogen therapy require 900-1000 mg total daily elemental calcium intake. Women not receiving estrogens require 1500 mg elemental calcium daily to maintain calcium balance.

Special Geriatric Considerations Constipation and gas can be significant in the elderly but are usually mild and may be eliminated by switching to another salt form. Calcium carbonate has been associated with the highest incidence of side effects, probably due to its high calcium content. Calcium carbonate absorption is impaired in achlorhydria. Since achlorhydria is common in the elderly, calcium carbonate may not be the ideal calcium supplement for dietary or treatment use. Administration with food helps this problem.

Dosage Forms Elemental calcium listed in brackets:

Calcium carbonate:
Capsule: 1500 mg [600 mg]
  Calci-Mix™: 1250 mg [500 mg]
  Florical®: 364 mg [145.6 mg] with sodium fluoride 8.3 mg
Liquid (Tums® Extra Strength): 1000 mg/5 mL (360 mL)
Lozenge (Mylanta® Soothing Antacids): 600 mg [240 mg]
Powder (Cal Carb-HD®): 6.5 g/packet [2.6 g]
Suspension, oral: 1250 mg/5 mL [500 mg]
Tablet: 650 mg [260 mg], 1500 mg [600 mg]
  Calciday-667®: 667 mg [267 mg]
  Florical®: 364 mg [145.6 mg] with sodium fluoride 8.3 mg
  Os-Cal® 500, Oyst-Cal 500, Oystercal® 500: 1250 mg [500 mg]
  Cal-Plus®, Caltrate® 600, Gencalc® 600, Nephro-Calci®: 1500 mg [600 mg]
  Chewable:
    Alka-Mints®: 850 mg [340 mg]
    Amitone®: 350 mg [140 mg]
    Calci-Chew™, Os-Cal®: 750 mg [300 mg]
    Chooz®, Dicarbosil®, Equilet®, Tums®: 500 mg [200 mg]

Mallamint® : 420 mg [168 mg]
Rolaids® Calcium Rich: 550 mg [220 mg]
Tums® E-X Extra Strength: 750 mg [300 mg]
Tums® Ultra®: 1000 mg [400 mg]

Calcium carbonate and simethicone (Titralac® Plus Liquid):
Liquid: Calcium carbonate 500 mg [200 mg] and simethicone 20 mg per 5 mL

Calcium citrate (Citracal®):
Tablet: 950 mg [200 mg]
Tablet, effervescent: 2376 mg [500 mg]

Calcium glubionate (Neo-Calglucon®):
Syrup: 1.8 g/5 mL [115 mg/5 mL] (480 mL)

Calcium gluconate:
Tablet: 500 mg [45 mg], 650 mg [58.5 mg], 975 mg [87.75 mg], 1 g [90 mg]

Calcium lactate:
Tablet: 325 mg [42.25 mg], 650 mg [84.5 mg]

Calcium phosphate, tribasic (Posture®):
Tablet, sugar free: 1565.2 mg [600 mg]

Candesartan (kan de SAR tan)

Related Information
Angiotensin Agents *on page* 1985
Medication Safety Issues
Sound-alike/look-alike issues:
Atacand® may be confused with antacid
Brand Names: U.S. Atacand®
Brand Names: Canada Apo-Candesartan; Atacand®; Sandoz-Candesartan
Index Terms Candesartan Cilexetil
Generic Availability (U.S.) No
Pharmacologic Category Angiotensin II Receptor Blocker
Use Alone or in combination with other antihypertensive agents in treating essential hypertension; treatment of heart failure (NYHA class II-IV)
Contraindications Hypersensitivity to candesartan or any component of the formulation; severe hepatic impairment and/or cholestasis
Warnings/Precautions May cause hyperkalemia; avoid potassium supplementation unless specifically required by healthcare provider. Avoid use or use a smaller dose in patients who are volume depleted; correct depletion first. May be associated with deterioration of renal function and/or increases in serum creatinine, particularly in patients with low renal blood flow (eg, renal artery stenosis, heart failure) whose glomerular filtration rate (GFR) is dependent on efferent arteriolar vasoconstriction by angiotensin II. Use with caution in unstented unilateral/bilateral renal artery stenosis, pre-existing renal insufficiency, or significant aortic/mitral stenosis. Use with caution in patients with moderate hepatic impairment. Contraindicated with severe hepatic impairment and/or cholestasis. Use caution when initiating in heart failure; may need to adjust dose, and/or concurrent diuretic therapy, because of candesartan-induced hypotension. Hypotension may occur during major surgery and anesthesia; use cautiously before, during, and immediately after such interventions. Although concurrent therapy with an ▶

◀ ACE inhibitor may be rational in select patients, concurrent use of ACE inhibitors may increase the risk of clinically-significant adverse events (eg, renal dysfunction, hyperkalemia).

Adverse Reactions (Reflective of adult population; not specific for elderly)

Cardiovascular: Angina, hypotension (CHF 19%), MI, palpitation, tachycardia

Central nervous system: Dizziness, lightheadedness, drowsiness, headache, vertigo, anxiety, depression, somnolence, fever

Dermatologic: Angioedema, rash

Endocrine & metabolic: Hyperglycemia, hyperkalemia (CHF <1% to 6%), hypertriglyceridemia, hyperuricemia

Gastrointestinal: Dyspepsia, gastroenteritis

Neuromuscular & skeletal: Back pain, CPK increased, myalgia, paresthesia, weakness

Renal: Serum creatinine increased (up to 13% in patients with CHF with drug discontinuation required in 6%), hematuria

Respiratory: Dyspnea, epistaxis, pharyngitis, rhinitis, upper respiratory tract infection

Miscellaneous: Diaphoresis increased

Drug Interactions

Metabolism/Transport Effects Substrate of CYP2C9 (minor); **Inhibits** CYP2C8 (weak), 2C9 (weak)

Avoid Concomitant Use There are no known interactions where it is recommended to avoid concomitant use.

Increased Effect/Toxicity

Candesartan may increase the levels/effects of: ACE Inhibitors; Amifostine; Antihypertensives; Hypotensive Agents; Lithium; Nonsteroidal Anti-Inflammatory Agents; Potassium-Sparing Diuretics; RiTUXimab; Sodium Phosphates

The levels/effects of Candesartan may be increased by: Alfuzosin; Diazoxide; Eplerenone; Herbs (Hypotensive Properties); MAO Inhibitors; Pentoxifylline; Phosphodiesterase 5 Inhibitors; Potassium Salts; Prostacyclin Analogues; Tolvaptan; Trimethoprim

Decreased Effect

The levels/effects of Candesartan may be decreased by: Herbs (Hypertensive Properties); Methylphenidate; Nonsteroidal Anti-Inflammatory Agents; Yohimbine

Ethanol/Nutrition/Herb Interactions Herb/Nutraceutical: Avoid dong quai if using for hypertension (has estrogenic activity). Avoid ephedra, yohimbe, ginseng (may worsen hypertension). Avoid garlic (may have increased antihypertensive effect).

Mechanism of Action Candesartan is an angiotensin receptor antagonist. Angiotensin II acts as a vasoconstrictor. In addition to causing direct vasoconstriction, angiotensin II also stimulates the release of aldosterone. Once aldosterone is released, sodium as well as water are reabsorbed. The end result is an elevation in blood pressure. Candesartan binds to the AT1 angiotensin II receptor. This binding prevents angiotensin II from binding to the receptor thereby blocking the vasoconstriction and the aldosterone secreting effects of angiotensin II.

Pharmacodynamics/Kinetics

Onset of action: 2-3 hours

Peak effect: 6-8 hours

Duration: >24 hours

Distribution: V_d: 0.13 L/kg

Protein binding: 99%

Metabolism: To candesartan by the intestinal wall cells

Bioavailability: 15%

Half-life elimination (dose dependent): 5-9 hours

Time to peak: 3-4 hours

Excretion: Urine (26%)

Clearance: Total body: 0.37 mL/kg/minute; Renal: 0.19 mL/kg/minute

Dosage

Geriatric Refer to adult dosing. No initial dosage adjustment is necessary for elderly patients (although higher concentrations (C_{max}) and AUC were observed in these populations), for patients with mildly impaired renal function, or for patients with mildly impaired hepatic function.

Adult

Hypertension: Oral: 4-32 mg once daily. Dosage must be individualized. Blood pressure response is dose related over the range of 2-32 mg. The usual recommended starting dose is 16 mg once daily when it is used as monotherapy in patients who are not volume depleted. It can be administered once or twice daily with total daily doses ranging from 8-32 mg; larger doses do not appear to have a greater effect and there is relatively little experience with such doses.

Congestive heart failure: Oral: Initial: 4 mg once daily; double the dose at 2-week intervals, as tolerated; target dose: 32 mg
  Note: In selected cases, concurrent therapy with an ACE inhibitor may provide additional benefit.
Hepatic Impairment
  Mild hepatic impairment: No initial dosage adjustment required.
  Moderate hepatic impairment: Consider initiation at lower dosages (AUC increased by 145%).
  Severe hepatic impairment and/or cholestasis: Contraindicated
Monitoring Parameters Supine blood pressure, electrolytes, serum creatinine, BUN, urinalysis, symptomatic hypotension, and tachycardia; in CHF, serum potassium during dose escalation and periodically thereafter
Pharmacotherapy Pearls May have an advantage over losartan due to minimal metabolism requirements and consequent use in mild-to-moderate hepatic impairment
Special Geriatric Considerations High concentrations occur in the elderly compared to younger subjects. AUC may be doubled in patients with renal impairment. No initial dose adjustment necessary since repeated dose did not demonstrate accumulation of drug or metabolites in elderly.
Dosage Forms Excipient information presented when available (limited, particularly for generics); consult specific product labeling.
  Tablet, oral, as cilexetil:
    Atacand®: 4 mg, 8 mg, 16 mg, 32 mg [scored]
Selected References
Granger CB, McMurray JJ, Yusuf S, et al, "Effects of Candesartan in Patients With Chronic Heart Failure and Reduced Left-Ventricular Systolic Function Intolerant to Angiotensin-Converting-Enzyme Inhibitors: The CHARM-Alternative Trial," *Lancet*, 2003, 362(9386):772-6.

Candesartan and Hydrochlorothiazide
(kan de SAR tan & hye droe klor oh THYE a zide)

Related Information
  Candesartan *on page 257*
  Hydrochlorothiazide *on page 876*
Brand Names: U.S. Atacand HCT®
Brand Names: Canada Atacand® Plus
Index Terms Candesartan Cilexetil and Hydrochlorothiazide; Hydrochlorothiazide and Candesartan
Generic Availability (U.S.) No
Pharmacologic Category Angiotensin II Receptor Blocker; Diuretic, Thiazide
Use Treatment of hypertension; combination product should not be used for initial therapy
Dosage
  Geriatric & Adult Hypertension, replacement therapy: Oral: Combination product can be substituted for individual agents; maximum therapeutic effect would be expected within 4 weeks

  Usual dosage range:
    Candesartan: 16-32 mg/day, given once daily or twice daily in divided doses
    Hydrochlorothiazide: 12.5-25 mg once daily
  Renal Impairment Serum levels of candesartan are increased and the half-life of hydrochlorothiazide is prolonged in patients with renal impairment. Contraindicated with severe renal impairment (Cl_{cr} <30 mL/minute).
  Hepatic Impairment Use with caution with moderate hepatic impairment. Contraindicated with severe hepatic impairment and/or cholestasis.
Special Geriatric Considerations No initial dosage adjustment is recommended in patients with normal renal and hepatic function; some patients may have increased sensitivity. Hydrochlorothiazide is not effective in patients with a Cl_{cr} <30 mL/minute; therefore, it may not be a useful agent in many elderly patients.
Dosage Forms Excipient information presented when available (limited, particularly for generics); consult specific product labeling.
  Tablet:
    Atacand HCT®:
      16/12.5: Candesartan cilexetil 16 mg and hydrochlorothiazide 12.5 mg
      32/12.5: Candesartan cilexetil 32 mg and hydrochlorothiazide 12.5 mg
      32/25: Candesartan cilexetil 32 mg and hydrochlorothiazide 25 mg

◆ **Candesartan Cilexetil** *see* Candesartan *on page 257*
◆ **Candesartan Cilexetil and Hydrochlorothiazide** *see* Candesartan and Hydrochlorothiazide *on page 259*

- **Cankaid® [OTC]** *see* Carbamide Peroxide *on page 272*
- **Capastat® Sulfate** *see* Capreomycin *on page 260*
- **Capex®** *see* Fluocinolone (Topical) *on page 748*
- **Caphosol®** *see* Saliva Substitute *on page 1652*
- **Capital® and Codeine** *see* Acetaminophen and Codeine *on page 37*

Capreomycin (kap ree oh MYE sin)

Medication Safety Issues
Sound-alike/look-alike issues:
Capastat® may be confused with Cepastat®
Brand Names: U.S. Capastat® Sulfate
Index Terms Capreomycin Sulfate
Generic Availability (U.S.) No
Pharmacologic Category Antibiotic, Miscellaneous; Antitubercular Agent
Use Treatment of tuberculosis in conjunction with at least one other antituberculosis agent
Contraindications Hypersensitivity to capreomycin or any component of the formulation
Warnings/Precautions [U.S. Boxed Warnings]: Use in patients with renal insufficiency or pre-existing auditory impairment must be undertaken with great caution, and the risk of additional eighth nerve impairment or renal injury should be weighed against the benefits to be derived from therapy. Since other parenteral antituberculous agents (eg, streptomycin) also have similar and sometimes irreversible toxic effects, particularly on eighth cranial nerve and renal function, simultaneous administration of these agents with capreomycin is not recommended. Use with nonantituberculous drugs (ie, aminoglycoside antibiotics) having ototoxic or nephrotoxic potential should be undertaken only with great caution. Use caution with renal dysfunction and in the elderly; dosage reductions are recommended for known or suspected renal impairment. Electrolyte imbalances (hypocalcemia, hypokalemia, and hypomagnesemia) have been reported with use. Prolonged use may result in fungal or bacterial superinfection, including *C. difficile*-associated diarrhea (CDAD) and pseudomembranous colitis; CDAD has been observed >2 months postantibiotic treatment.
Adverse Reactions (Reflective of adult population; not specific for elderly)
>10%:
Otic: Ototoxicity (subclinical hearing loss: 11%; clinical loss: 3%)
Renal: Nephrotoxicity (36%, increased BUN)
1% to 10%: Hematologic: Eosinophilia (dose related, mild)
Drug Interactions
Avoid Concomitant Use
Avoid concomitant use of Capreomycin with any of the following: BCG
Increased Effect/Toxicity
Capreomycin may increase the levels/effects of: Aminoglycosides; Colistimethate; Neuromuscular-Blocking Agents; Polymyxin B
Decreased Effect
Capreomycin may decrease the levels/effects of: BCG
Stability Powder for injection should be stored at room temperature of 15°C to 30°C (59°F to 86°F). Dissolve powder with 2 mL of NS or SWFI; allow 2-3 minutes for dissolution.
For I.V. administration: Further dilute in NS 100 mL.
For I.M. administration:
1 g dose: Administer contents of reconstituted vial
<1 g dose: See table:

Capreomycin Dilution for Doses <1 g (I.M. Administration)

Diluent Volume (mL)	Capreomycin Solution Volume (mL)	Final Concentration (approximate)
2.15	2.85	370 mg/mL
2.63	3.33	315 mg/mL
3.3	4	260 mg/mL
4.3	5	210 mg/mL

Following reconstitution, may store under refrigeration for up to 24 hours.
Mechanism of Action Capreomycin is a cyclic polypeptide antimicrobial. It is administered as a mixture of capreomycin IA and capreomycin IB. The mechanism of action of capreomycin is not well understood. Mycobacterial species that have become resistant to other agents are

usually still sensitive to the action of capreomycin. However, significant cross-resistance with viomycin, kanamycin, and neomycin occurs.

Pharmacodynamics/Kinetics

Half-life elimination: Normal renal function: 4-6 hours; Cl_{cr} 100-110 mL/minute: 5-6 hours; Cl_{cr} 50-80 mL/minute: 7-10 hours; Cl_{cr} 20-40 mL/minute: 12-20 hours; Cl_{cr} 10 mL/minute: 29 hours; Cl_{cr} 0 mL/minute: 55 hours

Time to peak, serum: I.M.: 1-2 hours

Excretion: Urine (52% within 12 hours)

Dosage

Geriatric Refer to adult dosing. Use with caution due to the increased potential for pre-existing renal dysfunction or impaired hearing. The manufacturer recommends initiating at lower end of dosing range. Adults >59 years of age: 10 mg/kg (maximum: 750 mg/dose) for 5-7 days per week for 2-4 months, followed by 10 mg/kg (maximum: 750 mg/dose) 2-3 times/week (*MMWR*, 2003).

Adult Tuberculosis: I.M., I.V.: 1 g/day (maximum: 20 mg/kg/day) for 60-120 days, followed by 1 g 2-3 times/week **or** 15 mg/kg/day (maximum: 1 g/dose) for 2-4 months, followed by 15 mg/kg (maximum: 1 g/dose) 2-3 times/week (*MMWR*, 2003)

Renal Impairment Adults:

The FDA-approved labeling contains the following renal dosing adjustment guidelines (maximum: 1 g/dose):

Cl_{cr} 110 mL/minute: Administer 13.9 mg/kg every 24 hours

Cl_{cr} 100 mL/minute: Administer 12.7 mg/kg every 24 hours

Cl_{cr} 80 mL/minute: Administer 10.4 mg/kg every 24 hours

Cl_{cr} 60 mL/minute: Administer 8.2 mg/kg every 24 hours

Cl_{cr} 50 mL/minute: Administer 7 mg/kg every 24 hours **or** 14 mg/kg every 48 hours

Cl_{cr} 40 mL/minute: Administer 5.9 mg/kg every 24 hours **or** 11.7 mg/kg every 48 hours

Cl_{cr} 30 mL/minute: Administer 4.7 mg/kg every 24 hours **or** 9.5 mg/kg every 48 hours **or** 14.2 mg/kg every 72 hours

Cl_{cr} 20 mL/minute: Administer 3.6 mg/kg every 24 hours **or** 7.2 mg/kg every 48 hours **or** 10.7 mg/kg every 72 hours

Cl_{cr} 10 mL/minute: Administer 2.4 mg/kg every 24 hours **or** 4.9 mg/kg every 48 hours **or** 7.3 mg/kg every 72 hours

Cl_{cr} 0 mL/minute: Administer 1.3 mg/kg every 24 hours **or** 2.6 mg/kg every 48 hours **or** 3.9 mg/kg every 72 hours

The following (unlabeled) guidelines may also be used:

MMWR, 2003:

Cl_{cr} ≥30 mL/minute: No adjustment required

Cl_{cr} <30 mL/minute and hemodialysis: 12-15 mg/kg (maximum: 1 g/dose) 2-3 days per week (**NOT** daily)

Aronoff, 2007:

Cl_{cr} ≥10 mL/minute: 1 g every 24 hours

Cl_{cr} <10 mL/minute: 1 g every 48 hours

Hemodialysis: Administer dose after hemodialysis only

Continuous renal replacement therapy (CRRT): 5 mg/kg every 24 hours

Administration Administer by deep I.M. injection into large muscle mass

Monitoring Parameters Audiometric measurements and vestibular function at baseline and during therapy; renal function at baseline and weekly during therapy; frequent assessment of serum electrolytes (including calcium, magnesium, and potassium), liver function tests

Reference Range Recommended concentration for susceptibility testing: 10 mcg/mL

Special Geriatric Considerations Has not been studied in the elderly. I.M. administration may limit use due to painful injection or lack of sites in patients with decreased muscle mass. Use with caution in patients with pre-existing hearing impairment due to potential ototoxicity.

Dosage Forms Excipient information presented when available (limited, particularly for generics); consult specific product labeling.

Injection, powder for reconstitution, as sulfate:

Capastat® Sulfate: 1 g

Selected References

Aronoff GR, Bennett WM, Berns JS, et al, *Drug Prescribing in Renal Failure: Dosing Guidelines for Adults and Children*, 5th ed. Philadelphia, PA: American College of Physicians; 2007.

◆ **Capreomycin Sulfate** *see* Capreomycin *on page 260*

Capsaicin (kap SAY sin)

Medication Safety Issues

Sound-alike/look-alike issues:

Zostrix® may be confused with Zestril®, Zovirax®

CAPSAICIN

◄ **Brand Names: U.S.** Capzasin-HP® [OTC]; Capzasin-P® [OTC]; DiabetAid® Pain and Tingling Relief [OTC]; Qutenza™; Salonpas® Hot [OTC]; Zostrix® Diabetic Foot Pain [OTC]; Zostrix® [OTC]; Zostrix®-HP [OTC]

Brand Names: Canada Zostrix®; Zostrix® H.P.

Index Terms NGX-4010

Generic Availability (U.S.) Yes: Cream

Pharmacologic Category Analgesic, Topical; Topical Skin Product; Transient Receptor Potential Vanilloid 1 (TRPV1) Agonist

Use
Topical patch (Qutenza™): Management of postherpetic neuralgia (PHN)
OTC labeling: Temporary treatment of minor pain associated with muscles and joints due to backache, strains, sprains, bruises, cramps or arthritis; temporary relief of pain associated with diabetic neuropathy

Unlabeled/Investigational Use Diabetic neuropathy; treatment of pain associated with psoriasis and intractable pruritus. Potential use as topical agent in burning mouth syndrome and oral mucositis.

Contraindications There are no contraindications listed in the manufacturer's labeling.

Warnings/Precautions
Topical high-concentration capsaicin patch (Qutenza™): Do not apply to face, scalp, or allow contact with eyes or mucous membranes. If an unintended area of skin is inadvertently exposed, the cleansing gel should be used. Post-application pain should be treated with local cooling methods and/or analgesics (opioids may be necessary). Avoid rapid removal of patches to decrease risk of aerosolization of capsaicin; inhalation of airborne capsaicin may result in coughing or sneezing; if shortness of breath occurs, medical care is required; remove patches gently and slowly to decrease risk of aerosolization. Use with caution in patients with uncontrolled hypertension, or a history of cardiovascular or cerebrovascular events; transient increases in blood pressure due to treatment-related pain have occurred during and after application of patch.

Topical OTC products: Apply externally; avoid contact with eyes or mucous membranes. Should not be applied to broken or irritated skin. Treated area should not be exposed to heat or direct sunlight. Affected area should not be bandaged. Transient burning may occur and generally disappears after several days; discontinue use if severe burning develops. Stop use and consult a healthcare provider if redness or irritation develops, symptoms get worse, or symptoms resolve and then recur.

Adverse Reactions (Reflective of adult population; not specific for elderly) Topical patch (Qutenza™, capsaicin 8%):
>10%: Local: Erythema (63%), pain (42%)
1% to 10%:
Cardiovascular: Hypertension (2%; transient)
Dermatologic: Pruritus (2%)
Gastrointestinal: Nausea (5%), vomiting (3%)
Local: Pruritus (6%), papules (6%), edema (4%), dryness (2%), swelling (2%)
Respiratory: Nasopharyngitis (4%), sinusitis (3%), bronchitis (2%)

Drug Interactions
Metabolism/Transport Effects Substrate of CYP2E1 (minor)
Avoid Concomitant Use There are no known interactions where it is recommended to avoid concomitant use.
Increased Effect/Toxicity There are no known significant interactions involving an increase in effect.
Decreased Effect
The levels/effects of Capsaicin may be decreased by: Cyproterone

Stability Qutenza™: Store at room temperature between 20°C to 25°C (68°F to 77°F).

Mechanism of Action Capsaicin, a transient receptor potential vanilloid 1 receptor (TRPV1) agonist, activates TRPV1 ligand-gated cation channels on nociceptive nerve fibers, resulting in depolarization, initiation of action potential, and pain signal transmission to the spinal cord; capsaicin exposure results in subsequent desensitization of the sensory axons and inhibition of pain transmission initiation. In arthritis, capsaicin induces release of substance P, the principal chemomediator of pain impulses from the periphery to the CNS, from peripheral sensory neurons; after repeated application, capsaicin depletes the neuron of substance P and prevents reaccumulation. The functional link between substance P and the capsaicin receptor, TRPV1, is not well understood.

Pharmacodynamics/Kinetics
Absorption: Topical patch (capsaicin 8%): Systemic absorption is transient and low (<5 ng/mL) in approximately one-third of patients when measured following 60-minute application. In patients with quantifiable levels, most fell below the limit of quantitation at 3-6 hours post application.

CAPSAICIN

Half-life elimination: Topical patch (capsaicin 8%): 1.64 hours (Babbar, 2009)

Dosage

Geriatric & Adult

Pain relief: OTC labeling:

Patch (Salonpas®-Hot): Apply patch to affected area up to 3-4 times/day for 7 days. Patch may remain in place for up to 8 hours.

Topical products (cream, gel, liquid, lotion): Apply to affected area 3-4 times/day; efficacy may be decreased if used less than 3 times/day; best results seen after 2-4 weeks of continuous use

Postherpetic neuralgia: Patch (Qutenza™ [capsaicin 8%]): Apply patch to most painful area for 60 minutes. Up to 4 patches may be applied in a single application. Treatment may be repeated ≥3 months as needed for return of pain (do not apply more frequently than every 3 months). Area should be pretreated with a topical anesthetic prior to patch application.

Diabetic neuropathy (unlabeled use): Cream (0.075%): Apply 4 times/day (Bril, 2011)

Administration

Topical products (cream, gel, liquid, lotion): Wear gloves to apply; wash hands with soap and water after applying to avoid spreading to eyes or other sensitive areas of the body.

Topical patch (Salonpas®-Hot): Apply patch externally to clean and dry affected area. Backing film should be removed prior to application. Do not use within 1 hour prior to a bath or immediately after bathing. Do not use with a heating pad.

Topical patch (Qutenza™ [capsaicin 8%]): Patch should only be applied by a physician or by a healthcare professional under the close supervision of a physician. The treatment area must be identified and marked by a physician. The patch can be cut to match size/shape of treatment area. If necessary, excessive hair present on and surrounding the treatment area, may be clipped (not shaved) to promote adherence. Prior to application, the treatment area should be cleansed with mild soap and water and dried thoroughly. The treatment area should be anesthetized with a topical anesthetic prior to patch application. Anesthetic should be removed with a dry wipe, and area should be cleansed again with soap/water, and dried. Patch may then be applied to dry, intact skin within 2 hours of opening the patch; apply patch using nitrile gloves (latex gloves should **not** be used). During application, slowly peel back the release liner under the patch. Patch should remain in place for 60 minutes. Remove patches gently and slowly. Following patch removal, apply cleansing gel to the treatment area and leave in place for at least 1 minute. All treatment materials should be disposed of according to biomedical waste procedures.

Special Geriatric Considerations Capsaicin products are available over-the-counter. Counsel patients about the appropriate use of these products. The American College of Rheumatology recommends capsaicin for the symptomatic treatment of osteoarthritis of the knee.

Dosage Forms Excipient information presented when available (limited, particularly for generics); consult specific product labeling. [DSC] = Discontinued product

Cream, topical: 0.025% (60 g); 0.075% (60 g [DSC])

Capzasin-HP®: 0.1% (42.5 g) [contains benzyl alcohol]

Capzasin-P®: 0.035% (42.5 g) [contains benzyl alcohol]

Zostrix®: 0.025% (60 g) [contains benzyl alcohol]

Zostrix® Diabetic Foot Pain: 0.075% (60 g) [contains benzyl alcohol]

Zostrix®-HP: 0.075% (60 g) [contains benzyl alcohol]

Gel, topical:

Capzasin-P®: 0.025% (42.5 g) [contains menthol]

Liquid, topical:

Capzasin-P®: 0.15% (29.5 mL)

Lotion, topical:

DiabetAid® Pain and Tingling Relief: 0.025% (120 mL)

Patch, topical:

Qutenza™: 8% (1s, 2s) [contains metal; supplied with cleansing gel]

Salonpas® Hot: 0.025% (1s) [contains metal, natural rubber/natural latex in packaging]

Selected References

"Recommendations for the Medical Management of Osteoarthritis of the Hip and Knee: 2000 Update. American College of Rheumatology Subcommittee on Osteoarthritis Guidelines," *Arthritis Rheum* 2000, 43(9):1905-15.

Captopril (KAP toe pril)

Related Information
Angiotensin Agents *on page 1985*

Medication Safety Issues
Sound-alike/look-alike issues:
Captopril may be confused with calcitriol, Capitrol®, carvedilol
International issues:
Acepril [Great Britain] may be confused with Accupril which is a brand name for quinapril in the U.S.
Acepril: Brand name for captopril [Great Britain], but also the brand name for enalapril [Hungary, Switzerland]; lisinopril [Malaysia]

Brand Names: Canada Apo-Capto®; Capoten®; Dom-Captopril; Mylan-Captopril; Nu-Capto; PMS-Captopril; Teva-Captopril

Index Terms ACE

Generic Availability (U.S.) Yes

Pharmacologic Category Angiotensin-Converting Enzyme (ACE) Inhibitor

Use Management of hypertension; treatment of heart failure, left ventricular dysfunction after myocardial infarction, diabetic nephropathy

Unlabeled/Investigational Use To delay the progression of nephropathy and reduce risks of cardiovascular events in hypertensive patients with type 1 or 2 diabetes mellitus; treatment of hypertensive crisis, rheumatoid arthritis; diagnosis of anatomic renal artery stenosis, hypertension secondary to scleroderma renal crisis; diagnosis of aldosteronism, idiopathic edema, Bartter's syndrome, postmyocardial infarction for prevention of ventricular failure; increase circulation in Raynaud's phenomenon, hypertension secondary to Takayasu's disease

Contraindications Hypersensitivity to captopril, any other ACE inhibitor, or any component of the formulation; angioedema related to previous treatment with an ACE inhibitor

Warnings/Precautions Anaphylactic reactions may occur rarely with ACE inhibitors. At any time during treatment (especially following first dose) angioedema may occur rarely with ACE inhibitors; may involve the head and neck (potentially compromising airway) or the intestine (presenting with abdominal pain). African-Americans and patients with idiopathic or hereditary angioedema may be at an increased risk. Prolonged frequent monitoring may be required especially if tongue, glottis, or larynx are involved as they are associated with airway obstruction. Patients with a history of airway surgery may have a higher risk of airway obstruction. Aggressive early and appropriate management is critical. Use in patients with previous angioedema associated with ACE inhibitor therapy is contraindicated. Severe anaphylactoid reactions may be seen during hemodialysis (eg, CVVHD) with high-flux dialysis membranes (eg, AN69), and rarely, during low density lipoprotein apheresis with dextran sulfate cellulose. Rare cases of anaphylactoid reactions have been reported in patients undergoing sensitization treatment with hymenoptera (bee, wasp) venom while receiving ACE inhibitors.

Symptomatic hypotension with or without syncope can occur with ACE inhibitors (usually with the first several doses); effects are most often observed in volume depleted patients; close monitoring of patient is required especially with initial dosing and dosing increases; blood pressure must be lowered at a rate appropriate for the patient's clinical condition. Initiation of therapy in patients with ischemic heart disease or cerebrovascular disease warrants close observation due to the potential consequences posed by falling blood pressure (eg, MI, stroke). Use with caution in hypertrophic cardiomyopathy with outflow tract obstruction, severe aortic stenosis, or before, during, or immediately after major surgery.

Hyperkalemia may occur with ACE inhibitors; risk factors include renal dysfunction, diabetes mellitus, concomitant use of potassium-sparing diuretics, potassium supplements and/or potassium containing salts. Use cautiously, if at all, with these agents and monitor potassium closely. Cough may occur with ACE inhibitors. Other causes of cough should be considered (eg, pulmonary congestion in patients with heart failure) and excluded prior to discontinuation.

May be associated with deterioration of renal function and/or increases in serum creatinine, particularly in patients with low renal blood flow (eg, renal artery stenosis, heart failure) whose glomerular filtration rate (GFR) is dependent on efferent arteriolar vasoconstriction by angiotensin II; deterioration may result in oliguria, acute renal failure, and progressive azotemia. Small increases in serum creatinine may occur following initiation; consider discontinuation only in patients with progressive and/or significant deterioration in renal function. Use with caution in patients with unstented unilateral/bilateral renal artery stenosis. When unstented bilateral renal artery stenosis is present, use is generally avoided due to the elevated risk of deterioration in renal function unless possible benefits outweigh risks.

Concurrent use of angiotensin receptor blockers may increase the risk of clinically-significant adverse events (eg, renal dysfunction, hyperkalemia).

Rare toxicities associated with ACE inhibitors include cholestatic jaundice (which may progress to fulminant hepatic necrosis), agranulocytosis, neutropenia, or leukopenia with myeloid hypoplasia. Patients with collagen vascular diseases (especially with concomitant renal impairment) or renal impairment alone may be at increased risk for hematologic toxicity; closely monitor CBC with differential for the first 3 months of therapy and periodically thereafter in these patients.

Adverse Reactions (Reflective of adult population; not specific for elderly)
Frequency not defined:
Cardiovascular: Angioedema, cardiac arrest, cerebrovascular insufficiency, rhythm disturbances, orthostatic hypotension, syncope, flushing, pallor, angina, MI, Raynaud's syndrome, CHF

Central nervous system: Ataxia, confusion, depression, nervousness, somnolence

Dermatologic: Bullous pemphigus, erythema multiforme, Stevens-Johnson syndrome, exfoliative dermatitis

Endocrine & metabolic: Alkaline phosphatase increased, bilirubin increased, gynecomastia

Gastrointestinal: Pancreatitis, glossitis, dyspepsia

Genitourinary: Urinary frequency, impotence

Hematologic: Anemia, thrombocytopenia, pancytopenia, agranulocytosis, anemia

Hepatic: Jaundice, hepatitis, hepatic necrosis (rare), cholestasis, hyponatremia (symptomatic), transaminases increased

Neuromuscular & skeletal: Asthenia, myalgia, myasthenia

Ocular: Blurred vision

Renal: Renal insufficiency, renal failure, nephrotic syndrome, polyuria, oliguria

Respiratory: Bronchospasm, eosinophilic pneumonitis, rhinitis

Miscellaneous: Anaphylactoid reactions

1% to 10%:
Cardiovascular: Hypotension (1% to 3%), tachycardia (1%), chest pain (1%), palpitation (1%)

Dermatologic: Rash (maculopapular or urticarial) (4% to 7%), pruritus (2%); in patients with rash, a positive ANA and/or eosinophilia has been noted in 7% to 10%.

Endocrine & metabolic: Hyperkalemia (1% to 11%)

Hematologic: Neutropenia may occur in up to 4% of patients with renal insufficiency or collagen-vascular disease.

Renal: Proteinuria (1%), serum creatinine increased, worsening of renal function (may occur in patients with bilateral renal artery stenosis or hypovolemia)

Respiratory: Cough (<1% to 2%)

Miscellaneous: Hypersensitivity reactions (rash, pruritus, fever, arthralgia, and eosinophilia) have occurred in 4% to 7% of patients (depending on dose and renal function); dysgeusia - loss of taste or diminished perception (2% to 4%)

Drug Interactions
Metabolism/Transport Effects Substrate of CYP2D6 (major)

Avoid Concomitant Use There are no known interactions where it is recommended to avoid concomitant use.

Increased Effect/Toxicity
Captopril may increase the levels/effects of: Allopurinol; Amifostine; Antihypertensives; AzaTHIOprine; CycloSPORINE; CycloSPORINE (Systemic); Ferric Gluconate; Gold Sodium Thiomalate; Hypotensive Agents; Iron Dextran Complex; Lithium; Nonsteroidal Anti-Inflammatory Agents; RiTUXimab; Sodium Phosphates

The levels/effects of Captopril may be increased by: Abiraterone Acetate; Alfuzosin; Angiotensin II Receptor Blockers; CYP2D6 Inhibitors (Moderate); CYP2D6 Inhibitors (Strong); Darunavir; Diazoxide; DPP-IV Inhibitors; Eplerenone; Everolimus; Herbs (Hypotensive Properties); Loop Diuretics; MAO Inhibitors; Pentoxifylline; Phosphodiesterase 5 Inhibitors; Potassium Salts; Potassium-Sparing Diuretics; Prostacyclin Analogues; Sirolimus; Temsirolimus; Thiazide Diuretics; TiZANidine; Tolvaptan; Trimethoprim

Decreased Effect
The levels/effects of Captopril may be decreased by: Antacids; Aprotinin; Herbs (Hypertensive Properties); Icatibant; Lanthanum; Methylphenidate; Nonsteroidal Anti-Inflammatory Agents; Peginterferon Alfa-2b; Salicylates; Yohimbine

Ethanol/Nutrition/Herb Interactions
Food: Captopril serum concentrations may be decreased if taken with food. Long-term use of captopril may result in a zinc deficiency which can result in a decrease in taste perception.

◄

Herb/Nutraceutical: Avoid bayberry, blue cohosh, cayenne, ephedra, ginger, ginseng (American), kola, licorice (may worsen hypertension). Avoid black cohosh, california poppy, coleus, golden seal, hawthorn, mistletoe, periwinkle, quinine, shepherd's purse (may have increased antihypertensive effect).

Mechanism of Action Competitive inhibitor of angiotensin-converting enzyme (ACE); prevents conversion of angiotensin I to angiotensin II, a potent vasoconstrictor; results in lower levels of angiotensin II which causes an increase in plasma renin activity and a reduction in aldosterone secretion

Pharmacodynamics/Kinetics

Onset of action: Peak effect: Blood pressure reduction: 1-1.5 hours after dose

Duration: Dose related, may require several weeks of therapy before full hypotensive effect

Absorption: 60% to 75%; reduced 30% to 40% by food

Protein binding: 25% to 30%

Metabolism: 50%

Half-life elimination (renal and cardiac function dependent):

Adults, healthy volunteers: 1.9 hours; Heart failure: 2.06 hours; Anuria: 20-40 hours

Time to peak: 1 hour

Excretion: Urine (>95%) within 24 hours (40% to 50% as unchanged drug)

Dosage

Geriatric Refer to adult dosing. In the management of hypertension, consider lower initial doses and titrate to response (Aronow, 2011).

Adult Note: Titrate dose according to patient's response; use lowest effective dose.

Acute hypertension (urgency/emergency): Oral: 12.5-25 mg, may repeat as needed (may be given sublingually, but no therapeutic advantage demonstrated)

Heart failure: Oral:

Initial dose: 6.25-12.5 mg 3 times/day in conjunction with cardiac glycoside and diuretic therapy; initial dose depends upon patient's fluid/electrolyte status

Target dose: 50 mg 3 times/day

Hypertension: Oral: Initial: 12.5-25 mg 2-3 times/day; may increase by 12.5-25 mg/dose at 1- to 2-week intervals up to 50 mg 3 times/day. Maximum: 150 mg 3 times/day. Add diuretic before further dosage increases.

Usual dose range (JNC 7): 25-100 mg/day in 2 divided doses

LV dysfunction following MI: Oral: Initial: 6.25 mg; followed by 12.5 mg 3 times/day; increase to 25 mg 3 times/day over the next few days; followed by gradual increase to a goal of 50 mg 3 times/day (some dose schedules are more aggressive to achieve an increased goal dose within the first few days of initiation).

Diabetic nephropathy: Oral: 25 mg 3 times/day. May be taken with other antihypertensive therapy if required to further lower blood pressure

Renal Impairment

Cl_{cr} 10-50 mL/minute: Administer 75% of normal dose.

Cl_{cr} <10 mL/minute: Administer 50% of normal dose.

Note: Smaller dosages given every 8-12 hours are indicated in patients with renal dysfunction. Renal function and leukocyte count should be carefully monitored during therapy.

Hemodialysis effects: Moderately dialyzable (20% to 50%); administer dose postdialysis or administer 25% to 35% supplemental dose.

Peritoneal dialysis: Supplemental dose is not necessary.

Administration Unstable in aqueous solutions; to prepare solution for oral administration, mix prior to administration and use within 10 minutes.

Monitoring Parameters BUN, electrolytes, serum creatinine; blood pressure. In patients with renal impairment and/or collagen vascular disease, closely monitor CBC with differential for the first 3 months of therapy and periodically thereafter.

Test Interactions Positive Coombs' [direct]; may cause false-positive results in urine acetone determinations using sodium nitroprusside reagent

Pharmacotherapy Pearls Watch for hypotensive effect within 1-3 hours of first dose or new higher dose. Many patients complain of transient cough during early therapy; food decreases absorption of captopril 30% to 40%; administer captopril 1 hour before meals; clinical significance not known; therefore, observe for loss of effect. Newer data demonstrate that lower doses of ACE inhibitors are effective and toxic reactions are decreased.

Special Geriatric Considerations Due to frequent decreases in glomerular filtration (also Cl_{cr}) with aging, elderly patients may have exaggerated responses to ACE inhibitors; differences in clinical response due to hepatic changes are not observed. ACE inhibitors may be preferred agents in elderly patients with congestive heart failure and diabetes mellitus. Diabetic proteinuria is reduced and insulin sensitivity is enhanced. In general, the side effect profile is favorable in the elderly and causes little or no CNS confusion; use lowest dose recommendations initially. Many elderly may be volume depleted due to diuretic use and/or blunted thirst reflex resulting in inadequate fluid intake.

Dosage Forms Excipient information presented when available (limited, particularly for generics); consult specific product labeling.

Tablet, oral: 12.5 mg, 25 mg, 50 mg, 100 mg

Selected References

American Diabetes Association, "Standards of Medical Care in Diabetes Mellitus – 2009," *Diabetes Care*, 2009, 32 (Suppl 1):13-61.

Chobanian AV, Bakris GL, Black HR, et al, "The Seventh Report of the Joint National Committee on Prevention, Detection, Evaluation, and Treatment of High Blood Pressure: The JNC 7 Report," *JAMA*, 2003, 289(19):2560-71.

Miller DR, Oliveria SA, Berlowitz DR, et al, "Angioedema Incidence in US Veterens Initiating Angiotensin-Converting Enzyme Inhibitors," *Hypertension*, 2008, 51(6):1-7.

Captopril and Hydrochlorothiazide (KAP toe pril & hye droe klor oh THYE a zide)

Related Information

Captopril *on page 264*

Hydrochlorothiazide *on page 876*

Medication Safety Issues

International issues:

Ecazide [France, Spain] may be confused with Eskazine, a brand name for trifluoperazine [Spain]

Index Terms Hydrochlorothiazide and Captopril

Generic Availability (U.S.) Yes

Pharmacologic Category Angiotensin-Converting Enzyme (ACE) Inhibitor; Diuretic, Thiazide

Use Management of hypertension

Dosage

Geriatric Refer to dosing in individual monographs.

Adult Hypertension, CHF: May be substituted for previously titrated dosages of the individual components; alternatively, may initiate as follows: Oral:

Initial: Single tablet (captopril 25 mg/hydrochlorothiazide 15 mg) taken once daily; daily dose of captopril should not exceed 150 mg; daily dose of hydrochlorothiazide should not exceed 50 mg

Renal Impairment May respond to smaller or less frequent doses.

Special Geriatric Considerations Divided doses of diuretics may increase the incidence of nocturia in the elderly. Hydrochlorothiazide is not effective in patients with a Cl$_{cr}$ <30 mL/minute; therefore, it may not be a useful agent in many elderly patients.

Dosage Forms Excipient information presented when available (limited, particularly for generics); consult specific product labeling.

Tablet: 25/15: Captopril 25 mg and hydrochlorothiazide 15 mg; 25/25: Captopril 25 mg and hydrochlorothiazide 25 mg; 50/15: Captopril 50 mg and hydrochlorothiazide 15 mg; 50/25: Captopril 50 mg and hydrochlorothiazide 25 mg

◆ **Capzasin-HP® [OTC]** *see* Capsaicin *on page 261*

◆ **Capzasin-P® [OTC]** *see* Capsaicin *on page 261*

◆ **Carafate®** *see* Sucralfate *on page 1711*

Carbachol (KAR ba kole)

Related Information

Glaucoma Drug Therapy *on page 2008*

Medication Safety Issues

Sound-alike/look-alike issues:

Isopto® Carbachol may be confused with Isopto® Carpine

Brand Names: U.S. Isopto® Carbachol; Miostat®

Brand Names: Canada Isopto® Carbachol; Miostat®

Index Terms Carbacholine; Carbamylcholine Chloride

Generic Availability (U.S.) No

Pharmacologic Category Cholinergic Agonist; Ophthalmic Agent, Antiglaucoma; Ophthalmic Agent, Miotic

Use Lowers intraocular pressure in the treatment of glaucoma; cause miosis during surgery

Contraindications Hypersensitivity to carbachol or any component of the formulation; acute iritis, acute inflammatory disease of the anterior chamber

Warnings/Precautions Use with caution in patients undergoing general anesthesia and in presence of corneal abrasion. Use caution with acute cardiac failure, asthma, peptic ulcer, hyperthyroidism, gastrointestinal spasm, urinary tract obstruction, and Parkinson's disease.

◀ **Adverse Reactions (Reflective of adult population; not specific for elderly)** Frequency not defined.
Cardiovascular: Arrhythmia, flushing, hypotension, syncope
Central nervous system: Headache
Gastrointestinal: Abdominal cramps, diarrhea, epigastric distress, salivation, vomiting
Genitourinary: Urinary bladder tightness
Ocular: Bullous keratopathy, burning (transient), ciliary spasm, conjunctival injection, corneal clouding, irritation, postoperative iritis (following cataract extraction), retinal detachment, stinging (transient)
Respiratory: Asthma
Miscellaneous: Diaphoresis

Drug Interactions
Avoid Concomitant Use There are no known interactions where it is recommended to avoid concomitant use.
Increased Effect/Toxicity
The levels/effects of Carbachol may be increased by: Acetylcholinesterase Inhibitors
Decreased Effect There are no known significant interactions involving a decrease in effect.

Stability
Intraocular: Store at room temperature of 15°C to 30°C (59°F to 86°F).
Topical: Store at 8°C to 27°C (46°F to 80°F).

Mechanism of Action Synthetic direct-acting cholinergic agent that causes miosis by stimulating muscarinic receptors in the eye

Pharmacodynamics/Kinetics
Ophthalmic instillation:
Onset of action: Miosis: 10-20 minutes
Duration: Reduction in intraocular pressure: 4-8 hours
Intraocular administration:
Onset of action: Miosis: 2-5 minutes
Duration: 24 hours

Dosage
Geriatric & Adult
Glaucoma: Ophthalmic: Instill 1-2 drops up to 3 times/day
Ophthalmic surgery (miosis): Intraocular: 0.5 mL instilled into anterior chamber before or after securing sutures

Administration Finger pressure should be applied on the lacrimal sac for 1-2 minutes following topical instillation; remove excess around the eye with a tissue

Special Geriatric Considerations Evaluate the patient's or caregiver's ability to safely administer the correct dose of ophthalmic medication.

Dosage Forms Excipient information presented when available (limited, particularly for generics); consult specific product labeling.
Solution, intraocular:
Miostat®: 0.01% (1.5 mL)
Solution, ophthalmic:
Isopto® Carbachol: 1.5% (15 mL); 3% (15 mL) [contains benzalkonium chloride]

◆ **Carbacholine** *see* Carbachol *on page* 267

CarBAMazepine (kar ba MAZ e peen)

Related Information
Liquid Compatibility of Antidepressants, Antipsychotics, and Mood Stabilizers *on page* 2111
Medication Safety Issues
Sound-alike/look-alike issues:
CarBAMazepine may be confused with OXcarbazepine
Carbatrol® may be confused with Cartrol®
Epitol® may be confused with Epinal®
TEGretol®, TEGretol®-XR may be confused with Mebaral®, Toprol-XL®, Toradol®, TRENtal®
Brand Names: U.S. Carbatrol®; Epitol®; Equetro®; TEGretol®; TEGretol®-XR
Brand Names: Canada Apo-Carbamazepine®; Dom-Carbamazepine; Mapezine®; Mylan-Carbamazepine CR; Nu-Carbamazepine; PMS-Carbamazepine; Sandoz-Carbamazepine; Taro-Carbamazepine Chewable; Tegretol®; Teva-Carbamazepine
Index Terms CBZ; SPD417
Generic Availability (U.S.) Yes: Excludes capsule (extended release)
Pharmacologic Category Anticonvulsant, Miscellaneous

Use

Carbatrol®, Tegretol®, Tegretol®-XR: Partial seizures with complex symptomatology (psychomotor, temporal lobe), generalized tonic-clonic seizures (grand mal), mixed seizure patterns, trigeminal neuralgia

Equetro®: Acute manic and mixed episodes associated with bipolar 1 disorder

Unlabeled/Investigational Use Treatment of restless leg syndrome and post-traumatic stress disorders

Medication Guide Available Yes

Contraindications Hypersensitivity to carbamazepine, tricyclic antidepressants, or any component of the formulation; bone marrow depression; with or within 14 days of MAO inhibitor use; concurrent use of nefazodone

Warnings/Precautions [U.S. Boxed Warning]: Potentially fatal blood cell abnormalities have been reported. Patients with a previous history of adverse hematologic reaction to any drug may be at increased risk.

Antiepileptics are associated with an increased risk of suicidal behavior/thoughts with use (regardless of indication); patients should be monitored for signs/symptoms of depression, suicidal tendencies, and other unusual behavior changes during therapy and instructed to inform their healthcare provider immediately if symptoms occur.

Administer carbamazepine with caution to patients with history of cardiac damage, ECG abnormalities (or at risk for ECG abnormalities), hepatic or renal disease. When used to treat bipolar disorder, the smallest effective dose is suggested to reduce the risk for overdose/suicide; high-risk patients should be monitored for suicidal ideations. Prescription should be written for the smallest quantity consistent with good patient care. May activate latent psychosis and/or cause confusion or agitation; elderly patients may be at an increased risk for psychiatric effects. Potentially serious, sometimes fatal multiorgan hypersensitivity reactions have been reported with some antiepileptic drugs; monitor for signs and symptoms of possible disparate manifestations associated with lymphatic, hepatic, renal, and/or hematologic organ systems; gradual discontinuation and conversion to alternate therapy may be required.

Carbamazepine is not effective in absence, myoclonic, or akinetic seizures; exacerbation of certain seizure types have been seen after initiation of carbamazepine therapy in children with mixed seizure disorders. Abrupt discontinuation is not recommended in patients being treated for seizures. Dizziness or drowsiness may occur; caution should be used when performing tasks which require alertness until the effects are known. Effects with other sedative drugs or ethanol may be potentiated. Carbamazepine has a high potential for drug interactions; use caution in patients taking strong CYP3A4 inducers or inhibitors or medications significantly metabolized via CYP1A2, 2B6, 2C9, 2C19, and 3A4. Coadministration of carbamazepine and nefazodone may lead to insufficient plasma levels of nefazodone; combination is contraindicated. Carbamazepine has mild anticholinergic activity; use with caution in patients with increased intraocular pressure, or sensitivity to anticholinergic effects. Severe dermatologic reactions, including toxic epidermal necrolysis and Stevens-Johnson syndrome, although rarely reported, have resulted in fatalities. **[U.S. Boxed Warning]: Use caution and screen for the genetic susceptibility genotype (*HLA-B*1502* allele) in Asian patients. Patients with a positive result should not be started on carbamazepine.** Discontinue if there are any signs of hypersensitivity. Elderly patients may have an increased risk of SIADH-like syndrome.

Administration of the suspension will yield higher peak and lower trough serum levels than an equal dose of the tablet form; consider a lower starting dose given more frequently (same total daily dose) when using the suspension.

Adverse Reactions (Reflective of adult population; not specific for elderly) Frequency not defined, unless otherwise specified.

Cardiovascular: Arrhythmias, AV block, bradycardia, chest pain (bipolar use), CHF, edema, hyper-/hypotension, lymphadenopathy, syncope, thromboembolism, thrombophlebitis

Central nervous system: Amnesia (bipolar use), anxiety (bipolar use; case report), ataxia (bipolar use 15%), aseptic meningitis (case report), confusion, depression (bipolar use), dizziness (bipolar use 44%), fatigue, headache (bipolar use 22%), sedation, slurred speech, somnolence (bipolar use 32%)

Dermatologic: Alopecia, alterations in skin pigmentation, erythema multiforme, exfoliative dermatitis, photosensitivity reaction, pruritus (bipolar use 8%), purpura, rash, Stevens-Johnson syndrome, toxic epidermal necrolysis, urticaria

Endocrine & metabolic: Chills, fever, hyponatremia, syndrome of inappropriate ADH secretion (SIADH)

Gastrointestinal: Abdominal pain, anorexia, constipation, diarrhea, dyspepsia (bipolar use), gastric distress, nausea (bipolar use 29%), pancreatitis, vomiting (bipolar use 18%), xerostomia (bipolar use)

◄ Genitourinary: Azotemia, impotence, renal failure, urinary frequency, urinary retention

Hematologic: Acute intermittent porphyria, agranulocytosis, aplastic anemia, bone marrow suppression, eosinophilia, leukocytosis, leukopenia, pancytopenia, thrombocytopenia

Hepatic: Abnormal liver function tests, hepatic failure, hepatitis, jaundice

Neuromuscular & skeletal: Back pain, pain (bipolar use 12%), peripheral neuritis, weakness

Ocular: Blurred vision, conjunctivitis, lens opacities, nystagmus

Otic: Hyperacusis, tinnitus

Miscellaneous: Diaphoresis, hypersensitivity (including multiorgan reactions, may include disorders mimicking lymphoma, eosinophilia, hepatosplenomegaly, vasculitis); infection (bipolar use 12%)

Drug Interactions

Metabolism/Transport Effects Substrate of CYP2C8 (minor), 3A4 (major); **Induces** CYP1A2 (strong), 2B6 (strong), 2C8 (strong), 2C9 (strong), 2C19 (strong), 3A4 (strong), P-glycoprotein

Avoid Concomitant Use

Avoid concomitant use of CarBAMazepine with any of the following: Boceprevir; Conivaptan; Crizotinib; Dabigatran Etexilate; Dronedarone; Etravirine; Everolimus; Lapatinib; Lurasidone; MAO Inhibitors; Nefazodone; Nilotinib; Pazopanib; Praziquantel; Ranolazine; Rilpivirine; Roflumilast; RomiDEPsin; Telaprevir; Ticagrelor; Tolvaptan; Vandetanib; Voriconazole

Increased Effect/Toxicity

CarBAMazepine may increase the levels/effects of: Adenosine; Alcohol (Ethyl); ClomiPR-AMINE; CNS Depressants; Desmopressin; Fosphenytoin; Lithium; MAO Inhibitors; Methotrimeprazine; Phenytoin

The levels/effects of CarBAMazepine may be increased by: Allopurinol; Antifungal Agents (Azole Derivatives, Systemic); Calcium Channel Blockers (Nondihydropyridine); Carbonic Anhydrase Inhibitors; Cimetidine; Conivaptan; CYP3A4 Inhibitors (Moderate); CYP3A4 Inhibitors (Strong); Danazol; Darunavir; Dasatinib; Droperidol; Fluconazole; Grapefruit Juice; HydrOXYzine; Isoniazid; LamoTRIgine; Macrolide Antibiotics; Methotrimeprazine; Nefazodone; Propoxyphene; Protease Inhibitors; QuiNINE; Selective Serotonin Reuptake Inhibitors; Telaprevir; Thiazide Diuretics; Zolpidem

Decreased Effect

CarBAMazepine may decrease the levels/effects of: Acetaminophen; ARIPiprazole; Bendamustine; Benzodiazepines (metabolized by oxidation); Boceprevir; Brentuximab Vedotin; Calcium Channel Blockers (Dihydropyridine); Calcium Channel Blockers (Nondihydropyridine); Caspofungin; CloZAPine; Contraceptives (Estrogens); Contraceptives (Progestins); Crizotinib; CycloSPORINE; CycloSPORINE (Systemic); CYP1A2 Substrates; CYP2B6 Substrates; CYP2C19 Substrates; CYP2C8 Substrates (High risk); CYP2C9 Substrates (High risk); CYP3A4 Substrates; Dabigatran Etexilate; Diclofenac; Divalproex; Doxycycline; Dronedarone; Etravirine; Everolimus; Exemestane; Felbamate; Flunarizine; Fosphenytoin; Gefitinib; GuanFACINE; Haloperidol; Imatinib; Irinotecan; Ixabepilone; Lacosamide; LamoTRIgine; Lapatinib; Linagliptin; Lopinavir; Lurasidone; Maraviroc; Mebendazole; Methadone; Nefazodone; Nilotinib; Paliperidone; Pazopanib; P-Glycoprotein Substrates; Phenytoin; Praziquantel; Protease Inhibitors; QuiNINE; Ranolazine; Rilpivirine; RisperiDONE; Rivaroxaban; Roflumilast; RomiDEPsin; Rufinamide; Saxagliptin; Selective Serotonin Reuptake Inhibitors; SORAfenib; Tadalafil; Telaprevir; Temsirolimus; Theophylline Derivatives; Thyroid Products; Ticagrelor; Tolvaptan; Topiramate; Treprostinil; Tricyclic Antidepressants; Ulipristal; Valproic Acid; Vandetanib; Vecuronium; Vemurafenib; Vitamin K Antagonists; Voriconazole; Ziprasidone; Zolpidem

The levels/effects of CarBAMazepine may be decreased by: CYP3A4 Inducers (Strong); Deferasirox; Divalproex; Felbamate; Fosphenytoin; Herbs (CYP3A4 Inducers); Ketorolac; Ketorolac (Nasal); Ketorolac (Systemic); Mefloquine; Methylfolate; Phenytoin; Rufinamide; Theophylline Derivatives; Tocilizumab; Valproic Acid

Ethanol/Nutrition/Herb Interactions

Ethanol: May increase CNS depression; monitor for increased effects with coadministration. Caution patients about effects.

Food: Carbamazepine serum levels may be increased if taken with food. Carbamazepine serum concentration may be increased if taken with grapefruit juice; avoid concurrent use.

Herb/Nutraceutical: Avoid evening primrose (seizure threshold decreased). Avoid valerian, St John's wort, kava kava, gotu kola (may increase CNS depression).

Mechanism of Action In addition to anticonvulsant effects, carbamazepine has anticholinergic, antineuralgic, antidiuretic, muscle relaxant, antimanic, antidepressive, and antiarrhythmic properties; may depress activity in the nucleus ventralis of the thalamus or decrease synaptic transmission or decrease summation of temporal stimulation leading to neural discharge by limiting influx of sodium ions across cell membrane or other unknown mechanisms; stimulates the release of ADH and potentiates its action in promoting reabsorption of water; chemically related to tricyclic antidepressants

Pharmacodynamics/Kinetics

Absorption: Slow

Distribution: V_d: Adults: 0.59-2 L/kg

Protein binding: Carbamazepine: 75% to 90%; Epoxide metabolite: 50%

Metabolism: Hepatic via CYP3A4 to active epoxide metabolite; induces hepatic enzymes to increase metabolism

Bioavailability: 85%

Half-life elimination: **Note:** Half-life is variable because of autoinduction which is usually complete 3-5 weeks after initiation of a fixed carbamazepine regimen.

Carbamazepine: Initial: 25-65 hours; Extended release: 35-40 hours; Multiple doses: Adults: 12-17 hours

Epoxide metabolite: Initial: 25-43 hours

Time to peak, serum: Unpredictable:

Immediate release: Suspension: 1.5 hour; tablet: 4-5 hours

Extended release: Carbatrol®, Equetro®: 12-26 hours (single dose), 4-8 hours (multiple doses); Tegretol®-XR: 3-12 hours

Excretion: Urine 72% (1% to 3% as unchanged drug); feces (28%)

Dosage

Geriatric & Adult Dosage must be adjusted according to patient's response and serum concentrations. Administer tablets (chewable or conventional) in 2-3 divided doses daily and suspension in 4 divided doses daily. Oral:

Epilepsy: Initial: 400 mg/day in 2 divided doses (tablets or extended release tablets) or 4 divided doses (oral suspension); increase by up to 200 mg/day at weekly intervals using a twice daily regimen of extended release tablets or capsules, or a 3-4 times/day regimen of other formulations until optimal response and therapeutic levels are achieved; usual dose: 800-1200 mg/day

Maximum recommended dose: 1600 mg/day; however, some patients have required up to 1.6-2.4 g/day

Trigeminal or glossopharyngeal neuralgia: Initial: 200 mg/day in 2 divided doses (tablets, extended release tablets, or extended release capsules) or 4 divided doses (oral suspension) with food, gradually increasing in increments of 200 mg/day as needed.

Maintenance: Usual: 400-800 mg daily in 2 divided doses (tablets, extended release tablets, or extended release capsules) or 4 divided doses (oral suspension); maximum dose: 1200 mg/day

Bipolar disorder: Initial: 400 mg/day in 2 divided doses (tablets, extended release tablets, or extended release capsules) or 4 divided doses (oral suspension), may adjust by 200 mg/day increments; maximum dose: 1600 mg/day.

Note: Equetro® is the only formulation specifically approved by the FDA for the management of bipolar disorder.

Renal Impairment Dosage adjustments are not required or recommended in the manufacturer's labeling; however, the following guidelines have been used by some clinicians (Aronoff, 2007):

Adults:

GFR <10 mL/minute: Administer 75% of dose.

Hemodialysis, peritoneal dialysis: Administer 75% of dose.

Continuous renal replacement therapy (CRRT): Adults: No dosage adjustment recommended.

Hepatic Impairment Use with caution in hepatic impairment; metabolized primarily in the liver.

Administration

Suspension: Must be given on a 3-4 times/day schedule versus tablets which can be given 2-4 times/day. Since a single dose of suspension will produce higher peak and lower trough levels than the same dose given as the tablet form, patients given the suspension should be started on lower doses given more frequently (same total daily dose) and increased slowly to avoid unwanted side effects. When carbamazepine suspension has been combined with chlorpromazine or thioridazine solutions, a precipitate forms which may result in loss of effect. Therefore, it is recommended that the carbamazepine suspension dosage form not be administered at the same time with other liquid medicinal agents or diluents. Should be administered with meals.

Extended release capsule (Carbatrol®, Equetro®): Consists of three different types of beads: Immediate release, extended-release, and enteric release. The bead types are combined in a ratio to allow twice daily dosing. May be opened and contents sprinkled over food such as a teaspoon of applesauce; may be administered with or without food; do not crush or chew.

Extended release tablet: Should be inspected for damage. Damaged extended release tablets (without release portal) should not be administered. Should be administered with meals; swallow whole, do not crush or chew.

◀ **Monitoring Parameters** CBC with platelet count, reticulocytes, serum iron, lipid panel, liver function tests, urinalysis, BUN, serum carbamazepine levels, thyroid function tests, serum sodium; ophthalmic exams (pupillary reflexes); observe patient for excessive sedation, especially when instituting or increasing therapy; signs of rash; *HLA-B*1502* genotype screening prior to therapy initiation in patients of Asian descent; suicidality (eg, suicidal thoughts, depression, behavioral changes)

Reference Range

Timing of serum samples: Absorption is slow, peak levels occur 6-8 hours after ingestion of the first dose; the half-life ranges from 8-60 hours, therefore, steady-state is achieved in 2-5 days

Therapeutic levels: 4-12 mcg/mL (SI: 17-51 µmol/L)

Toxic concentration: >15 mcg/mL; patients who require higher levels of 8-12 mcg/mL (SI: 34-51 µmol/L) should be watched closely. Side effects including CNS effects occur commonly at higher dosage levels. If other anticonvulsants are given therapeutic range is 4-8 mcg/mL.

Test Interactions May cause false-positive serum TCA screen. Increased BUN, AST, ALT, bilirubin, alkaline phosphatase (S); decreased calcium, T_3, T_4, sodium (S)

Special Geriatric Considerations Elderly may have increased risk of SIADH-like syndrome. Elderly are more susceptible to carbamazepine-induced confusion and agitation, AV block, and bradycardia.

Dosage Forms Excipient information presented when available (limited, particularly for generics); consult specific product labeling.

Capsule, extended release, oral:

Carbatrol®: 100 mg, 200 mg, 300 mg

Equetro®: 100 mg, 200 mg, 300 mg

Suspension, oral: 100 mg/5 mL (5 mL, 10 mL, 450 mL)

TEGretol®: 100 mg/5 mL (450 mL) [contains propylene glycol; citrus-vanilla flavor]

Tablet, oral: 200 mg

Epitol®: 200 mg [scored]

TEGretol®: 200 mg [scored]

Tablet, chewable, oral: 100 mg

TEGretol®: 100 mg [scored]

Tablet, extended release, oral: 200 mg, 400 mg

TEGretol®-XR: 100 mg, 200 mg, 400 mg

Selected References

Ketter TA, Kalali AH, and Weisler RH, "A 6-Month, Multicenter, Open-Label Evaluation of Beaded, Extended-Release Carbamazepine Capsule Monotherapy in Bipolar Disorder Patients With Manic or Mixed Episodes: SPD417 Study Group," *J Clin Psychiatry*, 2004, 65(5):668-73.

Rabins PV, Blacker D, Rovner BW, et al, "Practice Guidelines for the Treatment of Patients With Alzheimer's Disease and Other Dementias," *Am J Psychiatry*, 2007, 164(12 Suppl):5-56. Available at http://www.psych.org/psych_pract/treatg/pg/prac_guide.cfm.

Weisler RH, Kalali AH, and Ketter TA, "A Multicenter, Randomized, Double-Blind, Placebo-Controlled Trial of Extended-Release Carbamazepine Capsules as Monotherapy for Bipolar Disorder Patients With Manic or Mixed Episodes: SPD417 Study Group," *J Clin Psychiatry*, 2004, 65(4):478-84.

Carbamide Peroxide (KAR ba mide per OKS ide)

Brand Names: U.S. Auraphene B® [OTC]; Auro® [OTC]; Cankaid® [OTC]; Debrox® [OTC]; E-R-O® [OTC]; Gly-Oxide® [OTC]; Murine® Ear Wax Removal Kit [OTC]; Murine® Ear [OTC]; Otix® [OTC]

Index Terms Urea Peroxide

Generic Availability (U.S.) Yes

Pharmacologic Category Anti-inflammatory, Locally Applied; Otic Agent, Cerumenolytic

Use Relief of minor inflammation of gums, oral mucosal surfaces, and lips including canker sores and dental irritation; emulsify and disperse ear wax

Dosage

Geriatric & Adult

Minor inflammation of gums, oral mucosal surfaces, and lips: Topical: Oral solution (should not be used for >7 days): Apply several drops undiluted on affected area 4 times/day after meals and at bedtime; expectorate after 2-3 minutes **or** place 10 drops onto tongue, mix with saliva, swish for several minutes, expectorate

Ear wax removal: Otic: Tilt head sideways and instill 5-10 drops twice daily up to 4 days, tip of applicator should not enter ear canal; keep drops in ear for several minutes by keeping head tilted and placing cotton in ear

Special Geriatric Considerations Avoid contact with hearing aids.

Dosage Forms Excipient information presented when available (limited, particularly for generics); consult specific product labeling.

Liquid, oral: 10% (60 mL)
  Cankaid®: 10% (15 mL)
  Gly-Oxide®: 10% (15 mL, 60 mL)
Solution, otic [drops]: 6.5% (15 mL)
  Auraphene B®: 6.5% (15 mL)
  Auro®: 6.5% (22.2 mL)
  Debrox®: 6.5% (15 mL, 30 mL)
  E-R-O®: 6.5% (15 mL) [ethanol free]
  Murine® Ear: 6.5% (15 mL) [contains ethanol 6.3%]
  Murine® Ear Wax Removal Kit: 6.5% (15 mL) [contains ethanol 6.3%]
  Otix®: 6.5% (15 mL)

◆ **Carbamylcholine Chloride** see Carbachol on page 267
◆ **Carbatrol®** see CarBAMazepine on page 268

Carbidopa (kar bi DOE pa)

Medication Safety Issues
  International issues:
  Lodosyn [U.S.] may be confused with Lidosen brand name for lidocaine [Italy]
Brand Names: U.S. Lodosyn®
Generic Availability (U.S.) No
Pharmacologic Category Anti-Parkinson's Agent, Decarboxylase Inhibitor
Use Given with levodopa in the treatment of parkinsonism to enable a lower dosage of levodopa to be used and a more rapid response to be obtained and to decrease side effects; has no effect without levodopa
Contraindications Hypersensitivity to carbidopa or levodopa, or any component of the formulation; use of nonselective MAO antagonists; narrow-angle glaucoma; history of melanoma or undiagnosed skin lesions
Warnings/Precautions Use with caution in patients with history of cardiovascular disease (including myocardial infarction and arrhythmias), psychosis, pulmonary dieases (such as asthma), endocrine disease, peptic ulcer disease, as well as in severe renal and hepatic dysfunction. Observe patients closely for development of depression with concomitant suicidal tendencies. Use with extreme caution in patients with psychotic disorders; observe patients closely for development of depression with concomitant suicidal tendencies.

Dopamine agonists have been associated with compulsive behaviors and/or loss of impulse control, which has manifested as pathological gambling, libido increases (hypersexuality), and/or binge eating. Causality has not been established, and controversy exists as to whether this phenomenon is related to the underlying disease, prior behaviors/addictions and/or drug therapy. Dose reduction or discontinuation of therapy has been reported to reverse these behaviors in some, but not all cases. Risk for melanoma development is increased in Parkinson's disease patients; drug causation or factors contributing to risk have not been established. Patients should be monitored closely and periodic skin examinations should be performed. Dopaminergic agents have been associated with a syndrome resembling neuro-leptic malignant syndrome on abrupt withdrawal or significant dosage reduction after long-term use. Protein in the diet should be distributed throughout the day to avoid fluctuations in levodopa absorption. Carbidopa has no antiparkinsonian activity when administered alone.
Adverse Reactions (Reflective of adult population; not specific for elderly) Adverse reactions are associated with concomitant administration with levodopa

>10%: Central nervous system: Anxiety, confusion, nervousness, mental depression
1% to 10%:
  Cardiovascular: Orthostatic hypotension, palpitation, cardiac arrhythmia
  Central nervous system: Memory loss, insomnia, fatigue, hallucinations, ataxia, dystonic movements
  Gastrointestinal: Nausea, vomiting, GI bleeding
  Ocular: Blurred vision
Drug Interactions
  Avoid Concomitant Use There are no known interactions where it is recommended to avoid concomitant use.
  Increased Effect/Toxicity There are no known significant interactions involving an increase in effect.
  Decreased Effect There are no known significant interactions involving a decrease in effect. ▶

◀ **Mechanism of Action** Carbidopa is a peripheral decarboxylase inhibitor with little or no pharmacological activity when given alone in usual doses. It inhibits the peripheral decarboxylation of levodopa to dopamine; and as it does not cross the blood-brain barrier, unlike levodopa, effective brain concentrations of dopamine are produced with lower doses of levodopa. At the same time, reduced peripheral formation of dopamine reduces peripheral side-effects, notably nausea and vomiting, and cardiac arrhythmias, although the dyskinesias and adverse mental effects associated with levodopa therapy tend to develop earlier.

Pharmacodynamics/Kinetics
Absorption: 40% to 70%
Distribution: Does not cross the blood-brain barrier
Protein binding: 36%
Half-life elimination: 1-2 hours
Excretion: Urine (as unchanged drug and metabolites)

Dosage
Geriatric & Adult Parkinson's disease (adjunct to levodopa): Oral: 70-100 mg/day; maximum daily dose: 200 mg

Administration Administer with meals to decrease GI upset.

Pharmacotherapy Pearls Usually used in combination with levodopa (Sinemet®); plain carbidopa tablets are available from Merck & Co to physicians for use in patients requiring individual titration of carbidopa and levodopa.

Dosage Forms Excipient information presented when available (limited, particularly for generics); consult specific product labeling.
Tablet, oral:
Lodosyn®: 25 mg [scored]

Selected References
Olanow CW, Watts RL, and Koller WC, "An Algorithm (Decision Tree) for the Management of Parkinson's Disease (2001): Treatment Guidelines," *Neurology*, 2001, 56(11 Suppl 5):S1-S88.

Carbidopa and Levodopa (kar bi DOE pa & lee voe DOE pa)

Related Information
Antiparkinsonian Agents *on page 1995*
Carbidopa *on page 273*

Medication Safety Issues
Sound-alike/look-alike issues:
Sinemet® may be confused with Serevent®
International issues:
Zimox: Brand name for carbidopa and levodopa [Greece], but also the brand name for amoxicillin [Italy]
Zimox [Greece] may be confused with Diamox which is a brand name for acetazolamide [Canada and multiple international markets]

Brand Names: U.S. Parcopa®; Sinemet®; Sinemet® CR
Brand Names: Canada Apo-Levocarb®; Apo-Levocarb® CR; Dom-Levo-Carbidopa; Duodopa™; Endo®-Levodopa/Carbidopa; Levocarb CR; Novo-Levocarbidopa; Nu-Levocarb; PRO-Levocarb; Sinemet®; Sinemet® CR
Index Terms Levodopa and Carbidopa
Generic Availability (U.S.) Yes
Pharmacologic Category Anti-Parkinson's Agent, Decarboxylase Inhibitor; Anti-Parkinson's Agent, Dopamine Precursor
Use Idiopathic Parkinson's disease; postencephalitic parkinsonism; symptomatic parkinsonism

Duodopa™ intestinal gel: Canadian labeling (not available in U.S.): Treatment of advanced levodopa-responsive Parkinson's disease in which severe motor symptoms are not controlled by other Parkinson's agents

Unlabeled/Investigational Use Restless leg syndrome

Prescribing and Access Restrictions Duodopa™ intestinal gel (Canadian labeling; product not available in U.S.): In Canada, the Duodopa™ Education Program is a risk mitigation program established to provide safe and effective use of Duodopa™ in advanced Parkinson's patients. The program involves:
- Education of prescribing neurologists and other healthcare providers on suitable candidates for treatment, surgical procedures (PEG tube placement), and follow-up care including infusion device education.
- Distribution of educational materials to patients and caregivers describing Duodopa™ intestinal gel and its proper use, PEG tube placement, and complications associated with the mode of administration and/or PEG tube placement.

Contraindications Hypersensitivity to levodopa, carbidopa, or any component of the formulation; narrow-angle glaucoma; use of MAO inhibitors within prior 14 days (however, may be administered concomitantly with the manufacturer's recommended dose of an MAO inhibitor with selectivity for MAO type B); history of melanoma or undiagnosed skin lesions

Canadian labeling: Additional contraindications: Clinical or laboratory evidence of uncompensated cardiovascular, cerebrovascular, endocrine, renal, hepatic, hematologic or pulmonary disease; when administration of a sympathomimetic amine (eg, epinephrine, norepinephrine or isoproterenol) is contraindicated; intestinal gel therapy in patients with any condition preventing the required placement of a PEG tube for administration.

Warnings/Precautions Use with caution in patients with history of cardiovascular disease (including myocardial infarction and arrhythmias), pulmonary diseases (such as asthma), psychosis, wide-angle glaucoma, peptic ulcer disease, seizure disorder or prone to seizures, and in severe renal and hepatic dysfunction. Use with caution when interpreting plasma/urine catecholamine levels; falsely diagnosed pheochromocytoma has been rarely reported. Severe cases or rhabdomyolysis have been reported. Sudden discontinuation of levodopa may cause a worsening of Parkinson's disease. Elderly may be more sensitive to CNS effects of levodopa. May cause or exacerbate dyskinesias. Patients have reported falling asleep while engaging in activities of daily living; this has been reported to occur without significant warning signs. May cause orthostatic hypotension; Parkinson's disease patients appear to have an impaired capacity to respond to a postural challenge; use with caution in patients at risk of hypotension (such as those receiving antihypertensive drugs) or where transient hypotensive episodes would be poorly tolerated (cardiovascular disease or cerebrovascular disease). Observe patients closely for development of depression with concomitant suicidal tendencies.

Dopamine agonists have been associated with compulsive behaviors and/or loss of impulse control, which has manifested as pathological gambling, libido increases (hypersexuality), and/or binge eating. Causality has not been established, and controversy exists as to whether this phenomenon is related to the underlying disease, prior behaviors/addictions and/or drug therapy. Dose reduction or discontinuation of therapy has been reported to reverse these behaviors in some, but not all cases. Risk for melanoma development is increased in Parkinson's disease patients; drug causation or factors contributing to risk have not been established. Patients should be monitored closely and periodic skin examinations should be performed. Dopaminergic agents have been associated with a syndrome resembling neuroleptic malignant syndrome on abrupt withdrawal or significant dosage reduction after long-term use. Protein in the diet should be distributed throughout the day to avoid fluctuations in levodopa absorption.

Intestinal gel (available in Canada, not available in U.S.): Product should be prescribed only by neurologists experienced in the treatment of Parkinson's disease and who have completed the Duodopa™ Education Program. Response to levodopa/carbidopa intestinal gel therapy should be assessed with a test period (~3 days) of administration via a temporary nasoduodenal tube prior to placement of a percutaneous endoscopic gastrostomy (PEG) tube for permanent access and administration. Sudden deterioration in therapy response with recurring motor symptoms may indicate PEG tube complications (eg, displacement) or obstruction of the infusion device. Tube or infusion device complications may require initiation of oral levodopa/carbidopa therapy until complications are resolved. Discontinue therapy 2-3 hours prior to surgical procedures requiring general anesthesia, if possible. May resume therapy postoperatively when oral fluid intake is permitted.

Adverse Reactions (Reflective of adult population; not specific for elderly) Frequency not defined.

Cardiovascular: Arrhythmia, chest pain, edema, flushing, hypotension, hypertension, MI, orthostatic hypotension, palpitation, phlebitis, syncope

Central nervous system: Agitation, anxiety, ataxia, confusion, delusions, dementia, depression (with or without suicidal tendencies), disorientation, dizziness, dreams abnormal, EPS, euphoria, faintness, falling, fatigue, gait abnormalities, headache, hallucinations, impulse control symptoms, insomnia, malaise, memory impairment, mental acuity decreased, nervousness, neuroleptic malignant syndrome, nightmares, on-off phenomena, paranoid ideation, pathological gambling, psychosis, seizure (causal relationship not established), somnolence

Dermatologic: Alopecia, malignant melanoma, rash

Endocrine & metabolic: Hot flashes, hyperglycemia, hypokalemia, libido increased (including hypersexuality), uric acid increased

Gastrointestinal: Abdominal pain, abdominal distress, anorexia, bruxism, constipation, diarrhea, discoloration of saliva, duodenal ulcer, dyspepsia, dysphagia, flatulence, GI bleeding, heartburn, nausea, sialorrhea, taste alterations, tongue burning sensation, weight gain/loss, vomiting, xerostomia

CARBIDOPA AND LEVODOPA

Genitourinary: Discoloration of urine, glycosuria, urinary frequency, priapism, proteinuria, urinary incontinence, urinary retention, urinary tract infection

Hematologic: Agranulocytosis, anemia, Coombs' test abnormal, hematocrit decreased, hemoglobin decreased, hemolytic anemia, leukopenia

Hepatic: Alkaline phosphatase abnormal, ALT abnormal, AST abnormal, bilirubin abnormal, LDH abnormal

Neuromuscular & skeletal: Back pain, dyskinesias (including choreiform, dystonic and other involuntary movements), leg pain, muscle cramps, muscle twitching, numbness, paresthesia, peripheral neuropathy, shoulder pain, tremor increased, trismus, weakness

Ocular: Blepharospasm, blurred vision, diplopia, Horner's syndrome reactivation, mydriasis, oculogyric crises (may be associated with acute dystonic reactions)

Renal: Difficult urination

Respiratory: Cough, dyspnea, hoarseness, pharyngeal pain, upper respiratory infection

Miscellaneous: Discoloration of sweat, diaphoresis increased, hiccups, hypersensitivity reactions (angioedema, pruritus, urticaria, bullous lesions [including pemphigus-like reactions], Henoch-Schönlein purpura)

Drug Interactions

Avoid Concomitant Use There are no known interactions where it is recommended to avoid concomitant use.

Increased Effect/Toxicity

Carbidopa and Levodopa may increase the levels/effects of: MAO Inhibitors

The levels/effects of Carbidopa and Levodopa may be increased by: Antipsychotics (Typical); MAO Inhibitors; Methylphenidate; Sapropterin

Decreased Effect

Carbidopa and Levodopa may decrease the levels/effects of: Antipsychotics (Typical)

The levels/effects of Carbidopa and Levodopa may be decreased by: Antipsychotics (Atypical); Fosphenytoin; Glycopyrrolate; Iron Salts; Methionine; Metoclopramide; Phenytoin; Pyridoxine

Ethanol/Nutrition/Herb Interactions

Ethanol: Avoid ethanol (due to CNS depression).

Food: Avoid high protein diets due to potential for impaired levodopa absorption; levodopa competes with certain amino acids for transport across the gut wall or across the blood brain barrier.

Herb/Nutraceutical: Avoid kava kava (may decrease effects). Pyridoxine (vitamin B_6) in doses >10-25 mg (for levodopa alone) may decrease efficacy. Iron supplements or iron-containing multivitamins may reduce absorption of levodopa.

Stability

Tablet: Store at 20°C to 25°C (68°F to 77°F); excursions permitted between 15°C to 30°C (59°F to 86°F). Protect from light and moisture.

Intestinal gel (Canadian labeling; not available in U.S.): Store in refrigerator at 2°C to 8°C (36°F to 46°F). Keep in outer carton to protect from light. Cassettes are for single use only and should be discarded daily following infusion (up to 16 hours).

Mechanism of Action Parkinson's symptoms are due to a lack of striatal dopamine; levodopa circulates in the plasma to the blood-brain-barrier (BBB), where it crosses, to be converted by striatal enzymes to dopamine; carbidopa inhibits the peripheral plasma breakdown of levodopa by inhibiting its decarboxylation, and thereby increases available levodopa at the BBB

Pharmacodynamics/Kinetics

Carbidopa:
  Absorption: Oral: 40% to 70%
  Protein binding: 36%
  Half-life: 1-2 hours
  Elimination: Excreted unchanged
Levodopa:
  Absorption: May be decreased if given with a high protein meal
  Half-life: 1.2-2.3 hours
  Elimination: Primarily in urine (80%) as dopamine, norepinephrine, and homovanillic acid

Dosage

Geriatric & Adult

Parkinson's disease:

Oral:
  Immediate release tablet, orally-disintegrating tablet:
    Initial: Carbidopa 25 mg/levodopa 100 mg 3 times/day
    Dosage adjustment: Alternate tablet strengths may be substituted according to individual carbidopa/levodopa requirements. Increase by 1 tablet every 1-2 days as necessary, except when using the carbidopa 25 mg/levodopa 250 mg tablets where increases

276

should be made using 1/2-1 tablet every 1-2 days. Use of more than 1 dosage strength or dosing 4 times/day may be required (maximum: 8 tablets of any strength/day or 200 mg of carbidopa and 2000 mg of levodopa)

Controlled release tablet:

Patients not currently receiving levodopa: Initial: Carbidopa 50 mg/levodopa 200 mg 2 times/day, at intervals not <6 hours

Patients converting from immediate release formulation to controlled release: Initial: Dosage should be substituted at an amount that provides ~10% more of levodopa/day; total calculated dosage is administered in divided doses 2-3 times/day (or ≥3 times/day for patients maintained on levodopa ≥700 mg/day). Intervals between doses should be 4-8 hours while awake; when divided doses are not equal, smaller doses should be given toward the end of the day. Depending on clinical response, dosage may need to be increased to provide up to 30% more levodopa/day.

Dosage adjustment: May adjust every 3 days; intervals should be between 4-8 hours during the waking day (maximum dose: 8 tablets/day)

Intestinal infusion via PEG tube: Intestinal gel (Canadian labeling; not available in U.S.): **Note:** Conversion to/from oral levodopa tablet formulations and the intestinal gel formulation can be done on a 1:1 ratio. Total daily dose (expressed in terms of levodopa) consists of a morning bolus dose, a continuous maintenance dose, and additional bolus doses when necessary. Nighttime dosing may be necessary in certain rare situations (eg, nocturnal akinesia). Dosage adjustments should be carried out over a period of a few weeks.

Morning bolus dose (based on previous morning levodopa intake and volume to fill intestinal tubing): Usual: Levodopa 100-200 mg (5-10 mL); Maximum: Levodopa 300 mg (15 mL)

Continuous maintenance dose: Adjustable in increments of 2 mg/hour (0.1 mL/hour) and based on previous daily intake of levodopa: Usual: Levodopa 40-120 mg/hour (2-6 mL/hour) infused up to 16 hours; Range: Levodopa 20-200 mg/hour (1-10 mL/hour)

Additional bolus dose: Usual: Levodopa: 10-40 mg (0.5-2 mL), if needed for daytime hypokinesia; in patients requiring >5 additional boluses/day, the maintenance dose should be increased

Restless leg syndrome (RLS) (unlabeled use; Silber, 2004): Oral:

Immediate release tablet: Carbidopa 25 mg/levodopa 100 mg (0.5-1 tablet) given in the evening, at bedtime, or upon waking during the night with RLS symptoms

Controlled release tablet: Carbidopa 25 mg/levodopa 100 mg (1 tablet) before bedtime for RLS symptoms that awaken patient during the night

Renal Impairment Use with caution; manufacturer labeling makes no specific dosing recommendations.

Hepatic Impairment Use with caution; manufacturer labeling makes no specific dosing recommendations.

Administration

Oral tablet formulations: Space doses evenly over the waking hours. Give with meals to decrease GI upset. Controlled release product should not be chewed or crushed. Orally-disintegrating tablets do not require water; the tablet should disintegrate on the tongue's surface before swallowing.

Intestinal gel (Canadian labeling; not available in U.S.): Gel is administered directly to the duodenum via a portable infusion pump (CADD-legacy Duodopa™ pump). Administer through a temporary nasoduodenal tube for at least 3 days to evaluate patient response and for dose optimization. Long-term administration requires placement of PEG tube for intestinal infusion. Continuous maintenance dose is infused throughout the day for up to 16 hours.

Monitoring Parameters Periodic hepatic function tests, BUN, creatinine, and CBC; periodic skin examinations; blood pressure, standing and sitting/supine; symptoms of parkinsonism, dyskinesias, mental status

Test Interactions False-positive reaction for urinary glucose with Clinitest®; false-negative reaction using Clinistix®; false-positive urine ketones with Acetest®, Ketostix®, Labstix®

Pharmacotherapy Pearls To block the peripheral conversion of levodopa to dopamine, ≥70 mg/day of carbidopa is needed. "On-off" (a clinical syndrome characterized by sudden periods of drug activity/inactivity), can be managed by giving smaller, more frequent doses of Sinemet® or adding a dopamine agonist or selegiline; when adding a new agent, doses of Sinemet® can usually be decreased. Protein in the diet should be distributed throughout the day to avoid fluctuations in levodopa absorption. Levodopa is the drug of choice when rigidity is the predominant presenting symptom.

Conversion from levodopa to carbidopa/levodopa: **Note:** Levodopa must be discontinued at least 12 hours prior to initiation of levodopa/carbidopa:

Initial dose: Levodopa portion of carbidopa/levodopa should be at least 25% of previous levodopa therapy.

◀

Levodopa <1500 mg/day: Sinemet® or Parcopa™ (levodopa 25 mg/carbidopa 100 mg) 3-4 times/day

Levodopa ≥1500 mg/day: Sinemet® or Parcopa™ (levodopa 25 mg/carbidopa 250 mg) 3-4 times/day

Conversion from immediate release carbidopa/levodopa (Sinemet® or Parcopa™) to Sinemet® CR (50/200):

Sinemet® or Parcopa™ [total daily dose of levodopa]/Sinemet® CR:

Sinemet® or Parcopa™ (levodopa 300-400 mg/day): Sinemet® CR (50/200) 1 tablet twice daily

Sinemet® or Parcopa™ (levodopa 500-600 mg/day): Sinemet® CR (50/200) 1 1/2 tablets twice daily or 1 tablet 3 times/day

Sinemet® or Parcopa™ (levodopa 700-800 mg/day): Sinemet® CR (50/200) 4 tablets in 3 or more divided doses

Sinemet® or Parcopa™ (levodopa 900-1000 mg/day): Sinemet® CR (50/200) 5 tablets in 3 or more divided doses

Intervals between doses of Sinemet® CR should be 4-8 hours while awake; when divided doses are not equal, smaller doses should be given toward the end of the day

Special Geriatric Considerations The elderly may be more sensitive to the CNS effects of levodopa.

Dosage Forms Excipient information presented when available (limited, particularly for generics); consult specific product labeling.

Tablet: 10/100: Carbidopa 10 mg and levodopa 100 mg; 25/100: Carbidopa 25 mg and levodopa 100 mg; 25/250: Carbidopa 25 mg and levodopa 250 mg

Sinemet®:

10/100: Carbidopa 10 mg and levodopa 100 mg

25/100: Carbidopa 25 mg and levodopa 100 mg

25/250: Carbidopa 25 mg and levodopa 250 mg

Tablet, extended release: 25/100: Carbidopa 25 mg and levodopa 100 mg; 50/200: Carbidopa 50 mg and levodopa 200 mg

Tablet, orally disintegrating: 10/100: Carbidopa 10 mg and levodopa 100 mg; 25/100: Carbidopa 25 mg and levodopa 100 mg; 25/250: Carbidopa 25 mg and levodopa 250 mg

Parcopa®:

10/100: Carbidopa 10 mg and levodopa 100 mg [contains phenylalanine 3.4 mg/tablet; mint flavor]

25/100: Carbidopa 25 mg and levodopa 100 mg [contains phenylalanine 3.4 mg/tablet; mint flavor]

25/250: Carbidopa 25 mg and levodopa 250 mg [contains phenylalanine 8.4 mg/tablet; mint flavor]

Tablet, sustained release: 25/100: Carbidopa 25 mg and levodopa 100 mg; 50/200: Carbidopa 50 mg and levodopa 200 mg

Sinemet® CR:

25/100: Carbidopa 25 mg and levodopa 100 mg

50/200: Carbidopa 50 mg and levodopa 200 mg

Dosage Forms: Canada Excipient information presented when available (limited, particularly for generics); consult specific product labeling.

Intestinal gel:

Duodopa™: Carbidopa 5 mg and levodopa 20 mg/1 mL (100 mL)

Selected References

Factor SA, "Current Status of Symptomatic Medical Therapy in Parkinson's Disease," *Neurotherapeutics*, 2008, 5 (2):164-80.

Olanow CW, Watts RL, and Koller WC, "An Algorithm (Decision Tree) for the Management of Parkinson's Disease (2001): Treatment Guidelines," *Neurology*, 2001, 56(11 Suppl 5):S1-S88.

Weintraub D, Siderowf AD, Potenza MN, et al, "Association of Dopamine Agonist Use With Impulse Control Disorders in Parkinson Disease," *Arch Neurol*, 2006, 63(7):969-73.

Carisoprodol (kar eye soe PROE dole)

Related Information
  Beers Criteria – Potentially Inappropriate Medications for Geriatrics *on page 2089*
Medication Safety Issues
  BEERS Criteria medication:
    This drug may be inappropriate for use in geriatric patients (high severity risk).
Brand Names: U.S. Soma®
Index Terms Carisoprodate; Isobamate
Generic Availability (U.S.) Yes
Pharmacologic Category Skeletal Muscle Relaxant
Use Short-term (2-3 weeks) treatment of acute musculoskeletal pain
Contraindications Hypersensitivity to carisoprodol, meprobamate, or any component of the formulation; acute intermittent porphyria
Warnings/Precautions Can cause CNS depression, which may impair physical or mental abilities. Patients must be cautioned about performing tasks which require mental alertness (eg, operating machinery or driving); postmarketing reports of motor vehicle accidents have been associated with use. Effects with other CNS-depressant drugs or ethanol may be potentiated. Use with caution in patients with hepatic/renal dysfunction. Tolerance or drug dependence may result from extended use. Limit use to 2-3 weeks; use caution in patients who may be prone to addiction. May precipitate withdrawal after abrupt cessation of prolonged use.

Idiosyncratic reactions and/or severe allergic reactions may occur. Idiosyncratic reactions occur following the initial dose and may include severe weakness, transient quadriplegia, euphoria, or vision loss (temporary). Has been associated (rarely) with seizures in patients with and without seizure history. Carisoprodol should be used with caution in patients who are poor CYP2C19 metabolizers; poor metabolizers have been shown to have a fourfold increase in exposure to carisoprodol and a 50% reduced exposure to the metabolite meprobamate compared to normal metabolizers. This class of medication is poorly tolerated by the elderly due to anticholinergic effects, sedation, and weakness. Efficacy is questionable at dosages tolerated by elderly patients (Beers Criteria).

Adverse Reactions (Reflective of adult population; not specific for elderly)
  >10%: Central nervous system: Drowsiness (13% to 17%)
  1% to 10%: Central nervous system: Dizziness (7% to 8%), headache (3% to 5%)
Drug Interactions
  Metabolism/Transport Effects Substrate of CYP2C19 (major)
  Avoid Concomitant Use There are no known interactions where it is recommended to avoid concomitant use.
  Increased Effect/Toxicity
    Carisoprodol may increase the levels/effects of: Alcohol (Ethyl); CNS Depressants; Methotrimeprazine; Selective Serotonin Reuptake Inhibitors

    The levels/effects of Carisoprodol may be increased by: CYP2C19 Inhibitors (Moderate); CYP2C19 Inhibitors (Strong); Droperidol; HydrOXYzine; Methotrimeprazine
  Decreased Effect
    The levels/effects of Carisoprodol may be decreased by: CYP2C19 Inducers (Strong)
Ethanol/Nutrition/Herb Interactions Ethanol: May increase CNS depression; monitor for increased effects with coadministration. Caution patients about effects.
Stability Store at controlled room temperature of 20°C to 25°C (68°F to 77°F).
Mechanism of Action Precise mechanism is not yet clear, but many effects have been ascribed to its central depressant actions. In animals, carisoprodol blocks interneuronal activity and depresses polysynaptic neuron transmission in the spinal cord and reticular formation of the brain. It is also metabolized to meprobamate, which has anxiolytic and sedative effects.
Pharmacodynamics/Kinetics
  Onset of action: ~30 minutes
  Duration: 4-6 hours
  Metabolism: Hepatic, via CYP2C19 to active metabolite (meprobamate)
  Half-life elimination: ~2 hours; Meprobamate: 10 hours
  Time to peak, plasma: 1.5-2 hours
  Excretion: Urine, as metabolite
Dosage
  Geriatric Not recommended for use in the elderly.

◄ **Adult Note:** Carisoprodol should only be used for short periods (2-3 weeks) due to lack of evidence of effectiveness with prolonged use.

Acute musculoskeletal pain: Oral: 250-350 mg 3 times/day and at bedtime

Renal Impairment Use in renal impairment has not been studied; use with caution.

Dialysis: Removed by hemo- and peritoneal dialysis

Hepatic Impairment Use in hepatic impairment has not been studied; use with caution.

Administration Administer with or without food.

Monitoring Parameters CNS effects (eg, mental status, excessive drowsiness); relief of pain and/or muscle spasm; signs of drug abuse in addiction-prone individuals

Special Geriatric Considerations Avoid or use with caution in the elderly; not considered a drug of choice because of the risk of orthostatic hypotension and CNS depression; no data available on the use of skeletal muscle relaxants in the geriatric population.

This medication is considered to be potentially inappropriate in this patient population (Beers Criteria severity: High).

Dosage Forms Excipient information presented when available (limited, particularly for generics); consult specific product labeling.

Tablet, oral: 350 mg

Soma®: 250 mg, 350 mg

◆ **Carmol® Scalp Treatment** see Sulfacetamide (Topical) on page 1713
◆ **Carrington® Antifungal [OTC]** see Miconazole on page 1206
◆ **Carrington® Oral Wound Rinse [OTC]** see Maltodextrin on page 1114

Carteolol (Ophthalmic) (KAR tee oh lole)

Related Information

Glaucoma Drug Therapy on page 2008

Medication Safety Issues

Sound-alike/look-alike issues:

Carteolol may be confused with carvedilol

Index Terms Carteolol Hydrochloride

Generic Availability (U.S.) Yes

Pharmacologic Category Ophthalmic Agent, Antiglaucoma

Use Treatment of chronic open-angle glaucoma and intraocular hypertension

Contraindications Hypersensitivity to carteolol or any component of the formulation; sinus bradycardia; heart block greater than first-degree (except in patients with a functioning artificial pacemaker); cardiogenic shock; bronchial asthma, bronchospasm, or COPD; uncompensated cardiac failure; pulmonary edema

Warnings/Precautions Consider pre-existing conditions such as sick sinus syndrome before initiating. Use caution in patients with PVD (can aggravate arterial insufficiency) or myasthenia gravis. In general, patients with bronchospastic disease should not receive beta-blockers; if used at all, should be used cautiously with close monitoring. Use cautiously in diabetics because it can mask prominent hypoglycemic symptoms. Systemic absorption and adverse effects may occur with ophthalmic product, including bradycardia and/or hypotension. Should not be used alone in angle-closure glaucoma (has no effect on pupillary constriction). Adequate alpha-blockade is required prior to use of any beta-blocker for patients with untreated pheochromocytoma.

Adverse Reactions (Reflective of adult population; not specific for elderly)

>10%: Ocular: Conjunctival hyperemia

1% to 10%: Ocular: Anisocoria, corneal punctate keratitis, corneal sensitivity decreased, corneal staining, eye pain, vision disturbances

Drug Interactions

Metabolism/Transport Effects Substrate of CYP2D6 (minor)

Avoid Concomitant Use

Avoid concomitant use of Carteolol (Ophthalmic) with any of the following: Floctafenine; Methacholine

Increased Effect/Toxicity

Carteolol (Ophthalmic) may increase the levels/effects of: Alpha-/Beta-Agonists (Direct-Acting); Alpha1-Blockers; Alpha2-Agonists; Amifostine; Antihypertensives; Antipsychotic Agents (Phenothiazines); Bupivacaine; Cardiac Glycosides; Fingolimod; Hypotensive Agents; Insulin; Lidocaine; Lidocaine (Systemic); Lidocaine (Topical); Mepivacaine; Methacholine; Midodrine; RiTUXimab; Sulfonylureas

The levels/effects of Carteolol (Ophthalmic) may be increased by: Acetylcholinesterase Inhibitors; Amiodarone; Anilidopiperidine Opioids; Antipsychotic Agents (Phenothiazines); Calcium Channel Blockers (Dihydropyridine); Calcium Channel Blockers

(Nondihydropyridine); Diazoxide; Dipyridamole; Disopyramide; Dronedarone; Floctafenine; Herbs (Hypotensive Properties); MAO Inhibitors; Pentoxifylline; Phosphodiesterase 5 Inhibitors; Prostacyclin Analogues; Reserpine

Decreased Effect

Carteolol (Ophthalmic) may decrease the levels/effects of: Beta2-Agonists; Theophylline Derivatives

The levels/effects of Carteolol (Ophthalmic) may be decreased by: Barbiturates; Herbs (Hypertensive Properties); Methylphenidate; Nonsteroidal Anti-Inflammatory Agents; Yohimbine

Mechanism of Action Blocks both beta$_1$- and beta$_2$-receptors and has mild intrinsic sympathomimetic activity; reduces intraocular pressure by decreasing aqueous humor production

Dosage

Geriatric & Adult Glaucoma or intraocular hypertension: Ophthalmic: Instill 1 drop in affected eye(s) twice daily

Administration Intended for twice daily dosing. Keep eye open and do not blink for 30 seconds after instillation. Wear sunglasses to avoid photophobic discomfort. Apply gentle pressure to lacrimal sac during and immediately following instillation (1 minute).

Monitoring Parameters Intraocular pressure

Pharmacotherapy Pearls When treating glaucoma/intraocular hypertension, if the desired IOP is not achieved, consider adding concomitant therapy with pilocarpine, dipivefrin, etc.

Special Geriatric Considerations Evaluate the patient's ability to self-administer the ophthalmic product.

Dosage Forms Excipient information presented when available (limited, particularly for generics); consult specific product labeling.

Solution, ophthalmic, as hydrochloride [drops]: 1% (5 mL, 10 mL, 15 mL) [contains benzalkonium chloride]

◆ **Carteolol Hydrochloride** *see* Carteolol (Ophthalmic) *on page 280*
◆ **Cartia XT®** *see* Diltiazem *on page 514*

Carvedilol (KAR ve dil ole)

Related Information

Beta-Blockers *on page 2001*

Medication Safety Issues

Sound-alike/look-alike issues:

Carvedilol may be confused with atenolol, captopril, carbidopa, carteolol

Coreg® may be confused with Corgard®, Cortef®, Cozaar®

Brand Names: U.S. Coreg CR®; Coreg®

Brand Names: Canada Apo-Carvedilol®; Coreg®; Dom-Carvedilol; JAMP-Carvedilol; Mylan-Carvedilol; Novo-Carvedilol; PHL-Carvedilol; PMS-Carvedilol; RAN™-Carvedilol; ratio-Carvedilol; ZYM-Carvedilol

Generic Availability (U.S.) Yes: Tablet

Pharmacologic Category Beta Blocker With Alpha-Blocking Activity

Use Mild-to-severe heart failure of ischemic or cardiomyopathic origin (usually in addition to standard therapy); left ventricular dysfunction following myocardial infarction (MI) (clinically stable with LVEF ≤40%); management of hypertension

Unlabeled/Investigational Use Angina pectoris

Contraindications Serious hypersensitivity to carvedilol or any component of the formulation; decompensated cardiac failure requiring intravenous inotropic therapy; bronchial asthma or related bronchospastic conditions; second- or third-degree AV block, sick sinus syndrome, and severe bradycardia (except in patients with a functioning artificial pacemaker); cardiogenic shock; severe hepatic impairment

Warnings/Precautions Consider pre-existing conditions such as sick sinus syndrome before initiating. Heart failure patients may experience a worsening of renal function (rare); risk factors include ischemic heart disease, diffuse vascular disease, underlying renal dysfunction, and systolic BP <100 mm Hg. Initiate cautiously and monitor for possible deterioration in patient status (eg, symptoms of HF). Worsening heart failure or fluid retention may occur during upward titration; dose reduction or temporary discontinuation may be necessary. Adjustment of other medications (ACE inhibitors and/or diuretics) may also be required. Bradycardia may be observed more frequently in elderly patients (>65 years of age); dosage reductions may be necessary.

Symptomatic hypotension with or without syncope may occur with carvedilol (usually within the first 30 days of therapy); close monitoring of patient is required especially with initial dosing and dosing increases; blood pressure must be lowered at a rate appropriate for the patient's

◀ clinical condition. Initiation with a low dose, gradual up-titration, and administration with food may help to decrease the occurrence of hypotension or syncope. Patients should be advised to avoid driving or other hazardous tasks during initiation of therapy due to the risk of syncope. Beta-blocker therapy should not be withdrawn abruptly (particularly in patients with CAD), but gradually tapered to avoid acute tachycardia, hypertension, and/or ischemia. Chronic beta-blocker therapy should not be routinely withdrawn prior to major surgery.

In general, patients with bronchospastic disease should not receive beta-blockers; if used at all, should be used cautiously with close monitoring. May precipitate or aggravate symptoms of arterial insufficiency in patients with PVD and Raynaud's disease; use with caution and monitor for progression of arterial obstruction. Use caution with concurrent use of digoxin, verapamil or diltiazem; bradycardia or heart block can occur. Use with caution in patients receiving inhaled anesthetic agents known to depress myocardial contractility. Use cautiously in patients with diabetes because it can mask prominent hypoglycemic symptoms. In patients with heart failure and diabetes, use of carvedilol may worsen hyperglycemia; may require adjustment of antidiabetic agents. May mask signs of hyperthyroidism (eg, tachycardia); if hyperthyroidism is suspected, carefully manage and monitor; abrupt withdrawal may exacerbate symptoms of hyperthyroidism or precipitate thyroid storm. May induce or exacerbate psoriasis. Use with caution in patients with myasthenia gravis or psychiatric disease (may cause CNS depression). Use with caution in patients with mild-to-moderate hepatic impairment; use is contraindicated in patients with severe impairment. Manufacturer recommends discontinuation of therapy if liver injury occurs (confirmed by laboratory testing). Adequate alpha-blockade is required prior to use of any beta-blocker for patients with untreated pheochromocytoma. Use caution with history of severe anaphylaxis to allergens; patients taking beta-blockers may become more sensitive to repeated challenges. Treatment of anaphylaxis (eg, epinephrine) in patients taking beta-blockers may be ineffective or promote undesirable effects.

Intraoperative floppy iris syndrome has been observed in cataract surgery patients who were on or were previously treated with alpha$_1$-blockers; causality has not been established and there appears to be no benefit in discontinuing alpha-blocker therapy prior to surgery. Instruct patients to inform ophthalmologist of carvedilol use when considering eye surgery.

Adverse Reactions (Reflective of adult population; not specific for elderly) Note: Frequency ranges include data from hypertension and heart failure trials. Higher rates of adverse reactions have generally been noted in patients with heart failure. However, the frequency of adverse effects associated with placebo is also increased in this population.

>10%:
  Cardiovascular: Hypotension (9% to 20%)
  Central nervous system: Dizziness (2% to 32%), fatigue (4% to 24%)
  Endocrine & metabolic: Hyperglycemia (5% to 12%)
  Gastrointestinal: Diarrhea (1% to 12%), weight gain (10% to 12%)
  Neuromuscular & skeletal: Weakness (7% to 11%)
1% to 10%:
  Cardiovascular: Bradycardia (2% to 10%), syncope (3% to 8%), peripheral edema (1% to 7%), generalized edema (5% to 6%), angina (1% to 6%), dependent edema (≤4%), AV block, cerebrovascular accident, hypertension, hyper-/hypovolemia, postural hypotension, palpitation
  Central nervous system: Headache (5% to 8%), depression, fever, hypoesthesia, hypotonia, insomnia, malaise, somnolence, vertigo
  Endocrine & metabolic: Hypercholesterolemia (1% to 4%), hypertriglyceridemia (1%), diabetes mellitus, gout, hyperkalemia, hyperuricemia, hypoglycemia, hyponatremia
  Gastrointestinal: Nausea (2% to 9%), vomiting (1% to 6%), abdominal pain, melena, periodontitis, weight loss
  Genitourinary: Impotence
  Hematologic: Anemia, prothrombin decreased, purpura, thrombocytopenia
  Hepatic: Alkaline phosphatase increased (1% to 3%), GGT increased, transaminases increased
  Neuromuscular & skeletal: Back pain (2% to 7%), arthralgia (1% to 6%), arthritis, muscle cramps, paresthesia
  Ocular: Blurred vision (1% to 5%)
  Renal: BUN increased (≤6%), nonprotein nitrogen increased (6%), albuminuria, creatinine increased, glycosuria, hematuria, renal insufficiency
  Respiratory: Cough (5% to 8%), nasopharyngitis (4%), rales (4%), dyspnea (>3%), pulmonary edema (>3%), rhinitis (2%), nasal congestion (1%), sinus congestion (1%)
  Miscellaneous: Injury (3% to 6%), allergy, flu-like syndrome, sudden death

Drug Interactions
  Metabolism/Transport Effects Substrate of CYP1A2 (minor), CYP2C9 (major), CYP2D6 (major), CYP2E1 (minor), CYP3A4 (minor), P-glycoprotein; **Inhibits** P-glycoprotein

Avoid Concomitant Use

Avoid concomitant use of Carvedilol with any of the following: Floctafenine; Methacholine; Topotecan

Increased Effect/Toxicity

Carvedilol may increase the levels/effects of: Alpha-/Beta-Agonists (Direct-Acting); Alpha1-Blockers; Alpha2-Agonists; Amifostine; Antihypertensives; Antipsychotic Agents (Phenothiazines); Bupivacaine; Cardiac Glycosides; Colchicine; CycloSPORINE; CycloSPORINE (Systemic); Dabigatran Etexilate; Digoxin; Everolimus; Fingolimod; Hypotensive Agents; Insulin; Lidocaine; Lidocaine (Systemic); Lidocaine (Topical); Mepivacaine; Methacholine; Midodrine; P-Glycoprotein Substrates; RiTUXimab; Rivaroxaban; Sulfonylureas; Topotecan

The levels/effects of Carvedilol may be increased by: Abiraterone Acetate; Acetylcholinesterase Inhibitors; Aminoquinolines (Antimalarial); Amiodarone; Anilidopiperidine Opioids; Antipsychotic Agents (Phenothiazines); Calcium Channel Blockers (Dihydropyridine); Calcium Channel Blockers (Nondihydropyridine); Cimetidine; Conivaptan; CYP2C9 Inhibitors (Moderate); CYP2C9 Inhibitors (Strong); CYP2D6 Inhibitors (Moderate); CYP2D6 Inhibitors (Strong); Darunavir; Diazoxide; Dipyridamole; Disopyramide; Dronedarone; Floctafenine; Herbs (Hypotensive Properties); MAO Inhibitors; Pentoxifylline; P-Glycoprotein Inhibitors; Phosphodiesterase 5 Inhibitors; Propafenone; Propoxyphene; Prostacyclin Analogues; QuiNIDine; Reserpine; Selective Serotonin Reuptake Inhibitors

Decreased Effect

Carvedilol may decrease the levels/effects of: Beta2-Agonists; Theophylline Derivatives

The levels/effects of Carvedilol may be decreased by: Barbiturates; Cyproterone; Herbs (Hypertensive Properties); Methylphenidate; Nonsteroidal Anti-Inflammatory Agents; Peginterferon Alfa-2b; P-Glycoprotein Inducers; Rifamycin Derivatives; Tocilizumab; Yohimbine

Ethanol/Nutrition/Herb Interactions

Food: Food decreases rate but not extent of absorption. Administration with food minimizes risks of orthostatic hypotension.

Herb/Nutraceutical: Avoid herbs with hypertensive properties (bayberry, blue cohosh, cayenne, ephedra, ginger, ginseng [American], kola, licorice); may diminish the antihypertensive effect of carvedilol. Avoid herbs with hypotensive properties (black cohosh, California poppy, coleus, golden seal, hawthorn, mistletoe, periwinkle, quinine, shepherd's purse); may enhance the hypotensive effect of carvedilol.

Stability

Coreg®: Store at <30°C (<86°F). Protect from moisture.

Coreg CR®: Store at 25°C (77°F); excursions permitted to 15°C to 30°C (59°F to 86°F).

Mechanism of Action As a racemic mixture, carvedilol has nonselective beta-adrenoreceptor and alpha-adrenergic blocking activity. No intrinsic sympathomimetic activity has been documented. Associated effects in hypertensive patients include reduction of cardiac output, exercise- or beta-agonist-induced tachycardia, reduction of reflex orthostatic tachycardia, vasodilation, decreased peripheral vascular resistance (especially in standing position), decreased renal vascular resistance, reduced plasma renin activity, and increased levels of atrial natriuretic peptide. In CHF, associated effects include decreased pulmonary capillary wedge pressure, decreased pulmonary artery pressure, decreased heart rate, decreased systemic vascular resistance, increased stroke volume index, and decreased right arterial pressure (RAP).

Pharmacodynamics/Kinetics

Onset of action: 1-2 hours

Peak antihypertensive effect: ~1-2 hours

Absorption: Rapid and extensive

Distribution: V_d: 115 L

Protein binding: >98%, primarily to albumin

Metabolism: Extensively hepatic, via CYP2C9, 2D6, 3A4, and 2C19 (2% excreted unchanged); three active metabolites (4-hydroxyphenyl metabolite is 13 times more potent than parent drug for beta-blockade); first-pass effect; plasma concentrations in the elderly and those with cirrhotic liver disease are 50% and 4-7 times higher, respectively

Bioavailability: Immediate release: 25% to 35% (due to significant first-pass metabolism); Extended release: 85% of immediate release

Half-life elimination: 7-10 hours

Time to peak, plasma: Extended release: 5 hours

Excretion: Primarily feces

Dosage

Geriatric Refer to adult dosing. In the management of hypertension, consider lower initial doses and titrate to response (Aronow, 2011).

◀ **Adult** Reduce dosage if heart rate drops to <55 beats/minute.
Hypertension: Oral:

Immediate release: 6.25 mg twice daily; if tolerated, dose should be maintained for 1-2 weeks, then increased to 12.5 mg twice daily. If necessary, dosage may be increased to a maximum of 25 mg twice daily after 1-2 weeks.

Extended release: Initial: 20 mg once daily, if tolerated, dose should be maintained for 1-2 weeks then increased to 40 mg once daily if necessary; maximum dose: 80 mg once daily

Heart failure: Oral:

Immediate release: 3.125 mg twice daily for 2 weeks; if this dose is tolerated, may increase to 6.25 mg twice daily. Double the dose every 2 weeks to the highest dose tolerated by patient. (Prior to initiating therapy, other heart failure medications should be stabilized and fluid retention minimized.)

Maximum recommended dose:
Mild-to-moderate heart failure:
<85 kg: 25 mg twice daily
>85 kg: 50 mg twice daily
Severe heart failure: 25 mg twice daily

Extended release: Initial: 10 mg once daily for 2 weeks; if the dose is tolerated, increase dose to 20 mg, 40 mg, and 80 mg over successive intervals of at least 2 weeks. Maintain on lower dose if higher dose is not tolerated.

Left ventricular dysfunction following MI: Oral: **Note:** Should be initiated only after patient is hemodynamically stable and fluid retention has been minimized.

Immediate release: Initial 3.125-6.25 mg twice daily; increase dosage incrementally (ie, from 6.25-12.5 mg twice daily) at intervals of 3-10 days, based on tolerance, to a target dose of 25 mg twice daily.

Extended release: Initial: Extended release: Initial: 10-20 mg once daily; increase dosage incrementally at intervals of 3-10 days, based on tolerance, to a target dose of 80 mg once daily.

Angina pectoris (unlabeled use): Oral: *Immediate release:* 25-50 mg twice daily

Conversion from immediate release to extended release (Coreg CR®):
Current dose immediate release tablets 3.125 mg twice daily: Convert to extended release capsules 10 mg once daily
Current dose immediate release tablets 6.25 mg twice daily: Convert to extended release capsules 20 mg once daily
Current dose immediate release tablets 12.5 mg twice daily: Convert to extended release capsules 40 mg once daily
Current dose immediate release tablets 25 mg twice daily: Convert to extended release capsules 80 mg once daily

Renal Impairment None necessary

Hepatic Impairment Use is contraindicated in severe liver dysfunction.

Administration Administer with food. Extended release capsules should not be crushed or chewed. Capsules may be opened and sprinkled on applesauce for immediate use.

Monitoring Parameters Heart rate, blood pressure (base need for dosage increase on trough blood pressure measurements and for tolerance on standing systolic pressure 1 hour after dosing); renal studies, BUN, liver function; in patient with increase risk for developing renal dysfunction, monitor during dosage titration.

Pharmacotherapy Pearls Fluid retention during therapy should be treated with an increase in diuretic dosage.

Special Geriatric Considerations Due to alterations in the beta-adrenergic autonomic nervous system, beta-adrenergic blockade may result in less hemodynamic response than seen in younger adults. In U.S. trials conducted by the manufacturer, hypertension patients who were elderly (>65%) had a higher incidence of dizziness (8.8% vs 6%) than seen in younger patients. No other differences noted between young and old in these trials.

Dosage Forms Excipient information presented when available (limited, particularly for generics); consult specific product labeling.
Capsule, extended release, oral, as phosphate:
Coreg CR®: 10 mg, 20 mg, 40 mg, 80 mg
Tablet, oral: 3.125 mg, 6.25 mg, 12.5 mg, 25 mg
Coreg®: 3.125 mg, 6.25 mg, 12.5 mg, 25 mg

Selected References
Hunt HA, Baker DW, Chin MH, et al, "ACC/AHA Guidelines for the Evaluation and Management of Chronic Heart Failure in the Adult: Executive Summary A Report of the American College of Cardiology/American Heart Association Task Force on Practice Guidelines (Committee to Revise the 1995 Guidelines for the Evaluation and Management of Heart Failure): Developed in Collaboration With the International Society for Heart and Lung Transplantation; Endorsed by the Heart Failure Society of America," *Circulation* 2001, 104(24):2996-3007.

Packer M, Coats AJ, Fowler MB, et al, "Effect of Carvedilol on Survival in Severe Chronic Heart Failure," *N Engl J Med*, 2001, 344(22):1651-8.

◆ **Casodex®** *see* Bicalutamide *on page 201*

Caspofungin (kas poe FUN jin)

Brand Names: U.S. Cancidas®
Brand Names: Canada Cancidas®
Index Terms Caspofungin Acetate
Generic Availability (U.S.) No
Pharmacologic Category Antifungal Agent, Parenteral; Echinocandin
Use Treatment of invasive *Aspergillus* infections in patients who are refractory or intolerant of other therapy; treatment of candidemia and other *Candida* infections (intra-abdominal abscesses, esophageal, peritonitis, pleural space); empirical treatment for presumed fungal infections in febrile neutropenic patient
Contraindications Hypersensitivity to caspofungin or any component of the formulation
Warnings/Precautions Concurrent use of cyclosporine should be limited to patients for whom benefit outweighs risk, due to a high frequency of hepatic transaminase elevations observed during concurrent use. Use caution in hepatic impairment; increased transaminases and rare cases of liver impairment have been reported in pediatric and adult patients. Dosage reduction required in adults with moderate hepatic impairment; safety and efficacy have not been established in adults with severe hepatic impairment.
Adverse Reactions (Reflective of adult population; not specific for elderly)
>10%:
  Cardiovascular: Hypotension (3% to 20%), peripheral edema (6% to 11%), tachycardia (4% to 11%)
  Central nervous system: Fever (6% to 30%), chills (9% to 23%), headache (5% to 15%)
  Dermatologic: Rash (4% to 23%)
  Endocrine & metabolic: Hypokalemia (5% to 23%)
  Gastrointestinal: Diarrhea (6% to 27%), vomiting (6% to 17%), nausea (4% to 15%)
  Hematologic: Hemoglobin decreased (18% to 21%), hematocrit decreased (13% to 18%), WBC decreased (12%), anemia (2% to 11%)
  Hepatic: Serum alkaline phosphatase increased (9% to 22%), transaminases increased (2% to 18%), bilirubin increased (5% to 13%)
  Local: Phlebitis/thrombophlebitis (18%)
  Renal: Serum creatinine increased (3% to 11%)
  Respiratory: Respiratory failure (2% to 20%), cough (6% to 11%), pneumonia (4% to 11%)
  Miscellaneous: Infusion reactions (20% to 35%), septic shock (11% to 14%)
5% to 10%:
  Cardiovascular: Hypertension (5% to 6%; children 9% to 10%)
  Dermatologic: Erythema (4% to 9%), pruritus (6% to 7%)
  Endocrine & metabolic: Hypomagnesemia (7%), hyperglycemia (6%)
  Gastrointestinal: Mucosal inflammation (4% to 10%), abdominal pain (4% to 9%)
  Hepatic: Albumin decreased (7%)
  Local: Infection (1% to 9%, central line)
  Renal: Hematuria (10%), blood urea nitrogen increased (4% to 9%)
  Respiratory: Dyspnea (9%), pleural effusion (9%), respiratory distress (≤8%), rales (7%)
  Miscellaneous: Sepsis (5% to 7%)
Drug Interactions
  Avoid Concomitant Use There are no known interactions where it is recommended to avoid concomitant use.
  Increased Effect/Toxicity
    The levels/effects of Caspofungin may be increased by: CycloSPORINE; CycloSPORINE (Systemic)
  Decreased Effect
    Caspofungin may decrease the levels/effects of: Saccharomyces boulardii; Tacrolimus; Tacrolimus (Systemic)

    The levels/effects of Caspofungin may be decreased by: Inducers of Drug Clearance; Rifampin
Stability Store vials at 2°C to 8°C (36°F to 46°F). Reconstituted solution may be stored at ≤25°C (≤77°F) for 1 hour prior to preparation of infusion solution. Infusion solutions may be stored at ≤25°C (≤77°F) and should be used within 24 hours; up to 48 hours if stored at 2°C to 8°C (36°F to 46°F).

Bring refrigerated vial to room temperature. Reconstitute vials using 0.9% sodium chloride for injection, SWFI, or bacteriostatic water for injection. Mix gently until clear solution is formed; do not use if cloudy or contains particles. Solution should be further diluted with 0.9%, 0.45%, or 0.225% sodium chloride or LR (do not exceed final concentration of 0.5 mg/mL).

◀ **Mechanism of Action** Inhibits synthesis of β(1,3)-D-glucan, an essential component of the cell wall of susceptible fungi. Highest activity in regions of active cell growth. Mammalian cells do not require β(1,3)-D-glucan, limiting potential toxicity.

Pharmacodynamics/Kinetics

Protein binding: ~97% to albumin

Metabolism: Slowly, via hydrolysis and N-acetylation as well as by spontaneous degradation, with subsequent metabolism to component amino acids. Overall metabolism is extensive.

Half-life elimination: Beta (distribution): 9-11 hours; Terminal: 40-50 hours

Excretion: Urine (41%; primarily as metabolites, ~1% of total dose as unchanged drug); feces (35%; primarily as metabolites)

Dosage

Geriatric & Adult Note: Duration of caspofungin treatment should be determined by patient status and clinical response. Empiric therapy should be given until neutropenia resolves. In patients with positive cultures, treatment should continue until 14 days after last positive culture. In neutropenic patients, treatment should be given at least 7 days after both signs and symptoms of infection **and** neutropenia resolve.

Aspergillosis, invasive: Initial dose: 70 mg on day 1; subsequent dosing: 50 mg/day. If clinical response inadequate, may increase up to 70 mg/day if tolerated, but increased efficacy not demonstrated. **Note:** Duration of therapy should be a minimum of 6-12 weeks or throughout period of immunosuppression.

Candidiasis: Initial dose: 70 mg on day 1; subsequent dosing: 50 mg/day; higher doses (150 mg once daily infused over ~2 hours) compared to the standard adult dosing regimen (50 mg once daily) have not demonstrated additional benefit or toxicity in patients with invasive candidiasis (Betts, 2009)

Esophageal: 50 mg/day; **Note:** The majority of patients studied for this indication also had oropharyngeal involvement.

Empiric therapy: Initial dose: 70 mg on day 1; subsequent dosing: 50 mg/day; if clinical response inadequate, may increase up to 70 mg/day if tolerated, but increased efficacy not demonstrated

Dosage adjustment with concomitant use of an enzyme inducer:

Patients receiving rifampin: 70 mg caspofungin daily

Patients receiving carbamazepine, dexamethasone, efavirenz, nevirapine, or phenytoin (and possibly other enzyme inducers) may require an increased daily dose of caspofungin (70 mg/day).

Renal Impairment No dosage adjustment required in renal impairment.

Poorly dialyzed; no supplemental dose or dosage adjustment necessary, including patients on intermittent hemodialysis, peritoneal dialysis, or continuous renal replacement therapy (eg, CVVHD).

Hepatic Impairment Adults:

Mild hepatic insufficiency (Child-Pugh score 5-6): No adjustment necessary.

Moderate hepatic insufficiency (Child-Pugh score 7-9): 70 mg on day 1 (where recommended), followed by 35 mg once daily.

Severe hepatic insufficiency (Child-Pugh score >9): No information available.

Administration Infuse slowly, over 1 hour (manufacturer); recent study, using doses of 50-150 mg, infused over ~2 hours (Betts, 2009); monitor during infusion. Isolated cases of possible histamine-related reactions have occurred during clinical trials (rash, flushing, pruritus, facial edema).

Monitoring Parameters Liver function

Special Geriatric Considerations The number of patients >65 years of age in clinical studies was not sufficient to establish whether a difference in response may be anticipated.

Dosage Forms Excipient information presented when available (limited, particularly for generics); consult specific product labeling.

Injection, powder for reconstitution, as acetate:

Cancidas® 50 mg [contains sucrose 39 mg]

Cancidas® 70 mg [contains sucrose 54 mg]

Selected References

Betts RF, Nucci M, Talwar D, et al, "A Multicenter, Double-Blind Trial of a High-Dose Caspofungin Treatment Regimen Versus a Standard Caspofungin Treatment Regimen for Adult Patients With Invasive Candidiasis," *Clin Infect Dis*, 2009, 48(12):1676-84.

Pappas PG, Kauffman CA, Andes D, et al, "Clinical Practice Guidelines for the Management of Candidiasis: 2009 Update by the Infectious Diseases Society of America," *Clin Infect Dis*, 2009, 48(5):503-35.

Walsh TJ, Anaissie EJ, Denning DW, et al, "Treatment of Aspergillosis: Clinical Practice Guidelines of the Infectious Diseases Society of America," *Clin Infect Dis*, 2008, 46(3):327-60.

◆ **Caspofungin Acetate** *see* Caspofungin *on page 285*

Castor Oil (KAS tor oyl)

Related Information
Laxatives, Classification and Properties *on page 2012*
Index Terms Oleum Ricini
Generic Availability (U.S.) Yes: Oil
Pharmacologic Category Laxative, Miscellaneous
Use Preparation for rectal or bowel examination or surgery; rarely used to relieve constipation; also applied to skin as emollient and protectant
Dosage
 Geriatric & Adult Bowel evacuation, constipation: Oil: Oral: 15-60 mL as a single dose
Special Geriatric Considerations Elderly are often predisposed to constipation due to disease, immobility, drugs, low residue diets, and a decreased fluid intake usually due to a decreased "thirst reflex" with age. Avoid stimulant cathartic use on a chronic basis if possible. Use osmotic, lubricant, stool softeners, and bulk agents as prophylaxis. Patients should be instructed for proper dietary fiber and fluid intake as well as regular exercise. Monitor closely for fluid/electrolyte imbalance, CNS signs of fluid/electrolyte loss, and hypotension. Strong and chronic purging may cause severe fluid and electrolyte loss which may affect mental function (CNS). Not a drug of first choice for constipation in the elderly.
Dosage Forms Excipient information presented when available (limited, particularly for generics); consult specific product labeling.
 Oil, oral: 100% (60 mL, 120 mL, 180 mL, 480 mL, 3840 mL)

◆ **Castor Oil, Trypsin, and Balsam Peru** *see* Trypsin, Balsam Peru, and Castor Oil *on page 1876*
◆ **Cataflam®** *see* Diclofenac (Systemic) *on page 496*
◆ **Catapres®** *see* CloNIDine *on page 388*
◆ **Catapres-TTS®-1** *see* CloNIDine *on page 388*
◆ **Catapres-TTS®-2** *see* CloNIDine *on page 388*
◆ **Catapres-TTS®-3** *see* CloNIDine *on page 388*
◆ **Cathflo® Activase®** *see* Alteplase *on page 75*
◆ **Caverject®** *see* Alprostadil *on page 73*
◆ **Caverject Impulse®** *see* Alprostadil *on page 73*
◆ **CaviRinse™** *see* Fluoride *on page 751*
◆ **Cayston®** *see* Aztreonam *on page 178*
◆ **CB-1348** *see* Chlorambucil *on page 331*
◆ **CB7630** *see* Abiraterone Acetate *on page 24*
◆ **CBZ** *see* CarBAMazepine *on page 268*
◆ **CDP870** *see* Certolizumab Pegol *on page 324*
◆ **CDX** *see* Bicalutamide *on page 201*
◆ **CE** *see* Estrogens (Conjugated/Equine, Systemic) *on page 658*
◆ **CE** *see* Estrogens (Conjugated/Equine, Topical) *on page 661*
◆ **Cedax®** *see* Ceftibuten *on page 311*
◆ **CEE** *see* Estrogens (Conjugated/Equine, Systemic) *on page 658*
◆ **CEE** *see* Estrogens (Conjugated/Equine, Topical) *on page 661*

Cefaclor (SEF a klor)

Medication Safety Issues
 Sound-alike/look-alike issues:
 Cefaclor may be confused with cephalexin
Brand Names: Canada Apo-Cefaclor®; Ceclor®; Novo-Cefaclor; Nu-Cefaclor; PMS-Cefaclor
Generic Availability (U.S.) Yes
Pharmacologic Category Antibiotic, Cephalosporin (Second Generation)
Use Treatment of susceptible bacterial infections including otitis media, lower respiratory tract infections, acute exacerbations of chronic bronchitis, pharyngitis and tonsillitis, urinary tract infections, skin and skin structure infections
Contraindications Hypersensitivity to cefaclor, any component of the formulation, or other cephalosporins

◀ **Warnings/Precautions** Modify dosage in patients with severe renal impairment. Prolonged use may result in fungal or bacterial superinfection, including *C. difficile*-associated diarrhea (CDAD) and pseudomembranous colitis; CDAD has been observed >2 months postantibiotic treatment. Use with caution in patients with a history of penicillin allergy, especially IgE-mediated reactions (eg, anaphylaxis, urticaria). Beta-lactamase-negative, ampicillin-resistant (BLNAR) strains of *H. influenzae* should be considered resistant to cefaclor. Some products may contain phenylalanine.

Adverse Reactions (Reflective of adult population; not specific for elderly)

1% to 10%:

Dermatologic: Rash (maculopapular, erythematous, or morbilliform) (1% to 2%)

Gastrointestinal: Diarrhea (3%)

Genitourinary: Vaginitis (2%)

Hematologic: Eosinophilia (2%)

Hepatic: Transaminases increased (3%)

Miscellaneous: Moniliasis (2%)

Reactions reported with other cephalosporins: Fever, abdominal pain, superinfection, renal dysfunction, toxic nephropathy, hemorrhage, cholestasis

Drug Interactions

Avoid Concomitant Use

Avoid concomitant use of Cefaclor with any of the following: BCG

Increased Effect/Toxicity

The levels/effects of Cefaclor may be increased by: Probenecid

Decreased Effect

Cefaclor may decrease the levels/effects of: BCG; Typhoid Vaccine

Ethanol/Nutrition/Herb Interactions Food: Cefaclor serum levels may be decreased slightly if taken with food. The bioavailability of cefaclor extended release tablets is decreased 23% and the maximum concentration is decreased 67% when taken on an empty stomach.

Stability Store at controlled room temperature. Refrigerate suspension after reconstitution. Discard after 14 days. Do not freeze.

Mechanism of Action Inhibits bacterial cell wall synthesis by binding to one or more of the penicillin-binding proteins (PBPs) which in turn inhibits the final transpeptidation step of peptidoglycan synthesis in bacterial cell walls, thus inhibiting cell wall biosynthesis. Bacteria eventually lyse due to ongoing activity of cell wall autolytic enzymes (autolysins and murein hydrolases) while cell wall assembly is arrested.

Pharmacodynamics/Kinetics

Absorption: Well absorbed, acid stable

Distribution: Widely throughout the body and reaches therapeutic concentration in most tissues and body fluids, including synovial, pericardial, pleural, peritoneal fluids; bile, sputum, and urine; bone, myocardium, gallbladder, skin and soft tissue

Protein binding: 25%

Metabolism: Partially hepatic

Half-life elimination: 0.5-1 hour; prolonged with renal impairment

Time to peak: Capsule: 60 minutes; Suspension: 45 minutes

Excretion: Urine (80% as unchanged drug)

Dosage

Geriatric & Adult Treatment of infections: Oral: Dosing range: 250-500 mg every 8 hours

Renal Impairment

Cl_{cr} 10-50 mL/minute: Administer 50% to 100% of dose

Cl_{cr} <10 mL/minute: Administer 50% of dose

Hemodialysis: Moderately dialyzable (20% to 50%)

Administration Administer around-the-clock to promote less variation in peak and trough serum levels.

Chewable tablet: Should be chewed before swallowing; should not be swallowed whole

Extended release tablet: Should not be cut, crushed, or chewed; should be administered with food

Oral suspension: Shake well before using.

Monitoring Parameters Assess patient at beginning and throughout therapy for infection; monitor for signs of anaphylaxis during first dose

Test Interactions Positive direct Coombs', false-positive urinary glucose test using cupric sulfate (Benedict's solution, Clinitest®, Fehling's solution), false-positive serum or urine creatinine with Jaffé reaction

Special Geriatric Considerations Has not been studied in the elderly. Adjust dose for renal function in elderly. Considered to be one of the drugs of choice in the outpatient treatment of community-acquired pneumonia in elderly.

Dosage Forms Excipient information presented when available (limited, particularly for generics); consult specific product labeling.

Capsule, oral: 250 mg, 500 mg

Powder for suspension, oral: 125 mg/5 mL (75 mL, 150 mL); 250 mg/5 mL (75 mL, 150 mL); 375 mg/5 mL (50 mL, 100 mL)

Tablet, extended release, oral: 500 mg

Selected References

Mandell LA, Wunderink RG, Anzueto A, et al, "Infectious Diseases Society of America/American Thoracic Society Consensus Guidelines on the Management of Community-Acquired Pneumonia in Adults," *Clin Infect Dis*, 2007, 44 (Suppl 2):27-72.

Cefadroxil (sef a DROKS il)

Related Information

Prevention of Infective Endocarditis *on page 2064*

Brand Names: Canada Apo-Cefadroxil®; Novo-Cefadroxil; PRO-Cefadroxil

Index Terms Cefadroxil Monohydrate; Duricef

Generic Availability (U.S.) Yes

Pharmacologic Category Antibiotic, Cephalosporin (First Generation)

Use Treatment of susceptible bacterial infections, including those caused by group A beta-hemolytic *Streptococcus*

Contraindications Hypersensitivity to cefadroxil, any component of the formulation, or other cephalosporins

Warnings/Precautions Modify dosage in patients with severe renal impairment. Use with caution in patients with a history of penicillin allergy, especially IgE-mediated reactions (eg, anaphylaxis, angioedema, urticaria). Prolonged use may result in fungal or bacterial super-infection, including *C. difficile*-associated diarrhea (CDAD) and pseudomembranous colitis; CDAD has been observed >2 months postantibiotic treatment.

Adverse Reactions (Reflective of adult population; not specific for elderly)

1% to 10%: Gastrointestinal: Diarrhea

Reactions reported with other cephalosporins: Toxic epidermal necrolysis, abdominal pain, superinfection, renal dysfunction, toxic nephropathy, aplastic anemia, hemolytic anemia, hemorrhage, prothrombin time prolonged, BUN increased, creatinine increased, eosinophilia, pancytopenia, seizure

Drug Interactions

Avoid Concomitant Use

Avoid concomitant use of Cefadroxil with any of the following: BCG

Increased Effect/Toxicity

The levels/effects of Cefadroxil may be increased by: Probenecid

Decreased Effect

Cefadroxil may decrease the levels/effects of: BCG; Typhoid Vaccine

Ethanol/Nutrition/Herb Interactions Food: Concomitant administration with food or cow's milk does **not** significantly affect absorption.

Stability Refrigerate suspension after reconstitution; discard after 14 days.

Mechanism of Action Inhibits bacterial cell wall synthesis by binding to one or more of the penicillin-binding proteins (PBPs) which in turn inhibits the final transpeptidation step of peptidoglycan synthesis in bacterial cell walls, thus inhibiting cell wall biosynthesis. Bacteria eventually lyse due to ongoing activity of cell wall autolytic enzymes (autolysins and murein hydrolases) while cell wall assembly is arrested.

Pharmacodynamics/Kinetics

Absorption: Rapid and well absorbed

Distribution: Widely throughout the body and reaches therapeutic concentrations in most tissues and body fluids, including synovial, pericardial, pleural, and peritoneal fluids; bile, sputum, and urine; bone, myocardium, gallbladder, skin, and soft tissue

Protein binding: 20%

Half-life elimination: 1-2 hours; Renal failure: 20-24 hours

Time to peak, serum: 70-90 minutes

Excretion: Urine (>90% as unchanged drug)

Dosage

Geriatric & Adult

Susceptible infections: Oral: 1-2 g/day in 2 divided doses

Orofacial infections: Oral: 250-500 mg every 8 hours

Renal Impairment

Cl_{cr} 10-25 mL/minute: Administer every 24 hours.

Cl_{cr} <10 mL/minute: Administer every 36 hours.

◀ **Administration** Administer around-the-clock to promote less variation in peak and trough serum levels.

Monitoring Parameters Observe for signs and symptoms of anaphylaxis during first dose.

Test Interactions Positive direct Coombs', false-positive urinary glucose test using cupric sulfate (Benedict's solution, Clinitest®, Fehling's solution), false-positive serum or urine creatinine with Jaffé reaction

Special Geriatric Considerations Adjust dose for renal function in the elderly.

Dosage Forms Excipient information presented when available (limited, particularly for generics); consult specific product labeling.

Capsule, oral, as hemihydrate [strength expressed as base]: 500 mg

Capsule, oral, as monohydrate [strength expressed as base]: 500 mg

Powder for suspension, oral, as monohydrate [strength expressed as base]: 250 mg/5 mL (50 mL, 100 mL); 500 mg/5 mL (75 mL, 100 mL)

Tablet, oral, as hemihydrate [strength expressed as base]: 1 g

Tablet, oral, as monohydrate [strength expressed as base]: 1 g

Selected References
Cutler RE, Blair AD, and Kelly MR, "Cefadroxil Kinetics in Patients With Renal Insufficiency," *Clin Pharmacol Ther,* 1979, 25(5 Pt 1):514-21.

◆ **Cefadroxil Monohydrate** *see* Cefadroxil *on page* 289

CeFAZolin (sef A zoe lin)

Related Information
Antibiotic Treatment of Adults With Infective Endocarditis *on page* 2053
Prevention of Infective Endocarditis *on page* 2064

Medication Safety Issues
Sound-alike/look-alike issues:
CeFAZolin may be confused with cefoTEtan, cefOXitin, cefprozil, cefTAZidime, cefTRIAXone, cephalexin, cephalothin
Kefzol® may be confused with Cefzil®

Index Terms Ancef; Cefazolin Sodium

Generic Availability (U.S.) Yes

Pharmacologic Category Antibiotic, Cephalosporin (First Generation)

Use Treatment of respiratory tract, skin, genital, urinary tract, biliary tract, bone and joint infections, and septicemia due to susceptible gram-positive cocci (except *Enterococcus*); some gram-negative bacilli including *E. coli*, *Proteus*, and *Klebsiella* may be susceptible; surgical prophylaxis

Unlabeled/Investigational Use Prophylaxis against bacterial endocarditis

Contraindications Hypersensitivity to cefazolin sodium, any component of the formulation, or other cephalosporins

Warnings/Precautions Modify dosage in patients with severe renal impairment. Use with caution in patients with a history of penicillin allergy, especially IgE-mediated reactions (eg, anaphylaxis, angioedema, urticaria). Prolonged use may result in fungal or bacterial superinfection, including *C. difficile*-associated diarrhea (CDAD) and pseudomembranous colitis; CDAD has been observed >2 months postantibiotic treatment. May be associated with increased INR, especially in nutritionally-deficient patients, prolonged treatment, hepatic or renal disease. Use with caution in patients with a history of seizure disorder; high levels, particularly in the presence of renal impairment, may increase risk of seizures.

Adverse Reactions (Reflective of adult population; not specific for elderly) Frequency not defined.

Central nervous system: Fever, seizure

Dermatologic: Rash, pruritus, Stevens-Johnson syndrome

Gastrointestinal: Diarrhea, nausea, vomiting, abdominal cramps, anorexia, pseudomembranous colitis, oral candidiasis

Genitourinary: Vaginitis

Hepatic: Transaminases increased, hepatitis

Hematologic: Eosinophilia, neutropenia, leukopenia, thrombocytopenia, thrombocytosis

Local: Pain at injection site, phlebitis

Renal: BUN increased, serum creatinine increased, renal failure

Miscellaneous: Anaphylaxis

Reactions reported with other cephalosporins: Toxic epidermal necrolysis, abdominal pain, cholestasis, superinfection, toxic nephropathy, aplastic anemia, hemolytic anemia, hemorrhage, prothrombin time prolonged, pancytopenia

Drug Interactions
Avoid Concomitant Use
Avoid concomitant use of CeFAZolin with any of the following: BCG

Increased Effect/Toxicity

CeFAZolin may increase the levels/effects of: Fosphenytoin; Phenytoin; Vitamin K Antagonists

The levels/effects of CeFAZolin may be increased by: Probenecid

Decreased Effect

CeFAZolin may decrease the levels/effects of: BCG; Typhoid Vaccine

Stability Store intact vials at room temperature and protect from temperatures exceeding 40°C. Dilute large vial with 2.5 mL SWFI; 10 g vial may be diluted with 45 mL to yield 1 g/5 mL or 96 mL to yield 1 g/10 mL. May be injected or further dilution for I.V. administration in 50-100 mL compatible solution. Standard diluent is 1 g/50 mL D_5W or 2 g/50 mL D_5W.

Reconstituted solutions of cefazolin are light yellow to yellow. Protection from light is recommended for the powder and for the reconstituted solutions. Reconstituted solutions are stable for 24 hours at room temperature and for 10 days under refrigeration. Stability of parenteral admixture at room temperature (25°C) is 48 hours. Stability of parenteral admixture at refrigeration temperature (4°C) is 14 days.

DUPLEX™: Store at 20°C to 25°C (68°F to 77°F); excursions permitted to 15°C to 30°C (59°F to 86°F) prior to activation. Following activation, stable for 24 hours at room temperature and for 7 days under refrigeration.

Mechanism of Action Inhibits bacterial cell wall synthesis by binding to one or more of the penicillin-binding proteins (PBPs) which in turn inhibits the final transpeptidation step of peptidoglycan synthesis in bacterial cell walls, thus inhibiting cell wall biosynthesis. Bacteria eventually lyse due to ongoing activity of cell wall autolytic enzymes (autolysins and murein hydrolases) while cell wall assembly is arrested.

Pharmacodynamics/Kinetics

Distribution: Widely into most body tissues and fluids including gallbladder, liver, kidneys, bone, sputum, bile, pleural, and synovial; CSF penetration is poor

Protein binding: 74% to 86%

Metabolism: Minimally hepatic

Half-life elimination: 90-150 minutes; prolonged with renal impairment

Time to peak, serum: I.M.: 0.5-2 hours

Excretion: Urine (80% to 100% as unchanged drug)

Dosage

Geriatric & Adult

Usual dosage range: I.M., I.V.: 1-1.5 g every 8 hours, depending on severity of infection; maximum: 12 g/day

Cholecystitis, mild-to-moderate: I.V.: 1-2 g every 8 hours for 4-7 days (provided source controlled)

Endocarditis due to MSSA (without prosthesis) (unlabeled use): I.V.: 2 g every 8 hours; **Note:** Recommended for penicillin-allergic (nonanaphylactoid) patients (Baddour, 2005)

Intra-abdominal infection, complicated, community-acquired, mild-to-moderate (in combination with metronidazole): I.V.: 1-2 g every 8 hours for 4-7 days (provided source controlled)

Moderate-to-severe infections: 500 mg to 1 g every 6-8 hours

Mild infection with gram-positive cocci: 250-500 mg every 8 hours

Perioperative prophylaxis: 1-2 g within 60 minutes prior to surgery (may repeat in 2-5 hours intraoperatively); followed by 500 mg to 1 g every 6-8 hours for 24 hours postoperatively

Cardiothoracic surgery: 1 g within 60 minutes prior to incision, followed by 1 g at sternotomy and 1 g after cardiopulmonary bypass; may continue 1 g every 6 hours for 24-48 hours postoperatively (Eagle, 2004)

Cholecystectomy: 1-2 g every 8 hours, discontinue within 24 hours unless infection outside gallbladder suspected

Total joint replacement: 1 g 1 hour prior to the procedure

Pneumococcal pneumonia: 500 mg every 12 hours

Severe infection: 1-1.5 g every 6 hours

Prophylaxis against infective endocarditis (unlabeled use): 1 g 30-60 minutes before procedure. **Note:** Intramuscular injections should be avoided in patients who are receiving anticoagulant therapy. In these circumstances, orally administered regimens should be given whenever possible. Intravenously administered antibiotics should be used for patients who are unable to tolerate or absorb oral medications.

Note: American Heart Association (AHA) guidelines now recommend prophylaxis only in patients undergoing invasive procedures and in whom underlying cardiac conditions may predispose to a higher risk of adverse outcomes should infection occur. As of April 2007, routine prophylaxis for GI/GU procedures is no longer recommended by the AHA.

UTI (uncomplicated): 1 g every 12 hours

◀ **Renal Impairment**

Cl$_{cr}$ 35-54 mL/minute: Administer full dose in intervals of ≥8 hours

Cl$_{cr}$ 11-34 mL/minute: Administer 1/2 usual dose every 12 hours

Cl$_{cr}$ ≤10 mL/minute: Administer 1/2 usual dose every 18-24 hours

Intermittent hemodialysis (IHD) (administer after hemodialysis on dialysis days): Dialyzable (20% to 50%): 0.5-1 g every 24 hours **or** use 1-2 g every 48-72 hours (Heintz, 2009); **Note:** Dosing dependent on the assumption of 3 times/week, complete IHD sessions. Alternatively, may administer 15-20 mg/kg (maximum dose: 2 g) after dialysis without regularly scheduled dosing (Ahern, 2003; Sowinski, 2001).

Peritoneal dialysis (PD): 0.5 g every 12 hours

Continuous renal replacement therapy (CRRT) (Heintz, 2009; Trotman, 2005): Drug clearance is highly dependent on the method of renal replacement, filter type, and flow rate. Appropriate dosing requires close monitoring of pharmacologic response, signs of adverse reactions due to drug accumulation, as well as drug concentrations in relation to target trough (if appropriate). The following are general recommendations only (based on dialysate flow/ultrafiltration rates of 1-2 L/hour and minimal residual renal function) and should not supersede clinical judgment:

CVVH: Loading dose of 2 g followed by 1-2 g every 12 hours

CVVHD/CVVHDF: Loading dose of 2 g followed by either 1 g every 8 hours **or** 2 g every 12 hours. **Note:** Dosage of 1 g every 8 hours results in similar steady-state concentrations as 2 g every 12 hours and is more cost effective (Heintz, 2009).

Administration

I.M.: Inject deep I.M. into large muscle mass.

I.V.: Inject direct I.V. over 5 minutes. Infuse intermittent infusion over 30-60 minutes.

Some penicillins (eg, carbenicillin, ticarcillin and piperacillin) have been shown to inactivate aminoglycosides *in vitro*. This has been observed to a greater extent with tobramycin and gentamicin, while amikacin has shown greater stability against inactivation. Concurrent use of these agents may pose a risk of reduced antibacterial efficacy *in vivo*, particularly in the setting of profound renal impairment. However, definitive clinical evidence is lacking. If combination penicillin/aminoglycoside therapy is desired in a patient with renal dysfunction, separation of doses (if feasible), and routine monitoring of aminoglycoside levels, CBC, and clinical response should be considered.

Monitoring Parameters Renal function periodically when used in combination with other nephrotoxic drugs, hepatic function tests, CBC; monitor for signs of anaphylaxis during first dose

Test Interactions Positive direct Coombs', false-positive urinary glucose test using cupric sulfate (Benedict's solution, Clinitest®, Fehling's solution), false-positive serum or urine creatinine with Jaffé reaction.

Some penicillin derivatives may accelerate the degradation of aminoglycosides *in vitro*, leading to a potential underestimation of aminoglycoside serum concentration.

Pharmacotherapy Pearls Sodium content of 1 g: 48 mg (2 mEq)

Special Geriatric Considerations Adjust dose for renal function.

Dosage Forms Excipient information presented when available (limited, particularly for generics); consult specific product labeling.

Infusion, premixed iso-osmotic dextrose solution: 1 g (50 mL) [contains sodium 46 mg/g]

Injection, powder for reconstitution: 500 mg [contains sodium 48 mg (2 mEq)/g], 1 g [contains sodium 48 mg (2 mEq)/g], 10 g [contains sodium 48 mg (2 mEq)/g], 20 g [contains sodium 48 mg (2 mEq)/g], 100 g [contains sodium 48 mg (2 mEq)/g], 300 g [contains sodium 48 mg (2 mEq)/g]

Selected References

Simon VC, Malerczyk V, Tenscherf B, et al, "Die Geriatrische Pharmakologie von Cefazolin, Cefradin, und Sulfisomidin," *Arzneim Forsch*, 1976, 26(7):1377-82.

◆ **Cefazolin Sodium** *see* CeFAZolin *on page 290*

Cefdinir (SEF di ner)

Brand Names: U.S. Omnicef®

Brand Names: Canada Omnicef®

Index Terms CFDN

Generic Availability (U.S.) Yes

Pharmacologic Category Antibiotic, Cephalosporin (Third Generation)

Use Treatment of community-acquired pneumonia, acute exacerbations of chronic bronchitis, acute bacterial otitis media, acute maxillary sinusitis, pharyngitis/tonsillitis, and uncomplicated skin and skin structure infections.

Contraindications Hypersensitivity to cefdinir, any component of the formulation, other cephalosporins, or related antibiotics

Warnings/Precautions Administer cautiously to penicillin-sensitive patients, especially IgE-mediated reactions (eg, anaphylaxis, urticaria). Prolonged use may result in fungal or bacterial superinfection, including *C. difficile*-associated diarrhea (CDAD) and pseudomembranous colitis; CDAD has been observed >2 months postantibiotic treatment. Use caution with renal dysfunction (Cl_{cr} <30 mL/minute); dose adjustment may be required.

Adverse Reactions (Reflective of adult population; not specific for elderly)
>10%: Gastrointestinal: Diarrhea (8% to 15%)
1% to 10%:
  Central nervous system: Headache (2%)
  Dermatologic: Rash (≤3%)
  Endocrine & metabolic: Bicarbonate decreased (≤1%), hyperglycemia (≤1%), hyperphosphatemia (≤1%)
  Gastrointestinal: Nausea (≤3%), abdominal pain (≤1%), vomiting (≤1%)
  Genitourinary: Vaginal moniliasis (≤4%), urine leukocytes increased (≤2%), urine pH increased (≤1%), urine specific gravity increased (≤1%), vaginitis (≤1%)
  Hematologic: Lymphocytes increased (≤2%), eosinophils increased (1%), lymphocytes decreased (1%), platelets increased (≤1%), PMN changes (≤1%), WBC decreased/increased (≤1%)
  Hepatic: Alkaline phosphatase increased (≤1%), ALT increased (≤1%)
  Renal: Proteinuria (1% to 2%), microhematuria (≤1%), glycosuria (≤1%)
  Miscellaneous: GGT increased (≤1%), lactate dehydrogenase increased (≤1%)
  Additional reactions reported with other cephalosporins: Agranulocytosis, angioedema, aplastic anemia, asterixis, encephalopathy, hemorrhage, interstitial nephritis, neuromuscular excitability, PT prolonged, seizure, superinfection, and toxic nephropathy

Drug Interactions
  Avoid Concomitant Use
    Avoid concomitant use of Cefdinir with any of the following: BCG
  Increased Effect/Toxicity
    The levels/effects of Cefdinir may be increased by: Probenecid
  Decreased Effect
    Cefdinir may decrease the levels/effects of: BCG; Typhoid Vaccine

    The levels/effects of Cefdinir may be decreased by: Iron Salts

Stability Capsules and unmixed powder should be stored at 25°C (77°F); excursions permitted to 15°C to 30°C (59°F to 86°F). Oral suspension should be mixed with 38 mL water for the 60 mL bottle and 63 mL of water for the 100 mL bottle. After mixing, the suspension can be stored at room temperature of 25°C (77°F) for 10 days.

Mechanism of Action Inhibits bacterial cell wall synthesis by binding to one or more of the penicillin-binding proteins (PBPs) which in turn inhibits the final transpeptidation step of peptidoglycan synthesis in bacterial cell walls, thus inhibiting cell wall biosynthesis. Bacteria eventually lyse due to ongoing activity of cell wall autolytic enzymes (autolysins and murein hydrolases) while cell wall assembly is arrested.

Pharmacodynamics/Kinetics
  Distribution: V_d: Adults: 0.06-0.64 L/kg
  Protein binding: 60% to 70%
  Metabolism: Minimally hepatic
  Bioavailability: Capsule: 16% to 21%; suspension 25%
  Half-life elimination: 100 minutes
  Excretion: Primarily urine

Dosage
  Geriatric & Adult
    Acute exacerbations of chronic bronchitis, pharyngitis/tonsillitis: Oral: 300 mg twice daily for 5-10 days **or** 600 mg once daily for 10 days
    Acute maxillary sinusitis: Oral: 300 mg twice daily **or** 600 mg once daily for 10 days
    Community-acquired pneumonia, uncomplicated skin and skin structure infections: Oral: 300 mg twice daily for 10 days
  Renal Impairment Adults: 300 mg once daily
  Hepatic Impairment No adjustment necessary.

Administration Twice daily doses should be given every 12 hours. May be administered with or without food. Manufacturer recommends administering at least 2 hours before or after antacids or iron supplements. Shake suspension well before use.

Monitoring Parameters Observe for signs and symptoms of anaphylaxis during first dose.

Test Interactions False-positive reaction for urinary ketones may occur with nitroprusside-but not nitroferricyanide-based tests. False-positive urine glucose results may occur when using Clinitest®, Benedict's solution, or Fehling's solution; glucose-oxidase-based reaction systems (eg, Clinistix®, Tes-Tape®) are recommended. May cause positive direct Coombs' test.

Special Geriatric Considerations Cefdinir has not been studied exclusively in the elderly. Patients ≥65 years of age have been included in clinical. No information is available on their response or tolerance.

Dosage Forms Excipient information presented when available (limited, particularly for generics); consult specific product labeling.

Capsule, oral: 300 mg
  Omnicef®: 300 mg
Powder for suspension, oral: 125 mg/5 mL (60 mL, 100 mL); 250 mg/5 mL (60 mL, 100 mL)
  Omnicef®: 125 mg/5 mL (60 mL, 100 mL); 250 mg/5 mL (60 mL, 100 mL) [contains sodium benzoate, sucrose 2.86 g/5 mL; strawberry flavor]

Cefditoren (sef de TOR en)

Medication Safety Issues
International issues:
Spectracef [U.S., Great Britain, Mexico, Portugal, Spain] may be confused with Spectrocef brand name for cefotaxime [Italy]

Brand Names: U.S. Spectracef®
Index Terms Cefditoren Pivoxil
Generic Availability (U.S.) Yes
Pharmacologic Category Antibiotic, Cephalosporin (Third Generation)
Use Treatment of acute bacterial exacerbation of chronic bronchitis or community-acquired pneumonia (due to susceptible organisms including *Haemophilus influenzae*, *Haemophilus parainfluenzae*, *Streptococcus pneumoniae*-penicillin susceptible only, *Moraxella catarrhalis*); pharyngitis or tonsillitis (*Streptococcus pyogenes*); and uncomplicated skin and skin-structure infections (*Staphylococcus aureus* - not MRSA, *Streptococcus pyogenes*)
Contraindications Hypersensitivity to cefditoren, any component of the formulation, other cephalosporins, or milk protein; carnitine deficiency
Warnings/Precautions Use with caution in patients with a history of penicillin allergy, especially IgE-mediated reactions (eg, anaphylaxis, urticaria). Prolonged use may result in fungal or bacterial superinfection, including *C. difficile*-associated diarrhea (CDAD) and pseudomembranous colitis; CDAD has been observed >2 months postantibiotic treatment. Caution in individuals with seizure disorders; high levels, particularly in the presence of renal impairment, may increase risk of seizures. Use caution in patients with renal or hepatic impairment; modify dosage in patients with severe renal impairment. Cefditoren causes renal excretion of carnitine; do not use in patients with carnitine deficiency; not for long-term therapy due to the possible development of carnitine deficiency over time. May prolong prothrombin time; use with caution in patients with a history of bleeding disorder. Cefditoren tablets contain sodium caseinate, which may cause hypersensitivity reactions in patients with milk protein hypersensitivity; this does not affect patients with lactose intolerance.
Adverse Reactions (Reflective of adult population; not specific for elderly)
>10%: Gastrointestinal: Diarrhea (11% to 15%)
1% to 10%:
  Central nervous system: Headache (2% to 3%)
  Endocrine & metabolic: Glucose increased (1% to 2%)
  Gastrointestinal: Nausea (4% to 6%), abdominal pain (2%), dyspepsia (1% to 2%), vomiting (1%)
  Genitourinary: Vaginal moniliasis (3% to 6%)
  Hematologic: Hematocrit decreased (2%)
  Renal: Hematuria (3%), urinary white blood cells increased (2%)
Reactions reported with other cephalosporins: Anaphylaxis, aplastic anemia, cholestasis, hemorrhage, hemolytic anemia, renal dysfunction, reversible hyperactivity, serum sickness-like reaction, toxic nephropathy
Drug Interactions
Avoid Concomitant Use There are no known interactions where it is recommended to avoid concomitant use.
Increased Effect/Toxicity
The levels/effects of Cefditoren may be increased by: Probenecid
Decreased Effect
The levels/effects of Cefditoren may be decreased by: Antacids; H2-Antagonists; Proton Pump Inhibitors
Ethanol/Nutrition/Herb Interactions Food: Moderate- to high-fat meals increase bioavailability and maximum plasma concentration.
Stability Store at controlled room temperature of 15°C to 30°C (59°F to 86°F). Protect from light and moisture.

Mechanism of Action Inhibits bacterial cell wall synthesis by binding to one or more of the penicillin-binding proteins (PBPs) which in turn inhibits the final transpeptidation step of peptidoglycan synthesis in bacterial cell walls, thus inhibiting cell wall biosynthesis. Bacteria eventually lyse due to ongoing activity of cell wall autolytic enzymes (autolysins and murein hydrolases) while cell wall assembly is arrested.

Pharmacodynamics/Kinetics
Distribution: 9.3 ± 1.6 L
Protein binding: 88% (*in vitro*), primarily to albumin
Metabolism: Cefditoren pivoxil is hydrolyzed to cefditoren (active) and pivalate
Bioavailability: ~14% to 16%, increased by moderate- to high-fat meal
Half-life elimination: 1.6 ± 0.4 hours
Time to peak: 1.5-3 hours
Excretion: Urine (as cefditoren and pivaloylcarnitine)

Dosage
Geriatric & Adult
Acute bacterial exacerbation of chronic bronchitis: Oral: 400 mg twice daily for 10 days
Community-acquired pneumonia: Oral: 400 mg twice daily for 14 days
Dental infections (unlabeled use): Oral: 400 mg twice daily for 10 days
Pharyngitis, tonsillitis, uncomplicated skin and skin structure infections: Oral: 200 mg twice daily for 10 days
Renal Impairment
Cl_{cr} 30-49 mL/minute/1.73 m^2: Maximum dose: 200 mg twice daily
Cl_{cr} <30 mL/minute/1.73 m^2: Maximum dose: 200 mg once daily
End-stage renal disease: Appropriate dosing not established
Hepatic Impairment
Mild-to-moderate impairment: Adjustment not required
Severe impairment (Child-Pugh class C): Specific guidelines not available

Administration Should be administered with meals.

Monitoring Parameters Assess patient at beginning and throughout therapy for infection; monitor for signs of anaphylaxis during first dose.

Test Interactions May induce a positive direct Coomb's test. May cause a false-negative ferricyanide test. Glucose oxidase or hexokinase methods recommended for blood/plasma glucose determinations. False-positive urine glucose test when using copper reduction based assays (eg, Clinitest®).

Special Geriatric Considerations No dose adjustment is necessary for patients with normal age-adjusted renal function.

Dosage Forms Excipient information presented when available (limited, particularly for generics); consult specific product labeling.
Tablet, oral: 200 mg, 400 mg
Spectracef®: 200 mg, 400 mg [contains sodium caseinate]

♦ **Cefditoren Pivoxil** *see* Cefditoren *on page 294*

Cefepime (SEF e pim)

Medication Safety Issues
Sound-alike/look-alike issues:
Cefepime may be confused with cefixime, cefTAZidime
Brand Names: U.S. Maxipime®
Brand Names: Canada Maxipime®
Index Terms Cefepime Hydrochloride
Generic Availability (U.S.) Yes
Pharmacologic Category Antibiotic, Cephalosporin (Fourth Generation)
Use Treatment of uncomplicated and complicated urinary tract infections, including pyelonephritis caused by typical urinary tract pathogens; monotherapy for febrile neutropenia; uncomplicated skin and skin structure infections caused by *Streptococcus pyogenes*; moderate-to-severe pneumonia caused by pneumococcus, *Pseudomonas aeruginosa*, and other gram-negative organisms; complicated intra-abdominal infections (in combination with metronidazole). Also active against methicillin-susceptible staphylococci, *Enterobacter* sp, and many other gram-negative bacilli.
Unlabeled/Investigational Use Brain abscess (postneurosurgical prevention); malignant otitis externa; septic lateral/cavernous sinus thrombosis
Contraindications Hypersensitivity to cefepime, other cephalosporins, penicillins, other beta-lactam antibiotics, or any component of the formulation
Warnings/Precautions Modify dosage in patients with renal impairment (Cl_{cr} ≤60 mL/minute); may increase risk of encephalopathy, myoclonus, and seizures. Use with caution in patients with a history of penicillin or cephalosporin allergy, especially IgE-mediated

reactions (eg, anaphylaxis, urticaria). Prolonged use may result in fungal or bacterial super-infection, including *C. difficile*-associated diarrhea (CDAD) and pseudomembranous colitis; CDAD has been observed >2 months postantibiotic treatment. Use with caution in patients with a history of gastrointestinal disease, especially colitis. May be associated with increased INR, especially in nutritionally-deficient patients, prolonged treatment, hepatic or renal disease. Use with caution in patients with a history of seizure disorder; high levels, particularly in the presence of renal impairment, may increase risk of seizures.

Adverse Reactions (Reflective of adult population; not specific for elderly)
>10%: Hematologic: Positive Coombs' test without hemolysis (16%)
1% to 10%:
  Central nervous system: Fever (1%), headache (1%)
  Dermatologic: Rash (1% to 4%), pruritus (1%)
  Endocrine & metabolic: Hypophosphatemia (3%)
  Gastrointestinal: Diarrhea (≤3%), nausea (≤2%), vomiting (≤1%)
  Hematologic: Eosinophils (2%)
  Hepatic: ALT increased (3%), AST increased (2%), PTT abnormal (2%), PT abnormal (1%)
  Local: Inflammation, phlebitis, and pain (1%)
Reactions reported with other cephalosporins: Aplastic anemia, erythema multiforme, hemolytic anemia, hemorrhage, pancytopenia, PT prolonged, renal dysfunction, Stevens-Johnson syndrome, superinfection, toxic epidermal necrolysis, toxic nephropathy, vaginitis

Drug Interactions
  Avoid Concomitant Use
  Avoid concomitant use of Cefepime with any of the following: BCG
  Increased Effect/Toxicity
  The levels/effects of Cefepime may be increased by: Probenecid
  Decreased Effect
  Cefepime may decrease the levels/effects of: BCG; Typhoid Vaccine

Stability
  Vials: Store at 20°C to 25°C (68°F to 77°F). Protect from light. After reconstitution, stable in normal saline, D_5W, and a variety of other solutions for 24 hours at room temperature and 7 days refrigerated.
  Premixed solution: Store frozen at -20°C (-4°F). Thawed solution is stable for 24 hours at room temperature or 7 days under refrigeration; do not refreeze.

Mechanism of Action Inhibits bacterial cell wall synthesis by binding to one or more of the penicillin-binding proteins (PBPs) which in turn inhibits the final transpeptidation step of peptidoglycan synthesis in bacterial cell walls, thus inhibiting cell wall biosynthesis. Bacteria eventually lyse due to ongoing activity of cell wall autolytic enzymes (autolysis and murein hydrolases) while cell wall assembly is arrested.

Pharmacodynamics/Kinetics Note: A longer half-life (mean 3 hours) and reduced renal and total clearances have been reported in older adults compared to younger subjects
  Absorption: I.M.: Rapid and complete
  Distribution: V_d: Adults: 16-20 L; penetrates into inflammatory fluid at concentrations ~80% of serum levels and into bronchial mucosa at levels ~60% of those reached in the plasma; crosses blood-brain barrier
  Protein binding, plasma: ~20%
  Metabolism: Minimally hepatic
  Half-life elimination: 2 hours
  Time to peak: I.M.: 1-2 hours; I.V.: 0.5 hours
  Excretion: Urine (85% as unchanged drug)

Dosage
  Geriatric & Adult
    Brain abscess, postneurosurgical prevention (unlabeled use): I.V.: 2 g every 8 hours with vancomycin
    Febrile neutropenia, monotherapy: I.V: 2 g every 8 hours for 7 days or until the neutropenia resolves
    Intra-abdominal infections, complicated, severe (in combination with metronidazole): I.V.: 2 g every 12 hours for 7-10 days. **Note:** 2010 IDSA guidelines recommend 2 g every 8-12 hours for 4-7 days (provided source controlled). Not recommended for hospital-acquired intra-abdominal infections (IAI) associated with multidrug-resistant gram negative organisms or in mild-to-moderate community-acquired IAIs due to risk of toxicity and the development of resistant organisms (Solomkin, 2010).
    Otitis externa, malignant (unlabeled use): I.V.: 2 g every 12 hours
    Pneumonia: I.V.:
      Nosocomial (HAP/VAP): 1-2 g every 8-12 hours; **Note:** Duration of therapy may vary considerably (7-21 days); usually longer courses are required if *Pseudomonas*. In absence of *Pseudomonas*, and if appropriate empiric treatment used and patient

responsive, it may be clinically appropriate to reduce duration of therapy to 7-10 days (American Thoracic Society Guidelines, 2005).

Community-acquired (including pseudomonal): 1-2 g every 12 hours for 10 days

Septic lateral/cavernous sinus thrombosis (unlabeled use): I.V.: 2 g every 8-12 hours; with metronidazole for lateral

Skin and skin structure, uncomplicated: I.V.: 2 g every 12 hours for 10 days

Urinary tract infections, complicated and uncomplicated:

Mild-to-moderate: I.M., I.V.: 0.5-1 g every 12 hours for 7-10 days

Severe: I.V.: 2 g every 12 hours for 10 days

Renal Impairment

Cefepime Hydrochloride

Creatinine Clearance (mL/minute)	Recommended Maintenance Schedule			
>60 (normal recommended dosing schedule)	500 mg every 12 hours	1 g every 12 hours	2 g every 12 hours	2 g every 8 hours
30-60	500 mg every 24 hours	1 g every 24 hours	2 g every 24 hours	2 g every 12 hours
11-29	500 mg every 24 hours	500 mg every 24 hours	1 g every 24 hours	2 g every 24 hours
<11	250 mg every 24 hours	250 mg every 24 hours	500 mg every 24 hours	1 g every 24 hours

Intermittent hemodialysis (IHD) (administer after hemodialysis on dialysis days): I.V.: Initial: 1 g (single dose) on day 1. Maintenance: 0.5-1 g every 24 hours **or** 1-2 g every 48-72 hours (Heintz, 2009). **Note:** Dosing dependent on the assumption of 3 times/week, complete IHD sessions.

Peritoneal dialysis (PD): Removed to a lesser extent than hemodialysis; administer normal recommended dose every 48 hours

Continuous renal replacement therapy (CRRT) (Heintz, 2009; Trotman, 2005): Drug clearance is highly dependent on the method of renal replacement, filter type, and flow rate. Appropriate dosing requires close monitoring of pharmacologic response, signs of adverse reactions due to drug accumulation, as well as drug concentrations in relation to target trough (if appropriate). The following are general recommendations only (based on dialysate flow/ultrafiltration rates of 1-2 L/hour and minimal residual renal function) and should not supersede clinical judgment:

CVVH: Loading dose of 2 g followed by 1-2 g every 12 hours

CVVHD/CVVHDF: Loading dose of 2 g followed by either 1 g every 8 hours **or** 2 g every 12 hours. **Note:** Dosage of 1 g every 8 hours results in similar steady-state concentrations as 2 g every 12 hours and is more cost effective (Heintz, 2009).

Note: Consider higher dosage of 4 g/day if treating *Pseudomonas* or life-threatening infections in order to maximize time above MIC (Trotman, 2005). Dosage of 2 g every 8 hours may be needed for gram-negative rods with MIC ≥4 mg/L (Heintz, 2009).

Administration May be administered either I.M. or I.V.

Inject deep I.M. into large muscle mass. Inject direct I.V. over 5 minutes. Infuse intermittent infusion over 30 minutes.

Monitoring Parameters Obtain specimen for culture and susceptibility prior to the first dose. Monitor for signs of anaphylaxis during first dose.

Test Interactions Positive direct Coombs', false-positive urinary glucose test using cupric sulfate (Benedict's solution, Clinitest®, Fehling's solution), false-positive serum or urine creatinine with Jaffé reaction, false-positive urinary proteins and steroids

Special Geriatric Considerations Adjust dose for changes in renal function.

Dosage Forms Excipient information presented when available (limited, particularly for generics); consult specific product labeling.

Infusion, premixed iso-osmotic dextrose solution, as hydrochloride: 1 g (50 mL); 2 g (100 mL)

Injection, powder for reconstitution, as hydrochloride: 1 g, 2 g

Maxipime®: 500 mg, 1 g, 2 g

Selected References

Barbhaiya RH, Knupp CA, and Pittman KA, "Effects of Age and Gender on Pharmacokinetics of Cefepime," *J Antimicrob Chemother*, 1992, 36(6):1181-5.

Mandell LA, Wunderink RG, Anzueto A, et al, "Infectious Diseases Society of America/American Thoracic Society Consensus Guidelines on the Management of Community-Acquired Pneumonia in Adults," *Clin Infect Dis*, 2007, 44 Suppl 2:S27-72.

Yahav D, Paul M, Fraser A, et al, "Efficacy and Safety of Cefepime: A Systematic Review and Meta-Analysis," *Lancet Infect Dis*, 2007, 7(5):338-48.

◆ **Cefepime Hydrochloride** *see* Cefepime *on page 295*

Cefixime (sef IKS eem)

Medication Safety Issues
Sound-alike/look-alike issues:
Cefixime may be confused with cefepime
Suprax® may be confused with Sporanox®, Surbex®
International issues:
Cefiton: Brand name for cefixime [Portugal] may be confused with Ceftim brand name for ceftazidime [Italy, Portugal]; Ceftime brand name for ceftazidime [Thailand]; Ceftin brand name for cefuroxime [U.S., Canada]

Brand Names: U.S. Suprax®

Brand Names: Canada Suprax®

Index Terms Cefixime Trihydrate

Generic Availability (U.S.) No

Pharmacologic Category Antibiotic, Cephalosporin (Third Generation)

Use Treatment of urinary tract infections, otitis media, respiratory infections due to susceptible organisms including *S. pneumoniae* and *S. pyogenes*, *H. influenzae*, and many Enterobacteriaceae; uncomplicated cervical/urethral gonorrhea due to *N. gonorrhoeae*

Contraindications Hypersensitivity to cefixime, any component of the formulation, or other cephalosporins

Warnings/Precautions Prolonged use may result in fungal or bacterial superinfection, including *C. difficile*-associated diarrhea (CDAD) and pseudomembranous colitis; CDAD has been observed >2 months postantibiotic treatment. Modify dosage in patients with renal impairment. Use with caution in patients with a history of penicillin allergy, especially IgE-mediated reactions (eg, anaphylaxis, urticaria).

Adverse Reactions (Reflective of adult population; not specific for elderly)
>10%: Gastrointestinal: Diarrhea (16%)
2% to 10%: Gastrointestinal: Abdominal pain, nausea, dyspepsia, flatulence, loose stools
Reactions reported with other cephalosporins: Interstitial nephritis, aplastic anemia, hemolytic anemia, hemorrhage, pancytopenia, agranulocytosis, colitis, superinfection

Drug Interactions
Avoid Concomitant Use
Avoid concomitant use of Cefixime with any of the following: BCG
Increased Effect/Toxicity
The levels/effects of Cefixime may be increased by: Probenecid
Decreased Effect
Cefixime may decrease the levels/effects of: BCG; Typhoid Vaccine

Ethanol/Nutrition/Herb Interactions Food: Delays cefixime absorption.

Stability After reconstitution, suspension may be stored for 14 days at room temperature or under refrigeration.

Mechanism of Action Inhibits bacterial cell wall synthesis by binding to one or more of the penicillin-binding proteins (PBPs); which in turn inhibits the final transpeptidation step of peptidoglycan synthesis in bacterial cell walls, thus inhibiting cell wall biosynthesis. Bacteria eventually lyse due to ongoing activity of cell wall autolytic enzymes (autolysins and murein hydrolases) while cell wall assembly is arrested.

Pharmacodynamics/Kinetics
Absorption: 40% to 50%
Distribution: Widely throughout the body and reaches therapeutic concentration in most tissues and body fluids, including synovial, pericardial, pleural, peritoneal; bile, sputum, and urine; bone, myocardium, gallbladder, and skin and soft tissue
Protein binding: 65%
Half-life elimination: Normal renal function: 3-4 hours; Renal failure: Up to 11.5 hours
Time to peak, serum: 2-6 hours; delayed with food
Excretion: Urine (50% of absorbed dose as active drug); feces (10%)

Dosage
Geriatric & Adult
Susceptible infections: Oral: 400 mg/day divided every 12-24 hours
***S. pyogenes* infections:** Treat for 10 days
Typhoid fever (unlabeled use): Oral: 20-30 mg/kg/day in 2 divided doses for 7-14 days after I.V. therapy
Uncomplicated cervical/urethral gonorrhea due to *N. gonorrhoeae*: Oral: 400 mg as a single dose
Renal Impairment
Cl_{cr} 21-60 mL/minute: Administer 75% of the standard dose.
Cl_{cr} <20 mL/minute: Administer 50% of the standard dose.
10% removed by hemodialysis

Administration May be administered with or without food; administer with food to decrease GI distress. Shake oral suspension well before use.

Monitoring Parameters With prolonged therapy, monitor renal and hepatic function periodically. Observe for signs and symptoms of anaphylaxis during first dose.

Test Interactions Positive direct Coombs', false-positive urinary glucose test using cupric sulfate (Benedict's solution, Clinitest®, Fehling's solution), false-positive serum or urine creatinine with Jaffé reaction; false-positive urine ketones using tests with nitroprusside

Pharmacotherapy Pearls Otitis media should be treated with the suspension since it results in higher peak blood levels than the tablet

Special Geriatric Considerations Adjust dose for renal impairment.

Dosage Forms Excipient information presented when available (limited, particularly for generics); consult specific product labeling.
  Powder for suspension, oral, as trihydrate:
    Suprax®: 100 mg/5 mL (50 mL, 100 mL); 200 mg/5 mL (50 mL, 75 mL) [contains sodium benzoate; strawberry flavor]
  Tablet, oral, as trihydrate:
    Suprax®: 400 mg [scored]

Selected References
Faulkner RD, Bohaycheck W, Lanc RA, et al, "Pharmacokinetics of Cefixime in Young and Elderly," *J Antimicrob Chemother*, 1988, 21(6):787-94.

◆ **Cefixime Trihydrate** *see* Cefixime *on page 298*
◆ **Cefotan** *see* CefoTEtan *on page 301*

Cefotaxime (sef oh TAKS eem)

Related Information
  Community-Acquired Pneumonia in Adults *on page 2059*

Medication Safety Issues
  Sound-alike/look-alike issues:
    Cefotaxime may be confused with cefOXitin, cefuroxime
  International issues:
    Spectrocef [Italy] may be confused with Spectracef brand name for cefditoren [U.S., Great Britain, Mexico, Portugal, Spain]

Brand Names: U.S. Claforan®

Brand Names: Canada Claforan®

Index Terms Cefotaxime Sodium

Generic Availability (U.S.) Yes: Powder

Pharmacologic Category Antibiotic, Cephalosporin (Third Generation)

Use Treatment of susceptible infection in respiratory tract, skin and skin structure, bone and joint, urinary tract, gynecologic as well as septicemia, and documented or suspected meningitis. Active against most gram-negative bacilli (not *Pseudomonas*) and gram-positive cocci (not enterococcus). Active against many penicillin-resistant pneumococci.

Contraindications Hypersensitivity to cefotaxime, any component of the formulation, or other cephalosporins

Warnings/Precautions Modify dosage in patients with severe renal impairment. Prolonged use may result in superinfection. A potentially life-threatening arrhythmia has been reported in patients who received a rapid bolus injection via central line. Granulocytopenia and more rarely agranulocytosis may develop during prolonged treatment (>10 days). Minimize tissue inflammation by changing infusion sites when needed. Use with caution in patients with a history of penicillin allergy, especially IgE-mediated reactions (eg, anaphylaxis, urticaria). Prolonged use may result in fungal or bacterial superinfection, including *C. difficile*-associated diarrhea (CDAD) and pseudomembranous colitis; CDAD has been observed >2 months postantibiotic treatment.

Adverse Reactions (Reflective of adult population; not specific for elderly)
  1% to 10%:
    Dermatologic: Rash, pruritus
    Gastrointestinal: Diarrhea, nausea, vomiting, colitis
    Local: Pain at injection site
  Reactions reported with other cephalosporins: Agranulocytosis, aplastic anemia, cholestasis, hemolytic anemia, hemorrhage, nephropathy, pancytopenia, renal dysfunction, seizure, superinfection.

Drug Interactions
  Avoid Concomitant Use
    Avoid concomitant use of Cefotaxime with any of the following: BCG
  Increased Effect/Toxicity
    The levels/effects of Cefotaxime may be increased by: Probenecid

CEFOTAXIME

◀ **Decreased Effect**
Cefotaxime may decrease the levels/effects of: BCG; Typhoid Vaccine

Stability Reconstituted solution is stable for 12-24 hours at room temperature and 7-10 days when refrigerated and for 13 weeks when frozen. For I.V. infusion in NS or D$_5$W, solution is stable for 24 hours at room temperature, 5 days when refrigerated, or 13 weeks when frozen in Viaflex® plastic containers. Thawed solutions previously of frozen premixed bags are stable for 24 hours at room temperature or 10 days when refrigerated.

Mechanism of Action Inhibits bacterial cell wall synthesis by binding to one or more of the penicillin-binding proteins (PBPs) which in turn inhibits the final transpeptidation step of peptidoglycan synthesis in bacterial cell walls, thus inhibiting cell wall biosynthesis. Bacteria eventually lyse due to ongoing activity of cell wall autolytic enzymes (autolysins and murein hydrolases) while cell wall assembly is arrested.

Pharmacodynamics/Kinetics

Distribution: Widely to body tissues and fluids including aqueous humor, ascitic and prostatic fluids, bone; penetrates CSF best when meninges are inflamed

Metabolism: Partially hepatic to active metabolite, desacetylcefotaxime

Half-life elimination: 1-1.5 hours; prolonged with renal and/or hepatic impairment
Desacetylcefotaxime: 1.5-1.9 hours; prolonged with renal impairment

Time to peak, serum: I.M.: Within 30 minutes

Excretion: Urine (as unchanged drug and metabolites)

In patients 60-80 years of age, the serum half-life was prolonged, the clearance decreased, and AUC increased for cefotaxime and less so for its desacetyl metabolite. A significantly greater increase in half-life and decrease in clearance in patients >80 years of age has been reported.

Dosage

Geriatric & Adult

Arthritis (septic): I.V.: 1 g every 8 hours

Brain abscess and meningitis: I.V.: 2 g every 4-6 hours

C-section: 1 g as soon as the umbilical cord is clamped, then 1 g I.M., I.V. at 6- and 12-hours intervals

Epiglottitis: I.V.: 2 g every 4-8 hours

Gonorrhea: I.M.: 1 g as a single dose; disseminated 1 g every 8 hours

Intra-abdominal infection, complicated, community-acquired, mild-to-moderate (in combination with metronidazole): I.V.: 1-2 g every 6 -8 hours for 4-7 days (provided source controlled)

Life-threatening infections: I.V.: 2 g every 4 hours

Liver abscess: I.V.: 1-2 g every 6 hours

Lyme disease:
Cardiac manifestations: I.V.: 2 g every 4 hours
CNS manifestations: I.V.: 2 g every 8 hours for 14-28 days

Moderate/severe infections: I.M., I.V.: 1-2 g every 8 hours

Orbital cellulitis: I.V.: 2 g every 4 hours

Peritonitis (spontaneous): I.V.: 2 g every 8 hours, unless life-threatening then 2 g every 4 hours

Septicemia: I.V.: 2 g every 6-8 hours

Skin and soft tissue:
Mixed, necrotizing: I.V.: 2 g every 6 hours, with metronidazole or clindamycin
Bite wounds (animal): I.V.: 2 g every 6 hours

Surgical prophylaxis: I.M., I.V.: 1 g 30-90 minutes before surgery

Uncomplicated infections: I.M., I.V.: 1 g every 12 hours

Renal Impairment

Cl$_{cr}$ 10-50 mL/minute: Administer every 8-12 hours.

Cl$_{cr}$ <10 mL/minute: Administer every 24 hours.

Intermittent hemodialysis (IHD) (administer after hemodialysis on dialysis days): Dialyzable (20% to 50%): 1-2 g every 24 hours (Heintz, 2009). **Note:** Dosing dependent on the assumption of 3 times/week, complete IHD sessions.

Peritoneal dialysis (PD): 0.5-1 g every 24 hours

Continuous renal replacement therapy (CRRT) (Heintz, 2009; Trotman, 2005): Drug clearance is highly dependent on the method of renal replacement, filter type, and flow rate. Appropriate dosing requires close monitoring of pharmacologic response, signs of adverse reactions due to drug accumulation, as well as drug concentrations in relation to target trough (if appropriate). The following are general recommendations only (based on dialysate flow/ultrafiltration rates of 1-2 L/hour and minimal residual renal function) and should not supersede clinical judgment:

CVVH: 1-2 g every 8-12 hours
CVVHD: 1-2 g every 8 hours
CVVHDF: 1-2 g every 6-8 hours

Hepatic Impairment Dosage reduction generally not necessary unless concurrent severe renal impairment. Consider dose reduction to 0.5 g every 12 hours in patients with Cl_{cr} <5 mL/minute (Wise, 1985).

Administration Cefotaxime can be administered IVP over 3-5 minutes, or I.V. retrograde or I.V. intermittent infusion over 15-30 minutes; final concentration for I.V. administration should not exceed 100 mg/mL; I.M. dosing should be in a large muscle mass (ie, gluteus maximus)

Monitoring Parameters Observe for signs and symptoms of anaphylaxis during first dose; CBC with differential (especially with long courses)

Test Interactions Positive direct Coombs', false-positive urinary glucose test using cupric sulfate (Benedict's solution, Clinitest®, Fehling's solution), false-positive serum or urine creatinine with Jaffé reaction

Special Geriatric Considerations Adjust dose for renal impairment.

Dosage Forms Excipient information presented when available (limited, particularly for generics); consult specific product labeling.

Infusion, premixed iso-osmotic solution:
Claforan®: 1 g (50 mL); 2 g (50 mL) [contains sodium ~50.5 mg (2.2 mEq) per cefotaxime 1 g]

Injection, powder for reconstitution: 500 mg, 1 g, 2 g, 10 g, 20 g
Claforan®: 500 mg, 1 g, 2 g, 10 g [contains sodium ~50.5 mg (2.2 mEq) per cefotaxime 1 g]

Selected References

Deeter RG, Weinstein MP, Swanson KA, et al, "Crossover Assessment of Serum Bactericidal Activity and Pharmacokinetics of Five Broad-Spectrum Cephalosporins in the Elderly," *Antimicrob Agents Chemother*, 1990, 34(6):1007-13.

Ludwig E, Székely É, Csiba A, et al, "Pharmacokinetics of Cefotaxime and Desacetylcefotaxime in Elderly Patients," *Drugs*, 1988, 35(Suppl 2):51-6.

Mandell LA, Wunderink RG, Anzueto A, et al, "Infectious Diseases Society of America/American Thoracic Society Consensus Guidelines on the Management of Community-Acquired Pneumonia in Adults," *Clin Infect Dis*, 2007, 44 Suppl 2:S27-72.

◆ **Cefotaxime Sodium** *see* Cefotaxime *on page 299*

CefoTEtan (SEF oh tee tan)

Medication Safety Issues

Sound-alike/look-alike issues:

CefoTEtan may be confused with ceFAZolin, cefOXitin, cefTAZidime, Ceftin®, cefTRIAXone

CefoTEtan may be confused with Ceftin®

International issues:

Cefotan may be confused with Lexotan® which is a brand name for bromazepam in multiple international markets

Cefotan may be confused with Cefiton® which is a brand name for cefixime in Portugal

Index Terms Cefotan; Cefotetan Disodium

Generic Availability (U.S.) Yes

Pharmacologic Category Antibiotic, Cephalosporin (Second Generation)

Use Surgical prophylaxis; intra-abdominal infections and other mixed infections; respiratory tract, skin and skin structure, bone and joint, urinary tract and gynecologic as well as septicemia; active against gram-negative enteric bacilli including *E. coli*, *Klebsiella*, and *Proteus*; less active against staphylococci and streptococci than first generation cephalosporins, but active against anaerobes including *Bacteroides fragilis*

Contraindications Hypersensitivity to cefotetan, any component of the formulation, or other cephalosporins; previous cephalosporin-associated hemolytic anemia

Warnings/Precautions Modify dosage in patients with severe renal impairment. Although cefotetan contains the methyltetrazolethiol side chain, bleeding has not been a significant problem. Use with caution in patients with a history of penicillin allergy, especially IgE-mediated reactions (eg, anaphylaxis, urticaria). Cefotetan has been associated with a higher risk of hemolytic anemia relative to other cephalosporins (approximately threefold); monitor carefully during use and consider cephalosporin-associated immune anemia in patients who have received cefotetan within 2-3 weeks (either as treatment or prophylaxis). Prolonged use may result in fungal or bacterial superinfection, including *C. difficile*-associated diarrhea (CDAD) and pseudomembranous colitis; CDAD has been observed >2 months postantibiotic treatment. May be associated with increased INR, especially in nutritionally-deficient patients, prolonged treatment, hepatic or renal disease.

Adverse Reactions (Reflective of adult population; not specific for elderly)

1% to 10%:
Gastrointestinal: Diarrhea (1%)
Hepatic: Transaminases increased (1%)
Miscellaneous: Hypersensitivity reactions (1%)

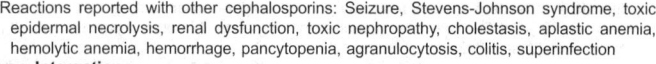

Reactions reported with other cephalosporins: Seizure, Stevens-Johnson syndrome, toxic epidermal necrolysis, renal dysfunction, toxic nephropathy, cholestasis, aplastic anemia, hemolytic anemia, hemorrhage, pancytopenia, agranulocytosis, colitis, superinfection

Drug Interactions

Avoid Concomitant Use

Avoid concomitant use of CefoTEtan with any of the following: BCG

Increased Effect/Toxicity

CefoTEtan may increase the levels/effects of: Alcohol (Ethyl); Vitamin K Antagonists

The levels/effects of CefoTEtan may be increased by: Probenecid

Decreased Effect

CefoTEtan may decrease the levels/effects of: BCG; Typhoid Vaccine

Ethanol/Nutrition/Herb Interactions Ethanol: Avoid ethanol (may cause a disulfiram-like reaction).

Stability Reconstituted solution is stable for 24 hours at room temperature and 96 hours when refrigerated. For I.V. infusion in NS or D_5W solution and after freezing, thawed solution is stable for 24 hours at room temperature or 96 hours when refrigerated. Frozen solution is stable for 12 weeks.

Mechanism of Action Inhibits bacterial cell wall synthesis by binding to one or more of the penicillin-binding proteins (PBPs) which in turn inhibits the final transpeptidation step of peptidoglycan synthesis in bacterial cell walls, thus inhibiting cell wall biosynthesis. Bacteria eventually lyse due to ongoing activity of cell wall autolytic enzymes (autolysins and murein hydrolases) while cell wall assembly is arrested.

Pharmacodynamics/Kinetics

Distribution: Widely to body tissues and fluids including bile, sputum, prostatic, peritoneal; low concentrations enter CSF

Protein binding: 76% to 90%

Half-life elimination: 3-5 hours

Time to peak, serum: I.M.: 1.5-3 hours

Excretion: Primarily urine (as unchanged drug); feces (20%)

Dosage

Geriatric & Adult

Susceptible infections: I.M., I.V.: 1-6 g/day in divided doses every 12 hours; usual dose: 1-2 g every 12 hours for 5-10 days; 1-2 g may be given every 24 hours for urinary tract infection; **Note:** Due to high rates of *B. fragilis* group resistance, not recommended for the treatment of community-acquired intra-abdominal infections (Solomkin, 2010)

Orbital cellulitis, odontogenic infections: I.V.: 2 g every 12 hours

Pelvic inflammatory disease: I.V.: 2 g every 12 hours; used in combination with doxycycline

Preoperative prophylaxis: I.M., I.V.: 1-2 g 30-60 minutes prior to surgery; when used for cesarean section, dose should be given as soon as umbilical cord is clamped

Urinary tract infection: I.M., I.V.: 1-2 g may be given every 24 hours

Renal Impairment I.M., I.V.:

Cl_{cr} 10-30 mL/minute: Administer every 24 hours

Cl_{cr} <10 mL/minute: Administer every 48 hours

Hemodialysis: Dialyzable (5% to 20%); administer 1/4 the usual dose every 24 hours on days between dialysis; administer 1/2 the usual dose on the day of dialysis.

Continuous arteriovenous or venovenous hemodiafiltration effects: Administer 750 mg every 12 hours

Administration I.M. doses should be given in a large muscle mass (ie, gluteus maximus)

Monitoring Parameters Observe for signs and symptoms of anaphylaxis during first dose; monitor for signs and symptoms of hemolytic anemia, including hematologic parameters where appropriate.

Test Interactions Positive direct Coombs', false-positive urinary glucose test using cupric sulfate (Benedict's solution, Clinitest®, Fehling's solution), false-positive serum or urine creatinine with Jaffé reaction

Pharmacotherapy Pearls Sodium content of 1 g: 3.5 mEq

Special Geriatric Considerations Cefotetan has not been studied in the elderly. Adjust dose for renal function in the elderly.

Dosage Forms Excipient information presented when available (limited, particularly for generics); consult specific product labeling.

Injection, powder for reconstitution: 1 g [contains sodium 80 mg (3.5 mEq)/g], 2 g [contains sodium 80 mg (3.5 mEq)/g], 10 g [contains sodium 80 mg (3.5 mEq)/g]

◆ **Cefotetan Disodium** *see* CefoTEtan *on page 301*

CefOXitin (se FOKS i tin)

Medication Safety Issues
Sound-alike/look-alike issues:
CefOXitin may be confused with ceFAZolin, cefotaxime, cefoTEtan, cefTAZidime, cefTRIAX-one, Cytoxan

Mefoxin® may be confused with Lanoxin®

Brand Names: U.S. Mefoxin®

Brand Names: Canada Apo-Cefoxitin®

Index Terms Cefoxitin Sodium

Generic Availability (U.S.) Yes: Excludes infusion

Pharmacologic Category Antibiotic, Cephalosporin (Second Generation)

Use Less active against staphylococci and streptococci than first generation cephalosporins, but active against anaerobes including *Bacteroides fragilis*; active against gram-negative enteric bacilli including *E. coli*, *Klebsiella*, and *Proteus*; used predominantly for respiratory tract, skin, bone and joint, urinary tract and gynecologic as well as septicemia; surgical prophylaxis; intra-abdominal infections and other mixed infections; indicated for bacterial *Eikenella corrodens* infections

Contraindications Hypersensitivity to cefoxitin, any component of the formulation, or other cephalosporins

Warnings/Precautions Modify dosage in patients with severe renal impairment. Prolonged use may result in superinfection. Use with caution in patients with a history of penicillin allergy, especially IgE-mediated reactions (eg, anaphylaxis, urticaria). Prolonged use may result in fungal or bacterial superinfection, including *C. difficile*-associated diarrhea (CDAD) and pseudomembranous colitis; CDAD has been observed >2 months postantibiotic treatment.

Adverse Reactions (Reflective of adult population; not specific for elderly)

1% to 10%: Gastrointestinal: Diarrhea

Reactions reported with other cephalosporins: Agranulocytosis, aplastic anemia, cholestasis, colitis, erythema multiforme, hemolytic anemia, hemorrhage, pancytopenia, renal dysfunction, serum-sickness reactions, seizure, Stevens-Johnson syndrome, superinfection, toxic nephropathy, vaginitis

Drug Interactions
Avoid Concomitant Use
Avoid concomitant use of CefOXitin with any of the following: BCG

Increased Effect/Toxicity
CefOXitin may increase the levels/effects of: Vitamin K Antagonists

The levels/effects of CefOXitin may be increased by: Probenecid

Decreased Effect
CefOXitin may decrease the levels/effects of: BCG; Typhoid Vaccine

Stability Reconstitute vials with SWFI, bacteriostatic water for injection, NS, or D_5W. For I.V. infusion, solutions may be further diluted in NS, $D_5^{1/4}NS$, $D_5^{1/2}NS$, D_5NS, D_5W, $D_{10}W$, LR, D_5LR, mannitol 10%, or sodium bicarbonate 5%. Reconstituted solution is stable for 6 hours at room temperature or 7 days when refrigerated; I.V. infusion in NS or D_5W solution is stable for 18 hours at room temperature or 48 hours when refrigerated. Premixed frozen solution, when thawed, is stable for 24 hours at room temperature or 21 days when refrigerated.

Mechanism of Action Inhibits bacterial cell wall synthesis by binding to one or more of the penicillin-binding proteins (PBPs) which in turn inhibits the final transpeptidation step of peptidoglycan synthesis in bacterial cell walls, thus inhibiting cell wall biosynthesis. Bacteria eventually lyse due to ongoing activity of cell wall autolytic enzymes (autolysins and murein hydrolases) while cell wall assembly is arrested.

Pharmacodynamics/Kinetics
Distribution: Widely to body tissues and fluids including pleural, synovial, ascitic, bile; poorly penetrates into CSF even with inflammation of the meninges

Protein binding: 65% to 79%

Half-life elimination: 45-60 minutes; significantly prolonged with renal impairment

Time to peak, serum: I.M.: 20-30 minutes

Excretion: Urine (85% as unchanged drug)

Compared to younger patients (<55 years), older patients (66-94 years) have been reported to have a reduced total body clearance, prolonged half-life, increased volume of distribution, and reduced protein binding.

Dosage
Geriatric & Adult
Susceptible infections: I.M., I.V.: 1-2 g every 6-8 hours (I.M. injection is painful); up to 12 g/day

Amnionitis and endomyometritis: I.M., I.V.: 2 g every 6-8 hours

◄

Aspiration pneumonia, empyema, orbital cellulitis, parapharyngeal space, and human bites: I.M., I.V.: 2 g every 8 hours

Intra-abdominal infection, complicated, community acquired, mild-to-moderate: I.V.: 2 g every 6 hours for 4-7 days (provided source controlled)

Liver abscess: I.V.: 1 g every 4 hours

Mycobacterium species, not MTB or MAI: I.V.: 12 g/day with amikacin

Pelvic inflammatory disease:

Inpatients: I.V.: 2 g every 6 hours **plus** doxycycline 100 mg I.V. or 100 mg orally every 12 hours until improved, followed by doxycycline 100 mg orally twice daily to complete 14 days

Outpatients: I.M.: 2 g **plus** probenecid 1 g orally as a single dose, followed by doxycycline 100 mg orally twice daily for 14 days

Perioperative prophylaxis: I.M., I.V.: 1-2 g 30-60 minutes prior to surgery (may repeat in 2-5 hours intraoperatively) followed by 1-2 g every 6-8 hours for no more than 24 hours after surgery depending on the procedure

Renal Impairment I.M., I.V.:

Cl_{cr} 30-50 mL/minute: Administer 1-2 g every 8-12 hours

Cl_{cr} 10-29 mL/minute: Administer 1-2 g every 12-24 hours

Cl_{cr} 5-9 mL/minute: Administer 0.5-1 g every 12-24 hours

Cl_{cr} <5 mL/minute: Administer 0.5-1 g every 24-48 hours

Hemodialysis: Moderately dialyzable (20% to 50%); administer a loading dose of 1-2 g after each hemodialysis; maintenance dose as noted above based on Cl_{cr}

Continuous arteriovenous or venovenous hemodiafiltration effects: Dose as for Cl_{cr} 10-50 mL/minute

Administration

I.M.: Inject deep I.M. into large muscle mass.

I.V.: Can be administered IVP over 3-5 minutes at a maximum concentration of 100 mg/mL or I.V. intermittent infusion over 10-60 minutes at a final concentration for I.V. administration not to exceed 40 mg/mL

Monitoring Parameters Monitor renal function periodically when used in combination with other nephrotoxic drugs; observe for signs and symptoms of anaphylaxis during first dose

Test Interactions Positive direct Coombs', false-positive urinary glucose test using cupric sulfate (Benedict's solution, Clinitest®, Fehling's solution), false-positive serum or urine creatinine with Jaffé reaction

Pharmacotherapy Pearls Sodium content of 1 g: 53 mg (2.3 mEq)

Special Geriatric Considerations Adjust dose for renal function in the elderly.

Dosage Forms Excipient information presented when available (limited, particularly for generics); consult specific product labeling.

Infusion, premixed iso-osmotic dextrose solution:

Mefoxin®: 1 g (50 mL); 2 g (50 mL) [contains sodium 53.8 mg (2.3 mEq)/g]

Injection, powder for reconstitution: 1 g, 2 g, 10 g

Selected References

Garcia MJ, Garcia A, Nieto MJ, et al, "Disposition of Cefoxitin in the Elderly," *Int J Clin Pharmacol Ther Toxicol*, 1980, 18(11):503-9.

◆ **Cefoxitin Sodium** *see* CefOXitin *on page 303*

Cefpodoxime (sef pode OKS eem)

Related Information

Community-Acquired Pneumonia in Adults *on page 2059*

Medication Safety Issues

Sound-alike/look-alike issues:

Vantin may be confused with Ventolin®

Index Terms Cefpodoxime Proxetil; Vantin

Generic Availability (U.S.) Yes

Pharmacologic Category Antibiotic, Cephalosporin (Third Generation)

Use Treatment of susceptible acute, community-acquired pneumonia caused by *S. pneumoniae* or nonbeta-lactamase producing *H. influenzae*; acute uncomplicated gonorrhea caused by *N. gonorrhoeae*; uncomplicated skin and skin structure infections caused by *S. aureus* or *S. pyogenes*; acute otitis media caused by *S. pneumoniae, H. influenzae,* or *M. catarrhalis*; pharyngitis or tonsillitis; and uncomplicated urinary tract infections caused by *E. coli, Klebsiella,* and *Proteus*

Contraindications Hypersensitivity to cefpodoxime, any component of the formulation, or other cephalosporins

Warnings/Precautions Modify dosage in patients with severe renal impairment. Prolonged use may result in fungal or bacterial superinfection, including *C. difficile*-associated diarrhea (CDAD) and pseudomembranous colitis; CDAD has been observed >2 months postantibiotic treatment. Use with caution in patients with a history of penicillin allergy, especially IgE-mediated reactions (eg, anaphylaxis, urticaria).

Adverse Reactions (Reflective of adult population; not specific for elderly)
>10%:
  Dermatologic: Diaper rash (12%)
  Gastrointestinal: Diarrhea in infants and toddlers (15%)
1% to 10%:
  Central nervous system: Headache (1%)
  Dermatologic: Rash (1%)
  Gastrointestinal: Diarrhea (7%), nausea (4%), abdominal pain (2%), vomiting (1% to 2%)
  Genitourinary: Vaginal infection (3%)
Reactions reported with other cephalosporins: Seizure, Stevens-Johnson syndrome, toxic epidermal necrolysis, erythema multiforme, urticaria, serum-sickness reactions, renal dysfunction, interstitial nephritis toxic nephropathy, cholestasis, aplastic anemia, hemolytic anemia, hemorrhage, pancytopenia, agranulocytosis, colitis, vaginitis, superinfection

Drug Interactions
  Avoid Concomitant Use
    Avoid concomitant use of Cefpodoxime with any of the following: BCG
  Increased Effect/Toxicity
    The levels/effects of Cefpodoxime may be increased by: Probenecid
  Decreased Effect
    Cefpodoxime may decrease the levels/effects of: BCG; Typhoid Vaccine

    The levels/effects of Cefpodoxime may be decreased by: Antacids; H2-Antagonists

Ethanol/Nutrition/Herb Interactions Food: Food delays absorption; cefpodoxime serum levels may be increased if taken with food.

Stability Shake well before using. After mixing, keep suspension in refrigerator. Discard unused portion after 14 days.

Mechanism of Action Inhibits bacterial cell wall synthesis by binding to one or more of the penicillin-binding proteins (PBPs) which in turn inhibits the final transpeptidation step of peptidoglycan synthesis in bacterial cell walls, thus inhibiting cell wall biosynthesis. Bacteria eventually lyse due to ongoing activity of cell wall autolytic enzymes (autolysins and murein hydrolases) while cell wall assembly is arrested.

Pharmacodynamics/Kinetics
  Absorption: Rapid and well absorbed (50%), acid stable; enhanced in the presence of food or low gastric pH
  Distribution: Good tissue penetration, including lung and tonsils; penetrates into pleural fluid
  Protein binding: 18% to 23%
  Metabolism: De-esterified in GI tract to active metabolite, cefpodoxime
  Half-life elimination: 2.2 hours; prolonged with renal impairment
  Time to peak: Within 1 hour
  Excretion: Urine (80% as unchanged drug) in 24 hours

Dosage
  Geriatric & Adult
    Acute community-acquired pneumonia and bacterial exacerbations of chronic bronchitis: Oral: 200 mg every 12 hours for 14 days and 10 days, respectively
    Acute maxillary sinusitis: Oral: 200 mg every 12 hours for 10 days
    Pharyngitis/tonsillitis: Oral: 100 mg every 12 hours for 5-10 days
    Skin and skin structure: Oral: 400 mg every 12 hours for 7-14 days
    Uncomplicated gonorrhea (male and female) and rectal gonococcal infections (female): Oral: 200 mg as a single dose
    Uncomplicated urinary tract infection: Oral: 100 mg every 12 hours for 7 days
  Renal Impairment
    Cl_{cr} <30 mL/minute: Administer every 24 hours.
    Hemodialysis: Dose 3 times/week following dialysis.
  Hepatic Impairment Dose adjustment is not necessary in patients with cirrhosis.

Administration Administer around-the-clock to promote less variation in peak and trough serum levels.

Monitoring Parameters Observe for signs and symptoms of anaphylaxis during first dose

Test Interactions Positive direct Coombs', false-positive urinary glucose test using cupric sulfate (Benedict's solution, Clinitest®, Fehling's solution), false-positive serum or urine creatinine with Jaffé reaction

Pharmacotherapy Pearls Dose adjustment is not necessary in patients with cirrhosis

CEFPODOXIME

Special Geriatric Considerations Considered one of the drugs of choice for outpatient treatment of community-acquired pneumonia in the elderly. Adjust dosage with renal impairment.

Dosage Forms Excipient information presented when available (limited, particularly for generics); consult specific product labeling.

Granules for suspension, oral: 50 mg/5 mL (50 mL, 100 mL); 100 mg/5 mL (50 mL, 100 mL)

Tablet, oral: 100 mg, 200 mg

Selected References

Backhouse C, Wade A, Williamson P, et al, "Multiple Dose Pharmacokinetics of Cefpodoxime in Young Adult and Elderly Patients," *J Antimicrob Chemother*, 1990, 26(Suppl E):29-34.

Mandell LA, Wunderink RG, Anzueto A, et al, "Infectious Diseases Society of America/American Thoracic Society Consensus Guidelines on the Management of Community-Acquired Pneumonia in Adults," *Clin Infect Dis*, 2007, 44 Suppl 2:S27-72.

◆ **Cefpodoxime Proxetil** see Cefpodoxime on page 304

Cefprozil (sef PROE zil)

Medication Safety Issues

Sound-alike/look-alike issues:

Cefprozil may be confused with ceFAZolin, cefuroxime

Cefzil may be confused with Cefol®, Ceftin®, Kefzol®

Brand Names: Canada Apo-Cefprozil®; Cefzil®; Mint-Cefprozil; RAN™-Cefprozil; Sandoz-Cefprozil

Index Terms Cefzil

Generic Availability (U.S.) Yes

Pharmacologic Category Antibiotic, Cephalosporin (Second Generation)

Use Treatment of otitis media and infections involving the respiratory tract and skin and skin structure; active against methicillin-sensitive staphylococci, many streptococci, and various gram-negative bacilli including *E. coli*, some *Klebsiella*, *P. mirabilis*, *H. influenzae*, and *Moraxella*.

Contraindications Hypersensitivity to cefprozil, any component of the formulation, or other cephalosporins

Warnings/Precautions Modify dosage in patients with severe renal impairment. Use with caution in patients with a history of penicillin allergy, especially IgE-mediated reactions (eg, anaphylaxis, urticaria). Prolonged use may result in fungal or bacterial superinfection, including *C. difficile*-associated diarrhea (CDAD) and pseudomembranous colitis; CDAD has been observed >2 months postantibiotic treatment. Some products may contain phenylalanine.

Adverse Reactions (Reflective of adult population; not specific for elderly)

1% to 10%:

Central nervous system: Dizziness (1%)

Dermatologic: Diaper rash (2%)

Gastrointestinal: Diarrhea (3%), nausea (4%), vomiting (1%), abdominal pain (1%)

Genitourinary: Vaginitis, genital pruritus (2%)

Hepatic: Transaminases increased (2%)

Miscellaneous: Superinfection

Reactions reported with other cephalosporins: Seizure, toxic epidermal necrolysis, renal dysfunction, interstitial nephritis, toxic nephropathy, aplastic anemia, hemolytic anemia, hemorrhage, pancytopenia, agranulocytosis, colitis, vaginitis, superinfection

Drug Interactions

Avoid Concomitant Use

Avoid concomitant use of Cefprozil with any of the following: BCG

Increased Effect/Toxicity

The levels/effects of Cefprozil may be increased by: Probenecid

Decreased Effect

Cefprozil may decrease the levels/effects of: BCG; Typhoid Vaccine

Ethanol/Nutrition/Herb Interactions Food: Food delays cefprozil absorption.

Mechanism of Action Inhibits bacterial cell wall synthesis by binding to one or more of the penicillin-binding proteins (PBPs) which in turn inhibits the final transpeptidation step of peptidoglycan synthesis in bacterial cell walls, thus inhibiting cell wall biosynthesis. Bacteria eventually lyse due to ongoing activity of cell wall autolytic enzymes (autolysins and murein hydrolases) while cell wall assembly is arrested.

Pharmacodynamics/Kinetics A mixture of *cis*- (90%) and *trans*- (10%) isomers; well absorbed from the GI tract (90%); food does not delay or reduce absorption; distribution is to most body tissues including the aqueous humor, bone, soft tissues, and the CSF. Elimination is primarily renal with 60% to 70% of the drug excreted in the urine in 24 hours; hepatic dysfunction does not appear to significantly alter elimination. Significantly greater peak concentrations and area under the curve is found in patients with Cl_{cr} <30 mL/minute; also, the half-life is prolonged 1.7 vs 5.9 hours and renal clearance reduced 198 mL/minute vs 18.8 mL/minute compared to patients with normal renal function.

Dosage

Geriatric & Adult

Pharyngitis/tonsillitis: Oral: 500 mg every 24 hours for 10 days

Secondary bacterial infection of acute bronchitis or acute bacterial exacerbation of chronic bronchitis: Oral: 500 mg every 12 hours for 10 days

Uncomplicated skin and skin structure infections: Oral: 250 mg every 12 hours, or 500 mg every 12-24 hours for 10 days

Renal Impairment

Cl_{cr} <30 mL/minute: Reduce dose by 50%.

Hemodialysis effects: 55% is removed by hemodialysis.

Administration Administer around-the-clock to promote less variation in peak and trough serum levels. Chilling the reconstituted oral suspension improves flavor (do not freeze).

Monitoring Parameters Assess patient at beginning and throughout therapy for infection; monitor for signs of anaphylaxis during first dose

Test Interactions Positive direct Coombs', false-positive urinary glucose test using cupric sulfate (Benedict's solution, Clinitest®, Fehling's solution), false-positive serum or urine creatinine with Jaffé reaction

Special Geriatric Considerations Has not been studied exclusively in the elderly. Adjust dose for estimated renal function.

Dosage Forms Excipient information presented when available (limited, particularly for generics); consult specific product labeling.

Powder for suspension, oral: 125 mg/5 mL (50 mL, 75 mL, 100 mL); 250 mg/5 mL (50 mL, 75 mL, 100 mL)

Tablet, oral: 250 mg, 500 mg

Selected References
Shukla UA, Pittman KA, and Barbhaiya RH, "Pharmacokinetic Interactions of Cefprozil With Food, Propantheline, Metoclopramide, and Probenecid in Healthy Volunteers," *J Clin Pharmacol*, 1992, 32(8):725-31.
Shyu WC, Pittman KA, Wilber RB, et al, "Pharmacokinetics of Cefprozil in Healthy Subjects and Patients With Hepatic Impairment," *J Clin Pharmacol*, 1991, 31(4):372-6.

Ceftaroline Fosamil (sef TAR oh leen FOS a mil)

Brand Names: U.S. Teflaro™

Index Terms PPI-0903; PPI-0903M; T-91825; TAK-599

Generic Availability (U.S.) No

Pharmacologic Category Antibiotic, Cephalosporin (Fifth Generation)

Use Treatment of acute bacterial skin and skin structure infections (ABSSSI) caused by susceptible isolates of *Staphylococcus aureus* (including methicillin-susceptible and –resistant isolates), *Streptococcus pyogenes, Streptococcus agalactiae, Escherichia coli, Klebsiella pneumoniae,* and *Klebsiella oxytoca,* and community-acquired pneumonia (CAP) caused by *Streptococcus pneumoniae* (including cases with concurrent bacteremia), *Staphylococcus aureus* (methicillin-susceptible isolates only), *Haemophilus influenzae, Klebsiella pneumoniae, Klebsiella oxytoca,* and *Escherichia coli*

Contraindications Hypersensitivity to ceftaroline, other cephalosporins, or any component of the formulation

Warnings/Precautions Use with caution in patients with a history of penicillin allergy, especially IgE-mediated reactions (eg, anaphylaxis, angioedema, urticaria). Prolonged use may result in fungal or bacterial superinfection, including *C. difficile*-associated diarrhea (CDAD) and pseudomembranous colitis; CDAD has been observed >2 months postantibiotic treatment. Use with caution in patients with renal impairment (Cl_{cr} ≤50 mL/minute); dosage adjustments recommended.

Adverse Reactions (Reflective of adult population; not specific for elderly)

>10%: Hematologic: Positive Coombs' test without hemolysis (~11%)

2% to 10%:

Central nervous system: Headache (3% to 5%), insomnia (3% to 4%)

Dermatologic: Pruritus (3% to 4%), rash (3%)

Endocrine & metabolic: Hypokalemia (2%)

Gastrointestinal: Diarrhea (5%), nausea (4%), constipation (2%), vomiting (2%)

Hepatic: Transaminases increased (2%)

Local: Phlebitis (2%)

Drug Interactions

Avoid Concomitant Use

Avoid concomitant use of Ceftaroline Fosamil with any of the following: BCG

◀ **Increased Effect/Toxicity**

The levels/effects of Ceftaroline Fosamil may be increased by: Probenecid

Decreased Effect

Ceftaroline Fosamil may decrease the levels/effects of: BCG; Typhoid Vaccine

Stability Store unused vials at 2°C to 8°C (36°F to 46°F); unused vials may be stored at room temperature, up to 25ºC (77ºF), for ≤7 days. Reconstitute 400 mg or 600 mg vial with 20 mL SWFI; mix gently; reconstituted solution should be further diluted for I.V. administration in >250 mL of a compatible solution (eg, D_5W, NS); use within 6 hours at room temperature or within 24 hours if refrigerated; color of infusion solutions ranges from clear and light to dark yellow depending on concentration and storage conditions.

Mechanism of Action Inhibits bacterial cell wall synthesis by binding to penicillin-binding proteins (PBPs) 1 through 3. This action blocks the final transpeptidation step of peptidoglycan synthesis in bacterial cell walls and inhibits cell wall biosynthesis. Bacteria eventually lyse due to ongoing activity of cell wall autolytic enzymes (autolysins and murein hydrolases) while cell wall assembly is arrested. Ceftaroline has a strong affinity for PBP2a, a modified PBP in MRSA, and PBP2x in *S. pneumoniae*, contributing to its spectrum of activity against these bacteria.

Pharmacodynamics/Kinetics

Distribution: V_d: 18.3-21.6 L

Protein binding: ~20%

Metabolism: Ceftaroline fosamil (inactive prodrug) undergoes rapid conversion to bioactive ceftaroline in plasma by phosphatase enzyme; ceftaroline is hydrolyzed to form inactive ceftaroline M-1 metabolite

Half-life elimination: Normal renal function: 2.4 hours; Moderate renal impairment (Cl_{cr} 30-50 mL/minute): 4.5 hours

Time to peak: 1 hour

Excretion: Urine (~88%); feces (~6%)

Dosage

Geriatric & Adult

Usual dosage range: I.V.: 600 mg every 12 hours

Indication-specific dosage: I.V.:

Pneumonia, community-acquired: 600 mg every 12 hours for 5-7 days

Skin and skin structure, complicated: 600 mg every 12 hours for 5-14 days

Renal Impairment

Cl_{cr} 31-50 mL/minute: Administer 400 mg every 12 hours

Cl_{cr} 15-30 mL/minute: Administer 300 mg every 12 hours

Cl_{cr} <15mL/minute and ESRD patients receiving hemodialysis: Administer 200 mg every 12 hours; should be given after hemodialysis, if applicable

Administration Administer by slow I.V. infusion over 60 minutes.

Monitoring Parameters Obtain specimen for culture and susceptibility prior to the first dose. Monitor for signs of anaphylaxis during first dose. Monitor renal function.

Pharmacotherapy Pearls Considered to be ineffective against *Pseudomonas aeruginosa*, *Enterococcus* species (including vancomycin-susceptible and –resistant isolates), extended-spectrum beta-lactamase (ESBL) producing or AmpC overexpressing Enterobacteriaceae.

Special Geriatric Considerations Persons 65 years and older accounted for 30.5% of the participants (n=397) in the clinical trials leading to FDA's approval of ceftaroline. Similar cure rates for ABSSI and CABP were reported for those 65 years and older compared to younger adults. Adverse drug events were reported in 52.4% of older participants compared to 42.8% in patients less than 65 years of age. A 33% increase in ceftaroline's AUC was found in healthy older adults (65 and older) compared to younger adults. The increase in AUC was attributed to age-related decrease in kidney function.

Dosage Forms Excipient information presented when available (limited, particularly for generics); consult specific product labeling.

Injection, powder for reconstitution:

Teflaro™: 600 mg

Selected References

Biek D, Critchley IA, Riccobene TA, et al, "Ceftaroline Fosamil: A Novel Broad-Spectrum Cephalosporin With Expanded Anti-Gram-Positive Activity," *J Antimicrob Chemother*, 2010, 65(Suppl 4):iv9-16.

Corey GR, Wilcox M, Talbot GH, et al, "Integrated Analysis of CANVAS 1 and 2: Phase 3,Multicenter, Randomized, Double-Blind Studies to Evaluate the Safety and Efficacy of Ceftaroline Versus Vancomycin Plus Aztreonam in Complicated Skin and Skin-Structure Infection," *Clin Infect Dis*, 2010, 51(6):641-50.

File TM Jr, Low DE, Eckburg PB, et al, "Integrated Analysis of FOCUS 1and FOCUS 2: Randomized, Double-Blinded, Multicenter Phase 3 Trials of the Efficacy and Safety of Ceftaroline Fosamil Versus Ceftriaxone in Patients With Community-Acquired Pneumonia," *Clin Infect Dis*, 2010, 51(12):1395-405.

Steed ME and Rybak MJ, "Ceftaroline: A New Cephalosporin With Activity Against Resistant Gram-Positive Pathogens," *Pharmacotherapy*, 2010 30(4):375-89.

CefTAZidime (SEF tay zi deem)

Medication Safety Issues
Sound-alike/look-alike issues:
CefTAZidime may be confused with ceFAZolin, cefepime, cefoTEtan, cefOXitin, cefTRIAXone

Ceptaz® may be confused with Septra®

Tazicef® may be confused with Tazidime®

Tazidime® may be confused with Tazicef®

International issues:
Ceftim [Italy, Portugal] and Ceftime [Thailand] brand names for ceftazidime may be confused with Ceftin brand name for cefuroxime [U.S., Canada]; Cefiton brand name for cefixime [Portugal]

Brand Names: U.S. Fortaz®; Tazicef®

Brand Names: Canada Fortaz®

Generic Availability (U.S.) Yes: Injection

Pharmacologic Category Antibiotic, Cephalosporin (Third Generation)

Use Treatment of documented susceptible *Pseudomonas aeruginosa* infection and infections due to other susceptible aerobic gram-negative organisms; empiric therapy of a febrile, granulocytopenic patient

Unlabeled/Investigational Use Bacterial endophthalmitis

Contraindications Hypersensitivity to ceftazidime, any component of the formulation, or other cephalosporins

Warnings/Precautions Modify dosage in patients with severe renal impairment. Use with caution in patients with a history of penicillin allergy, especially IgE-mediated reactions (eg, anaphylaxis, urticaria). Prolonged use may result in fungal or bacterial superinfection, including *C. difficile*-associated diarrhea (CDAD) and pseudomembranous colitis; CDAD has been observed >2 months postantibiotic treatment. May be associated with increased INR, especially in nutritionally-deficient patients, prolonged treatment, hepatic or renal disease. Use with caution in patients with a history of seizure disorder; high levels, particularly in the presence of renal impairment, may increase risk of seizures.

Adverse Reactions (Reflective of adult population; not specific for elderly)
1% to 10%:
Gastrointestinal: Diarrhea (1%)
Local: Pain at injection site (1%)
Miscellaneous: Hypersensitivity reactions (2%)

Reactions reported with other cephalosporins: Seizure, urticaria, serum-sickness reactions, renal dysfunction, interstitial nephritis, toxic nephropathy, BUN increased, creatinine increased, cholestasis, aplastic anemia, hemolytic anemia, pancytopenia, agranulocytosis, colitis, prolonged PT, hemorrhage, superinfection

Drug Interactions
Avoid Concomitant Use
Avoid concomitant use of CefTAZidime with any of the following: BCG

Increased Effect/Toxicity
The levels/effects of CefTAZidime may be increased by: Probenecid

Decreased Effect
CefTAZidime may decrease the levels/effects of: BCG; Typhoid Vaccine

Stability
Fortaz®: Store dry vials at 15°C to 30°C (59°F to 86°F). Protect from light. Reconstituted solution and solution further diluted for I.V. infusion are stable for 12 hours at room temperature, for 3 days when refrigerated, or for 12 weeks when frozen at -20°C (-4°F). After freezing, thawed solution in SWFI for I.M. administration is stable for 3 hours at room temperature or for 3 days when refrigerated; thawed solution in NS in a Viaflex® small volume container for I.V. administration is stable for 12 hours at room temperature or for 3 days when refrigerated; and thawed solution in SWFI in the original container is stable for 8 hours at room temperature or for 3 days when refrigerated.

Premixed frozen solution: Store frozen at -20°C (-4°F). Thawed solution is stable for 8 hours at room temperature or for 3 days under refrigeration; do not refreeze.

Fortaz®, Tazicef®: ADD-Vantage® vials: Diluted in 50 or 100 mL of D$_5$W, NS, or 0.45% sodium chloride in an ADD-Vantage® flexible diluent container only, may be stored for up to 12 hours at room temperature or for 3 days under refrigeration. Freezing solutions in the ADD-Vantage® system is not recommended. Joined vials that have not been activated may be used within 14 days.

◀ Tazicef® vials: Store dry vials at 20°C to 25°C (68°F to 77°F). Protect from light. Reconstituted vials and solution further diluted for I.V. infusion are stable for 24 hours at room temperature, for 7 days when refrigerated, or for 12 weeks when frozen at -20°C (-4°F). When thawed, solution is stable for 8 hours at room temperature and 4 days when refrigerated.

Reconstitution:
I.M.: Using SWFI, bacteriostatic water, lidocaine 0.5%, or lidocaine 1%, reconstitute the 500 mg vials with 1.5 mL or the 1 g vials with 3 mL; final concentration of ~*280 mg/mL*
I.V.: Using SWFI, reconstitute as follows (**Note:** After reconstitution, may dilute further with a compatible solution to administer via I.V. infusion):
Fortaz®:
  ~*100 mg/mL solution:*
    500 mg vial: 5.3 mL SWFI (withdraw 5 mL from the reconstituted vial to obtain a 500 mg dose)
    1 g vial: 10 mL SWFI (withdraw 10 mL from the reconstituted vial to obtain a 1 g dose)
    6 g vial: 56 mL SWFI (withdraw 10 mL from the reconstituted vial to obtain a 1 g dose)
  ~*170 mg/mL solution:* 2 g vial: 10 mL SWFI (withdraw 11.5 mL from the reconstituted vial to obtain a 2 g dose)
  ~*200 mg/mL solution:* 6 g vial: 26 mL SWFI (withdraw 5 mL from the reconstituted vial to obtain a 1 g dose)
Tazicef®:
  ~*95 mg/mL solution:* 1 g vial: 10 mL SWFI (withdraw 10.6 mL from the reconstituted vial to obtain a 1 g dose)
  ~*180 mg/mL solution:* 2 g vial: 10 mL SWFI (withdraw 11.2 mL from the reconstituted vial to obtain a 2 g dose)
Fortaz®, Tazicef®: ADD-Vantage® vials: Dilute in 50 or 100 mL of D_5W, NS, or 0.45% sodium chloride in an ADD-Vantage® flexible diluent container only.

Mechanism of Action Inhibits bacterial cell wall synthesis by binding to one or more of the penicillin-binding proteins (PBPs) which in turn inhibits the final transpeptidation step of peptidoglycan synthesis in bacterial cell walls, thus inhibiting cell wall biosynthesis. Bacteria eventually lyse due to ongoing activity of cell wall autolytic enzymes (autolysins and murein hydrolases) while cell wall assembly is arrested.

Pharmacodynamics/Kinetics
Distribution: Widely throughout the body including bone, bile, skin, CSF (diffuses into CSF with higher concentrations when the meninges are inflamed) endometrium, heart, pleural and lymphatic fluids
Protein binding: 17%, <10% protein binding in older adults; in older adults half-life increased, volume of distribution decreased, and AUC increased
Half-life: 1-2 hours (prolonged with renal impairment)
Time to peak serum concentration: I.M.: Within 60 minutes
Elimination: By glomerular filtration with 80% to 90% of the dose excreted as unchanged drug within 24 hours

Dosage
Geriatric I.M., I.V.: Dosage should be based on renal function with a dosing interval not more frequent then every 12 hours.
Adult
Bacterial arthritis (gram negative bacilli): I.V.: 1-2 g every 8 hours
Bone and joint infections: I.V.: 2 g every 12 hours
Cystic fibrosis, lung infection caused by *Pseudomonas* **spp:** I.V.: 30-50 mg/kg every 8 hours (maximum: 6 g/day)
Endophthalmitis, bacterial (unlabeled use): Intravitreal: 2.25 mg/0.1 mL NS in combination with vancomycin
Intra-abdominal infection, severe (in combination with metronidazole): I.V.: 2 g every 8 hours for 4-7 days (provided source controlled). Not recommended for hospital-acquired intra-abdominal infections (IAI) associated with multidrug-resistant gram negative organisms or in mild-to-moderate community-acquired IAIs due to risk of toxicity and the development of resistant organisms (Solomkin, 2010).
Melioidosis: I.V.: 40 mg/kg every 8 hours for 10 days, followed by oral therapy with doxycycline or TMP/SMX
Otitis externa: I.V.: 2 g every 8 hours
Peritonitis (CAPD):
  Anuric, intermittent: 1000-1500 mg/day
  Anuric, continuous (per liter exchange): Loading dose: 250 mg; maintenance dose: 125 mg
Pneumonia: I.V.:
  Uncomplicated: 500 mg to 1 g every 8 hours
  Complicated or severe: 2 g every 8 hours
Skin and soft tissue infections: I.V., I.M.: 500 mg to 1 g every 8 hours

Severe infections, including meningitis, complicated pneumonia, endophthalmitis, CNS infection, osteomyelitis, gynecological, skin and soft tissue: I.V.: 2 g every 8 hours

Urinary tract infections: I.V., I.M.:
Uncomplicated: 250 mg every 12 hours
Complicated: 500 mg every 8-12 hours

Renal Impairment

Cl_{cr} 30-50 mL/minute: Administer every 12 hours

Cl_{cr} 10-30 mL/minute: Administer every 24 hours

Cl_{cr} <10 mL/minute: Administer every 48-72 hours

Intermittent hemodialysis (IHD) (administer after hemodialysis on dialysis days): Dialyzable (50% to 100%): 0.5-1 g every 24 hours **or** 1-2 g every 48-72 hours (Heintz, 2009). **Note:** Dosing dependent on the assumption of 3 times/week, complete IHD sessions.

Peritoneal dialysis (PD): Loading dose of 1 g, followed by 500 mg every 24 hours

Continuous renal replacement therapy (CRRT) (Heintz, 2009; Trotman, 2005): Drug clearance is highly dependent on the method of renal replacement, filter type, and flow rate. Appropriate dosing requires close monitoring of pharmacologic response, signs of adverse reactions due to drug accumulation, as well as drug concentrations in relation to target trough (if appropriate). The following are general recommendations only (based on dialysate flow/ultrafiltration rates of 1-2 L/hour and minimal residual renal function) and should not supersede clinical judgment:

CVVH: Loading dose of 2 g followed by 1-2 g every 12 hours

CVVHD/CVVHDF: Loading dose of 2 g followed by either 1g every 8 hours **or** 2 g every 12 hours. **Note:** Dosage of 1 g every 8 hours results in similar steady-state concentrations as 2 g every 12 hours and is more cost effective. Dosage of 2 g every 8 hours may be needed for gram-negative rods with MIC ≥4 mg/L (Heintz, 2009).

Note: For patients receiving CVVHDF, some recommend giving a loading dose of 2 g followed by 3 g over 24 hours as a continuous I.V. infusion to maintain concentrations ≥4 times the MIC for susceptible pathogens (Heintz, 2009).

Administration Any carbon dioxide bubbles that may be present in the withdrawn solution should be expelled prior to injection. Ceftazidime can be administered IVP over 3-5 minutes, or I.V. retrograde or I.V. intermittent infusion over 15-30 minutes; final concentration for I.V. administration should not exceed 100 mg/mL; can be reconstituted for I.M. administration with 0.5% or 1% lidocaine if volume tolerated.

Monitoring Parameters Observe for signs and symptoms of anaphylaxis during first dose

Test Interactions Positive direct Coombs', false-positive urinary glucose test using cupric sulfate (Benedict's solution, Clinitest®, Fehling's solution), false-positive serum or urine creatinine with Jaffé reaction

Pharmacotherapy Pearls Sodium content of 1 g: 54 mg (2.3 mEq). For most older adults; weak third generation cephalosporin strongest against anaerobes and gram-positive bacteria; *Pseudomonas* sp.

Special Geriatric Considerations Changes in renal function associated with aging and corresponding alterations in pharmacokinetics result in every 12-hour dosing being an adequate dosing interval. Adjust dose based on renal function.

Dosage Forms Excipient information presented when available (limited, particularly for generics); consult specific product labeling.

Infusion, premixed iso-osmotic solution, as sodium [strength expressed as base]:
Fortaz®: 1 g (50 mL); 2 g (50 mL) [contains sodium ~54 mg (2.3 mEq)/g]

Injection, powder for reconstitution: 500 mg, 1 g, 2 g, 6 g
Fortaz®: 500 mg, 1 g, 2 g, 6 g [contains sodium ~54 mg (2.3 mEq)/g]
Tazicef®: 1 g, 2 g, 6 g [contains sodium ~54 mg (2.3 mEq)/g]

Selected References

Sirgo MA and Norris S, "Ceftazidime in the Elderly: Appropriateness of Twice-Daily Dosing," *DICP Ann Pharmacother*, 1991, 25(3):284-8.

Slaker RA and Danielson B, "Neurotoxicity Associated With Ceftazidime Therapy in Geriatric Patients With Renal Dysfunction," *Pharmacotherapy*, 1991, 11(4):351-2.

Ceftibuten (sef TYE byoo ten)

Medication Safety Issues

Sound-alike/look-alike issues:
Cedax® may be confused with Cidex®

International issues:
Cedax [U.S. and multiple international markets] may be confused with Codex brand name for acetaminophen/codeine [Brazil] and *Saccharomyces boulardii* [Italy]

Brand Names: U.S. Cedax®

Generic Availability (U.S.) No

CEFTIBUTEN

Pharmacologic Category Antibiotic, Cephalosporin (Third Generation)

Use Treatment of acute exacerbations of chronic bronchitis, acute bacterial otitis media, and pharyngitis/tonsillitis

Contraindications Hypersensitivity to ceftibuten, any component of the formulation, or other cephalosporins

Warnings/Precautions Modify dosage in patients with moderate-to-severe renal impairment. Prolonged use may result in fungal or bacterial superinfection, including *C. difficile*-associated diarrhea (CDAD) and pseudomembranous colitis; CDAD has been observed >2 months postantibiotic treatment. Use with caution in patients with a history of colitis and other gastrointestinal diseases. Use with caution in patients with a history of penicillin allergy, especially IgE-mediated reactions (eg, anaphylaxis, urticaria). Oral suspension formulation contains sucrose.

Adverse Reactions (Reflective of adult population; not specific for elderly)

1% to 10%:

Central nervous system: Headache (≤3%), dizziness (≤1%)

Gastrointestinal: Nausea (≤4%), diarrhea (3% to 4%), dyspepsia (≤2%), loose stools (≤2%), abdominal pain (1% to 2%), vomiting (1% to 2%)

Hematologic: Eosinophils increased (3%), hemoglobin decreased (1% to 2%), platelets increased (≤1%)

Hepatic: ALT increased (≤1%), bilirubin increased (≤1%)

Renal: BUN increased (2% to 4%)

Additional reactions reported with other cephalosporins: Allergic reaction, agranulocytosis, angioedema, aplastic anemia, anaphylaxis, asterixis, cholestasis, drug fever, encephalopathy, erythema multiforme, hemolytic anemia, hemorrhage, interstitial nephritis, neuromuscular excitability, neutropenia, pancytopenia, prolonged PT, renal dysfunction, seizure, superinfection, toxic nephropathy

Drug Interactions

Avoid Concomitant Use

Avoid concomitant use of Ceftibuten with any of the following: BCG

Increased Effect/Toxicity

The levels/effects of Ceftibuten may be increased by: Probenecid

Decreased Effect

Ceftibuten may decrease the levels/effects of: BCG; Typhoid Vaccine

Stability Store capsules and powder for suspension at 2°C to 25°C (36°F to 77°F). Reconstituted suspension is stable for 14 days when refrigerated at 2°C to 8°C (36°F to 46°F).

Mechanism of Action Inhibits bacterial cell wall synthesis by binding to one or more of the penicillin-binding proteins (PBPs) which in turn inhibits the final transpeptidation step of peptidoglycan synthesis in bacterial cell walls, thus inhibiting cell wall biosynthesis. Bacteria eventually lyse due to ongoing activity of cell wall autolytic enzymes (autolysins and murein hydrolases) while cell wall assembly is arrested.

Pharmacodynamics/Kinetics

Absorption: Rapid; food decreases peak concentrations, delays T_{max}, and lowers AUC

Distribution: V_d: Adults: 0.21 L/kg

Protein binding: 65%

Half-life elimination: 2 hours; Cl_{cr} 30-49 mL/minute: 7 hours; Cl_{cr} 5-29 mL/minute: 13 hours; Cl_{cr} <5 mL/minute: 22 hours

Time to peak: 2-3 hours

Excretion: Urine (~56%); feces (39%)

Dosage

Geriatric & Adult Susceptible infections: Oral: 400 mg once daily for 10 days

Renal Impairment

Cl_{cr} ≥50 mL/minute: No adjustment needed

Cl_{cr} 30-49 mL/minute: Administer 4.5 mg/kg or 200 mg every 24 hours.

Cl_{cr} 5-29 mL/minute: Administer 2.25 mg/kg or 100 mg every 24 hours.

Hemodialysis: Administer 400 mg or 9 mg/kg (maximum: 400 mg) after each hemodialysis session.

Administration

Capsule: Administer without regard to food.

Suspension: Administer 2 hours before or 1 hour after meals. Shake well before use.

Monitoring Parameters Observe for signs and symptoms of anaphylaxis during first dose; with prolonged therapy, monitor renal, hepatic, and hematologic function periodically

Test Interactions Positive direct Coombs', false-positive urinary glucose test using cupric sulfate (Benedict's solution, Clinitest®, Fehling's solution), false-positive serum or urine creatinine with Jaffé reaction

Special Geriatric Considerations Has not been studied specifically in the elderly. Adjust dose for renal function.

Dosage Forms Excipient information presented when available (limited, particularly for generics); consult specific product labeling.

Capsule, oral:
  Cedax®: 400 mg
Powder for suspension, oral:
  Cedax®: 90 mg/5 mL (60 mL, 90 mL, 120 mL); 180 mg/5 mL (60 mL) [contains sodium benzoate, sucrose ~1 g/5 mL; cherry flavor]

◆ **Ceftin®** see Cefuroxime on page 316

CefTRIAXone (sef trye AKS one)

Related Information
  Antibiotic Treatment of Adults With Infective Endocarditis on page 2053
  Community-Acquired Pneumonia in Adults on page 2059
  Prevention of Infective Endocarditis on page 2064
Medication Safety Issues
  Sound-alike/look-alike issues:
    CefTRIAXone may be confused with CeFAZolin, cefoTEtan, cefOXitin, cefTAZidime, Cetraxal®
    Rocephin® may be confused with Roferon®
Brand Names: U.S. Rocephin®
Brand Names: Canada Ceftriaxone for Injection; Ceftriaxone Sodium for Injection BP; Rocephin®
Index Terms Ceftriaxone Sodium
Generic Availability (U.S.) Yes
Pharmacologic Category Antibiotic, Cephalosporin (Third Generation)
Use Treatment of lower respiratory tract infections, acute bacterial otitis media, skin and skin structure infections, bone and joint infections, intra-abdominal and urinary tract infections, pelvic inflammatory disease (PID), uncomplicated gonorrhea, bacterial septicemia, and meningitis; used in surgical prophylaxis
Unlabeled/Investigational Use Treatment of chancroid, epididymitis, complicated gonococcal infections; sexually-transmitted diseases (STD); periorbital or buccal cellulitis; salmonellosis or shigellosis; atypical community-acquired pneumonia; epiglottitis, Lyme disease; used in chemoprophylaxis for high-risk contacts (close exposure to patients with invasive meningococcal disease); sexual assault; typhoid fever, Whipple's disease
Contraindications Hypersensitivity to ceftriaxone sodium, any component of the formulation, or other cephalosporins.
Warnings/Precautions Use with caution in patients with a history of penicillin allergy, especially IgE-mediated reactions (eg, anaphylaxis, urticaria). Abnormal gallbladder sonograms have been reported, possibly due to cetriaxone-calcium precipitates; discontinue in patients with signs and symptoms of gallbladder disease. Secondary to biliary obstruction, pancreatitis has been reported rarely. Use with caution in patients with a history of GI disease, especially colitis. Severe cases (including some fatalities) of immune-related hemolytic anemia have been reported in patients receiving cephalosporins, including ceftriaxone. Prolonged use may result in fungal or bacterial superinfection, including C. difficile-associated diarrhea (CDAD) and pseudomembranous colitis; CDAD has been observed >2 months postantibiotic treatment.

May be associated with increased INR (rarely), especially in nutritionally-deficient patients, prolonged treatment, hepatic or renal disease. No adjustment is generally necessary in patients with renal impairment; use with caution in patients with concurrent hepatic dysfunction and significant renal disease, dosage should not exceed 2 g/day. Ceftriaxone may complex with calcium causing precipitation. Fatal lung and kidney damage associated with calcium-ceftriaxone precipitates has been observed in premature and term neonates. Do not reconstitute, admix, or coadminister with calcium-containing solutions, even via separate infusion lines/sites or at different times in any neonatal patient. Ceftriaxone should not be diluted or administered simultaneously with any calcium-containing solution via a Y-site in any patient. However, ceftriaxone and calcium-containing solution may be administered sequentially of one another for use in patients **other than neonates** if infusion lines are thoroughly flushed, with a compatible fluid, between infusions
Adverse Reactions (Reflective of adult population; not specific for elderly)
>10%: Local: Induration (I.M. 5% to 17%), warmth (I.M.), tightness (I.M.)
1% to 10%:
  Dermatologic: Rash (2%)
  Gastrointestinal: Diarrhea (3%)
  Hematologic: Eosinophilia (6%), thrombocytosis (5%), leukopenia (2%)

Hepatic: Transaminases increased (3%)
Local: Tenderness at injection site (I.V. 1%), pain
Renal: BUN increased (1%)

Reactions reported with other cephalosporins: Angioedema, allergic reaction, aplastic anemia, asterixis, cholestasis, encephalopathy, hemorrhage, hepatic dysfunction, hyperactivity (reversible), hypertonia, interstitial nephritis, LDH increased, neuromuscular excitability, pancytopenia, paresthesia, renal dysfunction, superinfection, toxic nephropathy

Drug Interactions

Avoid Concomitant Use
Avoid concomitant use of CefTRIAXone with any of the following: BCG

Increased Effect/Toxicity
CefTRIAXone may increase the levels/effects of: Vitamin K Antagonists

The levels/effects of CefTRIAXone may be increased by: Calcium Salts (Intravenous); Probenecid; Ringer's Injection (Lactated)

Decreased Effect
CefTRIAXone may decrease the levels/effects of: BCG; Typhoid Vaccine

Stability

Powder for injection: Prior to reconstitution, store at room temperature ≤25°C (≤77°F). Protect from light.

Premixed solution (manufacturer premixed): Store at -20°C. Once thawed, solutions are stable for 3 days at room temperature of 25°C (77°F) or for 21 days refrigerated at 5°C (41°F). Do not refreeze.

Stability of reconstituted solutions:

10-40 mg/mL: Reconstituted in D_5W, $D_{10}W$, NS, or SWFI: Stable for 2 days at room temperature of 25°C (77°F) or for 10 days when refrigerated at 4°C (39°F). Stable for 26 weeks when frozen at -20°C when reconstituted with D_5W or NS. Once thawed (at room temperature), solutions are stable for 2 days at room temperature of 25°C (77°F) or for 10 days when refrigerated at 4°C (39°F); does not apply to manufacturer's premixed bags. Do not refreeze.

100 mg/mL:
  Reconstituted in D_5W, SWFI, or NS: Stable for 2 days at room temperature of 25°C (77°F) or for 10 days when refrigerated at 4°C (39°F).
  Reconstituted in lidocaine 1% solution or bacteriostatic water: Stable for 24 hours at room temperature of 25°C (77°F) or for 10 days when refrigerated at 4°C (39°F).

250-350 mg/mL: Reconstituted in D_5W, NS, lidocaine 1% solution, bacteriostatic water, or SWFI: Stable for 24 hours at room temperature of 25°C (77°F) or for 3 days when refrigerated at 4°C (39°F).

Reconstitution:

I.M. injection: Vials should be reconstituted with appropriate volume of diluent (including D_5W, NS, SWFI, bacteriostatic water, or 1% lidocaine) to make a final concentration of 250 mg/mL or 350 mg/mL.

Volume to add to create a **250 mg/mL** solution:
  250 mg vial: 0.9 mL
  500 mg vial: 1.8 mL
  1 g vial: 3.6 mL
  2 g vial: 7.2 mL

Volume to add to create a **350 mg/mL** solution:
  500 mg vial: 1.0 mL
  1 g vial: 2.1 mL
  2 g vial: 4.2 mL

I.V. infusion: Infusion is prepared in two stages: Initial reconstitution of powder, followed by dilution to final infusion solution.

Vials: Reconstitute powder with appropriate I.V. diluent (including SWFI, D_5W, $D_{10}W$, NS) to create an initial solution of ~100 mg/mL. Recommended volume to add:
  250 mg vial: 2.4 mL
  500 mg vial: 4.8 mL
  1 g vial: 9.6 mL
  2 g vial: 19.2 mL

  Note: After reconstitution of powder, further dilution into a volume of compatible solution (eg, 50-100 mL of D_5W or NS) is recommended.

Piggyback bottle: Reconstitute powder with appropriate I.V. diluent (D_5W or NS) to create a resulting solution of ~100 mg/mL. Recommended initial volume to add:
  1 g bottle: 10 mL
  2 g bottle: 20 mL

Note: After reconstitution, to prepare the final infusion solution, further dilution to 50 mL or 100 mL volumes with the appropriate I.V. diluent (including D$_5$W or NS) is recommended.

Mechanism of Action Inhibits bacterial cell wall synthesis by binding to one or more of the penicillin-binding proteins (PBPs) which in turn inhibits the final transpeptidation step of peptidoglycan synthesis in bacterial cell walls, thus inhibiting cell wall biosynthesis. Bacteria eventually lyse due to ongoing activity of cell wall autolytic enzymes (autolysins and murein hydrolases) while cell wall assembly is arrested.

Pharmacodynamics/Kinetics

Absorption: I.M.: Well absorbed

Distribution: V$_d$: 6-14 L; widely throughout the body including gallbladder, lungs, bone, bile, CSF (higher concentrations achieved when meninges are inflamed)

Protein binding: 85% to 95%

Half-life elimination: Normal renal and hepatic function: 5-9 hours; Renal impairment (mild-to-severe): 12-16 hours

Time to peak, serum: I.M.: 2-3 hours

Excretion: Urine (33% to 67% as unchanged drug); feces (as inactive drug)

Dosage

Geriatric & Adult

Dosage range: Usual: 1-2 g every 12-24 hours, depending on the type and severity of infection

Arthritis, septic (unlabeled use): I.V.: 1-2 g once daily

Brain abscess (unlabeled use): I.V.: 2 g every 12 hours with metronidazole

Cavernous sinus thrombosis (unlabeled use): I.V.: 2 g once daily with vancomycin or linezolid

Chancroid (unlabeled use): I.M.: 250 mg as single dose (CDC, 2010)

Chemoprophylaxis for high-risk contacts (close exposure to patients with invasive meningococcal disease) (unlabeled use): I.M.: 250 mg in a single dose

Cholecystitis, mild-to-moderate: 1-2 g every 12-24 hours for 4-7 days (provided source controlled)

Gonococcal infections (CDC, 2010):

Conjunctivitis, complicated (unlabeled use): I.M., I.V.: 1 g in a single dose

Disseminated (unlabeled use): I.M., I.V.: 1 g once daily for 24-48 hours may switch to cefixime (after improvement noted) to complete a total of 7 days of therapy

Endocarditis (unlabeled use): I.M., I.V.: 1-2 g every 24 hours for at least 28 days

Epididymitis, acute (unlabeled use): I.M.: 250 mg in a single dose with doxycycline

Meningitis: I.M., I.V.: 1-2 g every 12 hours for 10-14 days

Proctitis (unlabeled use): I.M.: 250 mg in a single dose with doxycycline

Prostatitis (unlabeled use): I.M.: 125-250 mg in a single dose with doxycycline

Uncomplicated cervicitis, pharyngitis, urethritis (unlabeled use): I.M.: 250 mg in a single dose with doxycycline or azithromycin

Infective endocarditis: I.M., I.V.:

Native valve: 2 g once daily for 2-4 weeks; **Note:** If using 2-week regimen, concurrent gentamicin is recommended

Prosthetic valve: I.M., I.V.: 2 g once daily for 6 weeks (with or without 2 weeks of gentamicin [dependent on penicillin MIC]); **Note:** For HACEK organisms, duration of therapy is 4 weeks

Enterococcus faecalis (resistant to penicillin, aminoglycoside, and vancomycin), native or prosthetic valve: 2 g twice daily for ≥8 weeks administered concurrently with ampicillin

Prophylaxis: I.M., I.V.: 1 g 30-60 minutes before procedure. Intramuscular injections should be avoided in patients who are receiving anticoagulant therapy. In these circumstances, orally administered regimens should be given whenever possible. Intravenously administered antibiotics should be used for patients who are unable to tolerate or absorb oral medications.

Note: American Heart Association (AHA) guidelines now recommend prophylaxis only in patients undergoing invasive procedures and in whom underlying cardiac conditions may predispose to a higher risk of adverse outcomes should infection occur. As of April 2007, routine prophylaxis for GI/GU procedures is no longer recommended by the AHA.

Intra-abdominal infection, complicated, community-acquired, mild-to-moderate (in combination with metronidazole): 1-2 g every 12-24 hours for 4-7 days (provided source controlled)

Lyme disease (unlabeled use): I.V.: 2 g once daily for 14-28 days

Mastoiditis (hospitalized; unlabeled use): I.V.: 2 g once daily; >60 years old: 1 g once daily

Meningitis: I.V.: 2 g every 12 hours for 7-14 days (longer courses may be necessary for selected organisms)

Orbital cellulitis (unlabeled use) and endophthalmitis: I.V.: 2 g once daily

Pelvic inflammatory disease: I.M.: 250 mg in a single dose plus doxycycline (with or without metronidazole) (CDC, 2010)

Pneumonia, community-acquired: I.V.: 1 g once daily, usually in combination with a macrolide; consider 2 g/day for patients at risk for more severe infection and/or resistant organisms (ICU status, age >65 years, disseminated infection)

Prophylaxis against sexually-transmitted diseases following sexual assault: I.M.: 250 mg as a single dose (in combination with azithromycin and metronidazole) (CDC, 2010)

Pyelonephritis (acute, uncomplicated): Females: I.V.: 1-2 g once daily (Stamm, 1993). Many physicians administer a single parenteral dose before initiating oral therapy (Warren, 1999).

Septic/toxic shock/necrotizing fasciitis (unlabeled use): I.V.: 2 g once daily; with clindamycin for toxic shock

Surgical prophylaxis: I.V.: 1 g 30 minutes to 2 hours before surgery

Cholecystectomy: 1-2 g every 12-24 hours, discontinue within 24 hours unless infection outside gallbladder suspected

Syphilis (unlabeled use): I.M., I.V.: 1 g once daily for 10-14 days; **Note:** Alternative treatment for early syphilis, optimal dose, and duration have not been defined (CDC, 2010)

Typhoid fever (unlabeled use): I.V.: 2 g once daily for 14 days

Whipple's disease (unlabeled use): Initial: 2 g once daily for 10-14 days, then oral therapy for ~1 year.

Renal Impairment No dosage adjustment is generally necessary in renal impairment; **Note:** Concurrent renal and hepatic dysfunction: Maximum dose: ≤2 g/day

Poorly dialyzed; no supplemental dose or dosage adjustment necessary, including patients on intermittent hemodialysis, peritoneal dialysis, or continuous renal replacement therapy (eg, CVVHD).

Hepatic Impairment No adjustment necessary unless there is concurrent renal dysfunction (see Dosage: Renal Impairment).

Administration Do not admix with aminoglycosides in same bottle/bag. Do not reconstitute, admix, or coadminister with calcium-containing solutions. Infuse intermittent infusion over 30 minutes.

I.M.: Inject deep I.M. into large muscle mass; a concentration of 250 mg/mL or 350 mg/mL is recommended for all vial sizes except the 250 mg size (250 mg/mL is suggested); can be diluted with 1:1 water and 1% lidocaine for I.M. administration.

I.V.: Infuse intermittent infusion over 30 minutes.

Monitoring Parameters Observe for signs and symptoms of anaphylaxis

Test Interactions Positive direct Coombs', false-positive urinary glucose test using cupric sulfate (Benedict's solution, Clinitest®, Fehling's solution), false-positive serum or urine creatinine with Jaffé reaction

Special Geriatric Considerations No adjustment for changes in renal function necessary.

Dosage Forms Excipient information presented when available (limited, particularly for generics); consult specific product labeling.

Infusion, premixed in D_5W: 1 g (50 mL); 2 g (50 mL)

Injection, powder for reconstitution: 250 mg, 500 mg, 1 g, 2 g, 10 g

Rocephin®: 500 mg, 1 g [contains sodium ~83 mg (3.6 mEq) per ceftriaxone 1 g]

Selected References

Deeter RG, Weinstein MP, Swanson KA, et al, "Crossover Assessment of Serum Bactericidal Activity and Pharmacokinetics of Five Broad-Spectrum Cephalosporins in the Elderly," *Antimicrob Agents Chemother*, 1990, 34(6):1007-13.

Hayton WL and Stoeckel K, "Age-Associated Changes in Ceftriaxone Pharmacokinetics," *Clin Pharmacokinet*, 1986, 11(1):76-82.

Mandell LA, Wunderink RG, Anzueto A, et al, "Infectious Diseases Society of America/American Thoracic Society Consensus Guidelines on the Management of Community-Acquired Pneumonia in Adults," *Clin Infect Dis*, 2007, 44 Suppl 2:S27-72.

◆ **Ceftriaxone Sodium** *see* CefTRIAXone *on page 313*

Cefuroxime (se fyoor OKS eem)

Related Information

Community-Acquired Pneumonia in Adults *on page 2059*

Medication Safety Issues

Sound-alike/look-alike issues:

Cefuroxime may be confused with cefotaxime, cefprozil, deferoxamine

Ceftin® may be confused with Cefzil®, Cipro®

Zinacef® may be confused with Zithromax®

International issues:
Ceftin [U.S., Canada] may be confused with Cefiton brand name for cefixime [Portugal]; Ceftim brand name for ceftazidime [Italy, Portugal]; Ceftime brand name for ceftazidime [Thailand]

Brand Names: U.S. Ceftin®; Zinacef®

Brand Names: Canada Apo-Cefuroxime®; Ceftin®; Cefuroxime For Injection; PRO-Cefuroxime; ratio-Cefuroxime

Index Terms Cefuroxime Axetil; Cefuroxime Sodium

Generic Availability (U.S.) Yes

Pharmacologic Category Antibiotic, Cephalosporin (Second Generation)

Use Treatment of infections caused by staphylococci, group B streptococci, *H. influenzae* (type A and B), *E. coli*, *Enterobacter*, *Salmonella*, and *Klebsiella*; treatment of susceptible infections of the upper and lower respiratory tract, otitis media, urinary tract, uncomplicated skin and soft tissue, bone and joint, sepsis, uncomplicated gonorrhea, and early Lyme disease; surgical prophylaxis

Contraindications Hypersensitivity to cefuroxime, any component of the formulation, or other cephalosporins

Warnings/Precautions Modify dosage in patients with severe renal impairment. Use with caution in patients with a history of penicillin allergy, especially IgE-mediated reactions (eg, anaphylaxis, urticaria). Prolonged use may result in fungal or bacterial superinfection, including *C. difficile*-associated diarrhea (CDAD) and pseudomembranous colitis; CDAD has been observed >2 months postantibiotic treatment. May be associated with increased INR, especially in nutritionally-deficient patients, prolonged treatment, hepatic or renal disease. Tablets and oral suspension are not bioequivalent (do not substitute on a mg-per-mg basis). Some products may contain phenylalanine.

Adverse Reactions (Reflective of adult population; not specific for elderly)
>10%: Gastrointestinal: Diarrhea (4% to 11%, duration-dependent)
1% to 10%:
Dermatologic: Diaper rash (3%)
Endocrine & metabolic: Alkaline phosphatase increased (2%), lactate dehydrogenase increased (1%)
Gastrointestinal: Nausea/vomiting (3% to 7%)
Genitourinary: Vaginitis (≤5%)
Hematologic: Eosinophilia (7%), hemoglobin and hematocrit decreased (10%)
Hepatic: Transaminases increased (2% to 4%)
Local: Thrombophlebitis (2%)
Reactions reported with other cephalosporins: Agranulocytosis, aplastic anemia, asterixis, encephalopathy, hemorrhage, neuromuscular excitability, serum-sickness reactions, superinfection, toxic nephropathy

Drug Interactions

Avoid Concomitant Use
Avoid concomitant use of Cefuroxime with any of the following: BCG

Increased Effect/Toxicity
The levels/effects of Cefuroxime may be increased by: Probenecid

Decreased Effect
Cefuroxime may decrease the levels/effects of: BCG; Typhoid Vaccine

The levels/effects of Cefuroxime may be decreased by: Antacids; H2-Antagonists

Ethanol/Nutrition/Herb Interactions Food: Bioavailability is increased with food; cefuroxime serum levels may be increased if taken with food or dairy products.

Stability
Injection: Reconstituted solution is stable for 24 hours at room temperature and 48 hours when refrigerated. I.V. infusion in NS or D_5W solution is stable for 24 hours at room temperature, 7 days when refrigerated, or 26 weeks when frozen. After freezing, thawed solution is stable for 24 hours at room temperature or 21 days when refrigerated.
Oral suspension: Prior to reconstitution, store at 2°C to 30°C (36°F to 86°F). Reconstituted suspension is stable for 10 days at 2°C to 8°C (36°F to 46°F).
Tablet: Store at 15°C to 30°C (59°F to 86°F).

Mechanism of Action Inhibits bacterial cell wall synthesis by binding to one or more of the penicillin-binding proteins (PBPs) which in turn inhibits the final transpeptidation step of peptidoglycan synthesis in bacterial cell walls, thus inhibiting cell wall biosynthesis. Bacteria eventually lyse due to ongoing activity of cell wall autolytic enzymes (autolysins and murein hydrolases) while cell wall assembly is arrested.

◀ **Pharmacodynamics/Kinetics**
Absorption: Oral (cefuroxime axetil): Increases with food
Distribution: Widely to body tissues and fluids; crosses blood-brain barrier; therapeutic concentrations achieved in CSF even when meninges are not inflamed
Protein binding: 33% to 50%
Bioavailability: Tablet: Fasting: 37%; Following food: 52%
Half-life elimination: 1-2 hours; prolonged with renal impairment
Time to peak, serum: I.M.: ~15-60 minutes; I.V.: 2-3 minutes; Oral: 2-3 hours
Excretion: Urine (66% to 100% as unchanged drug)

Dosage

Geriatric & Adult Note: Cefuroxime axetil film-coated tablets and oral suspension are not bioequivalent and are not substitutable on a mg/mg basis. All oral doses listed are for tablet formulation:

Bronchitis, acute (and exacerbations of chronic bronchitis):
Oral: 250-500 mg every 12 hours for 10 days
I.V.: 500-750 mg every 8 hours (complete therapy with oral dosing)

Cellulitis, orbital: I.V.: 1.5 g every 8 hours

Cholecystitis, mild-to-moderate: 1.5 g every 8 hours for 4-7 days (provided source controlled)

Gonorrhea:
Disseminated: I.M., I.V.: 750 mg every 8 hours
Uncomplicated:
Oral: 1 g as a single dose
I.M.: 1.5 g as single dose (administer in two different sites with probenecid)

Intra-abdominal infection, complicated, community-acquired, mild-to-moderate (in combination with metronidazole): 1.5 g every 8 hours for 4-7 days (provided source controlled)

Lyme disease (early): Oral: 500 mg twice daily for 20 days

Pharyngitis/tonsillitis and sinusitis: Oral: 250 mg twice daily for 10 days

Skin/skin structure infection, uncomplicated:
Oral: 250-500 mg every 12 hours for 10 days
I.M., I.V.: 750 mg every 8 hours

Pneumonia, uncomplicated: I.M., I.V.: 750 mg every 8 hours

Severe or complicated infections: I.M., I.V.: 1.5 g every 8 hours (up to 1.5 g every 6 hours in life-threatening infections)

Surgical prophylaxis: I.V.: 1.5 g 30 minutes to 1 hour prior to procedure (if procedure is prolonged can give 750 mg every 8 hours I.M.)
Cholecystectomy: I.V.: 1.5 g every 8 hours, discontinue within 24 hours unless infection outside gallbladder suspected
Open heart: I.V.: 1.5 g every 12 hours to a total of 6 g

Urinary tract infection, uncomplicated:
Oral: 125-250 mg twice daily for 7-10 days
I.V., I.M.: 750 mg every 8 hours

Renal Impairment
Cl_{cr} 10-20 mL/minute: Administer every 12 hours.
Cl_{cr} <10 mL/minute: Administer every 24 hours.
Hemodialysis: Dialyzable (25%)
Peritoneal dialysis: Dose every 24 hours
Continuous renal replacement therapy (CRRT): 1 g every 12 hours
Note: Cefuroxime axetil film-coated tablets and oral suspension are not bioequivalent and are not substitutable on a mg/mg basis.

Administration Tablets can be crushed and given with soft foods to mask the bitter taste; I.M. doses should be given deep into a large muscle (ie, gluteus maximus)

Monitoring Parameters Observe for signs and symptoms of anaphylaxis during first dose; with prolonged therapy, monitor renal, hepatic, and hematologic function periodically; monitor prothrombin time in patients at risk of prolongation during cephalosporin therapy (nutritionally-deficient, prolonged treatment, renal or hepatic disease)

Test Interactions Positive direct Coombs', false-positive urinary glucose test using cupric sulfate (Benedict's solution, Clinitest®, Fehling's solution); false-negative may occur with ferricyanide test. Glucose oxidase or hexokinase-based methods should be used.

Pharmacotherapy Pearls Sodium content of 1 g: 54.2 mg (2.4 mEq)

Special Geriatric Considerations Adjust dose for renal function in the elderly. Considered one of the drugs of choice for outpatient treatment of community-acquired pneumonia in the elderly.

Dosage Forms Excipient information presented when available (limited, particularly for generics); consult specific product labeling.

Infusion, premixed iso-osmotic solution, as sodium [strength expressed as base]:

Zinacef®: 750 mg (50 mL); 1.5 g (50 mL) [contains sodium 4.8 mEq (111 mg) per 750 mg]

Injection, powder for reconstitution, as sodium [strength expressed as base]: 750 mg, 1.5 g, 7.5 g, 75 g

Zinacef®: 750 mg, 1.5 g, 7.5 g [contains sodium ~1.8 mEq (41 mg) per 750 mg]

Powder for suspension, oral, as axetil [strength expressed as base]: 125 mg/5 mL (100 mL); 250 mg/5 mL (100 mL)

Ceftin®: 125 mg/5 mL (100 mL) [contains phenylalanine 11.8 mg/5 mL; tutti frutti flavor]

Ceftin®: 250 mg/5 mL (50 mL, 100 mL) [contains phenylalanine 25.2 mg/5 mL; tutti frutti flavor]

Tablet, oral, as axetil [strength expressed as base]: 250 mg, 500 mg

Ceftin®: 250 mg, 500 mg

Selected References

Broekhuysen J, Deger F, Douchamps J, et al, "Pharmacokinetic Study of Cefuroxime in the Elderly," *Br J Clin Pharmacol*, 1981, 21(6):801-5.

Douglas JG, Bax RP, and Munro JF, "The Pharmacokinetics of Cefuroxime in the Elderly," *J Antimicrob Chemother*, 1980, 6(4):543-9.

Mandell LA, Wunderink RG, Anzueto A, et al, "Infectious Diseases Society of America/American Thoracic Society Consensus Guidelines on the Management of Community-Acquired Pneumonia in Adults," *Clin Infect Dis*, 2007, 44 Suppl 2:S27-72.

◆ **Cefuroxime Axetil** *see* Cefuroxime *on page 316*
◆ **Cefuroxime Sodium** *see* Cefuroxime *on page 316*
◆ **Cefzil** *see* Cefprozil *on page 306*
◆ **CeleBREX®** *see* Celecoxib *on page 319*

Celecoxib (se le KOKS ib)

Medication Safety Issues

Sound-alike/look-alike issues:

CeleBREX® may be confused with CeleXA®, cerebra, Cerebyx®, Cervarix®, Clarinex

Brand Names: U.S. CeleBREX®

Brand Names: Canada Celebrex®

Generic Availability (U.S.) No

Pharmacologic Category Nonsteroidal Anti-inflammatory Drug (NSAID), COX-2 Selective

Use Relief of the signs and symptoms of osteoarthritis, ankylosing spondylitis, and rheumatoid arthritis; management of acute pain

Medication Guide Available Yes

Contraindications Hypersensitivity to celecoxib, sulfonamides, aspirin, other NSAIDs, or any component of the formulation; perioperative pain in the setting of coronary artery bypass graft (CABG) surgery

Canadian labeling: Additional contraindications (not in U.S. labeling): Severe, uncontrolled heart failure; active gastrointestinal ulcer (gastric, duodenal, peptic) or bleeding; inflammatory bowel disease; cerebrovascular bleeding; severe liver impairment or active hepatic disease; severe renal impairment (Cl$_{cr}$ <30 mL/minute) or deteriorating renal disease; known hyperkalemia

Warnings/Precautions [U.S. Boxed Warning]: NSAIDs are associated with an increased risk of serious (and potentially fatal) adverse cardiovascular thrombotic events, including MI and stroke. Risk may be increased with duration of use or pre-existing cardiovascular risk factors or disease. Carefully evaluate individual cardiovascular risk profiles prior to prescribing. New-onset or exacerbation of hypertension may occur (NSAIDS may impair response to thiazide or loop diuretics); may contribute to cardiovascular events; monitor blood pressure; use with caution in patients with hypertension. May cause sodium and fluid retention; use with caution in patients with edema, cerebrovascular disease, or ischemic heart disease. Avoid use in heart failure.

[U.S. Boxed Warning]: Celecoxib is contraindicated for treatment of perioperative pain in the setting of coronary artery bypass graft (CABG) surgery. Risk of MI and stroke may be increased with use following CABG surgery.

[U.S. Boxed Warning]: NSAIDs may increase risk of serious gastrointestinal ulceration, bleeding, and perforation (may be fatal). These events may occur at any time during therapy and without warning. Use caution with a history of GI disease (bleeding or ulcers), concurrent therapy with aspirin, anticoagulants and/or corticosteroids, smoking, use of alcohol, the elderly or debilitated patients. When used concomitantly with ≤325 mg of aspirin, a substantial increase in the risk of gastrointestinal complications (eg, ulcer) occurs; concomitant gastroprotective therapy (eg, proton pump inhibitors) is recommended (Bhatt, 2008).

Use the lowest effective dose for the shortest duration of time, consistent with individual patient goals, to reduce risk of cardiovascular or GI adverse events. Alternate therapies should be considered for patients at high risk.

NSAIDs may cause serious skin adverse events including exfoliative dermatitis, Stevens-Johnson syndrome (SJS), and toxic epidermal necrolysis (TEN); may occur without warning and in patients without prior known sulfa allergy. Anaphylactoid reactions may occur, even without prior exposure; patients with "aspirin triad" (bronchial asthma, aspirin intolerance, rhinitis) may be at increased risk. Do not use in patients who experience bronchospasm, asthma, rhinitis, or urticaria with NSAID or aspirin therapy. Use with caution in other forms of asthma.

Use with caution in patients with decreased hepatic (dosage adjustments are recommended for moderate hepatic impairment; not recommended for patients with severe hepatic impairment) or renal function. Transaminase elevations have been reported with use; closely monitor patients with any abnormal LFT. Severe hepatic reactions (eg, fulminant hepatitis, liver failure) have occurred with NSAID use, rarely; discontinue if signs or symptoms of liver disease develop, if systemic manifestations occur, or with persistent or worsening abnormal hepatic function tests. NSAID use may compromise existing renal function; dose-dependent decreases in prostaglandin synthesis may result from NSAID use, causing a reduction in renal blood flow which may cause renal decompensation (usually reversible). Patients with impaired renal function, dehydration, heart failure, liver dysfunction, those taking diuretics, ACE inhibitors, angiotensin II receptor blockers, and the elderly are at greater risk for renal toxicity. Rehydrate patient before starting therapy; monitor renal function closely. Not recommended for use in patients with advanced renal disease or severe renal insufficiency; discontinue use with persistent or worsening abnormal renal function tests. Long-term NSAID use may result in renal papillary necrosis. Should not be considered a treatment or replacement of corticosteroid-dependent diseases.

Anaphylactoid reactions may occur, even with no prior exposure to celecoxib. Use with caution in patients with known or suspected deficiency of cytochrome P450 isoenzyme 2C9; poor metabolizers may have higher plasma levels due to reduced metabolism; consider reduced initial doses.

Anemia may occur with use; monitor hemoglobin or hematocrit in patients on long-term treatment. Celecoxib does not affect PT, PTT or platelet counts; does not inhibit platelet aggregation at approved doses.

Adverse Reactions (Reflective of adult population; not specific for elderly)

≥2%
  Cardiovascular: Peripheral edema
  Central nervous system: Dizziness, fever, headache, insomnia
  Dermatologic: Rash
  Gastrointestinal: Abdominal pain, diarrhea, dyspepsia, flatulence, nausea, vomiting
  Neuromuscular & skeletal: Arthralgia, back pain
  Respiratory: Cough, nasopharyngitis, pharyngitis, rhinitis, sinusitis, upper respiratory tract infection

0.1% to 1.9%:
  Cardiovascular: Angina, aortic valve incompetence, chest pain, coronary artery disorder, edema, facial edema, hypertension (aggravated), MI, palpitation, sinus bradycardia, tachycardia, ventricular hypertrophy
  Central nervous system: Anxiety, depression, fatigue, hypoesthesia, migraine, nervousness, pain, somnolence, vertigo
  Dermatologic: Alopecia, bruising, cellulitis, dermatitis, dry skin, photosensitivity, pruritus, rash (erythematous), rash (maculopapular), urticaria
  Endocrine & metabolic: Hot flashes, hypercholesterolemia, hyperglycemia, hypokalemia, ovarian cyst, testosterone decreased
  Gastrointestinal: Anorexia, appetite increased, constipation, diverticulitis, dysphagia, eructation, esophagitis, gastritis, gastroenteritis, gastroesophageal reflux, gastrointestinal ulcer, hemorrhoids, hiatal hernia, melena, stomatitis, tenesmus, weight gain, xerostomia
  Genitourinary: Cystitis, dysuria, urinary frequency
  Hematologic: Anemia, thrombocythemia
  Hepatic: Alkaline phosphatase increased, transaminases increased
  Neuromuscular & skeletal: Arthrosis, CPK increased, hypertonia, leg cramps, myalgia, paresthesia, synovitis, tendonitis
  Ocular: Conjunctival hemorrhage, vitreous floaters
  Otic: Deafness, labyrinthitis, tinnitus
  Renal: Albuminuria, BUN increased, creatinine increased, hematuria, nonprotein nitrogen increased, renal calculi

Respiratory: Bronchitis, bronchospasm, dyspnea, epistaxis, laryngitis, pneumonia
Miscellaneous: Allergic reactions, allergy aggravated, cyst, diaphoresis, flu-like syndrome

Drug Interactions

Metabolism/Transport Effects Substrate of CYP2C9 (major), 3A4 (minor); **Inhibits** CYP2C8 (moderate), 2D6 (weak)

Avoid Concomitant Use

Avoid concomitant use of Celecoxib with any of the following: Floctafenine; Ketorolac; Ketorolac (Nasal); Ketorolac (Systemic); Thioridazine

Increased Effect/Toxicity

Celecoxib may increase the levels/effects of: Aminoglycosides; Anticoagulants; Antiplatelet Agents; Bisphosphonate Derivatives; CycloSPORINE; CycloSPORINE (Systemic); CYP2C8 Substrates (High risk); CYP2D6 Substrates; Deferasirox; Desmopressin; Digoxin; Eplerenone; Fesoterodine; Haloperidol; Lithium; Methotrexate; Nebivolol; Nonsteroidal Anti-Inflammatory Agents; Porfimer; Potassium-Sparing Diuretics; PRALAtrexate; Quinolone Antibiotics; Tamoxifen; Thioridazine; Thrombolytic Agents; Vancomycin; Vitamin K Antagonists

The levels/effects of Celecoxib may be increased by: ACE Inhibitors; Angiotensin II Receptor Blockers; Antidepressants (Tricyclic, Tertiary Amine); Conivaptan; Corticosteroids (Systemic); CYP2C9 Inhibitors (Moderate); CYP2C9 Inhibitors (Strong); Floctafenine; Herbs (Anticoagulant/Antiplatelet Properties); Ketorolac; Ketorolac (Nasal); Ketorolac (Systemic); Probenecid; Selective Serotonin Reuptake Inhibitors; Sodium Phosphates; Treprostinil

Decreased Effect

Celecoxib may decrease the levels/effects of: ACE Inhibitors; Angiotensin II Receptor Blockers; Antiplatelet Agents; Beta-Blockers; Codeine; Eplerenone; HydrALAZINE; Potassium-Sparing Diuretics; Thiazide Diuretics; TraMADol

The levels/effects of Celecoxib may be decreased by: Bile Acid Sequestrants; CYP2C9 Inducers (Highly Effective); Peginterferon Alfa-2b; Tocilizumab

Ethanol/Nutrition/Herb Interactions

Ethanol: Avoid ethanol (increased GI irritation).

Food: Peak concentrations are delayed and AUC is increased by 10% to 20% when taken with a high-fat meal.

Herb/Nutraceutical: Avoid concomitant use with herbs possessing anticoagulation/antiplatelet properties, including alfalfa, anise, bilberry, bladderwrack, bromelain, cat's claw, celery, chamomile, coleus, cordyceps, dong quai, evening primrose, fenugreek, feverfew, garlic, ginger, ginkgo biloba, ginseng (American, Panax, Siberian), grapeseed, green tea, guggul, horse chestnuts, horseradish, licorice, prickly ash, red clover, reishi, SAMe (S-adenosylmethionine), sweet clover, turmeric, white willow.

Stability Store at 25°C (77°F); excursions permitted to 15°C to 30°C (59°F to 86°F).

Mechanism of Action Inhibits prostaglandin synthesis by decreasing the activity of the enzyme, cyclooxygenase-2 (COX-2), which results in decreased formation of prostaglandin precursors; has antipyretic, analgesic, and anti-inflammatory properties. Celecoxib does not inhibit cyclooxygenase-1 (COX-1) at therapeutic concentrations.

Pharmacodynamics/Kinetics

Distribution: V_d (apparent): ~400 L

Protein binding: ~97% primarily to albumin

Metabolism: Hepatic via CYP2C9; forms inactive metabolites

Bioavailability: Absolute: Unknown

Half-life elimination: ~11 hours (fasted)

Time to peak: ~3 hours

Excretion: Feces (~57% as metabolites, <3% as unchanged drug); urine (27% as metabolites, <3% as unchanged drug)

Dosage

Geriatric Refer to adult dosing. No specific adjustment based on age is recommended. However, the AUC in elderly patients may be increased by 50% as compared to younger subjects. Initiate at the lowest recommended dose in patients weighing <50 kg.

Adult Note: Use the lowest effective dose for the shortest duration of time, consistent with individual patient treatment goals.

Osteoarthritis: Oral: 200 mg/day as a single dose or in divided doses twice daily

Ankylosing spondylitis: Oral: 200 mg/day as a single dose or in divided doses twice daily; if no effect after 6 weeks, may increase to 400 mg/day. If no response following 6 weeks of treatment with 400 mg/day, consider discontinuation and alternative treatment.

Canadian labeling; Recommended maximum dose: 200 mg/day

Rheumatoid arthritis: Oral: 100-200 mg twice daily

Acute pain: Oral: Initial dose: 400 mg, followed by an additional 200 mg if needed on day 1; maintenance dose: 200 mg twice daily as needed

Canadian labeling; Recommended maximum dose for treatment of acute pain: 400 mg/day up to 7 days

Dosing adjustment in poor CYP2C9 metabolizers (eg, CYP2C9*3/*3): Consider reducing initial dose by 50%

Canadian labeling: Recommended maximum dose: 100 mg/day.

Renal Impairment

Advanced renal disease: Use is not recommended, however, if celecoxib treatment cannot be avoided, monitor renal function closely.

Severe renal insufficiency: Use is not recommended.

Canadian labeling: Cl_{cr} <30 mL/minute: Use is contraindicated.

Abnormal renal function tests (persistent or worsening): Discontinue use.

Hepatic Impairment

Moderate hepatic impairment (Child-Pugh class B): Reduce dose by 50%.

Severe hepatic impairment (Child-Pugh class C): Use is not recommended.

Canadian labeling: Use is contraindicated.

Abnormal liver function tests (persistent or worsening): Discontinue use.

Administration May be administered without regard to meals. Capsules may be swallowed whole or the entire contents emptied onto a teaspoon of cool or room temperature applesauce. The contents of the capsules sprinkled onto applesauce may be stored under refrigeration for up to 6 hours.

Monitoring Parameters CBC; blood chemistry profile; occult blood loss and periodic liver function tests; monitor renal function (urine output, serum BUN and creatinine; monitor response (pain, range of motion, grip strength, mobility, ADL function), inflammation; blood pressure (baseline and during treatment); observe for weight gain, edema; observe for bleeding, bruising; evaluate gastrointestinal effects (abdominal pain, bleeding, dyspepsia)

Special Geriatric Considerations The elderly are at increased risk for adverse effects from NSAIDs. As many as 60% of elderly can develop peptic ulceration and/or hemorrhage asymptomatically; however, elderly patients may demonstrate these adverse effects at lower doses than younger adults. The elderly are also at increased risk of renal toxicity. Although celecoxib is associated with a decreased incidence of GI side effects, use the lowest recommended dose in patients weighing <50 kg.

Dosage Forms Excipient information presented when available (limited, particularly for generics); consult specific product labeling.

Capsule, oral:

CeleBREX®: 50 mg, 100 mg, 200 mg, 400 mg

Selected References

Bertagnolli MM, Eagle CJ, Zauber AG, et al, "Celecoxib for the Prevention of Sporadic Colorectal Adenomas," *N Engl J Med*, 2006, 355(9):873-84.

Steinbach G, Lynch PM, Phillips RK, et al, "The Effect of Celecoxib, a Cyclooxygenase-2 Inhibitor, in Familial Adenomatous Polyposis," *N Engl J Med*, 2000, 342(26):1946-52.

◆ **Celestone®** *see* Betamethasone *on page 195*
◆ **Celestone® Soluspan®** *see* Betamethasone *on page 195*
◆ **CeleXA®** *see* Citalopram *on page 365*
◆ **Celontin®** *see* Methsuximide *on page 1174*
◆ **Cemill 500 [OTC]** *see* Ascorbic Acid *on page 149*
◆ **Cemill 1000 [OTC]** *see* Ascorbic Acid *on page 149*
◆ **Cenestin®** *see* Estrogens (Conjugated A/Synthetic) *on page 652*
◆ **Centany®** *see* Mupirocin *on page 1250*
◆ **Centany® AT** *see* Mupirocin *on page 1250*

Cephalexin (sef a LEKS in)

Related Information

Prevention of Infective Endocarditis *on page 2064*

Medication Safety Issues

Sound-alike/look-alike issues:

Cephalexin may be confused with cefaclor, ceFAZolin, cephalothin, ciprofloxacin

Keflex® may be confused with Keppra®, Valtrex®

Brand Names: U.S. Keflex®

Brand Names: Canada Apo-Cephalex®; Dom-Cephalexin; Keflex®; Keftab®; Novo-Lexin; Nu-Cephalex; PMS-Cephalexin

Index Terms Cephalexin Monohydrate

Generic Availability (U.S.) Yes

Pharmacologic Category Antibiotic, Cephalosporin (First Generation)

Use Treatment of susceptible bacterial infections including respiratory tract infections, otitis media, skin and skin structure infections, bone infections, and genitourinary tract infections, including acute prostatitis; alternative therapy for acute infective endocarditis prophylaxis

Contraindications Hypersensitivity to cephalexin, any component of the formulation, or other cephalosporins

Warnings/Precautions Modify dosage in patients with severe renal impairment. Use with caution in patients with a history of penicillin allergy, especially IgE-mediated reactions (eg, anaphylaxis, urticaria). Prolonged use may result in fungal or bacterial superinfection, including *C. difficile*-associated diarrhea (CDAD) and pseudomembranous colitis; CDAD has been observed >2 months postantibiotic treatment. May be associated with increased INR, especially in nutritionally-deficient patients, prolonged treatment, hepatic or renal disease.

Adverse Reactions (Reflective of adult population; not specific for elderly) Frequency not defined.

Central nervous system: Agitation, confusion, dizziness, fatigue, hallucinations, headache

Dermatologic: Angioedema, erythema multiforme (rare), rash, Stevens-Johnson syndrome (rare), toxic epidermal necrolysis (rare), urticaria

Gastrointestinal: Abdominal pain, diarrhea, dyspepsia, gastritis, nausea (rare), pseudomembranous colitis, vomiting (rare)

Genitourinary: Genital pruritus, genital moniliasis, vaginitis, vaginal discharge

Hematologic: Eosinophilia, hemolytic anemia, neutropenia, thrombocytopenia

Hepatic: ALT increased, AST increased, cholestatic jaundice (rare), transient hepatitis (rare)

Neuromuscular & skeletal: Arthralgia, arthritis, joint disorder

Renal: Interstitial nephritis (rare)

Miscellaneous: Allergic reactions, anaphylaxis

Drug Interactions

Avoid Concomitant Use

Avoid concomitant use of Cephalexin with any of the following: BCG

Increased Effect/Toxicity

Cephalexin may increase the levels/effects of: MetFORMIN

The levels/effects of Cephalexin may be increased by: Probenecid

Decreased Effect

Cephalexin may decrease the levels/effects of: BCG; Typhoid Vaccine

Ethanol/Nutrition/Herb Interactions Food: Peak antibiotic serum concentration is lowered and delayed, but total drug absorbed is not affected. Cephalexin serum levels may be decreased if taken with food.

Stability

Capsule: Store at 15°C to 30°C (59°F to 86°F).

Powder for oral suspension: Refrigerate suspension after reconstitution; discard after 14 days.

Mechanism of Action Inhibits bacterial cell wall synthesis by binding to one or more of the penicillin-binding proteins (PBPs) which in turn inhibits the final transpeptidation step of peptidoglycan synthesis in bacterial cell walls, thus inhibiting cell wall biosynthesis. Bacteria eventually lyse due to ongoing activity of cell wall autolytic enzymes (autolysins and murein hydrolases) while cell wall assembly is arrested.

Pharmacodynamics/Kinetics

Absorption: Rapid (90%)

Distribution: Widely into most body tissues and fluids, including gallbladder, liver, kidneys, bone, sputum, bile, and pleural and synovial fluids; CSF penetration is poor

Protein binding: 6% to 15%

Half-life elimination: Adults: 0.5-1.2 hours; prolonged with renal impairment

Time to peak, serum: ~1 hour

Excretion: Urine (80% to 100% as unchanged drug) within 8 hours

Dosage

Geriatric & Adult

Dosing range: Oral: 250-1000 mg every 6 hours (maximum: 4 g/day)

Cellulitis and mastitis: Oral: 500 mg every 6 hours

Furunculosis/skin abscess: Oral: 250 mg 4 times/day

Prophylaxis against infective endocarditis (dental, oral, or respiratory tract procedures): Oral: 2 g 30-60 minutes prior to procedure. **Note:** American Heart Association (AHA) guidelines now recommend prophylaxis only in patients undergoing invasive procedures and in whom underlying cardiac conditions may predispose to a higher risk of adverse outcomes should infection occur.

Prophylaxis in total joint replacement patients undergoing dental procedures which produce bacteremia: Oral: 2 g 1 hour prior to procedure

Streptococcal pharyngitis, skin and skin structure infections: Oral: 500 mg every 12 hours

Uncomplicated cystitis: Oral: 500 mg every 12 hours for 7-14 days

Renal Impairment Adults:

Cl_{cr} 10-50 mL/minute: 500 mg every 8-12 hours

Cl_{cr} <10: 250-500 mg every 12-24 hours

Hemodialysis: 250 mg every 12-24 hours; moderately dialyzable (20% to 50%); give dose after dialysis session

Administration Take without regard to food. If GI distress, take with food. Give around-the-clock to promote less variation in peak and trough serum levels.

Panixine DisperDose™: Tablets should be mixed in ~10 mL of water immediately prior to administration. Drink entire solution, then rinse glass with additional water and drink contents to ensure entire dose has been taken. Tablets should not be chewed or swallowed whole.

Monitoring Parameters With prolonged therapy monitor renal, hepatic, and hematologic function periodically; monitor for signs of anaphylaxis during first dose

Test Interactions Positive direct Coombs', false-positive urinary glucose test using cupric sulfate (Benedict's solution, Clinitest®, Fehling's solution), false-positive serum or urine creatinine with Jaffé reaction, false-positive urinary proteins and steroids

Special Geriatric Considerations Adjust dose for renal function.

Dosage Forms Excipient information presented when available (limited, particularly for generics); consult specific product labeling.

Capsule, oral: 250 mg, 500 mg

Keflex®: 250 mg, 500 mg, 750 mg

Powder for suspension, oral: 125 mg/5 mL (100 mL, 200 mL); 250 mg/5 mL (100 mL, 200 mL)

Tablet, oral: 250 mg, 500 mg

◆ **Cephalexin Monohydrate** see Cephalexin on page 322

◆ **Cerebyx®** see Fosphenytoin on page 793

◆ **Cerefolin® NAC** see Methylfolate, Methylcobalamin, and Acetylcysteine on page 1178

Certolizumab Pegol (cer to LIZ u mab PEG ol)

Brand Names: U.S. Cimzia®

Brand Names: Canada Cimzia®

Index Terms CDP870

Generic Availability (U.S.) No

Pharmacologic Category Antirheumatic, Disease Modifying; Gastrointestinal Agent, Miscellaneous; Tumor Necrosis Factor (TNF) Blocking Agent

Use Treatment of moderately- to severely-active Crohn's disease in patients who have inadequate response to conventional therapy; moderately- to severely-active rheumatoid arthritis (as monotherapy or in combination with nonbiological disease-modifying antirheumatic drugs [DMARDS])

Medication Guide Available Yes

Contraindications There are no contraindications listed within the manufacturer's labeling.

Warnings/Precautions [U.S. Boxed Warning]: Patients receiving certolizumab are at increased risk for serious infections which may result in hospitalization and/or fatality; infections usually developed in patients receiving concomitant immunosuppressive agents (eg, methotrexate or corticosteroids). Active tuberculosis (or reactivation of latent tuberculosis), invasive fungal (including aspergillosis, blastomycosis, candidiasis, coccidioidomycosis, histoplasmosis, and pneumocystosis) and other opportunistic infections have been reported in patients receiving TNF-blocking agents, including certolizumab. Monitor closely for signs/symptoms of infection. Discontinue for serious infection or sepsis. Consider risks versus benefits prior to use in patients with a history of chronic or recurrent infection. Caution should be exercised when considering the use in patients with concomitant immunosuppressive therapy or predisposition to infection (eg, diabetes or residence/travel from areas of endemic mycoses). Do not administer to patients with an active chronic or localized infection. Patients who develop a new infection while undergoing treatment should be monitored closely. If a patient develops a serious infection, therapy should be discontinued. **[U.S. Boxed Warning]: Lymphoma and other malignancies have been reported in children and adolescent patients receiving other TNF-blocking agents.** Use of TNF blockers may affect defenses against malignancies; impact on the development and course of malignancies is not fully defined. Lymphoma has been noted in clinical trials. Chronic immunosuppressant therapy use may be a predisposing factor for malignancy development; rheumatoid arthritis alone has been previously associated with an increased rate of lymphoma.

Tuberculosis has been reported with certolizumab treatment. **[U.S. Boxed Warnings]: Patients should be evaluated for tuberculosis risk factors and for latent tuberculosis infection (with a tuberculin skin test) prior to therapy. Treatment of latent tuberculosis should be initiated before use. Patients with initial negative tuberculin skin tests should receive continued monitoring for tuberculosis throughout treatment;** active tuberculosis has developed in this population during treatment. Use with caution in patients who have resided in regions where tuberculosis is endemic. If appropriate, antituberculosis therapy should be considered (prior to certolizumab treatment) in patients with several or with highly significant risk factors for tuberculosis development.

Rare and sometimes fatal reactivation of hepatitis B virus (HBV) has occurred in chronic virus carriers (usually in patients receiving concomitant immunosuppressive agents); evaluate prior to initiation, during, and for several months after treatment. Evaluate patients at risk for HBV infection prior to therapy to determine HBV status. Use with extreme caution in patients identified as HBV carriers, use has not been evaluated in this population. Discontinue certolizumab treatment (and initiate appropriate antiviral therapy) if HBV reactivation occurs if resumption of therapy is deemed necessary, use caution and monitor closely.

Hypersensitivity reactions, including angioedema, dyspnea, rash, serum sickness and urticaria have been reported (rarely) with treatment; discontinue and do not resume therapy if hypersensitivity occurs. Use with caution in patients who have experienced hypersensitivity with other TNF blockers. Use with caution in heart failure patients; worsening heart failure and new onset heart failure have been reported with TNF blockers, including certolizumab pegol; monitor closely. Rare cases of pancytopenia and other significant cytopenias, including aplastic anemia and have been reported with TNF-blocking agents. Leukopenia and thrombocytopenia have occurred with certolizumab; use with caution in patients with underlying hematologic disorders; consider discontinuing therapy with significant hematologic abnormalities. Autoantibody formation may develop; rarely resulting in autoimmune disorder, including lupus-like syndrome; monitor and discontinue if symptoms develop. A small number of patients (8%) develop antibodies to certolizumab during therapy. Antibody-positive patients may have an increased incidence of adverse events (including injection site pain/erythema, abdominal pain and erythema nodosum). Use with caution in patients with pre-existing or recent-onset CNS demyelinating disorders; rare cases of optic neuritis, seizure, peripheral neuropathy, and demyelinating disease (new onset or exacerbation) have been reported.

The manufacturer does not recommend concurrent use with anakinra or other tumor necrosis factor (TNF) blocking agents due to the risk of serious infections. Do not use in combination with biologic DMARDS. Patients should be up to date with all immunizations before initiating therapy; live vaccines should not be given concurrently. There is no data available concerning the effects of therapy on vaccination or secondary transmission of live vaccines in patients receiving therapy. Use has not been studied in patients with renal impairment; however, the pharmacokinetics of the pegylated (polyethylene glycol) component may be dependent on renal function. Use with caution in the elderly, may be at higher risk for infections.

Adverse Reactions (Reflective of adult population; not specific for elderly)
>10%:
  Central nervous system: Headache (5% to 18%)
  Gastrointestinal: Nausea (≤11%)
  Respiratory: Upper respiratory infection (6% to 20%), nasopharyngitis (4% to 13%)
  Miscellaneous: Infection (14% to 38%; serious: 3%)
1% to 10%:
  Cardiovascular: Hypertension (≤5%)
  Central nervous system: Dizziness (≤6%), fever (≤5%), fatigue (≤3%)
  Dermatologic: Rash (9%)
  Gastrointestinal: Abdominal pain (≤6%), vomiting (5%)
  Genitourinary: Urinary tract infection (≤8%)
  Local: Injection site reactions (includes bleeding, burning, erythema, inflammation, pain, rash: ≤7%; incidence higher with placebo)
  Neuromuscular & skeletal: Arthralgia (6% to 7%), back pain (≤4%)
  Respiratory: Cough (≤6%), bronchitis (≤3%), pharyngitis (≤3%)
  Miscellaneous: Antibody formation (7% to 8%), positive ANA (≤4%)

Drug Interactions
  Avoid Concomitant Use
    Avoid concomitant use of Certolizumab Pegol with any of the following: Abatacept; Anakinra; Anti-TNF Agents; BCG; Canakinumab; Natalizumab; Pimecrolimus; Rilonacept; RiTUXimab; Tacrolimus (Topical); Vaccines (Live)

Increased Effect/Toxicity

Certolizumab Pegol may increase the levels/effects of: Abatacept; Anakinra; Canakinumab; Leflunomide; Natalizumab; Rilonacept; Vaccines (Live)

The levels/effects of Certolizumab Pegol may be increased by: Anti-TNF Agents; Denosumab; Pimecrolimus; RiTUXimab; Roflumilast; Tacrolimus (Topical); Trastuzumab

Decreased Effect

Certolizumab Pegol may decrease the levels/effects of: BCG; Sipuleucel-T; Vaccines (Inactivated); Vaccines (Live)

The levels/effects of Certolizumab Pegol may be decreased by: Echinacea; Pegloticase

Ethanol/Nutrition/Herb Interactions Herb/Nutraceutical: Echinacea may decrease the therapeutic effects of certolizumab; avoid concurrent use.

Stability Prior to reconstitution, store refrigerated at 2°C to 8°C (36°F to 46°F); do not freeze. Bring to room temperature prior to administration.

Prefilled syringe: Protect from light.

Vials: Allow to reach room temperature prior to reconstitution. Using aseptic technique, reconstitute each vial with 1 mL sterile water for injection (provided) to a concentration of ~200 mg/mL; the manufacturer recommends using a 20-gauge needle (provided). Gently swirl to facilitate wetting of powder; do not shake. Allow vials to set undisturbed (may take up to 30 minutes) until fully reconstituted. Reconstituted solutions should not contain visible particles or gels in the solution. Reconstituted vials may be retained at room temperature for ≤2 hours or refrigerated (do not freeze) for ≤24 hours prior to administration.

Mechanism of Action Certolizumab pegol is a pegylated humanized antibody Fab' fragment of tumor necrosis factor alpha (TNF-alpha) monoclonal antibody. Certolizumab pegol binds to and selectively neutralizes human TNF-alpha activity. (Elevated levels of TNF-alpha have a role in the inflammatory process associated with Crohn's disease and in joint destruction associated with rheumatoid arthritis.) Since it is not a complete antibody (lacks Fc region), it does not induce complement activation, antibody-dependent cell-mediated cytotoxicity, or apoptosis. Pegylation of certolizumab allows for delayed elimination and therefore an extended half-life.

Pharmacodynamics/Kinetics

Distribution: V_{ss}: 6-8 L

Bioavailability: SubQ: ~80% (range: 76% to 88%)

Half-life elimination: ~14 days

Time to peak, plasma: 54-171 hours

Dosage

Geriatric & Adult Note: Each 400 mg dose should be administered as 2 injections of 200 mg each

Crohn's disease: SubQ: Initial: 400 mg, repeat dose 2 and 4 weeks after initial dose; Maintenance: 400 mg every 4 weeks

Rheumatoid arthritis: SubQ: Initial: 400 mg, repeat dose 2 and 4 weeks after initial dose; Maintenance: 200 mg every other week. May consider maintenance dose of 400 mg every 4 weeks.

Renal Impairment Moderate-to-severe renal impairment: The pharmacokinetics of the pegylated (polyethylene glycol) component may be dependent on renal function; however, data is insufficient to provide a dosing recommendation.

Administration SubQ: Bring to room temperature prior to administration. Total dose requires 2 vials **or** 2 prefilled syringes. After reconstitution (of vials), draw each vial into separate syringes (using 20-gauge needles).

Administer each syringe subcutaneously (using provided 23-gauge needle) to separate sites on abdomen or thigh. Rotate injections sites; do not administer to areas where skin is tender, bruised, red, or hard.

Monitoring Parameters Signs and symptoms of infection, signs and symptoms of hypersensitivity reaction, symptoms of lupus-like syndrome; hepatitis B virus and TB screening prior to therapy initiation

Test Interactions Tests for latent tuberculosis may be falsely negative while on certolizumab pegol treatment. Falsely elevated aPTT assays have been reported with PTT-Lupus Anticoagulant (LA) and Standard Target Activated Partial Thromboplastin time (STA-PTT) tests from Diagnostica Stago, and with HemosIL APTT-SP liquid and HemosIL lyophilized silica tests from Instrumentation Laboratories.

Special Geriatric Considerations Studies to date have insufficient data to make conclusions for use in elderly. Anecdotal reports in clinical settings do not demonstrate any clinical difference between elderly and younger adults. Since elderly have a higher incidence of infection, use with caution and close monitoring.

Dosage Forms Excipient information presented when available (limited, particularly for generics); consult specific product labeling.

Injection, powder for reconstitution [preservative free]:

Cimzia® 200 mg [contains sucrose 100 mg]

Injection, solution [preservative free]:

Cimzia® 200 mg/mL (1 mL)

Selected References

Fleischmann R, Vencovsky J, van Vollenhoven RF, et al, "Efficacy and Safety of Certolizumab Pegol Monotherapy Every 4 Weeks in Patients With Rheumatoid Arthritis Failing Previous Disease-Modifying Antirheumatic Therapy: The FAST4WARD Study," *Ann Rheum Dis*, 2009, 68(6):805-11.

Keystone E, Heijde D, Mason D Jr, et al, "Certolizumab Pegol Plus Methotrexate is Significantly More Effective Than Placebo Plus Methotrexate in Active Rheumatoid Arthritis: Findings of a Fifty-Two-Week, Phase III, Multicenter, Randomized, Double-Blind, Placebo-Controlled, Parallel-Group Study," *Arthritis Rheum*, 2008, 58(11):3319-29.

Rutgeerts P, Schreiber S, Feagan B, et al, "Certolizumab Pegol, a Monthly Subcutaneously Administered Fc-Free Anti-TNFalpha, Improves Health-Related Quality of Life in Patients With Moderate to Severe Crohn's Disease," *Int J Colorectal Dis*, 2008, 23(3):289-96.

Sandborn WJ, Feagan BG, Stoinov S, et al, "Certolizumab Pegol for the Treatment of Crohn's Disease," *N Engl J Med*, 2007, 357(3):228-38.

Schreiber S, Khaliq-Kareemi M, Lawrence IC, et al, "Maintenance Therapy With Certolizumab Pegol for Crohn's Disease," *N Engl J Med*, 2007, 357(3):239-50.

Schreiber S, Rutgeerts P, Fedorak RN, et al, "A Randomized, Placebo-Controlled Trial of Certolizumab Pegol (CDP870) for Treatment of Crohn's Disease," *Gastroenterology*, 2005, 129(1):807-18.

Smolen J, Landewé RB, Mease P, "Efficacy and Safety of Certolizumab Pegol Plus Methotrexate in Active Rheumatoid Arthritis: The RAPID 2 Study. A Randomised Controlled Trial," *Ann Rheum Dis*, 2009, 68(6):797-804.

◆ **C.E.S.** see Estrogens (Conjugated/Equine, Systemic) *on page* 658
◆ **C.E.S.** see Estrogens (Conjugated/Equine, Topical) *on page* 661
◆ **Cetafen® [OTC]** see Acetaminophen *on page* 33
◆ **Cetafen Cold® [OTC]** see Acetaminophen and Phenylephrine *on page* 38
◆ **Cetafen® Extra [OTC]** see Acetaminophen *on page* 33

Cetirizine (se TI ra zeen)

Medication Safety Issues

Sound-alike/look-alike issues:

ZyrTEC® may be confused with Lipitor©, serax, Xanax®, Zantac®, Zerit®, Zocor®, ZyPREXA®, ZyrTEC-D®

ZyrTEC® (cetirizine) may be confused with ZyrTEC® Itchy Eye (ketotifen)

Brand Names: U.S. All Day Allergy [OTC]; ZyrTEC® Allergy [OTC]; ZyrTEC® Children's Allergy [OTC]; ZyrTEC® Children's Hives Relief [OTC]

Brand Names: Canada Apo-Cetirizine®; PMS-Cetirizine; Reactine™

Index Terms Cetirizine Hydrochloride; P-071; UCB-P071

Generic Availability (U.S.) Yes

Pharmacologic Category Histamine H_1 Antagonist; Histamine H_1 Antagonist, Second Generation; Piperazine Derivative

Use Perennial and seasonal allergic rhinitis and other allergic symptoms including urticaria; chronic idiopathic urticaria

Contraindications Hypersensitivity to cetirizine, hydroxyzine, or any component of the formulation

Warnings/Precautions Cetirizine should be used cautiously in patients with hepatic or renal dysfunction; dosage adjustment recommended. Use with caution in the elderly; may be more sensitive to adverse effects. May cause drowsiness; use caution performing tasks which require alertness (eg, operating machinery or driving). Effects may be potentiated when used with other sedative drugs or ethanol.

Adverse Reactions (Reflective of adult population; not specific for elderly)

>10%: Central nervous system: Headache (children 11% to 14%, placebo 12%), somnolence (adults 14%, children 2% to 4%)

2% to 10%:

Central nervous system: Insomnia (children 9%, adults <2%), fatigue (adults 6%), malaise (4%), dizziness (adults 2%)

Gastrointestinal: Abdominal pain (children 4% to 6%), dry mouth (adults 5%), diarrhea (children 2% to 3%), nausea (children 2% to 3%, placebo 2%), vomiting (children 2% to 3%)

Respiratory: Epistaxis (children 2% to 4%, placebo 3%), pharyngitis (children 3% to 6%, placebo 3%), bronchospasm (children 2% to 3%, placebo 2%)

Drug Interactions

Metabolism/Transport Effects Substrate of CYP3A4 (minor), P-glycoprotein

Avoid Concomitant Use There are no known interactions where it is recommended to avoid concomitant use.

◀ **Increased Effect/Toxicity**

Cetirizine may increase the levels/effects of: Alcohol (Ethyl); Anticholinergics; CNS Depressants; Selective Serotonin Reuptake Inhibitors

The levels/effects of Cetirizine may be increased by: Conivaptan; Droperidol; HydrOXYzine; P-Glycoprotein Inhibitors; Pramlintide

Decreased Effect

Cetirizine may decrease the levels/effects of: Acetylcholinesterase Inhibitors (Central); Benzylpenicilloyl Polylysine; Betahistine

The levels/effects of Cetirizine may be decreased by: Acetylcholinesterase Inhibitors (Central); Amphetamines; P-Glycoprotein Inducers; Tocilizumab

Ethanol/Nutrition/Herb Interactions Ethanol: May increase CNS depression; monitor for increased effects with coadministration. Caution patients about effects.

Stability Store at room temperature.

Syrup: Store at room temperature of 15°C to 30°C (59°F to 86°F), or under refrigeration at 2°C to 8°C (36°F to 46°F).

Mechanism of Action Competes with histamine for H_1-receptor sites on effector cells in the gastrointestinal tract, blood vessels, and respiratory tract

Pharmacodynamics/Kinetics

Distribution: Minimal penetration into central nervous system

Protein binding: 93%

Metabolism: **Not** extensively metabolized by the liver

Half-life: 7.4-9 hours; in mild-moderate renal failure the half-life is increased to 19-21 hours

Time to peak: 0.5-1 hour; food may delay time to peak and decrease C_{max}

Elimination: 60% of dose is excreted unchanged in urine within 24 hours

Note: In older adults, there was a 50% increase in half-life and a 40% decrease in clearance, most likely due to change in renal function; not removed by hemodialysis

Dosage

Geriatric Oral: Initial: 5 mg once daily; may increase to 10 mg/day

Note: Manufacturer recommends 5 mg/day in patients ≥77 years of age.

Adult Perennial or seasonal allergic rhinitis, chronic urticaria: Oral: 5-10 mg once daily, depending upon symptom severity

Renal Impairment Adults:

Cl_{cr} 11-31 mL/minute or hemodialysis: Administer 5 mg once daily

Cl_{cr} <11 mL/minute, not on dialysis: Cetirizine use not recommended.

Hepatic Impairment Adults: Administer 5 mg once daily

Administration May be administered with or without food.

Monitoring Parameters Relief of symptoms, sedation and anticholinergic effects

Test Interactions May cause false-positive serum TCA screen.

Special Geriatric Considerations Adjust dose for renal function. Because of its OTC status, counsel patients on appropriate use.

Dosage Forms Excipient information presented when available (limited, particularly for generics); consult specific product labeling.

Capsule, liquid gel, oral, as hydrochloride:

ZyrTEC® Allergy: 10 mg

Syrup, oral, as hydrochloride: 5 mg/5 mL (5 mL, 118 mL, 120 mL, 473 mL, 480 mL)

ZyrTEC® Children's Allergy: 5 mg/5 mL (118 mL) [contains propylene glycol; grape flavor]

ZyrTEC® Children's Allergy: 5 mg/5 mL (118 mL) [dye free; sugar free; contains propylene glycol, sodium benzoate; bubblegum flavor]

ZyrTEC® Children's Hives Relief: 5 mg/5 mL (118 mL) [contains propylene glycol; grape flavor]

Tablet, oral, as hydrochloride: 5 mg, 10 mg

All Day Allergy: 10 mg

ZyrTEC® Allergy: 10 mg

Tablet, chewable, oral, as hydrochloride: 5 mg, 10 mg

All Day Allergy: 5 mg [fruit flavor]

ZyrTEC® Children's Allergy: 5 mg, 10 mg [grape flavor]

◆ **Cetirizine Hydrochloride** *see* Cetirizine *on page 327*

◆ **Cetraxal®** *see* Ciprofloxacin (Otic) *on page 364*

Cevimeline (se vi ME leen)

Medication Safety Issues

Sound-alike/look-alike issues:

Cevimeline may be confused with Savella®

Evoxac® may be confused with Eurax®

Brand Names: U.S. Evoxac®
Brand Names: Canada Evoxac®
Index Terms Cevimeline Hydrochloride
Generic Availability (U.S.) No
Pharmacologic Category Cholinergic Agonist
Use Treatment of symptoms of dry mouth in patients with Sjögren's syndrome
Contraindications Hypersensitivity to cevimeline or any component of the formulation; uncontrolled asthma; narrow-angle glaucoma; acute iritis; other conditions where miosis is undesirable
Warnings/Precautions May alter cardiac conduction and/or heart rate; use caution in patients with significant cardiovascular disease, including angina, myocardial infarction, or conduction disturbances. Cevimeline has the potential to increase bronchial smooth muscle tone, airway resistance, and bronchial secretions; use with caution in patients with controlled asthma, COPD, or chronic bronchitis. May cause decreased visual acuity (particularly at night and in patients with central lens changes) and impaired depth perception. Patients should be cautioned about driving at night or performing hazardous activities in reduced lighting. May cause a variety of parasympathomimetic effects, which may be particularly dangerous in elderly patients; excessive sweating may lead to dehydration in some patients.

Use with caution in patients with a history of biliary stones or nephrolithiasis; cevimeline may induce smooth muscle spasms, precipitating cholangitis, cholecystitis, biliary obstruction, renal colic, or ureteral reflux in susceptible patients. Patients with a known or suspected deficiency of CYP2D6 may be at higher risk of adverse effects.
Adverse Reactions (Reflective of adult population; not specific for elderly)
>10%:
  Central nervous system: Headache (14%; placebo 20%)
  Gastrointestinal: Nausea (14%), diarrhea (10%)
  Respiratory: Rhinitis (11%), sinusitis (12%), upper respiratory infection (11%)
  Miscellaneous: Diaphoresis increased (19%)
1% to 10%:
  Cardiovascular: Peripheral edema, chest pain, edema, palpitation
  Central nervous system: Dizziness (4%), fatigue (3%), pain (3%), insomnia (2%), anxiety (1%), fever, depression, migraine, hypoesthesia, vertigo
  Dermatologic: Rash (4%; placebo 6%), pruritus, skin disorder, erythematous rash
  Endocrine & metabolic: Hot flashes (2%)
  Gastrointestinal: Dyspepsia (8%; placebo 9%), abdominal pain (8%), vomiting (5%), excessive salivation (2%), constipation, salivary gland pain, dry mouth, sialoadenitis, gastroesophageal reflux, flatulence, ulcerative stomatitis, eructation, amylase increased, anorexia, toothache
  Genitourinary: Urinary tract infection (6%), vaginitis, cystitis
  Hematologic: Anemia
  Local: Abscess
  Neuromuscular & skeletal: Back pain (5%), arthralgia (4%), skeletal pain (3%), rigors (1%), hypertonia, tremor, myalgia, hyporeflexia, leg cramps
  Ocular: Conjunctivitis (4%), abnormal vision, eye pain, eye abnormality, xerophthalmia
  Otic: Earache, otitis media
  Respiratory: Coughing (6%), bronchitis (4%), pneumonia, epistaxis
  Miscellaneous: Flu-like syndrome, infection, fungal infection, allergy, hiccups
Drug Interactions
  Metabolism/Transport Effects Substrate (minor) of CYP2D6, CYP3A4
  Avoid Concomitant Use There are no known interactions where it is recommended to avoid concomitant use.
  Increased Effect/Toxicity
  The levels/effects of Cevimeline may be increased by: Acetylcholinesterase Inhibitors; Conivaptan
  Decreased Effect
  The levels/effects of Cevimeline may be decreased by: Peginterferon Alfa-2b; Tocilizumab
Stability Store at 25°C (77°F).
Mechanism of Action Binds to muscarinic (cholinergic) receptors, causing an increase in secretion of exocrine glands (including salivary glands)
Pharmacodynamics/Kinetics
  Distribution: V_d: 6 L/kg
  Protein binding: <20%
  Metabolism: Hepatic via CYP2D6 and CYP3A4
  Half-life elimination: 5 hours
  Time to peak: 1.5-2 hours
  Excretion: Urine (as metabolites and unchanged drug)

◀ **Dosage**

Geriatric Refer to adult dosing. No specific dosage adjustment is recommended; however, use caution when initiating due to potential for increased sensitivity.

Adult Xerostomia (in Sjögren's syndrome): Oral: 30 mg 3 times/day

Renal Impairment Not studied; no specific dosage adjustment is recommended

Hepatic Impairment Not studied; no specific dosage adjustment is recommended

Administration Administer with or without food.

Monitoring Parameters Vital signs, visual changes

Special Geriatric Considerations No specific studies in the elderly are available. However, elderly often have cardiovascular, pulmonary, and gastrointestinal diseases which may restrict or contraindicate the use of this agent. The use of saliva substitutes should be considered initially. Although the clinical studies included elderly patients (>65 years of age), the number of elderly was insufficient to determine any significant differences between young adults and elderly.

Dosage Forms Excipient information presented when available (limited, particularly for generics); consult specific product labeling.

Capsule, oral, as hydrochloride:

Evoxac®: 30 mg

◆ **Cevimeline Hydrochloride** see Cevimeline on page 328
◆ **CFDN** see Cefdinir on page 292
◆ **CG5503** see Tapentadol on page 1736
◆ **C-Gel [OTC]** see Ascorbic Acid on page 149
◆ **CGP 33101** see Rufinamide on page 1644
◆ **CGP-39393** see Desirudin on page 474
◆ **CGP-42446** see Zoledronic Acid on page 1952
◆ **C-Gram [OTC]** see Ascorbic Acid on page 149
◆ **CGS-20267** see Letrozole on page 1037
◆ **Chantix®** see Varenicline on page 1902
◆ **Cheracol® D [OTC]** see Guaifenesin and Dextromethorphan on page 848
◆ **Cheracol® Plus [OTC]** see Guaifenesin and Dextromethorphan on page 848
◆ **Cheratussin** see GuaiFENesin on page 846
◆ **Chew-C [OTC]** see Ascorbic Acid on page 149
◆ **Chew-Cal [OTC]** see Calcium and Vitamin D on page 248
◆ **Children's Nasal Decongestant [OTC]** see Pseudoephedrine on page 1545
◆ **Chloral** see Chloral Hydrate on page 330

Chloral Hydrate (KLOR al HYE drate)

Medication Safety Issues

High alert medication:

The Institute for Safe Medication Practices (ISMP) includes this medication among its list of drugs which have a heightened risk of causing significant patient harm when used in error.

Brand Names: U.S. Somnote®

Brand Names: Canada PMS-Chloral Hydrate

Index Terms Chloral; Hydrated Chloral; Trichloroacetaldehyde Monohydrate

Generic Availability (U.S.) Yes: Syrup

Pharmacologic Category Hypnotic, Nonbenzodiazepine

Use Short-term sedative and hypnotic (<2 weeks); sedative/hypnotic for diagnostic procedures; sedative prior to EEG evaluations

Dosage

Geriatric Hypnotic: Initial: Oral: 250 mg at bedtime; adjust for renal impairment.

Adult

Sedation, anxiety: Oral: 250 mg 3 times/day

Hypnotic: Oral: 500-1000 mg at bedtime or 30 minutes prior to procedure, not to exceed 2 g/24 hours

Discontinuation: Withdraw gradually over 2 weeks if patient has been maintained on high doses for prolonged period of time. Do not stop drug abruptly; sudden withdrawal may result in delirium.

Renal Impairment

Cl_{cr} <50 mL/minute: Avoid use.

Hemodialysis effects: Supplemental dose is not necessary; dialyzable (50% to 100%).

Hepatic Impairment Avoid use in patients with severe hepatic impairment.

Special Geriatric Considerations Chloral hydrate is not a hypnotic agent of choice in the elderly. Guidelines from the Centers for Medicare and Medicaid Services (CMS) discourage the use of chloral hydrate in residents of long-term care facilities.

Controlled Substance C-IV

Dosage Forms Excipient information presented when available (limited, particularly for generics); consult specific product labeling.

Capsule, oral:

Somnote®: 500 mg

Syrup, oral: 500 mg/5 mL (5 mL, 473 mL)

Chlorambucil (klor AM byoo sil)

Medication Safety Issues

Sound-alike/look-alike issues:

Chlorambucil may be confused with Chloromycetin®

Leukeran® may be confused with Alkeran®, leucovorin, Leukine®, Myleran®

High alert medication:

The Institute for Safe Medication Practices (ISMP) includes this medication among its list of drugs which have a heightened risk of causing significant patient harm when used in error.

Brand Names: U.S. Leukeran®

Brand Names: Canada Leukeran®

Index Terms CB-1348; Chlorambucilum; Chloraminophene; Chlorbutinum; WR-139013

Generic Availability (U.S.) No

Pharmacologic Category Antineoplastic Agent, Alkylating Agent

Use Management of chronic lymphocytic leukemia (CLL), Hodgkin's lymphoma, non-Hodgkin's lymphoma (NHL)

Unlabeled/Investigational Use Nephrotic syndrome, Waldenström's macroglobulinemia

Contraindications Hypersensitivity to chlorambucil or any component of the formulation; hypersensitivity to other alkylating agents (may have cross-hypersensitivity)

Warnings/Precautions Hazardous agent - use appropriate precautions for handling and disposal. Seizures have been observed; use with caution in patients with seizure disorder or head trauma; history of nephrotic syndrome and high pulse doses are at higher risk of seizures. **[U.S. Boxed Warning]: May cause bone marrow suppression;** reduce initial dosage if patient has received myelosuppressive or radiation therapy, or has a depressed baseline leukocyte or platelet count within the previous 4 weeks. Lymphopenia may occur. Avoid administration of live vaccines to immunocompromised patients. Rare instances of severe skin reactions (eg, erythema multiforme, Stevens-Johnson syndrome) have been reported; discontinue if a reaction occurs.

[U.S. Boxed Warning]: Affects human fertility; carcinogenic in humans and probably mutagenic and teratogenic as well; chromosomal damage has been documented. Fertility effects (reversible and irreversible sterility) include azoospermia (when administered to prepubertal and pubertal males) and amenorrhea. Secondary malignancies and acute myelocytic leukemia may be associated with chronic therapy.

Adverse Reactions (Reflective of adult population; not specific for elderly) Frequency not always defined.

Central nervous system: Agitation (rare), ataxia (rare), confusion (rare), drug fever, focal/ generalized seizure (rare), hallucinations (rare)

Dermatologic: Angioneurotic edema, erythema multiforme (rare), rash, skin hypersensitivity, Stevens-Johnson syndrome (rare), toxic epidermal necrolysis (rare), urticaria

Endocrine & metabolic: Amenorrhea, infertility, SIADH (rare)

Gastrointestinal: Diarrhea (infrequent), nausea (infrequent), oral ulceration (infrequent), vomiting (infrequent)

Genitourinary: Azoospermia, cystitis (sterile)

Hematologic: Neutropenia (25%; dose- and duration-related; onset: 3 weeks; recovery: 10 days after last dose), bone marrow failure (irreversible), bone marrow suppression, anemia, leukemia (secondary), leukopenia, lymphopenia, pancytopenia, thrombocytopenia

Hepatic: Hepatotoxicity, jaundice

Neuromuscular & skeletal: Flaccid paresis (rare), muscular twitching (rare), myoclonia (rare), peripheral neuropathy, tremor (rare)

Respiratory: Interstitial pneumonia, pulmonary fibrosis

Miscellaneous: Allergic reactions, malignancies (secondary)

Drug Interactions

Avoid Concomitant Use

Avoid concomitant use of Chlorambucil with any of the following: BCG; Natalizumab; Pimecrolimus; Tacrolimus (Topical); Vaccines (Live)

CHLORAMBUCIL

Increased Effect/Toxicity
Chlorambucil may increase the levels/effects of: Leflunomide; Natalizumab; Vaccines (Live)

The levels/effects of Chlorambucil may be increased by: Denosumab; Pimecrolimus; Roflumilast; Tacrolimus (Topical); Trastuzumab

Decreased Effect
Chlorambucil may decrease the levels/effects of: BCG; Sipuleucel-T; Vaccines (Inactivated); Vaccines (Live)

The levels/effects of Chlorambucil may be decreased by: Echinacea

Stability Store in refrigerator at 2°C to 8°C (36°F to 46°F). Protect from light.

Mechanism of Action Interferes with DNA replication and RNA transcription by alkylation and cross-linking the strands of DNA

Pharmacodynamics/Kinetics
Absorption: Rapid and complete
Distribution: V_d: 0.14-0.24 L/kg
Protein binding: ~99%
Metabolism: Hepatic; forms a major active metabolite (phenylacetic acid mustard) and inactive metabolites
Bioavailability: Reduced 10% to 20% with food
Half-life elimination: ~1.5 hours; Phenylacetic acid mustard: ~1.8 hours
Time to peak, plasma: Within 1 hour; Phenylacetic acid mustard: 1.2-2.6 hours
Excretion: Urine (15% to 60% primarily as inactive metabolites, <1% as unchanged drug or phenylacetic acid mustard)

Dosage
Geriatric
Refer to adult dosing. Begin at the lower end of dosing range(s)
Adult Refer to individual protocols.
CLL, NHL: Oral: 0.1 mg/kg/day for 3-6 weeks **or** 0.4 mg/kg (increased by 0.1mg/kg/dose until response/toxicity observed) biweekly **or** 0.4 mg/kg (increased by 0.1mg/kg/dose until response/toxicity observed) monthly **or** 0.03-0.1 mg/kg/day continuously
Hodgkin's lymphoma: Oral: 0.2 mg/kg/day for 3-6 weeks **or** 0.4 mg/kg (increased by 0.1 mg/kg/dose until response/toxicity observed) biweekly **or** 0.4 mg/kg (increased by 0.1 mg/kg/dose until response/toxicity observed) monthly **or** 0.03-0.1 mg/kg/day continuously
Waldenström's macroglobulinemia (unlabeled use): Oral: 0.1 mg/kg/day (continuously) for at least 6 months **or** 0.3 mg/kg/day for 7 days every 6 weeks for at least 6 months
Renal Impairment The FDA-approved labeling does not contain renal dosing adjustment guidelines. The following guidelines have been used by some clinicians (Aronoff, 2007): Adults:
Cl_{cr} 10-50 mL/minute: Administer 75% of dose
Cl_{cr} <10 mL/minute: Administer 50% of dose
Continuous ambulatory peritoneal dialysis (CAPD): Administer 50% of dose
Hepatic Impairment The FDA-approved labeling does not contain hepatic dosing adjustment guidelines. Chlorambucil is hepatically metabolized into active and inactive metabolites; dosage adjustment may be needed in patients with hepatic impairment.

Administration Usually administered as a single dose; preferably on an empty stomach

Monitoring Parameters Liver function tests, CBC with differential and platelets (weekly, with WBC monitored twice weekly during the first 3-6 weeks of treatment), serum uric acid

Special Geriatric Considerations Toxicity to immunosuppressives is increased in the elderly. Start with lowest recommended adult doses. Signs of infection, such as fever and rise in WBCs, may not occur. Lethargy and confusion may be more prominent signs of infection.

Dosage Forms Excipient information presented when available (limited, particularly for generics); consult specific product labeling.
Tablet, oral:
Leukeran®: 2 mg

♦ **Chlorambucilum** see Chlorambucil *on page 331*
♦ **Chloraminophene** see Chlorambucil *on page 331*

Chloramphenicol (klor am FEN i kole)

Medication Safety Issues
Sound-alike/look-alike issues:
Chloromycetin® may be confused with chlorambucil, Chlor-Trimeton®
Brand Names: Canada Chloromycetin®; Chloromycetin® Succinate; Diochloram®; Pentamycetin®

Generic Availability (U.S.) Yes

Pharmacologic Category Antibiotic, Miscellaneous

Use Treatment of serious infections due to organisms resistant to other less toxic antibiotics or when its penetrability into the site of infection is clinically superior to other antibiotics to which the organism is sensitive; useful in infections caused by *Bacteroides*, *H. influenzae*, *Neisseria meningitidis*, *Salmonella*, and *Rickettsia*; active against many vancomycin-resistant enterococci

Contraindications Hypersensitivity to chloramphenicol or any component of the formulation; treatment of trivial or viral infections; bacterial prophylaxis

Warnings/Precautions Hazardous agent - use appropriate precautions for handling and disposal. Gray syndrome characterized by circulatory collapse, cyanosis, acidosis, abdominal distention, myocardial depression, coma, and death has occurred. Use with caution in patients with impaired renal or hepatic function. Reduce dose with impaired liver function. Use with care in patients with glucose 6-phosphate dehydrogenase deficiency. **[U.S. Boxed Warning]: Serious and fatal blood dyscrasias (aplastic anemia, hypoplastic anemia, thrombocytopenia, and granulocytopenia) have occurred after both short-term and prolonged therapy. Monitor CBC frequently in all patients;** discontinue if evidence of myelosuppression. Irreversible bone marrow suppression may occur weeks or months after therapy. Avoid repeated courses of treatment. Should not be used for minor infections or when less potentially toxic agents are effective. Prolonged use may result in fungal or bacterial superinfection, including *C. difficile*-associated diarrhea (CDAD) and pseudomembranous colitis; CDAD has been observed >2 months postantibiotic treatment.

Adverse Reactions (Reflective of adult population; not specific for elderly) Frequency not defined.

Central nervous system: Confusion, delirium, depression, fever, headache

Dermatologic: Angioedema, rash, urticaria

Gastrointestinal: Diarrhea, enterocolitis, glossitis, nausea, stomatitis, vomiting

Hematologic: Aplastic anemia, bone marrow suppression, granulocytopenia, hypoplastic anemia, pancytopenia, thrombocytopenia

Ocular: Optic neuritis

Miscellaneous: Anaphylaxis, hypersensitivity reactions, Gray syndrome

Drug Interactions

Metabolism/Transport Effects Inhibits CYP2C9 (weak), 3A4 (weak)

Avoid Concomitant Use

Avoid concomitant use of Chloramphenicol with any of the following: BCG

Increased Effect/Toxicity

Chloramphenicol may increase the levels/effects of: Anticonvulsants (Hydantoin); Barbiturates; Sulfonylureas; Vitamin K Antagonists; Voriconazole

Decreased Effect

Chloramphenicol may decrease the levels/effects of: BCG; Cyanocobalamin; Typhoid Vaccine

The levels/effects of Chloramphenicol may be decreased by: Anticonvulsants (Hydantoin); Barbiturates; Rifampin

Ethanol/Nutrition/Herb Interactions Food: May decrease intestinal absorption of vitamin B_{12} may have increased dietary need for riboflavin, pyridoxine, and vitamin B_{12}.

Stability Store at room temperature prior to reconstitution. Reconstituted solutions remain stable for 30 days. Use only clear solutions. Frozen solutions remain stable for 6 months.

Mechanism of Action Reversibly binds to 50S ribosomal subunits of susceptible organisms preventing amino acids from being transferred to growing peptide chains thus inhibiting protein synthesis

Pharmacodynamics/Kinetics

Distribution: To most tissues and body fluids

Chloramphenicol: V_d: 0.5-1 L/kg

Chloramphenicol succinate: V_d: 0.2-3.1 L/kg; decreased with hepatic or renal dysfunction

Protein binding: Chloramphenicol: ~60%; decreased with hepatic or renal dysfunction

Metabolism:

Chloramphenicol: Hepatic to metabolites (inactive)

Chloramphenicol succinate: Hydrolyzed in the liver, kidney and lungs to chloramphenicol (active)

Bioavailability:

Chloramphenicol: Oral: ~80%

Chloramphenicol succinate: I.V.: ~70%; highly variable, dependant upon rate and extent of metabolism to chloramphenicol

Half-life elimination:
  Normal renal function:
    Chloramphenicol: Adults: ~4 hours
    Chloramphenicol succinate: Adults: ~3 hours
  End-stage renal disease: Chloramphenicol: 3-7 hours
  Hepatic disease: Prolonged
Excretion: Urine (~30% as unchanged chloramphenicol succinate in adults; 5% to 15% as chloramphenicol)

Dosage

Geriatric & Adult Systemic infections: I.V.: 50-100 mg/kg/day in divided doses every 6 hours; maximum daily dose: 4 g/day.

Renal Impairment Use with caution; monitor serum concentrations.

Hepatic Impairment Use with caution; monitor serum concentrations.

Administration Do not administer I.M.; can be administered IVP over at least 1 minute at a concentration of 100 mg/mL, or I.V. intermittent infusion over 15-30 minutes at a final concentration for administration of ≤20 mg/mL

Monitoring Parameters CBC with differential (baseline and every 2 days during therapy), periodic liver and renal function tests, serum drug concentration

Reference Range
Therapeutic levels:
  Meningitis:
    Peak: 15-25 mcg/mL; toxic concentration: >40 mcg/mL
    Trough: 5-15 mcg/mL
  Other infections:
    Peak: 10-20 mcg/mL
    Trough: 5-10 mcg/mL
Timing of serum samples: Draw levels 0.5-1.5 hours after completion of I.V. dose

Test Interactions May cause false-positive results in urine glucose tests when using cupric sulfate (Benedict's solution, Clinitest®).

Pharmacotherapy Pearls Sodium content of 1 g (injection): 51.8 mg (2.25 mEq)

Special Geriatric Considerations Chloramphenicol has not been studied in the elderly. It is not necessary to adjust the dose based upon the decrease in renal function associated with age. Chloramphenicol should be reserved for serious infections and the oral form avoided.

Dosage Forms Excipient information presented when available (limited, particularly for generics); consult specific product labeling.
Injection, powder for reconstitution: 1 g [contains sodium [~52 mg (2.25 mEq)/g]]

Selected References

Aronoff GR, Bennett WM, Berns JS, et al, *Drug Prescribing in Renal Failure: Dosing Guidelines for Adults and Children*, 5th ed. Philadelphia, PA: American College of Physicians; 2007.

Nahata MC and Powell DA, "Bioavailability and Clearance of Chloramphenicol After Intravenous Chloramphenicol Succinate," *Clin Pharmacol Ther*, 1981, 30(3):368-72.

Powell DA and Nahata MC, "Chloramphenicol: New Perspectives on an Old Drug," *Drug Intell Clin Pharm*, 1982, 16 (4):295-300.

Vozeh S, Schmidlin O, and Taeschner W, "Pharmacokinetic Drug Data," *Clin Pharmacokinet*, 1988, 15(4):254-82.

Yoshikawa TT, "Antimicrobial Therapy for the Elderly Patient," *J Am Geriatr Soc*, 1990, 38(12):1353-72.

◆ **Chlorbutinum** *see* Chlorambucil *on page 331*

ChlordiazePOXIDE (klor dye az e POKS ide)

Related Information

Anxiolytic, Sedative / Hypnotic, and Miscellaneous Benzodiazepines *on page 2000*
Beers Criteria – Potentially Inappropriate Medications for Geriatrics *on page 2089*

Medication Safety Issues
Sound-alike/look-alike issues:
  ChlordiazePOXIDE may be confused with chlorproMAZINE
  Librium may be confused with Librax®
BEERS Criteria medication:
  This drug may be inappropriate for use in geriatric patients (high severity risk).

Brand Names: Canada Apo-Chlordiazepoxide®

Index Terms Librium; Methaminodiazepoxide Hydrochloride

Generic Availability (U.S.) Yes

Pharmacologic Category Benzodiazepine

Use Management of anxiety disorder or for the short-term relief of symptoms of anxiety; withdrawal symptoms of acute alcoholism; preoperative apprehension and anxiety

Contraindications Hypersensitivity to chlordiazepoxide or any component of the formulation (cross-sensitivity with other benzodiazepines may also exist); narrow-angle glaucoma

Warnings/Precautions Active metabolites with extended half-lives may lead to delayed accumulation and adverse effects. Use with caution in elderly or debilitated patients, patients with hepatic disease (including alcoholics) or renal impairment, patients with respiratory disease or impaired gag reflex, patients with porphyria.

Parenteral administration should be avoided in comatose patients or shock. Adequate resuscitative equipment/personnel should be available, and appropriate monitoring should be conducted at the time of injection and for several hours following administration. The parenteral formulation should be diluted for I.M. administration with the supplied diluent only. This diluent should not be used when preparing the drug for intravenous administration.

Causes CNS depression (dose related) resulting in sedation, dizziness, confusion, or ataxia which may impair physical and mental capabilities. Patients must be cautioned about performing tasks which require mental alertness (eg, operating machinery or driving). Use with caution in patients receiving other CNS depressants or psychoactive agents (lithium, phenothiazines). Effects with other sedative drugs or ethanol may be potentiated. Benzodiazepines have been associated with falls and traumatic injury and should be used with extreme caution in patients who are at risk of these events (especially the elderly). Benzodiazepines with long half-lives may produce prolonged sedation and increase the risk of falls and fracture. Short- or intermediate-acting benzodiazepines are preferred in elderly patients (Beers Criteria).

Use caution in patients with depression, particularly if suicidal risk may be present. Use with caution in patients with a history of drug dependence. Benzodiazepines have been associated with dependence and acute withdrawal symptoms on discontinuation or reduction in dose. Acute withdrawal, including seizures, may be precipitated in patients after administration of flumazenil to patients receiving long-term benzodiazepine therapy.

Benzodiazepines have been associated with anterograde amnesia. Paradoxical reactions, including hyperactive or aggressive behavior have been reported with benzodiazepines, particularly in psychiatric patients. Does not have analgesic, antidepressant, or antipsychotic properties.

Adverse Reactions (Reflective of adult population; not specific for elderly)
>10%:
Central nervous system: Drowsiness, fatigue, ataxia, lightheadedness, memory impairment, dysarthria, irritability
Dermatologic: Rash
Endocrine & metabolic: Libido decreased, menstrual disorders
Gastrointestinal: Xerostomia, salivation decreased, appetite increased or decreased, weight gain/loss
Genitourinary: Micturition difficulties
1% to 10%:
Cardiovascular: Hypotension
Central nervous system: Confusion, dizziness, disinhibition, akathisia
Dermatologic: Dermatitis
Endocrine & metabolic: Libido increased
Gastrointestinal: Salivation increased
Genitourinary: Sexual dysfunction, incontinence
Neuromuscular & skeletal: Rigidity, tremor, muscle cramps
Otic: Tinnitus
Respiratory: Nasal congestion

Drug Interactions
Metabolism/Transport Effects Substrate of CYP3A4 (major)
Avoid Concomitant Use
Avoid concomitant use of ChlordiazePOXIDE with any of the following: Conivaptan; OLANZapine

Increased Effect/Toxicity
ChlordiazePOXIDE may increase the levels/effects of: Alcohol (Ethyl); CloZAPine; CNS Depressants; Fosphenytoin; Methotrimeprazine; Phenytoin; Selective Serotonin Reuptake Inhibitors

The levels/effects of ChlordiazePOXIDE may be increased by: Antifungal Agents (Azole Derivatives, Systemic); Aprepitant; Calcium Channel Blockers (Nondihydropyridine); Cimetidine; Conivaptan; Contraceptives (Estrogens); Contraceptives (Progestins); CYP3A4 Inhibitors (Moderate); CYP3A4 Inhibitors (Strong); Dasatinib; Disulfiram; Droperidol; Fluconazole; Fosaprepitant; Grapefruit Juice; HydrOXYzine; Isoniazid; Macrolide Antibiotics; MAO Inhibitors; Methotrimeprazine; Nefazodone; OLANZapine; Proton Pump Inhibitors; Selective Serotonin Reuptake Inhibitors

◀ **Decreased Effect**
The levels/effects of ChlordiazePOXIDE may be decreased by: CarBAMazepine; CYP3A4 Inducers (Strong); Deferasirox; Rifamycin Derivatives; St Johns Wort; Theophylline Derivatives; Tocilizumab; Yohimbine

Ethanol/Nutrition/Herb Interactions
Ethanol: May increase CNS depression; monitor for increased effects with coadministration. Caution patients about effects.
Food: Serum concentrations/effects may be increased with grapefruit juice, but unlikely because of high oral bioavailability of chlordiazepoxide.
Herb/Nutraceutical: Avoid valerian, St John's wort, kava kava, gotu kola (may increase CNS depression).

Stability Injection: Prior to reconstitution, store under refrigeration and protect from light. Solution should be used immediately following reconstitution.

I.M. use: Reconstitute by adding 2 mL of provided diluent; agitate gently until dissolved. Provided diluent is **not** for I.V. use.
I.V. use: Reconstitute by adding 5 mL NS or SWFI; agitate gently until dissolved; **do not administer this dilution I.M.**

Mechanism of Action Binds to stereospecific benzodiazepine receptors on the postsynaptic GABA neuron at several sites within the central nervous system, including the limbic system, reticular formation. Enhancement of the inhibitory effect of GABA on neuronal excitability results by increased neuronal membrane permeability to chloride ions. This shift in chloride ions results in hyperpolarization (a less excitable state) and stabilization.

Pharmacodynamics/Kinetics
Absorption: I.M.: Slow and erratic
Distribution: V_d: 3.3 L/kg
Protein binding: 90% to 98%
Metabolism: Extensive in the liver to desmethyldiazepam (active and long-acting)
Half-life: 5-30 hours; increased in older adults and in severe liver disease; desmethyldiazepam has a half-life of 50-100 hours and can be prolonged in older adults
Time to peak serum concentration: Oral: Within 2 hours. I.M.: Results in lower peak plasma concentrations than oral administration.

Dosage
Geriatric Anxiety: Oral: 5 mg 2-4 times/day; adjust for renal impairment. Avoid use if possible.
Adult
Anxiety:
Oral: 15-100 mg divided 3-4 times/day
I.M., I.V.: Initial: 50-100 mg followed by 25-50 mg 3-4 times/day as needed
Preoperative anxiety: I.M.: 50-100 mg prior to surgery
Ethanol withdrawal symptoms: Oral, I.V.: 50-100 mg to start, dose may be repeated in 2-4 hours as necessary to a maximum of 300 mg/24 hours
Note: Up to 300 mg may be given I.M. or I.V. during a 6-hour period, but not more than this in any 24-hour period.
Renal Impairment
Cl_{cr} <10 mL/minute: Administer 50% of dose.
Not dialyzable (0% to 5%)
Hepatic Impairment Avoid use.

Administration I.V. form is a powder and should be reconstituted with 5 mL of sterile water or saline prior to administration; do not use diluent provided with ampul for I.V. administration.

Monitoring Parameters Respiratory, cardiovascular and mental status; check for orthostasis

Reference Range Therapeutic: 0.1-3 mcg/mL (SI: 0-10 μmol/L); Toxic: >23 mcg/mL (SI: >77 μmol/L)

Pharmacotherapy Pearls Abrupt discontinuation after sustained use (generally >10 days) may cause withdrawal symptoms.

Special Geriatric Considerations Due to its long-acting metabolite, chlordiazepoxide is not considered a drug of choice in the elderly. Long-acting benzodiazepines have been associated with falls in the elderly; interpretive guidelines from the Centers for Medicare and Medicaid Services (CMS) discourage the use of this agent in residents of long-term care facilities.

This medication is considered to be potentially inappropriate in this patient population (Beers Criteria severity: High).

Controlled Substance C-IV

Dosage Forms Excipient information presented when available (limited, particularly for generics); consult specific product labeling.
Capsule, oral, as hydrochloride: 5 mg, 10 mg, 25 mg

Selected References

Hicks R, Dysken MW, Davis JM, et al, "The Pharmacokinetics of Psychotropic Medication in the Elderly: A Review," *J Clin Psychiatry*, 1981, 42(10):374-85.

Reidenberg MM, Levy M, Warner H, et al, "Relationship Between Diazepam Dose, Plasma Level, Age, and Central Nervous System Depression," *Clin Pharmacol Ther*, 1978, 23(4):371-4.

♦ **Chlordiazepoxide and Clidinium** *see* Clidinium and Chlordiazepoxide *on page 376*
♦ **Chlor Hist [OTC]** *see* Chlorpheniramine *on page 337*
♦ **Chlormeprazine** *see* Prochlorperazine *on page 1524*

Chlorothiazide (klor oh THYE a zide)

Medication Safety Issues
International issues:
Diuril: Brand name for chlorothiazide [U.S., Canada], but also the brand name for furosemide [Philippines]
Diuril [U.S., Canada] may be confused with Duorol brand name for acetaminophen [Spain]
Brand Names: U.S. Diuril®; Sodium Diuril®
Brand Names: Canada Diuril®
Generic Availability (U.S.) Yes: Excludes oral suspension
Pharmacologic Category Diuretic, Thiazide
Use Management of mild-to-moderate hypertension; adjunctive treatment of edema
Dosage
Geriatric Oral: 500 mg once daily **or** 1 g 3 times/week
Adult Note: The manufacturer states that I.V. and oral dosing are equivalent. Some clinicians may use lower I.V. doses; however, because of chlorothiazide's poor oral absorption.

Hypertension: Oral: 500-2000 mg/day divided in 1-2 doses (manufacturer labeling); doses of 125-500 mg/day have also been recommended (JNC 7)
Edema: Oral, I.V.: 500-1000 mg once or twice daily; intermittent treatment (eg, therapy on alternative days) may be appropriate for some patients
ACC/AHA 2009 Heart Failure guidelines:
Oral: 250-500 mg once or twice daily (maximum daily dose: 1000 mg)
I.V.: 500-1000 mg once or twice daily plus a loop diuretic
Renal Impairment Cl_{cr} <10 mL/minute: Avoid use. Ineffective with Cl_{cr} <30 mL/minute unless in combination with a loop diuretic (Aronoff, 2007)
Note: ACC/AHA 2009 Heart Failure Guidelines suggest that thiazides lose their efficacy when Cl_{cr} <40 mL/minute
Special Geriatric Considerations Chlorothiazide is minimally effective in patients with a Cl_{cr} <30 mL/minute. This may limit the usefulness of chlorothiazide in the elderly.
Dosage Forms Excipient information presented when available (limited, particularly for generics); consult specific product labeling.
Injection, powder for reconstitution, as sodium [strength expressed as base]: 500 mg
Sodium Diuril®: 0.5 g
Suspension, oral:
Diuril®: 250 mg/5 mL (237 mL) [contains benzoic acid, ethanol 0.5%]
Tablet, oral: 250 mg, 500 mg

♦ **Chlorphen [OTC]** *see* Chlorpheniramine *on page 337*

Chlorpheniramine (klor fen IR a meen)

Related Information
Beers Criteria – Potentially Inappropriate Medications for Geriatrics *on page 2089*
Medication Safety Issues
Sound-alike/look-alike issues:
Chlor-Trimeton® may be confused with Chloromycetin®
BEERS Criteria medication:
This drug may be inappropriate for use in geriatric patients (high severity risk).
Brand Names: U.S. Ahist™; Aller-Chlor® [OTC]; Chlor Hist [OTC]; Chlor-Trimeton® Allergy [OTC]; Chlorphen [OTC]; Diabetic Tussin® for Children Allergy Relief [OTC]; Ed Chlorped [DSC]; Ed-Chlortan; P-Tann [DSC]; Teldrin® HBP [OTC]
Brand Names: Canada Chlor-Tripolon®; Novo-Pheniram
Index Terms Chlorpheniramine Maleate; CTM
Generic Availability (U.S.) Yes: Syrup, tablet
Pharmacologic Category Alkylamine Derivative; Histamine H_1 Antagonist; Histamine H_1 Antagonist, First Generation
Use Perennial and seasonal allergic rhinitis and other allergic symptoms including urticaria

◀ **Contraindications** Hypersensitivity to chlorpheniramine maleate or any component of the formulation; narrow-angle glaucoma; bladder neck obstruction; symptomatic prostate hypertrophy; during acute asthmatic attacks; stenosing peptic ulcer; pyloroduodenal obstruction.

Warnings/Precautions Causes sedation, caution must be used in performing tasks which require alertness (eg, operating machinery or driving). Sedative effects of CNS depressants or ethanol are potentiated. Use with caution in patients with urinary tract obstruction, symptomatic prostatic hyperplasia, thyroid dysfunction, increased intraocular pressure, and cardiovascular disease (including hypertension and ischemic heart disease). May be inappropriate for use in elderly due to potent anticholinergic effects; nonanticholinergic antihistamines preferred for treating allergic reactions (Beers Criteria).

Adverse Reactions (Reflective of adult population; not specific for elderly)

>10%:

Central nervous system: Slight to moderate drowsiness

Respiratory: Thickening of bronchial secretions

1% to 10%:

Central nervous system: Headache, excitability, fatigue, nervousness, dizziness

Gastrointestinal: Nausea, xerostomia, diarrhea, abdominal pain, appetite increase, weight gain

Genitourinary: Urinary retention

Neuromuscular & skeletal: Arthralgia, weakness

Ocular: Diplopia

Renal: Polyuria

Respiratory: Pharyngitis

Drug Interactions

Metabolism/Transport Effects Substrate of CYP2D6 (minor), 3A4 (major); **Inhibits** CYP2D6 (weak)

Avoid Concomitant Use

Avoid concomitant use of Chlorpheniramine with any of the following: Conivaptan

Increased Effect/Toxicity

Chlorpheniramine may increase the levels/effects of: Alcohol (Ethyl); Anticholinergics; CNS Depressants; Selective Serotonin Reuptake Inhibitors

The levels/effects of Chlorpheniramine may be increased by: Conivaptan; CYP3A4 Inhibitors (Moderate); CYP3A4 Inhibitors (Strong); Dasatinib; Droperidol; HydrOXYzine; Pramlintide

Decreased Effect

Chlorpheniramine may decrease the levels/effects of: Acetylcholinesterase Inhibitors (Central); Benzylpenicilloyl Polylysine; Betahistine

The levels/effects of Chlorpheniramine may be decreased by: Acetylcholinesterase Inhibitors (Central); Amphetamines; Peginterferon Alfa-2b; Tocilizumab

Ethanol/Nutrition/Herb Interactions Ethanol: May increase CNS depression; monitor for increased effects with coadministration. Caution patients about effects.

Stability Protect from light.

Mechanism of Action Competes with histamine for H_1-receptor sites on effector cells in the gastrointestinal tract, blood vessels, and respiratory tract

Pharmacodynamics/Kinetics

Protein binding: 69% to 72%

Metabolism: In the liver

Half-life: 20-24 hours; one study found no significant difference in the half-life in older adult subjects though there was wide interindividual variation

Elimination: Metabolites and parent drug (3% to 4%) excreted in urine; 35% of total within 48 hours

Dosage

Geriatric Allergic symptoms, rhinitis: Oral: 4 mg once or twice daily, or 8 mg sustained release at bedtime. **Note:** Duration of action may be 36 hours or more when serum concentrations are low.

Adult Allergic symptoms, allergic rhinitis: Oral: 4 mg every 4-6 hours, not to exceed 24 mg/day or sustained release 8-12 mg every 8-12 hours, not to exceed 24 mg/day

Renal Impairment Hemodialysis: Supplemental dose is not necessary.

Administration Do not crush sustained release tablet

Monitoring Parameters Relief of symptoms

Pharmacotherapy Pearls Not effective for nasal stuffiness.

Special Geriatric Considerations Anticholinergic action may cause significant confusional symptoms, constipation, or problems voiding urine. If an antihistamine is indicated, a second generation nonsedating antihistamine would be a more appropriate choice.

This medication is considered to be potentially inappropriate in this patient population (Beers Criteria severity: High).

Dosage Forms Excipient information presented when available (limited, particularly for generics); consult specific product labeling. [DSC] = Discontinued product

Suspension, oral, as tannate:
  P-Tann: 8 mg/5 mL (473 mL [DSC]) [sugar free; contains sodium benzoate; bubblegum flavor]

Suspension, oral, as tannate [drops]:
  Ed Chlorped: 2 mg/mL (60 mL [DSC])

Syrup, oral, as maleate:
  Aller-Chlor®: 2 mg/5 mL (118 mL) [contains ethanol 5%, propylene glycol]
  Diabetic Tussin® for Children Allergy Relief: 2 mg/5 mL (118 mL) [dye free, ethanol free, sugar free; contains phenylalanine 8.4 mg/5 mL]

Tablet, oral, as maleate: 4 mg
  Aller-Chlor®: 4 mg [scored]
  Chlor Hist: 4 mg
  Chlor-Trimeton® Allergy: 4 mg
  Chlorphen: 4 mg
  Ed-Chlortan: 4 mg [scored]
  Teldrin® HBP: 4 mg

Tablet, extended release, oral, as maleate:
  Chlor-Trimeton® Allergy: 12 mg

Tablet, long acting, oral, as tannate:
  Ahist™: 12 mg [scored]

Selected References

Simons KJ, Martin TJ, Watson WT, et al, "Pharmacokinetics and Pharmacodynamics of Terfenadine and Chlorpheniramine in the Elderly," *J Allergy Clin Immunol*, 1990, 85(3):540-7.

◆ **Chlorpheniramine Maleate** *see* Chlorpheniramine *on page* 337

ChlorproMAZINE (klor PROE ma zeen)

Related Information
  Antipsychotic Agents *on page 1997*
  Beers Criteria – Potentially Inappropriate Medications for Geriatrics *on page 2089*
  Liquid Compatibility of Antidepressants, Antipsychotics, and Mood Stabilizers *on page 2111*
Medication Safety Issues
  Sound-alike/look-alike issues:
  ChlorproMAZINE may be confused with chlordiazePOXIDE, chlorproPAMIDE, clomiPRAMINE, prochlorperazine, promethazine
  Thorazine® may be confused with thiamine, thioridazine
Brand Names: Canada Largactil®; Novo-Chlorpromazine
Index Terms Chlorpromazine Hydrochloride; CPZ; Thorazine
Generic Availability (U.S.) Yes
Pharmacologic Category Antimanic Agent; Antipsychotic Agent, Typical, Phenothiazine
Use Control of mania; treatment of schizophrenia; control of nausea and vomiting; relief of restlessness and apprehension before surgery; acute intermittent porphyria; adjunct in the treatment of tetanus; intractable hiccups
Unlabeled/Investigational Use Management of psychotic disorders; behavioral symptoms associated with dementia (elderly); psychosis/agitation related to Alzheimer's dementia
Contraindications Hypersensitivity to chlorpromazine or any component of the formulation (cross-reactivity between phenothiazines may occur); severe CNS depression; coma
Warnings/Precautions [U.S. Boxed Warning]: Elderly patients with dementia-related psychosis treated with antipsychotics are at an increased risk of death compared to placebo. Most deaths appeared to be either cardiovascular (eg, heart failure, sudden death) or infectious (eg, pneumonia) in nature. Chlorpromazine is not approved for the treatment of dementia-related psychosis. Highly sedating, use with caution in disorders where CNS depression is a feature and in patients with Parkinson's disease. Use with caution in patients with hemodynamic instability, predisposition to seizures, subcortical brain damage, severe cardiac, hepatic, or renal disease. Use caution in respiratory disease (eg, severe asthma, emphysema) due to potential for CNS effects.

◀ Leukopenia, neutropenia, and agranulocytosis (sometimes fatal) have been reported in clinical trials and postmarketing reports with antipsychotic use; presence of risk factors (eg, pre-existing low WBC or history of drug-induced leuko/neutropenia) should prompt periodic blood count assessment. Discontinue therapy at first signs of blood dyscrasias or if absolute neutrophil count <1000/mm^3.

Esophageal dysmotility and aspiration have been associated with antipsychotic use; use with caution in patients at risk of aspiration pneumonia (ie, Alzheimer's disease). Use associated with increased prolactin levels; clinical significance of hyperprolactinemia in patients with breast cancer or other prolactin-dependent tumors is unknown. May alter temperature regulation or mask toxicity of other drugs due to antiemetic effects. May alter cardiac conduction; life-threatening arrhythmias have occurred with therapeutic doses of neuroleptics. May cause QT prolongation and subsequent torsade de pointes; avoid use in patients with diagnosed or suspected congenital long QT syndrome. Avoid concurrent use with other drugs known to prolong QT$_c$ interval.

Use with caution in patients at risk of hypotension (orthostasis is common) or those who would tolerate transient hypotensive episodes (cerebrovascular disease, cardiovascular disease, or other medications which may predispose). Significant hypotension may occur, particularly with parenteral administration. Injection contains sulfites.

Use with caution in patients with decreased gastrointestinal motility, urinary retention, BPH, xerostomia, or visual problems (ie, narrow-angle glaucoma), and myasthenia gravis. Relative to other neuroleptics, chlorpromazine has a moderate potency of cholinergic blockade. May cause pigmentary retinopathy, and lenticular and corneal deposits, particularly with prolonged therapy.

May cause extrapyramidal symptoms (EPS), including pseudoparkinsonism, acute dystonic reactions, akathisia, and tardive dyskinesia. Risk of dystonia (and possibly other EPS) may be greater with increased doses, use of conventional antipsychotics, males, and younger patients. May cause neuroleptic malignant syndrome (NMS). Use with caution in the elderly.

Adverse Reactions (Reflective of adult population; not specific for elderly) Frequency not defined.

Cardiovascular: Postural hypotension, tachycardia, dizziness, nonspecific QT changes

Central nervous system: Drowsiness, dystonias, akathisia, pseudoparkinsonism, tardive dyskinesia, neuroleptic malignant syndrome, seizure

Dermatologic: Photosensitivity, dermatitis, skin pigmentation (slate gray)

Endocrine & metabolic: Lactation, breast engorgement, false-positive pregnancy test, amenorrhea, gynecomastia, hyper- or hypoglycemia

Gastrointestinal: Xerostomia, constipation, nausea

Genitourinary: Urinary retention, ejaculatory disorder, impotence

Hematologic: Agranulocytosis, eosinophilia, leukopenia, hemolytic anemia, aplastic anemia, thrombocytopenic purpura

Hepatic: Jaundice

Ocular: Blurred vision, corneal and lenticular changes, epithelial keratopathy, pigmentary retinopathy

Drug Interactions

Metabolism/Transport Effects Substrate of CYP1A2 (minor), 2D6 (major), 3A4 (minor); **Inhibits** CYP2D6 (strong), 2E1 (weak)

Avoid Concomitant Use

Avoid concomitant use of ChlorproMAZINE with any of the following: Artemether; Dronedarone; Lumefantrine; Metoclopramide; Nilotinib; Pimozide; QUEtiapine; QuiNINE; Tetrabenazine; Thioridazine; Toremifene; Vandetanib; Vemurafenib; Ziprasidone

Increased Effect/Toxicity

ChlorproMAZINE may increase the levels/effects of: Alcohol (Ethyl); Analgesics (Opioid); Anticholinergics; Anti-Parkinson's Agents (Dopamine Agonist); Beta-Blockers; CNS Depressants; CYP2D6 Substrates; Desmopressin; Divalproex; Dronedarone; Fesoterodine; Haloperidol; Methylphenidate; Pimozide; Porfimer; QTc-Prolonging Agents; QuiNINE; Selective Serotonin Reuptake Inhibitors; Tamoxifen; Tetrabenazine; Thioridazine; Toremifene; Valproic Acid; Vandetanib; Vemurafenib; Ziprasidone

The levels/effects of ChlorproMAZINE may be increased by: Abiraterone Acetate; Acetylcholinesterase Inhibitors (Central); Alfuzosin; Antimalarial Agents; Artemether; Beta-Blockers; Chloroquine; Ciprofloxacin; Ciprofloxacin (Systemic); Conivaptan; CYP2D6 Inhibitors (Moderate); CYP2D6 Inhibitors (Strong); Darunavir; Gadobutrol; Haloperidol; Lithium formulations; Lumefantrine; Methylphenidate; Metoclopramide; Nilotinib; Pramlintide; QUEtiapine; QuiNINE; Tetrabenazine

Decreased Effect

ChlorproMAZINE may decrease the levels/effects of: Amphetamines; Quinagolide

The levels/effects of ChlorproMAZINE may be decreased by: Antacids; Anti-Parkinson's Agents (Dopamine Agonist); Cyproterone; Lithium formulations; Peginterferon Alfa-2b; Tocilizumab

Ethanol/Nutrition/Herb Interactions

Ethanol: May increase CNS depression; monitor for increased effects with coadministration. Caution patients about effects.

Herb/Nutraceutical: Avoid St John's wort (may decrease chlorpromazine levels, increase photosensitization, or enhance sedative effect). Avoid dong quai (may enhance photosensitization). Avoid kava kava, gotu kola, valerian (may increase CNS depression).

Stability Injection: Protect from light. A slightly yellowed solution does not indicate potency loss, but a markedly discolored solution should be discarded. Diluted injection (1 mg/mL) with NS and stored in 5 mL vials remains stable for 30 days.

Mechanism of Action Chlorpromazine is an aliphatic phenothiazine antipsychotic which blocks postsynaptic mesolimbic dopaminergic receptors in the brain; exhibits a strong alpha-adrenergic blocking effect and depresses the release of hypothalamic and hypophyseal hormones; believed to depress the reticular activating system, thus affecting basal metabolism, body temperature, wakefulness, vasomotor tone, and emesis

Pharmacodynamics/Kinetics

Onset of action: I.M.: 15 minutes; Oral: 30-60 minutes

Absorption: Rapid

Distribution: V_d: 20 L/kg

Protein binding: 92% to 97%

Metabolism: Extensively hepatic to active and inactive metabolites

Bioavailability: 20%

Half-life, biphasic: Initial: 2 hours; Terminal: 30 hours

Excretion: Urine (<1% as unchanged drug) within 24 hours

Dosage

Geriatric

Behavioral symptoms associated with dementia (unlabeled use): Initial: 10-25 mg 1-2 times/day; increase at 4- to 7-day intervals by 10-25 mg/day. Increase dose intervals (eg, twice daily, 3 times/day) as necessary to control behavior response or side effects; maximum daily dose: 800 mg; gradual increases (titration) may prevent some side effects or decrease their severity.

Other indications: Refer to adult dosing.

Adult

Schizophrenia/psychoses:

Oral: Range: 30-800 mg/day in 1-4 divided doses, initiate at lower doses and titrate as needed; usual dose: 200-600 mg/day; some patients may require 1-2 g/day

I.M., I.V.: Initial: 25 mg, may repeat (25-50 mg) in 1-4 hours, gradually increase to a maximum of 400 mg/dose every 4-6 hours until patient is controlled; usual dose: 300-800 mg/day

Intractable hiccups:

Oral, I.M.: 25-50 mg 3-4 times/day

I.V. (refractory to oral or I.M. treatment): 25-50 mg via slow I.V. infusion

Nausea and vomiting:

Oral: 10-25 mg every 4-6 hours

I.M., I.V.: 25-50 mg every 4-6 hours

Renal Impairment Not dialyzable (0% to 5%)

Hepatic Impairment Avoid use in severe hepatic dysfunction.

Administration Do not administer SubQ (tissue damage and irritation may occur); for direct I.V. injection: Dilute with normal saline to a maximum concentration of 1 mg/mL, administer slow I.V. at a rate not to exceed 1 mg/minute in adults. For treatment of intractable hiccups the manufacturer recommends diluting 25-50 mg of chlorpromazine in 500-1000 ml of normal saline. To reduce the risk of hypotension, patients receiving I.V. chlorpromazine must remain lying down during and for 30 minutes after the injection. **Note:** Avoid skin contact with solution; may cause contact dermatitis.

Monitoring Parameters Monitor orthostatic blood pressures 3-5 days after initiation of therapy or a dose increase; tremors, gait changes, abnormal movement in trunk, neck, buccal area, or extremities; monitor target behaviors for which the agent is given

Reference Range

Therapeutic: 50-300 ng/mL (SI: 157-942 nmol/L)

Toxic: >750 ng/mL (SI: >2355 nmol/L); serum concentrations poorly correlate with expected response

Test Interactions False-positives for phenylketonuria, amylase, uroporphyrins, urobilinogen.

◄ **Special Geriatric Considerations** Many elderly patients receive antipsychotic medications for inappropriate nonpsychotic behavior. Before initiating antipsychotic medication, the clinician should investigate any possible reversible cause; any stress or stress from any disease can cause acute "confusion" or worsening of baseline nonpsychotic behavior. Most commonly acute changes in behavior are due to increases in drug dose or addition of new drug to regimen; fluid electrolyte loss; infections; and changes in environment.

Any changes in disease status in any organ system can result in behavior changes.

In the treatment of agitated, demented, elderly patients, authors of meta-analysis of controlled trials of the response to the traditional antipsychotics (phenothiazines, butyrophenones) in controlling agitation have concluded that the use of neuroleptics results in a response rate of 18%. Clearly neuroleptic therapy for behavior control should be limited with frequent attempts to withdraw the agent given for behavior control.

Dosage Forms Excipient information presented when available (limited, particularly for generics); consult specific product labeling.

Injection, solution, as hydrochloride: 25 mg/mL (1 mL, 2 mL)

Tablet, oral, as hydrochloride: 10 mg, 25 mg, 50 mg, 100 mg, 200 mg

Selected References

Rabins PV, Blacker D, Rovner BW, et al, "Practice Guidelines for the Treatment of Patients With Alzheimer's Disease and Other Dementias," *Am J Psychiatry*, 2007, 164(12 Suppl):5-56. Available at http://www.psych.org/psych_pract/treatg/pg/prac_guide.cfm.

Saltz BL, Woerner MG, Kane JM, et al, "Prospective Study of Tardive Dyskinesia Incidence in the Elderly," *JAMA*, 1991, 266(17):2402-6.

Schneider LS, Tariot PN, Dagerman KS, et al, "Effectiveness of Atypical Antipsychotic Drugs in Patients With Alzheimer's Disease," *N Engl J Med*, 2006, 355(15):1525-38.

◆ **Chlorpromazine Hydrochloride** *see* ChlorproMAZINE *on page 339*

ChlorproPAMIDE (klor PROE pa mide)

Related Information

Beers Criteria – Potentially Inappropriate Medications for Geriatrics *on page 2089*

Diabetes Mellitus Management, Adults *on page 2073*

Medication Safety Issues

Sound-alike/look-alike issues:

ChlorproPAMIDE may be confused with chlorproMAZINE

Diabinese® may be confused with DiaBeta®, Dialume®, Diamox®

High alert medication:

The Institute for Safe Medication Practices (ISMP) includes this medication among its list of drugs which have a heightened risk of causing significant patient harm when used in error.

BEERS Criteria medication:

This drug may be inappropriate for use in geriatric patients (high severity risk).

Brand Names: Canada Apo-Chlorpropamide®; Novo-Propamide

Generic Availability (U.S.) Yes

Pharmacologic Category Antidiabetic Agent, Sulfonylurea

Use Management of blood sugar in type 2 diabetes mellitus (noninsulin dependent, NIDDM)

Unlabeled/Investigational Use Treatment of neurogenic diabetes insipidus

Contraindications Hypersensitivity to chlorpropamide, sulfonylureas, sulfonamides, or any component of the formulation; type 1 diabetes mellitus (insulin dependent, IDDM); diabetic ketoacidosis

Warnings/Precautions All sulfonylurea drugs are capable of producing severe hypoglycemia. Hypoglycemia is more likely to occur when caloric intake is deficient, after severe or prolonged exercise, when ethanol is ingested, or when more than one glucose-lowering drug is used. It is also more likely in elderly patients, malnourished patients and in patients with impaired renal or hepatic function; use with caution. May be inappropriate for use in the elderly due to prolonged half-life/hypoglycemia and risk of causing SIADH (Beers Criteria).

Loss of efficacy may be observed following prolonged use as a result of the progression of type 2 diabetes mellitus which results in continued beta cell destruction. In patients who were previously responding to sulfonylurea therapy, consider additional factors which may be contributing to decreased efficacy (eg, inappropriate dose, nonadherence to diet and exercise regimen). If no contributing factors can be identified, consider discontinuing use of the sulfonylurea due to secondary failure of treatment. Additional antidiabetic therapy (eg, insulin) will be required. It may be necessary to discontinue therapy and administer insulin if the patient is exposed to stress (fever, trauma, infection, surgery).

Chemical similarities are present among sulfonamides, sulfonylureas, carbonic anhydrase inhibitors, thiazides, and loop diuretics (except ethacrynic acid). Use in patients with sulfonylurea or sulfonamide allergy is specifically contraindicated in product labeling, however, a risk of cross-reaction exists in patients with allergy to any of these compounds; avoid use when previous reaction has been severe. Patients with G6PD deficiency may be at an increased risk of sulfonylurea-induced hemolytic anemia; however, cases have also been described in patients without G6PD deficiency during postmarketing surveillance. Use with caution and consider a nonsulfonylurea alternative in patients with G6PD deficiency.

Product labeling states oral hypoglycemic drugs may be associated with an increased cardiovascular mortality as compared to treatment with diet alone or diet plus insulin. Data to support this association are limited, and several studies, including a large prospective trial (UKPDS) have not supported an association.

Adverse Reactions (Reflective of adult population; not specific for elderly) Frequency not defined.
Central nervous system: Dizziness, headache
Dermatologic: Erythema multiforme, exfoliative dermatitis, maculopapular eruptions, photosensitivity, pruritus, urticaria
Endocrine & metabolic: Disulfiram-like reactions, hypoglycemia, SIADH
Gastrointestinal: Anorexia, diarrhea, hunger, nausea, proctocolitis, vomiting
Hematologic: Agranulocytosis, aplastic anemia, eosinophilia, hemolytic anemia, leukopenia, pancytopenia, porphyria cutanea tarda, thrombocytopenia
Hepatic: Cholestatic jaundice, hepatic porphyria, hepatitis, liver failure

Drug Interactions
Metabolism/Transport Effects Substrate of CYP2C9 (major)
Avoid Concomitant Use There are no known interactions where it is recommended to avoid concomitant use.
Increased Effect/Toxicity
ChlorproPAMIDE may increase the levels/effects of: Alcohol (Ethyl); Hypoglycemic Agents; Porfimer

The levels/effects of ChlorproPAMIDE may be increased by: Allopurinol; Beta-Blockers; Chloramphenicol; Cimetidine; Cyclic Antidepressants; CYP2C9 Inhibitors (Moderate); CYP2C9 Inhibitors (Strong); Fibric Acid Derivatives; Fluconazole; GLP-1 Agonists; Herbs (Hypoglycemic Properties); Pegvisomant; Quinolone Antibiotics; Ranitidine; Salicylates; Sulfonamide Derivatives; Voriconazole

Decreased Effect
The levels/effects of ChlorproPAMIDE may be decreased by: Corticosteroids (Orally Inhaled); Corticosteroids (Systemic); CYP2C9 Inducers (Highly Effective); Luteinizing Hormone-Releasing Hormone Analogs; Peginterferon Alfa-2b; Quinolone Antibiotics; Rifampin; Somatropin; Thiazide Diuretics

Ethanol/Nutrition/Herb Interactions
Ethanol: Avoid ethanol (possible disulfiram-like reaction).
Herb/Nutraceutical: Herbs with hypoglycemic properties may enhance the hypoglycemic effect of chlorpropamide. This includes alfalfa, aloe, bilberry, bitter melon, burdock, celery, damiana, fenugreek, garcinia, garlic, ginger, ginseng (American), gymnema, marshmallow, stinging nettle

Mechanism of Action Stimulates insulin release from the pancreatic beta cells; reduces glucose output from the liver; insulin sensitivity is increased at peripheral target sites

Pharmacodynamics/Kinetics
Onset of action: 1 hour
Peak effect: 3-6 hours
Duration: 24 hours
Absorption: Rapid
Distribution: V_d: 0.13-0.23 L/kg
Protein binding: 90%
Metabolism: Extensively hepatic (~80%), primarily via CYP2C9; forms metabolites
Half-life elimination: ~36 hours; prolonged in elderly or with renal impairment
End-stage renal disease: 50-200 hours
Time to peak, serum: 2-4 hours
Excretion: Urine

Dosage
Geriatric Reduce initial dose to 100-125 mg/day in older patients; subsequent dosages may be increased or decreased by 50-125 mg/day at 3- to 5-day intervals (slower upward titration may be appropriate in older patients)
Adult Type 2 diabetes: Oral: The dosage of chlorpropamide is variable and should be individualized based upon the patient's response

Initial dose: 250 mg/day in mild-to-moderate diabetes in middle-aged, stable diabetic; 100-125 mg/day in older patients

Titration: Subsequent dosages may be increased or decreased by 50-125 mg/day at 3- to 5-day intervals

Maintenance dose: 100-250 mg/day; severe patients with diabetes may require 500 mg/day; avoid doses >750 mg/day

Renal Impairment
Cl_{cr} <50 mL/minute: Avoid use.
Hemodialysis: Removed with hemoperfusion.
Peritoneal dialysis: Supplemental dose is not necessary.

Hepatic Impairment Dosage reduction is recommended. Conservative initial and maintenance doses are recommended in patients with liver impairment because chlorpropamide undergoes extensive hepatic metabolism.

Administration May be administered with food to reduce GI upset. Patients that are NPO or require decreased caloric intake may need doses held to avoid hypoglycemia.

Monitoring Parameters Blood glucose, Hgb A_{1c}; monitor for signs and symptoms of hypoglycemia (fatigue, sweating, numbness of extremities)

Reference Range
Recommendations for glycemic control in adults with diabetes:
Hb A_{1c}: <7%
Preprandial capillary plasma glucose: 70-130 mg/dL
Peak postprandial capillary blood glucose: <180 mg/dL
Blood pressure: <130/80 mm Hg
Recommendations for glycemic control in older adults with diabetes:
Relatively healthy, cognitively intact, and with a ≥5-year life expectancy: See Adults
Frail, life expectancy <5-years or those for whom the risks of intensive glucose control outweigh the benefits:
Hb A_{1c}: <8% to 9%
Blood pressure: <140/80 mm Hg or <130/80 mm Hg if tolerated

Pharmacotherapy Pearls Long half-life may complicate recovery from excess effects

Special Geriatric Considerations Because of chlorpropamide's long half-life, duration of action, drug interactions, and the increased risk for hypoglycemia, it is not considered a hypoglycemic agent of choice in the elderly. Intensive glucose control (HbA$_{1c}$ <6.5%) has been linked to increased all-cause and cardiovascular mortality, hypoglycemia requiring assistance, and weight gain in adult type 2 diabetes. How "tightly" to control a geriatric patient's blood glucose needs to be individualized. Such a decision should be based on several factors, including the patient's functional and cognitive status, how well he/she recognizes hypoglycemic or hyperglycemic symptoms, and how to respond to them and other disease states. An HbA$_{1c}$ <7.5% is an acceptable endpoint for a healthy older adult, while <8% is acceptable for frail elderly patients, those with a duration of illness >10 years, or those with comorbid conditions and requiring combination diabetes medications. Patients who are unable to accurately draw up their dose will need assistance, such as prefilled syringes. Initial doses may require considerations for renal function in the elderly with dosing adjusted subsequently based on blood glucose monitoring. For elderly patients with diabetes who are relatively healthy, attaining target goals for aspirin use, blood pressure, lipids, smoking cessation, and diet and exercise may be more important than normalized glycemic control.

This medication is considered to be potentially inappropriate in this patient population (Beers Criteria severity: High).

Dosage Forms Excipient information presented when available (limited, particularly for generics); consult specific product labeling.
Tablet, oral: 100 mg, 250 mg

Selected References
Action to Control Cardiovascular Risk in Diabetes Study Group, Gerstein HC, Miller ME, et al, "Effects of Intensive Glucose Lowering in Type 2 Diabetes," *N Engl J Med*, 2008, 358(24):2545-59.
ADVANCE Collaborative Group, Patel A, MacMahon S, et al, "Intensive Blood Glucose Control and Vascular Outcomes in Patients With Type 2 Diabetes," *N Engl J Med*, 2008, 358(24):2560-72.
American Diabetes Association, "Standards of Medical Care in Diabetes – 2011," *Diabetes Care*, 2011, 34(Suppl 1):11-61.
Brown AF, Mangione CM, Saliba D, et al, "Guidelines for Improving the Care of the Older Person With Diabetes Mellitus," *J Am Geriatr Soc*, 2003, 51(5 Suppl Guidelines):265-80.
"VA/DoD Clinical Practice Guideline for the Management of Diabetes Mellitus," 2010. Available at http://www.healthquality.va.gov/Diabetes_Mellitus.asp

Chlorthalidone (klor THAL i done)

Brand Names: U.S. Thalitone®
Brand Names: Canada Apo-Chlorthalidone®
Index Terms Hygroton
Generic Availability (U.S.) Yes
Pharmacologic Category Diuretic, Thiazide

Use Management of mild-to-moderate hypertension when used alone or in combination with other agents; treatment of edema associated with heart failure or nephrotic syndrome. Recent studies have found chlorthalidone effective in the treatment of isolated systolic hypertension in the elderly.

Dosage

Geriatric Oral: Initial: 12.5-25 mg/day or every other day; there is little advantage to using doses >25 mg/day.

Adult

Hypertension: Oral: 25-100 mg/day or 100 mg 3 times/week; usual dosage range (JNC 7): 12.5-25 mg/day

Edema: Initial: 50-100 mg/day or 100 mg on alternate days; maximum dose: 200 mg/day

Heart failure-associated edema: 12.5-25 mg once daily; maximum daily dose: 100 mg (ACC/AHA 2009 Heart Failure Guidelines)

Renal Impairment Cl_{cr} <10 mL/minute: Avoid use. Ineffective with low GFR (Aronoff, 2002)

Note: ACC/AHA 2009 Heart Failure Guidelines suggest that thiazides lose their efficacy when Cl_{cr} <40 mL/minute

Special Geriatric Considerations Studies have found chlorthalidone effective in the treatment of isolated systolic hypertension in the elderly. The use of chlorthalidone as a step 1 medication reduced the incidence of stroke in the SHEP trial.

Dosage Forms Excipient information presented when available (limited, particularly for generics); consult specific product labeling. [DSC] = Discontinued product

Tablet, oral: 25 mg, 50 mg, 100 mg [DSC]

Thalitone®: 15 mg

◆ **Chlor-Trimeton® Allergy [OTC]** *see* Chlorpheniramine *on page 337*

Chlorzoxazone (klor ZOKS a zone)

Related Information

Beers Criteria – Potentially Inappropriate Medications for Geriatrics *on page 2089*

Medication Safety Issues

Sound-alike/look-alike issues:

Parafon Forte® may be confused with Fam-Pren Forte

BEERS Criteria medication:

This drug may be inappropriate for use in geriatric patients (high severity risk).

Brand Names: U.S. Parafon Forte® DSC

Brand Names: Canada Parafon Forte®; Strifon Forte®

Generic Availability (U.S.) Yes

Pharmacologic Category Skeletal Muscle Relaxant

Use Symptomatic treatment of muscle spasm and pain associated with acute musculoskeletal conditions

Contraindications Hypersensitivity to chlorzoxazone or any component of the formulation; impaired liver function

Warnings/Precautions This class of medication is poorly tolerated by the elderly due to anticholinergic effects, sedation, and weakness. Efficacy is questionable at dosages tolerated by elderly patients (Beers Criteria).

Adverse Reactions (Reflective of adult population; not specific for elderly) Frequency not defined.

Central nervous system: Dizziness, drowsiness lightheadedness, paradoxical stimulation, malaise

Dermatologic: Rash, petechiae, ecchymoses (rare), angioneurotic edema

Gastrointestinal: Nausea, vomiting, stomach cramps

Genitourinary: Urine discoloration

Hepatic: Liver dysfunction

Miscellaneous: Anaphylaxis (very rare)

Drug Interactions

Metabolism/Transport Effects Substrate of CYP1A2 (minor), 2A6 (minor), 2D6 (minor), 2E1 (major), 3A4 (minor); **Inhibits** CYP2E1 (weak), 3A4 (weak)

Avoid Concomitant Use There are no known interactions where it is recommended to avoid concomitant use.

Increased Effect/Toxicity

Chlorzoxazone may increase the levels/effects of: Alcohol (Ethyl); CNS Depressants; Methotrimeprazine; Selective Serotonin Reuptake Inhibitors

The levels/effects of Chlorzoxazone may be increased by: Conivaptan; Disulfiram; Droperidol; HydrOXYzine; Isoniazid; Methotrimeprazine

◀ **Decreased Effect**

The levels/effects of Chlorzoxazone may be decreased by: Cyproterone; Peginterferon Alfa-2b; Tocilizumab

Ethanol/Nutrition/Herb Interactions Ethanol: May increase CNS depression; monitor for increased effects with coadministration. Caution patients about effects.

Mechanism of Action Acts on the spinal cord and subcortical levels by depressing polysynaptic reflexes

Pharmacodynamics/Kinetics

Onset of action: ~1 hour

Duration: 6-12 hours

Absorption: Readily absorbed

Metabolism: Extensively hepatic via glucuronidation

Excretion: Urine (as conjugates)

Dosage

Geriatric Oral: Initial: 250 mg 2-4 times/day; increase as necessary to 750 mg 3-4 times/day.

Adult Muscle spasm: Oral: 250-500 mg 3-4 times/day up to 750 mg 3-4 times/day

Monitoring Parameters Liver function tests, relief of symptoms, mental status

Pharmacotherapy Pearls Not useful in the chronic spasticity associated with stroke or Parkinson's disease

Special Geriatric Considerations No data available on the use of skeletal muscle relaxants in the elderly. Start dosing low and increase as necessary. Because it can cause unpredictable, fatal hepatic toxicity, the use of chlorzoxazone should be avoided.

This medication is considered to be potentially inappropriate in this patient population (Beers Criteria severity: High).

Dosage Forms Excipient information presented when available (limited, particularly for generics); consult specific product labeling. [DSC] = Discontinued product

Caplet, oral:

Parafon Forte® DSC: 500 mg [scored]

Tablet, oral: 250 mg [DSC], 500 mg

Cholecalciferol (kole e kal SI fer ole)

Medication Safety Issues

Sound-alike/look-alike issues:

Cholecalciferol may be confused with alfacalcidol, ergocalciferol

Administration issues:

Liquid vitamin D preparations have the potential for dosing errors when administered to infants. Droppers should be clearly marked to easily provide 400 international units. For products intended for infants, the FDA recommends that accompanying droppers deliver no more than 400 international units per dose.

Brand Names: U.S. Bio-D-Mulsion Forte® [OTC]; Bio-D-Mulsion® [OTC]; D-3 [OTC]; D3-50™ [OTC]; D3-5™ [OTC]; DDrops®; DDrops® Baby [OTC]; DDrops® Kids [OTC]; DDrops® [OTC]; Delta® D3 [OTC]; Enfamil® D-Vi-Sol™ [OTC]; Maximum D3® [OTC]; Vitamin D3 [OTC]

Brand Names: Canada D-Vi-Sol®

Index Terms D3

Generic Availability (U.S.) Yes

Pharmacologic Category Vitamin D Analog

Use Dietary supplement, treatment of vitamin D deficiency, or prophylaxis of deficiency

Unlabeled/Investigational Use Osteoporosis prevention

Contraindications Hypercalcemia; hypersensitivity to cholecalciferol or any component of the formulation; malabsorption syndrome; evidence of vitamin D toxicity

Adverse Reactions (Reflective of adult population; not specific for elderly) Frequency not defined: Endocrine & metabolic: Hypervitaminosis D (signs and symptoms include hypercalcemia, resulting in headache, nausea, vomiting, lethargy, confusion, sluggishness, abdominal pain, bone pain, polyuria, polydipsia, weakness, cardiac arrhythmias [eg, QT shortening, sinus tachycardia], soft tissue calcification, calciuria, and nephrocalcinosis)

Drug Interactions

Metabolism/Transport Effects Inhibits CYP2C9 (weak), 2C19 (weak), 2D6 (weak)

Avoid Concomitant Use

Avoid concomitant use of Cholecalciferol with any of the following: Aluminum Hydroxide; Sucralfate; Vitamin D Analogs

Increased Effect/Toxicity

Cholecalciferol may increase the levels/effects of: Aluminum Hydroxide; Cardiac Glycosides; Sucralfate; Vitamin D Analogs

The levels/effects of Cholecalciferol may be increased by: Calcium Salts; Thiazide Diuretics

Decreased Effect

The levels/effects of Cholecalciferol may be decreased by: Bile Acid Sequestrants; Mineral Oil; Orlistat

Ethanol/Nutrition/Herb Interactions Food: Olestra may impair the absorption of vitamin D.

Pharmacodynamics/Kinetics

Distribution: Primarily hepatic

Protein binding: Extensively to vitamin D-binding protein

Metabolism: Primary liver and kidney hydroxylation; glucuronidation (minimal)

Half-life elimination: 14 hours

Time to peak, plasma: 11 hours

Excretion: As metabolites, urine (2.4%) and feces (4.9%)

Dosage

Geriatric

Dietary Reference Intake for Vitamin D: Oral:

≤70 years: Refer to adult dosing.

>70 years: RDA: 800 int. units/day

Osteoporosis prevention (unlabeled use) Refer to adult dosing.

Vitamin D deficiency treatment (unlabeled dose): Refer to adult dosing.

Adult

Dietary Reference Intake for Vitamin D: Oral:

Adults: 19-70 years: RDA: 600 int. units/day

Osteoporosis prevention(unlabeled): Adults ≥50 years: Oral: 800-1000 int. units/day (NOF guidelines, 2010)

Monitoring Parameters Monitor renal function, serum calcium, and phosphate concentrations; if hypercalcemia is encountered, discontinue agent until serum calcium returns to normal

Reference Range

Serum calcium times phosphorus should not exceed 70 mg^2/dL^2 to avoid ectopic calcification

Vitamin D deficiency: There is no clear consensus on a reference range for total serum 25 (OH)D concentrations or the validity of this level as it relates clinically to bone health. In addition, there is significant variability in the reporting of serum 25 (OH)D levels as a result of different assay types in use. However, the following ranges have been suggested (NAS, 2011):

<30 nmol/L (12 ng/mL): At risk for deficiency

30-50 nmol/L (12-20 ng/mL): Potentially at risk for inadequacy

≥50 nmol/L (≥20 ng/mL): Sufficient levels in practically all persons

>125 nmol/L (>50 ng/mL): Concern for risk of toxicity

Pharmacotherapy Pearls 1 mg of cholecalciferol = 40,000 units of vitamin D activity

Special Geriatric Considerations Vitamin D, folate, and B_{12} (cyanocobalamin) have decreased absorption with age (clinical significance unknown); studies in ill geriatrics demonstrated that low serum concentrations of vitamin D result in greater bone loss. Calorie requirements decrease with age and therefore, nutrient density must be increased to ensure adequate nutrient intake, including vitamins and minerals. The use of a daily supplement with a multiple vitamin with minerals is recommended because elderly consume less vitamin D, absorption may be decreased, and many have decreased sun exposure. This is a recommendation of particular need to those with high risk for osteoporosis.

Vitamin D supplementation has been shown to increase muscle function and strength, as well as improve balance. Patients at risk for falls should have vitamin D serum concentrations measured and be evaluated for supplementation.

Dosage Forms Excipient information presented when available (limited, particularly for generics); consult specific product labeling.

Capsule, oral: 5000 int. units

D-3: 1000 int. units

D3-50™: 50,000 int. units

D3-5™: 5000 int. units

Maximum D3®: 10,000 int. units [contains soybean lecithin]

Capsule, softgel, oral:

D-3: 2000 int. units

Solution, oral [drops]:
Bio-D-Mulsion Forte®: 2000 int. units/drop (30 mL) [contains sesame oil]
Bio-D-Mulsion®: 400 int. units/drop (30 mL) [contains sesame oil]
DDrops®: 2000 int. units/drop (10 mL); 1000 units/drop (10 mL)
DDrops® Baby: 400 int. units/drop (10 mL)
DDrops® Kids: 400 int. units/drop (10 mL)
Enfamil® D-Vi-Sol™: 400 int. units/mL (50 mL) [gluten free, sugar free; citrus flavor]
Tablet, oral: 400 int. units, 1000 int. units
Delta® D3: 400 int. units [sugar free]
Vitamin D3: 1000 int. units [sugar free]

Selected References

Bischoff-Ferrari HA, Dawson-Hughes B, Staehelin HB, et al, "Fall Prevention With Supplemental and Active Forms of Vitamin D: A Meta-Analysis of Randomised Controlled Trials," *BMJ,* 2009, 339:b3692.

Bordelon P, Ghetu MV, and Langan RC, "Recognition and Management of Vitamin D Deficiency," *Am Fam Physician,* 2009, 80(8):841-6.

Fosnight SM, Zafirau WJ, and Hazelett SE, "Vitamin D Supplementation to Prevent Falls in the Elderly: Evidence and Practical Considerations," *Pharmacotherapy,* 2008, 28(2):225-34.

Holick MF, "Vitamin D Deficiency," *N Engl J Med,* 2007, 357(3):266-81.

Letsou AP and Price LS, "Health Aging and Nutrition: An Overview," *Clin Geriatr Med,* 1987, 3(2):253-60.

Myrianthopoulos M, "Dietary Treatment of Hyperlipidemia in the Elderly," *Clin Geriatr Med,* 1987, 3(2):343-59.

Riggs BL and Melton LJ, "The Prevention and Treatment of Osteoporosis," *N Engl J Med,* 1992, 327(9):620-7.

Vieth R, Bischoff-Ferrari H, Boucher BJ, et al, "The Urgent Need to Recommend an Intake of Vitamin D That is Effective," *Am J Clin Nutr,* 2007, 85(3):649-50.

◆ **Cholecalciferol and Alendronate** *see* Alendronate and Cholecalciferol *on page 56*

Cholestyramine Resin (koe LES teer a meen REZ in)

Related Information

Hyperlipidemia Management *on page 2021*

Brand Names: U.S. Prevalite®; Questran®; Questran® Light

Brand Names: Canada Novo-Cholamine; Novo-Cholamine Light; Olestyr; PMS-Cholestyramine; Questran®; Questran® Light Sugar Free; ZYM-Cholestyramine-Light; ZYM-Cholestyramine-Regular

Generic Availability (U.S.) Yes

Pharmacologic Category Antilipemic Agent, Bile Acid Sequestrant

Use Adjunct in the management of primary hypercholesterolemia; pruritus associated with elevated levels of bile acids; diarrhea associated with excess fecal bile acids; binding toxicologic agents; pseudomembranous colitis

Contraindications Hypersensitivity to bile acid sequestering resins or any component of the formulation; complete biliary obstruction; bowel obstruction

Warnings/Precautions Not to be taken simultaneously with many other medicines (decreased absorption). Treat any diseases contributing to hypercholesterolemia first. May interfere with fat-soluble vitamins (A, D, E, K) and folic acid. Chronic use may be associated with bleeding problems (especially in high doses). May produce or exacerbate constipation problems. Fecal impaction may occur. Hemorrhoids may be worsened. Questran® Light contains phenylalanine.

Adverse Reactions (Reflective of adult population; not specific for elderly)

>10%: Gastrointestinal: Constipation, heartburn, nausea, vomiting, stomach pain

1% to 10%:
Central nervous system: Headache
Gastrointestinal: Belching, bloating, diarrhea

Drug Interactions

Avoid Concomitant Use

Avoid concomitant use of Cholestyramine Resin with any of the following: Mycophenolate

Increased Effect/Toxicity There are no known significant interactions involving an increase in effect.

Decreased Effect

Cholestyramine Resin may decrease the levels/effects of: Acetaminophen; Amiodarone; Antidiabetic Agents (Thiazolidinedione); Cardiac Glycosides; Chenodiol; Contraceptives (Estrogens); Contraceptives (Progestins); Corticosteroids (Oral); Deferasirox; Ezetimibe; Fibric Acid Derivatives; Fluvastatin; Leflunomide; Loop Diuretics; Methotrexate; Methylfolate; Mycophenolate; Niacin; Nonsteroidal Anti-Inflammatory Agents; PHENobarbital; Pravastatin; Propranolol; Raloxifene; Tetracycline Derivatives; Thiazide Diuretics; Thyroid Products; Ursodiol; Vitamin D Analogs; Vitamin K Antagonists

Ethanol/Nutrition/Herb Interactions

Food: Cholestyramine (especially high doses or long-term therapy) may decrease the absorption of folic acid, calcium, and iron.

Herb/Nutraceutical: Cholestyramine (especially high doses or long-term therapy) may decrease the absorption of fat-soluble vitamins (vitamins A, D, E, and K).

Stability Store powder at controlled room temperature of 15°C to 30°C (59°F to 86°F). Mix contents of 1 packet or 1 level scoop of powder with 4-6 oz of beverage. Allow to stand 1-2 minutes prior to mixing. May also be mixed with highly-fluid soups, cereals, applesauce, etc. Suspension may be used for up to 48 hours after refrigeration.

Mechanism of Action Forms a nonabsorbable complex with bile acids in the intestine, releasing chloride ions in the process; inhibits enterohepatic reuptake of intestinal bile salts and thereby increases the fecal loss of bile salt-bound low density lipoprotein cholesterol

Pharmacodynamics/Kinetics
Onset of action: Peak effect: 21 days
Absorption: None
Excretion: Feces (as insoluble complex with bile acids)

Dosage
Geriatric & Adult Dyslipidemia: Oral (dosages are expressed in terms of anhydrous resin): 4 g 1-2 times/day to a maximum of 24 g/day (and a maximum of 6 times/day)
Renal Impairment Not removed by hemo- or peritoneal dialysis. Supplemental doses not necessary with dialysis or continuous arteriovenous or venovenous hemofiltration effects.

Administration Mix powder with water or other fluid prior to administration; not to be taken in dry form. Suspension should not be sipped or held in mouth for prolonged periods (may cause tooth discoloration or enamel decay).

Monitoring Parameters Bowel function, plasma cholesterol (LDL and VLDL fractions)

Test Interactions Increased prothrombin time; decreased cholesterol (S), iron (B)

Pharmacotherapy Pearls Overdose may result in GI obstruction; Questran® Light contains aspartame

Special Geriatric Considerations The definition of and, therefore, when to treat hyper-lipidemia in the elderly is a controversial issue. The National Cholesterol Education Program recommends that all adults maintain a plasma cholesterol <160 mg/dL. Elderly with one additional risk factor, goal LDL would be <130 mg/dL. It is the authors' belief that pharmacologic treatment be reserved for those who are unable to obtain a desirable plasma cholesterol concentration by diet alone and for whom the benefits of treatment are believed to outweigh the potential adverse effects, drug interactions, and cost of treatment.

Dosage Forms Excipient information presented when available (limited, particularly for generics); consult specific product labeling.
Powder for suspension, oral: Cholestyramine resin 4 g/5 g of powder (210 g); Cholestyramine resin 4 g/5.7 g of powder (239.4 g); Cholestyramine resin 4 g/9 g of powder (378 g); Cholestyramine resin 4 g/5 g packet (60s); Cholestyramine resin 4 g/5.7 g packet (60s); Cholestyramine resin 4 g/9 g packet (60s)
Prevalite®: Cholestyramine resin 4 g/5.5 g of powder (231 g); Cholestyramine resin 4 g/5.5 g packet (42s, 60s) [contains phenylalanine 14.1 mg/5.5 g; orange flavor]
Questran®: Cholestyramine resin 4 g/9 g of powder (378 g); Cholestyramine resin 4 g/9 g packet (60s) [orange flavor]
Questran® Light: Cholestyramine resin 4 g/5 g of powder (210 g); Cholestyramine resin 4 g/5 g packet (60s) [contains phenylalanine 14 mg/5 g; orange flavor]

Selected References
"Executive Summary of The Third Report of The National Cholesterol Education Program (NCEP) Expert Panel on Detection, Evaluation, and Treatment of High Blood Cholesterol in Adults (Adult Treatment Panel III)," *JAMA*, 2001, 285(19):2486-97.
Grundy SM, Cleeman JI, Merz CN, et al, "Implications of Recent Clinical Trials for the National Cholesterol Education Program Adult Treatment Panel III Guidelines," *J Am Coll Cardiol*, 2004, 44(3):720-32.
National Cholesterol Education Program (NCEP) Expert Panel on Detection, Evaluation, and Treatment of High Blood Cholesterol in Adults (Adult Treatment Panel III), "Third Report of the National Cholesterol Education Program (NCEP) Expert Panel on Detection, Evaluation, and Treatment of High Blood Cholesterol in Adults (Adult Treatment Panel III) Final Report," *Circulation*, 2002, 106(25):3143-421.

◆ **Choline Fenofibrate** see Fenofibric Acid *on page 704*

Choline Magnesium Trisalicylate (KOE leen mag NEE zhum trye sa LIS i late)

Index Terms Tricosal; Trilisate
Generic Availability (U.S.) Yes
Pharmacologic Category Salicylate
Use Management of osteoarthritis, rheumatoid arthritis, and other arthritis; acute painful shoulder
Contraindications Hypersensitivity to salicylates, other nonacetylated salicylates, other NSAIDs, or any component of the formulation; bleeding disorders

Warnings/Precautions Salicylate salts may not inhibit platelet aggregation and, therefore, should not be substituted for aspirin in the prophylaxis of thrombosis. Use with caution in patients with impaired hepatic or renal function, dehydration, erosive gastritis, asthma, or peptic ulcer.

Elderly are a high-risk population for adverse effects from NSAIDs. As many as 60% of elderly can develop peptic ulceration and/or hemorrhage asymptomatically. Use lowest effective dose for shortest period possible. Tinnitus or impaired hearing may indicate toxicity. Tinnitus may be a difficult and unreliable indication of toxicity due to age-related hearing loss or eighth cranial nerve damage. CNS adverse effects may be observed in the elderly at lower doses than younger adults.

Adverse Reactions (Reflective of adult population; not specific for elderly)
<20%:
Gastrointestinal: Nausea, vomiting, diarrhea, heartburn, dyspepsia, epigastric pain, constipation
Otic: Tinnitus
<2%:
Central nervous system: Headache, lightheadedness, dizziness, drowsiness, lethargy
Otic: Hearing impairment

Drug Interactions

Avoid Concomitant Use
Avoid concomitant use of Choline Magnesium Trisalicylate with any of the following: Influenza Virus Vaccine (Live/Attenuated)

Increased Effect/Toxicity
Choline Magnesium Trisalicylate may increase the levels/effects of: Anticoagulants; Carbonic Anhydrase Inhibitors; Corticosteroids (Systemic); Divalproex; Drotrecogin Alfa; Methotrexate; PRALAtrexate; Salicylates; Sulfonylureas; Thrombolytic Agents; Valproic Acid; Varicella Virus-Containing Vaccines; Vitamin K Antagonists

The levels/effects of Choline Magnesium Trisalicylate may be increased by: Antiplatelet Agents; Calcium Channel Blockers (Nondihydropyridine); Ginkgo Biloba; Herbs (Anticoagulant/Antiplatelet Properties); Influenza Virus Vaccine (Live/Attenuated); Loop Diuretics; Treprostinil

Decreased Effect
Choline Magnesium Trisalicylate may decrease the levels/effects of: ACE Inhibitors; Loop Diuretics; Probenecid

The levels/effects of Choline Magnesium Trisalicylate may be decreased by: Corticosteroids (Systemic)

Ethanol/Nutrition/Herb Interactions
Ethanol: Avoid ethanol (may enhance gastric mucosal irritation).
Food: May decrease the rate but not the extent of oral absorption.
Herb/Nutraceutical: Avoid cat's claw, dong quai, evening primrose, feverfew, garlic, ginger, ginkgo, red clover, horse chestnut, green tea, ginseng (all have additional antiplatelet activity). Limit curry powder, paprika, licorice, Benedictine liqueur, prunes, raisins, tea, and gherkins; may cause salicylate accumulation. These foods contain 6 mg salicylate/100 g.

Stability Store at controlled room temperature of 15°C to 30°C (59°F to 86°F).

Mechanism of Action Weakly inhibits cyclooxygenase enzymes, which results in decreased formation of prostaglandin precursors; antipyretic, analgesic, and anti-inflammatory properties.

Other proposed mechanisms not fully elucidated (and possibly contributing to the anti-inflammatory effect to varying degrees) include inhibiting chemotaxis, altering lymphocyte activity, inhibiting neutrophil aggregation/activation, and decreasing proinflammatory cytokine levels.

Pharmacodynamics/Kinetics
Absorption: From the stomach and small intestine
Distribution: Readily into most body fluids and tissues
Half-life: Dose-dependent ranging from 2-3 hours at low doses to 30 hours at high doses
Time to peak plasma concentrations: Within ~2 hours

Dosage
Geriatric Usual dose: 750 mg 3 times/day.
Adult Arthritis, pain: Oral (based on total salicylate content): 500 mg to 1.5 g 2-3 times/day **or** 3 g at bedtime; usual maintenance dose: 1-4.5 g/day
Renal Impairment Avoid use in severe renal impairment.
Administration Liquid may be mixed with fruit juice just before drinking. Do not administer with antacids. Take with a full glass of water and remain in an upright position for 15-30 minutes after administration.

Monitoring Parameters Serum concentrations, renal function; hearing changes or tinnitus; monitor for response (ie, pain, inflammation, range of motion, grip strength); observe for abnormal bleeding, bruising, weight gain

Reference Range Salicylate blood levels for anti-inflammatory effect: 150-300 mcg/mL; analgesia and antipyretic effect: 30-50 mcg/mL

Test Interactions False-negative results for glucose oxidase urinary glucose tests (Clinistix®); false-positives using the cupric sulfate method (Clinitest®); also, interferes with Gerhardt test (urinary ketone analysis), VMA determination; 5-HIAA, xylose tolerance test, and T_3 and T_4; increased PBI

Pharmacotherapy Pearls Salicylate salts do not inhibit platelet aggregation and, therefore, should not be substituted for aspirin in the prophylaxis of thrombosis; use caution in patients with renal failure or reduced renal function (ie, older adults - magnesium accumulation)

Special Geriatric Considerations Elderly are a high-risk population for adverse effects from nonsteroidal anti-inflammatory agents. As much as 60% of elderly can develop peptic ulceration and/or hemorrhage asymptomatically. The concomitant use of H_2 blockers and sucralfate is not effective as prophylaxis with the exception of NSAID-induced duodenal ulcers which may be prevented by the use of ranitidine. Misoprostol and proton pump inhibitors are the only agents proven to help prevent the development of NSAID-induced ulcers. Also, concomitant disease and drug use contribute to the risk for GI adverse effects. Avoid use of multiple drugs (OTCs) which contain salicylates (eg, bismuth subsalicylate with other salicylates). Use lowest effective dose for shortest period possible. Consider renal function decline with age. Use of NSAIDs can compromise existing renal function especially when Cl_{cr} is ≤30 mL/minute. There is the consideration that the use of choline magnesium salicylate may cause less gastrointestinal and renal adverse effects than ASA or other NSAIDs in the elderly. Tinnitus may be a difficult and unreliable indication of toxicity due to age-related hearing loss or eighth cranial nerve damage. CNS adverse effects such as confusion, agitation, and hallucination are generally seen in overdose or high dose situations, but elderly may demonstrate these adverse effects at lower doses than younger adults.

Dosage Forms Excipient information presented when available (limited, particularly for generics); consult specific product labeling. [DSC] = Discontinued product

Liquid, oral: 500 mg/5 mL (240 mL) [choline salicylate 293 mg and magnesium salicylate 362 mg per 5 mL]

Tablet, oral: 500 mg [DSC] [choline salicylate 293 mg and magnesium salicylate 362 mg], 750 mg [DSC] [choline salicylate 440 mg and magnesium salicylate 544 mg], 1000 mg [DSC] [choline salicylate 587 mg and magnesium salicylate 725 mg]

◆ **Choline Salicylate** see Salicylates (Various Salts) on page 1647
◆ **Chooz® [OTC]** see Calcium Salts (Oral) on page 256
◆ **CI-1008** see Pregabalin on page 1514
◆ **Cialis®** see Tadalafil on page 1727

Ciclesonide (Oral Inhalation) (sye KLES oh nide)

Brand Names: U.S. Alvesco®
Brand Names: Canada Alvesco®
Generic Availability (U.S.) No
Pharmacologic Category Corticosteroid, Inhalant (Oral)
Use Prophylactic management of bronchial asthma
Contraindications Hypersensitivity to ciclesonide or any component of the formulation; primary treatment of acute asthma or status asthmaticus; moderate-to-severe bronchiectasis

Canadian labeling: Additional contraindications (not in U.S. labeling): Untreated fungal, bacterial, or tuberculosis infections of the respiratory tract; moderate-to-severe bronchiectasis

Warnings/Precautions May cause hypercorticism or suppression of hypothalamic-pituitary-adrenal (HPA) axis, particularly in patients receiving high doses for prolonged periods. HPA axis suppression may lead to adrenal crisis. Withdrawal and discontinuation of a corticosteroid should be done slowly and carefully. Particular care is required when patients are transferred from systemic corticosteroids to inhaled products due to possible adrenal insufficiency or withdrawal from steroids, including an increase in allergic symptoms. Patients receiving >20 mg per day of prednisone (or equivalent) may be most susceptible. Fatalities have occurred due to adrenal insufficiency in asthmatic patients during and after transfer from systemic corticosteroids to aerosol steroids; aerosol steroids do **not** provide the systemic steroid needed to treat patients having trauma, surgery, or infections.

Bronchospasm may occur with wheezing after inhalation; if this occurs stop steroid and treat with a fast-acting bronchodilator. Supplemental steroids (oral or parenteral) may be needed during stress or severe asthma attacks. Not to be used in status asthmaticus or for the relief of

◄ acute bronchospasm. Oropharyngeal thrush due to candida albicans infection may occur with use. Prolonged use of corticosteroids may also increase the incidence of secondary infection, mask acute infection (including fungal infections), prolong or exacerbate viral infections, or limit response to vaccines. Exposure to chickenpox and measles should be avoided; corticosteroids should not be used to treat ocular herpes simplex. Close observation is required in patients with latent tuberculosis and/or TB reactivity; restrict use in active TB (only in conjunction with antituberculosis treatment). Use in patients with TB is contraindicated in the Canadian labeling. Prolonged treatment with corticosteroids has been associated with the development of Kaposi's sarcoma (case reports); if noted, discontinuation of therapy should be considered.

Use with caution in patients with thyroid disease, severe hepatic impairment, glaucoma, cataracts, patients at risk for osteoporosis, and patients at risk for seizures.

Adverse Reactions (Reflective of adult population; not specific for elderly)
>10%:
Central nervous system: Headache (≤11%)
Respiratory: Nasopharyngitis (≤11%)
1% to 10%:
Cardiovascular: Facial edema (≥3%)
Central nervous system: Dizziness (≥3%), fatigue (≥3%), dysphonia (1%)
Dermatologic: Urticaria (≥3%)
Gastrointestinal: Gastroenteritis (≥3%), oral candidiasis (≥3%)
Neuromuscular & skeletal: Arthralgia (≤4%), musculoskeletal chest pain (≥3%), back pain (≥3%), extremity pain (≥3%)
Ocular: Conjunctivitis (≥3%)
Otic: Ear pain (2%)
Respiratory: Upper respiratory infection (≤9%), epistaxis (≤8%), nasal congestion (≤6%), sinusitis (≤6%), pharyngolaryngeal pain (≤ 5%), hoarseness (≥3%), pneumonia (≥3%), paradoxical bronchospasm (2%)
Miscellaneous: Influenza (≥3%)

Drug Interactions
Metabolism/Transport Effects Substrate of CYP3A4 (major), 2D6 (minor)
Avoid Concomitant Use
Avoid concomitant use of Ciclesonide (Oral Inhalation) with any of the following: Aldesleukin
Increased Effect/Toxicity
Ciclesonide (Oral Inhalation) may increase the levels/effects of: Deferasirox

The levels/effects of Ciclesonide (Oral Inhalation) may be increased by: CYP3A4 Inhibitors (Moderate); Dasatinib; Telaprevir
Decreased Effect
Ciclesonide (Oral Inhalation) may decrease the levels/effects of: Aldesleukin; Corticorelin; Telaprevir

The levels/effects of Ciclesonide (Oral Inhalation) may be decreased by: Tocilizumab
Stability Store at 15°C to 30°C (59°F to 86°F); do not freeze.
Mechanism of Action Ciclesonide is a nonhalogenated, glucocorticoid prodrug that is hydrolyzed to the pharmacologically active metabolite des-ciclesonide following administration. Des-ciclesonide has a high affinity for the glucocorticoid receptor and exhibits anti-inflammatory activity. The mechanism of action for corticosteroids is believed to be a combination of three important properties − anti-inflammatory activity, immunosuppressive properties, and antiproliferative actions.
Pharmacodynamics/Kinetics
Absorption: 52% (lung deposition)
Protein binding: ≥99%
Metabolism: Ciclesonide hydrolyzed to active metabolite, des-ciclesonide via esterases in nasal mucosa and lungs; further metabolism via hepatic CYP3A4 and 2D6
Bioavailability: >50% (active metabolite)
Half-life elimination: ~5-7 hours
Time to peak: ~1 hour (active metabolite)
Excretion: Feces (78%)
Dosage
Geriatric & Adult Asthma: Oral inhalation (Alvesco®): **Note:** Titrate to the lowest effective dose once asthma stability is achieved:
U.S. labeling:
Prior therapy with bronchodilators alone: Initial: 80 mcg twice daily (maximum dose: 320 mcg/day)
Prior therapy with inhaled corticosteroids: Initial: 80 mcg twice daily (maximum dose: 640 mcg/day)

Prior therapy with oral corticosteroids: Initial: 320 mcg twice daily (maximum dose: 640 mcg/day)
Canadian labeling: Initial: 400 mcg once daily; maintenance: 100-800 mcg/day (1-2 puffs once or twice daily)

Conversion from oral to inhaled steroid: Initiation of oral inhalation therapy should begin in patients who have previously been stabilized on oral corticosteroids (OCS). A gradual dose reduction of OCS should begin ~7-10 days after starting inhaled therapy. U.S. labeling recommends reducing prednisone dose no more rapidly than ≤2.5 mg/day on a weekly basis. The Canadian labeling recommends decreasing the daily dose of prednisone by 1 mg (or equivalent of other OCS) every 7 days in closely monitored patients, and every 10 days in patients whom close monitoring is not possible. In the presence of withdrawal symptoms, resume previous OCS dose for 1 week before attempting further dose reductions.

Administration Remove mouthpiece cover, place inhaler in mouth, close lips around mouthpiece, and inhale slowly and deeply. Press down on top of inhaler after slow inhalation has begun. Remove inhaler while holding breath for approximately 10 seconds. Breathe out slowly and replace mouthpiece on inhaler. Do not wash or place inhaler in water. Clean mouthpiece using a dry cloth or tissue once weekly. Discard after the "discard by" date or after labeled number of doses has been used, even if container is not completely empty.

Shaking is not necessary since drug is formulated as a solution aerosol. Prime inhaler prior to initial use or if not in use for ≥1 week by releasing 3 puffs into the air.

Monitoring Parameters Signs/symptoms of HPA axis suppression/adrenal insufficiency; ocular effects (eg, cataracts, increased intraocular pressure, glaucoma)

Pharmacotherapy Pearls The incidence of oral candidiasis, as well as other localized oropharyngeal effects, observed with ciclesonide use has been reported to be approximately one-half of that seen with other commonly inhaled corticosteroids such as budesonide and fluticasone. Small particle size, minimal activation, and deposition in the oropharynx may explain this decreased incidence.

Special Geriatric Considerations Ensure proper use of inhaler.

Dosage Forms Excipient information presented when available (limited, particularly for generics); consult specific product labeling.

Aerosol, for oral inhalation:
Alvesco®: 80 mcg/inhalation (6.1 g); 160 mcg/inhalation (6.1 g) [60 metered actuations]

Dosage Forms: Canada Excipient information presented when available (limited, particularly for generics); consult specific product labeling.

Aerosol for oral inhalation:
Alvesco®: 50 mcg/inhalation [30-, 60-, and 120 metered actuations]; 100 mcg/inhalation [30-, 60-, and 120 metered actuations]; 200 mcg/inhalation [30-, 60-, and 120 metered actuations]

Ciclesonide (Nasal) (sye KLES oh nide)

Brand Names: U.S. Omnaris™
Brand Names: Canada Omnaris™
Generic Availability (U.S.) No
Pharmacologic Category Corticosteroid, Nasal
Use Management of seasonal and perennial allergic rhinitis
Dosage
  Geriatric & Adult
    Perennial allergic rhinitis: 2 sprays (50 mcg/spray) per nostril once daily; maximum: 200 mcg/day
    Seasonal allergic rhinitis: 2 sprays (50 mcg/spray) per nostril once daily; maximum: 200 mcg/day

Special Geriatric Considerations No specific information is available for the elderly patient.

Dosage Forms Excipient information presented when available (limited, particularly for generics); consult specific product labeling.

Suspension, intranasal [spray]:
Omnaris™: 50 mcg/inhalation (12.5 g) [120 metered actuations]

◆ **Ciclodan™** *see* Ciclopirox *on page 354*
◆ **Ciclodan™ Kit** *see* Ciclopirox *on page 354*

Ciclopirox (sye kloe PEER oks)

Medication Safety Issues
Sound-alike/look-alike issues:
Loprox® may be confused with Lonox®
Brand Names: U.S. Ciclodan™; Ciclodan™ Kit; Loprox®; Penlac®
Brand Names: Canada Loprox®; Penlac®; Stieprox®
Index Terms Ciclopirox Olamine
Generic Availability (U.S.) Yes
Pharmacologic Category Antifungal Agent, Topical
Use
Cream/suspension: Treatment of tinea pedis (athlete's foot), tinea cruris (jock itch), tinea corporis (ringworm), cutaneous candidiasis, and tinea versicolor (pityriasis)

Gel: Treatment of tinea pedis (athlete's foot), tinea corporis (ringworm); seborrheic dermatitis of the scalp

Lacquer (solution): Topical treatment of mild-to-moderate onychomycosis of the fingernails and toenails due to *Trichophyton rubrum* (not involving the lunula) and the immediately-adjacent skin

Shampoo: Treatment of seborrheic dermatitis of the scalp

Contraindications Hypersensitivity to ciclopirox or any component of the formulation; avoid occlusive wrappings or dressings

Warnings/Precautions For external use only; avoid contact with eyes. Nail lacquer is for topical use only and has not been studied in conjunction with systemic therapy or in patients with type 1 diabetes mellitus (insulin dependent, IDDM). Use has not been evaluated in immunosuppressed or immunocompromised patients. Discontinue treatment if signs and/or symptoms of hypersensitivity are noted.

Adverse Reactions (Reflective of adult population; not specific for elderly)
Central nervous system: Headache

Dermatologic: Alopecia, dry skin, erythema, facial edema, hair discoloration (rare; shampoo formulation in light-haired individuals), nail disorder (shape or color change with lacquer), pruritus, rash

Local: Burning sensation (gel: 34%; ≤1% with other forms), irritation, redness, or pain

Drug Interactions
Avoid Concomitant Use There are no known interactions where it is recommended to avoid concomitant use.

Increased Effect/Toxicity There are no known significant interactions involving an increase in effect.

Decreased Effect There are no known significant interactions involving a decrease in effect.

Stability
Cream, suspension: Store between 5°C to 25°C (41°F to 77°F).

Lacquer (solution): Store at room temperature of 15°C to 30°C (59°F to 86°F); protect from light. Flammable; keep away from heat and flame.

Gel, shampoo: Store at room temperature of 15°C to 30°C (59°F to 86°F).

Mechanism of Action Inhibiting transport of essential elements in the fungal cell disrupting the synthesis of DNA, RNA, and protein

Pharmacodynamics/Kinetics
Absorption: Cream, suspension: <2% through intact skin; increased with gel; <5% with lacquer

Distribution: Scalp application: To epidermis, corium (dermis), including hair, hair follicles, and sebaceous glands

Protein binding: 94% to 98%

Half-life elimination: Biologic: 1.7 hours (suspension); elimination: 5.5 hours (gel)

Excretion: Urine (gel: 3% to 10%); feces (small amounts)

Dosage
Geriatric & Adult
Tinea pedis, tinea corporis: Topical:
Cream and suspension: Apply twice daily, gently massage into affected areas; if no improvement after 4 weeks of treatment, re-evaluate the diagnosis.

Gel: Apply twice daily, gently massage into affected areas and surrounding skin; if no improvement after 4 weeks of treatment, re-evaluate diagnosis

Tinea cruris, cutaneous candidiasis, and tinea versicolor: Topical: *Cream and suspension:* Apply twice daily, gently massage into affected areas; if no improvement after 4 weeks of treatment, re-evaluate the diagnosis.

Onychomycosis of the fingernails and toenails: Topical: *Lacquer (solution):* Apply to adjacent skin and affected nails daily (as a part of a comprehensive management program for onychomycosis). Remove with alcohol every 7 days.

Seborrheic dermatitis of the scalp: Topical:
Gel: Apply twice daily, gently massage into affected areas and surrounding skin; if no improvement after 4 weeks of treatment, re-evaluate diagnosis.
Shampoo: Apply ~5 mL (1 teaspoonful) to wet hair; lather, and leave in place ~3 minutes; rinse. May use up to 10 mL for longer hair. Repeat twice weekly for 4 weeks; allow a minimum of 3 days between applications.

Administration Topical:
Cream, suspension: Gently massage into affected areas.
Gel: Gently massage into affected areas and adjacent skin.
Lacquer (solution): Apply evenly over nail and surrounding skin at bedtime (or allow 8 hours before washing); apply daily over previous coat for 7 days; after 7 days, may remove with alcohol and continue cycle.
Shampoo: Apply to wet hair; lather and leave in place for ~3 minutes; rinse.

Dosage Forms Excipient information presented when available (limited, particularly for generics); consult specific product labeling.
Cream, topical, as olamine: 0.77% (15 g, 30 g, 90 g)
Gel, topical: 0.77% (30 g, 45 g, 100 g)
Loprox®: 0.77% (30 g, 45 g, 100 g) [contains isopropyl alcohol]
Shampoo, topical: 1% (120 mL)
Loprox®: 1% (120 mL)
Solution, topical [nail lacquer]: 8% (6.6 mL)
Ciclodan™: 8% (6.6 mL) [contains isopropyl alcohol]
Ciclodan™ Kit: 8% (6.6 mL) [contains isopropyl alcohol; packaged with Toetal Fresh™]
Penlac®: 8% (6.6 mL) [contains isopropyl alcohol]
Suspension, topical, as olamine: 0.77% (30 mL, 60 mL)

♦ **Ciclopirox Olamine** see Ciclopirox on page 354
♦ **Cidecin** see DAPTOmycin on page 454

Cilostazol (sil OH sta zol)

Medication Safety Issues
Sound-alike/look-alike issues:
Pletal® may be confused with Plendil®
Brand Names: U.S. Pletal®
Index Terms OPC-13013
Generic Availability (U.S.) Yes
Pharmacologic Category Antiplatelet Agent; Phosphodiesterase Enzyme Inhibitor
Use Symptomatic management of peripheral vascular disease, primarily intermittent claudication
Unlabeled/Investigational Use Investigational: Treatment of acute coronary syndromes and for graft patency improvement in percutaneous coronary interventions with or without stenting
Contraindications Hypersensitivity to cilostazol or any component of the formulation; heart failure (HF) of any severity; hemostatic disorders or active bleeding
Warnings/Precautions [U.S. Boxed Warning]: The use of this drug is contraindicated in patients with heart failure. Use with caution in severe underlying heart disease. Use with caution in patients receiving other platelet aggregation inhibitors or in patients with thrombocytopenia. Discontinue therapy if thrombocytopenia or leukopenia occur; progression to agranulocytosis (reversible) has been reported when cilostazol was not immediately stopped. When cilostazol and clopidogrel are used concurrently, manufacturer recommends checking bleeding times. Withhold for at least 4-6 half-lives prior to elective surgical procedures. Use with caution in patients receiving CYP3A4 inhibitors (eg, ketoconazole or erythromycin) or CYP2C19 inhibitors (eg, omeprazole). If concurrent use is warranted, consider dosage adjustment of cilostazol. Use caution in moderate-to-severe hepatic impairment. Use cautiously in severe renal impairment (Cl$_{cr}$ <25 mL/minute).
Adverse Reactions (Reflective of adult population; not specific for elderly)
>10%:
Central nervous system: Headache (27% to 34%)
Gastrointestinal: Abnormal stools (12% to 15%), diarrhea (12% to 19%)
Respiratory: Rhinitis (7% to 12%)
Miscellaneous: Infection (10% to 14%)
2% to 10%:
Cardiovascular: Peripheral edema (7% to 9%), palpitation (5% to 10%), tachycardia (4%)
Central nervous system: Dizziness (9% to 10%), vertigo (up to 3%)
Gastrointestinal: Dyspepsia (6%), nausea (6% to 7%), abdominal pain (4% to 5%), flatulence (2% to 3%)

CILOSTAZOL

Neuromuscular & skeletal: Back pain (6% to 7%), myalgia (2% to 3%)
Respiratory: Pharyngitis (7% to 10%), cough (3% to 4%)

Drug Interactions

Metabolism/Transport Effects Substrate of CYP1A2 (minor), 2C19 (minor), 2D6 (minor), 3A4 (major)

Avoid Concomitant Use

Avoid concomitant use of Cilostazol with any of the following: Conivaptan

Increased Effect/Toxicity

Cilostazol may increase the levels/effects of: Anticoagulants; Antiplatelet Agents; Collagenase (Systemic); Drotrecogin Alfa; Ibritumomab; Rivaroxaban; Salicylates; Thrombolytic Agents; Tositumomab and Iodine I 131 Tositumomab

The levels/effects of Cilostazol may be increased by: Antifungal Agents (Azole Derivatives, Systemic); Conivaptan; CYP2C19 Inhibitors (Moderate); CYP2C19 Inhibitors (Strong); CYP3A4 Inhibitors (Moderate); CYP3A4 Inhibitors (Strong); Dasatinib; Esomeprazole; Glucosamine; Herbs (Anticoagulant/Antiplatelet Properties); Macrolide Antibiotics; Nonsteroidal Anti-Inflammatory Agents; Omega-3-Acid Ethyl Esters; Omeprazole; Pentosan Polysulfate Sodium; Pentoxifylline; Prostacyclin Analogues; Vitamin E

Decreased Effect

The levels/effects of Cilostazol may be decreased by: CYP3A4 Inducers (Strong); Cyproterone; Deferasirox; Herbs (CYP3A4 Inducers); Nonsteroidal Anti-Inflammatory Agents; Peginterferon Alfa-2b; Tocilizumab

Ethanol/Nutrition/Herb Interactions

Food: Taking cilostazol with a high-fat meal may increase peak concentration by 90%. Avoid concurrent ingestion of grapefruit juice due to the potential to inhibit CYP3A4.

Herb/Nutraceutical: St John's wort may decrease the levels/effects of cilostazol. Avoid alfalfa, anise, bilberry, bladderwrack, bromelain, cat's claw, chamomile, coleus, cordyceps, dong quai, evening primrose oil, fenugreek, feverfew, garlic, ginger, ginkgo biloba, ginseng (American), ginseng (Panax), ginseng (Siberian), grape seed, green tea, guggul, horse chestnut seed, horseradish, licorice, prickly ash, red clover, reishi, SAMe (S-adenosylmethionine), sweet clover, turmeric, white willow (all have additional antiplatelet activity).

Stability Store at 25°C (77°F); excursions permitted to 15°C to 30°C (59°F to 86°F).

Mechanism of Action Cilostazol and its metabolites are inhibitors of phosphodiesterase III. As a result, cyclic AMP is increased leading to reversible inhibition of platelet aggregation, vasodilation, and inhibition of vascular smooth muscle cell proliferation.

Pharmacodynamics/Kinetics

Onset of action: 2-4 weeks; may require up to 12 weeks

Protein binding: Cilostazol 95% to 98%; active metabolites 66% to 97%

Metabolism: Hepatic via CYP3A4 (primarily), 1A2, 2C19, and 2D6; at least one metabolite has significant activity

Half-life elimination: 11-13 hours

Excretion: Urine (74%) and feces (20%) as metabolites

Dosage

Geriatric & Adult Peripheral vascular disease: Oral: 100 mg twice daily

Dosage adjustment for cilostazol with concomitant medications:

CYP2C19 inhibitors (see Drug Interactions): Dosage of cilostazol should be reduced to 50 mg twice daily

CYP3A4 inhibitors (see Drug Interactions): Dosage of cilostazol should be reduced to 50 mg twice daily

Administration Administer cilostazol 30 minutes before or 2 hours after meals.

Monitoring Parameters Monitor response (increased walking distance, increased mobility)

Special Geriatric Considerations Elderly must be evaluated for cardiac status. Since CHF is common, this disease cannot be overlooked.

Dosage Forms Excipient information presented when available (limited, particularly for generics); consult specific product labeling.

Tablet, oral: 50 mg, 100 mg

Pletal®: 50 mg, 100 mg

◆ **Ciloxan®** *see* Ciprofloxacin (Ophthalmic) *on page 363*

Cimetidine (sye MET i deen)

Related Information
Beers Criteria – Potentially Inappropriate Medications for Geriatrics *on page 2089*

Medication Safety Issues
Sound-alike/look-alike issues:
Cimetidine may be confused with simethicone
BEERS Criteria medication:
This drug may be inappropriate for use in geriatric patients (low severity risk).

Brand Names: U.S. Tagamet HB 200® [OTC]

Brand Names: Canada Apo-Cimetidine®; Dom-Cimetidine; Mylan-Cimetidine; Novo-Cime-tidine; Nu-Cimet; PMS-Cimetidine; Tagamet® HB

Generic Availability (U.S.) Yes

Pharmacologic Category Histamine H_2 Antagonist

Use Short-term treatment of active duodenal ulcers and benign gastric ulcers; maintenance therapy of duodenal ulcer; treatment of gastric hypersecretory states; treatment of gastro-esophageal reflux disease (GERD)

OTC labeling: Prevention or relief of heartburn, acid indigestion, or sour stomach

Unlabeled/Investigational Use Part of a multidrug regimen for *H. pylori* eradication to reduce the risk of duodenal ulcer recurrence

Contraindications Hypersensitivity to cimetidine, any component of the formulation, or other H_2 antagonists

Warnings/Precautions Reversible confusional states, usually clearing within 3-4 days after discontinuation, have been linked to use. Increased age (>50 years) and renal or hepatic impairment are thought to be associated. May be inappropriate for use in the elderly due to risk of confusion and other CNS effects (Beers Criteria). Dosage should be adjusted in renal/hepatic impairment or in patients receiving drugs metabolized through the P450 system. Rapid intravenous administration has been associated with rare cases of arrhythmia and/or hypotension.

Over the counter (OTC) cimetidine should not be taken by individuals experiencing painful swallowing, vomiting with blood, or bloody or black stools; medical attention should be sought. A physician should be consulted prior to use when pain in the stomach, shoulder, arms or neck is present; if heartburn has occurred for >3 months; or if unexplained weight loss, or nausea and vomiting occur. Frequent wheezing, shortness of breath, lightheadedness, or sweating, especially with chest pain or heartburn, should also be reported. Consultation of a healthcare provider should occur by patients if also taking theophylline, phenytoin, or warfarin; if heartburn or stomach pain continues or worsens; or if use is required for >14 days. Symptoms of GI distress may be associated with a variety of conditions; symptomatic response to H_2 antagonists does not rule out the potential for significant pathology (eg, malignancy).

Adverse Reactions (Reflective of adult population; not specific for elderly)
1% to 10%:
Central nervous system: Headache (2% to 4%), dizziness (1%), somnolence (1%), agitation
Endocrine & metabolic: Gynecomastia (<1% to 4%)
Gastrointestinal: Diarrhea (1%)
Frequency not defined:
Cardiovascular: AV block, bradycardia, hypotension, tachycardia, vasculitis
Central nervous system: Confusion, fever
Dermatologic: Alopecia, erythema multiforme, exfoliative dermatitis, Stevens-Johnson syndrome, toxic epidermal necrolysis, rash
Endocrine & metabolic: Edema of the breasts, sexual ability decreased
Gastrointestinal: Nausea, pancreatitis, vomiting
Hematologic: Agranulocytosis, aplastic anemia, hemolytic anemia (immune-based), neutropenia, pancytopenia, thrombocytopenia
Hepatic: ALT increased, AST increased, hepatic fibrosis (case report)
Neuromuscular & skeletal: Arthralgia, myalgia, polymyositis
Renal: Creatinine increased, interstitial nephritis
Miscellaneous: Anaphylaxis, pneumonia (causal relationship not established)

Drug Interactions
Metabolism/Transport Effects Substrate of P-glycoprotein; **Inhibits** CYP1A2 (moderate), 2C9 (weak), 2C19 (moderate), 2D6 (moderate), 2E1 (weak), 3A4 (moderate)
Avoid Concomitant Use
Avoid concomitant use of Cimetidine with any of the following: Clopidogrel; Delavirdine; Dofetilide; Epirubicin; Thioridazine; Tolvaptan

◄ **Increased Effect/Toxicity**

Cimetidine may increase the levels/effects of: Alfentanil; Amiodarone; Anticonvulsants (Hydantoin); Benzodiazepines (metabolized by oxidation); Bromazepam; Budesonide (Systemic, Oral Inhalation); Calcium Channel Blockers; CarBAMazepine; Carmustine; Carvedilol; Cisapride; CloZAPine; Colchicine; CYP1A2 Substrates; CYP2C19 Substrates; CYP2D6 Substrates; CYP3A4 Substrates; Dexmethylphenidate; Dofetilide; Epirubicin; Eplerenone; Everolimus; Fesoterodine; Halofantrine; Lurasidone; MetFORMIN; Methylphenidate; Moclobemide; Nebivolol; Nicotine; Pentoxifylline; Pimecrolimus; Pramipexole; Praziquantel; Procainamide; Propafenone; QuiNIDine; QuiNINE; Ranolazine; Roflumilast; Salmeterol; Saquinavir; Saxagliptin; Selective Serotonin Reuptake Inhibitors; Sulfonylureas; Tamoxifen; Theophylline Derivatives; Thioridazine; Tolvaptan; Tricyclic Antidepressants; Varenicline; Vitamin K Antagonists; Zaleplon; ZOLMitriptan

The levels/effects of Cimetidine may be increased by: P-Glycoprotein Inhibitors

Decreased Effect

Cimetidine may decrease the levels/effects of: Atazanavir; Cefditoren; Cefpodoxime; Cefuroxime; Clopidogrel; Dasatinib; Delavirdine; Erlotinib; Fosamprenavir; Gefitinib; Indinavir; Iron Salts; Itraconazole; Ketoconazole; Ketoconazole (Systemic); Mesalamine; Nelfinavir; Posaconazole; Rilpivirine

The levels/effects of Cimetidine may be decreased by: P-Glycoprotein Inducers

Ethanol/Nutrition/Herb Interactions

Ethanol: Avoid ethanol (may enhance gastric mucosal irritation).

Food: Cimetidine may increase serum caffeine levels if taken with caffeine. Cimetidine peak serum levels may be decreased if taken with food.

Herb/Nutraceutical: St John's wort may decrease cimetidine levels.

Stability Tablet: Store between 15°C and 30°C (59°F to 86°F). Protect from light.

Mechanism of Action Competitive inhibition of histamine at H_2 receptors of the gastric parietal cells resulting in reduced gastric acid secretion, gastric volume and hydrogen ion concentration reduced

Pharmacodynamics/Kinetics

Absorption: Rapid

Protein binding: 13% to 25%

Bioavailability: 60% to 70%

Metabolism: Hepatic

Half-life: Adults with normal renal function: 2 hours

Time to peak serum concentrations: Oral: Within 1-2 hours

Excretion: Primarily urine (48% as unchanged drug); feces (some)

Dosage

Geriatric & Adult

Short-term treatment of active ulcers: Oral: 300 mg 4 times/day or 800 mg at bedtime or 400 mg twice daily for up to 8 weeks

Note: Higher doses of 1600 mg at bedtime for 4 weeks may be beneficial for a subpopulation of patients with larger duodenal ulcers (>1 cm defined endoscopically) who are also heavy smokers (≥1 pack/day).

Duodenal ulcer prophylaxis: 400 mg at bedtime

Gastric hypersecretory conditions: 300-600 mg every 6 hours; dosage not to exceed 2.4 g/day

Gastroesophageal reflux disease: 400 mg 4 times/day or 800 mg twice daily for 12 weeks

Peptic ulcer disease eradication of *Helicobacter pylori* (unlabeled use): 400 mg twice daily; requires combination therapy with antibiotics

Heartburn, acid indigestion, sour stomach (OTC labeling): 200 mg up to twice daily; may take 30 minutes prior to eating foods or beverages expected to cause heartburn or indigestion

Renal Impairment

Cl_{cr} 10-50 mL/minute: Administer 50% of normal dose

Cl_{cr} <10 mL/minute: Administer 25% of normal dose

Slightly dialyzable (5% to 20%); administer after dialysis

Hepatic Impairment Usual dose is safe in mild liver disease but use with caution and in reduced dosage in severe liver disease. Increased risk of CNS toxicity in cirrhosis suggested by enhanced penetration of CNS.

Administration

Oral: Administer with meals so that the drug's peak effect occurs at the proper time (peak inhibition of gastric acid secretion occurs at 1 and 3 hours after dosing in fasting subjects and approximately 2 hours in nonfasting subjects; this correlates well with the time food is no longer in the stomach offering a buffering effect)

Injection: May be administered as a slow I.V. push or preferably as an I.V. intermittent or I.V. continuous infusion. Administer each 300 mg (or fraction thereof) over a minimum of 5 minutes when giving I.V. push. Give intermittent infusion over 15-30 minutes for each 300 mg dose. Intermittent infusions are administered over 15-30 minutes at a final concentration not to exceed 6 mg/mL; for patients with an active bleed, preferred method of administration is continuous infusion.

Monitoring Parameters CBC, gastric pH, occult blood with GI bleeding; monitor renal function to correct dose.

Special Geriatric Considerations Patients diagnosed with PUD should be evaluated for *Helicobacter pylori*. H$_2$ blockers are the preferred drugs for treating PUD in elderly due to cost and ease of administration. These agents are no less or more effective than any other therapy. The preferred agents, due to favorable pharmacokinetic, side effect and drug interaction profiles are ranitidine, famotidine, and nizatidine. Due to the potential for confusion and drug interactions, cimetidine has been identified by a panel of experts as a drug to avoid in the elderly. Consider evaluating creatinine clearance before initiating H$_2$-blocker therapy.

This medication is considered to be potentially inappropriate in this patient population (Beers Criteria severity: Low).

Dosage Forms Excipient information presented when available (limited, particularly for generics); consult specific product labeling.
Solution, oral, as hydrochloride [strength expressed as base]: 300 mg/5 mL (237 mL, 473 mL)
Tablet, oral: 200 mg, 300 mg, 400 mg, 800 mg
  Tagamet HB 200®: 200 mg

Selected References
Fick DM, Cooper JW, Wade WE, et al "Updating the Beers Criteria for Potentially Inappropriate Medication Use in Older Adults," *Intern Med*, 2003, 163(22):2716-24.

◆ **Cimzia®** see Certolizumab Pegol *on page 324*
◆ **Cipro®** see Ciprofloxacin (Systemic) *on page 359*
◆ **Ciprodex®** see Ciprofloxacin and Dexamethasone *on page 364*

Ciprofloxacin (Systemic) (sip roe FLOKS a sin)

Related Information
Antibiotic Treatment of Adults With Infective Endocarditis *on page 2053*
Community-Acquired Pneumonia in Adults *on page 2059*
Medication Safety Issues
Sound-alike/look-alike issues:
Ciprofloxacin may be confused with cephalexin
Cipro® may be confused with Ceftin®

Brand Names: U.S. Cipro®; Cipro® I.V.; Cipro® XR

Brand Names: Canada Apo-Ciproflox®; Cipro®; Cipro® XL; CO Ciprofloxacin; Dom-Ciprofloxacin; Mint-Ciprofloxacin; Mylan-Ciprofloxacin; Novo-Ciprofloxacin; PHL-Ciprofloxacin; PMS-Ciprofloxacin; PRO-Ciprofloxacin; RAN™-Ciprofloxacin; ratio-Ciprofloxacin; Riva-Ciprofloxacin; Sandoz-Ciprofloxacin; Taro-Ciprofloxacin

Index Terms Ciprofloxacin Hydrochloride

Generic Availability (U.S.) Yes: Excludes suspension

Pharmacologic Category Antibiotic, Quinolone

Use
To reduce incidence or progression of disease following exposure to aerolized *Bacillus anthracis*.
Treatment of the following infections when caused by susceptible bacteria: Urinary tract infections; acute uncomplicated cystitis in females; chronic bacterial prostatitis; lower respiratory tract infections (including acute exacerbations of chronic bronchitis); acute sinusitis; skin and skin structure infections; bone and joint infections; complicated intra-abdominal infections (in combination with metronidazole); infectious diarrhea; typhoid fever due to *Salmonella typhi* (eradication of chronic typhoid carrier state has not been proven); uncomplicated cervical and urethra gonorrhea (due to *N. gonorrhoeae*); nosocomial pneumonia; empirical therapy for febrile neutropenic patients (in combination with piperacillin)

Note: As of April 2007, the CDC no longer recommends the use of fluoroquinolones for the treatment of gonococcal disease.

Unlabeled/Investigational Use Cutaneous/gastrointestinal/oropharyngeal anthrax (treatment); disseminated gonococcal infection; chancroid; prophylaxis to *Neisseria meningitidis* following close contact with an infected person; empirical therapy (oral) for febrile neutropenia in low-risk cancer patients; HACEK group endocarditis

Medication Guide Available Yes

Contraindications Hypersensitivity to ciprofloxacin, any component of the formulation, or other quinolones; concurrent administration of tizanidine

◄ **Warnings/Precautions [U.S. Boxed Warning]: There have been reports of tendon inflammation and/or rupture with quinolone antibiotics; risk may be increased with concurrent corticosteroids, organ transplant recipients, and in patients >60 years of age.** Rupture of the Achilles tendon sometimes requiring surgical repair has been reported most frequently; but other tendon sites (eg, rotator cuff, biceps) have also been reported. Strenuous physical activity, rheumatoid arthritis, and renal impairment may be an independent risk factor for tendonitis. Discontinue at first sign of tendon inflammation or pain. May occur even after discontinuation of therapy. Use with caution in patients with rheumatoid arthritis; may increase risk of tendon rupture. CNS stimulation may occur (tremor, restlessness, confusion, and very rarely hallucinations or seizures). Use with caution in patients with known or suspected CNS disorder. Potential for seizures, although very rare, may be increased with concomitant NSAID therapy. Use with caution in individuals at risk of seizures. Fluoroquinolones may prolong QT_c interval; avoid use in patients with a history of QT_c prolongation, uncorrected hypokalemia, hypomagnesemia, or concurrent administration of other medications known to prolong the QT interval (including Class Ia and Class III antiarrhythmics, cisapride, erythromycin, antipsychotics, and tricyclic antidepressants). Prolonged use may result in fungal or bacterial superinfection, including *C. difficile*-associated diarrhea (CDAD) and pseudomembranous colitis; CDAD has been observed >2 months postantibiotic treatment. Rarely crystalluria has occurred; urine alkalinity may increase the risk. Ensure adequate hydration during therapy. Rare cases of peripheral neuropathy may occur.

Fluoroquinolones have been associated with the development of serious, and sometimes fatal, hypoglycemia, most often in elderly diabetics but also in patients without diabetes. This occurred most frequently with gatifloxacin (no longer available systemically), but may occur at a lower frequency with other quinolones.

Severe hypersensitivity reactions, including anaphylaxis, have occurred with quinolone therapy. Reactions may present as typical allergic symptoms after a single dose, or may manifest as severe idiosyncratic dermatologic, vascular, pulmonary, renal, hepatic, and/or hematologic events, usually after multiple doses. Prompt discontinuation of drug should occur if skin rash or other symptoms arise. **[U.S. Boxed Warning]: Quinolones may exacerbate myasthenia gravis; avoid use (rare, potentially life-threatening weakness of respiratory muscles may occur).** Use caution in renal impairment. Avoid excessive sunlight and take precautions to limit exposure (eg, loose fitting clothing, sunscreen); may cause moderate-to-severe phototoxicity reactions. Discontinue use if photosensitivity occurs. Since ciprofloxacin is ineffective in the treatment of syphilis and may mask symptoms, all patients should be tested for syphilis at the time of gonorrheal diagnosis and 3 months later. Hemolytic reactions may (rarely) occur with quinolone use in patients with latent or actual G6PD deficiency.

Ciprofloxacin is a potent inhibitor of CYP1A2. Coadministration of drugs which depend on this pathway may lead to substantial increases in serum concentrations and adverse effects.

Adverse Reactions (Reflective of adult population; not specific for elderly)
1% to 10%:
Central nervous system: Neurologic events (children 2%, includes dizziness, insomnia, nervousness, somnolence); fever (children 2%); headache (I.V. administration); restlessness (I.V. administration)
Dermatologic: Rash (children 2%, adults 1%)
Gastrointestinal: Nausea (3%); diarrhea (children 5%, adults 2%); vomiting (children 5%, adults 1%); abdominal pain (children 3%, adults <1%); dyspepsia (children 3%)
Hepatic: ALT increased, AST increased (adults 1%)
Local: Injection site reactions (I.V. administration)
Respiratory: Rhinitis (children 3%)

Drug Interactions
Metabolism/Transport Effects Substrate of P-glycoprotein; **Inhibits** CYP1A2 (strong), 3A4 (weak)

Avoid Concomitant Use
Avoid concomitant use of Ciprofloxacin (Systemic) with any of the following: BCG; TiZANidine

Increased Effect/Toxicity
Ciprofloxacin (Systemic) may increase the levels/effects of: Bendamustine; Caffeine; Corticosteroids (Systemic); CYP1A2 Substrates; Erlotinib; Methotrexate; Pentoxifylline; Porfimer; QTc-Prolonging Agents; ROPINIRole; Ropivacaine; Sulfonylureas; Theophylline Derivatives; TiZANidine; Vitamin K Antagonists

The levels/effects of Ciprofloxacin (Systemic) may be increased by: Insulin; Nonsteroidal Anti-Inflammatory Agents; P-Glycoprotein Inhibitors; Probenecid

Decreased Effect

Ciprofloxacin (Systemic) may decrease the levels/effects of: BCG; Fosphenytoin; Mycophenolate; Phenytoin; Sulfonylureas; Typhoid Vaccine

The levels/effects of Ciprofloxacin (Systemic) may be decreased by: Antacids; Calcium Salts; Didanosine; Iron Salts; Lanthanum; Magnesium Salts; P-Glycoprotein Inducers; Quinapril; Sevelamer; Sucralfate; Zinc Salts

Ethanol/Nutrition/Herb Interactions

Food: Food decreases rate, but not extent, of absorption. Ciprofloxacin serum levels may be decreased if taken with dairy products or calcium-fortified juices. Ciprofloxacin may increase serum caffeine levels if taken with caffeine.

Enteral feedings may decrease plasma concentrations of ciprofloxacin probably by >30% inhibition of absorption. Ciprofloxacin should not be administered with enteral feedings. The feeding would need to be discontinued for 1-2 hours prior to and after ciprofloxacin administration. Nasogastric administration produces a greater loss of ciprofloxacin bioavailability than does nasoduodenal administration.

Herb/Nutraceutical: Avoid dong quai, St John's wort (may also cause photosensitization).

Stability

Injection:

Premixed infusion: Store between 5°C to 25°C (41°F to 77°F); avoid freezing. Protect from light.

Vial: Store between 5°C to 30°C (41°F to 86°F); avoid freezing. Protect from light. May be diluted with NS, D$_5$W, SWFI, D$_{10}$W, D$_5$1/4NS, D$_5$1/2NS, LR. Diluted solutions of 0.5-2 mg/mL are stable for up to 14 days refrigerated or at room temperature.

Microcapsules for oral suspension: Prior to reconstitution, store below 25°C (77°F); protect from freezing. Following reconstitution, store below 30°C (86°F) for up to 14 days; protect from freezing.

Tablet:

Immediate release: Store below 30°C (86°F).

Extended release: Store at room temperature of 15°C to 30°C (59°F to 86°F).

Mechanism of Action Inhibits DNA-gyrase in susceptible organisms; inhibits relaxation of supercoiled DNA and promotes breakage of double-stranded DNA

Pharmacodynamics/Kinetics

Absorption: Oral: Immediate release tablet: Rapid (~50% to 85%)

Distribution: V$_d$: 2.1-2.7 L/kg; tissue concentrations often exceed serum concentrations especially in kidneys, gallbladder, liver, lungs, gynecological tissue, and prostatic tissue; CSF concentrations: 10% of serum concentrations (noninflamed meninges), 14% to 37% (inflamed meninges)

Protein binding: 20% to 40%

Metabolism: Partially hepatic; forms 4 metabolites (limited activity)

Half-life elimination: Adults: Normal renal function: 3-5 hours

Time to peak: Oral:

Immediate release tablet: 0.5-2 hours

Extended release tablet: Cipro® XR: 1-2.5 hours; Proquin® XR: 3.5-8.7 hours

Excretion: Urine (30% to 50% as unchanged drug); feces (15% to 43%)

Dosage

Geriatric Refer to adult dosing. Adjust dose carefully based on renal function.

Adult Note: Extended release tablets and immediate release formulations are not interchangeable. Unless otherwise specified, oral dosing reflects the use of immediate release formulations.

Anthrax:

Inhalational (postexposure prophylaxis):

Oral: 500 mg every 12 hours for 60 days

I.V.: 400 mg every 12 hours for 60 days

Cutaneous (treatment, CDC guidelines): Oral: Immediate release formulation: 500 mg every 12 hours for 60 days. **Note:** In the presence of systemic involvement, extensive edema, lesions on head/neck, refer to I.V. dosing for treatment of inhalational/gastrointestinal/oropharyngeal anthrax.

Inhalational/gastrointestinal/oropharyngeal (treatment, CDC guidelines): I.V.: 400 mg every 12 hours. **Note:** Initial treatment should include two or more agents predicted to be effective (per CDC recommendations). Continue combined therapy for 60 days.

Bone/joint infections:

Oral: 500-750 mg twice daily for 4-6 weeks

I.V.:

Mild/moderate: 400 mg every 12 hours for 4-6 weeks

Severe/complicated: 400 mg every 8 hours for 4-6 weeks

Chancroid (unlabeled use): Oral: 500 mg twice daily for 3 days (CDC, 2010)

◀ **Endocarditis due to HACEK organisms (AHA guidelines, unlabeled use): Note:** Not first-line option; use only if intolerant of beta-lactam therapy:

Oral: 500 mg every 12 hours for 4 weeks

I.V.: 400 mg every 12 hours for 4 weeks

Febrile neutropenia: I.V.: 400 mg every 8 hours for 7-14 days (combination therapy generally recommended)

Gonococcal infections:

Urethral/cervical gonococcal infections: Oral: 250-500 mg as a single dose (CDC recommends concomitant doxycycline or azithromycin due to possible coinfection with *Chlamydia*; **Note:** As of April 2007, the CDC no longer recommends the use of fluoroquinolones for the treatment of uncomplicated gonococcal disease.

Disseminated gonococcal infection (CDC guidelines): Oral: 500 mg twice daily to complete 7 days of therapy (initial treatment with ceftriaxone 1 g I.M./I.V. daily for 24-48 hours after improvement begins); **Note:** As of April 2007, the CDC no longer recommends the use of fluoroquinolones for the treatment of more serious gonococcal disease, unless no other options exist and susceptibility can be confirmed via culture.

Granuloma inguinale (donovanosis) (unlabeled use): Oral: 750 mg twice daily for at least 3 weeks (and until lesions have healed) (CDC, 2010)

Infectious diarrhea: Oral:

Salmonella: 500 mg twice daily for 5-7 days

Shigella: 500 mg twice daily for 3 days

Traveler's diarrhea: Mild: 750 mg for one dose; Severe: 500 mg twice daily for 3 days

Vibrio cholerae: 1 g for one dose

Intra-abdominal, complicated, community-acquired (in combination with metronidazole): Note: Avoid using in settings where *E. coli* susceptibility to fluoroquinolones is <90%:

Oral: 500 mg every 12 hours for 7-14 days

I.V.: 400 mg every 12 hours for 7-14 days; **Note:** 2010 IDSA guidelines recommend treatment duration of 4-7 days (provided source controlled)

Lower respiratory tract, skin/skin structure infections:

Oral: 500-750 mg twice daily for 7-14 days

I.V.:

Mild/moderate: 400 mg every 12 hours for 7-14 days

Severe/complicated: 400 mg every 8 hours for 7-14 days

Nosocomial pneumonia: I.V.: 400 mg every 8 hours for 10-14 days

Periodontitis (unlabeled use): Oral: 500 mg every 12 hours for 8-10 days

Prostatitis (chronic, bacterial): Oral: 500 mg every 12 hours for 28 days

Sinusitis (acute): Oral: 500 mg every 12 hours for 10 days

Typhoid fever: Oral: 500 mg every 12 hours for 10 days

Urinary tract infection:

Acute uncomplicated, cystitis:

Oral:

Immediate release formulation: 250 mg every 12 hours for 3 days

Extended release formulation (Cipro® XR): 500 mg every 24 hours for 3 days

I.V.: 200 mg every 12 hours for 7-14 days

Complicated (including pyelonephritis):

Oral:

Immediate release formulation: 500 mg every 12 hours for 7-14 days

Extended release formulation (Cipro® XR): 1000 mg every 24 hours for 7-14 days

I.V.: 400 mg every 12 hours for 7-14 days

Renal Impairment Adults:

Cl_{cr} 30-50 mL/minute: Oral: Administer 250-500 mg every 12 hours.

Cl_{cr} <30 mL/minute: Acute uncomplicated pyelonephritis or complicated UTI: Oral: Extended release formulation: 500 mg every 24 hours

Cl_{cr} 5-29 mL/minute:

Oral: Administer 250-500 mg every 18 hours.

I.V.: Administer 200-400 mg every 18-24 hours.

Intermittent hemodialysis (IHD) (administer after hemodialysis on dialysis days): Minimally dialyzable (<10%): Oral: 250-500 mg every 24 hours **or** I.V.: 200-400 mg every 24 hours (Heintz, 2009). **Note:** Dosing dependent on the assumption of 3 times/week, complete IHD sessions.

Continuous renal replacement therapy (CRRT) (Heintz, 2009; Trotman, 2005): Drug clearance is highly dependent on the method of renal replacement, filter type, and flow rate. Appropriate dosing requires close monitoring of pharmacologic response, signs of adverse reactions due to drug accumulation, as well as drug concentrations in relation to target trough (if appropriate). The following are general recommendations only (based on dialysate flow/ultrafiltration rates of 1-2 L/hour and minimal residual renal function) and should not supersede clinical judgment:

CVVH/CVVHD/CVVHDF: I.V.: 200-400 mg every 12-24 hours

Administration

Oral: May administer with food to minimize GI upset; avoid antacid use; maintain proper hydration and urine output. Administer immediate release ciprofloxacin and Cipro® XR at least 2 hours before or 6 hours after antacids or other products containing calcium, iron, or zinc (including dairy products or calcium-fortified juices). Separate oral administration from drugs which may impair absorption (see Drug Interactions).

Oral suspension: Should not be administered through feeding tubes (suspension is oil-based and adheres to the feeding tube). Patients should avoid chewing on the microcapsules.

Nasogastric/orogastric tube: Crush immediate-release tablet and mix with water. Flush feeding tube before and after administration. Hold tube feedings at least 1 hour before and 2 hours after administration.

Tablet, extended release: Do not crush, split, or chew. May be administered with meals containing dairy products (calcium content <800 mg), but not with dairy products alone.

Parenteral: Administer by slow I.V. infusion over 60 minutes to reduce the risk of venous irritation (burning, pain, erythema, and swelling); final concentration for administration should not exceed 2 mg/mL.

Monitoring Parameters CBC, renal and hepatic function during prolonged therapy

Reference Range Therapeutic: 2.6-3 mcg/mL; Toxic: >5 mcg/mL

Test Interactions Some quinolones may produce a false-positive urine screening result for opiates using commercially-available immunoassay kits. This has been demonstrated most consistently for levofloxacin and ofloxacin, but other quinolones have shown cross-reactivity in certain assay kits. Confirmation of positive opiate screens by more specific methods should be considered.

Pharmacotherapy Pearls No geriatric-specific information.

Special Geriatric Considerations See Warnings/Precautions regarding tendon rupture in patients >60 years of age. Ciprofloxacin should not be used as first-line therapy unless the culture and sensitivity findings show resistance to usual therapy. The interactions with caffeine and theophylline can result in serious toxicity in the elderly. Adjust dose for renal function.

Dosage Forms Excipient information presented when available (limited, particularly for generics); consult specific product labeling.

Infusion, premixed in D_5W: 200 mg (100 mL); 400 mg (200 mL)
Cipro® I.V.: 200 mg (100 mL); 400 mg (200 mL)
Infusion, premixed in D_5W [preservative free]: 200 mg (100 mL); 400 mg (200 mL)
Injection, solution: 10 mg/mL (20 mL, 40 mL)
Injection, solution [preservative free]: 10 mg/mL (20 mL, 40 mL)
Microcapsules for suspension, oral:
Cipro®: 250 mg/5 mL (100 mL); 500 mg/5 mL (100 mL) [strawberry flavor]
Tablet, oral, as hydrochloride [strength expressed as base]: 100 mg, 250 mg, 500 mg, 750 mg
Cipro®: 250 mg, 500 mg
Tablet, extended release, oral, as base and hydrochloride [strength expressed as base]: 500 mg, 1000 mg
Cipro® XR: 500 mg, 1000 mg

Selected References

Bayer A, Gajewska A, Stephens M, et al, "Pharmacokinetics of Ciprofloxacin in the Elderly," *Respiration*, 1987, 51 (4):292-5.

Guay DRP, Awni WM, Peterson PK, et al, "Single and Multiple Dose Pharmacokinetics of Oral Ciprofloxacin in Elderly Patients," *Int J Clin Pharmacol Ther Toxicol*, 1988, 26(6):279-84.

Mandell LA, Wunderink RG, Anzueto A, et al, "Infectious Diseases Society of America/American Thoracic Society Consensus Guidelines on the Management of Community-Acquired Pneumonia in Adults," *Clin Infect Dis*, 2007, 44 Suppl 2:S27-72.

Ciprofloxacin (Ophthalmic) (sip roe FLOKS a sin)

Medication Safety Issues

Sound-alike/look-alike issues:

Ciprofloxacin may be confused with cephalexin

Ciloxan® may be confused with cinoxacin, Cytoxan

Brand Names: U.S. Ciloxan®

Brand Names: Canada Ciloxan®

◀ **Index Terms** Ciprofloxacin Hydrochloride
Generic Availability (U.S.) Yes: Excludes ointment
Pharmacologic Category Antibiotic, Ophthalmic; Antibiotic, Quinolone
Use Treatment of superficial ocular infections (corneal ulcers, conjunctivitis) due to susceptible strains
Dosage
  Geriatric & Adult
    Bacterial conjunctivitis:
      Ophthalmic solution: Instill 1-2 drops in eye(s) every 2 hours while awake for 2 days and 1-2 drops every 4 hours while awake for the next 5 days
      Ophthalmic ointment: Apply a 1/2" ribbon into the conjunctival sac 3 times/day for the first 2 days, followed by a 1/2" ribbon applied twice daily for the next 5 days
    Corneal ulcer: *Ophthalmic solution:* Instill 2 drops into affected eye every 15 minutes for the first 6 hours, then 2 drops into the affected eye every 30 minutes for the remainder of the first day. On day 2, instill 2 drops into the affected eye hourly. On days 3-14, instill 2 drops into affected eye every 4 hours. Treatment may continue after day 14 if re-epithelialization has not occurred.
Dosage Forms Excipient information presented when available (limited, particularly for generics); consult specific product labeling.
Ointment, ophthalmic, as hydrochloride:
  Ciloxan®: 3.33 mg/g (3.5 g) [equivalent to ciprofloxacin base 0.3%]
Solution, ophthalmic, as hydrochloride [drops]: 3.5 mg/mL (2.5 mL, 5 mL, 10 mL) [equivalent to ciprofloxacin base 0.3%]
  Ciloxan®: 3.5 mg/mL (5 mL) [contains benzalkonium chloride; equivalent to ciprofloxacin base 0.3%]

Ciprofloxacin (Otic) (sip roe FLOKS a sin)

Medication Safety Issues
  Sound-alike/look-alike issues:
    Cetraxal® may be confused with cefTRIAXone
    Ciprofloxacin may be confused with cephalexin
Brand Names: U.S. Cetraxal®
Index Terms Ciprofloxacin Hydrochloride
Generic Availability (U.S.) No
Pharmacologic Category Antibiotic, Otic; Antibiotic, Quinolone
Use Treatment of acute otitis externa due to susceptible strains of *Pseudomonas aeruginosa* or *Staphylococcus aureus*
Dosage
  Geriatric & Adult Acute otitis externa: Otic solution: Instill 0.25 mL (contents of 1 single-dose container) into affected ear twice daily for 7 days
Dosage Forms Excipient information presented when available (limited, particularly for generics); consult specific product labeling.
Solution, otic, as hydrochloride [preservative free]:
  Cetraxal®: 0.5 mg/0.25 mL (14s) [equivalent to ciprofloxacin base 0.2%]

Ciprofloxacin and Dexamethasone (sip roe FLOKS a sin & deks a METH a sone)

Related Information
  Ciprofloxacin (Otic) *on page 364*
Brand Names: U.S. Ciprodex®
Brand Names: Canada Ciprodex®
Index Terms Ciprofloxacin Hydrochloride and Dexamethasone; Dexamethasone and Ciprofloxacin
Generic Availability (U.S.) No
Pharmacologic Category Antibiotic, Otic; Antibiotic/Corticosteroid, Otic; Corticosteroid, Otic
Use Treatment of acute otitis externa
Dosage
  Geriatric & Adult Acute otitis externa: Otic: Instill 4 drops into affected ear(s) twice daily for 7 days
Dosage Forms Excipient information presented when available (limited, particularly for generics); consult specific product labeling.
Suspension, otic:
  Ciprodex®: Ciprofloxacin 0.3% and dexamethasone 0.1% (7.5 mL) [contains benzalkonium chloride]

Ciprofloxacin and Hydrocortisone (sip roe FLOKS a sin & hye droe KOR ti sone)

Related Information
  Ciprofloxacin (Otic) *on page 364*
Brand Names: U.S. Cipro® HC
Brand Names: Canada Cipro® HC
Index Terms Ciprofloxacin Hydrochloride and Hydrocortisone; Hydrocortisone and Ciprofloxacin
Generic Availability (U.S.) No
Pharmacologic Category Antibiotic/Corticosteroid, Otic
Use Treatment of acute otitis externa, sometimes known as "swimmer's ear"
Dosage
  Geriatric & Adult Otitis externa: Otic: The recommended dosage for all patients is three drops of the suspension in the affected ear twice daily for 7 days; twice-daily dosing schedule is more convenient for patients than that of existing treatments with hydrocortisone, which are typically administered three or four times a day
Dosage Forms Excipient information presented when available (limited, particularly for generics); consult specific product labeling.
  Suspension, otic:
    Cipro® HC: Ciprofloxacin hydrochloride 0.2% and hydrocortisone 1% (10 mL) [contains benzyl alcohol]

♦ **Ciprofloxacin Hydrochloride** *see* Ciprofloxacin (Ophthalmic) *on page 363*
♦ **Ciprofloxacin Hydrochloride** *see* Ciprofloxacin (Otic) *on page 364*
♦ **Ciprofloxacin Hydrochloride** *see* Ciprofloxacin (Systemic) *on page 359*
♦ **Ciprofloxacin Hydrochloride and Dexamethasone** *see* Ciprofloxacin and Dexamethasone *on page 364*
♦ **Ciprofloxacin Hydrochloride and Hydrocortisone** *see* Ciprofloxacin and Hydrocortisone *on page 365*
♦ **Cipro® HC** *see* Ciprofloxacin and Hydrocortisone *on page 365*
♦ **Cipro® I.V.** *see* Ciprofloxacin (Systemic) *on page 359*
♦ **Cipro® XR** *see* Ciprofloxacin (Systemic) *on page 359*

Citalopram (sye TAL oh pram)

Related Information
  Antidepressant Agents *on page 1991*
  Beers Criteria – Potentially Inappropriate Medications for Geriatrics *on page 2089*
  Liquid Compatibility of Antidepressants, Antipsychotics, and Mood Stabilizers *on page 2111*
Medication Safety Issues
  Sound-alike/look-alike issues:
    CeleXA® may be confused with CeleBREX®, Cerebra®, Cerebyx®, Ranexa™, ZyPREXA®
Brand Names: U.S. CeleXA®
Brand Names: Canada Apo-Citalopram®; Celexa®; Citalopram-Odan; CO Citalopram; CTP 30; Dom-Citalopram; JAMP-Citalopram; Mint-Citalopram; Mylan-Citalopram; NG-Citalopram; Novo-Citalopram; PHL-Citalopram; PMS-Citalopram; RAN™-Citalo; ratio-Citalopram; Riva-Citalopram; Sandoz-Citalopram; Septa-Citalopram; Teva-Citalopram
Index Terms Citalopram Hydrobromide; Nitalapram
Generic Availability (U.S.) Yes
Pharmacologic Category Antidepressant, Selective Serotonin Reuptake Inhibitor
Use Treatment of depression
Unlabeled/Investigational Use Treatment of mild dementia-associated agitation in non-psychotic patients; smoking cessation; ethanol abuse; diabetic neuropathy
Medication Guide Available Yes
Contraindications Hypersensitivity to citalopram or any component of the formulation; concomitant use with MAO inhibitors or within 2 weeks of discontinuing MAO inhibitors; concomitant use with pimozide; patients with congenital long QT syndrome
Warnings/Precautions [U.S. Boxed Warning]: Antidepressants increase the risk of suicidal thinking and behavior in children, adolescents, and young adults (18-24 years of age) with major depressive disorder (MDD) and other psychiatric disorders; consider risk prior to prescribing. Short-term studies did not show an increased risk in patients >24 years of age and showed a decreased risk in patients ≥65 years. Closely monitor patients for clinical worsening, suicidality, or unusual changes in behavior, particularly during the initial 1-2 months of therapy or during periods of dosage adjustments (increases or decreases); the patient's family or caregiver should be instructed to closely observe the patient and

communicate condition with healthcare provider. A medication guide concerning the use of antidepressants should be dispensed with each prescription. **Citalopram is not FDA approved for use in children.**

The possibility of a suicide attempt is inherent in major depression and may persist until remission occurs. Use caution in high-risk patients. Worsening depression and severe abrupt suicidality that are not part of the presenting symptoms may require discontinuation or modification of drug therapy. The patient's family or caregiver should be alerted to monitor patients for the emergence of suicidality and associated behaviors (such as agitation, irritability, hostility, impulsivity, and hypomania) and call healthcare provider.

May worsen psychosis in some patients or precipitate a shift to mania or hypomania in patients with bipolar disorder. Patients presenting with depressive symptoms should be screened for bipolar disorder. Monotherapy in patients with bipolar disorder should be avoided. **Citalopram is not FDA approved for the treatment of bipolar depression.**

Serotonin syndrome and neuroleptic malignant syndrome (NMS)-like reactions have occurred with serotonin/norepinephrine reuptake inhibitors (SNRIs) and selective serotonin reuptake inhibitors (SSRIs) when used alone, and particularly when used in combination with serotonergic agents (eg, triptans) or antidopaminergic agents (eg, antipsychotics). Concurrent use with MAO inhibitors is contraindicated. May increase the risks associated with electro-convulsive therapy. Has a low potential to impair cognitive or motor performance; caution operating hazardous machinery or driving.

Use with caution in patients with hepatic or renal dysfunction, in elderly patients, and concomitant CNS depressants. Use caution with concomitant use of aspirin, NSAIDs, warfarin, or other drugs that affect coagulation; the risk of bleeding may be potentiated. May cause hyponatremia/SIADH (elderly at increased risk); volume depletion and diuretics may increase risk. May cause or exacerbate sexual dysfunction. Upon discontinuation of citalopram therapy, gradually taper dose. If intolerable symptoms occur following a decrease in dosage or upon discontinuation of therapy, then resuming the previous dose with a more gradual taper should be considered.

Adverse Reactions (Reflective of adult population; not specific for elderly)

>10%:

Central nervous system: Somnolence (18%; dose related), insomnia (15%; dose related)

Gastrointestinal: Nausea (21%), xerostomia (20%)

Miscellaneous: Diaphoresis (11%; dose related)

1% to 10%:

Cardiovascular: Postural hypotension, tachycardia

Central nervous system: Fatigue (5%; dose related), anorexia (4%), anxiety (4%), agitation (3%), fever (2%), yawning (2%; dose related), amnesia, apathy, concentration impaired, confusion, depression, migraine, suicide attempt

Dermatologic: Rash, pruritus

Endocrine & metabolic: Libido decreased (1% to 4%), dysmenorrhea (3%), amenorrhea, sexual dysfunction

Gastrointestinal: Diarrhea (8%), dyspepsia (5%), vomiting (4%), abdominal pain (3%), flatulence, salivation increased, taste perversion, weight gain/loss

Genitourinary: Ejaculation disorder (6%), impotence (3%; dose related), polyuria

Neuromuscular & skeletal: Tremor (8%), arthralgia (2%), myalgia (2%), paresthesia

Ocular: Abnormal accommodation

Respiratory: Rhinitis (5%), upper respiratory tract infection (5%), sinusitis (3%), cough

Drug Interactions

Metabolism/Transport Effects Substrate of CYP2C19 (major), 2D6 (minor), 3A4 (major); **Inhibits** CYP1A2 (weak), 2B6 (weak), 2C19 (weak), 2D6 (weak)

Avoid Concomitant Use

Avoid concomitant use of Citalopram with any of the following: Artemether; Conivaptan; Dronedarone; Iobenguane I 123; Lumefantrine; MAO Inhibitors; Methylene Blue; Nilotinib; Pimozide; QUEtiapine; QuiNINE; Sibutramine; Tetrabenazine; Thioridazine; Toremifene; Tryptophan; Vandetanib; Vemurafenib; Ziprasidone

Increased Effect/Toxicity

Citalopram may increase the levels/effects of: Alpha-/Beta-Blockers; Anticoagulants; Anti-depressants (Serotonin Reuptake Inhibitor/Antagonist); Antiplatelet Agents; Aspirin; Bus-PIRone; CarBAMazepine; CloZAPine; Collagenase (Systemic); Desmopressin; Dextromethorphan; Dronedarone; Drotrecogin Alfa; Haloperidol; Ibritumomab; Lithium; Methadone; Methylene Blue; Mexiletine; NSAID (COX-2 Inhibitor); NSAID (Nonselective); Pimozide; QTc-Prolonging Agents; QuiNINE; RisperiDONE; Rivaroxaban; Salicylates; Sero-tonin Modulators; Tetrabenazine; Thioridazine; Thrombolytic Agents; Toremifene; Tositumo-mab and Iodine I 131 Tositumomab; TraMADol; Tricyclic Antidepressants; Vandetanib; Vemurafenib; Vitamin K Antagonists; Ziprasidone

The levels/effects of Citalopram may be increased by: Alcohol (Ethyl); Alfuzosin; Analgesics (Opioid); Artemether; BusPIRone; Chloroquine; Cimetidine; Ciprofloxacin; Ciprofloxacin (Systemic); CNS Depressants; Conivaptan; CYP2C19 Inhibitors (Moderate); CYP2C19 Inhibitors (Strong); CYP3A4 Inhibitors (Moderate); CYP3A4 Inhibitors (Strong); Fluconazole; Gadobutrol; Glucosamine; Herbs (Anticoagulant/Antiplatelet Properties); Lumefantrine; Macrolide Antibiotics; MAO Inhibitors; Metoclopramide; Nilotinib; Omega-3-Acid Ethyl Esters; Pentosan Polysulfate Sodium; Pentoxifylline; Prostacyclin Analogues; QUEtiapine; QuiNINE; Sibutramine; TraMADol; Tryptophan; Vitamin E

Decreased Effect

Citalopram may decrease the levels/effects of: Iobenguane I 123

The levels/effects of Citalopram may be decreased by: CarBAMazepine; CYP2C19 Inducers (Strong); CYP3A4 Inducers (Strong); Cyproheptadine; Deferasirox; NSAID (Nonselective); Peginterferon Alfa-2b; Tocilizumab

Ethanol/Nutrition/Herb Interactions

Ethanol: May increase CNS depression; monitor for increased effects with coadministration. Caution patients about effects.

Herb/Nutraceutical: Avoid valerian, St John's wort, SAMe, kava kava, and gotu kola (may increase CNS depression).

Stability Store at 20°C to 25°C (68°F to 77°F); excursions permitted to 15°C to 30°C (59°F to 86°F). Protect from light.

Mechanism of Action A racemic bicyclic phthalane derivative, citalopram selectively inhibits serotonin reuptake in the presynaptic neurons and has minimal effects on norepinephrine or dopamine. Uptake inhibition of serotonin is primarily due to the *S*-enantiomer of citalopram. Displays little to no affinity for serotonin, dopamine, adrenergic, histamine, GABA, or muscarinic receptor subtypes.

Pharmacodynamics/Kinetics

Onset of action: Depression: The onset of action is within a week; however, individual response varies greatly and full response may not be seen until 8-12 weeks after initiation of treatment.

Distribution: V_d: 12 L/kg

Protein binding, plasma: ~80%

Metabolism: Extensively hepatic, via CYP3A4 and 2C19 (major pathways), and 2D6 (minor pathway); forms metabolites, N-demethylcitalopram (DCT) and didemethylcitalopram (DDCT) which are at least eight times less potent than citalopram

Bioavailability: 80%

Half-life elimination: 24-48 hours (average: 35 hours); doubled with hepatic impairment

Time to peak, serum: 1-6 hours, average within 4 hours

Excretion: Urine (Citalopram 10% and DCT 5%)

> **Note:** Clearance was decreased, while AUC and half-life were significantly increased in elderly patients and in patients with hepatic impairment. Mild-to-moderate renal impairment may reduce clearance (17%) and prolong half-life of citalopram. No pharmacokinetic information is available concerning patients with severe renal impairment.

Dosage

Geriatric

Refer to adult dosing. **Note:** Due to increased serum concentrations in patients ≥60 years and the risk of QT prolongation, the maximum recommended dose in elderly patients is 20 mg/day.

Alzheimer's dementia-related depression (unlabeled use): Oral: Initial: 5-10 mg/day; may increase at multi-week intervals to maximum of 40 mg/day (Rabins, 2007)

Adult Depression: Oral: Initial: 20 mg/day, generally with an increase to 40 mg/day; maximum dose in adults <60 years: 40 mg/day; maximum dose in adults ≥60 years: 20 mg/day

Poor metabolizers of CYP2C19 or concurrent use of CYP2C19 inhibitors (eg, cimetidine): Maximum dose: 20 mg/day

Renal Impairment

Mild-to-moderate impairment: No dosage adjustment needed.

Severe impairment: Cl_{cr} <20 mL/minute: Use with caution.

Hepatic Impairment Oral: 20 mg once daily; maximum dose: 20 mg/day due to increased serum concentrations and the risk of QT prolongation

Administration May be administered without regard to food.

Monitoring Parameters ECG; liver function tests and CBC with continued therapy; monitor patient periodically for symptom resolution; mental status for depression, suicidal ideation (especially at the beginning of therapy or when doses are increased or decreased), anxiety, social functioning, mania, panic attacks; akathisia

◀ **Special Geriatric Considerations** A seven- to eightfold variation in citalopram S(+) (active) and R(-) enantiomer concentrations have been reported in the elderly. The racemic citalopram concentration-to-dose ratio was 1.8 times greater in elderly patients compared to younger patients.

Clearance was decreased, while AUC and half-life were significantly increased in elderly patients and in patients with hepatic impairment. Mild-to-moderate renal impairment may reduce clearance of citalopram (17% reduction noted in trials). No pharmacokinetic information is available concerning patients with severe renal impairment. The elderly are more prone to SSRI/SNRI-induced hyponatremia.

Dosage Forms Excipient information presented when available (limited, particularly for generics); consult specific product labeling.

Solution, oral: 10 mg/5 mL (240 mL)

Tablet, oral: 10 mg, 20 mg, 40 mg

CeleXA®: 10 mg

CeleXA®: 20 mg, 40 mg [scored]

Selected References

Foglia JP, Pollock BG, Kirshner MA, et al, "Plasma Levels of Citalopram Enantiomers and Metabolites in Elderly Patients," *Psychopharmacol Bull*, 1997, 33(1):109-12.

Rabins PV, Blacker D, Rovner BW, et al, "Practice Guidelines for the Treatment of Patients With Alzheimer's Disease and Other Dementias," *Am J Psychiatry*, 2007, 164(12 Suppl):5-56. Available at http://www.psych.org/psych_pract/treatg/pg/prac_guide.cfm.

◆ **Citalopram Hydrobromide** *see* Citalopram *on page 365*
◆ **Citracal® [OTC]** *see* Calcium Salts (Oral) *on page 256*
◆ **Citracal® Maximum [OTC]** *see* Calcium and Vitamin D *on page 248*
◆ **Citracal® Petites [OTC]** *see* Calcium and Vitamin D *on page 248*
◆ **Citracal® Regular [OTC]** *see* Calcium and Vitamin D *on page 248*
◆ **Citrate of Magnesia** *see* Magnesium Citrate *on page 1107*
◆ **Citric Acid and Sodium Citrate** *see* Sodium Citrate and Citric Acid *on page 1693*

Citric Acid, Sodium Citrate, and Potassium Citrate
(SIT rik AS id, SOW dee um SIT rate, & poe TASS ee um SIT rate)

Medication Safety Issues

Sound-alike/look-alike issues:

Polycitra may be confused with Bicitra

Brand Names: U.S. Cytra-3; Tricitrates

Index Terms Polycitra; Potassium Citrate, Citric Acid, and Sodium Citrate; Sodium Citrate, Citric Acid, and Potassium Citrate

Generic Availability (U.S.) Yes

Pharmacologic Category Alkalinizing Agent, Oral

Use Conditions where long-term maintenance of an alkaline urine is desirable as in control and dissolution of uric acid and cystine calculi of the urinary tract

Contraindications Severe renal impairment with oliguria or azotemia; untreated Addison's disease; severe myocardial damage.

Warnings/Precautions Use with caution in patients with heart failure, peripheral or pulmonary edema, and renal impairment; contains sodium. Conversion to bicarbonate may be impaired in patients who are severely ill, in shock, or with hepatic failure. Use with caution in digitalized patients or those who are receiving concomitant medications that increase potassium.

Adverse Reactions (Reflective of adult population; not specific for elderly) Frequency not defined.

Cardiovascular: Cardiac abnormalities

Endocrine & metabolic: Metabolic alkalosis, calcium levels, hyperkalemia, hypernatremia

Gastrointestinal: Diarrhea

Neuromuscular & skeletal: Tetany

Drug Interactions

Avoid Concomitant Use There are no known interactions where it is recommended to avoid concomitant use.

Increased Effect/Toxicity

Citric Acid, Sodium Citrate, and Potassium Citrate may increase the levels/effects of: ACE Inhibitors; Aluminum Hydroxide; Angiotensin II Receptor Blockers; Potassium-Sparing Diuretics

The levels/effects of Citric Acid, Sodium Citrate, and Potassium Citrate may be increased by: Eplerenone

Decreased Effect There are no known significant interactions involving a decrease in effect.

Stability Store at controlled room temperature of 20°C to 25°C (68°F to 77°F); do not freeze. Protect from excessive heat.

Dosage

Geriatric & Adult Alkalinizing agent/bicarbonate precursor/potassium supplement: Oral: 15-30 mL diluted in water after meals and at bedtime

Administration Administer after meals. Dilute with water prior to administration. Chilling solution prior to dosing helps to enhance palatability. May follow dose with additional water.

Monitoring Parameters Blood gas (pH and bicarbonate); serum bicarbonate

Dosage Forms Excipient information presented when available (limited, particularly for generics); consult specific product labeling. [DSC] = Discontinued product

Solution, oral:

Cytra-3: Citric acid 334 mg, sodium citrate 500 mg, and potassium citrate 550 mg per 5 mL (480 mL) [equivalent to potassium 1 mEq, sodium 1 mEq, and bicarbonate 2 mEq per 1 mL; alcohol free, sugar free; contains sodium benzoate and propylene glycol; raspberry flavor]

Tricitrates: Citric acid 334 mg, sodium citrate 500 mg, and potassium citrate 550 mg per 5 mL (480 mL) [equivalent to potassium 1 mEq, sodium 1 mEq, and bicarbonate 2 mEq per 1 mL; alcohol free; contains sodium benzoate; raspberry flavor]

Tricitrates: Citric acid 334 mg, sodium citrate 500 mg, and potassium citrate 550 mg per 5 mL (15 mL [DSC]; 30 mL [DSC]; 480 mL) [equivalent to potassium 1 mEq, sodium 1 mEq, and bicarbonate 2 mEq per 1 mL; alcohol free, sugar free; contains sodiuim benzoate and propylene glycol; raspberry flavor]

◆ **Citroma® [OTC]** see Magnesium Citrate *on page 1107*
◆ **CL-118,532** see Triptorelin *on page 1872*
◆ **CI-719** see Gemfibrozil *on page 812*
◆ **Claforan®** see Cefotaxime *on page 299*
◆ **Clarinex®** see Desloratadine *on page 476*

Clarithromycin (kla RITH roe mye sin)

Related Information

Helicobacter pylori Treatment in Adult Patients *on page 2009*
Prevention of Infective Endocarditis *on page 2064*

Medication Safety Issues

Sound-alike/look-alike issues:

Clarithromycin may be confused with Claritin®, clindamycin, erythromycin

Brand Names: U.S. Biaxin®; Biaxin® XL

Brand Names: Canada Apo-Clarithromycin®; Biaxin®; Biaxin® XL; Dom-Clarithromycin; Mylan-Clarithromycin; PMS-Clarithromycin; RAN™-Clarithromycin; ratio-Clarithromycin; Riva-Clarithromycin; Sandoz-Clarithromycin

Generic Availability (U.S.) Yes

Pharmacologic Category Antibiotic, Macrolide

Use

Pharyngitis/tonsillitis due to susceptible *S. pyogenes*

Acute maxillary sinusitis due to susceptible *H. influenzae, M. catarrhalis,* or *S. pneumoniae*

Acute exacerbation of chronic bronchitis due to susceptible *H. influenzae, H. parainfluenzae, M. catarrhalis,* or *S. pneumoniae*

Community-acquired pneumonia due to susceptible *H. influenzae, H. parainfluenzae, Mycoplasma pneumoniae, S. pneumoniae,* or *Chlamydia pneumoniae* (TWAR), *Moraxella catarrhalis*

Uncomplicated skin/skin structure infections due to susceptible *S. aureus, S. pyogenes*

Disseminated mycobacterial infections due to *M. avium* or *M. intracellulare*

Prevention of disseminated mycobacterial infections due to *M. avium* complex (MAC) disease (eg, patients with advanced HIV infection)

Duodenal ulcer disease due to *H. pylori* in regimens with other drugs including amoxicillin and lansoprazole or omeprazole, ranitidine bismuth citrate, bismuth subsalicylate, tetracycline, and/or an H$_2$ antagonist

Unlabeled/Investigational Use Pertussis (CDC guidelines); alternate antibiotic for prophylaxis of infective endocarditis in patients who are allergic to penicillin and undergoing surgical or dental procedures (ACC/AHA guidelines)

Contraindications Hypersensitivity to clarithromycin, erythromycin, or any macrolide antibiotic; use with ergot derivatives, pimozide, cisapride, astemizole, terfenadine, colchicine (if patient has concomitant renal or hepatic impairment); history of cholestatic jaundice or hepatic dysfunction with prior clarithromycin use

◀ **Warnings/Precautions** Dosage adjustment required with severe renal impairment; decreased dosage or prolonged dosing interval may be appropriate. May cause hepatotoxicity (elevated liver function tests, hepatitis, jaundice, hepatic failure); use caution with preexisting hepatic disease or hepatotoxic medications. Use with caution in patients with myasthenia gravis. Colchicine toxicity (including fatalities) has been reported with concomitant use; concomitant use is contraindicated in patients with renal or hepatic impairment. Prolonged use may result in fungal or bacterial superinfection, including *C. difficile*-associated diarrhea (CDAD) and pseudomembranous colitis; CDAD has been observed >2 months postantibiotic treatment. Macrolides (including clarithromycin) have been associated with rare QT prolongation and ventricular arrhythmias, including torsade de pointes. Use caution in patients with coronary artery disease. Avoid use of extended release tablets (Biaxin® XL) in patients with known stricture/narrowing of the GI tract.

Adverse Reactions (Reflective of adult population; not specific for elderly)
1% to 10%:
Central nervous system: Headache (adults and children 2%)
Dermatologic: Rash (children 3%)
Gastrointestinal: Abnormal taste (adults 3% to 7%), diarrhea (adults 3% to 6%; children 6%), vomiting (children 6%), nausea (adults 3%), abdominal pain (adults 2%; children 3%), dyspepsia (adults 2%)
Hepatic: Prothrombin time increased (adults 1%)
Renal: BUN increased (4%)

Drug Interactions

Metabolism/Transport Effects Substrate of CYP3A4 (major); **Inhibits** CYP1A2 (weak), CYP3A4 (strong), P-glycoprotein

Avoid Concomitant Use
Avoid concomitant use of Clarithromycin with any of the following: Alfuzosin; Artemether; BCG; Cisapride; Conivaptan; Crizotinib; Dihydroergotamine; Disopyramide; Dronedarone; Eplerenone; Ergotamine; Everolimus; Fluticasone (Oral Inhalation); Halofantrine; Lapatinib; Lovastatin; Lumefantrine; Lurasidone; Nilotinib; Nisoldipine; Pimozide; QUEtiapine; QuiNINE; Ranolazine; Rivaroxaban; RomiDEPsin; Salmeterol; Silodosin; Simvastatin; Tamsulosin; Terfenadine; Tetrabenazine; Thioridazine; Ticagrelor; Tolvaptan; Topotecan; Toremifene; Vandetanib; Vemurafenib; Ziprasidone

Increased Effect/Toxicity
Clarithromycin may increase the levels/effects of: Alfentanil; Alfuzosin; Almotriptan; Alosetron; Antifungal Agents (Azole Derivatives, Systemic); Antineoplastic Agents (Vinca Alkaloids); Benzodiazepines (metabolized by oxidation); Bortezomib; Brentuximab Vedotin; Brinzolamide; Budesonide (Nasal); Budesonide (Systemic, Oral Inhalation); BusPIRone; Calcium Channel Blockers; CarBAMazepine; Cardiac Glycosides; Ciclesonide; Cilostazol; Cisapride; CloZAPine; Colchicine; Conivaptan; Corticosteroids (Orally Inhaled); Corticosteroids (Systemic); Crizotinib; CycloSPORINE; CycloSPORINE (Systemic); CYP3A4 Inducers (Strong); CYP3A4 Substrates; Dabigatran Etexilate; Dienogest; Dihydroergotamine; Disopyramide; Dronedarone; Dutasteride; Eletriptan; Eplerenone; Ergot Derivatives; Ergotamine; Everolimus; FentaNYL; Fesoterodine; Fluticasone (Nasal); Fluticasone (Oral Inhalation); GlipiZIDE; GlyBURIDE; GuanFACINE; Halofantrine; HMG-CoA Reductase Inhibitors; Iloperidone; Ixabepilone; Lapatinib; Lovastatin; Lumefantrine; Lurasidone; Maraviroc; MethylPREDNISolone; Nilotinib; Nisoldipine; Paricalcitol; Pazopanib; P-Glycoprotein Substrates; Pimecrolimus; Pimozide; Protease Inhibitors; QTc-Prolonging Agents; QuiNIDine; QuiNINE; Ranolazine; Repaglinide; Rifamycin Derivatives; Rivaroxaban; RomiDEPsin; Salmeterol; Saxagliptin; Selective Serotonin Reuptake Inhibitors; Sildenafil; Silodosin; Simvastatin; Sirolimus; SORAfenib; Tacrolimus; Tacrolimus (Systemic); Tacrolimus (Topical); Tadalafil; Tamsulosin; Telaprevir; Temsirolimus; Terfenadine; Tetrabenazine; Theophylline Derivatives; Thioridazine; Ticagrelor; Tolterodine; Tolvaptan; Topotecan; Toremifene; Vandetanib; Vardenafil; Vemurafenib; Vilazodone; Vitamin K Antagonists; Zidovudine; Ziprasidone; Zopiclone

The levels/effects of Clarithromycin may be increased by: Alfuzosin; Antifungal Agents (Azole Derivatives, Systemic); Artemether; Chloroquine; Ciprofloxacin; Ciprofloxacin (Systemic); CYP3A4 Inducers (Strong); CYP3A4 Inhibitors (Moderate); CYP3A4 Inhibitors (Strong); Gadobutrol; Lumefantrine; Nilotinib; Protease Inhibitors; QUEtiapine; QuiNINE; Telaprevir

Decreased Effect
Clarithromycin may decrease the levels/effects of: BCG; Clopidogrel; Prasugrel; Ticagrelor; Typhoid Vaccine; Zidovudine

The levels/effects of Clarithromycin may be decreased by: CYP3A4 Inducers (Strong); Deferasirox; Etravirine; Herbs (CYP3A4 Inducers); Protease Inhibitors; Tocilizumab

Ethanol/Nutrition/Herb Interactions

Food: Immediate release: Food delays rate, but not extent of absorption; Extended release: Food increases clarithromycin AUC by ~30% relative to fasting conditions.

Herb/Nutraceutical: St John's wort may decrease clarithromycin levels.

Stability

Immediate release 250 mg tablets and granules for oral suspension: Store at controlled room temperature of 15°C to 30°C (59°F to 86°F). Reconstituted oral suspension should not be refrigerated because it might gel; microencapsulated particles of clarithromycin in suspension are stable for 14 days when stored at room temperature. Protect tablets from light.

Immediate release 500 mg tablets and Biaxin® XL: Store at controlled room temperature of 20°C to 25°C (68°F to 77°F); excursions permitted to 15°C to 30°C (59°F to 86°F).

Mechanism of Action Exerts its antibacterial action by binding to 50S ribosomal subunit resulting in inhibition of protein synthesis. The 14-OH metabolite of clarithromycin is twice as active as the parent compound against certain organisms.

Pharmacodynamics/Kinetics

Absorption: Immediate release: Rapid; food delays rate, but not extent of absorption

Distribution: Widely into most body tissues except CNS

Protein binding: 42% to 50%

Metabolism: Partially hepatic via CYP3A4; converted to 14-OH clarithromycin (active metabolite)

Bioavailability: ~50%

Half-life elimination: Immediate release: Clarithromycin: 3-7 hours; 14-OH-clarithromycin: 5-9 hours

Time to peak: Immediate release: 2-3 hours

Excretion: Primarily urine (20% to 40% as unchanged drug; additional 10% to 15% as metabolite)

Clearance: Approximates normal GFR

Dosage

Geriatric & Adult

Usual dosage range: Oral: 250-500 mg every 12 hours **or** 1000 mg (two 500 mg extended release tablets) once daily for 7-14 days

Acute exacerbation of chronic bronchitis: Oral:

M. catarrhalis and *S. pneumoniae*: 250 mg every 12 hours for 7-14 days **or** 1000 mg (two 500 mg extended release tablets) once daily for 7 days

H. influenzae: 500 mg every 12 hours for 7-14 days **or** 1000 mg (two 500 mg extended release tablets) once daily for 7 days

H. parainfluenzae: 500 mg every 12 hours for 7 days **or** 1000 mg (two 500 mg extended release tablets) once daily for 7 days

Acute maxillary sinusitis: Oral: 500 mg every 12 hours **or** 1000 mg (two 500 mg extended release tablets) once daily for 14 days

Mycobacterial infection (prevention and treatment): Oral: 500 mg twice daily (use with other antimycobacterial drugs, eg, ethambutol or rifampin)

Peptic ulcer disease: Eradication of *Helicobacter pylori*: Dual or triple combination regimens with bismuth subsalicylate, amoxicillin, an H_2-receptor antagonist, or proton-pump inhibitor: 500 mg every 8-12 hours for 10-14 days

Pertussis (unlabeled use; CDC, 2005): Oral: 500 mg twice daily for 7 days

Pharyngitis, tonsillitis: Oral: 250 mg every 12 hours for 10 days

Pneumonia: Oral:

C. pneumoniae, *M. pneumoniae*, and *S. pneumoniae*: 250 mg every 12 hours for 7-14 days **or** 1000 mg (two 500 mg extended release tablets) once daily for 7 days

H. influenzae: 250 mg every 12 hours for 7 days **or** 1000 mg (two 500 mg extended release tablets) once daily for 7 days

H. parainfluenzae and *M. catarrhalis*: 1000 mg (two 500 mg extended release tablets) once daily for 7 days

Prophylaxis against infective endocarditis (unlabeled use): Oral: 500 mg 30-60 minutes prior to procedure. **Note:** American Heart Association (AHA) guidelines now recommend prophylaxis only in patients undergoing invasive procedures and in whom underlying cardiac conditions may predispose to a higher risk of adverse outcomes should infection occur. As of April 2007, routine prophylaxis for GI/GU procedures is no longer recommended by the AHA.

Skin and skin structure infection, uncomplicated: Oral: 250 mg every 12 hours for 7-14 days

Renal Impairment
Cl$_{cr}$ <30 mL/minute: Decrease clarithromycin dose by 50%
Hemodialysis: Administer after HD session is completed (Aronoff, 2007).
In combination with atazanavir or ritonavir:
Cl$_{cr}$ 30-60 mL/minute: Decrease clarithromycin dose by 50%.
Cl$_{cr}$ <30 mL/minute: Decrease clarithromycin dose by 75%.

Hepatic Impairment No dosing adjustment is needed as long as renal function is normal.

Administration Clarithromycin immediate release tablets and oral suspension may be administered with or without meals. Give every 12 hours rather than twice daily to avoid peak and trough variation. Shake suspension well before each use.

Extended release tablets: Should be given with food. Do not crush or chew extended release tablet.

Monitoring Parameters CBC with differential, BUN, creatinine; perform culture and sensitivity studies prior to initiating drug therapy

Special Geriatric Considerations Considered one of the drugs of choice in the outpatient treatment of community-acquired pneumonia in elderly. After doses of 500 mg every 12 hours for 5 days, 12 healthy elderly subjects had significantly increased C$_{max}$ and C$_{min}$, elimination half-lives of clarithromycin and 14-OH clarithromycin compared to 12 healthy young subjects. These changes were attributed to a significant decrease in renal clearance; at a dose of 1000 mg twice daily, 100% of 13 elderly subjects experienced an adverse event compared to only 10% taking 500 mg twice daily.

Dosage Forms Excipient information presented when available (limited, particularly for generics); consult specific product labeling.
Granules for suspension, oral: 125 mg/5 mL (50 mL, 100 mL); 250 mg/5 mL (50 mL, 100 mL)
Biaxin®: 125 mg/5 mL (50 mL, 100 mL); 250 mg/5 mL (50 mL, 100 mL) [fruit-punch flavor]
Tablet, oral: 250 mg, 500 mg
Biaxin®: 250 mg, 500 mg
Tablet, extended release, oral: 500 mg
Biaxin® XL: 500 mg

Selected References
Chu SY, Wilson DS, Guay DR, et al, "Clarithromycin Pharmacokinetics in Healthy Young and Elderly Volunteers," *J Clin Pharmacol*, 1992, 32(11):1045-9.
Mandell LA, Wunderink RG, Anzueto A, et al, "Infectious Diseases Society of America/American Thoracic Society Consensus Guidelines on the Management of Community-Acquired Pneumonia in Adults," *Clin Infect Dis*, 2007, 44 Suppl 2:S27-72.
Wallace RJ Jr, Brown BA, and Griffith DE, "Drug Intolerance to High-Dose Clarithromycin Among Elderly Patients," *Diagn Microbiol Infect Dis*, 1993, 16(3):215-21.

◆ **Claritin® 24 Hour Allergy [OTC]** *see* Loratadine *on page 1087*
◆ **Claritin® Children's Allergy [OTC]** *see* Loratadine *on page 1087*
◆ **Claritin™ Eye [OTC]** *see* Ketotifen *on page 1013*
◆ **Claritin® Liqui-Gels® 24 Hour Allergy [OTC]** *see* Loratadine *on page 1087*
◆ **Claritin® RediTabs® 24 Hour Allergy [OTC]** *see* Loratadine *on page 1087*
◆ **Clavulanic Acid and Amoxicillin** *see* Amoxicillin and Clavulanate Potassium *on page 116*
◆ **Clean & Clear® Advantage® Acne Cleanser [OTC]** *see* Salicylic Acid *on page 1648*
◆ **Clean & Clear® Advantage® Acne Spot Treatment [OTC]** *see* Salicylic Acid *on page 1648*
◆ **Clean & Clear® Advantage® Invisible Acne Patch [OTC]** *see* Salicylic Acid *on page 1648*
◆ **Clean & Clear® Advantage® Oil-Free Acne [OTC]** *see* Salicylic Acid *on page 1648*
◆ **Clean & Clear® Blackhead Clearing Daily Cleansing [OTC]** *see* Salicylic Acid *on page 1648*
◆ **Clean & Clear® Blackhead Clearing Scrub [OTC]** *see* Salicylic Acid *on page 1648*
◆ **Clean & Clear® Continuous Control® Acne Wash [OTC]** *see* Salicylic Acid *on page 1648*
◆ **Clean & Clear® Deep Cleaning [OTC]** *see* Salicylic Acid *on page 1648*
◆ **Clean & Clear® Dual Action Moisturizer [OTC]** *see* Salicylic Acid *on page 1648*
◆ **Clean & Clear® Invisible Blemish Treatment [OTC]** *see* Salicylic Acid *on page 1648*
◆ **Clear eyes® for Dry Eyes Plus ACR Relief [OTC]** *see* Naphazoline (Ophthalmic) *on page 1262*
◆ **Clear eyes® for Dry Eyes plus Redness Relief [OTC]** *see* Naphazoline (Ophthalmic) *on page 1262*
◆ **Clear eyes® Redness Relief [OTC]** *see* Naphazoline (Ophthalmic) *on page 1262*
◆ **Clear eyes® Seasonal Relief [OTC]** *see* Naphazoline (Ophthalmic) *on page 1262*

Clemastine (KLEM as teen)

Brand Names: U.S. Tavist® Allergy [OTC]
Index Terms Clemastine Fumarate
Generic Availability (U.S.) Yes

Pharmacologic Category Ethanolamine Derivative; Histamine H_1 Antagonist; Histamine H_1 Antagonist, First Generation

Use Perennial and seasonal allergic rhinitis and other allergic symptoms including urticaria

Contraindications Hypersensitivity to clemastine or any component of the formulation; narrow-angle glaucoma

Warnings/Precautions Use caution with bladder neck obstruction, symptomatic prostate hypertrophy, asthmatic attacks, stenosing peptic ulcer, increased intraocular pressure, hyperthyroidism, cardiovascular disease, hypertension, and in the elderly. May cause drowsiness; use caution in performing tasks which require alertness. Effects may be potentiated when used with other sedative drugs or ethanol.

Adverse Reactions (Reflective of adult population; not specific for elderly) Frequency not defined.

Cardiovascular: Palpitation, hypotension, tachycardia

Central nervous system: Dyscoordination, sedation, somnolence slight to moderate, sleepiness, confusion, restlessness, nervousness, insomnia, irritability, fatigue, headache, dizziness increased

Dermatologic: Rash, photosensitivity

Gastrointestinal: Diarrhea, nausea, xerostomia, epigastric distress, vomiting, constipation

Genitourinary: Urinary frequency, difficult urination, urinary retention

Hematologic: Hemolytic anemia, thrombocytopenia, agranulocytosis

Ocular: Blurred vision

Otic: Tinnitus

Respiratory: Thickening of bronchial secretions

Miscellaneous: Anaphylaxis

Drug Interactions

Metabolism/Transport Effects Inhibits CYP2D6 (weak), 3A4 (weak)

Avoid Concomitant Use There are no known interactions where it is recommended to avoid concomitant use.

Increased Effect/Toxicity

Clemastine may increase the levels/effects of: Alcohol (Ethyl); Anticholinergics; CNS Depressants; Selective Serotonin Reuptake Inhibitors

The levels/effects of Clemastine may be increased by: Droperidol; HydrOXYzine; Pramlintide

Decreased Effect

Clemastine may decrease the levels/effects of: Acetylcholinesterase Inhibitors (Central); Benzylpenicilloyl Polylysine; Betahistine

The levels/effects of Clemastine may be decreased by: Acetylcholinesterase Inhibitors (Central); Amphetamines

Ethanol/Nutrition/Herb Interactions Ethanol: May increase CNS depression; monitor for increased effects with coadministration. Caution patients about effects.

Mechanism of Action Competes with histamine for H_1-receptor sites on effector cells in the gastrointestinal tract, blood vessels, and respiratory tract

Pharmacodynamics/Kinetics

Onset of action: Peak effect: Therapeutic: 5-7 hours

Duration: 8-16 hours

Absorption: Almost complete

Metabolism: Hepatic

Excretion: Urine

Dosage

Geriatric Lower doses should be considered in patients >60 years of age.

Adult

Rhinitis or allergic symptoms (including urticaria): Oral:

1.34 mg clemastine fumarate (1 mg base) twice daily to 2.68 mg (2 mg base) 3 times/day; do not exceed 8.04 mg/day (6 mg base)

OTC labeling: 1.34 mg clemastine fumarate (1 mg base) twice daily; do not exceed 2 mg base/24 hours

Monitoring Parameters Look for a reduction of rhinitis, urticaria, eczema, pruritus, or other allergic symptoms

Pharmacotherapy Pearls 1.34 mg of clemastine fumarate = 1 mg clemastine base. Clemastine offers no significant benefit over other antihistamines except that it may be dosed twice daily (in adults) as compared to other antihistamines with more frequent dosing.

Special Geriatric Considerations Elderly patients may be more susceptible to adverse effects.

◄ **Dosage Forms** Excipient information presented when available (limited, particularly for generics); consult specific product labeling.

Syrup, oral, as fumarate: 0.67 mg/5 mL (120 mL) [equivalent to clemastine base 0.5 mg/5 mL; prescription formulation]

Tablet, oral, as fumarate: 1.34 mg [equivalent to clemastine base 1 mg; OTC], 2.68 mg [equivalent to clemastine base 2 mg; prescription formulation]

Tavist® Allergy: 1.34 mg [scored; equivalent to clemastine base 1 mg]

◆ **Clemastine Fumarate** *see* Clemastine *on page* 372
◆ **Cleocin®** *see* Clindamycin (Topical) *on page* 379
◆ **Cleocin HCl®** *see* Clindamycin (Systemic) *on page* 376
◆ **Cleocin Pediatric®** *see* Clindamycin (Systemic) *on page* 376
◆ **Cleocin Phosphate®** *see* Clindamycin (Systemic) *on page* 376
◆ **Cleocin T®** *see* Clindamycin (Topical) *on page* 379
◆ **Cleocin® Vaginal Ovule** *see* Clindamycin (Topical) *on page* 379

Clevidipine (klev ID i peen)

Related Information

Calcium Channel Blockers *on page* 2003

Medication Safety Issues

Sound-alike/look-alike issues:

Clevidipine may be confused with cladribine, clofarabine, clomiPRAMINE

Cleviprex™ may be confused with Claravis™

Brand Names: U.S. Cleviprex™

Index Terms Clevidipine Butyrate

Generic Availability (U.S.) No

Pharmacologic Category Calcium Channel Blocker; Calcium Channel Blocker, Dihydropyridine

Use Management of hypertension

Contraindications Hypersensitivity to clevidipine or any component of the formulation (soybeans, soy products, eggs, egg products); hypertriglyceridemia or complications of hypertriglyceridemia (eg, acute pancreatitis); lipid nephrosis; severe aortic stenosis

Warnings/Precautions Symptomatic hypotension with or without syncope and reflex tachycardia may rarely occur. Blood pressure must be lowered at a rate appropriate for the patient's clinical condition; dosage reductions may be necessary. Treatment of clevidipine-induced tachycardia with beta-blockers is **not** recommended. After prolonged use, discontinuation may cause rebound hypertension; monitor closely for ≥8 hours after discontinuation. Use with caution in patients with heart failure (may worsen symptoms). Clevidipine is formulated within a 20% fat emulsion (0.2 g/mL); hypertriglyceridemia is an expected side effect with high-dose or extended treatment periods; median infusion duration in clinical trials was approximately 6.5 hours (Aronson, 2008). Patients who develop hypertriglyceridemia (eg, >500 mg/dL) are at risk of developing pancreatitis. A reduction in the quantity of concurrently administered lipids may be necessary. Use is contraindicated in patients with hypertriglyceridemia or complications associated with hypertriglyceridemia (eg, acute pancreatitis) and lipid nephrosis. Withdrawal from concomitant beta-blocker therapy should be done gradually. Initiate therapy at the low end of the dosage range in the elderly, with careful upward titration if needed. Vials may support microbial growth; maintain aseptic technique while handling.

Adverse Reactions (Reflective of adult population; not specific for elderly)

>10%:

Central nervous system: Fever (19%), insomnia (12%)

Gastrointestinal: Nausea (5% to 21%)

1% to 10%:

Central nervous system: Headache (6%)

Gastrointestinal: Vomiting (3%)

Hematologic: Postprocedural hemorrhage (3%)

Renal: Acute renal failure (9%)

Respiratory: Pneumonia (3%), respiratory failure (3%)

Drug Interactions

Avoid Concomitant Use There are no known interactions where it is recommended to avoid concomitant use.

Increased Effect/Toxicity

Clevidipine may increase the levels/effects of: Amifostine; Antihypertensives; Beta-Blockers; Calcium Channel Blockers (Nondihydropyridine); Hypotensive Agents; Magnesium Salts; Neuromuscular-Blocking Agents (Nondepolarizing); Nitroprusside; QuiNIDine; RiTUXimab

CLEVIDIPINE

The levels/effects of Clevidipine may be increased by: Alpha1-Blockers; Calcium Channel Blockers (Nondihydropyridine); Diazoxide; Herbs (Hypotensive Properties); Magnesium Salts; MAO Inhibitors; Pentoxifylline; Phosphodiesterase 5 Inhibitors; Prostacyclin Analogues; QuiNIDine

Decreased Effect

Clevidipine may decrease the levels/effects of: QuiNIDine

The levels/effects of Clevidipine may be decreased by: Calcium Salts; Herbs (Hypertensive Properties); Methylphenidate; Yohimbine

Ethanol/Nutrition/Herb Interactions Herb/Nutraceutical: Avoid bayberry, blue cohosh, cayenne, ephedra, ginger, ginseng (American), kola, licorice (may worsen hypertension). Avoid black cohosh, California poppy, coleus, golden seal, hawthorn, mistletoe, periwinkle, quinine, shepherd's purse (may have increased antihypertensive effect).

Stability Store in refrigerator at 2°C to 8°C (36°F to 46°F). Unopened vials are stable for 2 months at room temperature. Vials are stable for 4 hours once opened. Protect from light during storage. Do not freeze.

Mechanism of Action Dihydropyridine calcium channel blocker with potent arterial vasodilating activity. Inhibits calcium ion influx through the L-type calcium channels during depolarization in arterial smooth muscle, producing a decrease in mean arterial pressure (MAP) by reducing systemic vascular resistance.

Pharmacodynamics/Kinetics

Onset of action: 2-4 minutes after start of infusion

Duration: I.V.: 5-15 minutes

Distribution: V_{dss}: 0.17 L/kg

Protein binding: >99.5%

Metabolism: Rapid hydrolysis primarily by esterases in blood and extravascular tissues to an inactive carboxylic acid metabolite and formaldehyde

Half-life elimination: Biphasic: Initial: 1 minute (predominant); Terminal: 15 minutes

Excretion: Urine (63% to 74% as metabolites); feces (7% to 22% as metabolites)

Dosage

Geriatric Refer to adult dosing. Initiate at the low end of the dosage range.

Adult Management of hypertension: I.V.: Initial: 1-2 mg/hour

Titration: Initial: dose may be doubled at 90-second intervals toward blood pressure goal. As blood pressure approaches goal, dose may be increased by less than double every 5-10 minutes. Note: For every 1-2 mg/hour increase in dose, an approximate reduction of 2-4 mm Hg in systolic blood pressure may occur.

Usual maintenance: 4-6 mg/hour; maximum: 21 mg/hour (1000 mL within a 24-hour period due to lipid load restriction). There is limited short-term experience with doses up to 32 mg/hour. Data is limited beyond 72 hours.

Renal Impairment No adjustment required with initial infusion rate.

Hepatic Impairment No adjustment required with initial infusion rate.

Administration I.V.: Maintain aseptic technique. Do not use if contamination is suspected. Do not dilute. Invert vial gently several times to ensure uniformity of emulsion prior to administration. Administer as a slow continuous infusion via central or peripheral line, using infusion device allowing for calibrated infusion rates. Use within 4 hours of puncturing vial; discard any tubing and unused portion, including that currently being infused.

Monitoring Parameters Blood pressure, heart rate; patients who receive prolonged infusions of clevidipine and are not transitioned to other antihypertensive therapy should be monitored for at least 8 hours after discontinuation

Special Geriatric Considerations No overall differences in safety or efficacy noted in the initial studies in elderly. Doses should be started at low end of dosage range and titrated slowly since elderly may experience a greater hypotensive response, reflecting their greater frequency of renal and cardiac disease with decreased function and concomitant drug therapy.

Dosage Forms Excipient information presented when available (limited, particularly for generics); consult specific product labeling.

Injection, emulsion:

Cleviprex™: 0.5 mg/mL (50 mL, 100 mL) [contains egg yolk phospholipid, soybean oil]

Selected References

Chobanian AV, Bakris GL, Black HR, et al, "The Seventh Report of the Joint National Committee on Prevention, Detection, Evaluation, and Treatment of High Blood Pressure: The JNC 7 Report," *JAMA*, 2003, 289(19):2560-71.

Levy JH, Mancao MY, Gitter R, et al, "Clevidipine Effectively and Rapidly Controls Blood Pressure Preoperatively in Cardiac Surgery Patients: The Results of the Randomized, Placebo-Controlled Efficacy Study of Clevidipine Assessing Its Preoperative Antihypertensive Effect in Cardiac Surgery-1," *Anesth Analg*, 2007, 105(4):918-25.

Marik PE and Varon J, "Hypertensive Crises: Challenges and Management," *Chest*, 2007, 131(6); 1949-62. Available at http://chestjournal.org/cgi/content/abstract/131/6/1949

Peacock WF, Varon J, Garrison N, et al, "IV Clevidipine for Hypertension: Safety, Efficacy, and Transition to Oral Therapy," *Ann Emerg Med*, 2007, 50(3 Suppl 1):8-9.

Singla N, Warltier DC, Gandhi SD, et al, "Treatment of Acute Postoperative Hypertension in Cardiac Surgery Patients: An Efficacy Study of Clevidipine Assessing Its Postoperative Antihypertensive Effect in Cardiac Surgery-2 (ESCAPE-2), a Randomized, Double- Blind, Placebo-Controlled Trial," *Anesth Analg*, 2008, 107(1):59-67.

Varon J, "Treatment of Acute Severe Hypertension: Current and Newer Agents," *Drugs*, 2008, 68(3):283-97.

Zhang JG, Dehal SS, Ho T, et al, "Human Cytochrome P450 Induction and Inhibition Potential of Clevidipine and Its Primary Metabolite H152/81," *Drug Metab Dispos*, 2006, 34(5):734-37.

◆ **Clevidipine Butyrate** *see Clevidipine on page 374*
◆ **Cleviprex™** *see Clevidipine on page 374*

Clidinium and Chlordiazepoxide (kli DI nee um & klor dye az e POKS ide)

Related Information
Beers Criteria – Potentially Inappropriate Medications for Geriatrics *on page 2089*
ChlordiazePOXIDE *on page 334*
Medication Safety Issues
Sound-alike/look-alike issues:
Librax® may be confused with Librium
Librax® formulation may be cause for confusion:
In November 2004, Valeant Pharmaceuticals licensed the Librax® trademark to Victory Pharmaceuticals. Subsequently, the product was reformulated to contain chlordiazepoxide and methscopolamine. In January 2006, Valeant Pharmaceuticals began redistributing the original formulation of Librax®, containing clidinium and chlordiazepoxide. Victory Pharmaceuticals has discontinued their product. **Note:** The formulation of Librax® distributed in Canada (Valeant Canada Ltd) always contained clidinium and chlordiazepoxide.
BEERS Criteria medication:
This drug may be inappropriate for use in geriatric patients (high severity risk).
Brand Names: U.S. Librax® *[original formulation]*
Brand Names: Canada Apo-Chlorax®; Librax®
Index Terms Chlordiazepoxide and Clidinium
Generic Availability (U.S.) Yes
Pharmacologic Category Antispasmodic Agent, Gastrointestinal; Benzodiazepine
Use Adjunct treatment of peptic ulcer; treatment of irritable bowel syndrome
Dosage
Geriatric & Adult Adjunct treatment of peptic ulcer; treatment of IBS: Oral: 1-2 capsules 3-4 times/day, before meals or food and at bedtime. **Caution:** Do not abruptly discontinue after prolonged use; taper dose gradually.
Special Geriatric Considerations The use of anticholinergic agents may cause problems with bladder emptying, constipation, or confusion. The addition of chlordiazepoxide may enhance confusion potential. Avoid use in the elderly; if it must be used, monitor closely.

This medication is considered to be potentially inappropriate in this patient population (Beers Criteria severity: High).
Dosage Forms Excipient information presented when available (limited, particularly for generics); consult specific product labeling.
Capsule: Clidinium bromide 2.5 mg and chlordiazepoxide hydrochloride 5 mg
Librax® [original formulation]: Clidinium bromide 2.5 mg and chlordiazepoxide hydrochloride 5 mg

◆ **Climara®** *see Estradiol (Systemic) on page 641*
◆ **Clindagel®** *see Clindamycin (Topical) on page 379*
◆ **ClindaMax®** *see Clindamycin (Topical) on page 379*

Clindamycin (Systemic) (klin da MYE sin)

Related Information
Community-Acquired Pneumonia in Adults *on page 2059*
Prevention of Infective Endocarditis *on page 2064*
Medication Safety Issues
Sound-alike/look-alike issues:
Cleocin® may be confused with bleomycin, Clinoril®, Cubicin®, Lincocin®
Clindamycin may be confused with clarithromycin, Claritin®, vancomycin
Brand Names: U.S. Cleocin HCl®; Cleocin Pediatric®; Cleocin Phosphate®
Brand Names: Canada Alti-Clindamycin; Apo-Clindamycin®; Clindamycin Injection, USP; Clindamycine; Gen-Clindamycin; Mylan-Clindamycin; Novo-Clindamycin; NV-Clindamycin; PMS-Clindamycin; ratio-Clindamycin; Riva-Clindamycin; Teva-Clindamycin
Index Terms Clindamycin Hydrochloride; Clindamycin Palmitate
Generic Availability (U.S.) Yes

Pharmacologic Category Antibiotic, Lincosamide

Use Treatment of susceptible bacterial infections, mainly those caused by anaerobes, streptococci, pneumococci, and staphylococci; pelvic inflammatory disease (I.V.)

Unlabeled/Investigational Use May be useful in PCP; alternate treatment for toxoplasmosis; bacterial vaginosis (oral); alternate treatment for MRSA infections; alternate antibiotic for prophylaxis of infective endocarditis in patients who are allergic to penicillin and undergoing surgical or dental procedures (ACC/AHA guidelines); treatment of severe or uncomplicated malaria; treatment of babesiosis

Contraindications Hypersensitivity to clindamycin, lincomycin, or any component of the formulation

Warnings/Precautions Dosage adjustment may be necessary in patients with severe hepatic dysfunction. **[U.S. Boxed Warning]: Can cause severe and possibly fatal colitis.** Prolonged use may result in fungal or bacterial superinfection, including *C. difficile*-associated diarrhea (CDAD) and pseudomembranous colitis; CDAD has been observed >2 months postantibiotic treatment. Use with caution in patients with a history of gastrointestinal disease. Discontinue drug if significant diarrhea, abdominal cramps, or passage of blood and mucus occurs. Some dosage forms contain benzyl alcohol or tartrazine. Use caution in atopic patients. Not appropriate for use in the treatment of meningitis due to inadequate penetration into the CSF.

Adverse Reactions (Reflective of adult population; not specific for elderly) Frequency not defined.

Cardiovascular: Cardiac arrest (rare; I.V. administration), hypotension (rare; I.V. administration)

Dermatologic: Erythema multiforme (rare), exfoliative dermatitis (rare), pruritus, rash, Stevens-Johnson syndrome (rare), urticaria

Gastrointestinal: Abdominal pain, diarrhea, esophagitis, nausea, pseudomembranous colitis, vomiting

Genitourinary: Vaginitis

Hematologic: Agranulocytosis, eosinophilia (transient), neutropenia (transient), thrombocytopenia

Hepatic: Jaundice, liver function test abnormalities

Local: Induration/pain/sterile abscess (I.M.), thrombophlebitis (I.V.)

Neuromuscular & skeletal: Polyarthritis (rare)

Renal: Renal dysfunction (rare)

Miscellaneous: Anaphylactoid reactions (rare)

Drug Interactions

Avoid Concomitant Use

Avoid concomitant use of Clindamycin (Systemic) with any of the following: BCG; Erythromycin; Erythromycin (Systemic)

Increased Effect/Toxicity

Clindamycin (Systemic) may increase the levels/effects of: Neuromuscular-Blocking Agents

Decreased Effect

Clindamycin (Systemic) may decrease the levels/effects of: BCG; Erythromycin (Systemic); Typhoid Vaccine

The levels/effects of Clindamycin (Systemic) may be decreased by: Erythromycin; Kaolin

Ethanol/Nutrition/Herb Interactions

Food: Peak concentrations may be delayed with food.

Herb/Nutraceutical: St John's wort may decrease clindamycin levels.

Stability

Capsule: Store at room temperature of 20°C to 25°C (68°F to 77°F).

I.V.: Infusion solution in NS or D₅W solution is stable for 16 days at room temperature, 32 days refrigerated, or 8 weeks frozen. Prior to use, store vials and premixed bags at controlled room temperature 20°C to 25°C (68°F to 77°F). After initial use, discard any unused portion of vial after 24 hours.

Oral solution: Do not refrigerate reconstituted oral solution (it will thicken); following reconstitution, oral solution is stable for 2 weeks at room temperature of 20°C to 25°C (68°F to 77°F).

Mechanism of Action Reversibly binds to 50S ribosomal subunits preventing peptide bond formation thus inhibiting bacterial protein synthesis; bacteriostatic or bactericidal depending on drug concentration, infection site, and organism

Pharmacodynamics/Kinetics

Absorption: Oral, hydrochloride: Rapid (90%)

Distribution: High concentrations in bone and urine; no significant levels in CSF, even with inflamed meninges

V_d: ~2 L/kg

◄ Metabolism: Hepatic; forms metabolites (variable activity); Clindamycin phosphate is converted to clindamycin HCl (active)

Half-life elimination: ~2-3 hours; Elderly: 4 hours (range 3.4-5.1 hours)

Time to peak, serum: Oral: Within 60 minutes; I.M.: 1-3 hours

Excretion: Urine (10%) and feces (~4%) as active drug and metabolites

Dosage

Geriatric & Adult

Usual dose:

Oral: 150-450 mg/dose every 6-8 hours; maximum dose: 1.8 g/day

I.M., I.V.: 1.2-2.7 g/day in 2-4 divided doses; maximum dose: 4.8 g/day

Amnionitis: *I.V.:* 450-900 mg every 8 hours

Anthrax (unlabeled use): *I.V.:* 900 mg every 8 hours with ciprofloxacin or doxycycline

Babesiosis (unlabeled use):

Oral: 600 mg 3 times/day for 7-10 days with quinine (*Medical Letter*, 2007)

I.V.: 1.2 g twice daily for 7-10 days with quinine (*Medical Letter*, 2007)

Bacterial vaginosis (unlabeled use): *Oral:* 300 mg twice daily for 7 days (CDC, 2010)

Bite wounds (canine): *Oral:* 300 mg 4 times/day with a fluoroquinolone

Cellulitis due to MRSA (unlabeled use): Oral: 300-450 mg 3 times/day for 5-10 days (Liu, 2011)

Complicated skin/soft tissue infection due to MRSA (unlabeled use): I.V., Oral: 600 mg 3 times/day for 7-14 days (Liu, 2011)

Gangrenous pyomyositis: *I.V.:* 900 mg every 8 hours with penicillin G

Group B streptococcus (neonatal prophylaxis): *I.V.:* 900 mg every 8 hours until delivery

Malaria, severe (unlabeled use): I.V.: Load: 10 mg/kg followed by 15 mg/kg/day divided every 8 hours *plus* I.V. quinidine gluconate; switch to oral therapy (clindamycin *plus* quinine) when able for total clindamycin treatment duration of 7 days (**Note:** Quinine duration is region specific, consult CDC for current recommendations) (CDC, 2009)

Malaria, uncomplicated treatment (unlabeled use): Oral: 20 mg/kg/day divided every 8 hours for 7 days *plus* quinine (CDC, 2009)

Orofacial/parapharyngeal space infections:

Oral: 150-450 mg every 6 hours for at least 7 days; maximum dose: 1.8 g/day

I.V.: 600-900 mg every 8 hours

Osteomyelitis due to MRSA (unlabeled use): *I.V., Oral:* 600 mg 3 times/day for a minimum of 8 weeks (some experts combine with rifampin) (Liu, 2011)

Pelvic inflammatory disease: *I.V.:* 900 mg every 8 hours with gentamicin (conventional or single daily dosing); 24 hours after clinical improvement may convert to oral doxycycline 100 mg twice daily **or** clindamycin 450 mg 4 times/day to complete 14 days of total therapy. Avoid doxycycline if tubo-ovarian abscess is present. (CDC, 2010)

Pneumocystis jirovecii **pneumonia (unlabeled use):**

I.V.: 600-900 mg every 6-8 hours with primaquine for 21 days (CDC, 2009)

Oral: 300-450 mg every 6-8 hours with primaquine for 21 days (CDC, 2009)

Pneumonia due to MRSA (unlabeled use): *I.V., Oral:* 600 mg 3 times/day for 7-21 days (Liu, 2011)

Prophylaxis against infective endocarditis (unlabeled use):

Oral: 600 mg 30-60 minutes before procedure with no follow-up dose needed (Wilson, 2007)

I.M., I.V.: 600 mg 30-60 minutes before procedure. Intramuscular injections should be avoided in patients who are receiving anticoagulant therapy. In these circumstances, orally administered regimens should be given whenever possible. Intravenously administered antibiotics should be used for patients who are unable to tolerate or absorb oral medications (Wilson, 2007).

Note: American Heart Association (AHA) guidelines now recommend prophylaxis only in patients undergoing invasive procedures and in whom underlying cardiac conditions may predispose to a higher risk of adverse outcomes should infection occur. As of April 2007, routine prophylaxis for GI/GU procedures is no longer recommended by the AHA.

Prophylaxis in total joint replacement patients undergoing dental procedures which produce bacteremia (unlabeled use):

Oral: 600 mg 1 hour prior to procedure (ADA, 2003)

I.V.: 600 mg 1 hour prior to procedure (for patients unable to take oral medication) (ADA, 2003)

Septic arthritis due to MRSA (unlabeled use): *I.V., Oral:* 600 mg 3 times/day for 3-4 weeks (Liu, 2011)

Toxic shock syndrome: *I.V.:* 900 mg every 8 hours with penicillin G or ceftriaxone

Toxoplasmosis (HIV-exposed/positive; secondary prevention [unlabeled use]): *Oral:* 600 mg every 8 hours (with pyrimethamine and leucovorin calcium) (CDC, 2009)

Renal Impairment No dosage adjustment required in renal impairment.

Poorly dialyzed; no supplemental dose or dosage adjustment necessary, including patients on intermittent hemodialysis, peritoneal dialysis, or continuous renal replacement therapy (eg, CVVHD).

Hepatic Impairment Systemic use: No adjustment required. Use caution with severe hepatic impairment.

Administration

I.M.: Deep I.M. sites, rotate sites; do not exceed 600 mg in a single injection.

I.V.: **Never administer as bolus**; administer by I.V. intermittent infusion over at least 10-60 minutes, at a rate **not** to exceed 30 mg/minute (do not exceed 1200 mg/hour); final concentration for administration should not exceed 18 mg/mL.

Oral: Administer with a full glass of water to minimize esophageal ulceration; give around-the-clock to promote less variation in peak and trough serum levels.

Monitoring Parameters Observe for changes in bowel frequency. Monitor for colitis and resolution of symptoms. During prolonged therapy monitor CBC, liver and renal function tests periodically.

Pharmacotherapy Pearls *In vitro* susceptibility rates to clindamycin are higher in community acquired versus hospital acquired MRSA, although this may vary by geographic region. The D-zone test is recommended for detection of inducible resistance to clindamycin in erythromycin-resistant but clindamycin-susceptible isolates (Liu, 2011).

Special Geriatric Considerations Clindamycin has not been studied in the elderly; however, since it is eliminated principally by nonrenal mechanisms, major alteration in its pharmacokinetics are not expected. Elderly patients are often at a higher risk for developing serious colitis and require close monitoring.

Dosage Forms Excipient information presented when available (limited, particularly for generics); consult specific product labeling.

Capsule, oral, as hydrochloride [strength expressed as base]: 75 mg, 150 mg, 300 mg
Cleocin HCl®: 75 mg, 150 mg [contains tartrazine]
Cleocin HCl®: 300 mg

Granules for solution, oral, as palmitate hydrochloride [strength expressed as base]: 75 mg/5 mL (100 mL)
Cleocin Pediatric®: 75 mg/5 mL (100 mL) [cherry flavor]

Infusion, premixed in D_5W, as phosphate [strength expressed as base]:
Cleocin Phosphate®: 300 mg (50 mL); 600 mg (50 mL); 900 mg (50 mL) [contains edetate disodium]

Injection, solution, as phosphate [strength expressed as base]: 150 mg/mL (2 mL, 4 mL, 6 mL, 60 mL)
Cleocin Phosphate®: 150 mg/mL (2 mL, 4 mL, 6 mL, 60 mL) [contains benzyl alcohol, edetate disodium]

Selected References

del Carmen Carrasco-Portugal M, Lujan M, and Flores-Murrieta FJ, "Evaluation of Gender in the Oral Pharmacokinetics of Clindamycin in Humans," *Biopharm Drug Dispos*, 2008, 29(7):427-30.

Yoshikawa TT, "Antimicrobial Therapy for the Elderly Patient," *J Am Geriatr Soc*, 1990, 38(12):1353-72.

Clindamycin (Topical) (klin da MYE sin)

Medication Safety Issues

Sound-alike/look-alike issues:

Cleocin® may be confused with bleomycin, Clinoril®, Cubicin®, Lincocin®

Clindamycin may be confused with clarithromycin, Claritin®, vancomycin

Brand Names: U.S. Cleocin T®; Cleocin®; Cleocin® Vaginal Ovule; Clindagel®; Clinda-Max®; ClindaReach®; Clindesse®; Evoclin®

Brand Names: Canada Clinda-T; Clindasol™; Clindets; Dalacin® C; Dalacin® T; Dalacin® Vaginal; Taro-Clindamycin

Index Terms Clindamycin Phosphate

Generic Availability (U.S.) Yes: Excludes foam, vaginal suppositories

Pharmacologic Category Antibiotic, Lincosamide; Topical Skin Product, Acne

Use Treatment of bacterial vaginosis (vaginal cream, vaginal suppository); topically in treatment of severe acne

Dosage

Geriatric & Adult

Acne: *Topical:*

Gel, pledget, lotion, solution: Apply a thin film twice daily

Foam (Evoclin®): Apply once daily

◄ **Bacterial vaginosis:** *Intravaginal:*
Suppositories: Insert one ovule (100 mg clindamycin) daily into vagina at bedtime for 3 days
Cream:
Cleocin®: One full applicator inserted intravaginally once daily before bedtime for 3 or 7 consecutive days in nonpregnant patients or for 7 consecutive days in pregnant patients
Clindesse®: One full applicator inserted intravaginally as a single dose at anytime during the day in nonpregnant patients

Special Geriatric Considerations This formulation has not been studied in a sufficient number of elderly patients to draw conclusions.

Dosage Forms Excipient information presented when available (limited, particularly for generics); consult specific product labeling. [DSC] = Discontinued product
Aerosol, topical, as phosphate [strength expressed as base, foam]: 1% (50 g, 100 g)
Evoclin®: 1% (50 g, 100 g) [contains ethanol 58%]
Cream, vaginal, as phosphate [strength expressed as base]: 2% (40 g)
Cleocin®: 2% (40 g) [contains benzyl alcohol, mineral oil]
Clindesse®: 2% (5 g) [contains mineral oil]
Gel, topical, as phosphate [strength expressed as base]: 1% (30 g, 60 g)
Cleocin T®: 1% (30 g, 60 g)
Clindagel®: 1% (40 mL, 75 mL)
ClindaMax®: 1% (30 g, 60 g)
Lotion, topical, as phosphate [strength expressed as base]: 1% (60 mL)
Cleocin T®: 1% (60 mL)
ClindaMax®: 1% (60 mL)
Pledget, topical, as phosphate [strength expressed as base]: 1% (60s, 69s [DSC])
Cleocin T®: 1% (60s) [contains isopropyl alcohol 50%]
ClindaReach®: 1% (120s) [contains isopropyl alcohol 50%]
Solution, topical, as phosphate [strength expressed as base]: 1% (30 mL, 60 mL)
Cleocin T®: 1% (30 mL, 60 mL) [contains isopropyl alcohol 50%]
Suppository, vaginal, as phosphate [strength expressed as base]:
Cleocin® Vaginal Ovule: 100 mg (3s) [contains oleaginous base]

Clindamycin and Tretinoin (klin da MYE sin & TRET i noyn)

Brand Names: U.S. Veltin™; Ziana™
Index Terms Clindamycin Phosphate and Tretinoin; Tretinoin and Clindamycin; Veltin™
Generic Availability (U.S.) No
Pharmacologic Category Acne Products; Retinoic Acid Derivative; Topical Skin Product; Topical Skin Product, Acne
Use Treatment of acne vulgaris
Dosage
Adult Acne: Topical: Apply once daily
Special Geriatric Considerations This formulation has not been studied in a sufficient number of elderly patients to draw conclusions.
Dosage Forms Excipient information presented when available (limited, particularly for generics); consult specific product labeling.
Gel, topical:
Veltin™: Clindamycin phosphate 1.2% and tretinoin 0.025% (30 g, 60 g)
Ziana™: Clindamycin phosphate 1.2% and tretinoin 0.025% (30 g, 60 g)

◆ **Clindamycin Hydrochloride** *see* Clindamycin (Systemic) *on page 376*
◆ **Clindamycin Palmitate** *see* Clindamycin (Systemic) *on page 376*
◆ **Clindamycin Phosphate** *see* Clindamycin (Topical) *on page 379*
◆ **Clindamycin Phosphate and Tretinoin** *see* Clindamycin and Tretinoin *on page 380*
◆ **ClindaReach®** *see* Clindamycin (Topical) *on page 379*
◆ **Clindesse®** *see* Clindamycin (Topical) *on page 379*
◆ **Clinoril®** *see* Sulindac *on page 1720*
◆ **Clinpro™ 5000** *see* Fluoride *on page 751*

Clobetasol (kloe BAY ta sol)

Related Information
Corticosteroids *on page 2005*
Medication Safety Issues
International issues:
Clobex [U.S., Canada, and multiple international markets] may be confused with Codex brand name for *Saccharomyces boulardii* [Italy]

Cloderm: Brand name for clobetasol [China, India, Malaysia, Singapore, Thailand], but also brand name for alclometasone [Indonesia]; clocortolone [U.S., Canada]; clotrimazole [Germany]

Brand Names: U.S. Clobex®; Cormax®; Olux-E™; Olux®; Olux®/Olux-E™ CP [DSC]; Temovate E®; Temovate®

Brand Names: Canada Clobex®; Dermovate®; Gen-Clobetasol; Mylan-Clobetasol Cream; Mylan-Clobetasol Ointment; Mylan-Clobetasol Scalp Application; Novo-Clobetasol; PMS-Clobetasol; ratio-Clobetasol; Taro-Clobetasol

Index Terms Clobetasol Propionate

Generic Availability (U.S.) Yes: Excludes lotion, shampoo, spray

Pharmacologic Category Corticosteroid, Topical

Use Short-term relief of inflammation of moderate-to-severe corticosteroid-responsive dermatoses (very high potency topical corticosteroid)

Contraindications Hypersensitivity to clobetasol or any component of the formulation; viral, fungal, or tubercular skin lesions

Warnings/Precautions Systemic absorption of topical corticosteroids may cause hypothalamic-pituitary-adrenal (HPA) axis suppression (reversible). HPA axis suppression may lead to adrenal crisis. Risk is increased when used over large surface areas, for prolonged periods, or with occlusive dressings. Allergic contact dermatitis can occur, it is usually diagnosed by failure to heal rather than clinical exacerbation. Prolonged treatment with corticosteroids has been associated with the development of Kaposi's sarcoma (case reports); if noted, discontinuation of therapy should be considered. Adverse systemic effects including hyperglycemia, glycosuria, fluid and electrolyte changes, and HPA suppression may occur when used on large surface areas, for prolonged periods, or with an occlusive dressing. Do not use on the face, axillae, or groin.

Adverse Reactions (Reflective of adult population; not specific for elderly) Frequency not defined; may depend upon formulation used, length of application, surface area covered, and the use of occlusive dressings.

Endocrine & metabolic: Adrenal suppression, Cushing's syndrome, hyperglycemia
Local: Application site: Burning, cracking/fissuring of the skin, dryness, erythema, folliculitis, irritation, numbness, pruritus, skin atrophy, stinging, telangiectasia
Renal: Glucosuria
Effects reported with other high-potency topical steroids: Acneiform eruptions, allergic contact dermatitis, hypertrichosis, hypopigmentation, maceration of the skin, miliaria, perioral dermatitis, secondary infection

Drug Interactions
  Avoid Concomitant Use
  Avoid concomitant use of Clobetasol with any of the following: Aldesleukin
  Increased Effect/Toxicity
  Clobetasol may increase the levels/effects of: Deferasirox

  The levels/effects of Clobetasol may be increased by: Telaprevir
  Decreased Effect
  Clobetasol may decrease the levels/effects of: Aldesleukin; Corticorelin; Telaprevir

Stability
Cream, emollient cream, ointment: Store at room temperature, between 15°C to 30°C (59°F to 86°F); do not refrigerate.
Foam: Store at room temperature; do not expose to temperatures >49°C (120°F). Avoid fire, flame, or smoking during and immediately following application.
Gel: Store between 2°C to 30°C (36°F to 86°F).
Lotion, shampoo, spray: Store at room temperature of 20°C to 25°C (68°F to 77°F). Spray is flammable; do not use near open flame.
Solution: Store between 4°C to 25°C (39°F to 77°F). Do not use near an open flame.

Mechanism of Action Stimulates the synthesis of enzymes needed to decrease inflammation, suppress mitotic activity, and cause vasoconstriction

Pharmacodynamics/Kinetics
Absorption: Percutaneous absorption is variable and dependent upon many factors including vehicle used, integrity of epidermis, dose, and use of occlusive dressings
Metabolism: Hepatic
Excretion: Urine and feces

Dosage
  Geriatric & Adult Note: Discontinue when control achieved; if improvement not seen within 2 weeks, reassessment of diagnosis may be necessary
    Oral mucosal inflammation (unlabeled use): Topical: Cream: Apply twice daily for up to 2 weeks (maximum dose: 50 g/week); discontinue application when control is achieved; if no improvement is seen, reassessment of diagnosis may be necessary

Steroid-responsive dermatoses: Topical:

Cream, emollient cream, gel, lotion, ointment: Apply twice daily for up to 2 weeks (maximum dose: 50 g/week)

Foam (Olux-E™): Apply to affected area twice daily for up to 2 weeks (maximum dose: 50 g/week); do not apply to face or intertriginous areas

Steroid-responsive dermatoses of the scalp: Topical: Foam (Olux®), solution: Apply to affected scalp twice daily for up to 2 weeks (maximum dose: 50 g or 50 mL/week)

Mild-to-moderate plaque-type psoriasis of nonscalp areas: Topical: Foam (Olux®): Apply to affected area twice daily for up to 2 weeks (maximum dose: 50 g/week); do not apply to face or intertriginous areas

Moderate-to-severe plaque-type psoriasis: Topical:

Emollient cream, lotion: Apply twice daily for up to 2 weeks, has been used for up to 4 weeks when application is <10% of body surface area; use with caution (maximum dose: 50 g/week)

Spray: Apply by spraying directly onto affected area twice daily; should be gently rubbed into skin. Should be used for not longer than 4 weeks; treatment beyond 2 weeks should be limited to localized lesions which have not improved sufficiently. Total dose should not exceed 50 g/week or 59 mL/week.

Scalp psoriasis: Topical: Shampoo: Apply thin film to dry scalp once daily; leave in place for 15 minutes, then add water, lather; rinse thoroughly

Administration

Cream, gel, lotion, ointment, solution: Apply the smallest amount that will cover affected area. Do not apply to face or intertriginous areas. Total dose should not exceed 50 g/week (or 50 mL/week of lotion or solution).

Foam: Turn can upside down and spray a small amount (golf ball size) of foam into the cap or another cool surface. If fingers are warm, rinse with cool water and dry prior to handling (foam will melt on contact with warm skin). Massage foam into affected area. If the can is warm or the foam is runny, run can under cold water.

Monitoring Parameters Adrenal suppression with extensive/prolonged use (ACTH stimulation test, morning plasma cortisol test, urinary free cortisol test)

Pharmacotherapy Pearls Considered a super high potency steroid; avoid use on face

Special Geriatric Considerations Due to age-related changes in skin, limit use of topical corticosteroids.

Dosage Forms Excipient information presented when available (limited, particularly for generics); consult specific product labeling. [DSC] = Discontinued product

Aerosol, topical, as propionate [combination package/foam]:

Olux®/Olux-E™ CP: Olux-E™: 0.05% (50 g) and Olux® 0.05% (50 g) [contains ethanol 60%] (1s [DSC]); Olux-E™: 0.05% (10 g) and Olux® 0.05% (100 g) [contains ethanol 60%] (1s [DSC])

Aerosol, topical, as propionate [foam]: 0.05% (50 g, 100 g)

Olux-E™: 0.05% (50 g, 100 g) [ethanol free]

Olux®: 0.05% (50 g, 100 g) [contains ethanol 60%; for scalp application]

Cream, topical, as propionate: 0.05% (15 g, 30 g, 45 g, 60 g)

Temovate®: 0.05% (30 g [DSC], 60 g [DSC])

Cream, topical, as propionate [emollient-based]: 0.05% (15 g, 30 g, 60 g)

Temovate E®: 0.05% (60 g)

Cream, topical, as propionate [emulsion-based]: 0.05% (15 g [DSC], 30 g [DSC], 60 g [DSC])

Gel, topical, as propionate: 0.05% (15 g, 30 g, 60 g)

Temovate®: 0.05% (60 g)

Lotion, topical, as propionate:

Clobex®: 0.05% (30 mL, 59 mL, 118 mL)

Ointment, topical, as propionate: 0.05% (15 g, 30 g, 45 g, 60 g)

Cormax®: 0.05% (15 g, 45 g)

Temovate®: 0.05% (15 g, 30 g)

Shampoo, topical, as propionate:

Clobex®: 0.05% (118 mL) [contains ethanol]

Solution, topical, as propionate [for scalp application]: 0.05% (25 mL, 50 mL)

Cormax®: 0.05% (25 mL, 50 mL) [contains isopropyl alcohol 40%]

Temovate®: 0.05% (50 mL) [contains isopropyl alcohol 39.3%]

Solution, topical, as propionate [spray]:

Clobex®: 0.05% (59 mL, 125 mL) [contains ethanol]

◆ **Clobetasol Propionate** *see* Clobetasol *on page 380*

◆ **Clobex®** *see* Clobetasol *on page 380*

ClomiPRAMINE (kloe MI pra meen)

Related Information

Antidepressant Agents *on page 1991*

Medication Safety Issues

Sound-alike/look-alike issues:

ClomiPRAMINE may be confused with chlorproMAZINE, clevidipine, clomiPHENE, desipramine, Norpramin®

Anafranil® may be confused with alfentanil, enalapril, nafarelin

Brand Names: U.S. Anafranil®

Brand Names: Canada Anafranil®; Apo-Clomipramine®; CO Clomipramine; Gen-Clomipramine

Index Terms Clomipramine Hydrochloride

Generic Availability (U.S.) Yes

Pharmacologic Category Antidepressant, Tricyclic (Tertiary Amine)

Use Treatment of obsessive-compulsive disorder (OCD)

Unlabeled/Investigational Use Treatment of depression, panic attacks, chronic pain

Medication Guide Available Yes

Contraindications Hypersensitivity to clomipramine, other tricyclic agents, or any component of the formulation; use of MAO inhibitors within 14 days; use in a patient during the acute recovery phase of MI

Warnings/Precautions [U.S. Boxed Warning]: Antidepressants increase the risk of suicidal thinking and behavior in children, adolescents, and young adults (18-24 years of age) with major depressive disorder (MDD) and other psychiatric disorders; consider risk prior to prescribing. Short-term studies did not show an increased risk in patients >24 years of age and showed a decreased risk in patients ≥65 years. Closely monitor for clinical worsening, suicidality, or unusual changes in behavior; the patient's family or caregiver should be instructed to closely observe the patient and communicate condition with healthcare provider. A medication guide should be dispensed with each prescription. **Clomipramine is FDA approved for the treatment of OCD in children ≥10 years of age.**

The possibility of a suicide attempt is inherent in major depression and may persist until remission occurs. Monitor for worsening of depression or suicidality, especially during initiation of therapy (generally first 1-2 months) or with dose increases or decreases. Use caution in high-risk patients. Worsening depression and severe abrupt suicidality that are not part of the presenting symptoms may require discontinuation or modification of drug therapy. The patient's family or caregiver should be alerted to monitor patients for the emergence of suicidality and associated behaviors (such as agitation, irritability, hostility, impulsivity, and hypomania) and notify the healthcare provider.

May worsen psychosis in some patients or precipitate a shift to mania or hypomania in patients with bipolar disorder. Patients presenting with depressive symptoms should be screened for bipolar disorder. Monotherapy in patients with bipolar disorder should be avoided. **Clomipramine is not FDA approved for bipolar depression.**

TCAs may rarely cause bone marrow suppression; monitor for any signs of infection and obtain CBC if symptoms (eg, fever, sore throat) evident. May cause seizures (relationship to dose and/or duration of therapy) - do not exceed maximum doses. Use caution in patients with a previous seizure disorder or condition predisposing to seizures such as brain damage, alcoholism, or concurrent therapy with other drugs which lower the seizure threshold. May increase the risks associated with electroconvulsive therapy. Has been associated with a high incidence of sexual dysfunction. Weight gain may occur. Hyperpyrexia has been observed with TCAs in combination with anticholinergics and/or neuroleptics, particularly during hot weather.

The degree of sedation, anticholinergic effects, and conduction abnormalities are high relative to other antidepressants. Clomipramine often causes drowsiness/sedation, resulting in impaired performance of tasks requiring alertness (eg, operating machinery or driving). Sedative effects may be additive with other CNS depressants and/or ethanol. The risk of orthostasis is moderate to high relative to other antidepressants. Use with caution in patients with a history of cardiovascular disease (including previous MI, stroke, tachycardia, or conduction abnormalities). Use with caution in patients with urinary retention, benign prostatic hyperplasia, narrow-angle glaucoma, xerostomia, visual problems, constipation, or a history of bowel obstruction.

Consider discontinuing, when possible, prior to elective surgery. Therapy should not be abruptly discontinued in patients receiving high doses for prolonged periods. Use with caution

◀ in hyperthyroid patients or those receiving thyroid supplementation. Use with caution in patients with hepatic or renal dysfunction and in elderly patients.

Adverse Reactions (Reflective of adult population; not specific for elderly) Data shown for children reflects both children and adolescents studied in clinical trials.

>10%:

Central nervous system: Dizziness (54%), somnolence (54%), drowsiness, headache (52%; children 28%), fatigue (39%), insomnia (25%; children 11%), malaise, nervousness (18%; children 4%)

Endocrine & metabolic: Libido changes (21%), hot flushes (5%)

Gastrointestinal: Xerostomia (84%, children 63%) constipation (47%; children 22%), nausea (33%; children 9%), dyspepsia (22%; children 13%), weight gain (18%; children 2%), diarrhea (13%; children 7%), anorexia (12%; children 22%), abdominal pain (11%), appetite increased (11%)

Genitourinary: Ejaculation failure (42%), impotence (20%), micturition disorder (14%; children 4%)

Neuromuscular & skeletal: Tremor (54%), myoclonus (13%; children 2%), myalgia (13%)

Ocular: Abnormal vision (18%; children 7%)

Respiratory: Pharyngitis (14%), rhinitis (12%)

Miscellaneous: Diaphoresis increased (29%; children 9%)

1% to 10%:

Cardiovascular: Flushing (8%), postural hypotension (6%), palpitation (4%), tachycardia (4%; children 2%), chest pain (4%), edema (2%)

Central nervous system: Anxiety (9%), memory impairment (9%), twitching (7%), depression (5%), concentration impaired (5%), fever (4%), hypertonia (4%), abnormal dreaming (3%), agitation (3%), confusion (3%), migraine (3%), pain (3%), psychosomatic disorder (3%), speech disorder (3%), yawning (3%), aggressiveness (children 2%), chills (2%), depersonalization (2%), emotional lability (2%), irritability (2%), panic reaction (1%)

Dermatologic: Rash (8%), pruritus (6%), purpura (3%), dermatitis (2%), acne (2%), dry skin (2%), urticaria (1%)

Endocrine & metabolic: Amenorrhea (1%), breast enlargement (2%), breast pain (1%), hot flushes (5%), lactation (nonpuerperal) (4%)

Gastrointestinal: Taste disturbance (8%), vomiting (7%), flatulence (6%), dental caries and teeth grinding (5%), dysphagia (2%), esophagitis (1%)

Genitourinary: UTI (2% to 6%), micturition frequency (5%), dysuria (2%), leucorrhea (2%), vaginitis (2%), urinary retention (2%)

Neuromuscular & skeletal: Paresthesia (9%), back pain (6%), arthralgia (3%), paresis (children 2%), weakness (1%)

Ocular: Lacrimation abnormal (3%), mydriasis (2%), conjunctivitis (1%)

Otic: Tinnitus (6%)

Respiratory: Sinusitis (6%), coughing (6%), bronchospasm (2%; children 7%), epistaxis (2%)

Drug Interactions

Metabolism/Transport Effects Substrate of CYP1A2 (major), 2C19 (major), 2D6 (major), 3A4 (minor); **Inhibits** CYP2D6 (moderate)

Avoid Concomitant Use

Avoid concomitant use of ClomiPRAMINE with any of the following: Artemether; Dronedarone; Iobenguane I 123; Lumefantrine; MAO Inhibitors; Methylene Blue; Nilotinib; Pimozide; QUEtiapine; QuiNINE; Sibutramine; Tetrabenazine; Thioridazine; Toremifene; Vandetanib; Vemurafenib; Ziprasidone

Increased Effect/Toxicity

ClomiPRAMINE may increase the levels/effects of: Alpha-/Beta-Agonists (Direct-Acting); Alpha1-Agonists; Amphetamines; Anticholinergics; Aspirin; Beta2-Agonists; CYP2D6 Substrates; Desmopressin; Dronedarone; Fesoterodine; Methylene Blue; Milnacipran; Nebivolol; NSAID (COX-2 Inhibitor); NSAID (Nonselective); Pimozide; QTc-Prolonging Agents; QuiNIDine; QuiNINE; Serotonin Modulators; Sodium Phosphates; Sulfonylureas; Tamoxifen; Tetrabenazine; Thioridazine; Toremifene; TraMADol; Vandetanib; Vemurafenib; Vitamin K Antagonists; Yohimbine; Ziprasidone

The levels/effects of ClomiPRAMINE may be increased by: Abiraterone Acetate; Alfuzosin; Altretamine; Artemether; BuPROPion; CarBAMazepine; Chloroquine; Cimetidine; Cinacalcet; Ciprofloxacin; Ciprofloxacin (Systemic); Conivaptan; CYP1A2 Inhibitors (Moderate); CYP1A2 Inhibitors (Strong); CYP2C19 Inhibitors (Moderate); CYP2C19 Inhibitors (Strong); CYP2D6 Inhibitors (Moderate); CYP2D6 Inhibitors (Strong); Deferasirox; Dexmethylphenidate; Divalproex; DULoxetine; Gadobutrol; Grapefruit Juice; Lithium; Lumefantrine; MAO Inhibitors; Methylphenidate; Metoclopramide; Nilotinib; Pramlintide; Propoxyphene; Protease Inhibitors; QUEtiapine; QuiNIDine; QuiNINE; Selective Serotonin Reuptake Inhibitors; Sibutramine; Terbinafine; Terbinafine (Systemic); Valproic Acid

Decreased Effect

ClomiPRAMINE may decrease the levels/effects of: Acetylcholinesterase Inhibitors (Central); Alpha2-Agonists; Codeine; Iobenguane I 123

The levels/effects of ClomiPRAMINE may be decreased by: Acetylcholinesterase Inhibitors (Central); Barbiturates; CYP1A2 Inducers (Strong); CYP2C19 Inducers (Strong); Cyproterone; Peginterferon Alfa-2b; St Johns Wort; Tocilizumab

Ethanol/Nutrition/Herb Interactions

Ethanol: May increase CNS depression; monitor for increased effects with coadministration. Caution patients about effects.

Food: Serum concentrations/toxicity may be increased by grapefruit juice.

Herb/Nutraceutical: Avoid valerian, St John's wort, SAMe, kava kava.

Mechanism of Action Clomipramine appears to affect serotonin uptake while its active metabolite, desmethylclomipramine, affects norepinephrine uptake

Pharmacodynamics/Kinetics

Absorption: Rapid

Protein binding: 97%, primarily to albumin

Metabolism: Hepatic to desmethylclomipramine (DMI; active); extensive first-pass effect

Half-life elimination: Clomipramine: mean 32 hours (19-37 hours); DMI: mean 69 hours (range 54-77 hours)

Time to peak, plasma: 2-6 hours

Excretion: Urine and feces

Dosage

Geriatric & Adult Treatment of OCD: Oral: Initial: 25 mg/day; may gradually increase as tolerated over the first 2 weeks to 100 mg/day in divided doses; Maintenance: May further increase to recommended maximum of 250 mg/day; may give as a single daily dose at bedtime once tolerated

Administration During titration, may divide doses and administer with meals to decrease gastrointestinal side effects. After titration, may administer total daily dose at bedtime to decrease daytime sedation.

Monitoring Parameters Pulse rate and blood pressure prior to and during therapy; ECG/cardiac status in older adults and patients with cardiac disease; suicidal ideation (especially at the beginning of therapy, after initiation, or when doses are increased or decreased)

Test Interactions Increased glucose; may interfere with urine detection of methadone (false-positive)

Special Geriatric Considerations Not approved as an antidepressant, clomipramine's anticholinergic and hypotensive effects limit its use versus other preferred antidepressants. Elderly patients were found to have higher dose-normalized plasma concentrations as a result of decreased demethylation (decreased 50%) and hydroxylation (25%).

Dosage Forms Excipient information presented when available (limited, particularly for generics); consult specific product labeling.

Capsule, oral, as hydrochloride: 25 mg, 50 mg, 75 mg

Anafranil®: 25 mg, 50 mg, 75 mg

Selected References

Bocksberger JP, Gex-Fabry M, Gauthey L, et al, "Clomipramine Therapy in the Geriatric Hospital: Experience With Therapeutic Drug Monitoring," *Ther Drug Monit*, 1994, 16(2):113-9.

◆ **Clomipramine Hydrochloride** *see* ClomiPRAMINE *on page 383*

ClonazePAM (kloe NA ze pam)

Related Information

Anxiolytic, Sedative / Hypnotic, and Miscellaneous Benzodiazepines *on page 2000*

Medication Safety Issues

Sound-alike/look-alike issues:

ClonazePAM may be confused with clofazimine, cloNIDine, clorazepate, cloZAPine, LORazepam

KlonoPIN® may be confused with clofazimine, cloNIDine, clorazepate, cloZAPine, LORazepam

Brand Names: U.S. KlonoPIN®

Brand Names: Canada Alti-Clonazepam; Apo-Clonazepam®; Clonapam; CO Clonazepam; Gen-Clonazepam; Klonopin®; Mylan-Clonazepam; Novo-Clonazepam; Nu-Clonazepam; PMS-Clonazepam; PRO-Clonazepam; Rho®-Clonazepam; Rivotril®; Sandoz-Clonazepam; ZYM-Clonazepam

Generic Availability (U.S.) Yes

Pharmacologic Category Benzodiazepine

CLONAZEPAM

Use Alone or as an adjunct in the treatment of petit mal variant (Lennox-Gastaut), akinetic, and myoclonic seizures; petit mal (absence) seizures unresponsive to succimides; panic disorder with or without agoraphobia

Unlabeled/Investigational Use Treatment of restless legs syndrome, neuralgia, multifocal tic disorder, parkinsonian dysarthria, bipolar disorder; adjunct therapy for schizophrenia

Medication Guide Available Yes

Contraindications Hypersensitivity to clonazepam or any component of the formulation (cross-sensitivity with other benzodiazepines may exist); significant liver disease; narrow-angle glaucoma

Warnings/Precautions Antiepileptics are associated with an increased risk of suicidal behavior/thoughts with use (regardless of indication); patients should be monitored for signs/symptoms of depression, suicidal tendencies, and other unusual behavior changes during therapy and instructed to inform their healthcare provider immediately if symptoms occur.

Use with caution in elderly or debilitated patients, patients with hepatic disease (including alcoholics), or renal impairment. Use with caution in patients with respiratory disease or impaired gag reflex or ability to protect the airway from secretions (salivation may be increased). Worsening of seizures may occur when added to patients with multiple seizure types. Concurrent use with valproic acid may result in absence status. Monitoring of CBC and liver function tests has been recommended during prolonged therapy.

Causes CNS depression (dose related) resulting in sedation, dizziness, confusion, or ataxia which may impair physical and mental capabilities. Patients must be cautioned about performing tasks which require mental alertness (eg, operating machinery or driving). Use with caution in patients receiving other CNS depressants or psychoactive agents. Effects with other sedative drugs or ethanol may be potentiated. Benzodiazepines have been associated with falls and traumatic injury and should be used with extreme caution in patients who are at risk of these events (especially the elderly).

Use caution in patients with depression, particularly if suicidal risk may be present. Use with caution in patients with a history of drug dependence. Benzodiazepines have been associated with dependence and acute withdrawal symptoms, including seizures, on discontinuation or reduction in dose. Acute withdrawal, including seizures, may be precipitated in patients after administration of flumazenil to patients receiving long-term benzodiazepine therapy.

Benzodiazepines have been associated with anterograde amnesia. Paradoxical reactions, including hyperactive or aggressive behavior, have been reported with benzodiazepines, particularly in psychiatric patients. Does not have analgesic, antidepressant, or antipsychotic properties.

Adverse Reactions (Reflective of adult population; not specific for elderly) Reactions reported in patients with seizure and/or panic disorder. Frequency not always defined.

Cardiovascular: Edema (ankle or facial), palpitation

Central nervous system: Amnesia, ataxia (seizure disorder ~30%; panic disorder 5%), behavior problems (seizure disorder ~25%), coma, confusion, depression, dizziness, drowsiness (seizure disorder ~50%), emotional lability, fatigue, fever, hallucinations, headache, hypotonia, hysteria, insomnia, intellectual ability reduced, memory disturbance, nervousness; paradoxical reactions (including aggressive behavior, agitation, anxiety, excitability, hostility, irritability, nervousness, nightmares, sleep disturbance, vivid dreams); psychosis, slurred speech, somnolence (panic disorder 37%), suicidal attempt, suicide ideation, vertigo

Dermatologic: Hair loss, hirsutism, skin rash

Endocrine & metabolic: Dysmenorrhea, libido increased/decreased

Gastrointestinal: Abdominal pain, anorexia, appetite increased/decreased, coated tongue, constipation, dehydration, diarrhea, gastritis, gum soreness, nausea, weight changes (loss/gain), xerostomia

Genitourinary: Colpitis, dysuria, ejaculation delayed, enuresis, impotence, micturition frequency, nocturia, urinary retention, urinary tract infection

Hematologic: Anemia, eosinophilia, leukopenia, thrombocytopenia

Hepatic: Alkaline phosphatase increased (transient), hepatomegaly, serum transaminases increased (transient)

Neuromuscular & skeletal: Choreiform movements, coordination abnormal, dysarthria, muscle pain, muscle weakness, myalgia, tremor

Ocular: Blurred vision, eye movements abnormal, diplopia, nystagmus

Respiratory: Chest congestion, cough, bronchitis, hypersecretions, pharyngitis, respiratory depression, respiratory tract infection, rhinitis, rhinorrhea, shortness of breath, sinusitis

Miscellaneous: Allergic reaction, aphonia, dysdiadochokinesis, encopresis, "glassy-eyed" appearance, hemiparesis, lymphadenopathy

Drug Interactions

Metabolism/Transport Effects Substrate of CYP3A4 (major)

Avoid Concomitant Use

Avoid concomitant use of ClonazePAM with any of the following: Conivaptan; OLANZapine

Increased Effect/Toxicity

ClonazePAM may increase the levels/effects of: Alcohol (Ethyl); CloZAPine; CNS Depressants; Fosphenytoin; Methotrimeprazine; Phenytoin; Selective Serotonin Reuptake Inhibitors

The levels/effects of ClonazePAM may be increased by: Antifungal Agents (Azole Derivatives, Systemic); Aprepitant; Calcium Channel Blockers (Nondihydropyridine); Cimetidine; Conivaptan; Contraceptives (Estrogens); Contraceptives (Progestins); CYP3A4 Inhibitors (Moderate); CYP3A4 Inhibitors (Strong); Dasatinib; Droperidol; Fluconazole; Fosaprepitant; Grapefruit Juice; HydrOXYzine; Isoniazid; Macrolide Antibiotics; Methotrimeprazine; Nefazodone; OLANZapine; Proton Pump Inhibitors; Selective Serotonin Reuptake Inhibitors

Decreased Effect

The levels/effects of ClonazePAM may be decreased by: CarBAMazepine; CYP3A4 Inducers (Strong); Deferasirox; Rifamycin Derivatives; St Johns Wort; Theophylline Derivatives; Tocilizumab; Yohimbine

Ethanol/Nutrition/Herb Interactions

Ethanol: May increase CNS depression; monitor for increased effects with coadministration. Caution patients about effects.

Food: Clonazepam serum concentration is unlikely to be increased by grapefruit juice because of clonazepam's high oral bioavailability.

Herb/Nutraceutical: St John's wort may decrease clonazepam levels. Avoid valerian, St John's wort, kava kava, gotu kola (may increase CNS depression).

Mechanism of Action The exact mechanism is unknown, but believed to be related to its ability to enhance the activity of GABA; suppresses the spike-and-wave discharge in absence seizures by depressing nerve transmission in the motor cortex

Pharmacodynamics/Kinetics

Onset of action: 20-60 minutes

Duration: ≤12 hours

Absorption: Well absorbed

Distribution: V_d: 1.5-4.4 L/kg

Protein binding: 85%

Metabolism: Extensively hepatic via glucuronide and sulfate conjugation

Half-life elimination: 19-50 hours

Time to peak, serum: 1-3 hours; Steady-state: 5-7 days

Excretion: Urine (<2% as unchanged drug); metabolites excreted as glucuronide or sulfate conjugates

Dosage

Geriatric Refer to adult dosing. Initiate with low doses and observe closely.

Adult

Burning mouth syndrome (unlabeled use): Oral: 0.25-3 mg/day in 2 divided doses, in morning and evening.

Seizure disorders: Oral:

Initial daily dose not to exceed 1.5 mg given in 3 divided doses; may increase by 0.5-1 mg every third day until seizures are controlled or adverse effects seen (maximum: 20 mg/day)

Usual maintenance dose: 0.05-0.2 mg/kg; do not exceed 20 mg/day

Panic disorder: Oral: 0.25 mg twice daily; increase in increments of 0.125-0.25 mg twice daily every 3 days; target dose: 1 mg/day (maximum: 4 mg/day)

Discontinuation of treatment: To discontinue, treatment should be withdrawn gradually. Decrease dose by 0.125 mg twice daily every 3 days until medication is completely withdrawn.

Renal Impairment Hemodialysis: Supplemental dose is not necessary.

Administration Orally-disintegrating tablet: Open pouch and peel back foil on the blister; do not push tablet through foil. Use dry hands to remove tablet and place in mouth. May be swallowed with or without water. Use immediately after removing from package.

Monitoring Parameters CBC, liver function tests; observe patient for excess sedation, respiratory depression; suicidality (eg, suicidal thoughts, depression, behavioral changes)

Reference Range Relationship between serum concentration and seizure control is not well established

Timing of serum samples: Peak serum levels occur 1-3 hours after oral ingestion; the half-life is 20-40 hours; therefore, steady-state occurs in 5-7 days

Therapeutic levels: 20-80 ng/mL; Toxic concentration: >80 ng/mL

Pharmacotherapy Pearls Ethosuximide or valproic acid may be preferred for treatment of absence (petit mal) seizures; clonazepam-induced behavioral disturbances may be more frequent in mentally handicapped patients; up to 30% of patients have demonstrated a loss of anticonvulsant control within several months which requires a dosage adjustment

Special Geriatric Considerations Hepatic clearance may be decreased allowing accumulation of active drug. Also, metabolites of clonazepam are renally excreted and may accumulate in the elderly as renal function declines with age. Observe for signs of CNS and pulmonary toxicity.

Controlled Substance C-IV

Dosage Forms Excipient information presented when available (limited, particularly for generics); consult specific product labeling.

Tablet, oral: 0.5 mg, 1 mg, 2 mg
  KlonoPIN®: 0.5 mg [scored]
  KlonoPIN®: 1 mg, 2 mg
Tablet, orally disintegrating, oral: 0.125 mg, 0.25 mg, 0.5 mg, 1 mg, 2 mg

---

CloNIDine (KLON i deen)

Related Information
  Beers Criteria − Potentially Inappropriate Medications for Geriatrics *on page 2089*

Medication Safety Issues

Sound-alike/look-alike issues:
  CloNIDine may be confused with Clomid®, clomiPHENE, clonazePAM, cloZAPine, KlonoPIN®, quiNIDine
  Catapres® may be confused with Cataflam®, Cetapred®, Combipres

High alert medication:
  The Institute for Safe Medication Practices (ISMP) includes this medication (epidural administration) among its list of drug classes which have a heightened risk of causing significant patient harm when used in error.

BEERS Criteria medication:
  This drug may be inappropriate for use in geriatric patients (low severity risk).

Administration issues:
  Use caution when interpreting dosing information. Pediatric dose for epidural infusion expressed as mcg/kg/**hour**.

Other safety concerns:
  Transdermal patch may contain conducting metal (eg, aluminum); remove patch prior to MRI. Errors have occurred when the inactive, optional adhesive cover has been applied instead of the active clonidine-containing patch.

Brand Names: U.S. Catapres-TTS®-1; Catapres-TTS®-2; Catapres-TTS®-3; Catapres®; Duraclon®; Kapvay™; Nexiclon™ XR

Brand Names: Canada Apo-Clonidine®; Carapres®; Dixarit®; Dom-Clonidine; Novo-Clonidine; Nu-Clonidine

Index Terms Clonidine Hydrochloride

Generic Availability (U.S.) Yes: Excludes extended release tablets, oral suspension

Pharmacologic Category Alpha$_2$-Adrenergic Agonist

Use

Oral:
  Immediate release: Management of hypertension (monotherapy or as adjunctive therapy)
  Extended release:
    Kapvay™: Treatment of attention-deficit/hyperactivity disorder (ADHD) (monotherapy or as adjunctive therapy)
    Nexiclon™ XR: Management of hypertension (monotherapy or as adjunctive therapy)
Epidural (Duraclon®): For continuous epidural administration as adjunctive therapy with opioids for treatment of severe cancer pain in patients tolerant to or unresponsive to opioids alone; epidural clonidine is generally more effective for neuropathic pain and less effective (or possibly ineffective) for somatic or visceral pain
Transdermal patch: Management of hypertension (monotherapy or as adjunctive therapy)

Unlabeled/Investigational Use Heroin or nicotine withdrawal; severe pain; dysmenorrhea; vasomotor symptoms associated with menopause; ethanol dependence; prophylaxis of migraines; glaucoma; diabetes-associated diarrhea; impulse control disorder, clozapine-induced sialorrhea; aid in the diagnosis of growth hormone deficiency

Contraindications Hypersensitivity to clonidine hydrochloride or any component of the formulation

Epidural administration: Injection site infection; concurrent anticoagulant therapy; bleeding diathesis; administration above the C4 dermatome

Warnings/Precautions May cause CNS depression, which may impair physical or mental abilities; patients must be cautioned about performing tasks which require mental alertness (eg, operating machinery or driving). Sedating effects may be potentiated when used with other CNS-depressant drugs or ethanol. Use with caution in patients with severe coronary insufficiency; conduction disturbances; recent MI, CVA, or chronic renal insufficiency. May cause dose dependent reductions in heart rate; use with caution in patients with preexisting bradycardia or those predisposed to developing bradycardia. Caution in sinus node dysfunction. Use with caution in patients concurrently receiving agents known to reduce SA node function and/or AV nodal conduction (eg, digoxin, diltiazem, metoprolol, verapamil). May cause significant xerostomia. Clonidine may cause eye dryness in patients who wear contact lenses.

[U.S. Boxed Warning]: Must dilute concentrated epidural injectable (500 mcg/mL) solution prior to use. Epidural clonidine is not recommended for perioperative, obstetrical, or postpartum pain due to risk of hemodynamic instability. Clonidine injection should be administered via a continuous epidural infusion device. Monitor closely for catheter-related infection such as meningitis or epidural abscess. Epidural clonidine is not recommended for use in patients with severe cardiovascular disease or hemodynamic instability; may lead to cardiovascular instability (hypotension, bradycardia). Symptomatic hypotension may occur with use; in all patients, use epidural clonidine with caution due to the potential for severe hypotension especially in women and those of low body weight. Most hypotensive episodes occur within the first 4 days of initiation; however, episodes may occur throughout the duration of therapy.

Gradual withdrawal is needed (taper oral immediate release or epidural dose gradually over 2-4 days to avoid rebound hypertension) if drug needs to be stopped. Patients should be instructed about abrupt discontinuation (causes rapid increase in BP and symptoms of sympathetic overactivity). In patients on both a beta-blocker and clonidine where withdrawal of clonidine is necessary, withdraw the beta-blocker first and several days before clonidine withdrawal, then slowly decrease clonidine. Discontinue oral immediate release formulations within 4 hours of surgery then restart as soon as possible afterwards. Discontinue oral extended release formulations up to 28 hours prior to surgery, then restart the following day.

Oral formulations of clonidine (immediate release versus extended release) are not interchangeable on a mg:mg basis due to different pharmacokinetic profiles. This includes commercially available oral suspension (Nexiclon™ XR) which is an extended release preparation and should not be used interchangeably with any extemporaneously prepared clonidine oral suspension.

Transdermal patch may contain conducting metal (eg, aluminum); remove patch prior to MRI. Due to the potential for altered electrical conductivity, remove transdermal patch before cardioversion or defibrillation. Localized contact sensitization to the transdermal system has been reported; in these patients, allergic reactions (eg, generalized rash, urticaria, angioedema) have also occurred following subsequent substitution of oral therapy.

Clonidine may be inappropriate for use in the elderly due to CNS adverse events and orthostatic hypotension (Beers Criteria).

Adverse Reactions (Reflective of adult population; not specific for elderly) Frequency not always defined.

Oral, Transdermal: Incidence of adverse events may be less with transdermal compared to oral due to the lower peak/trough ratio.

Cardiovascular: Bradycardia (≤4%), palpitation (1%), tachycardia (1%), arrhythmia, atrioventricular block, chest pain, CHF, ECG abnormalities, flushing, orthostatic hypotension, pallor, Raynaud's phenomenon, syncope

Central nervous system: Drowsiness (12% to 38%), headache (1% to 29%), fatigue (4% to 16%), dizziness (2% to 16%), sedation (3% to 10%), insomnia (≤6%), lethargy (3%), nervousness (1% to 3%), mental depression (1%), aggression, agitation, anxiety, behavioral changes, CVA, delirium, delusional perception, fever, hallucinations (visual and auditory), irritability, malaise, nightmares, restlessness, vivid dreams

Dermatologic: Transient localized skin reactions characterized by pruritus and erythema (transdermal 15% to 50%), contact dermatitis (transdermal 8% to 34%), vesiculation (transdermal 7%), allergic contact sensitization (transdermal 5%), hyperpigmentation (transdermal 5%), burning (transdermal 3%), edema (3%), excoriation (transdermal 3%) blanching (transdermal 1%), generalized macular rash (1%), papules (transdermal 1%), throbbing (transdermal 1%), alopecia, angioedema, hives, localized hypopigmentation (transdermal), rash, urticaria

Endocrine & metabolic: Sexual dysfunction (3%), gynecomastia (1%), creatine phosphokinase increased (transient; oral), hyperglycemia (transient; oral), libido decreased

Gastrointestinal: Xerostomia (≤40%), constipation (2% to 10%), anorexia (1%), taste perversion (1%), weight gain (<1%), abdominal pain (oral), diarrhea, nausea, parotid gland pain (oral), parotitis (oral), pseudo-obstruction (oral), throat pain, vomiting

Genitourinary: Erectile dysfunction (2% to 3%), nocturia (1%), dysuria, enuresis, urinary retention

Hematologic: Thrombocytopenia (oral)

Hepatic: Liver function test (mild transient abnormalities; ≤1%), hepatitis

Neuromuscular & skeletal: Weakness (10%), arthralgia (1%), myalgia (1%), leg cramps (<1%), numbness (localized, transdermal), pain in extremities, paresthesia, tremor

Ocular: Accommodation disorder, blurred vision, burning eyes, dry eyes, lacrimation decreased, lacrimation increased

Otic: Ear pain, otitis media

Renal: Pollakiuria

Respiratory: Asthma, epistaxis, nasal congestion, nasal dryness, nasopharyngitis, respiratory tract infection, rhinorrhea

Miscellaneous: Withdrawal syndrome (1%), flu-like syndrome, thirst

Epidural: Note: The following adverse events occurred more often than placebo in cancer patients with intractable pain being treated with concurrent epidural morphine.

>10%:
Cardiovascular: Hypotension (45%), postural hypotension (32%)
Central nervous system: Confusion (13%), dizziness (13%)
Gastrointestinal: Xerostomia (13%)

1% to 10%:
Cardiovascular: Chest pain (5%)
Central nervous system: Hallucinations (5%)
Gastrointestinal: Nausea/vomiting (8%)
Otic: Tinnitus (5%)
Miscellaneous: Diaphoresis (5%)

Drug Interactions

Avoid Concomitant Use
Avoid concomitant use of CloNIDine with any of the following: Iobenguane I 123

Increased Effect/Toxicity
CloNIDine may increase the levels/effects of: Amifostine; Antihypertensives; Hypotensive Agents; RiTUXimab

The levels/effects of CloNIDine may be increased by: Alfuzosin; Beta-Blockers; Diazoxide; Herbs (Hypotensive Properties); MAO Inhibitors; Methylphenidate; Pentoxifylline; Phosphodiesterase 5 Inhibitors; Prostacyclin Analogues

Decreased Effect
CloNIDine may decrease the levels/effects of: Iobenguane I 123

The levels/effects of CloNIDine may be decreased by: Antidepressants (Alpha2-Antagonist); Herbs (Hypertensive Properties); Serotonin/Norepinephrine Reuptake Inhibitors; Tricyclic Antidepressants; Yohimbine

Ethanol/Nutrition/Herb Interactions
Ethanol: Avoid ethanol (may increase CNS depression). *In vitro* studies have shown high concentrations of alcohol may increase the rate of release of Nexiclon™ XR.

Herb/Nutraceutical: Avoid dong quai if using for hypertension (has estrogenic activity). Avoid ephedra, yohimbe, ginseng (may worsen hypertension). Avoid valerian, St John's wort, kava kava, gotu kola (may increase CNS depression).

Stability
Epidural formulation: Store at 25°C (77°F); excursions permitted to 15°C to 30°C (59°F to 86°F). **Preservative free;** discard unused portion. Prior to administration, the 500 mcg/mL concentration must be diluted in 0.9% sodium chloride for injection (preservative-free) to a final concentration of 100 mcg/mL.

Oral suspension, tablets: Store at 25°C (77°F); excursions permitted to 15°C to 30°C (59°F to 86°F). Protect from light.

Transdermal patches: Store below 30°C (86°F).

Mechanism of Action
Stimulates alpha$_2$-adrenoceptors in the brain stem, thus activating an inhibitory neuron, resulting in reduced sympathetic outflow from the CNS, producing a decrease in peripheral resistance, renal vascular resistance, heart rate, and blood pressure; epidural clonidine may produce pain relief at spinal presynaptic and postjunctional alpha$_2$-adrenoceptors by preventing pain signal transmission; pain relief occurs only for the body regions innervated by the spinal segments where analgesic concentrations of clonidine exist. For the treatment of ADHD, the mechanism of action is unknown; it has been proposed that postsynaptic alpha2-agonist stimulation regulates subcortical activity in the prefrontal cortex,

the area of the brain responsible for emotions, attentions, and behaviors and causes reduced hyperactivity, impulsiveness, and distractibility.

Pharmacodynamics/Kinetics

Onset of action: Oral: 0.5-1 hour; Transdermal: Initial application: 2-3 days

Duration: 6-10 hours

Absorption: Oral: Extended release tablets (Kapvay™) are not bioequivalent with immediate release formulations; peak plasma concentrations are 50% lower compared to immediate release formulations

Distribution: V_d: Adults: 2.1 L/kg; highly lipid soluble; distributes readily into extravascular sites

Note: Epidurally administered clonidine readily distributes into plasma via the epidural veins and attains clinically significant systemic concentrations.

Protein binding: 20% to 40%

Metabolism: Extensively hepatic to inactive metabolites; undergoes enterohepatic recirculation

Bioavailability: Oral: Immediate release: 75% to 85%; Extended release (Kapvay™): 89% (relative to immediate release formulation)

Half-life elimination: Adults: Normal renal function: 12-16 hours; Renal impairment: Up to 41 hours

Epidural administration: CSF half-life elimination: 0.8-1.8 hours

Time to peak: Oral: Immediate release: 3-5 hours; Extended release: 7-8 hours

Excretion: Urine (40% to 60%as unchanged drug)

Dosage

Geriatric Hypertension: Oral:

Immediate release: Initial: 0.1 mg once daily at bedtime, increase gradually as needed.

Extended release (Nexiclon™ XR): No specific recommendations are provided by the manufacturer although a lower initial dose is recommended.

Adult Note: Dosing is expressed as the salt (clonidine hydrochloride) unless otherwise noted. Formulations of clonidine (immediate release versus extended release) are not interchangeable on a mg:mg basis due to different pharmacokinetic profiles. This includes commercially available oral suspension (Nexiclon™ XR) which is an extended release preparation and should not be used interchangeably with any extemporaneously prepared clonidine oral suspension.

Hypertension:

Oral:

Immediate release: Initial dose: 0.1 mg twice daily (maximum recommended dose: 2.4 mg/day); usual dose range (JNC 7): 0.1-0.8 mg/day in 2 divided doses

Extended release (Nexiclon™ XR): Initial: 0.17 mg clonidine base once daily at bedtime; may increase increments of 0.09 mg/day every 7 days; maintenance: usual dose range: 0.17-0.52 mg clonidine base once daily; maximum: 0.52 mg/day clonidine base

Conversion between immediate release clonidine hydrochloride and extended release (Nexiclon™ XR) clonidine base:

Current dose immediate release tablets 0.05 mg twice daily: Convert to extended release tablet of 0.09 mg clonidine base once daily

Current dose immediate release tablets 0.1 mg twice daily: Convert to extended release tablet of 0.17 mg clonidine base once daily

Current dose immediate release tablets 0.2 mg twice daily: Convert to extended release tablet of 0.34 mg clonidine base once daily

Current dose immediate release tablets 0.3 mg twice daily: convert to extended release tablets of 0.52 mg clonidine base once daily

Transdermal: Initial: 0.1 mg/24 hour patch applied once every 7 days and increase by 0.1 mg at 1- to 2-week intervals (dosages >0.6 mg/24 hours do not improve efficacy); usual dose range (JNC 7): 0.1-0.3 mg/24 hour patch applied once every 7 days

Acute hypertension (urgency) (unlabeled use): Oral: Initial 0.1-0.2 mg; may be followed by additional doses of 0.1 mg every hour, if necessary, to a maximum total dose of 0.7 mg (Atkin, 1992; Jaker, 1989)

Unlabeled route of administration: Sublingual: Initial: 0.1-0.2 mg; followed by 0.05-0.1 mg every hour until blood pressure controlled or a cumulative dose of 0.7 mg is reached (Cunningham, 1994; Matuschka, 1999)

Nicotine withdrawal symptoms (unlabeled use; Fiore, 2008):

Oral: Initial: 0.1 mg twice daily; titrate by 0.1 mg/day every 7 days if needed; dosage range used in clinical trials: 0.15-0.75 mg/day; duration of therapy ranged from 3-10 weeks in clinical trials

Transdermal: Initial: 0.1 mg/24 hour patch applied once every 7 days and increase by 0.1 mg at 1-week intervals if necessary; dosage range used in clinical trials: 0.1-0.2 mg/24 hour patch applied once every 7 days; duration of therapy ranged from 3-10 weeks in clinical trials

CLONIDINE

Note: If transitioning from oral to transdermal therapy, overlap oral regimen for 1-2 days; transdermal route takes 2-3 days to achieve therapeutic effects.

Conversion from oral to transdermal:

Day 1: Place Catapres-TTS® 1; administer 100% of oral dose.

Day 2: Administer 50% of oral dose.

Day 3: Administer 25% of oral dose.

Day 4: Patch remains, no further oral supplement necessary.

Pain management: Epidural infusion: Reserved for cancer patients with severe intractable pain, unresponsive to other opioid analgesics: Starting dose: 30 mcg/hour; titrate as required for relief of pain or presence of side effects; experience with doses >40 mcg/hour is limited; should be considered an adjunct to opioid therapy

Renal Impairment Bradycardia, sedation, and hypotension may be more likely to occur in patients with renal failure; may consider using doses at the lower end of the dosing range and monitor closely.

Not dialyzable (0% to 5%) via hemodialysis; supplemental dose is not necessary; unclear how much is removed via peritoneal dialysis. Oral antihypertensive drugs given preferentially at night may reduce the nocturnal surge of blood pressure and minimize the intradialytic hypotension that may occur when taken the morning before a dialysis session (K/DOQI, 2005).

Oral: Extended release (Nexiclon™ XR):

Moderate-to-severe impairment (not on dialysis): No dosage adjustment recommended; titrate slowly

End-stage kidney disease (on maintenance dialysis): Initial: 0.09 mg clonidine base/day; titrate slowly

Administration

Epidural: Specialized techniques are required for continuous epidural administration; administration via this route should only be performed by qualified individuals familiar with the techniques of epidural administration and patient management problems associated with this route. Familiarization of the epidural infusion device is essential. Do not discontinue clonidine abruptly; if needed, gradually reduce dose over 2-4 days to avoid withdrawal symptoms.

Oral: May be taken with or without food. Do not discontinue clonidine abruptly. If needed, gradually reduce dose over 2-4 days to avoid rebound hypertension.

Extended release products:

Kapvay™: Swallow whole; do not crush, split, or chew.

Nexiclon™ XR: Tablets may be split. Shake suspension well before use.

Transdermal patch: Patches should be applied weekly at a consistent time to a clean, hairless area of the upper outer arm or chest. Rotate patch sites weekly. Redness under patch may be reduced if a topical corticosteroid spray is applied to the area before placement of the patch.

Monitoring Parameters Blood pressure, standing and sitting/supine, mental status, heart rate

When used for the treatment of ADHD, thoroughly evaluate for cardiovascular risk. Monitor heart rate, blood pressure (when started and weaned), and consider obtaining ECG prior to initiation (Vetter, 2008).

Clonidine tolerance test: In addition to growth hormone concentrations, monitor blood pressure and blood glucose (Huang, 2001).

Epidural: Carefully monitor infusion pump; inspect catheter tubing for obstruction or dislodgement to reduce risk of inadvertent abrupt withdrawal of infusion. Monitor closely for catheter-related infection (eg, meningitis or epidural abscess).

Test Interactions Positive Coombs' test

Pharmacotherapy Pearls Each 0.1 mg of clonidine hydrochloride (salt form) is equivalent to 0.087 mg of the free base.

Transdermal clonidine should only be used in patients unable to take oral medication. The transdermal product is much more expensive than oral clonidine and produces no better therapeutic effects.

When used for ADHD treatment, clonidine is recommended to be used as part of a comprehensive treatment program (eg, psychological, educational, and social) for attention-deficit disorder.

Special Geriatric Considerations Because of its potential CNS adverse effects, clonidine may not be considered a drug of choice in the elderly. If the decision is to use clonidine, adjust dose based on response and adverse reactions. In patients on the transdermal system, monitor for appropriate placement of the patch.

This medication is considered to be potentially inappropriate in this patient population (Beers Criteria severity: Low).

Dosage Forms Excipient information presented when available (limited, particularly for generics); consult specific product labeling.

Injection, solution, as hydrochloride [epidural, preservative free]: 100 mcg/mL (10 mL); 500 mcg/mL (10 mL)

   Duraclon®: 100 mcg/mL (10 mL); 500 mcg/mL (10 mL)

Patch, transdermal: 0.1 mg/24 hours (4s); 0.2 mg/24 hours (4s); 0.3 mg/24 hours (4s)

   Catapres-TTS®-1: 0.1 mg/24 hours (4s) [contains metal]

   Catapres-TTS®-2: 0.2 mg/24 hours (4s) [contains metal]

   Catapres-TTS®-3: 0.3 mg/24 hours (4s) [contains metal]

Suspension, extended release, oral, as base:

   Nexiclon™ XR: 0.09 mg/mL (118 mL)

Tablet, oral, as hydrochloride: 0.1 mg, 0.2 mg, 0.3 mg

   Catapres®: 0.1 mg, 0.2 mg, 0.3 mg [scored]

Tablet, extended release, oral, as base:

   Nexiclon™ XR: 0.17 mg [scored]

Tablet, extended release, oral, as hydrochloride:

   Kapvay™: 0.1 mg

Selected References

Chobanian AV, Bakris GL, Black HR, et al, "Seventh Report of the Joint National Committee on Prevention, Detection, Evaluation, and Treatment of High Blood Pressure," *Hypertension*, 2003, 42(6):1206-52.

"K/DOQI Clinical Practice Guidelines for Cardiovascular Disease in Dialysis Patients," *Am J Kidney Dis*, 2005, 45(4 Suppl 3):46-57.

◆ **Clonidine Hydrochloride** *see* CloNIDine *on page 388*

Clopidogrel (kloh PID oh grel)

Related Information

Beers Criteria – Potentially Inappropriate Medications for Geriatrics *on page 2089*

Medication Safety Issues

  Sound-alike/look-alike issues:

    Plavix® may be confused with Elavil®, Paxil®

Brand Names: U.S. Plavix®

Brand Names: Canada Plavix®

Index Terms Clopidogrel Bisulfate

Generic Availability (U.S.) No

Pharmacologic Category Antiplatelet Agent; Antiplatelet Agent, Thienopyridine

Use Reduces rate of atherothrombotic events (myocardial infarction, stroke, vascular deaths) in patients with recent MI or stroke, or established peripheral arterial disease; reduces rate of atherothrombotic events in patients with unstable angina (UA) or non-ST-segment elevation (NSTEMI) managed medically or with percutaneous coronary intervention (PCI) (with or without stent) or CABG; reduces rate of death and atherothrombotic events in patients with ST-segment elevation MI (STEMI) managed medically

Canadian labeling: Additional use (not in U.S. labeling): Prevention of atherothrombotic and thromboembolic events, including stroke, in patients with atrial fibrillation with at least 1 risk factor for vascular events who are not suitable for treatment with an anticoagulant and are at a low risk for bleeding.

Unlabeled/Investigational Use In patients with allergy or major gastrointestinal intolerance to aspirin, initial treatment of acute coronary syndromes (ACS) or prevention of coronary artery bypass graft closure (saphenous vein)

Medication Guide Available Yes

Contraindications Hypersensitivity to clopidogrel or any component of the formulation; active pathological bleeding such as peptic ulcer or intracranial hemorrhage

Canadian labeling: Additional contraindications (not in U.S. labeling): Significant liver impairment or cholestatic jaundice

Warnings/Precautions [U.S. Boxed Warning]: Patients with one or more copies of the variant *CYP2C19*2* and/or *CYP2C19*3* alleles (and potentially other reduced-function variants) may have reduced conversion of clopidogrel to its active thiol metabolite. Lower active metabolite exposure may result in reduced platelet inhibition and, thus, a higher rate of cardiovascular events following MI or stent thrombosis following PCI. Although evidence is insufficient to recommend routine genetic testing, tests are available to determine CYP2C19 genotype and may be used to determine therapeutic strategy; alternative treatment or treatment strategies may be considered if patient is identified as a CYP2C19 poor metabolizer. Genetic testing may be considered prior to initiating clopidogrel in patients at moderate or high risk for poor outcomes (eg, PCI in patients with extensive and/or very complex disease). The optimal dose for CYP2C19 poor metabolizers has yet to be

◀ determined. After initiation of clopidogrel, functional testing (eg, VerifyNow® P2Y12 assay) may also be done to determine clopidogrel responsiveness (Holmes, 2010).

Use with caution in patients who may be at risk of increased bleeding, including patients with PUD, trauma, or surgery. In patients with coronary stents, premature interruption of therapy may result in stent thrombosis with subsequent fatal and nonfatal MI. Duration of therapy, in general, is determined by the type of stent placed (bare metal or drug eluting) and whether an ACS event was ongoing at the time of placement. Consider discontinuing 5 days before elective surgery (except in patients with cardiac stents that have not completed their full course of dual antiplatelet therapy; patient-specific situations need to be discussed with cardiologist; AHA/ACC/SCAI/ACS/ADA Science Advisory provides recommendations). Use caution in concurrent treatment with anticoagulants (eg, heparin, warfarin) or other antiplatelet drugs; bleeding risk is increased. Concurrent use with drugs known to inhibit CYP2C19 (eg, proton pump inhibitors) may reduce levels of active metabolite and subsequently reduce clinical efficacy and increase the risk of cardiovascular events; if possible, avoid concurrent use of moderate-to-strong CYP2C19 inhibitors. In patients requiring antacid therapy, consider use of an acid-reducing agent lacking (eg, ranitidine) or with less CYP2C19 inhibition. If a PPI is necessary, the use of pantoprazole, a weak CYP2C19 inhibitor, has been shown to have less of an effect on the pharmacologic activity of clopidogrel. Of the PPIs, lansoprazole exhibits the most potent CYP2C19 inhibitory effects (Li, 2004).Use with caution in patients with severe liver or renal disease (experience is limited). Cases of TTP (usually occurring within the first 2 weeks of therapy), resulting in some fatalities, have been reported; urgent plasmapheresis is required. Use in patients with severe hepatic impairment or cholestatic jaundice is contraindicated in the Canadian labeling. Cases of TTP (usually occurring within the first 2 weeks of therapy), resulting in some fatalities, have been reported; urgent plasmapheresis is required. Concurrent use of aspirin and clopidogrel is not recommended for secondary prevention of ischemic stroke or TIA in patients unable to take oral anti-coagulants due to hemorrhagic risk (Furie, 2011).

Assess bleeding risk carefully prior to initiating therapy in patients with atrial fibrillation (Canadian labeling; not an approved use in U.S. labeling); in clinical trials, a significant increase in major bleeding events (including intracranial hemorrhage and fatal bleeding events) were observed in patients receiving clopidogrel plus aspirin versus aspirin alone. Vitamin K antagonist (VKA) therapy (in suitable patients) has demonstrated a greater benefit in stroke reduction than aspirin (with or without clopidogrel).

Adverse Reactions (Reflective of adult population; not specific for elderly) As with all drugs which may affect hemostasis, bleeding is associated with clopidogrel. Hemorrhage may occur at virtually any site. Risk is dependent on multiple variables, including the concurrent use of multiple agents which alter hemostasis and patient susceptibility.

3% to 10%:
    Dermatologic: Rash (4%), pruritus (3%)
    Hematologic: Bleeding (major 4%; minor 5%), purpura/bruising (5%), epistaxis (3%)
1% to 3%:
    Gastrointestinal: GI hemorrhage (2%)
    Hematologic: Hematoma

Drug Interactions

Metabolism/Transport Effects Substrate of CYP2C19, 3A4, 1A2 (minor); **Inhibits** CYP2B6 (moderate), 2C9 (weak)

Avoid Concomitant Use

Avoid concomitant use of Clopidogrel with any of the following: CYP2C19 Inhibitors (Moderate); CYP2C19 Inhibitors (Strong); Omeprazole

Increased Effect/Toxicity

Clopidogrel may increase the levels/effects of: Anticoagulants; Antiplatelet Agents; Collagenase (Systemic); CYP2B6 Substrates; Drotrecogin Alfa; Ibritumomab; Rivaroxaban; Salicylates; Thrombolytic Agents; Tositumomab and Iodine I 131 Tositumomab; Warfarin

The levels/effects of Clopidogrel may be increased by: Dasatinib; Glucosamine; Herbs (Anticoagulant/Antiplatelet Properties); Nonsteroidal Anti-Inflammatory Agents; Omega-3-Acid Ethyl Esters; Pentosan Polysulfate Sodium; Pentoxifylline; Prostacyclin Analogues; Rifamycin Derivatives; Vitamin E

Decreased Effect

The levels/effects of Clopidogrel may be decreased by: Amiodarone; Calcium Channel Blockers; CYP2C19 Inhibitors (Moderate); CYP2C19 Inhibitors (Strong); Dexlansoprazole; Esomeprazole; Lansoprazole; Macrolide Antibiotics; Nonsteroidal Anti-Inflammatory Agents; Omeprazole; Pantoprazole; RABEprazole

Ethanol/Nutrition/Herb Interactions Herb/Nutraceutical: Avoid alfalfa, anise, bilberry, bladderwrack, bromelain, cat's claw, chamomile, coleus, cordyceps, dong quai, evening primrose oil, fenugreek, feverfew, garlic, ginger, ginkgo biloba, ginseng (American), ginseng (Panax), ginseng (Siberian), grape seed, green tea, guggul, horse chestnut seed, horse-radish, licorice, prickly ash, red clover, reishi, SAMe (S-adenosylmethionine), sweet clover, turmeric, white willow (all have additional antiplatelet activity).

Stability Store at 25°C (77°F); excursions permitted to 15°C to 30°C (59°F to 86°F).

Mechanism of Action Clopidogrel requires *in vivo* biotransformation to an active thiol metabolite. The active metabolite irreversibly blocks the $P2Y_{12}$ component of ADP receptors on the platelet surface, which prevents activation of the GPIIb/IIIa receptor complex, thereby reducing platelet aggregation. Platelets blocked by clopidogrel are affected for the remainder of their lifespan (~7-10 days).

Pharmacodynamics/Kinetics

Onset of action: Inhibition of platelet aggregation (IPA): Dose-dependent:

300-600 mg loading dose: Detected within 2 hours

50-100 mg/day: Detected by the second day of treatment

Peak effect: Time to maximal IPA: Dose-dependent: **Note:** Degree of IPA based on adenosine diphosphate (ADP) concentration used during light aggregometry:

300-600 mg loading dose:

ADP 5 μmol/L: 20% to 30% IPA at 6 hours post administration (Montelescot, 2006)

ADP 20 μmol/L: 30% to 37% IPA at 6 hours post administration (Montelescot, 2006)

50-100 mg/day: ADP 5 μmol/L: 50% to 60% IPA at 5-7 days (Herbert, 1993)

Absorption: Well absorbed

Protein binding: Parent drug: 98%; Inactive metabolite: 94%

Metabolism: Extensively hepatic via esterase-mediated hydrolysis to a carboxylic acid derivative (inactive) and via CYP450-mediated (CYP2C19 primarily) oxidation to a thiol metabolite (active)

Half-life elimination: Parent drug: ~6 hours; Active metabolite: ~30 minutes

Time to peak, serum: ~0.75 hours

Excretion: Urine (50%); feces (46%)

Dosage

Geriatric & Adult

Recent MI, recent stroke, or established arterial disease: Oral: 75 mg once daily

Acute coronary syndrome:

Unstable angina, non-ST-segment elevation myocardial infarction (UA/NSTEMI): Initial: 300 mg loading dose, followed by 75 mg once daily for at least 1 month and ideally up to 12 months (in combination with aspirin 75-162 mg once daily indefinitely) (Wright, 2011).

ST-segment elevation myocardial infarction (STEMI): 75 mg once daily (in combination with aspirin 162-325 mg initially followed by 81-162 mg/day). **Note:** CLARITY-TIMI 28 used a 300 mg loading dose (with thrombolysis) demonstrating an improvement in the patency rate of the infarct related artery and reduction in ischemic complications. The duration of therapy was <28 days (usually until hospital discharge) unless nonprimary percutaneous coronary intervention (PCI) was performed (Sabatine, 2005).

The American College of Chest Physicians (Goodman, 2008) recommends:

Patients ≤75 years: Initial: 300 mg loading dose, followed by 75 mg once daily for up to 28 days (in combination with aspirin)

Patients >75 years: 75 mg once daily for up to 28 days (with or without thrombolysis)

Percutaneous coronary intervention (PCI) for UA/NSTEMI or STEMI: Loading dose: 300-600 mg (600 mg may be preferred for early invasive strategy with UA/NSTEMI) given as early as possible before or at the time of PCI, followed by 75 mg once daily. **Note:** If an initial loading dose of 300 mg was given prior to PCI, a supplemental loading dose of 300 mg (total loading dose of 600 mg) may be administered (Kushner, 2009). For patients with UA/NSTEMI, it has been recommended that the loading dose be given at least 2 hours (or 24 hours in patients unable to take aspirin) prior to PCI (*Chest* guidelines, 2008).

Higher versus standard maintenance dosing: May consider a maintenance dose of 150 mg once daily for 6 days, then 75 mg once daily thereafter in patients not at high risk for bleeding (CURRENT-OASIS 7 Investigators, 2010; Wright, 2011); however, in another study, in patients with high on-treatment platelet reactivity, the use of 150 mg once daily for 6 months did not demonstrate a difference in 6-month incidence of death from cardiovascular causes, nonfatal MI, or stent thrombosis compared to standard dose therapy (Price, 2011).

Duration of clopidogrel (in combination with aspirin) after stent placement: **Premature interruption of therapy may result in stent thrombosis with subsequent fatal and nonfatal MI.** With STEMI, clopidogrel for at least 12 months regardless of stent type (ie, either bare metal or drug eluting stent) is recommended (Kushner, 2009). With UA/NSTEMI, at least 12 months of clopidogrel is recommended in patients receiving a drug eluting stent (DES) unless the risk of bleeding outweighs the benefits. For bare metal stent (BMS) placement, at least 1 month and ideally up to 12 months duration is recommended unless the risk of bleeding outweighs the benefits then a minimum of 2 weeks is recommended (Wright, 2011). In either setting, a duration >15 months may be considered in patients with DES placement (Kushner, 2009; Wright 2011). For patients without ongoing ACS, clopidogrel should be continued for at least 1 month (for BMS) or at least 12 months (for DES) (Becker, 2008).

CYP2C19 poor metabolizers (ie, *CYP2C19*2* or **3* carriers): An appropriate regimen for this patient population has not been established in clinical outcome trials. Although the manufacturer suggests a 600 mg loading dose, followed by 150 mg once daily, it does not appear that this dosing strategy improves outcomes for this patient population (Price, 2011).

Atrial fibrillation (in patients not candidates for warfarin and at a low risk of bleeding) (Canadian labeling; not in U.S. labeling): Oral: 75 mg once daily (in combination with aspirin 75-100 mg once daily)

Prevention of coronary artery bypass graft closure (saphenous vein) [*Chest* guidelines, 2008]: Aspirin-allergic patients (unlabeled use): Oral: Loading dose: 300 mg administered 6 hours following procedure; maintenance: 75 mg once daily

Renal Impairment No adjustment is necessary.

Hepatic Impairment Use with caution; experience is limited. **Note:** Inhibition of ADP-induced platelet aggregation and mean bleeding time prolongation were similar in patients with severe hepatic impairment compared to healthy subjects after repeated doses of 75 mg once daily for 10 days.

Administration May be administered without regard to meals.

Monitoring Parameters Signs of bleeding; hemoglobin and hematocrit periodically. Consider platelet function testing to determine platelet inhibitory response if results of testing may alter management (Wright, 2011).

Special Geriatric Considerations Plasma concentrations of the main metabolite of clopidogrel were significantly higher in the elderly (≥75 years). This was not associated with changes in bleeding time or platelet aggregation. No dosage adjustment is recommended.

Dosage Forms Excipient information presented when available (limited, particularly for generics); consult specific product labeling.
Tablet, oral:
Plavix®: 75 mg, 300 mg

Selected References

Bal dit Sollier C, Mahe I, Berge N, et al, "Reduced Thrombus Cohesion in an *ex vivo* Human Model of Arterial Thrombosis Induced by Clopidogrel Treatment: Kinetics of the Effect and Influence of Single and Double Loading-Dose Regimens," *Thromb Res*, 2003, 111(1-2):19-27.

Goodman SG, Menon V, Cannon CP, et al, "Acute ST-Segment Elevation Myocardial Infarction: American College of Chest Physicians Evidence-Based Clinical Practice Guidelines (8th Edition)," *Chest*, 2008, 133(6 Suppl):707-75.

Kushner FG, Hand M, Smith SC, et al, "2009 Focused Updates: ACC/AHA Guidelines for the Management of Patients With ST-Elevation Myocardial Infarction (Updating the 2004 Guideline and 2007 Focused Update) and ACC/AHA/SCAI Guidelines on Percutaneous Coronary Intervention (Updating the 2005 Guideline and 2007 Focused Update): A Report of the American College of Cardiology Foundation/American Heart Association Task Force on Practice Guidelines," *J Am Coll Cardiol*, 2009, 54(23):2205-41.

Smith SC, Feldman TE, Hirshfeld JW, et al, "ACC/AHA/SCAI 2005 Guideline Update for Percutaneous Coronary Intervention. A Report of the American College of Cardiology/American Heart Association Task Force on Practice Guidelines (ACC/AHA/SCAI Writing Committee to Update the 2001 Guidelines for Percutaneous Coronary Intervention)," *J Am Coll Cardiol*, 2006, 47(1):216-235.

◆ **Clopidogrel Bisulfate** *see* Clopidogrel *on page 393*

Clorazepate (klor AZ e pate)

Related Information
Anxiolytic, Sedative / Hypnotic, and Miscellaneous Benzodiazepines *on page 2000*

Medication Safety Issues
Sound-alike/look-alike issues:
Clorazepate may be confused with clofibrate, clonazepam, KlonoPIN®
BEERS Criteria medication:
This drug may be inappropriate for use in geriatric patients (high severity risk).

Brand Names: U.S. Tranxene® T-Tab®
Brand Names: Canada Apo-Clorazepate®; Novo-Clopate
Index Terms Clorazepate Dipotassium; Tranxene T-Tab
Generic Availability (U.S.) Yes
Pharmacologic Category Benzodiazepine
Use Treatment of generalized anxiety disorder; management of ethanol withdrawal; adjunct anticonvulsant in management of partial seizures
Medication Guide Available Yes

Contraindications Hypersensitivity to clorazepate or any component of the formulation (cross-sensitivity with other benzodiazepines may exist); narrow-angle glaucoma

Warnings/Precautions Antiepileptics are associated with an increased risk of suicidal behavior/thoughts with use (regardless of indication); patients should be monitored for signs/symptoms of depression, suicidal tendencies, and other unusual behavior changes during therapy and instructed to inform their healthcare provider immediately if symptoms occur.

Not recommended for use in patients <9 years of age or patients with depressive or psychotic disorders. Use with caution in elderly or debilitated patients, patients with hepatic disease (including alcoholics), or renal impairment. Active metabolites with extended half-lives may lead to delayed accumulation and adverse effects. Use with caution in patients with respiratory disease or impaired gag reflex. Avoid use in patients with sleep apnea.

Causes CNS depression (dose related) resulting in sedation, dizziness, confusion, or ataxia which may impair physical and mental capabilities. Patients must be cautioned about performing tasks which require mental alertness (eg, operating machinery or driving). Use with caution in patients receiving other CNS depressants or psychoactive agents. Effects with other sedative drugs or ethanol may be potentiated. Benzodiazepines have been associated with falls and traumatic injury and should be used with extreme caution in patients who are at risk of these events. Benzodiazepines with long half-lives may produce prolonged sedation and increase the risk of falls and fracture; short- or intermediate-acting benzodiazepines are preferred in elderly patients (Beers Criteria).

Use caution in patients with depression, particularly if suicidal risk may be present. Use with caution in patients with a history of drug dependence. Benzodiazepines have been associated with dependence and acute withdrawal symptoms on discontinuation or reduction in dose. Acute withdrawal, including seizures, may be precipitated in patients after administration of flumazenil to patients receiving long-term benzodiazepine therapy.

Benzodiazepines have been associated with anterograde amnesia. Paradoxical reactions, including hyperactive or aggressive behavior, have been reported with benzodiazepines, particularly in psychiatric patients. Does not have analgesic, antidepressant, or antipsychotic properties.

Adverse Reactions (Reflective of adult population; not specific for elderly) Frequency not defined.

Cardiovascular: Hypotension

Central nervous system: Drowsiness, fatigue, ataxia, lightheadedness, memory impairment, insomnia, anxiety, headache, depression, slurred speech, confusion, nervousness, dizziness, irritability

Dermatologic: Rash

Endocrine & metabolic: Libido decreased

Gastrointestinal: Xerostomia, constipation, diarrhea, nausea, salivation decreased, vomiting, appetite increased or decreased

Hepatic: Jaundice, transaminase increased

Neuromuscular & skeletal: Dysarthria, tremor

Ocular: Blurred vision, diplopia

Drug Interactions

Metabolism/Transport Effects Substrate of CYP3A4 (major)

Avoid Concomitant Use

Avoid concomitant use of Clorazepate with any of the following: Conivaptan; OLANZapine

Increased Effect/Toxicity

Clorazepate may increase the levels/effects of: Alcohol (Ethyl); CloZAPine; CNS Depressants; Fosphenytoin; Methotrimeprazine; Phenytoin; Selective Serotonin Reuptake Inhibitors

The levels/effects of Clorazepate may be increased by: Antifungal Agents (Azole Derivatives, Systemic); Aprepitant; Calcium Channel Blockers (Nondihydropyridine); Cimetidine; Conivaptan; Contraceptives (Estrogens); Contraceptives (Progestins); CYP3A4 Inhibitors (Moderate); CYP3A4 Inhibitors (Strong); Dasatinib; Droperidol; Fluconazole; Fosamprenavir; Fosaprepitant; Grapefruit Juice; HydrOXYzine; Isoniazid; Macrolide Antibiotics; MAO Inhibitors; Methotrimeprazine; Nefazodone; OLANZapine; Proton Pump Inhibitors; Ritonavir; Saquinavir; Selective Serotonin Reuptake Inhibitors

Decreased Effect

The levels/effects of Clorazepate may be decreased by: CarBAMazepine; CYP3A4 Inducers (Strong); Deferasirox; Rifamycin Derivatives; St Johns Wort; Theophylline Derivatives; Tocilizumab; Yohimbine

◀ **Ethanol/Nutrition/Herb Interactions**

Ethanol: May increase CNS depression; monitor for increased effects with coadministration. Caution patients about effects.

Food: Serum concentrations/toxicity may be increased by grapefruit juice.

Herb/Nutraceutical: Avoid valerian, St John's wort, kava kava, gotu kola (may increase CNS depression).

Stability Store at controlled room temperature at 20° to 25°C (68° to 77°F). Protect from moisture; keep bottle tightly closed; dispense in tightly closed, light-resistant container.

Mechanism of Action Binds to stereospecific benzodiazepine receptors on the postsynaptic GABA neuron at several sites within the central nervous system, including the limbic system, reticular formation. Enhancement of the inhibitory effect of GABA on neuronal excitability results by increased neuronal membrane permeability to chloride ions. This shift in chloride ions results in hyperpolarization (a less excitable state) and stabilization.

Pharmacodynamics/Kinetics

Onset of action: 1-2 hours

Duration: Variable, 8-24 hours

Distribution: Appears in urine

Protein binding: Nordiazepam 97% to 98%

Metabolism: Rapidly decarboxylated to nordiazepam (active) in acidic stomach prior to absorption; hepatically to oxazepam (active)

Half-life elimination: Adults: Nordiazepam: 40-50 hours; Oxazepam: 6-8 hours

Time to peak, serum: ~1 hour

Excretion: Primarily urine

Dosage

Geriatric Oral: Anxiety: 7.5 mg 1-2 times/day; use is not recommended in the elderly.

Adult

Anxiety: Oral: 7.5-15 mg 2-4 times/day

Ethanol withdrawal: Oral: Initial: 30 mg, then 15 mg 2-4 times/day on first day; maximum daily dose: 90 mg; gradually decrease dose over subsequent days.

Seizures (anticonvulsant): Oral: Initial: Up to 7.5 mg/dose 2-3 times/day; increase dose by 7.5 mg at weekly intervals; not to exceed 90 mg/day

Monitoring Parameters Respiratory and cardiovascular status, excess CNS depression; suicidality (eg, suicidal thoughts, depression, behavioral changes)

Reference Range Therapeutic: 0.12-1 mcg/mL (SI: 0.36-3.01 µmol/L)

Test Interactions Decreased hematocrit; abnormal liver and renal function tests

Pharmacotherapy Pearls Abrupt discontinuation after sustained use (generally >10 days) may cause withdrawal symptoms.

Special Geriatric Considerations Due to its long-acting metabolite, clorazepate is not considered a drug of choice in the elderly. Long-acting benzodiazepines have been associated with falls in the elderly. Interpretive guidelines from the Centers for Medicare and Medicaid Services (CMS) discourage the use of this agent in residents of long-term care facilities.

This medication is considered to be potentially inappropriate in this patient population (Beers Criteria severity: High).

Controlled Substance C-IV

Dosage Forms Excipient information presented when available (limited, particularly for generics); consult specific product labeling.

Tablet, oral, as dipotassium: 3.75 mg, 7.5 mg, 15 mg

Tranxene® T-Tab®: 3.75 mg, 7.5 mg, 15 mg [scored]

◆ **Clorazepate Dipotassium** *see* Clorazepate *on page 396*

Clotrimazole (Oral) (kloe TRIM a zole)

Medication Safety Issues

Sound-alike/look-alike issues:

Clotrimazole may be confused with co-trimoxazole

Mycelex may be confused with Myoflex®

International issues:

Cloderm: Brand name for clotrimazole [Germany], but also brand name for alclomethasone [Indonesia]; clobetasol [China, India, Malaysia, Singapore, Thailand]; clocortolone [U.S., Canada]

Canesten: Brand name for clotrimazole [multiple international markets] may be confused with Canesten Bifonazol Comp brand name for bifonazole/urea [Austria]; Canesten Extra brand name for bifonazole [China, Germany]; Canesten Extra Nagelset brand name for bifonazole/urea [Denmark]; Canesten Fluconazole brand name for fluconazole [New

Zealand]; Canesten Oasis brand name for sodium citrate [Great Britain]; Canesten Once Daily brand name for bifonazole [Australia]; Canesten Oral brand name for fluconazole [United Kingdom]; Cenestin® brand name for estrogens (conjugated A/synthetic) [U.S., Canada]

Mycelex: Brand name for clotrimazole [U.S.] may be confused with Mucolex brand name for carbocysteine [Ireland, Portugal, Thailand]; guaifenesin [China]

Index Terms Mycelex

Generic Availability (U.S.) Yes

Pharmacologic Category Antifungal Agent, Oral Nonabsorbed

Use Treatment of susceptible fungal infections, including oropharyngeal candidiasis; limited data suggest that clotrimazole troches may be effective for prophylaxis against oropharyngeal candidiasis in neutropenic patients

Contraindications Hypersensitivity to clotrimazole or any component of the formulation

Warnings/Precautions Clotrimazole should not be used for treatment of systemic fungal infection.

Adverse Reactions (Reflective of adult population; not specific for elderly)
>10%: Hepatic: Abnormal liver function tests
Frequency not defined:
Dermatologic: Pruritus
Gastrointestinal: Nausea, vomiting

Drug Interactions
Metabolism/Transport Effects Inhibits CYP1A2 (weak), 2A6 (weak), 2B6 (weak), 2C8 (weak), 2C9 (weak), 2C19 (weak), 2D6 (weak), 2E1 (weak), 3A4 (moderate)
Avoid Concomitant Use
Avoid concomitant use of Clotrimazole (Oral) with any of the following: Tolvaptan
Increased Effect/Toxicity
Clotrimazole (Oral) may increase the levels/effects of: Budesonide (Systemic, Oral Inhalation); Colchicine; CYP3A4 Substrates; Eplerenone; Everolimus; FentaNYL; Halofantrine; Lurasidone; Pimecrolimus; Ranolazine; Salmeterol; Saxagliptin; Tacrolimus; Tacrolimus (Systemic); Tolvaptan; Vilazodone
Decreased Effect
Clotrimazole (Oral) may decrease the levels/effects of: Saccharomyces boulardii

Mechanism of Action Binds to phospholipids in the fungal cell membrane altering cell wall permeability resulting in loss of essential intracellular elements

Pharmacodynamics/Kinetics
Distribution: Oral (troche): Inhibitory concentrations remain in the saliva for up to 3 hours after dissolution of the troche
Excretion: Feces (as metabolites)

Dosage
Geriatric & Adult Oropharyngeal candidiasis: Oral:
Prophylaxis: 10 mg troche dissolved 3 times/day for the duration of chemotherapy or until steroids are reduced to maintenance levels
Treatment: 10 mg troche dissolved slowly 5 times/day for 14 consecutive days

Administration Oral: Allow troche to dissolve slowly over 15-30 minutes.

Monitoring Parameters Periodic liver function tests during oral therapy with clotrimazole troche

Special Geriatric Considerations Localized fungal infections frequently follow broad-spectrum antimicrobial therapy. Specifically, oral and vaginal infections due to *Candida*.

Dosage Forms Excipient information presented when available (limited, particularly for generics); consult specific product labeling.
Troche, oral: 10 mg

Clotrimazole (Topical) (kloe TRIM a zole)

Medication Safety Issues
Sound-alike/look-alike issues:
Clotrimazole may be confused with co-trimoxazole
Lotrimin® may be confused with Lotrisone®, Otrivin®
International issues:
Cloderm: Brand name for clotrimazole [Germany], but also brand name for alclomethasone [Indonesia]; clobetasol [China, India, Malaysia, Singapore, Thailand]; clocortolone [U.S., Canada]
Canesten: Brand name for clotrimazole [multiple international markets] may be confused with Canesten Bifonazol Comp brand name for bifonazole/urea [Austria]; Canesten Extra brand name for bifonazole [China, Germany]; Canesten Extra Nagelset brand name for bifonazole/urea [Denmark]; Canesten Fluconazole brand name for fluconazole [New

Zealand]; Canesten Oasis brand name for sodium citrate [Great Britain]; Canesten Once Daily brand name for bifonazole [Australia]; Canesten Oral brand name for fluconazole [United Kingdom]; Cenestin® brand name for estrogens (conjugated A/synthetic) [U.S., Canada]

Brand Names: U.S. Anti-Fungal™ [OTC]; Cruex® [OTC]; Gyne-Lotrimin® 3 [OTC]; Gyne-Lotrimin® 7 [OTC]; Lotrimin® AF Athlete's Foot [OTC]; Lotrimin® AF for Her [OTC]; Lotrimin® AF Jock Itch [OTC]

Brand Names: Canada Canesten® Topical; Canesten® Vaginal; Clotrimaderm; Trivagizole-3®

Generic Availability (U.S.) Yes

Pharmacologic Category Antifungal Agent, Topical; Antifungal Agent, Vaginal

Use Treatment of susceptible fungal infections, including dermatophytoses, superficial mycoses, and cutaneous candidiasis, as well as vulvovaginal candidiasis

Dosage

Geriatric & Adult

Dermatophytosis, cutaneous candidiasis: Topical (cream, solution): Apply twice daily; if no improvement occurs after 4 weeks of therapy, re-evaluate diagnosis.

Vulvovaginal candidiasis: Intravaginal:

Cream (1%): Insert 1 applicatorful of 1% vaginal cream daily (preferably at bedtime) for 7 consecutive days.

Cream (2%): Insert 1 applicatorful of 2% vaginal cream daily (preferably at bedtime) for 3 consecutive days.

Dermatologic infection (superficial): Topical (cream, solution): Apply to affected area twice daily (morning and evening) for 7 consecutive days.

Special Geriatric Considerations Localized fungal infections frequently follow broad-spectrum antimicrobial therapy. Specifically, oral and vaginal infections due to *Candida*.

Dosage Forms Excipient information presented when available (limited, particularly for generics); consult specific product labeling.

Cream, topical: 1% (15 g, 30 g, 45 g)

Anti-Fungal™: 1% (113 g)

Cruex®: 1% (15 g) [contains benzyl alcohol]

Lotrimin® AF Athlete's Foot: 1% (12 g) [contains benzyl alcohol]

Lotrimin® AF for Her: 1% (24 g) [contains benzyl alcohol]

Lotrimin® AF Jock Itch: 1% (12 g) [contains benzyl alcohol]

Cream, vaginal: 1% (45 g); 2% (21 g)

Gyne-Lotrimin® 7: 1% (45 g) [contains benzyl alcohol]

Gyne-Lotrimin® 3: 2% (21 g) [contains benzyl alcohol]

Solution, topical: 1% (10 mL, 30 mL)

Cloxacillin (kloks a SIL in)

Brand Names: Canada Apo-Cloxi®; Novo-Cloxin; Nu-Cloxi

Index Terms Cloxacillin Sodium

Pharmacologic Category Antibiotic, Penicillin

Use Treatment of bacterial infections including endocarditis, pneumonia, bone and joint infections, skin and soft-tissue infections, and sepsis that are caused by susceptible strains of penicillinase-producing staphylococci. **Note:** Exhibits good activity against *Staphylococcus aureus*; has activity against many streptococci, but is less active than penicillin and is generally not used in clinical practice to treat streptococcal infections.

Contraindications Hypersensitivity to cloxacillin, other penicillins, cephalosporins, or any component of the formulation

Warnings/Precautions Serious and occasionally severe or fatal hypersensitivity (anaphylactoid) reactions have been reported in patients on penicillin therapy, especially with a history of beta-lactam hypersensitivity, history of sensitivity to multiple allergens, or previous IgE-mediated reactions (eg, anaphylaxis, angioedema, urticaria). Use with caution in renal impairment as the rate of elimination is decreased. Use with caution in asthmatic patients. Prolonged use may result in fungal or bacterial superinfection, including *C. difficile*-associated diarrhea (CDAD) and pseudomembranous colitis; CDAD has been observed >2 months postantibiotic treatment. Use with caution in patients with a history of seizure disorders, particularly in the presence of renal impairment as increased serum levels may increase risk for seizures. Penicillin transport across the blood-brain barrier may be enhanced by inflamed meninges or during cardiopulmonary bypass increasing the risk of myoclonia, seizures, or reduced consciousness especially in patients with renal failure. Penicillin use has been associated with hematologic disorders (eg, agranulocytosis, neutropenia, thrombocytopenia) believed to be a hypersensitivity phenomena. Reactions are most often reversible upon discontinuing therapy.

Adverse Reactions (Reflective of adult population; not specific for elderly) Frequency not defined.

Cardiovascular: Hypotension

Central nervous system: Confusion, fever, lethargy, seizure (high doses and/or renal failure)

Dermatologic: Pruritus, rash, urticaria

Gastrointestinal: Abdominal pain, black or hairy tongue, diarrhea, flatulence, nausea, oral candidiasis, pseudomembranous colitis, stomatitis, vomiting

Hematologic: Agranulocytosis, bone marrow depression, eosinophilia, granulocytopenia, hemolytic anemia, leukopenia, neutropenia, thrombocytopenia

Hepatic: Alkaline phosphatase increased, ALT increased, AST increased, hepatotoxicity

Local: Thrombophlebitis

Neuromuscular & skeletal: Arthralgia, myalgia, myoclonus

Renal: Hematuria, interstitial nephritis, proteinuria, renal insufficiency, renal tubular damage

Respiratory: Bronchospasm, laryngeal edema, laryngospasm, sneezing, wheezing

Miscellaneous: Anaphylaxis, angioedema, allergic reaction, serum sickness-like reaction

Drug Interactions

Avoid Concomitant Use

Avoid concomitant use of Cloxacillin with any of the following: BCG

Increased Effect/Toxicity

Cloxacillin may increase the levels/effects of: Methotrexate

The levels/effects of Cloxacillin may be increased by: Probenecid

Decreased Effect

Cloxacillin may decrease the levels/effects of: BCG; Mycophenolate; Typhoid Vaccine

The levels/effects of Cloxacillin may be decreased by: Fusidic Acid; Tetracycline Derivatives

Ethanol/Nutrition/Herb Interactions Food: Decreases cloxacillin absorption; serum levels are reduced by ~50%.

Stability

Capsule: Store at room temperature not exceeding 25°C (77°F).

Powder for injection: Store at controlled room temperature not exceeding 25°C (77°F). Upon reconstitution the resulting solution is stable for up to 24 hours at controlled room temperature and 48 hours under refrigeration.

I.M. injection: Vials should be reconstituted with appropriate volume of SWFI to make a final concentration of 125 mg/mL or 250 mg/mL

I.V. injection: Vials should be reconstituted with appropriate volume of SWFI to make a final concentration of 50 mg/mL or 100 mg/mL

I.V. infusion: Infusion is prepared in 2 stages: Initial reconstitution of powder, followed by dilution to final infusion solution.

Note: After reconstitution of powder with appropriate volume of sterile water for injection, the manufacturer suggests further dilution to concentrations of 1-2 mg/mL in a compatible solution (eg, D_5W, NS); solutions are stable for up to 12 hours at controlled room temperature.

Powder for oral solution: Prior to mixing, store powder at room temperature not exceeding 25°C (77°F). Refrigerate oral solution after reconstitution; discard after 14 days.

Mechanism of Action Inhibits bacterial cell wall synthesis by binding to one or more of the penicillin-binding proteins (PBPs) which in turn inhibit the final transpeptidation step of peptidoglycan synthesis in bacterial cell walls, thus inhibiting cell wall biosynthesis. Bacteria eventually lyse due to ongoing activity of cell wall autolytic enzymes (autolysins and murein hydrolases) while cell wall assembly is arrested.

Pharmacodynamics/Kinetics

Absorption: Oral: ~50%; reduced by food

Protein binding: ~94% (primarily albumin)

Metabolism: Significant in the liver to active and inactive metabolites

Half-life: 30-90 minutes (prolonged with renal impairment); reported to be longer in older adults, but is not considered clinically significant

Time to peak serum concentration: Oral: Within 0.5-2 hours

Elimination: In urine and through bile

Dosage

Geriatric & Adult Note: Dose and duration of therapy can vary depending on infecting organism, severity of infection, and clinical response of patient. Treat severe staphylococcal infections for at least 14 days; endocarditis and osteomyelitis require an extended duration of therapy for 4-6 weeks. The intravenous route should be used for severe infections.

Susceptible infections:

Oral: 250-500 mg every 6 hours (manufacturer recommended maximum adult dose: 6 g/day)

◀ I.M., I.V.: 250-500 mg every 6 hours (manufacturer recommended maximum adult dose: 6 g/day)

Dosing recommendations of World Health Organization unless otherwise noted:

Arthritis (septic), methicillin-sensitive *Staphylococcus aureus* (MSSA) (unlabeled dosing): I.M., I.V.: 2 g every 6 hours for 2-3 weeks; **Note:** Oral therapy of 1 g every 6 hours may be used to complete therapy if parenteral therapy is discontinued prior to 2-3 week duration

Endocarditis (MSSA) (unlabeled dosing): I.V.:

Native valve: 2 g every 4 hours for 6 weeks; may give with gentamicin for initial 5 days (Choudri, 2000)

Prosthetic valve: 2 g every 4 hours for 6 weeks; give with gentamicin for 2 weeks and rifampin for 6 weeks (Choudri, 2000)

Uncomplicated endocarditis in I.V. drug users: 2 g every 4 hours for 4 weeks and gentamicin for initial 5 days **or** 2 g every 4 hours and gentamicin both given for 2 weeks total (Choudri, 2000)

Osteomyelitis (MSSA) (unlabeled dosing): I.M., I.V.: 2 g every 6 hours for 4-6 weeks (preferred) **or** for a minimum of 14 days, **followed by** 1 g every 6 hours orally to complete 4-6 weeks of therapy

Pneumonia (MSSA) (unlabeled dosing): I.M., I.V.: 1-2 g every 6 hours for 10-14 days

Renal Impairment No dosage adjustment necessary.

Administration

Oral: Administer with water 1 hour before or 2 hours after meals

I.M.: Administer slowly over 2-4 minutes

I.V.:

I.V. push: Administer slowly over 2-4 minutes

I.V. infusion: Administer over 30-40 minutes

Monitoring Parameters Observe for signs and symptoms of anaphylaxis during first dose; CBC with differential (prior to initiating therapy and weekly thereafter), periodic BUN, creatinine, hepatic function

Test Interactions May interfere with urinary glucose tests using cupric sulfate (Benedict's solution, Clinitest®); may inactivate aminoglycosides *in vitro*; false-positive urine and serum proteins; false-positive in uric acid, urinary steroids

Special Geriatric Considerations Dosage change for renal function is not necessary.

Product Availability Not available in U.S.

Dosage Forms: Canada Excipient information presented when available (limited, particularly for generics); consult specific product labeling.

Capsule, oral, as sodium: 250 mg, 500 mg

Injection, powder for reconstitution: 250 mg, 500 mg, 1000 mg, 2000 mg

Powder for suspension, oral, as sodium: 125 mg/5 mL (60 mL, 100 mL, 200 mL)

◆ **Cloxacillin Sodium** *see* Cloxacillin *on page 400*

CloZAPine (KLOE za peen)

Related Information

Antipsychotic Agents *on page 1997*

Atypical Antipsychotics *on page 1999*

Beers Criteria − Potentially Inappropriate Medications for Geriatrics *on page 2089*

Medication Safety Issues

Sound-alike/look-alike issues:

CloZAPine may be confused with clonazePAM, cloNIDine, KlonoPIN®

Clozaril® may be confused with Clinoril®, Colazal®

Brand Names: U.S. Clozaril®; FazaClo®

Brand Names: Canada Apo-Clozapine®; Clozaril®; Gen-Clozapine

Generic Availability (U.S.) Yes: Excludes orally-disintegrating tablet

Pharmacologic Category Antipsychotic Agent, Atypical

Use Treatment-refractory schizophrenia; to reduce risk of recurrent suicidal behavior in schizophrenia or schizoaffective disorder

Unlabeled/Investigational Use Schizoaffective disorder, bipolar disorder, severe obsessive-compulsive disorder; psychosis/agitation related to Alzheimer's dementia

Prescribing and Access Restrictions

U.S.: Clozaril® is deemed to have an approved REMS program. As a requirement of the REMS program, access to this medication is restricted. Patient-specific registration is required to dispense clozapine. Monitoring systems for individual clozapine manufacturers are independent. If a patient is switched from one brand/manufacturer of clozapine to another, the patient must be entered into a new registry (must be completed by the prescriber and delivered to the dispensing pharmacy). Healthcare providers, including pharmacists dispensing clozapine, should verify the patient's hematological status and qualification to receive clozapine with all existing registries. The manufacturer of Clozaril® requests that healthcare providers submit all WBC/ANC values following discontinuation of therapy to the Clozaril National Registry for all nonrechallengable patients until WBC is ≥3500/mm³ and ANC is ≥2000/mm³.

Canada: Distribution of clozapine is available only through the Clozaril Support and Assistance Network (CSAN). Details regarding CSAN are available to Canadian practitioners at (800-267-2726).

Contraindications Hypersensitivity to clozapine or any component of the formulation; history of agranulocytosis or severe granulocytopenia with clozapine; uncontrolled epilepsy, severe central nervous system depression or comatose state; paralytic ileus; myeloproliferative disorders or use with other agents which have a well-known risk of agranulocytosis or bone marrow suppression

Canadian labeling: Additional contraindications (not in U.S. labeling): Active hepatic disease associated with nausea, anorexia, or jaundice; progressive hepatic disease or hepatic failure; severe renal impairment; severe cardiac disease (eg, myocarditis); patients unable to undergo blood testing

Warnings/Precautions [U.S. Boxed Warning]: Elderly patients with dementia-related psychosis treated with antipsychotics are at an increased risk of death compared to placebo. Most deaths appeared to be either cardiovascular (eg, heart failure, sudden death) or infectious (eg, pneumonia) in nature. Clozapine is not approved for the treatment of dementia-related psychosis.

[U.S. Boxed Warning]: Significant risk of agranulocytosis, potentially life-threatening. Therapy should not be initiated in patients with WBC <3500 cells/mm³ or ANC <2000 cells/mm³ or history of myeloproliferative disorder. WBC testing should occur periodically on an ongoing basis (see prescribing information for monitoring details) to ensure that acceptable WBC/ANC counts are maintained. Initial episodes of moderate leukopenia or granulopoietic suppression confer up to a 12-fold increased risk for subsequent episodes of agranulocytosis. WBCs must be monitored weekly for at least 4 weeks after therapy discontinuation or until WBC is ≥3500/mm³ and ANC is ≥2000/mm³. Use with caution in patients receiving other marrow suppressive agents. Eosinophilia has been reported to occur with clozapine. Interrupt therapy for eosinophil count >4000/mm³. May resume therapy when eosinophil count <3000/mm³. (**Note:** The Canadian labeling recommends discontinuing therapy for eosinophil count >3000/mm³; may resume therapy when eosinophil count <1000/mm³). Due to the significant risk of agranulocytosis, it is strongly recommended that a patient must fail at least two trials of other primary medications for the treatment of schizophrenia (of adequate dose and duration) before initiating therapy with clozapine.

Cognitive and/or motor impairment (sedation) is common with clozapine, resulting in impaired performance of tasks requiring alertness (eg, operating machinery or driving); use caution in patients receiving general anesthesia. **[U.S. Boxed Warning]: Seizures have been associated with clozapine use in a dose-dependent manner;** use with caution in patients at risk of seizures, including those with a history of seizures, head trauma, brain damage, alcoholism, or concurrent therapy with medications which may lower seizure threshold. Benign transient temperature elevation (>100.4°F) may occur; peaking within the first 3 weeks of treatment. Rule out infection, agranulocytosis, and neuroleptic malignant syndrome (NMS) in patients presenting with fever. However, clozapine may also be associated with severe febrile reactions, including neuroleptic malignant syndrome (NMS). Clozapine's potential for extrapyramidal symptoms (including tardive dyskinesia) appears to be extremely low. Risk of dystonia (and probably other EPS) may be greater with increased doses, use of conventional antipsychotics, males, and younger patients.

Deep vein thrombosis, myocarditis, pericarditis, pericardial effusion, cardiomyopathy, and HF have also been associated with clozapine. **[U.S. Boxed Warning]: Fatalities due to myocarditis have been reported; highest risk in the first month of therapy, however, later cases also reported.** Myocarditis or cardiomyopathy should be considered in patients who present with signs/symptoms of heart failure (dyspnea, fatigue, orthopnea, paroxysmal nocturnal dyspnea, peripheral edema), chest pain, palpitations, new electrocardiographic abnormalities (arrhythmias, ST-T wave abnormalities), or unexplained fever. Patients with tachycardia during the first month of therapy should be closely monitored for other signs of myocarditis. Discontinue clozapine if myocarditis is suspected; do not rechallenge in patients with clozapine-related myocarditis. The reported rate of myocarditis in clozapine-treated patients appears to be 17-322 times greater than in the general population. Clozapine should be discontinued in patients with confirmed cardiomyopathy unless benefit clearly outweighs risk. Rare cases of thromboembolism, including pulmonary embolism and stroke resulting in fatalities, have been associated with clozapine.

An increased incidence of cerebrovascular effects (eg, transient ischemic attack, stroke), including fatalities, has been reported in placebo-controlled trials of atypical antipsychotics in elderly patients with dementia-related psychosis.

May cause anticholinergic effects; use with caution in patients with urinary retention, benign prostatic hyperplasia, narrow-angle glaucoma, xerostomia, visual problems, constipation, or history of bowel obstruction. May cause hyperglycemia; in some cases may be extreme and associated with ketoacidosis, hyperosmolar coma, or death. Use with caution in patients with diabetes or other disorders of glucose regulation; monitor for worsening of glucose control. Antipsychotic use has been associated with esophageal dysmotility and aspiration; use with caution in patients at risk of pneumonia (eg, Alzheimer's disease). Use with caution in patients with hepatic disease or impairment; monitor hepatic function regularly. Hepatitis has been reported as a consequence of therapy. Discontinuation of therapy may be necessary with significant elevations in liver function tests; may reinitiate with close monitoring and if values return to normal. Use with caution in patients with renal disease.

Use caution with cardiovascular or pulmonary disease; gradually increase dose. **[U.S. Boxed Warning]: May cause orthostatic hypotension (with or without syncope);** generally occurs more frequently with initial titration and in association with rapid dose increases; use with caution in patients at risk of hypotension or in patients where transient hypotensive episodes would be poorly tolerated (cardiovascular disease or cerebrovascular disease). Concurrent use with benzodiazepines may increase the risk of severe cardiopulmonary reactions. May cause tachycardia (including sustained); sustained tachycardia is not limited to a reflex response to orthostatic hypotension, and is present in all positions.

The possibility of a suicide attempt is inherent in psychotic illness or bipolar disorder; use caution in high-risk patients during initiation of therapy. Prescriptions should be written for the smallest quantity consistent with good patient care.

Medication should not be stopped abruptly; taper off over 1-2 weeks. If conditions warrant abrupt discontinuation (leukopenia, myocarditis, cardiomyopathy), monitor patient for psychosis and cholinergic rebound (headache, nausea, vomiting, diarrhea). Significant weight gain has been observed with antipsychotic therapy; incidence varies with product. Monitor waist circumference and BMI. Elderly patients are more susceptible to adverse effects (including agranulocytosis, cardiovascular, anticholinergic, and tardive dyskinesia). Clozapine levels may be lower in patients who smoke. Smoking cessation may cause toxicity in a patient stabilized on clozapine. Monitor change in smoking. FazaClo® oral disintegrating tablets contain phenylalanine.

Adverse Reactions (Reflective of adult population; not specific for elderly)

>10%:
Cardiovascular: Tachycardia (25%)
Central nervous system: Drowsiness (39% to 46%), dizziness (19% to 27%), insomnia (2% to 20%)
Gastrointestinal: Sialorrhea (31% to 48%), weight gain (4% to 31%), constipation (14% to 25%), nausea/vomiting (3% to 17%)

1% to 10%:
Cardiovascular: Hypotension (9%), syncope (6%), hypertension (4%), angina (1%), ECG changes (1%)
Central nervous system: Headache (7%), agitation (4%), akinesia (4%), nightmares (4%), restlessness (4%), akathisia (3%), confusion (3%), seizure (3%), anxiety (1%), ataxia (1%), depression (1%), lethargy (1%), myoclonic jerks (1%), slurred speech (1%)
Dermatologic: Rash (2%)
Gastrointestinal: Abdominal discomfort/heartburn (4% to 14%), xerostomia (6%), diarrhea (2%), anorexia (1%), throat discomfort (1%)
Genitourinary: Urinary abnormalities (eg, abnormal ejaculation, retention, urgency, incontinence; 1% to 2%)
Hematologic: Agranulocytosis (1%), eosinophilia (1%), leukocytosis, leukopenia
Hepatic: Liver function tests abnormal (1%)
Neuromuscular & skeletal: Tremor (6%), hypokinesia (4%), rigidity (3%), hyperkinesia (1%), weakness (1%), pain (1%), spasm (1%)
Ocular: Visual disturbances (5%)
Respiratory: Dyspnea (1%), nasal congestion (1%)
Miscellaneous: Diaphoresis (6%), tongue numbness (1%)

Drug Interactions

Metabolism/Transport Effects Substrate of CYP1A2 (major), 2A6 (minor), 2C9 (minor), 2C19 (minor), 2D6 (minor), 3A4 (minor); **Inhibits** CYP1A2 (weak), 2C9 (weak), 2C19 (weak), 2D6 (moderate), 2E1 (weak), 3A4 (weak)

Avoid Concomitant Use

Avoid concomitant use of CloZAPine with any of the following: Metoclopramide; Thioridazine

Increased Effect/Toxicity

CloZAPine may increase the levels/effects of: Alcohol (Ethyl); Anticholinergics; CNS Depressants; CYP2D6 Substrates; Fesoterodine; Methotrimeprazine; Methylphenidate; Nebivolol; Tamoxifen; Thioridazine

The levels/effects of CloZAPine may be increased by: Abiraterone Acetate; Acetylcholinesterase Inhibitors (Central); Benzodiazepines; Cimetidine; Conivaptan; CYP1A2 Inhibitors (Moderate); CYP1A2 Inhibitors (Strong); Deferasirox; Droperidol; HydrOXYzine; Lithium formulations; Macrolide Antibiotics; MAO Inhibitors; Methotrimeprazine; Methylphenidate; Metoclopramide; Nefazodone; Omeprazole; Pramlintide; Selective Serotonin Reuptake Inhibitors; Tetrabenazine

Decreased Effect

CloZAPine may decrease the levels/effects of: Amphetamines; Anti-Parkinson's Agents (Dopamine Agonist); Codeine; Quinagolide; TraMADol

The levels/effects of CloZAPine may be decreased by: CarBAMazepine; CYP1A2 Inducers (Strong); Cyproterone; Fosphenytoin; Lithium formulations; Omeprazole; Peginterferon Alfa-2b; Phenytoin; Tocilizumab

Ethanol/Nutrition/Herb Interactions

Ethanol: May increase CNS depression; monitor for increased effects with coadministration. Caution patients about effects.

Herb/Nutraceutical: St John's wort may decrease clozapine levels. Avoid kava kava, gotu kola, valerian, St John's wort (may increase CNS depression).

Stability Store at ≤30°C (86°F).

FazaClo®: Store at 25°C (77°F); excursions permitted to 15°C to 30°C (59°F to 86°F). Protect from moisture; do not remove from package until ready to use.

Mechanism of Action Clozapine (dibenzodiazepine antipsychotic) exhibits weak antagonism of D_1, D_2, D_3, and D_5 dopamine receptor subtypes, but shows high affinity for D_4; in addition, it blocks the serotonin ($5HT_2$), alpha-adrenergic, histamine H_1, and cholinergic receptors

Pharmacodynamics/Kinetics

Protein binding: 97% to serum proteins

Metabolism: Extensively hepatic; forms metabolites with limited or no activity

Bioavailability: 50% to 60% (not affected by food)

Half-life elimination: Steady state: 12 hours (range: 4-66 hours)

Time to peak: 2.5 hours (range: 1-6 hours)

Excretion: Urine (~50%) and feces (30%) with trace amounts of unchanged drug

Dosage

Geriatric

Schizophrenia: Oral: Experience in the elderly is limited; initial dose should be 12.5-25 mg/day; increase as tolerated by 25 mg/day to desired response. Elderly may require slower titration and daily increases may not be tolerated.

Psychosis/agitation related to Alzheimer's dementia (unlabeled use): Oral: Initial: 12.5 mg/day; if necessary, gradually increase as tolerated not to exceed 75-100 mg/day (Rabins, 2007)

Adult

Schizophrenia: Initial: 12.5 mg once or twice daily; increased, as tolerated, in increments of 25-50 mg/day to a target dose of 300-450 mg/day after 2 weeks; may further titrate in increments not exceeding 100 mg and no more frequently than once or twice weekly. May require doses as high as 600-900 mg/day (maximum dose: 900 mg/day). **Note:** In some efficacy studies, total daily dosage was administered in 3 divided doses.

Suicidal behavior in schizophrenia or schizoaffective disorder: Initial: 12.5 mg once or twice daily; increased, as tolerated, in increments of 25-50 mg/day to a target dose of 300-450 mg/day after 2 weeks; mean dose is ~300 mg/day (range: 12.5-900 mg); treatment duration 2 years then reassess need. **Note:** If no longer a suicide risk, may resume prior antipsychotic therapy after gradually tapering off clozapine over 1-2 weeks.

Termination of therapy: If dosing is interrupted for ≥48 hours, therapy must be reinitiated at 12.5-25 mg/day; may be increased more rapidly than with initial titration, unless cardiopulmonary arrest occurred during initial titration.

In the event of planned termination of clozapine, gradual reduction in dose over a 1- to 2-week period is recommended. If conditions warrant abrupt discontinuation (leukopenia), monitor patient for psychosis and cholinergic rebound (headache, nausea, vomiting, diarrhea).

◀ **Administration** May be taken without regard to food. Total daily dose may be divided into uneven doses with larger dose administered at bedtime.

Canadian labeling: Maintenance dosing ≤200 mg/day may be administered as single dose in the evening.

Orally-disintegrating tablet: Should be removed from foil blister by peeling apart (do not push tablet through the foil). Remove immediately prior to use. Place tablet in mouth and allow to dissolve; swallow with saliva. If dosing requires splitting tablet, throw unused portion away.

Monitoring Parameters Note: The Canadian labeling recommends initiating treatment in an inpatient setting or an outpatient setting with medical supervision and monitoring of vital signs for at least 6-8 hours after the first few doses.

Mental status, ECG, WBC (see below), vital signs, fasting lipid profile and fasting blood glucose/Hgb A_{1c} (prior to treatment, at 3 months, then annually; liver function tests; BMI, personal/family history of obesity; waist circumference (weight should be assessed prior to treatment, at 4 weeks, 8 weeks, 12 weeks, and then at quarterly intervals. Consider titrating to a different antipsychotic agent for a weight gain ≥5% of the initial weight); blood pressure; abnormal involuntary movement scale (AIMS).

WBC and ANC should be obtained at baseline and at least weekly for the first 6 months (26 weeks) of continuous treatment. If counts remain acceptable (WBC ≥3500/mm^3, ANC ≥2000/mm^3) during this time period, then they may be monitored every other week for the next 6 months (26 weeks). If WBC/ANC continue to remain within these acceptable limits after the second 6 months (26 weeks) of therapy, monitoring can be decreased to every 4 weeks. If clozapine is discontinued, a weekly WBC should be conducted for an additional 4 weeks or until WBC is ≥3500/mm^3 and ANC is ≥2000/mm^3. If clozapine therapy is interrupted due to moderate leukopenia, weekly WBC/ANC monitoring is required for 12 months in patients restarted on clozapine treatment. (**Note:** When therapy is interrupted for >3 days, the Canadian labeling recommends weekly hematologic testing for an additional 6 weeks) If therapy is interrupted for reasons other than leukopenia/granulocytopenia, the 6-month time period for initiation of biweekly WBCs may need to be reset. **This determination depends upon the treatment duration, the length of the break in therapy, and whether or not an abnormal blood event occurred.**

Consult manufacturer prescribing information for determination of appropriate WBC/ANC monitoring interval.

Pharmacotherapy Pearls Medication should not be stopped abruptly; taper off over 1-2 weeks

Special Geriatric Considerations Not recommended for use in nonpsychotic patients (eg, dimentia-related psychotic symptoms). Studies in subjects >65 years of age have not been done. Orthostatic hypotension and sustained tachycardia have been noted in up to 25% of patients taking clozapine; therefore, elderly with cardiovascular disease may be at risk. The anticholinergic effects of clozapine may be prominent in elderly (eg, constipation, confusion, urinary retention).

Dosage Forms Excipient information presented when available (limited, particularly for generics); consult specific product labeling.

Tablet, oral: 25 mg, 50 mg, 100 mg, 200 mg
   Clozaril®: 25 mg, 100 mg [scored]
Tablet, orally disintegrating, oral:
   FazaClo®: 12.5 mg [contains phenylalanine 0.87 mg/tablet; mint flavor]
   FazaClo®: 25 mg [contains phenylalanine 1.74 mg/tablet; mint flavor]
   FazaClo®: 100 mg [contains phenylalanine 6.96 mg/tablet; mint flavor]
   FazaClo®: 150 mg [contains phenylalanine 10.44 mg/tablet; mint flavor]
   FazaClo®: 200 mg [contains phenylalanine 13.92 mg/tablet; mint flavor]

Selected References

American Diabetes Association; American Psychiatric Association; American Association of Clinical Endocrinologists; North American Association for the Study of Obesity, "Consensus Development Conference on Antipsychotic Drugs and Obesity and Diabetes," *Diabetes Care,* 2004, 27(2):596-601.

Hagg S, Spigset O, and Soderstrom TG, "Association of Venous Thromboembolism and Clozapine," *Lancet,* 2000, 355(9210):1155-6.

Rabins PV, Blacker D, Rovner BW, et al, "Practice Guidelines for the Treatment of Patients With Alzheimer's Disease and Other Dementias," *Am J Psychiatry,* 2007, 164(12 Suppl):5-56. Available at http://www.psych.org/psych_pract/treatg/pg/prac_guide.cfm.

Schneider LS, Tariot PN, Dagerman KS, et al, "Effectiveness of Atypical Antipsychotic Drugs in Patients With Alzheimer's Disease," *N Engl J Med,* 2006, 355(15):1525-38.

◆ **Clozaril®** see CloZAPine on page 402
◆ **CNTO-148** see Golimumab on page 837
◆ **CNTO 1275** see Ustekinumab on page 1884

Codeine (KOE deen)

Related Information
Opioid Analgesics *on page 2013*

Medication Safety Issues
Sound-alike/look-alike issues:
Codeine may be confused with Cardene®, Cophene®, Cordran®, iodine, Lodine®
High alert medication:
The Institute for Safe Medication Practices (ISMP) includes this medication among its list of drug classes which have a heightened risk of causing significant patient harm when used in error.

Brand Names: Canada Codeine Contin®

Index Terms Codeine Phosphate; Codeine Sulfate; Methylmorphine

Generic Availability (U.S.) Yes

Pharmacologic Category Analgesic, Opioid; Antitussive

Use Treatment of mild-to-moderate pain; antitussive in lower doses

Contraindications Hypersensitivity to codeine or any component of the formulation

Warnings/Precautions Use with caution in patients with hypersensitivity reactions to other phenanthrene-derivative opioid agonists (morphine, hydrocodone, hydromorphone, levorphanol, oxycodone, oxymorphone); respiratory diseases including asthma, emphysema, COPD, adrenal insufficiency, biliary tract impairment, CNS depression/coma, head trauma, morbid obesity, prostatic hyperplasia, urinary stricture, thyroid dysfunction, or severe liver or renal insufficiency; some preparations contain sulfites which may cause allergic reactions; tolerance or drug dependence may result from extended use. May obscure diagnosis or clinical course of patients with acute abdominal conditions. May cause CNS depression, which may impair physical or mental abilities; patients must be cautioned about performing tasks which require mental alertness (eg, operating machinery or driving). May cause hypotension; use with caution in patients with hypovolemia, cardiovascular disease (including acute MI), or drugs which may exaggerate hypotensive effects (including phenothiazines or general anesthetics). Use caution in patients with two or more copies of the variant CYP2D6*2 allele; may have extensive conversion to morphine and thus increased opioid-mediated effects.

Not recommended for use for cough control in patients with a productive cough; the elderly and debilitated patients may be particularly susceptible to adverse effects of narcotics

Not approved for I.V. administration (although this route has been used clinically). If given intravenously, must be given slowly and the patient should be lying down. Rapid intravenous administration of narcotics may increase the incidence of serious adverse effects, in part due to limited opportunity to assess response prior to administration of the full dose. Access to respiratory support should be immediately available.

Concurrent use of agonist/antagonist analgesics may precipitate withdrawal symptoms and/or reduced analgesic efficacy in patients following prolonged therapy with mu opioid agonists. Abrupt discontinuation following prolonged use may also lead to withdrawal symptoms.

Adverse Reactions (Reflective of adult population; not specific for elderly)
>10%:
Central nervous system: Drowsiness
Gastrointestinal: Constipation
1% to 10%:
Cardiovascular: Hypotension, tachycardia or bradycardia
Central nervous system: Confusion, dizziness, false feeling of well being, headache, lightheadedness, malaise, paradoxical CNS stimulation, restlessness
Dermatologic: Rash, urticaria
Gastrointestinal: Anorexia, nausea, vomiting, xerostomia
Genitourinary: Ureteral spasm, urination decreased
Hepatic: LFTs increased
Local: Burning at injection site
Neuromuscular & skeletal: Weakness
Ocular: Blurred vision
Respiratory: Dyspnea
Miscellaneous: Histamine release
Frequency not defined: ALT increased, AST increased

Drug Interactions
Metabolism/Transport Effects Substrate of CYP2D6 (major), 3A4 (minor); **Inhibits** CYP2D6 (weak)
Avoid Concomitant Use There are no known interactions where it is recommended to avoid concomitant use.

Increased Effect/Toxicity

Codeine may increase the levels/effects of: Alcohol (Ethyl); Alvimopan; CNS Depressants; Desmopressin; Selective Serotonin Reuptake Inhibitors; Thiazide Diuretics

The levels/effects of Codeine may be increased by: Amphetamines; Antipsychotic Agents (Phenothiazines); Droperidol; HydrOXYzine; Somatostatin Analogs; Succinylcholine

Decreased Effect

Codeine may decrease the levels/effects of: Pegvisomant

The levels/effects of Codeine may be decreased by: Ammonium Chloride; CYP2D6 Inhibitors (Moderate); CYP2D6 Inhibitors (Strong); Mixed Agonist / Antagonist Opioids

Ethanol/Nutrition/Herb Interactions

Ethanol: May increase CNS depression; monitor for increased effects with coadministration. Caution patients about effects.

Herb/Nutraceutical: St John's wort may decrease codeine levels. Avoid valerian, St John's wort, kava kava, gotu kola (may increase CNS depression).

Stability Store injection between 15°C to 30°C; avoid freezing. Do not use if injection is discolored or contains a precipitate. Protect injection from light.

Mechanism of Action Binds to opiate receptors in the CNS, causing inhibition of ascending pain pathways, altering the perception of and response to pain; causes cough supression by direct central action in the medulla; produces generalized CNS depression

Pharmacodynamics/Kinetics

Onset of action: Oral: 0.5-1 hour; I.M.: 10-30 minutes

Peak effect: Oral: 1-1.5 hours; I.M.: 0.5-1 hour

Duration: 4-6 hours

Absorption: Oral: Adequate

Protein binding: 7%

Metabolism: Hepatic to morphine (active)

Half-life elimination: 2.5-3.5 hours

Excretion: Urine (3% to 16% as unchanged drug, norcodeine, and free and conjugated morphine)

Dosage

Geriatric & Adult Note: These are guidelines and do not represent the maximum doses that may be required in all patients. Doses should be titrated to pain relief/prevention. Doses >1.5 mg/kg body weight are not recommended.

Pain management (analgesic):

Oral, regular release: 30 mg every 4-6 hours as needed; patients with prior opiate exposure may require higher initial doses. Usual range: 15-120 mg every 4-6 hours as needed. **Note:** The American Pain Society recommends an initial dose of 30-60 mg for adults with moderate pain.

Oral, controlled release formulation (Codeine Contin®, not available in U.S.): 50-300 mg every 12 hours. **Note:** A patient's codeine requirement should be established using prompt release formulations; conversion to long acting products may be considered when chronic, continuous treatment is required. Higher dosages should be reserved for use only in opioid-tolerant patients.

I.M., SubQ: 30 mg every 4-6 hours as needed; patients with prior opiate exposure may require higher initial doses. Usual range: 15-120 mg every 4-6 hours as needed; more frequent dosing may be needed

Cough (antitussive): Oral (for nonproductive cough): 10-20 mg/dose every 4-6 hours as needed; maximum: 120 mg/day

Renal Impairment

Cl$_{cr}$ 10-50 mL/minute: Administer 75% of dose.

Cl$_{cr}$ <10 mL/minute: Administer 50% of dose.

Hepatic Impairment Dosing adjustment is probably necessary in hepatic insufficiency.

Administration Not approved for I.V. administration (although this route has been used clinically). If given intravenously, must be given slowly and the patient should be lying down. Rapid intravenous administration of narcotics may increase the incidence of serious adverse effects, in part due to limited opportunity to assess response prior to administration of the full dose. Access to respiratory support should be immediately available.

Monitoring Parameters Pain relief, respiratory and mental status, blood pressure, heart rate

Reference Range Therapeutic: Not established; Toxic: >1.1 mcg/mL

Test Interactions Some quinolones may produce a false-positive urine screening result for opiates using commercially-available immunoassay kits. This has been demonstrated most consistently for levofloxacin and ofloxacin, but other quinolones have shown cross-reactivity in certain assay kits. Confirmation of positive opiate screens by more specific methods should be considered.

Pharmacotherapy Pearls May be habit-forming; dextromethorphan has equivalent anti-tussive activity but has much lower toxicity in accidental overdose

Special Geriatric Considerations The elderly may be particularly susceptible to CNS depression and confusion as well as the constipating effects of narcotics.

Controlled Substance C-II

Dosage Forms Excipient information presented when available (limited, particularly for generics); consult specific product labeling. [DSC] = Discontinued product

Injection, solution, as phosphate: 15 mg/mL (2 mL [DSC]) [contains sodium metabisulfite]; 30 mg/mL (2 mL [DSC]) [contains sodium metabisulfite]

Powder, for prescription compounding, as phosphate: USP: 100% (10 g, 25 g)

Tablet, oral, as phosphate: 30 mg, 60 mg

Tablet, oral, as sulfate: 15 mg, 30 mg, 60 mg

Dosage Forms: Canada Excipient information presented when available (limited, particularly for generics); consult specific product labeling.

Tablet, controlled release:

Codeine Contin®: 50 mg, 100 mg, 150 mg, 200 mg

Selected References

American Geriatrics Society Panel on Pharmacological Management of Persistent Pain in Older Persons, "Pharmacological Management of Persistent Pain in Older Persons," *J Am Geriatr Soc*, 2009, 57(8):1331-46.

◆ **Codeine and Acetaminophen** see Acetaminophen and Codeine on page 37
◆ **Codeine and Guaifenesin** see Guaifenesin and Codeine on page 848
◆ **Codeine Phosphate** see Codeine on page 407
◆ **Codeine Sulfate** see Codeine on page 407
◆ **Cogentin®** see Benztropine on page 192
◆ **Colace® [OTC]** see Docusate on page 547
◆ **ColBenemid** see Colchicine and Probenecid on page 412

Colchicine (KOL chi seen)

Medication Safety Issues

Sound-alike/look-alike issues:

Colchicine may be confused with Cortrosyn®

Brand Names: U.S. Colcrys®

Generic Availability (U.S.) No

Pharmacologic Category Antigout Agent

Use Prevention and treatment of acute gout flares; treatment of familial Mediterranean fever (FMF)

Unlabeled/Investigational Use Primary biliary cirrhosis; pericarditis

Medication Guide Available Yes

Contraindications Concomitant use of a P-glycoprotein (P-gp) or strong CYP3A4 inhibitor in presence of renal or hepatic impairment

Warnings/Precautions Hazardous agent - use appropriate precautions for handling and disposal. Myelosuppression (eg, thrombocytopenia, leukopenia, granulocytopenia, pancytopenia) and aplastic anemia have been reported in patients receiving therapeutic doses. Neuromuscular toxicity (including rhabdomyolysis) has been reported in patients receiving therapeutic doses; patients with renal dysfunction and elderly patients are at increased risk. Concomitant use of cyclosporine, diltiazem, verapamil, fibrates, and statins may increase the risk of myopathy. Clearance is decreased in renal or hepatic impairment; monitor closely for adverse effects/toxicity. Dosage adjustments may be required depending on degree of impairment or indication, and may be affected by the use of concurrent medication (CYP3A4 or P-gp inhibitors). Concurrent use of P-gp or strong CYP3A4 inhibitors is contraindicated in renal impairment; fatal toxicity has been reported. Colchicine does not have analgesic activity and should not be used to treat pain from other causes. Colchicine requires dosage adjustment when used concurrently with protease inhibitor regimens. Colchicine does not have analgesic activity and should not be used to treat pain from other causes.

Adverse Reactions (Reflective of adult population; not specific for elderly)

>10%: Gastrointestinal: Gastrointestinal disorders including abdominal pain, cramping, nausea, vomiting (up to 26%), diarrhea (up to 23%)

1% to 10%: Respiratory: Pharyngolaryngeal pain (3%)

Drug Interactions

Metabolism/Transport Effects Substrate of CYP3A4 (major), P-glycoprotein; **Induces** CYP2C8 (weak), 2C9 (weak), 2E1 (weak), 3A4 (weak)

Avoid Concomitant Use There are no known interactions where it is recommended to avoid concomitant use.

Increased Effect/Toxicity

Colchicine may increase the levels/effects of: HMG-CoA Reductase Inhibitors

The levels/effects of Colchicine may be increased by: CYP3A4 Inhibitors (Moderate); CYP3A4 Inhibitors (Strong); Dasatinib; Digoxin; Fibric Acid Derivatives; P-Glycoprotein Inhibitors; Telaprevir

Decreased Effect

Colchicine may decrease the levels/effects of: Cyanocobalamin; Saxagliptin

The levels/effects of Colchicine may be decreased by: P-Glycoprotein Inducers; Tocilizumab

Ethanol/Nutrition/Herb Interactions

Ethanol: Avoid ethanol.

Food: Cyanocobalamin (vitamin B_{12}): Malabsorption of the substrate. May result in macrocytic anemia or neurologic dysfunction. Grapefruit juice may increase colchicine serum concentrations.

Herb/Nutraceutical: Vitamin B_{12} absorption may be decreased by colchicine.

Stability Store at 20°C to 25°C (68°F to 77°F). Protect from light.

Mechanism of Action Disrupts cytoskeletal functions by inhibiting β-tubulin polymerization into microtubules, preventing activation, degranulation, and migration of neutrophils associated with mediating some gout symptoms. In familial Mediterranean fever, may interfere with intracellular assembly of the inflammasome complex present in neutrophils and monocytes that mediate activation of interleukin-1β.

Pharmacodynamics/Kinetics

Onset of action: Oral: Pain relief: ~18-24 hours

Distribution: Concentrates in leukocytes, kidney, spleen, and liver; does not distribute in heart, skeletal muscle, and brain

V_d: 5-8 L/kg

Protein binding: ~39%

Metabolism: Hepatic via CYP3A4; 3 metabolites (2 primary, 1 minor)

Bioavailability: ~45%

Half-life elimination: 27-31 hours (multiple oral doses; young, healthy volunteers)

Time to peak, serum: Oral: 0.5-3 hours

Excretion: Urine (40% to 65% as unchanged drug); enterohepatic recirculation and biliary excretion also possible

Dosage

Geriatric Use caution; reduce prophylactic daily dose by 50% in individuals >70 years (Terkeltaub, 2009)

Adult

Familial Mediterranean fever (FMF): Oral: 1.2-2.4 mg/day in 1-2 divided doses; titration: Increase or decrease dose in 0.3 mg increments based on efficacy or adverse effects; maximum: 2.4 mg/day

Gout: Oral:

Flare treatment: Initial: 1.2 mg at the first sign of flare, followed in 1 hour with a single dose of 0.6 mg (maximum: 1.8 mg within 1 hour). Patients receiving prophylaxis therapy may receive treatment dosing; wait 12 hours before resuming prophylaxis dose. **Note:** Current FDA-approved dose for gout flare is substantially lower than what has been historically used clinically. Doses larger than the currently recommended dosage for gout flare have not been proven to be more effective.

Prophylaxis: 0.6 mg once or twice daily; maximum: 1.2 mg/day

Pericarditis (unlabeled use): Oral: 0.6 mg twice daily (Antman, 2004)

Primary biliary cirrhosis (unlabeled use): Oral: 0.6 mg twice daily (Kaplan, 2005); **Note:** Use reserved for patients refractory to ursodiol.

Dosage adjustment for concomitant therapy with CYP3A4 or P-glycoprotein (P-gp) inhibitors: *Dosage adjustment also required in patients receiving CYP3A4 or P-gp inhibitors up to 14 days prior to initiation of colchicine.* **Note:** Treatment of gout flare with colchicine is not recommended in patients receiving prophylactic colchicine and CYP3A4 inhibitors.

Coadministration of **strong** CYP3A4 inhibitor (eg, atazanavir, clarithromycin, darunavir, indinavir, itraconazole, ketoconazole, lopinavir/ritonavir, nefazodone, nelfinavir, ritonavir, saquinavir, telithromycin, tipranavir):

FMF: Maximum dose: 0.6 mg/day (0.3 mg twice daily)

Gout prophylaxis:

If original dose is 0.6 mg twice daily, adjust dose to 0.3 mg once daily

If original dose is 0.6 mg once daily, adjust dose to 0.3 mg every other day

Gout flare treatment: Initial: 0.6 mg, followed in 1 hour by a single dose of 0.3 mg; do not repeat for at least 3 days

Coadministration of **moderate** CYP3A4 inhibitor (eg, aprepitant, diltiazem, erythromycin, fluconazole, fosamprenavir, grapefruit juice, verapamil):

FMF: Maximum dose: 1.2 mg/day (0.6 mg twice daily)

Gout prophylaxis:

If original dose is 0.6 mg twice daily, adjust dose to 0.3 mg twice daily **or** 0.6 mg once daily

If original dose is 0.6 mg once daily, adjust dose to 0.3 mg once daily

Gout flare treatment: 1.2 mg as a single dose; do not repeat for at least 3 days

Coadministration of P-gp inhibitor (eg, cyclosporine, ranolazine):

FMF: Maximum dose: 0.6 mg/day (0.3 mg twice daily)

Gout prophylaxis:

If original dose is 0.6 mg twice daily, adjust dose to 0.3 mg once daily

If original dose is 0.6 mg once daily, adjust dose to 0.3 mg every other day

Gout flare treatment: Initial: 0.6 mg as a single dose; do not repeat for at least 3 days

Renal Impairment Concurrent use of colchicine and P-gp or strong CYP3A4 inhibitors is **contraindicated** in renal impairment. Fatal toxicity has been reported. Treatment of gout flares is not recommended in patients with renal impairment receiving prophylactic colchicine.

FMF:

Cl_{cr} 30-80 mL/minute: Monitor closely for adverse effects; dose reduction may be necessary.

Cl_{cr} <30 mL/minute: Initial dose: 0.3 mg/day; use caution if dose titrated; monitor for adverse effects.

Dialysis: 0.3 mg as a single dose; use caution if dose titrated; dosing can be increased with close monitoring; monitor for adverse effects. Not removed by dialysis.

Gout prophylaxis:

Cl_{cr} 30-80 mL/minute: Dosage adjustment not required; monitor closely for adverse effects.

Cl_{cr} <30 mL/minute: Initial dose: 0.3 mg/day; use caution if dose titrated; monitor for adverse effects.

Dialysis: 0.3 mg twice weekly; monitor closely for adverse effects.

Gout flare treatment:

Cl_{cr} 30-80 mL/minute: Dosage adjustment not required; monitor closely for adverse effects.

Cl_{cr} <30 mL/minute: Dosage reduction not required but may be considered; treatment course should not be repeated more frequently than every 14 days.

Dialysis: 0.6 mg as a single dose; treatment course should not be repeated more frequently than every 14 days. Not removed by dialysis.

Hemodialysis: Avoid chronic use of colchicine.

Hepatic Impairment Concurrent use of colchicine and P-glycoprotein or strong CYP3A4 inhibitors is **contraindicated** in hepatic impairment. Fatal toxicity has been reported. Treatment of gout flare with colchicine is not recommended in patients with hepatic impairment receiving prophylactic colchicine.

FMF:

Mild-to-moderate impairment: Use caution; monitor closely for adverse effects.

Severe impairment: Consider dosage reduction.

Gout prophylaxis:

Mild-to-moderate impairment: Dosage adjustment not required; monitor closely for adverse effects.

Severe impairment: Dosage adjustment should be considered.

Gout flare treatment:

Mild-to-moderate impairment: Dosage adjustment not required; monitor closely for adverse effects.

Severe impairment: Dosage reduction not required but may be considered; treatment course should not be repeated more frequently than every 14 days.

Administration Administer orally with water and maintain adequate fluid intake. May be administered without regard to meals.

Monitoring Parameters CBC, renal and hepatic function tests

Test Interactions May cause false-positive results in urine tests for erythrocytes or hemoglobin

Pharmacotherapy Pearls Oral colchicine had been available as an unapproved medication without FDA-approved prescribing information. In August 2009, the FDA approved prescribing information for a brand name colchicine product. The currently approved prescribing information recommends a lower than historically used dosage for the treatment of acute gout. This recommendation is based on data from the AGREE trial. In this trial, low-dose colchicine (1.8 mg total) had similar efficacy to high dose colchicine (4.8 mg total). Additionally, the low dosage regimen was associated with a lower incidence (26% vs 77%) of GI adverse events.

COLCHICINE

Parenteral formulation of colchicine is no longer available in the U.S.; serious life-threatening complications (eg, neutropenia, acute renal failure, thrombocytopenia, heart failure) associated with intravenous colchicine have occurred prior to market withdrawal. The risks associated with oral colchicine are believed to be lower compared to intravenous use.

Special Geriatric Considerations Colchicine appears to be more toxic in older adults, particularly in the presence of renal, gastrointestinal, or cardiac disease. The most predictable oral side effects are gastrointestinal (eg, vomiting, abdominal pain, and nausea). If colchicine is stopped at this point, other more severe adverse effects may be avoided, such as bone marrow suppression, peripheral neuritis, etc.

Dosage Forms Excipient information presented when available (limited, particularly for generics); consult specific product labeling.
Tablet, oral: 0.6 mg
  Colcrys®: 0.6 mg [scored]

Dosage Forms: Canada Excipient information presented when available (limited, particularly for generics); consult specific product labeling.
Tablet, oral: 1 mg [scored]

Selected References
Antman EM, Anbe SC, Alpert JS, et al, "ACC/AHA Guidelines for the Management of Patients With ST-Elevation Myocardial Infarction - Executive Summary: A Report of the American College of Cardiology/American Heart Association Task Force on Practice Guidelines (Writing Committee to Revise the 1999 Guidelines for the Management of Patients With Acute Myocardial Infarction)," Circulation, 2004, 110:588-636. Available at: http://www.circulationaha.org/cgi/content/full/110/5/588. Last accessed October 26, 2004.
Centers for Disease Control and Prevention (CDC), "Deaths From Intravenous Colchicine Resulting From a Pharmacy Compounding Error - Oregon And Washington, 2007," MMWR Morb Mortal Wkly Rep, 2007, 56(40):1050-2.

Colchicine and Probenecid (KOL chi seen & proe BEN e sid)

Related Information
Colchicine on page 409
Probenecid on page 1519
Index Terms ColBenemid; Probenecid and Colchicine
Generic Availability (U.S.) Yes
Pharmacologic Category Anti-inflammatory Agent; Antigout Agent; Uricosuric Agent
Use Treatment of chronic gouty arthritis when complicated by frequent, recurrent acute attacks of gout
Dosage
  Geriatric & Adult Gout: Oral: One tablet/day for 1 week, then 1 tablet twice daily thereafter
    Note: Current prescribing information states a maximum dose of 4 tablets per day; however this exceeds the usual maximum dose of colchicine for gout prophylaxis (1.2 mg per day).
  Renal Impairment See individual agents.
Special Geriatric Considerations See individual agents.
Dosage Forms Excipient information presented when available (limited, particularly for generics); consult specific product labeling.
Tablet: Colchicine 0.5 mg and probenecid 0.5 g

♦ Colcrys® see Colchicine on page 409

Colesevelam (koh le SEV a lam)

Related Information
Diabetes Mellitus Management, Adults on page 2073
Hyperlipidemia Management on page 2021
Brand Names: U.S. Welchol®
Brand Names: Canada Welchol®
Generic Availability (U.S.) No
Pharmacologic Category Antilipemic Agent, Bile Acid Sequestrant
Use Management of elevated LDL in primary hypercholesterolemia (Fredrickson type IIa) when used alone or in combination with an HMG-CoA reductase inhibitor; management of heterozygous familial hypercholesterolemia (heFH) in adolescent patients (males and postmenarchal females 10-17 years of age) when used alone or in combination with an HMG-CoA reductase inhibitor, in patients who after an adequate trial of dietary therapy have LDL-C ≥190 mg/dL or LDL-C ≥160 mg/dL with positive family history of premature cardiovascular disease (CVD) or with two or more CVD risk factors; improve glycemic control in type 2 diabetes mellitus (noninsulin dependent, NIDDM) in conjunction with diet, exercise, and insulin or oral antidiabetic agents
Contraindications History of bowel obstruction; serum triglyceride concentration >500 mg/dL; history of hypertriglyceridemia-induced pancreatitis

Warnings/Precautions Use with caution in treating patients with serum triglyceride concentrations >300 mg/dL (may cause increased concentrations) or in patients susceptible to fat-soluble vitamin deficiencies. Discontinue if triglyceride concentrations exceed 500 mg/dL or hypertriglyceridemia-induced pancreatitis occurs. Use in patients with gastroparesis, other severe GI motility disorders, or a history of major GI tract surgery is not recommended due to constipating effects of colesevelam. Patients with dysphagia or swallowing disorders should use the oral suspension form of colesevelam due to large tablet size and risk for esophageal obstruction.

Minimal effects are seen on HDL-C and triglyceride levels. Secondary causes of hypercholesterolemia should be excluded before initiation. Colesevelam has not been studied in Fredrickson Type I, III, IV, or V dyslipidemias. Colesevelam is not indicated for the management of type 1 diabetes, particularly in the acute management (eg, DKA). It is also not indicated in type 2 diabetes mellitus as monotherapy and must be used as an adjunct to diet, exercise, and glycemic control with insulin or oral antidiabetic agents. Combination with dipeptidyl peptidase 4 inhibitors or thiazolidinediones has not been studied extensively.

Some products may contain phenylalanine.

Adverse Reactions (Reflective of adult population; not specific for elderly)
>10%: Gastrointestinal: Constipation (11%)
2% to 10%:
  Gastrointestinal: Dyspepsia (8%)
  Neuromuscular & skeletal: Weakness (4%), myalgia (2%)
  Respiratory: Pharyngitis (3%)
Incidence less than or equal to placebo: Infection, headache, pain, back pain, abdominal pain, flu syndrome, flatulence, diarrhea, nausea, sinusitis, rhinitis, cough

Drug Interactions
  Avoid Concomitant Use There are no known interactions where it is recommended to avoid concomitant use.
  Increased Effect/Toxicity There are no known significant interactions involving an increase in effect.
  Decreased Effect
    Colesevelam may decrease the levels/effects of: Amiodarone; Antidiabetic Agents (Thiazolidinedione); Chenodiol; Contraceptives (Estrogens); Contraceptives (Progestins); Corticosteroids (Oral); Ethinyl Estradiol; Ezetimibe; GlyBURIDE; Leflunomide; Loop Diuretics; Methotrexate; Niacin; Nonsteroidal Anti-Inflammatory Agents; Norethindrone; Phenytoin; Pravastatin; Propranolol; Raloxifene; Tetracycline Derivatives; Thiazide Diuretics; Thyroid Products; Ursodiol; Vitamin D Analogs; Vitamin K Antagonists

Stability Store at room temperature. Protect from moisture.

Mechanism of Action Colesevelam binds bile acids including glycocholic acid in the intestine, impeding their reabsorption. Increases the fecal loss of bile salt-bound LDL-C

Pharmacodynamics/Kinetics
  Onset of action: Peak effect: Therapeutic: ~2 weeks
  Absorption: Insignificant
  Excretion: Urine (0.05%) after 1 month of chronic dosing

Dosage
  Geriatric & Adult
    Dyslipidemia: Oral: 1.875 g (oral suspension or 3 tablets) twice daily **or** 3.75 g (oral suspension or 6 tablets) once daily
    Type 2 diabetes: *Combination therapy with insulin or oral antidiabetic agents:* Oral: 1.875 g (oral suspension or 3 tablets) twice daily **or** 3.75 g (oral suspension or 6 tablets) once daily

Administration Administer with meal(s) and a liquid. Make sure patient understands dietary guidelines.

Monitoring Parameters Serum cholesterol, LDL, and triglyceride levels should be obtained before initiating treatment and periodically thereafter (in accordance with NCEP guidelines)

Special Geriatric Considerations The definition of and, therefore, when to treat hyperlipidemia in elderly is a controversial issue. The National Cholesterol Education Program recommends that all adults maintain a plasma cholesterol <160 mg/dL. Elderly with one additional risk factor, goal LDL would be <130 mg/dL. It is the authors' belief that pharmacologic treatment be reserved for those who are unable to obtain a desirable plasma cholesterol concentration by diet alone and for whom the benefits of treatment are believed to outweigh the potential adverse effects, drug interactions, and cost of treatment.

Dosage Forms Excipient information presented when available (limited, particularly for generics); consult specific product labeling.
  Granules for suspension, oral, as hydrochloride:
    Welchol®: 3.75 g/packet (30s) [contains phenylalanine 48 mg/packet; citrus flavor]
  Tablet, oral, as hydrochloride:
    Welchol®: 625 mg

Selected References

Grundy SM, Cleeman JI, Merz CN, et al, "Implications of Recent Clinical Trials for the National Cholesterol Education Program Adult Treatment Panel III Guidelines," *J Am Coll Cardiol*, 2004, 44(3):720-32.

Staels B and Kuipers F, "Bile Acid Sequestrants and the Treatment of Type2 Diabetes Mellitus," *Drugs*, 2007, 67 (10):1383-92.

National Cholesterol Education Program (NCEP) Expert Panel on Detection, Evaluation, and Treatment of High Blood Cholesterol in Adults (Adult Treatment Panel III), "Third Report of the National Cholesterol Education Program (NCEP) Expert Panel on Detection, Evaluation, and Treatment of High Blood Cholesterol in Adults (Adult Treatment Panel III) Final Report," *Circulation*, 2002, 106(25):3143-421.

◆ **Colestid®** *see* Colestipol *on page* 414
◆ **Colestid® Flavored** *see* Colestipol *on page* 414

Colestipol (koe LES ti pole)

Related Information

Hyperlipidemia Management *on page 2021*

Medication Safety Issues

Sound-alike/look-alike issues:

Colestipol may be confused with calcitriol

Brand Names: U.S. Colestid®; Colestid® Flavored

Brand Names: Canada Colestid®

Index Terms Colestipol Hydrochloride

Generic Availability (U.S.) Yes

Pharmacologic Category Antilipemic Agent, Bile Acid Sequestrant

Use Adjunct in management of primary hypercholesterolemia; regression of arteriolosclerosis; relief of pruritus associated with elevated levels of bile acids; possibly used to decrease plasma half-life of digoxin in toxicity

Contraindications Hypersensitivity to bile acid sequestering resins or any component of the formulation; bowel obstruction

Warnings/Precautions Not to be taken simultaneously with many other medicines (decreased absorption). May interfere with fat soluble vitamins (A, D, E, K) and folic acid. Chronic use may be associated with bleeding problems. May produce or exacerbate constipation; fecal impaction may occur, hemorrhoids may be worsened. Some products may contain phenylalanine.

Adverse Reactions (Reflective of adult population; not specific for elderly)

>10%: Gastrointestinal: Constipation

1% to 10%:

Central nervous system: Headache, dizziness, anxiety, vertigo, drowsiness, fatigue

Gastrointestinal: Abdominal pain and distention, belching, flatulence, nausea, vomiting, diarrhea

Drug Interactions

Avoid Concomitant Use There are no known interactions where it is recommended to avoid concomitant use.

Increased Effect/Toxicity There are no known significant interactions involving an increase in effect.

Decreased Effect

Colestipol may decrease the levels/effects of: Amiodarone; Antidiabetic Agents (Thiazolidinedione); Cardiac Glycosides; Chenodiol; Contraceptives (Estrogens); Contraceptives (Progestins); Corticosteroids (Oral); Diltiazem; Ezetimibe; Fibric Acid Derivatives; Leflunomide; Loop Diuretics; Methotrexate; Methylfolate; Niacin; Nonsteroidal Anti-Inflammatory Agents; Pravastatin; Propranolol; Raloxifene; Tetracycline Derivatives; Thiazide Diuretics; Thyroid Products; Ursodiol; Vitamin D Analogs; Vitamin K Antagonists

Mechanism of Action Binds with bile acids to form an insoluble complex that is eliminated in feces; it thereby increases the fecal loss of bile acid-bound low density lipoprotein cholesterol

Pharmacodynamics/Kinetics Absorption: Oral: Not absorbed

Dosage

Geriatric & Adult Dyslipidemia: Oral:

Granules: 5-30 g/day given once or in divided doses 2-4 times/day; initial dose: 5 g 1-2 times/day; increase by 5 g at 1- to 2-month intervals

Tablets: 2-16 g/day; initial dose: 2 g 1-2 times/day; increase by 2 g at 1- to 2-month intervals

Administration Dry powder should be added to at least 90 mL of liquid and stirred until completely mixed; other drugs should be administered at least 1 hour before or 4 hours after colestipol

Monitoring Parameters Serum lipid profile; plasma cholesterol (LDL and VLDL fractions); observe for gastrointestinal side effects

Test Interactions Increased prothrombin time; decreased cholesterol (S)

Special Geriatric Considerations The definition of and, therefore, when to treat hyperlipidemia in the elderly is a controversial issue. The National Cholesterol Education Program recommends that all adults maintain a plasma cholesterol <160 mg/dL. Elderly with one additional risk factor, goal LDL would be <130 mg/dL. It is the authors' belief that pharmacologic treatment be reserved for those who are unable to obtain a desirable plasma cholesterol concentration by diet alone and for whom the benefits of treatment are believed to outweigh the potential adverse effects, drug interactions, and cost of treatment.

Dosage Forms Excipient information presented when available (limited, particularly for generics); consult specific product labeling.

Granules for suspension, oral, as hydrochloride: 5 g/scoop (500 g); 5 g/packet (30s, 90s)

Colestid®: 5 g/scoop (300 g, 500 g); 5 g/packet (30s, 90s) [unflavored]

Colestid® Flavored: 5 g/scoop (450 g) [contains phenylalanine 18.2 mg/scoop; orange flavor]

Colestid® Flavored: 5 g/packet (60s) [contains phenylalanine 18.2 mg/packet; orange flavor]

Tablet, oral, as hydrochloride: 1 g

Tablet, oral, as hydrochloride [micronized]: 1 g

Colestid®: 1 g

Selected References

Grundy SM, Cleeman JI, Merz CN, et al, "Implications of Recent Clinical Trials for the National Cholesterol Education Program Adult Treatment Panel III Guidelines," *J Am Coll Cardiol*, 2004, 44(3):720-32.

National Cholesterol Education Program (NCEP) Expert Panel on Detection, Evaluation, and Treatment of High Blood Cholesterol in Adults (Adult Treatment Panel III), "Third Report of the National Cholesterol Education Program (NCEP) Expert Panel on Detection, Evaluation, and Treatment of High Blood Cholesterol in Adults (Adult Treatment Panel III) Final Report," *Circulation*, 2002, 106(25):3143-421.

◆ **Colestipol Hydrochloride** see Colestipol on page 414
◆ **Colistin, Hydrocortisone, Neomycin, and Thonzonium** see Neomycin, Colistin, Hydrocortisone, and Thonzonium on page 1280

Collagenase (Topical) (KOL la je nase)

Medication Safety Issues

Sound-alike/look-alike issues:

Topical collagenase formulation (Santyl™) may be confused with the injectable collagenase clostridium histolyticum (Xiaflex™)

Brand Names: U.S. Santyl®

Generic Availability (U.S.) No

Pharmacologic Category Enzyme, Topical Debridement

Use Promotes debridement of necrotic tissue in dermal ulcers and severe burns

Contraindications Hypersensitivity to collagenase or any component of the formulation

Warnings/Precautions For external use only. Avoid contact with eyes. Monitor debilitated patients for systemic bacterial infections because debriding enzymes may increase the risk of bacteremia.

Adverse Reactions (Reflective of adult population; not specific for elderly) Frequency not defined.

Local: Irritation, pain and burning may occur at site of application

Drug Interactions

Avoid Concomitant Use There are no known interactions where it is recommended to avoid concomitant use.

Increased Effect/Toxicity There are no known significant interactions involving an increase in effect.

Decreased Effect There are no known significant interactions involving a decrease in effect.

Mechanism of Action Collagenase is an enzyme derived from the fermentation of *Clostridium histolyticum* and differs from other proteolytic enzymes in that its enzymatic action has a high specificity for native and denatured collagen. Collagenase will not attack collagen in healthy tissue or newly formed granulation tissue. In addition, it does not act on fat, fibrin, keratin, or muscle.

Dosage

Geriatric & Adult Dermal ulcers, burns: Topical: Apply once daily (or more frequently if the dressing becomes soiled).

Administration For external use only. Clean target area of all interfering agents listed above. If infection is persistent, apply powdered antibiotic first. Do not introduce into major body cavities. Monitor debilitated patients for systemic bacterial infections.

Special Geriatric Considerations Preventive skin care should be instituted in all older patients at high risk for pressure ulcers. Collagenase is indicated in stage 3 and 4 pressure ulcers.

COLLAGENASE (TOPICAL)

◀ **Dosage Forms** Excipient information presented when available (limited, particularly for generics); consult specific product labeling.
Ointment, topical:
Santyl®: 250 units/g (15 g, 30 g)

- ◆ **Colocort®** *see* Hydrocortisone (Topical) *on page 886*
- ◆ **Coly-Mycin® S** *see* Neomycin, Colistin, Hydrocortisone, and Thonzonium *on page 1280*
- ◆ **Combivent®** *see* Ipratropium and Albuterol *on page 975*
- ◆ **Commit® [OTC]** *see* Nicotine *on page 1297*
- ◆ **Compazine** *see* Prochlorperazine *on page 1524*
- ◆ **Compound E** *see* Cortisone *on page 418*
- ◆ **Compound F** *see* Hydrocortisone (Systemic) *on page 883*
- ◆ **Compound F** *see* Hydrocortisone (Topical) *on page 886*
- ◆ **Compound W® [OTC]** *see* Salicylic Acid *on page 1648*
- ◆ **Compound W® One Step Invisible Strip [OTC]** *see* Salicylic Acid *on page 1648*
- ◆ **Compound W® One-Step Wart Remover [OTC]** *see* Salicylic Acid *on page 1648*
- ◆ **Compound W® One Step Wart Remover for Feet [OTC]** *see* Salicylic Acid *on page 1648*
- ◆ **Compound W® One-Step Wart Remover for Kids [OTC]** *see* Salicylic Acid *on page 1648*
- ◆ **Compoz® [OTC]** *see* DiphenhydrAMINE (Systemic) *on page 520*
- ◆ **Compro®** *see* Prochlorperazine *on page 1524*
- ◆ **Comtan®** *see* Entacapone *on page 602*
- ◆ **Concerta®** *see* Methylphenidate *on page 1179*

Conivaptan (koe NYE vap tan)

Brand Names: U.S. Vaprisol®
Index Terms Conivaptan Hydrochloride; YM087
Generic Availability (U.S.) No
Pharmacologic Category Vasopressin Antagonist
Use Treatment of euvolemic and hypervolemic hyponatremia in hospitalized patients
Contraindications Hypersensitivity to conivaptan, corn or corn products, or any component of the formulation; use in hypovolemic hyponatremia; concurrent use with strong CYP3A4 inhibitors (eg, ketoconazole, itraconazole, ritonavir, indinavir, and clarithromycin); anuria
Warnings/Precautions Monitor closely for rate of serum sodium increase and neurological status; overly rapid serum sodium correction (>12 mEq/L/24 hours) can lead to seizures, permanent neurological damage, coma, or death. Discontinue use if rate of serum sodium increase is undesirable; may reinitiate infusion (at reduced dose) if hyponatremia persists in the absence of neurological symptoms typically associated with rapid sodium rise. Of note, raising serum sodium concentrations with conivaptan has not demonstrated symptomatic benefit. Discontinue if hypovolemia or hypotension occurs. Safety and efficacy in heart failure patients have not been established. Use in small numbers of hypervolemic, hyponatremic heart failure patients led to increased adverse events. In other heart failure studies, conivaptan did not show significant improvements in outcomes over placebo. Coadministration with digoxin may increase digoxin concentrations; monitor digoxin concentrations. Use with caution in patients with hepatic and renal impairment; dosage adjustment required. Do not use in patients with severe renal impairment (Cl_{cr} <30 mL/minute). Contraindicated in patients with anuria. May cause injection-site reactions.
Adverse Reactions (Reflective of adult population; not specific for elderly)
>10%:
Cardiovascular: Orthostatic hypotension (6% to 14%)
Central nervous system: Fever (5% to 11%)
Endocrine & metabolic: Hypokalemia (10% to 22%)
Local: Injection site reactions including pain, erythema, phlebitis, swelling (63% to 73%)
1% to 10%:
Cardiovascular: Hypertension (6% to 8%), hypotension (5% to 8%), peripheral edema (3% to 8%), phlebitis (5%), atrial fibrillation (2% to 5%), ECG abnormality (≤5%)
Central nervous system: Headache (8% to 10%), insomnia (4% to 5%), confusion (≤5%), pain (2%)
Dermatologic: Pruritus (1% to 5%), erythema (3%)
Endocrine & metabolic: Hyponatremia (6% to 8%), hypomagnesemia (2% to 5%), hyper-/hypoglycemia (3%)
Gastrointestinal: Constipation (6% to 8%), vomiting (5% to 7%), diarrhea (≤7%), nausea (3% to 5%), dry mouth (4%), dehydration (2%), oral candidiasis (2%)
Genitourinary: Urinary tract infection (4% to 5%)
Hematologic: Anemia (5% to 6%)
Renal: Polyuria (5% to 6%), hematuria (2%)

Respiratory: Pneumonia (2% to 5%), pharyngolaryngeal pain (1% to 5%)
Miscellaneous: Thirst (3% to 6%)

Drug Interactions

Metabolism/Transport Effects Substrate of CYP3A4 (major); **Inhibits** CYP3A4 (strong)

Avoid Concomitant Use

Avoid concomitant use of Conivaptan with any of the following: Alfuzosin; Antifungal Agents (Azole Derivatives, Systemic); Crizotinib; CYP3A4 Inhibitors (Strong); CYP3A4 Substrates; Dronedarone; Eplerenone; Everolimus; Fluticasone (Oral Inhalation); Halofantrine; Lapatinib; Lovastatin; Lurasidone; Nilotinib; Nisoldipine; Ranolazine; Rivaroxaban; RomiDEPsin; Salmeterol; Silodosin; Simvastatin; Tamsulosin; Ticagrelor; Tolvaptan; Toremifene

Increased Effect/Toxicity

Conivaptan may increase the levels/effects of: Alfuzosin; Almotriptan; Alosetron; Bortezomib; Brentuximab Vedotin; Brinzolamide; Budesonide (Nasal); Budesonide (Systemic, Oral Inhalation); Ciclesonide; Colchicine; Corticosteroids (Orally Inhaled); Crizotinib; CYP3A4 Substrates; CYP3A4 Substrates (Low risk); Dienogest; Digoxin; Dronedarone; Dutasteride; Eplerenone; Everolimus; FentaNYL; Fesoterodine; Fluticasone (Nasal); Fluticasone (Oral Inhalation); GuanFACINE; Halofantrine; Iloperidone; Ixabepilone; Lapatinib; Lovastatin; Lumefantrine; Lurasidone; Maraviroc; MethylPREDNISolone; Nilotinib; Nisoldipine; Paricalcitol; Pazopanib; Pimecrolimus; Ranolazine; Rivaroxaban; RomiDEPsin; Salmeterol; Saxagliptin; Sildenafil; Silodosin; Simvastatin; SORAfenib; Tadalafil; Tamsulosin; Ticagrelor; Tolterodine; Tolvaptan; Toremifene; Vardenafil; Vemurafenib; Vilazodone

The levels/effects of Conivaptan may be increased by: Antifungal Agents (Azole Derivatives, Systemic); CYP3A4 Inhibitors (Moderate); CYP3A4 Inhibitors (Strong); Dasatinib

Decreased Effect

Conivaptan may decrease the levels/effects of: Prasugrel; Ticagrelor

The levels/effects of Conivaptan may be decreased by: CYP3A4 Inducers (Strong); Deferasirox; Herbs (CYP3A4 Inducers); Tocilizumab

Ethanol/Nutrition/Herb Interactions Herb/Nutraceutical: St John's wort may decrease the levels/effects of conivaptan.

Stability Store at 25°C (77°F); brief excursions permitted up to 40°C (104°F). Protect from light and freezing. Do not remove protective overwrap until ready for use.

Mechanism of Action Conivaptan is an arginine vasopressin (AVP) receptor antagonist with affinity for AVP receptor subtypes V_{1A} and V_2. The antidiuretic action of AVP is mediated through activation of the V_2 receptor, which functions to regulate water and electrolyte balance at the level of the collecting ducts in the kidney. Serum levels of AVP are commonly elevated in euvolemic or hypervolemic hyponatremia, which results in the dilution of serum sodium and the relative hyponatremic state. Antagonism of the V_2 receptor by conivaptan promotes the excretion of free water (without loss of serum electrolytes) resulting in net fluid loss, increased urine output, decreased urine osmolality, and subsequent restoration of normal serum sodium concentrations.

Pharmacodynamics/Kinetics

Protein binding: 99%

Metabolism: Hepatic via CYP3A4 to four minimally-active metabolites

Half-life elimination: ~5-8 hours

Excretion: Feces (83%); urine (12%, primarily as metabolites)

Dosage

Geriatric & Adult Euvolemic or hypervolemic hyponatremia: I.V.: 20 mg infused over 30 minutes as a loading dose, followed by a continuous infusion of 20 mg over 24 hours (0.83 mg/hour); may increase to a maximum dose of 40 mg over 24 hours (1.7 mg/hour) if serum sodium not rising sufficiently; total duration of therapy not to exceed 4 days. **Note:** If patient requires 40 mg/24 hours, may administer two consecutive 20 mg/100 mL premixed solutions over 24 hours (ie, 20 mg over 12 hours followed by 20 mg over 12 hours).

Renal Impairment

Cl_{cr} >60 mL/minute: Dose adjustment is not necessary.

Moderate renal impairment (Cl_{cr} 30-60 mL/minute): 10 mg infused over 30 minutes as a loading dose, followed by a continuous infusion of 10 mg over 24 hours; may increase to a maximum dose of 20 mg over 24 hours if serum sodium not rising sufficiently; total duration of therapy not to exceed 4 days.

Severe renal impairment (Cl_{cr} <30 mL/minute): Use is not recommended.

Hepatic Impairment Child-Pugh classes A-C: 10 mg infused over 30 minutes as a loading dose, followed by a continuous infusion of 10 mg over 24 hours; may increase to a maximum dose of 20 mg over 24 hours if serum sodium not rising sufficiently; total duration of therapy not to exceed 4 days.

Administration For intravenous use only; infuse into large veins and change infusion site every 24 hours to minimize vascular irritation. Do not administer with any other product in the same intravenous line or container.

◀ **Monitoring Parameters** Rate of serum sodium increase, blood pressure, volume status, urine output

Special Geriatric Considerations Adverse events in elderly patients were generally similar to those seen in younger patients. In clinical studies, 52% of patients were >65 years of age and 34% were >75 years of age.

Dosage Forms Excipient information presented when available (limited, particularly for generics); consult specific product labeling.

Infusion, premixed in D_5W, as hydrochloride:
Vaprisol®: 20 mg (100 mL)

◆ **Conivaptan Hydrochloride** see Conivaptan on page 416
◆ **Conjugated Estrogen** see Estrogens (Conjugated/Equine, Systemic) on page 658
◆ **Conjugated Estrogen** see Estrogens (Conjugated/Equine, Topical) on page 661
◆ **Constulose** see Lactulose on page 1022
◆ **Contac® Cold + Flu Maximum Strength Non-Drowsy [OTC]** see Acetaminophen and Phenylephrine on page 38
◆ **ControlRx™** see Fluoride on page 751
◆ **ControlRx™ Multi** see Fluoride on page 751
◆ **Copegus®** see Ribavirin on page 1603
◆ **Cordarone®** see Amiodarone on page 97
◆ **Coreg®** see Carvedilol on page 281
◆ **Coreg CR®** see Carvedilol on page 281
◆ **Corgard®** see Nadolol on page 1254
◆ **Coricidin HBP® Chest Congestion and Cough [OTC]** see Guaifenesin and Dextromethorphan on page 848
◆ **Cormax®** see Clobetasol on page 380
◆ **Correctol® [OTC]** see Docusate on page 547
◆ **Correctol® Tablets [OTC]** see Bisacodyl on page 205
◆ **Cortaid® Advanced [OTC]** see Hydrocortisone (Topical) on page 886
◆ **Cortaid® Intensive Therapy [OTC]** see Hydrocortisone (Topical) on page 886
◆ **Cortaid® Maximum Strength [OTC]** see Hydrocortisone (Topical) on page 886
◆ **Cortef®** see Hydrocortisone (Systemic) on page 883
◆ **Cortenema®** see Hydrocortisone (Topical) on page 886
◆ **CortiCool® [OTC]** see Hydrocortisone (Topical) on page 886
◆ **Cortifoam®** see Hydrocortisone (Topical) on page 886
◆ **Cortisol** see Hydrocortisone (Systemic) on page 883
◆ **Cortisol** see Hydrocortisone (Topical) on page 886

Cortisone (KOR ti sone)

Related Information
Corticosteroids on page 2005
Medication Safety Issues
Sound-alike/look-alike issues:
Cortisone may be confused with Cardizem®, Cortizone®
Index Terms Compound E; Cortisone Acetate
Generic Availability (U.S.) Yes
Pharmacologic Category Corticosteroid, Systemic
Use Management of adrenocortical insufficiency
Contraindications Hypersensitivity to cortisone acetate or any component of the formulation; serious infections, except septic shock or tuberculous meningitis; administration of live virus vaccines
Warnings/Precautions Use with caution in patients with thyroid disease, hepatic impairment, renal impairment, cardiovascular disease, diabetes, glaucoma, cataracts, myasthenia gravis, patients at risk for osteoporosis, patients at risk for seizures, or GI diseases (diverticulitis, peptic ulcer, ulcerative colitis) due to perforation risk. Use caution following acute MI (corticosteroids have been associated with myocardial rupture). Because of the risk of adverse effects, systemic corticosteroids should be used cautiously in the elderly in the smallest possible effective dose for the shortest duration. May affect growth velocity. Withdraw therapy with gradual tapering of dose.

May cause hypercorticism or suppression of hypothalamic-pituitary-adrenal (HPA) axis, particularly in patients receiving high doses for prolonged periods. HPA axis suppression may lead to adrenal crisis. Withdrawal and discontinuation of a corticosteroid should be done slowly and carefully. Particular care is required when patients are transferred from systemic corticosteroids to inhaled products due to possible adrenal insufficiency or withdrawal from steroids, including an increase in allergic symptoms. Patients receiving >20 mg per day of prednisone (or equivalent) may be most susceptible. Fatalities have occurred due to adrenal insufficiency in asthmatic patients during and after transfer from systemic corticosteroids to aerosol steroids; aerosol steroids do not provide the systemic steroid needed to treat patients having trauma, surgery, or infections.

Acute myopathy has been reported with high dose corticosteroids, usually in patients with neuromuscular transmission disorders; may involve ocular and/or respiratory muscles; monitor creatine kinase; recovery may be delayed. Corticosteroid use may cause psychiatric disturbances, including depression, euphoria, insomnia, mood swings, and personality changes. Pre-existing psychiatric conditions may be exacerbated by corticosteroid use. Prolonged use of corticosteroids may also increase the incidence of secondary infection, mask acute infection (including fungal infections), prolong or exacerbate viral infections, or limit response to vaccines. Exposure to chickenpox should be avoided; corticosteroids should not be used to treat ocular herpes simplex. Corticosteroids should not be used for cerebral malaria or viral hepatitis. Close observation is required in patients with latent tuberculosis and/or TB reactivity; restrict use in active TB (only in conjunction with antituberculosis treatment). Prolonged treatment with corticosteroids has been associated with the development of Kaposi's sarcoma (case reports); if noted, discontinuation of therapy should be considered.

Adverse Reactions (Reflective of adult population; not specific for elderly)
>10%:
  Central nervous system: Insomnia, nervousness
  Gastrointestinal: Increased appetite, indigestion
1% to 10%:
  Dermatologic: Hirsutism
  Endocrine & metabolic: Diabetes mellitus
  Neuromuscular & skeletal: Arthralgia
  Ocular: Cataracts, glaucoma
  Respiratory: Epistaxis

Drug Interactions

Avoid Concomitant Use
  Avoid concomitant use of Cortisone with any of the following: Aldesleukin; BCG; Natalizumab; Pimecrolimus; Tacrolimus (Topical)

Increased Effect/Toxicity
  Cortisone may increase the levels/effects of: Acetylcholinesterase Inhibitors; Amphotericin B; Deferasirox; Leflunomide; Loop Diuretics; Natalizumab; NSAID (COX-2 Inhibitor); NSAID (Nonselective); Thiazide Diuretics; Vaccines (Live); Warfarin

  The levels/effects of Cortisone may be increased by: Antifungal Agents (Azole Derivatives, Systemic); Aprepitant; Calcium Channel Blockers (Nondihydropyridine); Denosumab; Estrogen Derivatives; Fluconazole; Fosaprepitant; Macrolide Antibiotics; Neuromuscular-Blocking Agents (Nondepolarizing); Pimecrolimus; Quinolone Antibiotics; Roflumilast; Salicylates; Tacrolimus (Topical); Telaprevir; Trastuzumab

Decreased Effect
  Cortisone may decrease the levels/effects of: Aldesleukin; Antidiabetic Agents; BCG; Calcitriol; Corticorelin; Isoniazid; Salicylates; Sipuleucel-T; Telaprevir; Vaccines (Inactivated)

  The levels/effects of Cortisone may be decreased by: Aminoglutethimide; Antacids; Barbiturates; Bile Acid Sequestrants; Echinacea; Mitotane; Primidone; Rifamycin Derivatives; Somatropin; Tesamorelin

Ethanol/Nutrition/Herb Interactions Food: Limit caffeine intake.

Mechanism of Action Decreases inflammation by suppression of migration of polymorphonuclear leukocytes and reversal of increased capillary permeability

Pharmacodynamics/Kinetics
  Onset of action: Peak effect: Oral: ~2 hours; I.M.: 20-48 hours
  Duration: 30-36 hours
  Absorption: Slow
  Distribution: Muscles, liver, skin, intestines, and kidneys
  Metabolism: Hepatic to inactive metabolites
  Half-life elimination: 0.5-2 hours; End-stage renal disease: 3.5 hours
  Excretion: Urine and feces

Dosage

  Geriatric & Adult If possible, administer glucocorticoids before 9 AM to minimize adrenocortical suppression; dosing depends upon the condition being treated and the response of the patient. **Note:** Supplemental doses may be warranted during times of stress in the course of withdrawing therapy.

  Anti-inflammatory or immunosuppressive: Oral: 25-300 mg/day in divided doses every 12-24 hours
  Physiologic replacement: Oral: 25-35 mg/day

Renal Impairment
Hemodialysis: Supplemental dose is not necessary.
Peritoneal dialysis: Supplemental dose is not necessary.
Administration Insoluble in water.
Monitoring Parameters Blood pressure, blood glucose, electrolytes, symptoms of fluid retention
Test Interactions May suppress the wheal and flare reactions to skin test antigens
Pharmacotherapy Pearls Approximately 80% the potency of cortisol; the maximum activity of the adrenal cortex is between 2 AM and 8 AM and it is minimal between 4 PM and midnight; if possible, administer glucocorticoids before 9 AM to minimize adrenocortical suppression; prolonged therapy (>5 days) of pharmacologic doses of corticosteroids may lead to hypothalamic-pituitary-adrenal suppression, the degree of adrenal suppression varies with the degree and duration of glucocorticoid therapy; this must be taken into consideration when taking patients off steroids; supplemental doses may be warranted during times of stress in the course of withdrawal therapy
Special Geriatric Considerations Because of the risk of adverse effects, systemic corticosteroids should be used cautiously in the elderly, in the smallest possible dose, and for the shortest possible time.
Dosage Forms Excipient information presented when available (limited, particularly for generics); consult specific product labeling.
Tablet, oral, as acetate: 25 mg

Cromolyn (Systemic, Oral Inhalation) (KROE moe lin)

Related Information
Asthma on page 2016
Inhalant Agents on page 2010
Brand Names: U.S. Gastrocrom®
Brand Names: Canada Nalcrom®; Nu-Cromolyn; PMS-Sodium Cromoglycate
Index Terms Cromoglycic Acid; Cromolyn Sodium; Disodium Cromoglycate; DSCG
Generic Availability (U.S.) No
Pharmacologic Category Mast Cell Stabilizer

Use
Inhalation: May be used as an adjunct in the prophylaxis of allergic disorders, including asthma; prevention of exercise-induced bronchospasm
Oral: Systemic mastocytosis

Unlabeled/Investigational Use Oral: Food allergy, treatment of inflammatory bowel disease

Contraindications Hypersensitivity to cromolyn or any component of the formulation; acute asthma attacks

Warnings/Precautions Severe anaphylactic reactions may occur rarely; cromolyn is a prophylactic drug with no benefit for acute situations; caution should be used when withdrawing the drug or tapering the dose as symptoms may reoccur; use with caution in patients with a history of cardiac arrhythmias. Dosage of oral product should be decreased with hepatic or renal dysfunction.

Adverse Reactions (Reflective of adult population; not specific for elderly) Frequency not defined.
Cardiovascular: Angioedema, chest pain, edema, flushing, palpitation, premature ventricular contractions, tachycardia
Central nervous system: Anxiety, behavior changes, convulsions, depression, dizziness, fatigue, hallucinations, headache, irritability, insomnia, lethargy, migraine, nervousness, hypoesthesia, postprandial lightheadedness, psychosis
Dermatologic: Erythema, photosensitivity, pruritus, purpura, rash, urticaria
Gastrointestinal: Abdominal pain, constipation, diarrhea, dyspepsia, dysphagia, esophagospasm, flatulence, glossitis, nausea, stomatitis, vomiting
Genitourinary: Dysuria, urinary frequency
Hematologic: Neutropenia, pancytopenia, polycythemia
Hepatic: Liver function test abnormal
Local: Burning
Neuromuscular & skeletal: Arthralgia, leg stiffness, leg weakness, myalgia, paresthesia
Otic: Tinnitus
Respiratory: Dyspnea, pharyngitis
Miscellaneous: Lupus erythematosus

Drug Interactions
Avoid Concomitant Use There are no known interactions where it is recommended to avoid concomitant use.
Increased Effect/Toxicity There are no known significant interactions involving an increase in effect.
Decreased Effect There are no known significant interactions involving a decrease in effect.

Stability Store at room temperature of 15°C to 30°C (59°F to 86°F). Protect from light. Do not use oral solution if solution becomes discolored or forms a precipitate.

Mechanism of Action Prevents the mast cell release of histamine, leukotrienes, and slow-reacting substance of anaphylaxis by inhibiting degranulation after contact with antigens

Pharmacodynamics/Kinetics
Onset: Response to treatment: Oral: May occur within 2-6 weeks
Absorption:
Inhalation: ~8% reaches lungs upon inhalation; well absorbed
Oral: <1% of dose absorbed
Half-life elimination: 80-90 minutes
Time to peak, serum: Inhalation: ~15 minutes
Excretion: Urine and feces (equal amounts as unchanged drug); exhaled gases (small amounts)

Dosage
Geriatric & Adult
Asthma: For chronic control of asthma, taper frequency to the lowest effective dose (ie, 4 times/day to 3 times/day to twice daily). **Note:** Not effective for immediate relief of symptoms in acute asthmatic attacks; must be used at regular intervals for 2-4 weeks to be effective.
Nebulization solution: Initial: 20 mg 4 times/day; usual dose: 20 mg 3-4 times/day
Prophylaxis of bronchospasm (allergen- or exercise-induced):
Note: Administer 10-15 minutes prior to exercise or allergen exposure but no longer than 1 hour before:
Nebulization solution: Single dose of 20 mg
Mastocytosis: Oral: 200 mg 4 times/day; given 1/2 hour prior to meals and at bedtime. If control of symptoms is not seen within 2-3 weeks, dose may be increased to a maximum 40 mg/kg/day
Food allergy (unlabeled use), inflammatory bowel disease (unlabeled use): Oral: Initial dose: 200 mg 4 times/day; may double the dose if effect is not satisfactory within 2-3 weeks; up to 400 mg 4 times/day
Renal Impairment Specific guidelines not available; consider lower dose of oral product.

◀ **Hepatic Impairment** Specific guidelines not available; consider lower dose of oral product.

Administration Oral solution: Open ampul and squeeze contents into glass of water; stir well; administer at least 30 minutes before meals and at bedtime

Monitoring Parameters Periodic pulmonary function tests

Special Geriatric Considerations Evaluate the patient's or caregiver's ability to safely administer the correct dose of medication.

Dosage Forms Excipient information presented when available (limited, particularly for generics); consult specific product labeling.
Solution, for nebulization, as sodium: 20 mg/2 mL (60s, 120s)
Solution, oral, as sodium [concentrate]:
Gastrocrom®: 100 mg/5 mL (96s)

Cromolyn (Nasal) (KROE moe lin)

Medication Safety Issues
  Sound-alike/look-alike issues:
    NasalCrom® may be confused with Nasacort®, Nasalide®
Brand Names: U.S. NasalCrom® [OTC]
Brand Names: Canada Rhinaris-CS Anti-Allergic Nasal Mist
Index Terms Cromoglycic Acid; Cromolyn Sodium; Disodium Cromoglycate; DSCG
Generic Availability (U.S.) Yes
Pharmacologic Category Mast Cell Stabilizer
Use Prevention and treatment of seasonal and perennial allergic rhinitis
Dosage
  Geriatric & Adult Allergic rhinitis (treatment and prophylaxis): Intranasal: Instill 1 spray in each nostril 3-4 times/day; may be increased to 6 times/day (symptomatic relief may require 2-4 weeks)
Dosage Forms Excipient information presented when available (limited, particularly for generics); consult specific product labeling.
Solution, intranasal, as sodium [spray]: 40 mg/mL (26 mL)
NasalCrom®: 40 mg/mL (13 mL, 26 mL) [contains benzalkonium chloride; 5.2 mg/inhalation]

Cromolyn (Ophthalmic) (KROE moe lin)

Brand Names: U.S. Crolom® [DSC]
Brand Names: Canada Opticrom®
Index Terms Cromoglycic Acid; Cromolyn Sodium; Disodium Cromoglycate; DSCG
Generic Availability (U.S.) Yes
Pharmacologic Category Mast Cell Stabilizer
Use Treatment of vernal keratoconjunctivitis, vernal conjunctivitis, and vernal keratitis
Dosage
  Geriatric & Adult Conjunctivitis and keratitis: Ophthalmic: 1-2 drops in each eye 4-6 times/day
Special Geriatric Considerations Evaluate the patient's or caregiver's ability to safely administer the correct dose of ophthalmic medication.
Dosage Forms Excipient information presented when available (limited, particularly for generics); consult specific product labeling. [DSC] = Discontinued product
Solution, ophthalmic, as sodium [drops]: 4% (10 mL)
Crolom®: 4% (10 mL [DSC]) [contains benzalkonium chloride]

♦ **Cromolyn Sodium** see Cromolyn (Nasal) on page 422
♦ **Cromolyn Sodium** see Cromolyn (Ophthalmic) on page 422
♦ **Cromolyn Sodium** see Cromolyn (Systemic, Oral Inhalation) on page 420

Crotamiton (kroe TAM i tonn)

Medication Safety Issues
  Sound-alike/look-alike issues:
    Eurax® may be confused with Efudex®, Eulexin, Evoxac™, serax, Urex
  International issues:
    Eurax [U.S., Canada, and multiple international markets] may be confused with Urex brand name for furosemide [Australia, China,Turkey] and methenamine [U.S., Canada]
Brand Names: U.S. Eurax®
Generic Availability (U.S.) No
Pharmacologic Category Scabicidal Agent

Use Treatment of scabies (*Sarcoptes scabiei*) and symptomatic treatment of pruritus

Contraindications Hypersensitivity to crotamiton or any component of the formulation; patients who manifest a primary irritation response to topical medications

Warnings/Precautions Avoid contact with face, eyes, mucous membranes, and urethral meatus. Do not apply to acutely inflamed or raw skin. For external use only.

Adverse Reactions (Reflective of adult population; not specific for elderly) Frequency not defined. Topical:
Dermatologic: Contact dermatitis, pruritus, rash
Local: Local irritation
Miscellaneous: Allergic sensitivity reactions, warm sensation

Drug Interactions
Avoid Concomitant Use There are no known interactions where it is recommended to avoid concomitant use.
Increased Effect/Toxicity There are no known significant interactions involving an increase in effect.
Decreased Effect There are no known significant interactions involving a decrease in effect.

Stability Store at room temperature.

Mechanism of Action Crotamiton has scabicidal activity against *Sarcoptes scabiei*; mechanism of action unknown

Dosage
Geriatric & Adult
Scabies: Topical: Wash thoroughly and scrub away loose scales, then towel dry; apply a thin layer and massage drug onto skin of the entire body from the neck to the toes (with special attention to skin folds, creases, and interdigital spaces). Repeat application in 24 hours. Take a cleansing bath 48 hours after the final application. Treatment may be repeated after 7-10 days if live mites are still present.
Pruritus: Topical: Massage into affected areas until medication is completely absorbed; repeat as necessary

Administration Lotion: Shake well before using; avoid contact with face, eyes, mucous membranes, and urethral meatus

Special Geriatric Considerations If cure is not achieved after 2 doses, use alternative therapy.

Dosage Forms Excipient information presented when available (limited, particularly for generics); consult specific product labeling.
Cream, topical:
Eurax®: 10% (60 g)
Lotion, topical:
Eurax®: 10% (60 mL, 480 mL)

Cyanocobalamin (sye an oh koe BAL a min)

Brand Names: U.S. CaloMist™; Ener-B® [OTC]; Nascobal®; Twelve Resin-K [OTC]
Index Terms Vitamin B$_{12}$
Generic Availability (U.S.) Yes: Excludes nasal spray
Pharmacologic Category Vitamin, Water Soluble

CYANOCOBALAMIN

Use Treatment of pernicious anemia; vitamin B_{12} deficiency due to dietary deficiencies or malabsorption diseases, inadequate secretion of intrinsic factor, and inadequate utilization of B_{12} (eg, during neoplastic treatment); increased B_{12} requirements due to thyrotoxicosis, hemorrhage, malignancy, liver or kidney disease

CaloMist™: Maintenance of vitamin B_{12} concentrations after initial correction in patients with B_{12} deficiency without CNS involvement

Contraindications Hypersensitivity to cyanocobalamin, cobalt, or any component of the formulation

Warnings/Precautions I.M./SubQ routes are used to treat pernicious anemia; oral and intranasal administration are not indicated until hematologic remission and no signs of nervous system involvement. Treatment of severe vitamin B_{12} megaloblastic anemia may result in thrombocytosis and severe hypokalemia, sometimes fatal, due to intracellular potassium shift upon anemia resolution. Vitamin B_{12} deficiency masks signs of polycythemia vera; use caution in other conditions where folic acid or vitamin B_{12} administration alone might mask true diagnosis, despite hematologic response. Vitamin B_{12} deficiency for >3 months results in irreversible degenerative CNS lesions; neurologic manifestations will not be prevented with folic acid unless vitamin B_{12} is also given. Spinal cord degeneration might also occur when folic acid used as a substitute for vitamin B_{12} in anemia prevention. Use caution in Leber's disease patients; B_{12} treatment may result in rapid optic atrophy. Some parenteral products contain aluminum; use caution in patients with impaired renal function. Some products contain benzyl alcohol. Avoid intravenous route; anaphylactic shock has occurred. Intradermal test dose of vitamin B_{12} is recommended for any patient suspected of cyanocobalamin sensitivity prior to intranasal or injectable administration. Efficacy of intranasal products in patients with nasal pathology or with other concomitant intranasal therapy has not been determined.

Adverse Reactions (Reflective of adult population; not specific for elderly) Frequency not defined.

Cardiovascular: CHF, peripheral vascular disorder, peripheral vascular thrombosis

Central nervous system: Anxiety, dizziness, headache, hypoesthesia, incoordination, pain, nervousness

Dermatologic: Itching, urticaria, exanthema (transient)

Gastrointestinal: Diarrhea, dyspepsia, glossitis, nausea, sore throat, vomiting

Hematologic: Polycythemia vera

Neuromuscular & skeletal: Abnormal gait, arthritis, back pain, myalgia, paresthesia, weakness

Respiratory: Dyspnea, pulmonary edema, rhinitis

Miscellaneous: Anaphylaxis (parenteral) and infection

Drug Interactions

Avoid Concomitant Use There are no known interactions where it is recommended to avoid concomitant use.

Increased Effect/Toxicity There are no known significant interactions involving an increase in effect.

Decreased Effect

The levels/effects of Cyanocobalamin may be decreased by: Chloramphenicol; Colchicine

Ethanol/Nutrition/Herb Interactions Ethanol: Heavy consumption >2 weeks may impair vitamin B_{12} absorption.

Stability

Injection: Clear pink to red solutions are stable at room temperature. Protect from light.

Intranasal spray: Store at 15°C to 30°C (59°F to 86°F); do not freeze. Protect from light.

Mechanism of Action Coenzyme for various metabolic functions, including fat and carbohydrate metabolism and protein synthesis, used in cell replication and hematopoiesis

Pharmacodynamics/Kinetics

Absorption: Oral: Variable from the terminal ileum; requires the presence of calcium and gastric "intrinsic factor" to transfer the compound across the intestinal mucosa

Distribution: Principally stored in the liver and bone marrow, also stored in the kidneys and adrenals

Protein binding: Transcobalamins

Metabolism: Converted in tissues to active coenzymes, methylcobalamin and deoxyadenosylcobalamin; undergoes some enterohepatic recycling

Bioavailability: Intranasal solution: Nascobal®: 6.1% (relative to I.M.)

Dosage

Geriatric & Adult

Recommended intake: 2.4 mcg/day

Vitamin B₁₂ deficiency:

Intranasal:

Nascobal®: 500 mcg in one nostril once weekly

CaloMist™: Maintenance therapy (following correction of vitamin B₁₂ deficiency): 25 mcg in each nostril daily (50 mcg/day). If inadequate response, 25 mcg in each nostril twice daily (100 mcg/day).

Oral: 250 mcg/day

I.M., deep SubQ: Initial: 30 mcg/day for 5-10 days; maintenance: 100-200 mcg/month

Pernicious anemia: I.M., deep SubQ (administer concomitantly with folic acid if needed, 1 mg/day for 1 month): 100 mcg/day for 6-7 days; if improvement, administer same dose on alternate days for 7 doses, then every 3-4 days for 2-3 weeks; once hematologic values have returned to normal, maintenance dosage: 100 mcg/month. **Note:** Alternative dosing of 1000 mcg/day for 5 days (followed by 500-1000 mcg/month) has been used.

Hematologic remission (without evidence of nervous system involvement):

Intranasal (Nascobal®): 500 mcg in one nostril once weekly

Oral: 1000-2000 mcg/day

I.M., SubQ: 100-1000 mcg/month

Schilling test: I.M.: 1000 mcg

Administration

I.M./SubQ: I.M. or deep SubQ are preferred routes of administration

Intranasal: Nasal spray:

Nascobal®: Prior to initial dose, activate (prime) spray nozzle by pumping unit quickly and firmly until first appearance of spray, then prime twice more. The unit must be reprimed once immediately before each subsequent use. Administer 1 hour before or after ingestion of hot foods/liquids.

CaloMist™: Prime unit by spraying 7 times. If ≥5 days since use, reprime with 2 sprays. Separate from other intranasal medications by several hours.

I.V.: Not recommended due to rapid elimination

Oral: Not recommended due to variable absorption; however, oral therapy of 1000-2000 mcg/day has been effective for anemia if I.M./SubQ routes refused or not tolerated.

Monitoring Parameters Vitamin B₁₂, hematocrit, reticulocyte count, folate and iron levels should be obtained prior to treatment; vitamin B₁₂ and peripheral blood counts should be monitored 1 month after beginning treatment, then every 3-6 months thereafter.

Megaloblastic anemia: In addition to normal hematological parameters, serum potassium and platelet counts should be monitored during therapy

CaloMist™: If vitamin B₁₂ levels declining despite maximum doses then should return to I.M. dosing

Reference Range Normal range of serum B₁₂ is 150-750 pg/mL; this represents 0.1% of total body content. Metabolic requirements are 2-5 mcg/day; years of deficiency required before hematologic and neurologic signs and symptoms are seen. Occasional patients with significant neuropsychiatric abnormalities may have no hematologic abnormalities and normal serum cobalamin levels, 200 pg/mL (SI: >150 pmol/L), or more commonly between 100-200 pg/mL (SI: 75-150 pmol/L).

Test Interactions Methotrexate, pyrimethamine, and most antibiotics invalidate folic acid and vitamin B₁₂ diagnostic blood assays

Special Geriatric Considerations There exists evidence that people, particularly elderly whose serum cobalamin concentrations are <500 pg/mL, should receive replacement parenteral therapy or oral replacement (1000 mcg daily). This recommendation is based upon neuropsychiatric disorders and cardiovascular disorders associated with lower sodium cobalamin concentrations.

Dosage Forms Excipient information presented when available (limited, particularly for generics); consult specific product labeling.

Injection, solution: 1000 mcg/mL (1 mL, 10 mL, 30 mL)

Lozenge, oral: 50 mcg (100s); 100 mcg (100s); 250 mcg (100s, 250s); 500 mcg (100s, 250s)

Lozenge, sublingual: 500 mcg (100s)

Solution, intranasal [spray]:

CaloMist™: 25 mcg/spray (10.7 mL) [contains benzalkonium chloride, benzyl alcohol; 60 metered sprays]

Nascobal®: 500 mcg/spray (2.3 mL) [contains benzalkonium chloride; delivers 8 doses]

Tablet, for buccal application/oral/sublingual:

Twelve Resin-K: 1000 mcg [gluten free]

Tablet, oral: 50 mcg, 100 mcg, 250 mcg, 500 mcg, 1000 mcg

Ener-B®: 100 mcg, 500 mcg, 1000 mcg

Tablet, sublingual: 1000 mcg, 2500 mcg, 5000 mcg

Tablet, timed release, oral: 1000 mcg

Ener-B®: 1500 mcg

Selected References

Andres E, Noel E, and Goichot B, "Metformin-Associated Vitamin B$_{12}$ Deficiency," *Arch Intern Med*, 2002, 162 (19):2251-2.

"Dietary Reference Intakes for Thiamin, Riboflavin, Niacin, Vitamin B$_6$, Folate, Vitamin B$_{12}$, Pantothenic Acid, Biotin, and Choline," (Chapter 9) available at http://books.nap.edu/openbook/0309065542/html/306.html. Last accessed February 22, 2005.

Lane LA and Rojas-Fernandez C, "Treatment of Vitamin B$_{12}$-Deficiency Anemia: Oral Versus Parenteral Therapy," *Ann Pharmacother*, 2002, 36(7-8):1268-72.

Schnyder G, Roffi M, Flammer Y, et al, "Effect of Homocysteine-Lowering Therapy With Folic Acid, Vitamin B12, and Vitamin B6 on Clinical Outcome After Percutaneous Coronary Intervention: The Swiss Heart Study: A Randomized Controlled Trial," *JAMA*, 2002, 288(8):973-9.

♦ **Cyanokit®** see Hydroxocobalamin *on page 893*

Cyclizine (SYE kli zeen)

Brand Names: U.S. Bonine® for Kids [OTC]; Marezine® [OTC]
Index Terms Cyclizine Hydrochloride; Cyclizine Lactate
Generic Availability (U.S.) No
Pharmacologic Category Histamine H$_1$ Antagonist; Histamine H$_1$ Antagonist, First Generation; Piperazine Derivative
Use Prevention and treatment of nausea, vomiting, and vertigo associated with motion sickness
Dosage
Geriatric & Adult Motion sickness (prophylaxis and treatment): Oral: 50 mg taken 30 minutes before departure; may repeat in 4-6 hours if needed, up to 200 mg/day
Special Geriatric Considerations Due to anticholinergic action, use lowest dose in divided doses to avoid side effects and their inconvenience; limit use if possible; may cause confusion or aggravate symptoms of confusion in those with dementia; constipation and difficulty voiding urine may occur
Dosage Forms Excipient information presented when available (limited, particularly for generics); consult specific product labeling.
Tablet, oral, as hydrochloride:
 Marezine®: 50 mg
Tablet, chewable, oral, as hydrochloride:
 Bonine® for Kids: 25 mg [scored; berry blast flavor]

♦ **Cyclizine Hydrochloride** see Cyclizine *on page 426*
♦ **Cyclizine Lactate** see Cyclizine *on page 426*

Cyclobenzaprine (sye kloe BEN za preen)

Related Information
Beers Criteria – Potentially Inappropriate Medications for Geriatrics *on page 2089*
Medication Safety Issues
Sound-alike/look-alike issues:
Cyclobenzaprine may be confused with cycloSERINE, cyproheptadine
Flexeril® may be confused with Floxin®
BEERS Criteria medication:
This drug may be inappropriate for use in geriatric patients (high severity risk).
International issues:
Flexin: Brand name for cyclobenzaprine [Chile], but also the brand name for diclofenac [Argentina] and orphenadrine [Israel]
Flexin [Chile] may be confused with Floxin brand name for flunarizine [Thailand], norfloxacin [South Africa], ofloxacin [U.S., Canada], and perfloxacin [Philippines]; Fluoxin brand name for fluoxetine [Czech Republic]
Brand Names: U.S. Amrix®; Fexmid®; Flexeril®
Brand Names: Canada Apo-Cyclobenzaprine®; Dom-Cyclobenzaprine; Flexeril®; Flexitec; Gen-Cyclobenzaprine; Mylan-Cyclobenzaprine; Novo-Cycloprine; Nu-Cyclobenzaprine; PHL-Cyclobenzaprine; PMS-Cyclobenzaprine; ratio-Cyclobenzaprine; Riva-Cycloprine
Index Terms Cyclobenzaprine Hydrochloride
Generic Availability (U.S.) Yes
Pharmacologic Category Skeletal Muscle Relaxant
Use Treatment of muscle spasm associated with acute, painful musculoskeletal conditions
Unlabeled/Investigational Use Treatment of muscle spasm associated with acute temporomandibular joint pain (TMJ)
Contraindications Hypersensitivity to cyclobenzaprine or any component of the formulation; during or within 14 days of MAO inhibitors; hyperthyroidism; congestive heart failure; arrhythmias; heart block or conduction disturbances; acute recovery phase of MI

Warnings/Precautions May cause CNS depression, which may impair physical or mental abilities; patients must be cautioned about performing tasks which require mental alertness (eg, operating machinery or driving). Cyclobenzaprine shares the toxic potentials of the tricyclic antidepressants (including arrhythmias, tachycardia, and conduction time prolongation) and the usual precautions of tricyclic antidepressant therapy should be observed; use with caution in patients with urinary hesitancy or retention, angle-closure glaucoma or increased intraocular pressure, hepatic impairment, or in the elderly. This class of medication is poorly tolerated by the elderly due to anticholinergic effects, sedation, and weakness; efficacy is questionable at dosages tolerated by elderly patients (Beers Criteria). Extended release capsules not recommended for use in mild-to-severe hepatic impairment or in the elderly. Do not use concomitantly or within 14 days after MAO inhibitors; combination may cause hypertensive crisis, severe convulsions. Effects may be potentiated when used with other CNS depressants or ethanol.

Adverse Reactions (Reflective of adult population; not specific for elderly)
>10%:
  Central nervous system: Drowsiness (29% to 39%), dizziness (1% to 11%)
  Gastrointestinal: Xerostomia (21% to 32%)
1% to 10%:
  Central nervous system: Fatigue (1% to 6%), headache (1% to 5%), confusion (1% to 3%), irritability (1% to 3%), mental acuity decreased (1% to 3%), nervousness (1% to 3%), somnolence (1% to 2%)
  Gastrointestinal: Dyspepsia (≤4%), abdominal pain (1% to 3%), constipation (1% to 3%), diarrhea (1% to 3%), nausea (1% to 3%), unpleasant taste (1% to 3%)
  Neuromuscular & skeletal: Weakness (1% to 3%)
  Ocular: Blurred vision (1% to 3%)
  Respiratory: Pharyngitis (1% to 3%), upper respiratory infection (1% to 3%)

Drug Interactions
  Metabolism/Transport Effects Substrate of CYP1A2 (major), 2D6 (minor), 3A4 (minor)
  Avoid Concomitant Use
    Avoid concomitant use of Cyclobenzaprine with any of the following: MAO Inhibitors
  Increased Effect/Toxicity
    Cyclobenzaprine may increase the levels/effects of: Alcohol (Ethyl); Anticholinergics; CNS Depressants; MAO Inhibitors; Methotrimeprazine; Selective Serotonin Reuptake Inhibitors

    The levels/effects of Cyclobenzaprine may be increased by: Abiraterone Acetate; Conivaptan; CYP1A2 Inhibitors (Moderate); CYP1A2 Inhibitors (Strong); Deferasirox; HydrOXYzine; Methotrimeprazine; Pramlintide
  Decreased Effect
    Cyclobenzaprine may decrease the levels/effects of: Acetylcholinesterase Inhibitors (Central)

    The levels/effects of Cyclobenzaprine may be decreased by: Acetylcholinesterase Inhibitors (Central); Cyproterone; Peginterferon Alfa-2b; Tocilizumab

Ethanol/Nutrition/Herb Interactions
  Ethanol: May increase CNS depression; monitor for increased effects with coadministration. Caution patients about effects.
  Food: Food increases bioavailability (peak plasma concentrations increased by 35% and area under the curve by 20%) of the extended release capsule.
  Herb/Nutraceutical: Avoid valerian, kava kava, gotu kola (may increase CNS depression).

Stability
  Amrix®, Flexeril®: Store at 25°C (77°F); excursions permitted to 15°C to 30°C (59°F to 86°F). Fexmid®: Store at 20°C to 25°C (68°F to 77°F).

Mechanism of Action Centrally-acting skeletal muscle relaxant pharmacologically related to tricyclic antidepressants; reduces tonic somatic motor activity influencing both alpha and gamma motor neurons

Pharmacodynamics/Kinetics
  Metabolism: Hepatic via CYP3A4, 1A2, and 2D6; may undergo enterohepatic recirculation
  Bioavailability: 33% to 55%
  Half-life elimination: Range: 8-37 hours; Immediate release tablet: 18 hours; Extended release capsule: 32-33 hours
  Time to peak, serum: Extended release capsule: 7-8 hours
  Excretion: Urine (as inactive metabolites); feces (as unchanged drug)

Dosage
  Geriatric
    Capsule, extended release: Use not recommended
    Tablet, immediate release: Initial: 5 mg; titrate dose slowly and consider less frequent dosing

◀ **Adult Muscle spasm:** Oral: **Note:** Do not use longer than 2-3 weeks

Capsule, extended release: Usual: 15 mg once daily; some patients may require up to 30 mg once daily

Tablet, immediate release: Initial: 5 mg 3 times/day; may increase up to 10 mg 3 times/day if needed

Hepatic Impairment

Capsule, extended release: Mild-to-severe impairment: Use not recommended.

Tablet, immediate release:

Mild impairment: Initial: 5 mg; use with caution; titrate slowly and consider less frequent dosing

Moderate-to-severe impairment: Use not recommended

Administration Oral: Extended release capsules: Administer at the same time each day. Do not crush or chew.

Monitoring Parameters Relief of pain and muscle spasm, liver function tests, mental status

Test Interactions May cause false-positive serum TCA screen.

Special Geriatric Considerations High doses in the elderly caused drowsiness and dizziness; therefore, use the lowest dose possible. Because cyclobenzaprine causes anticholinergic effects, it may not be the skeletal muscle relaxant of choice in the elderly.

This medication is considered to be potentially inappropriate in this patient population (Beers Criteria severity: High).

Dosage Forms Excipient information presented when available (limited, particularly for generics); consult specific product labeling.

Capsule, extended release, oral, as hydrochloride: 15 mg, 30 mg

Amrix®: 15 mg, 30 mg

Tablet, oral, as hydrochloride: 5 mg, 10 mg

Fexmid®: 7.5 mg

Flexeril®: 5 mg, 10 mg

Selected References

Winchell GA, King JD, Chavez-Eng CM, et al, "Cyclobenzaprine Pharmacokinetics, Including the Effects of Age, Gender, and Hepatic Insufficiency," *J Clin Pharmacol*, 2002, 42(1):61-9.

◆ **Cyclobenzaprine Hydrochloride** see Cyclobenzaprine on page 426

Cyclophosphamide (sye kloe FOS fa mide)

Medication Safety Issues

Sound-alike/look-alike issues:

Cyclophosphamide may be confused with cycloSPORINE, ifosfamide

Cytoxan may be confused with cefOXitin, Centoxin®, Ciloxan®, cytarabine, CytoGam®, Cytosar®, Cytosar-U®, Cytotec®

High alert medication:

This medication is in a class the Institute for Safe Medication Practices (ISMP) includes among its list of drugs which have a heightened risk of causing significant patient harm when used in error.

Brand Names: Canada Procytox®

Index Terms CPM; CTX; CYT; Cytoxan; Neosar

Generic Availability (U.S.) Yes

Pharmacologic Category Antineoplastic Agent, Alkylating Agent

Use Treatment of Hodgkin's lymphoma, non-Hodgkin's lymphoma (including Burkitt's lymphoma), chronic lymphocytic leukemia (CLL), chronic myelocytic leukemia (CML), acute myelocytic leukemia (AML), acute lymphocytic leukemia (ALL), mycosis fungoides, multiple myeloma, neuroblastoma, retinoblastoma; breast cancer; ovarian adenocarcinoma

Unlabeled/Investigational Use

Oncology-related uses: Ewing's sarcoma, rhabdomyosarcoma, Wilms tumor, ovarian germ cell tumors, small cell lung cancer, testicular cancer, pheochromocytoma, bone marrow transplantation conditioning regimen

Nononcology uses: Severe rheumatoid disorders, Wegener's granulomatosis, myasthenia gravis, multiple sclerosis, systemic lupus erythematosus, lupus nephritis, autoimmune hemolytic anemia, idiopathic thrombocytic purpura (ITP), and antibody-induced pure red cell aplasia; juvenile idiopathic arthritis (JIA)

Contraindications Hypersensitivity to cyclophosphamide or any component of the formulation

Warnings/Precautions Hazardous agent - use appropriate precautions for handling and disposal. Dosage adjustment may be needed for renal or hepatic failure. Hemorrhagic cystitis may occur; increased hydration and frequent voiding is recommended. Immunosuppression may occur; monitor for infections. May cause cardiotoxicity (HF, usually with higher doses); may potentiate the cardiotoxicity of anthracyclines. May impair fertility; interferes with oogenesis and spermatogenesis. Secondary malignancies (usually delayed) have been reported

Adverse Reactions (Reflective of adult population; not specific for elderly)

>10%:

Dermatologic: Alopecia (40% to 60%) but hair will usually regrow although it may be a different color and/or texture. Hair loss usually begins 3-6 weeks after the start of therapy.

Endocrine & metabolic: Fertility: May cause sterility; interferes with oogenesis and spermatogenesis; may be irreversible in some patients; gonadal suppression (amenorrhea)

Gastrointestinal: Nausea and vomiting (usually beginning 6-10 hours after administration; severe with high-dose therapy); anorexia, diarrhea, mucositis, and stomatitis are also seen

Genitourinary: Severe, potentially fatal, acute hemorrhagic cystitis or urinary fibrosis (7% to 40%)

Hematologic: Anemia, leukopenia (dose-related; recovery: 7-10 days after cessation), thrombocytopenia

1% to 10%:

Cardiovascular: Facial flushing

Central nervous system: Headache

Dermatologic: Skin rash

Respiratory: Nasal congestion occurs when I.V. doses are administered too rapidly; patients experience runny eyes, rhinorrhea, sinus congestion, and sneezing during or immediately after the infusion

Drug Interactions

Metabolism/Transport Effects Substrate of CYP2A6 (minor), 2B6 (major), 2C9 (minor), 2C19 (minor), 3A4 (minor); **Inhibits** CYP3A4 (weak); **Induces** CYP2B6 (weak), 2C8 (weak), 2C9 (weak)

Avoid Concomitant Use

Avoid concomitant use of Cyclophosphamide with any of the following: BCG; Belimumab; Etanercept; Natalizumab; Pimecrolimus; Tacrolimus (Topical); Vaccines (Live)

Increased Effect/Toxicity

Cyclophosphamide may increase the levels/effects of: Leflunomide; Natalizumab; Succinylcholine; Vaccines (Live); Vitamin K Antagonists

The levels/effects of Cyclophosphamide may be increased by: Allopurinol; Belimumab; Conivaptan; CYP2B6 Inhibitors (Moderate); CYP2B6 Inhibitors (Strong); Denosumab; Etanercept; Pentostatin; Pimecrolimus; Quazepam; Roflumilast; Tacrolimus (Topical); Trastuzumab

Decreased Effect

Cyclophosphamide may decrease the levels/effects of: BCG; Cardiac Glycosides; Sipuleucel-T; Vaccines (Inactivated); Vaccines (Live); Vitamin K Antagonists

The levels/effects of Cyclophosphamide may be decreased by: CYP2B6 Inducers (Strong); Echinacea; Tocilizumab

Ethanol/Nutrition/Herb Interactions Herb/Nutraceutical: Avoid black cohosh, dong quai in estrogen-dependent tumors.

Stability Store intact vials of powder at room temperature of 15°C to 30°C (59°F to 86°F). Reconstitute vials with sterile water, normal saline, or 5% dextrose to a concentration of 20 mg/mL. Reconstituted solutions are stable for 24 hours at room temperature and 6 days under refrigeration at 2°C to 8°C (36°F to 46°F). Further dilutions in D_5W or NS are stable for 24 hours at room temperature and 6 days at refrigeration.

Mechanism of Action Cyclophosphamide is an alkylating agent that prevents cell division by cross-linking DNA strands and decreasing DNA synthesis. It is a cell cycle phase nonspecific agent. Cyclophosphamide also possesses potent immunosuppressive activity. Cyclophosphamide is a prodrug that must be metabolized to active metabolites in the liver.

Pharmacodynamics/Kinetics

Absorption: Oral: Well absorbed

Distribution: V_d: 0.48-0.71 L/kg; crosses into CSF (not in high enough concentrations to treat meningeal leukemia)

Protein binding: 10% to 60%

Metabolism: Hepatic to active metabolites acrolein, 4-aldophosphamide, 4-hydroperoxycyclophosphamide, and nor-nitrogen mustard; A large fraction of cyclophosphamide is eliminated by hepatic metabolism.

Half-life elimination: 3-12 hours

Time to peak, serum: Oral: ~1 hour

Elimination: Urine (<30% as unchanged drug, 85% to 90% as metabolites)

Dosage

Geriatric Details concerns dosing in combination regimens should also be consulted: Initial and maintenance for induction: 1-2 mg/kg/day; adjust for renal clearance.

CYCLOPHOSPHAMIDE

◀ **Adult** Details concerns dosing in combination regimens should also be consulted.

Single I.V. doses: 400-1800 mg/m^2 (30-50 mg/kg) per treatment course (1-5 days) which can be repeated at 2-4 week intervals

Continuous I.V. daily doses: 60-120 mg/m^2 (1-2.5 mg/kg) per day

Malignancy: Oral: Usual range (in the manufacturer's labeling): 1-5 mg/kg/day (initial and maintenance dosing)

Breast cancer (unlabeled dosing; combination chemotherapy): Oral:

CEF: 75 mg/m^2/day days 1-14 every 28 days (Levine, 1998)

CMF: 100 mg/m^2/day days 1-14 every 28 days (Bonadonna, 1995; Levine, 1998)

Nephrotic syndrome (refractory; unlabeled use): Oral: 2.5-3 mg/kg/day every day for 60-90 days (when refractory or intolerant to corticosteroid treatment)

JIA/vasculitis (unlabeled use): I.V.: 10 mg/kg every 2 weeks

SLE (unlabeled use): I.V.: 500 mg/m^2 every month; may increase up to a maximum dose of 1 g/m^2 every month (Austin, 1986)

Autologous BMT (unlabeled use): IVPB: 50 mg/kg/dose x 4 days **or** 60 mg/kg/dose for 2 days; total dose is usually divided over 2-4 days

High-dose BMT (unlabeled use):

I.V.:

60 mg/kg/day for 2 days (total dose: 120 mg/kg)

50 mg/kg/day for 4 days (total dose: 200 mg/kg)

1.8 g/m^2/day for 4 days (total dose: 7.2 g/m^2)

Continuous I.V.:

1.5 g/m^2/24 hours for 96 hours (total dose: 6 g/m^2)

1875 mg/m^2/24 hours for 72 hours (total dose: 5625 mg/m^2)

Note: Duration of infusion is 1-24 hours; generally combined with other high-dose chemotherapeutic drugs, lymphocyte immune globulin, or total body irradiation (TBI).

Renal Impairment The FDA-approved labeling states there is insufficient evidence to recommend dosage adjustment and therefore, does not contain renal dosing adjustment guidelines. The following guidelines have been used by some clinicians (Aronoff, 2007):

Cl$_{cr}$ <10 mL/minute: Administer 75% of normal dose

Hemodialysis effects: Moderately dialyzable (20% to 50%)

Administer 50% of dose posthemodialysis

Continuous ambulatory peritoneal dialysis (CAPD): Administer 75% of normal dose

Continuous renal replacement therapy (CRRT): Administer 100% of normal dose

Hepatic Impairment The pharmacokinetics of cyclophosphamide are not significantly altered in the presence of hepatic insufficiency. The FDA-approved labeling does not contain hepatic dosing adjustment guidelines. The following guidelines have been used by some clinicians (Floyd, 2006):

Serum bilirubin 3.1-5 mg/dL or transaminases >3 times ULN: Administer 75% of dose

Serum bilirubin >5 mg/mL: Avoid use

Administration May be administered I.P., intrapleurally, IVPB, or continuous I.V. infusion; may also be administered slow IVP in doses ≤1 g.

I.V. infusions may be administered over 1-24 hours

Doses >500 mg to approximately 2 g may be administered over 20-30 minutes

To minimize bladder toxicity, increase normal fluid intake during and for 1-2 days after cyclophosphamide dose. Most adult patients will require a fluid intake of at least 2 L/day. High-dose regimens should be accompanied by vigorous hydration with or without mesna therapy.

Oral: Tablets are not scored and should not be cut or crushed. To minimize the risk of bladder irritation, do not administer tablets at bedtime.

Monitoring Parameters CBC with differential and platelet count, BUN, UA, serum electrolytes, serum creatinine

Pharmacotherapy Pearls In patients with CYP2B6 G516T variant allele, cyclophosphamide metabolism is markedly increased; metabolism is not influenced by CYP2C9 and CYP2C19 isotypes.

Special Geriatric Considerations Toxicity to immunosuppressives is increased in the elderly. Start with lowest recommended adult doses. Signs of infection, such as fever and WBC rise, may not occur. Lethargy and confusion may be more prominent signs of infection; adjust dose for renal function.

Dosage Forms Excipient information presented when available (limited, particularly for generics); consult specific product labeling.

Injection, powder for reconstitution: 500 mg, 1 g, 2 g

Tablet, oral: 25 mg, 50 mg

Extemporaneously Prepared A 2 mg/mL oral elixir was stable for 14 days when refrigerated when made as follows: Reconstitute a 200 mg vial with aromatic elixir, withdraw the solution, and add sufficient aromatic elixir to make a final volume of 100 mL (store in amber glass container).

Brook D, Davis RE, and Bequette RJ, "Chemical Stability of Cyclophosphamide in Aromatic Elixir U.S.P.," *Am J Health Syst Pharm*, 1973, 30:618-20.

Selected References
Hutchins LF and Lipschitz DA, "Cancer, Clinical Pharmacology, and Aging," *Clin Geriatr Med*, 1987, 3(3):483-503.

Kaplan HG, "Use of Cancer Chemotherapy in the Elderly," *Drug Treatment in the Elderly*, Vestal RE, ed, Boston, MA: ADIS Health Science Press, 1984, 338-49.

Xie H, Griskevicius L, Stahle L, et al, "Pharmacogenetics of Cyclophosphamide in Patients With Hematologic Malignancies," *Eur J Pharm Sci*, 2006, 27(1):54-61.

CycloSERINE (sye kloe SER een)

Medication Safety Issues
Sound-alike/look-alike issues:
CycloSERINE may be confused with cyclobenzaprine, cycloSPORINE
Brand Names: U.S. Seromycin®
Generic Availability (U.S.) No
Pharmacologic Category Antibiotic, Miscellaneous; Antitubercular Agent
Use Adjunctive treatment in pulmonary or extrapulmonary tuberculosis
Unlabeled/Investigational Use Treatment of Gaucher's disease
Contraindications Hypersensitivity to cycloserine or any component of the formulation
Warnings/Precautions Has been associated with CNS toxicity, including seizures, psychosis, depression, and confusion; decrease dosage or discontinue use if occurs. Use with caution in patients with epilepsy, depression, severe anxiety, psychosis, severe renal insufficiency, chronic alcoholism and patients with potential folate deficiency (malnourished, chronic anticonvulsant therapy, or elderly). Prolonged use may result in fungal or bacterial superinfection, including *C. difficile*-associated diarrhea (CDAD) and pseudomembranous colitis; CDAD has been observed >2 months postantibiotic treatment.
Adverse Reactions (Reflective of adult population; not specific for elderly) Frequency not defined.
Cardiovascular: Cardiac arrhythmia
Central nervous system: Drowsiness, headache, dizziness, vertigo, seizure, confusion, psychosis, paresis, coma
Dermatologic: Rash
Endocrine & metabolic: Vitamin B_{12} deficiency
Hematologic: Folate deficiency
Hepatic: Liver enzymes increased
Neuromuscular & skeletal: Tremor
Drug Interactions
Avoid Concomitant Use
Avoid concomitant use of CycloSERINE with any of the following: Alcohol (Ethyl); BCG
Increased Effect/Toxicity
The levels/effects of CycloSERINE may be increased by: Alcohol (Ethyl); Ethionamide; Isoniazid
Decreased Effect
CycloSERINE may decrease the levels/effects of: BCG; Typhoid Vaccine
Ethanol/Nutrition/Herb Interactions
Ethanol: Avoid ethanol (may increase CNS depression).
Food: May increase vitamin B_{12} and folic acid dietary requirements.
Mechanism of Action Inhibits bacterial cell wall synthesis by competing with amino acid (D-alanine) for incorporation into the bacterial cell wall; bacteriostatic or bactericidal
Pharmacodynamics/Kinetics
Absorption: ~70% to 90%
Distribution: Widely to most body fluids and tissues including CSF, breast milk, bile, sputum, lymph tissue, lungs, and ascitic, pleural, and synovial fluids; crosses placenta
Metabolism: Hepatic
Half-life elimination: Normal renal function: 10 hours
Time to peak, serum: 3-4 hours
Excretion: Urine (60% to 70% as unchanged drug) within 72 hours; feces (small amounts); remainder metabolized
Dosage
Geriatric & Adult Note: Some of the neurotoxic effects may be relieved or prevented by the concomitant administration of pyridoxine.

Tuberculosis: Oral: Initial: 250 mg every 12 hours for 14 days, then give 500 mg to 1 g/day in 2 divided doses for 18-24 months (maximum daily dose: 1 g)

◀ **Renal Impairment**
Cl$_{cr}$ 10-50 mL/minute: Administer every 12-24 hours.
Cl$_{cr}$ <10 mL/minute: Administer every 24 hours.
Monitoring Parameters Periodic renal, hepatic, hematological tests, and plasma cycloserine concentrations
Reference Range Toxicity is greatly increased at levels >30 mcg/mL
Special Geriatric Considerations Adjust dose for renal function.
Dosage Forms Excipient information presented when available (limited, particularly for generics); consult specific product labeling.
Capsule, oral:
Seromycin®: 250 mg

◆ **Cycloset®** see Bromocriptine on page 214
◆ **Cycloset®** see Bromocriptine on page 214
◆ **Cyclosporin A** see CycloSPORINE (Ophthalmic) on page 438
◆ **Cyclosporin A** see CycloSPORINE (Systemic) on page 432

CycloSPORINE (Systemic) (SYE kloe spor een)

Medication Safety Issues
Sound-alike/look-alike issues:
CycloSPORINE may be confused with cyclophosphamide, Cyklokapron®, cycloSERINE
CycloSPORINE modified (Neoral®, Gengraf®) may be confused with cycloSPORINE non-modified (SandIMMUNE®)
Gengraf® may be confused with Prograf®
Neoral® may be confused with Neurontin®, Nizoral®
SandIMMUNE® may be confused with SandoSTATIN®
Brand Names: U.S. Gengraf®; Neoral®; SandIMMUNE®
Brand Names: Canada Apo-Cyclosporine®; Neoral®; Rhoxal-cyclosporine; Sandimmune® I.V.; Sandoz-Cyclosporine
Index Terms CsA; CyA; Cyclosporin A
Generic Availability (U.S.) Yes
Pharmacologic Category Calcineurin Inhibitor; Immunosuppressant Agent
Use Prophylaxis of organ rejection in kidney, liver, and heart transplants, has been used with azathioprine and/or corticosteroids; severe, active rheumatoid arthritis (RA) not responsive to methotrexate alone; severe, recalcitrant plaque psoriasis in nonimmunocompromised adults unresponsive to or unable to tolerate other systemic therapy
Unlabeled/Investigational Use Allogenic stem cell transplants for prevention and treatment of graft-versus-host disease; also used in some cases of severe autoimmune disease (eg, SLE) that are resistant to corticosteroids and other therapy; focal segmental glomerulosclerosis; severe ulcerative colitis
Contraindications Hypersensitivity to cyclosporine or any component of the formulation. I.V. cyclosporine is contraindicated in hypersensitivity to polyoxyethylated castor oil (Cremophor® EL).
Rheumatoid arthritis and psoriasis: Abnormal renal function, uncontrolled hypertension, malignancies. Concomitant treatment with PUVA or UVB therapy, methotrexate, other immunosuppressive agents, coal tar, or radiation therapy are also contraindications for use in patients with psoriasis.
Warnings/Precautions [U.S. Boxed Warning]: Renal impairment, including structural kidney damage has occurred (when used at high doses); monitor renal function closely. Use caution with other potentially nephrotoxic drugs (eg, acyclovir, aminoglycoside antibiotics, amphotericin B, ciprofloxacin). **[U.S. Boxed Warning]: Increased risk of lymphomas and other malignancies, particularly those of the skin;** risk is related to intensity/duration of therapy and the use of >1 immunosuppressive agent; all patients should avoid excessive sun/ UV light exposure. **[U.S. Boxed Warning]: Increased risk of infection; fatal infections have been reported.** Latent viral infections may be activated (including BK virus which is associated with nephropathy) and result in serious adverse effects. **[U.S. Boxed Warning]: May cause hypertension.** Use caution when changing dosage forms. **[U.S. Boxed Warning]: Cyclosporine (modified) has increased bioavailability as compared to cyclosporine (non-modified) and cannot be used interchangeably without close monitoring.** Monitor cyclosporine concentrations closely following the addition, modification, or deletion of other medications; live, attenuated vaccines may be less effective; use should be avoided. Increased hepatic enzymes and bilirubin have occurred (when used at high doses); improvement usually seen with dosage reduction.

Transplant patients: To be used initially with corticosteroids. May cause significant hyperkalemia and hyperuricemia, seizures (particularly if used with high dose corticosteroids), and encephalopathy. Make dose adjustments based on cyclosporine blood concentrations. **[U.S. Boxed Warning]: Adjustment of dose should only be made under the direct supervision of an experienced physician.** Anaphylaxis has been reported with I.V. use; reserve for patients who cannot take oral form. **[U.S. Boxed Warning]: Risk of skin cancer may be increased in transplant patients.**

Psoriasis: Patients should avoid excessive sun exposure. **[U.S. Boxed Warning]: Risk of skin cancer may be increased with a history of PUVA and possibly methotrexate or other immunosuppressants, UVB, coal tar, or radiation.**

Rheumatoid arthritis: Safety and efficacy for use in juvenile rheumatoid arthritis have not been established. If receiving other immunosuppressive agents, radiation or UV therapy, concurrent use of cyclosporine is not recommended.

Products may contain corn oil, ethanol, or propylene glycol; injection also contains Cremophor® EL (polyoxyethylated castor oil), which has been associated with rare anaphylactic reactions.

Adverse Reactions (Reflective of adult population; not specific for elderly) Adverse reactions reported with systemic use, including rheumatoid arthritis, psoriasis, and transplantation (kidney, liver, and heart). Percentages noted include the highest frequency regardless of indication/dosage. Frequencies may vary for specific conditions or formulation.

>10%:
Cardiovascular: Hypertension (8% to 53%), edema (5% to 14%)
Central nervous system: Headache (2% to 25%)
Dermatologic: Hirsutism (21% to 45%), hypertrichosis (5% to 19%)
Endocrine & metabolic: Triglycerides increased (15%), female reproductive disorder (9% to 11%)
Gastrointestinal: Nausea (23%), diarrhea (3% to 13%), gum hyperplasia (2% to 16%), abdominal discomfort (<1% to 15%), dyspepsia (2% to 12%)
Neuromuscular & skeletal: Tremor (7% to 55%), paresthesia (1% to 11%), leg cramps/ muscle contractions (2% to 12%)
Renal: Renal dysfunction/nephropathy (10% to 38%), creatinine increased (16% to ≥50%)
Respiratory: Upper respiratory infection (1% to 14%)
Miscellaneous: Infection (3% to 25%)
Kidney, liver, and heart transplant only (≤2% unless otherwise noted):
Cardiovascular: Flushes (<1% to 4%), MI
Central nervous system: Convulsions (1% to 5%), anxiety, confusion, fever, lethargy
Dermatologic: Acne (1% to 6%), brittle fingernails, hair breaking, pruritus
Endocrine & metabolic: Gynecomastia (<1% to 4%), hyperglycemia
Gastrointestinal: Nausea (2% to 10%), vomiting (2% to 10%), diarrhea (3% to 8%), abdominal discomfort (<1% to 7%), cramps (0% to 4%), anorexia, constipation, gastritis, mouth sores, pancreatitis, swallowing difficulty, upper GI bleed, weight loss
Hematologic: Leukopenia (<1% to 6%), anemia, thrombocytopenia
Hepatic: Hepatotoxicity (<1% to 7%)
Neuromuscular & skeletal: Paresthesia (1% to 3%), joint pain, muscle pain, tingling, weakness
Ocular: Conjunctivitis, visual disturbance
Otic: Hearing loss, tinnitus
Renal: Hematuria
Respiratory: Sinusitis (<1% to 7%)
Miscellaneous: Lymphoma (<1% to 6%), allergic reactions, hiccups, night sweats
Rheumatoid arthritis only (1% to <3% unless otherwise noted):
Cardiovascular: Hypertension (8%), edema (5%), chest pain (4%), arrhythmia (2%), abnormal heart sounds, cardiac failure, MI, peripheral ischemia
Central nervous system: Dizziness (8%), pain (6%), insomnia (4%), depression (3%), migraine (2%), anxiety, hypoesthesia, emotional lability, impaired concentration, malaise, nervousness, paranoia, somnolence, vertigo
Dermatologic: Purpura (3%), abnormal pigmentation, angioedema, cellulitis, dermatitis, dry skin, eczema, folliculitis, nail disorder, pruritus, skin disorder, urticaria
Endocrine & metabolic: Menstrual disorder (3%), breast fibroadenosis, breast pain, diabetes mellitus, goiter, hot flashes, hyperkalemia, hyperuricemia, hypoglycemia, libido increased/ decreased
Gastrointestinal: Vomiting (9%), flatulence (5%), gingivitis (4%), gum hyperplasia (2%), constipation, dry mouth, dysphagia, enanthema, eructation, esophagitis, gastric ulcer, gastritis, gastroenteritis, gingival bleeding, glossitis, peptic ulcer, salivary gland enlargement, taste perversion, tongue disorder, gum hyperplasia, weight loss/gain
Genitourinary: Leukorrhea (1%), abnormal urine, micturition urgency, nocturia, polyuria, pyelonephritis, urinary incontinence, uterine hemorrhage
Hematologic: Anemia, leukopenia

◄ Hepatic: Bilirubinemia

Neuromuscular & skeletal: Paresthesia (8%), tremor (8%), leg cramps/muscle contractions (2%), arthralgia, bone fracture, joint dislocation, myalgia, neuropathy, stiffness, synovial cyst, tendon disorder, weakness

Ocular: Abnormal vision, cataract, conjunctivitis, eye pain

Otic: Tinnitus, deafness, vestibular disorder

Renal: BUN increased, hematuria, renal abscess

Respiratory: Cough (5%), dyspnea (5%), sinusitis (4%), abnormal chest sounds, bronchospasm, epistaxis

Miscellaneous: Infection (9%), abscess, allergy, bacterial infection, carcinoma, fungal infection, herpes simplex, herpes zoster, lymphadenopathy, moniliasis, diaphoresis increased, tonsillitis, viral infection

Psoriasis only (1% to <3% unless otherwise noted):

Cardiovascular: Chest pain, flushes

Central nervous system: Psychiatric events (4% to 5%), pain (3% to 4%), dizziness, fever, insomnia, nervousness, vertigo

Dermatologic: Hypertrichosis (5% to 7%), acne, dry skin, folliculitis, keratosis, pruritus, rash, skin malignancies

Endocrine & metabolic: Hot flashes

Gastrointestinal: Nausea (5% to 6%), diarrhea (5% to 6%), gum hyperplasia (4% to 6%), abdominal discomfort (3% to 6%), dyspepsia (2% to 3%), abdominal distention, appetite increased, constipation, gingival bleeding

Genitourinary: Micturition increased

Hematologic: Bleeding disorder, clotting disorder, platelet disorder, red blood cell disorder

Hepatic: Hyperbilirubinemia

Neuromuscular & skeletal: Paresthesia (5% to 7%), arthralgia (1% to 6%)

Ocular: Abnormal vision

Respiratory: Bronchospasm (5%), cough (5%), dyspnea (5%), rhinitis (5%), respiratory infection

Miscellaneous: Flu-like syndrome (8% to 10%)

Drug Interactions

Metabolism/Transport Effects Substrate of CYP3A4 (major), P-glycoprotein; **Inhibits** CYP2C9 (weak), CYP3A4 (moderate), P-glycoprotein

Avoid Concomitant Use

Avoid concomitant use of CycloSPORINE (Systemic) with any of the following: Aliskiren; BCG; Bosentan; Conivaptan; Crizotinib; Dronedarone; Natalizumab; Pimecrolimus; Pitavastatin; Silodosin; Sitaxentan; Tacrolimus; Tacrolimus (Systemic); Tacrolimus (Topical); Tolvaptan; Topotecan; Vaccines (Live)

Increased Effect/Toxicity

CycloSPORINE (Systemic) may increase the levels/effects of: Aliskiren; Ambrisentan; Bosentan; Budesonide (Systemic, Oral Inhalation); Calcium Channel Blockers (Dihydropyridine); Calcium Channel Blockers (Nondihydropyridine); Cardiac Glycosides; Caspofungin; Colchicine; CYP3A4 Substrates; Dabigatran Etexilate; Dexamethasone; Dexamethasone (Systemic); DOXOrubicin; Dronedarone; Eplerenone; Etoposide; Etoposide Phosphate; Everolimus; Ezetimibe; FentaNYL; Fibric Acid Derivatives; Halofantrine; HMG-CoA Reductase Inhibitors; Imipenem; Leflunomide; Loop Diuretics; Lurasidone; Methotrexate; MethylPREDNISolone; Minoxidil; Minoxidil (Systemic); Minoxidil (Topical); Natalizumab; P-Glycoprotein Substrates; Pitavastatin; PredniSOLONE; PredniSOLONE (Systemic); PredniSONE; Protease Inhibitors; Ranolazine; Repaglinide; Rivaroxaban; Salmeterol; Saxagliptin; Silodosin; Sirolimus; Sitaxentan; Tacrolimus; Tacrolimus (Systemic); Tacrolimus (Topical); Tolvaptan; Topotecan; Vaccines (Live); Vilazodone

The levels/effects of CycloSPORINE (Systemic) may be increased by: ACE Inhibitors; Aminoglycosides; Amiodarone; Amphotericin B; Androgens; Antifungal Agents (Azole Derivatives, Systemic); Bromocriptine; Calcium Channel Blockers (Nondihydropyridine); Carvedilol; Conivaptan; Crizotinib; CYP3A4 Inhibitors (Moderate); CYP3A4 Inhibitors (Strong); Dasatinib; Denosumab; Dexamethasone; Dexamethasone (Systemic); Ezetimibe; Fluconazole; GlyBURIDE; Grapefruit Juice; Imatinib; Imipenem; Macrolide Antibiotics; Melphalan; Methotrexate; MethylPREDNISolone; Metoclopramide; MetroNIDAZOLE; MetroNIDAZOLE (Systemic); Nonsteroidal Anti-Inflammatory Agents; Norfloxacin; Omeprazole; P-Glycoprotein Inhibitors; Pimecrolimus; PredniSOLONE; PredniSOLONE (Systemic); PredniSONE; Protease Inhibitors; Pyrazinamide; Quinupristin; Roflumilast; Sirolimus; Sulfonamide Derivatives; Tacrolimus; Tacrolimus (Systemic); Tacrolimus (Topical); Telaprevir; Temsirolimus; Trastuzumab

Decreased Effect

CycloSPORINE (Systemic) may decrease the levels/effects of: BCG; GlyBURIDE; Myco-phenolate; Sipuleucel-T; Vaccines (Inactivated); Vaccines (Live)

The levels/effects of CycloSPORINE (Systemic) may be decreased by: Armodafinil; Ascorbic Acid; Barbiturates; Bosentan; CarBAMazepine; CYP3A4 Inducers (Strong); Defer-asirox; Dexamethasone; Dexamethasone (Systemic); Echinacea; Efavirenz; Fibric Acid Derivatives; Fosphenytoin; Griseofulvin; Imipenem; MethylPREDNISolone; Modafinil; Naf-cillin; Orlistat; P-Glycoprotein Inducers; Phenytoin; PrednisoLONE; PrednisoLONE (Sys-temic); PredniSONE; Rifamycin Derivatives; Somatostatin Analogs; St Johns Wort; Sulfinpyrazone [Off Market]; Sulfonamide Derivatives; Terbinafine; Tocilizumab; Vitamin E

Ethanol/Nutrition/Herb Interactions

Food: Grapefruit juice increases cyclosporine serum concentrations.

Herb/Nutraceutical: Avoid St John's wort; as an enzyme inducer, it may increase the metabolism of and decrease plasma levels of cyclosporine; organ rejection and graft loss have been reported. Avoid cat's claw, echinacea (have immunostimulant properties).

Stability

Capsule: Store at controlled room temperature.

Injection: Store at controlled room temperature; do not refrigerate. Ampuls and vials should be protected from light. Stability of injection of parenteral admixture at room temperature (25°C) is 6 hours in PVC; 12-24 hours in Excel®, PAB® containers, or glass. To minimize leaching of DEHP, non-PVC containers and sets should be used for preparation and administration. Sandimmune® injection: Injection should be further diluted [1 mL (50 mg) of concentrate in 20-100 mL of D_5W or NS] for administration by intravenous infusion.

Oral solution: Store at controlled room temperature; do not refrigerate. Use within 2 months after opening; should be mixed in glass containers.

Neoral® oral solution: Orange juice, apple juice; avoid changing diluents frequently; mix thoroughly and drink at once.

Sandimmune® oral solution: Milk, chocolate milk, orange juice; avoid changing diluents frequently; mix thoroughly and drink at once.

Mechanism of Action Inhibition of production and release of interleukin II and inhibits interleukin II-induced activation of resting T-lymphocytes.

Pharmacodynamics/Kinetics

Absorption: Oral:

Cyclosporine (non-modified): Erratic and incomplete; dependent on presence of food, bile acids, and GI motility

Cyclosporine (modified): Erratic and incomplete; increased absorption, up to 30% when compared to cyclosporine (non-modified); less dependent on food, bile acids, or GI motility when compared to cyclosporine (non-modified)

Distribution: Widely in tissues and body fluids including the liver, pancreas, and lungs

V_{dss}: 4-6 L/kg in renal, liver, and marrow transplant recipients (slightly lower values in cardiac transplant patients)

Protein binding: 90% to 98% to lipoproteins

Metabolism: Extensively hepatic via CYP3A4; forms at least 25 metabolites; extensive first-pass effect following oral administration

Bioavailability: Oral:

Cyclosporine (non-modified): Dependent on patient population and transplant type (<10% in adult liver transplant patients and as high as 89% in renal transplant patients); bioavail-ability of Sandimmune® capsules and oral solution are equivalent; bioavailability of oral solution is ~30% of the I.V. solution

Cyclosporine (modified): Bioavailability of Neoral® capsules and oral solution are equivalent: Adults: 23% greater than with cyclosporine (non-modified) in renal transplant patients; 50% greater in liver transplant patients

Half-life elimination: Oral: May be prolonged in patients with hepatic impairment and shorter in pediatric patients due to the higher metabolism rate

Cyclosporine (non-modified): Biphasic: Alpha: 1.4 hours; Terminal: 19 hours (range: 10-27 hours)

Cyclosporine (modified): Biphasic: Terminal: 8.4 hours (range: 5-18 hours)

Time to peak, serum: Oral:

Cyclosporine (non-modified): 2-6 hours; some patients have a second peak at 5-6 hours

Cyclosporine (modified): Renal transplant: 1.5-2 hours

Excretion: Primarily feces; urine (6%, 0.1% as unchanged drug and metabolites)

Dosage

Geriatric Refer to adult dosing. **Sandimmune® and Neoral®/Genraf® are not bioequiva-lent and cannot be used interchangeably.**

Adult Neoral®/Genraf® and Sandimmune® are not bioequivalent and cannot be used interchangeably.

◀ **Newly-transplanted patients:** Adjunct therapy with corticosteroids is recommended. Initial dose should be given 4-12 hours prior to transplant or may be given postoperatively; adjust initial dose to achieve desired plasma concentration.

Oral: Dose is dependent upon type of transplant and formulation:

Cyclosporine (modified):

Renal: 9 ± 3 mg/kg/day, divided twice daily

Liver: 8 ± 4 mg/kg/day, divided twice daily

Heart: 7 ± 3 mg/kg/day, divided twice daily

Cyclosporine (non-modified): Initial doses of 10-14 mg/kg/day have been used for renal transplants (the manufacturer's labeling includes dosing from initial clinical trials of 15 mg/kg/day [range: 14-18 mg/kg/day]; however, this higher dosing level is rarely used any longer). Continue initial dose daily for 1-2 weeks; taper by 5% per week to a maintenance dose of 5-10 mg/kg/day; some renal transplant patients may be dosed as low as 3 mg/kg/day

Note: When using the non-modified formulation, cyclosporine levels may increase in liver transplant patients when the T-tube is closed; dose may need decreased

I.V.: Cyclosporine (non-modified): Manufacturer's labeling: Initial dose: 5-6 mg/kg/day or one-third of the oral dose as a single dose, infused over 2-6 hours; use should be limited to patients unable to take capsules or oral solution; patients should be switched to an oral dosage form as soon as possible

Note: Many transplant centers administer cyclosporine as "divided dose" infusions (in 2-3 doses/day) or as a continuous (24-hour) infusion; dosages range from 3-7.5 mg/kg/day. Specific institutional protocols should be consulted.

Note: Conversion to cyclosporine (modified) from cyclosporine (non-modified): Start with daily dose previously used and adjust to obtain preconversion cyclosporine trough concentration. Plasma concentrations should be monitored every 4-7 days and dose adjusted as necessary, until desired trough level is obtained. When transferring patients with previously poor absorption of cyclosporine (non-modified), monitor trough levels at least twice weekly (especially if initial dose exceeds 10 mg/kg/day); high plasma levels are likely to occur.

Rheumatoid arthritis: Oral: Cyclosporine (modified): Initial dose: 2.5 mg/kg/day, divided twice daily; salicylates, NSAIDs, and oral glucocorticoids may be continued (refer to Drug Interactions); dose may be increased by 0.5-0.75 mg/kg/day if insufficient response is seen after 8 weeks of treatment; additional dosage increases may be made again at 12 weeks (maximum dose: 4 mg/kg/day). Discontinue if no benefit is seen by 16 weeks of therapy.

Note: Increase the frequency of blood pressure monitoring after each alteration in dosage of cyclosporine. Cyclosporine dosage should be decreased by 25% to 50% in patients with no history of hypertension who develop sustained hypertension during therapy and, if hypertension persists, treatment with cyclosporine should be discontinued.

Psoriasis: Oral: Cyclosporine (modified): Initial dose: 2.5 mg/kg/day, divided twice daily; dose may be increased by 0.5 mg/kg/day if insufficient response is seen after 4 weeks of treatment; additional dosage increases may be made every 2 weeks if needed (maximum dose: 4 mg/kg/day). Discontinue if no benefit is seen by 6 weeks of therapy. Once patients are adequately controlled, the dose should be decreased to the lowest effective dose. Doses <2.5 mg/kg/day may be effective. Treatment longer than 1 year is not recommended.

Note: Increase the frequency of blood pressure monitoring after each alteration in dosage of cyclosporine. Cyclosporine dosage should be decreased by 25% to 50% in patients with no history of hypertension who develop sustained hypertension during therapy and, if hypertension persists, treatment with cyclosporine should be discontinued.

Focal segmental glomerulosclerosis (unlabeled use): Oral: Initial: 3.5-5 mg/kg/day divided every 12 hours (in combination with oral prednisone) (Braun, 2008; Cattran, 1999)

Lupus nephritis (unlabeled use): Oral: Initial: 4 mg/kg/day for 1 month (reduce dose if trough concentrations >200 ng/mL); reduce dose by 0.5 mg/kg every 2 weeks to a maintenance dose of 2.5-3 mg/kg/day (Moroni, 2006)

Severe ulcerative colitis (steroid-refractory) (unlabeled use):

I.V.: Cyclosporine (non-modified): 2-4 mg/kg/day, infused continuously over 24 hours. (Lichtiger, 1994; Van Assche, 2003). **Note:** Some studies suggest no therapeutic difference between low-dose (2 mg/kg) and high-dose (4 mg/kg) cyclosporine regimens (Van Assche, 2003).

Oral: Cyclosporine (modified): 2.3-3 mg/kg every 12 hours (Weber 2006; De Saussure 2005)

Note: Patients responsive to I.V. therapy should be switched to oral therapy when possible.

Renal Impairment For severe psoriasis:

Serum creatinine levels ≥25% above pretreatment levels: Take another sample within 2 weeks; if the level remains ≥25% above pretreatment levels, decrease dosage of cyclosporine (modified) by 25% to 50%. If two dosage adjustments do not reverse the increase in serum creatinine levels, treatment should be discontinued.

Serum creatinine levels ≥50% above pretreatment levels: Decrease cyclosporine dosage by 25% to 50%. If two dosage adjustments do not reverse the increase in serum creatinine levels, treatment should be discontinued.

Hemodialysis: Supplemental dose is not necessary.

Peritoneal dialysis: Supplemental dose is not necessary.

Hepatic Impairment Dosage adjustment is probably necessary; monitor levels closely

Administration

Oral solution: Do not administer liquid from plastic or styrofoam cup. May dilute Neoral® oral solution with orange juice or apple juice. May dilute Sandimmune® oral solution with milk, chocolate milk, or orange juice. Avoid changing diluents frequently. Mix thoroughly and drink at once. Use syringe provided to measure dose. Mix in a glass container and rinse container with more diluent to ensure total dose is taken. Do not rinse syringe before or after use (may cause dose variation).

Combination therapy with renal transplantation:

Everolimus: Administer cyclosporine at the same time as everolimus

Sirolimus: Administer cyclosporine 4 hours prior to sirolimus

I.V.: The manufacturer recommends that following dilution, intravenous admixture be administered over 2-6 hours. However, many transplant centers administer as divided doses (2-3 doses/day) or as a 24-hour continuous infusion. Discard solution after 24 hours. Anaphylaxis has been reported with I.V. use; reserve for patients who cannot take oral form. Patients should be under continuous observation for at least the first 30 minutes of the infusion, and should be monitored frequently thereafter. Maintain patent airway; other supportive measures and agents for treating anaphylaxis should be present when I.V. drug is given. To minimize leaching of DEHP, non-PVC sets should be used for administration.

Monitoring Parameters Monitor blood pressure and serum creatinine after any cyclosporine dosage changes or addition, modification, or deletion of other medications. Monitor plasma concentrations periodically.

Transplant patients: Cyclosporine trough levels, serum electrolytes, renal function, hepatic function, blood pressure, lipid profile

Psoriasis therapy: Baseline blood pressure, serum creatinine (2 levels each), BUN, CBC, serum magnesium, potassium, uric acid, lipid profile. Biweekly monitoring of blood pressure, complete blood count, and levels of BUN, uric acid, potassium, lipids, and magnesium during the first 3 months of treatment for psoriasis. Monthly monitoring is recommended after this initial period. Also evaluate any atypical skin lesions prior to therapy. Increase the frequency of blood pressure monitoring after each alteration in dosage of cyclosporine. Cyclosporine dosage should be decreased by 25% to 50% in patients with no history of hypertension who develop sustained hypertension during therapy and, if hypertension persists, treatment with cyclosporine should be discontinued.

Rheumatoid arthritis: Baseline blood pressure, and serum creatinine (2 levels each); serum creatinine every 2 weeks for first 3 months, then monthly if patient is stable. Increase the frequency of blood pressure monitoring after each alteration in dosage of cyclosporine. Cyclosporine dosage should be decreased by 25% to 50% in patients with no history of hypertension who develop sustained hypertension during therapy and, if hypertension persists, treatment with cyclosporine should be discontinued.

Reference Range Reference ranges are method dependent and specimen dependent; use the same analytical method consistently

Method-dependent and specimen-dependent: Trough levels should be obtained:

Oral: 12-18 hours after dose (chronic usage)

I.V.: 12 hours after dose **or** immediately prior to next dose

Therapeutic range: Not absolutely defined, dependent on organ transplanted, time after transplant, organ function and CsA toxicity:

General range of 100-400 ng/mL

Toxic level: Not well defined, nephrotoxicity may occur at any level

Recommend cyclosporine therapeutic ranges when administered in combination with everolimus for renal transplant (Zortress® product labeling, 2010):

Month 1 post-transplant: 100-200 ng/mL

Months 2 and 3 post-transplant: 75-150 ng/mL

Months 4 and 5 post-transplant: 50-100 ng/mL

Months 6-12 post-transplant: 25-50 ng/mL

Test Interactions Specific whole blood assay for cyclosporine may be falsely elevated if sample is drawn from the same central venous line through which dose was administered (even if flush has been administered and/or dose was given hours before); cyclosporine metabolites cross-react with radioimmunoassay and fluorescence polarization immunoassay

Pharmacotherapy Pearls Cyclosporine (modified): Refers to the capsule dosage formulation of cyclosporine in an aqueous dispersion (previously referred to as "microemulsion"). Cyclosporine (modified) has increased bioavailability as compared to cyclosporine (non-modified) and cannot be used interchangeably without close monitoring.

◀ **Special Geriatric Considerations** Cyclosporine has not been specifically studied in the elderly. Cyclosporine is being used in combination therapy for the treatment of severe rheumatoid arthritis.

Dosage Forms Excipient information presented when available (limited, particularly for generics); consult specific product labeling.

Capsule, oral [modified]:

Gengraf®: 25 mg, 100 mg [contains ethanol 12.8%]

Capsule, oral [non-modified]: 25 mg, 100 mg

Capsule, softgel, oral [modified]: 25 mg, 50 mg, 100 mg

Neoral®: 25 mg, 100 mg [contains corn oil, dehydrated ethanol 11.9%]

Capsule, softgel, oral [non-modified]:

SandIMMUNE®: 25 mg, 100 mg [contains corn oil, dehydrated ethanol 12.7%]

Injection, solution [non-modified]: 50 mg/mL (5 mL)

SandIMMUNE®: 50 mg/mL (5 mL) [contains ethanol 32.9%, polyoxyethylated castor oil]

Injection, solution [non-modified, preservative free]: 50 mg/mL (5 mL)

Solution, oral [modified]: 100 mg/mL (50 mL)

Gengraf®: 100 mg/mL (50 mL) [contains propylene glycol]

Neoral®: 100 mg/mL (50 mL) [contains corn oil, dehydrated ethanol 11.9%, propylene glycol]

Solution, oral [non-modified]: 100 mg/mL (50 mL)

SandIMMUNE®: 100 mg/mL (50 mL) [contains ethanol 12.5%]

CycloSPORINE (Ophthalmic) (SYE kloe spor een)

Medication Safety Issues

Sound-alike/look-alike issues:

CycloSPORINE may be confused with cyclophosphamide, Cyklokapron®, cycloSERINE

Brand Names: U.S. Restasis®

Index Terms CsA; CyA; Cyclosporin A

Generic Availability (U.S.) No

Pharmacologic Category Immunosuppressant Agent

Use Increase tear production when suppressed tear production is presumed to be due to keratoconjunctivitis sicca-associated ocular inflammation (in patients not already using topical anti-inflammatory drugs or punctal plugs)

Dosage

Geriatric & Adult Keratoconjunctivitis sicca: Ophthalmic (Restasis®): Instill 1 drop in each eye every 12 hours

Dosage Forms Excipient information presented when available (limited, particularly for generics); consult specific product labeling.

Emulsion, ophthalmic [drops, preservative free]:

Restasis®: 0.05% (0.4 mL) [contains castor oil]

◆ **Cymbalta®** see DULoxetine on page 583

Cyproheptadine (si proe HEP ta deen)

Related Information

Beers Criteria – Potentially Inappropriate Medications for Geriatrics on page 2089

Medication Safety Issues

Sound-alike/look-alike issues:

Cyproheptadine may be confused with cyclobenzaprine

Periactin may be confused with Perative®, Percodan®, Persantine®

BEERS Criteria medication:

This drug may be inappropriate for use in geriatric patients (high severity risk).

Index Terms Cyproheptadine Hydrochloride; Periactin

Generic Availability (U.S.) Yes

Pharmacologic Category Histamine H_1 Antagonist; Histamine H_1 Antagonist, First Generation; Piperidine Derivative

Use Perennial and seasonal allergic rhinitis and other allergic symptoms including urticaria

Unlabeled/Investigational Use Migraine headache prophylaxis, pruritus, spasticity associated with spinal cord damage

Contraindications Hypersensitivity to cyproheptadine or any component of the formulation; narrow-angle glaucoma; bladder neck obstruction; pyloroduodenal obstruction; symptomatic prostatic hyperplasia; stenosing peptic ulcer; concurrent use of MAO inhibitors; use in debilitated elderly patients

Warnings/Precautions May cause CNS depression, which may impair physical or mental abilities; patients must be cautioned about performing tasks which require mental alertness (eg, operating machinery or driving). Effects may be potentiated when used with other sedative drugs or ethanol. Use with caution in patients with cardiovascular disease; increased intraocular pressure; respiratory disease; or thyroid dysfunction. May be inappropriate for use in the elderly due to potent anticholinergic effects (Beers Criteria).

Adverse Reactions (Reflective of adult population; not specific for elderly) Frequency not defined.

Cardiovascular: Extrasystoles, hypotension, palpitation, tachycardia

Central nervous system: Confusion, coordination disturbed, dizziness, excitation, euphoria, faintness, hallucinations, headache, hysteria, insomnia, irritability, nervousness, neuritis, restlessness, sedation, seizure, sleepiness, tremor, vertigo

Dermatologic: Angioedema, photosensitivity, rash, urticaria

Gastrointestinal: Abdominal pain, anorexia, appetite increased, constipation, diarrhea, nausea, vomiting, xerostomia

Genitourinary: Difficult urination, urinary frequency, urinary retention

Hematologic: Agranulocytosis, hemolytic anemia, leukopenia, thrombocytopenia

Hepatic: Cholestasis, hepatic failure, hepatitis, jaundice

Neuromuscular & skeletal: Paresthesia

Ocular: Blurred vision, diplopia

Otic: Labyrinthitis (acute), tinnitus

Respiratory: Bronchial secretions (thickening), nasal congestion, pharyngitis

Miscellaneous: Allergic reactions, anaphylactic shock, chills, diaphoresis, fatigue

Drug Interactions

Avoid Concomitant Use There are no known interactions where it is recommended to avoid concomitant use.

Increased Effect/Toxicity

Cyproheptadine may increase the levels/effects of: Alcohol (Ethyl); Anticholinergics; CNS Depressants

The levels/effects of Cyproheptadine may be increased by: Droperidol; HydrOXYzine; Pramlintide

Decreased Effect

Cyproheptadine may decrease the levels/effects of: Acetylcholinesterase Inhibitors (Central); Benzylpenicilloyl Polylysine; Betahistine; Selective Serotonin Reuptake Inhibitors

The levels/effects of Cyproheptadine may be decreased by: Acetylcholinesterase Inhibitors (Central); Amphetamines

Ethanol/Nutrition/Herb Interactions Ethanol: May increase CNS depression; monitor for increased effects with coadministration. Caution patients about effects.

Mechanism of Action A potent antihistamine and serotonin antagonist, competes with histamine for H_1-receptor sites on effector cells in the gastrointestinal tract, blood vessels, and respiratory tract

Pharmacodynamics/Kinetics

Absorption: Completely

Metabolism: Almost completely hepatic

Time to peak, plasma: 6-9 hours (Hintze, 1975)

Excretion: Urine (~40% primarily as metabolites); feces (2% to 20%)

Dosage

Geriatric Initiate therapy at the lower end of the dosage range.

Adult

Allergic conditions: Oral: 4-20 mg/day divided every 8 hours (not to exceed 0.5 mg/kg/day); some patients may require up to 32 mg/day for adequate control of symptoms

Spasticity associated with spinal cord damage (unlabeled use): Oral: Initial: 2-4 mg every 8 hours; maximum: 8 mg every 8 hours (Barbeau, 1982; Wainberg, 1990)

Test Interactions Diagnostic antigen skin test results may be suppressed; false positive serum TCA screen

Special Geriatric Considerations Elderly patients may not tolerate the anticholinergic effects of cyproheptadine.

This medication is considered to be potentially inappropriate in this patient population (Beers Criteria severity: High).

Dosage Forms Excipient information presented when available (limited, particularly for generics); consult specific product labeling.

Syrup, oral, as hydrochloride: 2 mg/5 mL (473 mL, 480 mL)

Tablet, oral, as hydrochloride: 4 mg

◆ **Cyproheptadine Hydrochloride** see Cyproheptadine on page 438

◆ **CYT** see Cyclophosphamide on page 428

- **Cytomel®** *see* Liothyronine *on page 1072*
- **Cytotec®** *see* Misoprostol *on page 1225*
- **Cytovene®-IV** *see* Ganciclovir (Systemic) *on page 809*
- **Cytoxan** *see* Cyclophosphamide *on page 428*
- **Cytra-2** *see* Sodium Citrate and Citric Acid *on page 1693*
- **Cytra-3** *see* Citric Acid, Sodium Citrate, and Potassium Citrate *on page 368*
- **D2** *see* Ergocalciferol *on page 618*
- **D2E7** *see* Adalimumab *on page 46*
- **D3** *see* Cholecalciferol *on page 346*
- **D-3 [OTC]** *see* Cholecalciferol *on page 346*
- **D3-5™ [OTC]** *see* Cholecalciferol *on page 346*
- **D3-50™ [OTC]** *see* Cholecalciferol *on page 346*
- **D-3-Mercaptovaline** *see* Penicillamine *on page 1412*

Dabigatran Etexilate (da BIG a tran ett EX ill ate)

Brand Names: U.S. Pradaxa®
Brand Names: Canada Pradax™
Index Terms Dabigatran Etexilate Mesylate
Pharmacologic Category Anticoagulant, Thrombin Inhibitor
Use Prevention of stroke and systemic embolism in patients with nonvalvular atrial fibrillation
2011 ACCF/AHA/HRS atrial fibrillation guidelines: Not recommended for patients with coexisting prosthetic heart valve or hemodynamically significant valve disease, severe renal failure (Cl_{cr} <15 mL/minute), or advanced liver disease (impaired baseline clotting function)

Canadian labeling: Additional uses (not in U.S. labeling): Postoperative thromboprophylaxis in patients who have undergone total hip or knee replacement procedures
Medication Guide Available Yes
Contraindications Serious hypersensitivity (eg, anaphylaxis) to dabigatran or any component of the formulation; active pathological bleeding

Canadian labeling: Additional contraindications (not in U.S. labeling): Severe renal impairment (Cl_{cr} <30 mL/minute); bleeding diathesis or patients with spontaneous or pharmacological hemostatic impairment; lesions at risk of clinically significant bleeding (eg, hemorrhagic or ischemic cerebral infarction) within previous 6 months; concomitant therapy with oral ketoconazole
Warnings/Precautions The most common complication is bleeding, and sometimes fatal bleeding. Risk factors for bleeding include concurrent use of drugs that increase the risk of bleeding (eg, antiplatelet agents, heparin) and labor and delivery. Monitor for signs and symptoms of bleeding; discontinue in patients with active pathological bleeding; **no specific antidote exists for dabigatran reversal.** Therapy for severe hemorrhage may include transfusions of fresh frozen plasma, packed red blood cells, or surgical intervention when appropriate (Wann, 2011). The use of a PCC (Cofact ®, not available in the U.S.) has been shown **not** to be effective for dabigatran reversal (Eerenberg, 2011). Use in patients with moderate hepatic impairment (Child-Pugh class B) demonstrated large inter-subject variability; however no consistent change in exposure or pharmacodynamics was seen. Use in patients with advanced liver disease (impaired baseline clotting function) is not recommended (Wann, 2011). Use in patients with a coexisting prosthetic heart valve or hemodynamically significant valve disease is not recommended (Wann, 2011).

Due to an increased risk of bleeding, avoid use with other direct thrombin inhibitors (eg, bivalirudin), unfractionated heparin or heparin derivatives, low molecular weight heparins (eg, enoxaparin), fondaparinux, thienopyridines (eg, clopidogrel, ticlodipine), GPIIb/IIIa antagonists (eg, eptifibatide), aspirin, coumarin derivatives, and sulfinpyrazone. NSAIDs should be used cautiously. Appropriate doses of unfractionated heparin may be used to maintain catheter patency. The concomitant use of P-gp inducers (eg, rifampin) may reduce dabigatran bioavailability and should be avoided. Concurrent use of certain P-gp inhibitors (ie, ketoconazole, verapamil, amiodarone, quinidine, and clarithromycin) does not require dosage adjustment; however, this should not be extrapolated to other P-gp inhibitors. Despite this, concurrent use of oral ketoconazole is contraindicated in the Canadian labeling.

Evaluate renal function prior to and during therapy. Discontinue therapy in patients who develop acute renal failure. Use dabigatran with caution in patients with severe renal impairment (Cl_{cr} 15-30 mL/minute); dosage reduction required. Use in patients with Cl_{cr} <15 mL/minute is not recommended due to insufficient evidence to support use. Canadian labeling contraindicates use in severe renal impairment (Cl_{cr} <30 mL/minute) and recommends indication-specific dose reductions in patients with moderate impairment (Cl_{cr} 30-50 mL/minute). According to the manufacturer, risk of bleeding and stroke increases with age; however, the risk-benefit profile was similar in all age groups in the RE-LY trial, therefore, no dosage adjustment is recommended in the U.S. labeling (unless renal impairment coexists). However, case reports of serious bleeding including fatality has occurred in the elderly with low body weight and mild-moderate renal impairment; the risk is expected to be higher in patients receiving other interacting drugs (eg, amiodarone) (Legrand, 2011). Canadian labeling recommends a dose reduction for patients ≥80 years of age with atrial fibrillation and suggests that dose reductions may be considered in patients >75 years receiving postoperative thromboprophylaxis.

If possible, discontinue dabigatran 1-2 days (Cl_{cr} ≥50 mL/minute) or 3-5 days (Cl_{cr} <50 mL/minute) before invasive or surgical procedures due to the risk of bleeding; consider longer times for patients undergoing major surgery, spinal puncture, or insertion of a spinal or epidural catheter or port. If surgery cannot be delayed, the risk of bleeding is elevated; weigh risk of bleeding with urgency of procedure. Bleeding risk can be assessed by the ecarin clotting time (ECT) if available; if ECT is not available, use of aPTT may provide an approximation of dabigatran's anticoagulant activity. When temporarily discontinuing anticoagulants, including dabigatran, for active bleeding, elective surgery, or invasive procedures, the risk of stroke may increase (dependent on amount of elapsed time); avoid lapses in therapy and reinitiate therapy as soon as possible if discontinuation is warranted.

Adverse Reactions (Reflective of adult population; not specific for elderly) Adverse reactions listed below are reflective of both the U.S. and Canadian product information. **Important:** No specific antidote exists for dabigatran reversal. Therapy for severe hemorrhage may include transfusions of fresh frozen plasma, packed red blood cells, or surgical intervention when appropriate (Wann, 2011).

>10%:
Gastrointestinal: Dyspepsia (11%; includes abdominal discomfort/pain, epigastric discomfort)
Hematologic: Bleeding (8% to 33%; major: ≤6%)
1% to 10%:
Gastrointestinal: GI hemorrhage (≤6%), gastritis-like symptoms (eg, GERD, esophagitis, erosive gastritis, GI ulcer)
Hematologic: Anemia (1% to 4%), hematoma (1% to 2%), hemoglobin decreased (1% to 2%), hemorrhage (postprocedural or wound: 1% to 2%)
Hepatic: ALT increased (≥3 x ULN: 2% to 3%)
Renal: Hematuria (1%)
Miscellaneous: Wound secretion (5%), postprocedural discharge (1%)

Drug Interactions
Avoid Concomitant Use
Avoid concomitant use of Dabigatran Etexilate with any of the following: P-Glycoprotein Inducers; Rivaroxaban
Increased Effect/Toxicity
Dabigatran Etexilate may increase the levels/effects of: Anticoagulants; Collagenase (Systemic); Deferasirox; Ibritumomab; Rivaroxaban; Tositumomab and Iodine I 131 Tositumomab

The levels/effects of Dabigatran Etexilate may be increased by: Amiodarone; Antiplatelet Agents; Dasatinib; Herbs (Anticoagulant/Antiplatelet Properties); Nonsteroidal Anti-Inflammatory Agents; Pentosan Polysulfate Sodium; P-Glycoprotein Inhibitors; Prostacyclin Analogues; QuiNIDine; Salicylates; Thrombolytic Agents; Verapamil
Decreased Effect
The levels/effects of Dabigatran Etexilate may be decreased by: Antacids; Atorvastatin; P-Glycoprotein Inducers; Proton Pump Inhibitors
Ethanol/Nutrition/Herb Interactions
Food: Food has no affect on the bioavailability of dabigatran, but delays the time to peak plasma concentrations by 2 hours.
Herb/Nutraceutical: St John's wort may decrease levels/effects of dabigatran (concomitant use is not recommended). Concomitant use of dabigatran with herbs possessing anticoagulant/antiplatelet properties may increase the risk for bleeding.
Stability
Blister: Store at 25°C (77°F); excursions permitted between 15°C to 30°C (59°F to 86°F). Protect from moisture.
Bottle: Store at 25°C (77°F); excursions permitted between 15°C to 30°C (59°F to 86°F). Dispense and store in original manufacturer's bottle to protect from moisture; discard 60 days after opening original container.
Mechanism of Action Prodrug lacking anticoagulant activity that is converted *in vivo* to the active dabigatran, a specific, reversible, direct thrombin inhibitor that inhibits both free and fibrin-bound thrombin. Inhibits coagulation by preventing thrombin-mediated effects, including

cleavage of fibrinogen to fibrin monomers, activation of factors V, VIII, XI, and XIII, and inhibition of thrombin-induced platelet aggregation.

Pharmacodynamics/Kinetics

Absorption: Rapid; initially slow postoperatively

Distribution: V_d: 50-70 L

Protein binding: 35%

Metabolism: Hepatic; dabigatran etexilate is rapidly and completely hydrolyzed to dabigatran (active form) by plasma and hepatic esterases; dabigatran undergoes hepatic glucuronidation to active acylglucuronide isomers (similar activity to parent compound; accounts for <10% of total dabigatran in plasma)

Bioavailability: 3% to 7%

Half-life elimination: 12-17 hours; Elderly: 14-17 hours; Mild-to-moderate renal impairment: 15-18 hours; Severe renal impairment: 28 hours (Stangier, 2010)

Time to peak, plasma: Dabigatran: 1 hour; delayed 2 hours by food (no effect on bioavailability)

Excretion: Urine (80%)

Dosage

Geriatric

Nonvalvular atrial fibrillation (to prevent stroke and systemic embolism): Oral:

U.S. labeling: Patients >65 years: Refer to adult dosing. No dosage adjustment required unless renal impairment exists.

Canadian labeling:

Patients <80 years: 150 mg twice daily; **Note:** The manufacturer labeling suggests that a dose reduction to 110 mg twice daily may be considered in patients >75 years with at least one other risk factor for bleeding, however, efficacy in stroke prevention may be lessened with this dose reduction.

Patients ≥80 years: 110 mg twice daily

Postoperative thromboprophylaxis (Canadian labeling): Oral: Patients >75 years: 220 mg/day. Manufacturer labeling suggests that a dose reduction to 150 mg/day may be considered.

Adult

Nonvalvular atrial fibrillation (to prevent stroke and systemic embolism): Oral: 150 mg twice daily

Conversion from a parenteral anticoagulant: Initiate dabigatran ≤2 hours prior to the time of the next scheduled dose of the parenteral anticoagulant (eg, enoxaparin) or at the time of discontinuation for a continuously administered parenteral drug (eg, I.V. heparin); discontinue parenteral anticoagulant at the time of dabigatran initiation.

Conversion to a parenteral anticoagulant: Wait 12 hours (Cl_{cr} ≥30 mL/minute) or 24 hours (Cl_{cr} <30 mL/minute) after the last dose of dabigatran before initiating a parenteral anticoagulant.

Conversion from warfarin: Discontinue warfarin and initiate dabigatran when INR <2.0

Conversion to warfarin: Start time must be adjusted based on Cl_{cr}:

Cl_{cr} >50 mL/minute: Initiate warfarin 3 days before discontinuation of dabigatran

Cl_{cr} 31-50 mL/minute: Initiate warfarin 2 days before discontinuation of dabigatran

Cl_{cr} 15-30 mL/minute: Initiate warfarin 1 day before discontinuation of dabigatran

Cl_{cr} <15 mL/minute: No recommendations provided

Note: Since dabigatran contributes to INR elevation, warfarin's effect on the INR will be better reflected after dabigatran has been stopped for ≥2 days

Postoperative thromboprophylaxis (Canadian labeling): Oral: **Note:** Therapy should not be initiated until hemostasis has been established. When transitioning from parenteral anticoagulation therapy, initiate oral dabigatran therapy ≤2 hours prior to the time of next regularly scheduled dose of intermittent parenteral anticoagulant or at the time of discontinuation for continuously administered parenteral anticoagulation therapy. When transitioning from dabigatran to I.V. anticoagulation therapy, allow 24 hours after the last dabigatran dose before initiating I.V. anticoagulation therapy.

Knee replacement: Initial: 110 mg given 1-4 hours after completion of surgery and establishment of hemostasis **OR** 220 mg as 1 dose in postoperative patients in whom therapy is not initiated on day of surgery regardless of reason; maintenance: 220 mg once daily (total duration of therapy: 10 days)

Hip replacement: Initial: 110 mg given 1-4 hours after completion of surgery and establishment of hemostasis **OR** 220 mg as 1 dose in postoperative patients in whom therapy is not initiated on day of surgery regardless of reason; maintenance: 220 mg once daily (total duration of therapy: 28-35 days)

Renal Impairment

Nonvalvular atrial fibrillation (to prevent stroke and systemic embolism):

U.S. labeling:

Mild-to-moderate renal impairment (Cl_{cr} >30 mL/minute): No dosage adjustment recommended.

Severe renal impairment (Cl_{cr} 15-30 mL/minute): 75 mg twice daily; **Note:** Patients with Cl_{cr} <30 mL/minute were excluded from the RE-LY trial (Connolly, 2009)

Cl_{cr} <15 mL/minute or hemodialysis dependent: No recommendation provided due to insufficient evidence; **Note:** Hemodialysis removes ~60% over 2-3 hours

Canadian labeling:

Cl_{cr} ≥30 mL/minute: No dosage adjustment recommended.

Severe renal impairment (Cl_{cr} <30 mL/minute): Use is contraindicated.

Postoperative thromboprophylaxis: Canadian labeling:

Moderate renal impairment (Cl_{cr} 30-50 mL/minute): Initial: 75 mg given 1-4 hours after completion of surgery and establishment of hemostasis; Maintenance: 150 mg/day

Severe renal impairment (Cl_{cr} < 30 mL/minute): Use is contraindicated.

Hepatic Impairment Nonvalvular atrial fibrillation (to prevent stroke and systemic embolism): No dosage adjustment required.

Administration Do not break, chew, or open capsules, as this will lead to 75% increase in absorption and potentially serious adverse reactions. Administer with water. May be taken without regard to meals.

Monitoring Parameters Activated partial thromboplastin time (aPTT) (values >2.5 x control may indicate overanticoagulation), ecarin clotting test (ECT) if available, thrombin time (TT), CBC with differential, renal function

Reference Range

At therapeutic dabigatran doses, aPTT, ECT (ecarin clotting time), and TT (thrombin time) are prolonged. A median peak aPTT of ~2 x control and a median trough aPTT of 1.5 x control were observed in subjects taking dabigatran 150 mg twice daily in the RE-LY trail

A therapeutic range has not been established for aPTT or for other tests of anticoagulant activity

Dosage Forms Excipient information presented when available (limited, particularly for generics); consult specific product labeling.

Capsule, oral:

Pradaxa®: 75 mg, 150 mg

Dosage Forms: Canada Excipient information presented when available (limited, particularly for generics); consult specific product labeling.

Capsule, oral:

Pradax™: 75 mg, 110 mg, 150 mg

Selected References

Alban S, "Pharmacological Strategies for Inhibition of Thrombin Activity," *Curr Pharm Des*, 2008, 14(12):1152-75.

Blech S, Ebner T, Ludwig-Schwellinger E, et al, "The Metabolism and Disposition of The Oral Direct Thrombin Inhibitor, Dabigatran, in Humans," *Drug Metab Dispos*, 2008, 36(2):386-99.

Connolly SJ, Ezekowitz MD, Yusuf S, et al, "Dabigatran Versus Warfarin in Patients With Atrial Fibrillation," *N Engl J Med*, 2009, 361(12):1139-51

Eikelboom JW, Wallentin L, Connolly SJ, et al, "Risk of Bleeding With 2 Doses of Dabigatran Compared With Warfarin in Older and Younger Patients With Atrial Fibrillation: An Analysis of the Randomized Evaluation of Long-Term Anticoagulant Therapy (RE-LY) Trial," *Circulation*, 2011, 123(21):2363-72.

Ezekowitz MD, Reilly PA, Nehmiz G, et al, "Dabigatran With or Without Concomitant Aspirin Compared With Warfarin Alone in Patients With Nonvalvular Atrial Fibrillation (PETRO Study)," *Am J Cardiol*, 2007, 100(9):1419-26.

Eriksson BI, Dahl OE, Kurth AA, et al, "Oral Dabigatran Etexilate Versus Subcutaneous Enoxaparin for the Prevention of Venous Thromboembolism after Total Knee Replacement: The RE-MODEL Randomized Trial," *J Thromb Haemost*, 2007, 5(11):2178-85.

Eriksson BI, Dahl OE, Rosencher N, et al, "Dabigatran Etexilate Versus Enoxaparin for Prevention of Venous Thromboembolism after Total Hip Replacement: A Randomised, Double-Blind, Non-Inferiority Trial," *Lancet*, 2007, 370(9591):949-56.

Hirsh J, Guyatt G, Albers GW, et al, "Executive Summary: American College of Chest Physicians Evidence-Based Clinical Practice Guidelines (8th Edition)," *Chest*, 2008, 133(6 Suppl):71-109.

Nutescu EA, Shapiro NL, and Chevalier A, "New Anticoagulant Agents: Direct Thrombin Inhibitors," *Cardiol Clin*, 2008, 26(2): 169-87.

Stangier J, Eriksson BI, Dahl OE, et al, "Pharmacokinetic Profile of the Oral Direct Thrombin Inhibitor Dabigatran Etexilate in Healthy Volunteers and Patients Undergoing Total Hip Replacement," *J Clin Pharmacol*, 2005, 45(5): 555-63.

Stangier J, Rathgen K, Stähle H, et al, "Influence of Renal Impairment on the Pharmacokinetics and Pharmacodynamics of Oral Dabigatran Etexilate," *Clin Pharmacokinet*, 2010, 49(4):259-68.

van Ryn J, Stangier J, Haertter S, et al, "Dabigatran Etexilate – A Novel, Reversible, Oral Direct Thrombin Inhibitor: Interpretation of Coagulation Assays and Reversal of Anticoagulant Activity," *Thromb Haemost*, 2010, 103 (6):1116-27.

Wallentin L, Yusuf S, Ezekowitz MD, et al, "Efficacy and Safety of Dabigatran Compared With Warfarin at Different Levels of International Normalised Ratio Control for Stroke Prevention in Atrial Fibrillation: An Analysis of the RE-LY Trial," *Lancet*, 2010, 376(9745):975-83.

Wann SL, Curtis AB, Ellenbogen KA, et al, "2011 ACCF/AHA/HRS Focused Update on the Management of Patients With Atrial Fibrillation (Update on Dabigatran): A Report of the American College of Cardiology Foundation/American Heart Association Task Force on Practice Guidelines," *Circulation*, 2011, 123(10):1144-50.

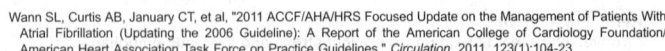

Wann SL, Curtis AB, January CT, et al, "2011 ACCF/AHA/HRS Focused Update on the Management of Patients With Atrial Fibrillation (Updating the 2006 Guideline): A Report of the American College of Cardiology Foundation/ American Heart Association Task Force on Practice Guidelines," *Circulation*, 2011, 123(1):104-23.

◆ **Dabigatran Etexilate Mesylate** *see* Dabigatran Etexilate *on page* 440
◆ **Dacodyl™ [OTC]** *see* Bisacodyl *on page* 205

Dalfampridine (dal FAM pri deen)

Medication Safety Issues
Sound-alike/look-alike issues:
Ampyra™ may be confused with anakinra
Dalfampridine may be confused with delavirdine, desipramine
Brand Names: U.S. Ampyra™
Index Terms 4-aminopyridine; 4-AP; EL-970; Fampridine-SR
Pharmacologic Category Potassium Channel Blocker
Use Treatment to improve walking in multiple sclerosis (MS) patients
Medication Guide Available Yes
Contraindications History of seizure; moderate or severe renal impairment (Cl_{cr} ≤50 mL/minute)
Warnings/Precautions Dalfampridine administration is associated with a dose-dependent risk of seizure; discontinue use and do not reinitiate therapy if seizure occurs during treatment. Use is contraindicated in patients with a history of seizures. Use with caution in patients with mild renal impairment. No specific dosage adjustment is recommended by the manufacturer; however, risk of seizure may be increased secondary to reduced clearance in these patients. Use is contraindicated in moderate-to-severe renal impairment (Cl_{cr} ≤50 mL/minute). To avoid adverse reactions, dalfampridine should not be administered with other 4-aminopyridine formulations (eg, compounded immediate release fampridine)
Adverse Reactions (Reflective of adult population; not specific for elderly)
>10%: Genitourinary: Urinary tract infection (12%)
1% to 10%:
Central nervous system: Insomnia (9%), dizziness (7%), headache (7%), multiple sclerosis relapse (4%), seizures (up to 4%; dose-dependent)
Gastrointestinal: Nausea (7%), constipation (3%), dyspepsia (2%)
Neuromuscular & skeletal: Weakness (7%), back pain (5%), balance disorder (5%), paresthesia (4%)
Respiratory: Nasopharyngitis (4%), pharyngolaryngeal pain (2%)
Drug Interactions
Avoid Concomitant Use There are no known interactions where it is recommended to avoid concomitant use.
Increased Effect/Toxicity There are no known significant interactions involving an increase in effect.
Decreased Effect
The levels/effects of Dalfampridine may be decreased by: Cyproterone
Stability Store at 25°C (77°F); excursions permitted to 15°C to 30°C (59°F to 86°F).
Mechanism of Action Nonspecific potassium channel blocker which improves conduction in focally demyelinated axons by delaying repolarization and prolonging the duration of action potentials. Enhanced neuronal conduction is thought to strengthen skeletal muscle fiber twitch activity, thereby, improving peripheral motor neurologic function.
Pharmacodynamics/Kinetics
Absorption: Rapid and complete
Distribution: V_d: 2.6 L/kg
Protein binding: Negligible
Metabolism: No active metabolites detected
Bioavailability: 96% (relative to aqueous solution)
Half-life elimination: 5-7 hours; prolonged in severe renal impairment (~3 times longer)
Time to peak, plasma: 3-4 hours
Excretion: Urine (96%; 90% of total dose as unchanged drug); feces (0.5%)
Dosage
Geriatric & Adult Multiple sclerosis: Oral: 10 mg every 12 hours (maximum daily dose: 20 mg); no additional benefit seen with doses >20 mg/day
Renal Impairment
Mild renal impairment (Cl_{cr} 51-80 mL/minute): No specific adjustment recommended by the manufacturer; however, risk of seizure may be increased secondary to reduced clearance.
Moderate-to-severe renal impairment (Cl_{cr} ≤50 mL/minute): Contraindicated.
Administration May be administered with or without food. Do not chew, crush, dissolve, or divide tablet.

Monitoring Parameters Renal function; EEG; walking ability

Special Geriatric Considerations Dalfampridine is contraindicated in patients with a Cl_{cr} ≤50 mL/minute. Because many older patients have impaired renal function, this medication should be used with caution and only when the renal function is known to be Cl_{cr} >50 mL/ minute.

Dosage Forms Excipient information presented when available (limited, particularly for generics); consult specific product labeling.

Tablet, extended release, oral:

Ampyra™: 10 mg

Selected References

Feret B, "Fampridine-SR: A Potassium-Channel Blocker for the Improvement of Walking Ability in Patients With MS," *Formulary*, 2009, 44:293-9.

Goodman AD, Brown TR, Krupp LB, et al, "Sustained-Release Oral Fampridine in Multiple Sclerosis: A Randomised, Double-Blind, Controlled Trial," *Lancet*, 2009, 373(9665):732-8.

Korenke AR, Rivey MP, and Allington DR. "Sustained-Release Fampridine for Symptomatic Treatment of Multiple Sclerosis," *Ann Pharmacother*, 2008, 42(10):1458-65.

◆ **Dalfopristin and Quinupristin** *see* Quinupristin and Dalfopristin *on page* 1570

◆ **d-Alpha Gems™ [OTC]** *see* Vitamin E *on page* 1921

◆ *d*-Alpha Tocopherol *see* Vitamin E *on page* 1921

Dalteparin (dal TE pa rin)

Related Information

Anticoagulants, Injectable *on page* 1989

Medication Safety Issues

High alert medication:

The Institute for Safe Medication Practices (ISMP) includes this medication among its list of drugs which have a heightened risk of causing significant patient harm when used in error.

2009 National Patient Safety Goals:

The Joint Commission (TJC) requires healthcare organizations that provide anticoagulant therapy to have a process in place to reduce the risk of anticoagulant-associated patient harm. Patients receiving anticoagulants should receive individualized care through a defined process that includes standardized ordering, dispensing, administration, monitoring and education. This does not apply to routine short-term use of anticoagulants for prevention of venous thromboembolism when the expectation is that the patient's laboratory values will remain within or close to normal values (NPSG.03.05.01).

Brand Names: U.S. Fragmin®

Brand Names: Canada Fragmin®

Index Terms Dalteparin Sodium; NSC-714371

Generic Availability (U.S.) No

Pharmacologic Category Low Molecular Weight Heparin

Use Prevention of deep vein thrombosis (DVT) which may lead to pulmonary embolism, in patients requiring abdominal surgery who are at risk for thromboembolic complications (eg, patients >40 years of age, obesity, patients with malignancy, history of DVT or pulmonary embolism, and surgical procedures requiring general anesthesia and lasting >30 minutes); prevention of DVT in patients undergoing hip-replacement surgery; patients immobile during an acute illness; prevention of ischemic complications in patients with unstable angina or non-Q-wave myocardial infarction on concurrent aspirin therapy; in patients with cancer, extended treatment (6 months) of acute symptomatic venous thromboembolism (DVT and/or PE) to reduce the recurrence of venous thromboembolism

Unlabeled/Investigational Use Active treatment of deep vein thrombosis (noncancer patients)

Contraindications Hypersensitivity to dalteparin or any component of the formulation; history of heparin-induced thrombocytopenia (HIT) or HIT with thrombosis; hypersensitivity to heparin or pork products; patients with active major bleeding; patients with unstable angina, non-Q-wave MI, or acute venous thromboembolism undergoing epidural/neuraxial anesthesia

Warnings/Precautions [U.S. Boxed Warning]: Spinal or epidural hematomas, including subsequent paralysis, may occur with recent or anticipated neuraxial anesthesia (epidural or spinal) or spinal puncture in patients anticoagulated with LMWH or heparinoids. Consider risk versus benefit prior to spinal procedures; risk is increased by the use of concomitant agents which may alter hemostasis, the use of indwelling epidural catheters for analgesia, a history of spinal deformity or spinal surgery, as well as traumatic or repeated epidural or spinal punctures. Patient should be observed closely for bleeding if enoxaparin is administered during or immediately following diagnostic lumbar puncture, epidural anesthesia, or spinal anesthesia.

Use with caution in patients with pre-existing thrombocytopenia, recent childbirth, subacute bacterial endocarditis, peptic ulcer disease, pericarditis or pericardial effusion, liver or renal function impairment, recent lumbar puncture, vasculitis, concurrent use of aspirin (increased bleeding risk), previous hypersensitivity to heparin, heparin-associated thrombocytopenia. Monitor platelet count closely. Rare thrombocytopenia may occur. Consider discontinuation of dalteparin in any patient developing significant thrombocytopenia related to initiation of dalteparin. Rare cases of thrombocytopenia with thrombosis have occurred. Use caution in patients with congenital or drug-induced thrombocytopenia or platelet defects. Cancer patients with thrombocytopenia may require dose adjustments for treatment of acute venous thromboembolism.

Use with caution in patients with known hypersensitivity to methylparaben or propylparaben. Monitor patient closely for signs or symptoms of bleeding. Certain patients are at increased risk of bleeding. Risk factors include bacterial endocarditis; congenital or acquired bleeding disorders; active ulcerative or angiodysplastic GI diseases; severe uncontrolled hypertension; hemorrhagic stroke; or use shortly after brain, spinal, or ophthalmology surgery; in patient treated concomitantly with platelet inhibitors; recent GI bleeding; thrombocytopenia or platelet defects; severe liver disease; hypertensive or diabetic retinopathy; or in patients undergoing invasive procedures.

Use with caution in patients with severe renal failure (has not been studied). Rare cases of thrombocytopenia with thrombosis have occurred. Heparin can cause hyperkalemia by affecting aldosterone. Similar reactions could occur with dalteparin. Monitor for hyperkalemia. Do **not** administer intramuscularly. Not to be used interchangeably (unit for unit) with heparin or any other low molecular weight heparins.

There is no consensus for adjusting/correcting the weight-based dosage of LMWH for patients who are morbidly obese (BMI ≥40 kg/m^2). For patients undergoing inpatient bariatric surgery, the American College of Chest Physicians Practice Guidelines suggest using a higher thromboprophylaxis dose of LMWH for obese patients (Geerts, 2008).

Adverse Reactions (Reflective of adult population; not specific for elderly) Note: As with all anticoagulants, bleeding is the major adverse effect of dalteparin. Hemorrhage may occur at virtually any site. Risk is dependent on multiple variables.

>10%: Hematologic: Bleeding (3% to 14%), thrombocytopenia (including heparin-induced thrombocytopenia), <1%; cancer clinical trials: ~11%)

1% to 10%:

Hematologic: Major bleeding (up to 6%), wound hematoma (up to 3%)

Hepatic: AST >3 times upper limit of normal (5% to 9%), ALT >3 times upper limit of normal (4% to 10%)

Local: Pain at injection site (up to 12%), injection site hematoma (up to 7%)

Drug Interactions

Avoid Concomitant Use

Avoid concomitant use of Dalteparin with any of the following: Rivaroxaban

Increased Effect/Toxicity

Dalteparin may increase the levels/effects of: Anticoagulants; Collagenase (Systemic); Deferasirox; Drotrecogin Alfa; Ibritumomab; Rivaroxaban; Tositumomab and Iodine I 131 Tositumomab

The levels/effects of Dalteparin may be increased by: 5-ASA Derivatives; Antiplatelet Agents; Dasatinib; Herbs (Anticoagulant/Antiplatelet Properties); Nonsteroidal Anti-Inflammatory Agents; Pentosan Polysulfate Sodium; Pentoxifylline; Prostacyclin Analogues; Salicylates; Thrombolytic Agents

Decreased Effect There are no known significant interactions involving a decrease in effect.

Ethanol/Nutrition/Herb Interactions Herb/Nutraceutical: Alfalfa, anise, bilberry, bladderwrack, bromelain, cat's claw, celery, chamomile, coleus, cordyceps, dong quai, evening primrose oil, fenugreek, feverfew, garlic, ginger, ginkgo biloba, ginseng (American), ginseng (panax), ginseng (Siberian), grapeseed, green tea, guggul, horse chestnut seed, horseradish, licorice, prickly ash, red clover, reishi, SAMe (s-adenosylmethionine), sweet clover, turmeric, white willow (all have additional antiplatelet/anticoagulant activity)

Stability Store at temperatures of 20°C to 25°C (68°F to 77°F). Multidose vials may be stored for up to 2 weeks at room temperature after entering.

Mechanism of Action Low molecular weight heparin analog with a molecular weight of 4000-6000 daltons; the commercial product contains 3% to 15% heparin with a molecular weight <3000 daltons, 65% to 78% with a molecular weight of 3000-8000 daltons and 14% to 26% with a molecular weight >8000 daltons; while dalteparin has been shown to inhibit both factor Xa and factor IIa (thrombin), the antithrombotic effect of dalteparin is characterized by a higher ratio of antifactor Xa to antifactor IIa activity (ratio = 4)

Pharmacodynamics/Kinetics Geriatrics: Pharmacokinetics not shown to be significantly altered by age.

Distribution: V_d: 40-60 mL/kg

Bioavailability: SubQ: 87%

Half-life:

Normal renal function: 1.82 hours

Patients with chronic renal insufficiency requiring hemodialysis: 5.7 hours

Elimination: Renal; clearance: 15-25 mL/minute

Dosage

Geriatric & Adult Note: Each 2500 int. units of anti-Xa activity is equal to 16 mg of dalteparin.

DVT prophylaxis: Note: In morbidly obese patients (BMI ≥40 kg/m^2), increasing the prophylactic dose by 30% may be appropriate (Nutescu, 2009):

Abdominal surgery:

Low-to-moderate DVT risk: SubQ: 2500 int. units 1-2 hours prior to surgery, then once daily for 5-10 days postoperatively

High DVT risk: SubQ: 5000 int. units the evening prior to surgery and then once daily for 5-10 days postoperatively. Alternatively in patients with malignancy: 2500 int. units 1-2 hours prior to surgery, 2500 int. units 12 hours later, then 5000 int. units once daily for 5-10 days postoperatively.

Total hip replacement surgery: SubQ: **Note:** Three treatment options are currently available. Dose is given for 5-10 days, although up to 14 days of treatment have been tolerated in clinical trials:

Postoperative regimen:

Initial: 2500 int. units 4-8 hours* after surgery

Maintenance: 5000 int. units once daily; start at least 6 hours after postsurgical dose

Preoperative regimen (starting day of surgery):

Initial: 2500 int. units within 2 hours before surgery

Adjustment: 2500 int. units 4-8 hours* after surgery

Maintenance: 5000 int. units once daily; start at least 6 hours after postsurgical dose

Preoperative regimen (starting evening prior to surgery):

Initial: 5000 int. units 10-14 hours before surgery

Adjustment: 5000 int. units 4-8 hours* after surgery

Maintenance: 5000 int. units once daily, allowing 24 hours between doses.

*Note: Dose may be delayed if hemostasis is not yet achieved.

Immobility during acute illness: 5000 int. units once daily

Unstable angina or non-Q-wave myocardial infarction: SubQ: 120 int. units/kg body weight (maximum dose: 10,000 int. units) every 12 hours for up to 8 days with concurrent aspirin therapy. Discontinue dalteparin once patient is clinically stable.

Obesity: Use actual body weight to calculate dose; dose capping at 10,000 int. units recommended (Nutescu, 2009)

Venous thromboembolism, extended treatment in cancer patients: SubQ:

Initial (month 1): 200 int. units/kg (maximum dose: 18,000 int. units) once daily for 30 days

Maintenance (months 2-6): ~150 int. units/kg (maximum dose: 18,000 int. units) once daily. If platelet count between 50,000-100,000/mm^3, reduce dose by 2,500 int. units until platelet count recovers to ≥100,000/mm^3. If platelet count <50,000/mm^3, discontinue dalteparin until platelet count recover to >50,000/mm^3.

Obesity: Use actual body weight to calculate dose; dose capping is not recommended (Nutescu, 2009). However, the manufacturer recommends a maximum dose of 18,000 units per day for the treatment of VTE in cancer patients.

DVT (with or without PE) treatment in noncancer patients (unlabeled use): SubQ: 200 int. units/kg once daily (Feissinger, 1996; Jaff, 2011; Wells, 2005) or 100 int. units/kg twice daily (Jaff, 2011)

Obesity: Use actual body weight to calculate dose; dose capping is not recommended (Nutescu, 2009). One study demonstrated similar anti-Xa levels after 3 days of therapy in obese patients (>40% above IBW; range: 82-190 kg) compared to those ≤20% above IBW or between 20% to 40% above IBW (Wilson, 2001).

Renal Impairment Half-life is increased in patients with chronic renal failure, use with caution, accumulation can be expected; specific dosage adjustments have not been recommended. Accumulation was not observed in critically ill patients with severe renal insufficiency (Cl$_{cr}$ <30 mL/minute) receiving prophylactic doses (5000 int. units) for a median of 7 days (Douketis, 2008). In cancer patients, receiving treatment for venous thromboembolism, if Cl$_{cr}$ <30 mL/minute, manufacturer recommends monitoring anti-Xa levels to determine appropriate dose.

Hepatic Impairment Use with caution in patients with hepatic insufficiency; specific dosage adjustments have not been recommended.

Administration For deep SubQ injection **only**. May be injected in a U-shape to the area surrounding the navel, the upper outer side of the thigh, or the upper outer quadrangle of the buttock. Use thumb and forefinger to lift a fold of skin when injecting dalteparin to the navel area or thigh. Insert needle at a 45- to 90-degree angle. The entire length of needle should be inserted. Do not expel air bubble from fixed-dose syringe prior to injection. Air bubble (and extra solution, if applicable) may be expelled from graduated syringes. In order to minimize bruising, do not rub injection site.

To convert from I.V. unfractionated heparin (UFH) infusion to SubQ dalteparin (Nutescu, 2007): Calculate specific dose for dalteparin based on indication, discontinue UFH and begin dalteparin within 1 hour

To convert from SubQ dalteparin to I.V. UFH infusion (Nutescu, 2007): Discontinue dalteparin; calculate specific dose for I.V. UFH infusion based on indication; omit heparin bolus/ loading dose

Converting from SubQ dalteparin dosed every 12 hours: Start I.V. UFH infusion 10-11 hours after last dose of dalteparin

Converting from SubQ dalteparin dosed every 24 hours: Start I.V. UFH infusion 22-23 hours after last dose of dalteparin

Monitoring Parameters Periodic CBC including platelet count; stool occult blood tests; monitoring of PT and PTT is not necessary. Once patient has received 3-4 doses, anti-Xa levels, drawn 4-6 hours after dalteparin administration, may be used to monitor effect in patients with severe renal dysfunction or if abnormal coagulation parameters or bleeding should occur. For patients >190 kg, if anti-Xa monitoring is available, adjusting dose based on anti-Xa levels is recommended; if anti-Xa monitoring is unavailable, reduce dose if bleeding occurs (Nutescu, 2009).

Reference Range Treatment: Venous thromboembolism: Target anti-Xa range: 0.5-1.5 int. units/mL

Special Geriatric Considerations No specific recommendations are necessary for the elderly.

Dosage Forms Excipient information presented when available (limited, particularly for generics); consult specific product labeling. [DSC] = Discontinued product

Injection, solution:
Fragmin®: 10,000 anti-Xa int. units/mL (9.5 mL [DSC]); 25,000 anti-Xa int. units/mL (3.8 mL) [contains benzyl alcohol]

Injection, solution [preservative free]:
Fragmin®: 10,000 anti-Xa int. units/mL (1 mL); 2500 anti-Xa int. units/0.2 mL (0.2 mL); 5000 anti-Xa int. units/0.2 mL (0.2 mL); 7500 anti-Xa int. units/0.3 mL (0.3 mL); 12,500 anti-Xa int. units/0.5 mL (0.5 mL); 15,000 anti-Xa int. units/0.6 mL (0.6 mL); 18,000 anti-Xa int. units/0.72 mL (0.72 mL)

Selected References

Mechanick JI, Kushner RF, Sugerman HJ, et al, "American Association of Clinical Endocrinologists, The Obesity Society, and American Society for Metabolic & Bariatric Surgery Medical Guidelines for Clinical Practice for the Perioperative Nutritional, Metabolic, and Nonsurgical Support of the Bariatric Surgery Patient," *Obesity*, 2009, 17 (Suppl 1):1-70.

Nutescu EA, Spinler SA, Wittkowsky A, et al, "Low-Molecular-Weight Heparins in Renal Impairment and Obesity: Available Evidence and Clinical Practice Recommendations Across Medical and Surgical Settings," *Ann Pharmacother*, 2009, 43(6):1064-83.

Simoneau G, Bergmann JF, Kher A, et al, "Pharmacokinetics of a Low Molecular Weight Heparin (Fragmin®) in Young and Elderly Subjects," *Thromb Res*, 1992, 66(5):603-7.

◆ **Dalteparin Sodium** *see* Dalteparin *on page 445*

Danaparoid (da NAP a roid)

Medication Safety Issues
  Sound-alike/look-alike issues:
  Orgaran® may be confused with argatroban
Brand Names: Canada Orgaran®
Index Terms Danaparoid Sodium
Pharmacologic Category Anticoagulant; Heparinoid
Use Prevention of postoperative deep vein thrombosis (DVT) following orthopedic or major abdominal and thoracic surgery; prevention of DVT in patients with confirmed diagnosis of non-hemorrhagic stroke; management of heparin-induced thrombocytopenia (HIT)
Unlabeled/Investigational Use Systemic anticoagulation for patients with heparin-induced thrombocytopenia: factor Xa inhibition is used to monitor degree of anticoagulation if necessary

Contraindications Hypersensitivity to danaparoid, or any component of the formulation (including sulfites); history of thrombocytopenia while receiving danaparoid or when associated with a positive *in vitro* test for antiplatelet antibodies in the presence of danaparoid; hemorrhagic stroke (without systemic emboli); acute hemorrhagic stroke; patients with active major bleeding; severe hemorrhagic diathesis (hemophilia, idiopathic thrombocytopenic purpura); acute or subacute bacterial endocarditis; active gastric or duodenal ulcer; surgery of CNS, eyes, or ears; diabetic or hemorrhagic retinopathy; severe uncontrolled hypertension; other conditions or diseases that increase risk of hemorrhage; not for I.M. use

Warnings/Precautions Hemorrhagic stroke should be ruled out by CT scan prior to initiating therapy. IV administration is recommended at least for initial therapy with suspected or confirmed HIT. SubQ administration for initial dosing and/or prophylactic dosing regimens may be associated with new/recurrent thrombosis in patients with acute HIT (Warkentin, 2008). Do not administer intramuscularly.

Spinal or epidural hematomas, including subsequent paralysis, may occur with recent or anticipated neuraxial anesthesia (epidural or spinal anesthesia) or spinal puncture in patients anticoagulated with LMWH or heparinoids. Consider risk versus benefit prior to spinal procedures; risk is increased by the use of concomitant agents which may alter hemostasis, the use of indwelling epidural catheters for analgesia, a history of spinal deformity or spinal surgery, as well as a history of traumatic or repeated epidural or spinal punctures. Spinal procedures should be avoided for 12 hours after the last danaparoid dose; allow at least 2 hours after procedure before resuming danaparoid therapy. Patient should be observed closely for bleeding and signs and symptoms of neurological impairment if therapy is administered during or immediately following diagnostic lumbar puncture, epidural anesthesia, or spinal anesthesia.

Use with caution in patients with history of peptic ulcer disease, hepatic impairment, and severe renal impairment. Monitor patient closely for signs or symptoms of bleeding. Certain patients are at increased risk of bleeding (eg, severe hepatic disease, patients undergoing knee surgery or other invasive procedures, concomitant therapy with platelet inhibitors, elderly). Discontinue use if bleeding occurs. Danaparoid is not effectively antagonized by protamine sulfate. No other antidote is available, so extreme caution is needed in monitoring dose given and resulting Xa inhibition effect.

Use caution in patients with or with a history of thrombocytopenia (heparin-induced, congenital) or platelet defects. The manufacturer labeling recommends that patients with a history of heparin-induced thrombocytopenia be tested for cross-reactivity with danaparoid prior to initiating therapy; if test is positive, alternative therapy should be employed unless otherwise not available. If danaparoid is administered, therapy must be discontinued immediately with clinical signs of positive cross-reactivity (eg, increased reduction in platelet counts, thrombosis, skin necrosis). May resume therapy (if needed) only after laboratory confirmed negative test for danaparoid activated antiplatelet antibodies. Cutaneous allergy tests may help detect the presence of cross-reactivity between heparins and danaparoid (Grassegger, 2001).

Safety and efficacy have not been established for use as thromboprophylaxis in patients with prosthetic heart valves. Heparin can cause hyperkalemia by affecting aldosterone. A similar reaction could occur with danaparoid. Monitor for hyperkalemia. Not to be used interchangeably (unit for unit) with heparin or any other low molecular weight heparins.

This product contains sodium sulfite which may cause allergic-type reactions, including anaphylactic symptoms and life-threatening asthmatic episodes in susceptible people; this is seen more frequently in asthmatics.

Adverse Reactions (Reflective of adult population; not specific for elderly) As with all anticoagulants, bleeding is the major adverse effect of danaparoid. Hemorrhage may occur at virtually any site. Risk is dependent on multiple variables.

Frequency not always defined.
Cardiovascular: Arterial pressure decreased, atrial fibrillation, cerebral infarction, DVT, hypotension, peripheral edema
Central nervous system: Pain (5%), fever (2% to 5%), confusion, fatigue, insomnia, loss of consciousness, restlessness
Dermatologic: Rash (1%), bruising
Gastrointestinal: Nausea (3%), constipation (2%)
Genitourinary: Urinary retention (1%), urinary incontinence
Hematologic: Cerebral hemorrhage, hematoma, hemorrhage, spinal or epidural hematomas (may occur following neuraxial anesthesia or spinal puncture, resulting in paralysis), thrombocytopenia
Hepatic: Alkaline phosphatase increased, ALT increased (transient), AST increased (transient)
Local: Injection site hematoma (≤5%)

◄ Neuromuscular & skeletal: Hemiparesis, involuntary muscle contractions, tremor
Renal: Hematuria
Respiratory: Apnea, asthma
Miscellaneous: Infection (2%), allergic reaction, sepsis

Drug Interactions

Avoid Concomitant Use
Avoid concomitant use of Danaparoid with any of the following: Rivaroxaban

Increased Effect/Toxicity
Danaparoid may increase the levels/effects of: Anticoagulants; Collagenase (Systemic); Deferasirox; Drotrecogin Alfa; Ibritumomab; Rivaroxaban; Tositumomab and Iodine I 131 Tositumomab

The levels/effects of Danaparoid may be increased by: Antiplatelet Agents; Dasatinib; Herbs (Anticoagulant/Antiplatelet Properties); Nonsteroidal Anti-Inflammatory Agents; Pentosan Polysulfate Sodium; Prostacyclin Analogues; Salicylates; Thrombolytic Agents

Decreased Effect There are no known significant interactions involving a decrease in effect.

Ethanol/Nutrition/Herb Interactions Herb/Nutraceutical: Avoid cat's claw, dong quai, evening primrose, feverfew, garlic, ginger, ginkgo, red clover, horse chestnut, green tea, and ginseng (all have additional antiplatelet activity).

Stability Store at 2°C to 30°C (36°F to 86°F). Protect from light. Stable for up to 48 hours in the following I.V. solutions: D_5NS, NS, Ringer's, LR, mannitol.

Mechanism of Action Inhibits factor Xa and IIa (anti-Xa effects >20 times anti-IIa effects). Prevents fibrin formation in the coagulation pathway via thrombin generation inhibition.

Pharmacodynamics/Kinetics
Onset of action: Peak effect: SubQ: Maximum antifactor Xa activities occur in 4-5 hours
Bioavailability: SubQ: ~100%
Half-life elimination: Anti-Xa activity: ~25 hours (renal impairment: 29-35 hours); Thrombin generation inhibition activity: ~7 hours
Excretion: Primarily urine

Dosage

Geriatric & Adult Note: Dosing recommendations per manufacturer labeling unless otherwise noted. Dose expressed as anti-Xa units.

Prevention of DVT following orthopedic, major abdominal, or thoracic surgery: SubQ: 750 units twice daily for up to 14 days; it is recommended that patients begin prophylactic therapy preoperatively and receive their last preoperative dose 1-4 hours before surgery.

Prevention of DVT in stroke (nonhemorrhagic):
Initial: I.V.: Up to 1000 units as single dose
Maintenance: SubQ: 750 units every 12 hours for 7-14 days

Heparin-induced thrombocytopenia (HIT):
Prevention of DVT (with current or past HIT): **Note:** May administer I.V. bolus of 1250 units if clinically necessary (ie, current HIT) or may initiate maintenance regimen without a bolus as follows:
SubQ:
≤90 kg: Current HIT or past HIT: 750 units every 8-12 hours for 7-10 days
>90 kg: Current HIT: 1250 units every 8-12 hours for 7-10 days; Past HIT: 1250 units every 12 hours or 750 units every 8 hours for 7-10 days

Treatment of DVT/PE (see also Warkentin, 2008):
Initial I.V. bolus: Thrombosis <5 days old: ≤55 kg: 1250-1500 units; 55-90 kg: 2250-2500 units; >90 kg: 3750 units; followed by a maintenance I.V. infusion or maintenance SubQ injections. **Note:** If thrombosis is ≥5 days old, administer an I.V. bolus dose of 1250 units followed by maintenance SubQ injections.
Maintenance: I.V. infusion (after I.V. bolus administered): Thrombosis <5 days old: 400 units/hour for 4 hours, then 300 units/hour for 4 hours, then 150-200 units/hour for 5-7 days; adjust rate according to target anti-Xa levels
or
Maintenance: SubQ injections (after I.V. bolus administered):
Thrombosis <5 days old: ≤55 kg: 1500 units every 12 hours; 55-90 kg: 2000 units every 12 hours; >90 kg: 1750 units every 8 hours for 4-7 days.
Thrombosis ≥5 days old: ≤90 kg: 750 units every 8-12 hours; >90 kg: 750 units every 8 hours or 1250 units every 8-12 hours

HIT/surgical thromboprophylaxis:
Nonvascular surgery: SubQ:
≤90 kg: 750 units 1-4 hours preoperatively and at ≥6 hours postop, followed by 750 units every 12 hours beginning day 1 post-op and continued for 7-10 days
>90 kg: 750 units 1-4 hours preoperatively and at ≥6 hours postop, followed by 750 units every 8 hours or 1250 units every 12 hours beginning day 1 post-op and continued for 7-10 days

Embolectomy:
  55-90 kg: I.V.: 2250-2500 units as a bolus preoperatively, followed by SubQ: 1250 units every 12 hours beginning ≥6 hours postop. **Note:** After several days of I.V. therapy, may switch to SubQ: 750 units every 8-12 hours or oral anticoagulant therapy.

  >90 kg: I.V.: 2250-2500 units as a bolus preoperatively, followed by 150-200 units/hour beginning ≥6 hours post-op for 5-7 days. **Note:** After several days of I.V. therapy, may switch to SubQ: 750 units every 8-12 hours or oral anticoagulant therapy.

HIT/cardiac procedures: Note: Other therapies may be preferred (eg, bivalirudin); long half-life and irreversibility of danaparoid make it a poor choice in these settings. Refer to product labeling for dosing recommendations.

Catheter patency: Mix 750 units with 50 mL normal saline. Flush catheter with 5-10 mL of resulting solution as needed.

Conversion to oral anticoagulant therapy (OAC): Establish adequate antithrombotic effect with danaparoid prior to initiation of oral anticoagulant (OAC) therapy. PT/INR should be therapeutic before discontinuing use of danaparoid. **Note:** Laboratory values taken within 5 hours of danaparoid administration may be unreliable.

Conversion of SubQ danaparoid to OAC (based on current danaparoid dose):
  Danaparoid 750 units every 12 hours: Initiate OAC and maintain danaparoid therapy until PT/INR is therapeutic; may take up to 5 days.

  Danaparoid 1250 units every 12 hours: Initiate OAC and decrease danaparoid to 750 units every 12 hours; maintain danaparoid therapy until PT/INR is therapeutic; may take up to 5 days.

Conversion of I.V. danaparoid to OAC: Initiate OAC with concurrent danaparoid I.V. infusion (maximum 300 units/hour); discontinue I.V. infusion once INR is therapeutic (maximum INR: 3.0). If bleeding risk is present, I.V. infusion should be reduced to 75 units/hour and OAC initiation withheld for 24 hours **or** danaparoid I.V. infusion may be switched to subcutaneous route at a dose of 1250 units every 12 hours and the recommended conversion of SubQ danaparoid to OAC regimen followed (ie, subsequent reduction to 750 units every 12 hours while OAC initiated).

Renal Impairment Note: Danaparoid half-life is significantly prolonged in renal impairment; anti-Xa levels should be closely monitored. Dosage reduction, especially with maintenance doses, may be required.

Mild or moderate impairment: There are no dosage adjustments provided in manufacturer's labeling.

Severe impairment (serum creatinine ≥220 micromol/L [≥2.5 mg/dL]): Following initial dose, dose reductions or temporary discontinuation of therapy may be necessary to prevent accumulation of plasma anti-Xa (indicated by consistent, steady state-plasma anti-Xa activity > 0.5 anti-Xa units).

Moderate-to severe impairment (unlabeled dosing): Adults: Treatment of suspected/confirmed HIT: Administer usual I.V. bolus dose (based on weight) followed by maintenance infusion: 400 units/hour x 4 hours, 300 units/hour x 4 hours, 150 units/hour (Warkentin, 2008)

Hemodialysis:
  Children: I.V.:
    First two dialysis sessions:
      <10 years: 30 units/kg *plus* 1000 units
      10-17 years: 30 units/kg *plus* 1500 units
    Third and subsequent sessions (based on predialysis anti-Xa levels):
      <300 units/L: Administer previous dialysis dose
      300-500 units/L: Reduce total dose by 250 units
      >500 units/L: No dose required with next dialysis
  Adults: I.V.: 1500-3750 units before dialysis session. **Note:** Dose depends on frequency of dialysis regimen (eg, daily dialysis vs every-other-day or less frequently) and weight of patient with the lower dose recommended for patients <55 kg. Do not administer prior to dialysis if plasma antifactor Xa levels >400 units/L and not receiving daily dialysis; however, if fibrin threads are present in bubble chamber may administer 1500 units.

Hemofiltration: Adults: I.V.: 55-90 kg: 2500 units as a bolus, followed by 600 units/hour for 4 hours, then 400 units/hour for 4 hours, then 200-600 units/hour to maintain adequate anti-Xa levels. **Note:** If patient is <55 kg, reduce bolus dose to 2000 units, followed by 400 units/hour for 4 hours, then 150-400 units/hour to maintain adequate anti-Xa levels.

Hepatic Impairment There are no dosage adjustments provided in manufacturer's labeling.

Administration Administer SubQ, not I.M.; have patient lie down and administer by deep SubQ injection using a fine needle (25-26 gauge); rotate sites of injection

Monitoring Parameters Platelets (baseline, every other day during week 1, twice weekly during weeks 2 and 3, and once weekly thereafter); occult blood or other signs of bleeding; anti-Xa activity (if available). See manufacturer's recommendations within labeling regarding anticipated anti-Xa levels.

◀ **Test Interactions** PT/INR, when measuring coumarin derivative activity, is not reliable within 5 hours following danaparoid administration.

Special Geriatric Considerations Evaluation of elderly's creatinine serum concentrations is important before initiating therapy.

Product Availability Not available in U.S.

Dosage Forms: Canada Excipient information presented when available (limited, particularly for generics); consult specific product labeling.

Injection, solution:
Organan®: 750 anti-Xa units/0.6 mL (0.6 mL)

◆ **Danaparoid Sodium** *see* Danaparoid *on page 448*
◆ **Dantrium®** *see* Dantrolene *on page 452*

Dantrolene (DAN troe leen)

Medication Safety Issues
Sound-alike/look-alike issues:
Dantrium® may be confused with danazol, Daraprim®
Revonto™ may be confused with Revatio®

Brand Names: U.S. Dantrium®; Revonto™
Brand Names: Canada Dantrium®
Index Terms Dantrolene Sodium
Generic Availability (U.S.) Yes: Capsule
Pharmacologic Category Skeletal Muscle Relaxant
Use Treatment of spasticity associated with upper motor neuron disorders (eg, spinal cord injury, stroke, cerebral palsy, or multiple sclerosis); management of malignant hyperthermia; prevention of malignant hyperthermia in susceptible individuals (preoperative/postoperative administration)
Unlabeled/Investigational Use Neuroleptic malignant syndrome (NMS)
Contraindications

I.V.: There are no contraindications listed within the manufacturers labeling.

Oral: Active hepatic disease; should not be used when spasticity is used to maintain posture/balance during locomotion or to obtain/maintain increased function

Warnings/Precautions [U.S. Boxed Warning]: Has potential for hepatotoxicity. Overt hepatitis has been most frequently observed between the third and twelfth month of therapy. Hepatic injury appears to be greater in females and in patients >35 years of age. Idiosyncratic and hypersensitivity reactions (sometimes fatal) of the liver have also occurred. Discontinue therapy if benefits not observed within 45 days when utilized for chronic spasticity.

Use oral therapy with caution in patients with impaired cardiac, hepatic, or pulmonary function (particularly in obstructive pulmonary disease). May cause photosensitivity. Patients should be cautioned about performing tasks which require mental alertness (eg, operating machinery or driving). The combination of I.V. dantrolene and calcium channel blockers is not recommended. Injection contains 3 g mannitol/vial; caution if additional mannitol required. Alkaline solution may cause tissue necrosis if extravasated. In addition to I.V. dantrolene, supportive measures must also be utilized for management of malignant hyperthermia.

Adverse Reactions (Reflective of adult population; not specific for elderly) Frequency not defined.

Cardiovascular: Blood pressure (altered), heart failure, tachycardia

Central nervous system: Chills, confusion, dizziness, drowsiness, fatigue, fever, headache, insomnia, lightheadedness, malaise, mental depression, nervousness, seizure, speech disturbance

Dermatologic: Eczematoid eruption, hair growth (abnormal), pruritus, rash, urticaria

Gastrointestinal: Abdominal cramps, anorexia, constipation, diarrhea, dysphagia, gastric irritation, gastrointestinal hemorrhage, nausea, taste change, vomiting

Genitourinary: Crystalluria, difficult erection, difficult urination, nocturia, polyuria, urinary frequency, urinary incontinence, urinary retention

Hematologic: Anemia (aplastic), leukopenia, thrombocytopenia

Hepatic: Hepatitis

Local: Injection site reaction (pain, erythema, swelling), thrombophlebitis, tissue necrosis

Neuromuscular & skeletal: Back pain, muscle weakness, myalgia

Ocular: Blurred vision, diplopia, tearing (excessive)

Renal: Hematuria

Respiratory: Feeling of suffocation, pleural effusion (associated with pericarditis), pulmonary edema, respiratory depression

Miscellaneous: Anaphylaxis, diaphoresis, lymphocytic lymphoma, sialorrhea

Drug Interactions
  Metabolism/Transport Effects Substrate of CYP3A4 (major)
  Avoid Concomitant Use
    Avoid concomitant use of Dantrolene with any of the following: Conivaptan
  Increased Effect/Toxicity
    Dantrolene may increase the levels/effects of: Alcohol (Ethyl); CNS Depressants; Metho-trimeprazine; Selective Serotonin Reuptake Inhibitors

    The levels/effects of Dantrolene may be increased by: Conivaptan; CYP3A4 Inhibitors (Moderate); CYP3A4 Inhibitors (Strong); Dasatinib; Droperidol; HydrOXYzine; Methotrimeprazine
  Decreased Effect
    The levels/effects of Dantrolene may be decreased by: CYP3A4 Inducers (Strong); Deferasirox; Herbs (CYP3A4 Inducers); Tocilizumab
  Ethanol/Nutrition/Herb Interactions
    Ethanol: May increase CNS depression; monitor for increased effects with coadministration. Caution patients about effects.
    Herb/Nutraceutical: Avoid valerian, St John's wort, kava kava, gotu kola (may increase CNS depression).
Stability Reconstitute vial by adding 60 mL of sterile water for injection USP (**not bacteriostatic water for injection**); incompatible with D_5W, NS, and other acidic solutions. Protect from light. Use reconstituted solution within 6 hours; avoid glass bottles for I.V. infusion due to potential for precipitate formation.
    Dantrium®: Store unreconstituted vials and reconstituted solutions at controlled room temperature of 15°C to 30°C (59°F to 86°F).
    Revonto™: Dissolution time reduced; shake vial for ~20 seconds or until solution is clear. Store unreconstituted vials and reconstituted solutions at controlled room temperature of 20°C to 25°C (68°F to 77°F).
Mechanism of Action Acts directly on skeletal muscle by interfering with release of calcium ion from the sarcoplasmic reticulum; prevents or reduces the increase in myoplasmic calcium ion concentration that activates the acute catabolic processes associated with malignant hyperthermia
Pharmacodynamics/Kinetics
    Absorption: Oral: Slow and incomplete
    Metabolism: Hepatic
    Half-life elimination: 4-8 hours
    Excretion: Feces (45% to 50%); urine (25% as unchanged drug and metabolites)
Dosage
  Geriatric & Adult
    Spasticity: Oral: Initial: 25 mg once daily for 7 days; increase to 25 mg 3 times/day for 7 days, increase to 50 mg 3 times/day for 7 days, and then increase to 100 mg 3 times/day; not to exceed 400 mg/day
    Malignant hyperthermia:
      Preoperative prophylaxis:
        Oral: 4-8 mg/kg/day in 4 divided doses, begin 1-2 days prior to surgery with last dose 3-4 hours prior to surgery
        I.V.: 2.5 mg/kg ~1¼ hours prior to anesthesia and infused over 1 hour with additional doses as needed and individualized
      Crisis: I.V.: 2.5 mg/kg; continuously repeat dose until symptoms subside or a cumulative dose of 10 mg/kg is reached; if physiologic and metabolic abnormalities reappear, repeat regimen (**Note:** Manufacturer's labeling suggests an initial dose of 1 mg/kg; however, guidelines recommend 2.5 mg/kg initially [www.mhaus.org]).
      Postcrisis follow-up: Oral: 4-8 mg/kg/day in 4 divided doses for 1-3 days; I.V. dantrolene may be used when oral therapy is not practical; individualize dosage beginning with 1 mg/kg or more as the clinical situation dictates
    Neuroleptic malignant syndrome (unlabeled use): I.V.: 1-2.5 mg/kg, may repeat dose up to maximum cumulative dose of 10 mg/kg/day, then switch to oral dosage (Strawn, 2007; Susman, 2001)
Administration I.V.: Therapeutic or emergency dose can be administered with rapid continuous I.V. push. Follow-up doses should be administered over 2-3 minutes.
Monitoring Parameters Motor performance should be monitored for therapeutic outcomes; nausea, vomiting, and liver function tests should be monitored for potential hepatotoxicity; intravenous administration requires cardiac monitor and blood pressure monitor
Pharmacotherapy Pearls Avoid glass bottles for I.V. infusion; exercise caution at meals on the day of administration because difficulty swallowing and choking has been reported
Special Geriatric Considerations There is little experience with this drug in the elderly.

Dosage Forms Excipient information presented when available (limited, particularly for generics); consult specific product labeling.

Capsule, oral, as sodium: 25 mg, 50 mg, 100 mg

Dantrium®: 25 mg, 50 mg, 100 mg

Injection, powder for reconstitution, as sodium:

Dantrium®: 20 mg [contains mannitol 3 g]

Revonto™: 20 mg [contains mannitol 3 g]

Selected References

Ward A, Chaffman MO, and Sorkin EM, "Dantrolene: A Review of Its Pharmacodynamic and Pharmacokinetic Properties and Therapeutic Use in Malignant Hyperthermia, the Neuroleptic Malignant Syndrome and an Update of Its Use in Muscle Spasticity," *Drugs*, 1986, 32(2):130-68.

◆ **Dantrolene Sodium** *see* Dantrolene *on page 452*
◆ **Dapcin** *see* DAPTOmycin *on page 454*
◆ **Daptacel®** *see* Diphtheria and Tetanus Toxoids, and Acellular Pertussis Vaccine *on page 531*

DAPTOmycin (DAP toe mye sin)

Medication Safety Issues

Sound-alike/look-alike issues:

Cubicin® may be confused with Cleocin®

DAPTOmycin may be confused with DACTINomycin

Brand Names: U.S. Cubicin®

Brand Names: Canada Cubicin®

Index Terms Cidecin; Dapcin; LY146032

Generic Availability (U.S.) No

Pharmacologic Category Antibiotic, Cyclic Lipopeptide

Use Treatment of complicated skin and skin structure infections caused by susceptible aerobic gram-positive organisms; *Staphylococcus aureus* bacteremia, including right-sided native valve infective endocarditis caused by MSSA or MRSA

Unlabeled/Investigational Use Treatment of severe infections caused by MRSA or VRE

Contraindications Hypersensitivity to daptomycin or any component of the formulation

Warnings/Precautions May be associated with an increased incidence of myopathy; discontinue in patients with signs and symptoms of myopathy in conjunction with an increase in CPK (>5 times ULN or 1000 units/L) or in asymptomatic patients with a CPK ≥10 times ULN. Myopathy may occur more frequently at dose and/or frequency in excess of recommended dosages. Use caution in patients receiving other drugs associated with myopathy (eg, HMG-CoA reductase inhibitors). Not indicated for the treatment of pneumonia (inactivation by pulmonary surfactant). Use caution in renal impairment (dosage adjustment required severe renal impairment [Cl$_{cr}$ <30 mL/minute]). Limited data (eg, subgroup analysis) from cSSSI and endocarditis trials suggest possibly reduced clinical efficacy (relative to comparators) in patients with baseline moderate renal impairment (<50 mL/minute). Symptoms suggestive of peripheral neuropathy have been observed with treatment; monitor for new-onset or worsening neuropathy. Prolonged use may result in fungal or bacterial superinfection, including *C. difficile*-associated diarrhea and pseudomembranous colitis. Hypersensitivity reactions and anaphylaxis have been reported with use; discontinue use immediately with signs/symptoms of hypersensitivity and initiate appropriate treatment. Use has been associated with eosinophilic pneumonia; generally develops 2-4 weeks after therapy initiation. Monitor for signs/symptoms of eosinophilic pneumonia, including new onset or worsening fever, dyspnea, difficulty breathing, new infiltrates on chest imaging studies, and/or >25% eosinophils present in bronchoalveolar lavage. Discontinue use immediately with signs/symptoms of eosinophilic pneumonia and initiate appropriate treatment (ie, corticosteroids). May reoccur with re-exposure.

Adverse Reactions (Reflective of adult population; not specific for elderly)

>10%:

Gastrointestinal: Diarrhea (5% to 12%), vomiting (3% to 12%), constipation (6% to 11%)

Hematologic: Anemia (2% to 13%)

1% to 10%:

Cardiovascular: Peripheral edema (7%), chest pain (7%), hypertension (1% to 6%), hypotension (2% to 5%)

Central nervous system: Insomnia (5% to 9%), headache (5% to 7%), fever (2% to 7%), dizziness (2% to 6%), anxiety (5%)

Dermatologic: Rash (4% to 7%), pruritus (3% to 6%), erythema (5%)

Endocrine & metabolic: Hypokalemia (9%), hyperkalemia (5%), hyperphosphatemia (3%)

Gastrointestinal: Nausea (6% to 10%), abdominal pain (6%), dyspepsia (1% to 4%), loose stool (4%), GI hemorrhage (2%)

Genitourinary: Urinary tract infection (2% to 7%)

Hematologic: INR increased (2%), eosinophilia (2%)

Hepatic: Transaminases increased (2% to 3%), alkaline phosphatase increased (2%)

Local: Injection site reaction (3% to 6%)

Neuromuscular & skeletal: CPK increased (3% to 9%), limb pain (2% to 9%), back pain (7%), weakness (5%), arthralgia (1% to 3%)

Renal: Renal failure (2% to 3%)

Respiratory: Pharyngolaryngeal pain (8%), pleural effusion (6%), cough (3%), pneumonia (3%), dyspnea (2% to 3%)

Miscellaneous: Osteomyelitis (6%), bacteremia (5%), diaphoresis (5%), sepsis (5%), infection (fungal, 2% to 3%)

Drug Interactions

Avoid Concomitant Use There are no known interactions where it is recommended to avoid concomitant use.

Increased Effect/Toxicity

The levels/effects of DAPTOmycin may be increased by: HMG-CoA Reductase Inhibitors

Decreased Effect There are no known significant interactions involving a decrease in effect.

Stability Store under refrigeration at 2°C to 8°C (36°F to 46°F). Intact vials may be stored at room temperature for up to 12 months (data on file [Cubist Pharmaceuticals, 2011]). However, the manufacturer recommends storage under refrigeration. Room temperature stability information should only be utilized in situations where the drug has been inadvertently exposed to prolonged room temperature.

Reconstitute vial with 10 mL NS. Add NS to vial and rotate gently to wet powder. Allow to stand for 10 minutes, then gently swirl to obtain completely reconstituted solution. Do not shake or agitate vial vigorously. If administering via IVPB, further dilute following reconstitution in an appropriate volume of NS. Reconstituted solution (either in vial or in infusion bag) is stable for a cumulative time of 12 hours at room temperature and 48 hours if refrigerated (2°C to 8°C). Incompatible with ReadyMED® elastomeric infusion pumps (Cardinal Health, Inc) due to an impurity (2-mercaptobenzothiazole) leaching from the pump system into the daptomycin solution.

Mechanism of Action Daptomycin binds to components of the cell membrane of susceptible organisms and causes rapid depolarization, inhibiting intracellular synthesis of DNA, RNA, and protein. Daptomycin is bactericidal in a concentration-dependent manner.

Pharmacodynamics/Kinetics

Distribution: V_{ss}: 0.1 L/kg; Critically-ill patients: V_{ss}: 0.23 ± 0.14 L/kg (Vilay, 2010)

Protein binding: 90% to 93%; 84% to 88% in patients with Cl_{cr}<30 mL/minute

Half-life elimination: 8-9 hours (up to 28 hours in renal impairment)

Excretion: Urine (78%; primarily as unchanged drug); feces (6%)

Dosage

Geriatric & Adult

Skin and/or skin structure infections (complicated): I.V.: 4 mg/kg once daily for 7-14 days

Bacteremia, right-sided native valve endocarditis caused by MSSA or MRSA: I.V.: 6 mg/kg once daily for 2-6 weeks (some experts recommend 8-10 mg/kg once daily for complicated bacteremia or infective endocarditis [Liu, 2011])

Osteomyelitis (unlabeled use): I.V.: 6 mg/kg once daily for a minimum of 8 weeks (some experts combine with rifampin) (Liu, 2011)

Septic arthritis (unlabeled use): I.V.: 6 mg/kg once daily for 3-4 weeks (Liu, 2011)

Renal Impairment

Cl_{cr} <30 mL/minute:

Skin and soft tissue infections: 4 mg/kg every 48 hours

Staphylococcal bacteremia: 6 mg/kg every 48 hours

Intermittent hemodialysis or peritoneal dialysis (PD): Dose as in Cl_{cr} <30 mL/minute (administer after hemodialysis on dialysis days) or (unlabeled dosing) may administer 6 mg/kg after hemodialysis 3 times weekly (Salama, 2010)

Note: High permeability intermittent hemodialysis removes ~50% during a 4-hour session (Salama, 2010).

Continuous renal replacement therapy (CRRT) (Heintz, 2009; Trotman, 2005): Drug clearance is highly dependent on the method of renal replacement, filter type, and flow rate. Appropriate dosing requires close monitoring of pharmacologic response, signs of adverse reactions due to drug accumulation, as well as drug concentrations in relation to target trough (if appropriate). The following are general recommendations only (based on dialysate flow/ultrafiltration rates of 1-2 L/hour and minimal residual renal function) and should not supersede clinical judgment:

Continuous veno-venous hemodialysis (CVVHD): 8 mg/kg every 48 hours (Vilay, 2010)

Note: For other forms of CRRT (eg, CVVH or CVVHDF), dosing as with Cl_{cr}<30 mL/minute may result in low C_{max}. May consider 4-6 mg/kg every 24 hours (or 8 mg/kg every 48 hours) depending on site or severity of infection or if not responding to standard dosing; therapeutic drug monitoring and/or more frequent serum CPK levels may be necessary (Heintz, 2009).

Slow extended daily dialysis (or extended dialysis): 6 mg/kg every 24 hours (Kielstein, 2010); **Note:** Dialysis should be initiated within 8 hours of administering daptomycin dose to avoid dose accumulation.

Hepatic Impairment No adjustment required for mild-to-moderate impairment (Child-Pugh class A or B). Not evaluated in severe hepatic impairment (Child-Pugh class C).

Administration May administer I.V. push over 2 minutes or infuse IVPB over 30 minutes. Do not use in conjunction with ReadyMED® elastomeric infusion pumps (Cardinal Health, Inc) due to an impurity (2-mercaptobenzothiazole) leaching from the pump system into the daptomycin solution.

Monitoring Parameters Monitor signs and symptoms of infection. CPK should be monitored at least weekly during therapy; more frequent monitoring if current or prior statin therapy, unexplained CPK increases, and/or renal impairment. Monitor for muscle pain or weakness, especially if noted in distal extremities. Canadian labeling recommends CPK monitoring every 48 hours with unexplained muscle pain, tenderness, weakness or cramps. Monitor for signs/symptoms of eosinophilic pneumonia.

Reference Range

Trough concentrations at steady-state:

4 mg/kg once daily: 5.9 ± 1.6 mcg/mL

6 mg/kg once daily: 6.7 ± 1.6 mcg/mL

Note: Trough concentrations are not predictive of efficacy/toxicity. Drug exhibits concentration-dependent bactericidal activity, so C_{max}:MIC ratios may be a more useful parameter.

Test Interactions Daptomycin may cause false prolongation of the PT and increase of INR with certain reagents. This appears to be a dose-dependent phenomenon. Therefore, it is recommended to obtain blood samples immediately prior to next daptomycin dose (eg, trough). If PT/INR elevated, clinicians should repeat PT/INR and evaluate for other causes of hypocoagulation.

Special Geriatric Considerations The manufacturer reports that in studies of complicated skin and skin structure infections, elderly patients had a lower clinical success rate and a higher incidence of adverse effects (no quantitative data provided in product labeling). Adjust dose in renal impairment.

Dosage Forms Excipient information presented when available (limited, particularly for generics); consult specific product labeling.

Injection, powder for reconstitution:

Cubicin®: 500 mg

Selected References

Tedesco KL and Rybak MJ, "Daptomycin," *Pharmacotherapy*, 2004, 24(1):41-57.

Darbepoetin Alfa (dar be POE e tin AL fa)

Medication Safety Issues

Sound-alike/look-alike issues:

Aranesp® may be confused with Aralast, Aricept®

Darbepoetin alfa may be confused with dalteparin, epoetin alfa, epoetin beta

Brand Names: U.S. Aranesp®; Aranesp® SingleJect®

Brand Names: Canada Aranesp®

Index Terms Erythropoiesis-Stimulating Agent (ESA); Erythropoiesis-Stimulating Protein; NESP; Novel Erythropoiesis-Stimulating Protein

Generic Availability (U.S.) No

Pharmacologic Category Colony Stimulating Factor; Growth Factor; Recombinant Human Erythropoietin

Use Treatment of anemia due to concurrent myelosuppressive chemotherapy in patients with cancer (nonmyeloid malignancies) receiving chemotherapy (palliative intent) for a planned minimum of 2 additional months of chemotherapy; treatment of anemia due to chronic kidney disease (including patients on dialysis and not on dialysis)

Note: Darbepoetin is **not** indicated for use under the following conditions:

- Cancer patients receiving hormonal therapy, therapeutic biologic products, or radiation therapy unless also receiving concurrent myelosuppressive chemotherapy
- Cancer patients receiving myelosuppressive chemotherapy when the expected outcome is curative
- As a substitute for RBC transfusion in patients requiring immediate correction of anemia

Note: In clinical trials, darbepoetin has not demonstrated improved quality of life, fatigue, or well-being.

Unlabeled/Investigational Use Treatment of symptomatic anemia in myelodysplastic syndrome (MDS)

Prescribing and Access Restrictions As a requirement of the REMS program, access to this medication is restricted. Healthcare providers and hospitals must be enrolled in the ESA APPRISE (Assisting Providers and Cancer Patients with Risk Information for the Safe use of ESAs) Oncology Program (866-284-8089; http://www.esa-apprise.com) to prescribe or dispense ESAs (ie, darbepoetin alfa, epoetin alfa) to patients with cancer.

Medication Guide Available Yes

Contraindications Hypersensitivity to darbepoetin or any component of the formulation; uncontrolled hypertension; pure red cell aplasia (due to darbepoetin or other erythropoietin protein drugs)

Warnings/Precautions [U.S. Boxed Warning]: Erythropoiesis-stimulating agents (ESAs) increased the risk of serious cardiovascular events, thromboembolic events, stroke, and/or tumor progression in clinical studies; a rapid rise in hemoglobin (>1 g/dL over 2 weeks) or maintaining higher hemoglobin levels may contribute to these risks. **[U.S. Boxed Warning]: A shortened overall survival and/or increased risk of tumor progression or recurrence has been reported in studies with breast, cervical, head and neck, lymphoid, and non small cell lung cancer patients.** It is of note that in these studies, patients received ESAs to a target hemoglobin of ≥12 g/dL; although risk has not been excluded when dosed to achieve a target hemoglobin of <12 g/dL. **[U.S. Boxed Warnings]: To decrease these risks, and risk of cardio- and thrombovascular events, use ESAs in cancer patients only for the treatment of anemia related to concurrent chemotherapy and use the lowest dose needed to avoid red blood cell transfusions. Discontinue ESA following completion of the chemotherapy course. ESAs are not indicated for patients receiving myelosuppressive therapy when the anticipated outcome is curative.** Use of ESAs has been associated with an increased risk of venous thromboembolism (VTE) without a reduction in transfusions in patients >65 years of age with cancer (Hershman, 2009). Improved anemia symptoms, quality of life, fatigue or well-being has not been demonstrated in controlled clinical trials. **[U.S. Boxed Warning]: Because of the risks of decreased survival and increased risk of tumor growth or progression, all healthcare providers and hospitals are required to enroll and comply with the ESA APPRISE (Assisting Providers and Cancer Patients with Risk Information for the Safe use of ESAs) Oncology Program prior to prescribing or dispensing ESAs to cancer patients.** Prescribers and patients will have to provide written documentation of discussed risks.

[U.S. Boxed Warning]: An increased risk of death, serious cardiovascular events, and stroke was reported in patients administered ESAs to target hemoglobin levels ≥13 g/dL; dosing should be individualized to achieve and maintain hemoglobin levels within 10-12 g/dL range. Hemoglobin rising >1 g/dL in a 2-week period may contribute to the risk. CRF patients who exhibit an inadequate hemoglobin response to ESA therapy may be at a higher risk for cardiovascular events and mortality compared to other patients. ESA therapy may reduce dialysis efficacy (due to increase in red blood cells and decrease in plasma volume); adjustments in dialysis parameters may be needed. CRF patients not requiring dialysis may have a better response to darbepoetin and may require lower doses. An increased risk of DVT has been observed in patients treated with epoetin undergoing surgical orthopedic procedures. Darbepoetin is **not** approved for reduction in allogeneic red blood cell transfusions in patients scheduled for surgical procedures. During therapy in any patient, hemoglobin levels should not exceed a target range of 10-12 g/dL and should not rise >1 g/dL per 2-week time period.

Use with caution in patients with hypertension or with a history of seizures; hypertensive encephalopathy and seizures have been reported. Use is contraindicated in patients with uncontrolled hypertension. If hypertension is difficult to control, reduce or hold darbepoetin alfa. Due to the delayed onset of erythropoiesis, darbepoetin alfa is **not** recommended for acute correction of severe anemia or as a substitute for emergency transfusion. Consider discontinuing in patients who receive a renal transplant.

Prior to treatment, correct or exclude deficiencies of iron, vitamin B_{12}, and/or folate, as well as other factors which may impair erythropoiesis (aluminum toxicity, inflammatory conditions, infections). Prior to and during therapy, iron stores must be evaluated. Supplemental iron is recommended if serum ferritin <100 mcg/L or serum transferrin saturation <20%. Poor response should prompt evaluation of these potential factors, as well as possible malignant processes, occult blood loss, hemolysis, and/or bone marrow fibrosis. Severe anemia and pure red cell aplasia (PRCA) with associated neutralizing antibodies to erythropoietin has been reported, predominantly in patients with CRF receiving SubQ darbepoetin (the I.V. route is preferred for hemodialysis patients). Cases have also been reported in patients with hepatitis C who were receiving ESAs, interferon, and ribavirin. Patients with a sudden loss of response to darbepoetin (with severe anemia and a low reticulocyte count) should be evaluated for PRCA with associated neutralizing antibodies to erythropoietin; discontinue treatment in patients with PRCA secondary to neutralizing antibodies to erythropoietin. Antibodies may cross-react; do not switch to another ESA in patients who develop antibody-mediated anemia.

Safety and efficacy in patients with underlying hematologic diseases (eg, porphyria, thalassemia, hemolytic anemia, and sickle cell disease) have not been established. Potentially serious allergic reactions have been reported (rarely). Discontinue immediately (and permanently) in patients who experience serious allergic/anaphylactic reactions. Some products may contain albumin and the packaging of some formulations may contain latex.

Adverse Reactions (Reflective of adult population; not specific for elderly)
>10%:
  Cardiovascular: Hypertension (31%), peripheral edema (17%), edema (6% to 13%)
  Gastrointestinal: Abdominal pain (10% to 13%)
  Respiratory: Dyspnea (17%), cough (12%)
1% to 10%:
  Cardiovascular: Angina, fluid overload, hypotension, MI, thromboembolic events
  Central nervous system: Cerebrovascular disorder
  Dermatologic: Rash/erythema
  Local: AV graft thrombosis, vascular access complications
  Respiratory: Pulmonary embolism

Drug Interactions
  Avoid Concomitant Use There are no known interactions where it is recommended to avoid concomitant use.
  Increased Effect/Toxicity There are no known significant interactions involving an increase in effect.
  Decreased Effect There are no known significant interactions involving a decrease in effect.

Ethanol/Nutrition/Herb Interactions Ethanol: Should be avoided due to adverse effects on erythropoiesis.

Stability Store at 2°C to 8°C (36°F to 46°F); do not freeze. Do not shake. Protect from light. Store in original carton until use. The following stability information has also been reported: May be stored at room temperature for up to 7 days (Cohen, 2007). Do not dilute or administer with other solutions.

Mechanism of Action Induces erythropoiesis by stimulating the division and differentiation of committed erythroid progenitor cells; induces the release of reticulocytes from the bone marrow into the bloodstream, where they mature to erythrocytes. There is a dose response relationship with this effect. This results in an increase in reticulocyte counts followed by a rise in hematocrit and hemoglobin levels. When administered SubQ or I.V., darbepoetin's half-life is ~3 times that of epoetin alfa concentrations.

Pharmacodynamics/Kinetics
  Onset of action: Increased hemoglobin levels not generally observed until 2-6 weeks after initiating treatment
  Absorption: SubQ: Slow
  Distribution: V_d: 0.06 L/kg
  Bioavailability: CRF: SubQ: Adults: ~37% (range: 30% to 50%)
  Half-life elimination:
    CRF: Adults:
      I.V.: 21 hours
      SubQ: Nondialysis patients: 70 hours (range: 35-139 hours); Dialysis patients: 46 hours (range: 12-89 hours)
    Cancer: Adults: SubQ: 74 hours (range: 24-144 hours)
    Note: Darbepoetin half-life is approximately threefold longer than epoetin alfa following I.V. administration
  Time to peak: SubQ:
    CRF: Adults: 48 hours (range: 12-72 hours; independent of dialysis)
    Cancer: Adults: 71-90 hours (range: 28-123 hours)

Dosage
  Geriatric & Adult Note: Hemoglobin levels should not exceed 12 g/dL and should not rise >1 g/dL per 2-week time period during therapy in any patient.

  Anemia associated with CRF: Individualize dosing to achieve and maintain hemoglobin levels to a target range of 10-12 g/dL. Hemoglobin levels should not exceed 12 g/dL.
    I.V., SubQ: Initial: 0.45 mcg/kg once weekly; alternative dose for nondialysis patients: 0.75 mcg/kg once every 2 weeks; Maintenance: titrate to maintain hemoglobin levels between 10-12 g/dL as described below (may be administered once weekly or every 2 weeks; nondialysis patients may require lower maintenance doses) **Note:** I.V. route is preferred in hemodialysis patients.

Dosage adjustment:

Decrease dose by ~25%: If hemoglobin approaches 12 g/dL **or** hemoglobin increases >1 g/dL in any 2-week period. If hemoglobin continues to increase, temporarily discontinue therapy until hemoglobin begins to decrease, then resume therapy with a ~25% reduction from previous dose.

Increase dose by ~25%: If hemoglobin does not increase by 1 g/dL after 4 weeks of therapy (with adequate iron stores). Do not increase dose more frequently than at 4-week intervals.

Inadequate or lack of response: If patient does not attain target hemoglobin range of 10-12 g/dL after appropriate dose titrations over 12 weeks:

Do not continue to increase dose and use the minimum effective dose that will maintain a hemoglobin level sufficient to avoid red blood cell transfusions **and** evaluate patient for other causes of anemia.

Monitor hemoglobin closely thereafter and if responsiveness improves, may resume making dosage adjustments as recommended above. If responsiveness does not improve and recurrent red blood cell transfusions continue to be needed, discontinue therapy.

Maintenance dose: Individualize to target hemoglobin range of 10-12 g/dL; limit additional dosage increase to every 4 weeks or longer. Patients generally require lower maintenance doses than initial doses to maintain target range.

Conversion from epoetin alfa: I.V., SubQ: Initial dose: Epoetin alfa doses may be converted to doses ranging from 6.25-200 mcg darbepoetin alfa per week (see conversion table below).

Anemia associated with chemotherapy: Titrate dosage to use the minimum effective dose that will maintain a hemoglobin level sufficient to avoid red blood cell transfusions. Do not initiate therapy if hemoglobin ≥10 g/dL. Discontinue darbepoetin following completion of chemotherapy.

SubQ: Initial: 2.25 mcg/kg once weekly **or** 500 mcg once every 3 weeks

Dosage adjustment:

Increase dose: If hemoglobin does not increase by 1 g/dL after 6 weeks of therapy (for patients receiving weekly therapy), the dose should be increased up to 4.5 mcg/kg once weekly

Decrease dose by 40%: If hemoglobin increases >1g/dL in any 2-week period **or** hemoglobin reaches a level sufficient to avoid red blood cell transfusion.

Withhold dose: If hemoglobin exceeds a level needed to avoid red blood cell transfusion. Resume treatment with a dose 40% below the previous dose when hemoglobin approaches a level where transfusions may be required.

Discontinue: On completion of chemotherapy or if after 8 weeks of therapy there is no hemoglobin response or transfusions still required

Symptomatic anemia associated with MDS (unlabeled use): Adults: SubQ: 150-300 mcg once weekly (NCCN MDS guidelines v.2.2010)

Conversion from epoetin alfa to darbepoetin alfa: See table.

Conversion From Epoetin Alfa to Darbepoetin Alfa (Initial Dose)

Previous Dosage of Epoetin Alfa (units/week)	Adults Darbepoetin Alfa Dosage (mcg/week)
<1500	6.25
1500-2499	6.25
2500-4999	12.5
5000-10,999	25
11,000-17,999	40
18,000-33,999	60
34,000-89,999	100
≥90,000	200

Note: In patients receiving epoetin alfa 2-3 times per week, darbepoetin alfa is administered once weekly. In patients receiving epoetin alfa once weekly, darbepoetin alfa is administered once every 2 weeks. The darbepoetin dose to be administered every 2 weeks is derived by adding together 2 weekly epoetin alfa doses and then converting to the appropriate darbepoetin dose. Titrate dose to hemoglobin response thereafter.

Administration May be administered by SubQ or I.V. injection. The I.V. route is recommended in hemodialysis patients. Do not shake; vigorous shaking may denature darbepoetin alfa,

◀ rendering it biologically inactive. Do not dilute or administer in conjunction with other drug solutions. Discard any unused portion of the vial; do not pool unused portions.

Monitoring Parameters Hemoglobin (at least once per week until maintenance dose established and after dosage changes; monitor less frequently once hemoglobin is stabilized); CKD patients should be also be monitored at least monthly following hemoglobin stability); iron stores (transferrin saturation and ferritin) prior to and during therapy; serum chemistry (CKD patients); blood pressure; fluid balance (CKD patients); seizures (CKD patients following initiation for first few months, includes new-onset or change in seizure frequency or premonitory symptoms)

Cancer patients: Examinations recommended by the ASCO/ASH guidelines (Rizzo, 2010) prior to treatment include peripheral blood smear (in some situations a bone marrow exam may be necessary), assessment for iron, folate, or vitamin B_{12} deficiency, reticulocyte count, renal function status, and occult blood loss; during ESA treatment, assess baseline and periodic iron, total iron-binding capacity, and transferrin saturation or ferritin levels.

Pharmacotherapy Pearls Oncology Comment: The American Society of Clinical Oncology (ASCO) and American Society of Hematology (ASH) 2010 updates to the clinical practice guidelines for the use of erythropoiesis-stimulating agents (ESAs) in patients with cancer indicate that ESAs are appropriate when used according to the parameters identified within the Food and Drug Administration (FDA) approved labeling for epoetin and darbepoetin (Rizzo, 2010). ESAs are an option for chemotherapy associated anemia when the hemoglobin has fallen to <10 g/dL to decrease the need for RBC transfusions. ESAs should only be used in conjunction with concurrent chemotherapy. Although the FDA label now limits ESA use to the palliative setting, the ASCO/ASH guidelines suggest using clinical judgment in weighing risks versus benefits as formal outcomes studies of ESA use defined by intent of chemotherapy treatment have not been conducted.

The ASCO/ASH guidelines continue to recommend following the FDA approved dosing (and dosing adjustment) guidelines as alternate dosing and schedules have not demonstrated consistent differences in effectiveness with regard to hemoglobin response. In patients who do not have a response within 6-8 weeks (hemoglobin rise <1-2 g/dL or no reduction in transfusions) ESA therapy should be discontinued.

Prior to the initiation of ESAs, other sources of anemia (in addition to chemotherapy or underlying hematologic malignancy) should be investigated. Examinations recommended prior to treatment include peripheral blood smear (in some situations a bone marrow exam may be necessary), assessment for iron, folate, or vitamin B_{12} deficiency, reticulocyte count, renal function status, and occult blood loss. During ESA treatment, assess baseline and periodic iron, total iron-binding capacity, and transferrin saturation or ferritin levels. Iron supplementation may be necessary.

The guidelines note that patients with an increased risk of thromboembolism (generally includes previous history of thrombosis, surgery, and/or prolonged periods of immobilization) and patients receiving concomitant medications that may increase thromboembolic risk, should begin ESA therapy only after careful consideration. With the exception of low-risk myelodysplasia-associated anemia (which has evidence supporting the use of ESAs without concurrent chemotherapy), the guidelines do not support the use of ESAs in the absence of concurrent chemotherapy.

Dosage Forms Excipient information presented when available (limited, particularly for generics); consult specific product labeling.

Injection, solution [preservative free]:

Aranesp®: 25 mcg/mL (1 mL); 40 mcg/mL (1 mL); 60 mcg/mL (1 mL); 100 mcg/mL (1 mL); 150 mcg/0.75 mL (0.75 mL); 200 mcg/mL (1 mL); 300 mcg/mL (1 mL) [contains polysorbate 80]

Aranesp® SingleJect®: 25 mcg/0.42 mL (0.42 mL); 40 mcg/0.4 mL (0.4 mL); 60 mcg/0.3 mL (0.3 mL); 100 mcg/0.5 mL (0.5 mL); 150 mcg/0.3 mL (0.3 mL); 200 mcg/0.4 mL (0.4 mL); 300 mcg/0.6 mL (0.6 mL); 500 mcg/mL (1 mL) [contains natural rubber/natural latex in packaging, polysorbate 80]

Darifenacin (dar i FEN a sin)

Related Information

Pharmacotherapy of Urinary Incontinence *on page 2032*

Brand Names: U.S. Enablex®

Brand Names: Canada Enablex®

Index Terms Darifenacin Hydrobromide; UK-88,525

Generic Availability (U.S.) No

Pharmacologic Category Anticholinergic Agent

Use Management of symptoms of bladder overactivity (urge incontinence, urgency, and frequency)

Contraindications Hypersensitivity to darifenacin or any component of the formulation; uncontrolled narrow-angle glaucoma; urinary retention, paralytic ileus, GI or GU obstruction

Warnings/Precautions May cause drowsiness and/or blurred vision, which may impair physical or mental abilities; patients must be cautioned about performing tasks which require mental alertness (eg, operating machinery or driving). May occur in the presence of increased environmental temperature; use caution in hot weather and/or exercise. Use with caution with hepatic impairment; dosage limitation is required in moderate hepatic impairment (Child-Pugh class B). Not recommended for use in severe hepatic impairment (Child-Pugh class C). Use with caution in patients with clinically-significant bladder outlet obstruction or prostatic hyperplasia (nonobstructive). Use caution in patients with decreased GI motility, constipation, hiatal hernia, reflux esophagitis, and ulcerative colitis. Use caution in patients with myasthenia gravis. In patients with controlled narrow-angle glaucoma, darifenacin should be used with extreme caution and only when the potential benefit outweighs risks of treatment. Use with caution in patients taking strong CYP3A4 inhibitors (see Drug Interactions); dosage limitation of darifenacin is required.

Adverse Reactions (Reflective of adult population; not specific for elderly)

>10%: Gastrointestinal: Xerostomia (19% to 35%), constipation (15% to 21%)

1% to 10%:

Cardiovascular: Hypertension (≥1%), peripheral edema (≥1%)

Central nervous system: Headache (7%), dizziness (<2%), pain (≥1%)

Dermatological: Dry skin (≥1%), pruritus (≥1%), rash (≥1%)

Gastrointestinal: Dyspepsia (3% to 8%), abdominal pain (2% to 4%), nausea (2% to 4%), vomiting (≥1%), weight gain (≥1%)

Genitourinary: Urinary tract infection (4% to 5%), vaginitis (≥1%), urinary retention (acute)

Neuromuscular & skeletal: Weakness (<3%), arthralgia (≥1%), back pain (≥1%)

Ocular: Dry eyes (2%), abnormal vision (≥1%)

Respiratory: Bronchitis (≥1%), pharyngitis (≥1%), rhinitis (≥1%), sinusitis (≥1%)

Miscellaneous: Flu-like syndrome (1% to 3%)

Drug Interactions

Metabolism/Transport Effects Substrate of CYP2D6 (minor), CYP3A4 (major); **Inhibits** CYP2D6 (moderate), 3A4 (weak)

Avoid Concomitant Use

Avoid concomitant use of Darifenacin with any of the following: Conivaptan; Thioridazine

Increased Effect/Toxicity

Darifenacin may increase the levels/effects of: AbobotulinumtoxinA; Anticholinergics; Cannabinoids; CYP2D6 Substrates; Fesoterodine; Nebivolol; OnabotulinumtoxinA; Potassium Chloride; RimabotulinumtoxinB; Tamoxifen; Thioridazine

The levels/effects of Darifenacin may be increased by: Conivaptan; CYP3A4 Inhibitors (Moderate); CYP3A4 Inhibitors (Strong); Dasatinib; Pramlintide

Decreased Effect

Darifenacin may decrease the levels/effects of: Acetylcholinesterase Inhibitors (Central); Codeine; Secretin; TraMADol

The levels/effects of Darifenacin may be decreased by: Acetylcholinesterase Inhibitors (Central); CYP3A4 Inducers (Strong); Deferasirox; Herbs (CYP3A4 Inducers); Peginterferon Alfa-2b; Tocilizumab

Ethanol/Nutrition/Herb Interactions Herb/Nutraceutical: Darifenacin serum concentration may be decreased by St John's wort (avoid concurrent use.)

Stability Store at 25°C (77°F); excursions permitted to 15°C to 30°C (59°F to 86°F). Protect from light.

Mechanism of Action Selective antagonist of the M3 muscarinic (cholinergic) receptor subtype. Blockade of the receptor limits bladder contractions, reducing the symptoms of bladder irritability/overactivity (urge incontinence, urgency and frequency).

Pharmacodynamics/Kinetics

Distribution: V_{dss}: ~163 L

Protein binding: ~98% (primarily alpha$_1$-acid glycoprotein)

Metabolism: Hepatic, via CYP3A4 (major) and CYP2D6 (minor)

Bioavailability: 15% to 19%

Half-life elimination: ~13-19 hours

Time to peak, plasma: ~7 hours

Excretion: As metabolites (inactive); urine (60%), feces (40%)

◄ **Dosage**
Geriatric & Adult
Symptoms of bladder overactivity: Oral: Initial: 7.5 mg once daily. If response is not adequate after a minimum of 2 weeks, dosage may be increased to 15 mg once daily.
Dosage adjustment with concomitant potent CYP3A4 inhibitors (eg, azole antifungals, erythromycin, isoniazid, protease inhibitors): Daily dosage should not exceed 7.5 mg/day
Renal Impairment No adjustment required.
Hepatic Impairment
Moderate impairment (Child-Pugh class B): Daily dosage should not exceed 7.5 mg/day
Severe impairment (Child-Pugh class C): Has not been evaluated; use is not recommended
Administration Tablet should be swallowed whole; may be taken without regard to food.

Special Geriatric Considerations There is a trend for decreased clearance of darifenacin with age, though no change in dose is recommended. The selectivity of darifenacin for the M3 receptor on the bladder may offer an advantage (less CNS and cardiovascular effects) over other anticholinergic agents used in the treatment of overactive bladder.

Dosage Forms Excipient information presented when available (limited, particularly for generics); consult specific product labeling.
Tablet, extended release, oral:
Enablex®: 7.5 mg, 15 mg

Selected References
Croom KF and Keating GM, "Darifenacin in the Treatment of Overactive Bladder," *Drugs Aging*, 2004, 21(13):885-92.

◆ **Darifenacin Hydrobromide** *see* Darifenacin *on page 460*
◆ **1-Day™ [OTC]** *see* Tioconazole *on page 1803*
◆ **Daypro®** *see* Oxaprozin *on page 1357*
◆ **Daytrana®** *see* Methylphenidate *on page 1179*
◆ **DDAVP®** *see* Desmopressin *on page 477*
◆ **DDrops®** *see* Cholecalciferol *on page 346*
◆ **DDrops® Baby [OTC]** *see* Cholecalciferol *on page 346*
◆ **DDrops® Kids [OTC]** *see* Cholecalciferol *on page 346*
◆ **1-Deamino-8-D-Arginine Vasopressin** *see* Desmopressin *on page 477*
◆ **Debrox® [OTC]** *see* Carbamide Peroxide *on page 272*
◆ **Decadron** *see* Dexamethasone (Systemic) *on page 483*
◆ **Decavac®** *see* Diphtheria and Tetanus Toxoids *on page 525*
◆ **Declomycin** *see* Demeclocycline *on page 467*
◆ **Deep Sea [OTC]** *see* Sodium Chloride *on page 1690*

Deferasirox (de FER a sir ox)

Medication Safety Issues
Sound-alike/look-alike issues:
Deferasirox may be confused with deferoxamine
International issues:
Deferasirox may be confused with deferiprone [Great Britain]
Brand Names: U.S. Exjade®
Brand Names: Canada Exjade®
Index Terms ICL670
Generic Availability (U.S.) No
Pharmacologic Category Antidote; Chelating Agent
Use Treatment of chronic iron overload due to blood transfusions (transfusional hemosiderosis)
Prescribing and Access Restrictions Deferasirox (Exjade®) is only available through a restricted distribution program called EPASS™ Complete Care. Prescribers must enroll patients in this program in order to obtain the medication. For patient enrollment, contact 1-888-90-EPASS (1-888-903-7277).
Contraindications Hypersensitivity to deferasirox or any component of the formulation; platelet counts (<50,000/mm^3); poor performance status and high-risk myelodysplastic syndromes or advanced malignancies; creatinine clearance <40 mL/minute or serum creatinine >2 x age-appropriate ULN

Canadian labeling: Additional contraindications (not in U.S. labeling): Cl_{cr} <60 mL/minute

Warnings/Precautions [U.S. Boxed Warning]: Acute renal failure (some fatal) and dose-related elevations in serum creatinine have been reported; fatalities generally observed more in patients with multiple comorbidities or advanced hematologic disorders. Monitor serum creatinine and/or creatinine clearance in all patients; monitor patients at risk for renal complications (eg, pre-existing renal conditions, elderly, comorbid conditions, and/or with concurrent medications that may affect renal function) more closely; dose reduction, interruption, or discontinuation may be required for serum creatinine elevations. May cause proteinuria; closely monitor. Renal tubulopathy has also been reported, primarily in pediatric patients with β-thalassemia and serum ferritin levels <1500 mcg/L.

[U.S. Boxed Warning]: Severe hepatic dysfunction or failure (including fatalities) have occurred (postmarketing reports), mostly in patients >55 years of age with underlying comorbidities (including hepatic cirrhosis and multiorgan failure). Hepatitis and elevated transaminases have also been reported; monitor transaminases and bilirubin closely and consider dose modification or interruption of therapy with severe or persistent hepatic function test abnormalities. Use with caution in patients with underlying hepatic disease. [U.S. Boxed Warning]: Gastrointestinal (GI) hemorrhage, including fatalities, has occurred with use, predominately in elderly patients with advanced hematologic malignancies and/or low platelet counts. Other GI effects including irritation and ulceration. Use caution with concurrent medications that may increase risk of adverse GI effects (eg, NSAIDs, corticosteroids, anticoagulants, oral bisphosphonates). Monitor patients closely for signs/symptoms of GI ulceration/bleeding.

May cause skin rash (dose-related), including erythema multiforme; mild-to-moderate rashes may resolve without treatment interruption; for severe rash, interrupt and consider restarting at a lower dose with dose escalation and oral steroids. Hypersensitivity reactions, including severe reactions (anaphylaxis and angioedema) have been reported, usually within the first month of treatment. Discontinuation of therapy may be necessary. Auditory (decreased hearing and high frequency hearing loss) or ocular disturbances (lens opacities, cataracts, intraocular pressure elevation, and retinal disorders) have been reported; monitor and consider dose reduction or treatment interruption. Cytopenias (including agranulocytosis, neutropenia, and thrombocytopenia) have been reported, predominately in patients with preexisting hematologic disorders; monitor closely; interrupt treatment for unexplained cytopenias. Potent UGT inducers (eg, rifampin) or cholestyramine may decrease the efficacy of deferasirox; avoid concomitant use. If coadministration necessary, dosage modifications may be needed; monitor serum ferritin and clinical response. Do not combine with other iron chelation therapies; safety of combinations has not been established. Treatment should be initiated with evidence of chronic iron overload (eg, transfusion of ~100 mL/kg of packed RBCs [~20 units for a 40 kg individual] and serum ferritin consistently >1000 mcg/L). Prior to use, consider risk versus anticipated benefit with respect to individual patient's life expectancy and prognosis. Use with caution in the elderly due to the higher incidence of hepatic, renal and cardiac dysfunction in the elderly.

Adverse Reactions (Reflective of adult population; not specific for elderly)
>10%:
  Central nervous system: Fever (19%), headache (16%)
  Dermatologic: Rash (dose related; 8% to 11%)
  Gastrointestinal: Abdominal pain (dose related; 21% to 28%), diarrhea (dose related; 12% to 20%), nausea (dose related; 11% to 23%), vomiting (dose related; 10% to 21%)
  Renal: Serum creatinine increased (dose related; 7% to 38%), proteinuria (19%)
  Respiratory: Cough (14%), nasopharyngitis (13%), pharyngolaryngeal pain (11%)
  Miscellaneous: Influenza (11%)
1% to 10%:
  Central nervous system: Fatigue (6%)
  Dermatologic: Urticaria (4%)
  Hepatic: ALT increased (2% to 8%), transaminitis (4%)
  Neuromuscular & skeletal: Arthralgia (7%), back pain (6%)
  Otic: Ear infection (5%)
  Respiratory: Respiratory tract infection (10%), bronchitis (9%), pharyngitis (8%), acute tonsillitis (6%), rhinitis (6%)

Drug Interactions
Metabolism/Transport Effects Substrate of UGT1A1 (major), 1A3; **Inhibits** CYP2C8 (moderate); **Induces** 3A4 (weak)

Avoid Concomitant Use
  Avoid concomitant use of Deferasirox with any of the following: Aluminum Hydroxide; Theophylline

Increased Effect/Toxicity
  Deferasirox may increase the levels/effects of: CYP1A2 Substrates; CYP2C8 Substrates (High risk); Theophylline

  The levels/effects of Deferasirox may be increased by: Anticoagulants; Bisphosphonate Derivatives; Corticosteroids; Corticosteroids (Systemic); Nonsteroidal Anti-Inflammatory Agents

DEFERASIROX

Decreased Effect

Deferasirox may decrease the levels/effects of: CYP3A4 Substrates

The levels/effects of Deferasirox may be decreased by: Aluminum Hydroxide; Cholestyramine Resin; Fosphenytoin; PHENobarbital; Phenytoin; Rifampin; Ritonavir

Stability Store at room temperature of 25°C (77°F); excursions permitted to 15°C and 30°C (59°F and 86°F). Protect from moisture.

Mechanism of Action Selectively binds iron, forming a complex which is excreted primarily through the feces.

Pharmacodynamics/Kinetics

Distribution: Adults: 11.7-17.1 L

Protein binding: ~99% to serum albumin

Metabolism: Hepatic via glucuronidation by UGT1A1(primarily) and UGT1A3; minor oxidation by CYP450; undergoes enterohepatic recirculation

Bioavailability: 70%

Half-life elimination: 8-16 hours

Time to peak, plasma: ~1.5-4 hours

Excretion: Feces (84%); urine (8%)

Dosage

Geriatric & Adult Chronic iron overload due to blood transfusion: Oral: **Note:** Baseline serum ferritin and iron levels should be obtained prior to therapy; toxicity may be increased in patients with low iron burden or with only slightly elevated serum ferritin.

Initial: 20 mg/kg daily (calculate dose to nearest whole tablet)

Maintenance: Adjust dose every 3-6 months based on serum ferritin levels; adjust by 5 or 10 mg/kg/day (calculate dose to nearest whole tablet); titrate. Usual range: 20-30 mg/kg/day; doses up to 40 mg/kg/day may be considered for serum ferritin levels persistently >2500 mcg/L (doses above 40 mg/kg/day are not recommended). In clinical trials, doses were individualized based on iron burden determined by liver iron concentrations (LIC); transfusional iron intake should be considered when individualizing maintenance dose. **Note:** Consider interrupting therapy for serum ferritin <500 mcg/L and dose reduction or interruption for hearing loss or visual disturbances.

Dosage adjustment with concomitant cholestyramine or potent UGT inducers (eg, rifampin, phenytoin, phenobarbital, ritonavir): Avoid concomitant use; if coadministration necessary, consider increasing the initial dose of deferasirox dose to 30 mg/kg; monitor serum ferritin and clinical response. Doses above 40 mg/kg are not recommended.

Renal Impairment

Cl$_{cr}$ ≥40 to <60 mL/minute: Use caution; monitor renal function closely, particularly in patients at increased risk for further renal impairment (eg, concomitant therapy, dehydration, severe infection)

Cl$_{cr}$ <40 mL/minute or serum creatinine >2 times age-appropriate ULN: Use is contraindicated

Progressive increase in serum creatinine: Consider dose reduction, interruption, or discontinuation. Interrupt treatment for progressive increase in serum creatinine above the age-appropriate ULN; once serum creatinine recovers to within the normal range, reinitiate treatment at a reduced dose; gradually escalate the dose if the clinical benefit outweighs potential risk.

Adults: For increase in serum creatinine >33% above the average pretreatment level at 2 consecutive levels (and cannot be attributed to other causes), reduce daily dose by 10 mg/kg

Hepatic Impairment Consider dose adjustment or discontinuation for severe or persistent elevations in liver function tests.

Administration Oral: **Do not chew or swallow whole tablets.** Disperse tablets in water, orange juice, or apple juice (use 3.5 ounces for total doses <1 g; 7 ounces for doses ≥1 g); stir to form suspension and drink entire contents. Rinse remaining residue with more fluid; drink. Administer at same time each day on an empty stomach, 30 minutes before food. Do not take simultaneously with aluminum-containing antacids.

Monitoring Parameters Serum ferritin (baseline, monthly thereafter), iron levels (baseline), CBC with differential, serum creatinine and/or creatinine clearance (2 baseline assessments then monthly thereafter; in patients who are at increased risk of complications [eg, pre-existing renal conditions, elderly, comorbid conditions, or receiving other potentially nephrotoxic medications]: weekly for the first month then monthly thereafter); urine protein (monthly); serum transaminases and bilirubin (baseline and annual auditory and ophthalmic function (including slit lamp examinations and dilated fundoscopy); number of RBC units received

Pharmacotherapy Pearls Deferasirox has a low affinity for binding with zinc and copper, may cause variable decreases in the serum concentration of these trace minerals.

Oncology Comment: The National Comprehensive Cancer Network (NCCN) guidelines for myelodysplastic syndromes (MDS) recommend considering iron chelation therapy in low- or intermediate-risk MDS patients to decrease iron overload due to multiple transfusions (v.2.2010). Treatment is generally recommended in MDS patients who have received ≥20 units of RBC transfusions and for those with serum ferritin levels >2500 mcg/L, with a goal to decrease ferritin levels to <1000 mcg/L. Although clinical trials in MDS are ongoing, deferasirox may be useful in the management of iron overload of these patients.

Special Geriatric Considerations Studies to date have not included sufficient numbers of subjects ≥65 years of age. Use caution in patients with liver dysfunction or low serum albumin. Monitor renal function. In general, this drug should be used with caution and close monitoring in elderly due to the greater incidence of decreased hepatic, renal, cardiac function, as well as concomitant disease and drug therapy.

Dosage Forms Excipient information presented when available (limited, particularly for generics); consult specific product labeling.

Tablet for suspension, oral:

Exjade®: 125 mg, 250 mg, 500 mg

Selected References

Cappellini MD, "Long-Term Efficacy and Safety of Deferasirox," *Blood Rev*, 2008, 22(Suppl 2):35-41.

National Comprehensive Cancer Network (NCCN), "Clinical Practice Guidelines in Oncology™: Myelodysplastic Syndromes," Version 2, 2008. Available at http://www.nccn.org/professionals/physician_gls/PDF/mds.pdf.

Degarelix (deg a REL ix)

Medication Safety Issues

Sound-alike/look-alike issues:

Degarelix may be confused with cetrorelix, ganirelix

Brand Names: U.S. Firmagon®

Brand Names: Canada Firmagon®

Index Terms Degarelix Acetate; FE200486

Generic Availability (U.S.) No

Pharmacologic Category Antineoplastic Agent, Gonadotropin-Releasing Hormone Antagonist; Gonadotropin Releasing Hormone Antagonist

Use Treatment of advanced prostate cancer

Contraindications Hypersensitivity to degarelix or any component of the formulation

Warnings/Precautions Hazardous agent - use appropriate precautions for handling and disposal. Long-term androgen deprivation therapy may prolong the QT interval; use with caution in patients with a known history of QT prolongation or other risk factors for QT prolongation (eg, concomitant use of medications known to prolong QT interval, heart failure, and/or electrolyte abnormalities). Androgen-deprivation therapy may increase the risk for cardiovascular disease (Levine, 2010) and decreased bone mineral density. Androgen deprivation therapy may cause obesity and insulin resistance; the risk for diabetes is increased.

Degarelix exposure is decreased in patients with hepatic impairment, dosage adjustment is not recommended in patients with mild-to-moderate hepatic impairment, although testosterone levels should be monitored. Has not been studied in patients with severe hepatic impairment; use with caution. Data for use in patients with moderate-to-severe renal impairment (Cl_{cr} <50 mL/minute) is limited; use with caution.

Adverse Reactions (Reflective of adult population; not specific for elderly)

>10%:

Endocrine & metabolic: Hot flashes (26%)

Local: Injections site reactions (35%, grade 3: ≤2%; pain 28%, erythema 17%, swelling 6%, induration 4%, nodule 3%)

1% to 10%:

Cardiovascular: Hypertension (6%)

Central nervous system: Chills (5%), dizziness (1% to 5%), fever (1% to 5%), headache (1% to 5%), insomnia (1% to 5%), fatigue (3%)

Dermatologic: Hyperhidrosis

Endocrine & metabolic: Hypercholesterolemia (3%), gynecomastia, testicular atrophy

Gastrointestinal: Weight gain (9%), constipation (5%), nausea (1% to 5%), diarrhea

Genitourinary: Urinary tract infection (5%), erectile dysfunction

Hepatic: ALT increased (10%; grade 3: <1%), AST increased (5%; grade 3: <1%), GGT increased

Neuromuscular & skeletal: Back pain (6%), arthralgia (5%), weakness (1% to 5%)

Miscellaneous: Antidegarelix antibody formation (10%), night sweats (1% to 5%)

◀ **Drug Interactions**
Avoid Concomitant Use
Avoid concomitant use of Degarelix with any of the following: Artemether; Dronedarone; Lumefantrine; Nilotinib; Pimozide; QUEtiapine; QuiNINE; Tetrabenazine; Thioridazine; Toremifene; Vandetanib; Vemurafenib; Ziprasidone

Increased Effect/Toxicity
Degarelix may increase the levels/effects of: Dronedarone; Pimozide; QTc-Prolonging Agents; QuiNINE; Tetrabenazine; Thioridazine; Toremifene; Vandetanib; Vemurafenib; Ziprasidone

The levels/effects of Degarelix may be increased by: Alfuzosin; Artemether; Chloroquine; Ciprofloxacin; Ciprofloxacin (Systemic); Gadobutrol; Lumefantrine; Nilotinib; QUEtiapine; QuiNINE

Decreased Effect There are no known significant interactions involving a decrease in effect.

Stability Store at 25°C (77°F); excursions permitted to 15°C to 30°C (59°F to 86°F). Use appropriate precautions (wear gloves for preparation and administration) for handling and disposal. Reconstitute with preservative free sterile water for injection (reconstitute each 120 mg vial with 3 mL; reconstitute the 80 mg vial with 4.2 mL). Swirl gently; do not shake (to prevent foaming). Dissolution may take up to 15 minutes. Keep vial upright at all times. Tilt vial slightly, keeping needle in lowest section of vial to withdraw for administration. Administer within 1 hour of reconstitution.

Mechanism of Action Gonadotropin-releasing hormone (GnRH) antagonist which reversibly binds to GnRH receptors in the anterior pituitary gland, blocking the receptor and decreasing secretion of luteinizing hormone (LH) and follicle stimulation hormone (FSH), resulting in rapid androgen deprivation by decreasing testosterone production, thereby decreasing testosterone levels. Testosterone levels do not exhibit an initial surge, or flare, as is typical with GnRH agonists.

Pharmacodynamics/Kinetics
Onset of action: Rapid; ~96% of patients had testosterone levels ≤50 ng/dL within 3 days (Klotz, 2008)
Distribution: V_d: >1000 L
Protein binding: ~90%
Metabolism: Hepatobiliary, via peptide hydrolysis
Bioavailability: Biphasic release: Rapid release initially, then slow release from depot formed after subcutaneous injection administration (Tornoe, 2007)
Half-life elimination: Loading dose: SubQ: ~53 days
Time to peak, plasma: Loading dose: SubQ: Within 2 days
Excretion: Feces (~70% to 80%, primarily as peptide fragments); urine (~20% to 30%)

Dosage
Geriatric & Adult Prostate cancer: SubQ:
Loading dose: 240 mg administered as two 120 mg (3 mL) injections
Maintenance dose: 80 mg every 28 days (beginning 28 days after initial loading dose)
Renal Impairment Cl_{cr} <50 mL/minute: Use with caution.
Hepatic Impairment
Mild-to-moderate hepatic impairment: No adjustment required; monitor serum testosterone levels.
Severe hepatic impairment: Has not been studied; use with caution.

Administration Not for I.V. use. Administer SubQ in the abdominal area by grasping skin and elevating SubQ tissue; inject at an angle ≤45 degrees. Avoid pressure exposed areas (eg, waistband, near ribs); rotate injection site. Inject loading dose as two 3 mL injections (40 mg/mL); maintenance dose should be administered as one 4 mL injection (20 mg/mL); begin maintenance dose 28 days after initial loading dose.

Monitoring Parameters Prostate-specific antigen (PSA) periodically, serum testosterone levels (if PSA increases; in patients with hepatic impairment: monitor testosterone levels monthly until achieve castration levels, then consider monitoring every other month), liver function tests (at baseline), serum electrolytes (calcium, magnesium, potassium, sodium); bone mineral density

Screen for diabetes and cardiovascular risk prior to initiating treatment.

Test Interactions Suppression of pituitary-gonadal function may affect diagnostic tests of pituitary gonadotropic and gonadal functions.

Special Geriatric Considerations No dosage adjustments are necessary in elderly. Monitor serum lipids and for hypertension.

Dosage Forms Excipient information presented when available (limited, particularly for generics); consult specific product labeling.
Injection, powder for reconstitution, as acetate:
Firmagon®: 80 mg, 120 mg

Selected References

Gittelman M, Pommerville JP, Persson BE, et al, "A 1-Year, Open Label, Randomized Phase II Dose Finding Study of Degarelix for the Treatment of Prostate Cancer in North America," *J Urol*, 2008, 180(5):1986-92.

Klotz L, Boccon-Gibod L, Shore ND, et al, "The Efficacy and Safety of Degarelix: A 12-month, Comparative, Randomized, Open-Label, Parallel-Group Phase III Study in Patients With Prostate Cancer," *BJU Int*, 2008, 102 (11):1531-8.

National Comprehensive Cancer Network® (NCCN), "Clinical Practice Guidelines in Oncology™: Prostate Cancer," Version 1, 2009. Available at http://www.nccn.org/professionals/physician_gls/PDF/prostate.pdf

Tornoe CW, Agerso H, Senderovitz T, et al, "Population Pharmacokinetic/Pharmacodynamic (PK/PD) Modelling of the Hypothalamic-Pituitary-Gonadal Axis Following Treatment With GnRH Analogues," *Br J Clin Pharmacol*, 2007, 63 (6):648-64.

- ◆ **Degarelix Acetate** *see Degarelix on page 465*
- ◆ **Dehydrobenzperidol** *see Droperidol on page 577*
- ◆ **Delatestryl®** *see Testosterone on page 1761*
- ◆ **Delestrogen®** *see Estradiol (Systemic) on page 641*
- ◆ **Delsym® [OTC]** *see Dextromethorphan on page 490*
- ◆ **Delta-9-tetrahydro-cannabinol** *see Dronabinol on page 574*
- ◆ **Delta-9 THC** *see Dronabinol on page 574*
- ◆ **Deltacortisone** *see PredniSONE on page 1511*
- ◆ **Delta® D3 [OTC]** *see Cholecalciferol on page 346*
- ◆ **Deltadehydrocortisone** *see PredniSONE on page 1511*
- ◆ **Demadex®** *see Torsemide on page 1837*

Demeclocycline (dem e kloe SYE kleen)

Index Terms Declomycin; Demeclocycline Hydrochloride; Demethylchlortetracycline
Generic Availability (U.S.) Yes
Pharmacologic Category Antibiotic, Tetracycline Derivative
Use Treatment of susceptible bacterial infections (acne, gonorrhea, pertussis, and urinary tract infections) caused by both gram-negative and gram-positive organisms
Unlabeled/Investigational Use Treatment of chronic syndrome of inappropriate secretion of antidiuretic hormone (SIADH)
Contraindications Hypersensitivity to demeclocycline, tetracyclines, or any component of the formulation; concomitant use with methoxyflurane
Warnings/Precautions Photosensitivity reactions occur frequently with this drug; avoid prolonged exposure to sunlight and do not use tanning equipment. Use caution in patients with renal or hepatic impairment (eg, elderly); dosage modification required in patients with renal impairment. May act as an antianabolic agent and increase BUN. Pseudotumor cerebri has been reported with tetracycline use (usually resolves with discontinuation). Outdated drug can cause nephropathy. Prolonged use may result in fungal or bacterial superinfection, including *C. difficile*-associated diarrhea (CDAD) and pseudomembranous colitis; CDAD has been observed >2 months postantibiotic treatment.
Adverse Reactions (Reflective of adult population; not specific for elderly) Frequency not defined.
Cardiovascular: Pericarditis
Central nervous system: Bulging fontanels (infants), dizziness, headache, pseudotumor cerebri (adults)
Dermatologic: Angioneurotic edema, erythema multiforme, erythematous rash, maculopapular rash, photosensitivity, pigmentation of skin, Stevens-Johnson syndrome (rare), urticaria
Endocrine & metabolic: Discoloration of thyroid gland (brown/black), nephrogenic diabetes insipidus
Gastrointestinal: Anorexia, diarrhea, dysphagia, enterocolitis, esophageal ulcerations, glossitis, nausea, pancreatitis, vomiting
Genitourinary: Balanitis
Hematologic: Eosinophilia, neutropenia, hemolytic anemia, thrombocytopenia
Hepatic: Hepatitis (rare), hepatotoxicity (rare), liver enzymes increased, liver failure (rare)
Neuromuscular & skeletal: Myasthenic syndrome, polyarthralgia, tooth discoloration (children <8 years, rarely in adults)
Ocular: Visual disturbances
Otic: Tinnitus
Renal: Acute renal failure
Respiratory: Pulmonary infiltrates
Miscellaneous: Anaphylaxis, anaphylactoid purpura, lupus-like syndrome, systemic lupus erythematosus exacerbation
Drug Interactions
Avoid Concomitant Use
Avoid concomitant use of Demeclocycline with any of the following: BCG; Retinoic Acid Derivatives

Increased Effect/Toxicity
Demeclocycline may increase the levels/effects of: Neuromuscular-Blocking Agents; Porfimer; Retinoic Acid Derivatives; Vitamin K Antagonists

Decreased Effect
Demeclocycline may decrease the levels/effects of: BCG; Desmopressin; Penicillins; Typhoid Vaccine

The levels/effects of Demeclocycline may be decreased by: Antacids; Bile Acid Sequestrants; Bismuth; Bismuth Subsalicylate; Calcium Salts; Iron Salts; Lanthanum; Magnesium Salts; Quinapril; Sucralfate; Zinc Salts

Ethanol/Nutrition/Herb Interactions
Food: Demeclocycline serum levels may be decreased if taken with food.
Herb/Nutraceutical: Avoid dong quai, St John's wort (may also cause photosensitization).

Stability Tetracyclines form toxic products when outdated or when exposed to light, heat, or humidity (Fanconi-like syndrome).

Mechanism of Action Inhibits protein synthesis by binding with the 30S and possibly the 50S ribosomal subunit(s) of susceptible bacteria; may also cause alterations in the cytoplasmic membrane; inhibits the action of ADH in patients with chronic SIADH

Pharmacodynamics/Kinetics
Onset of action: SIADH: Several days
Absorption: ~50% to 80%; reduced by food and dairy products
Protein binding: 41% to 50%
Metabolism: Hepatic (small amounts) to inactive metabolites; undergoes enterohepatic recirculation
Half-life elimination: 10-17 hours
Time to peak, serum: 3-6 hours
Excretion: Urine (42% to 50% as unchanged drug)

Dosage
Geriatric & Adult
Susceptible infections: Oral: 150 mg 4 times/day or 300 mg twice daily
SIADH (unlabeled use): Oral: 900-1200 mg/day or 13-15 mg/kg/day divided every 6-8 hours initially, then decrease to 600-900 mg/day
Renal Impairment Should be avoided in patients with renal dysfunction.
Hepatic Impairment Should be avoided in patients with hepatic dysfunction.

Administration Administer 1 hour before or 2 hours after food or milk with plenty of fluid; avoid administration within 2-3 hours of antacids

Monitoring Parameters CBC, renal and hepatic function

Test Interactions May interfere with tests for urinary glucose (false-negative urine glucose using Clinistix®, Tes-Tape®)

Special Geriatric Considerations Has not been studied exclusively in the elderly.

Dosage Forms Excipient information presented when available (limited, particularly for generics); consult specific product labeling.
Tablet, oral, as hydrochloride: 150 mg, 300 mg

◆ **Demeclocycline Hydrochloride** *see* Demeclocycline *on page 467*
◆ **Demerol®** *see* Meperidine *on page 1140*
◆ **Demethylchlortetracycline** *see* Demeclocycline *on page 467*
◆ **Denorex® Extra Strength Protection [OTC]** *see* Salicylic Acid *on page 1648*
◆ **Denorex® Extra Strength Protection 2-in-1 [OTC]** *see* Salicylic Acid *on page 1648*

Denosumab (den OH sue mab)

Related Information
Osteoporosis Management *on page 2027*
Brand Names: U.S. Prolia™; Xgeva™
Brand Names: Canada Prolia™; Xgeva™
Index Terms AMG-162
Generic Availability (U.S.) No
Pharmacologic Category Bone-Modifying Agent; Monoclonal Antibody
Use Treatment of osteoporosis in postmenopausal women at high risk for fracture; prevention of skeletal-related events (eg, fracture, spinal cord compression, bone pain requiring surgery/radiation therapy) in patients with bone metastases from solid tumors
Unlabeled/Investigational Use Prevention of bone loss due to androgen deprivation therapy in nonmetastatic prostate cancer; prevention of bone loss due to aromatase inhibitor therapy in nonmetastatic breast cancer; treatment of bone destruction caused by rheumatoid arthritis
Medication Guide Available Yes

Contraindications

Prolia™: Pre-existing hypocalcemia

Xgeva™: There are no contraindications listed in the manufacturer's labeling.

Warnings/Precautions Denosumab may cause or exacerbate hypocalcemia. Monitor calcium levels; correct pre-existing hypocalcemia prior to therapy. Use caution in patients with a history of hypoparathyroidism, thyroid surgery, parathyroid surgery, malabsorption syndromes, excision of small intestine, severe renal impairment/dialysis or other conditions which would predispose the patient to hypocalcemia; monitor calcium, phosphorus, and magnesium closely during therapy. Ensure adequate calcium and vitamin D intake; supplement with calcium and vitamin D; magnesium supplementation may also be necessary. Incidence of infections may be increased, including serious skin infections, abdominal, urinary, ear, or periodontal infections. Endocarditis has also been reported following use. Patients should be advised to contact healthcare provider if signs or symptoms of severe infection or cellulitis develop. Use with caution in patients with impaired immune systems or using concomitant immunosuppressive therapy; may be at increased risk for serious infections. Evaluate the need for continued treatment with serious infection. Osteonecrosis of the jaw (ONJ) has been reported in patients receiving denosumab. ONJ may manifest as jaw pain, osteomyelitis, osteitis, bone erosion, tooth/periodontal infection, toothache, gingival ulceration/erosion. Risk factors include invasive dental procedures (eg, tooth extraction, dental implants, boney surgery); a diagnosis of cancer, concomitant chemotherapy or corticosteroids, poor oral hygiene, ill-fitting dentures; and comorbid disorders (anemia, coagulopathy, infection, pre-existing dental disease). Patients should maintain good oral hygiene during treatment. A dental exam and preventative dentistry should be performed prior to therapy. The benefit/risk must be assessed by the treating physician and/or dentist/surgeon prior to any invasive dental procedure; avoid invasive procedures in patients with bone metastases receiving therapy for prevention of skeletal-related events. Patients developing ONJ while on denosumab therapy should receive care by a dentist or oral surgeon; extensive dental surgery to treat ONJ may exacerbate ONJ.

Postmenopausal osteoporosis: For use in women at high risk for fracture which is defined as a history of osteoporotic fracture or multiple risk factors for fracture. May also be used in women who failed or did not tolerate other therapies.

Bone metastases: Denosumab is not indicated for the prevention of skeletal-related events in patients with multiple myeloma. In trials with multiple myeloma patients, denosumab was noninferior to zoledronic acid in delaying time to first skeletal-related event and mortality was increased in a subset of the denosumab-treated group.

Denosumab therapy results in significant suppression of bone turnover; the long term effects of treatment are not known but may contribute to adverse outcomes such as ONJ, atypical fractures, or delayed fracture healing; monitor. Use with caution in patients with renal impairment (Cl_{cr} <30 mL/minute) or patients on dialysis; risk of hypocalcemia is increased. Dose adjustment is not needed. Dermatitis, eczema, and rash (which are not necessarily specific to the injection site) have been reported. Consider discontinuing use if symptoms occur. Packaging may contain natural latex rubber.

Adverse Reactions (Reflective of adult population; not specific for elderly) A postmarketing safety program for Prolia™ is available to collect information on adverse events; more information is available at http://www.proliasafety.com. To report adverse events for either Prolia™ or Xgeva™, prescribers may also call Amgen at 800-772-6436 or FDA at 800-332-1088. **Note:** Adverse events and frequencies occurred in patients with osteoporosis unless otherwise noted as occurring in patients with cancer.

>10%:

Central nervous system: Fatigue (cancer patients: 45%), headache (cancer patients: 13%)

Dermatologic: Dermatitis (11%), eczema (11%), rash (3% to 11%)

Endocrine & metabolic: Hypophosphatemia (cancer patients: 32%; grade 3: 15%), hypocalcemia (2%; cancer patients: 18%; grade 3: 3%)

Gastrointestinal: Nausea (cancer patients: 31%), diarrhea (cancer patients: 20%)

Neuromuscular & skeletal: Limb pain (12%), weakness (cancer patients: 45%; osteoporosis: 2%)

Respiratory: Dyspnea (cancer patients: 21%), cough (cancer patients: 15%)

1% to 10%:

Cardiovascular: Peripheral edema (5%), angina (3%)

Endocrine & metabolic: Hypercholesterolemia (7%)

Gastrointestinal: Flatulence (2%)

Neuromuscular & skeletal: Sciatica (5%), bone pain (4%), myalgia (3%), osteonecrosis of the jaw ([ONJ] cancer patients: 2%)

Respiratory: Upper respiratory tract infection (5%)

Miscellaneous: New malignancies (5%), infections (nonfatal, serious; 4%)

◀ **Drug Interactions**

Avoid Concomitant Use There are no known interactions where it is recommended to avoid concomitant use.

Increased Effect/Toxicity

Denosumab may increase the levels/effects of: Immunosuppressants

Decreased Effect There are no known significant interactions involving a decrease in effect.

Ethanol/Nutrition/Herb Interactions Ethanol: Avoid ethanol (may increase risk of osteoporosis).

Stability Prior to use, store in original carton under refrigeration, 2°C to 8°C (36°F to 46°F). Do not freeze. Prior to use, bring to room temperature of 25°C (77°F) in original container (usually takes 15-30 minutes). Use within 14 days once at room temperature. Protect from direct heat and light; do not expose to temperatures >25°C (77°F).

Mechanism of Action Denosumab is a monoclonal antibody with affinity for nuclear factor-kappa B ligand (RANKL). Osteoblasts secrete RANKL; RANKL activates osteoclast precursors and subsequent osteolysis which promotes release of bone-derived growth factors, such as insulin-like growth factor-1 (IGF1) and transforming growth factor-beta (TGF-beta), and increases serum calcium levels. Denosumab binds to RANKL, blocks the interaction between RANKL and RANK (a receptor located on osteoclast surfaces), and prevents osteoclast formation, leading to decreased bone resorption and increased bone mass in osteoporosis. In solid tumors with bony metastases, RANKL inhibition decreases osteoclastic activity leading to decreased skeletal related events and tumor-induced bone destruction.

Pharmacodynamics/Kinetics

Onset of action: Decreases markers of bone resorption by ~85% within 3 days; maximal reductions observed within 1 month

Duration: Markers of bone resorption return to baseline within 12 months of discontinuing therapy

Bioavailability: SubQ: 62%

Half-life elimination: ~25-28 days

Time to peak, serum: 10 days (range: 3-21 days)

Dosage

Geriatric & Adult

Prevention of skeletal-related events in bone metastases from solid tumors (Xgeva™): SubQ: 120 mg every 4 weeks

Treatment of osteoporosis in postmenopausal females (Prolia™): SubQ: 60 mg as a single dose, once every 6 months

Prevention of androgen-induced bone loss in nonmetastatic prostate cancer (unlabeled use): SubQ: 60 mg as a single dose, once every 6 months (Smith, 2009)

Prevention of aromatase inhibitor-induced bone loss in nonmetastatic breast cancer (unlabeled use): SubQ: 60 mg as a single dose, once every 6 months for 4 doses (Ellis, 2008)

Renal Impairment Dose adjustment is not needed; monitor patients with severe impairment (Cl_{cr} <30 mL/minute or on dialysis) due to increased risk of hypocalcemia.

Administration SubQ: Prior to administration, bring to room temperature in original container (allow to stand ~15-30 minutes); do not warm by any other method. Solution may contain trace amounts of translucent to white protein particles; do not use if cloudy, discolored (normal solution should be clear and colorless to pale yellow), or contains excessive particles or foreign matter. Avoid vigorous shaking. Administer via SubQ injection in the upper arm, upper thigh, or abdomen.

Osteoporosis: If a dose is missed, administer as soon as possible, then continue dosing every 6 months from the date of the last injection.

Monitoring Parameters Recommend monitoring of serum calcium, phosphorus and magnesium, signs and symptoms of hypocalcemia, especially in patients predisposed to hypocalcemia (severe renal impairment, thyroid/parathyroid surgery, malabsorption syndromes, hypoparathyroidism); infection, or dermatologic reactions; routine oral exam (prior to treatment); dental exam if risk factors for ONJ

Osteoporosis: Bone mineral density as measured by central dual-energy x-ray absorptiometry (DXA) of the hip or spine (prior to initiation of therapy and at least every 2 years; annual measurements of height and weight, assessment of chronic back pain; serum calcium and 25(OH)D; may consider monitoring biochemical markers of bone turnover (National Osteoporosis Foundation Guidelines, 2010)

Pharmacotherapy Pearls Oncology Comment: Metastatic breast cancer: The American Society of Clinical Oncology (ASCO) updated guidelines on the role of bone-modifying agents (BMAs) in the prevention and treatment of skeletal-related events for metastatic breast cancer patients (Van Poznak, 2011). The guidelines recommend initiating a BMA (denosumab, pamidronate, zoledronic acid) in patients with metastatic breast cancer to the bone. There is currently no literature indicating the superiority of one particular BMA. Optimal duration is not defined; however, the guidelines recommend continuing therapy until substantial decline in patient's performance status. In patients with normal creatinine clearance (Cl$_{cr}$ >60 mL/minute), no dosage/interval/infusion rate changes for pamidronate or zoledronic acid are necessary. For patients with Cl$_{cr}$ <30 mL/minute, pamidronate and zoledronic acid are not recommended. While no renal dose adjustments are recommended for denosumab, close monitoring is advised for risk of hypocalcemia in patients with Cl$_{cr}$ <30 mL/minute or on dialysis. The ASCO guidelines are in alignment with package insert guidelines for dosing, renal dose adjustments, infusion times, prevention and management of osteonecrosis of the jaw, and monitoring of laboratory parameter recommendations. BMAs are not the first-line therapy for pain. BMAs are to be used as adjunctive therapy for cancer-related bone pain associated with bone metastasis, demonstrating a modest pain control benefit. BMAs should be used in conjunction with agents such as NSAIDs, opioid and nonopioid analgesics, corticosteroids, radiation/surgery, and interventional procedures.

Dosage Forms Excipient information presented when available (limited, particularly for generics); consult specific product labeling.

Injection, solution [preservative free]:

Prolia™: 60 mg/mL (1 mL) [contains natural rubber/natural latex in packaging]

Xgeva™: 70 mg/mL (1.7 mL)

Selected References

Cummings SR, San Martin J, McClung MR, et al, "FREEDOM Trial. Denosumab for Prevention of Fractures in Postmenopausal Women With Osteoporosis," *N Engl J Med*, 2009, 361(8):756-65.

Kyrgidis A and Toulis KA, "Denosumab-Related Osteonecrosis of the Jaws," *Osteoporos Int*, 2010, [epub ahead of print].

National Osteoporosis Foundation, "Clinician's Guide to Prevention and Treatment of Osteoporosis," Washington, DC, 2010. Available at http://www.nof.org

Smith MR, Egerdie B, Hernández Toriz N, et al, "Denosumab in Men Receiving Androgen-Deprivation Therapy for Prostate Cancer," *N Engl J Med*, 2009, 361(8):745-55.

Desipramine (des IP ra meen)

Related Information

Antidepressant Agents *on page* 1991

Medication Safety Issues

Sound-alike/look-alike issues:

Desipramine may be confused with clomiPRAMINE, dalfampridine, diphenhydrAMINE, disopyramide, imipramine, nortriptyline

◄ Norpramin® may be confused with clomiPRAMINE, imipramine, Normodyne®, Norpace®, nortriptyline, Tenormin®

International issues:

Norpramin: Brand name for desipramine [U.S., Canada], but also the brand name for enalapril/hydrochlorothiazide [Portugal]; omeprazole [Spain]

Brand Names: U.S. Norpramin®

Brand Names: Canada Alti-Desipramine; Apo-Desipramine®; Norpramin®; Nu-Desipramine; PMS-Desipramine

Index Terms Desipramine Hydrochloride; Desmethylimipramine Hydrochloride

Generic Availability (U.S.) Yes

Pharmacologic Category Antidepressant, Tricyclic (Secondary Amine)

Use Treatment of depression

Unlabeled/Investigational Use Analgesic adjunct in chronic pain; peripheral neuropathies; substance-related disorders (eg, cocaine withdrawal); attention-deficit/hyperactivity disorder (ADHD)

Medication Guide Available Yes

Contraindications Hypersensitivity to desipramine, drugs of similar chemical class, or any component of the formulation; use of MAO inhibitors with or within 14 days; use in a patient during the acute recovery phase of MI

Warnings/Precautions [U.S. Boxed Warning]: Antidepressants increase the risk of suicidal thinking and behavior in children, adolescents, and young adults (18-24 years of age) with major depressive disorder (MDD) and other psychiatric disorders; consider risk prior to prescribing. Short-term studies did not show an increased risk in patients >24 years of age and showed a decreased risk in patients ≥65 years. Closely monitor for clinical worsening, suicidality, or unusual changes in behavior; the patient's family or caregiver should be instructed to closely observe the patient and communicate condition with healthcare provider. A medication guide should be dispensed with each prescription. **Desipramine is FDA approved for the treatment of depression in adolescents.**

The possibility of a suicide attempt is inherent in major depression and may persist until remission occurs. Monitor for worsening of depression or suicidality, especially during initiation of therapy (generally first 1-2 months) or with dose increases or decreases. Use caution in high-risk patients. Worsening depression and severe abrupt suicidality that are not part of the presenting symptoms may require discontinuation or modification of drug therapy. The patient's family or caregiver should be alerted to monitor patients for the emergence of suicidality and associated behaviors (such as agitation, irritability, hostility, impulsivity, and hypomania) and notify healthcare provider.

May worsen psychosis in some patients or precipitate a shift to mania or hypomania in patients with bipolar disorder. Patients presenting with depressive symptoms should be screened for bipolar disorder. Monotherapy in patients with bipolar disorder should be avoided. **Desipramine is not FDA approved for the treatment of bipolar depression.**

TCAs may rarely cause bone marrow suppression; monitor for any signs of infection and obtain CBC if symptoms (eg, fever, sore throat) evident. The degree of anticholinergic blockade produced by this agent is low relative to other cyclic antidepressants - however, extreme caution should be used in patients with urinary retention, benign prostatic hyperplasia, narrow-angle glaucoma, xerostomia, visual problems, constipation, or a history of bowel obstruction. The degree of sedation with desipramine are low relative to other antidepressants. However, desipramine may cause drowsiness/sedation, resulting in impaired performance of tasks requiring alertness (eg, operating machinery or driving). Sedative effects may be additive with other CNS depressants and/or ethanol. The risk of orthostasis is moderate relative to other antidepressants. Due to risk of conduction abnormalities, use with extreme caution in patients with a history of cardiovascular disease (including previous MI, stroke, tachycardia, or conduction abnormalities) or in patients with a family history of sudden death, dysrhythmias, or conduction abnormalities. Use with caution in patients with diabetes mellitus; may alter glucose regulation.

Consider discontinuing, when possible, prior to elective surgery. Therapy should not be abruptly discontinued. May lower seizure threshold - use extreme caution in patients with a previous seizure disorder or condition predisposing to seizures such as brain damage, alcoholism, or concurrent therapy with other drugs which lower the seizure threshold. In some patients, seizures may precede cardiac dysrhythmias and death. May increase the risks associated with electroconvulsive therapy. Use with extreme caution in hyperthyroid patients or those receiving thyroid supplementation. Use with caution in patients with glaucoma, hepatic or renal dysfunction and in elderly patients.

Adverse Reactions (Reflective of adult population; not specific for elderly) Frequency not defined.

Cardiovascular: Arrhythmias, edema, flushing, heart block, hyper-/hypotension, MI, palpitation, stroke, tachycardia

Central nervous system: Agitation, anxiety, ataxia, confusion, delusions, disorientation, dizziness, drowsiness, EEG alterations, exacerbation of psychosis, extrapyramidal symptoms, fatigue, fever, hallucinations, headache, hypomania, incoordination, insomnia, neuroleptic malignant syndrome, nightmares, restlessness, seizure, suicidal thinking and behavior

Dermatologic: Alopecia, itching, petechiae, photosensitivity, skin rash, urticaria

Endocrine & metabolic: Breast enlargement, galactorrhea, gynecomastia, hyper-/hypoglycemia, impotence, libido changes, SIADH

Gastrointestinal: Abdominal cramps, anorexia, black tongue, constipation, diarrhea, epigastric distress, nausea, parotid edema, paralytic ileus, stomatitis, sublingual adenitis, unpleasant taste, vomiting, weight gain/loss, xerostomia

Genitourinary: Micturition delayed, nocturia, painful ejaculation, polyuria, testicular edema, urinary retention

Hematologic: Agranulocytosis, eosinophilia, purpura, thrombocytopenia

Hepatic: Alkaline phosphatase increased, cholestatic jaundice, hepatitis, liver enzymes increased

Neuromuscular & skeletal: Falling, numbness, paresthesia of extremities, peripheral neuropathy, tingling, tremor, weakness

Ocular: Blurred vision, disturbances of accommodation, intraocular pressure increased, mydriasis

Otic: Tinnitus

Miscellaneous: Allergic reaction, diaphoresis (excessive), withdrawal symptoms

Drug Interactions

Metabolism/Transport Effects Substrate of CYP1A2 (minor), 2D6 (major); **Inhibits** CYP2A6 (moderate), 2B6 (moderate), 2D6 (moderate), 2E1 (weak), 3A4 (moderate)

Avoid Concomitant Use

Avoid concomitant use of Desipramine with any of the following: Artemether; Dronedarone; Iobenguane I 123; Lumefantrine; MAO Inhibitors; Methylene Blue; Nilotinib; Pimozide; QUEtiapine; QuiNINE; Sibutramine; Tetrabenazine; Thioridazine; Tolvaptan; Toremifene; Vandetanib; Vemurafenib; Ziprasidone

Increased Effect/Toxicity

Desipramine may increase the levels/effects of: Alpha-/Beta-Agonists (Direct-Acting); Alpha1-Agonists; Amphetamines; Anticholinergics; Beta2-Agonists; Budesonide (Systemic, Oral Inhalation); Colchicine; CYP2A6 Substrates; CYP2B6 Substrates; CYP2D6 Substrates; CYP3A4 Substrates; Desmopressin; Dronedarone; Eplerenone; Everolimus; FentaNYL; Fesoterodine; Lurasidone; Methylene Blue; Nebivolol; Pimecrolimus; Pimozide; QTc-Prolonging Agents; QuiNIDine; QuiNINE; Saxagliptin; Serotonin Modulators; Sodium Phosphates; Sulfonylureas; Tamoxifen; Tetrabenazine; Thioridazine; Tolvaptan; Toremifene; TraMADol; Vandetanib; Vemurafenib; Vitamin K Antagonists; Yohimbine; Ziprasidone

The levels/effects of Desipramine may be increased by: Abiraterone Acetate; Alfuzosin; Altretamine; Artemether; Boceprevir; BuPROPion; Chloroquine; Cimetidine; Cinacalcet; Ciprofloxacin; Ciprofloxacin (Systemic); CYP2D6 Inhibitors (Moderate); CYP2D6 Inhibitors (Strong); Dexmethylphenidate; Divalproex; DULoxetine; Gadobutrol; Lithium; Lumefantrine; MAO Inhibitors; Methylphenidate; Metoclopramide; Nilotinib; Propoxyphene; Protease Inhibitors; QUEtiapine; QuiNIDine; QuiNINE; Selective Serotonin Reuptake Inhibitors; Sibutramine; Telaprevir; Terbinafine; Terbinafine (Systemic); Valproic Acid

Decreased Effect

Desipramine may decrease the levels/effects of: Acetylcholinesterase Inhibitors (Central); Alpha2-Agonists; Codeine; Iobenguane I 123

The levels/effects of Desipramine may be decreased by: Acetylcholinesterase Inhibitors (Central); Barbiturates; CarBAMazepine; Cyproterone; Peginterferon Alfa-2b; St Johns Wort

Ethanol/Nutrition/Herb Interactions

Ethanol: May increase CNS depression; monitor for increased effects with coadministration. Caution patients about effects.

Food: Grapefruit juice may inhibit the metabolism of some TCAs and clinical toxicity may result.

Herb/Nutraceutical: Avoid valerian, St John's wort, SAMe, kava kava (may increase risk of serotonin syndrome and/or excessive sedation).

Stability Store at 20°C to 25°C (68°F to 77°F).

Mechanism of Action Traditionally believed to increase the synaptic concentration of norepinephrine (and to a lesser extent, serotonin) in the central nervous system by inhibition of its reuptake by the presynaptic neuronal membrane. However, additional receptor effects have been found including desensitization of adenyl cyclase, down regulation of beta-adrenergic receptors, and down regulation of serotonin receptors.

Pharmacodynamics/Kinetics
Onset of action: Earliest therapeutic effects: 2-5 days; Maximum antidepressant effect: >2 weeks

Metabolism: Hepatic

Half-life elimination: Adults: 15-24 hours (Weiner, 1981)

Time to peak, plasma: ~6 hours (Weiner, 1981)

Excretion: Urine (~70%)

Dosage
Geriatric Depression: Oral: Initial dose: Start at the lower range and increase based on tolerance and response to 100 mg/day in divided or single dose; usual maintenance dose: 25-100 mg/day, but doses up to 150 mg/day may be necessary in severely depressed patients

Adult
Depression: Oral: Initial dose: Start at the lower range and increase based on tolerance and response; usual maintenance dose: 100-200 mg/day, but doses up to 300 mg/day may be necessary in severely depressed patients

Neuropathic pain (unlabeled use): Oral: Initial: 10-25 mg/day; increase dose every 3 days as necessary until the desired effect is obtained; usual effective dose: 50-150 mg/day (maximum dose: 150 mg/day)

Renal Impairment Hemodialysis/peritoneal dialysis effects: Supplemental dose is not necessary.

Monitoring Parameters Monitor blood pressure and pulse rate prior to and during initial therapy; evaluate mental status, suicide ideation (especially at the beginning of therapy or when doses are increased or decreased); monitor weight; ECG in older adults and those patients with cardiac disease; blood levels are useful for therapeutic monitoring

Test Interactions Increased glucose; decreased glucose has also been reported. May interfere with urine detection of amphetamines/methamphetamines (false-positive).

Special Geriatric Considerations Preferred tricyclic antidepressant because of its milder side effect profile; patients may experience excitation or stimulation; in such cases, administer as a single morning dose or divided dose.

Dosage Forms Excipient information presented when available (limited, particularly for generics); consult specific product labeling.
Tablet, oral, as hydrochloride: 10 mg, 25 mg, 50 mg, 75 mg, 100 mg, 150 mg
Norpramin®: 10 mg, 25 mg, 50 mg, 75 mg, 100 mg, 150 mg [contains soybean oil]

Selected References
Nelson JC, Jatlow PI, and Mazure C, "Desipramine Plasma Levels and Response in Elderly Melancholic Patients," *J Clin Psychopharmacol*, 1985, 5(4):217-20.

Nies A, Robinson DS, Friedman MS, et al, "Relationship Between Age and Tricyclic Antidepressant Plasma Levels," *Am J Psychiatry*, 1977, 134:790-3.

◆ **Desipramine Hydrochloride** *see* Desipramine *on page 471*

Desirudin (des i ROO din)

Medication Safety Issues
High alert medication:
The Institute for Safe Medication Practices (ISMP) includes this medication among its list of drugs which have a heightened risk of causing significant patient harm when used in error.

Brand Names: U.S. Iprivask®

Index Terms CGP-39393; Desulfato-Hirudin; Desulfatohirudin; Desulphatohirudin; r-Hirudin; Recombinant Desulfatohirudin; Recombinant Hirudin

Generic Availability (U.S.) No

Pharmacologic Category Anticoagulant, Thrombin Inhibitor

Use Prophylaxis of deep vein thrombosis (DVT) in patients undergoing surgery for hip replacement

Contraindications Hypersensitivity to natural or recombinant hirudins; active bleeding and/or irreversible coagulation disorders

Warnings/Precautions [U.S. Boxed Warning]: Patients with recent or anticipated neuraxial anesthesia (epidural or spinal anesthesia) are at risk of epidural or spinal hematoma and subsequent paralysis. Consider risk versus benefit prior to neuraxial anesthesia; risk is increased by concomitant agents which may alter hemostasis, as well as traumatic or repeated epidural or spinal puncture. Patient should be observed closely for bleeding and signs and symptoms of neurological impairment if therapy is administered during or immediately following diagnostic lumbar puncture, epidural anesthesia, or spinal anesthesia.

Allergic and hypersensitivity reactions, including anaphylaxis and fatal anaphylactoid reactions have been reported with other hirudin derivatives. Exercise caution when re-exposing patients (anaphylaxis has been reported). Monitor patient closely for signs or symptoms of bleeding. Certain patients are at increased risk of bleeding. Risk factors include bacterial endocarditis; congenital or acquired bleeding disorders; active ulcerative or angiodysplastic GI diseases; severe uncontrolled hypertension; history of hemorrhagic stroke; use shortly after brain, spinal, or ophthalmology surgery; patients treated concomitantly with platelet inhibitors; recent GI bleeding; thrombocytopenia or platelet defects; renal impairment; hepatic impairment; hypertensive or diabetic retinopathy; or in patients undergoing invasive procedures. Do not administer with other agents that increase the risk of hemorrhage unless coadministration cannot be avoided. Discontinue if bleeding occurs. Contraindicated with active bleeding and/or irreversible coagulation disorders.

Do **not** administer intramuscularly (I.M.). Do not use interchangeably (unit-for-unit) with other hirudins. Use with caution in patients with moderate-to-severe renal dysfunction (Cl_{cr} <60 mL/minute/1.73 m^2); dosage reduction is necessary; monitor aPTT and renal function daily. The American College of Chest Physicians recommends against the use of desirudin in patients with Cl_{cr} <30 mL/minute (Hirsh, 2008). Use with caution in the elderly; elimination half-life prolonged in patients >75 years of age.

Adverse Reactions (Reflective of adult population; not specific for elderly) As with all anticoagulants, bleeding is the major adverse effect. Hemorrhage may occur at any site. 2% to 10%:

> Gastrointestinal: Nausea (2%)
> Hematologic: Hematoma (6%), hemorrhage (major, <1% to 3%; may include cases of intracranial, retroperitoneal, intraocular, intraspinal, or prosthetic joint hemorrhage), anemia (3%)
> Local: Injection site mass (4%), deep thrombophlebitis (2%)
> Miscellaneous: Wound secretion (4%)

Drug Interactions

Avoid Concomitant Use

Avoid concomitant use of Desirudin with any of the following: Rivaroxaban

Increased Effect/Toxicity

Desirudin may increase the levels/effects of: Anticoagulants; Collagenase (Systemic); Deferasirox; Ibritumomab; Rivaroxaban; Tositumomab and Iodine I 131 Tositumomab

The levels/effects of Desirudin may be increased by: Antiplatelet Agents; Dasatinib; Herbs (Anticoagulant/Antiplatelet Properties); Nonsteroidal Anti-Inflammatory Agents; Pentosan Polysulfate Sodium; Prostacyclin Analogues; Salicylates; Thrombolytic Agents

Decreased Effect There are no known significant interactions involving a decrease in effect.

Ethanol/Nutrition/Herb Interactions Herb/Nutraceutical: Avoid alfalfa, anise, bilberry, bladderwrack, bromelain, cat's claw, celery, coleus, cordyceps, dong quai, evening primrose oil, fenugreek, feverfew, garlic, ginger, ginkgo biloba, ginseng (American/Panax/Siberian), grapeseed, green tea, guggul, horse chestnut seed, horseradish, licorice, prickly ash, red clover, reishi, sweet clover, turmeric, white willow (all possess anticoagulant or antiplatelet activity and as such, may enhance the anticoagulant effects of desirudin).

Stability Store at 25°C (77°F); excursions permitted to 15°C to 30°C (59°F to 86°F). Protect from light. Following reconstitution, solution may be stored at room temperature for up to 24 hours. Discard unused solution after 24 hours.

Reconstitution: Attach enclosed vial adapter to vial containing desirudin. Remove syringe cap and attach provided syringe containing diluent to adapter on vial. Slowly push plunger down to transfer entire contents of syringe into vial. Do not remove syringe from vial adapter. Gently swirl solution; round tablet in vial will dissolve within 10 seconds. Resultant solution concentration is 31.5 mg/mL (15.75 mg/0.5 mL provides a 15 mg dose). Turn vial upside down; withdraw appropriate dose amount back into syringe. Remove syringe from vial. Attach enclosed Eclipse™ needle (or any needle appropriate for subcutaneous administration); pull pink lever down and uncap needle; ready for injection. After injection, flip up pink lever to cover needle until it snaps into place; dispose of syringe appropriately.

Mechanism of Action Desirudin is a direct, highly selective thrombin inhibitor. Reversibly binds to the active thrombin site of free and clot-associated thrombin. Inhibits fibrin formation, activation of coagulation factors V, VII, and XIII, and thrombin-induced platelet aggregation resulting in a dose-dependent prolongation of the activated partial thromboplastin time (aPTT).

Pharmacodynamics/Kinetics

> Absorption: Subcutaneous: Complete
> Distribution: V_{dss}: 0.25 L/kg
> Half-life elimination: ~2 hours; Prolonged with renal impairment (Cl_{cr} <31 mL/minute/1.73m^2: Up to 12 hours)

Time to peak, plasma: 1-3 hours
Excretion: Urine (40% to 50% as unchanged drug)

Dosage
  Geriatric & Adult DVT prophylaxis: SubQ: 15 mg every 12 hours; initial dose may be given up to 5-15 minutes prior to surgery (after induction of regional anesthesia, if used); has been administered for up to 12 days (average: 9-12 days) in clinical trials

  Renal Impairment
    Moderate renal impairment (Cl_{cr} ≥31-60 mL/minute/1.73 m^2): 5 mg every 12 hours
    Severe renal impairment (Cl_{cr} <31 mL/minute/1.73 m^2): 1.7 mg every 12 hours; **Note:** The American College of Chest Physicians recommends against the use of desirudin in patients with Cl_{cr} <30 mL/minute (Hirsh, 2008).

Administration Do **not** administer I.M.; for SubQ administration only. Administration should be alternated between the left and right anterolateral and left and right posterolateral thigh or abdominal wall. Insert needle into a skin fold held between the thumb and forefinger; the skin fold should be held throughout the injection. Do not rub injection site. Do not mix with other injections or infusions. Administer according to recommended regimen.

Monitoring Parameters Monitor aPTT, serum creatinine/creatinine clearance, CBC; stool occult blood tests. Serum creatinine and aPTT should be monitored daily in patients with moderate-to-severe renal insufficiency. Interrupt therapy if aPTT exceeds 2 times normal; resume at a reduced dose when aPTT is <2 times control.

Special Geriatric Considerations Serious adverse drug events are more common in persons ≥75 years of age. Dosage adjustment may be necessary based on kidney function.

Dosage Forms Excipient information presented when available (limited, particularly for generics); consult specific product labeling.
  Injection, powder for reconstitution [preservative free]:
    Iprivask®: 15 mg [supplied with prefilled diluent syringe]

Desloratadine (des lor AT a deen)

Medication Safety Issues
  Sound-alike/look-alike issues:
    Clarinex® may be confused with Celebrex®

Brand Names: U.S. Clarinex®

Brand Names: Canada Aerius®; Aerius® Kids

Generic Availability (U.S.) No

Pharmacologic Category Histamine H_1 Antagonist; Histamine H_1 Antagonist, Second Generation; Piperidine Derivative

Use Relief of nasal and non-nasal symptoms of seasonal allergic rhinitis (SAR) and perennial allergic rhinitis (PAR); treatment of chronic idiopathic urticaria (CIU)

Contraindications Hypersensitivity to desloratadine, loratadine, or any component of the formulation

Warnings/Precautions Dose should be adjusted in patients with liver or renal impairment. Use with caution in patients known to be slow metabolizers of desloratadine (incidence of side effects may be increased). Some products may contain phenylalanine.

Adverse Reactions (Reflective of adult population; not specific for elderly)
  >10%: Central nervous system: Headache (14%)
  1% to 10%:
    Central nervous system: Fatigue (2% to 5%), somnolence (2%), dizziness (4%)
    Endocrine & metabolic: Dysmenorrhea (2%)
    Gastrointestinal: Xerostomia (3%), nausea (5%), dyspepsia (3%)
    Neuromuscular & skeletal: Myalgia (2% to 3%)
    Respiratory: Pharyngitis (3% to 4%)

Drug Interactions
  Metabolism/Transport Effects Substrate of P-glycoprotein
  Avoid Concomitant Use There are no known interactions where it is recommended to avoid concomitant use.

  Increased Effect/Toxicity
    Desloratadine may increase the levels/effects of: Alcohol (Ethyl); Anticholinergics; CNS Depressants; Selective Serotonin Reuptake Inhibitors

    The levels/effects of Desloratadine may be increased by: Droperidol; HydrOXYzine; P-Glycoprotein Inhibitors; Pramlintide

  Decreased Effect
    Desloratadine may decrease the levels/effects of: Acetylcholinesterase Inhibitors (Central); Benzylpenicilloyl Polylysine; Betahistine

The levels/effects of Desloratadine may be decreased by: Acetylcholinesterase Inhibitors (Central); Amphetamines; P-Glycoprotein Inducers

Ethanol/Nutrition/Herb Interactions
Ethanol: May increase CNS depression; monitor for increased effects with coadministration. Caution patients about effects.
Food: Does not affect bioavailability.

Stability Syrup, tablet, orally-disintegrating tablet: Store at 25°C (77°F); excursions permitted between 15°C to 30°C (59°F to 86°F). Protect from moisture and excessive heat (85°F). Use orally-disintegrating tablet immediately after opening blister package. Syrup should be protected from light.

Mechanism of Action Desloratadine, a major metabolite of loratadine, is a long-acting tricyclic antihistamine with selective peripheral histamine H_1 receptor antagonistic activity and additional anti-inflammatory properties.

Pharmacodynamics/Kinetics
Onset of action: Within 1 hour
Duration: 24 hours
Protein binding: Desloratadine: 82% to 87%; 3-hydroxydesloratadine: 85% to 89%
Metabolism: Hepatic to active metabolite, 3-hydroxydesloratadine (specific enzymes not identified); undergoes glucuronidation. Decreased in slow metabolizers of desloratadine. Not expected to affect or be affected by medications metabolized by CYP with normal doses.
Half-life elimination: 27 hours
Time to peak: 3 hours
Excretion: Urine and feces (as metabolites)

Dosage
Geriatric & Adult Seasonal or perennial allergic rhinitis, chronic idiopathic urticaria: Oral: 5 mg once daily
Renal Impairment 5 mg every other day
Hepatic Impairment 5 mg every other day

Administration May be taken with or without food. RediTabs® should be placed on the tongue; tablet will disintegrate immediately. May be taken with or without water.

Monitoring Parameters Relief of symptoms, mental status

Test Interactions May suppress the wheal and flare reactions to skin test antigens

Dosage Forms Excipient information presented when available (limited, particularly for generics); consult specific product labeling.
Syrup, oral:
Clarinex®: 0.5 mg/mL (480 mL) [contains propylene glycol, sodium benzoate; bubblegum flavor]
Tablet, oral:
Clarinex®: 5 mg
Tablet, orally disintegrating, oral:
Clarinex®: 2.5 mg [contains phenylalanine 1.4 mg/tablet; tutti frutti flavor]
Clarinex®: 5 mg [contains phenylalanine 2.9 mg/tablet; tutti frutti flavor]

♦ **Desmethylimipramine Hydrochloride** *see* Desipramine *on page 471*

Desmopressin (des moe PRES in)

Brand Names: U.S. DDAVP®; Stimate®
Brand Names: Canada Apo-Desmopressin®; DDAVP®; DDAVP® Melt; Minirin®; Novo-Desmopressin; Octostim®; PMS-Desmopressin
Index Terms 1-Deamino-8-D-Arginine Vasopressin; Desmopressin Acetate
Generic Availability (U.S.) Yes
Pharmacologic Category Antihemophilic Agent; Hemostatic Agent; Vasopressin Analog, Synthetic

Use
Injection: Treatment of diabetes insipidus; maintenance of hemostasis and control of bleeding in hemophilia A with factor VIII coagulant activity levels >5% and mild-to-moderate classic von Willebrand's disease (type 1) with factor VIII coagulant activity levels >5%
Nasal solutions (DDAVP® Nasal Spray and DDAVP® Rhinal Tube): Treatment of central diabetes insipidus
Nasal spray (Stimate®): Maintenance of hemostasis and control of bleeding in hemophilia A with factor VIII coagulant activity levels >5% and mild-to-moderate classic von Willebrand's disease (type 1) with factor VIII coagulant activity levels >5%
Tablet: Treatment of central diabetes insipidus, temporary polyuria and polydipsia following pituitary surgery or head trauma, primary nocturnal enuresis

Unlabeled/Investigational Use Uremic bleeding associated with acute or chronic renal failure; prevention of surgical bleeding in patients with uremia

◀ **Contraindications** Hypersensitivity to desmopressin or any component of the formulation; hyponatremia or a history of hyponatremia; moderate-to-severe renal impairment (Cl_{cr}<50 mL/ minute)

Canadian labeling: Additional contraindications (not in U.S. labeling): Type 2B or platelet-type (pseudo) von Willebrand's disease (injection, intranasal, oral, sublingual); known hyponatremia, habitual or psychogenic polydipsia, cardiac insufficiency or other conditions requiring diuretic therapy (intranasal, sublingual); nephrosis, severe hepatic dysfunction (sublingual); primary nocturnal enuresis (intranasal)

Warnings/Precautions Allergic reactions and anaphylaxis have been reported rarely with both the I.V. and intranasal formulations. Fluid intake should be adjusted downward in the elderly and very young patients to decrease the possibility of water intoxication and hyponatremia. Use may rarely lead to extreme decreases in plasma osmolality, resulting in seizures, coma, and death. Use caution with cystic fibrosis, heart failure, renal dysfunction, polydipsia (habitual or psychogenic [contraindicated in Canadian labeling]), or other conditions associated with fluid and electrolyte imbalance due to potential hyponatremia. Use caution with coronary artery insufficiency or hypertensive cardiovascular disease; may increase or decrease blood pressure leading to changes in heart rate. Consider switching from nasal to intravenous solution if changes in the nasal mucosa (scarring, edema) occur leading to unreliable absorption. Use caution in patients predisposed to thrombus formation; thrombotic events (acute cerebrovascular thrombosis, acute myocardial infarction) have occurred (rare).

Desmopressin (intranasal and I.V.), when used for hemostasis in hemophilia, is not for use in hemophilia B, type 2B von Willebrand disease, severe classic von Willebrand disease (type 1), or in patients with factor VIII antibodies. In general, desmopressin is also not recommended for use in patients with ≤5% factor VIII activity level, although it may be considered in selected patients with activity levels between 2% and 5%.

Consider switching from nasal to intravenous administration if changes in the nasal mucosa (scarring, edema) occur leading to unreliable absorption. Consider alternative rout of administration (I.V. or intranasal) with inadequate therapeutic response at maximum recommended oral doses. Therapy should be interrupted if patient experiences an acute illness (eg, fever, recurrent vomiting or diarrhea), vigorous exercise, or any condition associated with an increase in water consumption. Some patients may demonstrate a change in response after long-term therapy (>6 months) characterized as decreased response or a shorter duration of response.

Adverse Reactions (Reflective of adult population; not specific for elderly) Frequency may not be defined (may be dose or route related).

Cardiovascular: Blood pressure increased/decreased (I.V.), facial flushing

Central nervous system: Headache (2% to 5%), dizziness (intranasal; ≤3%), chills (intranasal; 2%)

Dermatologic: Rash

Endocrine & metabolic: Hyponatremia, water intoxication

Gastrointestinal: Abdominal pain (intranasal; 2%), gastrointestinal disorder (intranasal; ≤2%), nausea (intranasal; ≤2%), abdominal cramps, sore throat

Hepatic: Transient increases in liver transaminases (associated primarily with tablets)

Local: Injection: Burning pain, erythema, and swelling at the injection site

Neuromuscular & Skeletal: Weakness (intranasal; ≤2%)

Ocular: Conjunctivitis (intranasal; ≤2%), eye edema (intranasal; ≤2%), lacrimation disorder (intranasal; ≤2%)

Respiratory: Rhinitis (intranasal; 3% to 8%), epistaxis (intranasal; ≤3%), nostril pain (intranasal; ≤2%), cough, nasal congestion, upper respiratory infection

Drug Interactions

Avoid Concomitant Use There are no known interactions where it is recommended to avoid concomitant use.

Increased Effect/Toxicity

Desmopressin may increase the levels/effects of: Lithium

The levels/effects of Desmopressin may be increased by: Analgesics (Opioid); CarBAMazepine; ChlorproMAZINE; LamoTRIgine; Nonsteroidal Anti-Inflammatory Agents; Selective Serotonin Reuptake Inhibitors; Tricyclic Antidepressants

Decreased Effect

The levels/effects of Desmopressin may be decreased by: Demeclocycline; Lithium

Ethanol/Nutrition/Herb Interactions Ethanol: Avoid ethanol (may decrease antidiuretic effect).

Stability

DDAVP®:

Nasal spray: Store at controlled room temperature of 20°C to 25°C (68°F to 77°F). Keep nasal spray in upright position.

Rhinal Tube solution: Store refrigerated at 2°C to 8°C (36°F to 46°F). May store at controlled room temperature of 20°C to 25°C (68°F to 77°F) for up to 3 weeks.

Solution for injection: Store refrigerated at 2°C to 8°C (36°F to 46°F). Dilute solution for injection in 10-50 mL NS for I.V. infusion (50 mL for adults).

Tablet: Store at controlled room temperature of 20°C to 25°C (68°F to 77°F).

DDAVP® Melt (CAN; not available in U.S.): Store at 15°C to 25°C (59°F to 77°F) in original container. Protect from moisture.

Stimate® nasal spray: Store at controlled room temperature of 20°C to 25°C (68°F to 77°F). Keep nasal spray in upright position. Discard 6 months after opening.

Mechanism of Action

In a dose dependent manner, desmopressin increases cyclic adenosine monophosphate (cAMP) in renal tubular cells which increases water permeability resulting in decreased urine volume and increased urine osmolality; increases plasma levels of von Willebrand factor, factor VIII, and t-PA contributing to a shortened activated partial thromboplastin time (aPTT) and bleeding time.

Pharmacodynamics/Kinetics

Onset of action:

Intranasal: Antidiuretic: 15-30 minutes; Increased factor VIII and von Willebrand factor (vWF) activity (dose related): 30 minutes

Peak effect: Antidiuretic: 1 hour; Increased factor VIII and vWF activity: 1.5 hours

I.V. infusion: Increased factor VIII and vWF activity: 30 minutes (dose related)

Peak effect: 1.5-2 hours

Oral tablet: Antidiuretic: ~1 hour

Peak effect: 4-7 hours

Duration: Intranasal, I.V. infusion, Oral tablet: ~6-14 hours

Absorption: Sublingual: Rapid

Bioavailability: Intranasal: ~3.5%; Oral tablet: 5% compared to intranasal, 0.16% compared to I.V.

Half-life elimination: Intranasal: ~3.5 hours; I.V. infusion: 3 hours; Oral tablet: 2-3 hours

Renal impairment: ≤9 hours

Excretion: Urine

Dosage

Geriatric & Adult

Diabetes insipidus:

I.V., SubQ: U.S. labeling: 2-4 mcg/day (0.5-1 mL) in 2 divided doses or one-tenth ($^{1}/_{10}$) of the maintenance intranasal dose. Fluid restriction should be observed.

I.M., I.V., SubQ: Canadian labeling (not in U.S. labeling): 1-4 mcg (0.25-1 mL) once daily or one-tenth ($^{1}/_{10}$) of the maintenance intranasal dose. Fluid restriction should be observed.

Intranasal (100 mcg/mL nasal solution): 10-40 mcg/day (0.1-0.4 mL) divided 1-3 times/day; adjust morning and evening doses separately for an adequate diurnal rhythm of water turnover. **Note:** The nasal spray pump can only deliver doses of 10 mcg (0.1 mL) or multiples of 10 mcg (0.1 mL); if doses other than these are needed, the rhinal tube delivery system is preferred. Fluid restriction should be observed.

Oral:

U.S. labeling: Initial: 0.05 mg twice daily; total daily dose should be increased or decreased as needed to obtain adequate antidiuresis (range: 0.1-1.2 mg divided 2-3 times/day). Fluid restriction should be observed.

Canadian labeling (not in U.S. labeling): Initial: 0.1 mg 3 times/day; total daily dose should be increased or decreased as needed to obtain adequate antidiuresis (range: 0.3-1.2 mg divided 3 times/day). Fluid restriction should be observed.

Sublingual formulation: Canadian labeling (not in U.S. labeling): Initial: 60 mcg 3 times/day; total daily dose should be increased or decreased as needed to obtain adequate antidiuresis. Usual maintenance: 60-120 mcg 3 times/day (range: 120-720 mcg divided 2-3 times/day). Fluid restriction should be observed.

Nocturnal enuresis: *Oral:* 0.2 mg at bedtime; dose may be titrated up to 0.6 mg to achieve desired response.

Hemophilia A and mild-to-moderate von Willebrand disease (type 1):

I.V.: 0.3 mcg/kg by slow infusion; if used preoperatively, administer 30 minutes before procedure

Canadian labeling (not in U.S. labeling): Maximum I.V. dose: 20 mcg

Intranasal (using high concentration spray [1.5 mg/mL]): <50 kg: 150 mcg (1 spray); >50 kg: 300 mcg (1 spray each nostril); repeat use is determined by the patient's clinical condition and laboratory work. If using preoperatively, administer 2 hours before surgery.

◀ **Uremic bleeding associated with acute or chronic renal failure (unlabeled use)** (Watson, 1984): I.V.: 0.4 mcg/kg over 10 minutes

Prevention of surgical bleeding in patients with uremia (unlabeled use) (Mannucci, 1983): I.V.: 0.3 mcg/kg over 30 minutes

Renal Impairment Cl_{cr} <50 mL/minute: Use is contraindicated according to the manufacturer; however, has been used in acute and chronic renal failure patients experiencing uremic bleeding or for prevention of surgical bleeding (unlabeled uses) (Mannucci, 1983; Watson, 1984).

Administration

I.M., I.V. push, SubQ injection: Central diabetes insipidus: Withdraw dose from ampul into appropriate syringe size (eg, insulin syringe). Further dilution is not required. Administer as direct injection.

I.V. infusion:
Hemophilia A, von Willebrand disease (type 1), and prevention of surgical bleeding in patients with uremia (unlabeled; Mannucci, 1983): Infuse over 15-30 minutes
Acute uremic bleeding (unlabeled; Watson, 1984): May infuse over 10 minutes

Intranasal:
DDAVP®: Nasal pump spray: Delivers 0.1 mL (10 mcg); for doses <10 mcg or for other doses which are not multiples, use rhinal tube. DDAVP® Nasal spray delivers fifty 10 mcg doses. For 10 mcg dose, administer in one nostril. Any solution remaining after 50 doses should be discarded. Pump must be primed prior to first use.
DDAVP® Rhinal tube: Insert top of dropper into tube (arrow marked end) in downward position. Squeeze dropper until solution reaches desired calibration mark. Disconnect dropper. Grasp the tube ³/₄ inch from the end and insert tube into nostril until the fingertips reach the nostril. Place opposite end of tube into the mouth (holding breath). Tilt head back and blow with a strong, short puff into the nostril. Reseal dropper after use.

Monitoring Parameters Blood pressure and pulse should be monitored during I.V. infusion

Note: For all indications, fluid intake, urine volume, and signs and symptoms of hyponatremia should be closely monitored especially in high-risk patient subgroups (eg, young children, elderly, patients with heart failure).
Diabetes insipidus: Urine specific gravity, plasma and urine osmolality, serum electrolytes
Hemophilia A: Factor VIII coagulant activity, factor VIII ristocetin cofactor activity, and factor VIII antigen levels, aPTT
von Willebrand disease: Factor VIII coagulant activity, factor VIII ristocetin cofactor activity, and factor VIII von Willebrand antigen levels, bleeding time
Nocturnal enuresis: Serum electrolytes if used for >7 days

Pharmacotherapy Pearls 10 mcg of desmopressin acetate is equivalent to 40 int. units

Special Geriatric Considerations Elderly patients should be cautioned not to increase their fluid intake beyond that sufficient to satisfy their thirst in order to avoid water intoxication and hyponatremia. Under experimental conditions, elderly have been shown to have a decreased responsiveness to vasopressin with respect to its effects on water homeostasis.

Dosage Forms Excipient information presented when available (limited, particularly for generics); consult specific product labeling.
Injection, solution, as acetate: 4 mcg/mL (1 mL, 10 mL)
DDAVP®: 4 mcg/mL (1 mL)
DDAVP®: 4 mcg/mL (10 mL) [contains chlorobutanol]
Solution, intranasal, as acetate: 0.1 mg/mL (2.5 mL)
DDAVP®: 0.1 mg/mL (2.5 mL) [contains benzalkonium chloride; with rhinal tube]
Solution, intranasal, as acetate [spray]: 0.1 mg/mL (5 mL)
DDAVP®: 0.1 mg/mL (5 mL) [contains benzalkonium chloride; delivers 10 mcg/spray]
Stimate®: 1.5 mg/mL (2.5 mL) [contains benzalkonium chloride; delivers 150 mcg/spray]
Tablet, oral, as acetate: 0.1 mg, 0.2 mg
DDAVP®: 0.1 mg, 0.2 mg [scored]

Dosage Forms: Canada Excipient information presented when available (limited, particularly for generics); consult specific product labeling.
Tablet, as acetate, sublingual:
DDAVP® Melt: 60 mcg, 120 mcg, 240 mcg

Selected References

Asplund R and Aberg H, "Desmopressin in Elderly Subjects With Increased Nocturnal Diuresis: A Two-Month Treatment Study," *Scand J Urol Nephrol*, 1993, 27(1):77-82.

Lindeman RD, Lee TD Jr, Yiengst MJ, et al, "Influence of Age, Renal Disease, Hypertension, Diuretics, and Calcium on the Antidiuretic Responses to Suboptimal Infusions of Vasopressin," *J Lab Clin Med*, 1966, 68(2):206-23.

Miller JH and Shock NW, "Age Differences in the Renal Tubular Response to Antidiuretic Hormone," *J Gerontol*, 1953, 8:446-50.

◆ **Desmopressin Acetate** see Desmopressin on page 477
◆ **Desoxyphenobarbital** see Primidone on page 1517
◆ **Desulfato-Hirudin** see Desirudin on page 474

♦ **Desulphatohirudin** *see* Desirudin *on page 474*

Desvenlafaxine (des ven la FAX een)

Related Information
Antidepressant Agents *on page 1991*
Brand Names: U.S. Pristiq®
Brand Names: Canada Pristiq®
Index Terms O-desmethylvenlafaxine; ODV
Generic Availability (U.S.) No
Pharmacologic Category Antidepressant, Serotonin/Norepinephrine Reuptake Inhibitor
Use Treatment of major depressive disorder
Unlabeled/Investigational Use Menopausal vasomotor symptoms
Medication Guide Available Yes
Contraindications Hypersensitivity to desvenlafaxine, venlafaxine or any component of the formulation; use of MAO inhibitors within 14 days; should not initiate MAO inhibitor within 7 days of discontinuing desvenlafaxine
Warnings/Precautions [U.S. Boxed Warning]: Antidepressants increase the risk of suicidal thinking and behavior in children, adolescents, and young adults (18-24 years of age) with major depressive disorder (MDD) and other psychiatric disorders; consider risk prior to prescribing. Short-term studies did not show an increased risk in patients >24 years of age and showed a decreased risk in patients ≥65 years. Closely monitor for clinical worsening, suicidality, or unusual changes in behavior; the patient's family or caregiver should be instructed to closely observe the patient and communicate condition with healthcare provider. A medication guide should be dispensed with each prescription. **Desvenlafaxine is not FDA approved for use in children.**

The possibility of a suicide attempt is inherent in major depression and may persist until remission occurs. Monitor for worsening of depression or suicidality, especially during initiation of therapy (generally first 1-2 months) or with dose increases or decreases. Use caution in high-risk patients. Worsening depression and severe abrupt suicidality that are not part of the presenting symptoms may require discontinuation or modification of drug therapy. The patient's family or caregiver should be alerted to monitor patients for the emergence of suicidality and associated behaviors (such as agitation, irritability, hostility, impulsivity, and hypomania) and call healthcare provider.

May worsen psychosis in some patients or precipitate a shift to mania or hypomania in patients with bipolar disorder. Patients presenting with depressive symptoms should be screened for bipolar disorder. Monotherapy in patients with bipolar disorder should be avoided. **Desvenlafaxine is not FDA approved for the treatment of bipolar depression.**

Serotonin syndrome and neuroleptic malignant syndrome (NMS)-like reactions have occurred with serotonin/norepinephrine reuptake inhibitors (SNRIs) and selective serotonin reuptake inhibitors (SSRIs) when used alone, and particularly when used in combination with serotonergic agents (eg, triptans) or antidopaminergic agents (eg, antipsychotics). Concurrent use with MAO inhibitors is contraindicated. Do not begin desvenlafaxine within 14 days of terminating MAO-I therapy; do not initiate MAO-I treatment within 7 days of discontinuing desvenlafaxine. May cause sustained increase in blood pressure or heart rate; dose related. Control pre-existing hypertension prior to initiation of desvenlafaxine. Use caution in patients with recent history of MI, unstable heart disease, or cerebrovascular disease; may cause increases in serum lipids (cholesterol, LDL, triglycerides). Use caution in patients with renal impairment; dose reduction required in severe renal impairment. Use caution in patients with hepatic impairment; clearance is decreased and average AUC is increased; dosage adjustment is recommended. May cause hyponatremia/SIADH (elderly at increased risk); volume depletion (diuretics may increase risk).

Interstitial lung disease and eosinophilic pneumonia have been rarely reported with venlafaxine (the parent drug of desvenlafaxine); may present as progressive dyspnea, cough, and/or chest pain. Prompt evaluation and possible discontinuation of therapy may be necessary. Use cautiously in patients with a history of seizures. The risks of cognitive or motor impairment are low. May cause or exacerbate sexual dysfunction. May impair platelet aggregation, resulting in bleeding.

Abrupt discontinuation or dosage reduction after extended (≥6 weeks) therapy may lead to agitation, dysphoria, nervousness, anxiety, and other symptoms; discontinuation symptoms may also occur when switching from another antidepressant. When discontinuing therapy or switching antidepressants, dosage should be tapered gradually over at least a 2-week period. If intolerable symptoms occur following a decrease in dosage or upon discontinuation of therapy, then resuming the previous dose with a more gradual taper should be considered. ▶

◄   Use caution in patients with increased intraocular pressure or at risk of acute narrow-angle glaucoma.

Adverse Reactions (Reflective of adult population; not specific for elderly)
Reported for 50-100 mg/day.

>10%:
  Central nervous system: Dizziness (10% to 13%), insomnia (9% to 12%)
  Gastrointestinal: Nausea (22% to 26%), xerostomia (11% to 17%), diarrhea (9% to 11%)
  Miscellaneous: Diaphoresis (10% to 11%)

1% to 10%:
  Cardiovascular: Palpitation (≤3%), orthostatic hypotension (<2%; elderly 8%), syncope (<2%), hypertension (dose related; ≤1% of patients taking 50-100 mg daily had sustained diastolic BP ≥90 mm Hg)
  Central nervous system: Somnolence (≤9%), fatigue (7%), anxiety (3% to 5%), abnormal dreams (2% to 3%), irritability (2%), vertigo (1% to 2%), feeling jittery (≤2%), depersonalization (<2%), extrapyramidal symptoms (<2%), hypomania (<2%), seizures (<2%), concentration decreased (≤1%)
  Dermatologic: Rash (1%)
  Endocrine & metabolic: Libido decreased (males 4% to 5%), cholesterol (increased by ≥50 mg/dL and ≥261 mg/dL: 3% to 4%), anorgasmia (females 1%; males ≤3%), hot flushes (1%), low density lipoprotein cholesterol (increased by ≥50 mg/dL and ≥190 mg/dL: ≤1%), sexual dysfunction (males ≤1%)
  Gastrointestinal: Constipation (9%), anorexia (5% to 8%), vomiting (≤4%), weight loss (≤2%), weight gain (<2%)
  Genitourinary: Urinary hesitancy (≤1%)
  Hepatic: Liver function tests abnormal (<2%)
  Neuromuscular & skeletal: Tremor (≤3%), paresthesia (2%), weakness (≤2%), stiffness (<2%)
  Ocular: Blurred vision (3% to 4%), mydriasis (2%)
  Otic: Tinnitus (≤2%)
  Renal: Proteinuria (6% to 8%)
  Respiratory: Epistaxis (<2%)
  Miscellaneous: Ejaculation retarded (1% to 5%), erectile dysfunction (3% to 6%), hypersensitivity reaction (<2%), yawning (1%), ejaculation failure (≤1%)

Class-wide adverse effects: Gastrointestinal hemorrhage, hallucinations, photosensitivity

Drug Interactions
  Metabolism/Transport Effects Substrate of 3A4 (minor); **Inhibits** 3A4 (weak)
  Avoid Concomitant Use
    Avoid concomitant use of Desvenlafaxine with any of the following: Iobenguane I 123; MAO Inhibitors; Methylene Blue; Sibutramine
  Increased Effect/Toxicity
    Desvenlafaxine may increase the levels/effects of: Alpha-/Beta-Agonists; Aspirin; Methylene Blue; NSAID (Nonselective); Serotonin Modulators; Vitamin K Antagonists

    The levels/effects of Desvenlafaxine may be increased by: Alcohol (Ethyl); MAO Inhibitors; Sibutramine
  Decreased Effect
    Desvenlafaxine may decrease the levels/effects of: Alpha2-Agonists; Iobenguane I 123

Ethanol/Nutrition/Herb Interactions
  Ethanol: May increase CNS depression; monitor for increased effects with coadministration. Caution patients about effects.
  Herb/Nutraceutical: Avoid St John's wort (may increase risk of serotonin syndrome and/or excessive sedation).

Mechanism of Action Desvenlafaxine is a potent and selective serotonin and norepinephrine reuptake inhibitor.

Pharmacodynamics/Kinetics
  Distribution: V_d: 3.4 L/kg
  Protein binding: 30%
  Metabolism: Hepatic via conjugation, and oxidation via CYP3A4 (minor pathway)
  Bioavailability: ~80%
  Half-life elimination: ~11 hours; prolonged in renal failure
  Time to peak, serum: ~7.5 hours
  Excretion: Urine (45% as unchanged drug; ~24% as metabolites)

Dosage
Geriatric & Adult
Depression: Oral: 50 mg once daily; up to 400 mg once daily have been studied, however, the manufacturer states there is no evidence that higher doses confer any additional benefit. A flat dose response curve for efficacy between 50-400 mg/day has been noted as well as an increase in adverse events.

Note: Gradually taper dose (by increasing dosing interval) if discontinuing.

Menopausal vasomotor symptoms (unlabled use): 100 mg daily

Renal Impairment
Cl_{cr} >50 mL/minute: No dosage adjustment required

Cl_{cr} 30-50 mL/minute: 50 mg once daily (maximum)

Cl_{cr} <30 mL/minute: 50 mg every other day (maximum)

Hemodialysis: 50 mg every other day (maximum). Supplemental doses not required after HD.

Hepatic Impairment 50 mg once daily; maximum dose: 100 mg/day

Administration May be taken with or without food. Swallow tablet whole; do not crush, chew, break, or dissolve. When discontinuing therapy, extend dosing interval to taper.

Monitoring Parameters Renal function for dosing purposes; blood pressure should be regularly monitored, especially in patients with a high baseline blood pressure; lipid panel (eg, total cholesterol, LDL, triglycerides); mental status for depression, suicide ideation (especially at the beginning of therapy or when doses are increased or decreased). Intraocular pressure should be monitored in those with baseline elevations or a history of glaucoma.

Special Geriatric Considerations No dose adjustment is necessary for age alone; adjust dose for renal function. According to desvenlafaxine's manufacturer, 5% of the 3292 patients in clinical trials were 65 years of age or older. No differences in safety or efficacy were reported between younger and older adults. The elderly are more prone to SSRI/SNRI-induced hyponatremia.

Dosage Forms Excipient information presented when available (limited, particularly for generics); consult specific product labeling.

Tablet, extended release, oral:

Pristiq®: 50 mg, 100 mg

Dexamethasone (Systemic) (deks a METH a sone)

Related Information
Corticosteroids on page 2005

Inhalant Agents on page 2010

Medication Safety Issues
Sound-alike/look-alike issues:

Dexamethasone may be confused with desoximetasone, dextroamphetamine

Decadron® may be confused with Percodan®

Brand Names: U.S. Baycadron™; Dexamethasone Intensol™; DexPak® 10 Day Taper-Pak®; DexPak® 13 Day TaperPak®; DexPak® 6 Day TaperPak®

Brand Names: Canada Apo-Dexamethasone®; Dexasone®

Index Terms Decadron; Dexamethasone Sodium Phosphate

Generic Availability (U.S.) Yes: Excludes concentrated oral solution

Pharmacologic Category Anti-inflammatory Agent; Antiemetic; Corticosteroid, Systemic

Use Primarily as an anti-inflammatory or immunosuppressant agent in the treatment of a variety of diseases including those of allergic, dermatologic, endocrine, hematologic, inflammatory, neoplastic, nervous system, renal, respiratory, rheumatic, and autoimmune origin; may be used in management of cerebral edema, chronic swelling, as a diagnostic agent, diagnosis of Cushing's syndrome, antiemetic

Unlabeled/Investigational Use Dexamethasone suppression test: General indicator consistent with depression and/or suicide

Contraindications Hypersensitivity to dexamethasone or any component of the formulation; systemic fungal infections, cerebral malaria

Warnings/Precautions Use with caution in patients with thyroid disease, hepatic impairment, renal impairment, cardiovascular disease, diabetes, glaucoma, cataracts, myasthenia gravis, patients at risk for osteoporosis, patients at risk for seizures, or GI diseases (diverticulitis, peptic ulcer, ulcerative colitis) due to perforation risk. Use caution following acute MI (corticosteroids have been associated with myocardial rupture). Because of the risk of adverse ▶

◄ effects, systemic corticosteroids should be used cautiously in the elderly in the smallest possible effective dose for the shortest duration. Withdraw therapy with gradual tapering of dose.

May cause hypercorticism or suppression of hypothalamic-pituitary-adrenal (HPA) axis, particularly in patients receiving high doses for prolonged periods. HPA axis suppression may lead to adrenal crisis. Withdrawal and discontinuation of a corticosteroid should be done slowly and carefully. Particular care is required when patients are transferred from systemic corticosteroids to inhaled products due to possible adrenal insufficiency or withdrawal from steroids, including an increase in allergic symptoms. Patients receiving >20 mg per day of prednisone (or equivalent) may be most susceptible. Fatalities have occurred due to adrenal insufficiency in asthmatic patients during and after transfer from systemic corticosteroids to aerosol steroids; aerosol steroids do not provide the systemic steroid needed to treat patients having trauma, surgery, or infections. Dexamethasone does not provide adequate mineralo-corticoid activity in adrenal insufficiency (may be employed as a single dose while cortisol assays are performed). The lowest possible dose should be used during treatment; discontin-uation and/or dose reductions should be gradual.

Acute myopathy has been reported with high dose corticosteroids, usually in patients with neuromuscular transmission disorders; may involve ocular and/or respiratory muscles; monitor creatine kinase; recovery may be delayed. Corticosteroid use may cause psychiatric disturbances, including depression, euphoria, insomnia, mood swings, and personality changes. Pre-existing psychiatric conditions may be exacerbated by corticosteroid use. Prolonged use of corticosteroids may also increase the incidence of secondary infection, mask acute infection (including fungal infections), prolong or exacerbate viral infections, or limit response to vaccines. Exposure to chickenpox should be avoided; corticosteroids should not be used to treat ocular herpes simplex. Corticosteroids should not be used for cerebral malaria or viral hepatitis. Close observation is required in patients with latent tuberculosis and/or TB reactivity; restrict use in active TB (only in conjunction with antituberculosis treatment). Prolonged treatment with corticosteroids has been associated with the development of Kaposi's sarcoma (case reports); if noted, discontinuation of therapy should be considered. High-dose corticosteroids should not be used to manage acute head injury.

Adverse Reactions (Reflective of adult population; not specific for elderly) Fre-quency not defined.

Cardiovascular: Arrhythmia, bradycardia, cardiac arrest, cardiomyopathy, CHF, circulatory collapse, edema, hypertension, myocardial rupture (post-MI), syncope, thromboembolism, vasculitis

Central nervous system: Depression, emotional instability, euphoria, headache, intracranial pressure increased, insomnia, malaise, mood swings, neuritis, personality changes, pseu-dotumor cerebri (usually following discontinuation), psychic disorders, seizure, vertigo

Dermatologic: Acne, allergic dermatitis, alopecia, angioedema, bruising, dry skin, erythema, fragile skin, hirsutism, hyper-/hypopigmentation, hypertrichosis, perianal pruritus (following I.V. injection), petechiae, rash, skin atrophy, skin test reaction impaired, striae, urticaria, wound healing impaired

Endocrine & metabolic: Adrenal suppression, carbohydrate tolerance decreased, Cushing's syndrome, diabetes mellitus, glucose intolerance decreased, growth suppression (children), hyperglycemia, hypokalemic alkalosis, menstrual irregularities, negative nitrogen balance, pituitary-adrenal axis suppression, protein catabolism, sodium retention

Gastrointestinal: Abdominal distention, appetite increased, gastrointestinal hemorrhage, gas-trointestinal perforation, nausea, pancreatitis, peptic ulcer, ulcerative esophagitis, weight gain

Genitourinary: Altered (increased or decreased) spermatogenesis

Hepatic: Hepatomegaly, transaminases increased

Local: Postinjection flare (intra-articular use), thrombophlebitis

Neuromuscular & skeletal: Arthropathy, aseptic necrosis (femoral and humoral heads), fractures, muscle mass loss, myopathy (particularly in conjunction with neuromuscular disease or neuromuscular-blocking agents), neuropathy, osteoporosis, parasthesia, tendon rupture, vertebral compression fractures, weakness

Ocular: Cataracts, exophthalmos, glaucoma, intraocular pressure increased

Renal: Glucosuria

Respiratory: Pulmonary edema

Miscellaneous: Abnormal fat deposition, anaphylactoid reaction, anaphylaxis, avascular necrosis, diaphoresis, hiccups, hypersensitivity, impaired wound healing, infections, Kapo-si's sarcoma, moon face, secondary malignancy

Drug Interactions

Metabolism/Transport Effects Substrate of CYP3A4 (major), P-glycoprotein; **Induces** CYP2A6 (weak), CYP2B6 (weak), CYP2C8 (weak), CYP2C9 (weak), CYP3A4 (strong), P-glycoprotein

Avoid Concomitant Use

Avoid concomitant use of Dexamethasone (Systemic) with any of the following: Aldesleukin; BCG; Conivaptan; Crizotinib; Dabigatran Etexilate; Dronedarone; Everolimus; Lapatinib; Lurasidone; Natalizumab; Nilotinib; Nisoldipine; Pazopanib; Pimecrolimus; Praziquantel; Ranolazine; Rilpivirine; RomiDEPsin; Tacrolimus (Topical); Ticagrelor; Tolvaptan; Vandetanib

Increased Effect/Toxicity

Dexamethasone (Systemic) may increase the levels/effects of: Acetylcholinesterase Inhibitors; Amphotericin B; CycloSPORINE; CycloSPORINE (Systemic); Deferasirox; Leflunomide; Lenalidomide; Loop Diuretics; Natalizumab; NSAID (COX-2 Inhibitor); NSAID (Nonselective); Thalidomide; Thiazide Diuretics; Vaccines (Live); Warfarin

The levels/effects of Dexamethasone (Systemic) may be increased by: Antifungal Agents (Azole Derivatives, Systemic); Aprepitant; Asparaginase; Calcium Channel Blockers (Nondihydropyridine); Conivaptan; CycloSPORINE; CycloSPORINE (Systemic); CYP3A4 Inhibitors (Moderate); CYP3A4 Inhibitors (Strong); Dasatinib; Denosumab; Estrogen Derivatives; Fluconazole; Fosaprepitant; Macrolide Antibiotics; Neuromuscular-Blocking Agents (Nondepolarizing); P-Glycoprotein Inhibitors; Pimecrolimus; Quinolone Antibiotics; Roflumilast; Salicylates; Tacrolimus (Topical); Telaprevir; Trastuzumab

Decreased Effect

Dexamethasone (Systemic) may decrease the levels/effects of: Aldesleukin; Antidiabetic Agents; BCG; Boceprevir; Brentuximab Vedotin; Calcitriol; Caspofungin; Corticorelin; Crizotinib; CycloSPORINE; CycloSPORINE (Systemic); CYP3A4 Substrates; Dabigatran Etexilate; Dronedarone; Everolimus; Exemestane; Gefitinib; GuanFACINE; Imatinib; Isoniazid; Ixabepilone; Lapatinib; Lurasidone; Maraviroc; NIFEdipine; Nilotinib; Nisoldipine; Pazopanib; P-Glycoprotein Substrates; Praziquantel; Ranolazine; Rilpivirine; Rivaroxaban; RomiDEPsin; Salicylates; Sipuleucel-T; SORAfenib; Tadalafil; Telaprevir; Ticagrelor; Tolvaptan; Ulipristal; Vaccines (Inactivated); Vandetanib; Vemurafenib

The levels/effects of Dexamethasone (Systemic) may be decreased by: Aminoglutethimide; Antacids; Barbiturates; Bile Acid Sequestrants; CYP3A4 Inducers (Strong); Echinacea; Herbs (CYP3A4 Inducers); Mitotane; P-Glycoprotein Inducers; Primidone; Rifamycin Derivatives; Tocilizumab

Ethanol/Nutrition/Herb Interactions

Ethanol: Avoid ethanol (may enhance gastric mucosal irritation).

Food: Dexamethasone interferes with calcium absorption. Limit caffeine.

Herb/Nutraceutical: Avoid cat's claw, echinacea (have immunostimulant properties).

Stability Injection solution: Store at room temperature; protect from light and freezing.

Stability of injection of parenteral admixture at room temperature (25°C): 24 hours

Stability of injection of parenteral admixture at refrigeration temperature (4°C): 2 days; protect from light and freezing.

Injection should be diluted in 50-100 mL NS or D_5W.

Mechanism of Action Decreases inflammation by suppression of neutrophil migration, decreased production of inflammatory mediators, and reversal of increased capillary permeability; suppresses normal immune response. Dexamethasone's mechanism of antiemetic activity is unknown.

Pharmacodynamics/Kinetics

Onset of action: Acetate: Prompt

Duration of metabolic effect: 72 hours; acetate is a long-acting repository preparation

Metabolism: Hepatic

Half-life elimination: Normal renal function: 1.8-3.5 hours; Biological half-life: 36-54 hours

Time to peak, serum: Oral: 1-2 hours; I.M.: ~8 hours

Excretion: Urine and feces

Dosage

Geriatric Refer to adult dosing. Use cautiously in the elderly in the smallest possible dose.

Adult

Anti-inflammatory:

Oral, I.M., I.V.: 0.75-9 mg/day in divided doses every 6-12 hours

Intra-articular, intralesional, or soft tissue: 0.4-6 mg/day

Extubation or airway edema: Oral, I.M., I.V.: 0.5-2 mg/kg/day in divided doses every 6 hours beginning 24 hours prior to extubation and continuing for 4-6 doses afterwards

Antiemetic:

Prophylaxis: Oral, I.V.: 10-20 mg 15-30 minutes before treatment on each treatment day

Continuous infusion regimen: Oral or I.V.: 10 mg every 12 hours on each treatment day

Mildly emetogenic therapy: Oral, I.M., I.V.: 4 mg every 4-6 hours

◀

Delayed nausea/vomiting: Oral: 4-10 mg 1-2 times/day for 2-4 days **or**
   8 mg every 12 hours for 2 days; then
   4 mg every 12 hours for 2 days **or**
   20 mg 1 hour before chemotherapy; then
   10 mg 12 hours after chemotherapy; then
   8 mg every 12 hours for 4 doses; then
   4 mg every 12 hours for 4 doses

Multiple myeloma: Oral, I.V.: 40 mg/day, days 1 to 4, 9 to 12, and 17 to 20, repeated every 4 weeks (alone or as part of a regimen)

Cerebral edema: I.V. 10 mg stat, 4 mg I.M./I.V. (should be given as sodium phosphate) every 6 hours until response is maximized, then switch to oral regimen, then taper off if appropriate; dosage may be reduced after 2-4 days and gradually discontinued over 5-7 days

Dexamethasone suppression test (depression/suicide indicator) (unlabeled use): Oral: 1 mg at 11 PM, draw blood at 8 AM the following day for plasma cortisol determination

Cushing's syndrome, diagnostic: Oral: 1 mg at 11 PM, draw blood at 8 AM; greater accuracy for Cushing's syndrome may be achieved by the following:
   Dexamethasone 0.5 mg by mouth every 6 hours for 48 hours (with 24-hour urine collection for 17-hydroxycorticosteroid excretion)
   Differentiation of Cushing's syndrome due to ACTH excess from Cushing's due to other causes: Oral: Dexamethasone 2 mg every 6 hours for 48 hours (with 24-hour urine collection for 17-hydroxycorticosteroid excretion)

Multiple sclerosis (acute exacerbation): Oral: 30 mg/day for 1 week, followed by 4-12 mg/day for 1 month

Treatment of shock:
   Addisonian crisis/shock (eg, adrenal insufficiency/responsive to steroid therapy): I.V.: 4-10 mg as a single dose, which may be repeated if necessary
   Unresponsive shock (eg, unresponsive to steroid therapy): I.V.: 1-6 mg/kg as a single I.V. dose or up to 40 mg initially followed by repeat doses every 2-6 hours while shock persists

Physiological replacement: Oral, I.M., I.V. (should be given as sodium phosphate): 0.03-0.15 mg/kg/day **or** 0.6-0.75 mg/m^2/day in divided doses every 6-12 hours

Renal Impairment Hemodialysis or peritoneal dialysis: Supplemental dose is not necessary.

Administration

Oral: Administer with meals to decrease GI upset.

I.V.: Administer as a 5-10 minute bolus; rapid injection is associated with a high incidence of perineal discomfort.

Monitoring Parameters Hemoglobin, occult blood loss, serum potassium, glucose

Reference Range Dexamethasone suppression test, overnight: 8 AM cortisol <6 mcg/100 mL (dexamethasone 1 mg); plasma cortisol determination should be made on the day after giving dose

Test Interactions May suppress the wheal and flare reactions to skin test antigens

Pharmacotherapy Pearls Effects of inhaled/intranasal steroids on growth have been observed in the absence of laboratory evidence of HPA axis suppression, suggesting that growth velocity is a more sensitive indicator of systemic corticosteroid exposure in pediatric patients than some commonly used tests of HPA axis function. The long-term effects of this reduction in growth velocity associated with orally-inhaled and intranasal corticosteroids, including the impact on final adult height, are unknown. The potential for "catch up" growth following discontinuation of treatment with inhaled corticosteroids has not been adequately studied.

Withdrawal/tapering of therapy: Corticosteroid tapering following short-term use is limited primarily by the need to control the underlying disease state; tapering may be accomplished over a period of days. Following longer-term use, tapering over weeks to months may be necessary to avoid signs and symptoms of adrenal insufficiency and to allow recovery of the HPA axis. Testing of HPA axis responsiveness may be of value in selected patients. Subtle deficits in HPA response may persist for months after discontinuation of therapy, and may require supplemental dosing during periods of acute illness or surgical stress.

Special Geriatric Considerations Because of the risk of adverse effects, systemic corticosteroids should be used cautiously in the elderly in the smallest possible dose, and for the shortest possible time.

Dosage Forms Excipient information presented when available (limited, particularly for generics); consult specific product labeling.

Elixir, oral: 0.5 mg/5 mL (237 mL)
   Baycadron™: 0.5 mg/5 mL (237 mL) [contains benzoic acid, ethanol 5.1%, propylene glycol; raspberry flavor]

Injection, solution, as sodium phosphate: 4 mg/mL (1 mL, 5 mL, 30 mL); 10 mg/mL (1 mL, 10 mL)

Injection, solution, as sodium phosphate [preservative free]: 10 mg/mL (1 mL)
Solution, oral: 0.5 mg/5 mL (240 mL, 500 mL)
Solution, oral [concentrate]:
Dexamethasone Intensol™: 1 mg/mL (30 mL) [dye free, sugar free; contains benzoic acid, ethanol 30%, propylene glycol]
Tablet, oral: 0.5 mg, 0.75 mg, 1 mg, 1.5 mg, 2 mg, 4 mg, 6 mg
DexPak® 6 Day TaperPak®: 1.5 mg [scored; 21 tablets on taper dose card]
DexPak® 10 Day TaperPak®: 1.5 mg [scored; 35 tablets on taper dose card]
DexPak® 13 Day TaperPak®: 1.5 mg [scored; 51 tablets on taper dose card]

Dexamethasone (Ophthalmic) (deks a METH a sone)

Medication Safety Issues
Sound-alike/look-alike issues:
Dexamethasone may be confused with desoximetasone, dextroamphetamine
Maxidex® may be confused with Maxzide®
Brand Names: U.S. Maxidex®; Ozurdex®
Brand Names: Canada Diodex®; Maxidex®
Index Terms Dexamethasone Sodium Phosphate
Generic Availability (U.S.) Yes: Ophthalmic solution
Pharmacologic Category Anti-inflammatory Agent, Ophthalmic; Corticosteroid, Ophthalmic
Use Management of steroid responsive inflammatory conditions such as allergic conjunctivitis, iritis, or cyclitis; symptomatic treatment of corneal injury from chemical, radiation, or thermal burns, or penetration of foreign bodies
Ophthalmic intravitreal implant (Ozurdex®): Treatment of macular edema following branch retinal vein occlusion (BRVO) or central retinal vein occlusion (CRVO); treatment of non-infective uveitis

Dosage
Geriatric Refer to adult dosing. Solution/suspension: Use cautiously in the elderly in the smallest possible dose.
Adult
Anti-inflammatory:
Ophthalmic solution: Instill 1-2 drops into conjunctival sac every hour during the day and every other hour during the night; gradually reduce dose to every 3-4 hours, then to 3-4 times/day.
Ophthalmic suspension: Instill 1-2 drops into conjunctival sac up to 4-6 times/day; may use hourly in severe disease; taper prior to discontinuation.
Macular edema (following BRVO or CRVO): *Ophthalmic injection:* Ocular implant (Ozurdex®): Intravitreal: 0.7 mg implant injected in affected eye
Noninfective uveitis: *Ophthalmic injection:* Ocular implant (Ozurdex®): Intravitreal: 0.7 mg implant injected in affected eye

Dosage Forms Excipient information presented when available (limited, particularly for generics); consult specific product labeling.
Implant, intravitreal:
Ozurdex®: 0.7 mg (1s)
Solution, ophthalmic, as phosphate [drops]: 0.1% (5 mL)
Suspension, ophthalmic [drops]:
Maxidex®: 0.1% (5 mL) [contains benzalkonium chloride]

◆ **Dexamethasone and Ciprofloxacin** *see* Ciprofloxacin and Dexamethasone *on page 364*
◆ **Dexamethasone and Tobramycin** *see* Tobramycin and Dexamethasone *on page 1815*
◆ **Dexamethasone Intensol™** *see* Dexamethasone (Systemic) *on page 483*
◆ **Dexamethasone, Neomycin, and Polymyxin B** *see* Neomycin, Polymyxin B, and Dexamethasone *on page 1280*
◆ **Dexamethasone Sodium Phosphate** *see* Dexamethasone (Ophthalmic) *on page 487*
◆ **Dexamethasone Sodium Phosphate** *see* Dexamethasone (Systemic) *on page 483*

Dexchlorpheniramine (deks klor fen EER a meen)

Related Information
Beers Criteria – Potentially Inappropriate Medications for Geriatrics *on page 2089*
Medication Safety Issues
BEERS Criteria medication:
This drug may be inappropriate for use in geriatric patients (high severity risk).
Index Terms Dexchlorpheniramine Maleate
Generic Availability (U.S.) Yes

◀ **Pharmacologic Category** Alkylamine Derivative; Histamine H_1 Antagonist; Histamine H_1 Antagonist, First Generation

Use Perennial and seasonal allergic rhinitis and other allergic symptoms including urticaria

Contraindications Hypersensitivity to dexchlorpheniramine or any component of the formulation; narrow-angle glaucoma

Warnings/Precautions Causes sedation, caution must be used in performing tasks which require alertness (eg, operating machinery or driving). Effects may be potentiated when used with other sedative drugs or ethanol. Use with caution in patients with angle-closure glaucoma, pyloroduodenal obstruction (including stenotic peptic ulcer), urinary tract obstruction (including bladder neck obstruction and symptomatic prostatic hyperplasia), hyperthyroidism, increased intraocular pressure, and cardiovascular disease (including hypertension and ischemic heart disease). May be inappropriate for use in the elderly due to potent anticholinergic effects (Beers Criteria).

Adverse Reactions (Reflective of adult population; not specific for elderly)

>10%:

Central nervous system: Slight to moderate drowsiness

Respiratory: Thickening of bronchial secretions

1% to 10%:

Central nervous system: Headache, fatigue, nervousness, dizziness

Gastrointestinal: Appetite increase, weight gain, nausea, diarrhea, abdominal pain, xerostomia

Neuromuscular & skeletal: Arthralgia

Respiratory: Pharyngitis

Drug Interactions

Avoid Concomitant Use There are no known interactions where it is recommended to avoid concomitant use.

Increased Effect/Toxicity

Dexchlorpheniramine may increase the levels/effects of: Alcohol (Ethyl); Anticholinergics; CNS Depressants; Selective Serotonin Reuptake Inhibitors

The levels/effects of Dexchlorpheniramine may be increased by: Droperidol; HydrOXYzine; Pramlintide

Decreased Effect

Dexchlorpheniramine may decrease the levels/effects of: Acetylcholinesterase Inhibitors (Central); Benzylpenicilloyl Polylysine; Betahistine

The levels/effects of Dexchlorpheniramine may be decreased by: Acetylcholinesterase Inhibitors (Central); Amphetamines

Ethanol/Nutrition/Herb Interactions Ethanol: May increase CNS depression; monitor for increased effects with coadministration. Caution patients about effects.

Mechanism of Action Competes with histamine for H_1-receptor sites on effector cells in the gastrointestinal tract, blood vessels, and respiratory tract. Dexchlorpheniramine is the predominant active isomer of chlorpheniramine and is approximately twice as active as the racemic compound.

Pharmacodynamics/Kinetics

Onset of action: ~1 hour

Duration: 3-6 hours

Absorption: Well absorbed

Metabolism: Hepatic

Dosage

Geriatric & Adult Allergy symptoms: Oral: 2 mg every 4-6 hours or 4-6 mg timed release at bedtime or every 8-10 hours

Administration May be administered without regard to meals.

Monitoring Parameters Monitor mental function, bowel function, and urinary retention

Special Geriatric Considerations Anticholinergic action may cause significant confusional symptoms, constipation, or problems voiding urine.

This medication is considered to be potentially inappropriate in this patient population (Beers Criteria severity: High).

Dosage Forms Excipient information presented when available (limited, particularly for generics); consult specific product labeling.

Syrup, oral, as maleate: 2 mg/5 mL (473 mL)

◆ **Dexchlorpheniramine Maleate** *see* Dexchlorpheniramine *on page 487*

◆ **Dexferrum®** *see* Iron Dextran Complex *on page 977*

◆ **Dexilant™** *see* Dexlansoprazole *on page 489*

Dexlansoprazole (deks lan SOE pra zole)

Medication Safety Issues
Sound-alike/look-alike issues:
Dexlansoprazole may be confused with aripiprazole, lansoprazole

Kapidex [DSC] may be confused with Casodex®, Kadian®

International issues:
Kapidex [DSC] may be confused with Capadex which is a brand name for propoxyphene/acetaminophen combination product in Australia and New Zealand

Brand Names: U.S. Dexilant™

Brand Names: Canada Dexilant™

Index Terms Kapidex; TAK-390MR

Generic Availability (U.S.) No

Pharmacologic Category Proton Pump Inhibitor; Substituted Benzimidazole

Use Short-term (4 weeks) treatment of heartburn associated with nonerosive GERD; short-term (up to 8 weeks) treatment of all grades of erosive esophagitis; to maintain healing of erosive esophagitis for up to 6 months

Contraindications Hypersensitivity to dexlansoprazole or any component of the formulation

Warnings/Precautions Use of proton pump inhibitors may increase the risk of gastrointestinal infections (eg, *Salmonella*, *Campylobacter*). Relief of symptoms does not preclude the presence of a gastric malignancy. Atrophic gastritis (by biopsy) has been noted with long-term omeprazole therapy; this may also occur with dexlansoprazole. No occurrences of enterochromaffin-like (ECL) cell carcinoids, dysplasia, or neoplasia, such as those seen in rodent studies, have been reported in humans. Patients with moderate hepatic impairment (Child-Pugh class B) may require dosage reductions; no studies have been conducted in patients with severe hepatic impairment. Proton pump inhibitors may diminish the therapeutic effect of clopidogrel, thought to be due to reduced formation of the active metabolite of clopidogrel; an increase in the risk of cardiovascular events may occur. The manufacturer of clopidogrel recommends avoidance of concomitant administration of another PPI (ie, omeprazole); given the potency of CYP2C19 inhibitory activity, similar recommendations with dexlansoprazole would appear prudent.

Increased incidence of osteoporosis-related bone fractures of the hip, spine, or wrist may occur with proton pump inhibitor therapy. Patients on high-dose (multiple daily doses) or long-term therapy (≥1 year) should be monitored. Use the lowest effective dose for the shortest duration of time, use vitamin D and calcium supplementation, and follow appropriate guidelines to reduce risk of fractures in patients at risk.

Hypomagnesemia, reported rarely, usually with prolonged PPI use of >3 months (most cases >1 year of therapy); may be symptomatic or asymptomatic; severe cases may cause tetany, seizures, and cardiac arrhythmias. Consider obtaining serum magnesium concentrations prior to beginning long-term therapy, especially if taking concomitant digoxin, diuretics, or other drugs known to cause hypomagnesemia; and periodically thereafter. Hypomagnesemia may be corrected by magnesium supplementation, although discontinuation of dexlansoprazole may be necessary; magnesium levels typically return to normal within 1 week of stopping.

Adverse Reactions (Reflective of adult population; not specific for elderly)
2% to 10%:

Gastrointestinal: Diarrhea (5%), abdominal pain (4%), nausea (3%), flatulence (1% to 3%), vomiting (1% to 2%)

Respiratory: Upper respiratory tract infection (2% to 3%)

Drug Interactions
Metabolism/Transport Effects Substrate of CYP2C9 (minor), 2C19 (major), 3A4 (major); **Inhibits** CYP2C9 (weak), 2C19 (moderate), 2D6 (weak), 3A4 (weak); **Induces** CYP1A2 (weak)

Avoid Concomitant Use
Avoid concomitant use of Dexlansoprazole with any of the following: Delavirdine; Erlotinib; Nelfinavir; Posaconazole; Rilpivirine

Increased Effect/Toxicity
Dexlansoprazole may increase the levels/effects of: Amphetamines; Benzodiazepines (metabolized by oxidation); Dexmethylphenidate; Methotrexate; Methylphenidate; Raltegravir; Saquinavir; Tacrolimus; Tacrolimus (Systemic); Voriconazole

The levels/effects of Dexlansoprazole may be increased by: Fluconazole; Ketoconazole; Ketoconazole (Systemic)

Decreased Effect

Dexlansoprazole may decrease the levels/effects of: Atazanavir; Bisphosphonate Derivatives; Cefditoren; Clopidogrel; Dabigatran Etexilate; Dasatinib; Delavirdine; Erlotinib; Gefitinib; Indinavir; Iron Salts; Itraconazole; Ketoconazole; Ketoconazole (Systemic); Mesalamine; Mycophenolate; Nelfinavir; Posaconazole; Rilpivirine

The levels/effects of Dexlansoprazole may be decreased by: Tipranavir

Ethanol/Nutrition/Herb Interactions Ethanol: Avoid ethanol (may cause gastric mucosal irritation).

Stability Store at 25°C (77°F); excursions permitted to 15°C to 30°C (59°F to 86°F).

Mechanism of Action Proton pump inhibitor; decreases acid secretion in gastric parietal cells through inhibition of (H+, K+)-ATPase enzyme system, blocking the final step in gastric acid production

Pharmacodynamics/Kinetics

Distribution: V_d: 40.3 L

Protein binding: ~96% to 99%

Metabolism: Hepatic via CYP2C19-mediated hydroxylation and CYP3A4-mediated oxidation; followed by reduction to sulfate, glucuronide, and glutathione conjugates (inactive)

Bioavailability: May be increased when administered with food

Half-life, elimination: ~1-2 hours

Time to peak, serum: **Note:** Two distinct peaks secondary to dual release formulation:

Peak 1: 1-2 hours

Peak 2: 4-5 hours

Excretion: Urine (~51% as metabolites); feces (~48% as metabolites)

Dosage

Geriatric & Adult

Erosive esophagitis: Oral: Short-term treatment: 60 mg once daily for up to 8 weeks; maintenance therapy: 30 mg once daily for up to 6 months

Symptomatic GERD: Oral: Short-term treatment: 30 mg once daily for 4 weeks

Renal Impairment No dosage adjustment is needed.

Hepatic Impairment

Mild hepatic impairment (Child-Pugh class A): No dosage adjustment is needed.

Moderate hepatic impairment (Child-Pugh class B): Consider a maximum dose of 30 mg/day.

Severe hepatic impairment (Child-Pugh class C): Use has not been studied in patients with severe hepatic impairment.

Administration May be administered without regard to meals; some patients may benefit from premeal administration if symptoms do not adequately respond to post-meal dosing. Capsules should be swallowed whole; alternatively, patients who are unable to swallow capsules may open the capsule, sprinkle the intact granules onto 1 tablespoon of applesauce, and swallow intact granules immediately.

Special Geriatric Considerations No dose adjustment is recommended based on age or renal function. An increased half-life (2.23 vs 1.5 hours) and greater AUC (34.5%) in elderly compared to younger subjects are not considered to be clinically significant.

An increased risk of fractures of the hip, spine, or wrist has been observed in epidemiologic studies with proton pump inhibitor (PPI) use, primarily in older adults ≥50 years of age. The greatest risk was seen in patients receiving high doses or on long-term therapy (≥1 year). Calcium and vitamin D supplementation and close monitoring are recommended to reduce the risk of fracture in high-risk patients.

Dosage Forms Excipient information presented when available (limited, particularly for generics); consult specific product labeling.

Capsule, delayed release, oral:

Dexilant™: 30 mg, 60 mg

Selected References

DeVault KR and Castell DO, "Updated Guidelines for the Diagnosis and Treatment of Gastroesophageal Reflux Disease," *Am J Gastroenterol*, 2005, 100(1):190-200.

◆ **DexPak® 6 Day TaperPak®** *see* Dexamethasone (Systemic) *on page 483*
◆ **DexPak® 10 Day TaperPak®** *see* Dexamethasone (Systemic) *on page 483*
◆ **DexPak® 13 Day TaperPak®** *see* Dexamethasone (Systemic) *on page 483*
◆ **Dextrin** *see* Wheat Dextrin *on page 1933*

Dextromethorphan (deks troe meth OR fan)

Medication Safety Issues

Sound-alike/look-alike issues:

Benylin® may be confused with Benadryl®, Ventolin®

Delsym® may be confused with Delfen®, Desyrel

Brand Names: U.S. Creo-Terpin® [OTC]; Creomulsion® Adult Formula [OTC]; Creomulsion® for Children [OTC]; Delsym® [OTC]; Father John's® [OTC]; Hold® DM [OTC]; Nycoff [OTC]; PediaCare® Children's Long-Acting Cough [OTC]; Robafen Cough [OTC]; Robitussin® Children's Cough Long-Acting [OTC]; Robitussin® Cough Long Acting [OTC]; Robitussin® CoughGels™ Long-Acting [OTC]; Scot-Tussin® Diabetes [OTC]; Silphen-DM [OTC]; Triaminic Thin Strips® Children's Long Acting Cough [OTC]; Triaminic® Children's Cough Long Acting [OTC]; Trocal® [OTC]; Vicks® 44® Cough Relief [OTC]; Vicks® DayQuil® Cough [OTC]

Generic Availability (U.S.) Yes: Excludes strip

Pharmacologic Category Antitussive; N-Methyl-D-Aspartate Receptor Antagonist

Use Symptomatic relief of coughs caused by the common cold or inhaled irritants

Unlabeled/Investigational Use N-methyl-D-aspartate (NMDA) antagonist

Contraindications Concurrent administration with or within 2 weeks of discontinuing an MAO inhibitor

Warnings/Precautions Symptoms of agitation, confusion, hallucinations, hyper-reflexia, myoclonus, shivering, and tachycardia may occur with concomitant proserotonergic drugs (ie, SSRIs/SNRIs or triptans); especially with higher dextromethorphan doses.

Some products may contain sodium benzoate which may cause allergic reactions in susceptible individuals.

Healthcare providers should be alert to problems of abuse or misuse. Abuse can cause death, brain damage, seizure, loss of consciousness and irregular heartbeat. Use with caution in patients who are sedated, debilitated or confined to a supine position. Some products may contain tartrazine.

Self-medication (OTC use): When used for self medication (OTC) notify healthcare provider if symptoms do not improve within 7 days, or are accompanied by fever, rash or persistent headache. Do not use for persistent or chronic cough (as with smoking, asthma, chronic bronchitis, emphysema) or if cough is accompanied by excessive phlegm unless directed to do so by healthcare provider.

Drug Interactions

Metabolism/Transport Effects Substrate of CYP2B6 (minor), 2C9 (minor), 2C19 (minor), 2D6 (major), 2E1 (minor), 3A4 (minor); **Inhibits** CYP2D6 (weak)

Avoid Concomitant Use

Avoid concomitant use of Dextromethorphan with any of the following: MAO Inhibitors; Sibutramine

Increased Effect/Toxicity

Dextromethorphan may increase the levels/effects of: Serotonin Modulators

The levels/effects of Dextromethorphan may be increased by: Abiraterone Acetate; Conivaptan; CYP2D6 Inhibitors (Moderate); CYP2D6 Inhibitors (Strong); Darunavir; MAO Inhibitors; QuiNIDine; Selective Serotonin Reuptake Inhibitors; Sibutramine

Decreased Effect

The levels/effects of Dextromethorphan may be decreased by: Cyproterone; Peginterferon Alfa-2b; Tocilizumab

Mechanism of Action Decreases the sensitivity of cough receptors and interrupts cough impulse transmission by depressing the medullary cough center through sigma receptor stimulation; structurally related to codeine

Pharmacodynamics/Kinetics

Onset of action: Antitussive: 15-30 minutes

Duration: ≤6 hours

Metabolism: Hepatic via demethylation via CYP2D6 to dextrorphan (active); CYP3A4 and CYP3A5 form smaller amounts of 3-hydroxy and 3-methoxy derivatives

Half-life elimination: Dextrorphan: Extensive metabolizers: 2-4 hours; poor metabolizers: 24 hours

Time to peak: 2-3 hours

Excretion: Primarily in urine as metabolites

Dosage

Geriatric & Adult Cough suppressant: Oral: 10-20 mg every 4 hours or 30 mg every 6-8 hours; extended release: 60 mg twice daily; maximum: 120 mg/day

Test Interactions False-positive phencyclidine (PCP), opiates, opioids and heroin urine drug screen

◀ **Dosage Forms** Excipient information presented when available (limited, particularly for generics); consult specific product labeling.
Capsule, liquid filled, oral, as hydrobromide:
Robafen Cough: 15 mg
Robitussin® CoughGels™ Long-Acting: 15 mg
Liquid, oral, as hydrobromide: 15 mg/5 mL (120 mL)
Creo-Terpin®: 10 mg/15 mL (120 mL) [contains ethanol 25%, tartrazine]
Scot-Tussin® Diabetes: 10 mg/5 mL (118 mL) [ethanol free, gluten free, sugar free; contains propylene glycol; cherry-strawberry flavor]
Vicks® 44® Cough Relief: 10 mg/5 mL (120 mL) [contains ethanol, propylene glycol, sodium 28 mg/15 mL, sodium benzoate]
Lozenge, oral, as hydrobromide:
Hold® DM: 5 mg (10s) [cherry flavor]
Hold® DM: 5 mg (10s) [original flavor]
Trocal®: 7.5 mg (50s, 300s) [cherry flavor]
Solution, oral, as hydrobromide:
PediaCare® Children's Long-Acting Cough: 7.5 mg/5 mL (118 mL) [ethanol free; contains sodium 15 mg/5 mL, sodium benzoate; grape flavor]
Vicks® DayQuil® Cough: 15 mg/15 mL (177 mL, 295 mL) [ethanol free; contains propylene glycol, sodium 15 mg/15 mL; citrus flavor]
Strip, orally disintegrating, oral, as hydrobromide:
Triaminic Thin Strips® Children's Long Acting Cough: 7.5 mg (14s, 16s) [contains ethanol; cherry flavor; equivalent to dextromethorphan 5.5 mg]
Suspension, extended release, oral:
Delsym®: Dextromethorphan polistirex [equivalent to dextromethorphan hydrobromide] 30 mg/5 mL (89 mL, 148 mL) [ethanol free; contains propylene glycol, sodium 7 mg/5 mL; grape flavor]
Delsym®: Dextromethorphan polistirex [equivalent to dextromethorphan hydrobromide] 30 mg/5 mL (89 mL, 148 mL) [ethanol free; contains propylene glycol, sodium 7 mg/5 mL; orange flavor]
Syrup, oral, as hydrobromide:
Creomulsion® Adult Formula: 20 mg/15 mL (120 mL) [ethanol free; contains sodium benzoate]
Creomulsion® for Children: 5 mg/5 mL (120 mL) [ethanol free; contains sodium benzoate; cherry flavor]
Father John's®: 10 mg/5 mL (118 mL, 236 mL) [ethanol free]
Robitussin® Children's Cough Long-Acting: 7.5 mg/5 mL (118 mL) [ethanol free; contains propylene glycol, sodium 5 mg/5 mL, sodium benzoate; fruit-punch flavor]
Robitussin® Cough Long Acting: 15 mg/5 mL (240 mL) [contains ethanol, sodium benzoate]
Silphen-DM: 10 mg/5 mL (120 mL) [strawberry flavor]
Triaminic® Children's Cough Long Acting: 7.5 mg/5 mL (118 mL) [contains benzoic acid, propylene glycol, sodium 7 mg/5 mL]
Tablet, oral, as hydrobromide:
Nycoff: 15 mg

◆ **Dextromethorphan and Guaifenesin** see Guaifenesin and Dextromethorphan on page 848
◆ **Dex-Tuss** see Guaifenesin and Codeine on page 848
◆ **DHE** see Dihydroergotamine on page 512
◆ **D.H.E. 45®** see Dihydroergotamine on page 512
◆ **DHPG Sodium** see Ganciclovir (Systemic) on page 809
◆ **DHS™ Sal [OTC]** see Salicylic Acid on page 1648
◆ **Diabeta** see GlyBURIDE on page 828
◆ **DiaBeta®** see GlyBURIDE on page 828
◆ **DiabetAid® Antifungal Foot Bath [OTC]** see Miconazole on page 1206
◆ **DiabetAid® Pain and Tingling Relief [OTC]** see Capsaicin on page 261
◆ **Diabetic Siltussin DAS-Na [OTC]** see GuaiFENesin on page 846
◆ **Diabetic Siltussin-DM DAS-Na [OTC]** see Guaifenesin and Dextromethorphan on page 848
◆ **Diabetic Siltussin-DM DAS-Na Maximum Strength [OTC]** see Guaifenesin and Dextromethorphan on page 848
◆ **Diabetic Tussin® DM [OTC]** see Guaifenesin and Dextromethorphan on page 848
◆ **Diabetic Tussin® DM Maximum Strength [OTC]** see Guaifenesin and Dextromethorphan on page 848
◆ **Diabetic Tussin® EX [OTC]** see GuaiFENesin on page 846
◆ **Diabetic Tussin® for Children Allergy Relief [OTC]** see Chlorpheniramine on page 337
◆ **Diamode [OTC]** see Loperamide on page 1085
◆ **Diamox® Sequels®** see AcetaZOLAMIDE on page 39
◆ **Diastat®** see Diazepam on page 493

◆ **Diastat® AcuDial™** *see* Diazepam *on page 493*

Diazepam (dye AZ e pam)

Related Information
Anxiolytic, Sedative / Hypnotic, and Miscellaneous Benzodiazepines *on page 2000*
Beers Criteria – Potentially Inappropriate Medications for Geriatrics *on page 2089*
Patient Information for Disposal of Unused Medications *on page 2125*

Medication Safety Issues
Sound-alike/look-alike issues:
Diazepam may be confused with diazoxide, diltiazem, Ditropan, LORazepam
Valium® may be confused with Valcyte®

BEERS Criteria medication:
This drug may be inappropriate for use in geriatric patients (high severity risk).

Brand Names: U.S. Diastat®; Diastat® AcuDial™; Diazepam Intensol™; Valium®

Brand Names: Canada Apo-Diazepam®; Diastat®; Diastat® Rectal Delivery System; Diazemuls®; Novo-Dipam®; Valium®

Generic Availability (U.S.) Yes

Pharmacologic Category Benzodiazepine

Use Management of anxiety disorders, ethanol withdrawal symptoms; skeletal muscle relaxant; treatment of convulsive disorders; preoperative or preprocedural sedation and amnesia
Rectal gel: Management of selected, refractory epilepsy patients on stable regimens of antiepileptic drugs requiring intermittent use of diazepam to control episodes of increased seizure activity

Unlabeled/Investigational Use Treatment of panic disorders

Contraindications Hypersensitivity to diazepam or any component of the formulation (cross-sensitivity with other benzodiazepines may exist); narrow-angle glaucoma

Warnings/Precautions Withdrawal has also been associated with an increase in the seizure frequency. Use with caution with drugs which may decrease diazepam metabolism. Use with caution in debilitated patients, obese patients, patients with hepatic disease (including alcoholics), or renal impairment. Active metabolites with extended half-lives may lead to delayed accumulation and adverse effects. Use with caution in patients with respiratory disease or impaired gag reflex.

Acute hypotension, muscle weakness, apnea, and cardiac arrest have occurred with parenteral administration. Acute effects may be more prevalent in patients receiving concurrent barbiturates, narcotics, or ethanol. Appropriate resuscitative equipment and qualified personnel should be available during administration and monitoring. Avoid use of the injection in patients with shock, coma, or acute ethanol intoxication. Intra-arterial injection or extravasation of the parenteral formulation should be avoided. Parenteral formulation contains propylene glycol, which has been associated with toxicity when administered in high dosages. Administration of rectal gel should only be performed by individuals trained to recognize characteristic seizure activity and monitor response.

Causes CNS depression (dose-related) resulting in sedation, dizziness, confusion, or ataxia which may impair physical and mental capabilities. Patients must be cautioned about performing tasks which require mental alertness (eg, operating machinery or driving). Use with caution in patients receiving other CNS depressants or psychoactive agents. Effects with other sedative drugs or ethanol may be potentiated. The dosage of narcotics should be reduced by approximately 1/3 when diazepam is added. Benzodiazepines have been associated with falls and traumatic injury and should be used with extreme caution in patients who are at risk of these events (especially the elderly). Benzodiazepines with long half-lives may produce prolonged sedation and increase the risk of falls and fracture. Short- or intermediate-acting benzodiazepines are preferred in elderly patients (Beers Criteria).

Use with caution in patients taking strong CYP3A4 inhibitors, moderate or strong CYP3A4 and CYP2C19 inducers and major CYP3A4 substrates.

Use caution in patients with depression or anxiety associated with depression, particularly if suicidal risk may be present. Use with caution in patients with a history of drug dependence. Benzodiazepines have been associated with dependence and acute withdrawal symptoms on discontinuation or reduction in dose. Acute withdrawal, including seizures, may be precipitated in patients after administration of flumazenil to patients receiving long-term benzodiazepine therapy.

Diazepam has been associated with anterograde amnesia. Psychiatric and paradoxical reactions, including hyperactive or aggressive behavior, have been reported with benzodiazepines, particularly in elderly patients. Does not have analgesic, antidepressant, or antipsychotic properties.

◀ **Adverse Reactions (Reflective of adult population; not specific for elderly)** Frequency not defined. Adverse reactions may vary by route of administration.

Cardiovascular: Hypotension, vasodilatation

Central nervous system: Amnesia, ataxia, confusion, depression, drowsiness, fatigue, headache, slurred speech, paradoxical reactions (eg, aggressiveness, agitation, anxiety, delusions, hallucinations, inappropriate behavior, increased muscle spasms, insomnia, irritability, psychoses, rage, restlessness, sleep disturbances, stimulation), vertigo

Dermatologic: Rash

Endocrine & metabolic: Libido changes

Gastrointestinal: Constipation, diarrhea, nausea, salivation changes (dry mouth or hypersalivation)

Genitourinary: Incontinence, urinary retention

Hepatic: Jaundice

Local: Phlebitis, pain with injection

Neuromuscular & skeletal: Dysarthria, tremor, weakness

Ocular: Blurred vision, diplopia

Respiratory: Apnea, asthma, respiratory rate decreased

Drug Interactions

Metabolism/Transport Effects Substrate of CYP1A2 (minor), 2B6 (minor), 2C9 (minor), 2C19 (major), 3A4 (major); **Inhibits** CYP2C19 (weak), 3A4 (weak)

Avoid Concomitant Use

Avoid concomitant use of Diazepam with any of the following: Conivaptan; OLANZapine

Increased Effect/Toxicity

Diazepam may increase the levels/effects of: Alcohol (Ethyl); CloZAPine; CNS Depressants; Fosphenytoin; Methotrimeprazine; Phenytoin; Selective Serotonin Reuptake Inhibitors

The levels/effects of Diazepam may be increased by: Antifungal Agents (Azole Derivatives, Systemic); Aprepitant; Calcium Channel Blockers (Nondihydropyridine); Cimetidine; Conivaptan; Contraceptives (Estrogens); Contraceptives (Progestins); CYP2C19 Inhibitors (Moderate); CYP2C19 Inhibitors (Strong); CYP3A4 Inhibitors (Moderate); CYP3A4 Inhibitors (Strong); Dasatinib; Disulfiram; Droperidol; Fluconazole; Fosamprenavir; Fosaprepitant; Grapefruit Juice; HydrOXYzine; Isoniazid; Macrolide Antibiotics; Methotrimeprazine; Nefazodone; OLANZapine; Proton Pump Inhibitors; Ritonavir; Saquinavir; Selective Serotonin Reuptake Inhibitors

Decreased Effect

The levels/effects of Diazepam may be decreased by: CarBAMazepine; CYP2C19 Inducers (Strong); CYP3A4 Inducers (Strong); Cyproterone; Deferasirox; Rifamycin Derivatives; St Johns Wort; Theophylline Derivatives; Tocilizumab; Yohimbine

Ethanol/Nutrition/Herb Interactions

Ethanol: May increase CNS depression; monitor for increased effects with coadministration. Caution patients about effects.

Food: Diazepam serum concentrations may be increased if taken with food. Grapefruit juice may increase diazepam serum concentrations; avoid concurrent use.

Herb/Nutraceutical: St John's wort may decrease diazepam levels. Avoid valerian, St John's wort, kava kava, gotu kola (may increase CNS depression).

Stability

Injection: Store at 20° to 25°C (68° to 77°F); excursions permitted to 15°C to 30°C (59°F to 86°F). Protect from light. Potency is retained for up to 3 months when kept at room temperature. Most stable at pH 4-8; hydrolysis occurs at pH <3. Per manufacturer, do not mix I.V. product with other medications.

Rectal gel: Store at 25°C (77°F); excursion permitted to 15°C to 30°C (59°F to 86°F).

Tablet: Store at 15°C to 30°C (59°F to 86°F).

Mechanism of Action Binds to stereospecific benzodiazepine receptors on the postsynaptic GABA neuron at several sites within the central nervous system, including the limbic system, reticular formation. Enhancement of the inhibitory effect of GABA on neuronal excitability results by increased neuronal membrane permeability to chloride ions. This shift in chloride ions results in hyperpolarization (a less excitable state) and stabilization.

Pharmacodynamics/Kinetics

I.V.: Status epilepticus:

Onset of action: Almost immediate

Duration: 20-30 minutes

Absorption: Oral: 85% to 100%, more reliable than I.M.

Protein binding: 98%

Metabolism: Hepatic

Half-life elimination: Parent drug: Adults: 20-50 hours; increased half-life in elderly, and those with severe hepatic disorders; Active major metabolite (desmethyldiazepam): 50-100 hours

Dosage

Geriatric Oral absorption is more reliable than I.M. Elderly and/or debilitated patients: *Oral:* 2-2.5 mg 1-2 times/day initially; increase gradually as needed and tolerated.

Rectal gel: Due to the increased half-life in elderly and debilitated patients, consider reducing dose.

Adult Note: Oral absorption is more reliable than I.M.

Acute ethanol withdrawal: *Oral:* 10 mg 3-4 times during first 24 hours, then decrease to 5 mg 3-4 times/day as needed

Anticonvulsant (acute treatment): *Rectal gel:* 0.2 mg/kg. **Note:** Dosage should be rounded upward to the next available dose, 2.5, 5, 7.5, 10, 12.5, 15, 17.5, and 20 mg/ dose; dose may be repeated in 4-12 hours if needed; do not use for more than 5 episodes per month or more than one episode every 5 days.

Anxiety (symptoms/disorders): *Oral, I.M, I.V.:* 2-10 mg 2-4 times/day if needed

Muscle spasm: *I.V., I.M.:* Initial: 5-10 mg; then 5-10 mg in 3-4 hours, if necessary. Larger doses may be required if associated with tetanus.

Sedation in the ICU patient: *I.V.:* 0.03-0.1 mg/kg every 30 minutes to 6 hours (Jacobi, 2002)

Skeletal muscle relaxant (adjunct therapy): *Oral:* 2-10 mg 3-4 times/day

Status epilepticus:

I.V.: 5-10 mg every 5-10 minutes given over ≤5 mg/minute (maximum dose: 30 mg)

Rectal gel: Premonitory/Out-of-hospital treatment: 10 mg once; may repeat once if necessary (Kälviäinen, 2007)

Rapid tranquilization of agitated patient (administer every 30-60 minutes): *Oral:* 5-10 mg; average total dose for tranquilization: 20-60 mg

Renal Impairment No dose adjustment recommended; decrease dose if administered for prolonged periods.

I.V.: Risk of propylene glycol toxicity; monitor closely if using for prolonged periods or at high doses.

Hemodialysis: Not dialyzable (0% to 5%); supplemental dose is not necessary.

Hepatic Impairment Decrease maintenance dose by 50%; half-life significantly prolonged.

Administration Intensol® should be diluted before use.

Adults: Do not exceed 5 mg/minute IVP

Rectal gel: Patient should be positioned on side (facing person responsible for monitoring), with top leg bent forward. Insert rectal tip (lubricated) into rectum and push in plunger gently over 3 seconds. Remove tip of rectal syringe after 3 additional seconds. Buttocks should be held together for 3 seconds after removal. Dispose of syringe appropriately.

Monitoring Parameters Respiratory, cardiovascular, and mental status; check for orthostasis

Reference Range Therapeutic: Diazepam: 0.2-1.5 mcg/mL (SI: 0.7-5.3 µmol/L); N-desmethyldiazepam (nordiazepam): 0.1-0.5 mcg/mL (SI: 0.35-1.8 µmol/L)

Test Interactions False-negative urinary glucose determinations when using Clinistix® or Diastix®

Pharmacotherapy Pearls Diazepam does not have any analgesic effects.

Diastat® AcuDial™: When dispensing, consult package information for directions on setting patient's dose; confirm green "ready" band is visible prior to dispensing product.

Special Geriatric Considerations Due to its long-acting metabolite, diazepam is not considered a drug of choice in the elderly. Long-acting benzodiazepines have been associated with falls in the elderly. Interpretive guidelines from the Centers for Medicare and Medicaid Services (CMS) strongly discourage the use of this agent in residents of long-term care facilities.

This medication is considered to be potentially inappropriate in this patient population (Beers Criteria severity: High).

Controlled Substance C-IV

Dosage Forms Excipient information presented when available (limited, particularly for generics); consult specific product labeling.

Gel, rectal [adult rectal tip (6 cm)]: 20 mg (4 mL) [delivers set doses of 12.5 mg, 15 mg, 17.5 mg, 20 mg]

Diastat® AcuDial™: 20 mg (4 mL) [contains benzoic acid, benzyl alcohol, ethanol 10%, propylene glycol, sodium benzoate; 5 mg/mL (delivers set doses of 12.5 mg, 15 mg, 17.5 mg, and 20 mg)]

Gel, rectal [pediatric rectal tip (4.4 cm)]: 5 mg/mL (0.5 mL)

Diastat®: 5 mg/mL (0.5 mL) [contains benzoic acid, benzyl alcohol, ethanol 10%, propylene glycol, sodium benzoate]

Gel, rectal [pediatric/adult rectal tip (4.4 cm)]: 10 mg (2 mL) [delivers set doses of 5 mg, 7.5 mg, 10 mg]
  Diastat® AcuDial™: 10 mg (2 mL) [contains benzoic acid, benzyl alcohol, ethanol 10%, propylene glycol, sodium benzoate; 5 mg/mL (delivers set doses of 5 mg, 7.5 mg, and 10 mg)]
Injection, solution: 5 mg/mL (2 mL, 10 mL)
Solution, oral: 5 mg/5 mL (5 mL, 500 mL)
Solution, oral [concentrate]:
  Diazepam Intensol™: 5 mg/mL (30 mL) [contains ethanol 19%, propylene glycol]
Tablet, oral: 2 mg, 5 mg, 10 mg
  Valium®: 5 mg, 10 mg [scored]
  Valium®: 2 mg [scored; dye free]

Selected References
Klotz U, Avant GR, Hoyumpa A, et al, "The Effects of Age and Liver Disease on the Disposition and Elimination of Diazepam in Adult Man," *J Clin Invest*, 1975, 55(2):347-59.
Pomara N, Stanley B, Block R, et al, "Increased Sensitivity of the Elderly to the Central Depressant Effects of Diazepam," *J Clin Psychiatry*, 1985, 46(5):185-7.
Reidenberg MM, Levy M, Warner H, et al, "Relationship Between Diazepam Dose, Plasma Level, Age, and Central Nervous System Depression," *Clin Pharmacol Ther*, 1978, 23(4):371-4.

◆ **Diazepam Intensol™** see Diazepam on page 493
◆ **Dibenzyline®** see Phenoxybenzamine on page 1440
◆ **Dicarbosil® [OTC]** see Calcium Salts (Oral) on page 256

Diclofenac (Systemic) (dye KLOE fen ak)

Medication Safety Issues
Sound-alike/look-alike issues:
  Diclofenac may be confused with Diflucan®, Duphalac®
  Cataflam® may be confused with Catapres®
  Voltaren may be confused with traMADol, Ultram®, Verelan®
International issues:
  Flexin: Brand name for diclofenac [Argentina], but also the brand name for cyclobenzaprine [Chile] and orphenadrine [Israel]
  Flexin [Argentina] may be confused with Floxin brand name for flunarizine [Thailand], norfloxacin [South Africa], ofloxacin [U.S., Canada], and perfloxacin [Philippines]; Fluoxin brand name for fluoxetine [Czech Republic]

Brand Names: U.S. Cambia™; Cataflam®; Voltaren®-XR; Zipsor™
Brand Names: Canada Apo-Diclo Rapide®; Apo-Diclo®; Apo-Diclo® SR®; Cataflam®; Diclofenac ECT; Diclofenac Sodium; Diclofenac Sodium SR; Diclofenac SR; Dom-Diclofenac; Dom-Diclofenac SR; Novo-Difenac ECT; Novo-Difenac K; Novo-Difenac Suppositories; Novo-Difenac-SR; Nu-Diclo; Nu-Diclo-SR; Pennsaid®; PMS-Diclofenac; PMS-Diclofenac SR; PMS-Diclofenac-K; PRO-Diclo-Rapide; Sandoz-Diclofenac; Sandoz-Diclofenac Rapide; Sandoz-Diclofenac SR; Voltaren Rapide®; Voltaren SR®; Voltaren®
Index Terms Diclofenac Potassium; Diclofenac Sodium; Voltaren
Generic Availability (U.S.) Yes: Excludes capsule, oral solution
Pharmacologic Category Nonsteroidal Anti-inflammatory Drug (NSAID); Nonsteroidal Anti-inflammatory Drug (NSAID), Oral
Use
  Capsule: Relief of mild-to-moderate acute pain
  Immediate-release tablet: Relief of mild-to-moderate pain; primary dysmenorrhea; acute and chronic treatment of rheumatoid arthritis, osteoarthritis
  Delayed-release tablet: Acute and chronic treatment of rheumatoid arthritis, osteoarthritis, ankylosing spondylitis
  Extended-release tablet: Chronic treatment of osteoarthritis, rheumatoid arthritis
  Oral solution: Treatment of acute migraine with or without aura
  Suppository (CAN; not available in U.S.): Symptomatic treatment of rheumatoid arthritis and osteoarthritis (including degenerative joint disease of hip)
Unlabeled/Investigational Use Juvenile idiopathic arthritis (JIA)
Medication Guide Available Yes
Contraindications Hypersensitivity to diclofenac or any component of the formulation; hypersensitivity to bovine protein (capsule formulation only); patients who exhibit asthma, urticaria, or other allergic-type reactions after taking aspirin or other NSAIDs; perioperative pain in the setting of coronary artery bypass graft (CABG) surgery

Additional contraindications in Canadian labeling (not in U.S. labeling): Uncontrolled heart failure, active gastric/duodenal/peptic ulcer; active GI bleed or perforation; regional ulcer, gastritis, or ulcerative colitis; cerebrovascular bleeding or other bleeding disorders; inflammatory bowel disease; severe hepatic impairment; active hepatic disease; severe renal impairment (Cl$_{cr}$ <30 mL/minute) or deteriorating renal disease; known hyperkalemia; use of diclofenac suppository if recent history of bleeding or inflammatory lesions of rectum/anus

Warnings/Precautions [U.S. Boxed Warning]: NSAIDs are associated with an increased risk of adverse cardiovascular thrombotic events, including MI and stroke. Risk may be increased with duration of use or pre-existing cardiovascular risk factors or disease. Carefully evaluate individual cardiovascular risk profiles prior to prescribing. May cause new-onset hypertension or worsening of existing hypertension. Monitor blood pressure closely. Use caution with fluid retention. Avoid use in heart failure. Concurrent administration of ibuprofen, and potentially other nonselective NSAIDs, may interfere with aspirin's cardioprotective effect. **[U.S. Boxed Warning]: Use is contraindicated for treatment of perioperative pain in the setting of coronary artery bypass graft (CABG) surgery.** Risk of MI and stroke may be increased with use following CABG surgery.

NSAID use may compromise existing renal function; dose-dependent decreases in prostaglandin synthesis may result from NSAID use, reducing renal blood flow which may cause renal decompensation. NSAID use may increase the risk for hyperkalemia. Patients with impaired renal function, dehydration, heart failure, liver dysfunction, those taking diuretics and ACEI, and the elderly are at greater risk of renal toxicity and hyperkalemia. Rehydrate patient before starting therapy; monitor renal function closely. Not recommended for use in patients with advanced renal disease. Long-term NSAID use may result in renal papillary necrosis while persistent urinary symptoms (eg, dysuria, bladder pain), cystitis, or hematuria may occur anytime after initiating NSAID therapy. Discontinue therapy with symptom onset and evaluate for origin.

[U.S. Boxed Warning]: NSAIDs may increase risk of gastrointestinal irritation, inflammation, ulceration, bleeding, and perforation. These events may occur at any time during therapy and without warning. Use caution with a history of GI disease (bleeding or ulcers), concurrent therapy with aspirin, anticoagulants and/or corticosteroids, smoking, use of alcohol, the elderly or debilitated patients. When used concomitantly with ≤325 mg of aspirin, a substantial increase in the risk of gastrointestinal complications (eg, ulcer) occurs; concomitant gastroprotective therapy (eg, proton pump inhibitors) is recommended (Bhatt, 2008).

Use the lowest effective dose for the shortest duration of time, consistent with individual patient goals, to reduce risk of cardiovascular or GI adverse events. Alternate therapies should be considered for patients at high risk.

NSAIDs may cause photosensitivity or serious skin adverse events including exfoliative dermatitis, Stevens-Johnson syndrome (SJS), and toxic epidermal necrolysis (TEN); discontinue use at first sign of skin rash or hypersensitivity. Anaphylactoid reactions may occur, even without prior exposure; patients with "aspirin triad" (bronchial asthma, aspirin intolerance, rhinitis) may be at increased risk. Do not use in patients who experience bronchospasm, asthma, rhinitis, or urticaria with NSAID or aspirin therapy. Use caution in other forms of asthma. Platelet adhesion and aggregation may be decreased; may prolong bleeding time; patients with coagulation disorders or who are receiving anticoagulants should be monitored closely. Anemia may occur; patients on long-term NSAID therapy should be monitored for anemia. Rarely, NSAID use may cause severe blood dyscrasias (eg, agranulocytosis, aplastic anemia, thrombocytopenia).

Use with caution in patients with impaired hepatic function. Closely monitor patients with any abnormal LFT. Diclofenac can cause transaminase elevations; initiate monitoring 4-8 weeks into therapy. Rarely, severe hepatic reactions (eg, fulminant hepatitis, liver failure) have occurred; discontinue all formulations if signs or symptoms of liver disease develop, or if systemic manifestations occur. Use with caution in hepatic porphyria (may trigger attack).

NSAIDS may cause drowsiness, dizziness, blurred vision and other neurologic effects which may impair physical or mental abilities; patients must be cautioned about performing tasks which require mental alertness (eg, operating machinery or driving). Discontinue use with blurred or diminished vision and perform ophthalmologic exam. Monitor vision with long-term therapy. The elderly are at increased risk for adverse effects (especially peptic ulceration, CNS effects, and renal toxicity) from NSAIDs even at low doses. May increase the risk of aseptic meningitis, especially in patients with systemic lupus erythematosus (SLE) and mixed connective tissue disorders.

Withhold for at least 4-6 half-lives prior to surgical or dental procedures.

Capsule: Contains gelatin; use is contraindicated in patients with history of hypersensitivity to bovine protein.

Oral solution: Only indicated for the acute treatment of migraine; not indicated for migraine prophylaxis or cluster headache. Not bioequivalent to other forms of diclofenac (even same dose); do not interchange products. Contains phenylalanine.

◀ **Adverse Reactions (Reflective of adult population; not specific for elderly)**

Oral:

1% to 10%:

Cardiovascular: Edema

Central nervous system: Dizziness, headache

Dermatologic: Pruritus, rash

Endocrine & metabolic: Fluid retention

Gastrointestinal: Abdominal distension, abdominal pain, constipation, diarrhea, dyspepsia, flatulence, GI perforation, heartburn, nausea, peptic ulcer/GI bleed, vomiting

Hematologic: Anemia, bleeding time increased

Hepatic: Liver enzyme abnormalities (>3 x ULN; ≤4%)

Otic: Tinnitus

Renal: Renal function abnormal

Miscellaneous: Diaphoresis increased

Rectal suppository (CAN; not available in U.S.): Also refer to adverse reactions associated with oral formulations.

Drug Interactions

Metabolism/Transport Effects Substrate (minor) of CYP1A2, 2B6, 2C8, 2C9, 2C19, 2D6, 3A4; **Inhibits** CYP1A2 (moderate), 2C9 (weak), 2E1 (weak), 3A4 (weak)

Avoid Concomitant Use

Avoid concomitant use of Diclofenac (Systemic) with any of the following: Floctafenine; Ketorolac; Ketorolac (Nasal); Ketorolac (Systemic)

Increased Effect/Toxicity

Diclofenac (Systemic) may increase the levels/effects of: Aminoglycosides; Anticoagulants; Antiplatelet Agents; Bisphosphonate Derivatives; Collagenase (Systemic); CycloSPORINE; CycloSPORINE (Systemic); CYP1A2 Substrates; Deferasirox; Desmopressin; Digoxin; Drotrecogin Alfa; Eplerenone; Haloperidol; Ibritumomab; Lithium; Methotrexate; Nonsteroidal Anti-Inflammatory Agents; PEMEtrexed; Porfimer; Potassium-Sparing Diuretics; PRALA-trexate; Quinolone Antibiotics; Rivaroxaban; Salicylates; Thrombolytic Agents; Tositumomab and Iodine I 131 Tositumomab; Vancomycin; Vitamin K Antagonists

The levels/effects of Diclofenac (Systemic) may be increased by: ACE Inhibitors; Angiotensin II Receptor Blockers; Antidepressants (Tricyclic, Tertiary Amine); Conivaptan; Corticosteroids (Systemic); Dasatinib; Floctafenine; Glucosamine; Herbs (Anticoagulant/Antiplatelet Properties); Ketorolac; Ketorolac (Nasal); Ketorolac (Systemic); Nonsteroidal Anti-Inflammatory Agents; Omega-3-Acid Ethyl Esters; Pentosan Polysulfate Sodium; Pentoxifylline; Probenecid; Prostacyclin Analogues; Selective Serotonin Reuptake Inhibitors; Serotonin/Norepinephrine Reuptake Inhibitors; Sodium Phosphates; Treprostinil; Vitamin E; Voriconazole

Decreased Effect

Diclofenac (Systemic) may decrease the levels/effects of: ACE Inhibitors; Angiotensin II Receptor Blockers; Antiplatelet Agents; Beta-Blockers; Eplerenone; HydrALAZINE; Potassium-Sparing Diuretics; Salicylates; Selective Serotonin Reuptake Inhibitors; Thiazide Diuretics

The levels/effects of Diclofenac (Systemic) may be decreased by: Bile Acid Sequestrants; Cyproterone; Nonsteroidal Anti-Inflammatory Agents; Peginterferon Alfa-2b; Salicylates; Tocilizumab

Ethanol/Nutrition/Herb Interactions

Ethanol: Avoid ethanol (may enhance gastric mucosal irritation).

Herb/Nutraceutical: Avoid alfalfa, anise, bilberry, bladderwrack, bromelain, cat's claw, celery, chamomile, coleus, cordyceps, dong quai, evening primrose, fenugreek, feverfew, garlic, ginger, ginkgo biloba, grapeseed, green tea, ginseng (Siberian), guggul, horse chestnut, horseradish, licorice, prickly ash, red clover, reishi, SAMe (s-adenosylmethionine), sweet clover, turmeric, white willow (all have additional antiplatelet activity).

Stability

Capsule, oral solution: Store at 25°C (77°F); excursions permitted to 15°C to 30°C (59°F to 86°F). Protect from moisture.

Suppository (CAN; not available in U.S.): Store at 15°C to 30°C (59°F to 86°F); protect from heat.

Tablet: Store below 30°C (86°F). Protect from moisture; store in tight container.

Mechanism of Action Reversibly inhibits cyclooxygenase-1 and 2 (COX-1 and 2) enzymes, which results in decreased formation of prostaglandin precursors; has antipyretic, analgesic, and anti-inflammatory properties

Other proposed mechanisms not fully elucidated (and possibly contributing to the anti-inflammatory effect to varying degrees), include inhibiting chemotaxis, altering lymphocyte activity, inhibiting neutrophil aggregation/activation, and decreasing proinflammatory cytokine levels.

Pharmacodynamics/Kinetics

Onset of action:

Cataflam® (potassium salt) is more rapid than the sodium salt because it dissolves in the stomach instead of the duodenum

Suppository: More rapid onset, but slower rate of absorption when compared to enteric coated tablet

Distribution: ~1.4 L/kg

Protein binding: >99%, primarily to albumin

Metabolism: Hepatic; undergoes first-pass metabolism; forms several metabolites (1 with weak activity)

Bioavailability: 55%

Half-life elimination: ~2 hours

Time to peak, serum:

Cambia™: ~0.25 hours

Cataflam®: ~1 hour

Voltaren® XR ~5 hours

Zipsor™: ~0.5 hour

Suppository: ≤1 hour; **Note:** Suppository: C_{max}: Approximately two-thirds of that observed with enteric coated tablet (equivalent 50 mg dose)

Tablet, delayed release (diclofenac sodium): ~2 hours

Excretion: Urine (~65%); feces (~35%)

Dosage

Geriatric Refer to adult dosing. No specific dosing recommendations; elderly may demonstrate adverse effects at lower doses than younger adults, and >60% may develop asymptomatic peptic ulceration with or without hemorrhage; monitor renal function.

Adult

Analgesia: Oral:

Immediate release tablet: Starting dose: 50 mg 3 times/day (maximum dose: 150 mg/day); may administer 100 mg loading dose, followed by 50 mg every 8 hours (maximum dose day 1: 200 mg/day; maximum dose day 2 and thereafter: 150 mg/day)

Immediate release capsule: 25 mg 4 times/day

Rheumatoid arthritis:

Oral: Immediate or delayed release tablet: 150-200 mg/day in 2-4 divided doses; Extended release tablet: 100-200 mg/day

Canadian labeling: 150 mg/day in 3 divided doses (75-150 mg/day of slow release tablet)

Rectal suppository (not available in U.S.): *Canadian labeling:* Insert 50mg or 100 mg rectally as single dose to substitute for final (third) oral daily dose (maximum combined dose [rectal and oral]: 150 mg/day

Osteoarthritis:

Oral: Immediate or delayed release tablet: 100-150 mg/day in 2-3 divided doses; Extended release tablet: 100 mg/day

Canadian labeling: 150 mg/day in 3 divided doses (75-150 mg/day of slow release tablet)

Rectal suppository (not available in U.S.): *Canadian labeling:* Insert 50mg or 100 mg rectally as single dose to substitute for final (third) oral daily dose (maximum combined dose [rectal and oral]: 150 mg/day

Ankylosing spondylitis: Oral: Delayed release tablet: 100-125 mg/day in 4-5 divided doses

Renal Impairment Not recommended in patients with advanced renal disease or significant renal impairment.

Hepatic Impairment May require dosage adjustment; use oral solution only if benefits outweigh risks.

Administration

Oral: Do not crush delayed or extended release tablets. Administer with food or milk to avoid gastric distress. Take with full glass of water to enhance absorption.

Oral solution: Empty contents of packet into 1-2 ounces (30-60 mL) of water (do not use other liquids), mix well and administer immediately; food may reduce effectiveness.

Rectal suppository: Remove entire plastic wrapping prior to inserting rectally.

Monitoring Parameters Monitor CBC, liver enzymes (periodically during chronic therapy starting 4-8 weeks after initiation), BUN/serum creatinine; monitor urine output; occult blood loss

Pharmacotherapy Pearls There are no clinical guidelines to predict which NSAID will give response in a particular patient. Trials with each must be initiated until response determined. Consider dose, patient convenience, and cost.

◀ **Special Geriatric Considerations** Elderly are a high-risk population for adverse effects from nonsteroidal anti-inflammatory agents. As much as 60% of the elderly can develop peptic ulceration and/or hemorrhage asymptomatically. The concomitant use of H_2 blockers and sucralfate is not effective as prophylaxis with the exception of NSAID-induced duodenal ulcers which may be prevented by the use of ranitidine. Misoprostol and proton pump inhibitors are the only agents proven to help prevent the development of NSAID-induced ulcers. Also, concomitant disease and drug use contribute to the risk for GI adverse effects. Use lowest effective dose for shortest period possible. Consider renal function decline with age. Use of NSAIDs can compromise existing renal function especially when Cl_{cr} is ≤30 mL/minute. CNS adverse effects such as confusion, agitation, and hallucination are generally seen in overdose or high dose situations, but elderly may demonstrate these adverse effects at lower doses than younger adults.

Dosage Forms Excipient information presented when available (limited, particularly for generics); consult specific product labeling.

Capsule, liquid filled, oral, as potassium:
Zipsor™: 25 mg [contains gelatin]
Powder for solution, oral, as potassium:
Cambia™: 50 mg/packet (1s) [contains phenylalanine 25 mg/packet; anise-mint flavor]
Tablet, oral, as potassium: 50 mg
Cataflam®: 50 mg
Tablet, delayed release, enteric coated, oral, as sodium: 25 mg, 50 mg, 75 mg
Tablet, extended release, oral, as sodium: 100 mg
Voltaren®-XR: 100 mg

Dosage Forms: Canada Excipient information presented when available (limited, particularly for generics); consult specific product labeling.

Suppository:
Voltaren®: 50 mg, 100mg

Diclofenac (Ophthalmic) (dye KLOE fen ak)

Medication Safety Issues
Sound-alike/look-alike issues:
Diclofenac may be confused with Diflucan®, Duphalac®
International Issues:
Flexin: Brand name for diclofenac [Argentina], but also the brand name for cyclobenzaprine [Chile] and orphenadrine [Israel]
Flexin [Argentina] may be confused with Floxin brand name for flunarizine [Thailand], norfloxacin [South Africa], ofloxacin [U.S., Canada], and pefloxacin [Philippines]; Fluoxin brand name for fluoxetine [Czech Republic]

Brand Names: U.S. Voltaren Ophthalmic®
Brand Names: Canada Voltaren Ophtha®
Index Terms Diclofenac Sodium
Generic Availability (U.S.) Yes
Pharmacologic Category Nonsteroidal Anti-inflammatory Drug (NSAID); Nonsteroidal Anti-inflammatory Drug (NSAID), Ophthalmic
Use Treatment of postoperative inflammation following cataract extraction; temporary relief of pain and photophobia in patients undergoing corneal refractive surgery

Dosage
Geriatric Refer to adult dosing. No specific dosing recommendations.
Adult
Cataract surgery: Ophthalmic: Instill 1 drop into affected eye 4 times/day beginning 24 hours after cataract surgery and continuing for 2 weeks
Corneal refractive surgery: Ophthalmic: Instill 1-2 drops into affected eye within the hour prior to surgery, within 15 minutes following surgery, and then continue for 4 times/day, up to 3 days

Dosage Forms Excipient information presented when available (limited, particularly for generics); consult specific product labeling.
Solution, ophthalmic, as sodium [drops]: 0.1% (2.5 mL, 5 mL)
Voltaren Ophthalmic®: 0.1% (2.5 mL, 5 mL) [contains sorbic acid]

Diclofenac (Topical) (dye KLOE fen ak)

Medication Safety Issues
Sound-alike/look-alike issues:
Diclofenac may be confused with Diflucan®, Duphalac®

Voltaren® may be confused with traMADol, Ultram®, Verelan®

Other safety concerns:

Transdermal patch (Flector®) contains conducting metal (eg, aluminum); remove patch prior to MRI.

International issues:

Flexin: Brand name for diclofenac [Argentina], but also the brand name for cyclobenzaprine [Chile] and orphenadirine [Israel]

Flexin [Argentina] may be confused with Floxin brand name for flunarizine [Thailand], norfloxacin [South Africa], ofloxacin [U.S., Canada], and perfloxacin [Philippines]; Fluoxin brand name for fluoxetine [Czech Republic]

Brand Names: U.S. Flector®; Pennsaid®; Solaraze®; Voltaren® Gel

Brand Names: Canada Voltaren® Emulgel™

Index Terms Diclofenac Diethylamine [CAN]; Diclofenac Epolamine; Diclofenac Sodium

Generic Availability (U.S.) No

Pharmacologic Category Nonsteroidal Anti-inflammatory Drug (NSAID); Nonsteroidal Anti-inflammatory Drug (NSAID), Topical

Use

Topical gel 1%: Relief of osteoarthritis pain in joints amenable to topical therapy (eg, ankle, elbow, foot, hand, knee, wrist)

Canadian labeling (not in U.S. labeling): Relief of pain associated with acute, localized joint/ muscle injuries (eg, sports injuries, strains) in patients ≥16 years of age

Topical gel 3%: Actinic keratosis (AK) in conjunction with sun avoidance

Topical patch: Acute pain due to minor strains, sprains, and contusions

Topical solution: Relief of osteoarthritis pain of the knee

Medication Guide Available Yes

Dosage

Geriatric Refer to adult dosing. No specific dosing recommendations; elderly may demonstrate adverse effects at lower doses than younger adults, and >60% may develop asymptomatic peptic ulceration with or without hemorrhage; monitor renal function.

Adult

Osteoarthritis:

Topical gel (Voltaren®): **Note:** Maximum total body dose of 1% gel should not exceed 32 g per day

Lower extremities: Apply 4 g of 1% gel to affected area 4 times daily (maximum: 16 g per joint per day)

Upper extremities: Apply 2 g of 1% gel to affected area 4 times daily (maximum: 8 g per joint per day)

Topical solution: Apply 40 drops to each affected knee(s) 4 times daily

Actinic keratosis (AK): Topical (Solaraze® Gel): Apply 3% gel to lesion area twice daily for 60-90 days

Acute pain (strains, sprains, contusions): Topical:

Patch: Apply 1 patch twice daily to most painful area of skin

Gel (Voltaren® Emulgel™ [CAN; not available in U.S.]): Apply to affected area(s) of skin 3 or 4 times daily for up to 7 days

Dosage Forms Excipient information presented when available (limited, particularly for generics); consult specific product labeling.

Gel, topical, as sodium:

Solaraze®: 3% (100 g) [contains benzyl alcohol]

Voltaren® Gel: 1% (100 g) [contains isopropyl alcohol]

Patch, transdermal, as epolamine:

Flector®: 1.3% (30s) [contains metal; 180 mg]

Solution, topical, as sodium:

Pennsaid®: 1.5% (150 mL)

Dosage Forms: Canada Excipient information presented when available (limited, particularly for generics); consult specific product labeling.

Gel, topical, as diethylamine:

Voltaren® Emulgel™: 1.16% (20 g, 50 g, 100 g)

Diclofenac and Misoprostol (dye KLOE fen ak & mye soe PROST ole)

Related Information

Diclofenac (Systemic) *on page 496*

Misoprostol *on page 1225*

Brand Names: U.S. Arthrotec®

Brand Names: Canada Arthrotec®

Index Terms Misoprostol and Diclofenac

◄ **Generic Availability (U.S.)** No

Pharmacologic Category Nonsteroidal Anti-inflammatory Drug (NSAID), Oral; Prostaglandin

Use Treatment of osteoarthritis and rheumatoid arthritis in patients at high risk for NSAID-induced gastric and duodenal ulceration

Medication Guide Available Yes

Dosage

Geriatric & Adult

Osteoarthritis: Oral: Arthotec® 50: 1 tablet 3 times/day

Rheumatoid arthritis: Oral: Arthotec® 50: 1 tablet 3 or 4 times/day

Note: For both indications, may administer Arthotec® 50 or Arthotec® 75 one tablet twice daily if recommended dose is not tolerated; however, these options are less effective in preventing GI ulceration. May adjust dose using individual agents in combination with Arthotec®. The maximum daily dose of misoprostal is 800 mcg and the maximum single dose of misoprostal is 200 mcg. The maximum daily dose of diclofenac is 150 mg/day (osteoarthritis) or 225 mg/day (rheumatoid arthritis).

Renal Impairment Not recommended for use in patients with advanced renal disease. In renal insufficiency, diclofenac should be used with caution due to potential detrimental effects on renal function, and misoprostol dosage reduction may be required if adverse effects occur (misoprostol is renally eliminated).

Hepatic Impairment May require dosage adjustment.

Special Geriatric Considerations Elderly are a high-risk population for adverse effects from nonsteroidal anti-inflammatory agents. As much as 60% of the elderly can develop peptic ulceration and/or hemorrhage asymptomatically. The concomitant use of H_2 blockers and sucralfate is not effective as prophylaxis with the exception of NSAID-induced duodenal ulcers which may be prevented by the use of ranitidine. Misoprostol and proton pump inhibitors are the only agents proven to help prevent the development of NSAID-induced ulcers. Also, concomitant disease and drug use contribute to the risk for GI adverse effects. Use lowest effective dose for shortest period possible. Consider renal function decline with age. Use of NSAIDs can compromise existing renal function especially when Cl_{cr} is ≤30 mL/minute. CNS adverse effects such as confusion, agitation, and hallucination are generally seen in overdose or high dose situations, but elderly may demonstrate these adverse effects at lower doses than younger adults.

Dosage Forms Excipient information presented when available (limited, particularly for generics); consult specific product labeling.

Tablet:

Arthotec® 50: Diclofenac sodium 50 mg and misoprostol 200 mcg

Arthotec® 75: Diclofenac sodium 75 mg and misoprostol 200 mcg

◆ **Diclofenac Diethylamine [CAN]** see Diclofenac (Topical) on page 500
◆ **Diclofenac Epolamine** see Diclofenac (Topical) on page 500
◆ **Diclofenac Potassium** see Diclofenac (Systemic) on page 496
◆ **Diclofenac Sodium** see Diclofenac (Ophthalmic) on page 500
◆ **Diclofenac Sodium** see Diclofenac (Systemic) on page 496
◆ **Diclofenac Sodium** see Diclofenac (Topical) on page 500

Dicloxacillin (dye kloks a SIL in)

Brand Names: Canada Dycill®; Pathocil®

Index Terms Dicloxacillin Sodium

Generic Availability (U.S.) Yes

Pharmacologic Category Antibiotic, Penicillin

Use Treatment of systemic infections such as pneumonia, skin and soft tissue infections, and osteomyelitis caused by penicillinase-producing staphylococci

Contraindications Hypersensitivity to dicloxacillin, penicillin, or any component of the formulation

Warnings/Precautions Monitor PT if patient concurrently on warfarin. Serious and occasionally severe or fatal hypersensitivity (anaphylactoid) reactions have been reported in patients on penicillin therapy, especially with a history of beta-lactam hypersensitivity, history of sensitivity to multiple allergens, or previous IgE-mediated reactions (eg, anaphylaxis, angioedema, urticaria). Use with caution in asthmatic patients. Prolonged use may result in fungal or bacterial superinfection, including *C. difficile*-associated diarrhea and pseudomembranous colitis.

Adverse Reactions (Reflective of adult population; not specific for elderly)

1% to 10%: Gastrointestinal: Nausea, diarrhea, abdominal pain

Drug Interactions

Metabolism/Transport Effects Induces CYP3A4 (weak)

Avoid Concomitant Use

Avoid concomitant use of Dicloxacillin with any of the following: BCG

Increased Effect/Toxicity

Dicloxacillin may increase the levels/effects of: Methotrexate

The levels/effects of Dicloxacillin may be increased by: Probenecid

Decreased Effect

Dicloxacillin may decrease the levels/effects of: BCG; Mycophenolate; Saxagliptin; Typhoid Vaccine; Vitamin K Antagonists

The levels/effects of Dicloxacillin may be decreased by: Fusidic Acid; Tetracycline Derivatives

Ethanol/Nutrition/Herb Interactions Food: Decreases drug absorption rate; decreases drug serum concentration.

Mechanism of Action Inhibits bacterial cell wall synthesis by binding to one or more of the penicillin-binding proteins (PBPs) which in turn inhibits the final transpeptidation step of peptidoglycan synthesis in bacterial cell walls, thus inhibiting cell wall biosynthesis. Bacteria eventually lyse due to ongoing activity of cell wall autolytic enzymes (autolysins and murein hydrolases) while cell wall assembly is arrested.

Pharmacodynamics/Kinetics

Absorption: 35% to 76% from GI tract

Half-life: 0.6-0.8 hours, half-life is slightly prolonged in patients with renal impairment Protein binding: 96%

Time to peak serum concentration: Within 0.5-2 hours

Elimination: Partially by the liver and excreted in bile, 56% to 70% is eliminated in urine as unchanged drug

The percent unbound has been reported to be increased in older adults compared to young healthy volunteers (8.8% vs 7.3%), but this is not felt to be clinically significant

Dosage

Geriatric & Adult

Susceptible infections: Oral: 125-500 mg every 6 hours

Erysipelas, furunculosis, mastitis, otitis externa, septic bursitis, skin abscess: Oral: 500 mg every 6 hours

Impetigo: 250 mg every 6 hours

Prosthetic joint (long-term suppression therapy): Oral: 250 mg twice daily

***Staphylococcus aureus,* methicillin susceptible infection if no I.V. access:** Oral: 500-1000 mg every 6-8 hours

Renal Impairment

Dosage adjustment is not necessary.

Not dialyzable (0% to 5%); supplemental dose is not necessary.

Peritoneal dialysis effects: Supplemental dose is not necessary.

Continuous arteriovenous or venovenous hemofiltration: Supplemental dose is not necessary.

Administration Administer 1 hour before or 2 hours after meals; administer around-the-clock rather than 4 times/day, 3 times/day, etc (ie, 12-6-12-6, not 9-1-5-9) to promote less variation in peak and trough serum concentrations

Monitoring Parameters Monitor prothrombin time if patient concurrently on warfarin; monitor for signs of anaphylaxis during first dose

Test Interactions False-positive urine and serum proteins; false-positive in uric acid, urinary steroids; may interfere with urinary glucose tests using cupric sulfate (Benedict's solution, Clinitest®); may inactivate aminoglycosides *in vitro*

Special Geriatric Considerations No dosage adjustment for renal function is necessary.

Dosage Forms Excipient information presented when available (limited, particularly for generics); consult specific product labeling.

Capsule, oral: 250 mg, 500 mg

Selected References

Pacifici GM, Viani A, Taddeucci-Brunelli G, et al, "Plasma Protein Binding of Dicloxacillin: Effects of Age and Diseases," *Int J Clin Pharmacol Ther Toxicol*, 1987, 25(11):622-6.

◆ **Dicloxacillin Sodium** see Dicloxacillin on page 502

Dicyclomine (dye SYE kloe meen)

Related Information
Beers Criteria – Potentially Inappropriate Medications for Geriatrics *on page 2089*
Pharmacotherapy of Urinary Incontinence *on page 2032*
Medication Safety Issues
  Sound-alike/look-alike issues:
    Dicyclomine may be confused with diphenhydrAMINE, doxycycline, dyclonine
    Bentyl® may be confused with Aventyl®, Benadryl®, Bontril®, Cantil®, Proventil®, Trental®
  BEERS Criteria medication:
    This drug may be inappropriate for use in geriatric patients (high severity risk).
Brand Names: U.S. Bentyl®
Brand Names: Canada Bentylol®; Formulex®; Lomine; Riva-Dicyclomine
Index Terms Dicyclomine Hydrochloride; Dicycloverine Hydrochloride
Generic Availability (U.S.) Yes: Excludes syrup
Pharmacologic Category Anticholinergic Agent
Use Treatment of functional bowel/irritable bowel syndrome
Unlabeled/Investigational Use Treatment of urinary incontinence
Dosage
  Geriatric 10-20 mg 4 times/day; increasing as necessary to 160 mg/day
  Adult Gastrointestinal motility disorders/irritable bowel:
    Oral: Initiate with 80 mg/day in 4 equally divided doses, then increase up to 160 mg/day
    I.M. **(should not be used I.V.):** 80 mg/day in 4 divided doses (20 mg/dose)
Special Geriatric Considerations Long-term use of antispasmodics should be avoided in the elderly. The potential for a toxic reaction is greater than the potential benefit. In addition, the anticholinergic effects of dicyclomine are not well tolerated in the elderly.

This medication is considered to be potentially inappropriate in this patient population (Beers Criteria severity: High).
Dosage Forms Excipient information presented when available (limited, particularly for generics); consult specific product labeling.
Capsule, oral, as hydrochloride: 10 mg
  Bentyl®: 10 mg
Injection, solution, as hydrochloride: 10 mg/mL (2 mL)
  Bentyl®: 10 mg/mL (2 mL)
Syrup, oral, as hydrochloride:
  Bentyl®: 10 mg/5 mL (480 mL) [contains propylene glycol]
Tablet, oral, as hydrochloride: 20 mg
  Bentyl®: 20 mg

◆ **Dicyclomine Hydrochloride** *see* Dicyclomine *on page 504*
◆ **Dicycloverine Hydrochloride** *see* Dicyclomine *on page 504*
◆ **Didronel®** *see* Etidronate *on page 680*
◆ **Dificid™** *see* Fidaxomicin (Systemic) *on page 732*
◆ **Difimicin** *see* Fidaxomicin (Systemic) *on page 732*
◆ **Diflucan®** *see* Fluconazole *on page 741*

Diflunisal (dye FLOO ni sal)

Medication Safety Issues
  Sound-alike/look-alike issues:
    Dolobid® (discontinued U.S. brand name [generics available]) may be confused with Slo-Bid®
  International issues:
    Dolobid® (brand name product available in multiple international markets) may be confused with Slo-Bid®
Brand Names: Canada Apo-Diflunisal®; Novo-Diflunisal; Nu-Diflunisal
Index Terms Dolobid
Generic Availability (U.S.) Yes
Pharmacologic Category Nonsteroidal Anti-inflammatory Drug (NSAID), Oral
Use Management of inflammatory disorders usually including rheumatoid arthritis and osteoarthritis; can be used as an analgesic for treatment of mild-to-moderate pain
Medication Guide Available Yes
Contraindications Hypersensitivity to diflunisal, aspirin, other NSAIDs, or any component of the formulation; perioperative pain in the setting of coronary artery bypass graft (CABG) surgery

Warnings/Precautions [U.S. Boxed Warning]: NSAIDs are associated with an increased risk of adverse cardiovascular thrombotic events, including MI and stroke. Risk may be increased with duration of use or pre-existing cardiovascular risk factors or disease. Carefully evaluate individual cardiovascular risk profiles prior to prescribing. May cause new-onset hypertension or worsening of existing hypertension. Use caution with fluid retention. Avoid use in heart failure. Concurrent administration of ibuprofen, and potentially other nonselective NSAIDs, may interfere with aspirin's cardioprotective effect. **[U.S. Boxed Warning]: Use is contraindicated for treatment of perioperative pain in the setting of coronary artery bypass graft (CABG) surgery.** Risk of MI and stroke may be increased with use following CABG surgery.

[U.S. Boxed Warning]: NSAIDs may increase risk of gastrointestinal irritation, inflammation, ulceration, bleeding, and perforation. Use caution with a history of GI disease (bleeding or ulcers), concurrent therapy with aspirin, anticoagulants and/or corticosteroids, smoking, use of alcohol, the elderly or debilitated patients. When used concomitantly with ≤325 mg of aspirin, a substantial increase in the risk of gastrointestinal complications (eg, ulcer) occurs; concomitant gastroprotective therapy (eg, proton pump inhibitors) is recommended (Bhatt, 2008).

Platelet adhesion and aggregation may be decreased; may prolong bleeding time; patients with coagulation disorders or who are receiving anticoagulants should be monitored closely. Anemia may occur; patients on long-term NSAID therapy should be monitored for anemia. Rarely, NSAID use may cause severe blood dyscrasias (eg, agranulocytosis, aplastic anemia, thrombocytopenia).

NSAID use may compromise existing renal function; dose-dependent decreases in prostaglandin synthesis may result from NSAID use, reducing renal blood flow which may cause renal decompensation. NSAID use may increase the risk for hyperkalemia. Patients with impaired renal function, dehydration, heart failure, liver dysfunction, those taking diuretics, and ACE inhibitors, and the elderly are at greater risk of renal toxicity and hyperkalemia. Rehydrate patient before starting therapy; monitor renal function closely. Not recommended for use in patients with advanced renal disease. Long-term NSAID use may result in renal papillary necrosis. Use with caution in patients with decreased hepatic function.

NSAIDS may cause drowsiness, dizziness, blurred vision and other neurologic effects which may impair physical or mental abilities; patients must be cautioned about performing tasks which require mental alertness (eg, operating machinery or driving). Discontinue use with blurred or diminished vision and perform ophthalmologic exam. Monitor vision with long-term therapy.

Use the lowest effective dose for the shortest duration of time, consistent with individual patient goals, to reduce risk of cardiovascular or GI adverse events.

NSAIDs may cause serious skin adverse events including exfoliative dermatitis, Stevens-Johnson syndrome (SJS), and toxic epidermal necrolysis (TEN); discontinue use at first sign of skin rash or hypersensitivity. Do not use in patients who experience bronchospasm, asthma, rhinitis, or urticaria with NSAID or aspirin therapy. Use caution in other forms of asthma.

A hypersensitivity syndrome has been reported; monitor for constitutional symptoms and cutaneous findings; other organ dysfunction may be involved.

Diflunisal is a derivative of acetylsalicylic acid and therefore may be associated with Reye's syndrome. Withhold for at least 4-6 half-lives prior to surgical or dental procedures.

Adverse Reactions (Reflective of adult population; not specific for elderly)
1% to 10%:
Central nervous system: Headache (3% to 9%), dizziness (1% to 3%), insomnia (1% to 3%), somnolence (1% to 3%), fatigue (1% to 3%)
Dermatologic: Rash (3% to 9%)
Gastrointestinal: Nausea (3% to 9%), dyspepsia (3% to 9%), GI pain (3% to 9%), diarrhea (3% to 9%), constipation (1% to 3%), flatulence (1% to 3%), vomiting (1% to 3%), GI ulceration
Otic: Tinnitus (1% to 3%)

Drug Interactions
Avoid Concomitant Use
Avoid concomitant use of Diflunisal with any of the following: Floctafenine; Ketorolac; Ketorolac (Nasal); Ketorolac (Systemic)
Increased Effect/Toxicity
Diflunisal may increase the levels/effects of: Aminoglycosides; Anticoagulants; Antiplatelet Agents; Bisphosphonate Derivatives; Collagenase (Systemic); CycloSPORINE; Cyclo-SPORINE (Systemic); Deferasirox; Desmopressin; Digoxin; Drotrecogin Alfa; Eplerenone; Haloperidol; Ibritumomab; Lithium; Methotrexate; Nonsteroidal Anti-Inflammatory Agents;

PEMEtrexed; Porfimer; Potassium-Sparing Diuretics; PRALAtrexate; Quinolone Antibiotics; Rivaroxaban; Salicylates; Thrombolytic Agents; Tositumomab and Iodine I 131 Tositumomab; Vancomycin; Vitamin K Antagonists

The levels/effects of Diflunisal may be increased by: ACE Inhibitors; Angiotensin II Receptor Blockers; Antidepressants (Tricyclic, Tertiary Amine); Corticosteroids (Systemic); Dasatinib; Floctafenine; Glucosamine; Herbs (Anticoagulant/Antiplatelet Properties); Ketorolac; Ketorolac (Nasal); Ketorolac (Systemic); Nonsteroidal Anti-Inflammatory Agents; Omega-3-Acid Ethyl Esters; Pentosan Polysulfate Sodium; Pentoxifylline; Probenecid; Prostacyclin Analogues; Selective Serotonin Reuptake Inhibitors; Serotonin/Norepinephrine Reuptake Inhibitors; Sodium Phosphates; Treprostinil; Vitamin E

Decreased Effect
Diflunisal may decrease the levels/effects of: ACE Inhibitors; Angiotensin II Receptor Blockers; Antiplatelet Agents; Beta-Blockers; Eplerenone; HydrALAZINE; Potassium-Sparing Diuretics; Salicylates; Selective Serotonin Reuptake Inhibitors; Thiazide Diuretics

The levels/effects of Diflunisal may be decreased by: Bile Acid Sequestrants; Nonsteroidal Anti-Inflammatory Agents; Salicylates

Ethanol/Nutrition/Herb Interactions
Ethanol: Avoid ethanol (may enhance gastric mucosal irritation).
Herb/Nutraceutical: Avoid alfalfa, anise, bilberry, bladderwrack, bromelain, cat's claw, celery, chamomile, coleus, cordyceps, dong quai, evening primrose, fenugreek, feverfew, garlic, ginger, ginkgo biloba, ginseng (American, Panax, Siberian), grapeseed, green tea, guggul, horse chestnut seed, horseradish, licorice, prickly ash, red clover, reishi, SAMe (S-adenosylmethionine), sweet clover, turmeric, white willow (all have additional antiplatelet activity).

Mechanism of Action Reversibly inhibits cyclooxygenase-1 and 2 (COX-1 and 2) enzymes, which results in decreased formation of prostaglandin precursors; has antipyretic, analgesic, and anti-inflammatory properties.

Other proposed mechanisms not fully elucidated (and possibly contributing to the anti-inflammatory effect to varying degrees) include inhibiting chemotaxis, altering lymphocyte activity, inhibiting neutrophil aggregation/activation, and decreasing proinflammatory cytokine levels.

Pharmacodynamics/Kinetics
Onset of action: Analgesic: ~1 hour; maximal effect: 2-3 hours
Duration: 8-12 hours
Absorption: Well absorbed
Protein binding: >99%
Distribution: 0.11 L/kg
Metabolism: Extensively hepatic; metabolic pathways are saturable
Half-life elimination: 8-12 hours; prolonged with renal impairment
Time to peak, serum: 2-3 hours
Excretion: Urine (~3% as unchanged drug, 90% as glucuronide conjugates) within 72-96 hours

Dosage
Geriatric & Adult
Mild-to-moderate pain: Oral: Initial: 500-1000 mg followed by 250-500 mg every 8-12 hours; maximum daily dose: 1.5 g
Arthritis: Oral: 500-1000 mg/day in 2 divided doses; maximum daily dose: 1.5 g
Renal Impairment
Use with caution; Cl_{cr} <50 mL/minute: Administer 50% of normal dose (Aronoff, 1998)
Hemodialysis: No supplement required
CAPD: No supplement require
CAVH: Dose for GFR 10-50

Administration Tablet should be swallowed whole; do not crush or chew.

Monitoring Parameters Fecal blood loss, renal function; hearing changes or tinnitus; monitor for response (ie, pain, inflammation, range of motion, grip strength); observe for abnormal bleeding, bruising, weight gain

Test Interactions Falsely elevated increase in serum salicylate levels

Pharmacotherapy Pearls Diflunisal is a salicylic acid derivative which is chemically different than aspirin and is not metabolized to salicylic acid. Diflunisal 500 mg is equal in analgesic efficacy to aspirin 650 mg, acetaminophen 650 mg, and acetaminophen 650 mg/propoxyphene napsylate 100 mg, but has a longer duration of effect (8-12 hours). Not recommended as an antipyretic. Not found to be clinically useful to treat fever; at doses of ≥2 g/day, platelets are reversibly inhibited in function. Diflunisal is uricosuric at 500-750 mg/day; causes less GI and renal toxicity than aspirin and other NSAIDs; fecal blood loss is $1/2$ that of aspirin at 2.6 g/day.

Special Geriatric Considerations The elderly are a high-risk population for adverse effects from nonsteroidal anti-inflammatory agents. As much as 60% of elderly can develop peptic ulceration and/or hemorrhage asymptomatically. The concomitant use of H_2 blockers and sucralfate is not effective as prophylaxis with the exception of NSAID-induced duodenal ulcers which may be prevented by the use of ranitidine. Misoprostol and proton pump inhibitors are the only agents proven to help prevent the development of NSAID-induced ulcers. Also, concomitant disease and drug use contribute to the risk for GI adverse effects. Use lowest effective dose for shortest period possible. Consider renal function decline with age. Use of NSAIDs can compromise existing renal function especially when Cl_{cr} is ≤30 mL/minute. Tinnitus may be a difficult and unreliable indication of toxicity due to age-related hearing loss or eighth cranial nerve damage. CNS adverse effects such as confusion, agitation, and hallucination are generally seen in overdose or high dose situations, but elderly may demonstrate these adverse effects at lower doses than younger adults.

Dosage Forms Excipient information presented when available (limited, particularly for generics); consult specific product labeling.

Tablet, oral: 500 mg

Selected References

Hunt SA, Abraham WT, Chin MH, et al, "ACC/AHA 2005 Guideline Update for the Diagnosis and Management of Chronic Heart Failure in the Adult-Summary Article A Report of the American College of Cardiology/American Heart Association Task Force on Practice Guidelines (Writing Committee to Update the 2001 Guidelines for the Evaluation and Management of Heart Failure)," *J Am Coll Cardiol*, 2005, 46(6):1116-43.

Difluprednate (dye floo PRED nate)

Medication Safety Issues

Sound-alike/look-alike issues:

Durezol™ may be confused with Durasal

Brand Names: U.S. Durezol®

Generic Availability (U.S.) No

Pharmacologic Category Corticosteroid, Ophthalmic

Use Treatment of inflammation and pain following ocular surgery

Contraindications Active viral (including herpes simplex keratitis, vaccinia, varicella) infections of the cornea or conjunctiva, fungal infection of ocular structures, or mycobacterial ocular infections

Warnings/Precautions For ophthalmic use only; not for intraocular administration. Steroids may mask infection or enhance existing ocular infection; prolonged use may result in secondary infections due to immunosuppression. Prolonged use has been associated with the development of corneal or scleral perforation and posterior subcapsular cataracts; may mask or enhance the establishment of acute purulent untreated infections of the eye; may delay healing after cataract surgery; intraocular pressure should be monitored if this product is used ≥10 days. Initial prescription and renewal of medication for >28 days should be made by healthcare provider only after examination with the aid of magnification such as slit lamp biomicroscopy or fluorescein staining (if appropriate). Contains sorbic acid which may be adsorbed by contact lenses; it is not recommended to wear contacts while using difluprednate.

Adverse Reactions (Reflective of adult population; not specific for elderly)

5% to 15%: Ocular: Anterior chamber cells/flare, blepharitis, ciliary and conjunctival hyperemia, conjunctival/corneal edema, pain, photophobia, posterior capsule opacification

1% to 5%: Ocular: Inflammation, iritis, punctuate keratitis, visual acuity reduced

Drug Interactions

Avoid Concomitant Use

Avoid concomitant use of Difluprednate with any of the following: Aldesleukin

Increased Effect/Toxicity

Difluprednate may increase the levels/effects of: Deferasirox

The levels/effects of Difluprednate may be increased by: Telaprevir

Decreased Effect

Difluprednate may decrease the levels/effects of: Aldesleukin; Corticorelin; Telaprevir

Stability Store at 15°C to 25°C (59°F to 77°F); do not freeze. Protect from light.

Mechanism of Action Corticosteroids inhibit the inflammatory response including edema, capillary dilation, leukocyte migration, and scar formation. Difluprednate penetrates cells readily to induce the production of lipocortins. These proteins modulate the activity of prostaglandins and leukotrienes.

Pharmacodynamics/Kinetics Absorption: Systemic: Limited

Dosage

Geriatric & Adult Anti-inflammatory: Ophthalmic: Adults: Instill 1 drop in conjunctival sac of the affected eye(s) 4 times/day beginning 24 hours after surgery, continue for 2 weeks, then decrease to 2 times/day for 1 week, then taper based on response

◀ **Monitoring Parameters** Intraocular pressure and periodic examination of lens (with prolonged use >28 days)

Special Geriatric Considerations Evaluate the patient's or caregiver's ability to safely
administer the correct dose of ophthalmic medication.

Dosage Forms Excipient information presented when available (limited, particularly for
generics); consult specific product labeling.

Emulsion, ophthalmic [drops]:

Durezol®: 0.05% (5 mL) [contains sorbic acid]

◆ **Digitalis** see Digoxin on page 508

Digoxin (di JOKS in)

Related Information

Beers Criteria − Potentially Inappropriate Medications for Geriatrics on page 2089

Medication Safety Issues

Sound-alike/look-alike issues:

Digoxin may be confused with Desoxyn®, doxepin

Lanoxin® may be confused with Lasix®, levothyroxine, Levoxyl®, Levsinex®, Lomotil®,
Lonox®, Mefoxin®, naloxone, Xanax®

High alert medication:

The Institute for Safe Medication Practices (ISMP) includes this medication among its list of
drugs which have a heightened risk of causing significant patient harm when used in error.

BEERS Criteria medication:

This drug may be inappropriate for use in geriatric patients (low severity risk).

International issues:

Lanoxin [U.S., Canada, and multiple international markets] may be confused with Limoxin
brand name for ambroxol [Indonesia] and amoxicillin [Mexico]

Brand Names: U.S. Lanoxin®

Brand Names: Canada Apo-Digoxin®; Digoxin CSD; Lanoxin®; Pediatric Digoxin CSD;
PMS-Digoxin; Toloxin®

Index Terms Digitalis

Generic Availability (U.S.) Yes

Pharmacologic Category Antiarrhythmic Agent, Miscellaneous; Cardiac Glycoside

Use Treatment of mild-to-moderate (or stage C as recommended by the ACCF/AHA) heart
failure (HF); atrial fibrillation (rate-control)

Note: In treatment of atrial fibrillation (AF), use is not considered first-line unless AF coexistent
with heart failure or in sedentary patients (Fuster, 2006).

Unlabeled/Investigational Use Fetal tachycardia with or without hydrops; to slow ventricular
rate in supraventricular tachyarrhythmias such as supraventricular tachycardia (SVT) excluding atrioventricular reciprocating tachycardia (AVRT)

Contraindications Hypersensitivity to digoxin (rare) or other forms of digitalis, or any
component of the formulation; ventricular fibrillation

Warnings/Precautions Watch for proarrhythmic effects (especially with digoxin toxicity).
Withdrawal in clinically stable patients with HF may lead to recurrence of HF symptoms.
During an episode of atrial fibrillation or flutter in patients with an accessory bypass tract (eg,
Wolff-Parkinson-White syndrome), use has been associated with increased anterograde
conduction down the accessory pathway leading to ventricular fibrillation; avoid use in such
patients. Avoid use in patients with second- or third-degree heart block (except in patients with
a functioning artificial pacemaker); incomplete AV block (eg, Stokes-Adams attack) may
progress to complete block with digoxin administration. HF patients with preserved left
ventricular function including patients with restrictive cardiomyopathy, constrictive pericarditis,
and amyloid heart disease may be susceptible to digoxin toxicity; avoid use unless used to
control ventricular response with atrial fibrillation. Digoxin should not be used in patients with
low EF, sinus rhythm, and no HF symptoms since the risk of harm may be greater than clinical
benefit. Avoid use in patients with hypertrophic cardiomyopathy (HCM) and outflow tract
obstruction unless used to control ventricular response with atrial fibrillation; outflow obstruction may worsen due to the positive inotropic effects of digoxin.

Use with caution in patients with hyperthyroidism, hypothyroidism, recent acute MI (within 6
months), sinus nodal disease (eg, sick sinus syndrome). Reduce dose with renal impairment
and when amiodarone, propafenone, quinidine, or verapamil are added to a patient on
digoxin; use with caution in patients taking strong inducers or inhibitors of P-glycoprotein
(eg, cyclosporine). Avoid rapid I.V. administration of calcium in digitalized patients; may
produce serious arrhythmias.

Atrial arrhythmias associated with hypermetabolic states are very difficult to treat; treat
underlying condition first; if digoxin is used, ensure digoxin toxicity does not occur. Patients

with beri beri heart disease may fail to adequately respond to digoxin therapy; treat underlying thiamine deficiency concomitantly. Correct electrolyte disturbances, especially hypokalemia or hypomagnesemia, prior to use and throughout therapy; toxicity may occur despite therapeutic digoxin concentrations. Hypercalcemia may increase the risk of digoxin toxicity; maintain normocalcemia. It is not necessary to routinely reduce or hold digoxin therapy prior to elective electrical cardioversion for atrial fibrillation; however, exclusion of digoxin toxicity (eg, clinical and ECG signs) is necessary prior to cardioversion. If signs of digoxin excess exist, withhold digoxin and delay cardioversion until toxicity subsides; usually >24 hours. Use with caution in the elderly; may develop exaggerated serum/tissue concentrations due to age-related alterations in clearance and pharmacodynamics differences; dosage reduction may be necessary; in general, avoid doses >0.125 mg/day (Beers Criteria).

Adverse Reactions (Reflective of adult population; not specific for elderly) Incidence not always reported.

Cardiovascular: Accelerated junctional rhythm, asystole, atrial tachycardia with or without block, AV dissociation, first-, second- (Wenckebach), or third-degree heart block, facial edema, PR prolongation, PVCs (especially bigeminy or trigeminy), ST segment depression, ventricular tachycardia or ventricular fibrillation

Central nervous system: Dizziness (6%), mental disturbances (5%), headache (4%), apathy, anxiety, confusion, delirium, depression, fever, hallucinations

Dermatologic: Rash (erythematous, maculopapular [most common], papular, scarlatiniform, vesicular or bullous), pruritus, urticaria, angioneurotic edema

Gastrointestinal: Nausea (4%), vomiting (2%), diarrhea (4%), abdominal pain, anorexia

Neuromuscular & skeletal: Weakness

Ocular: Visual disturbances (blurred or yellow vision)

Respiratory: Laryngeal edema

Children are more likely to experience cardiac arrhythmia as a sign of excessive dosing. The most common are conduction disturbances or tachyarrhythmia (atrial tachycardia with or without block) and junctional tachycardia. Ventricular tachyarrhythmias are less common. In infants, sinus bradycardia may be a sign of digoxin toxicity. Any arrhythmia seen in a child on digoxin should be considered as digoxin toxicity. The gastrointestinal and central nervous system symptoms are not frequently seen in children.

Drug Interactions

Metabolism/Transport Effects Substrate of CYP3A4 (minor), P-glycoprotein

Avoid Concomitant Use There are no known interactions where it is recommended to avoid concomitant use.

Increased Effect/Toxicity

Digoxin may increase the levels/effects of: Adenosine; Colchicine; Dronedarone; Midodrine

The levels/effects of Digoxin may be increased by: Aminoquinolines (Antimalarial); Amiodarone; Atorvastatin; Beta-Blockers; Boceprevir; Calcium Channel Blockers (Nondihydropyridine); Calcium Polystyrene Sulfonate; Carvedilol; Conivaptan; CycloSPORINE; CycloSPORINE (Systemic); Dronedarone; Etravirine; Glycopyrrolate; Itraconazole; Loop Diuretics; Macrolide Antibiotics; Milnacipran; Nefazodone; Neuromuscular-Blocking Agents; NIFEdipine; Nonsteroidal Anti-Inflammatory Agents; Paricalcitol; P-Glycoprotein Inhibitors; Posaconazole; Potassium-Sparing Diuretics; Propafenone; Protease Inhibitors; QuiNIDine; QuiNINE; Ranolazine; Reserpine; SitaGLIPtin; Sodium Polystyrene Sulfonate; Spironolactone; Telaprevir; Telmisartan; Ticagrelor; Tolvaptan; Vitamin D Analogs

Decreased Effect

Digoxin may decrease the levels/effects of: Antineoplastic Agents (Anthracycline)

The levels/effects of Digoxin may be decreased by: 5-ASA Derivatives; Acarbose; Aminoglycosides; Antineoplastic Agents; Antineoplastic Agents (Anthracycline); Bile Acid Sequestrants; Kaolin; Penicillamine; P-Glycoprotein Inducers; Potassium-Sparing Diuretics; St Johns Wort; Sucralfate; Tocilizumab

Ethanol/Nutrition/Herb Interactions

Food: Digoxin peak serum concentrations may be decreased if taken with food. Meals containing increased fiber (bran) or foods high in pectin may decrease oral absorption of digoxin.

Herb/Nutraceutical: Avoid ephedra (risk of cardiac stimulation). Avoid natural licorice (causes sodium and water retention and increases potassium loss).

Stability Store at 25°C (77°F); excursions permitted to 15°C to 30°C (59°F to 86°F). Protect elixir, injection, and tablets from light.

Mechanism of Action

Heart failure: Inhibition of the sodium/potassium ATPase pump in myocardial cells results in a transient increase of intracellular sodium, which in turn promotes calcium influx via the sodium-calcium exchange pump leading to increased contractility.

◀ Supraventricular arrhythmias: Direct suppression of the AV node conduction to increase effective refractory period and decrease conduction velocity - positive inotropic effect, enhanced vagal tone, and decreased ventricular rate to fast atrial arrhythmias. Atrial fibrillation may decrease sensitivity and increase tolerance to higher serum digoxin concentrations.

Pharmacodynamics/Kinetics

Distribution: V_d: Geriatrics: 194 L (range: 129-314 L)

Protein binding: 25%

Bioavailability: Dependent upon formulation:

Elixir: 70% to 85%

Tablets: 60% to 80% (76% in older adults)

Capsules: 90% to 100%

Half-life:

Geriatrics: 69 hours (average)

Adults: 38-48 hours

Anephric Adults: >4.5 days

Time to peak serum concentration:

Oral: 2-6 hours

I.V.: 1-5 hours

Elimination: Renal

Dosage

Geriatric Dose is based on lean body weight and normal renal function for age. Decrease dose in patients with decreased renal function (see Dosing: Renal Impairment).

Heart failure: If patient is >70 years of age, low doses (eg, 0.125 mg daily or every other day) should be used (Hunt, 2009).

Adult Note: When changing from oral (tablets or liquid) or I.M. to I.V. therapy, dosage should be reduced by 20% or 25%.

Atrial fibrillation (rate control) in patients with heart failure: Loading dose: I.V.: 0.25 mg every 2 hours, up to 1.5 mg within 24 hours; for nonacute situations, may administer 0.5 mg orally once daily for 2 days followed by oral maintenance dose. Maintenance dose: I.V., Oral: 0.125-0.375 mg once daily (Fuster, 2006)

Heart failure: Daily maintenance dose (**Note:** Loading dose not recommended): Oral: 0.125-0.25 mg once daily; higher daily doses (up to 0.5 mg/day) are rarely necessary. If patient is >70 years of age, has impaired renal function, or has a low lean body mass, low doses (eg, 0.125 mg daily or every other day) should be used (Hunt, 2009).

Supraventricular tachyarrhythmias (rate control):

Initial: Total digitalizing dose:

Oral: 0.75-1.5 mg

I.V., I.M.: 0.5-1 mg (**Note:** I.M. not preferred due to severe injection site pain.)

Give 1/2 (one-half) of the total digitalizing dose (TDD) as the initial dose, then give 1/4 (one-quarter) of the TDD in each of 2 subsequent doses at 6- to 8-hour intervals. Obtain ECG 6 hours after each dose to assess potential toxicity.

Daily maintenance dose:

Oral: 0.125-0.5 mg once daily

I.V., I.M.: 0.1-0.4 mg once daily (**Note:** I.M. not preferred due to severe injection site pain.)

Renal Impairment

Loading dose:

ESRD: If loading dose necessary, reduce dose by 50%

Acute renal failure: Based on expert opinion, if patient in acute renal failure requires ventricular rate control (eg, in atrial fibrillation), consider alternative therapy. If loading digoxin becomes necessary, patient volume of distribution may be increased and reduction in loading dose may not be necessary; however, maintenance dosing will require adjustment as long as renal failure persists.

Maintenance dose:

Cl_{cr} 10-50 mL/minute: Administer 25% to 75% of dose or every 36 hours.

Cl_{cr} <10 mL/minute: Administer 10% to 25% of dose or every 48 hours.

Not dialyzable

Administration

I.M.: I.V. route preferred. If I.M. injection necessary, administer by deep injection followed by massage at the injection site. Inject no more than 2 mL per injection site. May cause intense pain.

I.V.: May be administered undiluted or diluted fourfold in D_5W, NS, or SWFI for direct injection. Less than fourfold dilution may lead to drug precipitation. Inject slowly over ≥5 minutes.

Monitoring Parameters

Heart rate and rhythm should be monitored along with periodic ECGs to assess desired effects and signs of toxicity; baseline and periodic serum creatinine. Periodically monitor serum potassium, magnesium, and calcium especially if on medications where these electrolyte disturbances can occur (eg, diuretics), or if patient has a history of hypokalemia or hypomagnesemia. Observe patients for noncardiac signs of toxicity, confusion, and depression.

When to draw serum digoxin concentrations: Digoxin serum concentrations are monitored because digoxin possesses a narrow therapeutic serum range; the therapeutic endpoint is difficult to quantify and digoxin toxicity may be life-threatening. Digoxin serum concentrations should be drawn **at least 6-8 hours after last dose, regardless of route of administration (optimally 12-24 hours after a dose). Note:** Serum digoxin concentrations may decrease in response to exercise due to increased skeletal muscle uptake; a period of rest (eg, ~2 hours) after exercise may be necessary prior to drawing serum digoxin concentrations.

Initiation of therapy:

If a loading dose is given: Digoxin serum concentration may be drawn within 12-24 hours after the initial loading dose administration. Concentrations drawn this early may confirm the relationship of digoxin plasma concentrations and response but are of little value in determining maintenance doses.

If a loading dose is not given: Digoxin serum concentration should be obtained after 3-5 days of therapy.

Maintenance therapy:

Trough concentrations should be followed just prior to the next dose or at a minimum of 6-8 hours after last dose.

Digoxin serum concentrations should be obtained within 5-7 days (approximate time to steady-state) after any dosage changes. Continue to obtain digoxin serum concentrations 7-14 days after any change in maintenance dose. **Note:** In patients with end-stage renal disease, it may take 15-20 days to reach steady-state.

Patients who are receiving electrolyte-depleting medications such as diuretics, serum potassium, magnesium, and calcium should be monitored closely.

Digoxin serum concentrations should be obtained whenever any of the following conditions occur:

Questionable patient compliance or to evaluate clinical deterioration following an initial good response

Changing renal function

Suspected digoxin toxicity

Initiation or discontinuation of therapy with drugs (eg, amiodarone, quinidine, verapamil) which potentially interact with digoxin.

Any disease changes (eg, thyroid disease)

Reference Range

Digoxin therapeutic serum concentrations:

Heart failure: 0.5-0.8 ng/mL

Adults: <0.5 ng/mL; probably indicates underdigitalization unless there are special circumstances

Toxic: >2 ng/mL

Digoxin-like immunoreactive substance (DLIS) may cross-react with digoxin immunoassay. DLIS has been found in patients with renal and liver disease and heart failure

Test Interactions Spironolactone may interfere with digoxin radioimmunoassay.

Pharmacotherapy Pearls The AHCPR Clinical Practice Guideline for Heart Failure recommends that digoxin should be saved for patients who do not respond to ACE inhibitors and diuretics or who present with severe dyspnea on exertion. Digoxin is useful in systolic dysfunction, but not diastolic dysfunction.

Special Geriatric Considerations Digitalis preparations (primarily digoxin) are frequently used to treat common cardiac diseases in the elderly (heart failure, atrial fibrillation). Elderly are at risk for toxicity due to age-related changes; volume of distribution is diminished significantly; half-life is increased as a result of decreased total body clearance. Additionally, elderly frequently have concomitant diseases which affect the pharmacokinetics in digitalis glycosides; hypo- and hyperthyroidism and renal function decline will affect clearance of digoxin. Exercise in elderly will reduce serum concentrations of digoxin due to increased skeletal muscle uptake. Therefore, a knowledge of the physical activity of elderly helps interpret serum assays. Must be observant for noncardiac signs of toxicity in elderly such as anorexia, vision changes (blurred), confusion, and depression. Changes in dose may be necessary with declining renal function with age; monitor closely.

This medication is considered to be potentially inappropriate in this patient population (Beers Criteria severity: Low).

Dosage Forms Excipient information presented when available (limited, particularly for generics); consult specific product labeling. [DSC] = Discontinued product
Injection, solution: 250 mcg/mL (2 mL)
  Lanoxin®: 250 mcg/mL (2 mL) [contains ethanol 10%, propylene glycol 40%]
Injection, solution [pediatric]:
  Lanoxin®: 100 mcg/mL (1 mL) [contains ethanol 10%, propylene glycol 40%]
Solution, oral: 50 mcg/mL (2.5 mL [DSC], 60 mL)
Tablet, oral: 125 mcg, 250 mcg
  Lanoxin®: 125 mcg, 250 mcg [scored]

Dosage Forms: Canada Excipient information presented when available (limited, particularly for generics); consult specific product labeling.
Tablet, oral:
  Apo-Digoxin®: 62.5 mcg, 125 mcg, 250 mcg

Selected References

Adams KF, Lindenfeld J, Arnold JMO, et al, "HFSA 2006 Comprehensive Heart Failure Practice Guideline," *J Card Fail*, 2006, 12(1):e1-122. Available at http://www.heartfailureguideline.org

Antman EM, Anbe DT, Armstrong PW, et al, "ACC/AHA Guidelines for the Management of Patients With ST-Elevation Myocardial Infarction: A Report of the American College of Cardiology/American Heart Association Task Force on Practice Guidelines (Committee to Revise the 1999 Guidelines for the Management of Patients with Acute Myocardial Infarction)," *Circulation*, 2004, 110(9):e82-292.

Blomström-Lundqvist C, Scheinman MM, Aliot EM, et al, "ACC/AHA/ESC Guidelines for the Management of Patients With Supraventricular Arrhythmias–Executive Summary. A Report of the American College of Cardiology/American Heart Association Task Force on Practice Guidelines and the European Society of Cardiology Committee for Practice Guidelines (Writing Committee to Develop Guidelines for the Management of Patients With Supraventricular Arrhythmias) Developed in Collaboration With NASPE-Heart Rhythm Society)," *J Am Coll Cardiol*, 2003, 42 (8):1493-531.

Fuster V, Ryden LE, Cannom DS, et al, "ACC/AHA/ESC 2006 Guidelines for the Management of Patients With Atrial Fibrillation-Executive Summary. A Report of the American College of Cardiology/American Heart Association Task Force on Practice Guidelines and the European Society of Cardiology Committee for Practice Guidelines (Writing Committee to Revise the 2001 Guidelines for the Management of Patients With Atrial Fibrillation). Developed in Collaboration With the European Heart Rhythm Association and the Heart Rhythm Society)," *J Am Coll Cardiol*, 2006, 48(4):854-906.

Hunt SA, Abraham WT, Chin MH, et al, "2009 Focused Update Incorporated into the ACC/AHA 2005 Guidelines for the Diagnosis and Management of Heart Failure in Adults: A Report of the American College of Cardiology Foundation/ American Heart Association Task Force on Practice Guidelines Developed in Collaboration With the International Society for Heart and Lung Transplantation," *J Am Coll Cardiol*, 2009, 53(15):e1-90.

Rathore SS, Curtis JP, Wang Y, et al, "Association of Serum Digoxin Concentration and Outcomes in Patients With Heart Failure," *JAMA*, 2003, 289(7):871-8.

Siu CW, Lau CP, Lee WL, et al, "Intravenous Diltiazem is Superior to Intravenous Amiodarone or Digoxin for Achieving Ventricular Rate Control in Patients With Acute Uncomplicated Atrial Fibrillation," *Crit Care Med*, 2009, 37(7):2174-9.

Dihydroergotamine (dye hye droe er GOT a meen)

Brand Names: U.S. D.H.E. 45®; Migranal®
Brand Names: Canada Migranal®
Index Terms DHE; Dihydroergotamine Mesylate
Generic Availability (U.S.) Yes: Injection
Pharmacologic Category Antimigraine Agent; Ergot Derivative
Use Treatment of migraine headache with or without aura; injection also indicated for treatment of cluster headaches
Unlabeled/Investigational Use Adjunct for DVT prophylaxis for hip surgery, for orthostatic hypotension, xerostomia secondary to antidepressant use, and pelvic congestion with pain
Contraindications Hypersensitivity to dihydroergotamine or any component of the formulation; uncontrolled hypertension; ischemic heart disease, angina pectoris, history of MI, silent ischemia, or coronary artery vasospasm including Prinzmetal's angina; hemiplegic or basilar migraine; peripheral vascular disease; sepsis; severe hepatic or renal dysfunction; following vascular surgery; avoid use within 24 hours of sumatriptan, zolmitriptan, other serotonin agonists, or ergot-like agents; avoid during or within 2 weeks of discontinuing MAO inhibitors; concurrent use of peripheral and central vasoconstrictors; ergot alkaloids are contraindicated with potent inhibitors of CYP3A4 (includes protease inhibitors, azole antifungals, and some macrolide antibiotics)
Warnings/Precautions [U.S. Boxed Warning]: Ergot alkaloids are contraindicated with potent inhibitors of CYP3A4 (includes protease inhibitors, azole antifungals, and some macrolide antibiotics); concomitant use associated with an increased risk of vasospasm leading to cerebral ischemia and/or ischemia of the extremities. Do not give to patients with risk factors for CAD until a cardiovascular evaluation has been performed; if evaluation is satisfactory, the healthcare provider should administer the first dose and cardiovascular status should be periodically evaluated. May cause vasospastic reactions; persistent vasospasm may lead to gangrene or death in patients with compromised circulation. Discontinue if signs of vasoconstriction develop. Rare reports of increased blood pressure in patients without history of hypertension. Rare reports of adverse cardiac events

(acute MI, life-threatening arrhythmias, death) have been reported following use of the injection. Cerebral hemorrhage, subarachnoid hemorrhage, and stroke have also occurred following use of the injection. Not for prolonged use. Pleural and peritoneal fibrosis have been reported with prolonged daily use. Cardiac valvular fibrosis has also been associated with ergot alkaloids. Use with caution in the elderly.

Migranal® Nasal Spray: Local irritation to nose and throat (usually transient and mild-moderate in severity) can occur; long-term consequences on nasal or respiratory mucosa have not been extensively evaluated.

Adverse Reactions (Reflective of adult population; not specific for elderly)
>10%: Nasal spray: Respiratory: Rhinitis (26%)
1% to 10%: Nasal spray:
  Central nervous system: Dizziness (4%), somnolence (3%)
  Endocrine & metabolic: Hot flashes (1%)
  Gastrointestinal: Nausea (10%), taste disturbance (8%), vomiting (4%), diarrhea (2%)
  Local: Application site reaction (6%)
  Neuromuscular & skeletal: Weakness (1%), stiffness (1%)
  Respiratory: Pharyngitis (3%)

Drug Interactions
Metabolism/Transport Effects Substrate of CYP3A4 (major); **Inhibits** CYP3A4 (weak)

Avoid Concomitant Use
Avoid concomitant use of Dihydroergotamine with any of the following: Boceprevir; Clarithromycin; Conivaptan; Crizotinib; Efavirenz; Itraconazole; Nitroglycerin; Posaconazole; Protease Inhibitors; Serotonin 5-HT1D Receptor Agonists; Sibutramine; Telaprevir; Voriconazole

Increased Effect/Toxicity
Dihydroergotamine may increase the levels/effects of: Serotonin 5-HT1D Receptor Agonists; Serotonin Modulators

The levels/effects of Dihydroergotamine may be increased by: Boceprevir; Clarithromycin; Conivaptan; Crizotinib; CYP3A4 Inhibitors (Moderate); CYP3A4 Inhibitors (Strong); Dasatinib; Efavirenz; Itraconazole; Macrolide Antibiotics; Nitroglycerin; Posaconazole; Protease Inhibitors; Serotonin 5-HT1D Receptor Agonists; Sibutramine; Telaprevir; Voriconazole

Decreased Effect
Dihydroergotamine may decrease the levels/effects of: Nitroglycerin

The levels/effects of Dihydroergotamine may be decreased by: Tocilizumab

Stability
Injection: Store below 25°C (77°F); do not refrigerate or freeze; protect from heat. Protect from light.
Nasal spray: Prior to use, store below 25°C (77°F); do not refrigerate or freeze. Once spray applicator has been prepared, use within 8 hours; discard any unused solution.

Mechanism of Action Ergot alkaloid alpha-adrenergic blocker directly stimulates vascular smooth muscle to vasoconstrict peripheral and cerebral vessels; also has effects on serotonin receptors

Pharmacodynamics/Kinetics
Onset of action: I.M.: 15-30 minutes
Duration: I.M.: 3-4 hours
Distribution: V_d: ~800 L
Protein binding: 93%
Metabolism: Extensively hepatic
Half-life elimination: ~9-10 hours
Time to peak, serum: I.M.: 24 minutes; I.V.: 1-2 minutes; Intranasal: 30-60 minutes; SubQ 15-45 minutes
Excretion: Primarily feces; urine (6% to 7% as unchanged drug)

Dosage
Geriatric Refer to adult dosing. Patients >65 years of age were not included in controlled clinical studies.

Adult
Migraine, cluster headache:
  I.M., SubQ: 1 mg at first sign of headache; repeat hourly to a maximum dose of 3 mg/day; maximum dose: 6 mg/week
  I.V.: 1 mg at first sign of headache; repeat hourly up to a maximum dose of 2 mg/day; maximum dose: 6 mg/week
  Intranasal: 1 spray (0.5 mg) of nasal spray should be administered into each nostril; if needed, repeat after 15 minutes, up to a total of 4 sprays (2 mg). **Note:** Do not exceed 6 sprays (3 mg) in a 24-hour period and no more than 8 sprays (4 mg) in a week.

◀ **Intractable migraine (status migrainosus; >72 hours):** *I.V.:* Raskin protocol (unlabeled dosing): Initial test dose: 0.5 mg (following premedication with metoclopramide); subsequent dosing is titrated (range: 0.2-1 mg) every 8 hours for 2-3 days and administered with or without metoclopramide based on response and tolerance (Raskin, 1986; Raskin, 1990). **Note:** Some clinicians use modified versions of this protocol, with additional adjunctive medications and/or alternate antiemetic agents.

Renal Impairment Contraindicated in severe renal impairment

Hepatic Impairment Dosage reductions are probably necessary but specific guidelines are not available; contraindicated in severe hepatic dysfunction.

Administration

Intranasal: Prior to administration of nasal spray, the nasal spray applicator must be primed (pumped 4 times); in order to let the drug be absorbed through the skin in the nose, patients should not inhale deeply through the nose while spraying or immediately after spraying; for best results, treatment should be initiated at the first symptom or sign of an attack; however, nasal spray can be used at any stage of a migraine attack.

I.M., SubQ: May administer by intramuscular or subcutaneous injection.

I.V.: Administer slowly over 2-3 minutes (Raskin protocol)

Reference Range Minimum concentration for vasoconstriction is reportedly 0.06 ng/mL

Special Geriatric Considerations Monitor cardiac and peripheral effects closely in the elderly since they often have cardiovascular disease and peripheral vascular impairment (ie, diabetes mellitus, PVD) that will complicate therapy and monitoring for adverse effects.

Dosage Forms Excipient information presented when available (limited, particularly for generics); consult specific product labeling.

Injection, solution, as mesylate: 1 mg/mL (1 mL)

D.H.E. 45®: 1 mg/mL (1 mL) [contains ethanol 6.2%]

Solution, intranasal, as mesylate [spray]:

Migranal®: 4 mg/mL (1 mL) [contains caffeine 10 mg/mL; 0.5 mg/spray]

♦ **Dihydroergotamine Mesylate** *see* Dihydroergotamine *on page 512*
♦ **Dihydroergotoxine** *see* Ergoloid Mesylates *on page 620*
♦ **Dihydrogenated Ergot Alkaloids** *see* Ergoloid Mesylates *on page 620*
♦ **Dihydrohydroxycodeinone** *see* OxyCODONE *on page 1368*
♦ **Dihydromorphinone** *see* HYDROmorphone *on page 888*
♦ **1,25 Dihydroxycholecalciferol** *see* Calcitriol *on page 243*
♦ **Dihydroxypropyl Theophylline** *see* Dyphylline *on page 588*
♦ **Diiodohydroxyquin** *see* Iodoquinol *on page 972*
♦ **Dilacor XR®** *see* Diltiazem *on page 514*
♦ **Dilantin®** *see* Phenytoin *on page 1444*
♦ **Dilantin-125®** *see* Phenytoin *on page 1444*
♦ **Dilatrate®-SR** *see* Isosorbide Dinitrate *on page 987*
♦ **Dilaudid®** *see* HYDROmorphone *on page 888*
♦ **Dilaudid-HP®** *see* HYDROmorphone *on page 888*
♦ **Dilt-CD** *see* Diltiazem *on page 514*
♦ **Diltia XT®** *see* Diltiazem *on page 514*

Diltiazem (dil TYE a zem)

Related Information

Calcium Channel Blockers *on page 2003*

Medication Safety Issues

Sound-alike/look-alike issues:

Cardizem® may be confused with Cardene®, Cardene SR®, Cardizem CD®, Cardizem SR®, cardiem, cortisone

Cartia XT® may be confused with Procardia XL®

Diltiazem may be confused with Calan®, diazepam, Dilantin®

Tiazac® may be confused with Tigan®, Tiazac® XC [CAN], Ziac®

High alert medication:

The Institute for Safe Medication Practices (ISMP) includes this medication (I.V. formulation) among its list of drug classes which have a heightened risk of causing significant patient harm when used in error.

Administration issues:

Significant differences exist between oral and I.V. dosing. Use caution when converting from one route of administration to another.

International issues:

Cardizem [U.S., Canada, and multiple international markets] may be confused with Cardem brand name for celiprolol [Spain]

Cartia XT [U.S.] may be confused with Cartia brand name for aspirin [multiple international markets]

Dilacor XR [U.S.] may be confused with Dilacor brand name for verapamil [Brazil]

Dipen [Greece] may be confused with Depen brand name for penicillamine [U.S.]; Depin brand name for nifedipine [India]; Depon brand name for acetaminophen [Greece]

Tiazac: Brand name for diltiazem [U.S, Canada], but also the brand name for pioglitazone [Chile]

Brand Names: U.S. Cardizem®; Cardizem® CD; Cardizem® LA; Cartia XT®; Dilacor XR®; Dilt-CD; Dilt-XR; Diltia XT®; Diltzac; Matzim™ LA; Taztia XT®; Tiazac®

Brand Names: Canada Apo-Diltiaz CD®; Apo-Diltiaz SR®; Apo-Diltiaz TZ®; Apo-Diltiaz®; Apo-Diltiaz® Injectable; Cardizem® CD; Diltiazem HCl ER®; Diltiazem Hydrochloride Injection; Diltiazem TZ; Diltiazem-CD; Nu-Diltiaz; Nu-Diltiaz-CD; PMS-Diltiazem CD; ratio-Diltiazem CD; Sandoz-Diltiazem CD; Sandoz-Diltiazem T; Teva-Diltiazem; Teva-Diltiazem CD; Teva-Diltiazem HCL ER Capsules; Tiazac®; Tiazac® XC

Index Terms Diltiazem Hydrochloride

Generic Availability (U.S.) Yes

Pharmacologic Category Antiarrhythmic Agent, Class IV; Calcium Channel Blocker; Calcium Channel Blocker, Nondihydropyridine

Use

Oral: Essential hypertension; chronic stable angina or angina from coronary artery spasm

Injection: Control of rapid ventricular rate in patients with atrial fibrillation or atrial flutter; conversion of paroxysmal supraventricular tachycardia (PSVT)

Unlabeled/Investigational Use ACLS guidelines: Injection: Stable narrow-complex tachycardia uncontrolled or unconverted by adenosine or vagal maneuvers or if SVT is recurrent

Contraindications

Oral: Hypersensitivity to diltiazem or any component of the formulation; sick sinus syndrome (except in patients with a functioning artificial pacemaker); second- or third-degree AV block (except in patients with a functioning artificial pacemaker); severe hypotension (systolic <90 mm Hg); acute MI and pulmonary congestion

Intravenous (I.V.): Hypersensitivity to diltiazem or any component of the formulation; sick sinus syndrome (except in patients with a functioning artificial pacemaker); second- or third-degree AV block (except in patients with a functioning artificial pacemaker); severe hypotension (systolic <90 mm Hg); cardiogenic shock; administration concomitantly or within a few hours of the administration of I.V. beta-blockers; atrial fibrillation or flutter associated with accessory bypass tract (eg, Wolff-Parkinson-White syndrome); ventricular tachycardia (with wide-complex tachycardia, must determine whether origin is supraventricular or ventricular)

Warnings/Precautions Can cause first-, second-, and third-degree AV block or sinus bradycardia and risk increases with agents known to slow cardiac conduction. The most common side effect is peripheral edema; occurs within 2-3 weeks of starting therapy. Symptomatic hypotension with or without syncope can rarely occur; blood pressure must be lowered at a rate appropriate for the patient's clinical condition. Use caution when using diltiazem together with a beta-blocker; may result in conduction disturbances, hypotension, and worsened LV function. Simultaneous administration of I.V. diltiazem and an I.V. beta-blocker or administration within a few hours of each other may result in asystole and is contraindicated. Use with other agents known to either reduce SA node function and/or AV nodal conduction (eg, digoxin) or reduce sympathetic outflow (eg, clonidine) may increase the risk of serious bradycardia. Use caution in left ventricular dysfunction (may exacerbate condition). Avoid use of diltiazem in patients with heart failure and reduced ejection fraction (Hunt, 2009). Use with caution with hypertrophic obstructive cardiomyopathy; routine use is currently not recommended due to insufficient evidence (Maron, 2003). Use with caution in hepatic or renal dysfunction. Transient dermatologic reactions have been observed with use; if reaction persists, discontinue. May (rarely) progress to erythema multiforme or exfoliative dermatitis.

Adverse Reactions (Reflective of adult population; not specific for elderly) Note: Frequencies represent ranges for various dosage forms. Patients with impaired ventricular function and/or conduction abnormalities may have higher incidence of adverse reactions.

>10%:
Cardiovascular: Edema (2% to 15%)
Central nervous system: Headache (5% to 12%)

2% to 10%:
Cardiovascular: AV block (first degree 2% to 8%), edema (lower limb 2% to 8%), pain (6%), bradycardia (2% to 6%), hypotension (<2% to 4%), vasodilation (2% to 3%), extrasystoles (2%), flushing (1% to 2%), palpitation (1% to 2%)
Central nervous system: Dizziness (3% to 10%), nervousness (2%)
Dermatologic: Rash (1% to 4%)
Endocrine & metabolic: Gout (1% to 2%)

◄ Gastrointestinal: Dyspepsia (1% to 6%), constipation (<2% to 4%), vomiting (2%), diarrhea (1% to 2%)

Local: Injection site reactions: Burning, itching (4%)

Neuromuscular & skeletal: Weakness (1% to 4%), myalgia (2%)

Respiratory: Rhinitis (<2% to 10%), pharyngitis (2% to 6%), dyspnea (1% to 6%), bronchitis (1% to 4%), cough (≤3), sinus congestion (1% to 2%)

Drug Interactions

Metabolism/Transport Effects Substrate of CYP2C9 (minor), 2D6 (minor), 3A4 (major), P-glycoprotein; **Inhibits** CYP2C9 (weak), 2D6 (weak), 3A4 (moderate)

Avoid Concomitant Use

Avoid concomitant use of Diltiazem with any of the following: Conivaptan; Tolvaptan

Increased Effect/Toxicity

Diltiazem may increase the levels/effects of: Alfentanil; Amifostine; Amiodarone; Antihypertensives; Aprepitant; Atorvastatin; Benzodiazepines (metabolized by oxidation); Beta-Blockers; Budesonide (Systemic, Oral Inhalation); BusPIRone; Calcium Channel Blockers (Dihydropyridine); CarBAMazepine; Cardiac Glycosides; Colchicine; Corticosteroids (Systemic); CycloSPORINE; CycloSPORINE (Systemic); CYP3A4 Substrates; Dronedarone; Eletriptan; Eplerenone; Everolimus; Fingolimod; Fosaprepitant; Fosphenytoin; Halofantrine; Hypotensive Agents; Lithium; Lovastatin; Lurasidone; Magnesium Salts; Midodrine; Neuromuscular-Blocking Agents (Nondepolarizing); Nitroprusside; Phenytoin; Pimecrolimus; QuiNIDine; Ranolazine; Red Yeast Rice; RiTUXimab; Rivaroxaban; Salicylates; Salmeterol; Saxagliptin; Simvastatin; Tacrolimus; Tacrolimus (Systemic); Tacrolimus (Topical); Tolvaptan; Vilazodone

The levels/effects of Diltiazem may be increased by: Alpha1-Blockers; Anilidopiperidine Opioids; Antifungal Agents (Azole Derivatives, Systemic); Aprepitant; Atorvastatin; Calcium Channel Blockers (Dihydropyridine); Cimetidine; Conivaptan; CycloSPORINE; CycloSPORINE (Systemic); CYP3A4 Inhibitors (Moderate); CYP3A4 Inhibitors (Strong); Dasatinib; Diazoxide; Dronedarone; Fluconazole; Fosaprepitant; Grapefruit Juice; Herbs (Hypotensive Properties); Lovastatin; Macrolide Antibiotics; Magnesium Salts; MAO Inhibitors; Pentoxifylline; P-Glycoprotein Inhibitors; Phosphodiesterase 5 Inhibitors; Prostacyclin Analogues; Protease Inhibitors; Simvastatin

Decreased Effect

Diltiazem may decrease the levels/effects of: Clopidogrel

The levels/effects of Diltiazem may be decreased by: Barbiturates; Calcium Salts; CarBAMazepine; Colestipol; CYP3A4 Inducers (Strong); Deferasirox; Herbs (CYP3A4 Inducers); Herbs (Hypertensive Properties); Methylphenidate; Nafcillin; Peginterferon Alfa-2b; P-Glycoprotein Inducers; Rifamycin Derivatives; Tocilizumab; Yohimbine

Ethanol/Nutrition/Herb Interactions

Ethanol: Avoid ethanol (may increase risk of hypotension or vasodilation).

Food: Diltiazem serum levels may be elevated if taken with food. Serum concentrations were not altered by grapefruit juice in small clinical trials.

Herb/Nutraceutical: St John's wort may decrease diltiazem levels. Avoid bayberry, blue cohosh, cayenne, ephedra, ginger, ginseng (American), kola, licorice, yohimbe (may worsen hypertension). Avoid black cohosh, California poppy, coleus, garlic, golden seal, hawthorn, mistletoe, periwinkle, quinine, shepherd's purse (may have increased antihypertensive effect).

Stability

Capsule, tablet: Store at room temperature. Protect from light.

Solution for injection: Store in refrigerator at 2°C to 8°C (36°F to 46°F); do not freeze. May be stored at room temperature for up to 1 month. Following dilution to ≤1 mg/mL with $D_5^{1}/_{2}$NS, D_5W, or NS, solution is stable for 24 hours at room temperature or under refrigeration.

Mechanism of Action Nondihydropyridine calcium channel blocker which inhibits calcium ion from entering the "slow channels" or select voltage-sensitive areas of vascular smooth muscle and myocardium during depolarization, producing a relaxation of coronary vascular smooth muscle and coronary vasodilation; increases myocardial oxygen delivery in patients with vasospastic angina

Pharmacodynamics/Kinetics

Onset of action: Oral: Immediate release tablet: 30-60 minutes; I.V.: 3 minutes

Duration: I.V.: Bolus: 1-3 hours; Continuous infusion (after discontinuation): 0.5-10 hours

Absorption: Immediate release tablet: >90%; Extended release capsule: ~93%

Distribution: V_d: 3-13 L/kg

Protein binding: 70% to 80%

Metabolism: Hepatic (extensive first-pass effect); following single I.V. injection, plasma concentrations of N-monodesmethyldiltiazem and desacetyldiltiazem are typically undetectable; however, these metabolites accumulate to detectable concentrations following 24-hour constant rate infusion. N-monodesmethyldiltiazem appears to have 20% of the potency of diltiazem; desacetyldiltiazem is about 25% to 50% as potent as the parent compound.

Bioavailability: Oral: ~40% (undergoes extensive first-pass metabolism)

Half-life elimination: Immediate release tablet: 3-4.5 hours, may be prolonged with renal impairment; Extended release tablet: 6-9 hours; Extended release capsules: 5-10 hours; I.V.: single dose: ~3.4 hours; continuous infusion: 4-5 hours

Time to peak, serum: Immediate release tablet: 2-4 hours; Extended release tablet: 11-18 hours; Extended release capsule: 10-14 hours

Excretion: Urine (2% to 4% as unchanged drug; 6% to 7% as metabolites); feces

Dosage

Geriatric Refer to adult dosing. In the management of hypertension, consider lower initial doses (eg, 120 mg once daily using extended release capsule) and titrate to response (Aronow, 2011).

Adult

Angina: Oral:

Capsule, extended release:

Dilacor XR®, Dilt-XR, Diltia XT®: Initial: 120 mg once daily; titrate over 7-14 days; usual dose range: 120-320 mg/day: maximum: 480 mg/day

Cardizem® CD, Cartia XT®, Dilt-CD: Initial: 120-180 mg once daily; titrate over 7-14 days; usual dose range: 120-320 mg/day; maximum: 480 mg/day

Tiazac®, Taztia XT®: Initial: 120-180 mg once daily; titrate over 7-14 days; usual dose range: 120-320 mg/day; maximum: 540 mg/day

Tablet, extended release (Cardizem® LA, Matzim™ LA, Tiazac® XC [CAN; not available in U.S.]): 180 mg once daily; may increase at 7- to 14-day intervals; usual dose range: 120-320 mg/day; maximum: 360 mg/day

Tablet, immediate release (Cardizem®): Usual starting dose: 30 mg 4 times/day; titrate dose gradually at 1- to 2-day intervals; usual dose range: 120-320 mg/day

Hypertension: Oral:

Capsule, extended release (once-daily dosing):

Cardizem® CD, Cartia XT®, Dilt-CD: Initial: 180-240 mg once daily; dose adjustment may be made after 14 days; usual dose range (JNC 7): 180-420 mg/day; maximum: 480 mg/day

Dilacor® XR, Diltia XT®, Dilt-XR: Initial: 180-240 mg once daily; dose adjustment may be made after 14 days; usual dose range (JNC 7): 180-420 mg/day; maximum: 540 mg/day

Tiazac®, Taztia XT®: Initial: 120-240 mg once daily; dose adjustment may be made after 14 days; usual dose range (JNC 7): 180-420 mg/day; maximum: 540 mg/day

Capsule, extended release (twice-daily dosing): Initial: 60-120 mg twice daily; dose adjustment may be made after 14 days; usual dose range: 240-360 mg/day

Note: Diltiazem is available as a generic intended for either once- or twice-daily dosing, depending on the formulation; verify appropriate extended release capsule formulation is administered.

Tablet, extended release (Cardizem® LA, Matzim™ LA, Tiazac® XC [CAN; not available in U.S.]): Initial: 180-240 mg once daily; dose adjustment may be made after 14 days; usual dose range (JNC 7): 120-540 mg/day

Atrial fibrillation, atrial flutter, PSVT: I.V.:

Initial bolus dose: 0.25 mg/kg actual body weight over 2 minutes (average adult dose: 20 mg); ACLS guideline recommends 15-20 mg

Repeat bolus dose (may be administered after 15 minutes if the response is inadequate): 0.35 mg/kg actual body weight over 2 minutes (average adult dose: 25 mg); ACLS guideline recommends 20-25 mg

Continuous infusion (infusions >24 hours or infusion rates >15 mg/hour are not recommended): Initial infusion rate of 10 mg/hour; rate may be increased in 5 mg/hour increments up to 15 mg/hour as needed; some patients may respond to an initial rate of 5 mg/hour.

If diltiazem injection is administered by continuous infusion for >24 hours, the possibility of decreased diltiazem clearance, prolonged elimination half-life, and increased diltiazem and/or diltiazem metabolite plasma concentrations should be considered.

Conversion from I.V. diltiazem to oral diltiazem:

Oral dose (mg/day) is approximately equal to [rate (mg/hour) x 3 + 3] x 10.

3 mg/hour = 120 mg/day
5 mg/hour = 180 mg/day
7 mg/hour = 240 mg/day
11 mg/hour = 360 mg/day

Renal Impairment Use with caution; no dosing adjustments recommended.

Dialysis: Not removed by hemo- or peritoneal dialysis; supplemental dose is not necessary.

◀ **Hepatic Impairment** Use with caution; no specific dosing recommendations available; extensively metabolized by the liver; half-life is increased in patients with cirrhosis.

Administration

Oral:

Immediate release tablet (Cardizem®): Administer before meals and at bedtime.

Long acting dosage forms: Do not open, chew, or crush; swallow whole.

Cardizem® CD, Cardizem® LA, Cartia XT®, Dilt-CD, Matzim™ LA: May be administered without regards to meals.

Dilacor XR®, Dilt-XR, Diltia XT®: Administer on an empty stomach.

Taztia XT™, Tiazac®: Capsules may be opened and sprinkled on a spoonful of apple-sauce. Applesauce should not be hot and should be swallowed without chewing, followed by drinking a glass of water.

Tiazac® XC [CAN; not available in U.S.]: Administer at bedtime

I.V.: Bolus doses given over 2 minutes with continuous ECG and blood pressure monitoring. Continuous infusion should be via infusion pump.

Monitoring Parameters Liver function tests, blood pressure, ECG, heart rate

Special Geriatric Considerations Elderly may experience a greater hypotensive response; constipation may be encountered more often in elderly. Calcium channel blockers are no more effective in elderly than other therapies; however, they do not cause significant CNS effects which is an advantage over other antihypertensive agents (eg, beta-blockers, clonidine).

Dosage Forms Excipient information presented when available (limited, particularly for generics); consult specific product labeling.

Capsule, extended release, oral, as hydrochloride [once-daily dosing]: 120 mg, 180 mg, 240 mg, 300 mg, 360 mg, 420 mg

Cardizem® CD: 120 mg, 180 mg, 240 mg, 300 mg, 360 mg

Cartia XT®: 120 mg, 180 mg, 240 mg, 300 mg

Dilacor XR®: 240 mg

Dilt-CD: 120 mg, 180 mg, 240 mg, 300 mg

Dilt-XR: 120 mg, 180 mg, 240 mg

Diltia XT®: 120 mg, 180 mg, 240 mg

Diltzac: 120 mg, 180 mg, 240 mg, 300 mg, 360 mg

Taztia XT®: 120 mg, 180 mg, 240 mg, 300 mg, 360 mg

Tiazac®: 120 mg, 180 mg, 240 mg, 300 mg, 360 mg, 420 mg

Capsule, extended release, oral, as hydrochloride [twice-daily dosing]: 60 mg, 90 mg, 120 mg

Injection, powder for reconstitution, as hydrochloride: 100 mg

Injection, solution, as hydrochloride: 5 mg/mL (5 mL, 10 mL, 25 mL)

Tablet, oral, as hydrochloride: 30 mg, 60 mg, 90 mg, 120 mg

Cardizem®: 30 mg

Cardizem®: 60 mg, 90 mg, 120 mg [scored]

Tablet, extended release, oral, as hydrochloride [once-daily dosing]:

Cardizem® LA: 120 mg, 180 mg, 240 mg, 300 mg, 360 mg, 420 mg

Matzim™ LA: 180 mg, 240 mg, 300 mg, 360 mg, 420 mg

Dosage Forms: Canada Excipient information presented when available (limited, particularly for generics); consult specific product labeling.

Tablet, extended release, as hydrochloride:

Tiazac® XC: 120 mg, 180 mg, 240 mg, 300 mg, 360 mg

Selected References

Chobanian AV, Bakris GL, Black HR, et al, "The Seventh Report of the Joint National Committee on Prevention, Detection, Evaluation, and Treatment of High Blood Pressure: The JNC 7 Report," *JAMA*, 2003, 289(19):2560-71.

Hunt SA, Abraham WT, Chin MH, et al, "2009 Focused Update Incorporated into the ACC/AHA 2005 Guidelines for the Diagnosis and Management of Heart Failure in Adults: A Report of the American College of Cardiology Foundation/ American Heart Association Task Force on Practice Guidelines Developed in Collaboration With the International Society for Heart and Lung Transplantation," *J Am Coll Cardiol*, 2009, 53(15):e1-e90.

Maron BJ, McKenna WJ, Danielson GK, et al, "American College of Cardiology/European Society of Cardiology Clinical Expert Consensus Document on Hypertrophic Cardiomyopathy. A Report of the American College of Cardiology Foundation Task Force on Clinical Expert Consensus Documents and the European Society of Cardiology Committee for Practice Guidelines," *J Am Coll Cardiol*, 2003, 42(9):1687-713.

White WB, Lacourciere Y, Gana T, et al, "Effects of Graded-Release Diltiazem Versus Ramipril, Dosed at Bedtime, on Early Morning Blood Pressure, Heart Rate, and the Rate-Pressure Product," *Am Heart J*, 2004, 148(4):628-34.

♦ **Diltiazem Hydrochloride** see Diltiazem on page 514
♦ **Dilt-XR** see Diltiazem on page 514
♦ **Diltzac** see Diltiazem on page 514

DimenhyDRINATE (dye men HYE dri nate)

Medication Safety Issues

Sound-alike/look-alike issues:

DimenhyDRINATE may be confused with diphenhydrAMINE

Brand Names: U.S. Dramamine® [OTC]; Driminate [OTC]; TripTone® [OTC]

Brand Names: Canada Apo-Dimenhydrinate®; Children's Motion Sickness Liquid; Dimenhydrinate Injection; Dinate®; Gravol®; Nauseatol; Novo-Dimenate; PMS-Dimenhydrinate; Sandoz-Dimenhydrinate

Generic Availability (U.S.) Yes

Pharmacologic Category Ethanolamine Derivative; Histamine H_1 Antagonist; Histamine H_1 Antagonist, First Generation

Use Treatment and prevention of nausea, vertigo, and vomiting associated with motion sickness

Unlabeled/Investigational Use Treatment of Meniere's disease

Contraindications Hypersensitivity to dimenhydrinate or any component of the formulation

Warnings/Precautions Causes sedation, caution must be used in performing tasks which require alertness (eg, operating machinery or driving). May mask the symptoms of ototoxicity, use caution if used in conjuction with antibiotics that have the potential to cause ototoxicity. Effects may be potentiated when used with other sedative drugs or ethanol. Use with caution in patients with angle-closure glaucoma, asthma, pyloroduodenal obstruction (including stenotic peptic ulcer), urinary tract obstruction (including bladder neck obstruction and symptomatic prostatic hyperplasia), hyperthyroidism, increased intraocular pressure, and cardiovascular disease (including hypertension and tachycardia). Use with caution in the elderly; may be more sensitive to adverse effects. Some products may contain phenylalanine. Parenteral formulation should not be injected intra-arterially.

Adverse Reactions (Reflective of adult population; not specific for elderly) Frequency not defined.

Cardiovascular: Tachycardia

Central nervous system: Dizziness, drowsiness, excitation, headache, insomnia, lassitude, nervousness, restlessness

Dermatologic: Rash

Gastrointestinal: Anorexia, epigastric distress, nausea, xerostomia

Genitourinary: Dysuria

Ocular: Blurred vision

Respiratory: Thickening of bronchial secretions

Drug Interactions

Avoid Concomitant Use There are no known interactions where it is recommended to avoid concomitant use.

Increased Effect/Toxicity

DimenhyDRINATE may increase the levels/effects of: Alcohol (Ethyl); Anticholinergics; CNS Depressants; Selective Serotonin Reuptake Inhibitors

The levels/effects of DimenhyDRINATE may be increased by: Droperidol; HydrOXYzine; Pramlintide

Decreased Effect

DimenhyDRINATE may decrease the levels/effects of: Acetylcholinesterase Inhibitors (Central); Benzylpenicilloyl Polylysine; Betahistine

The levels/effects of DimenhyDRINATE may be decreased by: Acetylcholinesterase Inhibitors (Central); Amphetamines

Ethanol/Nutrition/Herb Interactions Ethanol: May increase CNS depression; monitor for increased effects with coadministration. Caution patients about effects.

Stability Injection: Store at 20°C to 25°C (68°F to 77°F). Protect from light.

Mechanism of Action Competes with histamine for H_1-receptor sites on effector cells in the gastrointestinal tract, blood vessels, and respiratory tract; blocks chemoreceptor trigger zone, diminishes vestibular stimulation, and depresses labyrinthine function through its central anticholinergic activity

Pharmacodynamics/Kinetics

Onset of action: Oral: ~15-30 minutes

Absorption: Oral: Well absorbed

Dosage

Geriatric & Adult Motion sickness (prevention/treatment):

Oral: 50-100 mg every 4-6 hours, not to exceed 400 mg/day

I.M., I.V.: 50 mg every 4 hours; maximum: 100 mg every 4 hours

Administration I.V. injection must be diluted to 10 mL with normal saline and given at 25 mg/minute

Monitoring Parameters Monitor for anticholinergic side effects; emetic episodes and nausea

Special Geriatric Considerations Monitor for anticholinergic side effects (confusion, constipation, etc); if possible, limit use to short-term therapy

◀ **Dosage Forms** Excipient information presented when available (limited, particularly for generics); consult specific product labeling. [DSC] = Discontinued product
Injection, solution: 50 mg/mL (1 mL) [contains benzyl alcohol]
Tablet, oral: 50 mg [DSC]
  Dramamine®: 50 mg [scored]
  Driminate: 50 mg [scored]
  TripTone®: 50 mg
Tablet, chewable, oral:
  Dramamine®: 50 mg [scored; contains phenylalanine 0.84 mg/tablet; orange flavor]

♦ **Diocto [OTC]** see Docusate on page 547
♦ **Dioctyl Calcium Sulfosuccinate** see Docusate on page 547
♦ **Dioctyl Sodium Sulfosuccinate** see Docusate on page 547
♦ **Diotame [OTC]** see Bismuth on page 207
♦ **Diovan®** see Valsartan on page 1892
♦ **Diovan HCT®** see Valsartan and Hydrochlorothiazide on page 1894
♦ **Dipentum®** see Olsalazine on page 1337
♦ **Diphen [OTC]** see DiphenhydrAMINE (Systemic) on page 520
♦ **Diphenhist® [OTC]** see DiphenhydrAMINE (Systemic) on page 520
♦ **Diphenhist® [OTC] [DSC]** see DiphenhydrAMINE (Topical) on page 523

DiphenhydrAMINE (Systemic) (dye fen HYE dra meen)

Related Information
Beers Criteria – Potentially Inappropriate Medications for Geriatrics on page 2089
Medication Safety Issues
Sound-alike/look-alike issues:
  DiphenhydrAMINE may be confused with desipramine, dicyclomine, dimenhyDRINATE
  Benadryl® may be confused with benazepril, Bentyl®, Benylin®, Caladryl®
BEERS Criteria medication:
  This drug may be inappropriate for use in geriatric patients (high severity risk).
International issues:
  Sominex®: Brand name for promethazine in Great Britain
Brand Names: U.S. Aler-Cap [OTC]; Aler-Dryl [OTC]; Aler-Tab [OTC]; AllerMax® [OTC]; Altaryl [OTC]; Anti-Hist [OTC]; Banophen™ [OTC]; Benadryl® Allergy Quick Dissolve [OTC]; Benadryl® Allergy [OTC]; Benadryl® Children's Allergy FastMelt® [OTC]; Benadryl® Children's Allergy Perfect Measure™ [OTC]; Benadryl® Children's Allergy [OTC]; Benadryl® Children's Dye Free Allergy [OTC]; Benadryl® Dye-Free Allergy [OTC]; Compoz® [OTC]; Diphen [OTC]; Diphenhist® [OTC]; Histaprin [OTC]; Nytol® Quick Caps [OTC]; Nytol® Quick Gels [OTC]; PediaCare® Children's Allergy [OTC]; PediaCare® Children's NightTime Cough [OTC]; Siladryl Allergy [OTC]; Silphen [OTC]; Simply Sleep® [OTC]; Sleep-ettes D [OTC]; Sleep-Tabs [OTC]; Sleepinal® [OTC]; Sominex® Maximum Strength [OTC]; Sominex® [OTC]; Theraflu® Thin Strips® Multi Symptom [OTC]; Triaminic Thin Strips® Children's Cough & Runny Nose [OTC]; Twilite® [OTC]; Unisom® SleepGels® Maximum Strength [OTC]; Unisom® SleepMelts™ [OTC]
Brand Names: Canada Allerdryl®; Allernix®; Benadryl®; Nytol®; Nytol® Extra Strength; PMS-Diphenhydramine; Simply Sleep®; Sominex®
Index Terms Diphenhydramine Citrate; Diphenhydramine Hydrochloride; Diphenhydramine Tannate
Generic Availability (U.S.) Yes: Excludes orally-disintegrating tablet, strip
Pharmacologic Category Ethanolamine Derivative; Histamine H$_1$ Antagonist; Histamine H$_1$ Antagonist, First Generation
Use Symptomatic relief of allergic symptoms caused by histamine release including nasal allergies and allergic dermatosis; adjunct to epinephrine in the treatment of anaphylaxis; nighttime sleep aid; prevention or treatment of motion sickness; antitussive; management of Parkinsonian syndrome including drug-induced extrapyramidal symptoms
Contraindications Hypersensitivity to diphenhydramine or any component of the formulation; acute asthma; use as a local anesthetic (injection)
Warnings/Precautions Causes sedation, caution must be used in performing tasks which require alertness (eg, operating machinery or driving). Sedative effects of CNS depressants or ethanol are potentiated. Should not be used as a hypnotic in the elderly; may cause excessive sedation and confusion; may be inappropriate in this age group when used as an antihistamine due to potent anticholinergic effects (nonanticholinergic antihistamines preferred); when used for emergency allergic reactions, use the smallest effective dose (Beers Criteria). Use with caution in patients with angle-closure glaucoma, pyloroduodenal obstruction (including stenotic peptic ulcer), urinary tract obstruction (including bladder neck obstruction and symptomatic prostatic hyperplasia), asthma, hyperthyroidism, increased intraocular

pressure, and cardiovascular disease (including hypertension and tachycardia). Some preparations contain soy protein; avoid use in patients with soy protein or peanut allergies. Some products may contain phenylalanine.

Self-medication (OTC use): Do not use with other products containing diphenhydramine, even ones used on the skin.

Adverse Reactions (Reflective of adult population; not specific for elderly) Frequency not defined.

Cardiovascular: Chest tightness, extrasystoles, hypotension, palpitation, tachycardia

Central nervous system: Chills, confusion, convulsion, disturbed coordination, dizziness, euphoria, excitation, fatigue, headache, insomnia, irritability, nervousness, paradoxical excitement, restlessness, sedation, sleepiness, vertigo

Endocrine & metabolic: Menstrual irregularities (early menses)

Gastrointestinal: Anorexia, constipation, diarrhea, dry mucous membranes, epigastric distress, nausea, throat tightness, vomiting, xerostomia

Genitourinary: Difficult urination, urinary frequency, urinary retention

Hematologic: Agranulocytosis, hemolytic anemia, thrombocytopenia

Neuromuscular & skeletal: Neuritis, paresthesia, tremor

Ocular: Blurred vision, diplopia

Otic: Labyrinthitis (acute), tinnitus

Respiratory: Nasal stuffiness, thickening of bronchial secretions, wheezing

Miscellaneous: Anaphylactic shock, diaphoresis

Drug Interactions

Metabolism/Transport Effects Inhibits CYP2D6 (moderate)

Avoid Concomitant Use There are no known interactions where it is recommended to avoid concomitant use.

Increased Effect/Toxicity

DiphenhydrAMINE (Systemic) may increase the levels/effects of: Alcohol (Ethyl); Anticholinergics; CNS Depressants; CYP2D6 Substrates; Fesoterodine; Nebivolol; Selective Serotonin Reuptake Inhibitors; Tamoxifen

The levels/effects of DiphenhydrAMINE (Systemic) may be increased by: Droperidol; HydrOXYzine; Pramlintide

Decreased Effect

DiphenhydrAMINE (Systemic) may decrease the levels/effects of: Acetylcholinesterase Inhibitors (Central); Benzylpenicilloyl Polylysine; Betahistine; Codeine; TraMADol

The levels/effects of DiphenhydrAMINE (Systemic) may be decreased by: Acetylcholinesterase Inhibitors (Central); Amphetamines

Ethanol/Nutrition/Herb Interactions

Ethanol: May increase CNS depression; monitor for increased effects with coadministration. Caution patients about effects.

Herb/Nutraceutical: Avoid valerian, St John's wort, kava kava, gotu kola (may increase CNS depression).

Stability Injection: Store at room temperature of 15°C to 30°C (59°F to 86°F); protect from freezing. Protect from light.

Mechanism of Action Competes with histamine for H_1-receptor sites on effector cells in the gastrointestinal tract, blood vessels, and respiratory tract; anticholinergic and sedative effects are also seen

Pharmacodynamics/Kinetics

Onset of action: Maximum sedative effect: 1-3 hours

Duration: 4-7 hours

Distribution: V_d: 3-22 L/kg

Protein binding: 78%

Metabolism: Extensively hepatic n-demethylation via CYP2D6; minor demethylation via CYP1A2, 2C9 and 2C19; smaller degrees in pulmonary and renal systems; significant first-pass effect

Bioavailability: Oral: ~40% to 70%

Half-life elimination: 2-10 hours; Elderly: 13.5 hours

Time to peak, serum: 2-4 hours

Excretion: Urine (as unchanged drug)

Dosage

Geriatric Initial: 25 mg 2-3 times/day increasing as needed

Adult Note: Dosages are expressed as the hydrochloride salt.

Allergic reactions or motion sickness:

Oral: 25-50 mg every 6-8 hours

I.M., I.V.: 10-50 mg per dose; single doses up to 100 mg may be used if needed; not to exceed 400 mg/day

Antitussive: Oral: 25 mg every 4 hours; maximum: 150 mg/24 hours
Night-time sleep aid: Oral: 50 mg at bedtime
Dystonic reaction: I.M., I.V.: 50 mg in a single dose; may repeat in 20-30 minutes if necessary

Administration When used to prevent motion sickness, first dose should be given 30 minutes prior to exposure. Injection solution is for I.V. or I.M. administration only; local necrosis may result with SubQ or intradermal use. For I.V. administration, inject at a rate ≤25 mg/minute.

Monitoring Parameters Relief of symptoms, mental alertness

Test Interactions May interfere with urine detection of methadone and PCP (false-positives); may cause false-positive serum TCA screen; may suppress the wheal and flare reactions to skin test antigens

Pharmacotherapy Pearls Diphenhydramine citrate 19 mg is equivalent to diphenhydramine hydrochloride 12.5 mg

Special Geriatric Considerations Diphenhydramine has high sedative and anticholinergic properties, so it may not be considered the antihistamine of choice for prolonged use in the elderly. Its use as a sleep aid is discouraged due to its anticholinergic effects; interpretive guidelines from the Centers for Medicare and Medicaid Services (CMS) discourage the use of diphenhydramine as a sedative or anxiolytic in long-term care facilities.

This medication is considered to be potentially inappropriate in this patient population (Beers Criteria severity: High).

Dosage Forms Excipient information presented when available (limited, particularly for generics); consult specific product labeling. [DSC] = Discontinued product
Caplet, oral, as hydrochloride: 25 mg [DSC]
  Aler-Dryl: 50 mg
  AllerMax®: 50 mg
  Anti-Hist: 25 mg
  Compoz®: 50 mg
  Histaprin: 25 mg
  Nytol® Quick Caps: 25 mg
  Simply Sleep®: 25 mg [contains calcium 20 mg/caplet]
  Sleep-ettes D: 50 mg
  Sominex® Maximum Strength: 50 mg
  Twilite®: 50 mg
Capsule, oral, as hydrochloride: 25 mg, 50 mg
  Aler-Cap: 25 mg
  Banophen™: 25 mg
  Benadryl® Allergy: 25 mg [contains calcium 35 mg/capsule]
  Diphen: 25 mg
  Diphenhist®: 25 mg
  Sleepinal®: 50 mg
Capsule, softgel, oral, as hydrochloride:
  Benadryl® Dye-Free Allergy: 25 mg [dye free]
  Compoz®: 50 mg
  Nytol® Quick Gels: 50 mg
  Unisom® SleepGels® Maximum Strength: 50 mg
Captab, oral, as hydrochloride:
  Diphenhist®: 25 mg
Elixir, oral, as hydrochloride:
  Altaryl: 12.5 mg/5 mL (120 mL, 480 mL, 3840 mL) [ethanol free; cherry flavor]
  Banophen™: 12.5 mg/5 mL (120 mL)
  Banophen™: 12.5 mg/5 mL (480 mL) [sugar free]
Injection, solution, as hydrochloride: 50 mg/mL (1 mL, 10 mL)
Injection, solution, as hydrochloride [preservative free]: 50 mg/mL (1 mL)
Liquid, oral, as hydrochloride:
  AllerMax®: 12.5 mg/5 mL (120 mL)
  Benadryl® Children's Allergy: 12.5 mg/5 mL (118 mL, 236 mL) [ethanol free; contains sodium 14 mg/5 mL, sodium benzoate; cherry flavor]
  Benadryl® Children's Allergy Perfect Measure™: 12.5 mg/5 mL (5 mL) [ethanol free; contains sodium 14 mg/5 mL, sodium benzoate; cherry flavor]
  Benadryl® Children's Dye Free Allergy: 12.5 mg/5 mL (118 mL) [dye free, ethanol free, sugar free; contains sodium 11 mg/5 mL, sodium benzoate; bubblegum flavor]
  Siladryl Allergy: 12.5 mg/5 mL (118 mL, 237 mL, 473 mL) [ethanol free, sugar free; black-cherry flavor]
Solution, oral, as hydrochloride: 12.5 mg/5 mL (5 mL, 10 mL, 20 mL [DSC])
  Diphenhist®: 12.5 mg/5 mL (120 mL, 480 mL) [ethanol free; contains sodium benzoate]

Strip, orally disintegrating, oral, as hydrochloride:
  Benadryl® Allergy Quick Dissolve: 25 mg (10s) [contains sodium 4 mg/strip; vanilla-mint flavor]
  Theraflu® Thin Strips® Multi Symptom: 25 mg (12s, 24s) [contains ethanol; cherry flavor]
  Triaminic Thin Strips® Children's Cough & Runny Nose: 12.5 mg (14s) [contains ethanol; grape flavor]
Syrup, oral, as hydrochloride:
  PediaCare® Children's Allergy: 12.5 mg/5 mL (118 mL) [contains sodium 14 mg/5 mL, sodium benzoate; cherry flavor]
  PediaCare® Children's NightTime Cough: 12.5 mg/5 mL (118 mL) [ethanol free; contains sodium 15 mg/5 mL, sodium benzoate; cherry flavor]
  Silphen: 12.5 mg/5 mL (118 mL, 237 mL, 473 mL) [contains ethanol 5%; strawberry flavor]
Tablet, oral, as hydrochloride: 25 mg, 50 mg
  Aler-Tab: 25 mg
  Banophen™: 25 mg
  Benadryl® Allergy: 25 mg
  Sleep-Tabs: 25 mg
  Sominex®: 25 mg
Tablet, orally dissolving, oral, as hydrochloride:
  Unisom® SleepMelts™: 25 mg [cherry flavor]
Tablet, orally dissolving, oral, as hydrochloride [strength expressed as base]:
  Benadryl® Children's Allergy FastMelt®: 12.5 mg [cherry flavor]
Selected References
Simons KJ, Watson WT, Martin TJ, et al, "Diphenhydramine: Pharmacokinetics and Pharmacodynamics in Elderly Adults, Young Adults, and Children," *J Clin Pharmacol*, 1990, 30(7):665-71.

DiphenhydrAMINE (Topical) (dye fen HYE dra meen)

Medication Safety Issues
  Sound-alike/look-alike issues:
    DiphenhydrAMINE may be confused with desipramine, dicyclomine, dimenhyDRINATE
    Benadryl® may be confused with benazepril, Bentyl®, Benylin®, Caladryl®
  Administration issues:
    Institute for Safe Medication Practices (ISMP) has reported cases of patients mistakenly *swallowing* Benadryl® Itch Stopping [OTC] gel intended for topical application. Unclear labeling and similar packaging of the topical gel in containers resembling an oral liquid are factors believed to be contributing to the administration errors. The topical gel contains camphor which can be toxic if swallowed. ISMP has requested the manufacturer to make the necessary changes to prevent further confusion.
Brand Names: U.S. Banophen™ Anti-Itch [OTC]; Benadryl® Extra Strength Itch Stopping [OTC]; Benadryl® Itch Relief Extra Strength [OTC]; Benadryl® Itch Stopping Extra Strength [OTC]; Benadryl® Itch Stopping [OTC]; Dermamycin® [OTC]; Diphenhist® [OTC] [DSC]
Brand Names: Canada Benadryl® Cream; Benadryl® Itch Relief Stick; Benadryl® Spray
Index Terms Diphenhydramine Hydrochloride
Generic Availability (U.S.) Yes: Excludes gel, liquid stick, spray
Pharmacologic Category Ethanolamine Derivative; Histamine H_1 Antagonist; Histamine H_1 Antagonist, First Generation; Topical Skin Product
Use Topically for relief of pain and itching associated with insect bites, minor cuts and burns, or rashes due to poison ivy, poison oak, and poison sumac
Dosage
  Adult Relief of pain and itching: Topical: Apply 1% or 2% to affected area up to 3-4 times/day
Dosage Forms Excipient information presented when available (limited, particularly for generics); consult specific product labeling. [DSC] = Discontinued product
Cream, topical, as hydrochloride: 2% (30 g)
  Banophen™ Anti-Itch: 2% (28.4 g) [contains zinc acetate 0.1%]
  Benadryl® Itch Stopping: 1% (14.2 g, 28.3 g) [contains zinc acetate 0.1%]
  Benadryl® Itch Stopping Extra Strength: 2% (14.2 g, 28.3 g) [contains zinc acetate 0.1%]
  Dermamycin®: 2% (28 g)
  Diphenhist®: 2% (28.4 g [DSC]) [contains zinc acetate 0.1%]
Gel, topical, as hydrochloride:
  Benadryl® Extra Strength Itch Stopping: 2% (120 mL)
Liquid, topical, as hydrochloride [spray]:
  Benadryl® Itch Stopping Extra Strength: 2% (59 mL) [contains ethanol; contains zinc acetate 0.1%]
  Dermamycin®: 2% (60 mL) [contains menthol]

Liquid, topical, as hydrochloride [stick]:
Benadryl® Itch Relief Extra Strength: 2% (14 mL) [contains ethanol; contains zinc acetate 0.1%]

Diphenoxylate and Atropine (dye fen OKS i late & A troe peen)

Related Information
Atropine *on page 165*
Medication Safety Issues
Sound-alike/look-alike issues:
Lomotil® may be confused with LaMICtal®, LamISIL®, lamoTRIgine, Lanoxin®, Lasix®
Lonox® may be confused with Lanoxin®, Loprox®
International issues:
Lomotil [U.S., Canada, and multiple international markets] may be confused with Lamictal brand name for lamotrigine [U.S., Canada, and multiple international markets]; lamotrigine [U.S., Canada, and multiple international markets]; Ludiomil brand name for maprotiline [multiple international markets]
Lomotil: Brand name for diphenoxylate [U.S., Canada, and multiple international markets], but also the brand name for loperamide [Mexico, Philippines]
Brand Names: U.S. Lomotil®
Brand Names: Canada Lomotil®
Index Terms Atropine and Diphenoxylate
Generic Availability (U.S.) Yes
Pharmacologic Category Antidiarrheal
Use Treatment of diarrhea
Contraindications Hypersensitivity to diphenoxylate, atropine, or any component of the formulation; obstructive jaundice; diarrhea associated with pseudomembranous enterocolitis or enterotoxin-producing bacteria
Warnings/Precautions Use in conjunction with fluid and electrolyte therapy when appropriate. In case of severe dehydration or electrolyte imbalance, withhold diphenoxylate/atropine treatment until corrective therapy has been initiated. Inhibiting peristalsis may lead to fluid retention in the intestine aggravating dehydration and electrolyte imbalance. Reduction of intestinal motility may be deleterious in diarrhea resulting from *Shigella, Salmonella*, toxigenic strains of *E. coli*, and pseudomembranous enterocolitis associated with broad-spectrum antibiotics; use is not recommended.

Use caution with acute ulcerative colitis, hepatic or renal dysfunction. If there is no response with 48 hours, this medication is unlikely to be effective and should be discontinued; if chronic diarrhea is not improved symptomatically within 10 days at maximum dosage, control is unlikely with further use. Physical and psychological dependence have been reported with higher than recommended dosing.
Adverse Reactions (Reflective of adult population; not specific for elderly) Frequency not defined.
Cardiovascular: Tachycardia
Central nervous system: Confusion, depression, dizziness, drowsiness, euphoria, flushing, headache, hyperthermia, lethargy, malaise, restlessness, sedation
Dermatologic: Angioneurotic edema, dry skin, pruritus, urticaria
Gastrointestinal: Abdominal discomfort, anorexia, gum swelling, nausea, pancreatitis, paralytic ileus, toxic megacolon, vomiting, xerostomia
Genitourinary: Urinary retention
Neuromuscular & skeletal: Numbness
Miscellaneous: Anaphylaxis
Drug Interactions
Avoid Concomitant Use There are no known interactions where it is recommended to avoid concomitant use.
Increased Effect/Toxicity
Diphenoxylate and Atropine may increase the levels/effects of: AbobotulinumtoxinA; Alcohol (Ethyl); Anticholinergics; Cannabinoids; CNS Depressants; Methotrimeprazine; OnabotulinumtoxinA; Potassium Chloride; RimabotulinumtoxinB; Selective Serotonin Reuptake Inhibitors

The levels/effects of Diphenoxylate and Atropine may be increased by: Droperidol; HydrOXYzine; Methotrimeprazine; Pramlintide

Decreased Effect

Diphenoxylate and Atropine may decrease the levels/effects of: Acetylcholinesterase Inhibitors (Central); Secretin

The levels/effects of Diphenoxylate and Atropine may be decreased by: Acetylcholinesterase Inhibitors (Central)

Ethanol/Nutrition/Herb Interactions Ethanol: May increase CNS depression; monitor for increased effects with coadministration. Caution patients about effects.

Mechanism of Action Diphenoxylate inhibits excessive GI motility and GI propulsion; commercial preparations contain a subtherapeutic amount of atropine to discourage abuse

Pharmacodynamics/Kinetics

Atropine: See Atropine monograph.

Diphenoxylate:

Onset of action: Antidiarrheal: 45-60 minutes

Duration: Antidiarrheal: 3-4 hours

Absorption: Well absorbed

Metabolism: Extensively hepatic via ester hydrolysis to diphenoxylic acid (active)

Half-life elimination: Diphenoxylate: 2.5 hours; Diphenoxylic acid: 12-14 hours

Time to peak, serum: 2 hours

Excretion: Primarily feces (49% as unchanged drug and metabolites); urine (~14%, <1% as unchanged drug)

Dosage

Geriatric & Adult Diarrhea: Oral: Diphenoxylate 5 mg 4 times/day until control achieved (maximum: 20 mg/day), then reduce dose as needed; some patients may be controlled on doses of 5 mg/day

Administration If there is no response within 48 hours of continuous therapy, this medication is unlikely to be effective and should be discontinued; if chronic diarrhea is not improved symptomatically within 10 days at maximum dosage, control is unlikely with further use.

Monitoring Parameters Watch for signs of atropinism (dryness of skin and mucous membranes, tachycardia, thirst, flushing); monitor number and consistency of stools; observe for signs of toxicity, fluid and electrolyte loss, hypotension, and respiratory depression

Pharmacotherapy Pearls If there is no response within 48 hours, the drug is unlikely to be effective and should be discontinued. If chronic diarrhea is not improved symptomatically within 10 days at maximum dosage of 20 mg/day, control is unlikely with further use. Diarrhea should also be treated with dietary measures (ie, clear liquids), and avoid milk products and high sodium foods such as bouillon and soups.

Special Geriatric Considerations Elderly are particularly sensitive to fluid and electrolyte loss. This generally results in lethargy, weakness, and confusion. Repletion and maintenance of electrolytes and water are essential in the treatment of diarrhea. Drug therapy must be limited in order to avoid toxicity with this agent.

Controlled Substance C-V

Dosage Forms Excipient information presented when available (limited, particularly for generics); consult specific product labeling. [DSC] = Discontinued product

Solution, oral: Diphenoxylate hydrochloride 2.5 mg and atropine sulfate 0.025 mg per 5 mL (5 mL, 10 mL, 60 mL)

Lomotil®: Diphenoxylate hydrochloride 2.5 mg and atropine sulfate 0.025 mg per 5 mL (60 mL) [contains alcohol 15%; cherry flavor] [DSC]

Tablet: Diphenoxylate hydrochloride 2.5 mg and atropine sulfate 0.025 mg

Lomotil®: Diphenoxylate hydrochloride 2.5 mg and atropine sulfate 0.025 mg

◆ **Diphenylhydantoin** *see* Phenytoin *on page 1444*

Diphtheria and Tetanus Toxoids (dif THEER ee a & TET a nus TOKS oyds)

Related Information

Immunization Administration Recommendations *on page 2037*

Immunization Recommendations *on page 2043*

Tetanus Toxoid (Adsorbed) *on page 1769*

Medication Safety Issues

Sound-alike/look-alike issues:

Diphtheria and Tetanus Toxoids (Td) may be confused with tuberculin purified protein derivative (PPD)

Pediatric diphtheria and tetanus (DT) may be confused with adult tetanus and diphtheria (Td)

Brand Names: U.S. Decavac®

Brand Names: Canada Td Adsorbed

Index Terms DT; Td; Tetanus and Diphtheria Toxoid

Generic Availability (U.S.) Yes

DIPHTHERIA AND TETANUS TOXOIDS

Pharmacologic Category Vaccine, Inactivated (Bacterial)
Use

Tetanus and diphtheria toxoids adsorbed for adult use (Td) (Decavac®): Adults: Active immunization against diphtheria and tetanus; tetanus prophylaxis in wound management

The Advisory Committee on Immunization Practices (ACIP) recommends routine vaccination for the following:
- Adults should receive a booster dose of Td every 10 years; may substitute a single Td booster dose with Tdap
- Adults and the elderly (≥65 years) who are wounded in bombings or similar mass casualty events who have penetrating injuries or nonintact skin exposure and who cannot confirm receipt of a tetanus booster within the previous 5 years, may also receive a single dose of Td; children ≥11 years and adults may also receive Td if Tdap is unavailable

Contraindications Hypersensitivity to diphtheria, tetanus toxoid, or any component of the formulation

Warnings/Precautions Do not confuse pediatric diphtheria and tetanus (DT) with adult tetanus and diphtheria (Td). Immediate treatment for anaphylactic/anaphylactoid reaction should be available during administration. Patients with a history of severe local reaction (Arthus-type) following a previous dose should not be given further routine or emergency doses of Td more frequently than every 10 years even if using for wound management with wounds that are not clean or minor; these patients generally have high serum antitoxin levels. Continue use with caution if Guillain-Barré syndrome occurs within 6 weeks of prior tetanus toxoid. For I.M. administration; use caution with history of bleeding disorders or anticoagulant therapy. Defer administration during moderate or severe illness (with or without fever). Immune response may be decreased in immunocompromised patients; in general, household and close contacts of persons with altered immunocompetence may receive all age appropriate vaccines. Some products may contain natural latex/natural rubber or thimerosal. In order to maximize vaccination rates, the ACIP recommends simultaneous administration of all age-appropriate vaccines (live or inactivated) for which a person is eligible at a single clinic visit, unless contraindications exist. The use of combination vaccines is generally preferred over separate injections, taking into consideration provider assessment, patient preference, and adverse events.

Adverse Reactions (Reflective of adult population; not specific for elderly) All serious adverse reactions must be reported to the U.S. Department of Health and Human Services (DHHS) Vaccine Adverse Event Reporting System (VAERS) 1-800-822-7967 or online at https://vaers.hhs.gov/esub/index. In Canada, adverse reactions may be reported to local provincial/territorial health agencies or to the Vaccine Safety Section at Public Health Agency of Canada (1-866-844-0018).

Note: Percentages noted within 2 weeks following booster dose of Decavac® in persons ≥11 years of age:
>10%:
Central nervous system: Headache (34% to 40%), tiredness (21% to 27%), chills (7% to 13%)
Gastrointestinal: Nausea (8% to 12%), diarrhea (10% to 11%)
Local: Injection site: Pain (63% to 71%), erythema (20% to 22%), swelling (17% to 18%)
Neuromuscular & skeletal: Body ache/muscle weakness (19% to 30%), sore/swollen joints (7% to 12%)
1% to 10%:
Central nervous system: Fever (1% to 3%)
Dermatologic: Rash (2%)
Endocrine & metabolic: Lymph node swelling (4% to 5%)
Gastrointestinal: Vomiting (2% to 3%)

Drug Interactions

Avoid Concomitant Use There are no known interactions where it is recommended to avoid concomitant use.

Increased Effect/Toxicity There are no known significant interactions involving an increase in effect.

Decreased Effect
The levels/effects of Diphtheria and Tetanus Toxoids may be decreased by: Belimumab; Fingolimod; Immunosuppressants

Stability Store at 2°C to 8°C (35°F to 46°F). Do not freeze; discard if product has been frozen.

Dosage

Geriatric & Adult

Primary immunization (Td): I.M.: Patients previously not immunized should receive 2 primary doses of 0.5 mL each, given at an interval of 4 weeks; third (reinforcing) dose of 0.5 mL 6 months later

Booster immunization (Td): I.M.: 0.5 mL every 10 years (for routine booster in patients who have completed primary immunization series). The ACIP prefers Tdap for use in in some situations if no contraindications exist; refer to Diphtheria and Tetanus Toxoids and Acellular Pertussis Vaccine monograph for additional information.

Tetanus prophylaxis in wound management: I.M.: Tetanus prophylaxis in patients with wounds should consider if the wound is clean or contaminated, the immunization status of the patient, proper use of tetanus toxoid and/or tetanus immune globulin (TIG), wound cleaning, and (if required) surgical debridement and the proper use of antibiotics. Patients with an uncertain or incomplete tetanus immunization status should have additional follow up to ensure a series is completed. Patients with a history of Arthus reaction following a previous dose of a tetanus toxoid-containing vaccine should not receive a tetanus toxoid-containing vaccine until >10 years after the most recent dose even if they have a wound that is neither clean nor minor. See table.

Tetanus Prophylaxis in Wound Management

History of Tetanus Immunization Doses	Clean, Minor Wounds		All Other Wounds[1]	
	Tetanus Toxoid[2]	TIG	Tetanus Toxoid[2]	TIG
Uncertain or <3 doses	Yes	No	Yes	Yes
3 or more doses	No[3]	No	No[4]	No

[1]Such as, but not limited to, wounds contaminated with dirt, feces, soil, and saliva; puncture wounds; wounds from crushing, tears, burns, and frostbite.

[2]Tetanus toxoid in this chart refers to a tetanus toxoid-containing vaccine. For children <7 years of age, DTaP (DT, if pertussis vaccine contraindicated) is preferred to tetanus toxoid alone. For children ≥7 years and Adults, Td preferred to tetanus toxoid alone; Tdap may be preferred if the patient has not previously been vaccinated with Tdap.

[3]Yes, if ≥10 years since last dose.

[4]Yes, if ≥5 years since last dose.

Adapted from CDC "Yellow Book" (*Health Information for International Travel 2010*), "Routine Vaccine-Preventable Diseases, Tetanus" (available at http://www.cdc.gov/yellowbook) and *MMWR* 2006, 55(RR-17).

Abbreviations: **DT** = Diphtheria and Tetanus Toxoids (formulation for age ≤6 years); **DTaP** = Diphtheria and Tetanus Toxoids, and Acellular Pertussis (formulation for age ≤6 years; Daptacel®, Infanrix®, Tripedia®); **Td** = Diphtheria and Tetanus Toxoids (formulation for age ≥7 years; Decavac®); **TT**= Tetanus toxoid (adsorbed [formulation for age ≥7 years]); **Tdap** = Diphtheria and Tetanus Toxoids, and Acellular Pertussis (Adacel® or Boostrix® [formulations for age ≥7 years]); **TIG** = Tetanus Immune Globulin

Administration For I.M. administration; prior to use, shake suspension well

Td: Administer in the deltoid muscle; do not inject in the gluteal area

DT: Administer in the anterolateral aspect of the thigh or the deltoid muscle; do not inject in the gluteal area

For patients at risk of hemorrhage following intramuscular injection, the ACIP recommends "it should be administered intramuscularly if, in the opinion of the physician familiar with the patients bleeding risk, the vaccine can be administered by this route with reasonable safety. If the patient receives antihemophilia or other similar therapy, intramuscular vaccination can be scheduled shortly after such therapy is administered. A fine needle (23 gauge or smaller) can be used for the vaccination and firm pressure applied to the site (without rubbing) for at least 2 minutes. The patient should be instructed concerning the risk of hematoma from the injection." Patients on anticoagulant therapy should be considered to have the same bleeding risks and treated as those with clotting factor disorders (CDC, 60[2], 2011).

Simultaneous administration of vaccines helps ensure the patients will be fully vaccinated by the appropriate age. Simultaneous administration of vaccines is defined as administering >1 vaccine on the same day at different anatomic sites. The use of licensed combination vaccines is generally preferred over separate injections of the equivalent components. Separate vaccines should not be combined in the same syringe unless indicated by product specific labeling. Separate needles and syringes should be used for each injection. The ACIP prefers each dose of a specific vaccine in a series come from the same manufacturer when possible. Adolescents and adults should be vaccinated while seated or lying down. In general, preterm infants should be vaccinated at the same chronological age as full-term infants (CDC, 60[2], 2011).

Antipyretics have not been shown to prevent febrile seizures. Antipyretics may be used to treat fever or discomfort following vaccination (CDC, 2011). One study reported that routine prophylactic administration of acetaminophen to prevent fever prior to vaccination decreased the immune response of some vaccines; the clinical significance of this reduction in immune response has not been established (Prymula, 2009).

Monitoring Parameters Monitor for syncope for ≥15 minutes following vaccination

◀ **Pharmacotherapy Pearls** Pediatric dosage form should only be used in patients ≤6 years of age. Federal law requires that the name of medication, date of administration, the vaccine manufacturer, lot number of vaccine, and the administering person's name, title, and address be entered into the patient's permanent medical record.

DT contains higher proportions of diphtheria toxoid than Td.

Special Geriatric Considerations Since protective tetanus and diphtheria antibodies decline with age (only 31% of persons >70 years of age in the U.S. are believed to be immune to tetanus) and older adults have a disproportionate burden of illness from tetanus, it is advisable to offer Td to the elderly concurrent with their influenza and other immunization programs if history of vaccination is unclear; boosters should be given at 10-year intervals (earlier for wounds). ACIP has issued recommendations for the use of Tdap in adults ≥65 years who previously may have not received a dose of Tdap. For patients who have or anticipate having close contact with an infant <12 months of age, a single dose of Tdap is recommended; for other adults ≥65 years, a single dose of Tdap may be given to replace a single dose of Td.

Dosage Forms Excipient information presented when available (limited, particularly for generics); consult specific product labeling. [DSC] = Discontinued product

Injection, suspension [Td, adult]: Diphtheria 2 Lf units and tetanus 2 Lf units per 0.5 mL (7.5 mL) [DSC]; Diphtheria 2 Lf units and tetanus 5 Lf units per 0.5 mL (5 mL) [DSC]

Injection, suspension [Td, adult; preservative free]: Diphtheria 2 Lf units and tetanus 2 Lf units per 0.5 mL (0.5 mL)

Decavac®: Diphtheria 2 Lf units and tetanus 5 Lf units per 0.5 mL (0.5 mL) [contains aluminum, may contain natural rubber/natural latex in prefilled syringe, thimerosal (may have trace amounts)]

Injection, suspension [DT, pediatric; preservative free]: Diphtheria 6.7 Lf units and tetanus 5 Lf units per 0.5 mL (0.5 mL)

Selected References

Centers for Disease Control and Prevention (CDC), "Preventing Tetanus, Diphtheria, and Pertussis Among Adults: Use of Tetanus Toxoid, Reduced Diphtheria Toxoid and Acellular Pertussis Vaccine, Recommendations of the Advisory Committee on Immunization Practices (ACIP) and Recommendation of ACIP, Supported by the Healthcare Infection Control Practices Advisory Committee (HICPAC), for Use of Tdap Among Health-Care Personnel,"*MMWR Recomm Rep*, 2006, 55(RR-17):1-37.

Centers for Disease Control and Prevention (CDC), "Recommendations for Postexposure Interventions to Prevent Infection With Hepatitis B Virus, Hepatitis C Virus, or Human Immunodeficiency Virus, and Tetanus in Persons Wounded During Bombings and Other Mass-Casualty Events – United States, 2008: Recommendations of the Centers For Disease Control And Prevention (CDC)," *MMWR Recomm Rep*, 2008, 57(RR-6):1-21.

Centers for Disease Control and Prevention (CDC), "Recommendations of the Advisory Committee on Immunization Practices (ACIP): General Recommendations on Immunization," *MMWR*, 2006, 55(RR-15):1-48.

Centers for Disease Control and Prevention (CDC), "Updated Recommendations for Use of Tetanus Toxoid, Reduced Diphtheria Toxoid and Acellular Pertussis (Tdap) Vaccine From the Advisory Committee on Immunization Practices, 2010," *MMWR Morb Mortal Wkly Rep*, 2011, 60(1):13-5.

McQuillan GM, Kruszon-Moran D, Deforest A, et al, "Serologic Immunity to Diphtheria and Tetanus in the United States," *Ann Intern Med*, 2002, 136(9):660-6.

Diphtheria and Tetanus Toxoids, Acellular Pertussis, and Poliovirus Vaccine

(dif THEER ee a & TET a nus TOKS oyds, ay CEL yoo lar per TUS sis & POE lee oh VYE rus vak SEEN)

Related Information

Immunization Administration Recommendations *on page 2037*

Immunization Recommendations *on page 2043*

Brand Names: U.S. Kinrix®

Index Terms Diphtheria and Tetanus Toxoids and Acellular Pertussis Adsorbed, and Inactivated Poliovirus Vaccine Combined; Diphtheria, Tetanus Toxoids, Acellular Pertussis (DTaP); DTaP-IPV; Poliovirus, Inactivated (IPV)

Generic Availability (U.S.) No

Pharmacologic Category Vaccine, Inactivated (Bacterial); Vaccine, Inactivated (Viral)

Use Active immunization against diphtheria, tetanus, pertussis, and poliomyelitis, used as the 5th dose in the DTaP series and the 4th dose in the IPV series

The Advisory Committee on Immunization Practices (ACIP) recommends routine vaccination for use as the fifth dose in the DTaP series and the fourth dose in the IPV series in children who received DTaP (Infanrix®) and/or DTaP-Hepatitis B-IPV (Pediarix®) as the first 3 doses and DTaP (Infanrix®) as the fourth dose. Whenever feasible, the same manufacturer should be used to provide the pertussis component; however, vaccination should not be deferred if a specific brand is not known or is not available.

DIPHTHERIA AND TETANUS TOXOIDS, ACELLULAR PERTUSSIS, AND POLIOVIRUS VACCINE

Contraindications Hypersensitivity to diphtheria and tetanus toxoids, pertussis, poliovirus vaccine, or any component of the vaccine; encephalopathy occurring within 7 days of a previous pertussis vaccine not (not attributable to another identifiable cause); progressive neurologic disorders (including uncontrolled epilepsy or progressive encephalopathy)

Warnings/Precautions Immediate treatment for anaphylactic/anaphylactoid reaction should be available during vaccine use. Use caution if one or more has occurred within 48 hours of whole-cell DTP or a vaccine containing acellular pertussis: Fever 40.5°C (≥105°F) within 48 hours not due to an identifiable cause; collapse or shock-like state (hypotonic-hyporesponsive episode [HHE]) occurring within 48 hours; persistent, inconsolable crying that occurs within 48 hours and lasts ≥3 hours; seizures with or without fever that occur within 3 days. Use caution if Guillain-Barré syndrome occurred within 6 weeks of prior vaccination with tetanus toxoid. May consider deferring administration in patients with moderate or severe acute illness (with or without fever); may administer to patients with mild acute illness (with or without fever).

Use with caution in patients with history of seizure disorder, progressive neurologic disease, or conditions predisposing to seizures; ACIP and AAP guidelines recommend deferring immunization until health status can be assessed and condition stabilized. Antipyretics may be considered at the time of and for 24 hours following vaccination to patients at high risk for seizures to reduce the possibility of postvaccination fever. Use caution with bleeding disorders. Use with caution in severely immunocompromised patients (eg, patients receiving chemo/radiation therapy or other immunosuppressive therapy [including high-dose corticosteroids]); may have a reduced response to vaccination. Contains aluminum, neomycin, polymyxin B, and polysorbate 80; packaging may contain latex. In order to maximize vaccination rates, the ACIP recommends simultaneous administration of all age-appropriate vaccines (live or inactivated) for which a person is eligible at a single clinic visit, unless contraindications exist. The use of combination vaccines is generally preferred over separate injections, taking into consideration provider assessment, patient preference, and adverse events.

Adverse Reactions (Reflective of adult population; not specific for elderly) All serious adverse reactions must be reported to the U.S. Department of Health and Human Services (DHHS) Vaccine Adverse Event Reporting System (VAERS) 1-800-822-7967 or online at https://vaers.hhs.gov/esub/index.

Adverse events reported within 4 days of vaccination: >10%:

Central nervous system: Drowsiness (19%, grade 3: 1%), fever (≥99.5°F: 16%, >100.4: 7%, >104: <1%)

Gastrointestinal: Loss of appetite (16%; grade 3: 1%)

Local: Injection site: Pain (57%; grade 3: 2%), redness (37%; ≥50 mm: 18%, ≥110 mm: 3%), arm circumference increase (36%, >20 mm: 7%, >30 mm: 2%), swelling (26%; ≥50 mm: 10%, ≥110 mm: 1%)

Drug Interactions

Avoid Concomitant Use There are no known interactions where it is recommended to avoid concomitant use.

Increased Effect/Toxicity There are no known significant interactions involving an increase in effect.

Decreased Effect

The levels/effects of Diphtheria and Tetanus Toxoids, Acellular Pertussis, and Poliovirus Vaccine may be decreased by: Belimumab; Fingolimod; Immunosuppressants

Stability Store under refrigeration of 2°C to 8°C (36°F to 46°F); do not freeze. Discard if frozen.

Mechanism of Action Promotes active immunity to diphtheria, tetanus, pertussis, and poliovirus (types 1, 2 and 3) by inducing production of specific antibodies and antitoxins.

Pharmacodynamics/Kinetics Onset of action: Immune response observed to all components ~1 month following vaccination

Administration For I.M. use only; do not administer intradermally, I.V., or SubQ. Shake well prior to use; do not use unless a homogeneous, turbid, white suspension forms. Discard if the suspension is discolored or if there are cracks in the vial or syringe. Administer in the deltoid muscle of the upper arm. Do not administer additional vaccines or immunoglobulins at the same site, or using the same syringe.

For patients at risk of hemorrhage following intramuscular injection, the ACIP recommends "it should be administered intramuscularly if, in the opinion of the physician familiar with the patients bleeding risk, the vaccine can be administered by this route with reasonable safety. If the patient receives antihemophilia or other similar therapy, intramuscular vaccination can be scheduled shortly after such therapy is administered. A fine needle (23 gauge or smaller) can be used for the vaccination and firm pressure applied to the site (without rubbing) for at least 2 minutes. The patient should be instructed concerning the risk of hematoma from the injection." Patients on anticoagulant therapy should be considered to have the same bleeding risks and treated as those with clotting factor disorders (CDC, 2011).

Simultaneous administration of vaccines helps ensure the patients will be fully vaccinated by the appropriate age. Simultaneous administration of vaccines is defined as administering >1 vaccine on the same day at different anatomic sites. The use of licensed combination vaccines is generally preferred over separate injections of the equivalent components. Separate vaccines should not be combined in the same syringe unless indicated by product specific labeling. Separate needles and syringes should be used for each injection. The ACIP prefers each dose of a specific vaccine in a series come from the same manufacturer when possible. Adolescents and adults should be vaccinated while seated or lying down. In general, preterm infants should be vaccinated at the same chronological age as full-term infants (CDC, 2011).

Antipyretics have not been shown to prevent febrile seizures. Antipyretics may be used to treat fever or discomfort following vaccination (CDC, 2011). One study reported that routine prophylactic administration of acetaminophen to prevent fever prior to vaccination decreased the immune response of some vaccines; the clinical significance of this reduction in immune response has not been established (Prymula, 2009).

Pharmacotherapy Pearls Federal law requires that the name of medication, date of administration, name of the vaccine manufacturer, lot number of vaccine, and the administering person's name, title, and address be entered into the patient's permanent medical record.

Contains the following three pertussis antigens: Inactivated pertussis toxin (PT), filamentous hemagglutinin (FHA), and pertactin. Contains the same diphtheria, tetanus toxoids, and pertussis antigens found in Infanrix® and Pediarix®. Contains the same poliovirus antigens found in Infanrix®.

Special Geriatric Considerations Since protective tetanus and diphtheria antibodies decline with age, only 28% of persons >70 years of age in the U.S. are believed to be immune to tetanus, and most of the tetanus-induced deaths occur in people >60 years of age, it is advisable to offer Td, especially to elderly, concurrent with their influenza and other immunization programs if history of vaccination is unclear; boosters should be given at 10-year intervals (earlier for wounds). For the elderly who cannot document a primary immunization series or at risk due to contact or travel, administer the initial series. Boosters may be necessary for travel since antibody titers may diminish with age.

Dosage Forms Excipient information presented when available (limited, particularly for generics); consult specific product labeling.

Injection, suspension [preservative free]:

Kinrix®: Diphtheria toxoid 25 Lf, tetanus toxoid 10 Lf, acellular pertussis antigens [inactivated pertussis toxin 25 mcg, filamentous hemagglutinin 25 mcg, pertactin 8 mcg], type 1 poliovirus 40 D-antigen units, type 2 poliovirus 8 D-antigen units, and type 3 poliovirus 32 D-antigen units per 0.5 mL (0.5 mL) [contains aluminum, neomycin sulfate, polymyxin B, polysorbate 80; may contain natural rubber/natural latex in prefilled syringe]

Selected References

Centers for Disease Control, "Recommendations of the Advisory Committee on Immunization Practices (ACIP): General Recommendations on Immunization," *MMWR Recomm Rep*, 2006, 55(RR-15):1-48.

Centers for Disease Control and Prevention (CDC), "Licensure of a Diphtheria and Tetanus Toxoids and Acellular Pertussis Adsorbed and Inactivated Poliovirus Vaccine and Guidance for Use as a Booster Dose," *MMWR Morb Mortal Wkly Rep*, 2008, 57(39):1078-9.

Diphtheria and Tetanus Toxoids, Acellular Pertussis, Hepatitis B (Recombinant), Poliovirus (Inactivated), and *Haemophilus influenzae* B Conjugate (Adsorbed) Vaccine

(dif THEER ee a & TET a nus TOKS oyds, ay CEL yoo lar per TUS sis, hep a TYE tis bee ree KOM be nant, POE lee oh VYE rus in ak ti VAY ted, & hem OF fi lus in floo EN za bee KON joo gate ad SORBED vak SEEN)

Medication Safety Issues

Sound-alike/look-alike issues:

Infanrix Hexa™ may be confused with Infanrix®

Brand Names: Canada Infanrix Hexa™

Index Terms Diphtheria and Tetanus Toxoids and Acellular Pertussis, Hepatitis B (Recombinant), Inactivated Poliovirus Vaccine, and *Haemophilus influenzae* Type B Combined; DTaP-HepB-IPV-Hib

Pharmacologic Category Vaccine, Inactivated (Bacterial, Viral)

DIPHTHERIA AND TETANUS TOXOIDS, AND ACELLULAR PERTUSSIS VACCINE

Use Active primary immunization against diphtheria, tetanus, pertussis, hepatitis B, polio-myelitis and disease caused by *Haemophilus influenzae* type b in infants and children 6 weeks to 2 years of age; booster immunization (at 18 months) in infants who previously received a full primary vaccination course of each component of the vaccine

Product Availability Not available in U.S.

Dosage Forms: Canada Excipient information presented when available (limited, particularly for generics); consult specific product labeling.

Injection, suspension:

Infanrix Hexa™: Diphtheria toxoid 25 Lf, tetanus toxoid 10 Lf, acellular pertussis antigens [inactivated pertussis toxin 25 mcg, filamentous hemagglutinin 25 mcg, pertactin 8 mcg], HBsAg 10 mcg, type 1 poliovirus 40 D antigen units, type 2 poliovirus 8 D antigen units and type 3 poliovirus 32 D antigen units, *Haemophilus* b capsular polysaccharide 10 mcg [bound to tetanus toxoid 20-40 mcg] per 0.5 mL (0.5 mL) [contains aluminum, neomycin sulfate (trace amounts), polymyxin B (trace amounts), polysorbate 20, polysorbate 80, and yeast protein ≤5%; Pediarix™ vaccine used to reconstitute Hib forms Infanrix Hexa™]

◆ **Diphtheria and Tetanus Toxoids and Acellular Pertussis Adsorbed, and Inactivated Poliovirus Vaccine Combined** *see* Diphtheria and Tetanus Toxoids, Acellular Pertussis, and Poliovirus Vaccine *on page 528*

◆ **Diphtheria and Tetanus Toxoids and Acellular Pertussis, Hepatitis B (Recombinant), Inactivated Poliovirus Vaccine, and *Haemophilus influenzae* Type B Combined** *see* Diphtheria and Tetanus Toxoids, Acellular Pertussis, Hepatitis B (Recombinant), Poliovirus (Inactivated), and *Haemophilus influenzae* B Conjugate (Adsorbed) Vaccine *on page 530*

Diphtheria and Tetanus Toxoids, and Acellular Pertussis Vaccine
(dif THEER ee a & TET a nus TOKS oyds & ay CEL yoo lar per TUS sis vak SEEN)

Related Information
Immunization Administration Recommendations *on page 2037*
Immunization Recommendations *on page 2043*
Medication Safety Issues
  Sound-alike/look-alike issues:
  Adacel® (Tdap) may be confused with Daptacel® (DTaP)
  Tdap (Adacel®, Boostrix®) may be confused with DTaP (Daptacel®, Infanrix®, Tripedia®)
  Administration issues:
  Carefully review product labeling to prevent inadvertent administration of Tdap when DTaP is indicated. Tdap contains lower amounts of diphtheria toxoid and some pertussis antigens than DTaP.
  Tdap is not indicated for use in children <10 years of age
  DTaP is not indicated for use in persons ≥7 years of age
  Guidelines are available in case of inadvertent administration of these products; refer to ACIP recommendations, February 2006 available at http://www.cdc.gov/mmwr/preview/mmwrhtml/rr55e223a1.htm
  Other safety concerns:
  DTaP: Diphtheria and tetanus toxoids and acellular pertussis vaccine
  DTP: Diphtheria and tetanus toxoids and pertussis vaccine (unspecified pertussis antigens)
  DTwP: Diphtheria and tetanus toxoids and whole-cell pertussis vaccine (no longer available on U.S. market)
  Tdap: Tetanus toxoid, reduced diphtheria toxoid, and acellular pertussis vaccine

Brand Names: U.S. Adacel®; Boostrix®; Daptacel®; Infanrix®; Tripedia® [DSC]

Brand Names: Canada Adacel®; Boostrix®

Index Terms DTaP; Tdap; Tetanus Toxoid, Reduced Diphtheria Toxoid, and Acellular Pertussis, Adsorbed

Generic Availability (U.S.) No

Pharmacologic Category Vaccine, Inactivated (Bacterial)

Use

Daptacel®, Infanrix®, Tripedia® (DTaP): Active immunization against diphtheria, tetanus, and pertussis from age 6 weeks through 6 years of age (prior to seventh birthday)

Adacel®, Boostrix® (Tdap): Active booster immunization against diphtheria, tetanus, and pertussis

DIPHTHERIA AND TETANUS TOXOIDS, AND ACELLULAR PERTUSSIS VACCINE

◀ The Advisory Committee on Immunization Practices (ACIP) recommends routine vaccination for the following:

Adolescents ≥11 years and Adults (Tdap):
- Persons wounded in bombings or similar mass casualty events and who cannot confirm receipt of a tetanus booster within the previous 5 years and who have penetrating injuries or nonintact skin exposure should receive a single dose of Tdap (CDC, 57 [RR6] 2008)

Adults 19-64 years (Tdap): A single dose of Tdap should be given to replace a single dose of the 10-year Td booster in patients who have not previously received Tdap or for whom vaccine status is not known, and as soon as feasible to all:
- Close contacts of children <12 months of age; Tdap should ideally be administered at least 2 weeks prior to beginning close contact (CDC, 60[4], 2011; CDC, 55[RR17], 2006)
- Healthcare providers with direct patient contact (CDC, 60[4], 2011; CDC, 55[RR17], 2006)

Adults ≥65 years who have not previously received Tdap:
- All adults ≥65 years may receive a single dose of Tdap in place of a dose of Td (CDC, 60 [1], 2011)
- Adults ≥65 years who anticipate close contact with children <12 months of age should receive a single dose of Tdap in place a of a dose of Td (CDC, 60[1], 2011)

Note: Tdap is currently recommended for a single dose only (all age groups) (CDC, 60 [1], 2011)

Contraindications Hypersensitivity to diphtheria, tetanus toxoids, pertussis, or any component of the formulation; history of any of the following effects from previous administration of pertussis-containing vaccine - progressive neurologic disorder, uncontrolled epilepsy or progressive epilepsy (postpone until condition stabilized); encephalopathy occurring within 7 days of administration and not attributable to another cause

Warnings/Precautions Defer administration during moderate or severe illness (with or without fever). Carefully consider use in patients with history of any of the following effects from previous administration of any pertussis-containing vaccine: Fever ≥105°F (40.5°C) within 48 hours of unknown cause; seizures with or without fever occurring within 3 days; shock or collapse within 48 hours. Carefully consider use in patients with history of Guillain-Barré syndrome occurring within 6 weeks of a vaccine containing tetanus toxoid. Td or Tdap vaccines and emergency doses of Td vaccine should not be given more frequently than every 10 years in patients who have experienced a serious Arthus-type hypersensitivity reaction following a prior use of tetanus toxoid even if using for wound management with wounds that are not clean or minor; these patients generally have high serum antitoxin levels.

Use caution in patients with coagulation disorders (including thrombocytopenia) where intramuscular injections should not be used. Patients who are immunocompromised may have reduced response; may be used in patients with HIV infection. In general, household and close contacts of persons with altered immunocompetence may receive all age appropriate vaccines. Use caution in patients with history of seizure disorder, progressive neurologic disease, or conditions predisposing to seizures; ACIP and APP guidelines recommend deferring immunization until health status can be assessed and condition stabilized. Antipyretics may be considered at the time of and for 24 hours following vaccination to patients at high risk for seizures to reduce the possibility of postvaccination fever. Products may contain thimerosal or gelatin; packaging may contain natural latex rubber. Immediate treatment for anaphylactic/anaphylactoid reaction should be available during vaccine use. In order to maximize vaccination rates, the ACIP recommends simultaneous administration of all age-appropriate vaccines (live or inactivated) for which a person is eligible at a single clinic visit, unless contraindications exist. The use of combination vaccines is generally preferred over separate injections, taking into consideration provider assessment, patient preference, and adverse events. When using combination vaccines, the minimum age for administration is the oldest minimum age for any individual component; the minimum interval between dosing is the greatest minimum interval between any individual component.

Adacel® is formulated with the same antigens found in Daptacel®, but with reduced quantities of tetanus and pertussis. Safety and efficacy have not been established in children <11 years of age.

Boostrix® is formulated with the same antigens found in Infanrix®, but in reduced quantities. Safety and efficacy have not been established in patients <10 years of age. Use of Adacel® or Boostrix® in the primary immunization series or to complete the primary series has not been evaluated.

Daptacel®, Infanrix®, Tripedia®: Safety and efficacy in children <6 weeks of age or ≥7 years of age have not been established.

Adverse Reactions (Reflective of adult population; not specific for elderly) All serious adverse reactions must be reported to the U.S. Department of Health and Human Services (DHHS) Vaccine Adverse Event Reporting System (VAERS) 1-800-822-7967 or online at https://vaers.hhs.gov/esub/index. In Canada, adverse reactions may be reported to local provincial/territorial health agencies or to the Vaccine Safety Section at Public Health Agency of Canada (1-866-844-0018).

Daptacel®, Infanrix®, Tripedia® (incidence of erythema, swelling, and fever increases with successive doses):
Frequency not defined:
Central nervous system: Drowsiness, fever, fussiness, irritability, lethargy
Gastrointestinal: Appetite decreased, vomiting
Local: Pain, redness, swelling, tenderness
Miscellaneous: Prolonged or persistent crying, refusal to play

Adacel®, Boostrix®: Note: Ranges presented, actual percent varies by product and age group
>10%:
Central nervous system: Fatigue, tiredness (24% to 37%; grade 3/severe: 1% to 4%), headache (12% to 44%; grade 3/severe: 1% to 4%), chills (8% to 15%; severe: <1%)
Gastrointestinal: Gastrointestinal symptoms, includes abdominal pain, diarrhea, nausea and/or vomiting (3% to 26%; grade 3/severe: ≤3%)
Local: Injection site pain (22% to 78%; grade 3/severe: ≤5%), arm circumference increased (28%; >40 mm: 0.5%), redness (11% to 25%; ≥50 mm: 2% to 4%), swelling (8% to 21%; ≥50 mm: ≤3%)
Neuromuscular & skeletal: Body aches/muscle weakness (22% to 30%; severe: 1%), soreness/swollen joints (9% to 11%; severe: <1%)
1% to 10%:
Central nervous system: Fever ≥38°C (≥100.4°F: 1% to 5%)
Dermatologic: Rash (2% to 3%)
Miscellaneous: Lymph node swelling (7%; severe: <1%)

Drug Interactions

Avoid Concomitant Use There are no known interactions where it is recommended to avoid concomitant use.

Increased Effect/Toxicity There are no known significant interactions involving an increase in effect.

Decreased Effect
The levels/effects of Diphtheria and Tetanus Toxoids, and Acellular Pertussis Vaccine may be decreased by: Belimumab; Fingolimod; Immunosuppressants

Stability Refrigerate at 2°C to 8°C (35°F to 46°F); do not freeze; discard if frozen. The following stability information has also been reported for Infanrix®: May be stored at room temperature for up to 72 hours (Cohen, 2007).

Mechanism of Action Promotes active immunity to diphtheria, tetanus, and pertussis by inducing production of specific antibodies.

Dosage

Geriatric & Adult Note: Tdap can be administered regardless of the interval between the last tetanus or diphtheria toxoid containing vaccine. Tdap is currently recommended for a single dose only (CDC, 60[1], 2011).

Booster Immunization: ACIP recommendations: I.M.:
Adults 19-64 years: 0.5 mL per dose. A single dose of Tdap should be given to replace a single dose of the 10 year Td booster in patients who have not previously received Tdap or for whom vaccine status is not known. A single dose of Tdap is recommended for health care personnel who have not previously received Tdap and who have direct patient contact (CDC, 55[17], 2006; CDC, 60[4], 2011).
Adults ≥65 years: 0.5 mL per dose. A single dose of Tdap may be given to older adults who have not previously received Tdap (CDC, 60[1], 2011)

Booster Immunization: Manufacturer's recommendations: I.M.:
Adults ≤64 years (Adacel®, Boostrix®): 0.5 mL as a single dose, administered 5 years after last dose of tetanus toxoid, diphtheria toxoid, and/or pertussis-containing vaccine
Adults ≥65 years (Boostrix®): 0.5 mL as a single dose, administered 5 years after last dose of tetanus toxoid, diphtheria toxoid, and/or pertussis-containing vaccine

Wound management: I.M.: Adacel® or Boostrix® may be used as an alternative to Td vaccine when a tetanus toxoid-containing vaccine is needed for wound management, and in whom the pertussis component is also indicated. Tetanus prophylaxis in patients with wounds should consider if the wound is clean or contaminated, the immunization status of the patient, proper use of tetanus toxoid and/or tetanus immune globulin (TIG), wound cleaning, and (if required) surgical debridement and the proper use of antibiotics. Patients with an uncertain or incomplete tetanus immunization status should have additional follow up to ensure a series is completed. Patients with a history of Arthus reaction following a previous dose of a tetanus toxoid-containing vaccine should not receive a tetanus toxoid-containing vaccine until >10 years after the most recent dose even if they have a wound that is neither clean nor minor. See table.

Tetanus Prophylaxis in Wound Management

History of Tetanus Immunization Doses	Clean, Minor Wounds		All Other Wounds[1]	
	Tetanus Toxoid[2]	TIG	Tetanus Toxoid[2]	TIG
Uncertain or <3 doses	Yes	No	Yes	Yes
3 or more doses	No[3]	No	No[4]	No

[1]Such as, but not limited to, wounds contaminated with dirt, feces, soil, and saliva; puncture wounds; wounds from crushing, tears, burns, and frostbite.

[2]Tetanus toxoid in this chart refers to a tetanus toxoid-containing vaccine. For children <7 years of age, DTaP (DT, if pertussis vaccine contraindicated) is preferred to tetanus toxoid alone. For children ≥7 years and Adults, Td preferred to tetanus toxoid alone; Tdap may be preferred if the patient has not previously been vaccinated with Tdap.

[3]Yes, if ≥10 years since last dose.

[4]Yes, if ≥5 years since last dose.

Adapted from CDC "Yellow Book" (*Health Information for International Travel 2010*), "Routine Vaccine-Preventable Diseases, Tetanus" (available at http://www.cdc.gov/yellowbook) and *MMWR* 2006, 55(RR-17).

Abbreviations: **DT** = Diphtheria and Tetanus Toxoids (formulation for age ≤6 years); **DTaP** = Diphtheria and Tetanus Toxoids, and Acellular Pertussis (formulation for age ≤6 years; Daptacel®, Infanrix®, Tripedia®); **Td** = Diphtheria and Tetanus Toxoids (formulation for age ≥7 years; Decavac®); **TT**= Tetanus toxoid (adsorbed [formulation for age ≥7 years]); **Tdap** = Diphtheria and Tetanus Toxoids, and Acellular Pertussis (Adacel® or Boostrix® [formulations for age ≥7 years]); **TIG** = Tetanus Immune Globulin

Administration Shake suspension well.
Adacel®, Boostrix®: Administer only I.M. in deltoid muscle of upper arm.
Daptacel®, Infanrix®, Tripedia®: Administer only I.M. in anterolateral aspect of thigh or deltoid muscle of upper arm.
If feasible, the same brand of DTaP should be used for all doses in the series (CDC, 60 [2], 2011).

For patients at risk of hemorrhage following intramuscular injection, the ACIP recommends "it should be administered intramuscularly if, in the opinion of the physician familiar with the patients bleeding risk, the vaccine can be administered by this route with reasonable safety. If the patient receives antihemophilia or other similar therapy, intramuscular vaccination can be scheduled shortly after such therapy is administered. A fine needle (23 gauge or smaller) can be used for the vaccination and firm pressure applied to the site (without rubbing) for at least 2 minutes. The patient should be instructed concerning the risk of hematoma from the injection." Patients on anticoagulant therapy should be considered to have the same bleeding risks and treated as those with clotting factor disorders (CDC, 60[2], 2011).

Simultaneous administration of vaccines helps ensure the patients will be fully vaccinated by the appropriate age. Simultaneous administration of vaccines is defined as administering >1 vaccine on the same day at different anatomic sites. The use of licensed combination vaccines is generally preferred over separate injections of the equivalent components. Separate vaccines should not be combined in the same syringe unless indicated by product specific labeling. Separate needles and syringes should be used for each injection. The ACIP prefers each dose of a specific vaccine in a series come from the same manufacturer when possible. Adolescents and adults should be vaccinated while seated or lying down. In general, preterm infants should be vaccinated at the same chronological age as full-term infants (CDC, 60[2], 2011).

Antipyretics have not been shown to prevent febrile seizures. Antipyretics may be used to treat fever or discomfort following vaccination (CDC, 2011). One study reported that routine prophylactic administration of acetaminophen to prevent fever prior to vaccination decreased the immune response of some vaccines; the clinical significance of this reduction in immune response has not been established (Prymula, 2009).

Monitoring Parameters Monitor for syncope for ≥15 minutes following vaccination

Pharmacotherapy Pearls DTaP may be given for the fourth and fifth doses in children who started immunization with DTP vaccine. In patients who cannot be given pertussis vaccine, DT for pediatric use should be given to complete the series.

TriHIBit® is Tripedia® vaccine used to reconstitute ActHIB® (*Haemophilus* b conjugate) vaccine. The combination can be used for the DTaP dose given at 15-18 months when Tripedia® was used for the initial doses and a primary series of HIB vaccine has been given.

Adacel® is formulated with the same antigens found in Daptacel® but with reduced quantities of pertussis and tetanus. It is intended for use as a booster dose in children and adults, 11-64 years of age, and **not** for primary immunization.

Boostrix® is formulated with the same antigens found in Infanrix® but in reduced quantities. It is intended for use as a booster dose in children and adults, 10-64 years of age, and is **not** for primary immunization.

Federal law requires that the name of medication, date of administration, the vaccine manufacturer, lot number of vaccine, and the administering person's name, title and address be entered into the patient's permanent medical record.

Special Geriatric Considerations Since protective tetanus and diphtheria antibodies decline with age (only 31% of persons >70 years of age in the U.S. are believed to be immune to tetanus) and older adults have a disproportionate burden of illness from tetanus, it is advisable to offer Td to the elderly concurrent with their influenza and other immunization programs if history of vaccination is unclear; boosters should be given at 10-year intervals; earlier for wounds. ACIP has issued recommendations for the use of Tdap in adults ≥65 years who previously have not received a dose of Tdap. For patients who have or anticipate having close contact with an infant <12 months of age, a single dose of Tdap is recommended; for other adults ≥65 years, a single dose of Tdap may be given to replace a single dose of Td.

Dosage Forms Excipient information presented when available (limited, particularly for generics); consult specific product labeling.

Injection, suspension [Tdap, booster formulation]:

Adacel®: Diphtheria 2 Lf units, tetanus 5 Lf units, and acellular pertussis antigens [detoxified pertussis toxin 2.5 mcg, filamentous hemagglutinin 5 mcg, pertactin 3 mcg, fimbriae (types 2 and 3) 5 mcg] per 0.5 mL (0.5 mL) [contains aluminum; may contain natural rubber/natural latex in prefilled syringe]

Boostrix®: Diphtheria 2.5 Lf units, tetanus 5 Lf units, and acellular pertussis antigens [inactivated pertussis toxin 8 mcg, filamentous hemagglutinin 8 mcg, pertactin 2.5 mcg] per 0.5 mL (0.5 mL) [contains aluminum and polysorbate 80; may contain natural rubber/natural latex in prefilled syringe]

Injection, suspension [DTaP, active immunization formulation]:

Daptacel®: Diphtheria 15 Lf units, tetanus 5 Lf units, and acellular pertussis antigens [detoxified pertussis toxin 10 mcg, filamentous hemagglutinin 5 mcg, pertactin 3 mcg, fimbriae (types 2 and 3) 5 mcg] per 0.5 mL (0.5 mL) [preservative free; contains aluminum]

Infanrix®: Diphtheria 25 Lf units, tetanus 10 Lf units, and acellular pertussis antigens [inactivated pertussis toxin 25 mcg, filamentous hemagglutinin 25 mcg, pertactin 8 mcg] per 0.5 mL (0.5 mL) [preservative free; contains aluminum and polysorbate 80]

Infanrix®: Diphtheria 25 Lf units, tetanus 10 Lf units, and acellular pertussis antigens [inactivated pertussis toxin 25 mcg, filamentous hemagglutinin 25 mcg, pertactin 8 mcg] per 0.5 mL (0.5 mL) [preservative free; contains aluminum and polysorbate 80; prefilled syringes contain natural rubber/natural latex] [DSC]

Tripedia®: Diphtheria 6.7 Lf units, tetanus 5 Lf units, and acellular pertussis antigens [inactivated pertussis toxin 23.4 mcg, filamentous hemagglutinin 23.4 mcg] per 0.5 mL (0.5 mL) [DSC] [contains aluminum, natural rubber/natural latex in packaging, polysorbate 80, and thimerosal (trace amounts)]

Note: Tripedia® vaccine is also used to reconstitute ActHIB® to prepare TriHIBit® vaccine (diphtheria, tetanus toxoids, and acellular pertussis and *Haemophilus influenzae* b conjugate vaccine combination)

Selected References

Centers for Disease Control and Prevention (CDC), "FDA Approval of Expanded Age Indication for a Tetanus Toxoid, Reduced Diphtheria Toxoid and Acellular Pertussis Vaccine," *MMWR Morb Mortal Wkly Rep*, 2009, 58(14):374-5.

Centers for Disease Control and Prevention (CDC), "Notice to Readers: Update: Supply of Diphtheria and Tetanus Toxoids and Acellular Pertussis Vaccine," *MMWR*, 2002, 50(51):1159.

Centers for Disease Control and Prevention (CDC), "Preventing Tetanus, Diphtheria, and Pertussis Among Adolescents: Use of Tetanus Toxoid, Reduced Diphtheria Toxoid and Acellular Pertussis Vaccine: Recommendations of the Advisory Committee on Immunization Practices (ACIP)," *MMWR Recomm Rep. 2006* , 2006, 55(RR-3);1-34.

Centers for Disease Control and Prevention (CDC), "Preventing Tetanus, Diphtheria, and Pertussis Among Adults: Use of Tetanus Toxoid, Reduced Diphtheria Toxoid and Acellular Pertussis Vaccine, Recommendations of the Advisory Committee on Immunization Practices (ACIP) and Recommendation of ACIP, Supported by the Healthcare Infection Control Practices Advisory Committee (HICPAC), for Use of Tdap Among Health-Care Personnel,"*MMWR Recomm Rep*, 2006, 55(RR-17):1-37.

Centers for Disease Control and Prevention (CDC), "Prevention of Pertussis, Tetanus, and Diphtheria Among Pregnant and Postpartum Women and Their Infants, Recommendations of the Advisory Committee on Immunization Practices (ACIP)," *MMWR Recomm Rep*, 2008, 57(RR-4):1-51.

Centers for Disease Control and Prevention (CDC), "Recommendations for Postexposure Interventions to Prevent Infection With Hepatitis B Virus, Hepatitis C Virus, or Human Immunodeficiency Virus, and Tetanus in Persons Wounded During Bombings and Other Mass-Casualty Events – United States, 2008: Recommendations of the Centers For Disease Control and Prevention (CDC)," *MMWR Recomm Rep*, 2008, 57(RR-6):1-21.

Centers for Disease Control and Prevention (CDC), "Recommendations of the Advisory Committee on Immunization Practices (ACIP): General Recommendations on Immunization," *MMWR Recomm Rep*, 2011, 60(2):1-64.

◀

Centers for Disease Control and Prevention (CDC), "Recommended Adult Immunization Schedule – United States, 2011," *MMWR Morb Mortal Wkly Rep*, 2011, 60(4):1-4.

Centers for Disease Control and Prevention (CDC), "Syncope After Vaccination – United States, January 2005-July 2007," *MMWR Morb Mortal Wkly Rep*, 2008, 57(17):457-60.

Centers for Disease Control and Prevention (CDC), "Updated Recommendations for Use of Tetanus Toxoid, Reduced Diphtheria Toxoid and Acellular Pertussis (Tdap) Vaccine From the Advisory Committee on Immunization Practices, 2010," *MMWR Morb Mortal Wkly Rep*, 2011, 60(1):13-5.

Centers For Disease Control and Prevention (CDC), "Use of Diphtheria Toxoid-Tetanus Toxoid-Acellular Pertussis Vaccine as a Five-Dose Series," *MMWR Recomm Rep*, 2000, 49(RR-13):1-8.

Cohen V, Jellinek SP, Teperikidis L, et al, "Room-Temperature Storage of Medications Labeled for Refrigeration," *Am J Health-Syst Pharm*, 2007, 64(16):1711-15.

McQuillan GM, Kruszon-Moran D, Deforest A, et al, "Serologic Immunity to Diphtheria and Tetanus in the United States," *Ann Intern Med*, 2002, 136(9):660-6.

Pichichero ME, Rennels MB, Edwards KM, et al, "Combined Tetanus, Diphtheria, and 5-Component Pertussis Vaccine for Use in Adolescents and Adults," *JAMA*, 2005, 293:3003-11.

Prymula R, Siegrist CA, Chlibek R, et al, "Effect of Prophylactic Paracetamol Administration at Time of Vaccination on Febrile Reactions and Antibody Responses in Children: Two Open-Label, Randomised Controlled Trials," *Lancet*, 2009, 374(9698):1339-50.

Steering Committee on Quality Improvement and Management, Subcommittee on Febrile Seizures American Academy of Pediatrics, "Febrile seizures: Clinical Practice Guideline for the Long-Term Management of the Child With Simple Febrile Seizures," *Pediatrics*, 2008, 121(6):1281-6.

◆ **Diphtheria, Tetanus Toxoids, Acellular Pertussis (DTaP)** *see* Diphtheria and Tetanus Toxoids, Acellular Pertussis, and Poliovirus Vaccine *on page 528*

◆ **Dipivalyl Epinephrine** *see* Dipivefrin *on page 536*

Dipivefrin (dye PI ve frin)

Related Information
Glaucoma Drug Therapy *on page 2008*

Brand Names: Canada Ophtho-Dipivefrin™; PMS-Dipivefrin; Propine®

Index Terms Dipivalyl Epinephrine; Dipivefrin Hydrochloride; DPE

Generic Availability (U.S.) No

Pharmacologic Category Alpha/Beta Agonist; Ophthalmic Agent, Antiglaucoma; Ophthalmic Agent, Vasoconstrictor

Use Reduces elevated intraocular pressure in chronic open-angle glaucoma; also used to treat ocular hypertension, low tension, and secondary glaucomas

Contraindications Hypersensitivity to dipivefrin, any component of the formulation, or epinephrine; angle-closure glaucoma

Warnings/Precautions Use with caution in patients with hypertension or cardiac disorders and in aphakic patients. Contains sodium metabisulfite.

Adverse Reactions (Reflective of adult population; not specific for elderly)
1% to 10%:
Central nervous system: Headache
Local: Burning, stinging
Ocular: Blepharoconjunctivitis, blurred vision, bulbar conjunctival follicles, cystoid macular edema, ocular congestion, ocular pain, mydriasis, photophobia

Drug Interactions
Avoid Concomitant Use
Avoid concomitant use of Dipivefrin with any of the following: Iobenguane I 123
Increased Effect/Toxicity
Dipivefrin may increase the levels/effects of: Sympathomimetics

The levels/effects of Dipivefrin may be increased by: Atomoxetine; Cannabinoids; Serotonin/Norepinephrine Reuptake Inhibitors
Decreased Effect
Dipivefrin may decrease the levels/effects of: Iobenguane I 123

The levels/effects of Dipivefrin may be decreased by: Spironolactone

Stability Avoid exposure to light and air. Discolored or darkened solutions indicate loss of potency.

Mechanism of Action Dipivefrin is a prodrug of epinephrine which is the active agent that stimulates alpha- and/or beta-adrenergic receptors increasing aqueous humor outflow

Pharmacodynamics/Kinetics
Ocular pressure effect:
Onset of action: ~30 minutes
Duration: ≥12 hours
Mydriasis:
Onset of action: ~30 minutes
Duration: Several hours

Absorption: Rapid into aqueous humor
Metabolism: Converted to epinephrine

Dosage
Geriatric & Adult Glaucoma: Ophthalmic: Instill 1 drop every 12 hours into the eyes

Monitoring Parameters Intraocular pressure; heart rate and blood pressure

Special Geriatric Considerations Use with caution in patients with heart disease. Evaluate the patient's or caregiver's ability to safely administer the correct dose of ophthalmic medication.

Dosage Forms Excipient information presented when available (limited, particularly for generics); consult specific product labeling. [DSC] = Discontinued product
Solution, ophthalmic, as hydrochloride [drops]:
Propine®: 0.1% (10 mL [DSC]) [contains benzalkonium chloride]

◆ **Dipivefrin Hydrochloride** *see* Dipivefrin *on page 536*
◆ **Diprolene®** *see* Betamethasone *on page 195*
◆ **Diprolene® AF** *see* Betamethasone *on page 195*
◆ **Dipropylacetic Acid** *see* Valproic Acid *on page 1888*

Dipyridamole (dye peer ID a mole)

Related Information
Beers Criteria – Potentially Inappropriate Medications for Geriatrics *on page 2089*

Medication Safety Issues
Sound-alike/look-alike issues:
Dipyridamole may be confused with disopyramide
Persantine® may be confused with Periactin®, Permitil®

BEERS Criteria medication:
This drug may be inappropriate for use in geriatric patients (low severity risk).

Brand Names: U.S. Persantine®

Brand Names: Canada Apo-Dipyridamole FC®; Dipyridamole For Injection; Persantine®

Generic Availability (U.S.) Yes

Pharmacologic Category Antiplatelet Agent; Vasodilator

Use
Oral: Used with warfarin to decrease thrombosis in patients after artificial heart valve replacement
I.V.: Diagnostic agent in CAD

Unlabeled/Investigational Use Stroke prevention (in combination with aspirin)

Contraindications Hypersensitivity to dipyridamole or any component of the formulation

Warnings/Precautions Use with caution in patients with hypotension, unstable angina, and/or recent MI. Use with caution in hepatic impairment. May be inappropriate for use in the elderly due to risk of orthostatic hypotension (Beers Criteria). Use caution in patients on other antiplatelet agents or anticoagulation. Severe adverse reactions have occurred with I.V. administration (rarely); use the I.V. form with caution in patients with bronchospastic disease or unstable angina. Aminophylline should be available in case of urgency or emergency with I.V. use.

Adverse Reactions (Reflective of adult population; not specific for elderly)
Oral:
>10%: Dizziness (14%)
1% to 10%:
Central nervous system: Headache (2%)
Dermatologic: Rash (2%)
Gastrointestinal: Abdominal distress (6%)
Frequency not defined: Diarrhea, vomiting, flushing, pruritus, angina pectoris, liver dysfunction
I.V.:
>10%:
Cardiovascular: Exacerbation of angina pectoris (20%)
Central nervous system: Dizziness (12%), headache (12%)
1% to 10%:
Cardiovascular: Hypotension (5%), hypertension (2%), blood pressure lability (2%), ECG abnormalities (ST-T changes, extrasystoles; 5% to 8%), pain (3%), tachycardia (3%)
Central nervous system: Flushing (3%), fatigue (1%)
Gastrointestinal: Nausea (5%)
Neuromuscular & skeletal: Paresthesia (1%)
Respiratory: Dyspnea (3%)

Drug Interactions
Metabolism/Transport Effects Inhibits ABCG2, P-glycoprotein

Avoid Concomitant Use

Avoid concomitant use of Dipyridamole with any of the following: Silodosin

Increased Effect/Toxicity

Dipyridamole may increase the levels/effects of: Adenosine; Anticoagulants; Antiplatelet Agents; Beta-Blockers; Colchicine; Collagenase (Systemic); Dabigatran Etexilate; Drotrecogin Alfa; Everolimus; Hypotensive Agents; Ibritumomab; P-Glycoprotein Substrates; Regadenoson; Rivaroxaban; Salicylates; Silodosin; Thrombolytic Agents; Topotecan; Tositumomab and Iodine I 131 Tositumomab

The levels/effects of Dipyridamole may be increased by: Dasatinib; Glucosamine; Herbs (Anticoagulant/Antiplatelet Properties); Nonsteroidal Anti-Inflammatory Agents; Omega-3-Acid Ethyl Esters; Pentosan Polysulfate Sodium; Pentoxifylline; Prostacyclin Analogues; Vitamin E

Decreased Effect

The levels/effects of Dipyridamole may be decreased by: Nonsteroidal Anti-Inflammatory Agents

Ethanol/Nutrition/Herb Interactions Herb/Nutraceutical: Avoid cat's claw, dong quai, evening primrose, feverfew, garlic, ginger, ginkgo, red clover, horse chestnut, green tea, ginseng (all have additional antiplatelet activity).

Stability I.V.: Store between 15°C to 25°C (59°F to 77°F); do not freeze. Protect from light. Prior to administration, dilute to a ≥1:2 ratio in NS, 1/2NS, or D_5W. Total volume should be ~20-50 mL.

Mechanism of Action Inhibits the activity of adenosine deaminase and phosphodiesterase, which causes an accumulation of adenosine, adenine nucleotides, and cyclic AMP; these mediators then inhibit platelet aggregation and may cause vasodilation; may also stimulate release of prostacyclin or PGD_2; causes coronary vasodilation

Pharmacodynamics/Kinetics

Absorption: Readily, but variable

Distribution: Adults: V_d: 2-3 L/kg

Protein binding: 91% to 99%

Metabolism: Hepatic

Half-life elimination: Terminal: 10-12 hours

Time to peak, serum: 2-2.5 hours

Excretion: Feces (as glucuronide conjugates and unchanged drug)

Dosage

Geriatric & Adult

Adjunctive therapy for prophylaxis of thromboembolism with cardiac valve replacement: Oral: 75-100 mg 4 times/day

Evaluation of coronary artery disease: I.V.: 0.14 mg/kg/minute for 4 minutes; maximum dose: 60 mg

Following dipyridamole infusion, inject thallium-201 within 5 minutes. **Note:** Aminophylline should be available for urgent/emergent use; dosing of 50-100 mg (range: 50-250 mg) I.V. push over 30-60 seconds.

Administration

I.V.: Infuse diluted solution over 4 minutes.

Tablet: Administer with water 1 hour before meals.

Monitoring Parameters Blood pressure, heart rate, ECG (stress test)

Test Interactions Concurrent caffeine or theophylline use may demonstrate a false-negative result with dipyridamole-thallium myocardial imaging.

Special Geriatric Considerations Since evidence suggests that clinically used doses are ineffective for prevention of platelet aggregation, consideration for low-dose aspirin (81-325 mg/day) alone may be necessary. This will decrease cost as well as inconvenience.

This medication is considered to be potentially inappropriate in this patient population (Beers Criteria severity: Low).

Dosage Forms Excipient information presented when available (limited, particularly for generics); consult specific product labeling. [DSC] = Discontinued product

Injection, solution: 5 mg/mL (2 mL [DSC], 10 mL)

Tablet, oral: 25 mg, 50 mg, 75 mg

Persantine®: 25 mg, 50 mg, 75 mg

◆ **Dipyridamole and Aspirin** *see* Aspirin and Dipyridamole *on page 158*

◆ **Disalicylic Acid** *see* Salsalate *on page 1656*

◆ **Disodium Cromoglycate** *see* Cromolyn (Nasal) *on page 422*

◆ **Disodium Cromoglycate** *see* Cromolyn (Ophthalmic) *on page 422*

◆ **Disodium Cromoglycate** *see* Cromolyn (Systemic, Oral Inhalation) *on page 420*

◆ **d-Isoephedrine Hydrochloride** *see* Pseudoephedrine *on page 1545*

Disopyramide (dye soe PEER a mide)

Related Information

Beers Criteria – Potentially Inappropriate Medications for Geriatrics *on page 2089*

Medication Safety Issues

Sound-alike/look-alike issues:

Disopyramide may be confused with desipramine, dipyridamole

Norpace® may be confused with Norpramin®

BEERS Criteria medication:

This drug may be inappropriate for use in geriatric patients (high severity risk).

Brand Names: U.S. Norpace®; Norpace® CR

Brand Names: Canada Norpace®; Rythmodan®; Rythmodan®-LA

Index Terms Disopyramide Phosphate

Generic Availability (U.S.) Yes

Pharmacologic Category Antiarrhythmic Agent, Class Ia

Use Suppression and prevention of unifocal and multifocal atrial and premature, ventricular premature complexes, coupled ventricular tachycardia; effective in the conversion of atrial fibrillation, atrial flutter, and paroxysmal atrial tachycardia to normal sinus rhythm and prevention of the recurrence of these arrhythmias after conversion by other methods

Unlabeled/Investigational Use Hypertrophic obstructive cardiomyopathy (HOCM)

Contraindications Hypersensitivity to disopyramide or any component of the formulation; cardiogenic shock; pre-existing second- or third-degree heart block (except in patients with a functioning artificial pacemaker); congenital QT syndrome; sick sinus syndrome

Warnings/Precautions Watch for proarrhythmic effects; may cause QT$_c$ prolongation and subsequent torsade de pointes; avoid use in patients with diagnosed or suspected congenital long QT syndrome. Monitor and adjust dose to prevent QT$_c$ prolongation. Avoid concurrent use with other medications that prolong QT interval or decrease myocardial contractility. Correct hypokalemia before initiating therapy; may worsen toxicity. **[U.S. Boxed Warning]: In the Cardiac Arrhythmia Suppression Trial (CAST), recent (>6 days but <2 years ago) myocardial infarction patients with asymptomatic, non-life-threatening ventricular arrhythmias did not benefit and may have been harmed by attempts to suppress the arrhythmia with flecainide or encainide. An increased mortality or nonfatal cardiac arrest rate (7.7%) was seen in the active treatment group compared with patients in the placebo group (3%). The applicability of the CAST results to other populations is unknown. Antiarrhythmic agents should be reserved for patients with life-threatening ventricular arrhythmias.** May precipitate or exacerbate HF. Due to significant anticholinergic effects, do not use in patients with urinary retention, BPH, glaucoma, or myasthenia gravis. Reduce dosage in renal or hepatic impairment. May be inappropriate for use in the elderly due to a risk of heart failure developing (potent negative inotrope) and potent anticholinergic properties; alternative antiarrhythmic agents preferred (Beers Criteria). The controlled release form is not recommended for Cl$_{cr}$ ≤40 mL/minute. In patients with atrial fibrillation or flutter, block the AV node before initiating. Use caution in Wolff-Parkinson-White syndrome or bundle branch block. Monitor closely for hypotension during the initiation of therapy.

Adverse Reactions (Reflective of adult population; not specific for elderly) The most common adverse effects are related to cholinergic blockade. The most serious adverse effects of disopyramide are hypotension and CHF.

>10%:

Gastrointestinal: Xerostomia (32%), constipation (11%)

Genitourinary: Urinary hesitancy (14% to 23%)

1% to 10%:

Cardiovascular: CHF, hypotension, cardiac conduction disturbance, edema, syncope, chest pain

Central nervous system: Fatigue, headache, malaise, dizziness, nervousness

Dermatologic: Rash, generalized dermatoses, pruritus

Endocrine & metabolic: Cholesterol increased, hypokalemia, triglycerides increased

Gastrointestinal: Dry throat, nausea, abdominal distension, flatulence, abdominal bloating, anorexia, diarrhea, vomiting, weight gain

Genitourinary: Urinary retention, urinary frequency, urinary urgency, impotence (1% to 3%)

Neuromuscular & skeletal: Muscle weakness, muscular pain

Ocular: Blurred vision, dry eyes

Respiratory: Dyspnea

Drug Interactions

Metabolism/Transport Effects Substrate of CYP3A4 (major)

◀ **Avoid Concomitant Use**
Avoid concomitant use of Disopyramide with any of the following: Artemether; Conivaptan; Dronedarone; Lumefantrine; Macrolide Antibiotics; Nilotinib; Pimozide; QUEtiapine; Qui-NINE; Tetrabenazine; Thioridazine; Toremifene; Vandetanib; Vemurafenib; Verapamil; Ziprasidone

Increased Effect/Toxicity
Disopyramide may increase the levels/effects of: AbobotulinumtoxinA; Anticholinergics; Beta-Blockers; Cannabinoids; Dronedarone; Lidocaine; Lidocaine (Systemic); OnabotulinumtoxinA; Pimozide; Potassium Chloride; QTc-Prolonging Agents; QuiNINE; RimabotulinumtoxinB; Tetrabenazine; Thioridazine; Toremifene; Vandetanib; Vemurafenib; Ziprasidone

The levels/effects of Disopyramide may be increased by: Alfuzosin; Amiodarone; Artemether; Chloroquine; Ciprofloxacin; Ciprofloxacin (Systemic); Conivaptan; CYP3A4 Inhibitors (Moderate); CYP3A4 Inhibitors (Strong); Eribulin; Fingolimod; Gadobutrol; Lumefantrine; Lurasidone; Macrolide Antibiotics; Nilotinib; Pramlintide; QUEtiapine; Qui-NINE; Verapamil

Decreased Effect
Disopyramide may decrease the levels/effects of: Acetylcholinesterase Inhibitors (Central); Secretin

The levels/effects of Disopyramide may be decreased by: Acetylcholinesterase Inhibitors (Central); Barbiturates; CYP3A4 Inducers (Strong); Deferasirox; Etravirine; Fosphenytoin; Herbs (CYP3A4 Inducers); Phenytoin; Rifamycin Derivatives; Tocilizumab

Ethanol/Nutrition/Herb Interactions
Ethanol: Avoid ethanol (may increase CNS depression).
Herb/Nutraceutical: St John's wort may decrease disopyramide levels. Avoid ephedra (may worsen arrhythmia).

Stability Extemporaneously prepared suspension is stable for 4 weeks refrigerated.

Mechanism of Action Class Ia antiarrhythmic: Decreases myocardial excitability and conduction velocity; reduces disparity in refractory between normal and infarcted myocardium; possesses anticholinergic, peripheral vasoconstrictive, and negative inotropic effects

Pharmacodynamics/Kinetics
Onset of action: 0.5-3.5 hours
Duration: 1.5-8.5 hours
Absorption: 60% to 83%
Distribution: V_d: 0.8-2 L/kg
Protein binding (concentration dependent): 20% to 60%
Metabolism: Hepatic to inactive metabolites
Half-life elimination: Adults: 4-10 hours; prolonged with hepatic or renal impairment
Time to peak, serum: Within 2 hours
Excretion: Urine (40% to 60% as unchanged drug); feces (10% to 15%)

Dosage
Geriatric & Adult
Dysrhythmia: Oral:
<50 kg: 100 mg every 6 hours or 200 mg every 12 hours (controlled release)
>50 kg: 150 mg every 6 hours or 300 mg every 12 hours (controlled release); if no response, may increase to 200 mg every 6 hours; maximum dose required for patients with severe refractory ventricular tachycardia is 400 mg every 6 hours.
Hypertrophic obstructive cardiomyopathy (unlabeled use): Oral: Initial: Controlled release: 200 mg twice daily. If symptoms do not improve, increase by 100 mg/day at 2-week intervals to a maximum daily dose of 600 mg.

Renal Impairment Oral: 100 mg (nonsustained release) given at the following intervals, based on creatinine clearance (mL/minute):
Cl_{cr} 30-40 mL/minute: Administer every 8 hours
Cl_{cr} 15-30 mL/minute: Administer every 12 hours
Cl_{cr} <15 mL/minute: Administer every 24 hours
or alter the dose as follows:
Cl_{cr} 30-<40 mL/minute: Reduce dose 50%
Cl_{cr} 15-30 mL/minute: Reduce dose 75%
Not dialyzable (0% to 5%) by hemo- or peritoneal methods; supplemental dose is not necessary.

Hepatic Impairment Administer 100 mg every 6 hours or 200 mg every 12 hours (controlled release).

Administration Administer around-the-clock rather than 4 times/day (ie, 12-6-12-6, not 9-1-5-9) to promote less variation in peak and trough serum levels

Monitoring Parameters ECG, blood pressure, urinary retention, CNS anticholinergic effects (confusion, agitation, hallucinations, etc)

Reference Range
Therapeutic concentration:
  Atrial arrhythmias: 2.8-3.2 mcg/mL
  Ventricular arrhythmias 3.3-7.5 mcg/mL
Toxic concentration: >7 mcg/mL

Special Geriatric Considerations Due to changes in total clearance (decreased) in the elderly, monitor closely; the anticholinergic action may be intolerable and require discontinuation; monitor for CNS anticholinergic effects (confusion, agitation, hallucinations, etc). **Note:** Dose needs to be altered with Cl_{cr} <40 mL/minute which may be found frequently in older adults.

Clinical studies of Norpace®/Norpace® CR did not include sufficient numbers of subjects ≥65 years of age to determine whether they respond differently from younger subjects. Other reported clinical experience has not identified differences in responses between elderly and younger patients. In general, dose selection for an elderly patient should be cautious, usually starting at the low end of the dosing range, reflecting the greater frequency of decreased hepatic, renal, or cardiac function, and of concomitant disease or other drug therapy.

Because of its anticholinergic activity, disopyramide phosphate should not be used in patients with glaucoma, urinary retention, or benign prostatic hyperplasia (medical conditions commonly associated with the elderly) unless adequate overriding measures are taken. In the event of increased anticholinergic side effects, plasma levels of disopyramide should be monitored and the dose of the drug adjusted accordingly. A reduction of the dose by one third, from the recommended 600 mg/day to 400 mg/day, would be reasonable, without changing the dosing interval. This drug is known to be substantially excreted by the kidney, and the risk of toxic reactions to this drug may be greater in patients with impaired renal function. Because elderly patients are more likely to have decreased renal function, care should be taken in dose selection, and it may be useful to monitor renal function.

This medication is considered to be potentially inappropriate in this patient population (Beers Criteria severity: High).

Dosage Forms Excipient information presented when available (limited, particularly for generics); consult specific product labeling.
Capsule, oral: 100 mg, 150 mg
  Norpace®: 100 mg, 150 mg
Capsule, controlled release, oral:
  Norpace® CR: 100 mg, 150 mg

Selected References
Fenster PE and Nolan PE, "Antiarrhythmic Drugs," *Geriatric Pharmacology*, Bressler R and Katz MD, eds, New York, NY: McGraw-Hill, 1993, 6:105-49.

◆ **Disopyramide Phosphate** see Disopyramide on page 539
◆ **Ditropan** see Oxybutynin on page 1365
◆ **Ditropan XL®** see Oxybutynin on page 1365
◆ **Diuril®** see Chlorothiazide on page 337

Divalproex (dye VAL proe ex)

Related Information
Liquid Compatibility of Antidepressants, Antipsychotics, and Mood Stabilizers on page 2111
Medication Safety Issues
  Sound-alike/look-alike issues:
    Depakote® may be confused with Depakene®, Depakote® ER, Senokot®
    Depakote® ER may be confused with Depakote®, divalproex enteric coated
Brand Names: U.S. Depakote®; Depakote® ER; Depakote® Sprinkle
Brand Names: Canada Apo-Divalproex®; Dom-Divalproex; Epival®; Mylan-Divalproex; Novo-Divalproex; Nu-Divalproex; PHL-Divalproex; PMS-Divalproex
Index Terms Divalproex Sodium; Valproate Semisodium; Valproic Acid Derivative
Generic Availability (U.S.) Yes
Pharmacologic Category Anticonvulsant, Miscellaneous; Antimanic Agent; Histone Deacetylase Inhibitor
Use Monotherapy and adjunctive therapy in the treatment of patients with complex partial seizures; monotherapy and adjunctive therapy of simple and complex absence seizures; adjunctive therapy in patients with multiple seizure types that include absence seizures
Depakote®, Depakote® ER: Mania associated with bipolar disorder; migraine prophylaxis
Unlabeled/Investigational Use Diabetic neuropathy
Contraindications Hypersensitivity to divalproex, derivatives, or any component of the formulation; hepatic disease or significant impairment; urea cycle disorders

DIVALPROEX

◀ **Warnings/Precautions**

[U.S. Boxed Warning]: Hepatic failure resulting in fatalities has occurred in patients. Other risk factors include organic brain disease, mental retardation with severe seizure disorders, congenital metabolic disorders, and patients on multiple anticonvulsants. Hepatotoxicity has usually been reported within 6 months of therapy initiation. Monitor patients closely for appearance of malaise, weakness, facial edema, anorexia, jaundice, and vomiting; discontinue immediately with signs/symptom of significant or suspected impairment. Liver function tests should be performed at baseline and at regular intervals after initiation of therapy, especially within the first 6 months. Hepatic dysfunction may progress despite discontinuing treatment. Should only be used as monotherapy in patients at high risk for hepatotoxicity. Contraindicated with severe impairment.

[U.S. Boxed Warning]: Cases of life-threatening pancreatitis, occurring at the start of therapy or following years of use, have been reported. Some cases have been hemorrhagic with rapid progression of initial symptoms to death. Promptly evaluate symptoms of abdominal pain, nausea, vomiting, and/or anorexia; should generally be discontinued if pancreatitis is diagnosed.

May cause severe thrombocytopenia, inhibition of platelet aggregation, and bleeding. Tremors may indicate overdosage; use with caution in patients receiving other anticonvulsants. Hypersensitivity reactions affecting multiple organs have been reported in association with divalproex use; may include dermatologic and/or hematologic changes (eosinophilia, neutropenia, thrombocytopenia) or symptoms of organ dysfunction.

Hyperammonemia and/or encephalopathy, sometimes fatal, have been reported following the initiation of divalproex therapy and may be present with normal transaminase levels. Ammonia levels should be measured in patients who develop unexplained lethargy and vomiting, changes in mental status, or in patients who present with hypothermia (unintentional drop in core body temperature to <35°C/95°F). Discontinue therapy if ammonia levels are increased and evaluate for possible urea cycle disorder (UCD); contraindicated in patients with UCD. Evaluation of UCD should be considered for the following patients prior to the start of therapy: History of unexplained encephalopathy or coma; encephalopathy associated with protein load; unexplained mental retardation; history of elevated plasma ammonia or glutamine; history of cyclical vomiting and lethargy; episodic extreme irritability, ataxia; low BUN or protein avoidance; family history of UCD or unexplained infant deaths (particularly male); or signs or symptoms of UCD (hyperammonemia, encephalopathy, respiratory alkalosis). Hypothermia has been reported with divalproex therapy; may or may not be associated with hyperammonemia; may also occur with concomitant topiramate therapy.

In vitro studies have suggested divalproex stimulates the replication of HIV and CMV viruses under experimental conditions. The clinical consequence of this is unknown, but should be considered when monitoring affected patients.

Antiepileptics are associated with an increased risk of suicidal behavior/thoughts with use (regardless of indication); patients should be monitored for signs/symptoms of depression, suicidal tendencies, and other unusual behavior changes during therapy and instructed to inform their healthcare provider immediately if symptoms occur.

Anticonvulsants should not be discontinued abruptly because of the possibility of increasing seizure frequency; divalproex should be withdrawn gradually to minimize the potential of increased seizure frequency, unless safety concerns require a more rapid withdrawal. Concomitant use with carbapenem antibiotics may reduce valproic acid levels to subtherapeutic levels; monitor levels frequently and consider alternate therapy if levels drop significantly or lack of seizure control occurs. Concomitant use with clonazepam may induce absence status. Patients treated for bipolar disorder should be monitored closely for clinical worsening or suicidality; prescriptions should be written for the smallest quantity consistent with good patient care.

CNS depression may occur with divalproex use. Patients must be cautioned about performing tasks which require mental alertness (operating machinery or driving). Effects with other sedative drugs or ethanol may be potentiated. Use with caution in the elderly.

Adverse Reactions (Reflective of adult population; not specific for elderly)

>10%:

Central nervous system: Headache (≤31%), somnolence (≤30%), dizziness (12% to 25%), insomnia (>1% to 15%), nervousness (>1% to 11%), pain (1% to 11%)

Dermatologic: Alopecia (>1% to 24%)

Gastrointestinal: Nausea (15% to 48%), vomiting (7% to 27%), diarrhea (7% to 23%), abdominal pain (7% to 23%), dyspepsia (7% to 23%), anorexia (>1% to 12%)

Hematologic: Thrombocytopenia (1% to 24%; dose related)

Neuromuscular & skeletal: Tremor (≤57%), weakness (6% to 27%)

Ocular: Diplopia (>1% to 16%), amblyopia/blurred vision (≤12%)

Miscellaneous: Infection (≤20%), flu-like syndrome (12%)

1% to 10%:

Cardiovascular: Peripheral edema (>1% to 8%), chest pain (>1% to <5%), edema (>1% to <5%), facial edema (>1% to <5%), hypertension (>1% to <5%), hypotension (>1% to <5%), palpitation (>1% to <5%), postural hypotension (>1% to <5%), tachycardia (>1% to <5%), vasodilation(>1% to <5%), arrhythmia

Central nervous system: Ataxia (>1% to 8%), amnesia (>1% to 7%), emotional lability (>1% to 6%), fever (>1% to 6%), abnormal thinking (≤6%), depression (>1% to 5%), abnormal dreams (>1% to <5%), agitation (>1% to <5%), anxiety (>1% to <5%), catatonia (>1% to <5%), chills (>1% to <5%), confusion (>1% to <5%), coordination abnormal (>1% to <5%), hallucination (>1% to <5%), malaise (>1% to <5%), personality disorder (>1% to <5%), speech disorder (>1% to <5%), tardive dyskinesia (>1% to <5%), vertigo (>1% to <5%), euphoria (1%), hypoesthesia (1%)

Dermatologic: Rash (>1% to 6%), bruising (>1% to 5%), discoid lupus erythematosus (>1% to <5%), dry skin (>1% to <5%), furunculosis (>1% to <5%), petechia (>1% to <5%), pruritus (>1% to <5), seborrhea (>1% to <5%)

Endocrine & metabolic: Amenorrhea (>1% to <5%), dysmenorrhea (>1% to <5%), metrorrhagia (>1% to <5%), hypoproteinemia

Gastrointestinal: Weight gain (4% to 9%), weight loss (6%), appetite increased (≤6%), constipation (>1% to 5%), xerostomia (>1% to 5%), eructation (>1% to <5%), fecal incontinence (>1% to <5%), flatulence (>1% to <5%), gastroenteritis (>1% to <5%), glossitis (>1% to <5%), hematemesis (>1% to <5%), pancreatitis (>1% to <5%), periodontal abscess (>1% to <5%), stomatitis (>1% to <5%), taste perversion (>1% to <5%), dysphagia, gum hemorrhage, mouth ulceration

Genitourinary: Cystitis (>1% to 5%), dysuria (>1% to 5%), urinary frequency (>1% to <5%), urinary incontinence (>1% to <5%), vaginal hemorrhage (>1% to 5%), vaginitis (>1% to <5%)

Hepatic: ALT increased (>1% to <5%), AST increased (>1% to <5%)

Local: Injection site pain (3%), injection site reaction (2%), injection site inflammation (1%)

Neuromuscular & skeletal: Back pain (≤8%), abnormal gait (>1% to <5%), arthralgia (>1% to <5%), arthrosis (>1% to <5%), dysarthria (>1% to <5%), hypertonia (>1% to <5%), hypokinesia (>1% to <5%), leg cramps (>1% to <5%), myalgia (>1% to <5%), myasthenia (>1% to <5%), neck pain (>1% to <5%), neck rigidity (>1% to <5%), paresthesia (>1% to <5%), reflex increased (>1% to <5%), twitching (>1% to <5%)

Ocular: Nystagmus (1% to 8%), dry eyes (>1% to 5%), eye pain (>1% to 5%), abnormal vision (>1% to <5%), conjunctivitis (>1% to <5%)

Otic: Tinnitus (1% to 7%), ear pain (>1% to 5%), deafness (>1% to <5%), otitis media (>1% to <5%)

Respiratory: Pharyngitis (2% to 8%), bronchitis (5%), rhinitis (>1% to 5%), dyspnea (1% to 5%), cough (>1% to <5%), epistaxis (>1% to <5%), pneumonia (>1% to <5%), sinusitis (>1% to <5%)

Miscellaneous: Diaphoresis (1%), hiccups

Drug Interactions

Metabolism/Transport Effects For divalproex: **Substrate** (minor) of CYP2A6, 2B6, 2C9, 2C19, 2E1; **Inhibits** CYP2C9 (weak), 2C19 (weak), 2D6 (weak), 3A4 (weak); **Induces** CYP2A6 (weak)

Avoid Concomitant Use There are no known interactions where it is recommended to avoid concomitant use.

Increased Effect/Toxicity

Divalproex may increase the levels/effects of: Barbiturates; Ethosuximide; LamoTRIgine; LORazepam; Paliperidone; Primidone; RisperiDONE; Rufinamide; Temozolomide; Topiramate; Tricyclic Antidepressants; Vorinostat; Zidovudine

The levels/effects of Divalproex may be increased by: ChlorproMAZINE; Felbamate; GuanFACINE; Salicylates

Decreased Effect

Divalproex may decrease the levels/effects of: CarBAMazepine; Fosphenytoin; OXcarbazepine; Phenytoin

The levels/effects of Divalproex may be decreased by: Barbiturates; CarBAMazepine; Carbapenems; Cyproterone; Ethosuximide; Fosphenytoin; Methylfolate; Phenytoin; Primidone; Protease Inhibitors; Rifampin

Ethanol/Nutrition/Herb Interactions

Ethanol: Avoid ethanol (may increase CNS depression).

Food: Food may delay but does not affect the extent of absorption. Valproic acid serum concentrations may be decreased if taken with food. Milk has no effect on absorption.

Herb/Nutraceutical: Avoid evening primrose (seizure threshold decreased).

DIVALPROEX

◀ **Stability**
Depakote® tablet: Store below 30°C (86°F).
Depakote® Sprinkles: Store below 25°C (77°F).
Depakote® ER: Store at controlled room temperature of 25°C (77°F).

Mechanism of Action Causes increased availability of gamma-aminobutyric acid (GABA), an inhibitory neurotransmitter, to brain neurons or may enhance the action of GABA or mimic its action at postsynaptic receptor sites

Pharmacodynamics/Kinetics
Distribution: Total valproate: 11 L/1.73 m²; Free valproate: 92 L/1.73 m²

Protein binding (dose dependent): 80% to 90%; decreased in the elderly and with hepatic or renal dysfunction

Metabolism: Extensively hepatic via glucuronide conjugation and mitochondrial beta-oxidation. The relationship between dose and total valproate concentration is nonlinear; concentration does not increase proportionally with the dose, but increases to a lesser extent due to saturable plasma protein binding. The kinetics of unbound drug are linear.

Bioavailability: Depakote® ER: ~90% relative to I.V. dose and ~89% relative to delayed release formulation

Half-life elimination (increased with liver disease): Adults: 9-16 hours

Time to peak, serum: Depakote® tablet: ~4 hours; Depakote® ER: 4-17 hours

Excretion: Urine (30% to 50% as glucuronide conjugate, 3% as unchanged drug)

Dosage
Geriatric Initiate at lower doses; dose escalation should be managed more slowly (in persons of advanced age). Refer to adult dosing.

Adult Equivalent oral dosages of divalproex and valproic acid deliver the same quantities of valproate ion.

Seizures: Oral: Administer doses >250 mg/day in divided doses.
Simple and complex absence seizure: Initial: 15 mg/kg/day; increase by 5-10 mg/kg/day at weekly intervals until therapeutic levels are achieved; maximum: 60 mg/kg/day.
Complex partial seizure: Initial: 10-15 mg/kg/day; increase by 5-10 mg/kg/day at weekly intervals until therapeutic levels are achieved; maximum: 60 mg/kg/day.

Note: Regular release and delayed release formulations are usually given in 2-4 divided doses/day; extended release formulation (Depakote® ER) is usually given once daily. Conversion to Depakote® ER from a stable dose of Depakote® may require an increase in the total daily dose between 8% and 20% to maintain similar serum concentrations.

Mania: Oral:
Depakote® tablet: Initial: 750 mg/day in divided doses; dose should be adjusted as rapidly as possible to desired clinical effect; maximum recommended dosage: 60 mg/kg/day
Depakote® ER: Initial: 25 mg/kg/day given once daily; dose should be adjusted as rapidly as possible to desired clinical effect; maximum recommended dose: 60 mg/kg/day.

Migraine prophylaxis: Oral:
Depakote® tablet: 250 mg twice daily; adjust dose based on patient response, up to 1000 mg/day
Depakote® ER: 500 mg once daily for 7 days, then increase to 1000 mg once daily; adjust dose based on patient response; usual dosage range: 500-1000 mg/day

Diabetic neuropathy (unlabeled use): Oral: 500-1200 mg/day (Bril, 2011)

Renal Impairment A 27% reduction in clearance of unbound valproate is seen in patients with Cl_cr <10 mL/minute. Hemodialysis reduces valproate concentrations by 20%, therefore, no dose adjustment is needed in patients with renal failure. Protein binding is reduced, monitoring only total valproate concentrations may be misleading.

Hepatic Impairment Dosage reduction is required. Clearance is decreased with liver impairment. Hepatic disease is also associated with decreased albumin concentrations and 2- to 2.6-fold increase in the unbound fraction. Free concentrations of valproate may be elevated while total concentrations appear normal. Use is contraindicated in severe impairment.

Administration
Depakote® ER: Swallow whole; do not crush or chew. Patients who need dose adjustments smaller than 500 mg/day for migraine prophylaxis should be changed to Depakote® delayed release tablets.

Depakote® Sprinkle capsules may be swallowed whole or open capsule and sprinkle on small amount (1 teaspoonful) of soft food and use immediately (do not store or chew).

Monitoring Parameters Liver enzymes (at baseline and during therapy), CBC with platelets (baseline and periodic intervals), PT/PTT (especially prior to surgery), serum ammonia (with symptoms of lethargy, mental status change), serum valproate levels; suicidality (eg, suicidal thoughts, depression, behavioral changes)

Test Interactions False-positive result for urine ketones

Pharmacotherapy Pearls Divalproex sodium is a compound of sodium valproate and valproic acid; divalproex dissociates to valproate in the GI tract.

Extended release tablets have 10% to 20% less fluctuation in serum concentration than delayed release tablets. Extended release tablets are not bioequivalent to delayed release tablets.

Special Geriatric Considerations Although there is little data in elderly for the use of divalproex in the treatment of seizures, there are a number of studies which demonstrate its benefit in the treatment of agitation and dementia and other psychiatric disorders. It is important that the clinician understand that serum concentrations do not correlate with behavior response; likewise, it is imperative to monitor LFTs and CBC during the first 6 months of therapy. See Warnings/Precautions, Monitoring Parameters, and Pharmacotherapy Pearls.

Elimination is decreased in elderly. Studies of older adults with dementia show a high incidence of somnolence (which is usually transient); cognitive side effects generally minimal. In some patients, this was associated with weight loss. Starting doses should be lower and increased slowly, with careful monitoring of nutritional intake and dehydration. Safety and efficacy for use in patients >65 years of age have not been studied for migraine prophylaxis.

Dosage Forms Excipient information presented when available (limited, particularly for generics); consult specific product labeling.

Capsule, sprinkle, oral: 125 mg [strength expressed as valproic acid]

Depakote® Sprinkle: 125 mg [strength expressed as valproic acid]

Tablet, delayed release, oral: 125 mg [strength expressed as valproic acid], 250 mg [strength expressed as valproic acid], 500 mg [strength expressed as valproic acid]

Depakote®: 125 mg, 250 mg, 500 mg [strength expressed as valproic acid]

Tablet, extended release, oral: 250 mg [strength expressed as valproic acid], 500 mg [strength expressed as valproic acid]

Depakote® ER: 250 mg, 500 mg [strength expressed as valproic acid]

Selected References

Loy R and Tariot PN, "Neuroprotective Properties of Valproate: Potential Benefit for AD and Tauopathies," *J Mol Neurosci*, 2002, 19(3):303-7.

Pratt CE and Davis SM, "Divalproex Sodium Therapy in Elderly With Dementia-Related Agitation," *Ann Pharmacother*, 2002, 36(10):1625-28.

Sink KM, Holden KF, and Yaffe K, "Pharmacological Treatment of Neuropsychiatric Symptoms of Dementia. A Review of Evidence," *JAMA*, 2005, 293(5):596-608.

Tariot PN, Raman R, Jakimovich L, et al, "Divalproex Sodium in Nursing Home Residents With Possible or Probable Alzheimer Disease Complicated by Agitation: A Randomized, Controlled Trial," *Am J Geriatr Psychiatry*, 2005, 13 (11):942-49.

◆ **Divalproex Sodium** *see* Divalproex *on page 541*

◆ **Divigel®** *see* Estradiol (Systemic) *on page 641*

◆ **5071-1DL(6)** *see* Megestrol *on page 1126*

◆ *dl*-Alpha Tocopherol *see* Vitamin E *on page 1921*

DOBUTamine (doe BYOO ta meen)

Medication Safety Issues

Sound-alike/look-alike issues:

DOBUTamine may be confused with DOPamine

High alert medication:

The Institute for Safe Medication Practices (ISMP) includes this medication among its list of drugs which have a heightened risk of causing significant patient harm when used in error.

Brand Names: Canada Dobutamine Injection, USP; Dobutrex®

Index Terms Dobutamine Hydrochloride

Generic Availability (U.S.) Yes

Pharmacologic Category Adrenergic Agonist Agent

Use Short-term management of patients with cardiac decompensation

Unlabeled/Investigational Use Positive inotropic agent for use in myocardial dysfunction related to sepsis; stress echocardiography

Contraindications Hypersensitivity to dobutamine or sulfites (some contain sodium metabisulfite), or any component of the formulation; idiopathic hypertrophic subaortic stenosis (IHSS)

Warnings/Precautions May increase heart rate. Patients with atrial fibrillation may experience an increase in ventricular response. An increase in blood pressure is more common, but occasionally a patient may become hypotensive. May exacerbate ventricular ectopy. If needed, correct hypovolemia first to optimize hemodynamics. Ineffective therapeutically in the presence of mechanical obstruction such as severe aortic stenosis. Use caution post-MI (can increase myocardial oxygen demand). Use cautiously in the elderly starting at lower end of the dosage range. Use with extreme caution in patients taking MAO inhibitors. Dobutamine

DOBUTAMINE

◄ in combination with stress echo may be used diagnostically. Product may contain sodium sulfite.

Adverse Reactions (Reflective of adult population; not specific for elderly) Incidence of adverse events is not always reported.

Cardiovascular: Increased heart rate, increased blood pressure, increased ventricular ectopic activity, hypotension, premature ventricular beats (5%, dose related), anginal pain (1% to 3%), nonspecific chest pain (1% to 3%), palpitation (1% to 3%)

Central nervous system: Fever (1% to 3%), headache (1% to 3%), paresthesia

Endocrine & metabolic: Slight decrease in serum potassium

Gastrointestinal: Nausea (1% to 3%)

Hematologic: Thrombocytopenia (isolated cases)

Local: Phlebitis, local inflammatory changes and pain from infiltration, cutaneous necrosis (isolated cases)

Neuromuscular & skeletal: Mild leg cramps

Respiratory: Dyspnea (1% to 3%)

Drug Interactions

Avoid Concomitant Use

Avoid concomitant use of DOBUTamine with any of the following: Iobenguane I 123

Increased Effect/Toxicity

DOBUTamine may increase the levels/effects of: Sympathomimetics

The levels/effects of DOBUTamine may be increased by: Atomoxetine; Cannabinoids; COMT Inhibitors

Decreased Effect

DOBUTamine may decrease the levels/effects of: Iobenguane I 123

The levels/effects of DOBUTamine may be decreased by: Calcium Salts

Stability Remix solution every 24 hours. Store reconstituted solution under refrigeration for 48 hours or 6 hours at room temperature. Pink discoloration of solution indicates slight oxidation but **no** significant loss of potency.

Stability of parenteral admixture at room temperature (25°C): 48 hours; at refrigeration (4°C): 7 days.

Standard adult diluent: 250 mg/500 mL D_5W; 500 mg/500 mL D_5W.

Mechanism of Action Stimulates beta$_1$-adrenergic receptors, causing increased contractility and heart rate, with little effect on beta$_2$- or alpha-receptors

Pharmacodynamics/Kinetics

Onset of action: I.V.: 1-10 minutes

Peak effect: 10-20 minutes

Metabolism: In tissues and hepatically to inactive metabolites

Half-life elimination: 2 minutes

Excretion: Urine (as metabolites)

Dosage

Geriatric & Adult Cardiac decompensation: I.V. infusion: 2.5-20 mcg/kg/minute; maximum: 40 mcg/kg/minute, titrate to desired response; see table.

Infusion Rates of Various Dilutions of Dobutamine

Desired Delivery Rate (mcg/kg/min)	Infusion Rate (mL/kg/min)	
	500 mcg/mL	1000 mcg/mL
2.5	0.005	0.0025
5	0.01	0.005
7.5	0.015	0.0075
10	0.02	0.01
12.5	0.025	0.0125
15	0.03	0.015

Administration Use infusion device to control rate of flow; administer into large vein. Do not administer through same I.V. line as heparin, hydrocortisone sodium succinate, cefazolin, or penicillin.

Monitoring Parameters Blood pressure, ECG, heart rate, CVP, RAP, MAP, urine output; if pulmonary artery catheter is in place, monitor CI, PCWP, and SVR

Pharmacotherapy Pearls Dobutamine lowers central venous pressure and wedge pressure but has little effect on pulmonary vascular resistance.

Dobutamine therapy should be avoided in patients with stable heart failure due to an increase in mortality. In patients with intractable heart failure, dobutamine may be used as a short-term infusion to provide symptomatic benefit. It is not known whether short-term dobutamine therapy in end-stage heart failure has any outcome benefit.

Dobutamine infusion during echocardiography is used as a cardiovascular stress. Wall motion abnormalities developing with increasing doses of dobutamine may help to identify ischemic and/or hibernating myocardium.

Special Geriatric Considerations One study demonstrated beneficial hemodynamic effects in elderly patients; monitor closely.

Dosage Forms Excipient information presented when available (limited, particularly for generics); consult specific product labeling. [DSC] = Discontinued product

Infusion, premixed in D_5W, as hydrochloride: 1 mg/mL (250 mL, 500 mL [DSC]); 2 mg/mL (250 mL); 4 mg/mL (250 mL)

Injection, solution, as hydrochloride: 12.5 mg/mL (20 mL, 40 mL)

Selected References

Dellinger RP, Levy MM, Carlet JM, et al, "Surviving Sepsis Campaign: International Guidelines for Management of Severe Sepsis and Septic Shock: 2008," *Intensive Care Med*, 2008, 34(1):17-60.

◆ **Dobutamine Hydrochloride** *see* DOBUTamine *on page 545*

Docusate (DOK yoo sate)

Related Information
Laxatives, Classification and Properties *on page 2012*

Medication Safety Issues
Sound-alike/look-alike issues:
Colace® may be confused with Calan®, Cozaar®
Docusate may be confused with Doxinate®
Dulcolax® (docusate) may be confused with Dulcolax® (bisacodyl)
Surfak® may be confused with Surbex®

Brand Names: U.S. Colace® [OTC]; Correctol® [OTC]; Diocto [OTC]; Docu-Soft [OTC]; DocuSoft S™ [OTC]; Dok™ [OTC]; DSS® [OTC]; Dulcolax® Stool Softener [OTC]; Dulcolax® [OTC]; Enemeez® Plus [OTC]; Enemeez® [OTC]; Fleet® Pedia-Lax™ Liquid Stool Softener [OTC]; Fleet® Sof-Lax® [OTC]; Kao-Tin [OTC]; Kaopectate® Stool Softener [OTC]; Phillips'® Liquid-Gels'® [OTC]; Phillips'® Stool Softener Laxative [OTC]; Silace [OTC]

Brand Names: Canada Apo-Docusate-Sodium®; Colace®; Colax-C®; Novo-Docusate Calcium; Novo-Docusate Sodium; PMS-Docusate Calcium; PMS-Docusate Sodium; Regulex®; Selax®; Soflax™

Index Terms Dioctyl Calcium Sulfosuccinate; Dioctyl Sodium Sulfosuccinate; Docusate Calcium; Docusate Potassium; Docusate Sodium; DOSS; DSS

Generic Availability (U.S.) Yes: Excludes enema, gelcap, tablet

Pharmacologic Category Stool Softener

Use Stool softener in patients who should avoid straining during defecation and constipation associated with hard, dry stools; prophylaxis for straining (Valsalva) following myocardial infarction. A safe agent to be used in elderly; some evidence that doses <200 mg are ineffective; stool softeners are unnecessary if stool is well hydrated or "mushy" and soft; shown to be ineffective used long-term.

Unlabeled/Investigational Use Ceruminolytic

Contraindications Hypersensitivity to docusate or any component of the formulation; concomitant use of mineral oil; intestinal obstruction, acute abdominal pain, nausea, or vomiting

Warnings/Precautions Prolonged, frequent or excessive use may result in dependence or electrolyte imbalance

Adverse Reactions (Reflective of adult population; not specific for elderly)
1% to 10%:
Gastrointestinal: Intestinal obstruction, diarrhea, abdominal cramping
Miscellaneous: Throat irritation

Drug Interactions
Avoid Concomitant Use There are no known interactions where it is recommended to avoid concomitant use.
Increased Effect/Toxicity There are no known significant interactions involving an increase in effect.
Decreased Effect There are no known significant interactions involving a decrease in effect.

Mechanism of Action Reduces surface tension of the oil-water interface of the stool resulting in enhanced incorporation of water and fat allowing for stool softening

Pharmacodynamics/Kinetics
Onset of action: 12-72 hours
Excretion: Feces

◀ **Dosage**

Geriatric & Adult Note: Docusate salts are interchangeable; the amount of sodium, calcium, or potassium per dosage unit is clinically insignificant.

Stool softener:

Oral: 50-500 mg/day in 1-4 divided doses

Rectal: Add 50-100 mg of docusate liquid to enema fluid (saline or water); give as retention or flushing enema

Administration Ensure adequate fluid intake. Docusate syrup should be administered with 6-8 ounces of milk, juice, or infant formula to mask the bitter taste.

Test Interactions Decreased potassium (S), decreased chloride (S)

Special Geriatric Considerations A safe agent to be used in the elderly. Some evidence that doses <200 mg are ineffective. Stool softeners are unnecessary if stool is well hydrated or "mushy" and soft; shown to be ineffective used long-term.

Dosage Forms Excipient information presented when available (limited, particularly for generics); consult specific product labeling. [DSC] = Discontinued product

Capsule, oral, as calcium: 240 mg [DSC]

Capsule, oral, as sodium: 100 mg [DSC]

Colace®: 50 mg [contains sodium 3 mg/capsule]

Colace®: 100 mg [contains sodium 5 mg/capsule]

Capsule, liquid, oral, as sodium:

DocuSoft S™: 100 mg [contains sodium 5 mg/capsule]

Capsule, softgel, oral, as calcium: 240 mg

Kao-Tin: 240 mg

Kaopectate® Stool Softener: 240 mg

Capsule, softgel, oral, as sodium: 100 mg, 250 mg

Correctol®: 100 mg

Docu-Soft: 100 mg

Dok™: 100 mg, 250 mg

DSS®: 100 mg, 250 mg

Dulcolax®: 100 mg [contains sodium 5 mg/capsule]

Dulcolax® Stool Softener: 100 mg [contains sodium 5 mg/capsule]

Fleet® Sof-Lax®: 100 mg [contains sodium 5 mg/capsule]

Phillips'® Liquid-Gels®: 100 mg [contains sodium 5.2 mg/capsule]

Phillips'® Stool Softener Laxative: 100 mg [contains sodium 5.2 mg/capsule]

Liquid, oral, as sodium: 50 mg/5 mL (10 mL, 25 mL, 473 mL); 150 mg/15 mL (480 mL)

Diocto: 150 mg/15 mL (480 mL)

Diocto: 150 mg/15 mL (480 mL) [vanilla flavor]

Fleet® Pedia-Lax™ Liquid Stool Softener: 50 mg/15 mL (118 mL) [contains propylene glycol, sodium 13 mg/15 mL; fruit-punch flavor]

Silace: 150 mg/15 mL (473 mL) [lemon-vanilla flavor]

Solution, rectal, as sodium [enema]:

Enemeez®: 283 mg/5 mL (5 mL)

Enemeez® Plus: 283 mg/5 mL (5 mL) [contains benzocaine]

Syrup, oral, as sodium: 20 mg/5 mL (25 mL, 473 mL)

Colace®: 60 mg/15 mL (473 mL) [ethanol free, sugar free; contains propylene glycol, sodium 34 mg/15 mL]

Diocto: 60 mg/15 mL (480 mL) [mint flavor]

Silace: 60 mg/15 mL (480 mL) [peppermint flavor]

Tablet, oral, as sodium:

Dok™: 100 mg [scored]

Docusate and Senna (DOK yoo sate & SEN na)

Related Information

Docusate *on page 547*
Laxatives, Classification and Properties *on page 2012*
Senna *on page 1667*
Treatment Options for Constipation *on page 2035*

Medication Safety Issues

Sound-alike/look-alike issues:

Senokot® may be confused with Depakote®

Brand Names: U.S. Dok™ Plus [OTC]; Peri-Colace® [OTC]; Senexon-S [OTC]; Senokot-S® [OTC]; SenoSol™-SS [OTC]

Index Terms Senna and Docusate; Senna-S

Generic Availability (U.S.) Yes

Pharmacologic Category Laxative, Stimulant; Stool Softener

Use Short-term treatment of constipation

Unlabeled/Investigational Use Evacuation of the colon for bowel or rectal examinations; management/prevention of opiate-induced constipation

Contraindications Hypersensitivity to any component; intestinal obstruction; acute intestinal inflammation (eg, Crohn's disease); ulcerative colitis; appendicitis; abdominal pain of unknown origin; concurrent use of mineral oil

Warnings/Precautions Not recommended for over-the-counter (OTC) use in patients experiencing stomach pain, nausea, vomiting, or a sudden change in bowel movements which lasts >2 weeks. OTC labeling does not recommend for use longer than 1 week.

Adverse Reactions (Reflective of adult population; not specific for elderly) Frequency not defined.

Gastrointestinal: Nausea, vomiting, diarrhea, abdominal cramps

Genitourinary: Urine discoloration (red/brown)

Mechanism of Action Docusate is a stool softener; sennosides are laxatives

Dosage

    Geriatric Constipation: OTC ranges: Oral: Consider half the initial dose in older, debilitated patients

    Adult Constipation: OTC ranges: Oral: Initial: 2 tablets (17.2 mg sennosides plus 100 mg docusate) once daily (maximum: 4 tablets twice daily)

Administration Oral: Once-daily doses should be taken at bedtime.

Pharmacotherapy Pearls Individual product labeling should be consulted prior to dosing.

Special Geriatric Considerations The chronic use of stimulant cathartics is inappropriate and should be avoided. Although the elderly commonly complain of constipation, such complaints require evaluation; short-term use of stimulant cathartics is best. If prophylaxis is desired, then the use of bulk agents (eg, psyllium), stool softeners, and hyperosmotic agents (eg, sorbitol 70%) is preferred. Stool softeners are unnecessary if stools are well-hydrated (as in use of hyperosmotics), soft or "mushy". Patients should be instructed for proper dietary fiber and fluid intake, as well as regular exercise. Monitor closely for fluid/electrolyte imbalance, CNS signs of fluid/electrolyte loss, and hypotension.

Dosage Forms Excipient information presented when available (limited, particularly for generics); consult specific product labeling.

Tablet, oral: Docusate sodium 50 mg and sennosides 8.6 mg

    Dok™ Plus: Docusate sodium 50 mg and sennosides 8.6 mg

    Peri-Colace®: Docusate sodium 50 mg and sennosides 8.6 mg

    Senexon-S: Docusate sodium 50 mg and sennosides 8.6 mg

    Senokot-S®: Docusate sodium 50 mg and sennosides 8.6 mg [sugar free; contains sodium 4 mg/tablet]

    SenoSol™-SS: Docusate sodium 50 mg and sennosides 8.6 mg [contains sodium 3 mg/tablet]

◆ **Docusate Calcium** see Docusate on page 547
◆ **Docusate Potassium** see Docusate on page 547
◆ **Docusate Sodium** see Docusate on page 547
◆ **Docu-Soft [OTC]** see Docusate on page 547
◆ **DocuSoft S™ [OTC]** see Docusate on page 547

Dofetilide (doe FET il ide)

Brand Names: U.S. Tikosyn®
Brand Names: Canada Tikosyn®
Generic Availability (U.S.) No
Pharmacologic Category Antiarrhythmic Agent, Class III

Use Maintenance of normal sinus rhythm in patients with chronic atrial fibrillation/atrial flutter of longer than 1-week duration who have been converted to normal sinus rhythm; conversion of atrial fibrillation and atrial flutter to normal sinus rhythm

Prescribing and Access Restrictions Tikosyn® is deemed to have an approved REMS program. As a requirement of the REMS program, access to this medication is restricted. Tikosyn® is only available to prescribers and hospitals that have confirmed their participation in a designated Tikosyn® Education Program. The program provides comprehensive education about the importance of in-hospital treatment initiation and individualized dosing.

T.I.P.S. is the Tikosyn® In Pharmacy System designated to allow retail pharmacies to stock and dispense Tikosyn® once they have been enrolled. A participating pharmacy must confirm receipt of the T.I.P.S. program materials and educate its pharmacy staff about the procedures required to fill an outpatient prescription for Tikosyn®. The T.I.P.S. enrollment form is available at www.tikosyn.com. Tikosyn® is only available from a special mail order pharmacy, and enrolled retail pharmacies. Pharmacists must verify that the hospital/prescriber is a confirmed participant before Tikosyn® is provided. For participant verification, the pharmacist may call 1-800-788-7353 or use the web site located at www.tikosynlist.com. Further details and directions on the program are provided at www.tikosyn.com.

Dofetilide therapy must be initiated/adjusted in a hospital setting with proper monitoring under the guidance of experienced personnel.

Medication Guide Available Yes

Contraindications Hypersensitivity to dofetilide or any component of the formulation; patients with congenital or acquired long QT syndromes, do not use if a baseline QT interval or QT_c is >440 msec (500 msec in patients with ventricular conduction abnormalities); severe renal impairment (estimated Cl_{cr} <20 mL/minute); concurrent use with verapamil, cimetidine, hydrochlorothiazide (alone or in combinations), trimethoprim (alone or in combination with sulfamethoxazole), itraconazole, ketoconazole, prochlorperazine, or megestrol; baseline heart rate <50 beats/minute; other drugs that prolong QT intervals (phenothiazines, cisapride, bepridil, tricyclic antidepressants, moxifloxacin); hypokalemia or hypomagnesemia; concurrent amiodarone, clarithromycin, or erythromycin

Warnings/Precautions [U.S. Boxed Warning]: Must be initiated (or reinitiated) in a setting with continuous monitoring and staff familiar with the recognition and treatment of life-threatening arrhythmias. Patients must be monitored with continuous ECG for a minimum of 3 days, or for a minimum of 12 hours after electrical or pharmacological cardioversion to normal sinus rhythm, whichever is greater. Patients should be readmitted for continuous monitoring if dosage is later increased.

Reserve for patients who are highly symptomatic with atrial fibrillation/atrial flutter; torsade de pointes significantly increases with doses >500 mcg twice daily; hold Class I or Class III antiarrhythmics for at least three half-lives prior to starting dofetilide; use in patients on amiodarone therapy only if serum amiodarone level is <0.3 mg/L or if amiodarone was stopped for >3 months previously; correct hypokalemia or hypomagnesemia before initiating dofetilide and maintain within normal limits during treatment. Risk of hypokalemia and/or hypomagnesemia may be increased by potassium-depleting diuretics, increasing the risk of torsade de pointes. Concurrent use with other drugs known to prolong QT_c interval is not recommended.

Patients with sick sinus syndrome or with second or third-degree heart block should not receive dofetilide unless a functional pacemaker is in place. Defibrillation threshold is reduced in patients with ventricular tachycardia or ventricular fibrillation undergoing implantation of a cardioverter-defibrillator device. Use with caution in renal impairment; not recommended in patients receiving drugs which may compete for renal secretion via cationic transport. Use with caution in patients with severe hepatic impairment.

In the Cardiac Arrhythmia Suppression Trial (CAST), recent (>6 days but <2 years ago) myocardial infarction patients with asymptomatic, non-life-threatening ventricular arrhythmias did not benefit and may have been harmed by attempts to suppress the arrhythmia with flecainide or encainide. An increased mortality or nonfatal cardiac arrest rate (7.7%) was seen in the active treatment group compared with patients in the placebo group (3%). The applicability of the CAST results to other populations is unknown. Antiarrhythmic agents should be reserved for patients with life-threatening ventricular arrhythmias.

Adverse Reactions (Reflective of adult population; not specific for elderly)
Supraventricular arrhythmia patients (incidence > placebo)
>10%: Central nervous system: Headache (11%)
2% to 10%:
  Central nervous system: Dizziness (8%), insomnia (4%)
  Cardiovascular: Ventricular tachycardia (2.6% to 3.7%), chest pain (10%), torsade de pointes (3.3% in CHF patients and 0.9% in patients with a recent MI; up to 10.5% in patients receiving doses in excess of those recommended). Torsade de pointes occurs most frequently within the first 3 days of therapy.
  Dermatologic: Rash (3%)
  Gastrointestinal: Nausea (5%), diarrhea (3%), abdominal pain (3%)
  Neuromuscular & skeletal: Back pain (3%)
  Respiratory: Respiratory tract infection (7%), dyspnea (6%)
  Miscellaneous: Flu syndrome (4%)
<2%:
  Central nervous system: CVA, facial paralysis, flaccid paralysis, migraine, paralysis
  Cardiovascular: AV block (0.4% to 1.5%), ventricular fibrillation (0% to 0.4%), bundle branch block, heart block, edema, heart arrest, myocardial infarct, sudden death, syncope
  Dermatologic: Angioedema
  Gastrointestinal: Liver damage
  Neuromuscular & skeletal: Paresthesia
  Respiratory: Cough

>2% (incidence ≤ placebo): Anxiety, pain, angina, atrial fibrillation, hypertension, palpitation, supraventricular tachycardia, peripheral edema, urinary tract infection, weakness, arthralgia, diaphoresis

Drug Interactions

Metabolism/Transport Effects Substrate of CYP3A4 (minor)

Avoid Concomitant Use

Avoid concomitant use of Dofetilide with any of the following: Antifungal Agents (Azole Derivatives, Systemic); Artemether; Cimetidine; Dronedarone; Lumefantrine; Megestrol; Nilotinib; Pimozide; Prochlorperazine; QUEtiapine; QuiNINE; Saquinavir; Tetrabenazine; Thiazide Diuretics; Thioridazine; Toremifene; Trimethoprim; Vandetanib; Vemurafenib; Verapamil; Ziprasidone

Increased Effect/Toxicity

Dofetilide may increase the levels/effects of: Dronedarone; Pimozide; QTc-Prolonging Agents; QuiNINE; Tetrabenazine; Thioridazine; Toremifene; Vandetanib; Vemurafenib; Ziprasidone

The levels/effects of Dofetilide may be increased by: Alfuzosin; AMILoride; Antifungal Agents (Azole Derivatives, Systemic); Artemether; Chloroquine; Cimetidine; Ciprofloxacin; Ciprofloxacin (Systemic); Conivaptan; Eribulin; Fingolimod; Gadobutrol; Loop Diuretics; Lumefantrine; Megestrol; MetFORMIN; Nilotinib; Prochlorperazine; QUEtiapine; QuiNINE; Saquinavir; Thiazide Diuretics; Triamterene; Trimethoprim; Verapamil

Decreased Effect

The levels/effects of Dofetilide may be decreased by: Tocilizumab

Ethanol/Nutrition/Herb Interactions Herb/Nutraceutical: St John's wort may decrease dofetilide levels. Avoid ephedra (may worsen arrhythmia).

Mechanism of Action Vaughan Williams Class III antiarrhythmic activity. Blockade of the cardiac ion channel carrying the rapid component of the delayed rectifier potassium current. Dofetilide has no effect on sodium channels, adrenergic alpha-receptors, or adrenergic beta-receptors. It increases the monophasic action potential duration due to delayed repolarization. The increase in the QT interval is a function of prolongation of both effective and functional refractory periods in the His-Purkinje system and the ventricles. Changes in cardiac conduction velocity and sinus node function have not been observed in patients with or without structural heart disease. PR and QRS width remain the same in patients with pre-existing heart block and or sick sinus syndrome.

Pharmacodynamics/Kinetics

Absorption: Well absorbed

Distribution: V_d: 3 L/kg

Protein binding: 60% to 70%

Metabolism: Hepatic via CYP3A4, but low affinity for it; metabolites formed by N-dealkylation and N-oxidation

Bioavailability: >90%

Half-life elimination: 10 hours

Time to peak, serum: Fasting: 2-3 hours

Excretion: Urine (80%; 80% as unchanged drug, 20% as inactive or minimally active metabolites); renal elimination consists of glomerular filtration and active tubular secretion via cationic transport system

Dosage

Geriatric Refer to adult dosing. No specific dosage adjustments are recommended based on age; however, careful assessment of renal function is particularly important in this population.

Adult Note: QT or QT_c must be determined prior to first dose. If QT_c >440 msec (>500 msec in patients with ventricular conduction abnormalities), dofetilide is contraindicated (see Contraindications and Warnings/Precautions).

Antiarrhythmic: Oral:

Initial: 500 mcg orally twice daily. Initial dosage must be adjusted in patients with estimated Cl_{cr} <60 mL/minute (see Dosage: Renal Impairment). Dofetilide may be initiated at lower doses than recommended based on physician discretion.

Modification of dosage in response to initial dose: QT_c interval should be measured 2-3 hours after the initial dose. If the QT_c >15% of baseline, or if the QT_c is >500 msec (550 msec in patients with ventricular conduction abnormalities), dofetilide should be adjusted. If the starting dose is 500 mcg twice daily, then adjust to 250 mcg twice daily. If the starting dose was 250 mcg twice daily, then adjust to 125 mcg twice daily. If the starting dose was 125 mcg twice daily, then adjust to 125 mcg every day.

◀ **Renal Impairment Note:** Using the Modification of Diet in Renal Disease (MDRD) equation and subsequent eGFR to determine dose may lead to overestimation of creatinine clearance and overdose of medication; use only the Cockcroft-Gault equation to estimate creatinine clearance (Denetclaw, 2011). The manufacturer recommends using actual body weight when using the Cockcroft-Gault equation to calculate creatinine clearance.

Cl_{cr} >60 mL/minute: Administer 500 mcg twice daily.

Cl_{cr} 40-60 mL/minute: Administer 250 mcg twice daily.

Cl_{cr} 20-39 mL/minute: Administer 125 mcg twice daily.

Cl_{cr} <20 mL/minute: Contraindicated in this group

Hepatic Impairment No dosage adjustments required in Child-Pugh class A and B; patients with severe hepatic impairment were not studied.

Administration Do not open capsules.

Monitoring Parameters ECG monitoring with attention to QT (if heart rate <60 beats per minute) or QT_c and occurrence of ventricular arrhythmias, baseline serum creatinine and changes in serum creatinine. Check serum potassium and magnesium levels if on medications where these electrolyte disturbances can occur, or if patient has a history of hypokalemia or hypomagnesemia. QT or QT_c must be monitored at baseline prior to the first dose and 2-3 hours afterwards. If at baseline, QT_c >440 msec (>500 msec in patients with ventricular conduction abnormalities), dofetilide is contraindicated. If dofetilide initiated, QT_c interval must be determined 2-3 hours after each subsequent dose of dofetilide for in-hospital doses 2-5. Thereafter, QT or QT_c and creatinine clearance should be evaluated every 3 months. If at any time during therapy the measured QT_c is >500 msec (550 msec in patients with ventricular conduction abnormalities), dofetilide should be discontinued.

Pharmacotherapy Pearls The management of atrial fibrillation deserves careful consideration in patients with heart failure, because the loss of atrial assistance to ventricular filling may have greater negative effects on cardiac output. The choice of antiarrhythmic is important because of the risk that antiarrhythmic therapy may increase mortality in this setting.

The two DIAMOND studies were 3-year trials comparing mortality between dofetilide and placebo in patients with left ventricular dysfunction. One study included patients with moderate to severe CHF (60% of participants were NYHA class III or IV) and the other study looked at patients with a recent MI (40% had NYHA class III or IV CHF). Dofetilide was an effective therapy for atrial fibrillation in carefully selected and monitored heart failure patients. Mortality was similar between those who received placebo and dofetilide; fewer patients of dofetilide were hospitalized for heart failure. It seems prudent, therefore, to carefully select and monitor patients in this situation.

Special Geriatric Considerations No specific dosage adjustments are recommended based on age; however, evaluation for use of this drug in the elderly is imperative. A complete review of medications, to assure there is no inadvertent use of contraindicated medications and those with potential drug interactions, can be re-evaluated for continued need. Laboratory values must be assessed prior to initiating medication; careful assessment of renal function is particularly important in the elderly population.

Dosage Forms Excipient information presented when available (limited, particularly for generics); consult specific product labeling.

Capsule, oral:

Tikosyn®: 125 mcg, 250 mcg, 500 mcg

Selected References

Fuster V, Rydén LE, Asinger RW, et al, "ACC/AHA/ESC Guidelines for the Management of Patients with Atrial Fibrillation: A Report of the American College of Cardiology/American Heart Association Task Force on Practice Guidelines and the European Society of Cardiology Committee for Practice Guidelines and Policy Conferences," *J Am Coll Cardiol*, 2001, 38(4):1231-66.

◆ **Dofus [OTC]** *see* Lactobacillus *on page 1020*

◆ **Dok™ [OTC]** *see* Docusate *on page 547*

◆ **Dok™ Plus [OTC]** *see* Docusate and Senna *on page 548*

Dolasetron (dol A se tron)

Medication Safety Issues

Sound-alike/look-alike issues:

Anzemet® may be confused with Aldomet®, Antivert®, Avandamet®

Dolasetron may be confused with granisetron, ondansetron, palonosetron

Brand Names: U.S. Anzemet®

Brand Names: Canada Anzemet®

Index Terms Dolasetron Mesylate; MDL 73,147EF

Generic Availability (U.S.) No

Pharmacologic Category Antiemetic; Selective 5-HT$_3$ Receptor Antagonist

DOLASETRON

Use

U.S. labeling:

Injection: Prevention and treatment of postoperative nausea and vomiting

Oral: Prevention of nausea and vomiting associated with emetogenic cancer chemotherapy (initial and repeat courses); prevention of postoperative nausea and vomiting

Canadian labeling: Oral: Prevention of nausea and vomiting associated with emetogenic cancer chemotherapy (initial and repeat courses)

Contraindications

U.S. labeling:

Injection: Hypersensitivity to dolasetron or any component of the formulation; use for the prevention of chemotherapy induced nausea and vomiting

Tablet: Hypersensitivity to dolasetron or any component of the formulation

Canadian labeling: Injection, tablet: Hypersensitivity to dolasetron or any component of the formulation; use for the prevention or treatment of postoperative nausea and vomiting

Warnings/Precautions

Dolasetron is associated with a number of dose-dependent increases in ECG intervals (eg, PR, QRS duration, QT/QT$_c$, JT), usually occurring 1-2 hours after I.V. administration and usually lasting 6-8 hours; however, may last ≥24 hours and rarely lead to heart block or arrhythmia. Clinically relevant QT-interval prolongation may occur resulting in torsade de pointes, when used in conjunction with other agents that prolong the QT interval (eg, Class I and III antiarrhythmics). Avoid use in patients at greater risk for QT prolongation (eg, patients with congenital long QT syndrome, medications known to prolong QT interval, electrolyte abnormalities, and cumulative high-dose anthracycline therapy) and/or ventricular arrhythmia. Correct potassium or magnesium abnormalities prior to initiating therapy. I.V. formulations of 5-HT$_3$ antagonists have more association with ECG interval changes, compared to oral formulations. Reduction in heart rate may also occur with the 5-HT$_3$ antagonists.

Use with caution in patients allergic to other 5-HT$_3$ receptor antagonists; cross-reactivity has been reported with other 5-HT$_3$ receptor antagonists. **For chemotherapy-associated nausea and vomiting, should be used on a scheduled basis, not on an "as needed" (PRN) basis,** since data support the use of this drug only in the prevention of nausea and vomiting (due to antineoplastic therapy) and not in the rescue of nausea and vomiting. Not intended for treatment of nausea and vomiting or for chronic continuous therapy.

Adverse Reactions (Reflective of adult population; not specific for elderly)

Adverse events may vary according to indication

>10%:

Central nervous system: Headache (7% to 24%)

Gastrointestinal: Diarrhea (2% to 12%)

1% to 10%:

Cardiovascular: Bradycardia (4% to 5%), hypertension (≤3%), tachycardia (2% to 3%)

Central nervous system: Dizziness (1% to 6%), fatigue (3% to 6%), fever (4%), pain (≤2%), chills/shivering (1% to 2%)

Gastrointestinal: Dyspepsia (≤3%), abdominal pain (≤3%)

Hepatic: Abnormal hepatic function (4%)

Renal: Oliguria (3%)

Drug Interactions

Metabolism/Transport Effects Substrate (minor) of CYP2C9, 3A4; **Inhibits** CYP2D6 (weak)

Avoid Concomitant Use

Avoid concomitant use of Dolasetron with any of the following: Apomorphine; Artemether; Dronedarone; Lumefantrine; Nilotinib; Pimozide; QUEtiapine; QuiNINE; Tetrabenazine; Thioridazine; Toremifene; Vandetanib; Vemurafenib; Ziprasidone

Increased Effect/Toxicity

Dolasetron may increase the levels/effects of: Apomorphine; Dronedarone; Pimozide; QTc-Prolonging Agents; QuiNINE; Tetrabenazine; Thioridazine; Toremifene; Vandetanib; Vemurafenib; Ziprasidone

The levels/effects of Dolasetron may be increased by: Alfuzosin; Artemether; Chloroquine; Ciprofloxacin; Ciprofloxacin (Systemic); Conivaptan; Gadobutrol; Lumefantrine; Nilotinib; QUEtiapine; QuiNINE

Decreased Effect

The levels/effects of Dolasetron may be decreased by: Tocilizumab

Ethanol/Nutrition/Herb Interactions Food: Food does not affect the bioavailability of oral doses.

◄ **Stability** Store intact vials and tablets at room temperature of 20°C to 25°C (68°F to 77°F). Protect from light. Dilute in 50 mL of a compatible solution (ie, 0.9% NS, D_5W, $D_5^{1/2}NS$, D_5LR, LR, and 10% mannitol injection). Solutions diluted for infusion are stable under normal lighting conditions at room temperature for 24 hours or under refrigeration for 48 hours.

Mechanism of Action Selective serotonin receptor (5-HT$_3$) antagonist, blocking serotonin both peripherally (primary site of action) and centrally at the chemoreceptor trigger zone

Pharmacodynamics/Kinetics
Absorption: Oral: Rapid and complete
Distribution: Hydrodolasetron: 5.8 L/kg
Protein binding: Hydrodolasetron: 69% to 77% (50% bound to alpha$_1$-acid glycoprotein)
Metabolism: Hepatic; rapid reduction by carbonyl reductase to hydrodolasetron (active metabolite); further metabolized by CYP2D6, CYP3A, and flavin monooxygenase
Bioavailability: Oral: ~75% (not affected by food)
Half-life elimination: Dolasetron: ≤10 minutes; hydrodolasetron: 6-8 hours; Severe renal impairment: 11 hours; Severe hepatic impairment: 11 hours
Time to peak, plasma: Hydrodolasetron: I.V.: 0.6 hours; Oral: ~1 hour
Excretion: Urine ~67% (53% to 61% of the total dose as active metabolite hydrodolasetron); feces ~33%

Dosage
Geriatric & Adult Note: Use of dolasetron injection is contraindicated for the prevention of chemotherapy induced nausea and vomiting. In Canada, use of dolasetron is also contraindicated in the prevention and treatment of postoperative nausea and vomiting in adults.

Prevention of chemotherapy-associated nausea and vomiting (including initial and repeat courses): Oral: 100 mg within 1 hour before chemotherapy
Postoperative nausea and vomiting: U.S. labeling:
Prevention:
Oral: 100 mg within 2 hours before surgery
I.V.: 12.5 mg ~15 minutes before cessation of anesthesia
Treatment: I.V.: 12.5 mg as soon as nausea or vomiting present
Renal Impairment No dosage adjustment necessary.
Hepatic Impairment No dosage adjustment necessary.

Administration
I.V. injection may be given either undiluted IVP over 30 seconds or diluted in 50 mL of compatible fluid and infused over 15 minutes. Flush line before and after dolasetron administration.
Oral: When unable to administer in tablet form, dolasetron injection may be diluted in apple or apple-grape juice and taken orally; this dilution is stable for 2 hours at room temperature.

Monitoring Parameters ECG (in patients with cardiovascular disease, elderly, renally impaired, those at risk of developing hypokalemia and/or hypomagnesemia); potassium, magnesium

Pharmacotherapy Pearls Efficacy of dolasetron, for chemotherapy treatment, is enhanced with concomitant administration of dexamethasone 20 mg (increases complete response by 10% to 20%). Oral administration of the intravenous solution is equivalent to tablets.

Special Geriatric Considerations In controlled trials, no difference in overall safety and efficacy were observed between elderly and younger adults. Pharmacokinetics are similar in younger adults and elderly. No dosage adjustment necessary.

Dosage Forms Excipient information presented when available (limited, particularly for generics); consult specific product labeling.
Injection, solution, as mesylate:
Anzemet®: 20 mg/mL (0.625 mL, 5 mL, 25 mL) [contains mannitol]
Tablet, oral, as mesylate:
Anzemet®: 50 mg, 100 mg

Extemporaneously Prepared Dolasetron injection may be diluted in apple or apple-grape juice and taken orally; this dilution is stable for 2 hours at room temperature.

♦ **Dolasetron Mesylate** *see* Dolasetron *on page* 552
♦ **Dolobid** *see* Diflunisal *on page* 504
♦ **Dolophine®** *see* Methadone *on page* 1158
♦ **Domeboro® [OTC]** *see* Aluminum Sulfate and Calcium Acetate *on page* 85

Donepezil (doh NEP e zil)

Medication Safety Issues
Sound-alike/look-alike issues:
Aricept® may be confused with AcipHex®, Ascriptin®, and Azilect®
Brand Names: U.S. Aricept®; Aricept® ODT

Brand Names: Canada Aricept®; Aricept® RDT
Index Terms E2020
Generic Availability (U.S.) Yes
Pharmacologic Category Acetylcholinesterase Inhibitor (Central)
Use Treatment of mild, moderate, or severe dementia of the Alzheimer's type
Unlabeled/Investigational Use Attention-deficit/hyperactivity disorder (ADHD); behavioral syndromes in dementia; mild-to-moderate dementia associated with Parkinson's disease; Lewy body dementia
Contraindications Hypersensitivity to donepezil, piperidine derivatives, or any component of the formulation
Warnings/Precautions Cholinesterase inhibitors may have vagotonic effects which may cause bradycardia and/or heart block with or without a history of cardiac disease; syncopal episodes have been associated with donepezil. Alzheimer's treatment guidelines consider bradycardia to be a relative contraindication for use of centrally-active cholinesterase inhibitors. Use with caution with sick sinus syndrome or other supraventricular cardiac conduction abnormalities, COPD, or asthma. Use with caution in patients with a history of seizure disorder; cholinomimetics may potentially cause generalized seizures, although seizure activity may also result from Alzheimer's disease. Use with caution in patients at risk of ulcer disease (eg, previous history or NSAID use), or in patients with bladder outlet obstruction. May cause dose-related diarrhea, nausea, and/or vomiting, which usually resolves in 1-3 weeks. May cause anorexia and/or weight loss (dose-related). May exaggerate neuromuscular blockade effects of depolarizing neuromuscular-blocking agents (eg, succinylcholine).

Adverse Reactions (Reflective of adult population; not specific for elderly)
>10%:
  Central nervous system: Insomnia (2% to 14%)
  Gastrointestinal: Nausea (3% to 19%; dose related), diarrhea (5% to 15%; dose related)
  Miscellaneous: Accident (7% to 13%), infection (11%)
1% to 10%:
  Cardiovascular: Hypertension (3%), chest pain (2%), hemorrhage (2%), syncope (2%), hypotension, atrial fibrillation, bradycardia, ECG abnormal, edema, heart failure, hot flashes, peripheral edema, vasodilation
  Central nervous system: Headache (3% to 10%), pain (3% to 9%), fatigue (1% to 8%), dizziness (2% to 8%), abnormal dreams (3%), hostility (3%), nervousness (1% to 3%), hallucinations (3%), depression (2% to 3%), confusion (2%), emotional lability (2%), personality disorder (2%), fever (2%), somnolence (2%), abnormal crying, aggression, agitation, anxiety, aphasia, delusions, irritability, restlessness, seizure, vertigo
  Dermatologic: Bruising (4% to 5%), eczema (3%), pruritus, rash, skin ulcer, urticaria
  Endocrine & metabolic: Dehydration (1% to 2%), hyperlipemia (2%), libido increased
  Gastrointestinal: Anorexia (2% to 8%), vomiting (3% to 9%; dose related), weight loss (3% to 5%; dose related), abdominal pain, bloating, constipation, dyspepsia, epigastric pain, fecal incontinence, gastroenteritis, GI bleeding, toothache
  Genitourinary: Urinary frequency (2%), urinary incontinence (1% to 3%), cystitis, hematuria, glycosuria, nocturia, UTI
  Hematologic: Contusion (≤2%), anemia
  Hepatic: Alkaline phosphatase increased
  Neuromuscular & skeletal: Muscle cramps (3% to 8%), back pain (3%), CPK increased (3%), arthritis (1% to 2%), ataxia, bone fracture, gait abnormal, lactate dehydrogenase increased, paresthesia, tremor, weakness (1% to 2%)
  Ocular: Blurred vision, cataract, eye irritation
  Respiratory: Bronchitis, cough increased, dyspnea, pharyngitis, pneumonia, sore throat
  Miscellaneous: Diaphoresis, fungal infection, flu symptoms, wandering
Drug Interactions
  Metabolism/Transport Effects Substrate (minor) of CYP2D6, 3A4
  Avoid Concomitant Use There are no known interactions where it is recommended to avoid concomitant use.
  Increased Effect/Toxicity
    Donepezil may increase the levels/effects of: Antipsychotics; Beta-Blockers; Cholinergic Agonists; Succinylcholine

    The levels/effects of Donepezil may be increased by: Conivaptan; Corticosteroids (Systemic)
  Decreased Effect
    Donepezil may decrease the levels/effects of: Anticholinergics; Neuromuscular-Blocking Agents (Nondepolarizing)

    The levels/effects of Donepezil may be decreased by: Anticholinergics; Peginterferon Alfa-2b; Tocilizumab

◀ **Ethanol/Nutrition/Herb Interactions** Herb/Nutraceutical: St John's wort may decrease donepezil levels. Ginkgo biloba may increase adverse effects/toxicity of acetylcholinesterase inhibitors.

Stability Store at 15°C to 30°C (59°F to 86°F).

Mechanism of Action Alzheimer's disease is characterized by cholinergic deficiency in the cortex and basal forebrain, which contributes to cognitive deficits. Donepezil reversibly and noncompetitively inhibits centrally-active acetylcholinesterase, the enzyme responsible for hydrolysis of acetylcholine. This appears to result in increased concentrations of acetylcholine available for synaptic transmission in the central nervous system.

Pharmacodynamics/Kinetics Geriatrics: No formal pharmacokinetic studies have been done in older adults; mean donepezil plasma concentrations were no different in older Alzheimer patients as compared to younger adults.

Absorption: Well absorbed

Distribution: V_{dss}: 12-16 L/kg

Protein binding: 96%, primarily to albumin (75%) and α_1-acid glycoprotein (21%)

Metabolism: Extensively to four major metabolites (two are active) via CYP2D6 and 3A4; undergoes glucuronidation

Bioavailability: 100%

Half-life elimination: 70 hours; time to steady-state: 15 days

Time to peak, plasma: Tablet, 10 mg: 3 hours; Tablet, 23 mg: ~8 hours; **Note:** Peak plasma concentrations almost twofold higher for the 23 mg tablet compared to the 10 mg tablet

Excretion: Urine 57% (17% as unchanged drug); feces 15%

Dosage

Geriatric Refer to adult dosing. **Note:** The Canadian labeling recommends a maximum dose of 5 mg once daily in elderly women of low body weight.

Adult Alzheimer's dementia: Oral:

Mild-to-moderate: Initial: 5 mg once daily; may increase to 10 mg once daily after 4-6 weeks; effective dosage range in clinical studies: 5-10 mg/day

Moderate-to-severe: Initial: 5 mg once daily; may increase to 10 mg once daily after 4-6 weeks; may increase further to 23 mg once daily after ≥3 months; effective dosage range in clinical studies: 10-23 mg/day

Administration Administer at bedtime without regard to food.

Aricept® 5 mg or 10 mg tablet: Swallow whole with water; do not split or crush per manufacturer's labeling. However, data available from the manufacturer showed that bioavailability was not affected by disintegration or dissolution when administered as a solution compared to a tablet during a bioequivalence study (data on file, Eisai Inc).

Aricept® 23 mg tablet: Swallow whole with water; do **NOT** crush or chew due to an increased rate of absorption. The 23 mg strength is provided in a unique film-coated formulation different from the 5 mg or 10 mg tablet strengths, which results in an altered pharmacokinetic profile.

Aricept® ODT: Allow tablet to dissolve completely on tongue and follow with water.

Monitoring Parameters Behavior, mood, bowel function, cognitive function, general function (eg, activities of daily living)

Dosage Forms Excipient information presented when available (limited, particularly for generics); consult specific product labeling.

Tablet, oral, as hydrochloride: 5 mg, 10 mg

Aricept®: 5 mg, 10 mg, 23 mg

Tablet, orally disintegrating, oral, as hydrochloride: 5 mg, 10 mg

Aricept® ODT: 5 mg, 10 mg

Selected References

Rabins PV, Blacker D, Rovner BW, et al, "Practice Guidelines for the Treatment of Patients With Alzheimer's Disease and Other Dementias," Am J Psychiatry, 2007, 164(12 Suppl):5-56. Available at http://www.psych.org/psych_pract/treatg/pg/prac_guide.cfm.

◆ **Donnatal®** see Hyoscyamine, Atropine, Scopolamine, and Phenobarbital *on page* 905

◆ **Donnatal Extentabs®** see Hyoscyamine, Atropine, Scopolamine, and Phenobarbital *on page* 905

DOPamine (DOE pa meen)

Medication Safety Issues

Sound-alike/look-alike issues:

DOPamine may be confused with DOBUTamine, Dopram®

High alert medication:

The Institute for Safe Medication Practices (ISMP) includes this medication among its list of drugs which have a heightened risk of causing significant patient harm when used in error.

Index Terms Dopamine Hydrochloride; Intropin

Generic Availability (U.S.) Yes

Pharmacologic Category Adrenergic Agonist Agent

Use Adjunct in the treatment of shock (eg, MI, open heart surgery, renal failure, cardiac decompensation) which persists after adequate fluid volume replacement

Unlabeled/Investigational Use Symptomatic bradycardia or heart block unresponsive to atropine or pacing

Contraindications Hypersensitivity to sulfites (commercial preparation contains sodium bisulfite); pheochromocytoma; ventricular fibrillation

Warnings/Precautions Use with caution in patients with cardiovascular disease or cardiac arrhythmias or patients with occlusive vascular disease. Correct hypovolemia and electrolytes when used in hemodynamic support. May cause increases in HR and arrhythmia. Use with caution in post-MI patients. Use with extreme caution in patients taking MAO inhibitors. Avoid extravasation; infuse into a large vein if possible. Avoid infusion into leg veins. Watch I.V. site closely. **[U.S. Boxed Warning]: If extravasation occurs, infiltrate the area with diluted phentolamine (5-10 mg in 10-15 mL of saline) with a fine hypodermic needle. Phentolamine should be administered as soon as possible after extravasation is noted.** Product may contain sodium metabisulfite.

Adverse Reactions (Reflective of adult population; not specific for elderly) Frequency not defined.

Cardiovascular: Ectopic beats, tachycardia, anginal pain, palpitation, hypotension, vaso-constriction

Central nervous system: Headache

Gastrointestinal: Nausea and vomiting

Respiratory: Dyspnea

Drug Interactions

Avoid Concomitant Use

Avoid concomitant use of DOPamine with any of the following: Inhalational Anesthetics; Iobenguane I 123; Lurasidone

Increased Effect/Toxicity

DOPamine may increase the levels/effects of: Lurasidone; Sympathomimetics

The levels/effects of DOPamine may be increased by: Atomoxetine; Cannabinoids; COMT Inhibitors; Inhalational Anesthetics

Decreased Effect

DOPamine may decrease the levels/effects of: Iobenguane I 123

Stability Protect from light; solutions that are darker than slightly yellow should not be used.

Mechanism of Action Stimulates both adrenergic and dopaminergic receptors, lower doses are mainly dopaminergic stimulating and produce renal and mesenteric vasodilation, higher doses also are both dopaminergic and beta$_1$-adrenergic stimulating and produce cardiac stimulation and renal vasodilation; large doses stimulate alpha-adrenergic receptors

Pharmacodynamics/Kinetics

Onset of action: Adults: 5 minutes

Duration: Adults: <10 minutes

Metabolism: Renal, hepatic, plasma; 75% to inactive metabolites by monoamine oxidase and 25% to norepinephrine

Half-life elimination: 2 minutes

Excretion: Urine (as metabolites)

Dosage

Geriatric & Adult

Hemodynamic support: I.V. infusion (administration requires the use of an infusion pump): 1-5 mcg/kg/minute up to 20 mcg/kg/minute; titrate to desired response (maximum: 50 mcg/kg/minute; however, doses >20 mcg/kg/minute may not have a beneficial effect on blood pressure and increase the risk of tachyarrhythmias); infusion may be increased by 1-4 mcg/kg/minute at 10- to 30-minute intervals until optimal response is obtained

Note: If dosages >20-30 mcg/kg/minute are needed, a more direct-acting vasopressor may be more beneficial (ie, epinephrine, norepinephrine).

Hemodynamic effects of dopamine are dose dependent (however, this is relative and there is overlap of clinical effects between dosing ranges):

Low-dose: 1-5 mcg/kg/minute, increased renal blood flow and urine output

Intermediate-dose: 5-15 mcg/kg/minute, increased renal blood flow, heart rate, cardiac contractility, and cardiac output

High-dose: >15 mcg/kg/minute, alpha-adrenergic effects begin to predominate, vaso-constriction, increased blood pressure

Administration Administer into large vein to prevent the possibility of extravasation (central line administration); monitor continuously for free flow; use infusion device to control rate of flow; administration into an umbilical arterial catheter is not recommended; when discontinuing the infusion, gradually decrease the dose of dopamine (sudden discontinuation may cause hypotension).

Extravasation management: Due to short half-life, withdrawal of drug is often only necessary treatment. Use phentolamine as antidote. Mix 5 mg with 9 mL of NS; inject a small amount of this dilution into extravasated area. Blanching should reverse immediately. Monitor site. If blanching should recur, additional injections of phentolamine may be needed.

Monitoring Parameters Blood pressure, ECG, heart rate, CVP, RAP, MAP, urine output; if pulmonary artery catheter is in place, monitor CI, PCWP, SVR, and PVR

Pharmacotherapy Pearls Dopamine is most frequently used for treatment of hypotension because of its peripheral vasoconstrictor action. In this regard, dopamine is often used together with dobutamine and minimizes hypotension secondary to dobutamine-induced vasodilation. Thus, pressure is maintained by increased cardiac output (from dobutamine) and vasoconstriction (by dopamine). It is critical neither dopamine nor dobutamine be used in patients in the absence of correcting any hypovolemia as a cause of hypotension.

Low-dose dopamine is often used in the intensive care setting for presumed beneficial effects on renal function. However, there is no clear evidence that low-dose dopamine confers any renal or other benefit. Indeed, dopamine may act on dopamine receptors in the carotid bodies causing chemoreflex suppression. In patients with heart failure, dopamine may inhibit breathing and cause pulmonary shunting. Both these mechanisms would act to decrease minute ventilation and oxygen saturation. This could potentially be deleterious in patients with respiratory compromise and patients being weaned from ventilators.

Special Geriatric Considerations Has not been specifically studied in the elderly; monitor closely, especially due to increase in cardiovascular disease with age.

Dosage Forms Excipient information presented when available (limited, particularly for generics); consult specific product labeling. [DSC] = Discontinued product

Infusion, premixed in D_5W, as hydrochloride: 0.8 mg/mL (250 mL, 500 mL); 1.6 mg/mL (250 mL, 500 mL); 3.2 mg/mL (250 mL)

Injection, solution, as hydrochloride: 40 mg/mL (5 mL, 10 mL); 80 mg/mL (5 mL, 10 mL [DSC]); 160 mg/mL (5 mL)

Selected References

Dellinger RP, Levy MM, Carlet JM, et al, "Surviving Sepsis Campaign: International Guidelines for Management of Severe Sepsis and Septic Shock: 2008," *Intensive Care Med*, 2007 [epub ahead of print].

◆ **Dopamine Hydrochloride** *see* DOPamine *on page 556*
◆ **Doral®** *see* Quazepam *on page 1554*
◆ **Doribax®** *see* Doripenem *on page 558*

Doripenem (dore i PEN em)

Medication Safety Issues
  Sound-alike/look-alike issues:
    Doribax® may be confused with Zovirax®
Brand Names: U.S. Doribax®
Brand Names: Canada Doribax®
Index Terms S-4661
Generic Availability (U.S.) No
Pharmacologic Category Antibiotic, Carbapenem
Use Treatment of complicated intra-abdominal infections and complicated urinary tract infections (including pyelonephritis) due to susceptible gram-positive, gram-negative (including *Pseudomonas aeruginosa*), and anaerobic bacteria

Canadian labeling: Additional use (not in U.S. labeling): Treatment of nosocomial pneumonia (including ventilator-associated pneumonia)

Contraindications Known serious hypersensitivity to doripenem or other carbapenems (eg, ertapenem, imipenem, meropenem); anaphylactic reactions to beta-lactam antibiotics

Warnings/Precautions Serious hypersensitivity reactions, including anaphylaxis, and skin reactions have been reported in patients receiving beta-lactams. Prolonged use may result in fungal or bacterial superinfection, including *C. difficile*-associated diarrhea (CDAD) and pseudomembranous colitis; CDAD has been observed >2 months postantibiotic treatment. Use with caution in patients with renal impairment; dosage adjustment required in patients with moderate-to-severe renal dysfunction. Carbapenems have been associated with CNS adverse effects, including confusional states and seizures (myoclonic); use caution with CNS disorders (eg, brain lesions and history of seizures) and adjust dose in renal impairment to avoid drug accumulation, which may increase seizure risk. May decrease divalproex sodium/ valproic acid concentrations leading to breakthrough seizures; concomitant use not recommended. Administer via intravenous infusion only. Per manufacturer's labeling, investigational experience of doripenem via inhalation resulted in pneumonitis.

Adverse Reactions (Reflective of adult population; not specific for elderly)
>10%:
  Central nervous system: Headache (4% to 16%)
  Gastrointestinal: Nausea (4% to 12%), diarrhea (6% to 11%)
1% to 10%:
  Dermatologic: Rash (1% to 5%; includes allergic/bullous dermatitis, erythema, macular/papular eruptions, urticaria, and erythema multiforme), pruritus (≤3%)
  Gastrointestinal: Oral candidiasis (1%)
  Hematologic: Anemia (2% to 10%)
  Hepatic: Transaminases increased (1% to 2%)
  Local: Phlebitis (4% to 8%)
  Renal: Renal impairment/failure (≤1%)
  Miscellaneous: Vulvomycotic infection (1% to 2%)

Drug Interactions
  Avoid Concomitant Use
    Avoid concomitant use of Doripenem with any of the following: BCG; Probenecid
  Increased Effect/Toxicity
    The levels/effects of Doripenem may be increased by: Probenecid
  Decreased Effect
    Doripenem may decrease the levels/effects of: BCG; Divalproex; Typhoid Vaccine; Valproic Acid

Stability Store dry powder vials at 15°C to 30°C (59°F to 86°F). Reconstitute 250 mg vial with 10 mL of SWFI or NS, and further dilute for infusion with 50 mL or 100 mL of NS or D_5W. Reconstitute 500 mg vial with 10 mL of SWFI or NS, and further dilute for infusion with 100 mL of NS or D_5W. Shake gently until clear. Reconstituted vial may be stored for up to 1 hour prior to preparation of infusion solution. Stability of solution when diluted in NS is 12 hours at room temperature or 72 hours under refrigeration; stability in D_5W is 4 hours at room temperature and 24 hours under refrigeration. To prepare a 250 mg dose using a 500 mg vial, reconstitute the 500 mg vial with 10 mL of SWFI or NS and further dilute with 100 mL of compatible solution as above, but remove and discard 55 mL from the infusion bag to leave the remaining solution containing the 250 mg dose.

Mechanism of Action Inhibits bacterial cell wall synthesis by binding to several of the penicillin-binding proteins, which in turn inhibits the final transpeptidation step of peptidoglycan synthesis in bacterial cell walls, thus inhibiting cell wall biosynthesis; bacteria eventually lyse due to ongoing activity of cell wall autolytic enzymes (autolysins and murein hydrolases) while cell wall assembly is arrested.

Pharmacodynamics/Kinetics
  Distribution: V_d: 16.8 L
  Protein binding: 8% to 9%
  Metabolism: Non-CYP-mediated metabolism via dehydropeptidase-I to doripenem-M1 (inactive metabolite)
  Half-life elimination: ~1 hour
  Excretion: Urine (70% as unchanged drug; 15% as doripenem-M1 metabolite); feces (<1%)

Dosage
  Geriatric & Adult
    Note: A switch to appropriate oral antimicrobial therapy may be considered after 3 days of parenteral therapy and demonstrated clinical improvement.
    Intra-abdominal infection, complicated, severe: 500 mg every 8 hours for 5-14 days. **Note:** 2010 IDSA guidelines recommend treatment duration of 4-7 days (provided source controlled). Not recommended for mild-to-moderate, community-acquired intra-abdominal infections due to risk of toxicity and the development of resistant organisms (Solomkin, 2010).
    Pneumonia (nosocomial, including ventilator-associated): Canadian labeling (not in U.S. labeling): I.V.: 500 mg every 8 hours for 7-14 days
    Urinary tract infection (complicated) or pyelonephritis: I.V.: 500 mg every 8 hours for 10-14 days
  Renal Impairment
    Cl_{cr} >50 mL/minute: No adjustment necessary.
    Cl_{cr} 30-50 mL/minute: 250 mg every 8 hours
    Cl_{cr} 11-29 mL/minute: 250 mg every 12 hours
    Hemodialysis: Dialyzable (~52% of dose removed during 4-hour session in ESRD patients)

Administration Infuse intravenously over 1 hour. **Note:** The Canadian labeling recommends a 4-hour infusion in late-onset ventilator-associated pneumonia (>5 days ventilation [not an approved indication in the U.S. labeling])

Monitoring Parameters Monitor for signs of anaphylaxis during first dose; periodic renal assessment; consider hematologic monitoring during prolonged therapy

◄ **Special Geriatric Considerations** Careful attention to dose adjustment based on renal function, as well as monitoring renal function during treatment is recommended. According to the manufacturer, 28% of clinical trial patients were ≥65 years and 12% were ≥75 years, with no differences in overall age-related safety findings.

Dosage Forms Excipient information presented when available (limited, particularly for generics); consult specific product labeling.
Injection, powder for reconstitution:
Doribax®: 250 mg, 500 mg

Selected References
Zhanel GG, Wiebe R, Dilay L, et al, "Comparative Review of the Carbapenems," *Drugs*, 2007, 67(7): 1027-52.

◆ **Doryx®** see Doxycycline *on page 570*

Dorzolamide (dor ZOLE a mide)

Related Information
Glaucoma Drug Therapy *on page 2008*
Brand Names: U.S. Trusopt®
Brand Names: Canada Trusopt®
Index Terms Dorzolamide Hydrochloride
Generic Availability (U.S.) Yes
Pharmacologic Category Carbonic Anhydrase Inhibitor; Ophthalmic Agent, Antiglaucoma
Use Treatment of elevated intraocular pressure in patients with ocular hypertension or open-angle glaucoma
Contraindications Hypersensitivity to dorzolamide or any component of the formulation
Warnings/Precautions Although administered topically, systemic absorption occurs. Similar adverse reactions attributed to sulfonamides may occur with topical administration. Chemical similarities are present among sulfonamides, sulfonylureas, carbonic anhydrase inhibitors, thiazides, and loop diuretics (except ethacrynic acid). In patients with allergy to one of these compounds, a risk of cross-reaction exists; avoid use when previous reaction has been severe.

Not recommended for use in patients with severe renal impairment (Cl_{cr} <30 mL/minute). Use with caution in patients with hepatic impairment. Concurrent use with oral carbonic anhydrase inhibitors is not recommended. Local ocular adverse effects (conjunctivitis and lid reactions) were reported with chronic administration. Many resolved with discontinuation of drug therapy. If such reactions occur, discontinue dorzolamide. Choriodal detachment has been reported after filtration procedures. Patients with low endothelial cell counts may have increased risk for corneal edema; use caution.

Inadvertent contamination of multiple-dose ophthalmic solutions, has caused bacterial keratitis. Some products contain benzalkonium chloride which may be absorbed by soft contact lenses. Dorzolamide should not be administered while wearing soft contact lenses.

Adverse Reactions (Reflective of adult population; not specific for elderly)
>10%:
Gastrointestinal: Bitter taste following administration (25%)
Ocular: Burning, stinging or discomfort immediately following administration (33%); superficial punctate keratitis (10% to 15%); signs and symptoms of ocular allergic reaction (10%)
1% to 5%: Ocular: Blurred vision, conjunctivitis, dryness, lid reactions, photophobia, redness, tearing

Drug Interactions
Metabolism/Transport Effects Substrate (minor) of CYP2C9, 3A4
Avoid Concomitant Use
Avoid concomitant use of Dorzolamide with any of the following: Carbonic Anhydrase Inhibitors
Increased Effect/Toxicity
Dorzolamide may increase the levels/effects of: Carbonic Anhydrase Inhibitors

The levels/effects of Dorzolamide may be increased by: Conivaptan
Decreased Effect
The levels/effects of Dorzolamide may be decreased by: Tocilizumab
Stability Store at room temperature 15°C to 30°C (59°F to 86°F). Protect from light.
Mechanism of Action Reversible inhibition of the enzyme carbonic anhydrase resulting in reduction of hydrogen ion secretion at renal tubule and an increased renal excretion of sodium, potassium, bicarbonate, and water to decrease production of aqueous humor; also inhibits carbonic anhydrase in central nervous system to retard abnormal and excessive discharge from CNS neurons

Pharmacodynamics/Kinetics
Onset of action: Peak effect: 2 hours
Duration: 8-12 hours
Absorption: Topical: Reaches systemic circulation where it accumulates in RBCs during chronic dosing as a result of binding to CA-II
Distribution: In RBCs during chronic administration
Protein binding: 33%
Metabolism: To N-desethyl metabolite (less potent than parent drug)
Half-life elimination: Terminal RBC: 147 days; washes out of RBCs nonlinearly, resulting in a rapid decline of drug concentration initially, followed by a slower elimination phase with a half-life of about 4 months
Excretion: Urine (as unchanged drug and metabolite, N-desethyl)

Dosage
Geriatric & Adult Reduction of intraocular pressure: Ophthalmic: Instill 1 drop in the affected eye(s) 3 times/day

Administration If more than one topical ophthalmic drug is being used, administer the drugs at least 10 minutes apart. Remove contact lens prior to administration and wait 15 minutes before reinserting. Instruct patients to avoid allowing the tip of the dispensing container to contact the eye or surrounding structures. Ocular solutions can become contaminated by common bacteria known to cause ocular infections. Serious damage to the eye and subsequent loss of vision may occur from using contaminated solutions.

Monitoring Parameters Ophthalmic exams and IOP periodically

Special Geriatric Considerations Evaluate the patient's or caregiver's ability to safely administer the correct dose of ophthalmic medication.

Dosage Forms Excipient information presented when available (limited, particularly for generics); consult specific product labeling.
Solution, ophthalmic [drops]: 2% (10 mL)
Trusopt®: 2% (10 mL) [contains benzalkonium chloride]

Dosage Forms: Canada Excipient information presented when available (limited, particularly for generics); consult specific product labeling.
Solution, ophthalmic [drops; preservative free]:
Trusopt®: 2% (0.2 mL)

Selected References
Biollaz J, Munafo A, Buclin T, et al, "Whole Blood Pharmacokinetics and Metabolic Affects of the Topical Carbonic Anhydrase Inhibitor Dorzolamide," *Eur J Clin Pharmacol*, 1995, 47(5):455-60.

Dorzolamide and Timolol (dor ZOLE a mide & TYE moe lole)

Related Information
Dorzolamide *on page 560*
Timolol (Ophthalmic) *on page 1799*

Brand Names: U.S. Cosopt®
Brand Names: Canada Apo-Dorzo-Timop; Cosopt®; Sandoz-Dorzolamide/Timolol
Index Terms Timolol and Dorzolamide
Generic Availability (U.S.) Yes
Pharmacologic Category Beta-Adrenergic Blocker, Nonselective; Carbonic Anhydrase Inhibitor; Ophthalmic Agent, Antiglaucoma
Use Treatment of elevated intraocular pressure in patients with ocular hypertension or open-angle glaucoma

Dosage
Geriatric & Adult Reduction of intraocular pressure: Ophthalmic: Instill 1 drop in affected eye(s) twice daily

Special Geriatric Considerations Evaluate the patient's or caregiver's ability to safely administer the correct dose of ophthalmic medication.

Dosage Forms Excipient information presented when available (limited, particularly for generics); consult specific product labeling. [DSC] = Discontinued product; **Note:** Strength expressed as base
Solution, ophthalmic [drops]: Dorzolamide hydrochloride 2% and timolol maleate 0.5% (10 mL)
Cosopt®: Dorzolamide hydrochloride 2% and timolol maleate 0.5% (5 mL [DSC]; 10 mL) [contains benzalkonium chloride]

Dosage Forms: Canada Excipient information presented when available (limited, particularly for generics); consult specific product labeling.
Solution, ophthalmic [drops; preservative free]:
Cosopt®: Dorzolamide hydrochloride 2% and timolol maleate 0.5% (0.2 mL) (15s)

◆ **Dorzolamide Hydrochloride** see Dorzolamide *on page 560*

◆ **DOSS** see Docusate on page 547
◆ **Double Tussin DM [OTC]** see Guaifenesin and Dextromethorphan on page 848
◆ **Dovonex®** see Calcipotriene on page 240

Doxazosin (doks AY zoe sin)

Related Information
Beers Criteria – Potentially Inappropriate Medications for Geriatrics on page 2089
Pharmacotherapy of Urinary Incontinence on page 2032
Medication Safety Issues
Sound-alike/look-alike issues:
Doxazosin may be confused with doxapram, doxepin, DOXOrubicin
Cardura® may be confused with Cardene®, Cordarone®, Cordran®, Coumadin®, K-Dur®, Ridaura®
BEERS Criteria medication:
This drug may be inappropriate for use in geriatric patients (low severity risk).
Brand Names: U.S. Cardura®; Cardura® XL
Brand Names: Canada Alti-Doxazosin; Apo-Doxazosin®; Cardura-1™; Cardura-2™; Cardura-4™; Gen-Doxazosin; Mylan-Doxazosin; Novo-Doxazosin
Index Terms Doxazosin Mesylate
Generic Availability (U.S.) Yes: Excludes extended release tablet
Pharmacologic Category Alpha$_1$ Blocker
Use
Immediate release formulation: Treatment of hypertension as monotherapy or in conjunction with diuretics, ACE inhibitors, beta-blockers, or calcium antagonists
Immediate release and extended release formulations: Treatment of urinary outflow obstruction and/or obstructive and irritative symptoms associated with benign prostatic hyperplasia (BPH)
Contraindications Hypersensitivity to quinazolines (prazosin, terazosin), doxazosin, or any component of the formulation
Warnings/Precautions Can cause significant orthostatic hypotension and syncope, especially with first dose; anticipate a similar effect if therapy is interrupted for a few days, if dosage is rapidly increased, or if another antihypertensive drug (particularly vasodilators) or a PDE-5 inhibitor is introduced. Discontinue if symptoms of angina occur or worsen. Patients should be cautioned about performing hazardous tasks when starting new therapy or adjusting dosage upward. Prostate cancer should be ruled out before starting for BPH. Use with caution in mild-to-moderate hepatic impairment; not recommended in severe dysfunction. Intraoperative floppy iris syndrome has been observed in cataract surgery patients who were on or were previously treated with alpha$_1$-blockers. Causality has not been established and there appears to be no benefit in discontinuing alpha-blocker therapy prior to surgery. May be inappropriate in the elderly due to potential for dry mouth, hypotension, and urinary problems (Beers Criteria).

The extended release formulation consists of drug within a nondeformable matrix; following drug release/absorption, the matrix/shell is expelled in the stool. The use of nondeformable products in patients with known stricture/narrowing of the GI tract has been associated with symptoms of obstruction. Use caution in patients with increased GI retention (eg, chronic constipation) as doxazosin exposure may be increased. Extended release formulation is not indicated for use in women or for the treatment of hypertension.
Adverse Reactions (Reflective of adult population; not specific for elderly) Note: Type and frequency of adverse reactions reflect combined data from BPH and hypertension trials and immediate release and extended release products.

>10%: Central nervous system: Dizziness (5% to 19%), headache (5% to 14%)
1% to 10%:
Cardiovascular: Orthostatic hypotension (dose related; 0.3% up to 2%), edema (3% to 4%), hypotension (1% to 2%), palpitation (1% to 2%), chest pain (1% to 2%), arrhythmia (1%), syncope (2%), flushing (1%)
Central nervous system: Fatigue (8% to 12%), somnolence (1% to 5%), nervousness (2%), pain (2%), vertigo (2% to 4%), insomnia (1%), anxiety (1%), paresthesia (1%), movement disorder (1%), ataxia (1%), hypertonia (1%), depression (1%)
Dermatologic: Rash (1%), pruritus (1%)
Endocrine & metabolic: Sexual dysfunction (2%)
Gastrointestinal: Abdominal pain (2%), diarrhea (2%), dyspepsia (1% to 2%), nausea (1% to 3%), xerostomia (1% to 2%), constipation (1%), flatulence (1%)
Genitourinary: Urinary tract infection (1%), impotence (1%), polyuria (2%), incontinence (1%)

Neuromuscular & skeletal: Back pain (2% to 3%), weakness (1% to 7%), arthritis (1%), muscle weakness (1%), myalgia (≤1%), muscle cramps (1%)

Ocular: Abnormal vision (1% to 2%), conjunctivitis (1%)

Otic: Tinnitus (1%)

Respiratory: Respiratory tract infection (5%), rhinitis (3%), dyspnea (1% to 3%), respiratory disorder (1%), epistaxis (1%)

Miscellaneous: Diaphoresis increased (1%), flu-like syndrome (1%)

Drug Interactions

Avoid Concomitant Use

Avoid concomitant use of Doxazosin with any of the following: Alpha1-Blockers

Increased Effect/Toxicity

Doxazosin may increase the levels/effects of: Alpha1-Blockers; Amifostine; Antihypertensives; Calcium Channel Blockers; Hypotensive Agents; RiTUXimab

The levels/effects of Doxazosin may be increased by: Beta-Blockers; Diazoxide; Herbs (Hypotensive Properties); MAO Inhibitors; Pentoxifylline; Phosphodiesterase 5 Inhibitors; Prostacyclin Analogues

Decreased Effect

The levels/effects of Doxazosin may be decreased by: Herbs (Hypertensive Properties); Methylphenidate; Yohimbine

Ethanol/Nutrition/Herb Interactions Herb/Nutraceutical: Avoid dong quai if using for hypertension (has estrogenic activity). Avoid ephedra, yohimbe, ginseng (may worsen hypertension). Avoid saw palmetto when used for BPH (due to limited experience with this combination). Avoid garlic (may have increased antihypertensive effect).

Stability Store at 25°C (77°F); excursions permitted to 15°C to 30°C (59°F to 86°F).

Mechanism of Action

Hypertension: Competitively inhibits postsynaptic alpha$_1$-adrenergic receptors which results in vasodilation of veins and arterioles and a decrease in total peripheral resistance and blood pressure; ~50% as potent on a weight by weight basis as prazosin.

BPH: Competitively inhibits postsynaptic alpha$_1$-adrenergic receptors in prostatic stromal and bladder neck tissues. This reduces the sympathetic tone-induced urethral stricture causing BPH symptoms.

Pharmacodynamics/Kinetics Increased age does not significantly affect pharmacokinetics of doxazosin. In studies of the extended-release tablets, the maximum plasma concentration was increased by 27% and the area under the curve was increased by 34% in the elderly.

Protein binding: Extended release: 98%

Metabolism: Extensively hepatic to active metabolites; primarily via CYP3A4; secondary pathways involve CYP2D6 and 2C19

Half-life elimination: 15-22 hours

Bioavailability: Extended release relative to immediate release: 54% to 59%

Time to peak, serum: Immediate release: 2-3 hours; extended release: 8-9 hours

Excretion: Feces (63% primarily as metabolites); urine (9%)

Dosage

Geriatric Refer to adult dosing. In the management of hypertension, consider lower initial doses (eg, immediate release: 0.5 mg once daily) and titrate to response (Aronow, 2011)

Adult

BPH: Oral:

Immediate release: 1 mg once daily in morning or evening; may be increased to 2 mg once daily. Thereafter titrate upwards, if needed, over several weeks, balancing therapeutic benefit with doxazosin-induced postural hypotension. Goal: 4-8 mg/day; maximum dose: 8 mg/day

Reinitiation of therapy: If therapy is discontinued for several days, restart at 1 mg dose and titrate as before

Extended release: 4 mg once daily with breakfast; titrate based on response and tolerability every 3-4 weeks to maximum recommended dose of 8 mg/day

Reinitiation of therapy: If therapy is discontinued for several days, restart at 4 mg dose and titrate as before

Note: Conversion to extended release from immediate release: Omit final evening dose of immediate release prior to starting morning dosing with extended release product; initiate extended release product using 4 mg once daily

Hypertension: Oral: *Immediate release:* 1 mg once daily in morning or evening; may be increased to 2 mg once daily. Thereafter titrate upwards, if needed, over several weeks, balancing therapeutic benefit with doxazosin-induced postural hypotension. Maximum dose: 16 mg/day

Reinitiation of therapy: If therapy is discontinued for several days, restart at 1 mg dose and titrate as before

Hepatic Impairment Use with caution in mild-to-moderate hepatic dysfunction. Do not use with severe impairment.

Administration Cardura ® XL: Tablets should be swallowed whole; do not crush, chew, or divide.

Monitoring Parameters Blood pressure, standing and sitting/supine; syncope may occur usually within 90 minutes of the initial dose

Pharmacotherapy Pearls First-dose hypotension occurs less frequently with doxazosin as compared to prazosin; this may be due to its slower onset of action

Special Geriatric Considerations Adverse reactions such as orthostatic hypotension, dry mouth, and urinary problems can be particularly bothersome in the elderly. In studies of the extended-release tablets, the incidence of hypotension was higher in the elderly compared to younger patients.

This medication is considered to be potentially inappropriate in this patient population (Beers Criteria severity: Low).

Dosage Forms Excipient information presented when available (limited, particularly for generics); consult specific product labeling.
Tablet, oral: 1 mg, 2 mg, 4 mg, 8 mg
  Cardura®: 1 mg, 2 mg, 4 mg, 8 mg [scored]
Tablet, extended release, oral:
  Cardura® XL: 4 mg, 8 mg

Selected References
  McConnell JD, Roehrborn CG, Bautista OM, et al, "The Long-Term Effect of Doxazosin, Finasteride, and Combination Therapy on the Clinical Progression of Benign Prostatic Hyperplasia. Medical Therapy of Prostatic Symptoms (MTOPS) Research Group," *N Engl J Med*, 2003, 349(25):2387-98.

◆ **Doxazosin Mesylate** *see* Doxazosin *on page 562*

Doxepin (Systemic) (DOKS e pin)

Related Information
  Antidepressant Agents *on page 1991*
  Beers Criteria – Potentially Inappropriate Medications for Geriatrics *on page 2089*
  Liquid Compatibility of Antidepressants, Antipsychotics, and Mood Stabilizers *on page 2111*

Medication Safety Issues
  Sound-alike/look-alike issues:
    Doxepin may be confused with digoxin, doxapram, doxazosin, Doxidan®, doxycycline
    SINEquan® may be confused with saquinavir, Serentil®, SEROquel®, Singulair®, Zonegran®
  BEERS Criteria medication:
    This drug may be inappropriate for use in geriatric patients (high severity risk).
  International issues:
    Doxal® [Finland] may be confused with Doxil® which is a brand name for doxorubicin in the U.S.
    Doxal® [Finland]: Brand name for doxycycline in Austria; brand name for pyridoxine/thiamine in Brazil

Brand Names: U.S. Silenor®
Brand Names: Canada Apo-Doxepin®; Doxepine; Novo-Doxepin; Sinequan®
Index Terms Doxepin Hydrochloride
Generic Availability (U.S.) Yes: Excludes tablet
Pharmacologic Category Antidepressant, Tricyclic (Tertiary Amine)
Use Depression; treatment of insomnia (with difficulty of sleep maintenance)
Unlabeled/Investigational Use Analgesic for certain chronic and neuropathic pain; anxiety
Medication Guide Available Yes
Contraindications Hypersensitivity to doxepin, drugs from similar chemical class, or any component of the formulation; narrow-angle glaucoma; urinary retention; use of MAO inhibitors within 14 days

Warnings/Precautions [U.S. Boxed Warning]: Antidepressants increase the risk of suicidal thinking and behavior in children, adolescents, and young adults (18-24 years of age) with major depressive disorder (MDD) and other psychiatric disorders; consider risk prior to prescribing. Short-term studies did not show an increased risk in patients >24 years of age and showed a decreased risk in patients ≥65 years. Closely monitor for clinical worsening, suicidality, or unusual changes in behavior; the patient's family or caregiver should be instructed to closely observe the patient and communicate condition with healthcare provider. A medication guide should be dispensed with each prescription. **Doxepin is approved for treatment of depression in adolescents.**

The possibility of a suicide attempt is inherent in major depression and may persist until remission occurs. Monitor for worsening of depression or suicidality, especially during initiation of therapy (generally first 1-2 months) or with dose increases or decreases. Use caution in high-risk patients. Worsening depression and severe abrupt suicidality that are not part of the presenting symptoms may require discontinuation or modification of drug therapy. The patient's family or caregiver should be alerted to monitor patients for the emergence of suicidality and associated behaviors (such as agitation, irritability, hostility, impulsivity, and hypomania) and call healthcare provider.

Risk of suicidal behavior may be increased regardless of doxepin dose; antidepressant doses of doxepin are 10- to 100-fold higher than doses for insomnia.

May worsen psychosis in some patients or precipitate a shift to mania or hypomania in patients with bipolar disorder. Patients presenting with depressive symptoms should be screened for bipolar disorder. Monotherapy in patients with bipolar disorder should be avoided. **Doxepin is not FDA approved for the treatment of bipolar depression.**

Should only be used for insomnia after evaluation of potential causes of sleep disturbance. Failure of sleep disturbance to resolve after 7-10 days may indicate psychiatric or medical illness. An increased risk for hazardous sleep-related activities has been noted; discontinue use with any sleep-related episodes. The risks of sedative and anticholinergic effects are high relative to other antidepressant agents. Doxepin frequently causes sedation, which may result in impaired performance of tasks requiring alertness (eg, operating machinery or driving). Sedative effects may be additive with other CNS depressants and/or ethanol. Also use caution in patients with benign prostatic hyperplasia, xerostomia, visual problems, constipation, or history of bowel obstruction.

May cause orthostatic hypotension or conduction disturbances (risks are moderate relative to other antidepressants). Use with caution in patients with a history of cardiovascular disease (including previous MI, stroke, tachycardia, or conduction abnormalities). Use with caution in patients with respiratory compromise or sleep apnea; use is generally not recommended with severe sleep apnea. Consider discontinuation, when possible, prior to elective surgery. Therapy should not be abruptly discontinued in patients receiving high doses for prolonged periods.

Use caution in patients with a previous seizure disorder or condition predisposing to seizures such as brain damage, alcoholism, or concurrent therapy with other drugs which lower the seizure threshold. Use with caution in hyperthyroid patients or those receiving thyroid supplementation. Use with caution in patients with hepatic or renal dysfunction. Use as an antidepressant in the elderly may be inappropriate due to potent anticholinergic and sedating effects (Beers Criteria).

Adverse Reactions (Reflective of adult population; not specific for elderly) Actual frequency may be dependent on diagnosis.

Cardiovascular: Flushing, hypertension (<3%), hypotension, tachycardia

Central nervous system: Ataxia, chills, confusion, disorientation, dizziness, drowsiness, fatigue, hallucinations, headache, seizure, somnolence/sedation (6% to 9%)

Dermatologic: Alopecia, photosensitivity, pruritus, rash

Endocrine & metabolic: Blood sugar increased/decreased, breast enlargement, galactorrhea, gynecomastia, libido increased/decreased, SIADH

Gastrointestinal: Anorexia, aphthous stomatitis, constipation, diarrhea, gastroenteritis (≤2%), indigestion, nausea (2%), trouble with gums, unpleasant taste, vomiting, weight gain, xerostomia; lower esophageal sphincter tone decrease may cause GE reflux

Genitourinary: Testicular edema, urinary retention

Hematologic: Agranulocytosis, eosinophilia, leukopenia, purpura, thrombocytopenia, purpura

Hepatic: Jaundice

Neuromuscular & skeletal: Extrapyramidal symptoms, numbness, paresthesia, tardive dyskinesia, tremor, weakness

Ocular: Blurred vision

Otic: Tinnitus

Respiratory: Asthma exacerbation, nasopharyngitis/upper respiratory tract infection (≤4%)

Miscellaneous: Allergic reactions, diaphoresis (excessive)

Drug Interactions

Metabolism/Transport Effects Substrate (major) of CYP1A2, 2D6, 3A4

Avoid Concomitant Use

Avoid concomitant use of Doxepin (Systemic) with any of the following: Artemether; Dronedarone; Iobenguane I 123; Lumefantrine; MAO Inhibitors; Methylene Blue; Nilotinib; Pimozide; QUEtiapine; QuiNINE; Sibutramine; Tetrabenazine; Thioridazine; Toremifene; Vandetanib; Vemurafenib; Ziprasidone

Increased Effect/Toxicity

Doxepin (Systemic) may increase the levels/effects of: Alpha-/Beta-Agonists (Direct-Acting); Alpha1-Agonists; Amphetamines; Anticholinergics; Aspirin; Beta2-Agonists; Desmopressin; Dronedarone; Methylene Blue; NSAID (COX-2 Inhibitor); NSAID (Nonselective); Pimozide; QTc-Prolonging Agents; QuiNIDine; QuiNINE; Serotonin Modulators; Sodium Phosphates; Sulfonylureas; Tetrabenazine; Thioridazine; Toremifene; TraMADol; Vandetanib; Vemurafenib; Vitamin K Antagonists; Yohimbine; Ziprasidone

The levels/effects of Doxepin (Systemic) may be increased by: Abiraterone Acetate; Alfuzosin; Altretamine; Artemether; BuPROPion; Chloroquine; Cimetidine; Cinacalcet; Ciprofloxacin; Ciprofloxacin (Systemic); Conivaptan; CYP2D6 Inhibitors (Moderate); CYP2D6 Inhibitors (Strong); Dexmethylphenidate; Divalproex; DULoxetine; Gadobutrol; Lithium; Lumefantrine; MAO Inhibitors; Methylphenidate; Metoclopramide; Nilotinib; Pramlintide; Propoxyphene; Protease Inhibitors; QUEtiapine; QuiNIDine; QuiNINE; Selective Serotonin Reuptake Inhibitors; Sibutramine; Terbinafine; Terbinafine (Systemic); Valproic Acid

Decreased Effect

Doxepin (Systemic) may decrease the levels/effects of: Acetylcholinesterase Inhibitors (Central); Alpha2-Agonists; Iobenguane I 123

The levels/effects of Doxepin (Systemic) may be decreased by: Acetylcholinesterase Inhibitors (Central); Barbiturates; CarBAMazepine; Cyproterone; Peginterferon Alfa-2b; St Johns Wort; Tocilizumab

Ethanol/Nutrition/Herb Interactions

Ethanol: May increase CNS depression; monitor for increased effects with coadministration. Caution patients about effects.

Food: A high-fat meal increases the bioavailability of Silenor® and delays the peak plasma concentration by ~3 hours

Herb/Nutraceutical: Avoid valerian, St John's wort, SAMe, kava kava (may increase risk of serotonin syndrome and/or excessive sedation).

Stability Store at 20°C to 25°C (68°F to 77°F). Protect from light.

Mechanism of Action Increases the synaptic concentration of serotonin and norepinephrine in the central nervous system by inhibition of their reuptake by the presynaptic neuronal membrane; antagonizes the histamine (H_1) receptor for sleep maintenance

Pharmacodynamics/Kinetics

Onset of action: Peak effect: Antidepressant: Usually >2 weeks; Anxiolytic: may occur sooner

Protein binding: ~80%

Metabolism: Hepatic via CYP2C19 and 2D6; metabolites include N-desmethyldoxepin (active)

Half-life elimination: Adults: Doxepin: ~15 hours; N-desmethyldoxepin: 31 hours

Time to peak, serum: Hypnotic: 3.5 hours

Excretion: Urine (<3% as unchanged drug or N-desmethyldoxepin)

Dosage

Geriatric

Depression and/or anxiety: Oral: Initial: 10-25 mg at bedtime; increase by 10-25 mg every 3 days for inpatients and weekly for outpatients if tolerated. Rarely does the maximum dose required exceed 75 mg/day; a single bedtime dose is recommended.

Insomnia: Oral: 3 mg once daily 30 minutes prior to bedtime; increase to 6 mg once daily if clinically needed

Adult

Depression and/or anxiety: Oral: Initial: 25-150 mg/day at bedtime or in 2-3 divided doses; may gradually increase up to 300 mg/day; single dose should not exceed 150 mg; select patients may respond to 25-50 mg/day

Insomnia (Silenor®): Oral: 3-6 mg once daily 30 minutes prior to bedtime; maximum dose: 6 mg/day

Hepatic Impairment Use a lower dose and adjust gradually.

Silenor®: Initial: 3 mg once daily

Administration Oral: Do not mix oral concentrate with carbonated beverages (physically incompatible).

Silenor®: Administer within 30 minutes prior to bedtime; do not take within 3 hours of food

Monitoring Parameters Monitor blood pressure and pulse rate prior to and during initial therapy; monitor mental status, suicidal ideation (especially at the beginning of therapy or when doses are increased or decreased); weight; ECG in older adults

Insomnia: Re-evaluate diagnosis if insomnia does not remit within 7-10 days of treatment.

Reference Range Proposed therapeutic concentration (doxepin plus desmethyldoxepin): 110-250 ng/mL. Toxic concentration (doxepin plus desmethyldoxepin): >500 ng/mL. Utility of serum level monitoring is controversial.

Test Interactions Increased glucose

Pharmacotherapy Pearls Entire daily dose may be given at bedtime; avoid unnecessary exposure to sunlight

Special Geriatric Considerations Less potential for anticholinergic effects than amitriptyline and less orthostatic hypotension than imipramine; however, dosing should be approached cautiously, initiated at the low end of the dosage range. Clinical trials with 3 mg and 6 mg to treat insomnia included patients 65 and 75 years of age and older. Confusion and oversedation remain a caution. The pharmacokinetics of doxepin have not been studied in elderly patients.

This medication is considered to be potentially inappropriate in this patient population (Beers Criteria severity: High).

Dosage Forms Excipient information presented when available (limited, particularly for generics); consult specific product labeling.

Capsule, oral: 10 mg, 25 mg, 50 mg, 75 mg, 100 mg, 150 mg

Solution, oral [concentrate]: 10 mg/mL (118 mL, 120 mL)

Tablet, oral:

Silenor®: 3 mg, 6 mg

Selected References

Lakshmanan M, Mion LC, and Frengley JD, "Effective Low Dose Tricyclic Antidepressant Treatment for Depressed Geriatric Rehabilitation Patients. A Double-Blind Study," *J Am Geriatr Soc,* 1986, 34(6):421-6.

Doxepin (Topical) (DOKS e pin)

Medication Safety Issues

Sound-alike/look-alike issues:

Doxepin may be confused with digoxin, doxapram, doxazosin, Doxidan®, doxycycline
Zonalon® may be confused with Zone-A Forte®

International issues:

Doxal® [Finland] may be confused with Doxil® which is a brand name for doxorubicin in the U.S.

Doxal® [Finland]: Brand name for doxycycline in Austria; brand name for pyridoxine/thiamine in Brazil

Brand Names: U.S. Prudoxin™; Zonalon®

Brand Names: Canada Zonalon®

Index Terms Doxepin Hydrochloride

Generic Availability (U.S.) No

Pharmacologic Category Topical Skin Product

Use Short-term (<8 days) management of moderate pruritus in adults with atopic dermatitis or lichen simplex chronicus

Unlabeled/Investigational Use Cream: Treatment of burning mouth syndrome and neuropathic pain

Dosage

Geriatric Pruritus: Topical: Refer to adult dosing.

Adult

Burning mouth syndrome (unlabeled use): Oral topical: Cream: Apply 3-4 times daily.

Pruritus: Topical: Apply a thin film 4 times/day with at least 3- to 4-hour interval between applications; not recommended for use >8 days. (Oral administration of doxepin 25-50 mg has also been used, but systemic adverse effects are increased.)

Special Geriatric Considerations Systemic absorption with plasma concentrations sufficient to result in anticholinergic effects, sedation, urinary retention, and delirium has been reported. Risk is likely related to the frequency of application and the surface area of application. Persons ≥65 years were not sufficiently represented in clinical trials.

Dosage Forms Excipient information presented when available (limited, particularly for generics); consult specific product labeling.

Cream, topical, as hydrochloride:

Prudoxin™: 5% (45 g) [contains benzyl alcohol]

Zonalon®: 5% (30 g, 45 g) [contains benzyl alcohol]

♦ **Doxepin Hydrochloride** see Doxepin (Systemic) on page 564

♦ **Doxepin Hydrochloride** see Doxepin (Topical) on page 567

Doxercalciferol (doks er kal si fe FEER ole)

Brand Names: U.S. Hectorol®

Brand Names: Canada Hectorol®

Index Terms 1α-Hydroxyergocalciferol

Generic Availability (U.S.) No

◀ **Pharmacologic Category** Vitamin D Analog

Use Treatment of secondary hyperparathyroidism in patients with chronic kidney disease

Contraindications History of hypercalcemia or evidence of vitamin D toxicity

Warnings/Precautions Other forms of vitamin D should be discontinued when doxercalciferol is started. Excessive administration may lead to over suppression of PTH, hypercalcemia, hypercalciuria, hyperphosphatemia and adynamic bone disease. Acute hypercalcemia may increase risk of cardiac arrhythmias and seizures; use caution with cardiac glycosides as digitalis toxicity may be increased. Chronic hypercalcemia may lead to generalized vascular and other soft-tissue calcification. Phosphate and vitamin D (and its derivatives) should be withheld during therapy to avoid hypercalcemia. Hyperphosphatemia should be corrected before initiating therapy. Use with caution in patients with hepatic impairment. Injection is intended for I.V. use only.

Adverse Reactions (Reflective of adult population; not specific for elderly)

Note: As reported in dialysis patients.

>10%:
  Cardiovascular: Edema (34%)
  Central nervous system: Headache (28%), malaise (28%), dizziness (12%)
  Gastrointestinal: Nausea/vomiting (21%)
  Respiratory: Dyspnea (12%)
1% to 10%:
  Cardiovascular: Bradycardia (7%)
  Central nervous system: Sleep disorder (3%)
  Dermatologic: Pruritus (8%)
  Endocrine & metabolic: Hypercalcemia (I.V. ~1%), hyperphosphatemia (I.V. 2% to 4%)
  Gastrointestinal: Anorexia (5%), dyspepsia (5%), weight gain (5%)
  Neuromuscular & skeletal: Arthralgia (5%)
  Miscellaneous: Abscess (3%)

Drug Interactions

Avoid Concomitant Use

Avoid concomitant use of Doxercalciferol with any of the following: Aluminum Hydroxide; Sucralfate; Vitamin D Analogs

Increased Effect/Toxicity

Doxercalciferol may increase the levels/effects of: Aluminum Hydroxide; Cardiac Glycosides; Sucralfate; Vitamin D Analogs

The levels/effects of Doxercalciferol may be increased by: Calcium Salts; Thiazide Diuretics

Decreased Effect

The levels/effects of Doxercalciferol may be decreased by: Bile Acid Sequestrants; Mineral Oil; Orlistat

Stability Store at controlled room temperature of 15°C to 30°C (59°F to 86°F). Protect injection from light.

Mechanism of Action Doxercalciferol is metabolized to the active form of vitamin D. The active form of vitamin D controls the intestinal absorption of dietary calcium, the tubular reabsorption of calcium by the kidneys, and in conjunction with PTH, the mobilization of calcium from the skeleton.

Pharmacodynamics/Kinetics

Metabolism: Hepatic via CYP27 to active metabolites

Half-life elimination: Active metabolite: 32-37 hours; up to 96 hours

Dosage

Geriatric & Adult Secondary hyperparathyroidism:

Oral:

Dialysis patients: Dose should be titrated to lower iPTH to 150-300 pg/mL; dose is adjusted at 8-week intervals (maximum dose: 20 mcg 3 times/week)

Initial dose: iPTH >400 pg/mL: 10 mcg 3 times/week at dialysis

Dose titration:

iPTH level decreased by 50% and >300 pg/mL: Dose can be increased to 12.5 mcg 3 times/week for 8 more weeks; this titration process can continue at 8-week intervals; each increase should be by 2.5 mcg/dose

iPTH level 150-300 pg/mL: Maintain current dose

iPTH level <100 pg/mL: Suspend doxercalciferol for 1 week; resume at a reduced dose; decrease each dose (not weekly dose) by at least 2.5 mcg

Predialysis patients: Dose should be titrated to lower iPTH to 35-70 pg/mL with stage 3 disease or to 70-110 pg/mL with stage 4 disease: Dose may be adjusted at 2-week intervals (maximum dose: 3.5 mcg/day)

Initial dose: 1 mcg/day

Dose titration:

iPTH level >70 pg/mL with stage 3 disease or >110 pg/mL with stage 4 disease: Increase dose by 0.5 mcg every 2 weeks as necessary

iPTH level 35-70 pg/mL with stage 3 disease or 70-110 pg/mL with stage 4 disease: Maintain current dose

iPTH level is <35 pg/mL with stage 3 disease or <70 pg/mL with stage 4 disease: Suspend doxercalciferol for 1 week, then resume at a reduced dose (at least 0.5 mcg lower)

I.V.:

Dialysis patients: Dose should be titrated to lower iPTH to 150-300 pg/mL; dose is adjusted at 8-week intervals (maximum dose: 18 mcg/week)

Initial dose: iPTH level >400 pg/mL: 4 mcg 3 times/week after dialysis, administered as a bolus dose

Dose titration:

iPTH level decreased by <50% and >300 pg/mL: Dose can be increased by 1-2 mcg at 8-week intervals, as necessary

iPTH level decreased by >50% and >300 pg/mL: Maintain current dose

iPTH level 150-300 pg/mL: Maintain current dose

iPTH level <100 pg/mL: Suspend doxercalciferol for 1 week; resume at a reduced dose (at least 1 mcg lower)

Hypercalcemia, hyperphosphatemia, or serum calcium times phosphorus product >55 mg^2/dL^2: Decrease or suspend dose and/or adjust dose of phosphate binders; if dose is suspended, resume at a reduced dose (at least 1 mcg lower)

Renal Impairment No adjustment is required.

Hepatic Impairment Use with caution; no guidelines for dosage adjustment.

Monitoring Parameters

Serum calcium and phosphorus: Frequency of measurement may be dependent upon the presence and magnitude of abnormalities, the rate of progression of CKD, and the use of treatments for CKD-mineral and bone disorders (KDIGO, 2009):

CKD stage 3: Every 6-12 months

CKD stage 4: Every 3-6 months

CKD stage 5 and 5D: Every 1-3 months

Periodic 24-hour urinary calcium and phosphorus; magnesium; alkaline phosphatase every 12 months or more frequently in the presence of elevated PTH; creatinine, BUN, albumin; intact parathyroid hormone (iPTH) every 3-12 months depending on CKD severity

Reference Range

Corrected total serum calcium (K/DOQI, 2003): CKD stages 3 and 4: 8.4-10.2 mg/dL (2.1-2.6 mmol/L); CKD stage 5: 8.4-9.5 mg/dL (2.1-2.37 mmol/L); KDIGO guidelines recommend maintaining normal ranges for all stages of CKD (3-5D) (KDIGO, 2009)

Phosphorus (K/DOQI, 2003): CKD stages 3 and 4: 2.7-4.6 mg/dL (0.87-1.48 mmol/L); CKD stage 5 (including those treated with dialysis): 3.5-5.5 mg/dL (1.13-1.78 mmol/L); KDIGO guidelines recommend maintaining normal ranges for CKD stages 3-5 and lowering elevated phosphorus levels toward the normal range for CKD stage 5D (KDIGO, 2009)

Serum calcium-phosphorus product (K/DOQI, 2003): CKD stage 3-5: <55 mg^2/dL^2

PTH: Whole molecule, immunochemiluminometric assay (ICMA): 1.0-5.2 pmol/L; whole molecule, radioimmunoassay (RIA): 10.0-65.0 pg/mL; whole molecule, immunoradiometric, double antibody (IRMA): 1.0-6.0 pmol/L

Target ranges by stage of chronic kidney disease (KDIGO, 2009): CKD stage 3-5: Optimal iPTH is unknown; maintain normal range (assay-dependent); CKD stage 5D: Maintain iPTH within 2-9 times the upper limit of normal for the assay used

Special Geriatric Considerations No special changes in dose are required. Caution should be used in the elderly using magnesium products (MOM, magnesium containing antacids, etc). These should be stopped if possible before initiating doxercalciferol.

Dosage Forms Excipient information presented when available (limited, particularly for generics); consult specific product labeling.

Capsule, softgel, oral:

Hectorol®: 0.5 mcg, 1 mcg, 2.5 mcg [contains coconut oil]

Injection, solution:

Hectorol®: 2 mcg/mL (1 mL, 2 mL) [contains edetate disodium, ethanol]

◆ **Doxidan® [OTC]** see Bisacodyl on page 205
◆ **Doxy 100™** see Doxycycline on page 570

Doxycycline (doks i SYE kleen)

Related Information
Community-Acquired Pneumonia in Adults *on page 2059*

Medication Safety Issues
Sound-alike/look-alike issues:
Doxycycline may be confused with dicyclomine, doxepin, doxylamine
Doxy100™ may be confused with Doxil®
Monodox® may be confused with Maalox®
Oracea® may be confused with Orencia®
Vibramycin® may be confused with vancomycin, Vibativ™

Brand Names: U.S. Adoxa®; Adoxa® Pak™ 1/150; Adoxa® Pak™ 1/75; Alodox™; Doryx®; Doxy 100™; Monodox®; Ocudox™; Oracea®; Oraxyl™; Periostat®; Vibramycin®

Brand Names: Canada Apo-Doxy Tabs®; Apo-Doxy®; Dom-Doxycycline; Doxycin; Doxytab; Novo-Doxylin; Nu-Doxycycline; Periostat®; PHL-Doxycycline; PMS-Doxycycline; Vibra-Tabs®; Vibramycin®

Index Terms Doxycycline Calcium; Doxycycline Hyclate; Doxycycline Monohydrate

Generic Availability (U.S.) Yes: Excludes capsule (variable release), powder for suspension, syrup

Pharmacologic Category Antibiotic, Tetracycline Derivative

Use Principally in the treatment of infections caused by susceptible *Rickettsia, Chlamydia,* and *Mycoplasma*; alternative to mefloquine for malaria prophylaxis; treatment for syphilis, uncomplicated *Neisseria gonorrhoeae, Listeria, Actinomyces israelii,* and *Clostridium* infections in penicillin-allergic patients; used for community-acquired pneumonia and other common infections due to susceptible organisms; anthrax due to *Bacillus anthracis,* including inhalational anthrax (postexposure); treatment of infections caused by uncommon susceptible gram-negative and gram-positive organisms including *Borrelia recurrentis, Ureaplasma urealyticum, Haemophilus ducreyi, Yersinia pestis, Francisella tularensis, Vibrio cholerae, Campylobacter fetus, Brucella* spp, *Bartonella bacilliformis,* and *Klebsiella granulomatis,* Q fever, Lyme disease; treatment of inflammatory lesions associated with rosacea; intestinal amebiasis; severe acne

Unlabeled/Investigational Use Sclerosing agent for pleural effusion injection; vancomycin-resistant enterococci (VRE); alternate treatment for MRSA infections; treatment of periodontitis (refractory)

Contraindications Hypersensitivity to doxycycline, tetracycline or any component of the formulation

Warnings/Precautions Photosensitivity reaction may occur with this drug; avoid prolonged exposure to sunlight or tanning equipment. Antianabolic effects of tetracyclines can increase BUN (dose-related). Autoimmune syndromes have been reported. Hepatotoxicity rarely occurs; if symptomatic, conduct LFT and discontinue drug. Pseudotumor cerebri has been (rarely) reported with tetracycline use; usually resolves with discontinuation. Prolonged use may result in fungal or bacterial superinfection, including *C. difficile*-associated diarrhea (CDAD) and pseudomembranous colitis; CDAD has been observed >2 months postantibiotic treatment. May cause tissue hyperpigmentation, enamel hypoplasia, or permanent tooth discoloration.

Additional specific warnings: Oracea™: Should not be used for the treatment or prophylaxis of bacterial infections, since the lower dose of drug per capsule may be subefficacious and promote resistance. Syrup contains sodium metabisulfite. Effectiveness of products intended for use in periodontitis has not been established in patients with coexistent oral candidiasis; use with caution in patients with a history or predisposition to oral candidiasis.

Adverse Reactions (Reflective of adult population; not specific for elderly) Frequency not defined.

Cardiovascular: Intracranial hypertension, pericarditis

Dermatologic: Angioneurotic edema, erythema multiforme, exfoliative dermatitis (rare), photosensitivity, rash, skin hyperpigmentation, Stevens-Johnson syndrome, toxic epidermal necrolysis, urticaria

Endocrine & metabolic: Brown/black discoloration of thyroid gland (no dysfunction reported), hypoglycemia

Gastrointestinal: Anorexia, diarrhea, dysphagia, enterocolitis, esophagitis (rare), esophageal ulcerations (rare), glossitis, inflammatory lesions in anogenital region, nausea, oral (mucosal) pigmentation, pseudomembranous colitis, tooth discoloration (children), vomiting

Hematologic: Eosinophilia, hemolytic anemia, neutropenia, thrombocytopenia

Hepatic: Hepatotoxicity (rare)

Renal: BUN increased (dose related)

Miscellaneous: Anaphylactoid purpura, anaphylaxis, bulging fontanels (infants), serum sickness, SLE exacerbation

Note: Adverse effects in clinical trials occurring at a frequency more than 1% greater than placebo:

Periostat®: Diarrhea, dyspepsia, joint pain, menstrual cramp, nausea, dyspepsia, pain

Oracea®: Abdominal distention, abdominal pain, anxiety, AST increased, back pain, fungal infection, hyperglycemia, influenza, LDH increased, nasal congestion, nasopharyngitis, pain, sinus headache, sinusitis, xerostomia

Drug Interactions

Metabolism/Transport Effects Inhibits CYP3A4 (moderate)

Avoid Concomitant Use

Avoid concomitant use of Doxycycline with any of the following: BCG; Retinoic Acid Derivatives

Increased Effect/Toxicity

Doxycycline may increase the levels/effects of: Neuromuscular-Blocking Agents; Porfimer; Retinoic Acid Derivatives; Vitamin K Antagonists

Decreased Effect

Doxycycline may decrease the levels/effects of: BCG; Penicillins; Typhoid Vaccine

The levels/effects of Doxycycline may be decreased by: Antacids; Barbiturates; Bile Acid Sequestrants; Bismuth; Bismuth Subsalicylate; Calcium Salts; CarBAMazepine; Fosphenytoin; Iron Salts; Lanthanum; Magnesium Salts; Phenytoin; Quinapril; Sucralfate

Ethanol/Nutrition/Herb Interactions

Ethanol: Chronic ethanol ingestion may reduce the serum concentration of doxycycline.

Food: Doxycycline serum levels may be slightly decreased if taken with food or milk. Administration with iron or calcium may decrease doxycycline absorption. May decrease absorption of calcium, iron, magnesium, zinc, and amino acids.

Herb/Nutraceutical: St John's wort may decrease doxycycline levels. Avoid dong quai, St John's wort (may also cause photosensitization).

Stability

Capsule, tablet: Store at controlled room temperature of 25°C (77°F); excursions permitted to 15°C to 30°C (59°F to 86°F). Protect from light.

I.V. infusion: Following reconstitution with sterile water for injection, dilute to a final concentration of 0.1-1 mg/mL using a compatible solution. Solutions for I.V. infusion may be prepared using 0.9% sodium chloride, D_5W, Ringer's injection, lactated Ringer's, D_5LR. Protect from light. Stability varies based on solution.

Mechanism of Action Inhibits protein synthesis by binding with the 30S and possibly the 50S ribosomal subunit(s) of susceptible bacteria; may also cause alterations in the cytoplasmic membrane

Periostat® capsules (proposed mechanism): Has been shown to inhibit collagenase activity *in vitro*. Also has been noted to reduce elevated collagenase activity in the gingival crevicular fluid of patients with periodontal disease. Systemic levels do not reach inhibitory concentrations against bacteria.

Pharmacodynamics/Kinetics

Absorption: Oral: Almost complete

Distribution: Widely into body tissues and fluids including synovial, pleural, prostatic, seminal fluids, and bronchial secretions; saliva, aqueous humor, and CSF penetration is poor

Protein binding: 90%

Metabolism: Not hepatic; partially inactivated in GI tract by chelate formation

Bioavailability: Reduced at high pH; may be clinically significant in patients with gastrectomy, gastric bypass surgery or who are otherwise deemed achlorhydric

Half-life elimination: 12-15 hours (usually increases to 22-24 hours with multiple doses); End-stage renal disease: 18-25 hours; Oracea®: 21 hours

Time to peak, serum: 1.5-4 hours

Excretion: Feces (30%); urine (23%)

Dosage

Geriatric & Adult

Usual dosage range: Oral, I.V.: 100-200 mg/day in 1-2 divided doses

Anthrax:

Inhalational (postexposure prophylaxis): Oral, I.V. (use oral route when possible): 100 mg every 12 hours for 60 days (ACIP, 2010)

Cutaneous (treatment): Oral: 100 mg every 12 hours for 60 days. **Note:** In the presence of systemic involvement, extensive edema, lesions on head/neck, refer to I.V. dosing for treatment of inhalational/gastrointestinal/oropharyngeal anthrax

Inhalational/gastrointestinal/oropharyngeal (treatment): I.V.: Initial: 100 mg every 12 hours; switch to oral therapy when clinically appropriate; some recommend initial loading dose of 200 mg, followed by 100 mg every 8-12 hours (Franz, 1997). **Note:** Initial treatment should include two or more agents predicted to be effective (CDC, 2001). Agents suggested for use in conjunction with doxycycline or ciprofloxacin include rifampin, vancomycin, imipenem, penicillin, ampicillin, chloramphenicol, clindamycin, and clarithromycin. May switch to oral antimicrobial therapy when clinically appropriate. Continue combined therapy for 60 days

Brucellosis: Oral: 100 mg twice daily for 6 weeks with rifampin or streptomycin

Cellulitis (purulent) due to community-acquired MRSA (unlabeled use): Oral: 100 mg twice daily for 5-10 days (Liu, 2011)

Chlamydial infections, uncomplicated: Oral: 100 mg twice daily for ≥7 days

Community-acquired pneumonia, bronchitis: Oral, I.V.: 100 mg twice daily (Ailani, 1999; Mandell, 2007)

Epididymitis: Oral: 100 mg twice daily for 10 days (in combination with ceftriaxone) (CDC, 2010)

Gonococcal infection, uncomplicated (cervix, pharynx, rectum, urethra): Oral: 100 mg twice daily for 7 days (in combination with a cephalosporin) (CDC, 2010)

Alternatively, the manufacturer recommends a single-visit dose in nonanorectal infections in men: 300 mg initially, repeat dose in 1 hour (total dose: 600 mg)

Granuloma inguinale (donovanosis): Oral: 100 mg twice daily for at least 3 weeks (and until lesions have healed) (CDC, 2010)

Lyme disease: Oral (Halperin, 2007; Wormser, 2006):

Prevention: Initiate within 72 hours of tick removal: 200 mg administered as a single dose

Treatment (early lyme disease without neurologic manifestations): 100 mg twice daily for 10-21 days

Treatment (meningitis or other early neurologic manifestations): 100-200 mg twice daily for 14 days (range: 10-28 days)

Lymphogranuloma venereum: Oral: 100 mg twice daily for 21 days (CDC, 2010)

Malaria prophylaxis: 100 mg/day. Start 1-2 days prior to travel to endemic area; continue daily during travel and for 4 weeks after leaving endemic area

Nongonococcal urethritis: Oral: 100 mg twice daily for 7 days (CDC, 2010)

Pelvic inflammatory disease:

Treatment, inpatient: Oral, I.V.: 100 mg twice daily (in combination with cefoxitin or cefotetan); may transition to oral doxycycline (add clindamycin or metronidazole if tubo-ovarian abscess present) to complete 14 days of treatment (CDC, 2010)

Treatment, outpatient: Oral: 100 mg twice daily for 14 days (with or without metronidazole); preceded by a single I.M. dose of cefoxitin (plus oral probenecid) or ceftriaxone (CDC, 2010)

Periodontitis: Oral (Periostat®): 20 mg twice daily as an adjunct following scaling and root planing

Periodontitis, refractory (unlabeled use): Oral: 100-200 mg daily

Proctitis: Oral: 100 mg twice daily for 7 days (in combination with ceftriaxone) (CDC, 2010)

Q fever: Oral: 100 mg every 12 hours for 15-21days (CDC, 2009)

Rosacea (Oracea®): Oral: 40 mg once daily in the morning

Sclerosing agent for pleural effusion (unlabeled use): Intrapleural: 500 mg as a single dose in 100 mL NS (Porcel, 2006); may require a repeat dose (Kvale, 2007)

Syphilis:

Primary/secondary syphilis: Oral: 100 mg twice daily for 14 days (CDC, 2010)

Latent syphilis: Oral: 100 mg twice daily for 28 days (CDC, 2010)

Tickborne rickettsial disease: Oral, I.V.: 100 mg twice daily for 5-7 days; severe or complicated disease may require longer treatment; human granulocytotropic anaplasmosis (HGA) should be treated for 10-14 days

Tularemia: I.V. (may transition to oral if clinically appropriate): Initial: 100 mg every 12 hours for 14-21 days (Dennis, 2001)

Vibrio cholerae: Oral: 300 mg as a single dose (WHO, 2004)

Yersinia pestis **(plague):** Oral, I.V.: 200 mg initially then 100 mg twice daily **or** 200 mg once daily for 10 days (Daya, 2005; Inglesby, 2000)

Renal Impairment No dosage adjustment necessary in renal impairment.

Poorly dialyzed; no supplemental dose or dosage adjustment necessary, including patients on intermittent hemodialysis, peritoneal dialysis, or continuous renal replacement therapy (eg, CVVHD).

Administration Oral administration is preferable unless patient has significant nausea and vomiting; I.V. and oral routes are bioequivalent.

Oral: May give with meals to decrease GI upset. Capsule and tablet: Administer with at least 8 ounces of water and have patient sit up for at least 30 minutes after taking to reduce the risk of esophageal irritation and ulceration.

Oracea®: Take on an empty stomach 1 hour before or 2 hours after meals.

Doryx®: May be administered by carefully breaking up the tablet and sprinkling tablet contents on a spoonful of cold applesauce. The delayed release pellets must not be crushed or damaged when breaking up tablet. Should be administered immediately after preparation and without chewing.

I.V.: Infuse I.V. doxycycline over 1-4 hours; avoid extravasation

Intrapleural (unlabeled route): Add to 100 mL NS and instill into chest tube (Porcel, 2006)

Monitoring Parameters Perform culture and sensitivity testing prior to initiating therapy. CBC, renal and liver function tests periodically with prolonged therapy.

Test Interactions False-negative urine glucose using Clinistix®, Tes-Tape®; false-positive urine glucose using Clinitest®; false elevations of urinary catecholamines with fluorescence test

Pharmacotherapy Pearls Oracea® capsules are not bioequivalent to other doxycycline products.

Special Geriatric Considerations Dose adjustment for renal function is not necessary.

Dosage Forms Excipient information presented when available (limited, particularly for generics); consult specific product labeling. [DSC] = Discontinued product

Capsule, oral, as hyclate [strength expressed as base]: 50 mg, 100 mg
    Ocudox™: 50 mg [kit includes Ocudox™ capsules (60s), Ocusoft® Lid Scrub™ Plus eyelid cleanser pads, and Tears Again® advanced spray]
    Oraxyl™: 20 mg
    Vibramycin®: 100 mg

Capsule, oral, as monohydrate [strength expressed as base]: 50 mg, 100 mg, 150 mg
    Adoxa®: 150 mg
    Monodox®: 50 mg, 75 mg, 100 mg

Capsule, variable release, oral [strength expressed as base]:
    Oracea®: 40 mg [30 mg (immediate release) and 10 mg (delayed release)]

Injection, powder for reconstitution, as hyclate [strength expressed as base]: 100 mg
    Doxy 100™: 100 mg

Powder for suspension, oral, as monohydrate [strength expressed as base]:
    Vibramycin®: 25 mg/5 mL (60 mL) [raspberry flavor]

Syrup, oral, as calcium [strength expressed as base]:
    Vibramycin®: 50 mg/5 mL (473 mL) [contains propylene glycol, sodium metabisulfite; raspberry-apple flavor]

Tablet, oral, as hyclate [strength expressed as base]: 20 mg, 100 mg
    Alodox™: 20 mg [kit includes Alodox™ tablets (60s), Ocusoft® Lid Scrub™ pads, eyelid cleanser, and goggles]
    Periostat®: 20 mg

Tablet, oral, as monohydrate [strength expressed as base]: 50 mg, 75 mg, 100 mg, 150 mg
    Adoxa®: 50 mg, 75 mg [DSC], 100 mg [DSC]
    Adoxa® Pak™ 1/150: 150 mg [scored]
    Adoxa® Pak™ 1/75: 75 mg

Tablet, delayed release coated beads, oral, as hyclate [strength expressed as base]: 75 mg, 100 mg

Tablet, delayed release coated pellets, oral, as hyclate [strength expressed as base]:
    Doryx®: 75 mg [scored; contains sodium 4.5 mg (0.196 mEq)/tablet]
    Doryx®: 100 mg [scored; contains sodium 6 mg (0.261 mEq)/tablet]
    Doryx®: 150 mg [scored; contains sodium 9 mg (0.392 mEq)/tablet]

Selected References

Böcker R, Mühlberg W, Platt D, et al, "Serum Level, Half-Life and Apparent Volume of Distribution of Doxycycline in Geriatric Patients," *Eur J Clin Pharmacol*, 1986, 30(1):105-8.

Centers for Disease Control and Prevention, "Update: Investigation of Anthrax Associated With Intentional Exposure and Interim Public Health Guidelines, October 2001," *MMWR*, 2001, 50(41):889-93. Accessed October 19, 2001, at http://www.cdc.gov/mmwr/preview/mmwrhtml/mm5041a1.htm.

Ljungberg B and Nilsson-Ehle I, "Pharmacokinetics of Antimicrobial Agents in the Elderly," *Rev Infect Dis*, 1987, 9 (2):250-64.

Mandell LA, Wunderink RG, Anzueto A, et al, "Infectious Diseases Society of America/American Thoracic Society Consensus Guidelines on the Management of Community-Acquired Pneumonia in Adults," *Clin Infect Dis*, 2007, 44 Suppl 2:S27-72.

Dronabinol (droe NAB i nol)

Medication Safety Issues
Sound-alike/look-alike issues:
Dronabinol may be confused with droperidol

Brand Names: Canada Marinol®

Index Terms Delta-9 THC; Delta-9-tetrahydro-cannabinol; Tetrahydrocannabinol; THC

Generic Availability (U.S.) Yes

Pharmacologic Category Antiemetic; Appetite Stimulant

Use Chemotherapy-associated nausea and vomiting refractory to other antiemetic(s); AIDS-related anorexia

Unlabeled/Investigational Use Cancer-related anorexia

Contraindications Hypersensitivity to dronabinol, cannabinoids, sesame oil, or any component of the formulation, or marijuana; should be avoided in patients with a history of schizophrenia

Warnings/Precautions Use with caution in patients with hepatic disease or seizure disorders. Reduce dosage in patients with severe hepatic impairment. May cause additive CNS effects with sedatives, hypnotics or other psychoactive agents; patients must be cautioned about performing tasks which require mental alertness (eg, operating machinery or driving).

May have potential for abuse; drug is psychoactive substance in marijuana; use caution in patients with a history of substance abuse or potential. May cause withdrawal symptoms upon abrupt discontinuation. Use with caution in patients with mania, depression, or schizophrenia; careful psychiatric monitoring is recommended. Use caution in elderly; they are more sensitive to adverse effects.

Adverse Reactions (Reflective of adult population; not specific for elderly) Frequency not always specified.
>1%:
Cardiovascular: Palpitations, tachycardia, vasodilation/facial flushing
Central nervous system: Euphoria (8% to 24%, dose related), abnormal thinking (3% to 10%), dizziness (3% to 10%), paranoia (3% to 10%), somnolence (3% to 10%), amnesia, anxiety, ataxia, confusion, depersonalization, hallucination
Gastrointestinal: Abdominal pain (3% to 10%), nausea (3% to 10%), vomiting (3% to 10%)
Neuromuscular & skeletal: Weakness

Drug Interactions
Avoid Concomitant Use There are no known interactions where it is recommended to avoid concomitant use.

Increased Effect/Toxicity
Dronabinol may increase the levels/effects of: Alcohol (Ethyl); CNS Depressants; Methotrimeprazine; Selective Serotonin Reuptake Inhibitors; Sympathomimetics

The levels/effects of Dronabinol may be increased by: Anticholinergic Agents; Cocaine; Droperidol; HydrOXYzine; MAO Inhibitors; Methotrimeprazine; Ritonavir

Decreased Effect There are no known significant interactions involving a decrease in effect.

Ethanol/Nutrition/Herb Interactions
Ethanol: May increase CNS depression; monitor for increased effects with coadministration. Caution patients about effects.
Food: Administration with high-lipid meals may increase absorption.
Herb/Nutraceutical: St John's wort may decrease dronabinol levels.

Stability Store under refrigeration (or in a cool environment) between 8°C and 15°C (46°F and 59°F); protect from freezing.

Mechanism of Action Unknown, may inhibit endorphins in the brain's emetic center, suppress prostaglandin synthesis, and/or inhibit medullary activity through an unspecified cortical action. Some pharmacologic effects appear to involve sympathimometic activity; tachyphylaxis to some effect (eg, tachycardia) may occur, but appetite-stimulating effects do not appear to wane over time. Antiemetic activity may be due to effect on cannabinoid receptors (CB1) within the central nervous system.

Pharmacodynamics/Kinetics
Onset of action: Within 1 hour
Peak effect: 2-4 hours
Duration: 24 hours (appetite stimulation)
Absorption: Oral: 90% to 95%; 10% to 20% of dose gets into systemic circulation
Distribution: V_d: 10 L/kg; dronabinol is highly lipophilic and distributes to adipose tissue
Protein binding: 97% to 99%
Metabolism: Hepatic to at least 50 metabolites, some of which are active; 11-hydroxy-delta-9-tetrahydrocannabinol (11-OH-THC) is the major metabolite; extensive first-pass effect
Half-life elimination: Dronabinol: 25-36 hours (terminal); Dronabinol metabolites: 44-59 hours

Time to peak, serum: 0.5-4 hours

Excretion: Feces (50% as unconjugated metabolites, 5% as unchanged drug); urine (10% to 15% as acid metabolites and conjugates)

Dosage

Geriatric & Adult

Antiemetic: Oral: 5 mg/m² 1-3 hours before chemotherapy, then give 5 mg/m²/dose every 2-4 hours after chemotherapy for a total of 4-6 doses/day; dose may be increased up to a maximum of 15 mg/m²/dose if needed (dosage may be increased by 2.5 mg/m² increments).

Appetite stimulant (AIDS-related): Oral: Initial: 2.5 mg twice daily (before lunch and dinner); titrate up to a maximum of 20 mg/day.

Hepatic Impairment Usual dose should be reduced in patients with severe liver failure.

Monitoring Parameters CNS effects, heart rate, blood pressure, behavioral profile

Reference Range Antinauseant effects: 5-10 ng/mL

Test Interactions Decreased FSH, LH, and testosterone

Special Geriatric Considerations Elderly patients may be more sensitive to the CNS effects and postural hypotensive effects of dronabinol. Titrate the dose slowly and monitor for adverse effects.

Controlled Substance C-III

Dosage Forms Excipient information presented when available (limited, particularly for generics); consult specific product labeling.

Capsule, soft gelatin, oral: 2.5 mg [contains sesame oil], 5 mg [contains sesame oil], 10 mg [contains sesame oil]

Dronedarone (droe NE da rone)

Brand Names: U.S. Multaq®

Brand Names: Canada Multaq®

Index Terms Dronedarone Hydrochloride; SR33589

Generic Availability (U.S.) No

Pharmacologic Category Antiarrhythmic Agent, Class III

Use To reduce the risk of hospitalization related to paroxysmal or persistent atrial fibrillation (AF) or atrial flutter (AFL) in patients with a recent episode of AF/AFL and associated cardiovascular risk factors (eg, age >70 years, hypertension, diabetes, prior cerebrovascular accident, left atrial diameter ≥50 mm or left ventricular ejection fraction <40%), who are in normal sinus rhythm or will be cardioverted

Medication Guide Available Yes

Contraindications NYHA Class IV heart failure (HF); NYHA Class II-III HF with recent decompensation requiring hospitalization or referral to a specialized HF clinic; second- or third-degree heart block, or sick sinus syndrome (except in patients with a functioning artificial pacemaker); bradycardia <50 bpm; concomitant use of strong CYP3A4 inhibitors (eg, ketoconazole, itraconazole, voriconazole, cyclosporine, telithromycin, clarithromycin, nefazodone, or ritonavir); concomitant use of drugs or herbal products known to prolong the QT interval increasing the risk for torsade de pointes (eg, phenothiazine antipsychotics, tricyclic antidepressants, certain oral macrolide antibiotics, or class I and III antiarrhythmics); QT$_c$ (Bazett) interval ≥500 msec or PR interval >280 msec; severe hepatic impairment

Warnings/Precautions [U.S. Boxed Warning]: In patients with severe HF requiring recent hospitalization or referral to a specialized HF clinic for worsening symptoms, patients receiving dronedarone had a greater than twofold increase in mortality; use is contraindicated in patients with NYHA Class IV HF or NYHA Class II-III HF with recent decompensation requiring hospitalization or referral to a specialized HF clinic. If patients develop new or worsening HF symptoms (eg, weight gain, dependent edema, or increasing shortness of breath) while on therapy, consider suspension or discontinuation of dronedarone.

Dronedarone induces a moderate prolongation of the QT interval (average ~10 msec); much greater effects have been observed. Use in patients with QT$_c$ (Bazett) interval ≥500 msec is contraindicated; discontinue use of dronedarone if this occurs during therapy. Following initiation, dronedarone may produce a slight increase in serum creatinine (~0.1 mg/dL) due to inhibition of tubular secretion; glomerular filtration rate is not affected; effect is reversible upon discontinuation.

Severe liver injury, including acute liver failure leading to liver transplant, has been rarely reported. If liver injury is suspected, discontinue therapy and evaluate liver enzymes/bilirubin. Appropriate treatment should be started and therapy should not be reinitiated if liver injury is confirmed. Advise patients to report any signs or symptoms of hepatic injury (unusual fatigue, jaundice, nausea, vomiting, abdominal pain, and/or fever). Consider periodic monitoring of serum liver enzymes and bilirubin, especially during the first 6 months of therapy. Use with caution in patients with mild-to-moderate hepatic impairment; use is contraindicated in severe hepatic impairment.

Chronic administration of antiarrhythmic drugs may affect defibrillation or pacing thresholds; assess when initiating dronedarone and during therapy. Correct electrolyte disturbances, especially hypokalemia or hypomagnesemia, prior to use and throughout therapy. Dronedarone is a moderate inhibitor of CYP3A4 and CYP2D6 enzymes and has potential to inhibit p-glycoprotein, which may lead to increased serum concentrations/toxicity of a number of medications. Use caution when initiating dronedarone in patients on warfarin. Cases of increased INR with or without bleeding have occurred in patients treated with warfarin; monitor INR closely after initiating dronedarone in these patients.

Adverse Reactions (Reflective of adult population; not specific for elderly)
>10%:
  Cardiovascular: QT_c (Bazett) prolongation (28% [placebo: 19%]; defined as >450 msec in males or >470 msec in females)
  Renal: Serum creatinine increased ≥10% (51%; occurred 5 days after initiation)
1% to 10%:
  Cardiovascular: Bradycardia (3%)
  Dermatologic: Allergic dermatitis (≤5%), dermatitis (≤5%), eczema (≤5%), pruritus (≤5%), rash (≤5%; described as generalized, macular, maculopapular, erythematous)
  Gastrointestinal: Diarrhea (9%), nausea (5%), abdominal pain (4%), dyspepsia (2%), vomiting (2%)
  Neuromuscular & skeletal: Weakness (7%)

Drug Interactions
  Metabolism/Transport Effects Inhibits P-glycoprotein
  Avoid Concomitant Use
  Avoid concomitant use of Dronedarone with any of the following: Artemether; Cyclo-SPORINE; CycloSPORINE (Systemic); CYP3A4 Inducers (Strong); CYP3A4 Inhibitors (Strong); Grapefruit Juice; Lumefantrine; Nilotinib; Pimozide; QTc-Prolonging Agents; QUEtiapine; QuiNINE; Silodosin; St Johns Wort; Tetrabenazine; Thioridazine; Tolvaptan; Topotecan; Toremifene; Vandetanib; Vemurafenib; Ziprasidone
  Increased Effect/Toxicity
  Dronedarone may increase the levels/effects of: Atorvastatin; Beta-Blockers; Budesonide (Systemic, Oral Inhalation); Calcium Channel Blockers (Nondihydropyridine); Colchicine; CYP2D6 Substrates; CYP3A4 Substrates; Dabigatran Etexilate; Digoxin; DOCEtaxel; Eplerenone; Everolimus; FentaNYL; Fesoterodine; Lovastatin; Lurasidone; P-Glycoprotein Substrates; Pimecrolimus; Pimozide; QTc-Prolonging Agents; QuiNINE; Red Yeast Rice; Rivaroxaban; Salmeterol; Saxagliptin; Silodosin; Simvastatin; Tamoxifen; Tetrabenazine; Thioridazine; Tolvaptan; Topotecan; Toremifene; Vandetanib; Vemurafenib; Vilazodone; Vitamin K Antagonists; Ziprasidone

  The levels/effects of Dronedarone may be increased by: Alfuzosin; Artemether; Calcium Channel Blockers (Nondihydropyridine); Chloroquine; Ciprofloxacin; Ciprofloxacin (Systemic); CycloSPORINE; CycloSPORINE (Systemic); CYP3A4 Inhibitors (Moderate); CYP3A4 Inhibitors (Strong); Digoxin; Eribulin; Fingolimod; Gadobutrol; Grapefruit Juice; Lumefantrine; Nilotinib; QTc-Prolonging Agents; QUEtiapine; QuiNINE
  Decreased Effect
  Dronedarone may decrease the levels/effects of: Codeine; TraMADol

  The levels/effects of Dronedarone may be decreased by: CYP3A4 Inducers (Strong); Deferasirox; St Johns Wort; Tocilizumab
Ethanol/Nutrition/Herb Interactions
  Food: Increases the rate and extent of absorption of dronedarone. Grapefruit juice increases bioavailability of dronedarone threefold; altered effects are possible; use should be avoided during therapy.
  Herb/Nutraceutical: St John's wort may decrease dronedarone levels. Avoid ephedra (may worsen arrhythmia). Avoid dong quai.
Stability Store at 25°C (77°F); excursions permitted to 15°C to 30°C (59°F to 86°F).
Mechanism of Action A noniodinated antiarrhythmic agent structurally related to amiodarone exhibiting properties of all 4 antiarrhythmic classes. Dronedarone inhibits sodium (I_{Na}) and potassium (I_{Kr}, I_{KS}, I_{k1}, and I_{k-ACh}) channels resulting in prolongation of the action potential and refractory period in myocardial tissue without reverse-use dependent effects; decreases AV conduction and sinus node function through inhibition of calcium (I_{Ca-L}) channels and beta$_1$-receptor blocking activity. Similar to amiodarone, dronedarone also inhibits alpha$_1$-receptor mediated increases in blood pressure.

Pharmacodynamics/Kinetics

Distribution: V_d: ~20 L/kg (based on a 70 kg patient)

Protein binding: >98%

Metabolism: Hepatic via CYP3A4 to active N-debutyl metabolite ($^1/_{10}$ to $^1/_3$ as potent as dronedarone) and other inactive metabolites

Bioavailability: Oral: Without food: 4%; With high-fat meal: 15%

Half-life elimination: 13-19 hours

Time to peak, plasma: 3-6 hours

Excretion: Feces (84% mainly as metabolites); urine (~6% mainly as metabolites)

Dosage

Geriatric & Adult Atrial fibrillation/atrial flutter: Oral: 400 mg twice daily

Renal Impairment No dosage adjustment necessary.

Hepatic Impairment No dosage adjustment necessary for moderate hepatic impairment. Contraindicated with severe hepatic impairment.

Administration Administer with morning and evening meal.

Monitoring Parameters Blood pressure, heart rate (ECG) and rhythm throughout therapy; assess patient for signs of lethargy, edema of the hands or feet; monitor serum electrolytes, especially potassium and magnesium; serum liver enzymes and bilirubin (periodically, especially during the first 6 months of therapy)

Patients with implantable cardiac devices: Monitor pacing or defibrillation thresholds with initiation of dronedarone and during treatment.

Special Geriatric Considerations Clinical studies, involving over 2000 patients 75 years of age and older, did not demonstrate any difference in safety and efficacy between younger adults and elderly. No dosage adjustments necessary for age.

Dosage Forms Excipient information presented when available (limited, particularly for generics); consult specific product labeling.

Tablet, oral:

Multaq®: 400 mg

Selected References

Hohnloser SH, Crijns HJ, van Eickels M, et al, "Effect of Dronedarone on Cardiovascular Events in Atrial Fibrillation," N Engl J Med, 2009, 360(7):668-78.

Kober L, Torp-Pedersen C, McMurray JJV, et al, "Increased Mortality After Dronedarone Therapy for Severe Heart Failure," N Engl J Med, 2008, 358(25):2678-87.

Singh BN, Connolly SJ, Crijns HJ, et al, "Dronedarone for Maintenance of Sinus Rhythm in Atrial Fibrillation or Flutter," N Engl J Med, 2007, 357(10):987-99.

Tschuppert Y, Buclin T, Rothuizen LE, et al, "Effect of Dronedarone on Renal Function in Healthy Subjects," Br J Clin Pharmacol, 2007, 64(6):785-91.

Wegener FT, Ehrlich JR, and Hohnloser SH, "Dronedarone: An Emerging Agent With Rhythm- and Rate-Controlling Effects," J Cardiovasc Electrolphysiol, 2006, 17(Suppl 2):17-20.

◆ **Dronedarone Hydrochloride** see Dronedarone on page 575

Droperidol (droe PER i dole)

Medication Safety Issues

Sound-alike/look-alike issues:

Droperidol may be confused with dronabinol

Brand Names: Canada Droperidol Injection, USP

Index Terms Dehydrobenzperidol

Generic Availability (U.S.) Yes

Pharmacologic Category Antiemetic; Antipsychotic Agent, Typical

Use Prevention and/or treatment of nausea and vomiting from surgical and diagnostic procedures

Contraindications Hypersensitivity to droperidol or any component of the formulation; known or suspected QT prolongation, including congenital long QT syndrome (prolonged QT_c is defined as >440 msec in males or >450 msec in females)

Warnings/Precautions May alter cardiac conduction. **[U.S. Boxed Warning]: Cases of QT prolongation and torsade de pointes, including some fatal cases, have been reported.** Use extreme caution in patients with bradycardia (<50 bpm), cardiac disease, concurrent MAO inhibitor therapy, Class I and Class III antiarrhythmics or other drugs known to prolong QT interval, and electrolyte disturbances (hypokalemia or hypomagnesemia), including concomitant drugs which may alter electrolytes (diuretics).

Use with caution in patients with seizures or severe liver disease. May be sedating, use with caution in disorders where CNS depression is a feature. Caution in patients with hemodynamic instability, predisposition to seizures, subcortical brain damage, pheochromocytoma or renal disease. Esophageal dysmotility and aspiration have been associated with antipsychotic use - use with caution in patients at risk of pneumonia (ie, Alzheimer's disease). Caution in breast cancer or other prolactin-dependent tumors (may elevate prolactin levels). May alter temperature regulation or mask toxicity of other drugs due to antiemetic effects. May cause orthostatic hypotension - use with caution in patients at risk of this effect or those who would tolerate transient hypotensive episodes (cerebrovascular disease, cardiovascular disease, or other medications which may predispose). Significant hypotension may occur.

May cause anticholinergic effects (confusion, agitation, constipation, xerostomia, blurred vision, urinary retention). Therefore, they should be used with caution in patients with decreased gastrointestinal motility, urinary retention, BPH, xerostomia, or visual problems. Conditions which also may be exacerbated by cholinergic blockade include narrow-angle glaucoma (screening is recommended) and worsening of myasthenia gravis. Relative to other neuroleptics, droperidol has a low potency of cholinergic blockade.

May cause extrapyramidal symptoms (EPS), including pseudoparkinsonism, acute dystonic reactions, akathisia, and tardive dyskinesia. Risk of dystonia (and possibly other EPS) may be greater with increased doses, use of conventional antipsychotics, males, and younger patients. May be associated with neuroleptic malignant syndrome (NMS). May mask toxicity of other drugs or conditions (eg, intestinal obstruction, Reye's syndrome, brain tumor) due to antiemetic effects. Use with caution in the elderly; reduce initial dose.

Adverse Reactions (Reflective of adult population; not specific for elderly) Frequency not defined.

Cardiovascular: Cardiac arrest, hypertension, hypotension (especially orthostatic), QT_c prolongation (dose dependent), tachycardia, torsade de pointes, ventricular tachycardia

Central nervous system: Anxiety, chills, depression (postoperative, transient), dizziness, drowsiness (postoperative) increased, dysphoria, extrapyramidal symptoms (akathisia, dystonia, oculogyric crisis), hallucinations (postoperative), hyperactivity, neuroleptic malignant syndrome (NMS) (rare), restlessness

Respiratory: Bronchospasm, laryngospasm

Miscellaneous: Anaphylaxis, shivering

Drug Interactions

Avoid Concomitant Use

Avoid concomitant use of Droperidol with any of the following: Artemether; Dronedarone; Lumefantrine; Metoclopramide; Nilotinib; Pimozide; QUEtiapine; QuiNINE; Tetrabenazine; Thioridazine; Toremifene; Vandetanib; Vemurafenib; Ziprasidone

Increased Effect/Toxicity

Droperidol may increase the levels/effects of: Alcohol (Ethyl); Anticholinergics; Anti-Parkinson's Agents (Dopamine Agonist); CNS Depressants; Dronedarone; Methylphenidate; Metoclopramide; Pimozide; QTc-Prolonging Agents; QuiNINE; Selective Serotonin Reuptake Inhibitors; Tetrabenazine; Thioridazine; Toremifene; Vandetanib; Vemurafenib; Ziprasidone

The levels/effects of Droperidol may be increased by: Acetylcholinesterase Inhibitors (Central); Alfuzosin; Artemether; Chloroquine; Ciprofloxacin; Ciprofloxacin (Systemic); Gadobutrol; HydrOXYzine; Lithium formulations; Lumefantrine; MAO Inhibitors; Methylphenidate; Metoclopramide; Nilotinib; Pramlintide; QUEtiapine; QuiNINE; Tetrabenazine

Decreased Effect

Droperidol may decrease the levels/effects of: Amphetamines; Quinagolide

The levels/effects of Droperidol may be decreased by: Anti-Parkinson's Agents (Dopamine Agonist); Lithium formulations

Stability Store at 20°C to 25°C (68° to 77°F); excursions permitted to 15°C to 30°C (59°F to 86°F). Protect from light. Solutions diluted in NS or D_5W are stable at room temperature for up to 7 days in PVC bags or glass bottles. Solutions diluted in LR are stable at room temperature for 24 hours in PVC bags and up to 7 days in glass bottles.

Mechanism of Action Droperidol is a butyrophenone antipsychotic; antiemetic effect is a result of blockade of dopamine stimulation of the chemoreceptor trigger zone. Other effects include alpha-adrenergic blockade, peripheral vascular dilation, and reduction of the pressor effect of epinephrine resulting in hypotension and decreased peripheral vascular resistance; may also reduce pulmonary artery pressure

Pharmacodynamics/Kinetics

Onset of action: 3-10 minutes

Peak effect: ~30 minutes

Duration: 2-4 hours, may extend to 12 hours

Absorption: I.M.: Rapid

Distribution: Crosses blood-brain barrier and placenta

Adults: ~1.5 L/kg

Protein binding: 85% to 90%

Metabolism: Hepatic, to *p*-fluorophenylacetic acid, benzimidazolone, *p*-hydroxypiperidine

Half-life elimination: ~2.3 hours

Excretion: Urine (75%, <1% as unchanged drug); feces (22%, 11% as unchanged drug)

Dosage

Geriatric & Adult Note: Titrate carefully to desired effect

Prevention of PONV: I.M., I.V.:

Manufacturer labeling: Maximum initial dose: 2.5 mg; additional doses of 1.25 mg may be administered with caution to achieve desired effect

Consensus guideline recommendations: 0.625-1.25 mg I.V. administered at the end of surgery (Gan, 2007)

Canadian labeling:

Prevention and treatment of PONV: I.V.: 0.625-1.25 mg 30 minutes prior to anticipated end of surgery, and then every 6 hours as needed for breakthrough PONV

Renal Impairment

U.S. labeling: Specific dosing recommendations are not provided; use with caution.

Canadian labeling: I.V.: 0.625 mg; additional dosing should be administered with caution.

Hepatic Impairment

U.S. labeling: Specific dosing recommendations are not provided; use with caution.

Canadian labeling: I.V.: 0.625 mg; additional dosing should be administered with caution.

Administration Administer I.M. or I.V.; according to the manufacturer, I.V. push administration should be slow (generally regarded as 2-5 minutes); however, many clinicians administer I.V. doses rapidly (over 30-60 seconds) in an effort to reduce the incidence of EPS. The effect, if any, of rapid administration on QT prolongation is unclear. For I.V. infusion, dilute in 50-100 mL NS or D_5W; ECG monitoring for 2-3 hours after administration is recommended regardless of rate of infusion.

Monitoring Parameters To identify QT prolongation, a 12-lead ECG prior to use is recommended; continued ECG monitoring for 2-3 hours following administration is recommended. Vital signs; serum magnesium and potassium; mental status, abnormal involuntary movement scale (AIMS); observe for dystonias, extrapyramidal side effects, and temperature changes

Pharmacotherapy Pearls Has good antiemetic effect as well as sedative and antianxiety effects

Special Geriatric Considerations Many elderly patients receive antipsychotic medications for inappropriate nonpsychotic behavior although the use of droperidol is seldom used for this indication. Since elderly frequently have cardiac disease which may result in QT prolongation, evaluation should be made prior to considering use of this agent.

Dosage Forms Excipient information presented when available (limited, particularly for generics); consult specific product labeling.

Injection, solution: 2.5 mg/mL (2 mL)

Injection, solution [preservative free]: 2.5 mg/mL (2 mL)

Selected References

Rabins PV, Blacker D, Rovner BW, et al, "Practice Guidelines for the Treatment of Patients With Alzheimer's Disease and Other Dementias," *Am J Psychiatry*, 2007, 164(12 Suppl):5-56. Available at http://www.psych.org/psych_pract/treatg/pg/prac_guide.cfm.

Schneider LS, Tariot PN, Dagerman KS, et al, "Effectiveness of Atypical Antipsychotic Drugs in Patients With Alzheimer's Disease," *N Engl J Med*, 2006, 355(15):1525-38.

Drospirenone and Estradiol (droh SPYE re none & es tra DYE ole)

Brand Names: U.S. Angeliq®

Brand Names: Canada Angeliq®

Index Terms E2 and DRSP; Estradiol and Drospirenone

Generic Availability (U.S.) No

Pharmacologic Category Estrogen and Progestin Combination

Use Treatment of moderate-to-severe vasomotor symptoms associated with menopause; treatment of vulvar and vaginal atrophy associated with menopause

Contraindications Hypersensitivity to drospirenone, estradiol, or any component of the formulation; undiagnosed abnormal vaginal bleeding; history of current thrombophlebitis or venous thromboembolic disorders (including DVT, PE); active or recent (within 1 year) arterial thromboembolic disease (eg, stroke, MI); carcinoma of the breast; estrogen-dependent tumor; hepatic or renal dysfunction or disease; adrenal insufficiency

Warnings/Precautions Drospirenone has antimineralocorticoid activity that may lead to hyperkalemia in patients with renal insufficiency, hepatic dysfunction, or adrenal insufficiency. Use caution with medications that may increase serum potassium.

Cardiovascular-related considerations: Estrogens with or without progestin should not be used to prevent coronary heart disease. Use caution with cardiovascular disease or dysfunction. May increase the risks of hypertension, myocardial infarction (MI), stroke, pulmonary emboli (PE), and deep vein thrombosis; incidence of these effects was shown to be significantly increased in postmenopausal women using conjugated equine estrogens (CEE) in combination with medroxyprogesterone acetate (MPA). Nonfatal MI, PE, and thrombophlebitis have also been reported in males taking high doses of CEE (eg, for prostate cancer). Estrogen compounds are generally associated with lipid effects such as increased HDL-cholesterol and decreased LDL-cholesterol. Triglycerides may also be increased; use with caution in patients with familial defects of lipoprotein metabolism. Whenever possible, estrogens should be discontinued at least 4 weeks prior to and for 2 weeks following elective surgery associated with an increased risk of thromboembolism or during periods of prolonged immobilization.

Neurological considerations: The risk of dementia may be increased in postmenopausal women; increased incidence was observed in women ≥65 years of age taking CEE alone or in combination with MPA.

Cancer-related considerations: Unopposed estrogens may increase the risk of endometrial carcinoma in postmenopausal women. Estrogens may exacerbate endometriosis. Malignant transformation of residual endometrial implants has been reported posthysterectomy with estrogen only therapy. Estrogens may increase the risk of breast cancer. An increased risk of invasive breast cancer was observed in postmenopausal women using CEE in combination with MPA; a smaller increase in risk was seen with estrogen therapy alone in observational studies. An increase in abnormal mammograms has also been reported with estrogen and progestin therapy. Estrogen use may lead to severe hypercalcemia in patients with breast cancer and bone metastases; discontinue estrogen if hypercalcemia occurs. Postmenopausal estrogen therapy and combined estrogen/progesterone therapy may increase the risk of ovarian cancer; however, the absolute risk to an individual woman is small. Although results from various studies are not consistent, risk does not appear to be significantly associated with the duration, route, or dose of therapy. In one study, the risk decreased after 2 years following discontinuation of therapy.

Estrogens may cause retinal vascular thrombosis; discontinue permanently if papilledema or retinal vascular lesions are observed on examination. Use with caution in patients with diseases which may be exacerbated by fluid retention, including asthma, epilepsy, migraine, diabetes, or renal dysfunction. Use with caution in patients with a history of severe hypocalcemia, SLE, hepatic hemangiomas, porphyria, endometriosis, and gallbladder disease. Use caution with history of cholestatic jaundice associated with past estrogen use.

Before prescribing estrogen therapy to postmenopausal women, the risks and benefits must be weighed for each patient. Women should be informed of these risks and benefits, as well as possible effects of progestin when added to estrogen therapy. Estrogens with or without progestin should be used for shortest duration possible consistent with treatment goals. Conduct periodic risk:benefit assessments. When used solely for the treatment of vulvar and vaginal atrophy, topical vaginal products should be considered. Not for use prior to menopause.

Adverse Reactions (Reflective of adult population; not specific for elderly)

>10%:
  Endocrine & metabolic: Breast pain (19%)
  Gastrointestinal: Abdominal pain (11%)
  Respiratory: Upper respiratory tract infection (19%)
1% to 10%:
  Cardiovascular: Peripheral edema (2%)
  Central nervous system: Headache (10%), pain (8%)
  Gastrointestinal: Abdomen enlarged (7%)
  Genitourinary: Vaginal hemorrhage (9%), endometrial disorder (2%), leukorrhea (1%)
  Neuromuscular & skeletal: Back pain (7%)
  Respiratory: Flu-like syndrome (7%), sinusitis (5%)
Additional adverse effects reported with estrogens and/or progestins: Abdominal cramps, acne, abnormal uterine bleeding, aggravation of porphyria, amenorrhea, anaphylactoid reactions, anaphylaxis, antifactor Xa decreased, antithrombin III decreased, appetite changes, bloating, breast enlargement, breast tenderness, cerebral embolism, cerebral thrombosis, chloasma, cholestatic jaundice, cholecystitis, cholelithiasis, chorea, contact lens intolerance, corneal curvature steepening, cystitis-like syndrome, decreased carbohydrate tolerance, depression, dementia, dizziness, dysmenorrhea; factors VII, VIII, IX, X, XII, VII-X complex, and II-VII-X complex increased; endometrial hyperplasia, erythema multiforme, erythema nodosum, galactorrhea, hemorrhagic eruption, fatigue, fibrinogen increased, impaired glucose tolerance, HDL-cholesterol increased, hirsutism, hypertension, gallbladder disease, insomnia, LDL-cholesterol decreased, libido changes, melasma, migraine, mood disturbances, nausea, nervousness, optic neuritis, pancreatitis, platelet aggregability and

platelet count increased, premenstrual-like syndrome, PT and PTT accelerated, pulmonary embolism, pyrexia, retinal thrombosis, scalp hair loss, somnolence, stroke, thrombophlebitis, thyroid-binding globulin increased, total thyroid hormone (T_4) increased, triglycerides increased, urticaria, uterine leiomyomata size increased, vaginal candidiasis, vomiting, weight gain/loss

Drug Interactions

Metabolism/Transport Effects

Drospirenone: **Substrate** of CYP3A4 (minor); **Inhibits** CYP1A2 (weak), 2C9 (weak), 2C19 (weak), 3A4 (weak)

Estradiol: **Substrate** of CYP1A2 (major), CYP2A6 (minor), CYP2B6 (minor), CYP2C9 (minor), CYP2C19 (minor), CYP2D6 (minor), CYP2E1 (minor), CYP3A4 (major), P-glycoprotein; **Inhibits** CYP1A2 (weak), 2C8 (weak); **Induces** CYP3A4 (weak)

Avoid Concomitant Use

Avoid concomitant use of Drospirenone and Estradiol with any of the following: Anastrozole; Boceprevir; Griseofulvin; Tacrolimus

Increased Effect/Toxicity

Drospirenone and Estradiol may increase the levels/effects of: ACE Inhibitors; Amifostine; Ammonium Chloride; Antihypertensives; Benzodiazepines (metabolized by oxidation); Cardiac Glycosides; Corticosteroids (Systemic); Hypotensive Agents; Potassium-Sparing Diuretics; RiTUXimab; ROPINIRole; Selegiline; Sodium Phosphates; Tacrolimus; Tipranavir; Tranexamic Acid; Voriconazole

The levels/effects of Drospirenone and Estradiol may be increased by: Alfuzosin; Angiotensin II Receptor Blockers; Ascorbic Acid; Boceprevir; Conivaptan; Diazoxide; Eplerenone; Herbs (Estrogenic Properties); Herbs (Hypotensive Properties); Herbs (Progestogenic Properties); MAO Inhibitors; Nonsteroidal Anti-Inflammatory Agents; Pentoxifylline; P-Glycoprotein Inhibitors; Phosphodiesterase 5 Inhibitors; Potassium Salts; Prostacyclin Analogues; Tolvaptan; Voriconazole

Decreased Effect

Drospirenone and Estradiol may decrease the levels/effects of: Anastrozole; Cardiac Glycosides; Chenodiol; QuiNIDine; Saxagliptin; Somatropin; Thyroid Products; Ursodiol; Vitamin K Antagonists

The levels/effects of Drospirenone and Estradiol may be decreased by: Acitretin; Aminoglutethimide; Aprepitant; Artemether; Barbiturates; Bexarotene; Bexarotene (Systemic); Bile Acid Sequestrants; Bosentan; CarBAMazepine; CYP1A2 Inducers (Strong); CYP3A4 Inducers (Strong); Cyproterone; Deferasirox; Felbamate; Fosaprepitant; Fosphenytoin; Griseofulvin; Herbs (Hypertensive Properties); LamoTRIgine; Methylphenidate; Mycophenolate; Nonsteroidal Anti-Inflammatory Agents; OXcarbazepine; Peginterferon Alfa-2b; P-Glycoprotein Inducers; Phenytoin; Retinoic Acid Derivatives; Rifamycin Derivatives; St Johns Wort; Telaprevir; Tipranavir; Tocilizumab; Topiramate; Yohimbine

Ethanol/Nutrition/Herb Interactions Ethanol: Avoid ethanol (routine use increases estrogen level and risk of breast cancer). Ethanol may also increase the risk of osteoporosis.

Stability Store at controlled room temperature of 15°C to 30°C (59°F to 86°F).

Mechanism of Action

Drospirenone is a synthetic progestin and spironolactone analog with antimineralocorticoid and antiandrogenic activity. Counteracts estrogen effects causing endometrial thinning.

Estrogens are responsible for the development and maintenance of the female reproductive system and secondary sexual characteristics. Estradiol is the principal intracellular human estrogen and is more potent than estrone and estriol at the receptor level; it is the primary estrogen secreted prior to menopause. Following menopause, estrone and estrone sulfate are more highly produced. Estrogens modulate the pituitary secretion of gonadotropins, luteinizing hormone, and follicle-stimulating hormone through a negative feedback system; estrogen replacement reduces elevated levels of these hormones in postmenopausal women.

Pharmacodynamics/Kinetics

Distribution: Drospirenone: 4.2 L/kg

Protein binding:

Drospirenone: 97%; does not bind to sex hormone binding globulin or corticosteroid binding globulin

Estradiol: 37% bound to sex hormone binding globulin; 61% bound to albumin

Metabolism: Hepatic

Drospirenone forms two metabolites (inactive)

Estradiol: Converted to estrone and estriol; also undergoes enterohepatic recirculation; estrone sulfite is the main metabolite in postmenopausal women

Bioavailability: Drospirenone: 76% to 85%

Time to peak, plasma: Drospirenone: 1 hour; Estradiol: 6-8 hours

◀ **Dosage**
   Geriatric & Adult
     Moderate-to-severe vasomotor symptoms associated with menopause: Oral: One tablet daily; re-evaluate patients at 3- and 6-month intervals to determine if treatment is still necessary.
     Atrophic vaginitis in females with an intact uterus: Oral: One tablet daily; re-evaluate patients at 3- and 6-month intervals to determine if treatment is still necessary.
     Note: The lowest dose of estrogen/progestin that will control symptoms should be used; medication should be discontinued as soon as possible.
   Renal Impairment Use in contraindicated.
   Hepatic Impairment Use in contraindicated.
Monitoring Parameters Yearly physical examination that includes blood pressure and Papanicolaou smear, breast exam, mammogram. Monitor for signs of endometrial cancer. Adequate diagnostic measures, including endometrial sampling, if indicated, should be performed to rule out malignancy in all cases of undiagnosed abnormal vaginal bleeding. Monitor for loss of vision, sudden onset of proptosis, diplopia, migraine; signs and symptoms of thromboembolic disorders; glycemic control in patients with diabetes; lipid profiles in patients being treated for hyperlipidemias; thyroid function in patients on thyroid hormone replacement therapy.
Menopausal symptoms: Assess need for therapy at 3- to 6-month intervals.
Test Interactions Pathologist should be advised of estrogen/progesterone therapy when specimens are submitted. Reduced response to metyrapone test.
Special Geriatric Considerations Before prescribing estrogen therapy to postmenopausal women, the risks and benefits must be weighed for each patient. Women should be informed of these risks and benefits, as well as possible side effects and the return of menstrual bleeding (when cycled with a progestin), and be involved in the decision to prescribe. A higher incidence of stroke and invasive breast cancer was observed in women >75 years in a WHI substudy. Oral therapy may be more convenient for vaginal atrophy and urinary incontinence.
Dosage Forms Excipient information presented when available (limited, particularly for generics); consult specific product labeling.
Tablet:
   Angeliq®: Drospirenone 0.5 mg and estradiol 1 mg
Selected References
Rossouw JE, Anderson GL, Prentice RL, et al, "Risks and Benefits of Estrogen Plus Progestin in Healthy Postmenopausal Women: Principle Results From the Women's Health Initiative Randomized Controlled Trial,"- *JAMA*, 2002, 288(3):321-33.
Shumaker SA, Legault C, Rapp SR, et al, "WHIMS Investigators. Estrogen Plus Progestin and the Incidence of Dementia and Mild Cognitive Impairment in Postmenopausal Women: The Women's Health Initiative Memory Study: A Randomized Controlled Trial," *JAMA*, 2003, 289(20):2651-62.
Wassertheil-Smoller S, Hendrix S, Limacher M, et al, "Effect of Estrogen Plus Progestin on Stroke in Postmenopausal Women: The Women's Health Initiative: A Randomized Trial," *JAMA*, 2003, 289:2673-84.

◆ **Droxia®** *see* Hydroxyurea *on page 897*
◆ **Dr. Scholl's® Callus Removers [OTC]** *see* Salicylic Acid *on page 1648*
◆ **Dr. Scholl's® Clear Away® One Step Wart Remover [OTC]** *see* Salicylic Acid *on page 1648*
◆ **Dr. Scholl's® Clear Away® Plantar Wart Remover For Feet [OTC]** *see* Salicylic Acid *on page 1648*
◆ **Dr. Scholl's® Clear Away® Wart Remover [OTC]** *see* Salicylic Acid *on page 1648*
◆ **Dr. Scholl's® Clear Away® Wart Remover Fast-Acting [OTC]** *see* Salicylic Acid *on page 1648*
◆ **Dr. Scholl's® Clear Away® Wart Remover Invisible Strips [OTC]** *see* Salicylic Acid *on page 1648*
◆ **Dr. Scholl's® Corn/Callus Remover [OTC]** *see* Salicylic Acid *on page 1648*
◆ **Dr. Scholl's® Corn Removers [OTC]** *see* Salicylic Acid *on page 1648*
◆ **Dr. Scholl's® Extra-Thick Callus Removers [OTC]** *see* Salicylic Acid *on page 1648*
◆ **Dr. Scholl's® Extra Thick Corn Removers [OTC]** *see* Salicylic Acid *on page 1648*
◆ **Dr. Scholl's® For Her Corn Removers [OTC]** *see* Salicylic Acid *on page 1648*
◆ **Dr. Scholl's® OneStep Callus Removers [OTC]** *see* Salicylic Acid *on page 1648*
◆ **Dr. Scholl's® OneStep Corn Removers [OTC]** *see* Salicylic Acid *on page 1648*
◆ **Dr. Scholl's® Small Corn Removers [OTC]** *see* Salicylic Acid *on page 1648*
◆ **Dr. Scholl's® Ultra-Thin Corn Removers [OTC]** *see* Salicylic Acid *on page 1648*
◆ **DSCG** *see* Cromolyn (Nasal) *on page 422*
◆ **DSCG** *see* Cromolyn (Ophthalmic) *on page 422*
◆ **DSCG** *see* Cromolyn (Systemic, Oral Inhalation) *on page 420*
◆ **DSS** *see* Docusate *on page 547*
◆ **DSS® [OTC]** *see* Docusate *on page 547*
◆ **DT** *see* Diphtheria and Tetanus Toxoids *on page 525*
◆ **DTaP** *see* Diphtheria and Tetanus Toxoids, and Acellular Pertussis Vaccine *on page 531*

- **DTaP-HepB-IPV-Hib** *see* Diphtheria and Tetanus Toxoids, Acellular Pertussis, Hepatitis B (Recombinant), Poliovirus (Inactivated), and *Haemophilus influenzae* B Conjugate (Adsorbed) Vaccine *on page 530*
- **DTaP-IPV** *see* Diphtheria and Tetanus Toxoids, Acellular Pertussis, and Poliovirus Vaccine *on page 528*
- **D-Trp(6)-LHRH** *see* Triptorelin *on page 1872*
- **Duetact™** *see* Pioglitazone and Glimepiride *on page 1460*
- **Dulcolax® [OTC]** *see* Bisacodyl *on page 205*
- **Dulcolax® [OTC]** *see* Docusate *on page 547*
- **Dulcolax Balance® [OTC]** *see* Polyethylene Glycol 3350 *on page 1480*
- **Dulcolax® Stool Softener [OTC]** *see* Docusate *on page 547*
- **Dulera®** *see* Mometasone and Formoterol *on page 1234*
- **Dull-C® [OTC]** *see* Ascorbic Acid *on page 149*

DULoxetine (doo LOX e teen)

Related Information
Antidepressant Agents *on page 1991*
Medication Safety Issues
Sound-alike/look-alike issues:
Cymbalta® may be confused with Symbyax®
DULoxetine may be confused with FLUoxetine
Brand Names: U.S. Cymbalta®
Brand Names: Canada Cymbalta®
Index Terms (+)-(S)-N-Methyl-γ-(1-naphthyloxy)-2-thiophenepropylamine Hydrochloride; Duloxetine Hydrochloride; LY248686
Generic Availability (U.S.) No
Pharmacologic Category Antidepressant, Serotonin/Norepinephrine Reuptake Inhibitor
Use Acute and maintenance treatment of major depressive disorder (MDD); treatment of generalized anxiety disorder (GAD); management of diabetic peripheral neuropathic pain (DPNP); management of fibromyalgia (FM); chronic musculoskeletal pain (eg, chronic low back pain, osteoarthritis)
Unlabeled/Investigational Use Treatment of stress incontinence
Medication Guide Available Yes
Contraindications Concomitant use or within 2 weeks of MAO inhibitors; uncontrolled narrow-angle glaucoma
  Note: MAO inhibitor therapy must be stopped for 14 days before duloxetine is initiated. Treatment with MAO inhibitors should not be initiated until 5 days after the discontinuation of duloxetine.

Canadian labeling: Additional contraindications (not in U.S. labeling): Hypersensitivity to duloxetine or any component of the formulation; hepatic impairment; severe renal impairment (eg, Cl_{cr} <30 mL/minute) or end-stage renal disease (ESRD); concomitant use with thioridazine or with CYP1A2 inhibitors
Warnings/Precautions [U.S. Boxed Warning]: Antidepressants increase the risk of suicidal thinking and behavior in children, adolescents, and young adults (18-24 years of age) with major depressive disorder (MDD) and other psychiatric disorders; consider risk prior to prescribing. Short-term studies did not show an increased risk in patients >24 years of age and showed a decreased risk in patients ≥65 years. Closely monitor for clinical worsening, suicidality, or unusual changes in behavior; the patient's family or caregiver should be instructed to closely observe the patient and communicate condition with healthcare provider. A medication guide concerning the use of antidepressants in children and teenagers should be dispensed with each prescription. **Duloxetine is not FDA approved for use in children.**

The possibility of a suicide attempt is inherent in major depression and may persist until remission occurs. Patients treated with antidepressants should be observed for clinical worsening and suicidality, especially during the initial (generally first 1-2 months) few months of a course of drug therapy, or at times of dose changes, either increases or decreases. Use caution in high-risk patients. Worsening depression and severe abrupt suicidality that are not part of the presenting symptoms may require discontinuation or modification of drug therapy. The patient's family or caregiver should be alerted to monitor patients for the emergence of suicidality and associated behaviors (such as agitation, irritability, hostility, impulsivity, and hypomania) and call healthcare provider.

May worsen psychosis in some patients or precipitate a shift to mania or hypomania in patients with bipolar disorder. Patients presenting with depressive symptoms should be screened for bipolar disorder. Monotherapy in patients with bipolar disorder should be avoided. **Duloxetine is not FDA approved for the treatment of bipolar depression.**

May cause orthostatic hypotension/syncope at therapeutic doses especially within the first week of therapy and after dose increases. Monitor blood pressure with initiation of therapy, dose increases (especially in patients receiving >60 mg/day), or with concomitant use of vasodilators, CYP2D6 inhibitors/substrates, or CYP1A2 inhibitors. Use caution in patients with hypertension. May increase blood pressure. Rare cases of hypertensive crisis have been reported in patients with pre-existing hypertension; evaluate blood pressure prior to initiating therapy and periodically thereafter; consider dose reduction or gradual discontinuation of therapy in individuals with sustained hypertension during therapy.

Modest increases in serum glucose and hemoglobin A_{1c} (Hb A_{1c}) levels have been observed in some diabetic patients receiving duloxetine therapy for diabetic peripheral neuropathic pain (DPNP). Duloxetine may cause increased urinary resistance; advise patient to report symptoms of urinary hesitation/difficulty. Has a low potential to impair cognitive or motor performance. Use caution with a previous seizure disorder or condition predisposing to seizures such as brain damage or alcoholism. Avoid use in patients with substantial ethanol intake, evidence of chronic liver disease, or hepatic impairment (contraindicated in Canadian labeling). Rare cases of hepatic failure (including fatalities) have been reported with use. Hepatitis with abdominal pain, hepatomegaly, elevated transaminase levels >20 times the upper limit of normal (ULN) with and without jaundice have all been observed. Discontinue therapy with the presentation of jaundice or other signs of hepatic dysfunction and do not reinitiate therapy unless another source or cause is identified. Use caution in patients with impaired gastric motility (eg, some diabetics) may affect stability of the capsule's enteric coating.

May cause hyponatremia/SIADH (elderly at increased risk); volume depletion (diuretics may increase risk). Use with caution in patients with controlled narrow angle glaucoma. May cause or exacerbate sexual dysfunction. Use caution in patients with renal impairment (contraindicated in Canadian labeling for severe renal impairment or ESRD). Use caution with concomitant CNS depressants. May impair platelet aggregation; use caution with concomitant use of NSAIDs, ASA, or other drugs that affect coagulation; the risk of bleeding may be potentiated.

Serotonin syndrome and neuroleptic malignant syndrome (NMS)-like reactions have occurred with serotonin/norepinephrine reuptake inhibitors (SNRIs) and selective serotonin reuptake inhibitors (SSRIs) when used alone, and particularly when used in combination with serotonergic agents (eg, triptans) or antidopaminergic agents (eg, antipsychotics). Concurrent use with MAO inhibitors is contraindicated. Use caution during concurrent therapy with triptans and drugs which lower the seizure threshold; concurrent use of serotonin precursors (eg, tryptophan) is not recommended. To discontinue therapy with duloxetine, gradually taper dose. If intolerable symptoms occur following a decrease in dosage or upon discontinuation of therapy, then resuming the previous dose with a more gradual taper should be considered. May increase the risks associated with electroconvulsive therapy. Consider discontinuing, when possible, prior to elective surgery. Formulation contains sucrose; patients with fructose intolerance, glucose-galactose malabsorption, or sucrose-isomaltase deficiency should avoid use.

Adverse Reactions (Reflective of adult population; not specific for elderly)

>10%:

Central nervous system: Headache (13% to 14%), somnolence (10% to 12%; dose related), fatigue (10 to 11%)

Gastrointestinal: Nausea (23% to 25%), xerostomia (11% to 15%; dose related)

1% to 10%:

Cardiovascular: Palpitation (1% to 2%)

Central nervous system: Dizziness (10%), insomnia (10%; dose related), agitation (3% to 5%), anxiety (3%), dreams abnormal (1% to 2%), yawning (1% to 2%), hypoesthesia (≥1%), lethargy (≥1%), vertigo (≥1%), chills (1%), sleep disorder (1%)

Dermatologic: Hyperhidrosis (6% to 7%)

Endocrine & metabolic: Libido decreased (2% to 4%), hot flushes (1% to 3%), orgasm abnormality (1% to 3%)

Gastrointestinal: Constipation (10%; dose related), diarrhea (9% to 10%), appetite decreased (7% to 9%; dose related), abdominal pain (4% to 6%), vomiting (3% to 5%), dyspepsia (2%), weight loss (2%), flatulence (≥1%), taste abnormal (≥1%), weight gain (≥1%)

Genitourinary: Erectile dysfunction (4% to 5%), ejaculation delayed (3%; dose related), ejaculatory dysfunction (2%)

Hepatic: ALT >3x ULN (1%)

Neuromuscular & skeletal: Muscle spasms (3%), tremor (2% to 3%; dose related), musculoskeletal pain (≥1%), paresthesia (≥1%), rigors (≥1%)

Ocular: Blurred vision (1% to 3%)
Respiratory: Nasopharyngitis (5%), cough (3%)
Miscellaneous: Influenza (3%)

Drug Interactions

Metabolism/Transport Effects Substrate (major) of CYP1A2, 2D6; **inhibits** CYP2D6 (moderate)

Avoid Concomitant Use

Avoid concomitant use of DULoxetine with any of the following: Iobenguane I 123; MAO Inhibitors; Methylene Blue; Sibutramine; Thioridazine

Increased Effect/Toxicity

DULoxetine may increase the levels/effects of: Alpha-/Beta-Agonists; Aspirin; CYP2D6 Substrates; Fesoterodine; Methylene Blue; Nebivolol; NSAID (Nonselective); Serotonin Modulators; Tamoxifen; Thioridazine; Tricyclic Antidepressants

The levels/effects of DULoxetine may be increased by: Abiraterone Acetate; Alcohol (Ethyl); CYP1A2 Inhibitors (Moderate); CYP1A2 Inhibitors (Strong); CYP2D6 Inhibitors (Moderate); CYP2D6 Inhibitors (Strong); Darunavir; Deferasirox; FluvoxaMINE; MAO Inhibitors; PARoxetine; Sibutramine

Decreased Effect

DULoxetine may decrease the levels/effects of: Alpha2-Agonists; Codeine; Iobenguane I 123

The levels/effects of DULoxetine may be decreased by: CYP1A2 Inducers (Strong); Cyproterone; Peginterferon Alfa-2b

Ethanol/Nutrition/Herb Interactions

Ethanol: Ethanol may increase hepatotoxic potential of duloxetine. Ethanol may also increase CNS depression; monitor for increased effects with coadministration. Caution patients about effects.

Herb/Nutraceutical: Avoid valerian, St John's wort, SAMe, kava kava, and gotu kola (may increase CNS depression).

Stability Store at 25°C (77°F); excursions permitted to 15°C to 30°C (59°F to 86°F)

Mechanism of Action Duloxetine is a potent inhibitor of neuronal serotonin and norepinephrine reuptake and a weak inhibitor of dopamine reuptake. Duloxetine has no significant activity for muscarinic cholinergic, H_1-histaminergic, or alpha$_2$-adrenergic receptors. Duloxetine does not possess MAO-inhibitory activity.

Pharmacodynamics/Kinetics

Absorption: Well absorbed, 2-hour delay in absorption after ingestion; food decreases extent of absorption ~10% (no effect on C_{max})

Distribution: 1640 L (range: 701-3800 L)

Protein binding: >90%; primarily to albumin and α_1-acid glycoprotein

Metabolism: Hepatic, via CYP1A2 and CYP2D6; forms multiple metabolites (inactive)

Half-life elimination: 12 hours (range: 8-17 hours)

Time to peak: 6 hours; 10 hours when ingested with food

Excretion: Urine (~70%; <1% of total dose as unchanged drug); feces (~20%)

Dosage

Geriatric

Major depressive disorder: Oral: Manufacturer does not recommend specific dosage adjustment. Conservatively, may initiate at a dose of 20 mg 1-2 times/day; increase to 40-60 mg/day as a single daily dose or in divided doses **or** initiate therapy at 30 mg/day for 1 week then increase to 60 mg/day as tolerated.

Other indications: Refer to adult dosing.

Adult

Major depressive disorder: Oral: Initial: 40-60 mg/day; dose may be divided (ie, 20 or 30 mg twice daily) or given as a single daily dose of 60 mg; maintenance: 60 mg once daily; for doses >60 mg/day, titrate dose in increments of 30 mg/day over 1 week as tolerated to a maximum dose: 120 mg/day. **Note:** Doses >60 mg/day have not been demonstrated to be more effective.

Diabetic neuropathy: Oral: 60 mg once daily; lower initial doses may be considered in patients where tolerability is a concern and/or renal impairment is present. **Note:** Doses up to 120 mg/day administered in clinical trials offered no additional benefit and were less well tolerated than dose of 60 mg/day.

Fibromyalgia: Oral: 30 mg once daily for 1 week, then increase to 60 mg once daily as tolerated. **Note:** Doses up to 120 mg/day administered in clinical trials offered no additional benefit and were less well tolerated than dose of 60 mg/day.

Generalized anxiety disorder: Oral: Initial: 30-60 mg/day as a single daily dose; patients initiated at 30 mg/day should be titrated to 60 mg/day after 1 week; maximum dose: 120 mg/day. **Note:** Doses >60 mg/day have not been demonstrated to be more effective than 60 mg/day.

◄ **Chronic musculoskeletal pain:** Oral: 30 mg once daily for 1 week, then increase to 60 mg once daily as tolerated

Stress incontinence (unlabeled use): Oral: 40 mg twice daily (Dmochowski, 2003)

Note: Upon discontinuation of duloxetine therapy, gradually taper dose. If intolerable symptoms occur following a dose reduction, consider resuming the previously prescribed dose and/or decrease dose at a more gradual rate.

Renal Impairment Not recommended for use in Cl_{cr} <30 mL/minute or ESRD (contraindicated in Canadian labeling). In mild-moderate impairment, lower initial doses may be considered with titration guided by response and tolerability.

Hepatic Impairment Not recommended for use in hepatic impairment (contraindicated in Canadian labeling).

Administration Capsule should be swallowed whole; do not crush or chew. Although the manufacturer does not recommend opening the capsule to facilitate administration; the contents of capsule may be sprinkled on applesauce or in apple juice and swallowed (without chewing) immediately. Do not sprinkle contents on chocolate pudding (Wells, 2008). Administer without regard to meals.

Monitoring Parameters Blood pressure should be checked prior to initiating therapy and then regularly monitored, especially in patients with a high baseline blood pressure; mental status for depression, suicidal ideation (especially at the beginning of therapy or when doses are increased or decreased), anxiety, social functioning, mania, panic attacks; glucose levels and Hb A_{1c} levels in diabetic patients, creatinine, BUN, transaminases

For musculoskeletal pain: Pain relief

Special Geriatric Considerations In an 8-week study of elderly patients with a history of recurrent major depressive disorder, improvements in verbal learning and memory, and depression response and remission rates were significantly greater in subjects randomized to duloxetine 60 mg per day compared to placebo. Duloxetine was well tolerated by older patients in clinical trials who accounted for nearly one-third of subjects. Response rate did not differ between younger and older subjects. No dose adjustment is necessary for age alone; adjust dose for renal function in the elderly. Higher doses are generally required for treatment of general anxiety disorder, neuropathic pain and stress urinary incontinence (unlabeled use). The elderly are more prone to SSRI/SNRI-induced hyponatremia.

Dosage Forms Excipient information presented when available (limited, particularly for generics); consult specific product labeling.

Capsule, delayed release, enteric coated pellets, oral:

Cymbalta®: 20 mg, 30 mg, 60 mg

Selected References

Dmochowski RR, Miklos JR, Norton PA, et al, "Duloxetine Versus Placebo for the Treatment of North American Women With Stress Urinary Incontinence," *J Urol*, 2003, 170(4 Pt 1):1259-63.

Millard RJ, Moore K, Rencken R, et al, "Duloxetine vs Placebo in the Treatment of Stress Urinary Incontinence: A Four-Continent Randomized Clinical Trial," *BJU Int*, 2004, 93(3):311-8.

Raskin J, Wiltse CG, Siegal A, et al, "Efficacy of Duloxetine on Cognition, Depression, and Pain in Elderly Patients With Major Depressive Disorder: An 8-Week, Double-Blind, Placebo-Controlled Trial," *Am J Psychiatry*, 2007, 164 (6):900-9.

van Kerrebroeck P, Abrams P, Lange R, et al, "Duloxetine Versus Placebo in the Treatment of European and Canadian Women With Stress Urinary Incontinence," *BJOG*, 2004, 111(3):249-57.

◆ **Duloxetine Hydrochloride** *see* DULoxetine *on page 583*
◆ **DuoFilm® [OTC]** *see* Salicylic Acid *on page 1648*
◆ **DuoNeb®** *see* Ipratropium and Albuterol *on page 975*
◆ **DuP 753** *see* Losartan *on page 1092*
◆ **Duraclon®** *see* CloNIDine *on page 388*
◆ **Duragesic®** *see* FentaNYL *on page 709*
◆ **Duramist Plus [OTC]** *see* Oxymetazoline (Nasal) *on page 1374*
◆ **Duramorph** *see* Morphine (Systemic) *on page 1238*
◆ **Durasal™** *see* Salicylic Acid *on page 1648*
◆ **Durezol®** *see* Difluprednate *on page 507*
◆ **Duricef** *see* Cefadroxil *on page 289*

Dutasteride (doo TAS teer ide)

Brand Names: U.S. Avodart®
Brand Names: Canada Avodart®
Generic Availability (U.S.) No
Pharmacologic Category 5 Alpha-Reductase Inhibitor
Use Treatment of symptomatic benign prostatic hyperplasia (BPH) as monotherapy or combination therapy with tamsulosin
Unlabeled/Investigational Use Treatment of male pattern baldness

Contraindications Hypersensitivity to dutasteride, other 5α-reductase inhibitors (eg, finasteride), or any component of the formulation; not indicated for use in women; pregnant women or women trying to conceive should not handle the product

Warnings/Precautions Hazardous agent - use appropriate precautions for handling and disposal. Pregnant women or women trying to conceive should not handle the product; active ingredient can be absorbed through the skin and may negatively impact fetal development. Urological diseases, including prostate cancer, and/or obstructive uropathy should be ruled out before initiating. Avoid donating blood during or for 6 months following treatment due to risk of administration to a pregnant female transfusion recipient. Use caution in hepatic impairment and with concurrent use of potent, chronic CYP3A4 inhibitors. Reduces PSA by ~50% within 3-6 months of use; if following serial PSAs, re-establish a new baseline ≥3 months after treatment initiation and monitor PSA periodically thereafter. If interpreting an isolated PSA value in a patient treated for ≥3 months, then double the PSA value for comparison to a normal PSA value in an untreated man. Failure to demonstrate a meaningful PSA decrease (<50%) or a PSA increase while on this medication may be associated with an increased risk for prostate cancer (NCCN Prostate Cancer Early Detection Guidelines, v.1.2011). Patients on a 5-alpha-reductase inhibitor (5-ARI) with any increase in PSA levels, even if within normal limits, should be evaluated; may indicate presence of prostate cancer. When compared to placebo, 5-ARIs have been shown to reduce the overall incidence of prostate cancer, although an increase in the incidence of high-grade prostate cancers has been observed; 5-ARIs are not FDA-approved for the prevention of prostate cancer.

Adverse Reactions (Reflective of adult population; not specific for elderly)
1% to 10%: Endocrine & metabolic: Impotence (1% to 5%), libido decreased (≤3%), ejaculation disorders (≤1%), gynecomastia (including breast tenderness, breast enlargement; ≤1%)
Note: Frequency of adverse events (except gynecomastia) tends to decrease with continued use (>6 months).

Drug Interactions
Metabolism/Transport Effects Substrate of CYP3A4 (minor)
Avoid Concomitant Use There are no known interactions where it is recommended to avoid concomitant use.
Increased Effect/Toxicity
The levels/effects of Dutasteride may be increased by: CYP3A4 Inhibitors (Strong)
Decreased Effect
The levels/effects of Dutasteride may be decreased by: Tocilizumab

Ethanol/Nutrition/Herb Interactions
Ethanol: No effect or interaction noted.
Food: Maximum serum concentrations reduced by 10% to 15% when taken with food; not clinically significant.
Herb/Nutraceutical: St John's wort may decrease dutasteride levels. Avoid saw palmetto (concurrent use has not been adequately studied).

Stability Store at controlled room temperature of 25°C (77°F); excursions permitted to 15°C to 30°C (59°F to 86°F).

Mechanism of Action Dutasteride is a 4-azo analog of testosterone and is a competitive, selective inhibitor of both reproductive tissues (type 2) and skin and hepatic (type 1) 5α-reductase. This results in inhibition of the conversion of testosterone to dihydrotestosterone and markedly suppresses serum dihydrotestosterone levels.

Pharmacodynamics/Kinetics
Absorption: Absorbed via skin when handling capsules
Distribution: V_d: 300-500 L, ~12% of serum concentrations partitioned into semen
Protein binding: 99% to albumin; ~97% to $α_1$-acid glycoprotein; >96% to semen protein
Metabolism: Hepatic via CYP3A4 isoenzyme; forms metabolites: 6-hydroxydutasteride has activity similar to parent compound, 4'-hydroxydutasteride and 1,2-dihydrodutasteride are much less potent than parent *in vitro*
Bioavailability: ~60% (range: 40% to 94%)
Half-life elimination: Terminal: ~5 weeks
Time to peak: 2-3 hours
Excretion: Feces (40% as metabolites, ~5% as unchanged drug); urine (<1% as unchanged drug); ~55% of dose unaccounted for

Dosage
Geriatric & Adult Males: **Benign prostatic hyperplasia (BPH):** Oral: 0.5 mg once daily alone or in combination with tamsulosin
Renal Impairment No adjustment is required.
Hepatic Impairment Use caution; no specific adjustments recommended.

Administration May be administered without regard to meals. Capsule should be swallowed whole; do not chew or open; contact with opened capsule can cause oropharyngeal irritation. Should not be touched or handled by women who are pregnant or are of childbearing age.

◀ **Monitoring Parameters** Objective and subjective signs of relief of benign prostatic hyper-plasia, including improvement in urinary flow, reduction in symptoms of urgency, and relief of difficulty in micturition; for serial PSA monitoring, establish a new baseline PSA level after 3 months of therapy and monitor PSA periodically thereafter.

Test Interactions PSA levels decrease in treated patients. After 3 months of therapy, PSA levels stabilize to a new baseline that is ~50% of pretreatment values. If following serial PSAs in a patient, re-establish a new baseline after ≥3 months of use. If interpreting an isolated PSA value in a patient treated for ≥3 months, then double the PSA value for comparison.

Special Geriatric Considerations No dosage adjustment necessary.

Dosage Forms Excipient information presented when available (limited, particularly for generics); consult specific product labeling.

Capsule, softgel, oral:
Avodart®: 0.5 mg

Dutasteride and Tamsulosin (doo TAS teer ide & tam SOO loe sin)

Related Information
Dutasteride on page 586
Tamsulosin on page 1734
Brand Names: U.S. Jalyn™
Index Terms Tamsulosin and Dutasteride; Tamsulosin Hydrochloride and Dutasteride
Generic Availability (U.S.) No
Pharmacologic Category 5 Alpha-Reductase Inhibitor; Alpha₁ Blocker
Use Treatment of symptomatic benign prostatic hyperplasia (BPH)
Dosage
Geriatric & Adult Males:
Benign prostatic hyperplasia (BPH): Oral: One capsule (0.5 mg dutasteride/0.4 mg tamsulosin) once daily ~30 minutes after the same meal each day
Renal Impairment
Cl_{cr} 10-30 mL/minute/1.73 m²: No adjustment needed
Cl_{cr} <10 mL/minute/1.73 m²: Not studied
Hepatic Impairment Use caution; no specific adjustments recommended
Dosage Forms Excipient information presented when available (limited, particularly for generics); consult specific product labeling.
Capsule, oral:
Jalyn™: Dutasteride 0.5 mg and tamsulosin hydrochloride 0.4 mg

◆ **DW286** see Gemifloxacin on page 814
◆ **Dyazide®** see Hydrochlorothiazide and Triamterene on page 879
◆ **DynaCirc CR®** see Isradipine on page 992

Dyphylline (DYE fi lin)

Medication Safety Issues
International issues:
Dilor® [Canada] may be confused with Dilar® which is a brand name for paramethasone in France and Mexico
Brand Names: U.S. Lufyllin®
Index Terms Dihydroxypropyl Theophylline
Generic Availability (U.S.) No
Pharmacologic Category Theophylline Derivative
Use Bronchodilator in reversible airway obstruction due to asthma, chronic bronchitis, or emphysema
Dosage
Geriatric & Adult Bronchoconstriction (asthma, COPD): Oral: Up to 15 mg/kg 4 times/day, individualize dosage
Renal Impairment
Cl_{cr} 50-80 mL/minute: Administer 75% of normal dose.
Cl_{cr} 10-50 mL/minute: Administer 50% of normal dose.
Cl_{cr} <10 mL/minute: Administer 25% of normal dose.
Dosage Forms Excipient information presented when available (limited, particularly for generics); consult specific product labeling.
Tablet, oral:
Lufyllin®: 200 mg, 400 mg [scored]

◆ **Dyrenium®** see Triamterene on page 1858

◆ **Dysport™** *see* AbobotulinumtoxinA *on page* 26
◆ **E2 and DRSP** *see* Drospirenone and Estradiol *on page* 579
◆ **E2020** *see* Donepezil *on page* 554
◆ **E 2080** *see* Rufinamide *on page* 1644

Echothiophate Iodide (ek oh THYE oh fate EYE oh dide)

Related Information
Glaucoma Drug Therapy *on page* 2008
Brand Names: U.S. Phospholine Iodide®
Index Terms Ecostigmine Iodide
Generic Availability (U.S.) No
Pharmacologic Category Acetylcholinesterase Inhibitor; Ophthalmic Agent, Antiglaucoma; Ophthalmic Agent, Miotic
Use Used as miotic in treatment of chronic, open-angle glaucoma; may be useful in specific cases of angle-closure glaucoma (postiridectomy or where surgery refused/contraindicated); postcataract surgery-related glaucoma; accommodative esotropia
Contraindications Hypersensitivity to echothiophate or any component of the formulation; most cases of angle-closure glaucoma; active uveal inflammation
Warnings/Precautions If general anesthesia required, use succinylcholine with great caution due to potential for respiratory or cardiovascular collapse. Use caution in patients on concomitant anticholinesterase agents; warn patients of possible additive effects if chronically exposed to organophosphate/carbamate pesticides/insecticides. Baseline measurement of anterior chamber angle recommended; routine lens examinations (for opacities) should be conducted. Do not use for tonometric glaucoma, or with active or history of uveitis, or retinal detachment. Discontinue if cardiac irregularities or symptoms of excess cholinergic activity (eg, salivation, sweating, urinary incontinence). Not generally recommended for use in patients with any of the following: Vagotonia, asthma GI disturbances, PUD, bradycardia or hypotension, recent MI, epilepsy, parkinsonism. Use cautiously prior to ophthalmic surgery due to risk of blood in the anterior chamber. May depress plasma and erythrocyte cholinesterase levels after a few weeks of therapy. Tolerance may develop after prolonged use; a rest period restores response to the drug.
Adverse Reactions (Reflective of adult population; not specific for elderly) Frequency not defined.
Cardiovascular: Bradycardia, cardiac irregularities, flushing, hypotension
Gastrointestinal: Diarrhea, nausea, vomiting
Neurologic & skeletal: Muscle weakness
Ocular: Blurred vision, browache, burning eyes, ciliary redness, conjunctival redness/thickening, intraocular pressure increases (paradoxical), iris cysts, lacrimation, lid muscle twitching, miosis, myopia, latent iritis or uveitis activation, lens opacities, retinal detachment, stinging
Respiratory: Dyspnea
Miscellaneous: Diaphoresis, nasolacrimal canal obstruction
Drug Interactions
Avoid Concomitant Use There are no known interactions where it is recommended to avoid concomitant use.
Increased Effect/Toxicity
Echothiophate Iodide may increase the levels/effects of: Succinylcholine
Decreased Effect There are no known significant interactions involving a decrease in effect.
Stability Store undiluted vials at 2°C to 8°C (36°F to 46°F). Reconstituted solutions remain stable for 30 days at room temperature; do not refrigerate.
Mechanism of Action Long-acting inhibition of cholinesterase enhances activity of endogenous acetylcholine. Reduced degradation of acetylcholine leads to continuous stimulation of the ciliary muscle producing miosis; other effects include potentiation of accommodation and facilitation of aqueous humor outflow, with attendant reduction in intraocular pressure.
Pharmacodynamics/Kinetics
Onset of action: Miosis: 10-30 minutes; Intraocular pressure decrease: 4-8 hours
Peak effect: Intraocular pressure decrease: 24 hours
Duration: Miosis: 1-4 weeks
Dosage
Geriatric & Adult Open-angle or secondary glaucoma: Ophthalmic:
Initial: Instill 1 drop (0.03%) twice daily into eyes with 1 dose just prior to bedtime
Maintenance: Some patients have been treated with 1 dose daily or every other day
Conversion from other ophthalmic agents: If IOP control was unsatisfactory, patients may be expected to require higher doses of echothiophate (eg, ≥0.06%); however, patients should be initially started on the 0.03% strength for a short period to better tolerance.

◀ **Administration** Proper administration technique is required for maximal benefit. The nasolacrimal duct(s) should be compressed for 1-2 minutes after instillation of the drops. Excess fluid around the eye should be blotted with tissue, and any contact of medication to the hands should be immediately washed off.

Monitoring Parameters Intraocular pressure

Pharmacotherapy Pearls Tolerance may develop after prolonged use; a rest period restores response to the drug.

Special Geriatric Considerations Evaluate the patient's or caregiver's ability to safely administer the correct dose of ophthalmic medication.

Dosage Forms Excipient information presented when available (limited, particularly for generics); consult specific product labeling.

Powder for reconstitution, ophthalmic:

Phospholine Iodide®: 6.25 mg (5 mL) [0.125%]

◆ **EC-Naprosyn®** see Naproxen on page 1263
◆ **Econopred** see PrednisoLONE (Ophthalmic) on page 1510
◆ **Ecostigmine Iodide** see Echothiophate Iodide on page 589
◆ **Ecotrin® [OTC]** see Aspirin on page 153
◆ **Ecotrin® Arthritis Strength [OTC]** see Aspirin on page 153
◆ **Ecotrin® Low Strength [OTC]** see Aspirin on page 153
◆ **Edarbi™** see Azilsartan on page 173
◆ **Ed Chlorped [DSC]** see Chlorpheniramine on page 337
◆ **Ed-Chlortan** see Chlorpheniramine on page 337
◆ **Edecrin®** see Ethacrynic Acid on page 675
◆ **Edex®** see Alprostadil on page 73
◆ **Edluar™** see Zolpidem on page 1960

Edrophonium (ed roe FOE nee um)

Brand Names: U.S. Enlon®
Brand Names: Canada Enlon®; Tensilon®
Index Terms Edrophonium Chloride
Generic Availability (U.S.) No
Pharmacologic Category Acetylcholinesterase Inhibitor; Antidote; Diagnostic Agent
Use Diagnosis of myasthenia gravis; differentiation of cholinergic crises from myasthenia crises; reversal of nondepolarizing neuromuscular blockers
Contraindications Hypersensitivity to edrophonium, sulfites, or any component of the formulation; GI or GU obstruction
Warnings/Precautions Use with caution in patients with bronchial asthma and those receiving a cardiac glycoside; atropine sulfate should always be readily available as an antagonist. Overdosage can cause cholinergic crisis which may be fatal. I.V. atropine should be readily available for treatment of cholinergic reactions. Use with caution in patients with cardiac arrhythmias (eg, bradyarrhythmias). Avoid use in myasthenia gravis; may exacerbate muscular weakness. Products may contain sodium sulfite.
Adverse Reactions (Reflective of adult population; not specific for elderly) Frequency not defined.

Cardiovascular: Arrhythmias (especially bradycardia), AV block, carbon monoxide decreased, cardiac arrest, ECG changes (nonspecific), flushing, hypotension, nodal rhythm, syncope, tachycardia

Central nervous system: Convulsions, dizziness, drowsiness, dysarthria, dysphonia, headache, loss of consciousness

Dermatologic: Skin rash, thrombophlebitis (I.V.), urticaria

Gastrointestinal: Diarrhea, dysphagia, flatulence, hyperperistalsis, nausea, salivation, stomach cramps, vomiting

Genitourinary: Urinary urgency

Neuromuscular & skeletal: Arthralgias, fasciculations, muscle cramps, spasms, weakness

Ocular: Lacrimation, small pupils

Respiratory: Bronchiolar constriction, bronchospasm, dyspnea, bronchial secretions increased, laryngospasm, respiratory arrest, respiratory depression, respiratory muscle paralysis

Miscellaneous: Allergic reactions, anaphylaxis, diaphoresis increased

Drug Interactions

Avoid Concomitant Use There are no known interactions where it is recommended to avoid concomitant use.

Increased Effect/Toxicity

Edrophonium may increase the levels/effects of: Beta-Blockers; Cholinergic Agonists; Succinylcholine

The levels/effects of Edrophonium may be increased by: Corticosteroids (Systemic)

Decreased Effect

Edrophonium may decrease the levels/effects of: Neuromuscular-Blocking Agents (Non-depolarizing)

Mechanism of Action Inhibits destruction of acetylcholine by acetylcholinesterase. This facilitates transmission of impulses across myoneural junction and results in increased cholinergic responses such as miosis, increased tonus of intestinal and skeletal muscles, bronchial and ureteral constriction, bradycardia, and increased salivary and sweat gland secretions.

Pharmacodynamics/Kinetics

Onset of action: I.M.: 2-10 minutes; I.V.: 30-60 seconds

Duration: I.M.: 5-30 minutes: I.V.: 10 minutes

Distribution: V_d: Adults: 1.1 L/kg

Half-life elimination: Adults: 1.2-2.4 hours; Anephric patients: 2.4-4.4 hours

Excretion: Adults: Primarily urine (67%)

Dosage

Geriatric & Adult Usually administered I.V., however, if not possible, I.M. or SubQ may be used.

Diagnosis of Myasthenia gravis:

I.V.: 2 mg test dose administered over 15-30 seconds; 8 mg given 45 seconds later if no response is seen. Test dose may be repeated after 30 minutes.

I.M.: Initial: 10 mg; if no cholinergic reaction occurs, give 2 mg 30 minutes later to rule out false-negative reaction.

Titration of oral anticholinesterase therapy: 1-2 mg given 1 hour after oral dose of anticholinesterase; if strength improves, an increase in neostigmine or pyridostigmine dose is indicated.

Differentiation of cholinergic from myasthenic crisis: I.V.: 1 mg; may repeat after 1 minute. **Note:** Intubation and controlled ventilation may be required if patient has cholinergic crisis.

Reversal of nondepolarizing neuromuscular blocking agents (neostigmine with atropine usually preferred): I.V.: 10 mg over 30-45 seconds; may repeat every 5-10 minutes up to 40 mg.

Termination of paroxysmal atrial tachycardia: I.V. rapid injection: 5-10 mg

Renal Impairment Dose may need to be reduced in patients with chronic renal failure.

Administration Edrophonium is administered by direct I.V. injection; see Dosage

Monitoring Parameters Pre- and postinjection strength (cranial musculature is most useful); heart rate, respiratory rate, blood pressure

Test Interactions Increased aminotransferase [ALT/AST] (S), amylase (S)

Pharmacotherapy Pearls In the diagnosis of myasthenia gravis, all anticholinesterase medications should be discontinued for at least 8 hours before administering neostigmine; monitor for signs of cholinergic crisis

Special Geriatric Considerations Many elderly will have diseases which may influence the use of edrophonium. Also, many elderly will need doses reduced 50% due to creatinine clearances in the 10-50 mL/minute range (common in the aged). Side effects or concomitant disease may warrant use of pyridostigmine.

Dosage Forms Excipient information presented when available (limited, particularly for generics); consult specific product labeling.

Injection, solution, as chloride:

Enlon®: 10 mg/mL (15 mL) [contains natural rubber/natural latex in packaging, sodium sulfite]

ELETRIPTAN

- ◆ **EL-970** *see* Dalfampridine *on page 444*
- ◆ **Elavil** *see* Amitriptyline *on page 103*
- ◆ **Eldepryl®** *see* Selegiline *on page 1663*
- ◆ **Electrolyte Lavage Solution** *see* Polyethylene Glycol-Electrolyte Solution and Bisacodyl *on page 1481*
- ◆ **Elestat®** *see* Epinastine *on page 605*
- ◆ **Elestrin®** *see* Estradiol (Systemic) *on page 641*

Eletriptan (el e TRIP tan)

Brand Names: U.S. Relpax®
Brand Names: Canada Relpax®
Index Terms Eletriptan Hydrobromide
Generic Availability (U.S.) No
Pharmacologic Category Antimigraine Agent; Serotonin 5-HT$_{1B, 1D}$ Receptor Agonist
Use Acute treatment of migraine, with or without aura
Contraindications Hypersensitivity to eletriptan or any component of the formulation; ischemic heart disease (angina pectoris, history of myocardial infarction, or proven silent ischemia) or in patients with symptoms consistent with ischemic heart disease, coronary artery vasospasm, or Prinzmetal's angina; cerebrovascular syndromes (including strokes, transient ischemic attacks); peripheral vascular syndromes (including ischemic bowel disease); uncontrolled hypertension; use within 24 hours of ergotamine derivatives; use within 24 hours of another 5-HT$_1$ agonist; management of hemiplegic or basilar migraine; severe hepatic impairment
Warnings/Precautions Only indicated for treatment of acute migraine; not indicated for migraine prophylaxis, or for the treatment of cluster headache, hemiplegic or basilar migraine. If a patient does not respond to the first dose, the diagnosis of migraine should be reconsidered. Do not give to patients with risk factors for CAD until a cardiovascular evaluation has been performed; if evaluation is satisfactory, the healthcare provider should administer the first dose (consider ECG monitoring) and cardiovascular status should be periodically evaluated. Cardiac events (coronary artery vasospasm, transient ischemia, MI, ventricular tachycardia/fibrillation, cardiac arrest, and death), cerebral/subarachnoid hemorrhage, stroke, peripheral vascular ischemia, and colonic ischemia have been reported with 5-HT$_1$ agonist administration. Patients who experience sensations of chest pain/pressure/tightness or symptoms suggestive of angina following dosing should be evaluated for coronary artery disease or Prinzmetal's angina before receiving additional doses; if dosing is resumed and similar symptoms recur, monitor with ECG. Significant elevation in blood pressure, including hypertensive crisis, has also been reported on rare occasions in patients with and without a history of hypertension. Use with caution with mild-to-moderate hepatic impairment. Symptoms of agitation, confusion, hallucinations, hyper-reflexia, myoclonus, shivering, and tachycardia (serotonin syndrome) may occur with concomitant proserotonergic drugs (ie, SSRIs/SNRIs or triptans) or agents which reduce eletriptan's metabolism. Concurrent use of serotonin precursors (eg, tryptophan) is not recommended. If concomitant administration with SSRIs is warranted, monitor closely, especially at initiation and with dose increases. Use not recommended within 72 hours in patients taking strong CYP3A4 inhibitors.
Adverse Reactions (Reflective of adult population; not specific for elderly)
1% to 10%:
Cardiovascular: Chest pain/tightness (1% to 4%; placebo 1%), palpitation
Central nervous system: Dizziness (3% to 7%; placebo 3%), somnolence (3% to 7%; placebo 4%), headache (3% to 4%; placebo 3%), chills, pain, vertigo
Gastrointestinal: Nausea (4% to 8%; placebo 5%), xerostomia (2% to 4%, placebo 2%), dysphagia (1% to 2%), abdominal pain/discomfort (1% to 2%; placebo 1%), dyspepsia (1% to 2%; placebo 1%)
Neuromuscular & skeletal: Weakness (4% to 10%), paresthesia (3% to 4%), back pain, hypertonia, hypoesthesia
Respiratory: Pharyngitis
Miscellaneous: Diaphoresis
Drug Interactions
Metabolism/Transport Effects Substrate of CYP3A4 (major)
Avoid Concomitant Use
Avoid concomitant use of Eletriptan with any of the following: Conivaptan; Ergot Derivatives; Sibutramine

Increased Effect/Toxicity

Eletriptan may increase the levels/effects of: Ergot Derivatives; Serotonin Modulators

The levels/effects of Eletriptan may be increased by: Antifungal Agents (Azole Derivatives, Systemic); Calcium Channel Blockers (Nondihydropyridine); Conivaptan; CYP3A4 Inhibitors (Moderate); CYP3A4 Inhibitors (Strong); Dasatinib; Ergot Derivatives; Fluconazole; Macrolide Antibiotics; Sibutramine

Decreased Effect

The levels/effects of Eletriptan may be decreased by: Tocilizumab

Ethanol/Nutrition/Herb Interactions Food: High-fat meal increases bioavailability.

Stability Store at 25°C (77°F); excursions permitted to 15°C to 30°C (59°F to 86°F).

Mechanism of Action Selective agonist for serotonin (5-HT$_{1B}$ and 5-HT$_{1D}$ receptors) in cranial arteries; causes vasoconstriction and reduces sterile inflammation associated with antidromic neuronal transmission correlating with relief of migraine

Pharmacodynamics/Kinetics

Absorption: Well absorbed

Distribution: V$_d$: 138 L

Protein binding: ~85%

Metabolism: Hepatic via CYP3A4; forms one metabolite (active)

Bioavailability: ~50%, increased with high-fat meal

Half-life elimination: ~4 hours (Elderly: 4.4-5.7 hours); Metabolite: ~13 hours

Time to peak, plasma: 1.5-2 hours

Dosage

Geriatric & Adult Acute migraine: Oral: Initial: 20-40 mg (maximum: 40 mg/dose); if the headache improves but returns, dose may be repeated after 2 hours have elapsed since first dose (maximum: 80 mg/day)

Note: If the first dose is ineffective, diagnosis needs to be re-evaluated. Safety of treating >3 headaches/month has not been established.

Renal Impairment No dosing adjustment needed; monitor for increased blood pressure.

Hepatic Impairment

Mild-to-moderate impairment: No adjustment necessary.

Severe impairment: Use is contraindicated.

Special Geriatric Considerations Since elderly often have cardiovascular disease, careful evaluation of the use of 5-HT agonists is needed to avoid complications with the use of these agents. Safety and efficacy in elderly >65 years of age have not been established, however, pharmacokinetic disposition is similar to that in younger adults. Use lowest recommended doses initially.

Dosage Forms Excipient information presented when available (limited, particularly for generics); consult specific product labeling.

Tablet, oral:

Relpax®: 20 mg, 40 mg

◆ **Eletriptan Hydrobromide** *see* Eletriptan *on page 592*
◆ **Eligard®** *see* Leuprolide *on page 1039*
◆ **Elimite** *see* Permethrin *on page 1429*
◆ **Eliphos™** *see* Calcium Acetate *on page 247*
◆ **Elixophyllin® Elixir** *see* Theophylline *on page 1775*
◆ **Elocon®** *see* Mometasone (Topical) *on page 1233*
◆ **Emadine®** *see* Emedastine *on page 593*
◆ **EMD 68843** *see* Vilazodone *on page 1919*

Emedastine (em e DAS teen)

Brand Names: U.S. Emadine®

Index Terms Emedastine Difumarate

Pharmacologic Category Histamine H$_1$ Antagonist; Histamine H$_1$ Antagonist, Second Generation

Use Treatment of allergic conjunctivitis

Dosage

Geriatric & Adult Allergic conjunctivitis: Ophthalmic: Instill 1 drop in affected eye up to 4 times/day

Dosage Forms Excipient information presented when available (limited, particularly for generics); consult specific product labeling.

Solution, ophthalmic, as difumarate [drops]:

Emadine®: 0.05% (5 mL) [contains benzalkonium chloride]

◆ **Emedastine Difumarate** *see* Emedastine *on page 593*

♦ **Emend®** see Aprepitant on page 139
♦ **Emend® for Injection** see Fosaprepitant on page 788
♦ **Emsam®** see Selegiline on page 1663
♦ **ENA 713** see Rivastigmine on page 1627
♦ **Enablex®** see Darifenacin on page 460

Enalapril (e NAL a pril)

Related Information
Angiotensin Agents on page 1985
Medication Safety Issues
Sound-alike/look-alike issues:
Enalapril may be confused with Anafranil®, Elavil®, Eldepryl®, ramipril
Administration issues:
Significant differences exist between oral and I.V. dosing. Use caution when converting from one route of administration to another.
International issues:
Acepril [Hungary, Switzerland] may be confused with Accupril which is a brand name for quinapril [U.S.]

Acepril: Brand name for enalapril [Hungary, Switzerland], but also brand name for captopril [Great Britain]; lisinopril [Malaysia]
Brand Names: U.S. Vasotec®
Brand Names: Canada Apo-Enalapril®; CO Enalapril; Mylan-Enalapril; Novo-Enalapril; PMS-Enalapril; PRO-Enalapril; RAN™-Enalapril; ratio-Enalapril; Riva-Enalapril; Sandoz-Enalapril; Sig-Enalapril; Taro-Enalapril; Teva-Enalapril; Vasotec®; Vasotec® I.V.
Index Terms Enalapril Maleate; Enalaprilat
Generic Availability (U.S.) Yes
Pharmacologic Category Angiotensin-Converting Enzyme (ACE) Inhibitor
Use Treatment of hypertension; treatment of symptomatic heart failure; treatment of asymptomatic left ventricular dysfunction
Unlabeled/Investigational Use
Unlabeled: To delay the progression of nephropathy and reduce risks of cardiovascular events in hypertensive patients with type 1 or 2 diabetes mellitus; hypertensive crisis, diabetic nephropathy, hypertension secondary to scleroderma renal crisis, diagnosis of aldosteronism, idiopathic edema, Bartter's syndrome, postmyocardial infarction for prevention of ventricular failure

Investigational: Acute cardiogenic pulmonary edema (enalaprilat)
Contraindications Hypersensitivity to enalapril or enalaprilat; angioedema related to previous treatment with an ACE inhibitor; patients with idiopathic or hereditary angioedema
Warnings/Precautions Anaphylactic reactions may occur rarely with ACE inhibitors. At any time during treatment (especially following first dose) angioedema may occur rarely with ACE inhibitors; it may involve the head and neck (potentially compromising airway) or the intestine (presenting with abdominal pain). African-Americans may be at an increased risk. Prolonged frequent monitoring may be required especially if tongue, glottis, or larynx are involved as they are associated with airway obstruction. Patients with a history of airway surgery may have a higher risk of airway obstruction. Aggressive early and appropriate management is critical. Use in patients with idiopathic or hereditary angioedema or previous angioedema associated with ACE inhibitor therapy is contraindicated. Severe anaphylactoid reactions may be seen during hemodialysis (eg, CVVHD) with high-flux dialysis membranes (eg, AN69), and rarely, during low density lipoprotein apheresis with dextran sulfate cellulose. Rare cases of anaphylactoid reactions have been reported in patients undergoing sensitization treatment with hymenoptera (bee, wasp) venom while receiving ACE inhibitors.

Symptomatic hypotension with or without syncope can occur with ACE inhibitors (usually with the first several doses); effects are most often observed in volume depleted patients; correct volume depletion prior to initiation; close monitoring of patient is required especially with initial dosing and dosing increases; blood pressure must be lowered at a rate appropriate for the patient's clinical condition. Initiation of therapy in patients with ischemic heart disease or cerebrovascular disease warrants close observation due to the potential consequences posed by falling blood pressure (eg, MI, stroke). Use with caution in hypertrophic cardiomyopathy with outflow tract obstruction, severe aortic stenosis, or before, during, or immediately after major surgery.

Hyperkalemia may occur with ACE inhibitors; risk factors include renal dysfunction, diabetes mellitus, concomitant use of potassium-sparing diuretics, potassium supplements, and/or potassium-containing salts. Use cautiously, if at all, with these agents and monitor potassium closely. Cough may occur with ACE inhibitors. Other causes of cough should be considered (eg, pulmonary congestion in patients with heart failure) and excluded prior to discontinuation.

May be associated with deterioration of renal function and/or increases in serum creatinine, particularly in patients with low renal blood flow (eg, renal artery stenosis, heart failure) whose glomerular filtration rate (GFR) is dependent on efferent arteriolar vasoconstriction by angiotensin II; deterioration may result in oliguria, acute renal failure, and progressive azotemia. Small increases in serum creatinine may occur following initiation; consider discontinuation only in patients with progressive and/or significant deterioration in renal function. Use with caution in patients with unstented unilateral/bilateral renal artery stenosis. When unstented bilateral renal artery stenosis is present, use is generally avoided due to the elevated risk of deterioration in renal function unless possible benefits outweigh risks. Concurrent use of angiotensin receptor blockers may increase the risk of clinically-significant adverse events (eg, renal dysfunction, hyperkalemia).

Rare toxicities associated with ACE inhibitors include cholestatic jaundice (which may progress to fulminant hepatic necrosis), agranulocytosis, neutropenia or leukopenia with myeloid hypoplasia. Patients with collagen vascular diseases (especially with concomitant renal impairment) or renal impairment alone may be at increased risk for hematologic toxicity; periodically monitor CBC with differential in these patients.

Adverse Reactions (Reflective of adult population; not specific for elderly) Note: Frequency ranges include data from hypertension and heart failure trials. Higher rates of adverse reactions have generally been noted in patients with CHF. However, the frequency of adverse effects associated with placebo is also increased in this population.

1% to 10%:
   Cardiovascular: Hypotension (0.9% to 7%), chest pain (2%), syncope (0.5% to 2%), orthostasis (2%), orthostatic hypotension (2%)
   Central nervous system: Headache (2% to 5%), dizziness (4% to 8%), fatigue (2% to 3%)
   Dermatologic: Rash (2%)
   Gastrointestinal: Abnormal taste, abdominal pain, vomiting, nausea, diarrhea, anorexia, constipation
   Neuromuscular & skeletal: Weakness
   Renal: Serum creatinine increased (0.2% to 20%), worsening of renal function (in patients with bilateral renal artery stenosis or hypovolemia)
   Respiratory (1% to 2%): Bronchitis, cough, dyspnea

Drug Interactions
   Metabolism/Transport Effects Substrate of CYP3A4 (minor)
   Avoid Concomitant Use There are no known interactions where it is recommended to avoid concomitant use.
   Increased Effect/Toxicity
   Enalapril may increase the levels/effects of: Allopurinol; Amifostine; Antihypertensives; AzaTHIOprine; CycloSPORINE; CycloSPORINE (Systemic); Ferric Gluconate; Gold Sodium Thiomalate; Hypotensive Agents; Iron Dextran Complex; Lithium; Nonsteroidal Anti-Inflammatory Agents; RiTUXimab; Sodium Phosphates

   The levels/effects of Enalapril may be increased by: Alfuzosin; Angiotensin II Receptor Blockers; Conivaptan; Diazoxide; DPP-IV Inhibitors; Eplerenone; Everolimus; Herbs (Hypotensive Properties); Loop Diuretics; MAO Inhibitors; Pentoxifylline; Phosphodiesterase 5 Inhibitors; Potassium Salts; Potassium-Sparing Diuretics; Prostacyclin Analogues; Sirolimus; Temsirolimus; Thiazide Diuretics; TiZANidine; Tolvaptan; Trimethoprim
   Decreased Effect
   The levels/effects of Enalapril may be decreased by: Antacids; Aprotinin; CYP3A4 Inducers (Strong); Deferasirox; Herbs (CYP3A4 Inducers); Herbs (Hypertensive Properties); Icatibant; Lanthanum; Methylphenidate; Nonsteroidal Anti-Inflammatory Agents; Salicylates; Tocilizumab; Yohimbine

Ethanol/Nutrition/Herb Interactions Herb/Nutraceutical: Avoid bayberry, blue cohosh, cayenne, ephedra, ginger, ginseng (American), kola, licorice (may worsen hypertension). Avoid black cohosh, california poppy, coleus, golden seal, hawthorn, mistletoe, periwinkle, quinine, shepherd's purse (may have increased antihypertensive effect).

Stability Enalaprilat: Clear, colorless solution which should be stored at <30°C. I.V. is 24 hours at room temperature in D_5W or NS.

Mechanism of Action Competitive inhibitor of angiotensin-converting enzyme (ACE); prevents conversion of angiotensin I to angiotensin II, a potent vasoconstrictor; results in lower levels of angiotensin II which causes an increase in plasma renin activity and a reduction in aldosterone secretion

◀ **Pharmacodynamics/Kinetics**
Onset of action: Oral: ~1 hour; I.V.: ≤15 minutes
  Peak effect: Oral: 4-6 hours; I.V.: 1-4 hours
Duration: Oral: 12-24 hours; I.V.: ~6 hours
Absorption: Oral: 55% to 75%
Protein binding: 50% to 60%
Metabolism: Prodrug, undergoes hepatic biotransformation to enalaprilat
Half-life elimination:
  Enalapril: Adults: Healthy: 2 hours; Congestive heart failure: 3.4-5.8 hours
  Enalaprilat: Adults: 35-38 hours
Time to peak, serum: Oral: Enalapril: 0.5-1.5 hours; Enalaprilat (active): 3-4.5 hours
Excretion: Urine (60% to 80%); some feces

Dosage

Geriatric & Adult Use lower listed initial dose in patients with hyponatremia, hypovolemia, severe congestive heart failure, decreased renal function, or in those receiving diuretics.

Asymptomatic left ventricular dysfunction: Oral: 2.5 mg twice daily, titrated as tolerated to 20 mg/day

Heart failure:
  Oral: Initial: 2.5 mg once or twice daily (usual range: 5-40 mg/day in 2 divided doses). Titrate slowly at 1- to 2-week intervals. Target dose: 10-20 mg twice daily (ACC/AHA 2009 Heart Failure Guidelines)
  I.V.: Avoid I.V. administration in patients with unstable heart failure or those suffering acute myocardial infarction.

Hypertension:
  Oral: 2.5-5 mg/day then increase as required, usually at 1- to 2-week intervals; usual dose range (JNC 7): 2.5-40 mg/day in 1-2 divided doses. **Note:** Initiate with 2.5 mg if patient is taking a diuretic which cannot be discontinued. May add a diuretic if blood pressure cannot be controlled with enalapril alone.
  I.V. (Enalaprilat): 1.25 mg/dose, given over 5 minutes every 6 hours; doses as high as 5 mg/dose every 6 hours have been tolerated for up to 36 hours. **Note:** If patients are concomitantly receiving diuretic therapy, begin with 0.625 mg I.V. over 5 minutes; if the effect is not adequate after 1 hour, repeat the dose and administer 1.25 mg at 6-hour intervals thereafter; if adequate, administer 0.625 mg I.V. every 6 hours.

Conversion from I.V. to oral therapy: If not concurrently receiving diuretics, initiate 5 mg once daily; if concurrently receiving diuretics and responding to 0.625 mg I.V. every 6 hours, initiate with 2.5 mg once daily; subsequent titration as needed.

Renal Impairment
Oral: Enalapril: Hypertension:
  Cl_{cr} 30-80 mL/minute: Administer 5 mg/day titrated upwards to maximum of 40 mg.
  Cl_{cr} <30 mL/minute: Administer 2.5 mg day titrated upward until blood pressure is controlled up to a maximum of 40 mg.
  For heart failure patients with sodium <130 mEq/L or serum creatinine >1.6 mg/dL, initiate dosage with 2.5 mg/day, increasing to twice daily as needed; increase further in increments of 2.5 mg/dose at >4-day intervals to a maximum daily dose of 40 mg.
I.V.: Enalaprilat:
  Cl_{cr} >30 mL/minute: Initiate with 1.25 mg every 6 hours and increase dose based on response.
  Cl_{cr} <30 mL/minute: Initiate with 0.625 mg every 6 hours and increase dose based on response.
Moderately dialyzable (20% to 50%)
  Administer dose postdialysis (eg, 0.625 mg I.V. every 6 hours) or administer 20% to 25% supplemental dose following dialysis; Clearance: 62 mL/minute
Peritoneal dialysis effects: Supplemental dose is not necessary, although some removal of drug occurs.

Hepatic Impairment Hydrolysis of enalapril to enalaprilat may be delayed and/or impaired in patients with severe hepatic impairment, but the pharmacodynamic effects of the drug do not appear to be significantly altered. No dosage adjustment is necessary.

Administration Administer direct IVP over at least 5 minutes or dilute up to 50 mL and infuse; discontinue diuretic, if possible, for 2-3 days before beginning enalapril therapy

Monitoring Parameters Blood pressure; serum creatinine and potassium; if patient has collagen vascular disease and/or renal impairment, periodically monitor CBC with differential

Test Interactions Positive Coombs' [direct]; may cause false-positive results in urine acetone determinations using sodium nitroprusside reagent

Pharmacotherapy Pearls Severe hypotension may occur in patients who are sodium and/or volume depleted; initiate lower doses and watch for hypotensive effect within 1-3 hours of first dose or new higher dose.

Special Geriatric Considerations Due to frequent decreases in glomerular filtration (also creatinine clearance) with aging, elderly patients may have exaggerated responses to ACE inhibitors; differences in clinical response due to hepatic changes are not observed. ACE inhibitors may be preferred agents in elderly patients with congestive heart failure and diabetes mellitus. Diabetic proteinuria is reduced and insulin sensitivity is enhanced. In general, the side effect profile is favorable in the elderly and causes little or no CNS confusion; use lowest dose recommendations initially; adjust dose for renal function in the elderly. Many elderly may be volume depleted due to diuretic use and/or blunted thirst reflex resulting in inadequate fluid intake.

Dosage Forms Excipient information presented when available (limited, particularly for generics); consult specific product labeling.

Injection, solution, as enalaprilat: 1.25 mg/mL (1 mL, 2 mL)

Tablet, oral, as maleate: 2.5 mg, 5 mg, 10 mg, 20 mg

  Vasotec®: 2.5 mg, 5 mg, 10 mg, 20 mg [scored]

Extemporaneously Prepared An enalapril oral suspension (1 mg/mL) has been made using 20 mg tablets and Bicitra®. Add 50 mL Bicitra® to a polyethylene terephthalate (PET) bottle containing ten 20 mg tablets and shake for at least 2 minutes. Let concentrate stand for 60 minutes. Following the 60-minute hold time, shake the concentration for an additional minute. Add 150 mL Bicitra® to the concentrate and shake the suspension to disperse the ingredients. The suspension should refrigerated at 2°C to 8°C (36°F to 46°F); it can be stored for up to 30 days. Shake suspension well before use.

  Package labeling, Merck & Co, Inc, issued October 2000.

Selected References

American Diabetes Association, "Standards of Medical Care in Diabetes Mellitus – 2009," *Diabetes Care*, 2009, 32 (Suppl 1):13-61.

Chobanian AV, Bakris GL, Black HR, et al, "The Seventh Report of the Joint National Committee on Prevention, Detection, Evaluation, and Treatment of High Blood Pressure: The JNC 7 Report," *JAMA*, 2003, 289(19):2560-72.

Miller DR, Oliveria SA, Berlowitz DR, et al, "Angioedema Incidence in US Veterens Initiating Angiotensin-Converting Enzyme Inhibitors," *Hypertension*, 2008, 51(6):1-7.

Enalapril and Hydrochlorothiazide (e NAL a pril & hye droe klor oh THYE a zide)

Related Information

  Enalapril *on page 594*

  Hydrochlorothiazide *on page 876*

Medication Safety Issues

  International issues:

  Norpramin: Brand name for enalapril/hydrochlorothiazide [Portugal], but also the brand name for desipramine [U.S., Canada]; omeprazole [Spain]

Brand Names: U.S. Vaseretic®

Brand Names: Canada Vaseretic®

Index Terms Enalapril Maleate and Hydrochlorothiazide; Hydrochlorothiazide and Enalapril

Generic Availability (U.S.) Yes

Pharmacologic Category Angiotensin-Converting Enzyme (ACE) Inhibitor; Diuretic, Thiazide

Use Treatment of hypertension

Dosage

  Geriatric Refer to dosing in individual monographs; adjust for renal impairment.

  Adult Hypertension: Oral: Enalapril 5-10 mg and hydrochlorothiazide 12.5-25 mg once daily (maximum: 40 mg/day [enalapril]; 50 mg/day [hydrochlorothiazide])

  Renal Impairment

   Cl_{cr} >30 mL/minute: Administer usual dose.

   Severe renal failure: Avoid; loop diuretics are recommended.

Dosage Forms Excipient information presented when available (limited, particularly for generics); consult specific product labeling.

Tablet:

  5/12.5: Enalapril maleate 5 mg and hydrochlorothiazide 12.5 mg

  10/25: Enalapril maleate 10 mg and hydrochlorothiazide 25 mg

  Vaseretic®:

   10/25: Enalapril maleate 10 mg and hydrochlorothiazide 25 mg

◆ **Enalaprilat** *see* Enalapril *on page 594*

◆ **Enalapril Maleate** *see* Enalapril *on page 594*

◆ **Enalapril Maleate and Hydrochlorothiazide** *see* Enalapril and Hydrochlorothiazide *on page 597*

◆ **Enbrel®** *see* Etanercept *on page 672*

◆ **Enbrel® SureClick®** *see* Etanercept *on page 672*

◆ **Endocet®** *see* Oxycodone and Acetaminophen *on page 1371*

Enoxaparin (ee noks a PA rin)

Related Information
Anticoagulants, Injectable *on page 1989*

Medication Safety Issues

Sound-alike/look-alike issues:
Lovenox® may be confused with Lasix®, Levaquin®, Lotronex®, Protonix®

High alert medication:
The Institute for Safe Medication Practices (ISMP) includes this medication among its list of drugs which have a heightened risk of causing significant patient harm when used in error.

2009 National Patient Safety Goals:
The Joint Commission (TJC) requires healthcare organizations that provide anticoagulant therapy to have a process in place to reduce the risk of anticoagulant-associated patient harm. Patients receiving anticoagulants should receive individualized care through a defined process that includes standardized ordering, dispensing, administration, monitoring, and education. This does not apply to routine short-term use of anticoagulants for prevention of venous thromboembolism when the expectation is that the patient's laboratory values will remain within or close to normal values (NPSG.03.05.01).

Brand Names: U.S. Lovenox®

Brand Names: Canada Enoxaparin Injection; Lovenox®; Lovenox® HP

Index Terms Enoxaparin Sodium

Generic Availability (U.S.) Yes: Injection solution (preservative free)

Pharmacologic Category Low Molecular Weight Heparin

Use
Acute coronary syndromes: Unstable angina (UA), non-ST-elevation (NSTEMI), and ST-elevation myocardial infarction (STEMI)

DVT prophylaxis: Following hip or knee replacement surgery, abdominal surgery, or in medical patients with severely-restricted mobility during acute illness who are at risk for thromboembolic complications

DVT treatment (acute): Inpatient treatment (patients with and without pulmonary embolism) and outpatient treatment (patients without pulmonary embolism)

Note: High-risk patients include those with one or more of the following risk factors: >40 years of age, obesity, general anesthesia lasting >30 minutes, malignancy, history of deep vein thrombosis or pulmonary embolism

Unlabeled/Investigational Use Anticoagulant bridge therapy during temporary interruption of vitamin K antagonist therapy in patients at high risk for thromboembolism; DVT prophylaxis following moderate-risk general surgery, major gynecologic surgery and following higher-risk general surgery for cancer

Contraindications Hypersensitivity to enoxaparin, heparin, or any component of the formulation; thrombocytopenia associated with a positive *in vitro* test for antiplatelet antibodies in the presence of enoxaparin; hypersensitivity to pork products; active major bleeding; not for I.M. use

Warnings/Precautions [U.S. Boxed Warning]: Spinal or epidural hematomas, including subsequent paralysis, may occur with recent or anticipated neuraxial anesthesia (epidural or spinal anesthesia) or spinal puncture in patients anticoagulated with LMWH or heparinoids. Consider risk versus benefit prior to spinal procedures; risk is increased by the use of concomitant agents which may alter hemostasis, the use of indwelling epidural catheters for analgesia, a history of spinal deformity or spinal surgery, as well as a history of traumatic or repeated epidural or spinal punctures. Patient should be observed closely for bleeding and signs and symptoms of neurological impairment if therapy is administered during or immediately following diagnostic lumbar puncture, epidural anesthesia, or spinal anesthesia.

Do not administer intramuscularly. Not recommended for thromboprophylaxis in patients with prosthetic heart valves. Not to be used interchangeably (unit for unit) with heparin or any other low molecular weight heparins. Use caution in patients with history of heparin-induced thrombocytopenia. Monitor patient closely for signs or symptoms of bleeding. Certain patients are at increased risk of bleeding. Risk factors include bacterial endocarditis; congenital or acquired bleeding disorders; active ulcerative or angiodysplastic GI diseases; severe uncontrolled hypertension; history of hemorrhagic stroke; use shortly after brain, spinal, or ophthalmic surgery; patients treated concomitantly with platelet inhibitors; recent GI bleeding; thrombocytopenia or platelet defects; severe liver disease; hypertensive or diabetic retinopathy; or in patients undergoing invasive procedures. Monitor platelet count closely. Rare cases of thrombocytopenia have occurred. Discontinue therapy and consider alternative treatment if platelets are <100,000/mm^3 and/or thrombosis develops. Rare cases of thrombocytopenia with thrombosis have occurred. Use caution in patients with congenital or drug-induced thrombocytopenia or platelet defects. Risk of bleeding may be increased in women <45 kg and in men <57 kg. Use caution in patients with renal impairment; dosage adjustment needed if Cl$_{cr}$ <30 mL/minute. Use with caution in the elderly (delayed elimination may occur); dosage alteration/adjustment may be required (eg, omission of I.V. bolus in acute STEMI in patients ≥75 years of age). Monitor for hyperkalemia; can cause hyperkalemia possibly by suppressing aldosterone production.

There is no consensus for adjusting/correcting the weight-based dosage of LMWH for patients who are morbidly obese (BMI ≥40 kg/m^2). For patients undergoing inpatient bariatric surgery, the American College of Chest Physicians Practice Guidelines suggest using a higher thromboprophylaxis dose of LMWH for obese patients (Geerts, 2008).

Adverse Reactions (Reflective of adult population; not specific for elderly) As with all anticoagulants, bleeding is the major adverse effect of enoxaparin. Hemorrhage may occur at virtually any site. Risk is dependent on multiple variables. At the recommended doses, single injections of enoxaparin do not significantly influence platelet aggregation or affect global clotting time (ie, PT or aPTT).

1% to 10%:
  Central nervous system: Fever (5% to 8%), confusion, pain
  Dermatologic: Erythema, bruising
  Gastrointestinal: Nausea (3%), diarrhea
  Hematologic: Hemorrhage (major, <1% to 4%; includes cases of intracranial, retroperitoneal, or intraocular hemorrhage; incidence varies with indication/population), thrombocytopenia (moderate 1%; severe 0.1% - see **"Note"** below), anemia (<2%)
  Hepatic: ALT increased, AST increased
  Local: Injection site hematoma (9%), local reactions (irritation, pain, ecchymosis, erythema)
  Renal: Hematuria (<2%)
Note: Thrombocytopenia with thrombosis: Cases of heparin-induced thrombocytopenia (some complicated by organ infarction, limb ischemia, or death) have been reported.
Drug Interactions
  Avoid Concomitant Use
    Avoid concomitant use of Enoxaparin with any of the following: Rivaroxaban
  Increased Effect/Toxicity
    Enoxaparin may increase the levels/effects of: Anticoagulants; Collagenase (Systemic); Deferasirox; Drotrecogin Alfa; Ibritumomab; Rivaroxaban; Tositumomab and Iodine I 131 Tositumomab

    The levels/effects of Enoxaparin may be increased by: 5-ASA Derivatives; Antiplatelet Agents; Dasatinib; Herbs (Anticoagulant/Antiplatelet Properties); Nonsteroidal Anti-Inflammatory Agents; Pentosan Polysulfate Sodium; Pentoxifylline; Prostacyclin Analogues; Salicylates; Thrombolytic Agents
  Decreased Effect There are no known significant interactions involving a decrease in effect.
Ethanol/Nutrition/Herb Interactions Herb/Nutraceutical: Avoid cat's claw, dong quai, evening primrose, feverfew, garlic, ginger, ginkgo, red clover, horse chestnut, green tea, ginseng (all have additional antiplatelet activity).
Stability Store at 25°C (77°F); excursions permitted to 15°C to 30°C (59°F to 86°F); do not freeze.
Mechanism of Action Standard heparin consists of components with molecular weights ranging from 4000-30,000 daltons with a mean of 16,000 daltons. Heparin acts as an anticoagulant by enhancing the inhibition rate of clotting proteases by antithrombin III impairing normal hemostasis and inhibition of factor Xa. Low molecular weight heparins have a small effect on the activated partial thromboplastin time and strongly inhibit factor Xa. Enoxaparin is derived from porcine heparin that undergoes benzylation followed by alkaline depolymerization. The average molecular weight of enoxaparin is 4500 daltons which is distributed as (≤20%) 2000 daltons, (≥68%) 2000-8000 daltons, and (≤15%) >8000 daltons.

◄ Enoxaparin has a higher ratio of antifactor Xa to antifactor IIa activity than unfractionated heparin.

Pharmacodynamics/Kinetics

Onset of action: Peak effect: SubQ: Antifactor Xa and antithrombin (antifactor IIa): 3-5 hours

Duration: 40 mg dose: Antifactor Xa activity: ~12 hours

Distribution: 4.3 L (based on antifactor Xa activity)

Protein binding: Does not bind to heparin binding proteins

Metabolism: Hepatic, to lower molecular weight fragments (little activity)

Half-life elimination, plasma: 2-4 times longer than standard heparin, independent of dose; based on anti-Xa activity: 4.5-7 hours

Excretion: Urine (40% of dose; 10% as active fragments)

Dosage

Geriatric SubQ: Refer to adult dosing. Increased incidence of bleeding with doses of 1.5 mg/kg/day or 1 mg/kg every 12 hours; injection-associated bleeding and serious adverse reactions are also increased in the elderly. Careful attention should be paid to elderly patients, particularly those <45 kg. **Note:** Dosage alteration/adjustment may be required.

Adult One mg of enoxaparin is equal to 100 int. units of anti-Xa activity (World Health Organization First International Low Molecular Weight Heparin Reference Standard).

DVT prophylaxis: Note: In morbidly obese patients (BMI ≥40 kg/m^2), increasing the prophylactic dose by 30% may be appropriate for some indications (Nutescu, 2009). For bariatric surgery, dose increases may be >30% based on clinical trial data. SubQ:

Hip replacement surgery:
Twice-daily dosing: 30 mg every 12 hours, with initial dose within 12-24 hours after surgery, and every 12 hours for at least 10 days or until risk of DVT has diminished or the patient is adequately anticoagulated on warfarin.
Once-daily dosing: 40 mg once daily, with initial dose within 9-15 hours before surgery, and daily for at least 10 days (or up to 35 days postoperatively) or until risk of DVT has diminished or the patient is adequately anticoagulated on warfarin.

Knee replacement surgery: 30 mg every 12 hours, with initial dose within 12-24 hours after surgery, and every 12 hours for at least 10 days or until risk of DVT has diminished or the patient is adequately anticoagulated on warfarin.

Abdominal surgery: 40 mg once daily, with initial dose given 2 hours prior to surgery; continue until risk of DVT has diminished (usually 7-10 days).

Bariatric surgery: Roux-en-Y gastric bypass: Appropriate dosing strategies have not been clearly defined (Borkgren-Okonek, 2008; Scholten, 2002):
BMI ≤50 kg/m^2: 40 mg every 12 hours
BMI >50 kg/m^2: 60 mg every 12 hours
Note: Bariatric surgery guidelines suggest initiation 30-120 minutes before surgery and postoperatively until patient is fully mobile (Mechanick, 2009). Alternatively, limiting administration to the postoperative period may reduce perioperative bleeding.

Medical patients with severely-restricted mobility during acute illness: 40 mg once daily; continue until risk of DVT has diminished (usually 6-11 days).

DVT treatment (acute): SubQ: **Note:** Start warfarin on the first treatment day and continue enoxaparin until INR is between 2 and 3 (usually 5-7 days).

Inpatient treatment (with or without pulmonary embolism): 1 mg/kg/dose every 12 hours or 1.5 mg/kg once daily.

Outpatient treatment (without pulmonary embolism): 1 mg/kg/dose every 12 hours.

Obesity: Use actual body weight to calculate dose; dose capping not recommended; use of twice daily dosing preferred (Nutescu, 2009)

Percutaneous coronary intervention (PCI), adjunctive therapy: In enoxaparin-treated patients undergoing PCI, if balloon inflation occurs ≤8 hours after the last SubQ enoxaparin dose, no additional dosing is needed. If balloon inflation occurs 8-12 hours after the last SubQ enoxaparin dose, a single I.V. dose of 0.3 mg/kg should be administered (Hirsh, 2008; King, 2007)

ST-elevation MI (STEMI):

Patients <75 years of age: Initial: 30 mg I.V. single bolus plus 1 mg/kg (maximum 100 mg for the first 2 doses only) SubQ every 12 hours. The first SubQ dose should be administered with the I.V. bolus. Maintenance: After first 2 doses, administer 1 mg/kg SubQ every 12 hours.

Patients ≥75 years of age: Initial: SubQ: 0.75 mg/kg every 12 hours (**Note:** No I.V. bolus is administered in this population); a maximum dose of 75 mg is recommended for the first 2 doses. Maintenance: After first 2 doses, administer 0.75 mg/kg SubQ every 12 hours

Obesity: Use weight-based dosing; a maximum dose of 100 mg is recommended for the first 2 doses (Nutescu, 2009)

Additional notes on STEMI treatment: Therapy was continued for 8 days or until hospital discharge; optimal duration not defined. Unless contraindicated, all patients received aspirin (75-325 mg daily) in clinical trials. In patients with STEMI receiving thrombolytics, initiate enoxaparin dosing between 15 minutes before and 30 minutes after fibrinolytic therapy. In patients undergoing PCI, if balloon inflation occurs ≤8 hours after the last SubQ enoxaparin dose, no additional dosing is needed. If balloon inflation occurs 8-12 hours after last SubQ enoxaparin dose, a single I.V. dose of 0.3 mg/kg should be administered (Hirsh, 2008; King, 2007).

Unstable angina or non-ST-elevation MI (NSTEMI): 1 mg/kg every 12 hours in conjunction with oral aspirin therapy (100-325 mg once daily); continue until clinical stabilization (a minimum of at least 2 days)

Obesity: Use actual body weight to calculate dose; dose capping not recommended (Nutescu, 2009)

Renal Impairment

Cl$_{cr}$ ≥30 mL/minute: No specific adjustment recommended (per manufacturer); monitor closely for bleeding.

Cl$_{cr}$ <30 mL/minute:

DVT prophylaxis in abdominal surgery, hip replacement, knee replacement, or in medical patients during acute illness: SubQ: 30 mg once daily

DVT treatment (inpatient or outpatient treatment in conjunction with warfarin): SubQ: 1 mg/kg once daily

STEMI:

<75 years: Initial: I.V.: 30 mg as a single dose with the first dose of the SubQ maintenance regimen administered at the same time as the I.V. bolus; Maintenance: SubQ: 1 mg/kg every 24 hours

≥75 years of age: Omit I.V. bolus; Maintenance: SubQ: 1 mg/kg every 24 hours

Unstable angina, NSTEMI: SubQ: 1 mg/kg once daily

Dialysis: Enoxaparin has not been FDA approved for use in dialysis patients. It's elimination is primarily via the renal route. Serious bleeding complications have been reported with use in patients who are dialysis dependent or have severe renal failure. LMWH administration at fixed doses without monitoring has greater unpredictable anticoagulant effects in patients with chronic kidney disease. If used, dosages should be reduced and anti-Xa levels frequently monitored, as accumulation may occur with repeated doses. Many clinicians would not use enoxaparin in this population especially without timely anti-Xa levels.

Hemodialysis: Supplemental dose is not necessary.

Peritoneal dialysis: Significant drug removal is unlikely based on physiochemical characteristics.

Administration Do **not** administer I.M.; should be administered by deep SubQ injection to the left or right anterolateral and left or right posterolateral abdominal wall. A single dose may be administered I.V. as part of treatment for ST-elevation myocardial infarction (STEMI) to patients <75 years of age; no I.V. bolus is given to patients ≥75 years of age. To avoid loss of drug from the 30 mg and 40 mg syringes, do not expel the air bubble from the syringe prior to injection. In order to minimize bruising, do not rub injection site. An automatic injector (Lovenox EasyInjector™) is available with the 30 mg and 40 mg syringes to aid the patient with self-injections. **Note:** Enoxaparin is available in 100 mg/mL and 150 mg/mL concentrations.

To convert from I.V. unfractionated heparin (UFH) infusion to SubQ enoxaparin (Nutescu, 2007): Calculate specific dose for enoxaparin based on indication, discontinue UFH and begin enoxaparin within 1 hour.

To convert from SubQ enoxaparin to I.V. UFH infusion (Nutescu, 2007): Discontinue enoxaparin, calculate specific dose for I.V. UFH infusion based on indication, omit heparin bolus/loading dose:

Converting from SubQ enoxaparin dosed every 12 hours: Start I.V. UFH infusion 10-11 hours after last dose of enoxaparin

Converting from SubQ enoxaparin dosed every 24 hours: Start I.V. UFH infusion 22-23 hours after last dose of enoxaparin

Monitoring Parameters Platelets, occult blood, anti-Xa levels, serum creatinine; monitoring of PT and/or aPTT is not necessary. Routine monitoring of anti-Xa levels is not required, but has been utilized in patients with obesity and/or renal insufficiency.

Reference Range The following therapeutic ranges for anti-Xa levels have been suggested, but have not been validated in a controlled trial. Anti-Xa level measured 4 hours postdose.

DVT treatment (every-12-hour dosing): 0.6-1 units/mL

DVT treatment (once-daily dosing): 1-2 units/mL

Special Geriatric Considerations No specific dosage adjustment recommendations for most indications, however, total clearance is lower and elimination is delayed in patients with renal failure. Adjustment may be necessary if renal impairment is present. In the treatment of STEMI, a lower dosage (0.75 mg/kg every 12 hours) and omission of the I.V. bolus, are recommended in patients ≥75 years of age.

ENOXAPARIN

In clinical trials, the efficacy of enoxaparin injection in elderly (≥65 years) was similar to that seen in younger patients (<65 years). The incidence of bleeding complications was similar between elderly and younger patients when 30 mg every 12 hours or 40 mg once daily doses of enoxaparin injection was administered at doses of 1.5 mg/kg/day or 1 mg/kg every 12 hours. The risk of enoxaparin injection associated bleeding increased with age. Serious adverse events increased with age for patients receiving enoxaparin injections. Other clinical experience has not revealed additional differences in the safety of enoxaparin injection between elderly and younger patients. Careful attention to dosing intervals and concomitant medications (especially antiplatelet medications) is advised. Monitoring of elderly patients with low body weight (<45 kg) and those predisposed to decreased renal function should be considered.

Dosage Forms Excipient information presented when available (limited, particularly for generics); consult specific product labeling.

Injection, solution, as sodium:

Lovenox®: 100 mg/mL (3 mL) [contains benzyl alcohol; vial]

Injection, solution, as sodium [preservative free]: 30 mg/0.3 mL (0.3 mL); 40 mg/0.4 mL (0.4 mL); 60 mg/0.6 mL (0.6 mL); 80 mg/0.8 mL (0.8 mL); 100 mg/mL (1 mL); 120 mg/0.8 mL (0.8 mL); 150 mg/mL (1 mL)

Lovenox®: 30 mg/0.3 mL (0.3 mL); 40 mg/0.4 mL (0.4 mL); 60 mg/0.6 mL (0.6 mL); 80 mg/0.8 mL (0.8 mL); 100 mg/mL (1 mL); 120 mg/0.8 mL (0.8 mL); 150 mg/mL (1 mL) [prefilled syringe]

♦ **Enoxaparin Sodium** *see* Enoxaparin *on page 598*

Entacapone (en TA ka pone)

Related Information

Antiparkinsonian Agents *on page 1995*

Brand Names: U.S. Comtan®

Brand Names: Canada Comtan®

Generic Availability (U.S.) No

Pharmacologic Category Anti-Parkinson's Agent, COMT Inhibitor

Use Adjunct to levodopa/carbidopa therapy in patients with idiopathic Parkinson's disease who experience "wearing-off" symptoms at the end of a dosing interval

Contraindications Hypersensitivity to entacapone or any of component of the formulation

Warnings/Precautions May cause orthostatic hypotension and syncope; Parkinson's disease patients appear to have an impaired capacity to respond to a postural challenge; use with caution in patients at risk of hypotension (such as those receiving antihypertensive drugs) or where transient hypotensive episodes would be poorly tolerated (cardiovascular disease or cerebrovascular disease). Parkinson's patients being treated with dopaminergic agonists ordinarily require careful monitoring for signs and symptoms of postural hypotension, especially during dose escalation, and should be informed of this risk. May cause hallucinations, which may improve with reduction in levodopa therapy. Use with caution in patients with pre-existing dyskinesias; exacerbation of pre-existing dyskinesia and severe rhabdomyolysis has been reported. Levodopa dosage reduction may be required, particularly in patients with levodopa dosages >600 mg daily or with moderate-to-severe dyskinesia prior to initiation. Entacapone, in conjunction with other drug therapy that alters brain biogenic amine concentrations (eg, MAO inhibitors, SSRIs), has been associated with a syndrome resembling neuroleptic malignant syndrome (hyperpyrexia and confusion - some fatal) on abrupt withdrawal or dosage reduction. Concomitant use of entacapone and nonselective MAO inhibitors should be avoided. Selegiline is a selective MAO type B inhibitor (when given orally at ≤10 mg/day) and can be taken with entacapone.

Dopaminergic agents have been associated with compulsive behaviors and/or loss of impulse control, which has manifested as pathological gambling, libido increases (hypersexuality), and/or binge eating. Causality has not been established, and controversy exists as to whether this phenomenon is related to the underlying disease, prior behaviors/addictions and/or drug therapy. Dose reduction or discontinuation of therapy has been reported to reverse these behaviors in some, but not all cases. Risk for melanoma development is increased in Parkinson's disease patients; drug causation or factors contributing to risk have not been established. Patients should be monitored closely and periodic skin examinations should be performed. Dopaminergic agents from the ergot class have also been associated with fibrotic complications, such as retroperitoneal fibrosis, pulmonary infiltrates or effusion and pleural thickening. It is unknown whether non-ergot, pro-dopaminergic agents like entacapone confer this risk. Use caution in patients with hepatic impairment or severe renal impairment. Do not withdraw therapy abruptly. Discoloration of urine, saliva, or sweat to dark colors (red, brown, black) may be observed during therapy. Use with caution in patients with lower gastrointestinal disease or an increased risk of dehydration; has been associated with delayed development of diarrhea (usual onset after 4-12 weeks). Diarrhea may be a sign of drug-induced colitis. Discontinue use with prolonged diarrhea.

Adverse Reactions (Reflective of adult population; not specific for elderly)
>10%:
Gastrointestinal: Nausea (14%)
Neuromuscular & skeletal: Dyskinesia (25%), placebo (15%)
1% to 10%:
Cardiovascular: Orthostatic hypotension (4%), syncope (1%)
Central nervous system: Dizziness (8%), fatigue (6%), hallucinations (4%), anxiety (2%), somnolence (2%), agitation (1%)
Dermatologic: Purpura (2%)
Gastrointestinal: Diarrhea (10%), abdominal pain (8%), constipation (6%), vomiting (4%), dry mouth (3%), dyspepsia (2%), flatulence (2%), gastritis (1%), taste perversion (1%)
Genitourinary: Brown-orange urine discoloration (10%)
Neuromuscular & skeletal: Hyperkinesia (10%), hypokinesia (9%), back pain (4%), weakness (2%)
Respiratory: Dyspnea (3%)
Miscellaneous: Diaphoresis increased (2%), bacterial infection (1%)

Drug Interactions
Metabolism/Transport Effects Inhibits CYP1A2 (weak), 2A6 (weak), 2C9 (weak), 2C19 (weak), 2D6 (weak), 2E1 (weak), 3A4 (weak)
Avoid Concomitant Use There are no known interactions where it is recommended to avoid concomitant use.

Increased Effect/Toxicity
Entacapone may increase the levels/effects of: Alcohol (Ethyl); CNS Depressants; COMT Substrates; MAO Inhibitors; Methotrimeprazine; Selective Serotonin Reuptake Inhibitors

The levels/effects of Entacapone may be increased by: Droperidol; HydrOXYzine; Methotrimeprazine
Decreased Effect There are no known significant interactions involving a decrease in effect.

Ethanol/Nutrition/Herb Interactions
Ethanol: May increase CNS depression; monitor for increased effects with coadministration. Caution patients about effects.
Food: Entacapone has been reported to chelate iron and decreasing serum iron levels were noted in clinical trials; however, clinically significant anemia has not been observed.

Mechanism of Action Entacapone is a reversible and selective inhibitor of catechol-O-methyltransferase (COMT). When entacapone is taken with levodopa, the pharmacokinetics are altered, resulting in more sustained levodopa serum levels compared to levodopa taken alone. The resulting levels of levodopa provide for increased concentrations available for absorption across the blood-brain barrier, thereby providing for increased CNS levels of dopamine, the active metabolite of levodopa.

Pharmacodynamics/Kinetics
Onset of action: Rapid
Peak effect: 1 hour
Absorption: Rapid
Distribution: I.V.: V_{dss}: 20 L
Protein binding: 98%, primarily to albumin
Metabolism: Isomerization to the *cis*-isomer, followed by direct glucuronidation of the parent and *cis*-isomer
Bioavailability: 35%
Half-life elimination: B phase: 0.4-0.7 hours; Y phase: 2.4 hours
Time to peak, serum: 1 hour
Excretion: Feces (90%); urine (10%)

Dosage
Geriatric & Adult Parkinson's disease: Oral: 200 mg with each dose of levodopa/carbidopa, up to a maximum of 8 times/day (maximum daily dose: 1600 mg/day). To optimize therapy, the dosage of levodopa may need reduced or the dosing interval may need extended. Patients taking levodopa ≥800 mg/day or who had moderate-to-severe dyskinesias prior to therapy required an average decrease of 25% in the daily levodopa dose.
Renal Impairment No adjustment is required; dialysis patients were not studied.
Hepatic Impairment Dosage adjustment in chronic therapy with standard treatment has not been studied.
Administration Always administer in association with levodopa/carbidopa; can be combined with both the immediate and sustained release formulations of levodopa/carbidopa. May be administered without regard to meals. Should not be abruptly withdrawn from patient's therapy due to significant worsening of symptoms.

◀ **Monitoring Parameters** Signs and symptoms of Parkinson's disease; liver function tests, blood pressure, patient's mental status; serum iron (if signs of anemia)

Pharmacotherapy Pearls No increase in LFTs has been noted; therefore, does not require LFT monitoring. Because of this, entacapone may be preferred over the other COMT inhibitor, tolcapone, in patients with "wearing off". Entacapone has not been studied in patients with stable Parkinson's disease.

Special Geriatric Considerations No difference in adverse effects was noted in the elderly. Monitor levodopa dose.

Dosage Forms Excipient information presented when available (limited, particularly for generics); consult specific product labeling.

Tablet, oral:

Comtan®: 200 mg

Selected References

Holm KJ and Spencer CM, "Entacapone. A Review of Its Use in Parkinson's Disease," *Drugs*, 1999, 58(1):159-77.

Olanow CW, Watts RL, and Koller WC, "An Algorithm (Decision Tree) for the Management of Parkinson's Disease (2001): Treatment Guidelines," *Neurology*, 2001, 56(11 Suppl 5):S1-S88.

Pahwa R, Factor SA, Lyons KE, et al, "Practice Parameter: Treatment of Parkinson Disease With Motor Fluctuations and Dyskinesia (An Evidence-Based Review): Report of the Quality Standards Subcommittee of the American Academy of Neurology," *Neurology*, 2006, 66(7):983-95.

◆ **Entacapone, Carbidopa, and Levodopa** *see* Levodopa, Carbidopa, and Entacapone *on page 1051*

◆ **Entertainer's Secret® [OTC]** *see* Saliva Substitute *on page 1652*

◆ **Entocort® EC** *see* Budesonide (Systemic, Oral Inhalation) *on page 219*

◆ **Entsol® [OTC]** *see* Sodium Chloride *on page 1690*

◆ **Enulose** *see* Lactulose *on page 1022*

EPHEDrine (Systemic) (e FED rin)

Medication Safety Issues

Sound-alike/look-alike issues:

EPHEDrine may be confused with Epifrin®, EPINEPHrine

Index Terms Ephedrine Sulfate

Generic Availability (U.S.) Yes

Pharmacologic Category Alpha/Beta Agonist

Use Treatment of nasal congestion, anesthesia-induced hypotension

Unlabeled/Investigational Use Postoperative nausea and vomiting (PONV) refractory to traditional antiemetics; idiopathic orthostatic hypotension

Contraindications Hypersensitivity to ephedrine or any component of the formulation; angle-closure glaucoma; concurrent use of other sympathomimetic agents

Warnings/Precautions Blood volume depletion should be corrected before injectable ephedrine therapy is instituted; use caution in patients with unstable vasomotor symptoms, diabetes, hyperthyroidism, prostatic hyperplasia or a history of seizures; also use caution in the elderly and those patients with cardiovascular disorders such as coronary artery disease, arrhythmias, and hypertension. Ephedrine may cause hypertension. Long-term use may cause anxiety and symptoms of paranoid schizophrenia. Use with caution in the elderly, since it crosses the blood-brain barrier and may cause confusion. Use with extreme caution in patients taking MAO inhibitors.

Adverse Reactions (Reflective of adult population; not specific for elderly) Frequency not defined.

Cardiovascular: Arrhythmias, chest pain, elevation or depression of blood pressure, hypertension, palpitation, tachycardia, unusual pallor

Central nervous system: Agitation, anxiety, apprehension, CNS stimulating effects, dizziness, excitation, fear, headache hyperactivity, insomnia, irritability, nervousness, restlessness, tension

Gastrointestinal: Anorexia, GI upset, nausea, vomiting, xerostomia

Genitourinary: Painful urination

Neuromuscular & skeletal: Trembling, tremor (more common in the elderly), weakness

Respiratory: Dyspnea

Miscellaneous: Diaphoresis increased

Drug Interactions

Avoid Concomitant Use

Avoid concomitant use of EPHEDrine (Systemic) with any of the following: Iobenguane I 123; MAO Inhibitors

Increased Effect/Toxicity

EPHEDrine (Systemic) may increase the levels/effects of: Bromocriptine; Sympathomimetics

The levels/effects of EPHEDrine (Systemic) may be increased by: Antacids; Atomoxetine; Cannabinoids; Carbonic Anhydrase Inhibitors; MAO Inhibitors; Serotonin/Norepinephrine Reuptake Inhibitors

Decreased Effect

EPHEDrine (Systemic) may decrease the levels/effects of: Benzylpenicilloyl Polylysine; Iobenguane I 123

The levels/effects of EPHEDrine (Systemic) may be decreased by: Spironolactone

Ethanol/Nutrition/Herb Interactions Herb/Nutraceutical: Avoid ephedra, yohimbe (may cause CNS stimulation).

Stability Protect all dosage forms from light.

Injection: Store at room temperature. **Note:** Storage guidelines vary; check product labeling for exact temperature range.

Mechanism of Action Releases tissue stores of norepinephrine and thereby produces an alpha- and beta-adrenergic stimulation; longer-acting and less potent than epinephrine

Pharmacodynamics/Kinetics

Duration: Oral: 3-6 hours

Metabolism: Minimally hepatic; metabolites include p-hydroxyephedrine, p-hydroxynorephedrine, norephedrine

Half-life elimination: 2.5-3.6 hours

Excretion: Urine (60% to 77% as unchanged drug) within 24 hours

Dosage

Geriatric & Adult

Hypotension induced by anesthesia: I.V.: 5-25 mg/dose slow I.V. push repeated after 5-10 minutes as needed, then every 3-4 hours (maximum: 150 mg/24 hours)

Idiopathic orthostatic hypotension (unlabeled use): Oral: 25-50 mg 3 times/day; maximum: 150 mg/day. **Note:** Not considered first-line for this indication.

PONV refractory to traditional antiemetics (unlabeled use): I.M.: 0.5 mg/kg at the end of surgery (Gan, 2007; Hagemann, 2000)

Administration Injection solution: Dilute to 5 or 10 mg/mL. Administer as a slow I.V. push. Do not administer unless solution is clear.

Monitoring Parameters Injection solution: Monitor blood pressure, pulse

Test Interactions Can cause a false-positive amphetamine EMIT assay

Special Geriatric Considerations Avoid as a bronchodilator. Use caution since it crosses the blood-brain barrier and may cause confusion.

Dosage Forms Excipient information presented when available (limited, particularly for generics); consult specific product labeling. [DSC] = Discontinued product

Capsule, oral, as sulfate: 25 mg

Injection, solution, as sulfate: 50 mg/mL (1 mL [DSC], 10 mL [DSC])

Injection, solution, as sulfate [preservative free]: 50 mg/mL (1 mL)

◆ **Ephedrine Sulfate** *see* EPHEDrine (Systemic) *on page 604*
◆ **Epiflur™** *see* Fluoride *on page 751*
◆ **Epiklor™** *see* Potassium Chloride *on page 1487*
◆ **Epiklor™/25** *see* Potassium Chloride *on page 1487*

Epinastine (ep i NAS teen)

Brand Names: U.S. Elestat®

Index Terms Epinastine Hydrochloride

Generic Availability (U.S.) Yes

Pharmacologic Category Histamine H_1 Antagonist; Histamine H_1 Antagonist, Second Generation

Use Treatment of allergic conjunctivitis

Dosage

Geriatric & Adult Allergic conjunctivitis: Ophthalmic: Instill 1 drop into each eye twice daily. Continue throughout period of exposure, even in the absence of symptoms.

Special Geriatric Considerations No difference in safety and efficacy was observed between elderly and younger patients.

Dosage Forms Excipient information presented when available (limited, particularly for generics); consult specific product labeling.

Solution, ophthalmic, as hydrochloride [drops]: 0.05% (5 mL)

Elestat®: 0.05% (5 mL) [contains benzalkonium chloride]

♦ **Epinastine Hydrochloride** *see* Epinastine *on page 605*

EPINEPHrine (Systemic, Oral Inhalation) (ep i NEF rin)

Medication Safety Issues

Sound-alike/look-alike issues:

EPINEPHrine may be confused with ePHEDrine

Epifrin® may be confused with ephedrine, EpiPen®

EpiPen® may be confused with Epifrin®

High alert medication:

The Institute for Safe Medication Practices (ISMP) includes this medication among its list of drugs which have a heightened risk of causing significant patient harm when used in error.

Administration issues:

Medication errors have occurred due to confusion with epinephrine products expressed as ratio strengths (eg, 1:1000 vs 1:10,000).

Epinephrine 1:1000 = 1 mg/mL and is most commonly used I.M.

Epinephrine 1:10,000 = 0.1 mg/mL and is used I.V.

Medication errors have occurred when topical epinephrine 1 mg/mL (1:1000) has been inadvertently injected. Vials of injectable and topical epinephrine look very similar. Epinephrine should always be appropriately labeled with the intended administration.

International issues:

EpiPen [U.S., Canada, and multiple international markets] may be confused with Epigen brand name for glycyrrhizinic acid [Argentina, Mexico, Russia] and Epopen brand name for epoetin alfa [Spain]

Brand Names: U.S. Adrenaclick™ [DSC]; Adrenalin®; EpiPen 2-Pak®; EpiPen Jr 2-Pak®; EpiPen® Jr. [DSC]; EpiPen® [DSC]; Primatene® Mist [OTC]; S2® [OTC]; Twinject®

Brand Names: Canada Adrenalin®; Epi E-Z Pen®; EpiPen®; EpiPen® Jr; Twinject®

Index Terms Adrenaline; Epinephrine Bitartrate; Epinephrine Hydrochloride; Racemic Epinephrine; Racepinephrine

Generic Availability (U.S.) Yes: Solution for injection

Pharmacologic Category Alpha/Beta Agonist

Use Treatment of bronchospasms, bronchial asthma, viral croup, anaphylactic reactions, cardiac arrest; added to local anesthetics to decrease systemic absorption of intraspinal and local anesthetics and increase duration of action; decrease superficial hemorrhage

Unlabeled/Investigational Use ACLS guidelines: Ventricular fibrillation (VF) or pulseless ventricular tachycardia (VT) unresponsive to initial defibrillatory shocks; pulseless electrical activity; asystole; hypotension/shock unresponsive to volume resuscitation; symptomatic bradycardia unresponsive to atropine or pacing; inotropic support

Contraindications There are no absolute contraindications to the use of injectable epinephrine (including EpiPen®, EpiPen® Jr, and Twinject®) in a life-threatening situation.

Oral inhalation: Concurrent use or within 2 weeks of MAO inhibitors

Injectable solution: Per the manufacturer, contraindicated in narrow-angle glaucoma; shock; during general anesthesia with halogenated hydrocarbons or cyclopropane (currently not available in U.S.); individuals with organic brain damage; with local anesthesia of the digits; during labor; heart failure; coronary insufficiency

Warnings/Precautions Use with caution in elderly patients, patients with diabetes mellitus, cardiovascular diseases (eg, coronary artery disease, hypertension), thyroid disease, cerebrovascular disease, Parkinson's disease, or patients taking tricyclic antidepressants. Some products contain sulfites as preservatives; the presence of sulfites in some products (eg, EpiPen® and Twinject®) should not deter administration during a serious allergic or other emergency situation even if the patient is sulfite-sensitive. Accidental injection into digits, hands, or feet may result in local reactions, including injection site pallor, coldness and hypoesthesia or injury, resulting in bruising, bleeding, discoloration, erythema or skeletal injury; patient should seek immediate medical attention if this occurs. Rapid I.V. administration may cause death from cerebrovascular hemorrhage or cardiac arrhythmias; however, rapid I.V. administration during pulseless arrest is necessary.

Oral inhalation: Use with caution in patients with prostate enlargement or urinary retention; may cause temporary worsening of symptoms.

Self medication (OTC use): Oral inhalation: Prior to self-medication, patients should contact healthcare provider. The product should only be used in persons with a diagnosis of asthma. If symptoms are not relieved in 20 minutes or become worse do not continue to use the product - seek immediate medical assistance. The product should not be used more frequently or at higher doses than recommended unless directed by a healthcare provider. This product should not be used in patients who have required hospitalization for asthma or if a patient is taking prescription medication for asthma. Do not use if you have taken a MAO inhibitor (certain drugs used for depression, Parkinson's disease, or other conditions) within 2 weeks.

Adverse Reactions (Reflective of adult population; not specific for elderly) Frequency not defined.

Cardiovascular: Angina, cardiac arrhythmia, chest pain, flushing, hypertension, pallor, palpitation, sudden death, tachycardia (parenteral), vasoconstriction, ventricular ectopy

Central nervous system: Anxiety (transient), apprehensiveness, cerebral hemorrhage, dizziness, headache, insomnia, lightheadedness, nervousness, restlessness

Gastrointestinal: Dry throat, loss of appetite, nausea, vomiting, xerostomia

Genitourinary: Acute urinary retention in patients with bladder outflow obstruction

Neuromuscular & skeletal: Tremor, weakness

Ocular: Allergic lid reaction, burning, eye pain, ocular irritation, precipitation of or exacerbation of narrow-angle glaucoma, transient stinging

Respiratory: Dyspnea, pulmonary edema

Miscellaneous: Diaphoresis

Drug Interactions

Avoid Concomitant Use

Avoid concomitant use of EPINEPHrine (Systemic, Oral Inhalation) with any of the following: Iobenguane I 123; Lurasidone

Increased Effect/Toxicity

EPINEPHrine (Systemic, Oral Inhalation) may increase the levels/effects of: Bromocriptine; Lurasidone; Sympathomimetics

The levels/effects of EPINEPHrine (Systemic, Oral Inhalation) may be increased by: Antacids; Atomoxetine; Beta-Blockers; Cannabinoids; Carbonic Anhydrase Inhibitors; COMT Inhibitors; Inhalational Anesthetics; MAO Inhibitors; Serotonin/Norepinephrine Reuptake Inhibitors; Tricyclic Antidepressants

Decreased Effect

EPINEPHrine (Systemic, Oral Inhalation) may decrease the levels/effects of: Benzylpenicilloyl Polylysine; Iobenguane I 123

The levels/effects of EPINEPHrine (Systemic, Oral Inhalation) may be decreased by: Spironolactone

Ethanol/Nutrition/Herb Interactions Herb/Nutraceutical: Avoid ephedra, yohimbe (may cause CNS stimulation).

Stability Epinephrine is sensitive to light and air; protection from light is recommended. Oxidation turns drug pink, then a brown color. **Solutions should not be used if they are discolored or contain a precipitate.**

Adrenalin®: Store between 15°C to 25°C (59°F to 77°F); do not freeze. Protect from light. The 1:1000 solution should be discarded 30 days after initial use.

EpiPen® and EpiPen® Jr: Store at 25°C (77°F); excursions permitted to 15°C to 30°C (59°F to 86°F); do not freeze or refrigerate. Protect from light by storing in carrier tube provided.

Twinject®: Store between 20°C to 25°C (68°F to 77°F); excursions permitted to 15°C to 30°C (59°F to 86°F); do not freeze or refrigerate. Protect from light.

Primatene® Mist: Store between 20°C to 25°C (68°F to 77°F).

S2®: Store between 2°C to 20°C (36°F to 68°F). Protect from light. Dilution not required when administered via hand-bulb nebulizer; dilute with NS 3-5 mL if using jet nebulizer

Stability of injection of parenteral admixture at room temperature (25°C) or refrigeration (4°C) is 24 hours.

Standard I.V. diluent: 1 mg/250 mL NS.

Preparation of adult I.V. infusion: Dilute 1 mg in 250 mL of D_5W or NS (4 mcg/mL).

Mechanism of Action Stimulates alpha-, beta$_1$-, and beta$_2$-adrenergic receptors resulting in relaxation of smooth muscle of the bronchial tree, cardiac stimulation (increasing myocardial oxygen consumption), and dilation of skeletal muscle vasculature; small doses can cause vasodilation via beta$_2$-vascular receptors; large doses may produce constriction of skeletal and vascular smooth muscle

Pharmacodynamics/Kinetics

Onset of action: Bronchodilation: SubQ: ~5-10 minutes; Inhalation: ~1 minute

Metabolism: Taken up into the adrenergic neuron and metabolized by monoamine oxidase and catechol-o-methyltransferase; circulating drug hepatically metabolized

Excretion: Urine (as inactive metabolites, metanephrine, and sulfate and hydroxy derivatives of mandelic acid, small amounts as unchanged drug)

Dosage

Geriatric & Adult

Asystole/pulseless arrest, pulseless VT/VF (ACLS, 2010):

I.V., I.O.: 1 mg every 3-5 minutes until return of spontaneous circulation; if this approach fails, higher doses of epinephrine (up to 0.2 mg/kg) have been used for treatment of specific problems (eg, beta-blocker or calcium channel blocker overdose)

Endotracheal: 2-2.5 mg every 3-5 minutes until I.V./I.O access established or return of spontaneous circulation; dilute in 5-10 mL NS or sterile water. **Note:** Absorption may be greater with sterile water (Naganobu, 2000). May cause false-negative reading with exhaled CO_2 detectors; use second method to confirm tube placement if CO_2 is not detected (Neumar, 2010).

Bradycardia (symptomatic; unresponsive to atropine or pacing): *I.V. infusion:* 2-10 mcg/minute **or** 0.1-0.5 mcg/kg/minute (7-35 mcg/minute in a 70 kg patient); titrate to desired effect (ACLS, 2010)

Bronchodilator:

SubQ: 0.3-0.5 mg (**1:1000** [1 mg/mL] solution) every 20 minutes for 3 doses

Nebulization: S2® (racepinephrine, OTC labeling)

Hand-bulb nebulizer: Add 0.5 mL (~10 drops) to nebulizer; 1-3 inhalations up to every 3 hours if needed

Jet nebulizer: Add 0.5 mL (~10 drops) to nebulizer and dilute with 3 mL of NS; administer over ~15 minutes every 3-4 hours as needed

Inhalation: Primatene® Mist (OTC labeling): One inhalation, wait at least 1 minute; if not relieved, may use once more. Do not use again for at least 3 hours.

Hypersensitivity reaction: Note: SubQ administration results in slower absorption and is less reliable. I.M. administration in the anterolateral aspect of the middle third of the thigh is preferred in the setting of anaphylaxis (ACLS guidelines, 2010; Kemp, 2008).

I.M., SubQ: 0.2-0.5 mg (**1:1000** [1 mg/mL] solution) every 5-15 minutes in the absence of clinical improvement (ACLS 2010; Kemp, 2008; Lieberman, 2010). If clinician deems appropriate, the 5-minute interval between injections may be shortened to allow for more frequent administration (Lieberman, 2010).

I.V.: 0.1 mg (**1:10,000** [0.1 mg/mL] solution) over 5 minutes; may infuse at 1-4 mcg/minute to prevent the need to repeat injections frequently **or** may initiate with an infusion at 5-15 mcg/minute (with crystalloid administration) (ACLS, 2010; Brown, 2004). In general, I.V. administration should only be done in patients who are profoundly hypotensive or are in cardiopulmonary arrest refractory to volume resuscitation and several epinephrine injections (Lieberman, 2010).

Self-administration following severe allergic reactions (eg, insect stings, food): **Note:** The World Health Organization (WHO) and Anaphylaxis Canada recommend the availability of one dose for every 10-20 minutes of travel time to a medical emergency facility. More than 2 doses should only be administered under direct medical supervision.

Twinject®: I.M., SubQ: 0.3 mg; if anaphylactic symptoms persist, dose may be repeated in 5-15 minutes using the same device after partial disassembly

EpiPen®: I.M., SubQ: 0.3 mg; if anaphylactic symptoms persist, dose may be repeated in 5-15 minutes using an additional EpiPen®

Hypotension/shock, severe and fluid resistant (unlabeled use): *I.V. infusion:* Initial: 0.1-0.5 mcg/kg/minute (7-35 mcg/minute in a 70 kg patient); titrate to desired response (ACLS, 2010)

Administration When administering as a continuous infusion, central line administration is preferred. I.V. infusions require an infusion pump. Epinephrine solutions for injection can be administered I.M., I.O., endotracheally, I.V., or SubQ. **Note:** EpiPen® and EpiPen® Jr Auto-Injectors contain a single, fixed-dose of epinephrine. Twinject® Auto-Injectors contain two doses; the first fixed-dose is available for auto-injection; the second dose is available for manual injection following partial disassembly of device.

Subcutaneous: SubQ administration results in slower absorption and is less reliable.

I.M.: I.M. administration into the buttocks should be avoided. I.M. administration in the anterolateral aspect of the middle third of the thigh is preferred in the setting of anaphylaxis (ACLS guidelines, 2010; Kemp, 2008). EpiPen®, EpiPen® Jr, and Twinject® Auto-Injectors should only be injected into the anterolateral aspect of the thigh, through clothing if necessary.

Endotracheal: Dilute in NS or sterile water. Absorption may be greater with sterile water (Naganobu, 2000). Pass catheter beyond tip of tracheal tube, stop compressions, spray drug quickly down tube. Follow immediately with several quick insufflations and continue chest compressions. May cause false-negative reading with exhaled CO_2 detectors; use second method to confirm tube placement if CO_2 is not detected (Neumar, 2010).

Oral inhalation: S2®: If using jet nebulizer: Administer over ~15 minutes; must be diluted. If using hand-held rubber bulb nebulizer, dilution is not required.

Extravasation management: Use phentolamine as antidote. Mix 5 mg phentolamine with 9 mL of NS. Inject a small amount of this dilution into extravasated area. Blanching should reverse immediately. Monitor site. If blanching should recur, additional injections of phentolamine may be needed.

Monitoring Parameters Pulmonary function, heart rate, blood pressure, site of infusion for blanching, extravasation; cardiac monitor and blood pressure monitor required during continuous infusion. If using to treat hypotension, assess intravascular volume and support as needed.

Pharmacotherapy Pearls Twinject® and EpiPen® are not interchangeable due to packaging considerations.

Special Geriatric Considerations The use of epinephrine in the treatment of acute exacerbations of asthma was studied in the elderly. A dose of 0.3 mg SubQ every 20 minutes for three doses was well tolerated in elderly patients with no history of angina or recent myocardial infarction. There was no significant difference in the incidence of ventricular arrhythmias in elderly versus younger adults.

Dosage Forms Excipient information presented when available (limited, particularly for generics); consult specific product labeling. [DSC] = Discontinued product

Aerosol, for oral inhalation:

Primatene® Mist: 0.22 mg/inhalation (15 mL) [contains chlorofluorocarbon, dehydrated ethanol 34%]

Injection, solution: 0.1 mg/mL (10 mL); 0.15 mg/0.15 mL (1.1 mL) [1:1000 solution; delivers 0.15 mg per injection]; 0.3 mg/0.3 mL (1.1 mL) [1:1000 solution; delivers 0.3 mg per injection]; 1 mg/mL (1 mL)

Adrenaclick™: 0.15 mg/0.15 mL (1.1 mL [DSC]) [contains chlorobutanol, sodium bisulfite; 1:1000 solution; delivers 0.15 mg per injection]

Adrenaclick™: 0.3 mg/0.3 mL (1.1 mL [DSC]) [contains chlorobutanol, sodium bisulfite; 1:1000 solution; delivers 0.3 mg per injection]

EpiPen 2-Pak®: 0.3 mg/0.3 mL (2 mL) [contains sodium metabisulfite; 1:1000 solution; delivers 0.3 mg per injection]

EpiPen Jr 2-Pak®: 0.15 mg/0.3 mL (2 mL) [contains sodium metabisulfite; 1:2000 solution; delivers 0.15 mg per injection]

EpiPen®: 0.3 mg/0.3 mL (2 mL [DSC]) [contains sodium metabisulfite; 1:1000 solution; delivers 0.3 mg per injection]

EpiPen® Jr.: 0.15 mg/0.3 mL (2 mL [DSC]) [contains sodium metabisulfite; 1:2000 solution; delivers 0.15 mg per injection]

Twinject®: 0.15 mg/0.15 mL (1.1 mL) [contains chlorobutanol, sodium bisulfite; 1:1000 solution; delivers 0.15 mg per injection]

Twinject®: 0.3 mg/0.3 mL (1.1 mL) [contains chlorobutanol, sodium bisulfite; 1:1000 solution; delivers 0.3 mg per injection]

Injection, solution, as hydrochloride: 1 mg/mL (30 mL)

Adrenalin®: 1 mg/mL (30 mL) [contains chlorobutanol, sodium bisulfite; 1:1000 solution]

Adrenalin®: 1 mg/mL (1 mL) [contains sodium bisulfite; 1:1000 solution]

Injection, solution, as hydrochloride [preservative free]: 1 mg/mL (1 mL)

Solution, for oral inhalation [racepinephrine, preservative free]:

S2®: 2.25% (0.5 mL) [as d-epinephrine 1.125% and l-epinephrine 1.125%]

Selected References

Cydulka R, Davison R, Grammer L, et al, "The Use of Epinephrine in the Treatment of Older Adult Asthmatics," *Ann Emerg Med*, 1988, 17(4):322-6.

Field JM, Hazinski MF, Sayre MR, et al, "Part 1: Executive Summary: 2010 American Heart Association Guidelines for Cardiopulmonary Resuscitation and Emergency Cardiovascular Care," *Circulation*, 2010, 122(18 Suppl 3):640-56.

National Asthma Education and Prevention Program, "Expert Panel Report 3 (EPR-3): Guidelines for the Diagnosis and Management of Asthma-Summary Report 2007," *J Allergy Clin Immunol*, 2007, 120(5 Suppl):94-138.

♦ **Epinephrine Bitartrate** *see* EPINEPHrine (Systemic, Oral Inhalation) *on page 606*
♦ **Epinephrine Hydrochloride** *see* EPINEPHrine (Systemic, Oral Inhalation) *on page 606*
♦ **EpiPen® [DSC]** *see* EPINEPHrine (Systemic, Oral Inhalation) *on page 606*
♦ **EpiPen 2-Pak®** *see* EPINEPHrine (Systemic, Oral Inhalation) *on page 606*
♦ **EpiPen® Jr. [DSC]** *see* EPINEPHrine (Systemic, Oral Inhalation) *on page 606*
♦ **EpiPen Jr 2-Pak®** *see* EPINEPHrine (Systemic, Oral Inhalation) *on page 606*
♦ **Epitol®** *see* CarBAMazepine *on page 268*

Eplerenone (e PLER en one)

Medication Safety Issues
Sound-alike/look-alike issues:
Inspra™ may be confused with Spiriva®
Brand Names: U.S. Inspra™
Generic Availability (U.S.) Yes

EPLERENONE

◀ **Pharmacologic Category** Diuretic, Potassium-Sparing; Selective Aldosterone Blocker

Use Treatment of hypertension (may be used alone or in combination with other antihypertensive agents); treatment of heart failure (HF) following acute MI

Contraindications Serum potassium >5.5 mEq/L at initiation; Cl_{cr} ≤30 mL/minute; concomitant use of strong CYP3A4 inhibitors (see Drug Interactions for details)

The following additional contraindications apply to patients with hypertension: Type 2 diabetes mellitus (noninsulin dependent, NIDDM) with microalbuminuria; serum creatinine >2.0 mg/dL in males or >1.8 mg/dL in females; Cl_{cr} <50 mL/minute; concomitant use with potassium supplements or potassium-sparing diuretics

Warnings/Precautions Dosage adjustment needed for patients on moderate CYP3A4 inhibitors. Monitor closely for hyperkalemia; increases in serum potassium were dose related during clinical trials and rates of hyperkalemia also increased with declining renal function. Safety and efficacy have not been established in patients with severe hepatic impairment. Use with caution in HF patients post-MI with diabetes (especially if patient has proteinuria); risk of hyperkalemia is increased. Risk of hyperkalemia is increased with declining renal function. Use with caution in patients with mild renal impairment; contraindicated with moderate-severe impairment (HTN: Cl_{cr} <50 mL/minute; other indications: Cl_{cr} ≤30 mL/minute).

Adverse Reactions (Reflective of adult population; not specific for elderly)

>10%: Endocrine & metabolic: Hyperkalemia ([HF post-MI: K >5.5 mEq/L: 16%; K ≥6 mEq/L: 6%] [HTN: K >5.5 mEq/L at doses ≤100 mg: ≤1%; doses >100 mg: 9%]), hypertriglyceridemia (1% to 15%, dose related)

1% to 10%:

Central nervous system: Dizziness (3%), fatigue (2%)

Endocrine & metabolic: Hyponatremia (2%, dose related), breast pain (males <1% to 1%), gynecomastia (males <1% to 1%), hypercholesterolemia (<1% to 1%)

Gastrointestinal: Diarrhea (2%), abdominal pain (1%)

Genitourinary: Abnormal vaginal bleeding (<1% to 2%)

Renal: Creatinine increased (HF post-MI: 6%), albuminuria (1%)

Respiratory: Cough (2%)

Miscellaneous: Flu-like syndrome (2%)

Drug Interactions

Metabolism/Transport Effects Substrate of CYP3A4 (major)

Avoid Concomitant Use

Avoid concomitant use of Eplerenone with any of the following: CYP3A4 Inhibitors (Strong); Itraconazole; Ketoconazole; Ketoconazole (Systemic); Posaconazole; Tacrolimus; Voriconazole

Increased Effect/Toxicity

Eplerenone may increase the levels/effects of: ACE Inhibitors; Amifostine; Angiotensin II Receptor Blockers; Antihypertensives; Hypotensive Agents; Potassium Salts; Potassium-Sparing Diuretics; RiTUXimab; Tacrolimus

The levels/effects of Eplerenone may be increased by: Alfuzosin; Calcium Channel Blockers (Nondihydropyridine); CYP3A4 Inhibitors (Moderate); CYP3A4 Inhibitors (Strong); Dasatinib; Diazoxide; Fluconazole; Herbs (Hypotensive Properties); Itraconazole; Ketoconazole; Ketoconazole (Systemic); Macrolide Antibiotics; MAO Inhibitors; Nonsteroidal Anti-Inflammatory Agents; Pentoxifylline; Phosphodiesterase 5 Inhibitors; Posaconazole; Prostacyclin Analogues; Protease Inhibitors; Voriconazole

Decreased Effect

The levels/effects of Eplerenone may be decreased by: CYP3A4 Inducers (Strong); Deferasirox; Herbs (CYP3A4 Inducers); Herbs (Hypertensive Properties); Methylphenidate; Nonsteroidal Anti-Inflammatory Agents; Tocilizumab; Yohimbine

Ethanol/Nutrition/Herb Interactions

Food: Grapefruit juice increases eplerenone AUC ~25%.

Herb/Nutraceutical: St John's wort may decrease levels of eplerenone. Avoid black cohosh, California poppy, coleus, golden seal, hawthorn, mistletoe, periwinkle, quinine, shepherd's purse (may have increased antihypertensive effect). Avoid bayberry, blue cohosh, cayenne, ephedra, ginger, ginseng (American), kola, licorice (may diminish the antihypertensive effect).

Stability Store at controlled room temperature of 25°C (77°F).

Mechanism of Action Aldosterone, a mineralocorticoid, increases blood pressure primarily by inducing sodium and water retention. Overexpression of aldosterone is thought to contribute to myocardial fibrosis (especially following myocardial infarction) and vascular fibrosis. Mineralocorticoid receptors are located in the kidney, heart, blood vessels, and brain. Eplerenone selectively blocks mineralocorticoid receptors reducing blood pressure in a dose-dependent manner and appears to prevent myocardial and vascular fibrosis.

Pharmacodynamics/Kinetics

Distribution: V_d: 43-90 L

Protein binding: ~50%; primarily to alpha$_1$-acid glycoproteins

Metabolism: Primarily hepatic via CYP3A4; metabolites inactive

Bioavailability: 69%

Half-life elimination: 4-6 hours

Time to peak, plasma: ~1.5 hours; may take up to 4 weeks for full antihypertensive effect

Excretion: Urine (~67%); feces (32%); <5% as unchanged drug in urine and feces

Dosage

Geriatric & Adult

Hypertension: Oral: Initial: 50 mg once daily; may increase to 50 mg twice daily if response is not adequate; may take up to 4 weeks for full therapeutic response. Doses >100 mg/day are associated with increased risk of hyperkalemia and no greater therapeutic effect.

Dose modification during concurrent use with moderate CYP3A4 inhibitors: Initial: 25 mg once daily

Heart failure (post-MI): Oral: Initial: 25 mg once daily; dosage goal: Titrate to 50 mg once daily within 4 weeks, as tolerated

Dosage adjustment per serum potassium concentrations for HF (post-MI):

<5.0 mEq/L:

Increase dose from 25 mg every other day to 25 mg daily **or**

Increase dose from 25 mg daily to 50 mg daily

5.0-5.4 mEq/L: No adjustment needed

5.5-5.9 mEq/L:

Decrease dose from 50 mg daily to 25 mg daily **or**

Decrease dose from 25 mg daily to 25 mg every other day **or**

Decrease dose from 25 mg every other day to withhold medication

≥6.0 mEq/L: Withhold medication until potassium <5.5 mEq/L, then restart at 25 mg every other day

Renal Impairment

Hypertension: Cl_{cr} <50 mL/minute or serum creatinine >2.0 mg/dL in males or >1.8 mg/dL in females: Use is contraindicated; risk of hyperkalemia increases with declining renal function

All other indications: Cl_{cr} ≤30 mL/minute: Use is contraindicated.

Hepatic Impairment No dosage adjustment needed for mild-to-moderate impairment. Safety and efficacy not established for severe impairment.

Administration May be administered with or without food.

Monitoring Parameters Blood pressure; serum potassium (levels monitored prior to therapy, within the first week, and at 1 month after start of treatment or dose adjustment, then periodically [monthly in clinical trials]); renal function

Special Geriatric Considerations Since this medication is contraindicated in the treatment of hypertension in patients with a Cl_{cr} <50 mL/minute, it may have limited use in the elderly. Due to physiologic changes, elderly may be at increased risk of hyperkalemia when using this medication.

Dosage Forms Excipient information presented when available (limited, particularly for generics); consult specific product labeling.

Tablet, oral: 25 mg, 50 mg

Inspra™: 25 mg, 50 mg

◆ **EPO** *see* Epoetin Alfa *on page 611*

Epoetin Alfa (e POE e tin AL fa)

Medication Safety Issues

Sound-alike/look-alike issues:

Epoetin alfa may be confused with darbepoetin alfa, epoetin beta

Epogen® may be confused with Neupogen®

International issues:

Epopen [Spain] may be confused with EpiPen brand name for epinephrine [U.S., Canada, and multiple international markets]

Brand Names: U.S. Epogen®; Procrit®

Brand Names: Canada Eprex®

Index Terms rHuEPO; rHuEPO-α; EPO; Erythropoiesis-Stimulating Agent (ESA); Erythropoietin

Generic Availability (U.S.) No

Pharmacologic Category Colony Stimulating Factor; Growth Factor; Recombinant Human Erythropoietin

Use Treatment of anemia due to concurrent myelosuppressive chemotherapy in patients with cancer (nonmyeloid malignancies) receiving chemotherapy (palliative intent) for a planned minimum of 2 additional months of chemotherapy; treatment of anemia due to chronic kidney disease (including patients on dialysis and not on dialysis) to decrease the need for RBC transfusion; treatment of anemia associated with HIV (zidovudine) therapy when endogenous erythropoietin levels ≤500 mUnits/mL; reduction of allogeneic RBC transfusion for elective, noncardiac, nonvascular surgery when perioperative hemoglobin is >10 to ≤13 g/dL and there is a high risk for blood loss

Note: Epoetin is **not** indicated for use under the following conditions:
- Cancer patients receiving hormonal therapy, therapeutic biologic products, or radiation therapy unless also receiving concurrent myelosuppressive chemotherapy
- Cancer patients receiving myelosuppressive chemotherapy when the expected outcome is curative
- Surgery patients who are willing to donate autologous blood
- Surgery patients undergoing cardiac or vascular surgery
- As a substitute for RBC transfusion in patients requiring immediate correction of anemia

Note: In clinical trials (and one meta analysis), epoetin has not demonstrated improved quality of life, fatigue, or well-being.

Unlabeled/Investigational Use Treatment of symptomatic anemia in myelodysplastic syndrome (MDS)

Prescribing and Access Restrictions As a requirement of the REMS program, access to this medication is restricted. Healthcare providers and hospitals must be enrolled in the ESA APPRISE (Assisting Providers and Cancer Patients with Risk Information for the Safe use of ESAs) Oncology Program (866-284-8089; http://www.esa-apprise.com) to prescribe or dispense ESAs (ie, epoetin alfa, darbepoetin alfa) to patients with cancer.

Medication Guide Available Yes

Contraindications Hypersensitivity to epoetin or any component of the formulation; uncontrolled hypertension; pure red cell aplasia (due to epoetin or other epoetin protein drugs); multidose vials contain benzyl alcohol and are contraindicated in neonates, infants, pregnant women, and nursing women

Warnings/Precautions [U.S. Boxed Warning]: Erythropoiesis-stimulating agents (ESAs) increased the risk of serious cardiovascular events, thromboembolic events, stroke, mortality, and/or tumor progression in clinical studies; a rapid rise in hemoglobin (>1 g/dL over 2 weeks) or maintaining higher hemoglobin levels may contribute to these risks. **[U.S. Boxed Warning]: A shortened overall survival and/or increased risk of tumor progression or recurrence has been reported in studies with breast, cervical, head and neck, lymphoid, and non small cell lung cancer patients.** It is of note that in these studies, patients received ESAs to a target hemoglobin of ≥12 g/dL; although risk has not been excluded when dosed to achieve a target hemoglobin of <12 g/dL. **[U.S. Boxed Warnings]: To decrease these risks, and risk of cardio- and thrombovascular events, use the lowest dose needed to avoid red blood cell transfusions. Use ESAs in cancer patients only for the treatment of anemia related to concurrent chemotherapy; discontinue ESA following completion of the chemotherapy course. ESAs are not indicated for patients receiving myelosuppressive therapy when the anticipated outcome is curative.** Use of ESAs has been associated with an increased risk of venous thromboembolism (VTE) without a reduction in transfusions in patients with cancer (Hershman, 2009). Improved anemia symptoms, quality of life, fatigue or well-being has not been demonstrated in controlled clinical trials. **[U.S. Boxed Warning]: Because of the risks of decreased survival and increased risk of tumor growth or progression, all healthcare providers and hospitals are required to enroll and comply with the ESA APPRISE (Assisting Providers and Cancer Patients with Risk Information for the Safe use of ESAs) Oncology Program prior to prescribing or dispensing ESAs to cancer patients.** Prescribers and patients will have to provide written documentation of discussed risks.

[U.S. Boxed Warning]: An increased risk of death, serious cardiovascular events, and stroke was reported in chronic renal failure patients administered ESAs to target hemoglobin levels ≥13 g/dL; dosing should be individualized to achieve and maintain hemoglobin levels within 10-12 g/dL range. Hemoglobin rising >1 g/dL in a 2-week period may contribute to the risk. Chronic renal failure patients who exhibit an inadequate hemoglobin response to ESA therapy may be at a higher risk for cardiovascular events and mortality compared to other patients. ESA therapy may reduce dialysis efficacy (due to increase in red blood cells and decrease in plasma volume); adjustments in dialysis parameters may be needed. Patients treated with epoetin may require increased heparinization during dialysis to prevent clotting of the artificial kidney. **[U.S. Boxed Warning]: Epoetin alfa increased the rate of DVT in perisurgery patients not receiving anticoagulant prophylaxis; consider DVT prophylaxis.** Increased mortality was also observed in patients undergoing coronary artery bypass surgery who received epoetin alfa; these deaths were associated with thrombotic events. Epoetin is not approved for reduction of red blood cell transfusion in patients undergoing cardiac or vascular surgery and is not indicated for anemic patients willing to donate autologous blood. During therapy in any patient, hemoglobin levels should not exceed a target range of 10-12 g/dL and should not rise >1 g/dL per 2-week time period.

Use with caution in patients with hypertension or with a history of seizures; hypertensive encephalopathy and seizures have been reported. If hypertension is difficult to control, reduce or hold epoetin alfa. An excessive rate of rise of hemoglobin is associated with hypertension or exacerbation of hypertension; decrease the epoetin dose if the hemoglobin increase exceeds 1 g/dL in any 2-week period. Blood pressure should be controlled prior to start of therapy and monitored closely throughout treatment. Due to the delayed onset of erythropoiesis, epoetin alfa is **not** recommended for acute correction of severe anemia or as a substitute for emergency transfusion.

Prior to treatment, correct or exclude deficiencies of iron, vitamin B_{12}, and/or folate, as well as other factors which may impair erythropoiesis (aluminum toxicity, inflammatory conditions, infections). Prior to and periodically during therapy, iron stores must be evaluated. Supplemental iron is recommended if serum ferritin <100 mcg/L or serum transferrin saturation <20%. Poor response should prompt evaluation of these potential factors, as well as possible malignant processes, occult blood loss, hemolysis, and/or bone marrow fibrosis. Severe anemia and pure red cell aplasia (PRCA) with associated neutralizing antibodies to erythropoietin has been reported, predominantly in patients with CRF receiving SubQ epoetin (the I.V. route is preferred for hemodialysis patients). Cases have also been reported in patients with hepatitis C who were receiving ESAs, interferon, and ribavirin. Patients with a sudden loss of response to epoetin alfa (with severe anemia and a low reticulocyte count) should be evaluated for PRCA with associated neutralizing antibodies to erythropoietin; discontinue treatment in patients with PRCA secondary to neutralizing antibodies to epoetin.

Safety and efficacy in patients with underlying hematologic diseases have not been established, including hypercoagulation disorders and sickle cell disease. Potentially serious allergic reactions have been reported (rarely). Discontinue immediately (and permanently) in patients who experience serious allergic/anaphylactic reactions. Use caution with porphyria, exacerbation of porphyria has been reported (rarely) in patients with chronic renal failure. Some products may contain albumin.

Adverse Reactions (Reflective of adult population; not specific for elderly)
>10%:
  Cardiovascular: Hypertension (3% to 28%)
  Central nervous system: Fever (10% to 42%), headache (5% to 18%)
  Dermatologic: Pruritus (12% to 21%), rash (2% to 19%)
  Gastrointestinal: Nausea (35% to 56%), vomiting (12% to 28%)
  Local: Injection site reaction (7% to 13%)
  Neuromuscular & skeletal: Arthralgia (10% to 16%)
  Respiratory: Cough (4% to 26%)
1% to 10%:
  Cardiovascular: Deep vein thrombosis, edema, thrombosis
  Central nervous system: Chills, depression, dizziness, insomnia
  Dermatologic: Urticaria
  Endocrine & metabolic: Hyperglycemia, hypokalemia
  Gastrointestinal: Dysphagia, stomatitis, weight loss
  Hematologic: Leukopenia
  Local: Clotted vascular access
  Neuromuscular & skeletal: Bone pain, muscle spasm, myalgia
  Respiratory: Pulmonary embolism, respiratory congestion, upper respiratory infection
Drug Interactions
  Avoid Concomitant Use There are no known interactions where it is recommended to avoid concomitant use.
  Increased Effect/Toxicity There are no known significant interactions involving an increase in effect.
  Decreased Effect There are no known significant interactions involving a decrease in effect.
Stability
  Vials should be stored at 2°C to 8°C (36°F to 46°F); **do not freeze or shake**. Protect from light.
  Single-dose 1 mL vial contains no preservative: Use one dose per vial. Do not re-enter vial; discard unused portions.
    Single-dose vials (except 40,000 units/mL vial) are stable for 2 weeks at room temperature (Cohen, 2007). Single-dose 40,000 units/mL vial is stable for 1 week at room temperature.

◄   **Multidose 1 mL or 2 mL vial** contains preservative. Store at 2°C to 8°C after initial entry and between doses. Discard 21 days after initial entry.

   Multidose vials (with preservative) are stable for 1 week at room temperature (Cohen, 2007).

   Prefilled syringes containing the 20,000 units/mL formulation with preservative are stable for 6 weeks refrigerated (2°C to 8°C) (Naughton, 2003).

   Dilutions of 1:10 and 1:20 (1 part epoetin:19 parts sodium chloride) are stable for 18 hours at room temperature (Ohls, 1996).

Prior to SubQ administration, preservative free solutions may be mixed with bacteriostatic NS containing benzyl alcohol 0.9% in a 1:1 ratio (Corbo, 1992). Dilutions of 1:10 in $D_{10}W$ with human albumin 0.05% or 0.1% are stable for 24 hours.

Mechanism of Action Induces erythropoiesis by stimulating the division and differentiation of committed erythroid progenitor cells; induces the release of reticulocytes from the bone marrow into the bloodstream, where they mature to erythrocytes. There is a dose response relationship with this effect. This results in an increase in reticulocyte counts followed by a rise in hematocrit and hemoglobin levels.

Pharmacodynamics/Kinetics

   Onset of action: Several days

   Peak effect: Hemoglobin level: 2-6 weeks

   Distribution: V_d: 9 L; rapid in the plasma compartment; concentrated in liver, kidneys, and bone marrow

   Metabolism: Some degradation does occur

   Bioavailability: SubQ: ~21% to 31%; intraperitoneal epoetin: 3% (Macdougall, 1989)

   Half-life elimination: Cancer: SubQ: 16-67 hours; Chronic kidney disease: I.V.: 4-13 hours

   Time to peak, serum: Chronic kidney disease: SubQ: 5-24 hours

   Excretion: Feces (majority); urine (small amounts, 10% unchanged in normal volunteers)

Dosage

Geriatric & Adult

   Anemia associated with chronic kidney disease: Individualize dosing and use the lowest dose necessary to reduce the need for RBC transfusions.

     Chronic kidney disease patients ON dialysis (I.V. route is preferred for hemodialysis patients; initiate treatment when hemoglobin is <10 g/dL; reduce dose or interrupt treatment if hemoglobin approaches or exceeds 11 g/dL): I.V., SubQ: Initial dose: 50-100 units/kg 3 times/week

     Chronic kidney disease patients NOT on dialysis (consider initiating treatment when hemoglobin is <10 g/dL; use only if rate of hemoglobin decline would likely result in RBC transfusion and desire is to reduce risk of alloimmunization or other RBC transfusion-related risks; reduce dose or interrupt treatment if hemoglobin exceeds 10 g/dL): I.V., SubQ: Initial dose: 50-100 units/kg 3 times/week

     Dosage adjustments for chronic kidney disease patients (either on dialysis or not on dialysis):

       If hemoglobin does not increase by >1 g/dL after 4 weeks: Increase dose by 25%; do not increase the dose more frequently than once every 4 weeks

       If hemoglobin increases >1 g/dL in any 2-week period: Reduce dose by ≥25%; dose reductions can occur more frequently than once every 4 weeks; avoid frequent dosage adjustments

       Inadequate or lack of response over a 12-week escalation period: Further increases are unlikely to improve response and may increase risks; use the minimum effective dose that will maintain a Hgb level sufficient to avoid RBC transfusions and evaluate patient for other causes of anemia. Discontinue therapy if responsiveness does not improve.

   Anemia due to chemotherapy in cancer patients: Initiate treatment only if hemoglobin <10 g/dL and anticipated duration of myelosuppressive chemotherapy is ≥2 months. Titrate dosage to use the minimum effective dose that will maintain a hemoglobin level sufficient to avoid red blood cell transfusions. Discontinue erythropoietin following completion of chemotherapy. SubQ: Initial dose: 150 units/kg 3 times/week or 40,000 units once weekly until completion of chemotherapy

     Dosage adjustments:

       If hemoglobin does not increase by >1 g/dL **and** remains below 10 g/dL after initial 4 weeks: Increase to 300 units/kg 3 times/week or 60,000 units weekly; discontinue after 8 weeks of treatment if RBC transfusions are still required or there is no hemoglobin response

       If hemoglobin exceeds a level needed to avoid red blood cell transfusion: Withhold dose; resume treatment with a 25% dose reduction when hemoglobin approaches a level where transfusions may be required.

       If hemoglobin increases >1 g/dL in any 2-week period **or** hemoglobin reaches a level sufficient to avoid red blood cell transfusion: Reduce dose by 25%.

Anemia due to zidovudine in HIV-infected patients: Titrate dosage to use the minimum effective dose that will maintain a hemoglobin level sufficient to avoid red blood cell transfusions. Hemoglobin levels should not exceed 12 g/dL.

Serum erythropoietin levels ≤500 mUnits/mL and zidovudine doses ≤4200 mg/week): I.V., SubQ: Initial: 100 units/kg 3 times/week; if hemoglobin does not increase after 8 weeks, increase dose by ~50-100 units/kg at 4-8 week intervals until hemoglobin reaches a level sufficient to avoid RBC transfusion; maximum dose: 300 units/kg. Withhold dose if hemoglobin exceeds 12 g/dL, may resume treatment with a 25% dose reduction once hemoglobin <11 g/dL. Discontinue if hemoglobin increase is not achieved with 300 units/kg for 8 weeks.

Surgery patients (perioperative hemoglobin should be >10 g/dL and ≤13 g/dL; DVT prophylactic anticoagulation is recommended): SubQ: Initial dose:

300 units/kg/day beginning 10 days before surgery, on the day of surgery, and for 4 days after surgery **or**

600 units/kg once weekly for 4 doses, beginning 21-, 14-, and 7 days before surgery, and on the day of surgery

Symptomatic anemia associated with myelodysplastic syndrome (unlabeled use): SubQ: 40,000-60,000 units 1-3 times/week (NCCN MDS guidelines v.2.2011)

Administration

SubQ is the preferred route of administration **except** in patients with CKD on hemodialysis; 1:1 dilution with bacteriostatic NS (containing benzyl alcohol) acts as a local anesthetic to reduce pain at the injection site

Patients with CKD on hemodialysis: I.V. route preferred; it may be administered into the venous line at the end of the dialysis procedure

Monitoring Parameters Transferrin saturation and serum ferritin (prior to and during treatment); hemoglobin (weekly after initiation and following dose adjustments until stable and sufficient to minimize need for RBC transfusion; CKD patients should be also be monitored at least monthly following hemoglobin stability); blood pressure; seizures (CKD patients following initiation for first few months, includes new-onset or change in seizure frequency or premonitory symptoms)

Cancer patients: Examinations recommended by the ASCO/ASH guidelines (Rizzo, 2010) prior to treatment include: peripheral blood smear (in some situations a bone marrow exam may be necessary), assessment for iron, folate, or vitamin B_{12} deficiency, reticulocyte count, renal function status, and occult blood loss; during ESA treatment, assess baseline and periodic iron, total iron-binding capacity, and transferrin saturation or ferritin levels.

Reference Range Zidovudine-treated HIV patients: Available evidence indicates patients with endogenous serum erythropoietin levels >500 mU/mL are unlikely to respond

Pharmacotherapy Pearls Oncology Comment: The American Society of Clinical Oncology (ASCO) and American Society of Hematology (ASH) 2010 updates to the clinical practice guidelines for the use of erythropoiesis-stimulating agents (ESAs) in patients with cancer indicate that ESAs are most appropriate when used according to the parameters identified within the Food and Drug Administration (FDA) approved labeling for epoetin and darbepoetin (Rizzo, 2010). ESAs are an option for chemotherapy associated anemia when the hemoglobin has fallen to <10 g/dL to decrease the need for RBC transfusions. ESAs should only be used in conjunction with concurrent chemotherapy. Although the FDA label now limits ESA use to the palliative setting, the ASCO/ASH guidelines suggest using clinical judgment in weighing risks versus benefits as formal outcomes studies of ESA use defined by intent of chemotherapy treatment have not been conducted.

The ASCO/ASH guidelines continue to recommend following the FDA approved dosing (and dosing adjustment) guidelines as alternate dosing and schedules have not demonstrated consistent differences in effectiveness with regard to hemoglobin response. In patients who do not have a response within 6-8 weeks (hemoglobin rise <1-2 g/dL or no reduction in transfusions) ESA therapy should be discontinued.

Prior to the initiation of ESAs, other sources of anemia (in addition to chemotherapy or underlying hematologic malignancy) should be investigated. Examinations recommended prior to treatment include peripheral blood smear (in some situations a bone marrow exam may be necessary), assessment for iron, folate, or vitamin B_{12} deficiency, reticulocyte count, renal function status, and occult blood loss. During ESA treatment, assess baseline and periodic iron, total iron-binding capacity, and transferrin saturation or ferritin levels. Iron supplementation may be necessary

The guidelines note that patients with an increased risk of thromboembolism (generally includes previous history of thrombosis, surgery, and/or prolonged periods of immobilization) and patients receiving concomitant medications that may increase thromboembolic risk, should begin ESA therapy only after careful consideration. With the exception of low-risk myelodysplasia-associated anemia (which has evidence supporting the use of ESAs without concurrent chemotherapy), the guidelines do not support the use of ESAs in the absence of concurrent chemotherapy.

Special Geriatric Considerations Endogenous erythropoietin secretion has been reported to be decreased in elderly with normocytic or iron deficiency anemias or those with a serum hemoglobin concentration <12 g/dL; one study did not find such a relationship in the elderly with chronic anemia. A blunted erythropoietin response to anemia has been reported in patients with cancer, rheumatoid arthritis, and AIDS.

Dosage Forms Excipient information presented when available (limited, particularly for generics); consult specific product labeling.

Injection, solution:

Epogen®: 10,000 units/mL (2 mL); 20,000 units/mL (1 mL) [contains albumin (human), benzyl alcohol]

Procrit®: 10,000 units/mL (2 mL); 20,000 units/mL (1 mL) [contains albumin (human), benzyl alcohol]

Injection, solution [preservative free]:

Epogen®: 2000 units/mL (1 mL); 3000 units/mL (1 mL); 4000 units/mL (1 mL); 10,000 units/mL (1 mL) [contains albumin (human)]

Procrit®: 2000 units/mL (1 mL); 3000 units/mL (1 mL); 4000 units/mL (1 mL); 10,000 units/mL (1 mL); 40,000 units/mL (1 mL) [contains albumin (human)]

Dosage Forms: Canada Excipient information presented when available (limited, particularly for generics); consult specific product labeling.

Injection, solution [preservative free]:

Eprex®: 1000 units/0.5 mL (0.5 mL); 2000 units/0.5 mL (0.5 mL); 3000 units/0.3 mL (0.3 mL); 4000 units/0.4 mL (0.4 mL); 5000 units/0.5 mL (0.5 mL); 6000 units/0.6 mL (0.6 mL); 8000 units/0.8 mL (0.8 mL); 10,000 units/mL (1 mL); 20,000 units/0.5 mL (0.5 mL); 30,000 units/0.75 mL (0.75 mL); 40,000 units/mL (1 mL) [contains polysorbate 80; prefilled syringe, free of human serum albumin]

Selected References

Carpenter MA, Kendall RG, O'Brien AE, et al, "Reduced Erythropoietin Response to Anaemia in Elderly Patients With Normocytic Anaemia," *Eur J Haematol*, 1992, 49(3):119-21.

Goodnough LT, Price TH, Parvin CA, "The Endogenous Erythropoietin Response and the Erythropoietic Response to Blood Loss Anemia: The Effects of Age and Gender," *J Lab Clin Med*, 1995, 126(1):57-64.

Joosten E, Van Hove L, Lesaffre E, et al, "Serum Erythropoietin Levels in Elderly Inpatients With Anemia of Chronic Disorders and Iron Deficiency Anemia," *J Am Geriatr Soc*, 1993, 41(12):1301-4.

Kario K, Matsuo T, and Nakao K, "Serum Erythropoietin Levels in the Elderly," *Gerontology*, 1991, 37(6):345-8.

Nafziger J, Pailla K, Luciani L, et al, "Decreased Erythropoietin Responsiveness to Iron Deficiency Anemia in the Elderly," *Am J Hematol*, 1993, 43(3):172-6.

National Kidney Foundation, "KDOQI Clinical Practice Guidelines and Clinical Practice Recommentaions for Anemia in Chronic Kidney Disease," *Am J Kidney Dis*, 2007, 50(3):529-30. Available at http://www.kidney.org/professionals/KDOQI/guidelines_anemiaUP/index.htm or http://www.kidney.org/professionals/KDOQI.

Powers JS, Krantz SB, Collins JC, et al, "Erythropoietin Response to Anemia as a Function of Age," *J Am Geriatr Soc*, 1991, 39(1):30-2.

♦ **Epogen®** *see* Epoetin Alfa *on page 611*

Eprosartan (ep roe SAR tan)

Related Information

Angiotensin Agents *on page 1985*

Brand Names: U.S. Teveten®

Brand Names: Canada Teveten®

Generic Availability (U.S.) No

Pharmacologic Category Angiotensin II Receptor Blocker

Use Treatment of hypertension; may be used alone or in combination with other antihypertensives

Contraindications Hypersensitivity to eprosartan or any component of the formulation

Warnings/Precautions May cause hyperkalemia; avoid potassium supplementation unless specifically required by healthcare provider. Avoid use or use a smaller dose in patients who are volume depleted; correct depletion first. May be associated with deterioration of renal function and/or increases in serum creatinine, particularly in patients with low renal blood flow (eg, renal artery stenosis, heart failure) whose glomerular filtration rate (GFR) is dependent on efferent arteriolar vasoconstriction by angiotensin II. Use with caution in unstented unilateral/bilateral renal artery stenosis. When unstented bilateral renal artery stenosis is present, use is generally avoided due to the elevated risk of deterioration in renal function unless possible benefits outweigh risks. Use with caution in pre-existing renal insufficiency; significant aortic/mitral stenosis. Concurrent use of ACE inhibitors may increase the risk of clinically-significant adverse events (eg, renal dysfunction, hyperkalemia).

Adverse Reactions (Reflective of adult population; not specific for elderly)
1% to 10%:
Central nervous system: Fatigue (2%), depression (1%)
Endocrine & metabolic: Hypertriglyceridemia (1%)
Gastrointestinal: Abdominal pain (2%)
Genitourinary: Urinary tract infection (1%)
Respiratory: Upper respiratory tract infection (8%), rhinitis (4%), pharyngitis (4%), cough (4%)
Miscellaneous: Viral infection (2%), injury (2%)

Drug Interactions

Metabolism/Transport Effects Inhibits CYP2C9 (weak)

Avoid Concomitant Use There are no known interactions where it is recommended to avoid concomitant use.

Increased Effect/Toxicity
Eprosartan may increase the levels/effects of: ACE Inhibitors; Amifostine; Antihypertensives; Hypotensive Agents; Lithium; Nonsteroidal Anti-Inflammatory Agents; Potassium-Sparing Diuretics; RiTUXimab; Sodium Phosphates

The levels/effects of Eprosartan may be increased by: Alfuzosin; Diazoxide; Eplerenone; Herbs (Hypotensive Properties); MAO Inhibitors; Pentoxifylline; Phosphodiesterase 5 Inhibitors; Potassium Salts; Prostacyclin Analogues; Tolvaptan; Trimethoprim

Decreased Effect
The levels/effects of Eprosartan may be decreased by: Herbs (Hypertensive Properties); Methylphenidate; Nonsteroidal Anti-Inflammatory Agents; Yohimbine

Ethanol/Nutrition/Herb Interactions Herb/Nutraceutical: Avoid dong quai if using for hypertension (has estrogenic activity). Avoid ephedra, yohimbe, ginseng (may worsen hypertension). Avoid garlic (may have increased antihypertensive effect).

Mechanism of Action Angiotensin II is formed from angiotensin I in a reaction catalyzed by angiotensin-converting enzyme (ACE, kininase II). Angiotensin II is the principal pressor agent of the renin-angiotensin system, with effects that include vasoconstriction, stimulation of synthesis and release of aldosterone, cardiac stimulation, and renal reabsorption of sodium. Eprosartan blocks the vasoconstrictor and aldosterone-secreting effects of angiotensin II by selectively blocking the binding of angiotensin II to the AT1 receptor in many tissues, such as vascular smooth muscle and the adrenal gland. Its action is therefore independent of the pathways for angiotensin II synthesis. Blockade of the renin-angiotensin system with ACE inhibitors, which inhibit the biosynthesis of angiotensin II from angiotensin I, is widely used in the treatment of hypertension. ACE inhibitors also inhibit the degradation of bradykinin, a reaction also catalyzed by ACE. Because eprosartan does not inhibit ACE (kininase II), it does not affect the response to bradykinin. Whether this difference has clinical relevance is not yet known. Eprosartan does not bind to or block other hormone receptors or ion channels known to be important in cardiovascular regulation.

Pharmacodynamics/Kinetics
Protein binding: 98%
Metabolism: Minimally hepatic
Bioavailability: 300 mg dose: 13%
Half-life elimination: Terminal: 5-9 hours
Time to peak, serum: Fasting: 1-2 hours
Excretion: Feces (90%); urine (7%, mostly as unchanged drug)
Clearance: 7.9 L/hour

Dosage
Geriatric & Adult Hypertension: Oral: Dosage must be individualized. Can administer once or twice daily with total daily doses of 400-800 mg. Usual starting dose is 600 mg once daily as monotherapy in patients who are euvolemic. Limited clinical experience with doses >800 mg.

Renal Impairment
Moderate-to-severe impairment: No initial starting dosage adjustment is necessary; however, carefully monitor the patient. Maximum dose: 600 mg daily.
Hemodialysis: Poorly removed (Cl_{HD} <1 L/hour)

Hepatic Impairment No starting dosage adjustment is necessary; however, carefully monitor the patient.

Monitoring Parameters Supine blood pressure, electrolytes, serum creatinine, BUN, urinalysis, symptomatic hypotension, tachycardia

Pharmacotherapy Pearls The angiotensin II receptor antagonists appear to have similar indications as the ACE inhibitors. While these drugs have been shown to be effective in treating hypertension, their efficacy in heart failure is being vigorously evaluated. The angiotensin II antagonists are especially useful in providing an alternative therapy in those patients who have intractable cough in response to ACE inhibitor therapy. Similar to ACE

◀ inhibitors, pre-existing volume depletion caused by diuretic therapy may potentiate hypotension in response to angiotensin II antagonists.

Because of the lack of effect on the response to bradykinin, angiotensin-receptor blockers are less likely to be associated with nonrenin-angiotensin effects such as cough and angioedema. Because of a different site of action in comparison to ACE inhibitors, the angiotensin II antagonists do not cause increases in levels of bradykinin. These different sites of action have lead to the supposition that the ACE inhibitors and the angiotensin II antagonists may be used in combination for enhanced response. This possibility is currently being evaluated.

Special Geriatric Considerations No specific dose adjustments are necessary in the elderly due to the drug's major route of elimination. However, since many elderly may be volume depleted due to their "blunted thirst reflex" and use of diuretics, care and monitoring of blood pressure and volume status are necessary upon initiation.

Dosage Forms Excipient information presented when available (limited, particularly for generics); consult specific product labeling.
Tablet, oral:
Teveten®: 400 mg, 600 mg

Eprosartan and Hydrochlorothiazide
(ep roe SAR tan & hye droe klor oh THYE a zide)

Related Information
Eprosartan on page 616
Hydrochlorothiazide on page 876
Brand Names: U.S. Teveten® HCT
Brand Names: Canada Teveten® HCT; Teveten® Plus
Index Terms Eprosartan Mesylate and Hydrochlorothiazide; Hydrochlorothiazide and Eprosartan
Generic Availability (U.S.) No
Pharmacologic Category Angiotensin II Receptor Blocker; Diuretic, Thiazide
Use Treatment of hypertension (not indicated for initial treatment)
Dosage
Geriatric & Adult Hypertension: Oral: Dose is individualized (combination substituted for individual components)
Usual recommended dose: Eprosartan 600 mg/hydrochlorothiazide 12.5 mg once daily (maximum dose: Eprosartan 600 mg/hydrochlorothiazide 25 mg once daily)
Renal Impairment Moderate-to-severe impairment: Initial dose adjustments are not necessary per manufacturer; however carefully monitor patient. Do not exceed a maximum dose of eprosartan 600 mg daily. Hydrochlorothiazide is ineffective in patients with Cl_{cr} <30 mL/minute.
Hepatic Impairment Initial dose adjustments not recommended by manufacturer; carefully monitor patient.
Dosage Forms Excipient information presented when available (limited, particularly for generics); consult specific product labeling.
Tablet:
600 mg/12.5 mg: Eprosartan 600 mg and hydrochlorothiazide 12.5 mg
600 mg/25 mg: Eprosartan 600 mg and hydrochlorothiazide 25 mg

◆ **Eprosartan Mesylate and Hydrochlorothiazide** see Eprosartan and Hydrochlorothiazide on page 618
◆ **Epsom Salt [OTC]** see Magnesium Salts (Various Salts) on page 1114
◆ **Equalactin® [OTC]** see Polycarbophil on page 1479
◆ **Equalizer Gas Relief [OTC]** see Simethicone on page 1679
◆ **Equanil** see Meprobamate on page 1144
◆ **Equetro®** see CarBAMazepine on page 268
◆ **Equilet® [OTC]** see Calcium Salts (Oral) on page 256

Ergocalciferol (er goe kal SIF e role)

Medication Safety Issues
Sound-alike/look-alike issues:
Calciferol™ may be confused with calcitriol
Drisdol® may be confused with Drysol™
Ergocalciferol may be confused with alfacalcidol, cholecalciferol

Pharmacologic Category Ergot Derivative

Use Treatment of cerebrovascular insufficiency in primary progressive dementia, Alzheimer's dementia, and senile onset

Contraindications Hypersensitivity to ergot or any component of the formulation; acute or chronic psychosis; ergot alkaloids are contraindicated with potent inhibitors of CYP3A4 (includes protease inhibitors, azole antifungals, and some macrolide antibiotics)

Warnings/Precautions Pleural and peritoneal fibrosis have been reported with prolonged daily use. Cardiac valvular fibrosis has also been associated with ergot alkaloids. Concomitant use with potent inhibitors of CYP3A4 (includes protease inhibitors, azole antifungals, and some macrolide antibiotics) and ergot alkaloids has been associated with acute ergot toxicity (ergotism); certain ergot alkaloids (eg, ergotamine and dihydroergotamine) are contraindicated by the manufacturer. May be inappropriate for use in the elderly; efficacy has not been demonstrated in the doses studied (Beers Criteria).

Adverse Reactions (Reflective of adult population; not specific for elderly) Adverse effects are minimal; most common include transient nausea, gastrointestinal disturbances and sublingual irritation with SL tablets; other common side effects include:

Cardiovascular: Bradycardia, orthostatic hypotension
Dermatologic: Flushing, skin rash
Ocular: Blurred vision
Respiratory: Nasal congestion

Drug Interactions

Metabolism/Transport Effects Substrate of CYP3A4 (major)

Avoid Concomitant Use

Avoid concomitant use of Ergoloid Mesylates with any of the following: Conivaptan; Efavirenz; Itraconazole; Nitroglycerin; Posaconazole; Protease Inhibitors; Serotonin 5-HT1D Receptor Agonists; Sibutramine; Telaprevir; Voriconazole

Increased Effect/Toxicity

Ergoloid Mesylates may increase the levels/effects of: Serotonin 5-HT1D Receptor Agonists; Serotonin Modulators

The levels/effects of Ergoloid Mesylates may be increased by: Conivaptan; CYP3A4 Inhibitors (Moderate); CYP3A4 Inhibitors (Strong); Dasatinib; Efavirenz; Itraconazole; Macrolide Antibiotics; Nitroglycerin; Posaconazole; Protease Inhibitors; Serotonin 5-HT1D Receptor Agonists; Sibutramine; Telaprevir; Voriconazole

Decreased Effect

Ergoloid Mesylates may decrease the levels/effects of: Nitroglycerin

The levels/effects of Ergoloid Mesylates may be decreased by: Tocilizumab

Mechanism of Action Ergoloid mesylates do not have the vasoconstrictor effects of the natural ergot alkaloids; exact mechanism in dementia is unknown; originally classed as peripheral and cerebral vasodilator, now considered a "metabolic enhancer"; there is no specific evidence which clearly establishes the mechanism by which ergoloid mesylate preparations produce mental effects, nor is there conclusive evidence that the drug particularly affects cerebral arteriosclerosis or cerebrovascular insufficiency

Pharmacodynamics/Kinetics

Absorption: Rapid yet incomplete
Half-life elimination, serum: 3.5 hours
Time to peak, serum: ~1 hour

Dosage

Geriatric & Adult Primary progressive dementia, Alzheimer's dementia: Oral: 1 mg 3 times/ day up to 4.5-12 mg/day; up to 6 months of therapy may be necessary

Monitoring Parameters Blood pressure, heart rate, mental status

Special Geriatric Considerations Ergoloid mesylates have no role in the treatment of dementia. Most clinicians regard it as no better than placebo and most patients do not experience significant benefits. Improvement in social function has been shown in some older studies, but no consistent improvement in memory or cognitive function was reported.

This medication is considered to be potentially inappropriate in this patient population (Beers Criteria severity: Low).

Dosage Forms Excipient information presented when available (limited, particularly for generics); consult specific product labeling.
Tablet, oral: 1 mg

♦ **Ergomar®** *see* Ergotamine *on page 622*

Ergotamine (er GOT a meen)

Brand Names: U.S. Ergomar®
Index Terms Ergotamine Tartrate
Generic Availability (U.S.) No
Pharmacologic Category Antimigraine Agent; Ergot Derivative
Use Abort or prevent vascular headaches, such as migraine, migraine variants, or so-called "histaminic cephalalgia"
Contraindications Hypersensitivity to ergotamine or any component of the formulation; peripheral vascular disease; hepatic or renal disease; coronary artery disease; hypertension; sepsis; ergot alkaloids are contraindicated with strong inhibitors of CYP3A4 (includes protease inhibitors, azole antifungals, and some macrolide antibiotics)
Warnings/Precautions Ergot alkaloids have been associated with fibrotic valve thickening (eg, aortic, mitral, tricuspid); usually associated with long-term, chronic use; vasospasm or vasoconstriction can occur; ergot alkaloid use may result in ergotism (intense vasoconstriction) resulting in peripheral vascular ischemia and possible gangrene; rare cases of pleural and/or retroperitoneal fibrosis have been reported with prolonged daily use. Discontinuation after extended use may result in withdrawal symptoms (eg, rebound headache). Use with caution in the elderly.

[U.S. Boxed Warning]: Ergot alkaloids are contraindicated with potent inhibitors of CYP3A4 (includes protease inhibitors, azole antifungals, and some macrolide antibiotics); concomitant use associated with acute ergot toxicity (ergotism).

Adverse Reactions (Reflective of adult population; not specific for elderly) Frequency not defined.

Cardiovascular: Absence of pulse, bradycardia, cardiac valvular fibrosis, cyanosis, edema, ECG changes, gangrene, hypertension, ischemia, precordial distress and pain, tachycardia, vasospasm

Central nervous system: Vertigo

Dermatologic: Itching

Gastrointestinal: Nausea, vomiting

Genitourinary: Retroperitoneal fibrosis

Neuromuscular & skeletal: Muscle pain, numbness, paresthesia, weakness

Respiratory: Pleuropulmonary fibrosis

Miscellaneous: Cold extremities

Drug Interactions

Metabolism/Transport Effects Substrate of CYP3A4 (major); Inhibits CYP3A4 (weak)

Avoid Concomitant Use

Avoid concomitant use of Ergotamine with any of the following: Boceprevir; Clarithromycin; Conivaptan; Crizotinib; Efavirenz; Itraconazole; Nitroglycerin; Posaconazole; Protease Inhibitors; Serotonin 5-HT1D Receptor Agonists; Sibutramine; Telaprevir; Voriconazole

Increased Effect/Toxicity

Ergotamine may increase the levels/effects of: Serotonin 5-HT1D Receptor Agonists; Serotonin Modulators

The levels/effects of Ergotamine may be increased by: Boceprevir; Clarithromycin; Conivaptan; Crizotinib; CYP3A4 Inhibitors (Moderate); CYP3A4 Inhibitors (Strong); Dasatinib; Efavirenz; Itraconazole; Macrolide Antibiotics; Nitroglycerin; Posaconazole; Protease Inhibitors; Serotonin 5-HT1D Receptor Agonists; Sibutramine; Telaprevir; Voriconazole

Decreased Effect

Ergotamine may decrease the levels/effects of: Nitroglycerin

The levels/effects of Ergotamine may be decreased by: Tocilizumab

Ethanol/Nutrition/Herb Interactions Food: Avoid tea, cola, and coffee (caffeine may increase GI absorption of ergotamine). Grapefruit juice may cause increased blood levels of ergotamine, leading to increased toxicity.

Stability Store sublingual tablet at room temperature; protect from heat. Protect from light.

Mechanism of Action Has partial agonist and/or antagonist activity against tryptaminergic, dopaminergic and alpha-adrenergic receptors depending upon their site; is a highly active uterine stimulant; it causes constriction of peripheral and cranial blood vessels and produces depression of central vasomotor centers

Pharmacodynamics/Kinetics

Absorption: Oral: Erratic; enhanced by caffeine coadministration

Metabolism: Extensively hepatic

Half-life elimination: 2 hours

Time to peak, serum: 0.5-3 hours

Excretion: Feces (90% as metabolites)

Dosage
Geriatric Not recommended for use in the elderly.
Adult Migraine: Sublingual: One tablet under tongue at first sign, then 1 tablet every 30 minutes if needed; maximum dose: 3 tablets/24 hours, 5 tablets/week
Administration Do not crush sublingual drug product.
Monitoring Parameters Relief of symptoms, blood pressure, pulse, peripheral circulation
Special Geriatric Considerations Not recommended for use in the elderly. May be harmful due to reduction in cerebral blood flow. May precipitate angina, myocardial infarction, or aggravate intermittent claudication.
Dosage Forms Excipient information presented when available (limited, particularly for generics); consult specific product labeling.
Tablet, sublingual, as tartrate:
Ergomar®: 2 mg [peppermint flavor]

Ergotamine and Caffeine (er GOT a meen & KAF een)

Related Information
Ergotamine on page 622
Medication Safety Issues
Sound-alike/look-alike issues:
Cafergot® may be confused with Carafate®
Brand Names: U.S. Cafergot®; Migergot®
Brand Names: Canada Cafergot®
Index Terms Caffeine and Ergotamine; Ergotamine Tartrate and Caffeine
Generic Availability (U.S.) Yes: Tablet
Pharmacologic Category Antimigraine Agent; Ergot Derivative; Stimulant
Use Abort or prevent vascular headaches, such as migraine, migraine variants, or so-called "histaminic cephalalgia"
Dosage
Adult Migraine:
Oral: Two tablets at onset of attack; then 1 tablet every 30 minutes as needed; maximum: 6 tablets per attack; do not exceed 10 tablets/week.
Rectal: One suppository rectally at first sign of an attack; follow with second dose after 1 hour, if needed; maximum: 2 per attack; do not exceed 5/week.
Special Geriatric Considerations Not recommended for use in the elderly. May be harmful due to reduction in cerebral blood flow. May precipitate angina, myocardial infarction, or aggravate intermittent claudication.
Dosage Forms Excipient information presented when available (limited, particularly for generics); consult specific product labeling.
Suppository, rectal:
Migergot®: Ergotamine tartrate 2 mg and caffeine 100 mg (12s)
Tablet, oral: Ergotamine tartrate 1 mg and caffeine 100 mg
Cafergot®: Ergotamine tartrate 1 mg and caffeine 100 mg

◆ **Ergotamine Tartrate** see Ergotamine on page 622
◆ **Ergotamine Tartrate and Caffeine** see Ergotamine and Caffeine on page 623
◆ **E-R-O® [OTC]** see Carbamide Peroxide on page 272

Ertapenem (er ta PEN em)

Medication Safety Issues
Sound-alike/look-alike issues:
Ertapenem may be confused with imipenem, meropenem
INVanz® may be confused with AVINza™, I.V. vancomycin
Brand Names: U.S. INVanz®
Brand Names: Canada Invanz®
Index Terms Ertapenem Sodium; L-749,345; MK0826
Generic Availability (U.S.) No
Pharmacologic Category Antibiotic, Carbapenem
Use Treatment of the following moderate-severe infections: Complicated intra-abdominal infections, complicated skin and skin structure infections (including diabetic foot infections without osteomyelitis), complicated UTI (including pyelonephritis), acute pelvic infections (including postpartum endomyometritis, septic abortion, postsurgical gynecologic infections), and community-acquired pneumonia. Prophylaxis of surgical site infection following elective colorectal surgery. Antibacterial coverage includes aerobic gram-positive organisms, aerobic gram-negative organisms, and anaerobic organisms.

ERTAPENEM

Note: Methicillin-resistant *Staphylococcus aureus, Enterococcus* spp, penicillin-resistant strains of *Streptococcus pneumoniae, Acinetobacter,* and *Pseudomonas aeruginosa,* are **resistant** to ertapenem..

Contraindications Hypersensitivity to ertapenem, other carbapenems (eg, doripenem, imipenem, meropenem), or any component of the formulation; anaphylactic reactions to beta-lactam antibiotics. If using intramuscularly, known hypersensitivity to local anesthetics of the amide type (lidocaine is the diluent).

Warnings/Precautions Use caution with renal impairment. Dosage adjustment required in patients with moderate-to-severe renal dysfunction; elderly patients often require lower doses (based upon renal function). Prolonged use may result in fungal or bacterial superinfection, including *C. difficile*-associated diarrhea (CDAD) and pseudomembranous colitis; CDAD has been observed >2 months postantibiotic treatment. Has been associated with CNS adverse effects, including confusional states and seizures; use caution with CNS disorders (eg, brain lesions, history of seizures, or renal impairment). Serious hypersensitivity reactions, including anaphylaxis, have been reported (some without a history of previous allergic reactions to beta-lactams). Doses for I.M. administration are mixed with lidocaine; consult Lidocaine (Systemic) on page 1061 information for associated Warnings/Precautions. Serum concentrations of valproic acid may be reduced to subtherapeutic levels with concomitant use; dose adjustment (of valproate) may not compensate; concurrent use not recommended.

Adverse Reactions (Reflective of adult population; not specific for elderly) Note: Percentages reported in adults.

1% to 10%:
Cardiovascular: Edema (3%), chest pain (1% to 2%), hypertension (1% to 2%), hypotension (1% to 2%), tachycardia (1% to 2%)
Central nervous system: Headache (6% to 7%); altered mental status (eg, agitation, confusion, disorientation, decreased mental acuity, changed mental status, somnolence, stupor) (3% to 5%); fever (2% to 5%), insomnia (3%), dizziness (2%), fatigue (1%), anxiety (1%)
Dermatologic: Rash (2% to 3%), pruritus (1% to 2%), erythema (1% to 2%)
Endocrine & metabolic: Hypokalemia (2%), hyperglycemia (1% to 2%), hyperkalemia (≤1%)
Gastrointestinal: Diarrhea (9% to 10%), nausea (6% to 9%), abdominal pain (4%), vomiting (4%), constipation (3% to 4%), acid regurgitation (1% to 2%), dyspepsia (1%), oral candidiasis (≤1%)
Genitourinary: Urine WBCs increased (2% to 3%), urine RBCs increased (1% to 3%), vaginitis (1% to 3%)
Hematologic: Thrombocytosis (4% to 7%), hematocrit/hemoglobin decreased (3% to 5%), eosinophils increased (1% to 2%), leukopenia (1% to 2%), neutrophils decreased (1% to 2%), thrombocytopenia (1%), prothrombin time increased (≤1%)
Hepatic: Hepatic enzyme increased (7% to 9%), alkaline phosphatase increase (4% to 7%), albumin decreased (1% to 2%), bilirubin (total) increased (1% to 2%)
Local: Infused vein complications (5% to 7%), phlebitis/thrombophlebitis (2%), extravasation (1% to 2%)
Neuromuscular & skeletal: Weakness (1%), leg pain (≤1%)
Renal: Serum creatinine increased (1%)
Respiratory: Dyspnea (1% to 3%), cough (1% to 2%), pharyngitis (1%), rales/rhonchi (1%), respiratory distress (≤1%)

Drug Interactions
Avoid Concomitant Use
Avoid concomitant use of Ertapenem with any of the following: BCG
Increased Effect/Toxicity
The levels/effects of Ertapenem may be increased by: Probenecid
Decreased Effect
Ertapenem may decrease the levels/effects of: BCG; Divalproex; Typhoid Vaccine; Valproic Acid

Stability Before reconstitution store at ≤25°C (77°F).
I.M.: Reconstitute 1 g vial with 3.2 mL of 1% lidocaine HCl injection (without epinephrine). Shake well. Use within 1 hour after preparation.
I.V.: Reconstitute 1 g vial with 10 mL of water for injection, 0.9% sodium chloride injection, or bacteriostatic water for injection. Shake well. For adults, transfer dose to 50 mL of 0.9% sodium chloride injection. Reconstituted I.V. solution may be stored at room temperature and must be used within 6 hours **or** refrigerated, stored for up to 24 hours and used within 4 hours after removal from refrigerator. Do not freeze.

Mechanism of Action Inhibits bacterial cell wall synthesis by binding to one or more of the penicillin-binding proteins; which in turn inhibits the final transpeptidation step of peptidoglycan synthesis in bacterial cell walls, thus inhibiting cell wall biosynthesis. Bacteria eventually lyse due to ongoing activity of cell wall autolytic enzymes (autolysins and murein hydrolases) while cell wall assembly is arrested.

Pharmacodynamics/Kinetics

Absorption: I.M.: Almost complete

Distribution: V_{dss}: Adults: ~0.12 L/kg

Protein binding (concentration dependent, primarily to albumin): 85% at 300 mcg/mL, 95% at <100 mcg/mL

Metabolism: Non-CYP-mediated hydrolysis to inactive metabolite

Bioavailability: I.M.: ~90%

Half-life elimination: Adults: ~4 hours

Time to peak: I.M.: ~2.3 hours

Excretion: Urine (~80% as unchanged drug and metabolite); feces (~10%)

Dosage

Geriatric & Adult Note: I.V. therapy may be administered for up to 14 days; I.M. for up to 7 days

Community-acquired pneumonia and complicated urinary tract infections (including pyelonephritis): I.M., I.V.: 1 g/day; duration of total antibiotic treatment: 10-14 days (**Note:** Duration includes possible switch to appropriate oral therapy after at least 3 days of parenteral treatment, once clinical improvement demonstrated.)

Intra-abdominal infection: I.M., I.V.: 1 g/day for 5-14 days; **Note:** 2010 IDSA guidelines recommend a treatment duration of 4-7 days (provided source controlled) for community-acquired, mild-to-moderate IAI

Pelvic infections (acute): I.M., I.V.: 1 g/day for 3-10 days

Prophylaxis of surgical site following colorectal surgery: I.V.: 1 g given 1 hour preoperatively

Skin and skin structure infections (including diabetic foot infections): I.M., I.V.: 1 g/day for 7-14 days

Renal Impairment

Adults:

Cl_{cr} >30 mL/minute/1.73 m^2: No adjustment required

Cl_{cr} ≤30 mL/minute/1.73 m^2 and ESRD: 500 mg/day

Hemodialysis: When the daily dose is given within 6 hours prior to hemodialysis, a supplementary dose of 150 mg is required following hemodialysis.

Hepatic Impairment Adjustments cannot be recommended (lack of experience and research in this patient population).

Administration

I.M.: Avoid injection into a blood vessel. Make sure patient does not have an allergy to lidocaine or another anesthetic of the amide type. Administer by deep I.M. injection into a large muscle mass (eg, gluteal muscle or lateral part of the thigh). Do not administer I.M. preparation or drug reconstituted for I.M. administration intravenously.

I.V.: Infuse over 30 minutes

Monitoring Parameters Periodic renal, hepatic, and hematopoietic assessment during prolonged therapy; neurological assessment

Special Geriatric Considerations According to the package insert, the total and unbound AUCs were increased 37% and 67%, respectively, in healthy men and women ≥65 years of age compared to younger adults. No dose adjustment is required for patients with normal age-adjusted renal function.

Dosage Forms Excipient information presented when available (limited, particularly for generics); consult specific product labeling.

Injection, powder for reconstitution:

INVanz®: 1 g [contains sodium ~137 mg (~6 mEq)/g]

- ◆ **Ertapenem Sodium** see Ertapenem on page 623
- ◆ **EryPed®** see Erythromycin (Systemic) on page 625
- ◆ **Ery-Tab®** see Erythromycin (Systemic) on page 625
- ◆ **Erythrocin®** see Erythromycin (Systemic) on page 625
- ◆ **Erythrocin® Lactobionate-I.V.** see Erythromycin (Systemic) on page 625

Erythromycin (Systemic) (er ith roe MYE sin)

Related Information

Community-Acquired Pneumonia in Adults on page 2059

Medication Safety Issues

Sound-alike/look-alike issues:

Erythromycin may be confused with azithromycin, clarithromycin, Ethmozine®

Akne-Mycin® may be confused with AK-Mycin®

E.E.S.® may be confused with DES®

Eryc® may be confused with Emcyt®, Ery-Tab®

Ery-Tab® may be confused with Eryc®
Erythrocin® may be confused with Ethmozine®

Brand Names: U.S. E.E.S.®; Ery-Tab®; EryPed®; Erythro-RX; Erythrocin®; Erythrocin® Lactobionate-I.V.; PCE®

Brand Names: Canada Apo-Erythro Base®; Apo-Erythro E-C®; Apo-Erythro-ES®; Apo-Erythro-S®; EES®; Erybid™; Eryc®; Novo-Rythro Estolate; Novo-Rythro Ethylsuccinate; Nu-Erythromycin-S; PCE®

Index Terms Erythromycin Base; Erythromycin Ethylsuccinate; Erythromycin Lactobionate; Erythromycin Stearate

Generic Availability (U.S.) Yes: Capsule, tablet (as base, ethylsuccinate, and stearate)

Pharmacologic Category Antibiotic, Macrolide

Use Treatment of susceptible bacterial infections including *S. pyogenes*, some *S. pneumoniae*, some *S. aureus*, *M. pneumoniae*, *Legionella pneumophila*, diphtheria, pertussis, *Chlamydia*, erythrasma, *N. gonorrhoeae*, *E. histolytica*, syphilis and nongonococcal urethritis, and *Campylobacter* gastroenteritis; used in conjunction with neomycin for decontaminating the bowel

Unlabeled/Investigational Use Treatment of gastroparesis, chancroid; preoperative gut sterilization

Contraindications Hypersensitivity to erythromycin, any macrolide antibiotics, or any component of the formulation

Concomitant use with pimozide, cisapride, ergotamine or dihydroergotamine, terfenadine, astemizole

Warnings/Precautions Use caution with hepatic impairment with or without jaundice has occurred, it may be accompanied by malaise, nausea, vomiting, abdominal colic, and fever; discontinue use if these occur. Use caution with other medication relying on CYP3A4 metabolism; high potential for drug interactions exists. Prolonged use may result in fungal or bacterial superinfection, including *C. difficile*-associated diarrhea (CDAD) and pseudomembranous colitis; CDAD has been observed >2 months postantibiotic treatment. Macrolides have been associated with rare QT_c prolongation and ventricular arrhythmias, including torsade de pointes. Use caution in elderly patients, as risk of adverse events may be increased. Use caution in myasthenia gravis patients; erythromycin may aggravate muscular weakness.

Adverse Reactions (Reflective of adult population; not specific for elderly) Frequency not defined. Incidence may vary with formulation.

Cardiovascular: QT_c prolongation, torsade de pointes, ventricular arrhythmia, ventricular tachycardia

Central nervous system: Seizure

Dermatologic: Erythema multiforme, pruritus, rash, Stevens-Johnson syndrome, toxic epidermal necrolysis

Gastrointestinal: Abdominal pain, anorexia, diarrhea, infantile hypertrophic pyloric stenosis, nausea, oral candidiasis, pancreatitis, pseudomembranous colitis, vomiting

Hepatic: Cholestatic jaundice (most common with estolate), hepatitis, liver function tests abnormal

Local: Phlebitis at the injection site, thrombophlebitis

Neuromuscular & skeletal: Weakness

Otic: Hearing loss

Miscellaneous: Allergic reactions, anaphylaxis, hypersensitivity reactions, interstitial nephritis, urticaria

Drug Interactions

Metabolism/Transport Effects Substrate of CYP2B6 (minor), CYP3A4 (major), P-glycoprotein; **Inhibits** CYP1A2 (weak), CYP3A4 (moderate), P-glycoprotein

Avoid Concomitant Use

Avoid concomitant use of Erythromycin (Systemic) with any of the following: Artemether; BCG; Cisapride; Conivaptan; Disopyramide; Dronedarone; Lincosamide Antibiotics; Lumefantrine; Nilotinib; Pimozide; QUEtiapine; QuiNINE; Silodosin; Terfenadine; Tetrabenazine; Thioridazine; Tolvaptan; Topotecan; Toremifene; Vandetanib; Vemurafenib; Ziprasidone

Increased Effect/Toxicity

Erythromycin (Systemic) may increase the levels/effects of: Alfentanil; Antifungal Agents (Azole Derivatives, Systemic); Antineoplastic Agents (Vinca Alkaloids); Benzodiazepines (metabolized by oxidation); Budesonide (Systemic, Oral Inhalation); BusPIRone; Calcium Channel Blockers; CarBAMazepine; Cardiac Glycosides; Cilostazol; Cisapride; CloZAPine; Colchicine; Corticosteroids (Systemic); CycloSPORINE; CycloSPORINE (Systemic); CYP3A4 Substrates; Dabigatran Etexilate; Disopyramide; Dronedarone; Eletriptan; Eplerenone; Ergot Derivatives; Everolimus; FentaNYL; Fexofenadine; HMG-CoA Reductase Inhibitors; Lurasidone; P-Glycoprotein Substrates; Pimecrolimus; Pimozide; QTc-Prolonging Agents; QuiNIDine; QuiNINE; Repaglinide; Rifamycin Derivatives; Rivaroxaban; Salmeterol; Saxagliptin; Selective Serotonin Reuptake Inhibitors; Silodosin; Sirolimus; Tacrolimus;

Tacrolimus (Systemic); Tacrolimus (Topical); Temsirolimus; Terfenadine; Tetrabenazine; Theophylline Derivatives; Thioridazine; Tolvaptan; Topotecan; Toremifene; Vandetanib; Vemurafenib; Vitamin K Antagonists; Ziprasidone; Zopiclone

The levels/effects of Erythromycin (Systemic) may be increased by: Alfuzosin; Antifungal Agents (Azole Derivatives, Systemic); Artemether; Chloroquine; Ciprofloxacin; Ciprofloxacin (Systemic); Conivaptan; CYP3A4 Inhibitors (Moderate); CYP3A4 Inhibitors (Strong); Gado-butrol; Lumefantrine; Nilotinib; P-Glycoprotein Inhibitors; QUEtiapine; QuiNINE

Decreased Effect

Erythromycin (Systemic) may decrease the levels/effects of: BCG; Clopidogrel; Typhoid Vaccine; Zafirlukast

The levels/effects of Erythromycin (Systemic) may be decreased by: CYP3A4 Inducers (Strong); Deferasirox; Etravirine; Herbs (CYP3A4 Inducers); Lincosamide Antibiotics; P-Glycoprotein Inducers; Tocilizumab

Ethanol/Nutrition/Herb Interactions

Ethanol: Avoid ethanol (may decrease absorption of erythromycin or enhance ethanol effects). Food: Erythromycin serum levels may be altered if taken with food (formulation-dependent). Herb/Nutraceutical: St John's wort may decrease erythromycin levels.

Stability

Injection:

Store unreconstituted vials at 15°C to 30°C (59°F to 86°F). Erythromycin lactobionate should be reconstituted with sterile water for injection without preservatives to avoid gel formation. The reconstituted solution is stable for 2 weeks when refrigerated or for 8 hours at room temperature.

Erythromycin I.V. infusion solution is stable at pH 6-8. Stability of lactobionate is pH dependent. I.V. form has the longest stability in 0.9% sodium chloride (NS) and should be prepared in this base solution whenever possible. Do not use D_5W as a diluent unless sodium bicarbonate is added to solution. If I.V. must be prepared in D_5W, 0.5 mL of the 8.4% sodium bicarbonate solution should be added per each 100 mL of D_5W.

Stability of parenteral admixture at room temperature (25°C) and at refrigeration temperature (4°C) is 24 hours.

Standard diluent: 500 mg/250 mL D_5W/NS; 750 mg/250 mL D_5W/NS; 1 g/250 mL D_5W/NS.

Oral suspension:

Granules: Prior to mixing, store at <30°C (<86°F). After mixing, store under refrigeration and use within 10 days.

Powder: Erythromycin ethylsuccinate may be stored at room temperature if used within 14 days. Refrigerate to preserve taste.

Tablet and capsule formulations: Store at <30°C (<86°F).

Mechanism of Action Inhibits RNA-dependent protein synthesis at the chain elongation step; binds to the 50S ribosomal subunit resulting in blockage of transpeptidation

Pharmacodynamics/Kinetics

Absorption: Oral: Variable but better with salt forms than with base form; 18% to 45%; ethylsuccinate may be better absorbed with food

Distribution:

Relative diffusion from blood into CSF: Minimal even with inflammation

CSF:blood level ratio: Normal meninges: 2% to 13%; Inflamed meninges: 7% to 25%

Protein binding: Base: 73% to 81%

Metabolism: Demethylation primarily via hepatic CYP3A4

Half-life elimination: Peak: 1.5-2 hours; End-stage renal disease: 5-6 hours

Time to peak, serum: Base: 4 hours; Ethylsuccinate: 0.5-2.5 hours; delayed with food due to differences in absorption

Excretion: Primarily feces; urine (2% to 15% as unchanged drug)

Dosage

Geriatric & Adult Note: Due to differences in absorption, 400 mg erythromycin ethyl-succinate produces the same serum levels as 250 mg erythromycin base or stearate.

Usual dosage range:

Oral:

Base: 250-500 mg every 6-12 hours

Ethylsuccinate: 400-800 mg every 6-12 hours

I.V.: Lactobionate: 15-20 mg/kg/day divided every 6 hours or 500 mg to 1 g every 6 hours, or given as a continuous infusion over 24 hours (maximum: 4 g/24 hours)

Indication-specific dosing:

***Bartonella sp* infections (bacillary angiomatosis [BA], peliosis hepatis [PH]) (unla-beled use):** Oral: 500 mg 4 times/day for 3 months (BA) or 4 months (PH)

Chancroid (unlabeled use): Oral: 500 mg (base) 3 times/day for 7 days; **Note:** Not a preferred agent; isolates with intermediate resistance have been documented (CDC, 2010)

Gastrointestinal prokinetic (unlabeled use): I.V.: 200 mg initially followed by 250 mg (base) orally 3 times/day 30 minutes before meals. Lower dosages have been used in some trials.

Granuloma inguinale (donovanosis) (unlabeled use): Oral: 500 mg (base) 4 times/day for 21 days (CDC, 2010)

Legionnaires' disease: Oral: 1.6-4 g (ethylsuccinate)/day or 1-4 g (base)/day in divided doses for 21 days. **Note:** No longer preferred therapy and only used in nonhospitalized patients.

Lymphogranuloma venereum: Oral: 500 mg (base) 4 times/day for 21 days; **Note:** Preferred therapy for pregnant or lactating women (CDC, 2010)

Nongonococcal urethritis (including coinfection with *C. trachomatis*): Oral: 500 mg (base) 4 times/day for 7 days or 800 mg (ethylsuccinate) 4 times/day for 7 days. **Note:** May use 250 mg (base) or 400 mg (ethylsuccinate) 4 times/day for 14 days if gastrointestinal intolerance.

Pertussis: Oral: 500 mg (base) every 6 hours for 14 days

Preop bowel preparation: Oral: 1 g erythromycin base at 1, 2, and 11 PM on the day before surgery combined with mechanical cleansing of the large intestine and oral neomycin

Renal Impairment Slightly dialyzable (5% to 20%); supplemental dose is not necessary in hemo- or peritoneal dialysis or in continuous arteriovenous or venovenous hemofiltration.

Administration

Oral: Do not crush enteric coated drug product. GI upset, including diarrhea, is common. May be administered with food to decrease GI upset. Do not give with milk or acidic beverages.

I.V.: Infuse 1 g over 20-60 minutes. I.V. infusion may be very irritating to the vein. If phlebitis/pain occurs with used dilution, consider diluting further (eg, 1:5) if fluid status of the patient will tolerate, or consider administering in larger available vein. The addition of lidocaine or bicarbonate does not decrease the irritation of erythromycin infusions.

Test Interactions False-positive urinary catecholamines, 17-hydroxycorticosteroids and 17-ketosteroids

Special Geriatric Considerations Dose does not need to be adjusted unless there is severe renal or hepatic impairment. Elderly may be at an increased risk for torsade de pointes, ototoxicity (particularly when dose is ≥4 g/day in conjunction with renal or hepatic impairment).

Dosage Forms Excipient information presented when available (limited, particularly for generics); consult specific product labeling. [DSC] = Discontinued product

Capsule, delayed release, enteric coated pellets, oral, as base: 250 mg

Granules for suspension, oral, as ethylsuccinate [strength expressed as base]:

E.E.S.®: 200 mg/5 mL (100 mL, 200 mL) [contains sodium 25.9 mg (1.1 mEq)/5 mL; cherry flavor]

E.E.S.®: 200 mg/5 mL (100 mL) [contains sodium 25.9 mg (1.1 mEq)/5 mL; cherry flavor]

Injection, powder for reconstitution, as lactobionate [strength expressed as base]:

Erythrocin® Lactobionate-I.V.: 500 mg

Powder, for prescription compounding:

Erythro-RX: USP: 100% (50 g)

Powder for suspension, oral, as ethylsuccinate [strength expressed as base]:

EryPed®: 200 mg/5 mL (100 mL) [contains sodium 117.5 mg (5.1 mEq)/5 mL; fruit flavor]

EryPed®: 400 mg/5 mL (100 mL) [contains sodium 117.5 mg (5.1 mEq)/5 mL; banana flavor]

Tablet, oral, as base: 250 mg, 500 mg

Tablet, oral, as ethylsuccinate [strength expressed as base]: 400 mg

E.E.S.®: 400 mg [contains potassium 10 mg (0.3 mEq)/tablet, sodium 47 mg (2 mEq)/tablet]

Tablet, oral, as stearate [strength expressed as base]:

Erythrocin®: 250 mg [contains potassium 5 mg (0.1 mEq)/tablet, sodium 56.7 mg (2.5 mEq)/tablet]

Erythrocin®: 500 mg [sodium free; contains potassium 7 mg (0.2 mEq)/tablet]

Tablet, delayed release, enteric coated, oral, as base:

Ery-Tab®: 250 mg [contains sodium 8.3 mg (0.4 mEq)/tablet]

Ery-Tab®: 333 mg [contains sodium 11.2 mg (0.5 mEq)/tablet]

Ery-Tab®: 500 mg [contains sodium 16.7 mg (0.7 mEq)/tablet]

Tablet, polymer coated particles, oral, as base:

PCE®: 333 mg [contains sodium 0.5 mg (0.02mEq)/tablet]

PCE®: 500 mg [dye free, sodium free]

Erythromycin and Sulfisoxazole (er ith roe MYE sin & sul fi SOKS a zole)

Related Information
Erythromycin (Systemic) *on page 625*
Medication Safety Issues
Sound-alike/look-alike issues:
Pediazole® may be confused with Pediapred®
Brand Names: U.S. E.S.P.®
Brand Names: Canada Pediazole®
Index Terms Sulfisoxazole and Erythromycin
Generic Availability (U.S.) Yes
Pharmacologic Category Antibiotic, Macrolide; Antibiotic, Macrolide Combination; Antibiotic, Sulfonamide Derivative
Use Treatment of susceptible bacterial infections of the upper and lower respiratory tract and many other infections in patients allergic to penicillin
Contraindications Hypersensitivity to erythromycin, sulfonamides, or any component of the formulation; hepatic dysfunction; porphyria; concurrent use with pimozide or cisapride
Warnings/Precautions Use with caution in patients with impaired renal or hepatic function, myasthenia gravis, G6PD deficiency (hemolysis may occur). Macrolides have been associated with rare QT_c prolongation and ventricular arrhythmias, including torsade de pointes; use with caution in patients at risk of prolonged cardiac repolarization. Chemical similarities are present among sulfonamides, sulfonylureas, carbonic anhydrase inhibitors, thiazides, and loop diuretics (except ethacrynic acid). In patients with allergy to one of these compounds, a risk of cross-reaction exists; avoid use when previous reaction has been severe. Prolonged use may result in fungal or bacterial superinfection, including *C. difficile*-associated diarrhea (CDAD) and pseudomembranous colitis; CDAD has been observed >2 months postantibiotic treatment.
Adverse Reactions (Reflective of adult population; not specific for elderly) Frequency not defined.
Cardiovascular: Ventricular arrhythmia,
Central nervous system: Headache, fever
Dermatologic: Rash, Stevens-Johnson syndrome, toxic epidermal necrolysis
Gastrointestinal: Abdominal pain, cramping, nausea, vomiting, oral candidiasis, hypertrophic pyloric stenosis, diarrhea, pseudomembranous colitis
Hematologic: Agranulocytosis, aplastic anemia, eosinophilia
Hepatic: Hepatic necrosis, cholestatic jaundice
Local: Phlebitis at the injection site, thrombophlebitis
Renal: Toxic nephrosis, crystalluria
Miscellaneous: Hypersensitivity reactions
Drug Interactions
Metabolism/Transport Effects
Erythromycin: **Substrate** of CYP2B6 (minor), CYP3A4 (major), P-glycoprotein; **Inhibits** CYP1A2 (weak), CYP3A4 (moderate), P-glycoprotein
Sulfisoxazole: **Substrate** of CYP2C9 (major); **Inhibits** CYP2C8/9 (strong)
Avoid Concomitant Use
Avoid concomitant use of Erythromycin and Sulfisoxazole with any of the following: Artemether; BCG; Cisapride; Conivaptan; Disopyramide; Dronedarone; Lincosamide Antibiotics; Lovastatin; Lumefantrine; Methenamine; Nilotinib; Pimozide; Potassium P-Aminobenzoate; Procaine; QUEtiapine; QuiNINE; Silodosin; Simvastatin; Terfenadine; Tetrabenazine; Thioridazine; Tolvaptan; Topotecan; Toremifene; Vandetanib; Vemurafenib; Ziprasidone
Increased Effect/Toxicity
Erythromycin and Sulfisoxazole may increase the levels/effects of: Alfentanil; Antifungal Agents (Azole Derivatives, Systemic); Antineoplastic Agents (Vinca Alkaloids); Benzodiazepines (metabolized by oxidation); Budesonide (Systemic, Oral Inhalation); BusPIRone; Calcium Channel Blockers; CarBAMazepine; Cardiac Glycosides; Carvedilol; Cilostazol; Cisapride; CloZAPine; Colchicine; Corticosteroids (Systemic); CycloSPORINE; CycloSPORINE (Systemic); CYP2C9 Substrates (High risk); CYP3A4 Substrates; Dabigatran Etexilate; Diclofenac; Disopyramide; Dronedarone; Eletriptan; Eplerenone; Ergot Derivatives; Everolimus; FentaNYL; Fexofenadine; Fosphenytoin; HMG-CoA Reductase Inhibitors; Lovastatin; Lurasidone; Methotrexate; P-Glycoprotein Substrates; Phenytoin; Pimecrolimus; Pimozide; Porfimer; QTc-Prolonging Agents; QuiNIDine; QuiNINE; Repaglinide; Rifamycin Derivatives; Rivaroxaban; Salmeterol; Saxagliptin; Selective Serotonin Reuptake Inhibitors; Sildenafil; Silodosin; Simvastatin; Sirolimus; Sulfonylureas; Tacrolimus; Tacrolimus (Systemic); Tacrolimus (Topical); Telaprevir; Temsirolimus; Terfenadine; Tetrabenazine;

629

Theophylline Derivatives; Thioridazine; Tolvaptan; Topotecan; Toremifene; Vandetanib; Vardenafil; Vemurafenib; Vitamin K Antagonists; Ziprasidone; Zopiclone

The levels/effects of Erythromycin and Sulfisoxazole may be increased by: Alfuzosin; Antifungal Agents (Azole Derivatives, Systemic); Artemether; Chloroquine; Ciprofloxacin; Ciprofloxacin (Systemic); Conivaptan; CYP2C9 Inhibitors (Moderate); CYP2C9 Inhibitors (Strong); CYP3A4 Inhibitors (Moderate); CYP3A4 Inhibitors (Strong); Gadobutrol; Lumefantrine; Methenamine; Nilotinib; P-Glycoprotein Inhibitors; QUEtiapine; QuiNINE; Telaprevir

Decreased Effect

Erythromycin and Sulfisoxazole may decrease the levels/effects of: BCG; Clopidogrel; CycloSPORINE; CycloSPORINE (Systemic); Lincosamide Antibiotics; Typhoid Vaccine; Zafirlukast

The levels/effects of Erythromycin and Sulfisoxazole may be decreased by: CYP2C9 Inducers (Highly Effective); CYP3A4 Inducers (Strong); Deferasirox; Etravirine; Herbs (CYP3A4 Inducers); Peginterferon Alfa-2b; P-Glycoprotein Inducers; Potassium P-Aminobenzoate; Procaine; Tocilizumab

Stability Reconstituted suspension is stable for 14 days when refrigerated.

Mechanism of Action Erythromycin inhibits bacterial protein synthesis; sulfisoxazole competitively inhibits bacterial synthesis of folic acid from para-aminobenzoic acid

Pharmacodynamics/Kinetics See individual agents.

Dosage

Geriatric Not recommended for use in the elderly.

Adult Susceptible infections: Oral (dosage recommendation is based on the product's erythromycin content): 400 mg erythromycin and 1200 mg sulfisoxazole every 6 hours

Renal Impairment Sulfisoxazole must be adjusted in renal impairment.

Cl_{cr} 10-50 mL/minute: Administer every 8-12 hours.

Cl_{cr} <10 mL/minute: Administer every 12-24 hours.

Monitoring Parameters CBC and periodic liver function test

Test Interactions False-positive urinary protein; false-positive urinary catecholamines, 17-hydroxycorticosteroids and 17-ketosteroids

Dosage Forms Excipient information presented when available (limited, particularly for generics); consult specific product labeling.

Powder for oral suspension: Erythromycin ethylsuccinate 200 mg and sulfisoxazole acetyl 600 mg per 5 mL (100 mL, 150 mL, 200 mL)

E.S.P.®: Erythromycin ethylsuccinate 200 mg and sulfisoxazole acetyl 600 mg per 5 mL (100 mL, 150 mL, 200 mL) [cheri beri flavor]

♦ **Erythromycin Base** *see* Erythromycin (Systemic) *on page 625*
♦ **Erythromycin Ethylsuccinate** *see* Erythromycin (Systemic) *on page 625*
♦ **Erythromycin Lactobionate** *see* Erythromycin (Systemic) *on page 625*
♦ **Erythromycin Stearate** *see* Erythromycin (Systemic) *on page 625*
♦ **Erythropoiesis-Stimulating Agent (ESA)** *see* Darbepoetin Alfa *on page 456*
♦ **Erythropoiesis-Stimulating Agent (ESA)** *see* Epoetin Alfa *on page 611*
♦ **Erythropoiesis-Stimulating Protein** *see* Darbepoetin Alfa *on page 456*
♦ **Erythropoietin** *see* Epoetin Alfa *on page 611*
♦ **Erythro-RX** *see* Erythromycin (Systemic) *on page 625*

Escitalopram (es sye TAL oh pram)

Related Information

Antidepressant Agents *on page 1991*

Liquid Compatibility of Antidepressants, Antipsychotics, and Mood Stabilizers *on page 2111*

Medication Safety Issues

Sound-alike/look-alike issues:

Lexapro® may be confused with Loxitane®

International issues:

Zavesca: Brand name for escitalopram [in multiple international markets; ISMP April 21, 2010], but also brand name for miglustat [Canada, U.S., and multiple international markets]

Brand Names: U.S. Lexapro®

Brand Names: Canada Cipralex®

Index Terms Escitalopram Oxalate; Lu-26-054; S-Citalopram

Generic Availability (U.S.) No

Pharmacologic Category Antidepressant, Selective Serotonin Reuptake Inhibitor

Use Treatment of major depressive disorder; generalized anxiety disorders (GAD)

Unlabeled/Investigational Use Treatment of mild dementia-associated agitation in non-psychotic patients

Medication Guide Available Yes

Contraindications Hypersensitivity to escitalopram, citalopram, or any component of the formulation; concomitant use with pimozide; concomitant use or within 2 weeks of MAO inhibitors

Warnings/Precautions [U.S. Boxed Warning]: Antidepressants increase the risk of suicidal thinking and behavior in children, adolescents, and young adults (18-24 years of age) with major depressive disorder (MDD) and other psychiatric disorders; consider risk prior to prescribing. Short-term studies did not show an increased risk in patients >24 years of age and showed a decreased risk in patients ≥65 years. Closely monitor patients for clinical worsening, suicidality, or unusual changes in behavior, particularly during the initial 1-2 months of therapy or during periods of dosage adjustments (increases or decreases); the patient's family or caregiver should be instructed to closely observe the patient and communicate condition with healthcare provider. A medication guide concerning the use of antidepressants should be dispensed with each prescription. **Escitalopram is not FDA approved for use in children <12 years of age.**

The possibility of a suicide attempt is inherent in major depression and may persist until remission occurs. Use caution in high-risk patients. Worsening depression and severe abrupt suicidality that are not part of the presenting symptoms may require discontinuation or modification of drug therapy. The patient's family or caregiver should be alerted to monitor patients for the emergence of suicidality and associated behaviors (such as agitation, irritability, hostility, impulsivity, and hypomania) and call healthcare provider.

May worsen psychosis in some patients or precipitate a shift to mania or hypomania in patients with bipolar disorder. Patients presenting with depressive symptoms should be screened for bipolar disorder. Monotherapy in patients with bipolar disorder should be avoided. Escitalopram is not FDA approved for the treatment of bipolar depression. Escitalopram is not FDA approved for the treatment of bipolar depression.

Serotonin syndrome and neuroleptic malignant syndrome (NMS)-like reactions have occurred with serotonin/norepinephrine reuptake inhibitors (SNRIs) and selective serotonin reuptake inhibitors (SSRIs) when used alone, and particularly when used in combination with serotonergic agents (eg, triptans) or antidopaminergic agents (eg, antipsychotics). Concurrent use or within 2 weeks of an MAO inhibitor is contraindicated. May increase the risks associated with electroconvulsive therapy. Has a low potential to impair cognitive or motor performance; caution operating hazardous machinery or driving.

Use caution with a previous seizure disorder or condition predisposing to seizures such as brain damage, alcoholism, or concurrent therapy with other drugs which lower the seizure threshold. May cause hyponatremia/SIADH (elderly at increased risk); volume depletion (diuretics may increase risk) may occur. May cause or exacerbate sexual dysfunction. Use caution with severe renal impairment or liver impairment; concomitant CNS depressants. Use caution with concomitant use of aspirin, NSAIDs, warfarin, or other drugs that affect coagulation; the risk of bleeding may be potentiated.

Upon discontinuation of escitalopram therapy, gradually taper dose. If intolerable symptoms occur following a decrease in dosage or upon discontinuation of therapy, then resuming the previous dose with a more gradual taper should be considered.

Adverse Reactions (Reflective of adult population; not specific for elderly)

>10%:

Central nervous system: Headache (24%), somnolence (6% to 13%), insomnia (9% to 12%)

Gastrointestinal: Nausea (15% to 18%)

Genitourinary: Ejaculation disorder (9% to 14%)

1% to 10%:

Central nervous system: Fatigue (5% to 8%), dizziness (5%), abnormal dreaming (3%), lethargy (3%), yawning (2%)

Endocrine & metabolic: Libido decreased (3% to 7%), anorgasmia (2% to 6%), menstrual disorder (2%)

Gastrointestinal: Xerostomia (6% to 9%), diarrhea (8%), constipation (3% to 5%), appetite decreased (3%), indigestion (3%), vomiting (3%), abdominal pain (2%), flatulence (2%), toothache (2%)

Genitourinary: Impotence (2% to 3%)

Neuromuscular & skeletal: Neck/shoulder pain (3%), paresthesia (2%)

Respiratory: Rhinitis (5%), sinusitis (3%)

Miscellaneous: Diaphoresis (4% to 5%), flu-like syndrome (5%)

Drug Interactions

Metabolism/Transport Effects Substrate (major) of CYP2C19, 3A4; **Inhibits** CYP2D6 (weak)

◀ **Avoid Concomitant Use**
Avoid concomitant use of Escitalopram with any of the following: Artemether; Conivaptan; Dronedarone; Iobenguane I 123; Lumefantrine; MAO Inhibitors; Methylene Blue; Nilotinib; Pimozide; QUEtiapine; QuiNINE; Sibutramine; Tetrabenazine; Thioridazine; Toremifene; Tryptophan; Vandetanib; Vemurafenib; Ziprasidone

Increased Effect/Toxicity
Escitalopram may increase the levels/effects of: Alpha-/Beta-Blockers; Anticoagulants; Antidepressants (Serotonin Reuptake Inhibitor/Antagonist); Antiplatelet Agents; Aspirin; BusPIRone; CarBAMazepine; CloZAPine; Collagenase (Systemic); Desmopressin; Dextromethorphan; Dronedarone; Drotrecogin Alfa; Haloperidol; Ibritumomab; Lithium; Methadone; Methylene Blue; Mexiletine; NSAID (COX-2 Inhibitor); NSAID (Nonselective); Pimozide; QTc-Prolonging Agents; QuiNINE; RisperiDONE; Rivaroxaban; Salicylates; Serotonin Modulators; Tetrabenazine; Thioridazine; Thrombolytic Agents; Toremifene; Tositumomab and Iodine I 131 Tositumomab; TraMADol; Tricyclic Antidepressants; Vandetanib; Vemurafenib; Vitamin K Antagonists; Ziprasidone

The levels/effects of Escitalopram may be increased by: Alcohol (Ethyl); Alfuzosin; Analgesics (Opioid); Artemether; BusPIRone; Chloroquine; Cimetidine; Ciprofloxacin; Ciprofloxacin (Systemic); CNS Depressants; Conivaptan; CYP2C19 Inhibitors (Moderate); CYP2C19 Inhibitors (Strong); CYP3A4 Inhibitors (Moderate); CYP3A4 Inhibitors (Strong); Gadobutrol; Glucosamine; Herbs (Anticoagulant/Antiplatelet Properties); Lumefantrine; Macrolide Antibiotics; MAO Inhibitors; Metoclopramide; Nilotinib; Omega-3-Acid Ethyl Esters; Pentosan Polysulfate Sodium; Pentoxifylline; Prostacyclin Analogues; QUEtiapine; QuiNINE; Sibutramine; TraMADol; Tryptophan; Vitamin E

Decreased Effect
Escitalopram may decrease the levels/effects of: Iobenguane I 123

The levels/effects of Escitalopram may be decreased by: CarBAMazepine; CYP2C19 Inducers (Strong); CYP3A4 Inducers (Strong); Cyproheptadine; Deferasirox; NSAID (Nonselective); Telaprevir; Tocilizumab

Ethanol/Nutrition/Herb Interactions
Ethanol: May increase CNS depression; monitor for increased effects with coadministration. Caution patients about effects.
Herb/Nutraceutical: Avoid valerian, St John's wort, SAMe, kava kava, and gotu kola (may increase CNS depression).

Stability Store at 25°C (77°F); excursions permitted to 15°C to 30°C (59°F to 86°F).

Mechanism of Action Escitalopram is the S-enantiomer of the racemic derivative citalopram, which selectively inhibits the reuptake of serotonin with little to no effect on norepinephrine or dopamine reuptake. It has no or very low affinity for 5-HT$_{1-7}$, alpha- and beta-adrenergic, D$_{1-5}$, H$_{1-3}$, M$_{1-5}$, and benzodiazepine receptors. Escitalopram does not bind to or has low affinity for Na$^+$, K$^+$, Cl$^-$, and Ca^{++} ion channels.

Pharmacodynamics/Kinetics
Onset of action: Depression: The onset of action is within a week; however, individual response varies greatly and full response may not be seen until 8-12 weeks after initiation of treatment.
Protein binding: ~56% to plasma proteins
Metabolism: Hepatic via CYP2C19 and 3A4 to an active metabolite, S-desmethylcitalopram (S-DCT; 1/7 the activity of escitalopram); S-DCT is metabolized to S-didesmethylcitalopram (S-DDCT; active; 1/27 the activity of escitalopram) via CYP2D6
Half-life elimination: Escitalopram: 27-32 hours; S-DCT: 59 hours
Time to peak: Escitalopram: ~5 hours; S-DCT: 14 hours
Excretion: Urine (Escitalopram: 8%; S-DCT: 10%)

Dosage
Geriatric Major depressive disorder, generalized anxiety disorder: Oral: 10 mg once daily
Adult Major depressive disorder, generalized anxiety disorder: Oral: Initial: 10 mg once daily; dose may be increased to 20 mg once daily after at least 1 week
Renal Impairment
Mild-to-moderate impairment: No dosage adjustment needed.
Severe impairment: Cl$_{cr}$ <20 mL/minute: Use with caution.
Hepatic Impairment 10 mg once daily

Administration Administer once daily (morning or evening), with or without food.

Monitoring Parameters Mental status for depression, suicidal ideation (especially at the beginning of therapy or when doses are increased or decreased); anxiety, social functioning, mania, panic attacks; akathisia

Pharmacotherapy Pearls The tablet and oral solution dosage forms are bioequivalent. Clinically, escitalopram 20 mg is equipotent to citalopram 40 mg. Do not coadminister with citalopram.

Special Geriatric Considerations Bioavailability and half-life are increased by 50% in the elderly. Clinical trials comparing escitalopram to placebo found no difference in the change in depression scales scores from baseline or relief of symptoms with either treatment. Escitalopram has been shown to delay the time to relapse compared to placebo over 6 months. The elderly are more prone to SSRI/SNRI-induced hyponatremia.

Dosage Forms Excipient information presented when available (limited, particularly for generics); consult specific product labeling.

Solution, oral:
Lexapro®: 1 mg/mL (240 mL) [contains propylene glycol; peppermint flavor]
Tablet, oral:
Lexapro®: 5 mg
Lexapro®: 10 mg, 20 mg [scored]

Dosage Forms: Canada Excipient information presented when available (limited, particularly for generics); consult specific product labeling.

Tablet:
Cipralex®: 10 mg, 20 mg

Selected References
Bose A, Li D, and Gandhi C, "Escitalopram in the Acute Treatment of Depressed Patients Aged 60 Years or Older," *Am J Geriatr Psychiatry*, 2008, 16(1):14-20.

Dunkley EJ, Isbister GK, Sibbritt D, et al, "The Hunter Serotonin Toxicity Criteria: Simple and Accurate Diagnostic Decision Rules for Serotonin Toxicity," *QJM*, 2003, 96(9):635-42.

Gorwood P, Weiller E, Lemming O, et al, "Escitalopram Prevents Relapse in Older Patients With Major Depressive Disorder," *Am J Geriatr Psychiatry*, 2007, 15(7):581-93.

Rabins PV, Blacker D, Rovner BW, et al, "Practice Guidelines for the Treatment of Patients With Alzheimer's Disease and Other Dementias," *Am J Psychiatry*, 2007, 164(12 Suppl):5-56. Available at http://www.psych.org/psych_pract/treatg/pg/prac_guide.cfm.

Stevens DL, "Association Between Selective Serotonin-Reuptake Inhibitors, Second-Generation Antipsychotics, and Neuroleptic Malignant Syndrome," *Ann Pharmacother*, 2008, 42(9):1290-7.

◆ **Escitalopram Oxalate** see Escitalopram *on page 630*
◆ **Eserine Salicylate** see Physostigmine *on page 1449*
◆ **Eskalith** see Lithium *on page 1082*

Esmolol (ES moe lol)

Related Information
Beta-Blockers *on page 2001*

Medication Safety Issues
Sound-alike/look-alike issues:
Esmolol may be confused with Osmitrol®
Brevibloc® may be confused with Brevital®, Bumex®, Buprenex®
High alert medication:
The Institute for Safe Medication Practices (ISMP) includes this medication among its list of drugs which have a heightened risk of causing significant patient harm when used in error.

Brand Names: U.S. Brevibloc

Brand Names: Canada Brevibloc®

Index Terms Esmolol Hydrochloride

Generic Availability (U.S.) Yes: Excludes infusion

Pharmacologic Category Antiarrhythmic Agent, Class II; Beta Blocker, Beta-1 Selective

Use Treatment of supraventricular tachycardia (SVT) and atrial fibrillation/flutter (control ventricular rate); treatment of intraoperative and postoperative tachycardia and/or hypertension; treatment of noncompensatory sinus tachycardia

Unlabeled/Investigational Use Arrhythmia/rate control during acute coronary syndrome (eg, acute myocardial infarction, unstable angina), aortic dissection, intubation, thyroid storm, pheochromocytoma, electroconvulsive therapy

Contraindications Hypersensitivity to esmolol or any component of the formulation; sinus bradycardia; heart block greater than first degree (except in patients with a functioning artificial pacemaker); cardiogenic shock; bronchial asthma (relative); uncompensated cardiac failure; hypotension

Warnings/Precautions Consider pre-existing conditions such as sick sinus syndrome before initiating. Hypotension is common; patients need close blood pressure monitoring. Administer cautiously in compensated heart failure and monitor for a worsening of the condition. Can precipitate or aggravate symptoms of arterial insufficiency in patients with PVD and Raynaud's disease. Use with caution and monitor for progression of arterial obstruction. Use caution with concurrent use of digoxin, verapamil or diltiazem; bradycardia or heart block can occur. Use with caution in patients receiving inhaled anesthetic agents known to depress myocardial contractility. Use beta-blockers cautiously in patients with bronchospastic disease; monitor pulmonary status closely. Use cautiously in patients with diabetes because it can mask prominent hypoglycemic symptoms. Bradycardia may be observed more frequently in elderly

◀ patients (>65 years of age); dosage reductions may be necessary. May mask signs of hyperthyroidism (eg, tachycardia); if hyperthyroidism is suspected, carefully manage and monitor; abrupt withdrawal may exacerbate symptoms of hyperthyroidism or precipitate thyroid storm. Use with caution in patients with myasthenia gravis. Use caution in patients with renal dysfunction (active metabolite retained). Adequate alpha-blockade is required prior to use of any beta-blocker for patients with untreated pheochromocytoma. Use caution with history of severe anaphylaxis to allergens; patients taking beta-blockers may become more sensitive to repeated challenges. Treatment of anaphylaxis (eg, epinephrine) in patients taking beta-blockers may be ineffective or promote undesirable effects. Beta-blocker therapy should not be withdrawn abruptly (particularly in patients with CAD), but gradually tapered to avoid acute tachycardia, hypertension, and/or ischemia. Do not use in the treatment of hypertension associated with vasoconstriction related to hypothermia. Extravasation can lead to skin necrosis and sloughing.

Adverse Reactions (Reflective of adult population; not specific for elderly)

>10%:
 Cardiovascular: Asymptomatic hypotension (dose related: 25% to 38%), symptomatic hypotension (dose related: 12%)
 Miscellaneous: Diaphoresis (10%)

1% to 10%:
 Cardiovascular: Peripheral ischemia (1%)
 Central nervous system: Dizziness (3%), somnolence (3%), confusion (2%), headache (2%), agitation (2%), fatigue (1%)
 Gastrointestinal: Nausea (7%), vomiting (1%)
 Local: Pain on injection (8%), infusion site reaction

Drug Interactions

Avoid Concomitant Use

 Avoid concomitant use of Esmolol with any of the following: Floctafenine; Methacholine

Increased Effect/Toxicity

 Esmolol may increase the levels/effects of: Alpha-/Beta-Agonists (Direct-Acting); Alpha1-Blockers; Alpha2-Agonists; Amifostine; Antihypertensives; Antipsychotic Agents (Phenothiazines); Bupivacaine; Cardiac Glycosides; Fingolimod; Hypotensive Agents; Insulin; Lidocaine; Lidocaine (Systemic); Lidocaine (Topical); Mepivacaine; Methacholine; Midodrine; RiTUXimab; Sulfonylureas

 The levels/effects of Esmolol may be increased by: Acetylcholinesterase Inhibitors; Aminoquinolines (Antimalarial); Amiodarone; Anilidopiperidine Opioids; Antipsychotic Agents (Phenothiazines); Calcium Channel Blockers (Dihydropyridine); Calcium Channel Blockers (Nondihydropyridine); Diazoxide; Dipyridamole; Disopyramide; Dronedarone; Floctafenine; Herbs (Hypotensive Properties); MAO Inhibitors; Pentoxifylline; Phosphodiesterase 5 Inhibitors; Propafenone; Propoxyphene; Prostacyclin Analogues; QuiNIDine; Reserpine

Decreased Effect

 Esmolol may decrease the levels/effects of: Beta2-Agonists; Theophylline Derivatives

 The levels/effects of Esmolol may be decreased by: Barbiturates; Herbs (Hypertensive Properties); Methylphenidate; Nonsteroidal Anti-Inflammatory Agents; Rifamycin Derivatives; Yohimbine

Stability Clear, colorless to light yellow solution which should be stored at 25°C (77°F); excursions permitted to 15°C to 30°C (59°F to 86°F); do not freeze. Protect from excessive heat.
Stability of parenteral admixture at room temperature (25°C) is 24 hours.

Mechanism of Action Class II antiarrhythmic: Competitively blocks response to beta$_1$-adrenergic stimulation with little or no effect of beta$_2$-receptors except at high doses, no intrinsic sympathomimetic activity, no membrane stabilizing activity

Pharmacodynamics/Kinetics

Onset of action: Beta-blockade: I.V.: 2-10 minutes (quickest when loading doses are administered)

Duration of hemodynamic effects: 10-30 minutes; prolonged following higher cumulative doses, extended duration of use

Distribution: V_d: Esmolol: ~3.4 L/kg; Acid metabolite: ~0.4 L/kg

Protein binding: Esmolol: 55%; Acid metabolite: 10%

Metabolism: In blood by red blood cell esterases; forms acid metabolite (negligible activity; produces no clinically important effects) and methanol (does not achieve concentrations associated with methanol toxicity)

Half-life elimination: Adults: Esmolol: 9 minutes; Acid metabolite: 3.7 hours; elimination of metabolite decreases with end-stage renal disease

Excretion: Urine (~73% to 88% as acid metabolite, <2% unchanged drug)

Dosage

Geriatric & Adult

Intraoperative tachycardia and/or hypertension (immediate control): I.V.: Initial bolus: 80 mg (1 mg/kg) over 30 seconds, followed by a 150 mcg/kg/minute infusion, if necessary. Adjust infusion rate as needed to maintain desired heart rate and/or blood pressure, up to 300 mcg/kg/minute.

For control of postoperative hypertension, as many as one-third of patients may require higher doses (250-300 mcg/kg/minute) to control blood pressure; the safety of doses >300 mcg/kg/minute has not been studied.

Supraventricular tachycardia (SVT), gradual control of postoperative tachycardia/hypertension: I.V.: Loading dose: 500 mcg/kg over 1 minute; follow with a 50 mcg/kg/minute infusion for 4 minutes; response to this initial infusion rate may be a rough indication of the responsiveness of the ventricular rate.

Infusion may be continued at 50 mcg/kg/minute or, if the response is inadequate, titrated upward in 50 mcg/kg/minute increments (increased no more frequently than every 4 minutes) to a maximum of 200 mcg/kg/minute.

Note: To achieve more rapid response, following the initial loading dose and 50 mcg/kg/minute infusion, rebolus with a second 500 mcg/kg loading dose over 1 minute, and increase the maintenance infusion to 100 mcg/kg/minute for 4 minutes. If necessary, a third (and final) 500 mcg/kg loading dose may be administered, prior to increasing to an infusion rate of 150 mcg/kg/minute. After 4 minutes of the 150 mcg/kg/minute infusion, the infusion rate may be increased to a maximum rate of 200 mcg/kg/minute (without a bolus dose).

Acute coronary syndromes (when relative contraindications to beta-blockade exist; unlabeled use): 500 mcg/kg over 1 minute; follow with a 50 mcg/kg/minute infusion; if tolerated and response inadequate, may titrate upward in 50 mcg/kg/minute increments every 5-15 minutes to a maximum of 300 mcg/kg/minute (Mitchell, 2002); an additional bolus (500 mcg/kg over 1 minute) may be administered prior to each increase in infusion rate (Mooss, 1994)

Electroconvulsive therapy (unlabeled use): 1 mg/kg administered 1 minute prior to induction of anesthesia (Weinger, 1991)

Intubation (unlabeled use): 1-2 mg/kg I.V. given 1.5-3 minutes prior to intubation (Kindler, 1996)

Guidelines for transfer to oral therapy (beta-blocker, calcium channel blocker):

Infusion should be reduced by 50% 30 minutes following the first dose of the alternative agent

Manufacturer suggests following the second dose of the alternative drug, patient's response should be monitored and if control is adequate for the first hour, esmolol may be discontinued.

Renal Impairment Not removed by hemo- or peritoneal dialysis. Supplemental dose is not necessary.

Administration Infusions must be administered with an infusion pump. The concentrate (250 mg/mL ampul) is **not** for direct I.V. injection, but rather must first be diluted to a final concentration of 10 mg/mL (ie, 2.5 g in 250 mL or 5 g in 500 mL). Concentrations >10 mg/mL or infusion into small veins or through a butterfly catheter should be avoided (can cause thrombophlebitis). Decrease or discontinue infusion if hypotension or congestive heart failure occur. Medication port of premixed bags should be used to withdraw only the initial bolus, if necessary (not to be used for withdrawal of additional bolus doses).

Monitoring Parameters Blood pressure, MAP, heart rate, continuous ECG, respiratory rate, I.V. site

Special Geriatric Considerations Due to alterations in the beta-adrenergic autonomic nervous system, beta-adrenergic blockade may result in less hemodynamic response than seen in younger adults. Studies indicate that despite decreased sensitivity to the chronotropic effects of beta-blockade with age, there appears to be an increased myocardial sensitivity to the negative inotropic effect during stress (ie, exercise). Controlled trials have shown the overall response rate for propranolol to be only 20% to 50% in elderly populations. Therefore, all beta-adrenergic blocking drugs may result in a decreased response as compared to younger adults.

Dosage Forms Excipient information presented when available (limited, particularly for generics); consult specific product labeling. [DSC] = Discontinued product

Infusion, premixed in NS, as hydrochloride [preservative free]:

Brevibloc: 2000 mg (100 mL) [20 mg/mL; double strength]

Brevibloc: 2500 mg (250 mL) [10 mg/mL]

Injection, solution, as hydrochloride [preservative free]: 10 mg/mL (10 mL)

Brevibloc: 10 mg/mL (10 mL)

Brevibloc: 20 mg/mL (5 mL [DSC]) [double strength]

♦ **Esmolol Hydrochloride** *see* Esmolol *on page 633*

Esomeprazole (es oh ME pray zol)

Related Information
Helicobacter pylori Treatment in Adult Patients *on page 2009*
Medication Safety Issues
Sound-alike/look-alike issues:
Esomeprazole may be confused with ARIPiprazole
NexIUM® may be confused with NexAVAR®
Brand Names: U.S. NexIUM®; NexIUM® I.V.
Brand Names: Canada Apo-Esomeprazole®; Nexium®
Index Terms Esomeprazole Magnesium; Esomeprazole Sodium
Generic Availability (U.S.) No
Pharmacologic Category Proton Pump Inhibitor; Substituted Benzimidazole
Use
Oral: Short-term (4-8 weeks) treatment of erosive esophagitis; maintaining symptom resolution and healing of erosive esophagitis; treatment of symptomatic gastroesophageal reflux disease (GERD); as part of a multidrug regimen for *Helicobacter pylori* eradication in patients with duodenal ulcer disease (active or history of within the past 5 years); prevention of gastric ulcers in patients at risk (age ≥60 years and/or history of gastric ulcer) associated with continuous NSAID therapy; long-term treatment of pathological hypersecretory conditions including Zollinger-Ellison syndrome
Canadian labeling: Additional use (not in U.S. labeling): Oral: Treatment of nonerosive reflux disease (NERD)

I.V.: Short-term (≤10 days) treatment of gastroesophageal reflux disease (GERD) when oral therapy is not possible or appropriate
Unlabeled/Investigational Use I.V.: Prevention of recurrent peptic ulcer bleeding postendoscopy
Contraindications Hypersensitivity to esomeprazole, substituted benzimidazoles (eg, omeprazole, lansoprazole), or any component of the formulation
Warnings/Precautions Use of proton pump inhibitors may increase the risk of gastrointestinal infections (eg, *Salmonella, Campylobacter*). Relief of symptoms does not preclude the presence of a gastric malignancy. Atrophic gastritis (by biopsy) has been noted with long-term omeprazole therapy; this may also occur with esomeprazole. No reports of enterochromaffin-like (ECL) cell carcinoids, dysplasia, or neoplasia have occurred. Severe liver dysfunction may require dosage reductions. Safety and efficacy of I.V. therapy >10 days have not been established; transition from I.V. to oral therapy as soon possible. Bioavailability may be increased in Asian populations, the elderly, and patients with hepatic dysfunction. Decreased *H. pylori* eradication rates have been observed with short-term (≤7 days) combination therapy. The American College of Gastroenterology recommends 10-14 days of therapy (triple or quadruple) for eradication of *H. pylori* (Chey, 2007). Proton pump inhibitors may diminish the therapeutic effect of clopidogrel, thought to be due to reduced formation of the active metabolite of clopidogrel; an increase in the risk of cardiovascular events may occur. The manufacturer of clopidogrel recommends avoidance of concomitant administration of another PPI (ie, omeprazole); similar recommendations with esomeprazole would appear prudent. Avoid concurrent use of CYP3A4 and 2C19 inducers (eg, St John's wort, rifampin) as esomeprazole's efficacy may be reduced.

Increased incidence of osteoporosis-related bone fractures of the hip, spine, or wrist may occur with proton pump inhibitor therapy. Patients on high-dose or long-term therapy should be monitored. Use the lowest effective dose for the shortest duration of time, use vitamin D and calcium supplementation, and follow appropriate guidelines to reduce risk of fractures in patients at risk.

Hypomagnesemia, reported rarely, usually with prolonged PPI use of >3 months (most cases >1 year of therapy); may be symptomatic or asymptomatic; severe cases may cause tetany, seizures, and cardiac arrhythmias. Consider obtaining serum magnesium concentrations prior to beginning long-term therapy, especially if taking concomitant digoxin, diuretics, or other drugs known to cause hypomagnesemia; and periodically thereafter. Hypomagnesemia may be corrected by magnesium supplementation, although discontinuation of esomeprazole may be necessary; magnesium levels typically return to normal within 1 week of stopping. Serum chromogranin A levels may be increased if assessed while patient on esomeprazole; may lead to diagnostic errors related to neuroendocrine tumors.

Adverse Reactions (Reflective of adult population; not specific for elderly) Unless otherwise specified, percentages represent adverse reactions identified in clinical trials evaluating the oral formulation.

>10%: Central nervous system: Headache (I.V. 11%; oral ≤8%)

1% to 10%:

Cardiovascular: Hypertension (≤3%), chest pain (>1%)

Central nervous system: Pain (4%), dizziness (oral >1%; I.V. 3%), anxiety (2%), insomnia (2%), pyrexia (2%), fatigue (>1%)

Dermatologic: Rash (>1%), pruritus (I.V. ≤1%)

Endocrine & metabolic: Hypercholesterolemia (2%)

Gastrointestinal: Flatulence (oral ≤5%; I.V. 10%), diarrhea (oral ≤7%; I.V. 4%), abdominal pain (oral ≤6%; I.V. 6%), nausea (oral 5%; I.V. 6%), dyspepsia (oral >1%; I.V. 6%), gastritis (≤6%), constipation (oral 2%; I.V. 3%), vomiting (≤3%), benign GI neoplasm (>1%), dyspepsia (>1%), duodenitis (>1%), epigastric pain (>1%), esophageal disorder (>1%), gastroenteritis (>1%), GI mucosal discoloration (>1%), serum gastrin increased (>1%), xerostomia (1%)

Genitourinary: Urinary tract infection (4%)

Hematologic: Anemia (>1%)

Hepatic: Transaminases increased (>1%)

Local: Injection site reaction (I.V. 2%)

Neuromuscular & skeletal: Arthralgia (3%), back pain (>1%), fracture (>1%), arthropathy (1%), myalgia (1%)

Respiratory: Respiratory infection (oral ≤9%; I.V. 1%), bronchitis (4%), sinusitis (oral ≤4%; I.V. 2%), coughing (>1%), rhinitis (>1%), dyspnea (1%)

Miscellaneous: Accident/injury (≤8%), viral infection (4%), allergy (2%), ear infection (2%), hernia (>1%), flu-like syndrome (1%)

Drug Interactions

Metabolism/Transport Effects Substrate of CYP2C19 (major), 3A4 (major); **Inhibits** CYP2C19 (moderate)

Avoid Concomitant Use

Avoid concomitant use of Esomeprazole with any of the following: Delavirdine; Erlotinib; Nelfinavir; Posaconazole; Rifampin; Rilpivirine; St Johns Wort

Increased Effect/Toxicity

Esomeprazole may increase the levels/effects of: Amphetamines; Benzodiazepines (metabolized by oxidation); Cilostazol; CYP2C19 Substrates; Dexmethylphenidate; Methotrexate; Methylphenidate; Raltegravir; Saquinavir; Tacrolimus; Tacrolimus (Systemic); Vitamin K Antagonists; Voriconazole

The levels/effects of Esomeprazole may be increased by: Conivaptan; Fluconazole; Ketoconazole; Ketoconazole (Systemic)

Decreased Effect

Esomeprazole may decrease the levels/effects of: Atazanavir; Bisphosphonate Derivatives; Cefditoren; Clopidogrel; Dabigatran Etexilate; Dasatinib; Delavirdine; Erlotinib; Gefitinib; Indinavir; Iron Salts; Itraconazole; Ketoconazole; Ketoconazole (Systemic); Mesalamine; Mycophenolate; Nelfinavir; Posaconazole; Rilpivirine

The levels/effects of Esomeprazole may be decreased by: CYP2C19 Inducers (Strong); Rifampin; St Johns Wort; Tipranavir; Tocilizumab

Ethanol/Nutrition/Herb Interactions

Food: Absorption is decreased by 43% to 53% when taken with food.

Herb/Nutraceutical: Avoid use of St John's wort (may decrease efficacy of esomeprazole).

Stability

Capsule, granules: Store at 15°C to 30°C (59°F to 86°F). Keep container tightly closed.

Powder for injection: Store at 25°C (77°F); excursions permitted to 15°C to 30°C (59°F to 86°F). Protect from light.

For I.V. injection: Adults: Reconstitute powder with 5 mL NS.

For I.V. infusion: Adults: Initially reconstitute powder with 5 mL of NS, LR, or D_5W, then further dilute to a final volume of 50 mL.

Per the manufacturer, following reconstitution, solution for injection prepared in NS, and solution for infusion prepared in NS or LR should be used within 12 hours. Following reconstitution, solution for infusion prepared in D_5W should be used within 6 hours. Refrigeration is not required following reconstitution.

Additional stability data: Following reconstitution, solutions for infusion prepared in D_5W, NS, or LR in PVC bags are chemically and physically stable for 48 hours at room temperature (25°C) and for at least 120 hours under refrigeration (4°C) (Kupiec, 2008).

Mechanism of Action Proton pump inhibitor suppresses gastric acid secretion by inhibition of the H^+/K^+-ATPase in the gastric parietal cell. Esomeprazole is the S-isomer of omeprazole. ▶

◀ **Pharmacodynamics/Kinetics**
Distribution: V_{dss}: 16 L
Protein binding: 97%
Metabolism: Hepatic via CYP2C19 primarily and (to a lesser extent) via 3A4 to hydroxy, desmethyl, and sulfone metabolites (all inactive)
Bioavailability: Oral: 90% with repeat dosing
Half-life elimination: ~1-1.5 hours
Time to peak: Oral: 1.5-2 hours
Excretion: Urine (80%, primarily as inactive metabolites; <1% as active drug); feces (20%)

Dosage

Geriatric Refer to adult dosing. No dosage adjustment needed.

Adult

Erosive esophagitis (healing): Oral: Initial: 20-40 mg once daily for 4-8 weeks; if incomplete healing, may continue for an additional 4-8 weeks; maintenance: 20 mg once daily (controlled studies did not extend beyond 6 months)

Nonerosive reflux disease (NERD) (Canadian labeling): Initial: 20 mg once daily for 2-4 weeks; lack of symptom control after 4 weeks warrants further evaluation; maintenance (in patients with successful initial therapy): 20 mg once daily as needed

Symptomatic gastroesophageal reflux: Oral: 20 mg once daily for 4 weeks; may consider an additional 4 weeks of treatment if symptoms do not resolve

Treatment of GERD (short-term): I.V.: 20 mg or 40 mg once daily. **Note:** Indicated only in cases where oral therapy is inappropriate or not possible;safety/efficacy ≥10 days has not been established.

Prevention of recurrent peptic ulcer bleeding postendoscopy (unlabeled use; Sung, 2009): I.V. 80 mg over 30 minutes, followed by 8 mg/hour infusion for 72 hours, then 40 mg *orally* once daily for 27 additional days

Helicobacter pylori **eradication:** Oral:
Manufacturer labeling: 40 mg once daily administered with amoxicillin 1000 mg *and* clarithromycin 500 mg twice daily for 10 days
American College of Gastroenterology guidelines (Chey, 2007):
Nonpenicillin allergy: 40 mg once daily administered with amoxicillin 1000 mg *and* clarithromycin 500 mg twice daily for 10-14 days
Penicillin allergy: 40 mg once daily administered with clarithromycin 500 mg *and* metronidazole 500 mg twice daily for 10-14 days **or** 40 mg once daily administered with bismuth subsalicylate 525 mg *and* metronidazole 250 mg *plus* tetracycline 500 mg 4 times/day for 10-14 days
Canadian labeling: 20 mg twice daily for 7 days; requires combination therapy

Prevention of NSAID-induced gastric ulcers: 20-40 mg once daily for up to 6 months

Treatment of NSAID-induced gastric ulcers (Canadian labeling): 20 mg once daily for 4-8 weeks.

Pathological hypersecretory conditions (Zollinger-Ellison syndrome): 40 mg twice daily; adjust regimen to individual patient needs; doses up to 240 mg/day have been administered

Renal Impairment No adjustment is necessary.

Hepatic Impairment
Mild-to-moderate hepatic impairment (Child-Pugh class A or B): No dosage adjustment needed.
Severe hepatic impairment (Child-Pugh class C): Dose should not exceed 20 mg/day.

Administration
Oral:
Capsule: Should be swallowed whole and taken at least 1 hour before eating (best if taken before breakfast). Capsule can be opened and contents mixed with 1 tablespoon of applesauce. Swallow immediately; mixture should not be chewed or warmed. For patients with difficulty swallowing, use of granules may be more appropriate.
Granules: Empty into container with 1 tablespoon of water and stir; leave 2-3 minutes to thicken. Stir and drink within 30 minutes. If any medicine remains after drinking, add more water, stir and drink immediately.
Tablet (Canadian formulation, not available in U.S.): Swallow whole or may be dispersed in a half a glass of noncarbonated water. Stir until tablets disintegrate, leaving a liquid containing pellets. Drink contents within 30 minutes. Do not chew or crush pellets. After drinking, rinse glass with water and drink.
I.V.: Flush line prior to and after administration with NS, LR, or D_5W: Adults: May be administered by injection (≥3 minutes), intermittent infusion (10-30 minutes), or continuous infusion for up to 72 hours (Sung, 2009).

Nasogastric tube:

Capsule: Open capsule and place intact granules into a 60 mL catheter-tip syringe; mix with 50 mL of water. Replace plunger and shake vigorously for 15 seconds. Ensure that no granules remain in syringe tip. Do not administer if pellets dissolve or disintegrate. Use immediately after preparation. After administration, flush nasogastric tube with additional water.

Granules: Delayed release oral suspension granules can also be given by nasogastric or gastric tube. Add 15 mL of water to a catheter-tip syringe, add granules from packet. Shake the syringe, leave 2-3 minutes to thicken. Shake the syringe and administer through nasogastric or gastric tube (size 6 French or greater) within 30 minutes. Refill the syringe with 15 mL of water, shake and flush nasogastric/gastric tube.

Tablet (Canadian formulation, not available in U.S.): Disperse tablets in 50 mL of non-carbonated water. Stir until tablets disintegrate leaving a liquid containing pellets. After administration, flush with additional 25-50 mL of water to clear the syringe and tube.

Monitoring Parameters Susceptibility testing recommended in patients who fail *H. pylori* eradication regimen. Monitor for rebleeding in patients with peptic ulcer bleed.

Test Interactions Esomeprazole may falsely elevate serum chromogranin A (CgA) levels. The increased CgA level may cause false-positive results in the diagnosis of a neuroendocrine tumor. Temporarily stop esomeprazole if assessing CgA level; repeat level if initially elevated; use the same laboratory for all testing of CgA levels.

Special Geriatric Considerations Dose adjustment is not necessary.

An increased risk of fractures of the hip, spine, or wrist has been observed in epidemiologic studies with proton pump inhibitor (PPI) use, primarily in older adults ≥50 years of age. The greatest risk was seen in patients receiving high doses or on long-term therapy (≥1 year). Calcium and vitamin D supplementation and close monitoring are recommended to reduce the risk of fracture in high-risk patients.

Dosage Forms Excipient information presented when available (limited, particularly for generics); consult specific product labeling.

Capsule, delayed release, oral, as magnesium [strength expressed as base]:
NexIUM®: 20 mg, 40 mg

Granules for suspension, delayed release, oral, as magnesium [strength expressed as base]:
NexIUM®: 10 mg/packet (30s); 20 mg/packet (30s); 40 mg/packet (30s)

Injection, powder for reconstitution, as sodium [strength expressed as base]:
NexIUM® I.V.: 20 mg, 40 mg [contains edetate disodium]

Dosage Forms: Canada Excipient information presented when available (limited, particularly for generics); consult specific product labeling.

Note: Strength expressed as base

Granules, for oral suspension, delayed release, as magnesium:
Nexium®: 10 mg/packet (28s)

Tablet, extended release, as magnesium:
Nexium®: 20 mg, 40 mg

Selected References

Chey WD, Wong BC, et al, "American College of Gastroenterology Guideline on the Management of *Helicobacter pylori* Infection," *Am J Gastroent*, 2007, 102(8):1808-25.

Kupiec TC, Aloumanis V, Ben M, et al, "Physical and Chemical Stability of Esomeprazole Sodium Solutions," *Ann Pharmacother*, 2008, 42(9):1247-51.

◆ **Esomeprazole and Naproxen** see Naproxen and Esomeprazole *on page 1267*
◆ **Esomeprazole Magnesium** see Esomeprazole *on page 636*
◆ **Esomeprazole Sodium** see Esomeprazole *on page 636*
◆ **E.S.P.®** see Erythromycin and Sulfisoxazole *on page 629*

Estazolam (es TA zoe lam)

Related Information
Anxiolytic, Sedative / Hypnotic, and Miscellaneous Benzodiazepines *on page 2000*

Medication Safety Issues
Sound-alike/look-alike issues:
ProSom® may be confused with PhosLo®, Proscar®, Pro-Sof® Plus, PROzac®, Psorcon®

Index Terms ProSom

Generic Availability (U.S.) Yes

Pharmacologic Category Benzodiazepine

Use Short-term management of insomnia

Contraindications Hypersensitivity to estazolam or any component of the formulation (cross-sensitivity with other benzodiazepines may exist)

Note: Manufacturer states concurrent therapy with itraconazole or ketoconazole is contraindicated.

◀ **Warnings/Precautions** As a hypnotic, should be used only after evaluation of potential causes of sleep disturbance. Failure of sleep disturbance to resolve after 7-10 days may indicate psychiatric or medical illness. Use is not recommended in patients with depressive disorders or psychoses. Avoid use in patients with sleep apnea. Postmarketing studies have indicated that the use of hypnotic/sedative agents for sleep has been associated with hypersensitivity reactions including anaphylaxis as well as angioedema. An increased risk for hazardous sleep-related activities such as sleep-driving; cooking and eating food, and making phone calls while asleep have also been noted. Use with caution in patients receiving concurrent CYP3A4 inhibitors, particularly when these agents are added to therapy. Use with caution in elderly or debilitated patients, patients with hepatic disease (including alcoholics), renal impairment, respiratory disease, impaired gag reflex, or obese patients. Rebound or withdrawal symptoms may occur following abrupt discontinuation or large decreases in dose. Use caution when reducing dose or withdrawing therapy; decrease slowly and monitor for withdrawal symptoms.

Causes CNS depression (dose related) which may impair physical and mental capabilities. Use with caution in patients receiving other CNS depressants or psychoactive agents. Benzodiazepines have been associated with falls and traumatic injury and should be used with extreme caution in patients who are at risk of these events (especially the elderly). May cause physical or psychological dependence - use with caution in patients with a history of drug dependence.

Benzodiazepines have been associated with anterograde amnesia. Paradoxical reactions, including hyperactive or aggressive behavior, have been reported with benzodiazepines, particularly in psychiatric patients. Does not have analgesic, antidepressant, or antipsychotic properties.

Adverse Reactions (Reflective of adult population; not specific for elderly)
>10%:
Central nervous system: Somnolence
Neuromuscular & skeletal: Weakness
1% to 10%:
Cardiovascular: Flushing, palpitation
Central nervous system: Anxiety, confusion, dizziness, hypokinesia, abnormal coordination, hangover effect, agitation, amnesia, apathy, emotional lability, euphoria, hostility, seizure, sleep disorder, stupor, twitch
Dermatologic: Dermatitis, pruritus, rash, urticaria
Gastrointestinal: Xerostomia, constipation, appetite increased/decreased, flatulence, gastritis, perverse taste
Genitourinary: Frequent urination, menstrual cramps, urinary hesitancy, urinary frequency, vaginal discharge/itching
Neuromuscular & skeletal: Paresthesia
Ocular: Photophobia, eye pain, eye swelling
Respiratory: Cough, dyspnea, asthma, rhinitis, sinusitis
Miscellaneous: Diaphoresis

Drug Interactions
Metabolism/Transport Effects Substrate of CYP3A4 (minor)
Avoid Concomitant Use
Avoid concomitant use of Estazolam with any of the following: OLANZapine
Increased Effect/Toxicity
Estazolam may increase the levels/effects of: Alcohol (Ethyl); CloZAPine; CNS Depressants; Fosphenytoin; Methotrimeprazine; Phenytoin; Selective Serotonin Reuptake Inhibitors

The levels/effects of Estazolam may be increased by: Antifungal Agents (Azole Derivatives, Systemic); Aprepitant; Calcium Channel Blockers (Nondihydropyridine); Cimetidine; Conivaptan; Contraceptives (Estrogens); Contraceptives (Progestins); Droperidol; Fluconazole; Fosaprepitant; Grapefruit Juice; HydrOXYzine; Isoniazid; Macrolide Antibiotics; Methotrimeprazine; Nefazodone; OLANZapine; Proton Pump Inhibitors; Ritonavir; Selective Serotonin Reuptake Inhibitors
Decreased Effect
The levels/effects of Estazolam may be decreased by: CarBAMazepine; Rifamycin Derivatives; St Johns Wort; Theophylline Derivatives; Tocilizumab; Yohimbine
Ethanol/Nutrition/Herb Interactions
Ethanol: May increase CNS depression; monitor for increased effects with coadministration. Caution patients about effects.
Food: Serum levels and/or toxicity may be increased by grapefruit juice.

Mechanism of Action Binds to stereospecific benzodiazepine receptors on the postsynaptic GABA neuron at several sites within the central nervous system, including the limbic system, reticular formation. Enhancement of the inhibitory effect of GABA on neuronal excitability results by increased neuronal membrane permeability to chloride ions. This shift in chloride ions results in hyperpolarization (a less excitable state) and stabilization.

Pharmacodynamics/Kinetics
Onset of action: ~1 hour
Duration: Variable
Metabolism: Extensively hepatic
Half-life elimination: 10-24 hours (no significant changes in elderly)
Time to peak, serum: 0.5-1.6 hours
Excretion: Urine (<5% as unchanged drug)

Dosage
Geriatric Start at doses of 0.5 mg in small elderly patients.
Adult Insomnia: Oral: 1 mg at bedtime, some patients may require 2 mg; start at doses of 0.5 mg in debilitated patients.
Hepatic Impairment Adjustment may be necessary.

Monitoring Parameters Respiratory, cardiovascular, and mental status

Pharmacotherapy Pearls Abrupt discontinuation after sustained use (generally >10 days) may cause withdrawal symptoms.

Special Geriatric Considerations Because of its lack of active metabolites, estazolam could be considered for elderly patients when a benzodiazepine hypnotic is indicated.

Controlled Substance C-IV

Dosage Forms Excipient information presented when available (limited, particularly for generics); consult specific product labeling.
Tablet, oral: 1 mg, 2 mg

◆ **Ester-E™ [OTC]** *see* Vitamin E *on page* *1921*
◆ **Esterified Estrogens** *see* Estrogens (Esterified) *on page* *667*
◆ **Estrace®** *see* Estradiol (Systemic) *on page* *641*
◆ **Estrace®** *see* Estradiol (Topical) *on page* *648*
◆ **Estraderm®** *see* Estradiol (Systemic) *on page* *641*
◆ **Estradiol** *see* Estradiol (Systemic) *on page* *641*
◆ **17β-estradiol** *see* Estradiol (Topical) *on page* *648*

Estradiol (Systemic) (es tra DYE ole)

Medication Safety Issues
Sound-alike/look-alike issues:
Alora® may be confused with Aldara®
Elestrin™ may be confused with alosetron
Estraderm® may be confused with Testoderm®
BEERS Criteria medication:
This drug may be inappropriate for use in geriatric patients (low severity risk).
Other safety issues:
Transdermal patch may contain conducting metal (eg, aluminum); remove patch prior to MRI.
International issues:
Vivelle®: Brand name for ethinyl estradiol and norgestimate in Austria

Brand Names: U.S. Alora®; Climara®; Delestrogen®; Depo®-Estradiol; Divigel®; Elestrin®; Estrace®; Estraderm®; Estrasorb®; EstroGel®; Evamist™; Femring®; Femtrace®; Menostar®; Vivelle-Dot®

Brand Names: Canada Climara®; Depo®-Estradiol; Estraderm®; Estradot®; EstroGel®; Menostar®; Oesclim®; Sandoz-Estradiol Derm 100; Sandoz-Estradiol Derm 50; Sandoz-Estradiol Derm 75

Index Terms Estradiol; Estradiol Acetate; Estradiol Transdermal; Estradiol Valerate

Generic Availability (U.S.) Yes: Oral tablet, patch, valerate oil for injection

Pharmacologic Category Estrogen Derivative

Use Treatment of moderate-to-severe vasomotor symptoms associated with menopause; treatment of moderate-to-severe vulvar and vaginal atrophy associated with menopause; hypoestrogenism (due to hypogonadism, castration, or primary ovarian failure); advanced prostatic cancer (palliation); metastatic breast cancer (palliation) in men and postmenopausal women; postmenopausal osteoporosis (prophylaxis)

Contraindications Hypersensitivity to estradiol or any component of the formulation; undiagnosed abnormal vaginal bleeding; DVT or PE (current or history of); active or recent (within 1 year) arterial thromboembolic disease (eg, stroke, MI); carcinoma of the breast (known, suspected or history of), except in appropriately selected patients being treated for metastatic disease; estrogen-dependent tumor; hepatic dysfunction or disease

Warnings/Precautions

[U.S. Boxed Warning]: Unopposed estrogens may increase the risk of endometrial carcinoma in postmenopausal women with an intact uterus. Adequate diagnostic measures, including endometrial sampling, if indicated, should be performed to rule out malignancy in all cases of undiagnosed abnormal vaginal bleeding. The use of a progestin should be considered when administering estrogens to postmenopausal women with an intact uterus. When indicated, oral progestins should be used. The use of a progestin is not generally required when low doses of estrogen are used locally for vaginal atrophy or when ultralow doses are used transdermally to prevent osteoporosis (NAMS, 2010). Estrogens may exacerbate endometriosis. Malignant transformation of residual endometrial implants has been reported posthysterectomy with estrogen only therapy. Consider adding a progestin in women with residual endometriosis posthysterectomy. Postmenopausal estrogen therapy and combined estrogen/progesterone therapy may increase the risk of ovarian cancer; however, the absolute risk to an individual woman is small. Although results from various studies are not consistent, risk does not appear to be significantly associated with the duration, route, or dose of therapy. In one study, the risk decreased after 2 years following discontinuation of therapy (Mørch, 2009). Although the risk of ovarian cancer is rare, women who are at an increased risk (eg, family history) should be counseled about the association (NAMS, 2010). Estrogens may increase the risk of breast cancer. An increased risk of invasive breast cancer was observed in postmenopausal women using conjugated equine estrogens (CEE) in combination with medroxyprogesterone acetate (MPA); a smaller increase in risk was seen with estrogen therapy alone in observational studies. An increase in abnormal mammograms has also been reported with estrogen and progestin therapy. Estrogen use may lead to severe hypercalcemia in patients with breast cancer and bone metastases; discontinue estrogen if hypercalcemia occurs.

[U.S. Boxed Warning]: Estrogens with or without progestin should not be used to prevent coronary heart disease. Use caution with cardiovascular disease or dysfunction. May increase the risks of myocardial infarction (MI), stroke, pulmonary emboli (PE), and deep vein thrombosis (DVT); incidence of these effects was shown to be significantly increased in postmenopausal women using CEE in combination with MPA. Nonfatal MI, PE, and thrombophlebitis have also been reported in males taking high doses of CEE (eg, for prostate cancer). Risk factors include diabetes mellitus, hypercholesterolemia, hypertension, SLE, obesity, and/or venous thromboembolism (VTE). Use caution in patients with known inherited thrombophilias (eg, protein C or S deficiency); may have increased risk of VTE (DeSancho, 2010). Use is contraindicated in patients with DVT or PE (current or history of).

[U.S. Boxed Warning]: The risk of dementia may be increased in postmenopausal women; increased incidence was observed in women ≥65 years of age taking CEE alone or in combination with MPA.

[U.S. Boxed Warning]: Estrogens with or without progestin should be used for shortest duration possible at the lowest effective dose consistent with treatment goals. Before prescribing estrogen therapy to postmenopausal women, the risks and benefits must be weighed for each patient. Women should be informed of these risks and benefits, as well as possible effects of progestin when added to estrogen therapy. Conduct periodic risk:benefit assessments. Outcomes reported from clinical trials using CEE should be assumed to be similar for estradiol until comparable data becomes available. In addition, risks associated with oral CEE should be assumed to be similar for other dosage forms (eg, vaginal, transdermal) until additional information is available.

Estrogen compounds are generally associated with lipid effects such as increased HDL-cholesterol and decreased LDL-cholesterol. Triglycerides may also be increased; use with caution in patients with familial defects of lipoprotein metabolism. Estrogens may increase thyroid-binding globulin (TBG) levels leading to increased circulating total thyroid hormone levels. Women on thyroid replacement therapy may require higher doses of thyroid hormone while receiving estrogens.

Estrogens may cause retinal vascular thrombosis; discontinue if migraine, loss of vision, proptosis, diplopia, or other visual disturbances occur; discontinue permanently if papilledema or retinal vascular lesions are observed on examination. Estrogens are poorly metabolized in patients with hepatic dysfunction. Use caution with a history of cholestatic jaundice associated with prior estrogen use or pregnancy. Discontinue if jaundice develops or if acute or chronic hepatic disturbances occur. Use is contraindicated with hepatic disease. Use caution in patients with asthma, epilepsy, hepatic hemangiomas, migraine, porphyria, or SLE; may exacerbate disease. May have adverse effects on glucose tolerance; use caution in women with diabetes. Use with caution in patients with diseases which may be exacerbated by fluid retention, including cardiac or renal dysfunction. Use of postmenopausal estrogen may be associated with an increased risk of gallbladder disease requiring surgery. Use with caution in patients with severe hypocalcemia. May be inappropriate in for use in the elderly due to potential of increased risk of breast and endometrial cancers and lack of proven cardioprotection (Beers Criteria). Prior to puberty, estrogens may cause premature closure of the epiphyses, premature breast development in girls or gynecomastia in boys. Vaginal bleeding and vaginal cornification may also be induced in girls. Whenever possible, estrogens should be discontinued at least 4-6 weeks prior to elective surgery associated with an increased risk of thromboembolism or during periods of prolonged immobilization.

Some products may contain chlorobutanol (a chloral derivative) as a preservative, which may be habit forming; some products may contain tartrazine.

Topical emulsion, gel, spray: Absorption of the topical emulsion (Estrasorb®) and topical gel (Elestrin®) is increased by application of sunscreen; do not apply sunscreen within close proximity of estradiol. When sunscreen is applied ~1 hour prior to the topical spray (Evamist™), no change in absorption was observed (estradiol absorption was decreased when sunscreen is applied 1 hour after Evamist™). Application of Divigel® or EstroGel® with sunscreen has not been evaluated. Patients should make sure that children do not come in contact with any skin area where the spray is applied.

Transdermal patch: May contain conducting metal (eg, aluminum); remove patch prior to MRI.

Vaginal ring: Use may not be appropriate in women with narrow vagina, vaginal stenosis, vaginal infections, cervical prolapse, rectoceles, cystoceles, or other conditions which may increase the risk of vaginal irritation, ulceration, or increase the risk of expulsion. Ring should be removed in case of ulceration, erosion, or adherence to vaginal wall; do not reinsert until healing is complete. Ensure proper vaginal placement of the ring to avoid inadvertent urinary bladder insertion.

Osteoporosis: For use only in women at significant risk of osteoporosis and for who other nonestrogen medications are not considered appropriate.

Vulvar and vaginal atrophy: When used solely for the treatment of vulvar and vaginal atrophy, topical vaginal products should be considered. Use caution applying topical products to severely atrophic vaginal mucosa. Use of a progestin is normally not required when low-dose estrogen is applied locally and only for this purpose (NAMS, 2007).

Adverse Reactions (Reflective of adult population; not specific for elderly) Frequency not defined. Some adverse reactions observed with estrogen and/or progestin combination therapy.

Cardiovascular: Chest pain, DVT, edema, hypertension, MI, stroke, syncope, TIA, vasodilation, venous thromboembolism

Central nervous system: Anxiety, dementia, dizziness, epilepsy exacerbation, headache, insomnia, irritability, mental depression, migraine, mood disturbances, nervousness

Dermatologic: Angioedema, chloasma, dermatitis, erythema multiforme, erythema nodosum, hemorrhagic eruption, hirsutism, loss of scalp hair, melasma, rash, pruritus, urticaria

Endocrine & metabolic: Breast cancer, breast enlargement, breast pain, breast tenderness, carbohydrate intolerance, fibrocystic breast changes, fluid retention, galactorrhea, hot flashes, hypocalcemia, libido changes, nipple discharge, nipple pain

Gastrointestinal: Abdominal cramps, abdominal pain, bloating, cholecystitis, cholelithiasis, constipation, diarrhea, dyspepsia, flatulence, gallbladder disease, gastritis, nausea, pancreatitis, vomiting, weight gain/loss

Genitourinary: Alterations in frequency and flow of bleeding patterns, breakthrough bleeding, cervical ectropion changes, cervical secretion changes, cystitis, dysmenorrhea, endometrial cancer, endometrial hyperplasia, genital eruption, menorrhagia, metrorrhagia, ovarian cancer, ovarian cyst, Pap smear suspicious, spotting, uterine leiomyomata size increased, leukorrhea, uterine cancer, uterine enlargement, uterine pain, urinary incontinence, urogenital pruritus, vaginal candidiasis, vaginal discharge, vaginal moniliasis, vaginitis

Hematologic: Aggravation of porphyria

Hepatic: Cholestatic jaundice, hepatic hemangioma enlargement

Local: Thrombophlebitis
   Gel, spray: Application site reaction
   Transdermal patches: Erythema, irritation

Neuromuscular & skeletal: Arthralgia, back pain, chorea, leg cramps, myalgia, muscle cramps, skeletal pain, weakness

Ocular: Blindness, contact lens intolerance, corneal curvature steepening, retinal vascular thrombosis

◀ Respiratory: Asthma exacerbation, pulmonary thromboembolism

Miscellaneous: Anaphylactoid/anaphylactic reactions, hypersensitivity reactions

Drug Interactions

Metabolism/Transport Effects Substrate of CYP1A2 (major), CYP2A6 (minor), CYP2B6 (minor), CYP2C9 (minor), CYP2C19 (minor), CYP2D6 (minor), CYP2E1 (minor), CYP3A4 (major), P-glycoprotein; **Inhibits** CYP1A2 (weak), 2C8 (weak); **Induces** CYP3A4 (weak)

Avoid Concomitant Use

Avoid concomitant use of Estradiol (Systemic) with any of the following: Anastrozole

Increased Effect/Toxicity

Estradiol (Systemic) may increase the levels/effects of: Corticosteroids (Systemic); ROPINIRole; Tipranavir

The levels/effects of Estradiol (Systemic) may be increased by: Ascorbic Acid; Conivaptan; Herbs (Estrogenic Properties); P-Glycoprotein Inhibitors

Decreased Effect

Estradiol (Systemic) may decrease the levels/effects of: Anastrozole; Chenodiol; Saxagliptin; Somatropin; Thyroid Products; Ursodiol

The levels/effects of Estradiol (Systemic) may be decreased by: CYP1A2 Inducers (Strong); CYP3A4 Inducers (Strong); Cyproterone; Deferasirox; Herbs (CYP3A4 Inducers); Peginterferon Alfa-2b; P-Glycoprotein Inducers; Tipranavir; Tocilizumab

Ethanol/Nutrition/Herb Interactions

Ethanol: Avoid ethanol (routine use increases estrogen level and risk of breast cancer). Ethanol may also increase the risk of osteoporosis.

Food: Folic acid absorption may be decreased

Herb/Nutraceutical: St John's wort may decrease levels. Herbs with estrogenic properties may enhance the adverse/toxic effect of estrogen derivatives; examples include alfalfa, black cohosh, bloodroot, hops, kudzu, licorice, red clover, saw palmetto, soybean, thyme, wild yam, yucca.

Stability Store all products at controlled room temperature. In addition:

Climara®, Estraderm®, Menostar®: Do not store >30°C (>86°F); store in protective pouch.

Mechanism of Action Estrogens are responsible for the development and maintenance of the female reproductive system and secondary sexual characteristics. Estradiol is the principle intracellular human estrogen and is more potent than estrone and estriol at the receptor level; it is the primary estrogen secreted prior to menopause. Following menopause, estrone and estrone sulfate are more highly produced. Estrogens modulate the pituitary secretion of gonadotropins, luteinizing hormone, and follicle-stimulating hormone through a negative feedback system; estrogen replacement reduces elevated levels of these hormones in postmenopausal women.

Pharmacodynamics/Kinetics

Absorption: Well absorbed from the gastrointestinal tract, mucous membranes, and the skin. Average serum estradiol concentrations (C_{avg}) vary by product

Oral: Femtrace®: C_{avg}: 23.5-92.1 pg/mL

Injection: Estradiol valerate and estradiol cypionate are absorbed over several weeks following I.M. injection

Topical:

Alora®: C_{avg}: 41-98 pg/mL

Climara®: C_{avg}: 22-106 pg/mL

Divigel®: C_{avg}: 9.8-30.5 pg/mL

Elestrin®: C_{avg}: 15.4-39.2 pg/mL; Exposure increased by 55% with application of sunscreen 10 minutes prior to dose

Estraderm® 0.1 mg/day: C_{avg}: 73 pg/mL

Estrasorb®: Mean serum concentration on day 22 of therapy: ~35-65 pg/mL; Exposure increased by 35% with application of sunscreen 10 minutes prior to dose

Estrogel®: C_{avg} on day 14 of therapy: 28.3 pg/mL

Evamist®: C_{avg}: 19.6-30.9 pg/mL

Menostar®: C_{avg}: 13.7 pg/mL

Vivelle-Dot®: C_{avg}: 34-104 pg/mL

Vaginal: Femring®: Rapid during the first hour following application, then declines to a steady rate over 3 months; C_{avg}: 40.6-76 pg/mL

Distribution: Widely distributed; high concentrations in the sex hormone target organs

Protein binding: Bound to sex hormone-binding globulin and albumin

Metabolism: Hepatic; partial metabolism via CYP3A4 enzymes; estradiol is reversibly converted to estrone and estriol; oral estradiol also undergoes enterohepatic recirculation by conjugation in the liver, followed by excretion of sulfate and glucuronide conjugates into the bile, then hydrolysis in the intestine and estrogen reabsorption. Sulfate conjugates are the primary form found in postmenopausal women. With transdermal application, less estradiol is metabolized leading to higher circulating concentrations of estradiol and lower concentrations of estrone and conjugates.

Half-life elimination: Femtrace®: 21-26 hours

Time to peak, plasma: Oral: Femtrace®: 0.4-0.75 hours

Excretion: Primarily urine (as estradiol, estrone, estriol and their glucuronide and sulfate conjugates)

Dosage

Geriatric & Adult All dosage needs to be adjusted based upon the patient's response:

Vulvar and vaginal atrophy associated with menopause:

I.M.: Valerate (Delestrogen®): 10-20 mg every 4 weeks

Intravaginal: Vaginal ring (Femring®): 0.05 mg intravaginally; following insertion, ring should remain in place for 3 months; dose may be increased to 0.1 mg if needed

Oral (Estrace®): 1-2 mg/day; administration should be cyclic (3 weeks on, 1 week off)

Topical gel (EstroGel®): 1.25 g/day applied at the same time each day

Transdermal (Alora®, Climara®, Estraderm®, Vivelle-Dot®): Refer to product-specific dosing.

Breast cancer, metastatic (appropriately selected patients): Oral (Estrace®): Males and postmenopausal females: 10 mg 3 times/day **or** (unlabeled dosing) postmenopausal women: 2 mg 3 times/day (Ellis, 2009)

Hypoestrogenism (female) due to hypogonadism, castration, or primary ovarian failure:

Oral (Estrace®): 1-2 mg/day; titrate as necessary to control symptoms using minimal effective dose for maintenance therapy

I.M: Valerate (Delestrogen®): 10-20 mg every 4 weeks

Transdermal (Alora®, Climara®, Estraderm®, Vivelle-Dot®): Refer to product-specific dosing.

Hypoestrogenism (female) due to hypogonadism: *I.M: Cypionate* (Depo®- Estradiol): 1.5-2 mg monthly

Osteoporosis prevention (females):

Oral (Estrace®): Lowest effective dose has not been determined; doses of 0.5 mg/day in a cyclic regimen for 23 days of a 28-week cycle were used in clinical studies

Transdermal (Alora®, Climara®, Estraderm®, Menostar®, Vivelle-Dot®): Refer to product-specific dosing (below)

Prostate cancer, advanced (androgen-dependent):

I.M.: Valerate (Delestrogen®): 30 mg or more every 1-2 weeks

Oral (Estrace®): 1-2 mg 3 times/day

Vasomotor symptoms associated with menopause:

Oral:

Estrace®: 1-2 mg daily, adjusted as necessary to limit symptoms; administration should be cyclic (3 weeks on, 1 week off)

Femtrace®: Initial dose: 0.45 mg/day; dosage range 0.45-1.8 mg/day

I.M. Cypionate (Depo®-Estradiol): 1-5 mg every 3-4 weeks

I.M. Valerate (Delestrogen®): 10-20 mg every 4 weeks

Topical emulsion (Estrasorb®): 3.48 g applied once daily in the morning

Topical gel:

Divigel®: 0.25 g/day; adjust dose based on patient response. Dosing range: 0.25-1 g/day

Elestrin®: 0.87 g/day applied at the same time each day; adjust dose based on patient response. Dosing range: 0.87-1.7 g/day.

EstroGel®: 1.25 g/day applied at the same time each day

Topical spray (Evamist™): Initial: One spray (1.53 mg) per day. Adjust dose based on patient response. Dosing range: 1-3 sprays per day.

Transdermal (Alora®, Climara®, Estraderm®, Vivelle-Dot®): See product-specific dosing (below)

Vaginal ring (Femring®): Initial: 0.05 mg intravaginally; following insertion, ring should remain in place for 3 months; dose may be increased to 0.1 mg if needed

Transdermal product-specific dosing:

Note: Indicated dose may be used continuously in patients without an intact uterus. May be given continuously or cyclically (3 weeks on, 1 week off) in patients with an intact uterus **(exception - Menostar®, see specific dosing instructions).** When changing patients from oral to transdermal therapy, start transdermal patch 1 week after discontinuing oral hormone (may begin sooner if symptoms reappear within 1 week):

Transdermal once-weekly patch:

Vasomotor symptoms associated with menopause, vulvar and vaginal atrophy associated with menopause, female hypoestrogenism (due to hypogonadism, castration, or primary ovarian failure):

Climara®: Initial: Apply 0.025 mg/day patch once weekly. Adjust dose as necessary to control symptoms.

Prevention of osteoporosis in postmenopausal women:

Climara®: Apply patch once weekly; minimum effective dose 0.025 mg/day; adjust dosage based on response to therapy as indicated by biological markers and bone mineral density.

Menostar®: Apply patch once weekly (0.014 mg/day). In women with a uterus, also administer a progestin for 14 days every 6-12 months.

Transdermal twice-weekly patch:

Vasomotor symptoms associated with menopause, vulvar and vaginal atrophy associated with menopause, female hypoestrogenism (due to hypogonadism, castration, or primary ovarian failure): Titrate to lowest dose possible to control symptoms, adjusting initial dose after the first month of therapy:

Alora®, Estraderm®: Apply 0.05 mg patch twice weekly

Vivelle-Dot®: Apply 0.0375 mg patch twice weekly

Prevention of osteoporosis in postmenopausal women:

Alora®, Vivelle-Dot®: Apply 0.025 mg patch twice weekly; increase dose as necessary

Estraderm®: Apply 0.05 mg patch twice weekly; increase dose as necessary

Administration The use of a progestin should be considered when administering estrogens to postmenopausal women with an intact uterus.

Injection formulation: Intramuscular use only. Estradiol valerate should be injected into the upper outer quadrant of the gluteal muscle; administer with a dry needle (solution may become cloudy with wet needle).

Emulsion (Estrasorb®): Apply to clean, dry skin while in a sitting position. Contents of two pouches (total 3.48 g) are to be applied individually, once daily in the morning. Apply contents of first pouch to left thigh; massage into skin of left thigh and calf until thoroughly absorbed (~3 minutes). Apply excess from both hands to the buttocks. Apply contents of second pouch to the right thigh; massage into skin of right thigh and calf until thoroughly absorbed (~3 minutes). Apply excess from both hands to buttocks. Wash hands with soap and water. Allow skin to dry before covering legs with clothing. Do not apply to other areas of body. Do not apply to red or irritated skin.

Gel: Apply to clean, dry, unbroken skin at the same time each day. Allow to dry for 5 minutes prior to dressing. Gel is flammable; avoid fire or flame until dry. After application, wash hands with soap and water. Prior to the first use, pump must be primed. Do not apply gel to breast.

Divigel®: Apply entire contents of packet to right or left upper thigh each day (alternate sites). Do not apply to face, breasts, vaginal area or irritated skin. Apply over an area ~5x7 inches. Do not wash application site for 1 hour. Allow gel to dry before dressing

Elestrin®: Apply to upper arm and shoulder area using two fingers to spread gel. Apply after bath or shower; allow at least 2 hours between applying gel and going swimming. Wait at least 25 minutes before applying sunscreen to application area. Do not apply sunscreen to application area for ≥7 days (may increase absorption of gel).

EstroGel®: Apply gel to the arm, from the wrist to the shoulder. Spread gel as thinly as possible over one arm.

Spray: Evamist™: Prior to first use, prime pump by spraying 3 sprays with the cover on. To administer dose, hold container upright and vertical and rest the plastic cone flat against the skin while spraying. Spray to the inner surface of the forearm, starting near the elbow. If more than one spray is needed, apply to adjacent but not overlapping areas. Apply at the same time each day. Allow spray to dry for ~2 minutes. Do not wash application site for 30 minutes. Apply to clean, dry, unbroken skin. Do not apply to skin other than that of the forearm. Make sure that children do not come in contact with any skin area where the drug was applied. If contact with children is unavoidable, wear a garment with long sleeves that covers the site of application. If direct exposure should occur, wash the child in the area of exposure with soap and water as soon as possible. Solution contained in the spray is flammable; avoid fire, flame, or smoking until spray has dried. If needed, sunscreen should be applied ~1 hour prior to application of Evamist™.

Transdermal patch: Do not apply transdermal system to breasts, but place on trunk of body (preferably abdomen). Rotate application sites allowing a 1-week interval between applications at a particular site. Do not apply to oily, damaged or irritated skin; avoid waistline or other areas where tight clothing may rub the patch off. Apply patch immediately after removing from protective pouch. In general, if patch falls off, the same patch may be reapplied or a new system may be used for the remainder of the dosing interval (not recommended with all products). When replacing patch, reapply to a new site. Swimming, bathing or showering are not expected to affect use of the patch. Note the following exceptions:

Estraderm®: Do not apply to an area exposed to direct sunlight.

Climara®, Menostar®: Swimming, bathing, or wearing patch while in a sauna have not been studied; adhesion of patch may be decreased or delivery of estradiol may be affected. Remove patch slowly after use to avoid skin irritation. If any adhesive remains on the skin after removal, first allow skin to dry for 15 minutes, then gently rub area with an oil-based cream or lotion. If patch falls off, a new patch should be applied for the remainder of the dosing interval.

Vaginal ring: Exact positioning is not critical for efficacy; however, patient should not feel anything once inserted. In case of discomfort, ring should be pushed further into vagina. If ring is expelled prior to 90 days, it may be rinsed off and reinserted. Ensure proper vaginal placement of the ring to avoid inadvertent urinary bladder insertion. If vaginal infection develops, Femring® may remain in place during local treatment of a vaginal infection.

Monitoring Parameters Routine physical examination that includes blood pressure and Papanicolaou smear, breast exam, mammogram. Monitor for signs of endometrial cancer in female patients with uterus. Adequate diagnostic measures, including endometrial sampling, if indicated, should be performed to rule out malignancy in all cases of undiagnosed abnormal vaginal bleeding. Monitor for loss of vision, sudden onset of proptosis, diplopia, migraine; signs and symptoms of thromboembolic disorders; glycemic control in patients with diabetes; lipid profiles in patients being treated for hyperlipidemias; thyroid function in patients on thyroid hormone replacement therapy.

Menostar®: When used in a woman with a uterus, endometrial sampling is recommended at yearly intervals or when clinically indicated.

Menopausal symptoms, vulvar and vaginal atrophy: Assess need for therapy at 3- to 6-month intervals

Prevention of osteoporosis: Bone density measurement

Reference Range

Male: 10-50 pg/mL (SI: 37-184 pmol/L)

Female:

Premenopausal: 30-400 pg/mL (SI: 110-1468 pmol/L)

Postmenopausal: 0-30 pg/mL (SI: 0-110 pmol/L)

Test Interactions Thyroid function tests: Estrogens may increase thyroid binding globulin and circulating total thyroid hormone (when measured by T_4 RIA, T_4 by column, or by PBI); decreases free T_3 resin uptake; concentration of free T_4 is not altered; metyrapone test: Response may be reduced

Special Geriatric Considerations Before prescribing estrogen therapy to postmenopausal women, the risks and benefits must be weighed for each patient. Data in women ≥80 years are minimal and it is unclear if the reduced risk is applicable to women in this age group. Women should be informed of these risks and benefits, as well as possible side effects and the return of menstrual bleeding (when cycled with a progestin), and be involved in the decision to prescribe.

This medication is considered to be potentially inappropriate in this patient population (Beers Criteria severity: Low).

Dosage Forms Excipient information presented when available (limited, particularly for generics); consult specific product labeling.

Emulsion, topical, as hemihydrate:

Estrasorb®: 2.5 mg/g (56s) [each pouch contains estradiol hemihydrate 4.35 mg; contents of two pouches delivers estradiol 0.05 mg/day]

Gel, topical:

Divigel®: 0.1% (30s) [delivers estradiol 0.25 mg/0.25 g packet]

Divigel®: 0.1% (30s) [delivers estradiol 0.5 mg/0.5 g packet]

Divigel®: 0.1% (30s) [delivers estradiol 1 mg/1 g packet]

Elestrin®: 0.06% (35 g) [delivers estradiol 0.52 mg/0.87 g; 30 actuations]

Elestrin®: 0.06% (70 g) [delivers estradiol 0.52 mg/0.87 g; 60 actuations; packaged as 2x35 g]

EstroGel®: 0.06% (50 g) [contains ethanol; delivers estradiol 0.75 mg/1.25 g; 32 actuations]

Injection, oil, as cypionate:

Depo®-Estradiol: 5 mg/mL (5 mL) [contains chlorobutanol, cottonseed oil]

Injection, oil, as valerate: 20 mg/mL (5 mL); 40 mg/mL (5 mL)

Delestrogen®: 10 mg/mL (5 mL) [contains chlorobutanol, sesame oil]

Delestrogen®: 20 mg/mL (5 mL); 40 mg/mL (5 mL) [contains benzyl alcohol, benzyl benzoate, castor oil]

Patch, transdermal [once-weekly patch]: 0.025 mg/24 hours (4s); 0.0375 mg/24 hours (4s); 0.05 mg/24 hours (4s); 0.06 mg/24 hours (4s); 0.075 mg/24 hours (4s); 0.1 mg/24 hours (4s)

Climara®: 0.025 mg/24 hours (4s) [6.5 cm², total estradiol 2.04 mg]

Climara®: 0.0375 mg/24 hours (4s) [9.375 cm², total estradiol 2.85 mg]

Climara®: 0.05 mg/24 hours (4s) [12.5 cm², total estradiol 3.8 mg]

Climara®: 0.06 mg/24 hours (4s) [15 cm², total estradiol 4.55 mg]

Climara®: 0.075 mg/24 hours (4s) [18.75 cm², total estradiol 5.7 mg]

Climara®: 0.1 mg/24 hours (4s) [25 cm², total estradiol 7.6 mg]

Menostar®: 0.014 mg/24 hours (4s) [3.25 cm², total estradiol 1 mg]

Patch, transdermal [twice-weekly patch]:
Alora®: 0.025 mg/24 hours (8s) [9 cm², total estradiol 0.77 mg]
Alora®: 0.05 mg/24 hours (8s) [18 cm², total estradiol 1.5 mg]
Alora®: 0.075 mg/24 hours (8s) [27 cm², total estradiol 2.3 mg]
Alora®: 0.1 mg/24 hours (8s) [36 cm², total estradiol 3.1 mg]
Estraderm®: 0.05 mg/24 hours (8s) [10 cm², total estradiol 4 mg]
Estraderm®: 0.1 mg/24 hours (8s) [20 cm², total estradiol 8 mg]
Vivelle-Dot®: 0.025 mg/24 hours (24s) [2.5 cm², total estradiol 0.39 mg]
Vivelle-Dot®: 0.0375 mg/24 hours (24s) [3.75 cm², total estradiol 0.585 mg]
Vivelle-Dot®: 0.05 mg/24 hours (24s) [5 cm², total estradiol 0.78 mg]
Vivelle-Dot®: 0.075 mg/24 hours (24s) [7.5 cm², total estradiol 1.17 mg]
Vivelle-Dot®: 0.1 mg/24 hours (24s) [10 cm², total estradiol 1.56 mg]
Ring, vaginal, as acetate:
Femring®: 0.05 mg/24 hours (1s) [total estradiol 12.4 mg; releases 0.05 mg/24 hours over 3 months]
Femring®: 0.1 mg/24 hours (1s) [total estradiol 24.8 mg; releases 0.1 mg/24 hours over 3 months]
Solution, topical [spray]:
Evamist™: 1.53 mg/spray (8.1 mL) [contains ethanol; contains 56 sprays after priming]
Tablet, oral [micronized]: 0.5 mg, 1 mg, 2 mg
Estrace®: 0.5 mg, 1 mg [scored]
Estrace®: 2 mg [scored; contains tartrazine]
Tablet, oral, as acetate:
Femtrace®: 0.45 mg, 0.9 mg, 1.8 mg

Selected References

Mørch LS, Løkkegaard E, Andreasen AH, et al, "Hormone Therapy and Ovarian Cancer," *JAMA*, 2009, 302 (3):298-305.

Estradiol (Topical) (es tra DYE ole)

Medication Safety Issues
International issues:
Estring [U.S., Canada, and multiple international markets] may be confused with Estrena [Finland]
Brand Names: U.S. Estrace®; Estring®; Vagifem®
Brand Names: Canada Estrace®; Estring®; Vagifem®; Vagifem® 10
Index Terms 17β-estradiol
Generic Availability (U.S.) No
Pharmacologic Category Estrogen Derivative
Use Treatment of moderate-to-severe vulvar and vaginal atrophy associated with menopause
Dosage
Geriatric & Adult All dosage needs to be adjusted based upon the patient's response:
Vulvar and vaginal atrophy associated with menopause: Intravaginal:
Vaginal cream (Estrace®): Insert 2-4 g/day intravaginally for 1-2 weeks, then gradually reduce to ½ the initial dose for 1-2 weeks, followed by a maintenance dose of 1 g 1-3 times/week
Vaginal ring (Estring®): 2 mg intravaginally; following insertion, ring should remain in place for 90 days
Vaginal tablet (Vagifem®): Initial: Insert 1 tablet (10 mcg) once daily for 2 weeks; Maintenance: Insert 1 tablet twice weekly
Special Geriatric Considerations Topical estrogen is beneficial in the management of urogenital atrophy and prevention of recurrent urinary tract infections in postmenopausal women. Topical estrogens are not void of the risks associated with oral and transdermal forms; thus, the risks and benefits must be weighed for each patient.
Dosage Forms Excipient information presented when available (limited, particularly for generics); consult specific product labeling. [DSC] = Discontinued product
Cream, vaginal:
Estrace®: 0.1 mg/g (42.5 g)
Ring, vaginal, as base:
Estring®: 2 mg (1s) [total estradiol 2 mg; releases 7.5 mcg/day over 90 days]
Tablet, vaginal, as base:
Vagifem®: 10 mcg, 25 mcg [DSC]

◆ **Estradiol Acetate** see Estradiol (Systemic) on page 641
◆ **Estradiol and Drospirenone** see Drospirenone and Estradiol on page 579
◆ **Estradiol and NGM** see Estradiol and Norgestimate on page 649

Estradiol and Norgestimate (es tra DYE ole & nor JES ti mate)

Related Information
Estradiol (Systemic) *on page 641*
Brand Names: U.S. Prefest™
Index Terms Estradiol and NGM; Norgestimate and Estradiol; Ortho Prefest
Generic Availability (U.S.) No
Pharmacologic Category Estrogen and Progestin Combination
Use Women with an intact uterus: Treatment of moderate-to-severe vasomotor symptoms associated with menopause; treatment of atrophic vaginitis; prevention of osteoporosis
Contraindications Hypersensitivity to estradiol, norgestimate, or any component of the formulation; undiagnosed abnormal vaginal bleeding; history of or current thrombophlebitis or venous thromboembolic disorders (including DVT, PE); active or recent (within 1 year) arterial thromboembolic disease (eg, stroke, MI); carcinoma of the breast; estrogen-dependent tumor; hepatic dysfunction or disease
Warnings/Precautions
Cardiovascular-related considerations: **[U.S. Boxed Warning]: Estrogens with or without progestin should not be used to prevent coronary heart disease.** Use caution with cardiovascular disease or dysfunction. May increase the risks of myocardial infarction (MI), stroke, pulmonary emboli (PE), and deep vein thrombosis (DVT); incidence of these effects was shown to be significantly increased in postmenopausal women using CEE in combination with MPA. Nonfatal MI, PE, and thromboplebitis have also been reported in males taking high doses of CEE (eg, for prostate cancer). Risk factors include diabetes mellitus, hypercholesterolemia, hypertension, SLE, obesity, and/or venous thromboembolism (VTE). Estrogen compounds are generally associated with lipid effects such as increased HDL-cholesterol and decreased LDL-cholesterol. Triglycerides may be increased; use with caution in patients with familial defects of lipoprotein metabolism. Whenever possible, combination hormonal contraceptives should be discontinued at least 4 weeks prior to and for 2 weeks following elective surgery associated with an increased risk of thromboembolism or during periods of prolonged immobilization. Use caution in patients with known inherited thrombophilias (eg, protein C or S deficiency); may have increased risk of VTE (DeSancho, 2010); use is contraindicated in patients with DVT or PE (current or history of).

Neurological considerations: **[U.S. Boxed Warning]: The risk of dementia may be increased in postmenopausal women;** increased incidence was observed in women ≥65 years of age taking CEE alone or in combination with MPA.

Cancer-related considerations: Unopposed estrogens may increase the risk of endometrial carcinoma in postmenopausal women. Estrogens may exacerbate endometriosis. Malignant transformation of residual endometrial implants has been reported posthysterectomy with estrogen only therapy. Estrogens may increase the risk of breast cancer. An increased risk of invasive breast cancer was observed in postmenopausal women using CEE in combination with MPA; a smaller increase in risk was seen with estrogen therapy alone in observational studies. An increase in abnormal mammograms has also been reported with estrogen and progestin therapy. Estrogen use may lead to severe hypercalcemia in patients with breast cancer and bone metastases; discontinue estrogen if hypercalcemia occurs. Postmenopausal estrogen therapy and combined estrogen/progesterone therapy may increase the risk of ovarian cancer; however, the absolute risk to an individual woman is small. Although results from various studies are not consistent, risk does not appear to be significantly associated with the duration, route, or dose of therapy. In one study, the risk decreased after 2 years following discontinuation of therapy.

Estrogens may cause retinal vascular thrombosis; discontinue permanently if papilledema or retinal vascular lesions are observed on examination. Use with caution in patients with diseases which may be exacerbated by fluid retention, including asthma, epilepsy, migraine, diabetes or renal dysfunction. Use with caution in patients with a history of severe hypocalcemia, SLE, hepatic hemangiomas, porphyria, endometriosis, and gallbladder disease. Use caution with history of cholestatic jaundice associated with past estrogen use or pregnancy. Not for use prior to menopause.

Before prescribing estrogen therapy to postmenopausal women, the risks and benefits must be weighed for each patient. Women should be informed of these risks and benefits, as well as possible effects of progestin when added to estrogen therapy. Estrogens with or without progestin should be used for shortest duration possible consistent with treatment goals. Conduct periodic risk:benefit assessments.

Osteoporosis use: For use only in women at significant risk of osteoporosis and for who other nonestrogen medications are not considered appropriate.

◀ Vulvar and vaginal atrophy use: When used solely for the treatment of vulvar and vaginal atrophy, topical vaginal products should be considered.

Adverse Reactions (Reflective of adult population; not specific for elderly)

>10%:

Central nervous system: Headache (23%)

Endocrine & metabolic: Breast pain (16%)

Gastrointestinal: Abdominal pain (12%)

Neuromuscular & skeletal: Back pain (12%)

Respiratory: Upper respiratory tract infection (21%)

Miscellaneous: Flu-like syndrome (11%)

1% to 10%:

Central nervous system: Fatigue (6%), pain (6%), depression (5%), dizziness (5%)

Endocrine & metabolic: Vaginal bleeding (9%), dysmenorrhea (8%), vaginitis (7%)

Gastrointestinal: Nausea (6%), flatulence (5%)

Neuromuscular & skeletal: Arthralgia (9%), myalgia (5%)

Respiratory: Sinusitis (8%), pharyngitis (7%), cough (5%)

Miscellaneous: Viral infection (6%)

Additional adverse effects associated with **estrogens and progestins**; frequency not defined:

Cardiovascular: Edema, hypertension, MI, stroke, venous thrombosis

Central nervous system: Anxiety, epilepsy exacerbation, insomnia, irritability, migraine, mood disturbances, nervousness, pyrexia, somnolence

Dermatologic: Acne, chloasma, erythema multiforme, erythema nodosum, hemorrhagic eruptions, hirsutism, itching, melasma, pruritus, rash, scalp hair loss, urticaria

Endocrine & metabolic: Amenorrhea, breast cancer, breast discharge, breast enlargement, Breast tenderness, carbohydrate tolerance decreased, endometrial cancer, endometrial hyperplasia, fibrocystic breast changes, galactorrhea, hypocalcemia, libido changes, ovarian cancer, triglycerides increased

Gastrointestinal: Abdominal cramps, appetite changes, bloating, gallbladder disease, pancreatitis, vomiting, weight gain/loss

Genitourinary: Abnormal withdrawal bleeding/flow, breakthrough bleeding, cervical secretion changes, cystitis syndrome, uterine leiomyomata size increased, vaginal candidiasis, vaginal bleeding/spotting

Hematologic: Anemia, porphyria

Hepatic: Cholestatic jaundice

Local: Thrombophlebitis

Neuromuscular & skeletal: Chorea

Ocular: Contact lens intolerance, corneal curvature steepening, neuro-ocular lesions

Respiratory: Asthma exacerbation, pulmonary embolism

Miscellaneous: Anaphylaxis

Drug Interactions

Metabolism/Transport Effects Estradiol: **Substrate** of CYP1A2 (major), CYP2A6 (minor), CYP2B6 (minor), CYP2C9 (minor), CYP2C19 (minor), CYP2D6 (minor), CYP2E1 (minor), CYP3A4 (major), P-glycoprotein; **Inhibits** CYP1A2 (weak), 2C8 (weak); **Induces** CYP3A4 (weak)

Avoid Concomitant Use

Avoid concomitant use of Estradiol and Norgestimate with any of the following: Anastrozole; Griseofulvin

Increased Effect/Toxicity

Estradiol and Norgestimate may increase the levels/effects of: Benzodiazepines (metabolized by oxidation); Corticosteroids (Systemic); ROPINIRole; Selegiline; Tipranavir; Tranexamic Acid; Voriconazole

The levels/effects of Estradiol and Norgestimate may be increased by: Ascorbic Acid; Boceprevir; Conivaptan; Herbs (Estrogenic Properties); Herbs (Progestogenic Properties); P-Glycoprotein Inhibitors; Voriconazole

Decreased Effect

Estradiol and Norgestimate may decrease the levels/effects of: Anastrozole; Chenodiol; Saxagliptin; Somatropin; Thyroid Products; Ursodiol; Vitamin K Antagonists

The levels/effects of Estradiol and Norgestimate may be decreased by: Acitretin; Aminoglutethimide; Aprepitant; Artemether; Barbiturates; Bexarotene; Bexarotene (Systemic); Bile Acid Sequestrants; Bosentan; CarBAMazepine; CYP1A2 Inducers (Strong); CYP3A4 Inducers (Strong); Cyproterone; Deferasirox; Efavirenz; Felbamate; Fosaprepitant; Fosphenytoin; Griseofulvin; LamoTRIgine; Mycophenolate; OXcarbazepine; Peginterferon Alfa-2b; P-Glycoprotein Inducers; Phenytoin; Retinoic Acid Derivatives; Rifamycin Derivatives; St Johns Wort; Telaprevir; Tipranavir; Tocilizumab; Topiramate

Ethanol/Nutrition/Herb Interactions

Ethanol: Avoid ethanol (routine use increases estrogen level and risk of breast cancer). Ethanol may also increase the risk of osteoporosis.

Food: CNS effects of caffeine may be enhanced if combination estrogen/progestins are used concurrently with caffeine. Grapefruit juice increases ethinyl estradiol concentrations and would be expected to increase progesterone serum levels as well; clinical implications are unclear.

Herb/Nutraceutical: St John's wort may decrease the plasma levels of combination estrogen/progestin combinations by inducing hepatic enzymes. Avoid dong quai and black cohosh (have estrogen activity). Avoid saw palmetto, red clover, ginseng.

Stability Store at 25°C (77°F).

Mechanism of Action Estrogens are responsible for the development and maintenance of the female reproductive system and secondary sexual characteristics. Estradiol is the principle intracellular human estrogen and is more potent than estrone and estriol at the receptor level; it is the primary estrogen secreted prior to menopause. Following menopause, estrone and estrone sulfate are more highly produced. Estrogens modulate the pituitary secretion of gonadotropins, luteinizing hormone, and follicle-stimulating hormone through a negative feedback system; estrogen replacement reduces elevated levels of these hormones in postmenopausal women.

Progestins inhibit gonadotropin production which then prevents follicular maturation and ovulation. In women with adequate estrogen, progestins transform a proliferative endometrium into a secretory endometrium; when administered with estradiol, reduces the incidence of endometrial hyperplasia and risk of adenocarcinoma.

Pharmacodynamics/Kinetics

Estradiol: See Estradiol (Systemic) monograph.

Norgestimate:

Protein binding: 17-deacetylnorgestimate: 99%

Metabolism: Forms 17-deacetylnorgestimate (major active metabolite) and other metabolites; first-pass effect

Half-life elimination: 17-deacetylnorgestimate: 37 hours

Excretion: Norgestimate metabolites: Urine and feces

Dosage

Geriatric & Adult Females with an intact uterus:

Treatment of menopausal symptoms, atrophic vaginitis, prevention of osteoporosis:

Oral: Treatment is cyclical and consists of the following: One tablet of estradiol 1 mg (pink tablet) once daily for 3 days, followed by 1 tablet of estradiol 1 mg and norgestimate 0.09 mg (white tablet) once daily for 3 days; repeat sequence continuously. **Note:** This dose may not be the lowest effective combination for these indications. In case of a missed tablet, restart therapy with next available tablet in sequence (taking only 1 tablet each day).

Administration In case of a missed tablet, restart therapy with next available tablet in sequence (taking only 1 tablet each day).

Monitoring Parameters Yearly physical examination that includes blood pressure and Papanicolaou smear, breast exam, mammogram. Monitor for signs of endometrial cancer. Adequate diagnostic measures, including endometrial sampling, if indicated, should be performed to rule out malignancy in all cases of undiagnosed abnormal vaginal bleeding. Monitor for loss of vision, sudden onset of proptosis, diplopia, migraine; signs and symptoms of thromboembolic disorders; glycemic control in patients with diabetes; lipid profiles in patients being treated for hyperlipidemias; thyroid function in patients on thyroid hormone replacement therapy.

Menopausal symptoms: Assess need for therapy at 3- to 6-month intervals

Prevention of osteoporosis: Bone density measurement

Test Interactions Pathologist should be advised of estrogen/progesterone therapy when specimens are submitted. Reduced response to metyrapone test.

Special Geriatric Considerations See Estradiol (Systemic) monograph on page 641.

Dosage Forms Excipient information presented when available (limited, particularly for generics); consult specific product labeling.

Tablet, oral:

Prefest™: Estradiol 1 mg [15 peach tablets] and estradiol 1 mg and norgestimate 0.09 mg [15 white tablets]

Selected References

Mørch LS, Løkkegaard E, Andreasen AH, et al, "Hormone Therapy and Ovarian Cancer," *JAMA*, 2009, 302 (3):298-305.

♦ **Estradiol Transdermal** *see* Estradiol (Systemic) *on page 641*

♦ **Estradiol Valerate** *see* Estradiol (Systemic) *on page 641*

♦ **Estrasorb®** *see* Estradiol (Systemic) *on page 641*

♦ **Estring®** *see* Estradiol (Topical) *on page 648*

◆ **EstroGel®** *see* Estradiol (Systemic) *on page 641*
◆ **Estrogenic Substances, Conjugated** *see* Estrogens (Conjugated/Equine, Systemic) *on page 658*
◆ **Estrogenic Substances, Conjugated** *see* Estrogens (Conjugated/Equine, Topical) *on page 661*

Estrogens (Conjugated A/Synthetic)
(ES troe jenz, KON joo gate ed, aye, sin THET ik)

Related Information
Osteoporosis Management *on page 2027*
Pharmacotherapy of Urinary Incontinence *on page 2032*
Medication Safety Issues
Sound-alike/look-alike issues:
Cenestin® may be confused with Senexon®
BEERS Criteria medication:
This drug may be inappropriate for use in geriatric patients (low severity risk).
International issues:
Cenestin [U.S., Canada] may be confused with Canesten which is a brand name for clotrimazole [multiple international markets] and a brand name for fluconazole [Great Britain]
Brand Names: U.S. Cenestin®
Brand Names: Canada Cenestin
Generic Availability (U.S.) No
Pharmacologic Category Estrogen Derivative
Use Treatment of moderate-to-severe vasomotor symptoms of menopause; treatment of vulvar and vaginal atrophy
Contraindications Hypersensitivity to estrogens or any component of the formulation; undiagnosed abnormal vaginal bleeding; history of or current thrombophlebitis or venous thromboembolic disorders (including DVT, PE); active or recent (within 1 year) arterial thromboembolic disease (eg, stroke, MI); carcinoma of the breast; estrogen-dependent tumor; hepatic dysfunction or disease
Warnings/Precautions
Cardiovascular-related considerations: **[U.S. Boxed Warning]: Estrogens with or without progestin should not be used to prevent coronary heart disease.** Use caution with cardiovascular disease or dysfunction. May increase the risks of myocardial infarction (MI), stroke, pulmonary emboli (PE), and deep vein thrombosis (DVT); incidence of these effects was shown to be significantly increased in postmenopausal women using CEE in combination with MPA. Nonfatal MI, PE, and thrombophlebitis have also been reported in males taking high doses of CEE (eg, for prostate cancer). Risk factors include diabetes mellitus, hypercholesterolemia, hypertension, SLE, obesity, and/or venous thromboembolism (VTE). Estrogen compounds are generally associated with lipid effects such as increased HDL-cholesterol and decreased LDL-cholesterol. Triglycerides may also be increased; use with caution in patients with familial defects of lipoprotein metabolism. Whenever possible, estrogens should be discontinued at least 4 weeks prior to and for 2 weeks following elective surgery associated with an increased risk of thromboembolism or during periods of prolonged immobilization. Use caution in patients with known inherited thrombophilias (eg, protein C or S deficiency); may have increased risk of VTE (DeSancho, 2010); use is contraindicated in patients with DVT or PE (current or history of).

Neurological considerations: **[U.S. Boxed Warning]: The risk of dementia may be increased in postmenopausal women;** increased incidence was observed in women ≥65 years of age taking CEE alone or in combination with MPA.

Cancer-related considerations: **[U.S. Boxed Warning]: Unopposed estrogens may increase the risk of endometrial carcinoma in postmenopausal women.** Estrogens may exacerbate endometriosis. Malignant transformation of residual endometrial implants has been reported posthysterectomy with estrogen only therapy. Consider adding a progestin in women with residual endometriosis posthysterectomy. Estrogens may increase the risk of breast cancer. An increased risk of invasive breast cancer was observed in postmenopausal women using CEE in combination with MPA; a smaller increase in risk was seen with estrogen therapy alone in observational studies. An increase in abnormal mammograms has also been reported with estrogen and progestin therapy. Estrogen use may lead to severe hypercalcemia in patients with breast cancer and bone metastases; discontinue estrogen if hypercalcemia occurs. Postmenopausal estrogen therapy and combined estrogen/progesterone therapy may increase the risk of ovarian cancer; however, the absolute risk to an individual woman is small. Although results from various studies are not consistent, risk does not appear to be significantly associated with the duration, route, or dose of therapy. In one study, the risk decreased after 2 years following discontinuation of therapy.

Estrogens may cause retinal vascular thrombosis; discontinue permanently if papilledema or retinal vascular lesions are observed on examination. Use with caution in patients with diseases which may be exacerbated by fluid retention, including asthma, epilepsy, migraine, diabetes or renal dysfunction. Use with caution in patients with a history of severe hypocalcemia, SLE, hepatic hemangiomas, porphyria, endometriosis, and gallbladder disease. Use caution with history of cholestatic jaundice associated with past estrogen use or pregnancy. May be inappropriate for use in the elderly due to potential of increased risk of breast and endometrial cancers and lack of proven cardioprotection (Beers Criteria).

Before prescribing estrogen therapy to postmenopausal women, the risks and benefits must be weighed for each patient. Women should be informed of these risks and benefits, as well as possible effects of progestin when added to estrogen therapy. Estrogens with or without progestin should be used for shortest duration possible consistent with treatment goals. Conduct periodic risk:benefit assessments.

Vulvar and vaginal atrophy use: When used solely for the treatment of vulvar and vaginal atrophy, topical vaginal products should be considered.

Adverse Reactions (Reflective of adult population; not specific for elderly)
>10%:
Central nervous system: Headache (11% to 68%), dizziness (11%), pain (11%)
Endocrine & metabolic: Breast pain (29%), endometrial thickening (19%), metrorrhagia (14%)
Gastrointestinal: Abdominal pain (9% to 28%), nausea (9% to 18%)
Neuromuscular & skeletal: Paresthesia (8% to 33%), back pain (14%)
Respiratory: Upper respiratory tract infection (13%)
Miscellaneous: Infection (2% to 14%)
1% to 10%:
Central nervous system: Anxiety (6%), fever (1%)
Gastrointestinal: Dyspepsia (10%), vomiting (7%), constipation (6%), diarrhea (6%), weight gain (6%)
Genitourinary: Vaginitis (8%)
Neuromuscular & skeletal: Leg cramps (10%), hypertonia (6%)
Respiratory: Rhinitis (6% to 8%), cough (6%)

In addition, the following have been reported with estrogen and/or progestin therapy:
Cardiovascular: Edema, hypertension, MI, stroke, venous thromboembolism
Central nervous system: Epilepsy exacerbation, irritability, mental depression, migraine, mood disturbances, nervousness
Dermatologic: Angioedema, chloasma, erythema multiforme, erythema nodosum, hemorrhagic eruption, hirsutism, melasma, pruritus, rash, scalp hair loss, urticaria
Endocrine & metabolic: Breast cancer, breast enlargement, breast tenderness, glucose tolerance impaired, HDL-cholesterol increased, hyper-/hypocalcemia, LDL-cholesterol decreased, libido changes, serum triglycerides/phospholipids increased, thyroid-binding globulin increased, total thyroid hormone (T_4) increased
Gastrointestinal: Abdominal cramps, bloating, cholecystitis, cholelithiasis, gallbladder disease, pancreatitis, weight gain/loss
Genitourinary: Alterations in frequency and flow of menses, cervical secretion changes, endometrial cancer, endometrial hyperplasia, uterine leiomyomata size increased, vaginal candidiasis
Hematologic: Aggravation of porphyria, antithrombin III and antifactor Xa decreased, fibrinogen levels increased, platelet aggregability and platelet count increased; prothrombin and factors VII, VIII, IX, X increased
Hepatic: Cholestatic jaundice, hepatic hemangiomas enlarged
Neuromuscular & skeletal: Arthralgias, chorea, leg cramps
Local: Thrombophlebitis
Ocular: Contact lens intolerance, retinal vascular thrombosis, corneal curvature steepening
Respiratory: Asthma exacerbation, pulmonary thromboembolism
Miscellaneous: Anaphylactoid/anaphylactic reactions, carbohydrate intolerance

Drug Interactions
Metabolism/Transport Effects Based on estradiol and estrone: **Substrate** of CYP1A2 (major), 2A6 (minor), 2B6 (minor), 2C9 (minor), 2C19 (minor), 2D6 (minor), 2E1 (minor), 3A4 (major); **Inhibits** CYP1A2 (weak); **Induces** CYP3A4 (weak)
Avoid Concomitant Use
Avoid concomitant use of Estrogens (Conjugated A/Synthetic) with any of the following: Anastrozole

Increased Effect/Toxicity

Estrogens (Conjugated A/Synthetic) may increase the levels/effects of: Corticosteroids (Systemic); ROPINIRole; Tipranavir

The levels/effects of Estrogens (Conjugated A/Synthetic) may be increased by: Ascorbic Acid; Conivaptan; Herbs (Estrogenic Properties)

Decreased Effect

Estrogens (Conjugated A/Synthetic) may decrease the levels/effects of: Anastrozole; Chenodiol; Saxagliptin; Somatropin; Thyroid Products; Ursodiol

The levels/effects of Estrogens (Conjugated A/Synthetic) may be decreased by: CYP1A2 Inducers (Strong); CYP3A4 Inducers (Strong); Cyproterone; Deferasirox; Herbs (CYP3A4 Inducers); Peginterferon Alfa-2b; Tipranavir; Tocilizumab

Ethanol/Nutrition/Herb Interactions

Ethanol: Avoid ethanol (routine use increases estrogen plasma concentrations and risk of breast cancer).

Food: Grapefruit juice may increase estrogen plasma concentrations, leading to increased adverse effects.

Herb/Nutraceutical: St John's wort may decrease levels. Herbs with estrogenic properties may enhance the adverse/toxic effect of estrogen derivatives; examples include alfalfa, black cohosh, bloodroot, hops, kudzu, licorice, red clover, saw palmetto, soybean, thyme, wild yam, yucca.

Stability Store at room temperature of 25°C (77°F).

Mechanism of Action Conjugated A/synthetic estrogens contain a mixture of 9 synthetic estrogen substances, including sodium estrone sulfate, sodium equilin sulfate, sodium 17 alpha-dihydroequilin, sodium 17 alpha-estradiol and sodium 17 beta-dihydroequilin. Estrogens are responsible for the development and maintenance of the female reproductive system and secondary sexual characteristics. Estradiol is the principle intracellular human estrogen and is more potent than estrone and estriol at the receptor level; it is the primary estrogen secreted prior to menopause. Following menopause, estrone and estrone sulfate are more highly produced. Estrogens modulate the pituitary secretion of gonadotropins, luteinizing hormone, and follicle-stimulating hormone through a negative feedback system; estrogen replacement reduces elevated levels of these hormones in postmenopausal women.

Pharmacodynamics/Kinetics

Absorption: Well absorbed over a period of several hours

Protein-binding: Sex hormone-binding globulin (SHBG) and albumin

Metabolism: Hepatic via CYP3A4; estradiol is converted to estrone and estriol; also undergoes enterohepatic recirculation; estrone sulfate is the main metabolite in postmenopausal women

Excretion: Urine (primarily estriol, also as estradiol, estrone, and conjugates)

Dosage

Geriatric Refer to adult dosing. A higher incidence of stroke and invasive breast cancer were observed in women >75 years in a WHI substudy using conjugated equine estrogen.

Adult The lowest dose that will control symptoms should be used. Medication should be discontinued as soon as possible.

Menopause, moderate-to-severe vasomotor symptoms: Oral: 0.45 mg/day; may be titrated up to 1.25 mg/day; attempts to discontinue medication should be made at 3- to 6-month intervals

Vulvar and vaginal atrophy: Oral: 0.3 mg/day

Monitoring Parameters Yearly physical examination that includes blood pressure and Papanicolaou smear, breast exam, mammogram. Monitor for signs of endometrial cancer in female patients with uterus. Adequate diagnostic measures, including endometrial sampling, if indicated, should be performed to rule out malignancy in all cases of undiagnosed abnormal vaginal bleeding. Monitor for loss of vision, sudden onset of proptosis, diplopia, migraine; signs and symptoms of thromboembolic disorders; glycemic control in patients with diabetes; lipid profiles in patients being treated for hyperlipidemias; thyroid function in patients on thyroid hormone replacement therapy.

Menopausal symptoms: Assess need for therapy at 3- to 6-month intervals

Test Interactions Pathologist should be advised of estrogen/progesterone therapy when specimens are submitted. Reduced response to metyrapone test observed with conjugated estrogens (equine).

Pharmacotherapy Pearls Not biologically equivalent to conjugated estrogens from equine source. Contains 9 unique estrogenic compounds (equine source contains at least 10 active estrogenic compounds).

Special Geriatric Considerations Before prescribing estrogen therapy to postmenopausal women, the risks and benefits must be weighed for each patient. Women should be informed of these risks and benefits, as well as possible side effects and the return of menstrual bleeding (when cycled with a progestin), and be involved in the decision to prescribe. A higher incidence of stroke and invasive breast cancer were observed in women >75 years in a WHI substudy using conjugated equine estrogen.

This medication is considered to be potentially inappropriate in this patient population (Beers Criteria severity: Low).

Dosage Forms Excipient information presented when available (limited, particularly for generics); consult specific product labeling.

Tablet, oral:

Cenestin®: 0.3 mg, 0.45 mg, 0.625 mg, 0.9 mg, 1.25 mg

Estrogens (Conjugated B/Synthetic)
(ES troe jenz, KON joo gate ed, bee, sin THET ik)

Medication Safety Issues

Sound-alike/look-alike issues:

Enjuvia™ may be confused with Januvia®

BEERS Criteria medication:

This drug may be inappropriate for use in geriatric patients (low severity risk).

Brand Names: U.S. Enjuvia™

Generic Availability (U.S.) No

Pharmacologic Category Estrogen Derivative

Use Treatment of moderate-to-severe vasomotor symptoms of menopause; treatment of vulvar and vaginal atrophy associated with menopause; treatment of moderate-to-severe vaginal dryness and pain with intercourse associated with menopause

Contraindications Hypersensitivity to estrogens or any component of the formulation; undiagnosed abnormal vaginal bleeding; history of or current thrombophlebitis or venous thromboembolic disorders (including DVT, PE); active or recent (within 1 year) arterial thromboembolic disease (eg, stroke, MI); carcinoma of the breast; estrogen-dependent tumor; hepatic dysfunction or disease

Warnings/Precautions

Cardiovascular-related considerations: **[U.S. Boxed Warning]: Estrogens with or without progestin should not be used to prevent coronary heart disease.** Use caution in patients with cardiovascular disease or dysfunction. May increase the risks of myocardial infarction (MI), stroke, pulmonary emboli (PE), and deep vein thrombosis (DVT); incidence of these effects was shown to be significantly increased in postmenopausal women using CEE in combination with MPA. Nonfatal MI, PE, and thrombophlebitis have also been reported in males taking high doses of CEE (eg, for prostate cancer). Risk factors include diabetes mellitus, hyper-cholesterolemia, hypertension, SLE, obesity, and/or venous thromboembolism (VTE). Estro-gen compounds are generally associated with lipid effects such as increased HDL-cholesterol and decreased LDL-cholesterol. Triglycerides may also be increased; use with caution in patients with familial defects of lipoprotein metabolism. Whenever possible, estrogens should be discontinued at least 4 weeks prior to and for 2 weeks following elective surgery associated with an increased risk of thromboembolism or during periods of prolonged immobilization. Use caution in patients with known inherited thrombophilias (eg, protein C or S deficiency); may have increased risk of VTE (DeSancho, 2010); use is contraindicated in patients with DVT or PE (current or history of).

Neurological considerations: **[U.S. Boxed Warning]: The risk of dementia may be increased in postmenopausal women;** increased incidence was observed in women ≥65 years of age taking CEE alone or in combination with MPA.

Cancer-related considerations: **[U.S. Boxed Warning]: Unopposed estrogens may increase the risk of endometrial carcinoma in postmenopausal women.** Estrogens may exacerbate endometriosis. Malignant transformation of residual endometrial implants has been reported posthysterectomy with estrogen only therapy. Consider adding a progestin in women with residual endometriosis posthysterectomy. Estrogens may increase the risk of breast cancer. An increased risk of invasive breast cancer was observed in postmenopausal women using CEE in combination with MPA; a smaller increase in risk was seen with estrogen therapy alone in observational studies. An increase in abnormal mammograms has also been reported with estrogen and progestin therapy. Estrogen use may lead to severe hyper-calcemia in patients with breast cancer and bone metastases; discontinue estrogen if hypercalcemia occurs. Postmenopausal estrogen therapy and combined estrogen/progester-one therapy may increase the risk of ovarian cancer; however, the absolute risk to an individual woman is small. Although results from various studies are not consistent, risk does not appear to be significantly associated with the duration, route, or dose of therapy. In one study, the risk decreased after 2 years following discontinuation of therapy.

Estrogens may cause retinal vascular thrombosis; discontinue permanently if papilledema or retinal vascular lesions are observed on examination. Use with caution in patients with diseases which may be exacerbated by fluid retention, including asthma, epilepsy, migraine, diabetes or renal dysfunction. Use with caution in patients with a history of severe hypocalcemia, SLE, hepatic hemangiomas, porphyria, endometriosis, and gallbladder disease. Use caution with history of cholestatic jaundice associated with past estrogen use or pregnancy. May be inappropriate for use in the elderly due to potential of increased risk of breast and endometrial cancers and lack of proven cardioprotection (Beers Criteria).

Before prescribing estrogen therapy to postmenopausal women, the risks and benefits must be weighed for each patient. Women should be informed of these risks and benefits, as well as possible effects of progestin when added to estrogen therapy. Estrogens with or without progestin should be used for shortest duration possible consistent with treatment goals. Conduct periodic risk:benefit assessments. When used solely for the treatment of vaginal dryness and pain with intercourse, or vulvar and vaginal atrophy, topical vaginal products should be considered.

Adverse Reactions (Reflective of adult population; not specific for elderly)
>10%:
  Central nervous system: Headache (15% to 25%), pain (10% to 19%)
  Endocrine & metabolic: Breast pain (up to 14%)
  Gastrointestinal: Abdominal pain (4% to 15%), nausea (7% to 12%)
1% to 10%:
  Central nervous system: Dizziness (1% to 7%)
  Endocrine & metabolic: Dysmenorrhea (1% to 8%)
  Gastrointestinal: Flatulence (4% to 7%)
  Genitourinary: Vaginitis (2% to 7%)
  Neuromuscular & skeletal: Paresthesia (up to 6%)
  Respiratory: Bronchitis (up to 7%), rhinitis (4% to 7%), sinusitis (3% to 7%)
  Miscellaneous: Flu-like syndrome (4% to 7%)
In addition, the following have been reported with estrogen and/or progestin therapy:
  Cardiovascular: Edema, hypertension, MI, stroke, venous thromboembolism
  Central nervous system: Epilepsy exacerbation, irritability, mental depression, migraine, mood disturbances, nervousness
  Dermatologic: Angioedema, chloasma, erythema multiforme, erythema nodosum, hemorrhagic eruption, hirsutism, loss of scalp hair, melasma, pruritus, rash, urticaria
  Endocrine & metabolic: Breast cancer, breast enlargement, breast tenderness, HDL-cholesterol increased, hyper-/hypocalcemia, impaired glucose tolerance, LDL-cholesterol decreased, libido (changes in), serum triglycerides/phospholipids increased, thyroid-binding globulin increased, total thyroid hormone (T_4) increased
  Gastrointestinal: Abdominal cramps, bloating, cholecystitis, cholelithiasis, gallbladder disease, pancreatitis, weight gain/loss
  Genitourinary: Alterations in frequency and flow of menses, changes in cervical secretions, endometrial cancer, endometrial hyperplasia, increased size of uterine leiomyomata, vaginal candidiasis
  Hematologic: Aggravation of porphyria; antithrombin III and antifactor Xa decreased; fibrinogen levels increased; platelet aggregability and platelet count increased; prothrombin and factors VII, VIII, IX, X increased
  Hepatic: Cholestatic jaundice, hepatic hemangiomas enlarged
  Local: Thrombophlebitis
  Neuromuscular & skeletal: Arthralgias, chorea, leg cramps
  Ocular: Contact lens intolerance, corneal curvature steepening, retinal vascular thrombosis
  Respiratory: Asthma exacerbation, pulmonary thromboembolism
  Miscellaneous: Anaphylactoid/anaphylactic reactions, carbohydrate intolerance
Drug Interactions
  Metabolism/Transport Effects Based on estradiol and estrone: **Substrate** of CYP1A2 (major), 2A6 (minor), 2B6 (minor), 2C9 (minor), 2C19 (minor), 2D6 (minor), 2E1 (minor), 3A4 (major); **Inhibits** CYP1A2 (weak); **Induces** CYP3A4 (weak)
  Avoid Concomitant Use
  Avoid concomitant use of Estrogens (Conjugated B/Synthetic) with any of the following: Anastrozole
  Increased Effect/Toxicity
  Estrogens (Conjugated B/Synthetic) may increase the levels/effects of: Corticosteroids (Systemic); ROPINIRole; Tipranavir

  The levels/effects of Estrogens (Conjugated B/Synthetic) may be increased by: Ascorbic Acid; Conivaptan; Herbs (Estrogenic Properties)

Decreased Effect

Estrogens (Conjugated B/Synthetic) may decrease the levels/effects of: Anastrozole; Chenodiol; Somatropin; Thyroid Products; Ursodiol

The levels/effects of Estrogens (Conjugated B/Synthetic) may be decreased by: CYP3A4 Inducers (Strong); Deferasirox; Herbs (CYP3A4 Inducers); Tipranavir; Tocilizumab

Ethanol/Nutrition/Herb Interactions

Ethanol: Avoid ethanol (routine use increases estrogen plasma concentrations and risk of breast cancer).

Food: Grapefruit juice may increase estrogen plasma concentrations, leading to increased adverse effects.

Herb/Nutraceutical: St John's wort may decrease levels. Herbs with estrogenic properties may enhance the adverse/toxic effect of estrogen derivatives; examples include alfalfa, black cohosh, bloodroot, hops, kudzu, licorice, red clover, saw palmetto, soybean, thyme, wild yam, and yucca.

Stability Store at room temperature of 25°C (77°F).

Mechanism of Action Conjugated B/synthetic estrogens contain a mixture of 10 synthetic estrogen substances, including sodium estrone sulfate, sodium equilin sulfate, sodium 17-alpha-dihydroequilin, sodium 17-alpha-estradiol, and sodium 17-beta-dihydroequilin. Estrogens are responsible for the development and maintenance of the female reproductive system and secondary sexual characteristics. Estradiol is the principle intracellular human estrogen and is more potent than estrone and estriol at the receptor level; it is the primary estrogen secreted prior to menopause. Following menopause, estrone and estrone sulfate are more highly produced. Estrogens modulate the pituitary secretion of gonadotropins, luteinizing hormone, and follicle-stimulating hormone through a negative feedback system; estrogen replacement reduces elevated levels of these hormones in postmenopausal women.

Pharmacodynamics/Kinetics

Absorption: Well absorbed over a period of several hours

Protein-binding: Sex hormone-binding globulin (SHBG) and albumin

Metabolism: Hepatic via CYP3A4; estradiol is converted to estrone and estriol; also undergoes enterohepatic recirculation; estrone sulfate is the main metabolite in postmenopausal women

Half-life elimination: Conjugated estrone: 8-20 hours; conjugated equilin: 5-17 hours

Excretion: Urine (primarily estriol, also as estradiol, estrone, and conjugates)

Dosage

Geriatric Refer to adult dosing. A higher incidence of stroke and invasive breast cancer were observed in women >75 years in a WHI substudy using conjugated equine estrogen.

Adult The lowest dose that will control symptoms should be used. Medication should be discontinued as soon as possible.

Menopause, moderate-to-severe vasomotor symptoms: Oral: 0.3 mg/day; may be titrated up to 1.25 mg/day. Attempts to discontinue medication should be made at 3- to 6-month intervals.

Vaginal dryness/vulvar and vaginal atrophy associated with menopause: Oral: 0.3 mg/day. Attempts to discontinue medication should be made at 3- to 6-month intervals.

Monitoring Parameters Yearly physical examination that may include blood pressure and Papanicolaou smear, breast exam, mammogram. Monitor for signs of endometrial cancer in female patients with uterus. Adequate diagnostic measures, including endometrial sampling, if indicated, should be performed to rule out malignancy in all cases of undiagnosed abnormal vaginal bleeding. Monitor for loss of vision, sudden onset of proptosis, diplopia, migraine; signs and symptoms of thromboembolic disorders; glycemic control in patients with diabetes; lipid profiles in patients being treated for hyperlipidemias; thyroid function in patients on thyroid hormone replacement therapy.

Test Interactions Pathologist should be advised of estrogen/progesterone therapy when specimens are submitted. Reduced response to metyrapone test observed with conjugated estrogens (equine).

Pharmacotherapy Pearls Not biologically equivalent to conjugated estrogens from equine source. Contains 10 unique estrogenic compounds (equine source contains at least 10 active estrogenic compounds).

Special Geriatric Considerations Enjuvia™ has not been studied in an elderly population. Before prescribing estrogen therapy to postmenopausal women, the risks and benefits must be weighed for each patient. Women should be informed of these risks and benefits, as well as possible side effects and the return of menstrual bleeding (when cycled with a progestin), and be involved in the decision to prescribe. A higher incidence of stroke and invasive breast cancer was observed in women >75 years of age in a WHI substudy.

This medication is considered to be potentially inappropriate in this patient population (Beers Criteria severity: Low).

◀ **Dosage Forms** Excipient information presented when available (limited, particularly for generics); consult specific product labeling.
Tablet, oral:
Enjuvia™: 0.3 mg, 0.45 mg, 0.625 mg, 0.9 mg, 1.25 mg

Estrogens (Conjugated/Equine, Systemic)
(ES troe jenz KON joo gate ed, EE kwine)

Medication Safety Issues
Sound-alike/look-alike issues:
Premarin® may be confused with Primaxin®, Provera®, Remeron®
BEERS Criteria medication:
This drug may be inappropriate for use in geriatric patients (low severity risk).
Brand Names: U.S. Premarin®
Brand Names: Canada C.E.S.®; Premarin®
Index Terms C.E.S.; CE; CEE; Conjugated Estrogen; Estrogenic Substances, Conjugated
Generic Availability (U.S.) No
Pharmacologic Category Estrogen Derivative
Use Treatment of moderate-to-severe vasomotor symptoms associated with menopause; treatment of vulvar and vaginal atrophy; hypoestrogenism (due to hypogonadism, castration, or primary ovarian failure); prostatic cancer (palliation); breast cancer (palliation); osteoporosis (prophylaxis, postmenopausal women at significant risk only); abnormal uterine bleeding; moderate-to-severe dyspareunia (pain during intercourse) due to vaginal/vulvar atrophy of menopause
Unlabeled/Investigational Use Uremic bleeding
Contraindications Hypersensitivity to estrogens or any component of the formulation; undiagnosed abnormal vaginal bleeding; history of current thrombophlebitis or venous thromboembolic disorders (including DVT, PE); active or recent (within 1 year) arterial thromboembolic disease (eg, stroke, MI); carcinoma of the breast (except in appropriately selected patients being treated for metastatic disease); estrogen-dependent tumor; hepatic dysfunction or disease

Warnings/Precautions
Cardiovascular-related considerations: **[U.S. Boxed Warning]: Estrogens with or without progestin should not be used to prevent cardiovascular disease.** Use caution with cardiovascular disease or dysfunction. May increase the risks of myocardial infarction (MI), stroke, pulmonary emboli (PE), and deep vein thrombosis (DVT); incidence of these effects was shown to be significantly increased in postmenopausal women using CEE in combination with MPA. Nonfatal MI, PE, and thrombophlebitis have also been reported in males taking high doses of CEE (eg, for prostate cancer). Risk factors include diabetes mellitus, hyper-cholesterolemia, hypertension, SLE, obesity, and/or venous thromboembolism (VTE). Estrogen compounds are generally associated with lipid effects such as increased HDL-cholesterol and decreased LDL-cholesterol. Triglycerides may also be increased; use with caution in patients with familial defects of lipoprotein metabolism. Whenever possible, estrogens should be discontinued at least 4 weeks prior to and for 2 weeks following elective surgery associated with an increased risk of thromboembolism or during periods of prolonged immobilization. Use caution in patients with known inherited thrombophilias (eg, protein C or S deficiency); may have increased risk of VTE (DeSancho, 2010); use is contraindicated in patients with DVT or PE (current or history of).

Neurological considerations: **[U.S. Boxed Warning]: The risk of dementia may be increased in postmenopausal women;** increased incidence was observed in women ≥65 years of age taking CE alone or in combination with MPA.

Cancer-related considerations: **[U.S. Boxed Warning]: Adequate diagnostic measures, including endometrial sampling, if indicated, should be performed to rule out malignancy in all cases of undiagnosed abnormal vaginal bleeding. Unopposed estrogens may increase the risk of endometrial carcinoma in postmenopausal women with an intact uterus.** Risk appears to be associated with long-term use The use of a progestin should be considered when administering estrogens to postmenopausal women with an intact uterus. Estrogens may exacerbate endometriosis. Malignant transformation of residual endometrial implants has been reported posthysterectomy with estrogen only therapy. Consider adding a progestin in women with residual endometriosis posthysterectomy. Presentation of irregular, unresolving vaginal bleeding warrants further evaluation including endometrial sampling, if indicated, to rule out malignancy. Estrogens may increase the risk of breast cancer. An increased risk of invasive breast cancer was observed in postmenopausal women using CE in combination with MPA; a smaller increase in risk was seen with estrogen therapy alone in observational studies. An increase in abnormal mammograms has also been reported with estrogen and progestin therapy. Estrogen use may lead to severe hypercalcemia in patients with breast cancer and bone metastases; discontinue estrogen if hypercalcemia occurs.

Estrogens may cause retinal vascular thrombosis; discontinue permanently if papilledema or retinal vascular lesions are observed on examination. Use with caution in patients with diseases which may be exacerbated by fluid retention, including asthma, epilepsy, migraine, diabetes, heart failure, or renal dysfunction. Use with caution in patients with a history of severe hypocalcemia, SLE, hepatic hemangiomas, porphyria, endometriosis, and gallbladder disease. Use caution with history of cholestatic jaundice associated with past estrogen use or pregnancy. May be inappropriate for use in the elderly due to potential of increased risk of breast and endometrial cancers and lack of proven cardioprotection (Beers Criteria). Prior to puberty, estrogens may cause premature closure of the epiphyses, premature breast development in girls or gynecomastia in boys. Vaginal bleeding and vaginal cornification may also be induced in girls.

[U.S. Boxed Warning]: Estrogens with or without progestin should be used for shortest duration possible at the lowest effective dose consistent with treatment goals. Before prescribing estrogen therapy to postmenopausal women, the risks and benefits must be weighed for each patient. Women should be informed of these risks and benefits, as well as possible effects of progestin when added to estrogen therapy. Estrogens with or without progestin should be used for shortest duration possible consistent with treatment goals. Conduct periodic risk:benefit assessments.

Osteoporosis use: For use only in women at significant risk of osteoporosis and for who other nonestrogen medications are not considered appropriate.

Adverse Reactions (Reflective of adult population; not specific for elderly)
Note: Percentages reported in postmenopausal women following oral use.
>10%:
 Central nervous system: Headache (26% to 32%; placebo 28%)
 Endocrine & metabolic: Breast pain (7% to 12%; placebo 9%)
 Gastrointestinal: Abdominal pain (15% to 17%)
 Genitourinary: Vaginal hemorrhage (2% to 14%)
 Neuromuscular & skeletal: Back pain (13% to 14%)
1% to 10%:
 Central nervous system: Nervousness (2% to 5%)
 Dermatologic: Pruritus (4% to 5%)
 Gastrointestinal: Flatulence (6% to 7%)
 Genitourinary: Vaginitis (5% to 7%), leukorrhea (4% to 7%), vaginal moniliasis (5% to 6%)
 Neuromuscular & skeletal: Weakness (7% to 8%), leg cramps (3% to 7%)
Additional adverse reactions reported with injection or vaginal cream; frequency not defined:
 Genitourinary: Cystis-like syndrome, genital pruritus, vulvovaginal discomfort
 Local: injection site: Edema, pain, phlebitis

In addition, the following have been reported with estrogen and/or progestin therapy:
Cardiovascular: DVT, edema, hypertension, MI, stroke, superficial venous thrombosis
Central nervous system: Dementia, dizziness, epilepsy exacerbation, headache, irritability, mental depression, migraine, mood disturbances, nervousness
Dermatologic: Angioedema, chloasma, erythema multiforme, erythema nodosum, hemorrhagic eruption, hirsutism, loss of scalp hair, melasma, pruritus, rash, urticaria
Endocrine & metabolic: Breast cancer, breast discharge, breast enlargement, breast tenderness, dysmenorrhea, fibrocystic breast changes, galactorrhea, glucose intolerance, HDL-cholesterol increased, hyper-/hypocalcemia, LDL-cholesterol decreased, libido (changes in), ovarian cancer, serum triglycerides/phospholipids increased, thyroid-binding globulin increased, total thyroid hormone (T_4) increased
Gastrointestinal: Abdominal cramps, bloating, cholecystitis, cholelithiasis, gallbladder disease, ischemic colitis, nausea, pancreatitis, vomiting, weight gain/loss
Genitourinary: Abnormal uterine bleeding/spotting, changes in cervical ectropion, changes in cervical secretions, endometrial cancer, endometrial hyperplasia, increased size of uterine leiomyomata, vaginal candidiasis
Hematologic: Aggravation of porphyria, antithrombin III and antifactor Xa decreased; factors II, II-VII-X complex, VII, VIII, VII-X complex, IX, X, and XII increased; increased beta-thromboglobulin, fibrinogen levels, plasminogen/plasminogen activity, platelet aggregability, platelet count, and prothrombin
Hepatic: Cholestatic jaundice, hepatic hemangiomas enlarged
Neuromuscular & skeletal: Arthralgias, chorea, leg cramps
Local: Thrombophlebitis
Ocular: Contact lens intolerance, corneal curvature steepening, retinal vascular thrombosis
Respiratory: Asthma exacerbation, pulmonary thromboembolism
Miscellaneous: Anaphylactoid/anaphylactic reactions, benign meningioma growth potentiation

◄ **Drug Interactions**
Metabolism/Transport Effects
Based on estradiol and estrone: **Substrate** of CYP1A2 (major), 2A6 (minor), 2B6 (minor), 2C9 (minor), 2C19 (minor), 2D6 (minor), 2E1 (minor), 3A4 (major); Inhibits CYP1A2 (weak), 2C8 (weak); Induces CYP3A4 (weak)

Avoid Concomitant Use
Avoid concomitant use of Estrogens (Conjugated/Equine, Systemic) with any of the following: Anastrozole

Increased Effect/Toxicity
Estrogens (Conjugated/Equine, Systemic) may increase the levels/effects of: Corticosteroids (Systemic); ROPINIRole; Tipranavir

The levels/effects of Estrogens (Conjugated/Equine, Systemic) may be increased by: Ascorbic Acid; Conivaptan; Herbs (Estrogenic Properties)

Decreased Effect
Estrogens (Conjugated/Equine, Systemic) may decrease the levels/effects of: Anastrozole; Chenodiol; Saxagliptin; Somatropin; Thyroid Products; Ursodiol

The levels/effects of Estrogens (Conjugated/Equine, Systemic) may be decreased by: CYP1A2 Inducers (Strong); CYP3A4 Inducers (Strong); Cyproterone; Deferasirox; Herbs (CYP3A4 Inducers); Peginterferon Alfa-2b; Tipranavir; Tocilizumab

Ethanol/Nutrition/Herb Interactions
Ethanol: Avoid ethanol (routine use increases estrogen plasma concentrations and risk of breast cancer). Ethanol may also increase the risk of osteoporosis.
Food: Folic acid absorption may be decreased.
Herb/Nutraceutical: St John's wort may decrease levels. Herbs with estrogenic properties may enhance the adverse/toxic effect of estrogen derivatives; examples include alfalfa, black cohosh, bloodroot, hops, kudzu, licorice, red clover, saw palmetto, soybean, thyme, wild yam, yucca.

Stability
Injection: Refrigerate at 2°C to 8°C (36°F to 46°F) prior to reconstitution. Reconstitute with sterile water for injection; slowly inject diluent against side wall of the vial. Agitate gently; do not shake violently. Use immediately following reconstitution.
Tablets: Store at room temperature 20°C to 25°C (68°F to 77°F).

Mechanism of Action Conjugated estrogens contain a mixture of estrone sulfate, equilin sulfate, 17 alpha-dihydroequilin, 17 alpha-estradiol and 17 beta-dihydroequilin. Estrogens are responsible for the development and maintenance of the female reproductive system and secondary sexual characteristics. Estradiol is the principle intracellular human estrogen and is more potent than estrone and estriol at the receptor level; it is the primary estrogen secreted prior to menopause. Following menopause, estrone and estrone sulfate are more highly produced. Estrogens modulate the pituitary secretion of gonadotropins, luteinizing hormone, and follicle-stimulating hormone through a negative feedback system; estrogen replacement reduces elevated levels of these hormones in postmenopausal women.

Pharmacodynamics/Kinetics
Absorption: Well absorbed
Protein binding: Binds to sex-hormone-binding globulin and albumin
Metabolism: Hepatic via CYP3A4; estradiol is converted to estrone and estriol; also undergoes enterohepatic recirculation (avoided with vaginal administration); estrone sulfate is the main metabolite in postmenopausal women
Half-life elimination: Total estrone: 27 hours
Time to peak, plasma: Total estrone: 7 hours
Excretion: Urine (primarily estriol, also as estradiol, estrone, and conjugates

Dosage
Geriatric Refer to adult dosing. A higher incidence of stroke and breast cancer was observed in women >75 years in a WHI substudy.

Adult
Breast cancer palliation, metastatic disease in selected patients (male and female): Oral: 10 mg 3 times/day for at least 3 months
Uremic bleeding (unlabeled use): I.V.: 0.6 mg/kg/day for 5 days
Androgen-dependent prostate cancer palliation (males): Oral: 1.25-2.5 mg 3 times/day
Prevention of postmenopausal osteoporosis: Oral: Initial: 0.3 mg/day, cyclically* or daily, depending on medical assessment of patient. Dose may be adjusted based on bone mineral density and clinical response. The lowest effective dose should be used.
Menopause (moderate-to-severe vasomotor symptoms): Oral: Initial: 0.3 mg/day. May be given cyclically* or daily, depending on medical assessment of patient. The lowest dose that will control symptoms should be used. Medication should be discontinued as soon as possible.

Vulvar and vaginal atrophy: Oral: Initial: 0.3 mg/day. The lowest dose that will control symptoms should be used. May be given cyclically* or daily, depending on medical assessment of patient. Medication should be discontinued as soon as possible.

Female hypogonadism: Oral: 0.3-0.625 mg/day given cyclically*; dose may be titrated in 6- to 12-month intervals; progestin treatment should be added to maintain bone mineral density once skeletal maturity is achieved.

Female castration, primary ovarian failure: Oral: 1.25 mg/day given cyclically*; adjust according to severity of symptoms and patient response. For maintenance, adjust to the lowest effective dose.

Abnormal uterine bleeding:

Acute/heavy bleeding:

Oral (unlabeled route): 1.25 mg, may repeat every 4 hours for 24 hours, followed by 1.25 mg once daily for 7-10 days

I.M., I.V.: 25 mg, may repeat in 6-12 hours if needed

Note: Treatment should be followed by a low-dose oral contraceptive; medroxyprogesterone acetate along with or following estrogen therapy can also be given

Nonacute/lesser bleeding: Oral (unlabeled route): 1.25 mg once daily for 7-10 days

*Cyclic administration: Either 3 weeks on, 1 week off **or** 25 days on, 5 days off

Hepatic Impairment

Mild-to-moderate liver impairment: Dosage reduction of estrogens is recommended.

Severe liver impairment: **Not recommended.**

Administration

Injection: May also be administered intramuscularly; when administered I.V., drug should be administered slowly to avoid the occurrence of a flushing reaction

Oral tablet: Administer at bedtime to minimize adverse effects. May be administered without regard to meals.

Monitoring Parameters Routine physical examination that includes blood pressure and Papanicolaou smear, breast exam, mammogram. Monitor for signs of endometrial cancer in female patients with uterus. Adequate diagnostic measures, including endometrial sampling, if indicated, should be performed to rule out malignancy in all cases of undiagnosed abnormal vaginal bleeding. Monitor for loss of vision, sudden onset of proptosis, diplopia, migraine; signs and symptoms of thromboembolic disorders; glycemic control in patients with diabetes; lipid profiles in patients being treated for hyperlipidemias; thyroid function in patients on thyroid hormone replacement therapy.

Menopausal symptoms: Assess need for therapy at 3- to 6-month intervals

Prevention of osteoporosis: Bone density measurement

Uremic bleeding: Bleeding time

Reference Range Adults:

Male: 15-40 mcg/24 hours (SI: 52-139 µmol/day)

Female: Postmenopausal: <20 mcg/24 hours (SI: <69 µmol/day)

Test Interactions Thyroid function tests: Estrogens may increase thyroid binding globulin and circulating total thyroid hormone (when measured by T_4 RIA, T_4 by column, or by PBI); decreases free T_3 resin uptake; concentration of free T_4 is not altered; metyrapone test: Response may be reduced

Special Geriatric Considerations Before prescribing estrogen therapy to postmenopausal women, the risks and benefits must be weighed for each patient. Women should be informed of these risks and benefits, as well as possible side effects and the return of menstrual bleeding (when cycled with a progestin), and be involved in the decision to prescribe. A higher incidence of stroke and invasive breast cancer was observed in women >75 years in a WHI substudy.

This medication is considered to be potentially inappropriate in this patient population (Beers Criteria severity: Low).

Dosage Forms Excipient information presented when available (limited, particularly for generics); consult specific product labeling.

Injection, powder for reconstitution:

Premarin®: 25 mg [contains benzyl alcohol (in diluent), lactose 200 mg]

Tablet, oral:

Premarin®: 0.3 mg, 0.45 mg, 0.625 mg, 0.9 mg, 1.25 mg

Estrogens (Conjugated/Equine, Topical)

(ES troe jenz KON joo gate ed, EE kwine)

Medication Safety Issues

Sound-alike/look-alike issues:

Premarin® may be confused with Primaxin®, Provera®, Remeron®

Brand Names: U.S. Premarin®

ESTROGENS (CONJUGATED/EQUINE, TOPICAL)

Brand Names: Canada Premarin®

Index Terms C.E.S.; CE; CEE; Conjugated Estrogen; Estrogenic Substances, Conjugated

Generic Availability (U.S.) No

Pharmacologic Category Estrogen Derivative

Use Treatment of vulvar and vaginal atrophy; moderate-to-severe dyspareunia (pain during intercourse) due to vaginal/vulvar atrophy of menopause

Contraindications Hypersensitivity to estrogens or any component of the formulation; undiagnosed abnormal vaginal bleeding; history of or current thrombophlebitis or venous thromboembolic disorders (including DVT, PE); active or recent (within 1 year) arterial thromboembolic disease (eg, stroke, MI); carcinoma of the breast (except in appropriately selected patients being treated for metastatic disease); estrogen-dependent tumor; hepatic dysfunction or disease

Warnings/Precautions

Cardiovascular-related considerations: **[U.S. Boxed Warning]: Estrogens with or without progestin should not be used to prevent cardiovascular disease.** Use caution with cardiovascular disease or dysfunction. May increase the risks of myocardial infarction (MI), stroke, pulmonary emboli (PE), and deep vein thrombosis (DVT); incidence of these effects was shown to be significantly increased in postmenopausal women using CEE in combination with MPA. Nonfatal MI, PE, and thrombophlebitis have also been reported in males taking high doses of CEE (eg, for prostate cancer). Risk factors include diabetes mellitus, hyper-cholesterolemia, hypertension, SLE, obesity, and/or venous thromboembolism (VTE). Estrogen compounds are generally associated with lipid effects such as increased HDL-cholesterol and decreased LDL-cholesterol. Triglycerides may also be increased; use with caution in patients with familial defects of lipoprotein metabolism. Whenever possible, estrogens should be discontinued at least 4 weeks prior to and for 2 weeks following elective surgery associated with an increased risk of thromboembolism or during periods of prolonged immobilization. Use caution in patients with known inherited thrombophilias (eg, protein C or S deficiency); may have increased risk of VTE (DeSancho, 2010); use is contraindicated in patients with DVT or PE (current or history of).

Neurological considerations: **[U.S. Boxed Warning]: The risk of dementia may be increased in postmenopausal women;** increased incidence was observed in women ≥65 years of age taking CE alone or in combination with MPA.

Cancer-related considerations: **[U.S. Boxed Warning]: Adequate diagnostic measures, including endometrial sampling, if indicated, should be performed to rule out malignancy in all cases of undiagnosed abnormal vaginal bleeding. Unopposed estrogens may increase the risk of endometrial carcinoma in postmenopausal women with an intact uterus.** Risk appears to be associated with long-term use The use of a progestin should be considered when administering estrogens to postmenopausal women with an intact uterus. Estrogens may exacerbate endometriosis. Malignant transformation of residual endometrial implants has been reported posthysterectomy with estrogen only therapy. Consider adding a progestin in women with residual endometriosis posthysterectomy. Presentation of irregular, unresolving vaginal bleeding warrants further evaluation including endometrial sampling, if indicated, to rule out malignancy. Estrogens may increase the risk of breast cancer. An increased risk of invasive breast cancer was observed in postmenopausal women using CE in combination with MPA; a smaller increase in risk was seen with estrogen therapy alone in observational studies. An increase in abnormal mammograms has also been reported with estrogen and progestin therapy. Estrogen use may lead to severe hyper-calcemia in patients with breast cancer and bone metastases; discontinue estrogen if hypercalcemia occurs. Postmenopausal estrogen therapy and combined estrogen/progester-one therapy may increase the risk of ovarian cancer; however, the absolute risk to an individual woman is small. Although results from various studies are not consistent, risk does not appear to be significantly associated with the duration, route, or dose of therapy. In one study, the risk decreased after 2 years following discontinuation of therapy.

Estrogens may cause retinal vascular thrombosis; discontinue permanently if papilledema or retinal vascular lesions are observed on examination. Use with caution in patients with diseases which may be exacerbated by fluid retention, including asthma, epilepsy, migraine, diabetes, heart failure, or renal dysfunction. Use with caution in patients with a history of severe hypocalcemia, SLE, hepatic hemangiomas, porphyria, endometriosis, and gallbladder disease. Use caution with history of cholestatic jaundice associated with past estrogen use or pregnancy. Prior to puberty, estrogens may cause premature closure of the epiphyses, premature breast development in girls or gynecomastia in boys. Vaginal bleeding and vaginal cornification may also be induced in girls.

[U.S. Boxed Warning]: Estrogens with or without progestin should be used for shortest duration possible at the lowest effective dose consistent with treatment goals. Before prescribing estrogen therapy to postmenopausal women, the risks and benefits must be weighed for each patient. Women should be informed of these risks and benefits, as well as possible effects of progestin when added to estrogen therapy. Estrogens with or without progestin should be used for shortest duration possible consistent with treatment goals. Conduct periodic risk:benefit assessments.

Vulvar and vaginal atrophy use: When used solely for the treatment of vulvar and vaginal atrophy, topical vaginal products should be considered. Use caution applying topical products to severely atrophic vaginal mucosa.

Vaginal cream: Use of the vaginal cream may weaken latex found in condoms, diaphragms or cervical caps.

Adverse Reactions (Reflective of adult population; not specific for elderly) Due to systemic absorption, other adverse effects associated with systemic therapy may also occur. Frequency not defined:

Genitourinary: Cystis-like syndrome, genital pruritus, vulvovaginal discomfort

Drug Interactions

Metabolism/Transport Effects

Based on estradiol and estrone: **Substrate** of CYP1A2 (major), 2A6 (minor), 2B6 (minor), 2C9 (minor), 2C19 (minor), 2D6 (minor), 2E1 (minor), 3A4 (major); Inhibits CYP1A2 (weak), 2C8 (weak); Induces CYP3A4 (weak)

Avoid Concomitant Use

Avoid concomitant use of Estrogens (Conjugated/Equine, Topical) with any of the following: Anastrozole

Increased Effect/Toxicity

Estrogens (Conjugated/Equine, Topical) may increase the levels/effects of: Corticosteroids (Systemic); ROPINIRole; Tipranavir

The levels/effects of Estrogens (Conjugated/Equine, Topical) may be increased by: Ascorbic Acid; Conivaptan; Herbs (Estrogenic Properties)

Decreased Effect

Estrogens (Conjugated/Equine, Topical) may decrease the levels/effects of: Anastrozole; Chenodiol; Saxagliptin; Somatropin; Thyroid Products; Ursodiol

The levels/effects of Estrogens (Conjugated/Equine, Topical) may be decreased by: CYP1A2 Inducers (Strong); CYP3A4 Inducers (Strong); Cyproterone; Deferasirox; Herbs (CYP3A4 Inducers); Peginterferon Alfa-2b; Tipranavir; Tocilizumab

Stability Vaginal cream: Store at room temperature 20°C to 25°C (68°F to 77°F).

Mechanism of Action Conjugated estrogens contain a mixture of estrone sulfate, equilin sulfate, 17 alpha-dihydroequilin, 17 alpha-estradiol and 17 beta-dihydroequilin. Estrogens are responsible for the development and maintenance of the female reproductive system and secondary sexual characteristics. Estradiol is the principle intracellular human estrogen and is more potent than estrone and estriol at the receptor level; it is the primary estrogen secreted prior to menopause. Following menopause, estrone and estrone sulfate are more highly produced. Estrogens modulate the pituitary secretion of gonadotropins, luteinizing hormone, and follicle-stimulating hormone through a negative feedback system; estrogen replacement reduces elevated levels of these hormones in postmenopausal women.

Pharmacodynamics/Kinetics

Absorption: Systemic absorption occurs

Protein binding: Binds to sex-hormone-binding globulin and albumin

Metabolism: Hepatic via CYP3A4; estradiol is converted to estrone and estriol; also under-goes enterohepatic recirculation (avoided with vaginal administration); estrone sulfate is the main metabolite in postmenopausal women

Half-life elimination: Total estrone: 27 hours

Time to peak, plasma: Total estrone: 7 hours

Excretion: Urine (primarily estriol, also as estradiol, estrone, and conjugates

Dosage

Geriatric Refer to adult dosing. A higher incidence of stroke and breast cancer was observed in women >75 years in a WHI substudy.

Adult

Moderate-to-severe dyspareunia: Intravaginal: 0.5 g twice weekly (eg, Monday and Thursday) **or** once daily cyclically*

Vulvar and vaginal atrophy: Intravaginal: 0.5-2 g/day given cyclically*

*Cyclic administration: Either 3 weeks on, 1 week off **or** 25 days on, 5 days off

Administration Administer at bedtime to minimize adverse effects. Applicator calibrated in 0.5 g increments up to 2 g. To clean applicator, remove plunger from barrel. Wash with mild soap and warm water; do not boil or use hot water.

◀ **Monitoring Parameters** Routine physical examination that includes blood pressure and Papanicolaou smear, breast exam, mammogram. Monitor for signs of endometrial cancer in female patients with uterus. Adequate diagnostic measures, including endometrial sampling, if indicated, should be performed to rule out malignancy in all cases of undiagnosed abnormal vaginal bleeding. Monitor for loss of vision, sudden onset of proptosis, diplopia, migraine; signs and symptoms of thromboembolic disorders; glycemic control in patients with diabetes; lipid profiles in patients being treated for hyperlipidemias; thyroid function in patients on thyroid hormone replacement therapy.

Test Interactions Thyroid function tests: Estrogens may increase thyroid binding globulin and circulating total thyroid hormone (when measured by T_4 RIA, T_4 by column, or by PBI); decreases free T_3 resin uptake; concentration of free T_4 is not altered; metyrapone test: Response may be reduced

Special Geriatric Considerations Topical estrogen is beneficial in the management of urogenital atrophy and prevention of recurrent urinary tract infections in postmenopausal women. Topical estrogens are not void of the risks associated with oral and transdermal forms; thus, the risks and benefits must be weighed for each patient.

Dosage Forms Excipient information presented when available (limited, particularly for generics); consult specific product labeling.
Cream, vaginal:
Premarin®: 0.625 mg/g (42.5 g)

Estrogens (Conjugated/Equine) and Medroxyprogesterone
(ES troe jenz KON joo gate ed/EE kwine & me DROKS ee proe JES te rone)

Related Information
Estrogens (Conjugated/Equine, Systemic) *on page 658*
MedroxyPROGESTERone *on page 1122*

Medication Safety Issues
Sound-alike/look-alike issues:
Premphase® may be confused with Prempro®
Prempro® may be confused with Premphase®

Brand Names: U.S. Premphase®; Prempro®
Brand Names: Canada Premphase®; Premplus®; Prempro®
Index Terms Medroxyprogesterone and Estrogens (Conjugated); MPA and Estrogens (Conjugated)
Generic Availability (U.S.) No
Pharmacologic Category Estrogen and Progestin Combination
Use Women with an intact uterus: Treatment of moderate-to-severe vasomotor symptoms associated with menopause; treatment of moderate-to-severe vulvar and vaginal atrophy due to menopause; postmenopausal osteoporosis (prophylaxis)
Contraindications Undiagnosed abnormal vaginal bleeding; history of or current thrombophlebitis or venous thromboembolic disorders (including DVT, PE); active or history of arterial thromboembolic disease (eg, stroke, MI); known, suspected, or history of carcinoma of the breast; estrogen-dependent tumor; hepatic dysfunction or disease

Warnings/Precautions
Cardiovascular-related considerations: **[U.S. Boxed Warning]: Estrogens with or without progestin should not be used to prevent coronary heart disease.** Use caution with cardiovascular disease or dysfunction. May increase the risks of myocardial infarction (MI), stroke, pulmonary emboli (PE), and deep vein thrombosis (DVT); incidence of these effects was shown to be significantly increased in postmenopausal women using CEE in combination with MPA. Nonfatal MI, PE, and thrombophlebitis have also been reported in males taking high doses of CEE (eg, for prostate cancer). Risk factors include diabetes mellitus, hypercholesterolemia, hypertension, SLE, obesity, and/or venous thromboembolism (VTE). Estrogen compounds are generally associated with lipid effects such as increased HDL-cholesterol and decreased LDL-cholesterol. Triglycerides may also be increased; use with caution in patients with familial defects of lipoprotein metabolism. Discontinue if pancreatitis occurs. Whenever possible, estrogens should be discontinued at least 4-6 weeks prior to and for 2 weeks following elective surgery associated with an increased risk of thromboembolism or during periods of prolonged immobilization. Use caution in patients with known inherited thrombophilias (eg, protein C or S deficiency); may have increased risk of VTE (DeSancho, 2010); use is contraindicated in patients with DVT or PE (current or history of).

Neurological considerations: **[U.S. Boxed Warning]: The risk of dementia may be increased in postmenopausal women;** increased incidence was observed in women ≥65 years of age taking CE alone or in combination with MPA.

Cancer-related considerations: **[U.S. Boxed Warning]: Adequate diagnostic measures, including endometrial sampling (if indicated), should be performed to rule out malignancy in all cases of undiagnosed abnormal vaginal bleeding. Unopposed estrogens may increase the risk of endometrial carcinoma in postmenopausal women with an intact uterus.** Risk appears to be associated with long-term use. The use of a progestin should be considered when administering estrogens to postmenopausal women with an intact uterus. Estrogens may exacerbate endometriosis. Malignant transformation of residual endometrial implants has been reported posthysterectomy with estrogen only therapy. Consider adding a progestin in women with residual endometriosis posthysterectomy. **[U.S. Boxed Warning]: Estrogen plus progestin may increase the risk of invasive breast cancer.** An increased risk of invasive breast cancer was observed in postmenopausal women using CE in combination with MPA; a smaller increase in risk was seen with estrogen therapy alone in observational studies. An increase in abnormal mammograms has also been reported with estrogen and progestin therapy. Estrogen use may lead to severe hypercalcemia in patients with breast cancer and bone metastases; discontinue estrogen if hypercalcemia occurs. Postmenopausal estrogen therapy and combined estrogen/progesterone therapy may increase the risk of ovarian cancer; however, the absolute risk to an individual woman is small. Although results from various studies are not consistent, risk does not appear to be significantly associated with the duration, route, or dose of therapy. In one study, the risk decreased after 2 years following discontinuation of therapy.

Estrogens may cause retinal vascular thrombosis; discontinue pending exam if loss of vision or other visual disturbances occur; discontinue permanently if papilledema or retinal vascular lesions are observed. Use with caution in patients with diseases which may be exacerbated by fluid retention, including asthma, epilepsy, migraine, diabetes, or renal dysfunction. Use with caution in patients with a history of severe hypocalcemia, SLE, hepatic hemangiomas, porphyria, endometriosis, and gallbladder disease. Use caution with history of cholestatic jaundice associated with past estrogen use or pregnancy. Presentation of irregular, unresolving vaginal bleeding warrants further evaluation including endometrial sampling, if indicated, to rule out malignancy.

[U.S. Boxed Warning]: Estrogens with or without progestin should be used for shortest duration possible at the lowest effective dose consistent with treatment goals. Before prescribing estrogen therapy to postmenopausal women, the risks and benefits must be weighed for each patient. Women should be informed of these risks and benefits, as well as possible effects of progestin when added to estrogen therapy. Conduct periodic risk:benefit assessments.

Osteoporosis use: For use only in women at significant risk of osteoporosis and for who other nonestrogen medications are not considered appropriate.

When used solely for the treatment of vulvar and vaginal atrophy, topical vaginal products should be considered.

Adverse Reactions (Reflective of adult population; not specific for elderly)
>10%:
Central nervous system: Headache (28% to 37%), pain (11% to 13%), depression (6% to 11%)
Endocrine & metabolic: Breast pain (32% to 38%), dysmenorrhea (5% to 13%)
Gastrointestinal: Abdominal pain (16% to 23%), nausea (9% to 11%)
Neuromuscular & skeletal: Back pain (13% to 16%)
Respiratory: Pharyngitis (11% to 13%)
Miscellaneous: Infection (16% to 18%), flu-like syndrome (10% to 13%)
1% to 10%:
Cardiovascular: Peripheral edema (3% to 4%)
Central nervous system: Dizziness (3% to 5%)
Dermatologic: Pruritus (5% to 10%), rash (4% to 6%)
Endocrine & metabolic: Leukorrhea (5% to 9%)
Gastrointestinal: Flatulence (8% to 9%), diarrhea (5% to 6%), dyspepsia (5% to 6%)
Genitourinary: Vaginitis (5% to 7%), cervical changes (4% to 5%), pelvic pain (4 to 5%), vaginal hemorrhage (1% to 3%)
Neuromuscular & skeletal: Weakness (6% to 10%), arthralgia (7% to 9%), leg cramps (3% to 5%), hypertonia (3% to 4%)
Respiratory: Sinusitis (7% to 8%), rhinitis (6% to 8%)

Drug Interactions
Metabolism/Transport Effects
Based on estradiol and estrone: **Substrate** of CYP1A2 (major), 2A6 (minor), 2B6 (minor), 2C9 (minor), 2C19 (minor), 2D6 (minor), 2E1 (minor), 3A4 (major); **Inhibits** CYP1A2 (weak), 2C8 (weak); **Induces** CYP3A4 (weak)
Medroxyprogesterone: **Substrate** of CYP3A4 (major); **Induces** CYP3A4 (weak)

ESTROGENS (CONJUGATED/EQUINE) AND MEDROXYPROGESTERONE

◀ **Avoid Concomitant Use**

Avoid concomitant use of Estrogens (Conjugated/Equine) and Medroxyprogesterone with any of the following: Anastrozole; Griseofulvin

Increased Effect/Toxicity

Estrogens (Conjugated/Equine) and Medroxyprogesterone may increase the levels/effects of: Benzodiazepines (metabolized by oxidation); Corticosteroids (Systemic); ROPINIRole; Selegiline; Tipranavir; Tranexamic Acid; Voriconazole

The levels/effects of Estrogens (Conjugated/Equine) and Medroxyprogesterone may be increased by: Ascorbic Acid; Boceprevir; Conivaptan; Herbs (Estrogenic Properties); Herbs (Progestogenic Properties); Voriconazole

Decreased Effect

Estrogens (Conjugated/Equine) and Medroxyprogesterone may decrease the levels/effects of: Anastrozole; Chenodiol; Saxagliptin; Somatropin; Thyroid Products; Ursodiol; Vitamin K Antagonists

The levels/effects of Estrogens (Conjugated/Equine) and Medroxyprogesterone may be decreased by: Acitretin; Aminoglutethimide; Aprepitant; Artemether; Barbiturates; Bexarotene; Bexarotene (Systemic); Bile Acid Sequestrants; Bosentan; CarBAMazepine; CYP1A2 Inducers (Strong); CYP3A4 Inducers (Strong); Cyproterone; Deferasirox; Felbamate; Fosaprepitant; Fosphenytoin; Griseofulvin; LamoTRIgine; Mycophenolate; OXcarbazepine; Peginterferon Alfa-2b; Phenytoin; Retinoic Acid Derivatives; Rifamycin Derivatives; St Johns Wort; Telaprevir; Tipranavir; Tocilizumab; Topiramate

Ethanol/Nutrition/Herb Interactions

Ethanol: Avoid ethanol (routine use increases estrogen plasma concentrations and risk of breast cancer). Ethanol may also increase the risk of osteoporosis.

Food: Folic acid absorption may be decreased.

Herb/Nutraceutical: St John's wort may decrease levels. Avoid black cohosh, dong quai (has estrogenic activity). Avoid red clover, saw palmetto, ginseng (due to potential hormonal effects).

Stability Store at room temperature 20°C to 25°C (68°F to 77°F).

Mechanism of Action

Conjugated estrogens contain a mixture of estrone sulfate, equilin sulfate, 17 alpha-dihydroequilin, 17 alpha-estradiol, and 17 beta-dihydroequilin. Estrogens are responsible for the development and maintenance of the female reproductive system and secondary sexual characteristics. Estradiol is the principle intracellular human estrogen and is more potent than estrone and estriol at the receptor level; it is the primary estrogen secreted prior to menopause. Following menopause, estrone and estrone sulfate are more highly produced. Estrogens modulate the pituitary secretion of gonadotropins, luteinizing hormone, and follicle-stimulating hormone through a negative feedback system; estrogen replacement reduces elevated levels of these hormones in postmenopausal women.

MPA inhibits gonadotropin production which then prevents follicular maturation and ovulation. In women with adequate estrogen, MPA transforms a proliferative endometrium into a secretory endometrium; when administered with conjugated estrogens, reduces the incidence of endometrial hyperplasia and risk of adenocarcinoma.

Pharmacodynamics/Kinetics

Absorption: Well absorbed

Protein binding:

Conjugated estrogens: Albumin

Unconjugated estrogens: Albumin and sex-hormone-binding globulin (SHBG)

MPA: Plasma proteins (90%), but not SHBG

Metabolism:

Conjugated estrogens and MPA are both metabolized in the liver

MPA is hydroxylated and conjugated

Half-life: Conjugated estrogens: 10-24 hours; MPA: 38-46 hours

Time to peak: Conjugated estrogens: 4-10 hours; MPA: 2-4 hours

Elimination:

Conjugated estrogens: Urine, bile

MPA: Urine as glucuronide conjugates (major) and sulfates (minor)

Dosage

Geriatric Refer to adult dosing. A higher incidence of stroke and breast cancer was observed in women >75 years in a WHI substudy.

Adult

Treatment of moderate-to-severe vasomotor symptoms associated with menopause; treatment of vulvar and vaginal atrophy due to menopause in women with a uterus; osteoporosis prophylaxis in females with an intact uterus (**Note:** The lowest dose that will control symptoms should be used; medication should be discontinued as soon as possible):

Premphase®: Oral: One maroon conjugated estrogen 0.625 mg tablet daily on days 1 through 14 and 1 light blue conjugated estrogen 0.625 mg/mPA 5 mg tablet daily on days 15 through 28

Prempro®: Oral: One conjugated estrogen/MPA tablet once daily; maximum dose: 1 conjugated estrogen 0.625 mg/mPA 5 mg tablet daily

Monitoring Parameters Routine physical examination that includes blood pressure and Papanicolaou smear, breast exam, mammogram. Monitor for signs of endometrial cancer. Adequate diagnostic measures, including endometrial sampling, if indicated, should be performed to rule out malignancy in all cases of undiagnosed abnormal vaginal bleeding. Monitor for loss of vision, sudden onset of proptosis, diplopia, migraine; signs and symptoms of thromboembolic disorders; glycemic control in patients with diabetes; lipid profiles in patients being treated for hyperlipidemias; thyroid function in patients on thyroid hormone replacement therapy.

Menopausal symptoms: Assess need for therapy at 3- to 6-month intervals

Prevention of osteoporosis: Bone density measurement

Test Interactions Pathologist should be advised of estrogen/progesterone therapy when specimens are submitted. Reduced response to metyrapone test.

Special Geriatric Considerations Before prescribing estrogen therapy to postmenopausal women, the risks and benefits must be weighed for each patient. Women should be informed of these risks and benefits, as well as possible side effects and the return of menstrual bleeding (when cycled with a progestin), and be involved in the decision to prescribe. A higher incidence of stroke and invasive breast cancer was observed in women >75 years in a WHI substudy.

Dosage Forms Excipient information presented when available (limited, particularly for generics); consult specific product labeling.

Tablet:

Premphase® [therapy pack contains 2 separate tablet formulations]: Conjugated estrogens 0.625 mg [14 maroon tablets] and conjugated estrogen 0.625 mg/medroxyprogesterone acetate 5 mg [14 light blue tablets] (28s)

Prempro®:

0.3/1.5: Conjugated estrogens 0.3 mg and medroxyprogesterone acetate 1.5 mg (28s)

0.45/1.5: Conjugated estrogens 0.45 mg and medroxyprogesterone acetate 1.5 mg (28s)

0.625/2.5: Conjugated estrogens 0.625 mg and medroxyprogesterone acetate 2.5 mg (28s)

0.625/5: Conjugated estrogens 0.625 mg and medroxyprogesterone acetate 5 mg (28s)

Estrogens (Esterified) (ES troe jenz, es TER i fied)

Related Information

Osteoporosis Management *on page 2027*

Medication Safety Issues

Sound-alike/look-alike issues:

Estratab® may be confused with Estratest®, Estratest® H.S.

Beers Criteria medication:

This drug may be inappropriate for use in geriatric patients (low severity risk).

Brand Names: U.S. Menest®

Brand Names: Canada Estragyn; Estratab®; Menest®

Index Terms Esterified Estrogens

Generic Availability (U.S.) No

Pharmacologic Category Estrogen Derivative

Use Treatment of moderate-to-severe vasomotor symptoms associated with menopause; treatment of moderate-to-severe vulvar and vaginal atrophy associated with menopause; hypoestrogenism (due to hypogonadism, castration, or primary ovarian failure); advanced prostatic cancer (palliation), metastatic breast cancer (palliation) in men and postmenopausal women

Contraindications Hypersensitivity to estrogens or any component of the formulation; undiagnosed abnormal vaginal bleeding; DVT or PE (current or history of); active or recent (within 1 year) arterial thromboembolic disease (eg, stroke, MI); carcinoma of the breast (known, suspected or history of), except in appropriately selected patients being treated for metastatic disease; estrogen-dependent tumor; hepatic dysfunction or disease

ESTROGENS (ESTERIFIED)

◀ **Warnings/Precautions**

[U.S. Boxed Warning]: Unopposed estrogens may increase the risk of endometrial carcinoma in postmenopausal women with an intact uterus. Adequate diagnostic measures, including endometrial sampling, if indicated, should be performed to rule out malignancy in all cases of undiagnosed abnormal vaginal bleeding. The use of a progestin should be considered when administering estrogens to postmenopausal women with an intact uterus. When indicated, oral progestins should be used (NAMS, 2010). Estrogens may exacerbate endometriosis. Malignant transformation of residual endometrial implants has been reported posthysterectomy with estrogen only therapy. Consider adding a progestin in women with residual endometriosis posthysterectomy. Postmenopausal estrogen therapy and combined estrogen/progesterone therapy may increase the risk of ovarian cancer; however, the absolute risk to an individual woman is small. Although results from various studies are not consistent, risk does not appear to be significantly associated with the duration, route, or dose of therapy. In one study, the risk decreased after 2 years following discontinuation of therapy (Mørch, 2009). Although the risk of ovarian cancer is rare, women who are at an increased risk (eg, family history) should be counseled about the association (NAMS, 2010). Estrogens may increase the risk of breast cancer. An increased risk of invasive breast cancer was observed in postmenopausal women using conjugated equine estrogens (CEE) in combination with medroxyprogesterone acetate (MPA); a smaller increase in risk was seen with estrogen therapy alone in observational studies. An increase in abnormal mammograms has also been reported with estrogen and progestin therapy. Estrogen use may lead to severe hypercalcemia in patients with breast cancer and bone metastases; discontinue estrogen if hypercalcemia occurs.

[U.S. Boxed Warning]: Estrogens with or without progestin should not be used to prevent coronary heart disease. Use caution with cardiovascular disease or dysfunction. May increase the risks of myocardial infarction (MI), stroke, pulmonary emboli (PE), and deep vein thrombosis (DVT); incidence of these effects was shown to be significantly increased in postmenopausal women using CEE in combination with MPA. Nonfatal MI, PE, and thrombophlebitis have also been reported in males taking high doses of CEE (eg, for prostate cancer). Risk factors include diabetes mellitus, hypercholesterolemia, hypertension, SLE, obesity, and/or venous thromboembolism (VTE). Use caution in patients with known inherited thrombophilias (eg, protein C or S deficiency); may have increased risk of VTE (DeSancho, 2010); use is contraindicated in patients with DVT or PE (current or history of).

[U.S. Boxed Warning]: The risk of dementia may be increased in postmenopausal women; increased incidence was observed in women ≥65 years of age taking CEE alone or in combination with MPA.

[U.S. Boxed Warning]: Estrogens with or without progestin should be used for shortest duration possible at the lowest effective dose consistent with treatment goals. Before prescribing estrogen therapy to postmenopausal women, the risks and benefits must be weighed for each patient. Women should be informed of these risks and benefits, as well as possible effects of progestin when added to estrogen therapy. Conduct periodic risk:benefit assessments. Outcomes reported from clinical trials using CEE should be assumed to be similar for estradiol until comparable data becomes available. Moderate to severe symptoms of vulvar and vaginal atrophy include vaginal dryness, dyspareunia, and atrophic vaginitis. When used solely for the treatment of vulvar and vaginal atrophy, topical vaginal products should be considered

Estrogen compounds are generally associated with lipid effects such as increased HDL-cholesterol and decreased LDL-cholesterol. Triglycerides may also be increased; use with caution in patients with familial defects of lipoprotein metabolism. Estrogens may increase thyroid-binding globulin (TBG) levels leading to increased circulating total thyroid hormone levels. Women on thyroid replacement therapy may require higher doses of thyroid hormone while receiving estrogens.

Estrogens may cause retinal vascular thrombosis; discontinue if migraine, loss of vision, proptosis, diplopia or other visual disturbances occur; discontinue permanently if papilledema or retinal vascular lesions are observed on examination. Estrogens are poorly metabolized in patients with hepatic dysfunction. Use caution with a history of cholestatic jaundice associated with prior estrogen use or pregnancy. Discontinue if jaundice develops or if acute or chronic hepatic disturbances occur. Use is contraindicated with hepatic disease. Use caution in patients with asthma, epilepsy, hepatic hemangiomas, migraine, porphyria, or SLE; may exacerbate disease. May have adverse effects on glucose tolerance; use caution in women with diabetes. Use with caution in patients with diseases which may be exacerbated by fluid retention, including cardiac or renal dysfunction. Use of postmenopausal estrogen may be associated with an increased risk of gallbladder disease requiring surgery. Use with caution in patients with severe hypocalcemia. May be inappropriate in for use in the elderly due to potential of increased risk of breast and endometrial cancers and lack of proven cardioprotection (Beers Criteria). Prior to puberty, estrogens may cause premature closure of the epiphyses, premature breast development in girls or gynecomastia in boys. Vaginal bleeding and vaginal cornification may also be induced in girls. Whenever possible, estrogens should be discontinued at least 4-6 weeks prior to elective surgery associated with an increased risk of thromboembolism or during periods of prolonged immobilization.

Adverse Reactions (Reflective of adult population; not specific for elderly) Frequency not defined.

Cardiovascular: Edema, hypertension, MI, stroke, venous thromboembolism

Central nervous system: Dementia exacerbation, dizziness, epilepsy exacerbation, headache, irritability, mental depression, migraine, mood disturbances, nervousness

Dermatologic: Angioedema, chloasma, erythema multiforme, erythema nodosum, hemorrhagic eruption, hirsutism, pruritus, loss of scalp hair, melasma, rash, urticaria

Endocrine & metabolic: Breast cancer, breast enlargement, breast tenderness, carbohydrate intolerance, fibrocystic breast changes, galactorrhea, hypocalcemia, libido (changes in), nipple discharge, premenstrual like syndrome

Gastrointestinal: Abdominal cramps, bloating, gallbladder disease, nausea, pancreatitis, vomiting, weight gain/loss

Genitourinary: Alterations in frequency and flow of menstrual patterns, breakthrough bleeding, changes in cervical secretions, cervical ectropion changes, cystitis-like syndrome, dysmenorrhea, endometrial hyperplasia, endometrial cancer, increased size of uterine leiomyomata, ovarian cancer, vaginal candidiasis, vaginitis

Hematologic: Aggravation of porphyria

Hepatic: Cholestatic jaundice, hemangioma enlargement

Local: Thrombophlebitis

Neuromuscular & skeletal: Arthralgia, chorea, leg cramps

Ocular: Contact lens intolerance, corneal curvature steepening, retinal vascular thrombosis

Respiratory: Asthma exacerbation, pulmonary embolism

Miscellaneous: Anaphylactoid/anaphylactic reactions

Drug Interactions

Metabolism/Transport Effects Based on estrone: **Substrate** of CYP1A2 (major), 2B6 (minor), 2C9 (minor), 2E1 (minor), 3A4 (major)

Avoid Concomitant Use

Avoid concomitant use of Estrogens (Esterified) with any of the following: Anastrozole

Increased Effect/Toxicity

Estrogens (Esterified) may increase the levels/effects of: Corticosteroids (Systemic); ROPINIRole; Tipranavir

The levels/effects of Estrogens (Esterified) may be increased by: Ascorbic Acid; Conivaptan; Herbs (Estrogenic Properties)

Decreased Effect

Estrogens (Esterified) may decrease the levels/effects of: Anastrozole; Chenodiol; Somatropin; Thyroid Products; Ursodiol

The levels/effects of Estrogens (Esterified) may be decreased by: CYP1A2 Inducers (Strong); CYP3A4 Inducers (Strong); Cyproterone; Deferasirox; Herbs (CYP3A4 Inducers); Tipranavir; Tocilizumab

Ethanol/Nutrition/Herb Interactions

Ethanol: Avoid ethanol (routine use increases estrogen plasma concentrations and risk of breast cancer). Ethanol may also increase the risk of osteoporosis.

Food: Folic acid absorption may be decreased.

Herb/Nutraceutical: St John's wort may decrease levels. Herbs with estrogenic properties may enhance the adverse/toxic effect of estrogen derivatives; examples include alfalfa, black cohosh, bloodroot, hops, kudzu, licorice, red clover, saw palmetto, soybean, thyme, wild yam, yucca.

Mechanism of Action Esterified estrogens contain a mixture of estrogenic substances; the principle component is estrone. Preparations contain 75% to 85% sodium estrone sulfate and 6% to 15% sodium equilin sulfate such that the total is not <90%. Estrogens are responsible for the development and maintenance of the female reproductive system and secondary sexual characteristics. Estradiol is the principle intracellular human estrogen and is more potent than estrone and estriol at the receptor level; it is the primary estrogen secreted prior to menopause. In males and following menopause in females, estrone and estrone sulfate are more highly produced. Estrogens modulate the pituitary secretion of gonadotropins, luteinizing hormone, and follicle-stimulating hormone through a negative feedback system; estrogen replacement reduces elevated levels of these hormones.

Pharmacodynamics/Kinetics

Absorption: Readily

Distribution: Widely distributed; high concentrations in the sex hormone target organs

Protein binding: Bound to sex hormone-binding globulin and albumin

◀ Metabolism: Hepatic; partial metabolism via CYP3A4 enzymes; estradiol is reversibly converted to estrone and estriol; oral estradiol also undergoes enterohepatic recirculation by conjugation in the liver, followed by excretion of sulfate and glucuronide conjugates into the bile, then hydrolysis in the intestine and estrogen reabsorption. Sulfate conjugates are the primary form found in postmenopausal women.

Excretion: Primarily urine (as estradiol, estrone, estriol, and their glucuronide and sulfate conjugates)

Dosage

Geriatric & Adult

Prostate cancer, advanced: Oral: 1.25-2.5 mg 3 times/day

Female hypoestrogenism due to hypogonadism: Oral: 2.5-7.5 mg/day in divided doses for 20 days followed by a 10-day rest period. Administer cyclically (3 weeks on and 1 week off). If bleeding does not occur by the end of the 10-day period, repeat the same dosing schedule; the number of courses dependent upon the responsiveness of the endometrium. If bleeding occurs before the end of the 10-day period, begin an estrogen-progestin cyclic regimen of 2.5-7.5 mg/day in divided doses for 20 days; during the last 5 days of estrogen therapy, give an oral progestin. If bleeding occurs before regimen is concluded, discontinue therapy and resume on the fifth day of bleeding.

Female hypoestrogenism due to castration and primary ovarian failure: Oral: 1.25 mg/day, cyclically. Adjust dosage upward or downward, according to the severity of symptoms and patient response. For maintenance, adjust dosage to lowest level that will provide effective control.

Vasomotor symptoms associated with menopause: Oral: 1.25 mg/day administered cyclically (3 weeks on and 1 week off). If patient has not menstruated within the last 2 months or more, cyclic administration is started arbitrary. If the patient is menstruating, cyclical administration is started on day 5 of the bleeding. For short-term use only and should be discontinued as soon as possible. Re-evaluate at 3- to 6-month intervals for tapering or discontinuation of therapy.

Vulvar and vaginal atrophy associated with menopause: Oral: 0.3 to ≥1.25 mg/day, depending on the tissue response of the individual patient. Administer cyclically. For short-term use only and should be discontinued as soon as possible. Re-evaluate at 3- to 6-month intervals for tapering or discontinuation of therapy.

Breast cancer, metastatic (appropriately selected patients): Males and postmenopausal females: Oral: 10 mg 3 times/day for at least 3 months

Administration Administer with food at same time each day.

Monitoring Parameters Routine physical examination that includes blood pressure and Papanicolaou smear, breast exam, mammogram. Monitor for signs of endometrial cancer in female patients with uterus. Adequate diagnostic measures, including endometrial sampling, if indicated, should be performed to rule out malignancy in all cases of undiagnosed abnormal vaginal bleeding. Monitor for loss of vision, sudden onset of proptosis, diplopia, migraine; signs and symptoms of thromboembolic disorders; glycemic control in patients with diabetes; lipid profiles in patients being treated for hyperlipidemias; thyroid function in patients on thyroid hormone replacement therapy.

Menopausal symptoms; vulvar and vaginal atrophy: Assess need for therapy at 3- to 6-month intervals

Test Interactions Pathologist should be advised of estrogen/progesterone therapy when specimens are submitted. Reduced response to metyrapone test.

Prothrombin time, partial thromboplastin time, and platelet aggregation time may be accelerated; platelet count may be increased; factors II, VII antigen, VIII antigen, VII coagulant activity, IX, V, VII, VII-X complex, II-VII-X complex, and beta-thromboglobulin may be increased; antifactor Xa and antithrombin III levels may be decreased; antithrombin III activity may be decreased; fibrinogen and fibrinogen activity may be increased; plasminogen and plasminogen activity may be increased

Thyroid-binding globulin levels may be increased; HDL and triglyceride plasma levels may be increased; LDL levels may be decreased

Special Geriatric Considerations Before prescribing estrogen therapy to postmenopausal women, the risks and benefits must be weighed for each patient. Women should be informed of these risks and benefits, as well as possible side effects and the return of menstrual bleeding (when cycled with a progestin), and be involved in the decision to prescribe. A higher incidence of stroke and invasive breast cancer were observed in women >75 years in a WHI substudy using conjugated equine estrogen.

This medication is considered to be potentially inappropriate in this patient population (Beers Criteria severity: Low).

Dosage Forms Excipient information presented when available (limited, particularly for generics); consult specific product labeling.
Tablet, oral:
  Menest®: 0.3 mg, 0.625 mg, 1.25 mg, 2.5 mg

Eszopiclone (es zoe PIK lone)

Medication Safety Issues
  Sound-alike/look-alike issues:
    Lunesta® may be confused with Neulasta®
Brand Names: U.S. Lunesta®
Generic Availability (U.S.) No
Pharmacologic Category Hypnotic, Nonbenzodiazepine
Use Treatment of insomnia
Medication Guide Available Yes
Contraindications There are no contraindications listed within the manufacturer's labeling.
Warnings/Precautions Symptomatic treatment of insomnia should be initiated only after careful evaluation of potential causes of sleep disturbance. Tolerance did not develop over 6 months of use. Use with caution in patients with depression or a history of drug dependence. Abrupt discontinuance may lead to withdrawal symptoms. Use with caution in patients receiving other CNS depressants or psychoactive medications. Hypnotics/sedatives have been associated with abnormal thinking and behavior changes including decreased inhibition, aggression, bizarre behavior, agitation, hallucinations, and depersonalization. These changes may occur unpredictably and may indicate previously unrecognized psychiatric disorders; evaluate appropriately. Amnesia may occur. May impair physical and mental capabilities. Postmarketing studies have indicated that the use of hypnotic/sedative agents for sleep has been associated with hypersensitivity reactions including anaphylaxis as well as angioedema. An increased risk for hazardous sleep-related activities such as sleep-driving (as well as cooking and eating food and making phone calls while asleep) has also been noted. Use caution in patients with respiratory compromise, hepatic dysfunction, elderly or those taking strong CYP3A4 inhibitors. Because of the rapid onset of action, administer immediately prior to bedtime or after the patient has gone to bed and is having difficulty falling asleep.
Adverse Reactions (Reflective of adult population; not specific for elderly)
  >10%:
    Central nervous system: Headache (15% to 21%)
    Gastrointestinal: Unpleasant taste (8% to 34%)
  1% to 10%:
    Cardiovascular: Chest pain, peripheral edema
    Central nervous system: Somnolence (8% to 10%), dizziness (5% to 7%), pain (4% to 5%), nervousness (up to 5%), depression (1% to 4%), confusion (up to 3%), hallucinations (1% to 3%), anxiety (1% to 3%), abnormal dreams (1% to 3%), migraine
    Dermatologic: Rash (3% to 4%), pruritus (1% to 4%)
    Endocrine & metabolic: Libido decreased (up to 3%), dysmenorrhea (up to 3%), gynecomastia (males up to 3%)
    Gastrointestinal: Xerostomia (3% to 7%), dyspepsia (2% to 6%), nausea (4% to 5%), diarrhea (2% to 4%), vomiting (up to 3%)
    Genitourinary: Urinary tract infection (up to 3%)
    Neuromuscular & skeletal: Neuralgia (up to 3%)
    Miscellaneous: Infection (5% to 10%), viral infection (3%), accidental injury (up to 3%)
Drug Interactions
  Metabolism/Transport Effects Substrate of CYP2E1 (minor), 3A4 (major)
  Avoid Concomitant Use
    Avoid concomitant use of Eszopiclone with any of the following: Conivaptan
  Increased Effect/Toxicity
    Eszopiclone may increase the levels/effects of: Alcohol (Ethyl); CNS Depressants; Methotrimeprazine; Selective Serotonin Reuptake Inhibitors

    The levels/effects of Eszopiclone may be increased by: Antifungal Agents (Azole Derivatives, Systemic); Conivaptan; CYP3A4 Inhibitors (Moderate); CYP3A4 Inhibitors (Strong); Dasatinib; Droperidol; HydrOXYzine; Methotrimeprazine
  Decreased Effect
    The levels/effects of Eszopiclone may be decreased by: CYP3A4 Inducers (Strong); Cyproterone; Deferasirox; Flumazenil; Herbs (CYP3A4 Inducers); Tocilizumab

▶

◀ **Ethanol/Nutrition/Herb Interactions**
Ethanol: Ethanol: May increase CNS depression; monitor for increased effects with coadministration. Caution patients about effects.
Food: Onset of action may be reduced if taken with or immediately after a heavy meal.
Herb/Nutraceutical: Avoid valerian, St John's wort, kava kava, gotu kola (may increase CNS depression).

Stability Store at controlled room temperature of 25°C (77°F).

Mechanism of Action May interact with GABA-receptor complexes at binding domains located close to or allosterically coupled to benzodiazepine receptors.

Pharmacodynamics/Kinetics
Absorption: Rapid; high-fat/heavy meal may delay absorption
Protein binding: 52% to 59%
Metabolism: Hepatic via oxidation and demethylation (CYP2E1, 3A4); 2 primary metabolites; one with activity less than parent.
Half-life elimination: ~6 hours; Elderly (≥65 years): ~9 hours
Time to peak, plasma: ~1 hour
Excretion: Urine (up to 75%, primarily as metabolites; <10% as parent drug)

Dosage
Geriatric
Difficulty **falling** asleep: Initial: 1 mg before immediately bedtime; maximum dose: 2 mg.
Difficulty **staying** asleep: 2 mg immediately before bedtime.
Adult
Insomnia: Oral: Initial: 2 mg immediately before bedtime (maximum dose: 3 mg)
Concurrent use with strong CYP3A4 inhibitor: 1 mg immediately before bedtime; if needed, dose may be increased to 2 mg
Renal Impairment No adjustment required.
Hepatic Impairment
Mild-to-moderate: Use with caution; dosage adjustment unnecessary
Severe: Initial dose: 1 mg; maximum dose: 2 mg

Administration Because of the rapid onset of action, eszopiclone should be administered immediately prior to bedtime or after the patient has gone to bed and is having difficulty falling asleep. Do not take with, or immediately following, a high-fat meal; do not crush or break tablet.

Special Geriatric Considerations In subjects >65 years of age, the AUC was increased by 41%. The manufacturer reports that in studies, the pattern of adverse reactions in elderly subjects was not different from that seen in younger adults.

Controlled Substance C-IV

Dosage Forms Excipient information presented when available (limited, particularly for generics); consult specific product labeling.
Tablet, oral:
Lunesta®: 1 mg, 2 mg, 3 mg

Etanercept (et a NER sept)

Medication Safety Issues
Sound-alike/look-alike issues:
Enbrel® may be confused with Levbid®
Brand Names: U.S. Enbrel®; Enbrel® SureClick®
Brand Names: Canada Enbrel®
Generic Availability (U.S.) No
Pharmacologic Category Antirheumatic, Disease Modifying; Tumor Necrosis Factor (TNF) Blocking Agent
Use Treatment of moderately- to severely-active rheumatoid arthritis (RA); moderately- to severely-active polyarticular juvenile idiopathic arthritis (JIA); psoriatic arthritis; active ankylosing spondylitis (AS); moderate-to-severe chronic plaque psoriasis
Medication Guide Available Yes
Contraindications Hypersensitivity to etanercept or any component of the formulation; patients with sepsis (mortality may be increased)
Warnings/Precautions [U.S. Boxed Warning]: Serious and potentially fatal infections have been reported including bacterial, mycobacterial, viral, and invasive fungal infections; usually in patients taking concomitant immunosuppressive medication; infection may be disseminated, rather than localized, upon presentation. Cases of unrecognized invasive fungal infections (eg, histoplasmosis, blastomycosis, coccidioidomycosis, listeriosis, candidiasis, aspergillosis, pneumocystosis) have also been reported with anti-TNF agent use. Discontinue administration if patient develops a serious infection or sepsis. Caution should be exercised when considering the use in patients with chronic infection, history of recurrent

infection, or predisposition to infection (eg, poorly-controlled diabetes or residence/travel from areas of endemic mycoses). Do not give to patients with an active chronic or localized infection. Patients should be educated about the symptoms of infection and closely monitored for signs and symptoms while undergoing treatment. **[U.S. Boxed Warning]: Tuberculosis (disseminated or extrapulmonary) has been reported in patients receiving etanercept; both reactivation of latent infection and new infections have been reported.** Patients should be evaluated for tuberculosis risk factors and for latent tuberculosis infection with a tuberculin skin test prior to starting therapy. Treatment of latent tuberculosis should be initiated before etanercept therapy; consider antituberculosis treatment if adequate course of treatment cannot be confirmed in patients with a history of latent or active tuberculosis or with risk factors despite negative skin test. Some patients who tested negative prior to therapy have developed active infection; monitor for signs and symptoms of tuberculosis in all patients. Rare reactivation of hepatitis B has occurred in chronic carriers of the virus; evaluate prior to initiation and during treatment in patients at risk for hepatitis B infection. Patients should be brought up to date with all immunizations before initiating therapy. Live vaccines should not be given concurrently with etanercept. Patients with a significant exposure to varicella virus should temporarily discontinue etanercept. Treatment with varicella zoster immune globulin should be considered.

[U.S. Boxed Warning]: Lymphoma and other malignancies have been reported in children and adolescent patients receiving TNF-blocking agents, including etanercept. Half of the malignancies reported in children were lymphomas (Hodgkin's and non-Hodgkin's) while other cases varied and included malignancies not typically observed in this population. The impact of etanercept on the development and course of malignancy is not fully defined. Compared to the general population, an increased risk of lymphoma has been noted in clinical trials; however, rheumatoid arthritis alone has been previously associated with an increased rate of lymphoma. Lymphomas and other malignancies were also observed (at rates higher than expected for the general population) in adult patients receiving etanercept. Etanercept is not recommended for use in patients with Wegener's granulomatosis who are receiving immunosuppressive therapy. Treatment may result in the formation of autoimmune antibodies; cases of autoimmune disease have not been described. Non-neutralizing antibodies to etanercept may also be formed. Rarely, a reversible lupus-like syndrome has occurred.

Allergic reactions may occur; if an anaphylactic reaction or other serious allergic reaction occurs, administration should be discontinued immediately and appropriate therapy initiated. Use with caution in patients with pre-existing or recent onset CNS demyelinating disorders; rare cases of new onset or exacerbation of CNS demyelinating disorders have occurred; may present with mental status changes and some may be associated with permanent disability. Optic neuritis, transverse myelitis, multiple sclerosis, and new onset or exacerbation of seizures have been reported. Use with caution in patients with heart failure or decreased left ventricular function; worsening and new-onset heart failure has been reported. Use caution in patients with a history of significant hematologic abnormalities; has been associated with pancytopenia and aplastic anemia (rare). Discontinue if significant hematologic abnormalities are confirmed. Use with caution in patients with moderate to severe alcoholic hepatitis. Compared to placebo, the mortality rate in patients treated with etanercept was similar at one month but significantly higher after 6 months

Due to a higher incidence of serious infections, concomitant use with anakinra is not recommended. Some dosage forms may contain dry natural rubber (latex).

Adverse Reactions (Reflective of adult population; not specific for elderly) Percentages reported for adults except where specified.

>10%:
  Central nervous system: Headache (17%; children 19%)
  Dermatologic: Rash (3% to 13%)
  Gastrointestinal: Abdominal pain (5%; children 19%), vomiting (3%; children 13%)
  Local: Injection site reaction (14% to 43%; bleeding, bruising, erythema, itching, pain or swelling)
  Respiratory: Respiratory tract infection (upper; 38% to 65%), rhinitis (12%)
  Miscellaneous: Infection (50% to 81%; children 62%), positive ANA (11%), positive anti-double-stranded DNA antibodies (15% by RIA, 3% by *Crithidia luciliae* assay)
≥3% to 10%:
  Central nervous system: Dizziness (7%)
  Dermatologic: Pruritus (2% to 5%)
  Gastrointestinal: Nausea (children 9%), dyspepsia (4%), diarrhea (3%)
  Neuromuscular & skeletal: Weakness (5%)
  Respiratory: Pharyngitis (7%), cough (6%), respiratory disorder (5%), sinusitis (3%)

◀ **Drug Interactions**

Avoid Concomitant Use

Avoid concomitant use of Etanercept with any of the following: Abatacept; Anakinra; BCG; Belimumab; Canakinumab; Certolizumab Pegol; Cyclophosphamide; Natalizumab; Pimecrolimus; Rilonacept; Tacrolimus (Topical); Vaccines (Live)

Increased Effect/Toxicity

Etanercept may increase the levels/effects of: Abatacept; Anakinra; Belimumab; Canakinumab; Certolizumab Pegol; Cyclophosphamide; Leflunomide; Natalizumab; Rilonacept; Vaccines (Live)

The levels/effects of Etanercept may be increased by: Denosumab; Pimecrolimus; Roflumilast; Tacrolimus (Topical); Trastuzumab

Decreased Effect

Etanercept may decrease the levels/effects of: BCG; Sipuleucel-T; Vaccines (Inactivated); Vaccines (Live)

The levels/effects of Etanercept may be decreased by: Echinacea

Ethanol/Nutrition/Herb Interactions Herb/Nutraceutical: Echinacea may decrease the therapeutic effects of etanercept (avoid concurrent use).

Stability

Prefilled syringes, autoinjectors: Store prefilled syringes and autoinjectors at 2°C to 8°C (36°F to 46°F); do not freeze. Protect from light; do not shake. The following stability information has also been reported: May be stored at room temperature for up to 4 days (Cohen, 2007).

Powder for reconstitution: Must be refrigerated at 2°C to 8°C (36°F to 46°F); do not freeze. The following stability information has also been reported: May be stored at room temperature for up to 7 days (Cohen, 2007). Reconstitute lyophilized powder aseptically with 1 mL sterile bacteriostatic water for injection, USP (supplied); swirl gently, do not shake. Do not filter reconstituted solution during preparation or administration. Upon reconstitution of vial, administer immediately. If not administered immediately after reconstitution, vial may be stored at 2°C to 8°C (36°F to 46°F) for up to 14 days.

Mechanism of Action Etanercept is a recombinant DNA-derived protein composed of tumor necrosis factor receptor (TNFR) linked to the Fc portion of human IgG1. Etanercept binds tumor necrosis factor (TNF) and blocks its interaction with cell surface receptors. TNF plays an important role in the inflammatory processes and the resulting joint pathology of rheumatoid arthritis (RA), polyarticular-course juvenile idiopathic arthritis (JIA), ankylosing spondylitis (AS), and plaque psoriasis.

Pharmacodynamics/Kinetics

Onset of action: ~2-3 weeks; RA: 1-2 weeks

Half-life elimination: RA: SubQ: 72-132 hours

Time to peak: RA: SubQ: 35-103 hours

Dosage

Geriatric SubQ: Refer to adult dosing. Although greater sensitivity of some elderly patients cannot be ruled out, no overall differences in safety or effectiveness were observed.

Adult

Rheumatoid arthritis, psoriatic arthritis, ankylosing spondylitis: SubQ:

Once-weekly dosing: 50 mg once weekly

Twice-weekly dosing: 25 mg given twice weekly (individual doses should be separated by 72-96 hours)

Plaque psoriasis: SubQ:

Initial: 50 mg twice weekly, 72-96 hours apart; maintain initial dose for 3 months (starting doses of 25 or 50 mg once weekly have also been used successfully)

Maintenance dose: 50 mg once weekly

Administration Administer subcutaneously. Rotate injection sites. New injections should be given at least one inch from an old site and never into areas where the skin is tender, bruised, red, or hard. **Note:** If the physician determines that it is appropriate, patients may self-inject after proper training in injection technique.

Powder for reconstitution: Follow package instructions carefully for reconstitution. The maximum amount injected at any single site should not exceed 25 mg.

Solution for injection: May be allowed to reach room temperature prior to injection.

Monitoring Parameters Monitor for response (inflammation, pain, grip strength), mobility, ADLs; observe for infections, allergic reactions. Monitor injection site for signs of reaction (swelling, pain, itching); latent TB screening prior to therapy initiation

Special Geriatric Considerations Clinical trials including those ≥65 years of age with rheumatoid arthritis have not demonstrated any differences in safety and efficacy between elderly and younger adults to date. Since elderly have a higher incidence of infections in general, caution should be used, with close monitoring and patient education.

Dosage Forms Excipient information presented when available (limited, particularly for generics); consult specific product labeling.
Injection, powder for reconstitution:
Enbrel® 25 mg [contains benzyl alcohol (in diluent), sucrose 10 mg]
Injection, solution [preservative free]:
Enbrel® 50 mg/mL (0.51 mL, 0.98 mL) [contains natural rubber/natural latex in packaging, sucrose 1%; prefilled syringe]
Enbrel® SureClick®: 50 mg/mL (0.98 mL) [contains natural rubber/natural latex in packaging, sucrose 1%; autoinjector]

Selected References
Mease PJ, Goffe BS, Metz J, et al, "Etanercept in the Treatment of Psoriatic Arthritis and Psoriasis: A Randomised Trial," *Lancet*, 2000, 356(9227):385-90.

◆ **Ethacrynate Sodium** *see* Ethacrynic Acid *on page 675*

Ethacrynic Acid (eth a KRIN ik AS id)

Related Information
Beers Criteria – Potentially Inappropriate Medications for Geriatrics *on page 2089*
Medication Safety Issues
Sound-alike/look-alike issues:
Edecrin® may be confused with Eulexin, Ecotrin®
BEERS Criteria medication:
This drug may be inappropriate for use in geriatric patients (low severity risk).
Brand Names: U.S. Edecrin®; Sodium Edecrin®
Brand Names: Canada Edecrin®
Index Terms Ethacrynate Sodium
Generic Availability (U.S.) No
Pharmacologic Category Diuretic, Loop
Use Management of edema associated with congestive heart failure; hepatic cirrhosis or renal disease; short-term management of ascites due to malignancy, idiopathic edema, and lymphedema
Dosage
Geriatric Oral: Initial: 25-50 mg/day
Adult I.V. formulation should be diluted in D_5W or NS (1 mg/mL) and infused over several minutes.

Edema:
Oral: 50-200 mg/day in 1-2 divided doses; may increase in increments of 25-50 mg at intervals of several days to a maximum of 400 mg/24 hours.
I.V.: 0.5-1 mg/kg/dose (maximum: 100 mg/dose); repeat doses not routinely recommended; however, if indicated, repeat doses every 8-12 hours.
Renal Impairment
Cl_{cr} <10 mL/minute: Avoid use.
Not removed by hemo- or peritoneal dialysis; supplemental dose is not necessary.
Special Geriatric Considerations Ethacrynic acid is rarely used because of its increased incidence of ototoxicity as compared to the other loop diuretics.

This medication is considered to be potentially inappropriate in this patient population (Beers Criteria severity: Low).
Dosage Forms Excipient information presented when available (limited, particularly for generics); consult specific product labeling.
Injection, powder for reconstitution, as ethacrynate sodium:
Sodium Edecrin®: 50 mg
Tablet, oral:
Edecrin®: 25 mg [scored]

Ethambutol (e THAM byoo tole)

Medication Safety Issues
Sound-alike/look-alike issues:
Myambutol® may be confused with Nembutal®
Brand Names: U.S. Myambutol®
Brand Names: Canada Etibi®
Index Terms Ethambutol Hydrochloride
Generic Availability (U.S.) Yes
Pharmacologic Category Antitubercular Agent

ETHAMBUTOL

◄ **Use** Treatment of pulmonary tuberculosis in conjunction with other antituberculosis agents

Unlabeled/Investigational Use Other mycobacterial diseases in conjunction with other antimycobacterial agents

Contraindications Hypersensitivity to ethambutol or any component of the formulation; optic neuritis (risk vs benefit decision); use in unconscious patients or any other patient who may be unable to discern and report visual changes

Warnings/Precautions May cause optic neuritis (unilateral or bilateral), resulting in decreased visual acuity or other vision changes. Discontinue promptly in patients with changes in vision, color blindness, or visual defects (effects normally reversible, but reversal may require up to a year). Irreversible blindness has been reported. Monitor visual acuity prior to and during therapy. Evaluation of visual acuity changes may be more difficult in patients with cataracts, optic neuritis, diabetic retinopathy, and inflammatory conditions of the eye; consideration should be given to whether or not visual changes are related to disease progression or effects of therapy. Dosage modification is required in patients with renal insufficiency; monitor renal function prior to and during treatment. Hepatic toxicity has been reported, possibly due to concurrent therapy; monitor liver function prior to and during treatment.

Adverse Reactions (Reflective of adult population; not specific for elderly) Frequency not defined.

Cardiovascular: Myocarditis, pericarditis

Central nervous system: Confusion, disorientation, dizziness, fever, hallucinations, headache, malaise

Dermatologic: Dermatitis, erythema multiforme, exfoliative dermatitis, pruritus, rash

Endocrine & metabolic: Acute gout or hyperuricemia

Gastrointestinal: Abdominal pain, anorexia, GI upset, nausea, vomiting

Hematologic: Eosinophilia, leukopenia, lymphadenopathy, neutropenia, thrombocytopenia

Hepatic: Hepatitis, hepatotoxicity (possibly related to concurrent therapy), LFTs abnormal

Neuromuscular & skeletal: Arthralgia, peripheral neuritis

Ocular: Optic neuritis; symptoms may include decreased acuity, scotoma, color blindness, or visual defects (usually reversible with discontinuation, irreversible blindness has been described)

Renal: Nephritis

Respiratory: Infiltrates (with or without eosinophilia), pneumonitis

Miscellaneous: Anaphylaxis, anaphylactoid reaction; hypersensitivity syndrome (cutaneous reactions, eosinophilia, and organ-specific inflammation)

Drug Interactions

Avoid Concomitant Use There are no known interactions where it is recommended to avoid concomitant use.

Increased Effect/Toxicity There are no known significant interactions involving an increase in effect.

Decreased Effect
The levels/effects of Ethambutol may be decreased by: Aluminum Hydroxide

Stability Store at controlled room temperature of 20°C to 25°C (68°F to 77°F).

Mechanism of Action Inhibits arabinosyl transferase resulting in impaired mycobacterial cell wall synthesis

Pharmacodynamics/Kinetics

Absorption: ~80%

Distribution: Widely throughout body; concentrated in kidneys, lungs, saliva, and red blood cells

Relative diffusion from blood into CSF: Adequate with or without inflammation (exceeds usual MICs)

CSF:blood level ratio: Normal meninges: 0%; Inflamed meninges: 25%

Protein binding: 20% to 30%

Metabolism: Hepatic (20%) to inactive metabolite

Half-life elimination: 2.5-3.6 hours; End-stage renal disease: 7-15 hours

Time to peak, serum: 2-4 hours

Excretion: Urine (~50% as unchanged drug, 8% to 15% as metabolites); feces (~20% as unchanged drug)

Dosage

Geriatric & Adult

Disseminated *Mycobacterium avium* (MAC) treatment in patients with advanced HIV infection (unlabeled use; ATS/IDSA guidelines, 2007): Oral: 15 mg/kg ethambutol in combination with clarithromycin or azithromycin with/without rifabutin

Tuberculosis, active: Oral: FDA-approved labeling: Adolescents ≥13 years and Adults: Initial: 15 mg/kg once daily (maximum dose: 1.5 g); Retreatment (previous antituberculosis therapy): 25 mg/kg once daily (maximum dose: 2.5 g) for 60 days or until bacteriologic smears and cultures become negative, followed by 15 mg/kg daily.

Suggested doses by lean body weight (CDC, 2003):

Daily therapy: 15-25 mg/kg (maximum dose: 1.6 g)
    40-55 kg: 800 mg
    56-75 kg: 1200 mg
    76-90 kg: 1600 mg

Twice weekly directly observed therapy (DOT): 50 mg/kg (maximum dose: 4 g)
    40-55 kg: 2000 mg
    56-75 kg: 2800 mg
    76-90 kg: 4000 mg

Three times/week DOT: 25-30 mg/kg (maximum dose: 2.4 g)
    40-55 kg: 1200 mg
    56-75 kg: 2000 mg
    76-90 kg: 2400 mg

Note: Used as part of a multidrug regimen. Treatment regimens consist of an initial 2 month phase, followed by a continuation phase of 4 or 7 additional months; frequency of dosing may differ depending on phase of therapy.

Nontuberculous mycobacterium *(M. kansasii)* (unlabeled use; ATS/IDSA guidelines, 2007): Oral: 15 mg/kg/day ethambutol for duration to include 12 months of culture-negative sputum; typically used in combination with rifampin and isoniazid; **Note:** Previous recommendations stated to use 25 mg/kg/day for the initial 2 months of therapy; however, IDSA guidelines state this may be unnecessary given the success of rifampin-based regimens with ethambutol 15 mg/kg/day or omitted altogether.

Renal Impairment
MMWR, 2003: Cl$_{cr}$ <30 mL/minute and hemodialysis: 15-25 mg/kg/dose 3 times weekly
Aronoff, 2007
    Cl$_{cr}$ 10-50 mL/minute: Administer every 24-36 hours
    Cl$_{cr}$ <10 mL/minute: Administer every 48 hours
Hemodialysis: Slightly dialyzable (5% to 20%); Administer dose postdialysis
Peritoneal dialysis: Dose for Cl$_{cr}$ <10 mL/minute: Administer every 48 hours
Continuous arteriovenous or venovenous hemofiltration: Dose for Cl$_{cr}$ 10-50 mL/minute: Administer every 24-36 hours

Monitoring Parameters Baseline and periodic (monthly) visual testing (each eye individually, as well as both eyes tested together) in patients receiving >15 mg/kg/day; baseline and periodic renal, hepatic, and hematopoietic tests

Special Geriatric Considerations Since most elderly patients acquired their tuberculosis before current antituberculin regimens were available, ethambutol is only indicated when patients are from areas where drug resistant *M. tuberculosis* is endemic, in HIV-infected elderly patients, and when drug resistant *M. tuberculosis* is suspected (see Dosage: Renal Impairment).

Dosage Forms Excipient information presented when available (limited, particularly for generics); consult specific product labeling.

Tablet, oral, as hydrochloride: 100 mg, 400 mg
    Myambutol®: 100 mg
    Myambutol®: 400 mg [scored]

Selected References
American Thoracic Society, "Treatment of Tuberculosis," *MMWR Recomm Rep*, 2003, 52(RR-11):1-77. Available at http://www.cdc.gov/mmwr/preview/mmwrhtml/rr5211a1.htm
Aronoff GR, Bennett WM, Berns JS, et al, *Drug Prescribing in Renal Failure: Dosing Guidelines for Adults and Children*, 5th ed. Philadelphia, PA: American College of Physicians; 2007.

◆ **Ethambutol Hydrochloride** *see* Ethambutol *on page 675*

Ethionamide (e thye on AM ide)

Brand Names: U.S. Trecator®
Brand Names: Canada Trecator®
Generic Availability (U.S.) No
Pharmacologic Category Antitubercular Agent
Use Treatment of tuberculosis and other mycobacterial diseases, in conjunction with other antituberculosis agents, when first-line agents have failed or resistance has been demonstrated
Contraindications Hypersensitivity to ethionamide or any component of the formulation; severe hepatic impairment

Warnings/Precautions Use with caution in patients with diabetes mellitus or thyroid dysfunction; use with caution in patients receiving cycloserine or isoniazid. Cross-resistance to isoniazid has been reported if inhA mutation is present. May cause hepatotoxicity; monitor liver function tests monthly. Use not recommended in patients with porphyria; animal and *in vitro* studies have shown porphyria-inducing effects. Periodic eye exams are recommended. Drug-resistant tuberculosis develops rapidly if ethionamide is used alone; must administer with at least one other antituberculosis agent.

Adverse Reactions (Reflective of adult population; not specific for elderly) Frequency not defined.

Cardiovascular: Postural hypotension

Central nervous system: Depression, dizziness, drowsiness, headache, psychiatric disturbances, restlessness, seizure

Dermatologic: Acne, alopecia, photosensitivity, purpura, rash

Endocrine & metabolic: Gynecomastia, hypoglycemia, hypothyroidism or goiter, menstrual irregularities, pellagra-like syndrome

Gastrointestinal: Abdominal pain, anorexia, diarrhea, excessive salivation, metallic taste, nausea, stomatitis, vomiting, weight loss

Genitourinary: Impotence

Hematologic: Leukopenia, thrombocytopenia

Hepatic: Bilirubin increased, hepatitis, jaundice, liver function tests increased

Neuromuscular & skeletal: Arthralgia, peripheral neuritis

Ocular: Blurred vision, diplopia, optic neuritis

Respiratory: Olfactory disturbances

Miscellaneous: Hypersensitivity reaction

Drug Interactions

Avoid Concomitant Use There are no known interactions where it is recommended to avoid concomitant use.

Increased Effect/Toxicity

Ethionamide may increase the levels/effects of: CycloSERINE; Isoniazid

The levels/effects of Ethionamide may be increased by: Alcohol (Ethyl)

Decreased Effect There are no known significant interactions involving a decrease in effect.

Ethanol/Nutrition/Herb Interactions Ethanol: Avoid excessive ethanol ingestion; psychotic reaction may occur.

Stability Store at 20°C to 25°C (68°F to 77°F). Keep containers tightly closed.

Mechanism of Action Inhibits peptide synthesis; bacteriostatic

Pharmacodynamics/Kinetics

Absorption: Rapid, complete

Distribution: Crosses placenta; V_d: 93.5 L

Protein binding: ~30%

Metabolism: Prodrug; extensively hepatic to active and inactive metabolites

Bioavailability: 80%

Half-life elimination: 2 hours

Time to peak, serum: 1 hour

Excretion: Urine (<1% as unchanged drug; as active and inactive metabolites)

Dosage

Geriatric & Adult Tuberculosis: Oral: 15-20 mg/kg/day; initiate dose at 250 mg/day for 1-2 days, then increase to 250 mg twice daily for 1-2 days, with gradual increases to highest tolerated dose; average adult dose: 750 mg/day (maximum: 1 g/day in 3-4 divided doses)

Renal Impairment Cl_{cr} <30 mL/minute: 250-500 mg/day

Administration Neurotoxic effects may be relieved by the administration of pyridoxine (6-100 mg daily, lower doses are more common). May be taken with or without meals. Gastrointestinal adverse effects may be decreased by administration at bedtime, decreased dose, or giving antiemetics.

Monitoring Parameters Initial and periodic serum ALT and AST; blood glucose; TSH every 6 months; initial and periodic ophthalmic exams

Pharmacotherapy Pearls Neurotoxic effects may be relieved by the administration of pyridoxine.

Special Geriatric Considerations Since many elderly have Cl_{cr} <50 mL/minute, adjust dose for renal function.

Dosage Forms Excipient information presented when available (limited, particularly for generics); consult specific product labeling.

Tablet, oral:

Trecator®: 250 mg

Ethosuximide (eth oh SUKS i mide)

Medication Safety Issues
  Sound-alike/look-alike issues:
    Ethosuximide may be confused with methsuximide
    Zarontin® may be confused with Neurontin®, Xalatan®, Zantac®, Zaroxolyn®
Brand Names: U.S. Zarontin®
Brand Names: Canada Zarontin®
Generic Availability (U.S.) Yes
Pharmacologic Category Anticonvulsant, Succinimide
Use Management of absence (petit mal) seizures
Medication Guide Available Yes
Contraindications History of hypersensitivity to succinimides
Warnings/Precautions Antiepileptics are associated with an increased risk of suicidal behavior/thoughts with use (regardless of indication); patients should be monitored for signs/symptoms of depression, suicidal tendencies, and other unusual behavior changes during therapy and instructed to inform their healthcare provider immediately if symptoms occur. Use with caution in patients with hepatic or renal disease; abrupt withdrawal of the drug may precipitate absence status; ethosuximide may increase tonic-clonic seizures when used alone in patients with mixed seizure disorders; ethosuximide must be used in combination with other anticonvulsants in patients with both absence and tonic-clonic seizures. Succinimides have been associated with severe blood dyscrasias and cases of systemic lupus erythematosus. Consider evaluation of blood counts in patients with signs/symptoms of infection. May cause CNS depression, which may impair physical or mental abilities; patients must be cautioned about performing tasks which require mental alertness (eg, operating machinery or driving). Effects with other sedative drugs or ethanol may be potentiated.
Adverse Reactions (Reflective of adult population; not specific for elderly) Frequency not defined.
  Central nervous system: Aggressiveness, ataxia, concentration impaired, dizziness, drowsiness, euphoria, fatigue, headache, hyperactivity, inability to concentrate, irritability, lethargy, mental depression (with cases of overt suicidal intentions), night terrors, paranoid psychosis, sleep disturbance
  Dermatologic: Hirsutism, pruritus, rash, Stevens-Johnson syndrome, urticaria
  Endocrine & metabolic: Libido increased
  Gastrointestinal: Abdominal pain, anorexia, cramps, diarrhea, epigastric pain, gastric upset, gum hypertrophy, nausea, tongue swelling, vomiting, weight loss
  Genitourinary: Hematuria (microscopic), vaginal bleeding
  Hematologic: Agranulocytosis, eosinophilia, leukopenia, pancytopenia
  Ocular: Myopia
  Miscellaneous: Allergic reaction, hiccups, systemic lupus erythematosus
Drug Interactions
  Metabolism/Transport Effects Substrate of CYP3A4 (major)
  Avoid Concomitant Use
    Avoid concomitant use of Ethosuximide with any of the following: Conivaptan
  Increased Effect/Toxicity
    Ethosuximide may increase the levels/effects of: Alcohol (Ethyl); CNS Depressants; Methotrimeprazine; Selective Serotonin Reuptake Inhibitors

    The levels/effects of Ethosuximide may be increased by: Conivaptan; CYP3A4 Inhibitors (Moderate); CYP3A4 Inhibitors (Strong); Dasatinib; Divalproex; Droperidol; HydrOXYzine; Methotrimeprazine; Valproic Acid
  Decreased Effect
    Ethosuximide may decrease the levels/effects of: Divalproex; Valproic Acid

    The levels/effects of Ethosuximide may be decreased by: Amphetamines; CYP3A4 Inducers (Strong); Deferasirox; Herbs (CYP3A4 Inducers); Ketorolac; Ketorolac (Nasal); Ketorolac (Systemic); Mefloquine; Tocilizumab
Ethanol/Nutrition/Herb Interactions
  Ethanol: May increase CNS depression; monitor for increased effects with coadministration. Caution patients about effects.
  Herb/Nutraceutical: St John's wort may decrease ethosuximide levels.
Stability
  Capsules: Store at 25°C (77°F); excursions permitted to 15°C to 30°C (59°F to 86°F).
  Solution: Store below 30°C (86°F); do not freeze. Protect from light.
Mechanism of Action Increases the seizure threshold and suppresses paroxysmal spike-and-wave pattern in absence seizures; depresses nerve transmission in the motor cortex

◄ **Pharmacodynamics/Kinetics**
Distribution: Adults: V_d: 0.62-0.72 L/kg
Metabolism: Hepatic (~80% to 3 inactive metabolites)
Half-life elimination, serum: Adults: 50-60 hours
Time to peak, serum: Capsule: ~2-4 hours; Syrup: <2-4 hours
Excretion: Urine, slowly (50% as metabolites, 10% to 20% as unchanged drug); feces (small amounts)
Dosage
Geriatric & Adult Management of absence (petit mal) seizures: Oral: Initial: 500 mg/day; increase by 250 mg as needed every 4-7 days up to 1.5 g/day in divided doses
Renal Impairment Use with caution.
Hepatic Impairment Use with caution.
Administration Administer with food or milk to avoid GI upset
Monitoring Parameters Seizure frequency; trough serum concentrations, CBC, platelets, liver enzymes, urinalysis; suicidality (eg, suicidal thoughts, depression, behavioral changes)
Reference Range Therapeutic: 40-100 mcg/mL
Pharmacotherapy Pearls Considered to be drug of choice for simple absence seizures
Special Geriatric Considerations No specific studies with the use of this medication in the elderly. Consider renal function and proceed slowly with dosing increases; monitor closely.
Dosage Forms Excipient information presented when available (limited, particularly for generics); consult specific product labeling.
Capsule, softgel, oral: 250 mg
  Zarontin®: 250 mg
Solution, oral: 250 mg/5 mL (473 mL)
  Zarontin®: 250 mg/5 mL (480 mL) [contains sodium benzoate; raspberry flavor]
Syrup, oral: 250 mg/5 mL (473 mL)

◆ **Ethoxynaphthamido Penicillin Sodium** see Nafcillin on page 1256
◆ **Ethyl Esters of Omega-3 Fatty Acids** see Omega-3-Acid Ethyl Esters on page 1338

Etidronate (e ti DROE nate)

Medication Safety Issues
Sound-alike/look-alike issues:
  Etidronate may be confused with etidocaine, etomidate, etretinate
Brand Names: U.S. Didronel®
Brand Names: Canada Co-Etidronate; Mylan-Etidronate
Index Terms EHDP; Etidronate Disodium; Sodium Etidronate
Generic Availability (U.S.) Yes
Pharmacologic Category Bisphosphonate Derivative
Use Symptomatic treatment of Paget's disease; prevention and treatment of heterotopic ossification due to spinal cord injury or after total hip replacement
Unlabeled/Investigational Use Postmenopausal osteoporosis
Contraindications Hypersensitivity to bisphosphonates or any component of the formulation; overt osteomalacia; patients with abnormalities of the esophagus which delay esophageal emptying, such as stricture or achalasia
Warnings/Precautions Ensure adequate calcium and vitamin D intake. Etidronate may retard mineralization of bone; treatment may need delayed or interrupted until callus is present. Use caution in patients with renal impairment. Use caution with enterocolitis; diarrhea has been reported at high doses and therapy may need to be withheld.

Osteonecrosis of the jaw (ONJ) has been reported in patients receiving bisphosphonates. Risk factors include invasive dental procedures (eg, tooth extraction, dental implants, boney surgery); a diagnosis of cancer, with concomitant chemotherapy or corticosteroids; poor oral hygiene, ill-fitting dentures; and comorbid disorders (anemia, coagulopathy, infection, pre-existing dental disease). Most reported cases occurred after I.V. bisphosphonate therapy; however, cases have been reported following oral therapy. A dental exam and preventative dentistry should be performed prior to placing patients with risk factors on chronic bisphosphonate therapy. The manufacturer's labeling states that discontinuing bisphosphonates in patients requiring invasive dental procedures may reduce the risk of ONJ. However, other experts suggest that there is no evidence that discontinuing therapy reduces the risk of developing ONJ (Assael, 2009). The benefit/risk must be assessed by the treating physician and/or dentist/surgeon prior to any invasive dental procedure. Patients developing ONJ while on bisphosphonates should receive care by an oral surgeon.

Infrequently, severe (and occasionally debilitating) bone, joint, and/or muscle pain have been reported during bisphosphonate treatment. The onset of pain ranged from a single day to several months. Consider discontinuing therapy in patients who experience severe symptoms; symptoms usually resolve upon discontinuation. Some patients experienced recurrence when rechallenged with same drug or another bisphosphonate; avoid use in patients with a history of these symptoms in association with bisphosphonate therapy. Do not exceed recommended dose or use continuously for >6 months in patients with Paget's disease; risk of osteomalacia or fractures may be increased. Long bones with predominantly lytic lesions may be prone to fracture, particularly in patients unresponsive to treatment.

Adverse Reactions (Reflective of adult population; not specific for elderly) Frequency not defined.

Gastrointestinal: Diarrhea, nausea

Neuromuscular & skeletal: Bone pain

Drug Interactions

Avoid Concomitant Use There are no known interactions where it is recommended to avoid concomitant use.

Increased Effect/Toxicity

Etidronate may increase the levels/effects of: Deferasirox; Phosphate Supplements

The levels/effects of Etidronate may be increased by: Aminoglycosides; Nonsteroidal Anti-Inflammatory Agents

Decreased Effect

The levels/effects of Etidronate may be decreased by: Antacids; Calcium Salts; Iron Salts; Magnesium Salts; Proton Pump Inhibitors

Ethanol/Nutrition/Herb Interactions Food: Food decreases the absorption and bioavailability of the drug.

Stability Store at controlled room temperature of 15°C to 30°C (59°F to 86°F).

Mechanism of Action Decreases bone resorption by inhibiting osteocystic osteolysis; decreases mineral release and matrix or collagen breakdown in bone

Pharmacodynamics/Kinetics

Onset of action: 1-3 months

Duration: Can persist for 12 months without continuous therapy

Absorption: ~3%

Metabolism: None

Half-life elimination: 1-6 hours

Excretion: Primarily urine (as unchanged drug); feces (as unabsorbed drug)

Dosage

Geriatric & Adult

Paget's disease: Oral:

Initial: 5-10 mg/kg/day (not to exceed 6 months) or 11-20 mg/kg/day (not to exceed 3 months). Doses >20 mg/kg/day are **not** recommended.

Retreatment: Initiate only after etidronate-free period ≥90 days. Monitor patients every 3-6 months. Retreatment regimens are the same as for initial treatment.

Heterotopic ossification: Oral:

Caused by spinal cord injury: 20 mg/kg/day for 2 weeks, then 10 mg/kg/day for 10 weeks; total treatment period: 12 weeks

Complicating total hip replacement: 20 mg/kg/day for 1 month preoperatively then 20 mg/kg/day for 3 months postoperatively; total treatment period is 4 months

Postmenopausal osteoporosis (unlabeled use): Oral: 400 mg/day orally for 2 weeks followed by a 13-week period with no etidronate, then repeat cycle; maintain adequate calcium and vitamin D intake during entire 15-week treatment cycle

Renal Impairment Use with caution; specific guidelines are not available, however consider dose reduction.

Administration Administer tablet on an empty stomach 2 hours before food.

Monitoring Parameters Paget's disease: Alkaline phosphatase; pain; serum calcium and 25 (OH)D

Reference Range Calcium (total): Adults: 9.0-11.0 mg/dL

Test Interactions Bisphosphonates may interfere with diagnostic imaging agents such as technetium-99m-diphosphonate in bone scans.

Special Geriatric Considerations The elderly are frequently treated long-term for osteoporosis. Elderly patients should be advised to report any lower extremity, jaw (osteonecrosis), or muscle pain that cannot be explained or lasts longer than 2 weeks. Additionally, elderly often receive concomitant diuretic therapy and therefore their electrolyte status (eg, calcium, phosphate) should be periodically evaluated.

Dosage Forms Excipient information presented when available (limited, particularly for generics); consult specific product labeling.

Tablet, oral, as disodium: 200 mg, 400 mg

Didronel® : 400 mg [scored]

◀ **Selected References**
Hillner BE, Ingle JN, Chlebowski RT, et al, "American Society of Clinical Oncology 2003 Update on the Role of Bisphosphonates and Bone Health Issues in Women With Breast Cancer," *J Clin Oncol*, 2003, 21(21):4042-57.

Storm T, Thamsborg G, Steiniche T, et al, "Effect of Intermittent Cyclical Etidronate Therapy on Bone Mass and Fracture Rate in Women With Postmenopausal Osteoporosis," *N Engl J Med*, 1990, 322(18):1265-71.

Watts NB, Harris ST, Genant HK, et al, "Intermittent Cyclical Etidronate Treatment of Postmenopausal Osteoporosis," *N Engl J Med*, 1990, 323(2):73-9.

◆ **Etidronate Disodium** *see* Etidronate *on page 680*

Etodolac (ee toe DOE lak)

Medication Safety Issues
Sound-alike/look-alike issues:
Lodine® may be confused with codeine, iodine, Iopidine®, Lopid®
Brand Names: Canada Apo-Etodolac®; Utradol™
Index Terms Etodolic Acid; Lodine
Generic Availability (U.S.) Yes
Pharmacologic Category Nonsteroidal Anti-inflammatory Drug (NSAID), Oral
Use Acute and long-term use in the management of signs and symptoms of osteoarthritis; rheumatoid arthritis and juvenile idiopathic arthritis (JIA); management of acute pain
Unlabeled/Investigational Use Treatment of rheumatoid arthritis
Medication Guide Available Yes
Contraindications Hypersensitivity to etodolac, aspirin, other NSAIDs, or any component of the formulation; perioperative pain in the setting of coronary artery bypass graft (CABG) surgery
Warnings/Precautions [U.S. Boxed Warning]: NSAIDs are associated with an increased risk of adverse cardiovascular thrombotic events, including MI and stroke. Risk may be increased with duration of use or pre-existing cardiovascular risk factors or disease. Carefully evaluate individual cardiovascular risk profiles prior to prescribing. May cause new-onset hypertension or worsening of existing hypertension. Use caution with fluid retention. Avoid use in heart failure. Concurrent administration of ibuprofen, and potentially other nonselective NSAIDs, may interfere with aspirin's cardioprotective effect. **[U.S. Boxed Warning]: Use is contraindicated for treatment of perioperative pain in the setting of coronary artery bypass graft (CABG) surgery.** Risk of MI and stroke may be increased with use following CABG surgery.

[U.S. Boxed Warning]: NSAIDs may increase risk of gastrointestinal irritation, inflammation, ulceration, bleeding, and perforation. These events may occur at any time during therapy and without warning. Use caution with a history of GI disease (bleeding or ulcers), concurrent therapy with aspirin, anticoagulants and/or corticosteroids, smoking, use of alcohol, the elderly or debilitated patients. When used concomitantly with ≤325 mg of aspirin, a substantial increase in the risk of gastrointestinal complications (eg, ulcer) occurs; concomitant gastroprotective therapy (eg, proton pump inhibitors) is recommended (Bhatt, 2008).

Platelet adhesion and aggregation may be decreased; may prolong bleeding time; patients with coagulation disorders or who are receiving anticoagulants should be monitored closely. Anemia may occur; patients on long-term NSAID therapy should be monitored for anemia. Rarely, NSAID use may cause severe blood dyscrasias (eg, agranulocytosis, aplastic anemia, thrombocytopenia).

NSAID use may compromise existing renal function; dose-dependent decreases in prostaglandin synthesis may result from NSAID use, reducing renal blood flow which may cause renal decompensation. NSAID use may increase the risk for hyperkalemia. Patients with impaired renal function, dehydration, heart failure, liver dysfunction, those taking diuretics and ACE inhibitors, and the elderly are at greater risk for renal toxicity and hyperkalemia. Rehydrate patient before starting therapy; monitor renal function closely. Not recommended for use in patients with advanced renal disease. Long-term NSAID use may result in renal papillary necrosis.

Use the lowest effective dose for the shortest duration of time, consistent with individual patient goals, to reduce risk of cardiovascular or GI adverse events. Alternate therapies should be considered for patients at high risk.

NSAIDs may cause serious skin adverse events including exfoliative dermatitis, Stevens-Johnson syndrome (SJS), and toxic epidermal necrolysis (TEN); discontinue use at first sign of skin rash or hypersensitivity. Anaphylactoid reactions may occur, even without prior exposure; patients with "aspirin triad" (bronchial asthma, aspirin intolerance, rhinitis) may be at increased risk. Do not use in patients who experience bronchospasm, asthma, rhinitis, or urticaria with NSAID or aspirin therapy. Use caution in other forms of asthma.

Use with caution in patients with decreased hepatic function. Closely monitor patients with any abnormal LFT. Severe hepatic reactions (eg, fulminant hepatitis, liver failure) have occurred with NSAID use, rarely; discontinue if signs or symptoms of liver disease develop, or if systemic manifestations occur.

NSAIDS may cause drowsiness, dizziness, blurred vision and other neurologic effects which may impair physical or mental abilities; patients must be cautioned about performing tasks which require mental alertness (eg, operating machinery or driving). Discontinue use with blurred or diminished vision and perform ophthalmologic exam. Monitor vision with long-term therapy. The elderly are at increased risk for adverse effects (especially peptic ulceration, CNS effects, renal toxicity) from NSAIDs even at low doses.

Withhold for at least 4-6 half-lives prior to surgical or dental procedures.

Use of extended release product consisting of a nondeformable matrix should be avoided in patients with stricture/narrowing of the GI tract; symptoms of obstruction have been associated with nondeformable products.

Adverse Reactions (Reflective of adult population; not specific for elderly)
1% to 10%:
Central nervous system: Dizziness (3% to 9%), chills/fever (1% to 3%), depression (1% to 3%), nervousness (1% to 3%)
Dermatologic: Rash (1% to 3%), pruritus (1% to 3%)
Gastrointestinal: Dyspepsia (10%), abdominal cramps (3% to 9%), diarrhea (3% to 9%), flatulence (3% to 9%), nausea (3% to 9%), vomiting (1% to 3%), constipation (1% to 3%), melena (1% to 3%), gastritis (1% to 3%)
Genitourinary: Dysuria (1% to 3%)
Neuromuscular & skeletal: Weakness (3% to 9%)
Ocular: Blurred vision (1% to 3%)
Otic: Tinnitus (1% to 3%)
Renal: Polyuria (1% to 3%)

Drug Interactions
Avoid Concomitant Use
Avoid concomitant use of Etodolac with any of the following: Floctafenine; Ketorolac; Ketorolac (Nasal); Ketorolac (Systemic)

Increased Effect/Toxicity
Etodolac may increase the levels/effects of: Aminoglycosides; Anticoagulants; Antiplatelet Agents; Bisphosphonate Derivatives; Collagenase (Systemic); CycloSPORINE; CycloSPORINE (Systemic); Deferasirox; Desmopressin; Digoxin; Drotrecogin Alfa; Eplerenone; Haloperidol; Ibritumomab; Lithium; Methotrexate; Nonsteroidal Anti-Inflammatory Agents; PEMEtrexed; Porfimer; Potassium-Sparing Diuretics; PRALAtrexate; Quinolone Antibiotics; Rivaroxaban; Salicylates; Thrombolytic Agents; Tositumomab and Iodine I 131 Tositumomab; Vancomycin; Vitamin K Antagonists

The levels/effects of Etodolac may be increased by: ACE Inhibitors; Angiotensin II Receptor Blockers; Antidepressants (Tricyclic, Tertiary Amine); Corticosteroids (Systemic); Dasatinib; Floctafenine; Glucosamine; Herbs (Anticoagulant/Antiplatelet Properties); Ketorolac; Ketorolac (Nasal); Ketorolac (Systemic); Nonsteroidal Anti-Inflammatory Agents; Omega-3-Acid Ethyl Esters; Pentosan Polysulfate Sodium; Pentoxifylline; Probenecid; Prostacyclin Analogues; Selective Serotonin Reuptake Inhibitors; Serotonin/Norepinephrine Reuptake Inhibitors; Sodium Phosphates; Treprostinil; Vitamin E

Decreased Effect
Etodolac may decrease the levels/effects of: ACE Inhibitors; Angiotensin II Receptor Blockers; Antiplatelet Agents; Beta-Blockers; Eplerenone; HydrALAZINE; Potassium-Sparing Diuretics; Salicylates; Selective Serotonin Reuptake Inhibitors; Thiazide Diuretics

The levels/effects of Etodolac may be decreased by: Bile Acid Sequestrants; Nonsteroidal Anti-Inflammatory Agents; Salicylates

Ethanol/Nutrition/Herb Interactions
Ethanol: Avoid ethanol (may enhance gastric mucosal irritation).
Food: Etodolac peak serum levels may be decreased if taken with food.
Herb/Nutraceutical: Avoid alfalfa, anise, bilberry, bladderwrack, bromelain, cat's claw, celery, chamomile, coleus, cordyceps, dong quai, evening primrose, fenugreek, feverfew, garlic, ginger, ginkgo biloba, ginseng (American, Panax, Siberian), grapeseed, green tea, guggul, horse chestnut seed, horseradish, licorice, prickly ash, red clover, reishi, SAMe (S-adenosylmethionine), sweet clover, turmeric, white willow (all have additional antiplatelet activity).

Stability Store at 20°C to 25°C (68°F to 77°F). Protect from moisture.

◀ **Mechanism of Action** Reversibly inhibits cyclooxygenase-1 and 2 (COX-1 and 2) enzymes, which results in decreased formation of prostaglandin precursors; has antipyretic, analgesic, and anti-inflammatory properties

Other proposed mechanisms not fully elucidated (and possibly contributing to the anti-inflammatory effect to varying degrees), include inhibiting chemotaxis, altering lymphocyte activity, inhibiting neutrophil aggregation/activation, and decreasing proinflammatory cytokine levels.

Pharmacodynamics/Kinetics
Onset of action: Analgesic: 2-4 hours; Maximum anti-inflammatory effect: A few days
Absorption: ≥80%
Distribution: V_d:
  Immediate release: Adults:0.4 L/kg
  Extended release: Adults: 0.57 L/kg
Protein binding: ≥99%, primarily albumin
Metabolism: Hepatic
Bioavailability: 100%
Half-life elimination: Terminal: Adults: 5-8 hours
Time to peak, serum:
  Immediate release: Adults: 1-2 hours
  Extended release: Extended release: 5-7 hours, increased 1.4-3.8 hours with food
Excretion: Urine 73% (1% unchanged); feces 16%

Dosage
  Geriatric & Adult Note: For chronic conditions, response is usually observed within 2 weeks.
    Acute pain: Oral: Immediate release formulation: 200-400 mg every 6-8 hours, as needed, not to exceed total daily doses of 1000 mg
    Rheumatoid arthritis, osteoarthritis: Oral:
      Immediate release formulation: 400 mg 2 times/day **or** 300 mg 2-3 times/day **or** 500 mg 2 times/day (doses >1000 mg/day have not been evaluated)
      Extended release formulation: 400-1000 mg once daily
  Renal Impairment
    Mild-to-moderate: No adjustment required
    Severe: Use not recommended; use with caution
    Hemodialysis: Not removed
  Hepatic Impairment No adjustment required.

Administration May be administered with food to decrease GI upset.

Monitoring Parameters Monitor CBC, liver enzymes; monitor BUN/serum creatinine in patients receiving diuretics; monitor response (pain, range of motion, grip strength, mobility, ADL function), inflammation; observe for weight gain, edema; monitor renal function; observe for bleeding, bruising; evaluate gastrointestinal effects (abdominal pain, bleeding, dyspepsia); mental confusion, disorientation

Test Interactions False-positive for urinary bilirubin and ketone

Pharmacotherapy Pearls Single dose of 76-100 mg is comparable to the analgesic effect of aspirin 650 mg; there are no clinical guidelines to predict which NSAID will give response in a particular patient. Trials with each must be initiated until response determined. Consider dose, patient convenience, and cost.

Special Geriatric Considerations The elderly are a high-risk population for adverse effects from nonsteroidal anti-inflammatory agents. As much as 60% of older adults who experience GI side effects can develop peptic ulceration and/or hemorrhage asymptomatically. The concomitant use of H_2 blockers and sucralfate is not effective as prophylaxis with the exception of NSAID-induced duodenal ulcers which may be prevented by the use of ranitidine. Misoprostol and proton pump inhibitors are the only agents proven to help prevent the development of NSAID-induced ulcers. Also, concomitant disease and drug use contribute to the risk for GI adverse effects. Use lowest effective dose for shortest period possible. Consider renal function decline with age. Use of NSAIDs can compromise existing renal function especially when Cl_{cr} is ≤30 mL/minute.
Tinnitus may be a difficult and unreliable indication of toxicity due to age-related hearing loss or eighth cranial nerve damage. CNS adverse effects such as confusion, agitation, and hallucination are generally seen in overdose or high dose situations, but older adults may demonstrate these adverse effects at lower doses than younger adults. In patients ≥65 years, no substantial differences in the pharmacokinetics or side-effects profile were seen compared with the general population. Studies with etodolac in elderly demonstrated no difference in safety or efficacy compared to younger adults. No dosing adjustment necessary in elderly.

Dosage Forms Excipient information presented when available (limited, particularly for generics); consult specific product labeling.

Capsule, oral: 200 mg, 300 mg

Tablet, oral: 400 mg, 500 mg

Tablet, extended release, oral: 400 mg, 500 mg, 600 mg

Selected References

Clinch D, Banerjee AK, and Ostick G, "Absence of Abdominal Pain in Elderly Patients With Peptic Ulcer," *Age Ageing*, 1984, 13(2):120-3.

Clive DM and Stoff JS, "Renal Syndromes Associated With Nonsteroidal Anti-inflammatory Drugs," *N Engl J Med*, 1984, 310(9):563-72.

Gurwitz JH, Avorn J, Ross-Degnan D, et al, "Nonsteroidal Anti-inflammatory Drug-Associated Azotemia in the Very Old," *JAMA*, 1990, 264(4):471-5.

Pounder R, "Silent Peptic Ulceration: Deadly Silence or Golden Silence?" *Gastroenterology*, 1989, 96(2 Pt 2 Suppl):626-31.

Exemestane (ex e MES tane)

Medication Safety Issues
Sound-alike/look-alike issues:
Aromasin® may be confused with Arimidex®
Exemestane may be confused with estramustine.

Brand Names: U.S. Aromasin®

Brand Names: Canada Aromasin®

Generic Availability (U.S.) Yes

Pharmacologic Category Antineoplastic Agent, Aromatase Inactivator

Use Treatment of advanced breast cancer in postmenopausal women whose disease has progressed following tamoxifen therapy; adjuvant treatment of postmenopausal estrogen receptor-positive early breast cancer following 2-3 years of tamoxifen (for a total of 5 years of adjuvant therapy)

Contraindications Hypersensitivity to exemestane or any component of the formulation

Warnings/Precautions Hazardous agent - use appropriate precautions for handling and disposal. Due to decreased circulating estrogen levels, exemestane is associated with a reduction in bone mineral density; decreases (from baseline) in lumbar spine and femoral neck density have been observed. Grade 3 or 4 lymphocytopenia has been observed with exemestane use, although most patients had preexisting lower grade lymphopenia. Increases in bilirubin, alkaline phosphatase and serum creatinine have been observed. Not to be given with estrogen-containing agents. Dose adjustment recommended with concomitant CYP3A4 inducers.

Adverse Reactions (Reflective of adult population; not specific for elderly)
>10%:
Cardiovascular: Hypertension (5% to 15%)
Central nervous system: Fatigue (8% to 22%), insomnia (11% to 14%), pain (13%), headache (7% to 13%), depression (6% to 13%)
Dermatological: Hyperhidrosis (4% to 18%), alopecia (15%)
Endocrine & metabolic: Hot flashes (13% to 33%)
Gastrointestinal: Nausea (9% to 18%), abdominal pain (6% to 11%)
Hepatic: Alkaline phosphatase increased (14% to 15%)
Neuromuscular & skeletal: Arthralgia (15% to 29%)
1% to 10%:
Cardiovascular: Edema (6% to 7%); cardiac ischemic events (2%: MI, angina, myocardial ischemia); chest pain
Central nervous system: Dizziness (8% to 10%), anxiety (4% to 10%), fever (5%), confusion, hypoesthesia
Dermatologic: Dermatitis (8%), itching, rash

◄

    Endocrine & metabolic: Weight gain (8%)

    Gastrointestinal: Diarrhea (4% to 10%), vomiting (7%), anorexia (6%), constipation (5%), appetite increased (3%), dyspepsia

    Genitourinary: Urinary tract infection (2% to 5%)

    Hepatic: Bilirubin increased (5% to 7%)

    Neuromuscular & skeletal: Back pain (9%), limb pain (9%), myalgia (6%), osteoarthritis (6%), weakness (6%), osteoporosis (5%), pathological fracture (4%), paresthesia (3%), carpal tunnel syndrome (2%), cramps (2%)

    Ocular: Visual disturbances (5%)

    Renal: Creatinine increased (6%)

    Respiratory: Dyspnea (10%), cough (6%), bronchitis, pharyngitis, rhinitis, sinusitis, upper respiratory infection

    Miscellaneous: Flu-like syndrome (6%), lymphedema, infection

A dose-dependent decrease in sex hormone-binding globulin has been observed with daily doses of ≥2.5 mg. Serum luteinizing hormone and follicle-stimulating hormone levels have increased with this medicine.

Drug Interactions

    Metabolism/Transport Effects Substrate of CYP3A4 (major)

    Avoid Concomitant Use There are no known interactions where it is recommended to avoid concomitant use.

    Increased Effect/Toxicity

    The levels/effects of Exemestane may be increased by: Conivaptan

    Decreased Effect

    Exemestane may decrease the levels/effects of: Saxagliptin

    The levels/effects of Exemestane may be decreased by: CYP3A4 Inducers (Strong); Deferasirox; Herbs (CYP3A4 Inducers); Rifampin; Tocilizumab

Ethanol/Nutrition/Herb Interactions

    Food: Plasma levels increased by 40% when exemestane was taken with a fatty meal.

    Herb/Nutraceutical: St John's wort may decrease exemestane levels. Avoid black cohosh, dong quai in estrogen-dependent tumors.

Stability Store at 25°C (77°F); excursions permitted to 15°C to 30°C (59°F to 86°F).

Mechanism of Action Exemestane is an irreversible, steroidal aromatase inactivator. It is structurally related to androstenedione, and is converted to an intermediate that irreversibly blocks the active site of the aromatase enzyme, leading to inactivation ("suicide inhibition") and thus preventing conversion of androgens to estrogens in peripheral tissues. In post-menopausal breast cancers where growth is estrogen-dependent, this medicine will lower circulating estrogens.

Pharmacodynamics/Kinetics

    Absorption: Rapid and moderate (~42%) following oral administration; absorption increases ~40% following high-fat meal

    Distribution: Extensive into tissues

    Protein binding: 90%, primarily to albumin and α_1-acid glycoprotein

    Metabolism: Extensively hepatic; oxidation (CYP3A4) of methylene group, reduction of 17-keto group with formation of many secondary metabolites; metabolites are inactive

    Half-life elimination: 24 hours

    Time to peak: Women with breast cancer: 1.2 hours

    Excretion: Urine (<1% as unchanged drug, 39% to 45% as metabolites); feces (36% to 48%)

Dosage

    Geriatric & Adult Females: Postmenopausal:

        Breast cancer, advanced: Oral: 25 mg once daily; continue until tumor progression

        Breast cancer, early (adjuvant treatment): Oral: 25 mg once daily (following 2-3 years of tamoxifen therapy) for a total duration of 5 years of endocrine therapy (in the absence of recurrence or contralateral breast cancer)

        Dosage adjustment with CYP3A4 inducers: 50 mg once daily when used with potent inducers (eg, rifampin, phenytoin)

    Renal Impairment Safety of chronic dosing in renal impairment has not been studied, although dosage adjustment does not appear necessary.

    Hepatic Impairment Safety of chronic dosing in hepatic impairment has not been studied, although dosage adjustment does not appear necessary.

Administration Administer after a meal.

Pharmacotherapy Pearls Oncology Comment: The American Society of Clinical Oncology (ASCO) guidelines for adjuvant endocrine therapy in postmenopausal women with HR-positive breast cancer (Burstein, 2010) recommend considering aromatase inhibitor (AI) therapy at some point in the treatment course (primary, sequentially, or extended). Optimal duration at this time is not known; however, treatment with an AI should not exceed 5 years in primary and extended therapies, and 2-3 years if followed by tamoxifen in sequential therapy (total of 5 years). If initial therapy with AI has been discontinued before the 5 years, consideration should be taken to receive tamoxifen for a total of 5 years. The optimal time to switch to an AI is also not known, but data supports switching after 2-3 years of tamoxifen (sequential) or after 5 years of tamoxifen (extended). If patient becomes intolerant or has poor adherence, consideration should be made to switch to another AI or initiate tamoxifen.

Special Geriatric Considerations In pharmacokinetic trials, no significant changes were seen in women <68 years of age.

Dosage Forms Excipient information presented when available (limited, particularly for generics); consult specific product labeling.
Tablet, oral: 25 mg
    Aromasin®: 25 mg

Exenatide (ex EN a tide)

Related Information
Diabetes Mellitus Management, Adults *on page 2073*
Brand Names: U.S. Byetta®
Index Terms AC 2993; AC002993; Exendin-4; LY2148568
Generic Availability (U.S.) No
Pharmacologic Category Antidiabetic Agent, Glucagon-Like Peptide-1 (GLP-1) Receptor Agonist
Use Treatment of type 2 diabetes mellitus (noninsulin dependent, NIDDM) to improve glycemic control
Medication Guide Available Yes
Contraindications Hypersensitivity to exenatide or any component of the formulation
Warnings/Precautions Mechanism requires the presence of insulin, therefore use in type 1 diabetes (insulin dependent, IDDM) or diabetic ketoacidosis is not recommended; it is not a substitute for insulin in insulin-requiring patients. Concurrent use with insulin therapy has not been evaluated. May increase the risk of hypoglycemia in patients receiving concomitant insulin secretagogues (eg, sulfonylureas, meglitinides); dosage reduction of sulfonylureas may be required. Clinicians should note that the risk of hypoglycemia is not increased when exenatide is added to metformin monotherapy.

Exenatide is frequently associated with gastrointestinal adverse effects and is not recommended for use in patients with gastroparesis or severe gastrointestinal disease. Gastrointestinal effects may be dose-related and may decrease in frequency/severity with gradual titration and continued use. Due to its effects on gastric emptying, exenatide may reduce the rate and extent of absorption of orally-administered drugs; use with caution in patients receiving medications with a narrow therapeutic window or require rapid absorption from the GI tract. Administer medications 1 hour prior to the use of exenatide when optimal drug absorption and peak levels are important to the overall therapeutic effect (eg, antibiotics, oral contraceptives). Cases of acute pancreatitis (including hemorrhagic and necrotizing with some fatalities) have been reported; monitor for unexplained severe abdominal pain and if pancreatitis suspected, discontinue use. Do not resume unless an alternative etiology of pancreatitis is confirmed. Consider alternative antidiabetic therapy in patients with a history of pancreatitis. Use may be associated with the development of anti-exenatide antibodies. Low titers are not associated with a loss of efficacy; however, high titers (observed in 6% of patients in clinical studies) may result in an attenuation of response. May be associated with weight loss (due to reduced intake) independent of the change in hemoglobin A_{1c}. Not recommended in severe renal impairment (Cl_{cr} <30 mL/minute) or end-stage renal disease (ESRD). Patients with ESRD receiving dialysis may be more susceptible to GI effects (eg, nausea, vomiting) which may result in hypovolemia and further reductions in renal function. Use with caution in patients with renal transplantation and when initiating or escalating doses in patients with moderate renal impairment (Cl_{cr} 30-50 mL/minute).

Adverse Reactions (Reflective of adult population; not specific for elderly) Percentages as reported for combination therapy (sulfonylurea and/or metformin; thiazolidinedione and/or metformin) unless otherwise noted:
>10%:
    Endocrine & metabolic: Hypoglycemia (monotherapy 4% to 5%; combination therapy: sulfonylurea - 14% to 36%; metformin - similar to placebo; thiazolidinedione - 11%)
    Gastrointestinal: Nausea (monotherapy 8%; combination therapy 40% to 44%; dose-dependent), vomiting (monotherapy 4%; combination therapy 13%), diarrhea (monotherapy <2%; combination therapy 6% to 13%)
    Miscellaneous: Anti-exenatide antibodies (low titers 38%, high titers 6%)
1% to 10%:
    Central nervous system: Dizziness (monotherapy <2%; combination therapy 9%), headache (9%)

◄ Dermatologic: Hyperhidrosis (3%)
Endocrine & metabolic: Appetite decreased (<2%)
Gastrointestinal: Dyspepsia (monotherapy 3%; combination therapy 6% to 7%), GERD (3%)
Neuromuscular & skeletal: Weakness (4%)
Miscellaneous: Feeling jittery (9%)

Drug Interactions

Avoid Concomitant Use There are no known interactions where it is recommended to avoid concomitant use.

Increased Effect/Toxicity
Exenatide may increase the levels/effects of: Sulfonylureas; Vitamin K Antagonists

The levels/effects of Exenatide may be increased by: Pegvisomant

Decreased Effect
The levels/effects of Exenatide may be decreased by: Corticosteroids (Orally Inhaled); Corticosteroids (Systemic); Luteinizing Hormone-Releasing Hormone Analogs; Somatropin; Thiazide Diuretics

Ethanol/Nutrition/Herb Interactions Ethanol: Caution with ethanol (may cause hypoglycemia)

Stability Prior to initial use, store under refrigeration at 2°C to 8°C (36°F to 46°F); after initial use, may be stored at a temperature ≤25°C (≤77°F). Do not freeze (discard if freezing occurs). Protect from light. Pen should be discarded 30 days after initial use.

Mechanism of Action Exenatide is an analog of the hormone incretin (glucagon-like peptide 1 or GLP-1) which increases glucose-dependent insulin secretion, decreases inappropriate glucagon secretion, increases B-cell growth/replication, slows gastric emptying, and decreases food intake. Exenatide administration results in decreases in hemoglobin A_{1c} by approximately 0.5% to 1%.

Pharmacodynamics/Kinetics
Distribution: V_d: 28.3 L
Metabolism: Minimal systemic metabolism; proteolytic degradation may occur following glomerular filtration
Half-life elimination: 2.4 hours
Time to peak, plasma: SubQ: 2.1 hours
Excretion: Urine (majority of dose)

Dosage

Geriatric & Adult Adjunctive therapy of type 2 diabetes: SubQ: Initial: 5 mcg twice daily within 60 minutes prior to a meal; after 1 month, may be increased to 10 mcg twice daily (based on response)

Renal Impairment
Cl_{cr} ≥50 mL/minute: No adjustment necessary.
Cl_{cr} 30-50 mL/minute: Use caution when initiating or escalating doses.
Cl_{cr} <30 mL/minute: Not recommended.

Administration SubQ: Use only if clear, colorless, and free of particulate matter. Administer via injection in the upper arm, thigh, or abdomen. Administer within 60 minutes prior to morning and evening meal (or prior to the 2 main meals of the day, approximately ≥6 hours apart). Set up each new pen before the first use by priming it. See pen user manual for further details. Dial the dose into the dose window before each administration.

Monitoring Parameters Serum glucose, hemoglobin A_{1c}, and renal function

Reference Range Recommendations for glycemic control in adults with diabetes (ADA, 2010):
Hb A_{1c}: <7%
Preprandial capillary plasma glucose: 70-130 mg/dL
Peak postprandial capillary blood glucose: <180 mg/dL

Pharmacotherapy Pearls A dosing strategy which employs progressive dose escalation of exenatide (initiating at 0.02 mcg/kg 3 times daily and increasing in increments of 0.02 mcg/kg every 3 days) has been described, limiting the frequency and severity of gastrointestinal adverse effects. The complexity of this regimen may limit its clinical application.

In animal models, exenatide has been a useful adjunctive therapy when added to immunotherapy protocols, resulting in recovery of beta cell function and sustained remission.

Special Geriatric Considerations Intensive glucose control (HbA$_{1c}$ <6.5%) has been linked to increased all-cause and cardiovascular mortality, hypoglycemia requiring assistance, and weight gain in adult type 2 diabetes. How "tightly" to control a geriatric patient's blood glucose needs to be individualized. Such a decision should be based on several factors, including the patient's functional and cognitive status, how well he/she recognizes hypoglycemic or hyperglycemic symptoms, and how to respond to them and other disease states. An HbA$_{1c}$ <7.5% is an acceptable endpoint for a healthy older adult, while <8% is acceptable for frail elderly patients, those with a duration of illness >10 years, or with those with comorbid conditions and requiring combination diabetes medications. Patients who are unable to accurately draw up their dose will need assistance, such as prefilled syringes. Initial doses may require considerations for renal function in the elderly with dosing adjusted subsequently based on blood glucose monitoring. For elderly patients with diabetes who are relatively healthy, attaining target goals for aspirin use, blood pressure, lipids, smoking cessation, and diet and exercise may be more important than normalized glycemic control.

Dosage Forms Excipient information presented when available (limited, particularly for generics); consult specific product labeling.

Injection, solution:

Byetta®: 250 mcg/mL (2.4 mL) [10 mcg/0.04 mL; 60 doses]

Byetta®: 250 mcg/mL (1.2 mL) [5 mcg/0.02 mL; 60 doses]

Selected References

Action to Control Cardiovascular Risk in Diabetes Study Group, Gerstein HC, Miller ME, et al, "Effects of Intensive Glucose Lowering in Type 2 Diabetes," *N Engl J Med*, 2008, 358(24):2545-59.

ADVANCE Collaborative Group, Patel A, MacMahon S, et al, "Intensive Blood Glucose Control and Vascular Outcomes in Patients With Type 2 Diabetes," *N Engl J Med*, 2008, 358(24):2560-72.

American Diabetes Association, "Standards of Medical Care in Diabetes – 2011," *Diabetes Care*, 2011, 34(Suppl 1):11-61.

Brown AF, Mangione CM, Saliba D, et al, "Guidelines for Improving the Care of the Older Person With Diabetes Mellitus," *J Am Geriatr Soc*, 2003, 51(5 Suppl Guidelines):265-80.

"VA/DoD Clinical Practice Guideline for the Management of Diabetes Mellitus," 2010. Available at http://www.-healthquality.va.gov/Diabetes_Mellitus.asp

Ezetimibe (ez ET i mibe)

Related Information

Hyperlipidemia Management on page 2021

Medication Safety Issues

Sound-alike/look-alike issues:

Zetia® may be confused with Zebeta®, Zestril®

Brand Names: U.S. Zetia®

Brand Names: Canada Ezetrol®

Generic Availability (U.S.) No

Pharmacologic Category Antilipemic Agent, 2-Azetidinone

Use Use in combination with dietary therapy for the treatment of primary hypercholesterolemia (as monotherapy or in combination with HMG-CoA reductase inhibitors); homozygous sitosterolemia; homozygous familial hypercholesterolemia (in combination with atorvastatin or simvastatin); mixed hyperlipidemia (in combination with fenofibrate)

Contraindications Hypersensitivity to ezetimibe or any component of the formulation; concomitant use with an HMG-CoA reductase inhibitor in patients with active hepatic disease, unexplained persistent elevations in serum transaminases

Warnings/Precautions Secondary causes of hyperlipidemia should be ruled out prior to therapy. Use caution with severe renal (Cl_{cr} <30 mL/minute) or mild hepatic impairment (Child-Pugh class A); not recommended for use with moderate or severe hepatic impairment (Child-Pugh classes B and C). Concurrent use of ezetimibe and fibric acid derivatives may increase the risk of cholelithiasis.

Adverse Reactions (Reflective of adult population; not specific for elderly)

1% to 10%:

Central nervous system: Fatigue (2%)

Gastrointestinal: Diarrhea (4%)

Hepatic: Transaminases increased (with HMG-CoA reductase inhibitors) (≥3 x ULN, 1%)

Neuromuscular & skeletal: Arthralgia (3%), pain in extremity (3%)

Respiratory: Upper respiratory tract infection (4%), sinusitis (3%)

Miscellaneous: Influenza (2%)

Drug Interactions

Metabolism/Transport Effects Substrate of SLCO1B1

◀ **Avoid Concomitant Use** There are no known interactions where it is recommended to avoid concomitant use.

Increased Effect/Toxicity

Ezetimibe may increase the levels/effects of: CycloSPORINE; CycloSPORINE (Systemic)

The levels/effects of Ezetimibe may be increased by: CycloSPORINE; CycloSPORINE (Systemic); Eltrombopag; Fibric Acid Derivatives

Decreased Effect

The levels/effects of Ezetimibe may be decreased by: Bile Acid Sequestrants

Ethanol/Nutrition/Herb Interactions Food: Ezetimibe did not cause meaningful reductions in fat-soluble vitamin concentrations during a 2-week clinical trial. Effects of long-term therapy have not been evaluated.

Stability Store at controlled room temperature of 25°C (77°F). Protect from moisture.

Mechanism of Action Inhibits absorption of cholesterol at the brush border of the small intestine via the sterol transporter, Niemann-Pick C1-Like1 (NPC1L1). This leads to a decreased delivery of cholesterol to the liver, reduction of hepatic cholesterol stores and an increased clearance of cholesterol from the blood; decreases total C, LDL-cholesterol (LDL-C), ApoB, and triglycerides (TG) while increasing HDL-cholesterol (HDL-C).

Pharmacodynamics/Kinetics

Protein binding: >90% to plasma proteins

Metabolism: Undergoes glucuronide conjugation in the small intestine and liver; forms metabolite (active); may undergo enterohepatic recycling

Bioavailability: Variable

Half-life elimination: 22 hours (ezetimibe and metabolite)

Time to peak, plasma: 4-12 hours

Excretion: Feces (78%, 69% as ezetimibe); urine (11%, 9% as metabolite)

Dosage

Geriatric & Adult Hyperlipidemias, sitosterolemia: Oral: 10 mg/day

Renal Impairment AUC increased with severe impairment (Cl_{cr} <30 mL/minute); no dosing adjustment recommended.

Hepatic Impairment AUC increased with hepatic impairment:

Mild impairment (Child-Pugh class A): No dosing adjustment necessary.

Moderate-to-severe impairment (Child-Pugh classes B and C): Use of ezetimibe not recommended.

Administration May be administered without regard to meals. May be taken at the same time as HMG-CoA reductase inhibitors. Administer ≥2 hours before or ≥4 hours after bile acid sequestrants.

Monitoring Parameters Total cholesterol profile prior to therapy, and when clinically indicated and/or periodically thereafter. When used in combination with fenofibrate, monitor LFTs and signs and symptoms of cholelithiasis.

Pharmacotherapy Pearls When studied in combination with fenofibrate for mixed hyperlipidemia, the dose of fenofibrate was 160 mg daily.

Special Geriatric Considerations The definition of and, therefore, when to treat hyperlipidemia in the elderly is a controversial issue. The National Cholesterol Education Program recommends that all adults maintain a plasma cholesterol <160 mg/dL. For elderly patients with one additional risk factor, goal LDL would be <130 mg/dL. It is the authors' belief that pharmacologic treatment be reserved for those who are unable to obtain a desirable plasma cholesterol concentration by diet alone and for whom the benefits of treatment are believed to outweigh the potential adverse effects, drug interactions, and cost of treatment.

Dosage Forms Excipient information presented when available (limited, particularly for generics); consult specific product labeling.

Tablet, oral:

Zetia®: 10 mg

Selected References

Grundy SM, Cleeman JI, Merz CN, et al, "Implications of Recent Clinical Trials for the National Cholesterol Education Program Adult Treatment Panel III Guidelines," *J Am Coll Cardiol*, 2004, 44(3):720-32.

National Cholesterol Education Program (NCEP) Expert Panel on Detection, Evaluation, and Treatment of High Blood Cholesterol in Adults (Adult Treatment Panel III), "Third Report of the National Cholesterol Education Program (NCEP) Expert Panel on Detection, Evaluation, and Treatment of High Blood Cholesterol in Adults (Adult Treatment Panel III) Final Report," *Circulation*, 2002, 106(25):3143-421.

Ezetimibe and Simvastatin (ez ET i mibe & SIM va stat in)

Related Information
Ezetimibe *on page 689*
Hyperlipidemia Management *on page 2021*
Simvastatin *on page 1681*
Medication Safety Issues
Sound-alike/look-alike issues:
Vytorin® may be confused with Vyvanse™
Brand Names: U.S. Vytorin®
Index Terms Simvastatin and Ezetimibe
Generic Availability (U.S.) No
Pharmacologic Category Antilipemic Agent, 2-Azetidinone; Antilipemic Agent, HMG-CoA Reductase Inhibitor
Use Used in combination with dietary modification for the treatment of primary hypercholesterolemia and homozygous familial hypercholesterolemia
Dosage
Geriatric & Adult
Note: Dosing limitation: Simvastatin 80 mg is limited to patients that have been taking this dose for >12 consecutive months without evidence of myopathy and are not currently taking or beginning to take a simvastatin dose-limiting or contraindicated interacting medication.
Homozygous familial hypercholesterolemia: Oral: Ezetimibe 10 mg and simvastatin 40 mg once daily in the evening. Dosing range: Ezetimibe 10 mg and simvastatin 10-40 mg once daily.
Hyperlipidemias: Oral: Initial: Ezetimibe 10 mg and simvastatin 20 mg once daily in the evening
Patients who require less aggressive reduction in LDL-C: Initial: Ezetimibe 10 mg and simvastatin 10 mg once daily in the evening
Patients who require >55% reduction in LDL-C: Initial: Ezetimibe 10 mg and simvastatin 40 mg once daily in the evening
Dosage adjustment with concomitant medications: Oral:
Amiodarone, diltiazem, or verapamil: Dose should **not** exceed ezetimibe 10 mg and simvastatin 10 mg once daily
Amlodipine or ranolazine: Dose should **not** exceed ezetimibe 10 mg and simvastatin 20 mg once daily
Dosage adjustment in Chinese patients on niacin doses ≥1 g/day: Oral: Use caution with simvastatin doses exceeding 20 mg/day; because of an increased risk of myopathy, do not administer ezetimibe 10 mg and simvastatin 80 mg
Renal Impairment Dosage adjustment unnecessary in mild-to-moderate renal dysfunction. In severe dysfunction, start only if patient tolerates 5 mg daily of simvastatin; monitor closely.
Hepatic Impairment
Mild impairment: No dosage adjustment required.
Moderate-to-severe impairment: Use not recommended.
Special Geriatric Considerations According to the manufacturer, 32% (3242/10,189) of the patients in the clinical trials were >65 years of age, including 8% who were ≥75 years. The safety observed in this group was similar to the younger patients, although age ≥65 is a risk factor for myopathy. Adding ezetimibe to a statin will decrease LDL-C; however, benefit in event outcomes has not been demonstrated. No dose adjustment is necessary for initiation of treatment in the elderly.
Dosage Forms Excipient information presented when available (limited, particularly for generics); consult specific product labeling.
Tablet:
Vytorin® 10/10: Ezetimibe 10 mg and simvastatin 10 mg
Vytorin® 10/20: Ezetimibe 10 mg and simvastatin 20 mg
Vytorin® 10/40: Ezetimibe 10 mg and simvastatin 40 mg
Vytorin® 10/80: Ezetimibe 10 mg and simvastatin 80 mg

♦ **F₃T** *see* Trifluridine *on page 1864*
♦ **Factive®** *see* Gemifloxacin *on page 814*

Famciclovir (fam SYE kloe veer)

Medication Safety Issues
Sound-alike/look-alike issues:
Famvir® may be confused with Femara®

FAMCICLOVIR

◀ **Brand Names: U.S.** Famvir®

Brand Names: Canada Apo-Famciclovir®; CO Famciclovir; Famvir®; PMS-Famciclovir; Sandoz-Famciclovir

Generic Availability (U.S.) Yes

Pharmacologic Category Antiviral Agent

Use Treatment of acute herpes zoster (shingles); treatment and suppression of recurrent episodes of genital herpes in immunocompetent patients; treatment of herpes labialis (cold sores) in immunocompetent patients; treatment of recurrent mucocutaneous/genital herpes simplex in HIV-infected patients

Contraindications Hypersensitivity to famciclovir, penciclovir, or any component of the formulation

Warnings/Precautions Has not been studied in immunocompromised patients or patients with ophthalmic, disseminated zoster, or with initial episode of genital herpes. Dosage adjustment is required in patients with renal insufficiency. Tablets contain lactose; do not use with galactose intolerance, severe lactase deficiency, or glucose-galactose malabsorption syndromes.

Adverse Reactions (Reflective of adult population; not specific for elderly) Note: Frequencies vary with dose and duration. Single-dose treatment (herpes labialis) was associated only with headache (10%), diarrhea (2%), fatigue (1%), and dysmenorrhea (1%).

>10%:
Central nervous system: Headache (14% to 39%)
Gastrointestinal: Nausea (3% to 13%)
1% to 10%:
Central nervous system: Fatigue (1% to 5%), migraine (1% to 3%)
Dermatologic: Pruritus (≤4%), rash (≤3%)
Endocrine & metabolic: Dysmenorrhea (≤8%)
Gastrointestinal: Diarrhea (5% to 9%), abdominal pain (≤8%), flatulence (1% to 5%), vomiting (1% to 5%)
Hematologic: Neutropenia (3%)
Hepatic: Transaminases increased (2% to 3%), bilirubin increased (2%)
Neuromuscular & skeletal: Paresthesia (≤3%)

Drug Interactions

Avoid Concomitant Use
Avoid concomitant use of Famciclovir with any of the following: Zoster Vaccine

Increased Effect/Toxicity There are no known significant interactions involving an increase in effect.

Decreased Effect
Famciclovir may decrease the levels/effects of: Zoster Vaccine

Ethanol/Nutrition/Herb Interactions Food: Rate of absorption and/or conversion to penciclovir and peak concentration are reduced with food, but bioavailability is not affected.

Stability Store at 25°C (77°F); excursions permitted to 15°C to 30°C (59°F to 86°F).

Mechanism of Action Famciclovir undergoes rapid biotransformation to the active compound, penciclovir (prodrug), which is phosphorylated by viral thymidine kinase in HSV-1, HSV-2, and VZV-infected cells to a monophosphate form; this is then converted to penciclovir triphosphate and competes with deoxyguanosine triphosphate to inhibit HSV-2 polymerase, therefore, herpes viral DNA synthesis/replication is selectively inhibited.

Pharmacodynamics/Kinetics
Absorption: Food decreases maximum peak penciclovir concentration and delays time to penciclovir peak; AUC remains the same
Distribution: V_d: Penciclovir: 0.91-1.25 L/kg
Protein binding: Penciclovir: ≤20%
Metabolism: Famciclovir is rapidly deacetylated and oxidized to penciclovir (active prodrug); not via CYP
Bioavailability: Penciclovir: 69% to 85%
Half-life elimination: Penciclovir: 2-4 hours; Prolonged in renal impairment: Cl_{cr} 20-39 mL/minute: 5-8 hours, Cl_{cr} <20 mL/minute: 3-24 hours
Time to peak: Penciclovir: 0.9 hours; C_{max} and T_{max} are decreased and prolonged with noncompensated hepatic impairment
Excretion: Urine (73% primarily as penciclovir); feces (27%)

Dosage

Geriatric & Adult

Acute herpes zoster: Oral: 500 mg every 8 hours for 7 days (**Note:** Initiate therapy within 72 hours of rash onset.)

Genital herpes simplex virus (HSV) infection in immunocompetent patients: Oral:
Initial episode: 250 mg 3 times/day for 7-10 days (CDC, 2010)
Recurrence: 1000 mg twice daily for 1 day (**Note:** Initiate therapy within 6 hours of symptoms/lesions)
Alternatively, the following regimens are also recommended: 125 mg twice daily for 5 days or 500 mg as a single dose, followed by 250 mg twice daily for 2 days (CDC, 2010)
Suppressive therapy: 250 mg twice daily for up to 1 year; **Note:** Duration not established, but efficacy/safety have been demonstrated for 1 year (CDC, 2010)

Recurrent herpes labialis (cold sores): Oral: 1500 mg as a single dose; initiate therapy at first sign or symptom such as tingling, burning, or itching (initiated within 1 hour in clinical studies)

Recurrent mucocutaneous/genital HSV infection in HIV patients: Oral: 500 mg twice daily for 7 days or 5-10 days (CDC, 2010)

Prevention of HSV reactivation in HIV patients: Oral: 500 mg twice daily (CDC, 2010)

Renal Impairment
Herpes zoster:
Cl_{cr} 40-59 mL/minute: Administer 500 mg every 12 hours
Cl_{cr} 20-39 mL/minute: Administer 500 mg every 24 hours
Cl_{cr} <20 mL/minute: Administer 250 mg every 24 hours
Hemodialysis: Administer 250 mg after each dialysis session.
Recurrent genital herpes: Treatment (single day regimen):
Cl_{cr} 40-59 mL/minute: Administer 500 mg every 12 hours for 1 day
Cl_{cr} 20-39 mL/minute: Administer 500 mg as a single dose
Cl_{cr} <20 mL/minute: Administer 250 mg as a single dose
Hemodialysis: Administer 250 mg as a single dose after dialysis session.
Recurrent genital herpes: Suppression:
Cl_{cr} 20-39 mL/minute: Administer 125 mg every 12 hours
Cl_{cr} <20 mL/minute: Administer 125 mg every 24 hours
Hemodialysis: Administer 125 mg after each dialysis session.
Recurrent herpes labialis: Treatment (single dose regimen):
Cl_{cr} 40-59 mL/minute: Administer 750 mg as a single dose
Cl_{cr} 20-39 mL/minute: Administer 500 mg as a single dose
Cl_{cr} <20 mL/minute: Administer 250 mg as a single dose
Hemodialysis: Administer 250 mg as a single dose after dialysis session.
Recurrent orolabial or genital herpes in HIV-infected patients:
Cl_{cr} 20-39 mL/minute: Administer 500 mg every 24 hours
Cl_{cr} <20 mL/minute: Administer 250 mg every 24 hours
Hemodialysis: Administer 250 mg after each dialysis session.

Administration May be administered without regard to meals.

Monitoring Parameters Periodic CBC during long-term therapy

Pharmacotherapy Pearls Most effective for herpes zoster if therapy is initiated within 48 hours of initial lesion. Resistance may occur by alteration of thymidine kinase, resulting in loss of or reduced penciclovir phosphorylation (cross-resistance occurs between acyclovir and famciclovir). When treatment for herpes labialis is initiated within 1 hour of symptom onset, healing time is reduced by ~2 days.

Special Geriatric Considerations For herpes zoster (shingles) infections, famciclovir should be started within 72 hours of the appearance of the rash to be effective. Famciclovir has been shown to accelerate healing, reduce the duration of viral shedding, and resolve posthepatic neuralgia faster than placebo. Adjust dose for estimated renal function.

Dosage Forms Excipient information presented when available (limited, particularly for generics); consult specific product labeling.
Tablet, oral: 125 mg, 250 mg, 500 mg
Famvir®: 125 mg [contains lactose 26.9 mg/tablet]
Famvir®: 250 mg [contains lactose 53.7 mg/tablet]
Famvir®: 500 mg [contains lactose 107.4 mg/tablet]

Selected References

Pue MA and Benet LZ, "Pharmacokinetics of Famciclovir in Man," *Antivir Chem Chemother*, 1993, 4(Suppl 1):47-55.
Spruance SL, Bodsworth N, Resnick H, et al, "Single-Dose, Patient-Initiated Famciclovir: A Randomized, Double-Blind, Placebo-Controlled Trial for Episodic Treatment of Herpes Labialis," *J Am Acad Dermatol*, 2006, 55(1):47-53.
Tyring S, Barbarash RA, Nahlik JE, et al, "Famciclovir for the Treatment of Acute Herpes Zoster: Effects on Acute Disease and Postherpetic Neuralgia," *Ann Intern Med*, 1995, 123(2):89-96.

Famotidine (fa MOE ti deen)

Medication Safety Issues
Sound-alike/look-alike issues:
Famotidine may be confused with FLUoxetine, furosemide

◀ **Brand Names: U.S.** Heartburn Relief Maximum Strength [OTC]; Heartburn Relief [OTC]; Pepcid®; Pepcid® AC Maximum Strength [OTC]; Pepcid® AC [OTC]

Brand Names: Canada Acid Control; Apo-Famotidine®; Apo-Famotidine® Injectable; Famotidine Omega; Mylan-Famotidine; Novo-Famotidine; Nu-Famotidine; Pepcid®; Pepcid® AC; Pepcid® I.V.; Ulcidine

Generic Availability (U.S.) Yes: Infusion, Injection, oral suspension, tablet

Pharmacologic Category Histamine H$_2$ Antagonist

Use Maintenance therapy and treatment of duodenal ulcer; treatment of gastroesophageal reflux disease (GERD), active benign gastric ulcer; pathological hypersecretory conditions

OTC labeling: Relief of heartburn, acid indigestion, and sour stomach

Unlabeled/Investigational Use Part of a multidrug regimen for *H. pylori* eradication to reduce the risk of duodenal ulcer recurrence; stress ulcer prophylaxis in critically-ill patients; symptomatic relief in gastritis

Contraindications Hypersensitivity to famotidine, other H$_2$ antagonists, or any component of the formulation

Warnings/Precautions Modify dose in patients with moderate-to-severe renal impairment. Prolonged QT interval has been reported in patients with renal dysfunction. The FDA has received reports of torsade de pointes occurring with famotidine (Poluzzi, 2009). Relief of symptoms does not preclude the presence of a gastric malignancy. Reversible confusional states, usually clearing within 3-4 days after discontinuation, have been linked to use. Increased age (>50 years) and renal or hepatic impairment are thought to be associated. Multidose vials for injection contain benzyl alcohol.

OTC labeling: When used for self-medication, patients should be instructed not to use if they have difficulty swallowing, are vomiting blood, or have bloody or black stools. Not for use with other acid reducers.

Adverse Reactions (Reflective of adult population; not specific for elderly)

1% to 10%:

Central nervous system: Headache (5%), dizziness (1%)

Gastrointestinal: Diarrhea (2%), constipation (1%)

Drug Interactions

Avoid Concomitant Use

Avoid concomitant use of Famotidine with any of the following: Delavirdine

Increased Effect/Toxicity

Famotidine may increase the levels/effects of: Dexmethylphenidate; Methylphenidate; Saquinavir; Varenicline

Decreased Effect

Famotidine may decrease the levels/effects of: Atazanavir; Cefditoren; Cefpodoxime; Cefuroxime; Dasatinib; Delavirdine; Erlotinib; Fosamprenavir; Gefitinib; Indinavir; Iron Salts; Itraconazole; Ketoconazole; Ketoconazole (Systemic); Mesalamine; Nelfinavir; Posaconazole; Rilpivirine

Ethanol/Nutrition/Herb Interactions

Ethanol: Avoid ethanol (may cause gastric mucosal irritation).

Food: Famotidine bioavailability may be increased if taken with food.

Stability

Oral:

Powder for oral suspension: Prior to mixing, dry powder should be stored at controlled room temperature of 25°C (77°F). Reconstituted oral suspension is stable for 30 days at room temperature; do not freeze.

Tablet: Store at controlled room temperature. Protect from moisture.

I.V.:

Solution for injection: Prior to use, store at 2°C to 8°C (36°F to 46°F). If solution freezes, allow to solubilize at controlled room temperature. May be stored at room temperature for up to 3 months (data on file [Bedford Laboratories, 2011]).

I.V. push: Dilute famotidine with NS (or another compatible solution) to a total of 5-10 mL (some centers also administer undiluted). Following preparation, solutions for I.V. push should be used immediately, or may be stored in refrigerator and used within 48 hours.

Infusion: Dilute with D$_5$W 100 mL or another compatible solution. Following preparation, the manufacturer states may be stored for up to 48 hours under refrigeration; however, solutions for infusion have been found to be physically and chemically stable for 7 days at room temperature.

Solution for injection, premixed bags: Store at controlled room temperature of 25°C (77°F); avoid excessive heat.

Mechanism of Action Competitive inhibition of histamine at H$_2$ receptors of the gastric parietal cells, which inhibits gastric acid secretion

Pharmacodynamics/Kinetics

Onset of action: Antisecretory effect: Oral: Within 1 hour; I.V.: Within 30 minutes
  Peak effect: Antisecretory effect: Oral: Within 1-3 hours (dose-dependent)
Duration: Antisecretory effect: I.V., Oral: 10-12 hours
Absorption: Oral: Incompletely absorbed
Distribution: V_d: ~1 L/kg
Protein binding: 15% to 20%
Metabolism: Minimal first-pass metabolism; forms one metabolite (S-oxide)
Bioavailability: Oral: 40% to 45%
Half-life elimination: 2.5-3.5 hours; prolonged with renal impairment; Oliguria: >20 hours
Time to peak, serum: Oral: ~1-3 hours
Excretion: Urine (25% to 30% [oral], 65% to 70% [I.V.] as unchanged drug)

Dosage

Geriatric & Adult

Duodenal ulcer: Oral: Acute therapy: 40 mg/day at bedtime (or 20 mg twice daily) for 4-8 weeks; maintenance therapy: 20 mg/day at bedtime

Gastric ulcer: Oral: Acute therapy: 40 mg/day at bedtime

Hypersecretory conditions: Oral: Initial: 20 mg every 6 hours, may increase in increments up to 160 mg every 6 hours

GERD: Oral: 20 mg twice daily for 6 weeks

Esophagitis and accompanying symptoms due to GERD: Oral: 20 mg or 40 mg twice daily for up to 12 weeks

Peptic ulcer disease: Eradication of *Helicobacter pylori* (unlabeled use): Oral: 40 mg once daily; requires combination therapy with antibiotics

Patients unable to take oral medication: I.V.: 20 mg every 12 hours

Heartburn, indigestion, sour stomach: OTC labeling: Oral: 10-20 mg every 12 hours; dose may be taken 15-60 minutes before eating foods known to cause heartburn

Renal Impairment Cl_{cr} <50 mL/minute: Manufacturer recommendation: Administer 50% of dose **or** increase the dosing interval to every 36-48 hours (to limit potential CNS adverse effects).

Administration

I.V. push: Inject over at least 2 minutes
Solution for infusion: Administer over 15-30 minutes

Monitoring Parameters Signs and symptoms of peptic ulcer disease, occult blood with GI bleeding, gastric pH where necessary; monitor renal function to correct dose; monitor for side effects

Pharmacotherapy Pearls The expensive parenteral route should only be used when a patient is unable to take oral medication

Special Geriatric Considerations H_2 blockers are the preferred drugs for treating PUD in the elderly due to cost and ease of administration. They are no less or more effective than any other therapy. Famotidine is one of the preferred agents (due to side effects, drug interaction profile, and pharmacokinetics). Treatment for PUD in the elderly is recommended for 12 weeks since their lesions are typically larger; therefore, take longer to heal. Always adjust dose based upon creatinine clearance, since slight accumulation may result in CNS side effects, mainly confusion.

Dosage Forms Excipient information presented when available (limited, particularly for generics); consult specific product labeling.

Infusion, premixed in NS [preservative free]: 20 mg (50 mL)
Injection, solution: 10 mg/mL (4 mL, 20 mL, 50 mL)
Injection, solution [preservative free]: 10 mg/mL (2 mL)
Powder for suspension, oral: 40 mg/5 mL (50 mL)
  Pepcid®: 40 mg/5 mL (50 mL) [contains sodium benzoate; cherry-banana-mint flavor]
Tablet, oral: 10 mg, 20 mg, 40 mg
  Heartburn Relief: 10 mg
  Heartburn Relief Maximum Strength: 20 mg
  Pepcid®: 20 mg, 40 mg
  Pepcid® AC: 10 mg
  Pepcid® AC Maximum Strength: 20 mg
Tablet, chewable, oral:
  Pepcid® AC Maximum Strength: 20 mg [berries 'n' cream flavor]
  Pepcid® AC Maximum Strength: 20 mg [cool mint flavor]

Famotidine, Calcium Carbonate, and Magnesium Hydroxide
(fa MOE ti deen, KAL see um KAR bun ate, & mag NEE zhum hye DROKS ide)

Related Information
  Famotidine *on page 693*
  Magnesium Hydroxide *on page 1109*
Brand Names: U.S. Pepcid® Complete® [OTC]; Tums® Dual Action [OTC]
Brand Names: Canada Pepcid® Complete® [OTC]
Index Terms Calcium Carbonate, Magnesium Hydroxide, and Famotidine; Magnesium Hydroxide, Famotidine, and Calcium Carbonate
Generic Availability (U.S.) No
Pharmacologic Category Antacid; Histamine H_2 Antagonist
Use Relief of heartburn due to acid indigestion
Dosage
  Geriatric & Adult Relief of heartburn due to acid indigestion: Oral: Pepcid® Complete: 1 tablet as needed; no more than 2 tablets in 24 hours; do **not** swallow whole, chew tablet completely before swallowing; do not use for longer than 14 days
  Special Geriatric Considerations Use with caution in the elderly with reduced renal function (Cl_{cr} <30 mL/minute), since accumulation of magnesium and famotidine may occur and potentiate side effects
  Dosage Forms Excipient information presented when available (limited, particularly for generics); consult specific product labeling.
  Tablet, chewable, oral:
    Pepcid® Complete®: Famotidine 10 mg, calcium carbonate 800 mg, and magnesium hydroxide 165 mg [contains calcium 320 mg/tablet, magnesium 70 mg/tablet; berry flavor]
    Pepcid® Complete®: Famotidine 10 mg, calcium carbonate 800 mg, and magnesium hydroxide 165 mg [contains calcium 320 mg/tablet, magnesium 70 mg/tablet; mint flavor]
    Pepcid® Complete®: Famotidine 10 mg, calcium carbonate 800 mg, and magnesium hydroxide 165 mg [contains calcium 320 mg/tablet, magnesium 70 mg/tablet, tartrazine; tropical fruit flavor]
    Tums® Dual Action: Famotidine 10 mg, calcium carbonate 800 mg, and magnesium hydroxide 165 mg [contains calcium 320 mg/tablet, magnesium 65 mg/tablet, phenylalanine 2.2 mg/tablet; berry flavor]
    Tums® Dual Action: Famotidine 10 mg, calcium carbonate 800 mg, and magnesium hydroxide 165 mg [contains calcium 320 mg/tablet, magnesium 65 mg/tablet, phenylalanine 2.2 mg/tablet; mint flavor]

◆ **Fampridine-SR** *see* Dalfampridine *on page 444*
◆ **Famvir®** *see* Famciclovir *on page 691*
◆ **Fanapt®** *see* Iloperidone *on page 913*
◆ **Fareston®** *see* Toremifene *on page 1835*
◆ **Faslodex®** *see* Fulvestrant *on page 799*
◆ **Father John's® [OTC]** *see* Dextromethorphan *on page 490*
◆ **FazaClo®** *see* CloZAPine *on page 402*
◆ **5-FC** *see* Flucytosine *on page 744*
◆ **FC1157a** *see* Toremifene *on page 1835*
◆ **FE200486** *see* Degarelix *on page 465*

Febuxostat (feb UX oh stat)

Brand Names: U.S. Uloric®
Brand Names: Canada Uloric®
Index Terms TEI-6720; TMX-67
Generic Availability (U.S.) No
Pharmacologic Category Antigout Agent; Xanthine Oxidase Inhibitor
Use Chronic management of hyperuricemia in patients with gout
Contraindications Concurrent use with azathioprine or mercaptopurine

  Canadian labeling: Additional contraindications (not in U.S. labeling): Hypersensitivity to febuxostat or any component of the formulation; concomitant administration with theophylline
Warnings/Precautions Administer concurrently with an NSAID or colchicine (up to 6 months) to prevent gout flare upon initiation of therapy. Do not use to treat asymptomatic or secondary hyperuricemia. Significant hepatic transaminase elevations (>3 x ULN), MI, stroke and cardiovascular deaths have been reported in controlled trials (causal relationship not established). Monitor patients for signs/symptoms of MI and stroke. Liver function tests should be monitored 2 and 4 months after initiation of therapy and then periodically. Use with caution in

patients with severe hepatic impairment (Child-Pugh class C); not studied. Use with caution in patients with severe renal impairment (Cl$_{cr}$ <30 mL/minute); insufficient data.

Adverse Reactions (Reflective of adult population; not specific for elderly)
1% to 10%:
Dermatologic: Rash (1% to 2%)
Hepatic: Liver function abnormalities (5% to 7%)
Neuromuscular & skeletal: Arthralgia (1%)

Drug Interactions

Avoid Concomitant Use
Avoid concomitant use of Febuxostat with any of the following: AzaTHIOprine; Didanosine; Mercaptopurine

Increased Effect/Toxicity
Febuxostat may increase the levels/effects of: AzaTHIOprine; Didanosine; Mercaptopurine; Theophylline Derivatives

Decreased Effect There are no known significant interactions involving a decrease in effect.

Stability Store at 25°C (77°F); excursions permitted to 15°C to 30°C (59°F to 86°F). Protect from light.

Mechanism of Action Selectively inhibits xanthine oxidase, the enzyme responsible for the conversion of hypoxanthine to xanthine to uric acid thereby decreasing uric acid. At therapeutic concentration does not inhibit other enzymes involved in purine and pyrimidine synthesis.

Pharmacodynamics/Kinetics
Absorption: ≥49%
Distribution: V$_{ss}$: ~50 L
Protein binding: ~99%, primarily to albumin
Metabolism: Extensive conjugation via uridine diphosphate glucuronosyltransferases (UGTs) 1A1, 1A3, 1A9, and 2B7 and oxidation via cytochrome P450 (CYP) 1A2, 2C8, and 2C9 as well as non-P450 enzymes. Oxidation leads to formation of active metabolites (67M-1, 67M-2, 67M-4)
Half-life elimination: ~5-8 hours
Time to peak, plasma: 1-1.5 hours
Excretion: Urine (~49% mostly as metabolites, 3% as unchanged drug); feces (~45% mostly as metabolites, 12% as unchanged drug)

Dosage

Geriatric & Adult Management of hyperuricemia in patients with gout: Note: It is recommended to take an NSAID or colchicine with initiation of therapy and may continue for up to 6 months to help prevent gout flares. If a gout flare occurs, febuxostat does not need to be discontinued.
Oral:
U.S. labeling: Initial: 40 mg once daily; may increase to 80 mg once daily in patients who do not achieve a serum uric acid level <6 mg/dL after 2 weeks
Canadian labeling: 80 mg once daily

Renal Impairment
Mild-to-moderate impairment (Cl$_{cr}$ 30-89 mL/minute): No adjustment needed
Severe impairment (Cl$_{cr}$ <30 mL/minute): Insufficient data; use caution (use not recommended in the Canadian labeling)
Dialysis: Not studied (use not recommended in the Canadian labeling)

Hepatic Impairment
Mild-to-moderate impairment (Child-Pugh classes A and B): No adjustment needed
Severe impairment (Child-Pugh class C): Not studied; use caution (use not recommended in the Canadian labeling)

Administration Administer with or without meals or antacids.

Monitoring Parameters Liver function tests 2 and 4 months after initiation and then periodically, serum uric acid levels (as early as 2 weeks after initiation)

Reference Range Uric acid, serum:
Adults:
Male: 3.4-7 mg/dL or slightly more
Female: 2.4-6 mg/dL or slightly more
Target: <6 mg/dL
Values >7 mg/dL are sometimes arbitrarily regarded as hyperuricemia, but there is no sharp line between normals on the one hand, and the serum uric acid of those with clinical gout. Normal ranges cannot be adjusted for purine ingestion, but high purine diet increases uric acid. Uric acid may be increased with body size, exercise, and stress.

Special Geriatric Considerations In clinical trials, no clinically significant differences in safety or effectiveness were observed in elderly subjects. See Dosage: Renal Impairment.

◀ **Dosage Forms** Excipient information presented when available (limited, particularly for generics); consult specific product labeling.
Tablet, oral:
Uloric® 40 mg, 80 mg
Selected References
Bruce SP, "Febuxostat: A Selective Xanthine Oxidase Inhibitor for the Treatment of Hyperuricemia and Gout," *Ann Pharmacother,* 2006, 40(12):2187-94.

Felbamate (FEL ba mate)

Brand Names: U.S. Felbatol®
Generic Availability (U.S.) No
Pharmacologic Category Anticonvulsant, Miscellaneous
Use Not as a first-line antiepileptic treatment; only in those patients who respond inadequately to alternative treatments and whose epilepsy is so severe that a substantial risk of aplastic anemia and/or liver failure is deemed acceptable in light of the benefits conferred by its use. Patient must be fully advised of risk and provide signed written informed consent. Felbamate can be used as either monotherapy or adjunctive therapy in the treatment of partial seizures (with and without generalization) and in adults with epilepsy.
Prescribing and Access Restrictions A patient "informed consent" form should be completed and signed by the patient and physician. Copies are available from MEDA Pharmaceuticals by calling 800-526-3840.
Contraindications Hypersensitivity to felbamate any component of the formulation; or known sensitivity to other carbamates; history of any blood dyscrasia; hepatic dysfunction
Warnings/Precautions Use with caution in patients allergic to other carbamates (eg, meprobamate); antiepileptic drugs should not be suddenly discontinued because of the possibility of increasing seizure frequency. Antiepileptics are associated with an increased risk of suicidal behavior/thoughts with use (regardless of indication); patients should be monitored for signs/symptoms of depression, suicidal tendencies, and other unusual behavior changes during therapy and instructed to inform their healthcare provider immediately if symptoms occur. **[U.S. Boxed Warning]: Felbamate is associated with an increased risk of aplastic anemia. [U.S. Boxed Warning]: Felbamate has been associated with rare cases of hepatic failure (estimated >6 cases per 75,000 patients per year).** Do not initiate treatment in patients with pre-existing hepatic dysfunction. Use caution in renal impairment (dose adjustment recommended). "Informed consent" (concerning hematological/hepatic risks) should be documented prior to initiation of therapy. Effects with other sedative drugs or ethanol may be potentiated.
Adverse Reactions (Reflective of adult population; not specific for elderly)
>10%:
Central nervous system: Somnolence (children 48%; adults 19%), headache (children 7%; adults 7% to 37%), fever (children 23%; adults 3%), dizziness (18%), insomnia (9% to 18%), fatigue (7% to 17%), nervousness (7% to 16%)
Dermatologic: Purpura (children 13%)
Gastrointestinal: Anorexia (children 55%; adults 19%), vomiting (children 39%; adults 9% to 17%), nausea (children 7%; adults 34%), constipation (7% to 13%), dyspepsia (7% to 12%)
Respiratory: Upper respiratory infection (children 45%; adults 5% to 9%)
1% to 10%:
Cardiovascular: Chest pain (3%), facial edema (3%), palpitation (≥1%), tachycardia (≥1%)
Central nervous system: Nervousness (7% to 16%), abnormal thinking (7%), emotional lability (children 7%), ataxia (4% to 7%), depression (5%), anxiety (5%), stupor (3%), malaise (≥1%), agitation (≥1%), psychological disturbances (≥1%), aggressive reaction (≥1%), euphoria (≤1%), hallucination (≤1%), migraine (≤1%), suicide attempt (≤1%)
Dermatologic: Skin rash (children 10%; adults 3% to 4%), acne (3%), pruritus (≥1%), bullous eruption (≤1%), urticaria (≤1%)
Endocrine and metabolic: Hypophosphatemia (≤1% to 3%), intramenstrual bleeding (3%), hypokalemia (≤1%), hyponatremia (≤1%)
Gastrointestinal: Hiccup (children 10%), weight loss (3% to 7%), taste perversion (6%), diarrhea (5%), abdominal pain (5%), xerostomia (3%), weight gain (≥1%), appetite increased (≤1%), esophagitis (≤1%)
Genitourinary: Urinary tract infection (3%)
Hematologic: Leukopenia (1% to 7%), granulocytopenia (≤1%), lymphadenopathy (≤1%), leukocytosis (≤1%), thrombocytopenia (≤1%)
Hepatic: Liver function tests increased (1% to 4%), alkaline phosphatase increased (≤1%)
Neuromuscular & skeletal: Abnormal gait (children 10%; adults 5%), pain (children 7%), tremor (6%), paresthesia (4%), myalgia (3%), weakness (≥1%), dystonia (≤1%)
Ocular: Miosis (7%), diplopia (3% to 6%), abnormal vision (5%)

Otic: Otitis media (children 10%; adults 3%)
Respiratory: Pharyngitis (children 10%; adults 3%), cough (children 7%), rhinitis (7%), sinusitis (4%)
Miscellaneous: Flu-like syndrome (≥1%), lymphadenopathy (≥1%)

Drug Interactions

Metabolism/Transport Effects Substrate of CYP2E1 (minor), 3A4 (major); **Inhibits** CYP2C19 (weak); **Induces** CYP3A4 (weak)

Avoid Concomitant Use

Avoid concomitant use of Felbamate with any of the following: Conivaptan

Increased Effect/Toxicity

Felbamate may increase the levels/effects of: Alcohol (Ethyl); Barbiturates; CNS Depressants; Divalproex; Fosphenytoin; Methotrimeprazine; PHENobarbital; Phenytoin; Primidone; Selective Serotonin Reuptake Inhibitors; Valproic Acid

The levels/effects of Felbamate may be increased by: Conivaptan; CYP3A4 Inhibitors (Moderate); CYP3A4 Inhibitors (Strong); Dasatinib; Droperidol; HydrOXYzine; Methotrimeprazine

Decreased Effect

Felbamate may decrease the levels/effects of: CarBAMazepine; Contraceptives (Estrogens); Contraceptives (Progestins); Saxagliptin

The levels/effects of Felbamate may be decreased by: Barbiturates; CarBAMazepine; CYP3A4 Inducers (Strong); Cyproterone; Deferasirox; Fosphenytoin; Herbs (CYP3A4 Inducers); Ketorolac; Ketorolac (Nasal); Ketorolac (Systemic); Mefloquine; PHENobarbital; Phenytoin; Primidone; Tocilizumab

Ethanol/Nutrition/Herb Interactions

Ethanol: May increase CNS depression; monitor for increased effects with coadministration. Caution patients about effects.
Food: Food does not affect absorption.
Herb/Nutraceutical: Avoid evening primrose (seizure threshold decreased).

Stability Store in tightly closed container at controlled room temperature of 20°C to 25°C (68°F to 77°F).

Mechanism of Action Mechanism of action is unknown but has properties in common with other marketed anticonvulsants; has weak inhibitory effects on GABA-receptor binding, benzodiazepine receptor binding, and is devoid of activity at the MK-801 receptor binding site of the NMDA receptor-ionophore complex.

Pharmacodynamics/Kinetics Geriatrics: Reduced clearance and prolonged half-life have been reported in persons 66-78 years of age, compared to persons 18-45 years of age.

Absorption: Rapid and almost complete; food has no effect upon the tablet's absorption
Distribution: V_d: 0.7-0.8 L/kg
Protein binding: 22% to 25%, primarily to albumin
Half-life: 20-23 hours (average); prolonged in renal dysfunction
Time to peak, serum: 3-5 hours
Elimination: Urine (40% to 50% as unchanged drug, 40% as inactive metabolites)

Dosage

Geriatric & Adult

Anticonvulsant, monotherapy: Oral:

Initial: 1200 mg/day in divided doses 3 or 4 times/day; titrate previously untreated patients under close clinical supervision, increasing the dosage in 600 mg increments every 2 weeks to 2400 mg/day based on clinical response and thereafter to 3600 mg/day as clinically indicated

Conversion to monotherapy: Initiate at 1200 mg/day in divided doses 3 or 4 times/day, reduce the dosage of the concomitant anticonvulsant(s) by 20% to 33% at the initiation of felbamate therapy; at week 2, increase the felbamate dosage to 2400 mg/day while reducing the dosage of the other anticonvulsant(s) up to an additional 33% of their original dosage; at week 3, increase the felbamate dosage up to 3600 mg/day and continue to reduce the dosage of the other anticonvulsant(s) as clinically indicated

Anticonvulsant, adjunctive therapy: Oral: Initial: 1200 mg/day in divided doses 3 or 4 times/day; may increase once per week by 1200 mg/day increments up to 3600 mg/day in divided doses 3 or 4 times/day.

Note: Dose of concomitant carbamazepine, phenobarbital, phenytoin, or valproic acid should be decreased by 20% to 33% when initiating felbamate therapy. Further dosage reductions may be necessary as dose of felbamate is increased.

Renal Impairment Use caution; reduce initial and maintenance doses by 50% (half-life prolonged by 9-15 hours)

Administration Administer on an empty stomach for best absorption.

◀ **Monitoring Parameters** Monitor serum levels of concomitant anticonvulsant therapy; obtain transaminases (AST, ALT) levels before initiation of therapy and periodically thereafter and bilirubin weekly. Hematologic evaluations before therapy begins, frequently during therapy, and for a significant period after discontinuation. Monitor for suicidality (eg, suicidal thoughts, depression, behavioral changes).

Reference Range Not necessary to routinely monitor serum drug levels, since dose should be titrated to clinical response

Pharmacotherapy Pearls Monotherapy has not been associated with gingival hyperplasia, impaired concentration, weight gain, or abnormal thinking. Because felbamate is the only drug shown effective in Lennox-Gastaut syndrome, it is considered an orphan drug for this indication.

Special Geriatric Considerations Clinical studies have not included large numbers of patients >65 years of age. Due to decreased hepatic and renal function, dosing should start at the lower end of the dosage range.

Dosage Forms Excipient information presented when available (limited, particularly for generics); consult specific product labeling.
Suspension, oral:
Felbatol®: 600 mg/5 mL (240 mL, 960 mL)
Tablet, oral:
Felbatol®: 400 mg, 600 mg [scored]

◆ **Felbatol®** see Felbamate on page 698
◆ **Feldene®** see Piroxicam on page 1469

Felodipine (fe LOE di peen)

Related Information
Calcium Channel Blockers on page 2003
Medication Safety Issues
Sound-alike/look-alike issues:
Plendil may be confused with Isordil®, pindolol, Pletal®, PriLOSEC®, Prinivil®
Brand Names: Canada Plendil®; Renedil®; Sandoz-Felodipine
Index Terms Plendil
Generic Availability (U.S.) Yes
Pharmacologic Category Calcium Channel Blocker; Calcium Channel Blocker, Dihydropyridine
Use Treatment of hypertension
Contraindications Hypersensitivity to felodipine, any component of the formulation, or other calcium channel blocker
Warnings/Precautions Increased angina and/or MI has occurred with initiation or dosage titration of dihydropyridine calcium channel blockers, reflex tachycardia may occur resulting in angina and/or MI in patients with obstructive coronary disease especially in the absence of concurrent beta-blockade. Use with extreme caution in patients with severe aortic stenosis. Use caution in patients with heart failure and/or hypertrophic cardiomyopathy with outflow tract obstruction. Elderly patients and patients with hepatic impairment should start off with a lower dose. Peripheral edema (dose dependent) is the most common side effect (occurs within 2-3 weeks of starting therapy). Symptomatic hypotension with or without syncope can rarely occur; blood pressure must be lowered at a rate appropriate for the patient's clinical condition. Dosage titration should occur after 14 days on a given dose.
Adverse Reactions (Reflective of adult population; not specific for elderly)
>10%: Central nervous system: Headache (11% to 15%)
2% to 10%: Cardiovascular: Peripheral edema (2% to 17%), tachycardia (0.4% to 2.5%), flushing (4% to 7%)
Drug Interactions
Metabolism/Transport Effects Substrate of CYP3A4 (major); **Inhibits** CYP2C8 (moderate), 2C9 (weak), 2D6 (weak), 3A4 (weak)
Avoid Concomitant Use
Avoid concomitant use of Felodipine with any of the following: Conivaptan
Increased Effect/Toxicity
Felodipine may increase the levels/effects of: Amifostine; Antihypertensives; Beta-Blockers; Calcium Channel Blockers (Nondihydropyridine); CYP2C8 Substrates (High risk); Fosphenytoin; Hypotensive Agents; Magnesium Salts; Neuromuscular-Blocking Agents (Nondepolarizing); Nitroprusside; Phenytoin; RiTUXimab; Tacrolimus; Tacrolimus (Systemic)

The levels/effects of Felodipine may be increased by: Alpha1-Blockers; Antifungal Agents (Azole Derivatives, Systemic); Calcium Channel Blockers (Nondihydropyridine); Cimetidine; Conivaptan; CycloSPORINE; CycloSPORINE (Systemic); CYP3A4 Inhibitors (Moderate);

CYP3A4 Inhibitors (Strong); Dasatinib; Diazoxide; Fluconazole; Grapefruit Juice; Herbs (Hypotensive Properties); Macrolide Antibiotics; Magnesium Salts; MAO Inhibitors; Pentoxifylline; Phosphodiesterase 5 Inhibitors; Prostacyclin Analogues; Protease Inhibitors

Decreased Effect

Felodipine may decrease the levels/effects of: Clopidogrel

The levels/effects of Felodipine may be decreased by: Barbiturates; Calcium Salts; CarBAMazepine; CYP3A4 Inducers (Strong); Deferasirox; Herbs (CYP3A4 Inducers); Herbs (Hypertensive Properties); Methylphenidate; Nafcillin; Rifamycin Derivatives; Tocilizumab; Yohimbine

Ethanol/Nutrition/Herb Interactions

Ethanol: Increases felodipine's absorption; watch for a greater hypotensive effect.

Food: Increased therapeutic and vasodilator side effects, including severe hypotension and myocardial ischemia, may occur if felodipine is taken with grapefruit juice; avoid concurrent use. High-fat/carbohydrate meals will increase C_{max} by 60%; grapefruit juice will increase C_{max} by twofold.

Herb/Nutraceutical: St John's wort may decrease felodipine levels. Avoid dong quai if using for hypertension (has estrogenic activity). Avoid ephedra, yohimbe, ginseng (may worsen hypertension). Avoid garlic (may have increased antihypertensive effect).

Mechanism of Action Inhibits calcium ions from entering the "slow channels" or select voltage-sensitive areas of vascular smooth muscle and myocardium during depolarization, producing a relaxation of coronary vascular smooth muscle and coronary vasodilation; increases myocardial oxygen delivery in patients with vasospastic angina

Pharmacodynamics/Kinetics

Onset of action: Antihypertensive: 2-5 hours

Duration of antihypertensive effect: 24 hours

Absorption: 100%; Absolute: 20% due to first-pass effect

Protein binding: >99%

Metabolism: Hepatic; CYP3A4 substrate (major); extensive first-pass effect

Half-life elimination: Immediate release: 11-16 hours

Excretion: Urine (70% as metabolites); feces 10%

Dosage

Geriatric Refer to adult dosing. In the management of hypertension, consider lower initial doses (eg, 2.5 mg once daily) and titrate to response (Aronow, 2011).

Adult Hypertension: Oral: 2.5-10 mg once daily; increase by 5 mg at 2-week intervals, as needed, to a maximum of 20 mg/day; usual dose range (JNC 7): 2.5-20 mg once daily.

Hepatic Impairment Initial: 2.5 mg/day; monitor blood pressure

Administration Do not crush or chew extended release tablets; swallow whole.

Monitoring Parameters Heart rate, blood pressure

Pharmacotherapy Pearls Felodipine maintains renal and mesenteric blood flow during hemorrhagic shock in animals.

Special Geriatric Considerations Elderly may experience a greater hypotensive response. Constipation may be more of a problem in the elderly. Calcium channel blockers are no more effective in the elderly than other therapies; however, they do not cause significant CNS effects which is an advantage over some antihypertensive agents.

Dosage Forms Excipient information presented when available (limited, particularly for generics); consult specific product labeling.

Tablet, extended release, oral: 2.5 mg, 5 mg, 10 mg

Selected References

Chobanian AV, Bakris GL, Black HR, et al, "The Seventh Report of the Joint National Committee on Prevention, Detection, Evaluation, and Treatment of High Blood Pressure: The JNC 7 Report," *JAMA*, 2003, 289(19):2560-71.

Fenofibrate (fen oh FYE brate)

Related Information

Hyperlipidemia Management *on page 2021*

Medication Safety Issues

Sound-alike/look-alike issues:

TriCor® may be confused with Fibricor®, Tracleer®

Brand Names: U.S. Antara®; Fenoglide®; Lipofen®; Lofibra®; TriCor®; Triglide®

◀ **Brand Names: Canada** Apo-Feno-Micro®; Apo-Feno-Super®; Apo-Fenofibrate®; Dom-Fenofibrate Micro; Feno-Micro-200; Fenofibrate Micro; Fenofibrate-S; Fenomax; Lipidil EZ®; Lipidil Micro®; Lipidil Supra®; Mylan-Fenofibrate Micro; Novo-Fenofibrate; Novo-Fenofibrate Micronized; Novo-Fenofibrate-S; Nu-Fenofibrate; PHL-Fenofibrate Micro; PHL-Fenofibrate Supra; PMS-Fenofibrate Micro; PRO-Feno-Super; ratio-Fenofibrate MC; Riva-Fenofibrate Micro; Sandoz-Fenofibrate S

Index Terms Procetofene; Proctofene

Generic Availability (U.S.) Yes: Micronized capsule and tablet

Pharmacologic Category Antilipemic Agent, Fibric Acid

Use Adjunct to dietary therapy for the treatment of adults with elevations of serum triglyceride levels (types IV and V hyperlipidemia); adjunct to dietary therapy for the reduction of low density lipoprotein cholesterol (LDL-C), total cholesterol (total-C), triglycerides, and apolipoprotein B (apo B), and to increase high density lipoprotein cholesterol (HDL-C) in adult patients with primary hypercholesterolemia or mixed dyslipidemia (Fredrickson types IIa and IIb)

Contraindications Hypersensitivity to fenofibrate or any component of the formulation; hepatic dysfunction including primary biliary cirrhosis and unexplained persistent liver function abnormalities; severe renal dysfunction; pre-existing gallbladder disease

Canadian labeling: Additional contraindications (not in U.S. labeling): Known photoallergy or phototoxic reaction during treatment with fibrates or ketoprofen; allergy to soya lecithin or peanut or arachis oil

Warnings/Precautions Secondary causes of hyperlipidemia should be ruled out prior to therapy. Hepatic transaminases can become significantly elevated (dose-related); hepatocellular, chronic active, and cholestatic hepatitis have been reported. Regular monitoring of liver function tests is required. Increases in serum creatinine (>2 mg/dL) have been observed with use; monitor renal function in patients with renal impairment and consider monitoring patients with increased risk for developing renal impairment. May cause cholelithiasis. Use with caution in patient taking oral anticoagulants (eg, warfarin); adjustments in anticoagulation therapy may be required. Use caution with HMG-CoA reductase inhibitors (may lead to myopathy, rhabdomyolysis). In combination with HMG-CoA reductase inhibitors, fenofibrate is generally regarded as safer than gemfibrozil due to limited pharmacokinetic interaction with statins. Therapy should be withdrawn if an adequate response is not obtained after 2-3 months of therapy at the maximal daily dose. The occurrence of pancreatitis may represent a failure of efficacy in patients with severely elevated triglycerides. May cause mild-to-moderate decreases in hemoglobin, hematocrit, and WBC upon initiation of therapy which usually stabilizes with long-term therapy. Agranulocytosis and thrombocytopenia have rarely been reported. Periodic monitoring of blood counts is recommended during the first year of therapy.

Rare hypersensitivity reactions may occur. Use has been associated with pulmonary embolism (PE) and deep vein thrombosis (DVT). Use with caution in patients with risk factors for VTE. Dose adjustment is required for renal impairment and may be required for elderly patients.

Adverse Reactions (Reflective of adult population; not specific for elderly)
>10%: Hepatic: Liver function tests increased (dose related; 3% to 13%)
1% to 10%:
  Central nervous system: Headache (3%)
  Gastrointestinal: Abdominal pain (5%), constipation (2%), nausea (2%)
  Neuromuscular & skeletal: Back pain (3%), CPK increased (3%)
  Respiratory: Respiratory disorder (6%), rhinitis (2%)

Drug Interactions

  Metabolism/Transport Effects Substrate of CYP3A4 (minor); **Inhibits** CYP2A6 (weak), 2C8 (weak), 2C9 (weak), 2C19 (weak)

  Avoid Concomitant Use There are no known interactions where it is recommended to avoid concomitant use.

  Increased Effect/Toxicity

    Fenofibrate may increase the levels/effects of: Colchicine; Ezetimibe; HMG-CoA Reductase Inhibitors; Sulfonylureas; Vitamin K Antagonists; Warfarin

    The levels/effects of Fenofibrate may be increased by: Conivaptan; CycloSPORINE; CycloSPORINE (Systemic)

  Decreased Effect

    Fenofibrate may decrease the levels/effects of: Chenodiol; CycloSPORINE; CycloSPORINE (Systemic); Ursodiol

    The levels/effects of Fenofibrate may be decreased by: Bile Acid Sequestrants; Tocilizumab

Stability Store at 15°C to 30°C (59°F to 86°F). Protect from light and moisture. Store tablets in moisture-protective container.

Mechanism of Action Fenofibric acid, an agonist for the nuclear transcription factor peroxisome proliferator-activated receptor-alpha (PPAR-alpha), downregulates apoprotein C-III (an inhibitor of lipoprotein lipase) and upregulates the synthesis of apolipoprotein A-I, fatty acid transport protein, and lipoprotein lipase resulting in an increase in VLDL catabolism, fatty acid oxidation, and elimination of triglyceride-rich particles; as a result of a decrease in VLDL levels, total plasma triglycerides are reduced by 30% to 60%; modest increase in HDL occurs in some hypertriglyceridemic patients.

Pharmacodynamics/Kinetics

Absorption: Increased when taken with meals

Distribution: Widely to most tissues

Protein binding: >99%

Metabolism: Tissue and plasma via esterases to active form, fenofibric acid; undergoes inactivation by glucuronidation hepatically or renally

Half-life elimination: Fenofibric acid: Mean: 20 hours (range: 10-35 hours)

Time to peak: 3-8 hours

Excretion: Urine (60% as metabolites); feces (25%); hemodialysis has no effect on removal of fenofibric acid from plasma

Dosage

Geriatric Oral: Initial:

Antara® (micronized): 43 mg/day

Fenoglide®: Adjust dosage based on creatinine clearance

Lipidil EZ® [CAN; not available in U.S.]: 48 mg/day

Lipidil Micro® [CAN; not available in U.S.]: Adjust dosage based on creatinine clearance

Lipidil Supra® [CAN; not available in U.S.]: Adjust dosage based on creatinine clearance

Lipofen®: 50 mg/day

Lofibra® (micronized): 67 mg/day

Lofibra® (tablets): 54 mg/day

TriCor®: Adjust dosage based on creatinine clearance

Triglide®: 50 mg/day

Adult

Hypertriglyceridemia: Oral Initial:

Antara® (micronized): 43-130 mg/day; maximum dose: 130 mg/day

Fenoglide®: 40-120 mg/day; maximum dose: 120 mg/day

Lipidil EZ® [CAN; not available in U.S.]: 145 mg/day; maximum dose: 145 mg/day

Lipidil Micro® [CAN; not available in U.S.]: 200 mg/day; maximum dose: 200 mg/day

Lipidil Supra® [CAN; not available in U.S.]: 160 mg/day; maximum dose: 200 mg/day

Lipofen®: 50-150 mg/day; maximum dose: 150 mg/day

Lofibra® (micronized): 67-200 mg/day with meals; maximum dose: 200 mg/day

Lofibra® (tablets): 54-160 mg/day; maximum dose: 160 mg/day

TriCor®: 48-145 mg/day; maximum dose: 145 mg/day

Triglide®: 50-160 mg/day; maximum dose: 160 mg/day

Hypercholesterolemia or mixed hyperlipidemia: Oral:

Antara® (micronized): 130 mg/day

Fenoglide®: 120 mg/day

Lipidil EZ® [CAN; not available in U.S.]: 145 mg/day; maximum dose: 145 mg/day

Lipidil Micro® [CAN; not available in U.S.]: 200 mg/day; maximum dose: 200 mg/day

Lipidil Supra® [CAN; not available in U.S.]: 160 mg/day; maximum dose: 200 mg/day

Lipofen®: 150 mg/day

Lofibra® (micronized): 200 mg/day

Lofibra® (tablets): 160 mg/day

TriCor®: 145 mg/day

Triglide®: 160 mg/day

Renal Impairment Monitor renal function and lipid panel before adjusting. Decrease dose or increase dosing interval for patients with renal failure: **Note:** Use in severe renal impairment is contraindicated (see specific product labeling):

Antara® (micronized): 43 mg/day

Fenoglide®: Cl_{cr} 31-80 mL/minute: 40 mg/day

Lipidil EZ® [CAN; not available in U.S.]: Cl_{cr} ≥20-50 mL/minute: 48 mg/day

Lipidil Micro® [CAN; not available in U.S.]: Cl_{cr} ≥20-100 mL/minute: 67 mg/day; **Note:** Lipidil Micro® 67 mg capsules are discontinued in Canada. Micronized formulation at this dosage strength is available through other manufacturers in Canada.

Lipidil Supra® [CAN; not available in U.S.]: Cl_{cr} ≥20-100 mL/minute: 100 mg/day

Lipofen®: 50 mg/day

Lofibra® (micronized): 67 mg/day

Lofibra® (tablets): 54 mg/day

TriCor®: Cl_{cr} 31-80 mL/minute: 48 mg/day

Triglide®: 50 mg/day

◀ **Administration** 6-8 weeks of therapy is required to determine efficacy.

Fenoglide®, Lofibra® (capsules [micronized] and tablets), Lipofen®: Administer with meals.

Antara®, TriCor®: May be administered with or without food.

Triglide®: Do not consume chipped or broken tablets. May be administered with or without food.

Canadian products [not available in U.S.]:

Lipidil Micro®, Lipidil Supra®: Administer with meals.

Lipidil EZ®: May be administered with or without food.

Monitoring Parameters Periodic blood counts during first year of therapy. Total cholesterol, LDL-C, triglycerides, and HDL-C should be measured periodically; If only marginal changes are noted in 6-8 weeks, the drug should be discontinued. Monitor LFTs regularly and discontinue therapy if levels remain >3 times normal limits.

Special Geriatric Considerations The definition of and, therefore, when to treat hyperlipidemia in the elderly is a controversial issue. The National Cholesterol Education Program recommends that all adults maintain a plasma cholesterol <160 mg/dL. Older adults with one additional risk factor, goal LDL would be <130 mg/dL. It is the authors' belief that pharmacologic treatment be reserved for those who are unable to obtain a desirable plasma cholesterol concentration by diet alone and for whom the benefits of treatment are believed to outweigh the potential adverse effects, drug interactions, and cost of treatment.

Dosage Forms Excipient information presented when available (limited, particularly for generics); consult specific product labeling.

Capsule, oral:

Lipofen®: 50 mg, 150 mg

Capsule, oral [micronized]: 67 mg, 134 mg, 200 mg

Antara®: 43 mg, 130 mg

Lofibra®: 67 mg, 134 mg, 200 mg

Tablet, oral: 54 mg, 160 mg

Fenoglide®: 40 mg, 120 mg

Lofibra®: 54 mg, 160 mg

TriCor®: 48 mg, 145 mg [contains soybean lecithin]

Triglide®: 50 mg, 160 mg [contains egg lecithin]

Selected References

"Executive Summary of The Third Report of The National Cholesterol Education Program (NCEP) Expert Panel on Detection, Evaluation, and Treatment of High Blood Cholesterol in Adults (Adult Treatment Panel III)," *JAMA*, 2001, 285(19):2486-97.

Grundy SM, Cleeman JI, Merz CN, et al, "Implications of Recent Clinical Trials for the National Cholesterol Education Program Adult Treatment Panel III Guidelines," *J Am Coll Cardiol*, 2004, 44(3):720-32.

National Cholesterol Education Program (NCEP) Expert Panel on Detection, Evaluation, and Treatment of High Blood Cholesterol in Adults (Adult Treatment Panel III), "Third Report of the National Cholesterol Education Program (NCEP) Expert Panel on Detection, Evaluation, and Treatment of High Blood Cholesterol in Adults (Adult Treatment Panel III) Final Report," *Circulation*, 2002, 106(25):3143-421.

Fenofibric Acid (fen oh FYE brik AS id)

Medication Safety Issues

Sound-alike/look-alike issues:

Fibricor® may be confused with Tricor®

TriLipix™ may be confused with Trileptal®, TriLyte®

Brand Names: U.S. Fibricor®; TriLipix®

Index Terms ABT-335; Choline Fenofibrate

Generic Availability (U.S.) Yes

Pharmacologic Category Antilipemic Agent, Fibric Acid

Use Adjunct to dietary therapy for the treatment of severely elevated serum triglyceride levels; adjunct to dietary therapy for the reduction of low density lipoprotein cholesterol (LDL-C), total cholesterol (total-C), triglycerides, and apolipoprotein B (apo B) and to increase high density lipoprotein cholesterol (HDL-C) in patients with primary hypercholesterolemia or mixed dyslipidemia

TriLipix™ is also indicated as adjunct to dietary therapy concomitantly with a statin to reduce triglyceride levels and increase HDL-C levels in patients with mixed dyslipidemia and coronary heart disease (CHD) or at risk for CHD

Medication Guide Available Yes

Contraindications Hypersensitivity to fenofibric acid, choline fenofibrate, fenofibrate, or any component of the formulation; hepatic dysfunction including primary biliary cirrhosis and unexplained persistent liver function abnormalities; severe renal dysfunction (including patients on dialysis); pre-existing gallbladder disease

Warnings/Precautions Secondary causes of hyperlipidemia should be ruled out prior to therapy. Has been associated with rare myositis or rhabdomyolysis; patients should be monitored closely. Risk increased in the elderly, patients with diabetes mellitus, renal failure, or hypothyroidism. Patients should be instructed to report unexplained muscle pain, tenderness, weakness, or brown urine. Hepatic transaminases can become significantly elevated (dose-related); hepatocellular, chronic active, and cholestatic hepatitis have been reported. Regular monitoring of liver function tests is required. Increases in serum creatinine (>2 mg/dL) have been observed with use; monitor renal function in patients with renal impairment and consider monitoring patients with increased risk for developing renal impairment. May cause cholelithiasis discontinue if gallstones found upon gallbladder studies. Use caution with oral anticoagulants; adjustments in therapy may be required.

Use caution with HMG-CoA reductase inhibitors (may lead to myopathy, rhabdomyolysis). In combination with HMG-CoA reductase inhibitors, fenofibric acid derivatives are generally regarded as safer than gemfibrozil due to limited pharmacokinetic interaction. Therapy should be withdrawn if an adequate response is not obtained after 2-3 months of therapy at the maximal daily dose. The occurrence of pancreatitis may represent a failure of efficacy in patients with severely elevated triglycerides. May cause mild-to-moderate decreases in hemoglobin, hematocrit, and WBC upon initiation of therapy, which usually stabilizes with long-term therapy. Rare hypersensitivity reactions may occur. Use has been associated with pulmonary embolism (PE) and deep vein thrombosis (DVT). Use with caution in patients with risk factors for VTE. Dose adjustment is required for renal impairment and elderly patients.

Adverse Reactions (Reflective of adult population; not specific for elderly) Adverse reactions and frequency reported as observed during monotherapy and concurrent administration with a statin (HMG-CoA reductase inhibitor).

>10%: Central nervous system: Headache (12% to 13%)

1% to 10%:
Central nervous system: Dizziness (3% to 4%), pain (1% to 4%), fatigue (2% to 3%)
Gastrointestinal: Nausea (4% to 6%), dyspepsia (3% to 5%), diarrhea (3% to 4%), constipation (3%)
Hepatic: ALT increased (monotherapy: 1%; coadministered with statin: 3%)
Neuromuscular & skeletal: Back pain (4% to 6%), pain in extremities (3% to 5%), arthralgia (4%), myalgia (3% to 4%), muscle spasm (2% to 3%)
Respiratory: Nasopharyngitis (4% to 5%), upper respiratory infection (4% to 5%), sinusitis (3% to 4%)

Additional adverse reactions when fenofibric acid coadministered with a statin (frequency not defined): AST increased, bronchitis, cough, CPK increased, hepatic enzymes increased, hypertension, influenza, insomnia, musculoskeletal pain, pharyngolaryngeal pain, urinary tract infection

Drug Interactions

Avoid Concomitant Use There are no known interactions where it is recommended to avoid concomitant use.

Increased Effect/Toxicity
Fenofibric Acid may increase the levels/effects of: Carvedilol; Colchicine; CYP2C9 Substrates (High risk); Ezetimibe; HMG-CoA Reductase Inhibitors; Sulfonylureas; Vitamin K Antagonists; Warfarin

The levels/effects of Fenofibric Acid may be increased by: CycloSPORINE; CycloSPORINE (Systemic)

Decreased Effect
Fenofibric Acid may decrease the levels/effects of: Chenodiol; CycloSPORINE; Cyclo-SPORINE (Systemic); Ursodiol

The levels/effects of Fenofibric Acid may be decreased by: Bile Acid Sequestrants

Stability Store at 25°C (77°F); excursions permitted to 15°C to 30°C (59°F to 86°F). Protect from light and moisture.

Mechanism of Action Fenofibric acid, an agonist for the nuclear transcription factor peroxisome proliferator-activated receptor-alpha (PPAR-alpha), downregulates apoprotein C-III (an inhibitor of lipoprotein lipase) and upregulates the synthesis of apolipoprotein A-I, fatty acid transport protein, and lipoprotein lipase resulting in an increase in VLDL catabolism, fatty acid oxidation, and elimination of triglyceride-rich particles; as a result of a decrease in VLDL levels, total plasma triglycerides are reduced by 30% to 60%; modest increased in HDL occurs in some hypertriglyceridemia patients.

Pharmacodynamics/Kinetics
Absorption: Well absorbed
Protein binding: ~99%
Metabolism: Fenofibric acid (active form) undergoes inactivation by glucuronidation. The choline salt dissociates in the GI tract to form fenofibric acid (free acid)

◀ Bioavailability: TriLipix™: ~81%
Half-life elimination: ~20 hours
Time to peak, plasma: Fibricor®: ~2.5 hours; TriLipix™: 4-5 hours
Excretion: Urine (as fenofibric acid and fenofibric acid glucuronide)

Dosage

Geriatric Oral: Dosage based on renal function

Adult

Mixed dyslipidemia (coadministered with a statin): Oral: TriLipix™: 135 mg once daily (maximum: 135 mg/day)

Hypertriglyceridemia: Oral:
Fibricor®: Initial: 35-105 mg once daily; Maintenance: Individualize according to patient response (maximum: 105 mg/day)
TriLipix™: Initial: 45-135 mg once daily; Maintenance: Individualize according to patient response (maximum: 135 mg/day)

Primary hypercholesterolemia or mixed dyslipidemia: Oral:
Fibricor®: 105 mg once daily (maximum: 105 mg/day)
TriLipix™: 135 mg once daily (maximum: 135 mg/day)

Renal Impairment
Mild-to-moderate impairment (Cl$_{cr}$ 30-80 mL/minute): Initial: Fibricor®: 35 mg once daily or TriLipix™: 45 mg once daily; only increase once effects on lipids and renal function evaluated
Severe impairment (Cl$_{cr}$ <30 mL/minute; with or without dialysis): Contraindicated

Administration May be administered with or without food.

Monitoring Parameters Periodic blood counts during first year of therapy; total cholesterol, LDL-C, triglycerides, and HDL-C should be measured periodically; monitor LFTs (including ALT) regularly and discontinue therapy if levels remain >3 times normal limits; serum creatinine (in patients with or at risk for renal impairment)

Special Geriatric Considerations The definition of and, therefore, when to treat hyperlipidemia in the elderly is a controversial issue. The National Cholesterol Education Program recommends that all adults maintain a plasma cholesterol <160 mg/dL. Older adults with one additional risk factor, goal LDL would be <130 mg/dL. It is the authors' belief that pharmacologic treatment be reserved for those who are unable to obtain a desirable plasma cholesterol concentration by diet alone and for whom the benefits of treatment are believed to outweigh the potential adverse effects, drug interactions, and cost of treatment.

Dosage Forms Excipient information presented when available (limited, particularly for generics); consult specific product labeling.
Capsule, delayed release, oral:
TriLipix®: 45 mg, 135 mg
Tablet, oral: 35 mg, 105 mg
Fibricor®: 35 mg, 105 mg

Selected References
National Cholesterol Education Program (NCEP) Expert Panel on Detection, Evaluation, and Treatment of High Blood Cholesterol in Adults (Adult Treatment Panel III), "Third Report of the National Cholesterol Education Program (NCEP) Expert Panel on Detection, Evaluation, and Treatment of High Blood Cholesterol in Adults (Adult Treatment Panel III) Final Report," *Circulation*, 2002, 106(25):3143-421.

◆ **Fenoglide®** see Fenofibrate *on page 701*

Fenoprofen (fen oh PROE fen)

Medication Safety Issues
Sound-alike/look-alike issues:
Fenoprofen may be confused with flurbiprofen
Nalfon® may be confused with Naldecon®

Brand Names: U.S. Nalfon®

Brand Names: Canada Nalfon®

Index Terms Fenoprofen Calcium

Generic Availability (U.S.) Yes: Tablet

Pharmacologic Category Nonsteroidal Anti-inflammatory Drug (NSAID), Oral

Use Symptomatic treatment of acute and chronic rheumatoid arthritis and osteoarthritis; relief of mild-to-moderate pain

Medication Guide Available Yes

Contraindications Hypersensitivity to fenoprofen, aspirin, or other NSAIDs, or any component of the formulation; perioperative pain in the setting of coronary artery bypass graft (CABG) surgery; significant renal dysfunction

Warnings/Precautions [U.S. Boxed Warning]: NSAIDs are associated with an increased risk of adverse cardiovascular thrombotic events, including MI and stroke. Risk may be increased with duration of use or pre-existing cardiovascular risk factors or disease. Carefully evaluate individual cardiovascular risk profiles prior to prescribing. May cause new-onset hypertension or worsening of existing hypertension. Use caution with fluid retention. Avoid use in heart failure. Concurrent administration of ibuprofen, and potentially other nonselective NSAIDs, may interfere with aspirin's cardioprotective effect. **[U.S. Boxed Warning]: Use is contraindicated for treatment of perioperative pain in the setting of coronary artery bypass graft (CABG) surgery.** Risk of MI and stroke may be increased with use following CABG surgery.

NSAID use may compromise existing renal function; dose-dependent decreases in prostaglandin synthesis may result from NSAID use, reducing renal blood flow which may cause renal decompensation. NSAID use may increase the risk for hyperkalemia. Patients with impaired renal function, dehydration, heart failure, liver dysfunction, those taking diuretics, and ACE inhibitors, and the elderly are at greater risk of renal toxicity and hyperkalemia. Rehydrate patient before starting therapy; monitor renal function closely. Not recommended for use in patients with advanced renal disease. Long-term NSAID use may result in renal papillary necrosis.

[U.S. Boxed Warning]: NSAIDs may increase risk of gastrointestinal irritation, inflammation, ulceration, bleeding, and perforation. These events may occur at any time during therapy and without warning. Use caution with a history of GI disease (bleeding or ulcers), concurrent therapy with aspirin, anticoagulants and/or corticosteroids, smoking, use of alcohol, the elderly or debilitated patients. When used concomitantly with ≤325 mg of aspirin, a substantial increase in the risk of gastrointestinal complications (eg, ulcer) occurs; concomitant gastroprotective therapy (eg, proton pump inhibitors) is recommended (Bhatt, 2008).

Platelet adhesion and aggregation may be decreased; may prolong bleeding time; patients with coagulation disorders or who are receiving anticoagulants should be monitored closely. Anemia may occur; patients on long-term NSAID therapy should be monitored for anemia. Rarely, NSAID use has been associated with potentially severe blood dyscrasias (eg, agranulocytosis, thrombocytopenia, aplastic anemia).

Use the lowest effective dose for the shortest duration of time, consistent with individual patient goals, to reduce risk of cardiovascular or GI adverse events. Alternate therapies should be considered for patients at high risk.

NSAIDs may cause serious skin adverse events including exfoliative dermatitis, Stevens-Johnson syndrome (SJS), and toxic epidermal necrolysis (TEN); discontinue use at first sign of skin rash or hypersensitivity. Anaphylactoid reactions may occur, even without prior exposure; patients with "aspirin triad" (bronchial asthma, aspirin intolerance, rhinitis) may be at increased risk. Do not use in patients who experience bronchospasm, asthma, rhinitis, or urticaria with NSAID or aspirin therapy. Use caution in other forms of asthma.

Use with caution in patients with decreased hepatic function. Closely monitor patients with any abnormal LFT. Severe hepatic reactions (eg, fulminant hepatitis, liver failure) have occurred with NSAID use, rarely; discontinue if signs or symptoms of liver disease develop, or if systemic manifestations occur.

NSAIDS may cause drowsiness, dizziness, blurred vision and other neurologic effects which may impair physical or mental abilities; patients must be cautioned about performing tasks which require mental alertness (eg, operating machinery or driving). Discontinue use with blurred or diminished vision and perform ophthalmologic exam. Monitor vision with long-term therapy. The elderly are at increased risk for adverse effects (especially peptic ulceration, CNS effects, renal toxicity) from NSAIDs even at low doses.

Withhold for at least 4-6 half-lives prior to surgical or dental procedures.

Adverse Reactions (Reflective of adult population; not specific for elderly)
1% to 10%:
Cardiovascular: Peripheral edema (5%), palpitation (3%)
Central nervous system: Headache (9%), somnolence (9%), dizziness (7%), nervousness (6%), fatigue (2%), confusion (1%)
Dermatologic: Itching (4%), rash (4%)
Gastrointestinal: Dyspepsia (10%), nausea (8%), constipation (7%), vomiting (3%), abdominal pain (2%)
Neuromuscular & skeletal: Weakness (5%), tremor (2%)
Ocular: Blurred vision (2%)
Otic: Tinnitus (5%), hearing decreased (2%)
Respiratory: Dyspnea (3%), nasopharyngitis (1%)
Miscellaneous: Diaphoresis (5%)

◀ **Drug Interactions**

Avoid Concomitant Use

Avoid concomitant use of Fenoprofen with any of the following: Floctafenine; Ketorolac; Ketorolac (Nasal); Ketorolac (Systemic)

Increased Effect/Toxicity

Fenoprofen may increase the levels/effects of: Aminoglycosides; Anticoagulants; Antiplatelet Agents; Bisphosphonate Derivatives; Collagenase (Systemic); CycloSPORINE; CycloSPORINE (Systemic); Deferasirox; Desmopressin; Digoxin; Drotrecogin Alfa; Eplerenone; Haloperidol; Ibritumomab; Lithium; Methotrexate; Nonsteroidal Anti-Inflammatory Agents; PEMEtrexed; Porfimer; Potassium-Sparing Diuretics; PRALAtrexate; Quinolone Antibiotics; Rivaroxaban; Salicylates; Thrombolytic Agents; Tositumomab and Iodine I 131 Tositumomab; Vancomycin; Vitamin K Antagonists

The levels/effects of Fenoprofen may be increased by: ACE Inhibitors; Angiotensin II Receptor Blockers; Antidepressants (Tricyclic, Tertiary Amine); Corticosteroids (Systemic); Dasatinib; Floctafenine; Glucosamine; Herbs (Anticoagulant/Antiplatelet Properties); Ketorolac; Ketorolac (Nasal); Ketorolac (Systemic); Nonsteroidal Anti-Inflammatory Agents; Omega-3-Acid Ethyl Esters; Pentosan Polysulfate Sodium; Pentoxifylline; Probenecid; Prostacyclin Analogues; Selective Serotonin Reuptake Inhibitors; Serotonin/Norepinephrine Reuptake Inhibitors; Sodium Phosphates; Treprostinil; Vitamin E

Decreased Effect

Fenoprofen may decrease the levels/effects of: ACE Inhibitors; Angiotensin II Receptor Blockers; Antiplatelet Agents; Beta-Blockers; Eplerenone; HydrALAZINE; Potassium-Sparing Diuretics; Salicylates; Selective Serotonin Reuptake Inhibitors; Thiazide Diuretics

The levels/effects of Fenoprofen may be decreased by: Bile Acid Sequestrants; Nonsteroidal Anti-Inflammatory Agents; Salicylates

Ethanol/Nutrition/Herb Interactions

Ethanol: Avoid ethanol (may enhance gastric mucosal irritation).

Food: Fenoprofen peak serum levels may be decreased if taken with food; total amount absorbed is not affected.

Herb/Nutraceutical: Avoid alfalfa, anise, bilberry, bladderwrack, bromelain, cat's claw, celery, chamomile, coleus, cordyceps, dong quai, evening primrose, fenugreek, feverfew, garlic, ginger, ginkgo biloba, ginseng (American, Panax, Siberian), grapeseed, green tea, guggul, horse chestnut seed, horseradish, licorice, prickly ash, red clover, reishi, SAMe (S-adenosylmethionine), sweet clover, turmeric, white willow (all have additional antiplatelet activity).

Stability Store at controlled room temperature of 20°C to 25°C (67°F to 77°F).

Mechanism of Action Reversibly inhibits cyclooxygenase-1 and 2 (COX-1 and 2) enzymes, which results in decreased formation of prostaglandin precursors; has antipyretic, analgesic, and anti-inflammatory properties

Other proposed mechanisms not fully elucidated (and possibly contributing to the anti-inflammatory effect to varying degrees), include inhibiting chemotaxis, altering lymphocyte activity, inhibiting neutrophil aggregation/activation, and decreasing proinflammatory cytokine levels.

Pharmacodynamics/Kinetics

Onset of action: A few days; full benefit: up to 2-3 weeks

Absorption: Rapid, 80%

Protein binding: 99%; to albumin

Metabolism: Extensively hepatic

Half-life elimination: 2.5-3 hours

Time to peak, serum: ~2 hours

Excretion: Urine (2% to 5% as unchanged drug); feces (small amounts)

Dosage

Geriatric & Adult

Rheumatoid arthritis, osteoarthritis: Oral: 300-600 mg 3-4 times/day; maximum dose: 3.2 g/day

Mild-to-moderate pain: Oral: 200 mg every 4-6 hours as needed; maximum dose: 3.2 g/day

Renal Impairment Not recommended in patients with advanced renal disease.

Administration Do not crush tablets. Swallow whole with a full glass of water. Take with food to minimize stomach upset.

Monitoring Parameters Monitor CBC, liver enzymes; monitor urine output and BUN/serum creatinine in patients receiving diuretics; monitor blood pressure in patients receiving antihypertensives; audiogram (in patients with baseline hearing impairment)

Reference Range Therapeutic: 20-65 mcg/mL (SI: 82-268 μmol/L)

Test Interactions Fenoprofen may interfere with Amerlex-M kit assay values; falsely elevated values of total and free triiodothyronine have been reported.

Pharmacotherapy Pearls There are no clinical guidelines to predict which NSAID will give response in a particular patient. Trials with each must be initiated until response determined. Consider dose, patient convenience, and cost.

Special Geriatric Considerations Elderly are a high-risk population for adverse effects from NSAIDs. As much as 60% of elderly can develop peptic ulceration and/or hemorrhage asymptomatically. The concomitant use of H_2 blockers and sucralfate is not effective as prophylaxis with the exception of NSAID-induced duodenal ulcers which may be prevented by the use of ranitidine. Misoprostol and proton pump inhibitors are the only agents proven to help prevent the development of NSAID-induced ulcers. Also, concomitant disease and drug use contribute to the risk for GI adverse effects. Use lowest effective dose for shortest period possible. Consider renal function decline with age. Use of NSAIDs can compromise existing renal function especially when Cl_{cr} is ≤30 mL/minute. Tinnitus may be a difficult and unreliable indication of toxicity due to age-related hearing loss or eighth cranial nerve damage. CNS adverse effects such as confusion, agitation, and hallucination are generally seen in overdose or high-dose situations, but elderly may demonstrate these adverse effects at lower doses than younger adults.

Dosage Forms Excipient information presented when available (limited, particularly for generics); consult specific product labeling.

Capsule, oral:

Nalfon®: 200 mg, 400 mg

Tablet, oral: 600 mg

Selected References

Capone ML, Sciulli MG, Tacconelli S, et al, "Pharmacodynamic Interaction of Naproxen With Low-dose Aspirin in Healthy Subjects," *J Am Coll Cardiol*, 2005, 45 (8):1295-1301.

Catella-Lawson F, Reilly MP, Kapoor SC, et al, "Cyclooxygenase Inhibitors and the Antiplatelet Effects of Aspirin," *N Engl J Med*, 2001, 345(25):1809-17.

Conlin P, Moore T, Swartz S, et al, "Effect of Indomethacin on Blood Pressure Lowering by Captopril and Losartan in Hypertensive Patients," *Hypertension*, 2000, 36(3):461-5.

"Drugs for Pain," *Med Lett Drugs Ther*, 2000, 42(1085):73-8.

Jacobi J, Fraser GL, Coursin DB, et al, "Clinical Practice Guidelines for the Sustained Use of Sedatives and Analgesics in the Critically Ill Adult," *Crit Care Med*, 2002, 30(1):119-41. Available at: http://www.sccm.org/pdf/sedatives.pdf. Accessed August 2, 2003.

Morgan TO, Anderson A, and Bertram D, "Effect of Indomethacin on Blood Pressure in Elderly People With Essential Hypertension Well Controlled on Amlodipine or Enalapril," *Am J Hypertens*, 2000, 13(11):1161-7.

Page J and Henry D, "Consumption of NSAIDs and the Development of Congestive Heart Failure in Elderly Patients: An Underrecognized Public Health Problem," *Arch Intern Med*, 2000, 160(6):777-84.

◆ **Fenoprofen Calcium** *see Fenoprofen on page 706*

FentaNYL (FEN ta nil)

Related Information

Opioid Analgesics *on page 2013*

Patient Information for Disposal of Unused Medications *on page 2125*

Medication Safety Issues

Sound-alike/look-alike issues:

FentaNYL may be confused with alfentanil, SUFentanil

High alert medication:

The Institute for Safe Medication Practices (ISMP) includes this medication among its list of drug classes which have a heightened risk of causing significant patient harm when used in error.

Administration issues:

Fentanyl transdermal system patches: Leakage of fentanyl gel from the patch has been reported; patch may be less effective; do not use. Thoroughly wash any skin surfaces coming into direct contact with gel with water (do not use soap). May contain conducting metal (eg, aluminum); remove patch prior to MRI.

Other safety concerns:

Dosing of transdermal fentanyl patches may be confusing. Transdermal fentanyl patches should always be prescribed in mcg/hour, not size. Patch dosage form of Duragesic®-12 actually delivers 12.5 mcg/hour of fentanyl. Use caution, as orders may be written as "Duragesic 12.5" which can be erroneously interpreted as a 125 mcg dose.

Fentora®, Onsolis™, Abstral®, and Actiq® are not interchangeable; do not substitute doses on a mcg-per-mcg basis.

Brand Names: U.S. Abstral®; Actiq®; Duragesic®; Fentora®; Onsolis™

Brand Names: Canada Abstral™; Actiq®; Duragesic®; Duragesic® MAT; Fentanyl Citrate Injection, USP; Novo-Fentanyl; PMS-Fentanyl MTX; RAN™-Fentanyl Matrix Patch; RAN™-Fentanyl Transdermal System; ratio-Fentanyl

Index Terms Fentanyl Citrate; Fentanyl Hydrochloride; Fentanyl Patch; Lazanda®; OTFC (Oral Transmucosal Fentanyl Citrate)

Generic Availability (U.S.) Yes: Excludes buccal film, buccal tablet, sublingual tablet

◄ **Pharmacologic Category** Analgesic, Opioid; Anilidopiperidine Opioid; General Anesthetic

Use

Injection: Relief of pain, preoperative medication, adjunct to general or regional anesthesia

Iontophoretic transdermal system (Ionsys™): Short-term, in-hospital management of acute postoperative pain

Transdermal patch (eg, Duragesic®): Management of persistent moderate-to-severe chronic pain

Transmucosal lozenge (eg, Actiq®), buccal tablet (Fentora®), buccal film (Onsolis™), sublingual tablet (Abstral®): Management of breakthrough cancer pain in opioid-tolerant patients

Prescribing and Access Restrictions As a requirement of the REMS program, access is restricted.

Abstral® (fentanyl sublingual tablet) is only available through the ABSTRAL REMS (Risk Evaluation and Mitigation Strategy) program. For outpatient use, enrollment in the ABSTRAL REMS program is required for prescribers, outpatient pharmacies, and patients. For inpatient use, enrollment in the ABSTRAL REMS program is required for inpatient pharmacies; patient and prescriber enrollment is not required for inpatient use. Distributors must also be enrolled in the program. Further information may be obtained by calling the ABSTRAL REMS program at 1-888-227-8725 or online at www.abstralrems.com

Actiq® (fentanyl lozenge) is only available through the ACTIQ REMS program. Enrollment in the ACTIQ REMS program is required for prescribers for outpatient use, pharmacies (inpatient and outpatient), outpatients, and distributors. Further information may be obtained by calling the ACTIQ REMS program at 1-888-688-6885 or online at www.-actiqandfentorarems.com.

Fentora® (fentanyl buccal tablet) is only available through the FENTORA REMS program. Enrollment in the FENTORA REMS program is required for prescribers for outpatient use, pharmacies (inpatient and outpatient), outpatients, and distributors. Further information may be obtained by calling the FENTORA REMS program at 1-888-688-6885 or online at www.actiqandfentorarems.com.

Onsolis™ (fentanyl buccal film) is only available through the restricted distribution program (FOCUS™). Enrollment in the FOCUS™ program is required for prescribers, pharmacies, and patients. Further information may be obtained from the manufacturer, Meda Pharmaceuticals, Inc (1-877-466-7654).

Medication Guide Available Yes

Contraindications Hypersensitivity to fentanyl or any component of the formulation

Transdermal system: Severe respiratory disease or depression including acute asthma (unless patient is mechanically ventilated); paralytic ileus; patients requiring short-term therapy, management of intermittent pain

Transmucosal buccal tablets (Fentora®), buccal films (Onsolis™), lozenges (eg, Actiq®), sublingual tablets (Abstral®), and/or transdermal patches (eg, Duragesic®): Contraindicated in the management of acute or postoperative pain (including headache, migraine, dental pain, or use in emergency room), and in patients who are not opioid tolerant

Canadian labeling: Additional contraindication (not in U.S. labeling): Sublingual tablets (Abstral™): Severe respiratory depression or severe obstructive lung diseaseStability

Warnings/Precautions An opioid-containing analgesic regimen should be tailored to each patient's needs and based upon the type of pain being treated (acute versus chronic), the route of administration, degree of tolerance for opioids (naive versus chronic user), age, weight, and medical condition. The optimal analgesic dose varies widely among patients. Doses should be titrated to pain relief/prevention. May cause CNS depression, which may impair physical or mental abilities; patients must be cautioned about performing tasks which require mental alertness (eg, operating machinery or driving). When using with other CNS depressants, reduce dose of one or both agents. Fentanyl shares the toxic potentials of opiate agonists, and precautions of opiate agonist therapy should be observed; use with caution in patients with bradycardia or bradyarrhythmias; rapid I.V. infusion may result in skeletal muscle and chest wall rigidity leading to respiratory distress and/or apnea, bronchoconstriction, laryngospasm; inject slowly over 3-5 minutes. **[U.S. Boxed Warning]: Healthcare provider should be alert to problems of abuse, misuse, and diversion.** Tolerance or drug dependence may result from extended use. The elderly may be particularly susceptible to the CNS depressant and constipating effects of narcotics. Use extreme caution in patients with COPD or other chronic respiratory conditions. Use caution with head injuries, morbid obesity, renal impairment, or hepatic dysfunction. **[U.S. Boxed Warning]: Use with strong or moderate CYP3A4 inhibitors may result in increased effects and potentially fatal respiratory depression.** Use is not recommended with MAO inhibitors or within 14 days of MAO inhibitor use; severe and unpredictable adverse effects may result. Concurrent use of agonist/antagonist analgesics may precipitate withdrawal symptoms and/or reduced analgesic efficacy in patients following prolonged therapy with mu opioid agonists. Abrupt discontinuation following prolonged use may also lead to withdrawal symptoms.

[U.S. Boxed Warning] Abstral®, Actiq®, Duragesic®, Fentora®, Onsolis™: May cause potentially life-threatening hypoventilation, respiratory depression, and/or death; Abstral®, Actiq®, Duragesic®, Fentora®, or Onsolis™ should only be prescribed for opioid-tolerant patients. Risk of respiratory depression increased in elderly patients, debilitated patients, and patients with conditions associated with hypoxia or hypercapnia; usually occurs after administration of initial dose in nontolerant patients or when given with other drugs that depress respiratory function.

Transmucosal: Lozenge (eg, Actiq®), buccal tablet (Fentora®), buccal film (Onsolis™), sublingual tablet (Abstral®): **[U.S. Boxed Warning]: Should be used only for the care of opioid-tolerant cancer patients with breakthrough pain and is intended for use by specialists who are knowledgeable in treating cancer pain.** Not approved for use in management of acute or postoperative pain.

Transmucosal: Buccal film (eg, Onsolis™): **[U.S. Boxed Warning]: Available only through the FOCUS Program, a restricted distribution program with prescriber, pharmacy, and patient required enrollment. [U.S. Boxed Warning]: Onsolis™ is contraindicated in the management of acute or postoperative pain, including headache/migraine. [U.S. Boxed Warning]: Due to higher bioavailability of fentanyl in the buccal film formulation, do not substitute Onsolis™ on a mcg-per-mcg basis for any other fentanyl product. Serious adverse events, including death, may occur when used inappropriately (improper dose or patient selection). All patients must begin therapy with a 200 mcg dose and titrate, if needed. During therapy, patients must wait at least 2 hours before taking another dose.**

Transmucosal: Buccal tablet (Fentora®): **[U.S. Boxed Warning]: Due to the higher bioavailability of fentanyl in Fentora®, when converting patients from oral transmucosal fentanyl citrate (OTFC, Actiq®) to Fentora®, do not substitute Fentora®: on a mcg-per-mcg basis for any other fentanyl product. [U.S. Boxed Warning]: Fentora® is contraindicated in the management of acute or postoperative pain, including headache/migraine. Serious adverse events, including death, have been reported when used inappropriately (improper dose or patient selection). [U.S. Boxed Warning]: Patients using Fentora® who experience breakthrough pain may only take one additional dose using the same strength and must wait four hours before taking another dose.**

Transmucosal: Lozenge (Actiq®): **[U.S. Boxed Warning]: The substitution of Actiq® for any other fentanyl product may result in a fatal overdose. Do not convert patients on a mcg-per-mcg basis to Actiq® from other fentanyl products. Do not substitute Actiq® for any other fentanyl product. [U.S. Boxed Warning]: Patients using fentanyl lozenges who experience breakthrough may only take 1 additional dose using the same strength and must wait 4 hours before taking another dose.**

Transmucosal: Sublingual tablet (Abstral®): **[U.S. Boxed Warning]: Available only through the ABSTRAL REMS program. Prescribers who prescribe to outpatients, outpatients, pharmacies, and distributors are required to enroll in the program. [U.S. Boxed Warning]: Abstral® is contraindicated in opioid nontolerant patients. [U.S. Boxed Warning]: Due to differing pharmacokinetics of fentanyl in the sublingual tablet formulation, do not substitute Abstral® on a mcg-per-mcg basis for any other fentanyl product. Serious adverse events, including death, may occur when used inappropriately (improper dose or patient selection). All patients must begin therapy with a 100 mcg dose. During therapy, patients must wait at least 2 hours before treating another episode of breakthrough pain.**

Transdermal patches (eg, Duragesic®): **[U.S. Boxed Warning]: Indicated for the management of persistent moderate-to-severe pain when around the clock pain control is needed for an extended time period. Should only be used in patients who are already receiving opioid therapy, are opioid tolerant, and who require a total daily dose equivalent to 25 mcg/hour transdermal patch. Contraindicated in patients who are not opioid tolerant, in the management of short-term analgesia, or in the management of postoperative pain. Should be applied only to intact skin. Use of a patch that has been cut, damaged, or altered in any way may result in overdosage.** Serum fentanyl concentrations may increase approximately one-third for patients with a body temperature of 40°C secondary to a temperature-dependent increase in fentanyl release from the patch and increased skin permeability. **[U.S. Boxed Warning]: Avoid exposure of application site and surrounding area to direct external heat sources.** Patients who experience fever or increase in core temperature should be monitored closely. Patients who experience adverse reactions should be monitored for at least 24 hours after removal of the patch. Transdermal patch may contain conducting metal (eg, aluminum); remove patch prior to MRI.

◀ **Adverse Reactions (Reflective of adult population; not specific for elderly)**

>10%:

Cardiovascular: Bradycardia, edema

Central nervous system: CNS depression, confusion, dizziness, drowsiness, fatigue, headache, sedation

Endocrine & metabolic: Dehydration

Gastrointestinal: Constipation, nausea, vomiting, xerostomia

Local: Application-site reaction erythema

Neuromuscular & skeletal: Chest wall rigidity (high dose I.V.), muscle rigidity, weakness

Ocular: Miosis

Respiratory: Dyspnea, respiratory depression

Miscellaneous: Diaphoresis

1% to 10%:

Cardiovascular: Cardiac arrhythmia, chest pain, DVT, flushing, hyper-/hypotension, orthostatic hypotension, pallor, palpitation, peripheral edema, syncope, tachycardia, vasodilation

Central nervous system: Abnormal dreams, abnormal thinking, agitation, amnesia, anxiety, attention disturbance, DVT, depression, dysphoria, euphoria, fever, hallucinations, hypoesthesia, insomnia, lethargy, malaise, mental status change, migraine, nervousness, paranoid reaction, somnolence, stupor, vertigo

Dermatologic: Alopecia, bruising, cellulitis, erythema, hyperhidrosis, papules, pruritus, rash

Endocrine & metabolic: Breast pain, hot flashes, hyper-/hypocalcemia, hyper-/hypoglycemia, hypoalbuminemia, hypokalemia, hypomagnesemia

Gastrointestinal: Abdominal pain, abnormal taste, anorexia, appetite decreased, biliary tract spasm, diarrhea, dyspepsia, dysphagia (buccal tablet/film), flatulence, GI hemorrhage, gingival pain (buccal tablet), gingivitis (lozenge), glossitis (lozenge), ileus, intestinal obstruction (buccal film), periodontal abscess (lozenge/buccal tablet), stomatitis (lozenge/buccal tablet/sublingual tablet), tongue disorder (sublingual tablet), ulceration (gingival, lip, mouth; transmucosal use), weight loss

Genitourinary: Dysuria, erectile dysfunction, urinary incontinence, urinary retention, vaginitis, vaginal hemorrhage

Hematologic: Anemia, leukopenia, neutropenia, thrombocytopenia

Hepatic: Ascites, jaundice

Local: Application site pain, application site irritation

Neuromuscular & skeletal: Abnormal coordination, abnormal gait, arthralgia, back pain, myalgia, neuropathy, paresthesia, rigors, tremor

Ocular: Blurred vision, diplopia

Renal: Renal failure

Respiratory: Apnea, asthma, bronchitis, cough, epistaxis, hemoptysis, hypoventilation, hypoxia, nasopharyngitis, pharyngolaryngeal pain, pharyngitis, pneumonia, rhinitis, sinusitis, upper respiratory infection, wheezing

Miscellaneous: Flu-like syndrome, hiccups, hypersensitivity, lymphadenopathy, night sweats, parosmia, speech disorder, withdrawal syndrome

Drug Interactions

Metabolism/Transport Effects Substrate of CYP3A4 (major); **Inhibits** CYP3A4 (weak)

Avoid Concomitant Use

Avoid concomitant use of FentaNYL with any of the following: Crizotinib; MAO Inhibitors

Increased Effect/Toxicity

FentaNYL may increase the levels/effects of: Alcohol (Ethyl); Alvimopan; Beta-Blockers; Calcium Channel Blockers (Nondihydropyridine); CNS Depressants; Desmopressin; MAO Inhibitors; Selective Serotonin Reuptake Inhibitors; Thiazide Diuretics

The levels/effects of FentaNYL may be increased by: Amphetamines; Antipsychotic Agents (Phenothiazines); Crizotinib; CYP3A4 Inhibitors (Moderate); CYP3A4 Inhibitors (Strong); Dasatinib; Droperidol; HydrOXYzine; MAO Inhibitors; Succinylcholine

Decreased Effect

FentaNYL may decrease the levels/effects of: Pegvisomant

The levels/effects of FentaNYL may be decreased by: Ammonium Chloride; Mixed Agonist / Antagonist Opioids; Rifamycin Derivatives; Tocilizumab

Ethanol/Nutrition/Herb Interactions

Ethanol: May increase CNS depression; monitor for increased effects with coadministration. Caution patients about effects.

Food: Fentanyl concentrations may be increased by grapefruit juice; avoid concurrent intake of large quantities (>1 quart/day).

Herb/Nutraceutical: St John's wort may decrease fentanyl levels. Avoid valerian, St John's wort, kava kava, gotu kola (may increase CNS depression).

Stability

Injection formulation: Store at controlled room temperature of 20°C to 25°C (68°F to 77°F). Protect from light.

Transdermal patch: Do not store above 25°C (77°F).

Transmucosal (buccal film, buccal tablet, lozenge, sublingual tablet): Store at controlled room temperature of 20°C to 25°C (68°F to 77°F). Protect from freezing and moisture. Keep out of the reach of children.

Mechanism of Action Binds with stereospecific receptors at many sites within the CNS, increases pain threshold, alters pain reception, inhibits ascending pain pathways

Pharmacodynamics/Kinetics

Onset of action: Analgesic: I.M.: 7-8 minutes; I.V.: Almost immediate; Transdermal (initial placement): 6 hours; Transmucosal: 5-15 minutes

Peak effect: Analgesic: Transdermal (initial placement): 12 hours; Transmucosal: 15-30 minutes

Duration: I.M.: 1-2 hours; I.V.: 0.5-1 hour; Transdermal (removal of patch/no replacement): 12 hours; Transmucosal: Related to blood level; respiratory depressant effect may last longer than analgesic effect

Absorption:

Transdermal: Initial application: Gradually absorbed for the first 12-24 hours, followed by a constant absorption for the remainder of the dosing interval. Absorption is decreased in cachectic patients (compared to normal size patients).

Transmucosal, buccal tablet and buccal film: Rapid, ~50% from the buccal mucosa; remaining 50% swallowed with saliva and slowly absorbed from GI tract.

Transmucosal, lozenge: Rapid, ~25% from the buccal mucosa; 75% swallowed with saliva and slowly absorbed from GI tract

Distribution: 4-6 L/kg; Highly lipophilic, redistributes into muscle and fat

Protein binding: 80% to 85%

Metabolism: Hepatic, primarily via CYP3A4

Bioavailability:

Buccal film: 71% (mucositis did not have a clinically significant effect on C_{max} and AUC; however, bioavailability is expected to decrease if film is inappropriately chewed and swallowed)

Buccal tablet: 65% (range: 45% to 85%)

Lozenge: 47% (range: 37% to 57%)

Sublingual tablet: 54%

Half-life elimination:

I.V.: 2-4 hours

Transdermal patch: 17 hours (13-22 hours, half-life is influenced by absorption rate)

Transmucosal: Lozenge: 7 hours; Buccal film: ~14 hours; Buccal tablet: 100-200 mcg: 3-4 hours, 400-800 mcg: 11-12 hours; Sublingual tablet: 100-200 mcg: 5-7 hours; 400-800 mcg: 10-14 hours

Time to peak:

Buccal film: 0.75-4 hours (median: 1 hour)

Buccal tablet: 20-240 minutes (median: 47 minutes)

Lozenge: 20-480 minutes (median: 20-40 minutes)

Sublingual tablet: 15-240 minutes (median: 30-60 minutes)

Transdermal patch: 24-72 hours, after several sequential 72-hour applications, steady state serum concentrations are reached

Excretion: Urine 75% (primarily as metabolites, <7% to 10% as unchanged drug); feces ~9%

Dosage

Geriatric Elderly have been found to be twice as sensitive as younger patients to the effects of fentanyl. A wide range of doses may be used. When choosing a dose, take into consideration the following patient factors: age, weight, physical status, underlying disease states, other drugs used, type of anesthesia used, and the surgical procedure to be performed.

Transmucosal lozenge (eg, Actiq®): In clinical trials, patients who were >65 years of age were titrated to a mean dose that was 200 mcg less than that of younger patients.

Adult Note: These are guidelines and do not represent the maximum doses that may be required in all patients. Doses and dosage intervals should be titrated to pain relief/prevention. Monitor vital signs routinely. Single I.M. doses have duration of 1-2 hours, single I.V. doses last 0.5-1 hour.

Surgery:

Premedication: I.M., slow I.V.: 50-100 mcg/dose 30-60 minutes prior to surgery

Adjunct to regional anesthesia: Slow I.V.: 25-100 mcg/dose over 1-2 minutes. **Note:** An I.V. should be in place with regional anesthesia so the I.M. route is rarely used but still maintained as an option in the package labeling.

◀

    Adjunct to general anesthesia: Slow I.V.:

      Low dose: 0.5-2 mcg/kg/dose depending on the indication.

      Moderate dose: Initial: 2-20 mcg/kg/dose; Maintenance (bolus or infusion): 1-2 mcg/kg/**hour**. Discontinuing fentanyl infusion 30-60 minutes prior to the end of surgery will usually allow adequate ventilation upon emergence from anesthesia. For "fast-tracking" and early extubation following major surgery, total fentanyl doses are limited to 10-15 mcg/kg.

      High dose: 20-50 mcg/kg/dose; **Note:** High-dose fentanyl as an adjunct to general anesthesia is rarely used, but is still described in the manufacturer's label.

Pain management: Adults:

    I.V. (unlabeled use): Bolus at start of infusion: 1-2 mcg/kg **or** 25-100 mcg/dose; continuous infusion rate: 1-2 mcg/kg/**hour or** 25-200 mcg/hour

    Severe (unlabeled use): I.M, I.V.: 50-100 mcg/dose every 1-2 hours as needed; patients with prior opiate exposure may tolerate higher initial doses

    Patient-controlled analgesia (PCA) (unlabeled use): I.V.:

      Usual concentration: 10 mcg/mL

      Demand dose: Usual: 20 mcg; range: 10-50 mcg

      Lockout interval: 5-8 minutes

      Usual basal rate: ≤50 mcg/hour

    Critically-ill patients (unlabeled dose): Slow I.V.: 25-100 mcg (based on ~70 kg patient) **or** 0.35-1.5 mcg/kg every 30-60 minutes as needed. **Note:** More frequent dosing may be needed (eg, mechanically-ventilated patients).

      Continuous infusion: 50-700 mcg/hour (based on ~70 kg patient) **or** 0.7-10 mcg/kg/**hour**

    Intrathecal (I.T.) (unlabeled use; American Pain Society, 2008): **Must be preservative-free.** Doses must be adjusted for age, injection site, and patient's medical condition and degree of opioid tolerance.

      Single dose: 5-25 mcg/dose; may provide adequate relief for up to 6 hours

      Continuous infusion: Not recommended in acute pain management due to risk of excessive accumulation. For chronic cancer pain, infusion of very small doses may be practical (American Pain Society, 2008).

    Epidural (unlabeled use; American Pain Society, 2008): **Must be preservative-free.** Doses must be adjusted for age, injection site, and patient's medical condition and degree of opioid tolerance

      Single dose: 25-100 mcg/dose; may provide adequate relief for up to 8 hours

      Continuous infusion: 25-100 mcg/hour

Breakthrough cancer pain: For patients who are tolerant to and currently receiving opioid therapy for persistent cancer pain; dosing should be individually titrated to provide adequate analgesia with minimal side effects. Dose titration should be done if patient requires more than 1 dose/breakthrough pain episode for several consecutive episodes. Patients experiencing >4 breakthrough pain episodes/day should have the dose of their long-term opioid re-evaluated.

    Lozenge: Initial dose: 200 mcg; the second dose may be started 15 minutes after completion of the first dose if pain unrelieved. A maximum of 1 additional dose can be given per pain episode; must wait at least 4 hours before treating another episode. Consumption should be limited to ≤4 units/day. Additional requirements suggest need for improved baseline therapy.

    Buccal film (Onsolis™): Initial dose: 200 mcg for all patients **Note:** Patients previously using another transmucosal product should be initiated at doses of 200 mcg; do **not** switch patients using any other fentanyl product on a mcg-per-mcg basis.

    Dose titration: If titration required, increase dose in 200 mcg increments once per episode using multiples of the 200 mcg film; do not redose within a single episode of break-through pain and separate single doses by ≥2 hours. During titration, do not exceed 4 simultaneous applications of the 200 mcg films (800 mcg). If >800 mcg required, treat next episode with one 1200 mcg film (maximum dose: 1200 mcg). Once maintenance dose is determined, all other unused films should be disposed of and that strength (using a single film) should be used. During any pain episode, if adequate relief is not achieved after 30 minutes following buccal film application, a rescue medication (as determined by healthcare provider) may be used.

    Maintenance: Determined dose applied as a single film once per episode and separated by ≥2 hours (dose range: 200-1200 mcg); limit to 4 applications/day. Consider increasing the around-the-clock opioid therapy in patients experiencing >4 break-through pain episodes/day.

    Buccal tablet (Fentora®): Initial dose: 100 mcg; a second 100 mcg dose, if needed, may be started 30 minutes after the start of the first dose. **Note:** For patients previously using the transmucosal lozenge (Actiq®), the initial dose should be selected using the conversions listed below (maximum: 2 doses per breakthrough pain episode every 4 hours).

Dose titration, if required, should be done using multiples of the 100 mcg tablets. Patient can take two 100 mcg tablets (one on each side of mouth). If that dose is not successful, can use four 100 mcg tablets (two on each side of mouth). If titration requires >400 mcg/dose, then use 200 mcg tablets.

Conversion from lozenge to buccal tablet (Fentora®):

Lozenge dose 200-400 mcg, then buccal tablet 100 mcg

Lozenge dose 600-800 mcg, then buccal tablet 200 mcg

Lozenge dose 1200-1600 mcg, then buccal tablet 400 mcg

Note: Four 100 mcg buccal tablets deliver approximately 12% and 13% higher values of C_{max} and AUC, respectively, compared to one 400 mcg buccal tablet. To prevent confusion, patient should only have one strength available at a time. Using more than four buccal tablets at a time has not been studied.

Sublingual tablet (Abstral®):

Initial dose:

U.S. labeling: 100 mcg for all patients; if pain is unrelieved, a second dose may be given 30 minutes after administration of the first dose. A maximum of 2 doses can be given per breakthrough pain episode; must wait at least 2 hours before treating another episode.

Canadian labeling: 100 mcg for all patients; if pain is unrelieved 30 minutes after administration of Abstral™, an alternative rescue medication (other than Abstral™) may be given. Administer only 1 dose of Abstral™ per breakthrough pain episode; must wait at least 2 hours before treating another episode.

Note: Patients previously using another fentanyl product should be initiated at a dose of 100 mcg; do not convert patients from other fentanyl products to Abstral® on a mcg-per-mcg basis.

Dose titration: If titration required, increase in 100 mcg increments (up to 400 mcg) over consecutive breakthrough episodes. If titration requires >400 mcg/dose, increase in increments of 200 mcg, starting with 600 mcg dose. During titration, patients may use multiples of 100 mcg and/or 200 mcg tablets for any single dose; do not exceed 4 tablets at one time; safety and efficacy of doses >800 mcg have not been evaluated.

Maintenance dose: Once maintenance dose for breakthrough pain episode has been determined, use only 1 tablet in the appropriate strength per episode; if pain is unrelieved with maintenance dose:

U.S. labeling recommendations: A second dose may be given after 30 minutes; maximum of 2 doses/episode of breakthrough pain; separate treatment of subsequent episodes by ≥2 hours; limit treatment to ≤4 breakthrough episodes/day.

Canadian labeling recommendations: Administer alternative rescue medication after 30 minutes; maximum of 1 Abstral™ dose/episode of breakthrough pain; separate treatment of subsequent episodes by ≥2 hours; limit treatment to ≤4 breakthrough episodes/day.

Consider increasing the around-the-clock long-acting opioid therapy in patients experiencing >4 breakthrough pain episodes/day; if long-acting opioid therapy dose altered, re-evaluate and retitrate Abstral® dose as needed.

Chronic pain management: Adults (opioid-tolerant patients): Transdermal patch (Duragesic®):

Initial: To convert patients from oral or parenteral opioids to transdermal patch, a 24-hour analgesic requirement should be calculated (based on prior opiate use). Using the tables, the appropriate initial dose can be determined. The initial fentanyl dosage may be approximated from the 24-hour morphine dosage equivalent and titrated to minimize adverse effects and provide analgesia. With the initial application, the absorption of transdermal fentanyl requires several hours to reach plateau; therefore transdermal fentanyl is inappropriate for management of acute pain. Change patch every 72 hours.

Conversion from continuous infusion of fentanyl: In patients who have adequate pain relief with a fentanyl infusion, fentanyl may be converted to transdermal dosing at a rate equivalent to the intravenous rate. A two-step taper of the infusion to be completed over 12 hours has been recommended (Kornick, 2001) after the patch is applied. The infusion is decreased to 50% of the original rate six hours after the application of the first patch, and subsequently discontinued twelve hours after application.

Titration: Short-acting agents may be required until analgesic efficacy is established and/or as supplements for "breakthrough" pain. The amount of supplemental doses should be closely monitored. Appropriate dosage increases may be based on daily supplemental dosage using the ratio of 45 mg/24 hours of oral morphine to a 12.5 mcg/hour increase in fentanyl dosage.

Frequency of adjustment: The dosage should not be titrated more frequently than every 3 days after the initial dose or every 6 days thereafter. Patients should wear a consistent fentanyl dosage through two applications (6 days) before dosage increase based on supplemental opiate dosages can be estimated. **Note:** Upon discontinuation, ~17 hours are required for a 50% decrease in fentanyl levels.

Frequency of application: The majority of patients may be controlled on every 72-hour administration; however, a small number of patients require every 48-hour administration.

Dose conversion guidelines for transdermal fentanyl (see tables).
Note: U.S. and Canadian dose conversion guidelines differ. Consult appropriate table.

U.S. Labeling: Dose Conversion Guidelines: Recommended Initial Duragesic® Dose Based Upon Daily Oral Morphine Dose[1,2]

Oral 24-Hour Morphine (mg/day)	Duragesic® Dose[3] (mcg/h)
60-134	25
135-224	50
225-314	75
315-404	100
405-494	125
495-584	150
585-674	175
675-764	200
765-854	225
855-944	250
945-1034	275
1035-1124	300

[1]The table should NOT be used to convert from transdermal fentanyl (Duragesic®) to other opioid analgesics. Rather, following removal of the patch, titrate the dose of the new opioid until adequate analgesia is achieved.

[2]Recommendations are based on U.S. product labeling for Duragesic®.

[3]Pediatric patients initiating therapy on a 25 mcg/hour Duragesic® system should be opioid-tolerant and receiving at least 60 mg oral morphine equivalents per day.

U.S. Labeling: Dose Conversion Guidelines[1,2]

Current Analgesic	Daily Dosage (mg/day)			
Morphine (I.M./I.V.)	10-22	23-37	38-52	53-67
Oxycodone (oral)	30-67	67.5-112	112.5-157	157.5-202
Oxycodone (I.M./I.V.)	15-33	33.1-56	56.1-78	78.1-101
Codeine (oral)	150-447	448-747	748-1047	1048-1347
Hydromorphone (oral)	8-17	17.1-28	28.1-39	39.1-51
Hydromorphone (I.V.)	1.5-3.4	3.5-5.6	5.7-7.9	8-10
Meperidine (I.M.)	75-165	166-278	279-390	391-503
Methadone (oral)	20-44	45-74	75-104	105-134
Methadone (I.M.)	10-22	23-37	38-52	53-67
Fentanyl transdermal recommended dose (mcg/h)	25 mcg/h	50 mcg/h	75 mcg/h	100 mcg/h

[1]The table should NOT be used to convert from transdermal fentanyl (Duragesic®) to other opioid analgesics. Rather, following removal of the patch, titrate the dose of the new opioid until adequate analgesia is achieved.

[2]Recommendations are based on U.S. product labeling for Duragesic®.

Transdermal patch (Duragesic® MAT [Canada; not available in U.S.]): Adults:

Canadian Labeling: Dose Conversion Guidelines (Adults): Recommended Initial Duragesic® MAT Dose Based Upon Daily Oral Morphine Dose[1,2]

Oral 24-Hour Morphine (Current Dose in mg/day)	Duragesic® MAT Dose (Initial Dose in mcg/h)
45-59	12
60-134	25
135-179	37
180-224	50
225-269	62
270-314	75
315-359	87
360-404	100
405-494	125
495-584	150
585-674	175
675-764	200
765-854	225
855-944	250
945-1034	275
1035-1124	300

[1]The table should NOT be used to convert from transdermal fentanyl (Duragesic® MAT) to other opioid analgesics. Rather, following removal of the patch, titrate the dose of the new opioid until adequate analgesia is achieved.

[2]Recommendations are based on Canadian product labeling for Duragesic® MAT.

Note: The 12 mcg/hour dose included in this table is to be used for incremental dose adjustment and is generally not recommended for initial dosing, except for patients in whom lower starting doses are deemed clinically appropriate.

Canadian Labeling: Dosing Conversion Guidelines (Adults)[1,2]

Current Analgesic	Daily Dosage (mg/day)						
Morphine[3] (I.M./I.V.)	20-44	45-60	61-75	76-90	n/a[4]	n/a[4]	n/a[4]
Oxycodone (oral)	30-66	67-90	91-112	113-134	135-157	158-179	180-202
Codeine (oral)	150-447	448-597	598-747	748-897	898-1047	1048-1197	1198-1347
Hydromorphone (oral)	8-16	17-22	23-28	29-33	34-39	40-45	46-51
Hydromorphone (I.V.)	4-8.4	8.5-11.4	11.5-14.4	14.5-16.5	16.6-19.5	19.6-22.5	22.6-25.5
Fentanyl transdermal recommended dose (mcg/h)	25 mcg/h	37 mcg/h	50 mcg/h	62 mcg/h	75 mcg/h	87 mcg/h	100 mcg/h

[1]The table should NOT be used to convert from transdermal fentanyl (Duragesic® MAT) to other opioid analgesics. Rather, following removal of the patch, titrate the dose of the new opioid until adequate analgesia is achieved.

[2]Recommendations are based on Canadian product labeling for Duragesic® MAT.

[3]Morphine dose conversion based upon I.M to oral dose ratio of 1:3.

[4]Insufficient data available to provide specific dosing recommendations. Use caution; adjust dose conservatively.

Hepatic Impairment Fentanyl kinetics may be altered in hepatic disease.

◀ **Administration**
I.V.: Administer as slow I.V. infusion over 1-2 minutes. May also be administered as continuous infusion or PCA (unlabeled use) routes. Muscular rigidity may occur with rapid I.V. administration.

Transdermal patch (eg, Duragesic®): Apply to nonirritated and nonirradiated skin, such as chest, back, flank, or upper arm. Do not shave skin; hair at application site should be clipped. Prior to application, clean site with clear water and allow to dry completely. Do not use damaged, cut or leaking patches; patch may be less effective. Skin exposure from fentanyl gel leaking from patch may lead to serious adverse effects; thoroughly wash affected skin surfaces with water (do not use soap). Firmly press in place and hold for 30 seconds. Change patch every 72 hours. Do **not** use soap, alcohol, or other solvents to remove transdermal gel if it accidentally touches skin; use copious amounts of water. Avoid exposing application site to external heat sources (eg, heating pad, electric blanket, heat lamp, hot tub). If there is difficulty with patch adhesion, the edges of the system may be taped in place with first-aid tape. If there is continued difficulty with adhesion, an adhesive film dressing (eg, Bioclusive®, Tegaderm®) may be applied over the system.

Lozenge: Foil overwrap should be removed just prior to administration. Place the unit in mouth between the cheek and gum and allow it to dissolve. Do not chew. Lozenge may be moved from one side of the mouth to the other. The unit should be consumed over a period of 15 minutes. Handle should be removed after the lozenge is consumed; early removal should be considered if the patient has achieved an adequate response and/or shows signs of respiratory depression.

Buccal film: Foil overwrap should be removed just prior to administration. Prior to placing film, wet inside of cheek using tongue or by rinsing with water. Place film inside mouth with the pink side of the unit against the inside of the moistened cheek. With finger, press the film against cheek and hold for 5 seconds. The film should stick to the inside of cheek after 5 seconds. The film should be left in place until it dissolves (usually within 15-30 minutes after application). Liquids may be consumed after 5 minutes of application. Food can be eaten after film dissolves. If using more than 1 film simultaneously (during titration period), apply films on either side of mouth (do not apply on top of each other). Do not chew or swallow film. Do not cut or tear the film. All patients must initiate therapy using the 200 mcg film.

Buccal tablet: Patient should not open blister until ready to administer. The blister backing should be peeled back to expose the tablet; tablet should not be pushed out through the blister. Immediately use tablet once removed from blister. Place entire tablet in the buccal cavity (above a rear molar, between the upper cheek and gum). Tablet should not be broken, sucked, chewed, or swallowed. Should dissolve in about 14-25 minutes when left between the cheek and the gum. If remnants remain they may be swallowed with water.

Sublingual tablet: Remove from the blister unit immediately prior to administration. Place tablet directly under the tongue on the floor of the mouth and allow to completely dissolve; do not chew, suck, or swallow. Do not eat or drink anything until tablet is completely dissolved. In patients with a dry mouth, water may be used to moisten the buccal mucosa just before administration. All patients must initiate therapy using the 100 mcg tablet.

Monitoring Parameters Respiratory and cardiovascular status, blood pressure, heart rate; signs of misuse, abuse, or addiction
Transdermal patch: Monitor for 24 hours after application of first dose

Pharmacotherapy Pearls Fentanyl is 50-100 times as potent as morphine; morphine 10 mg I.M. is equivalent to fentanyl 0.1-0.2 mg I.M.; fentanyl has less hypotensive effects than morphine due to lack of histamine release. However, fentanyl may cause rigidity with high doses. If the patient has required high-dose analgesia or has used for a prolonged period (~7 days), taper dose to prevent withdrawal; monitor for signs and symptoms of withdrawal.

Transmucosal (oral lozenge, Actiq®): Disposal of lozenge units: After consumption of a complete unit, the handle may be disposed of in a trash container that is out of the reach of children. For a partially-consumed unit, or a unit that still has any drug matrix remaining on the handle, the handle should be placed under hot running tap water until the drug matrix has dissolved. Special child-resistant containers are available to temporarily store partially consumed units that cannot be disposed of immediately.

Transmucosal (buccal film, Onsolis™): Disposal of film: Remove foil overwrap from any unused, unneeded films and dispose by flushing in the toilet.

Transmucosal (sublingual tablet, Abstral®): Disposal of tablets: Remove any unused tablets from the blister cards and dispose by flushing in the toilet.

Transdermal patch (Duragesic®): Upon removal of the patch, ~17 hours are required before serum concentrations fall to 50% of their original values. Opioid withdrawal symptoms are possible. Gradual downward titration (potentially by the sequential use of lower-dose patches) is recommended. Keep transdermal patch (both used and unused) out of the reach of children. Do **not** use soap, alcohol, or other solvents to remove transdermal gel if it accidentally touches skin as they may increase transdermal absorption, use copious amounts of water. Avoid exposure of direct external heat sources (eg, heating pads, electric blankets, heat lamps, saunas, hot tubs, heated water beds) to application site.

Special Geriatric Considerations The elderly may be particularly susceptible to the CNS depressant and constipating effects of narcotics; therefore, use with caution. The effect of age on the pharmacokinetics of Fentora® (oral transmucosal buccal tablets) has not been studied. Instruct patients on proper use of the transdermal patch.

Product Availability

Lazanda®: FDA approved June 2011; availability expected in the second half of 2011

Lazanda® is a fentanyl nasal spray formulation indicated for the management of breakthrough cancer pain in opioid-tolerant patients.

Controlled Substance C-II

Dosage Forms Excipient information presented when available (limited, particularly for generics); consult specific product labeling.

Film, for buccal application, as citrate [strength expressed as base]:

Onsolis™: 200 mcg (30s); 400 mcg (30s); 600 mcg (30s); 800 mcg (30s); 1200 mcg (30s)

Injection, solution, as citrate [strength expressed as base, preservative free]: 0.05 mg/mL (2 mL, 5 mL, 10 mL, 20 mL, 50 mL)

Lozenge, oral, as citrate [strength expressed as base, transmucosal]: 200 mcg (30s); 400 mcg (30s); 600 mcg (30s); 800 mcg (30s); 1200 mcg (30s); 1600 mcg (30s)

Actiq®: 200 mcg (30s); 400 mcg (30s); 600 mcg (30s); 800 mcg (30s); 1200 mcg (30s); 1600 mcg (30s) [contains sugar 2 g/lozenge; berry flavor]

Patch, transdermal, as base: 12 [delivers 12.5 mcg/hr] (5s); 25 [delivers 25 mcg/hr] (5s); 50 [delivers 50 mcg/hr] (5s); 75 [delivers 75 mcg/hr] (5s); 100 [delivers 100 mcg/hr] (5s)

Duragesic®: 12 [delivers 12.5 mcg/hr] (5s) [contains ethanol 0.1mL/10 cm^2; 5 cm^2]

Duragesic®: 25 [delivers 25 mcg/hr] (5s) [contains ethanol 0.1 mL/10 cm^2; 10 cm^2]

Duragesic®: 50 [delivers 50 mcg/hr] (5s) [contains ethanol 0.1 mL/10 cm^2; 20 cm^2]

Duragesic®: 75 [delivers 75 mcg/hr] (5s) [contains ethanol 0.1 mL/10 cm^2; 30 cm^2]

Duragesic®: 100 [delivers 100 mcg/hr] (5s) [contains ethanol 0.1 mL/10 $cm^{2;}$ 40 cm^2]

Powder, for prescription compounding, as citrate: USP: 100% (1 g)

Tablet, for buccal application, as citrate [strength expressed as base]:

Fentora®: 100 mcg (28s); 200 mcg (28s); 400 mcg (28s); 600 mcg (28s); 800 mcg (28s)

Tablet, sublingual, as citrate [strength expressed as base]:

Abstral®: 100 mcg (12s, 32s); 200 mcg (12s, 32s); 300 mcg (12s, 32s); 400 mcg (12s, 32s); 600 mcg (12s, 32s); 800 mcg (32s)

Dosage Forms: Canada Excipient information presented when available (limited, particularly for generics); consult specific product labeling.

Patch, transdermal, as base: 12 mcg/hr (5s); 25 mcg/hr (5s); 50 mcg/hr (5s); 75 mcg/hr (5s); 100 mcg/hr (5s)

Duragesic® MAT: 12 mcg/hr (5s) [contains ethanol 0.1 mL/10 cm^2; 5 cm^2]

Duragesic® MAT: 25 mcg/hr (5s) [contains ethanol 0.1 mL/10 cm^2; 10 cm^2]

Duragesic® MAT: 50 mcg/hr (5s) [contains ethanol 0.1 mL/10 cm^2; 20 cm^2]

Duragesic® MAT: 75 mcg/hr (5s) [contains ethanol 0.1 mL/10 cm^2; 30 cm^2]

Duragesic® MAT: 100 mcg/hr (5s) [contains ethanol 0.1 mL/10 cm^2; 40 cm^2]

Selected References

American Geriatrics Society Panel on Pharmacological Management of Persistent Pain in Older Persons, "Pharmacological Management of Persistent Pain in Older Persons," *J Am Geriatr Soc*, 2009, 57(8):1331-46.

Heiskanen T, Matzke S, Haakana S, et al, "Transdermal Fentanyl in Cachetic Cancer Patients," *Pain*, 2009, 144 (1-2):218-22.

Ferric Gluconate (FER ik GLOO koe nate)

Medication Safety Issues
Sound-alike/look-alike issues:
Ferric gluconate may be confused with ferumoxytol
Ferrlecit® may be confused with Ferralet®

Brand Names: U.S. Ferrlecit®; Nulecit™

Brand Names: Canada Ferrlecit®

Index Terms Sodium Ferric Gluconate

Generic Availability (U.S.) No

Pharmacologic Category Iron Salt

Use Repletion of total body iron content in patients with iron-deficiency anemia who are undergoing hemodialysis in conjunction with erythropoietin therapy

Unlabeled/Investigational Use Cancer-/chemotherapy-associated anemia

Contraindications Hypersensitivity to ferric gluconate or any component of the formulation; use in any anemia not caused by iron deficiency; iron overload

Warnings/Precautions Potentially serious hypersensitivity reactions may occur. Fatal immediate hypersensitivity reactions have occurred with other iron carbohydrate complexes. Avoid rapid administration. Flushing and transient hypotension may occur. May augment hemodialysis-induced hypotension. Use with caution in elderly patients. Use only in patients with documented iron deficiency; caution with hemoglobinopathies or other refractory anemias.

Adverse Reactions (Reflective of adult population; not specific for elderly) Frequency not defined.
Cardiovascular: Angina, bradycardia, chest pain, edema, hyper-/hypotension, hypervolemia, MI, pulmonary edema, syncope, tachycardia, thrombosis, vasodilation
Central nervous system: Agitation, chills, dizziness, fatigue, fever, headache, insomnia, malaise, pain, somnolence
Dermatologic: Pruritus, rash
Endocrine & metabolic: Hyper-/hypokalemia, hypoglycemia
Gastrointestinal: Abdominal pain, anorexia, diarrhea, dyspepsia, epigastric pain, eructation, flatulence, melena, nausea, vomiting
Genitourinary: Urinary tract infection
Hematologic: Abnormal erythrocytes, leukocytosis, lymphadenopathy
Local: Injection site reactions, injection site pain
Neuromuscular & skeletal: Arthralgia, back pain, cramps, groin pain, leg cramps, myalgia, paresthesia, rigors, weakness
Ocular: Blurred vision, conjunctivitis
Respiratory: Cough, dyspnea, pneumonia, rhinitis, upper respiratory infection
Miscellaneous: Carcinoma, diaphoresis increased, flu-like syndrome, hypersensitivity reactions, infection, sepsis

Drug Interactions
Avoid Concomitant Use
Avoid concomitant use of Ferric Gluconate with any of the following: Dimercaprol
Increased Effect/Toxicity
The levels/effects of Ferric Gluconate may be increased by: ACE Inhibitors; Dimercaprol
Decreased Effect
Ferric Gluconate may decrease the levels/effects of: Cefdinir; Eltrombopag; Levothyroxine; Phosphate Supplements; Trientine

The levels/effects of Ferric Gluconate may be decreased by: Pancrelipase; Trientine

Stability Store at 20°C to 25°C (68°F to 77°F). Do not freeze. For I.V. infusion, dilute 10 mL ferric gluconate in 0.9% sodium chloride (100 mL NS); use immediately after dilution.

Mechanism of Action Supplies a source to elemental iron necessary to the function of hemoglobin, myoglobin and specific enzyme systems; allows transport of oxygen via hemoglobin

Pharmacodynamics/Kinetics Half-life elimination: Bound: 1 hour

Dosage
Geriatric & Adult
Repletion of iron in hemodialysis patients: I.V.: 125 mg elemental iron per 10 mL (either by I.V. infusion or slow I.V. injection). Most patients will require a cumulative dose of 1 g elemental iron over approximately 8 sequential dialysis treatments to achieve a favorable response.
Note: A test dose of 2 mL diluted in NS 50 mL administered over 60 minutes was previously recommended (not in current manufacturer labeling). Doses >125 mg are associated with increased adverse events.

Cancer-/chemotherapy-associated anemia (unlabeled use): I.V. infusion: 125 mg over 1 hour; maximum: 250 mg/infusion. Repeat dose every week for 8 doses. Test doses (25 mg slow I.V. push or infusion) are recommended in patients with iron dextran hypersensitivity or those with other drug allergies (NCCN guidelines, v.2.2010)

Administration I.V.: Monitor patient for hypotension or hypersensitivity reactions during infusion.

Adults: May be diluted prior to administration; avoid rapid administration. Infusion rate should not exceed 2.1 mg/minute. If administered undiluted, infuse slowly at a rate of up to 12.5 mg/minute.

Monitoring Parameters Hemoglobin and hematocrit, serum ferritin, iron saturation; vital signs

NKF K/DOQI guidelines recommend that iron status should be monitored monthly during initiation through the percent transferrin saturation (TSAT) and serum ferritin.

Reference Range CKD patients should have sufficient iron to achieve and maintain hemoglobin of 11-12 g/dL. To achieve and maintain this target Hgb, sufficient iron should be administered to maintain a TSAT of 20%, and a serum ferritin level >100 ng/mL (non-dialysis chronic kidney disease and peritoneal dialysis chronic kidney disease) or serum ferritin level >200 ng/mL (hemodialysis chronic kidney disease).

Test Interactions Serum or transferrin bound iron levels may be falsely elevated if assessed within 24 hours of ferric gluconate administration. Serum ferritin levels may be falsely elevated for 5 days after ferric gluconate administration.

Special Geriatric Considerations Anemia in the elderly is often caused by "anemia of chronic disease," a result of aging changes in the bone marrow, or associated with inflammation rather than blood loss. Iron stores are usually normal or increased, with a serum ferritin >50 ng/mL and a decreased total iron binding capacity; hence, the anemia is not secondary to iron deficiency but the inability of the reticuloendothelial system to use available iron stores. Timed release iron preparations should be avoided due to their erratic absorption. Products combined with a laxative or stool softener should not be used unless the need for the combination is demonstrated.

Dosage Forms Excipient information presented when available (limited, particularly for generics); consult specific product labeling.

Injection, solution:

Ferrlecit®: Elemental iron 12.5 mg/mL (5 mL) [contains benzyl alcohol, sucrose 20%]

Nulecit™: Elemental iron 12.5 mg/mL (5 mL) [contains benzyl alcohol, sucrose ~20%]

Selected References

National Kidney Foundation, "KDOQI Clinical Practice Guidelines and Clinical Practice Recommentaions for Anemia in Chronic Kidney Disease." Available at www.kidney.org/professionals/KDOQI/guidelines_anemia/cpr32.htm. Last accessed November 20, 2006.

◆ **Ferrlecit®** see Ferric Gluconate on page 720
◆ **Ferrocite™ [OTC]** see Ferrous Fumarate on page 721
◆ **Ferro-Sequels® [OTC]** see Ferrous Fumarate on page 721

Ferrous Fumarate (FER us FYOO ma rate)

Brand Names: U.S. Femiron® [OTC]; Ferretts® [OTC]; Ferro-Sequels® [OTC]; Ferrocite™ [OTC]; Hemocyte® [OTC]; Ircon® [OTC]

Brand Names: Canada Palafer®

Index Terms Iron Fumarate

Generic Availability (U.S.) Yes: Tablet

Pharmacologic Category Iron Salt

Use Prevention and treatment of iron-deficiency anemias

Contraindications Hypersensitivity to iron salts or any component of the formulation; hemochromatosis, hemolytic anemia

Warnings/Precautions Avoid in patients with peptic ulcer, enteritis, or ulcerative colitis. Administration of iron for >6 months should be avoided except in patients with continuous bleeding or menorrhagia. Anemia in the elderly is often caused by "anemia of chronic disease" or associated with inflammation rather than blood loss. Iron stores are usually normal or increased, with a serum ferritin >50 ng/mL and a decreased total iron binding capacity. Hence, the "anemia of chronic disease" is not secondary to iron deficiency but the inability of the reticuloendothelial system to reclaim available iron stores. Avoid in patients receiving frequent blood transfusions. **[U.S. Boxed Warning]: Severe iron toxicity may occur in overdose, particularly when ingested by children; iron is a leading cause of fatal poisoning in children; store out of children's reach and in child-resistant containers.**

Adverse Reactions (Reflective of adult population; not specific for elderly)
>10%: Gastrointestinal: Constipation, dark stools, nausea, stomach cramping, vomiting
1% to 10%:
Gastrointestinal: Diarrhea, heartburn, staining of teeth
Genitourinary: Discoloration of urine
Drug Interactions
Avoid Concomitant Use
Avoid concomitant use of Ferrous Fumarate with any of the following: Dimercaprol
Increased Effect/Toxicity
The levels/effects of Ferrous Fumarate may be increased by: Dimercaprol
Decreased Effect
Ferrous Fumarate may decrease the levels/effects of: Bisphosphonate Derivatives; Cefdinir; Eltrombopag; Levodopa; Levothyroxine; Methyldopa; Penicillamine; Phosphate Supplements; Quinolone Antibiotics; Tetracycline Derivatives; Trientine

The levels/effects of Ferrous Fumarate may be decreased by: Antacids; H2-Antagonists; Pancrelipase; Proton Pump Inhibitors; Trientine
Ethanol/Nutrition/Herb Interactions Food: Cereals, dietary fiber, tea, coffee, eggs, and milk may decrease absorption.
Stability Iron is a leading cause of fatal poisoning in children. Store out of children's reach and in child-resistant containers.
Mechanism of Action Replaces iron found in hemoglobin, myoglobin, and enzymes; allows the transportation of oxygen via hemoglobin
Pharmacodynamics/Kinetics
Absorption: Iron is absorbed in the duodenum and upper jejunum; in persons with normal iron stores 10% of an oral dose is absorbed, this is increased to 20% to 30% in persons with inadequate iron stores. Food and achlorhydria will decrease absorption; aging has not been shown to affect absorption, but the percent uptake by red cells decreases from 91.2% in healthy young adults to 60% in healthy older adults.
Elimination: Iron is largely bound to serum transferrin and excreted in the urine, sweat, and sloughing of intestinal mucosa.
Dosage
Geriatric Lower doses (15-50 mg elemental iron/day) may have similar efficacy and less GI adverse events (eg, nausea,constipation) as compared to higher doses (eg, 150 mg elemental iron/day) (Rimon, 2005).
Adult
Dietary Reference Intake: Dose is RDA presented as elemental iron unless otherwise noted:
19-50 years: Male: 8 mg/day; Female: 18 mg/day
≥50 years: 8 mg/day

Doses expressed in terms of elemental iron; elemental iron content of ferrous fumarate is 33%.
Treatment of iron deficiency: Oral: Usual range: 150-200 mg elemental iron/day in divided doses; 60-100 mg elemental iron twice daily, up to 60 mg elemental iron 4 times/day
Prophylaxis of iron deficiency: Oral: 60-100 mg elemental iron/day
Note: To avoid GI upset, start with a single daily dose and increase by 1 tablet/day each week or as tolerated until desired daily dose is achieved
Administration Should be administered with water or juice on an empty stomach. Administer 2 hours prior to or 4 hours after antacids.
Monitoring Parameters Hemoglobin, hematocrit, ferritin, reticulocyte count
Reference Range
Serum iron:
Male: 75-175 mcg/dL (SI: 13.4-31.3 µmol/L)
Female: 65-165 mcg/dL (SI: 11.6-29.5 µmol/L)
Total iron binding capacity: 230-430 mcg/dL
Transferrin: 204-360 mg/dL
Percent transferrin saturation: 20% to 50%
Iron levels >300 mcg/dL can be considered toxic, should be treated as an overdose
Pharmacotherapy Pearls The elemental iron content in ferrous fumarate is 33% (ie, 200 mg ferrous fumarate is equivalent to 66 mg ferrous iron). Administration of iron for longer than 6 months should be avoided except in patients with continuous bleeding or menorrhagia.
Special Geriatric Considerations Anemia in the elderly is often caused by "anemia of chronic disease," a result of aging changes in the bone marrow, or associated with inflammation rather than blood loss. Iron stores are usually normal or increased, with a serum ferritin >50 ng/mL and a decreased total iron binding capacity. Hence, the anemia is not

secondary to iron deficiency but the inability of the reticuloendothelial system to use available iron stores. Timed release iron preparations should be avoided due to their erratic absorption. Products combined with a laxative or stool softener should not be used unless the need for the combination is demonstrated.

Dosage Forms Excipient information presented when available (limited, particularly for generics); consult specific product labeling.

Tablet, oral: 324 mg [elemental iron 106 mg]
Femiron®: 63 mg [elemental iron 20 mg]
Ferretts®: 325 mg [scored; elemental iron 106 mg]
Ferrocite™: 324 mg [elemental iron 106 mg]
Hemocyte®: 324 mg [elemental iron 106 mg]
Ircon®: 200 mg [elemental iron 66 mg]
Tablet, timed release, oral:
Ferro-Sequels®: 150 mg [contains sodium benzoate; elemental iron 50 mg; with docusate sodium]

Selected References

Lipschitz DA, "The Anemia of Chronic Disease," *J Am Geriatr Soc*, 1990, 38(11):1258-64.
Marx JJ, "Normal Iron Absorption and Decreased Red Cell Iron Uptake in the Aged," *Blood*, 1979, 53(2):204-11.
Rimon E, Kagansky N, Kagansky M, et al, "Are We Giving Too Much Iron? Low-Dose Iron Therapy is Effective in Octogenarians," *Am J Med*, 2005, 118(10):1142-7.

Ferrous Gluconate (FER us GLOO koe nate)

Brand Names: U.S. Ferate [OTC]; Fergon® [OTC]
Brand Names: Canada Apo-Ferrous Gluconate®; Novo-Ferrogluc
Index Terms Iron Gluconate
Generic Availability (U.S.) Yes
Pharmacologic Category Iron Salt
Use Prevention and treatment of iron-deficiency anemias
Contraindications Hypersensitivity to iron salts or any component of the formulation; hemochromatosis, hemolytic anemia
Warnings/Precautions Avoid in patients with peptic ulcer, enteritis, or ulcerative colitis. Administration of iron for >6 months should be avoided except in patients with continuous bleeding or menorrhagia. Anemia in the elderly is often caused by "anemia of chronic disease" or associated with inflammation rather than blood loss. Iron stores are usually normal or increased, with a serum ferritin >50 ng/mL and a decreased total iron binding capacity. Hence, the "anemia of chronic disease" is not secondary to iron deficiency but the inability of the reticuloendothelial system to reclaim available iron stores. Avoid in patients receiving frequent blood transfusions. **[U.S. Boxed Warning]: Severe iron toxicity may occur in overdose, particularly when ingested by children; iron is a leading cause of fatal poisoning in children; store out of children's reach and in child-resistant containers.**
Adverse Reactions (Reflective of adult population; not specific for elderly)
>10%: Gastrointestinal: Constipation, dark stools, nausea, stomach cramping, vomiting
1% to 10%:
Gastrointestinal: Diarrhea, heartburn, staining of teeth
Genitourinary: Discoloration of urine
Drug Interactions
Avoid Concomitant Use
Avoid concomitant use of Ferrous Gluconate with any of the following: Dimercaprol
Increased Effect/Toxicity
The levels/effects of Ferrous Gluconate may be increased by: Dimercaprol
Decreased Effect
Ferrous Gluconate may decrease the levels/effects of: Bisphosphonate Derivatives; Cefdinir; Eltrombopag; Levodopa; Levothyroxine; Methyldopa; Penicillamine; Phosphate Supplements; Quinolone Antibiotics; Tetracycline Derivatives; Trientine

The levels/effects of Ferrous Gluconate may be decreased by: Antacids; H2-Antagonists; Pancrelipase; Proton Pump Inhibitors; Trientine
Ethanol/Nutrition/Herb Interactions Food: Cereals, dietary fiber, tea, coffee, eggs, and milk may decrease absorption.
Stability Iron is a leading cause of fatal poisoning in children. Store out of children's reach and in child-resistant containers.
Mechanism of Action Replaces iron found in hemoglobin, myoglobin, and enzymes; allows the transportation of oxygen via hemoglobin

◀ **Pharmacodynamics/Kinetics**

Absorption: Iron is absorbed in the duodenum and upper jejunum; in persons with normal iron stores 10% of an oral dose is absorbed, this is increased to 20% to 30% in persons with inadequate iron stores. Food and achlorhydria will decrease absorption; aging has not been shown to affect absorption, but the percent uptake by red cells decreases from 91.2% in healthy young adults to 60% in healthy older adults.

Elimination: Iron is largely bound to serum transferrin and excreted in the urine, sweat, and sloughing of intestinal mucosa

Dosage

Geriatric Lower doses (15-50 mg elemental iron/day) may have similar efficacy and less GI adverse events (eg, nausea, constipation) as compared to higher doses (eg, 150 mg elemental iron/day) (Rimon, 2005).

Adult

Dietary Reference Intake: Dose is RDA presented as elemental iron unless otherwise noted:

19-50 years: Male: 8 mg/day; Female: 18 mg/day

≥50 years: 8 mg/day

Dose expressed in terms of elemental iron:

Treatment of iron deficiency anemia: Oral: 60 mg twice daily up to 60 mg 4 times/day

Prophylaxis of iron deficiency: Oral: 60 mg/day

Administration Administer 2 hours before or 4 hours after antacids

Monitoring Parameters Serum iron, total iron binding capacity, reticulocyte count, hemoglobin

Reference Range Therapeutic: Male: 75-175 mcg/dL (SI: 13.4-31.3 μmol/L); Female: 65-165 mcg/dL (SI: 11.6-29.5 μmol/L); serum iron level >300 mcg/dL usually requires treatment of overdose due to severe toxicity

Test Interactions False-positive for blood in stool by the guaiac test

Pharmacotherapy Pearls Gluconate contains 12% elemental iron (ie, 300 mg ferrous gluconate is equivalent to 34 mg ferrous iron); administration of iron for longer than 6 months should be avoided except in patients with continued bleeding or menorrhagia

Special Geriatric Considerations Anemia in the elderly is often caused by "anemia of chronic disease," a result of aging changes in the bone marrow, or associated with inflammation rather than blood loss. Iron stores are usually normal or increased, with a serum ferritin >50 ng/mL and a decreased total iron binding capacity. Hence, the anemia is not secondary to iron deficiency but the inability of the reticuloendothelial system to use available iron stores. Timed release iron preparations should be avoided due to their erratic absorption. Products combined with a laxative or stool softener should not be used unless the need for the combination is demonstrated.

Dosage Forms Excipient information presented when available (limited, particularly for generics); consult specific product labeling.

Tablet, oral: 246 mg [elemental iron 28 mg], 324 mg [elemental iron 38 mg], 325 mg [elemental iron 36 mg]

Ferate: 240 mg [elemental iron 27 mg]

Fergon®: 240 mg [elemental iron 27 mg]

Selected References

Lipschitz DA, "The Anemia of Chronic Disease," *J Am Geriatr Soc*, 1990, 38(11):1258-64.

Marx JJ, "Normal Iron Absorption and Decreased Red Cell Iron Uptake in the Aged," *Blood*, 1979, 53(2):204-11.

Rimon E, Kagansky N, Kagansky M, et al, "Are We Giving Too Much Iron? Low-Dose Iron Therapy is Effective in Octogenarians," *Am J Med*, 2005, 118(10):1142-7.

Ferrous Sulfate (FER us SUL fate)

Related Information

Beers Criteria – Potentially Inappropriate Medications for Geriatrics *on page 2089*

Medication Safety Issues

Sound-alike/look-alike issues:

Feosol® may be confused with Fer-In-Sol®

Fer-In-Sol® may be confused with Feosol®

Slow FE® may be confused with Slow-K®

BEERS Criteria medication:

This drug may be inappropriate for use in geriatric patients (dosage dependent, low severity risk).

Administration issues:
Fer-In-Sol® (manufactured by Mead Johnson) and a limited number of generic products are available at a concentration of 15 mg/mL. However, many other generics and brand name products of ferrous sulfate oral liquid drops are available at a concentration of 15 mg/0.6 mL. Check concentration closely prior to dispensing. Prescriptions written in milliliters (mL) should be clarified.

Brand Names: U.S. Feosol® [OTC]; Fer-In-Sol® [OTC]; Fer-iron [OTC]; MyKidz Iron 10™ [OTC]; Slow FE® [OTC]; Slow Release [OTC]

Brand Names: Canada Apo-Ferrous Sulfate®; Fer-In-Sol®; Ferodan™

Index Terms FeSO$_4$; Iron Sulfate

Generic Availability (U.S.) Yes

Pharmacologic Category Iron Salt

Use Prevention and treatment of iron-deficiency anemias

Contraindications Hypersensitivity to iron salts or any component of the formulation; hemochromatosis, hemolytic anemia

Warnings/Precautions Avoid in patients with peptic ulcer, enteritis, or ulcerative colitis. Administration of iron for >6 months should be avoided except in patients with continuous bleeding or menorrhagia. Anemia in the elderly is often caused by "anemia of chronic disease" or associated with inflammation rather than blood loss. Iron stores are usually normal or increased, with a serum ferritin >50 ng/mL and a decreased total iron binding capacity. Hence, the "anemia of chronic disease" is not secondary to iron deficiency but the inability of the reticuloendothelial system to reclaim available iron stores. Avoid using doses >325 mg daily of ferrous sulfate, as this may increase potential for constipation, but not significantly increase absorption (Beers Criteria). Avoid in patients receiving frequent blood transfusions. **[U.S. Boxed Warning]: Severe iron toxicity may occur in overdose, particularly when ingested by children; iron is a leading cause of fatal poisoning in children; store out of children's reach and in child-resistant containers.**

Adverse Reactions (Reflective of adult population; not specific for elderly)
>10%: Gastrointestinal: Constipation, dark stools, epigastric pain, GI irritation, nausea, stomach cramping, vomiting
1% to 10%:
Gastrointestinal: Diarrhea, heartburn
Genitourinary: Discoloration of urine
Miscellaneous: Liquid preparations may temporarily stain the teeth

Drug Interactions
Avoid Concomitant Use
Avoid concomitant use of Ferrous Sulfate with any of the following: Dimercaprol
Increased Effect/Toxicity
The levels/effects of Ferrous Sulfate may be increased by: Dimercaprol
Decreased Effect
Ferrous Sulfate may decrease the levels/effects of: Bisphosphonate Derivatives; Cefdinir; Eltrombopag; Levodopa; Levothyroxine; Methyldopa; Penicillamine; Phosphate Supplements; Quinolone Antibiotics; Tetracycline Derivatives; Trientine

The levels/effects of Ferrous Sulfate may be decreased by: Antacids; H2-Antagonists; Pancrelipase; Proton Pump Inhibitors; Trientine

Ethanol/Nutrition/Herb Interactions Food: Cereals, dietary fiber, tea, coffee, eggs, and milk may decrease absorption.

Stability Iron is a leading cause of fatal poisoning in children. Store out of children's reach and in child-resistant containers.

Mechanism of Action Replaces iron, found in hemoglobin, myoglobin, and other enzymes; allows the transportation of oxygen via hemoglobin

Pharmacodynamics/Kinetics
Absorption: Iron is absorbed in the duodenum and upper jejunum; in persons with normal serum iron stores, 10% of an oral dose is absorbed; this is increased to 20% to 30% in persons with inadequate iron stores. Food and achlorhydria will decrease absorption; aging has not been shown to affect absorption, but the percent uptake by red cells decreases from 91.2% in healthy young adults to 60% in healthy older adults.
Elimination: Iron is largely bound to serum transferrin and excreted in the urine, sweat, and sloughing of the intestinal mucosa

Dosage
Geriatric Lower doses (15-50 mg elemental iron/day) may have similar efficacy and less GI adverse events (eg, nausea, constipation) as compared to higher doses (eg, 150 mg elemental iron/day) (Rimon, 2005).

◀ **Adult Note:** Multiple concentrations of ferrous sulfate oral liquid exist; close attention must be paid to the concentration when ordering and administering ferrous sulfate; incorrect selection or substitution of one ferrous sulfate liquid for another without proper dosage volume adjustment may result in serious over- or underdosing.

Dietary Reference Intake: Dose is RDA presented as elemental iron unless otherwise noted:
19-50 years: Male: 8 mg/day; Female: 18 mg/day
≥50 years: 8 mg/day

Dose expressed in terms of ferrous sulfate:
Treatment of iron deficiency anemia: Oral: 300 mg twice daily up to 300 mg 4 times/day or 250 mg (extended release) 1-2 times/day
Prophylaxis of iron deficiency: Oral: 300 mg/day

Administration Should be taken with water or juice on an empty stomach; administer ferrous sulfate 2 hours prior to, or 4 hours after antacids

Monitoring Parameters Serum iron, total iron binding capacity, reticulocyte count, hemoglobin

Reference Range
Serum iron:
Male: 75-175 mcg/dL (SI: 13.4-31.3 µmol/L)
Female: 65-165 mcg/dL (SI: 11.6-29.5 µmol/L)
Total iron binding capacity: 230-430 mcg/dL
Transferrin: 204-360 mg/dL
Percent transferrin saturation: 20% to 50%

Test Interactions False-positive for blood in stool by the guaiac test

Pharmacotherapy Pearls The elemental iron content of ferrous sulfate is 20% (ie, 300 mg ferrous sulfate is equivalent to 60 mg ferrous iron). Administration of iron for longer than 6 months should be avoided except in patients with continued bleeding, or menorrhagia.

Special Geriatric Considerations Anemia in the elderly is often caused by "anemia of chronic disease," a result of aging changes in the bone marrow, or associated with inflammation rather than blood loss. Iron stores are usually normal or increased, with a serum ferritin >50 ng/mL and a decreased total iron binding capacity. Hence, the anemia is not secondary to iron deficiency but the inability of the reticuloendothelial system to use available iron stores. Timed release iron preparations should be avoided due to their erratic absorption. Products combined with a laxative or stool softener should not be used unless the need for the combination is demonstrated. This medication is considered to be potentially inappropriate in this patient population (Beers Criteria severity: Low, dosage dependent).

Dosage Forms Excipient information presented when available (limited, particularly for generics); consult specific product labeling. [DSC] = Discontinued product
Elixir, oral: 220 mg/5 mL (473 mL, 480 mL) [elemental iron 44 mg/5 mL]
Liquid, oral: 300 mg/5 mL (5 mL) [elemental iron ~60 mg/5 mL]
Liquid, oral [drops]: 75 mg/mL (50 mL) [elemental iron 15 mg/mL]; 75 mg/0.6 mL (50 mL [DSC]) [elemental iron 15 mg/0.6 mL]
Fer-In-Sol®: 75 mg/mL (50 mL) [gluten free; contains ethanol 0.2%, sodium bisulfite; elemental iron 15 mg/mL]
Fer-iron: 75 mg/mL (50 mL) [contains ethanol 0.2%, sodium bisulfite; lemon flavor; elemental iron 15 mg/mL]
Suspension, oral [drops]:
MyKidz Iron 10™: 75 mg/1.5 mL (118 mL) [dye free, ethanol free; contains propylene glycol, sodium 12 mg/1.5 mL; strawberry-banana flavor; elemental iron 15 mg/1.5 mL]
Tablet, oral: 324 mg [elemental iron 65 mg], 325 mg [elemental iron 65 mg]
Tablet, oral [exsiccated]:
Feosol®: 200 mg [elemental iron 65 mg]
Tablet, enteric coated, oral: 324 mg [elemental iron 65 mg], 325 mg [elemental iron 65 mg]
Tablet, extended release, oral: 140 mg [elemental iron 45 mg], 160 mg [DSC] [elemental iron 50 mg]
Tablet, slow release, oral: 160 mg [elemental iron 50 mg]
Slow FE®: 142 mg [elemental iron 45 mg]
Slow Release: 140 mg [elemental iron 45 mg]

Selected References
Lipschitz DA, "The Anemia of Chronic Disease," *J Am Geriatr Soc*, 1990, 38(11):1258-64.
Marx JJ, "Normal Iron Absorption and Decreased Red Cell Iron Uptake in the Aged," *Blood*, 1979, 53(2):204-11.
Rimon E, Kagansky N, Kagansky M, et al, "Are We Giving Too Much Iron? Low-Dose Iron Therapy is Effective in Octogenarians," *Am J Med*, 2005, 118(10):1142-7.

Ferumoxytol (fer ue MOX i tol)

Medication Safety Issues
Sound-alike/look-alike issues:
Ferumoxytol may be confused with ferric gluconate, iron dextran complex, iron sucrose
Brand Names: U.S. Feraheme®
Generic Availability (U.S.) No
Pharmacologic Category Iron Salt
Use Treatment of iron-deficiency anemia in chronic kidney disease
Contraindications Hypersensitivity to ferumoxytol or any component of the formulation
Warnings/Precautions Serious hypersensitivity reactions, including rare anaphylactic and anaphylactoid reactions, may occur, presenting with cardiac/cardiorespiratory arrest, clinically significant hypotension, syncope, or unresponsiveness; equipment for resuscitation and trained personnel experienced in handling emergencies should be immediately available during use. Monitor patients for signs/symptoms of hypersensitivity reactions for ≥30 minutes and until clinically stable following administration.

Do not administer in the presence of tissue iron overload; periodic monitoring of hemoglobin, serum ferritin, serum iron, and transferrin saturation is recommended. Serum iron and transferrin-bound iron may be overestimated in laboratory assays if level is drawn during the first 24 hours following administration. Administration may alter magnetic resonance (MR) imaging; conduct anticipated MRI studies prior to use. MR imaging alterations may persist for ≤3 months following use, with peak alterations anticipated in the first 2 days following administration. If MR imaging is required within 3 months after administration, use T1- or proton density-weighted MR pulse sequences to decrease effect on imagining. Do not use T2-weighted sequence MR imaging prior to 4 weeks following ferumoxytol administration. Ferumoxytol does not interfere with X-ray, computed tomography (CT), positron emission tomography (PET), single photon emission computed tomography (SPECT), ultrasound or nuclear medicine imaging.

Adverse Reactions (Reflective of adult population; not specific for elderly)
1% to 10%:
Cardiovascular: Hypotension (≤3%), edema (2%), peripheral edema (2%), chest pain (1%), hypertension (1%)
Central nervous system: Dizziness (3%), headache (2%), fever (1%)
Dermatologic: Pruritus (1%), rash (1%)
Gastrointestinal: Diarrhea (4%), nausea (3%), constipation (2%), vomiting (2%), abdominal pain (1%)
Neuromuscular & skeletal: Back pain (1%), muscle spasms (1%)
Respiratory: Cough (1%), dyspnea (1%)
Miscellaneous: Hypersensitivity reactions (≤4%; serious reactions: <1%)

Drug Interactions
Avoid Concomitant Use
Avoid concomitant use of Ferumoxytol with any of the following: Dimercaprol
Increased Effect/Toxicity
The levels/effects of Ferumoxytol may be increased by: Dimercaprol
Decreased Effect There are no known significant interactions involving a decrease in effect.
Stability Store vials at controlled room temperature of 20°C to 25°C (68°F to 77°F); excursions permitted to 15°C to 30°C (59°F to 86°F). Do not freeze.
Mechanism of Action Superparamagnetic iron oxide coated with a low molecular weight semisynthetic carbohydrate; iron-carbohydrate complex enters the reticuloendothelial system macrophages of the liver, spleen, and bone marrow where the iron is released from the complex. The released iron is either transported into storage pools or is transported via plasma transferrin for incorporation into hemoglobin.
Pharmacodynamics/Kinetics
Distribution: V_d: 3.16 L
Metabolism: Iron released from iron-carbohydrate complex after uptake in the reticuloendo-thelial system macrophages of the liver, spleen, and bone marrow
Half-life elimination: ~15 hours
Dialysis: Ferumoxytol is not removed by hemodialysis
Dosage
Geriatric & Adult Doses expressed in mg of **elemental** iron. **Note:** Test dose: Product labeling does not indicate need for a test dose.
Iron-deficiency anemia in chronic kidney disease: I.V.: 510 mg (17 mL) as a single dose, followed by a second 510 mg dose 3-8 days after initial dose. Recommended dose may be readministered in patients with persistent or recurrent iron deficiency anemia.

◀ **Renal Impairment** Hemodialysis patients should receive injection after at least 1 hour of hemodialysis has been completed and once blood pressure has stabilized.

Administration Administer intravenously as an undiluted injection at a rate ≤1 mL/second (30 mg of elemental iron/second). Do not administer if solution has particulate matter or is discolored (solution is black to reddish-brown).

Hemodialysis patients should receive injection after at least 1 hour of hemodialysis has been completed and once blood pressure has stabilized.

Monitoring Parameters Hemoglobin, serum ferritin, serum iron, transferrin saturation (for at least 1 month following second injection and periodically); signs/symptoms of hypotension following administration; signs/symptoms of hypersensitivity reactions (≥30 minutes following administration)

Reference Range
Hemoglobin: Adults:
Males: 13.5-16.5 g/dL
Females: 12.0-15.0 g/dL
Serum iron: 40-160 mcg/dL
Total iron-binding capacity: 230-430 mcg/dL
Transferrin: 204-360 mg/dL
Percent transferrin saturation: 20% to 50%

Test Interactions May interfere with MR imaging; alterations may persist for ≤3 months following use, with peak alterations anticipated in the first 2 days following administration. If MR imaging is required within 3 months after administration, use T1- or proton density-weighted MR pulse sequences to decrease effect on imaging. Do not use T2-weighted sequence MR imaging prior to 4 weeks following administration.

Serum iron and transferrin-bound iron may be overestimated in laboratory assays if level is drawn during the first 24 hours following administration (due to contribution of iron in ferumoxytol).

Special Geriatric Considerations The manufacturer states that in clinical trials, ferumoxytol was reportedly as safe and effective in patients 65 years and older as younger patients. Anemia in the elderly is most often caused by "anemia of chronic disease", a result of aging effect in bone marrow, or associated with inflammation rather than blood loss. Iron stores are usually normal or increased, with a serum ferritin >50 ng/mL and a decreased total iron binding capacity. Hence, the anemia is not secondary to iron deficiency but the inability of the reticuloendothelial system to use available iron stores. I.V. administration of iron is often preferred over I.M. in the elderly secondary to a decreased muscle mass and the need for daily injections.

Dosage Forms Excipient information presented when available (limited, particularly for generics); consult specific product labeling.
Injection, solution:
Feraheme®: Elemental iron 30 mg/mL (17 mL)

◆ **FESO** see Fesoterodine on page 728
◆ **FeSO₄** see Ferrous Sulfate on page 724

Fesoterodine (fes oh TER oh deen)

Related Information
Pharmacotherapy of Urinary Incontinence on page 2032

Medication Safety Issues
Sound-alike/look-alike issues:
Fesoterodine may be confused with fexofenadine, tolterodine

Brand Names: U.S. Toviaz™

Index Terms FESO; Fesoterodine Fumarate

Generic Availability (U.S.) No

Pharmacologic Category Anticholinergic Agent

Use Treatment of patients with an overactive bladder with symptoms of urinary frequency, urgency, or urge incontinence.

Contraindications Hypersensitivity to fesoterodine or any component of the formulation; urinary retention; gastric retention; uncontrolled narrow-angle glaucoma

Warnings/Precautions Cases of angioedema involving the face, lips, tongue, and/or larynx have been reported. Immediately discontinue if tongue, hypopharynx, or larynx are involved. May cause drowsiness and/or blurred vision, which may impair physical or mental abilities; patients must be cautioned about performing tasks which require mental alertness (eg, operating machinery or driving). Patients may experience decreased sweating; caution use in hot weather or during exercise. Use is not recommended in patients with severe hepatic impairment (Child-Pugh class C). Doses >4 mg are not recommended for patients with severe renal impairment (Cl$_{cr}$ <30 mL/minute) or patients receiving concurrent therapy with potent CYP3A4 inhibitors. Use caution in patients with bladder flow obstruction, gastrointestinal obstructive disorders, myasthenia gravis, and treated narrow-angle glaucoma. Risk of adverse effects may be increased in elderly patients.

Adverse Reactions (Reflective of adult population; not specific for elderly)
>10%: Gastrointestinal: Xerostomia (19% to 35%; dose related)
1% to 10%:
  Central nervous system: Insomnia (1%)
  Dermatological: Rash (1%)
  Gastrointestinal: Constipation (4% to 6%), dyspepsia (2%), nausea (1% to 2%), abdominal pain (1%)
  Genitourinary: Urinary tract infection (3% to 4%), dysuria (1% to 2%), urinary retention (1%)
  Hepatic: ALT increased (1%), GGT increased (1%)
  Neuromuscular & skeletal: Back pain (1% to 2%)
  Ocular: Dry eyes (1% to 4%)
  Respiratory: Upper respiratory tract infection (2% to 3%), cough (1% to 2%), dry throat (1% to 2%)
  Miscellaneous: Peripheral edema (1%)

Drug Interactions
  Avoid Concomitant Use There are no known interactions where it is recommended to avoid concomitant use.
  Increased Effect/Toxicity
  Fesoterodine may increase the levels/effects of: AbobotulinumtoxinA; Anticholinergics; Cannabinoids; OnabotulinumtoxinA; Potassium Chloride; RimabotulinumtoxinB

  The levels/effects of Fesoterodine may be increased by: CYP2D6 Inhibitors; CYP3A4 Inhibitors (Moderate); CYP3A4 Inhibitors (Strong); Dasatinib; Pramlintide
  Decreased Effect
  Fesoterodine may decrease the levels/effects of: Acetylcholinesterase Inhibitors (Central); Secretin

  The levels/effects of Fesoterodine may be decreased by: Acetylcholinesterase Inhibitors (Central); CYP3A4 Inducers (Strong); Deferasirox; Herbs (CYP3A4 Inducers); Peginterferon Alfa-2b; Tocilizumab

Ethanol/Nutrition/Herb Interactions Ethanol: Adverse effects may be potentiated
Stability Store at 20°C to 25°C (68°F to 77°F); excursions permitted between 15°C to 30°C (59°F to 86°F). Protect from moisture.
Mechanism of Action Fesoterodine acts as a prodrug and is converted to an active metabolite, 5-hydroxymethyl tolterodine (5-HMT); 5-HMT is responsible for fesoterodine's antimuscarinic activity and acts as a competitive antagonist of muscarinic receptors.

Urinary bladder contractions are mediated by muscarinic receptors; fesoterodine inhibits the receptors in the bladder preventing symptoms of urgency and frequency.

Pharmacodynamics/Kinetics
Absorption: Well absorbed
Distribution: I.V.: 5-HMT: V$_d$: 169 L
Protein binding: 5-HMT: ~50% (primarily to albumin and alpha$_1$-acid glycoprotein)
Metabolism: Fesoterodine is rapidly and extensively metabolized to its active metabolite (5-hydroxymethyl tolterodine; 5-HMT) by nonspecific esterases; 5-HMT is further metabolized via CYP2D6 and CYP3A4 to inactive metabolites.
Bioavailability: 5-HMT: 52%
Half-life elimination: ~7 hours
Time to peak, plasma: 5-HMT: ~5 hours; C$_{max}$ higher in poor CYP2D6 metabolizers
Excretion: Urine (~70%; 16% as 5-HMT, ~53% as inactive metabolites); feces (7%)

Dosage
  Geriatric & Adult Overactive bladder: Oral: 4 mg once daily; dose may be increased to 8 mg once daily based on individual response and tolerability
    Dosing adjustment for concomitant CYP3A4 inhibitors: Maximum dose: 4 mg/day when administered concomitantly with potent CYP3A4 inhibitors including (but not limited to) ketoconazole, itraconazole, and clarithromycin. Concurrent therapy of weak or moderate CYP3A4 inhibitors and fesoterodine should be limited to 4 mg/day and increased to 8 mg/day after assessing tolerability.
  Renal Impairment
    Mild-to-moderate renal impairment (Cl$_{cr}$ 30-80 mL/minute): No dose adjustment is recommended.
    Severe renal impairment (Cl$_{cr}$ <30 mL/minute): Maximum dose: 4 mg.

Hepatic Impairment

Moderate hepatic impairment (Child-Pugh class B): No dose adjustment is recommended.

Severe hepatic impairment (Child-Pugh class C): Use is not recommended; not studied in severe impairment.

Administration May be administered with or without food. Swallow whole; do not chew, crush, or divide.

Special Geriatric Considerations See Dosage: Renal Impairment. In clinical trials, patients >75 years of age experienced more anticholinergic side effects than younger patients.

Dosage Forms Excipient information presented when available (limited, particularly for generics); consult specific product labeling.

Tablet, extended release, oral, as fumarate:

Toviaz™: 4 mg, 8 mg [contains soya lecithin]

Selected References

Nitti VW, Dmochowski R, Sand PK, et al, "Efficacy, Safety and Tolerability of Fesoterodine for Overactive Bladder Syndrome," *J Urol*, 2007, 178(5):2488-94.

◆ **Fesoterodine Fumarate** *see* Fesoterodine *on page 728*

◆ **Feverall® [OTC]** *see* Acetaminophen *on page 33*

◆ **Fexmid®** *see* Cyclobenzaprine *on page 426*

Fexofenadine (feks oh FEN a deen)

Medication Safety Issues

Sound-alike/look-alike issues:

Fexofenadine may be confused with fesoterodine

Allegra® may be confused with Viagra®

International issues:

Allegra [U.S, Canada, and multiple international markets] may be confused with Allegro brand name for fluticasone [Israel] and frovatriptan [Germany]

Brand Names: U.S. Allegra®; Allegra® Allergy 12 Hour [OTC]; Allegra® Allergy 24 Hour [OTC]; Allegra® Children's Allergy ODT [OTC]; Allegra® Children's Allergy [OTC]; Allegra® ODT [DSC]

Brand Names: Canada Allegra®

Index Terms Fexofenadine Hydrochloride

Generic Availability (U.S.) Yes: Excludes orally disintegrating tablet and suspension

Pharmacologic Category Histamine H_1 Antagonist; Histamine H_1 Antagonist, Second Generation; Piperidine Derivative

Use Relief of symptoms associated with seasonal allergic rhinitis; treatment of chronic idiopathic urticaria

OTC labeling: Relief of symptoms associated with allergic rhinitis

Contraindications Hypersensitivity to fexofenadine or any component of the formulation

Warnings/Precautions Use with caution in patients with renal impairment; dosage adjustment recommended. Orally disintegrating tablet contains phenylalanine.

Adverse Reactions (Reflective of adult population; not specific for elderly)

>10%:

Central nervous system: Headache (5% to 11%)

Gastrointestinal: Vomiting (children 6 months to 5 years: 4% to 12%)

1% to 10%:

Central nervous system: Fatigue (1% to 3%), somnolence (1% to 3%), dizziness (2%), fever (2%), pain (2%), drowsiness (1%)

Endocrine & metabolic: Dysmenorrhea (2%)

Gastrointestinal: Diarrhea (3% to 4%), nausea (2%), dyspepsia (1% to 2%)

Neuromuscular & skeletal: Myalgia (3%), back pain (2% to 3%), pain in extremities (2%)

Otic: Otitis media (2% to 4%)

Respiratory: Upper respiratory tract infection (3% to 4%), cough (2% to 4%), rhinorrhea (1% to 2%)

Miscellaneous: Viral infection (3%)

Drug Interactions

Metabolism/Transport Effects Substrate of CYP3A4 (minor), P-glycoprotein, SLCO1B1; Inhibits CYP2D6 (weak)

Avoid Concomitant Use There are no known interactions where it is recommended to avoid concomitant use.

Increased Effect/Toxicity

Fexofenadine may increase the levels/effects of: Alcohol (Ethyl); Anticholinergics; CNS Depressants; Selective Serotonin Reuptake Inhibitors

The levels/effects of Fexofenadine may be increased by: Conivaptan; Droperidol; Eltrombopag; Erythromycin; Erythromycin (Systemic); HydrOXYzine; Itraconazole; Ketoconazole; Ketoconazole (Systemic); P-Glycoprotein Inhibitors; Pramlintide; Verapamil

Decreased Effect

Fexofenadine may decrease the levels/effects of: Acetylcholinesterase Inhibitors (Central); Benzylpenicilloyl Polylysine; Betahistine

The levels/effects of Fexofenadine may be decreased by: Acetylcholinesterase Inhibitors (Central); Amphetamines; Antacids; Grapefruit Juice; P-Glycoprotein Inducers; Rifampin; Tocilizumab

Ethanol/Nutrition/Herb Interactions

Ethanol: May increase CNS depression; monitor for increased effects with coadministration. Caution patients about effects.

Food: Fruit juice (apple, grapefruit, orange) may decrease bioavailability of fexofenadine by ~36%.

Herb/Nutraceutical: St John's wort may decrease fexofenadine levels.

Stability Store at controlled room temperature of 20°C to 25°C (68°F to 77°F). Protect from excessive moisture.

Mechanism of Action Fexofenadine is an active metabolite of terfenadine and like terfenadine it competes with histamine for H_1-receptor sites on effector cells in the gastrointestinal tract, blood vessels and respiratory tract; it appears that fexofenadine does not cross the blood brain barrier to any appreciable degree, resulting in a reduced potential for sedation

Pharmacodynamics/Kinetics

Onset of action: 60 minutes

Duration: Antihistaminic effect: ≥12 hours

Absorption: Rapid

Protein binding: 60% to 70%, primarily albumin and alpha$_1$-acid glycoprotein

Metabolism: Minimal (Hepatic ~5%)

Half-life elimination: 14.4 hours (31% to 72% longer in renal impairment)

Time to peak, serum: ODT: 2 hours (4 hours with high-fat meal); Tablet: ~2.6 hours; Suspension: ~1 hour

Excretion: Feces (~80%) and urine (~11%) as unchanged drug

Dosage

Geriatric Chronic idiopathic urticaria, seasonal allergic rhinitis: Oral: Use caution; adjust dose for renal impairment.

Adult Seasonal allergic rhinitis, idiopathic urticaria, allergic rhinitis (OTC labeling): Oral: 60 mg twice daily **or** 180 mg once daily

Renal Impairment Cl_{cr} <80 mL/minute: Initial: 60 mg once daily

Not effectively removed by hemodialysis

Administration

Suspension, tablet: Administer with water only; do not administer with fruit juices. Shake suspension well before use.

Orally disintegrating tablet: Take on an empty stomach. Do not remove from blister pack until administered. Using dry hands, place immediately on tongue. Tablet will dissolve within seconds, and may be swallowed with or without liquid (do not administer with fruit juices). Do not split or chew.

Monitoring Parameters Relief of symptoms

Test Interactions May suppress the wheal and flare reactions to skin test antigens

Special Geriatric Considerations Plasma levels in the elderly are generally higher than those observed in other age groups. Once daily dosing is recommended when starting therapy in elderly patients or patients with decreased renal function.

Dosage Forms Excipient information presented when available (limited, particularly for generics); consult specific product labeling. [DSC] = Discontinued product

Suspension, oral, as hydrochloride:

Allegra®: 6 mg/mL (300 mL) [contains propylene glycol; raspberry cream flavor]

Allegra® Children's Allergy: 6 mg/mL (120 mL) [contains propylene glycol, sodium 18 mg/5 mL; berry flavor]

Tablet, oral, as hydrochloride: 30 mg, 60 mg, 180 mg

Allegra®: 60 mg [DSC], 180 mg [DSC]

Allegra® Allergy 12 Hour: 60 mg

Allegra® Allergy 24 Hour: 180 mg

Allegra® Children's Allergy: 30 mg

◀ Tablet, orally disintegrating, oral, as hydrochloride:
Allegra® Children's Allergy ODT: 30 mg [contains phenylalanine 5.3 mg/tablet, sodium 5 mg/tablet; orange cream flavor]
Allegra® ODT: 30 mg [DSC] [contains phenylalanine 5.3 mg/tablet; orange cream flavor]

◆ **Fexofenadine Hydrochloride** *see* Fexofenadine *on page 730*
◆ **Fiberall® [OTC]** *see* Psyllium *on page 1547*
◆ **FiberCon® [OTC]** *see* Polycarbophil *on page 1479*
◆ **Fiber-Lax [OTC]** *see* Polycarbophil *on page 1479*
◆ **Fiber-Tabs™ [OTC]** *see* Polycarbophil *on page 1479*
◆ **Fibricor®** *see* Fenofibric Acid *on page 704*
◆ **Fibro-XL [OTC]** *see* Psyllium *on page 1547*
◆ **Fibro-Lax [OTC]** *see* Psyllium *on page 1547*
◆ **Fidaxomicin** *see* Fidaxomicin (Systemic) *on page 732*

Fidaxomicin (Systemic) (fye DAX oh mye sin)

Brand Names: U.S. Dificid™
Index Terms Difimicin; Fidaxomicin; Lipiarrmycin; OPT-80; PAR-101; Tiacumicin B
Generic Availability (U.S.) No
Pharmacologic Category Antibiotic, Macrolide
Use Treatment of *Clostridium difficile*-associated diarrhea (CDAD)
Contraindications There are no contraindications listed in the manufacturer's labeling.
Warnings/Precautions Do not use for systemic infections; fidaxomicin systemic absorption is negligible. Use only in patients with proven or strongly suspected *Clostridium difficile (C. difficile)* infections.
Adverse Reactions (Reflective of adult population; not specific for elderly)
>10%: Gastrointestinal: Nausea (11%)
2% to 10%:
  Gastrointestinal: Gastrointestinal hemorrhage (4%), abdominal pain, vomiting
  Hematologic: Anemia (2%), neutropenia (2%)
Drug Interactions
  Avoid Concomitant Use There are no known interactions where it is recommended to avoid concomitant use.
  Increased Effect/Toxicity There are no known significant interactions involving an increase in effect.
  Decreased Effect There are no known significant interactions involving a decrease in effect.
Stability Store at 20°C to 25°C (68°F to 77°F); excursions permitted to 15°C to 30°C (59°F to 86°F).
Mechanism of Action Inhibits RNA polymerase sigma subunit resulting in inhibition of protein synthesis and cell death in susceptible organisms including *C. difficile*; bactericidal
Pharmacodynamics/Kinetics
Absorption: Oral: Minimal systemic absorption
Distribution: Largely confined to the gastrointestinal tract; in single- and multiple-dose studies, fecal concentrations of fidaxomicin and its active metabolite (OP-1118) are very high while serum concentrations are minimally detectable to undetectable
Metabolism: Intestinal hydrolysis to less active metabolite (OP-1118)
Excretion: Feces (>92% as unchanged drug and metabolites); urine (<1% as metabolite)
Dosage
  Geriatric & Adult Treatment of diarrhea due to *Clostridium difficile* (CDAD): Oral: 200 mg twice daily for 10 days
  Renal Impairment Minimal systemic absorption; no dosage adjustment needed
  Hepatic Impairment Not studied; minimally absorbed, so no dosage adjustment predicted
Administration May be administered with or without food.
Pharmacotherapy Pearls Fidaxomicin is bactericidal against gram-positive anaerobes (including *C. difficile* NAP1/B1/027 strain) and gram-positive aerobes. Fidaxomicin spectrum does **not** include gram-negative aerobes or gram-negative anaerobes (eg, *Bacteroides spp*). At the approved dose, concentrations in feces substantially exceed the 90% MIC of *C. difficile*. Postantibiotic effects against *C. difficile* in clinical studies range from 6–10 hours. Clinical studies excluded patients with a history of >1 recurrent *C. difficile*-associated diarrhea (CDAD) episode within 3 months.
Special Geriatric Considerations Fifty percent of subjects in fidaxomicin's pivotal trial were ≥65 years; 31% were ≥75 years. No difference in safety or efficacy vs vancomycin was noted between younger and older subjects. Clinical studies excluded patients with life-threatening or fulminant *C. difficile* infections or a history of more than one recurrent *C. difficile*-associated diarrhea episode in the preceding 3 months; hence, its efficacy in these patients has not been established.

Dosage Forms Excipient information presented when available (limited, particularly for generics); consult specific product labeling.

Tablet, oral:

Dificid™: 200 mg [contains soy lecithin]

Selected References

Cohen SH, Gerding DN, Johnson S, et al, "Clinical Practice Guidelines for *Clostridium difficile* Infection in Adults: 2010 Update by the Society for Healthcare Epidemiology of America (SHEA) and the Infectious Diseases Society of America (IDSA)," *Infect Control Hosp Epidemiol*, 2010, 31(5):431-55.

Louie TJ, Emery J, Krulicki W, et al, "OPT-80 Eliminates *Clostridium difficile* and Is Sparing of Bacteroides Species During Treatment of *C. difficile* Infection," *Antimicrob Agents Chemother*, 2009, 53(1):261-3.

Louie TJ, Miller MA, Mullane KM, et al, "Fidaxomicin Versus Vancomycin for *Clostridium difficile* Infection," *N Engl J Med*, 2011, 364(5):422-31.

Louie T, Miller M, Donskey C, et al, "Clinical Outcomes, Safety, and Pharmacokinetics of OPT-80 in a Phase 2 Trial With Patients With *Clostridium difficile* Infection," *Antimicrob Agents Chemother*, 2009, 53(1):223-8.

Shue YK, Sears PS, Shangle S, et al, "Safety, Tolerance, and Pharmacokinetic Studies of OPT-80 in Healthy Volunteers Following Single and Multiple Oral Doses," *Antimicrob Agents Chemother*, 2008, 52(4):1391-5.

Sullivan KM and Spooner LM, "Fidaxomicin: A Macrocyclic Antibiotic for the Management of *Clostridium difficile* Infection," *Ann Pharmacother*, 2010, 44(2):352-9.

Tannock GW, Munro K, Taylor C, et al, "A New Macrocyclic Antibiotic, Fidaxomicin (OPT-80), Causes Less Alteration to the Bowel Microbiota of *Clostridium difficile*-Infected Patients Than Does Vancomycin," *Microbiology*, 2010, 156(Pt 11):3354-9.

Filgrastim (fil GRA stim)

Medication Safety Issues

Sound-alike/look-alike issues:

Neupogen® may be confused with Epogen®, Neulasta®, Neumega®, Neupro®, Nutramigen®

Brand Names: U.S. Neupogen®

Brand Names: Canada Neupogen®

Index Terms G-CSF; Granulocyte Colony Stimulating Factor

Generic Availability (U.S.) No

Pharmacologic Category Colony Stimulating Factor

Use

Cancer patients (nonmyeloid malignancies) receiving myelosuppressive chemotherapy to decrease the incidence of infection (febrile neutropenia) in regimens associated with a high incidence of neutropenia with fever

Acute myelogenous leukemia (AML) following induction or consolidation chemotherapy to shorten time to neutrophil recovery and reduce the duration of fever

Cancer patients (nonmyeloid malignancies) receiving bone marrow transplant to shorten the duration of neutropenia and neutropenia-related events (eg, neutropenic fever)

Peripheral stem cell transplantation to mobilize hematopoietic progenitor cells for leukapheresis collection

Severe chronic neutropenia (SCN; chronic administration) to reduce the incidence and duration of neutropenic complications (fever, infections, oropharyngeal ulcers) in symptomatic patients with congenital, cyclic, or idiopathic neutropenia

Unlabeled/Investigational Use Treatment of anemia in myelodysplastic syndrome; mobilization of hematopoietic stem cells (HSC) for collection and subsequent autologous transplantation (in combination with plerixafor) in patients with non-Hodgkin's lymphoma (NHL) and multiple myeloma (MM); treatment of neutropenia in HIV-infected patients receiving zidovudine; hepatitis C treatment-associated neutropenia

Contraindications Hypersensitivity to filgrastim, *E. coli*-derived proteins, or any component of the formulation

Warnings/Precautions Do not use filgrastim in the period 24 hours before to 24 hours after administration of cytotoxic chemotherapy because of the potential sensitivity of rapidly dividing myeloid cells to cytotoxic chemotherapy. May potentially act as a growth factor for any tumor type, particularly myeloid malignancies; caution should be exercised in the usage of filgrastim in any malignancy with myeloid characteristics. Increases circulating leukocytes when used in conjunction with plerixafor for stem cell mobilization; monitor WBC; use with caution in patients with neutrophil count >50,000/mm^3; tumor cells released from marrow could be collected in leukapheresis product; potential effect of tumor cell reinfusion is unknown. Reports of alveolar hemorrhage, manifested as pulmonary infiltrates and hemoptysis, have occurred in healthy donors undergoing PBPC collection (not FDA approved for use in healthy donors); hemoptysis resolved upon discontinuation. Safety and efficacy have not been established with patients receiving radiation therapy (avoid concurrent radiation therapy with filgrastim), or chemotherapy associated with delayed myelosuppression (eg, nitrosoureas, mitomycin C).

◄ Allergic-type reactions (rash, urticaria, facial edema, wheezing, dyspnea, tachycardia, and/or hypotension) have occurred with first or subsequent doses. Reactions tended to involve ≥2 body systems and occur more frequently with intravenous administration and generally within 30 minutes of administration; may recur with rechallenge. Rare cases of acute respiratory distress syndrome (ARDS) have been reported (possibly due to influx of neutrophils to sites of lung inflammation); withhold or discontinue filgrastim if ARDS occurs; patients must be instructed to report respiratory distress; monitor for fever, infiltrates, or respiratory distress. Rare cases of splenic rupture have been reported (may be fatal); patients must be instructed to report left upper quadrant pain or shoulder tip pain. Cutaneous vasculitis has been reported, generally occurring in severe chronic neutropenia (SCN) patients on long-term therapy; symptoms generally developed with increasing absolute neutrophil count (ANC) and subsided when the ANC decreased; dose reductions may improve symptoms to allow for continued therapy. Use caution in patients with sickle cell disorders; severe sickle cell crises (sometimes resulting in fatalities) have been reported following filgrastim therapy. Filgrastim use prior to appropriate diagnosis of SCN may impair proper evaluation and treatment for neutropenia not due to SCN. Cytogenetic abnormalities, transformation to myelodysplastic syndrome (MDS) and acute myeloid leukemia (AML) have been observed in patients treated with filgrastim for congenital neutropenia; a longer duration of treatment and poorer ANC response appear to increase the risk. Carefully consider the risk of continuing filgrastim in patients who develop abnormal cytogenetics or MDS. The packaging of some forms may contain latex.

Adverse Reactions (Reflective of adult population; not specific for elderly)

>10%:

Central nervous system: Fever (12%)

Dermatologic: Petechiae (≤17%), rash (≤12%)

Endocrine & metabolic: LDH increased, uric acid increased

Gastrointestinal: Splenomegaly (severe chronic neutropenia: 30%; rare in other patients)

Hepatic: Alkaline phosphatase increased (21%)

Neuromuscular & skeletal: Bone/skeletal pain (22% to 33%; dose related), commonly in the lower back, posterior iliac crest, and sternum

Respiratory: Epistaxis (9% to 15%)

1% to 10%:

Cardiovascular: Hyper-/hypotension (4%), myocardial infarction/arrhythmias (3%)

Central nervous system: Headache (7%)

Gastrointestinal: Nausea (10%), vomiting (7%), peritonitis (≤2%)

Hematologic: Leukocytosis (2%)

Miscellaneous: Transfusion reaction (≤10%)

Drug Interactions

Avoid Concomitant Use There are no known interactions where it is recommended to avoid concomitant use.

Increased Effect/Toxicity

Filgrastim may increase the levels/effects of: Bleomycin; Topotecan

Decreased Effect There are no known significant interactions involving a decrease in effect.

Stability Intact vials and prefilled syringes should be stored under refrigeration at 2°C to 8°C (36°F to 46°F) and protected from direct sunlight. Filgrastim should be protected from freezing and temperatures >30°C to avoid aggregation. Do not shake.

Filgrastim vials and prefilled syringes are stable for 24 hours at 9°C to 30°C (47°F to 86°F).

Undiluted filgrastim is stable for 24 hours at 15°C to 30°C (59°F to 86°F) and for up to 14 days at 2°C to 8°C (36°F to 46°F) (data on file, Amgen Medical Information) in BD tuberculin syringes; however, sterility has only been assessed and maintained for up to 7 days when prepared under strict aseptic conditions (Jacobson, 1996; Singh, 1994). The manufacturer recommends using syringes within 24 hours due to the potential for bacterial contamination.

Do not dilute with saline at any time; product may precipitate. Filgrastim may be diluted with D_5W for I.V. infusion administration (5-15 mcg/mL; minimum concentration is 5 mcg/mL). This diluted solution is stable for 7 days at 2°C to 8°C (36°F to 46°F), however, should be used within 24 hours due to the possibility for bacterial contamination. Concentrations 5-15 mcg/mL require addition of albumin (final albumin concentration of 2 mg/mL) to prevent adsorption to plastics. Dilution to <5 mcg/mL is not recommended.

Mechanism of Action Stimulates the production, maturation, and activation of neutrophils; filgrastim activates neutrophils to increase both their migration and cytotoxicity.

Pharmacodynamics/Kinetics

Onset of action: ~24 hours; plateaus in 3-5 days

Duration: Neutrophil counts generally return to baseline within 4 days

Absorption: SubQ: 100%

Distribution: V_d: 150 mL/kg; no evidence of drug accumulation over a 11- to 20-day period

Metabolism: Systemically degraded

Half-life elimination: 1.8-3.5 hours

Time to peak, serum: SubQ: 2-8 hours

Dosage

Geriatric & Adult Details concerning dosing in combination regimens and institution protocols should also be consulted. Rounding doses to the nearest vial size may enhance patient convenience and reduce costs without compromising clinical response.

Chemotherapy-induced neutropenia SubQ, I.V.: 5 mcg/kg/day; doses may be increased by 5 mcg/kg (for each chemotherapy cycle) according to the duration and severity of the neutropenia; continue for up to 14 days or until the ANC reaches 10,000/mm^3

Bone marrow transplantation (in patients with cancer; to shorten the duration of neutropenia and neutropenia-related events): SubQ, I.V.: 10 mcg/kg/day (administer ≥24 hours after chemotherapy and ≥24 hours after bone marrow infusion); adjust the dose according to the duration and severity of neutropenia; recommended steps based on neutrophil response:

When ANC >1000/mm^3 for 3 consecutive days: Reduce filgrastim dose to 5 mcg/kg/day

If ANC remains >1000/mm^3 for 3 more consecutive days: Discontinue filgrastim

If ANC decreases to <1000/mm^3: Resume at 5 mcg/kg/day.

If ANC decreases to <1000/mm^3 during the 5 mcg/kg/day dose: Increase filgrastim to 10 mcg/kg/day and follow the above steps.

Peripheral blood progenitor cell (PBPC) collection: SubQ: 10 mcg/kg daily, usually for 6-7 days. Begin at least 4 days before the first leukapheresis and continue until the last leukapheresis; consider dose adjustment for WBC >100,000/mm^3

Severe chronic neutropenia: SubQ:

Congenital: Initial: 6 mcg/kg twice daily; adjust the dose based on ANC and clinical response

Idiopathic/cyclic: Initial: 5 mcg/kg/day; adjust the dose based on ANC and clinical response

Anemia in myelodysplastic syndrome (unlabeled use; in combination with epoetin): SubQ: 30 mcg, 75 mcg, or 150 mcg once daily (Hellstrom-Lindberg, 1998) **or** 1 mcg/kg once daily (Greenberg, 2009) **or** 75 mcg, 150 mcg or 300 mcg/dose 3 times/week (Hellstrom-Lindberg, 2003) **or** 1-2 mcg/kg/dose 1-3 times/week (NCCN MDS guidelines v.2.2011)

Hematopoietic stem cell mobilization in autologous transplantation in patients with non-Hodgkin's lymphoma or multiple myeloma (in combination with plerixafor; unlabeled use): SubQ: 10 mcg/kg once daily; begin 4 days before initiation of plerixafor; continue G-CSF on each day prior to apheresis for up to 8 days (DiPersio, *JCO* 2009; DiPersio, *Blood* 2009)

Hepatitis C treatment-associated neutropenia (unlabeled use): SubQ: 150 mcg once weekly to 300 mcg 3 times/week; titrate to maintain ANC between 750-10,000/mm^3 (Younossi, 2008)

Administration May be administered undiluted by SubQ injection. May also be administered by I.V. bolus, or a short infusion over 15-30 minutes in D_5W, or by continuous SubQ or I.V. infusion. Do not administer earlier than 24 hours after or in the 24 hours prior to cytotoxic chemotherapy.

Monitoring Parameters CBC with differential and platelets prior to treatment and twice weekly during filgrastim treatment for chemotherapy-induced neutropenia (3 times/week following marrow transplantation). For severe chronic neutropenia, monitor CBC with differential and platelets twice weekly during the first month of therapy and for 2 weeks following dose adjustments; once clinically stable, monthly for 1 year and quarterly thereafter; for congenital neutropenia also monitor bone marrow and karyotype prior to treatment; and monitor marrow and cytogenetics annually throughout treatment. Monitor temperature.

Reference Range No additional clinical benefit seen when filgrastim is used with ANC >10,000/mm^3

Test Interactions May interfere with bone imaging studies; increased hematopoietic activity of the bone marrow may appear as transient positive bone imaging changes

Special Geriatric Considerations Out of 855 participants in randomized, placebo-controlled clinical trials who had received myelosuppressive chemotherapy, a total of 232 subjects were ≥65 years and 22 subjects were ≥75 years. No overall differences in safety or effectiveness were observed between these older and younger subjects; other clinical experience has not identified differences in the responses between elderly and younger patients.

Dosage Forms Excipient information presented when available (limited, particularly for generics); consult specific product labeling.

Injection, solution [preservative free]:

Neupogen®: 300 mcg/mL (1 mL, 1.6 mL) [contains polysorbate 80, sodium 0.035 mg/mL, sorbitol; vial]

Neupogen®: 600 mcg/mL (0.5 mL, 0.8 mL) [contains natural rubber/natural latex in packaging, polysorbate 80, sodium 0.035 mg/mL, sorbitol; prefilled syringe]

◀ **Selected References**
  Andres E, Kurtz JE, Martin-Hunyadi C, et al, "Nonchemotherapy Drug-Induced Agranulocytosis in Elderly Patients:
    The Effects of Granulocyte Colony-Stimulating Factor," *Am J Med*, 2002, 112(6):460-4.
  Rosenberg PS, Alter BP, Bolyard AA, et al, "The Incidence of Leukemia and Mortality From Sepsis in Patients With
    Severe Congenital Neutropenia Receiving Long-Term G-CSF Therapy," *Blood*, 2006, 107(12): 4628-35.

Finasteride (fi NAS teer ide)

Medication Safety Issues
Sound-alike/look-alike issues:
  Finasteride may be confused with furosemide
  Proscar® may be confused with ProSom®, Provera®, PROzac®, Psorcon®
Brand Names: U.S. Propecia®; Proscar®
Brand Names: Canada CO Finasteride; JAMP-Finasteride; Mylan-Finasteride; Novo-Finas-
  teride; PMS-Finasteride; Propecia®; Proscar®; ratio-Finasteride; Sandoz-Finasteride
Generic Availability (U.S.) Yes
Pharmacologic Category 5 Alpha-Reductase Inhibitor
Use
  Propecia®: Treatment of male pattern hair loss in **men only**. Safety and efficacy were
    demonstrated in men between 18-41 years of age.
  Proscar®: Treatment of symptomatic benign prostatic hyperplasia (BPH); can be used in
    combination with an alpha-blocker, doxazosin
Unlabeled/Investigational Use Adjuvant monotherapy after radical prostatectomy in the
  treatment of prostatic cancer; treatment of female hirsutism
Contraindications Hypersensitivity to finasteride or any component of the formulation
Warnings/Precautions Hazardous agent - use appropriate precautions for handling and
  disposal. Other urological diseases (including prostate cancer) should be ruled out before
  initiating. For BPH, a minimum of 6 months of treatment may be necessary to determine
  whether an individual will respond to finasteride; for male pattern hair loss, daily use for 3
  months or longer may be required before benefit is observed. Reduces prostate specific
  antigen (PSA) by ~50%; in patients treated for ≥6 months the PSA value should be doubled
  when comparing to normal ranges in untreated patients (for interpretation of serial PSAs, a
  new PSA baseline should be established ≥6 months after treatment initiation and PSA
  monitored periodically thereafter). Failure to demonstrate a meaningful PSA decrease
  (<50%) or a PSA increase while on this medication may be associated with an increased
  risk for prostate cancer (NCCN prostate cancer early detection guidelines, v.1.2011). Patients
  on a 5-alpha-reductase inhibitor (5-ARI) with any increase in PSA levels, even if within normal
  limits, should be evaluated; may indicate presence of prostate cancer. Use with caution in
  patients with hepatic dysfunction; finasteride is extensively metabolized in the liver. When
  compared to placebo, 5-ARIs have been shown to reduce the overall incidence of prostate
  cancer, although an increase in the incidence of high-grade prostate cancers has been
  observed; 5-ARIs are not FDA-approved for the prevention of prostate cancer. Carefully
  monitor patients with a large residual urinary volume or severely diminished urinary flow for
  obstructive uropathy; these patients may not be candidates for finasteride therapy. Patients
  should promptly report any breast changes, including lumps, pain, or nipple discharge. Active
  ingredient can be absorbed through the skin; women should always use caution whenever
  handling. Pregnant women or women trying to conceive should not handle the product;
  finasteride may negatively impact fetal development.
Adverse Reactions (Reflective of adult population; not specific for elderly) Note:
  "Combination therapy" refers to finasteride and doxazosin.
  >10%:
    Endocrine & metabolic: Impotence (5% to 19%; combination therapy 23%), libido decreased
      (2% to 10%; combination therapy 12%)
    Neuromuscular & skeletal: Weakness (5%; combination therapy 17%)
  1% to 10%:
    Cardiovascular: Postural hypotension (9%; combination therapy 18%), edema (1%; combi-
      nation therapy 3%)
    Central nervous system: Dizziness (7%; combination therapy 23%), somnolence (2%;
      combination therapy 3%)
    Dermatologic: Rash (1%)
    Genitourinary: Ejaculation disturbances (<1% to 7%; combination therapy 14%), decreased
      volume of ejaculate (2% to 4%)
    Endocrine & metabolic: Gynecomastia (1% to 2%), breast tenderness (≤1%)
    Respiratory: Dyspnea (1%; combination therapy 2%), rhinitis (1%; combination therapy 2%)
Drug Interactions
Metabolism/Transport Effects Substrate of CYP3A4 (minor)

Avoid Concomitant Use There are no known interactions where it is recommended to avoid concomitant use.

Increased Effect/Toxicity
The levels/effects of Finasteride may be increased by: Conivaptan

Decreased Effect
The levels/effects of Finasteride may be decreased by: Tocilizumab

Ethanol/Nutrition/Herb Interactions Herb/Nutraceutical: St John's wort may decrease finasteride levels. Avoid saw palmetto (concurrent use has not been adequately studied).

Stability
Propecia®: Store at 15°C to 30°C (59°F to 86°F). Protect from moisture.
Proscar®: Store below 30°C (86°F). Protect from light.

Mechanism of Action Finasteride is a competitive inhibitor of both tissue and hepatic 5-alpha reductase. This results in inhibition of the conversion of testosterone to dihydrotestosterone and markedly suppresses serum dihydrotestosterone levels

Pharmacodynamics/Kinetics
Onset of action: BPH: 6 months; Male pattern hair loss: ≥3 months of daily use
Duration:
After a single oral dose as small as 0.5 mg: 65% depression of plasma dihydrotestosterone levels persists 5-7 days
After 6 months of treatment with 5 mg/day: Circulating dihydrotestosterone levels are reduced to castrate levels without significant effects on circulating testosterone; levels return to normal within 14 days of discontinuation of treatment
Distribution: V_{dss}: 76 L
Protein binding: ~90%
Metabolism: Hepatic via CYP3A4; two active metabolites (<20% activity of finasteride)
Bioavailability: Mean: 65%
Half-life elimination, serum: 6 hours (range: 3-16 hours); Elderly: 8 hours (range: 6-15 hours)
Time to peak, serum: 1-2 hours
Excretion: Feces (57%) and urine (39%) as metabolites

Dosage
Geriatric & Adult
Benign prostatic hyperplasia (Proscar®): Oral: 5 mg once daily as a single dose; clinical responses occur within 12 weeks to 6 months of initiation of therapy; long-term administration is recommended for maximal response
Male pattern baldness (Propecia®): Oral: 1 mg daily
Renal Impairment No adjustment is necessary.
Hepatic Impairment Use with caution in patients with liver function abnormalities because finasteride is metabolized extensively in the liver

Administration May be administered without regard to meals. Women of childbearing age should not touch or handle broken tablets.

Monitoring Parameters Objective and subjective signs of relief of benign prostatic hyperplasia, including improvement in urinary flow, reduction in symptoms of urgency, and relief of difficulty in micturition; for interpretation of serial PSAs, establish a new PSA baseline ≥6 months after treatment initiation and monitor PSA periodically thereafter.

Test Interactions PSA levels decrease in treated patients. After 6 months of therapy, PSA levels stabilize to a new baseline that is ~50% of pretreatment values. If following serial PSAs in a patient, re-establish a new baseline after ≥6 months of use.

Special Geriatric Considerations Clearance of finasteride is decreased in the elderly, but no dosage reductions are necessary.

Dosage Forms Excipient information presented when available (limited, particularly for generics); consult specific product labeling.
Tablet, oral: 5 mg
Propecia®: 1 mg
Proscar®: 5 mg

Selected References
Lepor H, Williford WO, Barry MJ, et al, "The Efficacy of Terazosin, Finasteride, or Both in Benign Prostatic Hyperplasia," *N Engl J Med*, 1996, 335(8):533-9.
McConnell JD, Roehrborn CG, Bautista OM, et al, "The Long-Term Effect of Doxazosin, Finasteride, and Combination Therapy on the Clinical Progression of Benign Prostatic Hyperplasia. Medical Therapy of Prostatic Symptoms (MTOPS) Research Group," *N Engl J Med*, 2003, 349(25):2387-98.
Thompson IM, Goodman PJ, Tangen CM, et al, "The Influence of Finasteride on the Development of Prostate Cancer," *N Engl J Med*, 2003, Jul 349(3):215-24.

- ◆ **First®-Testosterone** *see* Testosterone *on page 1761*
- ◆ **First®-Testosterone MC** *see* Testosterone *on page 1761*
- ◆ **Fisalamine** *see* Mesalamine *on page 1150*
- ◆ **Fish Oil** *see* Omega-3-Acid Ethyl Esters *on page 1338*
- ◆ **Flagyl®** *see* MetroNIDAZOLE (Systemic) *on page 1200*
- ◆ **Flagyl® 375** *see* MetroNIDAZOLE (Systemic) *on page 1200*
- ◆ **Flagyl® ER** *see* MetroNIDAZOLE (Systemic) *on page 1200*

FlavoxATE (fla VOKS ate)

Related Information
Beers Criteria – Potentially Inappropriate Medications for Geriatrics *on page 2089*

Medication Safety Issues
Sound-alike/look-alike issues:
FlavoxATE may be confused with fluvoxaMINE
Urispas may be confused with Urised®

Brand Names: Canada Apo-Flavoxate®; Urispas®

Index Terms Flavoxate Hydrochloride; Urispas

Generic Availability (U.S.) Yes

Pharmacologic Category Antispasmodic Agent, Urinary

Use Antispasmodic to provide symptomatic relief of dysuria, nocturia, suprapubic pain, urgency, and incontinence due to detrusor instability and hyper-reflexia in elderly with cystitis, urethritis, urethrocystitis, urethrotrigonitis, and prostatitis

Contraindications Hypersensitivity to flavoxate; pyloric or duodenal obstruction; GI hemorrhage; GI obstruction; ileus; achalasia; obstructive uropathies of lower urinary tract (BPH)

Warnings/Precautions May cause drowsiness, vertigo, and ocular disturbances. Give cautiously in patients with suspected glaucoma.

Adverse Reactions (Reflective of adult population; not specific for elderly) Frequency not defined.
Cardiovascular: Palpitations, tachycardia
Central nervous system: Confusion (especially in the elderly), drowsiness, fatigue, headache, hyperpyrexia, nervousness, vertigo
Dermatologic: Rash, urticaria
Gastrointestinal: Constipation, dry throat, nausea, vomiting, xerostomia
Genitourinary: Dysuria
Hematologic: Leukopenia
Ocular: Blurred vision, intraocular pressure increased

Drug Interactions
Avoid Concomitant Use There are no known interactions where it is recommended to avoid concomitant use.

Increased Effect/Toxicity
FlavoxATE may increase the levels/effects of: AbobotulinumtoxinA; Anticholinergics; Cannabinoids; OnabotulinumtoxinA; Potassium Chloride; RimabotulinumtoxinB

The levels/effects of FlavoxATE may be increased by: Pramlintide

Decreased Effect
FlavoxATE may decrease the levels/effects of: Acetylcholinesterase Inhibitors (Central); Secretin

The levels/effects of FlavoxATE may be decreased by: Acetylcholinesterase Inhibitors (Central)

Ethanol/Nutrition/Herb Interactions Ethanol: Avoid ethanol (may increase CNS depression).

Mechanism of Action Synthetic antispasmotic with similar actions to that of propantheline; it exerts a direct relaxant effect on smooth muscles via phosphodiesterase inhibition, providing relief to a variety of smooth muscle spasms; it is especially useful for the treatment of bladder spasticity, whereby it produces an increase in urinary capacity

Pharmacodynamics/Kinetics
Onset of action: 55-60 minutes
Metabolism: To methyl; flavone carboxylic acid active
Excretion: Urine (10% to 30%) within 6 hours

Dosage
Geriatric & Adult Urinary spasms: Oral: 100-200 mg 3-4 times/day; reduce the dose when symptoms improve.

Administration Should be administered with water on an empty stomach.

Monitoring Parameters Monitor incontinence episodes; postvoid residual (PVR); monitor for anticholinergic side effects

Special Geriatric Considerations Caution should be used in the elderly due to anticholinergic activity (eg, confusion, constipation, blurred vision, and tachycardia).

Dosage Forms Excipient information presented when available (limited, particularly for generics); consult specific product labeling.

Tablet, oral, as hydrochloride: 100 mg

◆ **Flavoxate Hydrochloride** *see* FlavoxATE *on page* 738
◆ **Flebogamma® DIF** *see* Immune Globulin *on page* 922

Flecainide (fle KAY nide)

Medication Safety Issues
Sound-alike/look-alike issues:
Flecainide may be confused with fluconazole
Tambocor™ may be confused with Pamelor®, Temodar®, tamoxifen, Tamiflu®

Brand Names: U.S. Tambocor™
Brand Names: Canada Apo-Flecainide®; Tambocor™
Index Terms Flecainide Acetate
Generic Availability (U.S.) Yes
Pharmacologic Category Antiarrhythmic Agent, Class Ic

Use Prevention and suppression of documented life-threatening ventricular arrhythmias (eg, sustained ventricular tachycardia); controlling symptomatic, disabling supraventricular tachycardias in patients without structural heart disease in whom other agents fail

Contraindications Hypersensitivity to flecainide or any component of the formulation; pre-existing second- or third-degree AV block or with right bundle branch block when associated with a left hemiblock (bifascicular block) (except in patients with a functioning artificial pacemaker); cardiogenic shock; coronary artery disease (based on CAST study results); concurrent use of ritonavir or amprenavir

Warnings/Precautions [U.S. Boxed Warning]: In the Cardiac Arrhythmia Suppression Trial (CAST), recent (>6 days but <2 years ago) myocardial infarction patients with asymptomatic, non-life-threatening ventricular arrhythmias did not benefit and may have been harmed by attempts to suppress the arrhythmia with flecainide or encainide. An increased mortality or nonfatal cardiac arrest rate (7.7%) was seen in the active treatment group compared with patients in the placebo group (3%). The applicability of the CAST results to other populations is unknown. The risks of class 1C agents and the lack of improved survival make use in patients without life-threatening arrhythmias generally unacceptable. **[U.S. Boxed Warning]: Watch for proarrhythmic effects;** monitor and adjust dose to prevent QT$_c$ prolongation. Not recommended for patients with chronic atrial fibrillation. **[U.S. Boxed Warning]: When treating atrial flutter, 1:1 atrioventricular conduction may occur; pre-emptive negative chronotropic therapy (eg, digoxin, beta-blockers) may lower the risk.** Pre-existing hypokalemia or hyperkalemia should be corrected before initiation (can alter drug's effect). A worsening or new arrhythmia may occur (proarrhythmic effect). Use caution in heart failure (may precipitate or exacerbate HF). Dose-related increases in PR, QRS, and QT intervals occur. Use with caution in sick sinus syndrome or with permanent pacemakers or temporary pacing wires (can increase endocardial pacing thresholds). Cautious use in significant hepatic impairment.

Adverse Reactions (Reflective of adult population; not specific for elderly)
>10%:
Central nervous system: Dizziness (19% to 30%)
Ocular: Visual disturbances (16%)
Respiratory: Dyspnea (~10%)
1% to 10%:
Cardiovascular: Palpitation (6%), chest pain (5%), edema (3.5%), tachycardia (1% to 3%), proarrhythmic (4% to 12%), sinus node dysfunction (1.2%)
Central nervous system: Headache (4% to 10%), fatigue (8%), nervousness (5%) additional symptoms occurring at a frequency between 1% and 3%: fever, malaise, hypoesthesia, paresis, ataxia, vertigo, syncope, somnolence, tinnitus, anxiety, insomnia, depression
Dermatologic: Rash (1% to 3%)
Gastrointestinal: Nausea (9%), constipation (1%), abdominal pain (3%), anorexia (1% to 3%), diarrhea (0.7% to 3%)
Neuromuscular & skeletal: Tremor (5%), weakness (5%), paresthesia (1%)
Ocular: Diplopia (1% to 3%), blurred vision

Drug Interactions
Metabolism/Transport Effects Substrate of CYP1A2 (minor), 2D6 (major); Inhibits CYP2D6 (weak)

Avoid Concomitant Use

Avoid concomitant use of Flecainide with any of the following: Artemether; Dronedarone; Lumefantrine; Nilotinib; Pimozide; QUEtiapine; QuiNINE; Ritonavir; Saquinavir; Tetrabenazine; Thioridazine; Tipranavir; Toremifene; Vandetanib; Vemurafenib; Ziprasidone

Increased Effect/Toxicity

Flecainide may increase the levels/effects of: Dronedarone; Pimozide; QTc-Prolonging Agents; QuiNINE; Tetrabenazine; Thioridazine; Toremifene; Vandetanib; Vemurafenib; Ziprasidone

The levels/effects of Flecainide may be increased by: Abiraterone Acetate; Alfuzosin; Amiodarone; Artemether; Boceprevir; Carbonic Anhydrase Inhibitors; Chloroquine; Ciprofloxacin; Ciprofloxacin (Systemic); CYP2D6 Inhibitors (Moderate); CYP2D6 Inhibitors (Strong); Darunavir; Gadobutrol; Lumefantrine; Nilotinib; QUEtiapine; QuiNINE; Ritonavir; Saquinavir; Sodium Bicarbonate; Sodium Lactate; Telaprevir; Tipranavir; Tromethamine; Verapamil

Decreased Effect

The levels/effects of Flecainide may be decreased by: Cyproterone; Etravirine; Peginterferon Alfa-2b; Sodium Bicarbonate

Ethanol/Nutrition/Herb Interactions Food: Clearance may be decreased in patients following strict vegetarian diets due to urinary pH ≥8.

Mechanism of Action Class Ic antiarrhythmic; slows conduction in cardiac tissue by altering transport of ions across cell membranes; causes slight prolongation of refractory periods; decreases the rate of rise of the action potential without affecting its duration; increases electrical stimulation threshold of ventricle, His-Purkinje system; possesses local anesthetic and moderate negative inotropic effects

Pharmacodynamics/Kinetics

Absorption: Oral: Rapid

Distribution: V_d: Adults: 5-13.4 L/kg

Protein binding: 40% to 50% (alpha$_1$ glycoprotein)

Metabolism: In the liver

Bioavailability: 85% to 90%

Half-life: Adults: 7-22 hours (average: 14 hours); increased half-life with congestive heart failure or renal dysfunction

Time to peak serum concentrations: Within 1.5-3 hours

Elimination: 80% to 90% in urine as unchanged drug and metabolites (10% to 50%)

Dosage

Geriatric & Adult

Life-threatening ventricular arrhythmias: Oral:

Initial: 100 mg every 12 hours; increase by 50-100 mg/day (given in 2 doses/day) every 4 days; maximum: 400 mg/day

For patients receiving 400 mg/day who are not controlled and have trough concentrations <0.6 mcg/mL, dosage may be increased to 600 mg/day.

Prevention of paroxysmal supraventricular arrhythmias: Oral: (**Note:** In patients with disabling symptoms but no structural heart disease): Initial: 50 mg every 12 hours; increase by 50 mg twice daily at 4-day intervals; maximum: 300 mg/day

Paroxysmal atrial fibrillation: Outpatient "Pill-in-the-pocket" dose (unlabeled dose): Oral: 200 mg (weight <70 kg), 300 mg (weight ≥70 kg). May not repeat in ≤24 hours. **Note:** An initial inpatient conversion trial should have been successful before sending patient home on this approach. Patient must be taking an AV nodal-blocking agent (eg, beta-blocker, nondihydropyridine calcium channel blocker) prior to initiation of antiarrhythmic.

Renal Impairment GFR ≤50 mL/minute: Decrease dose by 50%; dose increases should be made cautiously at intervals >4 days and serum levels monitored frequently.

Hemodialysis: No supplemental dose recommended.

Peritoneal dialysis: No supplemental dose recommended.

Hepatic Impairment Monitoring of plasma levels is recommended because half-life is significantly increased. When transferring from another antiarrhythmic agent, allow for 2-4 half-lives of the agent to pass before initiating flecainide therapy.

Administration Administer around-the-clock to promote less variation in peak and trough serum levels

Monitoring Parameters ECG, blood pressure, pulse, periodic serum concentrations, especially in patients with renal or hepatic impairment

Reference Range Therapeutic: 0.2-1 mcg/mL

Special Geriatric Considerations Decreased clearance and, therefore, prolonged half-life is possible; however, studies have shown no difference in response to usual doses in the elderly despite slight decrease in clearance; calculate or measure GFR since elderly patients may have GFR ≤50 mL/minute.

Dosage Forms Excipient information presented when available (limited, particularly for generics); consult specific product labeling.

Tablet, oral, as acetate: 50 mg, 100 mg, 150 mg

Tambocor™: 50 mg

Tambocor™: 100 mg, 150 mg [scored]

Selected References

Fuster V, Ryden LE, Cannom DS, et al, "ACC/AHA/ESC 2006 Guidelines for the Management of Patients With Atrial Fibrillation-Executirve Summary. A Report of the American College of Cardiology/American Heart Association Task Force on Practice Guidelines and the European Society of Cardiology Committee for Practice Guidelines (Writing Committee to Revise the 2001 Guidelines for the Management of Patients With Atrial Fibrillation). Developed in Collaboration With the European Heart Rhythm Association and the Heart Rhythm Society," *J Am Coll Cardiol*, 2006, 48(4):854-906.

Fluconazole (floo KOE na zole)

Medication Safety Issues

Sound-alike/look-alike issues:

Fluconazole may be confused with flecainide, FLUoxetine, furosemide, itraconazole

Diflucan® may be confused with diclofenac, Diprivan®, disulfiram

International issues:

Canesten [Great Britain] may be confused with Canesten brand name for clotrimazole [multiple international markets]; Cenestin brand name estrogens (conjugated A/synthetic) [U.S., Canada]

Brand Names: U.S. Diflucan®

Brand Names: Canada Apo-Fluconazole®; CanesOral®; CO Fluconazole; Diflucan®; Dom-Fluconazole; Fluconazole Injection; Fluconazole Omega; Mylan-Fluconazole; Novo-Fluconazole; PHL-Fluconazole; PMS-Fluconazole; PRO-Fluconazole; Riva-Fluconazole; Taro-Fluconazole; ZYM-Fluconazole

Generic Availability (U.S.) Yes

Pharmacologic Category Antifungal Agent, Oral; Antifungal Agent, Parenteral

◀ **Use** Treatment of candidiasis (vaginal, oropharyngeal, esophageal, urinary tract infections, peritonitis, pneumonia, and systemic infections); cryptococcal meningitis; antifungal prophylaxis in allogeneic bone marrow transplant recipients

Unlabeled/Investigational Use Cryptococcal pneumonia; candidal intertrigo

Contraindications Hypersensitivity to fluconazole or any component of the formulation (cross-reaction with other azole antifungal agents may occur, but has not been established; use caution); concomitant administration with cisapride or terfenadine

Warnings/Precautions Should be used with caution in patients with renal and hepatic dysfunction or previous hepatotoxicity from other azole derivatives. Patients who develop abnormal liver function tests during fluconazole therapy should be monitored closely and discontinued if symptoms consistent with liver disease develop. Rare exfoliative skin disorders have been observed; monitor closely if rash develops and discontinue if lesions progress. The manufacturer reports rare cases of QT$_c$ prolongation and torsade de pointes associated with fluconazole use and advises caution in patients with concomitant medications or conditions which are arrhythmogenic. However, given the limited number of cases and the presence of multiple confounding variables, the likelihood that fluconazole causes conduction abnormalities appears remote.

Adverse Reactions (Reflective of adult population; not specific for elderly) Frequency not always defined.

Cardiovascular: Angioedema, pallor, QT prolongation (rare, case reports), torsade de pointes (rare, case reports)

Central nervous system: Headache (2% to 13%), dizziness (1%), seizure

Dermatologic: Rash (2%), alopecia, toxic epidermal necrolysis, Stevens-Johnson syndrome

Endocrine & metabolic: Hypercholesterolemia, hypertriglyceridemia, hypokalemia

Gastrointestinal: Nausea (2% to 7%), abdominal pain (2% to 6%), vomiting (2% to 5%), diarrhea (2% to 3%), dyspepsia (1%), taste perversion (1%)

Hematologic: Agranulocytosis, leukopenia, neutropenia, thrombocytopenia

Hepatic: Alkaline phosphatase increased, ALT increased, AST increased, cholestasis, hepatic failure (rare), hepatitis, jaundice

Respiratory: Dyspnea

Miscellaneous: Anaphylactic reactions (rare)

Drug Interactions

Metabolism/Transport Effects Inhibits CYP1A2 (weak), 2C9 (strong), 2C19 (strong), 3A4 (moderate)

Avoid Concomitant Use

Avoid concomitant use of Fluconazole with any of the following: Artemether; Cisapride; Clopidogrel; Conivaptan; Dofetilide; Dronedarone; Lumefantrine; Nilotinib; Pimozide; QUEtiapine; QuiNIDine; QuiNINE; Ranolazine; Tetrabenazine; Thioridazine; Tolvaptan; Toremifene; Vandetanib; Vemurafenib; Voriconazole; Ziprasidone

Increased Effect/Toxicity

Fluconazole may increase the levels/effects of: Alfentanil; Aprepitant; Benzodiazepines (metabolized by oxidation); Bosentan; Budesonide (Systemic, Oral Inhalation); BusPIRone; Busulfan; Calcium Channel Blockers; CarBAMazepine; Carvedilol; Cilostazol; Cinacalcet; Cisapride; Citalopram; Colchicine; Conivaptan; Corticosteroids (Systemic); CycloSPORINE; CycloSPORINE (Systemic); CYP2C19 Substrates; CYP2C9 Substrates (High risk); CYP3A4 Substrates; Diclofenac; DOCEtaxel; Dofetilide; Dronedarone; Eletriptan; Eplerenone; Erlotinib; Eszopiclone; Etravirine; Everolimus; FentaNYL; Fosaprepitant; Fosphenytoin; Gefitinib; HMG-CoA Reductase Inhibitors; Imatinib; Irbesartan; Irinotecan; Losartan; Lurasidone; Macrolide Antibiotics; Methadone; Phenytoin; Phosphodiesterase 5 Inhibitors; Pimecrolimus; Pimozide; Protease Inhibitors; Proton Pump Inhibitors; QTc-Prolonging Agents; QuiNIDine; QuiNINE; Ramelteon; Ranolazine; Repaglinide; Rifamycin Derivatives; Salmeterol; Saxagliptin; Sirolimus; Solifenacin; SUNItinib; Tacrolimus; Tacrolimus (Systemic); Tacrolimus (Topical); Temsirolimus; Tetrabenazine; Thioridazine; Tolterodine; Tolvaptan; Toremifene; Vandetanib; Vemurafenib; Vilazodone; Vitamin K Antagonists; Voriconazole; Zidovudine; Ziprasidone; Zolpidem

The levels/effects of Fluconazole may be increased by: Alfuzosin; Artemether; Chloroquine; Ciprofloxacin; Ciprofloxacin (Systemic); Etravirine; Gadobutrol; Grapefruit Juice; Lumefantrine; Macrolide Antibiotics; Nilotinib; Protease Inhibitors; QUEtiapine; QuiNINE

Decreased Effect

Fluconazole may decrease the levels/effects of: Amphotericin B; Clopidogrel; Saccharomyces boulardii

The levels/effects of Fluconazole may be decreased by: Didanosine; Etravirine; Fosphenytoin; Phenytoin; Rifamycin Derivatives; Sucralfate

Stability
Tablet: Store at <30°C (86°F).
Powder for oral suspension: Store dry powder at <30°C (86°F). Following reconstitution, store at 5°C to 30°C (41°F to 86°F). Discard unused portion after 2 weeks. Do not freeze.
Injection: Store injection in glass at 5°C to 30°C (41°F to 86°F). Store injection in Viaflex® at 5°C to 25°C (41°F to 77°F). Do not freeze. Do not unwrap unit until ready for use.

Mechanism of Action Interferes with fungal cytochrome P450 activity (lanosterol 14-α-demethylase), decreasing ergosterol synthesis (principal sterol in fungal cell membrane) and inhibiting cell membrane formation

Pharmacodynamics/Kinetics
Distribution: Widely throughout body with good penetration into CSF, eye, peritoneal fluid, sputum, skin, and urine
Relative diffusion blood into CSF: Adequate with or without inflammation (exceeds usual MICs)
CSF:blood level ratio: Normal meninges: 70% to 80%; Inflamed meninges: >70% to 80%
Protein binding, plasma: 11% to 12%
Bioavailability: Oral: >90%
Half-life elimination: Normal renal function: ~30 hours
Time to peak, serum: Oral: 1-2 hours
Excretion: Urine (80% as unchanged drug)

Dosage
Geriatric & Adult The daily dose of fluconazole is the same for both oral and I.V. administration
Usual dosage range: 150 mg once or 200-800 mg/day; duration and dosage depends on severity of infection

Indication-specific dosing:
Candidiasis (Pappas, 2009):
Candidemia (neutropenic and non-neutropenic): Loading dose: 800 mg on first day, then 400 mg/day for 14 days after first negative blood culture and resolution of signs/symptoms; **Note:** Not recommended for neutropenic patients with recent azole exposure and critical illness
Chronic, disseminated: 400 mg/day until calcification or lesion resolution
CNS candidemia: 400-800 mg/day until CSF/radiological abnormalities resolved
Oropharyngeal: 100-200 mg/day for 7-14 days for uncomplicated, moderate-to-severe disease; chronic therapy of 100 mg 3 times weekly is recommended in immunocompromised patients with history of oropharyngeal candidiasis (OPC)
Osteoarticular: 400 mg/day for 6-12 months (osteomyelitis) or 6 weeks (septic arthritis)
Esophageal: 200-400 mg/day for 14-21 days
Prophylaxis:
  Solid organ: 200-400 mg/day for 7-14 days
  Neutropenic patients: 400 mg/day for duration of neutropenia
Urinary tract:
  Fungus balls: 200-400 mg/day
  Pyelonephritis: 200-400 mg/day for 2 weeks
  Symptomatic cystitis: 200 mg/day for 2 weeks
Vaginal:
  Uncomplicated: 150 mg as a single dose
  Complicated: 150 mg every 72 hours for 3 doses
  Recurrent: 150 mg daily for 10-14 days, followed by 150 mg once weekly for 6 months
Candidal intertrigo (unlabeled use; Coldiron, 1991; Nozickova, 1998; Stengel, 1994): 50 mg/day or 150 mg once weekly
Coccidioidomycosis (unlabeled use; Galgiani, 2005): 400-800 mg/day; doses of 800-1000 mg/day have been used for meningeal disease; usual duration of therapy ranges from 3-6 months for primary uncomplicated infections and up to 1 year for pulmonary (chronic and diffuse) infection
Endocarditis, prosthetic valve, early (unlabeled use; Pappas, 2009): 400-800 mg/day for 6 weeks after valve replacement (as step-down in stable, culture-negative patients); long-term suppression in absence of valve replacement: 400-800 mg/day
Endophthalmitis (Pappas, 2009): 400-800 mg/day for 4-6 weeks until examination indicates resolution
Meningitis, cryptococcal (Perfect, 2010):
Induction therapy: Typically consists of an amphotericin product and flucytosine for 2-6 weeks
Consolidation therapy: Fluconazole 400-800 mg/day for 8 weeks
Maintenance therapy: 200 mg/day for 6-12 months (post-transplant patients; non-HIV infected patients) or ≥1 year (HIV-infected patients may require lifelong therapy; CDC, 2009)

◀

Pericarditis or myocarditis (Pappas, 2009): 400-800 mg/day

Pneumonia, cryptococcal (mild-to-moderate) (unlabeled use; Perfect, 2010): 400 mg/day for 6-12 months (HIV-infected patients may require lifelong therapy; CDC, 2009)

Renal Impairment

No adjustment for vaginal candidiasis single-dose therapy

For multiple dosing, administer usual load then adjust daily doses as follows:

Cl_{cr} ≤50 mL/minute (no dialysis): Administer 50% of recommended dose or administer every 48 hours.

Intermittent hemodialysis (IHD): Dialyzable (50%): May administer 100% of daily dose (according to indication) after each dialysis session. Alternatively, doses of 200-400 mg every 48-72 hours **or** 100- 200 mg every 24 hours have been recommended (Heintz, 2009). **Note:** Dosing dependent on the assumption of 3 times/week, complete IHD sessions.

Continuous renal replacement therapy (CRRT) (Heintz, 2009; Trotman, 2005): Drug clearance is highly dependent on the method of renal replacement, filter type, and flow rate. Appropriate dosing requires close monitoring of pharmacologic response, signs of adverse reactions due to drug accumulation, as well as drug concentrations in relation to target trough (if appropriate). The following are general recommendations only (based on dialysate flow/ultrafiltration rates of 1-2 L/hour and minimal residual renal function) and should not supersede clinical judgment:

CVVH: Loading dose of 400-800 mg followed by 200-400 mg every 24 hours

CVVHD/CVVHDF: Loading dose of 400-800 mg followed by 400-800 mg every 24 hours (CVVHD or CVVHDF) **or** 800 mg every 24 hours (CVVHDF)

Note: Higher maintenance doses of 400 mg every 24 hours (CVVH), 800 mg every 24 hours (CVVHD), and 500-600 mg every 12 hours (CVVHDF) may be considered when treating resistant organisms and/or when employing combined ultrafiltration and dialysis flow rates of ≥2 L/hour for CVVHD/CVVHDF (Heintz, 2009; Trotman, 2005).

Administration Parenteral fluconazole must be administered by I.V. infusion over ~1-2 hours; do not exceed 200 mg/hour when giving I.V. infusion

Monitoring Parameters Periodic liver function tests (AST, ALT, alkaline phosphatase) and renal function tests, potassium

Pharmacotherapy Pearls An expensive oral alternative to I.V. amphotericin B infusions; in some clinical studies it has been as effective as amphotericin B, but is less likely to cause serious adverse reactions

Special Geriatric Considerations Has not been specifically studied in the elderly.

Dosage Forms Excipient information presented when available (limited, particularly for generics); consult specific product labeling. [DSC] = Discontinued product

Infusion, premixed iso-osmotic dextrose solution: 200 mg (100 mL); 400 mg (200 mL)

Diflucan®: 400 mg (200 mL [DSC])

Infusion, premixed iso-osmotic sodium chloride solution: 100 mg (50 mL); 200 mg (100 mL); 400 mg (200 mL)

Diflucan®: 200 mg (100 mL); 400 mg (200 mL)

Infusion, premixed iso-osmotic sodium chloride solution [preservative free]: 200 mg (100 mL); 400 mg (200 mL)

Powder for suspension, oral: 10 mg/mL (35 mL); 40 mg/mL (35 mL)

Diflucan®: 10 mg/mL (35 mL); 40 mg/mL (35 mL) [contains sodium benzoate, sucrose; orange flavor]

Tablet, oral: 50 mg, 100 mg, 150 mg, 200 mg

Diflucan®: 50 mg, 100 mg, 150 mg, 200 mg

Selected References

Grant SM and Clissold SP, "Fluconazole: A Review of Its Pharmacodynamic and Pharmacokinetic Properties and Therapeutic Potential in Superficial and Systemic Mycoses," *Drugs*, 1990, 39(6):877-916.

Pappas PG, Rex JH, Sobel JD, et al, "Guidelines for Treatment of Candidiasis. Infectious Diseases Society of America," *Clin Infect Dis*, 2004, 38(2):161-89.

Flucytosine (floo SYE toe seen)

Medication Safety Issues

Sound-alike/look-alike issues:

Flucytosine may be confused with fluorouracil

Ancobon® may be confused with Oncovin®

High alert medication:

The Institute for Safe Medication Practices (ISMP) includes this medication among its list of drugs which have a heightened risk of causing significant patient harm when used in error.

Brand Names: U.S. Ancobon®

Brand Names: Canada Ancobon®

Index Terms 5-FC; 5-Fluorocytosine; 5-Flurocytosine
Generic Availability (U.S.) No
Pharmacologic Category Antifungal Agent, Oral
Use Adjunctive treatment of systemic fungal infections (eg, septicemia, endocarditis, UTI, meningitis, or pulmonary) caused by susceptible strains of *Candida* or *Cryptococcus*
Contraindications Hypersensitivity to flucytosine or any component of the formulation
Warnings/Precautions [U.S. Boxed Warning]: Use with extreme caution in patients with renal dysfunction; dosage adjustment required. Avoid use as monotherapy; resistance rapidly develops. Use with caution in patients with bone marrow depression; patients with hematologic disease or who have been treated with radiation or drugs that suppress the bone marrow may be at greatest risk. Bone marrow toxicity can be irreversible. **[U.S. Boxed Warning]: Closely monitor hematologic, renal, and hepatic status.** Hepatotoxicity and bone marrow toxicity appear to be dose related; monitor levels closely and adjust dose accordingly.
Adverse Reactions (Reflective of adult population; not specific for elderly) Frequency not defined.
Cardiovascular: Cardiac arrest, myocardial toxicity, ventricular dysfunction, chest pain
Central nervous system: Ataxia, confusion, dizziness, drowsiness, fatigue, hallucinations, headache, parkinsonism, psychosis, pyrexia, sedation, seizure, vertigo
Dermatologic: Rash, photosensitivity, pruritus, toxic epidermal necrolysis, urticaria
Endocrine & metabolic: Hypoglycemia, hypokalemia
Gastrointestinal: Abdominal pain, diarrhea, dry mouth, duodenal ulcer, hemorrhage, loss of appetite, nausea, ulcerative colitis, vomiting
Hematologic: Agranulocytosis, anemia, aplastic anemia, eosinophilia, leukopenia, pancytopenia, thrombocytopenia
Hepatic: Acute hepatic injury, bilirubin increased, hepatic dysfunction, jaundice, liver enzymes increased
Neuromuscular & skeletal: Paresthesia, peripheral neuropathy, weakness
Otic: Hearing loss
Renal: Azotemia, BUN increased, crystalluria, renal failure, serum creatinine increased
Respiratory: Dyspnea, respiratory arrest
Miscellaneous: Allergic reaction
Drug Interactions
  Avoid Concomitant Use There are no known interactions where it is recommended to avoid concomitant use.
  Increased Effect/Toxicity
  The levels/effects of Flucytosine may be increased by: Amphotericin B
  Decreased Effect
  Flucytosine may decrease the levels/effects of: Saccharomyces boulardii

  The levels/effects of Flucytosine may be decreased by: Cytarabine
Ethanol/Nutrition/Herb Interactions Food: Food decreases the rate, but not the extent of absorption.
Stability Store at room temperature of 15°C to 30°C (59°F to 86°F). Protect from light.
Mechanism of Action Penetrates fungal cells and is converted to fluorouracil which competes with uracil interfering with fungal RNA and protein synthesis
Pharmacodynamics/Kinetics
Absorption: 76% to 89%
Distribution: Into CSF, aqueous humor, joints, peritoneal fluid, and bronchial secretions; V_d: 0.6 L/kg
Protein binding: 3% to 4%
Metabolism: Minimally hepatic; deaminated, possibly via gut bacteria, to 5-fluorouracil
Half-life elimination:
  Normal renal function: 2-5 hours
  Anuria: 85 hours (range: 30-250)
  End stage renal disease: 75-200 hours
Time to peak, serum: ~1-2 hours
Excretion: Urine (>90% as unchanged drug)
Dosage
  Geriatric & Adult
    Endocarditis: Oral: 25-37.5 mg/kg every 6 hours (with amphotericin B) for at least 6 weeks after valve replacement
    Meningoencephalitis, cryptococcal: Induction: Oral: 25 mg/kg/dose (with amphotericin B) every 6 hours for 2 weeks; if clinical improvement, may discontinue both amphotericin and flucytosine and follow with an extended course of fluconazole (400 mg/day); alternatively, may continue flucytosine for 6-10 weeks (with amphotericin B) without conversion to fluconazole treatment

Renal Impairment Use lower initial dose:
  Cl_{cr} 20-40 mL/minute: Administer 37.5 mg/kg every 12 hours
  Cl_{cr} 10-20 mL/minute: Administer 37.5 mg/kg every 24 hours
  Cl_{cr} <10 mL/minute: Administer 37.5 mg/kg every 24-48 hours, but monitor drug concentrations frequently
  Hemodialysis: Dialyzable (50% to 100%); administer dose posthemodialysis
  Peritoneal dialysis: Adults: Administer 0.5-1 g every 24 hours
  Continuous arteriovenous or venovenous hemodiafiltration effects: Change dosing frequency to every 12-24 hours (monitor serum concentrations and adjust)

Administration Administer around-the-clock to promote less variation in peak and trough serum levels. To avoid nausea and vomiting, administer a few capsules at a time over 15 minutes until full dose is taken.

Monitoring Parameters
  Pretreatment: Electrolytes (especially potassium), CBC with differential, BUN, renal function, blood culture
  During treatment: CBC with differential, and LFTs (eg, alkaline phosphatase, AST/ALT) frequently, serum flucytosine concentration, renal function

Reference Range
  Therapeutic: Trough: 25-50 mcg/mL; peak: 50-100 mcg/mL; peak levels should not exceed 100 mcg/mL to avoid toxic bone marrow depressive and hepatic effects
  Trough: Draw just prior to dose administration
  Peak: Draw 2 hours after an oral dose administration

Test Interactions Flucytosine causes markedly false elevations in serum creatinine values when the Ektachem® analyzer is used. The Jaffé reaction is recommended for determining serum creatinine.

Special Geriatric Considerations Adjust for renal function.

Dosage Forms Excipient information presented when available (limited, particularly for generics); consult specific product labeling.
  Capsule, oral:
  Ancobon®: 250 mg, 500 mg

Fludrocortisone (floo droe KOR ti sone)

Related Information
  Corticosteroids on page 2005

Medication Safety Issues
  Sound-alike/look-alike issues:
  Florinef® may be confused with Fioricet®, Fiorinal®

Brand Names: Canada Florinef®

Index Terms 9α-Fluorohydrocortisone Acetate; Florinef; Fludrocortisone Acetate; Fluohydrisone Acetate; Fluohydrocortisone Acetate

Generic Availability (U.S.) Yes

Pharmacologic Category Corticosteroid, Systemic

Use Partial replacement therapy for primary and secondary adrenocortical insufficiency in Addison's disease; treatment of salt-losing adrenogenital syndrome

Contraindications Hypersensitivity to fludrocortisone or any component of the formulation; systemic fungal infections

Warnings/Precautions May cause hypercorticism or suppression of hypothalamic-pituitary-adrenal (HPA) axis, particularly in patients receiving high doses for prolonged periods. HPA axis suppression may lead to adrenal crisis. Withdrawal and discontinuation of a corticosteroid should be done slowly and carefully. Fludrocortisone is primarily a mineralocorticoid agonist, but may also inhibit the HPA axis. May increase risk of infection and/or limit response to vaccinations; close observation is required in patients with latent tuberculosis and/or TB reactivity. Restrict use in active TB (only in conjunction with antituberculosis treatment). Use with caution in patients with sodium retention and potassium loss, hepatic impairment, myocardial infarction, osteoporosis, and/or renal impairment. Use with caution in the elderly. Withdraw therapy with gradual tapering of dose.

Adverse Reactions (Reflective of adult population; not specific for elderly) Frequency not defined.
  Cardiovascular: CHF, edema, hypertension
  Central nervous system: Dizziness, headache, seizures
  Dermatologic: Acne, bruising, rash
  Endocrine & metabolic: HPA suppression, hyperglycemia, hypokalemic alkalosis, suppression of growth
  Gastrointestinal: Peptic ulcer
  Neuromuscular & skeletal: Muscle weakness

Ocular: Cataracts

Miscellaneous: Anaphylaxis (generalized), diaphoresis

Drug Interactions

Avoid Concomitant Use

Avoid concomitant use of Fludrocortisone with any of the following: Aldesleukin; BCG; Natalizumab; Pimecrolimus; Tacrolimus (Topical)

Increased Effect/Toxicity

Fludrocortisone may increase the levels/effects of: Acetylcholinesterase Inhibitors; Amphotericin B; Deferasirox; Leflunomide; Loop Diuretics; Natalizumab; NSAID (COX-2 Inhibitor); NSAID (Nonselective); Thiazide Diuretics; Vaccines (Live); Warfarin

The levels/effects of Fludrocortisone may be increased by: Antifungal Agents (Azole Derivatives, Systemic); Aprepitant; Calcium Channel Blockers (Nondihydropyridine); Denosumab; Estrogen Derivatives; Fluconazole; Fosaprepitant; Macrolide Antibiotics; Neuromuscular-Blocking Agents (Nondepolarizing); Pimecrolimus; Quinolone Antibiotics; Roflumilast; Salicylates; Tacrolimus (Topical); Telaprevir; Trastuzumab

Decreased Effect

Fludrocortisone may decrease the levels/effects of: Aldesleukin; Antidiabetic Agents; BCG; Calcitriol; Corticorelin; Isoniazid; Salicylates; Sipuleucel-T; Telaprevir; Vaccines (Inactivated)

The levels/effects of Fludrocortisone may be decreased by: Aminoglutethimide; Antacids; Barbiturates; Bile Acid Sequestrants; Echinacea; Mitotane; Primidone; Rifamycin Derivatives

Mechanism of Action Promotes increased reabsorption of sodium and loss of potassium from renal distal tubules

Pharmacodynamics/Kinetics

Absorption: Rapid and complete

Protein binding: 42%

Metabolism: Hepatic

Half-life elimination, plasma: 30-35 minutes; Biological: 18-36 hours

Time to peak, serum: ~1.7 hours

Dosage

Geriatric & Adult Mineralocorticoid deficiency: Oral: 0.05-0.2 mg/day with ranges of 0.1 mg 3 times/week to 0.2 mg/day

Administration Administration in conjunction with a glucocorticoid is preferable

Monitoring Parameters Monitor blood pressure and signs of edema when patient is on chronic therapy; very potent mineralocorticoid with high glucocorticoid activity; monitor serum electrolytes, serum renin activity, and blood pressure; monitor for evidence of infection; stop treatment if a significant increase in weight or blood pressure, edema, or cardiac enlargement occurs

Pharmacotherapy Pearls Very potent mineralocorticoid with high glucocorticoid activity

Special Geriatric Considerations The most common use of fludrocortisone in the elderly is orthostatic hypotension that is unresponsive to more conservative measures. Attempt nonpharmacologic measures (hydration, support stockings etc) before starting drug therapy.

Dosage Forms Excipient information presented when available (limited, particularly for generics); consult specific product labeling.

Tablet, oral, as acetate: 0.1 mg

◆ **Fludrocortisone Acetate** *see* Fludrocortisone *on page 746*

◆ **FluLaval®** *see* Influenza Virus Vaccine (Inactivated) *on page 936*

◆ **Flumadine®** *see* Rimantadine *on page 1616*

◆ **FluMist®** *see* Influenza Virus Vaccine (Live/Attenuated) *on page 940*

Flunisolide (Nasal) (floo NISS oh lide)

Related Information

Inhalant Agents *on page 2010*

Medication Safety Issues

Sound-alike/look-alike issues:

Flunisolide may be confused with Flumadine®, fluocinonide

Nasarel may be confused with Nizoral®

Brand Names: Canada Apo-Flunisolide®; Nasalide®; Rhinalar®

Generic Availability (U.S.) Yes

Pharmacologic Category Corticosteroid, Nasal

Use Seasonal or perennial rhinitis

◀ **Dosage**
   Geriatric & Adult Seasonal allergic rhinitis: Intranasal: 2 sprays each nostril twice daily
   (morning and evening); may increase to 2 sprays 3 times daily; maximum dose: 8 sprays/
   day in each nostril (400 mcg/day)
Dosage Forms Excipient information presented when available (limited, particularly for
generics); consult specific product labeling.
   Solution, intranasal [spray]: 25 mcg/actuation (25 mL); 29 mcg/actuation (25 mL)

Fluocinolone (Ophthalmic) (floo oh SIN oh lone)

Related Information
   Corticosteroids on page 2005
Medication Safety Issues
   Sound-alike/look-alike issues:
   Fluocinolone may be confused with fluocinonide
Brand Names: U.S. Retisert®
Index Terms Fluocinolone Acetonide
Generic Availability (U.S.) No
Pharmacologic Category Corticosteroid, Ophthalmic
Use Treatment of chronic, noninfectious uveitis affecting the posterior segment of the eye
Dosage
   Geriatric & Adult Chronic uveitis: Ocular implant: One silicone-encased tablet (0.59 mg)
   surgically implanted into the posterior segment of the eye is designed to initially release 0.6
   mcg/day, decreasing over 30 days to a steady-state release rate of 0.3-0.4 mcg/day for 30
   months. Recurrence of uveitis denotes depletion of tablet, requiring reimplantation.
Dosage Forms Excipient information presented when available (limited, particularly for
generics); consult specific product labeling.
   Implant, intravitreal, as acetonide:
   Retisert®: 0.59 mg (1s) [enclosed in silicone elastomer]

Fluocinolone (Otic) (floo oh SIN oh lone)

Related Information
   Corticosteroids on page 2005
Medication Safety Issues
   Sound-alike/look-alike issues:
   Fluocinolone may be confused with fluocinonide
Brand Names: U.S. DermOtic®
Index Terms Fluocinolone Acetonide
Generic Availability (U.S.) No
Pharmacologic Category Corticosteroid, Otic
Use Relief of chronic eczematous external otitis
Dosage
   Geriatric & Adult Chronic eczematous external otitis: Otic: 5 drops into the affected ear
   twice daily for 1-2 weeks
Dosage Forms Excipient information presented when available (limited, particularly for
generics); consult specific product labeling.
   Oil, otic, as acetonide [drops]:
   DermOtic®: 0.01% (20 mL) [contains peanut oil]

Fluocinolone (Topical) (floo oh SIN oh lone)

Related Information
   Corticosteroids on page 2005
Medication Safety Issues
   Sound-alike/look-alike issues:
   Fluocinolone may be confused with fluocinonide
Brand Names: U.S. Capex®; Derma-Smoothe/FS®
Brand Names: Canada Capex®; Derma-Smoothe/FS®; Synalar®
Index Terms Fluocinolone Acetonide
Generic Availability (U.S.) Yes: Excludes oil, shampoo
Pharmacologic Category Corticosteroid, Topical
Use Relief of susceptible inflammatory dermatosis [low, medium corticosteroid]; dermatitis or
psoriasis of the scalp; atopic dermatitis

Dosage
Geriatric & Adult
Atopic dermatitis (Derma-Smoothe/FS® body oil): Apply thin film to affected area 3 times/day
Corticosteroid-responsive dermatoses: Topical: Cream, ointment, solution: Apply a thin layer to affected area 2-4 times/day; may use occlusive dressings to manage psoriasis or recalcitrant conditions
Inflammatory and pruritic manifestations (dental use): Topical: Apply to oral lesion 4 times/day, after meals and at bedtime
Scalp psoriasis (Derma-Smoothe/FS® scalp oil): Topical: Massage thoroughly into wet or dampened hair/scalp; cover with shower cap. Leave on overnight (or for at least 4 hours). Remove by washing hair with shampoo and rinsing thoroughly.
Seborrheic dermatitis of the scalp (Capex®): Topical: Apply no more than 1 ounce to scalp once daily; work into lather and allow to remain on scalp for ~5 minutes. Remove from hair and scalp by rinsing thoroughly with water.
Special Geriatric Considerations Due to age-related changes in skin, limit use of topical corticosteroids.
Dosage Forms Excipient information presented when available (limited, particularly for generics); consult specific product labeling.
Cream, topical, as acetonide: 0.01% (15 g, 60 g); 0.025% (15 g, 60 g)
Oil, topical, as acetonide [body oil]:
Derma-Smoothe/FS®: 0.01% (120 mL) [contains peanut oil]
Oil, topical, as acetonide [scalp oil]:
Derma-Smoothe/FS®: 0.01% (120 mL) [contains peanut oil]
Ointment, topical, as acetonide: 0.025% (15 g, 60 g)
Shampoo, topical, as acetonide:
Capex®: 0.01% (120 mL)
Solution, topical, as acetonide: 0.01% (60 mL)

♦ **Fluocinolone Acetonide** see Fluocinolone (Ophthalmic) on page 748
♦ **Fluocinolone Acetonide** see Fluocinolone (Otic) on page 748
♦ **Fluocinolone Acetonide** see Fluocinolone (Topical) on page 748

Fluocinonide (floo oh SIN oh nide)

Related Information
Corticosteroids on page 2005
Medication Safety Issues
Sound-alike/look-alike issues:
Fluocinonide may be confused with flunisolide, fluocinolone
Lidex® may be confused with Lasix®, Videx®, Wydase®
Brand Names: U.S. Vanos®
Brand Names: Canada Lidemol®; Lidex®; Lyderm®; Tiamol®; Topactin; Topsyn®
Index Terms Lidex
Generic Availability (U.S.) Yes
Pharmacologic Category Corticosteroid, Topical
Use Anti-inflammatory, antipruritic; treatment of plaque-type psoriasis (up to 10% of body surface area) [high-potency topical corticosteroid]
Contraindications Hypersensitivity to fluocinonide or any component of the formulation; viral, fungal, or tubercular skin lesions, herpes simplex
Warnings/Precautions Systemic absorption of topical corticosteroids may cause hypothalamic-pituitary-adrenal (HPA) axis suppression (reversible). HPA axis suppression may lead to adrenal crisis. Risk is increased when used over large surface areas, for prolonged periods, or with occlusive dressings. Allergic contact dermatitis can occur, it is usually diagnosed by failure to heal rather than clinical exacerbation. Prolonged treatment with corticosteroids has been associated with the development of Kaposi's sarcoma (case reports); if noted, discontinuation of therapy should be considered. Adverse systemic effects including hyperglycemia, glycosuria, fluid and electrolyte changes, and HPA suppression may occur when used on large surface areas, for prolonged periods, or with an occlusive dressing. Lower-strength cream (0.05%) may be used cautiously on face or opposing skin surfaces that may rub or touch (eg, skin folds of the groin, axilla, and breasts); higher-strength (0.1%) should not be used on the face, groin, or axillae. Use of the 0.1% cream for >2 weeks is not recommended.

◀ **Adverse Reactions (Reflective of adult population; not specific for elderly)** Frequency not defined.

Cardiovascular: Intracranial hypertension

Dermatologic: Acne, allergic dermatitis, contact dermatitis, dry skin, folliculitis, hypertrichosis, hypopigmentation, maceration of the skin, miliaria, perioral dermatitis, pruritus, skin atrophy, striae, telangiectasia

Endocrine & metabolic: Cushing's syndrome, growth retardation, HPA suppression, hyperglycemia

Local: Burning, irritation

Renal: Glycosuria

Miscellaneous: Secondary infection

Drug Interactions

Avoid Concomitant Use

Avoid concomitant use of Fluocinonide with any of the following: Aldesleukin

Increased Effect/Toxicity

Fluocinonide may increase the levels/effects of: Deferasirox

The levels/effects of Fluocinonide may be increased by: Telaprevir

Decreased Effect

Fluocinonide may decrease the levels/effects of: Aldesleukin; Corticorelin; Telaprevir

Mechanism of Action Fluorinated topical corticosteroid considered to be of high potency. The mechanism of action for all topical corticosteroids is not well defined, however, is felt to be a combination of three important properties: anti-inflammatory activity, immunosuppressive properties, and antiproliferative actions.

Pharmacodynamics/Kinetics

Absorption: Dependent on strength of product, amount applied, and nature of skin at application site; ranges from ~1% in areas of thick stratum corneum (palms, soles, elbows, etc) to 36% in areas of thin stratum corneum (face, eyelids, etc); increased in areas of skin damage, inflammation, or occlusion

Distribution: Throughout local skin; absorbed drug into muscle, liver, skin, intestines, and kidneys

Metabolism: Primarily in skin; small amount absorbed into systemic circulation is primarily hepatic to inactive compounds

Excretion: Urine (primarily as glucuronide and sulfate, also as unconjugated products); feces (small amounts as metabolites)

Dosage

Geriatric & Adult

Pruritus and inflammation: Topical (0.05% cream): Apply thin layer to affected area 2-4 times/day depending on the severity of the condition. Therapy should be discontinued when control is achieved; if no improvement is seen, reassessment of diagnosis may be necessary.

Plaque-type psoriasis (Vanos™): Topical (0.1% cream): Apply a thin layer once or twice daily to affected areas (limited to <10% of body surface area). **Note:** Not recommended for use >2 consecutive weeks or >60 g/week total exposure. Discontinue when control is achieved.

Monitoring Parameters Relief of symptoms

Pharmacotherapy Pearls Considered a high potency steroid; avoid prolonged use on the face; may cause atrophic changes

Special Geriatric Considerations Due to age-related changes in skin, limit use of topical corticosteroids.

Dosage Forms Excipient information presented when available (limited, particularly for generics); consult specific product labeling.

Cream, topical:

Vanos®: 0.1% (30 g, 60 g, 120 g)

Cream, anhydrous, emollient, topical: 0.05% (15 g, 30 g, 60 g, 120 g)

Cream, aqueous, emollient, topical: 0.05% (15 g, 30 g, 60 g)

Gel, topical: 0.05% (15 g, 30 g, 60 g)

Ointment, topical: 0.05% (15 g, 30 g, 60 g)

Solution, topical: 0.05% (20 mL, 60 mL)

◆ **Fluohydrisone Acetate** *see* Fludrocortisone *on page 746*

◆ **Fluohydrocortisone Acetate** *see* Fludrocortisone *on page 746*

◆ **Fluorabon™** *see* Fluoride *on page 751*

◆ **Fluor-A-Day®** *see* Fluoride *on page 751*

Fluoride (FLOR ide)

Medication Safety Issues
Sound-alike/look-alike issues:
Phos-Flur® may be confused with PhosLo®
International issues:
Fluorex [France] may be confused with Flarex brand name for fluorometholone [U.S., Canada, and multiple international markets] and Fluarix brand name for influenza virus vaccine (inactivated) [U.S., and multiple international markets]

Brand Names: U.S. Act® Kids [OTC]; Act® Restoring™ [OTC]; Act® Total Care™ [OTC]; Act® [OTC]; CaviRinse™; Clinpro™ 5000; ControlRx™; ControlRx™ Multi; Denta 5000 Plus™; DentaGel™; Epiflur™; Fluor-A-Day®; Fluorabon™; Fluorinse®; Fluoritab; Flura-Drops®; Gel-Kam® Rinse; Gel-Kam® [OTC]; Just For Kids™ [OTC]; Lozi-Flur™; Neutra-Care®; NeutraGard® Advanced; Omni Gel™ [OTC]; OrthoWash™; PerioMed™; Phos-Flur®; Phos-Flur® Rinse [OTC]; PreviDent®; PreviDent® 5000 Booster; PreviDent® 5000 Dry Mouth; PreviDent® 5000 Plus®; PreviDent® 5000 Sensitive; StanGard® Perio; Stop®

Brand Names: Canada Fluor-A-Day

Index Terms Acidulated Phosphate Fluoride; Sodium Fluoride; Stannous Fluoride

Generic Availability (U.S.) Yes: Excludes lozenge, gel drops

Pharmacologic Category Nutritional Supplement

Use Prevention of dental caries

Contraindications Hypersensitivity to fluoride, tartrazine, or any component of the formulation; when fluoride content of drinking water exceeds 0.7 ppm; low sodium or sodium-free diets

Warnings/Precautions Prolonged ingestion with excessive doses may result in dental fluorosis and osseous changes; do **not** exceed recommended dosage. Some products contain tartrazine.

Drug Interactions
Avoid Concomitant Use There are no known interactions where it is recommended to avoid concomitant use.

Increased Effect/Toxicity There are no known significant interactions involving an increase in effect.

Decreased Effect There are no known significant interactions involving a decrease in effect.

Stability Store in tight plastic containers (not glass).

Mechanism of Action Promotes remineralization of decalcified enamel; inhibits the cariogenic microbial process in dental plaque; increases tooth resistance to acid dissolution

Pharmacodynamics/Kinetics
Absorption: Oral: Rapid and complete; sodium fluoride; other soluble fluoride salts; calcium, iron, or magnesium may delay absorption

Distribution: 50% of fluoride is deposited in teeth and bone after ingestion; topical application works superficially on enamel and plaque

Excretion: Urine and feces

Dosage
Geriatric & Adult Prevention of dental caries: Oral:
Dental rinse or gel: 10 mL rinse or apply to teeth and spit daily after brushing
Product-specific dosing:
PreviDent® rinse: Once weekly, rinse 10 mL vigorously around and between teeth for 1 minute, then spit; this should be done preferably at bedtime, after thoroughly brushing teeth; for maximum benefit, do not eat, drink, or rinse mouth for at least 30 minutes after treatment; do not swallow
Fluorinse®: Once weekly, vigorously swish 5-10 mL in mouth for 1 minute, then spit

Pharmacotherapy Pearls 2.2 mg of sodium fluoride is equivalent to 1 mg of fluoride ion

Special Geriatric Considerations Postmenopausal women taking high doses of sodium fluoride have increased their bone density in the lumbar spine by 35% with a smaller increase in the femoral neck. In spite of these increases, the overall rate of vertebral fracture did not decline significantly while the rate of hip fracture increased. The results of a randomized, placebo-controlled trial using an investigational slow-release fluoride formulation at a lower dose (50 mg/day) are encouraging. Patients who received fluoride for 1 year or more had a lower vertebral fracture rate and substantial increase in L2-L4 bone mass and femoral neck bone density compared to placebo. Both groups took calcium. At the present time, restricted to investigational protocols.

Dosage Forms Excipient information presented when available (limited, particularly for generics); consult specific product labeling.

Cream, oral, as sodium [toothpaste]: 1.1% (51 g) [equivalent to fluoride 2.5 mg/dose]
  Denta 5000 Plus™: 1.1% (51 g) [spearmint flavor; equivalent to fluoride 2.5 mg/dose]
  PreviDent® 5000 Plus®: 1.1% (51 g) [contains sodium benzoate; fruitastic™ flavor; equivalent to fluoride 2.5 mg/dose]
  PreviDent® 5000 Plus®: 1.1% (51 g) [contains sodium benzoate; spearmint flavor; equivalent to fluoride 2.5 mg/dose]
Gel, topical, as acidulated phosphate:
  Phos-Flur®: 1.1% (51 g) [contains propylene glycol, sodium benzoate; mint flavor; equivalent to fluoride 0.5%]
Gel, oral, as sodium [toothpaste]:
  PreviDent® 5000 Booster: 1.1% (100 mL, 106 mL) [contains sodium benzoate; fruitastic™ flavor; equivalent to fluoride 2.5 mg/dose]
  PreviDent® 5000 Booster: 1.1% (100 mL, 106 mL) [contains sodium benzoate; spearmint flavor; equivalent to fluoride 2.5 mg/dose]
  PreviDent® 5000 Dry Mouth: 1.1% (100 mL) [mint flavor; equivalent to fluoride 2.5 mg/dose]
  PreviDent® 5000 Sensitive: 1.1% (100 mL) [mild mint flavor; equivalent to fluoride 2.5 mg/dose]
Gel, topical, as sodium: 1.1% (56 g) [equivalent to fluoride 2 mg/dose]
  DentaGel™: 1.1% (56 g) [fresh mint flavor; neutral pH; equivalent to fluoride 2 mg/dose]
  NeutraCare®: 1.1% (60 g) [grape flavor; neutral pH]
  NeutraCare®: 1.1% (60 g) [mint flavor; neutral pH]
  NeutraGard® Advanced: 1.1% (60 g) [mint flavor; neutral pH]
  NeutraGard® Advanced: 1.1% (60 g) [mixed berry flavor; neutral pH]
  PreviDent®: 1.1% (56 g) [mint flavor; equivalent to fluoride 2 mg/dose]
  PreviDent®: 1.1% (56 g) [very berry flavor; equivalent to fluoride 2 mg/dose]
Gel, topical, as stannous flouride:
  Gel-Kam®: 0.4% (129 g) [cinnamon flavor]
  Gel-Kam®: 0.4% (129 g) [fruit & berry flavor]
  Gel-Kam®: 0.4% (129 g) [mint flavor]
  Just For Kids™: 0.4% (122 g) [bubblegum flavor]
  Just For Kids™: 0.4% (122 g) [fruit-punch flavor]
  Just For Kids™: 0.4% (122 g) [grapey grape flavor]
  Omni Gel™: 0.4% (122 g) [cinnamon flavor]
  Omni Gel™: 0.4% (122 g) [grape flavor]
  Omni Gel™: 0.4% (122 g) [mint flavor]
  Omni Gel™: 0.4% (122 g) [natural flavor]
  Omni Gel™: 0.4% (122 g) [raspberry flavor]
  Stop®: 0.4% (120 g) [bubblegum flavor]
  Stop®: 0.4% (120 g) [cinnamon flavor]
  Stop®: 0.4% (120 g) [grape flavor]
  Stop®: 0.4% (120 g) [mint flavor]
Liquid, oral, as base:
  Fluoritab: 0.125 mg/drop [dye free]
Lozenge, oral, as sodium:
  Lozi-Flur™: 2.21 mg (90s) [sugar free; cherry flavor; equivalent to fluoride 1 mg]
Paste, oral, as sodium [toothpaste]:
  Clinpro™ 5000: 1.1% (113 g) [vanilla-mint flavor]
  ControlRx™: 1.1% (57 g) [berry flavor]
  ControlRx™: 1.1% (57 g) [vanilla-mint flavor]
  ControlRx™ Multi: 1.1% (57 g) [vanilla-mint flavor]
Solution, oral, as fluoride [rinse]:
  Act® Total Care™: 0.02% (1000 mL) [ethanol free; contains menthol, propylene glycol, sodium benzoate, tartrazine; fresh mint flavor; equivalent to fluoride 0.009%]
Solution, oral, as sodium [drops]: 1.1 mg/mL (50 mL) [equivalent to fluoride 0.5 mg/mL]
  Fluor-A-Day®: 0.278 mg/drop (30 mL) [equivalent to fluoride 0.125 mg/drop]
  Fluorabon™: 0.55 mg/0.6 mL (60 mL) [dye free, sugar free; equivalent to fluoride 0.25 mg/0.6 mL]
  Flura-Drops®: 0.55 mg/drop (24 mL) [dye free, sugar free; equivalent to fluoride 0.25 mg/drop]
Solution, oral, as sodium [rinse]: 0.2% (473 mL)
  Act®: 0.05% (532 mL) [contains benzyl alcohol, propylene glycol, sodium benzoate, tartrazine; cinnamon flavor; equivalent to fluoride 0.02%]
  Act®: 0.05% (532 mL) [contains propylene glycol, sodium benzoate, tartrazine; mint flavor; equivalent to fluoride 0.02%]
  Act® Kids: 0.05% (532 mL) [ethanol free; contains benzyl alcohol, propylene glycol, sodium benzoate; bubblegum flavor; equivalent to fluoride 0.02%]

Act® Kids: 0.05% (500 mL) [ethanol free; contains benzyl alcohol, propylene glycol, sodium benzoate; ocean berry flavor; equivalent to fluoride 0.02%]

Act® Restoring™: 0.02% (1000 mL) [contains ethanol 11%, propylene glycol, sodium benzoate; Cool Splash™ mint flavor; equivalent to fluoride 0.009%]

Act® Restoring™: 0.02% (1000 mL) [contains ethanol 11%, propylene glycol, sodium benzoate; Cool Splash™ spearmint flavor; equivalent to fluoride 0.009%]

Act® Restoring™: 0.05% (532 mL) [contains ethanol 11%, propylene glycol, sodium benzoate; Cool Splash™ mint flavor; equivalent to fluoride 0.02%]

Act® Restoring™: 0.05% (532 mL) [contains ethanol 11%, propylene glycol, sodium benzoate; Cool Splash™ spearmint flavor; equivalent to fluoride 0.02%]

Act® Restoring™: 0.05% (532 mL) [contains ethanol 11%, propylene glycol, sodium benzoate; Cool Splash™ vanilla-mint flavor; equivalent to fluoride 0.02%]

Act® Total Care™: 0.02% (1000 mL) [contains ethanol 11%, propylene glycol, sodium benzoate; icy clean mint flavor; equivalent to fluoride 0.009%]

Act® Total Care™: 0.05% (88 mL, 532 mL) [contains ethanol 11%, propylene glycol, sodium benzoate; icy clean mint flavor; equivalent to fluoride 0.02%]

Act® Total Care™: 0.05% (88 mL, 532 mL) [ethanol free; contains menthol, propylene glycol, sodium benzoate, tartrazine; fresh mint flavor; equivalent to fluoride 0.02%]

CaviRinse™: 0.2% (240 mL) [mint flavor]

Fluorinse®: 0.2% (480 mL) [ethanol free; cinnamon flavor]

Fluorinse®: 0.2% (480 mL) [ethanol free; mint flavor]

OrthoWash™: 0.044% (480 mL) [contains sodium benzoate; grape flavor]

OrthoWash™: 0.044% (480 mL) [contains sodium benzoate; strawberry flavor]

Phos-Flur® Rinse: 0.044% (473 mL) [ethanol free, sugar free; bubblegum flavor]

Phos-Flur® Rinse: 0.044% (473 mL) [ethanol free, sugar free; gushing grape flavor]

Phos-Flur® Rinse: 0.044% (500 mL) [sugar free; cool mint flavor]

PreviDent®: 0.2% (473 mL) [contains benzoic acid, ethanol 6%, sodium benzoate; cool mint flavor]

Solution, oral, as stannous flouride [concentrated rinse]: 0.63% (300 mL) [equivalent to fluoride 7 mg/30 mL dose]

Gel-Kam® Rinse: 0.63% (300 mL) [mint flavor; equivalent to fluoride 7 mg/30 mL dose]

PerioMed™: 0.63% (284 mL) [ethanol free; cinnamon flavor; equivalent to fluoride 7 mg/30 mL dose]

PerioMed™: 0.63% (284 mL) [ethanol free; mint flavor; equivalent to fluoride 7 mg/30 mL dose]

PerioMed™: 0.63% (284 mL) [ethanol free; tropical fruit flavor; equivalent to fluoride 7 mg/30 mL dose]

StanGard® Perio: 0.63% (284 mL) [mint flavor]

Tablet, chewable, oral, as sodium: 0.55 mg [equivalent to fluoride 0.25 mg], 1.1 mg [equivalent to fluoride 0.5 mg], 2.2 mg [equivalent to fluoride 1 mg]

Epiflur™: 0.55 mg [sugar free; vanilla flavor; equivalent to fluoride 0.25 mg]

Epiflur™: 1.1 mg [sugar free; vanilla flavor; equivalent to fluoride 0.5 mg]

Epiflur™: 2.2 mg [sugar free; vanilla flavor; equivalent to fluoride 1 mg]

Fluor-A-Day®: 1.1 mg [raspberry flavor; equivalent to fluoride 0.5 mg]

Fluor-A-Day®: 2.2 mg [raspberry flavor; equivalent to fluoride 1 mg]

Fluoritab: 2.2 mg [cherry flavor; equivalent to fluoride 1 mg]

Fluoritab: 1.1 mg [dye free; cherry flavor; equivalent to fluoride 0.5 mg]

Selected References

Pak CYS, Sakhaee K, Adams-Huet B, et al, "Treatment of Postmenopausal Osteoporosis With Slow-Release Sodium Fluoride: Final Report of a Randomized Controlled Trial," *Ann Intern Med*, 1995, 123(6):401-8.

Riggs BL, Hodgson SF, O'Fallon WM, et al, "Effect of Fluoride Treatment on the Fracture Rate in Postmenopausal Women With Osteoporosis," *N Engl J Med*, 1990, 322(12):802-9.

◆ **Fluorinse®** see Fluoride on page 751

◆ **Fluoritab** see Fluoride on page 751

◆ **5-Fluorocytosine** see Flucytosine on page 744

◆ **9α-Fluorohydrocortisone Acetate** see Fludrocortisone on page 746

FLUoxetine (floo OKS e teen)

Related Information

Antidepressant Agents on page 1991

Beers Criteria – Potentially Inappropriate Medications for Geriatrics on page 2089

Liquid Compatibility of Antidepressants, Antipsychotics, and Mood Stabilizers on page 2111

Medication Safety Issues

Sound-alike/look-alike issues:

FLUoxetine may be confused with DULoxetine, famotidine, Feldene®, fluconazole, fluvastatin, fluvoxaMINE, fosinopril, furosemide, PARoxetine, thiothixene

◀ PROzac® may be confused with Paxil®, Prelone®, PriLOSEC®, Prograf®, Proscar®, ProSom®, ProStep®, Provera®

Sarafem® may be confused with Serophene®

BEERS Criteria medication:
This drug may be inappropriate for use in geriatric patients (high severity risk).

International issues:
Reneuron [Spain] may be confused with Remeron brand name for mirtazapine [U.S., Canada, and multiple international markets]

Brand Names: U.S. PROzac®; PROzac® Weekly™; Sarafem®; Selfemra® [DSC]

Brand Names: Canada Apo-Fluoxetine®; CO Fluoxetine; Dom-Fluoxetine; Fluoxetine; FXT 40; Gen-Fluoxetine; Mylan-Fluoxetine; Novo-Fluoxetine; Nu-Fluoxetine; PHL-Fluoxetine; PMS-Fluoxetine; PRO-Fluoxetine; Prozac®; ratio-Fluoxetine; Riva-Fluoxetine; Sandoz-Fluoxetine; Teva-Fluoxetine; ZYM-Fluoxetine

Index Terms Fluoxetine Hydrochloride

Generic Availability (U.S.) Yes

Pharmacologic Category Antidepressant, Selective Serotonin Reuptake Inhibitor

Use Treatment of major depressive disorder (MDD); treatment of binge-eating and vomiting in patients with moderate-to-severe bulimia nervosa; obsessive-compulsive disorder (OCD); panic disorder with or without agoraphobia; in combination with olanzapine for treatment-resistant or bipolar I depression

Unlabeled/Investigational Use Selective mutism; treatment of mild dementia-associated agitation in nonpsychotic patients; post-traumatic stress disorder (PTSD); social anxiety disorder; chronic neuropathic pain, fibromyalgia; Raynaud's phenomenon

Medication Guide Available Yes

Contraindications Hypersensitivity to fluoxetine or any component of the formulation; patients currently receiving MAO inhibitors, pimozide, or thioridazine

Note: MAO inhibitor therapy must be stopped for 14 days before fluoxetine is initiated. Treatment with MAO inhibitors or thioridazine should not be initiated until 5 weeks after the discontinuation of fluoxetine.

Warnings/Precautions [U.S. Boxed Warning]: Antidepressants increase the risk of suicidal thinking and behavior in children, adolescents, and young adults (18-24 years of age) with major depressive disorder (MDD) and other psychiatric disorders; consider risk prior to prescribing. Short-term studies did not show an increased risk in patients >24 years of age and showed a decreased risk in patients ≥65 years. Closely monitor patients for clinical worsening, suicidality, or unusual changes in behavior, particularly during the initial 1-2 months of therapy or during periods of dosage adjustments (increases or decreases); the patient's family or caregiver should be instructed to closely observe the patient and communicate condition with healthcare provider. A medication guide concerning the use of antidepressants should be dispensed with each prescription. **Fluoxetine is FDA approved for the treatment of OCD in children ≥7 years of age and MDD in children ≥8 years of age.**

The possibility of a suicide attempt is inherent in major depression and may persist until remission occurs. Use caution in high-risk patients. Worsening depression and severe abrupt suicidality that are not part of the presenting symptoms may require discontinuation or modification of drug therapy. The patient's family or caregiver should be alerted to monitor patients for the emergence of suicidality and associated behaviors (such as agitation, irritability, hostility, impulsivity, and hypomania) and call healthcare provider.

May worsen psychosis in some patients or precipitate a shift to mania or hypomania in patients with bipolar disorder. Patients presenting with depressive symptoms should be screened for bipolar disorder. Monotherapy in patients with bipolar disorder should be avoided. **Fluoxetine monotherapy is not FDA approved for the treatment of bipolar depression.** May cause insomnia, anxiety, nervousness, or anorexia. Use with caution in patients where weight loss is undesirable. May impair cognitive or motor performance; caution operating hazardous machinery or driving.

Serotonin syndrome and neuroleptic malignant syndrome (NMS)-like reactions have occurred with serotonin/norepinephrine reuptake inhibitors (SNRIs) and selective serotonin reuptake inhibitors (SSRIs) when used alone, and particularly when used in combination with serotonergic agents (eg, triptans) or antidopaminergic agents (eg, antipsychotics). Concurrent use with MAO inhibitors is contraindicated. Fluoxetine may elevate plasma levels of thioridazine or pimozide and increase the risk of QT_c interval prolongation. This may lead to serious ventricular arrhythmias, such as torsade de pointes-type arrhythmias, and sudden death. Fluoxetine use has been associated with occurrences of significant rash and allergic events, including vasculitis, lupus-like syndrome, laryngospasm, anaphylactoid reactions, and pulmonary inflammatory disease. Discontinue if underlying cause of rash cannot be identified.

Use caution in patients with a previous seizure disorder or condition predisposing to seizures such as brain damage, alcoholism, or concurrent therapy with other drugs which lower the seizure threshold. Use with caution in patients with hepatic or severe renal dysfunction and in elderly patients. Fluoxetine (daily) may be inappropriate for use in the elderly due to risk of agitation, sleep disturbances, and excessive CNS stimulation, attributed to this drug's long half-life (Beers Criteria). May cause hyponatremia/SIADH (elderly at increased risk); volume depletion (diuretics may increase risk). May increase the risks associated with electro-convulsive treatment. Use caution with concomitant use of NSAIDs, ASA, or other drugs that affect coagulation; the risk of bleeding may be potentiated. Use caution with history of MI or unstable heart disease; use in these patients is limited. May alter glycemic control in patients with diabetes. Due to the long half-life of fluoxetine and its metabolites, the effects and interactions noted may persist for prolonged periods following discontinuation. May cause or exacerbate sexual dysfunction. May cause mydriasis; use caution in patients at risk of acute narrow-angle glaucoma or with increased intraocular pressure. Discontinuation symptoms (eg, dysphoric mood, irritability, agitation, confusion, anxiety, insomnia, hypomania) may occur upon abrupt discontinuation. Taper dose when discontinuing therapy.

Adverse Reactions (Reflective of adult population; not specific for elderly) Percentages listed for adverse effects as reported in placebo-controlled trials and were generally similar in adults and children; actual frequency may be dependent upon diagnosis and in some cases the range presented may be lower than or equal to placebo for a particular disorder.

>10%:
  Central nervous system: Insomnia (10% to 33%), headache (21%), somnolence (5% to 17%), anxiety (6% to 15%), nervousness (8% to 14%)
  Endocrine & metabolic: Libido decreased (1% to 11%)
  Gastrointestinal: Nausea (12% to 29%), diarrhea (8% to 18%), anorexia (4% to 17%), xerostomia (4% to 12%)
  Neuromuscular & skeletal: Weakness (7% to 21%), tremor (3% to 13%)
  Respiratory: Pharyngitis (3% to 11%), yawn (≤11%)
1% to 10%:
  Cardiovascular: Vasodilation (1% to 5%), chest pain, hemorrhage, hypertension, palpitation
  Central nervous system: Dizziness (9%), abnormal dreams (1% to 5%), abnormal thinking (2%), agitation, amnesia, chills, confusion, emotional lability, sleep disorder
  Dermatologic: Rash (2% to 6%), pruritus (4%)
  Endocrine & metabolic: Ejaculation abnormal (≤7%), impotence (≤7%), menorrhagia (≥2%)
  Gastrointestinal: Dyspepsia (6% to 10%), constipation (5%), flatulence (3%), vomiting (3%), thirst (≥2%), weight loss (2%), appetite increased, taste perversion, weight gain
  Genitourinary: Urinary frequency
  Neuromuscular & skeletal: Hyperkinesia (≥2%)
  Ocular: Vision abnormal (2%)
  Otic: Ear pain, tinnitus
  Respiratory: Sinusitis (1% to 6%)
  Miscellaneous: Flu-like syndrome (3% to 10%), diaphoresis (2% to 8%), epistaxis (≥2%)
Drug Interactions
  Metabolism/Transport Effects Substrate of CYP1A2 (minor), 2B6 (minor), 2C9 (major), 2C19 (minor), 2D6 (major), 2E1 (minor), 3A4 (minor); **Inhibits** CYP1A2 (moderate), 2B6 (weak), 2C9 (weak), 2C19 (moderate), 2D6 (strong), 3A4 (weak)
  Avoid Concomitant Use
    Avoid concomitant use of FLUoxetine with any of the following: Artemether; Clopidogrel; Dronedarone; Iobenguane I 123; Lumefantrine; MAO Inhibitors; Methylene Blue; Nilotinib; Pimozide; QUEtiapine; QuiNINE; Sibutramine; Tamoxifen; Tetrabenazine; Thioridazine; Toremifene; Tryptophan; Vandetanib; Vemurafenib; Ziprasidone
  Increased Effect/Toxicity
    FLUoxetine may increase the levels/effects of: Alpha-/Beta-Blockers; Anticoagulants; Antidepressants (Serotonin Reuptake Inhibitor/Antagonist); Antiplatelet Agents; Aspirin; Atomoxetine; Benzodiazepines (metabolized by oxidation); Beta-Blockers; BusPIRone; CarBAMazepine; CloZAPine; Collagenase (Systemic); CYP1A2 Substrates; CYP2C19 Substrates; CYP2D6 Substrates; Desmopressin; Dextromethorphan; Dronedarone; Drotrecogin Alfa; Fesoterodine; Fosphenytoin; Galantamine; Haloperidol; Ibritumomab; Lithium; Methadone; Methylene Blue; Mexiletine; NIFEdipine; NiMODipine; NSAID (COX-2 Inhibitor); NSAID (Nonselective); Phenytoin; Pimozide; Propafenone; QTc-Prolonging Agents; QuiNIDine; QuiNINE; RisperiDONE; Rivaroxaban; Salicylates; Serotonin Modulators; Tamoxifen; Tetrabenazine; Thioridazine; Thrombolytic Agents; Toremifene; Tositumomab and Iodine I 131 Tositumomab; TraMADol; Tricyclic Antidepressants; Vandetanib; Vemurafenib; Vitamin K Antagonists; Ziprasidone

◀ *The levels/effects of FLUoxetine may be increased by:* Abiraterone Acetate; Alcohol (Ethyl); Alfuzosin; Analgesics (Opioid); Artemether; BusPIRone; Chloroquine; Cimetidine; Ciprofloxacin; Ciprofloxacin (Systemic); CNS Depressants; Conivaptan; CYP2C9 Inhibitors (Moderate); CYP2C9 Inhibitors (Strong); CYP2D6 Inhibitors (Moderate); CYP2D6 Inhibitors (Strong); Darunavir; Gadobutrol; Glucosamine; Herbs (Anticoagulant/Antiplatelet Properties); Lumefantrine; Macrolide Antibiotics; MAO Inhibitors; Metoclopramide; Nilotinib; Omega-3-Acid Ethyl Esters; Pentosan Polysulfate Sodium; Pentoxifylline; Prostacyclin Analogues; QUEtiapine; QuiNINE; Sibutramine; TraMADol; Tryptophan; Vitamin E

Decreased Effect

FLUoxetine may decrease the levels/effects of: Clopidogrel; Iobenguane I 123

The levels/effects of FLUoxetine may be decreased by: CarBAMazepine; CYP2C9 Inducers (Highly Effective); Cyproheptadine; Cyproterone; NSAID (Nonselective); Peginterferon Alfa-2b; Tocilizumab

Ethanol/Nutrition/Herb Interactions

Ethanol: May increase CNS depression; monitor for increased effects with coadministration. Caution patients about effects.

Herb/Nutraceutical: Avoid valerian, St John's wort, kava kava, gotu kola (may increase CNS depression).

Stability All dosage forms should be stored at controlled room temperature of 15°C to 30°C (50°F to 86°F). Oral liquid should be dispensed in a light-resistant container.

Mechanism of Action Inhibits CNS neuron serotonin reuptake; minimal or no effect on reuptake of norepinephrine or dopamine; does not significantly bind to alpha-adrenergic, histamine, or cholinergic receptors

Pharmacodynamics/Kinetics

Onset of action: Depression: The onset of action is within a week; however, individual response varies greatly and full response may not be seen until 8-12 weeks after initiation of treatment.

Absorption: Well absorbed; delayed 1-2 hours with weekly formulation

Distribution: V_d: 12-43 L/kg

Protein binding: 95% to albumin and alpha$_1$ glycoprotein

Metabolism: Hepatic, via CYP2C19 and 2D6, to norfluoxetine (activity equal to fluoxetine)

Half-life elimination: Adults:

Parent drug: 1-3 days (acute), 4-6 days (chronic), 7.6 days (cirrhosis)

Metabolite (norfluoxetine): 9.3 days (range: 4-16 days), 12 days (cirrhosis)

Time to peak, serum: 6-8 hours

Excretion: Urine (10% as norfluoxetine, 2.5% to 5% as fluoxetine)

Note: Weekly formulation results in greater fluctuations between peak and trough concentrations of fluoxetine and norfluoxetine compared to once-daily dosing (24% daily/164% weekly; 17% daily/43% weekly, respectively). Trough concentrations are 76% lower for fluoxetine and 47% lower for norfluoxetine than the concentrations maintained by 20 mg once-daily dosing. Steady-state fluoxetine concentrations are ~50% lower following the once-weekly regimen compared to 20 mg once daily. Average steady-state concentrations of once-daily dosing were highest in children ages 6 to <13 (fluoxetine 171 ng/mL; norfluoxetine 195 ng/mL), followed by adolescents ages 13 to <18 (fluoxetine 86 ng/mL; norfluoxetine 113 ng/mL); concentrations were considered to be within the ranges reported in adults (fluoxetine 91-302 ng/mL; norfluoxetine 72-258 ng/mL).

Dosage

Geriatric Oral: Some patients may require an initial dose of 10 mg/day with dosage increases of 10 mg and 20 mg every several weeks as tolerated; should not be taken at night unless patient experiences sedation.

Adult

Depression, obsessive-compulsive disorder, bulimia: Oral: 20 mg/day in the morning; may increase after several weeks by 20 mg/day increments; maximum: 80 mg/day; doses >20 mg may be given once daily or divided twice daily. **Note:** Lower doses of 5-10 mg/day have been used for initial treatment.

Usual dosage range:

Bulimia nervosa: Oral:60 mg/day

Depression: Oral: Initial: 20 mg/day; may increase after several weeks if inadequate response (maximum: 80 mg/day). Patients maintained on Prozac® 20 mg/day may be changed to Prozac® Weekly™ 90 mg/week, starting dose 7 days after the last 20 mg/day dose

Depression associated with bipolar disorder (in combination with olanzapine): Oral: Initial: 20 mg in the evening; adjust as tolerated to usual range of 20-50 mg/day. See **"Note."**

Fibromyalgia (unlabeled use): Oral: Range: 20-80 mg/day (Arnold, 2002)

Obsessive-compulsive disorder: Oral: Initial: 20 mg/day; may increase after several weeks if inadequate response; recommended range: 20-60 mg/day (maximum: 80 mg/day)

Panic disorder: Oral: Initial: 10 mg/day; after 1 week, increase to 20 mg/day; may increase after several weeks; doses >60 mg/day have not been evaluated

Post-traumatic stress disorder (PTSD) (unlabeled use): Oral: 20-40 mg/day

Raynaud's phenomena (unlabeled use): Oral: 20 mg/day (Coleiro, 2001)

Social anxiety disorder (unlabeled use): Oral: Target dose: 40 mg/day; range 30-60 mg/day (Davidson, 2004)

Treatment-resistant depression (in combination with olanzapine): Oral: Initial: 20 mg in the evening; adjust as tolerated to usual range of 20-50 mg/day. See **"Note."**

Note: When using individual components of fluoxetine with olanzapine rather than fixed dose combination product (Symbyax®), approximate dosage correspondence is as follows:

Olanzapine 2.5 mg + fluoxetine 20 mg = Symbyax® 3/25
Olanzapine 5 mg + fluoxetine 20 mg = Symbyax® 6/25
Olanzapine 12.5 mg + fluoxetine 20 mg = Symbyax® 12/25
Olanzapine 5 mg + fluoxetine 50 mg = Symbyax® 6/50
Olanzapine 12.5 mg + fluoxetine 50 mg = Symbyax® 12/50

Note: Upon discontinuation of fluoxetine therapy, gradually taper dose. If intolerable symptoms occur following a dose reduction, consider resuming the previously prescribed dose and/or decrease dose at a more gradual rate.

Renal Impairment

Single dose studies: Pharmacokinetics of fluoxetine and norfluoxetine were similar among subjects with all levels of impaired renal function, including anephric patients on chronic hemodialysis.

Chronic administration: Additional accumulation of fluoxetine or norfluoxetine may occur in patients with severely impaired renal function.

Not removed by hemodialysis; use of lower dose or less frequent dosing is not usually necessary.

Hepatic Impairment Elimination half-life of fluoxetine is prolonged in patients with hepatic impairment. A lower dose or less frequent dosing of fluoxetine should be used in these patients.

Cirrhosis patient: Administer a lower dose or less frequent dosing interval.

Compensated cirrhosis without ascites: Administer 50% of normal dose.

Administration Administer without regard to meals.

Bipolar I disorder and treatment-resistant depression: Take once daily in the evening.

Major depressive disorder and obsessive compulsive disorder: Once daily doses should be taken in the morning, or twice daily (morning and noon).

Bulimia: Take once daily in the morning.

Monitoring Parameters Mental status for depression, suicidal ideation (especially at the beginning of therapy or when doses are increased or decreased), anxiety, social functioning, mania, panic attacks; akathisia, sleep status; blood glucose (for diabetic patients), baseline liver function

Reference Range Therapeutic levels have not been well established

Therapeutic: Fluoxetine: 100-800 ng/mL (SI: 289-2314 nmol/L); Norfluoxetine: 100-600 ng/mL (SI: 289-1735 nmol/L)

Toxic: Fluoxetine plus norfluoxetine: >2000 ng/mL

Pharmacotherapy Pearls ECG may reveal S-T segment depression. Not shown to be teratogenic in rodents; 15-60 mg/day, buspirone and cyproheptadine, may be useful in treatment of sexual dysfunction during treatment with a selective serotonin reuptake inhibitor.

Weekly capsules are a delayed release formulation containing enteric-coated pellets of fluoxetine hydrochloride, equivalent to 90 mg fluoxetine. Therapeutic equivalence of weekly formulation with daily formulation for delaying time to relapse has not been established.

Special Geriatric Considerations Fluoxetine's potential stimulating and anorexic effects may be bothersome to some patients and has not been shown to be superior in efficacy to other SSRIs. The long half-life in the elderly makes it less attractive compared to other SSRIs. The elderly are more prone to SSRI/SNRI-induced hyponatremia.

Daily fluoxetine is considered to be potentially inappropriate in this patient population (Beers Criteria severity: High).

Dosage Forms Excipient information presented when available (limited, particularly for generics); consult specific product labeling. [DSC] = Discontinued product

Capsule, oral: 10 mg, 20 mg, 40 mg
PROzac®: 10 mg, 20 mg, 40 mg
Selfemra®: 10 mg [DSC], 20 mg [DSC] [contains soya lecithin]

Capsule, delayed release, enteric coated pellets, oral: 90 mg
PROzac® Weekly™: 90 mg
Solution, oral: 20 mg/5 mL (5 mL, 120 mL)
Tablet, oral: 10 mg, 20 mg
Sarafem®: 10 mg, 15 mg, 20 mg
Extemporaneously Prepared A 20 mg capsule may be mixed with 4 oz of water, apple juice, or Gatorade® to provide a solution that is stable for 14 days under refrigeration

Selected References

Feighner JP and Cohn JB, "Double-Blind Comparative Trials of Fluoxetine and Doxepin in Geriatric Patients With Major Depressive Disorder," *J Clin Psychiatry*, 1985, 46(3 Pt 2):20-5.

Harvey AT and Preskorn SH, "Fluoxetine Pharmacokinetics and Effect on CYP2C19 in Young and Elderly Volunteers," *J Clin Psychopharmacol*, 2001, 21(2):161-6.

Roose SP, Glassman AH, Attia E, et al, "Comparative Efficacy of Selective Serotonin Reuptake Inhibitors and Tricyclics in the Treatment of Melancholia," *Am J Psychiatry*, 1994, 151(12):1735-9.

Schone W and Ludwig M, "A Double-Blind Study of Paroxetine Compared With Fluoxetine in Geriatric Patients With Major Depression," *J Clin Psychopharmacol*, 1993, 13(6 Suppl 2):34S-9S.

♦ **Fluoxetine Hydrochloride** *see* FLUoxetine *on page 753*

FluPHENAZine (floo FEN a zeen)

Related Information
Antipsychotic Agents *on page 1997*
Liquid Compatibility of Antidepressants, Antipsychotics, and Mood Stabilizers *on page 2111*

Medication Safety Issues
Sound-alike/look-alike issues:
FluPHENAZine may be confused with fluvoxaMINE
International issues:
Prolixin [Turkey] may be confused with Prolixan brand name for azapropazone [Greece]

Brand Names: Canada Apo-Fluphenazine Decanoate®; Apo-Fluphenazine®; Modecate®; Modecate® Concentrate; PMS-Fluphenazine Decanoate

Index Terms Fluphenazine Decanoate; Fluphenazine Hydrochloride

Generic Availability (U.S.) Yes

Pharmacologic Category Antipsychotic Agent, Typical, Phenothiazine

Use Management of manifestations of psychotic disorders and schizophrenia; depot formulation may offer improved outcome in individuals with psychosis who are nonadherent with oral antipsychotics

Unlabeled/Investigational Use Psychosis/agitation related to Alzheimer's dementia

Contraindications Hypersensitivity to fluphenazine or any component of the formulation (cross-reactivity between phenothiazines may occur); severe CNS depression; coma; subcortical brain damage; in patients receiving large doses of hypnotics; blood dyscrasias; hepatic disease

Warnings/Precautions [U.S. Boxed Warning]: Elderly patients with dementia-related psychosis treated with antipsychotics are at an increased risk of death compared to placebo. Most deaths appeared to be either cardiovascular (eg, heart failure, sudden death) or infectious (eg, pneumonia) in nature. Fluphenazine is not approved for the treatment of dementia-related psychosis. May be sedating; use with caution in disorders where CNS depression is a feature. Use with caution in Parkinson's disease. Caution in patients with hemodynamic instability; predisposition to seizures; or severe cardiac disease. Use caution in renal impairment; discontinue therapy if BUN abnormal. Use caution in hepatic impairment; use contraindicated in patients with liver damage. Esophageal dysmotility and aspiration have been associated with antipsychotic use; use with caution in patients at risk of pneumonia (ie, Alzheimer's disease). May alter temperature regulation or mask toxicity of other drugs due to antiemetic effects. May alter cardiac conduction; life-threatening arrhythmias have occurred with therapeutic doses of phenothiazines. Hypotension may occur, particularly with I.M. administration. May cause orthostatic hypotension; use with caution in patients at risk of this effect or those who would not tolerate transient hypotensive episodes (cerebrovascular disease, cardiovascular disease, or other medications which may predispose). Adverse effects of depot injections may be prolonged. Use associated with increased prolactin levels; clinical significance of hyperprolactinemia in patients with breast cancer or other prolactin-dependent tumors is unknown. May cause pigmentary retinopathy, and lenticular and corneal deposits, particularly with prolonged therapy.

Leukopenia, neutropenia, and agranulocytosis (sometimes fatal) have been reported in clinical trials and postmarketing reports with antipsychotic use; presence of risk factors (eg, pre-existing low WBC or history of drug-induced leuko-/neutropenia) should prompt periodic blood count assessment. Discontinue therapy at first signs of blood dyscrasias or if absolute neutrophil count <1000/mm^3.

Due to anticholinergic effects, use caution in patients with decreased gastrointestinal motility, urinary retention, BPH, xerostomia, visual problems, narrow-angle glaucoma, and myasthenia gravis. Relative to other antipsychotics, fluphenazine has a low potency of cholinergic blockade.

May cause extrapyramidal symptoms, including pseudoparkinsonism, acute dystonic reactions, akathisia, and tardive dyskinesia (risk of these reactions is high relative to other antipsychotics). Risk of dystonia (and possibly other EPS) may be greater with increased doses, use of conventional antipsychotics, males, and younger patients. May also be associated with neuroleptic malignant syndrome (NMS). Use caution in the elderly.

Adverse Reactions (Reflective of adult population; not specific for elderly) Frequency not defined.

Cardiovascular: Hyper-/hypotension, tachycardia, fluctuations in blood pressure, arrhythmia, edema

Central nervous system: Parkinsonian symptoms, akathisia, dystonias, tardive dyskinesia, dizziness, hyper-reflexia, headache, cerebral edema, drowsiness, lethargy, restlessness, excitement, bizarre dreams, EEG changes, depression, seizure, NMS, altered central temperature regulation

Dermatologic: Dermatitis, eczema, erythema, itching, photosensitivity, rash, seborrhea, skin pigmentation, urticaria

Endocrine & metabolic: Menstrual cycle changes, breast pain, amenorrhea, galactorrhea, gynecomastia, libido changes, prolactin increased, SIADH

Gastrointestinal: Weight gain, appetite loss, salivation, xerostomia, constipation, paralytic ileus, laryngeal edema

Genitourinary: Ejaculatory disturbances, impotence, polyuria, bladder paralysis, enuresis

Hematologic: Agranulocytosis, leukopenia, thrombocytopenia, nonthrombocytopenic purpura, eosinophilia, pancytopenia

Hepatic: Cholestatic jaundice, hepatotoxicity

Neuromuscular & skeletal: Trembling of fingers, SLE, facial hemispasm

Ocular: Pigmentary retinopathy, cornea and lens changes, blurred vision, glaucoma

Respiratory: Nasal congestion, asthma

Drug Interactions

Metabolism/Transport Effects Substrate of CYP2D6 (major); **Inhibits** CYP1A2 (weak), 2C9 (weak), 2D6 (weak), 2E1 (weak)

Avoid Concomitant Use

Avoid concomitant use of FluPHENAZine with any of the following: Metoclopramide

Increased Effect/Toxicity

FluPHENAZine may increase the levels/effects of: Alcohol (Ethyl); Analgesics (Opioid); Anticholinergics; Anti-Parkinson's Agents (Dopamine Agonist); Beta-Blockers; CNS Depressants; Methotrimeprazine; Methylphenidate; Porfimer; Selective Serotonin Reuptake Inhibitors

The levels/effects of FluPHENAZine may be increased by: Abiraterone Acetate; Acetylcholinesterase Inhibitors (Central); Antimalarial Agents; Beta-Blockers; CYP2D6 Inhibitors (Moderate); CYP2D6 Inhibitors (Strong); Darunavir; Droperidol; Lithium formulations; Methotrimeprazine; Methylphenidate; Metoclopramide; Pramlintide; Tetrabenazine

Decreased Effect

FluPHENAZine may decrease the levels/effects of: Amphetamines; Quinagolide

The levels/effects of FluPHENAZine may be decreased by: Antacids; Anti-Parkinson's Agents (Dopamine Agonist); Lithium formulations; Peginterferon Alfa-2b

Ethanol/Nutrition/Herb Interactions

Ethanol: May increase CNS depression; monitor for increased effects with coadministration. Caution patients about effects.

Herb/Nutraceutical: Avoid dong quai, St John's wort (may also cause photosensitization). Avoid kava kava, gotu kola, valerian, St John's wort (may increase CNS depression).

Stability Store at room temperature; avoid freezing and excessive heat. Protect all dosage forms from light. Clear or slightly yellow solutions may be used. Should be dispensed in amber or opaque vials/bottles. Solutions may be diluted or mixed with fruit juices or other liquids, but must be administered immediately after mixing. Do not prepare bulk dilutions or store bulk dilutions.

Mechanism of Action Fluphenazine is a piperazine phenothiazine antipsychotic which blocks postsynaptic mesolimbic dopaminergic D_1 and D_2 receptors in the brain; depresses the release of hypothalamic and hypophyseal hormones; believed to depress the reticular activating system, thus affecting basal metabolism, body temperature, wakefulness, vasomotor tone, and emesis

◀ **Pharmacodynamics/Kinetics**

Absorption: Oral: May be affected by the inherent anticholinergic action on the gastrointestinal tissue causing variable absorption. Absorption from tablets is erratic with less variation seen with solutions. These agents are widely distributed in tissues with CNS concentrations exceeding that of plasma due to their lipophilic characteristics.

Protein binding: Antipsychotic agents are bound 90% to 99% to plasma or proteins; highly bound to brain and lung tissue and other tissues with a high blood perfusion

Metabolism: Hepatic

Half-life (derivative dependent):

Enanthate: 84-96 hours

Hydrochloride: 33 hours

Decanoate: 163-232 hours

Time to peak serum concentrations: 2-4 hours

Elimination: Excretion occurs through hepatic metabolism (oxidation) where numerous active metabolites are produced; active metabolites excreted in urine; elimination half-lives of antipsychotics ranges from 20-40 hours which may be extended in older adults due to decline in oxidative hepatic reactions (phase I) with age.

The biologic effect of a single dose persists for 24 hours. When the patient has accommodated to initial side effects (sedation), once daily dosing is possible due to the long half-life of antipsychotics.

Steady-state plasma concentrations are achieved in 4-7 days; therefore, if possible, do not make dose adjustments more than once in a 7-day period.

Due to the long half-lives of antipsychotics, as needed (prn) use is ineffective since repeated doses are necessary to achieve therapeutic tissue concentrations in the CNS.

Dosage

Geriatric Oral: Initial: 1-2.5 mg daily; titrated gradually based on patient response.

Adult

Psychosis:

Oral: Initial: 2.5-10 mg/day in divided doses at 6- to 8-hour intervals; Maintenance: 1-5 mg/day; **Note:** Some patients may require up to 40 mg/day for symptom control (long-term safety of higher doses not established)

PORT guidelines: Acute therapy: 6-20 mg/day for up to 6 weeks; Maintenance: 6-12 mg/day (Buchanan, 2009)

I.M. (hydrochloride): Initial: 1.25 mg as a single dose; depending on severity and duration, may need 2.5-10 mg/day in divided doses at 6- to 8-hour intervals (4 mg I.M. fluphenazine HCl is approximately equivalent to 10 mg oral fluphenazine HCl); use caution with doses >10 mg/day; once symptoms stabilized, transition to oral maintenance therapy

Long-acting maintenance injections (decanoate):

I.M., SubQ (decanoate): Initial: 12.5-25 mg every 2-4 weeks; response may last up to 6 weeks in some patients; titrate dose cautiously, if doses >50 mg are needed, increase in 12.5 mg increments (maximum dose: 100 mg)

Conversion from hydrochloride dosage forms to decanoate I.M.: 12.5 mg of decanoate every 2-4 weeks is approximately equivalent to 10 mg of oral hydrochloride/day; **Note:** Clinically, an every-2-week interval is frequently utilized

PORT guidelines: 6.25-25 mg every 2 weeks (Buchanan, 2009)

Renal Impairment Use with caution; not dialyzable (0% to 5%).

Hepatic Impairment Use with caution.

Administration

I.M., SubQ: The hydrochloride or decanoate formulation may be administered intramuscularly. Watch for hypotension when administering I.M. Only the decanoate formulation may be administered subcutaneously. When administering fluphenazine decanoate, use a dry syringe and needle of ≥21 gauge to administer the fluphenazine decanoate; a wet needle/syringe may cause the solution to become cloudy.

Oral: Avoid contact of oral solution or injection with skin (contact dermatitis). Oral liquid should be diluted into at least 60 mL (2 fl oz) of the following **only**: Water, saline, homogenized milk, carbonated orange beverages, pineapple, apricot, prune, orange, tomato, and grapefruit juices. Do **not** dilute in beverages containing caffeine, tannics (eg, tea), or pectinate (eg, apple juice).

Monitoring Parameters Monitor orthostatic blood pressures 3-5 days after initiation of therapy or a dose increase; tremors, gait changes, abnormal movement in trunk, neck, buccal area, or extremities; monitor target behaviors for which the agent is given

Reference Range Therapeutic: 0.3-3 ng/mL (SI: 0.6-6.0 nmol/L); correlation of serum concentrations and efficacy is controversial; most often dosed to best response

Pharmacotherapy Pearls Oral liquid to be diluted in the following **only**: water, saline, 7-UP, homogenized milk, carbonated orange beverages, pineapple, apricot, prune, orange, V-8 juice, tomato, and grapefruit juices; do not mix with beverages containing caffeine, tannins, or pectin (ie, coffee, tea, apple juice)

Special Geriatric Considerations Any changes in disease status in any organ system can result in behavior changes.

Many elderly patients receive antipsychotic medications for inappropriate nonpsychotic behavior. Before initiating antipsychotic medication, the clinician should investigate any possible reversible cause; any stress or stress from any disease can cause acute "confusion" or worsening of baseline nonpsychotic behavior. Most commonly, acute changes in behavior are due to increases in drug dose or addition of a new drug to regimen, fluid electrolyte loss, infections, and changes in environment.

In the treatment of agitated, demented, and elderly patients, authors of meta-analysis of controlled trials of the response to the traditional antipsychotics (phenothiazines, butyrophenones) in controlling agitation have concluded that the use of neuroleptics results in a response rate of 18%. Clearly, neuroleptic therapy for behavior control should be limited with frequent attempts to withdraw the agent given for behavior control.

Dosage Forms Excipient information presented when available (limited, particularly for generics); consult specific product labeling.
Elixir, oral, as hydrochloride: 2.5 mg/5 mL (60 mL, 473 mL)
Injection, oil, as decanoate: 25 mg/mL (5 mL)
Injection, solution, as hydrochloride: 2.5 mg/mL (10 mL)
Solution, oral, as hydrochloride [concentrate]: 5 mg/mL (118 mL)
Tablet, oral, as hydrochloride: 1 mg, 2.5 mg, 5 mg, 10 mg

Selected References

Rabins PV, Blacker D, Rovner BW, et al, "Practice Guidelines for the Treatment of Patients With Alzheimer's Disease and Other Dementias," *Am J Psychiatry*, 2007, 164(12 Suppl):5-56. Available at http://www.psych.org/psych_pract/treatg/pg/prac_guide.cfm.

Schneider LS, Tariot PN, Dagerman KS, et al, "Effectiveness of Atypical Antipsychotic Drugs in Patients With Alzheimer's Disease," *N Engl J Med*, 2006, 355(15):1525-38.

♦ **Fluphenazine Decanoate** *see* FluPHENAZine *on page 758*
♦ **Fluphenazine Hydrochloride** *see* FluPHENAZine *on page 758*
♦ **Flura-Drops®** *see* Fluoride *on page 751*

Flurazepam (flure AZ e pam)

Related Information
Anxiolytic, Sedative / Hypnotic, and Miscellaneous Benzodiazepines *on page 2000*
Beers Criteria – Potentially Inappropriate Medications for Geriatrics *on page 2089*

Medication Safety Issues
Sound-alike/look-alike issues:
Flurazepam may be confused with temazepam
Dalmane® may be confused with Demulen®, Dialume®

BEERS Criteria medication:
This drug may be inappropriate for use in geriatric patients (high severity risk).

Brand Names: Canada Apo-Flurazepam®; Dalmane®; Som Pam
Index Terms Flurazepam Hydrochloride
Generic Availability (U.S.) Yes
Pharmacologic Category Hypnotic, Benzodiazepine
Use Short-term treatment of insomnia
Medication Guide Available Yes
Contraindications Hypersensitivity to flurazepam or any component of the formulation (cross-sensitivity with other benzodiazepines may exist); narrow-angle glaucoma
Warnings/Precautions Use with caution in elderly or debilitated patients, patients with hepatic disease (including alcoholics), or renal impairment. Use with caution in patients with respiratory disease or impaired gag reflex. Avoid use in patients with sleep apnea.

Causes CNS depression (dose related); patients must be cautioned about performing tasks which require mental alertness (eg, operating machinery or driving). Use with caution in patients receiving other CNS depressants or psychoactive agents. Benzodiazepines have been associated with falls and traumatic injury and should be used with extreme caution in patients who are at risk of these events. Benzodiazepines with long half-lives may produce prolonged sedation and increase the risk of falls and fracture. Short- or medium-acting benzodiazepines are preferred in elderly patients (Beers Criteria).

Use caution in patients with depression, particularly if suicidal risk may be present. Use with caution in patients with a history of drug dependence. Benzodiazepines have been associated with dependence and acute withdrawal symptoms on discontinuation or reduction in dose (may occur after as little as 10 days of use).

As a hypnotic, should be used only after evaluation of potential causes of sleep disturbance. Failure of sleep disturbance to resolve after 7-10 days may indicate psychiatric or medical illness. A worsening of insomnia or the emergence of new abnormalities of thought or behavior may represent unrecognized psychiatric or medical illness and requires immediate and careful evaluation. Postmarketing studies have indicated that the use of hypnotic/sedative agents for sleep has been associated with hypersensitivity reactions including anaphylaxis as well as angioedema. An increased risk for hazardous sleep-related activities such as sleep-driving; cooking and eating food, and making phone calls while asleep have also been noted.

Benzodiazepines have been associated with anterograde amnesia. Paradoxical reactions have been reported, particularly in psychiatric patients. Does not have analgesic, antidepressant, or antipsychotic properties.

Adverse Reactions (Reflective of adult population; not specific for elderly) Frequency not defined.

Cardiovascular: Chest pain, flushing, hypotension, palpitation

Central nervous system: Apprehension, ataxia, confusion, depression, dizziness, drowsiness, euphoria, faintness, falling, hallucinations, hangover effect, headache, irritability, lightheadedness, memory impairment, nervousness, paradoxical reactions, restlessness, slurred speech, staggering, talkativeness

Dermatologic: Pruritus, rash

Gastrointestinal: Appetite increased/decreased, bitter taste, constipation, diarrhea, GI pain, heartburn, nausea, salivation increased/excessive, upset stomach, vomiting, weight gain/loss, xerostomia

Hematologic: Granulocytopenia, leukopenia

Hepatic: Alkaline phosphatase increased, ALT increased, AST increased, cholestatic jaundice, total bilirubin increased

Neuromuscular & skeletal: Body/joint pain, dysarthria, reflex slowing, weakness

Ocular: Blurred vision, burning eyes, difficulty focusing

Respiratory: Apnea, dyspnea

Miscellaneous: Diaphoresis, drug dependence

Postmarketing and/or case reports: Anaphylaxis, angioedema, complex sleep-related behavior (sleep-driving, cooking or eating food, making phone calls)

Drug Interactions

Metabolism/Transport Effects Substrate of CYP3A4 (major); **Inhibits** CYP2E1 (weak)

Avoid Concomitant Use

Avoid concomitant use of Flurazepam with any of the following: Conivaptan; OLANZapine

Increased Effect/Toxicity

Flurazepam may increase the levels/effects of: Alcohol (Ethyl); CloZAPine; CNS Depressants; Fosphenytoin; Methotrimeprazine; Phenytoin; Selective Serotonin Reuptake Inhibitors

The levels/effects of Flurazepam may be increased by: Antifungal Agents (Azole Derivatives, Systemic); Aprepitant; Calcium Channel Blockers (Nondihydropyridine); Cimetidine; Conivaptan; Contraceptives (Estrogens); Contraceptives (Progestins); CYP3A4 Inhibitors (Moderate); CYP3A4 Inhibitors (Strong); Dasatinib; Droperidol; Fluconazole; Fosamprenavir; Fosaprepitant; Grapefruit Juice; HydrOXYzine; Isoniazid; Macrolide Antibiotics; Methotrimeprazine; Nefazodone; OLANZapine; Proton Pump Inhibitors; Ritonavir; Saquinavir; Selective Serotonin Reuptake Inhibitors

Decreased Effect

The levels/effects of Flurazepam may be decreased by: CarBAMazepine; CYP3A4 Inducers (Strong); Deferasirox; Rifamycin Derivatives; St Johns Wort; Theophylline Derivatives; Tocilizumab; Yohimbine

Ethanol/Nutrition/Herb Interactions

Ethanol: May increase CNS depression; monitor for increased effects with coadministration. Caution patients about effects.

Food: Serum levels and response to flurazepam may be increased by grapefruit juice, but unlikely because of flurazepam's high oral bioavailability.

Herb/Nutraceutical: Avoid valerian, St John's wort, kava kava, gotu kola (may increase CNS depression).

Stability Store at 15°C to 30°C (59°F to 86°F).

Mechanism of Action Binds to stereospecific benzodiazepine receptors on the postsynaptic GABA neuron at several sites within the central nervous system, including the limbic system, reticular formation. Enhancement of the inhibitory effect of GABA on neuronal excitability results by increased neuronal membrane permeability to chloride ions. This shift in chloride ions results in hyperpolarization (a less excitable state) and stabilization.

Pharmacodynamics/Kinetics
Onset of action: Hypnotic: 15-20 minutes
  Peak effect: 3-6 hours
Duration: 7-8 hours
Distribution: V_d: 3.4 L/kg
Protein binding: ~97%
Metabolism: Hepatic to N-desalkylflurazepam (active) and N-hydroxyethylflurazepam
Half-life elimination:
  Flurazepam: 2.3 hours
  N-desalkylflurazepam:
    Adults: Single dose: 74-90 hours; Multiple doses: 111-113 hours
    Elderly (61-85 years): Single dose: 120-160 hours; Multiple doses: 126-158 hours
Time to peak, serum:
  N-desalkylflurazepam: 10.6 hours (range: 7.6-13.6 hours)
  N-hydroxyethylflurazepam: ~1 hour
Excretion: Urine: N-hydroxyethylflurazepam (22% to 55%); N-desalkylflurazepam (<1%)

Dosage
  Geriatric Oral: 15 mg at bedtime. Avoid use if possible.
  Adult Insomnia (short-term treatment): Oral: 15-30 mg at bedtime

Monitoring Parameters Respiratory, cardiovascular, and mental status

Reference Range Therapeutic: 0-4 ng/mL (SI: 0-9 nmol/L); Metabolite N-desalkylflurazepam: 20-110 ng/mL (SI: 43-240 nmol/L); Toxic: >0.12 mcg/mL

Special Geriatric Considerations Due to its long-acting metabolite, flurazepam is not considered a drug of choice in the elderly. Long-acting benzodiazepines have been associated with falls in the elderly. Interpretive guidelines from the Centers for Medicare and Medicaid Services (CMS) discourage the use of this agent in residents of long-term care facilities.

This medication is considered to be potentially inappropriate in this patient population (Beers Criteria severity: High).

Controlled Substance C-IV

Dosage Forms Excipient information presented when available (limited, particularly for generics); consult specific product labeling.
Capsule, oral, as hydrochloride: 15 mg, 30 mg

Selected References
  Reidenberg MM, Levy M, Warner H, et al, "Relationship Between Diazepam Dose, Plasma Level, Age, and Central Nervous System Depression," *Clin Pharmacol Ther*, 1978, 23(4):371-4.

◆ **Flurazepam Hydrochloride** *see* Flurazepam *on page 761*

Flurbiprofen (Systemic) (flure BI proe fen)

Medication Safety Issues
  Sound-alike/look-alike issues:
    Flurbiprofen may be confused with fenoprofen
    Ansaid® may be confused with Asacol®, Axid®

Brand Names: Canada Alti-Flurbiprofen; Ansaid®; Apo-Flurbiprofen®; Froben-SR®; Froben®; Novo-Flurprofen; Nu-Flurprofen

Index Terms Flurbiprofen Sodium

Generic Availability (U.S.) Yes

Pharmacologic Category Nonsteroidal Anti-inflammatory Drug (NSAID), Oral

Use Treatment of rheumatoid arthritis and osteoarthritis

Unlabeled/Investigational Use Management of postoperative pain

Medication Guide Available Yes

Contraindications Hypersensitivity to flurbiprofen, aspirin, other NSAIDs, or any component of the formulation; perioperative pain in the setting of coronary artery bypass (CABG) surgery

Warnings/Precautions [U.S. Boxed Warning]: NSAIDs are associated with an increased risk of adverse cardiovascular thrombotic events, including MI and stroke. Risk may be increased with duration of use or pre-existing cardiovascular risk factors or disease. Carefully evaluate individual cardiovascular risk profiles prior to prescribing. May cause new-onset hypertension or worsening of existing hypertension. Use caution with fluid retention. Avoid use in heart failure. Concurrent administration of ibuprofen, and potentially other nonselective NSAIDs, may interfere with aspirin's cardioprotective effect. **[U.S. Boxed Warning]: Use is contraindicated for treatment of perioperative pain in the setting of coronary artery bypass graft (CABG) surgery.** Risk of MI and stroke may be increased with use following CABG surgery.

Platelet adhesion and aggregation may be decreased; may prolong bleeding time; patients with coagulation disorders or who are receiving anticoagulants should be monitored closely. Anemia may occur; patients on long-term NSAID therapy should be monitored for anemia. NSAID use may compromise existing renal function; dose-dependent decreases in prosta-glandin synthesis may result from NSAID use, reducing renal blood flow which may cause renal decompensation. Patients with impaired renal function, dehydration, heart failure, liver dysfunction, those taking diuretics, and ACE inhibitors, and the elderly are at greater risk of renal toxicity. Rehydrate patient before starting therapy; monitor renal function closely. Not recommended for use in patients with advanced renal disease. Long-term NSAID use may result in renal papillary necrosis.

[U.S. Boxed Warning]: NSAIDs may increase risk of gastrointestinal irritation, inflam-mation, ulceration, bleeding, and perforation. These events may occur at any time during therapy and without warning. Use caution with a history of GI disease (bleeding or ulcers), concurrent therapy with aspirin, anticoagulants and/or corticosteroids, smoking, use of alcohol, the elderly, or debilitated patients. When used concomitantly with ≤325 mg of aspirin, a substantial increase in the risk of gastrointestinal complications (eg, ulcer) occurs; con-comitant gastroprotective therapy (eg, proton pump inhibitors) is recommended (Bhatt, 2008).

Use the lowest effective dose for the shortest duration of time, consistent with individual patient goals, to reduce risk of cardiovascular or GI adverse events. Alternate therapies should be considered for patients at high risk.

NSAIDs may cause serious skin adverse events including exfoliative dermatitis, Stevens-Johnson syndrome (SJS), and toxic epidermal necrolysis (TEN); discontinue use at first sign of skin rash or hypersensitivity. Anaphylactoid reactions may occur, even without prior exposure; patients with "aspirin triad" (bronchial asthma, aspirin intolerance, rhinitis) may be at increased risk. Do not use in patients who experience bronchospasm, asthma, rhinitis, or urticaria with NSAID or aspirin therapy. Use caution in other forms of asthma.

Use with caution in patients with decreased hepatic function. Closely monitor patients with any abnormal LFT. Severe hepatic reactions (eg, fulminant hepatitis, liver failure) have occurred with NSAID use, rarely; discontinue if signs or symptoms of liver disease develop, or if systemic manifestations occur.

The elderly are at increased risk for adverse effects (especially peptic ulceration, CNS effects, renal toxicity) from NSAIDs even at low doses.

Withhold for at least 4-6 half-lives prior to surgical or dental procedures.

Adverse Reactions (Reflective of adult population; not specific for elderly)
>1%:
Cardiovascular: Edema
Central nervous system: Amnesia, anxiety, depression, dizziness, headache, insomnia, malaise, nervousness, somnolence, vertigo
Dermatologic: Rash
Gastrointestinal: Abdominal pain, constipation, diarrhea, dyspepsia, flatulence, GI bleeding, nausea, vomiting, weight changes
Hepatic: Liver enzymes increased
Neuromuscular & skeletal: Reflexes increased, tremor, weakness
Ocular: Vision changes
Otic: Tinnitus
Respiratory: Rhinitis

Drug Interactions
Metabolism/Transport Effects Substrate of CYP2C9 (minor); **Inhibits** CYP2C9 (strong)
Avoid Concomitant Use
Avoid concomitant use of Flurbiprofen (Systemic) with any of the following: Floctafenine; Ketorolac; Ketorolac (Nasal); Ketorolac (Systemic)

Increased Effect/Toxicity
Flurbiprofen (Systemic) may increase the levels/effects of: Aminoglycosides; Anticoagu-lants; Antiplatelet Agents; Bisphosphonate Derivatives; Collagenase (Systemic); Cyclo-SPORINE; CycloSPORINE (Systemic); Deferasirox; Desmopressin; Digoxin; Drotrecogin Alfa; Eplerenone; Haloperidol; Ibritumomab; Lithium; Methotrexate; Nonsteroidal Anti-Inflam-matory Agents; PEMEtrexed; Porfimer; Potassium-Sparing Diuretics; PRALAtrexate; Qui-nolone Antibiotics; Rivaroxaban; Salicylates; Thrombolytic Agents; Tositumomab and Iodine I 131 Tositumomab; Vancomycin; Vitamin K Antagonists

The levels/effects of Flurbiprofen (Systemic) may be increased by: ACE Inhibitors; Angio-tensin II Receptor Blockers; Antidepressants (Tricyclic, Tertiary Amine); Corticosteroids (Systemic); Dasatinib; Floctafenine; Glucosamine; Herbs (Anticoagulant/Antiplatelet Proper-ties); Ketorolac; Ketorolac (Nasal); Ketorolac (Systemic); Nonsteroidal Anti-Inflammatory Agents; Omega-3-Acid Ethyl Esters; Pentosan Polysulfate Sodium; Pentoxifylline;

Probenecid; Prostacyclin Analogues; Selective Serotonin Reuptake Inhibitors; Serotonin/ Norepinephrine Reuptake Inhibitors; Sodium Phosphates; Treprostinil; Vitamin E

Decreased Effect

Flurbiprofen (Systemic) may decrease the levels/effects of: ACE Inhibitors; Angiotensin II Receptor Blockers; Antiplatelet Agents; Beta-Blockers; Eplerenone; HydrALAZINE; Potassium-Sparing Diuretics; Salicylates; Selective Serotonin Reuptake Inhibitors; Thiazide Diuretics

The levels/effects of Flurbiprofen (Systemic) may be decreased by: Bile Acid Sequestrants; Nonsteroidal Anti-Inflammatory Agents; Salicylates

Ethanol/Nutrition/Herb Interactions

Ethanol: Avoid ethanol (may enhance gastric mucosal irritation).

Food: Food may decrease the rate but not the extent of absorption.

Herb/Nutraceutical: Avoid alfalfa, anise, bilberry, bladderwrack, bromelain, cat's claw, celery, chamomile, coleus, cordyceps, dong quai, evening primrose, fenugreek, feverfew, garlic, ginger, ginkgo biloba, ginseng (American, Panax, Siberian), grapeseed, green tea, guggul, horse chestnut seed, horseradish, licorice, prickly ash, red clover, reishi, SAMe (S-adenosylmethionine), sweet clover, turmeric, white willow (all have additional antiplatelet activity).

Mechanism of Action Reversibly inhibits cyclooxygenase-1 and 2 (COX-1 and 2) enzymes, which results in decreased formation of prostaglandin precursors; has antipyretic, analgesic, and anti-inflammatory properties

Other proposed mechanisms not fully elucidated (and possibly contributing to the anti-inflammatory effect to varying degrees), include inhibiting chemotaxis, altering lymphocyte activity, inhibiting neutrophil aggregation/activation, and decreasing proinflammatory cytokine levels.

Pharmacodynamics/Kinetics

Onset of action: ~1-2 hours

Distribution: V_d: 0.12 L/kg

Protein binding: 99%, primarily albumin

Metabolism: Hepatic via CYP2C9; forms metabolites such as 4-hydroxy-flurbiprofen (inactive)

Half-life elimination: 5.7 hours

Time to peak: 1.5 hours

Excretion: Urine (primarily as metabolites)

Dosage

Geriatric & Adult

Rheumatoid arthritis and osteoarthritis: Oral: 200-300 mg/day in 2, 3, or 4 divided doses; do not administer more than 100 mg for any single dose; maximum: 300 mg/day

Management of postoperative dental pain (unlabeled use): Oral: 100 mg every 12 hours

Renal Impairment Not recommended in patients with advanced renal disease.

Administration Administer with a full glass of water.

Monitoring Parameters Monitor response (pain, range of motion, grip strength, mobility, ADL function), inflammation; observe for weight gain, edema; monitor renal function; observe for bleeding, bruising; evaluate gastrointestinal effects (abdominal pain, bleeding, dyspepsia); mental confusion, disorientation, CBC, serum creatinine, BUN, liver function tests

Pharmacotherapy Pearls There are no clinical guidelines to predict which NSAID will give response in a particular patient. Trials with each must be initiated until response is determined. Consider dose, patient convenience, and cost.

Special Geriatric Considerations Elderly are a high-risk population for adverse effects from NSAIDs. As much as 60% of the elderly can develop peptic ulceration and/or hemorrhage asymptomatically. The concomitant use of H_2 blockers, omeprazole, and sucralfate is not effective as prophylaxis with the exception of NSAID-induced duodenal ulcers which may be prevented by the use of ranitidine. Misoprostol and proton pump inhibitors are the only agents proven to help prevent the development of NSAID-induced ulcers. Also, concomitant disease and drug use contribute to the risk for GI adverse effects. Use lowest effective dose for shortest period possible. Consider renal function decline with age. Use of NSAIDs can compromise existing renal function, especially when Cl_{cr} is ≤30 mL/minute. Tinnitus may be a difficult and unreliable indication of toxicity due to age-related hearing loss or eighth cranial nerve damage. CNS adverse effects, such as confusion, agitation, and hallucinations, are generally seen in overdose or high-dose situations, but elderly may demonstrate these adverse effects at lower doses than younger adults.

Dosage Forms Excipient information presented when available (limited, particularly for generics); consult specific product labeling.

Tablet, oral: 50 mg, 100 mg

Flurbiprofen (Ophthalmic) (flure BI proe fen)

Medication Safety Issues
 Sound-alike/look-alike issues:
  Flurbiprofen may be confused with fenoprofen
  Ocufen® may be confused with Ocuflox®, Ocupress®
Brand Names: U.S. Ocufen®
Brand Names: Canada Ocufen®
Index Terms Flurbiprofen Sodium
Generic Availability (U.S.) Yes
Pharmacologic Category Nonsteroidal Anti-inflammatory Drug (NSAID), Ophthalmic
Use Inhibition of intraoperative miosis
Dosage
 Geriatric & Adult Ophthalmic anti-inflammatory/surgical aid: Ophthalmic: Instill 1 drop every 30 minutes, beginning 2 hours prior to surgery (total of 4 drops in each affected eye)
Dosage Forms Excipient information presented when available (limited, particularly for generics); consult specific product labeling.
 Solution, ophthalmic, as sodium [drops]: 0.03% (2.5 mL)
  Ocufen®: 0.03% (2.5 mL)

◆ **Flurbiprofen Sodium** see Flurbiprofen (Ophthalmic) on page 766
◆ **Flurbiprofen Sodium** see Flurbiprofen (Systemic) on page 763
◆ **5-Flurocytosine** see Flucytosine on page 744

Flutamide (FLOO ta mide)

Medication Safety Issues
 Sound-alike/look-alike issues:
  Flutamide may be confused with Flumadine®, thalidomide
  Eulexin may be confused with Edecrin®, Eurax®
Brand Names: Canada Apo-Flutamide®; Euflex®; Eulexin®; Novo-Flutamide; PMS-Flutamide; Teva-Flutamide
Index Terms 4'-Nitro-3'-Trifluoromethylisobutyrantide; Eulexin; Niftolid; NSC-147834; SCH 13521
Generic Availability (U.S.) Yes
Pharmacologic Category Antineoplastic Agent, Antiandrogen
Use Treatment of metastatic prostatic carcinoma in combination therapy with LHRH agonist analogues
Unlabeled/Investigational Use Treatment of female hirsutism
Contraindications Hypersensitivity to flutamide or any component of the formulation; severe hepatic impairment
Warnings/Precautions Hazardous agent - use appropriate precautions for handling and disposal. **[U.S. Boxed Warning]: Hospitalization and, rarely, death due to liver failure have been reported in patients taking flutamide.** Elevated serum transaminase levels, jaundice, hepatic encephalopathy, and acute hepatic failure have been reported. Androgen-deprivation therapy may increase the risk for cardiovascular disease (Levine, 2010). Product labeling states flutamide is not for use in women, particularly for non-life-threatening conditions. In some patients, the toxicity reverses after discontinuation of therapy. About 50% of the cases occur within the first 3 months of treatment. Serum transaminase levels should be measured prior to starting treatment, monthly for 4 months, and periodically thereafter. Liver function tests should be obtained at the first suggestion of liver dysfunction (nausea, vomiting, abdominal pain, fatigue, anorexia, "flu-like" symptoms, hyperbilirubinuria, jaundice, or right upper quadrant tenderness). Flutamide should be immediately discontinued any time a patient has jaundice, and/or an ALT level greater than twice the upper limit of normal. Flutamide should not be used in patients whose ALT values are greater than twice the upper limit of normal.

Patients with glucose-6 phosphate dehydrogenase deficiency or hemoglobin M disease or smokers are at risk of toxicities associated with aniline exposure, including methemoglobinemia, hemolytic anemia, and cholestatic jaundice. Monitor methemoglobin levels.
Adverse Reactions (Reflective of adult population; not specific for elderly)
 >10%:
  Endocrine & metabolic: Gynecomastia, hot flashes, breast tenderness, galactorrhea (9% to 42%), impotence, libido decreased, tumor flare
  Gastrointestinal: Nausea, vomiting (11% to 12%)
  Hepatic: AST increased (transient; mild), LDH increased (transient; mild)

1% to 10%:
Cardiovascular: Hypertension (1%), edema
Central nervous system: Drowsiness, confusion, depression, anxiety, nervousness, headache, dizziness, insomnia
Dermatologic: Ecchymosis, photosensitivity, pruritus
Gastrointestinal: Anorexia, appetite increased, constipation, indigestion, upset stomach (4% to 6%); diarrhea
Hematologic: Anemia (6%), leukopenia (3%), thrombocytopenia (1%)
Neuromuscular & skeletal: Weakness (1%)
Miscellaneous: Herpes zoster

Drug Interactions
Metabolism/Transport Effects Substrate (major) of CYP1A2, 3A4; **Inhibits** CYP1A2 (weak)
Avoid Concomitant Use
Avoid concomitant use of Flutamide with any of the following: Conivaptan
Increased Effect/Toxicity
The levels/effects of Flutamide may be increased by: Abiraterone Acetate; Conivaptan; CYP1A2 Inhibitors (Moderate); CYP1A2 Inhibitors (Strong); CYP3A4 Inhibitors (Moderate); CYP3A4 Inhibitors (Strong); Dasatinib; Deferasirox
Decreased Effect
The levels/effects of Flutamide may be decreased by: CYP1A2 Inducers (Strong); CYP3A4 Inducers (Strong); Cyproterone; Deferasirox; Herbs (CYP3A4 Inducers); Tocilizumab

Ethanol/Nutrition/Herb Interactions
Food: No effect on bioavailability of flutamide.
Herb/Nutraceutical: St John's wort may decrease flutamide levels.

Stability Store at room temperature.
Mechanism of Action Nonsteroidal antiandrogen that inhibits androgen uptake or inhibits binding of androgen in target tissues

Pharmacodynamics/Kinetics
Absorption: Oral: Rapid and complete
Protein binding: Parent drug: 94% to 96%; 2-hydroxyflutamide: 92% to 94%
Metabolism: Extensively hepatic to more than 10 metabolites, primarily 2-hydroxyflutamide (active)
Half-life elimination: 5-6 hours (2-hydroxyflutamide)
Excretion: Primarily urine (as metabolites)

Dosage
Geriatric & Adult Refer to individual protocols.
Prostate carcinoma: Oral: 250 mg 3 times/day; alternatively, once-daily doses of 0.5-1.5 g have been used (unlabeled dosing)
Female hirsutism (unlabeled use): Oral: 250 mg daily

Administration Usually administered orally in 3 divided doses; contents of capsule may be opened and mixed with applesauce, pudding, or other soft foods; mixing with a beverage is not recommended

Monitoring Parameters Serum transaminase levels should be measured prior to starting treatment and should be repeated monthly for the first 4 months of therapy, and periodically thereafter. LFTs should be checked at the first sign or symptom of liver dysfunction (eg, nausea, vomiting, abdominal pain, fatigue, anorexia, flu-like symptoms, hyperbilirubinuria, jaundice, or right upper quadrant tenderness). Other parameters include tumor reduction, testosterone/estrogen, and phosphatase serum levels.

Special Geriatric Considerations No specific dose alterations are necessary in the elderly.
Dosage Forms Excipient information presented when available (limited, particularly for generics); consult specific product labeling.
Capsule, oral: 125 mg

Fluticasone (Oral Inhalation) (floo TIK a sone)

Related Information
Asthma *on page 2016*
Inhalant Agents *on page 2010*
Medication Safety Issues
Sound-alike/look-alike issues:
Flovent® may be confused with Flonase®
International issues:
Allegro: Brand name for fluticasone [Israel], but also the brand name for frovatriptan [Germany]

FLUTICASONE (ORAL INHALATION)

◄

Allegro [Israel] may be confused with Allegra and Allegra-D brand names for fexofenadine and fexofenadine/pseudoephedrine, respectively, [U.S., Canada, and multiple international markets]

Flovent® [U.S., Canada] may be confused with Flogen brand name for naproxen [Mexico]

Brand Names: U.S. Flovent® Diskus®; Flovent® HFA

Brand Names: Canada Flovent® Diskus®; Flovent® HFA

Index Terms Flovent; Fluticasone Propionate

Generic Availability (U.S.) No

Pharmacologic Category Corticosteroid, Inhalant (Oral)

Use Maintenance treatment of asthma as prophylactic therapy; also indicated for patients requiring oral corticosteroid therapy for asthma to assist in total discontinuation or reduction of total oral dose

Contraindications Hypersensitivity to fluticasone or any component of the formulation; primary treatment of status asthmaticus or acute bronchospasm

Warnings/Precautions May cause hypercorticism or suppression of hypothalamic-pituitary-adrenal (HPA) axis, particularly in patients receiving high doses for prolonged periods. HPA axis suppression may lead to adrenal crisis. Withdrawal and discontinuation of a corticosteroid should be done slowly and carefully. Particular care is required when patients are transferred from systemic corticosteroids to inhaled products due to possible adrenal insufficiency or withdrawal from steroids, including an increase in allergic symptoms. Patients receiving ≥20 mg per day of prednisone (or equivalent) may be most susceptible. Concurrent use of ritonavir (and potentially other strong inhibitors of CYP3A4) may increase fluticasone levels and effects on HPA suppression. Fatalities have occurred due to adrenal insufficiency in asthmatic patients during and after transfer from systemic corticosteroids to aerosol steroids; aerosol steroids do **not** provide the systemic steroid needed to treat patients having trauma, surgery, or infections.

Bronchospasm may occur with wheezing after inhalation; if this occurs, stop steroid and treat with a fast-acting bronchodilator. Supplemental steroids (oral or parenteral) may be needed during stress or severe asthma attacks. Corticosteroid use may cause psychiatric disturbances, including depression, euphoria, insomnia, mood swings, and personality changes. Pre-existing psychiatric conditions may be exacerbated by corticosteroid use. Prolonged use of corticosteroids may also increase the incidence of secondary infection, mask acute infection (including fungal infections), prolong or exacerbate viral infections, or limit response to vaccines. Exposure to chickenpox should be avoided; corticosteroids should not be used to treat ocular herpes simplex. Corticosteroids should not be used for cerebral malaria. Close observation is required in patients with latent tuberculosis and/or TB reactivity; restrict use in active TB (only in conjunction with antituberculosis treatment). Rare cases of vasculitis (Churg-Strauss syndrome) or other eosinophilic conditions can occur. Prolonged treatment with corticosteroids have been associated with the development of Kaposi's sarcoma (case reports); if noted, discontinuation of therapy should be considered.

Use with caution in patients with thyroid disease, hepatic impairment, renal impairment, cardiovascular disease, diabetes, glaucoma, cataracts, myasthenia gravis, patients at risk for osteoporosis, patients at risk for seizures, or GI diseases (diverticulitis, peptic ulcer, ulcerative colitis) due to perforation risk. Use caution following acute MI (corticosteroids have been associated with myocardial rupture). Because of the risk of adverse effects, systemic corticosteroids should be used cautiously in the elderly in the smallest possible effective dose for the shortest duration.

Not to be used in status asthmaticus or for the relief of acute bronchospasm. Flovent® Diskus® contains lactose; very rare anaphylactic reactions have been reported in patients with severe milk protein allergy. There have been reports of systemic corticosteroid withdrawal symptoms (eg, joint/muscle pain, lassitude, depression) when withdrawing oral inhalation therapy. Local yeast infections (eg, oral pharyngeal candidiasis) may occur. Lower respiratory tract infections, including pneumonia, have been reported in patients with COPD with an even higher incidence in the elderly.

Adverse Reactions (Reflective of adult population; not specific for elderly)

>10%:

Central nervous system: Headache (2% to 14%)

Respiratory: Upper respiratory tract infection (14% to 21%), throat irritation (3% to 22%)

3% to 10%:

Central nervous system: Fever (1% to 7%)

Gastrointestinal: Oral candidiasis (≤9%), nausea/vomiting (1% to 8%), gastrointestinal infection (including viral; 1% to 5%), gastrointestinal discomfort/pain (1% to 4%)

Neuromuscular & skeletal: Musculoskeletal pain (2% to 5%), muscle injury (1% to 5%)

Respiratory: Sinusitis/sinus infection (4% to 10%), lower respiratory tract infections/pneumonia (1% to 7%; COPD diagnosis and age >65 years increase risk), cough (1% to 6%), bronchitis (≤8%), hoarseness/dysphonia (2% to 6%), upper respiratory tract inflammation (≤5%), viral respiratory infection (1% to 5%), rhinitis (1% to 4%)

Miscellaneous: Viral infection (≤5%)

1% to 3%:

Cardiovascular: Chest symptoms, edema, palpitation

Central nervous system: Cranial nerve paralysis, dizziness, fatigue, malaise, migraine, mood disorders, pain, sleep disorder

Dermatologic: Acne, dermatitis/dermatosis, eczema, folliculitis, photodermatitis, infection (fungal, viral), pruritus, rash, urticaria

Endocrine & metabolic: Fluid disturbance, goiter, uric acid metabolism disturbance

Gastrointestinal: Abdominal discomfort/pain, appetite changes, dental discomfort/pain, diarrhea, dyspepsia, gastroenteritis, hyposalivation, oral discomfort/pain, oral erythema/rash, oral ulcerations, oropharyngeal plaques, tooth decay, weight gain

Genitourinary: Reproductive organ infections (bacterial), urinary tract infection

Hematologic: Hematoma

Hepatic: Cholecystitis

Neuromuscular & skeletal: Arthralgia, articular rheumatism, muscle cramps/spasms, muscle pain, muscle stiffness/tightness/rigidity, musculoskeletal inflammation

Ocular: Blepharoconjunctivitis, conjunctivitis, keratitis

Otic: Otitis

Respiratory: Epistaxis, hoarseness/dysphonia, laryngitis, nasal sinus disorder, pharyngitis/throat infection, rhinorrhea/postnasal drip, throat constriction

Miscellaneous: Infection (bacterial, fungal); injuries (including muscle, soft tissue); polyps (ear, nose, throat); tonsillitis

Drug Interactions

Metabolism/Transport Effects Substrate of CYP3A4 (major)

Avoid Concomitant Use

Avoid concomitant use of Fluticasone (Oral Inhalation) with any of the following: Aldesleukin; BCG; CYP3A4 Inhibitors (Strong); Natalizumab; Pimecrolimus; Tacrolimus (Topical)

Increased Effect/Toxicity

Fluticasone (Oral Inhalation) may increase the levels/effects of: Amphotericin B; Deferasirox; Leflunomide; Loop Diuretics; Natalizumab; Thiazide Diuretics

The levels/effects of Fluticasone (Oral Inhalation) may be increased by: CYP3A4 Inhibitors (Moderate); CYP3A4 Inhibitors (Strong); Dasatinib; Denosumab; Pimecrolimus; Tacrolimus (Topical); Telaprevir; Trastuzumab

Decreased Effect

Fluticasone (Oral Inhalation) may decrease the levels/effects of: Aldesleukin; Antidiabetic Agents; BCG; Corticorelin; Sipuleucel-T; Telaprevir; Vaccines (Inactivated)

The levels/effects of Fluticasone (Oral Inhalation) may be decreased by: Echinacea; Tocilizumab

Ethanol/Nutrition/Herb Interactions Herb/Nutraceutical: In theory, St John's wort may decrease serum levels of fluticasone by inducing CYP3A4 isoenzymes.

Stability

Flovent® HFA: Store at 15°C to 30°C (59°F to 86°F). Discard device when the dose counter reads "000". Store with mouthpiece down.

Flovent® Diskus®: Store at 20°C to 25°C (68°F to 77°F) in a dry place away from direct heat or sunlight. Discard after 6 weeks from removal from protective foil pouch or when the dose counter reads "0" (whichever comes first); device is not reusable.

Mechanism of Action Fluticasone belongs to a group of corticosteroids which utilizes a fluorocarbothioate ester linkage at the 17 carbon position; extremely potent vasoconstrictive and anti-inflammatory activity. The effectiveness of inhaled fluticasone is due to its direct local effect.

Pharmacodynamics/Kinetics

Onset of action: Maximal benefit may take 1-2 weeks or longer

Absorption: Absorbed systemically (Flovent® Diskus®: ~18%) primarily via lungs, minimal GI absorption (<1%) due to presystemic metabolism

Distribution: 4.2 L/kg

Protein binding: 91% to >99%

Metabolism: Hepatic via CYP3A4 to 17β-carboxylic acid (negligible activity)

Bioavailability: ~18% to 21%

Excretion: Feces (as parent drug and metabolites); urine (<5% as metabolites)

FLUTICASONE (ORAL INHALATION)

◄ **Dosage**
Geriatric & Adult Asthma: Inhalation, oral: **Note:** Titrate to the lowest effective dose once asthma stability is achieved

Flovent® HFA: Manufacturers labeling: Dosing based on previous therapy
Bronchodilator alone: Recommended starting dose: 88 mcg twice daily; highest recommended dose: 440 mcg twice daily
Inhaled corticosteroids: Recommended starting dose: 88-220 mcg twice daily; highest recommended dose: 440 mcg twice daily; a higher starting dose may be considered in patients previously requiring higher doses of inhaled corticosteroids
Oral corticosteroids:
Recommended starting dose: 440 mcg twice daily
Highest recommended dose: 880 mcg twice daily; starting dose is patient dependent. In patients on chronic oral corticosteroids therapy, reduce prednisone dose no faster than 2.5-5 mg/day on a weekly basis; begin taper after 1 week of fluticasone therapy.
NIH Asthma Guidelines (NIH, 2007) (administer in divided doses twice daily):
"Low" dose: 88-264 mcg/day
"Medium" dose: 264-440 mcg/day
"High" dose: >440 mcg/day
Flovent® Diskus® *(U.S. labeling)*: **Note:** May increase dose after 2 weeks of therapy in patients not adequately controlled. Higher starting doses may be considered in patients with poorer asthma control or those requiring high ranges of inhaled corticosteroids. Titrate to the lowest effective dose once asthma stability is achieved.
Bronchodilator alone: Recommended starting dose: 100 mcg twice daily; maximum recommended dose: 500 mcg twice daily
Inhaled corticosteroids: Recommended starting dose: 100-250 mcg twice daily; maximum recommended dose: 500 mcg twice daily
Oral corticosteroids: Recommended starting dose: 500-1000 mcg twice daily; maximum recommended dose: 1000 mcg twice daily. Starting dose is patient dependent. In patients on chronic oral corticosteroids therapy, reduce prednisone dose no faster than 2.5 mg/day on a weekly basis; begin taper after 1 week of fluticasone therapy.
Flovent® Diskus® *(Canadian labeling)*:
Mild asthma: 100-250 mcg twice daily
Moderate asthma: 250-500 mcg twice daily
Severe asthma: 500 mcg twice daily; may increase to 1000 mcg twice daily in very severe patients requiring high doses of corticosteroids
Hepatic Impairment Fluticasone is primarily cleared in the liver. Fluticasone plasma levels may be increased in patients with hepatic impairment, use with caution; monitor.
Administration
Aerosol inhalation: Flovent® HFA: Shake container thoroughly before using. Take 3-5 deep breaths. Use inhaler on inspiration. Allow 1 full minute between inhalations. Rinse mouth with water after use to reduce aftertaste and incidence of candidiasis; do not swallow. Inhaler must be primed before first use, when not used for 7 days, or if dropped. To prime the first time, release 4 sprays into air; shake well before each spray and spray away from face. If dropped or not used for 7 days, prime by releasing a single test spray. Patient should contact pharmacy for refill when the dose counter reads "020". Discard device when the dose counter reads "000". Do not use "float" test to determine contents.
Powder for oral inhalation: Flovent® Diskus®: Do not use with a spacer device. Do not exhale into Diskus®. Do not wash or take apart. Use in horizontal position. Mouth should be rinsed with water after use (do not swallow). Discard after 6 weeks once removed from protective pouch or when the dose counter reads "0", whichever comes first (device is not reusable).
Monitoring Parameters Signs/symptoms of HPA axis suppression/adrenal insufficiency; possible eosinophilic conditions (including Churg-Strauss syndrome); FEV_1, peak flow, and/or other pulmonary function tests; asthma symptoms
Pharmacotherapy Pearls In the United States, dosage for the metered dose inhaler (Flovent® HFA) is expressed as the amount of drug which leaves the actuator and is delivered to the patient. This differs from other countries, which express the dosage as the amount of drug which leaves the valve.
Special Geriatric Considerations No specific geriatric information is available. No differences in safety have been observed in the elderly when compared to younger patients. Based on current data, no dosage adjustment is needed based on age.
Dosage Forms Excipient information presented when available (limited, particularly for generics); consult specific product labeling.
Aerosol, for oral inhalation, as propionate:
Flovent® HFA: 44 mcg/inhalation (10.6 g); 110 mcg/inhalation (12 g); 220 mcg/inhalation (12 g) [chlorofluorocarbon free; 120 metered actuations]
Powder, for oral inhalation, as propionate:
Flovent® Diskus®: 50 mcg (60s); 100 mcg (60s); 250 mcg (60s) [contains lactose]

Dosage Forms: Canada Excipient information presented when available (limited, particularly for generics); consult specific product labeling.

Powder, for oral inhalation, as propionate:

Flovent® Diskus®: 50 mcg (28s, 60s) [contains lactose; prefilled blister pack]

Flovent® Diskus®: 100 mcg (28s, 60s) [contains lactose; prefilled blister pack]

Flovent® Diskus®: 250 mcg (28s, 60s) [contains lactose; prefilled blister pack]

Flovent® Diskus®: 500 mcg (28s, 60s) [contains lactose; prefilled blister pack]

Selected References

National Asthma Education and Prevention Program, "Expert Panel Report 3 (EPR-3): Guidelines for the Diagnosis and Management of Asthma-Summary Report 2007," *J Allergy Clin Immunol*, 2007, 120(5 Suppl):94-138.

Fluticasone (Nasal) (floo TIK a sone)

Medication Safety Issues

Sound-alike/look-alike issues:

Flonase® may be confused with Flovent®

International issues:

Allegro: Brand name for fluticasone [Israel], but also the brand name for frovatriptan [Germany]

Allegro [Israel] may be confused with Allegra and Allegra-D brand names for fexofenadine and fexofenadine/pseudoephedrine, respectively, [U.S., Canada, and multiple international markets]

Brand Names: U.S. Flonase®; Veramyst®

Brand Names: Canada Apo-Fluticasone®; Avamys®; Flonase®; ratio-Fluticasone

Index Terms Fluticasone Furoate; Fluticasone Propionate

Generic Availability (U.S.) Yes: Propionate spray

Pharmacologic Category Corticosteroid, Nasal

Use

Flonase®: Management of seasonal and perennial allergic rhinitis and nonallergic rhinitis

Veramyst®, Avamys® [CAN]: Management of seasonal and perennial allergic rhinitis

Dosage

Geriatric & Adult Rhinitis: Intranasal:

Flonase® (fluticasone propionate): Initial: 2 sprays (50 mcg/spray) per nostril once daily; may also be divided into 100 mcg twice a day. After the first few days, dosage may be reduced to 1 spray per nostril once daily for maintenance therapy.

Veramyst® (fluticasone furoate): Initial: 2 sprays (27.5 mcg/spray) per nostril once daily (110 mcg/day). Once symptoms are controlled, may reduce dosage to 1 spray per nostril once daily (55 mcg/day) for maintenance therapy.

Avamys® [CAN] (fluticasone furoate): 2 sprays (27.5 mcg/spray) in each nostril once daily (110 mcg/day). Total daily dosage should not exceed 2 sprays in each nostril (110 mcg)/day.

Special Geriatric Considerations No differences in safety have been observed in the elderly when compared to younger patients. Based on current data, no dosage adjustment is needed based on age.

Dosage Forms Excipient information presented when available (limited, particularly for generics); consult specific product labeling.

Suspension, intranasal, as furoate [spray]:

Veramyst®: 27.5 mcg/inhalation (10 g) [contains benzalkonium chloride; 120 metered actuations]

Suspension, intranasal, as propionate [spray]: 50 mcg/inhalation (16 g)

Flonase®: 50 mcg/inhalation (16 g) [contains benzalkonium chloride; 120 metered actuations]

Dosage Forms: Canada Excipient information presented when available (limited, particularly for generics); consult specific product labeling.

Suspension, intranasal, as furoate [spray]:

Avamys®: 27.5 mcg/inhalation (4.5 g) [30 metered actuations; contains benzalkonium chloride]; (10 g) [120 metered actuations; contains benzalkonium chloride]

Fluticasone (Topical) (floo TIK a sone)

Related Information
  Corticosteroids *on page 2005*
Medication Safety Issues
  Sound-alike/look-alike issues:
    Cutivate® may be confused with Ultravate®
  International issues:
    Allegro: Brand name for fluticasone [Israel], but also the brand name for frovatriptan [Germany]
    Allegro [Israel] may be confused with Allegra and Allegra-D brand names for fexofenadine and fexofenadine/pseudoephedrine, respectively, [U.S., Canada, and multiple international markets]
Brand Names: U.S. Cutivate®
Brand Names: Canada Cutivate™
Index Terms Fluticasone Propionate
Generic Availability (U.S.) Yes: Cream, ointment
Pharmacologic Category Corticosteroid, Topical
Use Relief of inflammation and pruritus associated with corticosteroid-responsive dermatoses; atopic dermatitis
Dosage
  Geriatric & Adult
    Corticosteroid-responsive dermatoses: Topical: Cream, lotion, ointment: Apply sparingly to affected area twice daily. If no improvement is seen within 2 weeks, reassessment of diagnosis may be necessary.
    Atopic dermatitis: Topical: Cream, lotion: Apply sparingly to affected area once or twice daily. If no improvement is seen within 2 weeks, reassessment of diagnosis may be necessary.
Dosage Forms Excipient information presented when available (limited, particularly for generics); consult specific product labeling.
  Cream, topical, as propionate: 0.05% (15 g, 30 g, 60 g)
    Cutivate®: 0.05% (30 g, 60 g)
  Lotion, topical, as propionate:
    Cutivate®: 0.05% (120 mL)
  Ointment, topical, as propionate: 0.005% (15 g, 30 g, 60 g)
    Cutivate®: 0.005% (30 g, 60 g)

Fluticasone and Salmeterol (floo TIK a sone & sal ME te role)

Related Information
  Fluticasone (Oral Inhalation) *on page 767*
  Salmeterol *on page 1653*
Medication Safety Issues
  Sound-alike/look-alike issues:
    Advair® may be confused with Adcirca®, Advicor®
Brand Names: U.S. Advair Diskus®; Advair® HFA
Brand Names: Canada Advair Diskus®; Advair®
Index Terms Fluticasone Propionate and Salmeterol Xinafoate; Salmeterol and Fluticasone
Generic Availability (U.S.) No
Pharmacologic Category Beta₂-Adrenergic Agonist; Beta₂-Adrenergic Agonist, Long-Acting; Corticosteroid, Inhalant (Oral)
Use Maintenance treatment of asthma; maintenance treatment of COPD
Medication Guide Available Yes
Contraindications Hypersensitivity to fluticasone, salmeterol, or any component of the formulation; status asthmaticus; acute episodes of asthma or COPD; severe hypersensitivity to milk proteins (Advair Diskus®)
Warnings/Precautions See individual agents.
Adverse Reactions (Reflective of adult population; not specific for elderly) Percentages reported in patients with asthma; also see individual agents:
  >10%:
    Central nervous system: Headache (12% to 21%)
    Respiratory: Upper respiratory tract infection (16% to 27%), pharyngitis (9% to 13%)
  >3% to 10%:
    Central nervous system: Dizziness (1% to 4%)
    Endocrine & metabolic: Menstruation symptoms (3% to 5%)

Gastrointestinal: Nausea/vomiting (3% to 6%), diarrhea (2% to 4%), pain/discomfort (1% to 4%), oral candidiasis (1% to 4%), gastrointestinal infections (including viral, ≤4%)

Neuromuscular & skeletal: Musculoskeletal pain (2% to 7%), muscle pain (≤4%)

Respiratory: Throat irritation (7% to 9%), bronchitis (2% to 8%), upper respiratory tract inflammation (4% to 7%), lower respiratory tract infections/pneumonia (1% to 7%; COPD diagnosis and age >65 years increase risk), cough (3% to 6%), sinusitis (4% to 5%), hoarseness/dysphonia (1% to 5%), viral respiratory tract infection (3% to 5%)

1% to 3%:

Cardiovascular: Arrhythmia, chest symptoms, fluid retention, MI, palpitation, syncope, tachycardia

Central nervous system: Compressed nerve syndromes, hypnagogic effects, migraine, pain, sleep disorders, tremor

Dermatologic: Dermatitis, dermatosis, eczema, hives, skin flakiness, urticaria, viral skin infection

Endocrine & metabolic: Hypothyroidism

Gastrointestinal: Constipation, dental discomfort/pain, gastrointestinal infection, hemorrhoids, oral discomfort/pain, oral erythema/rash, oral ulcerations, unusual taste, weight gain

Genitourinary: Urinary tract infection

Hematologic: Contusions/hematomas

Hepatic: Abnormal liver function tests

Neuromuscular & skeletal: Arthralgia, articular rheumatism, bone/cartilage disorders, bone pain, cramps, fractures, muscle injuries (≤3%), muscle spasm, muscle stiffness, tightness/rigidity

Ocular: Conjunctivitis, edema, eye redness, keratitis, xerophthalmia

Respiratory: Blood in nasal mucosa, congestion, ear/nose/throat infection, epistaxis, laryngitis, lower respiratory hemorrhage, nasal irritation, rhinitis, rhinorrhea/postnasal drip, sneezing

Miscellaneous: Allergies/allergic reactions, bacterial infection, burns, candidiasis (≤3%), diaphoresis, sweat/sebum disorders, viral infection, wounds and lacerations

Drug Interactions

Metabolism/Transport Effects Fluticasone: **Substrate** of CYP3A4 (major); Salmeterol: **Substrate** of CYP3A4 (major)

Avoid Concomitant Use

Avoid concomitant use of Fluticasone and Salmeterol with any of the following: Aldesleukin; BCG; CYP3A4 Inhibitors (Strong); Iobenguane I 123; Natalizumab; Pimecrolimus; Tacrolimus (Topical); Telaprevir

Increased Effect/Toxicity

Fluticasone and Salmeterol may increase the levels/effects of: Amphotericin B; Deferasirox; Leflunomide; Loop Diuretics; Natalizumab; Sympathomimetics; Thiazide Diuretics

The levels/effects of Fluticasone and Salmeterol may be increased by: Atomoxetine; Cannabinoids; CYP3A4 Inhibitors (Moderate); CYP3A4 Inhibitors (Strong); Dasatinib; Denosumab; MAO Inhibitors; Pimecrolimus; Roflumilast; Tacrolimus (Topical); Telaprevir; Trastuzumab; Tricyclic Antidepressants

Decreased Effect

Fluticasone and Salmeterol may decrease the levels/effects of: Aldesleukin; Antidiabetic Agents; BCG; Corticorelin; Iobenguane I 123; Sipuleucel-T; Telaprevir; Vaccines (Inactivated)

The levels/effects of Fluticasone and Salmeterol may be decreased by: Alpha-/Beta-Blockers; Beta-Blockers (Beta1 Selective); Beta-Blockers (Nonselective); Betahistine; Echinacea; Tocilizumab

Stability

Advair Diskus®: Store at controlled room temperature of 20°C to 25°C (68°F to 77°F). Store in a dry place out of direct heat or sunlight. Diskus® device should be discarded 1 month after removal from foil pouch, or when dosing indicator reads "0" (whichever comes first); device is not reusable.

Advair® HFA: Store at controlled room temperature of 25°C (77°F). Store with mouthpiece down. Discard after 120 inhalations. Discard device when the dose counter reads "000". Device is not reusable.

Mechanism of Action Combination of fluticasone (corticosteroid) and salmeterol (long-acting beta$_2$-agonist) designed to improve pulmonary function and control over what is produced by either agent when used alone. Because fluticasone and salmeterol act locally in the lung, plasma levels do not predict therapeutic effect.

Fluticasone: The mechanism of action for all topical corticosteroids is believed to be a combination of three important properties: Anti-inflammatory activity, immunosuppressive

◄ properties, and antiproliferative actions. Fluticasone has extremely potent vasoconstrictive and anti-inflammatory activity.

Salmeterol: Relaxes bronchial smooth muscle by selective action on beta$_2$-receptors with little effect on heart rate

Pharmacodynamics/Kinetics See individual agents.

Dosage

Geriatric & Adult Do not use to transfer patients from systemic corticosteroid therapy.

COPD: Oral Inhalation:

Advair Diskus®: Fluticasone 250 mcg/salmeterol 50 mcg twice daily, 12 hours apart. **Note:** This is the maximum dose.

Advair Diskus® [Canadian labeling; not in approved U.S. labeling]: Fluticasone 250 mcg/ salmeterol 50 mcg **or** fluticasone 500 mcg/salmeterol 50 mcg twice daily, 12 hours apart. Maximum dose: Fluticasone 500 mcg/salmeterol 50 mcg per inhalation (2 inhalations/day)

Asthma (maintenance): Oral inhalation:

Advair Diskus®: One inhalation twice daily, morning and evening, 12 hours apart

Maximum dose: Fluticasone 500 mcg/salmeterol 50 mcg per inhalation (2 inhalations/day)

Advair® HFA: Two inhalations twice daily, morning and evening, 12 hours apart

Maximum dose: Fluticasone 230 mcg/salmeterol 21 mcg per inhalation (4 inhalations/day)

Advair® 125 or Advair® 250 [Canadian labeling; not in approved U.S. labeling]: Two inhalations twice daily, morning and evening, 12 hours apart

Maximum dose: Fluticasone 250 mcg/salmeterol 25 mcg per inhalation (4 inhalations/day)

Note: Initial dose prescribed should be based upon previous dose of inhaled-steroid asthma therapy. Dose should be increased after 2 weeks if adequate response is not achieved. Patients should be titrated to lowest effective dose once stable. Each suggestion below specifies the product strength to use; remember to **use 1 inhalation for Diskus® and 2 inhalations for HFA.**

Patients not currently on inhaled corticosteroids:

Advair Diskus®: Fluticasone 100 mcg/salmeterol 50 mcg **or** fluticasone 250 mcg/ salmeterol 50 mcg

Advair® HFA: Fluticasone 45 mcg/salmeterol 21 mcg **or** fluticasone 115 mcg/salmeterol 21 mcg

Patients currently using inhaled beclomethasone dipropionate:

≤160 mcg/day: Fluticasone 100 mcg/salmeterol 50 mcg **or** Advair® HFA: Fluticasone 45 mcg/salmeterol 21 mcg

320 mcg/day: Fluticasone 250 mcg/salmeterol 50 mcg **or** Advair® HFA: Fluticasone 115 mcg/salmeterol 21 mcg

640 mcg/day: Fluticasone 500 mcg/salmeterol 50 mcg **or** Advair® HFA: Fluticasone 230 mcg/salmeterol 21 mcg

Patients currently using inhaled budesonide:

≤400 mcg/day: Fluticasone 100 mcg/salmeterol 50 mcg **or** Advair® HFA: Fluticasone 45 mcg/salmeterol 21 mcg

800-1200 mcg/day: Fluticasone 250 mcg/salmeterol 50 mcg **or** Advair® HFA: Fluticasone 115 mcg/salmeterol 21mcg

1600 mcg/day: Fluticasone 500 mcg/salmeterol 50 mcg **or** Advair® HFA: Fluticasone 230 mcg/salmeterol 21 mcg

Patients currently using inhaled flunisolide CFC aerosol:

≤1000 mcg/day: Fluticasone 100 mcg/salmeterol 50 mcg **or** Advair® HFA: Fluticasone 45 mcg/salmeterol 21 mcg

1250-2000 mcg/day: Fluticasone 250 mcg/salmeterol 50 mcg **or** Advair® HFA: Fluticasone 115 mcg/salmeterol 21 mcg

Patients currently using inhaled flunisolide HFA inhalation aerosol:

≤320 mcg/day: Fluticasone 100 mcg/salmeterol 50 mcg **or** Advair® HFA: Fluticasone 45 mcg/salmeterol 21 mcg

640 mcg/day: Fluticasone 250 mcg/salmeterol 50 mcg **or** Advair® HFA: Fluticasone 115 mcg/salmeterol 21 mcg

Patients currently using inhaled fluticasone HFA aerosol:

≤176 mcg/day: Fluticasone 100 mcg/salmeterol 50 mcg **or** Advair® HFA: Fluticasone 45 mcg/salmeterol 21 mcg

440 mcg/day: Fluticasone 250 mcg/salmeterol 50 mcg **or** Advair® HFA: Fluticasone 115 mcg/salmeterol 21 mcg

660-880 mcg/day: Fluticasone 500 mcg/salmeterol 50 mcg **or** Advair® HFA: Fluticasone 230 mcg/salmeterol 21 mcg

Patients currently using inhaled fluticasone propionate powder:

≤200 mcg/day: Fluticasone 100 mcg/salmeterol 50 mcg **or** Advair® HFA: Fluticasone 45 mcg/salmeterol 21 mcg

500 mcg/day: Fluticasone 250 mcg/salmeterol 50 mcg **or** Advair® HFA: Fluticasone 115 mcg/salmeterol 21 mcg

1000 mcg/day: Fluticasone 500 mcg/salmeterol 50 mcg **or** Advair® HFA: Fluticasone 230 mcg/salmeterol 21 mcg

Patients currently using inhaled mometasone furoate powder:

220 mcg/day: Fluticasone 100 mcg/salmeterol 50 mcg **or** Advair® HFA: Fluticasone 45 mcg/salmeterol 21 mcg

440 mcg/day: Fluticasone 250 mcg/salmeterol 50 mcg **or** Advair® HFA: Fluticasone 115 mcg/salmeterol 21 mcg

880 mcg/day: Fluticasone 500 mcg/salmeterol 50 mcg **or** Advair® HFA: Fluticasone 230 mcg/salmeterol 21 mcg

Patients currently using inhaled triamcinolone acetonide:

≤1000 mcg/day: Fluticasone 100 mcg/salmeterol 50 mcg **or** Advair® HFA: Fluticasone 45 mcg/salmeterol 21 mcg

1100-1600 mcg/day: Fluticasone 250 mcg/salmeterol 50 mcg **or** Advair® HFA: Fluticasone 115 mcg/salmeterol 21 mcg

Hepatic Impairment No dosage adjustment required; manufacturer suggests close monitoring of patients with hepatic impairment.

Administration

Advair Diskus®: After removing from box and foil pouch, write the "Pouch opened" and "Use by" dates on the label on top of the Diskus®. The "Use by" date is 1 month from date of opening the pouch. Every time the lever is pushed back, a dose is ready to be inhaled. Do not close or tilt the Diskus® after the lever is pushed back. Do not play with the lever or move the lever more than once. The dose indicator tells you how many doses are left. When the numbers 5 to 0 appear in red, only a few doses remain. Discard device 1 month after you remove it from the foil pouch or when the dose counter reads "0" (whichever comes first). Rinse mouth with water after use and spit to reduce risk of oral candidiasis.

Advair® HFA: Shake well for 5 seconds before each spray. Prime with 4 test sprays (into air and away from face) before using for the first time. If canister is dropped or not used for >4 weeks, prime with 2 sprays. Patient should contact pharmacy for refill when the dose counter reads "020". Discard device when the dose counter reads "000". Do not spray in eyes. Rinse mouth with water after use and spit to reduce risk of oral candidiasis.

Monitoring Parameters FEV$_1$, peak flow, and/or other pulmonary function tests; blood pressure, heart rate; CNS stimulation. Monitor for increased use of short-acting beta$_2$-agonist inhalers; may be marker of a deteriorating asthma condition.

Pharmacotherapy Pearls Effects of inhaled/intranasal steroids on growth have been observed in the absence of laboratory evidence of HPA axis suppression, suggesting that growth velocity is a more sensitive indicator of systemic corticosteroid exposure in pediatric patients than some commonly used tests of HPA axis function. The long-term effects of this reduction in growth velocity associated with orally-inhaled and intranasal corticosteroids, including the impact on final adult height, are unknown. The potential for "catch up" growth following discontinuation of treatment with inhaled corticosteroids has not been adequately studied.

Advair® HFA: Salmeterol (base) 21 mcg is equivalent to 30.45 mcg of salmeterol xinafoate.

Special Geriatric Considerations No differences in safety or effectiveness have been seen in studies of patients ≥65 years of age. However, increased sensitivity may be seen in the elderly. Use with caution in patients with concomitant cardiovascular disease.

Dosage Forms Excipient information presented when available (limited, particularly for generics); consult specific product labeling. [DSC] = Discontinued product

Aerosol, for oral inhalation:

Advair® HFA:

45/21: Fluticasone propionate 45 mcg and salmeterol 21 mcg per inhalation (8 g) [chlorofluorocarbon free; 60 metered actuations]

45/21: Fluticasone propionate 45 mcg and salmeterol 21 mcg per inhalation (12 g) [chlorofluorocarbon free; 120 metered actuations]

115/21: Fluticasone propionate 115 mcg and salmeterol 21 mcg per inhalation (8 g) [chlorofluorocarbon free; 60 metered actuations]

115/21: Fluticasone propionate 115 mcg and salmeterol 21 mcg per inhalation (12 g) [chlorofluorocarbon free; 120 metered actuations]

230/21: Fluticasone propionate 230 mcg and salmeterol 21 mcg per inhalation (8 g) [chlorofluorocarbon free; 60 metered actuations]

230/21: Fluticasone propionate 230 mcg and salmeterol 21 mcg per inhalation (12 g) [chlorofluorocarbon free; 120 metered actuations]

FLUTICASONE AND SALMETEROL

Powder, for oral inhalation:
Advair Diskus®:
100/50: Fluticasone propionate 100 mcg and salmeterol 50 mcg (14s, 28s [DSC], 60s) [contains lactose]
250/50: Fluticasone propionate 250 mcg and salmeterol 50 mcg (14s [DSC], 60s) [contains lactose]
500/50: Fluticasone propionate 500 mcg and salmeterol 50 mcg (14s [DSC], 60s) [contains lactose]

Dosage Forms: Canada Excipient information presented when available (limited, particularly for generics); consult specific product labeling.
Aerosol, for oral inhalation:
Advair®;
125/25: Fluticasone propionate 125 mcg and salmeterol 25 mcg per inhalation (12 g) [120 metered actuations]
250/25: Fluticasone propionate 250 mcg and salmeterol 25 mcg per inhalation (12 g) [120 metered actuations]

Selected References

National Asthma Education and Prevention Program, "Expert Panel Report 3 (EPR-3): Guidelines for the Diagnosis and Management of Asthma-Summary Report 2007," *J Allergy Clin Immunol*, 2007, 120(5 Suppl):94-138.
Nelson HS, Weiss ST, Bleecker ER, et al, "The Salmeterol Multicenter Asthma Research Trial: A Comparison of Usual Pharmacotherapy for Asthma or Usual Pharmacotherapy Plus Salmeterol," *Chest*, 2006, 129(1):15-26.

◆ **Fluticasone Furoate** see Fluticasone (Nasal) on page 771
◆ **Fluticasone Propionate** see Fluticasone (Nasal) on page 771
◆ **Fluticasone Propionate** see Fluticasone (Oral Inhalation) on page 767
◆ **Fluticasone Propionate** see Fluticasone (Topical) on page 772
◆ **Fluticasone Propionate and Salmeterol Xinafoate** see Fluticasone and Salmeterol on page 772

Fluvastatin (FLOO va sta tin)

Related Information
Hyperlipidemia Management on page 2021

Medication Safety Issues
Sound-alike/look-alike issues:
Fluvastatin may be confused with fluoxetine, nystatin, pitavastatin

Brand Names: U.S. Lescol®; Lescol® XL
Brand Names: Canada Lescol®; Lescol® XL
Generic Availability (U.S.) No
Pharmacologic Category Antilipemic Agent, HMG-CoA Reductase Inhibitor
Use To be used as a component of multiple risk factor intervention in patients at risk for atherosclerosis vascular disease due to hypercholesterolemia

Adjunct to dietary therapy to reduce elevated total cholesterol (total-C), LDL-C, triglyceride, and apolipoprotein B (apo-B) levels and to increase HDL-C in primary hypercholesterolemia and mixed dyslipidemia (Fredrickson types IIa and IIb); to slow the progression of coronary atherosclerosis in patients with coronary heart disease; reduce risk of coronary revascularization procedures in patients with coronary heart disease

Contraindications Hypersensitivity to fluvastatin or any component of the formulation; active liver disease; unexplained persistent elevations of serum transaminases

Warnings/Precautions Secondary causes of hyperlipidemia should be ruled out prior to therapy. Liver function must be monitored by periodic laboratory assessment. Rhabdomyolysis with acute renal failure has occurred with fluvastatin and other HMG-CoA reductase inhibitors. Risk may be increased with concurrent use of other drugs which may cause rhabdomyolysis (including colchicine, gemfibrozil, fibric acid derivatives, or niacin at doses ≥1 g/day). The manufacturer recommends temporary discontinuation for elective major surgery, acute medical or surgical conditions, or in any patient experiencing an acute or serious condition predisposing to renal failure (eg, sepsis, hypotension, trauma, uncontrolled seizures). However, based upon current evidence, HMG-CoA reductase inhibitor therapy should be continued in the perioperative period unless risk outweighs cardioprotective benefit. Use with caution in patients with advanced age; these patients are predisposed to myopathy. Use caution in patients with previous liver disease or heavy ethanol use. Use caution in patients with concurrent medications or conditions which reduce steroidogenesis.

Adverse Reactions (Reflective of adult population; not specific for elderly) As reported with fluvastatin capsules; in general, adverse reactions reported with fluvastatin extended release tablet were similar, but the incidence was less.

1% to 10%:
Central nervous system: Headache (9%), fatigue (3%), insomnia (3%)

Gastrointestinal: Dyspepsia (8%), diarrhea (5%), abdominal pain (5%), nausea (3%)
Genitourinary: Urinary tract infection (2%)
Neuromuscular & skeletal: Myalgia (5%)
Respiratory: Sinusitis (3%), bronchitis (2%)

Drug Interactions

Metabolism/Transport Effects Substrate of CYP2C9 (major), CYP2C8 (minor), CYP2D6 (minor), CYP3A4 (minor), SLCO1B1; **Inhibits** CYP1A2 (weak), 2C8 (weak), 2C9 (moderate), 2D6 (weak), 3A4 (weak)

Avoid Concomitant Use

Avoid concomitant use of Fluvastatin with any of the following: Red Yeast Rice

Increased Effect/Toxicity

Fluvastatin may increase the levels/effects of: Carvedilol; CYP2C9 Substrates (High risk); DAPTOmycin; Trabectedin; Vitamin K Antagonists

The levels/effects of Fluvastatin may be increased by: Amiodarone; Colchicine; Conivaptan; Cyproterone; Eltrombopag; Fenofibrate; Fenofibric Acid; Fluconazole; Gemfibrozil; Niacin; Niacinamide; Red Yeast Rice; Rifamycin Derivatives

Decreased Effect

Fluvastatin may decrease the levels/effects of: Lanthanum

The levels/effects of Fluvastatin may be decreased by: Antacids; Cholestyramine Resin; Etravirine; Fosphenytoin; Peginterferon Alfa-2b; Phenytoin; Rifamycin Derivatives; Tocilizumab

Ethanol/Nutrition/Herb Interactions

Ethanol: Avoid excessive ethanol consumption (due to potential hepatic effects).
Food: Reduces rate but not the extent of absorption. Red yeast rice contains an estimated 2.4 mg lovastatin per 600 mg rice.

Stability Store at 15°C to 30°C (59°F to 86°F). Protect from light.

Mechanism of Action Acts by competitively inhibiting 3-hydroxyl-3-methylglutaryl-coenzyme A (HMG-CoA) reductase, the enzyme that catalyzes the reduction of HMG-CoA to mevalonate; this is an early rate-limiting step in cholesterol biosynthesis. HDL is increased while total, LDL, and VLDL cholesterols; apolipoprotein B; and plasma triglycerides are decreased.

Pharmacodynamics/Kinetics

Onset of action: Peak effect: Maximal LDL-C reductions achieved within 4 weeks
Distribution: V_d: 0.35 L/kg
Protein binding: >98%
Metabolism: To inactive and active metabolites (oxidative metabolism via CYP2C9 [75%], 2C8 [~5%], and 3A4 [~20%] isoenzymes); active forms do not circulate systemically; extensive (saturable) first-pass hepatic extraction
Bioavailability: Absolute: Capsule: 24%; Extended release tablet: 29%
Half-life elimination: Capsule: <3 hours; Extended release tablet: 9 hours
Time to peak: Capsule: 1 hour; Extended release tablet: 3 hours
Excretion: Feces (90%): urine (5%)

Dosage

Geriatric & Adult

Dyslipidemia (also delay in progression of CAD): Oral:

Patients requiring ≥25% decrease in LDL-C: 40 mg capsule once daily in the evening, 80 mg extended release tablet once daily (anytime), or 40 mg capsule twice daily

Patients requiring <25% decrease in LDL-C: Initial: 20 mg capsule once daily in the evening; may increase based on tolerability and response to a maximum recommended dose of 80 mg/day, given in 2 divided doses (immediate release capsule) or as a single daily dose (extended release tablet)

Renal Impairment Less than 6% is excreted renally. No dosage adjustment needed with mild-to-moderate renal impairment; use with caution in severe impairment.

Hepatic Impairment Levels may accumulate in patients with liver disease (increased AUC and C_{max}). Use caution with severe hepatic impairment or heavy ethanol ingestion. Contraindicated in active liver disease or unexplained transaminase elevations. Decrease dose and monitor effects carefully in patients with hepatic insufficiency.

Administration Patient should be placed on a standard cholesterol-lowering diet before and during treatment; fluvastatin may be taken without regard to meals; adjust dosage as needed in response to periodic lipid determinations during the first 4 weeks after a dosage change; lipid-lowering effects are additive when fluvastatin is combined with a bile-acid binding resin or niacin, however, it must be administered at least 2 hours following these drugs. Do not break, chew, or crush extended release tablets; do not open capsules.

Monitoring Parameters Obtain baseline LFTs and total cholesterol profile; repeat tests at 12 weeks after initiation of therapy or elevation in dose, and periodically thereafter; baseline CPK (recheck CPK in any patient with symptoms suggestive of myopathy). Monitor LDL-C at intervals no less than 4 weeks.

◀ **Special Geriatric Considerations** The definition of and, therefore, when to treat hyperlipidemia in the elderly is a controversial issue. The National Cholesterol Education Program recommends that all adults maintain a plasma cholesterol <160 mg/dL. In elderly patients with one additional risk factor, goal LDL would decrease to <130 mg/dL. Pharmacologic treatment should be reserved for those who are unable to obtain a desirable plasma cholesterol concentration by diet alone and for whom the benefits of treatment are believed to outweigh the potential adverse effects, drug interactions, and cost of treatment. Age ≥65 years is a risk factor for myopathy.

Dosage Forms Excipient information presented when available (limited, particularly for generics); consult specific product labeling.

Capsule, oral:

Lescol®: 20 mg, 40 mg

Tablet, extended release, oral:

Lescol® XL: 80 mg

Selected References

Fleisher LA, Beckman JA, Brown KA, et al, "ACC/AHA 2007 Guidelines on Perioperative Cardiovascular Evaluation and Care for Noncardiac Surgery: A Report of the American College of Cardiology/American Heart Association Task Force on Practice Guidelines (Writing Committee to Revise the 2002 Guidelines on Perioperative Cardiovascular Evaluation for Noncardiac Surgery) Developed in Collaboration With the American Society of Echocardiography, American Society of Nuclear Cardiology, Heart Rhythm Society, Society of Cardiovascular Anesthesiologists, Society for Cardiovascular Angiography and Interventions, Society for Vascular Medicine and Biology, and Society for Vascular Surgery," *J Am Coll Cardiol*, 2007, 50(17):e159-241.

Grundy SM, Cleeman JI, Merz CN, et al, "Implications of Recent Clinical Trials for the National Cholesterol Education Program Adult Treatment Panel III Guidelines," *J Am Coll Cardiol*, 2004, 44(3):720-32.

National Cholesterol Education Program (NCEP) Expert Panel on Detection, Evaluation, and Treatment of High Blood Cholesterol in Adults (Adult Treatment Panel III), "Third Report of the National Cholesterol Education Program (NCEP) Expert Panel on Detection, Evaluation, and Treatment of High Blood Cholesterol in Adults (Adult Treatment Panel III) Final Report," *Circulation*, 2002, 106(25):3143-421.

◆ **Fluvirin®** see Influenza Virus Vaccine (Inactivated) *on page 936*

FluvoxaMINE (floo VOKS a meen)

Related Information

Antidepressant Agents *on page 1991*

Beers Criteria – Potentially Inappropriate Medications for Geriatrics *on page 2089*

Medication Safety Issues

Sound-alike/look-alike issues:

FluvoxaMINE may be confused with flavoxATE, FLUoxetine, fluPHENAZine

Luvox may be confused with Lasix®, Levoxyl®, Lovenox®

Brand Names: U.S. Luvox® CR

Brand Names: Canada Alti-Fluvoxamine; Apo-Fluvoxamine®; Luvox®; Novo-Fluvoxamine; Nu-Fluvoxamine; PMS-Fluvoxamine; Rhoxal-fluvoxamine; Riva-Fluvox; Sandoz-Fluvoxamine

Index Terms Luvox

Generic Availability (U.S.) Yes: Excludes extended release capsule

Pharmacologic Category Antidepressant, Selective Serotonin Reuptake Inhibitor

Use Treatment of obsessive-compulsive disorder (OCD)

Unlabeled/Investigational Use Treatment of major depression; panic disorder; treatment of mild dementia-associated agitation in nonpsychotic patients; post-traumatic stress disorder (PTSD); social anxiety disorder (SAD)

Medication Guide Available Yes

Contraindications Hypersensitivity to fluvoxamine or any component of the formulation; concurrent use with alosetron, pimozide, ramelteon, thioridazine, or tizanidine; use with or within 14 days of MAO inhibitors

Warnings/Precautions [U.S. Boxed Warning]: Antidepressants increase the risk of suicidal thinking and behavior in children, adolescents, and young adults (18-24 years of age) with major depressive disorder (MDD) and other psychiatric disorders; consider risk prior to prescribing. Short-term studies did not show an increased risk in patients >24 years of age and showed a decreased risk in patients ≥65 years. Closely monitor patients for clinical worsening, suicidality, or unusual changes in behavior, particularly during the initial 1-2 months of therapy or during periods of dosage adjustments (increases or decreases); the patient's family or caregiver should be instructed to closely observe the patient and communicate condition with healthcare provider. A medication guide concerning the use of antidepressants should be dispensed with each prescription. **Fluvoxamine is FDA approved for the treatment of OCD in children ≥8 years of age; extended release capsules are not FDA approved for use in children.**

The possibility of a suicide attempt is inherent in major depression and may persist until remission occurs. Use caution in high-risk patients. Worsening depression and severe abrupt suicidality that are not part of the presenting symptoms may require discontinuation or modification of drug therapy. The patient's family or caregiver should be alerted to monitor patients for the emergence of suicidality and associated behaviors (such as agitation, irritability, hostility, impulsivity, and hypomania) and call healthcare provider.

May worsen psychosis in some patients or precipitate a shift to mania or hypomania in patients with bipolar disorder. Patients presenting with depressive symptoms should be screened for bipolar disorder. Monotherapy in patients with bipolar disorder should be avoided. **Fluvoxamine is not FDA approved for the treatment of bipolar depression.**

Serotonin syndrome and neuroleptic malignant syndrome (NMS)-like reactions have occurred with serotonin/norepinephrine reuptake inhibitors (SNRIs) and selective serotonin reuptake inhibitors (SSRIs) when used alone, and particularly when used in combination with serotonergic agents (eg, triptans) or antidopaminergic agents (eg, antipsychotics). Concurrent use with MAO inhibitors is contraindicated. Fluvoxamine has a low potential to impair cognitive or motor performance; caution operating hazardous machinery or driving. Use caution in patients with a previous seizure disorder or condition predisposing to seizures such as brain damage, alcoholism, or concurrent therapy with other drugs which lower the seizure threshold. Fluvoxamine may significantly increase alosetron concentrations; concurrent use **contra-indicated.** Potential for QT_c prolongation and arrhythmia with thioridazine and pimozide; concurrent use of fluvoxamine with either of these agents is **contraindicated.** Concomitant use with tizanidine may cause a significant decrease in blood pressure and increase in drowsiness; concurrent use is **contraindicated.** Fluvoxamine levels may be lower in patients who smoke.

May increase the risks associated with electroconvulsive therapy. Use with caution in patients with hepatic dysfunction and in elderly patients. May cause hyponatremia/SIADH (elderly at increased risk); volume depletion (diuretics may increase risk). Use with caution in patients at risk of bleeding or receiving concurrent anticoagulant therapy, although not consistently noted, fluvoxamine may cause impairment in platelet function. May cause or exacerbate sexual dysfunction.

Adverse Reactions (Reflective of adult population; not specific for elderly) Frequency varies by dosage form and indication. Adverse reactions reported as a composite of all indications.

>10%:
  Central nervous system: Headache (22% to 35%), insomnia (21% to 35%), somnolence (22% to 27%), dizziness (11% to 15%), nervousness (10% to 12%)
  Gastrointestinal: Nausea (34% to 40%), diarrhea (11% to 18%), xerostomia (10% to 14%), anorexia (6% to 14%)
  Genitourinary: Ejaculation abnormal (8% to 11%)
  Neuromuscular & skeletal: Weakness (14% to 26%)
1% to 10%:
  Cardiovascular: Chest pain (3%), palpitation (3%), vasodilation (2% to 3%), hypertension (1% to 2%), edema (≤1%), hypotension (≤1%), syncope (≤1%), tachycardia (≤1%)
  Central nervous system: Pain (10%), anxiety (5% to 8%), abnormal dreams (3%), abnormal thinking (3%), agitation (2% to 3%), apathy (≥1% to 3%), chills (2%), CNS stimulation (2%), depression (2%), neurosis (2%), amnesia, malaise, manic reaction, psychotic reaction
  Dermatologic: Bruising (4%), acne (2%)
  Endocrine & metabolic: Libido decreased (2% to 10%; incidence higher in males), anorgasmia (2% to 5%), sexual function abnormal (2% to 4%), menorrhagia (3%)
  Gastrointestinal: Dyspepsia (8% to 10%), constipation (4% to 10%), vomiting (4% to 6%), abdominal pain (5%), flatulence (4%), taste perversion (2% to 3%), toothache and dental caries (2% to 3%), dysphagia (2%), gingivitis (2%), weight loss (≤1% to 2%), weight gain
  Genitourinary: Polyuria (2% to 3%), impotence (2%), urinary tract infection (2%), urinary retention (1%)
  Hepatic: Liver function tests abnormal (≥1% to 2%)
  Neuromuscular & skeletal: Tremor (5% to 8%), myalgia (5%), paresthesia (3%), hypertonia (2%), twitching (2%), hyper-/hypokinesia, myoclonus
  Ocular: Amblyopia (2% to 3%)
  Respiratory: Upper respiratory infection (9%), pharyngitis (6%), yawn (2% to 5%), laryngitis (3%), bronchitis (2%), dyspnea (2%), epistaxis (2%), cough increased, sinusitis
  Miscellaneous: Diaphoresis (6% to 7%), flu-like syndrome (3%), viral infection (2%)

Drug Interactions
  Metabolism/Transport Effects Substrate (major) of CYP1A2, 2D6; **Inhibits** CYP1A2 (strong), 2B6 (weak), 2C9 (weak), 2C19 (strong), 2D6 (weak), 3A4 (weak)
  Avoid Concomitant Use
    Avoid concomitant use of FluvoxaMINE with any of the following: Alosetron; Clopidogrel; lobenguane I 123; MAO Inhibitors; Methylene Blue; Pimozide; Ramelteon; Sibutramine; Thioridazine; TiZANidine; Tryptophan

◀ **Increased Effect/Toxicity**

FluvoxaMINE may increase the levels/effects of: Alosetron; Anticoagulants; Antidepressants (Serotonin Reuptake Inhibitor/Antagonist); Antiplatelet Agents; Asenapine; Aspirin; Bendamustine; Benzodiazepines (metabolized by oxidation); Bromazepam; BusPIRone; CarBAMazepine; CloZAPine; Collagenase (Systemic); CYP1A2 Substrates; CYP2C19 Substrates; Desmopressin; Drotrecogin Alfa; DULoxetine; Erlotinib; Fosphenytoin; Haloperidol; Ibritumomab; Lithium; Methadone; Methylene Blue; Mexiletine; NSAID (COX-2 Inhibitor); NSAID (Nonselective); OLANZapine; Phenytoin; Pimozide; Propafenone; Propranolol; QuiNIDine; Ramelteon; Rivaroxaban; Roflumilast; Ropivacaine; Salicylates; Serotonin Modulators; Theophylline Derivatives; Thioridazine; Thrombolytic Agents; TiZANidine; Tositumomab; Tositumomab and Iodine I 131 Tositumomab; TraMADol; Tricyclic Antidepressants; Vitamin K Antagonists

The levels/effects of FluvoxaMINE may be increased by: Abiraterone Acetate; Alcohol (Ethyl); Analgesics (Opioid); BusPIRone; Cimetidine; CNS Depressants; CYP1A2 Inhibitors (Moderate); CYP1A2 Inhibitors (Strong); CYP2D6 Inhibitors (Moderate); CYP2D6 Inhibitors (Strong); Darunavir; Dasatinib; Deferasirox; Glucosamine; Herbs (Anticoagulant/Antiplatelet Properties); MAO Inhibitors; Metoclopramide; Omega-3-Acid Ethyl Esters; Pentosan Polysulfate Sodium; Pentoxifylline; Prostacyclin Analogues; Sibutramine; TraMADol; Tryptophan; Vitamin E

Decreased Effect

FluvoxaMINE may decrease the levels/effects of: Clopidogrel; Iobenguane I 123

The levels/effects of FluvoxaMINE may be decreased by: CarBAMazepine; CYP1A2 Inducers (Strong); Cyproheptadine; Cyproterone; NSAID (Nonselective); Peginterferon Alfa-2b

Ethanol/Nutrition/Herb Interactions

Ethanol: May increase CNS depression; monitor for increased effects with coadministration. Caution patients about effects.

Food: The bioavailability of melatonin has been reported to be increased by fluvoxamine.

Herb/Nutraceutical: Avoid valerian, St John's wort, SAMe, kava kava (may increase risk of serotonin syndrome and/or excessive sedation). Avoid alfalfa, anise, bilberry, bladderwrack, bromelain, cat's claw, celery, chamomile, coleus, cordyceps, dong quai, evening primrose, fenugreek, feverfew, garlic, ginger, ginkgo biloba, ginseng (American), ginseng (Panax), ginseng (Siberian), grape seed, green tea, guggul, horse chestnuts, horseradish, licorice, prickly ash, red clover, reishi, SAMe (S-adenosylmethionine), sweet clover, turmeric, white willow (all have additional antiplatelet activity).

Stability Protect from high humidity and store at controlled room temperature 25°C (77°F).

Mechanism of Action Inhibits CNS neuron serotonin uptake; minimal or no effect on reuptake of norepinephrine or dopamine; does not significantly bind to alpha-adrenergic, histamine or cholinergic receptors

Pharmacodynamics/Kinetics

Onset of action: Depression: The onset of action is within a week; however, individual response varies greatly and full response may not be seen until 8-12 weeks after initiation of treatment.

Absorption: Steady-state plasma concentrations have been noted to be 2-3 times higher in children than those in adolescents; female children demonstrated a significantly higher AUC than males

Distribution: V_d: ~25 L/kg

Protein binding: ~80%, primarily to albumin

Metabolism: Extensively hepatic via oxidative demethylation and deamination

Bioavailability: Immediate release: 53%; not significantly affected by food

Half-life elimination: 15-16 hours; 17-26 hours in the elderly

Time to peak, plasma: 3-8 hours

Excretion: Urine (~85% as metabolites; ~2% as unchanged drug)

Dosage

Geriatric Reduce dose; titrate slowly.

Adult

Obsessive-compulsive disorder: Oral:

Immediate release: Initial: 50 mg once daily at bedtime; may be increased in 50 mg increments at 4- to 7-day intervals, as tolerated; usual dose range: 100-300 mg/day; maximum dose: 300 mg/day. **Note:** When total daily dose exceeds 100 mg, the dose should be given in 2 divided doses with larger portion administered at bedtime.

Extended release: Initial: 100 mg once daily at bedtime; may be increased in 50 mg increments at intervals of at least 1 week; usual dosage range: 100-300 mg/day; maximum dose: 300 mg/day

Social anxiety disorder (unlabeled use): Oral: Extended release: Initial: 100 mg once daily at bedtime; may be increased in 50 mg increments at intervals of at least 1 week; usual dosage range: 100-300 mg/day; maximum dose: 300 mg/day (Davidson, 2004; Stein, 2003; Westenberg, 2004)

Post-traumatic stress disorder (PTSD) (unlabeled use): Immediate release: Oral: 75 mg twice daily (Spivak, 2006)

Hepatic Impairment Reduce dose; titrate slowly.

Administration May be administered with or without food. Do not crush, open, or chew extended release capsules.

Monitoring Parameters Mental status for depression, suicide ideation (especially at the beginning of therapy or when doses are increased or decreased), anxiety, social functioning, mania, panic attacks; akathisia, weight gain or loss, nutritional intake, sleep; liver function assessment prior to beginning drug therapy

Pharmacotherapy Pearls Abrupt withdrawal may result in CNS side effects (agitation, GI symptoms, "feelings of electrical shock").

Special Geriatric Considerations Given fluvoxamine's approved indication (OCD), the number of drug interactions, and the limited information available on its use in the elderly, it may be best to select a different agent when treating depression. The elderly are more prone to SSRI/SNRI-induced hyponatremia.

Dosage Forms Excipient information presented when available (limited, particularly for generics); consult specific product labeling.

Capsule, extended release, oral, as maleate:
  Luvox® CR: 100 mg, 150 mg [gluten free]
Tablet, oral, as maleate: 25 mg, 50 mg, 100 mg

Selected References
de Vries MH, Raghoebar M, Mathlener IS, et al, "Single and Multiple Oral Dose Fluvoxamine Kinetics in Young and Elderly Subjects," *Ther Drug Monit*, 1992, 14(6):493-8.

◆ **Fluzone®** see Influenza Virus Vaccine (Inactivated) *on page 936*
◆ **Fluzone® High-Dose** see Influenza Virus Vaccine (Inactivated) *on page 936*
◆ **Folacin** see Folic Acid *on page 781*
◆ **Folacin-800 [OTC]** see Folic Acid *on page 781*
◆ **Folate** see Folic Acid *on page 781*

Folic Acid (FOE lik AS id)

Medication Safety Issues
  Sound-alike/look-alike issues:
    Folic acid may be confused with folinic acid
Brand Names: U.S. Folacin-800 [OTC]
Brand Names: Canada Apo-Folic®
Index Terms Folacin; Folate; Pteroylglutamic Acid
Generic Availability (U.S.) Yes
Pharmacologic Category Vitamin, Water Soluble
Use Treatment of megaloblastic and macrocytic anemias due to folate deficiency; dietary supplement to prevent neural tube defects
Unlabeled/Investigational Use Adjunctive cofactor therapy in methanol toxicity (alternative to leucovorin calcium)
Contraindications Hypersensitivity to folic acid or any component of the formulation
Warnings/Precautions Not appropriate for monotherapy with pernicious, aplastic, or normocytic anemias when anemia is present with vitamin B_{12} deficiency. Doses >0.1 mg/day may obscure pernicious anemia with continuing irreversible nerve damage progression. Resistance to treatment may occur with depressed hematopoiesis, alcoholism, and deficiencies of other vitamins. Injection contains benzyl alcohol (1.5%) as preservative.
Adverse Reactions (Reflective of adult population; not specific for elderly) Frequency not defined.
Allergic reaction, bronchospasm, erythema, flushing (slight), malaise (general), pruritus, rash
Drug Interactions
  Avoid Concomitant Use
    Avoid concomitant use of Folic Acid with any of the following: Raltitrexed
  Increased Effect/Toxicity There are no known significant interactions involving an increase in effect.
  Decreased Effect
    Folic Acid may decrease the levels/effects of: Fosphenytoin; PHENobarbital; Phenytoin; Primidone; Raltitrexed

    The levels/effects of Folic Acid may be decreased by: Green Tea

◀ **Stability** Do not use with oxidizing and reducing agents or heavy metal ions.

Mechanism of Action Folic acid is necessary for formation of a number of coenzymes in many metabolic systems, particularly for purine and pyrimidine synthesis; required for nucleoprotein synthesis and maintenance in erythropoiesis; stimulates WBC and platelet production in folate deficiency anemia. Folic acid enhances the elimination of formic acid, the toxic metabolite of methanol (unlabeled use).

Pharmacodynamics/Kinetics
Onset of action: Peak effect: Oral: 0.5-1 hour
Absorption: Proximal part of small intestine
Metabolism: Hepatic
Excretion: Urine

Dosage

Geriatric Refer to adult dosing. Vitamin B_{12} deficiency must be ruled out before initiating folate therapy due to frequency of combined nutritional deficiencies: RDA requirements (1999): 400 mcg/day (0.4 mg) minimum.

Adult

Anemia: Oral, I.M., I.V., SubQ: 0.4 mg/day

RDA: Expressed as dietary folate equivalents: 400 mcg/day

Administration Oral preferred, but may also be administered by deep I.M., SubQ, or I.V. injection; a diluted solution for oral or for parenteral administration may be prepared by diluting 1 mL of folic acid injection (5 mg/mL), with 49 mL sterile water for injection; resulting solution is 0.1 mg folic acid per 1 mL

Monitoring Parameters Reticulocyte count within 5-10 days of initiation of therapy; hematocrit, hemoglobin, RBC count at monthly intervals; diarrheal episodes should stop in 2-3 days of therapy; monitor seizure activity, serum phenytoin concentration should be monitored more often

Reference Range Therapeutic: 0.005-0.015 mcg/mL

Test Interactions Falsely low serum concentrations may occur with the *Lactobacillus casei* assay method in patients on anti-infectives (eg, tetracycline)

Pharmacotherapy Pearls The RDA for folic acid is presented as dietary folate equivalents (DFE). DFE adjusts for the difference in bioavailability of folic acid from food as compared to dietary supplements.

Special Geriatric Considerations Elderly frequently have combined nutritional deficiencies. Must rule out vitamin B_{12} deficiency before initiating folate therapy. Elderly, due to decreased nutrient intake, may benefit from daily intake of a multiple vitamin with minerals.

Dosage Forms Excipient information presented when available (limited, particularly for generics); consult specific product labeling.
Injection, solution, as sodium folate: 5 mg/mL (10 mL)
Tablet, oral: 0.4 mg, 0.8 mg, 1 mg
Folacin-800: 0.8 mg [scored; gluten free, sugar free]

Fondaparinux (fon da PARE i nuks)

Related Information
Anticoagulants, Injectable *on page 1989*

Medication Safety Issues
High alert medication:
The Institute for Safe Medication Practices (ISMP) includes this medication among its list of drugs which have a heightened risk of causing significant patient harm when used in error.

Brand Names: U.S. Arixtra®

Brand Names: Canada Arixtra®

Index Terms Fondaparinux Sodium

Generic Availability (U.S.) Yes

Pharmacologic Category Factor Xa Inhibitor

Use Prophylaxis of deep vein thrombosis (DVT) in patients undergoing surgery for hip replacement, knee replacement, hip fracture (including extended prophylaxis following hip fracture surgery), or abdominal surgery (in patients at risk for thromboembolic complications); treatment of acute pulmonary embolism (PE); treatment of acute DVT without PE

Canadian labeling: Additional uses (not approved in U.S.): Unstable angina or non-ST segment elevation myocardial infarction (UA/NSTEMI) for the prevention of death and subsequent MI; ST segment elevation MI (STEMI) for the prevention of death and myocardial reinfarction

Unlabeled/Investigational Use Prophylaxis of DVT in patients with a history of heparin-induced thrombocytopenia (HIT)

Contraindications Hypersensitivity to fondaparinux or any component of the formulation; severe renal impairment (Cl$_{cr}$ <30 mL/minute); body weight <50 kg (prophylaxis); active major bleeding; bacterial endocarditis; thrombocytopenia associated with a positive *in vitro* test for antiplatelet antibody in the presence of fondaparinux

Warnings/Precautions [U.S. Boxed Warning]: Spinal or epidural hematomas, including subsequent paralysis, may occur with recent or anticipated neuraxial anesthesia (epidural or spinal anesthesia) or spinal puncture in patients anticoagulated with LMWH, heparinoids, or fondaparinux. Consider risk versus benefit prior to spinal procedures; risk is increased by the use of concomitant agents which may alter hemostasis, the use of indwelling epidural catheters for analgesia, a history of spinal deformity or spinal surgery, as well as a history of traumatic or repeated epidural or spinal punctures. Patient should be observed closely for bleeding and signs and symptoms of neurological impairment if therapy is administered during or immediately following diagnostic lumbar puncture, epidural anesthesia, or spinal anesthesia.

Not to be used interchangeably (unit-for-unit) with heparin, low molecular weight heparins (LMWHs), or heparinoids. Use caution in patients with moderate renal dysfunction (Cl$_{cr}$ 30-50 mL/minute); contraindicated in patients with Cl$_{cr}$ <30 mL/minute. Discontinue if severe dysfunction or labile function develops.

Use caution in congenital or acquired bleeding disorders; bacterial endocarditis; renal impairment; hepatic impairment; active ulcerative or angiodysplastic gastrointestinal disease; hemorrhagic stroke; shortly after brain, spinal, or ophthalmologic surgery; or in patients taking platelet inhibitors. Risk of major bleeding may be increased if initial dose is administered earlier than recommended (initiation recommended at 6-8 hours following surgery). Discontinue agents that may enhance the risk of hemorrhage if possible. Although considered an insensitive measure of fondaparinux activity, there have been postmarketing reports of bleeding associated with elevated aPTT. Thrombocytopenia has occurred with administration, including reports of thrombocytopenia with thrombosis similar to heparin-induced thrombocytopenia. Monitor patients closely and discontinue therapy if platelets fall to <100,000/mm^3.

For subcutaneous administration; not for I.M. administration. Do not use interchangeably (unit for unit) with low molecular weight heparins, heparin, or heparinoids. Use caution in patients <50 kg who are being treated for DVT/PE; dosage reduction recommended. Contraindicated in patients <50 kg when used for prophylactic therapy. Use with caution in the elderly. The needle guard contains natural latex rubber.

The administration of fondaparinux is **not recommended** prior to and during primary PCI in patients with STEMI, due to an increased risk for guiding-catheter thrombosis. Patients with UA/NSTEMI or STEMI undergoing any PCI should not receive fondaparinux as the sole anticoagulant. Use of an anticoagulant with antithrombin activity (eg, unfractionated heparin) is recommended as adjunctive therapy to PCI even if prior treatment with fondaparinux (must take into account whether GP IIb/IIIa antagonists have been administered) (King, 2008). Do not administer with other agents that increase the risk of hemorrhage unless they are essential for the management of the underlying condition (eg, warfarin for treatment of VTE).

Additional Canadian labeling warnings: Following sheath removal, fondaparinux therapy should not resume for at least 2 hours in patients with UA/NSTEMI and 3 hours in patients with STEMI. Avoid administration 24 hours before and 48 hours after coronary artery bypass graft (CABG) surgery.

Adverse Reactions (Reflective of adult population; not specific for elderly) As with all anticoagulants, bleeding is the major adverse effect. Hemorrhage may occur at any site. Risk appears increased by a number of factors including renal dysfunction, age (>75 years), and weight (<50 kg).

>10%:
  Central nervous system: Fever (4% to 14%)
  Gastrointestinal: Nausea (11%)
  Hematologic: Anemia (20%)
1% to 10%:
  Cardiovascular: Edema (9%), hypotension (4%), thrombosis PCI catheter (without heparin 1%)
  Central nervous system: Insomnia (5%), dizziness (4%), headache (2% to 5%), confusion (3%), pain (2%)
  Dermatologic: Rash (8%), purpura (4%), bullous eruption (3%)
  Endocrine & metabolic: Hypokalemia (1% to 4%)
  Gastrointestinal: Constipation (5% to 9%), nausea (3%), vomiting (6%), diarrhea (3%), dyspepsia (2%)
  Genitourinary: Urinary tract infection (4%), urinary retention (3%)

Hematologic: Moderate thrombocytopenia (50,000-100,000/mm^3: 3%), major bleeding (1% to 3%), minor bleeding (2% to 4%), hematoma (3%); risk of major bleeding increased as high as 5% in patients receiving initial dose <6 hours following surgery

Hepatic: ALT increased (≤3%), AST increased (≤2%)

Local: Injection site reaction (bleeding, rash, pruritus)

Miscellaneous: Wound drainage increased (5%)

Drug Interactions

Avoid Concomitant Use

Avoid concomitant use of Fondaparinux with any of the following: Rivaroxaban

Increased Effect/Toxicity

Fondaparinux may increase the levels/effects of: Anticoagulants; Collagenase (Systemic); Deferasirox; Ibritumomab; Rivaroxaban; Tositumomab and Iodine I 131 Tositumomab

The levels/effects of Fondaparinux may be increased by: Antiplatelet Agents; Dasatinib; Drotrecogin Alfa; Herbs (Anticoagulant/Antiplatelet Properties); Nonsteroidal Anti-Inflammatory Agents; Pentosan Polysulfate Sodium; Prostacyclin Analogues; Salicylates; Thrombolytic Agents

Decreased Effect There are no known significant interactions involving a decrease in effect.

Ethanol/Nutrition/Herb Interactions Herb/Nutraceutical: Avoid alfalfa, anise, bilberry, bladderwrack, bromelain, cat's claw, celery, coleus, cordyceps, dong quai, evening primrose oil, fenugreek, feverfew, garlic, ginger, ginkgo biloba, ginseng (American/Panax/Siberian), grapeseed, green tea, guggul, horse chestnut seed, horseradish, licorice, prickly ash, red clover, reishi, sweet clover, turmeric, white willow (all possess anticoagulant or antiplatelet activity and as such, may enhance the anticoagulant effects of fondaparinux).

Stability Store at 25°C (77°F); excursions permitted to 15°C to 30°C (59°F to 86°F).

Canadian labeling: For I.V. administration: May mix with 25 mL or 50 mL NS; manufacturer recommends immediate use once diluted in NS, but is stable for up to 24 hours at 15°C to 30°C (59°F to 86°F).

Mechanism of Action Fondaparinux is a synthetic pentasaccharide that causes an antithrombin III-mediated selective inhibition of factor Xa. Neutralization of factor Xa interrupts the blood coagulation cascade and inhibits thrombin formation and thrombus development.

Pharmacodynamics/Kinetics

Absorption: SubQ: Rapid and complete

Distribution: V_d: 7-11 L; mainly in blood

Protein binding: ≥94% to antithrombin III

Bioavailability: SubQ: 100%

Half-life elimination: 17-21 hours; prolonged with renal impairment

Time to peak: SubQ: 2-3 hours

Excretion: Urine (~77%, unchanged drug)

Dosage

Geriatric & Adult

DVT prophylaxis: SubQ: Adults ≥50 kg: 2.5 mg once daily. **Note:** Prophylactic use contraindicated in patients <50 kg. Initiate dose after hemostasis has been established, 6-8 hours postoperatively.

DVT prophylaxis with history of HIT (unlabeled use): 2.5 mg once daily.

Usual duration: 5-9 days (up to 10 days following abdominal surgery or up to 11 days following hip replacement or knee replacement).

Extended prophylaxis is recommended following hip fracture surgery (has been tolerated for up to 32 days total).

Acute DVT/PE treatment: SubQ: **Note:** Start warfarin on the first treatment day and continue fondaparinux until INR is between 2 and 3 (usually 5-7 days) (Hirsh, 2008):

<50 kg: 5 mg once daily

50-100 kg: 7.5 mg once daily

>100 kg: 10 mg once daily

Usual duration: 5-9 days (has been administered up to 26 days)

Canadian labeling only: Adults:

UA/NSTEMI: SubQ: 2.5 mg once daily; initiate as soon as possible after diagnosis; treat for up to 8 days or until hospital discharge.

STEMI: I.V.: 2.5 mg once; subsequent doses: SubQ: 2.5 mg once daily; treat for up to 8 days or until hospital discharge

Renal Impairment

Cl_{cr} 30-50 mL/minute: Use caution

Cl_{cr} <30 mL/minute: Contraindicated

Hepatic Impairment

Mild-to-moderate impairment: Dosage adjustment not required; monitor for signs of bleeding.

Severe impairment: No data.

Administration Do **not** administer I.M.; for SubQ administration only. Do not mix with other injections or infusions. Do not expel air bubble from syringe before injection. Administer according to recommended regimen; early initiation (before 6 hours after surgery) has been associated with increased bleeding.

To convert from I.V. unfractionated heparin (UFH) infusion to SubQ fondaparinux (Nutescu, 2007): Calculate specific dose for fondaparinux based on indication, discontinue UFH, and begin fondaparinux within 1 hour

To convert from SubQ fondaparinux to I.V. UFH infusion (Nutescu, 2007): Discontinue fondaparinux; calculate specific dose for I.V. UFH infusion based on indication; omit heparin bolus/loading dose

For subQ fondaparinux dosed every 24 hours: Start I.V. UFH infusion 22-23 hours after last dose of fondaparinux

Canadian labeling only: STEMI patients: I.V. push or mixed in 25-50 mL of NS and infused over 2 minutes. Flush tubing with NS after infusion to ensure complete administration of fondaparinux. Infusion bag should not be mixed with other agents.

Monitoring Parameters Periodic monitoring of CBC, serum creatinine, occult blood testing of stools recommended. Anti-Xa activity of fondaparinux can be measured by the assay if fondaparinux is used as the calibrator. PT and aPTT are insensitive measures of fondaparinux activity. If unexpected changes in coagulation parameters or major bleeding occur, discontinue fondaparinux (elevated aPTT associated with bleeding events have been reported in postmarketing data).

Test Interactions International standards of heparin or LMWH are not the appropriate calibrators for antifactor Xa activity of fondaparinux.

Special Geriatric Considerations Use with caution in patients with estimated or actual creatinine clearance between 30-50 mL/minute. Contraindicated in patients with Cl_{cr} <30 mL/minute.

Dosage Forms Excipient information presented when available (limited, particularly for generics); consult specific product labeling.

Injection, solution, as sodium [preservative free]: 2.5 mg/0.5 mL (0.5 mL); 5 mg/0.4 mL (0.4 mL); 7.5 mg/0.6 mL (0.6 mL); 10 mg/0.8 mL (0.8 mL)

Arixtra®: 2.5 mg/0.5 mL (0.5 mL); 5 mg/0.4 mL (0.4 mL); 7.5 mg/0.6 mL (0.6 mL); 10 mg/0.8 mL (0.8 mL)

◆ **Fondaparinux Sodium** *see* Fondaparinux *on page* 782
◆ **Foradil® Aerolizer®** *see* Formoterol *on page* 785

Formoterol (for MOH te rol)

Related Information
Inhalant Agents *on page* 2010
Medication Safety Issues
Sound-alike/look-alike issues:
Foradil® may be confused with Toradol®
Administration issues:
Foradil® capsules for inhalation are for administration via Aerolizer™ inhaler and are **not** for oral use.
International issues:
Foradil [U.S., Canada, and multiple international markets] may be confused with Theradol brand name for tramadol [Netherlands]
Brand Names: U.S. Foradil® Aerolizer®; Perforomist®
Brand Names: Canada Foradil®; Oxeze® Turbuhaler®
Index Terms Formoterol Fumarate; Formoterol Fumarate Dihydrate
Generic Availability (U.S.) No
Pharmacologic Category Beta$_2$-Adrenergic Agonist; Beta$_2$-Adrenergic Agonist, Long-Acting
Use Maintenance treatment of asthma and prevention of bronchospasm (as concomitant therapy) in patients ≥5 years of age with reversible obstructive airway disease, including patients with symptoms of nocturnal asthma; maintenance treatment of bronchoconstriction in patients with COPD; prevention of exercise-induced bronchospasm in patients ≥5 years of age (monotherapy may be indicated in patients without persistent asthma)

Canadian labeling: Oxeze®: Also approved for acute relief of symptoms ("on demand" treatment) in patients ≥6 years of age
Medication Guide Available Yes

◀ **Contraindications** Hypersensitivity to formoterol or any component of the formulation (Foradil® only); monotherapy in the treatment of asthma (ie, use without a concomitant long-term asthma control medication, such as an inhaled corticosteroid)

Canadian labeling: Oxeze®: Hypersensitivity to formoterol, inhaled lactose, or any component of the formulation; presence of tachyarrhythmias

Warnings/Precautions [U.S. Boxed Warning]: Long-acting beta$_2$-agonists (LABAs) increase the risk of asthma-related deaths. Formoterol should only be used in asthma patients as adjuvant therapy in patients who are currently receiving but are not adequately controlled on a long-term asthma control medication (ie, an inhaled cortico-steroid). Monotherapy with an LABA is contraindicated in the treatment of asthma. In a large, randomized, placebo-controlled U.S. clinical trial (SMART, 2006), salmeterol was associated with an increase in asthma-related deaths (when added to usual asthma therapy); risk is considered a class effect among all LABAs. Data are not available to determine if the addition of an inhaled corticosteroid lessens this increased risk of death associated with LABA use. Assess patients at regular intervals once asthma control is maintained on combination therapy to determine if step-down therapy is appropriate and the LABA can be discontinued (without loss of asthma control), and the patient can be maintained on an inhaled corticosteroid. LABAs are not appropriate in patients whose asthma is adequately controlled on low- or medium-dose inhaled corticosteroids. Do **not** use for acute bronchospasm. Short-acting beta$_2$-agonist (eg, albuterol) should be used for acute symptoms and symptoms occurring between treatments. Do **not** initiate in patients with significantly worsening or acutely deteriorating asthma; reports of severe (sometimes fatal) respiratory events have been reported when formoterol has been initiated in this situation. Corticosteroids should not be stopped or reduced when formoterol is initiated. Formoterol is not a substitute for inhaled or systemic corticosteroids and should not be used as monotherapy. During initiation, watch for signs of worsening asthma.

Because LABAs may disguise poorly controlled persistent asthma, frequent or chronic use of LABAs for exercise-induced bronchospasm is discouraged by the NIH Asthma Guidelines (NIH, 2007). The safety and efficacy of Perforomist™ in the treatment of asthma have not been established. Oxeze® is a formulation of formoterol (available outside the U.S. [eg, Canada]) approved for acute treatment of asthmatic symptoms. The labelings for U.S. approved formulations (Foradil®, Perforomist™) state that formoterol is not meant to relieve acute asthmatic symptoms.

Do **not** use for acute episodes of COPD. Do **not** initiate in patients with significantly worsening or acutely deteriorating COPD. Data are not available to determine if LABA use increases the risk of death in patients with COPD. Increased use and/or ineffectiveness of short-acting beta$_2$-agonists may indicate rapidly deteriorating disease and should prompt re-evaluation of the patient's condition.

Immediate hypersensitivity reactions (urticaria, angioedema, rash, bronchospasm) have been reported. Do not exceed recommended dose or frequency; serious adverse events (including serious asthma exacerbations and fatalities) have been associated with excessive use of inhaled sympathomimetics. Beta$_2$-agonists may increase risk of arrhythmias, decrease serum potassium, prolong QT$_c$ interval, or increase serum glucose. These effects may be exacerbated in hypoxemia. Use caution in patients with cardiovascular disease (arrhythmia, coronary insufficiency, hypertension, or HF), seizures, diabetes, hyperthyroidism, or hypokalemia. Beta-agonists may cause elevation in blood pressure and heart rate, and result in CNS stimulation/excitation. Tolerance to the bronchodilator effect, measured by FEV$_1$, has been observed in studies.

Powder for oral inhalation contains lactose; very rare anaphylactic reactions have been reported in patients with severe milk protein allergy. The contents of the Foradil® capsules are for inhalation via the Aerolizer™ device. There have been reports of incorrect administration (swallowing of the capsules).

Adverse Reactions (Reflective of adult population; not specific for elderly)

1% to 10%:

Cardiovascular: Chest pain (2% to 3%), palpitation

Central nervous system: Anxiety (2%), dizziness (2%), fever (2%), insomnia (2%), dysphonia (1%), headache

Dermatologic: Pruritus (2%), rash (1%)

Gastrointestinal: Diarrhea (5%), nausea (5%), xerostomia (1% to 3%), vomiting (2%), abdominal pain, dyspepsia, gastroenteritis

Neuromuscular & skeletal: Muscle cramps (2%), tremor

Respiratory: Infection (3% to 7%), asthma exacerbation (age 5-12 years: 5% to 6%; age >12 years: <4%), bronchitis (5%), pharyngitis (3% to 4%), sinusitis (3%), dyspnea (2%), tonsillitis (1%)

Drug Interactions
Metabolism/Transport Effects Substrate (minor) of CYP2A6, 2C9, 2C19, 2D6
Avoid Concomitant Use
Avoid concomitant use of Formoterol with any of the following: Iobenguane I 123
Increased Effect/Toxicity
Formoterol may increase the levels/effects of: Loop Diuretics; Sympathomimetics

The levels/effects of Formoterol may be increased by: Atomoxetine; Caffeine; Cannabinoids;
MAO Inhibitors; Theophylline Derivatives; Tricyclic Antidepressants
Decreased Effect
Formoterol may decrease the levels/effects of: Iobenguane I 123

The levels/effects of Formoterol may be decreased by: Alpha-/Beta-Blockers; Beta-Blockers
(Beta1 Selective); Beta-Blockers (Nonselective); Betahistine
Stability
Foradil®: Prior to dispensing, store in refrigerator at 2°C to 8°C (36°F to 46°F). After
dispensing, store at room temperature at 20°C to 25°C (68°F to 77°F). Protect from heat
and moisture. Capsules should always be stored in the blister and only removed immediately before use. Always check expiration date. Use within 4 months of purchase date or
product expiration date, whichever comes first.
Performomist™: Prior to dispensing, store in refrigerator at 2°C to 8°C (36°F to 46°F). After
dispensing, store at 2°C to 25°C (36°F to 77°F) for up to 3 months. Protect from heat. Unit-
dose vials should always be stored in the foil pouch and only removed immediately
before use.
Mechanism of Action Relaxes bronchial smooth muscle by selective action on beta$_2$
receptors with little effect on heart rate. Formoterol has a long-acting effect.
Pharmacodynamics/Kinetics
Onset of action: Powder for inhalation: Within 3 minutes
Peak effect: Powder for inhalation: 80% of peak effect within 15 minutes; Solution for
nebulization: 2 hours
Duration: Improvement in FEV$_1$ observed for 12 hours in most patients
Absorption: Rapidly into plasma
Protein binding: 61% to 64% *in vitro* at higher concentrations than achieved with usual dosing
Metabolism: Hepatic via direct glucuronidation and O-demethylation; CYP2D6, CYP2C8/9,
CYP2C19, CYP2A6 involved in O-demethylation
Half-life elimination: Powder: ~10-14 hours; Nebulized solution: ~7 hours
Time to peak: Maximum improvement in FEV$_1$ in 1-3 hours
Excretion: Urine (15% to 18% as direct glucuronide metabolites, 2% to 10% as
unchanged drug)
Dosage
Geriatric & Adult
Asthma, maintenance: Inhalation: **Note:** For asthma control, long-acting beta$_2$-agonists
(LABAs) should be used in combination with inhaled corticosteroids and **not** as mono-
therapy
Foradil®: 12 mcg capsule inhaled every 12 hours via Aerolizer™ device (maximum: 24
mcg/day)
Oxeze® (CAN): **Note:** Not labeled for use in the U.S.: Inhalation: 6 mcg or 12 mcg every 12
hours (maximum dose: 48 mcg/day)
Exercise-induced bronchospasm: Inhalation:
Foradil®: 12 mcg capsule inhaled via Aerolizer™ device at least 15 minutes before
exercise on an "as needed" basis; additional doses should not be used for another 12
hours. **Note:** If already using for asthma maintenance then should not use additional
doses for exercise-induced bronchospasm. Because LABAs may disguise poorly controlled persistent asthma, frequent or chronic use of LABAs for exercise-induced
bronchospasm is discouraged by the NIH Asthma Guidelines (NIH, 2007).
Oxeze® (CAN): **Note:** Not labeled for use in the U.S.: Inhalation: 6 mcg or 12 mcg at least
15 minutes before exercise.
COPD (maintenance): Inhalation:
Foradil®: 12 mcg capsule inhaled every 12 hours via Aerolizer™ device (maximum: 24
mcg/day)
Performomist™: 20 mcg twice daily (maximum dose: 40 mcg/day)
Acute ("on demand") relief of bronchoconstriction: *Indication for Oxeze® approved in
Canada:* 6 mcg or 12 mcg as a single dose (maximum dose: 72 mcg/24-hour period). The
prolonged use of high dosages (48 mcg/day for ≥3 consecutive days) may be a sign of
suboptimal control, and should prompt the re-evaluation of therapy.
Renal Impairment Not studied

◀ **Administration**
Foradil®: Remove capsule from foil blister **immediately** before use. Place capsule in the capsule-chamber in the base of the Aerolizer™ Inhaler. Must only use the Aerolizer™ Inhaler. Press both buttons **once only** and then release. Keep inhaler in a level, horizontal position. Exhale fully. Do not exhale into inhaler. Tilt head slightly back and inhale (rapidly, steadily, and deeply). Hold breath as long as possible. If any powder remains in capsule, exhale and inhale again. Repeat until capsule is empty. Throw away empty capsule; do not leave in inhaler. Do not use a spacer with the Aerolizer™ Inhaler. Always keep capsules and inhaler dry.

Perforomist™: Remove unit-dose vial from foil pouch **immediately** before use. Solution does not require dilution prior to administration; do not mix other medications with formoterol solution. Place contents of unit-dose vial into the reservoir of a standard jet nebulizer connected to an air compressor; assemble nebulizer based on the manufacturer's instructions and turn nebulizer on; breathe deeply and evenly until all of the medication has been inhaled. Discard any unused medication immediately; do not ingest contents of vial. Clean nebulizer after use.

Oxeze® Turbuhaler® [CAN; not available in U.S.]: Hold inhaler upright. Turn colored grip as far as it will go in one direction and then turn back to original position; a clicking sound should be heard which means the inhaler is ready for use. Exhale fully. Do not exhale into mouthpiece of inhaler. Place mouthpiece to lips and inhale forcefully and deeply. Do not chew or bite on mouthpiece. Clean outside of mouthpiece once weekly with a dry tissue. Avoid getting inhaler wet.

Monitoring Parameters FEV_1, peak flow, and/or other pulmonary function tests; blood pressure, heart rate; CNS stimulation; serum glucose, serum potassium

Special Geriatric Considerations Elderly patients should be specifically counseled about the proper use of this inhaler/spacing of doses and/or the proper use of a nebulizer system. No significant difference in both safety and effectiveness was seen between elderly and younger patients.

Dosage Forms Excipient information presented when available (limited, particularly for generics); consult specific product labeling.
Powder, for oral inhalation, as fumarate:
   Foradil® Aerolizer®: 12 mcg/capsule (12s, 60s) [contains lactose 25 mg/capsule]
Solution, for nebulization, as fumarate dihydrate:
   Perforomist®: 20 mcg/2 mL (60s)

Dosage Forms: Canada Excipient information presented when available (limited, particularly for generics); consult specific product labeling.
Powder for oral inhalation, as fumarate:
   Oxeze® Turbuhaler®: 6 mcg/inhalation [delivers 60 metered doses; contains lactose 600 mcg/dose]; 12 mcg/inhalation [delivers 60 metered doses; contains lactose 600 mcg/dose]

Selected References
Cazzola M and Donner CF, "Long-acting Beta2 Agonists in the Management of Stable Chronic Obstructive Pulmonary Disease," Drugs, 2000, 60:307-20.

◆ **Formoterol and Mometasone** see Mometasone and Formoterol on page 1234
◆ **Formoterol and Mometasone Furoate** see Mometasone and Formoterol on page 1234
◆ **Formoterol Fumarate** see Formoterol on page 785
◆ **Formoterol Fumarate Dihydrate** see Formoterol on page 785
◆ **Formoterol Fumarate Dihydrate and Mometasone** see Mometasone and Formoterol on page 1234
◆ **Formulation R™ [OTC]** see Phenylephrine (Topical) on page 1443
◆ **Fortamet®** see MetFORMIN on page 1155
◆ **Fortaz®** see CefTAZidime on page 309
◆ **Forteo®** see Teriparatide on page 1760
◆ **Fortesta™** see Testosterone on page 1761
◆ **Fortical®** see Calcitonin on page 241
◆ **Fosamax®** see Alendronate on page 53
◆ **Fosamax Plus D®** see Alendronate and Cholecalciferol on page 56

Fosaprepitant (fos a PRE pi tant)

Medication Safety Issues
   Sound-alike/look-alike issues:
   Fosaprepitant may be confused with aprepitant, fosamprenavir, fospropofol
   Emend® for Injection (fosaprepitant) may be confused with Emend® (aprepitant) which is an oral capsule formulation.
Brand Names: U.S. Emend® for Injection
Brand Names: Canada Emend® IV

Index Terms Aprepitant Injection; Fosaprepitant Dimeglumine; L-758,298; MK 0517

Generic Availability (U.S.) No

Pharmacologic Category Antiemetic; Substance P/Neurokinin 1 Receptor Antagonist

Use Prevention of acute and delayed nausea and vomiting associated with moderately- and highly-emetogenic chemotherapy (in combination with other antiemetics)

Contraindications Hypersensitivity to fosaprepitant, aprepitant, polysorbate 80, or any component of the formulation; concurrent use with pimozide or cisapride

Canadian labeling: Additional contraindications (not in U.S. labeling): Concurrent use with astemizole or terfenadine

Warnings/Precautions Fosaprepitant is rapidly converted to aprepitant, which has a high potential for drug interactions. Use caution with agents primarily metabolized via CYP3A4; aprepitant is a 3A4 inhibitor. Effect on orally administered 3A4 substrates is greater than those administered intravenously. Immediate hypersensitivity has been reported (rarely) with fosaprepitant; stop infusion with hypersensitivity symptoms (dyspnea, erythema, flushing, or anaphylaxis); do not reinitiate. Use caution with hepatic impairment; has not been studied in patients with severe hepatic impairment (Child-Pugh class C). Not studied for treatment of existing nausea and vomiting. Chronic continuous administration of fosaprepitant is not recommended.

Adverse Reactions (Reflective of adult population; not specific for elderly) Adverse reactions reported with aprepitant and fosaprepitant (as part of a combination chemotherapy regimen) occurring at a higher frequency than standard antiemetic therapy:

1% to 10%:

Central nervous system: Fatigue (1% to 3%), headache (2%)

Gastrointestinal: Anorexia (2%), constipation 2%), dyspepsia (2%), diarrhea (1%), eructation (1%)

Hepatic: ALT increased (1% to 3%), AST increased (1%)

Local: Injection site reactions (3%; includes erythema, induration, pain, pruritus, or thrombophlebitis)

Neuromuscular & skeletal: Weakness (3%)

Miscellaneous: Hiccups (5%)

Drug Interactions

Metabolism/Transport Effects Substrate of CYP1A2 (minor), 2C19 (minor), 3A4 (major); **Inhibits** CYP2C9 (weak), 2C19 (weak), 3A4 (moderate); **Induces** CYP2C9 (weak), 3A4 (weak)

Avoid Concomitant Use

Avoid concomitant use of Fosaprepitant with any of the following: Astemizole; Cisapride; Conivaptan; Pimozide; Terfenadine; Tolvaptan

Increased Effect/Toxicity

Fosaprepitant may increase the levels/effects of: Astemizole; Benzodiazepines (metabolized by oxidation); Budesonide (Systemic, Oral Inhalation); Cisapride; Colchicine; Corticosteroids (Systemic); CYP3A4 Substrates; Diltiazem; Eplerenone; Everolimus; FentaNYL; Halofantrine; Lurasidone; Pimecrolimus; Pimozide; Ranolazine; Salmeterol; Saxagliptin; Terfenadine; Tolvaptan; Vilazodone

The levels/effects of Fosaprepitant may be increased by: Antifungal Agents (Azole Derivatives, Systemic); Conivaptan; CYP3A4 Inhibitors (Moderate); CYP3A4 Inhibitors (Strong); Dasatinib; Diltiazem

Decreased Effect

Fosaprepitant may decrease the levels/effects of: Contraceptives (Estrogens); Contraceptives (Progestins); PARoxetine; Saxagliptin; TOLBUTamide; Warfarin

The levels/effects of Fosaprepitant may be decreased by: CYP3A4 Inducers (Strong); Cyproterone; Deferasirox; Herbs (CYP3A4 Inducers); PARoxetine; Rifampin; Tocilizumab

Ethanol/Nutrition/Herb Interactions

Food: Aprepitant serum concentration may be increased when taken with grapefruit juice; avoid concurrent use.

Herb/Nutraceutical: Avoid St John's wort (may decrease aprepitant levels).

Stability Store intact vials at 2°C to 8°C (36°F to 46°F). Reconstitute either vial size with 5 mL of sodium chloride 0.9%, directing diluent down side of vial to avoid foaming; swirl gently. Add reconstituted contents of the 150 mg vial to 145 mL sodium chloride 0.9% (add 115 mg vial to 110 mL), resulting in a final concentration of 1 mg/mL; gently invert bag to mix. Solutions diluted for infusion are stable for 24 hours at room temperature of ≤25°C (≤77°F).

Mechanism of Action Fosaprepitant is a prodrug of aprepitant, a substance P/neurokinin 1 (NK1) receptor antagonist. It is rapidly converted to aprepitant which prevents acute and delayed vomiting by inhibiting the substance P/neurokinin 1 (NK1) receptor; augments the antiemetic activity of the 5-HT$_3$ receptor antagonist and corticosteroid activity and inhibits chemotherapy-induced emesis.

◀ **Pharmacodynamics/Kinetics**

Distribution: Fosaprepitant: ~5 L; Aprepitant: V_d: ~70 L; crosses the blood brain barrier

Protein binding: Aprepitant: >95%

Metabolism:

Fosaprepitant: Hepatic and extrahepatic; rapidly (within 30 minutes after the end of infusion) converted to aprepitant (nearly complete conversion)

Aprepitant: Hepatic via CYP3A4 (major); CYP1A2 and CYP2C19 (minor); forms 7 weakly-active metabolites

Half-life elimination: Half-life elimination: Fosaprepitant: ~2 minutes; Aprepitant: ~9-13 hours

Time to peak, plasma: Fosaprepitant is converted to aprepitant within 30 minutes after the end of infusion

Excretion: Urine (57%); feces (45%)

Dosage

Geriatric & Adult Prevention of chemotherapy-induced nausea/vomiting: I.V.:

Single-dose regimen (for highly-emetogenic chemotherapy): 150 mg over 20-30 minutes ~30 minutes prior to chemotherapy on day 1 only (in combination with a 5-HT$_3$ antagonist on day 1 and dexamethasone on days 1 to 4)

3-day regimen (for highly-emetogenic chemotherapy): 115 mg over 15 minutes 30 minutes prior to chemotherapy on day 1, followed by aprepitant 80 mg orally on days 2 and 3 (in combination with a 5-HT$_3$ antagonist on day 1 and dexamethasone on days 1 to 4)

3-day regimen (for moderately-emetogenic chemotherapy): 115 mg over 15 minutes 30 minutes prior to chemotherapy on day 1, followed by aprepitant 80 mg orally on days 2 and 3 (in combination with a 5-HT$_3$ antagonist and dexamethasone on day 1)

Renal Impairment

Mild, moderate, or severe impairment: No adjustment required.

Dialysis-dependent end-stage renal disease (ESRD): No adjustment required.

Hepatic Impairment

Child-Pugh class A and B: No adjustment required.

Child-Pugh class C: Has not been evaluated; use with caution.

Administration

115 mg: Infuse over 15 minutes 30 minutes prior to chemotherapy

150 mg: Infuse over 20-30 minutes ~30 minutes prior to chemotherapy

Pharmacotherapy Pearls Oncology Comment: Fosaprepitant is recommended in the National Comprehensive Cancer Network® (NCCN) Clinical Practice Guidelines in Oncology for Antiemesis (version 1.2011) for use on day 1 in combination with a serotonin receptor antagonist and dexamethasone for chemotherapy with high emetic risk and for select moderately emetogenic regimens (carboplatin, cisplatin, doxorubicin, epirubicin, ifosfamide, irinotecan, or methotrexate). Either fosaprepitant 115 mg or aprepitant (125 mg orally) are administered on day 1; for day 2 and 3, patients should receive aprepitant 80 mg orally. The 1-day regimen (fosaprepitant 150 mg on day 1 only) is listed in the guidelines for highly emetogenic treatments.

Special Geriatric Considerations Prior studies with aprepitant by the manufacturer were demonstrated in a total of 544 patients, 31% were >65 years of age, while 5% were >75 years. No differences in safety and efficacy were noted between elderly subjects and younger adults. No dosing adjustment is necessary.

Dosage Forms Excipient information presented when available (limited, particularly for generics); consult specific product labeling. [DSC] = Discontinued product

Injection, powder for reconstitution:

Emend® for Injection: 115 mg [DSC] [contains edetate disodium, lactose 287.5 mg, polysorbate 80]

Emend® for Injection: 150 mg [contains edetate disodium, lactose 375 mg, polysorbate 80]

Selected References

Cocquyt V, Van Belle S, Reinhardt RR, et al, "Comparison of L-758,298, a Prodrug for the Selective Neurokinin-1 Antagonist, L-754,030, With Ondansetron for the Prevention of Cisplatin-Induced Emesis," *Eur J Cancer*, 2001, 37 (7):835-42.

Lasseter KC, Gambelle J, Jin B, et al, "Tolerability of Fosaprepitant and Bioequivalency to Aprepitant in Healthy Subjects," *J Clin Pharmacol*, 2007,47(7):834-40.

National Comprehensive Cancer Network® (NCCN), "Clinical Practice Guidelines in Oncology™: Antiemesis," Version 2.2010. Available at http://www.nccn.org/professionals/physician_gls/PDF/antiemesis.pdf.

Van Belle S, Lichinitser SR, Navari RM, et al," Prevention of Cisplatin-Induced Acute and Delayed Emesis by the Selective Neurokinin-1 Antagonists, L-758,298 and MK-869," *Cancer*, 2002, 94(11):3032-41.

◆ **Fosaprepitant Dimeglumine** *see* Fosaprepitant *on page 788*

Fosinopril (foe SIN oh pril)

Related Information
Angiotensin Agents *on page 1985*

Medication Safety Issues
Sound-alike/look-alike issues:
Fosinopril may be confused with FLUoxetine, Fosamax®, furosemide, lisinopril

Monopril may be confused with Accupril®, minoxidil, moexipril, Monoket®, Monurol®, ramipril

Brand Names: Canada Apo-Fosinopril®; Jamp-Fosinopril; Monopril®; Mylan-Fosinopril; PMS-Fosinopril; RAN™-Fosinopril; Riva-Fosinopril; Teva-Fosinopril

Index Terms Fosinopril Sodium; Monopril

Generic Availability (U.S.) Yes

Pharmacologic Category Angiotensin-Converting Enzyme (ACE) Inhibitor

Use Treatment of hypertension, either alone or in combination with other antihypertensive agents; treatment of heart failure (HF)

Contraindications Hypersensitivity to fosinopril, any other ACE inhibitor, or any component of the formulation; angioedema related to previous treatment with an ACE inhibitor

Warnings/Precautions Anaphylactic reactions may occur rarely with ACE inhibitors. At any time during treatment (especially following first dose), angioedema may occur rarely with ACE inhibitors; it may involve the head and neck (potentially compromising airway) or the intestine (presenting with abdominal pain). African-Americans may be at an increased risk and patients with idiopathic or hereditary angioedema may be at an increased risk. Prolonged frequent monitoring may be required especially if tongue, glottis, or larynx are involved as they are associated with airway obstruction. Patients with a history of airway surgery may have a higher risk of airway obstruction. Aggressive early and appropriate management is critical. Use in patients with previous angioedema associated with ACE inhibitor therapy is contraindicated. Severe anaphylactoid reactions may be seen during hemodialysis (eg, CVVHD) with high-flux dialysis membranes (eg, AN69), and rarely, during low density lipoprotein apheresis with dextran sulfate cellulose. Rare cases of anaphylactoid reactions have been reported in patients undergoing sensitization treatment with hymenoptera (bee, wasp) venom while receiving ACE inhibitors.

Symptomatic hypotension with or without syncope can occur with ACE inhibitors (usually with the first several doses); effects are most often observed in volume-depleted patients; correct volume depletion prior to initiation; close monitoring of patient is required especially with initial dosing and dosing increases; blood pressure must be lowered at a rate appropriate for the patient's clinical condition. Initiation of therapy in patients with ischemic heart disease or cerebrovascular disease warrants close observation due to the potential consequences posed by falling blood pressure (eg, MI, stroke). Use with caution in hypertrophic cardiomyopathy with outflow tract obstruction, severe aortic stenosis, or before, during, or immediately after major surgery.

Hyperkalemia may occur with ACE inhibitors; risk factors include renal dysfunction, diabetes mellitus, concomitant use of potassium-sparing diuretics, potassium supplements, and/or potassium-containing salts. Use cautiously, if at all, with these agents and monitor potassium closely. Cough may occur with ACE inhibitors. Other causes of cough should be considered (eg, pulmonary congestion in patients with heart failure) and excluded prior to discontinuation.

May be associated with deterioration of renal function and/or increases in serum creatinine, particularly in patients with low renal blood flow (eg, renal artery stenosis, heart failure) whose glomerular filtration rate (GFR) is dependent on efferent arteriolar vasoconstriction by angiotensin II; deterioration may result in oliguria, acute renal failure, and progressive azotemia. Small increases in serum creatinine may occur following initiation; consider discontinuation only in patients with progressive and/or significant deterioration in renal function. Use with caution in patients with unstented unilateral/bilateral renal artery stenosis. When unstented bilateral renal artery stenosis is present, use is generally avoided due to the elevated risk of deterioration in renal function unless possible benefits outweigh risks. Concurrent use of angiotensin receptor blockers may increase the risk of clinically-significant adverse events (eg, renal dysfunction, hyperkalemia).

Rare toxicities associated with ACE inhibitors include cholestatic jaundice (which may progress to fulminant hepatic necrosis), agranulocytosis, neutropenia or leukopenia with myeloid hypoplasia. Patients with collagen vascular diseases (especially with concomitant renal impairment) or renal impairment alone may be at increased risk for hematologic toxicity; periodically monitor CBC with differential in these patients.

◀ **Adverse Reactions (Reflective of adult population; not specific for elderly)** Note: Frequency ranges include data from hypertension and heart failure trials. Higher rates of adverse reactions have generally been noted in patients with CHF. However, the frequency of adverse effects associated with placebo is also increased in this population.

>10%: Central nervous system: Dizziness (2% to 12%)

1% to 10%:

Cardiovascular: Orthostatic hypotension (1% to 2%), palpitation (1%)

Central nervous system: Dizziness (1% to 2%; up to 12% in CHF patients), headache (3%), fatigue (1% to 2%)

Endocrine & metabolic: Hyperkalemia (2.6%)

Gastrointestinal: Diarrhea (2%), nausea/vomiting (1.2% to 2.2%)

Hepatic: Transaminases increased

Neuromuscular & skeletal: Musculoskeletal pain (<1% to 3%), noncardiac chest pain (<1% to 2%), weakness (1%)

Renal: Serum creatinine increased, renal function worsening (in patients with bilateral renal artery stenosis or hypovolemia)

Respiratory: Cough (2% to 10%)

Miscellaneous: Upper respiratory infection (2%)

>1% but ≤ frequency in patients receiving placebo: Sexual dysfunction, fever, flu-like syndrome, dyspnea, rash, headache, insomnia

Other events reported with ACE inhibitors: Neutropenia, agranulocytosis, eosinophilic pneumonitis, cardiac arrest, pancytopenia, hemolytic anemia, anemia, aplastic anemia, thrombocytopenia, acute renal failure, hepatic failure, jaundice, symptomatic hyponatremia, bullous pemphigus, exfoliative dermatitis, Stevens-Johnson syndrome. In addition, a syndrome which may include fever, myalgia, arthralgia, interstitial nephritis, vasculitis, rash, eosinophilia and positive ANA, and elevated ESR has been reported for other ACE inhibitors.

Drug Interactions

Avoid Concomitant Use There are no known interactions where it is recommended to avoid concomitant use.

Increased Effect/Toxicity

Fosinopril may increase the levels/effects of: Allopurinol; Amifostine; Antihypertensives; AzaTHIOprine; CycloSPORINE; CycloSPORINE (Systemic); Ferric Gluconate; Gold Sodium Thiomalate; Hypotensive Agents; Iron Dextran Complex; Lithium; Nonsteroidal Anti-Inflammatory Agents; RiTUXimab; Sodium Phosphates

The levels/effects of Fosinopril may be increased by: Alfuzosin; Angiotensin II Receptor Blockers; Diazoxide; DPP-IV Inhibitors; Eplerenone; Everolimus; Herbs (Hypotensive Properties); Loop Diuretics; MAO Inhibitors; Pentoxifylline; Phosphodiesterase 5 Inhibitors; Potassium Salts; Potassium-Sparing Diuretics; Prostacyclin Analogues; Sirolimus; Temsirolimus; Thiazide Diuretics; TiZANidine; Tolvaptan; Trimethoprim

Decreased Effect

The levels/effects of Fosinopril may be decreased by: Antacids; Aprotinin; Herbs (Hypertensive Properties); Icatibant; Lanthanum; Methylphenidate; Nonsteroidal Anti-Inflammatory Agents; Salicylates; Yohimbine

Ethanol/Nutrition/Herb Interactions Herb/Nutraceutical: Avoid bayberry, blue cohosh, cayenne, ephedra, ginger, ginseng (American), kola, licorice (may worsen hypertension). Avoid black cohosh, california poppy, coleus, golden seal, hawthorn, mistletoe, periwinkle, quinine, shepherd's purse (may have increased antihypertensive effect).

Stability Store at 25°C (77°F); excursions permitted to 15°C to 30°C (59°F to 86°F). Protect from moisture by keeping bottle tightly closed.

Mechanism of Action Competitive inhibitor of angiotensin-converting enzyme (ACE); prevents conversion of angiotensin I to angiotensin II, a potent vasoconstrictor; results in lower levels of angiotensin II which causes an increase in plasma renin activity and a reduction in aldosterone secretion; a CNS mechanism may also be involved in hypotensive effect as angiotensin II increases adrenergic outflow from CNS; vasoactive kallikreins may be decreased in conversion to active hormones by ACE inhibitors, thus reducing blood pressure

Pharmacodynamics/Kinetics

Onset of action: 1 hour

Duration: 24 hours

Absorption: 36%

Protein binding: 95%

Metabolism: Prodrug, hydrolyzed to its active metabolite fosinoprilat by intestinal wall and hepatic esterases

Bioavailability: 36%

Half-life elimination, serum (fosinoprilat): 12 hours

Time to peak, serum: ~3 hours

Excretion: Urine and feces (as fosinoprilat and other metabolites in roughly equal proportions, 45% to 50%)

Dosage

Geriatric & Adult

Heart failure: Oral: Initial: 10 mg/day (5 mg if renal dysfunction present) and increase, as needed, to a maximum of 40 mg once daily over several weeks. Usual dose: 20-40 mg/day. If hypotension, orthostasis, or azotemia occurs during titration, consider decreasing concomitant diuretic dose, if any.

Hypertension: Oral: Initial: 10 mg/day; increase to a maximum dose of 80 mg/day. Most patients are maintained on 20-40 mg/day. May need to divide the dose into two if trough effect is inadequate. Discontinue the diuretic, if possible 2-3 days before initiation of therapy. Resume diuretic therapy carefully, if needed.

Renal Impairment None needed since hepatobiliary elimination compensates adequately diminished renal elimination.

Hemodialysis: Moderately dialyzable (20% to 50%)

Hepatic Impairment Decrease dose and monitor effects

Monitoring Parameters Blood pressure; serum creatinine and potassium; if patient has collagen vascular disease and/or renal impairment, periodically monitor CBC with differential

Test Interactions Positive Coombs' (direct); may cause false-positive results in urine acetone determinations using sodium nitroprusside reagent; may cause false low serum digoxin levels with the Digi-Tab RIA kit for digoxin

Pharmacotherapy Pearls Watch for hypotensive effect within 1-3 hours of first dose or new higher dose. Some patients may have a decreased hypotensive effect between 12-16 hours; consider dividing total daily dose into 2 doses 12 hours apart; if patient is receiving a diuretic, a potential for first-dose hypotension is increased; to decrease this potential, stop diuretic for 2-3 days prior to initiating fosinopril if possible; continue diuretic if needed to control blood pressure

Special Geriatric Considerations Due to frequent decreases in glomerular filtration (also creatinine clearance) with aging, elderly patients may have exaggerated responses to ACE inhibitors. Differences in clinical response due to hepatic changes are not observed. ACE inhibitors may be preferred agents in elderly patients with congestive heart failure and diabetes mellitus. Diabetic proteinuria is reduced and insulin sensitivity is enhanced. In general, the side effect profile is favorable in the elderly and causes little or no CNS confusion; use lowest dose recommendations initially. Many elderly may be volume depleted due to diuretic use and/or blunted thirst reflex resulting in inadequate fluid intake.

Dosage Forms Excipient information presented when available (limited, particularly for generics); consult specific product labeling.

Tablet, oral, as sodium: 10 mg, 20 mg, 40 mg

◆ **Fosinopril Sodium** *see* Fosinopril *on page* 791

Fosphenytoin (FOS fen i toyn)

Medication Safety Issues

Sound-alike/look-alike issues:

Cerebyx® may be confused with Celebrex®, Celexa™, Cerezyme®, Cervarix®

Fosphenytoin may be confused with fospropofol

Administration issues:

Overdoses have occurred due to confusion between the **mg per mL concentration** of fosphenytoin (50 mg PE/mL) and **total drug content per vial** (either 100 mg PE/2 mL vial or 500 mg PE/10 mL vial). ISMP recommends that the total drug content per container is identified instead of the concentration in mg per mL to avoid confusion and potential overdosages. Additionally, since most errors have occurred with overdoses in children, they recommend that pediatric hospitals should consider stocking only the 2 mL vial.

Brand Names: U.S. Cerebyx®

Brand Names: Canada Cerebyx®

Index Terms Fosphenytoin Sodium

Generic Availability (U.S.) Yes

Pharmacologic Category Anticonvulsant, Hydantoin

Use Used for the control of generalized convulsive status epilepticus and prevention and treatment of seizures occurring during neurosurgery; indicated for short-term parenteral administration when other means of phenytoin administration are unavailable, inappropriate, or deemed less advantageous (the safety and effectiveness of fosphenytoin use for more than 5 days has not been systematically evaluated)

◄ **Contraindications** Hypersensitivity to phenytoin, other hydantoins, or any component of the formulation; patients with sinus bradycardia, sinoatrial block, second- and third-degree AV block, or Adams-Stokes syndrome; occurrence of rash during treatment (should not be resumed if rash is exfoliative, purpuric, or bullous); treatment of absence seizures

Warnings/Precautions Doses of fosphenytoin are expressed as their phenytoin sodium equivalent (PE). Antiepileptic drugs should not be abruptly discontinued. Hypotension may occur, especially after I.V. administration at high doses and high rates of administration. Administration of phenytoin has been associated with atrial and ventricular conduction depression and ventricular fibrillation. Careful cardiac monitoring is needed when administering I.V. loading doses of fosphenytoin. Acute hepatotoxicity associated with a hypersensitivity syndrome characterized by fever, skin eruptions, and lymphadenopathy has been reported to occur within the first 2 months of treatment. Discontinue if skin rash or lymphadenopathy occurs. A spectrum of hematologic effects have been reported with use (eg, neutropenia, leukopenia, thrombocytopenia, pancytopenia, and anemias). Use with caution in patients with hypotension, severe myocardial insufficiency, diabetes mellitus, porphyria, hypoalbuminemia, hypothyroidism, fever, or hepatic or renal dysfunction. Effects with other sedative drugs or ethanol may be potentiated. Severe reactions, including toxic epidermal necrolysis and Stevens-Johnson syndromes, although rarely reported, have resulted in fatalities; drug should be discontinued if there are any signs of rash. Patients of Asian descent with the variant *HLA-B*1502* may be at an increased risk of developing Stevens-Johnson syndrome and/or toxic epidermal necrolysis.

Adverse Reactions (Reflective of adult population; not specific for elderly) The more important adverse clinical events caused by the I.V. use of fosphenytoin or phenytoin are cardiovascular collapse and/or central nervous system depression. Hypotension can occur when either drug is administered rapidly by the I.V. route. Do not exceed a rate of 150 mg phenytoin equivalent/minute when administering fosphenytoin.

The adverse clinical events most commonly observed with the use of fosphenytoin in clinical trials were nystagmus, dizziness, pruritus, paresthesia, headache, somnolence, and ataxia. Paresthesia and pruritus were seen more often following fosphenytoin (versus phenytoin) administration and occurred more often with I.V. fosphenytoin than with I.M. administration. These events were dose and rate related (doses ≥15 mg/kg at a rate of 150 mg/minute). These sensations, generally described as itching, burning, or tingling are usually not at the infusion site. The location of the discomfort varied with the groin mentioned most frequently. The paresthesia and pruritus were transient events that occurred within several minutes of the start of infusion and generally resolved within 10 minutes after completion of infusion.

Transient pruritus, tinnitus, nystagmus, somnolence, and ataxia occurred 2-3 times more often at doses ≥15 mg/kg and rates ≥150 mg/minute.

I.V. administration (maximum dose/rate):
>10%:
 Central nervous system: Nystagmus, dizziness, somnolence, ataxia
 Dermatologic: Pruritus
1% to 10%:
 Cardiovascular: Hypotension, vasodilation, tachycardia
 Central nervous system: Stupor, incoordination, paresthesia, extrapyramidal syndrome, tremor, agitation, hypoesthesia, dysarthria, vertigo, brain edema, headache
 Gastrointestinal: Nausea, tongue disorder, dry mouth, vomiting
 Neuromuscular & skeletal: Pelvic pain, muscle weakness, back pain
 Ocular: Diplopia, amblyopia
 Otic: Tinnitus, deafness
 Miscellaneous: Taste perversion

I.M. administration (substitute for oral phenytoin):
1% to 10%:
 Central nervous system: Nystagmus, tremor, ataxia, headache, incoordination, somnolence, dizziness, paresthesia, reflexes decreased
 Dermatologic: Pruritus
 Gastrointestinal: Nausea, vomiting
 Hematologic/lymphatic: Ecchymosis
 Neuromuscular & skeletal: Muscle weakness

Drug Interactions
Metabolism/Transport Effects As phenytoin: **Substrate** of CYP2C9 (major), 2C19 (major), 3A4 (minor); **Induces** CYP2B6 (strong), 2C8 (strong), 2C9 (strong), 2C19 (strong), 3A4 (strong)

Avoid Concomitant Use
Avoid concomitant use of Fosphenytoin with any of the following: Crizotinib; Darunavir; Dronedarone; Etravirine; Everolimus; Lapatinib; Lurasidone; Nilotinib; Pazopanib; Praziquantel; Ranolazine; Roflumilast; RomiDEPsin; Ticagrelor; Tolvaptan; Vandetanib

Increased Effect/Toxicity

Fosphenytoin may increase the levels/effects of: Alcohol (Ethyl); Clarithromycin; CNS Depressants; Fosamprenavir; Lithium; Methotrimeprazine; Selective Serotonin Reuptake Inhibitors; Vecuronium; Vitamin K Antagonists

The levels/effects of Fosphenytoin may be increased by: Allopurinol; Amiodarone; Antifungal Agents (Azole Derivatives, Systemic); Benzodiazepines; Calcium Channel Blockers; Capecitabine; CarBAMazepine; Carbonic Anhydrase Inhibitors; CeFAZolin; Chloramphenicol; Cimetidine; Clarithromycin; Conivaptan; CYP2C19 Inhibitors (Moderate); CYP2C19 Inhibitors (Strong); CYP2C9 Inhibitors (Moderate); CYP2C9 Inhibitors (Strong); Dexmethylphenidate; Disulfiram; Droperidol; Efavirenz; Felbamate; Floxuridine; Fluconazole; Fluorouracil; Fluorouracil (Systemic); Fluorouracil (Topical); FLUoxetine; FluvoxaMINE; HydrOXYzine; Isoniazid; Methotrimeprazine; Methylphenidate; MetroNIDAZOLE; MetroNIDAZOLE (Systemic); Proton Pump Inhibitors; Sertraline; Sulfonamide Derivatives; Tacrolimus (Systemic); Ticlopidine; Topiramate; Trimethoprim; Vitamin K Antagonists

Decreased Effect

Fosphenytoin may decrease the levels/effects of: Acetaminophen; Amiodarone; Antifungal Agents (Azole Derivatives, Systemic); Brentuximab Vedotin; CarBAMazepine; Chloramphenicol; Clarithromycin; CloZAPine; Contraceptives (Estrogens); Contraceptives (Progestins); Crizotinib; CycloSPORINE; CycloSPORINE (Systemic); CYP2B6 Substrates; CYP2C19 Substrates; CYP2C8 Substrates (High risk); CYP2C9 Substrates (High risk); CYP3A4 Substrates; Darunavir; Deferasirox; Diclofenac; Disopyramide; Divalproex; Doxycycline; Dronedarone; Efavirenz; Etoposide; Etoposide Phosphate; Etravirine; Everolimus; Exemestane; Felbamate; Flunarizine; Gefitinib; GuanFACINE; HMG-CoA Reductase Inhibitors; Imatinib; Irinotecan; Ixabepilone; Lacosamide; LamoTRIgine; Lapatinib; Levodopa; Linagliptin; Loop Diuretics; Lopinavir; Lurasidone; Maraviroc; Mebendazole; Meperidine; Methadone; MetroNIDAZOLE; MetroNIDAZOLE (Systemic); Metyrapone; Mexiletine; Nilotinib; Pazopanib; Praziquantel; QUEtiapine; QuiNIDine; QuiNINE; Ranolazine; Ritonavir; Rivaroxaban; Roflumilast; RomiDEPsin; Saxagliptin; Sertraline; SORAfenib; Tacrolimus (Systemic); Tadalafil; Teniposide; Theophylline Derivatives; Thyroid Products; Ticagrelor; Tipranavir; Tolvaptan; Topiramate; Treprostinil; Ulipristal; Valproic Acid; Vandetanib; Vecuronium; Vemurafenib; Zonisamide

The levels/effects of Fosphenytoin may be decreased by: Antacids; Barbiturates; CarBAMazepine; Ciprofloxacin; Ciprofloxacin (Systemic); CISplatin; CYP2C19 Inducers (Strong); CYP2C9 Inducers (Highly Effective); Diazoxide; Divalproex; Folic Acid; Fosamprenavir; Ketorolac; Ketorolac (Nasal); Ketorolac (Systemic); Leucovorin Calcium-Levoleucovorin; Levomefolate; Lopinavir; Mefloquine; Methylfolate; Peginterferon Alfa-2b; Pyridoxine; Rifamycin Derivatives; Ritonavir; Theophylline Derivatives; Tipranavir; Tocilizumab; Valproic Acid; Vigabatrin

Ethanol/Nutrition/Herb Interactions Ethanol:

Acute use: Avoid or limit ethanol (inhibits metabolism of phenytoin). Ethanol may also increase CNS depression; monitor for increased effects with coadministration. Caution patients about effects.

Chronic use: Avoid or limit ethanol (stimulates metabolism of phenytoin).

Stability Refrigerate at 2°C to 8°C (36°F to 46°F). Do not store at room temperature for more than 48 hours. Do not use vials that develop particulate matter. Must be diluted to concentrations of 1.5-25 mg PE/mL, in normal saline or D_5W, for I.V. infusion.

Mechanism of Action Diphosphate ester salt of phenytoin which acts as a water soluble prodrug of phenytoin; after administration, plasma esterases convert fosphenytoin to phosphate, formaldehyde, and phenytoin as the active moiety; phenytoin works by stabilizing neuronal membranes and decreasing seizure activity by increasing efflux or decreasing influx of sodium ions across cell membranes in the motor cortex during generation of nerve impulses

Pharmacodynamics/Kinetics Also refer to Phenytoin monograph for additional information.

Protein binding: Fosphenytoin: 95% to 99% to albumin; can displace phenytoin and increase free fraction (up to 30% unbound) during the period required for conversion of fosphenytoin to phenytoin

Metabolism: Fosphenytoin is rapidly converted via hydrolysis to phenytoin; phenytoin is metabolized in the liver and forms metabolites

Bioavailability: I.M.: Fosphenytoin: 100%

Half-life elimination:

Fosphenytoin: 15 minutes

Phenytoin: Variable (mean: 12-29 hours); kinetics of phenytoin are saturable

Time to peak: Conversion to phenytoin: Following I.V. administration (maximum rate of administration): 15 minutes; following I.M. administration, peak phenytoin levels are reached in 3 hours

Excretion: Phenytoin: Urine (as inactive metabolites)

FOSPHENYTOIN

◄ **Dosage**

Geriatric Phenytoin clearance is decreased in geriatric patients; lower doses may be required. In addition, older adults may have lower serum albumin which may increase the free fraction and, therefore, pharmacologic response. Refer to adult dosing.

Adult

The dose, concentration in solutions, and infusion rates for fosphenytoin are expressed as phenytoin sodium equivalents (PE); fosphenytoin should always be prescribed and dispensed in phenytoin sodium equivalents (PE)

Status epilepticus: I.V.: Loading dose: 15-20 mg PE/kg I.V. administered at 100-150 mg PE/minute

Nonemergent loading and maintenance dosing: I.V. or I.M.:

Loading dose: 10-20 mg PE/kg (I.V. rate: Infuse over 30 minutes; maximum rate: 150 mg PE/minute)

Initial daily maintenance dose: 4-6 mg PE/kg/day

Substitution for oral phenytoin therapy: I.M. or I.V.: May be substituted for oral phenytoin sodium at the same total daily dose; however, Dilantin® capsules are ~90% bioavailable by the oral route; phenytoin, supplied as fosphenytoin, is 100% bioavailable by both the I.M. and I.V. routes; for this reason, plasma phenytoin concentrations may increase when I.M. or I.V. fosphenytoin is substituted for oral phenytoin sodium therapy; in clinical trials, I.M. fosphenytoin was administered as a single daily dose utilizing either 1 or 2 injection sites; some patients may require more frequent dosing

Renal Impairment Free phenytoin levels should be monitored closely in patients with renal disease or in those with hypoalbuminemia; furthermore, fosphenytoin clearance to phenytoin may be increased without a similar increase in phenytoin clearance in these patients leading to increase frequency and severity of adverse events.

Hepatic Impairment Phenytoin clearance may be substantially reduced in cirrhosis and plasma level monitoring with dose adjustment advisable. Free phenytoin levels should be monitored closely in patients with hepatic disease or in those with hypoalbuminemia; furthermore, fosphenytoin clearance to phenytoin may be increased without a similar increase in phenytoin clearance in these patients leading to increased frequency and severity of adverse events.

Administration Since there is no precipitation problem with fosphenytoin, no I.V. filter is required; I.V. administration rate should not exceed 150 mg/minute

Monitoring Parameters Continuous blood pressure, ECG, and respiratory function monitoring with loading dose and for 10-20 minutes following infusion; vital signs, CBC, liver function tests, plasma level monitoring (plasma levels should not be measured until conversion to phenytoin is complete, ~2 hours after an I.V. infusion or ~4 hours after an I.M. injection)

Reference Range

Therapeutic: 10-20 mcg/mL (SI: 40-79 µmol/L); toxicity is measured clinically, and some patients require levels outside the suggested therapeutic range

Toxic: 30-50 mcg/mL (SI: 120-200 µmol/L)

Lethal: >100 mcg/mL (SI: >400 µmol/L)

Manifestations of toxicity:

Nystagmus: 20 mcg/mL (SI: 79 µmol/L)

Ataxia: 30 mcg/mL (SI: 118.9 µmol/L)

Decreased mental status: 40 mcg/mL (SI: 159 µmol/L)

Coma: 50 mcg/mL (SI: 200 µmol/L)

Peak serum phenytoin level after a 375 mg I.M. fosphenytoin dose in healthy males: 5.7 mcg/mL

Peak serum fosphenytoin levels and phenytoin levels after a 1.2 g infusion (I.V.) in healthy subjects over 30 minutes were 129 mcg/mL and 17.2 mcg/mL, respectively

Test Interactions Falsely high plasma phenytoin concentrations (due to cross-reactivity with fosphenytoin) when measured by immunoanalytical techniques (eg, TD_x®, TD_xFL_x™, Emit® 2000) prior to complete conversion of fosphenytoin to phenytoin. Phenytoin may produce falsely low results for dexamethasone or metyrapone tests.

Pharmacotherapy Pearls 1.5 mg fosphenytoin is approximately equivalent to 1 mg phenytoin; equimolar fosphenytoin dose is 375 mg (75 mg/mL solution) to phenytoin 250 mg (50 mg/mL); 0.0037 mmol phosphate/mg PE fosphenytoin

Water solubility: 142 mg/mL at pH of 9

Antiarrhythmic effects may be similar to phenytoin; parenteral product contains no propylene sterol; this should allow for rapid intravenous bolus dosing without cardiovascular complications; formaldehyde production is not expected to be clinically consequential (about 200 mg) if used for one week

Special Geriatric Considerations No significant changes in fosphenytoin pharmacokinetics with age have been noted. Phenytoin clearance is decreased in the elderly and lower doses may be needed. Elderly may have reduced hepatic clearance due to age decline in Phase I metabolism. Elderly may have low albumin which will increase free fraction and, therefore, pharmacologic response. Monitor closely in those who are hypoalbuminemic. Free fraction measurements advised, also elderly may display a higher incidence of adverse effects (cardiovascular) when using the I.V. loading regimen; therefore, it is recommended to decrease loading I.V. dose to 25 mg/minute.

Dosage Forms Excipient information presented when available (limited, particularly for generics); consult specific product labeling.

Injection, solution, as sodium: 75 mg/mL (2 mL, 10 mL) [equivalent to phenytoin sodium 50 mg/mL]

Cerebyx®: 75 mg/mL (2 mL) [equivalent to phenytoin sodium 50 mg/mL]

Injection, solution, as sodium [preservative free]: 75 mg/mL (2 mL)

◆ **Fosphenytoin Sodium** see Fosphenytoin on page 793
◆ **Fosrenol®** see Lanthanum on page 1032
◆ **Fragmin®** see Dalteparin on page 445
◆ **Freezone® [OTC]** see Salicylic Acid on page 1648
◆ **Frova®** see Frovatriptan on page 797

Frovatriptan (froe va TRIP tan)

Medication Safety Issues
International issues:

Allegro: Brand name for frovatriptan [Germany], but also the brand name for fluticasone [Israel]

Allegro [Germany] may be confused with Allegra and Allegra-D brand names for fexofenadine and fexofenadine/pseudoehedrine, respectively, in the [U.S., Canada, and multiple international markets]

Brand Names: U.S. Frova®
Brand Names: Canada Frova®
Index Terms Frovatriptan Succinate
Generic Availability (U.S.) No
Pharmacologic Category Antimigraine Agent; Serotonin 5-HT$_{1B, 1D}$ Receptor Agonist
Use Acute treatment of migraine with or without aura
Contraindications Hypersensitivity to frovatriptan or any component of the formulation; patients with ischemic heart disease or signs or symptoms of ischemic heart disease (including Prinzmetal's angina, angina pectoris, myocardial infarction, silent myocardial ischemia); cerebrovascular syndromes (including strokes, transient ischemic attacks); peripheral vascular syndromes (including ischemic bowel disease); uncontrolled hypertension; use within 24 hours of ergotamine derivatives; use within 24 hours of another 5-HT$_1$ agonist; management of hemiplegic or basilar migraine

Canadian labeling: Additional contraindications (not in U.S. labeling): Cardiac arrhythmias, valvular heart disease, congenital heart disease, atherosclerotic disease; management of ophthalmoplegic migraine; severe hepatic impairment

Warnings/Precautions Not intended for migraine prophylaxis, or treatment of cluster headaches, hemiplegic or basilar migraines. Rule out underlying neurologic disease in patients with atypical headache, migraine (with no prior history of migraine) or inadequate clinical response to initial dosing. Cardiac events (coronary artery vasospasm, transient ischemia, MI, ventricular tachycardia/fibrillation, cardiac arrest, and death), cerebral/subarachnoid hemorrhage, stroke, peripheral vascular ischemia, and colonic ischemia have been reported with 5-HT$_1$ agonist administration. May cause vasospastic reactions resulting in colonic, peripheral, or coronary ischemia. Do not give to patients with risk factors for CAD until a cardiovascular evaluation has been performed; if evaluation is satisfactory, the healthcare provider should administer the first dose and cardiovascular status should be periodically evaluated. Significant elevation in blood pressure, including hypertensive crisis, has also been reported on rare occasions in patients using other 5-HT$_{1D}$ agonists with and without a history of hypertension. May lower seizure threshold, use caution in epilepsy or structural brain lesions. Symptoms of agitation, confusion, hallucinations, hyper-reflexia, myoclonus, shivering, and tachycardia (serotonin syndrome) may occur with concomitant proserotonergic drugs (ie, SSRIs/SNRIs or triptans) or agents which reduce frovatriptan's metabolism.

Adverse Reactions (Reflective of adult population; not specific for elderly)
1% to 10%:

Cardiovascular: Flushing (4%), chest pain (2%), palpitation (1%)

Central nervous system: Dizziness (8%), fatigue (5%), headache (4%), hot or cold sensation (3%), somnolence (≥2%), anxiety (1%), dysesthesia (1%), hypoesthesia (1%), insomnia (1%), pain (1%)

Gastrointestinal: Xerostomia (3%), nausea (≥2%), dyspepsia (2%), abdominal pain (1%), diarrhea (1%), vomiting (1%)

Neuromuscular & skeletal: Paresthesia (4%), skeletal pain (3%)

Ocular: Vision abnormal (1%)

Otic: Tinnitus (1%)

Respiratory: Rhinitis (1%), sinusitis (1%)

Miscellaneous: Diaphoresis (1%)

Drug Interactions

Metabolism/Transport Effects Substrate of CYP1A2 (minor)

Avoid Concomitant Use
Avoid concomitant use of Frovatriptan with any of the following: Ergot Derivatives; Sibutramine

Increased Effect/Toxicity
Frovatriptan may increase the levels/effects of: Ergot Derivatives; Serotonin Modulators

The levels/effects of Frovatriptan may be increased by: Ergot Derivatives; Sibutramine

Decreased Effect
The levels/effects of Frovatriptan may be decreased by: Cyproterone

Ethanol/Nutrition/Herb Interactions Food: Food does not affect frovatriptan bioavailability.

Stability Store at controlled room temperature of 25°C (77°F); excursions permitted to 15°C to 30°C (59°F to 86°F). Protect from moisture.

Mechanism of Action Selective agonist for serotonin (5-HT$_{1B}$ and 5-HT$_{1D}$ receptors) in cranial arteries; causes vasoconstriction and reduces sterile inflammation associated with antidromic neuronal transmission correlating with relief of migraine.

Pharmacodynamics/Kinetics
Distribution: Male: 4.2 L/kg; Female: 3.0 L/kg

Protein binding: ~15%

Metabolism: Primarily hepatic via CYP1A2

Bioavailability: Male: ~20%; Female: ~30%

Half-life elimination: ~26 hours

Time to peak: 2-4 hours

Excretion: Feces (62%); urine (32%; <10% as unchanged drug)

Dosage

Geriatric & Adult Migraine: Oral:
U.S. labeling: 2.5 mg; if headache recurs, a second dose may be given if first dose provided relief and at least 2 hours have elapsed since the first dose (maximum daily dose: 7.5 mg)

Canadian labeling: 2.5 mg; if headache recurs, a second dose may be given if first dose provided relief and at least 4 hours have elapsed since the first dose (maximum daily dose: 5 mg)

Note: The safety of treating more than 4 migraines/month has not been established.

Renal Impairment No adjustment necessary.

Hepatic Impairment No adjustment necessary in mild-to-moderate hepatic impairment; use with caution in severe impairment (has not been studied in severe impairment).
Canadian labeling (not in U.S. labeling): Use is contraindicated in severe hepatic impairment.

Administration Administer with fluids.

Pharmacotherapy Pearls Blocks 5-HT$_{1B}$ and 5-HT$_{1D}$ receptors. Relieves symptoms of migraine by blocking vasoconstrictive and other effects of serotonin.

Special Geriatric Considerations Migraine headaches occur infrequently in elderly; however, since elderly often have cardiovascular disease, careful evaluation of the use of 5-HT agonists is needed to avoid complications with the use of these agents. The pharmacokinetic disposition of these agents is similar to that seen in younger adults.

Dosage Forms Excipient information presented when available (limited, particularly for generics); consult specific product labeling.
Tablet, oral:
Frova®: 2.5 mg

◆ **Frovatriptan Succinate** see Frovatriptan on page 797
◆ **Frusemide** see Furosemide on page 800

Fulvestrant (fool VES trant)

Brand Names: U.S. Faslodex®
Brand Names: Canada Faslodex®
Index Terms ICI-182,780; ZD9238
Generic Availability (U.S.) No
Pharmacologic Category Antineoplastic Agent, Estrogen Receptor Antagonist
Use Treatment of hormone receptor positive metastatic breast cancer in postmenopausal women with disease progression following antiestrogen therapy
Contraindications Hypersensitivity to fulvestrant or any component of the formulation
Warnings/Precautions Hazardous agent - use appropriate precautions for handling and disposal. Use caution in hepatic impairment; dosage adjustment is recommended in patients with moderate hepatic impairment. Safety and efficacy have not been established in severe hepatic impairment. Use with caution in patients with a history of bleeding disorders (including thrombocytopenia) and/or patients on anticoagulant therapy; bleeding/hematoma may occur from I.M. administration.
Adverse Reactions (Reflective of adult population; not specific for elderly) Adverse reactions reported with 500 mg dose.

>10%:
  Endocrine & metabolic: Hot flushes (7% to 13%)
  Hepatic: Alkaline phosphatase increased (>15%; grades 3/4: 1 to 2%), transaminases increased (>15%; grades 3/4: 1 to 2%)
  Local: Injection site pain (12% to 14%)
  Neuromuscular & skeletal: Joint disorders (14% to 19%)
1% to 10%:
  Cardiovascular: Ischemic disorder (1%)
  Central nervous system: Fatigue (8%), headache (8%)
  Gastrointestinal: Nausea (10%), anorexia (6%), vomiting (6%), constipation (5%), weight gain (≤1%)
  Genitourinary: Urinary tract infection (2% to 4%)
  Neuromuscular & skeletal: Bone pain (9%), arthralgia (8%), back pain (8%), extremity pain (7%), musculoskeletal pain (6%), weakness (6%)
  Respiratory: Cough (5%), dyspnea (4%)
<1%, postmarketing, and/or case reports (reported with 250 mg or 500 mg dose): Angioedema, hypersensitivity reactions, leukopenia, myalgia, osteoporosis, thrombosis, urticaria, vaginal bleeding, vertigo

Drug Interactions
  Metabolism/Transport Effects Substrate of CYP3A4 (minor)
  Avoid Concomitant Use There are no known interactions where it is recommended to avoid concomitant use.
  Increased Effect/Toxicity
  The levels/effects of Fulvestrant may be increased by: Conivaptan
  Decreased Effect
  The levels/effects of Fulvestrant may be decreased by: Tocilizumab
Stability Store in original carton under refrigeration at 2°C to 8°C (36°F to 46°F). Protect from light.
Mechanism of Action Estrogen receptor antagonist; competitively binds to estrogen receptors on tumors and other tissue targets, producing a nuclear complex that causes a dose-related down-regulation of estrogen receptors and inhibits tumor growth.
Pharmacodynamics/Kinetics
  Duration: I.M.: Steady state concentrations reached within first month, when administered with additional dose given 2 weeks following the initial dose; plasma levels maintained for at least 1 month
  Distribution: V_d: ~3-5 L/kg
  Protein binding: 99%; to plasma proteins (VLDL, LDL and HDL lipoprotein fractions)
  Metabolism: Hepatic via multiple biotransformation pathways (CYP3A4 substrate involved in oxidation pathway, although relative contribution to metabolism unknown); metabolites formed are either less active or have similar activity to parent compound
  Half-life elimination: 250 mg: ~40 days
  Excretion: Feces (~90%); urine (<1%)
Dosage
  Geriatric & Adult Breast cancer, metastatic (postmenopausal women): I.M.: Initial: 500 mg on days 1, 15, and 29; Maintenance: 500 mg once monthly

◀ **Hepatic Impairment**
Moderate impairment (Child-Pugh class B): Decrease initial and maintenance dose to 250 mg
Severe impairment (Child-Pugh class C): Use has not been evaluated.
Administration For I.M. administration only; do not administer I.V., SubQ, or intra-arterially. Administer 500 mg dose as two 5 mL injections (one in each buttocks) slowly over 1-2 minutes per injection.
Dosage Forms Excipient information presented when available (limited, particularly for generics); consult specific product labeling.
Injection, solution:
Faslodex®: 50 mg/mL (5 mL) [contains benzyl alcohol, benzyl benzoate, castor oil, ethanol 10% w/v]

◆ **Fung-O® [OTC]** see Salicylic Acid on page 1648
◆ **Fungoid® [OTC]** see Miconazole on page 1206
◆ **Furadantin®** see Nitrofurantoin on page 1309
◆ **Furazosin** see Prazosin on page 1505

Furosemide (fyoor OH se mide)

Medication Safety Issues
Sound-alike/look-alike issues:
Furosemide may be confused with famotidine, finasteride, fluconazole, FLUoxetine, fosinopril, loperamide, torsemide
Lasix® may be confused with Esidrix®, Lanoxin®, Lidex®, Lomotil®, Lovenox®, Luvox®, Luxiq®
International issues:
Diuril: Brand name for furosemide [Philippines], but also the brand name for chlorothiazide [U.S., Canada]
Urex: Brand name for furosemide [Australia], but is also brand name for methenamine [multiple international markets]
Urex [Australia] may be confused with Eurax brand name for crotamiton [U.S., Canada, and multiple international markets]
Brand Names: U.S. Lasix®
Brand Names: Canada Apo-Furosemide®; Bio-Furosemide; Dom-Furosemide; Furosemide Injection, USP; Furosemide Special; Lasix®; Lasix® Special; Novo-Semide; Nu-Furosemide; PMS-Furosemide
Index Terms Frusemide
Generic Availability (U.S.) Yes
Pharmacologic Category Diuretic, Loop
Use Management of edema associated with heart failure and hepatic or renal disease; acute pulmonary edema; treatment of hypertension (alone or in combination with other antihypertensives)
Contraindications Hypersensitivity to furosemide or any component of the formulation; anuria
Warnings/Precautions [U.S. Boxed Warning]: If given in excessive amounts, furosemide, similar to other loop diuretics, can lead to profound diuresis, resulting in fluid and electrolyte depletion; close medical supervision and dose evaluation are required. Watch for and correct electrolyte disturbances; adjust dose to avoid dehydration. When electrolyte depletion is present, therapy should not be initiated unless serum electrolytes, especially potassium, are normalized. In cirrhosis, avoid electrolyte and acid/base imbalances that might lead to hepatic encephalopathy; correct electrolyte and acid/base imbalances prior to initiation when hepatic coma is present. Coadministration of antihypertensives may increase the risk of hypotension.

Monitor fluid status and renal function in an attempt to prevent oliguria, azotemia, and reversible increases in BUN and creatinine; close medical supervision of aggressive diuresis is required. May increase risk of contrast-induced nephropathy. Rapid I.V. administration, renal impairment, excessive doses, hypoproteinemia, and concurrent use of other ototoxins is associated with ototoxicity. Asymptomatic hyperuricemia has been reported with use; rarely, gout may precipitate. Photosensitization may occur.

Use with caution in patients with prediabetes or diabetes mellitus; may see a change in glucose control. Use with caution in patients with systemic lupus erythematosus (SLE); may cause SLE exacerbation or activation. Use with caution in patients with prostatic hyperplasia/ urinary stricture; may cause urinary retention. Chemical similarities are present among sulfonamides, sulfonylureas, carbonic anhydrase inhibitors, thiazides, and loop diuretics (except ethacrynic acid). A risk of cross-reaction exists in patients with allergy to any of these compounds; avoid use when previous reaction has been severe. Discontinue if signs of hypersensitivity are noted.

Adverse Reactions (Reflective of adult population; not specific for elderly) Frequency not defined.

Cardiovascular: Acute hypotension, chronic aortitis, necrotizing angiitis, orthostatic hypotension, vasculitis

Central nervous system: Dizziness, fever, headache, hepatic encephalopathy, lightheadedness, restlessness, vertigo

Dermatologic: Bullous pemphigoid, cutaneous vasculitis, erythema multiforme, exfoliative dermatitis, photosensitivity, pruritus, purpura, rash, Stevens-Johnson syndrome, toxic epidermal necrolysis, urticaria

Endocrine & metabolic: Cholesterol and triglycerides increased, glucose tolerance test altered, gout, hyperglycemia, hyperuricemia, hypocalcemia, hypochloremia, hypokalemia, hypomagnesemia, hyponatremia, metabolic alkalosis

Gastrointestinal: Anorexia, constipation, cramping, diarrhea, nausea, oral and gastric irritation, pancreatitis, vomiting

Genitourinary: Urinary bladder spasm, urinary frequency

Hematological: Agranulocytosis (rare), anemia, aplastic anemia (rare), eosinophilia, hemolytic anemia, leukopenia, thrombocytopenia

Hepatic: Intrahepatic cholestatic jaundice, ischemic hepatitis, liver enzymes increased

Local: Injection site pain (following I.M. injection), thrombophlebitis

Neuromuscular & skeletal: Muscle spasm, paresthesia, weakness

Ocular: Blurred vision, xanthopsia

Otic: Hearing impairment (reversible or permanent with rapid I.V. or I.M. administration), tinnitus

Renal: Allergic interstitial nephritis, fall in glomerular filtration rate and renal blood flow (due to overdiuresis), glycosuria, transient rise in BUN

Miscellaneous: Anaphylaxis (rare), exacerbate or activate systemic lupus erythematosus

Drug Interactions

Avoid Concomitant Use

Avoid concomitant use of Furosemide with any of the following: Chloral Hydrate; Ethacrynic Acid

Increased Effect/Toxicity

Furosemide may increase the levels/effects of: ACE Inhibitors; Allopurinol; Amifostine; Aminoglycosides; Antihypertensives; Cardiac Glycosides; Chloral Hydrate; CISplatin; Dofetilide; Ethacrynic Acid; Hypotensive Agents; Lithium; Methotrexate; Neuromuscular-Blocking Agents; RisperiDONE; RiTUXimab; Salicylates; Sodium Phosphates

The levels/effects of Furosemide may be increased by: Alfuzosin; Beta2-Agonists; Corticosteroids (Orally Inhaled); Corticosteroids (Systemic); CycloSPORINE (Systemic); Diazoxide; Herbs (Hypotensive Properties); Licorice; MAO Inhibitors; Methotrexate; Pentoxifylline; Phosphodiesterase 5 Inhibitors; Probenecid; Prostacyclin Analogues

Decreased Effect

Furosemide may decrease the levels/effects of: Lithium; Neuromuscular-Blocking Agents

The levels/effects of Furosemide may be decreased by: Aliskiren; Bile Acid Sequestrants; Fosphenytoin; Herbs (Hypertensive Properties); Methotrexate; Methylphenidate; Phenytoin; Probenecid; Salicylates; Sucralfate; Yohimbine

Ethanol/Nutrition/Herb Interactions

Food: Furosemide serum levels may be decreased if taken with food.

Herb/Nutraceutical: Avoid bayberry, blue cohosh, cayenne, ephedra, ginger, ginseng (American), kola, licorice (may worsen hypertension). Avoid black cohosh, California poppy, coleus, golden seal, hawthorn, mistletoe, periwinkle, quinine, shepherd's purse (may increase antihypertensive effect). Licorice may also cause or worsen hypokalemia.

Stability

Injection: Store at room temperature of 15°C to 30°C (59°F to 86°F). Protect from light. Exposure to light may cause discoloration; do not use furosemide solutions if they have a yellow color. Furosemide solutions are unstable in acidic media, but very stable in basic media. Refrigeration may result in precipitation or crystallization; however, resolubilization at room temperature or warming may be performed without affecting the drug's stability.

I.V. infusion solution mixed in NS or D_5W solution is stable for 24 hours at room temperature. May also be diluted for infusion to 1-2 mg/mL (maximum: 10 mg/mL).

Tablet: Store at 25°C (77°F); excursions permitted to 15°C to 30°C (59°F to 89°F). Protect from light.

Mechanism of Action Inhibits reabsorption of sodium and chloride in the ascending loop of Henle and distal renal tubule, interfering with the chloride-binding cotransport system, thus causing increased excretion of water, sodium, chloride, magnesium, and calcium

◀ **Pharmacodynamics/Kinetics**
Onset of action: Diuresis: Oral, S.L.: 30-60 minutes; I.M.: 30 minutes; I.V.: ~5 minutes
Symptomatic improvement with acute pulmonary edema: Within 15-20 minutes; occurs prior to diuretic effect
Peak effect: Oral, S.L.: 1-2 hours
Duration: Oral, S.L.: 6-8 hours; I.V.: 2 hours
Protein binding: 91% to 99%; primarily to albumin
Metabolism: Minimally hepatic
Bioavailability: Oral tablet: 47% to 64%; Oral solution: 50%; S.L. administration of oral tablet: ~60%; results of a small comparative study (n=11) showed bioavailability of S.L. administration of tablet was ~12% higher than oral administration of tablet (Haegeli, 2007)
Half-life elimination: Normal renal function: 0.5-2 hours; End-stage renal disease: 9 hours
Excretion: Urine (Oral: 50%, I.V.: 80%) within 24 hours; feces (as unchanged drug); nonrenal clearance prolonged in renal impairment

Dosage
Geriatric Oral, I.M., I.V.: Initial: 20 mg/day; increase slowly to desired response.
Adult
Edema, heart failure:
Oral: Initial: 20-80 mg/dose; if response not adequate, may repeat the same dose or increase dose in increments of 20-40 mg/dose at intervals of 6-8 hours; may be titrated up to 600 mg/day with severe edematous states; usual maintenance dose interval is once or twice daily. **Note:** Dosing frequency may be adjusted based on patient-specific diuretic needs.
I.M., I.V.: Initial: 20-40 mg/dose; if response not adequate, may repeat the same dose or increase dose in increments of 20 mg/dose and administer 1-2 hours after previous dose (maximum dose: 200 mg/dose). Individually determined dose should then be given once or twice daily although some patients may initially require dosing as frequent as every 6 hours. **Note:** ACC/AHA 2009 guidelines for heart failure recommend a maximum single dose of 160-200 mg.
Continuous I.V. infusion (Howard, 2001; Hunt, 2009): Initial: I.V. bolus dose 20-40 mg over 1-2 minutes, followed by continuous I.V. infusion doses of 10-40 mg/hour. If urine output is <1 mL/kg/hour, double as necessary to a maximum of 80-160 mg/hour. The risk associated with higher infusion rates (80-160 mg/hour) must be weighed against alternative strategies. **Note:** ACC/AHA 2009 guidelines for heart failure recommend 40 mg I.V. load, then 10-40 mg/hour infusion.
Acute pulmonary edema: *I.V.:* 40 mg over 1-2 minutes. If response not adequate within 1 hour, may increase dose to 80 mg. **Note:** ACC/AHA 2009 guidelines for heart failure recommend a maximum single dose of 160-200 mg.
Hypertension, resistant (Chobanian, 2003; JNC 7): *Oral:* 20-80 mg/day in 2 divided doses
Refractory heart failure: *Oral, I.V.:* Doses up to 8 g/day have been used.
Renal Impairment
Acute renal failure: Doses up to 1-3 g/day may be necessary to initiate desired response; avoid use in oliguric states.
Not removed by hemo- or peritoneal dialysis; supplemental dose is not necessary.
Hepatic Impairment Diminished natriuretic effect with increased sensitivity to hypokalemia and volume depletion in cirrhosis. Monitor effects, particularly with high doses.
Administration
I.V.: I.V. injections should be given slowly. Undiluted direct I.V. injections may be administered at a rate of 20-40 mg per minute; maximum rate of administration for short-term intermittent infusion is 4 mg/minute; exceeding this rate increases the risk of ototoxicity.
Oral: Administer on an empty stomach (Bard, 2004). May be administered with food or milk if GI distress occurs; however, this may reduce diuretic efficacy.
Note: When I.V. or oral administration is not possible, the sublingual route may be used. Place 1 tablet under tongue for at least 5 minutes to allow for maximal absorption. Patients should be advised not to swallow during disintegration time (Haegeli, 2007).
Monitoring Parameters Monitor weight and I & O daily; blood pressure, orthostasis; serum electrolytes, renal function; monitor hearing with high doses or rapid I.V. administration
Special Geriatric Considerations Loop diuretics are potent diuretics; excess amounts can lead to profound diuresis with fluid and electrolyte loss; close medical supervision and dose evaluation is required, particularly in the elderly. Severe loss of sodium and/or increase in BUN can cause confusion. For any change in mental status in patients on furosemide, monitor electrolytes and renal function.
Dosage Forms Excipient information presented when available (limited, particularly for generics); consult specific product labeling.
Injection, solution [preservative free]: 10 mg/mL (2 mL, 4 mL, 10 mL)
Solution, oral: 40 mg/5 mL (5 mL, 500 mL); 10 mg/mL (4 mL, 60 mL, 120 mL)

Tablet, oral: 20 mg, 40 mg, 80 mg
   Lasix®: 20 mg
   Lasix®: 40 mg, 80 mg [scored]

Selected References

Chaudhry AY, Bing RF, Castleden CM, et al, "The Effect of Aging on the Response to Frusemide in Normal Subjects," *Eur J Clin Pharmacol*, 1984, 27(3):303-6.

Mühlberg W, "Pharmacokinetics of Diuretics in Geriatric Patients." *Arch Gerontol Geriatr*, 1989, 9(3):283-90.

Murray MD, Haag, KM, Black PK, et al, "Variable Furosemide Absorption and Poor Predictability of Response in Elderly Patients," *Pharmacotherapy*, 1997, 17(1):98-106.

Gabapentin (GA ba pen tin)

Medication Safety Issues

Sound-alike/look-alike issues:
   Neurontin® may be confused with Motrin®, Neoral®, nitrofurantoin, Noroxin®, Zarontin®

Brand Names: U.S. Neurontin®

Brand Names: Canada Apo-Gabapentin®; CO Gabapentin; Dom-Gabapentin; Mylan-Gabapentin; Neurontin®; PHL-Gabapentin; PMS-Gabapentin; PRO-Gabapentin; RAN™-Gabapentin; ratio-Gabapentin; Riva-Gabapentin; Teva-Gabapentin

Generic Availability (U.S.) Yes

Pharmacologic Category Anticonvulsant, Miscellaneous; GABA Analog

Use Adjunct for treatment of partial seizures with and without secondary generalized seizures in patients with epilepsy; management of postherpetic neuralgia (PHN)

Unlabeled/Investigational Use Neuropathic pain, diabetic peripheral neuropathy, fibromyalgia, postoperative pain, bipolar disorder, restless legs syndrome (RLS), social phobia, vasomotor symptoms

Medication Guide Available Yes

Contraindications Hypersensitivity to gabapentin or any component of the formulation

Warnings/Precautions Antiepileptics are associated with an increased risk of suicidal behavior/thoughts with use (regardless of indication); patients should be monitored for signs/symptoms of depression, suicidal tendencies, and other unusual behavior changes during therapy and instructed to inform their healthcare provider immediately if symptoms occur. Avoid abrupt withdrawal, may precipitate seizures; use cautiously in patients with severe renal dysfunction; male rat studies demonstrated an association with pancreatic adenocarcinoma (clinical implication unknown). May cause CNS depression, which may impair physical or mental abilities. Patients must be cautioned about performing tasks which require mental alertness (eg, operating machinery or driving). Effects with other sedative drugs or ethanol may be potentiated. Gabapentin products are not interchangeable with gabapentin encarbil (Horizant™) due to differences in formulation, indications, and pharmacokinetics.

Adverse Reactions (Reflective of adult population; not specific for elderly)

>10%:
   Central nervous system: Somnolence (20%), dizziness (17% to 28%), ataxia (13%), fatigue (11%)
   Miscellaneous: Viral infection

1% to 10%:
   Cardiovascular: Peripheral edema (2% to 8%), vasodilatation (1%)
   Central nervous system: Fever, hostility, emotional lability, fatigue, headache (3%), ataxia (3%), abnormal thinking (2% to 3%), amnesia (2%), depression (2%), dysarthria (2%), nervousness (2%), abnormal coordination (1% to 2%), twitching (1%), hyperesthesia (1%)
   Dermatologic: Pruritus (1%), rash (1%)
   Endocrine & metabolic: Hyperglycemia (1%)
   Gastrointestinal: Diarrhea (6%), Nausea/vomiting (3% to 4%), abdominal pain (3%), weight gain (2% to 3%), dyspepsia (2%), flatulence (2%), dry throat (2%), xerostomia (2% to 5%), constipation (2% to 4%), dental abnormalities (2%), appetite stimulation (1%)
   Genitourinary: Impotence (2%)
   Hematologic: Leukopenia (1%), decreased WBC (1%)
   Neuromuscular & skeletal: Tremor (7%), weakness (6%), hyperkinesia, abnormal gait (2%), back pain (2%), myalgia (2%), fracture (1%)
   Ocular: Nystagmus (8%), diplopia (1% to 6%), blurred vision (3% to 4%), conjunctivitis (1%)
   Otic: Otitis media (1%)
   Respiratory: Rhinitis (4%), bronchitis (3%), respiratory infection (3%), pharyngitis (1% to 3%), cough (2%)
   Miscellaneous: Infection (5%)

GABAPENTIN

◀ **Drug Interactions**

Avoid Concomitant Use There are no known interactions where it is recommended to avoid concomitant use.

Increased Effect/Toxicity

Gabapentin may increase the levels/effects of: Alcohol (Ethyl); CNS Depressants; Methotrimeprazine; Selective Serotonin Reuptake Inhibitors

The levels/effects of Gabapentin may be increased by: Droperidol; HydrOXYzine; Methotrimeprazine

Decreased Effect

The levels/effects of Gabapentin may be decreased by: Antacids; Ketorolac; Ketorolac (Nasal); Ketorolac (Systemic); Mefloquine

Ethanol/Nutrition/Herb Interactions

Ethanol: May increase CNS depression; monitor for increased effects with coadministration. Caution patients about effects.

Food: Does not change rate or extent of absorption.

Herb/Nutraceutical: Avoid evening primrose (seizure threshold decreased). Avoid valerian, St John's wort, kava kava, gotu kola (may increase CNS depression).

Stability Store at 25°C (77°F); excursions permitted to 15°C to 30°C (59°F to 86°F).

Mechanism of Action Gabapentin is structurally related to GABA. However, it does not bind to $GABA_A$ or $GABA_B$ receptors, and it does not appear to influence synthesis or uptake of GABA. High affinity gabapentin binding sites have been located throughout the brain; these sites correspond to the presence of voltage-gated calcium channels specifically possessing the alpha-2-delta-1 subunit. This channel appears to be located presynaptically, and may modulate the release of excitatory neurotransmitters which participate in epileptogenesis and nociception.

Pharmacodynamics/Kinetics

Absorption: 50% to 60% from proximal small bowel by L-amino transport system

Distribution: V_d: 0.6-0.8 L/kg

Protein binding: <3%

Bioavailability: Inversely proportional to dose due to saturable absorption:

900 mg/day: 60%
1200 mg/day: 47%
2400 mg/day: 34%
3600 mg/day: 33%
4800 mg/day: 27%

Half-life elimination: 5-7 hours; anuria 132 hours; during dialysis 3.8 hours

Excretion: Proportional to renal function; urine (as unchanged drug)

Dosage

Geriatric Studies in elderly patients have shown a decrease in clearance as age increases. This is most likely due to age-related decreases in renal function; dose reductions may be needed.

Adult

Anticonvulsant: Oral:

Initial: 300 mg 3 times/day, if necessary the dose may be increased up to 1800 mg/day

Maintenance: 900-1800 mg/day administered in 3 divided doses; doses of up to 2400 mg/day have been tolerated in long-term clinical studies; up to 3600 mg/day has been tolerated in short-term studies

Note: If gabapentin is discontinued or if another anticonvulsant is added to therapy, it should be done slowly over a minimum of 1 week.

Chronic pain (unlabeled use): Oral: 300-1800 mg/day given in 3 divided doses has been the most common dosage range

Diabetic neuropathy (unlabeled use): Oral: 900-3600 mg/day (Bril, 2011)

Postoperative pain (unlabeled use): Oral: 300-1200 mg 1-2 hours before surgery

Postherpetic neuralgia: Day 1: 300 mg, Day 2: 300 mg twice daily, Day 3: 300 mg 3 times/day; dose may be titrated as needed for pain relief (range: 1800-3600 mg/day, daily doses >1800 mg do not generally show greater benefit)

Restless legs syndrome (RLS) (unlabeled use): Oral: Initial: 300 mg once daily 2 hours before bedtime. Doses ≥600 mg/day have been given in 2 divided doses (late afternoon and 2 hours before bedtime). Dose may be titrated every 2 weeks until symptom relief achieved (range: 300-1800 mg/day). Suggested maintenance dosing schedule: One-third of total daily dose given at 12 pm, remaining two-thirds total daily dose given at 8 pm. (Garcia-Borreguero, 2002; Happe, 2003; Saletu, 2010; Vignatelli, 2006)

Vasomotor symptoms associated with menopause (unlabeled use; Butt, 2008): 300 mg 3 times/day

Renal Impairment Adults: See table on next page.

Hemodialysis: Dialyzable

Gabapentin Dosing Adjustments in Renal Impairment

Creatinine Clearance (mL/min)	Daily Dose Range
≥60	300-1200 mg tid
>30-59	200-700 mg bid
>15-29	200-700 mg daily
15[1]	100-300 mg daily
Hemodialysis[2]	125-350 mg

[1]Cl_{cr}<15 mL/minute: Reduce daily dose in proportion to creatinine clearance.

[2]Single supplemental dose administered after each 4 hours of hemodialysis

Administration Administer first dose on first day at bedtime to avoid somnolence and dizziness. Dosage must be adjusted for renal function; when given 3 times daily, the maximum time between doses should not exceed 12 hours.

Monitoring Parameters Monitor serum levels of concomitant anticonvulsant therapy; suicidality (eg, suicidal thoughts, depression, behavioral changes)

Test Interactions False positives have been reported with the Ames N-Multistix SG® dipstick test for urine protein

Special Geriatric Considerations Studies in the elderly have shown a decrease in clearance as age increases. This is most likely due to age-related decreases in renal function; calculations of Cl_{cr} recommended since dose reductions may be needed.

Product Availability

Gralise™: FDA approved January 2011; availability expected in late 2011
Gralise™ is a once-daily formulation of gabapentin approved for the treatment of postherpetic neuralgia.

Dosage Forms Excipient information presented when available (limited, particularly for generics); consult specific product labeling.

Capsule, oral: 100 mg, 300 mg, 400 mg
  Neurontin®: 100 mg, 300 mg, 400 mg
Solution, oral: 250 mg/5 mL (470 mL)
  Neurontin®: 250 mg/5 mL (470 mL) [cool strawberry-anise flavor]
Tablet, oral: 600 mg, 800 mg
  Neurontin®: 600 mg, 800 mg [scored]

Gabapentin Enacarbil (gab a PEN tin en a KAR bil)

Brand Names: U.S. Horizant™
Index Terms GSK 1838262; Horizant™; Solzira; XP13512
Generic Availability (U.S.) No
Pharmacologic Category Anticonvulsant, Miscellaneous
Use Treatment of moderate-to-severe restless leg syndrome (RLS)
Medication Guide Available Yes
Contraindications There are no contraindication listed within the manufacturer's labeling.
Warnings/Precautions Gabapentin and other antiepileptics are associated with an increased risk of suicidal behavior/thoughts with use (regardless of indication); gabapentin enacarbil is a prodrug of gabapentin and may also increase patient's risk. Patients should be monitored for signs/symptoms of depression, suicidal tendencies, and other unusual behavior changes during therapy and instructed to inform their healthcare provider immediately if symptoms occur. Doses >600 mg/day (not included in approved labeling) should be reduced to 600 mg daily for 1 week prior to stopping. Rat studies demonstrated an association with pancreatic adenocarcinoma (clinical implication unknown). May cause CNS depression, which may impair physical or mental abilities. Patients must be cautioned about performing tasks which require mental alertness (eg, operating machinery or driving). Effects with other sedative drugs or ethanol may be potentiated. Use with caution in patients with renal impairment; use not recommended in patients with severe impairment (Cl_{cr} <30 mL/minute). Gabapentin enacarbil (Horizant™) and other gabapentin products are not interchangeable due to differences in formulation, indications and pharmacokinetics.
Adverse Reactions (Reflective of adult population; not specific for elderly) Percentages reported are for 600 mg/day dosing.
>10%: Central nervous system: Sedation/somnolence (20%), dizziness (13%), headache (12%)
1% to 10%:
  Central nervous system: Fatigue (6%), irritability (4%), balance disorder (<2%), disorientation (<2%), lethargy (<2%), drunk feeling (1%), vertigo (1%)

Gastrointestinal: Nausea (6%), flatulence (3%), xerostomia (3%), appetite increased (2%), weight gain (2%)

Ocular: Blurred vision (<2%)

Drug Interactions

Avoid Concomitant Use There are no known interactions where it is recommended to avoid concomitant use.

Increased Effect/Toxicity

Gabapentin Enacarbil may increase the levels/effects of: Alcohol (Ethyl); CNS Depressants; Methotrimeprazine; Selective Serotonin Reuptake Inhibitors

The levels/effects of Gabapentin Enacarbil may be increased by: Droperidol; HydrOXYzine; Methotrimeprazine

Decreased Effect

The levels/effects of Gabapentin Enacarbil may be decreased by: Ketorolac; Ketorolac (Nasal); Ketorolac (Systemic); Mefloquine

Ethanol/Nutrition/Herb Interactions

Ethanol: Avoid ethanol (may increase CNS depression).

Herb/Nutraceutical: Avoid evening primrose (seizure threshold decreased). Avoid valerian, St John's wort, kava kava, gotu kola (may increase CNS depression).

Stability Store at 25°C (77°F); excursions permitted to 15°C to 30°C (59°F to 86°F). Protect from moisture. Do not remove from original container.

Mechanism of Action Gabapentin enacarbil is a prodrug of gabapentin. Gabapentin is structurally related to GABA. However, it does not bind to GABA_A or GABA_B receptors, and it does not appear to influence synthesis or uptake of GABA. High affinity gabapentin binding sites have been located throughout the brain; these sites correspond to the presence of voltage-gated calcium channels specifically possessing the alpha-2-delta-1 subunit. This channel appears to be located presynaptically, and may modulate the release of excitatory neurotransmitters. These effects on RLS are unknown.

Pharmacodynamics/Kinetics

Absorption: Mediated by active transport via proton-linked monocarboxylate transporter, MCT-1

Distribution: V_d: 76 L

Protein binding: <3%

Bioavailability: With food: ~75%; Fasting: 42% to 65%

Metabolism: Prodrug hydrolyzed primarily in the intestines to active metabolite

Time to peak, plasma: With food: 7.3 hours; Fasting: 5 hours

Half-life elimination: 5-6 hours

Excretion: Urine (94%); feces (5%)

Dosage

Geriatric & Adult Restless legs syndrome (RLS): Oral: 600 mg once daily (at ~5:00 pm); increasing to 1200 mg/day provided no additional benefit and increased side effects

Renal Impairment Note: Estimation of renal function for the purpose of drug dosing should be done using the Cockcroft-Gault formula.

Cl_{cr} >30-59 mL/minute: 600 mg/day on day 1 and day 3, then every day thereafter.

Cl_{cr} <30 mL/minute: Not recommended.

Administration Administer with food at ~5:00 pm daily; tablet should be swallowed whole; do not break, chew, cut, or crush.

Monitoring Parameters Suicidality (eg, suicidal thoughts, depression, behavioral changes)

Special Geriatric Considerations Since many elderly may have a creatinine clearance of <60 mL/minute due to age-related renal function decline, it is advised to estimate (calculate) the creatinine clearance before initiating gabapentin enacarbil.

Dosage Forms Excipient information presented when available (limited, particularly for generics); consult specific product labeling.

Tablet, extended release, oral:

Horizant™: 600 mg

Selected References

Bogan RK, Bornemann MA, Kushida CA, et al, "Long-term Maintenance Treatment of Restless Legs Syndrome With Gabapentin Enacarbil: A Randomized Controlled Study," *Mayo Clin Proc*, 2010, 85(6):512-21.

Garcia-Borreguero D, Stillman P, Benes H, et al, "Algorithms for the Diagnosis and Treatment of Restless Legs Syndrome in Primary Care," *BMC Neurology*, 2011, 11(28): 2-13.

Kushida CA, Becker PM, Ellenbogen AL, et al, "Randomized, Double-Blind, Placebo-Controlled Study of XP13512/GSK1838262 in Patients With RLS," *Neurology*, 2009, 72(5):439-46.

Kushida CA, Walters AS, Becker P, et al, "A Randomized, Double-Blind, Placebo-Controlled, Crossover Study of XP13512/GSK1838262 in the Treatment of Patients With Primary Restless Legs Syndrome," *Sleep*, 2009, 32 (2):159-68.

Vignatelli L, Billiard M, Clarenbach P, et al, "EFNS Guidelines on Management of Restless Leg Syndrome and Periodic Limb Movement Disorder in Sleep," *Eur J Neurol*, 2006, 13(10):1049-65.

Yaltho TC and Ondo WG, "The Use of Gabapentin Enacarbil in the Treatement of Restless Legs Syndrome," *Ther Adv Neurol Disord*, 2010, 3(5):269-75.

◆ **Gabitril®** *see* TiaGABine *on page 1787*
◆ **Gablofen®** *see* Baclofen *on page 181*

Galantamine (ga LAN ta meen)

Medication Safety Issues
Sound-alike/look-alike issues:
Razadyne® may be confused with Rozerem™
Reminyl® may be confused with Amaryl®, Robinul®
Due to patient safety concerns regarding prescribing and dispensing errors between Reminyl® and Amaryl®, Reminyl® (galantamine) is being renamed to Razadyne® (immediate-release) and Razadyne® ER (extended-release). The brand name Reminyl® was discontinued with the July, 2005 distribution of Razadyne®.
International issues:
Reminyl [multiple international markets] may be confused with Amarel [France] and Amaryl [U.S., Canada, and multiple international markets], brand names for glimepiride

Brand Names: U.S. Razadyne®; Razadyne® ER
Brand Names: Canada Mylan-Galantamine ER; PAT-Galantamine ER; Reminyl®; Reminyl® ER
Index Terms Galantamine Hydrobromide
Generic Availability (U.S.) Yes
Pharmacologic Category Acetylcholinesterase Inhibitor (Central)
Use Treatment of mild-to-moderate dementia of Alzheimer's disease
Unlabeled/Investigational Use Severe dementia associated with Alzheimer's disease; mild-to-moderate dementia associated with Parkinson's disease; Lewy body dementia
Contraindications Hypersensitivity to galantamine or any component of the formulation; severe liver dysfunction (Child-Pugh score 10-15); severe renal dysfunction (Cl_{cr} <9 mL/minute)
Warnings/Precautions Use caution in patients with supraventricular conduction delays (without a functional pacemaker in place); Alzheimer's treatment guidelines consider bradycardia to be a relative contraindication for use of centrally-active cholinesterase inhibitors. Use caution in patients taking medicines that slow conduction through SA or AV node. Use caution in peptic ulcer disease (or in patients at risk); seizure disorder; asthma; COPD; mild-to-moderate liver dysfunction; moderate renal dysfunction. May cause bladder outflow obstruction. May exaggerate neuromuscular blockade effects of succinylcholine and like agents. May cause nausea, vomiting, diarrhea, weight loss, and anorexia.
Adverse Reactions (Reflective of adult population; not specific for elderly)
>10%: Gastrointestinal: Nausea (6% to 24%), vomiting (4% to 13%), diarrhea (6% to 12%)
1% to 10%:
Cardiovascular: Bradycardia (2% to 3%), syncope (0.4% to 2.2%: dose related), chest pain (≥1%)
Central nervous system: Dizziness (9%), headache (8%), depression (7%), fatigue (5%), insomnia (5%), somnolence (4%)
Gastrointestinal: Anorexia (7% to 9%), weight loss (5% to 7%), abdominal pain (5%), dyspepsia (5%), flatulence (≥1%)
Genitourinary: Urinary tract infection (8%), hematuria (<1% to 3%), incontinence (≥1%)
Hematologic: Anemia (3%)
Neuromuscular & skeletal: Tremor (3%)
Respiratory: Rhinitis (4%)
Drug Interactions
Metabolism/Transport Effects Substrate (minor) of CYP2D6, 3A4
Avoid Concomitant Use There are no known interactions where it is recommended to avoid concomitant use.
Increased Effect/Toxicity
Galantamine may increase the levels/effects of: Antipsychotics; Beta-Blockers; Cholinergic Agonists; Succinylcholine

The levels/effects of Galantamine may be increased by: Conivaptan; Corticosteroids (Systemic); Selective Serotonin Reuptake Inhibitors
Decreased Effect
Galantamine may decrease the levels/effects of: Anticholinergics; Neuromuscular-Blocking Agents (Nondepolarizing)

The levels/effects of Galantamine may be decreased by: Anticholinergics; Peginterferon Alfa-2b; Tocilizumab

◀ **Ethanol/Nutrition/Herb Interactions**
Ethanol: Avoid ethanol (may increase CNS adverse events).
Herb/Nutraceutical: St John's wort may decrease galantamine serum levels; avoid concurrent use.

Stability Store at 15°C to 30°C (59°F to 86°F). Do not freeze oral solution; protect from light.

Mechanism of Action Centrally-acting cholinesterase inhibitor (competitive and reversible). It elevates acetylcholine in cerebral cortex by slowing the degradation of acetylcholine. Modulates nicotinic acetylcholine receptor to increase acetylcholine from surviving presynaptic nerve terminals. May increase glutamate and serotonin levels.

Pharmacodynamics/Kinetics
Duration: 3 hours; maximum inhibition of erythrocyte acetylcholinesterase ~40% at 1 hour post 8 mg oral dose; levels return to baseline at 30 hours
Absorption: Rapid and complete
Distribution: 175 L; levels in the brain are 2-3 times higher than in plasma
Protein binding: 18%
Metabolism: Hepatic; linear, CYP2D6 and 3A4; metabolized to epigalanthaminone and galanthaminone both of which have acetylcholinesterase inhibitory activity 130 times less than galantamine
Bioavailability: ~90%
Half-life elimination: 7 hours
Time to peak: Immediate release: 1 hour (2.5 hours with food); extended release: 4.5-5 hours
Excretion: Urine (25%)

Dosage
Geriatric & Adult
Alzheimer's dementia (mild-to-moderate): Oral:
Immediate release tablet or solution: Mild-to-moderate dementia of Alzheimer's: Initial: 4 mg twice a day for 4 weeks; if tolerated, increase to 8 mg twice daily for ≥4 weeks; if tolerated, increase to 12 mg twice daily
Range: 16-24 mg/day in 2 divided doses
Extended-release capsule: Initial: 8 mg once daily for 4 weeks; if tolerated, increase to 16 mg once daily for ≥4 weeks; if tolerated, increase to 24 mg once daily
Range: 16-24 mg once daily
Note: Oral solution and tablet should be taken with breakfast and dinner; capsule should be taken with breakfast. If therapy is interrupted for ≥3 days, restart at the lowest dose and increase to current dose.

Conversion to galantamine from other cholinesterase inhibitors: Patients experiencing poor tolerability with donepezil or rivastigmine should wait until side effects subside or allow a 7-day washout period prior to beginning galantamine. Patients not experiencing side effects with donepezil or rivastigmine may begin galantamine therapy the day immediately following discontinuation of previous therapy (Morris, 2001).

Renal Impairment
Moderate renal impairment: Maximum dose: 16 mg/day.
Severe renal dysfunction (Cl_{cr} <9 mL/minute): Use is not recommended

Hepatic Impairment
Moderate liver dysfunction (Child-Pugh score 7-9): Maximum dose: 16 mg/day
Severe liver dysfunction (Child-Pugh score 10-15): Use is not recommended

Administration Administer oral solution or tablet with breakfast and dinner; administer extended release capsule with breakfast. If therapy is interrupted for ≥3 days, restart at the lowest dose and increase to current dose. If using oral solution, mix dose with 3-4 ounces of any nonalcoholic beverage; mix well and drink immediately.

Monitoring Parameters Mental status

Special Geriatric Considerations No dosage adjustment needed.

Dosage Forms Excipient information presented when available (limited, particularly for generics); consult specific product labeling.
Capsule, extended release, oral, as hydrobromide [strength expressed as base]: 8 mg, 16 mg, 24 mg
Razadyne® ER: 8 mg, 16 mg, 24 mg [contains gelatin]
Solution, oral, as hydrobromide: 4 mg/mL (100 mL)
Razadyne®: 4 mg/mL (100 mL)
Tablet, oral, as hydrobromide [strength expressed as base]: 4 mg, 8 mg, 12 mg
Razadyne®: 4 mg, 8 mg, 12 mg

Selected References
Rabins PV, Blacker D, Rovner BW, et al, "Practice Guidelines for the Treatment of Patients With Alzheimer's Disease and Other Dementias," *Am J Psychiatry*, 2007, 164(12 Suppl):5-56. Available at http://www.psych.org/psych_pract/treatg/pg/prac_guide.cfm.

◆ **Galantamine Hydrobromide** *see* Galantamine *on page 807*

♦ **GamaSTAN™ S/D** *see* Immune Globulin *on page 922*
♦ **Gamma Benzene Hexachloride** *see* Lindane *on page 1068*
♦ **Gamma E-Gems® [OTC]** *see* Vitamin E *on page 1921*
♦ **Gamma-E PLUS [OTC]** *see* Vitamin E *on page 1921*
♦ **Gammagard® Liquid** *see* Immune Globulin *on page 922*
♦ **Gammagard S/D®** *see* Immune Globulin *on page 922*
♦ **Gamma Globulin** *see* Immune Globulin *on page 922*
♦ **Gammaplex®** *see* Immune Globulin *on page 922*
♦ **Gamunex® [DSC]** *see* Immune Globulin *on page 922*
♦ **Gamunex®-C** *see* Immune Globulin *on page 922*

Ganciclovir (Systemic) (gan SYE kloe veer)

Medication Safety Issues
Sound-alike/look-alike issues:
Cytovene® may be confused with Cytosar®, Cytosar-U®
Ganciclovir may be confused with acyclovir

Brand Names: U.S. Cytovene®-IV
Brand Names: Canada Cytovene®
Index Terms DHPG Sodium; GCV Sodium; Nordeoxyguanosine
Generic Availability (U.S.) Yes
Pharmacologic Category Antiviral Agent
Use Treatment of CMV retinitis in immunocompromised individuals, including patients with acquired immunodeficiency syndrome; prophylaxis of CMV infection in transplant patients
Unlabeled/Investigational Use CMV retinitis: May be given in combination with foscarnet in patients who relapse after monotherapy with either drug
Contraindications Hypersensitivity to ganciclovir, acyclovir, or any component of the formulation
Warnings/Precautions Hazardous agent - use appropriate precautions for handling and disposal. **[U.S. Boxed Warning]: Granulocytopenia (neutropenia), anemia, and thrombocytopenia may occur.** Dosage adjustment or interruption of ganciclovir therapy may be necessary in patients with neutropenia and/or thrombocytopenia and patients with impaired renal function. **[U.S. Boxed Warning]: Animal studies have demonstrated carcinogenic and teratogenic effects, and inhibition of spermatogenesis;** contraceptive precautions for female and male patients need to be followed during and for at least 90 days after therapy with the drug; take care to administer only into veins with good blood flow. **[U.S. Boxed Warning]: Indicated only for treatment of CMV retinitis in the immunocompromised patient and CMV prevention in transplant patients at risk.**
Adverse Reactions (Reflective of adult population; not specific for elderly)
>10%:
Central nervous system: Fever (48%)
Gastrointestinal: Diarrhea (44%), anorexia (14%), vomiting (13%)
Hematologic: Thrombocytopenia (57%), leukopenia (41%), anemia (16% to 26%), neutropenia with ANC <500/mm^3 (12% to 14%)
Ocular: Retinal detachment (11%; relationship to ganciclovir not established)
Renal: Serum creatinine increased (2% to 14%)
Miscellaneous: Sepsis (15%), diaphoresis (12%)
1% to 10%:
Central nervous system: Chills (10%), neuropathy (9%)
Dermatologic: Pruritus (5%)
<1%, postmarketing, and/or case reports (limited to important or life-threatening): Allergic reaction (including anaphylaxis), alopecia, arrhythmia, bronchospasm, cardiac arrest, cataracts, cholestasis, coma, dyspnea, edema, encephalopathy, exfoliative dermatitis, extrapyramidal symptoms, hepatitis, hepatic failure, pancreatitis, pancytopenia, pulmonary fibrosis, psychosis, rhabdomyolysis, seizure, alopecia, urticaria, eosinophilia, hemorrhage, Stevens-Johnson syndrome, torsade de pointes, renal failure, SIADH, visual loss
Drug Interactions
Avoid Concomitant Use
Avoid concomitant use of Ganciclovir (Systemic) with any of the following: Imipenem
Increased Effect/Toxicity
Ganciclovir (Systemic) may increase the levels/effects of: Imipenem; Mycophenolate; Reverse Transcriptase Inhibitors (Nucleoside); Tenofovir

The levels/effects of Ganciclovir (Systemic) may be increased by: Mycophenolate; Probenecid; Tenofovir
Decreased Effect There are no known significant interactions involving a decrease in effect. ▶

◄ **Stability** Intact vials should be stored at room temperature and protected from temperatures >40°C Reconstitute powder with unpreserved sterile water **not** bacteriostatic water because parabens may cause precipitation; dilute in 250-1000 mL D_5W or NS to a concentration ≤10 mg/mL for infusion.

Reconstituted solution is stable for 12 hours at room temperature, however, conflicting data indicates that reconstituted solution is stable for 60 days under refrigeration (4°C). Stability of parenteral admixture at room temperature (25°C) and at refrigeration temperature (4°C) is 5 days.

Mechanism of Action Ganciclovir is phosphorylated to a substrate which competitively inhibits the binding of deoxyguanosine triphosphate to DNA polymerase resulting in inhibition of viral DNA synthesis

Pharmacodynamics/Kinetics

Distribution: V_d: 15.26 L/1.73 m^2; widely to all tissues including CSF and ocular tissue

Protein binding: 1% to 2%

Half-life elimination: 1.7-5.8 hours; prolonged with renal impairment; End-stage renal disease: 5-28 hours

Excretion: Urine (80% to 99% as unchanged drug)

Dosage

Geriatric Refer to adult dosing. In general, dose selection should be cautious, reflecting greater frequency of organ impairment.

Adult

CMV retinitis: *I.V. (slow infusion):*

Induction therapy: 5 mg/kg/dose every 12 hours for 14-21 days followed by maintenance therapy

Maintenance therapy: 5 mg/kg/day as a single daily dose for 7 days/week or 6 mg/kg/day for 5 days/week

Prevention of CMV disease in transplant patients: *I.V. (slow infusion):* Same initial and maintenance dose as CMV retinitis except duration of initial course is 7-14 days, duration of maintenance therapy is dependent on clinical condition and degree of immunosuppression

Renal Impairment

I.V. (Induction):

Cl_{cr} 50-69 mL/minute: Administer 2.5 mg/kg/dose every 12 hours.

Cl_{cr} 25-49 mL/minute: Administer 2.5 mg/kg/dose every 24 hours.

Cl_{cr} 10-24 mL/minute: Administer 1.25 mg/kg/dose every 24 hours.

Cl_{cr} <10 mL/minute: Administer 1.25 mg/kg/dose 3 times/week following hemodialysis.

I.V. (Maintenance):

Cl_{cr} 50-69 mL/minute: Administer 2.5 mg/kg/dose every 24 hours.

Cl_{cr} 25-49 mL/minute: Administer 1.25 mg/kg/dose every 24 hours.

Cl_{cr} 10-24 mL/minute: Administer 0.625 mg/kg/dose every 24 hours

Cl_{cr} <10 mL/minute: Administer 0.625 mg/kg/dose 3 times/week following hemodialysis.

Intermittent hemodialysis (IHD) (administer after hemodialysis on dialysis days): Dialyzable (50%): CMV Infection: I.V.: Induction: 1.25 mg/kg every 48-72 hours; Maintenance: 0.625 mg/kg every 48-72 hours. **Note:** Dosing dependent on the assumption of 3 times/week, complete IHD sessions.

Peritoneal dialysis (PD): Dose as for Cl_{cr} <10 mL/minute.

Continuous renal replacement therapy (CRRT) (Heintz, 2009; Trotman, 2005): Drug clearance is highly dependent on the method of renal replacement, filter type, and flow rate. Appropriate dosing requires close monitoring of pharmacologic response, signs of adverse reactions due to drug accumulation, as well as drug concentrations in relation to target trough (if appropriate). The following are general recommendations only (based on dialysate flow/ultrafiltration rates of 1-2 L/hour and minimal residual renal function) and should not supersede clinical judgment: CMV Infection:

CVVH: I.V.: Induction: 2.5 mg/kg every 24 hours; Maintenance: 1.25 mg/kg every 24 hours

CVVHD/CVVHDF: I.V.: Induction: 2.5 mg/kg every 12 hours; Maintenance: 2.5 mg/kg every 24 hours

Administration Should not be administered by I.M., SubQ, or rapid IVP; administer by slow I.V. infusion over at least 1 hour. Too rapid infusion can cause increased toxicity and excessive plasma levels.

Monitoring Parameters CBC with differential and platelet count, serum creatinine

Pharmacotherapy Pearls Sodium content of 500 mg vial: 46 mg

Special Geriatric Considerations Adjust dose based upon renal function.

Dosage Forms Excipient information presented when available (limited, particularly for generics); consult specific product labeling.

Injection, powder for reconstitution: 500 mg

Cytovene®-IV: 500 mg

Ganciclovir (Ophthalmic) (gan SYE kloe veer)

Medication Safety Issues
  Sound-alike/look-alike issues:
    Ganciclovir may be confused with acyclovir
Brand Names: U.S. Vitrasert®; Zirgan®
Brand Names: Canada Vitrasert®
Index Terms Nordeoxyguanosine
Generic Availability (U.S.) No
Pharmacologic Category Antiviral Agent, Ophthalmic
Use
  Intravitreal implant: Treatment of CMV retinitis in patients with acquired immunodeficiency syndrome
  Ophthalmic gel: Treatment of acute herpetic keratitis (dendritic ulcers)
Dosage
  Geriatric & Adult
    CMV retinitis: *Intravitreal implant:* One implant for 5- to 8-month period; following depletion of ganciclovir, as evidenced by progression of retinitis, implant may be removed and replaced
    Herpetic keratitis: *Ophthalmic gel:* Apply 1 drop in affected eye 5 times/day (approximately every 3 hours while awake) until corneal ulcer heals, then 1 drop 3 times/day for 7 days
Dosage Forms Excipient information presented when available (limited, particularly for generics); consult specific product labeling.
  Gel, ophthalmic [drops]:
    Zirgan®: 0.15% (5 g) [contains benzalkonium chloride]
  Implant, intravitreal:
    Vitrasert®: 4.5 mg (1s) [released gradually over 5-8 months]

◆ **Ganidin® NR [OTC] [DSC]** *see* GuaiFENesin *on page* 846
◆ **Gani-Tuss DM NR [DSC]** *see* Guaifenesin and Dextromethorphan *on page* 848
◆ **Gani-Tuss® NR** *see* Guaifenesin and Codeine *on page* 848
◆ **GAR-936** *see* Tigecycline *on page* 1794
◆ **Garamycin®** *see* Gentamicin (Ophthalmic) *on page* 820
◆ **Gas-X® [OTC]** *see* Simethicone *on page* 1679
◆ **Gas-X® Children's Tongue Twisters™ [OTC]** *see* Simethicone *on page* 1679
◆ **Gas-X® Extra Strength [OTC]** *see* Simethicone *on page* 1679
◆ **Gas-X® Maximum Strength [OTC]** *see* Simethicone *on page* 1679
◆ **Gas-X® Thin Strips™ [OTC]** *see* Simethicone *on page* 1679
◆ **Gas Free Extra Strength [OTC]** *see* Simethicone *on page* 1679
◆ **Gas Relief Ultra Strength [OTC]** *see* Simethicone *on page* 1679
◆ **Gastrocrom®** *see* Cromolyn (Systemic, Oral Inhalation) *on page* 420

Gatifloxacin (gat i FLOKS a sin)

Brand Names: U.S. Zymar® [DSC]; Zymaxid™
Brand Names: Canada Zymar®
Generic Availability (U.S.) No
Pharmacologic Category Antibiotic, Ophthalmic; Antibiotic, Quinolone
Use Treatment of bacterial conjunctivitis
Contraindications
  Zymar®: Hypersensitivity to gatifloxacin, other quinolone antibiotics, or any component of the formulation
  Zymaxid™: There are no contraindications listed in the manufacturer's labeling.
Warnings/Precautions Severe hypersensitivity reactions, including anaphylaxis, have occurred with systemic quinolone therapy. Reactions may present as typical allergic symptoms after a single dose, or may manifest as severe idiosyncratic dermatologic, vascular, pulmonary, renal, hepatic, and/or hematologic events, usually after multiple doses. Prompt discontinuation of drug should occur if skin rash or other symptoms arise. Prolonged use may result in fungal or bacterial superinfection. For topical ophthalmic use only. Do not inject ophthalmic solution subconjunctivally or introduce directly into the anterior chamber of the eye. Contact lenses should not be worn during treatment of ophthalmic infections.
Adverse Reactions (Reflective of adult population; not specific for elderly)
  1% to 10%:
  Central nervous system: Headache
  Gastrointestinal: Taste disturbance

◄ Ocular: Chemosis, conjunctival hemorrhage, conjunctival irritation, discharge, dry eye, edema, irritation, keratitis, lacrimation increased, pain, papillary conjunctivitis, visual acuity decreased

Drug Interactions

Avoid Concomitant Use There are no known interactions where it is recommended to avoid concomitant use.

Increased Effect/Toxicity There are no known significant interactions involving an increase in effect.

Decreased Effect There are no known significant interactions involving a decrease in effect.

Stability Store between 15°C to 25°C (59°F to 77°F); do not freeze.

Mechanism of Action Gatifloxacin is a DNA gyrase inhibitor, and also inhibits topoisomerase IV. DNA gyrase (topoisomerase II) is an essential bacterial enzyme that maintains the superhelical structure of DNA. DNA gyrase is required for DNA replication and transcription, DNA repair, recombination, and transposition; inhibition is bactericidal.

Pharmacodynamics/Kinetics Absorption: Ophthalmic: Not measurable

Dosage

Geriatric & Adult Bacterial conjunctivitis: Ophthalmic:

Zymar®:

Days 1 and 2: Instill 1 drop into affected eye(s) every 2 hours while awake (maximum: 8 times/day)

Days 3-7: Instill 1 drop into affected eye(s) up to 4 times/day while awake

Zymaxid™:

Day 1: Instill 1 drop into affected eye(s) every 2 hours while awake (maximum: 8 times/day)

Days 2-7: Instill 1 drop into affected eye(s) 2-4 times/day while awake

Administration Concentrated injection (10 mg/mL) must be diluted to 2 mg/mL prior to administration. No further dilution is required for premixed 100 mL and 200 mL solutions. Suspension may be administered through a gastric feeding tube.

Monitoring Parameters Signs of infection

Test Interactions Some quinolones may produce a false-positive urine screening result for opiates using commercially-available immunoassay kits. This has been demonstrated most consistently for levofloxacin and ofloxacin, but other quinolones have shown cross-reactivity in certain assay kits. Confirmation of positive opiate screens by more specific methods should be considered.

Special Geriatric Considerations Evaluate the patient's or caregiver's ability to safely administer the correct dose of ophthalmic medication.

Dosage Forms Excipient information presented when available (limited, particularly for generics); consult specific product labeling. [DSC] = Discontinued product

Solution, ophthalmic [drops]:

Zymar®: 0.3% (5 mL [DSC]) [contains benzalkonium chloride]

Zymaxid™: 0.5% (2.5 mL) [contains benzalkonium chloride]

♦ **Gaviscon® Extra Strength [OTC]** *see* Aluminum Hydroxide and Magnesium Carbonate *on page 80*

♦ **Gaviscon® Liquid [OTC]** *see* Aluminum Hydroxide and Magnesium Carbonate *on page 80*

♦ **Gaviscon® Tablet [OTC]** *see* Aluminum Hydroxide and Magnesium Trisilicate *on page 83*

♦ **Gax-X® Infant [OTC]** *see* Simethicone *on page 1679*

♦ **G-CSF** *see* Filgrastim *on page 733*

♦ **G-CSF (PEG Conjugate)** *see* Pegfilgrastim *on page 1402*

♦ **GCV Sodium** *see* Ganciclovir (Systemic) *on page 809*

♦ **Gelclair®** *see* Mucosal Barrier Gel, Oral *on page 1250*

♦ **Gel-Kam® [OTC]** *see* Fluoride *on page 751*

♦ **Gel-Kam® Rinse** *see* Fluoride *on page 751*

♦ **Gelnique®** *see* Oxybutynin *on page 1365*

♦ **Gelusil® [OTC]** *see* Aluminum Hydroxide, Magnesium Hydroxide, and Simethicone *on page 84*

Gemfibrozil (jem FI broe zil)

Related Information

Hyperlipidemia Management *on page 2021*

Medication Safety Issues

Sound-alike/look-alike issues:

Lopid® may be confused with Levbid®, Lipitor®, Lodine®, Lorabid®, Slo-bid™

Brand Names: U.S. Lopid®

Brand Names: Canada Apo-Gemfibrozil®; Gen-Gemfibrozil; GMD-Gemfibrozil; Lopid®; Mylan-Gemfibrozil; Novo-Gemfibrozil; Nu-Gemfibrozil; PMS-Gemfibrozil

Index Terms CI-719

Generic Availability (U.S.) Yes

Pharmacologic Category Antilipemic Agent, Fibric Acid

Use Treatment of hypertriglyceridemia in Fredrickson types IV and V hyperlipidemia for patients who are at greater risk for pancreatitis and who have not responded to dietary intervention; to reduce the risk of CHD development in Fredrickson type IIb patients without a history or symptoms of existing CHD who have not responded to dietary and other interventions (including pharmacologic treatment) and who have decreased HDL, increased LDL, and increased triglycerides

Contraindications Hypersensitivity to gemfibrozil or any component of the formulation; hepatic or severe renal dysfunction; primary biliary cirrhosis; pre-existing gallbladder disease; concurrent use with repaglinide

Warnings/Precautions Secondary causes of hyperlipidemia should be ruled out prior to therapy. Possible increased risk of malignancy and cholelithiasis. Anemia, leukopenia, thrombocytopenia, and bone marrow hypoplasia have rarely been reported. Periodic monitoring recommended during the first year of therapy. Elevations in serum transaminases can be seen. Discontinue if lipid response not seen. Be careful in patient selection; this is not a first- or second-line choice. Other agents may be more suitable. Adjustments in warfarin therapy may be required with concurrent use. Has been associated with rare myositis or rhabdomyolysis; patients should be monitored closely. Patients should be instructed to report unexplained muscle pain, tenderness, weakness, or brown urine. Use caution when combining gemfibrozil with HMG-CoA reductase inhibitors (may lead to myopathy, rhabdomyolysis). Use with caution in patients with mild-to-moderate renal impairment; contraindicated in patients with severe impairment. Renal function deterioration has been seen when used in patients with a serum creatinine >2 mg/dL.

Adverse Reactions (Reflective of adult population; not specific for elderly)
>10%: Gastrointestinal: Dyspepsia (20%)
1% to 10%:
  Cardiovascular: Atrial fibrillation (1%)
  Central nervous system: Fatigue (4%), vertigo (2%)
  Dermatologic: Eczema (2%), rash (2%)
  Gastrointestinal: Abdominal pain (10%), nausea/vomiting (3%)

Reports where causal relationship has not been established: Alopecia, anaphylaxis, cataracts, colitis, confusion, decreased fertility (male), drug-induced lupus-like syndrome, extrasystoles, hepatoma, intracranial hemorrhage, pancreatitis, peripheral vascular disease, photosensitivity, positive ANA, renal dysfunction, retinal edema, seizure, syncope, thrombocytopenia, vasculitis, weight loss

Drug Interactions
Metabolism/Transport Effects Substrate of CYP3A4 (minor); **Inhibits** CYP1A2 (moderate), 2C8 (strong), 2C9 (strong), 2C19 (strong)
Avoid Concomitant Use
Avoid concomitant use of Gemfibrozil with any of the following: Bexarotene; Bexarotene (Systemic); Clopidogrel; Repaglinide; Simvastatin
Increased Effect/Toxicity
Gemfibrozil may increase the levels/effects of: Antidiabetic Agents (Thiazolidinedione); Atorvastatin; Bexarotene; Bexarotene (Systemic); Carvedilol; Colchicine; CYP1A2 Substrates; CYP2C19 Substrates; CYP2C8 Substrates (High risk); CYP2C9 Substrates (High risk); Diclofenac; Ezetimibe; Fluvastatin; Lovastatin; Pitavastatin; Pravastatin; Repaglinide; Rosuvastatin; Simvastatin; Sulfonylureas; Treprostinil; Vitamin K Antagonists

The levels/effects of Gemfibrozil may be increased by: Conivaptan; CycloSPORINE; CycloSPORINE (Systemic)
Decreased Effect
Gemfibrozil may decrease the levels/effects of: Chenodiol; Clopidogrel; CycloSPORINE; CycloSPORINE (Systemic); Ursodiol

The levels/effects of Gemfibrozil may be decreased by: Bile Acid Sequestrants; Tocilizumab
Ethanol/Nutrition/Herb Interactions
Ethanol: Avoid ethanol to decrease triglycerides.
Food: When given after meals, the AUC of gemfibrozil is decreased.
Stability Store at controlled room temperature of 20°C to 25°C (68°F to 77°F). Protect from light and moisture.
Mechanism of Action The exact mechanism of action of gemfibrozil is unknown, however, several theories exist regarding the VLDL effect; it can inhibit lipolysis and decrease subsequent hepatic fatty acid uptake as well as inhibit hepatic secretion of VLDL; together these actions decrease serum VLDL levels; increases HDL-cholesterol; the mechanism behind HDL elevation is currently unknown

Pharmacodynamics/Kinetics
Onset of action: May require several days
Absorption: Well absorbed
Protein binding: 99%
Metabolism: Hepatic via oxidation to two inactive metabolites; undergoes enterohepatic recycling
Half-life elimination: 1.5 hours
Time to peak, serum: 1-2 hours
Excretion: Urine (~70% primarily as conjugated drug); feces (6%)

Dosage
Geriatric & Adult Hyperlipidemia/hypertriglyceridemia: Oral: 600 mg twice daily; administer 30 minutes before breakfast and dinner
Renal Impairment
Mild-to-moderate impairment: Use caution; deterioration of renal function has been reported in patients with baseline serum creatinine >2 mg/dL
Severe impairment: Use is contraindicated
Hemodialysis: Not removed by hemodialysis; supplemental dose is not necessary
Hepatic Impairment Use is contraindicated.

Administration Administer 30 minutes prior to breakfast and dinner.
Monitoring Parameters Serum cholesterol, LFTs periodically, CBC periodically (first year)
Pharmacotherapy Pearls If no appreciable triglyceride or cholesterol lowering effect occurs after 3 months, the drug should be discontinued
Special Geriatric Considerations Gemfibrozil is the drug of choice for the treatment of hypertriglyceridemia and hypoalphaproteinemia in the elderly; it is usually well tolerated; myositis may be more common in patients with poor renal function. The definition of and, therefore, when to treat hyperlipidemia in the elderly is a controversial issue. The National Cholesterol Education Program recommends that all adults maintain a plasma cholesterol <160 mg/dL. Older adults with one additional risk factor, goal LDL would be <130 mg/dL. It is the authors' belief that pharmacologic treatment be reserved for those who are unable to obtain a desirable plasma cholesterol concentration by diet alone and for whom the benefits of treatment are believed to outweigh the potential adverse effects, drug interactions, and cost of treatment.
Dosage Forms Excipient information presented when available (limited, particularly for generics); consult specific product labeling.
Tablet, oral: 600 mg
Lopid®: 600 mg [scored]

Selected References
Grundy SM, Cleeman JI, Merz CN, et al, "Implications of Recent Clinical Trials for the National Cholesterol Education Program Adult Treatment Panel III Guidelines," *J Am Coll Cardiol*, 2004, 44(3):720-32.
National Cholesterol Education Program (NCEP) Expert Panel on Detection, Evaluation, and Treatment of High Blood Cholesterol in Adults (Adult Treatment Panel III), "Third Report of the National Cholesterol Education Program (NCEP) Expert Panel on Detection, Evaluation, and Treatment of High Blood Cholesterol in Adults (Adult Treatment Panel III) Final Report," *Circulation*, 2002, 106(25):3143-421.

Gemifloxacin (je mi FLOKS a sin)

Brand Names: U.S. Factive®
Brand Names: Canada Factive®
Index Terms DW286; Gemifloxacin Mesylate; LA 20304a; SB-265805
Generic Availability (U.S.) No
Pharmacologic Category Antibiotic, Quinolone; Respiratory Fluoroquinolone
Use Treatment of acute exacerbation of chronic bronchitis; treatment of community-acquired pneumonia (CAP), including pneumonia caused by multidrug-resistant strains of *S. pneumoniae* (MDRSP)
Unlabeled/Investigational Use Acute sinusitis
Medication Guide Available Yes
Contraindications Hypersensitivity to gemifloxacin, other fluoroquinolones, or any component of the formulation
Warnings/Precautions [U.S. Boxed Warning]: There have been reports of tendon inflammation and/or rupture with quinolone antibiotics; risk may be increased with concurrent corticosteroids, organ transplant recipients, and in patients >60 years of age. Rupture of the Achilles tendon sometimes requiring surgical repair has been reported most frequently; but other tendon sites (eg, rotator cuff, biceps) have also been reported. Strenuous physical activity, rheumatoid arthritis, and renal impairment may be an independent risk factor for tendonitis. Discontinue at first sign of tendon inflammation or pain. May occur even after discontinuation of therapy. Use with caution in patients with rheumatoid arthritis; may increase risk of tendon rupture. Fluoroquinolones may prolong QT_c interval; avoid use of

gemifloxacin in patients with a history of QT$_c$ prolongation, uncorrected hypokalemia, hypomagnesemia, or concurrent administration of other medications known to prolong the QT interval (including Class Ia and Class III antiarrhythmics, cisapride, erythromycin, antipsychotics, and tricyclic antidepressants). Use with caution in patients with significant bradycardia or acute myocardial ischemia. Use with caution in individuals at risk of seizures (CNS disorders or concurrent therapy with medications which may lower seizure threshold). Potential for seizures, although very rare, may be increased with concomitant NSAID therapy. Discontinue in patients who experience significant CNS adverse effects (dizziness, hallucinations, suicidal ideation or actions). Use caution in renal dysfunction; dosage adjustment required for Cl$_{cr}$ ≤40 mL/minute.

Fluoroquinolones have been associated with the development of serious, and sometimes fatal, hypoglycemia, most often in elderly diabetics, but also in patients without diabetes. This occurred most frequently with gatifloxacin (no longer available systemically) but may occur at a lower frequency with other quinolones.

Severe hypersensitivity reactions, including anaphylaxis, have occurred with quinolone therapy. Reactions may present as typical allergic symptoms after a single dose, or may manifest as severe idiosyncratic dermatologic, vascular, pulmonary, renal, hepatic, and/or hematologic events, usually after multiple doses. May cause maculopapular rash, usually 8-10 days after treatment initiation; risk factors may include age <40 years, female gender (including postmenopausal women on HRT), and treatment duration >7 days. Prompt discontinuation of drug should occur if skin rash or other symptoms arise. **[U.S. Boxed Warning]: Quinolones may exacerbate myasthenia gravis; avoid use (rare, potentially life-threatening weakness of respiratory muscles may occur).** Avoid excessive sunlight and take precautions to limit exposure (eg, loose fitting clothing, sunscreen); may cause moderate-to-severe phototoxicity reactions. Discontinue use if photosensitivity occurs. Prolonged use may result in fungal or bacterial superinfection, including C. difficile-associated diarrhea (CDAD) and pseudomembranous colitis; CDAD has been observed >2 months postantibiotic treatment. Peripheral neuropathy has been linked to the use of quinolones; these cases were rare. Hemolytic reactions may (rarely) occur with quinolone use in patients with latent or actual G6PD deficiency.

Adverse Reactions (Reflective of adult population; not specific for elderly)
1% to 10%:
Central nervous system: Headache (4%), dizziness (2%)
Dermatologic: Rash (4%)
Gastrointestinal: Diarrhea (5%), nausea (4%), abdominal pain (2%), vomiting (2%)
Hepatic: Transaminases increased (1% to 4%)

Important adverse effects reported with other agents in this drug class include (not reported for gemifloxacin): Allergic reactions, CNS stimulation, hepatitis, jaundice, peripheral neuropathy, pneumonitis (eosinophilic); seizure; sensorimotor-axonal neuropathy (paresthesia, hypoesthesias, dysesthesias, weakness); severe dermatologic reactions (toxic epidermal necrolysis, Stevens-Johnson syndrome); torsade de pointes, vasculitis

Drug Interactions
Avoid Concomitant Use
Avoid concomitant use of Gemifloxacin with any of the following: BCG
Increased Effect/Toxicity
Gemifloxacin may increase the levels/effects of: Corticosteroids (Systemic); Porfimer; Sulfonylureas; Vitamin K Antagonists

The levels/effects of Gemifloxacin may be increased by: Insulin; Nonsteroidal Anti-Inflammatory Agents; Probenecid
Decreased Effect
Gemifloxacin may decrease the levels/effects of: BCG; Mycophenolate; Sulfonylureas; Typhoid Vaccine

The levels/effects of Gemifloxacin may be decreased by: Antacids; Calcium Salts; Didanosine; Iron Salts; Magnesium Salts; Quinapril; Sevelamer; Sucralfate; Zinc Salts

Ethanol/Nutrition/Herb Interactions Herb/Nutraceutical: Avoid dong quai, St John's wort (may also cause photosensitization).

Stability Store at 25°C (77°F). Protect from light.

Mechanism of Action Gemifloxacin is a DNA gyrase inhibitor and also inhibits topoisomerase IV. DNA gyrase (topoisomerase IV) is an essential bacterial enzyme that maintains the superhelical structure of DNA. DNA gyrase is required for DNA replication and transcription, DNA repair, recombination, and transposition; bactericidal

◀ **Pharmacodynamics/Kinetics**
Absorption: Well absorbed from the GI tract
Distribution: V_{dss}: 4.2 L/kg
Protein binding: ~60% to 70%
Metabolism: Hepatic (minor); forms metabolites (CYP isoenzymes are not involved)
Bioavailability: ~71%
Half-life elimination: 7 hours (range 4-12 hours)
Time to peak, plasma: 0.5-2 hours
Excretion: Feces (61%); urine (36%)

Dosage

Geriatric & Adult
Susceptible infections: Oral: 320 mg once daily
Acute exacerbations of chronic bronchitis: Oral: 320 mg once daily for 5 days
Community-acquired pneumonia (mild-to-moderate): Oral: 320 mg once daily for 5 or 7 days (decision to use 5- or 7-day regimen should be guided by initial sputum culture; 7 days are recommended for MDRSP, *Klebsiella*, or *M. catarrhalis* infection)
Sinusitis (unlabeled use): Oral: 320 mg once daily for 10 days

Renal Impairment
Cl_{cr} >40 mL/minute: No adjustment required.
Cl_{cr} ≤40 mL/minute (or patients on hemodialysis/CAPD): 160 mg once daily (administer dose following hemodialysis).

Hepatic Impairment No adjustment required.

Administration May be administered with or without food, milk, or calcium supplements. Gemifloxacin should be taken 3 hours before or 2 hours after supplements (including multivitamins) containing iron, zinc, or magnesium.

Monitoring Parameters WBC, signs/symptoms of infection, renal function

Special Geriatric Considerations The risk of torsade de pointes and tendon inflammation and/or rupture associated with the concomitant use of corticosteroids and quinolones is increased in the elderly population. See Warnings/Precautions regarding tendon rupture in patients >60 years of age.

Dosage Forms Excipient information presented when available (limited, particularly for generics); consult specific product labeling.
Tablet, oral:
Factive®: 320 mg [scored]

Selected References
Khaliq Y and Zhanel GG, "Fluoroquinolone-Associated Tendinopathy: A Critical Review of the Literature," *Clin Infect Dis*, 2003, 36(11):1404-10.

◆ **Gemifloxacin Mesylate** *see* Gemifloxacin *on page 814*
◆ **Genac™ [OTC] [DSC]** *see* Triprolidine and Pseudoephedrine *on page 1872*
◆ **Genaphed™ [OTC] [DSC]** *see* Pseudoephedrine *on page 1545*
◆ **Genaton™ [OTC]** *see* Aluminum Hydroxide and Magnesium Carbonate *on page 80*
◆ **Gencalc® 600 [OTC]** *see* Calcium Salts (Oral) *on page 256*
◆ **Generlac** *see* Lactulose *on page 1022*
◆ **Genfiber™ [OTC] [DSC]** *see* Psyllium *on page 1547*
◆ **Gengraf®** *see* CycloSPORINE (Systemic) *on page 432*
◆ **Gentak®** *see* Gentamicin (Ophthalmic) *on page 820*

Gentamicin (Systemic) (jen ta MYE sin)

Related Information
Aminoglycoside Dosing and Monitoring *on page 2050*
Antibiotic Treatment of Adults With Infective Endocarditis *on page 2053*
Community-Acquired Pneumonia in Adults *on page 2059*

Medication Safety Issues
Sound-alike/look-alike issues:
Gentamicin may be confused with gentian violet, kanamycin, vancomycin
High alert medication:
The Institute for Safe Medication Practices (ISMP) includes this medication (intrathecal administration) among its list of drug classes which have a heightened risk of causing significant patient harm when used in error.

Brand Names: Canada Gentamicin Injection, USP
Index Terms Gentamicin Sulfate
Generic Availability (U.S.) Yes
Pharmacologic Category Antibiotic, Aminoglycoside

Use Treatment of susceptible bacterial infections, normally gram-negative organisms, including *Pseudomonas*, *Proteus*, *Serratia*, and gram-positive *Staphylococcus*; treatment of bone infections, respiratory tract infections, skin and soft tissue infections, as well as abdominal and urinary tract infections, and septicemia; treatment of infective endocarditis

Contraindications Hypersensitivity to gentamicin or other aminoglycosides

Warnings/Precautions [U.S. Boxed Warning]: Aminoglycosides may cause neurotoxicity and/or nephrotoxicity; usual risk factors include pre-existing renal impairment, concomitant neuro-/nephrotoxic medications, advanced age and dehydration. Ototoxicity may be directly proportional to the amount of drug given and the duration of treatment; tinnitus or vertigo are indications of vestibular injury and impending hearing loss; renal damage is usually reversible. May cause neuromuscular blockade and respiratory paralysis; especially when given soon after anesthesia or muscle relaxants.

Not intended for long-term therapy due to toxic hazards associated with extended administration; use caution in pre-existing renal insufficiency, vestibular or cochlear impairment, myasthenia gravis, hypocalcemia, conditions which depress neuromuscular transmission. Dosage modification required in patients with impaired renal function. Prolonged use may result in fungal or bacterial superinfection, including *C. difficile*-associated diarrhea (CDAD) and pseudomembranous colitis; CDAD has been observed >2 months postantibiotic treatment.

Adverse Reactions (Reflective of adult population; not specific for elderly)
>10%:
  Central nervous system: Neurotoxicity (vertigo, ataxia)
  Neuromuscular & skeletal: Gait instability
  Otic: Ototoxicity (auditory), ototoxicity (vestibular)
  Renal: Nephrotoxicity, decreased creatinine clearance
1% to 10%: Cardiovascular: Edema

Drug Interactions
  Avoid Concomitant Use
    Avoid concomitant use of Gentamicin (Systemic) with any of the following: Agalsidase Alfa; Agalsidase Beta; BCG; Gallium Nitrate
  Increased Effect/Toxicity
    Gentamicin (Systemic) may increase the levels/effects of: AbobotulinumtoxinA; Bisphosphonate Derivatives; CARBOplatin; Colistimethate; CycloSPORINE; CycloSPORINE (Systemic); Gallium Nitrate; Neuromuscular-Blocking Agents; OnabotulinumtoxinA; RimabotulinumtoxinB

    The levels/effects of Gentamicin (Systemic) may be increased by: Amphotericin B; Capreomycin; CISplatin; Loop Diuretics; Nonsteroidal Anti-Inflammatory Agents; Vancomycin
  Decreased Effect
    Gentamicin (Systemic) may decrease the levels/effects of: Agalsidase Alfa; Agalsidase Beta; BCG; Typhoid Vaccine

    The levels/effects of Gentamicin (Systemic) may be decreased by: Penicillins

Stability
  Gentamicin is a colorless to slightly yellow solution which should be stored between 2°C to 30°C, but refrigeration is not recommended.
  I.V. infusion solutions mixed in NS or D_5W solution are stable for 24 hours at room temperature and refrigeration.
  Premixed bag: Manufacturer expiration date.
  Out of overwrap stability: 30 days.

Mechanism of Action Interferes with bacterial protein synthesis by binding to 30S and 50S ribosomal subunits resulting in a defective bacterial cell membrane

Pharmacodynamics/Kinetics
  Absorption:
    Intramuscular: Rapid and complete
    Oral: None
  Distribution: Primarily into extracellular fluid (highly hydrophilic); high concentration in the renal cortex; minimal penetration to ocular tissues via I.V. route
    V_d: Increased by edema, ascites, fluid overload; decreased with dehydration
      Adults: 0.2-0.3 L/kg
  Relative diffusion from blood into CSF: Minimal even with inflammation
  CSF:blood level ratio: Normal meninges: Nil; Inflamed meninges: 10% to 30%
  Protein binding: <30%
  Half-life elimination: Adults: 1.5-3 hours; End-stage renal disease: 36-70 hours
  Time to peak, serum: I.M.: 30-90 minutes; I.V.: 30 minutes after 30-minute infusion
  Excretion: Urine (as unchanged drug)
    Clearance: Directly related to renal function

◀ **Dosage**

Geriatric & Adult Individualization is **critical** because of the low therapeutic index.

Use of ideal body weight (IBW) for determining the mg/kg/dose appears to be more accurate than dosing on the basis of total body weight (TBW). In morbid obesity, dosage requirement may best be estimated using a dosing weight of IBW + 0.4 (TBW - IBW).

Initial and periodic plasma drug levels (eg, peak and trough with conventional dosing) should be determined, particularly in critically-ill patients with serious infections or in disease states known to significantly alter aminoglycoside pharmacokinetics (eg, cystic fibrosis, burns, or major surgery).

Usual dosage ranges:

I.M., I.V.:

Conventional: 1-2.5 mg/kg/dose every 8-12 hours; to ensure adequate peak concentrations early in therapy, higher initial dosage may be considered in selected patients when extracellular water is increased (edema, septic shock, postsurgical, or trauma)

Once daily: 4-7 mg/kg/dose once daily; some clinicians recommend this approach for all patients with normal renal function; this dose is at least as efficacious with similar, if not less, toxicity than conventional dosing

Intrathecal: 4-8 mg/day

Indication-specific dosing: I.M., I.V.:

Brucellosis: 240 mg (I.M.) daily or 5 mg/kg (I.V.) daily for 7 days; either regimen recommended in combination with doxycycline

Cholangitis: 4-6 mg/kg once daily with ampicillin

Diverticulitis (complicated): 1.5-2 mg/kg every 8 hours (with ampicillin and metronidazole)

Endocarditis: Treatment: 3 mg/kg/day in 1-3 divided doses

Meningitis *Enterococcus* sp or *Pseudomonas aeruginosa:* I.V.: Loading dose 2 mg/kg, then 1.7 mg/kg/dose every 8 hours (administered with another bacteriocidal drug)

Pelvic inflammatory disease: Loading dose: 2 mg/kg, then 1.5 mg/kg every 8 hours Alternate therapy: 4.5 mg/kg once daily

Plague (*Yersinia pestis***):** Treatment: 5 mg/kg/day, followed by postexposure prophylaxis with doxycycline

Pneumonia, hospital- or ventilator-associated: 7 mg/kg/day (with antipseudomonal beta-lactam or carbapenem)

Synergy (for gram-positive infections): 3 mg/kg/day in 1-3 divided doses (with ampicillin)

Tularemia: 5 mg/kg/day divided every 8 hours for 1-2 weeks

Urinary tract infection: 1.5 mg/kg/dose every 8 hours

Renal Impairment

Conventional dosing:

Cl_{cr} ≥60 mL/minute: Administer every 8 hours

Cl_{cr} 40-60 mL/minute: Administer every 12 hours

Cl_{cr} 20-40 mL/minute: Administer every 24 hours

Cl_{cr} <20 mL/minute: Loading dose, then monitor levels

High-dose therapy: Interval may be extended (eg, every 48 hours) in patients with moderate renal impairment (Cl_{cr} 30-59 mL/minute) and/or adjusted based on serum level determinations.

Intermittent hemodialysis (IHD) (administer after hemodialysis on dialysis days) (Heintz, 2009): Dialyzable (~50%; variable; dependent on filter, duration, and type of IHD):

Loading dose of 2-3 mg/kg loading dose followed by:

Mild UTI or synergy: 1 mg/kg every 48-72 hours; consider redosing for pre-HD or post-HD concentrations <1 mg/L

Moderate-to-severe UTI: 1-1.5 mg/kg every 48-72 hours; consider redosing for pre-HD concentrations <1.5-2 mg/L or post-HD concentrations <1 mg/L

Systemic gram-negative rod infection: 1.5-2 mg/kg every 48-72 hours; consider redosing for pre-HD concentrations <3-5 mg/L or post-HD concentrations <2 mg/L

Note: Dosing dependent on the assumption of 3 times/week, complete IHD sessions.

Peritoneal dialysis (PD):

Administration via PD fluid:

Gram-positive infection (eg, synergy): 3-4 mg/L (3-4 mcg/mL) of PD fluid

Gram-negative infection: 4-8 mg/L (4-8 mcg/mL) of PD fluid

Administration via I.V., I.M. route during PD: Dose as for Cl_{cr} <10 mL/minute and follow levels

Continuous renal replacement therapy (CRRT) (Heintz, 2009; Trotman, 2005): Drug clearance is highly dependent on the method of renal replacement, filter type, and flow rate. Appropriate dosing requires close monitoring of pharmacologic response, signs of adverse reactions due to drug accumulation, as well as drug concentrations in relation to target trough (if appropriate). The following are general recommendations only (based on dialysate flow/ultrafiltration rates of 1-2 L/hour and minimal residual renal function) and should not supersede clinical judgment:

CVVH/CVVHD/CVVHDF: Loading dose of 2-3 mg/kg followed by:

Mild UTI or synergy: 1 mg/kg every 24-36 hours (redose when concentration <1 mg/L)

Moderate-to-severe UTI: 1-1.5 mg/kg every 24-36 hours (redose when concentration <1.5-2 mg/L)

Systemic gram-negative infection: 1.5-2.5 mg/kg every 24-48 hours (redose when concentration <3-5 mg/L)

Hepatic Impairment Monitor plasma concentrations.

Administration

I.M.: Administer by deep I.M. route if possible. Slower absorption and lower peak concentrations, probably due to poor circulation in the atrophic muscle, may occur following I.M. injection; in paralyzed patients, suggest I.V. route.

Some penicillins (eg, carbenicillin, ticarcillin, and piperacillin) have been shown to inactivate aminoglycosides *in vitro*. This has been observed to a greater extent with tobramycin and gentamicin, while amikacin has shown greater stability against inactivation. Concurrent use of these agents may pose a risk of reduced antibacterial efficacy *in vivo*, particularly in the setting of profound renal impairment. However, definitive clinical evidence is lacking. If combination penicillin/aminoglycoside therapy is desired in a patient with renal dysfunction, separation of doses (if feasible), and routine monitoring of aminoglycoside levels, CBC, and clinical response should be considered.

Monitoring Parameters Urinalysis, urine output, BUN, serum creatinine; hearing should be tested before, during, and after treatment; particularly in those at risk for ototoxicity or who will be receiving prolonged therapy (>2 weeks)

Some penicillin derivatives may accelerate the degradation of aminoglycosides *in vitro*. This may be clinically-significant for certain penicillin (ticarcillin, piperacillin, carbenicillin) and aminoglycoside (gentamicin, tobramycin) combination therapy in patients with significant renal impairment. Close monitoring of aminoglycoside levels is warranted.

Reference Range

Timing of serum samples: Draw peak 30 minutes after 30-minute infusion has been completed or 1 hour after I.M. injection; draw trough immediately before next dose

Sample size: 0.5-2 mL blood (red top tube) or 0.1-1 mL serum (separated)

Therapeutic levels:

Peak:

Serious infections: 6-8 mcg/mL (12-17 µmol/L)

Life-threatening infections: 8-10 mcg/mL (17-21 µmol/L)

Urinary tract infections: 4-6 mcg/mL

Synergy against gram-positive organisms: 3-5 mcg/mL

Trough:

Serious infections: 0.5-1 mcg/mL

Life-threatening infections: 1-2 mcg/mL

The American Thoracic Society (ATS) recommends trough levels of <1 mcg/mL for patients with hospital-acquired pneumonia.

Obtain drug levels after the third dose unless renal dysfunction/toxicity suspected

Test Interactions Some penicillin derivatives may accelerate the degradation of aminoglycosides *in vitro*, leading to a potential underestimation of aminoglycoside serum concentration.

Special Geriatric Considerations The aminoglycosides are important therapeutic interventions for infections due to susceptible organisms and as empiric therapy in seriously ill patients. Their use is not without risk of toxicity, however, these risks can be minimized if initial dosing is adjusted for estimated renal function and appropriate monitoring performed. High dose, once daily aminoglycosides have been advocated as an alternative to traditional dosing regimens. Once daily or extended interval dosing is as effective and may be safer than traditional dosing. The interval must be adjusted for renal function.

Dosage Forms Excipient information presented when available (limited, particularly for generics); consult specific product labeling. [DSC] = Discontinued product

Infusion, premixed in NS: 40 mg (50 mL [DSC]); 60 mg (50 mL, 100 mL); 80 mg (50 mL, 100 mL); 100 mg (50 mL, 100 mL); 120 mg (100 mL)

Injection, solution: 40 mg/mL (2 mL, 20 mL)

Injection, solution [pediatric]: 10 mg/mL (2 mL [DSC])

Injection, solution [pediatric, preservative free]: 10 mg/mL (2 mL)

Selected References

Matzke GR, Jameson JJ, and Halstenson CE, "Gentamicin Disposition in Young and Elderly Patients With Various Degrees of Renal Function," *J Clin Pharmacol*, 1987, 27(3):216-20.

◄
Nicolau DP, Freeman CD, Belliveau PP, et al, "Experience With a Once-Daily Aminoglycoside Program Administered to 2184 Adult Patients," *Antimicrob Agents Chemother*, 1995, 39(3):650-5.

Gentamicin (Ophthalmic) (jen ta MYE sin)

Medication Safety Issues
Sound-alike/look-alike issues:
Gentamicin may be confused with gentian violet, kanamycin, vancomycin
Brand Names: U.S. Garamycin®; Gentak®
Brand Names: Canada Diogent®; Garamycin®; Garasone; Gentak®; Gentocin; PMS-Gentamicin
Index Terms Gentamicin Sulfate
Generic Availability (U.S.) Yes
Pharmacologic Category Antibiotic, Aminoglycoside; Antibiotic, Ophthalmic
Use Treatment of ophthalmic infections caused by susceptible bacteria
Dosage
Geriatric & Adult Ophthalmic infections: Ophthalmic:
Ointment: Instill ¹/₂" (1.25 cm) 2-3 times/day to every 3-4 hours
Solution: Instill 1-2 drops every 4 hours, up to 2 drops every hour for severe infections
Dosage Forms Excipient information presented when available (limited, particularly for generics); consult specific product labeling.
Ointment, ophthalmic:
Gentak®: 0.3% (3.5 g)
Ointment, ophthalmic [preservative free]:
Garamycin®: 0.3% (3.5 g)
Solution, ophthalmic [drops]: 0.3% (5 mL, 15 mL)
Garamycin®: 0.3% (5 mL) [contains benzalkonium chloride]
Gentak®: 0.3% (5 mL) [contains benzalkonium chloride]

Gentamicin (Topical) (jen ta MYE sin)

Medication Safety Issues
Sound-alike/look-alike issues:
Gentamicin may be confused with gentian violet, kanamycin, vancomycin
Brand Names: Canada PMS-Gentamicin; ratio-Gentamicin
Generic Availability (U.S.) Yes
Pharmacologic Category Antibiotic, Aminoglycoside; Antibiotic, Topical
Use Used topically to treat superficial infections of the skin
Dosage
Geriatric & Adult Dermatologic infections: Topical: Apply 3-4 times/day to affected area
Dosage Forms Excipient information presented when available (limited, particularly for generics); consult specific product labeling.
Cream, topical: 0.1% (15 g, 30 g)
Ointment, topical: 0.1% (15 g, 30 g)

Glimepiride (GLYE me pye ride)

Related Information
Diabetes Mellitus Management, Adults *on page 2073*
Medication Safety Issues
Sound-alike/look-alike issues:
Glimepiride may be confused with glipiZIDE

Amaryl® may be confused with Altace®, Amerge®, Reminyl®

High alert medication:
The Institute for Safe Medication Practices (ISMP) includes this medication among its list of drugs which have a heightened risk of causing significant patient harm when used in error.

International issues:
Amarel [France], Amaryl [U.S., Canada, and multiple international markets] may be confused with Reminyl brand name for galantamine [multiple international markets]

Amaryl [U.S., Canada, and multiple international markets] may be confused with Almarl brand name for arotinolol [Japan]

Brand Names: U.S. Amaryl®

Brand Names: Canada Amaryl®; Apo-Glimepiride®; CO Glimepiride; Novo-Glimepiride; PMS-Glimepiride; ratio-Glimepiride; Rhoxal-glimepiride; Sandoz-Glimepiride

Generic Availability (U.S.) Yes

Pharmacologic Category Antidiabetic Agent, Sulfonylurea

Use Management of type 2 diabetes mellitus (noninsulin dependent, NIDDM) as an adjunct to diet and exercise to lower blood glucose; may be used in combination with metformin or insulin in patients whose hyperglycemia cannot be controlled by diet and exercise in conjunction with a single oral hypoglycemic agent

Contraindications Hypersensitivity to glimepiride, any component of the formulation, or sulfonamides; diabetic ketoacidosis (with or without coma)

Warnings/Precautions All sulfonylurea drugs are capable of producing severe hypoglycemia. Hypoglycemia is more likely to occur when caloric intake is deficient, after severe or prolonged exercise, when ethanol is ingested, or when more than one glucose-lowering drug is used. It is also more likely in elderly patients, malnourished patients and in patients with impaired renal or hepatic function; use with caution. Autonomic neuropathy, advanced age, and concomitant use of beta-blockers or other sympatholytic agents may impair the patient's ability to recognize the signs and symptoms of hypoglycemia; use with caution.

Loss of efficacy may be observed following prolonged use as a result of the progression of type 2 diabetes mellitus which results in continued beta cell destruction. In patients who were previously responding to sulfonylurea therapy, consider additional factors which may be contributing to decreased efficacy (eg, inappropriate dose, nonadherence to diet and exercise regimen). If no contributing factors can be identified, consider discontinuing use of the sulfonylurea due to secondary failure of treatment. Additional antidiabetic therapy (eg, insulin) will be required. It may be necessary to discontinue therapy and administer insulin if the patient is exposed to stress (fever, trauma, infection, surgery).

Chemical similarities are present among sulfonamides, sulfonylureas, carbonic anhydrase inhibitors, thiazides, and loop diuretics (except ethacrynic acid). Use in patients with sulfonamide allergy is not specifically contraindicated in product labeling, however, a risk of cross-reaction exists in patients with allergy to any of these compounds; avoid use when previous reaction has been severe. Patients with G6PD deficiency may be at an increased risk of sulfonylurea-induced hemolytic anemia; however, cases have also been described in patients without G6PD deficiency during postmarketing surveillance. Use with caution and consider a nonsulfonylurea alternative in patients with G6PD deficiency.

Product labeling states oral hypoglycemic drugs may be associated with an increased cardiovascular mortality as compared to treatment with diet alone or diet plus insulin. Data to support this association are limited, and several studies, including a large prospective trial (UKPDS) have not supported an association.

Adverse Reactions (Reflective of adult population; not specific for elderly)
1% to 10%:
Central nervous system: Dizziness (2%), headache (2%)
Endocrine & metabolic: Hypoglycemia (1% to 2%)
Gastrointestinal: Nausea (1%)
Neuromuscular & skeletal: Weakness (2%)

Drug Interactions
Metabolism/Transport Effects Substrate of CYP2C9 (major)
Avoid Concomitant Use There are no known interactions where it is recommended to avoid concomitant use.
Increased Effect/Toxicity
Glimepiride may increase the levels/effects of: Alcohol (Ethyl); Hypoglycemic Agents; Porfimer

The levels/effects of Glimepiride may be increased by: Beta-Blockers; Chloramphenicol; Cimetidine; Cyclic Antidepressants; CYP2C9 Inhibitors (Moderate); CYP2C9 Inhibitors (Strong); Fibric Acid Derivatives; Fluconazole; GLP-1 Agonists; Herbs (Hypoglycemic Properties); Pegvisomant; Quinolone Antibiotics; Ranitidine; Salicylates; Sulfonamide Derivatives; Voriconazole

◀ **Decreased Effect**
The levels/effects of Glimepiride may be decreased by: Corticosteroids (Orally Inhaled); Corticosteroids (Systemic); CYP2C9 Inducers (Highly Effective); Luteinizing Hormone-Releasing Hormone Analogs; Peginterferon Alfa-2b; Quinolone Antibiotics; Rifampin; Somatropin; Thiazide Diuretics

Ethanol/Nutrition/Herb Interactions
Ethanol: Caution with ethanol (may cause hypoglycemia).
Herb/Nutraceutical: Caution with chromium, garlic, gymnema (may cause hypoglycemia).

Mechanism of Action Stimulates insulin release from the pancreatic beta cells; reduces glucose output from the liver; insulin sensitivity is increased at peripheral target sites

Pharmacodynamics/Kinetics
Onset of action: Peak effect: Blood glucose reductions: 2-3 hours
Duration: 24 hours
Absorption: 100%; delayed when given with food
Distribution: V_d: 8.8 L
Protein binding: >99.5%
Metabolism: Hepatic oxidation via CYP2C9 to M1 metabolite (~33% activity of parent compound); further oxidative metabolism to inactive M2 metabolite
Half-life elimination: 5-9 hours
Time to peak, plasma: 2-3 hours
Excretion: Urine (60%, 80% to 90% as M1 and M2); feces (40%, 70% as M1 and M2)

Dosage
Geriatric Initial: 1 mg/day; dose titration and maintenance dosing should be conservative to avoid hypoglycemia

Adult
Type 2 diabetes: Oral:
Initial: 1-2 mg once daily, administered with breakfast or the first main meal
Adjustment: Allow several days between dose titrations: usual maintenance dose: 1-4 mg once daily; after a dose of 2 mg once daily, increase in increments of 2 mg at 1- to 2-week intervals based upon the patient's blood glucose response to a maximum of 8 mg once daily. If inadequate response to maximal dose, combination therapy with metformin may be considered.

Combination with insulin therapy:
Note: Fasting glucose level for instituting combination therapy is in the range of >150 mg/dL in plasma or serum depending on the patient)
Initial: 8 mg once daily with the first main meal
Adjustment: After starting with low-dose insulin, upward adjustments of insulin can be done approximately weekly as guided by frequent measurements of fasting blood glucose. Once stable, combination-therapy patients should monitor their capillary blood glucose on an ongoing basis, preferably daily.

Conversion from therapy with long half-life agents: Observe patient carefully for 1-2 weeks when converting from a longer half-life agent (eg, chlorpropamide) to glimepiride due to overlapping hypoglycemic effects.

Renal Impairment Cl_{cr} <22 mL/minute: Initial starting dose should be 1 mg and dosage increments should be based on fasting blood glucose levels.

Administration Administer once daily with breakfast or first main meal of the day. Patients that are NPO or require decreased caloric intake may need doses held to avoid hypoglycemia.

Monitoring Parameters Monitor for signs and symptoms of hypoglycemia (fatigue, excessive hunger, profuse sweating, numbness of extremities), fasting blood glucose, hemoglobin A_{1c}

Reference Range
Recommendations for glycemic control in adults with diabetes:
Hb A_{1c}: <7%
Preprandial capillary plasma glucose: 70-130 mg/dL
Peak postprandial capillary blood glucose: <180 mg/dL
Blood pressure: <130/80 mm Hg
Recommendations for glycemic control in older adults with diabetes:
Relatively healthy, cognitively intact, and with a ≥5-year life expectancy: See Adults
Frail, life expectancy <5-years or those for whom the risks of intensive glucose control outweigh the benefits:
Hb A_{1c}: <8% to 9%
Blood pressure: <140/80 mm Hg or <130/80 mm Hg if tolerated

Special Geriatric Considerations Rapid and prolonged hypoglycemia (>12 hours) despite hypertonic glucose injections have been reported with glimepiride. Age, hepatic impairment, and renal impairment are independent risk factors for hypoglycemia; dosage titration should be made at weekly intervals. Intensive glucose control (HbA$_{1c}$ <6.5%) has been linked to increased all-cause and cardiovascular mortality, hypoglycemia requiring assistance, and weight gain in adult type 2 diabetes. How "tightly" to control a geriatric patient's blood glucose needs to be individualized. Such a decision should be based on several factors, including the patient's functional and cognitive status, how well he/she recognizes hypoglycemic or hyperglycemic symptoms, and how to respond to them and other disease states. An HbA_{1c} <7.5% is an acceptable endpoint for a healthy older adult, while <8% is acceptable for frail elderly patients, those with a duration of illness >10 years, or those with comorbid conditions and requiring combination diabetes medications. Patients who are unable to accurately draw up their dose will need assistance, such as prefilled syringes. Initial doses may require considerations for renal function in the elderly with dosing adjusted subsequently based on blood glucose monitoring. For elderly patients with diabetes who are relatively healthy, attaining target goals for aspirin use, blood pressure, lipids, smoking cessation, and diet and exercise may be more important than normalized glycemic control.

Dosage Forms Excipient information presented when available (limited, particularly for generics); consult specific product labeling.

Tablet, oral: 1 mg, 2 mg, 4 mg

Amaryl®: 1 mg, 2 mg, 4 mg [scored]

Selected References

Action to Control Cardiovascular Risk in Diabetes Study Group, Gerstein HC, Miller ME, et al, "Effects of Intensive Glucose Lowering in Type 2 Diabetes," *N Engl J Med*, 2008, 358(24):2545-59.

ADVANCE Collaborative Group, Patel A, MacMahon S, et al, "Intensive Blood Glucose Control and Vascular Outcomes in Patients With Type 2 Diabetes," *N Engl J Med*, 2008, 358(24):2560-72.

American Diabetes Association, "Standards of Medical Care in Diabetes – 2011," *Diabetes Care*, 2011, 34(Suppl 1):11-61.

Brown AF, Mangione CM, Saliba D, et al, "Guidelines for Improving the Care of the Older Person With Diabetes Mellitus," *J Am Geriatr Soc*, 2003, 51(5 Suppl Guidelines):265-80.

"VA/DoD Clinical Practice Guideline for the Management of Diabetes Mellitus," 2010. Available at http://www.healthquality.va.gov/Diabetes_Mellitus.asp

◆ **Glimepiride and Pioglitazone** *see* Pioglitazone and Glimepiride *on page 1460*

◆ **Glimepiride and Pioglitazone Hydrochloride** *see* Pioglitazone and Glimepiride *on page 1460*

◆ **Glimepiride and Rosiglitazone Maleate** *see* Rosiglitazone and Glimepiride *on page 1638*

GlipiZIDE (GLIP i zide)

Related Information

Diabetes Mellitus Management, Adults *on page 2073*

Medication Safety Issues

Sound-alike/look-alike issues:

GlipiZIDE may be confused with glimepiride, glyBURIDE

Glucotrol® may be confused with Glucophage®, Glucotrol® XL, glyBURIDE

Glucotrol XL® may be confused with Glucotrol®

High alert medication:

The Institute for Safe Medication Practices (ISMP) includes this medication among its list of drugs which have a heightened risk of causing significant patient harm when used in error.

Brand Names: U.S. Glucotrol XL®; Glucotrol®

Index Terms Glydiazinamide

Generic Availability (U.S.) Yes

Pharmacologic Category Antidiabetic Agent, Sulfonylurea

Use Management of type 2 diabetes mellitus (noninsulin dependent, NIDDM)

Contraindications Hypersensitivity to glipizide or any component of the formulation, other sulfonamides; type 1 diabetes mellitus (insulin dependent, IDDM); diabetic ketoacidosis

Warnings/Precautions All sulfonylurea drugs are capable of producing severe hypoglycemia. Hypoglycemia is more likely to occur when caloric intake is deficient, after severe or prolonged exercise, when ethanol is ingested, or when more than one glucose-lowering drug is used. It is also more likely in elderly patients, malnourished patients and in patients with impaired renal or hepatic function; use with caution.

Use with caution in patients with severe hepatic disease. It may be necessary to discontinue therapy and administer insulin if the patient is exposed to stress (fever, trauma, infection, surgery). Loss of efficacy may be observed following prolonged use as a result of the progression of type 2 diabetes mellitus which results in continued beta cell destruction. In patients who were previously responding to sulfonylurea therapy, consider additional factors which may be contributing to decreased efficacy (eg, inappropriate dose, nonadherence to diet and exercise regimen). If no contributing factors can be identified, consider discontinuing use of the sulfonylurea due to secondary failure of treatment. Additional antidiabetic therapy (eg, insulin) will be required. Chemical similarities are present among sulfonamides, sulfonylureas, carbonic anhydrase inhibitors, thiazides, and loop diuretics (except ethacrynic acid). Use in patients with sulfonamide allergy is specifically contraindicated in product labeling, however, a risk of cross-reaction exists in patients with allergy to any of these compounds; avoid use when previous reaction has been severe. Patients with G6PD deficiency may be at an increased risk of sulfonylurea-induced hemolytic anemia; however, cases have also been described in patients without G6PD deficiency during postmarketing surveillance. Use with caution and consider a nonsulfonylurea alternative in patients with G6PD deficiency.

Product labeling states oral hypoglycemic drugs may be associated with an increased cardiovascular mortality as compared to treatment with diet alone or diet plus insulin. Data to support this association are limited, and several studies, including a large prospective trial (UKPDS) have not supported an association. Avoid use of extended release tablets (Glucotrol XL®) in patients with known stricture/narrowing of the GI tract.

Adverse Reactions (Reflective of adult population; not specific for elderly) Frequency not defined.

Cardiovascular: Edema, syncope

Central nervous system: Anxiety, depression, dizziness, drowsiness, headache, hypoesthesia, insomnia, nervousness, pain

Dermatologic: Eczema, erythema, maculopapular eruptions, morbilliform eruptions, photosensitivity, pruritus, rash, urticaria

Endocrine & metabolic: Disulfiram-like reaction, hypoglycemia, hyponatremia, SIADH (rare)

Gastrointestinal: Anorexia, constipation, diarrhea, epigastric fullness, flatulence, gastralgia, heartburn, nausea, vomiting

Hematologic: Agranulocytopenia, aplastic anemia, blood dyscrasias, hemolytic anemia, leukopenia, pancytopenia, porphyria cutanea tarda, thrombocytopenia

Hepatic: Hepatic porphyria

Neuromuscular & skeletal: Arthralgia, leg cramps, myalgia, paresthesia, tremor

Ocular: Blurred vision

Renal: Diuretic effect (minor)

Respiratory: Rhinitis

Miscellaneous: Diaphoresis

Drug Interactions

Metabolism/Transport Effects Substrate of 2C9 (major)

Avoid Concomitant Use There are no known interactions where it is recommended to avoid concomitant use.

Increased Effect/Toxicity

GlipiZIDE may increase the levels/effects of: Alcohol (Ethyl); Hypoglycemic Agents; Porfimer

The levels/effects of GlipiZIDE may be increased by: Beta-Blockers; Chloramphenicol; Cimetidine; Clarithromycin; Cyclic Antidepressants; CYP2C9 Inhibitors (Moderate); CYP2C9 Inhibitors (Strong); Fibric Acid Derivatives; Fluconazole; GLP-1 Agonists; Herbs (Hypoglycemic Properties); Pegvisomant; Posaconazole; Quinolone Antibiotics; Ranitidine; Salicylates; Sulfonamide Derivatives; Voriconazole

Decreased Effect

The levels/effects of GlipiZIDE may be decreased by: Corticosteroids (Orally Inhaled); Corticosteroids (Systemic); CYP2C9 Inducers (Highly Effective); Luteinizing Hormone-Releasing Hormone Analogs; Peginterferon Alfa-2b; Quinolone Antibiotics; Rifampin; Somatropin; Thiazide Diuretics

Ethanol/Nutrition/Herb Interactions

Ethanol: Caution with ethanol (may cause hypoglycemia or rare disulfiram reaction).

Food: A delayed release of insulin may occur if glipizide is taken with food. Immediate release tablets should be administered 30 minutes before meals to avoid erratic absorption.

Herb/Nutraceutical: Herbs with hypoglycemic properties may enhance the hypoglycemic effect of glipizide. This includes alfalfa, aloe, bilberry, bitter melon, burdock, celery, damiana, fenugreek, garcinia, garlic, ginger, ginseng (American), gymnema, marshmallow, stinging nettle

Mechanism of Action Stimulates insulin release from the pancreatic beta cells; reduces glucose output from the liver; insulin sensitivity is increased at peripheral target sites

Pharmacodynamics/Kinetics

Duration: 12-24 hours

Absorption: Rapid and complete; delayed with food

Distribution: 10-11 L

Protein binding: 98% to 99%; primarily to albumin

Bioavailability: 90% to 100%

Metabolism: Hepatic via CYP2C9; forms metabolites (inactive)

Half-life elimination: 2-5 hours

Time to peak: 1-3 hours; extended release tablets: 6-12 hours

Excretion: Urine (60% to 80%, 91% to 97% as metabolites); feces (11%)

Dosage

Geriatric & Adult

Type 2 diabetes: Oral:

Immediate release tablet: Initial: 5 mg once daily; titrate in 2.5-5 mg increments no more frequently than every few days based on blood glucose response; if once-daily dose is ineffective, may divide the dose; doses >15 mg/day should be administered in divided doses. Maximum recommended once-daily dose: 15 mg; maximum recommended total daily dose: 40 mg (some clinicians recommend a maximum total daily dose of 20 mg [Defronzo, 1999]).

Extended release tablet (Glucotrol XL®): Initial: 5 mg once daily; usual dose: 5-10 mg once daily; maximum recommended dose: 20 mg/day; preferred method for monitoring response to therapy and adjusting dosage is hemoglobin A_{1c} level at initiation and at ~3-month intervals; alternatively, dosage adjustments based on blood glucose monitoring should be made no more frequently than every 7 days

When transferring from immediate release to extended release glipizide: May switch the total daily dose of immediate release to the nearest equivalent daily dose of the extended release tablet and administer once daily; alternatively, may initiate extended release at 5 mg once daily and titrate accordingly.

When transferring from insulin to glipizide immediate release or extended release tablet:

Current insulin requirement ≤20 units: Discontinue insulin and initiate glipizide at usual dose

Current insulin requirement >20 units: Decrease insulin by 50% and initiate glipizide at usual dose; gradually decrease insulin dose based on patient response.

Renal Impairment The FDA-approved labeling recommends that caution should be used with initial and maintenance dosing in patients with renal impairment; however, no specific dosage adjustment guidelines are provided. The following guidelines have been used by some clinicians (Aronoff, 2007): GFR ≤50 mL/minute: Decrease dose by 50%.

Hepatic Impairment

Immediate release tablet: Initial: 2.5 mg/day

Extended release tablet: There are no dosage adjustments provided in manufacturer's labeling; use of a lower initial and maintenance dose should be considered.

Administration Administer immediate release tablets 30 minutes before a meal to achieve greatest reduction in postprandial hyperglycemia. Extended release tablets should be given with breakfast. Patients that are NPO or require decreased caloric intake may need doses held to avoid hypoglycemia.

Monitoring Parameters Signs and symptoms of hypoglycemia (fatigue, excessive hunger, profuse sweating, numbness of extremities), blood glucose, hemoglobin A_{1c}

Reference Range

Recommendations for glycemic control in adults with diabetes:

Hb A_{1c}: <7%

Preprandial capillary plasma glucose: 70-130 mg/dL

Peak postprandial capillary blood glucose: <180 mg/dL

Blood pressure: <130/80 mm Hg

Recommendations for glycemic control in older adults with diabetes:

Relatively healthy, cognitively intact, and with a ≥5-year life expectancy: See Adults

Frail, life expectancy <5-years or those for whom the risks of intensive glucose control outweigh the benefits:

Hb A_{1c}: <8% to 9%

Blood pressure: <140/80 mm Hg or <130/80 mm Hg if tolerated

Special Geriatric Considerations Glipizide is a useful agent since there are few drug-to-drug interactions and elimination of the active drug is not dependent upon renal function. Intensive glucose control (HbA$_{1c}$ <6.5%) has been linked to increased all-cause and cardiovascular mortality, hypoglycemia requiring assistance, and weight gain in adult type 2 diabetes. How "tightly" to control a geriatric patient's blood glucose needs to be individualized. Such a decision should be based on several factors, including the patient's functional and cognitive status, how well he/she recognizes hypoglycemic or hyperglycemic symptoms, and how to respond to them and other disease states. An HbA$_{1c}$ <7.5% is an acceptable endpoint for a healthy older adult, while <8% is acceptable for frail elderly patients, those with a duration of illness >10 years, or those with comorbid conditions and requiring combination diabetes medications. Patients who are unable to accurately draw up their dose will need assistance, such as prefilled syringes. Initial doses may require considerations for renal function in the elderly with dosing adjusted subsequently based on blood glucose monitoring. For elderly patients with diabetes who are relatively healthy, attaining target goals for aspirin use, blood pressure, lipids, smoking cessation, and diet and exercise may be more important than normalized glycemic control.

◀ **Dosage Forms** Excipient information presented when available (limited, particularly for generics); consult specific product labeling.

Tablet, oral: 5 mg, 10 mg

Glucotrol®: 5 mg, 10 mg [scored; dye free]

Tablet, extended release, oral: 2.5 mg, 5 mg, 10 mg

Glucotrol XL®: 2.5 mg, 5 mg, 10 mg

Selected References

Action to Control Cardiovascular Risk in Diabetes Study Group, Gerstein HC, Miller ME, et al, "Effects of Intensive Glucose Lowering in Type 2 Diabetes," *N Engl J Med*, 2008, 358(24):2545-59.

ADVANCE Collaborative Group, Patel A, MacMahon S, et al, "Intensive Blood Glucose Control and Vascular Outcomes in Patients With Type 2 Diabetes," *N Engl J Med*, 2008, 358(24):2560-72.

American Diabetes Association, "Standards of Medical Care in Diabetes – 2011," *Diabetes Care*, 2011, 34(Suppl 1):11-61.

Brown AF, Mangione CM, Saliba D, et al, "Guidelines for Improving the Care of the Older Person With Diabetes Mellitus," *J Am Geriatr Soc*, 2003, 51(5 Suppl Guidelines):265-80.

"VA/DoD Clinical Practice Guideline for the Management of Diabetes Mellitus," 2010. Available at http://www.healthquality.va.gov/Diabetes_Mellitus.asp

---

Glipizide and Metformin (GLIP i zide & met FOR min)

Related Information

GlipiZIDE *on page 823*

MetFORMIN *on page 1155*

Medication Safety Issues

High alert medication:

The Institute for Safe Medication Practices (ISMP) includes this medication among its list of drugs which have a heightened risk of causing significant patient harm when used in error.

Brand Names: U.S. Metaglip™

Index Terms Glipizide and Metformin Hydrochloride; Metformin and Glipizide

Generic Availability (U.S.) Yes

Pharmacologic Category Antidiabetic Agent, Biguanide; Antidiabetic Agent, Sulfonylurea

Use Indicated as an adjunct to diet and exercise to improve glycemic control in adults with type 2 diabetes mellitus (noninsulin dependent, NIDDM)

Dosage

Geriatric Conservative doses are recommended in the elderly due to potentially decreased renal function; **do not titrate to maximum dose**; should not be used in patients ≥80 years unless renal function is verified as normal

Adult Type 2 diabetes:

Patients inadequately controlled on diet and exercise alone: Initial dose: Glipizide 2.5 mg/metformin 250 mg once daily with a meal. In patients with fasting plasma glucose (FPG) 280-320 mg/dL, initiate therapy with glipizide 2.5 mg/metformin 500 mg twice daily.

Note: Increase dose by 1 tablet/day every 2 weeks (maximum daily dose: Glipizide 10 mg/metformin 2000 mg in divided doses)

Patients inadequately controlled on a sulfonylurea and/or metformin: Initial dose: Glipizide 2.5 mg/metformin 500 mg or glipizide 5 mg/metformin 500 mg twice daily with morning and evening meals; starting dose should not exceed current daily dose of glipizide (or sulfonylurea equivalent) and/or metformin.

Note: Increase dose in increments of no more than glipizide 5 mg/metformin 500 mg (maximum daily dose: Glipizide 20 mg/metformin 2000 mg)

Renal Impairment Contraindicated in the presence of renal disease or renal dysfunction (serum creatinine ≥1.5 mg/dL [males], ≥1.4 mg/dL [females], or abnormal creatinine clearance).

Hepatic Impairment Avoid use in patients with impaired liver function.

Special Geriatric Considerations Metformin should not be used in patients ≥80 years of age unless renal function is verified as normal. **Do not titrate to maximum dose.** Intensive glucose control (HbA$_{1c}$ <6.5%) has been linked to increased all-cause and cardiovascular mortality, hypoglycemia requiring assistance, and weight gain in adult type 2 diabetes. How "tightly" to control a geriatric patient's blood glucose needs to be individualized. Such a decision should be based on several factors, including the patient's functional and cognitive status, how well he/she recognizes hypoglycemic or hyperglycemic symptoms, and how to respond to them and other disease states. An HbA$_{1c}$ <7.5% is an acceptable endpoint for a healthy older adult, while <8% is acceptable for frail elderly patients, those with a duration of illness >10 years, or those with comorbid conditions and requiring combination diabetes medications. Patients who are unable to accurately draw up their dose will need assistance, such as prefilled syringes. Initial doses may require considerations for renal function in the elderly with dosing adjusted subsequently based on blood glucose monitoring. For elderly patients with diabetes who are relatively healthy, attaining target goals for aspirin use, blood pressure, lipids, smoking cessation, and diet and exercise may be more important than normalized glycemic control.

Dosage Forms Excipient information presented when available (limited, particularly for generics); consult specific product labeling. [DSC] = Discontinued product

Tablet, oral: 2.5/250: Glipizide 2.5 mg and metformin hydrochloride 250 mg; 2.5/500: Glipizide 2.5 mg and metformin hydrochloride 500 mg; 5/500: Glipizide 5 mg and metformin hydrochloride 500 mg

Metaglip™ 2.5/250: Glipizide 2.5 mg and metformin hydrochloride 250 mg [DSC]

Metaglip™ 2.5/500: Glipizide 2.5 mg and metformin hydrochloride 500 mg

Metaglip™ 5/500: Glipizide 5 mg and metformin hydrochloride 500 mg

◆ **Glipizide and Metformin Hydrochloride** see Glipizide and Metformin on page 826
◆ **GlucaGen®** see Glucagon on page 827
◆ **GlucaGen® Diagnostic Kit** see Glucagon on page 827
◆ **GlucaGen® HypoKit®** see Glucagon on page 827

Glucagon (GLOO ka gon)

Medication Safety Issues

Sound-alike/look-alike issues:

Glucagon may be confused with Glaucon®

Brand Names: U.S. GlucaGen®; GlucaGen® Diagnostic Kit; GlucaGen® HypoKit®; Glucagon Emergency Kit

Index Terms Glucagon Hydrochloride

Generic Availability (U.S.) No

Pharmacologic Category Antidote; Antidote, Hypoglycemia; Diagnostic Agent

Use Management of hypoglycemia; diagnostic aid in radiologic examinations to temporarily inhibit GI tract movement

Unlabeled/Investigational Use Used with some success as a cardiac stimulant in management of severe cases of beta-adrenergic blocking agent overdosage; treatment of myocardial depression due to calcium channel blocker overdose

Contraindications Hypersensitivity to glucagon or any component of the formulation; insulinoma; pheochromocytoma

Warnings/Precautions Use of glucagon is contraindicated in insulinoma; exogenous glucagon may cause an initial rise in blood glucose followed by rebound hypoglycemia. Use of glucagon is contraindicated in pheochromocytoma; exogenous glucagon may cause the release of catecholamines, resulting in an increase in blood pressure. Use caution with prolonged fasting, starvation, adrenal insufficiency or chronic hypoglycemia; levels of glucose stores in liver may be decreased. Supplemental carbohydrates should be given to patients who respond to glucagon for severe hypoglycemia to prevent secondary hypoglycemia. Monitor blood glucose levels closely.

In patients with hypoglycemia secondary to insulin or sulfonylurea overdose, dextrose should be immediately administered; if I.V. access cannot be established or if dextrose is not available, glucagon may be considered as alternative acute treatment until dextrose can be administered.

May contain lactose; avoid administration in hereditary galactose intolerance, Lapp lactase deficiency, or glucose-galactose malabsorption.

Adverse Reactions (Reflective of adult population; not specific for elderly) Frequency not defined.

Cardiovascular: Hypotension (up to 2 hours after GI procedures), hypertension, tachycardia

Gastrointestinal: Nausea, vomiting (high incidence with rapid administration of high doses)

Miscellaneous: Hypersensitivity reactions, anaphylaxis

Drug Interactions

Avoid Concomitant Use There are no known interactions where it is recommended to avoid concomitant use.

Increased Effect/Toxicity

Glucagon may increase the levels/effects of: Vitamin K Antagonists

Decreased Effect There are no known significant interactions involving a decrease in effect.

Ethanol/Nutrition/Herb Interactions Glucagon depletes glycogen stores.

Stability Prior to reconstitution, store at controlled room temperature of 20°C to 25°C (69°F to 77°F); do not freeze. Reconstitute powder for injection by adding 1 mL of sterile diluent to a vial containing 1 unit of the drug, to provide solutions containing 1 mg of glucagon/mL. Gently roll vial to dissolve. Use immediately after reconstitution. May be kept at 5°C for up to 48 hours if necessary.

◄ **Mechanism of Action** Stimulates adenylate cyclase to produce increased cyclic AMP, which promotes hepatic glycogenolysis and gluconeogenesis, causing a raise in blood glucose levels

Pharmacodynamics/Kinetics

Onset of action: Peak effect: Blood glucose levels: Parenteral:

I.V.: 5-20 minutes

I.M.: 30 minutes

SubQ: 30-45 minutes

Duration: Glucose elevation:

SubQ: 60-90 minutes

I.V.: 30 minutes

Metabolism: Primarily hepatic; some inactivation occurring renally and in plasma

Half-life elimination, plasma: 8-18 minutes

Dosage

Geriatric & Adult

Hypoglycemia: I.M., I.V., SubQ: 1 mg; may repeat in 20 minutes as needed

Note: I.V. dextrose should be administered as soon as it is available; if patient fails to respond to glucagon, I.V. dextrose must be given.

Beta-blocker- or calcium channel blocker-induced myocardial depression (with or without hypotension) unresponsive to standard measures (unlabeled use): I.V.: 3-10 mg (or 0.05-0.15 mg/kg) bolus followed by an infusion of 3-5 mg/hour (or 0.05-0.1 mg/kg/hour); titrate infusion rate to achieve adequate hemodynamic response (ACLS, 2010)

Diagnostic aid:

I.M.: 1-2 mg 10 minutes prior to gastrointestinal procedure

I.V.: 0.25-2 mg 10 minutes prior to gastrointestinal procedure

Administration I.V.: Bolus may be associated with nausea and vomiting. Continuous infusions may be used in beta-blocker overdose/toxicity.

Monitoring Parameters Blood pressure, blood glucose, ECG, heart rate, mentation

Pharmacotherapy Pearls 1 unit = 1 mg

Special Geriatric Considerations No specific recommendations needed.

Dosage Forms Excipient information presented when available (limited, particularly for generics); consult specific product labeling.

Injection, powder for reconstitution:

Glucagon Emergency Kit: 1 mg [contains glycerin (in diluent), lactose 49 mg; equivalent to 1 unit]

Injection, powder for reconstitution, as hydrochloride:

GlucaGen®: 1 mg [contains lactose 107 mg; equivalent to 1 unit]

GlucaGen® Diagnostic Kit: 1 mg [contains lactose 107 mg; equivalent to 1 unit]

GlucaGen® HypoKit®: 1 mg [contains lactose 107 mg; equivalent to 1 unit]

◆ **Glucagon Emergency Kit** see Glucagon on page 827
◆ **Glucagon Hydrochloride** see Glucagon on page 827
◆ **Glucophage®** see MetFORMIN on page 1155
◆ **Glucophage® XR** see MetFORMIN on page 1155
◆ **Glucotrol®** see GlipiZIDE on page 823
◆ **Glucotrol XL®** see GlipiZIDE on page 823
◆ **Glucovance®** see Glyburide and Metformin on page 832
◆ **Glulisine Insulin** see Insulin Glulisine on page 952
◆ **Glumetza®** see MetFORMIN on page 1155
◆ **Glybenclamide** see GlyBURIDE on page 828
◆ **Glybenzcyclamide** see GlyBURIDE on page 828

GlyBURIDE (GLYE byoor ide)

Related Information

Diabetes Mellitus Management, Adults on page 2073

Medication Safety Issues

Sound-alike/look-alike issues:

GlyBURIDE may be confused with glipiZIDE, Glucotrol®

Diaβeta® may be confused with Diabinese®, Zebeta®

Micronase may be confused with microK®, miconazole, Micronor®, Microzide™

High alert medication:

The Institute for Safe Medication Practices (ISMP) includes this medication among its list of drugs which have a heightened risk of causing significant patient harm when used in error.

Brand Names: U.S. DiaBeta®; Glynase® PresTab®

Brand Names: Canada Apo-Glyburide®; Diaβeta®; Dom-Glyburide; Euglucon®; Med-Glybe; Mylan-Glybe; Novo-Glyburide; Nu-Glyburide; PMS-Glyburide; PRO-Glyburide; ratio-Glyburide; Riva-Glyburide; Sandoz-Glyburide; Teva-Glyburide

Index Terms Diabeta; Glibenclamide; Glybenclamide; Glybenzcyclamide; Micronase

Generic Availability (U.S.) Yes

Pharmacologic Category Antidiabetic Agent, Sulfonylurea

Use Adjunct to diet and exercise for the management of type 2 diabetes mellitus (noninsulin dependent, NIDDM)

Unlabeled/Investigational Use Alternative to insulin in women for the treatment of gestational diabetes mellitus (GDM) (11-33 weeks gestation)

Contraindications Hypersensitivity to glyburide or any component of the formulation; type 1 diabetes mellitus (insulin dependent, IDDM), diabetic ketoacidosis; concomitant use with bosentan

Warnings/Precautions All sulfonylurea drugs are capable of producing severe hypoglycemia. Hypoglycemia is more likely to occur when caloric intake is deficient, after severe or prolonged exercise, when ethanol is ingested, or when more than one glucose-lowering drug is used. It is also more likely in elderly patients, malnourished patients and in patients with impaired renal or hepatic function; use with caution.

It may be necessary to discontinue therapy and administer insulin if the patient is exposed to stress (fever, trauma, infection, surgery). Loss of efficacy may be observed following prolonged use as a result of the progression of type 2 diabetes mellitus which results in continued beta cell destruction. In patients who were previously responding to sulfonylurea therapy, consider additional factors which may be contributing to decreased efficacy (eg, inappropriate dose, nonadherence to diet and exercise regimen). If no contributing factors can be identified, consider discontinuing use of the sulfonylurea due to secondary failure of treatment. Additional antidiabetic therapy (eg, insulin) will be required.

Elderly: Rapid and prolonged hypoglycemia (>12 hours) despite hypertonic glucose injections have been reported; age and hepatic and renal impairment are independent risk factors for hypoglycemia; dosage titration should be made at weekly intervals.

Chemical similarities are present among sulfonamides, sulfonylureas, carbonic anhydrase inhibitors, thiazides, and loop diuretics (except ethacrynic acid). Use in patients with sulfonamide allergy is not specifically contraindicated in product labeling, however, a risk of cross-reaction exists in patients with allergy to any of these compounds; avoid use when previous reaction has been severe.

Product labeling states oral hypoglycemic drugs may be associated with an increased cardiovascular mortality as compared to treatment with diet alone or diet plus insulin. Data to support this association are limited, and several studies, including a large prospective trial (UKPDS) have not supported an association.

Patients with G6PD deficiency may be at an increased risk of sulfonylurea-induced hemolytic anemia; however, cases have also been described in patients without G6PD deficiency during postmarketing surveillance. Use with caution and consider a nonsulfonylurea alternative in patients with G6PD deficiency.

Micronized glyburide tablets are **not** bioequivalent to *conventional* glyburide tablets; retitration should occur if patients are being transferred to a different glyburide formulation (eg, micronized-to-conventional or vice versa) or from other hypoglycemic agents.

Adverse Reactions (Reflective of adult population; not specific for elderly) Frequency not defined.

Cardiovascular: Vasculitis

Central nervous system: Dizziness, headache

Dermatologic: Angioedema, erythema, maculopapular eruptions, morbilliform eruptions, photosensitivity reaction, pruritus, purpura, rash, urticaria

Endocrine & metabolic: Disulfiram-like reaction, hypoglycemia, hyponatremia (SIADH reported with other sulfonylureas)

Gastrointestinal: Anorexia, constipation, diarrhea, epigastric fullness, heartburn, nausea

Genitourinary: Nocturia

Hematologic: Agranulocytosis, aplastic anemia, hemolytic anemia, leukopenia, pancytopenia, porphyria cutanea tarda, thrombocytopenia

Hepatic: Cholestatic jaundice, hepatitis, liver failure, transaminase increased

Neuromuscular & skeletal: Arthralgia, myalgia, paresthesia

Ocular: Blurred vision

Renal: Diuretic effect (minor)

Miscellaneous: Allergic reaction

Drug Interactions

Metabolism/Transport Effects **Substrate** of CYP2C9 (major), 3A4 (minor);**Inhibits** CYP2C8 (weak), 3A4 (weak)

Avoid Concomitant Use

Avoid concomitant use of GlyBURIDE with any of the following: Bosentan

Increased Effect/Toxicity

GlyBURIDE may increase the levels/effects of: Alcohol (Ethyl); Bosentan; CycloSPORINE; CycloSPORINE (Systemic); Hypoglycemic Agents; Porfimer

The levels/effects of GlyBURIDE may be increased by: Beta-Blockers; Chloramphenicol; Cimetidine; Clarithromycin; Cyclic Antidepressants; CYP2C9 Inhibitors (Moderate); CYP2C9 Inhibitors (Strong); Fibric Acid Derivatives; Fluconazole; GLP-1 Agonists; Herbs (Hypoglycemic Properties); Pegvisomant; Quinolone Antibiotics; Ranitidine; Salicylates; Sulfonamide Derivatives; Voriconazole

Decreased Effect

GlyBURIDE may decrease the levels/effects of: Bosentan

The levels/effects of GlyBURIDE may be decreased by: Bosentan; Colesevelam; Corticosteroids (Orally Inhaled); Corticosteroids (Systemic); CycloSPORINE; CycloSPORINE (Systemic); CYP2C9 Inducers (Highly Effective); Luteinizing Hormone-Releasing Hormone Analogs; Peginterferon Alfa-2b; Quinolone Antibiotics; Rifampin; Somatropin; Thiazide Diuretics

Ethanol/Nutrition/Herb Interactions

Ethanol: Caution with ethanol (may cause hypoglycemia).

Herb/Nutraceutical: Herbs with hypoglycemic properties may enhance the hypoglycemic effect of glyburide. This includes alfalfa, aloe, bilberry, bitter melon, burdock, celery, damiana, fenugreek, garcinia, garlic, ginger, ginseng (American), gymnema, marshmallow, stinging nettle

Mechanism of Action Stimulates insulin release from the pancreatic beta cells; reduces glucose output from the liver; insulin sensitivity is increased at peripheral target sites

Pharmacodynamics/Kinetics

Onset of action: Serum insulin levels begin to increase 15-60 minutes after a single dose

Duration: ≤24 hours

Absorption: Significant within 1 hour

Distribution: 9-10 L

Protein binding, plasma: >99% primarily to albumin

Metabolism: Hepatic; forms metabolites (weakly active)

Bioavailability: Variable among oral dosage forms

Half-life elimination: Diabeta®: 10 hours; Glynase® PresTab®: ~4 hours; may be prolonged with renal or hepatic impairment

Time to peak, serum: Adults: 2-4 hours

Excretion: Feces (50%) and urine (50%) as metabolites

Dosage

Geriatric Regular tablets (Diaβeta®): Oral: Initial: 1.25-2.5 mg/day, increase by 1.25-2.5 mg/day every 1-3 weeks. Refer to adult dosing.

Adult Micronized glyburide tablets are **not** bioequivalent to conventional glyburide tablets; retitration should occur if patients are being transferred to a different glyburide formulation (eg, micronized-to-conventional or vice versa) or from other hypoglycemic agents.

Type 2 diabetes: Oral:

Note: Regular tablets cannot be used interchangeably with micronized tablet formulations

Regular tablets (Diaβeta®):

Initial: 2.5-5 mg/day, administered with breakfast or the first main meal of the day. In patients who are more sensitive to hypoglycemic drugs, start at 1.25 mg/day.

Adjustment: Increase in increments of no more than 2.5 mg/day at weekly intervals based on the patient's blood glucose response

Maintenance: 1.25-20 mg/day given as single or divided doses. Some patients (especially those receiving >10 mg/day) may have a more satisfactory response with twice-daily dosing. Maximum: 20 mg/day

Micronized tablets (Glynase® PresTab®):

Initial: 1.5-3 mg/day, administered with breakfast or the first main meal of the day in patients who are more sensitive to hypoglycemic drugs, start at 0.75 mg/day. Increase in increments of no more than 1.5 mg/day in weekly intervals based on the patient's blood glucose response.

Maintenance: 0.75-12 mg/day given as a single dose or in divided doses. Some patients (especially those receiving >6 mg/day) may have a more satisfactory response with twice-daily dosing. Maximum: 12 mg/day

Management of noninsulin-dependent diabetes mellitus in patients previously maintained on insulin: Oral: Initial dosage dependent upon previous insulin dosage, see table.

Dose Conversion: Insulin to Glyburide

Previous Daily Insulin Dosage (units/day)	Initial Glyburide Dosage *Conventional Formulation* (mg/day)	Initial Glyburide Dosage *Micronized Formulation* (mg/day)	Insulin Dosage Change (after glyburide started)
<20	2.5-5	1.5-3	Discontinue
20-40	5	3	Discontinue
>40	5 (increase in increments of 1.25-2.5 mg every 2-10 days)	3 (increase in increments of 0.75-1.5 mg every 2-10 days)	Reduce insulin dosage by 50% (gradually taper off insulin as glyburide dosage increased)

Renal Impairment Cl_{cr} <50 mL/minute: Not recommended

Hepatic Impairment Use conservative initial and maintenance doses and avoid use in severe disease.

Administration Administer with meals at the same time each day (twice-daily dosing may be beneficial if conventional glyburide doses are >10 mg or micronized glyburide doses are >6 mg). Patients that are NPO or require decreased caloric intake may need doses held to avoid hypoglycemia.

Monitoring Parameters Signs and symptoms of hypoglycemia, fasting blood glucose, hemoglobin A_{1c}

Reference Range Recommendations for glycemic control in adults with diabetes:
Hb A_{1c}: <7%
Preprandial capillary plasma glucose: 70-130 mg/dL
Peak postprandial capillary blood glucose: <180 mg/dL
Blood pressure: <130/80 mm Hg

Special Geriatric Considerations Glyburide is not a drug of choice for the elderly because of its association with severe hypoglycemia. Rapid and prolonged hypoglycemia (>12 hours) despite hypertonic glucose injections has been reported; age, hepatic, and renal impairment are independent risk factors for hypoglycemia; dosage titration should be made at weekly intervals. **Do not titrate to maximum dose.** Intensive glucose control (HbA$_{1c}$ <6.5%) has been linked to increased all-cause and cardiovascular mortality, hypoglycemia requiring assistance, and weight gain in adult type 2 diabetes. How "tightly" to control a geriatric patient's blood glucose needs to be individualized. Such a decision should be based on several factors, including the patient's functional and cognitive status, how well he/she recognizes hypoglycemic or hyperglycemic symptoms, and how to respond to them and other disease states. An HbA$_{1c}$ <7.5% is an acceptable endpoint for a healthy older adult, while <8% is acceptable for frail elderly patients, those with a duration of illness >10 years, or those with comorbid conditions and requiring combination diabetes medications. Patients who are unable to accurately draw up their dose will need assistance, such as prefilled syringes. Initial doses may require considerations for renal function in the elderly with dosing adjusted subsequently based on blood glucose monitoring. For elderly patients with diabetes who are relatively healthy, attaining target goals for aspirin use, blood pressure, lipids, smoking cessation, and diet and exercise may be more important than normalized glycemic control.

Dosage Forms Excipient information presented when available (limited, particularly for generics); consult specific product labeling.
Tablet, oral: 1.25 mg, 2.5 mg, 5 mg
 DiaBeta®: 1.25 mg, 2.5 mg, 5 mg [scored]
Tablet, oral [micronized]: 1.5 mg, 3 mg, 5 mg, 6 mg
 Glynase® PresTab®: 1.5 mg, 3 mg, 6 mg [scored]

Selected References

Action to Control Cardiovascular Risk in Diabetes Study Group, Gerstein HC, Miller ME, et al, "Effects of Intensive Glucose Lowering in Type 2 Diabetes," *N Engl J Med*, 2008, 358(24):2545-59.

ADVANCE Collaborative Group, Patel A, MacMahon S, et al, "Intensive Blood Glucose Control and Vascular Outcomes in Patients With Type 2 Diabetes," *N Engl J Med*, 2008, 358(24):2560-72.

American Diabetes Association, "Standards of Medical Care in Diabetes – 2011," *Diabetes Care*, 2011, 34(Suppl 1):11-61.

Brodows RG, "Benefits and Risks With Glyburide and Glipizide in Elderly NIDDM Patients," *Diabetes Care*, 1992, 15 (1):75-80.

Brown AF, Mangione CM, Saliba D, et al, "Guidelines for Improving the Care of the Older Person With Diabetes Mellitus," *J Am Geriatr Soc*, 2003, 51(5 Suppl Guidelines):265-80.

Rosenstock J, Corrao PJ, Goldberg RB, et al, "Diabetes Control in the Elderly: A Randomized, Comparative Study of Glyburide Versus Glipizide in Non-insulin-Dependent Diabetes Mellitus," *Clin Ther*, 1993, 15(6):1031-40.

Sonnenblick M and Shilo S, "Glibenclamide Induced Prolonged Hypoglycaemia," *Age Ageing*, 1986, 15(3):185-9.

"VA/DoD Clinical Practice Guideline for the Management of Diabetes Mellitus," 2010. Available at http://www.-healthquality.va.gov/Diabetes_Mellitus.asp

Glyburide and Metformin (GLYE byoor ide & met FOR min)

Related Information
GlyBURIDE *on page 828*
MetFORMIN *on page 1155*

Medication Safety Issues
Sound-alike/look-alike issues:
Glucovance® may be confused with Vyvanse™
High alert medication:
The Institute for Safe Medication Practices (ISMP) includes this medication among its list of drugs which have a heightened risk of causing significant patient harm when used in error.

Brand Names: U.S. Glucovance®

Index Terms Glyburide and Metformin Hydrochloride; Metformin and Glyburide

Generic Availability (U.S.) Yes

Pharmacologic Category Antidiabetic Agent, Biguanide; Antidiabetic Agent, Sulfonylurea

Use Adjunct to diet and exercise for the management of type 2 diabetes mellitus (noninsulin dependent, NIDDM)

Dosage
Geriatric Refer to adult dosing. Adjust carefully to renal function. Should not be used in patients ≥80 years of age unless renal function is verified as normal. Do not titrate to maximum dose.

Adult Note: Dose must be individualized. All doses should be taken with a meal. Twice daily dosage should be taken with the morning and evening meals. Dosages expressed as glyburide/metformin components.

Type 2 diabetes: Oral:
No prior treatment with sulfonylurea or metformin: Initial: 1.25 mg/250 mg once daily with a meal; patients with Hb A$_{1c}$ >9% or fasting plasma glucose (FPG) >200 mg/dL may start with 1.25 mg/250 mg twice daily with meals. Adjustment: Dosage may be increased in increments of 1.25 mg/250 mg, at intervals of not less than 2 weeks; maximum daily dose: 10 mg/2000 mg (limited experience with higher doses); **Note:** Doses of 5 mg/500 mg should not be used as initial therapy, due to risk of hypoglycemia.

Previously treated with a sulfonylurea or metformin alone: Initial: 2.5 mg/500 mg or 5 mg/500 mg twice daily with meals; increase in increments no greater than 5 mg/500 mg; maximum daily dose: 20 mg/2000 mg

Note: When switching patients previously on a sulfonylurea and metformin together, do not exceed the daily dose of glyburide (or glyburide equivalent) or metformin. When adding thiazolidinedione, continue glyburide and metformin at current dose and initiate thiazolidinedione at recommended starting dose.

Combination with thiazolidinedione: May be combined with a thiazolidinedione in patients with an inadequate response to glyburide/metformin therapy, however the risk of hypoglycemia may be increased.

Special Geriatric Considerations Glyburide is not a drug of choice for the elderly because of its association with severe hypoglycemia. Metformin should not be used in patients ≥80 years of age unless renal function is verified as normal. **Do not titrate to maximum dose.** Intensive glucose control (HbA$_{1c}$ <6.5%) has been linked to increased all-cause and cardiovascular mortality, hypoglycemia requiring assistance, and weight gain in adult type 2 diabetes. How "tightly" to control a geriatric patient's blood glucose needs to be individualized. Such a decision should be based on several factors, including the patient's functional and cognitive status, how well he/she recognizes hypoglycemic or hyperglycemic symptoms, and how to respond to them and other disease states. An HbA$_{1c}$ <7.5% is an acceptable endpoint for a healthy older adult, while <8% is acceptable for frail elderly patients, those with a duration of illness >10 years, or those with comorbid conditions and requiring combination diabetes medications. Patients who are unable to accurately draw up their dose will need assistance, such as prefilled syringes. Initial doses may require considerations for renal function in the elderly with dosing adjusted subsequently based on blood glucose monitoring. For elderly patients with diabetes who are relatively healthy, attaining target goals for aspirin use, blood pressure, lipids, smoking cessation, and diet and exercise may be more important than normalized glycemic control.

Dosage Forms Excipient information presented when available (limited, particularly for generics); consult specific product labeling. [DSC] = Discontinued product
Tablet: 1.25 mg/250 mg: Glyburide 1.25 mg and metformin hydrochloride 250 mg; 2.5 mg/500 mg: Glyburide 2.5 mg and metformin hydrochloride 500 mg; 5 mg/500 mg: Glyburide 5 mg and metformin hydrochloride 500 mg

Glucovance®: 1.25 mg/250 mg: Glyburide 1.25 mg and metformin hydrochloride 250 mg [DSC]
Glucovance®: 2.5 mg/500 mg: Glyburide 2.5 mg and metformin hydrochloride 500 mg
Glucovance®: 5 mg/500 mg: Glyburide 5 mg and metformin hydrochloride 500 mg

◆ **Glyburide and Metformin Hydrochloride** see Glyburide and Metformin on page 832

Glycerin (GLIS er in)

Related Information
Laxatives, Classification and Properties on page 2012
Brand Names: U.S. Fleet® Glycerin Maximum Strength [OTC]; Fleet® Glycerin Suppositories [OTC]; Fleet® Liquid Glycerin [OTC]; Fleet® Pedia-Lax™ Glycerin Suppositories [OTC]; Fleet® Pedia-Lax™ Liquid Glycerin Suppositories [OTC]; Orajel® Dry Mouth [OTC]; Sani-Supp® [OTC]
Index Terms Glycerol
Generic Availability (U.S.) Yes: Suppositories
Pharmacologic Category Laxative, Osmotic; Ophthalmic Agent, Miscellaneous
Use Constipation; reduction of intraocular pressure; reduction of corneal edema; glycerin has been administered orally to reduce intracranial pressure
Adverse Reactions (Reflective of adult population; not specific for elderly) Frequency not defined.
Cardiovascular: Arrhythmias
Central nervous system: Confusion, dizziness, headache, hyperosmolar nonketotic coma
Endocrine & metabolic: Dehydration, hyperglycemia, polydipsia
Gastrointestinal: Cramping pain, diarrhea, dry mouth, nausea, rectal irritation, tenesmus, vomiting
Drug Interactions
  Avoid Concomitant Use There are no known interactions where it is recommended to avoid concomitant use.
  Increased Effect/Toxicity There are no known significant interactions involving an increase in effect.
  Decreased Effect There are no known significant interactions involving a decrease in effect.
Stability
Refrigerate suppositories; avoid freezing. Protect from heat.
Ophthalmic: Store at room temperature. Keep bottle tightly closed. Discard 6 months after dropper is first placed in the solution.
Mechanism of Action Osmotic dehydrating agent which increases osmotic pressure; draws fluid into colon and thus stimulates evacuation
Pharmacodynamics/Kinetics
Onset of action:
  Decrease in intraocular pressure: Oral: 10-30 minutes
  Reduction of intracranial pressure: Oral: 10-60 minutes
  Constipation: Suppository: 15-30 minutes
Peak effect:
  Decrease in intraocular pressure: Oral: 60-90 minutes
  Reduction of intracranial pressure: Oral: 60-90 minutes
Duration:
  Decrease in intraocular pressure: Oral: 4-8 hours
  Reduction of intracranial pressure: Oral: ~2-3 hours
Absorption: Oral: Well absorbed; Rectal: Poorly absorbed
Half-life elimination, serum: 30-45 minutes
Dosage
  Geriatric & Adult
  Constipation: Rectal: 1 adult suppository 1-2 times/day as needed or 5-15 mL as an enema
  Reduction of intracranial pressure: Oral: 1.5 g/kg/day divided every 4 hours; 1 g/kg/dose every 6 hours has also been used
  Reduction of corneal edema: Ophthalmic solution: Instill 1-2 drops in eye(s) prior to examination OR for lubricant effect, instill 1-2 drops in eye(s) every 3-4 hours
  Reduction of intraocular pressure: Oral: 1-1.8 g/kg 1-1½ hours preoperatively; additional doses may be administered at 5-hour intervals
Administration Apply topical anesthetic before instilling ophthalmic drops
Pharmacotherapy Pearls Suppository needs to melt to provide laxative effect
Special Geriatric Considerations The primary use of glycerin in the elderly is as a laxative, although it is not recommended as a first-line treatment

◀ **Dosage Forms** Excipient information presented when available (limited, particularly for generics); consult specific product labeling.
Gel, oral:
  Orajel® Dry Mouth: 18% (42 g) [contains benzalkonium chloride]
Liquid, for prescription compounding: USP: 100% (3840 mL)
Liquid, topical: USP: 100% (120 mL, 180 mL, 480 mL, 3840 mL)
Solution, rectal:
  Fleet® Liquid Glycerin: 5.6 g/5.5 mL (7.5 mL) [4 units per box]
  Fleet® Pedia-Lax™ Liquid Glycerin Suppositories: 2.3 g/2.3 mL (4 mL) [6 units per box]
Suppository, rectal [adult]: 80.7% (25s, 100s); 82.5% (12s, 25s, 50s, 100s)
  Fleet® Glycerin Maximum Strength: 3 g (18s)
  Fleet® Glycerin Suppositories: 2 g (12s, 50s)
  Sani-Supp®: 82.5% (10s, 25s)
Suppository, rectal [pediatric]: 1.5 g (12s, 25s); 82.5% (12s, 25s)
  Fleet® Pedia-Lax™ Glycerin Suppositories: 1 g (12s)
  Sani-Supp®: 82.5% (10s, 25s)

◆ **Glycerol** see Glycerin on page 833
◆ **Glycerol Guaiacolate** see GuaiFENesin on page 846
◆ **Glyceryl Trinitrate** see Nitroglycerin on page 1311

Glycopyrrolate (glye koe PYE roe late)

Medication Safety Issues
Sound-alike/look-alike issues:
Robinul® may be confused with Reminyl®
Brand Names: U.S. Cuvposa™; Robinul®; Robinul® Forte
Brand Names: Canada Glycopyrrolate Injection, USP
Index Terms Glycopyrronium Bromide
Generic Availability (U.S.) Yes: Excludes oral solution
Pharmacologic Category Anticholinergic Agent
Use Inhibit salivation and excessive secretions of the respiratory tract preoperatively; control of upper airway secretions; intraoperatively to counteract drug-induced or vagal mediated bradyarrhythmias; adjunct in treatment of peptic ulcer (indication listed in product labeling but currently has no place in management of peptic ulcer disease)

Cuvposa™: Reduce chronic, severe drooling in those with neurologic conditions (eg, cerebral palsy) associated with drooling
Unlabeled/Investigational Use Adjunct with acetylcholinesterase inhibitors (eg, neostigmine, edrophonium, pyridostigmine) to antagonize cholinergic effects
Contraindications Hypersensitivity to glycopyrrolate or any component of the formulation; medical conditions that preclude use of anticholinergic medication; severe ulcerative colitis, toxic megacolon complicating ulcerative colitis, paralytic ileus, obstructive disease of GI tract (eg, pyloric stenosis), intestinal atony in the elderly or debilitated patient; unstable cardiovascular status in acute hemorrhage; narrow-angle glaucoma; acute hemorrhage; tachycardia; obstructive uropathy; myasthenia gravis

Oral solution: Additional contraindication: Concomitant use of potassium chloride in a solid oral dosage form
Warnings/Precautions Diarrhea may be a sign of incomplete intestinal obstruction, treatment should be discontinued if this occurs. Use caution in elderly and in patients with autonomic neuropathy, hepatic or renal disease, or ulcerative colitis; may precipitate/aggravate toxic megacolon, hyperthyroidism, CAD, CHF, arrhythmias, tachycardia, BPH, or hiatal hernia with reflux. Use of anticholinergics in gastric ulcer treatment may cause a delay in gastric emptying due to antral statis. Caution should be used in individuals demonstrating decreased pigmentation (skin and iris coloration, dark versus light) since there has been some evidence that these individuals have an enhanced sensitivity to the anticholinergic response. May cause drowsiness, eye sensitivity to light, or blurred vision; caution should be used when performing tasks which require mental alertness, such as driving. Thr risk of heat stroke with this medication may be increased during exercise or hot weather.
Adverse Reactions (Reflective of adult population; not specific for elderly)
>10% (as reported with Cuvposa™):
  Cardiovascular: Flushing (30%)
  Central nervous system: Headache (15%)
  Gastrointestinal: Vomiting (40%), xerostomia (40%), constipation (35%)
  Genitourinary: Urinary retention (15%)
  Respiratory: Nasal congestion (30%), sinusitis (15%), upper respiratory tract infection (15%)

<10% (frequency not always defined):

Cardiovascular: Pallor (≤2%), arrhythmias, cardiac arrest, heart block, hyper-/hypotension, malignant hyperthermia, palpitation, QT_c-interval prolongation, tachycardia

Central nervous system: Aggressiveness (≤2%), agitation (≤2%), crying (abnormal; ≤2%), irritability (≤2%), mood changes (≤2%), pain (≤2%), restlessness (≤2%), confusion, dizziness, drowsiness, excitement, insomnia, nervousness, seizure

Dermatologic: Dry skin (≤2%), pruritus (≤2%), rash (≤2%), urticaria

Endocrine & metabolic: Dehydration (≤2%), lactation suppression

Gastrointestinal: Abdominal distention (≤2%), abdominal pain (≤2%), flatulence (≤2%), retching (≤2%), bloated feeling, intestinal obstruction, loss of taste, nausea, pseudo-obstruction

Genitourinary: Urinary tract infection (≤2%), impotence, urinary hesitancy

Local: Injection site reactions (edema, erythema, pain)

Neuromuscular & skeletal: Weakness

Ocular: Nystagmus (≤2%), blurred vision, cycloplegia, mydriasis, ocular tension increased, photophobia, sensitivity to light increased

Respiratory: Bronchial secretion (thickening; ≤2%), nasal dryness (≤2%), pneumonia (≤2%), respiratory depression

Miscellaneous: Anaphylactoid reactions, diaphoresis decreased, hypersensitivity reactions

Drug Interactions

Avoid Concomitant Use
Avoid concomitant use of Glycopyrrolate with any of the following: Potassium Chloride

Increased Effect/Toxicity
Glycopyrrolate may increase the levels/effects of: AbobotulinumtoxinA; Anticholinergics; Atenolol; Cannabinoids; Digoxin; MetFORMIN; OnabotulinumtoxinA; Potassium Chloride; RimabotulinumtoxinB

The levels/effects of Glycopyrrolate may be increased by: Amantadine; MAO Inhibitors; Pramlintide

Decreased Effect
Glycopyrrolate may decrease the levels/effects of: Acetylcholinesterase Inhibitors (Central); Haloperidol; Levodopa; Secretin

The levels/effects of Glycopyrrolate may be decreased by: Acetylcholinesterase Inhibitors (Central)

Ethanol/Nutrition/Herb Interactions Food: Administration with a high-fat meal significantly reduced absorption; administer on an empty stomach.

Stability Store at 20°C to 25°C (68°F to 77°F).

Mechanism of Action Blocks the action of acetylcholine at parasympathetic sites in smooth muscle, secretory glands, and the CNS; indirectly reduces the rate of salivation by preventing the stimulation of acetylcholine receptors

Pharmacodynamics/Kinetics
Absorption: Oral: Poor and erratic

Distribution: V_d: 0.2-0.62 L/kg

Metabolism: Hepatic (minimal)

Bioavailability: ~10%

Half-life elimination: Adults: ~30-75 minutes

Excretion: Urine (as unchanged drug, I.M.: 80%, I.V.: 85%); bile (as unchanged drug)

Dosage

Geriatric & Adult
Reduction of secretions:
Preoperative: I.M.: 4 mcg/kg 30-60 minutes before procedure

Intraoperative: I.V.: 0.1 mg repeated as needed at 2- to 3-minute intervals

Reversal of neuromuscular blockade: I.V.: 0.2 mg for each 1 mg of neostigmine or 5 mg of pyridostigmine administered or 5-15 mcg/kg glycopyrrolate with 25-70 mcg/kg of neostigmine or 0.1-0.3 mg/kg of pyridostigmine (agents usually administered simultaneously, but glycopyrrolate may be administered first if bradycardia is present)

Administration For I.V. administration, glycopyrrolate may also be administered via the tubing of a running I.V. infusion of a compatible solution; may be administered in the same syringe with neostigmine or pyridostigmine.

Monitoring Parameters Heart rate; anticholinergic effects; bowel sounds; bowel movements; effects on drooling

Pharmacotherapy Pearls Because of its bothersome and potentially dangerous side effects, glycopyrrolate is rarely used for the treatment of peptic ulcer disease

Special Geriatric Considerations Anticholinergic agents are generally not well tolerated in the elderly and their use should be avoided when possible.

Dosage Forms Excipient information presented when available (limited, particularly for generics); consult specific product labeling.

Injection, solution: 0.2 mg/mL (1 mL, 2 mL, 5 mL, 20 mL)
  Robinul®: 0.2 mg/mL (1 mL, 2 mL, 5 mL, 20 mL) [contains benzyl alcohol]
Solution, oral:
  Cuvposa™: 1 mg/5 mL (473 mL) [contains propylene glycol; cherry flavor]
Tablet, oral: 1 mg, 2 mg
  Robinul®: 1 mg [scored]
  Robinul® Forte: 2 mg [scored]

Selected References
Friedl KE, Hannan CJ, Mader TH, et al, "Effect of Eye Color on Heart Rate Response to Intramuscular Administration of Atropine," *J Auton Nerv Syst*, 1988, 24(1-2):51-6.

◆ **Glycopyrronium Bromide** *see* Glycopyrrolate *on page 834*
◆ **Glydiazinamide** *see* GlipiZIDE *on page 823*
◆ **Glynase® PresTab®** *see* GlyBURIDE *on page 828*
◆ **Gly-Oxide® [OTC]** *see* Carbamide Peroxide *on page 272*
◆ **Glyset®** *see* Miglitol *on page 1213*

Gold Sodium Thiomalate (gold SOW dee um thye oh MAL ate)

Brand Names: U.S. Myochrysine®
Brand Names: Canada Myochrysine®
Index Terms Sodium Aurothiomalate
Generic Availability (U.S.) No
Pharmacologic Category Gold Compound
Use Adjunctive treatment of active rheumatoid arthritis
Contraindications Hypersensitivity to gold compounds or any component of the formulation; history of severe toxicity to gold compounds or heavy metals; systemic lupus erythematosus; severe debilitation
Warnings/Precautions Frequent monitoring of patients for signs and symptoms of toxicity will prevent/limit serious adverse reactions. Must not be administered by I.V. injection. In patients with hematologic abnormalities (blood dyscrasias, hemorrhagic diathesis), renal impairment, hepatic impairment, SLE or dermatitis: Consider alternative therapy (these conditions may be considered relative contraindications); may increase risk and/or symptoms of gold toxicity may be more difficult to detect.

[U.S. Boxed Warning]: May cause significant toxicity involving dermatologic, gastrointestinal, hematologic, pulmonary, renal and hepatic systems; patient education is required. Dermatitis and lesions of the mucous membranes are common and may be serious; pruritus may precede the early development of a skin reaction. Signs of toxicity include hematologic depression (depressed hemoglobin, leukocytes, granulocytes, or platelets); stomatitis, persistent diarrhea, enterocolitis, cholestatic jaundice; proteinuria (nephritic syndrome), and interstitial pulmonary fibrosis. Use caution in patients with HF, hypertension, or cerebrovascular disease. Avoid use in patients with prior inflammatory bowel disease. Injection contains benzyl alcohol.

In general, NSAIDS and corticosteroids may be discontinued after initiation of therapy (corticosteroid tapering may be required). Concurrent ACE inhibitors may be associated with a higher risk of nitritoid reactions.

Adverse Reactions (Reflective of adult population; not specific for elderly) Frequency not defined.
Cardiovascular: Bradycardia, syncope
Central nervous system: Confusion, fever, Guillain-Barré syndrome, hallucinations, seizure
Dermatologic: Alopecia, angioedema, dermatitis, nail shedding, pruritus, rash, urticaria
Gastrointestinal: Anorexia, abdominal cramps, diarrhea, dysphagia, enterocolitis (ulcerative), gingivitis, glossitis, nausea, stomatitis, taste disturbance (metallic), thick tongue, vomiting
Hematologic: Agranulocytosis, aplastic anemia, eosinophilia, leukopenia, purpura, thrombocytopenia
Hepatic: Cholestasis, hepatitis, hepatotoxicity, jaundice
Neuromuscular & skeletal: Arthralgia, peripheral neuropathy
Ocular: Conjunctivitis, corneal ulcers, gold deposits in ocular tissues, iritis
Respiratory: Dyspnea, gold bronchitis, interstitial pneumonitis, pulmonary fibrosis
Renal: Glomerulitis, hematuria, nephrotic syndrome, proteinuria
Miscellaneous: Anaphylactoid reaction, anaphylaxis, nitritoid reaction
Drug Interactions
Avoid Concomitant Use There are no known interactions where it is recommended to avoid concomitant use.

Increased Effect/Toxicity
The levels/effects of Gold Sodium Thiomalate may be increased by: ACE Inhibitors
Decreased Effect There are no known significant interactions involving a decrease in effect.
Stability Should not be used if solution is darker than pale yellow.
Mechanism of Action Unknown, may decrease prostaglandin synthesis or may alter cellular mechanisms by inhibiting sulfhydryl systems
Pharmacodynamics/Kinetics
Onset of action: Delayed; may require up to 3 months
Half-life elimination: 5 days; may be prolonged with multiple doses
Time to peak, serum: 4-6 hours
Excretion: Urine (60% to 90%); feces (10% to 40%)
Dosage
Geriatric & Adult Rheumatoid arthritis: I.M.: 10 mg first week; 25 mg second week; then 25-50 mg/week until development of toxicity or 1 g cumulative dose has been given; if improvement occurs without adverse reactions, the dose may be decreased or the dosing interval increased; Maintenance: 25-50 mg every other week for 2-20 weeks, then every 3-4 weeks indefinitely
Note: Failure to improve during initial therapy may warrant continuation of 25-50 mg for additional 10 weeks or a dose increase in increments of 10 mg every 1-4 weeks (maximum: 100 mg/injection). Discontinue therapy if no improvement or toxicity develops.
Renal Impairment Aronoff, 2007:
Cl_{cr} 50-80 mL/minute: Administer 50% of normal dose.
Cl_{cr} <50 mL/minute: Avoid use.
Administration Deep I.M. injection into the upper outer quadrant of the gluteal region addition of 0.1 mL of 1% lidocaine to each injection may reduce the discomfort associated with I.M. administration
Monitoring Parameters Patients should have a CBC with differential, platelet count, hemoglobin determination and urinalysis for protein, white cells, red cells and casts; at baseline and prior to each injection. Skin and oral mucosa should be inspected for skin rash, bruising or oral ulceration/stomatitis. Specific questioning for symptoms such as pruritus, rash, stomatitis or metallic taste should be included. Dosing should be withheld in patients with significant gastrointestinal, renal, dermatologic, or hematologic effects (platelet count falls to <100,000/mm^3, WBC <4000, granulocytes <1500/mm^3
Reference Range Gold: Normal: 0-0.1 mcg/mL (SI: 0-0.0064 µmol/L); Therapeutic: 1-3 mcg/mL (SI: 0.06-0.18 µmol/L); Urine: <0.1 mcg/24 hour
Pharmacotherapy Pearls Approximately 50% gold
Special Geriatric Considerations Tolerance to gold decreases with advanced age; use cautiously only after traditional therapy and other disease-modifying antirheumatic drugs (DMARDs) have been attempted. Since elderly frequently have Cl_{cr} <50 mL/minute, it is advisable to measure or calculate creatinine clearance before use.
Dosage Forms Excipient information presented when available (limited, particularly for generics); consult specific product labeling. [DSC] = Discontinued product
Injection, solution:
Myochrysine®: 50 mg/mL (1 mL, 10 mL [DSC]) [contains benzyl alcohol]

Golimumab (goe LIM ue mab)

Brand Names: U.S. Simponi®
Brand Names: Canada Simponi®
Index Terms CNTO-148
Generic Availability (U.S.) No
Pharmacologic Category Antipsoriatic Agent; Antirheumatic, Disease Modifying; Monoclonal Antibody; Tumor Necrosis Factor (TNF) Blocking Agent
Use Treatment of active rheumatoid arthritis (moderate-to-severe), active psoriatic arthritis, and active ankylosing spondylitis
Medication Guide Available Yes
Contraindications There are no contraindications listed in the FDA-approved manufacturer's labeling.

Canadian labeling: Hypersensitivity to golimumab, latex, or any other component of formulation or packaging; patients with severe infections (eg, sepsis, tuberculosis, opportunistic infections)
Warnings/Precautions [U.S. Boxed Warning]: Patients receiving golimumab are at increased risk for serious infections which may result in hospitalization and/or fatality; infections usually developed in patients receiving concomitant immunosuppressive agents (eg, methotrexate or corticosteroids); infection may be disseminated, rather

◀ than localized, upon presentation. **Active tuberculosis (or reactivation of latent tuberculosis), invasive fungal (including aspergillosis, candidiasis, coccidioidomycosis, histoplasmosis, and pneumocystosis), bacterial, viral, and other opportunistic infections have been reported in patients receiving TNF-blocking agents, including golimumab. Monitor closely for signs/symptoms of infection.** Discontinue for serious infection, opportunistic infection, or sepsis. Consider risks versus benefits prior to use in patients with a history of chronic or recurrent infection. Caution should be exercised when considering the use in patients with concomitant immunosuppressive therapy or predisposition to infection (eg, diabetes or residence/travel from areas of endemic mycoses). Do not administer to patients with an active chronic or localized infection. Patients who develop a new infection while undergoing treatment should be monitored closely. If a patient develops a serious infection, therapy should be discontinued.

[U.S. Boxed Warning]: Tuberculosis (disseminated or extrapulmonary) has been reported in patients receiving golimumab; both reactivation of latent infection and new infections have been reported. Patients should be evaluated for tuberculosis risk factors and latent tuberculosis infection (with a tuberculin skin test) prior to therapy. Treatment of latent tuberculosis should be initiated before use. Patients with initial negative tuberculin skin tests should receive continued monitoring for tuberculosis throughout treatment; active tuberculosis has developed in this population during treatment with TNF-blocking agents. Use with caution in patients who have resided in regions where tuberculosis is endemic. Consider antituberculosis therapy if an adequate course of treatment cannot be confirmed in patients with a history of latent or active tuberculosis or for patients with risk factors despite negative skin test.

Rare reactivation of HBV has occurred in chronic carriers of the virus usually in patients receiving concomitant immunosuppressants; evaluate prior to initiation and during treatment in patients at risk for HBV infection. If resumption of therapy is deemed necessary, exercise caution and monitor closely. Patients should be brought up to date with all immunizations before initiating therapy. Live vaccines should not be given concurrently. In clinical trials, humoral response to pneumococcal vaccine was not suppressed in psoriatic arthritis patients.

[U.S. Boxed Warning]: Lymphoma and other malignancies have been reported in children and adolescent patients receiving TNF-blocking agents. Half of the malignancies reported in children were lymphomas (Hodgkin's and non-Hodgkin's) while other cases varied and included malignancies not typically observed in this population. The impact of golimumab on the development and course of malignancy is not fully defined. Compared to the general population, an increased risk of lymphoma has been noted in clinical trials; however, rheumatoid arthritis alone has been previously associated with an increased rate of lymphoma. Lymphomas and other malignancies were also observed (at rates higher than expected for the general population) in adult patients receiving TNF-blocking agents. Treatment may result in the formation of autoimmune antibodies; cases of autoimmune disease have not been described. Neutralizing antibodies to golimumab may also be formed. Rarely, a reversible lupus-like syndrome has occurred with use of TNF blockers.

Use with caution in patients with peripheral or central nervous system demyelinating disorders; rare cases of new onset or exacerbation of demyelinating disorders (eg, multiple sclerosis, Guillain-Barré syndrome) have occurred with use of TNF-blockers, including golimumab. Consider discontinuing use in patients who develop peripheral or central nervous system demyelinating disorders during treatment. Optic neuritis, transverse myelitis, multiple sclerosis, and new onset or exacerbation of seizures has been reported. Use with caution in patients with heart failure or decreased left ventricular function and discontinue use with new onset or worsening of symptoms. Use caution in patients with a history of significant hematologic abnormalities (cytopenias).

Avoid concomitant use with abatacept (increased incidence of serious infections) or anakinra (increased incidence of neutropenia and serious infection). Use caution when switching between biological disease-modifying antirheumatic drugs (DMARDs); overlapping of biological activity may increase the risk for infection. Use with caution in the elderly (general incidence of infection is higher). Packaging (prefilled syringe and needle cover) contains dry natural rubber (latex). Some dosage forms may contain dry natural rubber (latex) and/or polysorbate 80.

Adverse Reactions (Reflective of adult population; not specific for elderly)
>10%:
  Respiratory: Upper respiratory tract infection (16%; includes laryngitis, nasopharyngitis, pharyngitis, and rhinitis)
  Miscellaneous: Infection (28%)
1% to 10%:
  Cardiovascular: Hypertension (3%)

Central nervous system: Dizziness (2%), fever (1%)
Gastrointestinal: Constipation (1%)
Hepatic: ALT increased (4%), AST increased (3%)
Local: Injection site reactions (6%)
Neuromuscular & skeletal: Paresthesia (2%)
Respiratory: Bronchitis (2%), sinusitis (2%)
Miscellaneous: Viral infection (5%; includes herpes and influenza), antibody formation (4%), fungal infection (superficial; 2%)

Drug Interactions

Avoid Concomitant Use

Avoid concomitant use of Golimumab with any of the following: Abatacept; Anakinra; BCG; Belimumab; Canakinumab; Certolizumab Pegol; Natalizumab; Pimecrolimus; Rilonacept; Tacrolimus (Topical); Vaccines (Live)

Increased Effect/Toxicity

Golimumab may increase the levels/effects of: Abatacept; Anakinra; Belimumab; Canakinumab; Certolizumab Pegol; Leflunomide; Natalizumab; Rilonacept; Vaccines (Live)

The levels/effects of Golimumab may be increased by: Abciximab; Denosumab; Pimecrolimus; Roflumilast; Tacrolimus (Topical); Trastuzumab

Decreased Effect

Golimumab may decrease the levels/effects of: BCG; Sipuleucel-T; Vaccines (Inactivated); Vaccines (Live)

The levels/effects of Golimumab may be decreased by: Echinacea

Stability Store under refrigeration at 2°C to 8°C (36°F to 46°F); do not freeze. Do not shake. Protect from light.

Mechanism of Action Human monoclonal antibody that binds to human tumor necrosis factor alpha (TNFα), thereby interfering with endogenous TNFα activity. Biological activities of TNFα include the induction of proinflammatory cytokines (interleukin [IL]-6, IL-8, Granulocyte-colony stimulating factor, granulocyte-macrophage colony stimulating factor), expression of adhesion molecules (E-selectin, vascular cell adhesion molecule [VCAM]-1, intercellular adhesion molecule [ICAM]-1) necessary for leukocyte infiltration, activation of neutrophils and eosinophils.

Pharmacodynamics/Kinetics

Distribution: V_d: I.V.: 0.058-0.126 L/kg
Bioavailability: SubQ: ~53%
Half-life elimination: ~2 weeks
Time to peak, serum: SubQ: 2-6 days

Dosage

Geriatric & Adult Note: Should be administered in conjunction with methotrexate in rheumatoid arthritis; may administer with or without methotrexate or other nonbiologic disease-modifying antirheumatic drugs (DMARDs) in psoriatic arthritis or ankylosing spondylitis.

Rheumatoid arthritis, psoriatic arthritis, ankylosing spondylitis: SubQ: 50 mg once per month

Administration Subcutaneous injection: Prior to administration, allow syringe to sit at room temperature for 30 minutes. Solution should be clear to slightly opalescent and colorless to light yellow. Discard if solution is cloudy, discolored, or has foreign particles. Hold autoinjector firmly against skin and inject subcutaneously into thigh, lower abdomen (below navel), or upper arm. A loud click is heard when injection has begun. Continue to hold autoinjector against skin until second click is heard (may take 3-15 seconds). Following second click, lift autoinjector from injection site. Discard any unused portion. Rotate injection sites and avoid injecting into tender, red, hard, or bruised skin.

Monitoring Parameters Latent TB screening prior to initiating and during therapy; signs/symptoms of infection (prior to, during, and following therapy); CBC with differential; signs/symptoms/worsening of heart failure; HBV screening (for patients at risk), HBV carriers (during and for several months following therapy)

Special Geriatric Considerations Phase three trials did not demonstrate any significant differences in adverse drug reactions, infections, or in the side effects profile in elderly compared to younger adults. However, since elderly experience a higher incidence of infections, use with caution and close monitoring in the elderly patient.

Dosage Forms Excipient information presented when available (limited, particularly for generics); consult specific product labeling.

Injection, solution [preservative free]:
Simponi®: 50 mg/0.5 mL (0.5 mL) [contains natural rubber/natural latex in packaging, polysorbate 80; autoinjector]

Simponi®: 50 mg/0.5 mL (0.5 mL) [contains natural rubber/natural latex in packaging, polysorbate 80; prefilled syringe]

Selected References

Inman RD, Davis JC Jr, van der Heijde D, et al, "Efficacy and Safety of Golimumab in Patients With Ankylosing Spondylitis, Results of a Randomized, Double-Blind, Placebo-Controlled, Phase III Trial," *Arthritis Rheum*, 2008, 58 (11):3402-12.

Kavanaugh A, Mcinnes I, Mease P, et al, "Golimumab, a New Human Tumor Necrosis Factor α Antibody, Administered Every Four Weeks as a Subcutaneous Injection in Psoriatic Arthritis, Twenty-Four-Week Efficacy and Safety Results of a Randomized, Placebo-Controlled Study," *Arthritis Rheum*, 2009, 60(4):976-86.

Kay J, Matteson EL, Dasgupta B, et al, "Golimumab in Patients With Active Rheumatoid Arthritis Despite Treatment With Methotrexate, A Randomized, Double-Blind, Placebo-Controlled, Dose-Ranging Study," *Arthritis Rheum*, 2008, 58(4):964-75.

Keystone EC, Genovese MC, Klareskog L, et al, "Golimumab, a Human Antibody to TNF- α Given by Monthly Subcutaneous Injections, in Active Rheumatoid Arthritis Despite Methotrexate: The GO-FORWARD Study," *Ann Rheum Dis,*, 2009, 68(6):789-96.

◆ **Gordofilm [OTC]** *see* Salicylic Acid *on page 1648*
◆ **Gordon Boro-Packs [OTC]** *see* Aluminum Sulfate and Calcium Acetate *on page 85*

Goserelin (GOE se rel in)

Brand Names: U.S. Zoladex®
Brand Names: Canada Zoladex®; Zoladex® LA
Index Terms Goserelin Acetate; ICI-118630; ZDX
Generic Availability (U.S.) No
Pharmacologic Category Antineoplastic Agent, Gonadotropin-Releasing Hormone Agonist; Gonadotropin Releasing Hormone Agonist
Use Treatment of locally confined prostate cancer; palliative treatment of advanced prostate cancer; palliative treatment of advanced breast cancer in pre- and perimenopausal women; treatment of endometriosis, including pain relief and reduction of endometriotic lesions; endometrial thinning agent as part of treatment for dysfunctional uterine bleeding
Contraindications Hypersensitivity to goserelin, GnRH, GnRH agonist analogues, or any component of the formulation
Warnings/Precautions Hazardous agent - use appropriate precautions for handling and disposal. Allergic hypersensitivity reactions (including anaphylaxis) and antibody formation may occur; monitor. Androgen-deprivation therapy may increase the risk for cardiovascular disease (Levine, 2010). Transient increases in serum testosterone (in men with prostate cancer) and estrogen (in women with breast cancer) may result in a worsening of disease signs and symptoms (tumor flare) during the first few weeks of treatment. Urinary tract obstruction or spinal cord compression have been reported when used for prostate cancer; closely observe patients for weakness, paresthesias, and urinary tract obstruction in first few weeks of therapy. Decreased bone density has been reported in women and may be irreversible; use caution if other risk factors are present; evaluate and institute preventative treatment if necessary. Cervical resistance may be increased; use caution when dilating the cervix. The 3-month implant currently has no approved indications for use in women. Rare cases of pituitary apoplexy (frequently secondary to pituitary adenoma) have been observed with leuprolide administration (onset from 1 hour to usually <2 weeks); may present as sudden headache, vomiting, visual or mental status changes, and infrequently cardiovascular collapse; immediate medical attention required. Hyperglycemia has been reported in males and may manifest as diabetes or worsening of pre-existing diabetes. Decreased bioavailability may be observed when using the 3-month implant in obese patients. Monitor testosterone levels if desired clinical response is not observed.
Adverse Reactions (Reflective of adult population; not specific for elderly) Percentages reported with the 1-month implant:
>10%:
  Cardiovascular: Peripheral edema (female 21%)
  Central nervous system: Headache (female 32% to 75%; male 1% to 5%), emotional lability (female 60%), depression (female 54%; male 1% to 5%), pain (female 17%; male 8%), insomnia (female 11%; male 5%)
  Dermatologic: Acne (female 42%), seborrhea (female 26%)
  Endocrine & metabolic: Hot flashes (female 57% to 96%; male 62%), libido decreased (female 48% to 61%), sexual dysfunction (male 21%), breast atrophy (female 33%), breast enlargement (female 18%), erections decreased (18%), libido increased (female 12%)
  Gastrointestinal: Nausea (female 8% to 11%; male 5%), abdominal pain (female 7% to 11%)
  Genitourinary: Vaginitis (75%), pelvic symptoms (female 9% to 18%), dyspareunia (female 14%), lower urinary symptoms (male 13%)
  Neuromuscular & skeletal: Bone mineral density decreased (female 23%; ~4% decrease from baseline in 6 months; postmarketing reports in males), weakness (female 11%)

Miscellaneous: Diaphoresis (female 16% to 45%; male 6%), tumor flare (female: 23%), infection (female 13%)

1% to 10%:

Cardiovascular: Arrhythmia, cerebrovascular accident, chest pain, edema, heart failure, hypertension, MI, palpitation, peripheral vascular disorder, tachycardia

Central nervous system: Abnormal thinking, anxiety, chills, dizziness, fever, lethargy, malaise, migraine, nervousness, somnolence

Dermatologic: Alopecia, bruising, dry skin, hair disorder, hirsutism, pruritus, rash, skin discoloration

Endocrine & metabolic: Breast pain, breast swelling/tenderness, dysmenorrhea, gout, hyperglycemia

Gastrointestinal: Anorexia, appetite increased, constipation, diarrhea, dyspepsia, flatulence, ulcer, vomiting, weight gain/loss, xerostomia

Genitourinary: Urinary frequency, urinary obstruction, urinary tract infection, vaginal hemorrhage, vulvovaginitis

Hematologic: Anemia, hemorrhage

Local: Application site reaction

Neuromuscular & skeletal: Arthralgia, back pain, hypertonia, joint disorder, leg cramps, myalgia, paresthesia

Ocular: Amblyopia, dry eyes

Renal: Renal insufficiency

Respiratory: Bronchitis, COPD, cough, epistaxis, pharyngitis, rhinitis, sinusitis, upper respiratory tract infection

Miscellaneous: Allergic reaction, flu-like syndrome, voice alteration

Drug Interactions

Avoid Concomitant Use There are no known interactions where it is recommended to avoid concomitant use.

Increased Effect/Toxicity There are no known significant interactions involving an increase in effect.

Decreased Effect

Goserelin may decrease the levels/effects of: Antidiabetic Agents

Stability Zoladex® should be stored at room temperature not to exceed 25°C or 77°F. Protect from light.

Mechanism of Action Goserelin (a gonadotropin-releasing hormone [GnRH] analog) causes an initial increase in luteinizing hormone (LH) and follicle stimulating hormone (FSH), chronic administration of goserelin results in a sustained suppression of pituitary gonadotropins. Serum testosterone falls to levels comparable to surgical castration. The exact mechanism of this effect is unknown, but may be related to changes in the control of LH or down-regulation of LH receptors.

Pharmacodynamics/Kinetics

Onset:

Females: Estradiol suppression reaches postmenopausal levels within 3 weeks and FSH and LH are suppressed to follicular phase levels within 4 weeks of initiation

Males: Testosterone suppression reaches castrate levels within 2-4 weeks after initiation

Duration:

Females: Estradiol, LH and FSH generally return to baseline levels within 12 weeks following the last monthly implant.

Males: Testosterone levels maintained at castrate levels throughout the duration of therapy.

Absorption: SubQ: Rapid and can be detected in serum in 30-60 minutes; 3.6 mg: released slowly in first 8 days, then rapid and continuous release for 28 days

Distribution: V_d: Male: 44.1 L; Female: 20.3 L

Protein binding: 27%

Time to peak, serum: SubQ: Male: 12-15 days, Female: 8-22 days

Half-life elimination: SubQ: Male: ~4 hours, Female: ~2 hours; Renal impairment: Male: 12 hours

Excretion: Urine (>90%; 20% as unchanged drug)

Dosage

Geriatric & Adult

Prostate cancer, advanced: SubQ:

28-day implant: 3.6 mg every 28 days

12-week implant: 10.8 mg every 12 weeks

Prostate cancer, locally confined (in combination with an antiandrogen and radiotherapy; begin 8 weeks prior to radiotherapy): SubQ:

Combination 28-day/12-week implant: 3.6 mg implant, followed in 28 days by 10.8 mg implant

28-day implant (alternate dosing): 3.6 mg; repeated every 28 days for a total of 4 doses

Breast cancer, advanced: SubQ: 3.6 mg every 28 days

◄ **Endometriosis:** SubQ: 3.6 mg every 28 days for 6 months
Endometrial thinning: SubQ: 3.6 mg every 28 days for 1 or 2 doses
Renal Impairment No adjustment is necessary.
Hepatic Impairment No adjustment is necessary.
Administration SubQ: Administer implant by inserting needle at a 30-45 degree angle into the anterior abdominal wall below the navel line. Goserelin is an implant; therefore, do not attempt to eliminate air bubbles prior to injection (may displace implant). Do not attempt to aspirate prior to injection; if a large vessel is penetrated, blood will be visualized in the syringe chamber (if vessel is penetrated, withdraw needle and inject elsewhere with a new syringe). Do not penetrate into muscle or peritoneum. Implant may be detected by ultrasound if removal is required.
Monitoring Parameters Bone mineral density, serum calcium, cholesterol/lipids
Prostate cancer: Weakness, paresthesias, and urinary tract obstruction in first few weeks of therapy; screen for diabetes
Test Interactions Interferes with pituitary gonadotropic and gonadal function tests during and for up to 12 weeks after discontinued
Pharmacotherapy Pearls If removal is necessary, implant may be located by ultrasound.
Special Geriatric Considerations No dosage adjustments are needed in the elderly. Monitoring for bone density changes, serum lipid, hemoglobin A_{1c}, blood pressure, and serum calcium changes is recommended.
Dosage Forms Excipient information presented when available (limited, particularly for generics); consult specific product labeling.
Implant, subcutaneous:
Zoladex®: 3.6 mg (1s) [1 month implant]
Zoladex®: 10.8 mg (1s) [3 month implant]

◆ **Goserelin Acetate** *see* Goserelin *on page 840*
◆ **GP 47680** *see* OXcarbazepine *on page 1362*
◆ **GR38032R** *see* Ondansetron *on page 1347*
◆ **Gramicidin, Neomycin, and Polymyxin B** *see* Neomycin, Polymyxin B, and Gramicidin *on page 1282*

Granisetron (gra NI se tron)

Medication Safety Issues
Sound-alike/look-alike issues:
Granisetron may be confused with dolasetron, ondansetron, palonosetron
Brand Names: U.S. Granisol™; Kytril®; Sancuso®
Brand Names: Canada Granisetron Hydrochloride Injection; Kytril®
Index Terms BRL 43694
Generic Availability (U.S.) Yes: Injection, tablet
Pharmacologic Category Antiemetic; Selective 5-HT₃ Receptor Antagonist
Use Prophylaxis of nausea and vomiting associated with emetogenic chemotherapy and radiation therapy; prophylaxis and treatment of postoperative nausea and vomiting (PONV)
Unlabeled/Investigational Use Breakthrough treatment of nausea and vomiting associated with chemotherapy
Contraindications Hypersensitivity to granisetron or any component of the formulation
Warnings/Precautions Use with caution in patients with congenital long QT syndrome or other risk factors for QT prolongation (eg, medications known to prolong QT interval, electrolyte abnormalities, and cumulative high-dose anthracycline therapy). 5-HT₃ antagonists have been associated with a number of dose-dependent increases in ECG intervals (eg, PR, QRS duration, QT/QTc, JT), usually occurring 1-2 hours after I.V. administration. In general, these changes are not clinically relevant, however, when used in conjunction with other agents that prolong these intervals, arrhythmia may occur. When used with agents that prolong the QT interval (eg, Class I and III antiarrhythmics), clinically relevant QT interval prolongation may occur resulting in torsade de pointes. I.V. formulations of 5-HT₃ antagonists have more association with ECG interval changes, compared to oral formulations.

For chemotherapy-related emesis, **granisetron should be used on a scheduled basis, not on an "as needed" (PRN) basis**, since data support the use of this drug in the prevention of nausea and vomiting and not in the rescue of nausea and vomiting. Granisetron should be used only in the first 24-48 hours of receiving chemotherapy or radiation. Data do not support any increased efficacy of granisetron in delayed nausea and vomiting.

Use with caution in patients allergic to other 5-HT₃ receptor antagonists; cross-reactivity has been reported. Routine prophylaxis for PONV is not recommended in patients where there is little expectation of nausea and vomiting postoperatively. In patients where nausea and vomiting must be avoided postoperatively, administer to all patients even when expected incidence of nausea and vomiting is low. Use caution following abdominal surgery or in chemotherapy-induced nausea and vomiting; may mask progressive ileus or gastric distention. Application site reactions, generally mild, have occurred with transdermal patch use; if skin reaction is severe or generalized, remove patch. Cover patch application site with clothing to protect from natural or artificial sunlight exposure while patch is applied and for 10 days following removal; granisetron may potentially be affected by natural or artificial sunlight. Do not apply patch to red, irritated, or damaged skin.

Adverse Reactions (Reflective of adult population; not specific for elderly)
>10%:
  Central nervous system: Headache (3% to 21%; transdermal patch: 1%)
  Gastrointestinal: Constipation (3% to 18%)
  Neuromuscular & skeletal: Weakness (5% to 18%)
1% to 10%:
  Cardiovascular: QT_c prolongation (1% to 3%), hypertension (1% to 2%)
  Central nervous system: Pain (10%), fever (3% to 9%), dizziness (4% to 5%), insomnia (<2% to 5%), somnolence (1% to 4%), anxiety (2%), agitation (<2%), CNS stimulation (<2%)
  Dermatologic: Rash (1%)
  Gastrointestinal: Diarrhea (3% to 9%), abdominal pain (4% to 6%), dyspepsia (3% to 6%), taste perversion (2%)
  Hepatic: Liver enzymes increased (5% to 6%)
  Renal: Oliguria (2%)
  Respiratory: Cough (2%)
  Miscellaneous: Infection (3%)

Drug Interactions
  Metabolism/Transport Effects Substrate of CYP3A4 (minor)
  Avoid Concomitant Use
    Avoid concomitant use of Granisetron with any of the following: Apomorphine; Artemether; Dronedarone; Lumefantrine; Nilotinib; Pimozide; QUEtiapine; QuiNINE; Tetrabenazine; Thioridazine; Toremifene; Vandetanib; Vemurafenib; Ziprasidone
  Increased Effect/Toxicity
    Granisetron may increase the levels/effects of: Apomorphine; Dronedarone; Pimozide; QTc-Prolonging Agents; QuiNINE; Tetrabenazine; Thioridazine; Toremifene; Vandetanib; Vemurafenib; Ziprasidone

    The levels/effects of Granisetron may be increased by: Alfuzosin; Artemether; Chloroquine; Ciprofloxacin; Ciprofloxacin (Systemic); Conivaptan; Gadobutrol; Lumefantrine; Nilotinib; QUEtiapine; QuiNINE
  Decreased Effect
    The levels/effects of Granisetron may be decreased by: Tocilizumab

Stability
  I.V.: Store at 15°C to 30°C (59°F to 86°F). Stable when mixed in NS or D_5W for 7 days under refrigeration and for 3 days at room temperature. Protect from light. Do not freeze vials.
  Oral: Store tablet or oral solution at 15°C to 30°C (59°F to 86°F). Protect from light.
  Transdermal patch: Store at 20°C to 25°C (68°F to 77°F). Keep patch in original packaging until immediately prior to use.

Mechanism of Action Selective 5-HT$_3$-receptor antagonist, blocking serotonin, both peripherally on vagal nerve terminals and centrally in the chemoreceptor trigger zone

Pharmacodynamics/Kinetics
  Duration: Oral, I.V.: Generally up to 24 hours
  Absorption: Oral: Tablets and oral solution are bioequivalent; Transdermal patch: ~66% over 7 days
  Distribution: V_d: 2-4 L/kg; widely throughout body
  Protein binding: 65%
  Metabolism: Hepatic via N-demethylation, oxidation, and conjugation; some metabolites may have 5-HT$_3$ antagonist activity
  Half-life elimination: Oral: 6 hours; I.V.: 9 hours
  Time to peak, plasma: Transdermal patch: Maximum systemic concentrations: ~48 hours after application (range: 24-168 hours)
  Excretion: Urine (12% as unchanged drug, 48% to 49% as metabolites); feces (34% to 38% as metabolites)

Dosage
  Geriatric & Adult
    Prophylaxis of chemotherapy-related emesis:
      Oral: 2 mg once daily up to 1 hour before chemotherapy or 1 mg twice daily; the first 1 mg dose should be given up to 1 hour before chemotherapy.

I.V.:

Within U.S.: 10 mcg/kg/dose (maximum: 1 mg/dose) given 30 minutes prior to chemotherapy; for some drugs (eg, carboplatin, cyclophosphamide) with a later onset of emetic action, 10 mcg/kg every 12 hours may be necessary.

Outside U.S.: 40 mcg/kg/dose (or 3 mg/dose); maximum: 9 mg/24 hours

Breakthrough: Granisetron has not been shown to be effective in terminating nausea or vomiting once it occurs and should not be used for this purpose.

Transdermal patch: Prophylaxis of chemotherapy-related emesis: Apply 1 patch at least 24 hours prior to chemotherapy; do not apply ≥48 hours before chemotherapy. Remove patch a minimum of 24 hours after chemotherapy completion. Maximum duration: Patch may be worn up to 7 days, depending on chemotherapy regimen duration.

Prophylaxis of radiation therapy-associated emesis: Oral: 2 mg once daily given 1 hour before radiation therapy.

Postoperative nausea and vomiting (PONV): I.V.:

Prevention: 1 mg given undiluted over 30 seconds; the manufacturer recommends administration before induction of anesthesia or immediately before reversal of anesthesia. **Note:** The Society for Ambulatory Anesthesia (SAMBA) Guidelines recommend a dosage range of 0.35-1.5 mg administered at the end of surgery (Gan, 2007). However, doses ≤1 mg are generally used since doses >1 mg are not more effective. Of note, 5 mcg/kg (~0.35 mg in a 70 kg adult) has been shown to be effective; doses >5 mcg/kg were not more effective (Mikawa, 1997).

Treatment: 1 mg given undiluted over 30 seconds

Renal Impairment No dosage adjustment required.

Hepatic Impairment Kinetic studies in patients with hepatic impairment showed that total clearance was approximately halved; however, standard doses were very well tolerated, and dose adjustments are not necessary.

Administration

Oral: Doses should be given up to 1 hour prior to initiation of chemotherapy/radiation

I.V.: Administer I.V. push over 30 seconds or as a 5-10 minute-infusion

Prevention of PONV: Administer before induction of anesthesia or immediately before reversal of anesthesia.

Treatment of PONV: Administer undiluted over 30 seconds.

Transdermal (Sancuso®): Apply patch to clean, dry, intact skin on upper outer arm. Do not use on red, irritated or damaged skin. Remove patch from pouch immediately before application. Do not cut patch.

Monitoring Parameters Monitor for control of nausea and vomiting

Special Geriatric Considerations Clinical trials with patients older than 65 years of age are limited; however, the data indicates that safety and efficacy are similar to that observed in younger adults. No adjustment in dose necessary for elderly.

Dosage Forms Excipient information presented when available (limited, particularly for generics); consult specific product labeling. [DSC] = Discontinued product

Injection, solution: 0.1 mg/mL (1 mL [DSC]); 1 mg/mL (1 mL, 4 mL)

Kytril®: 1 mg/mL (4 mL [DSC]) [contains benzyl alcohol]

Injection, solution [preservative free]: 0.1 mg/mL (1 mL); 1 mg/mL (1 mL)

Patch, transdermal:

Sancuso®: 3.1 mg/24 hours (1s) [52 cm^2, total granisetron 34.3 mg]

Solution, oral:

Granisol™: 2 mg/10 mL (30 mL) [contains sodium benzoate; orange flavor]

Tablet, oral: 1 mg

Kytril®: 1 mg

Extemporaneously Prepared A 0.2 mg/mL oral suspension may be prepared by crushing twelve (12) 1 mg tablets and mixing with 30 mL water and enough cherry syrup to provide a final volume of 60 mL; this preparation is stable for 14 days at room temperature or when refrigerated

Quercia RA, Zhang JH, Fan C, et al, "Stability of Granisetron (Kytril®) in an Extemporaneously Prepared Oral Liquid," *International Pharmaceutical Abstracts*, 1996, May 15, Vol 33.

Selected References

Gill D and Howell J, "Pharmacokinetics and Bioavailability of Transdermal Granisetron After a Six-Day Application of Three Patch Sizes, Compared to 2 mg Once-Daily Oral Dose of Granisetron for Five Days," *Support Care Cancer*, 2008, 16(6):619-756 [abstract from 2008 International MASCC/ISOO Symposium].

◆ **Granisol™** *see* Granisetron *on page 842*
◆ **Granulex®** *see* Trypsin, Balsam Peru, and Castor Oil *on page 1876*
◆ **Granulocyte Colony Stimulating Factor** *see* Filgrastim *on page 733*
◆ **Granulocyte Colony Stimulating Factor (PEG Conjugate)** *see* Pegfilgrastim *on page 1402*
◆ **Grifulvin V®** *see* Griseofulvin *on page 845*

Griseofulvin (gri see oh FUL vin)

Medication Safety Issues
International issues:
Fulvicin® (brand name used in international markets) may be confused with Furacin®
Brand Names: U.S. Grifulvin V®; Gris-PEG®
Index Terms Griseofulvin Microsize; Griseofulvin Ultramicrosize
Generic Availability (U.S.) Yes: Suspension, ultramicrosized product
Pharmacologic Category Antifungal Agent, Oral
Use Treatment of susceptible tinea infections of the skin, hair, and nails
Contraindications Hypersensitivity to griseofulvin or any component of the formulation; severe liver disease; porphyria (interferes with porphyrin metabolism)
Warnings/Precautions During long-term therapy, periodic assessment of hepatic, renal, and hematopoietic functions should be performed; avoid exposure to intense sunlight to prevent photosensitivity reactions; hypersensitivity cross reaction between penicillins and griseofulvin is possible
Adverse Reactions (Reflective of adult population; not specific for elderly) Frequency not defined.
Central nervous system: Dizziness, fatigue, headache, insomnia, mental confusion
Dermatologic: Angioneurotic edema (rare), erythema multiforme-like drug reaction, photosensitivity, rash (most common), urticaria (most common),
Gastrointestinal: Diarrhea, epigastric distress, GI bleeding, nausea, vomiting
Genitourinary: Menstrual irregularities (rare)
Hematologic: Granulocytopenia, leukopenia
Hepatic: Hepatotoxicity
Neuromuscular & skeletal: Paresthesia (rare)
Renal: Nephrosis, proteinuria
Miscellaneous: Drug-induced lupus-like syndrome (rare), oral thrush

Drug Interactions
Metabolism/Transport Effects Induces CYP1A2 (weak), 2C8 (weak), 2C9 (weak), 3A4 (weak)
Avoid Concomitant Use
Avoid concomitant use of Griseofulvin with any of the following: Contraceptives (Progestins)
Increased Effect/Toxicity
Griseofulvin may increase the levels/effects of: Alcohol (Ethyl); Porfimer
Decreased Effect
Griseofulvin may decrease the levels/effects of: Contraceptives (Estrogens); Contraceptives (Progestins); CycloSPORINE; CycloSPORINE (Systemic); Saccharomyces boulardii; Saxagliptin; Vitamin K Antagonists

The levels/effects of Griseofulvin may be decreased by: Barbiturates
Ethanol/Nutrition/Herb Interactions
Ethanol: Avoid ethanol (may increase CNS depression). Concomitant use with ethanol will cause "disulfiram"-type reaction consisting of tachycardia, flushing, headache, nausea, and in some patients, vomiting and chest and/or abdominal pain.
Food: Griseofulvin concentrations may be increased if taken with food, especially with high-fat meals.
Mechanism of Action Inhibits fungal cell mitosis at metaphase; binds to human keratin making it resistant to fungal invasion

Pharmacodynamics/Kinetics
Absorption: Ultramicrosize griseofulvin is almost complete; absorption of microsize griseofulvin is variable (25% to 70% of an oral dose); absorption is enhanced by ingestion of a fatty meal
Distribution: Deposited in varying concentrations in the keratin layer of the skin, hair, and nails; only a very small fraction is distributed in the body fluids and tissues
Metabolism: Extensive in the liver
Half-life: 9-22 hours
Time to peak serum concentration: ~4 hours
Elimination: <1% excreted unchanged in urine; also excreted in feces and perspiration

Dosage
Geriatric & Adult
Tinea infections: Oral:
Microsize: 500-1000 mg/day in single or divided doses
Ultramicrosize: 375 mg/day in single or divided doses; doses up to 750 mg/day have been used for infections more difficult to eradicate such as tinea unguium and tinea pedis.

Note: Duration of therapy depends on the site of infection:
Tinea corporis: 2-4 weeks
Tinea capitis: 4-6 weeks or longer (up to 8-12 weeks)
Tinea pedis: 4-8 weeks
Tinea unguium: 4-6 months

Administration Oral: Administer with a fatty meal (peanuts or ice cream) to increase absorption, or with food or milk to avoid GI upset

Gris-PEG® tablets: May be swallowed whole or crushed and sprinkled onto 1 tablespoonful of applesauce and swallowed immediately without chewing.

Monitoring Parameters Periodic renal, hepatic, and hematopoietic function tests

Test Interactions False-positive urinary VMA levels

Special Geriatric Considerations No specific changes in dosing are needed.

Dosage Forms Excipient information presented when available (limited, particularly for generics); consult specific product labeling.
Suspension, oral [microsize]: 125 mg/5 mL (120 mL)
Tablet, oral [microsize]:
Grifulvin V®: 500 mg [scored]
Tablet, oral [ultramicrosize]:
Gris-PEG®: 125 mg, 250 mg [scored]

♦ **Griseofulvin Microsize** see Griseofulvin on page 845
♦ **Griseofulvin Ultramicrosize** see Griseofulvin on page 845
♦ **Gris-PEG®** see Griseofulvin on page 845
♦ **GSK 1838262** see Gabapentin Enacarbil on page 805
♦ **Guaiatussin AC** see Guaifenesin and Codeine on page 848
♦ **Guaicon DM [OTC] [DSC]** see Guaifenesin and Dextromethorphan on page 848
♦ **Guaicon DMS [OTC]** see Guaifenesin and Dextromethorphan on page 848

GuaiFENesin (gwye FEN e sin)

Medication Safety Issues
Sound-alike/look-alike issues:
GuaiFENesin may be confused with guanFACINE
Mucinex® may be confused with Mucomyst®
Naldecon® may be confused with Nalfon®
International issues:
Mucolex® [Hong Kong] may be confused with Mycelex® which is a brand name for clotrimazole in the U.S.

Brand Names: U.S. Allfen [OTC]; Bidex®-400 [OTC]; Diabetic Siltussin DAS-Na [OTC]; Diabetic Tussin® EX [OTC]; Fenesin IR [OTC]; Ganidin® NR [OTC] [DSC]; Geri-Tussin [OTC]; Humibid® Maximum Strength [OTC]; Mucinex® Kid's Mini-Melts™ [OTC]; Mucinex® Kid's [OTC]; Mucinex® Maximum Strength [OTC]; Mucinex® [OTC]; Mucus Relief [OTC]; Organidin® NR [OTC] [DSC]; Refenesen™ 400 [OTC]; Refenesen™ [OTC]; Robafen [OTC]; Scot-Tussin® Expectorant [OTC]; Siltussin DAS [OTC] [DSC]; Siltussin SA [OTC]; Vicks® Casero™ Chest Congestion Relief [OTC]; Vicks® DayQuil® Mucus Control [OTC]; Xpect™ [OTC]

Brand Names: Canada Balminil Expectorant; Benylin® E Extra Strength; Koffex Expectorant; Robitussin®

Index Terms Cheratussin; GG; Glycerol Guaiacolate

Generic Availability (U.S.) Yes; Excludes extended release and granules

Pharmacologic Category Expectorant

Use Help loosen phlegm and thin bronchial secretions to make coughs more productive

Contraindications Hypersensitivity to guaifenesin or any component of the formulation

Warnings/Precautions When used for self medication (OTC) notify healthcare provider if symptoms do not improve within 7 days, or are accompanied by fever, rash, or persistent headache. Do not use for persistent or chronic cough (as with smoking, asthma, chronic bronchitis, emphysema) or if cough is accompanied by excessive phlegm unless directed to do so by healthcare provider. Some products may contain phenylalanine.

Adverse Reactions (Reflective of adult population; not specific for elderly) Frequency not defined.
Central nervous system: Dizziness, drowsiness, headache
Dermatologic: Rash
Endocrine & metabolic: Uric acid levels decreased
Gastrointestinal: Nausea, stomach pain, vomiting

Drug Interactions
Avoid Concomitant Use There are no known interactions where it is recommended to avoid concomitant use.

Increased Effect/Toxicity There are no known significant interactions involving an increase in effect.

Decreased Effect There are no known significant interactions involving a decrease in effect.

Mechanism of Action Thought to act as an expectorant by irritating the gastric mucosa and stimulating respiratory tract secretions, thereby increasing respiratory fluid volumes and decreasing mucous viscosity

Pharmacodynamics/Kinetics

Absorption: Well absorbed

Half-life elimination: ~1 hour

Excretion: Urine (as unchanged drug and metabolites)

Dosage

Geriatric & Adult

Cough (expectorant): Oral: 200-400 mg every 4 hours to a maximum of 2.4 g/day

Extended release tablet: 600-1200 mg every 12 hours, not to exceed 2.4 g/day

Administration Do not crush, chew, or break extended release tablets. Administer with a full glass of water.

Monitoring Parameters Cough, sputum consistency and volume

Test Interactions Possible color interference with determination of 5-HIAA and VMA; discontinue for 48 hours prior to test

Pharmacotherapy Pearls Should not be used for persistent or chronic cough such as that occurring with smoking, asthma, chronic bronchitis, or emphysema or for cough associated with excessive phlegm; there is lack of convincing studies to document the efficacy of guaifenesin.

Dosage Forms Excipient information presented when available (limited, particularly for generics); consult specific product labeling. [DSC] = Discontinued product

Caplet, oral:

Fenesin IR: 400 mg

Refenesen™ 400: 400 mg [dye free]

Granules, oral:

Mucinex® Kid's Mini-Melts™: 50 mg/packet (12s) [contains magnesium 6 mg/packet, phenylalanine 0.6 mg/packet, sodium 2 mg/packet; grape flavor]

Mucinex® Kid's Mini-Melts™: 100 mg/packet (12s) [contains magnesium 6 mg/packet, phenylalanine 1 mg/packet, sodium 3 mg/packet; bubblegum flavor]

Liquid, oral:

Diabetic Tussin® EX: 100 mg/5 mL (118 mL) [dye free, ethanol free, sugar free; contains phenylalanine 8.4 mg/5 mL]

Ganidin® NR: 100 mg/5 mL (473 mL [DSC]) [raspberry flavor]

Mucinex® Kid's: 100 mg/5 mL (118 mL) [contains propylene glycol, sodium 3 mg/5 mL; grape flavor]

Scot-Tussin® Expectorant: 100 mg/5 mL (120 mL) [dye free, ethanol free, sugar free; contains benzoic acid; grape flavor]

Siltussin DAS: 100 mg/5 mL (120 mL [DSC]) [dye free, ethanol free, sugar free; strawberry flavor]

Vicks® Casero™ Chest Congestion Relief: 100 mg/6.25 mL (120 mL, 240 mL) [contains phenylalanine 5.5 mg/12.5 mL, sodium 32 mg/12.5 mL, sodium benzoate; honey-menthol flavor]

Vicks® DayQuil® Mucus Control: 200 mg/15 mL (295 mL) [contains propylene glycol, sodium 25 mg/15 mL, sodium benzoate; citrus blend flavor]

Syrup, oral: 100 mg/5 mL (5 mL, 10 mL, 15 mL, 118 mL, 120 mL, 240 mL, 473 mL, 480 mL)

Diabetic Siltussin DAS-Na: 100 mg/5 mL (118 mL) [ethanol free, sugar free; contains benzoic acid, phenylalanine 3 mg/5 mL, propylene glycol; strawberry flavor]

Geri-Tussin: 100 mg/5 mL (120 mL, 240 mL, 480 mL) [ethanol free, sugar free; contains sodium benzoate]

Robafen: 100 mg/5 mL (120 mL, 240 mL, 480 mL) [ethanol free; contains sodium benzoate; cherry flavor]

Siltussin SA: 100 mg/5 mL (120 mL, 240 mL, 480 mL) [ethanol free, sugar free; strawberry flavor]

Tablet, oral: 200 mg [DSC], 400 mg

Allfen: 400 mg [scored]

Bidex®-400: 400 mg

Mucus Relief: 400 mg

Organidin® NR: 200 mg [DSC] [scored]

Refenesen™: 200 mg

Xpect™: 400 mg [sugar free]

◄ Tablet, extended release, oral:
Humibid® Maximum Strength: 1200 mg
Mucinex®: 600 mg
Mucinex® Maximum Strength: 1200 mg

Guaifenesin and Codeine (gwye FEN e sin & KOE deen)

Related Information
Codeine *on page 407*
GuaiFENesin *on page 846*
Brand Names: U.S. Allfen CD; Allfen CDX; Dex-Tuss; ExeClear-C; Gani-Tuss® NR;
Guaiatussin AC; Mar-Cof® CG; Robafen AC; Tusso-C™
Index Terms Codeine and Guaifenesin; Robitussin AC
Generic Availability (U.S.) Yes: Oral solution, syrup
Pharmacologic Category Antitussive; Cough Preparation; Expectorant
Use Temporary control of cough due to minor throat and bronchial irritation
Dosage
  Geriatric & Adult Cough (antitussive/expectorant): Oral:
    ExeClear-C: 10 mL every 4-6 hours; maximum: 60 mL/24 hours
    Dex-Tuss, Gani-Tuss® NR: 5 mL every 4-6 hours; maximum 40 mL/24 hours
    Note: Also refer to specific product labeling.
Special Geriatric Considerations Elderly may be more sensitive to the CNS depressant
effects of codeine; monitor closely for excessive sedation.
Controlled Substance C-V
Dosage Forms Excipient information presented when available (limited, particularly for
generics); consult specific product labeling.
  Liquid:
    Dex-Tuss: Guaifenesin 300 mg and codeine phosphate 10 mg per 5 mL (473 mL) [ethanol
      free, gluten free, sugar free; contains propylene glycol; grape flavor]
    Gani-Tuss® NR: Guaifenesin 100 mg and codeine phosphate 10 mg per 5 mL (480 mL)
      [raspberry flavor]
  Solution, oral: Guaifenesin 100 mg and codeine phosphate 10 mg per 5 mL (5 mL, 10 mL, 118
    mL, 473 mL)
    Mar-Cof® CG: Guaifenesin 225 mg and codeine phosphate 7.5 mg per 5 mL (473 ml)
      [ethanol free, sugar free; contains propylene glycol, sodium benzoate, sodium 6 mg/5 mL]
  Syrup: Guaifenesin 100 mg and codeine phosphate 10 mg per 5 mL (473 mL)
    ExeClear-C: Guaifenesin 200 mg and codeine phosphate 10 mg per 5 mL (473 mL) [dye
      free, ethanol free, sugar free; contains propylene glycol, sodium benzoate; fruit flavor]
    Guaiatussin AC: Guaifenesin 100 mg and codeine phosphate 10 mg per 5 mL (118 mL, 473
      mL) [contains ethanol 3.5%, sodium 1 mg/5 mL, sodium benzoate; cherry flavor]
    Robafen AC: Guaifenesin 100 mg and codeine phosphate 10 mg per 5 mL (120 mL, 480
      mL) [contains ethanol 3.5%, sodium 4 mg/5 mL, sodium benzoate; cherry flavor]
    Tusso-C™: Guaifenesin 200 mg and codeine phosphate 10 mg per 5 mL (480 mL) [ethanol
      free, dye free, sugar free; contains menthol, phenylalanine 0.03 mcg/5 mL; cherry vanilla
      flavor]
  Tablet:
    Allfen CD: Guaifenesin 400 mg and codeine phosphate 10 mg
    Allfen CDX: Guaifenesin 400 mg and codeine phosphate 20 mg

Guaifenesin and Dextromethorphan (gwye FEN e sin & deks troe meth OR fan)

Related Information
Dextromethorphan *on page 490*
GuaiFENesin *on page 846*
Medication Safety Issues
  Sound-alike/look-alike issues:
    Benylin® may be confused with Benadryl®, Ventolin®
Brand Names: U.S. Allfen DM [OTC] [DSC]; Cheracol® D [OTC]; Cheracol® Plus [OTC];
Coricidin HBP® Chest Congestion and Cough [OTC]; Diabetic Siltussin-DM DAS-Na Max-
imum Strength [OTC]; Diabetic Siltussin-DM DAS-Na [OTC]; Diabetic Tussin® DM Maximum
Strength [OTC]; Diabetic Tussin® DM [OTC]; Double Tussin DM [OTC]; Fenesin DM IR; Gani-
Tuss DM NR [DSC]; Guaicon DM [OTC] [DSC]; Guaicon DMS [OTC]; Guia-D [DSC];
Guiadrine™ DX [DSC]; Kolephrin® GG/DM [OTC]; Mintab DM [DSC]; Mucinex® DM Max-
imum Strength [OTC]; Mucinex® DM [OTC]; Mucinex® Kid's Cough Mini-Melts™ [OTC];
Mucinex® Kid's Cough [OTC]; Refenesen™ DM [OTC]; Robafen DM Clear [OTC]; Robafen

DM [OTC]; Robitussin® Cough & Chest Congestion DM Max [OTC]; Robitussin® Cough & Chest Congestion DM [OTC]; Robitussin® Cough & Chest Congestion Sugar-Free DM [OTC]; Safe Tussin® DM [OTC]; Scot-Tussin® Senior [OTC]; Silexin [OTC]; Siltussin DM DAS [OTC]; Siltussin DM [OTC]; Simuc-DM [DSC]; Su-Tuss DM [DSC]; Tussi-Bid®; Vicks® 44E [OTC]; Vicks® DayQuil® Mucus Control DM [OTC]; Vicks® Pediatric Formula 44E [OTC]

Brand Names: Canada Balminil DM E; Benylin® DM-E; Koffex DM-Expectorant; Robitussin® DM

Index Terms Dextromethorphan and Guaifenesin

Generic Availability (U.S.) Yes

Pharmacologic Category Antitussive; Cough Preparation; Expectorant

Use Temporary control of cough due to minor throat and bronchial irritation

Dosage

Geriatric & Adult Cough (antitussive/expectorant): Oral:

General dosing guidelines: Guaifenesin 200-400 mg and dextromethorphan 10-20 mg every 4 hours (maximum dose: Guaifenesin 2400 mg and dextromethorphan 120 mg per day)

Product-specific labeling:

Mucinex® DM: 1-2 tablets every 12 hours (maximum: 4 tablets/24 hours)

Vicks® 44E: 15 mL every 4 hours (maximum: 6 doses/24 hours)

Vicks® Pediatric Formula 44E: 30 mL every 4 hours (maximum: 6 doses/24 hours)

Dosage Forms Excipient information presented when available (limited, particularly for generics); consult specific product labeling. [DSC] = Discontinued product

Caplet, oral:

Fenesin DM IR: Guaifenesin 400 mg and dextromethorphan hydrobromide 15 mg

Refenesen™ DM: Guaifenesin 400 mg and dextromethorphan hydrobromide 20 mg

Capsule, softgel, oral:

Coricidin HBP® Chest Congestion and Cough: Guaifenesin 200 mg and dextromethorphan hydrobromide 10 mg

Elixir, oral:

Simuc-DM: Guaifenesin 225 mg and dextromethorphan hydrobromide 25 mg per 5 mL (480 mL) [grape flavor] [DSC]

Granules, oral:

Mucinex® Kid's Cough Mini-Melts™: Guaifenesin 100 mg and dextromethorphan hydrobromide 5 mg per packet (12s) [contains magnesium 6 mg/pack, phenylalanine 2 mg/packet, sodium 3 mg/packet; orange crème flavor]

Liquid, oral: Guaifenesin 100 mg and dextromethorphan hydrobromide 10 mg per 5 mL (480 mL); guaifenesin 300 mg and dextromethorphan hydrobromide 10 mg per 5 mL (120 mL, 480 mL)

Diabetic Tussin® DM: Guaifenesin 100 mg and dextromethorphan hydrobromide 10 mg per 5 mL (120 mL) [dye free, ethanol free, sugar free; contains phenylalanine 8.4 mg/5 mL]

Diabetic Tussin® DM Maximum Strength: Guaifenesin 200 mg and dextromethorphan hydrobromide 10 mg per 5 mL (120 mL) [dye free, ethanol free, sugar free; contains phenylalanine 8.4 mg/5 mL]

Double Tussin DM: Guaifenesin 300 mg and dextromethorphan hydrobromide 20 mg per 5 mL (120 mL, 480 mL) [dye free, ethanol free, sugar free]

Gani-Tuss NR: Guaifenesin 100 mg and dextromethorphan hydrobromide 10 mg per 5 mL (480 mL) [raspberry flavor] [DSC]

Guiadrine™ DX: Guaifenesin 225 mg and dextromethorphan hydrobromide 25 mg per 5 mL (473 mL) [ethanol free, sugar free; contains propylene glycol, sodium benzoate; grape flavor] [DSC]

Kolephrin® GG/DM: Guaifenesin 150 mg and dextromethorphan hydrobromide 10 mg per 5 mL (120 mL) [ethanol free; cherry flavor]

Mucinex® Kid's Cough: Guaifenesin 100 mg and dextromethorphan hydrobromide 5 mg per 5 mL (120 mL) [contains propylene glycol, sodium 3 mg/5 mL; cherry flavor]

Safe Tussin® DM: Guaifenesin 100 mg and dextromethorphan hydrobromide 15 mg per 5 mL (120 mL) [contains benzoic acid, phenylalanine 4.2 mg/5 mL, and propylene glycol; orange and mint flavors]

Scot-Tussin® Senior: Guaifenesin 200 mg and dextromethorphan hydrobromide 15 mg per 5 mL (120 mL) [ethanol free, sodium free, sugar free]

Vicks® 44E: Guaifenesin 200 mg and dextromethorphan hydrobromide 20 mg per 15 mL (120 mL, 235 mL) [contains ethanol, sodium 31 mg/15 mL, sodium benzoate]

Vicks® DayQuil® Mucus Control DM: Guaifenesin 200 mg and dextromethorphan hydrobromide 10 mg per 15 mL (295 mL) [contains propylene glycol, sodium 25 mg/15 mL, sodium benzoate; citrus blend flavor]

Vicks® Pediatric Formula 44E: Guaifenesin 100 mg and dextromethorphan hydrobromide 10 mg per 15 mL (120 mL) [ethanol free; contains sodium 30 mg/15 mL, sodium benzoate; cherry flavor]

GUAIFENESIN AND DEXTROMETHORPHAN

Syrup, oral: Guaifenesin 100 mg and dextromethorphan hydrobromide 10 mg per 5 mL (5 mL, 10 mL, 120 mL, 480 mL)

Cheracol® D: Guaifenesin 100 mg and dextromethorphan hydrobromide 10 mg per 5 mL (120 mL, 180 mL) [contains benzoic acid, ethanol 4.75%]

Cheracol® Plus: Guaifenesin 100 mg and dextromethorphan hydrobromide 10 mg per 5 mL (120 mL) [contains benzoic acid, ethanol 4.75%]

Diabetic Siltussin-DM DAS-Na: Guaifenesin 100 mg and dextromethorphan hydrobromide 10 mg per 5 mL (118 mL) [ethanol free, sugar free; contains benzoic acid, phenylalanine 3 mg/5 mL, propylene glycol; strawberry flavor]

Diabetic Siltussin-DM DAS-Na Maximum Strength: Guaifenesin 200 mg and dextromethorphan hydrobromide 10 mg per 5 mL (118 mL) [ethanol free, sugar free; contains benzoic acid, phenylalanine 3 mg/5 mL, propylene glycol; strawberry flavor]

Guaicon DM: Guaifenesin 100 mg and dextromethorphan hydrobromide 10 mg per 5 mL (10 mL) [ethanol free] [DSC]

Guaicon DMS: Guaifenesin 100 mg and dextromethorphan hydrobromide 10 mg per 5 mL (10 mL) [ethanol free, sugar free]

Mintab DM: Guaifenesin 200 mg and dextromethorphan hydrobromide 10 mg per 5 mL (480 mL) [dye free, ethanol free; cherry vanilla flavor] [DSC]

Robafen DM: Guaifenesin 100 mg and dextromethorphan hydrobromide 10 mg per 5 mL (120 mL, 240 mL, 480 mL) [cherry flavor]

Robafen DM Clear: Guaifenesin 100 mg and dextromethorphan hydrobromide 10 mg per 5 mL (120 mL)

Robitussin® Cough & Chest Congestion DM: Guaifenesin 100 mg and dextromethorphan hydrobromide 10 mg per 5 mL (120 mL, 240 mL, 360 mL) [ethanol free; contains propylene glycol, sodium 7 mg/5 mL, sodium benzoate]

Robitussin® Cough & Chest Congestion DM Max: Guaifenesin 200 mg and dextromethorphan hydrobromide 10 mg per 5 mL (120 mL, 240 mL) [ethanol free; contains propylene glycol, sodium 5 mg/5 mL, sodium benzoate]

Robitussin® Cough & Chest Congestion Sugar-Free DM: Guaifenesin 100 mg and dextromethorphan hydrobromide 10 mg per 5 mL (120 mL) [ethanol free, sugar free; contains propylene glycol, sodium 4 mg/5 mL, sodium benzoate]

Robitussin® Cough and Congestion: Guaifenesin 100 mg and dextromethorphan hydrobromide 10 mg per 5 mL (120 mL) [ethanol free; contains sodium benzoate]

Silexin: Guaifenesin 100 mg and dextromethorphan hydrobromide 10 mg per 5 mL (45 mL) [ethanol free, sugar free)]

Siltussin DM: Guaifenesin 100 mg and dextromethorphan hydrobromide 10 mg per 5 mL (120 mL, 240 mL, 480 mL) [strawberry flavor]

Siltussin DM DAS: Guaifenesin 100 mg and dextromethorphan hydrobromide 10 mg per 5 mL (120 mL) [dye free, ethanol free, sugar free; strawberry flavor]

Tablet, oral: Guaifenesin 1000 mg and dextromethorphan hydrobromide 60 mg; guaifenesin 1200 mg and dextromethorphan hydrobromide 60 mg

Allfen DM: Guaifenesin 400 mg and dextromethorphan hydrobromide 20 mg [DSC]

Silexin: Guaifenesin 100 mg and dextromethorphan hydrobromide 10 mg

Tablet, extended release, oral: Guaifenesin 800 mg and dextromethorphan hydrobromide 30 mg; Guaifenesin 1200 mg and dextromethorphan hydrobromide 20 mg

Mucinex® DM: Guaifenesin 600 mg and dextromethorphan hydrobromide 30 mg

Mucinex® DM Maximum Strength: Guaifenesin 1200 mg and dextromethorphan hydrobromide 60 mg

Tablet, long-acting, oral: Guaifenesin 1000 mg and dextromethorphan hydrobromide 60 mg

Tablet, sustained release, oral

Tussi-Bid®: Guaifenesin 1200 mg and dextromethorphan hydrobromide 60 mg

Tablet, timed release, oral [scored]: Guaifenesin 1200 mg and dextromethorphan hydrobromide 60 mg

Guia-D: Guaifenesin 1000 mg and dextromethorphan hydrobromide 60 mg [dye free] [DSC]

Guanabenz (GWAHN a benz)

Medication Safety Issues
Sound-alike/look-alike issues:
Guanabenz may be confused with guanadrel, guanfacine
Brand Names: Canada Wytensin®
Index Terms Guanabenz Acetate
Generic Availability (U.S.) Yes
Pharmacologic Category Alpha2-Adrenergic Agonist
Use Management of hypertension

Dosage

Geriatric Initial: 4 mg once daily, increase every 1-2 weeks

Adult Hypertension: Oral: Initial: 4 mg twice daily; increase in increments of 4-8 mg/day every 1-2 weeks to a maximum of 32 mg twice daily.

Hepatic Impairment Dosage adjustment is probably necessary; however, no specific guidelines are available.

Special Geriatric Considerations Because of its CNS adverse effects, guanabenz is not considered a drug of choice for the treatment of hypertension in the elderly.

Dosage Forms Excipient information presented when available (limited, particularly for generics); consult specific product labeling. [DSC] = Discontinued product

Tablet, oral: 4 mg, 8 mg [DSC]

◆ **Guanabenz Acetate** see Guanabenz on page 850

GuanFACINE (GWAHN fa seen)

Medication Safety Issues

Sound-alike/look-alike issues:

GuanFACINE may be confused with guaiFENesin, guanabenz, guanidine

Tenex® may be confused with Entex®, Ten-K®, Xanax®

International issues:

Tenex [U.S., Canada] may be confused with Kinex brand name for biperiden [Mexico]

Brand Names: U.S. Intuniv™; Tenex®

Index Terms Guanfacine Hydrochloride

Generic Availability (U.S.) Yes: Excludes extended release tablet

Pharmacologic Category Alpha$_2$-Adrenergic Agonist

Use

Tablet, immediate release: Management of hypertension

Tablet, extended release: Treatment of attention-deficit/hyperactivity disorder (ADHD) as monotherapy or adjunctive therapy to stimulants

Unlabeled/Investigational Use Tic disorder; aggression

Dosage

Geriatric Refer to adult dosing. In the management of hypertension, consider lower initial doses and titrate to response (Aronow, 2011).

Adult Hypertension: Oral: Immediate release: 1 mg usually at bedtime, may increase if needed at 3- to 4-week intervals; usual dose range (JNC 7): 0.5-2 mg once daily

Renal Impairment

No specific dosage adjustments are recommended by the manufacturer; consider using the lower end of the dosing range in patients with renal impairment.

Hemodialysis: Dialysis clearance is ~15% of total clearance; usual doses are recommended.

Hepatic Impairment No specific dosage adjustments are recommended by the manufacturer; however, dosage adjustments may be required.

Special Geriatric Considerations Because of adverse effects such as CNS depression, dry mouth, and constipation, guanfacine is not considered a drug of choice in the elderly.

Dosage Forms Excipient information presented when available (limited, particularly for generics); consult specific product labeling.

Tablet, oral: 1 mg, 2 mg

Tenex®: 1 mg, 2 mg

Tablet, extended release, oral:

Intuniv™: 1 mg, 2 mg, 3 mg, 4 mg

◆ **Guanfacine Hydrochloride** see GuanFACINE on page 851
◆ **Guia-D [DSC]** see Guaifenesin and Dextromethorphan on page 848
◆ **Guiadrine™ DX [DSC]** see Guaifenesin and Dextromethorphan on page 848
◆ **Gyne-Lotrimin® 3 [OTC]** see Clotrimazole (Topical) on page 399
◆ **Gyne-Lotrimin® 7 [OTC]** see Clotrimazole (Topical) on page 399
◆ **H1N1 Influenza Vaccine** see Influenza Virus Vaccine (Inactivated) on page 936
◆ **H1N1 Influenza Vaccine** see Influenza Virus Vaccine (Live/Attenuated) on page 940
◆ **H5N1 Influenza Vaccine** see Influenza Virus Vaccine (H5N1) on page 936
◆ **Habitrol** see Nicotine on page 1297

Halcinonide (hal SIN oh nide)

Related Information
Corticosteroids *on page 2005*
Medication Safety Issues
Sound-alike/look-alike issues:
Halcinonide may be confused with Halcion®
Halog® may be confused with Haldol®, Mycolog®
Brand Names: U.S. Halog®
Brand Names: Canada Halog®
Generic Availability (U.S.) No
Pharmacologic Category Corticosteroid, Topical
Use Inflammation of corticosteroid-responsive dermatoses [high potency topical corticosteroid]
Dosage
Geriatric & Adult Steroid-responsive dermatoses: Topical: Apply sparingly 1-3 times/day, occlusive dressing may be used for severe or resistant dermatoses; a thin film is effective; do not overuse. Therapy should be discontinued when control is achieved; if no improvement is seen, reassessment of diagnosis may be necessary.
Special Geriatric Considerations Due to age-related changes in skin, limit use of topical corticosteroids.
Dosage Forms Excipient information presented when available (limited, particularly for generics); consult specific product labeling.
Cream, topical:
Halog®: 0.1% (30 g, 60 g)
Ointment, topical:
Halog®: 0.1% (30 g, 60 g)

◆ **Halcion®** *see* Triazolam *on page 1859*
◆ **Haldol®** *see* Haloperidol *on page 853*
◆ **Haldol® Decanoate** *see* Haloperidol *on page 853*
◆ **Haley's M-O** *see* Magnesium Hydroxide and Mineral Oil *on page 1110*
◆ **HalfLytely® and Bisacodyl** *see* Polyethylene Glycol-Electrolyte Solution and Bisacodyl *on page 1481*
◆ **Halfprin® [OTC]** *see* Aspirin *on page 153*

Halobetasol (hal oh BAY ta sol)

Related Information
Corticosteroids *on page 2005*
Medication Safety Issues
Sound-alike/look-alike issues:
Ultravate® may be confused with Cutivate®
Brand Names: U.S. Ultravate®
Brand Names: Canada Ultravate®
Index Terms Halobetasol Propionate
Generic Availability (U.S.) Yes
Pharmacologic Category Corticosteroid, Topical
Use Relief of inflammatory and pruritic manifestations of corticosteroid-response dermatoses [super high potency topical corticosteroid]
Dosage
Geriatric & Adult
Inflammatory and pruritic manifestations (dental use): Cream: Apply sparingly to lesion twice daily. Treatment should not exceed 2 consecutive weeks and total dosage should not exceed 50 g/week. Therapy should be discontinued when control is achieved; if no improvement is seen, reassessment of diagnosis may be necessary.
Steroid-responsive dermatoses: Topical: Apply sparingly to skin twice daily, rub in gently and completely; treatment should not exceed 2 consecutive weeks and total dosage should not exceed 50 g/week. Therapy should be discontinued when control is achieved; if no improvement is seen, reassessment of diagnosis may be necessary.
Special Geriatric Considerations Due to age-related changes in skin, limit use of topical corticosteroids.

Dosage Forms Excipient information presented when available (limited, particularly for generics); consult specific product labeling.
Cream, topical, as propionate: 0.05% (15 g, 50 g)
   Ultravate®: 0.05% (15 g, 50 g)
Ointment, topical, as propionate: 0.05% (15 g, 50 g)
   Ultravate®: 0.05% (15 g, 50 g)

◆ **Halobetasol Propionate** see Halobetasol on page 852
◆ **Halog®** see Halcinonide on page 852

Haloperidol (ha loe PER i dole)

Related Information
Antipsychotic Agents on page 1997
Liquid Compatibility of Antidepressants, Antipsychotics, and Mood Stabilizers on page 2111

Medication Safety Issues
Sound-alike/look-alike issues:
Haloperidol may be confused Halotestin®
Haldol® may be confused with Halcion®, Halenol®, Halog®, Halotestin®, Stadol®

Brand Names: U.S. Haldol®; Haldol® Decanoate
Brand Names: Canada Apo-Haloperidol LA®; Apo-Haloperidol®; Haloperidol Injection, USP; Haloperidol Long Acting; Haloperidol-LA; Haloperidol-LA Omega; Novo-Peridol; PMS-Haloperidol; PMS-Haloperidol LA
Index Terms Haloperidol Decanoate; Haloperidol Lactate
Generic Availability (U.S.) Yes
Pharmacologic Category Antipsychotic Agent, Typical
Use Management of schizophrenia; control of tics and vocal utterances of Tourette's disorder
Unlabeled/Investigational Use Treatment of nonschizophrenia psychosis; may be used for the emergency sedation of severely-agitated or delirious patients; adjunctive treatment of ethanol dependence; postoperative nausea and vomiting (alternative therapy); psychosis/agitation related to Alzheimer's dementia
Contraindications Hypersensitivity to haloperidol or any component of the formulation; Parkinson's disease; severe CNS depression; coma
Warnings/Precautions [U.S. Boxed Warning]: Elderly patients with dementia-related psychosis treated with antipsychotics are at an increased risk of death compared to placebo. Most deaths appeared to be either cardiovascular (eg, heart failure, sudden death) or infectious (eg, pneumonia) in nature. Haloperidol is not approved for the treatment of dementia-related psychosis. Hypotension may occur, particularly with parenteral administration. Although the short-acting form (lactate) is used clinically, the I.V. use of the injection is not an FDA-approved route of administration; the decanoate form should never be administered intravenously.

May alter cardiac conduction and prolong QT interval; life-threatening arrhythmias have occurred with therapeutic doses of antipsychotics but risk may be increased with doses exceeding recommendations and/or intravenous administration (unlabeled route). Use caution or avoid use in patients with electrolyte abnormalities (eg, hypokalemia, hypomagnesemia), hypothyroidism, familial long QT syndrome, concomitant medications which may augment QT prolongation, or any underlying cardiac abnormality which may also potentiate risk. Monitor ECG closely for dose-related QT effects. Adverse effects of decanoate may be prolonged. Avoid in thyrotoxicosis.

Leukopenia, neutropenia, and agranulocytosis (sometimes fatal) have been reported in clinical trials and postmarketing reports with antipsychotic use; presence of risk factors (eg, pre-existing low WBC or history of drug-induced leuko-/neutropenia) should prompt periodic blood count assessment. Discontinue therapy at first signs of blood dyscrasias or if absolute neutrophil count <1000/mm^3.

May be sedating, use with caution in disorders where CNS depression is a feature. Effects may be potentiated when used with other sedative drugs or ethanol. Caution in patients with severe cardiovascular disease, predisposition to seizures, subcortical brain damage, or renal disease. Esophageal dysmotility and aspiration have been associated with antipsychotic use - use with caution in patients at risk of pneumonia (eg, Alzheimer's disease). Use associated with increased prolactin levels; clinical significance of hyperprolactinemia in patients with breast cancer or other prolactin-dependent tumors is unknown. May alter temperature regulation or mask toxicity of other drugs due to antiemetic effects. May cause orthostatic hypotension; use with caution in patients at risk of this effect or those who would tolerate transient hypotensive episodes (cerebrovascular disease, cardiovascular disease, or other

◀ medications which may predispose). Some tablets contain tartrazine. Antipsychotics have been associated with pigmentary retinopathy.

May cause anticholinergic effects (confusion, agitation, constipation, xerostomia, blurred vision, urinary retention). Therefore, they should be used with caution in patients with decreased gastrointestinal motility, urinary retention, BPH, xerostomia, or visual problems. Conditions which also may be exacerbated by cholinergic blockade include narrow-angle glaucoma and worsening of myasthenia gravis. Relative to other neuroleptics, haloperidol has a low potency of cholinergic blockade.

May cause extrapyramidal symptoms (EPS), including pseudoparkinsonism, acute dystonic reactions, akathisia, and tardive dyskinesia. Risk of dystonia (and possibly other EPS) may be greater with increased doses, use of conventional antipsychotics, males, and younger patients. May be associated with neuroleptic malignant syndrome (NMS). Use with caution in the elderly.

Adverse Reactions (Reflective of adult population; not specific for elderly) Frequency not defined.

Cardiovascular: Abnormal T waves with prolonged ventricular repolarization, arrhythmia, hyper-/hypotension, QT prolongation, sudden death, tachycardia, torsade de pointes

Central nervous system: Agitation, akathisia, altered central temperature regulation, anxiety, confusion, depression, drowsiness, dystonic reactions, euphoria, extrapyramidal reactions, headache, insomnia, lethargy, neuroleptic malignant syndrome (NMS), pseudoparkinsonian signs and symptoms, restlessness, seizure, tardive dyskinesia, tardive dystonia, vertigo

Dermatologic: Alopecia, contact dermatitis, hyperpigmentation, photosensitivity (rare), pruritus, rash

Endocrine & metabolic: Amenorrhea, breast engorgement, galactorrhea, gynecomastia, hyper-/hypoglycemia, hyponatremia, lactation, mastalgia, menstrual irregularities, sexual dysfunction

Gastrointestinal: Anorexia, constipation, diarrhea, dyspepsia, hypersalivation, nausea, vomiting, xerostomia

Genitourinary: Priapism, urinary retention

Hematologic: Cholestatic jaundice, obstructive jaundice

Ocular: Blurred vision

Respiratory: Bronchospasm, laryngospasm

Miscellaneous: Diaphoresis, heat stroke

Drug Interactions

Metabolism/Transport Effects Substrate of CYP1A2 (minor), 2D6 (major), 3A4 (major); **Inhibits** CYP2D6 (moderate), 3A4 (moderate)

Avoid Concomitant Use

Avoid concomitant use of Haloperidol with any of the following: Artemether; Conivaptan; Dronedarone; Lumefantrine; Metoclopramide; Nilotinib; Pimozide; QUEtiapine; QuiNINE; Tetrabenazine; Thioridazine; Tolvaptan; Toremifene; Vandetanib; Vemurafenib; Ziprasidone

Increased Effect/Toxicity

Haloperidol may increase the levels/effects of: Alcohol (Ethyl); Anticholinergics; Anti-Parkinson's Agents (Dopamine Agonist); Budesonide (Systemic, Oral Inhalation); ChlorproMAZINE; CNS Depressants; Colchicine; CYP2D6 Substrates; CYP3A4 Substrates; Dronedarone; Eplerenone; Everolimus; FentaNYL; Fesoterodine; Lurasidone; Methylphenidate; Nebivolol; Pimecrolimus; Pimozide; QTc-Prolonging Agents; QuiNIDine; QuiNINE; Salmeterol; Saxagliptin; Tamoxifen; Tetrabenazine; Thioridazine; Tolvaptan; Toremifene; Vandetanib; Vemurafenib; Ziprasidone

The levels/effects of Haloperidol may be increased by: Abiraterone Acetate; Acetylcholinesterase Inhibitors (Central); Alfuzosin; Artemether; Chloroquine; ChlorproMAZINE; Ciprofloxacin; Ciprofloxacin (Systemic); Conivaptan; CYP2D6 Inhibitors (Moderate); CYP2D6 Inhibitors (Strong); CYP3A4 Inhibitors (Moderate); CYP3A4 Inhibitors (Strong); Darunavir; Gadobutrol; HydrOXYzine; Lithium formulations; Lumefantrine; Metoclopramide; Nilotinib; Nonsteroidal Anti-Inflammatory Agents; Pramlintide; QUEtiapine; QuiNIDine; QuiNINE; Selective Serotonin Reuptake Inhibitors; Tetrabenazine

Decreased Effect

Haloperidol may decrease the levels/effects of: Amphetamines; Codeine; Quinagolide; TraMADol

The levels/effects of Haloperidol may be decreased by: Anti-Parkinson's Agents (Dopamine Agonist); CarBAMazepine; CYP3A4 Inducers (Strong); Cyproterone; Deferasirox; Glycopyrrolate; Herbs (CYP3A4 Inducers); Lithium formulations; Peginterferon Alfa-2b; Tocilizumab

Ethanol/Nutrition/Herb Interactions

Ethanol: May increase CNS depression; monitor for increased effects with coadministration. Caution patients about effects.

Herb/Nutraceutical: Avoid valerian, St John's wort, kava kava, gotu kola (may increase CNS depression).

Stability

Protect oral dosage forms from light.

Haloperidol lactate injection should be stored at controlled room temperature; do not freeze or expose to temperatures >40°C. Protect from light; exposure to light may cause discoloration and the development of a grayish-red precipitate over several weeks.

Haloperidol lactate may be administered IVPB or I.V. infusion in D_5W solutions. NS solutions should not be used due to reports of decreased stability and incompatibility.

Standardized dose: 0.5-100 mg/50-100 mL D_5W.

Stability of standardized solutions is 38 days at room temperature (24°C).

Mechanism of Action Haloperidol is a butyrophenone antipsychotic which blocks postsynaptic mesolimbic dopaminergic D_1 and D_2 receptors in the brain; depresses the release of hypothalamic and hypophyseal hormones; believed to depress the reticular activating system thus affecting basal metabolism, body temperature, wakefulness, vasomotor tone, and emesis

Pharmacodynamics/Kinetics

Onset of action: Sedation: I.M., I.V.: 30-60 minutes

Duration: Decanoate: 2-4 weeks

Distribution: V_d: 8-18 L/kg

Protein binding: 90%

Metabolism: Hepatic: 50% to 60% glucuronidation (inactive); 23% CYP3A4-mediated reduction to inactive metabolites (some back-oxidation to haloperidol); and 20% to 30% CYP3A4-mediated N-dealkylation, including minor oxidation pathway to toxic pyridinium derivative (Kudo, 1999)

Bioavailability: Oral: 60% to 70%

Half-life elimination: 18 hours; Decanoate: 21 days

Time to peak, serum: Oral: 2-6 hours; I.M.: 20 minutes; Decanoate: 7 days

Excretion: Urine (30%, 1% as unchanged drug); feces (15%)

Dosage

Geriatric Nonpsychotic patient, dementia behavior (unlabeled use): Initial: Oral: 0.25-0.5 mg 1-2 times/day; increase dose at 4- to 7-day intervals by 0.25-0.5 mg/day. Increase dosing intervals (twice daily, 3 times/day, etc) as necessary to control response or side effects.

Adult

Psychosis:

Oral: 0.5-5 mg 2-3 times/day; usual maximum: 30 mg/day

I.M. (as lactate): 2-5 mg every 4-8 hours as needed

I.M. (as decanoate): Initial: 10-20 times the daily oral dose administered at 4-week intervals. Maintenance dose: 10-15 times initial oral dose; used to stabilize psychiatric symptoms

Delirium in the intensive care unit (unlabeled use, unlabeled route; Jacobi, 2002): I.V.: Initial: 2-10 mg depending on degree of agitation; if inadequate response, may repeat bolus dose (with sequential doubling of initial bolus dose) every 15-30 minutes until calm achieved, then administer 25% of the last bolus dose every 6 hours; monitor ECG and QT_c interval. After the patient is controlled, haloperidol therapy should be tapered over several days. **Note:** QT_c prolongation may occur with cumulative doses ≥35 mg and torsade de pointes has been reported with single doses of ≥20 mg. The optimal dose and regimen of haloperidol for the treatment of severe agitation and/or delirium has not been established.

Rapid tranquilization of severely-agitated patient (unlabeled use; administer every 30-60 minutes):

Oral: 5-10 mg

I.M. (as lactate): 5 mg

Average total dose (oral or I.M.) for tranquilization: 10-20 mg

Postoperative nausea and vomiting (PONV) (unlabeled use): I.M., I.V.: 0.5-2 mg (Gan, 2007)

Renal Impairment Hemodialysis/peritoneal dialysis: Supplemental dose is not necessary.

Administration

Injection oil (decanoate): The decanoate injectable formulation should be administered I.M. only, **do not administer decanoate I.V.**

Injection solution (lactate): The lactate injectable formulation may be administered I.V. (unlabeled route) or I.M.

Oral solution (lactate): Dilute the oral concentrate with water or juice before administration. Avoid skin contact with oral solution; may cause contact dermatitis.

◀ **Monitoring Parameters** Vital signs; lipid profile, fasting blood glucose/Hgb A_{1c}; BMI; mental status, abnormal involuntary movement scale (AIMS), extrapyramidal symptoms (EPS); ECG (with off-label intravenous administration)

Reference Range

Therapeutic: 5-20 ng/mL (SI: 10-40 nmol/L) (psychotic disorders - less for Tourette's and mania)

Toxic: >42 ng/mL (SI: >84 nmol/L)

Special Geriatric Considerations Many elderly patients receive antipsychotic medications for inappropriate nonpsychotic behavior. Before initiating antipsychotic medication, the clinician should investigate any possible reversible cause; any stress or stress from any disease can cause acute "confusion" or worsening of baseline nonpsychotic behavior. Most commonly acute changes in behavior are due to increases in drug dose or addition of new drug to regimen; fluid electrolyte loss; infections; and changes in environment.

Any changes in disease status in any organ system can result in behavior changes.

In the treatment of agitated, demented, elderly patients, authors of meta-analysis of controlled trials of the response to the traditional antipsychotics (phenothiazines, butyrophenones) in controlling agitation have concluded that the use of neuroleptics results in a response rate of 18%. Clearly neuroleptic therapy for behavior control should be limited with frequent attempts to withdraw the agent given for behavior control.

Clinical studies of haloperidol did not include sufficient numbers of subjects ≥65 years of age to determine whether they respond differently from younger subjects. Other reported clinical experience has not consistently identified differences between the elderly and younger patients. However, the prevalence of tardive dyskinesia appears to be highest among the elderly, especially elderly women. Also, the pharmacokinetics of haloperidol in geriatric patients generally warrants the use of lower doses.

Dosage Forms Excipient information presented when available (limited, particularly for generics); consult specific product labeling.

Injection, oil, as decanoate [strength expressed as base]: 50 mg/mL (1 mL, 5 mL); 100 mg/mL (1 mL, 5 mL)

Haldol® Decanoate: 50 mg/mL (1 mL); 100 mg/mL (1 mL) [contains benzyl alcohol, sesame oil]

Injection, solution, as lactate [strength expressed as base]: 5 mg/mL (1 mL, 10 mL)

Haldol®: 5 mg/mL (1 mL)

Solution, oral, as lactate [strength expressed as base, concentrate]: 2 mg/mL (5 mL, 15 mL, 120 mL)

Tablet, oral: 0.5 mg, 1 mg, 2 mg, 5 mg, 10 mg, 20 mg

Selected References

Rabins PV, Blacker D, Rovner BW, et al, "Practice Guidelines for the Treatment of Patients With Alzheimer's Disease and Other Dementias," *Am J Psychiatry*, 2007, 164(12 Suppl):5-56. Available at http://www.psych.org/psych_pract/treatq/pl/prac_guide.cfm.

Schneider LS, Tariot PN, Dagerman KS, et al, "Effectiveness of Atypical Antipsychotic Drugs in Patients With Alzheimer's Disease," *N Engl J Med*, 2006, 355(15):1525-38.

Heparin (HEP a rin)

Related Information

Anticoagulants, Injectable *on page 1989*

Medication Safety Issues

Sound-alike/look-alike issues:

Heparin may be confused with Hespan®

High alert medication:

The Institute for Safe Medication Practices (ISMP) includes this medication among its list of drugs which have a heightened risk of causing significant patient harm when used in error.

2009 National Patient Safety Goals:

The Joint Commission (TJC) requires healthcare organizations that provide anticoagulant therapy to have a process in place to reduce the risk of anticoagulant-associated patient harm. Patients receiving anticoagulants should receive individualized care through a defined process that includes standardized ordering, dispensing, administration, monitoring and education. This does not apply to routine short-term use of anticoagulants for prevention of venous thromboembolism when the expectation is that the patient's laboratory values will remain within or close to normal values (NPSG.03.05.01).

Administration issues:

The 100 unit/mL concentration should not be used to flush heparin locks, I.V. lines, or intra-arterial lines in neonates or infants <10 kg (systemic anticoagulation may occur). The 10 unit/mL flush concentration may inadvertently cause systemic anticoagulation in infants <1 kg who receive frequent flushes.

Other safety concerns:

Heparin sodium injection 10,000 units/mL and Hep-Lock U/P 10 units/mL have been confused with each other. Fatal medication errors have occurred between the two whose labels are both blue. **Never rely on color as a sole indicator to differentiate product identity.**

Heparin lock flush solution is intended only to maintain patency of I.V. devices and is **not** to be used for anticoagulant therapy.

Brand Names: U.S. Hep-Lock; Hep-Lock U/P; HepFlush®-10

Brand Names: Canada Hepalean®; Hepalean® Leo; Hepalean®-LOK

Index Terms Heparin Calcium; Heparin Lock Flush; Heparin Sodium

Generic Availability (U.S.) Yes

Pharmacologic Category Anticoagulant

Use Prophylaxis and treatment of thromboembolic disorders; as an anticoagulant for extracorporeal and dialysis procedures

Note: Heparin lock flush solution is intended only to maintain patency of I.V. devices and is **not** to be used for systemic anticoagulant therapy.

Unlabeled/Investigational Use ST-elevation myocardial infarction (STEMI) as an adjunct to thrombolysis; unstable angina/non-STEMI (UA/NSTEMI); anticoagulant used during percutaneous coronary intervention (PCI)

Contraindications Hypersensitivity to heparin or any component of the formulation (unless a life-threatening situation necessitates use and use of an alternative anticoagulant is not possible); severe thrombocytopenia; uncontrolled active bleeding except when due to disseminated intravascular coagulation (DIC); not for use when appropriate blood coagulation tests cannot be obtained at appropriate intervals (applies to full-dose heparin only)

Warnings/Precautions Hypersensitivity reactions can occur. Only in life-threatening situations when use of an alternative anticoagulant is not possible should heparin be cautiously used in patients with a documented hypersensitivity reaction. Hemorrhage is the most common complication. Monitor for signs and symptoms of bleeding. Certain patients are at increased risk of bleeding. Risk factors for bleeding include bacterial endocarditis; congenital or acquired bleeding disorders; active ulcerative or angiodysplastic GI diseases; continuous GI tube drainage; severe uncontrolled hypertension; history of hemorrhagic stroke; or use shortly after brain, spinal, or ophthalmology surgery; patient treated concomitantly with platelet inhibitors; conditions associated with increased bleeding tendencies (hemophilia, vascular purpura); recent GI bleeding; thrombocytopenia or platelet defects; severe liver disease; hypertensive or diabetic retinopathy; renal failure; or in patients undergoing invasive procedures including spinal tap or spinal anesthesia. Many concentrations of heparin are available ranging from 1 unit/mL to 20,000 units/mL. Clinicians **must** carefully examine each prefilled syringe or vial prior to use ensuring that the correct concentration is chosen; fatal hemorrhages have occurred related to heparin overdose especially in pediatric patients. A higher incidence of bleeding has been reported in patients >60 years of age, particularly women. They are also more sensitive to the dose. Discontinue heparin if hemorrhage occurs; severe hemorrhage or overdosage may require protamine.

◀ May cause thrombocytopenia; monitor platelet count closely. Patients who develop HIT may be at risk of developing a new thrombus (heparin-induced thrombocytopenia and thrombosis [HITT]). Discontinue therapy and consider alternatives if platelets are <100,000/mm³ and/or thrombosis develops. HIT or HITT may be delayed and can occur up to several weeks after discontinuation of heparin. Osteoporosis may occur with prolonged use (>6 months) due to a reduction in bone mineral density. Monitor for hyperkalemia; can cause hyperkalemia by suppressing aldosterone production. Patients >60 years of age may require lower doses of heparin.

Some preparations contain sulfite which may cause allergic reactions.

Heparin resistance may occur in patients with antithrombin deficiency, increased heparin clearance, elevations in heparin-binding proteins, elevations in factor VIII and/or fibrinogen; frequently encountered in patients with fever, thrombosis, thrombophlebitis, infections with thrombosing tendencies, MI, cancer, and in postsurgical patients; measurement of anticoagulant effects using antifactor Xa levels may be of benefit.

Adverse Reactions (Reflective of adult population; not specific for elderly) Frequency not defined.

Cardiovascular: Allergic vasospastic reaction (possibly related to thrombosis), chest pain, hemorrhagic shock, shock, thrombosis

Central nervous system: Chills, fever, headache

Dermatologic: Alopecia (delayed, transient), bruising (unexplained), cutaneous necrosis, dysesthesia pedis, erythematous plaques (case reports), eczema, urticaria, purpura

Endocrine & metabolic: Adrenal hemorrhage, hyperkalemia (suppression of aldosterone synthesis), ovarian hemorrhage, rebound hyperlipidemia on discontinuation

Gastrointestinal: Constipation, hematemesis, nausea, tarry stools, vomiting

Genitourinary: Frequent or persistent erection

Hematologic: Bleeding from gums, epistaxis, hemorrhage, ovarian hemorrhage, retroperitoneal hemorrhage, thrombocytopenia (see note)

Hepatic: Liver enzymes increased

Local: Irritation, erythema, pain, hematoma, and ulceration have been rarely reported with deep SubQ injections; I.M. injection (not recommended) is associated with a high incidence of these effects

Neuromuscular & skeletal: Peripheral neuropathy, osteoporosis (chronic therapy effect)

Ocular: Conjunctivitis (allergic reaction), lacrimation

Renal: Hematuria

Respiratory: Asthma, bronchospasm (case reports), hemoptysis, pulmonary hemorrhage, rhinitis

Miscellaneous: Allergic reactions, anaphylactoid reactions, heparin resistance, hypersensitivity (including chills, fever, and urticaria)

Note: Thrombocytopenia has been reported to occur at an incidence between 0% and 30%. It is often of no clinical significance. However, immunologically mediated heparin-induced thrombocytopenia (HIT) has been estimated to occur in 1% to 2% of patients, and is marked by a progressive fall in platelet counts and, in some cases, thromboembolic complications (skin necrosis, pulmonary embolism, gangrene of the extremities, stroke, or MI). For recommendations regarding platelet monitoring during heparin therapy, see Monitoring Parameters.

Drug Interactions

Avoid Concomitant Use

Avoid concomitant use of Heparin with any of the following: Corticorelin; Rivaroxaban

Increased Effect/Toxicity

Heparin may increase the levels/effects of: Anticoagulants; Collagenase (Systemic); Corticorelin; Deferasirox; Drotrecogin Alfa; Ibritumomab; Rivaroxaban; Tositumomab and Iodine I 131 Tositumomab

The levels/effects of Heparin may be increased by: 5-ASA Derivatives; Antiplatelet Agents; Aspirin; Dasatinib; Herbs (Anticoagulant/Antiplatelet Properties); Nonsteroidal Anti-Inflammatory Agents; Pentosan Polysulfate Sodium; Pentoxifylline; Prostacyclin Analogues; Salicylates; Thrombolytic Agents

Decreased Effect

The levels/effects of Heparin may be decreased by: Nitroglycerin

Ethanol/Nutrition/Herb Interactions Herb/Nutraceutical: Avoid cat's claw, dong quai, evening primrose, feverfew, red clover, horse chestnut, garlic, green tea, ginseng, ginkgo (all have additional antiplatelet activity).

Stability

Heparin solutions are colorless to slightly yellow; minor color variations do not affect therapeutic efficacy.

Heparin should be stored at controlled room temperature. Protect from freezing and temperatures >40°C.

Stability at room temperature and refrigeration:

Prepared bag: 24-72 hours (specific to solution, concentration, and/or study conditions)

Premixed bag: After seal is broken, 4 days.

Out of overwrap stability: 30 days.

Standard concentration/diluent: 25,000 units/500 mL D_5W (premixed). If preparing solution, mix thoroughly prior to administration.

Minimum volume: 250 mL D_5W.

Mechanism of Action Potentiates the action of antithrombin III and thereby inactivates thrombin (as well as activated coagulation factors IX, X, XI, XII, and plasmin) and prevents the conversion of fibrinogen to fibrin; heparin also stimulates release of lipoprotein lipase (lipoprotein lipase hydrolyzes triglycerides to glycerol and free fatty acids)

Pharmacodynamics/Kinetics

Onset of action: Anticoagulation: I.V.: Immediate; SubQ: ~20-30 minutes

Absorption: Oral, rectal: Erratic at best from these routes of administration; SubQ absorption is also erratic, but considered acceptable for prophylactic use

Distribution: Does not cross placenta; does not enter breast milk

Metabolism: Hepatic; may be partially metabolized in the reticuloendothelial system

Half-life elimination:

Dose-dependent: I.V. bolus: 25 units/kg: 30 minutes; 100 units/kg: 60 minutes; 400 units/kg: 150 minutes (Hirsh, 2008)

Mean: 1.5 hours; Range: 1-2 hours; affected by obesity, renal function, malignancy, presence of pulmonary embolism, and infections

Note: At therapeutic doses, elimination occurs rapidly via nonrenal mechanisms. With very high doses, renal elimination may play more of a role; however, dosage adjustment remains unnecessary for patients with renal impairment (Hirsh, 2008).

Excretion: Urine (small amounts as unchanged drug)

Dosage

Geriatric Patients >60 years of age may have higher serum levels and clinical response (longer aPTTs) as compared to younger patients receiving similar dosages. Lower dosages may be required.

Adult Note: Many concentrations of heparin are available ranging from 1 unit/mL to 20,000 units/mL. Carefully examine each prefilled syringe or vial prior to use ensuring that the correct concentration is chosen. Heparin lock flush solution is intended only to maintain patency of I.V. devices and is not to be used for anticoagulant therapy.

DVT Prophylaxis (low-dose heparin): SubQ: 5000 units every 8-12 hours

Systemic anticoagulation: I.V. infusion (weight-based dosing per institutional nomogram recommended):

Acute coronary syndromes: I.V. infusion:

Percutaneous coronary intervention:

If no concurrent GPIIb/IIIa inhibitor: Initial bolus of 70-100 units/kg (target ACT 250-300 seconds for HemoTec®, 300-350 seconds for Hemochron®) (Kushner, 2009)

or

If receiving GPIIb/IIIa inhibitor: Initial bolus of 50-70 units/kg (target ACT 200-250 seconds)

STEMI: Fibrinolytic therapy:

Full-dose alteplase, reteplase, or tenecteplase with dosing as follows: Concurrent bolus of 60 units/kg (maximum: 4000 units), then 12 units/kg/hour (maximum: 1000 units/hour) as continuous infusion. Check aPTT every 4-6 hours; adjust to target of 1.5-2 times the upper limit of control (50-70 seconds in clinical trials); usual range: 10-30 units/kg/hour. Duration of heparin therapy depends on concurrent therapy and the specific patient risks for systemic or venous thromboembolism.

Combination regimen (unlabeled): Half-dose tenecteplase (15-25 mg based on weight) and abciximab 0.25 mg/kg bolus then 0.125 mcg/kg/minute (maximum: 10 mcg/minute) for 12 hours with heparin dosing as follows: Concurrent bolus of 40 units/kg (maximum: 3000 units), then 7 units/kg/hour (maximum: 800 units/hour) as continuous infusion. Adjust to a aPTT target of 50-70 seconds.

Unstable angina/Non-ST-elevation myocardial infarction (NSTEMI): Initial bolus of 60 units/kg (maximum: 4000 units), followed by an initial infusion of 12 units/kg/hour (maximum: 1000 units/hour). The American College of Chest Physicians consensus conference has recommended dosage adjustments to correspond to a therapeutic range equivalent to heparin levels of 0.3-0.7 units/mL by antifactor Xa determinations.

◄ **Treatment of venous thromboembolism:**
DVT/PE: I.V.: 80 units/kg (or alternatively 5000 units) I.V. push followed by continuous infusion of 18 units/kg/hour (or alternatively 1300 units/hour). The American College of Chest Physicians consensus conference has recommended dosage adjustments to correspond to a therapeutic range equivalent to heparin levels of 0.3-0.7 units/mL by antifactor Xa determinations.

DVT/PE: SubQ:
Monitored dosing regimen: Initial: 17,500 units or 250 units/kg then 250 units/kg every 12 hours. The American College of Chest Physicians consensus conference has recommended dosage adjustments to correspond to a therapeutic range equivalent to heparin levels of 0.3-0.7 units/mL by antifactor Xa determinations.

Unmonitored dosing regimen: Initial: 333 units/kg then 250 units/kg every 12 hours

Intermittent I.V. Anticoagulation: Intermittent I.V.: Initial: 10,000 units, then 50-70 units/kg (5000-10,000 units) every 4-6 hours

Maintenance of line patency (line flushing): When using daily flushes of heparin to maintain patency of single and double lumen central catheters, 10 units/mL is commonly used for younger infants (eg, <10 kg) while 100 units/mL is used for older infants, children, and adults. Capped PVC catheters and peripheral heparin locks require flushing more frequently (eg, every 6-8 hours). Volume of heparin flush is usually similar to volume of catheter (or slightly greater). Additional flushes should be given when stagnant blood is observed in catheter, after catheter is used for drug or blood administration, and after blood withdrawal from catheter.

Parenteral nutrition: Addition of heparin (0.5-3 unit/mL) to peripheral and central parenteral nutrition has not been shown to decrease catheter-related thrombosis. The final concentration of heparin used for TPN solutions may need to be decreased to 0.5 units/mL in small infants receiving larger amounts of volume in order to avoid approaching therapeutic amounts. Arterial lines are heparinized with a final concentration of 1 unit/mL.

Renal Impairment No dosage adjustment required; adjust therapeutic heparin according to aPTT or anti-Xa activity.

Hepatic Impairment No dosage adjustment required; adjust therapeutic heparin according to aPTT or anti-Xa activity.

Administration SubQ: Inject in subcutaneous tissue only (not muscle tissue). Injection sites should be rotated (usually left and right portions of the abdomen, above iliac crest).

Do not administer I.M. due to pain, irritation, and hematoma formation; central venous catheters must be flushed with heparin solution when newly inserted, daily (at the time of tubing change), after blood withdrawal or transfusion, and after an intermittent infusion through an injectable cap. A volume of at least 10 mL of blood should be removed and discarded from a heparinized line before blood samples are sent for coagulation testing.

Monitoring Parameters Hemoglobin, hematocrit, signs of bleeding; fecal occult blood test; aPTT (or antifactor Xa activity levels) or ACT depending upon indication

Platelet counts should be routinely monitored when the risk of HIT is >0.1% (eg, receiving therapeutic dose heparin, postoperative antithrombotic prophylaxis), if the patient has received heparin or low molecular weight heparin (eg, enoxaparin) within the past 100 days, if pre-exposure history is uncertain, or if anaphylactoid reaction to heparin occurs. When the risk of HIT is <0.1% (eg, medical/obstetrical patients receiving heparin flushes), routine platelet count monitoring is not recommended (Hirsh, 2008).

For intermittent I.V. injections, aPTT is measured 3.5-4 hours after I.V. injection.

For SubQ injections, when used for treatment (eg, monitored dosing regimen), aPTT is measured 6 hours after injection.

Note: Continuous I.V. infusion is preferred over I.V. intermittent injections. For full-dose heparin (ie, nonlow-dose), the dose should be titrated according to aPTT results. For anticoagulation, an aPTT 1.5-2.5 times normal is usually desired. Because of variation among hospitals in the control aPTT values, nomograms should be established at each institution, designed to achieve aPTT values in the target range (eg, for a control aPTT of 30 seconds, the target range [1.5-2.5 times control] would be 45-75 seconds). Measurements should be made prior to heparin therapy, 6 hours after initiation, and 6 hours after any dosage change, and should be used to adjust the heparin infusion until the aPTT exhibits a therapeutic level. When two consecutive aPTT values are therapeutic, subsequent measurements may be made every 24 hours, and if necessary, dose adjustment carried out. In addition, a significant change in the patient's clinical condition (eg, recurrent ischemia, bleeding, hypotension) should prompt an immediate aPTT determination, followed by dose adjustment if necessary. In general, may increase or decrease infusion by 2-4 units/kg/hour dependent upon aPTT.

Heparin infusion dose adjustment: A number of dose-adjustment nomograms have been developed which target an aPTT range of 1.5-2.5 times control (Cruickshank, 1991; Flaker, 1994; Hull, 1992; Raschke, 1993). However, institution-specific and indication-specific nomograms should be consulted for dose adjustment. **Note:** aPTT values vary throughout the day with maximum values occurring during the night (Decousus, 1985).

Reference Range Heparin: 0.3-0.7 unit/mL (by anti-Xa chromogenic assay) or 0.2-0.4 unit/mL (by protamine titration); aPTT: 1.5-2.5 times **the patient's baseline**

Test Interactions Increased thyroxine (competitive protein binding methods); increased PT

Aprotinin significantly increases aPTT and celite Activated Clotting Time (ACT) which may not reflect the actual degree of anticoagulation by heparin. Kaolin-based ACTs are not affected by aprotinin to the same degree as celite ACTs. While institutional protocols may vary, a minimal celite ACT of 750 seconds or kaolin-ACT of 480 seconds is recommended in the presence of aprotinin. Consult the manufacturer's information on specific ACT test interpretation in the presence of aprotinin.

Pharmacotherapy Pearls Heparin does not possess fibrinolytic activity and, therefore, cannot lyse established thrombi; discontinue heparin if hemorrhage occurs; severe hemorrhage or overdosage may require protamine; monitor platelet counts, signs of bleeding, PTT.

When using daily flushes of heparin to maintain patency of single and double lumen central catheters. Capped PVC catheters and peripheral heparin locks require flushing more frequently (eg, every 6-8 hours). Volume of heparin flush is usually similar to volume of catheter (or slightly greater) or may be standardized according to specific hospital's policy (eg, 2-5 mL/flush). Dose of heparin flush used should not approach therapeutic per kg dose. Additional flushes should be given when stagnant blood is observed in catheter, after catheter is used for drug or blood administration, and after blood withdrawal from catheter.

Heparin 1 unit/mL (final concentration) may be added to TPN solutions, both central and peripheral. (Addition of heparin to peripheral TPN has been shown to increase duration of line patency.)

Arterial lines are heparinized with a final concentration of 1 unit/mL.

Special Geriatric Considerations In the clinical setting, age has not been shown to be a reliable predictor of a patient's anticoagulant response to heparin. However, it is common for the elderly to have a "standard" response for the first 24-48 hours after a loading dose (5000 units) and a maintenance infusion of 800-1000 units/hour. After this period, they then have an exaggerated response (ie, elevated aPTT), requiring a lower infusion rate. Hence, monitor closely during this period of therapy. Elderly women are more likely to have bleeding complications and osteoporosis may be a problem when used >3 months or total daily dose exceeds 30,000 units.

Dosage Forms Excipient information presented when available (limited, particularly for generics); consult specific product labeling. [DSC] = Discontinued product

Infusion, premixed in 1/2 NS, as sodium [porcine intestinal mucosa source]: 25,000 units (250 mL, 500 mL)

Infusion, premixed in D$_5$W, as sodium [porcine intestinal mucosa source]: 10,000 units (250 mL); 12,500 units (250 mL); 20,000 units (500 mL); 25,000 units (250 mL, 500 mL)

Infusion, premixed in D$_5$W, as sodium [porcine intestinal mucosa source, preservative free]: 20,000 units (500 mL [DSC]); 25,000 units (250 mL [DSC], 500 mL [DSC])

Infusion, premixed in NS, as sodium [porcine intestinal mucosa source]: 1000 units (500 mL); 2000 units (1000 mL)

Infusion, premixed in NS, as sodium [porcine intestinal mucosa source, preservative free]: 1000 units (500 mL); 2000 units (1000 mL)

Injection, solution, as sodium [lock flush preparation; porcine intestinal mucosa source]: 10 units/mL (1 mL, 2 mL, 3 mL, 5 mL, 10 mL, 30 mL [DSC]); 100 units/mL (1 mL, 2 mL, 3 mL, 5 mL, 10 mL, 30 mL)

Hep-Lock: 10 units/mL (1 mL, 2 mL, 10 mL, 30 mL); 100 units/mL (1 mL, 2 mL, 10 mL, 30 mL) [contains benzyl alcohol]

Injection, solution, as sodium [lock flush preparation; porcine intestinal mucosa source, preservative free]: 1 units/mL (2 mL, 3 mL, 5 mL); 2 units/mL (3 mL); 10 units/mL (1 mL, 2 mL, 2.5 mL, 3 mL, 5 mL, 6 mL, 10 mL); 100 units/mL (1 mL, 2 mL, 2.5 mL, 3 mL, 5 mL, 10 mL)

Hep-Lock U/P: 10 units/mL (1 mL); 100 units/mL (1 mL)

HepFlush®-10: 10 units/mL (10 mL)

Injection, solution, as sodium [porcine intestinal mucosa source]: 1000 units/mL (1 mL, 10 mL, 30 mL); 5000 units/mL (1 mL, 10 mL); 10,000 units/mL (1 mL, 4 mL, 5 mL); 20,000 units/mL (1 mL)

Injection, solution, as sodium [porcine intestinal mucosa source, preservative free]: 1000 units/mL (2 mL); 5000 units/mL (0.5 mL); 10,000 units/mL (0.5 mL)

Injection, solution, oral, as sodium [porcine intestinal mucosa source]: 10,000 units/mL (1 mL)

Selected References

Bohannon AD and Lyles KW, "Drug-Induced Bone Disease," *Clin Geriatr Med*, 1994, 10(4):611-23.

Jick H, Slone D, Borda IT, et al, "Efficacy and Toxicity of Heparin in Relation to Age and Sex," *N Engl J Med*, 1968, 279 (6):284-6.

Kushner FG, Hand M, Smith SC, et al, "2009 Focused Updates: ACC/AHA Guidelines for the Management of Patients With ST-Elevation Myocardial Infarction (Updating the 2004 Guideline and 2007 Focused Update) and ACC/AHA/ SCAI Guidelines on Percutaneous Coronary Intervention (Updating the 2005 Guideline and 2007 Focused Update): A Report of the American College of Cardiology Foundation/American Heart Association Task Force on Practice Guidelines," *J Am Coll Cardiol*, 2009, 54(23):2205-41.

Smith SC, Feldman TE, Hirshfeld JW Jr, et al, "ACC/AHA/SCAI 2005 Guideline Update for Percutaneous Coronary Intervention. A Report of the American College of Cardiology/American Heart Association Task Force on Practice Guidelines (ACC/AHA/SCAI Writing Committee to Update the 2001 Guidelines for Percutaneous Coronary Intervention)," *Circulation*, 2006, 47(1):e1-121.

◆ **Heparin Calcium** *see* Heparin *on page 857*
◆ **Heparin Lock Flush** *see* Heparin *on page 857*
◆ **Heparin Sodium** *see* Heparin *on page 857*

Hepatitis A and Hepatitis B Recombinant Vaccine
(hep a TYE tis aye & hep a TYE tis bee ree KOM be nant vak SEEN)

Related Information
Hepatitis A Vaccine *on page 864*
Hepatitis B Vaccine (Recombinant) *on page 869*
Immunization Administration Recommendations *on page 2037*
Immunization Recommendations *on page 2043*
Brand Names: U.S. Twinrix®
Brand Names: Canada Twinrix®; Twinrix® Junior
Index Terms Engerix-B® and Havrix®; Havrix® and Engerix-B®; HepA-HepB; Hepatitis B and Hepatitis A Vaccine
Generic Availability (U.S.) No
Pharmacologic Category Vaccine, Inactivated (Viral)
Use Active immunization against disease caused by hepatitis A virus and hepatitis B virus (all known subtypes) in populations desiring protection against or at high risk of exposure to these viruses.

Populations include travelers or people living in or relocating to areas of intermediate/high endemicity for **both** HAV and HBV and are at increased risk of HBV infection due to behavioral or occupational factors; patients with chronic liver disease; laboratory workers who handle live HAV and HBV; healthcare workers, police, and other personnel who render first-aid or medical assistance; workers who come in contact with sewage; employees of day care centers and correctional facilities; patients/staff of hemodialysis units; men who have sex with men; patients frequently receiving blood products; military personnel; users of injectable illicit drugs; close household contacts of patients with hepatitis A and hepatitis B infection; residents of drug and alcohol treatment centers
Contraindications Hypersensitivity to hepatitis A vaccine, hepatitis B vaccine, or any component of the formulation
Warnings/Precautions Use caution in patients on anticoagulants, with thrombocytopenia, or bleeding disorders (bleeding may occur following intramuscular injection). Treatment for anaphylactic reactions should be immediately available. Postpone vaccination in moderate-to-severe acute illness (minor illness is not a contraindication). Use with caution in severely immunocompromised patients (eg, patients receiving chemo/radiation therapy or other immunosuppressive therapy (including high-dose corticosteroids)); may have a reduced response to vaccination. In general, household and close contacts of persons with altered immunocompetence may receive all age appropriate vaccines.

May contain yeast, aluminum, and trace amounts of neomycin; packaging may contain latex. In order to maximize vaccination rates, the ACIP recommends simultaneous administration of all age-appropriate vaccines (live or inactivated) for which a person is eligible at a single clinic visit, unless contraindications exist. The use of combination vaccines is generally preferred over separate injections, taking into consideration provider assessment, patient preference, and potential adverse events. When using combination vaccines, the minimum age for administration is the oldest minimum age for any individual component; the minimum interval between dosing is the greatest minimum interval between any individual component.

Unrecognized hepatitis A or B infection may be present, immunization may not prevent infection in these patients. Use hepatitis B vaccine with caution in patients with decreased cardiopulmonary function. Patients >65 years may have lower response rates to hepatitis B vaccine.

Adverse Reactions (Reflective of adult population; not specific for elderly) In the U.S., all serious adverse reactions must be reported to the U.S. Department of Health and Human Services (DHHS) Vaccine Adverse Event Reporting System (VAERS) 1-800-822-7967 or online at https://vaers.hhs.gov/esub/index.

Incidence of adverse effects of the combination product were similar to those occurring after administration of hepatitis A vaccine and hepatitis B vaccine alone. (Incidence reported is not versus placebo.)

Adults:
>10%:
  Central nervous system: Headache (13% to 22%), fatigue (11% to 14%)
  Local: Injection site reaction: Soreness (35% to 41%), redness (8% to 11%)
1% to 10%:
  Central nervous system: Fever (2% to 4%)
  Gastrointestinal: Diarrhea (4% to 6%), nausea (2% to 4%), vomiting (≤1%)
  Local: Injection site reaction: Swelling (4% to 6%), induration
  Respiratory: Upper respiratory tract infection
<1%: Abdominal pain, agitation, anorexia, arthralgia, back pain, bruising at the injection site, diaphoresis, dizziness, erythema, flu-like syndrome, flushing, insomnia, irritability, migraine, myalgia, paresthesia, petechiae, pruritus at the injection site, rash, respiratory tract illness, somnolence, syncope, urticaria, vertigo, weakness

Children (as reported in Canadian labeling):
>10%: Local: Injection site pain/redness
1% to 10%:
  Central nervous system: Fever (≥37.5°C), drowsiness, fatigue, headache, irritability, malaise
  Gastrointestinal: Appetite decreased, diarrhea, nausea, vomiting
  Local: Injection site edema

Drug Interactions
Avoid Concomitant Use There are no known interactions where it is recommended to avoid concomitant use.

Increased Effect/Toxicity There are no known significant interactions involving an increase in effect.

Decreased Effect There are no known significant interactions involving a decrease in effect.

Stability Store in refrigerator at 2°C to 8°C (36°F to 46°F); do not freeze (discard if frozen).

Mechanism of Action
Hepatitis A vaccine, an inactivated virus vaccine, offers active immunization against hepatitis A virus infection at an effective immune response rate in up to 99% of subjects.

Recombinant hepatitis B vaccine is a noninfectious subunit viral vaccine. The vaccine is derived from hepatitis B surface antigen (HB_sAg) produced through recombinant DNA techniques from yeast cells. The portion of the hepatitis B gene which codes for HB_sAg is cloned into yeast which is then cultured to produce hepatitis B vaccine.

In immunocompetent people, Twinrix® provides active immunization against hepatitis A virus infection (at an effective immune response rate >99% of subjects) and against hepatitis B virus infection (at an effective immune response rate of 93% to 97%) 30 days after completion of the 3-dose series. This is comparable to using hepatitis A vaccine and hepatitis B vaccine concomitantly.

Pharmacodynamics/Kinetics
Onset of action: Seroconversion for antibodies against HAV and HBV were detected 1 month after completion of the 3-dose series.

Duration: Patients remained seropositive for at least 4 years during clinical studies.

Dosage
Geriatric & Adult Primary immunization: I.M.: Three doses (1 mL each) given on a 0-, 1-, and 6-month schedule
  Alternative regimen: Accelerated regimen: Four doses (1 mL each) on day 0, 7, and 21-30, followed by a booster at 12 months

Administration I.M.: Shake well prior to use. Do not dilute prior to administration. Discard if the suspension is discolored or does not appear homogenous after shaking or if there are cracks in the vial or syringe. Administer in the deltoid region; do not administer in the gluteal region (may give suboptimal response). Do not administer at the same site, or using the same syringe, as additional vaccines or immunoglobulins.

For patients at risk of hemorrhage following intramuscular injection, the ACIP recommends "it should be administered intramuscularly if, in the opinion of the physician familiar with the patients bleeding risk, the vaccine can be administered by this route with reasonable safety. If the patient receives antihemophilia or other similar therapy, intramuscular vaccination can be scheduled shortly after such therapy is administered. A fine needle (23 gauge or smaller) can

◀ be used for the vaccination and firm pressure applied to the site (without rubbing) for at least 2 minutes. The patient should be instructed concerning the risk of hematoma from the injection." Patients on anticoagulant therapy should be considered to have the same bleeding risks and treated as those with clotting factor disorders (CDC, 2011).

Simultaneous administration of vaccines helps ensure the patients will be fully vaccinated by the appropriate age. Simultaneous administration of vaccines is defined as administering >1 vaccine on the same day at different anatomic sites. The use of licensed combination vaccines is generally preferred over separate injections of the equivalent components. Separate vaccines should not be combined in the same syringe unless indicated by product specific labeling. Separate needles and syringes should be used for each injection. The ACIP prefers each dose of a specific vaccine in a series come from the same manufacturer when possible. Adolescents and adults should be vaccinated while seated or lying down. In general, preterm infants should be vaccinated at the same chronological age as full-term infants (CDC, 2011).

Antipyretics have not been shown to prevent febrile seizures. Antipyretics may be used to treat fever or discomfort following vaccination (CDC, 2011). One study reported that routine prophylactic administration of acetaminophen to prevent fever prior to vaccination decreased the immune response of some vaccines; the clinical significance of this reduction in immune response has not been established (Prymula, 2009).

Monitoring Parameters Monitor for syncope for ≥15 minutes following vaccination.

Pharmacotherapy Pearls Federal law requires that the name of medication, date of administration, the vaccine manufacturer, lot number of vaccine, and the administering person's name, title, and address be entered into the patient's permanent medical record.

Special Geriatric Considerations No adjustment for age is necessary. Some studies with HBV demonstrate a lower antibody titer in the elderly as compared to younger adults.

Dosage Forms Excipient information presented when available (limited, particularly for generics); consult specific product labeling.

Injection, suspension [preservative free]:

Twinrix®: Hepatitis A virus antigen 720 ELISA units and hepatitis B surface antigen 20 mcg per mL (1 mL) [contains aluminum, yeast protein, and trace amounts of neomycin; may contain natural rubber/natural latex in prefilled syringe]

Dosage Forms: Canada Excipient information presented when available (limited, particularly for generics); consult specific product labeling.

Injection, suspension [preservative free]:

Twinrix® Junior: Hepatitis A virus antigen 360 ELISA units and hepatitis B surface antigen 10 mcg per 0.5 mL (0.5 mL) [contains aluminum and trace amounts of neomycin]

Hepatitis A Vaccine (hep a TYE tis aye vak SEEN)

Related Information

Immunization Administration Recommendations *on page 2037*
Immunization Recommendations *on page 2043*

Medication Safety Issues

International issues:

Avaxim [Canada and multiple international markets] may be confused with Avastin brand name for bevacizumab [U.S., Canada, and multiple international markets]

Brand Names: U.S. Havrix®; VAQTA®

Brand Names: Canada Avaxim®; Avaxim®-Pediatric; HAVRIX®; VAQTA®

Index Terms HepA

Generic Availability (U.S.) No

Pharmacologic Category Vaccine, Inactivated (Viral)

Use

Active immunization against disease caused by hepatitis A virus (HAV)

The Advisory Committee on Immunization Practices (ACIP) recommends routine vaccination for:

- All children ≥12 months of age
- All unvaccinated adults requesting protection from HAV infection
- All unvaccinated adults at risk for HAV infection, such as:

Behavioral risks: Men who have sex with men; injection drug users

Occupational risks: Persons who work with HAV-infected primates or with HAV in a research laboratory setting

Medical risks: Persons with chronic liver disease; patients who receive clotting-factor concentrates

- Other risks: International travelers to regions with high or intermediate levels of endemic HAV infection (a list of countries is available at http://wwwn.cdc.gov/travel/contentdiseases.aspx)
- Unvaccinated persons who anticipate close personal contact with international adoptee from a country of intermediate to high endemicity of HAV, during their first 60 days of arrival into the United States (eg, household contacts, babysitters)

Contraindications Hypersensitivity to hepatitis A vaccine or any component of the formulation

Warnings/Precautions Use caution in patients on anticoagulants, with thrombocytopenia, or bleeding disorders (bleeding may occur following intramuscular injection). Treatment for anaphylactic reactions should be immediately available. Postpone vaccination with acute infection or febrile illness. Use with caution in severely immunocompromised patients (eg, patients receiving chemo/radiation therapy or other immunosuppressive therapy (including high dose corticosteroids)); may have a reduced response to vaccination. In general, household and close contacts of persons with altered immunocompetence may receive all age appropriate vaccines. Unrecognized hepatitis A infection may be present; immunization may not prevent infection in these patients. Patients with chronic liver disease may have decreased antibody response. Packaging may contain natural latex rubber; some products may contain neomycin. In order to maximize vaccination rates, the ACIP recommends simultaneous administration of all age-appropriate vaccines (live or inactivated) for which a person is eligible at a single clinic visit, unless contraindications exist. The use of combination vaccines is generally preferred over separate injections, taking into consideration provider assessment, patient preference, and adverse events.

Adverse Reactions (Reflective of adult population; not specific for elderly) All serious adverse reactions must be reported to the U.S. Department of Health and Human Services (DHHS) Vaccine Adverse Event Reporting System (VAERS) at 1-800-822-7967 or online at https://vaers.hhs.gov/esub/index.

Frequency dependent upon age, product used, and concomitant vaccine administration. In general, headache and injection site reactions were less common in younger children.

>10%:

Central nervous system: Drowsiness, fever ≥100.4°F (1-5 days post vaccination), fever >98.6°C (1-14 days post vaccination), headache, irritability

Gastrointestinal: Appetite decreased

Local: Injection site: Erythema, pain, soreness, swelling, tenderness, warmth

1% to 10%:

Central nervous system: Chills, fatigue, fever ≥102°F (1-5 days postvaccination), insomnia, malaise

Dermatologic: Rash

Endocrine & metabolic: Menstrual disorder

Gastrointestinal: Abdominal pain, anorexia, constipation, diarrhea, gastroenteritis, nausea, vomiting

Local: Injection site bruising, induration

Neuromuscular & skeletal: Arm pain, back pain, myalgia, stiffness, weakness/fatigue

Ocular: Conjunctivitis

Otic: Otitis media

Respiratory: Asthma, cough, nasopharyngitis, nasal congestion, pharyngitis, rhinorrhea, rhinitis, upper respiratory tract infection

Miscellaneous: Crying

Drug Interactions

Avoid Concomitant Use There are no known interactions where it is recommended to avoid concomitant use.

Increased Effect/Toxicity There are no known significant interactions involving an increase in effect.

Decreased Effect

The levels/effects of Hepatitis A Vaccine may be decreased by: Belimumab; Fingolimod; Immunosuppressants

Stability Store under refrigeration at 2°C to 8°C (36°F to 46°F); do not freeze. The following stability information has also been reported for Havrix®: May be stored at room temperature for up to 72 hours (Cohen, 2007).

Mechanism of Action As an inactivated virus vaccine, hepatitis A vaccine offers active immunization against hepatitis A virus infection at an effective immune response rate in up to 99% of subjects

Pharmacodynamics/Kinetics

Onset of action (protection): 2-4 weeks after a single dose; 2 weeks after vaccine administration, 54% to 62% of patients develop neutralizing antibodies; this percentage increases to 94% to 100% at 1 month postvaccination (CDC, 2006)

◄ Duration: Neutralizing antibodies have persisted for up to 8 years; based on kinetic models, antibodies may be present ≥14-20 years in children and ≥25 years in adults who receive the complete vaccination series (CDC, 2006; Van Damme, 2003).

Dosage

Geriatric & Adult Immunization: I.M.: **Note:** When used for primary immunization, the vaccine should be given at least 2 weeks prior to expected HAV exposure. When used prior to an international adoption, the vaccination series should begin when adoption is being planned, but ideally ≥2 weeks prior to expected arrival of adoptee. When used for postexposure prophylaxis, the vaccine should be given as soon as possible.

HAVRIX®: 1440 ELISA units (1 mL) with a booster dose of 1440 ELISA units to be given 6-12 months following primary immunization

VAQTA®: 50 units (1 mL) with a booster dose of 50 units (1 mL) to be given 6-18 months after primary immunization (6-12 months if initial dose was with HAVRIX®)

Administration The deltoid muscle is the preferred site for injection for adults. Do not administer to the gluteal region; may decrease efficacy. Do not administer intravenously, intradermally, or subcutaneously. Shake well prior to use; discard if the suspension is discolored or does not appear homogenous after shaking, or if there are cracks in the vial or syringe. When used for primary immunization, the vaccine should be given at least 2 weeks prior to expected HAV exposure. When used for postexposure prophylaxis, the vaccine should be given as soon as possible. For patients at risk of hemorrhage following intramuscular injection, the ACIP recommends "it should be administered intramuscularly if, in the opinion of the physician familiar with the patients bleeding risk, the vaccine can be administered by this route with reasonable safety. If the patient receives antihemophilia or other similar therapy, intramuscular vaccination can be scheduled shortly after such therapy is administered. A fine needle (23 gauge or smaller) can be used for the vaccination and firm pressure applied to the site (without rubbing) for at least 2 minutes. The patient should be instructed concerning the risk of hematoma from the injection." Patients on anticoagulant therapy should be considered to have the same bleeding risks and treated as those with clotting factor disorders (CDC, 2011).

Simultaneous administration of vaccines helps ensure the patients will be fully vaccinated by the appropriate age. Simultaneous administration of vaccines is defined as administering >1 vaccine on the same day at different anatomic sites. The use of licensed combination vaccines is generally preferred over separate injections of the equivalent components. Separate vaccines should not be combined in the same syringe unless indicated by product specific labeling. Separate needles and syringes should be used for each injection. The ACIP prefers each dose of a specific vaccine in a series come from the same manufacturer when possible. Adolescents and adults should be vaccinated while seated or lying down. In general, preterm infants should be vaccinated at the same chronological age as full-term infants (CDC, 2011).

Antipyretics have not been shown to prevent febrile seizures. Antipyretics may be used to treat fever or discomfort following vaccination (CDC, 2011). One study reported that routine prophylactic administration of acetaminophen to prevent fever prior to vaccination decreased the immune response of some vaccines; the clinical significance of this reduction in immune response has not been established (Prymula, 2009).

Monitoring Parameters Liver function tests; monitor for syncope for ≥15 minutes following vaccination

Pharmacotherapy Pearls The ACIP currently recommends that older adults, the immuno-compromised, or persons with underlying medical conditions (including chronic liver disease) that are vaccinated <2 weeks from departure to an area with a high risk of hepatitis A infection also receive immune globulin (CDC, 2007).

Federal law requires that the name of medication, date of administration, the vaccine manufacturer, lot number of vaccine, and the administering person's name, title and address be entered into the patient's permanent medical record.

Special Geriatric Considerations There is no specific data to suggest dosing is different than it is for younger adults.

Dosage Forms Excipient information presented when available (limited, particularly for generics); consult specific product labeling. [DSC] = Discontinued product

Injection, suspension [adult, preservative free]:

Havrix®: Hepatitis A virus antigen 1440 ELISA units/mL (1 mL) [contains aluminum, neomycin (may have trace amounts); may contain natural rubber/natural latex in prefilled syringe]

VAQTA®: Hepatitis A virus antigen 50 units/mL (1 mL) [contains aluminum, natural rubber/natural latex in packaging]

Injection, suspension [pediatric, preservative free]:
  Havrix®: Hepatitis A virus antigen 720 ELISA units/0.5 mL (0.5 mL) [contains aluminum, neomycin (may have trace amounts); may contain natural rubber/natural latex in prefilled syringe]
Injection, suspension [pediatric/adolescent, preservative free]:
  VAQTA®: Hepatitis A virus antigen 25 units/0.5 mL (0.5 mL) [contains aluminum, natural rubber/natural latex in packaging]

Selected References

"Advisory Committee on Immunization Practices (ACIP) Centers for Disease Control and Prevention (CDC). Update: Prevention of Hepatitis A After Exposure to Hepatitis A Virus and in International Travelers. Updated Recommendations of the Advisory Committee on Immunization Practices (ACIP)," *MMWR Morb Mortal Wkly Rep*, 2007, 56 (41):1080-4.

♦ **Hepatitis B and Hepatitis A Vaccine** *see* Hepatitis A and Hepatitis B Recombinant Vaccine *on page 862*

Hepatitis B Immune Globulin (Human)
(hep a TYE tis bee i MYUN GLOB yoo lin YU man)

Related Information
Immunization Administration Recommendations *on page 2037*
Immunization Recommendations *on page 2043*

Medication Safety Issues
Sound-alike/look-alike issues:
HBIG may be confused with BabyBIG

Brand Names: U.S. HepaGam B®; HyperHEP B™ S/D; Nabi-HB®
Brand Names: Canada HepaGam B™; HyperHep B®
Index Terms HBIG
Generic Availability (U.S.) No
Pharmacologic Category Blood Product Derivative; Immune Globulin

Use
Passive prophylactic immunity to hepatitis B following: Acute exposure to blood containing hepatitis B surface antigen (HBsAg); sexual exposure to HBsAg-positive persons; household exposure to persons with acute HBV infection
Prevention of hepatitis B virus recurrence after liver transplantation in HBsAg-positive transplant patients
Note: Hepatitis B immune globulin is not indicated for treatment of active hepatitis B infection and is ineffective in the treatment of chronic active hepatitis B infection.

Contraindications Hypersensitivity to hepatitis B immune globulin or any component of the formulation; severe allergy to gamma globulin or anti-immunoglobulin therapies

Warnings/Precautions Hypersensitivity and anaphylactic reactions can occur; immediate treatment (including epinephrine 1:1000) should be available. Use with caution in patients with previous systemic hypersensitivity to human immunoglobulins. Use with caution in patients with thrombocytopenia or coagulation disorders; I.M. injections may be contraindicated. Use with caution in patients with IgA deficiency. Product of human plasma; may potentially contain infectious agents which could transmit disease. Screening of donors, as well as testing and/or inactivation or removal of certain viruses, reduces the risk. Infections thought to be transmitted by this product should be reported to the manufacturer. Some products may contain maltose, which may result in falsely-elevated blood glucose readings.

Adverse Reactions (Reflective of adult population; not specific for elderly)
Reported with postexposure prophylaxis; frequency not defined. Adverse events reported in liver transplant patients included tremor and hypotension, were associated with a single infusion during the first week of treatment, and did not recur with additional infusions.

Central nervous system: Fainting, headache, lightheadedness, malaise
Dermatologic: Angioedema, bruising, urticaria
Gastrointestinal: Nausea, vomiting
Hematologic: WBC decreased
Hepatic: Alkaline phosphatase increased, AST increased
Local: Ache, erythema, pain, and/or tenderness at injection site
Neuromuscular & skeletal: Arthralgia, joint stiffness, myalgia
Renal: Creatinine increased
Respiratory: Cold symptoms
Miscellaneous: Anaphylaxis, flu-like syndrome

Drug Interactions
Avoid Concomitant Use There are no known interactions where it is recommended to avoid concomitant use.

◄ **Increased Effect/Toxicity** There are no known significant interactions involving an increase in effect.

Decreased Effect

Hepatitis B Immune Globulin (Human) may decrease the levels/effects of: Vaccines (Live)

Stability Refrigerate at 2°C to 8°C (36°F to 46°F); do not freeze. Use within 6 hours of entering vial. Do not shake vial; avoid foaming. The following stability information has also been reported for HyperHEP B™ S/D: May be exposed to room temperature for a cumulative 7 days (Cohen, 2007).

Mechanism of Action Hepatitis B immune globulin (HBIG) is a nonpyrogenic sterile solution containing immunoglobulin G (IgG) specific to hepatitis B surface antigen (HB_sAg). HBIG differs from immune globulin in the amount of anti-HB_s. Immune globulin is prepared from plasma that is not preselected for anti-HB_s content. HBIG is prepared from plasma preselected for high titer anti-HB_s. In the U.S., HBIG has an anti-HB_s high titer >1:100,000 by IRA.

Pharmacodynamics/Kinetics

Duration: Postexposure prophylaxis: 3-6 months

Absorption: I.M.: Slow

Half-life: 17-25 days

Distribution: V_d: 7-15 L

Time to peak, serum: I.M.: 2-10 days

Dosage

Geriatric & Adult

Postexposure prophylaxis: I.M.: 0.06 mL/kg as soon as possible after exposure (ie, within 24 hours of needlestick, ocular, or mucosal exposure or within 14 days of sexual exposure); usual dose: 3-5 mL; repeat at 28-30 days after exposure in nonresponders to hepatitis B vaccine or in patients who refuse vaccination

Note: HBIG may be administered at the same time (but at a different site) or up to 1 month preceding hepatitis B vaccination without impairing the active immune response

Prevention of hepatitis B virus recurrence after liver transplantation (HepaGam B™):

I.V.: 20,000 int. units/dose according to the following schedule:

Anhepatic phase (Initial dose): One dose given with the liver transplant

Week 1 postop: One dose daily for 7 days (days 1-7)

Weeks 2-12 postop: One dose every 2 weeks starting day 14

Month 4 onward: One dose monthly starting on month 4

Dose adjustment: Adjust dose to reach anti-HBs levels of 500 int. units/L within the first week after transplantation. In patients with surgical bleeding, abdominal fluid drainage >500 mL or those undergoing plasmapheresis, administer 10,000 int. units/dose every 6 hours until target anti-HBs levels are reached.

Administration

I.M.: Postexposure prophylaxis: I.M. injection only in anterolateral aspect of upper thigh and deltoid muscle of upper arm; to prevent injury from injection, care should be taken when giving to patients with thrombocytopenia or bleeding disorders

I.V.:

HepaGam B™: Liver transplant: Administer at 2 mL/minute. Decrease infusion to ≤1 mL/minute for patient discomfort or infusion-related adverse events. Actual volume of infusion is dependent upon potency labeled on each individual vial.

Nabi-HB®: Although not FDA-approved for this purpose, Nabi-HB® has been administered intravenously in hepatitis B-positive liver transplant patients

Monitoring Parameters Liver transplant: Serum HBsAg; infusion-related adverse events

Test Interactions

Glucose testing: HepaGam B™ contains maltose. Falsely-elevated blood glucose levels may occur when glucose monitoring devices and test strips utilizing the glucose dehydrogenase pyrroloquinolinequinone (GDH-PQQ) based methods are used.

Serological testing: Antibodies transferred following administration of immune globulins may provide misleading positive test results (eg, Coombs' test)

Pharmacotherapy Pearls Hepatitis B immune globulin is not indicated for treatment of active hepatitis B infections and is ineffective in the treatment of chronic active hepatitis B infection. Administration of HBIG preceding or concomitantly with hepatitis B vaccine does not interfere with the immune response to vaccine; the two together provide more rapid protective antibodies to hepatitis B than when vaccine is used alone; rapid levels may be necessary in certain settings. Has been administered intravenously in hepatitis B-positive liver transplant patients.

Special Geriatric Considerations No data available to suggest different dosing in the elderly than in younger adults.

Dosage Forms Excipient information presented when available (limited, particularly for generics); consult specific product labeling.

Injection, solution [preservative free]:

HepaGam B®: Anti-HBs > 312 int. units/mL (1 mL, 5 mL) [contains maltose, polysorbate 80]

HyperHEP B™ S/D: Anti-HBs ≥ 220 int. units/mL (0.5 mL, 1 mL, 5 mL)

Nabi-HB®: Anti-HBs > 312 int. units/mL (1 mL, 5 mL) [contains polysorbate 80]

Selected References

Dickson RC, Terrault NA, Ishitani M, et al, "Protective Antibody Levels and Dose Requirements for IV 5% Nabi Hepatitis B Immune Globulin Combined With Lamivudine in Liver Transplantation for Hepatitis B-Induced End Stage Liver Disease," *Liver Transpl*, 2006, 12(1):124-33.

Mast EE, Weinbaum CM, Fiore AE, et al, "A Comprehensive Immunization Strategy to Eliminate Transmission of Hepatitis B Virus Infection in the United States: Recommendations of the Advisory Committee on Immunization Practices (ACIP) Part II: Immunization of Adults," *MMWR Recomm Rep*, 2006, 55(RR-16):1-33.

Tung BY and Kowdley KV, "Hepatitis B and Liver Transplantation," *Clin Infect Dis*, 2005, 41(10):1461-6.

◆ **Hepatitis B Inactivated Virus Vaccine (recombinant DNA)** *see* Hepatitis B Vaccine (Recombinant) *on page 869*

Hepatitis B Vaccine (Recombinant)
(hep a TYE tis bee vak SEEN ree KOM be nant)

Related Information
Immunization Administration Recommendations *on page 2037*
Immunization Recommendations *on page 2043*

Medication Safety Issues
Sound-alike/look-alike issues:
Engerix-B® adult may be confused with Engerix-B® pediatric/adolescent
Recombivax HB® may be confused with Comvax®

Brand Names: U.S. Engerix-B®; Recombivax HB®

Brand Names: Canada Engerix-B®; Recombivax HB®

Index Terms Hepatitis B Inactivated Virus Vaccine (recombinant DNA); HepB

Generic Availability (U.S.) No

Pharmacologic Category Vaccine, Inactivated (Viral)

Use Immunization against infection caused by all known subtypes of hepatitis B virus (HBV)

The Advisory Committee on Immunization Practices (ACIP) recommends routine vaccination for the following (CDC 2006; CDC 2005):
- All infants at birth
- All infants and children (post-birth dose; refer to recommended vaccination schedule)
- All unvaccinated adults requesting protection from HBV infection
- All unvaccinated adults at risk for HBV infection such as those with:
  Behavioral risks: Sexually-active persons with >1 partner in a 6-month period; persons seeking evaluation or treatment for a sexually-transmitted disease; men who have sex with men; injection drug users
  Occupational risks: Healthcare and public safety workers with reasonably anticipated risk for exposure to blood or blood contaminated body fluids
  Medical risks: Persons with end-stage renal disease (including predialysis, hemodialysis, peritoneal dialysis, and home dialysis); persons with HIV infection; persons with chronic liver disease
  Other risks: Household contacts and sex partners of persons with chronic HBV infection; residents and staff of facilities for developmentally disabled persons; international travelers to regions with high or intermediate levels of endemic HBV infection

In addition, the ACIP recommends vaccination for any persons who are wounded in bombings or similar mass casualty events who have penetrating injuries or nonintact skin exposure, or who have contact with mucous membranes (exception - superficial contact with intact skin), and who cannot confirm receipt of a hepatitis B vaccination (CDC, 2008).

Contraindications Hypersensitivity to yeast, hepatitis B vaccine, or any component of the formulation

Warnings/Precautions Immediate treatment for anaphylactic/anaphylactoid reaction should be available during vaccine use. Defer administration in patients with moderate or severe acute illness (with or without fever). Use caution with decreased cardiopulmonary function Unrecognized hepatitis B infection may be present prior to vaccination; immunization may not prevent infection in these patients. Patients >65 years of age may have lower response rates. Use with caution in severely immunocompromised patients (eg, patients receiving chemo/radiation therapy or other immunosuppressive therapy [including high-dose corticosteroids]); may have a reduced response to vaccination. In general, household and close contacts of persons with altered immunocompetence may receive all age appropriate vaccines. Use caution in multiple sclerosis patients; rare exacerbations of symptoms have been observed.

◀ Apnea has been reported following I.M. vaccine administration in premature infants; consider risk versus benefit in infants born prematurely. Some dosage forms contain dry natural latex rubber. In order to maximize vaccination rates, the ACIP recommends simultaneous administration of all age-appropriate vaccines (live or inactivated) for which a person is eligible at a single clinic visit, unless contraindications exist. The use of combination vaccines is generally preferred over separate injections, taking into consideration provider assessment, patient preference, and adverse events.

Adverse Reactions (Reflective of adult population; not specific for elderly) All serious adverse reactions must be reported to the U.S. Department of Health and Human Services (DHHS) Vaccine Adverse Event Reporting System (VAERS) at 1-800-822-7967 or online at https://vaers.hhs.gov/esub/index.

Frequency not defined. The most common adverse effects reported with both products included injection site reactions (>10%).

Cardiovascular: Flushing, hypotension

Central nervous system: Agitation, chills, dizziness, fatigue, fever (≥37.5°C/100°F), headache, insomnia, irritability, lightheadedness, malaise, somnolence, vertigo

Dermatologic: Angioedema, petechiae, pruritus, rash, urticaria

Gastrointestinal: Abdominal pain, anorexia, appetite decreased, constipation, cramps, diarrhea, dyspepsia, nausea, vomiting

Genitourinary: Dysuria

Local: Injection site reactions: Ecchymosis, erythema, induration, pain, nodule formation, soreness, swelling, tenderness, warmth

Neuromuscular & skeletal: Achiness, arthralgia, back pain, myalgia, neck pain, neck stiffness, paresthesia, shoulder pain, tingling, weakness

Otic: Earache

Respiratory: Cough, pharyngitis, rhinitis, upper respiratory tract infection

Miscellaneous: Diaphoresis, lymphadenopathy, flu-like syndrome

Drug Interactions

Avoid Concomitant Use There are no known interactions where it is recommended to avoid concomitant use.

Increased Effect/Toxicity There are no known significant interactions involving an increase in effect.

Decreased Effect

The levels/effects of Hepatitis B Vaccine (Recombinant) may be decreased by: Belimumab; Fingolimod; Immunosuppressants

Stability Refrigerate at 2°C to 8°C (36°F to 46°F); do not freeze. The following stability information has also been reported for Engerix-B®: May be stored at room temperature for up to 72 hours (Cohen, 2007).

Mechanism of Action Recombinant hepatitis B vaccine is a noninfectious subunit viral vaccine, which confers active immunity via formation of antihepatitis B antibodies. The vaccine is derived from hepatitis B surface antigen (HBsAg) produced through recombinant DNA techniques from yeast cells. The portion of the hepatitis B gene which codes for HBsAg is cloned into yeast which is then cultured to produce hepatitis B vaccine.

Pharmacodynamics/Kinetics Duration: Following a 3-dose series in children, up to 50% of patients will have low or undetectable anti-HB antibody 5-15 years postvaccination. However, anamnestic increases in anti-HB have been shown up to 23 years later suggesting a lifelong immune memory response.

Dosage

Geriatric & Adult

Primary immunization: I.M.: 1 mL/dose (adult formulation) for 3 total doses administered at 0, 1, and 6 months

Note: Adult formulations of hepatitis B vaccine products differ by concentration (mcg/mL) but when dosed in terms of volume (mL), the dose of Engerix-B® and Recombivax HB® are the same (both 1 mL).

Alternate dosing schedules (selection of schedule should optimize compliance with vaccination): All regimens use the adult formulation administered as one dose at the following intervals (three schedules presented):

0, 1, and 4 months (CDC, 2005)

0, 2, and 4 months (CDC, 2005)

0, 12, and 24 months (CDC, 2005)

Bombings or similar mass casualty events: I.M.: In persons without a reliable history of vaccination against HepB and who have no known contraindications to the vaccine, vaccination should begin within 24 hours (but no later than 7 days) following the event (CDC, 2008).

Renal Impairment Adults on dialysis:

Engerix-B® 20 mcg/mL: Administer 2 mL per dose at 0, 1, 2, and 6 months

Recombivax HB® 40 mcg/mL: Administer 1 mL per dose at 0, 1, and 6 months

Note: Serologic testing is recommended 1-2 months after the final dose of the primary vaccine series and annually to determine the need for booster doses. Persons with anti-HB$_s$ concentrations of <10 mIU/mL should be revaccinated with 3 doses of the vaccine (CDC, 2006).

Administration Pediatric/adolescent formulations of hepatitis B vaccine products differ by concentration (mcg/mL). However, when dosed in terms of volume (mL), the dose of Engerix-B® and Recombivax HB® are the same (both 0.5 mL). Adult formulations of hepatitis B vaccine products also differ by concentration (mcg/mL), but when dosed in terms of volume (mL), the dose of Engerix-B® and Recombivax HB® are the same (both 1 mL). It is possible to interchange the vaccines for completion of a series or for booster doses; the antibody produced in response to each type of vaccine is comparable, however, the quantity of the vaccine will vary.

I.M. injection only; in adults, the deltoid muscle is the preferred site. Not for gluteal administration. Shake well prior to withdrawal and use.

For patients at risk of hemorrhage following intramuscular injection, hepatitis B vaccine may be administered subcutaneously although lower titers and/or increased incidence of local reactions may result. The ACIP recommends "it should be administered intramuscularly if, in the opinion of the physician familiar with the patients bleeding risk, the vaccine can be administered by this route with reasonable safety. If the patient receives antihemophilia or other similar therapy, intramuscular vaccination can be scheduled shortly after such therapy is administered. A fine needle (23 gauge or smaller) can be used for the vaccination and firm pressure applied to the site (without rubbing) for at least 2 minutes. The patient should be instructed concerning the risk of hematoma from the injection." Patients on anticoagulant therapy should be considered to have the same bleeding risks and treated as those with clotting factor disorders (CDC, 2011).

Simultaneous administration of vaccines helps ensure the patients will be fully vaccinated by the appropriate age. Simultaneous administration of vaccines is defined as administering >1 vaccine on the same day at different anatomic sites. The use of licensed combination vaccines is generally preferred over separate injections of the equivalent components. Separate vaccines should not be combined in the same syringe unless indicated by product specific labeling. Separate needles and syringes should be used for each injection. The ACIP prefers each dose of a specific vaccine in a series come from the same manufacturer when possible. Adolescents and adults should be vaccinated while seated or lying down. In general, preterm infants should be vaccinated at the same chronological age as full-term infants (CDC, 2011).

Antipyretics have not been shown to prevent febrile seizures. Antipyretics may be used to treat fever or discomfort following vaccination (CDC, 2011). One study reported that routine prophylactic administration of acetaminophen to prevent fever prior to vaccination decreased the immune response of some vaccines; the clinical significance of this reduction in immune response has not been established (Prymula, 2009).

Vaccination at the time of HB$_s$Ag testing: For persons in whom vaccination is recommended, the first dose of hepatitis B vaccine can be given after blood is drawn to test for HB$_s$Ag.

Pharmacotherapy Pearls Federal law requires that the name of medication, date of administration, the vaccine manufacturer, lot number of vaccine, and the administering person's name, title, and address be entered into the patient's permanent medical record.

Special Geriatric Considerations No dose adjustments required based on age. Some studies demonstrate a lower antibody titer in the elderly as compared to young adults.

Dosage Forms Excipient information presented when available (limited, particularly for generics); consult specific product labeling. [DSC] = Discontinued product

Injection, suspension [adult, preservative free]:

Engerix-B®: Hepatitis B surface antigen 20 mcg/mL (1 mL) [contains aluminum, yeast protein, may contain natural rubber/natural latex in prefilled syringe]

Recombivax HB®: Hepatitis B surface antigen 10 mcg/mL (1 mL) [contains aluminum, natural rubber/natural latex in packaging, yeast protein]

Injection, suspension [dialysis formulation, preservative free]:

Recombivax HB®: Hepatitis B surface antigen 40 mcg/mL (1 mL) [contains aluminum, natural rubber/natural latex in packaging, yeast protein; dialysis]

Injection, suspension [pediatric/adolescent, preservative free]:

Engerix-B®: Hepatitis B surface antigen 10 mcg/0.5 mL (0.5 mL) [contains aluminum, yeast protein; may contain natural rubber/natural latex in prefilled syringe]

Recombivax HB®: Hepatitis B surface antigen 5 mcg/0.5 mL (0.5 mL) [contains aluminum, natural rubber/natural latex in packaging, yeast protein]

Selected References

Centers for Disease Control and Prevention, "A Comprehensive Immunization Strategy to Eliminate Transmission of Hepatitis B Virus Infection in the United States: Recommendations of the Advisory Committee on Immunization Practices (ACIP) Part II: Immunization of Adults," *MMWR Recomm Rep*, 2006, 54(RR16):1-25.

Centers for Disease Control, "Recommendations of the Advisory Committee on Immunization Practices (ACIP): General Recommendations on Immunization," *MMWR Recomm Rep*, 2006, 55(RR-15):1-48.

Chapman LE, Sullivent EE, Grohskopf LA, et al, "Recommendations for Postexposure Interventions to Prevent Infection With Hepatitis B Virus, Hepatitis C Virus, or Human Immunodeficiency Virus, and Tetanus in Persons Wounded During Bombings and Other Mass-Casualty Events – United States, 2008: Recommendations of the Centers for Disease Control and Prevention (CDC)," *MMWR Recomm Rep*, 2008, 57(RR-6):1-21.

Weinbaum CM, Williams I, Mast EE, et al, "Recommendations for Identification and Public Health Management of Persons With Chronic Hepatitis B Virus Infection," *MMWR Recomm Rep*, 2008, 57(RR-8):1-20.

◆ **HepB** see Hepatitis B Vaccine (Recombinant) *on page 869*
◆ **HepFlush®-10** see Heparin *on page 857*
◆ **Hep-Lock** see Heparin *on page 857*
◆ **Hep-Lock U/P** see Heparin *on page 857*
◆ **Hexachlorocyclohexane** see Lindane *on page 1068*
◆ **Hexamethylenetetramine** see Methenamine *on page 1164*
◆ **High Gamma Vitamin E Complete™ [OTC]** see Vitamin E *on page 1921*
◆ **High-Molecular-Weight Iron Dextran (DexFerrum®)** see Iron Dextran Complex *on page 977*
◆ **Hiprex®** see Methenamine *on page 1164*
◆ **Histaprin [OTC]** see DiphenhydrAMINE (Systemic) *on page 520*
◆ **Hizentra®** see Immune Globulin *on page 922*
◆ **HMR 3647** see Telithromycin *on page 1745*
◆ **Hold® DM [OTC]** see Dextromethorphan *on page 490*

Homatropine (hoe MA troe peen)

Medication Safety Issues

Sound-alike/look-alike issues:

Homatropine may be confused with Humatrope®, somatropin

Brand Names: U.S. Isopto® Homatropine

Index Terms Homatropine Hydrobromide

Generic Availability (U.S.) No

Pharmacologic Category Anticholinergic Agent, Ophthalmic; Ophthalmic Agent, Mydriatic

Use Producing cycloplegia and mydriasis for refraction; treatment of acute inflammatory conditions of the uveal tract; optical aid in axial lens opacities

Contraindications Hypersensitivity to homatropine or any component of the formulation; primary glaucoma or predisposition to glaucoma (eg, narrow-angle glaucoma)

Warnings/Precautions Excessive use may cause CNS disturbances, including confusion, delirium, agitation and coma (rare); may occur with any age group, although children and the elderly are more susceptible. May cause an increase in intraocular pressure. Use with caution in patients with keratoconus; may result in fixed pupil dilation. Use with caution in the elderly. May cause sensitivity to light; appropriate eye protection should be used. Some strengths may contain benzalkonium chloride which may be adsorbed by contact lenses; remove contacts prior to administration and wait 15 minutes before reinserting. To minimize systemic absorption, apply pressure over the nasolacrimal sac for 2-3 minutes after instillation. To avoid contamination, do not touch dropper tip to any surface. For topical ophthalmic use only.

Adverse Reactions (Reflective of adult population; not specific for elderly)

>10%: Ocular: Blurred vision, photophobia

1% to 10%:

Local: Stinging, local irritation

Ocular: Increased intraocular pressure

Respiratory: Congestion

Drug Interactions

Avoid Concomitant Use There are no known interactions where it is recommended to avoid concomitant use.

Increased Effect/Toxicity

Homatropine may increase the levels/effects of: AbobotulinumtoxinA; Anticholinergics; Cannabinoids; OnabotulinumtoxinA; Potassium Chloride; RimabotulinumtoxinB

The levels/effects of Homatropine may be increased by: Pramlintide

Decreased Effect

Homatropine may decrease the levels/effects of: Acetylcholinesterase Inhibitors (Central); Secretin

The levels/effects of Homatropine may be decreased by: Acetylcholinesterase Inhibitors (Central)

Stability Store at 8°C to 24°C (46°F to 75°F). Protect from light.

Mechanism of Action Blocks response of iris sphincter muscle and the accommodative muscle of the ciliary body to cholinergic stimulation resulting in dilation and loss of accommodation

Pharmacodynamics/Kinetics
Onset of action: Accommodation and pupil effect: Ophthalmic:
  Maximum mydriatic effect: Within 10-30 minutes
  Maximum cycloplegic effect: Within 30-90 minutes
Duration:
  Mydriasis: 6 hours to 4 days
  Cycloplegia: 10-48 hours

Dosage
  Geriatric & Adult
    Mydriasis and cycloplegia for refraction: Ophthalmic: Instill 1-2 drops of 2% solution or 1 drop of 5% solution before the procedure; repeat at 5- to 10-minute intervals as needed; maximum of 3 doses for refraction
    Uveitis: Ophthalmic: Instill 1-2 drops of 2% or 5% 2-3 times/day up to every 3-4 hours as needed

Administration Finger pressure should be applied to lacrimal sac for 1-2 minutes after instillation to decrease risk of absorption and systemic reactions

Special Geriatric Considerations Use with caution due to susceptibility to systemic effects. Evaluate the patient's or caregiver's ability to safely administer the correct dose of ophthalmic medication.

Dosage Forms Excipient information presented when available (limited, particularly for generics); consult specific product labeling.
Solution, ophthalmic, as hydrobromide [drops]:
  Isopto® Homatropine: 2% (5 mL); 5% (5 mL) [contains benzalkonium chloride]

Selected References
Barker DB and Solomon DA, "The Potential for Mental Status Changes Associated With Systemic Absorption of Anticholinergic Ophthalmic Medications: Concerns in the Elderly," *DICP Ann Pharmacother*, 1990, 24(9):847-50.

Hyaluronidase (hye al yoor ON i dase)

Medication Safety Issues
  Sound-alike/look-alike issues:
    Wydase may be confused with Lidex®, Wyamine®

HYALURONIDASE

Brand Names: U.S. Amphadase™; Hylenex; Vitrase®
Generic Availability (U.S.) No
Pharmacologic Category Enzyme
Use Increase the dispersion and absorption of other injected drugs; increase rate of absorption of parenteral fluids given by subcutaneous administration (hypodermoclysis)
Unlabeled/Investigational Use Management of drug extravasations
Dosage
  Geriatric & Adult
    Skin test: Intradermal: 0.02 mL (3 units) of a 150 units/mL solution. Positive reaction consists of a wheal with pseudopods appearing within 5 minutes and persisting for 20-30 minutes with localized itching.
    Dehydration: Hypodermoclysis: SubQ: Add 15 units to each 100 mL of I.V. fluid to be administered subcutaneously **or** 150 units followed by subcutaneous isotonic fluid administration ≥1000 mL; rate and volume of a single clysis should not exceed those used for infusion of I.V. fluids
    Extravasation (unlabeled use): SubQ: Inject 1 mL of a 150 unit/mL solution (as 5-10 injections of 0.1-0.2 mL) into affected area; doses of 15-250 units have been reported.
    Note: Do not use for extravasation of pressor agents (eg, dopamine, norepinephrine).
Special Geriatric Considerations The most common use of hyaluronidase in the elderly is in hypodermoclysis. Hypodermoclysis is very useful in dehydrated patients in whom oral intake is minimal and I.V. access is a problem.
Dosage Forms Excipient information presented when available (limited, particularly for generics); consult specific product labeling.
  Injection, solution [preservative free]:
    Hylenex: 150 units/mL (1 mL) [contains albumin (human), edetate disodium; recombinant]
  Injection, solution [bovine derived]:
    Amphadase™: 150 units/mL (1 mL) [contains edetate disodium, thimerosal]
  Injection, solution [ovine derived, preservative free]:
    Vitrase®: 200 units/mL (2 mL) [contains lactose 0.93 mg/mL]

◆ **hycet®** see Hydrocodone and Acetaminophen on page 880
◆ **Hydergine [DSC]** see Ergoloid Mesylates on page 620

HydrALAZINE (hye DRAL a zeen)

Medication Safety Issues
  Sound-alike/look-alike issues:
    HydrALAZINE may be confused with hydrOXYzine
Brand Names: Canada Apo-Hydralazine®; Apresoline®; Novo-Hylazin; Nu-Hydral
Index Terms Apresoline [DSC]; Hydralazine Hydrochloride
Generic Availability (U.S.) Yes
Pharmacologic Category Vasodilator
Use Management of moderate-to-severe hypertension
Unlabeled/Investigational Use Heart failure
Contraindications Hypersensitivity to hydralazine or any component of the formulation; mitral valve rheumatic heart disease
Warnings/Precautions May cause peripheral neuritis or a drug-induced lupus-like syndrome (more likely on larger doses, longer duration). Discontinue hydralazine in patients who develop SLE-like syndrome or positive ANA. Use with caution in patients with severe renal disease or cerebral vascular accidents or with known or suspected coronary artery disease; monitor blood pressure closely with I.V. use. Slow acetylators, patients with decreased renal function, and patients receiving >200 mg/day (chronically) are at higher risk for SLE. Titrate dosage cautiously to patient's response. Hypotensive effect after I.V. administration may be delayed and unpredictable in some patients. Usually administered with diuretic and a beta-blocker to counteract side effects of sodium and water retention and reflex tachycardia.

Adjust dose in severe renal dysfunction. Use with caution in CAD (increase in tachycardia may increase myocardial oxygen demand). Use with caution in pulmonary hypertension (may cause hypotension). Patients may be poorly compliant because of frequent dosing. Hydralazine-induced fluid and sodium retention may require addition or increased dosage of a diuretic.

Adverse Reactions (Reflective of adult population; not specific for elderly) Frequency not defined.

Cardiovascular: Angina pectoris, flushing, orthostatic hypotension, palpitations, paradoxical hypertension, peripheral edema, tachycardia, vascular collapse

Central nervous system: Anxiety, chills, depression, disorientation, dizziness, fever, headache, increased intracranial pressure (I.V.; in patient with pre-existing increased intracranial pressure), psychotic reaction

Dermatologic: Pruritus, rash, urticaria

Gastrointestinal: Anorexia, constipation, diarrhea, nausea, paralytic ileus, vomiting

Genitourinary: Dysuria, impotence

Hematologic: Agranulocytosis, eosinophilia, erythrocyte count reduced, hemoglobin decreased, hemolytic anemia, leukopenia, thrombocytopenia (rare)

Neuromuscular & skeletal: Muscle cramps, peripheral neuritis, rheumatoid arthritis, tremor, weakness

Ocular: Conjunctivitis, lacrimation

Respiratory: Dyspnea, nasal congestion

Miscellaneous: Diaphoresis, drug-induced lupus-like syndrome (dose related; fever, arthralgia, splenomegaly, lymphadenopathy, asthenia, myalgia, malaise, pleuritic chest pain, edema, positive ANA, positive LE cells, maculopapular facial rash, positive direct Coombs' test, pericarditis, pericardial tamponade)

Drug Interactions

Metabolism/Transport Effects Inhibits CYP3A4 (weak)

Avoid Concomitant Use There are no known interactions where it is recommended to avoid concomitant use.

Increased Effect/Toxicity

HydrALAZINE may increase the levels/effects of: Amifostine; Antihypertensives; Hypotensive Agents; RiTUXimab

The levels/effects of HydrALAZINE may be increased by: Alfuzosin; Diazoxide; Herbs (Hypotensive Properties); MAO Inhibitors; Pentoxifylline; Phosphodiesterase 5 Inhibitors; Prostacyclin Analogues

Decreased Effect

The levels/effects of HydrALAZINE may be decreased by: Herbs (Hypertensive Properties); Methylphenidate; Nonsteroidal Anti-Inflammatory Agents; Yohimbine

Ethanol/Nutrition/Herb Interactions

Ethanol: Avoid ethanol (may increase CNS depression).

Food: Food enhances bioavailability of hydralazine.

Herb/Nutraceutical: Avoid dong quai if using for hypertension (has estrogenic activity). Avoid ephedra, yohimbe, ginseng (may worsen hypertension). Avoid garlic (may have increased antihypertensive effect).

Stability Intact ampuls/vials of hydralazine should not be stored under refrigeration because of possible precipitation or crystallization. Hydralazine should be diluted in NS for IVPB administration due to decreased stability in D_5W. Stability of IVPB solution in NS is 4 days at room temperature.

Mechanism of Action Direct vasodilation of arterioles (with little effect on veins) with decreased systemic resistance

Pharmacodynamics/Kinetics

Onset of action: Oral: 20-30 minutes; I.V.: 5-20 minutes

Duration: Oral: Up to 8 hours; I.V.: 1-4 hours; **Note:** May vary depending on acetylator status of patient

Protein binding: 85% to 90%

Metabolism: Hepatically acetylated; extensive first-pass effect (oral)

Bioavailability: 30% to 50%; increased with food

Half-life elimination: Normal renal function: 2-8 hours; End-stage renal disease: 7-16 hours

Excretion: Urine (14% as unchanged drug)

Dosage

Geriatric Oral: Initial: 10 mg 2-3 times/day; increase by 10-25 mg/day every 2-5 days.

Adult

Hypertension: Oral:

Initial: 10 mg 4 times/day; increase by 10-25 mg/dose every 2-5 days (maximum: 300 mg/day); usual dose range (JNC 7): 25-100 mg/day in 2 divided doses

Acute hypertension: I.M., I.V.: Initial: 10-20 mg/dose every 4-6 hours as needed, may increase to 40 mg/dose; change to oral therapy as soon as possible.

Congestive heart failure: Oral:

Initial dose: 10-25 mg 3-4 times/day

Adjustment: Dosage must be adjusted based on individual response

Target dose: 225-300 mg/day in divided doses; use in combination with isosorbide dinitrate

◄ **Renal Impairment**
Cl$_{cr}$ 10-50 mL/minute: Administer every 8 hours.
Cl$_{cr}$ <10 mL/minute: Administer every 8-16 hours in fast acetylators and every 12-24 hours in slow acetylators.
Hemodialysis effects: Supplemental dose is not necessary.
Peritoneal dialysis effects: Supplemental dose is not necessary.

Administration Solution for injection: Administer as a slow I.V. push; maximum rate: 5 mg/minute

Monitoring Parameters Blood pressure (monitor closely with I.V. use), standing and sitting/ supine, heart rate, ANA titer

Pharmacotherapy Pearls Slow acetylators, patients with decreased renal function and patients receiving >200 mg/day (chronically) are at higher risk for SLE. Titrate dosage to patient's response. Usually administered with diuretic and a beta-blocker to counteract side effects of sodium and water retention and reflex tachycardia although the beta-blocker may not be necessary in older adults. For the treatment of CHF where hydralazine is used in place of an ACE inhibitor, it is necessary to use a combination of hydralazine and isosorbide.

Dosage Forms Excipient information presented when available (limited, particularly for generics); consult specific product labeling.
Injection, solution, as hydrochloride: 20 mg/mL (1 mL)
Tablet, oral, as hydrochloride: 10 mg, 25 mg, 50 mg, 100 mg

Selected References
Chobanian AV, Bakris GL, Black HR, et al, "The Seventh Report of the Joint National Committee on Prevention, Detection, Evaluation, and Treatment of High Blood Pressure: The JNC 7 Report," *JAMA*, 2003, 289(19):2560-71.

◆ **Hydralazine and Isosorbide Dinitrate** *see* Isosorbide Dinitrate and Hydralazine *on page 990*
◆ **Hydralazine Hydrochloride** *see* HydrALAZINE *on page 874*
◆ **Hydrated Chloral** *see* Chloral Hydrate *on page 330*
◆ **Hydrea®** *see* Hydroxyurea *on page 897*
◆ **Hydrisalic® [OTC]** *see* Salicylic Acid *on page 1648*

Hydrochlorothiazide (hye droe klor oh THYE a zide)

Medication Safety Issues
Sound-alike/look-alike issues:
Esidrix may be confused with Lasix®
HCTZ is an error-prone abbreviation (mistaken as hydrocortisone)
Hydrochlorothiazide may be confused with hydrocortisone, hydroflumethiazide, Viskazide® Microzide™ may be confused with Maxzide®, Micronase®

Brand Names: U.S. Microzide®
Brand Names: Canada Apo-Hydro®; Bio-Hydrochlorothiazide; Dom-Hydrochlorothiazide; Novo-Hydrazide; Nu-Hydro; PMS-Hydrochlorothiazide

Index Terms HCTZ (error-prone abbreviation); Hydrodiuril

Generic Availability (U.S.) Yes

Pharmacologic Category Diuretic, Thiazide

Use Management of mild-to-moderate hypertension; treatment of edema in heart failure and nephrotic syndrome

Unlabeled/Investigational Use Treatment of lithium-induced diabetes insipidus

Contraindications Hypersensitivity to hydrochlorothiazide or any component of the formulation, thiazides, or sulfonamide-derived drugs; anuria; renal decompensation

Warnings/Precautions Avoid in severe renal disease (ineffective as a diuretic). Electrolyte disturbances (hypokalemia, hypochloremic alkalosis, hyponatremia) can occur. Use with caution in severe hepatic dysfunction; hepatic encephalopathy can be caused by electrolyte disturbances. Gout may be precipitated in certain patients with a history of gout, a familial predisposition to gout, or chronic renal failure. Thiazide diuretics reduce calcium excretion; pathologic changes in the parathyroid glands with hypercalcemia and hypophosphatemia have been observed with prolonged use. Use with caution in patients with prediabetes and diabetes; may alter glucose control. May cause SLE exacerbation or activation. Use with caution in patients with moderate or high cholesterol concentrations. Photosensitization may occur. Correct hypokalemia before initiating therapy. Thiazide diuretics may decrease renal calcium excretion; consider avoiding use in patients with hypercalcemia. May cause acute transient myopia and acute angle-closure glaucoma, typically occurring within hours to weeks following initiation; discontinue therapy immediately in patients with acute decreases in visual acuity or ocular pain. Risk factors may include a history of sulfonamide or penicillin allergy.

Chemical similarities are present among sulfonamides, sulfonylureas, carbonic anhydrase inhibitors, thiazides, and loop diuretics (except ethacrynic acid). Use in patients with sulfonamide allergy is specifically contraindicated in product labeling, however, a risk of cross-reaction exists in patients with allergy to any of these compounds; avoid use when previous reaction has been severe. Discontinue if signs of hypersensitivity are noted.

Adverse Reactions (Reflective of adult population; not specific for elderly) Frequency not defined; adverse events reported were observed at doses ≥25 mg:

Cardiovascular: Hypotension, orthostatic hypotension

Central nervous system: Dizziness, fever, headache, vertigo

Dermatologic: Alopecia, erythema multiforme, exfoliative dermatitis, photosensitivity, purpura, rash, Stevens-Johnson syndrome, toxic epidermal necrolysis, urticaria

Endocrine & metabolic: Hyperglycemia, hypokalemia, hyperuricemia

Gastrointestinal: Anorexia, constipation, cramping, diarrhea, epigastric distress, gastric irritation, nausea, pancreatitis, sialadenitis, vomiting

Genitourinary: Glycosuria, impotence

Hematologic: Agranulocytosis, aplastic anemia, hemolytic anemia, leukopenia, thrombocytopenia

Hepatic: Jaundice

Neuromuscular & skeletal: Muscle spasm, paresthesia, restlessness, weakness

Ocular: Blurred vision (transient), xanthopsia

Renal: Interstitial nephritis, renal dysfunction, renal failure

Respiratory: Respiratory distress, pneumonitis, pulmonary edema

Miscellaneous: Anaphylactic reactions, necrotizing angiitis

Drug Interactions

Avoid Concomitant Use

Avoid concomitant use of Hydrochlorothiazide with any of the following: Dofetilide

Increased Effect/Toxicity

Hydrochlorothiazide may increase the levels/effects of: ACE Inhibitors; Allopurinol; Amifostine; Antihypertensives; Calcium Salts; CarBAMazepine; Dofetilide; Hypotensive Agents; Lithium; OXcarbazepine; Porfimer; RiTUXimab; Sodium Phosphates; Topiramate; Toremifene; Vitamin D Analogs

The levels/effects of Hydrochlorothiazide may be increased by: Alcohol (Ethyl); Alfuzosin; Analgesics (Opioid); Barbiturates; Corticosteroids (Orally Inhaled); Corticosteroids (Systemic); Herbs (Hypotensive Properties); Licorice; MAO Inhibitors; Pentoxifylline; Phosphodiesterase 5 Inhibitors; Prostacyclin Analogues

Decreased Effect

Hydrochlorothiazide may decrease the levels/effects of: Antidiabetic Agents

The levels/effects of Hydrochlorothiazide may be decreased by: Bile Acid Sequestrants; Herbs (Hypertensive Properties); Methylphenidate; Nonsteroidal Anti-Inflammatory Agents; Yohimbine

Ethanol/Nutrition/Herb Interactions

Food: Hydrochlorothiazide peak serum levels may be decreased if taken with food. This product may deplete potassium, sodium, and magnesium.

Herb/Nutraceutical: Avoid herbs with *hypertensive* properties (bayberry, blue cohosh, cayenne, ephedra, ginger, ginseng [American], kola, licorice); may diminish the antihypertensive effect of hydrochlorothiazide. Avoid herbs with *hypotensive* properties (black cohosh, California poppy, coleus, golden seal, hawthorn, mistletoe, periwinkle, quinine, shepherd's purse); may enhance the hypotensive effect of hydrochlorothiazide.

Mechanism of Action Inhibits sodium reabsorption in the distal tubules causing increased excretion of sodium and water as well as potassium and hydrogen ions

Pharmacodynamics/Kinetics

Onset of action: Diuresis: ~2 hours

Peak effect: 4-6 hours

Duration: 6-12 hours

Absorption: ~50% to 80%

Distribution: 3.6-7.8 L/kg

Protein binding: 68%

Metabolism: Not metabolized

Bioavailability: 50% to 80%

Half-life elimination: 5.6-14.8 hours

Time to peak: 1-2.5 hours

Excretion: Urine (as unchanged drug)

Dosage

Geriatric Oral: 12.5-25 mg once daily; minimal increase in response and more electrolyte disturbances are seen with doses >50 mg/day.

Adult

Edema (diuresis): Oral: 25-100 mg/day in 1-2 doses; maximum: 200 mg/day

Hypertension: Oral: 12.5-50 mg/day; minimal increase in response and more electrolyte disturbances are seen with doses >50 mg/day

◀ **Renal Impairment** Cl_{cr} <10 mL/minute: Avoid use. Usually ineffective with GFR <30 mL/minute. Effective at lower GFR in combination with a loop diuretic.

Note: ACC/AHA 2009 Heart Failure guidelines suggest that thiazides lose their efficacy when Cl_{cr} <40 mL/minute.

Administration May be administered with food or milk. Take early in day to avoid nocturia. Take the last dose of multiple doses no later than 6 PM unless instructed otherwise.

Monitoring Parameters Assess weight, I & O reports daily to determine fluid loss; blood pressure, serum electrolytes, BUN, creatinine

Test Interactions May interfere with parathyroid function tests. Tyramine and phentolamine tests, histamine tests for pheochromocytoma.

Pharmacotherapy Pearls If given the morning of surgery, hydrochlorothiazide may render the patient volume depleted and blood pressure may be labile during general anesthesia. Effect of drug may be decreased when used every day.

Special Geriatric Considerations Hydrochlorothiazide is not effective in patients with a Cl_{cr} <30 mL/minute, therefore, it may not be a useful agent in many elderly patients.

Dosage Forms Excipient information presented when available (limited, particularly for generics); consult specific product labeling.
Capsule, oral: 12.5 mg
  Microzide®: 12.5 mg
Tablet, oral: 12.5 mg, 25 mg, 50 mg

Selected References
Chobanian AV, Bakris GL, Black HR, et al, "Seventh Report of the Joint National Committee on Prevention, Detection, Evaluation, and Treatment of High Blood Pressure," *Hypertension*, 2003, 42(6):1206-52.

◆ **Hydrochlorothiazide, Aliskiren, and Amlodipine** *see* Aliskiren, Amlodipine, and Hydrochlorothiazide *on page 60*
◆ **Hydrochlorothiazide, Amlodipine, and Aliskiren** *see* Aliskiren, Amlodipine, and Hydrochlorothiazide *on page 60*
◆ **Hydrochlorothiazide, Amlodipine, and Valsartan** *see* Amlodipine, Valsartan, and Hydrochlorothiazide *on page 110*
◆ **Hydrochlorothiazide and Amiloride** *see* Amiloride and Hydrochlorothiazide *on page 93*
◆ **Hydrochlorothiazide and Benazepril** *see* Benazepril and Hydrochlorothiazide *on page 191*
◆ **Hydrochlorothiazide and Candesartan** *see* Candesartan and Hydrochlorothiazide *on page 259*
◆ **Hydrochlorothiazide and Captopril** *see* Captopril and Hydrochlorothiazide *on page 267*
◆ **Hydrochlorothiazide and Enalapril** *see* Enalapril and Hydrochlorothiazide *on page 597*
◆ **Hydrochlorothiazide and Eprosartan** *see* Eprosartan and Hydrochlorothiazide *on page 618*
◆ **Hydrochlorothiazide and Irbesartan** *see* Irbesartan and Hydrochlorothiazide *on page 977*
◆ **Hydrochlorothiazide and Lisinopril** *see* Lisinopril and Hydrochlorothiazide *on page 1082*
◆ **Hydrochlorothiazide and Losartan** *see* Losartan and Hydrochlorothiazide *on page 1095*
◆ **Hydrochlorothiazide and Metoprolol** *see* Metoprolol and Hydrochlorothiazide *on page 1199*
◆ **Hydrochlorothiazide and Metoprolol Tartrate** *see* Metoprolol and Hydrochlorothiazide *on page 1199*
◆ **Hydrochlorothiazide and Olmesartan Medoxomil** *see* Olmesartan and Hydrochlorothiazide *on page 1336*
◆ **Hydrochlorothiazide and Propranolol** *see* Propranolol and Hydrochlorothiazide *on page 1540*
◆ **Hydrochlorothiazide and Quinapril** *see* Quinapril and Hydrochlorothiazide *on page 1564*
◆ **Hydrochlorothiazide and Ramipril** *see* Ramipril and Hydrochlorothiazide *on page 1584*

Hydrochlorothiazide and Spironolactone
(hye droe klor oh THYE a zide & speer on oh LAK tone)

Related Information
Hydrochlorothiazide *on page 876*
Spironolactone *on page 1707*
Medication Safety Issues
Sound-alike/look-alike issues:
Aldactazide® may be confused with Aldactone®
Brand Names: U.S. Aldactazide®
Brand Names: Canada Aldactazide 25®; Aldactazide 50®; Novo-Spirozine
Index Terms Spironolactone and Hydrochlorothiazide
Generic Availability (U.S.) Yes
Pharmacologic Category Diuretic, Thiazide; Selective Aldosterone Blocker

Use Management of mild-to-moderate hypertension; treatment of edema in congestive heart failure and nephrotic syndrome, and cirrhosis of the liver accompanied by edema and/or ascites

Dosage

Geriatric Oral: Consider initiating therapy with the lowest available dose (usual initial doses of hydrochlorothiazide are 12.5-25 mg once daily); increase as necessary.

Adult Hypertension, edema: Oral: Hydrochlorothiazide 12.5-50 mg/day and spironolactone 12.5-50 mg/day; manufacturer labeling states hydrochlorothiazide maximum 200 mg/day, however, usual dose in JNC-7 is 12.5-50 mg/day

Renal Impairment Efficacy of hydrochlorothiazide is limited in patients with Cl_{cr} <30 mL/minute; contraindicated in patients with anuria

Special Geriatric Considerations The efficacy of hydrochlorothiazide is limited in patients with a Cl_{cr} <30 mL/minute; monitor serum potassium.

Dosage Forms Excipient information presented when available (limited, particularly for generics); consult specific product labeling.

Tablet: Hydrochlorothiazide 25 mg and spironolactone 25 mg

Aldactazide®:

25/25: Hydrochlorothiazide 25 mg and spironolactone 25 mg

50/50: Hydrochlorothiazide 50 mg and spironolactone 50 mg

◆ **Hydrochlorothiazide and Telmisartan** see Telmisartan and Hydrochlorothiazide on page 1750

Hydrochlorothiazide and Triamterene

(hye droe klor oh THYE a zide & trye AM ter een)

Related Information

Hydrochlorothiazide on page 876
Triamterene on page 1858

Medication Safety Issues

Sound-alike/look-alike issues:

Dyazide® may be confused with diazoxide, Dynacin®

Maxzide® may be confused with Maxidex®, Microzide®

Brand Names: U.S. Dyazide®; Maxzide®; Maxzide®-25

Brand Names: Canada Apo-Triazide®; Nu-Triazide; Pro-Triazide; Riva-Zide; Teva-Triamterene HCTZ

Index Terms Triamterene and Hydrochlorothiazide

Generic Availability (U.S.) Yes

Pharmacologic Category Diuretic, Potassium-Sparing; Diuretic, Thiazide

Use Treatment of hypertension or edema (not recommended for initial treatment) when hypokalemia has developed on hydrochlorothiazide alone or when the development of hypokalemia must be avoided

Dosage

Geriatric & Adult Hypertension, edema: Oral:

Hydrochlorothiazide 25 mg and triamterene 37.5 mg: 1-2 tablets/capsules once daily

Hydrochlorothiazide 50 mg and triamterene 75 mg: 1/2-1 tablet daily

Special Geriatric Considerations The efficacy of hydrochlorothiazide is limited in patients with a Cl_{cr} <30 mL/minute; monitor serum potassium.

Dosage Forms Excipient information presented when available (limited, particularly for generics); consult specific product labeling.

Capsule, oral: Hydrochlorothiazide 25 mg and triamterene 37.5 mg; hydrochlorothiazide 25 mg and triamterene 50 mg

Dyazide®: Hydrochlorothiazide 25 mg and triamterene 37.5 mg

Tablet: Hydrochlorothiazide 25 mg and triamterene 37.5 mg; hydrochlorothiazide 50 mg and triamterene 75 mg

Maxzide®: Hydrochlorothiazide 50 mg and triamterene 75 mg [scored]

Maxzide®-25: Hydrochlorothiazide 25 mg and triamterene 37.5 mg [scored]

◆ **Hydrochlorothiazide and Valsartan** see Valsartan and Hydrochlorothiazide on page 1894
◆ **Hydrochlorothiazide, Olmesartan, and Amlodipine** see Olmesartan, Amlodipine, and Hydrochlorothiazide on page 1335
◆ **Hydrocil® Instant [OTC]** see Psyllium on page 1547

Hydrocodone and Acetaminophen (hye droe KOE done & a seet a MIN oh fen)

Related Information
Acetaminophen *on page 33*
Opioid Analgesics *on page 2013*
Medication Safety Issues
  Sound-alike/look-alike issues:
    Lorcet® may be confused with Fioricet®
    Lortab® may be confused with Cortef®, Lorabid®
    Vicodin® may be confused with Hycodan®, Hycomine®, Indocin®, Uridon®
    Zydone® may be confused with Vytone®
  High alert medication:
    The Institute for Safe Medication Practices (ISMP) includes this medication among its list of drug classes which have a heightened risk of causing significant patient harm when used in error.
  Other safety concerns:
    Duplicate therapy issues: This product contains acetaminophen, which may be a component of other combination products. Do not exceed the maximum recommended daily dose of acetaminophen.
Brand Names: U.S. hycet®; Lorcet® 10/650; Lorcet® Plus; Lortab®; Margesic® H; Maxidone®; Norco®; Stagesic™; Vicodin®; Vicodin® ES; Vicodin® HP; Xodol® 10/300; Xodol® 5/300; Xodol® 7.5/300; Zamicet™; Zolvit™; Zydone®
Index Terms Acetaminophen and Hydrocodone
Generic Availability (U.S.) Yes: Oral solution, tablet
Pharmacologic Category Analgesic Combination (Opioid)
Use Relief of moderate-to-severe pain
Contraindications Hypersensitivity to hydrocodone, acetaminophen, or any component of the formulation; CNS depression; severe respiratory depression
Warnings/Precautions Use with caution in patients with hypersensitivity reactions to other phenanthrene derivative opioid agonists (morphine, hydromorphone, levorphanol, oxycodone, oxymorphone); tolerance or drug dependence may result from extended use. Concurrent use of agonist/antagonist analgesics may precipitate withdrawal symptoms and/or reduced analgesic efficacy in patients following prolonged therapy with mu opioid agonists. Abrupt discontinuation following prolonged use may also lead to withdrawal symptoms.

Respiratory depressant effects may be increased with head injuries. Use caution with acute abdominal conditions; clinical course may be obscured. Use caution with adrenal insufficiency, biliary tract impairment, morbidly obese patients, toxic psychosis, thyroid dysfunction, prostatic hyperplasia, respiratory disease, hepatic or renal disease, and in the debilitated or elderly. Causes sedation; caution must be used in performing tasks which require alertness (eg, operating machinery or driving). Effects may be potentiated when used with other sedative drugs or ethanol. May cause hypotension.

[U.S. Boxed Warning]: Acetaminophen may cause severe hepatotoxicity, potentially requiring liver transplant or resulting in death; hepatotoxicity is usually associated with excessive acetaminophen intake (>4 g/day). Risk is increased with alcohol use, pre-existing liver disease, and intake of more than one source of acetaminophen-containing medications. Chronic daily dosing in adults has also resulted in liver damage in some patients. Hypersensitivity and anaphylactic reactions have been reported with acetaminophen use; discontinue immediately if symptoms of allergic or hypersensitivity reactions occur. Use caution in patients with known G6PD deficiency.
Adverse Reactions (Reflective of adult population; not specific for elderly) Frequency not defined.
Cardiovascular: Bradycardia, cardiac arrest, circulatory collapse, coma, hypotension
Central nervous system: Anxiety, dizziness, drowsiness, dysphoria, euphoria, fear, lethargy, lightheadedness, malaise, mental clouding, mental impairment, mood changes, physiological dependence, sedation, somnolence, stupor
Dermatologic: Pruritus, rash
Endocrine & metabolic: Hypoglycemic coma
Gastrointestinal: Abdominal pain, constipation, gastric distress, heartburn, nausea, peptic ulcer, vomiting, xerostomia
Genitourinary: Ureteral spasm, urinary retention, vesical sphincter spasm
Hematologic: Agranulocytosis, bleeding time prolonged, hemolytic anemia, iron deficiency anemia, occult blood loss, thrombocytopenia
Hepatic: Hepatic necrosis, hepatitis

Neuromuscular & skeletal: Skeletal muscle rigidity

Otic: Hearing impairment or loss (chronic overdose)

Renal: Renal toxicity, renal tubular necrosis

Respiratory: Acute airway obstruction, apnea, dyspnea, respiratory depression (dose related)

Miscellaneous: Allergic reactions, clamminess, diaphoresis

Drug Interactions

Metabolism/Transport Effects

Hydrocodone: **Substrate** (minor) of CYP2D6, 3A

Acetaminophen: **Substrate** (minor) of CYP1A2, 2A6, 2C9, 2D6, 2E1, 3A4; **Inhibits** CYP3A4 (weak)

Avoid Concomitant Use There are no known interactions where it is recommended to avoid concomitant use.

Increased Effect/Toxicity

Hydrocodone and Acetaminophen may increase the levels/effects of: Alcohol (Ethyl); Alvimopan; CNS Depressants; Dasatinib; Desmopressin; Imatinib; Selective Serotonin Reuptake Inhibitors; SORAfenib; Thiazide Diuretics; Vitamin K Antagonists

The levels/effects of Hydrocodone and Acetaminophen may be increased by: Amphetamines; Antipsychotic Agents (Phenothiazines); Conivaptan; Dasatinib; Droperidol; HydrOXYzine; Imatinib; Isoniazid; MAO Inhibitors; Metyrapone; Probenecid; SORAfenib; Succinylcholine

Decreased Effect

Hydrocodone and Acetaminophen may decrease the levels/effects of: Pegvisomant

The levels/effects of Hydrocodone and Acetaminophen may be decreased by: Ammonium Chloride; Anticonvulsants (Hydantoin); Barbiturates; CarBAMazepine; Cholestyramine Resin; Cyproterone; Mixed Agonist / Antagonist Opioids; Peginterferon Alfa-2b; QuiNIDine; Tocilizumab

Ethanol/Nutrition/Herb Interactions

Ethanol: Consuming ≥3 alcoholic drinks/day may increase the risk of liver damage. Ethanol may also increase CNS depression; monitor for increased effects with coadministration. Caution patients about effects.

Herb/Nutraceutical: Avoid valerian, St John's wort, SAMe, kava kava (may increase risk of excessive sedation).

Mechanism of Action Hydrocodone, as with other narcotic (opiate) analgesics, blocks pain perception in the cerebral cortex by binding to specific receptor molecules (opiate receptors) within the neuronal membranes of synapses. This binding results in a decreased synaptic chemical transmission throughout the CNS thus inhibiting the flow of pain sensations into the higher centers. Mu and kappa are the two subtypes of the opiate receptor which hydrocodone binds to cause analgesia.

Acetaminophen inhibits the synthesis of prostaglandins in the CNS and peripherally blocks pain impulse generation; produces antipyresis from inhibition of hypothalamic heat-regulating center.

Pharmacodynamics/Kinetics

Acetaminophen: See Acetaminophen monograph.

Hydrocodone:

Onset of action: Narcotic analgesic: 10-20 minutes

Duration: 4-8 hours

Metabolism: Hepatic; O-demethylation; N-demethylation and 6-ketosteroid reduction

Half-life elimination: 3.3-4.4 hours

Excretion: Urine

Dosage

Geriatric Doses should be titrated to appropriate analgesic effect; 2.5-5 mg of the hydrocodone component every 4-6 hours. Do not exceed 4 g/day of acetaminophen.

Adult Pain management (analgesic): Oral (doses should be titrated to appropriate analgesic effect): Average starting dose in opioid naive patients: Hydrocodone 5-10 mg 4 times/day; the dosage of acetaminophen should be limited to ≤4 g/day (and possibly less in patients with hepatic impairment or ethanol use).

Dosage ranges (based on specific product labeling): Hydrocodone 2.5-10 mg every 4-6 hours (maximum dose of hydrocodone may be limited by the acetaminophen content of specific product)

Hepatic Impairment Use with caution. Limited, low-dose therapy usually well tolerated in hepatic disease/cirrhosis; however, cases of hepatotoxicity at daily acetaminophen dosages <4 g/day have been reported. Avoid chronic use in hepatic impairment.

◀ **Monitoring Parameters** Pain relief, respiratory and mental status, blood pressure

Special Geriatric Considerations Elderly may be particularly susceptible to the CNS depressant action (sedation, confusion) and constipating effects of narcotics.

Controlled Substance C-III

Dosage Forms Excipient information presented when available (limited, particularly for generics); consult specific product labeling.

Capsule, oral:

Margesic® H, Stagesic™: Hydrocodone bitartrate 5 mg and acetaminophen 500 mg

Elixir, oral:

Lortab®: Hydrocodone bitartrate 7.5 mg and acetaminophen 500 mg per 15 mL (480 mL) [contains ethanol 7%, propylene glycol; tropical fruit punch flavor]

Solution, oral: Hydrocodone bitartrate 7.5 mg and acetaminophen 325 mg per 15 mL; hydrocodone bitartrate 7.5 mg and acetaminophen 500 mg per 15 mL (5 mL, 10 mL, 15 mL, 118 mL, 473 mL); hydrocodone bitartrate 10 mg and acetaminophen 325 mg per 15 mL (7.5 mL, 15 mL)

hycet®: Hydrocodone bitartrate 7.5 mg and acetaminophen 325 mg per 15 mL (473 mL) [contains ethanol 7%, propylene glycol; fruit flavor]

Zamicet™: Hydrocodone bitartrate 10 mg and acetaminophen 325 mg per 15 mL (473 mL) [contains ethanol 6.7%, propylene glycol; fruit flavor]

Zolvit™: Hydrocodone bitartrate 10 mg and acetaminophen 300 mg per 15 mL (480 mL) [contains ethanol 7%, propylene glycol; tropical fruit-punch flavor]

Tablet, oral:

Hydrocodone bitartrate 2.5 mg and acetaminophen 500 mg

Hydrocodone bitartrate 5 mg and acetaminophen 300 mg

Hydrocodone bitartrate 5 mg and acetaminophen 325 mg

Hydrocodone bitartrate 5 mg and acetaminophen 500 mg

Hydrocodone bitartrate 7.5 mg and acetaminophen 300 mg

Hydrocodone bitartrate 7.5 mg and acetaminophen 325 mg

Hydrocodone bitartrate 7.5 mg and acetaminophen 500 mg

Hydrocodone bitartrate 7.5 mg and acetaminophen 650 mg

Hydrocodone bitartrate 7.5 mg and acetaminophen 750 mg

Hydrocodone bitartrate 10 mg and acetaminophen 300 mg

Hydrocodone bitartrate 10 mg and acetaminophen 325 mg

Hydrocodone bitartrate 10 mg and acetaminophen 500 mg

Hydrocodone bitartrate 10 mg and acetaminophen 650 mg

Hydrocodone bitartrate 10 mg and acetaminophen 660 mg

Hydrocodone bitartrate 10 mg and acetaminophen 750 mg

Lorcet® 10/650: Hydrocodone bitartrate 10 mg and acetaminophen 650 mg

Lorcet® Plus: Hydrocodone bitartrate 7.5 mg and acetaminophen 650 mg

Lortab®:

5/500: Hydrocodone bitartrate 5 mg and acetaminophen 500 mg

7.5/500: Hydrocodone bitartrate 7.5 mg and acetaminophen 500 mg

10/500: Hydrocodone bitartrate 10 mg and acetaminophen 500 mg

Maxidone®: Hydrocodone bitartrate 10 mg and acetaminophen 750 mg

Norco®:

Hydrocodone bitartrate 5 mg and acetaminophen 325 mg

Hydrocodone bitartrate 7.5 mg and acetaminophen 325 mg

Hydrocodone bitartrate 10 mg and acetaminophen 325 mg

Vicodin®: Hydrocodone bitartrate 5 mg and acetaminophen 500 mg

Vicodin® ES: Hydrocodone bitartrate 7.5 mg and acetaminophen 750 mg

Vicodin® HP: Hydrocodone bitartrate 10 mg and acetaminophen 660 mg

Xodol®:

5/300: Hydrocodone bitartrate 5 mg and acetaminophen 300 mg

7.5/300: Hydrocodone bitartrate 7.5 mg and acetaminophen 300 mg

10/300: Hydrocodone bitartrate 10 mg and acetaminophen 300 mg

Zydone®:

Hydrocodone bitartrate 5 mg and acetaminophen 400 mg

Hydrocodone bitartrate 7.5 mg and acetaminophen 400 mg

Hydrocodone bitartrate 10 mg and acetaminophen 400 mg

Selected References

American Geriatrics Society Panel on Pharmacological Management of Persistent Pain in Older Persons, "Pharmacological Management of Persistent Pain in Older Persons," *J Am Geriatr Soc*, 2009, 57(8):1331-46.

Hydrocortisone (Systemic) (hye droe KOR ti sone)

Related Information

Corticosteroids *on page 2005*

Medication Safety Issues

Sound-alike/look-alike issues:

Hydrocortisone may be confused with hydrocodone, hydroxychloroquine, hydrochlorothiazide

Cortef® may be confused with Coreg®, Lortab®

HCT (occasional abbreviation for hydrocortisone) is an error-prone abbreviation (mistaken as hydrochlorothiazide)

Solu-CORTEF® may be confused with Solu-MEDROL®

Brand Names: U.S. A-Hydrocort®; Cortef®; Solu-CORTEF®

Brand Names: Canada Cortef®; Solu-Cortef®

Index Terms A-hydroCort; Compound F; Cortisol; Hydrocortisone Sodium Succinate

Generic Availability (U.S.) Yes: Tablet

Pharmacologic Category Corticosteroid, Systemic

Use Management of adrenocortical insufficiency; anti-inflammatory or immunosuppressive

Unlabeled/Investigational Use Management of septic shock when blood pressure is poorly responsive to fluid resuscitation and vasopressor therapy

Contraindications Hypersensitivity to hydrocortisone or any component of the formulation; serious infections, except septic shock or tuberculous meningitis; viral, fungal, or tubercular skin lesions; I.M. administration contraindicated in idiopathic thrombocytopenia purpura; intrathecal administration of injection

Warnings/Precautions Use with caution in patients with thyroid disease, hepatic impairment, renal impairment, heart failure, hypertension, diabetes, glaucoma, cataracts, myasthenia gravis, patients at risk for osteoporosis, patients at risk for seizures, or GI diseases (diverticulitis, peptic ulcer, ulcerative colitis) due to perforation risk. Use caution following acute MI (corticosteroids have been associated with myocardial rupture). Because of the risk of adverse effects, systemic corticosteroids should be used cautiously in the elderly in the smallest possible effective dose for the shortest duration. Withdraw therapy with gradual tapering of dose.

May cause hypercorticism or suppression of hypothalamic-pituitary-adrenal (HPA) axis, particularly in patients receiving high doses for prolonged periods. HPA axis suppression may lead to adrenal crisis. Withdrawal and discontinuation of a corticosteroid should be done slowly and carefully. Particular care is required when patients are transferred from systemic corticosteroids to inhaled products due to possible adrenal insufficiency or withdrawal from steroids, including an increase in allergic symptoms. Patients receiving >20 mg per day of prednisone (or equivalent) may be most susceptible. Fatalities have occurred due to adrenal insufficiency in asthmatic patients during and after transfer from systemic corticosteroids to aerosol steroids; aerosol steroids do not provide the systemic steroid needed to treat patients having trauma, surgery, or infections.

Acute myopathy has been reported with high dose corticosteroids, usually in patients with neuromuscular transmission disorders; may involve ocular and/or respiratory muscles; monitor creatine kinase; recovery may be delayed. Corticosteroid use may cause psychiatric disturbances, including depression, euphoria, insomnia, mood swings, and personality changes. Pre-existing psychiatric conditions may be exacerbated by corticosteroid use. Prolonged use of corticosteroids may also increase the incidence of secondary infection, mask acute infection (including fungal infections), prolong or exacerbate viral infections, or limit response to vaccines. Exposure to chickenpox should be avoided; corticosteroids should not be used to treat ocular herpes simplex. Corticosteroids should not be used for cerebral malaria or viral hepatitis. Close observation is required in patients with latent tuberculosis and/or TB reactivity; restrict use in active TB (only in conjunction with antituberculosis treatment). Prolonged treatment with corticosteroids has been associated with the development of Kaposi's sarcoma (case reports); if noted, discontinuation of therapy should be considered. High-dose corticosteroids should not be used to manage acute head injury.

◄ **Adverse Reactions (Reflective of adult population; not specific for elderly)** Frequency not defined.

Cardiovascular: Arrhythmias, bradycardia, cardiac arrest, cardiomegaly, circulatory collapse, congestive heart failure, edema, fat embolism, hypertension, hypertrophic cardiomyopathy (premature infants), myocardial rupture (post MI), syncope, tachycardia, thromboembolism, vasculitis

Central nervous system: Delirium, depression, emotional instability, euphoria, hallucinations, headache, insomnia, intracranial pressure increased, malaise, mood swings, nervousness, neuritis, neuropathy, personality changes, pseudotumor cerebri, psychic disorders, psychoses, seizure, vertigo

Dermatologic: Acne, allergic dermatitis, alopecia, bruising, burning/tingling, dry scaly skin, edema, erythema, hirsutism, hyper-/hypopigmentation, impaired wound healing, petechiae, rash, skin atrophy, skin test reaction impaired, sterile abscess, striae, urticaria

Endocrine & metabolic: Adrenal suppression, alkalosis, amenorrhea, carbohydrate intolerance increased, Cushing's syndrome, diabetes mellitus, glucose intolerance, growth suppression, hyperglycemia, hyperlipidemia, hypokalemia, hypokalemic alkalosis, menstrual irregularities, negative nitrogen balance, pituitary-adrenal axis suppression, potassium loss, protein catabolism, sodium and water retention, sperm motility increased/decreased, spermatogenesis increased/decreased

Gastrointestinal: Abdominal distention, appetite increased, bowel dysfunction (intrathecal administration), indigestion, nausea, pancreatitis, peptic ulcer, gastrointestinal perforation, ulcerative esophagitis, vomiting, weight gain

Genitourinary: Bladder dysfunction (intrathecal administration)

Hematologic: Leukocytosis (transient)

Hepatic: Hepatomegaly, transaminases increased

Local: Atrophy (at injection site), postinjection flare (intra-articular use), thrombophlebitis

Neuromuscular & skeletal: Arthralgia, necrosis (femoral and humoral heads), Charcot-like arthropathy, fractures, muscle mass loss, muscle weakness, myopathy, osteoporosis, tendon rupture, vertebral compression fractures

Ocular: Cataracts, exophthalmoses, glaucoma, intraocular pressure increased

Miscellaneous: Abnormal fat deposits, anaphylaxis, avascular necrosis, diaphoresis, hiccups, hypersensitivity reactions, infection, secondary malignancy

Drug Interactions

Metabolism/Transport Effects Substrate of CYP3A4 (minor), P-glycoprotein; **Induces** CYP3A4 (weak)

Avoid Concomitant Use

Avoid concomitant use of Hydrocortisone (Systemic) with any of the following: Aldesleukin; BCG; Natalizumab; Pimecrolimus; Tacrolimus (Topical)

Increased Effect/Toxicity

Hydrocortisone (Systemic) may increase the levels/effects of: Acetylcholinesterase Inhibitors; Amphotericin B; Deferasirox; Leflunomide; Loop Diuretics; Natalizumab; NSAID (COX-2 Inhibitor); NSAID (Nonselective); Thiazide Diuretics; Vaccines (Live); Warfarin

The levels/effects of Hydrocortisone (Systemic) may be increased by: Antifungal Agents (Azole Derivatives, Systemic); Aprepitant; Calcium Channel Blockers (Nondihydropyridine); Conivaptan; Denosumab; Estrogen Derivatives; Fluconazole; Fosaprepitant; Macrolide Antibiotics; Neuromuscular-Blocking Agents (Nondepolarizing); P-Glycoprotein Inhibitors; Pimecrolimus; Quinolone Antibiotics; Roflumilast; Salicylates; Tacrolimus (Topical); Telaprevir; Trastuzumab

Decreased Effect

Hydrocortisone (Systemic) may decrease the levels/effects of: Aldesleukin; Antidiabetic Agents; BCG; Calcitriol; Corticorelin; Isoniazid; Salicylates; Sipuleucel-T; Telaprevir; Vaccines (Inactivated)

The levels/effects of Hydrocortisone (Systemic) may be decreased by: Aminoglutethimide; Antacids; Barbiturates; Bile Acid Sequestrants; Echinacea; Mitotane; P-Glycoprotein Inducers; Primidone; Rifamycin Derivatives; Tocilizumab

Ethanol/Nutrition/Herb Interactions

Ethanol: Avoid ethanol (may enhance gastric mucosal irritation).

Food: Hydrocortisone interferes with calcium absorption.

Herb/Nutraceutical: St John's wort may decrease hydrocortisone levels. Avoid cat's claw, echinacea (have immunostimulant properties).

Stability Store at controlled room temperature 20°C to 25°C (68°F to 77°F). Protect from light. Hydrocortisone sodium phosphate and hydrocortisone sodium succinate are clear, light yellow solutions which are heat labile.

Sodium succinate: Reconstitute 100 mg vials with bacteriostatic water (not >2 mL). Act-O-Vial (self-contained powder for injection plus diluent) may be reconstituted by pressing the activator to force diluent into the powder compartment. Following gentle agitation, solution may be withdrawn via syringe through a needle inserted into the center of the stopper. May be administered (I.V. or I.M.) without further dilution. After initial reconstitution, hydrocortisone sodium succinate solutions are stable for 3 days at room temperature or under refrigeration when protected from light. Stability of parenteral admixture (Solu-Cortef®) at room temperature (25°C) and at refrigeration temperature (4°C) is concentration-dependent: Stability of concentration 1 mg/mL: 24 hours.
Stability of concentration 2 mg/mL to 60 mg/mL: At least 4 hours.
Solutions for I.V. infusion: Reconstituted solutions may be added to an appropriate volume of compatible solution for infusion. Concentration should generally not exceed 1 mg/mL. However, in cases where administration of a small volume of fluid is desirable, 100-3000 mg may be added to 50 mL of D_5W or NS (stability limited to 4 hours).

Mechanism of Action Decreases inflammation by suppression of migration of polymorphonuclear leukocytes and reversal of increased capillary permeability

Pharmacodynamics/Kinetics
Onset of action: Hydrocortisone sodium succinate (water soluble): Rapid
Absorption: Rapid
Metabolism: Hepatic
Half-life elimination: Biologic: 8-12 hours
Excretion: Urine (primarily as 17-hydroxysteroids and 17-ketosteroids)

Dosage
Geriatric & Adult Dose should be based on severity of disease and patient response.
Adrenal hyperplasia (congenital): Oral: Initial: 10-20 mg/m^2/day in 3 divided doses; a variety of dosing schedules have been used. **Note:** Inconsistencies have occurred with liquid formulations; tablets may provide more reliable levels. Doses must be individualized by monitoring growth, bone age, and hormonal levels. Mineralocorticoid and sodium supplementation may be required based upon electrolyte regulation and plasma renin activity.
Adrenal insufficiency (acute): I.M., I.V.: Succinate: 100 mg I.V. bolus, then 300 mg/day in divided doses every 8 hours or as a continuous infusion for 48 hours. Once patient is stable change to oral, 50 mg every 8 hours for 6 doses, then taper to 30-50 mg/day in divided doses.
Adrenal insufficiency (chronic)/physiologic replacement: Oral: 20-30 mg/day
Anti-inflammatory or immunosuppressive: Oral, I.M., I.V.: Succinate: 15-240 mg every 12 hours
Septic shock (unlabeled use): I.V.: Succinate: 50 mg every 6 hours (Annane, 2002; Marik, 2008); not to exceed 300 mg/day (Dellinger, 2008). Practice guidelines also recommend alternative dosing of 100 mg bolus, followed by continuous infusion of 10 mg/hour (240 mg/day). Taper slowly (for total of 11 days) and do not stop abruptly. **Note:** Fludrocortisone is optional with use of hydrocortisone.
Status asthmaticus: I.V.: Succinate: 1-2 mg/kg/dose every 6 hours for 24 hours, then maintenance of 0.5-1 mg/kg every 6 hours
Stress dosing (surgery) in patients known to be adrenally-suppressed or on chronic systemic steroids: I.V.:
Minor stress (ie, inguinal herniorrhaphy): 25 mg/day for 1 day
Moderate stress (ie, joint replacement, cholecystectomy): 50-75 mg/day (25 mg every 8-12 hours) for 1-2 days
Major stress (pancreatoduodenectomy, esophagogastrectomy, cardiac surgery): 100-150 mg/day (50 mg every 8-12 hours) for 2-3 days

Administration
Oral: Administer with food or milk to decrease GI upset
Parenteral: Hydrocortisone sodium succinate may be administered by I.M. or I.V. routes. Dermal and/or subdermal skin depression may occur at the site of injection. Avoid injection into deltoid muscle (high incidence of subcutaneous atrophy).
I.V. bolus: Dilute to 50 mg/mL and administer over 30 seconds or over 10 minutes for doses ≥500 mg
I.V. intermittent infusion: Dilute to 1 mg/mL and administer over 20-30 minutes

Monitoring Parameters Serum glucose, electrolytes; blood pressure, weight, presence of infection; monitor IOP with therapy >6 weeks; bone mineral density

Reference Range Therapeutic: AM: 5-25 mcg/dL (SI: 138-690 nmol/L), PM: 2-9 mcg/dL (SI: 55-248 nmol/L) depending on test, assay

Test Interactions Interferes with skin tests

HYDROCORTISONE (SYSTEMIC)

◀ **Special Geriatric Considerations** Because of the risk of adverse effects, systemic corticosteroids should be used cautiously in the elderly, in the smallest possible dose, and for the
shortest possible time.

Dosage Forms Excipient information presented when available (limited, particularly for
generics); consult specific product labeling.

Injection, powder for reconstitution, as sodium succinate [strength expressed as base]:
  A-Hydrocort®: 100 mg
  Solu-CORTEF®: 100 mg

Injection, powder for reconstitution, as sodium succinate [strength expressed as base,
preservative free]:
  Solu-CORTEF®: 100 mg, 250 mg, 500 mg, 1000 mg [supplied with diluent]

Tablet, oral, as base: 5 mg, 10 mg, 20 mg
  Cortef®: 5 mg, 10 mg, 20 mg [scored]

Hydrocortisone (Topical) (hye droe KOR ti sone)

Medication Safety Issues
Sound-alike/look-alike issues:
Hydrocortisone may be confused with hydrocodone, hydroxychloroquine, hydrochlorothiazide

Anusol® may be confused with Anusol-HC, Aplisol®, Aquasol®

Anusol-HC® may be confused with Anusol®

Cortizone® may be confused with cortisone

HCT (occasional abbreviation for hydrocortisone) is an error-prone abbreviation (mistaken
as hydrochlorothiazide)

Hytone® may be confused with Vytone®

Proctocort® may be confused with ProctoCream®

ProctoCream® may be confused with Proctocort®

International issues:
Nutracort [U.S. and multiple international markets] may be confused with Nitrocor brand
name of nitroglycerin [Italy, Russia, and Venezuela]

Brand Names: U.S. Ala-Cort; Ala-Scalp; Anu-med HC; Anucort-HC™; Anusol-HC®; Aquanil
HC® [OTC]; Beta-HC® [OTC]; Caldecort® [OTC]; Colocort®; Cortaid® Advanced [OTC];
Cortaid® Intensive Therapy [OTC]; Cortaid® Maximum Strength [OTC]; Cortenema®; Corti-
Cool® [OTC]; Cortifoam®; Cortizone-10® Hydratensive Healing [OTC]; Cortizone-10® Hydra-
tensive Soothing [OTC]; Cortizone-10® Intensive Healing Eczema [OTC]; Cortizone-10®
Maximum Strength Cooling Relief [OTC]; Cortizone-10® Maximum Strength Easy Relief
[OTC]; Cortizone-10® Maximum Strength Intensive Healing Formula [OTC]; Cortizone-10®
Maximum Strength [OTC]; Cortizone-10® Plus Maximum Strength [OTC]; Dermarest®
Eczema Medicated [OTC]; Hemril® -30; Hydrocortisone Plus [OTC]; Hydroskin® [OTC];
Locoid Lipocream®; Locoid®; Pandel®; Pediaderm™ HC; Preparation H® Hydrocortisone
[OTC]; Procto-Pak™; Proctocort®; ProctoCream®-HC; Proctosol-HC®; Proctozone-HC
2.5%™; Recort [OTC]; Scalpana [OTC]; Texacort®; U-Cort®; Westcort®

Brand Names: Canada Aquacort®; Cortamed®; Cortenema®; Cortifoam™; Emo-Cort®;
Hycort™; Hyderm; HydroVal®; Locoid®; Prevex® HC; Sarna® HC; Westcort®

Index Terms A-hydroCort; Compound F; Cortisol; Hemorrhoidal HC; Hydrocortisone Acetate;
Hydrocortisone Butyrate; Hydrocortisone Probutate; Hydrocortisone Valerate

Generic Availability (U.S.) Yes: Excludes aerosol (acetate), cream (probutate), gel (base),
liquid (base), lotion (base), lotion (butyrate), solution (base)

Pharmacologic Category Corticosteroid, Rectal; Corticosteroid, Topical

Use Relief of inflammation of corticosteroid-responsive dermatoses (low and medium potency
topical corticosteroid); adjunctive treatment of ulcerative colitis

Dosage
Geriatric & Adult
Dermatosis: Topical: Apply to affected area 2-4 times/day.
Ulcerative colitis: Rectal: 10-100 mg 1-2 times/day for 2-3 weeks

Dosage Forms Excipient information presented when available (limited, particularly for
generics); consult specific product labeling. [DSC] = Discontinued product

Aerosol, rectal, as acetate [foam]:
  Cortifoam®: 10% (15 g) [90 mg/applicator]

Cream, topical, as acetate: 1% (28.4 g, 454 g); 2% (43 g)
  U-Cort®: 1% (28 g) [contains sodium metabisulfite]

Cream, topical, as acetate [strength expressed as base]: 1% (30 g)

Cream, topical, as base: 0.5% (28.4 g, 30 g); 1% (1 g, 1.5 g, 15 g, 28.35 g [DSC], 28.4 g,
  30 g, 114 g, 120 g [DSC], 454 g); 2.5% (20 g, 28 g, 28.35 g, 30 g, 454 g)
  Ala-Cort: 1% (28.4 g, 85.2 g)
  Anusol-HC®: 2.5% (30 g) [contains benzyl alcohol]

Caldecort®: 1% (28.4 g) [contains aloe]
Cortaid® Advanced: 1% (42 g) [contains aloe]
Cortaid® Intensive Therapy: 1% (37 g, 56 g)
Cortaid® Maximum Strength: 1% (14 g, 28 g, 37 g, 56 g) [contains aloe]
Cortizone-10® Maximum Strength: 1% (15 g, 28 g, 56 g) [contains aloe]
Cortizone-10® Maximum Strength Intensive Healing Formula: 1% (28 g, 56 g) [contains aloe, benzyl alcohol]
Cortizone-10® Plus Maximum Strength: 1% (28 g, 56 g) [contains aloe, vitamin A, vitamin E]
Hydrocortisone Plus: 1% (28.4 g) [contains aloe, vitamin A, vitamin D, vitamin E]
Hydroskin®: 1% (28 g)
Preparation H® Hydrocortisone: 1% (26 g) [contains sodium benzoate]
Procto-Pak™: 1% (28.4 g)
Proctocort®: 1% (28.35 g)
ProctoCream®-HC: 2.5% (30 g) [contains benzyl alcohol]
Proctosol-HC®: 2.5% (28.35 g)
Proctozone-HC 2.5%™: 2.5% (30 g)
Recort: 1% (30 g)
Cream, topical, as butyrate: 0.1% (15 g, 45 g)
 Locoid Lipocream®: 0.1% (15 g, 45 g, 60 g)
 Locoid®: 0.1% (15 g, 45 g)
Cream, topical, as probutate:
 Pandel®: 0.1% (15 g, 45 g, 80 g)
Cream, topical, as valerate: 0.2% (15 g, 45 g, 60 g)
Gel, topical, as base:
 CortiCool®: 1% (0.9 g, 42.5 g) [contains ethanol 20%]
 Cortizone-10® Maximum Strength Cooling Relief: 1% (28 g) [contains aloe, ethanol 15%]
Liquid, topical, as base:
 Cortizone-10® Maximum Strength Easy Relief: 1% (36 mL) [contains aloe, ethanol 45%]
 Scalpana: 1% (85.5 mL)
Lotion, topical, as base: 1% (114 g, 118 mL); 2.5% (59 mL, 60 mL [DSC], 118 mL)
 Ala-Scalp: 2% (29.6 mL)
 Aquanil HC®: 1% (120 mL) [contains benzyl alcohol]
 Beta-HC®: 1% (60 mL)
 Cortaid® Intensive Therapy: 1% (98 g)
 Cortizone-10® Hydratensive Healing: 1% (113 g) [contains aloe]
 Cortizone-10® Hydratensive Soothing: 1% (113 g) [contains aloe]
 Cortizone-10® Intensive Healing Eczema: 1% (99 g) [contains aloe, vitamin A, vitamin C, vitamin E]
 Dermarest® Eczema Medicated: 1% (118 mL)
 Hydroskin®: 1% (118 mL)
Lotion, topical, as base [kit]:
 Pediaderm™ HC: 2% (29.6 mL) [contains benzalkonium chloride, isopropyl alcohol; packaged with protective emollient]
Lotion, topical, as butyrate:
 Locoid®: 0.1% (60 mL)
Ointment, topical, as acetate [strength expressed as base]: 1% (30 g)
Ointment, topical, as base: 0.5% (30 g); 1% (25 g, 30 g, 110 g, 430 g, 454 g); 2.5% (20 g, 28.35 g [DSC], 30 g, 454 g)
 Cortaid® Maximum Strength: 1% (28 g, 37 g)
 Cortizone-10® Maximum Strength: 1% (28 g, 56 g)
Ointment, topical, as butyrate: 0.1% (15 g, 45 g)
 Locoid®: 0.1% (15 g, 45 g)
Ointment, topical, as valerate: 0.2% (15 g, 45 g, 60 g)
 Westcort®: 0.2% (15 g, 45 g, 60 g)
Powder, for prescription compounding, as acetate [micronized]: USP: 100% (10 g, 25 g, 100 g)
Solution, topical, as base:
 Texacort®: 2.5% (30 mL) [contains ethanol 48.8%]
Solution, topical, as base [spray]:
 Cortaid® Intensive Therapy: 1% (59 mL) [contains ethanol 45%]
Solution, topical, as butyrate: 0.1% (20 mL, 60 mL)
 Locoid®: 0.1% (20 mL, 60 mL) [contains isopropyl alcohol 50%]
Suppository, rectal, as acetate: 25 mg (12s); 30 mg (12s)
 Anu-med HC: 25 mg (12s)
 Anucort-HC™: 25 mg (12s, 24s, 100s)
 Anusol-HC®: 25 mg (12s, 24s)
 Hemril® -30: 30 mg (12s, 24s)
 Proctocort®: 30 mg (12s, 24s)

◄ Suspension, rectal, as base: 100 mg/60 mL (60 mL)
 Colocort®: 100 mg/60 mL (60 mL)
 Cortenema®: 100 mg/60 mL (60 mL)

♦ **Hydrocortisone Acetate** *see* Hydrocortisone (Topical) *on page 886*
♦ **Hydrocortisone and Ciprofloxacin** *see* Ciprofloxacin and Hydrocortisone *on page 365*
♦ **Hydrocortisone Butyrate** *see* Hydrocortisone (Topical) *on page 886*
♦ **Hydrocortisone, Neomycin, Colistin, and Thonzonium** *see* Neomycin, Colistin, Hydrocortisone, and Thonzonium *on page 1280*
♦ **Hydrocortisone Plus [OTC]** *see* Hydrocortisone (Topical) *on page 886*
♦ **Hydrocortisone Probutate** *see* Hydrocortisone (Topical) *on page 886*
♦ **Hydrocortisone Sodium Succinate** *see* Hydrocortisone (Systemic) *on page 883*
♦ **Hydrocortisone Valerate** *see* Hydrocortisone (Topical) *on page 886*
♦ **Hydrodiuril** *see* Hydrochlorothiazide *on page 876*

HYDROmorphone (hye droe MOR fone)

Related Information
Opioid Analgesics *on page 2013*
Patient Information for Disposal of Unused Medications *on page 2125*

Medication Safety Issues
Sound-alike/look-alike issues:
Dilaudid® may be confused with Demerol®, Dilantin®
HYDROmorphone may be confused with morphine; significant overdoses have occurred when hydromorphone products have been inadvertently administered instead of morphine sulfate. Commercially available prefilled syringes of both products looks similar and are often stored in close proximity to each other. **Note:** Hydromorphone 1 mg oral is approximately equal to morphine 4 mg oral; hydromorphone 1 mg I.V. is approximately equal to morphine 5 mg I.V.

High alert medication:
The Institute for Safe Medication Practices (ISMP) includes this medication among its list of drug classes which have a heightened risk of causing significant patient harm when used in error.

Administration issues:
Dilaudid®, Dilaudid-HP®: Extreme caution should be taken to avoid confusing the highly-concentrated (Dilaudid-HP®) injection with the less-concentrated (Dilaudid®) injectable product.
Exalgo™: Extreme caution should be taken to avoid confusing the extended release Exalgo™ 8 mg tablets with immediate release hydromorphone 8 mg tablets
Significant differences exist between oral and I.V. dosing. Use caution when converting from one route of administration to another.

Brand Names: U.S. Dilaudid-HP®; Dilaudid®; Exalgo™

Brand Names: Canada Dilaudid-HP-Plus®; Dilaudid-HP®; Dilaudid-XP®; Dilaudid®; Dilaudid® Sterile Powder; Hydromorph Contin®; Hydromorph-IR®; Hydromorphone HP; Hydromorphone HP® 10; Hydromorphone HP® 20; Hydromorphone HP® 50; Hydromorphone HP® Forte; Hydromorphone Hydrochloride Injection, USP; Jurnista™; PMS-Hydromorphone

Index Terms Dihydromorphinone; Hydromorphone Hydrochloride

Generic Availability (U.S.) Yes: Excludes extended release tablet, liquid, powder for injection

Pharmacologic Category Analgesic, Opioid

Use Management of moderate-to-severe pain
Exalgo™: Management of moderate-to-severe pain in opioid-tolerant patients (requiring around-the-clock analgesia for an extended period of time)

Prescribing and Access Restrictions Exalgo™: As a requirement of the REMS program, healthcare providers who prescribe Exalgo™ need to receive training on the proper use and potential risks of Exalgo™. For training, please refer to http://www.exalgorems.com. Prescribers will need retraining every 2 years or following any significant changes to the Exalgo™ REMS program.

Medication Guide Available Yes

Contraindications Hypersensitivity to hydromorphone, any component of the formulation; acute or severe asthma, severe respiratory depression (in absence of resuscitative equipment or ventilatory support); severe CNS depression; obstetrical analgesia

Warnings/Precautions Use with caution in patients with hypersensitivity reactions to other phenanthrene derivative opioid agonists (codeine, hydrocodone, levorphanol, oxycodone, oxymorphone). Hydromorphone shares toxic potential of opiate agonists, including CNS depression and respiratory depression. Precautions associated with opiate agonist therapy should be observed. May cause CNS depression, which may impair physical or mental abilities; patients must be cautioned about performing tasks which require mental alertness (eg, operating machinery or driving). Myoclonus and seizures have been reported with high doses. Critical respiratory depression may occur, even at therapeutic dosages, particularly in elderly or debilitated patients or in patients with pre-existing respiratory compromise (hypoxia and/or hypercapnia). Use caution in COPD or other obstructive pulmonary disease. Use with caution in patients with hypersensitivity to other phenanthrene opiates, kyphoscoliosis, cardiovascular disease, morbid obesity, adrenocortical insufficiency, hypothyroidism, acute alcoholism, delirium tremens, toxic psychoses, prostatic hyperplasia and/or urinary stricture, or severe liver or renal failure. Use with caution in patients with biliary tract dysfunction. Hydromorphone may increase biliary tract pressure following spasm in sphincter of Oddi. Use caution in patients with inflammatory or obstructive bowel disorder, acute pancreatitis secondary to biliary tract disease, and patients undergoing biliary surgery. Use extreme caution in patients with head injury, intracranial lesions, or elevated intracranial pressure; exaggerated elevation of ICP may occur (in addition, hydromorphone may complicate neurologic evaluation due to pupillary dilation and CNS depressant effects). Use with caution in patients with depleted blood volume or drugs which may exaggerate hypotensive effects (including phenothiazines or general anesthetics). May obscure diagnosis or clinical course of patients with acute abdominal conditions.

[U.S. Boxed Warning]: Hydromorphone has a high potential for abuse. Those at risk for opioid abuse include patients with a history of substance abuse or mental illness. Tolerance or drug dependence may result from extended use; however, concerns for abuse should not prevent effective management of pain. In general, abrupt discontinuation of therapy in dependent patients should be avoided.

An opioid-containing analgesic regimen should be tailored to each patient's needs and based upon the type of pain being treated (acute versus chronic), the route of administration, degree of tolerance for opioids (naive versus chronic user), age, weight, and medical condition. The optimal analgesic dose varies widely among patients. Doses should be titrated to pain relief/prevention. I.M. use may result in variable absorption and a lag time to peak effect.

Dosage form specific warnings:

[U.S. Boxed Warning]: Dilaudid-HP®: Extreme caution should be taken to avoid confusing the highly-concentrated (Dilaudid-HP®) injection with the less-concentrated (Dilaudid®) injectable product. Dilaudid-HP® should only be used in patients who are opioid-tolerant.

Controlled release: Capsules should only be used when continuous analgesia is required over an extended period of time. Controlled release products are not to be used on an "as needed" (PRN) basis.

Extended release tablets (Exalgo™): **[U.S. Boxed Warning]: For use in opioid tolerant patients only; fatal respiratory depression may occur in patient who are not opioid tolerant. Indicated for the management of moderate-to-severe pain when around the clock pain control is needed for an extended time period. Not for use as an as-needed analgesic or for the management of acute or postoperative pain. Tablets should be swallowed whole; do not crush, break, chew, dissolve or inject; doing so may lead to rapid release and absorption of a potentially fatal dose of hydromorphone. Accidental consumption may lead to fatal overdose, especially in children.** Exalgo™ tablets are nondeformable; do not administer to patients with preexisting severe gastrointestinal narrowing (eg, esophageal motility, small bowel inflammatory disease, short gut syndrome, history of peritonitis, cystic fibrosis, chronic intestinal pseudo-obstruction, Meckel's diverticulum); obstruction may occur. Exalgo™ is not recommended for use within 14 days of MAO inhibitors; severe and unpredictable potentiation by MAO inhibitors has been reported with opioid analgesics

Some dosage forms contain trace amounts of sodium metabisulfite which may cause allergic reactions in susceptible individuals.

Adverse Reactions (Reflective of adult population; not specific for elderly) Frequency not defined.

Cardiovascular: Bradycardia, extrasystoles, flushing of face, hyper-/hypotension, palpitation, peripheral edema, peripheral vasodilation, syncope, tachycardia

Central nervous system: Abnormal dreams, abnormal feelings, agitation, aggression, apprehension, attention disturbances, chills, coordination impaired, CNS depression, confusion, cognitive disorder, crying, dizziness, drowsiness, dysphoria, encephalopathy, euphoria, fatigue, hallucinations, headache, hyper-reflexia, hypo/hyperesthesia, hypothermia, increased intracranial pressure, insomnia, lightheadedness, listlessness, malaise, memory impairment, mental depression, mood alterations, nervousness, panic attacks, paranoia, psychomotor hyperactivity, restlessness, sedation, seizure, somnolence, suicide ideation, vertigo

Dermatologic: Hyperhidrosis, pruritus, rash, urticaria

HYDROMORPHONE

Endocrine & metabolic: Amylase decreased, dehydration, erectile dysfunction, fluid retention, hyperuricemia, hypogonadism, hypokalemia, libido decreased, sexual dysfunction, testosterone decreased

Gastrointestinal: Abdominal distention, anal fissure, anorexia, appetite increased, bezoar (Exalgo™), biliary tract spasm, constipation, diarrhea, diverticulum, diverticulitis, duodenitis, dysgeusia, dysphagia, eructation, flatulence, gastric emptying impaired, gastrointestinal motility disorder (Exalgo™), gastroenteritis, hematochezia, ileus, intestinal obstruction (Exalgo™), large intestine perforation (Exalgo™), nausea, painful defecation, paralytic ileus, stomach cramps, taste perversion, vomiting, weight loss, xerostomia

Genitourinary: Dysuria, micturition disorder, ureteral spasm, urinary frequency, urinary hesitation, urinary retention, urinary tract spasm, urination decreased

Hepatic: LFTs increased

Local: Pain at injection site (I.M.), wheal/flare over vein (I.V.)

Neuromuscular & skeletal: Arthralgia, dysarthria, dyskinesia, muscle rigidity, muscle spasms, myalgia, myoclonus, paresthesia, trembling, tremor, uncoordinated muscle movements, weakness

Ocular: Blurred vision, diplopia, dry eyes, miosis, nystagmus

Otic: Tinnitus

Respiratory: Apnea, bronchospasm, dyspnea, hyperventilation, hypoxia, laryngospasm, oxygen saturation decreased, respiratory depression/distress, rhinorrhea

Miscellaneous: Antidiuretic effects, balance disorder, diaphoresis, difficulty walking, histamine release, physical and psychological dependence

Drug Interactions

Avoid Concomitant Use

Avoid concomitant use of HYDROmorphone with any of the following: MAO Inhibitors

Increased Effect/Toxicity

HYDROmorphone may increase the levels/effects of: Alcohol (Ethyl); Alvimopan; CNS Depressants; Desmopressin; Selective Serotonin Reuptake Inhibitors; Thiazide Diuretics

The levels/effects of HYDROmorphone may be increased by: Amphetamines; Antipsychotic Agents (Phenothiazines); Droperidol; HydrOXYzine; MAO Inhibitors; Succinylcholine

Decreased Effect

HYDROmorphone may decrease the levels/effects of: Pegvisomant

The levels/effects of HYDROmorphone may be decreased by: Ammonium Chloride; Mixed Agonist / Antagonist Opioids

Ethanol/Nutrition/Herb Interactions

Ethanol: May increase CNS depression; monitor for increased effects with coadministration. Caution patients about effects.

Herb/Nutraceutical: Avoid valerian, St John's wort, kava kava, gotu kola (may increase CNS depression).

Stability Store injection and oral dosage forms at 15°C to 30°C (59°F to 86°F). Protect tablets from light. A slightly yellowish discoloration has not been associated with a loss of potency.

Mechanism of Action Binds to opiate receptors in the CNS, causing inhibition of ascending pain pathways, altering the perception of and response to pain; causes cough supression by direct central action in the medulla; produces generalized CNS depression

Pharmacodynamics/Kinetics

Onset of action: Analgesic: Immediate release formulations:
Oral: 15-30 minutes; Peak effect: 30-60 minutes
I.V.: 5 minutes; Peak effect: 10-20 minutes

Duration: Immediate release formulations: Oral, I.V.: 4-5 hours

Absorption: I.M.: Variable and delayed

Distribution: V_d: 4 L/kg

Protein binding: ~8% to 19%

Metabolism: Hepatic via glucuronidation; to inactive metabolites

Bioavailability: 62%

Half-life elimination:
Immediate release formulations: 2-3 hours
Extended release tablets (Exalgo™): ~11 hours

Excretion: Urine (primarily as glucuronide conjugates)

Dosage

Geriatric Doses should be titrated to appropriate analgesic effects. When changing routes of administration, oral doses and parenteral doses are **NOT** equivalent; parenteral doses are up to 5 times more potent. Therefore, when administered parenterally, one-fifth of the oral dose will provide similar analgesia.

Pain: Oral: 1-2 mg every 4-6 hours

Adult

Acute pain (moderate-to-severe): Note: These are guidelines and do not represent the maximum doses that may be required in all patients. Doses should be titrated to provide adequate pain relief. When changing routes of administration, oral doses and parenteral doses are **NOT** equivalent; parenteral doses are up to 5 times more potent. Therefore, when administered parenterally, one-fifth of the oral dose will provide similar analgesia.

Oral: Initial: Opiate-naive: 2-4 mg every 3-4 hours as needed; elderly/debilitated patients may require lower doses; patients with prior opiate exposure may require higher initial doses. **Note:** In adults with severe pain, the American Pain Society recommends an initial dose of 4-8 mg.

I.V.: Initial: Opiate-naive: 0.2-0.6 mg every 2-3 hours as needed; patients with prior opiate exposure may require higher initial doses.

Mechanically ventilated/critically ill patients (unlabeled use): 0.7-4 mg (based on 70 kg patient) every 4 hours as needed. **Note:** More frequent dosing may be needed (eg, every 1-2 hours); dose should be adjusted based on patient response; elderly patients may be more sensitive (Jacobi, 2002).

Continuous infusion: Usual dosage range: 0.5-1 mg/hour (based on 70 kg patient) or 7-15 mcg/kg/**hour**

Patient-controlled analgesia (PCA): **Note:** Opiate-naive: Consider lower end of dosing range:

Usual concentration: 0.2 mg/mL

Demand dose: Usual: 0.1-0.2 mg; range: 0.05-0.4 mg

Lockout interval: 5-10 minutes

Epidural PCA (de Leon-Casasola, 1996; Liu, 2010; Smith, 2009):

Bolus dose: 0.4-1 mg

Infusion rate: 0.03-0.3 mg/**hour**

Demand dose: 0.02-0.05 mg

Lockout interval: 10-15 minutes

I.M., SubQ: **Note:** I.M. use may result in variable absorption and lag time to peak effect.

Initial: Opiate-naive: 0.8-1 mg every 4-6 hours as needed; patients with prior opiate exposure may require higher initial doses

Usual dosage range: 1-2 mg every 4-6 hours as needed

Rectal: 3 mg every 6-8 hours as needed

Chronic pain: Note: Patients taking opioids chronically may become tolerant and require doses higher than the usual dosage range to maintain the desired effect. Tolerance can be managed by appropriate dose titration. There is no optimal or maximal dose for hydromorphone in chronic pain. The appropriate dose is one that relieves pain throughout its dosing interval without causing unmanageable side effects.

Controlled release formulation (Hydromorph Contin®, not available in U.S.): Oral: 3-30 mg every 12 hours. **Note:** A patient's hydromorphone requirement should be established using prompt release formulations; conversion to long acting products may be considered when chronic, continuous treatment is required. Higher dosages should be reserved for use only in opioid-tolerant patients.

Extended release formulation (Exalgo™): Dosing range: 8-64 mg every 24 hours. For use in opioid tolerant patients only; discontinue all other extended release opioids when starting therapy. Suggested recommendations for converting to Exalgo™ from other analgesics are presented, but when selecting the initial dose, other characteristics (eg, patient status, degree of opioid tolerance, concurrent medications, type of pain, risk factors for addiction or diversion, etc) should also be considered.

Individualization of dose: Pain relief and adverse events should be assessed frequently. Dose increases may occur not more often than every 3-4 days; consider titrating with increases of 25% to 50% of the current daily dose. If more than 2 doses of rescue medications are needed within 24 hours for 2 consecutive days, consider increasing the dose of Exalgo™. Do not administer more frequently than every 24 hours.

Discontinuing Exalgo™: Taper by gradually decreasing the dose by 25% to 50% every 2-3 days to a dose of 8 mg every 24 hours before discontinuing therapy.

Conversion from other oral hydromorphone formulations to Exalgo™: Start with the equivalent total daily dose of hydromorphone administered once daily. May titrate every 3-4 days until adequate pain relief with tolerable side effects have been achieved.

Conversion from other opioids to Exalgo™: In general, start Exalgo™ at 50% of the calculated total daily dose every 24 hours. Titrate until adequate pain relief with tolerable side effects has been achieved. The following conversion ratios may be used to convert from **oral** opioid therapy to Exalgo™.

Conversion ratios to Exalgo™ (see table on next page): Select the opioid, sum the total daily dose, then multiply by the conversion ratio to calculate the *approximate* oral hydromorphone equivalent; start Exalgo™ at 50% of the calculated total daily dose every 24 hours. (**Note:** The conversion ratios and approximate equivalent doses in this

◀ conversion table are only to be used for the conversion from current opioid therapy to Exalgo™).

Conversion Ratios to Exalgo™[1]

Previous Opioid	Approximate Equivalent Oral Dose	Oral Conversion Ratio[2]
Hydromorphone	12 mg	1
Codeine	200 mg	0.06
Hydrocodone	30 mg	0.4
Methadone[3]	20 mg	0.6
Morphine	60 mg	0.2
Oxycodone	30 mg	0.4
Oxymorphone	20 mg	0.6

[1] *Approximate* equivalent doses for conversion from current opioid therapy to Exalgo™.

[2] Ratio for converting oral opioid dose to approximate hydromorphone equivalent dose.

[3] Monitor closely; ratio between methadone and other opioid agonists may vary widely as a function of previous drug exposure. Methadone has a long half-life and may accumulate in the plasma.

Conversion from transdermal fentanyl to Exalgo™: Treatment with Exalgo™ can be started 18 hours after the removal of the transdermal fentanyl patch. For every fentanyl 25 mcg/hour transdermal dose, the equianalgesic dose of Exalgo™ is 12 mg every 24 hours. An appropriate starting dose is 50% of the calculated total daily dose given every 24 hours.

Renal Impairment Exalgo™:

Moderate impairment: Start with a reduced dose and monitor closely.

Severe impairment: Consider use of an alternate analgesic with better dosing flexibility.

Hepatic Impairment Dose adjustment should be considered.

Exalgo™: In patients with moderate and severe hepatic impairment, start with a reduced dose and monitor closely. Consider use of an alternate analgesic with better dosing flexibility.

Administration

Parenteral: May be given SubQ or I.M.; vial stopper contains latex

I.V.: For IVP, must be given slowly over 2-3 minutes (rapid IVP has been associated with an increase in side effects, especially respiratory depression and hypotension)

Oral: Hydromorph Contin®: Capsule should be swallowed whole; do not crush or chew; contents may be sprinkled on soft food and swallowed

Monitoring Parameters Pain relief, respiratory and mental status, blood pressure

Test Interactions Some quinolones may produce a false-positive urine screening result for opiates using commercially-available immunoassay kits. This has been demonstrated most consistently for levofloxacin and ofloxacin, but other quinolones have shown cross-reactivity in certain assay kits. Confirmation of positive opiate screens by more specific methods should be considered.

Pharmacotherapy Pearls Equianalgesic doses: Morphine 10 mg I.M. = hydromorphone 1.5 mg I.M.

Exalgo™ is indicated for the management of moderate-to-severe pain in opioid-tolerant patients (requiring around-the-clock analgesia for an extended period of time). Patients are considered to be opioid tolerant if they have been taking oral morphine ≥60 mg/day, fentanyl transdermal ≥25 mcg/hour, oral oxycodone ≥30 mg/day, oral hydromorphone ≥8 mg/day, oral oxymorphone ≥25 mg/day, or an equianalgesic dose of another opioid for ≥1 week.

Special Geriatric Considerations Elderly may be particularly susceptible to the CNS depressant and constipating effects of narcotics.

Controlled Substance C-II

Dosage Forms Excipient information presented when available (limited, particularly for generics); consult specific product labeling.

Injection, powder for reconstitution, as hydrochloride:

Dilaudid-HP®: 250 mg [contains natural rubber/natural latex in packaging, sodium meta-bisulfite]

Injection, solution, as hydrochloride: 1 mg/mL (1 mL); 2 mg/mL (1 mL, 20 mL); 4 mg/mL (1 mL); 10 mg/mL (1 mL, 5 mL, 50 mL)

Dilaudid-HP®: 10 mg/mL (50 mL) [contains natural rubber/natural latex in packaging, sodium metabisulfite]

Dilaudid-HP®: 10 mg/mL (1 mL, 5 mL) [contains sodium metabisulfite]

Dilaudid®: 1 mg/mL (1 mL); 2 mg/mL (1 mL); 4 mg/mL (1 mL) [contains sodium metabisulfite]

Injection, solution, as hydrochloride [preservative free]: 10 mg/mL (1 mL, 5 mL, 50 mL)

Liquid, oral, as hydrochloride:

Dilaudid®: 1 mg/mL (473 mL) [contains sodium metabisulfite (may have trace amounts)]

Powder, for prescription compounding, as hydrochloride: USP: 100% (972 mg)

Suppository, rectal, as hydrochloride: 3 mg (6s)

Tablet, oral, as hydrochloride: 2 mg, 4 mg, 8 mg

Dilaudid®: 2 mg, 4 mg [contains sodium metabisulfite (may have trace amounts)]

Dilaudid®: 8 mg [scored; contains sodium metabisulfite (may have trace amounts)]

Tablet, extended release, oral, as hydrochloride:

Exalgo™: 8 mg, 12 mg, 16 mg [contains sodium metabisulfite]

Dosage Forms: Canada Excipient information presented when available (limited, particularly for generics); consult specific product labeling.

Capsule, controlled release:

Hydromorph Contin®: 3 mg, 6 mg, 12 mg, 18 mg, 24 mg, 30 mg

Selected References

American Geriatrics Society Panel on Pharmacological Management of Persistent Pain in Older Persons, "Pharmacological Management of Persistent Pain in Older Persons," *J Am Geriatr Soc*, 2009, 57(8):1331-46.

◆ **Hydromorphone Hydrochloride** *see* HYDROmorphone *on page 888*
◆ **Hydroskin® [OTC]** *see* Hydrocortisone (Topical) *on page 886*

Hydroxocobalamin (hye droks oh koe BAL a min)

Brand Names: U.S. Cyanokit®
Brand Names: Canada Cyanokit®
Index Terms Vitamin B_{12a}
Generic Availability (U.S.) Yes: Excludes powder for injection
Pharmacologic Category Antidote; Vitamin, Water Soluble
Use Treatment of pernicious anemia, vitamin B_{12} deficiency due to dietary deficiencies or malabsorption diseases, inadequate secretion of intrinsic factor, and inadequate utilization of B_{12} (eg, during neoplastic treatment); diagnostic agent for Schilling test

Cyanokit®: Treatment of cyanide poisoning (known or suspected)

Unlabeled/Investigational Use Treatment of neuropathies, multiple sclerosis

Contraindications Hypersensitivity to hydroxocobalamin, cyanocobalamin, cobalt, or any component of the formulation

Warnings/Precautions

Solution for I.M. injection: Treatment of severe vitamin B_{12} megaloblastic anemia may result in thrombocytosis and severe hypokalemia, sometimes fatal, due to intracellular potassium shift upon anemia resolution. Use caution in folic acid deficient megaloblastic anemia; administration of vitamin B_{12} alone is not a substitute for folic acid and might mask true diagnosis. Vitamin B_{12} deficiency masks signs of polycythemia vera; vitamin B_{12} administration may unmask this condition. Neurologic manifestations of vitamin B_{12} deficiency will not be prevented with folic acid unless vitamin B_{12} is also given; spinal cord degeneration might also occur when folic acid is used as a substitute for vitamin B_{12} in anemia prevention. Blunted therapeutic response to vitamin B_{12} may occur in certain conditions (eg, infection, uremia, concurrent iron or folic acid deficiency) or in patients on medications with bone marrow suppressant properties (eg, chloramphenicol). Approved for use as I.M. injection only.

Cyanokit®: Use caution or consider alternatives in patients with known allergic reactions, including anaphylaxis, to hydroxocobalamin or cyanocobalamin. Increased blood pressure (≥180 mm Hg systolic or ≥110 mm Hg diastolic) is associated with infusion; elevations usually noted at beginning of infusion, peak toward the end of infusion and return to baseline within 4 hours of infusion. Collection of pretreatment blood cyanide concentrations does not preclude administration and should not delay administration in the emergency management of highly suspected or confirmed cyanide toxicity. Pretreatment levels may be useful as post infusion levels may be inaccurate. Treatment of cyanide poisoning should include decontamination and supportive therapy. Use caution with concurrent use of other cyanide antidotes; safety has not been established. Photosensitivity is a potential concern; avoid direct sunlight while skin remains discolored.

◀ **Adverse Reactions (Reflective of adult population; not specific for elderly)**

I.M. injection: Frequency not defined:

Dermatologic: Exanthema (transient), itching

Gastrointestinal: Diarrhea (mild, transient)

Local: Injection site pain

Miscellaneous: Anaphylaxis

I.V. infusion (Cyanokit®):

>10%:

Cardiovascular: Blood pressure increased (18% to 28%; systolic ≥180 mm Hg or diastolic ≥110 mm Hg)

Central nervous system: Headache (6% to 33%)

Dermatologic: Erythema (94% to 100%; may last up to 2 weeks), rash (predominantly acneiform; 20% to 44%; can appear 7-28 days after administration and usually resolves within a few weeks)

Gastrointestinal: Nausea (6% to 11%)

Genitourinary: Chromaturia (100%; may last up to 5 weeks after administration)

Hematologic: Lymphocytes decreased (8% to 17%)

Local: Infusion site reaction (6% to 39%)

Frequency not defined:

Cardiovascular: Chest discomfort, hot flashes, peripheral edema

Central nervous system: Dizziness, memory impairment, restlessness

Dermatologic: Pruritus, urticaria

Gastrointestinal: Abdominal discomfort, diarrhea, dyspepsia, dysphagia, hematochezia, vomiting

Ocular: Irritation, redness, swelling

Respiratory: Dry throat, dyspnea, throat tightness

Miscellaneous: Allergic reaction (including anaphylaxis)

Drug Interactions

Avoid Concomitant Use There are no known interactions where it is recommended to avoid concomitant use.

Increased Effect/Toxicity There are no known significant interactions involving an increase in effect.

Decreased Effect There are no known significant interactions involving a decrease in effect.

Stability

Solution for I.M. injection: Store at 20°C to 25°C (68°F to 77°F). Protect from light.

I.V. infusion (Cyanokit®): Prior to reconstitution, store at 25°C (77°F): excursions permitted to 15°C to 30°C (59°F to 86°F).

Temperature variation exposure allowed for transport of lyophilized form:

Usual transport: ≤15 days at 5°C to 40°C (41°F to 104°F)

Desert transport: ≤4 days at 5°C to 60°C (41°F to 140°F)

Freezing/defrosting cycles: ≤15 days at -20°C to 40°C (-4°F to 104°F)

Reconstitute each 2.5 g vial with 100 mL of NS using provided sterile transfer spike. If NS unavailable, may use LR or D_5W. Invert or rock each vial for at least 30 seconds prior to infusion; do not shake. Do not use if solution is **not** dark red. Following reconstitution, store up to 6 hours at ≤40°C (104°F); do not freeze. Discard any remaining solution after 6 hours.

Mechanism of Action Hydroxocobalamin (vitamin B_{12a}) is a precursor to cyanocobalamin (vitamin B_{12}). Cyanocobalamin acts as a coenzyme for various metabolic functions, including fat and carbohydrate metabolism and protein synthesis, used in cell replication and hematopoiesis. In the presence of cyanide, each hydroxocobalamin molecule can bind one cyanide ion by displacing it for the hydroxo ligand linked to the trivalent cobalt ion, forming cyanocobalamin.

Pharmacodynamics/Kinetics Following I.V. administration of Cyanokit®:

Protein binding: Significant; forms various cobalamin-(III) complexes

Half-life elimination: 26-31 hours

Excretion: Urine (50% to 60% within initial 72 hours)

Dosage

Geriatric & Adult

Vitamin B_{12} deficiency: I.M.: 30 mcg/day for 5-10 days, followed by 100-200 mcg/month

Note: Larger doses may be required in critically-ill patients or if patient has neurologic disease, an infectious disease, or hyperthyroidism.

Schilling test: I.M.: 1000 mcg

Cyanide toxicity (Cyanokit®): I.V.: Initial: 5 g as single infusion; may repeat a second 5 g dose depending on severity of poisoning and clinical response. Maximum cumulative dose: 10 g. **Note:** If suspected, antidotal therapy must be given immediately.

Administration

Solution for I.M. injection: Administer 1000 mcg/mL solution I.M. only

Cyanokit®: Administer by I.V. infusion over 15 minutes; if repeat dose needed, administer second dose over 15 minutes to 2 hours

Monitoring Parameters Vitamin B_{12}, hematocrit, hemoglobin, reticulocyte count, red blood cell counts, folate and iron levels should be obtained prior to treatment and periodically during treatment.

Cyanide toxicity: Blood pressure and heart rate during and after infusion, serum lactate levels, venous-arterial PO_2 gradient. Pretreatment levels may be useful as post infusion levels may be inaccurate.

Megaloblastic anemia: In addition to normal hematological parameters, serum potassium and platelet counts should be monitored during therapy, particularly in the first 48 hours of treatment.

Test Interactions The following values may be affected, *in vitro*, following hydroxocobalamin 5 g dose. Interference following hydroxocobalamin 10 g dose can be expected to last up to an additional 24 hours. **Note:** Extent and duration of interference dependent on analyzer used and patient variability.

Falsely elevated:

Basophils, hemoglobin, MCH, and MCHC [duration: 12-16 hours]

Albumin, alkaline phosphatase, cholesterol, creatinine, glucose, total protein, and triglycerides [duration: 24 hours]

Bilirubin [duration: up to 4 days]

Urinalysis: Glucose, protein, erythrocytes, leukocytes, ketones, bilirubin, urobilinogen, nitrite [duration: 2-8 days]

Falsely decreased: ALT and amylase [duration: 24 hours]

Unpredictable:

AST, CK, CKMB, LDH, phosphate, and uric acid [duration: 24 hours]

PT (quick or INR) and aPTT [duration: 24-48 hours]

Urine pH [duration: 2-8 days]

May also interfere with colorimetric tests and cause hemodialysis machines to shut down due to false detection of a blood leak from the blood-like appearance of the solution.

Pharmacotherapy Pearls Expert advice from a regional poison control center for appropriate use may be obtained (1-800-222-1222). Cyanide is a clear colorless gas or liquid with a faint bitter almond odor. Cyanide reacts with trivalent ions in cytochrome oxidase in the mitochondria leading to histotoxic hypoxia and lactic acidosis. Signs and symptoms of cyanide toxicity include headache, altered mental status, dyspnea, mydriasis, chest tightness, nausea, vomiting, tachycardia/hypertension (initially), bradycardia/hypotension (later), seizures, cardiovascular collapse, or coma.

Special Geriatric Considerations Evidence exists that people, particularly elderly, whose serum cobalamin concentrations are <500 pg/mL, should receive replacement parenteral therapy. This recommendation is based upon neuropsychiatric disorders and cardiovascular disorders associated with lower sodium cobalamin concentrations.

Dosage Forms Excipient information presented when available (limited, particularly for generics); consult specific product labeling.

Injection, powder for reconstitution:

Cyanokit®: 2.5 g

Injection, solution: 1000 mcg/mL (30 mL)

Selected References

Olszewski AJ, Szostak WB, Bialkowska M, et al, "Reduction of Plasma Lipid and Homocysteine Levels by Pyridoxine, Folate, Cobalamin, Choline, Riboflavin, and Troxerutin in Atherosclerosis," *Atherosclerosis*, 1989, 75(1):1-6.

Regland B, Gottfries CG, and Lindstedt G, "Dementia Patients With Low Serum Cobalamin Concentration: Relationship to Atrophic Gastritis," *Aging (Milano)*, 1992, 4(1):35-41.

Sauer SW and Keim ME, "Hydroxocobalamin: Improved Public Health Readiness for Cyanide Disasters," *Ann Emerg Med*, 2001, 37(6):635-41.

◆ **Hydroxycarbamide** *see* Hydroxyurea *on page* 897

Hydroxychloroquine (hye droks ee KLOR oh kwin)

Medication Safety Issues

Sound-alike/look-alike issues:

Hydroxychloroquine may be confused with hydrocortisone

Plaquenil® may be confused with Platinol®

Brand Names: U.S. Plaquenil®

Brand Names: Canada Apo-Hydroxyquine®; Gen-Hydroxychloroquine; Mylan-Hydroxychloroquine; Plaquenil®; PRO-Hydroxyquine

Index Terms Hydroxychloroquine Sulfate

Generic Availability (U.S.) Yes

◄ **Pharmacologic Category** Aminoquinoline (Antimalarial)
Use Suppression and treatment of acute attacks of malaria; treatment of systemic lupus erythematosus (SLE) and rheumatoid arthritis
Unlabeled/Investigational Use Treatment of porphyria cutanea tarda, polymorphous light eruptions
Contraindications Hypersensitivity to hydroxychloroquine, 4-aminoquinoline derivatives, or any component of the formulation; retinal or visual field changes attributable to 4-aminoquinolines
Warnings/Precautions May cause ophthalmic adverse effects (risk factors include daily doses >6.5 mg/kg lean body weight) or neuromyopathy; perform baseline and periodic (every 3 months) ophthalmologic examinations; test periodically for muscle weakness. Rare cardiomyopathy has been associated with long-term use of hydroxychloroquine. Aminoquinolines have been associated with rare hematologic reactions, including agranulocytosis, aplastic anemia, and thrombocytopenia; monitoring (CBC) is recommended in prolonged therapy. Use with caution in patients with hepatic disease, G6PD deficiency, psoriasis, and porphyria. Not effective in the treatment of malaria caused by chloroquine resistant *P. falciparum*. **[U.S. Boxed Warning]: Should be prescribed by physicians familiar with its use.**
Adverse Reactions (Reflective of adult population; not specific for elderly) Frequency not defined.
Cardiovascular: Cardiomyopathy (rare, relationship to hydroxychloroquine unclear)
Central nervous system: Ataxia, dizziness, emotional changes, headache, irritability, lassitude, nervousness, nightmares, psychosis, seizure, vertigo
Dermatologic: Alopecia, angioedema, bleaching of hair, pigmentation changes (skin and mucosal; black-blue color), rash (acute generalized exanthematous pustulosis, erythema annulare centrifugum, exfoliative dermatitis, lichenoid, maculopapular, morbilliform, purpuric, Stevens-Johnson syndrome, urticarial), urticaria
Gastrointestinal: Abdominal cramping, anorexia, diarrhea, nausea, vomiting, weight loss
Hematologic: Agranulocytosis, aplastic anemia, hemolysis (in patients with glucose-6-phosphate deficiency), leukopenia, thrombocytopenia
Hepatic: Abnormal liver function/hepatic failure (isolated cases)
Neuromuscular & skeletal: Myopathy, palsy, or neuromyopathy leading to progressive weakness and atrophy of proximal muscle groups (may be associated with mild sensory changes, loss of deep tendon reflexes, and abnormal nerve conduction)
Ocular: Abnormal color vision, abnormal retinal pigmentation, atrophy, attenuation of retinal arterioles, corneal changes/deposits (visual disturbances, blurred vision, photophobia [reversible on discontinuation]), decreased visual acuity, disturbance in accommodation, keratopathy, macular edema, nystagmus, optic disc pallor/atrophy, pigmentary retinopathy, retinopathy (early changes reversible [may progress despite discontinuation if advanced]), scotoma
Otic: Deafness, tinnitus
Miscellaneous: Exacerbation of porphyria and nonlight sensitive psoriasis
Respiratory: Bronchospasm, respiratory failure (myopathy-related)
Drug Interactions
  Avoid Concomitant Use
  Avoid concomitant use of Hydroxychloroquine with any of the following: Artemether; BCG; Lumefantrine; Mefloquine; Natalizumab; Pimecrolimus; Tacrolimus (Topical)
  Increased Effect/Toxicity
  Hydroxychloroquine may increase the levels/effects of: Antipsychotic Agents (Phenothiazines); Beta-Blockers; Cardiac Glycosides; Dapsone; Dapsone (Systemic); Dapsone (Topical); Leflunomide; Lumefantrine; Mefloquine; Natalizumab; Vaccines (Live)

  The levels/effects of Hydroxychloroquine may be increased by: Artemether; Dapsone; Dapsone (Systemic); Denosumab; Mefloquine; Pimecrolimus; Roflumilast; Tacrolimus (Topical); Trastuzumab
  Decreased Effect
  Hydroxychloroquine may decrease the levels/effects of: Anthelmintics; BCG; Sipuleucel-T; Vaccines (Inactivated)

  The levels/effects of Hydroxychloroquine may be decreased by: Echinacea
Ethanol/Nutrition/Herb Interactions Ethanol: Avoid ethanol (due to GI irritation).
Mechanism of Action Interferes with digestive vacuole function within sensitive malarial parasites by increasing the pH and interfering with lysosomal degradation of hemoglobin; inhibits locomotion of neutrophils and chemotaxis of eosinophils; impairs complement-dependent antigen-antibody reactions
Pharmacodynamics/Kinetics
Onset of action: Rheumatic disease: May require 4-6 weeks to respond
Absorption: Rapid and complete

Protein binding: 55%

Metabolism: Hepatic; metabolites include desethylhydroxychloroquine and desethylchloroquine

Half-life elimination: 32-50 days

Time to peak: Rheumatic disease: Several months

Excretion: Urine (as metabolites and unchanged drug [up to 60%]); may be enhanced by urinary acidification

Dosage

Geriatric & Adult Note: Hydroxychloroquine sulfate 200 mg is equivalent to 155 mg hydroxychloroquine base and 250 mg chloroquine phosphate. All doses below expressed as hydroxychloroquine sulfate. Second-line alternative treatment for malaria (chloroquine is preferred).

Malaria, chemoprophylaxis: Oral: 400 mg weekly on same day each week; begin 2 weeks before exposure; continue for 4 weeks (per CDC guidelines) after leaving endemic area; if suppressive therapy is not begun prior to the exposure, double the initial dose and give in 2 doses, 6 hours apart and continue treatment for 8 weeks

Malaria, acute attack: Oral: 800 mg initially, followed by 400 mg at 6, 24, and 48 hours

Rheumatoid arthritis: Oral: Initial: 400-600 mg/day taken with food or milk; increase dose gradually until optimum response level is reached; usually after 4-12 weeks dose should be reduced by 1/2 to a maintenance dose of 200-400 mg/day

Lupus erythematosus: Oral: 400 mg every day or twice daily for several weeks-months depending on response; 200-400 mg/day for prolonged maintenance therapy

Renal Impairment Use with caution; dosage adjustment may be necessary in severe dysfunction (Bernstein, 1992); specific guidelines not available.

Hepatic Impairment Use with caution; dosage adjustment may be necessary.

Administration Administer with food or milk.

Monitoring Parameters Ophthalmologic exam at baseline and every 3 months during prolonged therapy (including visual acuity, slit-lamp, fundoscopic, and visual field exam); CBC at baseline and periodically; muscle strength (especially proximal, as a symptom of neuromyopathy) during long-term therapy

Special Geriatric Considerations No specific recommendations for dosing.

Dosage Forms Excipient information presented when available (limited, particularly for generics); consult specific product labeling.

Tablet, oral, as sulfate: 200 mg [equivalent to 155 mg base]

Plaquenil®: 200 mg [equivalent to 155 mg base]

Selected References

Centers for Disease Control and Prevention, "Guidelines for the Treatment of Malaria in the United States," available at http://www.cdc.gov/malaria/diagnosis_treatment/tx_clinicians.htm and http://www.cdc.gov/malaria/pdf/treatmenttable.pdf; last accessed October 2, 2007.

- ◆ **Hydroxychloroquine Sulfate** see Hydroxychloroquine on page 895
- ◆ **Hydroxyethylcellulose** see Artificial Tears on page 148
- ◆ **9-hydroxy-risperidone** see Paliperidone on page 1378

Hydroxyurea (hye droks ee yoor EE a)

Medication Safety Issues

Sound-alike/look-alike issues:

Hydroxyurea may be confused with hydrOXYzine

High alert medication:

This medication is in a class the Institute for Safe Medication Practices (ISMP) includes among its list of drugs which have a heightened risk of causing significant patient harm when used in error.

International issues:

Hydrea [U.S., Canada, and multiple international markets] may be confused with Hydra brand name for isoniazid [Japan]

Brand Names: U.S. Droxia®; Hydrea®

Brand Names: Canada Apo-Hydroxyurea®; Gen-Hydroxyurea; Hydrea®; Mylan-Hydroxyurea

Index Terms Hydroxycarbamide; Hydurea

Generic Availability (U.S.) Yes

Pharmacologic Category Antineoplastic Agent, Antimetabolite

Use Treatment of melanoma, refractory chronic myelocytic leukemia (CML); recurrent, metastatic, or inoperable ovarian cancer; radiosensitizing agent in the treatment of squamous cell head and neck cancer (excluding lip cancer); adjunct in the management of sickle cell patients who have had at least three painful crises in the previous 12 months (to reduce frequency of these crises and the need for blood transfusions)

◀ **Unlabeled/Investigational Use** Treatment of HIV; treatment of psoriasis, treatment of hematologic conditions such as essential thrombocythemia, polycythemia vera, hypereosinophilia, and hyperleukocytosis due to acute leukemia; treatment of uterine, cervix and nonsmall cell lung cancers; radiosensitizing agent in the treatment of primary brain tumors; has shown activity against renal cell cancer and prostate cancer

Contraindications Hypersensitivity to hydroxyurea or any component of the formulation; severe anemia; severe bone marrow suppression; WBC <2500/mm^3 or platelet count <100,000/mm^3 (neutrophils <2000/mm^3, platelets <80,000/mm^3, and hemoglobin <4.5 g/dL for sickle cell anemia)

Warnings/Precautions Hazardous agent - use appropriate precautions for handling and disposal; to decrease risk of exposure, wear gloves when handling and wash hands before and after contact. Leukopenia may commonly occur (thrombocytopenia and anemia are less common; reversible with treatment interruption. Use with caution in patients with a history of prior chemotherapy or radiation therapy; myelosuppression is more common. Correct severe anemia prior to initiating treatment. Patients with a history of radiation therapy are also at risk for exacerbation of post irradiation erythema. Self-limiting megaloblastic erythropoiesis may be seen early in treatment (may resemble pernicious anemia, but is unrelated to vitamin B$_{12}$ or folic acid deficiency). Plasma iron clearance may be delayed and iron utilization rate (by erythrocytes) may be reduced. When treated concurrently with hydroxyurea and antiretroviral agents (including didanosine), HIV-infected patients are at higher risk for potentially fatal pancreatitis, hepatotoxicity, hepatic failure, and severe peripheral neuropathy. Hyperuricemia may occur with treatment; adequate hydration and initiation or dosage adjustment of uricosuric agents (eg, allopurinol) may be necessary.

In patients with sickle cell anemia, use is not recommended if neutrophils <2000/mm^3, platelets <80,000/mm^3, hemoglobin <4.5 g/dL, or reticulocytes <80,000/mm^3 when hemoglobin <9 g/dL. May cause macrocytosis, which can mask folic acid deficiency; prophylactic fold acid supplementation is recommended. **[U.S. Boxed Warning]: Hydroxyurea is mutagenic and clastogenic.** Treatment of myeloproliferative disorders (eg, polycythemia vera, thrombocythemia) with long-term hydroxyurea is associated with secondary leukemia; it is unknown if this is drug-related or disease-related. Cutaneous vasculitic toxicities (vasculitic ulceration and gangrene) have been reported with hydroxyurea treatment, most often in patients with a history of or receiving concurrent interferon therapy; discontinue hydroxyurea and consider alternate cytoreductive therapy if cutaneous vasculitic toxicity develops. Use caution with renal dysfunction; may require dose reductions. Elderly patients may be more sensitive to the effects of hydroxyurea; may require lower doses. **[U.S. Boxed Warning]: Should be administered under the supervision of a physician experienced in the treatment of sickle cell anemia** or in cancer chemotherapy.

Adverse Reactions (Reflective of adult population; not specific for elderly) Frequency not defined.

Cardiovascular: Edema

Central nervous system: Chills, disorientation, dizziness, drowsiness (dose-related), fever, hallucinations, headache, malaise, seizure

Dermatologic: Alopecia, cutaneous vasculitic toxicities, dermatomyositis-like skin changes, facial erythema, gangrene, hyperpigmentation, maculopapular rash, nail atrophy, nail discoloration, peripheral erythema, scaling - skin atrophy, skin cancer, skin ulcer, vasculitis ulcerations, violet papules

Endocrine & metabolic: Hyperuricemia

Gastrointestinal: Anorexia, constipation, diarrhea, gastrointestinal irritation and mucositis, (potentiated with radiation therapy), nausea, pancreatitis, stomatitis, vomiting

Genitourinary: Dysuria

Hematologic: Myelosuppression (anemia, leukopenia [common; reversal of WBC count occurs rapidly], thrombocytopenia); macrocytosis, megaloblastic erythropoiesis, secondary leukemias (long-term use)

Hepatic: Hepatic enzymes increased, hepatotoxicity

Neuromuscular & skeletal: Peripheral neuropathy, weakness

Renal: BUN increased, creatinine increased

Respiratory: Acute diffuse pulmonary infiltrates (rare), dyspnea, pulmonary fibrosis (rare)

Drug Interactions

  Avoid Concomitant Use

  Avoid concomitant use of Hydroxyurea with any of the following: BCG; Didanosine; Natalizumab; Pimecrolimus; Stavudine; Tacrolimus (Topical); Vaccines (Live)

  Increased Effect/Toxicity

  Hydroxyurea may increase the levels/effects of: Didanosine; Leflunomide; Natalizumab; Stavudine; Vaccines (Live)

  The levels/effects of Hydroxyurea may be increased by: Denosumab; Didanosine; Pimecrolimus; Roflumilast; Stavudine; Tacrolimus (Topical); Trastuzumab

Decreased Effect

Hydroxyurea may decrease the levels/effects of: BCG; Sipuleucel-T; Vaccines (Inactivated); Vaccines (Live)

The levels/effects of Hydroxyurea may be decreased by: Echinacea

Stability Store at room temperature of 25°C (77°F); excursions permitted between 15°C and 30°C (59°F and 86°F).

Mechanism of Action Antimetabolite which selectively inhibits ribonucleoside diphosphate reductase, preventing the conversion of ribonucleotides to deoxyribonucleotides, halting the cell cycle at the G1/S phase and therefore has radiation sensitizing activity by maintaining cells in the G_1 phase and interfering with DNA repair. In sickle cell anemia, hydroxyurea increases red blood cell (RBC) hemoglobin F levels, RBC water content, deformability of sickled cells, and alters adhesion of RBCs to endothelium.

Pharmacodynamics/Kinetics

Onset: Sickle cell anemia: Fetal hemoglobin increase: 4-12 weeks

Absorption: Readily (≥80%)

Distribution: Readily crosses blood-brain barrier; distributes into intestine, brain, lung, kidney tissues, effusions and ascites

Metabolism: 60% via hepatic and GI tract

Half-life elimination: 3-4 hours

Time to peak: 1-4 hours

Excretion: Urine (sickle cell anemia: 40% of administered dose)

Dosage

Geriatric & Adult

Antineoplastic uses: Titrate dose to patient response; if WBC count falls to <2500/mm^3, or the platelet count to <100,000/mm^3, therapy should be stopped for at least 3 days and resumed when values rise toward normal

Chronic myeloid leukemia (resistant): Oral: Continuous therapy: 20-30 mg/kg once daily

Solid tumors: Oral:

  Intermittent therapy: 80 mg/kg as a single dose every third day

  Continuous therapy: 20-30 mg/kg once daily

  Concomitant therapy with irradiation (head and neck cancer): 80 mg/kg as a single dose every third day starting at least 7 days before initiation of irradiation

Sickle cell anemia: Oral: Initial: 15 mg/kg/day; if blood counts are in an acceptable range, may increase by 5 mg/kg every 12 weeks until the maximum tolerated dose of 35 mg/kg/day is achieved or the dose that does not produce toxic effects (do not increase dose if blood counts are between acceptable and toxic ranges). Monitor for toxicity every 2 weeks; if toxicity occurs, withhold treatment until the bone marrow recovers, then restart with a dose reduction of 2.5 mg/kg/day; if no toxicity occurs over the next 12 weeks, then the subsequent dose may be increased by 2.5 mg/kg/day every 12 weeks to a maximum tolerated dose (dose which does not produce hematologic toxicity for 24 consecutive weeks). If hematologic toxicity recurs a second time at a specific dose, do not retry that dose.

  Acceptable hematologic ranges: Neutrophils ≥2500/mm^3; platelets ≥95,000/mm^3; hemoglobin >5.3 g/dL, and reticulocytes ≥95,000/mm^3 if the hemoglobin concentration is <9 g/dL

  Toxic hematologic ranges: Neutrophils <2000/mm^3; platelets <80,000/mm^3; hemoglobin <4.5 g/dL; and reticulocytes <80,000/mm^3 if the hemoglobin concentration is <9 g/dL

Cervical cancer (unlabeled use; with concurrent radiation therapy, cisplatin and fluorouracil): Oral: 2000 mg/m^2 (2 hours prior to radiation treatment) twice a week for 6 weeks (Rose, 2007)

Essential thrombocythemia, high-risk (unlabeled use): Oral: 500-1000 mg daily; adjust dose to maintain platelets <400,000/mm^3 (Harrison, 2005)

Head and neck cancer (unlabeled use; with concurrent radiation therapy and fluorouracil): Oral: 1000 mg every 12 hours for 11 doses (Garden, 2004)

Hypereosinophilic syndrome (unlabeled use): Oral: 1000-3000 mg/day (Klion, 2006)

Meningioma (unlabeled use): Oral: 20 mg/kg once daily (Newton, 2000; Rosenthal, 2002)

Polycythemia vera, high-risk (unlabeled use): Oral: 15-20 mg/kg/day (Finazzi, 2007)

Renal Impairment

The FDA-approved labeling recommends the following adjustment:

Sickle cell anemia:

  Cl_{cr} ≥60 mL/minute: No adjustment (of initial dose) required.

  Cl_{cr} <60 mL/minute: Reduce initial dose to 7.5 mg/kg/day; titrate to response/avoidance of toxicity (refer to Dosage: Geriatric & Adult).

  ESRD: Reduce initial dose to 7.5 mg/kg/dose (administer after dialysis on dialysis days); titrate to response/avoidance of toxicity.

Other approved indications: It is recommended to reduce the initial dose; however, no specific guidelines are available.

◀

The following guidelines have been used by some clinicians:

Aronoff, 2007: Adults:

Cl_{cr} 10-50 mL/minute: Administer 50% of dose.

Cl_{cr} <10 mL/minute: Administer 20% of dose.

Hemodialysis: Administer dose after dialysis on dialysis days; supplemental dose is not necessary. Hydroxyurea is a low molecular weight compound with high aqueous solubility that may be freely dialyzable, however, clinical studies confirming this hypothesis have not been performed.

Continuous renal replacement therapy (CRRT): Administer 50% of dose.

Kintzel, 1995:

Cl_{cr} 46-60 mL/minute: Administer 85% of dose.

Cl_{cr} 31-45 mL/minute: Administer 80% of dose.

Cl_{cr} <30 mL/minute: Administer 75% of dose.

Hepatic Impairment Specific guidelines are not available for dosage adjustment in hepatic impairment. The FDA-approved labeling recommends closely monitoring for bone marrow toxicity in patients with hepatic impairment.

Administration Capsules may be opened and emptied into water (will not dissolve completely); observe proper handling procedures

Monitoring Parameters CBC with differential and platelets, renal function and liver function tests, serum uric acid

Sickle cell disease: Monitor for toxicity every 2 weeks. If toxicity occurs, stop treatment until the bone marrow recovers; restart at 2.5 mg/kg/day less than the dose at which toxicity occurs. If no toxicity occurs over the next 12 weeks, then the subsequent dose should be increased by 2.5 mg/kg/day. Reduced dosage of hydroxyurea alternating with erythropoietin may decrease myelotoxicity and increase levels of fetal hemoglobin in patients who have not been helped by hydroxyurea alone.

Acceptable range: Neutrophils ≥2500 cells/mm^3, platelets ≥95,000/mm^3, hemoglobin >5.3 g/dL, and reticulocytes ≥95,000/mm^3 if the hemoglobin concentration is <9 g/dL

Toxic range: Neutrophils <2000 cells/mm^3, platelets <80,000/mm^3, hemoglobin <4.5 g/dL, and reticulocytes <80,000/mm^3 if the hemoglobin concentration is <9 g/dL

Test Interactions False-negative triglyceride measurement by a glycerol oxidase method

Pharmacotherapy Pearls Although I.V. use is reported, no parenteral product is commercially available in the U.S.

If WBC decreases to <2500/mm^3 or platelet count to <100,000/mm^3, interrupt therapy until values rise significantly toward normal. Treat anemia with whole blood replacement; do not interrupt therapy. Adequate trial period to determine the antineoplastic effectiveness is 6 weeks. Almost all patients receiving hydroxyurea in clinical trials needed to have their medication stopped for a time to allow their low blood count to return to acceptable levels.

Special Geriatric Considerations Elderly may be more sensitive to the effects of this drug and may require a lower dosage regimen; advance dose slowly and adjust dose for renal function with careful monitoring.

Dosage Forms Excipient information presented when available (limited, particularly for generics); consult specific product labeling.

Capsule, oral: 500 mg

Droxia®: 200 mg, 300 mg, 400 mg

Hydrea®: 500 mg

Selected References

Longhurst HJ and Pinching AJ, "Drug Points: Pancreatitis Associated With Hydroxyurea in Combination With Didanosine," *BMJ*, 2001, 322(7278):81.

HydrOXYzine (hye DROKS i zeen)

Related Information

Beers Criteria − Potentially Inappropriate Medications for Geriatrics *on page 2089*

Medication Safety Issues

Sound-alike/look-alike issues:

HydrOXYzine may be confused with hydrALAZINE, hydroxyurea

Atarax® may be confused with Ativan®

Vistaril® may be confused with Restoril™, Versed, Zestril®

BEERS Criteria medication:

This drug may be inappropriate for use in geriatric patients (high severity risk).

International issues:

Vistaril [U.S. and Turkey] may be confused with Vastarel brand name for trimetazidine [multiple international markets]

Brand Names: U.S. Vistaril®

Brand Names: Canada Apo-Hydroxyzine®; Atarax®; Hydroxyzine Hydrochloride Injection, USP; Novo-Hydroxyzin; Nu-Hydroxyzine; PMS-Hydroxyzine; Riva-Hydroxyzine

Index Terms Hydroxyzine Hydrochloride; Hydroxyzine Pamoate

Generic Availability (U.S.) Yes

Pharmacologic Category Antiemetic; Histamine H_1 Antagonist; Histamine H_1 Antagonist, First Generation; Piperazine Derivative

Use Treatment of anxiety/agitation (including adjunctive therapy in alcoholism); adjunct to pre- and postoperative analgesia and anesthesia; antipruritic; antiemetic

Contraindications Hypersensitivity to hydroxyzine or any component of the formulation; SubQ, intra-arterial, or I.V. administration of injection

Warnings/Precautions Causes sedation, caution must be used in performing tasks which require alertness (eg, operating machinery or driving). Sedative effects of CNS depressants or ethanol are potentiated. SubQ, I.V., and intra-arterial administration are contraindicated since tissue damage, intravascular hemolysis, thrombosis, and digital gangrene can occur. Use with caution with narrow-angle glaucoma, prostatic hyperplasia, bladder neck obstruction, asthma, or COPD. May be inappropriate for use in the elderly due to potent anticholinergic effects; nonanticholinergic antihistamines preferred for treating allergic reactions (Beers Criteria).

Adverse Reactions (Reflective of adult population; not specific for elderly) Frequency not defined.

Central nervous system: Dizziness, drowsiness, fatigue, hallucination, headache, nervousness, seizure

Dermatologic: Pruritus, rash, urticaria

Gastrointestinal: Xerostomia

Neuromuscular & skeletal: Involuntary movements, paresthesia, tremor

Ocular: Blurred vision

Respiratory: Respiratory depression (at higher than recommended doses)

Miscellaneous: Allergic reaction

Drug Interactions

Metabolism/Transport Effects Inhibits CYP2D6 (weak)

Avoid Concomitant Use There are no known interactions where it is recommended to avoid concomitant use.

Increased Effect/Toxicity

HydrOXYzine may increase the levels/effects of: Alcohol (Ethyl); Anticholinergics; Barbiturates; CNS Depressants; Meperidine; Selective Serotonin Reuptake Inhibitors

The levels/effects of HydrOXYzine may be increased by: Droperidol; Pramlintide

Decreased Effect

HydrOXYzine may decrease the levels/effects of: Acetylcholinesterase Inhibitors (Central); Benzylpenicilloyl Polylysine; Betahistine

The levels/effects of HydrOXYzine may be decreased by: Acetylcholinesterase Inhibitors (Central); Amphetamines

Ethanol/Nutrition/Herb Interactions

Ethanol: May increase CNS depression; monitor for increased effects with coadministration. Caution patients about effects.

Herb/Nutraceutical: Avoid valerian, St John's wort, kava kava, gotu kola (may increase CNS depression).

Stability

Injection: Store at 20°C to 25°C (68°F to 77°F); excursions permitted to 15°C to 30°C (59°F to 86°F). Protect from light.

Tablets: Store at 20°C to 25°C (68°F to 77°F).

Mechanism of Action Competes with histamine for H_1-receptor sites on effector cells in the gastrointestinal tract, blood vessels, and respiratory tract. Possesses skeletal muscle relaxing, bronchodilator, antihistamine, antiemetic, and analgesic properties.

Pharmacodynamics/Kinetics

Onset of action: Oral: 15-30 minutes; Injection: Rapid

Duration: Decreased histamine-induced wheal and flare areas: 2 to ≥36 hours; Suppression of pruritus: 1-12 hours (Simons, 1984)

Absorption: Oral: Rapid

Distribution: Adults: V_d ~16 L/kg (Simons, 1984); Elderly: ~23 L/kg (Simons K, 1989); Hepatic dysfunction: ~23 L/kg (Simons F, 1989)

Metabolism: Hepatic to multiple metabolites, including cetirizine (active) (Simons F, 1989)

Half-life elimination: Adults: ~20 hours (Simons, 1984); Elderly: ~29 hours (Simons K, 1989); Hepatic dysfunction: ~37 hours (Simons F, 1989)

Time to peak: Oral administration: Serum: ~2 hours; Peak suppression of antihistamine-induced wheal and flare: 4-12 hours (Simons, 1984)

Excretion: Urine

◀ **Dosage**

Geriatric Initiate dosing using the lower end of the recommended dosage range due to an increased potential for anticholinergic side effects. Refer to adult dosing.

Adult

Note: Adjust dose based on patient response.

Antiemetic: I.M.: 25-100 mg/dose

Anxiety:

Oral: 50-100 mg 4 times/day

I.M.: Initial: 50-100 mg, then every 4-6 hours as needed

Preoperative sedation:

Oral: 50-100 mg

I.M.: 25-100 mg

Pruritus: Oral: 25 mg 3-4 times/day

Hepatic Impairment Change dosing interval to every 24 hours in patients with primary biliary cirrhosis (Simons F, 1989)

Administration

Injection: For I. M. use only. Do not administer I.V., SubQ, or intra-arterially. Administer I.M. deep in large muscle. In adults, the preferred site is the upper outer quadrant of the buttock or midlateral thigh. The upper outer quadrant of the gluteal region should be used only when necessary to minimize potential damage to the sciatic nerve. With I.V. administration, extravasation can result in sterile abscess and marked tissue induration.

Oral: Shake suspension vigorously prior to use.

Monitoring Parameters Relief of symptoms, mental status, blood pressure

Test Interactions May cause false-positive serum TCA screen.

Special Geriatric Considerations Anticholinergic effects are not well tolerated in the elderly and frequently result in bowel, bladder, and mental status changes (ie, constipation, confusion, and urinary retention). Hydroxyzine may be useful as a short-term antipruritic, but it is not recommended for use as a sedative or anxiolytic in the elderly.

This medication is considered to be potentially inappropriate in this patient population (Beers Criteria severity: High).

Dosage Forms Excipient information presented when available (limited, particularly for generics); consult specific product labeling.

Capsule, oral, as pamoate: 25 mg, 50 mg, 100 mg

Vistaril®: 25 mg, 50 mg

Injection, solution, as hydrochloride: 25 mg/mL (1 mL); 50 mg/mL (1 mL, 2 mL, 10 mL)

Solution, oral, as hydrochloride: 10 mg/5 mL (473 mL)

Syrup, oral, as hydrochloride: 10 mg/5 mL (118 mL, 473 mL)

Tablet, oral, as hydrochloride: 10 mg, 25 mg, 50 mg

Selected References

Simons KJ, Watson WT, Chen XY, et al, "Pharmacokinetic and Pharmacodynamic Studies of the H_1-Receptor Antagonist Hydroxyzine in the Elderly," *Clin Pharmacol Ther*, 1989, 45(1):9-14.

Hyoscyamine (hye oh SYE a meen)

Related Information

Beers Criteria – Potentially Inappropriate Medications for Geriatrics *on page* 2089

Medication Safety Issues

Sound-alike/look-alike issues:

Anaspaz® may be confused with Anaprox®, Antispas®

Levbid® may be confused with Enbrel®, Lithobid®, Lopid®, Lorabid®

Levsinex® may be confused with Lanoxin®

Levsin/SL® maybe confused with Levaquin®

BEERS Criteria medication:

This drug may be inappropriate for use in geriatric patients (high severity risk).

Brand Names: U.S. Anaspaz®; HyoMax® -SR; HyoMax®-SL; HyoMax™-DT; HyoMax™-FT; Hyosyne; Levbid®; Levsin®; Levsin®/SL; Symax® DuoTab; Symax® FasTab; Symax® SL; Symax® SR

Brand Names: Canada Levsin®

Index Terms *l*-Hyoscyamine Sulfate; Hyoscyamine Sulfate

Generic Availability (U.S.) Yes: excludes Injection, solution, Tablet, chewable/disintegrating (oral), Tablet, variable release (oral)

Pharmacologic Category Anticholinergic Agent

Use

Oral: Adjunctive therapy for peptic ulcers, irritable bowel, neurogenic bladder/bowel; treatment of GI tract disorders caused by spasm; to reduce rigidity, tremors, sialorrhea, and hyperhidrosis associated with parkinsonism; as a drying agent in acute rhinitis

Injection: Preoperative antimuscarinic to reduce secretions and block cardiac vagal inhibitory reflexes; to improve radiologic visibility of the kidneys; symptomatic relief of biliary and renal colic; reduce GI motility to facilitate diagnostic procedures (ie, endoscopy, hypotonic duodenography); reduce pain and hypersecretion in pancreatitis, certain cases of partial heart block associated with vagal activity; reversal of neuromuscular blockade

Contraindications Hypersensitivity to belladonna alkaloids or any component of the formulation; glaucoma; obstructive uropathy; myasthenia gravis; obstructive GI tract disease, paralytic ileus, intestinal atony of elderly or debilitated patients, severe ulcerative colitis, toxic megacolon complicating ulcerative colitis; unstable cardiovascular status in acute hemorrhage, myocardial ischemia

Warnings/Precautions Heat prostration may occur in hot weather. Diarrhea may be a sign of incomplete intestinal obstruction, treatment should be discontinued if this occurs. May produce side effects as seen with other anticholinergic medications including drowsiness, dizziness, blurred vision, or psychosis. The elderly may be more susceptible to these effects. Use with caution in patients with autonomic neuropathy, coronary heart disease, CHF, cardiac arrhythmias, prostatic hyperplasia, hyperthyroidism, hypertension, renal disease, and hiatal hernia associated with reflux esophagitis. Avoid long-term use in the elderly due to anticholinergic adverse effects and uncertain effectiveness (Beers Criteria). May severely impair memory function (especially in those patients with previous memory problems). NuLev™ contains phenylalanine.

Adverse Reactions (Reflective of adult population; not specific for elderly) Frequency not defined.

Cardiovascular: Palpitation, tachycardia

Central nervous system: Ataxia, dizziness, drowsiness, headache, insomnia, mental confusion/excitement, nervousness, speech disorder

Dermatologic: Urticaria

Endocrine & metabolic: Lactation suppression

Gastrointestinal: Bloating, constipation, dry mouth, loss of taste, nausea, vomiting

Genitourinary: Impotence, urinary hesitancy, urinary retention

Neuromuscular & skeletal: Weakness

Ocular: Blurred vision, cycloplegia, increased ocular tension, mydriasis

Miscellaneous: Allergic reactions, sweating decreased

Drug Interactions

Avoid Concomitant Use There are no known interactions where it is recommended to avoid concomitant use.

Increased Effect/Toxicity

Hyoscyamine may increase the levels/effects of: AbobotulinumtoxinA; Anticholinergics; Cannabinoids; OnabotulinumtoxinA; Potassium Chloride; RimabotulinumtoxinB

The levels/effects of Hyoscyamine may be increased by: Pramlintide

Decreased Effect

Hyoscyamine may decrease the levels/effects of: Acetylcholinesterase Inhibitors (Central); Secretin

The levels/effects of Hyoscyamine may be decreased by: Acetylcholinesterase Inhibitors (Central)

Stability Store at controlled room temperature.

Mechanism of Action Blocks the action of acetylcholine at parasympathetic sites in smooth muscle, secretory glands and the CNS; increases cardiac output, dries secretions, antagonizes histamine and serotonin

Pharmacodynamics/Kinetics

Onset of action: 2-3 minutes

Duration: 4-6 hours

Absorption: Well absorbed

Protein binding: 50%

Metabolism: Hepatic

◀ Half-life elimination: 3-5 hours
Excretion: Urine
Dosage
Geriatric & Adult
Gastrointestinal spasms:
Oral or S.L.: 0.125-0.25 mg every 4 hours or as needed (before meals or food); maximum: 1.5 mg/24 hours
Oral, timed release: 0.375-0.75 mg every 12 hours; maximum: 1.5 mg/24 hours
I.M., I.V., SubQ: 0.25-0.5 mg; may repeat as needed up to 4 times/day, at 4-hour intervals
Diagnostic procedures: I.V.: 0.25-0.5 mg given 5-10 minutes prior to procedure
Preanesthesia: I.V.: 5 mcg/kg given 30-60 minutes prior to induction of anesthesia or at the time preoperative narcotics or sedatives are administered
To reduce drug-induced bradycardia during surgery: I.V.: 0.125 mg; repeat as needed
Reverse neuromuscular blockade: I.V.: 0.2 mg for every 1 mg neostigmine (or the physostigmine/pyridostigmine equivalent)
Administration
Oral: Tablets should be administered before meals or food.
Levbid®: Tablets are scored and may be broken in half for dose titration; do not crush or chew.
Levsin/SL®: Tablets may be used sublingually, chewed, or swallowed whole.
Symax® SL: Tablets may be used sublingually or swallowed whole.
I.M.: May be administered without dilution.
I.V.: Inject over at least 1 minute. May be administered without dilution.
Monitoring Parameters Pulse, anticholinergic effects, urine output, GI symptoms
Special Geriatric Considerations Avoid long-term use; the potential for toxic reactions is higher than the potential benefit, elderly are particularly prone to CNS side effects of anticholinergics (eg, confusion, delirium, hallucinations). Side effects often occur before clinical response is obtained.

This medication is considered to be potentially inappropriate in this patient population (Beers Criteria severity: High).
Dosage Forms Excipient information presented when available (limited, particularly for generics); consult specific product labeling.
Elixir, oral, as sulfate: 0.125 mg/5 mL (473 mL)
Hyosyne: 0.125 mg/5 mL (473 mL) [contains ethanol 20%, sodium benzoate; orange-lemon flavor]
Injection, solution, as sulfate:
Levsin®: 0.5 mg/mL (1 mL)
Solution, oral, as sulfate [drops]: 0.125 mg/mL (15 mL)
Hyosyne: 0.125 mg/mL (15 mL) [contains ethanol 5%, sodium benzoate; orange-lemon flavor]
Tablet, oral, as sulfate: 0.125 mg
Levsin®: 0.125 mg
Tablet, sublingual, as sulfate: 0.125 mg
HyoMax®-SL: 0.125 mg [peppermint flavor]
Levsin®/SL: 0.125 mg
Symax® SL: 0.125 mg
Tablet, chewable/disintegrating, oral, as sulfate:
HyoMax™-FT: 0.125 mg [mint flavor]
Symax® FasTab: 0.125 mg [mint flavor]
Tablet, extended release, oral, as sulfate: 0.375 mg
Levbid®: 0.375 mg
Tablet, orally disintegrating, oral, as sulfate: 0.125 mg
Anaspaz®: 0.125 mg [scored]
Tablet, sustained release, oral, as sulfate: 0.375 mg
HyoMax® -SR: 0.375 mg [scored]
Symax® SR: 0.375 mg
Tablet, variable release, oral:
HyoMax™-DT: Hyoscyamine sulfate 0.125 mg [immediate release] and hyoscyamine sulfate 0.25 mg [sustained release]
Symax® DuoTab: Hyoscyamine sulfate 0.125 mg [immediate release] and hyoscyamine sulfate 0.25 mg [sustained release]

Hyoscyamine, Atropine, Scopolamine, and Phenobarbital
(hye oh SYE a meen, A troe peen, skoe POL a meen, & fee noe BAR bi tal)

Related Information
Atropine *on page 165*
Hyoscyamine *on page 902*
PHENobarbital *on page 1437*
Scopolamine (Systemic) *on page 1661*

Medication Safety Issues
Sound-alike/look-alike issues:
Donnatal® may be confused with Donnagel®, Donnatal Extentabs®
BEERS Criteria medication:
This drug may be inappropriate for use in geriatric patients (high severity risk).

Brand Names: U.S. Donnatal Extentabs®; Donnatal®; Hyonatol

Index Terms Atropine, Hyoscyamine, Phenobarbital, and Scopolamine; Belladonna Alkaloids With Phenobarbital; Phenobarbital, Hyoscyamine, Atropine, and Scopolamine; Scopolamine, Hyoscyamine, Atropine, and Phenobarbital

Generic Availability (U.S.) Yes: Elixir, tablet

Pharmacologic Category Anticholinergic Agent; Antispasmodic Agent, Gastrointestinal

Use Adjunct in treatment of irritable bowel syndrome, acute enterocolitis, duodenal ulcer

Dosage
Geriatric & Adult Spasmolytic: Oral:
Donnatal®: 1-2 tablets or 5-10 mL of elixir 3-4 times/day
Donnatal Extentabs®: 1 tablet every 12 hours; may increase to 1 tablet every 8 hours if needed

Special Geriatric Considerations Because of the anticholinergic effects of this product, it is not recommended for use in the elderly.

This medication is considered to be potentially inappropriate in this patient population (Beers Criteria severity: High).

Dosage Forms Excipient information presented when available (limited, particularly for generics); consult specific product labeling. [DSC] = Discontinued product
Elixir: Hyoscyamine sulfate 0.1037 mg, atropine sulfate 0.0194 mg, scopolamine hydrobromide 0.0065 mg, and phenobarbital 16.2 mg per 5 mL (473 mL)
Donnatal®: Hyoscyamine sulfate 0.1037 mg, atropine sulfate 0.0194 mg, scopolamine hydrobromide 0.0065 mg, and phenobarbital 16.2 mg per 5 mL (120 mL, 480 mL) [contains ethanol <23.8%; citrus flavor] [DSC]
Donnatal®: Hyoscyamine sulfate 0.1037 mg, atropine sulfate 0.0194 mg, scopolamine hydrobromide 0.0065 mg, and phenobarbital 16.2 mg per 5 mL (120 mL, 480 mL) [contains ethanol <23.8%; grape flavor]
Tablet: Hyoscyamine sulfate 0.1037 mg, atropine sulfate 0.0194 mg, scopolamine hydrobromide 0.0065 mg, and phenobarbital 16.2 mg
Donnatal®: Hyoscyamine sulfate 0.1037 mg, atropine sulfate 0.0194 mg, scopolamine hydrobromide 0.0065 mg, and phenobarbital 16.2 mg
Hyonatol: Hyoscyamine sulfate 0.1037 mg, atropine sulfate 0.0194 mg, scopolamine hydrobromide 0.0065 mg, and phenobarbital 16.2 mg
Tablet, extended release:
Donnatal Extentabs®: Hyoscyamine sulfate 0.3111 mg, atropine sulfate 0.0582 mg, scopolamine hydrobromide 0.0195 mg, and phenobarbital 48.6 mg

◆ **Hyoscyamine Sulfate** *see* Hyoscyamine *on page 902*
◆ **Hyosyne** *see* Hyoscyamine *on page 902*
◆ **HyperHEP B™ S/D** *see* Hepatitis B Immune Globulin (Human) *on page 867*
◆ **HyperRAB™ S/D** *see* Rabies Immune Globulin (Human) *on page 1573*
◆ **Hyper-Sal™** *see* Sodium Chloride *on page 1690*
◆ **HyperTET™ S/D** *see* Tetanus Immune Globulin (Human) *on page 1767*
◆ **Hypertonic Saline** *see* Sodium Chloride *on page 1690*
◆ **HypoTears [OTC]** *see* Artificial Tears *on page 148*
◆ **HypoTears PF [OTC]** *see* Artificial Tears *on page 148*
◆ **Hytrin** *see* Terazosin *on page 1753*
◆ **Hyzaar®** *see* Losartan and Hydrochlorothiazide *on page 1095*

Ibandronate (eye BAN droh nate)

Related Information
Osteoporosis Management *on page 2027*
Brand Names: U.S. Boniva®
Index Terms Ibandronate Sodium; Ibandronic Acid
Generic Availability (U.S.) No
Pharmacologic Category Bisphosphonate Derivative
Use Treatment and prevention of osteoporosis in postmenopausal females
Unlabeled/Investigational Use Hypercalcemia of malignancy; corticosteroid-induced osteoporosis; Paget's disease; reduce bone pain and skeletal complications from metastatic bone disease
Medication Guide Available Yes
Contraindications Hypersensitivity to ibandronate or any component of the formulation; hypocalcemia; oral tablets are also contraindicated in patients unable to stand or sit upright for at least 60 minutes and in patients with abnormalities of the esophagus which delay esophageal emptying, such as stricture or achalasia
Warnings/Precautions Hypocalcemia must be corrected before therapy initiation. Ensure adequate calcium and vitamin D intake. Osteonecrosis of the jaw (ONJ) has been reported in patients receiving bisphosphonates. Risk factors include invasive dental procedures (eg, tooth extraction, dental implants, boney surgery); a diagnosis of cancer, with concomitant chemotherapy or corticosteroids; poor oral hygiene, ill-fitting dentures; and comorbid disorders (anemia, coagulopathy, infection, pre-existing dental disease). Most reported cases occurred after I.V. bisphosphonate therapy; however, cases have been reported following oral therapy. A dental exam and preventative dentistry should be performed prior to placing patients with risk factors on chronic bisphosphonate therapy. The manufacturer's labeling states that discontinuing bisphosphonates in patients requiring invasive dental procedures may reduce the risk of ONJ. However, other experts suggest that there is no evidence that discontinuing therapy reduces the risk of developing ONJ (Assael, 2009). The benefit/risk must be assessed by the treating physician and/or dentist/surgeon prior to any invasive dental procedure. Patients developing ONJ while on bisphosphonates should receive care by an oral surgeon.

Atypical femur fractures have been reported in patients receiving bisphosphonates for treatment/prevention of osteoporosis. The fractures include subtrochanteric femur (bone just below the hip joint) and diaphyseal femur (long segment of the thigh bone). Some patients experience prodromal pain weeks or months before the fracture occurs. It is unclear if bisphosphonate therapy is the cause for these fractures, although the majority have been reported in patients taking bisphosphonates. Patients receiving long-term (>3-5 years) therapy may be at an increased risk. Discontinue bisphosphonate therapy in patients who develop a femoral shaft fracture.

Infrequently, severe (and occasionally debilitating) bone, joint, and/or muscle pain have been reported during bisphosphonate treatment. The onset of pain ranged from a single day to several months. Consider discontinuing therapy in patients who experience severe symptoms; symptoms usually resolve upon discontinuation. Some patients experienced recurrence when rechallenged with same drug or another bisphosphonate; avoid use in patients with a history of these symptoms in association with bisphosphonate therapy.

Oral bisphosphonates may cause dysphagia, esophagitis, esophageal or gastric ulcer; risk may increase in patients unable to comply with dosing instructions; discontinue use if new or worsening symptoms develop. Intravenous bisphosphonates may cause transient decreases in serum calcium and have also been associated with renal toxicity.

Use not recommended with severe renal impairment (Cl_{cr} <30 mL/minute).
Adverse Reactions (Reflective of adult population; not specific for elderly) Percentages vary based on frequency of administration (daily vs monthly). Unless specified, percentages are reported with oral use.

>10%:
Gastrointestinal: Dyspepsia (6% to 12%)
Neuromuscular & skeletal: Back pain (4% to 14%)
1% to 10%:
Cardiovascular: Hypertension (6% to 7%)
Central nervous system: Headache (3% to 7%), dizziness (1% to 4%), insomnia (1% to 2%)
Dermatologic: Rash (1% to 2%)
Endocrine & metabolic: Hypercholesterolemia (5%)
Gastrointestinal: Abdominal pain (5% to 8%), diarrhea (4% to 7%), nausea (5%), constipation (3% to 4%), vomiting (3%)

Genitourinary: Urinary tract infection (2% to 6%)

Hepatic: Alkaline phosphatase decreased (frequency not defined)

Local: Injection site reaction (<2%)

Neuromuscular & skeletal: Pain in extremity (1% to 8%), arthralgia (4% to 6%), myalgia (1% to 6%), joint disorder (4%), osteonecrosis of the jaw (4%), weakness (4%), osteoarthritis (localized; 1% to 3%), muscle cramp (2%)

Respiratory: Bronchitis (3% to 10%), pneumonia (6%), pharyngitis/nasopharyngitis (3% to 4%), upper respiratory infection (2%)

Miscellaneous: Acute phase reaction (I.V. 10%; oral 3% to 9%), infection (4%), flu-like syndrome (1% to 4%), allergic reaction (3%)

Drug Interactions

Avoid Concomitant Use There are no known interactions where it is recommended to avoid concomitant use.

Increased Effect/Toxicity

Ibandronate may increase the levels/effects of: Deferasirox; Phosphate Supplements

The levels/effects of Ibandronate may be increased by: Aminoglycosides; Nonsteroidal Anti-Inflammatory Agents

Decreased Effect

The levels/effects of Ibandronate may be decreased by: Antacids; Calcium Salts; Iron Salts; Magnesium Salts; Proton Pump Inhibitors

Ethanol/Nutrition/Herb Interactions

Ethanol: Avoid ethanol (may increase risk of osteoporosis).

Food: May reduce absorption; mean oral bioavailability is decreased up to 90% when given with food.

Stability Store at controlled room temperature of 25°C (77°F); excursions permitted to 15°C to 30°C (59°F to 86°F).

Mechanism of Action A bisphosphonate which inhibits bone resorption via actions on osteoclasts or on osteoclast precursors; decreases the rate of bone resorption, leading to an indirect increase in bone mineral density.

Pharmacodynamics/Kinetics

Distribution: Terminal V_d: 90 L; 40% to 50% of circulating ibandronate binds to bone

Protein binding: 85.7% to 99.5%

Metabolism: Not metabolized

Bioavailability: Oral: 2.5 mg tablet: 0.6%; Reduced by 90% following standard breakfast

Half-life elimination:

Oral: 150 mg dose: Terminal: 37-157 hours

I.V.: Terminal: ~5-25 hours

Time to peak, plasma: Oral: 0.5-2 hours

Excretion: Urine (50% to 60% of absorbed dose, excreted as unchanged drug); feces (unabsorbed drug)

Dosage

Geriatric & Adult

Treatment of postmenopausal osteoporosis: Patients should receive supplemental calcium and vitamin D if dietary intake is inadequate

Oral: 2.5 mg once daily **or** 150 mg once a month

I.V.: 3 mg every 3 months

Prevention of postmenopausal osteoporosis: Patients should receive supplemental calcium and vitamin D if dietary intake is inadequate: Oral: 2.5 mg once daily **or** 150 mg once a month

Hypercalcemia of malignancy (unlabeled use): I.V.: 2-4 mg over 2 hours

Metastatic bone disease (unlabeled use):

Oral: 50 mg once daily

I.V.: 6 mg over 1 hour every 3-4 weeks

Renal Impairment

Mild or moderate impairment: Dosing adjustment not needed.

Severe impairment (Cl$_{cr}$ <30 mL/minute): Use not recommended.

Dosage adjustment in renal impairment for oncologic uses (unlabeled): Severe impairment (Cl$_{cr}$ <30 mL/minute):

Oral: 50 mg once weekly

I.V.: 2 mg over 1 hour every 3-4 weeks

Hepatic Impairment Dosing adjustment not needed.

Administration

Oral: Should be administered 60 minutes before the first food or drink of the day (other than water) and prior to taking any oral medications or supplements (eg, calcium, antacids, vitamins). Ibandronate should be taken in an upright position with a full glass (6-8 oz) of plain water and the patient should avoid lying down for 60 minutes to minimize the possibility of GI

◀ side effects. Mineral water with a high calcium content should be avoided. The tablet should be swallowed whole; do not chew or suck. Do not eat or drink anything (except water) for 60 minutes following administration of ibandronate.

Once-monthly dosing: The 150 mg tablet should be taken on the same date each month. In case of a missed dose, do not take two 150 mg tablets within the same week. If the next scheduled dose is 1-7 days away, wait until the next scheduled dose to take the tablet. If the next scheduled dose is >7 days away, take the dose the morning it is remembered, and then resume taking the once-monthly dose on the originally scheduled day.

I.V.: Administer as a 15-30 second bolus. Do not mix with calcium-containing solutions or other drugs. For osteoporosis, do not administer more frequently than every 3 months. Infuse over 1 hour for metastatic bone disease and over 2 hours for hypercalcemia of malignancy.

Monitoring Parameters

Osteoporosis: Bone mineral density as measured by central dual-energy x-ray absorptiometry (DXA) of the hip or spine (prior to initiation of therapy and at least every 2 years); annual measurements of height and weight, assessment of chronic back pain; serum calcium and 25(OH)D; may consider measuring biochemical markers of bone turnover

Serum creatinine prior to each I.V. dose

Test Interactions Bisphosphonates may interfere with diagnostic imaging agents such as technetium-99m-diphosphonate in bone scans.

Special Geriatric Considerations The elderly are frequently treated long-term for osteoporosis. Elderly patients should be advised to report any lower extremity, jaw (osteonecrosis), or muscle pain that cannot be explained or lasts longer than 2 weeks. Additionally, the elderly often receive concomitant diuretic therapy and therefore their electrolyte status (eg, calcium, phosphate) should be periodically evaluated. Since the elderly may have creatinine clearances <30 mL/minute, creatinine clearance should be measured or calculated before initiating therapy with ibandronate.

Dosage Forms Excipient information presented when available (limited, particularly for generics); consult specific product labeling. [DSC] = Discontinued product

Injection, solution:

Boniva®: 1 mg/mL (3 mL)

Tablet, oral:

Boniva®: 2.5 mg [DSC] [once-daily formulation]

Boniva®: 150 mg [once-monthly formulation]

Selected References

Barrett J, Worth E, Bauss F, et al, "Ibandronate: A Clinical Pharmacological and Pharmacokinetic Update," *J Clin Pharmacol*, 2004, 44(9):951-65.

Hillner BE, Ingle JN, Chlebowski RT, et al, "American Society of Clinical Oncology 2003 Update on the Role of Bisphosphonates and Bone Health Issues in Women With Breast Cancer," *J Clin Oncol*, 2003, 21(21):4042-57.

McCormack PL and Plosker GL, "Ibandronic Acid: A Review of Its Use in the Treatment of Bone Metastases of Breast Cancer," *Drugs*, 2006, 66(5):711-28.

Ruggiero SL, Mehrotra B, Rosenberg TJ, et al, "Osteonecrosis of the Jaws Associated With the Use of Bisphosphonates: A Review of 63 Cases," *J Oral Maxillofac Surg*, 2004, 62(5):527-34.

Tripathy D, Body JJ, and Bergstrom B, "Review of Ibandronate in the Treatment of Metastatic Bone Disease: Experience From Phase III Trials," *Clin Ther*, 2004, 26(12):1947-59.

Von Moos R, "Bisphosphonate Treatment Recommendations for Oncologists," *Oncologist*, 2005, 10(Suppl 1):19-24.

♦ **Ibandronate Sodium** *see* Ibandronate *on page 906*

♦ **Ibandronic Acid** *see* Ibandronate *on page 906*

♦ **Ibidomide Hydrochloride** *see* Labetalol *on page 1015*

♦ **Ibu®** *see* Ibuprofen *on page 908*

♦ **Ibu-200 [OTC]** *see* Ibuprofen *on page 908*

Ibuprofen (eye byoo PROE fen)

Medication Safety Issues

Sound-alike/look-alike issues:

Haltran® may be confused with Halfprin®

Motrin® may be confused with Neurontin®

Administration issues:

Injectable formulations: Both ibuprofen and ibuprofen lysine are available for parenteral use. Ibuprofen lysine is **only** indicated for closure of a clinically-significant patent ductus arteriosus.

Brand Names: U.S. Addaprin [OTC]; Advil® Children's [OTC]; Advil® Infants' [OTC]; Advil® Migraine [OTC]; Advil® [OTC]; Caldolor™; I-Prin [OTC]; Ibu-200 [OTC]; Ibu®; Midol® Cramps & Body Aches [OTC]; Motrin® Children's [OTC]; Motrin® IB [OTC]; Motrin® Infants' [OTC]; Motrin® Junior [OTC]; Proprinal® [OTC]; Ultraprin [OTC]

Brand Names: Canada Advil®; Apo-Ibuprofen®; Motrin® (Children's); Motrin® IB; Novo-Profen; Nu-Ibuprofen

Index Terms *p*-Isobutylhydratropic Acid

Generic Availability (U.S.) Yes: Caplet, softgel capsule, suspension, tablet

Pharmacologic Category Nonsteroidal Anti-inflammatory Drug (NSAID), Oral

Use

Oral: Inflammatory diseases and rheumatoid disorders including juvenile rheumatoid arthritis, mild-to-moderate pain, fever, dysmenorrhea, osteoarthritis

Ibuprofen injection (Caldolor™): Management of mild-to-moderate pain; management moderate-to-severe pain when used concurrently with an opioid analgesic; reduction of fever

Unlabeled/Investigational Use Cystic fibrosis, gout, ankylosing spondylitis, acute migraine headache

Medication Guide Available Yes

Contraindications Hypersensitivity to ibuprofen; history of asthma, urticaria, or allergic-type reaction to aspirin or other NSAIDs; aspirin triad (eg, bronchial asthma, aspirin intolerance, rhinitis); perioperative pain in the setting of coronary artery bypass graft (CABG) surgery

Warnings/Precautions [U.S. Boxed Warning: NSAIDs are associated with an increased risk of adverse cardiovascular thrombotic events, including fatal MI and stroke. Risk may be increased with duration of use or pre-existing cardiovascular risk factors or disease. Carefully evaluate individual cardiovascular risk profiles prior to prescribing. May cause new-onset hypertension or worsening of existing hypertension. Response to ACE inhibitors, thiazides, or loop diuretics may be impaired with concurrent use of NSAIDs. Use caution with fluid retention. Avoid use in heart failure. Concurrent administration of ibuprofen, and potentially other nonselective NSAIDs, may interfere with aspirin's cardioprotective effect. **[U.S. Boxed Warning]: Use is contraindicated for treatment of perioperative pain in the setting of coronary artery bypass graft (CABG) surgery.** Risk of MI and stroke may be increased with use following CABG surgery.

May increase the risk of aseptic meningitis, especially in patients with systemic lupus erythematosus (SLE) and mixed connective tissue disorders. Platelet adhesion and aggregation may be decreased; may prolong bleeding time; patients with coagulation disorders or who are receiving anticoagulants should be monitored closely. Anemia may occur; patients on long-term NSAID therapy should be monitored for anemia. Rarely, NSAID use may cause severe blood dyscrasias (eg, agranulocytosis, aplastic anemia, thrombocytopenia).

NSAID use may compromise existing renal function; dose-dependent decreases in prostaglandin synthesis may result from NSAID use, reducing renal blood flow which may cause renal decompensation. NSAID use may increase the risk for hyperkalemia. Patients with impaired renal function, dehydration, heart failure, liver dysfunction, those taking diuretics, and ACE inhibitors, and the elderly are at greater risk of renal toxicity and hyperkalemia. Rehydrate patient before starting therapy; monitor renal function closely. Not recommended for use in patients with advanced renal disease. Long-term NSAID use may result in renal papillary necrosis.

NSAIDs may increase risk of gastrointestinal irritation, inflammation, ulceration, bleeding, and perforation. These events can be fatal and may occur at any time during therapy and without warning. Use caution with a history of GI disease (bleeding or ulcers), concurrent therapy with aspirin, anticoagulants and/or corticosteroids, smoking, use of ethanol, the elderly or debilitated patients. When used concomitantly with ≤325 mg of aspirin, a substantial increase in the risk of gastrointestinal complications (eg, ulcer) occurs; concomitant gastroprotective therapy (eg, proton pump inhibitors) is recommended (Bhatt, 2008).

Use the lowest effective dose for the shortest duration of time, consistent with individual patient goals, to reduce risk of cardiovascular or GI adverse events. Alternate therapies should be considered for patients at high risk.

NSAIDs may cause serious skin adverse events including exfoliative dermatitis, Stevens-Johnson Syndrome (SJS) and toxic epidermal necrolysis (TEN); discontinue use at first sign of skin rash or hypersensitivity. Anaphylactoid reactions may occur, even without prior exposure; patients with "aspirin triad" (bronchial asthma, aspirin intolerance, rhinitis) may be at increased risk. Do not use in patients who experience bronchospasm, asthma, rhinitis, or urticaria with NSAID or aspirin therapy. Use caution in other forms of asthma.

NSAIDS may cause drowsiness, dizziness, blurred vision and other neurologic effects which may impair physical or mental abilities; patients must be cautioned about performing tasks which require mental alertness (eg, operating machinery or driving). Monitor vision with long-term therapy. Blurred/diminished vision, scotomata, and changes in color vision have been reported. Discontinue use with altered vision and perform ophthalmologic exam.

Use with caution in patients with decreased hepatic function. Closely monitor patients with any abnormal LFT. Severe hepatic reactions (eg, fulminant hepatitis, liver failure) have occurred

◄ with NSAID use, rarely; discontinue if signs or symptoms of liver disease develop, or if systemic manifestations occur.

The elderly are at increased risk for adverse effects (especially serious gastrointestinal events, CNS effects, renal toxicity) from NSAIDs even at low doses.

Withhold for at least 4-6 half-lives prior to surgical or dental procedures. Some products may contain phenylalanine. Ibuprofen injection (Caldolor™) must be diluted prior to administration; hemolysis can occur if not diluted.

Self medication (OTC use): Prior to self-medication, patients should contact healthcare provider if they have had recurring stomach pain or upset, ulcers, bleeding problems, high blood pressure, heart or kidney disease, other serious medical problems, are currently taking a diuretic, aspirin, anticoagulant, or are ≥60 years of age. If patients are using for migraines, they should also contact healthcare provider if they have not had a migraine diagnosis by healthcare provider, a headache that is different from usual migraine, worst headache of life, fever and neck stiffness, headache from head injury or coughing, first headache at ≥50 years of age, daily headache, or migraine requiring bed rest. Recommended dosages should not be exceeded, due to an increased risk of GI bleeding. Stop use and consult a healthcare provider if symptoms get worse, newly appear, fever lasts for >3 days or pain lasts >10 days (adults). Do not give for >10 days unless instructed by healthcare provider. Consuming ≥3 alcoholic beverages/day or taking longer than recommended may increase the risk of GI bleeding.

Adverse Reactions (Reflective of adult population; not specific for elderly)
Oral:
1% to 10%:
Cardiovascular: Edema (1% to 3%)
Central nervous system: Dizziness (3% to 9%), headache (1% to 3%), nervousness (1% to 3%)
Dermatologic: Rash (3% to 9%), itching (1% to 3%)
Endocrine & metabolic: Fluid retention (1% to 3%)
Gastrointestinal: Epigastric pain (3% to 9%), heartburn (3% to 9%), nausea (3% to 9%), abdominal pain/cramps/distress (1% to 3%), appetite decreased (1% to 3%), constipation (1% to 3%), diarrhea (1% to 3%), dyspepsia (1% to 3%), flatulence (1% to 3%), vomiting (1% to 3%)
Otic: Tinnitus (3% to 9%)

Injection: Ibuprofen (Caldolor™): Abdominal pain, anemia, BUN increased, cough, dizziness, dyspepsia, edema, flatulence, headache, hemorrhage, hypokalemia, hypernatremia, hypertension, nausea, neutropenia, pruritus, urinary retention, vomiting

Drug Interactions
Metabolism/Transport Effects Substrate (minor) of CYP2C9, 2C19; **Inhibits** CYP2C9 (strong)
Avoid Concomitant Use
Avoid concomitant use of Ibuprofen with any of the following: Floctafenine; Ketorolac; Ketorolac (Nasal); Ketorolac (Systemic)
Increased Effect/Toxicity
Ibuprofen may increase the levels/effects of: Aminoglycosides; Anticoagulants; Antiplatelet Agents; Bisphosphonate Derivatives; Collagenase (Systemic); CycloSPORINE; CycloSPORINE (Systemic); Deferasirox; Desmopressin; Digoxin; Drotrecogin Alfa; Eplerenone; Haloperidol; Ibritumomab; Lithium; Methotrexate; Nonsteroidal Anti-Inflammatory Agents; PEMEtrexed; Porfimer; Potassium-Sparing Diuretics; PRALAtrexate; Quinolone Antibiotics; Rivaroxaban; Salicylates; Thrombolytic Agents; Tositumomab and Iodine I 131 Tositumomab; Vancomycin; Vitamin K Antagonists

The levels/effects of Ibuprofen may be increased by: ACE Inhibitors; Angiotensin II Receptor Blockers; Antidepressants (Tricyclic, Tertiary Amine); Corticosteroids (Systemic); Dasatinib; Floctafenine; Glucosamine; Herbs (Anticoagulant/Antiplatelet Properties); Ketorolac; Ketorolac (Nasal); Ketorolac (Systemic); Nonsteroidal Anti-Inflammatory Agents; Omega-3-Acid Ethyl Esters; Pentosan Polysulfate Sodium; Pentoxifylline; Probenecid; Prostacyclin Analogues; Selective Serotonin Reuptake Inhibitors; Serotonin/Norepinephrine Reuptake Inhibitors; Sodium Phosphates; Treprostinil; Vitamin E; Voriconazole
Decreased Effect
Ibuprofen may decrease the levels/effects of: ACE Inhibitors; Angiotensin II Receptor Blockers; Antiplatelet Agents; Beta-Blockers; Eplerenone; HydrALAZINE; Potassium-Sparing Diuretics; Salicylates; Selective Serotonin Reuptake Inhibitors; Thiazide Diuretics

The levels/effects of Ibuprofen may be decreased by: Bile Acid Sequestrants; Nonsteroidal Anti-Inflammatory Agents; Salicylates
Ethanol/Nutrition/Herb Interactions
Ethanol: Avoid ethanol (may enhance gastric mucosal irritation).

Food: Ibuprofen peak serum levels may be decreased if taken with food.

Herb/Nutraceutical: Avoid alfalfa, anise, bilberry, bladderwrack, bromelain, cat's claw, celery, chamomile, coleus, cordyceps, dong quai, evening primrose, fenugreek, feverfew, garlic, ginger, ginkgo biloba, ginseng (American, Panax, Siberian), grapeseed, green tea, guggul, horse chestnut seed, horseradish, licorice, prickly ash, red clover, reishi, SAMe (S-adenosylmethionine), sweet clover, turmeric, white willow (all have additional antiplatelet activity).

Stability

Ibuprofen injection (Caldolor™): Store intact vials at room temperature of 20°C to 25°C (68°F to 77°F). Must be diluted prior to use. Dilute with D_5W, NS or LR to a final concentration ≤4 mg/mL. Diluted solutions stable for 24 hours at room temperature.

Suspension, tablet: Store at room temperature of 20°C to 25°C (68°F to 77°F).

Mechanism of Action Reversibly inhibits cyclooxygenase-1 and 2 (COX-1 and 2) enzymes, which results in decreased formation of prostaglandin precursors; has antipyretic, analgesic, and anti-inflammatory properties

Other proposed mechanisms not fully elucidated (and possibly contributing to the anti-inflammatory effect to varying degrees), include inhibiting chemotaxis, altering lymphocyte activity, inhibiting neutrophil aggregation/activation, and decreasing proinflammatory cytokine levels.

Pharmacodynamics/Kinetics

Onset of action: Oral: Analgesic: 30-60 minutes; Anti-inflammatory: ≤7 days

Peak effect: Oral: 1-2 weeks

Duration: Oral: 4-6 hours

Absorption: Oral: Rapid (85%)

Distribution: V_d: 6.35 L

Protein binding: 90% to 99%

Metabolism: Hepatic via oxidation

Half-life elimination: Adults: 2-4 hours; End-stage renal disease: Unchanged

Time to peak: Oral: ~1-2 hours

Excretion: Urine (primarily as metabolites; 1% as unchanged drug); some feces

Dosage

Geriatric & Adult

Inflammatory disease: Oral: 400-800 mg/dose 3-4 times/day (maximum: 3.2 g/day)

Analgesia/pain/fever/dysmenorrhea: Oral: 200-400 mg/dose every 4-6 hours (maximum daily dose: 1.2 g, unless directed by physician; under physician supervision daily doses ≤2.4 g may be used)

Analgesic: I.V. (Caldolor™): 400-800 mg every 6 hours as needed (maximum: 3.2 g/day). **Note:** Patients should be well hydrated prior to administration.

Antipyretic: I.V. (Caldolor™): Initial: 400 mg, then every 4-6 hours or 100-200 mg every 4 hours as needed (maximum: 3.2 g/day). **Note:** Patients should be well hydrated prior to administration.

OTC labeling (analgesic, antipyretic): Oral: 200 mg every 4-6 hours as needed (maximum: 1200 mg/24 hours); treatment for >10 days is not recommended unless directed by healthcare provider.

Migraine: 2 capsules at onset of symptoms (maximum: 400 mg/24 hours unless directed by healthcare provider)

Renal Impairment If anuria or oliguria evident, hold dose until renal function returns to normal.

Hepatic Impairment Avoid use in severe hepatic impairment.

Administration

Oral: Administer with food

I.V.:

Caldolor™: For I.V. administration only; must be diluted to a final concentration of ≤4 mg/mL prior to administration; infuse over at least 30 minutes

Monitoring Parameters Monitor response (pain, range of motion, grip strength, mobility, ADL function), inflammation; observe for weight gain, edema; monitor renal function; observe for bleeding, bruising; evaluate gastrointestinal effects (abdominal pain, bleeding, dyspepsia); mental confusion, disorientation, CBC, serum, creatinine, BUN, liver function tests

Reference Range Plasma concentrations >200 mcg/mL may be associated with severe toxicity

PDA: Minimum effective concentration: 10-12 mg/L

Test Interactions May interfere with urine detection of PCP, cannabinoids, and barbiturates (false-positives)

Pharmacotherapy Pearls There are no clinical guidelines to predict which NSAID will give response in a particular patient. Trials with each must be initiated until response determined. Consider dose, patient convenience, and cost.

◀ **Special Geriatric Considerations** Elderly are a high-risk population for adverse effects from NSAIDs. As much as 60% of elderly can develop peptic ulceration and/or hemorrhage asymptomatically. The concomitant use of H_2 blockers and sucralfate is not effective as prophylaxis with the exception of NSAID-induced duodenal ulcers which may be prevented by the use of ranitidine. Misoprostol and proton pump inhibitors are the only agents proven to help prevent the development of NSAID-induced ulcers. Also, concomitant disease and drug use contribute to the risk for GI adverse effects. Use lowest effective dose for shortest period possible. Consider renal function decline with age. Use of NSAIDs can compromise existing renal function especially when Cl_{cr} is ≤30 mL/minute. Tinnitus may be a difficult and unreliable indication of toxicity due to age-related hearing loss or eighth cranial nerve damage. CNS adverse effects such as confusion, agitation, and hallucination are generally seen in overdose or high dose situations, but the elderly may demonstrate these adverse effects at lower doses than younger adults.

Dosage Forms Excipient information presented when available (limited, particularly for generics); consult specific product labeling. [DSC] = Discontinued product
Caplet, oral: 200 mg
  Advil®: 200 mg [contains sodium benzoate]
  Ibu-200: 200 mg [DSC]
  Motrin® IB: 200 mg
  Motrin® Junior: 100 mg [scored]
Capsule, liquid filled, oral:
  Advil®: 200 mg [contains potassium 20 mg/capsule; solubilized ibuprofen]
  Advil® Migraine: 200 mg [contains potassium 20 mg/capsule; solubilized ibuprofen]
Capsule, softgel, oral: 200 mg
Gelcap, oral:
  Advil®: 200 mg [contains coconut oil]
Injection, solution:
  Caldolor™: 100 mg/mL (4 mL, 8 mL)
Suspension, oral: 100 mg/5 mL (5 mL, 10 mL, 120 mL, 240 mL [DSC], 480 mL)
  Advil® Children's: 100 mg/5 mL (120 mL) [contains propylene glycol, sodium 10 mg/5 mL, sodium benzoate; blue raspberry flavor]
  Advil® Children's: 100 mg/5 mL (120 mL) [contains propylene glycol, sodium 3 mg/5 mL, sodium benzoate; grape flavor]
  Advil® Children's: 100 mg/5 mL (120 mL) [contains sodium 3 mg/5 mL, sodium benzoate; fruit flavor]
  Motrin® Children's: 100 mg/5 mL (120 mL) [dye free, ethanol free; contains sodium 2 mg/5 mL, sodium benzoate; berry flavor]
  Motrin® Children's: 100 mg/5 mL (60 mL, 120 mL) [ethanol free; contains sodium 2 mg/5 mL, sodium benzoate; berry flavor]
  Motrin® Children's: 100 mg/5 mL (120 mL) [ethanol free; contains sodium 2 mg/5 mL, sodium benzoate; bubblegum flavor]
  Motrin® Children's: 100 mg/5 mL (120 mL) [ethanol free; contains sodium 2 mg/5 mL, sodium benzoate; grape flavor]
  Motrin® Children's: 100 mg/5 mL (120 mL) [ethanol free; contains sodium 2 mg/5 mL, sodium benzoate; tropical punch flavor]
Suspension, oral [concentrate/drops]: 40 mg/mL (15 mL)
  Advil® Infants': 40 mg/mL (15 mL) [contains sodium benzoate; grape flavor]
  Advil® Infants': 40 mg/mL (15 mL) [dye free; contains propylene glycol, sodium benzoate; white grape flavor]
  Motrin® Infants': 40 mg/mL (15 mL) [dye free, ethanol free; contains sodium benzoate; berry flavor]
  Motrin® Infants': 40 mg/mL (15 mL) [ethanol free; contains sodium benzoate; berry flavor]
Tablet, oral: 200 mg, 400 mg, 600 mg, 800 mg
  Addaprin: 200 mg
  Advil®: 200 mg [contains sodium benzoate]
  I-Prin: 200 mg
  Ibu-200: 200 mg
  Ibu®: 400 mg, 600 mg, 800 mg
  Midol® Cramps & Body Aches: 200 mg
  Motrin® IB: 200 mg
  Proprinal®: 200 mg [contains sodium benzoate]
  Ultraprin: 200 mg [sugar free]
Tablet, chewable, oral:
  Motrin® Junior: 100 mg [contains phenylalanine 2.8 mg/tablet; grape flavor]
  Motrin® Junior: 100 mg [contains phenylalanine 2.8 mg/tablet; orange flavor]

◆ **ICI-182,780** see Fulvestrant on page 799
◆ **ICI-204,219** see Zafirlukast on page 1937

- **ICI-46474** *see* Tamoxifen *on page 1731*
- **ICI-118630** *see* Goserelin *on page 840*
- **ICI-176334** *see* Bicalutamide *on page 201*
- **ICI-D1033** *see* Anastrozole *on page 134*
- **ICL670** *see* Deferasirox *on page 462*
- **IG** *see* Immune Globulin *on page 922*
- **IGIM** *see* Immune Globulin *on page 922*
- **IGIV** *see* Immune Globulin *on page 922*
- **IL-1Ra** *see* Anakinra *on page 132*

Iloperidone (eye loe PER i done)

Related Information
Antipsychotic Agents *on page 1997*
Atypical Antipsychotics *on page 1999*
Medication Safety Issues
Sound-alike/look-alike issues:
Fanapt® may be confused with Xanax®
Iloperidone may be confused with domperidone
Brand Names: U.S. Fanapt®
Generic Availability (U.S.) No
Pharmacologic Category Antipsychotic Agent, Atypical
Use Acute treatment of schizophrenia
Contraindications Hypersensitivity to iloperidone or any component of the formulation
Warnings/Precautions [U.S. Boxed Warning]: Elderly patients with dementia-related psychosis treated with antipsychotics are at an increased risk of death compared to placebo. Most deaths appeared to be either cardiovascular (eg, heart failure, sudden death) or infectious (eg, pneumonia) in nature. In addition, an increased incidence of cerebrovascular effects (eg, transient ischemic attack, cerebrovascular accidents) has been reported in studies of placebo-controlled trials of antipsychotics in elderly patients with dementia-related psychosis. Iloperidone is not approved for the treatment of dementia-related psychosis.

May be sedating; use with caution in disorders where CNS depression is a feature. Caution in patients with predisposition to seizures. Use is not recommended in patients with hepatic impairment. Esophageal dysmotility and aspiration have been associated with antipsychotic use; use with caution in patients at risk of aspiration pneumonia (ie, Alzheimer's disease). Use is associated with increased prolactin levels; clinical significance of hyperprolactinemia in patients with breast cancer or other prolactin-dependent tumors is unknown. May alter temperature regulation. Leukopenia, neutropenia, and agranulocytosis (sometimes fatal) have been reported in clinical trials and postmarketing reports; presence of risk factors (eg, pre-existing low WBC or history of drug-induced leuko-/neutropenia) should prompt periodic blood count assessment and discontinuation at first signs of blood dyscrasias.

May alter cardiac conduction and prolong the QT_c interval; life-threatening arrhythmias have occurred with therapeutic doses of antipsychotics. Risks may be increased by conditions or concomitant medications which cause bradycardia, hypokalemia, and/or hypomagnesemia. Avoid use in combination with QT_c-prolonging drugs and in patients with congenital long QT syndrome, history of cardiac arrhythmia, recent MI, or uncompensated heart failure. Discontinue treatment in patients found to have persistent QT_c intervals >500 msec. Further cardiac evaluation is warranted in patients with symptoms of dizziness, palpitations, or syncope. May cause orthostatic hypotension; use with caution in patients at risk of this effect (eg, concurrent medication use which may predispose to hypotension/bradycardia or presence of hypovolemia) or in those who would not tolerate transient hypotensive episodes. Use with caution in patients with cardiovascular diseases (eg, heart failure, history of myocardial infarction or ischemia, cerebrovascular disease, conduction abnormalities).

May cause anticholinergic effects (confusion, agitation, constipation, xerostomia, blurred vision, urinary retention); therefore, use with caution in patients with decreased gastrointestinal motility, urinary retention, BPH, xerostomia, or visual problems (including narrow-angle glaucoma). May cause extrapyramidal symptoms (EPS), including pseudoparkinsonism, acute dystonic reactions, akathisia, and tardive dyskinesia. Risk of dystonia (and probably other EPS) may be greater with increased doses, use of conventional antipsychotics, males, and younger patients. Risk of neuroleptic malignant syndrome (NMS) may be increased in patients with Parkinson's disease or Lewy body dementia. May cause hyperglycemia; in some cases may be extreme and associated with ketoacidosis, hyperosmolar coma, or death. Use with caution in patients with diabetes or other disorders of glucose regulation; monitor for worsening of glucose control. Significant weight gain has been observed with antipsychotic therapy; incidence varies with product. Monitor waist circumference and BMI. Rare cases of priapism have been reported.

Dosage adjustments are recommended for iloperidone when given concomitantly with strong CYP2D6 or CYP3A4 inhibitors or in poor metabolizers of CYP2D6. The possibility of a suicide attempt is inherent in psychotic illness; use caution in high-risk patients during initiation of therapy. Prescriptions should be written for the smallest quantity consistent with good patient care. Continued use for >6 weeks has not been evaluated.

Adverse Reactions (Reflective of adult population; not specific for elderly)

>10%:

Cardiovascular: Tachycardia (3% to 12%; dose related)

Central nervous system: Dizziness (10% to 20%; dose related), somnolence (9% to 15%)

1% to 10%:

Cardiovascular: Orthostatic hypotension (3% to 5%), hypotension (1% to 3%; dose related), palpitations (≥1%)

Central nervous system: Fatigue (4% to 6%), extrapyramidal symptoms (≤5%), tremor (3%), lethargy (≤3%), akathisia (2%), aggression (≥1%), delusion (≥1%), restlessness (≥1%)

Dermatologic: Rash (≤3%)

Gastrointestinal: Nausea (≤10%), xerostomia (8% to 10%), weight gain (1% to 9%; dose related), diarrhea (5% to 7%), abdominal discomfort (1% to 3%; dose related), weight loss (≥1%)

Genitourinary: Ejaculation failure (2%), urinary incontinence (≥1%), erectile dysfunction (≥1%)

Neuromuscular & skeletal: Arthralgia (3%), stiffness (1% to 3%; dose related), dyskinesia (<2%), muscle spasm (≥1%), myalgia (≥1%)

Ocular: Blurred vision (≤3%), conjunctivitis (≥1%)

Respiratory: Nasal congestion (5% to 8%), nasopharyngitis (≤4%), upper respiratory tract infection (2% to 3%), dyspnea (2%)

Drug Interactions

Metabolism/Transport Effects Substrate of CYP2D6 (major), 3A4 (minor)

Avoid Concomitant Use

Avoid concomitant use of Iloperidone with any of the following: Artemether; Dronedarone; Lumefantrine; Metoclopramide; Nilotinib; Pimozide; QUEtiapine; QuiNINE; Tetrabenazine; Thioridazine; Toremifene; Vandetanib; Vemurafenib; Ziprasidone

Increased Effect/Toxicity

Iloperidone may increase the levels/effects of: Alcohol (Ethyl); CNS Depressants; Dronedarone; Methylphenidate; Pimozide; QTc-Prolonging Agents; QuiNINE; Selective Serotonin Reuptake Inhibitors; Tetrabenazine; Thioridazine; Toremifene; Vandetanib; Vemurafenib; Ziprasidone

The levels/effects of Iloperidone may be increased by: Abiraterone Acetate; Acetylcholinesterase Inhibitors (Central); Alfuzosin; Artemether; Chloroquine; Ciprofloxacin; Ciprofloxacin (Systemic); CYP2D6 Inhibitors (Moderate); CYP2D6 Inhibitors (Strong); CYP3A4 Inhibitors (Strong); Gadobutrol; HydrOXYzine; Lithium formulations; Lumefantrine; MAO Inhibitors; Methylphenidate; Metoclopramide; Nilotinib; QUEtiapine; QuiNINE; Tetrabenazine

Decreased Effect

Iloperidone may decrease the levels/effects of: Amphetamines; Anti-Parkinson's Agents (Dopamine Agonist); Quinagolide

The levels/effects of Iloperidone may be decreased by: CYP2D6 Inhibitors (Strong); Lithium formulations; Peginterferon Alfa-2b; Tocilizumab

Ethanol/Nutrition/Herb Interactions

Ethanol: May increase CNS depression; monitor for increased effects with coadministration. Caution patients about effects.

Herb/Nutraceutical: Avoid St John's wort (may decrease serum levels of iloperidone). Avoid kava kava, gotu kola, valerian, St John's wort (may increase CNS depression).

Stability Store at 25°C (77°F); excursions permitted to 15°C to 30°C (59°F to 86°F). Protect from light and moisture.

Mechanism of Action Iloperidone is a piperidinyl-benzisoxazole atypical antipsychotic with mixed $D_2/5-HT_2$ antagonist activity. It exhibits high affinity for $5-HT_{2A}$, D_2, and D_3 receptors, low to moderate affinity for D_1, D_4, H_1, $5-HT_{1A}$, $5-HT_6$, $5HT_7$, and $NE_{\alpha 1}$ receptors, and no affinity for muscarinic receptors. The addition of serotonin antagonism to dopamine antagonism (classic neuroleptic mechanism) is thought to improve negative symptoms of psychoses and reduce the incidence of extrapyramidal side effects. Iloperidone's low affinity for histamine H_1 receptors may decrease the risk for weight gain and somnolence while its affinity for $NE_{\alpha 1/\alpha 2C}$ may provide antidepressant and anxiolytic activity and improved cognitive function.

Pharmacodynamics/Kinetics

Absorption: Well absorbed

Distribution: V_d: 1340-2800 L

Protein binding: ~95% (iloperidone and active metabolites)

Metabolism: Hepatic via carbonyl reduction, hydroxylation (CYP2D6) and O-demethylation (CYP3A4); forms active metabolites (P88 and P95)

Bioavailability: Oral: Tablet (relative to solution): 96%

Half-life elimination:

Extensive metabolizers: Iloperidone: 18 hours; P88: 26 hours; P95: 23 hours

Poor metabolizers: Iloperidone: 33 hours; P88: 37 hours; P95: 31 hours

Time to peak, plasma: 2-4 hours

Excretion: Urine (58% extensive metabolizers, 45% poor metabolizers); feces (20% extensive metabolizers, 22% poor metabolizers)

Dosage

Geriatric & Adult Schizophrenia: Oral: Initial: 1 mg twice daily; recommended dosage range: 6-12 mg twice daily (maximum: 24 mg/day)

Recommended titration schedule: Increase in 2 mg increments every 24 hours on days 2-7 (eg, Day 2: 2 mg twice daily; Day 3: 4 mg twice daily; Day 4: 6 mg twice daily; Day 5: 8 mg twice daily; Day 6: 10 mg twice daily; Day 7: 12 mg twice daily)

Note: Titrate dose to effect (to avoid orthostatic hypotensive effects); treatment >6 weeks has not been evaluated; when reinitiating treatment after discontinuation (>3 days), the initial titration schedule should be followed.

Dosage adjustment in patients receiving strong CYP2D6 inhibitors (eg, paroxetine, fluoxetine, quinidine): Decrease iloperidone dose by 50%; when the CYP2D6 inhibitor is discontinued, return to previous dose.

Dosage adjustment in patients receiving strong CYP3A4 inhibitors (eg, ketoconazole, clarithromycin): Decrease iloperidone dose by 50%; when the CYP3A4 inhibitor is discontinued, return to previous dose.

Dosage adjustment in poor metabolizers of CYP2D6: Decrease iloperidone dose by 50%.

Hepatic Impairment Not recommended in patients with hepatic impairment due to lack of data.

Administration May be administered with or without food.

Monitoring Parameters Vital signs; fasting blood glucose/Hgb A_{1c} (prior to treatment and periodically during treatment); signs and symptoms of hyperglycemia; signs and symptoms of cardiac arrhythmia; CBC (frequently during first few months of therapy); serum potassium and magnesium levels (prior to treatment and periodically during treatment); orthostatic blood pressure changes; assess weight prior to and periodically during treatment;

Special Geriatric Considerations Any change in disease status in any organ system may result in behavior changes. EPS appears significantly less than with the other agents in this class. Many elderly patients receive antipsychotic medications for inappropriate nonpsychotic behavior. Before initiating antipsychotic medication, the clinician should investigate any reversible cause; any stress or stress from any disease can cause acute "confusion" or worsening of baseline nonpsychotic behavior. Most commonly, acute changes in behavior are due to increases in drug dose or addition of a new medication to the regimen, fluid and electrolyte loss, infection, or changes in their environment.

Studies of elderly patients with psychosis associated with Alzheimer's disease, treated with antipsychotics, have demonstrated an increased risk of mortality and cardiovascular events as compared to younger patient populations.

Dosage Forms Excipient information presented when available (limited, particularly for generics); consult specific product labeling.

Tablet, oral:

Fanapt®: 1 mg, 2 mg, 4 mg, 6 mg, 8 mg, 10 mg, 12 mg

Tablet, oral [combination package (each titration pack contains)]:

Fanapt®: 1 mg (2s), 2 mg (2s), 4 mg (2s), and 6 mg (2s)

Selected References

Cutler AJ, Kalali AH, Weiden PJ, et al, "Four-Week, Double-Blind, Placebo and Ziprazidone-Controlled Trial of Iloperidone in Patients With Acute Exacerbations of Schizophrenia," *J Clin Psychopharmacol*, 2008;28(2 Suppl 1):20-8.

Dixon L, Perkins D, and Calmes C, *Guideline Watch (September 2009): Practice Guideline for the Treatment of Schizophrenia*, Arlington, Va: American Psychiatric Association, 2009. Available at http://www.psychiatryonline.com/content.aspx?aid=501001.

Kane JM, Lauriello J, Laska E, et al, "Long-Term Efficacy and Safety of Iloperidone: Results From 3 Clinical Trials for the Treatment of Schizophrenia," *J Clin Psychopharmacol*, 2008, 28(2 Suppl 1):29-35.

Potkin SG, Litman RE, Torres R, et al, "Efficacy of iloperidone in the Treatment of Schizophrenia: Initial Phase 3 Studies," *J Clin Psychopharmacol*, 2008, 28(2 Suppl 1):4-11.

Weiden PJ, Cutler AJ, Polymeropoulos MH, et al, "Safety Profile of iloperidone: A Pooled Analysis of 6-Week Acute-Phase pivotal Trials," *J Clin Psychopharmacol*, 2008, 28(2 Suppl 1):12-9.

◆ **Imdur®** see Isosorbide Mononitrate on page 990

- ◆ **Imferon** *see* Iron Dextran Complex *on page 977*
- ◆ **Imipemide** *see* Imipenem and Cilastatin *on page 916*

Imipenem and Cilastatin (i mi PEN em & sye la STAT in)

Related Information
Antibiotic Treatment of Adults With Infective Endocarditis *on page 2053*
Medication Safety Issues
Sound-alike/look-alike issues:
Imipenem may be confused with ertapenem, meropenem
Primaxin® may be confused with Premarin®, Primacor®
Brand Names: U.S. Primaxin® I.V.
Brand Names: Canada Imipenem and Cilastatin for Injection; Primaxin® I.V. Infusion; RAN™-Imipenem-Cilastatin
Index Terms Imipemide; Primaxin® I.M. [DSC]
Generic Availability (U.S.) No
Pharmacologic Category Antibiotic, Carbapenem
Use Treatment of lower respiratory tract, urinary tract, intra-abdominal, gynecologic, bone and joint, skin and skin structure, endocarditis (caused by *Staphylococcus aureus*) and polymicrobic infections as well as bacterial septicemia. Antibacterial activity includes gram-positive bacteria (methicillin-sensitive *S. aureus* and *Streptococcus* spp), resistant gram-negative bacilli (including extended spectrum beta-lactamase-producing *Escherichia coli* and *Klebsiella* spp, *Enterobacter* spp, and *Pseudomonas aeruginosa*), and anaerobes.
Unlabeled/Investigational Use Hepatic abscess; neutropenic fever; melioidosis
Contraindications Hypersensitivity to imipenem/cilastatin or any component of the formulation
Warnings/Precautions Dosage adjustment required in patients with impaired renal function; elderly patients often require lower doses (adjust carefully to renal function). Prolonged use may result in fungal or bacterial superinfection, including *C. difficile*-associated diarrhea (CDAD) and pseudomembranous colitis; CDAD has been observed >2 months postantibiotic treatment. Has been associated with CNS adverse effects, including confusional states and seizures (myoclonic); use with caution in patients with a history of seizures or hypersensitivity to beta-lactams (including penicillins and cephalosporins); patients with impaired renal function are at increased risk of seizures if not properly dose adjusted. May decrease divalproex sodium/valproic acid concentrations leading to breakthrough seizures; concomitant use not recommended. Serious hypersensitivity reactions, including anaphylaxis, have been reported (some without a history of previous allergic reactions to beta-lactams). Doses for I.M. administration are mixed with lidocaine; consult information on lidocaine for associated warnings/precautions. Two different imipenem/cilastatin products are available; due to differences in formulation, the I.V. and I.M. preparations **cannot** be interchanged.
Adverse Reactions (Reflective of adult population; not specific for elderly) Adverse reactions reported with use for both I.V. and I.M. formulations in adults, except where noted.
1% to 10%:
Cardiovascular: Tachycardia (infants 2%; adults <1%)
Central nervous system: Seizure (infants 6%; adults <1%)
Dermatologic: Rash (≤1%, children 2%)
Gastrointestinal: Nausea (1% to 2%), diarrhea (children 3% to 4%; adults 1% to 2%), vomiting (≤2%)
Genitourinary: Oliguria/anuria (infants 2%; adults <1%)
Local: Phlebitis/thrombophlebitis (3%), pain at I.M. injection site (1.2%)
Drug Interactions
Avoid Concomitant Use
Avoid concomitant use of Imipenem and Cilastatin with any of the following: BCG; Ganciclovir (Systemic); Ganciclovir-Valganciclovir
Increased Effect/Toxicity
Imipenem and Cilastatin may increase the levels/effects of: CycloSPORINE; CycloSPORINE (Systemic)

The levels/effects of Imipenem and Cilastatin may be increased by: CycloSPORINE; CycloSPORINE (Systemic); Ganciclovir (Systemic); Ganciclovir-Valganciclovir; Probenecid
Decreased Effect
Imipenem and Cilastatin may decrease the levels/effects of: BCG; CycloSPORINE; CycloSPORINE (Systemic); Divalproex; Typhoid Vaccine; Valproic Acid
Stability Imipenem/cilastatin powder for injection should be stored at <25°C (77°F).
I.V.: Prior to use, dilute dose into 100-250 mL of an appropriate solution. Imipenem is inactivated at acidic or alkaline pH. Final concentration should not exceed 5 mg/mL. The I.M. formulation is not buffered and cannot be used to prepare I.V. solutions. Reconstituted

I.V. solutions are stable for 4 hours at room temperature and 24 hours when refrigerated. Do not freeze.

Mechanism of Action Inhibits bacterial cell wall synthesis by binding to one or more of the penicillin-binding proteins (PBPs); which in turn inhibits the final transpeptidation step of peptidoglycan synthesis in bacterial cell walls, thus inhibiting cell wall biosynthesis. Bacteria eventually lyse due to ongoing activity of cell wall autolytic enzymes (autolysins and murein hydrolases) while cell wall assembly is arrested. Cilastatin prevents renal metabolism of imipenem by competitive inhibition of dehydropeptidase along the brush border of the renal tubules.

Pharmacodynamics/Kinetics

Distribution: Rapidly and widely to most tissues and fluids including sputum, pleural fluid, peritoneal fluid, interstitial fluid, bile, aqueous humor, and bone; highest concentrations in pleural fluid, interstitial fluid, and peritoneal fluid; low concentrations in CSF

Protein binding: Imipenem: 20%; cilastatin: 40%

Metabolism: Imipenem is metabolized in the kidney by dehydropeptidase I; cilastatin prevents imipenem metabolism by this enzyme; cilastatin is partially metabolized renally

Half-life elimination: I.V.: Both drugs: 60 minutes; prolonged with renal impairment

Excretion: Both drugs: Urine (~70% as unchanged drug)

Dosage

Geriatric & Adult Doses based on **imipenem** content.

Usual dosage range: Weight ≥70 kg: 250-1000 mg every 6-8 hours; maximum: 4 g/day. **Note:** For adults weighing <70 kg, refer to Dosage: Renal Impairment.

Indication-specific dosing:

Burkholderia pseudomallei **(melioidosis) (unlabeled use):** I.V.: Initial: 20 mg/kg every 8 hours for at least 10 days (White, 2003) **or** 25 mg/kg (up to 1 g) every 6 hours for at least 10 days (Currie, 2003); continue parenteral therapy until clinical improvement then switch to oral therapy if tolerated and/or appropriate.

Intra-abdominal infections: I.V.:

Mild infection: 250-500 mg every 6 hours

Severe infection: 500 mg every 6 hours **or** 1 g every 8 hours for 4-7 days (provided source controlled). **Note:** Not recommended for mild-to-moderate, community-acquired intra-abdominal infections due to risk of toxicity and the development of resistant organisms (Solomkin, 2010)

Liver abscess (unlabeled use): I.V.: 500 mg every 6 hours for 4-6 weeks (Ulug, 2010)

Moderate infections: I.V.:

Fully-susceptible organisms: 500 mg every 6-8 hours

Moderately-susceptible organisms: 500 mg every 6 hours or 1 g every 8 hours

Neutropenic fever (unlabeled use): I.V.: 500 mg every 6 hours (Paul, 2006)

Pseudomonas **infections:** I.V.: 500 mg every 6 hours; **Note:** Higher doses may be required based on organism sensitivity.

Severe infections: I.V.:

Fully-susceptible organisms: 500 mg every 6 hours

Moderately-susceptible organisms: 1 g every 6-8 hours

Maximum daily dose should not exceed 50 mg/kg or 4 g/day, whichever is lower

Urinary tract infection, uncomplicated: I.V.: 250 mg every 6 hours

Urinary tract infection, complicated: I.V.: 500 mg every 6 hours

Mild infections: Note: Rarely a suitable option in mild infections; normally reserved for moderate-severe cases: I.V.:

Fully-susceptible organisms: 250 mg every 6 hours

Moderately-susceptible organisms: 500 mg every 6 hours

Renal Impairment I.V.:

Patients with a Cl_{cr} ≤5 mL/minute/1.73 m^2 should not receive imipenem/cilastatin unless hemodialysis is instituted within 48 hours.

Patients weighing <30 kg with impaired renal function should not receive imipenem/cilastatin.

Reduced I.V. dosage regimen based on creatinine clearance and/or body weight: See table on next page.

Intermittent hemodialysis (IHD) (administer after hemodialysis on dialysis days): Use the dosing recommendation for patients with a Cl_{cr} 6-20 mL/minute; administer dose after dialysis session and every 12 hours thereafter **or** 250-500 mg every 12 hours (Heintz, 2009). **Note:** Dosing dependent on the assumption of 3 times/week, complete IHD sessions.

Peritoneal dialysis (unlabeled dosing): Dose as for Cl_{cr} 6-20 mL/minute (Somani, 1988)

Continuous renal replacement therapy (CRRT) (Heintz, 2009; Trotman, 2005): Drug clearance is highly dependent on the method of renal replacement, filter type, and flow rate. Appropriate dosing requires close monitoring of pharmacologic response, signs of adverse reactions due to drug accumulation, as well as drug concentrations in relation to target trough (if appropriate). The following are general recommendations only (based on dialysate flow/ultrafiltration rates of 1-2 L/hour and minimal residual renal function) and should not supersede clinical judgment:

CVVH: Loading dose of 1 g followed by either 250 mg every 6 hours **or** 500 mg every 8 hours

CVVHD: Loading dose of 1 g followed by either 250 mg every 6 hours **or** 500 mg every 6-8 hours

CVVHDF: Loading dose of 1 g followed by either 250 mg every 6 hours **or** 500 mg every 6 hours

Note: Data suggest that 500 mg every 8-12 hours may provide sufficient time above MIC to cover organisms with MIC values ≤2 mg/L; however, a higher dose of 500 mg every 6 hours is recommended for resistant organisms (particularly *Pseudomonas* spp) with MIC ≥4 mg/L or deep-seated infections (Fish, 2005).

Reduced I.V. dosage regimen based on creatinine clearance and/or body weight:
U.S. labeling: See table.

Imipenem and Cilastatin Dosage in Renal Impairment

Reduced I.V. Dosage Regimen Based on Creatinine Clearance (mL/minute/1.73 m^2) and/or Body Weight <70 kg				
Body Weight (kg)				
≥70	**60**	**50**	**40**	**30**
Total daily dose for normal renal function: 1 g/day				
Cl$_{cr}$ ≥71	250 mg q6h	250 mg q8h	125 mg q6h	125 mg q6h	125 mg q8h
Cl$_{cr}$ 41-70	250 mg q8h	125 mg q6h	125 mg q6h	125 mg q8h	125 mg q8h
Cl$_{cr}$ 21-40	250 mg q12h	250 mg q12h	125 mg q8h	125 mg q12h	125 mg q12h
Cl$_{cr}$ 6-20	250 mg q12h	125 mg q12h	125 mg q12h	125 mg q12h	125 mg q12h
Total daily dose for normal renal function: 1.5 g/day				
Cl$_{cr}$ ≥71	500 mg q8h	250 mg q6h	250 mg q6h	250 mg q8h	125 mg q6h
Cl$_{cr}$ 41-70	250 mg q6h	250 mg q8h	250 mg q8h	125 mg q6h	125 mg q8h
Cl$_{cr}$ 21-40	250 mg q8h	250 mg q8h	250 mg q12h	125 mg q8h	125 mg q8h
Cl$_{cr}$ 6-20	250 mg q12h	250 mg q12h	250 mg q12h	125 mg q12h	125 mg q12h
Total daily dose for normal renal function: 2 g/day				
Cl$_{cr}$ ≥71	500 mg q6h	500 mg q8h	250 mg q6h	250 mg q6h	250 mg q8h
Cl$_{cr}$ 41-70	500 mg q8h	250 mg q6h	250 mg q8h	250 mg q8h	125 mg q6h
Cl$_{cr}$ 21-40	250 mg q6h	250 mg q8h	250 mg q8h	250 mg q12h	125 mg q8h
Cl$_{cr}$ 6-20	250 mg q12h	250 mg q12h	250 mg q12h	250 mg q12h	125 mg q12h
Total daily dose for normal renal function: 3 g/day				
Cl$_{cr}$ ≥71	1000 mg q8h	750 mg q8h	500 mg q6h	500 mg q8h	250 mg q6h
Cl$_{cr}$ 41-70	500 mg q6h	500 mg q8h	500 mg q8h	250 mg q6h	250 mg q8h
Cl$_{cr}$ 21-40	500 mg q8h	500 mg q8h	250 mg q6h	250 mg q8h	250 mg q8h
Cl$_{cr}$ 6-20	500 mg q12h	500 mg q12h	250 mg q12h	250 mg q12h	250 mg q12h
Total daily dose for normal renal function: 4 g/day				
Cl$_{cr}$ ≥71	1000 mg q6h	1000 mg q8h	750 mg q8h	500 mg q6h	500 mg q8h
Cl$_{cr}$ 41-70	750 mg q8h	750 mg q8h	500 mg q6h	500 mg q8h	250 mg q6h
Cl$_{cr}$ 21-40	500 mg q6h	500 mg q8h	500 mg q8h	250 mg q6h	250 mg q8h
Cl$_{cr}$ 6-20	500 mg q12h	500 mg q12h	500 mg q12h	250 mg q12h	250 mg q12h

Canadian labeling: Reduced I.V. dosage regimen based on creatinine clearance (mL/minute/1.73 m^2) and body weight ≥70 kg (**Note:** The manufacturer labeling recommends further proportionate dose reductions for patients <70 kg, but does not provide specific dosing recommendations):
Mild renal impairment (Cl$_{cr}$ 31-70 mL/minute/1.73 m^2):
Fully-susceptible organisms: Maximum dosage: 500 mg every 8 hours

Less susceptible organisms (primarily some *Pseudomonas* strains): Maximum dosage: 500 mg every 6 hours

Moderate renal impairment (Cl_{cr} 21-30 mL/minute/1.73 m²):

Fully-susceptible organisms: Maximum dosage: 500 mg every 12 hours

Less susceptible organisms (primarily some *Pseudomonas* strains): Maximum dosage: 500 mg every 8 hours

Severe renal impairment (Cl_{cr} 0-20 mL/minute/1.73 m²):

Fully-susceptible organisms: Maximum dosage: 250 mg every 12 hours

Less susceptible organisms (primarily some *Pseudomonas* strains): Maximum dosage: 500 mg every 12 hours

Note: Patients with Cl_{cr} 6-20 mL/minute/1.73 m² should receive 250 mg every 12 hours or 3.5 mg/kg (whichever is lower) every 12 hours for most pathogens; seizure risk may increase with higher dosing.

Hepatic Impairment Hepatic dysfunction may further impair cilastatin clearance in patients receiving chronic renal replacement therapy; consider decreasing the dosing frequency.

Administration I.V.: Do not administer I.V. push. Infuse doses ≤500 mg over 20-30 minutes; infuse doses ≥750 mg over 40-60 minutes.

Monitoring Parameters Periodic renal, hepatic, and hematologic function tests; monitor for signs of anaphylaxis during first dose

Test Interactions Interferes with urinary glucose determination using Clinitest®; positive Coombs' [direct]

Special Geriatric Considerations Imipenem/cilastatin's role is limited to the treatment of infections caused by susceptible multiresistant organism(s) and in patients whose bacterial infection(s) have failed to respond to other appropriate antimicrobials; many of the seizures attributed to imipenem/cilastatin were in elderly patients; dose must be adjusted for creatinine clearance and body weight.

Dosage Forms Excipient information presented when available (limited, particularly for generics); consult specific product labeling.

Injection, powder for reconstitution:

Primaxin® I.V.: Imipenem 250 mg and cilastatin 250 mg [contains sodium 18.8 mg (0.8 mEq)]; imipenem 500 mg and cilastatin 500 mg [contains sodium 37.5 mg (1.6 mEq)]

Selected References

Finch RG, Craddock C, Kelly J, et al, "Pharmacokinetic Studies of Imipenem/Cilastatin in Elderly Patients," *J Antimicrob Chemother*, 1986, 18(Suppl E):103-7.

Toon S, Hopkins KJ, Garstang FM, et al, "Pharmacokinetics of Imipenem and Cilastatin After Their Simultaneous Administration to the Elderly," *Br J Clin Pharmacol*, 1987, 23(2):143-9.

Yoshikawa TT, "Antimicrobial Therapy for the Elderly Patient," *J Am Geriatr Soc*, 1990, 38(12):1353-72.

Imipramine (im IP ra meen)

Related Information

Antidepressant Agents *on page 1991*

Beers Criteria − Potentially Inappropriate Medications for Geriatrics *on page 2089*

Pharmacotherapy of Urinary Incontinence *on page 2032*

Medication Safety Issues

Sound-alike/look-alike issues:

Imipramine may be confused with amitriptyline, desipramine, Norpramin®

Brand Names: U.S. Tofranil-PM®; Tofranil®

Brand Names: Canada Apo-Imipramine®; Novo-Pramine; Tofranil®

Index Terms Imipramine Hydrochloride; Imipramine Pamoate

Generic Availability (U.S.) Yes

Pharmacologic Category Antidepressant, Tricyclic (Tertiary Amine)

Use Treatment of depression

Unlabeled/Investigational Use Analgesic for certain chronic and neuropathic pain; treatment of panic disorder, attention-deficit/hyperactivity disorder (ADHD)

Medication Guide Available Yes

Contraindications Hypersensitivity to imipramine (cross-reactivity with other dibenzodiazepines may occur) or any component of the formulation; concurrent use of MAO inhibitors (within 14 days); in a patient during acute recovery phase of MI

Warnings/Precautions [U.S. Boxed Warning]: Antidepressants increase the risk of suicidal thinking and behavior in children, adolescents, and young adults (18-24 years of age) with major depressive disorder (MDD) and other psychiatric disorders; consider risk prior to prescribing. Short-term studies did not show an increased risk in patients >24 years of age and showed a decreased risk in patients ≥65 years. Closely monitor for clinical worsening, suicidality, or unusual changes in behavior; the patient's family or caregiver should be instructed to closely observe the patient and communicate condition with healthcare provider. A medication guide should be dispensed with each prescription. **Imipramine is FDA approved for the treatment of nocturnal enuresis in children ≥6 years of age.**

The possibility of a suicide attempt is inherent in major depression and may persist until remission occurs. Monitor for worsening of depression or suicidality, especially during initiation of therapy (generally first 1-2 months) or with dose increases or decreases. Use caution in high-risk patients. Worsening depression and severe abrupt suicidality that are not part of the presenting symptoms may require discontinuation or modification of drug therapy. The patient's family or caregiver should be alerted to monitor patients for the emergence of suicidality and associated behaviors (such as agitation, irritability, hostility, impulsivity, and hypomania) and notify healthcare provider.

May worsen psychosis in some patients or precipitate a shift to mania or hypomania in patients with bipolar disorder. Patients presenting with depressive symptoms should be screened for bipolar disorder. Monotherapy in patients with bipolar disorder should be avoided. **Imipramine is not FDA approved for the treatment of bipolar depression.**

TCAs may rarely cause bone marrow suppression; monitor for any signs of infection and obtain CBC if symptoms (eg, fever, sore throat) evident. The degree of sedation, anticholinergic effects, orthostasis, and conduction abnormalities are high relative to other antidepressants. Imipramine often causes drowsiness/sedation, resulting in impaired performance of tasks requiring alertness (eg, operating machinery or driving). Sedative effects may be additive with other CNS depressants and/or ethanol. Use with caution in patients with a history of cardiovascular disease (including previous MI, stroke, tachycardia, or conduction abnormalities). Use with caution in patients with urinary retention, benign prostatic hyperplasia, narrow-angle glaucoma, xerostomia, visual problems, constipation, or a history of bowel obstruction.

Consider discontinuing, when possible, prior to elective surgery. Therapy should not be abruptly discontinued in patients receiving high doses for prolonged periods. May lower seizure threshold - use caution in patients with a previous seizure disorder or condition predisposing to seizures such as brain damage, alcoholism, or concurrent therapy with other drugs which lower the seizure threshold. May increase the risks associated with electroconvulsive therapy. Use with caution in hyperthyroid patients or those receiving thyroid supplementation. Use with caution in patients with diabetes mellitus; may alter glucose regulation. Use with caution in patients with hepatic or renal dysfunction and in elderly patients. Has been associated with photosensitization.

Adverse Reactions (Reflective of adult population; not specific for elderly)
Reported for tricyclic antidepressants in general. Frequency not defined.

Cardiovascular: Arrhythmia, CHF, ECG changes, heart block, hypertension, MI, orthostatic hypotension, palpitation, stroke, tachycardia

Central nervous system: Agitation, anxiety, confusion, delusions, disorientation, dizziness, drowsiness, fatigue, hallucination, headache, hypomania, insomnia, nightmares, psychosis, restlessness, seizure

Dermatologic: Alopecia, itching, petechiae, photosensitivity, purpura, rash, urticaria

Endocrine & metabolic: Breast enlargement, galactorrhea, gynecomastia, increase or decrease in blood sugar, increase or decrease in libido, SIADH

Gastrointestinal: Abdominal cramps, anorexia, black tongue, constipation, diarrhea, epigastric disorders, ileus, nausea, stomatitis, taste disturbance, vomiting, weight gain/loss, xerostomia

Genitourinary: Impotence, testicular swelling, urinary retention

Hematologic: Agranulocytosis, eosinophilia, thrombocytopenia

Hepatic: Cholestatic jaundice, transaminases increased

Neuromuscular & skeletal: Ataxia, extrapyramidal symptoms, incoordination, numbness, paresthesia, peripheral neuropathy, tingling, tremor, weakness

Ocular: Blurred vision, disturbances of accommodation, mydriasis

Otic: Tinnitus

Miscellaneous: Diaphoresis, falling, hypersensitivity (eg, drug fever, edema)

Drug Interactions

Metabolism/Transport Effects Substrate of CYP1A2 (minor), 2B6 (minor), 2C19 (major), 2D6 (major), 3A4 (minor); **Inhibits** CYP1A2 (weak), 2C19 (weak), 2D6 (moderate), 2E1 (weak)

Avoid Concomitant Use

Avoid concomitant use of Imipramine with any of the following: Artemether; Dronedarone; Iobenguane I 123; Lumefantrine; MAO Inhibitors; Methylene Blue; Nilotinib; Pimozide; QUEtiapine; QuiNINE; Sibutramine; Tetrabenazine; Thioridazine; Toremifene; Vandetanib; Vemurafenib; Ziprasidone

Increased Effect/Toxicity

Imipramine may increase the levels/effects of: Alpha-/Beta-Agonists (Direct-Acting); Alpha1-Agonists; Amphetamines; Anticholinergics; Aspirin; Beta2-Agonists; CYP2D6 Substrates; Desmopressin; Dronedarone; Fesoterodine; Methylene Blue; Nebivolol; NSAID (COX-2 Inhibitor); NSAID (Nonselective); Pimozide; QTc-Prolonging Agents; QuiNIDine; QuiNINE; Serotonin Modulators; Sodium Phosphates; Sulfonylureas; Tamoxifen; Tetrabenazine; Thioridazine; Toremifene; TraMADol; Vandetanib; Vemurafenib; Vitamin K Antagonists; Yohimbine; Ziprasidone

The levels/effects of Imipramine may be increased by: Abiraterone Acetate; Alfuzosin; Altretamine; Artemether; BuPROPion; Chloroquine; Cimetidine; Cinacalcet; Ciprofloxacin; Ciprofloxacin (Systemic); Conivaptan; CYP2C19 Inhibitors (Moderate); CYP2C19 Inhibitors (Strong); CYP2D6 Inhibitors (Moderate); CYP2D6 Inhibitors (Strong); Dexmethylphenidate; Divalproex; DULoxetine; Gadobutrol; Lithium; Lumefantrine; MAO Inhibitors; Methylphenidate; Metoclopramide; Nilotinib; Pramlintide; Propoxyphene; Protease Inhibitors; QUEtiapine; QuiNIDine; QuiNINE; Selective Serotonin Reuptake Inhibitors; Sibutramine; Terbinafine; Terbinafine (Systemic); Valproic Acid

Decreased Effect

Imipramine may decrease the levels/effects of: Acetylcholinesterase Inhibitors (Central); Alpha2-Agonists; Codeine; Iobenguane I 123

The levels/effects of Imipramine may be decreased by: Acetylcholinesterase Inhibitors (Central); Barbiturates; CarBAMazepine; CYP2C19 Inducers (Strong); Cyproterone; Peginterferon Alfa-2b; St Johns Wort; Tocilizumab

Ethanol/Nutrition/Herb Interactions

Ethanol: May increase CNS depression; monitor for increased effects with coadministration. Caution patients about effects.

Herb/Nutraceutical: St John's wort may decrease imipramine levels. Avoid valerian, St John's wort, SAMe, kava kava (may increase risk of serotonin syndrome and/or excessive sedation).

Mechanism of Action Traditionally believed to increase the synaptic concentration of serotonin and/or norepinephrine in the central nervous system by inhibition of their reuptake by the presynaptic neuronal membrane. However, additional receptor effects have been found including desensitization of adenyl cyclase, down regulation of beta-adrenergic receptors, and down regulation of serotonin receptors.

Pharmacodynamics/Kinetics

Onset of action: Peak antidepressant effect: Usually after ≥2 weeks

Absorption: Well absorbed

Metabolism: Hepatic, primarily via CYP2D6 to desipramine (active) and other metabolites; significant first-pass effect

Half-life elimination: 6-18 hours

Excretion: Urine (as metabolites)

Dosage

Geriatric

Depression: Initial: 25-50 mg at bedtime; may increase every 3 days for inpatients and weekly for outpatients if tolerated to a recommended maximum of 100 mg/day.

Adult

Depression:

Outpatients: Initial: 75 mg/day; may increase gradually to 150 mg/day. May be given in divided doses or as a single bedtime dose; maximum: 200 mg/day

Inpatients: Initial: 100-150 mg/day; may increase gradually to 200 mg/day; if no response after 2 weeks, may further increase to 250-300 mg/day. May be given in divided doses or as a single bedtime dose; maximum: 300 mg/day.

Note: Maximum antidepressant effect may not be seen for 2 or more weeks after initiation of therapy.

Post-traumatic stress disorder (PTSD) (unlabeled use): Oral: 75-200 mg/day

Monitoring Parameters Monitor blood pressure and pulse rate prior to and during initial therapy; ECG in older adults, with high doses, and/or in patients with pre-existing cardiovascular disease; evaluate mental status, suicide ideation (especially at the beginning of therapy or when doses are increased or decreased); blood levels are useful for therapeutic monitoring

Reference Range Therapeutic: Imipramine and desipramine: 150-250 ng/mL (SI: 530-890 nmol/L); desipramine: 150-300 ng/mL (SI: 560-1125 nmol/L); Toxic: >500 ng/mL (SI: 446-893 nmol/L); utility of serum level monitoring controversial

Special Geriatric Considerations Avoid in the elderly. Orthostatic hypotension is a concern with this agent, especially in patients taking other medications that may affect blood pressure. May precipitate arrhythmias in predisposed patients; may aggravate seizures. A less anticholinergic antidepressant may be a better choice.

◀ **Dosage Forms** Excipient information presented when available (limited, particularly for generics); consult specific product labeling.

Capsule, oral, as pamoate: 75 mg, 100 mg, 125 mg, 150 mg

Tofranil-PM®: 75 mg, 100 mg, 125 mg, 150 mg

Tablet, oral, as hydrochloride: 10 mg, 25 mg, 50 mg

Tofranil®: 10 mg, 25 mg, 50 mg

Selected References

Nies A, Robinson DS, Friedman MS, et al, "Relationship Between Age and Tricyclic Antidepressant Plasma Levels," *Am J Psychiatry*, 1977, 134:790-3.

◆ **Imipramine Hydrochloride** *see* Imipramine *on page 919*

◆ **Imipramine Pamoate** *see* Imipramine *on page 919*

◆ **Imitrex®** *see* SUMAtriptan *on page 1723*

Immune Globulin (i MYUN GLOB yoo lin)

Medication Safety Issues

Sound-alike/look-alike issues:

Gamimune® N may be confused with CytoGam®

Immune globulin (intravenous) may be confused with hepatitis B immune globulin

Brand Names: U.S. Carimune® NF; Flebogamma® DIF; GamaSTAN™ S/D; Gammagard S/D®; Gammagard® Liquid; Gammaplex®; Gamunex® [DSC]; Gamunex®-C; Hizentra®; Octagam®; Privigen®; Vivaglobin® [DSC]

Brand Names: Canada BayGam®; Gamimune® N; Gammagard Liquid; Gammagard S/D; Gamunex®; IGIVnex®; Privigen®; Vivaglobin®

Index Terms Gamma Globulin; IG; IGIM; IGIV; Immune Globulin Subcutaneous (Human); Immune Serum Globulin; ISG; IV Immune Globulin; IVIG; Panglobulin; SCIG

Generic Availability (U.S.) No

Pharmacologic Category Blood Product Derivative; Immune Globulin

Use

Treatment of primary humoral immunodeficiency syndromes (congenital agammaglobuline-mia, severe combined immunodeficiency syndromes [SCIDS], common variable immuno-deficiency, X-linked immunodeficiency, Wiskott-Aldrich syndrome) (Carimune® NF, Flebogamma® DIF, Gammagard® Liquid, Gammagard S/D®, Gammaplex®, Gamunex®, Gamunex®-C, Hizentra®, Octagam®, Privigen®, Vivaglobin®)

Treatment of acute and chronic immune (idiopathic) thrombocytopenic purpura (ITP) (Car-imune® NF, Gammagard S/D®, Gamunex®, Gamunex®-C, Privigen® [chronic only])

Treatment of chronic inflammatory demyelinating polyneuropathy (CIDP) (Gamunex®, Gamu-nex®-C)

Prevention of coronary artery aneurysms associated with Kawasaki syndrome (in combination with aspirin) (Gammagard S/D®)

Prevention of bacterial infection in patients with hypogammaglobulinemia and/or recurrent bacterial infections with B-cell chronic lymphocytic leukemia (CLL) (Gammagard S/D®)

Prevention of serious infection in immunoglobulin deficiency (select agammaglobulinemias) (GamaSTAN™ S/D)

Provision of passive immunity in the following susceptible individuals (GamaSTAN™ S/D):

Hepatitis A: Pre-exposure prophylaxis; postexposure: within 14 days and/or prior to manifestation of disease

Measles: For use within 6 days of exposure in an unvaccinated person, who has not previously had measles

Rubella: Postexposure prophylaxis (within 72 hours) to reduce the risk of infection and fetal damage in exposed pregnant women who will not consider therapeutic abortion

Varicella: For immunosuppressed patients when varicella zoster immune globulin is not available

Unlabeled/Investigational Use Acquired hypogammaglobulinemia secondary to malig-nancy; Guillain-Barré syndrome; hematopoietic stem cell transplantation (HSCT), to prevent bacterial infections among allogeneic recipients with severe hypogammaglobulinemia (IgG <400 mg/dL) at <100 days post transplant (CDC guidelines); HIV-associated thrombocytope-nia; multiple sclerosis (relapsing, remitting when other therapies cannot be used); myasthenia gravis; refractory dermatomyositis/polymyositis

Contraindications Hypersensitivity to immune globulin or any component of the formulation; selective IgA deficiency; hyperprolinemia (Hizentra®, Privigen®); severe thrombocytopenia or coagulation disorders; severe thrombocytopenia or coagulation disorders where IM injections are contraindicated

Warnings/Precautions [U.S. Boxed Warning]: I.V. formulation only: Acute renal dys-function (increased serum creatinine, oliguria, acute renal failure, osmotic nephrosis) can rarely occur; usually within 7 days of use (more likely with products stabilized with sucrose). Use with caution in the elderly, patients with renal disease, diabetes mellitus,

volume depletion, sepsis, paraproteinemia, and nephrotoxic medications due to risk of renal dysfunction. In patients at risk of renal dysfunction, the rate of infusion and concentration of solution should be minimized. Discontinue if renal function deteriorates. High-dose regimens (1 g/kg for 1-2 days) are not recommended for individuals with fluid overload or where fluid volume may be of concern. Hypersensitivity and anaphylaxis reactions can occur; a severe fall in blood pressure may rarely occur with anaphylactic reaction; immediate treatment (including epinephrine 1:1000) should be available. Product of human plasma; may potentially contain infectious agents which could transmit disease. Screening of donors, as well as testing and/or inactivation or removal of certain viruses, reduces the risk. Infections thought to be transmitted by this product should be reported to the manufacturer. Aseptic meningitis may occur with high doses (≥1-2 g/kg [product-dependent]) and/or rapid infusion; syndrome usually appears within several hours to 2 days following treatment; usually resolves within several days after IVIG is discontinued; patients with a migraine history may be at higher risk for AMS. Increased risk of hypersensitivity, especially in patients with anti-IgA antibodies. Increased risk of hematoma formation when administered subcutaneously for the treatment of ITP.

Intravenous immune globulin has been associated with antiglobulin hemolysis; monitor for signs of hemolytic anemia. Patients should be adequately hydrated prior to initiation of therapy. Hyperproteinemia, increased serum viscosity and hyponatremia may occur; distinguish hyponatremia from pseudohyponatremia to prevent volume depletion, a further increase in serum viscosity, and a higher risk of thrombotic events. Use caution in patients with a history of thrombotic events or a history of atherosclerosis or cardiovascular disease or patients with known/suspected hyperviscosity; there is clinical evidence of a possible association between thrombotic events and administration of intravenous immune globulin and subcutaneous immune globulin. Consider a baseline assessment of blood viscosity in patients at risk for hyperviscosity. Patients should be monitored for adverse events during and after the infusion. Stop administration with signs of infusion reaction (fever, chills, nausea, vomiting, and rarely shock). Risk may be increased with initial treatment, when switching brands of immune globulin, and with treatment interruptions of >8 weeks. Monitor for transfusion-related acute lung injury (TRALI); noncardiogenic pulmonary edema has been reported with intravenous immune globulin use. TRALI is characterized by severe respiratory distress, pulmonary edema, hypoxemia, and fever (in the presence of normal left ventricular function) and usually occurs within 1-6 hours after infusion. Response to live vaccinations may be impaired. Some clinicians may administer intravenous immune globulin products as a subcutaneous infusion based on patient tolerability and clinical judgment. SubQ infusion should begin 1 week after the last I.V. dose; dose should be individualized based on clinical response and serum IgG trough concentrations; consider premedicating with acetaminophen and diphenhydramine.

Some products may contain maltose, which may result in falsely-elevated blood glucose readings; maltose-containing products are contraindicated in patients with an allergy to corn. Some products may contain polysorbate 80, sodium, and/or sucrose. Some products may contain sorbitol; do not use in patients with fructose intolerance. Hizentra® and Privigen® contain the stabilizer L-proline and are contraindicated in patients with hyperprolinemia. Packaging of some products may contain natural latex/natural rubber; skin testing should not be performed with GamaSTAN™ S/D as local irritation can occur and be misinterpreted as a positive reaction.

Adverse Reactions (Reflective of adult population; not specific for elderly) Frequency not defined.

Cardiovascular: Angioedema, chest tightness, edema, flushing of the face, hyper-/hypotension, palpitation, tachycardia

Central nervous system: Anxiety, aseptic meningitis syndrome, chills, dizziness, drowsiness, fatigue, fever, headache, irritability, lethargy, lightheadedness, malaise, migraine, pain

Dermatologic: Bruising, contact dermatitis, eczema, erythema, hyperhidrosis, petechiae, pruritus, purpura, rash, urticaria

Gastrointestinal: Abdominal cramps, abdominal pain, diarrhea, discomfort, dyspepsia, gastroenteritis, nausea, sore throat, toothache, vomiting

Hematologic: Anemia, autoimmune hemolytic anemia, hematocrit decreased, hematoma, hemolysis (mild), hemorrhage, thrombocytopenia

Hepatic: Bilirubin increased, LDH increased, liver function test increased

Local: Muscle stiffness at I.M. site; pain, swelling, redness or irritation at the infusion site

Neuromuscular & skeletal: Arthralgia, back or hip pain, leg cramps, muscle cramps, myalgia, neck pain, rigors, weakness

Ocular: Conjunctivitis

Otic: Ear pain

Renal: Acute renal failure, acute tubular necrosis, anuria, BUN increased, creatinine increased, oliguria, proximal tubular nephropathy, osmotic nephrosis

Respiratory: Asthma aggravated, bronchitis, cough, dyspnea, epistaxis, nasal congestion, oropharyngeal pain, pharyngeal pain, pharyngitis, rhinitis, rhinorrhea, sinus headache, sinusitis, upper respiratory infection, wheezing

Miscellaneous: Anaphylaxis, diaphoresis, flu-like syndrome, hypersensitivity reactions, infusion reaction, thermal burn

Drug Interactions

Avoid Concomitant Use There are no known interactions where it is recommended to avoid concomitant use.

Increased Effect/Toxicity There are no known significant interactions involving an increase in effect.

Decreased Effect

Immune Globulin may decrease the levels/effects of: Vaccines (Live)

Stability Stability is dependent upon the manufacturer and brand. Do not freeze. Dilution is dependent upon the manufacturer and brand. Gently swirl; do not shake; avoid foaming. Do not mix products from different manufacturers together. Discard unused portion of vials.

Carimune® NF: Prior to reconstitution, store at or below 30°C (86°F). Reconstitute with NS, D_5W, or SWFI. Following reconstitution in a sterile laminar air flow environment, store under refrigeration. Begin infusion within 24 hours.

Flebogamma® DIF: Store at 2°C to 25°C (36°F to 77°F)); do not freeze. Dilution is not recommended.

GamaSTAN™ S/D: Store under refrigeration at 2°C to 8°C (36°F to 46°F). The following stability information has also been reported for GamaSTAN™ S/D: May be exposed to room temperature for a cumulative 7 days (Cohen, 2007).

Gammagard® Liquid: May dilute in D_5W only. Prior to use, store at 2°C to 8°C (36°F to 46°F); do not freeze. May store at room temperature of 25°C (77°F) within the first 24 months of manufacturing. Storage time at room temperature varies with length of time previously refrigerated; refer to product labeling for details.

Gammagard S/D®: Store at ≤25°C (≤77°F). Reconstitute with SWFI; may store diluted solution under refrigeration at 2°C to 8°C (36°F to 46°F) for up to 24 hours if originally prepared in a sterile laminar air flow environment.

Gammaplex®: Store at 2°C to 25°C (36°F to 77°F); do not freeze. Protect from light.

Gamunex®, Gamunex®-C: Store at 2°C to 8°C (36°F to 46°F); may be stored at ≤25°C (≤77°F) for up to 6 months. Dilute in D_5W only.

Hizentra®: Store at ≤25°C (≤77°F); do not freeze or use product if previously frozen. Do not shake.

Octagam®: Store at 2°C to 25°C (36°F to 77°F).

Privigen®: Store at ≤25°C (≤77°F); do not freeze (do not use if previously frozen). Protect from light. If necessary to further dilute, D_5W may be used.

Vivaglobin®: Store at 2°C to 8°C (36°F to 46°F); do not freeze or use product if previously frozen. Do not shake.

Mechanism of Action Replacement therapy for primary and secondary immunodeficiencies, and IgG antibodies against bacteria, viral, parasitic and mycoplasma antigens; interference with F_c receptors on the cells of the reticuloendothelial system for autoimmune cytopenias and ITP; provides passive immunity by increasing the antibody titer and antigen-antibody reaction potential

Pharmacodynamics/Kinetics

Onset of action: I.V.: Provides immediate antibody levels

Duration: I.M., I.V.: Immune effect: 3-4 weeks (variable)

Distribution: V_d: 0.09-0.13 L/kg

Intravascular portion (primarily): Healthy subjects: 41% to 57%; Patients with congenital humoral immunodeficiencies: ~70%

Bioavailability: SubQ: Vivaglobin®: 73%

Half-life elimination: I.M.: ~23 days; I.V.: IgG (variable among patients): Healthy subjects: 14-24 days; Patients with congenital humoral immunodeficiencies: 26-40 days; hypermetabolism associated with fever and infection have coincided with a shortened half-life

Time to peak:

Plasma: SubQ: Gammagard® Liquid: 2.9 days; Hizentra®: 2.9 days; Vivaglobin®: 2.5 days

Serum: I.M.: ~48 hours

Dosage

Geriatric & Adult According to manufacturer product labeling, intravenous formulations are for intravenous administration only. However, some clinicians may administer intravenous formulations as a subcutaneous infusion based on clinical judgment and patient tolerability. Some clinicians dose IVIG on ideal body weight or an adjusted ideal body weight in morbidly-obese patients (Siegel, 2010).

B-cell chronic lymphocytic leukemia (CLL) (Gammagard S/D®): I.V.: 400 mg/kg every 3-4 weeks

Chronic inflammatory demyelinating polyneuropathy (CIDP) (Gamunex®, Gamunex-C®): I.V.: Loading dose: 2000 mg/kg (given in divided doses over 2-4 consecutive days); Maintenance: 1000 mg/kg every 3 weeks. Alternatively, administer 500 mg/kg/day for 2 consecutive days every 3 weeks.

Hepatitis A (GamaSTAN™ S/D): I.M.:

Pre-exposure prophylaxis upon travel into endemic areas (hepatitis A vaccine preferred):
0.02 mL/kg for anticipated risk of exposure <3 months
0.06 mL/kg for anticipated risk of exposure ≥3 months; repeat every 4-6 months.

Postexposure prophylaxis: 0.02 mL/kg given within 14 days of exposure and/or prior to manifestation of disease; not needed if at least 1 dose of hepatitis A vaccine was given at ≥1 month before exposure

Immunoglobulin deficiency (GamaSTAN™ S/D): I.M.: 0.66 mL/kg (minimum dose should be 100 mg/kg) every 3-4 weeks. Administer a double dose at onset of therapy; some patients may require more frequent injections.

Immune (idiopathic) thrombocytopenic purpura (ITP):

Carimune® NF: I.V.: Initial: 400 mg/kg/day for 2-5 days; Maintenance: 400 mg/kg as needed to maintain platelet count ≥30,000/mm^3 and/or to control significant bleeding; may increase dose if needed (range: 800-1000 mg/kg)

Gammagard S/D®: I.V.: 1000 mg/kg; up to 3 additional doses may be given based on patient response and/or platelet count. **Note:** Additional doses should be given on alternate days.

Gamunex®, Gamunex-C®: I.V.: 1000 mg/kg/day for 2 consecutive days (second dose may be withheld if adequate platelet response in 24 hours) **or** 400 mg/kg once daily for 5 consecutive days

Privigen®: I.V.: 1000 mg/kg/day for 2 consecutive days

Kawasaki syndrome (Gammagard S/D®): I.V.:

Gammagard S/D®: 1000 mg/kg as a single dose **or** 400 mg/kg/day for 4 consecutive days. Begin within 7 days of onset of fever.

AHA guidelines (2004): 2000 mg/kg as a single dose within 10 days of disease onset

Note: Must be used in combination with aspirin: 80-100 mg/kg/day orally, divided every 6 hours for up to 14 days (until fever resolves for at least 48 hours); then decrease dose to 3-5 mg/kg/day once daily. In patients without coronary artery abnormalities, give lower dose for 6-8 weeks. In patients with coronary artery abnormalities, low-dose aspirin should be continued indefinitely.

Measles:

GamaSTAN™ S/D: I.M.: Immunocompetent: 0.25 mL/kg given within 6 days of exposure followed by live attenuated measles vaccine in 5-6 months when indicated (Watson, 1998)

Gamunex-C®, Octagam®: I.V.:

Prophylaxis in patients with primary humoral immunodeficiency (**ONLY** if routine dose is <400 mg/kg): ≥400 mg/kg immediately before expected exposure

Treatment in patients with primary immunodeficiency: 400 mg/kg administered as soon as possible after exposure

Hizentra®: SubQ infusion: Measles exposure in patients with primary humoral immunodeficiency: Weekly dose: ≥200 mg/kg for 2 consecutive weeks for patients at risk of measles exposure (eg, during an outbreak; travel to endemic area). In patients who have been exposed to measles, administer the minimum dose as soon as possible following exposure.

Primary humoral immunodeficiency disorders:

Carimune® NF: I.V.: 400-800 mg/kg every 3-4 weeks

Flebogamma® DIF, Gammagard® Liquid, Gammagard S/D®, Gamunex®, Gamunex-C®, Octagam®: I.V.: 300-600 mg/kg every 3-4 weeks; adjusted based on dosage and interval in conjunction with monitored serum IgG concentrations and clinical response

Gammaplex®: I.V.: 300-800 mg/kg every 3-4 weeks

Gamunex-C®: SubQ infusion: Begin 1 week after last I.V. dose. Use the following equation to calculate initial dose:

Initial weekly dose (grams) = [1.37 x IGIV dose (grams)] divided by [I.V. dose interval (weeks)]

Note: For subsequent dose adjustments, refer to product labeling.

Hizentra®: SubQ infusion: Begin 1 week after last I.V. dose. Use the following equation to calculate initial dose:

Initial weekly dose (grams) = [1.53 x IGIV dose (grams)] divided by [I.V. dose interval (weeks)]

Note: For subsequent dose adjustments, refer to product labeling.

Privigen®: I.V.: 200-800 mg/kg every 3-4 weeks; adjusted based on dosage and interval in conjunction with monitored serum IgG concentrations and clinical response

Vivaglobin®: SubQ infusion: Begin 1 week after last I.V. dose; **Note:** Patient should have received an I.V. immune globulin routinely for at least 3 months before switching to SubQ. Use the following equation to calculate initial dose:

Initial weekly dose (grams) = [1.37 x IGIV dose (grams)] divided by [I.V. dose interval (weeks)]

Note: For subsequent dose adjustments, refer to product labeling.

Rubella (GamaSTAN™ S/D): I.M.: Prophylaxis during pregnancy: 0.55 mL/kg within 72 hours of exposure (Watson, 1998)

Varicella (GamaSTAN™ S/D): I.M.: Prophylaxis: 0.6-1.2 mL/kg (varicella zoster immune globulin preferred) within 72 hours of exposure

Unlabeled uses: I.V.:

Acquired hypogammaglobulinemia secondary to malignancy (unlabeled use): Adults: 400 mg/kg/dose every 3 weeks; reevaluate every 4-6 months (Anderson, 2007)

Guillain-Barré syndrome (unlabeled use): Adults: Various regimens have been used, including:

400 mg/kg/day for 5 days (Hughes, 2003)

or

2000 mg/kg in divided doses administered over 2-5 days (Feasby, 2007)

Hematopoietic stem cell transplantation with hypogammaglobulinemia (CDC guidelines, 2000; unlabeled use): Adults: 500 mg/kg/week

HIV-associated thrombocytopenia (unlabeled use): Adults: 1000 mg/kg/day for 2 days (Anderson, 2007)

Multiple sclerosis (relapsing-remitting, when other therapies cannot be used) (unlabeled use): Adults: 1000 mg/kg per month, with or without an induction of 400 mg/kg/day for 5 days (Feasby, 2007)

Myasthenia gravis (severe exacerbation) (unlabeled use): Adults: Total dose of 2000 mg/kg over 2-5 days (Feasby, 2007)

Refractory dermatomyositis/polymyositis (unlabeled uses): Adults: 2000 mg/kg per treatment course administered over 2-5 days (Feasby, 2007)

Dosing adjustment/comments in renal impairment: Cl_{cr} <10 mL/minute: Avoid use; in patients at risk of renal dysfunction, consider infusion at a rate less than maximum.

Renal Impairment I.V.: Cl_{cr} <10 mL/minute: Avoid use; in patients at risk of renal dysfunction, consider infusion at a rate less than maximum.

Administration Note: If plasmapheresis employed for treatment of condition, administer immune globulin **after** completion of plasmapheresis session.

I.M.: Administer I.M. in the anterolateral aspects of the upper thigh or deltoid muscle of the upper arm. Avoid gluteal region due to risk of injury to sciatic nerve. Divide doses >10 mL and inject in multiple sites.

GamaSTAN™ S/D is for I.M. administration only.

I.V. infusion: Infuse over 2-24 hours; administer in separate infusion line from other medications; if using primary line, flush with saline prior to administration. Decrease dose, rate and/or concentration of infusion in patients who may be at risk of renal failure. Decreasing the rate or stopping the infusion may help relieve some adverse effects (flushing, changes in pulse rate, changes in blood pressure). Epinephrine should be available during administration. For initial treatment or in the elderly, a lower concentration and/or a slower rate of infusion should be used. Initial rate of administration and titration is specific to each IVIG product. Consult specific product prescribing information for detailed recommendations. Refrigerated product should be warmed to room temperature prior to infusion. Some products require filtration; refer to individual product labeling. Antecubital veins should be used, especially with concentrations ≥10% to prevent injection site discomfort.

SubQ infusion: Initial dose should be administered in a healthcare setting capable of providing monitoring and treatment in the event of hypersensitivity. Using aseptic technique, follow the infusion device manufacturer's instructions for filling the reservoir and preparing the pump. Remove air from administration set and needle by priming. Appropriate injection sites include the abdomen, thigh, upper arm, and/or lateral hip; dose may be infused into multiple sites (spaced ≥2 inches apart) simultaneously. After the sites are clean and dry, insert subcutaneous needle and prime administration set. Attach sterile needle to administration set, gently pull back on the syringe to assure a blood vessel has not been inadvertently accessed (do not use needle and tubing if blood present). Repeat for each injection site; deliver the dose following instructions for the infusion device. Rotate the site(s) weekly. Treatment may be transitioned to the home/home care setting in the absence of adverse reactions.

GamunexC®:
Injection sites: ≤8 simultaneous injection sites
Recommended infusion rate: 20 mL/hour per injection site

Hizentra®:
Injection sites: ≤4 simultaneous injection sites
Maximum infusion rate: First infusion: 15 mL/hour per injection site; subsequent infusions: 25 mL/hour per injection site (maximum: 50 mL/hour for all simultaneous sites combined)
Maximum infusion volume: First 4 infusions: 15 mL per injection site; subsequent infusions: 20 mL per injection site (maximum: 25 mL per site as tolerated)

Vivaglobin®:
Injection sites: Adults ≤65 years: ≤6 simultaneous injection sites; Adults >65 years: ≤4 simultaneous injection sites
Maximum infusion rate: 20 mL/hour per injection site (maximum: 3 mg/kg/minute [1.13 mL/kg/hour] for all simultaneous sites combined)
Maximum infusion volume: 15 mL per injection site

Monitoring Parameters Renal function, urine output, IgG concentrations, hemoglobin and hematocrit, platelets (in patients with ITP); infusion- or injection-related adverse reactions, anaphylaxis, signs and symptoms of hemolysis; blood viscosity (in patients at risk for hyperviscosity); presence of antineutrophil antibodies (if TRALI is suspected); volume status; neurologic symptoms (if AMS suspected); clinical response

SubQ infusion: Monitor IgG trough levels every 2-3 months before/after conversion from I.V.; subcutaneous infusions provide more constant IgG levels than usual I.V. immune globulin treatments.

Test Interactions Octagam® contains maltose. Falsely-elevated blood glucose levels may occur when glucose monitoring devices and test strips utilizing the glucose dehydrogenase pyrroloquinolinequinone (GDH-PQQ) based methods are used. Glucose monitoring devices and test strips which utilize the glucose-specific method are recommended. Passively-transferred antibodies may yield false-positive serologic testing results; may yield false-positive direct and indirect Coombs' test. Skin testing should not be performed with GamaSTAN™ S/D as local irritation can occur and be misinterpreted as a positive reaction.

Pharmacotherapy Pearls I.M.: When administering immune globulin for hepatitis A prophylaxis, use should be considered for the following close contacts of persons with confirmed hepatitis A: unvaccinated household and sexual contacts, persons who have shared illicit drugs, regular babysitters, staff and attendees of child care centers, food handlers within the same establishment (CDC, 2006).

All household contacts of measles patients should be evaluated to receive immune globulin unless the measles vaccine has been given on or after the first birthday, unless immunocompromised (CDC, 1998).

For travelers, immune globulin is not an alternative to careful selection of foods and water; immune globulin can interfere with the antibody response to parenterally administered live virus vaccines. Frequent travelers should be tested for hepatitis A antibody, immune hemolytic anemia, and neutropenia (with ITP, I.V. route is usually used).

IgA content:
Carimune® NF: 720 mcg/mL
Flebogamma® 5% DIF: 2.9 ± 0.1 mcg/mL
Flebogamma® 10% DIF: <100 mcg/mL
Gammagard® Liquid: 37 mcg/mL
Gammagard S/D® 5% solution: <1 mcg/mL or <2.2 mcg/mL(product dependent)
Gammaplex®: <10 mcg/mL
Gamunex-C®: 46 mcg/mL
Hizentra®: ≤50 mcg/mL
Octagam®: ≤200 mcg/mL
Privigen®: ≤25 mcg/mL
Vivaglobin®: ≤1700 mcg/mL

Dosage Forms Excipient information presented when available (limited, particularly for generics); consult specific product labeling. [DSC] = Discontinued product
Injection, powder for reconstitution [preservative free]:
Carimune® NF: 3 g, 6 g, 12 g [contains sucrose]
Gammagard S/D®: 2.5 g [contains albumin (human), glucose, glycine, natural rubber/natural latex in packaging, polyethylene glycol, polysorbate 80; IgA <2.2 mcg/mL]
Gammagard S/D®: 5 g [contains albumin (human), glucose, glycine, natural rubber/natural latex in packaging, polyethylene glycol, polysorbate 80; IgA <1 mcg/mL]
Gammagard S/D®: 5 g [contains albumin (human), glucose, glycine, natural rubber/natural latex in packaging, polyethylene glycol, polysorbate 80; IgA <2.2 mcg/mL]
Gammagard S/D®: 10 g [contains albumin (human), glucose, glycine, natural rubber/natural latex in packaging, polyethylene glycol, polysorbate 80; IgA <1 mcg/mL]
Gammagard S/D®: 10 g [contains albumin (human), glucose, glycine, natural rubber/natural latex in packaging, polyethylene glycol, polysorbate 80; IgA <2.2 mcg/mL]

◀ Injection, solution [preservative free]:
   Flebogamma® DIF: 5% [50 mg/mL] (10 mL, 50 mL, 100 mL, 200 mL, 400 mL); 10%
      [100 mg/mL] (100 mL, 200 mL) [contains polyethylene glycol, sorbitol]
   GamaSTAN™ S/D: 15% to 18% [150 to 180 mg/mL] (2 mL, 10 mL)
   Gammagard® Liquid: 10% [100 mg/mL] (10 mL, 25 mL, 50 mL, 100 mL, 200 mL) [sucrose
      free; contains glycine]
   Gammaplex®: 5% [50 mg/mL] (50 mL, 100 mL, 200 mL) [sucrose free; contains glycine,
      natural rubber/natural latex in packaging, polysorbate 80, sorbitol]
   Gamunex®: 10% [100 mg/mL] (10 mL [DSC], 25 mL [DSC], 50 mL [DSC], 100 mL [DSC],
      200 mL [DSC]) [contains glycine]
   Gamunex®-C: 10% [100 mg/mL] (10 mL, 25 mL, 50 mL, 100 mL, 200 mL) [contains glycine]
   Hizentra®: 200 mg/mL (5 mL, 10 mL, 20 mL) [contains L-proline, polysorbate 80]
   Octagam®: 5% [50 mg/mL] (20 mL, 50 mL, 100 mL, 200 mL) [sucrose free; contains
      maltose, sodium 30 mmol/L]
   Privigen®: 10% [100 mg/mL] (50 mL, 100 mL, 200 mL) [sucrose free; contains L-proline]
   Vivaglobin®: 160 mg/mL (3 mL [DSC], 10 mL [DSC], 20 mL [DSC])

◆ **Immune Globulin Subcutaneous (Human)** *see* Immune Globulin *on page 922*
◆ **Immune Serum Globulin** *see* Immune Globulin *on page 922*
◆ **Imodium® A-D [OTC]** *see* Loperamide *on page 1085*
◆ **Imodium® A-D for children [OTC]** *see* Loperamide *on page 1085*
◆ **Imodium® Multi-Symptom Relief [OTC]** *see* Loperamide and Simethicone *on page 1087*
◆ **Imogam® Rabies-HT** *see* Rabies Immune Globulin (Human) *on page 1573*
◆ **Imovax® Rabies** *see* Rabies Vaccine *on page 1575*
◆ **Imuran®** *see* AzaTHIOprine *on page 169*

Inamrinone (eye NAM ri none)

Medication Safety Issues
Sound-alike/look-alike issues:
   Amrinone (former name for inamrinone) may be confused with aMILoride, amiodarone
High alert medication:
   The Institute for Safe Medication Practices (ISMP) includes this medication among its list of
   drug classes which have a heightened risk of causing significant patient harm when used
   in error.
Index Terms Amrinone Lactate
Generic Availability (U.S.) Yes
Pharmacologic Category Phosphodiesterase Enzyme Inhibitor
Use Short-term therapy in patients with intractable heart failure
Contraindications Hypersensitivity to inamrinone, any component of the formulation, or
   bisulfites (contains sodium metabisulfite); patients with severe aortic or pulmonic valvular
   disease
Warnings/Precautions Due to a slight effect on AV conduction, may increase ventricular
   response rate in atrial fibrillation/atrial flutter; prior treatment with digoxin is recommended.
   Monitor liver function. Discontinue therapy if alteration in LFTs and clinical symptoms of
   hepatotoxicity occur. Observe for arrhythmias in this very high-risk patient population. Not
   recommended in acute MI treatment. Monitor fluid status closely; patients may require
   adjustment of diuretic and electrolyte replacement therapy. Can cause thrombocytopenia
   (dose dependent). Correct hypokalemia before initiating therapy. Increase risk of hospitalization and death with long-term therapy.
Adverse Reactions (Reflective of adult population; not specific for elderly)
1% to 10%:
Cardiovascular: Arrhythmias (3%; especially in high-risk patients), hypotension (1% to 2%;
   dose related)
Gastrointestinal: Nausea (1% to 2%), vomiting (1%)
Hematologic: Thrombocytopenia (~2%; dose related)
Drug Interactions
Avoid Concomitant Use There are no known interactions where it is recommended to
   avoid concomitant use.
Increased Effect/Toxicity There are no known significant interactions involving an increase
   in effect.
Decreased Effect There are no known significant interactions involving a decrease in effect.
Stability Store at 15°C to 30°C (59°F to 86°F). Protect from light. Store in carton until ready for
   use. For continuous infusion, dilute with 0.45% or 0.9% sodium chloride to final concentration
   of 1-3 mg/mL. Use within 24 hours. Do not directly dilute with dextrose-containing solutions;
   chemical interaction occurs. May be administered I.V. into running dextrose infusions.

Mechanism of Action Inhibits myocardial cyclic adenosine monophosphate (cAMP) phosphodiesterase activity and increases cellular levels of cAMP resulting in a positive inotropic effect and increased cardiac output; also possesses systemic and pulmonary vasodilator effects resulting in pre- and afterload reduction; slightly increases atrioventricular conduction

Pharmacodynamics/Kinetics
Onset of action: I.V.: 2-5 minutes
Peak effect: ~10 minutes
Duration (dose dependent): Low dose: ~30 minutes; Higher doses: ~2 hours
Half-life elimination, serum: Adults: Healthy volunteers: 3.6 hours, Congestive heart failure: 5.8 hours
Excretion: Urine (10% to 40% as parent drug)

Dosage
Geriatric & Adult Dosage is based on clinical response (**Note:** Dose should not exceed 10 mg/kg/24 hours).
Heart failure: 0.75 mg/kg I.V. bolus over 2-3 minutes followed by maintenance infusion of 5-10 mcg/kg/minute; I.V. bolus may need to be repeated in 30 minutes.
Renal Impairment Adults:
Cl_{cr} ≥10 mL/minute: Administer 100% of dose
Cl_{cr} <10 mL/minute: Administer 50% to 75% of dose

Administration May be administered undiluted for I.V. bolus doses. Dilute for use as continuous infusion.

Monitoring Parameters Platelet count, CBC, electrolytes (especially potassium and magnesium), liver function and renal function tests; ECG, CVP, SBP, DBP, heart rate; infusion site

If pulmonary artery catheter is in place, monitor cardiac index, stroke volume, systemic vascular resistance, pulmonary capillary wedge pressure and pulmonary vascular resistance.

Pharmacotherapy Pearls Normally prescribed for patients who have not responded well to therapy with digitalis, diuretics, and vasodilators; dosage is based on clinical response

Special Geriatric Considerations While inamrinone is not specifically arrhythmogenic, the elderly may be at high risk for ventricular and particularly atrial arrhythmias due to high incidence of arrhythmias in this population. Also, the elderly are often hypovolemic due to dehydration; therefore, monitor fluid status carefully (CVP line) in order to have effective falling pressure for maximal response. Found to be as effective as dobutamine in the elderly with heart failure in one study despite the decline in beta-adrenergic response with age.

Dosage Forms Excipient information presented when available (limited, particularly for generics); consult specific product labeling. [DSC] = Discontinued product
Injection, solution: 5 mg/mL (20 mL [DSC])

Selected References
Aronoff GR, Bennett WM, Berns JS, et al, *Drug Prescribing in Renal Failure: Dosing Guidelines for Adults and Children*, 5th ed. Philadelphia, PA: American College of Physicians; 2007, p 45, 145.
Heart Failure Society of America, "HFSA 2006 Comprehensive Heart Failure Practice Guideline," *J Card Fail*, 2006, 12 (1):e1-119. Available at http://www.heartfailureguideline.org.
Rich MW, Woods WL, Davila-Roman VG, et al, "A Randomized Comparison of Intravenous Amrinone Versus Dobutamine in Older Patients With Decompensated Congestive Heart Failure," *J Am Geriatr Soc*, 1995, 43(3):271-4.

IncobotulinumtoxinA (in kuh BOT yoo lin num TOKS in aye)

Medication Safety Issues
Other safety concerns:
Botulinum products are not interchangeable; potency differences may exist between the products.
Brand Names: U.S. Xeomin®
Brand Names: Canada Xeomin®
Index Terms Botulinum Toxin Type A
Generic Availability (U.S.) No
Pharmacologic Category Neuromuscular Blocker Agent, Toxin; Ophthalmic Agent, Toxin
Use Treatment of blepharospasm in patients previously treated with onabotulinumtoxinA (Botox®); treatment of cervical dystonia in botulinum toxin-naïve and previously treated patients; temporary improvement in the appearance of moderate-to-severe glabellar lines associated with corrugator and/or procerus muscle activity

Canadian labeling: Treatment of hypertonicity disorders of the seventh nerve (eg, blepharospasm, hemifacial spasm); treatment of poststroke spasticity of upper limb(s); treatment of cervical dystonia (spasmodic torticollis)
Medication Guide Available Yes

◀ **Dosage**

Geriatric Refer to adult dosing. Initiate therapy at lowest recommended dose.

Adult

Blepharospasm: I.M.:

U.S. labeling: Initial: Total dose should be the same as previously administered onabotulinumtoxinA dose. If prior onabotulinumtoxinA dose is not known: 1.25-2.5 units/injection site (maximum initial dose: 35 units/eye or 70 units/both eyes). Number and location of injection sites based on disease severity and previous dose/response to onabotulinumtoxinA (in clinical trials, a mean number of 6 injections per eye were administered). Cumulative dose should not exceed 35 units/eye or 70 units/both eyes administered no more frequently than every 3 months.

Canadian labeling: Initial: 1.25-2.5 units/injection site (maximum initial dose: 25 units/eye). Dose may be increased up to twice the previous dose if the response from the initial dose lasted ≤2 months; maximum dose per site: 5 units. Cumulative dose should not exceed 35 units/eye or 70 units/both eyes administered no more frequently than every 3 months.

Cervical dystonia: I.M.:

U.S. labeling: Initial total dose: 120 units (in clinical trials, similar efficacy was noted with initial total doses of 120 and 240 units and between treatment experienced and treatment naïve patients). Dose and number of injection sites should be individualized based on prior treatment, response, duration of effect, adverse events, number/location of muscle(s) to be treated and disease severity. In clinical trials most patients received a total of 2-10 injections into treated muscles. Administer no more frequently than every 3 months

Canadian labeling: Usual total dose: 200 units (maximum: 300 units; maximum dose per injection site: 50 units); administer no more frequently than every 3 months

Reduction of glabellar lines: I.M.: Inject 4 units into each of the 5 sites (2 injections in each corrugator muscle and 1 injection in the procerus muscle) for a total dose of 20 units per treatment session. Administer no more frequently than every 3 months.

Spasticity of upper limb (poststroke): *Canadian labeling (not in U.S. labeling):* I.M.: Individualize dose based on patient size, extent, and location of muscle involvement, degree of spasticity, local muscle weakness, and response to prior treatment. In clinical trials, total doses up to 400 units were administered as separate injections typically divided among selected muscles; may repeat therapy at ≥3 months with appropriate dosage based upon the clinical condition of patient at time of retreatment.

Suggested guidelines for the treatment of stroke-related upper limb spasticity: Note: The lowest recommended starting dose should be used. Dosage and number of injection sites should be individualized. Multiple injections may minimize adverse effects. Dose listed is total dose administered to site:

Biceps: 80 units

Brachialis: 50 units

Brachioradialis: 60 units

Flexor carpi radialis: 50 units

Flexor carpi ulnaris: 40 units

Flexor digitorum profundus: 40 units

Flexor digitorum superficialis: 40 units

Adductor pollicis: 10 units

Flexor pollicis brevis: 10 units

Flexor pollicis longus: 20 units

Pronator quadratus 25 units

Pronator teres: 40 units

Renal Impairment There are no dosage adjustments provided in manufacturer's labeling.

Hepatic Impairment There are no dosage adjustments provided in manufacturer's labeling.

Dosage Forms Excipient information presented when available (limited, particularly for generics); consult specific product labeling.

Injection, powder for reconstitution:

Xeomin®: 50 units, 100 units [contains albumin (human), sucrose 4.7 mg]

Indapamide (in DAP a mide)

Medication Safety Issues

Sound-alike/look-alike issues:

Indapamide may be confused with Iopidine®

International issues:

Pretanix [Hungary] may be confused with Protonix brand name for pantoprazole [U.S., Canada]

Brand Names: Canada Apo-Indapamide®; Dom-Indapamide; Lozide®; Lozol®; Mylan-Indapamide; Novo-Indapamide; Nu-Indapamide; PHL-Indapamide; PMS-Indapamide; PRO-Indapamide; Riva-Indapamide

Generic Availability (U.S.) Yes

Pharmacologic Category Diuretic, Thiazide-Related

Use Management of mild-to-moderate hypertension; treatment of edema in heart failure and nephrotic syndrome

Contraindications Hypersensitivity to indapamide or any component of the formulation, thiazides, or sulfonamide-derived drugs; anuria; renal decompensation

Warnings/Precautions Use with caution in severe renal disease. Electrolyte disturbances (hypokalemia, hypochloremic alkalosis, hyponatremia) can occur. Use with caution in severe hepatic dysfunction; hepatic encephalopathy can be caused by electrolyte disturbances. Gout may be precipitated in certain patients with a history of gout, a familial predisposition to gout, or chronic renal failure. Use caution in patients with prediabetes or diabetes; may alter glucose control. May cause SLE exacerbation or activation. Use with caution in patients with moderate or high cholesterol concentrations. Photosensitization may occur. Correct hypokalemia before initiating therapy.

Chemical similarities are present among sulfonamides, sulfonylureas, carbonic anhydrase inhibitors, thiazides, and loop diuretics (except ethacrynic acid). Use in patients with thiazide or sulfonamide allergy is specifically contraindicated in product labeling, however, a risk of cross-reaction exists in patients with allergy to any of these compounds; avoid use when previous reaction has been severe. Discontinue if signs of hypersensitivity are noted.

Adverse Reactions (Reflective of adult population; not specific for elderly)

1% to 10%:

Cardiovascular: Palpitation (<5%), flushing, orthostatic hypotension

Central nervous system: Headache (≥5%), nervousness (≥5%), dizziness (<5%), drowsiness (<5%), lightheadedness (<5%), restlessness (<5%), vertigo (<5%), agitation, anxiety, depression, fatigue, lassitude, lethargy, malaise

Dermatologic: Hives (<5%), pruritus (<5%), rash (<5%)

Endocrine & metabolic: Hyperglycemia (<5%), hyperuricemia (<5%)

Gastrointestinal: Abdominal pain, anorexia, bloating, constipation, cramping, diarrhea, dry mouth, gastric irritation, nausea, vomiting, weight loss

Genitourinary: Glycosuria (<5%), impotence (<5%), libido reduced (<5%), nocturia, polyuria, urinary frequency

Neuromuscular & skeletal: Weakness (≥5%), muscle cramps, spasm

Ocular: Blurred vision (<5%)

Renal: Cutaneous vasculitis (<5%), necrotizing angiitis, vasculitis

Respiratory: Rhinorrhea (<5%)

Drug Interactions

Avoid Concomitant Use

Avoid concomitant use of Indapamide with any of the following: Artemether; Dofetilide; Dronedarone; Lumefantrine; Nilotinib; Pimozide; QUEtiapine; QuiNINE; Tetrabenazine; Thioridazine; Toremifene; Vandetanib; Vemurafenib; Ziprasidone

Increased Effect/Toxicity

Indapamide may increase the levels/effects of: ACE Inhibitors; Allopurinol; Amifostine; Antihypertensives; Calcium Salts; CarBAMazepine; Dofetilide; Dronedarone; Hypotensive Agents; Lithium; OXcarbazepine; Pimozide; Porfimer; QTc-Prolonging Agents; QuiNINE; RiTUXimab; Sodium Phosphates; Tetrabenazine; Thioridazine; Topiramate; Toremifene; Vandetanib; Vemurafenib; Vitamin D Analogs; Ziprasidone

The levels/effects of Indapamide may be increased by: Alcohol (Ethyl); Alfuzosin; Analgesics (Opioid); Artemether; Barbiturates; Chloroquine; Ciprofloxacin; Ciprofloxacin (Systemic); Corticosteroids (Orally Inhaled); Corticosteroids (Systemic); Gadobutrol; Herbs (Hypotensive Properties); Licorice; Lumefantrine; MAO Inhibitors; Nilotinib; Pentoxifylline; Phosphodiesterase 5 Inhibitors; Prostacyclin Analogues; QUEtiapine; QuiNINE

Decreased Effect

Indapamide may decrease the levels/effects of: Antidiabetic Agents

The levels/effects of Indapamide may be decreased by: Bile Acid Sequestrants; Herbs (Hypertensive Properties); Methylphenidate; Nonsteroidal Anti-Inflammatory Agents; Yohimbine

Ethanol/Nutrition/Herb Interactions Herb/Nutraceutical: Avoid herbs with *hypertensive* properties (bayberry, blue cohosh, cayenne, ephedra, ginger, ginseng [American], kola, licorice); may diminish the antihypertensive effect of indapamide. Avoid herbs with *hypotensive* properties (black cohosh, California poppy, coleus, golden seal, hawthorn, mistletoe, periwinkle, quinine, shepherd's purse); may enhance the hypotensive effect of indapamide.

Mechanism of Action Diuretic effect is localized at the proximal segment of the distal tubule of the nephron; it does not appear to have significant effect on glomerular filtration rate nor renal blood flow; like other diuretics, it enhances sodium, chloride, and water excretion by interfering with the transport of sodium ions across the renal tubular epithelium

◀ **Pharmacodynamics/Kinetics**
Onset of action: 1-2 hours
Duration: ≤36 hours
Absorption: Complete
Protein binding, plasma: 71% to 79%
Metabolism: Extensively hepatic
Half-life elimination: 14-18 hours
Time to peak: 2-2.5 hours
Excretion: Urine (~60%) within 48 hours; feces (~16% to 23%)

Dosage
Geriatric & Adult
   Edema: Oral: 2.5-5 mg/day. **Note:** There is little therapeutic benefit to increasing the dose >5 mg/day; there is, however, an increased risk of electrolyte disturbances.
   Hypertension: Oral: 1.25 mg in the morning, may increase to 5 mg/day by increments of 1.25-2.5 mg; consider adding another antihypertensive and decreasing the dose if response is not adequate.

Administration May be taken with food or milk. Administer early in day to avoid nocturia. Administer the last dose of multiple doses no later than 6 PM unless instructed otherwise.

Monitoring Parameters Blood pressure (both standing and sitting/supine), serum electrolytes, renal function, assess weight, I & O reports daily to determine fluid loss

Special Geriatric Considerations Indapamide has the advantage over other related thiazide diuretics in that it may be effective when Cl_{cr} is <30 mL/minute.

Dosage Forms Excipient information presented when available (limited, particularly for generics); consult specific product labeling.
Tablet, oral: 1.25 mg, 2.5 mg

Selected References
Acchiardo SR and Skoutakis VA, "Clinical Efficacy, Safety, and Pharmacokinetics of Indapamide in Renal Impairment," *Am Heart J*, 1983, 106(1 Pt 2):237-44.
Beckett NS, Peters R, Fletcher AE, et al, "Treatment of Hypertension in Patients 80 Years of Age or Older," *N Engl J Med*, 2008, 358(18):1887-98.

◆ **Inderal® LA** see Propranolol *on page 1536*
◆ **Inderide** see Propranolol and Hydrochlorothiazide *on page 1540*
◆ **Indocin®** see Indomethacin *on page 932*
◆ **Indocin® I.V.** see Indomethacin *on page 932*
◆ **Indometacin** see Indomethacin *on page 932*

Indomethacin (in doe METH a sin)

Related Information
Beers Criteria − Potentially Inappropriate Medications for Geriatrics *on page 2089*

Medication Safety Issues
Sound-alike/look-alike issues:
   Indocin® may be confused with Imodium®, Lincocin®, Minocin®, Vicodin®
BEERS Criteria medication:
   This drug may be inappropriate for use in geriatric patients (high severity risk).
International issues:
   Flexin® [Great Britain] may be confused with Floxin® which is a brand name for ofloxacin in the U.S.
   Flexin® [Great Britain]: Brand name for orphenadrine in Israel

Brand Names: U.S. Indocin®; Indocin® I.V.

Brand Names: Canada Apo-Indomethacin®; Indocid® P.D.A.; Novo-Methacin; Nu-Indo; Pro-Indo; ratio-Indomethacin; Sandoz-Indomethacin

Index Terms Indometacin; Indomethacin Sodium Trihydrate

Generic Availability (U.S.) Yes: Excludes oral suspension

Pharmacologic Category Nonsteroidal Anti-inflammatory Drug (NSAID), Oral; Nonsteroidal Anti-inflammatory Drug (NSAID), Parenteral

Use Acute gouty arthritis, acute bursitis/tendonitis, moderate-to-severe osteoarthritis, rheumatoid arthritis, ankylosing spondylitis

Unlabeled/Investigational Use Management of preterm labor

Medication Guide Available Yes

Contraindications Hypersensitivity to indomethacin, aspirin, other NSAIDs, or any component of the formulation; perioperative pain in the setting of coronary artery bypass graft (CABG) surgery; patients with a history of proctitis or recent rectal bleeding (suppositories)

Warnings/Precautions [U.S. Boxed Warning]: NSAIDs are associated with an increased risk of adverse cardiovascular thrombotic events, including MI and stroke. Risk may be increased with duration of use or pre-existing cardiovascular risk factors or disease. May cause new-onset hypertension or worsening of existing hypertension. Use caution with fluid retention. Avoid use in heart failure. Concurrent administration of ibuprofen, and potentially other nonselective NSAIDs, may interfere with aspirin's cardioprotective effect. **[U.S. Boxed Warning]: Use is contraindicated for treatment of perioperative pain in the setting of coronary artery bypass graft (CABG) surgery.** Risk of MI and stroke may be increased with use following CABG surgery.

Platelet adhesion and aggregation may be decreased; may prolong bleeding time; patients with coagulation disorders or who are receiving anticoagulants should be monitored closely. Anemia may occur; patients on long-term NSAID therapy should be monitored for anemia. Rarely, NSAID use may cause severe blood dyscrasias (eg, agranulocytosis, aplastic anemia, thrombocytopenia).

NSAID use may compromise existing renal function; dose-dependent decreases in prostaglandin synthesis may result from NSAID use, reducing renal blood flow which may cause renal decompensation. NSAID use may increase the risk for hyperkalemia. Patients with impaired renal function, dehydration, heart failure, liver dysfunction, those taking diuretics, and ACE inhibitors are at greater risk of renal toxicity and hyperkalemia. Rehydrate patient before starting therapy; monitor renal function closely. Not recommended for use in patients with advanced renal disease. Long-term NSAID use may result in renal papillary necrosis.

The elderly are at increased risk for adverse effects (especially peptic ulceration, CNS effects, renal toxicity) from NSAIDs even at low doses. Risk of CNS adverse events may be higher with indomethacin compared to other NSAIDs; avoid use in this age group (Beers Criteria).

[U.S. Boxed Warning]: NSAIDs may increase risk of gastrointestinal irritation, inflammation, ulceration, bleeding, and perforation. Use caution with a history of GI disease (bleeding or ulcers), concurrent therapy with aspirin, anticoagulants and/or corticosteroids, smoking, use of alcohol, the elderly or debilitated patients. When used concomitantly with ≤325 mg of aspirin, a substantial increase in the risk of gastrointestinal complications (eg, ulcer) occurs; concomitant gastroprotective therapy (eg, proton pump inhibitors) is recommended (Bhatt, 2008).

Use the lowest effective dose for the shortest duration of time, consistent with individual patient goals, to reduce risk of cardiovascular or GI adverse events. Alternate therapies should be considered for patients at high risk.

NSAIDS may cause drowsiness, dizziness, blurred vision and other neurologic effects which may impair physical or mental abilities; patients must be cautioned about performing tasks which require mental alertness (eg, operating machinery or driving). Discontinue use with blurred or diminished vision and perform ophthalmologic exam. Monitor vision with long-term therapy.

NSAIDs may cause serious skin adverse events including exfoliative dermatitis, Stevens-Johnson syndrome (SJS) and toxic epidermal necrolysis (TEN); discontinue use at first sign of skin rash or hypersensitivity. Anaphylactoid reactions may occur, even without prior exposure; patients with "aspirin triad" (bronchial asthma, aspirin intolerance, rhinitis) may be at increased risk. Do not use in patients who experience bronchospasm, asthma, rhinitis, or urticaria with NSAID or aspirin therapy. Use caution in other forms of asthma.

Use with caution in patients with decreased hepatic function. Closely monitor patients with any abnormal LFT. Severe hepatic reactions (eg, fulminant hepatitis, liver failure) have occurred with NSAID use, rarely; discontinue if signs or symptoms of liver disease develop, or if systemic manifestations occur. The elderly are at increased risk for adverse effects (especially peptic ulceration, CNS effects, renal toxicity) from NSAIDs at low doses. Prolonged use may cause corneal deposits and retinal disturbances; discontinue if visual changes are observed. Use caution with depression, epilepsy, or Parkinson's disease.

Withhold for at least 4-6 half-lives prior to surgical or dental procedures.

Adverse Reactions (Reflective of adult population; not specific for elderly)
>10%: Central nervous system: Headache (12%)
1% to 10%:
  Central nervous system: Dizziness (3% to 9%), depression (<3%), fatigue (<3%), malaise (<3%), somnolence (<3%), vertigo (<3%)
  Gastrointestinal: Dyspepsia (3% to 9%), epigastric pain (3% to 9%), heartburn (3% to 9%), indigestion (3% to 9%), nausea (3% to 9%), abdominal pain/cramps/distress (<3%), constipation (<3%), diarrhea (<3%), rectal irritation (suppository), tenesmus (suppository), vomiting
  Otic: Tinnitus (<3%)

◀ **Drug Interactions**

Metabolism/Transport Effects Substrate (minor) of CYP2C9, 2C19; **Inhibits** CYP2C9 (strong), 2C19 (weak)

Avoid Concomitant Use

Avoid concomitant use of Indomethacin with any of the following: Floctafenine; Ketorolac; Ketorolac (Nasal); Ketorolac (Systemic)

Increased Effect/Toxicity

Indomethacin may increase the levels/effects of: Aminoglycosides; Anticoagulants; Antiplatelet Agents; Bisphosphonate Derivatives; Collagenase (Systemic); CycloSPORINE; CycloSPORINE (Systemic); Deferasirox; Desmopressin; Digoxin; Drotrecogin Alfa; Eplerenone; Haloperidol; Ibritumomab; Lithium; Methotrexate; Nonsteroidal Anti-Inflammatory Agents; PEMEtrexed; Porfimer; Potassium-Sparing Diuretics; PRALAtrexate; Quinolone Antibiotics; Rivaroxaban; Salicylates; Thrombolytic Agents; Tiludronate; Tositumomab and Iodine I 131 Tositumomab; Triamterene; Vancomycin; Vitamin K Antagonists

The levels/effects of Indomethacin may be increased by: ACE Inhibitors; Angiotensin II Receptor Blockers; Antidepressants (Tricyclic, Tertiary Amine); Corticosteroids (Systemic); Dasatinib; Floctafenine; Glucosamine; Herbs (Anticoagulant/Antiplatelet Properties); Ketorolac; Ketorolac (Nasal); Ketorolac (Systemic); Nonsteroidal Anti-Inflammatory Agents; Omega-3-Acid Ethyl Esters; Pentosan Polysulfate Sodium; Pentoxifylline; Probenecid; Prostacyclin Analogues; Selective Serotonin Reuptake Inhibitors; Serotonin/Norepinephrine Reuptake Inhibitors; Sodium Phosphates; Treprostinil; Vitamin E

Decreased Effect

Indomethacin may decrease the levels/effects of: ACE Inhibitors; Angiotensin II Receptor Blockers; Antiplatelet Agents; Beta-Blockers; Eplerenone; HydrALAZINE; Potassium-Sparing Diuretics; Salicylates; Selective Serotonin Reuptake Inhibitors; Thiazide Diuretics

The levels/effects of Indomethacin may be decreased by: Bile Acid Sequestrants; Nonsteroidal Anti-Inflammatory Agents; Salicylates

Ethanol/Nutrition/Herb Interactions

Ethanol: Avoid ethanol (may enhance gastric mucosal irritation).

Food: Food may decrease the rate but not the extent of absorption. Indomethacin peak serum levels may be delayed if taken with food.

Herb/Nutraceutical: Avoid alfalfa, anise, bilberry, bladderwrack, bromelain, cat's claw, celery, chamomile, coleus, cordyceps, dong quai, evening primrose, fenugreek, feverfew, garlic, ginger, ginkgo biloba, ginseng (American, Panax, Siberian), grapeseed, green tea, guggul, horse chestnut seed, horseradish, licorice, prickly ash, red clover, reishi, SAMe (S-adenosylmethionine), sweet clover, turmeric, white willow (all have additional antiplatelet activity).

Stability I.V.: Store below 30°C (86°F). Protect from light. Not stable in alkaline solution. Reconstitute with 1-2 mL preservative free NS or SWFI just prior to administration. Discard any unused portion. Do not use preservative-containing diluents for reconstitution.

Mechanism of Action Reversibly inhibits cyclooxygenase-1 and 2 (COX-1 and 2) enzymes, which results in decreased formation of prostaglandin precursors; has antipyretic, analgesic, and anti-inflammatory properties

Other proposed mechanisms not fully elucidated (and possibly contributing to the anti-inflammatory effect to varying degrees), include inhibiting chemotaxis, altering lymphocyte activity, inhibiting neutrophil aggregation/activation, and decreasing proinflammatory cytokine levels.

Pharmacodynamics/Kinetics

Onset of action: ~30 minutes

Duration: 4-6 hours

Absorption: Oral: Immediate release: Prompt and extensive; Extended release: 90% over 12 hours

Distribution: V_d: 0.34-1.57 L/kg; crosses blood brain barrier

Protein binding: 99%

Metabolism: Hepatic; significant enterohepatic recirculation

Bioavailability: 100%

Half-life elimination: 4.5 hours

Time to peak: Oral: Immediate release: 2 hours

Excretion: Urine (60%, primarily as glucuronide conjugates); feces (33%, primarily as metabolites)

Dosage

Geriatric Refer to adult dosing. Use lowest recommended dose and frequency in elderly to initiate therapy for indications listed in adult dosing.

Adult

Inflammatory/rheumatoid disorders (use lowest effective dose): Oral: 25-50 mg/dose 2-3 times/day; maximum dose: 200 mg/day; extended release capsule should be given on a 1-2 times/day schedule (maximum dose for extended release: 150 mg/day). In patients with arthritis and persistent night pain and/or morning stiffness, may give the larger portion (up to 100 mg) of the total daily dose at bedtime.

Bursitis/tendonitis: Oral: Initial dose: 75-150 mg/day in 3-4 divided doses **or** 1-2 divided doses for extended release; usual treatment is 7-14 days

Acute gouty arthritis: Oral: 50 mg 3 times daily until pain is tolerable then reduce dose; usual treatment <3-5 days

Renal Impairment Not recommended with advanced renal disease.

Administration Oral: Administer with food, milk, or antacids to decrease GI adverse effects. Extended release capsules must be swallowed whole; do not crush.

Monitoring Parameters Monitor response (pain, range of motion, grip strength, mobility, ADL function), inflammation; observe for weight gain, edema; monitor renal function (serum creatinine, BUN); observe for bleeding, bruising; evaluate gastrointestinal effects (abdominal pain, bleeding, dyspepsia); mental confusion, disorientation, CBC, liver function tests (particularly with pediatric use); ophthalmologic exams with prolonged therapy

Test Interactions False-negative dexamethasone suppression test

Pharmacotherapy Pearls There are no clinical guidelines to predict which NSAID will give response in a particular patient; trials with each must be initiated until response determined; consider dose, patient convenience, and cost

Special Geriatric Considerations Elderly are a high-risk population for adverse effects from NSAIDs. As much as 60% of elderly can develop peptic ulceration and/or hemorrhage asymptomatically. The concomitant use of H_2 blockers and sucralfate is not effective as prophylaxis with the exception of NSAID-induced duodenal ulcers which may be prevented by the use of ranitidine. Misoprostol and proton pump inhibitors are the only agents proven to help prevent the development of NSAID-induced ulcers. Also, concomitant disease and drug use contribute to the risk for GI adverse effects. Use lowest effective dose for shortest period possible. Consider renal function decline with age. Use of NSAIDs may compromise existing renal function especially when Cl_{cr} is ≤30 mL/minute. Tinnitus may be a difficult and unreliable indication of toxicity due to age-related hearing loss or eighth cranial nerve damage. CNS adverse effects such as confusion, agitation, and hallucination are generally seen in overdose or high-dose situations, but the elderly may demonstrate these adverse effects at lower doses than younger adults. Indomethacin frequently causes confusion at recommended doses in the elderly.

This medication is considered to be potentially inappropriate in this patient population (Beers Criteria severity: High).

Dosage Forms Excipient information presented when available (limited, particularly for generics); consult specific product labeling.

Capsule, oral: 25 mg, 50 mg

Capsule, extended release, oral: 75 mg

Injection, powder for reconstitution: 1 mg

Indocin® I.V.: 1 mg

Suppository, rectal: 50 mg (30s)

Suspension, oral:

Indocin®: 25 mg/5 mL (237 mL) [contains ethanol 1%; pineapple-coconut-mint flavor]

Selected References

Hunt SA, Abraham WT, Chin MH, et al, "ACC/AHA 2005 Guideline Update for the Diagnosis and Management of Chronic Heart Failure in the Adult: A Report of the American College of Cardiology/American Heart Association Task Force on Practice Guidelines (Writing Committee to Update the 2001 Guidelines for the Evaluation and Management of Heart Failure)," available at: http://www.acc.org/clinical/guidelines/failure//index.pdf

Influenza Virus Vaccine (H5N1) (in floo EN za VYE rus vak SEEN H5N1)

Related Information
Immunization Administration Recommendations *on page 2037*
Immunization Recommendations *on page 2043*
Medication Safety Issues
Sound-alike/look-alike issues:
Influenza virus vaccine (H5N1) may be confused with the nonavian strain of influenza virus vaccine
Index Terms Avian Influenza Virus Vaccine; Bird Flu Vaccine; H5N1 Influenza Vaccine; Influenza Virus Vaccine (Monovalent)
Generic Availability (U.S.) No
Pharmacologic Category Vaccine, Inactivated (Viral)
Use Active immunization of adults at increased risk of exposure to the H5N1 viral subtype of influenza
Prescribing and Access Restrictions Commercial distribution is not planned. The vaccine will be included as part of the U.S. Strategic National Stockpile. It will be distributed by public health officials if needed.
Dosage
Adult Immunization: Adults 18-64 years: I.M.: 1 mL, followed by second 1 mL dose given 28 days later (acceptable range: 21-35 days)
Special Geriatric Considerations No clinical studies in elderly have been done to date. Differences in immune response may be different than the titer response seen in younger adults.
Dosage Forms Excipient information presented when available (limited, particularly for generics); consult specific product labeling.
Injection, suspension [monovalent]: Hemagglutinin (H5N1strain) 90 mcg/mL (5 mL) [contains chicken, egg, and porcine protein, and thimerosal]

Influenza Virus Vaccine (Inactivated)
(in floo EN za VYE rus vak SEEN, in ak ti VAY ted)

Related Information
Immunization Administration Recommendations *on page 2037*
Immunization Recommendations *on page 2043*
Medication Safety Issues
Sound-alike/look-alike issues:
Fluarix® may be confused with Flarex®
Influenza virus vaccine may be confused with flumazenil
Influenza virus vaccine may be confused with tetanus toxoid and tuberculin products. Medication errors have occurred when tuberculin skin tests (PPD) have been inadvertently administered instead of tetanus toxoid products and influenza virus vaccine. These products are refrigerated and often stored in close proximity to each other.
International issues:
Fluarix [U.S., Canada, and multiple international markets] may be confused with Flarex brand name for fluorometholone [U.S. and multiple international markets] and Fluorex brand name for fluoride [France]
Brand Names: U.S. Afluria®; Fluarix®; FluLaval®; Fluvirin®; Fluzone®; Fluzone® High-Dose
Brand Names: Canada Fluviral S/F®; Vaxigrip®
Index Terms H1N1 Influenza Vaccine; Influenza Vaccine; Influenza Virus Vaccine (Purified Surface Antigen); Influenza Virus Vaccine (Split-Virus); TIV; Trivalent Inactivated Influenza Vaccine
Generic Availability (U.S.) No
Pharmacologic Category Vaccine, Inactivated (Viral)
Use Provide active immunity to influenza virus strains contained in the vaccine

The Advisory Committee on Immunization Practices (ACIP) recommends annual vaccination with the seasonal trivalent inactivated influenza vaccine (TIV) (injection) for all persons ≥6 months of age.
When vaccine supply is limited, target groups for vaccination (those at higher risk of complications from influenza infection and their close contacts) include the following:
• Persons ≥50 years of age
• Residents of nursing homes and other chronic-care facilities that house persons of any age with chronic medical conditions
• Adults with chronic disorders of the pulmonary or cardiovascular systems (except hypertension), including asthma

- Adults who have chronic metabolic diseases (including diabetes mellitus), hepatic disease, renal dysfunction, hematologic disorders, or immunosuppression (including immunosuppression caused by medications or HIV)
- Adults with cognitive or neurologic/neuromuscular conditions (including conditions such as spinal cord injuries or seizure disorders) which may compromise respiratory function, the handling of respiratory secretions, or that can increase the risk of aspiration
- Healthcare personnel
- Household contacts and caregivers of children <5 years (particularly children <6 months) and adults ≥50 years
- Household contacts and caregivers of persons with medical conditions which put them at high risk of complications from influenza infection
- American Indians/Alaska Natives
- Morbidly obese (BMI ≥40)

Contraindications Prior life-threatening reaction to previous influenza vaccination; hypersensitivity to any component of the formulation

Warnings/Precautions Anaphylactoid/hypersensitivity reactions: Immediate treatment (including epinephrine 1:1000) for anaphylactoid and/or hypersensitivity reactions should be available during vaccine use. Influenza vaccines from previous seasons must not be used. May consider deferring administration in patients with moderate or severe acute illness (with or without fever); may administer to patients with mild acute illness (with or without fever). Use with caution in patients with a history of bleeding disorders (including thrombocytopenia) and/or patients on anticoagulant therapy; bleeding/hematoma may occur from I.M. administration. Use with caution in patients with history of Guillain-Barré syndrome (GBS); patients with history of GBS have a greater likelihood of developing GBS than those without. As a precaution, the ACIP recommends that patients with a history of GBS and who are at low risk for severe influenza complications, and patients known to have experienced GBS within 6 weeks following previous vaccination should generally not be vaccinated (consider influenza antiviral chemoprophylaxis in these patients). The benefits of vaccination may outweigh the potential risks in persons with a history of GBS who are also at high risk for complications of influenza.

Use with caution in severely immunocompromised patients (eg, patients receiving chemo/radiation therapy or other immunosuppressive therapy [including high-dose corticosteroids]); may have a reduced response to vaccination. Inactivated vaccine is preferred over live virus vaccine for household members, healthcare workers and others coming in close contact with severely-immunosuppressed persons requiring care in a protected environment. Antigenic response may not be as great as expected in HIV-infected persons with CD4 cells <100/mm^3 and viral copies of HIV type 1 >30,000/mL. In order to maximize vaccination rates, the ACIP recommends simultaneous administration of all age-appropriate vaccines (live or inactivated) for which a person is eligible at a single clinic visit, unless contraindications exist. Some products are manufactured with chicken egg protein, gentamicin, kanamycin, neomycin, polymyxin, and/or thimerosal. Packaging may contain natural latex rubber.

Adverse Reactions (Reflective of adult population; not specific for elderly) All serious adverse reactions must be reported to the U.S. Department of Health and Human Services (DHHS) Vaccine Adverse Event Reporting System (VAERS) 1-800-822-7967 or online at https://vaers.hhs.gov/esub/index. In Canada, adverse reactions may be reported to local provincial/territorial health agencies or to the Vaccine Safety Section at Public Health Agency of Canada (1-866-844-0018).

Frequency not defined. Adverse reactions in adults ≥65 years of age may be greater using the high-dose vaccine, but are typically mild and transient.

Cardiovascular: Chest tightness, facial edema

Central nervous system: Chills, drowsiness, fatigue, fever, headache, irritability, malaise, migraine, shivering

Endocrine & metabolic: Dysmenorrhea

Gastrointestinal: Appetite decreased, diarrhea, nausea, sore throat, upper abdominal pain, vomiting

Local: Injection site reactions (including bruising, erythema, induration, inflammation, pain, soreness [10% to 64%; may last up to 2 days], swelling, tenderness)

Neuromuscular & skeletal: Arthralgia, back pain, myalgia (may start within 6-12 hours and last 1-2 days; incidence equal to placebo in adults; occurs more frequently than placebo in children)

Ocular: Red eyes

Otic: Earache

Respiratory: Cough, nasal congestion, nasopharyngitis, pharyngolaryngeal pain, rhinitis, upper respiratory tract infection, wheezing

Miscellaneous: Diaphoresis

Drug Interactions

Avoid Concomitant Use There are no known interactions where it is recommended to avoid concomitant use.

Increased Effect/Toxicity There are no known significant interactions involving an increase in effect.

Decreased Effect

The levels/effects of Influenza Virus Vaccine (Inactivated) may be decreased by: Belimumab; Fingolimod; Immunosuppressants

Stability Store all products between 2°C to 8°C (36°F to 46°F). Potency is destroyed by freezing; do not use if product has been frozen.

Fluarix®: Protect from light.

Afluria®, FluLaval®: Discard 28 days after initial entry. Protect from light.

Fluvirin®, Fluzone®, Fluzone® High Dose: Between uses, the multiple dose vial should be stored at 2°C to 8°C (36°F to 46°F).

Mechanism of Action Promotes immunity to seasonal influenza virus by inducing specific antibody production. Each year the formulation is standardized according to the U.S. Public Health Service. Preparations from previous seasons must not be used.

Pharmacodynamics/Kinetics

Onset of action: Protective antibody titers achieved ~3 weeks after vaccination

Duration: Protective antibody titers persist approximately ≥6 months. Elderly: Protective antibody titers may fall ≤4 months after vaccination.

Dosage

Geriatric It is important to note that influenza seasons vary in their timing and duration from year to year. In general, vaccination should begin soon after the vaccine becomes available and prior to onset of influenza activity in the community. However, vaccination should continue throughout the influenza season as long as vaccine is available.

Immunization: I.M.: Adults ≥ 65 years: *Afluria®, Fluarix®, FluLaval®, Fluvirin®, Fluzone®, Fluzone® High-Dose:* 0.5 mL/dose (1 dose per season) The ACIP considers Fluzone® High-Dose an alternative vaccine for this age group

Adult It is important to note that influenza seasons vary in their timing and duration from year to year. In general, vaccination should begin soon after the vaccine becomes available and prior to onset of influenza activity in the community. However, vaccination should continue throughout the influenza season as long as vaccine is available.

Immunization:

I.M.: *Afluria®, Fluarix®, FluLaval®, Fluvirin®, Fluzone®:* 0.5 mL/dose (1 dose per season)

Intradermal: Adults 18-64 years: *Fluzone® Intradermal:* 0.1 mL/dose (1 dose per season) The ACIP considers this an alternative vaccine for this age group.

Administration For I.M. administration only. Inspect for particulate matter and discoloration prior to administration. Adults should be vaccinated in the deltoid muscle using a ≥1 inch needle length. Do not inject into the gluteal region or areas where there may be a major nerve trunk. Suspensions should be shaken well prior to use.

If a pediatric vaccine (0.25 mL) is inadvertently administered to an adult, an additional 0.25 mL should be administered to provide the full adult dose (0.5 mL). If the error is discovered after the patient has left, an adult dose should be given as soon as the patient can return. If an adult vaccine (0.5 mL) is inadvertently given to a child, no action needs to be taken.

Note: For patients at risk of hemorrhage following intramuscular injection, the ACIP recommends "it should be administered intramuscularly if, in the opinion of the physician familiar with the patients bleeding risk, the vaccine can be administered by this route with reasonable safety. If the patient receives antihemophilia or other similar therapy, intramuscular vaccination can be scheduled shortly after such therapy is administered. A fine needle (23 gauge or smaller) can be used for the vaccination and firm pressure applied to the site (without rubbing) for at least 2 minutes. The patient should be instructed concerning the risk of hematoma from the injection." Patients on anticoagulant therapy should be considered to have the same bleeding risks and treated as those with clotting factor disorders (CDC, 2011).

Simultaneous administration of vaccines helps ensure the patients will be fully vaccinated by the appropriate age. Simultaneous administration of vaccines is defined as administering >1 vaccine on the same day at different anatomic sites. Separate vaccines should not be combined in the same syringe unless indicated by product specific labeling. Separate needles and syringes should be used for each injection. However, in general, vaccination should not be deferred if the brand name or route of the previous dose is not available or not known (CDC, 2011). Adolescents and adults should be vaccinated while seated or lying down. In general, preterm infants should be vaccinated at the same chronological age as full-term infants (CDC, 2011).

Antipyretics have not been shown to prevent febrile seizures. Antipyretics may be used to treat fever or discomfort following vaccination (CDC, 2011). One study reported that routine prophylactic administration of acetaminophen to prevent fever prior to vaccination decreased the immune response of some vaccines; the clinical significance of this reduction in immune response has not been established (Prymula, 2009).

Pharmacotherapy Pearls Pharmacies will stock the formulations(s) standardized according to the USPHS requirements for the season. Influenza vaccines from previous seasons must not be used. Federal law requires that the name of medication, date of administration, the vaccine manufacturer, lot number of vaccine, and the administering person's name, title, and address be entered into the patient's permanent medical record.

It is important to note that influenza seasons vary in their timing and duration from year to year. In general, vaccination should begin soon after the vaccine becomes available and if possible, prior to October. However, vaccination should continue throughout the influenza season as long as vaccine is available.

When vaccine supply is limited, administration should focus on the ACIP target groups. When TIV vaccine is in short supply, administering LAIV to eligible persons is encouraged to increase available TIV to those patients in whom LAIV cannot be used. During periods of inactivated influenza vaccine (TIV) shortage, the CDC and ACIP have recommended vaccination be prioritized based on the following three tiers. The grouping is based on influenza associated mortality and hospitalization rates. Those listed in group 1 should be vaccinated first, followed by persons in group 2, and then group 3. If the vaccine supply is extremely limited, group 1 has also been subdivided in three tiers, where those in group 1A should be vaccinated first, followed by 1B, then 1C.

Priority groups for vaccination with inactivated seasonal influenza vaccine during periods of vaccine shortage:
Tier 1A:
  Persons ≥65 years with comorbid conditions
  Residents of long-term-care facilities
Tier 1B:
  Persons 2-64 years with comorbid conditions
  Persons ≥65 years without comorbid conditions
  Children 6-23 months
  Pregnant women
Tier 1C:
  Healthcare personnel
  Household contacts and out-of-home caregivers of children <6 months
Tier 2:
  Household contacts of children and adults at increased risk of influenza-associated complications
  Healthy persons 50-64 years
Tier 3:
  Persons 2-49 years without high-risk conditions
Further information available at http://www.cdc.gov/mmwr/preview/mmwrhtml/mm5430a4.htm

Special Geriatric Considerations Limited data on the elderly exists due to ethical considerations precluding use of placebo and differences in studies and vaccines; 80% develop a 1:40 HA titer, 70% are completely protected, 90% protected from death.

Dosage Forms Excipient information presented when available (limited, particularly for generics); consult specific product labeling.
Injection, suspension [purified split-virus]:
  Afluria®: Hemagglutinin 45 mcg/0.5 mL (5 mL) [contains chicken egg protein, neomycin (may have trace amounts), polymyxin B (may have trace amounts), thimerosal]
  FluLaval®: Hemagglutinin 45 mcg/0.5 mL (5 mL) [contains chicken egg protein, thimerosal]
  Fluvirin®: Hemagglutinin 45 mcg/0.5 mL (5 mL) [contains chicken egg protein, neomycin (may have trace amounts), polymyxin B (may have trace amounts), thimerosal]
  Fluzone®: Hemagglutinin 45 mcg/0.5 mL (5 mL) [contains chicken egg protein, thimerosal]
Injection, suspension [purified split-virus, preservative free]:
  Afluria®: Hemagglutinin 45 mcg/0.5 mL (0.5 mL) [contains chicken egg protein, neomycin (may have trace amounts), polymyxin B (may have trace amounts)]
  Fluarix®: Hemagglutinin 45 mcg/0.5 mL (0.5 mL) [contains chicken egg protein, gentamicin (may have trace amounts), hydrocortisone (may have trace amounts), may contain natural rubber/natural latex in prefilled syringe, polysorbate 80]
  Fluvirin®: Hemagglutinin 45 mcg/0.5 mL (0.5 mL) [contains chicken egg protein, may contain natural rubber/natural latex in prefilled syringe, neomycin (may have trace amounts), polymyxin B (may have trace amounts)]
  Fluzone®: Hemagglutinin 22.5 mcg/0.25 mL (0.25 mL) [contains chicken egg protein, may contain natural rubber/natural latex in prefilled syringe]

INFLUENZA VIRUS VACCINE (INACTIVATED)

Fluzone®: Hemagglutinin 45 mcg/0.5 mL (0.5 mL) [contains chicken egg protein]

Fluzone®: Hemagglutinin 45 mcg/0.5 mL (0.5 mL) [contains chicken egg protein, may contain natural rubber/natural latex in prefilled syringe]

Fluzone® High-Dose: Hemagglutinin 180 mcg/0.5 mL (0.5 mL) [contains chicken egg protein, may contain natural rubber/natural latex in prefilled syringe]

Selected References

Centers for Disease Control and Prevention, "Prevention and Control of Seasonal Influenza With Vaccines," *MMWR Recomm Rep*, 2009, 58 (early release):1-52. Available at http://www.cdc.gov/mmwr/pdf/rr/rr58e0724.pdf.

Centers for Disease Control and Prevention, "Tiered Use of Inactivated Influenza Vaccine in the Event of a Vaccine Shortage," *MMWR Morb Mortal Wkly Rep*, 2005, 54(30):749-50.

Centers for Disease Control, "General Recommendations on Immunization. Recommendations of the Advisory Committee on Immunization Practices (ACIP)," *MMWR Recomm Rep*, 2006, 55(RR-15):1-48.

Influenza Virus Vaccine (Live/Attenuated) (in floo EN za VYE rus vak SEEN)

Related Information

Immunization Administration Recommendations *on page 2037*

Immunization Recommendations *on page 2043*

Medication Safety Issues

Sound-alike/look-alike issues:

Influenza virus vaccine may be confused with flumazenil

Brand Names: U.S. FluMist®

Brand Names: Canada FluMist®

Index Terms H1N1 Influenza Vaccine; Influenza Vaccine; Influenza Virus Vaccine (Trivalent, Live); LAIV; Live Attenuated Influenza Vaccine

Generic Availability (U.S.) No

Pharmacologic Category Vaccine, Live (Viral)

Use Provide active immunity to influenza virus strains contained in the vaccine

The Advisory Committee on Immunization Practices (ACIP) states that healthy, nonpregnant persons aged 2-49 years may receive vaccination with either the seasonal live, attenuated influenza vaccine (LAIV) (nasal spray) or the seasonal trivalent inactivated influenza vaccine (TIV) (injection).

Contraindications Prior life-threatening reaction to previous influenza vaccination; hypersensitivity to any component of the formulation

Warnings/Precautions Immediate treatment (including epinephrine 1:1000) for anaphylactoid and/or hypersensitivity reactions should be available during vaccine use. Influenza vaccines from previous seasons must not be used. May consider deferring administration in patients with moderate or severe acute illness (with or without fever); may administer to patients with mild acute illness (with or without fever). Defer immunization if nasal congestion is present which may impede delivery of vaccine. Use with caution in patients with history of Guillain-Barré syndrome (GBS); patients with history of GBS have a greater likelihood of developing GBS than those without. As a precaution, the ACIP recommends that patients with a history of GBS and who are at low risk for severe influenza complications, and patients known to have experienced GBS within 6 weeks following previous vaccination should generally not be vaccinated (consider influenza antiviral chemoprophylaxis in these patients). Use the nasal spray with caution in patients with asthma; risk of wheezing following vaccination is increased. Patients with severe asthma or active wheezing were not included in clinical trials. Because safety and efficacy information is limited, the ACIP does not recommend the use of LAIV in patients with chronic pulmonary disorders including asthma.

Because safety and efficacy information is limited, the ACIP does not recommend the use of LAIV in patients with chronic disorders of the cardiovascular system, diabetes, with hematologic disorders and hemoglobinopathies, hepatic disease, neurologic or neuromuscular disorders, or renal disease. Use with caution in severely-immunocompromised patients (eg, patients receiving chemo/radiation therapy or other immunosuppressive therapy [including high-dose corticosteroids]); may have a reduced response to vaccination. Data on the use of the nasal spray in immunocompromised patients is limited. **Avoid contact with severely-immunocompromised individuals for at least 7 days following vaccination.** Because safety and efficacy information is limited, the ACIP does not recommend the use of LAIV in immunosuppresed patients including patients with HIV. In order to maximize vaccination rates, the ACIP recommends simultaneous administration of all age-appropriate vaccines (live or inactivated) for which a person is eligible at a single clinic visit, unless contraindications exist. Safety and efficacy of the nasal spray have not been established in adults ≥50 years of age. Manufactured using arginine, chicken egg protein, gelatin, and gentamicin.

Adverse Reactions (Reflective of adult population; not specific for elderly) All serious adverse reactions must be reported to the U.S. Department of Health and Human Services (DHHS) Vaccine Adverse Event Reporting System (VAERS) 1-800-822-7967 or online at https://vaers.hhs.gov/esub/index. In Canada, adverse reactions may be reported to local provincial/territorial health agencies or to the Vaccine Safety Section at Public Health Agency of Canada (1-866-844-0018).

Frequency of events reported within 10 days.
>10%:
    Central nervous system: Headache (children 3% to 9%; adults 40%), irritability (children 12% to 21%), lethargy (children 6% to 14%)
    Gastrointestinal: Appetite decreased (children 13% to 21%), abdominal pain (children 2% to 12%)
    Neuromuscular & skeletal: Tiredness/weakness (adults 26%), muscle aches (children 2% to 6%; adults 17%)
    Respiratory: Cough (adults 14%), nasal congestion/ runny nose (children 51% to 58%; adults 9% to 44%), sore throat (children 5% to 11%; adults 28%)
1% to 10%:
    Central nervous system: Chills (children 2% to 4%, adults 9%), fever (100°F to 101°F: children 6% to 9%; >101°F: children 1% to 4%)
    Otic: Otitis media (children 3%)
    Respiratory: Sinusitis (adults 4%), sneezing (children 2%), wheezing (children 6-23 months 6%; children 24-59 months 2%)

Drug Interactions
  Avoid Concomitant Use
    Avoid concomitant use of Influenza Virus Vaccine (Live/Attenuated) with any of the following: Belimumab; Fingolimod; Immunosuppressants; Salicylates
  Increased Effect/Toxicity
    Influenza Virus Vaccine (Live/Attenuated) may increase the levels/effects of: Salicylates

    The levels/effects of Influenza Virus Vaccine (Live/Attenuated) may be increased by: AzaTHIOprine; Belimumab; Corticosteroids (Systemic); Fingolimod; Hydroxychloroquine; Immunosuppressants; Leflunomide; Mercaptopurine; Methotrexate
  Decreased Effect
    Influenza Virus Vaccine (Live/Attenuated) may decrease the levels/effects of: Tuberculin Tests

    The levels/effects of Influenza Virus Vaccine (Live/Attenuated) may be decreased by: Antiviral Agents (Influenza A and B); Fingolimod; Immune Globulins; Immunosuppressants
Stability Store in refrigerator at 2°C to 8°C (36°F to 46°F). **Do not freeze.**
Mechanism of Action Promotes immunity to seasonal influenza virus by inducing specific antibody production. Each year the formulation is standardized according to the U.S. Public Health Service. Preparations from previous seasons must not be used.
Pharmacodynamics/Kinetics
  Onset of action: Protective antibody titers achieved ~3 weeks after vaccination
  Duration: Protective antibody titers persist approximately ≥6 months. Elderly: Protective antibody titers may fall ≤4 months after vaccination.
  Distribution: Following nasal administration, vaccine is distributed in the nasal cavity (~90%), stomach (~3%), brain (~2%), and lung (0.4%)
Dosage
  Geriatric Not indicated for use in patients ≥50 years (U.S. labeling) or ≥60 years (Canadian labeling).
  Adult It is important to note that influenza seasons vary in their timing and duration from year to year. In general, vaccination should begin soon after the vaccine becomes available and prior to onset of influenza activity in the community. However, vaccination should continue throughout the influenza season as long as vaccine is available.

    Immunization: Intranasal (FluMist®):
      U.S. labeling: Adults ≤49 years: 0.2 mL/dose (1 dose per season)
      Canadian labeling: Adults ≤59 years: 0.2 mL/dose (1 dose per season)
Administration LAIV: Intranasal: Half the dose (0.1 mL) is administered to each nostril; patient should be in upright position. A dose divider clip is provided. Severely immunocompromised persons should not administer the live vaccine. If recipient sneezes following administration, the dose should not be repeated.

Simultaneous administration of vaccines helps ensure the patients will be fully vaccinated by the appropriate age. Simultaneous administration of vaccines is defined as administering >1 vaccine on the same day at different anatomic sites. The ACIP prefers each dose of a specific vaccine in a series come from the same manufacturer when possible. However, in general, vaccination should not be deferred if the brand name or route of the previous dose is not available or not known (CDC, 2011).

Antipyretics have not been shown to prevent febrile seizures. Antipyretics may be used to treat fever or discomfort following vaccination (CDC, 2011). One study reported that routine prophylactic administration of acetaminophen to prevent fever prior to vaccination decreased the immune response of some vaccines; the clinical significance of this reduction in immune response has not been established (Prymula, 2009).

Vaccine administration with oral influenza antiviral medications: Live influenza virus vaccine (LAIV) should not be given until 48 hours after the completion of influenza antiviral therapy (influenza A and B). Influenza antiviral therapy (influenza A and B) should not be administered for 2 weeks after receiving LAIV. If influenza antiviral therapy (influenza A and B) and LAIV are administered concomitantly, revaccination should be considered.

Test Interactions Administration of the intranasal influenza virus vaccine (live, LAIV) may cause a positive result on the rapid influenza diagnostic test for the 7 days after vaccine administration; for a person with influenza-like illness during this time, the positive test could be caused by either the live attenuated vaccine or wild-type influenza virus.

Pharmacotherapy Pearls Pharmacies will stock the formulations(s) standardized according to the USPHS requirements for the season. Influenza vaccines from previous seasons must not be used. Federal law requires that the name of medication, date of administration, the vaccine manufacturer, lot number of vaccine, and the administering person's name, title, and address, and documentation of the vaccine information statement (VIS; date on VIS and date given to patient) be entered into the patient's permanent medical record.

It is important to note that influenza seasons vary in their timing and duration from year to year. In general, vaccination should begin soon after the vaccine becomes available and prior to onset of influenza activity in the community. However, vaccination should continue throughout the influenza season as long as vaccine is available.

When vaccine supply is not limited, either TIV or LAIV can be used in healthy, nonpregnant persons aged 2-49 years of age.

When vaccine supply is limited, administration should focus on the ACIP target groups. When TIV vaccine is in short supply, administering LAIV to eligible persons is encouraged to increase available TIV to those patients in whom LAIV cannot be used. During periods of inactivated influenza vaccine (TIV) shortage, the CDC and ACIP have recommended vaccination be prioritized based on the following three tiers. The grouping is based on influenza-associated mortality and hospitalization rates. Those listed in group 1 should be vaccinated first, followed by persons in group 2, and then group 3. If the vaccine supply is extremely limited, group 1 has also been subdivided in three tiers, where those in group 1A should be vaccinated first, followed by 1B, then 1C.

Priority groups for vaccination with inactivated seasonal influenza vaccine during periods of vaccine shortage:
Tier 1A:
  Persons ≥65 years with comorbid conditions
  Residents of long-term-care facilities
Tier 1B:
  Persons 2-64 years with comorbid conditions
  Persons ≥65 years without comorbid conditions
  Children 6-23 months
  Pregnant women
Tier 1C:
  Healthcare personnel
  Household contacts and out-of-home caregivers of children <6 months
Tier 2:
  Household contacts of children and adults at increased risk of influenza-associated complications
  Healthy persons 50-64 years
Tier 3:
  Persons 2-49 years without high-risk conditions
Further information available at http://www.cdc.gov/mmwr/preview/mmwrhtml/mm5430a4.htm

Special Geriatric Considerations Limited data on the elderly exists due to ethical considerations precluding use of placebo and differences in studies and vaccines; 80% develop a 1:40 HA titer, 70% are completely protected, 90% protected from death.

Dosage Forms Excipient information presented when available (limited, particularly for generics); consult specific product labeling.

Solution, intranasal [spray, preservative free]:

FluMist®: (0.2 mL) [contains arginine, chicken egg protein, gelatin, gentamicin (may have trace amounts)]

Selected References

Centers for Disease Control and Prevention, "Prevention and Control of Seasonal Influenza With Vaccines," *MMWR Recomm Rep*, 2009, 58 (early release):1-52. Available at http://www.cdc.gov/mmwr/pdf/rr/rr58e0724.pdf.

Centers for Disease Control, "General Recommendations on Immunization. Recommendations of the Advisory Committee on Immunization Practices (ACIP)," *MMWR Recomm Rep*, 2006, 55(RR-15):1-48.

Centers for Disease Control, "Supplemental Recommendations of the Advisory Committee on Immunization Practices (ACIP): Using Live, Attenuated Influenza Vaccine for Prevention and Control of Influenza," *MMWR Recomm Rep*, 2003, 52(RR-13):1-8.

"H1N1 Clinicians Questions and Answers, October 8, 2009." Available at http://www.cdc.gov/h1n1flu/vaccination/clinicians_qa.htm

◆ **Influenza Virus Vaccine (Monovalent)** *see* Influenza Virus Vaccine (H5N1) *on page 936*
◆ **Influenza Virus Vaccine (Purified Surface Antigen)** *see* Influenza Virus Vaccine (Inactivated) *on page 936*
◆ **Influenza Virus Vaccine (Split-Virus)** *see* Influenza Virus Vaccine (Inactivated) *on page 936*
◆ **Influenza Virus Vaccine (Trivalent, Live)** *see* Influenza Virus Vaccine (Live/Attenuated) *on page 940*
◆ **Infumorph 200** *see* Morphine (Systemic) *on page 1238*
◆ **Infumorph 500** *see* Morphine (Systemic) *on page 1238*
◆ **INH** *see* Isoniazid *on page 984*
◆ **Innohep® [DSC]** *see* Tinzaparin *on page 1801*
◆ **InnoPran XL®** *see* Propranolol *on page 1536*
◆ **Inspra™** *see* Eplerenone *on page 609*

Insulin Aspart (IN soo lin AS part)

Related Information

Diabetes Mellitus Management, Adults *on page 2073*

Insulin Regular *on page 963*

Medication Safety Issues

Sound-alike/look-alike issues:

NovoLOG® may be confused with HumaLOG®, HumuLIN® R, NovoLIN® N, NovoLIN® R, NovoLOG® Mix 70/30

High alert medication:

The Institute for Safe Medication Practices (ISMP) includes this medication among its list of drugs which have a heightened risk of causing significant patient harm when used in error. *Due to the number of insulin preparations, it is essential to identify/clarify the type of insulin to be used.*

Other safety concerns:

Cross-contamination may occur if insulin pens are shared among multiple patients. Steps should be taken to prohibit sharing of insulin pens.

Brand Names: U.S. NovoLOG®; NovoLOG® FlexPen®; NovoLOG® Penfill®

Brand Names: Canada NovoRapid®

Index Terms Aspart Insulin

Generic Availability (U.S.) No

Pharmacologic Category Antidiabetic Agent, Insulin

Use Treatment of type 1 diabetes mellitus (insulin dependent, IDDM) and type 2 diabetes mellitus (noninsulin dependent, NIDDM) to improve glycemic control

Unlabeled/Investigational Use Mild-to-moderate diabetic ketoacidosis (DKA); mild-to-moderate hyperosmolar hyperglycemic state (HHS)

Contraindications Hypersensitivity to insulin aspart or any component of the formulation; during episodes of hypoglycemia

Warnings/Precautions Refer to Insulin Regular on page 963.

Due to the short duration of action of insulin aspart, a longer acting insulin or CSII via an external insulin pump is needed to maintain adequate glucose control in patients with type 1 diabetes mellitus. In both type 1 and type 2 diabetes, prandial administration of insulin aspart should be immediately followed by a meal within 5-10 minutes. May also be administered via CSII; do not dilute or mix with other insulin formulations when using an external insulin pump. Rule out pump failure if unexplained hyperglycemia or ketosis occurs; temporary SubQ insulin administration may be required until the problem is identified and corrected. Insulin aspart may also be administered I.V. in selected clinical situations to control hyperglycemia; close monitoring of blood glucose and serum potassium as well as medical supervision is required.

Drug Interactions

Metabolism/Transport Effects Induces CYP1A2 (weak)

Avoid Concomitant Use There are no known interactions where it is recommended to avoid concomitant use.

Increased Effect/Toxicity

Insulin Aspart may increase the levels/effects of: Antidiabetic Agents (Thiazolidinedione); Hypoglycemic Agents; Quinolone Antibiotics

The levels/effects of Insulin Aspart may be increased by: Beta-Blockers; Edetate CALCIUM Disodium; Edetate Disodium; Herbs (Hypoglycemic Properties); Pegvisomant

Decreased Effect

The levels/effects of Insulin Aspart may be decreased by: Corticosteroids (Orally Inhaled); Corticosteroids (Systemic); Luteinizing Hormone-Releasing Hormone Analogs; Somatropin; Thiazide Diuretics

Ethanol/Nutrition/Herb Interactions Refer to Insulin Regular on page 963.

Stability Unopened vials, cartridges, and prefilled pens may be stored under refrigeration between 2°C and 8°C (36°F to 46°F) until the expiration date or at room temperature <30°C (<86°F) for 28 days; do not freeze; keep away from heat and sunlight. Once punctured (in use), vials may be stored under refrigeration or at room temperature <30°C (<86°F); use within 28 days. Cartridges and prefilled pens that have been punctured (in use) should be stored at temperatures <30°C (<86°F) and used within 28 days; do not freeze or refrigerate. When used for CSII, insulin aspart contained within an external insulin pump reservoir should be replaced at least every 6 days; discard if exposed to temperatures >37°C (>98.6°F).

For SubQ administration: *NovoLog® vials:* May be diluted with Insulin Diluting Medium for NovoLog® to a concentration of 10 units/mL (U-10) or 50 units/mL (U-50). According to the manufacturer, diluted insulin should be stored at temperatures <30°C (<86°F) and used within 28 days; do not dilute insulin contained in a cartridge, prefilled pen, or external insulin pump.

For I.V. infusion: May be diluted in NS, D_5W, or $D_{10}W$ to concentrations of 0.05-1 unit/mL. Stable for 24 hours at room temperature.

Mechanism of Action Insulin aspart is a rapid-acting insulin analog.

Refer to Insulin Regular on page 963.

Pharmacodynamics/Kinetics Note: Rate of absorption, onset, and duration of activity may be affected by site of injection, exercise, presence of lipodystrophy, local blood supply, and/or temperature.

Onset of action: 0.2-0.3 hours

Peak effect: 1-3 hours

Duration: 3-5 hours

Protein binding: <10%

Half-life elimination: SubQ: 81 minutes

Time to peak, plasma: 40-50 minutes

Excretion: Urine

Dosage

Geriatric & Adult Note: When compared to insulin regular, insulin aspart has a more rapid onset and shorter duration of activity.

Diabetes mellitus, type 1 and type 2: SubQ: Refer to Insulin Regular on page 963.

Glycemic control in selected clinical situations and under appropriate medical supervision: I.V.: Refer to Insulin Regular on page 963.

Diabetic ketoacidosis (DKA), mild-to-moderate (unlabeled use): SubQ: Refer to Insulin Regular on page 963.

Hyperosmolar hyperglycemic state (HHS), mild-to-moderate (unlabeled use): SubQ: Refer to Insulin Regular on page 963.

Renal Impairment Refer to Insulin Regular on page 963.

Hepatic Impairment Refer to Insulin Regular on page 963.

Administration

SubQ administration: Do not use if solution is viscous or cloudy; use only if clear and colorless. Insulin aspart should be administered immediately (within 5-10 minutes) before a meal. Cold injections should be avoided. SubQ administration is usually made into the thighs, arms, buttocks, or abdomen; rotate injection sites. When mixing insulin aspart with other preparations of insulin (eg, insulin NPH), insulin aspart should be drawn into syringe first. Do not dilute or mix other insulin formulations with insulin aspart contained in a cartridge or prefilled pen.

CSII administration: Do not use if solution is viscous or cloudy; use only if clear and colorless. Patients should be trained in the proper use of their external insulin pump and in intensive insulin therapy. Infusion sets and infusion set insertion sites should be changed at least every 3 days; rotate infusion sites. Do not dilute or mix other insulin formulations with insulin aspart that is to be used in an external insulin pump.

I.V. administration: Do not use if solution is viscous or cloudy; use only if clear and colorless. May be administered I.V. with close monitoring of blood glucose and serum potassium; appropriate medical supervision is required. **Do not administer insulin mixtures intravenously.**

I.V. infusions: To minimize adsorption to I.V. solution bag: **Note:** Refer to institution-specific protocols where appropriate.

If new tubing is **not** needed: Wait a minimum of 30 minutes between the preparation of the solution and the initiation of the infusion

If new tubing is needed: After receiving the insulin drip solution, the administration set should be attached to the I.V. container and the entire line should be flushed with a priming infusion of 20-50 mL of the insulin solution (Goldberg, 2006; Hirsch, 2006). Wait 30 minutes, and then flush the line again with the insulin solution prior to initiating the infusion.

Because of adsorption, the actual amount of insulin being administered via I.V. infusion could be substantially less than the apparent amount. Therefore, adjustment of the I.V. infusion rate should be based on effect and not solely on the apparent insulin dose. The apparent dose may be used as a starting point for determining the subsequent SubQ dosing regimen (Moghissi, 2009); however, the transition to SubQ administration requires continuous medical supervision, frequent monitoring of blood glucose, and careful adjustment of therapy. In addition, SubQ insulin should be given 1-4 hours prior to the discontinuation of I.V. insulin to prevent hyperglycemia (Moghissi, 2009).

Monitoring Parameters

Diabetes mellitus: Plasma glucose, electrolytes, Hb A$_{1c}$

I.V. administration: Close monitoring of blood glucose and serum potassium

Reference Range Refer to Insulin Regular on page 963.

Pharmacotherapy Pearls Refer to Insulin Regular on page 963.

Special Geriatric Considerations Intensive glucose control (HbA$_{1c}$ <6.5%) has been linked to increased all-cause and cardiovascular mortality, hypoglycemia requiring assistance, and weight gain in adult type 2 diabetes. How "tightly" to control a geriatric patient's blood glucose needs to be individualized. Such a decision should be based on several factors, including the patient's functional and cognitive status, how well he/she recognizes hypoglycemic or hyperglycemic symptoms, and how to respond to them and other disease states. An HbA$_{1c}$ <7.5% is an acceptable endpoint for a healthy older adult, while <8% is acceptable for frail elderly patients, those with a duration of illness >10 years, or those with comorbid conditions and requiring combination diabetes medications. Patients who are unable to accurately draw up their dose will need assistance, such as prefilled syringes. Initial doses may require considerations for renal function in the elderly with dosing adjusted subsequently based on blood glucose monitoring. For elderly patients with diabetes who are relatively healthy, attaining target goals for aspirin use, blood pressure, lipids, smoking cessation, and diet and exercise may be more important than normalized glycemic control.

Dosage Forms Excipient information presented when available (limited, particularly for generics); consult specific product labeling.

Injection, solution:

NovoLOG®: 100 units/mL (10 mL) [vial]

NovoLOG® FlexPen®: 100 units/mL (3 mL)

NovoLOG® Penfill®: 100 units/mL (3 mL) [cartridge]

Selected References

Action to Control Cardiovascular Risk in Diabetes Study Group, Gerstein HC, Miller ME, et al, "Effects of Intensive Glucose Lowering in Type 2 Diabetes," *N Engl J Med*, 2008, 358(24):2545-59.

ADVANCE Collaborative Group, Patel A, MacMahon S, et al, "Intensive Blood Glucose Control and Vascular Outcomes in Patients With Type 2 Diabetes," *N Engl J Med*, 2008, 358(24):2560-72.

American Diabetes Association, "Standards of Medical Care in Diabetes – 2011," *Diabetes Care*, 2011, 34(Suppl 1):11-61.

Brown AF, Mangione CM, Saliba D, et al, "Guidelines for Improving the Care of the Older Person With Diabetes Mellitus," *J Am Geriatr Soc*, 2003, 51(5 Suppl Guidelines):265-80.

"VA/DoD Clinical Practice Guideline for the Management of Diabetes Mellitus," 2010. Available at http://www.-healthquality.va.gov/Diabetes_Mellitus.asp

◆ **Insulin Aspart and Insulin Aspart Protamine** see Insulin Aspart Protamine and Insulin Aspart on page 946

Insulin Aspart Protamine and Insulin Aspart
(IN soo lin AS part PROE ta meen & IN soo lin AS part)

Related Information
Diabetes Mellitus Management, Adults *on page 2073*
Insulin Regular *on page 963*
Medication Safety Issues
Sound-alike/look-alike issues:
NovoLOG® Mix 70/30 may be confused with HumaLOG® Mix 75/25™, HumuLIN® 70/30, NovoLIN® 70/30, NovoLOG®
High alert medication:
The Institute for Safe Medication Practices (ISMP) includes this medication among its list of drugs which have a heightened risk of causing significant patient harm when used in error. ***Due to the number of insulin preparations, it is essential to identify/clarify the type of insulin to be used.***
Other safety concerns:
Cross-contamination may occur if insulin pens are shared among multiple patients. Steps should be taken to prohibit sharing of insulin pens.
Brand Names: U.S. NovoLOG® Mix 70/30; NovoLOG® Mix 70/30 FlexPen®
Brand Names: Canada NovoMix® 30
Index Terms Insulin Aspart and Insulin Aspart Protamine; NovoLog 70/30
Generic Availability (U.S.) No
Pharmacologic Category Antidiabetic Agent, Insulin
Use Treatment of type 1 diabetes mellitus (insulin dependent, IDDM) and type 2 diabetes mellitus (noninsulin dependent, NIDDM) to improve glycemic control
Contraindications Hypersensitivity to any component of the formulation; during episodes of hypoglycemia
Warnings/Precautions Refer to Insulin Regular on page 963. Insulin aspart protamine and insulin aspart premixed combination products are **NOT** intended for I.V. or I.M. administration.
Adverse Reactions (Reflective of adult population; not specific for elderly) Refer to Insulin Regular on page 963.
Drug Interactions
Metabolism/Transport Effects Induces CYP1A2 (weak)
Avoid Concomitant Use There are no known interactions where it is recommended to avoid concomitant use.
Increased Effect/Toxicity
Insulin Aspart Protamine and Insulin Aspart may increase the levels/effects of: Antidiabetic Agents (Thiazolidinedione); Hypoglycemic Agents; Quinolone Antibiotics

The levels/effects of Insulin Aspart Protamine and Insulin Aspart may be increased by: Beta-Blockers; Edetate CALCIUM Disodium; Edetate Disodium; Herbs (Hypoglycemic Properties); Pegvisomant
Decreased Effect
The levels/effects of Insulin Aspart Protamine and Insulin Aspart may be decreased by: Corticosteroids (Orally Inhaled); Corticosteroids (Systemic); Luteinizing Hormone-Releasing Hormone Analogs; Somatropin; Thiazide Diuretics
Ethanol/Nutrition/Herb Interactions Refer to Insulin Regular on page 963.
Stability Unopened vials and prefilled pens may be stored under refrigeration between 2°C and 8°C (36°F to 46°F) until the expiration date or at room temperature <30°C (<86°F) for 14 days (prefilled pens) or 28 days (vials); do not freeze; keep away from heat and sunlight. Once punctured (in use), vials may be stored under refrigeration or at room temperature <30°C (<86°F); use within 28 days. Prefilled pens that have been punctured (in use) should be stored at room temperature <30°C (<86°F) and used within 14 days; do not freeze or refrigerate.
Mechanism of Action Insulin aspart protamine and insulin aspart is an intermediate-acting combination insulin product with a more rapid onset and similar duration of action as compared to that of insulin NPH and insulin regular combination products.
Refer to Insulin Regular on page 963.
Pharmacodynamics/Kinetics Note: Rate of absorption, onset, and duration of activity may be affected by site of injection, exercise, presence of lipodystrophy, local blood supply, and/or temperature.
Onset of action: 10-20 minutes
Peak effect: 1-4 hours
Duration: 18-24 hours
Protein binding: ≤9%
Half-life elimination: ~8-9 hours

Time to peak, plasma: 1-1.5 hours

Excretion: Urine

Dosage

Geriatric & Adult Note: Insulin aspart protamine and insulin aspart combination products are approximately equipotent to insulin NPH and insulin regular combination products but with a more rapid onset and similar duration of activity. The proportion of rapid-acting to long-acting insulin is fixed in the combination products; basal versus prandial dose adjustments cannot be made.

Diabetes mellitus, type 1 and type 2: SubQ: Refer to Insulin Regular on page 963.

Renal Impairment Refer to Insulin Regular on page 963.

Hepatic Impairment Refer to Insulin Regular on page 963.

Administration SubQ administration: In order to properly resuspend the insulin, vials and prefilled pens should be gently rolled between the palms ten times; in addition, prefilled pens should be inverted 180° ten times. Properly resuspended insulin should look uniformly cloudy or milky; do not use if any white insulin substance remains at the bottom of the container, if any clumps are present, if the insulin remains clear after adequate mixing, or if white particles are stuck to the bottom or wall of the container. Cold injections should be avoided. Insulin aspart protamine and insulin aspart combination products should be administered within 15 minutes before a meal (type 1 diabetes) or 15 minutes before or after a meal (type 2 diabetes); typically given twice daily. SubQ administration is usually made into the thighs, arms, buttocks, or abdomen; rotate injection sites. Do not dilute or mix with any other insulin formulation or solution; not recommended for use in external SubQ insulin infusion pump.

Monitoring Parameters Diabetes mellitus: Plasma glucose, electrolytes, Hb A$_{1c}$

Reference Range Refer to Insulin Regular on page 963.

Pharmacotherapy Pearls Refer to Insulin Regular on page 963.

Special Geriatric Considerations Intensive glucose control (HbA$_{1c}$ <6.5%) has been linked to increased all-cause and cardiovascular mortality, hypoglycemia requiring assistance, and weight gain in adult type 2 diabetes. How "tightly" to control a geriatric patient's blood glucose needs to be individualized. Such a decision should be based on several factors, including the patient's functional and cognitive status, how well he/she recognizes hypoglycemic or hyperglycemic symptoms, and how to respond to them and other disease states. An HbA$_{1c}$ <7.5% is an acceptable endpoint for a healthy older adult, while <8% is acceptable for frail elderly patients, those with a duration of illness >10 years, or those with comorbid conditions and requiring combination diabetes medications. Patients who are unable to accurately draw up their dose will need assistance, such as prefilled syringes. Initial doses may require considerations for renal function in the elderly with dosing adjusted subsequently based on blood glucose monitoring. For elderly patients with diabetes who are relatively healthy, attaining target goals for aspirin use, blood pressure, lipids, smoking cessation, and diet and exercise may be more important than normalized glycemic control.

Dosage Forms Excipient information presented when available (limited, particularly for generics); consult specific product labeling.

Injection, suspension:

NovoLOG® Mix 70/30: Insulin aspart protamine suspension 70% [intermediate acting] and insulin aspart solution 30% [rapid acting]: 100 units/mL (10 mL)

NovoLOG® Mix 70/30 FlexPen®: Insulin aspart protamine suspension 70% [intermediate acting] and insulin aspart solution 30% [rapid acting]: 100 units/mL (3 mL)

Selected References

Action to Control Cardiovascular Risk in Diabetes Study Group, Gerstein HC, Miller ME, et al, "Effects of Intensive Glucose Lowering in Type 2 Diabetes," *N Engl J Med*, 2008, 358(24):2545-59.

ADVANCE Collaborative Group, Patel A, MacMahon S, et al, "Intensive Blood Glucose Control and Vascular Outcomes in Patients With Type 2 Diabetes," *N Engl J Med*, 2008, 358(24):2560-72.

American Diabetes Association, "Standards of Medical Care in Diabetes – 2011," *Diabetes Care*, 2011, 34(Suppl 1):11-61.

Brown AF, Mangione CM, Saliba D, et al, "Guidelines for Improving the Care of the Older Person With Diabetes Mellitus," *J Am Geriatr Soc*, 2003, 51(5 Suppl Guidelines):265-80.

"VA/DoD Clinical Practice Guideline for the Management of Diabetes Mellitus," 2010. Available at http://www.healthquality.va.gov/Diabetes_Mellitus.asp

Insulin Detemir (IN soo lin DE te mir)

Related Information

Diabetes Mellitus Management, Adults *on page 2073*

Insulin Regular *on page 963*

Medication Safety Issues

High alert medication:

The Institute for Safe Medication Practices (ISMP) includes this medication among its list of drugs which have a heightened risk of causing significant patient harm when used in error.

◀ *Due to the number of insulin preparations, it is essential to identify/clarify the type of insulin to be used.*

Administration issues:
Insulin detemir is a clear solution, but it is NOT intended for I.V. or I.M. administration.

Other safety concerns:
Cross-contamination may occur if insulin pens are shared among multiple patients. Steps should be taken to prohibit sharing of insulin pens.

Brand Names: U.S. Levemir®; Levemir® FlexPen®

Brand Names: Canada Levemir®

Index Terms Detemir Insulin

Generic Availability (U.S.) No

Pharmacologic Category Antidiabetic Agent, Insulin

Use Treatment of type 1 diabetes mellitus (insulin dependent, IDDM) and type 2 diabetes mellitus (noninsulin dependent, NIDDM) to improve glycemic control

Contraindications Hypersensitivity to insulin detemir or any component of the formulation

Warnings/Precautions Refer to Insulin Regular on page 963.

The duration of action of insulin detemir is dose-dependent; consider this factor during dosage adjustment and titration. Insulin detemir is a clear solution but it is **NOT** intended for I.V. or I.M. administration.

Adverse Reactions (Reflective of adult population; not specific for elderly) Refer to Insulin Regular on page 963.

Drug Interactions

Metabolism/Transport Effects Induces CYP1A2 (weak)

Avoid Concomitant Use There are no known interactions where it is recommended to avoid concomitant use.

Increased Effect/Toxicity
Insulin Detemir may increase the levels/effects of: Antidiabetic Agents (Thiazolidinedione); Hypoglycemic Agents; Quinolone Antibiotics

The levels/effects of Insulin Detemir may be increased by: Beta-Blockers; Edetate CALCIUM Disodium; Edetate Disodium; Herbs (Hypoglycemic Properties); Pegvisomant

Decreased Effect
The levels/effects of Insulin Detemir may be decreased by: Corticosteroids (Orally Inhaled); Corticosteroids (Systemic); Luteinizing Hormone-Releasing Hormone Analogs; Somatropin; Thiazide Diuretics

Ethanol/Nutrition/Herb Interactions Refer to Insulin Regular on page 963.

Stability Unopened vials, cartridges, and prefilled pens may be stored under refrigeration between 2°C and 8°C (36°F to 46°F) until the expiration date or at room temperature <30°C (<86°F) for 42 days; do not freeze; keep away from heat and sunlight. Once punctured (in use), vials may be stored under refrigeration or at room temperature <30°C (<86°F); use within 42 days. Cartridges and prefilled pens that have been punctured (in use) should be stored at temperatures <30°C (<86°F) and used within 42 days; do not freeze or refrigerate.

Mechanism of Action Insulin detemir is an intermediate- to long-acting insulin analog. Refer to Insulin Regular on page 963.

Pharmacodynamics/Kinetics Note: Rate of absorption, onset, and duration of activity may be affected by site of injection, exercise, presence of lipodystrophy, local blood supply, and/or temperature.

Onset of action: 3-4 hours

Peak effect: 3-9 hours (Plank, 2005)

Duration: Dose dependent: 6-23 hours; **Note:** Duration is dose-dependent. At lower dosages (0.1-0.2 units/kg), mean duration is variable (5.7-12.1 hours). At 0.4 units/kg, the mean duration was 19.9 hours. At high dosages (≥0.8 units/kg) the duration is longer and less variable (mean of 22-23 hours) (Plank, 2005).

Distribution: V_d: 0.1 L/kg

Protein binding: >98% (albumin)

Bioavailability: 60%

Half-life elimination: 5-7 hours (dose-dependent)

Time to peak, plasma: 6-8 hours

Excretion: Urine

Dosage

Geriatric & Adult Note: When compared to insulin NPH, insulin detemir has a slower, more prolonged absorption; duration is dose-dependent. Insulin detemir may be given once or twice daily when used as the basal insulin component of therapy. Changing the basal insulin component from another insulin to insulin detemir can be done on a unit-to-unit basis.

Diabetes mellitus:

Type 1: SubQ: Refer to Insulin Regular on page 963.

Type 2: SubQ: Refer to Insulin Regular on page 963.

Initial basal insulin dose: Manufacturer recommendations: 0.1-0.2 units/kg once-daily **or** 10 units once- or twice daily.

Renal Impairment Refer to Insulin Regular on page 963.

Hepatic Impairment Refer to Insulin Regular on page 963.

Administration SubQ administration: Do not use if solution is viscous or cloudy; use only if clear and colorless with no visible particles. Insulin detemir should be administered once or twice daily. When given once daily, administer with the evening meal or at bedtime. When given twice daily, administer the evening dose with the evening meal, at bedtime, or 12 hours following the morning dose. Cold injections should be avoided. SubQ administration is usually made into the thighs, arms, buttocks, or abdomen; rotate injection sites. Do not dilute or mix insulin detemir with any other insulin formulation or solution; **not** recommended for use in external SubQ insulin infusion pump.

Monitoring Parameters Diabetes mellitus: Plasma glucose, electrolytes, Hb A$_{1c}$, lipid profile

Reference Range Refer to Insulin Regular on page 963.

Pharmacotherapy Pearls Insulin detemir differs from human insulin by a single amino acid omission (threonine at B30) and the addition of a 14-carbon fatty acid chain attached at the B29 position. On injection, the fatty acid chain facilitates self-association between the molecules as well as binding to albumin. The delayed release of insulin from the injection site and albumin binding sites result in more prolonged action and limits variability in the amount of free insulin at steady-state. Insulin detemir has a duration of action which is dose-dependent. The FDA-approved product labeling identifies this product as a long-acting insulin analog; however, at lower dosages (<0.4 units/kg) published data regarding its duration of action is consistent with an intermediate insulin form (12-20 hours) (Plank, 2005). In clinical trials it has been compared primarily with NPH insulin and dosed in a similar manner. In some patients, or at higher dosages, it may have a duration of action up to 24 hours, which is consistent with a long-acting insulin (Le Floch, 2009; Plank, 2005; Porcellati, 2007).

Refer to Insulin Regular on page 963

Special Geriatric Considerations Intensive glucose control (HbA$_{1c}$ <6.5%) has been linked to increased all-cause and cardiovascular mortality, hypoglycemia requiring assistance, and weight gain in adult type 2 diabetes. How "tightly" to control a geriatric patient's blood glucose needs to be individualized. Such a decision should be based on several factors, including the patient's functional and cognitive status, how well he/she recognizes hypoglycemic or hyperglycemic symptoms, and how to respond to them and other disease states. An HbA$_{1c}$ <7.5% is an acceptable endpoint for a healthy older adult, while <8% is acceptable for frail elderly patients, those with a duration of illness >10 years, or those with comorbid conditions and requiring combination diabetes medications. Patients who are unable to accurately draw up their dose will need assistance, such as prefilled syringes. Initial doses may require considerations for renal function in the elderly with dosing adjusted subsequently based on blood glucose monitoring. For elderly patients with diabetes who are relatively healthy, attaining target goals for aspirin use, blood pressure, lipids, smoking cessation, and diet and exercise may be more important than normalized glycemic control.

Dosage Forms Excipient information presented when available (limited, particularly for generics); consult specific product labeling.

Injection, solution:

Levemir®: 100 units/mL (10 mL)

Levemir® FlexPen®: 100 units/mL (3 mL)

Selected References

Action to Control Cardiovascular Risk in Diabetes Study Group, Gerstein HC, Miller ME, et al, "Effects of Intensive Glucose Lowering in Type 2 Diabetes," *N Engl J Med*, 2008, 358(24):2545-59.

ADVANCE Collaborative Group, Patel A, MacMahon S, et al, "Intensive Blood Glucose Control and Vascular Outcomes in Patients With Type 2 Diabetes," *N Engl J Med*, 2008, 358(24):2560-72.

American Diabetes Association, "Standards of Medical Care in Diabetes – 2011," *Diabetes Care*, 2011, 34(Suppl 1):11-61.

Brown AF, Mangione CM, Saliba D, et al, "Guidelines for Improving the Care of the Older Person With Diabetes Mellitus," *J Am Geriatr Soc*, 2003, 51(5 Suppl Guidelines):265-80.

"VA/DoD Clinical Practice Guideline for the Management of Diabetes Mellitus," 2010. Available at http://www.-healthquality.va.gov/Diabetes_Mellitus.asp

Insulin Glargine (IN soo lin GLAR jeen)

Related Information
Diabetes Mellitus Management, Adults *on page 2073*
Insulin Regular *on page 963*

Medication Safety Issues
Sound-alike/look-alike issues:
Insulin glargine may be confused with insulin glulisine
Lantus® may be confused with latanoprost, Latuda®, Xalatan®

High alert medication:
The Institute for Safe Medication Practices (ISMP) includes this medication among its list of drugs which have a heightened risk of causing significant patient harm when used in error.
Due to the number of insulin preparations, it is essential to identify/clarify the type of insulin to be used.

Administration issues:
Insulin glargine is a clear solution, but it is NOT intended for I.V. or I.M. administration.

Other safety concerns:
Cross-contamination may occur if insulin pens are shared among multiple patients. Steps should be taken to prohibit sharing of insulin pens.

International issues:
Lantus [U.S., Canada, and multiple international markets] may be confused with Lanvis brand name for thioguanine [Canada and multiple international markets]

Brand Names: U.S. Lantus®; Lantus® Solostar®

Brand Names: Canada Lantus®; Lantus® OptiSet®

Index Terms Glargine Insulin

Generic Availability (U.S.) No

Pharmacologic Category Antidiabetic Agent, Insulin

Use Treatment of type 1 diabetes mellitus (insulin dependent, IDDM) and type 2 diabetes mellitus (noninsulin dependent, NIDDM) to improve glycemic control

Contraindications Hypersensitivity to insulin glargine or any component of the formulation

Warnings/Precautions Refer to Insulin Regular on page 963. Insulin glargine is a clear solution, but it is **NOT** intended for I.V. or I.M. administration.

Adverse Reactions (Reflective of adult population; not specific for elderly) Refer to Insulin Regular on page 963.

Drug Interactions
Metabolism/Transport Effects Induces CYP1A2 (weak)

Avoid Concomitant Use There are no known interactions where it is recommended to avoid concomitant use.

Increased Effect/Toxicity
Insulin Glargine may increase the levels/effects of: Antidiabetic Agents (Thiazolidinedione); Hypoglycemic Agents; Quinolone Antibiotics

The levels/effects of Insulin Glargine may be increased by: Beta-Blockers; Edetate CALCIUM Disodium; Edetate Disodium; Herbs (Hypoglycemic Properties); Pegvisomant

Decreased Effect
The levels/effects of Insulin Glargine may be decreased by: Corticosteroids (Orally Inhaled); Corticosteroids (Systemic); Luteinizing Hormone-Releasing Hormone Analogs; Somatropin; Thiazide Diuretics

Ethanol/Nutrition/Herb Interactions Refer to Insulin Regular on page 963.

Stability Unopened vials, cartridges, and prefilled pens may be stored under refrigeration between 2°C and 8°C (36°F to 46°F) until the expiration date or at room temperature <30°C (<86°F) for 28 days; do not freeze; keep away from heat and sunlight. Once punctured (in use), vials may be stored under refrigeration or at room temperature <30°C (<86°F); use within 28 days. Cartridges within the OptiClik® system and prefilled pens (SoloStar®) that have been punctured (in use) should be stored at temperatures <30°C (<86°F) and used within 28 days; do not freeze or refrigerate.

Mechanism of Action Insulin glargine is a long-acting insulin analog.
Refer to Insulin Regular on page 963.

Pharmacodynamics/Kinetics Note: Rate of absorption, onset, and duration of activity may be affected by site of injection, exercise, presence of lipodystrophy, local blood supply, and/or temperature.

Onset of action: 3-4 hours
Peak effect: No pronounced peak
Duration: Generally 24 hours or longer; reported range: 10.8 to >24 hours (up to 32 hours documented in some studies)

Absorption: Slow; upon injection into the subcutaneous tissue, microprecipitates form which allow small amounts of insulin glargine to release over time

Metabolism: Partially metabolized in the skin to form two active metabolites

Time to peak, plasma: No pronounced peak

Excretion: Urine

Dosage

Geriatric & Adult Note: Insulin glargine is approximately equipotent to human insulin, but has a slower onset, no pronounced peak, and a longer duration of activity. Changing the basal insulin component from another insulin to insulin glargine can be done on a unit-to-unit basis.

Diabetes mellitus, type 1 and type 2: SubQ: Refer to Insulin Regular on page 963.

Renal Impairment Refer to Insulin Regular on page 963.

Hepatic Impairment Refer to Insulin Regular on page 963.

Administration SubQ administration: Do not use if solution is viscous or cloudy; use only if clear and colorless with no visible particles. Insulin glargine should be administered once daily, at any time of day; however, administer at the same time each day. Cold injections should be avoided. SubQ administration is usually made into the thighs, arms, buttocks, or abdomen; rotate injection sites. Do not dilute or mix insulin glargine with any other insulin formulation or solution.

Monitoring Parameters Diabetes mellitus: Plasma glucose, electrolytes, Hb A_{1c}

Reference Range Refer to Insulin Regular on page 963.

Pharmacotherapy Pearls The duration of action of insulin glargine is generally 24 hours or longer with a relatively flat action profile throughout this interval. Many pharmacokinetic and pharmacodynamic studies were terminated at 24 hours despite the fact that insulin glargine continued to exhibit hypoglycemic activity beyond 24 hours; therefore, it is difficult to determine the absolute duration of action.

Clinicians should be aware that, in rare cases, patients may exhibit hypoglycemic activity beyond 24 hours and that accumulation of insulin glargine is possible. Adequate monitoring and subsequent dosage adjustments should be made in patients who are requiring less insulin to maintain euglycemia after several days of therapy.

On the other hand, insulin glargine has a reported duration of action that ranges from 10.8 to >24 hours. On rare occasions, patients may require twice-daily injections of insulin glargine to deliver adequate basal insulin coverage over 24 hours. Some clinicians may also switch to twice-daily dosing in patients who require >100 units of insulin glargine per day to allow for complete absorption. Dosing insulin glargine 3 times daily is not recommended.

Also, refer to Insulin Regular on page 963.

Special Geriatric Considerations Intensive glucose control (HbA$_{1c}$ <6.5%) has been linked to increased all-cause and cardiovascular mortality, hypoglycemia requiring assistance, and weight gain in adult type 2 diabetes. How "tightly" to control a geriatric patient's blood glucose needs to be individualized. Such a decision should be based on several factors, including the patient's functional and cognitive status, how well he/she recognizes hypoglycemic or hyperglycemic symptoms, and how to respond to them and other disease states. An HbA$_{1c}$ <7.5% is an acceptable endpoint for a healthy older adult, while <8% is acceptable for frail elderly patients, those with a duration of illness >10 years, or those with comorbid conditions and requiring combination diabetes medications. Patients who are unable to accurately draw up their dose will need assistance, such as prefilled syringes. Initial doses may require considerations for renal function in the elderly with dosing adjusted subsequently based on blood glucose monitoring. For elderly patients with diabetes who are relatively healthy, attaining target goals for aspirin use, blood pressure, lipids, smoking cessation, and diet and exercise may be more important than normalized glycemic control.

Dosage Forms Excipient information presented when available (limited, particularly for generics); consult specific product labeling.

Injection, solution:

Lantus® 100 units/mL (3 mL) [cartridge]

Lantus® 100 units/mL (10 mL) [vial]

Lantus® Solostar®: 100 units/mL (3 mL) [prefilled pen]

Selected References

Action to Control Cardiovascular Risk in Diabetes Study Group, Gerstein HC, Miller ME, et al, "Effects of Intensive Glucose Lowering in Type 2 Diabetes," *N Engl J Med*, 2008, 358(24):2545-59.

ADVANCE Collaborative Group, Patel A, MacMahon S, et al, "Intensive Blood Glucose Control and Vascular Outcomes in Patients With Type 2 Diabetes," *N Engl J Med*, 2008, 358(24):2560-72.

American Diabetes Association, "Standards of Medical Care in Diabetes – 2011," *Diabetes Care*, 2011, 34(Suppl 1):11-61.

Brown AF, Mangione CM, Saliba D, et al, "Guidelines for Improving the Care of the Older Person With Diabetes Mellitus," *J Am Geriatr Soc*, 2003, 51(5 Suppl Guidelines):265-80.

"VA/DoD Clinical Practice Guideline for the Management of Diabetes Mellitus," 2010. Available at http://www.-healthquality.va.gov/Diabetes_Mellitus.asp

Insulin Glulisine (IN soo lin gloo LIS een)

Related Information
Diabetes Mellitus Management, Adults *on page 2073*
Insulin Regular *on page 963*

Medication Safety Issues
Sound-alike/look-alike issues:
Insulin glulisine may be confused with insulin glargine
High alert medication:
The Institute for Safe Medication Practices (ISMP) includes this medication among its list of drugs which have a heightened risk of causing significant patient harm when used in error. *Due to the number of insulin preparations, it is essential to identify/clarify the type of insulin to be used.*
Other safety concerns:
Cross-contamination may occur if insulin pens are shared among multiple patients. Steps should be taken to prohibit sharing of insulin pens.

Brand Names: U.S. Apidra®; Apidra® SoloStar®
Brand Names: Canada Apidra®
Index Terms Glulisine Insulin
Generic Availability (U.S.) No
Pharmacologic Category Antidiabetic Agent, Insulin
Use Treatment of type 1 diabetes mellitus (insulin dependent, IDDM) and type 2 diabetes mellitus (noninsulin dependent, NIDDM) to improve glycemic control
Contraindications Hypersensitivity to insulin glulisine or any component of the formulation; during episodes of hypoglycemia
Warnings/Precautions Refer to Insulin Regular on page 963.

Due to the short duration of action of insulin glulisine, a longer acting insulin or CSII via an external insulin pump is needed to maintain adequate glucose control in patients with type 1 diabetes mellitus. In both type 1 and type 2 diabetes, preprandial administration of insulin glulisine should be immediately followed by a meal within 15 minutes. May also be administered via CSII; do not dilute or mix with other insulin formulations when using an external insulin pump. Rule out pump failure if unexplained hyperglycemia or ketosis occurs; temporary SubQ insulin administration may be required until the problem is identified and corrected. Insulin glulisine may also be administered I.V. in selected clinical situations to control hyperglycemia; close monitoring of blood glucose and serum potassium as well as medical supervision is required.

Adverse Reactions (Reflective of adult population; not specific for elderly) Refer to Insulin Regular on page 963.

Drug Interactions
Metabolism/Transport Effects Induces CYP1A2 (weak)
Avoid Concomitant Use There are no known interactions where it is recommended to avoid concomitant use.
Increased Effect/Toxicity
Insulin Glulisine may increase the levels/effects of: Antidiabetic Agents (Thiazolidinedione); Hypoglycemic Agents; Quinolone Antibiotics

The levels/effects of Insulin Glulisine may be increased by: Beta-Blockers; Edetate CALCIUM Disodium; Edetate Disodium; Herbs (Hypoglycemic Properties); Pegvisomant
Decreased Effect
The levels/effects of Insulin Glulisine may be decreased by: Corticosteroids (Orally Inhaled); Corticosteroids (Systemic); Luteinizing Hormone-Releasing Hormone Analogs; Somatropin; Thiazide Diuretics
Ethanol/Nutrition/Herb Interactions Refer to Insulin Regular on page 963.
Stability Unopened vials, cartridges, and prefilled pens may be stored under refrigeration between 2°C and 8°C (36°F to 46°F) until the expiration date or at room temperature for 28 days; do not freeze; keep away from heat and sunlight. Once punctured (in use), vials may be stored under refrigeration or at room temperature ≤25°C (≤77°F); use within 28 days. Cartridges and prefilled pens that have been punctured (in use) should be stored at temperatures ≤25°C (≤77°F) and used within 28 days; do not freeze or refrigerate. When used for CSII, insulin glulisine contained within an external insulin pump reservoir should be replaced every 48 hours; discard if exposed to temperatures >37°C (>98.6°F).

For I.V. infusion: May be diluted in NS to concentrations of 0.05-1 unit/mL. Stable for 48 hours at room temperature.
Mechanism of Action Insulin glulisine is a rapid-acting insulin analog.
Refer to Insulin Regular on page 963.

Pharmacodynamics/Kinetics Note: Rate of absorption, onset, and duration of activity may be affected by site of injection, exercise, presence of lipodystrophy, local blood supply, and/or temperature.

Onset of action: 0.2-0.5 hours

Peak effect: 1.6-2.8 hours

Duration: 3-4 hours

Distribution: I.V.: 13 L

Bioavailability: SubQ: ~70%

Half-life elimination:

I.V.: 13 minutes

SubQ: 42 minutes

Time to peak, plasma: 0.6-2 hours

Excretion: Urine

Dosage

Geriatric & Adult Note: Insulin glulisine is equipotent to insulin regular, but has a more rapid onset and shorter duration of activity.

Diabetes mellitus, type 1 and type 2: SubQ: Refer to Insulin Regular on page 963.

Glycemic control in selected clinical situations and under appropriate medical supervision: I.V.: Refer to Insulin Regular on page 963.

Renal Impairment Refer to Insulin Regular on page 963.

Hepatic Impairment Refer to Insulin Regular on page 963.

Administration

SubQ administration: Do not use if solution is viscous or cloudy; use only if clear and colorless. Insulin glulisine should be administered within 15 minutes before or within 20 minutes after starting a meal. Cold injections should be avoided. SubQ administration is usually made into the thighs, arms, buttocks, or abdomen; rotate injection sites. When mixing insulin glulisine with other preparations of insulin (eg, insulin NPH), insulin glulisine should be drawn into syringe first. Do not mix other insulin formulations with insulin glulisine contained in a cartridge or prefilled pen.

CSII administration: Do not use if solution is viscous or cloudy; use only if clear and colorless. Patients should be trained in the proper use of their external insulin pump and in intensive insulin therapy. Infusion sets, reservoirs, and infusion set insertion sites should be changed every 48 hours; rotate infusion sites. Do not dilute or mix other insulin formulations with insulin glulisine that is to be used in an external insulin pump.

I.V. administration: Do not use if solution is viscous or cloudy; use only if clear and colorless. May be administered I.V. with close monitoring of blood glucose and serum potassium; appropriate medical supervision is required. **Do not administer insulin mixtures intravenously.**

I.V. infusions: To minimize adsorption to I.V. solution bag: **Note:** Refer to institution-specific protocols where appropriate.

If new tubing is not needed: Wait a minimum of 30 minutes between the preparation of the solution and the initiation of the infusion.

If new tubing is needed: After receiving the insulin drip solution, the administration set should be attached to the I.V. container and the entire line should be flushed with a priming infusion of 20-50 mL of the insulin solution (Goldberg, 2006; Hirsch, 2006). Wait 30 minutes, and then flush the line again with the insulin solution prior to initiating the infusion.

Because of adsorption, the actual amount of insulin being administered via I.V. infusion could be substantially less than the apparent amount. Therefore, adjustment of the I.V. infusion rate should be based on effect and not solely on the apparent insulin dose. The apparent dose may be used as a starting point for determining the subsequent SubQ dosing regimen (Moghissi, 2009); however, the transition to SubQ administration requires continuous medical supervision, frequent monitoring of blood glucose, and careful adjustment of therapy. In addition, SubQ insulin should be given 1-4 hours prior to the discontinuation of I.V. insulin to prevent hyperglycemia (Moghissi, 2009).

Monitoring Parameters

Diabetes mellitus: Plasma glucose, electrolytes, Hb A_{1c}

I.V. administration: Close monitoring of blood glucose and serum potassium

Reference Range Refer to Insulin Regular on page 963.

Pharmacotherapy Pearls Refer to Insulin Regular on page 963.

Special Geriatric Considerations Intensive glucose control (HbA$_{1c}$ <6.5%) has been linked to increased all-cause and cardiovascular mortality, hypoglycemia requiring assistance, and weight gain in adult type 2 diabetes. How "tightly" to control a geriatric patient's blood glucose needs to be individualized. Such a decision should be based on several factors, including the patient's functional and cognitive status, how well he/she recognizes hypoglycemic or hyperglycemic symptoms, and how to respond to them and other disease states. An HbA$_{1c}$ <7.5% is an acceptable endpoint for a healthy older adult, while <8% is acceptable for frail elderly patients, those with a duration of illness >10 years, or those with comorbid conditions and

◀ requiring combination diabetes medications. Patients who are unable to accurately draw up their dose will need assistance, such as prefilled syringes. Initial doses may require considerations for renal function in the elderly with dosing adjusted subsequently based on blood glucose monitoring. For elderly patients with diabetes who are relatively healthy, attaining target goals for aspirin use, blood pressure, lipids, smoking cessation, and diet and exercise may be more important than normalized glycemic control.

Dosage Forms Excipient information presented when available (limited, particularly for generics); consult specific product labeling.

Injection, solution:

Apidra®: 100 units/mL (3 mL) [cartridge]

Apidra®: 100 units/mL (10 mL) [vial]

Apidra® SoloStar®: 100 units/mL (3 mL) [prefilled pen]

Selected References

Action to Control Cardiovascular Risk in Diabetes Study Group, Gerstein HC, Miller ME, et al, "Effects of Intensive Glucose Lowering in Type 2 Diabetes," *N Engl J Med*, 2008, 358(24):2545-59.

ADVANCE Collaborative Group, Patel A, MacMahon S, et al, "Intensive Blood Glucose Control and Vascular Outcomes in Patients With Type 2 Diabetes," *N Engl J Med*, 2008, 358(24):2560-72.

American Diabetes Association, "Standards of Medical Care in Diabetes – 2011," *Diabetes Care*, 2011, 34(Suppl 1):11-61.

Brown AF, Mangione CM, Saliba D, et al, "Guidelines for Improving the Care of the Older Person With Diabetes Mellitus," *J Am Geriatr Soc*, 2003, 51(5 Suppl Guidelines):265-80.

"VA/DoD Clinical Practice Guideline for the Management of Diabetes Mellitus," 2010. Available at http://www.healthquality.va.gov/Diabetes_Mellitus.asp

Insulin Lispro (IN soo lin LYE sproe)

Related Information

Diabetes Mellitus Management, Adults *on page 2073*

Insulin Regular *on page 963*

Medication Safety Issues

Sound-alike/look-alike issues:

HumaLOG® may be confused with HumaLOG® Mix 50/50, Humira®, HumuLIN® N, HumuLIN® R, NovoLOG®

High alert medication:

The Institute for Safe Medication Practices (ISMP) includes this medication among its list of drugs which have a heightened risk of causing significant patient harm when used in error. *Due to the number of insulin preparations, it is essential to identify/clarify the type of insulin to be used.*

Other safety concerns:

Cross-contamination may occur if insulin pens are shared among multiple patients. Steps should be taken to prohibit sharing of insulin pens.

Brand Names: U.S. HumaLOG®; HumaLOG® KwikPen™

Brand Names: Canada Humalog®

Index Terms Lispro Insulin

Generic Availability (U.S.) No

Pharmacologic Category Antidiabetic Agent, Insulin

Use Treatment of type 1 diabetes mellitus (insulin dependent, IDDM) and type 2 diabetes mellitus (noninsulin dependent, NIDDM) to improve glycemic control

Unlabeled/Investigational Use Mild-to-moderate diabetic ketoacidosis (DKA); mild-to-moderate hyperosmolar hyperglycemic state (HHS)

Contraindications Hypersensitivity to insulin lispro or any component of the formulation; during episodes of hypoglycemia

Warnings/Precautions Refer to Insulin Regular on page 963.

Due to the short duration of action of insulin lispro, a longer acting insulin or CSII via an external insulin pump is needed to maintain adequate glucose control in patients with type 1 diabetes mellitus. In both type 1 and type 2 diabetes, preprandial administration of insulin lispro should be immediately followed by a meal within 15 minutes. May also be administered via CSII; do not dilute or mix with other insulin formulations when using an external insulin pump. Rule out pump failure if unexplained hyperglycemia or ketosis occurs; temporary SubQ insulin administration may be required until the problem is identified and corrected. Insulin lispro may also be administered I.V. in selected clinical situations to control hyperglycemia; close monitoring of blood glucose and serum potassium as well as medical supervision is required.

Adverse Reactions (Reflective of adult population; not specific for elderly) Refer to Insulin Regular on page 963.

Drug Interactions

Metabolism/Transport Effects Induces CYP1A2 (weak)

Avoid Concomitant Use There are no known interactions where it is recommended to avoid concomitant use.

Increased Effect/Toxicity

Insulin Lispro may increase the levels/effects of: Antidiabetic Agents (Thiazolidinedione); Hypoglycemic Agents; Quinolone Antibiotics

The levels/effects of Insulin Lispro may be increased by: Beta-Blockers; Edetate CALCIUM Disodium; Edetate Disodium; Herbs (Hypoglycemic Properties); Pegvisomant

Decreased Effect

The levels/effects of Insulin Lispro may be decreased by: Corticosteroids (Orally Inhaled); Corticosteroids (Systemic); Luteinizing Hormone-Releasing Hormone Analogs; Somatropin; Thiazide Diuretics

Ethanol/Nutrition/Herb Interactions Refer to Insulin Regular on page 963.

Stability Unopened vials, cartridges, and prefilled pens may be stored under refrigeration between 2°C and 8°C (36°F to 46°F) until the expiration date or at room temperature <30°C (<86°F) for 28 days; do not freeze; keep away from heat and sunlight. Once punctured (in use), vials may be stored under refrigeration or at room temperature <30°C (<86°F); use within 28 days. Cartridges and prefilled pens that have been punctured (in use) should be stored at temperatures <30°C (<86°F) and used within 28 days; do not freeze or refrigerate. When used for CSII, insulin lispro contained within an external insulin pump reservoir should be changed every 7 days and insulin lispro contained within a 3 mL cartridge should be discarded after 7 days; discard if exposed to temperatures >37°C (>98.6°F).

For SubQ administration: *Humalog® vials:* May be diluted with the universal diluent, Sterile Diluent for Humalog®, Humulin® N, Humulin® R, Humulin® 70/30, and Humulin® R U-500, to a concentration of 10 units/mL (U-10) or 50 units/mL (U-50). According to the manufacturer, diluted insulin should be stored at 30°C (86°F) and used within 14 days or 5°C (41°F) and used within 28 days; do not dilute insulin contained in a cartridge, prefilled pen, or external insulin pump.

For I.V. infusion (unlabeled use): May be diluted in NS or D_5W to concentrations of 0.025-2 units/mL. Stable for 48 hours at room temperature.

Mechanism of Action Insulin lispro is a rapid-acting insulin analog. Refer to Insulin Regular on page 963.

Pharmacodynamics/Kinetics Note: Rate of absorption, onset, and duration of activity may be affected by site of injection, exercise, presence of lipodystrophy, local blood supply, and/or temperature.

Onset of action: 0.25-0.5 hours

Peak effect: 0.5-2.5 hours

Duration: ≤5 hours

Distribution: V_d: 0.26-0.36 L/kg

Bioavailability: 55% to 77%

Half-life elimination:

I.V.: ~0.5-1 hour (dose-dependent)

SubQ: 1 hour

Time to peak, plasma: 0.5-1.5 hours

Excretion: Urine

Dosage

Geriatric & Adult Note: Insulin lispro is equipotent to insulin regular, but has a more rapid onset and shorter duration of activity.

Diabetes mellitus, type 1 and type 2: SubQ: Refer to Insulin Regular on page 963.

Diabetic ketoacidosis (DKA), mild-to-moderate (unlabeled use): SubQ: Refer to Insulin Regular on page 963.

Glycemic control in selected clinical situations and under appropriate medical supervision (unlabeled use): I.V.: Refer to Insulin Regular on page 963.

Hyperosmolar hyperglycemic state (HHS), mild-to-moderate (unlabeled use): SubQ: Refer to Insulin Regular on page 963.

Renal Impairment Refer to Insulin Regular on page 963.

Hepatic Impairment Refer to Insulin Regular on page 963.

Administration

SubQ administration: Do not use if solution is viscous or cloudy; use only if clear and colorless. Insulin lispro should be administered within 15 minutes before or immediately after a meal. Cold injections should be avoided. SubQ administration is usually made into the thighs, arms, buttocks, or abdomen; rotate injection sites. When mixing insulin lispro with other preparations of insulin (eg, insulin NPH), insulin lispro should be drawn into syringe first. Do not dilute or mix other insulin formulations with insulin lispro contained in a cartridge or prefilled pen.

◄ CSII administration: Do not use if solution is viscous or cloudy; use only if clear and colorless. Patients should be trained in the proper use of their external insulin pump and in intensive insulin therapy. Infusion sets and infusion set insertion sites should be changed every 3 days; rotate infusion sites. Insulin in reservoir should be changed every 7 days. Do not dilute or mix other insulin formulations with insulin lispro contained in an external insulin pump.

I.V. administration (unlabeled use): Do not use if solution is viscous or cloudy; use only if clear and colorless. May be administered I.V. with close monitoring of blood glucose and serum potassium; appropriate medical supervision is required. **Do not administer insulin mixtures intravenously.**

I.V. infusions: To minimize adsorption to I.V. solution bag: **Note:** Refer to institution-specific protocols where appropriate.

*If new tubing is **not** needed:* Wait a minimum of 30 minutes between the preparation of the solution and the initiation of the infusion. Wait a minimum of 30 minutes between the preparation of the solution and the initiation of the infusion.

If new tubing is needed: After receiving the insulin drip solution, the administration set should be attached to the I.V. container and the entire line should be flushed with a priming infusion of 20-50 mL of the insulin solution (Goldberg, 2006; Hirsch, 2006). Wait 30 minutes, and then flush the line again with the insulin solution prior to initiating the infusion.

Because of adsorption, the actual amount of insulin being administered via I.V. infusion could be substantially less than the apparent amount. Therefore, adjustment of the I.V. infusion rate should be based on effect and not solely on the apparent insulin dose. The apparent dose may be used as a starting point for determining the subsequent SubQ dosing regimen (Moghissi, 2009); however, the transition to SubQ administration requires continuous medical supervision, frequent monitoring of blood glucose, and careful adjustment of therapy. In addition, SubQ insulin should be given 1-4 hours prior to the discontinuation of I.V. insulin to prevent hyperglycemia (Moghissi, 2009).

Monitoring Parameters
Diabetes mellitus: Plasma glucose, electrolytes, Hb A_{1c}

I.V. administration (unlabeled use): Close monitoring of blood glucose and serum potassium

Reference Range Refer to Insulin Regular on page 963.

Pharmacotherapy Pearls Refer to Insulin Regular on page 963.

Special Geriatric Considerations Intensive glucose control (HbA_{1c} <6.5%) has been linked to increased all-cause and cardiovascular mortality, hypoglycemia requiring assistance, and weight gain in adult type 2 diabetes. How "tightly" to control a geriatric patient's blood glucose needs to be individualized. Such a decision should be based on several factors, including the patient's functional and cognitive status, how well he/she recognizes hypoglycemic or hyperglycemic symptoms, and how to respond to them and other disease states. An HbA_{1c} <7.5% is an acceptable endpoint for a healthy older adult, while <8% is acceptable for frail elderly patients, those with a duration of illness >10 years, or those with comorbid conditions and requiring combination diabetes medications. Patients who are unable to accurately draw up their dose will need assistance, such as prefilled syringes. Initial doses may require considerations for renal function in the elderly with dosing adjusted subsequently based on blood glucose monitoring. For elderly patients with diabetes who are relatively healthy, attaining target goals for aspirin use, blood pressure, lipids, smoking cessation, and diet and exercise may be more important than normalized glycemic control.

Dosage Forms Excipient information presented when available (limited, particularly for generics); consult specific product labeling.

Injection, solution:
HumaLOG®: 100 units/mL (3 mL) [cartridge]
HumaLOG®: 100 units/mL (3 mL, 10 mL) [vial]
HumaLOG® KwikPen™: 100 units/mL (3 mL)

Selected References

Action to Control Cardiovascular Risk in Diabetes Study Group, Gerstein HC, Miller ME, et al, "Effects of Intensive Glucose Lowering in Type 2 Diabetes," *N Engl J Med*, 2008, 358(24):2545-59.

ADVANCE Collaborative Group, Patel A, MacMahon S, et al, "Intensive Blood Glucose Control and Vascular Outcomes in Patients With Type 2 Diabetes," *N Engl J Med*, 2008, 358(24):2560-72.

American Diabetes Association, "Standards of Medical Care in Diabetes – 2011," *Diabetes Care*, 2011, 34(Suppl 1):11-61.

Brown AF, Mangione CM, Saliba D, et al, "Guidelines for Improving the Care of the Older Person With Diabetes Mellitus," *J Am Geriatr Soc*, 2003, 51(5 Suppl Guidelines):265-80.

"VA/DoD Clinical Practice Guideline for the Management of Diabetes Mellitus," 2010. Available at http://www.healthquality.va.gov/Diabetes_Mellitus.asp

◆ **Insulin Lispro and Insulin Lispro Protamine** *see* Insulin Lispro Protamine and Insulin Lispro *on page* 957

Insulin Lispro Protamine and Insulin Lispro
(IN soo lin LYE sproe PROE ta meen & IN soo lin LYE sproe)

Related Information
Diabetes Mellitus Management, Adults *on page 2073*
Insulin Regular *on page 963*

Medication Safety Issues
Sound-alike/look-alike issues:
HumaLOG® Mix 50/50™ may be confused with HumaLOG®
HumaLOG® Mix 75/25™ may be confused with HumuLIN® 70/30, NovoLIN® 70/30, and NovoLOG® Mix 70/30

High alert medication:
The Institute for Safe Medication Practices (ISMP) includes this medication among its list of drugs which have a heightened risk of causing significant patient harm when used in error. *Due to the number of insulin preparations, it is essential to identify/clarify the type of insulin to be used.*

Other safety concerns:
Cross-contamination may occur if insulin pens are shared among multiple patients. Steps should be taken to prohibit sharing of insulin pens.

Brand Names: U.S. HumaLOG® Mix 50/50™; HumaLOG® Mix 50/50™ KwikPen™; HumaLOG® Mix 75/25™; HumaLOG® Mix 75/25™ KwikPen™

Brand Names: Canada Humalog® Mix 25

Index Terms Insulin Lispro and Insulin Lispro Protamine

Generic Availability (U.S.) No

Pharmacologic Category Antidiabetic Agent, Insulin

Use Treatment of type 1 diabetes mellitus (insulin dependent, IDDM) and type 2 diabetes mellitus (noninsulin dependent, NIDDM) to improve glycemic control

Contraindications Hypersensitivity to any component of the formulation; during episodes of hypoglycemia

Warnings/Precautions Refer to Insulin Regular on page 963. Insulin lispro protamine and insulin lispro premixed combination products are **NOT** intended for I.V. or I.M. administration.

Adverse Reactions (Reflective of adult population; not specific for elderly) Refer to Insulin Regular on page 963.

Drug Interactions
Metabolism/Transport Effects Induces CYP1A2 (weak)
Avoid Concomitant Use There are no known interactions where it is recommended to avoid concomitant use.

Increased Effect/Toxicity
Insulin Lispro Protamine and Insulin Lispro may increase the levels/effects of: Antidiabetic Agents (Thiazolidinedione); Hypoglycemic Agents; Quinolone Antibiotics

The levels/effects of Insulin Lispro Protamine and Insulin Lispro may be increased by: Beta-Blockers; Edetate CALCIUM Disodium; Edetate Disodium; Herbs (Hypoglycemic Properties); Pegvisomant

Decreased Effect
The levels/effects of Insulin Lispro Protamine and Insulin Lispro may be decreased by: Corticosteroids (Orally Inhaled); Corticosteroids (Systemic); Luteinizing Hormone-Releasing Hormone Analogs; Somatropin; Thiazide Diuretics

Ethanol/Nutrition/Herb Interactions Refer to Insulin Regular on page 963.

Stability Unopened vials and prefilled pens may be stored under refrigeration between 2°C and 8°C (36°F to 46°F) until the expiration date or at room temperature <30°C (<86°F) for 10 days (prefilled pens) or 28 days (vials); do not freeze; keep away from heat and sunlight. Once punctured (in use), vials may be stored under refrigeration or at room temperature <30°C (<86°F); use within 28 days. Prefilled pens that have been punctured (in use) should be stored at room temperature <30°C (<86°F) and used within 10 days; do not freeze or refrigerate.

Mechanism of Action Insulin lispro protamine and insulin lispro is an intermediate-acting combination product with a more rapid onset and similar duration of action as compared to that of insulin NPH and insulin regular combination products.
Refer to Insulin Regular on page 963.

Pharmacodynamics/Kinetics Note: Rate of absorption, onset, and duration of activity may be affected by site of injection, exercise, presence of lipodystrophy, local blood supply, and/or temperature.
Onset of action: 0.25-0.5 hours
Peak effect:
Humalog® Mix 50/50™: 0.8-4.8 hours
Humalog® Mix 75/25™: 1-6.5 hours

Duration: 14-24 hours
Time to peak, plasma:
  Humalog® Mix 50/50™: 0.75-13.5 hours
  Humalog® Mix 75/25™: 0.5-4 hours
Excretion: Urine

Dosage

Geriatric & Adult Note: Insulin lispro protamine and insulin lispro combination products are approximately equipotent to insulin NPH and insulin regular combination products but with a more rapid onset and similar duration of activity.

Diabetes mellitus, type 1 and type 2: SubQ: Refer to Insulin Regular on page 963

Renal Impairment Refer to Insulin Regular on page 963.

Hepatic Impairment Refer to Insulin Regular on page 963.

Administration SubQ administration: In order to properly resuspend the insulin, vials should be carefully shaken or rolled several times and prefilled pens should be rolled between the palms ten times and inverted 180° ten times. Properly resuspended insulin should look uniformly cloudy or milky; do not use if any white insulin substance remains at the bottom of the container, if any clumps are present, if the insulin remains clear after adequate mixing, or if white particles are stuck to the bottom or wall of the container. Cold injections should be avoided. Insulin lispro protamine and insulin lispro combination products should be administered within 15 minutes before a meal; typically given once- or twice daily. SubQ administration is usually made into the thighs, arms, buttocks, or abdomen; rotate injection sites. Do not dilute or mix with any other insulin formulation or solution; **not** recommended for use in external SubQ insulin infusion pump.

Monitoring Parameters Diabetes mellitus: Plasma glucose, electrolytes, Hb A$_{1c}$

Reference Range Refer to Insulin Regular on page 963.

Pharmacotherapy Pearls Refer to Insulin Regular on page 963.

Special Geriatric Considerations Intensive glucose control (HbA$_{1c}$ <6.5%) has been linked to increased all-cause and cardiovascular mortality, hypoglycemia requiring assistance, and weight gain in adult type 2 diabetes. How "tightly" to control a geriatric patient's blood glucose needs to be individualized. Such a decision should be based on several factors, including the patient's functional and cognitive status, how well he/she recognizes hypoglycemic or hyperglycemic symptoms, and how to respond to them and other disease states. An HbA$_{1c}$ <7.5% is an acceptable endpoint for a healthy older adult, while <8% is acceptable for frail elderly patients, those with a duration of illness >10 years, or those with comorbid conditions and requiring combination diabetes medications. Patients who are unable to accurately draw up their dose will need assistance, such as prefilled syringes. Initial doses may require considerations for renal function in the elderly with dosing adjusted subsequently based on blood glucose monitoring. For elderly patients with diabetes who are relatively healthy, attaining target goals for aspirin use, blood pressure, lipids, smoking cessation, and diet and exercise may be more important than normalized glycemic control.

Dosage Forms Excipient information presented when available (limited, particularly for generics); consult specific product labeling.

Injection, suspension:
  HumaLOG® Mix 50/50™: Insulin lispro protamine suspension 50% [intermediate acting] and insulin lispro solution 50% [rapid acting]: 100 units/mL (10 mL)
  HumaLOG® Mix 50/50™ KwikPen™: Insulin lispro protamine suspension 50% [intermediate acting] and insulin lispro solution 50% [rapid acting]: 100 units/mL (3 mL)
  HumaLOG® Mix 75/25™: Insulin lispro protamine suspension 75% [intermediate acting] and insulin lispro solution 25% [rapid acting]: 100 units/mL (10 mL)
  HumaLOG® Mix 75/25™ KwikPen™: Insulin lispro protamine suspension 75% [intermediate acting] and insulin lispro solution 25% [rapid acting]: 100 units/mL (3 mL)

Selected References

Action to Control Cardiovascular Risk in Diabetes Study Group, Gerstein HC, Miller ME, et al, "Effects of Intensive Glucose Lowering in Type 2 Diabetes," *N Engl J Med*, 2008, 358(24):2545-59.

ADVANCE Collaborative Group, Patel A, MacMahon S, et al, "Intensive Blood Glucose Control and Vascular Outcomes in Patients With Type 2 Diabetes," *N Engl J Med*, 2008, 358(24):2560-72.

American Diabetes Association, "Standards of Medical Care in Diabetes – 2011," *Diabetes Care*, 2011, 34(Suppl 1):11-61.

Brown AF, Mangione CM, Saliba D, et al, "Guidelines for Improving the Care of the Older Person With Diabetes Mellitus," *J Am Geriatr Soc*, 2003, 51(5 Suppl Guidelines):265-80.

"VA/DoD Clinical Practice Guideline for the Management of Diabetes Mellitus," 2010. Available at http://www.healthquality.va.gov/Diabetes_Mellitus.asp

Insulin NPH (IN soo lin N P H)

Related Information
Diabetes Mellitus Management, Adults *on page 2073*
Insulin Regular *on page 963*

Medication Safety Issues
Sound-alike/look-alike issues:
HumuLIN® N may be confused with HumuLIN® R, HumaLOG®, Humira®
NovoLIN® N may be confused with NovoLIN® R, NovoLOG®

High alert medication:
The Institute for Safe Medication Practices (ISMP) includes this medication among its list of drugs which have a heightened risk of causing significant patient harm when used in error. *Due to the number of insulin preparations, it is essential to identify/clarify the type of insulin to be used.*

Other safety concerns:
Cross-contamination may occur if insulin pens are shared among multiple patients. Steps should be taken to prohibit sharing of insulin pens.

Brand Names: U.S. HumuLIN® N; NovoLIN® N

Brand Names: Canada Humulin® N; Novolin® ge NPH

Index Terms Isophane Insulin; NPH Insulin

Generic Availability (U.S.) No

Pharmacologic Category Antidiabetic Agent, Insulin

Use Treatment of type 1 diabetes mellitus (insulin dependent, IDDM) and type 2 diabetes mellitus (noninsulin dependent, NIDDM) to improve glycemic control

Contraindications Hypersensitivity to insulin NPH or any component of the formulation

Warnings/Precautions Refer to Insulin Regular on page 963. Insulin NPH is **NOT** intended for I.V. or I.M. administration.

Adverse Reactions (Reflective of adult population; not specific for elderly) Refer to Insulin Regular on page 963.

Drug Interactions
Metabolism/Transport Effects Induces CYP1A2 (weak)

Avoid Concomitant Use There are no known interactions where it is recommended to avoid concomitant use.

Increased Effect/Toxicity
Insulin NPH may increase the levels/effects of: Antidiabetic Agents (Thiazolidinedione); Hypoglycemic Agents; Quinolone Antibiotics

The levels/effects of Insulin NPH may be increased by: Beta-Blockers; Edetate CALCIUM Disodium; Edetate Disodium; Herbs (Hypoglycemic Properties); Pegvisomant

Decreased Effect
The levels/effects of Insulin NPH may be decreased by: Corticosteroids (Orally Inhaled); Corticosteroids (Systemic); Luteinizing Hormone-Releasing Hormone Analogs; Somatropin; Thiazide Diuretics

Ethanol/Nutrition/Herb Interactions Refer to Insulin Regular on page 963.

Stability Unopened vials, cartridges, and prefilled pens may be stored under refrigeration between 2°C and 8°C (36°F to 46°F) until the expiration date; do not freeze; keep away from heat and sunlight. If refrigeration is not possible, unopened Novolin® N vials may be kept at room temperature ≤25°C (≤77°F) for up to 42 days. Punctured (in use) Novolin® N vials may be stored at room temperature <25°C (<77°F); use within 42 days. Once punctured (in use) Humulin® N may be stored under refrigeration or at room temperature <30°C (<86°F); use within 28 days. Cartridges, and prefilled pens that have been punctured (in use) should be stored at room temperature between 15°C and 30°C (59°F to 86°F) and used within 14 days; do not freeze or refrigerate.

For SubQ administration:
Humulin® N vials: May be diluted with the universal diluent, Sterile Diluent for Humalog®, Humulin® N, Humulin® R, Humulin® 70/30, and Humulin® R U-500. According to the manufacturer, storage and stability information are not available for diluted Humulin® N; do not dilute insulin contained in a cartridge or prefilled pen.

Novolin® N: Insulin Diluting Medium for NovoLog® is not intended for use with Novolin® N or any insulin product other than insulin aspart.

Mechanism of Action Insulin NPH, an isophane suspension of human insulin, is an intermediate-acting insulin.
Refer to Insulin Regular on page 963.

◄ **Pharmacodynamics/Kinetics Note:** Rate of absorption, onset, and duration of activity may be affected by site of injection, exercise, presence of lipodystrophy, local blood supply, and/or temperature.

Onset of action: 1-2 hours

Peak effect: 4-12 hours

Duration: 14-24 hours

Time to peak, plasma: 6-10 hours

Excretion: Urine

Dosage

Geriatric & Adult Note: When compared to insulin regular, insulin NPH has a slower onset and longer duration of activity.

Diabetes mellitus, type 1 and type 2: SubQ: Refer to Insulin Regular on page 963.

Renal Impairment Refer to Insulin Regular on page 963.

Hepatic Impairment Refer to Insulin Regular on page 963.

Administration SubQ administration: In order to properly resuspend the insulin, vials should be carefully shaken or rolled several times, prefilled pens should be rolled between the palms ten times and inverted 180° ten times, and cartridges should be inverted 180° at least ten times. Properly resuspended insulin NPH should look uniformly cloudy or milky; do not use if any white insulin substance remains at the bottom of the container, if any clumps are present, or if white particles are stuck to the bottom or wall of the container. Cold injections should be avoided. SubQ administration is usually made into the thighs, arms, buttocks, or abdomen; rotate injection sites. When mixing insulin NPH with other preparations of insulin (eg, insulin aspart, insulin glulisine, insulin lispro, insulin regular), insulin NPH should be drawn into the syringe **after** the other insulin preparations. Do not dilute or mix other insulin formulations with insulin NPH contained in a cartridge or prefilled pen. Insulin NPH is **not** recommended for use in external SubQ insulin infusion pump.

Monitoring Parameters Diabetes mellitus: Plasma glucose, electrolytes, Hb A_{1c}

Reference Range Refer to Insulin Regular on page 963.

Pharmacotherapy Pearls Refer to Insulin Regular on page 963.

Special Geriatric Considerations Intensive glucose control (HbA$_{1c}$ <6.5%) has been linked to increased all-cause and cardiovascular mortality, hypoglycemia requiring assistance, and weight gain in adult type 2 diabetes. How "tightly" to control a geriatric patient's blood glucose needs to be individualized. Such a decision should be based on several factors, including the patient's functional and cognitive status, how well he/she recognizes hypoglycemic or hyperglycemic symptoms, and how to respond to them and other disease states. An HbA$_{1c}$ <7.5% is an acceptable endpoint for a healthy older adult, while <8% is acceptable for frail elderly patients, those with a duration of illness >10 years, or those with comorbid conditions and requiring combination diabetes medications. Patients who are unable to accurately draw up their dose will need assistance, such as prefilled syringes. Initial doses may require considerations for renal function in the elderly with dosing adjusted subsequently based on blood glucose monitoring. For elderly patients with diabetes who are relatively healthy, attaining target goals for aspirin use, blood pressure, lipids, smoking cessation, and diet and exercise may be more important than normalized glycemic control.

Dosage Forms Excipient information presented when available (limited, particularly for generics); consult specific product labeling.

Injection, suspension:

HumuLIN® N: 100 units/mL (3 mL) [prefilled pen]

HumuLIN® N: 100 units/mL (3 mL, 10 mL) [vial]

NovoLIN® N: 100 units/mL (10 mL) [vial]

Dosage Forms: Canada Excipient information presented when available (limited, particularly for generics); consult specific product labeling.

Injection, suspension:

Novolin® ge NPH: 100 units/mL (3 mL) [NovolinSet® prefilled syringe or PenFill® prefilled cartridge]; 10 mL [vial]

Selected References

Action to Control Cardiovascular Risk in Diabetes Study Group, Gerstein HC, Miller ME, et al, "Effects of Intensive Glucose Lowering in Type 2 Diabetes," *N Engl J Med*, 2008, 358(24):2545-59.

ADVANCE Collaborative Group, Patel A, MacMahon S, et al, "Intensive Blood Glucose Control and Vascular Outcomes in Patients With Type 2 Diabetes," *N Engl J Med*, 2008, 358(24):2560-72.

American Diabetes Association, "Standards of Medical Care in Diabetes – 2011," *Diabetes Care*, 2011, 34(Suppl 1):11-61.

Brown AF, Mangione CM, Saliba D, et al, "Guidelines for Improving the Care of the Older Person With Diabetes Mellitus," *J Am Geriatr Soc*, 2003, 51(5 Suppl Guidelines):265-80.

"VA/DoD Clinical Practice Guideline for the Management of Diabetes Mellitus," 2010. Available at http://www.-healthquality.va.gov/Diabetes_Mellitus.asp

Insulin NPH and Insulin Regular (IN soo lin N P H & IN soo lin REG yoo ler)

Related Information
Diabetes Mellitus Management, Adults *on page 2073*
Insulin Regular *on page 963*

Medication Safety Issues
Sound-alike/look-alike issues:
HumuLIN® 70/30 may be confused with HumaLOG® Mix 75/25, HumuLIN® R, NovoLIN® 70/30, NovoLOG® Mix 70/30
NovoLIN® 70/30 may be confused with HumaLOG® Mix 75/25, HumuLIN® 70/30, HumuLIN® R, NovoLIN® R, and NovoLOG® Mix 70/30

High alert medication:
The Institute for Safe Medication Practices (ISMP) includes this medication among its list of drugs which have a heightened risk of causing significant patient harm when used in error. *Due to the number of insulin preparations, it is essential to identify/clarify the type of insulin to be used.*

Other safety concerns:
Cross-contamination may occur if insulin pens are shared among multiple patients. Steps should be taken to prohibit sharing of insulin pens.

Brand Names: U.S. HumuLIN® 70/30; NovoLIN® 70/30

Brand Names: Canada Humulin® 20/80; Humulin® 70/30; Novolin® ge 30/70; Novolin® ge 40/60; Novolin® ge 50/50

Index Terms Insulin Regular and Insulin NPH; Isophane Insulin and Regular Insulin; NPH Insulin and Regular Insulin

Generic Availability (U.S.) No

Pharmacologic Category Antidiabetic Agent, Insulin

Use Treatment of type 1 diabetes mellitus (insulin dependent, IDDM) and type 2 diabetes mellitus (noninsulin dependent, NIDDM) to improve glycemic control

Contraindications Hypersensitivity to any component of the formulation; during episodes of hypoglycemia

Warnings/Precautions Refer to Insulin Regular on page 963. Insulin NPH and insulin regular combination products are **NOT** intended for I.V. or I.M. administration

Adverse Reactions (Reflective of adult population; not specific for elderly) Refer to Insulin Regular on page 963.

Drug Interactions
Metabolism/Transport Effects Induces CYP1A2 (weak)

Avoid Concomitant Use There are no known interactions where it is recommended to avoid concomitant use.

Increased Effect/Toxicity
Insulin NPH and Insulin Regular may increase the levels/effects of: Antidiabetic Agents (Thiazolidinedione); Hypoglycemic Agents; Quinolone Antibiotics

The levels/effects of Insulin NPH and Insulin Regular may be increased by: Beta-Blockers; Edetate CALCIUM Disodium; Edetate Disodium; Herbs (Hypoglycemic Properties); Pegvisomant

Decreased Effect
The levels/effects of Insulin NPH and Insulin Regular may be decreased by: Corticosteroids (Orally Inhaled); Corticosteroids (Systemic); Luteinizing Hormone-Releasing Hormone Analogs; Somatropin; Thiazide Diuretics

Ethanol/Nutrition/Herb Interactions Refer to Insulin Regular on page 963.

Stability Unopened vials, cartridges, and prefilled pens may be stored under refrigeration between 2°C and 8°C (36°F to 46°F) until the expiration date; do not freeze; keep away from heat and sunlight. Once punctured (in use), vials may be stored under refrigeration or at room temperature <30°C (<86°F); alternatively, punctured (in use) vials may be stored at room temperature <25°C (<77°F) for up to 4 weeks [Canadian labeling; not in U.S. labeling]. If refrigeration is not possible, unopened Novolin® 70/30 vials may be kept at room temperature ≤25°C (≤77°F) for up to 42 days. Punctured (in use) Novolin® 70/30 vials may be stored at room temperature <25°C (<77°F); use within 42 days. Cartridges and prefilled pens that have been punctured (in use) should be stored at room temperature <30°C (<86°F) and used within 10 days [U.S. labeling] or within 4 weeks [Canadian labeling; not in U.S. labeling]; do not freeze or refrigerate.

◀ For SubQ administration:
  Humulin® 70/30: May be diluted with the universal diluent, Sterile Diluent for Humalog®, Humulin® N, Humulin® R, Humulin® 70/30, and Humulin® R U-500. According to the manufacturer, storage and stability information are not available for diluted Humulin® 70/30; do not dilute insulin contained in a cartridge or prefilled pen.
  Novolin® 70/30: Insulin Diluting Medium for NovoLog® is not intended for use with Novolin® 70/30 or any insulin product other than insulin aspart.

Mechanism of Action Insulin NPH and insulin regular is an intermediate-acting combination insulin product with a more rapid onset than that of insulin NPH alone.
Refer to Insulin Regular on page 963.

Pharmacodynamics/Kinetics Note: Rate of absorption, onset, and duration of activity may be affected by site of injection, exercise, presence of lipodystrophy, local blood supply, and/or temperature.
Onset of action: 0.5 hours
Peak effect: 2-12 hours
Duration: 18-24 hours
Time to peak, plasma: Based on individual components:
  Insulin regular: 0.8-2 hours
  Insulin NPH: 6-10 hours
Excretion: Urine

Dosage
Geriatric & Adult Note: When compared to insulin NPH, the combination product (insulin NPH and insulin regular) has a more rapid onset of action and a similar duration of action.
  Diabetes mellitus, type 1 and type 2: SubQ: Refer to Insulin Regular on page 963.
Renal Impairment Refer to Insulin Regular on page 963.
Hepatic Impairment Refer to Insulin Regular on page 963.

Administration SubQ administration: In order to properly resuspend the insulin, vials should be carefully shaken or rolled several times, prefilled pens should be rolled between the palms ten times and inverted 180° ten times, and cartridges should be inverted 180° at least ten times. Properly resuspended insulin should look uniformly cloudy or milky; do not use if any white insulin substance remains at the bottom of the container, if any clumps are present, if the insulin remains clear after adequate mixing, or if white particles are stuck to the bottom or wall of the container. Cold injections should be avoided. Insulin NPH and insulin regular combination products should be administered within 30 minutes before a meal; typically given once- or twice daily. SubQ administration is usually made into the thighs, arms, buttocks, or abdomen; rotate injection sites. Do not mix with any other insulin formulation. Do not dilute combination product (insulin NPH and insulin regular) contained in a cartridge or prefilled pen. Combination insulin products are not recommended for use in an external SubQ insulin infusion pump.

Monitoring Parameters Diabetes mellitus: Plasma glucose, electrolytes, Hb A_{1c}
Reference Range Refer to Insulin Regular on page 963.
Pharmacotherapy Pearls Refer to Insulin Regular on page 963.

Special Geriatric Considerations Intensive glucose control (Hb A_{1c} <6.5%) has been linked to increased all cause and cardiovascular mortality, hypoglycemia requiring assistance, and weight gain in adult type 2 diabetes. For elderly patients with diabetes who are relatively healthy, attaining target goals for aspirin use, blood pressure, lipids, smoking cessation, and diet and exercise may be more important than normalized glycemic control.

Dosage Forms Excipient information presented when available (limited, particularly for generics); consult specific product labeling.
Injection, suspension:
  HumuLIN® 70/30: Insulin NPH suspension 70% [intermediate acting] and insulin regular solution 30% [short acting]: 100 units/mL (3 mL) [prefilled pen, vial]
  HumuLIN® 70/30: Insulin NPH suspension 70% [intermediate acting] and insulin regular solution 30% [short acting]: 100 units/mL (10 mL) [vial]
  NovoLIN® 70/30: Insulin NPH suspension 70% [intermediate acting] and insulin regular solution 30% [short acting]: 100 units/mL (10 mL) [vial]

Dosage Forms: Canada Excipient information presented when available (limited, particularly for generics); consult specific product labeling.
Injection, suspension:
  Humulin® 20/80: Insulin regular solution 20% [short acting] and insulin NPH suspension 80% [intermediate acting]: 100 units/mL (3 mL) [PenFill® prefilled cartridge]
  Novolin® ge 30/70: Insulin regular solution 30% [short acting] and insulin NPH suspension 70% [intermediate acting]: 100 units/mL (3 mL) [prefilled syringe or PenFill® prefilled cartridge]; (10 mL) [vial]
  Novolin® ge 40/60: Insulin regular solution 40% [short acting] and insulin NPH suspension 60% [intermediate acting]: 100 units/mL (3 mL) [PenFill® prefilled cartridge]

Novolin® ge 50/50: Insulin regular solution 50% [short acting] and insulin NPH suspension 50% [intermediate acting]: 100 units/mL (3 mL) [PenFill® prefilled cartridge]

Selected References

Action to Control Cardiovascular Risk in Diabetes Study Group, et al, "Effects of Intensive Glucose Lowering in Type 2 Diabetes," *N Engl J Med*, 2008, 358(24):2545-59.

ADVANCE Collaborative Group, et al, "Intensive Blood Glucose Control and Vascular Outcomes in Patients With Type 2 Diabetes," *N Engl J Med*, 2008, 358(24):2560-72.

American Diabetes Association, "Standards of Medical Care in Diabetes – 2008," *Diabetes Care*, 2008, 31(Suppl 1):12-54.

Brown AF, Mangione CM, Saliba D, et al, "Guidelines for Improving the Care of the Older Person With Diabetes Mellitus," *J Am Geriatr Soc*, 2003, 51(5 Suppl Guidelines):S265-80.

Insulin Regular (IN soo lin REG yoo ler)

Related Information

Diabetes Mellitus Management, Adults *on page 2073*
Insulin Aspart *on page 943*
Insulin Aspart Protamine and Insulin Aspart *on page 946*
Insulin Detemir *on page 947*
Insulin Glargine *on page 950*
Insulin Glulisine *on page 952*
Insulin Lispro *on page 954*
Insulin Lispro Protamine and Insulin Lispro *on page 957*
Insulin NPH *on page 959*
Insulin NPH and Insulin Regular *on page 961*

Medication Safety Issues

Sound-alike/look-alike issues:

HumuLIN® R may be confused with HumaLOG®, Humira®, HumuLIN® 70/30, HumuLIN® N, NovoLIN® 70/30, NovoLIN® R, NovoLOG®

NovoLIN® R may be confused with HumuLIN® R, NovoLIN® 70/30, NovoLIN® N, NovoLOG®

High alert medication:

The Institute for Safe Medication Practices (ISMP) includes this medication among its list of drugs which have a heightened risk of causing significant patient harm when used in error. *Due to the number of insulin preparations, it is essential to identify/clarify the type of insulin to be used.*

Administration issues:

Concentrated solutions (eg, U-500) should not be available in patient care areas. U-500 regular insulin should be stored, dispensed, and administered separately from U-100 regular insulin. For patients who receive U-500 insulin in the hospital setting, highlighting the strength prominently on the patient's medical chart and medication record may help to reduce dispensing errors.

Other safety concerns:

Cross-contamination may occur if insulin pens are shared among multiple patients. Steps should be taken to prohibit sharing of insulin pens.

Brand Names: U.S. HumuLIN® R; HumuLIN® R U-500; NovoLIN® R

Brand Names: Canada Humulin® R; Novolin® ge Toronto

Index Terms Regular Insulin

Generic Availability (U.S.) No

Pharmacologic Category Antidiabetic Agent, Insulin

Use Treatment of type 1 diabetes mellitus (insulin dependent, IDDM) and type 2 diabetes mellitus (noninsulin dependent, NIDDM) to improve glycemic control

Unlabeled/Investigational Use Hyperkalemia; diabetic ketoacidosis (DKA); hyperosmolar hyperglycemic state (HHS); adjunct of parenteral nutrition

Contraindications Hypersensitivity to regular insulin or any component of the formulation; during episodes of hypoglycemia

Warnings/Precautions Hypoglycemia is the most common adverse effect of insulin. The timing of hypoglycemia differs among various insulin formulations. Hypoglycemia may result from increased work or exercise without eating; use of long-acting insulin preparations (eg, insulin detemir, insulin glargine) may delay recovery from hypoglycemia. Profound and prolonged episodes of hypoglycemia may result in convulsions, unconsciousness, temporary or permanent brain damage or even death. Insulin requirements may be altered during illness, emotional disturbances or other stressors. Insulin may produce hypokalemia which, if left untreated, may result in respiratory paralysis, ventricular arrhythmia and even death. Use with caution in patients at risk for hypokalemia (eg, I.V. insulin use). Use with caution in renal or hepatic impairment.

◀ Human insulin differs from animal-source insulin. Any change of insulin should be made cautiously; changing manufacturers, type, and/or method of manufacture may result in the need for a change of dosage. U-500 regular insulin is a concentrated insulin formulation which contains 500 units of insulin per mL; for SubQ administration only using a U-100 insulin syringe or tuberculin syringe; **not for I.V. administration**. To avoid dosing errors when using a U-100 insulin syringe, the prescribed dose should be written in actual insulin units and as unit markings on the U-100 insulin syringe (eg, 50 units [10 units on a U-100 insulin syringe]). To avoid dosing errors when using a tuberculin syringe, the prescribed dose should be written in actual insulin units and as a volume (eg, 50 units [0.1 mL]). Mixing U-500 regular insulin with other insulin formulations is not recommended.

Regular insulin may be administered I.V. or I.M. in selected clinical situations; close monitoring of blood glucose and serum potassium, as well as medical supervision, is required.

The general objective of exogenous insulin therapy is to approximate the physiologic pattern of insulin secretion which is characterized by two distinct phases. Phase 1 insulin secretion suppresses hepatic glucose production and phase 2 insulin secretion occurs in response to carbohydrate ingestion; therefore, exogenous insulin therapy may consist of basal insulin (eg, intermediate- or long-acting insulin or via continuous subcutaneous insulin infusion [CSII]) and/or preprandial insulin (eg, short- or rapid-acting insulin) (see Related Information: Insulin Products). Patients with type 1 diabetes do not produce endogenous insulin; therefore, these patients require both basal and preprandial insulin administration. Patients with type 2 diabetes retain some beta-cell function in the early stages of their disease; however, as the disease progresses, phase 1 insulin secretion may become completely impaired and phase 2 insulin secretion becomes delayed and/or inadequate in response to meals. Therefore, patients with type 2 diabetes may be treated with oral antidiabetic agents, basal insulin, and/or preprandial insulin depending on the stage of disease and current glycemic control. Since treatment regimens often consist of multiple agents, dosage adjustments must address the specific phase of insulin release that is primarily contributing to the patient's impaired glycemic control. Diabetes self-management education (DSME) is essential to maximize the effectiveness of therapy. Treatment and monitoring regimens must be individualized.

Adverse Reactions (Reflective of adult population; not specific for elderly) Frequency not defined.

Cardiovascular: Palpitation, pallor, peripheral edema, tachycardia

Central nervous system: Fatigue, headache, hypothermia, loss of consciousness, mental confusion

Dermatologic: Pruritus, rash, redness, urticaria

Endocrine & metabolic: Hypoglycemia, hypokalemia

Gastrointestinal: Hunger, nausea, numbness of mouth, weight gain

Local: Injection site reaction (including edema, itching, pain or warmth, stinging), lipoatrophy, lipodystrophy

Neuromuscular & skeletal: Muscle weakness, paresthesia, tremor

Ocular: Transient presbyopia or blurred vision

Miscellaneous: Anaphylaxis, antibodies to insulin (no change in efficacy), diaphoresis, local allergy, systemic allergic symptoms

Drug Interactions

Metabolism/Transport Effects Induces CYP1A2 (weak)

Avoid Concomitant Use There are no known interactions where it is recommended to avoid concomitant use.

Increased Effect/Toxicity

Insulin Regular may increase the levels/effects of: Antidiabetic Agents (Thiazolidinedione); Hypoglycemic Agents; Quinolone Antibiotics

The levels/effects of Insulin Regular may be increased by: Beta-Blockers; Edetate CALCIUM Disodium; Edetate Disodium; Herbs (Hypoglycemic Properties); Pegvisomant

Decreased Effect

The levels/effects of Insulin Regular may be decreased by: Corticosteroids (Orally Inhaled); Corticosteroids (Systemic); Luteinizing Hormone-Releasing Hormone Analogs; Somatropin; Thiazide Diuretics

Ethanol/Nutrition/Herb Interactions

Ethanol: Use caution with ethanol; may increase risk of hypoglycemia.

Herb/Nutraceutical: Use caution with alfalfa, aloe, bilberry, bitter melon, burdock, celery, damiana, fenugreek, garcinia, garlic, ginger, ginseng (American), gymnema, marshmallow, stinging nettle; may increase risk of hypoglycemia.

Stability Store unopened vials in refrigerator between 2°C and 8°C (36°F to 46°F); do not freeze; keep away from heat and sunlight. Once punctured (in use), vials may be stored under refrigeration or at room temperature. If refrigeration is not possible, unopened Novolin® R vials may be kept at room temperature ≤25°C (≤77°F) for up to 42 days. Punctured (in use) Novolin® R vials may be stored at room temperature <25°C (<77°F); use within 42 days.
For SubQ administration:
  Humulin® R: May be diluted with the universal diluent, Sterile Diluent for Humalog®, Humulin® N, Humulin® R, Humulin® 70/30, and Humulin® R U-500, to a concentration of 10 units/mL (U-10) or 50 units/mL (U-50). According to the manufacturer, diluted insulin should be stored at 30°C (86°F) and used within 14 days **or** at 5°C (41°F) and used within 28 days.
  Novolin® R: Insulin Diluting Medium for NovoLog® is **not** intended for use with Novolin® R or any insulin product other than insulin aspart.
For I.V. infusion:
  Humulin® R: May be diluted in NS or D_5W to concentrations of 0.1-1 unit/mL. Stable for 48 hours at room temperature, 96 hours under refrigeration, or for 48 hours under refrigeration followed by 48 hours at room temperature.
  Novolin® R: May be diluted in NS, D_5W, or $D_{10}W$ with 40 mEq/L potassium chloride at concentrations of 0.05-1 unit/mL. Stable for 24 hours at room temperature

Mechanism of Action Insulin acts via specific membrane-bound receptors on target tissues to regulate metabolism of carbohydrate, protein, and fats. Target organs for insulin include the liver, skeletal muscle, and adipose tissue.

Within the liver, insulin stimulates hepatic glycogen synthesis. Insulin promotes hepatic synthesis of fatty acids, which are released into the circulation as lipoproteins. Skeletal muscle effects of insulin include increased protein synthesis and increased glycogen synthesis. Within adipose tissue, insulin stimulates the processing of circulating lipoproteins to provide free fatty acids, facilitating triglyceride synthesis and storage by adipocytes; also directly inhibits the hydrolysis of triglycerides. In addition, insulin stimulates the cellular uptake of amino acids and increases cellular permeability to several ions, including potassium, magnesium, and phosphate. By activating sodium-potassium ATPases, insulin promotes the intracellular movement of potassium.

Normally secreted by the pancreas, insulin products are manufactured for pharmacologic use through recombinant DNA technology using either *E. coli* or *Saccharomyces cerevisiae*. Insulins are categorized based on the onset, peak, and duration of effect (eg, rapid-, short-, intermediate-, and long-acting insulin).

Pharmacodynamics/Kinetics Note: Rate of absorption, onset, and duration of activity may be affected by site of injection, exercise, presence of lipodystrophy, local blood supply, and/or temperature.
Onset of action: SubQ: 0.5 hours
  Peak effect: SubQ: 2.5-5 hours
Duration: SubQ:
  U-100: 4-12 hours (may increase with dose)
  U-500: Up to 24 hours
Distribution: V_d: 0.26-0.36 L/kg
Bioavailability: SubQ: 55% to 77%
Half-life elimination: I.V.: ~0.5-1 hour (dose-dependent); SubQ: 1 hour
Time to peak, plasma: SubQ: 0.8-2 hours
Excretion: Urine

Dosage
  Geriatric & Adult
    Diabetes mellitus: SubQ: **Note:** Insulin requirements vary dramatically between patients and therapy requires dosage adjustments with careful medical supervision. Specific formulations may require distinct administration procedures; please see individual agents.
    Type 1: **Note:** Multiple daily injections (MDI) guided by blood glucose monitoring or the use of continuous subcutaneous insulin infusions (CSII) is the standard of care for patients with type 1 diabetes. Combinations of insulin formulations are commonly used.
      Initial dose: 0.5-1.0 units/kg/day in divided doses. Conservative initial doses of 0.2-0.4 units/kg/day may be recommended to avoid the potential for hypoglycemia.
      Division of daily insulin requirement: Generally, 50% to 75% of the total daily dose (TDD) is given as an intermediate- or long-acting form of insulin (in 1-2 daily injections). The remaining portion of the TDD is then divided and administered before or at mealtimes (depending on the formulation) as a rapid-acting or short-acting form of insulin. Premixed combinations are available that deliver the rapid- or short-acting component at the same time as the intermediate- or long-acting component. Some patients may benefit from the use of CSII which delivers rapid-acting insulin as a continuous infusion throughout the day and as boluses at mealtimes via an external pump device.

Adjustment of dose: Dosage must be titrated to achieve glucose control and avoid hypoglycemia. Adjust dose to maintain preprandial plasma glucose between 70-130 mg/dL for most patients. Since treatment regimens often consist of multiple formulations, dosage adjustments must address the specific phase of insulin release that is primarily contributing to the patient's impaired glycemic control. Treatment and monitoring regimens must be individualized. Also see Pharmacotherapy Pearls.

Usual maintenance range: 0.5-1.2 units/kg/day in divided doses. Insulin requirements are patient-specific and may vary based on age, body weight, and/or activity factors:

Adolescents: May require as much as 1.5 units/kg/day during puberty (Silverstein, 2005)

Prepuberty: 0.7-1 unit/kg/day

Type 2: The goal of therapy is to achieve an Hb A_{1c} <7% as quickly as possible using the safe titration of medications. According to a consensus statement by the ADA and European Association for the Study of Diabetes (EASD), basal insulin therapy (eg, intermediate- or long-acting insulin) should be considered in patients with type 2 diabetes who fail to achieve glycemic goals with lifestyle interventions and metformin ± a sulfonylurea. Pioglitazone or a GLP-1 agonist may also be considered prior to initiation of basal insulin therapy. In patients who continue to fail to achieve glycemic goals despite the addition of basal insulin, intensification of insulin therapy should be considered; this generally consists of multiple daily injections with a combination of insulin formulations (Nathan, 2009).

Initial basal insulin dose: 0.2 units/kg or 10 units/day (Nathan, 2009). **Note:** Current guidelines recommend that insulin therapy begin with intermediate- or long-acting insulin given at bedtime or long-acting insulin given in the morning (Nathan, 2009).

Adjustment of basal insulin dose: Increase dose by 2 units/day every 3 days until fasting glucose levels are consistently within target range (70-130 mg/dL); may increase dose in larger increments (eg, 4 units/day) if fasting glucose levels are >180 mg/dL (Nathan, 2009)

Note: If the patient experiences hypoglycemia following adjustment, reduce dose by 4 units/day or 10% of total daily dose, whichever is greater (Nathan, 2009). Additional algorithms, such as the "1-1-100", "2-4-6-8", "3-0-3", and "3-2-1" algorithms, exist to aid in the titration of basal insulin (Davies, 2005; Gerstein, 2006; Meneghini, 2007; Riddle, 2003); therapy should be individualized and based on patient-specific details.

Intensification of therapy: Add a second injection of a short-, rapid-, or intermediate-acting insulin as needed based on blood glucose monitoring; the timing of administration and type of insulin added for intensification of therapy depends on the blood glucose level that is consistently out of the target range (eg, preprandial glucose levels before lunch or dinner, postprandial glucose levels, and/or bedtime glucose levels). Additional injections and subsequent dosage adjustments must address the specific phase of insulin release that is primarily contributing to the patient's impaired glycemic control. Intensification of therapy can usually begin with a second injection of ~4 units/day followed by adjustments of ~2 units/day every 3 days until the targeted blood glucose is within range (Nathan, 2009).

In the setting of glucose toxicity (loss of beta-cell sensitivity to glucose concentrations), insulin therapy may be used for short-term management to restore sensitivity of beta-cells; in these cases, the dose may need to be rapidly reduced/withdrawn when sensitivity is re-established.

Diabetic ketoacidosis (DKA) (unlabeled use): Only I.V. regular insulin should be used for severe DKA; use of SubQ rapid-acting insulin analogs (eg, aspart, lispro) may be appropriate for mild-moderate DKA (Kitabchi, 2009). Treatment should continue until reversal of acid-base derangement/ketonemia. Serum glucose is not a direct indicator of these abnormalities, and may decrease more rapidly than correction of the metabolic abnormalities. Also, refer to institution-specific protocols where appropriate.

Adults <20 years (Kitabchi, 2004):

I.V. infusion: 0.1 units/kg/hour

Adjustment: If serum glucose does not fall by 50 mg/dL in the first hour, check hydration status; if acceptable, double insulin dose hourly until glucose levels fall at rate of 50-75 mg/dL per hour. Once serum glucose reaches 250 mg/dL, decrease dose to 0.05-0.1 units/kg/hour; dextrose-containing I.V. fluids should be administered to maintain serum glucose between 150-250 mg/dL until the acidosis clears. After resolution of DKA, supplement I.V. insulin with SubQ insulin as needed until the patient is able to eat and transition fully to a SubQ insulin regimen. An overlap of ~1-2 hours between discontinuation of I.V. insulin and administration of SubQ insulin is recommended to ensure adequate plasma insulin levels.

SubQ, I.M. (**Note:** Only use the SubQ and I.M route if I.V. infusion access is unavailable): 0.1-0.3 units/kg SubQ bolus, followed by 0.1 units/kg given every hour SubQ or I.M. or 0.15-0.2 units/kg every 2 hours SubQ; continue until acidosis clears, then decrease to 0.05 units/kg given every hour until SubQ replacement dosing can be initiated (Kitabchi, 2004; Wolfsdorf, 2007)

Adults ≥20 years (Kitabchi, 2009):

I.V.:

Bolus: 0.1 units/kg (optional)

Infusion: 0.1-0.14 units/kg/hour. **Note:** If no I.V. bolus was administered, patients should receive a continuous infusion of 0.14 units/kg/hour; lower doses may not achieve adequate insulin concentrations to suppress hepatic ketone body production.

Adjustment: If serum glucose does not fall by at least 10% in the first hour, give an I.V. bolus of 0.14 units/kg and continue previous regimen. In addition, if serum glucose does not fall by 50-70 mg/dL in the first hour, the insulin infusion dose should be increased hourly until a steady glucose decline is achieved Once serum glucose reaches 200 mg/dL, decrease infusion dose to 0.02-0.05 units/kg/hour or switch to SubQ rapid-acting insulin (eg, aspart, lispro) at 0.1 units/kg every 2 hours; dextrose-containing I.V. fluids should be administered to maintain serum glucose between 150-250 mg/dL until the acidosis clears. After resolution of DKA, supplement I.V. insulin with SubQ insulin as needed until the patient is able to eat and transition fully to a SubQ insulin regimen. An overlap of ~1-2 hours between discontinuation of I.V. insulin and administration of SubQ insulin is recommended to ensure adequate plasma insulin levels.

SubQ, I.M.: According to the 2009 ADA consensus statement on hyperglycemic crises, a rapid-acting insulin analog (eg, aspart, lispro) given every 1-2 hours via the SubQ route may be appropriate for mild-moderate DKA; however, specific dosing recommendations are not provided (Kitabchi, 2009). If using the I.V. route for severe DKA, consider switching to SubQ rapid-acting insulin once serum glucose reaches 200 mg/dL (Kitabchi, 2009). The following dosing regimen from the 2004 ADA position statement recommends regular insulin (Kitabchi, 2004):

Bolus: 0.4 units/kg; **Note:** Give half of the dose (0.2 units/kg) as an I.V. bolus and half of the dose (0.2 units/kg) as SubQ or I.M.

Intermittent: 0.1 units/kg given every hour SubQ or I.M.

Adjustment: If serum glucose does not fall by 50-70 mg/dL in the first hour, administer 10 units hourly by I.V. bolus until glucose levels fall at a rate of 50-70 mg/dL per hour. Once serum glucose reaches 250 mg/dL, decrease dose to 5-10 units SubQ every 2 hours; dextrose-containing I.V. fluids should be administered to maintain serum glucose between 150-250 mg/dL until the acidosis clears.

Hyperkalemia, moderate-to-severe (unlabeled use): I.V.: 10 units regular insulin mixed with 25 g dextrose (50 mL D_{50}W) given over 15-30 minutes (ACLS, 2005); alternatively, 50 mL D_{50}W over 5 minutes followed by 10 units regular insulin I.V. push over seconds may be administered in the setting of imminent cardiac arrest. In patients with ongoing cardiac arrest (eg, PEA with presumed hyperkalemia), administration of D_{50}W over <5 minutes is routine. Effects on potassium are temporary. As appropriate, consider methods of enhancing potassium removal/excretion.

Hyperosmolar hyperglycemic state (HHS) (unlabeled use): Only regular insulin should be used. Infusion should continue until reversal of mental status changes and hyperosmolality. Serum glucose is not a direct indicator of these abnormalities, and may decrease more rapidly than correction of the metabolic abnormalities. Also, refer to institution-specific protocols where appropriate.

Adults <20 years (Kitabchi, 2004):

I.V.:

Infusion: 0.1 units/kg/hour

Adjustment: If serum glucose does not fall by 50 mg/dL in the first hour, check hydration status; if acceptable, double insulin dose hourly until glucose levels fall at rate of 50-75 mg/dL per hour. Once serum glucose reaches 300 mg/dL, decrease dose to 0.05-0.1 units/kg/hour; dextrose-containing I.V. fluids should be administered to maintain serum glucose between 250-300 mg/dL until hyperosmolality clears and mental status returns to normal. After resolution of HHS, supplement I.V. insulin with SubQ insulin as needed until the patient is able to eat and transition fully to a SubQ insulin regimen. An overlap of ~1-2 hours between discontinuation of I.V. insulin and administration of SubQ insulin is recommended to ensure adequate plasma insulin levels.

SubQ, I.M. (**Note:** Only use the SubQ and I.M route if I.V. infusion access is unavailable): 0.1-0.3 units/kg SubQ bolus, followed by 0.1 units/kg given every hour SubQ or I.M. or 0.15-0.2 units/kg every 2 hours SubQ; continue until resolution of hyperosmolality, then decrease to 0.05 units/kg given every hour until SubQ replacement dosing can be initiated (Kitabchi, 2004; Wolfsdorf, 2007)

Adults ≥20 years (Kitabchi, 2009):

I.V.:

Bolus: 0.1 units/kg bolus (optional)

Infusion: 0.1-0.14 units/kg/hour. **Note:** If no I.V. bolus was administered, patients should receive a continuous infusion of 0.14 units/kg/hour.

Adjustment: If serum glucose does not fall by at least 10% in the first hour, give an I.V. bolus of 0.14 units/kg and continue previous regimen. In addition, if serum glucose does not fall by 50-70 mg/dL in the first hour, the insulin infusion dose should be increased hourly until a steady glucose decline is achieved. Once serum glucose reaches 300 mg/dL, decrease dose to 0.02-0.05 units/kg/hour; dextrose-containing I.V. fluids should be administered to maintain serum glucose between 200-300 mg/dL until the patient is mentally alert. After resolution of HHS, supplement I.V. insulin with SubQ insulin as needed until the patient is able to eat and transition fully to a SubQ insulin regimen. An overlap of ~1-2 hours between discontinuation of I.V. insulin and administration of SubQ insulin is recommended to ensure adequate plasma insulin levels.

Renal Impairment Insulin requirements are reduced due to changes in insulin clearance or metabolism. Close monitoring of blood glucose and adjustment of therapy is required in renal impairment.

Cl_{cr} 10-50 mL/minute: Administer at 75% of normal dose and monitor glucose closely

Cl_{cr} <10 mL/minute: Administer at 25% to 50% of normal dose and monitor glucose closely

Hemodialysis: Because of a large molecular weight (6000 daltons), insulin is not significantly removed by hemodialysis; supplemental dose is not necessary.

Peritoneal dialysis: Because of a large molecular weight (6000 daltons), insulin is not significantly removed by peritoneal dialysis; supplemental dose is not necessary.

Continuous renal replacement therapy: Administer 75% of normal dose and monitor glucose closely; supplemental dose is not necessary.

Hepatic Impairment Insulin requirements may be reduced. Close monitoring of blood glucose and adjustment of therapy is required in hepatic impairment.

Administration

SubQ administration: Do not use if solution is viscous or cloudy; use only if clear and colorless. Regular insulin should be administered within 30-60 minutes before a meal. Cold injections should be avoided. SubQ administration is usually made into the thighs, arms, buttocks, or abdomen; rotate injection sites. When mixing regular insulin with other preparations of insulin, regular insulin should be drawn into syringe first. Regular insulin is not recommended for use in external SubQ insulin infusion pump.

I.M. administration: Do not use if solution is viscous or cloudy; use only if clear and colorless. May be administered I.M. in selected clinical situations; close monitoring of blood glucose and serum potassium as well as medical supervision is required.

I.V. administration: Do not use if solution is viscous or cloudy; use only if clear and colorless. May be administered I.V. with close monitoring of blood glucose and serum potassium; appropriate medical supervision is required. If possible, avoid I.V. bolus administration in pediatric patients with DKA; may increase risk of cerebral edema. **Do not administer mixtures of insulin formulations intravenously.** I.V. administration of U-500 regular insulin is not recommended.

I.V. infusions: To minimize adsorption to I.V. solution bag (**Note:** Refer to institution-specific protocols where appropriate):

*If new tubing is **not** needed:* Wait a minimum of 30 minutes between the preparation of the solution and the initiation of the infusion.

If new tubing is needed: After receiving the insulin drip solution, the administration set should be attached to the I.V. container and the entire line should be flushed with a priming infusion of 20-50 mL of the insulin solution (Goldberg, 2006; Hirsch, 2006). Wait 30 minutes, then flush the line again with the insulin solution prior to initiating the infusion.

If insulin is required prior to the availability of the insulin drip, regular insulin should be administered by I.V. push injection.

Because of adsorption, the actual amount of insulin being administered via I.V. infusion could be substantially less than the apparent amount. Therefore, adjustment of the I.V. infusion rate should be based on effect and not solely on the apparent insulin dose. The apparent dose may be used as a starting point for determining the subsequent SubQ dosing regimen (Moghissi, 2009); however, the transition to SubQ administration requires continuous medical supervision, frequent monitoring of blood glucose, and careful adjustment of therapy. In addition, SubQ insulin should be given 1-4 hours prior to the discontinuation of I.V. insulin to prevent hyperglycemia (Moghissi, 2009).

Monitoring Parameters

Diabetes mellitus: Plasma glucose, electrolytes, Hb A_{1c}

DKA/HHS: Serum electrolytes, glucose, BUN, creatinine, osmolality, venous pH (repeat arterial blood gases are generally unnecessary), anion gap, urine output, urinalysis, mental status

Hyperkalemia: Serum potassium and glucose must be closely monitored to avoid hypokalemia, rebound hyperkalemia, and hypoglycemia.

Reference Range

Therapeutic, serum insulin (fasting): 5-20 µIU/mL (SI: 35-145 pmol/L)

Glucose, fasting:

Adults: 60-110 mg/dL

Elderly: 100-180 mg/dL

Recommendations for glycemic control, adults with type 1 diabetes:

Hb A_{1c}: <7%

Preprandial capillary plasma glucose: 70-130 mg/dL

Peak postprandial capillary blood glucose: <180 mg/dL

Blood pressure: <130/80 mm Hg

Recommendations for glycemic control in older adults with diabetes:

Relatively healthy, cognitively intact, and with a ≥5-year life expectancy: See Adults

Frail, life expectancy <5-years or those for whom the risks of intensive glucose control outweigh the benefits:

Hb A_{1c}: <8% to 9%

Blood pressure: <140/80 mm Hg or <130/80 mm Hg if tolerated

Criteria for diagnosis of DKA:

Serum glucose: >250 mg/dL

Arterial pH: <7.3

Bicarbonate: <15 mEq/L

Moderate ketonuria or ketonemia

Pharmacotherapy Pearls

Split-mixed or basal-bolus regimens: Combination regimens which optimize differences in the onset and duration of different insulin products are commonly used to approximate physiologic secretion. In split-mixed regimens, an intermediate-acting insulin (eg, NPH insulin) is administered once or twice daily and supplemented by short-acting (regular) or rapid-acting (lispro, aspart, or glulisine) insulin. Blood glucose measurements are completed several times daily. Dosages are adjusted emphasizing the individual component of the regimen which most directly influences the blood sugar in question (either the intermediate-acting component or the shorter-acting component). Fixed-ratio formulations (eg, 70/30 mix) may be used as twice daily injections in this scenario; however, the ability to titrate the dosage of an individual component is limited. An example of a "split-mixed" regimen would be 21 units of NPH plus 9 units of regular insulin in the morning and an evening meal dose consisting of 14 units of NPH plus 6 units of regular insulin.

Basal-bolus regimens are designed to more closely mimic physiologic secretion. These regimens employ a long-acting insulin (eg, glargine) to simulate basal insulin secretion. The basal component is frequently administered at bedtime or in the early morning. This is supplemented by multiple daily injections of rapid-acting products (lispro, aspart, or glulisine) immediately prior to a meal, which provides insulin at the time when nutrients are absorbed. An example of a basal-bolus regimen would be 30 units of glargine at bedtime and 12 units of lispro insulin prior to each meal.

Estimation of the effect per unit: A "Rule of 1500" has been frequently used as a means to estimate the change in blood sugar relative to each unit of insulin administered. In fact, the recommended values used in these calculations may vary from 1500-2200 (a value of 1500 is generally recommended for regular insulin while 1800 is recommended for "rapid-acting insulins"). The higher values lead to more conservative estimates of the effect per unit of insulin, and therefore lead to more cautious adjustments. The effect per unit of insulin is approximated by dividing the selected numerical value (eg, 1500-2200) by the number of units/day received by the patient. This may be used as a crude approximation of the patient's insulin sensitivity as adjustments to individual components of the regimen are made. Each additional unit of insulin added to the corresponding insulin dose may be expected to lower the blood glucose by this amount.

To illustrate, in the "basal-bolus" regimen example presented above, the rule of 1800 would indicate an expected change of 27 mg/dL per unit of lispro insulin (the total daily insulin dose is 66 units; using the formula: 1800/66 = 27). A patient may be instructed to add additional insulin if the preprandial glucose is >125 mg/dL. For a prelunch glucose of 195 mg/dL, this would mean the patient would administer the scheduled 12 units of lispro along with an additional "correctional" 3 units for a total of 15 units prior to the meal. If correctional doses are required on a consistent basis, an adjustment of the patients diet and/or scheduled insulin dose may be necessary.

◄ **Special Geriatric Considerations** Intensive glucose control (HbA_{1c} <6.5%) has been linked to increased all-cause and cardiovascular mortality, hypoglycemia requiring assistance, and weight gain in adult type 2 diabetes. How "tightly" to control a geriatric patient's blood glucose needs to be individualized. Such a decision should be based on several factors, including the patient's functional and cognitive status, how well he/she recognizes hypoglycemic or hyperglycemic symptoms, and how to respond to them and other disease states. An HbA_{1c} <7.5% is an acceptable endpoint for a healthy older adult, while <8% is acceptable for frail elderly patients, those with a duration of illness >10 years, or those with comorbid conditions and requiring combination diabetes medications. Patients who are unable to accurately draw up their dose will need assistance, such as prefilled syringes. Initial doses may require considerations for renal function in the elderly with dosing adjusted subsequently based on blood glucose monitoring. For elderly patients with diabetes who are relatively healthy, attaining target goals for aspirin use, blood pressure, lipids, smoking cessation, and diet and exercise may be more important than normalized glycemic control.

Dosage Forms Excipient information presented when available (limited, particularly for generics); consult specific product labeling.

Injection, solution:

HumuLIN® R: 100 units/mL (3 mL, 10 mL)

NovoLIN® R: 100 units/mL (10 mL)

Injection, solution [concentrate]:

HumuLIN® R U-500: 500 units/mL (20 mL)

Selected References

Action to Control Cardiovascular Risk in Diabetes Study Group, Gerstein HC, Miller ME, et al, "Effects of Intensive Glucose Lowering in Type 2 Diabetes," *N Engl J Med*, 2008, 358(24):2545-59.

ADVANCE Collaborative Group, Patel A, MacMahon S, et al, "Intensive Blood Glucose Control and Vascular Outcomes in Patients With Type 2 Diabetes," *N Engl J Med*, 2008, 358(24):2560-72.

American Diabetes Association, "Standards of Medical Care in Diabetes – 2011," *Diabetes Care*, 2011, 34(Suppl 1):11-61.

Brown AF, Mangione CM, Saliba D, et al, "Guidelines for Improving the Care of the Older Person With Diabetes Mellitus," *J Am Geriatr Soc*, 2003, 51(5 Suppl Guidelines):265-80.

"VA/DoD Clinical Practice Guideline for the Management of Diabetes Mellitus," 2010. Available at http://www.healthquality.va.gov/Diabetes_Mellitus.asp

◆ **Insulin Regular and Insulin NPH** *see* Insulin NPH and Insulin Regular *on page* 961
◆ **Interferon Alfa-2b (PEG Conjugate)** *see* Peginterferon Alfa-2b *on page* 1403

Interferon Beta-1b (in ter FEER on BAY ta won bee)

Brand Names: U.S. Betaseron®; Extavia®

Brand Names: Canada Betaseron®; Extavia®

Index Terms rIFN beta-1b

Generic Availability (U.S.) No

Pharmacologic Category Interferon

Use Treatment of relapsing forms of multiple sclerosis (MS); treatment of first clinical episode with MRI features consistent with MS

Canadian labeling: Additional use (not in U.S. labeling): Treatment of secondary-progressive MS

Medication Guide Available Yes

Contraindications Hypersensitivity to *E. coli*-derived products, natural or recombinant interferon beta, albumin human or any other component of the formulation

Warnings/Precautions Anaphylaxis has been reported rarely with use. Associated with a high incidence of flu-like adverse effects; improvement in symptoms occurs over time. Hepatotoxicity has been reported with beta interferons, including rare reports of hepatitis (autoimmune) and hepatic failure requiring transplant. Interferons have been associated with severe psychiatric adverse events (psychosis, mania, depression, suicidal behavior/ideation) in patients with and without previous psychiatric symptoms, avoid use in severe psychiatric disorders and use caution in patients with a history of depression; patients exhibiting symptoms of depression should be closely monitored and discontinuation of therapy should be considered. Use caution in patients with pre-existing cardiovascular disease, pulmonary disease, seizure disorders, renal impairment or hepatic impairment. Use caution in myelosuppression; routine monitoring for leukopenia is recommended; dose reduction may be required. Thyroid dysfunction has rarely been reported with use. Severe injection site reactions (necrosis) may occur, which may or may not heal with continued therapy; patient and/or caregiver competency in injection technique should be confirmed and periodically reevaluated. Contains albumin, which may carry a remote risk of transmitting viral diseases.

Adverse Reactions (Reflective of adult population; not specific for elderly) Note:
Flu-like syndrome (including at least two of the following - headache, fever, chills, malaise, diaphoresis, and myalgia) are reported in the majority of patients (60%) and decrease over time (average duration ~1 week).

>10%:
Cardiovascular: Peripheral edema (15%), chest pain (11%)
Central nervous system: Headache (57%), fever (36%), pain (51%), chills (25%), dizziness (24%), insomnia (24%)
Dermatologic: Rash (24%), skin disorder (12%)
Endocrine & metabolic: Metrorrhagia (11%)
Gastrointestinal: Nausea (27%), diarrhea (19%), abdominal pain (19%), constipation (20%), dyspepsia (14%)
Genitourinary: Urinary urgency (13%)
Hematologic: Lymphopenia (88%), neutropenia (14%), leukopenia (14%)
Local: Injection site reaction (85%), inflammation (53%), pain (18%)
Neuromuscular & skeletal: Weakness (61%), myalgia (27%), hypertonia (50%), myasthenia (46%), arthralgia (31%), incoordination (21%)
Miscellaneous: Flu-like syndrome (decreases over treatment course; 60%), neutralizing antibodies (≤45%; significance not known)
1% to 10%:
Cardiovascular: Palpitation (4%), vasodilation (8%), hypertension (7%), tachycardia (4%), peripheral vascular disorder (6%)
Central nervous system: Anxiety (10%), malaise (8%), nervousness (7%)
Dermatologic: Alopecia (4%)
Endocrine & metabolic: Menorrhagia (8%), dysmenorrhea (7%)
Gastrointestinal: Weight gain (7%)
Genitourinary: Impotence (9%), pelvic pain (6%), cystitis (8%), urinary frequency (7%), prostatic disorder (3%)
Hematologic: Lymphadenopathy (8%)
Hepatic: ALT increased >5x baseline (10%), AST increased >5x baseline (3%)
Local: Injection site necrosis (4% to 5%), edema (3%), mass (2%)
Neuromuscular & skeletal: Leg cramps (4%)
Respiratory: Dyspnea (7%)
Miscellaneous: Diaphoresis (8%), hypersensitivity (3%)

Drug Interactions
Avoid Concomitant Use There are no known interactions where it is recommended to avoid concomitant use.
Increased Effect/Toxicity
Interferon Beta-1b may increase the levels/effects of: Theophylline Derivatives; Zidovudine
Decreased Effect There are no known significant interactions involving a decrease in effect.

Stability Store at room temperature of 25°C (77°F); excursions permitted to 15°C to 30°C (59°F to 86°F). To reconstitute solution, inject 1.2 mL of diluent (provided); gently swirl to dissolve, do not shake. Reconstituted solution provides 0.25 mg/mL (8 million units). If not used immediately following reconstitution, refrigerate solution at 2°C to 8°C (36°F to 46°F) and use within 3 hours; do not freeze or shake solution. Discard unused portion of vial.

Mechanism of Action Interferon beta-1b differs from naturally occurring human protein by a single amino acid substitution and the lack of carbohydrate side chains; mechanism in the treatment of MS is unknown; however, immunomodulatory effects attributed to interferon beta-1b include enhancement of suppressor T cell activity, reduction of proinflammatory cytokines, down-regulation of antigen presentation, and reduced trafficking of lymphocytes into the central nervous system. Improves MRI lesions, decreases relapse rate, and disease severity in patients with secondary progressive MS.

Pharmacodynamics/Kinetics Limited data due to small doses used
Half-life elimination: 8 minutes to 4.3 hours
Time to peak, serum: 1-8 hours

Dosage
Geriatric & Adult Note: Gradual dose-titration, analgesics, and/or antipyretics may help decrease flu-like symptoms on treatment days.
Multiple sclerosis (relapsing): Initial: 0.0625 mg (2 million units [0.25 mL]) every other day; gradually increase dose by 0.0625 every 2 weeks
Target dose: 0.25 mg (8 million units [1 mL]) every other day
Multiple sclerosis (secondary-progressive) [Canadian labeling; not in U.S. labeling]:
Initial: 0.125 mg (4 million units [0.5 mL]) every other day for 2 weeks
Target dose: 0.25 mg (8 million units [1 mL]) every other day

◄ **Administration** Withdraw dose of reconstituted solution from the vial into a sterile syringe fitted with a 27-gauge needle and inject the solution subcutaneously; sites for self-injection include outer surface of the arms, abdomen, hips, and thighs. Rotate SubQ injection site. Patient should be well hydrated.

Monitoring Parameters Complete blood chemistries (including platelet count) and liver function tests are recommended at 1, 3, and 6 months following initiation of therapy and periodically thereafter. Thyroid function should be assessed every 6 months in patients with history of thyroid dysfunction.

Pharmacotherapy Pearls American Academy of Neurology and MS Council guidelines suggest that, based upon published data, 6 million units of Avonex® (interferon beta-1a) (30 mcg) is equivalent to approximately 7-9 million units of Betaseron® (220-280 mcg).

Special Geriatric Considerations No specific recommendations necessary for use in the elderly. Monitor for CNS adverse effects which may be significant in the elderly.

Dosage Forms Excipient information presented when available (limited, particularly for generics); consult specific product labeling.
Injection, powder for reconstitution:
Betaseron®: 0.3 mg [~9.6 million int. units] [contains albumin (human)]
Injection, powder for reconstitution [preservative free]:
Extavia®: 0.3 mg [~9.6 million int. units] [contains albumin (human)]

- ◆ **Interleukin-1 Receptor Antagonist** see Anakinra on page 132
- ◆ **Intropin** see DOPamine on page 556
- ◆ **Intuniv™** see GuanFACINE on page 851
- ◆ **INVanz®** see Ertapenem on page 623
- ◆ **Invega®** see Paliperidone on page 1378
- ◆ **Invega® Sustenna®** see Paliperidone on page 1378
- ◆ **Iodine and Potassium Iodide** see Potassium Iodide and Iodine on page 1491

Iodoquinol (eye oh doe KWIN ole)

Brand Names: U.S. Yodoxin®
Brand Names: Canada Diodoquin®
Index Terms Diiodohydroxyquin
Generic Availability (U.S.) No
Pharmacologic Category Amebicide
Use Treatment of acute and chronic intestinal amebiasis; asymptomatic cyst passers; Blastocystis hominis infections; ineffective for amebic hepatitis or hepatic abscess
Dosage
Geriatric This agent is no longer a drug of choice; use only if other therapy is contraindicated or has failed. Due to optic nerve damage, use cautiously in the elderly.
Adult Treatment of susceptible infections: Oral: 650 mg 3 times/day after meals for 20 days; not to exceed 2 g/day
Special Geriatric Considerations This agent is no longer a drug of choice; use only if other therapy is contraindicated or has failed. Due to optic nerve damage, use cautiously in the elderly.
Dosage Forms Excipient information presented when available (limited, particularly for generics); consult specific product labeling.
Tablet, oral:
Yodoxin®: 210 mg, 650 mg

- ◆ **Ionil® [OTC]** see Salicylic Acid on page 1648
- ◆ **Ionil Plus® [OTC]** see Salicylic Acid on page 1648
- ◆ **Iopidine®** see Apraclonidine on page 138

Ipecac Syrup (IP e kak SIR up)

Index Terms Syrup of Ipecac
Generic Availability (U.S.) Yes
Pharmacologic Category Antidote
Use Treatment of acute oral drug overdosage and in certain poisonings
Dosage
Geriatric & Adult Emetic: Oral: 15-30 mL followed by 200-300 mL of water; repeat dose one time if vomiting does not occur within 20 minutes.
Dosage Forms Excipient information presented when available (limited, particularly for generics); consult specific product labeling. [DSC] = Discontinued product
Syrup, oral: USP: 7% (30 mL [DSC])

♦ **IPOL®** *see* Poliovirus Vaccine (Inactivated) *on page 1477*

Ipratropium (Oral Inhalation) (i pra TROE pee um)

Related Information
Inhalant Agents *on page 2010*

Medication Safety Issues
Sound-alike/look-alike issues:
Atrovent® may be confused with Alupent®, Serevent®
Ipratropium may be confused with tiotropium

Brand Names: U.S. Atrovent® HFA

Brand Names: Canada Atrovent® HFA; Gen-Ipratropium; Mylan-Ipratropium Sterinebs; Novo-Ipramide; Nu-Ipratropium; PMS-Ipratropium

Index Terms Ipratropium Bromide

Generic Availability (U.S.) Yes: Solution for nebulization

Pharmacologic Category Anticholinergic Agent

Use Anticholinergic bronchodilator used in bronchospasm associated with COPD, bronchitis, and emphysema

Contraindications Hypersensitivity to ipratropium, atropine (and its derivatives), or any component of the formulation

Warnings/Precautions Immediate hypersensitivity reactions (urticaria, angioedema, rash, bronchospasm) have been reported. Rarely, paradoxical bronchospasm may occur with use of inhaled bronchodilating agents; this should be distinguished from inadequate response. Not indicated for the initial treatment of acute episodes of bronchospasm where rescue therapy is required for rapid response. Should only be used in acute exacerbations of asthma in conjunction with short-acting beta-adrenergic agonists for acute episodes. Use with caution in patients with myasthenia gravis, narrow-angle glaucoma, benign prostatic hyperplasia (BPH), or bladder neck obstruction

Adverse Reactions (Reflective of adult population; not specific for elderly)
>10%: Respiratory: Upper respiratory tract infection (9% to 34%), bronchitis (10% to 23%), sinusitis (1% to 11%)
1% to 10%:
Cardiovascular: Chest pain (3%), palpitation
Central nervous system: Headache (6% to 7%), dizziness (2% to 3%)
Gastrointestinal: Dyspepsia (1% to 5%), nausea (4%), xerostomia (2% to 4%)
Genitourinary: Urinary tract infection (2% to 10%)
Neuromuscular & skeletal: Back pain (2% to 7%)
Respiratory: Dyspnea (7% to 10%), rhinitis (2% to 6%), cough (3% to 5%), pharyngitis (4%), bronchospasm (2%), sputum increased (1%)
Miscellaneous: Flu-like syndrome (4% to 8%)

Drug Interactions
Avoid Concomitant Use There are no known interactions where it is recommended to avoid concomitant use.

Increased Effect/Toxicity
Ipratropium (Oral Inhalation) may increase the levels/effects of: AbobotulinumtoxinA; Anticholinergics; Cannabinoids; OnabotulinumtoxinA; Potassium Chloride; RimabotulinumtoxinB

The levels/effects of Ipratropium (Oral Inhalation) may be increased by: Pramlintide

Decreased Effect
Ipratropium (Oral Inhalation) may decrease the levels/effects of: Acetylcholinesterase Inhibitors (Central); Secretin

The levels/effects of Ipratropium (Oral Inhalation) may be decreased by: Acetylcholinesterase Inhibitors (Central)

Stability
Aerosol: Store at controlled room temperature of 25°C (77°F). Do not store near heat or open flame.
Solution: Store at 15°C to 30°C (59°F to 86°F). Protect from light.

Mechanism of Action Blocks the action of acetylcholine at parasympathetic sites in bronchial smooth muscle causing bronchodilation; local application to nasal mucosa inhibits serous and seromucous gland secretions.

Pharmacodynamics/Kinetics
Onset of action: Bronchodilation: Within 15 minutes
  Peak effect: 1-2 hours
Duration: 2-5 hours
Absorption: Negligible
Distribution: 15% of dose reaches lower airways
Protein Binding: ≤9%
Half-life elimination: 2 hours
Excretion: Urine

Dosage
Geriatric & Adult
Asthma exacerbation, acute (*NIH Asthma Guidelines, 2007*):
  Nebulization: 500 mcg every 20 minutes for 3 doses, then as needed. **Note:** Should be given in combination with a short-acting beta-adrenergic agonist.
  Metered-dose inhaler: 8 inhalations every 20 minutes as needed for up to 3 hours. **Note:** Should be given in combination with a short-acting beta-adrenergic agonist.
Bronchospasm associated with COPD:
  Nebulization: 500 mcg (one unit-dose vial) 3-4 times/day with doses 6-8 hours apart
  Metered-dose inhaler: 2 inhalations 4 times/day, up to 12 inhalations/24 hours

Administration Avoid spraying into the eyes.
Atrovent® HFA: Prior to initial use, prime inhaler by releasing 2 test sprays into the air. If the inhaler has not been used for >3 days, reprime.

Monitoring Parameters Pulmonary function tests

Special Geriatric Considerations The elderly may find it difficult to use the metered dose inhaler. A spacer device may be useful. Ipratropium has not been specifically studied in the elderly, but it is poorly absorbed from the airways and appears to be safe in this population.

Dosage Forms Excipient information presented when available (limited, particularly for generics); consult specific product labeling.
Aerosol, for oral inhalation, as bromide:
  Atrovent® HFA: 17 mcg/actuation (12.9 g) [chlorofluorocarbon free; 200 metered actuations]
Solution, for nebulization, as bromide: 0.02% [500 mcg/2.5 mL] (25s, 30s, 60s)
Solution, for nebulization, as bromide [preservative free]: 0.02% [500 mcg/2.5 mL] (25s, 30s, 60s)

Selected References
National Asthma Education and Prevention Program, "Expert Panel Report 3 (EPR-3): Guidelines for the Diagnosis and Management of Asthma-Summary Report 2007," *J Allergy Clin Immunol*, 2007, 120(5 Suppl):94-138.

Ipratropium (Nasal) (i pra TROE pee um)

Related Information
Inhalant Agents *on page 2010*

Medication Safety Issues
Sound-alike/look-alike issues:
Ipratropium may be confused with tiotropium
Atrovent® may be confused with Alupent®, Serevent®

Brand Names: U.S. Atrovent®

Brand Names: Canada Alti-Ipratropium; Apo-Ipravent®; Atrovent®; Mylan-Ipratropium Solution

Index Terms Ipratropium Bromide

Generic Availability (U.S.) Yes

Pharmacologic Category Anticholinergic Agent

Use Symptomatic relief of rhinorrhea associated with the common cold and allergic and nonallergic rhinitis

Dosage
Geriatric & Adult
Colds (symptomatic relief of rhinorrhea): Safety and efficacy of use beyond 4 days not established: *Intranasal:* Nasal spray (0.06%): 2 sprays in each nostril 3-4 times/day
Allergic/nonallergic rhinitis: *Intranasal:* Nasal spray (0.03%): 2 sprays in each nostril 2-3 times/day
Seasonal allergic rhinitis (safety and efficacy of use beyond 3 weeks in patients with seasonal allergic rhinitis has not been established): *Intranasal:* Nasal spray (0.06%): 2 sprays in each nostril 4 times/day

Special Geriatric Considerations Ipratropium has not been specifically studied in the elderly.

Dosage Forms Excipient information presented when available (limited, particularly for generics); consult specific product labeling.

Solution, intranasal, as bromide [spray]: 0.03% (30 mL); 0.06% (15 mL) [delivers 42 mcg/spray; 165 sprays]; 0.06% (15 mL)

Atrovent®: 0.03% (30 mL) [contains benzalkonium chloride; delivers 21 mcg/spray; 345 sprays]

Atrovent®: 0.06% (15 mL) [contains benzalkonium chloride; delivers 42 mcg/spray; 165 sprays]

Ipratropium and Albuterol (i pra TROE pee um & al BYOO ter ole)

Related Information
Albuterol on page 50
Ipratropium (Oral Inhalation) on page 973
Medication Safety Issues
Sound-alike/look-alike issues:
Combivent® may be confused with Combivir®, Serevent®
International issues:
DuoNeb® may be confused with DuoTrav™ which is a brand name for travoprost/timolol combination product in Canada or may be confused with Duovent® UDV which is a brand name for ipratropium/fenoterol combination product in Canada
Brand Names: U.S. Combivent®; DuoNeb®
Brand Names: Canada CO Ipra-Sal; Combivent UDV; Gen-Combo Sterinebs; ratio-Ipra Sal UDV
Index Terms Albuterol and Ipratropium; Salbutamol and Ipratropium
Generic Availability (U.S.) Yes: Solution for nebulization
Pharmacologic Category Anticholinergic Agent; Beta$_2$-Adrenergic Agonist
Use Treatment of COPD in those patients who are currently on a regular bronchodilator who continue to have bronchospasms and require a second bronchodilator
Dosage
Geriatric & Adult
COPD:
Aerosol for inhalation: 2 metered-dose inhalations 4 times/day; may receive additional doses as necessary, but total number of doses in 24 hours should not exceed 12 inhalations.
Solution for nebulization: Initial: 3 mL every 6 hours (maximum: 3 mL every 4 hours)
Dosage Forms Excipient information presented when available (limited, particularly for generics); consult specific product labeling.
Aerosol for oral inhalation:
Combivent®: Ipratropium bromide 18 mcg and albuterol (base) 90 mcg per inhalation (14.7 g) [contains chlorofluorocarbon, soya lecithin; 200 metered actuations]
Solution for nebulization: Ipratropium bromide 0.5 mg and albuterol (base) 2.5 mg per 3 mL (30s, 60s)
DuoNeb®: Ipratropium bromide 0.5 mg and albuterol (base) 2.5 mg per 3 mL (30s, 60s)

◆ **Ipratropium Bromide** see Ipratropium (Nasal) on page 974
◆ **Ipratropium Bromide** see Ipratropium (Oral Inhalation) on page 973
◆ **I-Prin [OTC]** see Ibuprofen on page 908
◆ **Iprivask®** see Desirudin on page 474
◆ **Iproveratril Hydrochloride** see Verapamil on page 1909
◆ **IPV** see Poliovirus Vaccine (Inactivated) on page 1477
◆ **Iquix®** see Levofloxacin (Ophthalmic) on page 1055

Irbesartan (ir be SAR tan)

Related Information
Angiotensin Agents on page 1985
Medication Safety Issues
Sound-alike/look-alike issues:
Avapro® may be confused with Anaprox®
Brand Names: U.S. Avapro®
Brand Names: Canada Avapro®; CO Irbesartan; PMS-Irbesartan; ratio-Irbesartan; Sandoz-Irbesartan; Teva-Irbesartan
Generic Availability (U.S.) No
Pharmacologic Category Angiotensin II Receptor Blocker

◀ **Use** Treatment of hypertension alone or in combination with other antihypertensives; treatment of diabetic nephropathy in patients with type 2 diabetes mellitus (noninsulin dependent, NIDDM) and hypertension

Contraindications Hypersensitivity to irbesartan or any component of the formulation

Warnings/Precautions May cause hyperkalemia; avoid potassium supplementation unless specifically required by healthcare provider. May be associated with deterioration of renal function and/or increases in serum creatinine, particularly in patients with low renal blood flow (eg, renal artery stenosis, heart failure) whose glomerular filtration rate (GFR) is dependent on efferent arteriolar vasoconstriction by angiotensin II. Avoid use or use a much smaller dose in patients who are intravascularly volume-depleted; use caution in patients with unstented unilateral or bilateral renal artery stenosis. When unstented bilateral renal artery stenosis is present, use is generally avoided due to the elevated risk of deterioration in renal function unless possible benefits outweigh risks. AUCs of irbesartan (not the active metabolite) are about 50% greater in patients with Cl$_{cr}$ <30 mL/minute and are doubled in hemodialysis patients. Concurrent use of ACE inhibitors may increase the risk of clinically-significant adverse events (eg, renal dysfunction, hyperkalemia).

Adverse Reactions (Reflective of adult population; not specific for elderly) Unless otherwise indicated, percentage of incidence is reported for patients with hypertension.

>10%: Endocrine & metabolic: Hyperkalemia (19%, diabetic nephropathy; rarely seen in HTN)

1% to 10%:

Cardiovascular: Orthostatic hypotension (5%, diabetic nephropathy)

Central nervous system: Fatigue (4%), dizziness (10%, diabetic nephropathy)

Gastrointestinal: Diarrhea (3%), dyspepsia (2%)

Respiratory: Upper respiratory infection (9%), cough (2.8% versus 2.7% in placebo)

>1% but frequency ≤ placebo: Abdominal pain, anxiety, chest pain, edema, headache, influenza, musculoskeletal pain, nausea, nervousness, pharyngitis, rash, rhinitis, sinus abnormality, syncope, tachycardia, urinary tract infection, vertigo, vomiting

Drug Interactions

Metabolism/Transport Effects Substrate of CYP2C9 (minor); **Inhibits** CYP2C8 (moderate), 2C9 (moderate), 2D6 (weak), 3A4 (weak)

Avoid Concomitant Use There are no known interactions where it is recommended to avoid concomitant use.

Increased Effect/Toxicity

Irbesartan may increase the levels/effects of: ACE Inhibitors; Amifostine; Antihypertensives; Carvedilol; CYP2C8 Substrates (High risk); CYP2C9 Substrates (High risk); Hypotensive Agents; Lithium; Nonsteroidal Anti-Inflammatory Agents; Potassium-Sparing Diuretics; RiTUXimab; Sodium Phosphates

The levels/effects of Irbesartan may be increased by: Alfuzosin; Diazoxide; Eplerenone; Fluconazole; Herbs (Hypotensive Properties); MAO Inhibitors; Pentoxifylline; Phosphodiesterase 5 Inhibitors; Potassium Salts; Prostacyclin Analogues; Tolvaptan; Trimethoprim

Decreased Effect

The levels/effects of Irbesartan may be decreased by: Herbs (Hypertensive Properties); Methylphenidate; Nonsteroidal Anti-Inflammatory Agents; Rifamycin Derivatives; Yohimbine

Ethanol/Nutrition/Herb Interactions Herb/Nutraceutical: Avoid dong quai if using for hypertension (has estrogenic activity). Avoid ephedra, yohimbe, ginseng (may worsen hypertension). Avoid garlic (may have increased antihypertensive effect).

Stability Store at room temperature of 15°C to 30°C (59°F to 86°F).

Mechanism of Action Irbesartan is an angiotensin receptor antagonist. Angiotensin II acts as a vasoconstrictor. In addition to causing direct vasoconstriction, angiotensin II also stimulates the release of aldosterone. Once aldosterone is released, sodium as well as water are reabsorbed. The end result is an elevation in blood pressure. Irbesartan binds to the AT1 angiotensin II receptor. This binding prevents angiotensin II from binding to the receptor thereby blocking the vasoconstriction and the aldosterone secreting effects of angiotensin II.

Pharmacodynamics/Kinetics

Onset of action: Peak effect: 1-2 hours

Duration: >24 hours

Distribution: V$_d$: 53-93 L

Protein binding, plasma: 90%

Metabolism: Hepatic, primarily CYP2C9

Bioavailability: 60% to 80%

Half-life elimination: Terminal: 11-15 hours

Time to peak, serum: 1.5-2 hours

Excretion: Feces (80%); urine (20%)

Dosage
Geriatric & Adult
Hypertension: Oral: 150 mg once daily; patients may be titrated to 300 mg once daily.
Note: Starting dose in volume-depleted patients should be 75 mg.

Nephropathy in patients with type 2 diabetes and hypertension: Oral: Target dose: 300 mg once daily

Renal Impairment No dosage adjustment necessary with mild to severe impairment unless the patient is also volume depleted.

Monitoring Parameters Baseline and periodic electrolyte panels, renal and liver function tests, urinalysis; symptoms of hypotension or hypersensitivity; monitor blood pressure and pulse

Special Geriatric Considerations No dosage adjustment is necessary when initiating angiotensin II receptor antagonists in the elderly. In clinical studies, no differences between younger adults and the elderly were demonstrated. Many elderly may be volume depleted due to diuretic use and/or blunted thirst reflex resulting in inadequate fluid intake.

Dosage Forms Excipient information presented when available (limited, particularly for generics); consult specific product labeling.
Tablet, oral:
Avapro®: 75 mg, 150 mg, 300 mg

Irbesartan and Hydrochlorothiazide
(ir be SAR tan & hye droe klor oh THYE a zide)

Related Information
Hydrochlorothiazide *on page 876*
Irbesartan *on page 975*

Medication Safety Issues
Sound-alike/look-alike issues:
Avalide® may be confused with Avandia®

Brand Names: U.S. Avalide®

Brand Names: Canada Avalide®; CO Irbesartan HCT; Irbesartan-HCTZ; PMS-Irbesartan HCTZ; Ran™-Irbesartan HCTZ; ratio-Irbesartan HCTZ; Sandoz-Irbesartan HCT; Teva-Irbesartan HCTZ

Index Terms Avapro® HCT; Hydrochlorothiazide and Irbesartan

Generic Availability (U.S.) No

Pharmacologic Category Angiotensin II Receptor Blocker; Diuretic, Thiazide

Use Combination therapy for the management of hypertension; may be used as initial therapy in patients likely to need multiple drugs to achieve blood pressure goals

Dosage
Geriatric & Adult Dose must be individualized.

Hypertension: Oral: **Note:** Maximum antihypertensive effects are attained within 2-4 weeks after initiation or a change in dose; however, if necessary, may carefully titrate dose as soon as after 1 week of treatment.

Add-on therapy: A patient who is not controlled with either agent alone may be switched to the combination product. The lowest dosage available is irbesartan 150 mg/hydrochlorothiazide 12.5 mg.

Initial therapy: Irbesartan 150 mg/hydrochlorothiazide 12.5 mg once daily. If initial response is inadequate, may titrate dose after 1-2 weeks, to a maximum dose of irbesartan 300 mg/hydrochlorothiazide 25 mg once daily.

Renal Impairment Not recommended in patients with Cl$_{cr}$ ≤30 mL/minute.

Hepatic Impairment Use with caution.

Dosage Forms Excipient information presented when available (limited, particularly for generics); consult specific product labeling.
Tablet:
Avalide® 150/12.5: Irbesartan 150 mg and hydrochlorothiazide 12.5 mg
Avalide® 300/12.5: Irbesartan 300 mg and hydrochlorothiazide 12.5 mg
Avalide® 300/25: Irbesartan 300 mg and hydrochlorothiazide 25 mg

◆ **Ircon® [OTC]** *see* Ferrous Fumarate *on page 721*
◆ **Iron Dextran** *see* Iron Dextran Complex *on page 977*

Iron Dextran Complex (EYE ern DEKS tran KOM pleks)

Medication Safety Issues
Sound-alike/look-alike issues:
Dexferrum® may be confused with Desferal®

◀ Iron dextran complex may be confused with ferumoxytol

Brand Names: U.S. Dexferrum®; INFeD®

Brand Names: Canada Dexiron™; Infufer®

Index Terms High-Molecular-Weight Iron Dextran (DexFerrum®); Imferon; Iron Dextran; Low-Molecular-Weight Iron Dextran (INFeD®)

Generic Availability (U.S.) No

Pharmacologic Category Iron Salt

Use Treatment of iron deficiency in patients in whom oral administration is infeasible or ineffective

Unlabeled/Investigational Use Cancer-/chemotherapy-associated anemia

Contraindications Hypersensitivity to iron dextran or any component of the formulation; any anemia not associated with iron deficiency

Warnings/Precautions [U.S. Boxed Warning]: Deaths associated with parenteral administration following anaphylactic-type reactions have been reported (use only where resuscitation equipment and personnel are available). A test dose should be administered to all patients prior to the first therapeutic dose. Fatal reactions have occurred even in patients who tolerated the test dose. Monitor patients for signs/symptoms of anaphylactic reactions during any iron dextran administration. A history of drug allergy (including multiple drug allergies) and/or the concomitant use of an ACE inhibitor may increase the risk of anaphylactic-type reactions. Adverse events (including life-threatening) associated with iron dextran usually occur with the high-molecular-weight formulation (Dexferrum®), compared to low-molecular-weight (INFeD®) (Chertow, 2006). Delayed (1-2 days) infusion reaction (including arthralgia, back pain, chills, dizziness, and fever) may occur with large doses (eg, total dose infusion) of I.V. iron dextran; usually subsides within 3-4 days. Delayed reaction may also occur (less commonly) with I.M. administration; subsiding within 3-7 days. Use with caution in patients with a history of significant allergies, asthma, serious hepatic impairment, pre-existing cardiac disease (may exacerbate cardiovascular complications), and rheumatoid arthritis (may exacerbate joint pain and swelling). Avoid use during acute kidney infection.

In patients with chronic kidney disease (CKD) requiring iron supplementation, the I.V. route is preferred for hemodialysis patients; either oral iron or I.V. iron may be used for nondialysis and peritoneal dialysis CKD patients. In patients with cancer-related anemia (either due to cancer or chemotherapy-induced) requiring iron supplementation, the I.V. route is superior to oral therapy; I.M. administration is not recommended for parenteral iron supplementation.

[U.S. Boxed Warning]: Use only in patients where the iron deficient state is not amenable to oral iron therapy. Discontinue oral iron prior to initiating parenteral iron therapy. Exogenous hemosiderosis may result from excess iron stores; patients with refractory anemias and/or hemoglobinopathies may be prone to iron overload with unwarranted iron supplementation. Anemia in the elderly is often caused by "anemia of chronic disease" or associated with inflammation rather than blood loss. Iron stores are usually normal or increased, with a serum ferritin >50 ng/mL and a decreased total iron binding capacity. I.V. administration of iron dextran is often preferred over I.M. in the elderly secondary to a decreased muscle mass and the need for daily injections. Intramuscular injections of iron-carbohydrate complexes may have a risk of delayed injection site tumor development. Iron dextran products differ in chemical characteristics. The high-molecular-weight formulation (Dexferrum®) and the low-molecular-weight formulation (INFeD®) are not clinically interchangeable.

Adverse Reactions (Reflective of adult population; not specific for elderly) Frequency not defined. **Note:** Adverse event risk is reported to be higher with the high-molecular-weight iron dextran formulation.

Cardiovascular: Arrhythmia, bradycardia, cardiac arrest, chest pain, chest tightness, cyanosis, flushing, hyper-/hypotension, shock, syncope, tachycardia

Central nervous system: Chills, disorientation, dizziness, fever, headache, malaise, seizure, unconsciousness, unresponsiveness

Dermatologic: Pruritus, purpura, rash, urticaria

Gastrointestinal: Abdominal pain, diarrhea, nausea, taste alteration, vomiting

Genitourinary: Discoloration of urine

Hematologic: Leukocytosis, lymphadenopathy

Local: Injection site reactions (cellulitis, inflammation, pain, phlebitis, soreness, swelling), muscle atrophy/fibrosis (with I.M. injection), skin/tissue staining (at the site of I.M. injection), sterile abscess

Neuromuscular & skeletal: Arthralgia, arthritis/arthritis exacerbation, back pain, myalgia, paresthesia, weakness

Respiratory: Bronchospasm, dyspnea, respiratory arrest, wheezing

Renal: Hematuria

Miscellaneous: Anaphylactic reactions (sudden respiratory difficulty, cardiovascular collapse), diaphoresis

Drug Interactions

Avoid Concomitant Use

Avoid concomitant use of Iron Dextran Complex with any of the following: Dimercaprol

Increased Effect/Toxicity

The levels/effects of Iron Dextran Complex may be increased by: ACE Inhibitors; Dimercaprol

Decreased Effect There are no known significant interactions involving a decrease in effect.

Stability Store at controlled room temperature. Solutions for infusion should be diluted in 250-1000 mL NS.

Mechanism of Action The released iron, from the plasma, eventually replenishes the depleted iron stores in the bone marrow where it is incorporated into hemoglobin

Pharmacodynamics/Kinetics

Onset of action: I.V.: Serum ferritin peak: 7-9 days after dose

Absorption:

I.M.: 50% to 90% is promptly absorbed, balance is slowly absorbed over month

I.V.: Uptake of iron by the reticuloendothelial system appears to be constant at about 10-20 mg/hour

Excretion: Urine and feces via reticuloendothelial system

Dosage

Geriatric & Adult

Note: A 0.5 mL test dose should be given prior to starting iron dextran therapy.

Iron-deficiency anemia: I.M. (INFeD®), I.V. (Dexferrum®, INFeD®):

Dose (mL) = 0.0442 (desired Hgb - observed Hgb) x LBW + (0.26 x LBW)

Desired hemoglobin: Usually 14.8 g/dL

LBW = Lean body weight in kg

Iron replacement therapy for blood loss: (INFeD®), I.V. (Dexferrum®, INFeD®): Replacement iron (mg) = blood loss (mL) x Hct

Maximum daily dosage: Manufacturer's labeling: **Note:** Replacement of larger estimated iron deficits may be achieved by serial administration of smaller incremental dosages. Daily dosages should be limited to 100 mg iron (2 mL)

Total dose infusion (unlabeled): The entire dose (estimated iron deficit) may be diluted and administered as a one-time I.V. infusion.

Cancer-/chemotherapy-associated anemia (NCCN guidelines v.2.2010) (unlabeled use): I.V.: Test dose: 25 mg slow I.V. slow push, followed 1 hour later by 100 mg over 5 minutes; larger doses (unlabeled), up to total dose infusion (over several hours) may be administered. Low-molecular-weight iron dextran preferred.

Administration Note: Test dose: A test dose should be given on the first day of therapy; patient should be observed for 1 hour for hypersensitivity reaction, then the remaining dose (dose minus test dose) should be given. Epinephrine should be available.

I.M. (INFeD®): Use Z-track technique (displacement of the skin laterally prior to injection); injection should be deep into the upper outer quadrant of buttock; alternate buttocks with subsequent injections. Administer test dose at same recommended site using the same technique.

I.V.: Test dose should be given gradually over at least 30 seconds (INFeD®) or 5 minutes (Dexferrum®). Subsequent dose(s) may be administered by I.V. bolus undiluted at a rate not to exceed 50 mg/minute or diluted in 250-1000 mL NS and infused over 1-6 hours (initial 25 mL should be given slowly and patient should be observed for allergic reactions); avoid dilutions with dextrose (increased incidence of local pain and phlebitis)

Monitoring Parameters Hemoglobin, hematocrit, reticulocyte count, serum ferritin, serum iron, TIBC; monitor for anaphylaxis/hypersensitivity reaction (during test dose and therapeutic dose)

Reference Range

Hemoglobin: Adults:

Males: 13.5-16.5 g/dL

Females: 12.0-15.0 g/dL

Serum iron: 40-160 mcg/dL

Total iron binding capacity: 230-430 mcg/dL

Transferrin: 204-360 mg/dL

Percent transferrin saturation: 20% to 50%

Test Interactions May cause falsely elevated values of serum bilirubin and falsely decreased values of serum calcium. Residual iron dextran may remain in reticuloendothelial cells; may affect accuracy of examination of bone marrow iron stores. Bone scans with 99m Tc-labeled bone seeking agents may show reduced bony uptake, marked renal activity, and excess blood

◀ pooling and soft tissue accumulation following I.V. iron dextran infusion or with high serum ferritin levels. Following I.M. iron dextran, bone scans with 99m Tc-diphosphonate may show dense activity in the buttocks.

Pharmacotherapy Pearls Avoid iron injection if oral intake is feasible; a test dose of 0.5 mL I.V. or I.M. should be given to observe for adverse reactions

Special Geriatric Considerations Anemia in the elderly is most often caused by "anemia of chronic disease," a result of aging effect in bone marrow, or associated with inflammation rather than blood loss. Iron stores are usually normal or increased, with a serum ferritin >50 ng/mL and a decreased total iron binding capacity. Hence, the anemia is not secondary to iron deficiency but the inability of the reticuloendothelial system to use available iron stores. I.V. administration of iron is often preferred over I.M. in the elderly secondary to a decreased muscle mass and the need for daily injections.

Dosage Forms Excipient information presented when available (limited, particularly for generics); consult specific product labeling.

Injection, solution:

Dexferrum®: Elemental iron 50 mg/mL (1 mL, 2 mL) [high-molecular-weight iron dextran]
INFeD®: Elemental iron 50 mg/mL (2 mL) [low-molecular-weight iron dextran]

Selected References

Lipschitz DA, "The Anemia of Chronic Disease," *J Am Geriatr Soc*, 1990, 38(11):1258-64.
National Comprehensive Cancer Network® (NCCN), "Practice Guidelines in Oncology™: Cancer- and Chemotherapy-Induced Anemia Version 2.2010." Available at http://www.nccn.org/professionals/physician_gls/PDF/anemia.pdf

◆ **Iron Fumarate** *see* Ferrous Fumarate *on page 721*
◆ **Iron Gluconate** *see* Ferrous Gluconate *on page 723*
◆ **Iron-Polysaccharide Complex, Vitamin B12, and Folic Acid** *see* Polysaccharide-Iron Complex, Vitamin B12, and Folic Acid *on page 1483*

Iron Sucrose (EYE ern SOO krose)

Medication Safety Issues
Sound-alike/look-alike issues:
Iron sucrose may be confused with ferumoxytol

Brand Names: U.S. Venofer®
Brand Names: Canada Venofer®
Generic Availability (U.S.) No
Pharmacologic Category Iron Salt
Use Treatment of iron-deficiency anemia in chronic renal failure, including nondialysis-dependent patients (with or without erythropoietin therapy) and dialysis-dependent patients receiving erythropoietin therapy

Unlabeled/Investigational Use Cancer-/chemotherapy-associated anemia

Contraindications Hypersensitivity to iron sucrose or any component of the formulation; evidence of iron overload; anemia not caused by iron deficiency

Warnings/Precautions Hypersensitivity reactions, including rare postmarketing anaphylactic and anaphylactoid reactions, have been reported. Hypotension has been reported frequently in hemodialysis-dependent patients. Hypotension has also been reported in peritoneal dialysis and nondialysis patients. Hypotension may be related to total dose or rate of administration (avoid rapid I.V. injection), follow recommended guidelines. Withhold iron in the presence of tissue iron overload; periodic monitoring of hemoglobin, hematocrit, serum ferritin, and transferrin saturation is recommended.

Adverse Reactions (Reflective of adult population; not specific for elderly)
>10%:
Cardiovascular: Hypotension (1% to 7%; 39% in hemodialysis patients; may be related to total dose or rate of administration), peripheral edema (2% to 17%)
Central nervous system: Headache (3% to 13%)
Gastrointestinal: Diarrhea (1% to 17%), nausea (1% to 15%), vomiting (3% to 12%)
Neuromuscular & skeletal: Muscle cramps (1% to 3%; 29% in hemodialysis patients)
1% to 10%:
Cardiovascular: Hypertension (6% to 8%), edema (1% to 7%), chest pain (1% to 6%), murmur (<1% to 3%), heart failure (2%), myocardial infarction (1%)
Central nervous system: Dizziness (1% to 10%), fatigue (2% to 5%), fever (1% to 3%), stroke (1%)
Dermatologic: Pruritus (1% to 7%), rash (≤1%)
Endocrine & metabolic: Gout (2% to 7%), hypoglycemia (<1% to 4%), hyperglycemia (3% to 4%), fluid overload (1% to 3%)
Gastrointestinal: Taste perversion (1% to 9%), peritoneal infection (≤8%), constipation (1% to 7%), abdominal pain (1% to 4%), positive fecal occult blood (1% to 3%)
Genitourinary: Urinary tract infection (≤1%)
Local: Injection site reaction (2% to 6%), catheter site infection (≤4%)

Neuromuscular & skeletal: Arthralgia (1% to 8%), back pain (1% to 8%), muscle pain (1% to 7%), extremity pain (3% to 6%), weakness (1% to 3%)

Ocular: Conjunctivitis (<1% to 3%)

Otic: Ear pain (1% to 7%)

Respiratory: Dyspnea (1% to 10%), pharyngitis (<1% to 7%), cough (1% to 7%), sinusitis (1% to 4%), nasopharyngitis (≤3%), upper respiratory infection (1% to 3%), nasal congestion (1%), pneumonia (1%), pulmonary edema (1%), rhinitis (≤1%)

Miscellaneous: Graft complication (1% to 10%), sepsis (2%)

Drug Interactions

Avoid Concomitant Use

Avoid concomitant use of Iron Sucrose with any of the following: Dimercaprol

Increased Effect/Toxicity

The levels/effects of Iron Sucrose may be increased by: Dimercaprol

Decreased Effect There are no known significant interactions involving a decrease in effect.

Stability Store vials at controlled room temperature of 25°C (77°F); do not freeze. May be administered via the dialysis line as an undiluted solution or by diluting 100 mg (5 mL) in a maximum of 100 mL normal saline. Doses ≥200 mg should be diluted in a maximum of 250 mL normal saline. Iron sucrose is stable for 7 days at room temperature or under refrigeration when undiluted in a plastic syringe or following dilution in normal saline in a plastic syringe (2-10 mg/mL) or I.V. bag (1-2 mg/mL) (data on file [American Regent, Inc, 2010]).

Mechanism of Action Iron sucrose is dissociated by the reticuloendothelial system into iron and sucrose. The released iron increases serum iron concentrations and is incorporated into hemoglobin.

Pharmacodynamics/Kinetics

Distribution: V_{dss}: Healthy adults: 7.9 L

Metabolism: Dissociated into iron and sucrose by the reticuloendothelial system

Half-life elimination: Healthy adults: 6 hours

Excretion: Healthy adults: Urine (5%) within 24 hours

Dosage

Geriatric Insufficient data to identify differences between elderly and other adults; use caution.

Adult Doses expressed in mg of **elemental** iron. **Note:** Test dose: Product labeling does not indicate need for a test dose in product-naive patients.

Iron-deficiency anemia in chronic renal disease: I.V.:

Hemodialysis-dependent patient: 100 mg over 2-5 minutes administered 1-3 times/week during dialysis; administer no more than 3 times/week to a cumulative total dose of 1000 mg (10 doses); may continue to administer at lowest dose necessary to maintain target hemoglobin, hematocrit, and iron storage parameters

Peritoneal dialysis-dependent patient: Two infusions of 300 mg each over 1.5 hours 14 days apart, followed by a single 400 mg infusion over 2.5 hours 14 days later (total cumulative dose of 1000 mg in 3 divided doses)

Nondialysis-dependent patient: 200 mg slow injection (over 2-5 minutes) on 5 different occasions within a 14-day period. Total cumulative dose: 1000 mg in 14-day period. **Note:** Dosage has also been administered as two infusions of 500 mg in a maximum of 250 mL normal saline infused over 3.5-4 hours on day 1 and day 14 (limited experience)

Cancer-/chemotherapy-associated anemia (unlabeled use): I.V. infusion: 200 mg over 1 hour; maximum 300-400 mg/infusion. Repeat dose every 2-3 weeks. Test doses (25 mg slow I.V. push) are recommended in patients with iron dextran hypersensitivity or those with other drug allergies (NCCN guidelines, v.2.2010)

Administration Not for rapid I.V. injection; inject slowly over 2-5 minutes. Can be administered through dialysis line. Do not mix with other medications or parenteral nutrient solutions.

Slow I.V. injection: May administer undiluted by slow I.V. injection (100 mg over 2-5 minutes in hemodialysis-dependent patients **or** 200 mg over 2-5 minutes in nondialysis-dependent patients)

Infusion: Dilute 100 mg in maximum of 100 mL normal saline; infuse over at least 15 minutes; 300 mg/250 mL should be infused over at least 1.5 hours; 400 mg/250 mL should be infused over at least 2.5 hours; 500 mg/250 mL should be infused over at least 3.5 hours

Monitoring Parameters Hematocrit, hemoglobin, serum ferritin, transferrin, percent transferrin saturation, TIBC; takes about 4 weeks of treatment to see increased serum iron and ferritin, and decreased TIBC. Serum iron concentrations should be drawn 48 hours after last dose.

Reference Range

Hemoglobin: Adults:

Males: 13.5-16.5 g/dL

Females: 12.0-15.0 g/dL

Serum iron: 40-160 mcg/dL

Total iron binding capacity: 230-430 mcg/dL

◀ Transferrin: 204-360 mg/dL

Percent transferrin saturation: 20% to 50%

Test Interactions May cause falsely elevated values of serum bilirubin and falsely decreased values of serum calcium.

Special Geriatric Considerations Anemia in the elderly is most often caused by "anemia of chronic disease," a result of aging effect in bone marrow, or associated with inflammation rather than blood loss. Iron stores are usually normal or increased, with a serum ferritin >50 ng/mL and a decreased total iron binding capacity. Hence, the anemia is not secondary to iron deficiency but the inability of the reticuloendothelial system to use available iron stores. I.V. administration of iron is often preferred over I.M. in the elderly secondary to a decreased muscle mass and the need for daily injections.

Dosage Forms Excipient information presented when available (limited, particularly for generics); consult specific product labeling.

Injection, solution [preservative free]:

Venofer®: Elemental iron 20 mg/mL (5 mL, 10 mL)

Selected References

National Comprehensive Cancer Network® (NCCN), "Practice Guidelines in Oncology™: Cancer- and Chemotherapy-Induced Anemia Version 2.2010." Available at http://www.nccn.org/professionals/physician_gls/PDF/anemia.pdf

- ◆ **Iron Sulfate** *see* Ferrous Sulfate *on page 724*
- ◆ **ISD** *see* Isosorbide Dinitrate *on page 987*
- ◆ **ISDN** *see* Isosorbide Dinitrate *on page 987*
- ◆ **ISG** *see* Immune Globulin *on page 922*
- ◆ **ISMN** *see* Isosorbide Mononitrate *on page 990*
- ◆ **Ismo®** *see* Isosorbide Mononitrate *on page 990*
- ◆ **Isobamate** *see* Carisoprodol *on page 279*

Isocarboxazid (eye soe kar BOKS a zid)

Related Information

Antidepressant Agents *on page 1991*

Brand Names: U.S. Marplan®

Generic Availability (U.S.) No

Pharmacologic Category Antidepressant, Monoamine Oxidase Inhibitor

Use Treatment of depression

Medication Guide Available Yes

Contraindications

Hypersensitivity to isocarboxazid or any component of the formulation; cardiovascular disease (including CHF, or HTN); cerebrovascular disease; history of hepatic disease or abnormal liver function tests; pheochromocytoma; renal disease or severe renal impairment

Concurrent use of sympathomimetics (including amphetamines, cocaine, dopamine, epinephrine, methylphenidate, norepinephrine, or phenylephrine) and related compounds (methyldopa, levodopa, phenylalanine, tryptophan, or tyrosine), as well as ophthalmic alpha₂-agonists (apraclonidine, brimonidine); may result in behavioral and neurologic symptoms

CNS depressants, cyclobenzaprine, dextromethorphan, ethanol, meperidine, bupropion, buspirone; may result in delirium, excitation, hyper-/hypotension, hyperpyrexia, seizures, and coma

Isocarboxazid **initiation**: At least 2 weeks should elapse between the discontinuation of serotoninergic agents (including SSRIs and tricyclics) and the initiation of isocarboxazid; at least 5 weeks should elapse between the discontinuation of fluoxetine and the initiation of isocarboxazid; at least 1 week should elapse between the discontinuation of other monoamine oxidase (MAO) inhibitors and the initiation of isocarboxazid (using half the normal starting dose). In all cases, a sufficient amount of time must be allowed for the clearance of the serotoninergic agent and any active metabolites prior to the initiation of isocarboxazid.

Isocarboxazid **discontinuation**: At least 2 weeks should elapse between the discontinuation of isocarboxazid and the initiation of the following agents: Serotoninergic agents (including SSRIs, fluoxetine, and tricyclics), bupropion, and other antidepressants. Two to 3 weeks should elapse between the discontinuation of isocarboxazid and the initiation of meperidine. At least 10 days should elapse between the discontinuation of isocarboxazid and initiation of buspirone. At least 1 week should elapse between the discontinuation of isocarboxazid and the initiation of other MAO inhibitors (see specific agent for details).

Antihypertensive agents (including thiazide diuretics): may result in potentiation of antihypertensive effects.

General anesthesia, spinal anesthesia (hypotension may be exaggerated). Use caution with local anesthetics containing sympathomimetic agents. Discontinue drug 10 days prior to elective surgery.

Foods high in tyramine or dopamine content; foods and/or supplements containing tyrosine, phenylalanine, tryptophan, or caffeine; may result in hypertensive reactions.

Warnings/Precautions [U.S. Boxed Warning]: Antidepressants increase the risk of suicidal thinking and behavior in children, adolescents, and young adults (18-24 years of age) with major depressive disorder (MDD) and other psychiatric disorders; consider risk prior to prescribing. Short-term studies did not show an increased risk in patients >24 years of age and showed a decreased risk in patients ≥65 years. Closely monitor for clinical worsening, suicidality, or unusual changes in behavior; the patient's family or caregiver should be instructed to closely observe the patient and communicate condition with healthcare provider. A medication guide should be dispensed with each prescription. **Isocarboxazid is FDA approved for the treatment of depression in children ≥16 years of age.**

The possibility of a suicide attempt is inherent in major depression and may persist until remission occurs. Monitor for worsening of depression or suicidality, especially during initiation of therapy (generally first 1-2 months) or with dose increases or decreases. Use caution in high-risk patients. Worsening depression and severe abrupt suicidality that are not part of the presenting symptoms may require discontinuation or modification of drug therapy. The patient's family or caregiver should be alerted to monitor patients for the emergence of suicidality and associated behaviors (such as agitation, irritability, hostility, impulsivity, and hypomania) and notify healthcare provider.

May worsen psychosis in some patients or precipitate a shift to mania or hypomania in patients with bipolar disorder. Patients presenting with depressive symptoms should be screened for bipolar disorder. Monotherapy in patients with bipolar disorder should be avoided. Isocarboxazid is not FDA approved for the treatment of bipolar depression. Isocarboxazid should not be used for initial therapy but reserved for patients who have not responded to other antidepressants.

Use with caution in patients who are hyperactive, hyperexcitable, have a seizure disorder, or who have glaucoma, hyperthyroidism, or diabetes, or renal impairment; avoid use in hepatic impairment or severe renal impairment. High potential for interactions; do not use with other MAO inhibitors or antidepressants. Avoid products containing sympathomimetic stimulants, dextromethorphan, disulfiram, and meperidine. Concurrent use with antihypertensive agents may lead to exaggeration of hypotensive effects. May cause orthostatic hypotension (especially at dosages >30 mg/day). Use with caution in patients with hypotension or patients who would not tolerate transient hypotensive episodes; effects may be additive when used with other agents known to cause orthostasis (phenothiazines). Hypertensive crisis may occur with foods/supplements high in tyramine, tryptophan, phenylalanine, or tyrosine content.

Discontinue at least 48 hours prior to myelography. May increase the risks associated with electroconvulsive therapy. Consider discontinuing, when possible, prior to elective surgery. Use with caution in patients receiving disulfiram.

Adverse Reactions (Reflective of adult population; not specific for elderly)
>10%: Central nervous system: Dizziness (29%), headache (15%)
1% to 10%:
 Cardiovascular: Orthostatic hypotension (4%), syncope (2%), palpitation (2%)
 Central nervous system: Sleep disturbance (5%), drowsiness (4%), anxiety (2%), chills (2%), forgetfulness (2%), hyperactivity (2%), lethargy (2%), sedation (2%)
 Gastrointestinal: Xerostomia (9%), constipation (7%), nausea (6%), diarrhea (2%)
 Genitourinary: Urinary frequency (2%), impotence (2%), urinary hesitancy (1%)
 Neuromuscular & skeletal: Tremor (4%), myoclonus (2%), paresthesia (2%)
 Miscellaneous: Diaphoresis (2%), heavy feeling (2%)

Drug Interactions

Avoid Concomitant Use
Avoid concomitant use of Isocarboxazid with any of the following: Alpha-/Beta-Agonists (Indirect-Acting); Alpha1-Agonists; Alpha2-Agonists (Ophthalmic); Amphetamines; Anilido-piperidine Opioids; Atomoxetine; Bezafibrate; Buprenorphine; BuPROPion; BusPIRone; CarBAMazepine; Cyclobenzaprine; Dexmethylphenidate; Dextromethorphan; Diethylpro-pion; HYDROmorphone; Linezolid; Maprotiline; Meperidine; Methyldopa; Methylene Blue; Methylphenidate; Mirtazapine; Oxymorphone; Pizotifen; Propoxyphene; Selective Serotonin Reuptake Inhibitors; Serotonin 5-HT1D Receptor Agonists; Serotonin/Norepinephrine Reup-take Inhibitors; Sibutramine; Tapentadol; Tetrabenazine; Tetrahydrozoline; Tetrahydrozoline (Nasal); Tricyclic Antidepressants; Tryptophan

Increased Effect/Toxicity
Isocarboxazid may increase the levels/effects of: Alpha-/Beta-Agonists (Direct-Acting); Alpha-/Beta-Agonists (Indirect-Acting); Alpha1-Agonists; Alpha2-Agonists (Ophthalmic); Amphetamines; Anticholinergics; Antihypertensives; Atomoxetine; Beta2-Agonists; Bezafi-brate; BuPROPion; Dexmethylphenidate; Dextromethorphan; Diethylpropion; Doxapram; HYDROmorphone; Linezolid; Lithium; Meperidine; Methadone; Methyldopa; Methylene

Blue; Methylphenidate; Mirtazapine; Orthostatic Hypotension Producing Agents; Pizotifen; Reserpine; Selective Serotonin Reuptake Inhibitors; Serotonin 5-HT1D Receptor Agonists; Serotonin Modulators; Serotonin/Norepinephrine Reuptake Inhibitors; Tetrahydrozoline; Tetrahydrozoline (Nasal); Tricyclic Antidepressants

The levels/effects of Isocarboxazid may be increased by: Altretamine; Anilidopiperidine Opioids; Buprenorphine; BusPIRone; CarBAMazepine; COMT Inhibitors; Cyclobenzaprine; Levodopa; MAO Inhibitors; Maprotiline; Oxymorphone; Pramlintide; Propoxyphene; Sibutramine; Tapentadol; Tetrabenazine; TraMADol; Tryptophan

Decreased Effect

Isocarboxazid may decrease the levels/effects of: Acetylcholinesterase Inhibitors (Central)

The levels/effects of Isocarboxazid may be decreased by: Acetylcholinesterase Inhibitors (Central)

Ethanol/Nutrition/Herb Interactions

Ethanol: May increase CNS depression; monitor for increased effects with coadministration. Caution patients about effects. Avoid beverages containing tyramine (hearty red wine and beer).

Food: Concurrent ingestion of foods rich in tyramine may cause sudden and severe high blood pressure (hypertensive crisis). Avoid tyramine-containing foods with MAO-Is.

Herb/Nutraceutical: Avoid valerian, St John's wort, SAMe, kava kava (may increase risk of serotonin syndrome and/or excessive sedation); Avoid supplements containing caffeine, tyrosine, tryptophan, or phenylalanine. Ingestion of large quantities may increase the risk of severe side effects (eg, hypertensive reactions, serotonin syndrome).

Mechanism of Action Thought to act by increasing endogenous concentrations of epinephrine, norepinephrine, dopamine, and serotonin through inhibition of the enzyme (monoamine oxidase) responsible for the breakdown of these neurotransmitters

Pharmacodynamics/Kinetics

Absorption: Oral: Well absorbed; undergoes acetylation in the liver; older patients have been reported to have higher blood concentrations than younger adults after 2 weeks of continuous treatment

Elimination: In urine primarily as metabolites and unchanged drug

Dosage

Geriatric & Adult Depression: Oral: Initial: 10 mg 2-4 times/day; may increase by 10 mg/day every 2-4 days to 40 mg/day by the end of the first week (divided into 3 doses). After first week, may increase by up to 20 mg/week to a maximum of 60 mg/day. May take 3-6 weeks to see effects. Dose should be reduced once maximum clinical effect is seen. If no response obtained within 6 weeks, additional titration is unlikely to be beneficial. **Note:** Use caution in patients on >40 mg/day; experience is limited.

Monitoring Parameters Blood pressure, heart rate; mood, suicidal ideation (especially at the beginning of therapy or when doses are increased or decreased)

Special Geriatric Considerations The MAO inhibitors are effective and generally well tolerated by elderly patients. It is their potential interactions with tyramine-containing foods and other drugs and their effects on blood pressure that have limited their use. The MAO inhibitors are usually reserved for patients who do not tolerate or respond to the traditional "cyclic" or "second generation" antidepressants. The brain activity of monoamine oxidase increases with age and even more so in patients with Alzheimer's disease. Therefore, the MAO inhibitor may have an increased role in patients with Alzheimer's disease who are depressed. Information on the use of isocarboxazid in the elderly is limited.

Dosage Forms Excipient information presented when available (limited, particularly for generics); consult specific product labeling.

Tablet, oral:

Marplan®: 10 mg [scored]

Isoniazid (eye soe NYE a zid)

Medication Safety Issues

International issues:

Hydra [Japan] may be confused with Hydrea brand name for hydroxyurea [U.S., Canada, and multiple international markets]

Brand Names: Canada Isotamine®; PMS-Isoniazid

Index Terms INH; Isonicotinic Acid Hydrazide

Generic Availability (U.S.) Yes

Pharmacologic Category Antitubercular Agent

Use Treatment of susceptible tuberculosis infections; treatment of latent tuberculosis infection (LTBI)

Contraindications Hypersensitivity to isoniazid or any component of the formulation; acute liver disease; previous history of hepatic damage during isoniazid therapy; previous severe adverse reaction (drug fever, chills, arthritis) to isoniazid

Warnings/Precautions Use with caution in patients with severe renal impairment and liver disease. **[U.S. Boxed Warning]: Severe and sometimes fatal hepatitis may occur; usually occurs within the first 3 months of treatment, although may develop even after many months of treatment.** The risk of developing hepatitis is age-related; daily ethanol consumption may also increase the risk. Patients must report any prodromal symptoms of hepatitis, such as fatigue, weakness, malaise, anorexia, nausea, abdominal pain, jaundice, or vomiting. Patients should be instructed to immediately discontinue therapy if any of these symptoms occur, even if a clinical evaluation has yet to be conducted. Treatment with isoniazid for latent tuberculosis infection should be deferred in patients with acute hepatic diseases. Periodic ophthalmic examinations are recommended even when usual symptoms do not occur. Pyridoxine (10-50 mg/day) is recommended in individuals at risk for development of peripheral neuropathies (eg, HIV infection, nutritional deficiency, diabetes). Multidrug regimens should be utilized for the treatment of active tuberculosis to prevent the emergence of drug resistance.

Adverse Reactions (Reflective of adult population; not specific for elderly) Frequency not defined.

Cardiovascular: Hypertension, palpitation, tachycardia, vasculitis

Central nervous system: Depression, dizziness, encephalopathy, fever, lethargy, memory impairment, psychosis, seizure, slurred speech, toxic encephalopathy

Dermatologic: Flushing, rash (morbilliform, maculopapular, pruritic, or exfoliative)

Endocrine & metabolic: Gynecomastia, hyperglycemia, metabolic acidosis, pellagra, pyridoxine deficiency

Gastrointestinal: Anorexia, epigastric distress, nausea, stomach pain, vomiting

Hematologic: Agranulocytosis, anemia (sideroblastic, hemolytic, or aplastic), eosinophilia, thrombocytopenia

Hepatic: LFTs mildly increased (10% to 20%), hyperbilirubinemia, bilirubinuria, jaundice, hepatic dysfunction, hepatitis (may involve progressive liver damage; risk increases with age; 2.3% in patients >50 years)

Neuromuscular & skeletal: Arthralgia, hyper-reflexia, paresthesia, peripheral neuropathy (dose-related incidence, 10% to 20% incidence with 10 mg/kg/day), weakness

Ocular: Blurred vision, loss of vision, optic neuritis and atrophy

Miscellaneous: Lupus-like syndrome, lymphadenopathy, rheumatic syndrome

Drug Interactions

Metabolism/Transport Effects Substrate of CYP2E1 (major); **Inhibits** CYP1A2 (weak), 2A6 (moderate), 2C9 (weak), 2C19 (strong), 2D6 (moderate), 2E1 (moderate), 3A4 (strong); **Induces** CYP2E1 (after discontinuation) (weak)

Avoid Concomitant Use

Avoid concomitant use of Isoniazid with any of the following: Clopidogrel; Thioridazine

Increased Effect/Toxicity

Isoniazid may increase the levels/effects of: Acetaminophen; Benzodiazepines (metabolized by oxidation); CarBAMazepine; Chlorzoxazone; CycloSERINE; CYP2A6 Substrates; CYP2C19 Substrates; CYP2D6 Substrates; CYP2E1 Substrates; Fesoterodine; Fosphenytoin; Nebivolol; Phenytoin; Tamoxifen; Theophylline Derivatives; Thioridazine

The levels/effects of Isoniazid may be increased by: Ethionamide; Rifamycin Derivatives

Decreased Effect

Isoniazid may decrease the levels/effects of: Clopidogrel; Codeine; TraMADol

The levels/effects of Isoniazid may be decreased by: Antacids; Corticosteroids (Systemic); Cyproterone

Ethanol/Nutrition/Herb Interactions

Ethanol: Avoid ethanol (increases the risk of hepatitis).

Food: Isoniazid should not be taken with food; serum levels may be decreased if taken with food. Has some ability to inhibit tyramine metabolism; several case reports of mild reactions (flushing, palpitations) after ingestion of cheese (with or without wine). Reactions resembling allergic symptoms following ingestion of fish high in histamine content have been reported. Isoniazid decreases folic acid absorption. Isoniazid alters pyridoxine metabolism.

Stability

Tablet: Store at 20°C to 25°C (68°F to 77°F). Protect from light.

Oral solution: Store at 15°C to 30°C (59°F to 86°F). Protect from light.

Mechanism of Action Unknown, but may include the inhibition of mycolic acid synthesis resulting in disruption of the bacterial cell wall

◀ **Pharmacodynamics/Kinetics**
Absorption: Rapid and complete; rate can be slowed with food
Distribution: All body tissues and fluids including CSF
Protein binding: 10% to 15%
Metabolism: Hepatic with decay rate determined genetically by acetylation phenotype
Half-life elimination: Fast acetylators: 30-100 minutes; Slow acetylators: 2-5 hours; may be prolonged with hepatic or severe renal impairment
Time to peak, serum: 1-2 hours
Excretion: Urine (75% to 95%); feces; saliva

Dosage
Geriatric & Adult Recommendations often change due to resistant strains and newly-developed information; consult *MMWR* for current CDC recommendations. Intramuscular injection is available for patients who are unable to either take or absorb oral therapy.
Nontuberculous mycobacterium *(M. kansasii)* (unlabeled use): Oral, I.M.: 5 mg/kg/day (maximum: 300 mg/day) for duration to include 12 months of culture-negative sputum; typically used in combination with ethambutol and rifampin
Treatment of latent tuberculosis infection (LTBI): Oral, I.M.: CDC recommendations: 5 mg/kg (maximum: 300 mg/dose) once daily or 15 mg/kg (maximum: 900 mg/dose) twice weekly by directly observed therapy (DOT) for 6-9 months in patients who do not have HIV infection (9 months is optimal, 6 months may be considered to reduce costs of therapy) and 9 months in patients who have HIV infection. Extend to 12 months of therapy if interruptions in treatment occur. (*MMWR*, 2000)
Treatment of active TB infection (drug susceptible): Oral, I.M.:
Daily therapy: CDC recommendations: 5 mg/kg/day once daily (usual dose: 300 mg/day) (*MMWR*, 2003)
Directly observed therapy (DOT): CDC recommendations: 15 mg/kg (maximum: 900 mg/dose) twice weekly or 3 times/week; **Note:** CDC guidelines state that once-weekly therapy (15 mg/kg/dose) may be considered, but only after the first 2 months of initial therapy in HIV-negative patients, and only in combination with rifapentine (*MMWR*, 2003).
Note: Treatment may be defined by the number of doses administered (eg, "six-month" therapy involves 182 doses of INH and rifampin, and 56 doses of pyrazinamide. Six months is the shortest interval of time over which these doses may be administered, assuming no interruption of therapy.
Note: Concomitant administration of 10-50 mg/day pyridoxine is recommended in malnourished patients or those prone to neuropathy (eg, alcoholics, patients with diabetes)
Renal Impairment No adjustment necessary
Hemodialysis: Dialyzable (50% to 100%); administer dose postdialysis
Hepatic Impairment No adjustment required, however, use with caution, may accumulate and additional liver damage may occur in patients with pre-existing liver disease. For ALT or AST >3 times the ULN: discontinue or temporarily withhold treatment. Treatment with isoniazid for latent tuberculosis infection should be deferred in patients with acute hepatic diseases.
Administration Should be administered 1 hour before or 2 hours after meals on an empty stomach.
Monitoring Parameters Baseline and periodic (more frequently in patients with higher risk for hepatitis) liver function tests (ALT and AST); sputum cultures monthly (until 2 consecutive negative cultures reported); monitoring for prodromal signs of hepatitis

LTBI therapy: American Thoracic Society/Centers for Disease Control (ATS/CDC) recommendations: Monthly clinical evaluation, including brief physical exam for adverse events. Baseline serum AST or ALT and bilirubin should be considered for patients at higher risk for adverse events (eg, history of liver disease, chronic ethanol use, HIV-infected patients, older adults with concomitant medications or diseases). Routine, periodic monitoring is recommended for any patient with an abnormal baseline or at increased risk for hepatotoxicity.
Test Interactions False-positive urinary glucose with Clinitest®
Pharmacotherapy Pearls Pyridoxine should be given concomitantly in persons with conditions in which neuropathy is common (eg, diabetes, alcoholism, malnutrition)
Special Geriatric Considerations Age has not been shown to affect the pharmacokinetics of INH since acetylation phenotype determines clearance and half-life, acetylation rate does not change significantly with age. Most strains of *M. tuberculosis* found the elderly should be susceptible to INH since most acquired their initial infection prior to INH's introduction.
Dosage Forms Excipient information presented when available (limited, particularly for generics); consult specific product labeling.
Injection, solution: 100 mg/mL (10 mL)
Solution, oral: 50 mg/5 mL (473 mL)
Tablet, oral: 100 mg, 300 mg

Selected References

American Thoracic Society, "Treatment of Tuberculosis," *MMWR Recomm Rep*, 2003, 52(RR-11):1-77. Available at http://www.cdc.gov/mmwr/preview/mmwrhtml/rr5211a1.htm

Kergueris MF, Bourin M, and Larousse C, "Pharmacokinetics of Isoniazid: Influence of Age," *Eur J Clin Pharmacol*, 1986, 30(3):335-40.

Yoshikawa TT, "Tuberculosis in Aging Adults," *J Am Geriatr Soc*, 1992, 40(2):178-87.

◆ **Isonicotinic Acid Hydrazide** *see* Isoniazid *on page 984*
◆ **Isonipecaine Hydrochloride** *see* Meperidine *on page 1140*
◆ **Isophane Insulin** *see* Insulin NPH *on page 959*
◆ **Isophane Insulin and Regular Insulin** *see* Insulin NPH and Insulin Regular *on page 961*

Isoproterenol (eye soe proe TER e nole)

Medication Safety Issues
 Sound-alike/look-alike issues:
  Isuprel® may be confused with Disophrol®, Ismelin®, Isordil®
Brand Names: U.S. Isuprel®
Index Terms Isoproterenol Hydrochloride
Generic Availability (U.S.) No
Pharmacologic Category Beta$_1$- & Beta$_2$-Adrenergic Agonist Agent
Use Manufacturer's labeled indications (see **"Note"**): Mild or transient episodes of heart block that do not require electric shock or pacemaker therapy; serious episodes of heart block and Adams-Stokes attacks (except when caused by ventricular tachycardia or fibrillation); cardiac arrest until electric shock or pacemaker therapy is available; bronchospasm during anesthesia; adjunct to fluid and electrolyte replacement therapy and other drugs and procedures in the treatment of hypovolemic or septic shock and low cardiac output states (eg, decompensated heart failure, cardiogenic shock)

Note: The use of isoproterenol in advanced cardiac life support (ACLS) has largely been supplanted by the use of other adrenergic agents (eg, epinephrine and dopamine). The use of isoproterenol for bronchospasm during anesthesia and cardiogenic, hypovolemic, or septic shock is no longer recommended. See *Unlabeled/Investigational Use* for more appropriate, yet unlabeled, uses.

Unlabeled/Investigational Use Pharmacologic overdrive pacing for refractory torsade de pointes; pharmacologic provocation during tilt table testing for syncope; temporary control of bradycardia in denervated heart transplant patients unresponsive to atropine; ventricular arrhythmias due to AV nodal block; beta-blocker overdose

Dosage
 Geriatric & Adult Note: Patients may exhibit dose-dependent vasodilation due to unopposed beta$_2$-agonism elicited by isoproterenol.
  Bradyarrhythmias, AV nodal block, or refractory torsade de pointes: Continuous I.V. infusion: Usual range: 2-10 mcg/minute; titrate to patient response.
  Brugada syndrome with electrical storm (unlabeled use): I.V. bolus: Initial: 1-2 mcg, followed by a continuous infusion of 0.15-0.3 mcg/minute for 1 day; may repeat sequence if ventricular tachycardia/fibrillation recurs (Watanabe, 2006; Zipes, 2006).
  Tilt table testing for syncope (Benditt, 1996; Brignole, 2004): Continuous I.V infusion: Initial: 1 mcg/minute; increase as necessary based on response; maximum dose: 5 mcg/minute. **Note:** Timing of initiation and dose adjustment during test may be institution-specific.

Dosage Forms Excipient information presented when available (limited, particularly for generics); consult specific product labeling.
 Injection, solution, as hydrochloride:
  Isuprel®: 0.2 mg/mL (1 mL, 5 mL) [contains sodium metabisulfite; 1:5000]

◆ **Isoproterenol Hydrochloride** *see* Isoproterenol *on page 987*
◆ **Isoptin® SR** *see* Verapamil *on page 1909*
◆ **Isopto® Atropine** *see* Atropine *on page 165*
◆ **Isopto® Carbachol** *see* Carbachol *on page 267*
◆ **Isopto® Carpine** *see* Pilocarpine (Ophthalmic) *on page 1452*
◆ **Isopto® Homatropine** *see* Homatropine *on page 872*
◆ **Isopto® Hyoscine** *see* Scopolamine (Ophthalmic) *on page 1663*
◆ **Isordil® Titradose™** *see* Isosorbide Dinitrate *on page 987*

Isosorbide Dinitrate (eye soe SOR bide dye NYE trate)

Medication Safety Issues
 Sound-alike/look-alike issues:
  Isordil® may be confused with Inderal®, Isuprel®, Plendil®

◀ **Brand Names: U.S.** Dilatrate®-SR; Isordil® Titradose™
Brand Names: Canada ISDN; Isosorbide; Novo-Sorbide; PMS-Isosorbide
Index Terms ISD; ISDN
Generic Availability (U.S.) Yes: Excludes capsule
Pharmacologic Category Vasodilator
Use Prevention and treatment of angina pectoris

Note: Due to slower onset of action, not the drug of choice to abort an acute anginal episode.

Unlabeled/Investigational Use Patients with heart failure (HF) who do not tolerate an ACE inhibitor or an angiotensin receptor blocker (ARB); African-American (self-identified) patients with HF remaining symptomatic despite optimal standard therapy; esophageal spastic disorders

Contraindications Hypersensitivity to isosorbide dinitrate or any component of the formulation; hypersensitivity to organic nitrates; concurrent use with phosphodiesterase-5 (PDE-5) inhibitors (sildenafil, tadalafil, or vardenafil)

Warnings/Precautions Severe hypotension can occur; paradoxical bradycardia and increased angina pectoris can accompany hypotension. Postural hypotension can also occur; ethanol may potentiate this effect. Use with caution in volume depletion and moderate hypotension, and use with extreme caution in inferior wall MI and suspected right ventricular infarctions. Nitrates may reduce preload, exacerbating obstruction and cause hypotension or syncope and/or worsening of heart failure (Gibbons, 2003). Avoid use in patients with hypertrophic cardiomyopathy (HCM).

Use of isosorbide dinitrate sublingual tablets to treat acute angina attacks is recommended only in patients unresponsive to sublingual nitroglycerin; however, current clinical practice guidelines do not recommend use during an acute anginal episode. Avoid use of extended release formulations in acute MI or acute HF; cannot easily reverse effects if adverse events develop. Nitrates may precipitate or aggravate increased intracranial pressure and subsequently may worsen clinical outcomes in patients with neurologic injury (eg, intracranial hemorrhage, traumatic brain injury). Appropriate dosing intervals are needed to minimize tolerance development. Tolerance can only be overcome by short periods of nitrate absence from the body. Dose escalation does not overcome this effect. When used for HF in combination with hydralazine, tolerance is less of a concern (Gogia, 1995).

Avoid concurrent use with PDE-5 inhibitors (eg, sildenafil, vardenafil, tadalafil). When nitrate administration becomes medically necessary, may administer nitrates only if 24 hours have elapsed after use of sildenafil or vardenafil (48 hours after tadalafil use) (Trujillo, 2007).

Adverse Reactions (Reflective of adult population; not specific for elderly) Frequency not defined.
   Cardiovascular: Crescendo angina (uncommon), hypotension, postural hypotension, rebound hypertension (uncommon), syncope (uncommon)
   Central nervous system: Headache (most common), lightheadedness (related to blood pressure changes)
   Hematologic: Methemoglobinemia (rare, overdose)
Drug Interactions
   Metabolism/Transport Effects Substrate of CYP3A4 (major)
   Avoid Concomitant Use
      Avoid concomitant use of Isosorbide Dinitrate with any of the following: Conivaptan; Phosphodiesterase 5 Inhibitors
   Increased Effect/Toxicity
      Isosorbide Dinitrate may increase the levels/effects of: Hypotensive Agents; Rosiglitazone

      The levels/effects of Isosorbide Dinitrate may be increased by: Conivaptan; CYP3A4 Inhibitors (Moderate); CYP3A4 Inhibitors (Strong); Dasatinib; Phosphodiesterase 5 Inhibitors
   Decreased Effect
      The levels/effects of Isosorbide Dinitrate may be decreased by: CYP3A4 Inducers (Strong); Deferasirox; Herbs (CYP3A4 Inducers); Tocilizumab
Ethanol/Nutrition/Herb Interactions
   Ethanol: Caution with ethanol (may increase risk of hypotension).
   Herb/Nutraceutical: Avoid black cohosh, California poppy, coleus, golden seal, hawthorn, mistletoe, periwinkle, quinine, shepherd's purse (may cause hypotension).
Mechanism of Action Stimulation of intracellular cyclic-GMP results in vascular smooth muscle relaxation of both arterial and venous vasculature with more prominent effects on the veins. Primarily reduces cardiac oxygen demand by decreasing preload (left ventricular end-diastolic pressure); may modestly reduce afterload. Additionally, coronary artery dilation improves collateral flow to ischemic regions.

Pharmacodynamics/Kinetics

Onset of action: Sublingual tablet: ~3 minutes; Oral tablet and capsule (includes extended-release formulations): ~1 hour

Duration: Sublingual tablet: 1-2 hours; Oral tablet and capsule (includes extended-release formulations): Up to 8 hours

Distribution: V_d: 2-4 L/kg

Metabolism: Extensively hepatic to conjugated metabolites, including isosorbide 5-mononitrate (active) and 2-mononitrate (active)

Bioavailability: Sublingual tablet: 40% to 50%; Oral immediate release formulations: Highly variable (10% to 90%); increases with chronic therapy

Half-life elimination: Parent drug: ~1 hour; Metabolites (5-mononitrate: 5 hours; 2-mononitrate: 2 hours)

Excretion: Urine and feces

Dosage

Geriatric Elderly patients should be given lowest recommended adult daily doses initially and titrate upward.

Adult

Angina:

Oral:

Immediate release: Initial: 5-20 mg 2-3 times/day; Maintenance: 10-40 mg 2-3 times/day **or** 5-80 mg 2-3 times/day (Anderson, 2007; Gibbons, 2002)

Sustained release: 40-160 mg/day has been used in clinical trials (a nitrate free interval of at least 18 hours is recommended; however, a clinically efficacious dosage interval has not been clearly established) **or** 40 mg 1-2 times/day (Anderson, 2007; Gibbons, 2002)

Sublingual:

Prophylactic use: 2.5-5 mg administered 15 minutes prior to activities which may provoke an anginal episode

Treatment of acute anginal episode (use only if patient has failed sublingual nitroglycerin): 2.5-5 mg every 5-10 minutes for maximum of 3 doses in 15-30 minutes

Heart failure (unlabeled use; Cohn, 1991; HFSA, 2010; Hunt, 2009): *Oral:*

Immediate release (**Note:** Use in combination with hydralazine):

Initial dose: 20 mg 3-4 times per day

Target dose: 160 mg/day in 4 divided doses

Esophageal spastic disorders (unlabeled use; Goyal, 1998): *Oral, sublingual:* Immediate release: 10-30 mg before meals

Renal Impairment

Hemodialysis: Supplemental dose is not necessary

Peritoneal dialysis: Supplemental dose is not necessary

Administration May consider administration of first dose in physician office; observe for maximal cardiovascular dynamic effects and adverse effects (orthostatic hypotension, headache). Do not administer around the clock; allow nitrate-free interval ≥14 hours (immediate release products) and >18 hours (sustained release products). Do not crush sublingual tablets or extended release formulations.

Immediate release products: When prescribed twice daily, consider administering at 8 AM and 1 PM. For 3 times/day dosing, consider 8 AM, 1 PM, and 6 PM.

Sustained release products: Consider once daily in morning or twice-daily dosing at 8 AM and between 1-2 PM.

Monitoring Parameters Blood pressure, heart rate

Special Geriatric Considerations The first dose of nitrates (sublingual, chewable, oral) should be taken in a physician's office to observe for maximal cardiovascular dynamic effects and adverse effects (eg, orthostatic blood pressure drop, headache). The use of nitrates for angina may occasionally promote reflux esophagitis. This may require dose adjustments or changing therapeutic agents to correct this adverse effect.

Dosage Forms Excipient information presented when available (limited, particularly for generics); consult specific product labeling.

Capsule, sustained release, oral:

Dilatrate®-SR: 40 mg

Tablet, oral: 5 mg, 10 mg, 20 mg, 30 mg

Isordil® Titradose™: 5 mg, 40 mg [scored]

Tablet, sublingual: 2.5 mg, 5 mg

Tablet, extended release, oral: 40 mg

Isosorbide Dinitrate and Hydralazine

(eye soe SOR bide dye NYE trate & hye DRAL a zeen)

Related Information

HydrALAZINE *on page 874*

Isosorbide Dinitrate *on page 987*

Brand Names: U.S. BiDil®

Index Terms Hydralazine and Isosorbide Dinitrate

Generic Availability (U.S.) No

Pharmacologic Category Vasodilator

Use Treatment of heart failure, adjunct to standard therapy, in self-identified African-Americans

Dosage

Geriatric & Adult Heart failure: Oral: Initial: 1 tablet 3 times/day; may titrate to a maximum dose of 2 tablets 3 times/day

Special Geriatric Considerations The pharmacokinetics of hydralazine and isosorbide dinitrate alone or in combination have not been studied. As with all antihypertensives and nitrate products, caution should be used on initiation of therapy, as hypotension may be encountered. Since many elderly are volume depleted, secondary to their blunted thirst reflex and/or use of diuretics, doses used initially should be at lowest recommended dose. The use of nitrates may occasionally promote reflux esophagitis. Monitor for these effects at start of therapy.

Dosage Forms

Tablet, oral:

BiDil®: Isosorbide dinitrate 20 mg and hydralazine 37.5 mg

Isosorbide Mononitrate (eye soe SOR bide mon oh NYE trate)

Medication Safety Issues

Sound-alike/look-alike issues:

Imdur® may be confused with Imuran®, Inderal LA®, K-Dur®

Monoket® may be confused with Monopril®

Brand Names: U.S. Imdur®; Ismo®; Monoket®

Brand Names: Canada Apo-ISMN®; Imdur®; PMS-ISMN; PRO-ISMN

Index Terms ISMN

Generic Availability (U.S.) Yes

Pharmacologic Category Vasodilator

Use Prevention of angina pectoris

Contraindications Hypersensitivity to isosorbide mononitrate or any component of the formulation; hypersensitivity to organic nitrates; concurrent use with phosphodiesterase-5 (PDE-5) inhibitors (sildenafil, tadalafil, or vardenafil)

Warnings/Precautions Avoid use in hypertrophic cardiomyopathy. Use with caution in volume depletion, moderate hypotension, and extreme caution with inferior wall MI and suspected right ventricular infarctions. Nitrates may precipitate or aggravate increased intra-cranial pressure and subsequently may worsen clinical outcomes in patients with neurologic injury (eg, intracranial hemorrhage, traumatic brain injury). Postural hypotension, transient episodes of weakness, dizziness, or syncope may occur even with small doses; ethanol accentuates these effects; tolerance and cross-tolerance to nitrate antianginal and hemody-namic effects may occur during prolonged isosorbide mononitrate therapy; (minimized by using the smallest effective dose, by alternating coronary vasodilators or offering drug-free intervals of as little as 12 hours). Excessive doses may result in severe headache, blurred vision, or xerostomia; increased anginal symptoms may be a result of dosage increases. Avoid concurrent use with PDE-5 inhibitors (eg, sildenafil, tadalafil, vardenafil). When nitrate administration becomes medically necessary, may administer nitrates only if 24 hours have elapsed after use of sildenafil or vardenafil (48 hours after tadalafil use) (O'Connor, 2010).

Adverse Reactions (Reflective of adult population; not specific for elderly)

>10%: Central nervous system: Headache (13% to 35%)

1% to 10%:

Cardiovascular: Angina (≤2%), flushing (≤2%)

Central nervous system: Dizziness (≤4%), fatigue (≤4%), pain (≤4%), emotional labil-ity (≤2%)

Dermatologic: Pruritus (≤2%), rash (≤2%)

Gastrointestinal: Nausea (≤3%), abdominal pain (≤2%), diarrhea (≤2%)

Respiratory: Upper respiratory infection (≤4%), cough increased (≤2%)

Miscellaneous: Allergic reaction (≤2%)

ISOSORBIDE MONONITRATE

Drug Interactions
Metabolism/Transport Effects Substrate of CYP3A4 (major)
Avoid Concomitant Use
Avoid concomitant use of Isosorbide Mononitrate with any of the following: Conivaptan; Phosphodiesterase 5 Inhibitors
Increased Effect/Toxicity
Isosorbide Mononitrate may increase the levels/effects of: Hypotensive Agents; Rosiglitazone

The levels/effects of Isosorbide Mononitrate may be increased by: Conivaptan; CYP3A4 Inhibitors (Moderate); CYP3A4 Inhibitors (Strong); Dasatinib; Phosphodiesterase 5 Inhibitors
Decreased Effect
The levels/effects of Isosorbide Mononitrate may be decreased by: CYP3A4 Inducers (Strong); Deferasirox; Herbs (CYP3A4 Inducers); Tocilizumab
Ethanol/Nutrition/Herb Interactions Ethanol: Caution with ethanol (may increase risk of hypotension).
Stability Tablets should be stored in a tight container at room temperature of 15°C to 30°C (59°F to 86°F).
Mechanism of Action Nitroglycerin and other nitrates form free radical nitric oxide. In smooth muscle, nitric oxide activates guanylate cyclase which increases guanosine 3'5' monophosphate (cGMP) leading to dephosphorylation of myosin light chains and smooth muscle relaxation. Produces a vasodilator effect on the peripheral veins and arteries with more prominent effects on the veins. Primarily reduces cardiac oxygen demand by decreasing preload (left ventricular end-diastolic pressure); may modestly reduce afterload; dilates coronary arteries and improves collateral flow to ischemic regions.
Pharmacodynamics/Kinetics
Onset of action: 30-60 minutes
Duration: Immediate release: ≥6 hours (Thadani, 1987); Extended release: ≥12-24 hours (Anderson, 2007)
Absorption: Nearly complete and low intersubject variability in its pharmacokinetic parameters and plasma concentrations
Distribution: V_d: ~0.6 L/kg
Protein binding: <5%
Metabolism: Hepatic
Bioavailability: ~100%
Half-life elimination: Mononitrate: ~5-6 hours
Excretion: Predominantly urine (2% as unchanged drug); feces (1% of dose)
Dosage
Geriatric Start with lowest recommended adult dose.
Adult
Angina: Oral:
Regular release tablet: Initial: 5-20 mg twice daily with the 2 doses given 7 hours apart (eg, 8 AM and 3 PM) to decrease tolerance development; patients initiating therapy with 5 mg twice daily (eg, small stature) should be titrated up to 10 mg twice daily in first 2-3 days.
Extended release tablet: Initial: 30-60 mg given once daily in the morning; titrate upward as needed, giving at least 3 days between increases; maximum daily single dose: 240 mg
Note: Tolerance to nitrate effects develops with chronic exposure. Dose escalation does not overcome this effect. Tolerance can only be overcome by short periods of nitrate absence from the body. Short periods of nitrate withdrawal may help minimize tolerance. Recommended twice daily dosage regimens incorporate this interval. Administer sustained release tablet once daily in the morning.
Renal Impairment Dose adjustment not necessary.
Hemodialysis: Dose supplementation is not necessary.
Peritoneal dialysis: Dose supplementation is not necessary.
Hepatic Impairment Dose adjustment not necessary.
Administration Do not administer around-the-clock. Immediate release tablet should be scheduled twice daily with doses 7 hours apart (8 AM and 3 PM); extended release tablet may be administered once daily in the morning upon rising with a half-glassful of fluid and should not be chewed or crushed.
Monitoring Parameters Monitor for orthostasis, increased hypotension
Special Geriatric Considerations The first dose of nitrates (sublingual, chewable, oral) should be taken in a physician's office to observe for maximal cardiovascular dynamic effects and adverse effects (eg, orthostatic blood pressure drop, headache). The use of nitrates for angina may occasionally promote reflux esophagitis. This may require dose adjustments or changing therapeutic agents to correct this adverse effect.

Dosage Forms Excipient information presented when available (limited, particularly for generics); consult specific product labeling.
Tablet, oral: 10 mg, 20 mg
  Ismo®: 20 mg [scored]
  Monoket®: 10 mg, 20 mg [scored]
Tablet, extended release, oral: 30 mg, 60 mg, 120 mg
  Imdur®: 30 mg, 60 mg [scored]
  Imdur®: 120 mg

Selected References

Gibbons RJ, Abrams J, Chatterjee K, et al, "ACC/AHA 2002 Guideline Update for the Management of Patients With Chronic Stable Angina - Summary Article: A Report of the American College of Cardiology/American Heart Association Task Force on Practice Guidelines (Committee on the Management of Patients With Chronic Stable Angina)," *J Am Coll Cardiol*, 2003, 41(1):159-68. Available at: http://http://www.acc.org/clinical/guidelines/stable/stable_clean.pdf. Accessed May 5, 2004.

Isoxsuprine (eye SOKS syoo preen)

Related Information
Beers Criteria – Potentially Inappropriate Medications for Geriatrics *on page 2089*

Medication Safety Issues
  Sound-alike/look-alike issues:
    Vasodilan® may be confused with Vasocidin®
  BEERS Criteria medication:
    This drug may be inappropriate for use in geriatric patients (low severity risk).

Index Terms Isoxsuprine Hydrochloride; Vasodilan

Generic Availability (U.S.) Yes

Pharmacologic Category Vasodilator

Use Treatment of peripheral vascular diseases, such as arteriosclerosis obliterans and Raynaud's disease

Dosage
  Geriatric & Adult Peripheral vascular disease: Oral: 10-20 mg 3-4 times/day; start with lower dose in elderly due to potential hypotension

Special Geriatric Considerations Vasodilators have been used to treat dementia upon the premise that dementia is secondary to a cerebral blood flow insufficiency. The hypothesis is that if blood flow could be increased, cognitive function would be increased. This hypothesis is no longer valid. The use of vasodilators for cognitive dysfunction is not recommended or proven by appropriate scientific study.

This medication is considered to be potentially inappropriate in this patient population (Beers Criteria severity: Low).

Dosage Forms Excipient information presented when available (limited, particularly for generics); consult specific product labeling.
Tablet, oral, as hydrochloride: 10 mg, 20 mg

◆ **Isoxsuprine Hydrochloride** *see* Isoxsuprine *on page 992*

Isradipine (iz RA di peen)

Related Information
Calcium Channel Blockers *on page 2003*

Medication Safety Issues
  Sound-alike/look-alike issues:
    DynaCirc® may be confused with Dynabac®, Dynacin®

Brand Names: U.S. DynaCirc CR®

Generic Availability (U.S.) Yes: Capsule

Pharmacologic Category Calcium Channel Blocker; Calcium Channel Blocker, Dihydropyridine

Use Treatment of hypertension

Contraindications Hypersensitivity to isradipine or any component of the formulation; hypotension (<90 mm Hg systolic)

Warnings/Precautions Increased angina and/or MI has occurred with initiation or dosage titration of calcium channel blockers. The most common side effect is peripheral edema; occurs within 2-3 weeks of starting therapy. Reflex tachycardia may occur with use. Symptomatic hypotension with or without syncope can rarely occur; blood pressure must be lowered at a rate appropriate for the patient's clinical condition. Use cautiously in HF, hypertrophic cardiomyopathy (IHSS), and in hepatic dysfunction. Use controlled release tablets with caution in patients with severe GI narrowing. Adjust doses at 2- to 4-week intervals.

Adverse Reactions (Reflective of adult population; not specific for elderly) Percentages reported with capsule formulation.

>10%: Central nervous system: Headache (dose related 2% to 22%)

1% to 10%:
   Cardiovascular: Edema (dose related 1% to 9%), palpitation (dose related 1% to 5%), flushing (dose related 1% to 5%), tachycardia (1% to 3%), chest pain (2% to 3%)
   Central nervous system: Dizziness (2% to 8%), fatigue (dose related 1% to 9%)
   Dermatologic: Rash (2%)
   Gastrointestinal: Nausea (1% to 5%), abdominal discomfort (≤3%), vomiting (≤1%), diarrhea (≤3%)
   Neuromuscular & skeletal: Weakness (≤1%)
   Renal: Urinary frequency (1% to 3%)
   Respiratory: Dyspnea (1% to 3%)

Drug Interactions

Metabolism/Transport Effects Substrate of CYP3A4 (major); **Inhibits** CYP3A4 (weak)

Avoid Concomitant Use
   Avoid concomitant use of Isradipine with any of the following: Artemether; Conivaptan; Dronedarone; Lumefantrine; Nilotinib; Pimozide; QUEtiapine; QuiNINE; Tetrabenazine; Thioridazine; Toremifene; Vandetanib; Vemurafenib; Ziprasidone

Increased Effect/Toxicity
   Isradipine may increase the levels/effects of: Amifostine; Antihypertensives; Beta-Blockers; Calcium Channel Blockers (Nondihydropyridine); Dronedarone; Fosphenytoin; Hypotensive Agents; Magnesium Salts; Neuromuscular-Blocking Agents (Nondepolarizing); Nitroprusside; Phenytoin; Pimozide; QTc-Prolonging Agents; QuiNIDine; QuiNINE; RiTUXimab; Tacrolimus; Tacrolimus (Systemic); Tetrabenazine; Thioridazine; Toremifene; Vandetanib; Vemurafenib; Ziprasidone

   The levels/effects of Isradipine may be increased by: Alfuzosin; Alpha1-Blockers; Antifungal Agents (Azole Derivatives, Systemic); Artemether; Calcium Channel Blockers (Nondihydropyridine); Chloroquine; Cimetidine; Ciprofloxacin; Ciprofloxacin (Systemic); Conivaptan; CycloSPORINE; CycloSPORINE (Systemic); CYP3A4 Inhibitors (Moderate); CYP3A4 Inhibitors (Strong); Diazoxide; Fluconazole; Gadobutrol; Herbs (Hypotensive Properties); Lumefantrine; Macrolide Antibiotics; Magnesium Salts; MAO Inhibitors; Nilotinib; Pentoxifylline; Phosphodiesterase 5 Inhibitors; Prostacyclin Analogues; Protease Inhibitors; QUEtiapine; QuiNIDine; QuiNINE

Decreased Effect
   Isradipine may decrease the levels/effects of: Clopidogrel; QuiNIDine

   The levels/effects of Isradipine may be decreased by: Barbiturates; Calcium Salts; CarBAMazepine; CYP3A4 Inducers (Strong); Deferasirox; Herbs (CYP3A4 Inducers); Herbs (Hypertensive Properties); Methylphenidate; Nafcillin; Rifamycin Derivatives; Tocilizumab; Yohimbine

Ethanol/Nutrition/Herb Interactions
   Food: Administration with food delays absorption, but does not affect availability
   Herb/Nutraceutical: St John's wort may decrease isradipine levels. Avoid dong quai if using for hypertension. Avoid bayberry, blue cohosh, cayenne, ephedra, ginger, ginseng (American), gotu kola, licorice (may worsen hypertension) Avoid garlic (may have increased antihypertensive effect).

Mechanism of Action Inhibits calcium ion from entering the "slow channels" or select voltage-sensitive areas of vascular smooth muscle and myocardium during depolarization, producing a relaxation of coronary vascular smooth muscle and coronary vasodilation; increases myocardial oxygen delivery in patients with vasospastic angina

Pharmacodynamics/Kinetics
   Onset of action: Immediate release: 2-3 hours
   Duration: Immediate release: >12 hours
   Absorption: 90% to 95%
   Distribution: V_d: 3 L/kg
   Protein binding: 95%
   Metabolism: Hepatic; CYP3A4 substrate (major); extensive first-pass effect; forms metabolites (inactive)
   Bioavailability: 15% to 24%
   Half-life elimination: Terminal: 8 hours
   Time to peak, serum: 1-1.5 hours
   Excretion: Urine (60% to 65% as metabolites); feces (25% to 30%)

Dosage

Geriatric

Capsule: Refer to adult dosing.

Controlled release tablet: Initial dose: 5 mg once daily

Adult Hypertension: Oral:

Capsule: 2.5 mg twice daily; antihypertensive response occurs in 2-3 hours; maximal response in 2-4 weeks; increase dose at 2- to 4-week intervals at 2.5-5 mg increments; usual dose range (JNC 7): 2.5-10 mg/day in 2 divided doses. **Note:** Most patients show no improvement with doses >10 mg/day except adverse reaction rate increases; therefore, maximal dose in older adults should be 10 mg/day.

Controlled release tablet: 5 mg once daily; antihypertensive response occurs in 2 hours. Adjust dose in increments of 5 mg at 2-4 week intervals. Maximum dose: 20 mg/day; adverse events are increased at doses >10 mg/day.

Renal Impairment

Cl_{cr} 30-80 mL/minute: Bioavailability increased by 45%

Cl_{cr} <10 mL/minute on hemodialysis: Bioavailability decreased by 20% to 50%

Capsule: Refer to adult dosing.

Controlled release tablet: Initial dose: 5 mg once daily

Hepatic Impairment

Peak serum concentrations are increased by 32% and bioavailability is increased by 52%.

Capsule: Refer to adult dosing.

Controlled release tablet: Initial dose: 5 mg once daily

Administration Controlled release tablets should be swallowed whole; do not divide or chew

Monitoring Parameters Blood pressure; renal, hepatic dysfunction

Special Geriatric Considerations Elderly may experience a greater hypotensive response. Constipation may be more of a problem in the elderly. Calcium channel blockers are no more effective in the elderly than other therapies; however, they do not cause significant CNS effects which is an advantage over some antihypertensive agents.

Dosage Forms Excipient information presented when available (limited, particularly for generics); consult specific product labeling.

Capsule, oral: 2.5 mg, 5 mg

Tablet, controlled release, oral:

DynaCirc CR®: 5 mg, 10 mg

Selected References

Chobanian AV, Bakris GL, Black HR, et al, "The Seventh Report of the Joint National Committee on Prevention, Detection, Evaluation, and Treatment of High Blood Pressure: The JNC 7 Report," *JAMA*, 2003, 289(19):2560-71.

◆ **Istalol®** *see* Timolol (Ophthalmic) *on page* 1799
◆ **Isuprel®** *see* Isoproterenol *on page* 987

Itraconazole (i tra KOE na zole)

Medication Safety Issues

Sound-alike/look-alike issues:

Itraconazole may be confused with fluconazole

Sporanox® may be confused with Suprax®, Topamax®

Brand Names: U.S. Sporanox®

Brand Names: Canada Sporanox®

Generic Availability (U.S.) Yes: Capsule

Pharmacologic Category Antifungal Agent, Oral

Use

Oral capsules: Treatment of susceptible fungal infections in immunocompromised and immunocompetent patients including blastomycosis and histoplasmosis; indicated for aspergillosis (in patients intolerant/refractory to amphotericin B), and onychomycosis of the toenail and fingernail (in nonimmunocompromised patients)

Oral solution: Treatment of oral and esophageal candidiasis

Contraindications Hypersensitivity to itraconazole (use caution in patients with a history of hypersensitivity to other azoles), any component of the formulation; concurrent administration with cisapride, dofetilide, ergot derivatives, levomethadyl, lovastatin, midazolam (oral), nisoldipine, pimozide, quinidine, simvastatin, or triazolam; treatment of onychomycosis (or other non-life-threatening indications) in patients with evidence of ventricular dysfunction, heart failure (HF) or a history of HF

Warnings/Precautions [U.S. Boxed Warning]: Negative inotropic effects have been observed following intravenous administration. Discontinue or reassess use if signs or symptoms of HF (heart failure) occur during treatment. [U.S. Boxed Warning]: Not recommended for treatment of onychomycosis in patients with ventricular dysfunction

or a history of HF. HF has been reported, particularly in patients receiving a total daily oral dose of 400 mg. Use with caution in patients with risk factors for HF (COPD, renal failure, edematous disorders, ischemic or valvular disease). Discontinue if signs or symptoms of HF or neuropathy occur during treatment. **[U.S. Boxed Warning]: Serious cardiovascular adverse events including, QT prolongation, ventricular tachycardia, torsade de pointes, cardiac arrest and/or sudden death have been observed due to increased cisapride, pimozide, quinidine or levomethadyl concentrations induced by itraconazole; concurrent use contraindicated.** Additionally, the following drugs metabolized by the CYP 3A4 isoenzyme system are also contraindicated: Ergot derivatives, lovastatin, midazolam (oral), simvastatin, and triazolam.

Calcium channel blockers (CCBs) may cause additive negative inotropic effects when used concurrently with itraconazole. Itraconazole may also inhibit the metabolism of CCBs. Use caution with concurrent use of itraconazole and CCBs due to an increased risk of HF. Concurrent use of itraconazole and nisoldipine is contraindicated.

Use with caution in patients with renal impairment. Rare cases of serious hepatotoxicity (including liver failure and death) have been reported (including some cases occurring within the first week of therapy); hepatotoxicity was reported in some patients without pre-existing liver disease or risk factors. Use with caution in patients with pre-existing hepatic impairment; monitor liver function closely and dosage adjustment may be warranted. Not recommended for use in patients with active liver disease, elevated liver enzymes, or prior hepatotoxic reactions to other drugs unless the expected benefit exceeds the risk of hepatotoxicity. Transient or permanent hearing loss has been reported. Quinidine (a contraindicated drug) was used concurrently in several of these cases. Hearing loss usually resolves after discontinuation, but may persist in some patients.

Large differences in itraconazole pharmacokinetic parameters have been observed in cystic fibrosis patients receiving the solution; if a patient with cystic fibrosis does not respond to therapy, alternate therapies should be considered. Due to differences in bioavailability, oral capsules and oral solution cannot be used interchangeably. Only the oral solution has proven efficacy for oral and esophageal candidiasis. Initiation of treatment with oral solution is not recommended in patients at immediate risk for systemic candidiasis (eg, patients with severe neutropenia).

Adverse Reactions (Reflective of adult population; not specific for elderly)
>10%: Gastrointestinal: Nausea (11%), diarrhea (3% to 11%)
1% to 10%:
Cardiovascular: Edema (4%), hypertension (3%), chest pain (3%)
Central nervous system: Fever (3% to 7%), headache (4%), fatigue (2% to 3%), dizziness (2%), depression (2%)
Dermatologic: Rash (4% to 9%), pruritus (3%)
Endocrine & metabolic: Hypokalemia (2%)
Gastrointestinal: Vomiting (5% to 7%), abdominal pain (2% to 6%), constipation (2%)
Hepatic: LFTs abnormal (3%)
Respiratory: Rhinitis (5% to 9%), cough (4%), dyspnea (2%), pneumonia (2%), sinusitis (2%), sputum increased (2%)
Miscellaneous: Diaphoresis increased (3%)

Drug Interactions
Metabolism/Transport Effects Substrate of CYP3A4 (major); **Inhibits** CYP3A4 (strong), P-glycoprotein
Avoid Concomitant Use
Avoid concomitant use of Itraconazole with any of the following: Alfuzosin; Aliskiren; Cisapride; Conivaptan; Crizotinib; Dofetilide; Dronedarone; Eplerenone; Ergot Derivatives; Everolimus; Fluticasone (Oral Inhalation); Halofantrine; Lapatinib; Lovastatin; Lurasidone; Nilotinib; Nisoldipine; Pimozide; QuiNIDine; Ranolazine; Rivaroxaban; RomiDEPsin; Salmeterol; Silodosin; Simvastatin; Tamsulosin; Ticagrelor; Tolvaptan; Topotecan; Toremifene
Increased Effect/Toxicity
Itraconazole may increase the levels/effects of: Alfentanil; Alfuzosin; Aliskiren; Almotriptan; Alosetron; Aprepitant; Benzodiazepines (metabolized by oxidation); Boceprevir; Bortezomib; Bosentan; Brentuximab Vedotin; Brinzolamide; Budesonide (Nasal); Budesonide (Systemic, Oral Inhalation); BusPIRone; Busulfan; Calcium Channel Blockers; CarBAMazepine; Cardiac Glycosides; Ciclesonide; Cilostazol; Cisapride; Colchicine; Conivaptan; Corticosteroids (Orally Inhaled); Corticosteroids (Systemic); Crizotinib; CycloSPORINE; CycloSPORINE (Systemic); CYP3A4 Substrates; Dabigatran Etexilate; Dienogest; DOCEtaxel; Dofetilide; Dronedarone; Dutasteride; Eletriptan; Ergot Derivatives; Erlotinib; Eszopiclone; Etravirine; Everolimus; FentaNYL; Fesoterodine; Fexofenadine; Fluticasone (Nasal); Fluticasone (Oral Inhalation); Fosaprepitant; Fosphenytoin; Gefitinib; GuanFACINE; Halofantrine; HMG-CoA Reductase Inhibitors; Iloperidone; Imatinib; Irinotecan; Ixabepilone; Lapatinib; Losartan; Lovastatin; Lumefantrine; Lurasidone; Macrolide Antibiotics; Maraviroc;

995

Methadone; MethylPREDNISolone; Nilotinib; Nisoldipine; Paliperidone; Paricalcitol; Pazopanib; P-Glycoprotein Substrates; Phenytoin; Phosphodiesterase 5 Inhibitors; Pimecrolimus; Pimozide; Protease Inhibitors; QuiNIDine; Ramelteon; Ranolazine; Repaglinide; Rifamycin Derivatives; Rivaroxaban; RomiDEPsin; Salmeterol; Saxagliptin; Sildenafil; Silodosin; Simvastatin; Sirolimus; Solifenacin; SORAfenib; SUNItinib; Tacrolimus; Tacrolimus (Systemic); Tacrolimus (Topical); Tadalafil; Tamsulosin; Telaprevir; Temsirolimus; Ticagrelor; Tolterodine; Tolvaptan; Topotecan; Toremifene; Vardenafil; Vemurafenib; Vilazodone; VinBLAStine; VinCRIStine; Vinorelbine; Vitamin K Antagonists; Ziprasidone; Zolpidem

The levels/effects of Itraconazole may be increased by: Boceprevir; Etravirine; Grapefruit Juice; Macrolide Antibiotics; Protease Inhibitors; Telaprevir

Decreased Effect

Itraconazole may decrease the levels/effects of: Amphotericin B; Prasugrel; Saccharomyces boulardii; Ticagrelor

The levels/effects of Itraconazole may be decreased by: Antacids; CYP3A4 Inducers (Strong); Deferasirox; Didanosine; Efavirenz; Etravirine; Fosphenytoin; H2-Antagonists; Herbs (CYP3A4 Inducers); Phenytoin; Proton Pump Inhibitors; Rifamycin Derivatives; Sucralfate; Tocilizumab

Ethanol/Nutrition/Herb Interactions

Food:

Capsules: Absorption enhanced by food and possibly by gastric acidity. Cola drinks have been shown to increase the absorption of the capsules in patients with achlorhydria or those taking H_2-receptor antagonists or other gastric acid suppressors. Avoid grapefruit juice.

Solution: Food decreases the bioavailability and increases the time to peak concentration.

Herb/Nutraceutical: St John's wort may decrease itraconazole levels.

Stability

Capsule: Store at room temperature, 15°C to 25°C (59°F to 77°F). Protect from light and moisture.

Oral solution: Store at ≤25°C (77°F); do not freeze.

Mechanism of Action Interferes with cytochrome P450 activity, decreasing ergosterol synthesis (principal sterol in fungal cell membrane) and inhibiting cell membrane formation

Pharmacodynamics/Kinetics

Absorption: Requires gastric acidity; capsule better absorbed with food, solution better absorbed on empty stomach

Distribution: V_d (average): 796 ± 185 L or 10 L/kg; highly lipophilic and tissue concentrations are higher than plasma concentrations. The highest concentrations: adipose, omentum, endometrium, cervical and vaginal mucus, and skin/nails. Aqueous fluids (eg, CSF and urine) contain negligible amounts.

Protein binding, plasma: 99.8%; metabolite hydroxy-itraconazole: 99.5%

Metabolism: Extensively hepatic via CYP3A4 into >30 metabolites including hydroxy-itraconazole (major metabolite); appears to have *in vitro* antifungal activity. Main metabolic pathway is oxidation; may undergo saturation metabolism with multiple dosing.

Bioavailability: Variable, ~55% (oral solution) in 1 small study; **Note:** Oral solution has a higher degree of bioavailability (149% ± 68%) relative to oral capsules; should not be interchanged

Half-life elimination: Oral: Single dose: ~21 hours, steady state: 64 hours; Cirrhosis (single dose): 37 hours (range 20-54 hours)

Time to peak, plasma: Capsules: 3-5 hours; Oral solution: 2-3 hours

Excretion: Urine (<0.03% active drug, 40% as inactive metabolites); feces (~3% to 18%)

Dosage

Geriatric & Adult

Aspergillosis, invasive (salvage therapy): Duration of therapy should be a minimum of 6-12 weeks or throughout period of immunosuppression: Oral: 200-400 mg/day; **Note:** 2008 IDSA guidelines recommend 600 mg/day for 3 days, followed by 400 mg/day.

Appropriate use: Itraconazole should **NOT** be used for voriconazole-refractory aspergillosis since the same antifungal and/or resistance mechanism(s) may be shared by both agents. Itraconazole oral solution and capsule formulations are not bioequivalent or interchangeable. Due to variable bioavailability of oral preparations, therapeutic drug monitoring advisable.

Aspergillosis, allergic (ABPA, sinusitis): Oral: 200 mg/day; may be used in conjunction with corticosteroids

Blastomycosis: Oral: 200 mg 3 times/day for 3 days, then 200 mg twice daily for 6-12 months; in moderately-severe to severe infection, therapy should be initiated with ~2 weeks of amphotericin B (Chapman, 2008)

Brain abscess: Cerebral phaeohyphomycosis (dematiaceous): Oral: 200 mg twice daily for at least 6 months with amphotericin

Candidiasis: Oral:
Oropharyngeal: Oral solution: 200 mg once daily for 1-2 weeks; in patients unresponsive or refractory to fluconazole: 100 mg twice daily (clinical response expected in 1-2 weeks)
Esophageal: Oral solution: 100-200 mg once daily for a minimum of 3 weeks; continue dosing for 2 weeks after resolution of symptoms

Coccidioidomycosis: Oral: 200 mg twice daily

Histoplasmosis: Oral: 200 mg 3 times/day for 3 days, then 200 mg twice daily (or once daily in mild-moderate disease) for 6-12 weeks in mild-moderate disease or ≥12 months in progressive disseminated or chronic cavitary pulmonary histoplasmosis; in moderately-severe to severe infection, therapy should be initiated with ~2 weeks of a lipid formation of amphotericin B (Wheat, 2007)
Long-term suppression therapy: 200 mg/day (AIDS*info* guidelines, 2008)

Meningitis: Oral:
Coccidioides: 400-800 mg/day
Coccidioides, HIV-positive (unlabeled use): 200 mg 3 times/day for 3 days, then 200 mg twice daily; maintenance: 200 mg twice daily life-long (AIDS*info* guidelines, 2008)
Appropriate use: Fluconazole is preferred for meningeal infections.

Onychomycosis: Oral: 200 mg once daily for 12 consecutive weeks; alternative "pulse-dosing" may be considering for fingernail involvement only: 200 mg twice daily for 1 week; repeat 1-week course after 3-week off-time

Penicilliosis, HIV-positive (unlabeled use): Oral: 200 mg twice daily for 8-10 weeks (in severely-ill patients, initiate therapy with 2 weeks of amphotericin B); maintenance: 200 mg/day (AIDS*info* guidelines, 2008)

Pneumonia: Oral:
Coccidioides: Mild-to-moderate: 200 mg twice daily
Coccidioides, HIV-positive (focal pneumonia): 200 mg 3 times/day for 3 days, then 200 mg twice daily (AIDS*info* guidelines, 2008)

Prototheca infection: Oral: 200 mg once daily for 2 months

Sporotrichosis: Oral:
Lymphocutaneous: 100-200 mg/day for 3-6 months
Osteoarticular and pulmonary: 200 mg twice daily for 1-2 years (may use amphotericin B initially for stabilization)

Renal Impairment The FDA-approved labeling states to use with caution in patients with renal impairment. The following guidelines have been used by some clinicians:
Aronoff, 2007:
Cl_{cr} >10 mL/minute: No adjustment recommended.
Cl_{cr} <10 mL/minute: Administer 50% of normal dose.
Poorly dialyzed; no supplemental dose or dosage adjustment necessary, including patients on intermittent hemodialysis, peritoneal dialysis, or continuous renal replacement therapy (eg, CVVHD).

Hepatic Impairment Use caution in patients with hepatic impairment.

Administration Doses >200 mg/day are given in 2 divided doses; do not administer with antacids. Capsule and oral solution formulations are not bioequivalent and thus are not interchangeable. Capsule absorption is best if taken with food, therefore, it is best to administer itraconazole after meals; solution should be taken on an empty stomach. When treating oropharyngeal and esophageal candidiasis, solution should be swished vigorously in mouth, then swallowed.

Monitoring Parameters Liver function in patients with pre-existing hepatic dysfunction, and in all patients being treated for longer than 1 month; serum concentrations particularly for oral therapy (due to erratic bioavailability with capsule formulation); renal function

Reference Range Serum concentrations may be performed to assure therapeutic levels. Itraconazole plus the metabolite hydroxyitraconazole concentrations should be >1 mcg/mL (not to exceed 10 mcg/mL).
Timing of serum samples: Obtain level after ~2 weeks of therapy, level may be drawn anytime during the dosing interval.

Pharmacotherapy Pearls Due to potential toxicity, the manufacturer recommends confirmation of diagnosis testing of nail specimens prior to treatment of onychomycosis.

Special Geriatric Considerations No specific data for the elderly. Transient or permanent hearing loss reported in the elderly; several reports include concurrent administration of quinidine.

Dosage Forms Excipient information presented when available (limited, particularly for generics); consult specific product labeling.
Capsule, oral: 100 mg
Sporanox®: 100 mg
Solution, oral:
Sporanox®: 10 mg/mL (150 mL) [contains propylene glycol; cherry-caramel flavor]

ITRACONAZOLE

Selected References

Aronoff GR, Bennett WM, Berns JS, et al, *Drug Prescribing in Renal Failure: Dosing Guidelines for Adults and Children*, 5th ed. Philadelphia, PA: American College of Physicians; 2007.

Chapman SW, Dismukes WE, Proia LA, et al, "Clinical Practice Guidelines for the Management of Blastomycosis: 2008 Update by the Infectious Diseases Society of America," *Clin Infect Dis*, 2008, 46(12):1801-12.

Walsh TJ, Anaissie EJ, Denning DW, et al, "Treatment of Aspergillosis: Clinical Practice Guidelines of the Infectious Diseases Society of America," *Clin Infect Dis*, 2008, 46(3):327-60.

Wheat J, Freifeld AG, Kleiman MB, et al, "Clinical Practice Guidelines for the Management of Patients With Histoplasmosis: 2007 Update by the Infectious Diseases Society of America," *Clin Infect Dis*, 2007, 45(7):807–25.

Kanamycin (kan a MYE sin)

Medication Safety Issues
Sound-alike/look-alike issues:
Kanamycin may be confused with Garamycin®, gentamicin

Index Terms Kanamycin Sulfate

Generic Availability (U.S.) Yes

Pharmacologic Category Antibiotic, Aminoglycoside

Use Treatment of serious infections caused by susceptible strains of *E. coli*, *Proteus* species, *Enterobacter aerogenes*, *Klebsiella pneumoniae*, *Serratia marcescens*, and *Acinetobacter* species; second-line treatment of *Mycobacterium tuberculosis*

Contraindications Hypersensitivity to kanamycin, any component of the formulation, or other aminoglycosides

Warnings/Precautions [U.S. Boxed Warning]: Aminoglycosides may cause neurotoxicity and/or nephrotoxicity; usual risk factors include pre-existing renal impairment, concomitant neuro-/nephrotoxic medications, advanced age, and dehydration. Ototoxicity may be directly proportional to the amount of drug given and the duration of treatment. Tinnitus or vertigo are indications of vestibular injury and impending hearing loss. Renal damage is usually reversible. May cause neuromuscular blockade and respiratory paralysis; especially when given soon after anesthesia or muscle relaxants.

Not intended for long-term therapy due to toxic hazards associated with extended administration. Use caution in pre-existing renal insufficiency, vestibular or cochlear impairment, myasthenia gravis, hypocalcemia, and conditions which depress neuromuscular transmission. Dosage modification required in patients with impaired renal function. Prolonged use may result in fungal or bacterial superinfection, including *C. difficile*-associated diarrhea (CDAD) and pseudomembranous colitis; CDAD has been observed >2 months postantibiotic treatment.

Adverse Reactions (Reflective of adult population; not specific for elderly) Frequency not defined.
Cardiovascular: Edema
Central nervous system: Neurotoxicity, drowsiness, headache, pseudomotor cerebri
Dermatologic: Skin itching, redness, rash, photosensitivity, erythema
Gastrointestinal: Nausea, vomiting, diarrhea, malabsorption syndrome (with prolonged and high-dose therapy of hepatic coma), anorexia, weight loss, salivation increased, enterocolitis
Hematologic: Granulocytopenia, agranulocytosis, thrombocytopenia
Local: Burning, stinging
Neuromuscular & skeletal: Weakness, tremor, muscle cramps
Otic: Ototoxicity (auditory), ototoxicity (vestibular)
Renal: Nephrotoxicity
Respiratory: Dyspnea

Drug Interactions
Avoid Concomitant Use
Avoid concomitant use of Kanamycin with any of the following: BCG; Gallium Nitrate

Increased Effect/Toxicity
Kanamycin may increase the levels/effects of: AbobotulinumtoxinA; Bisphosphonate Derivatives; CARBOplatin; Colistimethate; CycloSPORINE; CycloSPORINE (Systemic); Gallium Nitrate; Neuromuscular-Blocking Agents; OnabotulinumtoxinA; RimabotulinumtoxinB

The levels/effects of Kanamycin may be increased by: Amphotericin B; Capreomycin; CISplatin; Loop Diuretics; Nonsteroidal Anti-Inflammatory Agents; Vancomycin

Decreased Effect
Kanamycin may decrease the levels/effects of: BCG; Cardiac Glycosides; Typhoid Vaccine

The levels/effects of Kanamycin may be decreased by: Penicillins

Stability Store vial at controlled room temperature. Darkening of vials does not indicate loss of potency.
I.V.: Must be further diluted prior to I.V. infusion. For adults, dilute 500 mg in 100-200 mL of appropriate solution or 1 g in 200-400 mL.
Intraperitoneal: Dilute dose in 20 mL sterile distilled water.
Aerosol: Dilute 250 mg in 3 mL normal saline.

Mechanism of Action Interferes with protein synthesis in bacterial cell by binding to ribosomal subunit

Pharmacodynamics/Kinetics
Absorption:
I.M.: Rapid
Oral: Minimal
Distribution: V_d: ~0.3 L/kg:
Relative diffusion from blood into CSF: Good only with inflammation (exceeds usual MICs)
CSF:blood level ratio: Normal meninges: Nil; Inflamed meninges: 43%
Protein binding: 0%
Half-life elimination: 2-4 hours; Anuria: 80 hours; End-stage renal disease: 40-96 hours
Time to peak, serum: I.M.: 1-2 hours (decreased in burn patients)
Excretion: Urine (as unchanged drug)

Dosage
Geriatric I.M., I.V.: Initial dose should be 5-7.5 mg/kg based on ideal body weight (except in obese patients); maintenance dose and interval should be adjusted for estimated renal function; dosing interval in most older patients is every 12-24 hours (see Dosage: Renal Impairment).
Adult Note: Dosing should be based on ideal body weight
Susceptible systemic infections: I.M., I.V.: 5-7.5 mg/kg/dose in divided doses every 8-12 hours (<15 mg/kg/day)
Following surgical contamination, peritonitis: Intraperitoneal: 500 mg
Irrigating solution: 0.25%; maximum 1.5 g/day (via all administration routes)
Aerosol: 250 mg 2-4 times/day
Renal Impairment
Cl_{cr} 50-80 mL/minute: Administer 60% to 90% of dose or administer every 8-12 hours.
Cl_{cr} 10-50 mL/minute: Administer 30% to 70% of dose or administer every 12 hours.
Cl_{cr} <10 mL/minute: Administer 20% to 30% of dose or administer every 24-48 hours.

Administration Dilute to 100-200 mL and infuse over 30 minutes; I.M. doses should be given in a large muscle mass (ie, gluteus maximus).

Monitoring Parameters Serum creatinine and BUN every 2-3 days; peak and trough concentrations; hearing

Some penicillin derivatives may accelerate the degradation of aminoglycosides *in vitro*. This may be clinically-significant for certain penicillin (ticarcillin, piperacillin, carbenicillin) and aminoglycoside (gentamicin, tobramycin) combination therapy in patients with significant renal impairment. Close monitoring of aminoglycoside levels is warranted.

Reference Range Therapeutic: Peak: 15-30 mcg/mL; Trough: 5-10 mcg/mL; Toxic: Peak: >35 mcg/mL; Trough: >10 mcg/mL

Test Interactions Some penicillin derivatives may accelerate the degradation of aminoglycosides *in vitro*, leading to a potential underestimation of aminoglycoside serum concentration.

Pharmacotherapy Pearls Aminoglycoside levels in blood taken from silastic central catheters can sometime give falsely high readings.

Special Geriatric Considerations This is not a drug of choice since elderly may have increased adverse effects (renal).

Dosage Forms Excipient information presented when available (limited, particularly for generics); consult specific product labeling.
Injection, solution, as sulfate: 1 g/3 mL (3 mL)

Selected References
Yasuhara H, Kobayashi S, Sakamoto K, et al, "Pharmacokinetics of Amikacin and Cephalothin in Bedridden Elderly Patients," *J Clin Pharmacol*, 1982, 22(8-9):403-9.

Ketoconazole (Systemic) (kee toe KOE na zole)

Medication Safety Issues
Sound-alike/look-alike issues:
Nizoral® may be confused with Nasarel, Neoral®, Nitrol®
Brand Names: Canada Apo-Ketoconazole®; Novo-Ketoconazole
Generic Availability (U.S.) Yes
Pharmacologic Category Antifungal Agent, Oral
Use Treatment of susceptible fungal infections, including candidiasis, oral thrush, blastomycosis, histoplasmosis, paracoccidioidomycosis, coccidioidomycosis, chromomycosis, candiduria, chronic mucocutaneous candidiasis, as well as certain recalcitrant cutaneous dermatophytoses
Unlabeled/Investigational Use Treatment of prostate cancer (androgen synthesis inhibitor)
Contraindications Hypersensitivity to ketoconazole or any component of the formulation; CNS fungal infections (due to poor CNS penetration); coadministration with ergot derivatives, cisapride, or triazolam is contraindicated due to risk of potentially fatal cardiac arrhythmias
Warnings/Precautions [U.S. Boxed Warning]: Ketoconazole has been associated with hepatotoxicity, including some fatalities; use with caution in patients with impaired hepatic function and perform periodic liver function tests. **[U.S. Boxed Warning]: Concomitant use with cisapride is contraindicated due to the occurrence of ventricular arrhythmias.** High doses of ketoconazole may depress adrenocortical function.
Adverse Reactions (Reflective of adult population; not specific for elderly)
1% to 10%:
Dermatologic: Pruritus (2%)
Gastrointestinal: Nausea/vomiting (3% to 10%), abdominal pain (1%)
Drug Interactions
Metabolism/Transport Effects Substrate of CYP3A4 (major); **Inhibits** CYP1A2 (strong), CYP2A6 (moderate), CYP2B6 (weak), CYP2C8 (weak), CYP2C9 (strong), CYP2C19 (moderate), CYP2D6 (moderate), CYP3A4 (strong), P-glycoprotein
Avoid Concomitant Use
Avoid concomitant use of Ketoconazole (Systemic) with any of the following: Alfuzosin; Cisapride; Clopidogrel; Conivaptan; Crizotinib; Dofetilide; Dronedarone; Eplerenone; Everolimus; Fluticasone (Oral Inhalation); Halofantrine; Lapatinib; Lovastatin; Lurasidone; Nilotinib; Nisoldipine; Pimozide; QuiNIDine; Ranolazine; Rivaroxaban; RomiDEPsin; Salmeterol; Silodosin; Simvastatin; Tamsulosin; Thioridazine; Ticagrelor; Tolvaptan; Topotecan; Toremifene
Increased Effect/Toxicity
Ketoconazole (Systemic) may increase the levels/effects of: Alfentanil; Alfuzosin; Aliskiren; Almotriptan; Alosetron; Aprepitant; Bendamustine; Benzodiazepines (metabolized by oxidation); Boceprevir; Bortezomib; Bosentan; Brentuximab Vedotin; Brinzolamide; Budesonide (Nasal); Budesonide (Systemic, Oral Inhalation); BusPIRone; Busulfan; Calcium Channel Blockers; CarBAMazepine; Carvedilol; Ciclesonide; Cilostazol; Cinacalcet; Cisapride; Colchicine; Conivaptan; Corticosteroids (Orally Inhaled); Corticosteroids (Systemic); Crizotinib;

CycloSPORINE; CycloSPORINE (Systemic); CYP1A2 Substrates; CYP2A6 Substrates; CYP2C19 Substrates; CYP2C9 Substrates (High risk); CYP2D6 Substrates; CYP3A4 Substrates; Dabigatran Etexilate; Diclofenac; Dienogest; DOCEtaxel; Dofetilide; Dronedarone; Dutasteride; Eletriptan; Eplerenone; Erlotinib; Eszopiclone; Etravirine; Everolimus; FentaNYL; Fesoterodine; Fexofenadine; Fluticasone (Nasal); Fluticasone (Oral Inhalation); Fosaprepitant; Fosphenytoin; Gefitinib; GuanFACINE; Halofantrine; HMG-CoA Reductase Inhibitors; Iloperidone; Imatinib; Irinotecan; Ixabepilone; Lapatinib; Losartan; Lovastatin; Lumefantrine; Lurasidone; Macrolide Antibiotics; Maraviroc; Methadone; MethylPREDNISolone; Nebivolol; Nilotinib; Nisoldipine; Paricalcitol; Pazopanib; P-Glycoprotein Substrates; Phenytoin; Phosphodiesterase 5 Inhibitors; Pimecrolimus; Pimozide; Praziquantel; Protease Inhibitors; Proton Pump Inhibitors; QuiNIDine; Ramelteon; Ranolazine; Repaglinide; Rifamycin Derivatives; Rilpivirine; Rivaroxaban; RomiDEPsin; Salmeterol; Saxagliptin; Sildenafil; Silodosin; Simvastatin; Sirolimus; Solifenacin; SORAfenib; SUNItinib; Tacrolimus; Tacrolimus (Systemic); Tacrolimus (Topical); Tadalafil; Tamoxifen; Tamsulosin; Telaprevir; Temsirolimus; Thioridazine; Ticagrelor; Tolterodine; Tolvaptan; Topotecan; Toremifene; Vardenafil; Vemurafenib; Vilazodone; Vitamin K Antagonists; Ziprasidone; Zolpidem

The levels/effects of Ketoconazole (Systemic) may be increased by: Boceprevir; Etravirine; Grapefruit Juice; Macrolide Antibiotics; Protease Inhibitors; Telaprevir

Decreased Effect
Ketoconazole (Systemic) may decrease the levels/effects of: Amphotericin B; Clopidogrel; Codeine; Prasugrel; Saccharomyces boulardii; Ticagrelor; TraMADol

The levels/effects of Ketoconazole (Systemic) may be decreased by: Antacids; CYP3A4 Inducers (Strong); Deferasirox; Didanosine; Etravirine; Fosphenytoin; H2-Antagonists; Herbs (CYP3A4 Inducers); Phenytoin; Proton Pump Inhibitors; Rifamycin Derivatives; Rilpivirine; Sucralfate; Tocilizumab

Ethanol/Nutrition/Herb Interactions
Food: Ketoconazole peak serum levels may be prolonged if taken with food.
Herb/Nutraceutical: St John's wort may decrease ketoconazole levels.

Stability Store at 15°C to 25°C (59°F to 77°F).

Mechanism of Action Alters the permeability of the cell wall by blocking fungal cytochrome P450; inhibits biosynthesis of triglycerides and phospholipids by fungi; inhibits several fungal enzymes that results in a build-up of toxic concentrations of hydrogen peroxide; also inhibits androgen synthesis

Pharmacodynamics/Kinetics
Absorption: Rapid (~75%)
Distribution: Well into inflamed joint fluid, saliva, bile, urine, sebum, cerumen, feces, tendons, skin and soft tissue, and testes; crosses blood-brain barrier poorly; only negligible amounts reach CSF
Protein binding: 93% to 96%
Metabolism: Partially hepatic via CYP3A4 to inactive compounds
Bioavailability: Decreases as gastric pH increases
Half-life elimination: Biphasic: Initial: 2 hours; Terminal: 8 hours
Time to peak, serum: 1-2 hours
Excretion: Feces (57%); urine (13%)

Dosage
Geriatric & Adult
Fungal infections: Oral: 200-400 mg/day as a single daily dose
Prostate cancer (unlabeled use): Oral: 400 mg 3 times/day
Renal Impairment Hemodialysis: Not dialyzable (0% to 5%)
Hepatic Impairment Dose reductions should be considered in patients with severe liver disease.

Administration Administer oral tablets 2 hours prior to antacids to prevent decreased absorption due to the high pH of gastric contents.

Monitoring Parameters Liver function tests

Special Geriatric Considerations No specific recommendations.

Dosage Forms Excipient information presented when available (limited, particularly for generics); consult specific product labeling.
Tablet, oral: 200 mg

Ketoconazole (Topical) (kee toe KOE na zole)

Medication Safety Issues
Sound-alike/look-alike issues:
Nizoral® may be confused with Nasarel, Neoral®, Nitrol®
Brand Names: U.S. Extina®; Nizoral®; Nizoral® A-D [OTC]; Xolegel®

KETOCONAZOLE (TOPICAL)

Brand Names: Canada Ketoderm®; Xolegel®
Generic Availability (U.S.) Yes: Cream, shampoo
Pharmacologic Category Antifungal Agent, Topical
Use
Cream: Treatment of tinea corporis, tinea cruris, tinea versicolor, cutaneous candidiasis, seborrheic dermatitis
Foam, gel: Treatment of seborrheic dermatitis
Shampoo: Treatment of dandruff, seborrheic dermatitis, tinea versicolor
Unlabeled/Investigational Use Cream: Treatment of susceptible fungal infections in the oral cavity including candidiasis, oral thrush, and chronic mucocutaneous candidiasis
Dosage
Geriatric & Adult
Fungal infections: *Topical:*
Cream: Tinea infections: Rub gently into the affected area once daily. Duration of treatment: Tinea corporis, cruris: 2 weeks; tinea pedis: 6 weeks
Shampoo (ketoconazole 2%): Tinea versicolor: Apply to damp skin, lather, leave on 5 minutes, and rinse (one application should be sufficient)
Seborrheic dermatitis: *Topical:*
Cream: Rub gently into the affected area twice daily for 4 weeks or until clinical response is noted.
Foam: Apply to affected area twice daily for 4 weeks
Gel: Rub gently into the affected area once daily for 2 weeks.
Shampoo (ketoconazole 1%): Apply twice weekly for up to 8 weeks with at least 3 days between each shampoo
Susceptible fungal infections in the oral cavity (candidiasis, oral thrush, and chronic mucocutaneous candidiasis) (unlabeled use): *Topical:* Cream: Apply locally as directed with a thin coat to inner surface of denture and affected areas after meals
Dosage Forms Excipient information presented when available (limited, particularly for generics); consult specific product labeling. [DSC] = Discontinued product
Aerosol, topical [foam]:
Extina®: 2% (50 g, 100 g)
Cream, topical: 2% (15 g, 30 g, 60 g)
Gel, topical:
Xolegel®: 2% (15 g [DSC], 45 g) [contains dehydrated ethanol 34%]
Shampoo, topical: 2% (120 mL)
Nizoral®: 2% (120 mL)
Nizoral® A-D: 1% (6 mL [DSC], 120 mL, 210 mL)

Ketoprofen (kee toe PROE fen)

Medication Safety Issues
Sound-alike/look-alike issues:
Ketoprofen may be confused with ketotifen
Brand Names: Canada Apo-Keto SR®; Apo-Keto-E®; Apo-Keto®; Ketoprofen SR; Keto-profen-E; Nu-Ketoprofen; Nu-Ketoprofen-E; PMS-Ketoprofen; PMS-Ketoprofen-E
Generic Availability (U.S.) Yes
Pharmacologic Category Nonsteroidal Anti-inflammatory Drug (NSAID), Oral
Use Acute and long-term treatment of rheumatoid arthritis and osteoarthritis; mild-to-moderate pain
Medication Guide Available Yes
Contraindications Hypersensitivity to ketoprofen, aspirin, other NSAIDs, or any component of the formulation; perioperative pain in the setting of coronary artery bypass graft (CABG) surgery
Warnings/Precautions [U.S. Boxed Warning]: NSAIDs are associated with an increased risk of adverse cardiovascular thrombotic events, including MI and stroke Risk may be increased with duration of use or pre-existing cardiovascular risk factors or disease. Carefully evaluate individual cardiovascular risk profiles prior to prescribing. May cause new-onset hypertension or worsening of existing hypertension. Use caution with fluid retention. Avoid use in heart failure. Concurrent administration of ibuprofen, and potentially other nonselective NSAIDs, may interfere with aspirin's cardioprotective effect. **[U.S. Boxed Warning]: Use is contraindicated for treatment of perioperative pain in the setting of coronary artery bypass graft (CABG) surgery.** Risk of MI and stroke may be increased with use following CABG surgery.

NSAID use may compromise existing renal function; dose-dependent decreases in prostaglandin synthesis may result from NSAID use, reducing renal blood flow which may cause renal decompensation. NSAID use may increase the risk for hyperkalemia. Patients with impaired renal function, dehydration, heart failure, liver dysfunction, those taking diuretics, and ACE inhibitors, and the elderly are at greater risk of renal toxicity and hyperkalemia. Rehydrate patient before starting therapy; monitor renal function closely. Not recommended for use in patients with advanced renal disease. Long-term NSAID use may result in renal papillary necrosis.

[U.S. Boxed Warning]: NSAIDs may increase risk of gastrointestinal irritation, inflammation, ulceration, bleeding, and perforation. These events may occur at any time during therapy and without warning. Use caution with a history of GI disease (bleeding or ulcers), concurrent therapy with aspirin, anticoagulants and/or corticosteroids, smoking, use of alcohol, the elderly or debilitated patients. When used concomitantly with ≤325 mg of aspirin, a substantial increase in the risk of gastrointestinal complications (eg, ulcer) occurs; concomitant gastroprotective therapy (eg, proton pump inhibitors) is recommended (Bhatt, 2008). Platelet adhesion and aggregation may be decreased; may prolong bleeding time; patients with coagulation disorders or who are receiving anticoagulants should be monitored closely. Anemia may occur; patients on long-term NSAID therapy should be monitored for anemia. Rarely, NSAID use may cause severe blood dyscrasias (eg, agranulocytosis, aplastic anemia, thrombocytopenia).

Use the lowest effective dose for the shortest duration of time, consistent with individual patient goals, to reduce risk of cardiovascular or GI adverse events. Alternate therapies should be considered for patients at high risk.

NSAIDS may cause drowsiness, dizziness, blurred vision and other neurologic effects which may impair physical or mental abilities; patients must be cautioned about performing tasks which require mental alertness (eg, operating machinery or driving). Discontinue use with blurred or diminished vision and perform ophthalmologic exam. Monitor vision with long-term therapy.

NSAIDs may cause serious skin adverse events including exfoliative dermatitis, Stevens-Johnson syndrome (SJS), and toxic epidermal necrolysis (TEN); discontinue use at first sign of skin rash or hypersensitivity. Anaphylactoid reactions may occur, even without prior exposure; patients with "aspirin triad" (bronchial asthma, aspirin intolerance, rhinitis) may be at increased risk. Do not use in patients who experience bronchospasm, asthma, rhinitis, or urticaria with NSAID or aspirin therapy. Use caution in other forms of asthma.

Use with caution in patients with decreased hepatic function. Closely monitor patients with any abnormal LFT. Severe hepatic reactions (eg, fulminant hepatitis, liver failure) have occurred with NSAID use, rarely; discontinue if signs or symptoms of liver disease develop, or if systemic manifestations occur. The elderly are at increased risk for adverse effects (especially peptic ulceration, CNS effects, renal toxicity) from NSAIDs, even at low doses.

Withhold for at least 4-6 half-lives prior to surgical or dental procedures.

Adverse Reactions (Reflective of adult population; not specific for elderly)
>10%:
  Gastrointestinal: Dyspepsia (11%)
  Hepatic: Liver function test abnormal (≤15%)
1% to 10%:
  Cardiovascular: Peripheral edema (2%)
  Central nervous system: Headache (3% to 9%), depression, dizziness (>1%), dreams, insomnia, malaise, nervousness, somnolence
  Dermatologic: Rash (>1%)
  Gastrointestinal: Abdominal pain (3% to 9%), constipation (3% to 9%), diarrhea (3% to 9%), flatulence (3% to 9%), nausea (3% to 9%), gastrointestinal bleeding (>2%), peptic ulcer (>2%), anorexia (>1%), stomatitis (>1%), vomiting (>1%)
  Genitourinary: Urinary tract irritation (>1%)
  Ocular: Visual disturbances (>1%)
  Otic: Tinnitus (>1%)
  Renal: Renal dysfunction (3% to 9%)
Drug Interactions
  Metabolism/Transport Effects Inhibits CYP2C9 (weak)
  Avoid Concomitant Use
    Avoid concomitant use of Ketoprofen with any of the following: Floctafenine; Ketorolac; Ketorolac (Nasal); Ketorolac (Systemic)
  Increased Effect/Toxicity
    Ketoprofen may increase the levels/effects of: Aminoglycosides; Anticoagulants; Antiplatelet Agents; Bisphosphonate Derivatives; Collagenase (Systemic); CycloSPORINE; Cyclo-SPORINE (Systemic); Deferasirox; Desmopressin; Digoxin; Drotrecogin Alfa; Eplerenone; Haloperidol; Ibritumomab; Lithium; Methotrexate; Nonsteroidal Anti-Inflammatory Agents; PEMEtrexed; Porfimer; Potassium-Sparing Diuretics; PRALAtrexate; Quinolone Antibiotics;

◀ Rivaroxaban; Salicylates; Thrombolytic Agents; Tositumomab and Iodine I 131 Tositumomab; Vancomycin; Vitamin K Antagonists

The levels/effects of Ketoprofen may be increased by: ACE Inhibitors; Angiotensin II Receptor Blockers; Antidepressants (Tricyclic, Tertiary Amine); Corticosteroids (Systemic); Dasatinib; Floctafenine; Glucosamine; Herbs (Anticoagulant/Antiplatelet Properties); Ketorolac; Ketorolac (Nasal); Ketorolac (Systemic); Nonsteroidal Anti-Inflammatory Agents; Omega-3-Acid Ethyl Esters; Pentosan Polysulfate Sodium; Pentoxifylline; Probenecid; Prostacyclin Analogues; Selective Serotonin Reuptake Inhibitors; Serotonin/Norepinephrine Reuptake Inhibitors; Sodium Phosphates; Treprostinil; Vitamin E

Decreased Effect

Ketoprofen may decrease the levels/effects of: ACE Inhibitors; Angiotensin II Receptor Blockers; Antiplatelet Agents; Beta-Blockers; Eplerenone; HydrALAZINE; Potassium-Sparing Diuretics; Salicylates; Selective Serotonin Reuptake Inhibitors; Thiazide Diuretics

The levels/effects of Ketoprofen may be decreased by: Bile Acid Sequestrants; Nonsteroidal Anti-Inflammatory Agents; Salicylates

Ethanol/Nutrition/Herb Interactions

Ethanol: Avoid ethanol (due to GI irritation).

Food: Food slows rate of absorption resulting in delayed and reduced peak serum concentrations; total bioavailability is not affected by food.

Herb/Nutraceutical: Avoid alfalfa, anise, bilberry, bladderwrack, bromelain, cat's claw, celery, chamomile, coleus, cordyceps, dong quai, evening primrose, fenugreek, feverfew, garlic, ginger, ginkgo biloba, ginseng (American, Panax, Siberian), grapeseed, green tea, guggul, horse chestnut seed, horseradish, licorice, prickly ash, red clover, reishi, SAMe (S-adenosylmethionine), sweet clover, turmeric, and white willow (all have additional antiplatelet activity).

Stability Store at room temperature of 25°C (77°F). Protect from light; avoid excessive heat and humidity.

Mechanism of Action Reversibly inhibits cyclooxygenase-1 and 2 (COX-1 and 2) enzymes, which results in decreased formation of prostaglandin precursors; has antipyretic, analgesic, and anti-inflammatory properties

Other proposed mechanisms not fully elucidated (and possibly contributing to the anti-inflammatory effect to varying degrees), include inhibiting chemotaxis, altering lymphocyte activity, inhibiting neutrophil aggregation/activation, and decreasing proinflammatory cytokine levels.

Pharmacodynamics/Kinetics

Onset of action: Regular release: <30 minutes

Duration: Regular release: Up to 6 hours

Absorption: Almost complete

Distribution: 0.1 L/kg

Protein binding: >99%, primarily to albumin; Hepatic impairment: Unbound fraction is approximately doubled

Metabolism: Hepatic via glucuronidation; metabolite (inactive) can be converted back to parent compound; may have enterohepatic recirculation

Bioavailability: ~90%

Half-life elimination:

Regular release: 2-4 hours; Renal impairment: Mild: 3 hours; moderate-to-severe: 5-9 hours

Extended release: ~3-7.5 hours

Time to peak, serum:

Regular release: 0.5-2 hours

Extended release: 6-7 hours

Excretion: Urine (~80%, primarily as glucuronide conjugates)

Dosage

Geriatric Initial: 25-50 mg 3-4 times/day; increase up to 150-300 mg/day (maximum daily dose: 300 mg)

Adult Note: The extended release formulation is not recommended for the treatment of acute pain.

Rheumatoid arthritis or osteoarthritis: Oral:

Regular release: 50 mg 4 times/day **or** 75 mg 3 times/day; up to a maximum of 300 mg/day

Extended release: 200 mg once daily

Note: Lower doses may be used in small patients or in the elderly, or debilitated.

Mild-to-moderate pain: Oral: Regular release: 25-50 mg every 6-8 hours up to a maximum of 300 mg/day

Renal Impairment In general, NSAIDs are not recommended for use in patients with advanced renal disease, but the manufacturer of ketoprofen does provide some guidelines for adjustment in renal dysfunction:

Mild impairment: Maximum dose: 150 mg/day

Severe impairment: Cl_{cr} <25 mL/minute: Maximum dose: 100 mg/day

Hepatic Impairment Hepatic impairment and serum albumin <3.5 g/dL: Maximum dose: 100 mg/day

Administration May take with food to reduce GI upset. Do not crush or break extended release capsules.

Monitoring Parameters CBC, chemistry profile, occult blood loss, periodic liver function; renal function (urine output, serum BUN, creatinine)

Pharmacotherapy Pearls Dose must be lowest recommended in renal insufficiency. There are no clinical guidelines to predict which NSAID will give response in a particular patient. Trials with each must be initiated until response determined. Consider dose, patient convenience, and cost.

Special Geriatric Considerations Elderly are a high-risk population for adverse effects from NSAIDs. As much as 60% of the elderly can develop peptic ulceration and/or hemorrhage asymptomatically. The concomitant use of H_2 blockers and sucralfate is not effective as prophylaxis with the exception of NSAID-induced duodenal ulcers which may be prevented by the use of ranitidine. Misoprostol and proton pump inhibitors are the only agents proven to help prevent the development of NSAID-induced ulcers. Also, concomitant disease and drug use contribute to the risk for GI adverse effects. Use lowest effective dose for shortest period possible. Consider renal function decline with age. Use of NSAIDs can compromise existing renal function especially when Cl_{cr} is ≤30 mL/minute. Tinnitus may be a difficult and unreliable indication of toxicity due to age-related hearing loss or eighth cranial nerve damage. CNS adverse effects such as confusion, agitation, and hallucination are generally seen in overdose or high dose situations, but elderly may demonstrate these adverse effects at lower doses than younger adults.

Dosage Forms Excipient information presented when available (limited, particularly for generics); consult specific product labeling.

Capsule, oral: 50 mg, 75 mg

Capsule, extended release, oral: 200 mg

Selected References

Capone ML, Sciulli MG, Tacconelli S, et al, "Pharmacodynamic Interaction of Naproxen With Low-Dose Aspirin in Healthy Subjects," J Am Coll Cardiol, 2005, 45(8):1295-301.

Page J and Henry D, "Consumption of NSAIDs and the Development of Congestive Heart Failure in Elderly Patients: An Underrecognized Public Health Problem," Arch Intern Med, 2000, 160(6):777-84.

Ketorolac (Systemic) (KEE toe role ak)

Related Information

Beers Criteria – Potentially Inappropriate Medications for Geriatrics on page 2089

Medication Safety Issues

Sound-alike/look-alike issues:

Ketorolac may be confused with Ketalar®

Toradol® may be confused with Foradil®, Inderal®, TEGretol®, Torecan®, traMADol, tromethamine

Beers Criteria medication:

This drug may be inappropriate for use in geriatric patients (high severity risk).

International issues:

Toradol [Canada and multiple international markets] may be confused with Theradol brand name for tramadol [Netherlands]

Brand Names: Canada Apo-Ketorolac Injectable®; Apo-Ketorolac®; Ketorolac Tromethamine Injection, USP; Novo-Ketorolac; Nu-Ketorolac; Toradol®; Toradol® IM

Index Terms Ketorolac Tromethamine; Toradol

Generic Availability (U.S.) Yes

Pharmacologic Category Nonsteroidal Anti-inflammatory Drug (NSAID), Oral; Nonsteroidal Anti-inflammatory Drug (NSAID), Parenteral

Use Short-term (≤5 days) management of moderate-to-severe acute pain requiring analgesia at the opioid level

Medication Guide Available Yes

Contraindications Hypersensitivity to ketorolac, aspirin, other NSAIDs, or any component of the formulation; active or history of peptic ulcer disease; recent or history of GI bleeding or perforation; patients with advanced renal disease or risk of renal failure (due to volume depletion); prophylaxis before major surgery; suspected or confirmed cerebrovascular bleeding; hemorrhagic diathesis, incomplete hemostasis, or high risk of bleeding; concurrent ASA or other NSAIDs; concomitant probenecid or pentoxifylline; epidural or intrathecal administration; perioperative pain in the setting of coronary artery bypass graft (CABG) surgery

Warnings/Precautions [U.S. Boxed Warning]: May inhibit platelet function; contraindicated in patients with cerebrovascular bleeding (suspected or confirmed), hemorrhagic diathesis, incomplete hemostasis and patients at high risk for bleeding. Effects on platelet adhesion and aggregation may prolong bleeding time. Anemia may occur; patients on long-term NSAID therapy should be monitored for anemia. Rarely, NSAID use has been associated with potentially severe blood dyscrasias (eg, agranulocytosis, thrombocytopenia, aplastic anemia).

[U.S. Boxed Warning]: NSAIDs are associated with an increased risk of adverse cardiovascular thrombotic events, including MI and stroke. Risk may be increased with duration of use or pre-existing cardiovascular risk factors or disease. Carefully evaluate individual cardiovascular risk profiles prior to prescribing. May cause new-onset hypertension or worsening of existing hypertension. Use caution with fluid retention. Avoid use in heart failure. Concurrent administration of ibuprofen, and potentially other nonselective NSAIDs, may interfere with aspirin's cardioprotective effect. **[U.S. Boxed Warning]: Use is contraindicated as prophylactic analgesic before any major surgery and is contraindicated for treatment of perioperative pain in the setting of coronary artery bypass graft (CABG) surgery.** Risk of MI and stroke may be increased with use following CABG surgery. Wound bleeding and postoperative hematomas have been associated with ketorolac use in the perioperative setting. Withhold for at least 4-6 half-lives prior to surgical or dental procedures.

[U.S. Boxed Warning]: Ketorolac is contraindicated in patients with advanced renal impairment and in patients at risk for renal failure due to volume depletion. NSAID use may compromise existing renal function; dose-dependent decreases in prostaglandin synthesis may result from NSAID use, reducing renal blood flow which may cause renal decompensation. NSAID use may increase the risk for hyperkalemia. Patients with impaired renal function, dehydration, heart failure, liver dysfunction, those taking diuretics and ACE inhibitors, and the elderly are at greater risk of renal toxicity. Use with caution in patients with impaired renal function or history of kidney disease; dosage adjustment is required in patients with moderate elevation in serum creatinine. Monitor renal function closely. Acute renal failure, interstitial nephritis, and nephrotic syndrome have been reported with ketorolac use; papillary necrosis and renal injury have been reported with the use of NSAIDs. Use of NSAIDs can compromise existing renal function. Rehydrate patient before starting therapy.

[U.S. Boxed Warning]: NSAIDs may increase risk of gastrointestinal irritation, inflammation, ulceration, bleeding, and perforation. These events may occur at any time during therapy and without warning. Use caution with a history of GI disease (bleeding, ulcers, inflammatory bowel disease), concurrent therapy with aspirin, anticoagulants and/or corticosteroids, smoking, use of alcohol, the elderly, or debilitated patients. When used concomitantly with ≤325 mg of aspirin, a substantial increase in the risk of gastrointestinal complications (eg, ulcer) occurs; concomitant gastroprotective therapy (eg, proton pump inhibitors) is recommended (Bhatt, 2008).

NSAIDs may cause serious skin adverse events including exfoliative dermatitis, Stevens-Johnson syndrome (SJS), and toxic epidermal necrolysis (TEN); discontinue use at first sign of skin rash or hypersensitivity. Hypersensitivity or anaphylactoid reactions may occur, even without prior exposure; patients with "aspirin triad" (bronchial asthma, aspirin intolerance, rhinitis) may be at increased risk. Do not use in patients who experience bronchospasm, asthma, rhinitis, or urticaria with NSAID or aspirin therapy. **[U.S. Boxed Warning]: Ketorolac injection is contraindicated in patients with prior hypersensitivity reaction to aspirin or NSAIDs.** Use caution in other forms of asthma.

Use with caution in patients with hepatic impairment or a history of liver disease. Closely monitor patients with any abnormal LFT. Rarely, severe hepatic reactions (eg, fulminant hepatitis, hepatic necrosis, liver failure) have occurred with NSAID use; discontinue if signs or symptoms of liver disease develop, or if systemic manifestations occur.

[U.S. Boxed Warning]: Dosage adjustment is required for patients ≥65 years of age. The elderly are at increased risk for adverse effects (especially peptic ulceration, CNS effects, renal toxicity) from NSAIDs, even at low doses. **[U.S. Boxed Warning]: Dosage adjustment is required for patients weighing <50 kg (<110 pounds). [U.S. Boxed Warning]: Concurrent use of ketorolac with aspirin or other NSAIDs is contraindicated due to the increased risk of adverse reactions.**

[U.S. Boxed Warning]: Contraindicated for epidural or intrathecal administration. [U.S. Boxed Warning]: Systemic ketorolac is indicated for short term (≤5 days) use in adults for treatment of moderately severe acute pain requiring opioid-level analgesia. Low doses of narcotics may be needed for breakthrough pain. **[U.S. Boxed Warning]: Oral therapy is only indicated for use as continuation treatment, following parenteral**

ketorolac and is not indicated for minor or chronic painful conditions. **The maximum daily oral dose is 40 mg (adults); doses above 40 mg/day do not improve efficacy but may increase the risk of serious adverse effects.** The combined therapy duration (oral and parenteral) should not exceed 5 days. Use the lowest effective dose for the shortest duration of time, consistent with individual patient goals, to reduce risk of cardiovascular or GI adverse events. Alternate therapies should be considered for patients at high risk.

NSAIDS may cause drowsiness, dizziness, blurred vision and other neurologic effects which may impair physical or mental abilities; patients must be cautioned about performing tasks which require mental alertness (eg, operating machinery or driving). Discontinue use with blurred or diminished vision and perform ophthalmologic exam. Monitor vision with long-term therapy.

Adverse Reactions (Reflective of adult population; not specific for elderly)
Frequencies noted for parenteral administration:

>10%:

Central nervous system: Headache (17%)

Gastrointestinal: Gastrointestinal pain (13%), dyspepsia (12%), nausea (12%)

>1% to 10%:

Cardiovascular: Edema (4%), hypertension

Central nervous system: Dizziness (7%), drowsiness (6%)

Dermatologic: Pruritus, purpura, rash

Gastrointestinal: Diarrhea (7%), constipation, flatulence, GI bleeding, GI fullness, GI perfo-ration, GI ulcer, heartburn, stomatitis, vomiting

Hematologic: Anemia, bleeding time increased

Hepatic: Liver enzymes increased

Local: Injection site pain (2%)

Otic: Tinnitus

Renal: Renal function abnormal

Miscellaneous: Diaphoresis

Drug Interactions
Avoid Concomitant Use
Avoid concomitant use of Ketorolac (Systemic) with any of the following: Aspirin; Floctafe-nine; Ketorolac; Ketorolac (Nasal); Nonsteroidal Anti-Inflammatory Agents; Pentoxifylline; Probenecid

Increased Effect/Toxicity
Ketorolac (Systemic) may increase the levels/effects of: Aminoglycosides; Anticoagulants; Antiplatelet Agents; Aspirin; Bisphosphonate Derivatives; Collagenase (Systemic); Cyclo-SPORINE; CycloSPORINE (Systemic); Deferasirox; Desmopressin; Digoxin; Drotrecogin Alfa; Eplerenone; Haloperidol; Ibritumomab; Lithium; Methotrexate; Neuromuscular-Blocking Agents (Nondepolarizing); Nonsteroidal Anti-Inflammatory Agents; PEMEtrexed; Pentoxifyl-line; Porfimer; Potassium-Sparing Diuretics; PRALAtrexate; Quinolone Antibiotics; Rivarox-aban; Salicylates; Thrombolytic Agents; Tositumomab and Iodine I 131 Tositumomab; Vancomycin; Vitamin K Antagonists

The levels/effects of Ketorolac (Systemic) may be increased by: ACE Inhibitors; Angiotensin II Receptor Blockers; Antidepressants (Tricyclic, Tertiary Amine); Corticosteroids (Systemic); Dasatinib; Floctafenine; Glucosamine; Herbs (Anticoagulant/Antiplatelet Properties); Ketor-olac; Ketorolac (Nasal); Omega-3-Acid Ethyl Esters; Pentosan Polysulfate Sodium; Probe-necid; Prostacyclin Analogues; Selective Serotonin Reuptake Inhibitors; Serotonin/Norepinephrine Reuptake Inhibitors; Sodium Phosphates; Treprostinil; Vitamin E

Decreased Effect
Ketorolac (Systemic) may decrease the levels/effects of: ACE Inhibitors; Angiotensin II Receptor Blockers; Anticonvulsants; Antiplatelet Agents; Beta-Blockers; Eplerenone; HydrA-LAZINE; Potassium-Sparing Diuretics; Salicylates; Selective Serotonin Reuptake Inhibitors; Thiazide Diuretics

The levels/effects of Ketorolac (Systemic) may be decreased by: Bile Acid Sequestrants; Salicylates

Ethanol/Nutrition/Herb Interactions
Ethanol: Avoid ethanol (may enhance gastric mucosal irritation).

Food: Oral: High-fat meals may delay time to peak (by ~1 hour) and decrease peak concentrations.

Herb/Nutraceutical: Avoid alfalfa, anise, bilberry, bladderwrack, bromelain, cat's claw, celery, chamomile, coleus, cordyceps, dong quai, evening primrose, fenugreek, feverfew, garlic, ginger, ginkgo biloba, ginseng (American, Panax, Siberian), grapeseed, green tea, guggul, horse chestnut seed, horseradish, licorice, prickly ash, red clover, reishi, SAMe (S-adenosylmethionine), sweet clover, turmeric, and white willow (all have additional antipla-telet activity).

Stability
Injection: Store at room temperature of 15°C to 30°C (59°F to 86°F). Protect from light. Injection is clear and has a slight yellow color. Precipitation may occur at relatively low pH values.
Tablet: Store at room temperature of 15°C to 30°C (59°F to 86°F).
Mechanism of Action Reversibly inhibits cyclooxygenase-1 and 2 (COX-1 and 2) enzymes, which results in decreased formation of prostaglandin precursors; has antipyretic, analgesic, and anti-inflammatory properties

Other proposed mechanisms not fully elucidated (and possibly contributing to the anti-inflammatory effect to varying degrees), include inhibiting chemotaxis, altering lymphocyte activity, inhibiting neutrophil aggregation/activation, and decreasing proinflammatory cytokine levels.
Pharmacodynamics/Kinetics
Onset of action: Analgesic: I.M.: ~10 minutes
Peak effect: Analgesic: 2-3 hours
Duration: Analgesic: 6-8 hours
Absorption: Oral: Well absorbed (100%)
Distribution: ~13 L; poor penetration into CSF
Protein binding: 99%
Metabolism: Hepatic
Half-life elimination: 2-6 hours; prolonged 30% to 50% in elderly; up to 19 hours in renal impairment
Time to peak, serum: I.M.: 30-60 minutes
Excretion: Urine (92%, ~60% as unchanged drug); feces ~6%
Dosage
Geriatric Dosage adjustments in elderly (≥65 years), renal insufficiency, or low body weight (<50 kg): **Note:** These groups have an increased incidence of GI bleeding, ulceration, and perforation. The maximum combined duration of treatment (for parenteral and oral) is 5 days.
I.M.: 30 mg as a single dose or 15 mg every 6 hours (maximum daily dose: 60 mg)
I.V.: 15 mg as a single dose or 15 mg every 6 hours (maximum daily dose: 60 mg)
Oral: 10 mg, followed by 10 mg every 4-6 hours; do not exceed 40 mg/day; oral dosing is intended to be a continuation of I.M. or I.V. therapy only
Adult Pain management (acute; moderately-severe): Note: The maximum combined duration of treatment (for parenteral and oral) is 5 days; do not increase dose or frequency; supplement with low dose opioids if needed for breakthrough pain. For patients <50 kg and/or ≥65 years of age, see Dosage: Geriatric.
I.M.: 60 mg as a single dose or 30 mg every 6 hours (maximum daily dose: 120 mg)
I.V.: 30 mg as a single dose or 30 mg every 6 hours (maximum daily dose: 120 mg)
Oral: 20 mg, followed by 10 mg every 4-6 hours; do not exceed 40 mg/day; oral dosing is intended to be a continuation of I.M. or I.V. therapy only
Renal Impairment Contraindicated in patients with advanced renal impairment. Patients with moderately-elevated serum creatinine should use half the recommended dose, not to exceed 60 mg/day I.M./I.V.
Hepatic Impairment Use with caution, may cause elevation of liver enzymes; discontinue if clinical signs and symptoms of liver disease develop.
Administration
Oral: May take with food to reduce GI upset.
I.M.: Administer slowly and deeply into the muscle. Analgesia begins in 30 minutes and maximum effect within 2 hours.
I.V.: Administer I.V. bolus over a minimum of 15 seconds; onset within 30 minutes; peak analgesia within 2 hours.
Monitoring Parameters Monitor response (pain, range of motion, grip strength, mobility, ADL function), inflammation; observe for weight gain, edema; monitor renal function (serum creatinine, BUN, urine output); CBC and platelets, liver function tests; observe for bleeding, bruising; evaluate gastrointestinal effects (abdominal pain, bleeding, dyspepsia); mental confusion, disorientation
Reference Range Serum concentration: Therapeutic: 0.3-5 mcg/mL; Toxic: >5 mcg/mL
Pharmacotherapy Pearls First parenteral NSAID for analgesia; 30 mg provides the analgesia comparable to 12 mg of morphine or 100 mg of meperidine; pain relief usually begins within 10 minutes; there are no clinical guidelines to predict which NSAID will give response in a particular patient. Trials with each must be initiated until response determined. Consider dose, patient convenience, and cost.
Special Geriatric Considerations Ketorolac is cleared more slowly in the elderly. It is recommended to use lower doses in the elderly. Elderly are a high-risk population for adverse effects from NSAIDs. As much as 60% of elderly can develop peptic ulceration and/or hemorrhage asymptomatically. The concomitant use of H_2 blockers and sucralfate is not

effective as prophylaxis with the exception of NSAID-induced duodenal ulcers which may be prevented by the use of ranitidine. Misoprostol and proton pump inhibitors are the only agents proven to help prevent the development of NSAID-induced ulcers. Also, concomitant disease and drug use contribute to the risk for GI adverse effects. Use lowest effective dose for shortest period possible. Consider renal function decline with age. Use of NSAIDs can compromise existing renal function especially when Cl_{cr} is ≤30 mL/minute or weight <50 kg. Tinnitus may be a difficult and unreliable indication of toxicity due to age-related hearing loss or eighth cranial nerve damage. CNS adverse effects such as confusion, agitation, and hallucination are generally seen in overdose or high dose situations, but elderly may demonstrate these adverse effects at lower doses than younger adults.

This medication is considered to be potentially inappropriate in this patient population (Beers Criteria severity: High).

Dosage Forms Excipient information presented when available (limited, particularly for generics); consult specific product labeling.

Injection, solution, as tromethamine: 15 mg/mL (1 mL, 2 mL); 30 mg/mL (1 mL, 2 mL, 10 mL)

Tablet, oral, as tromethamine: 10 mg

Selected References

Obase Y, Matsuse H, Shimoda T, et al, "Pathogenesis and Management of Aspirin-Intolerant Asthma," *Treat Respir Med*, 2005, 4(5):325-36.

Ketorolac (Nasal) (KEE toe role ak)

Medication Safety Issues

Sound-alike/look-alike issues:

Ketorolac may be confused with Ketalar®

BEERS Criteria medication:

This drug may be inappropriate for use in geriatric patients (high severity risk).

Brand Names: U.S. Sprix®

Index Terms Ketorolac Tromethamine

Generic Availability (U.S.) No

Pharmacologic Category Nonsteroidal Anti-inflammatory Drug (NSAID), Nasal

Use Short-term (≤5 days) management of moderate-to-moderately-severe acute pain requiring analgesia at the opioid level

Medication Guide Available Yes

Contraindications Hypersensitivity to ketorolac, aspirin, other NSAIDs, or any component of the formulation; history of asthma, urticaria, or other allergic-type reactions following aspirin or other NSAID use; active or history of peptic ulcer disease; recent or history of GI bleeding or perforation); patients with advanced renal disease or risk of renal failure (due to volume depletion); prophylaxis before major surgery; suspected or confirmed cerebrovascular bleeding; hemorrhagic diathesis, incomplete hemostasis, or high risk of bleeding; concomitant probenecid or pentoxifylline; perioperative pain in the setting of coronary artery bypass graft (CABG) surgery

Warnings/Precautions [U.S. Boxed Warning]: May inhibit platelet function; contraindicated in patients with cerebrovascular bleeding (suspected or confirmed), hemorrhagic diathesis, incomplete hemostasis and patients at high risk for bleeding. Effects on platelet adhesion and aggregation may prolong bleeding time. Anemia may occur; patients on long-term NSAID therapy should be monitored for anemia. Rarely, NSAID use has been associated with potentially severe blood dyscrasias (eg, agranulocytosis, thrombocytopenia, aplastic anemia).

[U.S. Boxed Warning]: NSAIDs are associated with an increased risk of adverse cardiovascular thrombotic events, including MI and stroke. Risk may be increased with duration of use or pre-existing cardiovascular risk factors or disease. Carefully evaluate individual cardiovascular risk profiles prior to prescribing. Use caution with fluid retention. Avoid use in heart failure. Use may cause new-onset hypertension or worsening of existing hypertension. Concurrent administration of ibuprofen, and potentially other nonselective NSAIDs, may interfere with aspirin's cardioprotective effect. **[U.S. Boxed Warning]: Use is contraindicated for treatment of perioperative pain in the setting of coronary artery bypass graft (CABG) surgery.** Risk of MI and stroke may be increased with use following CABG surgery. Use is also contraindicated as prophylactic analgesic before any major surgery. Wound bleeding and postoperative hematomas have been associated with ketorolac use in the perioperative setting. Withhold for at least 4-6 half-lives prior to surgical or dental procedures.

[U.S. Boxed Warning]: Ketorolac is contraindicated in patients with advanced renal impairment and in patients at risk for renal failure due to volume depletion. NSAID use may compromise existing renal function; dose-dependent decreases in prostaglandin synthesis may result from NSAID use, reducing renal blood flow which may cause renal decompensation. NSAID use may increase the risk of hyperkalemia. Patients with impaired renal function, dehydration, heart failure, liver dysfunction, those taking diuretics and ACE inhibitors, and the elderly are at greater risk of renal toxicity. Use with caution in patients with impaired renal function or history of kidney disease. Dosage adjustment is required in patients with moderate elevation in serum creatinine. Acute renal failure, interstitial nephritis, and nephrotic syndrome have been reported with ketorolac use; papillary necrosis and renal injury have been reported with the use of NSAIDs. Rehydrate patient before starting therapy; monitor renal function closely.

[U.S. Boxed Warning]: NSAIDs may increase risk of gastrointestinal irritation, inflammation, ulceration, bleeding, and perforation. These events may occur at any time during therapy and without warning. Use caution with a history of GI disease (bleeding, ulcers, inflammatory bowel disease), concurrent therapy with aspirin, anticoagulants and/or corticosteroids, smoking, use of alcohol, the elderly, or debilitated patients.

NSAIDs may cause serious skin adverse events including exfoliative dermatitis, Stevens-Johnson syndrome (SJS), and toxic epidermal necrolysis (TEN); discontinue use at first sign of skin rash or hypersensitivity. Hypersensitivity or anaphylactoid reactions may occur, even without prior exposure. Ketorolac nasal spray is contraindicated in patients with prior hypersensitivity reaction to aspirin or NSAIDs. Use caution in patients with other forms of asthma.

Use with caution in patients with hepatic impairment or a history of liver disease. Closely monitor patients with any abnormal LFT. Rarely, severe hepatic reactions (eg, fulminant hepatitis, hepatic necrosis, liver failure) have occurred with NSAID use; discontinue if signs or symptoms of liver disease develop, or if systemic manifestations occur.

[U.S. Boxed Warning]: Ketorolac nasal spray is indicated for short term (≤5 days) use in adults for treatment of moderate to moderately severe acute pain requiring opioid-level analgesia. The combined therapy duration (nasal and other ketorolac formulations) should not exceed 5 days. Therapy is not appropriate for minor or chronic pain therapy. Use the lowest effective dose for the shortest duration of time, consistent with individual patient goals, to reduce risk of cardiovascular or GI adverse events. Alternate therapies should be considered for patients at high risk.

[U.S. Boxed Warning]: Nasal ketorolac is not indicated for use in children. Dosage adjustment is required for adults weighing <50 kg (<110 pounds) and/or for patients ≥65 years of age. The elderly are at increased risk for adverse effects (especially peptic ulceration, CNS effects, renal toxicity) from NSAIDs, even at low doses. Avoid immediate and long-term use (Beers Criteria). Avoid contact with the eyes; if eye exposure occurs, wash eye with water or saline; consult physician if irritation continues >1 hour. Preparation contains edetate sodium (EDTA); do not use in patients with hypersensitivity to EDTA.

Adverse Reactions (Reflective of adult population; not specific for elderly) Events reported with intranasal use; refer to Ketorolac (Systemic) monograph for other potential ketorolac-related adverse events.

>10%: Respiratory: Nasal discomfort (15%), rhinalgia (13%)

>1% to 10%:
Cardiovascular: Bradycardia (2%), hypertension (2%)
Dermatologic: Rash (3%)
Gastrointestinal: Throat irritation (4%)
Genitourinary: Urine output decreased (2%)
Hepatic: ALT/AST increased (2%)
Ocular: Lacrimation increased (5%)
Respiratory: Rhinitis (2%)
Renal: Oliguria (3%)

Drug Interactions

Avoid Concomitant Use

Avoid concomitant use of Ketorolac (Nasal) with any of the following: Aspirin; Floctafenine; Ketorolac; Ketorolac (Systemic); Nonsteroidal Anti-Inflammatory Agents; Pentoxifylline; Probenecid

Increased Effect/Toxicity

Ketorolac (Nasal) may increase the levels/effects of: Aminoglycosides; Anticoagulants; Antiplatelet Agents; Aspirin; Bisphosphonate Derivatives; Collagenase (Systemic); CycloSPORINE; CycloSPORINE (Systemic); Deferasirox; Desmopressin; Digoxin; Drotrecogin Alfa; Eplerenone; Haloperidol; Ibritumomab; Lithium; Methotrexate; Neuromuscular-Blocking Agents (Nondepolarizing); Nonsteroidal Anti-Inflammatory Agents; PEMEtrexed; Pentoxifylline; Porfimer; Potassium-Sparing Diuretics; PRALAtrexate; Quinolone Antibiotics; Rivaroxaban; Salicylates; Thrombolytic Agents; Tositumomab and Iodine I 131 Tositumomab; Vancomycin; Vitamin K Antagonists

The levels/effects of Ketorolac (Nasal) may be increased by: ACE Inhibitors; Angiotensin II Receptor Blockers; Antidepressants (Tricyclic, Tertiary Amine); Corticosteroids (Systemic); Dasatinib; Floctafenine; Glucosamine; Herbs (Anticoagulant/Antiplatelet Properties); Ketorolac; Ketorolac (Systemic); Omega-3-Acid Ethyl Esters; Pentosan Polysulfate Sodium; Probenecid; Prostacyclin Analogues; Selective Serotonin Reuptake Inhibitors; Serotonin/Norepinephrine Reuptake Inhibitors; Sodium Phosphates; Treprostinil; Vitamin E

Decreased Effect

Ketorolac (Nasal) may decrease the levels/effects of: ACE Inhibitors; Angiotensin II Receptor Blockers; Anticonvulsants; Antiplatelet Agents; Beta-Blockers; Eplerenone; HydrALAZINE; Potassium-Sparing Diuretics; Salicylates; Selective Serotonin Reuptake Inhibitors; Thiazide Diuretics

The levels/effects of Ketorolac (Nasal) may be decreased by: Bile Acid Sequestrants; Salicylates

Ethanol/Nutrition/Herb Interactions Herb/Nutraceutical: Avoid alfalfa, anise, bilberry, bladderwrack, bromelain, cat's claw, celery, chamomile, coleus, cordyceps, dong quai, evening primrose, fenugreek, feverfew, garlic, ginger, ginkgo biloba, ginseng (American, Panax, Siberian), grapeseed, green tea, guggul, horse chestnut seed, horseradish, licorice, prickly ash, red clover, reishi, SAMe (S-adenosylmethionine), sweet clover, turmeric, and white willow (all have additional antiplatelet activity).

Stability Store unopened nasal spray refrigerated at 2°C to 8°C (36°F to 46°F); protect from freezing. Protect from light. During use, store at room temperature of 15°C to 30°C (59°F to 86°F) and out of direct sunlight. Discard each nasal spray bottle within 24 hours of priming.

Mechanism of Action Reversibly inhibits cyclooxygenase-1 and 2 (COX-1 and 2) enzymes, which results in decreased formation of prostaglandin precursors; has antipyretic, analgesic, and anti-inflammatory properties

Other proposed mechanisms not fully elucidated (and possibly contributing to the anti-inflammatory effect to varying degrees), include inhibiting chemotaxis, altering lymphocyte activity, inhibiting neutrophil aggregation/activation, and decreasing proinflammatory cytokine levels.

Pharmacodynamics/Kinetics

Onset of analgesia: Within 20 minutes

Absorption: Rapid and well absorbed; C_{max}, t_{max} and AUC values were similar following multiple administrations for 5 days compared to the single-dose study in healthy volunteers.

Distribution: ~13 L following complete distribution; following intranasal administration, ketorolac is deposited primarily in the nasal cavity and pharynx; <20% deposited in the esophagus and stomach; <0.5% in the lungs

Protein binding: 99%

Metabolism: Hepatic to hydroxylated and conjugated forms

Bioavailability: ~60% to 70% relative to I.M. administration

Half-life elimination: ~5-6 hours (similar to I.M. administration); prolonged ~35% in elderly; up to 19 hours in renal impairment

Time to peak: 0.5-0.75 hours

Excretion: Urine (~92%, ~60% as unchanged drug); feces ~6%

Dosage

Geriatric Elderly (≥65 years): Intranasal: One spray (15.75 mg) in 1 nostril (total dose: 15.75 mg) every 6-8 hours; maximum dose: 4 doses (63 mg)/day

Adult Pain management (acute; moderate-to-moderately-severe): Note: The maximum combined duration of treatment (for nasal spray or other ketorolac formulations) is 5 days. Intranasal: Adults<65 years and ≥50 kg: One spray (15.75 mg) in each nostril (total dose: 31.5 mg) every 6-8 hours; maximum dose: 4 doses (126 mg)/day

Dosage adjustments in adults with low body weight (<50 kg): One spray (15.75 mg) in 1 nostril (total dose: 15.75 mg) every 6-8 hours; maximum dose: 4 doses (63 mg)/day

Renal Impairment

Renal insufficiency: Intranasal: One spray (15.75 mg) in 1 nostril (total dose: 15.75 mg) every 6-8 hours; maximum dose: 4 doses (63 mg)/day

Advanced renal impairment (or at risk for renal failure due to volume depletion): Use is contraindicated

Hepatic Impairment Use with caution with hepatic impairment or history of hepatic disease; use may cause elevation of liver enzymes; discontinue if clinical signs and symptoms of liver disease develop.

Administration Each nasal spray contains medication for 1 day of therapy. Before first use of a nasal spray container, prime by pressing pump 5 times. There is no need to prime the pump again if more doses are administered during the next 24 hours using the same nasal container. Repeat priming each day prior to first use of each new nasal spray. Blow nose to clear nostrils. Sit up straight or stand; tilt head slightly forward. Insert tip of container into nostril, keeping bottle upright, and point container away from the center of nose. Spray once, pressing down evenly on both sides of container.

Discard container within 24 hours of priming even if there is unused medication.

Monitoring Parameters Monitor for weight gain/edema; renal function (serum creatinine, BUN, urine output); observe for bleeding, bruising; evaluate gastrointestinal effects (abdominal pain, bleeding, dyspepsia); CBC and platelets, liver function tests

Reference Range Serum concentration: Therapeutic: 0.3-5 mcg/mL; Toxic: >5 mcg/mL

Special Geriatric Considerations Ketorolac is cleared more slowly in the elderly. It is recommended to use lower doses in the elderly. Elderly are a high-risk population for adverse effects from NSAIDs. As much as 60% of elderly can develop peptic ulceration and/or hemorrhage asymptomatically. The concomitant use of H_2 blockers and sucralfate is not effective as prophylaxis with the exception of NSAID-induced duodenal ulcers which may be prevented by the use of ranitidine. Misoprostol and proton pump inhibitors are the only agents proven to help prevent the development of NSAID-induced ulcers. Also, concomitant disease and drug use contribute to the risk for GI adverse effects. Use lowest effective dose for shortest period possible. Consider renal function decline with age. Use of NSAIDs can compromise existing renal function especially when Cl_{cr} is ≤30 mL/minute or weight <50 kg. Tinnitus may be a difficult and unreliable indication of toxicity due to age-related hearing loss or eighth cranial nerve damage. CNS adverse effects such as confusion, agitation, and hallucination are generally seen in overdose or high dose situations, but elderly may demonstrate these adverse effects at lower doses than younger adults.

This medication is considered to be potentially inappropriate in this patient population (Beers Criteria severity: High).

Dosage Forms Excipient information presented when available (limited, particularly for generics); consult specific product labeling.

Solution, intranasal, as tromethamine [spray, preservative free]:
Sprix®: 15.75 mg/spray (1.7 g) [delivers 8 metered sprays]

Selected References

Singla N, Singla S, Minkowitz HS, et al, "Intranasal Ketorolac for Acute Postoperative Pain," *Curr Med Res Opin*, 2010, 26(8): 1915-23.

McAleer SD, Majid O, Venables E, et al, "Pharmacokinetics and Safety of Ketorolac Following Single Intranasal and Intramuscular Administration in Healthy Volunteers," *J Clin Pharmacol*, 2007; 47(1):13-18.

Moodie JE, Brown CR, Bisley EJ, et al, "The Safety and Analgesic Efficacy of Intranasal Ketorolac in Patients With Postoperative Pain," *Anesth Analg*, 2008, 107(6):2025-31.

Ketorolac (Ophthalmic) (KEE toe role ak)

Medication Safety Issues
Sound-alike/look-alike issues:
Acular® may be confused with Acthar®, Ocular®
Ketorolac may be confused with Ketalar®

Brand Names: U.S. Acular LS®; Acular®; Acuvail®

Brand Names: Canada Acular LS®; Acular®; ratio-Ketorolac

Index Terms Ketorolac Tromethamine

Generic Availability (U.S.) Yes

Pharmacologic Category Nonsteroidal Anti-inflammatory Drug (NSAID), Ophthalmic

Use Temporary relief of ocular itching due to seasonal allergic conjunctivitis; postoperative inflammation following cataract extraction; reduction of ocular pain and photophobia following incisional refractive surgery; reduction of ocular pain, burning, and stinging following corneal refractive surgery

Dosage
Adult
Seasonal allergic conjunctivitis (relief of ocular itching) (Acular®): *Ophthalmic:* Instill 1 drop (0.25 mg) 4 times/day
Inflammation following cataract extraction (Acular®): *Ophthalmic:* Instill 1 drop (0.25 mg) to affected eye(s) 4 times/day beginning 24 hours after surgery; continue for 2 weeks
Pain following corneal refractive surgery (Acular LS®): *Ophthalmic:* Instill 1 drop 4 times/day as needed to affected eye for up to 4 days

Dosage Forms Excipient information presented when available (limited, particularly for generics); consult specific product labeling. [DSC] = Discontinued product

Solution, ophthalmic, as tromethamine [drops]: 0.4% (5 mL); 0.5% (3 mL, 5 mL, 10 mL)
Acular LS®: 0.4% (5 mL) [contains benzalkonium chloride]
Acular®: 0.5% (5 mL, 10 mL [DSC]) [contains benzalkonium chloride]
Solution, ophthalmic, as tromethamine [drops, preservative free]:
Acuvail®: 0.45% (0.4 mL)

♦ **Ketorolac Tromethamine** *see* Ketorolac (Nasal) *on page 1009*
♦ **Ketorolac Tromethamine** *see* Ketorolac (Ophthalmic) *on page 1012*
♦ **Ketorolac Tromethamine** *see* Ketorolac (Systemic) *on page 1005*

Ketotifen (kee toe TYE fen)

Medication Safety Issues
Sound-alike/look-alike issues:
Claritin™ Eye (ketotifen) may be confused with Claritin® (loratadine)
Ketotifen may be confused with ketoprofen
ZyrTEC® Itchy Eye (ketotifen) may be confused with ZyrTEC® (cetirizine)
Brand Names: U.S. Alaway™ [OTC]; Claritin™ Eye [OTC]; Zaditor® [OTC]; ZyrTEC® Itchy Eye [OTC]
Brand Names: Canada Novo-Ketotifen; Nu-Ketotifen®; Zaditen®; Zaditor®
Index Terms Ketotifen Fumarate
Generic Availability (U.S.) Yes
Pharmacologic Category Histamine H_1 Antagonist; Histamine H_1 Antagonist, Second Generation; Mast Cell Stabilizer; Piperidine Derivative
Use Ophthalmic: Temporary relief of eye itching due to allergic conjunctivitis
Contraindications Hypersensitivity to ketotifen or any component of the formulation
Warnings/Precautions Do not use to treat acute asthmatic attacks. Therapy for acute symptoms of asthma (eg, corticosteroids, beta$_2$-agonists, xanthine derivatives) should be maintained and gradually reduced. Several weeks of oral ketotifen therapy may be needed to observe clinical response while full therapeutic response is usually observed after 10 weeks of treatment. Patients with inadequate response to therapy should be maintained on therapy 2-3 months; then if no response, gradually discontinue therapy over 2-4 weeks. Oral dosage forms may cause sedation early in therapy. Sedative effects may be reduced by initiating therapy at one-half the recommended daily dose with gradual increase over 5 days to maintenance dose. Caution patients about performing tasks which require mental alertness (eg, driving or operating machinery). Thrombocytopenia has occurred rarely when used concomitantly with oral antidiabetic agents. Use caution in diabetics and individuals with benzoate allergies as the syrup preparation contains carbohydrates and benzoate compounds. Ophthalmic solution should not be used to treat contact lens-related irritation. After ketotifen use, soft contact lens wearers should wait at least 10 minutes before reinserting contact lenses. Do not wear contact lenses if eyes are red. Do not contaminate dropper tip or solution when placing drops in eyes.

When using ophthalmic solution for self-medication (OTC), notify healthcare provider if symptoms worsen or do not improve within 3 days. Contact healthcare provider if change in vision, eye pain, or redness occur. Do not use if solution is cloudy or changes color.

Adverse Reactions (Reflective of adult population; not specific for elderly)
Ophthalmic: 1% to 10%:
Ocular: Allergic reactions, burning or stinging, conjunctivitis, discharge, dry eyes, eye pain, eyelid disorder, itching, keratitis, lacrimation disorder, mydriasis, photophobia, rash
Respiratory: Pharyngitis
Miscellaneous: Flu syndrome

Oral: 1% to 10%:
Central nervous system: Sedation (8%; less than placebo), headache (1%), sleep disturbance (1%)
Dermatologic: Rash (4%), urticaria (1%)
Gastrointestinal: Weight gain (5%), abdominal pain (1%), appetite increased (1%)
Respiratory: Respiratory infection (4%), epistaxis (1%)
Miscellaneous: Flu (3%), puffy eyelid (1%)

Drug Interactions
Avoid Concomitant Use There are no known interactions where it is recommended to avoid concomitant use.
Increased Effect/Toxicity
Ketotifen may increase the levels/effects of: Alcohol (Ethyl); Anticholinergics; CNS Depressants; Selective Serotonin Reuptake Inhibitors

The levels/effects of Ketotifen may be increased by: Droperidol; HydrOXYzine; Pramlintide
Decreased Effect
Ketotifen may decrease the levels/effects of: Acetylcholinesterase Inhibitors (Central); Benzylpenicilloyl Polylysine; Betahistine

The levels/effects of Ketotifen may be decreased by: Acetylcholinesterase Inhibitors (Central); Amphetamines

◀ **Stability**
Ophthalmic solution: Store at 20°C to 25°C (68°F to 77°F).
Syrup: Store at up to 25°C (up to 77°F).
Tablet: Store at 15°C to 25°C (59°F to 77°F).

Mechanism of Action Exhibits noncompetitive H_1-receptor antagonist and mast cell stabilizer properties. Efficacy in conjunctivitis and asthma likely results from a combination of anti-inflammatory and antihistaminergic actions including interference with chemokine-induced migration of eosinophils into inflamed conjunctiva and airways, inhibition of airway hyperreactivity due to platelet activating factor (PAF), antagonism of leukotriene-induced bronchoconstriction.

Pharmacodynamics/Kinetics
Ophthalmic:
Onset of action: Minutes
Duration: 8-12 hours
Absorption: Minimally systemic
Oral:
Absorption: Rapid, ≥60%
Protein binding: 75%
Metabolism: Hepatic via N-glucuronidation to inactive metabolite ketotifen-N-glucuronide; N-demethylation to active metabolite nor-ketotifen; and keto-reduction to hydroxyl derivative
Bioavailability: ~50%
Half-life elimination: ~9-9.5 hours
Time to peak, plasma: 2-4 hours
Excretion: Urine (60% to 70% as metabolites, 1% as unchanged drug)

Dosage
Geriatric & Adult Allergic conjunctivitis: Ophthalmic: Instill 1 drop into the affected eye(s) twice daily, every 8-12 hours

Administration May administer without regard to meals.

Special Geriatric Considerations Instruct the patient on proper instillation of ophthalmic solution.

Dosage Forms Excipient information presented when available (limited, particularly for generics); consult specific product labeling.
Solution, ophthalmic [drops]: 0.025% (5 mL)
Alaway™: 0.025% (10 mL) [contains benzalkonium chloride]
Claritin™ Eye: 0.025% (5 mL) [contains benzalkonium chloride]
Zaditor®: 0.025% (5 mL) [contains benzalkonium chloride]
ZyrTEC® Itchy Eye: 0.025% (5 mL) [contains benzalkonium chloride]

Dosage Forms: Canada Excipient information presented when available (limited, particularly for generics); consult specific product labeling.
Syrup, oral: 1 mg/5 mL (250 mL)
Novo-Ketotifen®: 1 mg/5 mL (250 mL) [contains alcohol, benzoate compounds; strawberry flavor]
Nu-Ketotifen®: 1 mg/5 mL (250 mL)
Zaditen®: 1 mg/5 mL (250 mL)
Tablet:, oral 1 mg
Novo-Ketotifen®: 1 mg
Zaditen®: 1 mg

◆ **Ketotifen Fumarate** see Ketotifen on page 1013
◆ **Key-E® [OTC]** see Vitamin E on page 1921
◆ **Key-E® Kaps [OTC]** see Vitamin E on page 1921
◆ **Key-E® Powder [OTC]** see Vitamin E on page 1921
◆ **Kineret®** see Anakinra on page 132
◆ **Kinrix®** see Diphtheria and Tetanus Toxoids, Acellular Pertussis, and Poliovirus Vaccine on page 528
◆ **Kionex®** see Sodium Polystyrene Sulfonate on page 1697
◆ **Klaron®** see Sulfacetamide (Topical) on page 1713
◆ **KlonoPIN®** see ClonazePAM on page 385
◆ **Klor-Con®** see Potassium Chloride on page 1487
◆ **Klor-Con® 8** see Potassium Chloride on page 1487
◆ **Klor-Con® 10** see Potassium Chloride on page 1487
◆ **Klor-Con®/25** see Potassium Chloride on page 1487
◆ **Klor-Con® M10** see Potassium Chloride on page 1487
◆ **Klor-Con® M15** see Potassium Chloride on page 1487
◆ **Klor-Con® M20** see Potassium Chloride on page 1487
◆ **KMD 3213** see Silodosin on page 1677
◆ **Kolephrin® GG/DM [OTC]** see Guaifenesin and Dextromethorphan on page 848
◆ **Kombiglyze™ XR** see Saxagliptin and Metformin on page 1659

- ◆ **Kondremul® [OTC]** *see* Mineral Oil *on page 1217*
- ◆ **Konsyl® [OTC]** *see* Psyllium *on page 1547*
- ◆ **Konsyl-D™ [OTC]** *see* Psyllium *on page 1547*
- ◆ **Konsyl® Easy Mix™ [OTC]** *see* Psyllium *on page 1547*
- ◆ **Konsyl® Fiber [OTC]** *see* Polycarbophil *on page 1479*
- ◆ **Konsyl® Orange [OTC]** *see* Psyllium *on page 1547*
- ◆ **Konsyl® Original [OTC]** *see* Psyllium *on page 1547*
- ◆ **K-Phos® MF** *see* Potassium Phosphate and Sodium Phosphate *on page 1494*
- ◆ **K-Phos® Neutral** *see* Potassium Phosphate and Sodium Phosphate *on page 1494*
- ◆ **K-Phos® No. 2** *see* Potassium Phosphate and Sodium Phosphate *on page 1494*
- ◆ **K-Phos® Original** *see* Potassium Acid Phosphate *on page 1486*
- ◆ **Kristalose®** *see* Lactulose *on page 1022*
- ◆ **Krystexxa™** *see* Pegloticase *on page 1408*
- ◆ **K-Tab®** *see* Potassium Chloride *on page 1487*
- ◆ **Kytril®** *see* Granisetron *on page 842*
- ◆ **L-749,345** *see* Ertapenem *on page 623*
- ◆ **L-758,298** *see* Fosaprepitant *on page 788*
- ◆ **L-M-X® 4 [OTC]** *see* Lidocaine (Topical) *on page 1064*
- ◆ **L-M-X® 5 [OTC]** *see* Lidocaine (Topical) *on page 1064*
- ◆ **L 754030** *see* Aprepitant *on page 139*
- ◆ **LA 20304a** *see* Gemifloxacin *on page 814*

Labetalol (la BET a lole)

Related Information
Beta-Blockers *on page 2001*
Medication Safety Issues
Sound-alike/look-alike issues:
Labetalol may be confused with betaxolol, Hexadrol®, lamoTRIgine, Lipitor®
Normodyne® may be confused with Norpramin®
Trandate® may be confused with traMADol, Trendar®, Trental®, Tridrate®
High alert medication:
The Institute for Safe Medication Practices (ISMP) includes this medication among its list of drugs which have a heightened risk of causing significant patient harm when used in error.
Administration issues:
Significant differences exist between oral and I.V. dosing. Use caution when converting from one route of administration to another.
Brand Names: U.S. Trandate®
Brand Names: Canada Apo-Labetalol®; Labetalol Hydrochloride Injection, USP; Normodyne®; Trandate®
Index Terms Ibidomide Hydrochloride; Labetalol Hydrochloride
Generic Availability (U.S.) Yes
Pharmacologic Category Beta Blocker With Alpha-Blocking Activity
Use Treatment of mild-to-severe hypertension; I.V. for severe hypertension (eg, hypertensive emergencies)
Unlabeled/Investigational Use Hypertension during acute ischemic stroke
Contraindications Hypersensitivity to labetalol or any component of the formulation; severe bradycardia; heart block greater than first degree (except in patients with a functioning artificial pacemaker); cardiogenic shock; bronchial asthma; uncompensated cardiac failure; conditions associated with severe and prolonged hypotension
Warnings/Precautions Consider pre-existing conditions such as sick sinus syndrome before initiating. Symptomatic hypotension with or without syncope may occur with labetalol; close monitoring of patient is required especially with initial dosing and dosing increases; blood pressure must be lowered at a rate appropriate for the patient's clinical condition. Initiation with a low dose and gradual up-titration may help to decrease the occurrence of hypotension or syncope. Patients should be advised to avoid driving or other hazardous tasks during initiation of therapy due to the risk of syncope. Orthostatic hypotension may occur with I.V. administration; patient should remain supine during and for up to 3 hours after I.V. administration. Use with caution in impaired hepatic function; bioavailability is increased due to decreased first-pass metabolism. Severe hepatic injury including some fatalities have also been rarely reported with use: periodically monitor LFTs with prolonged use. Use with caution in patients with diabetes mellitus; may potentiate hypoglycemia and/or mask signs and symptoms. Bradycardia may be observed more frequently in elderly patients (>65 years of age); dosage reductions may be necessary. May also reduce release of insulin in response to hyperglycemia; dosage of antidiabetic agents may need to be adjusted. May mask signs of hyperthyroidism (eg, tachycardia); if hyperthyroidism is suspected, carefully manage and monitor; abrupt withdrawal may exacerbate symptoms of hyperthyroidism or precipitate

◀ thyroid storm. Elimination of labetalol is reduced in elderly patients; lower maintenance doses may be required.

Use only with extreme caution in compensated heart failure and monitor for a worsening of the condition. Beta-blocker therapy should not be withdrawn abruptly (particularly in patients with CAD), but gradually tapered to avoid acute tachycardia, hypertension, and/or ischemia. Chronic beta-blocker therapy should not be routinely withdrawn prior to major surgery. Use caution with concurrent use of digoxin, verapamil, or diltiazem; bradycardia or heart block can occur. Use with caution in patients receiving inhaled anesthetic agents known to depress myocardial contractility. Patients with bronchospastic disease should not receive beta-block-ers; if used at all, should be used cautiously with close monitoring. Use with caution in patients with myasthenia gravis or psychiatric disease (may cause or exacerbate CNS depression). Can precipitate or aggravate symptoms of arterial insufficiency in patients with PVD and Raynaud's disease; use with caution and monitor for progression of arterial obstruction. If possible, obtain diagnostic tests for pheochromocytoma prior to use. May induce or exacer-bate psoriasis. Labetalol has been shown to be effective in lowering blood pressure and relieving symptoms in patients with pheochromocytoma. However, some patients have experienced paradoxical hypertensive responses; use with caution in patients with pheochro-mocytoma. Additional alpha-blockade may be required during use of labetalol. Use caution with history of severe anaphylaxis to allergens; patients taking beta-blockers may become more sensitive to repeated challenges. Treatment of anaphylaxis (eg, epinephrine) in patients taking beta-blockers may be ineffective or promote undesirable effects.

Adverse Reactions (Reflective of adult population; not specific for elderly)

>10%:
   Cardiovascular: Postural hypotension (I.V. use; ≤58%)
   Central nervous system: Dizziness (1% to 20%), fatigue (1% to 11%)
   Gastrointestinal: Nausea (≤19%)
1% to 10%:
   Cardiovascular: Hypotension (1% to 5%), edema (≤2%), flushing (1%), ventricular arrhyth-mia (I.V. use; 1%)
   Central nervous system: Somnolence (3%), headache (2%), vertigo (1% to 2%)
   Dermatologic: Scalp tingling (≤7%), pruritus (1%), rash (1%)
   Gastrointestinal: Dyspepsia (≤4%), vomiting (≤3%), taste disturbance (1%)
   Genitourinary: Ejaculatory failure (≤5%), impotence (1% to 4%)
   Hepatic: Transaminases increased (4%)
   Neuromuscular & skeletal: Paresthesia (≤5%), weakness (1%)
   Ocular: Vision abnormal (1%)
   Renal: BUN increased (≤8%)
   Respiratory: Nasal congestion (1% to 6%), dyspnea (2%)
   Miscellaneous: Diaphoresis (≤4%)
Other adverse reactions noted with beta-adrenergic blocking agents include mental depres-sion, catatonia, disorientation, short-term memory loss, emotional lability, clouded senso-rium, intensification of pre-existing AV block, laryngospasm, respiratory distress, agranulocytosis, thrombocytopenic purpura, nonthrombocytopenic purpura, mesenteric artery thrombosis, and ischemic colitis.

Drug Interactions

Avoid Concomitant Use

Avoid concomitant use of Labetalol with any of the following: Floctafenine; Methacholine

Increased Effect/Toxicity

Labetalol may increase the levels/effects of: Alpha-/Beta-Agonists (Direct-Acting); Alpha1-Blockers; Alpha2-Agonists; Amifostine; Antihypertensives; Antipsychotic Agents (Phenothia-zines); Bupivacaine; Cardiac Glycosides; Fingolimod; Hypotensive Agents; Insulin; Lido-caine; Lidocaine (Systemic); Lidocaine (Topical); Mepivacaine; Methacholine; Midodrine; RiTUXimab; Sulfonylureas

The levels/effects of Labetalol may be increased by: Acetylcholinesterase Inhibitors; Amino-quinolines (Antimalarial); Amiodarone; Anilidopiperidine Opioids; Antipsychotic Agents (Phenothiazines); Calcium Channel Blockers (Dihydropyridine); Calcium Channel Blockers (Nondihydropyridine); Diazoxide; Dipyridamole; Disopyramide; Dronedarone; Floctafenine; Herbs (Hypotensive Properties); MAO Inhibitors; Pentoxifylline; Phosphodiesterase 5 Inhib-itors; Propafenone; Propoxyphene; Prostacyclin Analogues; QuiNIDine; Reserpine; Selec-tive Serotonin Reuptake Inhibitors

Decreased Effect

Labetalol may decrease the levels/effects of: Beta2-Agonists; Theophylline Derivatives

The levels/effects of Labetalol may be decreased by: Barbiturates; Herbs (Hypertensive Properties); Methylphenidate; Nonsteroidal Anti-Inflammatory Agents; Rifamycin Deriva-tives; Yohimbine

Ethanol/Nutrition/Herb Interactions

Food: Labetalol serum concentrations may be increased if taken with food.

Herb/Nutraceutical: Avoid dong quai if using for hypertension (has estrogenic activity). Avoid ephedra, yohimbe, ginseng (may worsen hypertension). Avoid natural licorice (causes sodium and water retention and increases potassium loss). Avoid garlic (may have increased antihypertensive effect).

Stability

Tablets: Store tablets at 2°C to 30°C (36°F to 86°F). Protect from light and excessive moisture.

Vials: Store unopened injectable vials at 20°C to 25°C (68°F to 77°F); do not freeze. Protect from light. The solution is clear to slightly yellow.

Parenteral admixture: Stability of parenteral admixture at room temperature (25°C) and refrigeration temperature (4°C): 3 days.

Standard concentration: 500 mg/250 mL D_5W.

Minimum volume: 250 mL D_5W.

Mechanism of Action Blocks alpha-, beta$_1$-, and beta$_2$-adrenergic receptor sites; elevated renins are reduced. The ratios of alpha- to beta-blockade differ depending on the route of administration: 1:3 (oral) and 1:7 (I.V.).

Pharmacodynamics/Kinetics

Onset of action: Oral: 20 minutes to 2 hours; I.V.: 2-5 minutes

Peak effect: Oral: 1-4 hours; I.V.: 5-15 minutes

Duration: Blood pressure response:

Oral: 8-12 hours (dose dependent)

I.V.: 2-18 hours (dose dependent; based on single and multiple sequential doses of 0.25-0.5 mg/kg with cumulative dosing up to 3.25 mg/kg)

Absorption: Complete

Distribution: V_d: Adults: 3-16 L/kg; mean: <9.4 L/kg; moderately lipid soluble, therefore, can enter CNS

Protein binding: 50%

Metabolism: Hepatic, primarily via glucuronide conjugation; extensive first-pass effect

Bioavailability: Oral: 25%; increased with liver disease, elderly, and concurrent cimetidine

Half-life elimination: Oral: 6-8 hours; I.V.: ~5.5 hours

Time to peak, plasma: Oral: 1-2 hours

Excretion: Urine (55% to 60% as glucuronide conjugates, <5% as unchanged drug)

Dosage

Geriatric & Adult

Hypertension: Oral: Initial: 100 mg twice daily, may increase as needed every 2-3 days by 100 mg twice daily (titration increments not to exceed 200 mg twice daily) until desired response is obtained; usual dose: 100-400 mg twice daily (JNC 7); may require up to 2.4 g/day.

Acute hypertension (hypertensive emergency/urgency):

I.V. bolus: Per the manufacturer: Initial: 20 mg I.V. push over 2 minutes; may administer 40-80 mg at 10-minute intervals, up to 300 mg total cumulative dose; as appropriate, follow with oral antihypertensive regimen

I.V. infusion (acute loading): Per the manufacturer: Initial: 2 mg/minute; titrate to response up to 300 mg total cumulative dose (eg, discontinue after 2.5 hours of 2 mg/minute); usual total dose required: 50-200 mg; as appropriate, follow with oral antihypertensive regimen

Note: Although loading infusions are well described in the product labeling, the labeling is silent in specific clinical situations, such as in the patient who has an initial response to labetalol infusions but cannot be converted to an oral route for subsequent dosing. There is limited documentation of prolonged continuous infusions (ie, >300 mg/day). In rare clinical situations, higher continuous infusion doses up to 6 mg/minute have been used in the critical care setting (eg, aortic dissection) and up to 8 mg/minute (eg, hypertension with ongoing acute ischemic stroke). At these doses, it may be best to consider an alternative agent if the labetalol infusion is not meeting the goals of therapy. At the other extreme, continuous infusions at relatively low doses (0.03-0.1 mg/minute) have been used in some settings (following loading infusion in patients who are unable to be converted to oral regimens or in some cases as a continuation of outpatient oral regimens). These prolonged infusions should not be confused with loading infusions. Because of wide variation in the use of infusions, an awareness of institutional policies and practices is extremely important. Careful clarification of orders and specific infusion rates/units is required to avoid confusion. Due to the prolonged duration of action, careful monitoring should be extended for the duration of the infusion and for several hours after the infusion. Excessive administration may result in prolonged hypotension and/or bradycardia.

◄

Arterial hypertension in acute ischemic stroke (unlabeled use [Adams, 2007; Jauch, 2010]): I.V.:

Patient otherwise eligible for reperfusion treatment (eg, alteplase): Blood pressure (BP): Systolic >185 mm Hg or diastolic >110 mm Hg: 10-20 mg over 1-2 minutes; may repeat once. If BP does not decline and remains >185/110 mm Hg, alteplase should not be administered.

Management of BP during and after reperfusion treatment (eg, alteplase): BP: Systolic ≥180 mm Hg or diastolic ≥105 mm Hg: 10 mg over 1-2 minutes; may repeat every 10-20 minutes (maximum dose: 300 mg) **or** 10 mg followed by an infusion of 2-8 mg/minute. If hypertension is refractory, consider other I.V. antihypertensives (eg, nitroprusside).

I.V. to oral conversion: Upon discontinuation of I.V. infusion, may initiate oral dose of 200 mg followed in 6-12 hours with an additional dose of 200-400 mg. Thereafter, dose patients with 400-2400 mg/day in divided doses depending on blood pressure response.

Renal Impairment Not removed by hemo- or peritoneal dialysis; supplemental dose is not necessary.

Hepatic Impairment Dosage reduction may be necessary.

Administration Bolus dose may be administered I.V. push at a rate of 10 mg/minute; may follow with continuous I.V. infusion

Monitoring Parameters Blood pressure, standing and sitting/supine, pulse, cardiac monitor and blood pressure monitor required for I.V. administration

Test Interactions False-positive urine catecholamines, vanillylmandelic acid (VMA) if measured by fluorometric or photometric methods; use HPLC or specific catecholamine radioenzymatic technique; false-positive amphetamine if measured by thin-layer chromatography or radioenzymatic assay (gas chromatographic-mass spectrometer technique should be used)

Special Geriatric Considerations Due to alterations in the beta-adrenergic autonomic nervous system, beta-adrenergic blockade may result in less hemodynamic response than seen in younger adults. Studies indicate that despite decreased sensitivity to the chronotropic effects of beta-blockade with age, there appears to be an increased myocardial sensitivity to the negative inotropic effect during stress (ie, exercise). Controlled trials have shown the overall response rate for propranolol to be only 20% to 50% in elderly populations. Therefore, all beta-adrenergic blocking drugs may result in a decreased response as compared to younger adults.

Dosage Forms Excipient information presented when available (limited, particularly for generics); consult specific product labeling.

Injection, solution, as hydrochloride: 5 mg/mL (4 mL, 20 mL, 40 mL)
  Trandate®: 5 mg/mL (20 mL, 40 mL) [contains edetate disodium]
Tablet, oral, as hydrochloride: 100 mg, 200 mg, 300 mg
  Trandate®: 100 mg [scored]
  Trandate®: 200 mg [scored; contains sodium benzoate]
  Trandate®: 300 mg [scored]

◆ **Labetalol Hydrochloride** *see* Labetalol *on page 1015*

Lacosamide (la KOE sa mide)

Medication Safety Issues
  Sound-alike/look-alike issues:
    Lacosamide may be confused with zonisamide
    Vimpat® may be confused with Vimovo™
Brand Names: U.S. Vimpat®
Brand Names: Canada Vimpat®
Index Terms ADD 234037; Harkoseride; LCM; SPM 927
Generic Availability (U.S.) No
Pharmacologic Category Anticonvulsant, Miscellaneous
Use Adjunctive therapy in the treatment of partial-onset seizures
Medication Guide Available Yes
Contraindications There are no contraindications listed in manufacturer's labeling.
Warnings/Precautions Antiepileptics are associated with an increased risk of suicidal behavior/thoughts with use (regardless of indication); patients should be monitored for signs/symptoms of depression, suicidal tendencies, and other unusual behavior changes during therapy and instructed to inform their healthcare provider immediately if symptoms occur. CNS effects may occur; patients should be cautioned about performing tasks which require alertness (eg, operating machinery or driving). Lacosamide may prolong PR interval; use caution in patients with conduction problems (eg, first/second degree atrioventricular block and sick sinus syndrome without pacemaker), myocardial ischemia, heart failure, or if concurrent use with other drugs that prolong the PR interval; ECG is recommended prior to

initiating therapy and when at steady state. During investigational trials, atrial fibrillation/flutter, or syncope occurred slightly more often in patients with diabetic neuropathy and/or cardiovascular disease. Use caution with renal or hepatic impairment; dosage adjustment may be necessary. Multiorgan hypersensitivity reactions can occur (rare); monitor patient and discontinue therapy if necessary. Withdraw therapy gradually (≥1 week) to minimize the potential of increased seizure frequency. Effects with ethanol may be potentiated. Some products may contain phenylalanine.

Adverse Reactions (Reflective of adult population; not specific for elderly)
>10%:
  Central nervous system: Dizziness (31%), headache (13%)
  Gastrointestinal: Nausea (11%)
  Ocular: Diplopia (11%)
1% to 10%:
  Cardiovascular: Syncope (1%; dose-related: >400 mg/day)
  Central nervous system: Fatigue (9%), ataxia (8%), somnolence (7%), coordination impaired (4%), vertigo (4%), depression (2%), memory impairment (2%)
  Dermatologic: Pruritus (2%)
  Gastrointestinal: Vomiting (9%), diarrhea (4%)
  Hepatic: ALT increased (1%)
  Local: Contusion (3%), skin laceration (3%), injection site pain/discomfort (2.5%), irritation (1%)
  Neuromuscular & skeletal: Tremor (7%), gait instability (2%), weakness (2%)
  Ocular: Blurred vision (8%), nystagmus (5%)

Drug Interactions
  Avoid Concomitant Use There are no known interactions where it is recommended to avoid concomitant use.
  Increased Effect/Toxicity There are no known significant interactions involving an increase in effect.
  Decreased Effect
    The levels/effects of Lacosamide may be decreased by: CarBAMazepine; Fosphenytoin; PHENobarbital; Phenytoin

Ethanol/Nutrition/Herb Interactions Ethanol: Avoid ethanol (may increase CNS depression).

Stability
  Injection: Store at 20°C to 25°C (68°F to 77°F); excursions permitted between 15°C to 30°C (59°F to 86°F). Do not freeze. Can be administered without further dilution or may be mixed with compatible diluents (NS, LR, D_5W). Reconstituted solution is stable for ≤24 hours in glass or PVC at room temperature of 15°C to 30°C (59°F to 86°F). Any unused portion should be discarded.
  Oral solution, tablets: Store at 20°C to 25°C (68°F to 77°F); excursions permitted between 15°C to 30°C (59°F to 86°F). Do not freeze oral solution. Discard any unused portion of oral solution after 7 weeks.

Mechanism of Action *In vitro* studies have shown that lacosamide stabilizes hyperexcitable neuronal membranes and inhibits repetitive neuronal firing by enhancing the slow inactivation of sodium channels (with no effects on fast inactivation of sodium channels).

Pharmacodynamics/Kinetics
  Absorption: Oral: Completely
  Distribution: V_d: ~0.6 L/kg
  Protein binding: <15%
  Metabolism: Hepatic; forms metabolite, O-desmethyl-lacosamide (inactive)
  Bioavailability: ~100%
  Half-life elimination: ~13 hours
  Time to peak, plasma: Oral: 1-4 hours postdose
  Excretion: Urine (95%; 40% as unchanged drug, 30% as inactive metabolite, 20% as uncharacterized metabolite); feces (<0.5%)

Dosage
  Geriatric & Adult Partial onset seizure: Oral, I.V.:
    Initial: 50 mg twice daily; may be increased at weekly intervals by 100 mg/day
    Maintenance dose: 200-400 mg/day
    Note: When switching from oral to I.V. formulations, the total daily dose and frequency should be the same; I.V. therapy should only be used temporarily.
  Renal Impairment Use caution when titrating dose.
    Mild-to-moderate renal impairment: No dose adjustment necessary.
    Severe renal impairment (Cl_{cr} ≤30 mL/minute): Maximum dose: 300 mg/day.
    Hemodialysis: Removed by hemodialysis; after 4-hour HD treatment, a supplemental dose of up to 50% should be considered.

◄ **Hepatic Impairment** Use caution when titrating dose.

Mild-to-moderate hepatic impairment: Maximum dose: 300 mg/day.

Severe hepatic impairment: Use is not recommended.

Administration

Injection: Administer over 30-60 minutes. Twice daily I.V. infusions have been used for up to 5 days.

Tablet: May be administered with or without food.

Monitoring Parameters Patients with conduction problems or severe cardiac disease should have ECG tracing prior to start of therapy and when at steady-state; suicidality (eg, suicidal thoughts, depression, behavioral changes)

Special Geriatric Considerations Elderly often have compromised renal function with creatinine clearance <30 mL/minute. Evaluate (calculate) creatinine clearance in the elderly before initiating lacosamide therapy. Monitor closely those elderly with cardiac disease and/or conduction disease. In healthy elderly patients, the AUC and C_{max} pharmacokinetic parameters were 20% higher than in younger adults. The higher serum concentrations may reflect differences in total body water (lean body mass) found in the elderly, as well as reduced renal function with aging.

Controlled Substance C-V

Dosage Forms Excipient information presented when available (limited, particularly for generics); consult specific product labeling.

Injection, solution:

Vimpat®: 10 mg/mL (20 mL)

Solution, oral:

Vimpat®: 10 mg/mL (20 mL) [contains phenylalanine 0.32 mg/20 mL, propylene glycol; strawberry flavor]

Tablet, oral:

Vimpat®: 50 mg, 100 mg, 150 mg, 200 mg

Selected References

Ben-Menachem E, Biton V, Jatuzis D, et al, "Efficacy and Safety of Oral Lacosamide as Adjunctive Therapy in Adults With Partial-Onset Seizures," Epilepsia, 2007, 48(7):1308-17.

Beyreuther BK, Freitag J, Heers C, et al, "Lacosamide: A Review of Preclinical Properties," CNS Drug Rev, 2007, 13 (1):21-42.

Biton V, Rosenfeld WE, Whitesides J, et al, "Intravenous Lacosamide as Replacement for Oral Lacosamide in Patients With Partial-Onset Seizures," Epilepsia, 2008, 49(3):418-24.

Doty P, Rudd GD, Stoehr T, et al, "Lacosamide," Neurotherapeutics, 2007, 4(1):145-8.

◆ **LaCrosse Complete [OTC]** see Sodium Phosphates on page 1694
◆ **Lactinex™ [OTC]** see Lactobacillus on page 1020

Lactobacillus (lak toe ba SIL us)

Brand Names: U.S. Bacid® [OTC]; Culturelle® [OTC]; Dofus [OTC]; Flora-Q™ [OTC]; Floranex™ [OTC]; Kala® [OTC]; Lactinex™ [OTC]; Lacto-Bifidus [OTC]; Lacto-Key [OTC]; Lacto-Pectin [OTC]; Lacto-TriBlend [OTC]; Megadophilus® [OTC]; MoreDophilus® [OTC]; RisaQuad®-2 [OTC]; RisaQuad™ [OTC]; Superdophilus® [OTC]; VSL #3® [OTC]; VSL #3®-DS

Brand Names: Canada Bacid®; Fermalac

Index Terms Lactobacillus acidophilus; Lactobacillus bifidus; Lactobacillus bulgaricus; Lactobacillus casei; Lactobacillus paracasei; Lactobacillus plantarum; Lactobacillus reuteri; Lactobacillus rhamnosus GG

Generic Availability (U.S.) Yes

Pharmacologic Category Dietary Supplement; Probiotic

Use Promote normal bacterial flora of the intestinal tract

Contraindications Hypersensitivity to any component of the formulation

Warnings/Precautions Lactobacillus species have been studied for various gastrointestinal disorders including diarrhea, inflammatory bowel disease, gastrointestinal infection. Effectiveness may be dependent upon actual species used; studies are ongoing. Currently, there are no FDA-approved disease-prevention or therapeutic indications for these products.

Adverse Reactions (Reflective of adult population; not specific for elderly) Gastrointestinal: Bloating (intestinal), flatulence

Drug Interactions

Avoid Concomitant Use There are no known interactions where it is recommended to avoid concomitant use.

Increased Effect/Toxicity There are no known significant interactions involving an increase in effect.

Decreased Effect There are no known significant interactions involving a decrease in effect.

Stability
Bacid®: Store at room temperature.
Flora-Q™: Store at or below room temperature; do not store in bathroom.
Kala®, MoreDophilus®: Refrigeration recommended after opening.
Lactinex™, Dofus: Store in refrigerator.
VSL #3®, VSL #3®-DS: Store in refrigerator; may be stored at room temperature for up to 1 week without loss in potency

Mechanism of Action Helps re-establish normal intestinal flora; suppresses the growth of potentially pathogenic microorganisms by producing lactic acid which favors the establishment of an aciduric flora.

Pharmacodynamics/Kinetics
Absorption: Oral: None
Distribution: Local, primarily colon
Excretion: Feces

Dosage
Geriatric & Adult Dietary supplement: Oral: Dosing varies by manufacturer; consult product labeling

Bacid®: 2 caplets/day
Culturelle®: 1 capsule daily; may increase to twice daily
Flora-Q™: 1 capsule/day
Lacto-Key 100 or 600: 1-2 capsules/day
Lactinex™: 1 packet or 4 tablets 3-4 times/day
VSL #3®: 1-8 sachets or 2-32 capsules/day
VSL #3®-DS: 1-4 packets/day

Administration
Culturelle®: Capsules may be opened and mixed in a cool beverage or sprinkled onto baby food or applesauce.
Flora-Q™: May be taken with or without food.
Lactinex™: Granules may be added to or administered with cereal, food, or milk.
Megadophilus®, Superdophilus®: Administer on an empty stomach; powder should be mixed in unchilled water.

Monitoring Parameters Monitor for decrease in frequency of stool and increased mass of stool

Special Geriatric Considerations No specific recommendations due to age; keep in mind that elderly suffer significantly with fluid and electrolyte loss (lethargy, confusion, etc) and diarrhea should be aggressively treated

Dosage Forms Excipient information presented when available (limited, particularly for generics); consult specific product labeling.
Capsule:
Culturelle®: *L. rhamnosus* GG 10 billion colony-forming units [contains casein and whey]
Dofus: *L. acidophilus* and *L. bifidus* 10:1 ratio [beet root powder base]
Flora-Q™: *L. acidophilus* and *L. paracasei* ≥8 billion colony-forming units [also contains *Bifidobacterium* and *S. thermophilus*]
Lacto-Key:
100: *L. acidophilus* 1 billion colony-forming units [milk, soy, and yeast free; rice derived]
600: *L. acidophilus* 6 billion colony-forming units [milk, soy, and yeast free; rice derived]
Lacto-Bifidus:
100: *L. bifidus* 1 billion colony-forming units [milk, soy, and yeast free; rice derived]
600: *L. bifidus* 6 billion colony-forming units [milk, soy, and yeast free; rice derived]
Lacto-Pectin: *L. acidophilus* and *L. casei* ≥5 billion colony-forming units [also contains *Bifidobacterium lactis* and citrus pectin cellulose complex]
Lacto-TriBlend:
100: *L. acidophilus*, *L. bifidus*, and *L. bulgaricus* 1 billion colony-forming units [milk, soy and yeast free; rice derived]
600: *L. acidophilus*, *L. bifidus*, and *L. bulgaricus* 6 billion colony-forming units [milk, soy, and yeast free; rice derived]
Megadophilus®, Superdophilus®: *L. acidophilus* 2 billion units [available in dairy based or dairy free formulations]
RisaQuad™: *L. acidophilus* and *L. paracasei* 8 billion colony-forming units [also includes *Bifidobacterium* and *Streptococcus thermophilus*]
VSL #3®: *L. acidophilus*, *L. plantarum*, *L. paracasei*, *L. bulgaricus* 112 billion live cells [also contains *Bifidobacterium breve*, *B. longum*, *B. infantis*, and *Streptococcus thermophilus*]
Capsule, double strength:
RisaQuad®-2: *L. acidophilus* and *L. paracasei* 16 billion colony-forming units [gluten free; also includes *Bifidobacterium* and *Streptococcus thermophilus*]
Capsule, softgel: *L. acidophilus* 100 active units

Caplet:
  Bacid®: *L. acidophilus* and *L. bulgaricus* [also contains *Bifidobacterium biffidum* and *Streptococcus thermophilus*
Granules:
  Floranex™: *L. acidophilus* and *L. bulgaricus* 100 million live cells per 1 g packet (12s) [contains milk, sodium 5 mg/packet, soy]
  Lactinex™: *L. acidophilus* and *L. bulgaricus* 100 million live cells per 1 g packet (12s) [gluten free; contains calcium 5 mg/packet, lactose 380 mg/packet, potassium 20 mg/packet, sodium 5 mg/packet, sucrose 34 mg/packet, whey, evaporated milk, and soy peptone]
Powder:
  Lacto-TriBlend: *L. acidophilus, L. bifidus,* and *L. bulgaricus* 10 billion colony-forming units per ¼ teaspoon (60 g) [milk, soy, and yeast free; rice derived]
  Megadophilus®, Superdophilus®: *L. acidophilus* 2 billion units per half-teaspoon (49 g, 70 g, 84 g, 126 g) [available in dairy based or dairy free (garbanzo bean) formulations]
  MoreDophilus®: *L. acidophilus* 12.4 billion units per teaspoon (30 g, 120 g) [dairy free, yeast free; soy and carrot derived]
  VSL #3®: *L. acidophilus, L. plantarum, L. paracasei, L. bulgaricus* 450 billion live cells per sachet (10s, 30s) [gluten free; also contains *Bifidobacterium breve, B. longum, B. infantis,* and *Streptococcus thermophilus*; lemon cream flavor and unflavored]
  VSL #3®-DS: *L. acidophilus, L. plantarum, L. paracasei, L. bulgaricus* 900 billion live cells per packet (20s,) [gluten free; also contains *Bifidobacterium breve, B. longum, B. infantis,* and *Streptococcus thermophilus*]
Tablet:
  Kala®: *L. acidophilus* 200 million units [dairy free, yeast free; soy based]
Tablet, chewable: *L. reuteri* 100 million organisms
  Floranex™: *L. acidophilus* and *L. bulgaricus* 1 million colony-forming units [contains lactose, nonfat dried milk, whey]
  Lactinex™: *L. acidophilus* and *L. bulgaricus* 1 million live cells [gluten free; contains calcium 5.2 mg/4 tablets, lactose 960 mg/4 tablets, potassium 20 mg/4 tablets, sodium 5.6 mg/4 tablets, and sucrose 500 sucrose/4 tablets; contains whey, evaporated milk, and soy peptone]
Wafer: *L. acidophilus* 90 mg and *L. bifidus* 25 mg (100s) [provides 1 billion organisms/wafer at time of manufacture; milk free]

Lactulose (LAK tyoo lose)

Related Information
Laxatives, Classification and Properties *on page 2012*
Treatment Options for Constipation *on page 2035*
Medication Safety Issues
Sound-alike/look-alike issues:
Lactulose may be confused with lactose
Brand Names: U.S. Constulose; Enulose; Generlac; Kristalose®
Brand Names: Canada Acilac; Apo-Lactulose®; Laxilose; PMS-Lactulose
Generic Availability (U.S.) Yes: Excludes crystals for solution
Pharmacologic Category Ammonium Detoxicant; Laxative, Osmotic
Use Prevention and treatment of portal-systemic encephalopathy (including hepatic precoma and coma); treatment of constipation
Contraindications Use in patients requiring a low galactose diet
Warnings/Precautions Use with caution in patients with diabetes mellitus; solution contains galactose and lactose. Monitor periodically for electrolyte imbalance when lactulose is used >6 months or in patients predisposed to electrolyte abnormalities (eg, elderly). Hepatic disease may predispose patients to electrolyte imbalance. Patients receiving lactulose and an oral anti-infective agent should be monitored for possible inadequate response to

lactulose. During proctoscopy or colonoscopy procedures involving electrocautery, a theoretical risk of reaction between H_2 gas accumulation and electrical spark may exist; thorough bowel cleansing with a nonfermentable solution is recommended.

Adverse Reactions (Reflective of adult population; not specific for elderly) Frequency not defined.

Endocrine & metabolic: Dehydration, hypernatremia, hypokalemia

Gastrointestinal: Abdominal discomfort, abdominal distention, belching, cramping, diarrhea (excessive dose), flatulence, nausea, vomiting

Drug Interactions

Avoid Concomitant Use There are no known interactions where it is recommended to avoid concomitant use.

Increased Effect/Toxicity There are no known significant interactions involving an increase in effect.

Decreased Effect There are no known significant interactions involving a decrease in effect.

Stability Store at room temperature; do not freeze. Protect from light. Discard solution if cloudy or very dark. Prolonged exposure to cold temperatures will cause thickening which will return to normal upon warming to room temperature.

Mechanism of Action The bacterial degradation of lactulose resulting in an acidic pH inhibits the diffusion of NH_3 into the blood by causing the conversion of NH_3 to NH_4+; also enhances the diffusion of NH_3 from the blood into the gut where conversion to NH_4+ occurs; produces an osmotic effect in the colon with resultant distention promoting peristalsis; reduces blood ammonia concentration to reduce the degree of portal systemic encephalopathy

Pharmacodynamics/Kinetics

Onset:

Constipation: Up to 24-48 hours to produce a normal bowel movement

Encephalopathy: At least 24-48 hours

Absorption: Not appreciable

Metabolism: Via colonic flora to lactic acid and acetic acid; requires colonic flora for drug activation

Excretion: Primarily feces; urine (≤3%)

Dosage

Geriatric & Adult

Constipation: Oral: 10-20 g (15-30 mL) daily; may increase to 40 g (60 mL) daily if necessary

Prevention of portal systemic encephalopathy (PSE): Oral: 20-30 g (30-45 mL) 3-4 times/day; adjust dose every 1-2 days to produce 2-3 soft stools/day

Treatment of acute PSE:

Oral: 20-30 g (30-45 mL) every 1 hour to induce rapid laxation; reduce to 20-30 g (30-45 mL) 3-4 times/day after laxation is achieved titrate to produce 2-3 soft stools/day

Rectal administration (retention enema): 200 g (300 mL) diluted with 700 mL of water or NS via rectal balloon catheter; retain for 30-60 minutes; may repeat every 4-6 hours; transition to oral treatment prior to discontinuing rectal administration

Administration

Oral solution: May mix with fruit juice, water or milk.

Crystals for oral solution: Dissolve contents of packet in 120 mL water.

Rectal: Mix with water or normal saline; administer as retention enema using a rectal balloon catheter; retain for 30-60 minutes. Transition to oral lactulose when appropriate (able to take oral medication and no longer a risk for aspiration) prior to discontinuing rectal administration

Monitoring Parameters Blood pressure, standing/supine; serum electrolytes, serum ammonia; bowel movement patterns, fluid status

Special Geriatric Considerations Elderly are more likely to show CNS signs of dehydration and electrolyte loss than younger adults. Therefore, monitor closely for fluid and electrolyte loss with chronic use. Sorbitol is equally effective as a laxative and less expensive. However, sorbitol **cannot be substituted** in the treatment of hepatic encephalopathy.

Dosage Forms Excipient information presented when available (limited, particularly for generics); consult specific product labeling. [DSC] = Discontinued product

Crystals for solution, oral:

Kristalose®: 10 g/packet (30s); 20 g/packet (30s)

Solution, oral: 10 g/15 mL (15 mL, 30 mL, 237 mL, 473 mL, 500 mL, 946 mL, 1892 mL)

Constulose: 10 g/15 mL (237 mL [DSC], 946 mL)

Enulose: 10 g/15 mL (473 mL)

Solution, oral/rectal: 10 g/15 mL (237 mL, 473 mL, 946 mL)

Generlac: 10 g/15 mL (473 mL, 1892 mL)

◆ **LAIV** see Influenza Virus Vaccine (Live/Attenuated) on page 940

◆ **LaMICtal®** see LamoTRIgine on page 1024

◆ **LaMICtal® ODT™** see LamoTRIgine on page 1024

♦ **LaMICtal® XR™** *see* LamoTRIgine *on page* 1024
♦ **LamISIL®** *see* Terbinafine (Systemic) *on page* 1754
♦ **LamISIL AT® [OTC]** *see* Terbinafine (Topical) *on page* 1756

LamoTRIgine (la MOE tri jeen)

Medication Safety Issues
Sound-alike/look-alike issues:
LamoTRIgine may be confused with labetalol, Lamisil®, lamiVUDine, levothyroxine, Lomotil®

LaMICtal® may be confused with LamISIL®, Lomotil®

Administration issues:
Potential exists for medication errors to occur among different formulations of Lamictal® (tablets, extended release tablets, orally disintegrating tablets, and chewable/dispersible tablets). Patients should be instructed to visually inspect tablets dispensed to verify receiving the correct medication and formulation. The medication guide includes illustrations to aid in tablet verification.

International issues:
Lamictal [U.S., Canada, and multiple international markets] may be confused with Ludiomil brand name for maprotiline [multiple international markets]

Lamotrigine [U.S., Canada, and multiple international markets] may be confused with Ludiomil brand name for maprotiline [multiple international markets]

Brand Names: U.S. LaMICtal®; LaMICtal® ODT™; LaMICtal® XR™

Brand Names: Canada Apo-Lamotrigine®; Lamictal®; Mylan-Lamotrigine; Novo-Lamotrigine; PMS-Lamotrigine; ratio-Lamotrigine; Teva-Lamotrigine

Index Terms BW-430C; LTG

Generic Availability (U.S.) Yes; excludes extended release tablet, orally disintegrating tablet

Pharmacologic Category Anticonvulsant, Miscellaneous

Use Adjunctive therapy in the treatment of generalized seizures of Lennox-Gastaut syndrome, primary generalized tonic-clonic seizures, and partial seizures; conversion to monotherapy in patients with partial seizures who are receiving treatment with valproic acid or a single enzyme-inducing antiepileptic drug (specifically carbamazepine, phenytoin, phenobarbital or primidone); maintenance treatment of bipolar I disorder

Medication Guide Available Yes

Contraindications Hypersensitivity to lamotrigine or any component of the formulation

Warnings/Precautions [U.S. Boxed Warning]: Severe and potentially life-threatening skin rashes requiring hospitalization have been reported; incidence of serious rash is higher in pediatric patients than adults; risk may be increased by coadministration with valproic acid, higher than recommended starting doses, and exceeding recommended dose titration. The majority of cases occur in the first 8 weeks; however, isolated cases may occur after prolonged treatment or in patients without these risk factors. Discontinue at first sign of rash and do not reinitiate therapy unless rash is clearly not drug related. Rare cases of Stevens-Johnson syndrome, toxic epidermal necrolysis, and angioedema have been reported.

Antiepileptics are associated with an increased risk of suicidal behavior/thoughts with use (regardless of indication); patients should be monitored for signs/symptoms of depression, suicidal tendencies, and other unusual behavior changes during therapy and instructed to inform their healthcare provider immediately if symptoms occur.

A spectrum of hematologic effects have been reported with use (eg, neutropenia, leukopenia, thrombocytopenia, pancytopenia, anemias, and rarely, aplastic anemia and pure red cell aplasia); patients with a previous history of adverse hematologic reaction to any drug may be at increased risk. Early detection of hematologic change is important; advise patients of early signs and symptoms including fever, sore throat, mouth ulcers, infections, easy bruising, petechial or purpuric hemorrhage. May be associated with hypersensitivity syndrome. Acute multiorgan failure has also been reported. Increased risk of developing aseptic meningitis has been reported; symptoms (eg, headache, nuchal rigidity, fever, nausea/vomiting, rash, photophobia) have generally occurred within 1-45 days following therapy initiation. Use caution in patients with renal or hepatic impairment. Avoid abrupt cessation, taper over at least 2 weeks if possible.

May cause CNS depression, which may impair physical or mental abilities. Patients must be cautioned about performing tasks which require mental alertness (eg, operating machinery or driving). Effects with other sedative drugs or ethanol may be potentiated. Binds to melanin and may accumulate in the eye and other melanin-rich tissues; the clinical significance of this is not known. Safety and efficacy have not been established for use as initial monotherapy, conversion to monotherapy from antiepileptic drugs (AED) other than carbamazepine, phenytoin, phenobarbital, primidone or valproic acid or conversion to monotherapy from two or more AEDs. Patients treated for bipolar disorder should be monitored closely for clinical worsening or suicidality; prescriptions should be written for the smallest quantity consistent with good patient care. Valproic acid may cause an increase in lamotrigine levels requiring dose adjustment. There is a potential for medication errors with similar-sounding medications and among different lamotrigine formulations; medication errors have occurred.

Adverse Reactions (Reflective of adult population; not specific for elderly) Percentages reported in adults on monotherapy for epilepsy or bipolar disorder.

>10%: Gastrointestinal: Nausea (7% to 14%)

1% to 10%:

Cardiovascular: Chest pain (5%), peripheral edema (2% to 5%), edema (1% to 5%)

Central nervous system: Insomnia (5% to 10%), somnolence (9%), fatigue (8%), coordination impaired (7%), dizziness (7%), anxiety (5%), pain (5%), ataxia (2% to 5%), irritability (2% to 5%), suicidal ideation (2% to 5%), agitation (1% to 5%), amnesia (1% to 5%), depression (1% to 5%), dream abnormality (1% to 5%), emotional lability (1% to 5%), fever (1% to 5%), hypoesthesia (1% to 5%), migraine (1% to 5%), thought abnormality (1% to 5%), confusion (1%)

Dermatologic: Rash (nonserious: 7%), dermatitis (2% to 5%), dry skin (2% to 5%)

Endocrine & metabolic: Dysmenorrhea (5%), libido increased (2% to 5%)

Gastrointestinal: Vomiting (5% to 9%), dyspepsia (7%), abdominal pain (6%), xerostomia (2% to 6%), constipation (5%), weight loss (5%), anorexia (2% to 5%), peptic ulcer (2% to 5%), rectal hemorrhage (2% to 5%), flatulence (1% to 5%), weight gain (1% to 5%)

Genitourinary: Urinary frequency (1% to 5%)

Neuromuscular & skeletal: Back pain (8%), weakness (2% to 5%), arthralgia (1% to 5%), myalgia (1% to 5%), neck pain (1% to 5%), paresthesia (1%)

Ocular: Nystagmus (2% to 5%), vision abnormal (2% to 5%), amblyopia (1%)

Respiratory: Rhinitis (7%), cough (5%), pharyngitis (5%), bronchitis (2% to 5%), dyspnea (2% to 5%), epistaxis (2% to 5%), sinusitis (1% to 5%)

Miscellaneous: Infection (5%), diaphoresis (2% to 5%), reflexes increased/decreased (2% to 5%), dyspraxia (1% to 5%)

Drug Interactions

Avoid Concomitant Use There are no known interactions where it is recommended to avoid concomitant use.

Increased Effect/Toxicity

LamoTRIgine may increase the levels/effects of: Alcohol (Ethyl); CarBAMazepine; CNS Depressants; Desmopressin; Methotrimeprazine; OLANZapine; Selective Serotonin Reuptake Inhibitors

The levels/effects of LamoTRIgine may be increased by: Divalproex; Droperidol; HydrOXYzine; Methotrimeprazine; Valproic Acid

Decreased Effect

LamoTRIgine may decrease the levels/effects of: Contraceptives (Progestins)

The levels/effects of LamoTRIgine may be decreased by: Barbiturates; CarBAMazepine; Contraceptives (Estrogens); Fosphenytoin; Ketorolac; Ketorolac (Nasal); Ketorolac (Systemic); Mefloquine; Phenytoin; Primidone; Rifampin; Ritonavir

Ethanol/Nutrition/Herb Interactions

Ethanol: May increase CNS depression; monitor for increased effects with coadministration. Caution patients about effects.

Food: Has no effect on absorption.

Herb/Nutraceutical: Avoid evening primrose (seizure threshold decreased).

Stability Store at 25°C (77°F); excursions permitted to 15°C to 30°C (59°F to 86°F). Protect from light.

Mechanism of Action A triazine derivative which inhibits release of glutamate (an excitatory amino acid) and inhibits voltage-sensitive sodium channels, which stabilizes neuronal membranes. Lamotrigine has weak inhibitory effect on the $5-HT_3$ receptor; *in vitro* inhibits dihydrofolate reductase.

Pharmacodynamics/Kinetics

Absorption: Immediate release: Rapid and complete

Distribution: V_d: 0.9-1.3 L/kg

Protein binding: ~55%

Metabolism: Hepatic and renal; metabolized primarily by glucuronic acid conjugation to inactive metabolites

Bioavailability: Immediate release: 98%; **Note:** AUCs were similar for immediate release and extended release preparations in patients receiving nonenzyme-inducing AEDs. In subjects receiving concomitant enzyme-inducing AEDs, bioavailability of extended release product was ~21% lower than immediate release product; in some of these subjects, a decrease in

◀ AUC of up to 70% was observed when switching from immediate release to extended release tablets.

Half-life elimination: Immediate release: Adults: 25-33 hours, Elderly: 25-43 hours; Extended release: Similar to immediate release

Concomitant valproic acid therapy: 48-70 hours

Concomitant phenytoin, phenobarbital, primidone, or carbamazepine therapy: 13-14 hours

Chronic renal failure: 43 hours

Hemodialysis: 13 hours during dialysis; 57 hours between dialysis (~20% of a dose is eliminated in a 4-hour dialysis session)

Hepatic impairment:

Mild: 26-66 hours

Moderate: 28-116 hours

Severe without ascites: 56-78 hours

Severe with ascites: 52-148 hours

Time to peak, plasma: Immediate release: 1-1.5 hours; Extended release: 4-11 hours (dependent on adjunct therapy)

Excretion: Urine (94%, ~90% as glucuronide conjugates and ~10% unchanged); feces (2%)

Dosage

Geriatric & Adult Note: Only whole tablets should be used for dosing, round calculated dose down to the nearest whole tablet. Enzyme-inducing regimens specifically refer to those containing carbamazepine, phenytoin, phenobarbital, or primidone.

Lennox-Gastaut (adjunctive), primary generalized tonic-clonic seizures (adjunctive) or partial seizures (adjunctive): Oral:

Immediate release formulations:

Regimens **not containing** carbamazepine, phenytoin, phenobarbital, primidone, or valproic acid: Initial: Week 1 and 2: 25 mg once daily; Week 3 and 4: 50 mg once daily; Week 5 and beyond: Increase by 50 mg/day every 1-2 weeks; Maintenance: 225-375 mg/day in 2 divided doses

Regimens **containing** valproic acid: Initial: Week 1 and 2: 25 mg every other day; Week 3 and 4: 25 mg once daily; Week 5 and beyond: Increase by 25-50 mg/day every 1-2 weeks; Maintenance: 100-200 mg/day (valproic acid alone) or 100-400 mg/day (valproic acid and other drugs that induce glucuronidation)

Regimens **containing** carbamazepine, phenytoin, phenobarbital, or primidone and without valproic acid: Initial: Week 1 and 2: 50 mg once daily; Week 3 and 4: 100 mg/day in 2 divided doses; Week 5 and beyond: Increase by 100 mg/day every 1-2 weeks; Maintenance: 300-500 mg/day in 2 divided doses; maximum daily dose: 700 mg

Partial seizures (adjunctive) and primary generalized tonic-clonic seizures (adjunctive):

Extended release formulation: **Note:** Dose increases after week 8 should not exceed 100 mg/day at weekly intervals:

Regimens **not containing** carbamazepine, phenytoin, phenobarbital, primidone, or valproic acid: Initial: Week 1 and 2: 25 mg once daily; Week 3 and 4: 50 mg once daily; Week 5: 100 mg once daily; Week 6: 150 mg once daily; Week 7: 200 mg once daily; Maintenance: 300-400 mg once daily

Regimens **containing** valproic acid: Initial: Week 1 and 2: 25 mg every other day; Week 3 and 4: 25 mg once daily; Week 5: 50 mg once daily; Week 6: 100 mg once daily; Week 7: 150 mg once daily; Maintenance: 200-250 mg once daily

Regimens **containing** carbamazepine, phenytoin, phenobarbital, or primidone and without valproic acid: Initial: Week 1 and 2: 50 mg once daily; Week 3 and 4: 100 mg once daily; Week 5: 200 mg once daily; Week 6: 300 mg once daily; Week 7: 400 mg once daily; Maintenance: 400-600 mg once daily

Conversion from adjunctive therapy with a single enzyme-inducing AED regimen for partial seizures to monotherapy with lamotrigine: **Note:** Goal is to achieve a lamotrigine monotherapy dose of 500 mg/day in 2 divided doses for immediate release formulations and a lamotrigine monotherapy dosage range of 250-300 mg once daily for the extended release formulation.

Conversion strategy from adjunctive therapy with valproic acid:

Immediate release formulations:

- Initiate and titrate as per escalation recommendations for adjunctive therapy to a lamotrigine dose of 200 mg/day.

- Then taper valproic acid dose in decrements of not >500 mg/day/week to a valproic acid dosage of 500 mg/day; this dosage should be maintained for 1 week. The lamotrigine dosage should then be increased to 300 mg/day while valproic acid is simultaneously decreased to 250 mg/day; this dosage should be maintained for 1 week.

- Valproic acid may then be discontinued, while the lamotrigine dose is increased by 100 mg/day at weekly intervals to achieve a lamotrigine maintenance dose of 500 mg/day in 2 divided doses.

Extended release formulation:

- Initiate and titrate as per escalation recommendations for adjunctive therapy to a lamotrigine dose of 150 mg/day.
- Then taper valproic acid dose in decrements of not >500 mg/day/week to a valproic acid dose of 500 mg/day; this dosage should be maintained for 1 week. The lamotrigine dosage should then be increased to 200 mg/day while valproic acid is simultaneously decreased to 250 mg/day; this dosage should be maintained for 1 week.
- Valproic acid may then be discontinued, while the lamotrigine dose is increased to achieve a maintenance dosage range of 250-300 mg once daily.

Conversion strategy from adjunctive therapy with carbamazepine, phenytoin, phenobarbital, or primidone: *Immediate release formulations and extended release formulation:*

- Initiate and titrate as per escalation recommendations for adjunctive therapy to a lamotrigine dose of 500 mg/day.
- Concomitant enzyme-inducing AED should then be withdrawn by 20% decrements each week over a 4-week period.
- Following withdrawal of the enzyme-inducing AED, the dosage of lamotrigine extended release may be tapered in decrements of not >100 mg/day at intervals of 1 week to achieve a maintenance dosage range of 250-300 mg once daily; no further dosage reduction is required for lamotrigine immediate release formulations.

Conversion strategy from adjunctive therapy with AED other than carbamazepine, phenytoin, phenobarbital, primidone or valproic acid:

Immediate release formulations: No specific guidelines available

Extended release formulation: Initiate and titrate as per escalation recommendations for adjunctive therapy to a lamotrigine dose of 250-300 mg/day. Concomitant AED should then be withdrawn by 20% decrements each week over a 4 week period.

Bipolar disorder: *Immediate release formulations:*

Regimens **not containing** carbamazepine, phenytoin, phenobarbital, primidone, or valproic acid: Initial: Week 1 and 2: 25 mg once daily; Week 3 and 4: 50 mg once daily; Week 5: 100 mg once daily; Week 6 and maintenance: 200 mg once daily

Regimens **containing** valproic acid: Initial: Week 1 and 2: 25 mg every other day; Week 3 and 4: 25 mg once daily; Week 5: 50 mg once daily; Week 6 and maintenance: 100 mg once daily

Regimens **containing** carbamazepine, phenytoin, phenobarbital, or primidone and without valproic acid: Initial: Week 1 and 2: 50 mg once daily; Week 3 and 4: 100 mg/day in divided doses; Week 5: 200 mg/day in divided doses; Week 6: 300 mg/day in divided doses; Maintenance: up to 400 mg/day in divided doses

Adjustment following discontinuation of psychotropic medication:

Discontinuing valproic acid with current dose of lamotrigine 100 mg/day: 150 mg/day for week 1, then increase to 200 mg/day beginning week 2

Discontinuing carbamazepine, phenytoin, phenobarbital, primidone, or rifampin with current dose of lamotrigine 400 mg/day: 400 mg/day for week 1, then decrease to 300 mg/day for week 2, then decrease to 200 mg/day beginning week 3

Conversion from immediate release to extended release (Lamictal® XR™): Initial dose of the extended release tablet should match the total daily dose of the immediate-release formulation. Adjust dose as needed within the recommended dosing guidelines.

Discontinuing therapy: Decrease dose by ~50% per week, over at least 2 weeks unless safety concerns require a more rapid withdrawal. Discontinuing carbamazepine, phenytoin, phenobarbital, primidone, or rifampin should prolong the half-life of lamotrigine; discontinuing valproic acid should shorten the half-life of lamotrigine

Restarting therapy after discontinuation: If lamotrigine has been withheld for >5 half-lives, consider restarting according to initial dosing recommendations. **Note:** Concomitant medications may affect the half-life of lamotrigine; consider pharmacokinetic interactions when restarting therapy.

Dosage adjustment with estrogen-containing hormonal contraceptives: Follow initial lamotrigine dosing guidelines, maintenance dose should be adjusted as follows, based on concomitant medications:

Patients taking concomitant carbamazepine, phenytoin, phenobarbital, primidone or rifampin: No dosing adjustment required

◀

Patients **not** taking concomitant carbamazepine, phenytoin, phenobarbital, primidone or rifampin: Lamotrigine maintenance dose may need increased by twofold over target dose. If already taking a stable dose of lamotrigine and starting contraceptive, maintenance dose may need increased by twofold. Dose increases should start when contraceptive is started and titrated to clinical response increasing no more rapidly than 50-100 mg/day every week. Gradual increases of lamotrigine plasma levels may occur during the inactive "pill-free" week and will be greater when dose increases are made the week before. If increased adverse events consistently occur during "pill-free" week, overall maintenance dose adjustments may be required. When discontinuing estrogen-containing hormonal contraceptive, dose of lamotrigine may need decreased by as much as 50%; do not decrease by more than 25% of total daily dose over a 2-week period unless clinical response or plasma levels indicate otherwise. Dose adjustments during "pill-free" week are not recommended.

Renal Impairment Decreased maintenance dosage may be effective in patients with significant renal impairment; has not been adequately studied; use with caution.

Hepatic Impairment

Mild impairment: No adjustment required.

Moderate-to-severe impairment without ascites: Decrease initial, escalation, and maintenance doses by ~25%; adjust according to clinical response.

Moderate-to-severe impairment with ascites: Decrease initial, escalation, and maintenance doses by ~50%; adjust according to clinical response.

Administration Doses should be rounded down to the nearest whole tablet.

Lamictal® chewable/dispersible tablets: May be chewed, dispersed in water or diluted fruit juice, or swallowed whole. To disperse tablets, add to a small amount of liquid (just enough to cover tablet); let sit ~1 minute until dispersed; swirl solution and consume immediately. Do not administer partial amounts of liquid. If tablets are chewed, a small amount of water or diluted fruit juice should be used to aid in swallowing.

Lamictal® ODT™: Place tablets on tongue and move around in the mouth. Tablets will dissolve rapidly and can be swallowed with or without food or water.

Lamictal® XR™: Administer without regard to meals. Swallow whole; do not chew, crush, or cut.

Monitoring Parameters Seizure, frequency and duration; serum levels of concurrent anticonvulsants, hypersensitivity reactions (especially rash); suicidality (eg, suicidal thoughts, depression, behavioral changes); signs/symptoms of aseptic meningitis

Reference Range A therapeutic serum concentration range has not been established for lamotrigine. Dosing should be based on therapeutic response. Lamotrigine plasma concentrations of 0.25-29.1 mcg/mL have been reported in the literature.

Special Geriatric Considerations No pharmacokinetic differences noted between young adults and the elderly. Use with caution in the elderly with significant renal decline.

Dosage Forms Excipient information presented when available (limited, particularly for generics); consult specific product labeling.

Tablet, oral: 25 mg, 100 mg, 150 mg, 200 mg

LaMICtal®: 25 mg, 100 mg, 150 mg, 200 mg [scored]

Tablet, oral [combination package (each unit-dose starter kit contains)]:

LaMICtal®: 25 mg (84s) [white tablets] and 100 mg (14s) [peach tablets] [scored; green kit; for patients taking carbamazepine, phenytoin, phenobarbital, primidone, or rifampin and **not** taking valproic acid]

LaMICtal®: 25 mg (42s) [white tablets] and 100 mg (7s) [peach tablets] [scored; orange kit; for patients **not** taking carbamazepine, phenytoin, phenobarbital, primidone, rifampin, or valproic acid]

Tablet, oral [each unit-dose starter kit contains]:

LaMICtal®: 25 mg [scored; blue kit; for patients taking valproic acid]

Tablet, chewable/dispersible, oral: 5 mg, 25 mg

LaMICtal®: 2 mg [black currant flavor]

LaMICtal®: 5 mg [scored; black currant flavor]

LaMICtal®: 25 mg [black currant flavor]

Tablet, extended release, oral:

LaMICtal® XR™: 25 mg, 50 mg, 100 mg, 200 mg, 300 mg

Tablet, extended release, oral [combination package (each partial titration kit contains)]:

LaMICtal® XR™: 25 mg (21s) [yellow/white tablets] and 50 mg (7s) [green/white tablets] [blue XR kit, for patients taking valproic acid]

LaMICtal® XR™: 50 mg (14s) [green/white tablets], 100 mg (14s) [orange/white tablets], and 200 mg (7s) [blue/white tablets] [green XR kit, for patients taking carbamazepine, phenytoin, phenobarbital, primidone, and **not** taking valproic acid]

LaMICtal® XR™: 25 mg (14s) [yellow/white tablets], 50 mg (14s) [green/white tablets], and 100 mg (7s) [orange/white tablets] [orange XR kit, for patients **not** taking carbamazepine, phenytoin, phenobarbital, primidone, or valproic acid]

Tablet, orally disintegrating, oral:
LaMICtal® ODT™: 25 mg, 50 mg, 100 mg, 200 mg [cherry flavor]
Tablet, orally disintegrating, oral [combination package (each patient titration kit contains)]:
LaMICtal® ODT™: 25 mg (21s) and 50 mg (7s) [cherry flavor; blue kit, for patients taking valproic acid]
LaMICtal® ODT™: 50 mg (42s) and 100 mg (14s) [cherry flavor; green kit, for patients taking carbamazepine, phenytoin, phenobarbital, primidone, or rifampin and **not** taking valproic acid]
LaMICtal® ODT™: 25 mg (14s), 50 mg (14s), and 100 mg (7s) [cherry flavor; orange kit, for patients **not** taking carbamazepine, phenytoin, phenobarbital, primidone, rifampin, or valproic acid]

Extemporaneously Prepared A 1 mg/mL oral suspension may be compounded as follows: Crush one 100 mg immediate release tablet and reduce to a fine powder. Add small amount of Ora-Sweet® or Ora-Plus® and mix to uniform paste. Transfer to graduate and qs to 100 mL. Shake well before using and refrigerate. Suspension is stable for 91 days.

Nahata M, Morosco R, Hipple T. "Stability of Lamotrigine in Two Extemporaneously Prepared Oral Suspensions at 4 and 25°C," *Am J Health Syst Pharm,* 1999, 56:240-2.

Selected References

Calabrese JR, Suppes T, Bowden CL, et al, "Double-Blind, Placebo-Controlled, Prophylaxis Study of Lamotrigine in Rapid-Cycling Bipolar Disorder," *J Clin Psychiatry,* 2000, 61:841-50.

Lofton AL and Klein-Schwartz W, "Evaluation of Lamotrigine Toxicity Reported to Poison Control Centers," *Ann Pharmacother,* 2004, 38(11):1811-5

♦ **Lanoxin®** see Digoxin *on page 508*

Lansoprazole (lan SOE pra zole)

Related Information
Helicobacter pylori Treatment in Adult Patients *on page 2009*
Medication Safety Issues
Sound-alike/look-alike issues:
Lansoprazole may be confused with aripiprazole, dexlansoprazole
Prevacid® may be confused with Pravachol®, Prevpac®, PriLOSEC®, Prinivil®
Brand Names: U.S. Prevacid®; Prevacid® 24 HR [OTC]; Prevacid® SoluTab™
Brand Names: Canada Apo-Lansoprazole®; Mylan-Lansoprazole®; Prevacid®; Prevacid® FasTab; Teva-Lansoprazole
Generic Availability (U.S.) Yes
Pharmacologic Category Proton Pump Inhibitor; Substituted Benzimidazole
Use Short-term treatment of active duodenal ulcers; maintenance treatment of healed duodenal ulcers; as part of a multidrug regimen for *H. pylori* eradication to reduce the risk of duodenal ulcer recurrence; short-term treatment of active benign gastric ulcer; treatment of NSAID-associated gastric ulcer; to reduce the risk of NSAID-associated gastric ulcer in patients with a history of gastric ulcer who require an NSAID; short-term treatment of symptomatic GERD; short-term treatment for all grades of erosive esophagitis; to maintain healing of erosive esophagitis; long-term treatment of pathological hypersecretory conditions, including Zollinger-Ellison syndrome

OTC labeling: Relief of frequent heartburn (≥2 days/week)
Contraindications Hypersensitivity to lansoprazole or any component of the formulation
Warnings/Precautions Use of proton pump inhibitors may increase the risk of gastrointestinal infections (eg, *Salmonella, Campylobacter*). Relief of symptoms does not preclude the presence of a gastric malignancy. Atrophic gastritis (by biopsy) has been noted with long-term omeprazole therapy; this may also occur with lansoprazole. No reports of enterochromaffin-like (ECL) cell carcinoids, dysplasia, or neoplasia have occurred. Severe liver dysfunction may require dosage reductions. Decreased *H. pylori* eradication rates have been observed with short-term (≤7 days) combination therapy. The American College of Gastroenterology recommends 10-14 days of therapy (triple or quadruple) for eradication of *H. pylori* (Chey, 2007). Proton pump inhibitors may diminish the therapeutic effect of clopidogrel thought to be due to reduced formation of the active metabolite of clopidogrel; an increase in the risk of cardiovascular events may occur. The manufacturer of clopidogrel recommends avoidance of concomitant administration of another PPI (ie, omeprazole); given the potency of lansoprazole's CYP2C19 inhibitory activity, similar recommendations would appear prudent.

Increased incidence of osteoporosis-related bone fractures of the hip, spine, or wrist may occur with proton pump inhibitor therapy. Patients on high-dose or long-term therapy should be monitored. Use the lowest effective dose for the shortest duration of time, use vitamin D and calcium supplementation, and follow appropriate guidelines to reduce risk of fractures in patients at risk.

Hypomagnesemia, reported rarely, usually with prolonged PPI use of >3 months (most cases >1 year of therapy); may be symptomatic or asymptomatic; severe cases may cause tetany, seizures, and cardiac arrhythmias. Consider obtaining serum magnesium concentrations prior to beginning long-term therapy, especially if taking concomitant digoxin, diuretics, or other drugs known to cause hypomagnesemia; and periodically thereafter. Hypomagnesemia may be corrected by magnesium supplementation, although discontinuation of lansoprazole may be necessary; magnesium levels typically return to normal within 1 week of stopping.

When used for self-medication, patients should be instructed not to use if they have difficulty swallowing, are vomiting blood, or have bloody or black stools. Prior to use, patients should contact healthcare provider if they have liver disease, heartburn for >3 months, heartburn with dizziness, lightheadedness, or sweating, MI symptoms, frequent chest pain, frequent wheezing (especially with heartburn), unexplained weight loss, nausea/vomiting, stomach pain, or are taking antifungals, atazanavir, digoxin, tacrolimus, theophylline, or warfarin. Patients should stop use and consult a healthcare provider if heartburn continues or worsens, or if they need to take for >14 days or more often than every 4 months. Patients should be informed that it may take 1-4 days for full effect to be seen; should not be used for immediate relief.

Adverse Reactions (Reflective of adult population; not specific for elderly)
1% to 10%:
Central nervous system: Headache (children 1-11 years 3%, 12-17 years 7%), dizziness (children 12-17 years 3%; adults <1%)
Gastrointestinal: Diarrhea (1% to 5%; 60 mg/day: 7%), abdominal pain (children 12-17 years 5%; adults 2%), constipation (children 1-11 years 5%; adults 1%), nausea (children 12-17 years 3%; adults 1%)

Drug Interactions
Metabolism/Transport Effects Substrate of CYP2C9 (minor), 2C19 (major), 3A4 (major); **Inhibits** CYP2C9 (weak), 2C19 (moderate), 2D6 (weak), 3A4 (weak); **Induces** CYP1A2 (weak)
Avoid Concomitant Use
Avoid concomitant use of Lansoprazole with any of the following: Delavirdine; Erlotinib; Nelfinavir; Posaconazole; Rilpivirine
Increased Effect/Toxicity
Lansoprazole may increase the levels/effects of: Amphetamines; CYP2C19 Substrates; Dexmethylphenidate; Imatinib; Methotrexate; Methylphenidate; Raltegravir; Saquinavir; Tacrolimus; Tacrolimus (Systemic); Vitamin K Antagonists; Voriconazole

The levels/effects of Lansoprazole may be increased by: Conivaptan; Fluconazole; Ketoconazole; Ketoconazole (Systemic)
Decreased Effect
Lansoprazole may decrease the levels/effects of: Atazanavir; Bisphosphonate Derivatives; Cefditoren; Clopidogrel; Dabigatran Etexilate; Dasatinib; Delavirdine; Erlotinib; Gefitinib; Indinavir; Iron Salts; Itraconazole; Ketoconazole; Ketoconazole (Systemic); Mesalamine; Mycophenolate; Nelfinavir; Posaconazole; Rilpivirine

The levels/effects of Lansoprazole may be decreased by: CYP2C19 Inducers (Strong); CYP3A4 Inducers (Strong); Deferasirox; Herbs (CYP3A4 Inducers); Tipranavir; Tocilizumab
Ethanol/Nutrition/Herb Interactions
Ethanol: Avoid ethanol (may cause gastric mucosal irritation).
Food: Lansoprazole serum concentrations may be decreased if taken with food.
Herb/Nutraceutical: Avoid St John's wort (may decrease the levels/effect of lansoprazole).
Stability Store at 25°C (77°F); excursions permitted to 15°C to 30°C (59°F to 86°F).
Mechanism of Action Decreases acid secretion in gastric parietal cells through inhibition of (H+, K+)-ATPase enzyme system, blocking the final step in gastric acid production.
Pharmacodynamics/Kinetics
Onset of action: Gastric acid suppression: Oral: 1-3 hours
Duration: Gastric acid suppression: Oral: >1 day
Absorption: Rapid
Distribution: V_d: 14-18 L
Protein binding: 97%
Metabolism: Hepatic via CYP2C19 and 3A4, and in parietal cells to two active metabolites that are not present in systemic circulation
Bioavailability: ≥80%; decreased 50% to 70% if given 30 minutes after food
Half-life elimination: 1.5 ± 1 hours; Elderly: 2-3 hours; Hepatic impairment: 3-7 hours
Time to peak, plasma: 1.7 hours
Excretion: Feces (67%); urine (33%)

Dosage
Geriatric & Adult
Symptomatic GERD: Oral: Short-term treatment: 15 mg once daily for up to 8 weeks

Erosive esophagitis: Oral: Short-term treatment: 30 mg once daily for up to 8 weeks; continued treatment for an additional 8 weeks may be considered for recurrence or for patients who do not heal after the first 8 weeks of therapy; maintenance therapy: 15 mg once daily

Hypersecretory conditions: Oral: Initial: 60 mg once daily; adjust dose based upon patient response and to reduce acid secretion to <10 mEq/hour (5 mEq/hour in patients with prior gastric surgery); doses of 90 mg twice daily have been used; administer doses >120 mg/day in divided doses

Duodenal ulcer: Oral: Short-term treatment: 15 mg once daily for 4 weeks; maintenance therapy: 15 mg once daily

***Helicobacter pylori* eradication:**

Manufacturer labeling: 30 mg 3 times/day administered with amoxicillin 1000 mg 3 times/day for 14 days **or** 30 mg twice daily administered with amoxicillin 1000 mg *and* clarithromycin 500 mg twice daily for 10-14 days

American College of Gastroenterology guidelines (Chey, 2007):

Nonpenicillin allergy: 30 mg twice daily administered with amoxicillin 1000 mg *and* clarithromycin 500 mg twice daily for 10-14 days

Penicillin allergy: 30 mg twice daily administered with clarithromycin 500 mg *and* metronidazole 500 mg twice daily for 10-14 days **or** 30 mg once or twice daily administered with bismuth subsalicylate 525 mg *and* metronidazole 250 mg *plus* tetracycline 500 mg 4 times/day for 10-14 days

Gastric ulcer: Oral: Short-term treatment: 30 mg once daily for up to 8 weeks

NSAID-associated gastric ulcer (healing): Oral: 30 mg once daily for 8 weeks; controlled studies did not extend past 8 weeks

NSAID-associated gastric ulcer (to reduce risk): Oral: 15 mg once daily for up to 12 weeks; controlled studies did not extend past 12 weeks

Heartburn (OTC labeling): Oral: 15 mg once daily for 14 days; may repeat 14 days of therapy every 4 months. Do not take for >14 days or more often than every 4 months, unless instructed by healthcare provider.

Renal Impairment No adjustment is necessary.

Hepatic Impairment Severe hepatic impairment: Consider a dose reduction.

Administration
Oral: Administer before food; best if taken before breakfast. The intact granules should not be chewed or crushed; however, several options are available for those patients unable to swallow capsules:

Capsules may be opened and the intact granules sprinkled on 1 tablespoon of applesauce, Ensure® pudding, cottage cheese, yogurt, or strained pears. The granules should then be swallowed immediately.

Capsules may be opened and emptied into ~60 mL orange juice, apple juice, or tomato juice; mix and swallow immediately. Rinse the glass with additional juice and swallow to assure complete delivery of the dose.

Orally-disintegrating tablets: Should not be swallowed whole, broken, cut, or chewed. Place tablet on tongue; allow to dissolve (with or without water) until particles can be swallowed. Orally-disintegrating tablets may also be administered via an oral syringe: Place the 15 mg tablet in an oral syringe and draw up ~4 mL water, or place the 30 mg tablet in an oral syringe and draw up ~10 mL water. After tablet has dispersed, administer within 15 minutes. Refill the syringe with water (2 mL for the 15 mg tablet; 5 mL for the 30 mg tablet), shake gently, then administer any remaining contents.

Nasogastric tube administration:

Capsule: Capsule can be opened, the granules mixed (not crushed) with 40 mL of apple juice and then injected through the NG tube into the stomach, then flush tube with additional apple juice. Do not mix with other liquids.

Orally-disintegrating tablet: Nasogastric tube ≥8 French: Place a 15 mg tablet in a syringe and draw up ~4 mL water, or place the 30 mg tablet in a syringe and draw up ~10 mL water. After tablet has dispersed, administer within 15 minutes. Refill the syringe with ~5 mL water, shake gently, and then flush the nasogastric tube.

Monitoring Parameters Patients with Zollinger-Ellison syndrome should be monitored for gastric acid output, which should be maintained at ≤10 mEq/hour during the last hour before the next lansoprazole dose; lab monitoring should include CBC, liver function, renal function, and serum gastrin levels

Special Geriatric Considerations The clearance of lansoprazole is decreased in the elderly; however, the half-life is only increased by 50% to 100%, resulting in a continued short half-life with no accumulation in the elderly. No dosage adjustment is required with normal hepatic function. The rate of healing and side effects are similar to younger adults.

◀ An increased risk of fractures of the hip, spine, or wrist has been observed in epidemiologic studies with proton pump inhibitor (PPI) use, primarily in older adults ≥50 years of age. The greatest risk was seen in patients receiving high doses or on long-term therapy (≥1 year). Calcium and vitamin D supplementation and close monitoring are recommended to reduce the risk of fracture in high-risk patients.

Dosage Forms Excipient information presented when available (limited, particularly for generics); consult specific product labeling.

Capsule, delayed release, oral: 15 mg, 30 mg

Prevacid®: 15 mg, 30 mg

Prevacid® 24 HR: 15 mg

Tablet, delayed release, orally disintegrating, oral: 15 mg, 30 mg

Prevacid® SoluTab™: 15 mg [contains phenylalanine 2.5 mg/tablet; strawberry flavor]

Prevacid® SoluTab™: 30 mg [contains phenylalanine 5.1 mg/tablet; strawberry flavor]

Selected References

Chey WD, Wong BC, and Practice Parameters Committee of the American College of Gastroenterology, "American College of Gastroenterology, Guideline on the Management of *Helicobacter pylori* Infection," *Am J Gastroenterol*, 2007, 102(8):1808-25.

DeVault KR and Castell DO, "Practice Guidelines. Updated Guidelines for the Diagnosis and Treatment of Gastroesophageal Reflux Disease", *Am J Gastroenterol*, 2005,100(1):190-200.

Natsch S, Vinks MH, Voogt AK, et al, "Anaphylactic Reactions to Proton-Pump Inhibitors," *Ann Pharmacother*, 2000, 34(4):474-6.

Paoluzi P, Iacopini F, Crispino P, et al, "2-Week Triple Therapy for *Helicobacter pylori* Infection Is Better Than 1-Week in Clinical Practice: a Large Prospective Single-Center Randomized Study," *Helicobacter*, 2006, 11(6):562-8.

Lanthanum (LAN tha num)

Medication Safety Issues

Sound-alike/look-alike issues:

Lanthanum may be confused with lithium

Brand Names: U.S. Fosrenol®

Brand Names: Canada Fosrenol®

Index Terms Lanthanum Carbonate

Generic Availability (U.S.) No

Pharmacologic Category Phosphate Binder

Use Reduction of serum phosphate in patients with stage 5 chronic kidney disease (end-stage renal disease [ESRD]; kidney failure: GFR <15 mL/minute/1.73 m^2 or dialysis)

Contraindications Bowel obstruction, fecal impaction, ileus

Warnings/Precautions Use caution with active peptic ulcer, ulcerative colitis, Crohn's disease, or bowel obstruction. Abdominal x-rays may have a radiopaque appearance in patients taking lanthanum.

Adverse Reactions (Reflective of adult population; not specific for elderly)

Reported in short-term (4-6 weeks) trials at frequency > placebo:

>10%: Gastrointestinal: Nausea (11%), vomiting (9%), abdominal pain (5%)

Drug Interactions

Avoid Concomitant Use There are no known interactions where it is recommended to avoid concomitant use.

Increased Effect/Toxicity There are no known significant interactions involving an increase in effect.

Decreased Effect

Lanthanum may decrease the levels/effects of: ACE Inhibitors; Ampicillin; Chloroquine; Halofantrine; Quinolone Antibiotics; Tetracycline Derivatives; Thyroid Products

The levels/effects of Lanthanum may be decreased by: HMG-CoA Reductase Inhibitors

Stability Store at 25°C (77°F); excursions permitted to 15°C to 30°C (59°F to 86°F). Protect from moisture.

Mechanism of Action Disassociates in the upper gastrointestinal tract to lanthanum ions (La^{3+}) which bind to dietary phosphate resulting in insoluble lanthanum phosphate complexes and a net decrease in serum phosphate and calcium levels.

Pharmacodynamics/Kinetics

Absorption: <0.002%

Protein binding: >99%

Metabolism: Not metabolized

Half-life elimination: Plasma: 53 hours; Bone: 2-3.6 years

Excretion: Feces primarily; urine <2%

Dosage

Geriatric & Adult Reduction of serum phosphorous: Oral: Initial: 1500 mg/day divided and taken with meals; typical increases of 750 mg/day every 2-3 weeks are suggested as needed to reduce the serum phosphate level <6 mg/dL; usual dosage range: 1500-3000 mg; doses of up to 4500 mg have been evaluated

Administration Administer with or immediately after meals; tablet should be chewed prior to swallowing; do not swallow whole

Monitoring Parameters Serum calcium and phosphorus: Frequency of measurement may be dependent upon the presence and magnitude of abnormalities, the rate of progression of CKD, and the use of treatments for CKD-mineral and bone disorders (KDIGO, 2009): CKD stage 5 and 5D: Every 1-3 months

Reference Range

Corrected total serum calcium (K/DOQI, 2003): CKD stage 5: 8.4-9.5 mg/dL (2.1-2.37 mmol/L); KDIGO guidelines recommend maintaining normal ranges for CKD stage 5 and 5D (KDIGO, 2009)

Phosphorus (K/DOQI, 2003): CKD stage 5 (including those treated with dialysis): 3.5-5.5 mg/dL (1.13-1.78 mmol/L); KDIGO guidelines recommend maintaining normal ranges for CKD stage 5 and lowering elevated phosphorus levels toward the normal range for CKD stage 5D (KDIGO, 2009)

Serum calcium-phosphorus product (K/DOQI, 2003): CKD stage 5: <55 mg^2/dL^2

Test Interactions Abdominal x-rays may have a radiopaque appearance.

Special Geriatric Considerations In initial studies, no overall clinical differences were noted in those >65 years of age compared to younger adults.

Dosage Forms Excipient information presented when available (limited, particularly for generics); consult specific product labeling.

Tablet, chewable, oral:

Fosrenol®: 500 mg, 750 mg, 1000 mg

Selected References

Behets GJ, Verberckmoes SC, D'Haese PC, et al, "Lanthanum Carbonate: A New Phosphate Binder," *Curr Opin Nephrol Hypertens*, 2004, 13:403-9.

- ◆ **Lanthanum Carbonate** see Lanthanum *on page 1032*
- ◆ **Lantus®** see Insulin Glargine *on page 950*
- ◆ **Lantus® Solostar®** see Insulin Glargine *on page 950*
- ◆ **Lasix®** see Furosemide *on page 800*
- ◆ **Lastacaft™** see Alcaftadine *on page 52*

Latanoprost (la TA noe prost)

Related Information

Glaucoma Drug Therapy *on page 2008*

Medication Safety Issues

Sound-alike/look-alike issues:

Latanoprost may be confused with Lantus®

Xalatan® may be confused with Lantus®, Travatan®, Xalacom™, Zarontin®

Brand Names: U.S. Xalatan®

Brand Names: Canada Xalatan®

Generic Availability (U.S.) Yes

Pharmacologic Category Ophthalmic Agent, Antiglaucoma; Prostaglandin, Ophthalmic

Use Reduction of elevated intraocular pressure in patients with open-angle glaucoma or ocular hypertension

Contraindications Hypersensitivity to latanoprost, benzalkonium chloride, or any component of the formulation

Warnings/Precautions May permanently change/increase brown pigmentation of the iris, the eyelid skin, and eyelashes. In addition, may increase the length and/or number of eyelashes (may vary between eyes); changes occur slowly and may not be noticeable for months or years. Long-term consequences and potential injury to eye are not known. Use with caution in patients with intraocular inflammation, aphakic patients, pseudophakic patients with a torn posterior lens capsule, or patients with risk factors for macular edema. Safety and efficacy have not been determined for use in patients with angle-closure-, inflammatory-, or neovascular glaucoma.

There have been reports of bacterial keratitis associated with the use of multiple-dose containers of topical ophthalmic products. Contains benzalkonium chloride which may be absorbed by contact lenses; remove contacts prior to administration and wait 15 minutes before reinserting.

Adverse Reactions (Reflective of adult population; not specific for elderly)
>10%: Ocular: Blurred vision, burning and stinging, conjunctival hyperemia, foreign body sensation, itching, increased pigmentation of the iris, and punctate epithelial keratopathy
1% to 10%:
Cardiovascular: Angina pectoris, chest pain
Dermatologic: Allergic skin reaction, rash
Neuromuscular & skeletal: Arthralgia, back pain, myalgia
Ocular: Dry eye, excessive tearing, eye pain, lid crusting, lid edema, lid erythema, lid discomfort/pain, photophobia
Respiratory: Cold, flu, upper respiratory tract infection

Drug Interactions
Avoid Concomitant Use There are no known interactions where it is recommended to avoid concomitant use.
Increased Effect/Toxicity
Latanoprost may increase the levels/effects of: Bimatoprost
Decreased Effect
The levels/effects of Latanoprost may be decreased by: NSAID (Ophthalmic)

Stability Store intact bottles under refrigeration (2°C to 8°C/36°F to 46°F). Protect from light. Once opened, the container may be stored at room temperature up to 25°C (77°F) for 6 weeks.

Mechanism of Action Latanoprost is a prostaglandin F_2-alpha analog believed to reduce intraocular pressure by increasing the outflow of the aqueous humor

Pharmacodynamics/Kinetics
Onset of action: 3-4 hours
Peak effect: Maximum: 8-12 hours
Absorption: Through the cornea where the isopropyl ester prodrug is hydrolyzed by esterases to the biologically active acid. Peak concentration is reached in 2 hours after topical administration in the aqueous humor.
Distribution: V_d: 0.16 L/kg
Metabolism: Primarily hepatic via fatty acid beta-oxidation
Half-life elimination: 17 minutes
Excretion: Urine (as metabolites)

Dosage
Geriatric & Adult Glaucoma: Ophthalmic: 1 drop (1.5 mcg) in the affected eye(s) once daily in the evening; do not exceed the once daily dosage because it has been shown that more frequent administration may decrease the IOP lowering effect
Note: A medication delivery device (Xal-Ease™) is available for use with Xalatan®.

Administration If more than one topical ophthalmic drug is being used, administer the drugs at least 5 minutes apart

Monitoring Parameters Intraocular pressure, funduscopic exam, visual field testing

Special Geriatric Considerations Evaluate the patient's or caregiver's ability to safely administer the correct dose of ophthalmic medication.

Dosage Forms Excipient information presented when available (limited, particularly for generics); consult specific product labeling.
Solution, ophthalmic [drops]: 0.005% (2.5 mL)
Xalatan®: 0.005% (2.5 mL) [contains benzalkonium chloride]

Selected References
Patel SS and Spencer CM, "Latanoprost: A Review of Its Pharmacological Properties, Clinical Efficacy and Tolerability in the Management of Primary Open-Angle Glaucoma and Ocular Hypertension," *Drugs Aging*, 1996, 9(5):363-78.

♦ **Latisse®** *see* Bimatoprost *on page 204*
♦ **Latuda®** *see* Lurasidone *on page 1104*
♦ **Lazanda®** *see* FentaNYL *on page 709*
♦ ***l*-Bunolol Hydrochloride** *see* Levobunolol *on page 1048*
♦ **LCM** *see* Lacosamide *on page 1018*
♦ **L-Deoxythymidine** *see* Telbivudine *on page 1744*
♦ **L-Deprenyl** *see* Selegiline *on page 1663*
♦ **LdT** *see* Telbivudine *on page 1744*

Leflunomide (le FLOO noh mide)

Brand Names: U.S. Arava®
Brand Names: Canada Apo-Leflunomide®; Arava®; Mylan-Leflunomide; Novo-Leflunomide; PHL-Leflunomide; PMS-Leflunomide; Sandoz-Leflunomide
Generic Availability (U.S.) Yes
Pharmacologic Category Antirheumatic, Disease Modifying

Use Treatment of active rheumatoid arthritis; indicated to reduce signs and symptoms, and to inhibit structural damage and improve physical function

Unlabeled/Investigational Use Treatment of cytomegalovirus (CMV) disease in transplant recipients resistant to standard antivirals; prevention of acute and chronic rejection in recipients of solid organ transplants

Contraindications Hypersensitivity to leflunomide or any component of the formulation

Warnings/Precautions Hazardous agent - use appropriate precautions for handling and disposal. **[U.S. Boxed Warning]: Use has been associated with rare reports of hepatotoxicity, hepatic failure, and death. Treatment should not be initiated in patients with pre-existing acute or chronic liver disease or ALT >2 x ULN. Use caution in patients with concurrent exposure to potentially hepatotoxic drugs. Monitor ALT levels during therapy; discontinue if ALT >3 x ULN occurs and, if hepatotoxicity is likely leflunomide-induced, start drug elimination procedures** (eg, cholestyramine, charcoal).

Use has been associated (rarely) with interstitial lung disease; discontinue in patients who develop new onset or worsening of pulmonary symptoms. Drug elimination procedures should be considered if interstitial lung disease occurs; fatal outcomes have been reported. May increase susceptibility to infection, including opportunistic pathogens. Severe infections, sepsis, and fatalities have been reported. Not recommended in patients with severe immunodeficiency, bone marrow dysplasia, or severe, uncontrolled infections. Caution should be exercised when considering the use in patients with a history of new/recurrent infections, with conditions that predispose them to infections, or with chronic, latent, or localized infections. Patients who develop a new infection while undergoing treatment should be monitored closely; consider discontinuation of therapy and drug elimination procedures if infection is serious.

Use may affect defenses against malignancies; impact on the development and course of malignancies is not fully defined. As compared to the general population, an increased risk of lymphoma has been noted in clinical trials; however, rheumatoid arthritis has been previously associated with an increased rate of lymphoma. Use with caution in patients with a prior history of significant hematologic abnormalities; avoid use with bone marrow dysplasia. Use has been associated with rare pancytopenia, agranulocytosis, and thrombocytopenia, generally when concurrently or recently with methotrexate or other immunosuppressive agents. Monitoring of hematologic function is required; discontinue if evidence of bone marrow suppression and begin drug elimination procedures (eg, cholestyramine or activated charcoal). Rare cases of dermatologic reactions (including Stevens-Johnson syndrome and toxic epidermal necrolysis) have been reported; discontinue if evidence of severe dermatologic reaction occurs, and begin drug elimination procedures (eg, cholestyramine or activated charcoal).

Safety has not been established in patients with latent tuberculosis infection. Patients should be screened for tuberculosis and if necessary, treated prior to initiating therapy. Use with caution in patients with renal impairment. Patients should be brought up to date with all immunizations before initiating therapy. Live vaccines should not be given concurrently; there is no data available concerning secondary transmission of live vaccines in patients receiving therapy. Due to variations in clearance, it may take up to 2 years to reach low levels of leflunomide metabolite serum concentrations. A drug elimination procedure using cholestyramine or activated charcoal is recommended when a more rapid elimination is needed.

Adverse Reactions (Reflective of adult population; not specific for elderly)
>10%:
  Gastrointestinal: Diarrhea (17%)
  Respiratory: Respiratory tract infection (4% to 15%)
1% to 10%:
  Cardiovascular: Hypertension (10%), chest pain (2%), edema (peripheral), palpitation, tachycardia, vasodilation, varicose vein, vasculitis
  Central nervous system: Headache (7%), dizziness (4%), pain (2%), anxiety, depression, fever, insomnia, malaise, migraine, sleep disorder, vertigo
  Dermatologic: Alopecia (10%), rash (10%), pruritus (4%), dry skin (2%), eczema (2%), acne, bruising, dermatitis, hair discoloration, hematoma, nail disorder, skin disorder/discoloration, skin ulcer, subcutaneous nodule
  Endocrine & metabolic: Hypokalemia (1%), diabetes mellitus, hyperglycemia, hyperlipidemia, hyperthyroidism, menstrual disorder
  Gastrointestinal: Nausea (9%), abdominal pain (5% to 6%), dyspepsia (5%), weight loss (4%), anorexia (3%), gastroenteritis (3%), mouth ulceration (3%), vomiting (3%), candidiasis (oral), colitis, constipation, esophagitis, flatulence, gastritis, gingivitis, melena, salivary gland enlarged, stomatitis, taste disturbance, xerostomia
  Genitourinary: Urinary tract infection (5%), albuminuria, cystitis, dysuria, prostate disorder, urinary frequency, vaginal candidiasis
  Hematologic: Anemia

◀ Hepatic: Abnormal LFTs (5%), cholelithiasis

Local: Abscess

Neuromuscular & skeletal: Back pain (5%), joint disorder (4%), weakness (3%), tenosynovitis (3%), synovitis (2%), paresthesia (2%), arthralgia (1%), leg cramps (1%), arthrosis, bone necrosis, bone pain, bursitis, CPK increased, myalgia, neck pain, neuralgia, neuritis, pelvic pain, tendon rupture

Ocular: Blurred vision, cataract, conjunctivitis, eye disorder

Renal: Hematuria

Respiratory: Bronchitis (7%), cough (3%), pharyngitis (3%), pneumonia (2%), rhinitis (2%), sinusitis (2%), asthma, dyspnea, epistaxis

Miscellaneous: Accidental injury (5%), allergic reactions (2%), flu-like syndrome (2%), cyst, diaphoresis, hernia, herpes infection

Drug Interactions

Metabolism/Transport Effects Inhibits CYP2C9 (weak)

Avoid Concomitant Use

Avoid concomitant use of Leflunomide with any of the following: BCG; Natalizumab; Pimecrolimus; Tacrolimus (Topical)

Increased Effect/Toxicity

Leflunomide may increase the levels/effects of: Carvedilol; CYP2C9 Substrates (High risk); Natalizumab; TOLBUTamide; Vaccines (Live); Vitamin K Antagonists

The levels/effects of Leflunomide may be increased by: Denosumab; Immunosuppressants; Methotrexate; Pimecrolimus; Rifampin; Roflumilast; Tacrolimus (Topical); TOLBUTamide; Trastuzumab

Decreased Effect

Leflunomide may decrease the levels/effects of: BCG; Sipuleucel-T; Vaccines (Inactivated)

The levels/effects of Leflunomide may be decreased by: Bile Acid Sequestrants; Charcoal, Activated; Echinacea

Ethanol/Nutrition/Herb Interactions

Food: No interactions with food have been noted.

Herb/Nutraceutical: Echinacea may diminish the therapeutic effect of leflunomide.

Stability Store at 25°C (77°F); excursions permitted to 15°C to 30°C (59°F to 86°F). Protect from light.

Mechanism of Action Leflunomide is an immunodulatory agent that inhibits pyrimidine synthesis, resulting in antiproliferative and anti-inflammatory effects. Leflunomide is a prodrug; the active metabolite is responsible for activity. For CMV, may interfere with virion assembly.

Pharmacodynamics/Kinetics

Distribution: V_d: M1: 0.13 L/kg

Protein binding: M1: >99% to albumin

Metabolism: Hepatic to an active metabolite M1 (also known as A77 1726 or teriflunomide), which accounts for nearly all pharmacologic activity; further metabolism to multiple inactive metabolites; undergoes enterohepatic recirculation

Bioavailability: 80% (relative to oral solution)

Half-life elimination: M1: Mean: 14-15 days; enterohepatic recycling appears to contribute to the long half-life of this agent, since activated charcoal and cholestyramine substantially reduce plasma half-life

Time to peak: M1: 6-12 hours

Excretion: Feces (48%); urine (43%)

Dosage

Geriatric & Adult

Rheumatoid arthritis: Oral: Loading dose: 100 mg/day for 3 days, followed by 20 mg/day; **Note:** The loading dose may be omitted in patients at increased risk of hepatic or hematologic toxicity (eg, recent concomitant methotrexate). Dosage may be decreased to 10 mg/day in patients who have difficulty tolerating the 20 mg dose. Due to the long half-life of the active metabolite, serum concentrations may require a prolonged period to decline after dosage reduction.

CMV disease, resistant to standard antivirals (unlabeled use): Oral: Some authors recommend 100-200 mg/day for 5-7 days, followed by 40-60 mg/day (Avery, 2004; Avery, 2010). Others have utilized the standard rheumatoid arthritis dosing (John, 2004). Adjust dose based on serum concentrations of metabolite and adverse events (Avery, 2008; Avery, 2010; Williams, 2002).

Renal Impairment No specific dosage adjustment is recommended. There is no clinical experience in the use of leflunomide in patients with renal impairment. The free fraction of M1 is doubled in dialysis patients. Patients should be monitored closely for adverse effects requiring dosage adjustment.

LETROZOLE

Hepatic Impairment Not recommended for use in patients with pre-existing liver disease or in patients with significant hepatic impairment (ALT >2 times ULN). Patients should have LFTs monitored closely. Discontinue leflunomide if ALT >3 times ULN.

Administration Administer without regard to meals.

Monitoring Parameters A complete blood count (WBC, platelet count, hemoglobin or hematocrit), serum phosphate, as well as serum transaminase determinations should be monitored at baseline and monthly during the initial 6 months of treatment; if stable, monitoring frequency may be decreased to every 6-8 weeks thereafter (continue monthly when used in combination with other immunosuppressive agents). ALT should be monitored at least monthly for the first 6 months of treatment, then every 6-8 weeks thereafter (discontinue if ALT >3 x ULN, treat with cholestyramine, and monitor liver function at least weekly until normal). In addition, monitor for signs/symptoms of severe infection, abnormalities in hepatic function tests, symptoms of hepatotoxicity, and blood pressure. If coadministered with methotrexate, monthly transaminases (ALT, AST) and serum albumin levels are recommended. Screen for tuberculosis prior to therapy.

When used for CMV disease, monitor serum trough concentrations of active metabolite (also see Reference Range).

Reference Range CMV disease:

Timing of serum samples: Initial: Obtain 24 hours after last dose of loading regimen and periodically thereafter

Therapeutic concentration: Active metabolite (A77 1726, M1, or teriflunomide): Trough: 50-80 mcg/mL (Avery, 2010) or up to 100 mcg/mL (Williams, 2002)

Special Geriatric Considerations In Phase III studies, no difference in safety and effectiveness were seen between older and younger adults. No dosage reduction necessary based on age alone; monitor in renal and hepatic impairment.

Dosage Forms Excipient information presented when available (limited, particularly for generics); consult specific product labeling.

Tablet, oral: 10 mg, 20 mg
Arava®: 10 mg, 20 mg

Selected References

Avery RK, "Update in Management of Ganciclovir-Resistant Cytomegalovirus Infection," *Curr Opin Infect Dis*, 2008, 21 (4):433-7.

♦ **Lescol®** *see* Fluvastatin *on page 776*
♦ **Lescol® XL** *see* Fluvastatin *on page 776*

Letrozole (LET roe zole)

Medication Safety Issues
Sound-alike/look-alike issues:
Femara® may be confused with Famvir®, femhrt®, Provera®
Letrozole may be confused with anastrozole

Brand Names: U.S. Femara®

Brand Names: Canada Femara®; MED-Letrozole; PMS-Letrozole; Sandoz-Letrozole

Index Terms CGS-20267

Generic Availability (U.S.) Yes

Pharmacologic Category Antineoplastic Agent, Aromatase Inhibitor

Use For use in postmenopausal women in the adjuvant treatment of hormone receptor positive early breast cancer, extended adjuvant treatment of early breast cancer after 5 years of tamoxifen, advanced breast cancer with disease progression following antiestrogen therapy, hormone receptor positive or hormone receptor unknown, locally-advanced, or first-line (or second-line) treatment of advanced or metastatic breast cancer

Unlabeled/Investigational Use Treatment of ovarian (epithelial) cancer, endometrial cancer

Warnings/Precautions Hazardous agent - use appropriate precautions for handling and disposal. Use caution with hepatic impairment; dose adjustment recommended in patients with cirrhosis or severe hepatic dysfunction. May cause dizziness, fatigue, and somnolence; patients should be cautioned before performing tasks which require mental alertness (eg, operating machinery or driving). May increase total serum cholesterol; in patients treated with adjuvant therapy and cholesterol levels within normal limits, an increase of >1.5 x ULN in total cholesterol has been demonstrated in 8.2% of letrozole-treated patients (25% requiring lipid-lowering medications) vs 3.2% of tamoxifen-treated patients (16% requiring medications); monitor cholesterol panel; may require antihyperlipidemics. May cause decreases in bone mineral density (BMD); a decrease in hip BMD by 3.8% from baseline in letrozole-treated patients vs 2% in placebo at 2 years has been demonstrated; however, there was no statistical difference in changes to the lumbar spine BMD scores; monitor BMD.

◀ **Adverse Reactions (Reflective of adult population; not specific for elderly)**
>10%:
Cardiovascular: Edema (7% to 18%)
Central nervous system: Headache (4% to 20%), dizziness (3% to 14%), fatigue (8% to 13%)
Endocrine & metabolic: Hypercholesterolemia (3% to 52%), hot flashes (6% to 50%)
Gastrointestinal: Nausea (9% to 17%), weight gain (2% to 13%), constipation (2% to 11%)
Neuromuscular & skeletal: Weakness (4% to 34%), arthralgia (8% to 25%), arthritis (7% to 25%), bone pain (5% to 22%), back pain (5% to 18%), bone mineral density decreased/osteoporosis (5% to 15%), bone fracture (10% to 14%)
Respiratory: Dyspnea (6% to 18%), cough (6% to 13%)
Miscellaneous: Diaphoresis (≤24%), night sweats (15%)
1% to 10%:
Cardiovascular: Chest pain (6% to 8%), hypertension (5% to 8%), chest wall pain (6%), peripheral edema (5%), cerebrovascular accident (2% to 3%), thromboembolic event (2% to 3%), MI (1% to 2%), angina (1%)
Central nervous system: Insomnia (6% to 7%), pain (5%), anxiety (<5%), depression (<5%), vertigo (<5%),somnolence (3%)
Dermatologic: Rash (5%), alopecia (3% to 5%), pruritus (1%)
Endocrine & metabolic: Breast pain (2% to 7%), hypercalcemia (<5%)
Gastrointestinal: Diarrhea (5% to 8%), vomiting (3% to 7%), weight loss (6% to 7%), abdominal pain (6%), anorexia (1% to 5%), dyspepsia (3%)
Genitourinary: Urinary tract infection (6%), vaginal bleeding (5%), vaginal dryness (5%), vaginal hemorrhage (5%), vaginal irritation (5%)
Neuromuscular & skeletal: Limb pain (4% to 10%), myalgia (7% to 9%)
Ocular: Cataract (2%)
Renal: Renal disorder (5%)
Respiratory: Pleural effusion (<5%)
Miscellaneous: Infection (7%), influenza (6%), viral infection (6%), secondary malignancy (2% to 4%)

Drug Interactions
Metabolism/Transport Effects Substrate (minor) of CYP2A6, 3A4; **Inhibits** CYP2A6 (strong), 2C19 (weak)
Avoid Concomitant Use There are no known interactions where it is recommended to avoid concomitant use.
Increased Effect/Toxicity
Letrozole may increase the levels/effects of: CYP2A6 Substrates

The levels/effects of Letrozole may be increased by: Conivaptan
Decreased Effect
The levels/effects of Letrozole may be decreased by: Tamoxifen; Tocilizumab

Stability Store at room temperature of 25°C (77°F); excursions permitted to 15°C to 30°C (59°F to 86°F).
Mechanism of Action Nonsteroidal competitive inhibitor of the aromatase enzyme system which binds to the heme group of aromatase, a cytochrome P450 enzyme which catalyzes conversion of androgens to estrogens (specifically, androstenedione to estrone and testosterone to estradiol). This leads to inhibition of the enzyme and a significant reduction in plasma estrogen (estrone, estradiol and estrone sulfate) levels. Does not affect synthesis of adrenal or thyroid hormones, aldosterone, or androgens.

Pharmacodynamics/Kinetics
Absorption: Rapid and well absorbed; not affected by food
Distribution: V_d: ~1.9 L/kg
Protein binding, plasma: Weak
Metabolism: Hepatic via CYP3A4 and 2A6 to an inactive carbinol metabolite
Half-life elimination: Terminal: ~2 days
Time to steady state, plasma: 2-6 weeks
Excretion: Urine (90%; 6% as unchanged drug, 75% as glucuronide carbinol metabolite, 9% as unidentified metabolites)

Dosage
Geriatric & Adult Females: Postmenopausal:
Breast cancer, advanced (first- or second-line treatment): Oral: 2.5 mg once daily; continue until tumor progression
Breast cancer, early (adjuvant treatment): Oral: 2.5 mg once daily; optimal duration unknown, duration in clinical trial is 5 years; discontinue at relapse
Breast cancer, early (extended adjuvant treatment): Oral: 2.5 mg once daily; optimal duration unknown, duration in clinical trials is 5 years (after 5 years of tamoxifen); discontinue at relapse

Ovarian (epithelial) cancer (unlabeled use): Oral: 2.5 mg once daily; continue until disease progression (Ramirez, 2008)

Renal Impairment No dosage adjustment is required in patients with renal impairment if Cl$_{cr}$ is ≥10 mL/minute.

Hepatic Impairment

Mild-to-moderate impairment (Child-Pugh class A and B): No adjustment recommended.

Severe impairment (Child-Pugh class C) and cirrhosis: 2.5 mg every other day.

Administration Administer with or without food.

Monitoring Parameters Monitor periodically during therapy: Complete blood counts, thyroid function tests; serum electrolytes, cholesterol, transaminases, and creatinine; blood pressure; bone density

Pharmacotherapy Pearls Oncology Comment: The American Society of Clinical Oncology (ASCO) guidelines for adjuvant endocrine therapy in postmenopausal women with HR-positive breast cancer (Burstein, 2010) recommend considering aromatase inhibitor (AI) therapy at some point in the treatment course (primary, sequentially, or extended). Optimal duration at this time is not known; however, treatment with an AI should not exceed 5 years in primary and extended therapies, and 2-3 years if followed by tamoxifen in sequential therapy (total of 5 years). If initial therapy with AI has been discontinued before the 5 years, consideration should be taken to receive tamoxifen for a total of 5 years. The optimal time to switch to an AI is also not known, but data supports switching after 2-3 years of tamoxifen (sequential) or after 5 years of tamoxifen (extended). If patient becomes intolerant or has poor adherence, consideration should be made to switch to another AI or initiate tamoxifen.

Special Geriatric Considerations No dosage adjustment recommended.

Dosage Forms Excipient information presented when available (limited, particularly for generics); consult specific product labeling.

Tablet, oral: 2.5 mg

Femara®: 2.5 mg

Selected References

Coates AS, Keshaviah A, Thurlimann B, et al, "Five Years of Letrozole Compared With Tamoxifen as Initial Adjuvant Therapy for Postmenopausal Women With Endocrine-Responsive Early Breast Cancer: Update of Study BIG 1-98," *J Clin Oncol*, 2007, 25(5):486-92.

National Comprehensive Cancer Network® (NCCN), "Clinical Practice Guidelines in Oncology™: Breast Cancer," Version 1.2009. Available at http://www.nccn.org/professionals/physician_gls/PDF/breast.pdf.

National Comprehensive Cancer Network® (NCCN), "Clinical Practice Guidelines in Oncology™: Breast Cancer Risk Reduction, Version 1.2009." Accessible at http://www.nccn.org/professionals/physician_gls/PDF/breast_risk.pdf

Smith IE and Dowsett M, "Aromatase Inhibitors in Breast Cancer," *N Engl J Med*, 2003, 348(24):2431-42.

Visvanathan K, Chlebowski RT, Hurley P, et al, "American Society of Clinical Oncology Clinical Practice Guideline Update on the Use of Pharmacologic Interventions Including Tamoxifen, Raloxifene, and Aromatase Inhibition for Breast Cancer Risk Reduction," *J Clin Oncol*, 2009, 27(19):3235-58.

◆ **Leukeran®** see Chlorambucil on page 331

Leuprolide (loo PROE lide)

Medication Safety Issues

Sound-alike/look-alike issues:

Lupron® may be confused with Nuprin®

Lupron Depot® (1-month or 3-month formulation) may be confused with Lupron Depot-Ped® (1-month or 3-month formulation)

Lupron Depot-Ped® is available in two formulations, a 1-month formulation and a 3-month formulation. Both formulations offer an 11.25 mg strength which may further add confusion.

Brand Names: U.S. Eligard®; Lupron Depot-Ped®; Lupron Depot®

Brand Names: Canada Eligard®; Lupron®; Lupron® Depot®

Index Terms Abbott-43818; Leuprolide Acetate; Leuprorelin Acetate; TAP-144

Generic Availability (U.S.) Yes: Injection (solution)

Pharmacologic Category Antineoplastic Agent, Gonadotropin-Releasing Hormone Agonist; Gonadotropin Releasing Hormone Agonist

Use Palliative treatment of advanced prostate cancer; management of endometriosis; treatment of anemia caused by uterine leiomyomata (fibroids)

Unlabeled/Investigational Use Treatment of breast cancer; prostatic hyperplasia

Contraindications Hypersensitivity to leuprolide, GnRH, GnRH-agonist analogs, or any component of the formulation; undiagnosed abnormal vaginal bleeding

Lupron Depot®-4 month (30 mg) is not indicated for use in women

Eligard® and Viadur® are contraindicated in women

Warnings/Precautions Hazardous agent - use appropriate precautions for handling and disposal. Transient increases in testosterone serum levels occur at the start of treatment. Androgen-deprivation therapy may increase the risk for cardiovascular disease (Levine, 2010). Tumor flare, bone pain, neuropathy, urinary tract obstruction, and spinal cord compression have been reported when used for prostate cancer; closely observe patients ►

for weakness, paresthesias, hematuria, and urinary tract obstruction in first few weeks of therapy. Observe patients with metastatic vertebral lesions or urinary obstruction closely. Exacerbation of endometriosis or uterine leiomyomata may occur initially. Decreased bone density has been reported when used for ≥6 months; use caution in patients with additional risk factors for bone loss (eg, chronic alcohol use, corticosteroid therapy). In patients with prostate cancer, androgen deprivation therapy may increase the risk for cardiovascular disease, diabetes, insulin resistance, obesity, alterations in lipids, and fractures. Use caution in patients with a history of psychiatric illness; alteration in mood, memory impairment, and depression have been associated with use. Rare cases of pituitary apoplexy (frequently secondary to pituitary adenoma) have been observed with leuprolide administration (onset from 1 hour to usually <2 weeks); may present as sudden headache, vomiting, visual or mental status changes, and infrequently cardiovascular collapse; immediate medical attention required. Females treated for precocious puberty may experience menses or spotting during the first 2 months of treatment; notify healthcare provider if bleeding continues after the second month.

Some dosage forms may contain benzyl alcohol; patients with benzyl alcohol allergy may demonstrate a hypersensitivity reaction (usually local) in the form of erythema and induration at the injection site. Vehicle used in injectable (polylactide-co-glycolide microspheres) has rarely been associated with retinal artery occlusion in patients with abnormal arteriovenous anastomosis.

Adverse Reactions (Reflective of adult population; not specific for elderly) Note:
For prostate cancer treatment, an initial rise in serum testosterone concentrations may cause "tumor flare" or worsening of symptoms, including bone pain, neuropathy, hematuria, or ureteral or bladder outlet obstruction during the first 2 weeks. Similarly, an initial increase in estradiol levels, with a temporary worsening of symptoms, may occur in women treated with leuprolide.

Delayed release formulations:
10%:
Cardiovascular: Edema (≤14%)
Central nervous system: Headache (≤65%), pain (<2% to 33%), depression (≤31%), insomnia (≤31%), fatigue (≤17%), dizziness/vertigo (≤16%)
Dermatologic: Skin reaction (≤12%)
Endocrine & metabolic: Hot flashes (25% to 98%), testicular atrophy (≤20%), hyperlipidemia (≤12%), libido decreased (≤11%)
Gastrointestinal: Nausea/vomiting (≤25%), bowel function altered (≤14%), weight gain/ loss (≤13%)
Genitourinary: Vaginitis (11% to 28%), urinary disorder (13% to 15%)
Local: Injection site burning/stinging (transient; ≤35%)
Neuromuscular & skeletal: Weakness (≤18%), joint disorder (≤12%)
Miscellaneous: Flu-like syndrome (≤12%)
1% to 10% (limited to important or life-threatening):
Cardiovascular: Angina (<5%), arrhythmia (<5%), atrial fibrillation (<5%), bradycardia (<5%), CHF (<5%), deep thrombophlebitis (<5%), hyper-/hypotension (<5%), palpitation (<5%), syncope (<5%), tachycardia (<5%)
Central nervous system: Nervousness (≤8%), anxiety (≤6%), confusion (<5%), delusions (<5%), dementia (<5%), fever (<5%), seizure (<5%)
Dermatologic: Acne (≤10%), alopecia (≤5%), bruising (≤5%), cellulitis (<5%), pruritus (≤3%), hirsutism (<2%), rash (<2%)
Endocrine & metabolic: Dehydration (≤8%), gynecomastia (≤7%), breast tenderness/pain (≤6%), bicarbonate decreased (≥5%), hyper-/hypocholesterolemia (≥5%), hyperglycemia (≥5%), hyperphosphatemia (≥5%), hyperuricemia (≥5%), hypoalbuminemia (≥5%), hypoproteinemia (≥5%), lactation (<5%), testicular pain (≤4%), menstrual disorder (≤2%)
Gastrointestinal: Dysphagia (<5%), gastrointestinal hemorrhage (<5%), intestinal obstruction (<5%), ulcer (<5%), gastroenteritis/colitis (≤3%), diarrhea (≤2%), constipation (≤2%)
Genitourinary: Prostatic acid phosphatase increased/decreased (≥5%), urine specific gravity increased/decreased (≥5%), impotence (≤5%), balanitis (<5%), incontinence (<5%), penile/testis disorder (<5%), urinary tract infection (<5%), nocturia (≤4%), polyuria (2% to 4%), bladder spasm (<2%), dysuria (<2%), erectile dysfunction (<2%), hematuria (<2%), urinary retention (<2%), urinary urgency (<2%)
Hematologic: Eosinophilia (≥5%), leukopenia (≥5%), platelets increased (≥5%), anemia
Hepatic: Liver function tests abnormal (≥5%), partial thromboplastin time increased (≥5%), prothrombin time increased (≥5%), hepatomegaly (<5%)
Local: Injection site pain (2% to 5%), injection site erythema (1% to 3%)
Neuromuscular & skeletal: Myalgia (≤8%), paresthesia (≤8%), neuropathy (<5%), paralysis (<5%), pathologic fracture (<5%), bone pain (<2%)
Renal: BUN increased (≥5%), creatinine increased (≥5%)

Respiratory: Emphysema (<5%), epistaxis (<5%), hemoptysis (<5%), pleural effusion (<5%), pulmonary edema (<5%), dyspnea (≤2%)

Miscellaneous: Diaphoresis (≤5%), allergic reaction (<5%), infection (5%), lymphadenopathy (<5%)

Immediate release formulation:

>10%:

Cardiovascular: ECG changes/ischemia (19%), peripheral edema (12%)

Central nervous system: Pain (13%)

Endocrine & metabolic: Hot flashes (55%)

1% to 10% (limited to important or life-threatening):

Cardiovascular: Hypertension (8%), murmur (3%), thrombosis/phlebitis (2%), CHF (1%), angina, arrhythmia, MI, syncope

Central nervous system: Headache (7%), insomnia (7%), dizziness/lightheadedness (5%), anxiety, depression, fatigue, fever, nervousness

Dermatologic: Dermatitis (5%), alopecia, bruising, itching, lesions, pigmentation

Endocrine & metabolic: Gynecomastia/breast tenderness/pain (7%), testicular size decreased (7%), diabetes, hypercalcemia, hypoglycemia, libido decreased, thyroid enlarged

Gastrointestinal: Constipation (7%), anorexia (6%), nausea/vomiting (5%), diarrhea, dysphagia, gastrointestinal bleeding, peptic ulcer, rectal polyps

Genitourinary: Urinary frequency/urgency (6%), impotence (4%), urinary tract infection (3%), bladder spasm, dysuria, incontinence, testicular pain, urinary obstruction

Hematologic: Anemia (5%)

Local: Injection site reaction

Neuromuscular & skeletal: Weakness (10%), bone pain (5%), peripheral neuropathy

Ocular: Blurred vision

Renal: Hematuria (6%), BUN increased, creatinine increased

Respiratory: Dyspnea (2%), cough, pneumonia, pulmonary embolus, pulmonary fibrosis

Miscellaneous: Infection, inflammation

Drug Interactions

Avoid Concomitant Use There are no known interactions where it is recommended to avoid concomitant use.

Increased Effect/Toxicity There are no known significant interactions involving an increase in effect.

Decreased Effect

Leuprolide may decrease the levels/effects of: Antidiabetic Agents

Stability

Eligard®: Store at 2°C to 8°C (36°F to 46°F). Allow to reach room temperature prior to using. Once mixed, must be administered within 30 minutes. Eligard® is packaged in two syringes; one contains the Atrigel® polymer system and the second contains leuprolide acetate powder. Follow package instructions for mixing.

Lupron Depot®, Lupron Depot-Ped®: Store at room temperature of 25°C (77°F); excursions permitted to 15°C to 30°C (59°F to 86°F). Upon reconstitution, the suspension does not contain a preservative and should be used immediately; discard if not used within 2 hours. Reconstitute only with diluent provided.

Leuprolide acetate 5 mg/mL solution: Store at 20°C to 25°C (68°F to 77°F); excursions permitted to 15°C to 30°C (59°F to 86°F). Protect from light and store vial in carton until use. Do not freeze.

Mechanism of Action Leuprolide, is an agonist of luteinizing hormone-releasing hormone (LHRH). Acting as a potent inhibitor of gonadotropin secretion; continuous administration results in suppression of ovarian and testicular steroidogenesis due to decreased levels of LH and FSH with subsequent decrease in testosterone (male) and estrogen (female) levels. In males, testosterone levels are reduced to below castrate levels. Leuprolide may also have a direct inhibitory effect on the testes, and act by a different mechanism not directly related to reduction in serum testosterone.

Pharmacodynamics/Kinetics

Onset of action: Following transient increase, testosterone suppression occurs in ~2-4 weeks of continued therapy

Distribution: Males: V_d: 27 L

Protein binding: 43% to 49%

Metabolism: Major metabolite, pentapeptide (M-1)

Bioavailability: SubQ: 94%

Excretion: Urine (<5% as parent and major metabolite)

◀ **Dosage**
Geriatric & Adult
Advanced prostate cancer:
I.M.:
Lupron Depot® 7.5 mg (monthly): 7.5 mg every month **or**
Lupron Depot® 22.5 mg (3 month): 22.5 mg every 12 weeks **or**
Lupron Depot® 30 mg (4 month): 30 mg every 16 weeks **or**
Lupron Depot® 45 mg (6 month): 45 mg every 24 weeks
SubQ:
Eligard®: 7.5 mg monthly **or** 22.5 mg every 3 months **or** 30 mg every 4 months **or** 45 mg every 6 months
Leuprolide acetate 5 mg/mL solution: 1 mg/day
Endometriosis: I.M.: Initial therapy may be with leuprolide alone or in combination with norethindrone; if retreatment for an additional 6 months is necessary, concomitant norethindrone should be used. Retreatment is not recommended for longer than one additional 6-month course.
Lupron Depot®: 3.75 mg every month for up to 6 months **or**
Lupron Depot®-3 month: 11.25 mg every 3 months for up to 2 doses (6 months total duration of treatment)
Uterine leiomyomata (fibroids): I.M. (in combination with iron):
Lupron Depot®: 3.75 mg every month for up to 3 months **or**
Lupron Depot®-3 month: 11.25 mg as a single injection
Breast cancer, premenopausal ovarian ablation (unlabeled use): I.M.:
Lupron Depot®: 3.75 mg every 28 days for up to 24 months (Boccardo, 1999) **or**
Lupron Depot®-3 month: 11.25 mg every 3 months for up to 24 months (Boccardo, 1999; Schmid, 2007)
Administration
I.M.: Lupron Depot®, Lupron Depot-Ped®: Administer as a single injection. Vary injection site periodically
SubQ:
Eligard®: Vary injection site; choose site with adequate subcutaneous tissue (eg, upper or mid-abdomen, upper buttocks); avoid areas that may be compressed or rubbed (eg, belt or waistband)
Leuprolide acetate 5 mg/mL solution: Vary injection site; if an alternate syringe from the syringe provided is required, insulin syringes should be used
Monitoring Parameters Bone mineral density
Prostatic cancer: LH and FSH levels, serum testosterone (2-4 weeks after initiation of therapy), PSA; weakness, paresthesias, and urinary tract obstruction in first few weeks of therapy. Screen for diabetes and cardiovascular risk prior to initiating treatment.
Test Interactions Interferes with pituitary gonadotropic and gonadal function tests during and up to 3 months after monthly administration of leuprolide therapy.
Pharmacotherapy Pearls
Eligard® Atrigel®: A nongelatin-based, biodegradable, polymer matrix

Oncology Comment: Guidelines from the American Society of Clinical Oncology (ASCO) for hormonal management of advanced prostate cancer which is androgen-sensitive (Loblaw, 2007) recommend either orchiectomy or luteinizing hormone-releasing hormone (LHRH) agonists as initial treatment for androgen deprivation.
Special Geriatric Considerations No dosage adjustments are needed in the elderly. Monitoring for bone density changes, serum lipid, hemoglobin A_{1c}, blood pressure, and serum calcium changes is recommended.
Product Availability
Lupron Depot-Ped® 3-month formulation: FDA approved August 2011; availability expected August 2011
Lupron Depot-Ped® 3-month formulation will be available in two strengths, 11.25 mg and 30 mg.
Dosage Forms Excipient information presented when available (limited, particularly for generics); consult specific product labeling.
Injection, powder for reconstitution, as acetate [depot formulation, preservative free]:
Eligard®: 7.5 mg (monthly), 22.5 mg (3 month), 30 mg (4 month), 45 mg (6 month) [contains polylactide-co-glycolide; supplied with diluent]
Lupron Depot-Ped®: 7.5 mg (monthly), 11.25 mg (3 month), 11.25 mg (monthly), 15 mg (monthly), 30 mg (3 month) [contains polylactide-co-glycolide, polysorbate 80]
Lupron Depot®: 3.75 mg (monthly), 7.5 mg (monthly), 11.25 mg (3 month), 22.5 mg (3 month), 30 mg (4 month), 45 mg (6 month) [contains polylactide-co-glycolide, polysorbate 80]
Injection, solution, as acetate: 5 mg/mL (2.8 mL)

Selected References

Adjuvant Breast Cancer Trials Collaborative Group, "Ovarian Ablation or Suppression in Premenopausal Early Breast Cancer: Results From the International Adjuvant Breast Cancer Ovarian Ablation or Suppression Randomized Trial," *J Natl Cancer Inst*, 2007, 99(7):516-25.

Boccardo F, Rubagotti A, Amoroso D, et al, "Endocrinological and Clinical Evaluation of Two Depot Formulations of Leuprolide Acetate in Pre- and Perimenopausal Breast Cancer Patients," *Cancer Chemother Pharmacol*, 1999, 43 (6):461-6.

National Comprehensive Cancer Network® (NCCN), "Clinical Practice Guidelines in Oncology™: Breast Cancer," Version 1.2009. Available at http://www.nccn.org/professionals/physician_gls/PDF/breast.pdf.

National Comprehensive Cancer Network® (NCCN), "Clinical Practice Guidelines in Oncology™: Ovarian Cancer," Version 2.2009. Available at http://www.nccn.org/professionals/physician_gls/PDF/ovarian.pdf

National Comprehensive Cancer Network® (NCCN), "Clinical Practice Guidelines in Oncology™: Prostate Carcinoma," Version 2.2009. Available at http://www.nccn.org/professionals/physician_gls/PDF/prostate.pdf

◆ **Leuprolide Acetate** *see* Leuprolide *on page 1039*
◆ **Leuprorelin Acetate** *see* Leuprolide *on page 1039*

Levalbuterol (leve al BYOO ter ole)

Related Information

Inhalant Agents *on page 2010*

Medication Safety Issues

Sound-alike/look-alike issues:

Xopenex® may be confused with Xanax®

Brand Names: U.S. Xopenex HFA™; Xopenex®

Brand Names: Canada Xopenex®

Index Terms Levalbuterol Hydrochloride; Levalbuterol Tartrate; R-albuterol

Generic Availability (U.S.) Yes: Excludes aerosol

Pharmacologic Category Beta$_2$-Adrenergic Agonist

Use Treatment or prevention of bronchospasm in adults with reversible obstructive airway disease

Contraindications Hypersensitivity to levalbuterol, albuterol, or any component of the formulation

Warnings/Precautions Optimize anti-inflammatory treatment before initiating maintenance treatment with levalbuterol. Do not use as a component of chronic therapy without an anti-inflammatory agent. Only the mildest form of asthma (Step 1 and/or exercise-induced) would not require concurrent use based upon asthma guidelines. Patient must be instructed to seek medical attention in cases where acute symptoms are not relieved or a previous level of response is diminished. The need to increase frequency of use may indicate deterioration of asthma, and treatment must not be delayed. A spacer device or valved holding chamber is recommended when using a metered-dose inhaler.

Use caution in patients with cardiovascular disease (arrhythmia or hypertension or HF), convulsive disorders, diabetes, glaucoma, hyperthyroidism, or hypokalemia. Beta-agonists may cause elevation in blood pressure, heart rate, and result in CNS stimulation/excitation. Beta$_2$-agonists may increase risk of arrhythmia, increase serum glucose, or decrease serum potassium.

Immediate hypersensitivity reactions (urticaria, angioedema, rash, bronchospasm) have been reported. Do not exceed recommended dose; serious adverse events including fatalities, have been associated with excessive use of inhaled sympathomimetics. Rarely, paradoxical bronchospasm may occur with use of inhaled bronchodilating agents; this should be distinguished from inadequate response.

Adverse Reactions (Reflective of adult population; not specific for elderly)

>10%:

Endocrine & metabolic: Serum glucose increased, serum potassium decreased
Neuromuscular & skeletal: Tremor (≤7%)
Respiratory: Rhinitis (3% to 11%)
Miscellaneous: Viral infection (7% to 12%)

>2% to 10%:

Central nervous system: Headache (8% to 12%), nervousness (3% to 10%), dizziness (1% to 3%), anxiety (≤3%), migraine (≤3%), weakness (3%)
Cardiovascular: Tachycardia (~3%)
Dermatologic: Rash (≤8%)
Gastrointestinal: Diarrhea (2% to 6%), dyspepsia (1% to 3%)
Neuromuscular & skeletal: Leg cramps (≤3%)

◄ Respiratory: Asthma (9%), pharyngitis (3% to 10%), cough (1% to 4%), sinusitis (1% to 4%), nasal edema (1% to 3%)

Miscellaneous: Flu-like syndrome (1% to 4%), accidental injury (≤3%)

Note: Immediate hypersensitivity reactions have occurred (including angioedema, oropharyngeal edema, urticaria, and anaphylaxis).

Drug Interactions

Avoid Concomitant Use

Avoid concomitant use of Levalbuterol with any of the following: Iobenguane I 123

Increased Effect/Toxicity

Levalbuterol may increase the levels/effects of: Loop Diuretics; Sympathomimetics

The levels/effects of Levalbuterol may be increased by: Atomoxetine; Cannabinoids; MAO Inhibitors; Tricyclic Antidepressants

Decreased Effect

Levalbuterol may decrease the levels/effects of: Iobenguane I 123

The levels/effects of Levalbuterol may be decreased by: Alpha-/Beta-Blockers; Beta-Blockers (Beta1 Selective); Beta-Blockers (Nonselective); Betahistine

Stability

Aerosol: Store at room temperature of 20°C to 25°C (68°F to 77°F); protect from freezing and direct sunlight. Store with mouthpiece down. Discard after 200 actuations.

Solution for nebulization: Store in protective foil pouch at room temperature of 20°C to 25°C (68°F to 77°F). Protect from light and excessive heat. Vials should be used within 2 weeks after opening protective pouch. Use within 1 week and protect from light if removed from pouch. Vials of concentrated solution should be used immediately after removing from protective pouch. Concentrated solution should be diluted with 2.5 mL NS prior to use.

Mechanism of Action Relaxes bronchial smooth muscle by action on beta$_2$-receptors with little effect on heart rate

Pharmacodynamics/Kinetics

Onset of action (as measured by a 15% increase in FEV$_1$):

Aerosol: 5.5-10.2 minutes

Peak effect: ~77 minutes

Nebulization: 10-17 minutes

Peak effect: 1.5 hours

Duration (as measured by a 15% increase in FEV$_1$):

Aerosol: 3-4 hours (up to 6 hours in some patients)

Nebulization: 5-6 hours (up to 8 hours in some patients)

Absorption: A portion of inhaled dose is absorbed to systemic circulation

Half-life elimination: 3.3-4 hours

Time to peak, serum:

Aerosol: 0.5 hours

Nebulization: 0.2 hours

Dosage

Geriatric Only a small number of patients have been studied. Although greater sensitivity of some elderly patients cannot be ruled out, no overall differences in safety or effectiveness were observed. An initial dose of 0.63 mg should be used in all patients >65 years of age.

Adult

Bronchospasm:

Metered-dose inhaler: 2 puffs every 4-6 hours

Solution for nebulization: 0.63 mg 3 times/day at intervals of 6-8 hours; dosage may be increased to 1.25 mg 3 times/day with close monitoring for adverse effects

Exacerbation of asthma (acute, severe) *(NIH Guidelines, 2007):*

Metered-dose inhaler: 4-8 puffs every 20 minutes for up to 4 hours, then every 1-4 hours as needed

Solution for nebulization: 1.25-2.5 mg every 20 minutes for 3 doses, then 1.25-5 mg every 1-4 hours as needed

Administration Inhalation:

Metered-dose inhaler: Shake well before use; prime with 4 test sprays prior to first use or if inhaler has not been use of more than 3 days. Clean actuator (mouthpiece) weekly. A spacer device or valved holding chamber is recommended when using a metered-dose inhaler.

Solution for nebulization: Safety and efficacy were established when administered with the following nebulizers: PARI LC Jet™, PARI LC Plus™, as well as the following compressors: PARI Master®, Dura-Neb® 2000, and Dura-Neb® 3000. Concentrated solution should be diluted prior to use. Blow-by administration is not recommended, use a mask device if patient unable to hold mouthpiece in mouth for administration.

Monitoring Parameters Asthma symptoms; FEV$_1$, peak flow, and/or other pulmonary function tests; heart rate, blood pressure, CNS stimulation; arterial blood gases (if condition warrants); serum potassium, serum glucose (in selected patients)

Pharmacotherapy Pearls Slightly smaller increase in heart rate and slightly lower incidence of nervousness were seen with levalbuterol compared to albuterol.

Special Geriatric Considerations For aerosol formulation, start with low end of dosage range. Refer to dosing information for nebulization dosing specifics.

Dosage Forms Excipient information presented when available (limited, particularly for generics); consult specific product labeling. [DSC] = Discontinued product

Aerosol, for oral inhalation, as tartrate [strength expressed as base]:
  Xopenex HFA™: 45 mcg/actuation (15 g) [chlorofluorocarbon free; 200 actuations]
Solution, for nebulization, as hydrochloride [strength expressed as base, preservative free]:
  Xopenex®: 0.31 mg/3 mL (24s); 0.63 mg/3 mL (24s); 1.25 mg/3 mL (24s)
Solution, for nebulization, as hydrochloride [strength expressed as base, concentrate, preservative free]: 1.25 mg/0.5 mL (30s)
  Xopenex®: 1.25 mg/0.5 mL (30s [DSC])

Selected References

National Asthma Education and Prevention Program, "Expert Panel Report 3 (EPR-3): Guidelines for the Diagnosis and Management of Asthma-Summary Report 2007," *J Allergy Clin Immunol*, 2007, 120(5 Suppl):94-138.

◆ **Levalbuterol Hydrochloride** see Levalbuterol on page *1043*
◆ **Levalbuterol Tartrate** see Levalbuterol on page *1043*
◆ **Levaquin®** see Levofloxacin (Systemic) on page *1052*
◆ **Levatol®** see Penbutolol on page *1410*
◆ **Levbid®** see Hyoscyamine on page *902*
◆ **Levemir®** see Insulin Detemir on page *947*
◆ **Levemir® FlexPen®** see Insulin Detemir on page *947*

LevETIRAcetam (lee va tye RA se tam)

Medication Safety Issues

Sound-alike/look-alike issues:
  Keppra® may be confused with Keflex®, Keppra XR™
  LevETIRAcetam may be confused with levOCARNitine, levofloxacin
  Potential for dispensing errors between Keppra® and Kaletra® (lopinavir/ritonavir)

Brand Names: U.S. Keppra XR™; Keppra®

Brand Names: Canada Apo-Levetiracetam®; CO Levetiracetam; Dom-Levetiracetam; Keppra®; PHL-Levetiracetam; PMS-Levetiracetam; PRO-Levetiracetam

Generic Availability (U.S.) Yes: Excludes extended release tablet

Pharmacologic Category Anticonvulsant, Miscellaneous

Use Adjunctive therapy in the treatment of partial onset, myoclonic, and/or primary generalized tonic-clonic seizures

Unlabeled/Investigational Use Bipolar disorder

Medication Guide Available Yes

Contraindications Hypersensitivity to levetiracetam or any component of the formulation

Warnings/Precautions Antiepileptics are associated with an increased risk of suicidal behavior/thoughts with use (regardless of indication); patients should be monitored for signs/symptoms of depression, suicidal tendencies, and other unusual behavior changes during therapy and instructed to inform their healthcare provider immediately if symptoms occur.

Psychotic symptoms (psychosis, hallucinations) and behavioral symptoms (including aggression, anger, anxiety, depersonalization, depression, personality disorder) may occur. Dose reduction may be required. Levetiracetam should be withdrawn gradually to minimize the potential of increased seizure frequency. Use caution with renal impairment; dosage adjustment may be necessary. Weakness, dizziness, and somnolence occur mostly during the first month of therapy. Although rare, decreases in red blood cell counts, hemoglobin, hematocrit, white blood cell counts and neutrophils have been observed.

Adverse Reactions (Reflective of adult population; not specific for elderly)
>10%:
  Central nervous system: Behavioral symptoms (agitation, aggression, anger, anxiety, apathy, depersonalization, depression, emotional lability, hostility, hyperkinesias, irritability, nervousness, neurosis and personality disorder: adults 5% to 13%; children 5% to 38%), somnolence (8% to 23%), headache (14%), hostility (2% to 12%)
  Gastrointestinal: Vomiting (15%), anorexia (3% to 13%)
  Neuromuscular & skeletal: Weakness (9% to 15%)
  Respiratory: Pharyngitis (6% to 14%), rhinitis (4% to 13%), cough (2% to 11%)
  Miscellaneous: Accidental injury (17%), infection (2% to 13%)

1% to 10%:
Cardiovascular: Facial edema (2%)
Central nervous system: Fatigue (10%), nervousness (4% to 10%), dizziness (5% to 9%), personality disorder (8%), pain (6% to 7%), agitation (6%), irritability (6% to 7%), emotional lability (2% to 6%), mood swings (5%), depression (3% to 5%), vertigo (3% to 5%), ataxia (3%), amnesia (2%), anxiety (2%), confusion (2%)
Dermatologic: Bruising (4%), pruritus (2%), rash (2%), skin discoloration (2%)
Endocrine & metabolic: Dehydration (2%)
Gastrointestinal: Diarrhea (8%), nausea (5%), gastroenteritis (4%), constipation (3%)
Genitourinary: Urine abnormality (2%)
Hematologic: Leukocytes decreased (2% to 3%)
Neuromuscular & skeletal: Neck pain (2% to 8%), paresthesia (2%), reflexes increased (2%)
Ocular: Conjunctivitis (3%), diplopia (2%), amblyopia (2%)
Otic: Ear pain (2%)
Renal: Albuminuria (4%)
Respiratory: Influenza (5%), asthma (2%), sinusitis (2%)
Miscellaneous: Flu-like syndrome (3% to 8%), viral infection (2%)

Drug Interactions

Avoid Concomitant Use There are no known interactions where it is recommended to avoid concomitant use.

Increased Effect/Toxicity
LevETIRAcetam may increase the levels/effects of: Alcohol (Ethyl); CNS Depressants; Methotrimeprazine; Selective Serotonin Reuptake Inhibitors

The levels/effects of LevETIRAcetam may be increased by: Droperidol; HydrOXYzine; Methotrimeprazine

Decreased Effect
The levels/effects of LevETIRAcetam may be decreased by: Ketorolac; Ketorolac (Nasal); Ketorolac (Systemic); Mefloquine

Ethanol/Nutrition/Herb Interactions

Ethanol: May increase CNS depression; monitor for increased effects with coadministration. Caution patients about effects.
Food: Food may delay, but does not affect the extent of absorption.

Stability

Oral solution, tablets: Store at 25°C (77°F); excursions permitted to 15°C to 30°C (59°F to 86°F).
Injection solution: Store at 25°C (77°F); excursions permitted to 15°C to 30°C (59°F to 86°F). Must dilute dose in 100 mL of NS, LR, or D_5W. Admixed solution is stable for 24 hours in PVC bags kept at room temperature.

Mechanism of Action

The precise mechanism by which levetiracetam exerts its antiepileptic effect is unknown. However, several studies have suggested the mechanism may involve one or more of the following central pharmacologic effects: inhibition of voltage-dependent N-type calcium channels; facilitation of GABA-ergic inhibitory transmission through displacement of negative modulators; reduction of delayed rectifier potassium current; and/or binding to synaptic proteins which modulate neurotransmitter release.

Pharmacodynamics/Kinetics

Absorption: Oral: Rapid and almost complete
Distribution: V_d: Similar to total body water
Protein binding: <10%
Metabolism: Not extensive; primarily by enzymatic hydrolysis; forms metabolites (inactive)
Bioavailability: 100%
Half-life elimination: ~6-8 hours; extended release tablet: ~7 hours; half-life increased in renal dysfunction
Time to peak, plasma: Oral: Immediate release: ~1 hour; Extended release: ~4 hours
Excretion: Urine (66% as unchanged drug)

Dosage

Geriatric & Adult

Myoclonic seizures: Oral: Immediate release: Initial: 500 mg twice daily; may increase every 2 weeks by 500 mg/dose to the recommended dose of 1500 mg twice daily. Efficacy of doses >3000 mg/day has not been established.

Partial onset seizures:
Oral:
Immediate release: Initial: 500 mg twice daily; may increase every 2 weeks by 500 mg/ dose to a maximum of 1500 mg twice daily. Doses >3000 mg/day have been used in trials; however, there is no evidence of increased benefit.
Extended release: Initial: 1000 mg once daily; may increase every 2 weeks by 1000 mg/day to a maximum of 3000 mg once daily.

I.V.: Initial: 500 mg twice daily; may increase every 2 weeks by 500 mg/dose to a maximum of 1500 mg twice daily. Doses >3000 mg/day have been used in trials; however, there is no evidence of increased benefit.

Note: When switching from oral to I.V. formulations, the total daily dose should be the same.

Tonic-clonic seizures: Oral: Immediate release: Initial: 500 mg twice daily; may increase every 2 weeks by 500 mg/dose to the recommended dose of 1500 mg twice daily. Efficacy of doses >3000 mg/day has not been established.

Bipolar disorder (unlabeled use): Oral: Immediate release: Initial: 500 mg twice daily; if tolerated, increase by 500 mg twice daily; dose may be increased every 3 days until target dose of 3000 mg/day is reached; maximum 4000 mg/day

Loading dose (unlabeled): Oral: Immediate release: Initial doses of 1500-2000 mg have been well-tolerated (Betts, 2000; Koubeissi, 2008), although the necessity of a loading dose has not been established

Refractory status epilepticus (unlabeled use): I.V.: 1000-3000 mg administered over 15 minutes (Meierkord, 2010); 2500 mg has been safely administered over 5 minutes in one report (Uges, 2009). **Note:** Levetiracetam has not been well studied in comparison to other agents routinely used in this setting.

Renal Impairment Adults:

Immediate release and I.V. formulations:
    Cl_{cr} >80 mL/minute: 500-1500 mg every 12 hours
    Cl_{cr} 50-80 mL/minute: 500-1000 mg every 12 hours
    Cl_{cr} 30-50 mL/minute: 250-750 mg every 12 hours
    Cl_{cr} <30 mL/minute: 250-500 mg every 12 hours
    End-stage renal disease patients using dialysis: 500-1000 mg every 24 hours; a supplemental dose of 250-500 mg following dialysis is recommended

Extended release tablets:
    Cl_{cr} >80 mL/minute: 1000-3000 mg every 24 hours
    Cl_{cr} 50-80 mL/minute: 1000-2000 mg every 24 hours
    Cl_{cr} 30-50 mL/minute: 500-1500 mg every 24 hours
    Cl_{cr} <30 mL/minute: 500-1000 mg every 24 hours

Hepatic Impairment No adjustment required

Administration

I.V.: Infuse over 15 minutes

Oral: may be taken with or without food.

Oral solution: Should be administered with a calibrated measuring device (not a household teaspoon or tablespoon)

Tablet (immediate release and extended release): Only administer as whole tablet; do not crush, break or chew.

Monitoring Parameters Suicidality (eg, suicidal thoughts, depression, behavioral changes)

Special Geriatric Considerations In a study of 16 older adults (61-88 years of age) receiving levetiracetam daily and with creatinine clearances ranging from 30-74 mL/minute, a decrease in creatinine clearance (38%) and a 2.5 hour longer half-life were recorded in the elderly compared to younger adults. The authors concluded that the difference was due to renal function. Other studies show no overall difference in safety and efficacy, although larger numbers in studies are needed to verify efficacy. Levetiracetam has demonstrated a low incidence of cognitive effects. When using the drug in elderly, it is essential to base the dose on estimated creatinine clearance and adjust appropriately.

Dosage Forms Excipient information presented when available (limited, particularly for generics); consult specific product labeling.

Injection, solution: 100 mg/mL (5 mL)
  Keppra®: 100 mg/mL (5 mL)

Solution, oral: 100 mg/mL (5 mL, 118 mL, 472 mL, 473 mL, 480 mL, 500 mL)
  Keppra®: 100 mg/mL (480 mL) [dye free; grape flavor]

Tablet, oral: 250 mg, 500 mg, 750 mg, 1000 mg
  Keppra®: 250 mg, 500 mg, 750 mg [scored; gluten free]

Tablet, extended release, oral:
  Keppra XR™: 500 mg, 750 mg

Selected References

Meador KJ, Gevins A, Loring DW, et al, "Neuropsychological and Neurophysiologic Effects of Carbamazepine and Levetiracetam," *Neurology*, 2007, 69(22):2076-84.

Roberts GM, Majoie HJ, Leenen LA, et al, "Ketter's Hypothesis of the Mood Effects of Antiepileptic Drugs Coupled to the Mechanism of Action of Topiramate and Levetiracetam," *Epilepsy Behav*, 2005, 6(3):366-72.

Sankar R and Holmes GL, "Mechanisms of Action for the Commonly Used Antiepileptic Drugs: Relevance to Antiepileptic Drug-Associated Neurobehavioral Adverse Effects," *J Child Neurol*, 2004, 19(Suppl 1):6-14.

Welty TE, Gidal BE, Ficker DM, et al, "Levetiracetam: A Different Approach to the Pharmacotherapy of Epilepsy," *Ann Pharmacother*, 2002, 36(2):296-304.

◆ **Levitra®** *see* Vardenafil *on page 1899*

Levobunolol (lee voe BYOO noe lole)

Related Information
Glaucoma Drug Therapy *on page 2008*
Medication Safety Issues
Sound-alike/look-alike issues:
Levobunolol may be confused with levocabastine
Betagan® may be confused with Betadine®, Betoptic® S
Brand Names: U.S. Betagan®
Brand Names: Canada Apo-Levobunolol®; Betagan®; Novo-Levobunolol; Optho-Bunolol®; PMS-Levobunolol; Sandoz-Levobunolol
Index Terms *l*-Bunolol Hydrochloride; Levobunolol Hydrochloride
Generic Availability (U.S.) Yes
Pharmacologic Category Beta-Adrenergic Blocker, Nonselective; Ophthalmic Agent, Antiglaucoma
Use To lower intraocular pressure in chronic open-angle glaucoma or ocular hypertension
Contraindications Hypersensitivity to levobunolol or any component of the formulation; bronchial asthma, severe COPD, sinus bradycardia, second- or third-degree AV block, cardiac failure, cardiogenic shock
Warnings/Precautions Consider pre-existing conditions such as sick sinus syndrome before initiating. Use with caution in patients with HF, diabetes mellitus, bronchospastic disease, myasthenia gravis, peripheral vascular disease, psychiatric disease, hyperthyroidism; contains metabisulfite. Because systemic absorption does occur with ophthalmic administration, the elderly with other disease states or syndromes that may be affected by a beta-blocker (HF, COPD, etc) should be monitored closely. Use caution with history of severe anaphylaxis to allergens; patients taking beta-blockers may become more sensitive to repeated challenges. Treatment of anaphylaxis (eg, epinephrine) in patients taking beta-blockers may be ineffective or promote undesirable effects. Product contains benzalkonium chloride which may be absorbed by soft contact lenses; do not administer while wearing soft contact lenses. Ophthalmic solutions contain metabisulfite.
Adverse Reactions (Reflective of adult population; not specific for elderly)
>10%: Ocular: Stinging/burning eyes
1% to 10%:
Cardiovascular: Bradycardia, arrhythmia, hypotension
Central nervous system: Dizziness, headache
Dermatologic: Alopecia, erythema
Local: Stinging, burning
Ocular: Blepharoconjunctivitis, conjunctivitis
Respiratory: Bronchospasm
Drug Interactions
Avoid Concomitant Use
Avoid concomitant use of Levobunolol with any of the following: Floctafenine; Methacholine
Increased Effect/Toxicity
Levobunolol may increase the levels/effects of: Alpha-/Beta-Agonists (Direct-Acting); Bupivacaine; Fingolimod; Hypotensive Agents; Lidocaine (Systemic); Lidocaine (Topical); Mepivacaine; Methacholine; Midodrine

The levels/effects of Levobunolol may be increased by: Anilidopiperidine Opioids; Dronedarone; Floctafenine; MAO Inhibitors; QuiNIDine; Reserpine
Decreased Effect
Levobunolol may decrease the levels/effects of: Beta2-Agonists; Theophylline Derivatives
Mechanism of Action A nonselective beta-adrenergic blocking agent that lowers intraocular pressure by reducing aqueous humor production and possibly increases the outflow of aqueous humor
Pharmacodynamics/Kinetics
Onset of action: ~1 hour
Peak effect: 2-6 hours
Duration: 1 day
Excretion: Not well defined
Dosage
Geriatric & Adult Glaucoma: Ophthalmic: Instill 1 drop in the affected eye(s) 1-2 times/day
Administration Apply finger pressure over nasolacrimal duct to decrease systemic absorption.
Monitoring Parameters Intraocular pressure, heart rate, funduscopic exam, visual field testing

Special Geriatric Considerations Because systemic absorption does occur with ophthalmic administration, the elderly with other disease states or syndromes that may be affected by a beta-blocker (CHF, COPD, etc) should be monitored closely. Evaluate the patient's or caregiver's ability to safely administer the correct dose of ophthalmic medication.

Dosage Forms Excipient information presented when available (limited, particularly for generics); consult specific product labeling. [DSC] = Discontinued product

Solution, ophthalmic, as hydrochloride [drops]: 0.25% (5 mL, 10 mL); 0.5% (5 mL, 10 mL, 15 mL)

Betagan®: 0.25% (5 mL [DSC], 10 mL [DSC]); 0.5% (2 mL [DSC], 5 mL, 10 mL, 15 mL) [contains benzalkonium chloride, sodium metabisulfite]

◆ **Levobunolol Hydrochloride** see Levobunolol on page 1048
◆ **Levocabastine Hydrochloride** see Levocabastine (Nasal) on page 1049
◆ **Levocabastine Hydrochloride** see Levocabastine (Ophthalmic) on page 1049

Levocabastine (Nasal) (LEE voe kab as teen)

Medication Safety Issues
Sound-alike/look-alike issues:
Levocabastine may be confused with levobunolol, levOCARNitine
Livostin® may be confused with lovastatin

Brand Names: Canada Livostin®

Index Terms Levocabastine Hydrochloride

Pharmacologic Category Histamine H_1 Antagonist; Histamine H_1 Antagonist, Second Generation; Piperidine Derivative

Use Symptomatic treatment of allergic rhinitis

Dosage

Adult Allergic rhinitis: Intranasal: Adults ≤65 years: Two sprays in each nostril twice daily; if necessary, may increase dose to 2 sprays 3-4 times daily; consider therapy discontinuation if no response within 3 days. Continuous treatment >10 weeks has not been evaluated.

Renal Impairment Use caution; manufacturer labeling provides no specific dosing recommendations.

Product Availability Not available in U.S.

Dosage Forms: Canada Excipient information presented when available (limited, particularly for generics); consult specific product labeling.

Microsuspension, intranasal, as hydrochloride [spray]:
Livostin®: 0.05% [50 mcg/spray] (15 mL) [contains benzalkonium chloride]

Levocabastine (Ophthalmic) (LEE voe kab as teen)

Medication Safety Issues
Sound-alike/look-alike issues:
Levocabastine may be confused with levobunolol, levOCARNitine
Livostin® may be confused with lovastatin

International issues:
Livostin [Canada and multiple international markets] may be confused with Limoxin brand name for ambroxol [Indonesia] and amoxicillin [Mexico]; Lovastin brand name for lovastatin [Malaysia, Poland, Singapore]

Brand Names: Canada Livostin® Eye Drops

Index Terms Levocabastine Hydrochloride

Pharmacologic Category Histamine H_1 Antagonist; Histamine H_1 Antagonist, Second Generation; Piperidine Derivative

Use Treatment of seasonal allergic conjunctivitis

Dosage

Adult Allergic conjunctivitis: Adults ≤65 years: Ophthalmic: Usual dose: Instill 1 drop in affected eye(s) 2 times/day; may increase to 1 drop 3-4 times/day. If no improvement within 3 days, consider discontinuation of therapy. Continuous therapy >16 weeks has not been studied.

Product Availability Not available in U.S.

Dosage Forms: Canada Excipient information presented when available (limited, particularly for generics); consult specific product labeling.

Suspension, ophthalmic:
Livostin®: 0.05% (5 mL, 10 mL) [contains benzalkonium chloride]

Levocetirizine (LEE vo se TI ra zeen)

Medication Safety Issues
Sound-alike/look-alike issues:
Levocetirizine may be confused with cetirizine

Brand Names: U.S. Xyzal®

Index Terms Levocetirizine Dihydrochloride

Generic Availability (U.S.) Yes: Tablet

Pharmacologic Category Histamine H_1 Antagonist; Histamine H_1 Antagonist, Second Generation; Piperazine Derivative

Use Relief of symptoms of perennial and seasonal allergic rhinitis; treatment of skin manifestations (uncomplicated) of chronic idiopathic urticaria

Contraindications Hypersensitivity to levocetirizine, cetirizine, or any component of the formulation; end-stage renal disease (Cl_{cr} <10 mL/minute); hemodialysis

Warnings/Precautions Use with caution in adults with mild-to-moderate renal impairment; dosage adjustments may be needed. Use is contraindicated in end-stage renal disease (Cl_{cr} <10 mL/minute), and patients undergoing hemodialysis. Use with caution in the elderly. May cause drowsiness; use caution performing tasks which require alertness (eg, operating machinery or driving). Effects may be potentiated when used with other sedative drugs or ethanol.

Adverse Reactions (Reflective of adult population; not specific for elderly)
>10%: Gastrointestinal: Diarrhea
1% to 10%:
Central nervous system: Somnolence (2% to 6%), fever, fatigue (1% to 4%)
Gastrointestinal: Constipation, vomiting, xerostomia (2% to 3%)
Neuromuscular & skeletal: Weakness (2%)
Otic: Otitis media
Respiratory: Nasopharyngitis (4% to 6%), cough, epistaxis, pharyngitis (1% to 2%)

The following potentially-severe adverse reactions have been reported with cetirizine and, therefore, may also occur with levocetirizine: Cholestasis, glomuleronephritis, hallucination, hypotension (severe), orofacial dyskinesia, suicidal ideation

Drug Interactions
Avoid Concomitant Use There are no known interactions where it is recommended to avoid concomitant use.

Increased Effect/Toxicity
Levocetirizine may increase the levels/effects of: Alcohol (Ethyl); Anticholinergics; CNS Depressants; Selective Serotonin Reuptake Inhibitors

The levels/effects of Levocetirizine may be increased by: Droperidol; HydrOXYzine; Pramlintide

Decreased Effect
Levocetirizine may decrease the levels/effects of: Acetylcholinesterase Inhibitors (Central); Benzylpenicilloyl Polylysine; Betahistine

The levels/effects of Levocetirizine may be decreased by: Acetylcholinesterase Inhibitors (Central); Amphetamines

Ethanol/Nutrition/Herb Interactions Ethanol: May increase CNS depression; monitor for increased effects with coadministration. Caution patients about effects.

Stability Store at room temperature of 20°C to 25°C (68°F to 77°F); excursions permitted to 15°C to 30°C (59°F to 86°F).

Mechanism of Action Levocetirizine is an antihistamine which selectively competes with histamine for H_1-receptor sites on effector cells in the gastrointestinal tract, blood vessels, and respiratory tract. Levocetirizine, the active enantiomer of cetirizine, has twice the binding affinity at the H1-receptor compared to cetirizine.

Pharmacodynamics/Kinetics
Absorption: Rapid and extensive
Distribution: 0.4 L/kg
Protein binding: 91% to 92%
Metabolism: Minimal (<14%); via aromatic oxidation, N and O-dealkylation (via CYPA4), and taurine conjugation
Half-life elimination: Adults: ~8 hours; Renal impairment: 11-34 hours; End-stage renal disease: 46 hours
Time to peak, plasma: Adults: 0.9 hours
Excretion: Urine (85%); feces (13%)

Dosage

Geriatric Refer to adult dosing; dosing should begin at the lower end of the dosing range.

Adult Allergic rhinitis, chronic urticaria: Oral: 5 mg once daily (in the evening); some patients may experience relief of symptoms with 2.5 mg once daily

Renal Impairment Adults:

Cl$_{cr}$ 50-80 mL/minute: 2.5 mg once daily

Cl$_{cr}$ 30-50 mL/minute: 2.5 mg once every other day

Cl$_{cr}$ 10-30 mL/minute: 2.5 mg twice weekly (every 3 or 4 days)

Cl$_{cr}$ <10 mL/minute, hemodialysis patients: Contraindicated

Hepatic Impairment No adjustment required.

Administration Administer in the evening. May be administered without regard to meals.

Monitoring Parameters Creatinine clearance (prior to treatment for dosing adjustment), relief of symptoms, mental status

Special Geriatric Considerations See Dosage: Renal Impairment.

Dosage Forms Excipient information presented when available (limited, particularly for generics); consult specific product labeling.

Solution, oral, as dihydrochloride:

Xyzal®: 0.5 mg/mL (150 mL)

Tablet, oral, as dihydrochloride: 5 mg

Xyzal®: 5 mg [scored]

Selected References

Nettis E, Colanardi MC, Barra L, et al, "Levocetirizine in the Treatment of Chronic Idiopathic Urticaria: A Randomized, Double-Blind, Placebo-Controlled Study," *Br J Dermatol*, 2006, 154(3):533-8.

◆ **Levocetirizine Dihydrochloride** *see* Levocetirizine *on page 1050*

◆ **Levodopa and Carbidopa** *see* Carbidopa and Levodopa *on page 274*

Levodopa, Carbidopa, and Entacapone

(lee voe DOE pa, kar bi DOE pa, & en TA ka pone)

Related Information

Antiparkinsonian Agents *on page 1995*

Carbidopa *on page 273*

Entacapone *on page 602*

Medication Safety Issues

Administration issues:

Strengths listed in Stalevo® brand names correspond to the **levodopa** component of the formulation only. All strengths of Stalevo® contain a levodopa/carbidopa ratio of 4:1 plus entacapone 200 mg.

Brand Names: U.S. Stalevo®

Brand Names: Canada Stalevo®

Index Terms Carbidopa, Entacapone, and Levodopa; Carbidopa, Levodopa, and Entacapone; Entacapone, Carbidopa, and Levodopa

Generic Availability (U.S.) No

Pharmacologic Category Anti-Parkinson's Agent, COMT Inhibitor; Anti-Parkinson's Agent, Decarboxylase Inhibitor; Anti-Parkinson's Agent, Dopamine Precursor

Use Treatment of idiopathic Parkinson's disease

Dosage

Geriatric & Adult

Note: All strengths of Stalevo® contain a carbidopa/levodopa ratio of 1:4 plus entacapone 200 mg.

Parkinson's disease: Oral: Dose should be individualized based on therapeutic response; doses may be adjusted by changing strength or adjusting interval. Fractionated doses are not recommended and only 1 tablet should be given at each dosing interval; maximum daily dose: 8 tablets of Stalevo® 50, 75, 100, 125, or 150, **or** 6 tablets of Stalevo® 200.

Patients previously treated with carbidopa/levodopa immediate release tablets (ratio of 1:4):

With current entacapone therapy: May switch directly to corresponding strength of combination tablet. No data available on transferring patients from controlled release preparations or products with a 1:10 ratio of carbidopa/levodopa.

Without entacapone therapy:

If current levodopa dose is >600 mg/day: Levodopa dose reduction may be required when adding entacapone to therapy; therefore, titrate dose using individual products first (carbidopa/levodopa immediate release with a ratio of 1:4 plus entacapone 200 mg); then transfer to combination product once stabilized.

If current levodopa dose is <600 mg without dyskinesias: May transfer to corresponding dose of combination product; monitor, dose reduction of levodopa may be required.

◀ **Patients previously treated with benserazide/levodopa immediate release tablets (Canadian labeling, not in U.S. labeling):** *With current entacapone therapy:* Prior to switching to combination product (carbidopa/levodopa/entacapone), withhold treatment for 1 night, then initiate (carbidopa/levodopa/entacapone) therapy the following morning at a dose that provides either an equivalent amount or ~5% to 10% more levodopa.

Renal Impairment Use caution with severe renal impairment; specific dosing recommendations not available.

Hepatic Impairment Use with caution; specific dosing recommendations not available.

Special Geriatric Considerations This combination product may be convenient for elderly patients to improve adherence.

Dosage Forms Excipient information presented when available (limited, particularly for generics); consult specific product labeling.

Tablet:
Stalevo® 50: Levodopa 50 mg, carbidopa 12.5 mg, and entacapone 200 mg
Stalevo® 75: Levodopa 75 mg, carbidopa 18.75 mg, and entacapone 200 mg
Stalevo® 100: Levodopa 100 mg, carbidopa 25 mg, and entacapone 200 mg
Stalevo® 125: Levodopa 125 mg, carbidopa 31.25 mg, and entacapone 200 mg
Stalevo® 150: Levodopa 150 mg, carbidopa 37.5 mg, and entacapone 200 mg
Stalevo® 200: Levodopa 200 mg, carbidopa 50 mg, and entacapone 200 mg

◆ **Levo-Dromoran** *see* Levorphanol *on page 1056*

Levofloxacin (Systemic) (lee voe FLOKS a sin)

Related Information
Community-Acquired Pneumonia in Adults *on page 2059*
Helicobacter pylori Treatment in Adult Patients *on page 2009*

Medication Safety Issues
Sound-alike/look-alike issues:
Levaquin® may be confused with Levoxyl®, Levsin/SL®, Lovenox®
Levofloxacin may be confused with levETIRAcetam, levodopa, Levophed®, levothyroxine

Brand Names: U.S. Levaquin®

Brand Names: Canada Levaquin®; Novo-Levofloxacin; PMS-Levofloxacin

Generic Availability (U.S.) Yes: Excludes injection solution

Pharmacologic Category Antibiotic, Quinolone; Respiratory Fluoroquinolone

Use Treatment of community-acquired pneumonia, including multidrug resistant strains of *S. pneumoniae* (MDRSP); nosocomial pneumonia; chronic bronchitis (acute bacterial exacerbation); acute bacterial sinusitis; prostatitis, urinary tract infection (uncomplicated or complicated); acute pyelonephritis; skin or skin structure infections (uncomplicated or complicated); reduce incidence or disease progression of inhalational anthrax (postexposure)

Unlabeled/Investigational Use Diverticulitis, enterocolitis (*Shigella* spp), epididymitis (nongonococcal), gonococcal infections, complicated intra-abdominal infections (in combination with metronidazole), Legionnaires' disease, peritonitis, PID

Note: As of April 2007, the CDC no longer recommends the use of fluoroquinolones for the treatment of gonococcal disease.

Medication Guide Available Yes

Contraindications Hypersensitivity to levofloxacin, any component of the formulation, or other quinolones

Warnings/Precautions
[U.S. Boxed Warning]: There have been reports of tendon inflammation and/or rupture with quinolone antibiotics; risk may be increased with concurrent corticosteroids, organ transplant recipients, and in patients >60 years of age. Rupture of the Achilles tendon sometimes requiring surgical repair has been reported most frequently; but other tendon sites (eg, rotator cuff, biceps) have also been reported. Strenuous physical activity, rheumatoid arthritis, and renal impairment may be an independent risk factor for tendonitis. Discontinue at first sign of tendon inflammation or pain. May occur even after discontinuation of therapy. Use with caution in patients with rheumatoid arthritis; may increase risk of tendon rupture. Potential for seizures, although very rare, may be increased with concomitant NSAID therapy. Use with caution in individuals at risk of seizures, with known or suspected CNS disorders or renal dysfunction. Avoid excessive sunlight and take precautions to limit exposure (eg, loose fitting clothing, sunscreen); may cause moderate-to-severe phototoxicity reactions. Discontinue use if photosensitivity occurs.

Rare cases of torsade de pointes have been reported in patients receiving levofloxacin. Use caution in patients with known prolongation of QT interval, bradycardia, hypokalemia, hypomagnesemia, or in those receiving concurrent therapy with Class Ia or Class III antiarrhythmics.

Severe hypersensitivity reactions, including anaphylaxis, have occurred with quinolone therapy. Reactions may present as typical allergic symptoms after a single dose, or may manifest as severe idiosyncratic dermatologic, vascular, pulmonary, renal, hepatic, and/or hematologic events, usually after multiple doses. Prompt discontinuation of drug should occur if skin rash or other symptoms arise. Prolonged use may result in fungal or bacterial superinfection, including *C. difficile*-associated diarrhea (CDAD) and pseudomembranous colitis; CDAD has been observed >2 months postantibiotic treatment. Peripheral neuropathies have been linked to levofloxacin use; discontinue if numbness, tingling, or weakness develops. **[U.S. Boxed Warning]: Quinolones may exacerbate myasthenia gravis; avoid use (rare, potentially life-threatening weakness of respiratory muscles may occur).** Unrelated to hypersensitivity, severe hepatotoxicity (including acute hepatitis and fatalities) has been reported. Elderly patients may be at greater risk. Discontinue therapy immediately if signs and symptoms of hepatitis occur. Hemolytic reactions may (rarely) occur with quinolone use in patients with latent or actual G6PD deficiency.

Fluoroquinolones have been associated with the development of serious, and sometimes fatal, hypoglycemia, most often in elderly diabetics, but also in patients without diabetes. This occurred most frequently with gatifloxacin (no longer available systemically) but may occur at a lower frequency with other quinolones.

Adverse Reactions (Reflective of adult population; not specific for elderly)
1% to 10%:
Cardiovascular: Chest pain (1%), edema (1%)
Central nervous system: Headache (6%), insomnia (4%), dizziness (3%), fatigue (1%), pain (1%)
Dermatologic: Rash (2%), pruritus (1%)
Gastrointestinal: Nausea (7%), diarrhea (5%), constipation (3%), abdominal pain (2%), dyspepsia (2%), vomiting (2%)
Genitourinary: Vaginitis (1%)
Local: Injection site reaction (1%)
Respiratory: Pharyngitis (4%), dyspnea (1%)
Miscellaneous: Moniliasis (1%)

Drug Interactions
Avoid Concomitant Use
Avoid concomitant use of Levofloxacin (Systemic) with any of the following: Artemether; BCG; Dronedarone; Lumefantrine; Nilotinib; Pimozide; QUEtiapine; QuiNINE; Tetrabenazine; Thioridazine; Toremifene; Vandetanib; Vemurafenib; Ziprasidone

Increased Effect/Toxicity
Levofloxacin (Systemic) may increase the levels/effects of: Corticosteroids (Systemic); Dronedarone; Pimozide; Porfimer; QTc-Prolonging Agents; QuiNINE; Sulfonylureas; Tetrabenazine; Thioridazine; Toremifene; Vandetanib; Vemurafenib; Vitamin K Antagonists; Ziprasidone

The levels/effects of Levofloxacin (Systemic) may be increased by: Alfuzosin; Artemether; Chloroquine; Ciprofloxacin; Ciprofloxacin (Systemic); Gadobutrol; Insulin; Lumefantrine; Nilotinib; Nonsteroidal Anti-Inflammatory Agents; Probenecid; QUEtiapine; QuiNINE

Decreased Effect
Levofloxacin (Systemic) may decrease the levels/effects of: BCG; Mycophenolate; Sulfonylureas; Typhoid Vaccine

The levels/effects of Levofloxacin (Systemic) may be decreased by: Antacids; Calcium Salts; Didanosine; Iron Salts; Lanthanum; Magnesium Salts; Quinapril; Sevelamer; Sucralfate; Zinc Salts

Stability
Solution for injection:
Vial: Store at room temperature. Protect from light. When diluted to 5 mg/mL in a compatible I.V. fluid, solution is stable for 72 hours when stored at room temperature; stable for 14 days when stored under refrigeration. When frozen, stable for 6 months; do not refreeze. Do not thaw in microwave or by bath immersion.
Premixed: Store at ≤25°C (77°F); do not freeze. Brief exposure to 40°C (104°F) does not affect product. Protect from light.
Tablet, oral solution: Store at 25°C (77°F); excursions permitted to 15°C to 30°C (59°F to 86°F).

Mechanism of Action As the S(-) enantiomer of the fluoroquinolone, ofloxacin, levofloxacin, inhibits DNA-gyrase in susceptible organisms thereby inhibits relaxation of supercoiled DNA and promotes breakage of DNA strands. DNA gyrase (topoisomerase II), is an essential bacterial enzyme that maintains the superhelical structure of DNA and is required for DNA replication and transcription, DNA repair, recombination, and transposition.

◀ **Pharmacodynamics/Kinetics**

Absorption: Rapid and complete

Distribution: V_d: 74-112 L; CSF concentrations ~15% of serum levels; high concentrations are achieved in prostate, lung, and gynecological tissues, sinus, saliva

Protein binding: ~24% to 38%; primarily to albumin

Metabolism: Minimally hepatic

Bioavailability: ~99%

Half-life elimination: ~6-8 hours

Time to peak, serum: Oral: 1-2 hours

Excretion: Urine (~87% as unchanged drug, <5% as metabolites); feces (<4%)

Dosage

Geriatric & Adult Note: Sequential therapy (intravenous to oral) may be instituted based on prescriber's discretion.

Anthrax (inhalational): 500 mg every 24 hours for 60 days, beginning as soon as possible after exposure

Chronic bronchitis (acute bacterial exacerbation): Oral, I.V.: 500 mg every 24 hours for at least 7 days

Diverticulitis, peritonitis (unlabeled use): Oral, I.V.: 750 mg every 24 hours for 7-10 days; use adjunctive metronidazole therapy

Dysenteric enterocolitis, *Shigella spp.* (unlabeled use): Oral, I.V.: 500 mg every 24 hours for 3-5 days

Epididymitis, nongonococcal (unlabeled use): 500 mg once daily for 10 days

Gonococcal infection (unlabeled use): Oral, I.V.:

Cervicitis, urethritis: 250 mg for one dose with azithromycin or doxycycline; **Note:** As of April 2007, the CDC no longer recommends the use of fluoroquinolones for the treatment of uncomplicated gonococcal disease.

Disseminated infection: 250 mg I.V. once daily; 24 hours after symptoms improve may change to 500 mg orally every 24 hours to complete total therapy of 7 days; **Note:** As of April 2007, the CDC no longer recommends the use of fluoroquinolones for the treatment of more serious gonococcal disease, unless no other options exist and susceptibility can be confirmed via culture.

Intra-abdominal infection, complicated, community-acquired (in combination with metronidazole) (unlabeled use): I.V.: 750 mg once daily for 4-7 days (provided source controlled). **Note:** Avoid using in settings where *E. coli* susceptibility to fluoroquinolones is <90%.

Pelvic inflammatory disease (unlabeled use): 500 mg once daily for 14 days with or without adjunctive metronidazole; **Note:** The CDC recommends use only if standard cephalosporin therapy is not feasible and community prevalence of quinolone-resistant gonococcal organisms is low. Culture sensitivity must be confirmed.

Pneumonia: Oral, I.V.:

Community-acquired: 500 mg every 24 hours for 7-14 days or 750 mg every 24 hours for 5 days (efficacy of 5-day regimen for MDRSP not established)

Nosocomial: 750 mg every 24 hours for 7-14 days

Prostatitis (chronic bacterial): Oral, I.V.: 500 mg every 24 hours for 28 days

Sinusitis (acute bacterial): Oral, I.V.: 500 mg every 24 hours for 10-14 days or 750 mg every 24 hours for 5 days

Skin and skin structure infections: Oral, I.V.:

Uncomplicated: 500 mg every 24 hours for 7-10 days

Complicated: 750 mg every 24 hours for 7-14 days

Traveler's diarrhea (unlabeled use): Oral, I.V.: 500 mg for one dose

Urinary tract infections: Oral, I.V.:

Uncomplicated: 250 mg once daily for 3 days

Complicated, including acute pyelonephritis: 250 mg once daily for 10 days **or** 750 mg once daily for 5 days

Renal Impairment

Normal renal function dosing of 750 mg/day:

Cl_{cr} 20-49 mL/minute: Administer 750 mg every 48 hours

Cl_{cr} 10-19 mL/minute: Administer 750 mg initial dose, followed by 500 mg every 48 hours

Hemodialysis (administer after hemodialysis on dialysis days)/peritoneal dialysis (PD): Administer 750 mg initial dose, followed by 500 mg every 48 hours

Normal renal function dosing of 500 mg/day:

Cl_{cr} 20-49 mL/minute: Administer 500 mg initial dose, followed by 250 mg every 24 hours

Cl_{cr} 10-19 mL/minute: Administer 500 mg initial dose, followed by 250 mg every 48 hours

Hemodialysis (administer after hemodialysis on dialysis days)/peritoneal dialysis (PD): Administer 500 mg initial dose, followed by 250 mg every 48 hours

Normal renal function dosing of 250 mg/day:

Cl_{cr} 20-49 mL/minute: No dosage adjustment required

Cl_{cr} 10-19 mL/minute: Administer 250 mg every 48 hours (except in uncomplicated UTI, where no dosage adjustment is required)

Hemodialysis (administer after hemodialysis on dialysis days)/peritoneal dialysis (PD): No information available.

Continuous renal replacement therapy (CRRT) (Heintz, 2009; Trotman, 2005): Drug clearance is highly dependent on the method of renal replacement, filter type, and flow rate. Appropriate dosing requires close monitoring of pharmacologic response, signs of adverse reactions due to drug accumulation, as well as drug concentrations in relation to target trough (if appropriate). The following are general recommendations only (based on dialysate flow/ultrafiltration rates of 1-2 L/hour and minimal residual renal function) and should not supersede clinical judgment:

CVVH: Loading dose of 500-750 mg followed by 250 mg every 24 hours

CVVHD: Loading dose of 500-750 mg followed by 250-500 mg every 24 hours

CVVHDF: Loading dose of 500-750 mg followed by 250-750 mg every 24 hours

Administration

Oral: Tablets may be administered without regard to meals. Oral solution should be administered 1 hour before or 2 hours after meals. Maintain adequate hydration of patient to prevent crystalluria.

I.V.: Infuse 250-500 mg I.V. solution over 60 minutes; infuse 750 mg I.V. solution over 90 minutes. Too rapid of infusion can lead to hypotension. Avoid administration through an intravenous line with a solution containing multivalent cations (eg, magnesium, calcium). Maintain adequate hydration of patient to prevent crystalluria.

Monitoring Parameters Evaluation of organ system functions (renal, hepatic, and hematopoietic) is recommended periodically during therapy; the possibility of crystalluria should be assessed; WBC and signs of infection

Test Interactions Some quinolones may produce a false-positive urine screening result for opiates using commercially-available immunoassay kits. This has been demonstrated most consistently for levofloxacin and ofloxacin, but other quinolones have shown cross-reactivity in certain assay kits. Confirmation of positive opiate screens by more specific methods should be considered.

Special Geriatric Considerations The risk of torsade de pointes and tendon inflammation and/or rupture associated with the concomitant use of corticosteroids and quinolones is increased in the elderly population. See Warnings/Precautions regarding tendon rupture in patients >60 years of age. Adjust dose for renal function.

Dosage Forms Excipient information presented when available (limited, particularly for generics); consult specific product labeling.

Infusion, premixed in D_5W [preservative free]: 250 mg (50 mL); 500 mg (100 mL); 750 mg (150 mL)

Levaquin® : 250 mg (50 mL); 500 mg (100 mL); 750 mg (150 mL)

Injection, solution [preservative free]:

Levaquin®: 25 mg/mL (20 mL, 30 mL)

Solution, oral: 25 mg/mL (100 mL, 200 mL, 480 mL)

Levaquin®: 25 mg/mL (480 mL) [contains benzyl alcohol, propylene glycol]

Tablet, oral: 250 mg, 500 mg, 750 mg

Levaquin®: 250 mg, 500 mg, 750 mg

Selected References

Nicolle LN, Bradley S, Colgan R et al, "Infectious Disease Society of America Guidelines for the Diagnosis and Treatment of Asymptomatic Bacteriuria in Adults," *Clinical Infectious Diseases*, 2005, 40:643-54.

Levofloxacin (Ophthalmic) (lee voe FLOKS a sin)

Medication Safety Issues

Sound-alike/look-alike issues:

Levofloxacin may be confused with levETIRAcetam, levodopa, levothyroxine

Brand Names: U.S. Iquix®; Quixin®

Generic Availability (U.S.) Yes

Pharmacologic Category Antibiotic, Ophthalmic; Antibiotic, Quinolone

Use Treatment of bacterial conjunctivitis caused by susceptible organisms (Quixin® 0.5% ophthalmic solution); treatment of corneal ulcer caused by susceptible organisms (Iquix® 1.5% ophthalmic solution)

◀ **Dosage**
Geriatric & Adult
Conjunctivitis (0.5% ophthalmic solution): Ophthalmic:
Treatment day 1 and day 2: Instill 1-2 drops into affected eye(s) every 2 hours while awake, up to 8 times/day
Treatment day 3 through day 7: Instill 1-2 drops into affected eye(s) every 4 hours while awake, up to 4 times/day
Corneal ulceration (1.5% ophthalmic solution): Ophthalmic:
Treatment day 1 through day 3: Instill 1-2 drops into affected eye(s) every 30 minutes to 2 hours while awake and 4-6 hours after retiring.
Treatment day 4 through completion: Instill 1-2 drops into affected eye(s) every 1-4 hours while awake.
Dosage Forms Excipient information presented when available (limited, particularly for generics); consult specific product labeling.
Solution, ophthalmic [drops]: 0.5% (5 mL)
Iquix®: 1.5% (5 mL)
Quixin®: 0.5% (5 mL) [contains benzalkonium chloride]

Levorphanol (lee VOR fa nole)

Related Information
Opioid Analgesics *on page 2013*
Medication Safety Issues
High alert medication:
The Institute for Safe Medication Practices (ISMP) includes this medication among its list of drug classes which have a heightened risk of causing significant patient harm when used in error.
Index Terms Levo-Dromoran; Levorphan Tartrate; Levorphanol Tartrate
Generic Availability (U.S.) Yes: Tablet
Pharmacologic Category Analgesic, Opioid
Use Relief of moderate-to-severe pain; preoperative sedation/analgesia; management of chronic pain (eg, cancer) requiring opioid therapy
Contraindications Hypersensitivity to levorphanol or any component of the formulation
Warnings/Precautions An opioid-containing analgesic regimen should be tailored to each patient's needs and based upon the type of pain being treated (acute versus chronic), the route of administration, degree of tolerance for opioids (naive versus chronic user), age, weight, and medical condition. The optimal analgesic dose varies widely among patients. Doses should be titrated to pain relief/prevention.

May cause CNS depression, which may impair physical or mental abilities; patients must be cautioned about performing tasks which require mental alertness (eg, operating machinery or driving). Effects may be potentiated when used with other sedative drugs or ethanol. Use with caution in patients with hypersensitivity reactions to other phenanthrene derivative opioid agonists (morphine, hydrocodone, hydromorphone, oxycodone, oxymorphone); respiratory diseases including asthma, emphysema, COPD, hypothyroidism, head trauma, morbid obesity, adrenal insufficiency, prostatic hyperplasia/urinary stricture, or severe liver or renal insufficiency. Use with caution in patients with biliary tract dysfunction; acute pancreatitis may cause constriction of sphincter of Oddi. May be habit-forming. May cause hypotension; use with caution in patients with depleted blood volume or drugs which may exaggerate hypotensive effects (including phenothiazines or general anesthetics). May obscure diagnosis or clinical course of patients with acute abdominal conditions. Concurrent use of agonist/ antagonist analgesics may precipitate withdrawal symptoms and/or reduced analgesic efficacy in patients following prolonged therapy with mu opioid agonists. Abrupt discontinuation following prolonged use may also lead to withdrawal symptoms. Elderly and debilitated patients may be particularly susceptible to the adverse effects of narcotics.
Adverse Reactions (Reflective of adult population; not specific for elderly) Frequency not defined.
Cardiovascular: Palpitation, hypotension, bradycardia, peripheral vasodilation, cardiac arrest, shock, tachycardia
Central nervous system: CNS depression, fatigue, drowsiness, dizziness, nervousness, headache, restlessness, anorexia, malaise, confusion, coma, convulsion, insomnia, amnesia, mental depression, hallucinations, paradoxical CNS stimulation, intracranial pressure (increased)
Dermatologic: Pruritus, urticaria, rash
Endocrine & metabolic: Antidiuretic hormone release
Gastrointestinal: Nausea, vomiting, dyspepsia, stomach cramps, xerostomia, constipation, abdominal pain, dry mouth, biliary tract spasm, paralytic ileus

Genitourinary: Decreased urination, urinary tract spasm, urinary retention

Neuromuscular & skeletal: Weakness

Ocular: Miosis, diplopia

Respiratory: Respiratory depression, apnea, hypoventilation, cyanosis

Miscellaneous: Histamine release, physical and psychological dependence

Drug Interactions

Avoid Concomitant Use There are no known interactions where it is recommended to avoid concomitant use.

Increased Effect/Toxicity

Levorphanol may increase the levels/effects of: Alcohol (Ethyl); Alvimopan; CNS Depressants; Desmopressin; Selective Serotonin Reuptake Inhibitors; Thiazide Diuretics

The levels/effects of Levorphanol may be increased by: Amphetamines; Antipsychotic Agents (Phenothiazines); Droperidol; HydrOXYzine; Succinylcholine

Decreased Effect

Levorphanol may decrease the levels/effects of: Pegvisomant

The levels/effects of Levorphanol may be decreased by: Ammonium Chloride; Mixed Agonist / Antagonist Opioids

Ethanol/Nutrition/Herb Interactions

Ethanol: May increase CNS depression; monitor for increased effects with coadministration. Caution patients about effects.

Herb/Nutraceutical: Avoid valerian, St John's wort, kava kava, gotu kola (may increase CNS depression).

Stability Store at 25°C (77°F); excursions permitted to 15°C to 30°C (59°F to 86°F).

Mechanism of Action Levorphanol tartrate is a synthetic opioid agonist that is classified as a morphinan derivative. Opioids interact with stereospecific opioid receptors in various parts of the central nervous system and other tissues. Analgesic potency parallels the affinity for these binding sites. These drugs do not alter the threshold or responsiveness to pain, but the perception of pain.

Pharmacodynamics/Kinetics

Onset of action: Oral: 10-60 minutes

Duration: 4-8 hours

Metabolism: Hepatic

Half-life elimination: 11-16 hours

Excretion: Urine (as inactive metabolite)

Dosage

Geriatric & Adult Note: These are guidelines and do not represent the maximum doses that may be required in all patients. Doses should be titrated to pain relief/prevention.

Acute pain (moderate-to-severe): *Oral:* Initial: Opiate-naive: 2 mg every 6-8 hours as needed; patients with prior opiate exposure may require higher initial doses; usual dosage range: 2-4 mg every 6-8 hours as needed

Note: The American Pain Society recommends an initial dose of 4 mg for severe pain in adults (APS, 6th ed)

Chronic pain: Patients taking opioids chronically may become tolerant and require doses higher than the usual dosage range to maintain the desired effect. Tolerance can be managed by appropriate dose titration. **There is no optimal or maximal dose for levorphanol in chronic pain. The appropriate dose is one that relieves pain throughout its dosing interval without causing unmanageable side effects.**

Renal Impairment Use with caution; initial dose should be reduced in severe renal impairment.

Hepatic Impairment Use with caution; initial dose should be reduced in severe hepatic impairment.

Monitoring Parameters Pain relief, respiratory and mental status, blood pressure

Pharmacotherapy Pearls 2 mg levorphanol I.M. produces analgesia comparable to that produced by 10 mg of morphine I.M.

Special Geriatric Considerations The elderly may be particularly susceptible to the CNS depressant and constipating effects of narcotics.

Controlled Substance C-II

Dosage Forms Excipient information presented when available (limited, particularly for generics); consult specific product labeling.

Tablet, oral, as tartrate: 2 mg

Selected References

American Geriatrics Society Panel on Pharmacological Management of Persistent Pain in Older Persons, "Pharmacological Management of Persistent Pain in Older Persons," *J Am Geriatr Soc,* 2009, 57(8):1331-46.

◆ **Levorphanol Tartrate** see Levorphanol *on page 1056*

◆ **Levorphan Tartrate** see Levorphanol *on page 1056*

◆ **Levothroid®** *see* Levothyroxine *on page* 1058

Levothyroxine (lee voe thye ROKS een)

Medication Safety Issues
Sound-alike/look-alike issues:
Levothyroxine may be confused with lamoTRIgine, Lanoxin®, levofloxacin, liothyronine
Levoxyl® may be confused with Lanoxin®, Levaquin®, Luvox®
Synthroid® may be confused with Symmetrel

Administration issues:
Significant differences exist between oral and I.V. dosing. Use caution when converting from one route of administration to another.

Other safety concerns:
To avoid errors due to misinterpretation of a decimal point, always express dosage in mcg (**not** mg).

Brand Names: U.S. Levothroid®; Levoxyl®; Synthroid®; Tirosint®; Unithroid®

Brand Names: Canada Eltroxin®; Euthyrox; Levothyroxine Sodium; Synthroid®

Index Terms *L*-Thyroxine Sodium; Levothyroxine Sodium; T_4

Generic Availability (U.S.) Yes

Pharmacologic Category Thyroid Product

Use Replacement or supplemental therapy in hypothyroidism; pituitary TSH suppression

Unlabeled/Investigational Use Management of hemodynamically unstable potential organ donors increasing the quantity of organs available for transplantation

Contraindications Hypersensitivity to levothyroxine sodium or any component of the formulation; acute MI; thyrotoxicosis of any etiology; uncorrected adrenal insufficiency
Capsule: Additional contraindication: Inability to swallow capsules

Warnings/Precautions [U.S. Boxed Warning]: Thyroid supplements are ineffective and potentially toxic when used for the treatment of obesity or for weight reduction, especially in euthyroid patients. High doses may produce serious or even life-threatening toxic effects particularly when used with some anorectic drugs (eg, sympathomimetic amines). Routine use of T_4 for TSH suppression is not recommended in patients with benign thyroid nodules. In patients deemed appropriate candidates, treatment should never be fully suppressive (TSH <0.1 mIU/L). Use with caution and reduce dosage in patients with angina pectoris or other cardiovascular disease; decrease initial dose. Use cautiously in the elderly since they may be more likely to have compromised cardiovascular functions. Patients with adrenal insufficiency, myxedema, diabetes mellitus and insipidus may have symptoms exaggerated or aggravated. Chronic hypothyroidism predisposes patients to coronary artery disease. Long-term therapy can decrease bone mineral density. Levoxyl® may rapidly swell and disintegrate causing choking or gagging (should be administered with a full glass of water); use caution in patients with dysphagia or other swallowing disorders.

Adverse Reactions (Reflective of adult population; not specific for elderly) Frequency not defined.
Cardiovascular: Angina, arrhythmia, cardiac arrest, flushing, heart failure, hypertension, MI, palpitation, pulse increased, tachycardia
Central nervous system: Anxiety, emotional lability, fatigue, fever, headache, hyperactivity, insomnia, irritability, nervousness, pseudotumor cerebri (children), seizure (rare)
Dermatologic: Alopecia
Endocrine & metabolic: Fertility impaired, menstrual irregularities
Gastrointestinal: Abdominal cramps, appetite increased, diarrhea, vomiting, weight loss
Hepatic: Liver function tests increased
Neuromuscular & skeletal: Bone mineral density decreased, muscle weakness, tremor, slipped capital femoral epiphysis (children)
Respiratory: Dyspnea
Miscellaneous: Diaphoresis, heat intolerance, hypersensitivity (to inactive ingredients, symptoms include urticaria, pruritus, rash, flushing, angioedema, GI symptoms, fever, arthralgia, serum sickness, wheezing)
Levoxyl®: Choking, dysphagia, gagging

Drug Interactions
Avoid Concomitant Use
Avoid concomitant use of Levothyroxine with any of the following: Sodium Iodide I131
Increased Effect/Toxicity
Levothyroxine may increase the levels/effects of: Vitamin K Antagonists

Decreased Effect

Levothyroxine may decrease the levels/effects of: Sodium Iodide I131; Theophylline Derivatives

The levels/effects of Levothyroxine may be decreased by: Aluminum Hydroxide; Bile Acid Sequestrants; Calcium Polystyrene Sulfonate; Calcium Salts; CarBAMazepine; Estrogen Derivatives; Fosphenytoin; Iron Salts; Lanthanum; Orlistat; Phenytoin; Raloxifene; Rifampin; Sevelamer; Sodium Polystyrene Sulfonate; Sucralfate

Ethanol/Nutrition/Herb Interactions Food: Taking levothyroxine with enteral nutrition may cause reduced bioavailability and may lower serum thyroxine levels leading to signs or symptoms of hypothyroidism. Soybean flour (infant formula), cottonseed meal, walnuts, and dietary fiber may decrease absorption of levothyroxine from the GI tract.

Stability

Capsules, tablets: Store at room temperature; excursions permitted to 15°C to 30°C (59°F to 86°F). Protect from light and moisture.

Injection: Store at room temperature; excursions permitted to 15°C to 30°C (59°F to 86°F). Dilute vials for injection with 5 mL normal saline. Reconstituted concentrations for the 200 mcg and 500 mcg vials are 40 mcg/mL and 100 mcg/mL, respectively. Shake well and use immediately after reconstitution (manufacturer recommendation); discard any unused portions.

Additional stability data:

Stability in polypropylene syringes (100 mcg/mL in NS) at 5°C ± 1°C is 7 days (Gupta, 2000). Stability in latex-free, PVC minibags protected from light and stored at 15°C to 30°C (59°F to 86°F) was 12 hours for a 2 mcg/mL concentration or 18 hours for a 0.4 mcg/mL concentration in NS. May be exposed to light; however, stability time is significantly reduced, especially for the 2 mcg/mL concentration (Strong, 2010).

Mechanism of Action Levothyroxine (T_4) is a synthetic form of thyroxine, an endogenous hormone secreted by the thyroid gland. T_4 is converted to its active metabolite, L-triiodothyronine (T_3). Thyroid hormones (T_4 and T_3) then bind to thyroid receptor proteins in the cell nucleus and exert metabolic effects through control of DNA transcription and protein synthesis; involved in normal metabolism, growth, and development; promotes gluconeogenesis, increases utilization and mobilization of glycogen stores, and stimulates protein synthesis, increases basal metabolic rate

Pharmacodynamics/Kinetics

Onset of action: Therapeutic: Oral: 3-5 days; I.V. 6-8 hours

Peak effect: I.V.: 24 hours

Absorption: Oral: Erratic (40% to 80% [per manufacturer]); may be decreased by age and specific foods and drugs

Protein binding: >99% bound to plasma proteins including thyroxine-binding globulin, thyroxine-binding prealbumin, and albumin

Metabolism: Hepatic to triiodothyronine (T_3; active); ~80% thyroxine (T_4) deiodinated in kidney and periphery; glucuronidation/conjugation also occurs; undergoes enterohepatic recirculation

Bioavailability: Oral tablets: 64% (nonfasting state) to 79% to 81% (fasting state)

Time to peak, serum: 2-4 hours

Half-life elimination: Euthyroid: 6-7 days; Hypothyroid: 9-10 days; Hyperthyroid: 3-4 days

Excretion: Urine (major route of elimination; decreases with age); feces (~20%)

Dosage

Geriatric Doses should be adjusted based on clinical response and laboratory parameters.

Hypothyroidism: Elderly patients may require <1 mcg/kg/day:

Oral:

>50 years without cardiac disease **or** <50 years with cardiac disease: Initial: 25-50 mcg/day; adjust dose by 12.5-25 mcg increments at 6- to 8-week intervals as needed

>50 years with cardiac disease: Initial: 12.5-25 mcg/day; adjust dose by 12.5-25 mcg increments at 4- to 6-week intervals (many clinicians prefer to adjust at 6- to 8-week intervals).

Note: Patients with combined hypothyroidism and cardiac disease should be monitored carefully for changes in stability.

I.M., I.V.: Refer to adult dosing.

Myxedema coma: *I.V.:* Refer to adult dosing; lower doses may be needed.

Adult Doses should be adjusted based on clinical response and laboratory parameters.

Hypothyroidism: Adults, healthy adults <50 years of age, and older adults who have been recently treated for hyperthyroidism or who have been hypothyroid for only a few months):

Oral: ~1.7 mcg/kg/day; usual doses are ≤200 mcg/day (range: 100-125 mcg/day for a 70 kg adult); doses ≥300 mcg/day are rare (consider poor compliance, malabsorption, and/or drug interactions). Titrate dose every 6 weeks.

Patients >50 years or patients with cardiac disease: Refer to geriatric dosing.

I.M., I.V.: 50% of the oral dose

◀ **Severe hypothyroidism:** Oral: Initial: 12.5-25 mcg/day; adjust dose by 25 mcg/day every 2-4 weeks as appropriate

Subclinical hypothyroidism (if treated): Oral: 1 mcg/kg/day

TSH suppression: Oral:

Well-differentiated thyroid cancer: Highly individualized; Doses >2 mcg/kg/day may be needed to suppress TSH to <0.1 mIU/mL. High-risk tumors may need a target level of <0.01 mIU/mL for TSH suppression.

Benign nodules and nontoxic multinodular goiter: Routine use of T_4 for TSH suppression is not recommended in patients with benign thyroid nodules. In patients deemed appropriate candidates, treatment should never be fully suppressive (TSH <0.1 mIU/mL) (Cooper, 2006; Gharib, 2006).

Note: Avoid use if TSH is already suppressed.

Myxedema coma or stupor: I.V.: 200-500 mcg, then 100-300 mcg the next day if necessary; smaller doses should be considered in patients with cardiovascular disease

Administration

Oral: Administer in the morning on an empty stomach, at least 30 minutes before food.

Capsule: Must be swallowed whole; do not cut, crush, or attempt to dissolve capsules in water to prepare a suspension

Tablet: May be crushed and suspended in 1-2 teaspoonfuls of water; suspension should be used immediately. Levoxyl® should be administered with a full glass of water to prevent gagging (due to tablet swelling).

Nasogastric tube: Bioavailability of levothyroxine is reduced if administered with enteral tube feeds. Since holding feedings for at least 1 hour before and after levothyroxine administration may not completely resolve the interaction, an increase in dose (eg, additional 25 mcg) may be necessary (Dickerson, 2010).

Parenteral: Dilute vial with 5 mL normal saline; use immediately after reconstitution; should not be admixed with other solutions

Monitoring Parameters Thyroid function test (serum thyroxine, thyrotropin concentrations), resin triiodothyronine uptake (rT_3U), free thyroxine index (FTI), T_4, TSH, heart rate, blood pressure, clinical signs of hypo- and hyperthyroidism; TSH is the most reliable guide for evaluating adequacy of thyroid replacement dosage. TSH may be elevated during the first few months of thyroid replacement despite patients being clinically euthyroid. In cases where T_4 remains low and TSH is within normal limits, an evaluation of "free" (unbound) T_4 is needed to evaluate further increase in dosage

Adults: Monitor TSH every 6-8 weeks until normalized; 8-12 weeks after dosage changes; every 6-12 months throughout therapy

Reference Range Approximate adult normal range: 4-12 mcg/dL (SI: 51-154 nmol/L). Borderline high: 11.1-13 mcg/dL (SI: 143-167 nmol/L); high: ≥13.1 mcg/dL (SI: 169 nmol/L). Normal range is increased in women on birth control pills (5.5-12 mcg/dL). TSH: 0.4-10 (for those ≥80 years) mIU/L; T_4: 4-12 mcg/dL (SI: 51-154 nmol/L); T_3 (RIA) (total T_3): 80-230 ng/dL (SI: 1.2-3.5 nmol/L); T_4 free (free T_4): 0.7-1.8 ng/dL (SI: 9-23 pmol/L).

Test Interactions Many drugs may have effects on thyroid function tests (see Pharmacotherapy Pearls). Infectious hepatitis and acute intermittent porphyria may increase TBG concentrations; nephrosis, severe hypoproteinemia, severe liver disease, and acromegaly may decrease TBG concentrations.

Pharmacotherapy Pearls Equivalent doses: The following statement on relative potency of thyroid products is included in a joint statement by American Thyroid Association (ATA), American Association of Clinical Endocrinologists (AACE) and The Endocrine Society (TES): For purposes of conversion, levothyroxine sodium (T_4) 100 mcg is usually considered equivalent to desiccated thyroid 60 mg, thyroglobulin 60 mg, or liothyronine sodium (T_3) 25 mcg. However, these are rough guidelines only and do not obviate the careful re-evaluation of a patient when switching thyroid hormone preparations, including a change from one brand of levothyroxine to another. Joint position statement is available at http://www.thyroid.org/professionals/advocacy/04_12_08_thyroxine.html.

Note: Several medications have effects on thyroid production or conversion. The impact in thyroid replacement has not been specifically evaluated, but patient response should be monitored:

Methimazole: Decreases thyroid hormone secretion, while propylthiouracil decrease thyroid hormone secretion and decreases conversion of T_4 to T_3.

Beta-adrenergic antagonists: Decrease conversion of T_4 to T_3 (dose related, propranolol ≥160 mg/day); patients may be clinically euthyroid.

Iodide, iodine-containing radiographic contrast agents may decrease thyroid hormone secretion; may also increase thyroid hormone secretion, especially in patients with Graves' disease.

Other agents reported to impact on thyroid production/conversion include aminoglutethimide, amiodarone, chloral hydrate, diazepam, ethionamide, interferon-alpha, interleukin-2, lithium, lovastatin (case report), glucocorticoids (dose-related), mercaptopurine, sulfonamides, thiazide diuretics, and tolbutamide.

In addition, a number of medications have been noted to cause transient depression in TSH secretion, which may complicate interpretation of monitoring tests for levothyroxine, including corticosteroids, octreotide, and dopamine. Metoclopramide may increase TSH secretion

Special Geriatric Considerations Elderly do not have a change in serum thyroxine associated with aging; however, plasma T_3 concentrations are decreased 25% to 40% in the elderly. There is not a compensatory rise in thyrotropin suggesting that lower T_3 is not reacted upon as a deficiency by the pituitary. This indicates a slightly lower than normal dosage of thyroid hormone replacement is usually sufficient in elderly patients than in younger adult patients. TSH must be monitored since insufficient thyroid replacement (elevated TSH) is a risk for coronary artery disease and excessive replacement (low TSH) may cause signs of hyperthyroidism and excessive bone loss. Some clinicians suggest levothyroxine is the drug of choice for replacement therapy.

Dosage Forms Excipient information presented when available (limited, particularly for generics); consult specific product labeling.

Capsule, soft gelatin, oral, as sodium:
Tirosint®: 13 mcg, 25 mcg, 50 mcg, 75 mcg, 88 mcg, 100 mcg, 112 mcg, 125 mcg, 137 mcg, 150 mcg

Injection, powder for reconstitution, as sodium: 200 mcg, 500 mcg

Tablet, oral, as sodium: 25 mcg, 50 mcg, 75 mcg, 88 mcg, 100 mcg, 112 mcg, 125 mcg, 137 mcg, 150 mcg, 175 mcg, 200 mcg, 300 mcg

Levothroid®: 25 mcg, 75 mcg, 88 mcg, 100 mcg, 112 mcg, 125 mcg, 137 mcg, 150 mcg, 175 mcg, 200 mcg, 300 mcg [scored]

Levothroid®: 50 mcg [scored; dye free]

Levoxyl®: 25 mcg, 75 mcg, 88 mcg, 100 mcg, 112 mcg, 125 mcg, 137 mcg, 150 mcg, 175 mcg, 200 mcg [scored]

Levoxyl®: 50 mcg [scored; dye free]

Synthroid®: 25 mcg, 75 mcg, 88 mcg, 100 mcg, 112 mcg, 125 mcg, 137 mcg, 150 mcg, 175 mcg, 200 mcg, 300 mcg [scored]

Synthroid®: 50 mcg [scored; dye free]

Unithroid®: 25 mcg, 75 mcg, 88 mcg, 100 mcg, 112 mcg, 125 mcg, 150 mcg, 175 mcg, 200 mcg, 300 mcg [scored]

Unithroid®: 50 mcg [scored; dye free]

Selected References
de Groot JW, Zonnenberg BA, Plukker JT, et al, "Imatinib Induces Hypothyroidism in Patients Receiving Levothyroxine," *Clin Pharmacol Ther*, 2005, 78(4):433-8.

Lidocaine (Systemic) (LYE doe kane)

Medication Safety Issues
High alert medication:
The Institute for Safe Medication Practices (ISMP) includes this medication (epidural administration; I.V. formulation) among its list of drugs which have a heightened risk of causing significant patient harm when used in error.

International issues:
Lidosen [Italy] may be confused with Lincocin brand name for lincomycin [U.S., Canada, and multiple international markets]; Linoten brand name for pamidronate [Spain]; Lodosyn brand name for carbidopa [U.S.]

◀ **Brand Names: U.S.** Xylocaine®; Xylocaine® Dental; Xylocaine® MPF
Brand Names: Canada Xylocard®
Index Terms Lidocaine Hydrochloride; Lignocaine Hydrochloride
Generic Availability (U.S.) Yes
Pharmacologic Category Antiarrhythmic Agent, Class Ib; Local Anesthetic
Use Local and regional anesthesia by infiltration, nerve block, epidural, or spinal techniques; acute treatment of ventricular arrhythmias from myocardial infarction or cardiac manipulation
Unlabeled/Investigational Use
  ACLS guidelines: Hemodynamically stable monomorphic ventricular tachycardia (VT) (preserved ventricular function); polymorphic VT (preserved ventricular function); drug-induced monomorphic VT; when amiodarone is not available, pulseless VT or ventricular fibrillation (VF) (unresponsive to defibrillation, CPR, and vasopressor administration)
  PALS guidelines: When amiodarone is not available, pulseless VT or VF (unresponsive to defibrillation, CPR, and epinephrine administration); consider in patients with cocaine overdose to prevent arrhythmias secondary to MI
  I.V. infusion for chronic pain syndrome
Contraindications Hypersensitivity to lidocaine or any component of the formulation; hypersensitivity to another local anesthetic of the amide type; Adam-Stokes syndrome; severe degrees of SA, AV, or intraventricular heart block (except in patients with a functioning artificial pacemaker); premixed injection may contain corn-derived dextrose and its use is contraindicated in patients with allergy to corn-related products
Warnings/Precautions Use caution in patients with severe hepatic dysfunction or pseudocholinesterase deficiency; may have increased risk of lidocaine toxicity.

Intravenous: Constant ECG monitoring is necessary during I.V. administration. Use cautiously in hepatic impairment, any degree of heart block, Wolff-Parkinson-White syndrome, HF, marked hypoxia, severe respiratory depression, hypovolemia, history of malignant hyperthermia, or shock. Increased ventricular rate may be seen when administered to a patient with atrial fibrillation. Correct electrolyte disturbances, especially hypokalemia or hypomagnesemia, prior to use and throughout therapy. Correct any underlying causes of ventricular arrhythmias. Monitor closely for signs and symptoms of CNS toxicity. The elderly may be prone to increased CNS and cardiovascular side effects. Reduce dose in hepatic dysfunction and CHF.

Injectable anesthetic: Follow appropriate administration techniques so as not to administer any intravascularly. Solutions containing antimicrobial preservatives should not be used for epidural or spinal anesthesia. Some solutions contain a bisulfite; avoid in patients who are allergic to bisulfite. Resuscitative equipment, medicine and oxygen should be available in case of emergency. Use products containing epinephrine cautiously in patients with significant vascular disease, compromised blood flow, or during or following general anesthesia (increased risk of arrhythmias). Adjust the dose for the elderly, acutely ill, and debilitated patients.

Adverse Reactions (Reflective of adult population; not specific for elderly) Effects vary with route of administration. Many effects are dose related.
  Frequency not defined.
    Cardiovascular: Arrhythmia, bradycardia, arterial spasms, cardiovascular collapse, defibrillator threshold increased, edema, flushing, heart block, hypotension, sinus node supression, vascular insufficiency (periarticular injections)
    Central nervous system: Agitation, anxiety, apprehension, coma, confusion, disorientation, dizziness, drowsiness, euphoria, hallucinations, headache, hyperesthesia, hypoesthesia, lethargy, lightheadedness, nervousness, psychosis, seizure, slurred speech, somnolence, unconsciousness
    Gastrointestinal: Metallic taste, nausea, vomiting
    Local: Thrombophlebitis
    Neuromuscular & skeletal: Paresthesia, transient radicular pain (subarachnoid administration; up to 1.9%), tremor, twitching, weakness
    Otic: Tinnitus
    Respiratory: Bronchospasm, dyspnea, respiratory depression or arrest
    Miscellaneous: Allergic reactions, anaphylactoid reaction, sensitivity to temperature extremes

  Following spinal anesthesia: Positional headache (3%), shivering (2%) nausea, peripheral nerve symptoms, respiratory inadequacy and double vision (<1%), hypotension, cauda equina syndrome
Drug Interactions
  Metabolism/Transport Effects Substrate of CYP1A2 (minor), CYP2A6 (minor), CYP2B6 (minor), CYP2C9 (minor), CYP2D6 (major), CYP3A4 (major), P-glycoprotein; **Inhibits** CYP1A2 (strong), 2D6 (moderate), 3A4 (moderate)

Avoid Concomitant Use

Avoid concomitant use of Lidocaine (Systemic) with any of the following: Conivaptan; Saquinavir; Thioridazine; Tolvaptan

Increased Effect/Toxicity

Lidocaine (Systemic) may increase the levels/effects of: Bendamustine; Budesonide (Systemic, Oral Inhalation); Colchicine; CYP1A2 Substrates; CYP2D6 Substrates; CYP3A4 Substrates; Eplerenone; Everolimus; Fesoterodine; Halofantrine; Lurasidone; Pimecrolimus; Ranolazine; Salmeterol; Saxagliptin; Tamoxifen; Thioridazine; Tolvaptan; Vilazodone

The levels/effects of Lidocaine (Systemic) may be increased by: Abiraterone Acetate; Amiodarone; Beta-Blockers; Conivaptan; CYP2D6 Inhibitors (Moderate); CYP2D6 Inhibitors (Strong); CYP3A4 Inhibitors (Moderate); CYP3A4 Inhibitors (Strong); Darunavir; Dasatinib; Disopyramide; P-Glycoprotein Inhibitors; Saquinavir; Telaprevir

Decreased Effect

The levels/effects of Lidocaine (Systemic) may be decreased by: CYP3A4 Inducers (Strong); Cyproterone; Deferasirox; Etravirine; Herbs (CYP3A4 Inducers); Peginterferon Alfa-2b; P-Glycoprotein Inducers; Tocilizumab

Ethanol/Nutrition/Herb Interactions Herb/Nutraceutical: St John's wort may decrease lidocaine levels; avoid concurrent use.

Stability Injection: Stable at room temperature. Stability of parenteral admixture at room temperature (25°C) is the expiration date on premixed bag; out of overwrap stability is 30 days.

Standard concentration/diluent: 2 g/250 mL D_5W.

Mechanism of Action Class Ib antiarrhythmic; suppresses automaticity of conduction tissue, by increasing electrical stimulation threshold of ventricle, His-Purkinje system, and spontaneous depolarization of the ventricles during diastole by a direct action on the tissues; blocks both the initiation and conduction of nerve impulses by decreasing the neuronal membrane's permeability to sodium ions, which results in inhibition of depolarization with resultant blockade of conduction

Pharmacodynamics/Kinetics

Onset of action: Single bolus dose: 45-90 seconds

Duration: 10-20 minutes

Distribution: V_d: 1.1-2.1 L/kg; alterable by many patient factors; decreased in CHF and liver disease; crosses blood-brain barrier

Protein binding: 60% to 80% to alpha$_1$ acid glycoprotein

Metabolism: 90% hepatic; active metabolites monoethylglycinexylidide (MEGX) and glycinexylidide (GX) can accumulate and may cause CNS toxicity

Half-life elimination: Biphasic: Prolonged with congestive heart failure, liver disease, shock, severe renal disease; Initial: 7-30 minutes; Terminal: 1.5-2 hours

Excretion: Urine (<10% as unchanged drug, ~90% as metabolites)

Dosage

Geriatric & Adult

Antiarrhythmic (ACLS, 2010):

VF or pulseless VT (after defibrillation attempts, CPR, and vasopressor administration) if amiodarone is not available: I.V., intraosseous (I.O.): Initial: 1-1.5 mg/kg. If refractory VF or pulseless VT, repeat 0.5-0.75 mg/kg bolus every 5-10 minutes (maximum cumulative dose: 3 mg/kg). Follow with continuous infusion (1-4 mg/minute) after return of perfusion. Reappearance of arrhythmia during constant infusion: 0.5 mg/kg bolus and reassessment of infusion (Zipes, 2000)

Intratracheal (loading dose only): 2-3.75 mg/kg (2-2.5 times the recommended I.V. dose); dilute in 5-10 mL NS or sterile water. **Note:** Absorption is greater with sterile water and results in less impairment of PaO$_2$.

Hemodynamically stable monomorphic VT: I.V.: 1-1.5 mg/kg; repeat with 0.5-0.75 mg/kg every 5-10 minutes as necessary (maximum cumulative dose: 3 mg/kg). Follow with continuous infusion of 1-4 mg/minute (or 14-57 mcg/kg/minute).

Note: Reduce maintenance infusion in patients with CHF, shock, or hepatic disease; initiate infusion at 10 mcg/kg/minute (maximum dose: 1.5 mg/minute or 20 mcg/kg/minute).

Anesthesia, local injectable: Varies with procedure, degree of anesthesia needed, vascularity of tissue, duration of anesthesia required, and physical condition of patient; maximum: 4.5 mg/kg/dose not to exceed 300 mg; do not repeat within 2 hours.

Renal Impairment Not dialyzable (0% to 5%) by hemo- or peritoneal dialysis; supplemental dose is not necessary.

Hepatic Impairment Reduce maintenance infusion. Initial: 0.75 mg/minute or 10 mcg/kg/minute; maximum dose: 1.5 mg/minute or 20 mcg/kg/minute. Monitor lidocaine concentrations closely and adjust infusion rate as necessary; consider alternative therapy.

Administration

Local infiltration: Buffered lidocaine for injectable local anesthetic may be prepared: Add 2 mL of sodium bicarbonate 8.4% to 18 mL of lidocaine 1% (Christoph, 1988)

Intratracheal (unlabeled administration route): Dilute in NS or sterile water. Absorption is greater with sterile water and results in less impairment of PaO_2 (Hahnel, 1990). Pass catheter beyond tip of tracheal tube, stop compressions, spray drug quickly down tube. Flush with 5 mL of NS and follow immediately with several quick insufflations and continue chest compressions.

Continuous I.V. infusion: **Infusion rates:** 2 g/250 mL D_5W
1 mg/minute: 7.5 mL/hour
2 mg/minute: 15 mL/hour
3 mg/minute: 22.5 mL/hour
4 mg/minute: 30 mL/hour

Intraosseous (I.O.; unlabeled administration route): Intraosseous administration is a safe and effective alternative to venous access in children with cardiac arrest; the onset for most medications is similar to that of I.V. administration (PALS, 2010). In adults, I.O. administration is a reasonable alternative when quick I.V. access is not feasible (ACLS, 2010).

Reference Range

Therapeutic: 1.5-5.0 mcg/mL (SI: 6-21 µmol/L)
Potentially toxic: >6 mcg/mL (SI: >26 µmol/L)
Toxic: >9 mcg/mL (SI: >38 µmol/L)

Special Geriatric Considerations Due to decreases in Phase I metabolism and possibly decrease in splanchnic perfusion with age, there may be a decreased clearance or increased half-life in the elderly and increased risk for CNS side effects and cardiac effects.

Dosage Forms Excipient information presented when available (limited, particularly for generics); consult specific product labeling. [DSC] = Discontinued product

Infusion, premixed in D_5W, as hydrochloride: 0.4% [4 mg/mL] (250 mL, 500 mL); 0.8% [8 mg/mL] (250 mL, 500 mL)

Injection, solution, as hydrochloride: 0.5% [5 mg/mL] (50 mL [DSC]); 1% [10 mg/mL] (2 mL, 10 mL, 20 mL, 30 mL, 50 mL); 2% [20 mg/mL] (2 mL, 5 mL, 20 mL, 50 mL)

Xylocaine®: 0.5% [5 mg/mL] (50 mL); 1% [10 mg/mL] (10 mL, 20 mL, 50 mL); 2% [20 mg/mL] (10 mL, 20 mL, 50 mL) [contains methylparaben]

Injection, solution, as hydrochloride [preservative free]: 0.5% [5 mg/mL] (50 mL); 1% [10 mg/mL] (2 mL, 5 mL, 30 mL); 1.5% [15 mg/mL] (20 mL); 2% [20 mg/mL] (2 mL, 5 mL, 10 mL); 4% [40 mg/mL] (5 mL)

Xylocaine®: 2% [20 mg/mL] (5 mL)

Xylocaine® MPF: 0.5% [5 mg/mL] (50 mL); 1% [10 mg/mL] (2 mL, 5 mL, 10 mL, 30 mL); 1.5% [15 mg/mL] (10 mL, 20 mL); 2% [20 mg/mL] (2 mL, 5 mL, 10 mL); 4% [40 mg/mL] (5 mL)

Injection, solution, as hydrochloride [for dental use]:
Xylocaine® Dental: 2% [20 mg/mL] (1.8 mL)

Injection, solution, premixed in $D_{7.5}W$, as hydrochloride [preservative free]: 5% [50 mg/mL] (2 mL)

Lidocaine (Ophthalmic) (LYE doe kane)

Brand Names: U.S. Akten™
Index Terms Lidocaine Hydrochloride; Lignocaine Hydrochloride
Generic Availability (U.S.) No
Pharmacologic Category Local Anesthetic; Local Anesthetic, Ophthalmic
Use To provide local anesthesia to ocular surface during ophthalmologic procedures
Dosage
 Geriatric & Adult Anesthesia, ocular: Apply 2 drops to ocular surface in area where procedure will occur; may reapply to maintain effect.
Dosage Forms Excipient information presented when available (limited, particularly for generics); consult specific product labeling.
 Gel, ophthalmic, as hydrochloride [drops, preservative free]:
 Akten™: 3.5% (5 mL)

Lidocaine (Topical) (LYE doe kane)

Brand Names: U.S. AneCream™ [OTC]; Anestafoam™ [OTC]; Band-Aid® Hurt Free® Antiseptic Wash [OTC]; Burn Jel Plus [OTC]; Burn Jel® [OTC]; L-M-X® 4 [OTC]; L-M-X® 5 [OTC]; LidaMantle®; Lidoderm®; LTA® 360; Premjact®; Regenecare®; Regenecare® HA [OTC]; Solarcaine® cool aloe Burn Relief [OTC]; Topicaine® [OTC]; Unburn® [OTC]; Xylocaine®

Brand Names: Canada Betacaine®; Lidodan™; Lidoderm®; Maxilene®; Xylocaine®
Index Terms Lidocaine Hydrochloride; Lidocaine Patch; Lignocaine Hydrochloride; Viscous Lidocaine; Xylocaine Viscous
Generic Availability (U.S.) Yes: Hydrochloride cream, jelly, ointment, solution
Pharmacologic Category Analgesic, Topical; Local Anesthetic
Use
Rectal: Temporary relief of pain and itching due to anorectal disorders
Topical: Local anesthetic for oral mucous membrane; use in laser/cosmetic surgeries; minor burns, cuts, and abrasions of the skin
Oral topical solution (viscous): Topical anesthesia of irritated oral mucous membranes and pharyngeal tissue
Patch (Lidoderm®): Relief of allodynia (painful hypersensitivity) and chronic pain in post-herpetic neuralgia
Dosage
Geriatric & Adult Anesthesia, topical:
Cream:
LidaMantle®: Skin irritation: Apply a thin film to affected area 2-3 times/day as needed
L-M-X® 4: Skin irritation: Apply up to 3-4 times daily to intact skin
L-M-X® 5: Relief of anorectal pain and itching: Apply to affected area up to 6 times/day
Gel, ointment: Apply to affected area ≤4 times/day as needed (maximum dose: 4.5 mg/kg, not to exceed 300 mg)
Topical solution: Apply 1-5 mL (40-200 mg) to affected area
Jelly: Maximum dose: 30 mL (600 mg) in any 12-hour period:
Anesthesia of male urethra: 5-30 mL (100-600 mg)
Anesthesia of female urethra: 3-5 mL (60-100 mg)
Oral topical solution (viscous):
Anesthesia of the mouth: 15 mL swished in the mouth and spit out no more frequently than every 3 hours (maximum: 8 doses per 24-hour period)
Anesthesia of the pharynx: 15 mL gargled no more frequently than every 3 hours (maximum: 8 doses per 24-hour period); may be swallowed
Patch: Postherpetic neuralgia: Apply patch to most painful area. Up to 3 patches may be applied in a single application. Patch(es) may remain in place for up to 12 hours in any 24-hour period.
Dosage Forms Excipient information presented when available (limited, particularly for generics); consult specific product labeling. [DSC] = Discontinued product
Aerosol, topical [foam]:
Anestafoam™: 4% (30 g) [contains benzalkonium chloride, benzyl alcohol]
Aerosol, topical [spray]:
Solarcaine® cool aloe Burn Relief: 0.5% (127 g) [contains aloe, vitamin E]
Cream, rectal:
L-M-X® 5: 5% (15 g, 30 g) [contains benzyl alcohol]
Cream, topical:
AneCream™: 4% (5 g, 15 g, 30 g) [contains benzyl alcohol, soybean lecithin]
L-M-X® 4: 4% (5 g, 15 g, 30 g) [contains benzyl alcohol]
Cream, topical, as hydrochloride: 0.5% (0.9 g)
LidaMantle®: 3% (85 g)
Gel, topical:
Topicaine®: 4% (10 g, 30 g, 113 g); 5% (10 g, 30 g, 113 g) [contains aloe, benzyl alcohol, ethanol 35%, jojoba]
Gel, topical, as hydrochloride:
Burn Jel Plus: 2.5% (118 mL) [contains vitamin E]
Burn Jel®: 2% (59 mL, 118 mL); 2% (3.5 g)
Regenecare®: 2% (14 g, 85 g) [contains aloe; contains calcium alginate]
Regenecare® HA: 2% (85 g) [contains aloe; contains hyaluronic acid]
Solarcaine® cool aloe Burn Relief: 0.5% (113 g, 226 g) [contains aloe, isopropyl alcohol, menthol, tartrazine]
Unburn®: 2.5% (59 mL) [contains vitamin E]
Jelly, topical, as hydrochloride: 2% (5 mL, 30 mL)
Xylocaine®: 2% (5 mL, 30 mL)
Jelly, topical, as hydrochloride [preservative free]: 2% (5 mL, 10 mL, 20 mL)
Lotion, topical, as hydrochloride:
LidaMantle®: 3% (177 mL)
Ointment, topical: 5% (35.4 g)
Patch, topical:
Lidoderm®: 5% (30s)
Solution, topical [spray]:
Premjact®: 9.6% (13 mL)

Solution, topical, as hydrochloride: 4% [40 mg/mL] (50 mL)
    Band-Aid® Hurt Free™ Antiseptic Wash: 2% [20 mg/mL] (177 mL) [contains aloe, benzal-konium chloride]
    LTA® 360: 4% [40 mg/mL] (4 mL)
    Xylocaine®: 4% (50 mL); 4% [40 mg/mL] (50 mL [DSC])
Solution, topical, as hydrochloride [preservative free]: 4% [40 mg/mL] (4 mL)
Solution, viscous, oral topical, as hydrochloride: 2% [20 mg/mL] (20 mL, 100 mL)

Lidocaine and Tetracaine (LYE doe kane & TET ra kane)

Medication Safety Issues
Other safety concerns:
Transdermal patch may contain conducting metal (eg, aluminum); remove patch prior to MRI.

Brand Names: U.S. Synera™

Index Terms Tetracaine and Lidocaine

Generic Availability (U.S.) No

Pharmacologic Category Analgesic, Topical; Local Anesthetic

Use Topical anesthetic for use on normal intact skin for minor procedures (eg, I.V. cannulation or venipuncture) and superficial dermatologic procedures

Dosage
Geriatric & Adult
Venipuncture or intravenous cannulation: Transdermal patch: Prior to procedure, apply to intact skin for 20-30 minutes; **Note:** Adults can use another patch at a new location to facilitate venous access after a failed attempt; remove previous patch.

Superficial dermatological procedures: Transdermal patch: Prior to procedure, apply to intact skin for 30 minutes

Hepatic Impairment Use caution in patients with severe hepatic dysfunction.

Special Geriatric Considerations The manufacturer reports that in clinical studies there were no significant differences in safety between geriatric adjustments and younger subjects.

Dosage Forms Excipient information presented when available (limited, particularly for generics); consult specific product labeling.

Patch, transdermal:
    Synera™: Lidocaine 70 mg and tetracaine 70 mg (10s) [contains heating component, metal; each patch is ~50 cm^2]

♦ **Lidocaine Hydrochloride** *see* Lidocaine (Ophthalmic) *on page 1064*
♦ **Lidocaine Hydrochloride** *see* Lidocaine (Systemic) *on page 1061*
♦ **Lidocaine Hydrochloride** *see* Lidocaine (Topical) *on page 1064*
♦ **Lidocaine Patch** *see* Lidocaine (Topical) *on page 1064*
♦ **Lidoderm®** *see* Lidocaine (Topical) *on page 1064*
♦ **Lignocaine Hydrochloride** *see* Lidocaine (Ophthalmic) *on page 1064*
♦ **Lignocaine Hydrochloride** *see* Lidocaine (Systemic) *on page 1061*
♦ **Lignocaine Hydrochloride** *see* Lidocaine (Topical) *on page 1064*

Linagliptin (lin a GLIP tin)

Related Information
Diabetes Mellitus Management, Adults *on page 2073*

Brand Names: U.S. Tradjenta™

Index Terms BI-1356; Trajenta

Pharmacologic Category Antidiabetic Agent, Dipeptidyl Peptidase IV (DPP-IV) Inhibitor

Use Management of type 2 diabetes mellitus (noninsulin dependent, NIDDM) as an adjunct to diet and exercise as monotherapy or in combination with other antidiabetic agents

Contraindications Hypersensitivity to linagliptin or any component of the formulation

Warnings/Precautions Avoid use in type 1 diabetes mellitus (insulin dependent, IDDM) and diabetic ketoacidosis (DKA) due to lack of efficacy in these populations. Use caution if used in conjunction with insulin or insulin secretagogues; risk of hypoglycemia is increased. Monitor blood glucose closely; dosage adjustments of insulin or insulin secretagogues may be necessary. Diabetes self-management education (DSME) is essential to maximize the effectiveness of therapy.

Adverse Reactions (Reflective of adult population; not specific for elderly)
>10%: Endocrine & metabolic: Hypoglycemia (combined with metformin/sulfonylurea [15%], metformin [<1%], pioglitazone [<1%]; monotherapy [<1%]) (Scott, 2011)
1% to 10%:
    Central nervous system: Headache (6%)

Endocrine & metabolic: Hyperuricemia (3%), lipids increased (3%), triglycerides increased (2%), weight gain (2%)

Neuromuscular & skeletal: Arthralgia (6%), back pain (6%)

Respiratory: Nasopharyngitis (6%), cough (2%)

Drug Interactions

Avoid Concomitant Use There are no known interactions where it is recommended to avoid concomitant use.

Increased Effect/Toxicity

Linagliptin may increase the levels/effects of: ACE Inhibitors; Hypoglycemic Agents

The levels/effects of Linagliptin may be increased by: Herbs (Hypoglycemic Properties); Pegvisomant; P-Glycoprotein Inhibitors; Ritonavir

Decreased Effect

The levels/effects of Linagliptin may be decreased by: Corticosteroids (Orally Inhaled); Corticosteroids (Systemic); CYP3A4 Inducers (Strong); Luteinizing Hormone-Releasing Hormone Analogs; P-Glycoprotein Inducers; Somatropin; Thiazide Diuretics

Ethanol/Nutrition/Herb Interactions

Ethanol: Caution with ethanol (may cause hypoglycemia).

Herb/Nutraceutical: Herbs with hypoglycemic properties may enhance the hypoglycemic effect of linagliptin. This includes alfalfa, aloe, bilberry, bitter melon, burdock, celery, damiana, fenugreek, garcinia, garlic, ginger, ginseng (American), gymnema, marshmallow, stinging nettle.

Stability Store at 25°C (77°F); excursions permitted between 15°C to 30°C (59°F to 86°F).

Mechanism of Action Linagliptin inhibits dipeptidyl peptidase IV (DPP-IV) enzyme resulting in prolonged active incretin levels. Incretin hormones (eg, glucagon-like peptide-1 [GLP-1] and glucose-dependent insulinotropic polypeptide [GIP]) regulate glucose homeostasis by increasing insulin synthesis and release from pancreatic beta cells and decreasing glucagon secretion from pancreatic alpha cells. Decreased glucagon secretion results in decreased hepatic glucose production. Under normal physiologic circumstances, incretin hormones are released by the intestine throughout the day and levels are increased in response to a meal; incretin hormones are rapidly inactivated by the DPP-IV enzyme.

Pharmacodynamics/Kinetics

Absorption: Rapid

Distribution: Extensive

Protein binding: 70% to 80%; concentration dependent

Metabolism: Not extensively metabolized

Bioavailability: 30%

Half-life elimination: Effective (therapeutic): ~12 hours; Terminal (DPP-IV saturable binding): >100 hours

Time to peak: 1.5 hours

Excretion: 80% feces unchanged; 5% urine unchanged

Dosage

Geriatric & Adult Type 2 diabetes: Oral: 5 mg once daily

Renal Impairment No adjustment recommended.

Hepatic Impairment No adjustment recommended.

Administration May be administered with or without food.

Monitoring Parameters Hb A_{1c}, serum glucose

Reference Range Recommendations for glycemic control in adults with diabetes:

Hb A_{1c}: <7%

Preprandial capillary plasma glucose: 70-130 mg/dL

Peak postprandial capillary blood glucose: <180 mg/dL

Special Geriatric Considerations According to the manufacturer, ~26% of participants in clinical trials were ≥65 years; ~3% were ≥75 years. No difference in efficacy or safety was noted between younger and older patients.

Dosage Forms Excipient information presented when available (limited, particularly for generics); consult specific product labeling.

Tablet, oral:

Tradjenta™: 5 mg

Selected References

American Diabetes Association, "Standards of Medical Care in Diabetes Mellitus – 2011," *Diabetes Care*, 2011, 34 (Suppl 1):11-61.

Handelsman Y, Mechanick JI, Blonde L, et al, "American Association of Clinical Endocrinologists Medical Guidelines for Clinical Practice for Developing a Diabetes Mellitus Comprehensive Care Plan," *Endocr Pract*, 2011, 17(Suppl 2):1-53.

Scott LJ, "Linagliptin: In Type 2 Diabetes Mellitus," *Drugs*, 2011, 71(5):611-24.

Lindane (LIN dane)

Brand Names: Canada Hexit™; PMS-Lindane

Index Terms Benzene Hexachloride; Gamma Benzene Hexachloride; Hexachlorocyclohexane

Generic Availability (U.S.) Yes

Pharmacologic Category Antiparasitic Agent, Topical; Pediculocide; Scabicidal Agent

Use Treatment of *Sarcoptes scabiei* (scabies), *Pediculus capitis* (head lice), and *Phthirus pubis* (crab lice); FDA recommends reserving lindane as a second-line agent or with inadequate response to other therapies

Medication Guide Available Yes

Contraindications Hypersensitivity to lindane or any component of the formulation; uncontrolled seizure disorders; crusted (Norwegian) scabies, acutely-inflamed skin or raw, weeping surfaces or other skin conditions which may increase systemic absorption

Warnings/Precautions [U.S. Boxed Warning]: Not considered a drug of first choice; use only in patients who have failed first-line treatments, or in patients who cannot tolerate these agents. Because of the potential for systemic absorption and CNS side effects, lindane should be used with caution; consider permethrin or crotamiton agent first. Oil-based hair dressing may increase toxic potential.

[U.S. Boxed Warning]: May be associated with severe neurologic toxicities (contraindicated in uncontrolled seizure disorders). Seizures and death have been reported with use; use with caution in patients <50 kg, or patients with a history of seizures; use caution with conditions which may increase risk of seizures or medications which decrease seizure threshold; use caution with hepatic impairment; avoid contact with face, eyes, mucous membranes, and urethral meatus.

[U.S. Boxed Warning]: A lindane medication use guide must be given to all patients along with instructions for proper use. Patients should be informed that itching may occur following successful killing of lice and re-treatment may not be indicated. Should be used as a part of an overall lice management program.

Adverse Reactions (Reflective of adult population; not specific for elderly) Frequency not defined (includes postmarketing and/or case reports).

Cardiovascular: Cardiac arrhythmia

Central nervous system: Ataxia, dizziness, headache, restlessness, seizure, pain

Dermatologic: Alopecia, contact dermatitis, skin and adipose tissue may act as repositories, eczematous eruptions, pruritus, urticaria

Gastrointestinal: Nausea, vomiting

Hematologic: Aplastic anemia

Hepatic: Hepatitis

Local: Burning and stinging

Neuromuscular & skeletal: Paresthesia

Renal: Hematuria

Respiratory: Pulmonary edema

Drug Interactions

Avoid Concomitant Use There are no known interactions where it is recommended to avoid concomitant use.

Increased Effect/Toxicity There are no known significant interactions involving an increase in effect.

Decreased Effect There are no known significant interactions involving a decrease in effect.

Mechanism of Action Directly absorbed by parasites and ova through the exoskeleton; stimulates the nervous system resulting in seizures and death of parasitic arthropods

Pharmacodynamics/Kinetics

Absorption: ≤13% systemically

Distribution: Stored in body fat; accumulates in brain; skin and adipose tissue may act as repositories

Metabolism: Hepatic

Excretion: Urine and feces

Dosage

Geriatric & Adult

Scabies: Topical: Apply a thin layer of lotion and massage it on skin from the neck to the toes; after 8-12 hours, bathe and remove the drug

Head lice, crab lice: Topical: Apply shampoo to dry hair and massage into hair for 4 minutes; add small quantities of water to hair until lather forms, then rinse hair thoroughly and comb with a fine tooth comb to remove nits. Amount of shampoo needed is based on length and density of hair; most patients will require 30 mL (maximum: 60 mL).

Administration For topical use only; never administer orally. Caregivers should apply with gloves (avoid natural latex, may be permeable to lindane). Rinse off with warm (not hot) water.

Lotion: Apply to dry, cool skin; do not apply to face or eyes. Wait at least 1 hour after bathing or showering (wet or warm skin increases absorption). Skin should be clean and free of any other lotions, creams, or oil prior to lindane application.

Shampoo: Apply to clean, dry hair. Wait at least 1 hour after washing hair before applying lindane shampoo. Hair should be washed with a shampoo not containing a conditioner; hair and skin of head and neck should be free of any lotions, oils, or creams prior to lindane application.

Special Geriatric Considerations Because of the potential for systemic absorption and CNS side effects, lindane should be used with caution. Not considered a drug of first choice; consider permethrin or crotamiton agent first.

Dosage Forms Excipient information presented when available (limited, particularly for generics); consult specific product labeling.

Lotion, topical: 1% (60 mL)

Shampoo, topical: 1% (60 mL)

Linezolid (li NE zoh lid)

Related Information

Antibiotic Treatment of Adults With Infective Endocarditis *on page 2053*

Community-Acquired Pneumonia in Adults *on page 2059*

Medication Safety Issues

Sound-alike/look-alike issues:

Zyvox® may be confused with Ziox™, Zosyn®, Zovirax®

Brand Names: U.S. Zyvox®

Brand Names: Canada Zyvoxam®

Generic Availability (U.S.) No

Pharmacologic Category Antibiotic, Oxazolidinone

Use Treatment of vancomycin-resistant *Enterococcus faecium* (VRE) infections, nosocomial pneumonia caused by *Staphylococcus aureus* (including MRSA) or *Streptococcus pneumoniae* (including multidrug-resistant strains [MDRSP]), complicated and uncomplicated skin and skin structure infections (including diabetic foot infections without concomitant osteomyelitis), and community-acquired pneumonia caused by susceptible gram-positive organisms

Contraindications Hypersensitivity to linezolid or any other component of the formulation; concurrent use or within 2 weeks of MAO inhibitors; patients with uncontrolled hypertension, pheochromocytoma, thyrotoxicosis, and/or taking sympathomimetics (eg, pseudoephedrine), vasopressive agents (eg, epinephrine, norepinephrine), or dopaminergic agents (eg, dopamine, dobutamine) unless closely monitored for increased blood pressure; patients with carcinoid syndrome and/or taking SSRIs, tricyclic antidepressants, serotonin 5-HT$_{1B,1D}$ receptor agonists, meperidine, or buspirone unless closely monitored for sign/symptoms of serotonin syndrome

Warnings/Precautions Myelosuppression has been reported and may be dependent on duration of therapy (generally >2 weeks of treatment); use with caution in patients with pre-existing myelosuppression, in patients receiving other drugs which may cause bone marrow suppression, or in chronic infection (previous or concurrent antibiotic therapy). Weekly CBC monitoring is recommended. Consider discontinuation in patients developing myelosuppression (or in whom myelosuppression worsens during treatment).

Lactic acidosis has been reported with use. Linezolid exhibits mild MAO inhibitor properties and has the potential to have the same interactions as other MAO inhibitors; use with caution and monitor closely in patients with uncontrolled hypertension, pheochromocytoma, carcinoid syndrome, or untreated hyperthyroidism; use is contraindicated in the absence of close monitoring. Symptoms of agitation, confusion, hallucinations, hyper-reflexia, myoclonus, shivering, and tachycardia may occur with concomitant proserotonergic drugs (eg, SSRIs/SNRIs or triptans) or agents which reduce linezolid's metabolism; concurrent use with these medications is contraindicated unless patient is closely monitored for signs/symptoms of serotonin syndrome. Unnecessary use may lead to the development of resistance to linezolid; consider alternatives before initiating outpatient treatment.

Peripheral and optic neuropathy (with vision loss) has been reported and may occur primarily with extended courses of therapy >28 days; any symptoms of visual change or impairment warrant immediate ophthalmic evaluation and possible discontinuation of therapy. Seizures have been reported; use with caution in patients with a history of seizures. Prolonged use may result in fungal or bacterial superinfection, including *C. difficile*-associated diarrhea (CDAD) and pseudomembranous colitis; CDAD has been observed >2 months postantibiotic treatment.

Due to inconsistent concentrations in the CSF, empiric use in pediatric patients with CNS infections is not recommended by the manufacturer; however, there are multiple case reports describing successful treatment of documented VRE and *Staphylococcus aureus* CNS and shunt infections in the literature. Linezolid should not be used in the empiric treatment of catheter-related bloodstream infection (CRBSI), but may be appropriate for targeted therapy (Mermel, 2009). Oral suspension contains phenylalanine.

Adverse Reactions (Reflective of adult population; not specific for elderly) Percentages as reported in adults; frequency similar in pediatric patients

>10%:
Central nervous system: Headache (<1% to 11%)
Gastrointestinal: Diarrhea (3% to 11%)

1% to 10%:
Central nervous system: Insomnia (3%), dizziness (≤2%), fever (2%)
Dermatologic: Rash (2%)
Gastrointestinal: Nausea (3% to 10%), lipase increased (3% to 4%), vomiting (1% to 4%), constipation (2%), taste alteration (1% to 2%), amylase increased (<1% to 2%), tongue discoloration (≤1%), oral moniliasis (≤1%), pancreatitis
Genitourinary: Vaginal moniliasis (1% to 2%)
Hematologic: Thrombocytopenia (<1% to 10%), hemoglobin decreased (1% to 7%), leukopenia (<1% to 2%), neutropenia (≤1%)
Hepatic: ALT increased (2% to 10%), AST increased (2% to 5%), alkaline phosphatase increased (<1% to 4%), bilirubin increased (≤1%)
Renal: BUN increased (≤2%)
Miscellaneous: Fungal infection (≤1% to 2%), lactate dehydrogenase increased (<1% to 2%)

Drug Interactions

Avoid Concomitant Use

Avoid concomitant use of Linezolid with any of the following: Alpha-/Beta-Agonists (Indirect-Acting); Alpha1-Agonists; Alpha2-Agonists (Ophthalmic); Amphetamines; Anilidopiperidine Opioids; Atomoxetine; Bezafibrate; Buprenorphine; BuPROPion; BusPIRone; CarBAMazepine; Cyclobenzaprine; Dexmethylphenidate; Dextromethorphan; Diethylpropion; HYDROmorphone; MAO Inhibitors; Maprotiline; Meperidine; Methyldopa; Methylene Blue; Methylphenidate; Mirtazapine; Oxymorphone; Pizotifen; Propoxyphene; Selective Serotonin Reuptake Inhibitors; Serotonin 5-HT1D Receptor Agonists; Serotonin/Norepinephrine Reuptake Inhibitors; Sibutramine; Tapentadol; Tetrabenazine; Tetrahydrozoline; Tetrahydrozoline (Nasal); Tricyclic Antidepressants; Tryptophan

Increased Effect/Toxicity

Linezolid may increase the levels/effects of: Alpha-/Beta-Agonists (Direct-Acting); Alpha-/Beta-Agonists (Indirect-Acting); Alpha1-Agonists; Alpha2-Agonists (Ophthalmic); Amphetamines; Antihypertensives; Atomoxetine; Beta2-Agonists; Bezafibrate; BuPROPion; Dexmethylphenidate; Dextromethorphan; Diethylpropion; Doxapram; HYDROmorphone; Lithium; Meperidine; Methadone; Methyldopa; Methylene Blue; Methylphenidate; Mirtazapine; Orthostatic Hypotension Producing Agents; Pizotifen; Reserpine; Selective Serotonin Reuptake Inhibitors; Serotonin 5-HT1D Receptor Agonists; Serotonin Modulators; Serotonin/Norepinephrine Reuptake Inhibitors; Tetrahydrozoline; Tetrahydrozoline (Nasal); Tricyclic Antidepressants

The levels/effects of Linezolid may be increased by: Altretamine; Anilidopiperidine Opioids; Buprenorphine; BusPIRone; CarBAMazepine; COMT Inhibitors; Cyclobenzaprine; Levodopa; MAO Inhibitors; Maprotiline; Oxymorphone; Propoxyphene; Sibutramine; Tapentadol; Tetrabenazine; TraMADol; Tryptophan

Decreased Effect There are no known significant interactions involving a decrease in effect.

Ethanol/Nutrition/Herb Interactions

Ethanol: Avoid ethanol (based on CNS depressant effects and potential tyramine content)
Food: Concurrent ingestion of foods rich in tyramine may cause sudden and severe high blood pressure (hypertensive crisis). Avoid tyramine-containing foods with MAOIs. Food's freshness is also an important concern; improperly stored or spoiled food can create an environment where tyramine concentrations may increase.
Herb/Nutraceutical: Avoid supplements containing caffeine, tyrosine, tryptophan or phenylalanine. Ingestion of large quantities may increase the risk of severe side effects (eg, hypertensive reactions, serotonin syndrome).

Stability

Infusion: Store at 25°C (77°F); excursions permitted to 15°C to 30°C (59°F to 86°F). Protect from light. Keep infusion bags in overwrap until ready for use. Protect infusion bags from freezing.

Oral suspension: Reconstitute with 123 mL of distilled water (in 2 portions); shake vigorously. Concentration is 100 mg/5 mL. Prior to administration mix gently by inverting bottle; do not shake. Following reconstitution, store at 25°C (77°F); excursions permitted to 15°C to 30°C (59°F to 86°F). Use reconstituted suspension within 21 days. Protect from light.

Tablet: Store at 25°C (77°F); excursions permitted to 15°C to 30°C (59°F to 86°F). Protect from light; protect from moisture.

Mechanism of Action Inhibits bacterial protein synthesis by binding to bacterial 23S ribosomal RNA of the 50S subunit. This prevents the formation of a functional 70S initiation complex that is essential for the bacterial translation process. Linezolid is bacteriostatic against enterococci and staphylococci and bactericidal against most strains of streptococci.

Pharmacodynamics/Kinetics

Absorption: Rapid and extensive

Distribution: V_{dss}: 40-50 L

Protein binding: 31%

Metabolism: Hepatic via oxidation of the morpholine ring, resulting in two inactive metabolites (aminoethoxyacetic acid, hydroxyethyl glycine); minimally metabolized, may be mediated by cytochrome P450

Bioavailability: Oral: ~100%

Half-life elimination: 4-5 hours

Time to peak: Oral: 1-2 hours

Excretion: Urine (~30% of total dose as parent drug, ~50% of total dose as metabolites); feces (~9% of total dose as metabolites)

Nonrenal clearance: ~65%

Dosage

Geriatric & Adult

Usual dosage: Oral, I.V.: 600 mg every 12 hours

Indication-specific dosing:

VRE infections including concurrent bacteremia: Oral, I.V.: 600 mg every 12 hours for 14-28 days

MRSA infections:

Brain abscess, subdural empyema, spinal epidural abscess (unlabeled use; Liu, 2011): Oral, I.V.: 600 mg every 12 hours for 4-6 weeks

Meningitis (unlabeled use; Liu, 2011): Oral, I.V.: 600 mg every 12 hours for 2 weeks

Osteomyelitis (unlabeled use; Liu, 2011): Oral, I.V.: 600 mg every 12 hours for a minimum of 8 weeks (some experts combine with rifampin)

Pneumonia (healthcare associated or community acquired) (Liu, 2011): Oral, I.V.: 600 mg every 12 hours for 7-21 days

Septic arthritis (unlabeled use; Liu, 2011): Oral, I.V.: 600 mg every 12 hours for 3-4 weeks

Septic thrombosis of cavernous or dural venous sinus (unlabeled use; Liu, 2011): Oral, I.V.: 600 mg every 12 hours for 4-6 weeks

Nosocomial pneumonia, complicated skin and skin structure infections, community-acquired pneumonia including concurrent bacteremia: Oral, I.V.: 600 mg every 12 hours for 10-14 days. **Note:** May consider 7-day treatment course (versus manufacturer recommended 10-14 days) in patients with healthcare-, hospital-, and ventilator- associated pneumonia who have demonstrated good clinical response (ATS/IDSA, 2005).

Uncomplicated skin and skin structure infections: Oral: 400 mg every 12 hours for 10-14 days. **Note:** 400 mg dose is recommended in the product labeling; however, 600 mg dose is commonly employed clinically (Stevens, 2005)

Renal Impairment No adjustment is recommended. The two primary metabolites may accumulate in patients with renal impairment but the clinical significance is unknown. Weigh the risk of accumulation of metabolites versus the benefit of therapy. Monitor for hematopoietic (eg, anemia, leukopenia, thrombocytopenia) and neuropathic (eg, peripheral neuropathy) adverse events when administering for extended periods.

Intermittent hemodialysis (administer after hemodialysis on dialysis days): Dialyzable (~30% removed during 3-hour dialysis session): If administration time is not immediately after dialysis session, may consider administration of a supplemental dose especially early in the treatment course to maintain levels above the MIC (Brier, 2003). Others have recommended no supplemental dose or dosage adjustment for patients on intermittent hemodialysis, peritoneal dialysis, or continuous renal replacement therapy (eg, CVVHD) (Heintz, 2009; Trotman, 2005).

Hepatic Impairment

Mild-to-moderate hepatic impairment (Child-Pugh class A or B): No dosage adjustment required.

Severe hepatic impairment (Child-Pugh class C): Use has not been adequately evaluated.

◀ **Administration**

I.V.: Administer intravenous infusion over 30-120 minutes. Do not mix or infuse with other medications. When the same intravenous line is used for sequential infusion of other medications, flush line with D_5W, NS, or LR before and after infusing linezolid. The yellow color of the injection may intensify over time without affecting potency.

Oral suspension: Invert gently to mix prior to administration, do not shake. Administer without regard to meals.

Monitoring Parameters Weekly CBC, particularly in patients at increased risk of bleeding, with pre-existing myelosuppression, on concomitant medications that cause bone marrow suppression, in those who require >2 weeks of therapy, or in those with chronic infection who have received previous or concomitant antibiotic therapy; visual function with extended therapy (≥3 months) or in patients with new onset visual symptoms, regardless of therapy length

Special Geriatric Considerations According to the manufacturer the pharmacokinetics of linezolid are not significantly altered in patients ≥65 years of age.

Dosage Forms Excipient information presented when available (limited, particularly for generics); consult specific product labeling.

Infusion, premixed:

Zyvox®: 200 mg (100 mL); 600 mg (300 mL) [contains sodium 0.38 mg/mL]

Powder for suspension, oral:

Zyvox®: 100 mg/5 mL (150 mL) [contains phenylalanine 20 mg/5 mL, sodium 8.52 mg (0.4 mEq)/5 mL, sodium benzoate; orange flavor]

Tablet, oral:

Zyvox®: 600 mg [contains sodium 2.92 mg (0.1 mEq)/tablet]

Selected References

Bain KT and Wittbrodt ET, "Linezolid for the Treatment of Resistant Gram-Positive Cocci," *Ann Pharmacother*, 2001, 35 (5):566-75.

Perry CM and Jarvis B, "Linezolid: A Review of Its Use in the Management of Serious Gram-Positive Infections," *Drugs*, 2001, 61(4):525-51.

◆ **Lioresal®** *see* Baclofen *on page 181*

Liothyronine (lye oh THYE roe neen)

Medication Safety Issues

Sound-alike/look-alike issues:

Liothyronine may be confused with levothyroxine

Other safety concerns:

T3 is an error-prone abbreviation (mistaken as acetaminophen and codeine [ie, Tylenol® #3])

Brand Names: U.S. Cytomel®; Triostat®

Brand Names: Canada Cytomel®

Index Terms Liothyronine Sodium; Sodium *L*-Triiodothyronine; T_3 Sodium (error-prone abbreviation)

Generic Availability (U.S.) Yes

Pharmacologic Category Thyroid Product

Use

Oral: Replacement or supplemental therapy in hypothyroidism; management of nontoxic goiter; a diagnostic aid

I.V.: Treatment of myxedema coma/precoma

Unlabeled/Investigational Use Management of hemodynamically unstable potential organ donors increasing the quantity of organs available for transplantation

Contraindications Hypersensitivity to liothyronine sodium or any component of the formulation; undocumented or uncorrected adrenal insufficiency; recent myocardial infarction or thyrotoxicosis; artificial rewarming (injection)

Warnings/Precautions [U.S. Boxed Warning]: Ineffective and potentially toxic for weight reduction. High doses may produce serious or even life-threatening toxic effects particularly when used with some anorectic drugs. Use with extreme caution in patients with angina pectoris or other cardiovascular disease (including hypertension) or coronary artery disease. Use with caution in elderly patients since they may be more likely to have compromised cardiovascular function. Patients with adrenal insufficiency, myxedema, diabetes mellitus and insipidus may have symptoms exaggerated or aggravated. Thyroid replacement requires periodic assessment of thyroid status. Chronic hypothyroidism predisposes patients to coronary artery disease.

Adverse Reactions (Reflective of adult population; not specific for elderly)

1% to 10%: Cardiovascular: Arrhythmia (6%), tachycardia (3%), cardiopulmonary arrest (2%), hypotension (2%), MI (2%)

Drug Interactions

Avoid Concomitant Use

Avoid concomitant use of Liothyronine with any of the following: Sodium Iodide I131

Increased Effect/Toxicity

Liothyronine may increase the levels/effects of: Vitamin K Antagonists

Decreased Effect

Liothyronine may decrease the levels/effects of: Sodium Iodide I131; Theophylline Derivatives

The levels/effects of Liothyronine may be decreased by: Bile Acid Sequestrants; Calcium Polystyrene Sulfonate; Calcium Salts; CarBAMazepine; Estrogen Derivatives; Fosphenytoin; Lanthanum; Phenytoin; Rifampin; Sodium Polystyrene Sulfonate

Stability Vials must be stored under refrigeration at 2°C to 8°C (36°F to 46°F). Store tablets at 15°C to 30°C (59°F to 86°F).

Mechanism of Action Exact mechanism of action is unknown; however, it is believed the thyroid hormone exerts its many metabolic effects through control of DNA transcription and protein synthesis; involved in normal metabolism, growth, and development; promotes gluconeogenesis, increases utilization and mobilization of glycogen stores, and stimulates protein synthesis, increases basal metabolic rate

Pharmacodynamics/Kinetics

Onset of action: ~3 hours

Peak response: 2-3 days

Absorption: Oral: Well absorbed (95% in 4 hours)

Half-life elimination: 2.5 days

Excretion: Urine

Dosage

Geriatric Oral: 5 mcg/day; increase by 5 mcg/day every 2 weeks

Adult

Hypothyroidism: Oral: 25 mcg/day increase by 12.5-25 mcg/day every 1-2 weeks to a maximum of 100 mcg/day; usual maintenance dose: 25-75 mcg/day

Patients with cardiovascular disease: Refer to geriatric dosing.

Suppression test: (T_3): Oral: 75-100 mcg/day for 7 days; use lowest dose for elderly

Myxedema: Oral: Initial: 5 mcg/day; increase in increments of 5-10 mcg/day every 1-2 weeks. When 25 mcg/day is reached, dosage may be increased at intervals of 5-25 mcg/day every 1-2 weeks. Usual maintenance dose: 50-100 mcg/day.

Myxedema coma: I.V.: 25-50 mcg

Patients with known or suspected cardiovascular disease: 10-20 mcg

Note: Normally, at least 4 hours should be allowed between doses to adequately assess therapeutic response and no more than 12 hours should elapse between doses to avoid fluctuations in hormone levels. Oral therapy should be resumed as soon as the clinical situation has been stabilized and the patient is able to take oral medication. If levothyroxine rather than liothyronine sodium is used in initiating oral therapy, the prescriber should bear in mind that there is a delay of several days in the onset of levothyroxine activity and that I.V. therapy should be discontinued gradually.

Simple (nontoxic) goiter: Oral: Initial: 5 mcg/day; increase by 5-10 mcg every 1-2 weeks; after 25 mcg/day is reached, may increase dose by 12.5-25 mcg. Usual maintenance dose: 75 mcg/day.

Administration I.V.: For I.V. use only; **do not administer I.M. or SubQ**

Administer doses at least 4 hours, and no more than 12 hours, apart

Resume oral therapy as soon as the clinical situation has been stabilized and the patient is able to take oral medication

When switching to tablets, discontinue the injectable, initiate oral therapy at a low dosage and increase gradually according to response

If **levothyroxine** is used for oral therapy, there is a delay of several days in the onset of activity; therefore, discontinue I.V. therapy gradually

Monitoring Parameters T_3, TSH, heart rate, blood pressure, renal function, clinical signs of hypo- and hyperthyroidism; TSH is the most reliable guide for evaluating adequacy of thyroid replacement dosage. TSH may be elevated during the first few months of thyroid replacement despite patients being clinically euthyroid. In cases where T_4 remains low and TSH is within normal limits, an evaluation of "free" (unbound) T_4 is needed to evaluate further increase in dosage.

Reference Range Free T_3, serum: 250-390 pg/dL; TSH: 0.4 and up to 10 (≥80 years) mIU/L

Test Interactions Many drugs may have effects on thyroid function tests (see Pharmacotherapy Pearls). Pregnancy, infectious hepatitis, and acute intermittent porphyria may increase TBG concentrations; nephrosis, severe hypoproteinemia, severe liver disease, and acromegaly may decrease TBG concentrations.

◀ **Pharmacotherapy Pearls** Equivalent doses: The following statement on relative potency of thyroid products is included in a joint statement by American Thyroid Association (ATA), American Association of Clinical Endocrinologists (AACE) and The Endocrine Society (TES): For purposes of conversion, levothyroxine sodium (T_4) 100 mcg is usually considered equivalent to desiccated thyroid 60 mg, thyroglobulin 60 mg, or liothyronine sodium (T_3) 25 mcg. However, these are rough guidelines only and do not obviate the careful re-evaluation of a patient when switching thyroid hormone preparations, including a change from one brand of levothyroxine to another. Joint position statement is available at http://www.thyroid.org/professionals/advocacy/04_12_08_thyroxine.html.

A synthetic form of *L*-Triiodothyronine (T_3) can be used in patients allergic to products derived from pork or beef.

Note: Several medications have effects on thyroid production or conversion. The impact in thyroid replacement has not been specifically evaluated, but patient response should be monitored:

Methimazole: Decreases thyroid hormone secretion, while propylthiouracil decrease thyroid hormone secretion and decreases conversion of T_4 to T_3.

Beta-adrenergic antagonists: Decrease conversion of T_4 to T_3 (dose related, propranolol ≥160 mg/day); patients may be clinically euthyroid.

Iodide, iodine-containing radiographic contrast agents may decrease thyroid hormone secretion; may also increase thyroid hormone secretion, especially in patients with Graves' disease.

Other agents reported to impact on thyroid production/conversion include aminoglutethimide, amiodarone, chloral hydrate, diazepam, ethionamide, interferon-alpha, interleukin-2, lithium, lovastatin (case report), glucocorticoids (dose-related), mercaptopurine, sulfonamides, thiazide diuretics, and tolbutamide.

In addition, a number of medications have been noted to cause transient depression in TSH secretion, which may complicate interpretation of monitoring tests for thyroid hormones, including corticosteroids, octreotide, and dopamine. Metoclopramide may increase TSH secretion.

Special Geriatric Considerations Elderly do not have a change in serum thyroxine associated with aging; however, plasma T_3 concentrations are decreased 25% to 40% in the elderly. There is not a compensatory rise in thyrotropin suggesting that lower T_3 is not reacted upon as a deficiency by the pituitary. This indicates a slightly lower than normal dosage of thyroid hormone replacement is usually sufficient in elderly patients than in younger adult patients. TSH must be monitored since insufficient thyroid replacement (elevated TSH) is a risk for coronary artery disease and excessive replacement (low TSH) may cause signs of hyperthyroidism and excessive bone loss.

Dosage Forms Excipient information presented when available (limited, particularly for generics); consult specific product labeling.

Injection, solution: 10 mcg/mL (1 mL)

Triostat®: 10 mcg/mL (1 mL) [contains ethanol 6.8%]

Tablet, oral: 5 mcg, 25 mcg, 50 mcg

Cytomel®: 5 mcg

Cytomel®: 25 mcg, 50 mcg [scored]

♦ **Liothyronine and Levothyroxine** see Liotrix on page 1074
♦ **Liothyronine Sodium** see Liothyronine on page 1072

Liotrix (LYE oh triks)

Medication Safety Issues

Sound-alike/look-alike issues:

Liotrix may be confused with Klotrix®

Thyrolar® may be confused with Thyrogen®, Thytropar®

Brand Names: U.S. Thyrolar®

Brand Names: Canada Thyrolar®

Index Terms Levothyroxine and Liothyronine; Liothyronine and Levothyroxine; T_3/T_4 Liotrix

Generic Availability (U.S.) No

Pharmacologic Category Thyroid Product

Use

Replacement or supplemental therapy in hypothyroidism (uniform mixture of T_4:T_3 in 4:1 ratio by weight)

Thyroid-stimulating hormone (TSH) suppressant therapy used in the management of thyroid cancer (levothyroxine is generally recommended for this indication); prevention or treatment of euthyroid goiters (eg, thyroid nodules, subacute or chronic lymphocytic thyroiditis [Hashimoto's], multinodular goiters)

Diagnostic agent in suppression tests to diagnose suspected mild hyperthyroidism or to demonstrate thyroid gland autonomy

Contraindications Hypersensitivity to liotrix or any component of the formulation; uncorrected adrenal insufficiency; untreated thyrotoxicosis

Warnings/Precautions [U.S. Boxed Warning]: In euthyroid patients, thyroid supplements are ineffective and potentially toxic for weight reduction (unapproved use); high doses may produce serious or even life-threatening toxic effects, particularly when used with some anorectic drugs. Use is not justified for the treatment of male or female infertility in euthyroid patients (unapproved use). Use with caution and reduce dosage in the elderly since they may be more likely to have compromised cardiovascular function and in patients with angina pectoris or other cardiovascular disease (chronic hypothyroidism predisposes patients to coronary artery disease). Suppressed TSH levels in the elderly may increase risk of atrial fibrillation and mortality secondary to cardiovascular disease (Gharib, 2010; Parle, 2001). Use with caution in patients with adrenal insufficiency, diabetes mellitus or insipidus, and myxedema; symptoms may be exaggerated or aggravated; initial dosage reduction is recommended in patients with long-standing myxedema.

Adverse Reactions (Reflective of adult population; not specific for elderly) Frequency not defined.

Cardiovascular: Blood pressure increased, cardiac arrhythmia, chest pain, palpitation, tachycardia

Central nervous system: Anxiety, ataxia, fever, headache, insomnia, nervousness

Dermatologic: Alopecia, hyperhydrosis, pruritus, urticaria

Endocrine & metabolic: Changes in menstrual cycle, increased appetite, weight loss

Gastrointestinal: Abdominal cramps, constipation, diarrhea, nausea, vomiting

Neuromuscular & skeletal: Hand tremor, myalgia, tremor

Respiratory: Dyspnea

Miscellaneous: Allergic skin reactions (rare), diaphoresis

Drug Interactions

Avoid Concomitant Use

Avoid concomitant use of Liotrix with any of the following: Sodium Iodide I131

Increased Effect/Toxicity

Liotrix may increase the levels/effects of: Vitamin K Antagonists

Decreased Effect

Liotrix may decrease the levels/effects of: Sodium Iodide I131; Theophylline Derivatives

The levels/effects of Liotrix may be decreased by: Bile Acid Sequestrants; Calcium Polystyrene Sulfonate; Calcium Salts; CarBAMazepine; Estrogen Derivatives; Fosphenytoin; Lanthanum; Phenytoin; Rifampin; Sodium Polystyrene Sulfonate

Stability Store at 2°C to 8°C (36°F to 46°F). Protect from light.

Mechanism of Action The primary active compound is T_3 (triiodothyronine), which may be converted from T_4 (thyroxine) and then circulates throughout the body to influence growth and maturation of various tissues. Liotrix is uniform mixture of synthetic T_4 and T_3 in 4:1 ratio; exact mechanism of action is unknown; however, it is believed the thyroid hormone exerts its many metabolic effects through control of DNA transcription and protein synthesis; involved in normal metabolism, growth, and development; promotes gluconeogenesis, increases utilization and mobilization of glycogen stores and stimulates protein synthesis, increases basal metabolic rate

Pharmacodynamics/Kinetics

Onset of action: Liothyronine (T_3): ~3 hours

Absorption: Thyroxine (T_4): 40% to 80%; T_3: 95%

Protein binding: T_4: >99% bound to plasma proteins including thyroxine-binding globulin, thyroxine-binding prealbumin, and albumin

Metabolism: Hepatic to triiodothyronine (active); ~80% T_4 deiodinated in kidney and periphery; glucuronidation/conjugation also occurs; undergoes enterohepatic recirculation

Half-life elimination:

T_4: Euthyroid: 6-7 days; Hyperthyroid: 3-4 days; Hypothyroid: 9-10 days

T_3: 2.5 days

Time to peak, serum: T_4: 2-4 hours; T_3: 2-3 days

Excretion: Urine (major route of elimination); partially feces

◀ **Dosage**

Geriatric Initial: Levothyroxine 12.5-25 mcg/Liothyronine 3.1-6.25 mcg once daily; may increase by levothyroxine 12.5 mcg/Liothyronine 3.1 mcg every 2-3 weeks

Adult Hypothyroidism: Oral: Initial: Levothyroxine 25 mcg/Liothyronine 6.25 mcg once daily; may increase by levothyroxine 12.5 mcg/Liothyronine 3.1 mcg every 2-3 weeks. A lower initial dose (levothyroxine 12.5 mcg/Liothyronine 3.1 mcg) is recommended in patients with long-standing myxedema, especially if cardiovascular impairment coexists. If angina occurs, reduce dose (usual maintenance dose: levothyroxine 50-100 mcg/Liothyronine 12.5-25 mcg)

Monitoring Parameters T_4, TSH, heart rate, blood pressure, clinical signs of hypo- and hyperthyroidism; TSH is the most reliable guide for evaluating adequacy of thyroid replacement dosage. TSH may be elevated during the first few months of thyroid replacement despite patients being clinically euthyroid. In cases where T_4 remains low and TSH is within normal limits, an evaluation of "free" (unbound) T_4 is needed to evaluate further increase in dosage.

Reference Range

TSH: Age 21-54 years: 0.4-4.2 mIU/L; Age 55-87 years: 0.5-8.9 mIU/L

T_4: 4-12 mcg/dL (SI: 51-154 nmol/L)

T_3 (RIA) (total T_3): 80-230 ng/dL (SI: 1.2-3.5 nmol/L)

T_4 free (free T_4): 0.7-1.8 ng/dL (SI: 9-23 pmol/L)

Test Interactions Many drugs may have effects on thyroid function tests; para-aminosalicylic acid, aminoglutethimide, amiodarone, barbiturates, carbamazepine, chloral hydrate, clofibrate, colestipol, corticosteroids, danazol, diazepam, estrogens, ethionamide, fluorouracil, I.V. heparin, insulin, lithium, methadone, methimazole, mitotane, nitroprusside, oxyphenbutazone, phenylbutazone, PTU, perphenazine, phenytoin, propranolol, salicylates, sulfonylureas, and thiazides

Pharmacotherapy Pearls Equivalent doses: The following statement on relative potency of thyroid products is included in a joint statement by American Thyroid Association (ATA), American Association of Clinical Endocrinologists (AACE) and The Endocrine Society (TES): For purposes of conversion, levothyroxine sodium (T_4) 100 mcg is usually considered equivalent to desiccated thyroid 60 mg, thyroglobulin 60 mg, or liothyronine sodium (T_3) 25 mcg. However, these are rough guidelines only and do not obviate the careful re-evaluation of a patient when switching thyroid hormone preparations, including a change from one brand of levothyroxine to another. Joint position statement is available at http://www.thyroid.org/professionals/advocacy/04_12_08_thyroxine.html.

Since T_3 is produced by monodeiodination of T_4 in peripheral tissues (80%) and since elderly have decreased T_3 (25% to 40%), little advantage to this product exists and cost is not justified; no advantage over synthetic levothyroxine sodium.

Special Geriatric Considerations Elderly do not have a change in serum thyroxine associated with aging; however, plasma T_3 concentrations are decreased 25% to 40% in older adults. There is not a compensatory rise in thyrotropin suggesting that lower T_3 is not reacted upon as a deficiency by the pituitary. This indicates a slightly lower than normal dosage of thyroid hormone replacement is usually sufficient in older patients than in younger adult patients. TSH must be monitored since insufficient thyroid replacement (elevated TSH) is a risk for coronary artery disease and excessive replacement (low TSH) may cause signs of hyperthyroidism and excessive bone loss.

Dosage Forms Excipient information presented when available (limited, particularly for generics); consult specific product labeling.

Tablet, oral:

Thyrolar®: ¼ [levothyroxine sodium 12.5 mcg and liothyronine sodium 3.1 mcg]

Thyrolar®: ½ [levothyroxine sodium 25 mcg and liothyronine sodium 6.25 mcg]

Thyrolar®: 1 [levothyroxine sodium 50 mcg and liothyronine sodium 12.5 mcg]

Thyrolar®: 2 [levothyroxine sodium 100 mcg and liothyronine sodium 25 mcg]

Thyrolar®: 3 [levothyroxine sodium 150 mcg and liothyronine sodium 37.5 mcg]

◆ **Lipancreatin** see Pancrelipase on page 1387

◆ **Lipase, Protease, and Amylase** see Pancrelipase on page 1387

◆ **Lipiarrmycin** see Fidaxomicin (Systemic) on page 732

◆ **Lipitor®** see Atorvastatin on page 162

◆ **Lipofen®** see Fenofibrate on page 701

◆ **Liqua-Cal [OTC]** see Calcium and Vitamin D on page 248

◆ **Liquid Paraffin** see Mineral Oil on page 1217

◆ **Liquifilm® Tears [OTC]** see Artificial Tears on page 148

Liraglutide (lir a GLOO tide)

Related Information
Diabetes Mellitus Management, Adults *on page 2073*

Medication Safety Issues
Other safety concerns:
Cross-contamination may occur if pens are shared among multiple patients. Steps should be taken to prohibit sharing of pens.

Brand Names: U.S. Victoza®

Brand Names: Canada Victoza®

Index Terms NN2211

Generic Availability (U.S.) No

Pharmacologic Category Antidiabetic Agent, Glucagon-Like Peptide-1 (GLP-1) Receptor Agonist

Use Treatment of type 2 diabetes mellitus (noninsulin dependent, NIDDM) to improve glycemic control

Medication Guide Available Yes

Contraindications History of or family history of medullary thyroid carcinoma (MTC); patients with multiple endocrine neoplasia syndrome type 2 (MEN2)

Warnings/Precautions [U.S. Boxed Warning] Dose and duration dependent thyroid C-cell tumors have developed in animal studies with liraglutide therapy; relevance in humans unknown. During clinical studies a few cases of thyroid C-cell hyperplasia were reported. Due to the finding in animal studies, patients were monitored with serum calcitonin or thyroid ultrasound during clinical trials; however it us unknown if this is beneficial in decreasing the risk of thyroid tumors. Consultation with an endocrinologist is recommended in patients who develop elevated calcitonin concentrations. Patients should be counseled on the risk and symptoms of thyroid tumors. Use is contraindicated in patients with or a family history of medullary thyroid cancer and in patients with multiple endocrine neoplasia syndrome type 2 (MEN2). Cases of acute and chronic pancreatitis (including one case of fatal necrotizing pancreatitis) have been reported although conclusive evidence to liraglutide therapy has not been established; monitor for unexplained severe abdominal pain, and if pancreatitis is suspected, discontinue use. Do not resume unless an alternative etiology of pancreatitis is confirmed. Use with caution in patients with a history of pancreatitis, cholelithiasis, and/or alcohol abuse. Most common reactions are gastrointestinal related; these symptoms may be dose-related and may decrease in frequency/severity with gradual titration and continued use. Use may be associated with weight loss (likely due to reduced intake) independent of the change in hemoglobin A_{1c}. Use with caution in patients with hepatic or renal impairment; cases of acute renal failure and chronic renal failure exacerbation have been reported.

Concurrent use with insulin therapy has not been evaluated. Concomitant use of an insulin secretagogue (eg, sulfonylurea, meglitinide) may increase the risk of hypoglycemia; dosage reduction of secretagogues may be required during initiation of liraglutide. Due to its effects on gastric emptying, liraglutide may reduce the rate and extent of absorption of orally-administered drugs; use with caution in patients receiving medications with a narrow therapeutic window or require rapid absorption from the GI tract. Not recommended for first-line therapy; use as adjunct to diet and exercise. Do not use in patients with type 1 diabetes mellitus or for the treatment of diabetic ketoacidosis; not a substitute for insulin. Diabetes self-management education (DSME) is essential to maximize the effectiveness of therapy.

Adverse Reactions (Reflective of adult population; not specific for elderly) Percentages are as reported for monotherapy.
>10%: Gastrointestinal: Nausea (28%), diarrhea (17%), vomiting (11%)
1% to 10%:
Cardiovascular: Hypertension (3%)
Central nervous system: Headache (9%), dizziness (6%)
Gastrointestinal: Constipation (10%)
Genitourinary: Urinary tract infection (6%)
Hepatic: Hyperbilirubinemia (4%)
Local: Injection site reactions (2%; includes rash, erythema)
Neuromuscular & skeletal: Back pain (5%)
Respiratory: Upper respiratory infection (10%), sinusitis (6%), nasopharyngitis (5%)
Miscellaneous: Anti-liraglutide antibodies (low titers 9%, cross-reacting 7%), influenza (7%)

Drug Interactions
Avoid Concomitant Use There are no known interactions where it is recommended to avoid concomitant use.

Increased Effect/Toxicity
Liraglutide may increase the levels/effects of: Sulfonylureas

The levels/effects of Liraglutide may be increased by: Pegvisomant

Decreased Effect
The levels/effects of Liraglutide may be decreased by: Corticosteroids (Orally Inhaled); Corticosteroids (Systemic); Luteinizing Hormone-Releasing Hormone Analogs; Somatropin; Thiazide Diuretics

Ethanol/Nutrition/Herb Interactions Ethanol: Caution with ethanol (may cause hypoglycemia).

Stability Prior to initial use, store under refrigeration at 2°C to 8°C (36°F to 46°F); after initial use, may be stored in refrigerator or at room temperature of 15°C to 30°C (59°F to 86°F). Do not freeze (discard if freezing occurs). Protect from heat and light. Pen should be discarded 30 days after initial use.

Mechanism of Action Liraglutide is a long acting analog of human glucagon-like peptide-1 (GLP-1) (an incretin hormone) which increases glucose-dependent insulin secretion, decreases inappropriate glucagon secretion, increases B-cell growth/replication, slows gastric emptying, and decreases food intake. Liraglutide administration results in decreases in hemoglobin A_{1c} by approximately 1%.

Pharmacodynamics/Kinetics
Distribution: V_d: SubQ: ~13 L; I.V.: 0.07 L/kg

Protein binding: >98%

Metabolism: Endogenously metabolized by dipeptidyl peptidase IV (DPP-IV) and endogenous endopeptidases (Croom, 2009); metabolism occurs slower than that seen with native GLP-1

Bioavailability: SubQ: ~55%

Half-life, elimination: ~13 hours

Time to peak, plasma: 8-12 hours

Excretion: Urine (6%, as metabolites); feces (5%, as metabolites)

Dosage
Geriatric & Adult Note: Initial dose is intended to reduce GI symptoms; does not provide effective glycemic control.

Treatment of type 2 diabetes: SubQ: Initial: 0.6 mg once daily for 1 week; then increase to 1.2 mg once daily; may increase further to 1.8 mg once daily if optimal glycemic response not achieved with 1.2 mg/day

Renal Impairment No dosage adjustment recommended; use caution, limited experience.

Hepatic Impairment No dosage adjustment recommended; use caution, limited experience.

Administration SubQ: Use only if clear, colorless, and free of particulate matter. Administer via injection in the upper arm, thigh, or abdomen. Administer without regard to meals or time of day. Change needle with each administration. Do not share pens between patients even if needle is changed.

Monitoring Parameters Plasma glucose, Hb A_{1c}

Reference Range
Recommendations for glycemic control in adults with diabetes (ADA, 2010):

Hb A_{1c}: <7%

Preprandial capillary plasma glucose: 70-130 mg/dL

Peak postprandial capillary blood glucose: <180 mg/dL

Special Geriatric Considerations In clinical trials liraglutide's pharmacokinetics did not differ between younger and older participants. The manufacturer reports that the safety and efficacy of liraglutide did not differ in older diabetics. Intensive glucose control (HbA$_{1c}$ <6.5%) has been linked to increased all-cause and cardiovascular mortality, hypoglycemia requiring assistance, and weight gain in adult type 2 diabetes. How "tightly" to control a geriatric patient's blood glucose needs to be individualized. Such a decision should be based on several factors, including the patient's functional and cognitive status, how well he/she recognizes hypoglycemic or hyperglycemic symptoms, and how to respond to them and other disease states. An HbA$_{1c}$ <7.5% is an acceptable endpoint for a healthy older adult, while <8% is acceptable for frail elderly patients, those with a duration of illness >10 years, or those with comorbid conditions and requiring combination diabetes medications. Patients who are unable to accurately draw up their dose will need assistance, such as prefilled syringes. Initial doses may require considerations for renal function in the elderly with dosing adjusted subsequently based on blood glucose monitoring. For elderly patients with diabetes who are relatively healthy, attaining target goals for aspirin use, blood pressure, lipids, smoking cessation, and diet and exercise may be more important than normalized glycemic control.

Dosage Forms Excipient information presented when available (limited, particularly for generics); consult specific product labeling.

Injection, solution [rDNA origin]:

Victoza®: 6 mg/mL (3 mL) [contains propylene glycol 14 mg/3 mL; prefilled pen]

Selected References

Action to Control Cardiovascular Risk in Diabetes Study Group, Gerstein HC, Miller ME, et al, "Effects of Intensive Glucose Lowering in Type 2 Diabetes," *N Engl J Med*, 2008, 358(24):2545-59.

ADVANCE Collaborative Group, Patel A, MacMahon S, et al, "Intensive Blood Glucose Control and Vascular Outcomes in Patients With Type 2 Diabetes," *N Engl J Med*, 2008, 358(24):2560-72.

American Diabetes Association, "Standards of Medical Care in Diabetes – 2011," *Diabetes Care*, 2011, 34(Suppl 1):11-61.

Brown AF, Mangione CM, Saliba D, et al, "Guidelines for Improving the Care of the Older Person With Diabetes Mellitus," *J Am Geriatr Soc*, 2003, 51(5 Suppl Guidelines):265-80.

"VA/DoD Clinical Practice Guideline for the Management of Diabetes Mellitus," 2010. Available at http://www.healthquality.va.gov/Diabetes_Mellitus.asp

Lisinopril (lyse IN oh pril)

Related Information

Angiotensin Agents *on page 1985*

Medication Safety Issues

Sound-alike/look-alike issues:

Lisinopril may be confused with fosinopril, Lioresal®, Lipitor®, RisperDAL®

Prinivil® may be confused with Plendil®, Pravachol®, Prevacid®, PriLOSEC®, Proventil®

Zestril® may be confused with Desyrel, Restoril™, Vistaril®, Zegerid®, Zerit®, Zetia®, Zostrix®, ZyPREXA®

International issues:

Acepril [Malaysia] may be confused with Accupril which is a brand name for quinapril [U.S.]

Acepril: Brand name for lisinopril [Malaysia], but also the brand name for captopril [Great Britain]; enalapril [Hungary, Switzerland]

Carace [Ireland] may be confused with Carac which is a brand name for fluorouracil [U.S.]

Brand Names: U.S. Prinivil®; Zestril®

Brand Names: Canada Apo-Lisinopril®; CO Lisinopril; Dom-Lisinopril; JAMP-Lisinopril; Mint-Lisinopril; Mylan-Lisinopril; PMS-Lisinopril; Prinivil®; PRO-Lisinopril; RAN™-Lisinopril; ratio-Lisinopril; ratio-Lisinopril P; ratio-Lisinopril Z; Riva-Lisinopril; Sandoz-Lisinopril; Teva-Lisinopril (Type P); Teva-Lisinopril (Type Z); Zestril®

Generic Availability (U.S.) Yes

Pharmacologic Category Angiotensin-Converting Enzyme (ACE) Inhibitor

Use Treatment of hypertension, either alone or in combination with other antihypertensive agents; adjunctive therapy in treatment of heart failure (afterload reduction); treatment of acute myocardial infarction within 24 hours in hemodynamically-stable patients to improve survival; treatment of left ventricular dysfunction after myocardial infarction

Contraindications Hypersensitivity to lisinopril or any component of the formulation; angioedema related to previous treatment with an ACE inhibitor; patients with idiopathic or hereditary angioedema

Warnings/Precautions Anaphylactic reactions may occur rarely with ACE inhibitors. At any time during treatment (especially following first dose), angioedema may occur rarely with ACE inhibitors; it may involve the head and neck (potentially compromising airway) or the intestine (presenting with abdominal pain). African-Americans may be at an increased risk. Prolonged frequent monitoring may be required especially if tongue, glottis, or larynx are involved as they are associated with airway obstruction. Patients with a history of airway surgery may have a higher risk of airway obstruction. Aggressive early and appropriate management is critical. Use in patients with idiopathic or hereditary angioedema or previous angioedema associated with ACE inhibitor therapy is contraindicated. Severe anaphylactoid reactions may be seen during hemodialysis (eg, CVVHD) with high-flux dialysis membranes (eg, AN69), and rarely, during low density lipoprotein apheresis with dextran sulfate cellulose. Rare cases of anaphylactoid reactions have been reported in patients undergoing sensitization treatment with hymenoptera (bee, wasp) venom while receiving ACE inhibitors.

Symptomatic hypotension with or without syncope can occur with ACE inhibitors (usually with the first several doses); effects are most often observed in volume depleted patients; correct volume depletion prior to initiation; close monitoring of patient is required especially with initial dosing and dosing increases; blood pressure must be lowered at a rate appropriate for the patient's clinical condition. Initiation of therapy in patients with ischemic heart disease or cerebrovascular disease warrants close observation due to the potential consequences posed by falling blood pressure (eg, MI, stroke). Use with caution in hypertrophic cardiomyopathy with outflow tract obstruction, severe aortic stenosis, or before, during, or immediately after major surgery.

Hyperkalemia may occur with ACE inhibitors; risk factors include renal dysfunction, diabetes mellitus, concomitant use of potassium-sparing diuretics, potassium supplements, and/or potassium-containing salts. Use cautiously, if at all, with these agents and monitor potassium closely. Cough may occur with ACE inhibitors. Other causes of cough should be considered (eg, pulmonary congestion in patients with heart failure) and excluded prior to discontinuation.

May be associated with deterioration of renal function and/or increases in serum creatinine, particularly in patients with low renal blood flow (eg, renal artery stenosis, heart failure) whose glomerular filtration rate (GFR) is dependent on efferent arteriolar vasoconstriction by angiotensin II; deterioration may result in oliguria, acute renal failure, and progressive azotemia. Small increases in serum creatinine may occur following initiation; consider discontinuation only in patients with progressive and/or significant deterioration in renal function. Use with caution in patients with unstented unilateral/bilateral renal artery stenosis. When unstented bilateral renal artery stenosis is present, use is generally avoided due to the elevated risk of deterioration in renal function unless possible benefits outweigh risks. Concurrent use of angiotensin receptor blockers may increase the risk of clinically-significant adverse events (eg, renal dysfunction, hyperkalemia).

Rare toxicities associated with ACE inhibitors include cholestatic jaundice (which may progress to fulminant hepatic necrosis), agranulocytosis, neutropenia, or leukopenia with myeloid hypoplasia. Patients with collagen vascular diseases (especially with concomitant renal impairment) or renal impairment alone may be at increased risk for hematologic toxicity; periodically monitor CBC with differential in these patients.

Adverse Reactions (Reflective of adult population; not specific for elderly) Note: Frequency ranges include data from hypertension and heart failure trials. Higher rates of adverse reactions have generally been noted in patients with CHF. However, the frequency of adverse effects associated with placebo is also increased in this population.

1% to 10%:
Cardiovascular: Orthostatic effects (1%), hypotension (1% to 4%)
Central nervous system: Headache (4% to 6%), dizziness (5% to 12%), fatigue (3%)
Dermatologic: Rash (1% to 2%)
Endocrine & metabolic: Hyperkalemia (2% to 5%)
Gastrointestinal: Diarrhea (3% to 4%), nausea (2%), vomiting (1%), abdominal pain (2%)
Genitourinary: Impotence (1%)
Hematologic: Decreased hemoglobin (small)
Neuromuscular & skeletal: Chest pain (3%), weakness (1%)
Renal: BUN increased (2%); deterioration in renal function (in patients with bilateral renal artery stenosis or hypovolemia); serum creatinine increased (often transient)
Respiratory: Cough (4% to 9%), upper respiratory infection (1% to 2%)

Drug Interactions

Avoid Concomitant Use There are no known interactions where it is recommended to avoid concomitant use.

Increased Effect/Toxicity

Lisinopril may increase the levels/effects of: Allopurinol; Amifostine; Antihypertensives; AzaTHIOprine; CycloSPORINE; CycloSPORINE (Systemic); Ferric Gluconate; Gold Sodium Thiomalate; Hypotensive Agents; Iron Dextran Complex; Lithium; Nonsteroidal Anti-Inflammatory Agents; RiTUXimab; Sodium Phosphates

The levels/effects of Lisinopril may be increased by: Alfuzosin; Angiotensin II Receptor Blockers; Diazoxide; DPP-IV Inhibitors; Eplerenone; Everolimus; Herbs (Hypotensive Properties); Loop Diuretics; MAO Inhibitors; Pentoxifylline; Phosphodiesterase 5 Inhibitors; Potassium Salts; Potassium-Sparing Diuretics; Prostacyclin Analogues; Sirolimus; Temsirolimus; Thiazide Diuretics; TiZANidine; Tolvaptan; Trimethoprim

Decreased Effect

The levels/effects of Lisinopril may be decreased by: Antacids; Aprotinin; Herbs (Hypertensive Properties); Icatibant; Lanthanum; Methylphenidate; Nonsteroidal Anti-Inflammatory Agents; Salicylates; Yohimbine

Ethanol/Nutrition/Herb Interactions

Food: Potassium-containing salt substitutes may increase risk of hyperkalemia.
Herb/Nutraceutical: Avoid bayberry, blue cohosh, cayenne, ephedra, ginger, ginseng (American), kola, licorice (may worsen hypertension). Avoid black cohosh, California poppy, coleus, golden seal, hawthorn, mistletoe, periwinkle, quinine, shepherd's purse (may have increased antihypertensive effect).

Mechanism of Action Competitive inhibitor of angiotensin-converting enzyme (ACE); prevents conversion of angiotensin I to angiotensin II, a potent vasoconstrictor; results in lower levels of angiotensin II which causes an increase in plasma renin activity and a reduction in aldosterone secretion; a CNS mechanism may also be involved in hypotensive effect as angiotensin II increases adrenergic outflow from CNS; vasoactive kallikreins may be decreased in conversion to active hormones by ACE inhibitors, thus reducing blood pressure

Pharmacodynamics/Kinetics
Onset of action: 1 hour
  Peak effect: Hypotensive: Oral: ~6 hours
Duration: 24 hours
Absorption: Well absorbed; unaffected by food
Protein binding: 25%
Metabolism: Not metabolized
Bioavailability: Decreased with NYHA Class II-IV heart failure
Half-life elimination: 11-12 hours
Time to peak: ~7 hours
Excretion: Primarily urine (as unchanged drug)

Dosage
  Geriatric Refer to adult dosing. In the management of hypertension, consider lower initial doses (eg, 2.5-5 mg/day) and titrate to response (Aronow, 2011).

  Adult
    Heart failure: Oral: Initial: 2.5-5 mg once daily; then increase by no more than 10 mg increments at intervals no less than 2 weeks to a maximum daily dose of 40 mg. Usual maintenance: 5-40 mg/day as a single dose. Target dose: 20-40 mg once daily (ACC/AHA 2009 Heart Failure Guidelines)
    Note: If patient has hyponatremia (serum sodium <130 mEq/L) or renal impairment (Cl_{cr} <30 mL/minute or creatinine >3 mg/dL), then initial dose should be 2.5 mg/day
    Hypertension: Oral: Usual dosage range (JNC 7): 10-40 mg/day
    Not maintained on diuretic: Initial: 10 mg/day
    Maintained on diuretic: Initial: 5 mg/day
    Note: Antihypertensive effect may diminish toward the end of the dosing interval especially with doses of 10 mg/day. An increased dose may aid in extending the duration of antihypertensive effect. Doses up to 80 mg/day have been used, but do not appear to give greater effect.
    Patients taking diuretics should have them discontinued 2-3 days prior to initiating lisinopril if possible. Restart diuretic after blood pressure is stable if needed. If diuretic cannot be discontinued prior to therapy, begin with 5 mg with close supervision until stable blood pressure. In patients with hyponatremia (<130 mEq/L), start dose at 2.5 mg/day.
    Acute myocardial infarction (within 24 hours in hemodynamically stable patients): Oral: 5 mg immediately, then 5 mg at 24 hours, 10 mg at 48 hours, and 10 mg every day thereafter for 6 weeks. Patients should continue to receive standard treatments such as thrombolytics, aspirin, and beta-blockers.
    Renal Impairment Adults: Initial doses should be modified and upward titration should be cautious, based on response (maximum: 40 mg/day)
    Cl_{cr} >30 mL/minute: Initial: 10 mg/day
    Cl_{cr} 10-30 mL/minute: Initial: 5 mg/day
    Hemodialysis: Initial: 2.5 mg/day; dialyzable (50%)

Administration Watch for hypotensive effects within 1-3 hours of first dose or new higher dose.

Monitoring Parameters BUN, serum creatinine, renal function, WBC, and potassium; if patient has collagen vascular disease and/or renal impairment, periodically monitor CBC with differential

Test Interactions May cause false-positive results in urine acetone determinations using sodium nitroprusside reagent

Special Geriatric Considerations Due to frequent decreases in glomerular filtration (also creatinine clearance) with aging, elderly patients may have exaggerated responses to ACE inhibitors. Differences in clinical response due to hepatic changes are not observed. ACE inhibitors may be preferred agents in elderly patients with congestive heart failure and diabetes mellitus. Diabetic proteinuria is reduced and insulin sensitivity is enhanced. In general, the side effect profile is favorable in the elderly and causes little or no CNS confusion. Use lowest dose recommendations initially. Many elderly may be volume depleted due to diuretic use and/or blunted thirst reflex resulting in inadequate fluid intake.

Dosage Forms Excipient information presented when available (limited, particularly for generics); consult specific product labeling.
Tablet, oral: 2.5 mg, 5 mg, 10 mg, 20 mg, 30 mg, 40 mg
  Prinivil®: 5 mg, 10 mg, 20 mg [scored]
  Zestril®: 2.5 mg
  Zestril®: 5 mg [scored]
  Zestril®: 10 mg, 20 mg, 30 mg, 40 mg

Lisinopril and Hydrochlorothiazide
(lyse IN oh pril & hye droe klor oh THYE a zide)

Related Information
Hydrochlorothiazide *on page 876*
Lisinopril *on page 1079*
Brand Names: U.S. Prinzide®; Zestoretic®
Brand Names: Canada Apo-Lisinopril®/Hctz; Mylan-Lisinopril/Hctz; Novo-Lisinopril/Hctz; Prinzide®; Sandoz-Lisinopril/Hctz; Teva-Lisinopril/Hctz (Type P); Teva-Lisinopril/Hctz (Type Z); Zestoretic®
Index Terms Hydrochlorothiazide and Lisinopril
Generic Availability (U.S.) Yes
Pharmacologic Category Angiotensin-Converting Enzyme (ACE) Inhibitor; Diuretic, Thiazide
Use Treatment of hypertension
Dosage
Geriatric & Adult Hypertension: Oral: Initial: Lisinopril 10 mg/hydrochlorothiazide 12.5 mg or lisinopril 20 mg/hydrochlorothiazide 12.5 mg with further increases of either or both components could depend on clinical response. Doses >80 mg/day lisinopril or >50 mg/day hydrochlorothiazide are not recommended.
Renal Impairment Dosage adjustments should be made with caution. Usual regimens of therapy need not be adjusted as long as patient's Cl$_{cr}$ >30 mL/minute. In patients with more severe renal impairment, loop diuretics are preferred.
Dosage Forms Excipient information presented when available (limited, particularly for generics); consult specific product labeling.
Tablet, oral: 10/12.5: Lisinopril 10 mg and hydrochlorothiazide 12.5 mg; 20/12.5: Lisinopril 20 mg and hydrochlorothiazide 12.5 mg; 20/25: Lisinopril 20 mg and hydrochlorothiazide 25 mg
Prinzide®:
10/12.5: Lisinopril 10 mg and hydrochlorothiazide 12.5 mg
20/12.5: Lisinopril 20 mg and hydrochlorothiazide 12.5 mg
Zestoretic®:
10/12.5: Lisinopril 10 mg and hydrochlorothiazide 12.5 mg
20/12.5: Lisinopril 20 mg and hydrochlorothiazide 12.5 mg
20/25: Lisinopril 20 mg and hydrochlorothiazide 25 mg

◆ **Lispro Insulin** *see* Insulin Lispro *on page 954*

Lithium (LITH ee um)

Related Information
Liquid Compatibility of Antidepressants, Antipsychotics, and Mood Stabilizers *on page 2111*
Medication Safety Issues
Sound-alike/look-alike issues:
Eskalith® may be confused with Estratest®
Lithium may be confused with lanthanum
Lithobid® may be confused with Levbid®, Lithostat®
Other safety concerns:
Do not confuse **mEq** (milliequivalent) with **mg** (milligram). **Note:** 300 mg lithium carbonate or citrate contain 8 mEq lithium. Dosage should be written in **mg** (milligrams) to avoid confusion.
Check prescriptions for unusually high volumes of the syrup for dosing errors.
Brand Names: U.S. Lithobid®
Brand Names: Canada Apo-Lithium® Carbonate; Apo-Lithium® Carbonate SR; Carbolith™; Duralith®; Euro-Lithium; Lithane™; Lithmax; PHL-Lithium Carbonate; PMS-Lithium Carbonate; PMS-Lithium Citrate
Index Terms Eskalith; Lithium Carbonate; Lithium Citrate
Generic Availability (U.S.) Yes
Pharmacologic Category Antimanic Agent
Use Management of bipolar disorders; treatment of mania in individuals with bipolar disorder (maintenance treatment prevents or diminishes intensity of subsequent episodes)
Unlabeled/Investigational Use Potential augmenting agent for antidepressants; treatment of aggression, post-traumatic stress disorder
Contraindications Hypersensitivity to lithium or any component of the formulation; avoid use in patients with severe cardiovascular or renal disease, or with severe debilitation, dehydration, or sodium depletion

Warnings/Precautions [U.S. Boxed Warning]: Lithium toxicity is closely related to serum levels and can occur at therapeutic doses; serum lithium determinations are required to monitor therapy. Use with caution in patients with thyroid disease, mild-moderate renal impairment, or mild-moderate cardiovascular disease. Use caution in patients receiving medications which alter sodium excretion (eg, diuretics, ACE inhibitors, NSAIDs), or in patients with significant fluid loss (protracted sweating, diarrhea, or prolonged fever); temporary reduction or cessation of therapy may be warranted. Some elderly patients may be extremely sensitive to the effects of lithium, see Dosage and Reference Range. Chronic therapy results in diminished renal concentrating ability (nephrogenic DI); this is usually reversible when lithium is discontinued. Changes in renal function should be monitored, and re-evaluation of treatment may be necessary. Use caution in patients at risk of suicide (suicidal thoughts or behavior).

Use with caution in patients receiving neuroleptic medications - a syndrome resembling NMS has been associated with concurrent therapy. Lithium may impair the patient's alertness, affecting the ability to operate machinery or driving a vehicle. Neuromuscular-blocking agents should be administered with caution; the response may be prolonged.

Higher serum concentrations may be required and tolerated during an acute manic phase; however, the tolerance decreases when symptoms subside. Normal fluid and salt intake must be maintained during therapy.

Adverse Reactions (Reflective of adult population; not specific for elderly) Frequency not defined.

Cardiovascular: Cardiac arrhythmia, hypotension, sinus node dysfunction, flattened or inverted T waves (reversible), edema, bradycardia, syncope

Central nervous system: Blackout spells, coma, confusion, dizziness, dystonia, fatigue, headache, lethargy, pseudotumor cerebri, psychomotor retardation, restlessness, sedation, seizure, slowed intellectual functioning, slurred speech, stupor, tics, vertigo

Dermatologic: Dry or thinning of hair, folliculitis, alopecia, exacerbation of psoriasis, rash

Endocrine & metabolic: Euthyroid goiter and/or hypothyroidism, hyperthyroidism, hyperglycemia, diabetes insipidus

Gastrointestinal: Polydipsia, anorexia, nausea, vomiting, diarrhea, xerostomia, metallic taste, weight gain, salivary gland swelling, excessive salivation

Genitourinary: Incontinence, polyuria, glycosuria, oliguria, albuminuria

Hematologic: Leukocytosis

Neuromuscular & skeletal: Tremor, muscle hyperirritability, ataxia, choreoathetoid movements, hyperactive deep tendon reflexes, myasthenia gravis (rare)

Ocular: Nystagmus, blurred vision, transient scotoma

Miscellaneous: Coldness and painful discoloration of fingers and toes

Postmarketing and/or case reports: Drug-induced Brugada syndrome

Drug Interactions

Avoid Concomitant Use

Avoid concomitant use of Lithium with any of the following: Sibutramine

Increased Effect/Toxicity

Lithium may increase the levels/effects of: Antipsychotics; Neuromuscular-Blocking Agents; Serotonin Modulators; Tricyclic Antidepressants

The levels/effects of Lithium may be increased by: ACE Inhibitors; Angiotensin II Receptor Blockers; Calcium Channel Blockers (Nondihydropyridine); CarBAMazepine; Desmopressin; Fosphenytoin; Loop Diuretics; MAO Inhibitors; Methyldopa; Nonsteroidal Anti-Inflammatory Agents; Phenytoin; Potassium Iodide; Selective Serotonin Reuptake Inhibitors; Sibutramine; Thiazide Diuretics; Topiramate

Decreased Effect

Lithium may decrease the levels/effects of: Amphetamines; Antipsychotics; Desmopressin

The levels/effects of Lithium may be decreased by: Calcitonin; Calcium Polystyrene Sulfonate; Carbonic Anhydrase Inhibitors; Loop Diuretics; Sodium Bicarbonate; Sodium Chloride; Sodium Polystyrene Sulfonate; Theophylline Derivatives

Ethanol/Nutrition/Herb Interactions Food: Limit caffeine.

Mechanism of Action Alters cation transport across cell membrane in nerve and muscle cells and influences reuptake of serotonin and/or norepinephrine; second messenger systems involving the phosphatidylinositol cycle are inhibited; postsynaptic D2 receptor supersensitivity is inhibited

Pharmacodynamics/Kinetics

Absorption: Rapid and complete

Distribution: V_d: Initial: 0.3-0.4 L/kg; V_{dss}: 0.7-1 L/kg; crosses placenta; enters breast milk at 35% to 50% the concentrations in serum; distribution is complete in 6-10 hours

CSF, liver concentrations: $1/3$ to $1/2$ of serum concentration

Erythrocyte concentration: ~$1/2$ of serum concentration

Heart, lung, kidney, muscle concentrations: Equivalent to serum concentration

Saliva concentration: 2-3 times serum concentration

Thyroid, bone, brain tissue concentrations: Increase 50% over serum concentrations

Protein binding: Not protein bound

Metabolism: Not metabolized

Bioavailability: Not affected by food; Capsule, immediate release tablet: 95% to 100%; Extended release tablet: 60% to 90%; Syrup: 100%

Half-life elimination: 18-24 hours; can increase to more than 36 hours in elderly or with renal impairment

Time to peak, serum: Immediate release: ~0.5-2 hours; extended release: 4-12 hours; syrup: 15-60 minutes

Excretion: Urine (90% to 98% as unchanged drug); sweat (4% to 5%); feces (1%)

Clearance: 80% of filtered lithium is reabsorbed in the proximal convoluted tubules; therefore, clearance approximates 20% of GFR or 20-40 mL/minute

Dosage

Geriatric Bipolar disorders: Oral: Initial: 300 mg twice daily; increase weekly in increments of 300 mg/day, monitoring levels; rarely need >900-1200 mg/day.

Adult

Bipolar disorders: Oral: 900-2400 mg/day in 3-4 divided doses or 900-1800 mg/day in two divided doses of extended release

Note: Monitor serum concentrations and clinical response (efficacy and toxicity) to determine proper dose

Renal Impairment

Cl_{cr} 10-50 mL/minute: Administer 50% to 75% of normal dose.

Cl_{cr} <10 mL/minute: Administer 25% to 50% of normal dose.

Dialyzable (50% to 100%); 4-7 times more efficient than peritoneal dialysis

Administration Administer with meals to decrease GI upset. Slow release tablets must be swallowed whole; do not crush or chew.

Monitoring Parameters Serum lithium every 4-5 days during initial therapy; draw lithium serum concentrations 12 hours postdose; renal, thyroid, and cardiovascular function; fluid status; serum electrolytes; CBC with differential, urinalysis; monitor for signs of toxicity

Reference Range Levels should be obtained twice weekly until both patient's clinical status and levels are stable then levels may be obtained every 1-3 months

Timing of serum samples: Draw trough just before next dose (8-12 hours after previous dose)

Therapeutic levels:

Acute mania: 0.6-1.2 mEq/L (SI: 0.6-1.2 mmol/L)

Protection against future episodes in most patients with bipolar disorder: 0.8-1 mEq/L (SI: 0.8-1.0 mmol/L); a higher rate of relapse is described in subjects who are maintained at <0.4 mEq/L (SI: 0.4 mmol/L)

Elderly patients can usually be maintained at lower end of therapeutic range (0.6-0.8 mEq/L)

Toxic concentration: >1.5 mEq/L (SI: >2 mmol/L)

Adverse effect levels:

GI complaints/tremor: 1.5-2 mEq/L

Confusion/somnolence: 2-2.5 mEq/L

Seizures/death: >2.5 mEq/L

Special Geriatric Considerations Some elderly patients may be extremely sensitive to the effects of lithium. Initial doses need to be adjusted for renal function in the elderly; thereafter, adjust doses based upon serum concentrations and response.

Dosage Forms Excipient information presented when available (limited, particularly for generics); consult specific product labeling. [DSC] = Discontinued product

Capsule, oral, as carbonate: 150 mg, 300 mg, 600 mg

Solution, oral, as citrate: 300 mg/5 mL (5 mL, 473 mL [DSC], 500 mL) [equivalent to amount of lithium in lithium carbonate]

Tablet, oral, as carbonate: 300 mg, 600 mg

Tablet, extended release, oral, as carbonate: 300 mg, 450 mg

Lithobid®: 300 mg

Selected References

Foster JF, Gershell WJ, and Goldfarb AI, "Lithium Treatment in the Elderly. I. Clinical Usage," *J Gerontol*, 1977, 32 (3):299-302.

Ward ME, Musa MN, Bailey L, "Clinical Pharmacokinetics of Lithium," *J Clin Pharmacol*, 1994, 34(4):280-5.

- **Little Phillips'® Milk of Magnesia [OTC]** *see* Magnesium Hydroxide *on page 1109*
- **Little Tummys® Gas Relief [OTC]** *see* Simethicone *on page 1679*
- **Little Tummys® Laxative [OTC]** *see* Senna *on page 1667*
- **Livalo®** *see* Pitavastatin *on page 1472*
- **Live Attenuated Influenza Vaccine** *see* Influenza Virus Vaccine (Live/Attenuated) *on page 940*
- **L-methylfolate** *see* Methylfolate *on page 1177*
- **L-methylfolate, Methylcobalamin, and N-acetylcysteine** *see* Methylfolate, Methylcobalamin, and Acetylcysteine *on page 1178*
- **Locoid®** *see* Hydrocortisone (Topical) *on page 886*
- **Locoid Lipocream®** *see* Hydrocortisone (Topical) *on page 886*
- **Lodine** *see* Etodolac *on page 682*
- **Lodosyn®** *see* Carbidopa *on page 273*

Lodoxamide (loe DOKS a mide)

Medication Safety Issues
International issues:
Thilomide [Greece, Turkey] may be confused with Thalomid brand name for thalidomide [U.S., Canada]

Brand Names: U.S. Alomide®
Brand Names: Canada Alomide®
Index Terms Lodoxamide Tromethamine
Generic Availability (U.S.) No
Pharmacologic Category Mast Cell Stabilizer
Use Treatment of vernal keratoconjunctivitis, vernal conjunctivitis, and vernal keratitis
Dosage
Geriatric & Adult Vernal conjunctivitis, keratitis: Ophthalmic: Instill 1-2 drops in eye(s) 4 times/day for up to 3 months
Special Geriatric Considerations Evaluate the patient's or caregiver's ability to safely administer the correct dose of ophthalmic medication.
Dosage Forms Excipient information presented when available (limited, particularly for generics); consult specific product labeling.
Solution, ophthalmic [drops]:
Alomide®: 0.1% (10 mL) [contains benzalkonium chloride]

- **Lodoxamide Tromethamine** *see* Lodoxamide *on page 1085*
- **Lodrane® 24 [DSC]** *see* Brompheniramine *on page 217*
- **Lofibra®** *see* Fenofibrate *on page 701*
- **LoHist-12** *see* Brompheniramine *on page 217*
- **Lomotil®** *see* Diphenoxylate and Atropine *on page 524*

Loperamide (loe PER a mide)

Medication Safety Issues
Sound-alike/look-alike issues:
Imodium® A-D may be confused with Indocin®
Loperamide may be confused with furosemide
International issues:
Indiaral [France] may be confused with Inderal and Inderal LA brand name for propranolol [U.S., Canada, and multiple international markets]
Lomotil: Brand name for loperamide [Mexico, Philippines], but also the brand name for diphenoxylate [U.S., Canada, and multiple international markets]
Lomotil [Mexico, Phillines] may be confused with Ludiomil brand name for maprotiline [multiple international markets]
Brand Names: U.S. Anti-Diarrheal [OTC]; Diamode [OTC]; Imodium® A-D for children [OTC]; Imodium® A-D [OTC]
Brand Names: Canada Apo-Loperamide®; Diarr-Eze; Dom-Loperamide; Imodium®; Loperacap; Novo-Loperamide; PMS-Loperamine; Rhoxal-loperamide; Rho®-Loperamine; Riva-Loperamide; Sandoz-Loperamide
Index Terms Loperamide Hydrochloride
Generic Availability (U.S.) Yes
Pharmacologic Category Antidiarrheal
Use Treatment of chronic diarrhea associated with inflammatory bowel disease; acute nonspecific diarrhea; increased volume of ileostomy discharge
OTC labeling: Control of symptoms of diarrhea, including Traveler's diarrhea

◀ **Unlabeled/Investigational Use** Cancer treatment-induced diarrhea (eg, irinotecan induced); chronic diarrhea caused by bowel resection

Contraindications Hypersensitivity to loperamide or any component of the formulation; abdominal pain without diarrhea

Avoid use as primary therapy in acute dysentery, acute ulcerative colitis, bacterial enterocolitis, pseudomembranous colitis

Warnings/Precautions Rare cases of anaphylaxis and anaphylactic shock have been reported. Should not be used if diarrhea is accompanied by high fever or blood in stool. Concurrent fluid and electrolyte replacement is often necessary in all age groups depending upon severity of diarrhea. Should not be used when inhibition of peristalsis is undesirable or dangerous. Discontinue if constipation, abdominal pain, or ileus develop. Use caution in treatment of AIDS patients; stop therapy at the sign of abdominal distention. Cases of toxic megacolon have occurred in this population. Loperamide is a symptom-directed treatment; if an underlying diagnosis is made, other disease-specific treatment may be indicated. Use caution in patients with hepatic impairment because of reduced first-pass metabolism; monitor for signs of CNS toxicity.

OTC labeling: If diarrhea lasts longer than 2 days, patient should stop taking loperamide and consult healthcare provider.

Adverse Reactions (Reflective of adult population; not specific for elderly)
1% to 10%:
Central nervous system: Dizziness (1%)
Gastrointestinal: Constipation (2% to 5%), abdominal cramping (<1% to 3%), nausea (<1% to 3%)
Postmarketing and/or case reports: Abdominal distention, abdominal pain, allergic reactions, anaphylactic shock, anaphylactoid reactions, angioedema, bullous eruption (rare), drowsiness, dry mouth, dyspepsia, erythema multiforme (rare), fatigue, flatulence, paralytic ileus, megacolon, pruritus, rash, Stevens-Johnson syndrome, toxic epidermal necrolysis, toxic megacolon, urinary retention, urticaria, vomiting

Drug Interactions
Metabolism/Transport Effects Substrate of CYP2B6 (minor), P-glycoprotein
Avoid Concomitant Use There are no known interactions where it is recommended to avoid concomitant use.
Increased Effect/Toxicity
The levels/effects of Loperamide may be increased by: P-Glycoprotein Inhibitors
Decreased Effect
The levels/effects of Loperamide may be decreased by: P-Glycoprotein Inducers

Stability Store at 15°C to 25°C (59°F to 77°F).

Mechanism of Action Acts directly on circular and longitudinal intestinal muscles, through the opioid receptor, to inhibit peristalsis and prolong transit time; reduces fecal volume, increases viscosity, and diminishes fluid and electrolyte loss; demonstrates antisecretory activity. Loperamide increases tone on the anal sphincter

Pharmacodynamics/Kinetics
Absorption: Poor
Distribution: Poor penetration into brain; low amounts enter breast milk
Metabolism: Hepatic via oxidative N-demethylation
Half-life elimination: 7-14 hours
Time to peak, plasma: Liquid: 2.5 hours; Capsule: 5 hours
Excretion: Urine and feces (1% as metabolites, 30% to 40% as unchanged drug)

Dosage
Geriatric & Adult
Acute diarrhea: Oral: Initial: 4 mg, followed by 2 mg after each loose stool, up to 16 mg/day
Chronic diarrhea: Oral: Initial: Follow acute diarrhea; maintenance dose should be slowly titrated downward to minimum required to control symptoms (typically, 4-8 mg/day in divided doses)
Traveler's diarrhea: Oral: Initial: 4 mg after first loose stool, followed by 2 mg after each subsequent stool (maximum dose: 8 mg/day)
Irinotecan-induced diarrhea (unlabeled use): Oral: 4 mg after first loose or frequent bowel movement, then 2 mg every 2 hours until 12 hours have passed without a bowel movement. If diarrhea recurs, then repeat administration
Hepatic Impairment No specific guidelines available.

Monitoring Parameters Monitor stool frequency and consistency; observe for toxicity with use more than 48 hours

Pharmacotherapy Pearls Therapy for chronic diarrhea should not exceed 10 days; if diarrhea persists longer than 48 hours for acute diarrhea, etiology should be examined

Special Geriatric Considerations Elderly are particularly sensitive to fluid and electrolyte loss. This generally results in lethargy, weakness, and confusion. Repletion and maintenance of electrolytes and water are essential in the treatment of diarrhea. Drug therapy must be limited in order to avoid toxicity with this agent.

Dosage Forms Excipient information presented when available (limited, particularly for generics); consult specific product labeling.

Caplet, oral, as hydrochloride: 2 mg
Anti-Diarrheal: 2 mg
Diamode: 2 mg
Imodium® A-D: 2 mg [scored]
Capsule, oral, as hydrochloride: 2 mg
Liquid, oral, as hydrochloride: 1 mg/5 mL (118 mL)
Anti-Diarrheal: 1 mg/5 mL (120 mL)
Imodium® A-D: 1 mg/5 mL (60 mL, 120 mL) [contains benzoic acid, ethanol 0.5%, sodium benzoate; cherry-mint flavor]
Imodium® A-D: 1 mg/7.5 mL (120 mL) [contains sodium 10 mg/30 mL, sodium benzoate; creamy-mint flavor]
Imodium® A-D for children: 1 mg/7.5 mL (120 mL) [contains sodium 16 mg/30 mL, sodium benzoate; creamy-mint flavor]
Solution, oral, as hydrochloride: 1 mg/5 mL (5 mL, 10 mL)

Selected References

Benson AB 3rd, Ajani JA, Catalano RB, et al, "Recommended Guidelines for the Treatment of Cancer Treatment-Induced Diarrhea," *J Clin Oncol*, 2004, 22(14):2918-26.

Ericsson CD, "Nonantimicrobial Agents in the Prevention and Treatment of Traveler's Diarrhea," *Clin Infect Dis*, 2005, 41(Suppl 8):557-63.

Loperamide and Simethicone (loe PER a mide & sye METH i kone)

Related Information
Loperamide *on page 1085*
Simethicone *on page 1679*
Brand Names: U.S. Imodium® Multi-Symptom Relief [OTC]
Brand Names: Canada Imodium® Advanced Multi-Symptom
Index Terms Simethicone and Loperamide Hydrochloride
Generic Availability (U.S.) No
Pharmacologic Category Antidiarrheal; Antiflatulent
Use Control of symptoms of diarrhea and gas (bloating, pressure, and cramps)
Dosage

Geriatric & Adult Acute diarrhea: Oral: 1 caplet or tablet after first loose stool, followed by 1 caplet or tablet with each subsequent loose stool (maximum: 4 caplets or tablets/24 hours)

Special Geriatric Considerations Elderly are particularly sensitive to fluid and electrolyte loss. This generally results in lethargy, weakness, and confusion. Repletion and maintenance of electrolytes and water are essential in the treatment of diarrhea. Drug therapy must be limited in order to avoid toxicity with this agent. Before treating excess gas or pain due to gas accumulation, a thorough evaluation must be made to determine cause since many bowel diseases may present with flatulence and bloating.

Dosage Forms Excipient information presented when available (limited, particularly for generics); consult specific product labeling.

Caplet:
Imodium® Multi-Symptom Relief: Loperamide hydrochloride 2 mg and simethicone 125 mg [contains calcium 65 mg/caplet, sodium 4 mg/caplet]
Tablet, chewable:
Imodium® Multi-Symptom Relief: Loperamide hydrochloride 2 mg and simethicone 125 mg [contains calcium 50 mg/tablet; mint flavor]

◆ **Loperamide Hydrochloride** *see* Loperamide *on page 1085*
◆ **Lopid®** *see* Gemfibrozil *on page 812*
◆ **Lopressor®** *see* Metoprolol *on page 1195*
◆ **Lopressor HCT®** *see* Metoprolol and Hydrochlorothiazide *on page 1199*
◆ **Loprox®** *see* Ciclopirox *on page 354*
◆ **Loradamed [OTC]** *see* Loratadine *on page 1087*

Loratadine (lor AT a deen)

Medication Safety Issues
Sound-alike/look-alike issues:
Claritin® may be confused with clarithromycin

LORATADINE

◄ Claritin® (loratadine) may be confused with Claritin™ Eye (ketotifen)

Brand Names: U.S. Alavert® Allergy 24 Hour [OTC]; Alavert® Children's Allergy [OTC]; Claritin® 24 Hour Allergy [OTC]; Claritin® Children's Allergy [OTC]; Claritin® Liqui-Gels® 24 Hour Allergy [OTC]; Claritin® RediTabs® 24 Hour Allergy [OTC]; Loradamed [OTC]; Tavist® ND Allergy [OTC]

Brand Names: Canada Apo-Loratadine®; Claritin®; Claritin® Kids

Generic Availability (U.S.) Yes: Excludes capsule, chewable tablet

Pharmacologic Category Histamine H_1 Antagonist; Histamine H_1 Antagonist, Second Generation; Piperidine Derivative

Use Relief of nasal and non-nasal symptoms of seasonal allergic rhinitis; treatment of chronic idiopathic urticaria

Contraindications Hypersensitivity to loratadine or any component of the formulation

Warnings/Precautions Use with caution in patients with liver or renal impairment; dosage adjustment recommended. Some products may contain phenylalanine.

Adverse Reactions (Reflective of adult population; not specific for elderly)

Adults:
Central nervous system: Headache (12%), somnolence (8%), fatigue (4%)
Gastrointestinal: Xerostomia (3%)

Children:
Central nervous system: Nervousness (4% ages 6-12 years), fatigue (3% ages 6-12 years, 2% to 3% ages 2-5 years), malaise (2% ages 6-12 years)
Dermatologic: Rash (2% to 3% ages 2-5 years)
Gastrointestinal: Abdominal pain (2% ages 6-12 years), stomatitis (2% to 3% ages 2-5 years)
Neuromuscular & skeletal: Hyperkinesia (3% ages 6-12 years)
Ocular: Conjunctivitis (2% ages 6-12 years)
Respiratory: Wheezing (4% ages 6-12 years), dysphonia (2% ages 6-12 years), upper respiratory infection (2% ages 6-12 years), epistaxis (2% to 3% ages 2-5 years), pharyngitis (2% to 3% ages 2-5 years)
Miscellaneous: Flu-like syndrome (2% to 3% ages 2-5 years), viral infection (2% to 3% ages 2-5 years)

Drug Interactions

Metabolism/Transport Effects Substrate of CYP2D6 (minor), CYP3A4 (minor), P-glycoprotein; **Inhibits** CYP2C8 (weak), 2C19 (moderate), 2D6 (weak)

Avoid Concomitant Use There are no known interactions where it is recommended to avoid concomitant use.

Increased Effect/Toxicity
Loratadine may increase the levels/effects of: Alcohol (Ethyl); Anticholinergics; CNS Depressants; Selective Serotonin Reuptake Inhibitors

The levels/effects of Loratadine may be increased by: Amiodarone; Conivaptan; Droperidol; HydrOXYzine; P-Glycoprotein Inhibitors; Pramlintide

Decreased Effect
Loratadine may decrease the levels/effects of: Acetylcholinesterase Inhibitors (Central); Benzylpenicilloyl Polylysine; Betahistine

The levels/effects of Loratadine may be decreased by: Acetylcholinesterase Inhibitors (Central); Amphetamines; Peginterferon Alfa-2b; P-Glycoprotein Inducers; Tocilizumab

Ethanol/Nutrition/Herb Interactions
Ethanol: May increase CNS depression; monitor for increased effects with coadministration. Caution patients about effects.
Food: Increases bioavailability and delays peak.
Herb/Nutraceutical: St John's wort may decrease loratadine levels.

Stability Store at 2°C to 25°C (36°F to 77°F).
Rapidly-disintegrating tablets: Use within 6 months of opening foil pouch, and immediately after opening individual tablet blister. Store in a dry place.

Mechanism of Action Long-acting tricyclic antihistamine with selective peripheral histamine H_1-receptor antagonistic properties

Pharmacodynamics/Kinetics
Onset of action: 1-3 hours
Peak effect: 8-12 hours
Duration: >24 hours
Absorption: Rapid
Metabolism: Extensively hepatic via CYP2D6 and 3A4 to active metabolite
Half-life elimination: 12-15 hours
Excretion: Urine (40%) and feces (40%) as metabolites

Dosage

Geriatric & Adult Seasonal allergic rhinitis, chronic idiopathic urticaria: Oral: 10 mg/day

Renal Impairment Cl_{cr} ≤30 mL/minute: 10 mg every other day

Hepatic Impairment

Elimination half-life increases with severity of disease.

Adults: 10 mg every other day

Administration May be administered without regard to meals.

Monitoring Parameters Relief of symptoms, mental status

Test Interactions May suppress the wheal and flare reactions to skin test antigens

Special Geriatric Considerations Loratadine is a nonsedating antihistamine. Because of its low incidence of side effects, it seems to be a good choice in the elderly; however, there is a wide variation in loratadine half-life reported in the elderly and this should be kept in mind when initiating dosing. Because of its OTC status, patients should be counseled on appropriate use.

Dosage Forms Excipient information presented when available (limited, particularly for generics); consult specific product labeling.

Capsule, liquid gel, oral:

Claritin® Liqui-Gels® 24 Hour Allergy: 10 mg

Solution, oral: 5 mg/5 mL (120 mL)

Syrup, oral: 5 mg/5 mL (120 mL)

Claritin® Children's Allergy: 5 mg/5 mL (60 mL, 120 mL) [dye free, ethanol free; contains propylene glycol, sodium benzoate; fruit flavor]

Claritin® Children's Allergy: 5 mg/5 mL (60 mL, 120 mL) [dye free, ethanol free, sugar free; contains propylene glycol, sodium 6 mg/5 mL, sodium benzoate; grape flavor]

Tablet, oral: 10 mg

Alavert® Allergy 24 Hour: 10 mg [dye free, gluten free, sucrose free]

Claritin® 24 Hour Allergy: 10 mg

Loradamed: 10 mg

Tavist® ND Allergy: 10 mg

Tablet, chewable, oral:

Claritin® Children's Allergy: 5 mg [contains phenylalanine 1.4 mg/tablet; grape flavor]

Tablet, orally disintegrating, oral: 10 mg

Alavert® Allergy 24 Hour: 10 mg [dye free, gluten free, sucrose free; contains phenylalanine 8.4 mg/tablet; Citrus Burst™ flavor]

Alavert® Allergy 24 Hour: 10 mg [dye free, gluten free, sucrose free; contains phenylalanine 8.4 mg/tablet; mint flavor]

Alavert® Children's Allergy: 10 mg [dye free, gluten free, sucrose free; contains phenylalanine 8.4 mg/tablet; Citrus Burst™ flavor]

Alavert® Children's Allergy: 10 mg [dye free, gluten free, sucrose free; contains phenylalanine 8.4 mg/tablet; bubblegum flavor]

Claritin® RediTabs® 24 Hour Allergy: 10 mg [mint flavor]

LORazepam (lor A ze pam)

Related Information

Anxiolytic, Sedative / Hypnotic, and Miscellaneous Benzodiazepines *on page 2000*

Beers Criteria − Potentially Inappropriate Medications for Geriatrics *on page 2089*

Medication Safety Issues

Sound-alike/look-alike issues:

LORazepam may be confused with ALPRAZolam, clonazePAM, diazepam, KlonoPIN®, Lovaza®, temazepam, zolpidem

Ativan® may be confused with Ambien®, Atarax®, Atgam®, Avitene®

BEERS Criteria medication:

This drug may be inappropriate for use in geriatric patients (high severity risk).

Administration issues:

Injection dosage form contains propylene glycol. Monitor for toxicity when administering continuous lorazepam infusions.

Brand Names: U.S. Ativan®; Lorazepam Intensol™

Brand Names: Canada Apo-Lorazepam®; Ativan®; Dom-Lorazepam; Lorazepam Injection, USP; Novo-Lorazem; Nu-Loraz; PHL-Lorazepam; PMS-Lorazepam; PRO-Lorazepam

Generic Availability (U.S.) Yes

Pharmacologic Category Benzodiazepine

◀ **Use**

Oral: Management of anxiety disorders or short-term (≤4 months) relief of the symptoms of anxiety, anxiety associated with depressive symptoms, or insomnia due to anxiety or transient stress

I.V.: Status epilepticus, amnesia, sedation

Unlabeled/Investigational Use Ethanol detoxification; treatment of insomnia, psychogenic catatonia, partial complex seizures, agitation (I.V.)

Contraindications Hypersensitivity to lorazepam or any component of the formulation (cross-sensitivity with other benzodiazepines may exist); acute narrow-angle glaucoma; sleep apnea (parenteral); intra-arterial injection of parenteral formulation; severe respiratory insufficiency (except during mechanical ventilation)

Warnings/Precautions Use with caution in elderly or debilitated patients, patients with hepatic disease (including alcoholics) or renal impairment. Due to increased sensitivity in the elderly, smaller doses of benzodiazepines may be safer and as effective; in this age group, avoid using doses >3 mg daily of lorazepam (Beers Criteria). Use with caution in patients with respiratory disease (COPD or sleep apnea) or limited pulmonary reserve, or impaired gag reflex. Initial doses in elderly or debilitated patients should be at the lower end of the dosing range. May worsen hepatic encephalopathy.

Causes CNS depression (dose-related) resulting in sedation, dizziness, confusion, or ataxia which may impair physical and mental capabilities. Patients must be cautioned about performing tasks which require mental alertness (eg, operating machinery or driving). Use with caution in patients receiving other CNS depressants or psychoactive agents. Effects with other sedative drugs or ethanol may be potentiated. Benzodiazepines have been associated with falls and traumatic injury and should be used with extreme caution in patients who are at risk of these events (especially the elderly).

Lorazepam may cause anterograde amnesia. Paradoxical reactions, including hyperactive or aggressive behavior have been reported with benzodiazepines, particularly in psychiatric patients. Does not have analgesic, antidepressant, or antipsychotic properties.

Use caution in patients with depression, particularly if suicidal risk may be present. Pre-existing depression may worsen or emerge during therapy. Not recommended for use in primary depressive or psychotic disorders. Use with caution in patients with a history of drug dependence, alcoholism, or significant personality disorders. Benzodiazepines have been associated with dependence and acute withdrawal symptoms on discontinuation or reduction in dose. Acute withdrawal, including seizures, may be precipitated after administration of flumazenil to patients receiving long-term benzodiazepine therapy.

As a hypnotic agent, should be used only after evaluation of potential causes of sleep disturbance. Failure of sleep disturbance to resolve after 7-10 days may indicate psychiatric or medical illness. A worsening of insomnia or the emergence of new abnormalities of thought or behavior may represent unrecognized psychiatric or medical illness and requires immediate and careful evaluation.

Parenteral formulation of lorazepam contains polyethylene glycol which has resulted in toxicity during high-dose and/or longer-term infusions. Parenteral formulation also contains propylene glycol (PG); may be associated with dose-related toxicity and can occur ≥48 hours after initiation of lorazepam. Limited data suggest increased risk of PG accumulation at doses of ≥6 mg/hour for 48 hours or more (Nelson, 2008). Consider monitoring for signs of toxicity which may include acute renal failure, lactic acidosis, and/or osmol gap. In high-risk patients requiring higher doses/extended treatment durations, use of enteral delivery of lorazepam tablets may be beneficial (Jacobi, 2002). Also contains benzyl alcohol.

Adverse Reactions (Reflective of adult population; not specific for elderly)

>10%:

Central nervous system: Sedation

Respiratory: Respiratory depression

1% to 10%:

Cardiovascular: Hypotension

Central nervous system: Akathisia, amnesia, ataxia, confusion, depression, disorientation, dizziness, headache

Dermatologic: Dermatitis, rash

Gastrointestinal: Changes in appetite, nausea, weight gain/loss

Neuromuscular & skeletal: Weakness

Ocular: Visual disturbances

Respiratory: Apnea, hyperventilation, nasal congestion

Drug Interactions

Avoid Concomitant Use

Avoid concomitant use of LORazepam with any of the following: OLANZapine

Increased Effect/Toxicity

LORazepam may increase the levels/effects of: Alcohol (Ethyl); CloZAPine; CNS Depressants; Fosphenytoin; Methotrimeprazine; Phenytoin; Selective Serotonin Reuptake Inhibitors

The levels/effects of LORazepam may be increased by: Divalproex; Droperidol; HydrOXYzine; Loxapine; Methotrimeprazine; OLANZapine; Probenecid; Valproic Acid

Decreased Effect

The levels/effects of LORazepam may be decreased by: Theophylline Derivatives; Yohimbine

Ethanol/Nutrition/Herb Interactions

Ethanol: May increase CNS depression; monitor for increased effects with coadministration. Caution patients about effects.

Herb/Nutraceutical: Avoid valerian, St John's wort, kava kava, gotu kola (may increase CNS depression).

Stability

I.V.: Intact vials should be refrigerated. Protect from light. Do not use discolored or precipitate-containing solutions. May be stored at room temperature for up to 3 months [data on file (Hospira Inc, 2010)]. Parenteral admixture is stable at room temperature (25°C) for 24 hours. Dilute I.V. dose with equal volume of compatible diluent (D_5W, NS, SWFI).

Infusion: Use 2 mg/mL injectable vial to prepare; there may be decreased stability when using 4 mg/mL vial. Dilute ≤1 mg/mL and mix in glass bottle. Precipitation may develop. Can also be administered undiluted via infusion.

Tablet: Store at room temperature.

Mechanism of Action Binds to stereospecific benzodiazepine receptors on the postsynaptic GABA neuron at several sites within the central nervous system, including the limbic system, reticular formation. Enhancement of the inhibitory effect of GABA on neuronal excitability results by increased neuronal membrane permeability to chloride ions. This shift in chloride ions results in hyperpolarization (a less excitable state) and stabilization.

Pharmacodynamics/Kinetics

Onset of action:
  Hypnosis: I.M.: 20-30 minutes
  Sedation: I.V.: 5-20 minutes
  Anticonvulsant: I.V.: 5 minutes, oral: 30-60 minutes
Duration: 6-8 hours
Absorption: Oral, I.M.: Prompt
Distribution: V_d: 1.3 L/kg
Protein binding: 85%; free fraction may be significantly higher in elderly
Metabolism: Hepatic to inactive compounds
Bioavailability: Oral: 90%
Half-life elimination: 12.9 hours; Elderly: 15.9 hours; End-stage renal disease: 32-70 hours
Time to peak: Oral: 2 hours
Excretion: Urine; feces (minimal)

Dosage

Geriatric

Anxiety, sedation, and procedural amnesia: Oral: Initial: 1-2 mg/day in divided doses; Beers Criteria: Avoid maintenance doses >3 mg/day

Other indications: Refer to adult dosing. Dose selection should generally be on the low end of the dosage range (ie, initial dose not to exceed 2 mg).

Adult

Antiemetic: Oral, I.V. (**Note:** May be administered sublingually; not a labeled route): 0.5-2 mg every 4-6 hours as needed

Anxiety, sedation, and procedural amnesia:
  Oral: 1-10 mg/day in 2-3 divided doses; usual dose: 2-6 mg/day in divided doses or 1-2 mg 1 hour before procedure
  I.M.: 0.05 mg/kg administered 2 hours before surgery (maximum: 4 mg/dose)
  I.V.: 0.044 mg/kg 15-20 minutes before surgery (usual dose 2 mg; maximum: 4 mg/dose)

Insomnia: Oral: 2-4 mg at bedtime

Status epilepticus: I.V.: 4 mg/dose slow I.V. (maximum rate: 2 mg/minute); may repeat in 10-15 minutes; usual maximum dose: 8 mg. May be given I.M, but I.V. preferred.

Rapid tranquilization of agitated patient (unlabeled use): Oral, I.M.: 1-2 mg administered every 30-60 minutes; may be administered with an antipsychotic (eg, haloperidol) (Battaglia, 2005; De Fruyt, 2004)
  Average total dose for tranquilization: 4-8 mg

Agitation in the ICU patient (unlabeled):
  I.V.: 0.02-0.06 mg/kg every 2-6 hours or 0.01-0.1 mg/kg/hour (Jacobi, 2002)
  Dosage adjustment for lorazepam with concomitant medications: *Probenecid or valproic acid:* Reduce lorazepam dose by 50%

◄ **Alcohol withdrawal syndrome (unlabeled use):** Oral: 2 mg every 6 hours for 4 doses, then 1 mg every 6 hours for 8 additional doses (Mayo-Smith, 1997)

Alcohol withdrawal delirium (unlabeled use) (Mayo-Smith, 2004):

I.V.: 1-4 mg every 5-15 minutes until calm, then every hour as needed to maintain light somnolence

I.M.: 1-40 mg every 30-60 minutes until calm, then every hour as needed to maintain light somnolence

Renal Impairment I.V.: Risk of propylene glycol toxicity. Monitor closely if using for prolonged periods or at high doses.

Hepatic Impairment No dose reduction necessary.

Administration See Warnings/Precautions.

Monitoring Parameters Respiratory and cardiovascular status, blood pressure, heart rate, symptoms of anxiety

Clinical signs of propylene glycol toxicity (for continuous high-dose and/or long duration intravenous use): Serum creatinine, BUN, serum lactate, osmol gap

Reference Range Therapeutic: 50-240 ng/mL (SI: 156-746 nmol/L)

Pharmacotherapy Pearls I.M. lorazepam is rapidly and completely absorbed and, therefore, may be more predictable as compared to I.M. chlordiazepoxide or diazepam

Special Geriatric Considerations Because lorazepam is relatively short-acting with an inactive metabolite, it is a preferred agent to use in elderly patients when a benzodiazepine is indicated.

This medication is considered to be potentially inappropriate in this patient population (Beers Criteria severity: High).

Controlled Substance C-IV

Dosage Forms Excipient information presented when available (limited, particularly for generics); consult specific product labeling. [DSC] = Discontinued product

Injection, solution: 2 mg/mL (1 mL, 10 mL); 4 mg/mL (1 mL, 10 mL)

Ativan®: 2 mg/mL (1 mL, 10 mL); 4 mg/mL (1 mL, 10 mL) [contains benzyl alcohol, polyethylene glycol 400, propylene glycol]

Injection, solution [preservative free]: 2 mg/mL (1 mL [DSC]); 4 mg/mL (1 mL [DSC])

Solution, oral [concentrate]: 2 mg/mL (30 mL)

Lorazepam Intensol™: 2 mg/mL (30 mL) [dye free, ethanol free, sugar free; contains propylene glycol]

Tablet, oral: 0.5 mg, 1 mg, 2 mg

Ativan®: 0.5 mg

Ativan®: 1 mg, 2 mg [scored]

Selected References

Divoll M and Greenblatt DJ, "Effect of Age and Sex on Lorazepam Protein Binding," *J Pharm Pharmacol*, 1982, 34 (2):122-3.

Greenblatt DJ, Allen MD, Locniskar A, et al, "Lorazepam Kinetics in the Elderly," *Clin Pharmacol Ther*, 1979, 26 (1):103-13.

Kälviäinen R, "Status Epilepticus Treatment Guidelines," *Epilepsia*, 2007, 48(Suppl 8):99-102.

◆ **Lorazepam Intensol™** see LORazepam *on page 1089*

◆ **Lorcet® 10/650** see Hydrocodone and Acetaminophen *on page 880*

◆ **Lorcet® Plus** see Hydrocodone and Acetaminophen *on page 880*

◆ **Lortab®** see Hydrocodone and Acetaminophen *on page 880*

Losartan (loe SAR tan)

Related Information

Angiotensin Agents *on page 1985*

Medication Safety Issues

Sound-alike/look-alike issues:

Cozaar® may be confused with Colace®, Coreg®, Hyzaar®, Zocor®

Losartan may be confused with valsartan

Brand Names: U.S. Cozaar®

Brand Names: Canada Cozaar®

Index Terms DuP 753; Losartan Potassium; MK594

Generic Availability (U.S.) Yes

Pharmacologic Category Angiotensin II Receptor Blocker

Use Treatment of hypertension (HTN); treatment of diabetic nephropathy in patients with type 2 diabetes mellitus (noninsulin dependent, NIDDM) and a history of hypertension; stroke risk reduction in patients with HTN and left ventricular hypertrophy (LVH)

Contraindications Hypersensitivity to losartan or any component of the formulation

Warnings/Precautions Avoid use or use a much smaller dose in patients who are volume-depleted; correct depletion first. Use with caution in patients with significant aortic/mitral stenosis. May cause hyperkalemia; avoid potassium supplementation unless specifically required by healthcare provider. May be associated with deterioration of renal function and/or increases in serum creatinine, particularly in patients with low renal blood flow (eg, renal artery stenosis, heart failure) whose glomerular filtration rate (GFR) is dependent on efferent arteriolar vasoconstriction by angiotensin II. Use caution in patients with unstented unilateral/bilateral renal artery stenosis. When unstented bilateral renal artery stenosis is present, use is generally avoided due to the elevated risk of deterioration in renal function unless possible benefits outweigh risks. Use with caution with pre-existing renal insufficiency. AUCs of losartan (not the active metabolite) are about 50% greater in patients with Cl_{cr} <30 mL/minute and are doubled in hemodialysis patients. Concurrent use of ACE inhibitors may increase the risk of clinically-significant adverse events (eg, renal dysfunction, hyperkalemia).

At any time during treatment (especially following first dose), angioedema may occur rarely; may involve the head and neck (potentially compromising airway) or the intestine (presenting with abdominal pain). Patients with idiopathic or hereditary angioedema or previous angioedema associated with ACE-inhibitor therapy may be at an increased risk. Prolonged frequent monitoring may be required, especially if tongue, glottis, or larynx are involved, as they are associated with airway obstruction. Patients with a history of airway surgery may have a higher risk of airway obstruction. Aggressive early management is critical; intramuscular (I.M.) administration of epinephrine may be necessary.

When used to reduce the risk of stroke in patients with HTN and LVH, may not be effective in African-American population. Use caution with hepatic dysfunction, dose adjustment may be needed.

Adverse Reactions (Reflective of adult population; not specific for elderly) Note: The incidence of some adverse reactions varied based on the underlying disease state. Notations are made, where applicable, for data derived from trials conducted in diabetic nephropathy and hypertensive patients, respectively.

>10%:
  Cardiovascular: Chest pain (12% diabetic nephropathy)
  Central nervous system: Fatigue (14% diabetic nephropathy)
  Endocrine: Hypoglycemia (14% diabetic nephropathy)
  Gastrointestinal: Diarrhea (2% hypertension to 15% diabetic nephropathy)
  Genitourinary: Urinary tract infection (13% diabetic nephropathy)
  Hematologic: Anemia (14% diabetic nephropathy)
  Neuromuscular & skeletal: Weakness (14% diabetic nephropathy), back pain (2% hypertension to 12% diabetic nephropathy)
  Respiratory: Cough (≤3% to 11%; similar to placebo; incidence higher in patients with previous cough related to ACE inhibitor therapy)
1% to 10%:
  Cardiovascular: Hypotension (7% diabetic nephropathy), orthostatic hypotension (4% hypertension to 4% diabetic nephropathy), first-dose hypotension (dose related: <1% with 50 mg, 2% with 100 mg)
  Central nervous system: Dizziness (4%), hypoesthesia (5% diabetic nephropathy), fever (4% diabetic nephropathy), insomnia (1%)
  Dermatology: Cellulitis (7% diabetic nephropathy)
  Endocrine: Hyperkalemia (<1% hypertension to 7% diabetic nephropathy)
  Gastrointestinal: Gastritis (5% diabetic nephropathy), weight gain (4% diabetic nephropathy), dyspepsia (1% to 4%), abdominal pain (2%), nausea (2%)
  Neuromuscular & skeletal: Muscular weakness (7% diabetic nephropathy), knee pain (5% diabetic nephropathy), leg pain (1% to 5%), muscle cramps (1%), myalgia (1%)
  Respiratory: Bronchitis (10% diabetic nephropathy), upper respiratory infection (8%), nasal congestion (2%), sinusitis (1% hypertension to 6% diabetic nephropathy)
  Miscellaneous: Infection (5% diabetic nephropathy), flu-like syndrome (10% diabetic nephropathy)

Drug Interactions

Metabolism/Transport Effects Substrate (major) of CYP2C9, 3A4; **Inhibits** CYP1A2 (weak), 2C8 (moderate), 2C9 (moderate), 2C19 (weak), 3A4 (weak)

Avoid Concomitant Use There are no known interactions where it is recommended to avoid concomitant use.

Increased Effect/Toxicity

Losartan may increase the levels/effects of: ACE Inhibitors; Amifostine; Antihypertensives; Carvedilol; CYP2C8 Substrates (High risk); CYP2C9 Substrates (High risk); Hypoglycemic Agents; Hypotensive Agents; Lithium; Nonsteroidal Anti-Inflammatory Agents; Potassium-Sparing Diuretics; RiTUXimab; Sodium Phosphates

◀

The levels/effects of Losartan may be increased by: Alfuzosin; Antifungal Agents (Azole Derivatives, Systemic); Conivaptan; CYP2C9 Inhibitors (Moderate); CYP2C9 Inhibitors (Strong); Diazoxide; Eplerenone; Fluconazole; Herbs (Hypoglycemic Properties); Herbs (Hypotensive Properties); MAO Inhibitors; Milk Thistle; Pentoxifylline; Phosphodiesterase 5 Inhibitors; Potassium Salts; Prostacyclin Analogues; Tolvaptan; Trimethoprim

Decreased Effect

The levels/effects of Losartan may be decreased by: CYP2C9 Inducers (Highly Effective); CYP3A4 Inducers (Strong); Deferasirox; Herbs (CYP3A4 Inducers); Herbs (Hypertensive Properties); Methylphenidate; Nonsteroidal Anti-Inflammatory Agents; Peginterferon Alfa-2b; Rifamycin Derivatives; Tocilizumab; Yohimbine

Ethanol/Nutrition/Herb Interactions Herb/Nutraceutical: St John's wort may decrease levels of losartan. Avoid bayberry, blue cohosh, ginseng (American), kola, licorice (may worsen hypertension). Avoid black cohosh; california poppy; coleus; golden seal; hawthorn; mistletoe; periwinkle; quinine; shepherd's purse (may increase risk for hypotension). Hypoglycemic effects of losartan may be enhanced by alfalfa; aloe; bilberry; bitter melon; burdock; celery; damiana; fenugreek; garcinia; garlic; ginger; ginseng (American); gymnema; marshmallow; stinging nettle.

Stability Store at 15°C to 30°C (59°F to 86°F). Protect from light.

Mechanism of Action As a selective and competitive, nonpeptide angiotensin II receptor antagonist, losartan blocks the vasoconstrictor and aldosterone-secreting effects of angiotensin II; losartan interacts reversibly at the AT1 and AT2 receptors of many tissues and has slow dissociation kinetics; its affinity for the AT1 receptor is 1000 times greater than the AT2 receptor. Angiotensin II receptor antagonists may induce a more complete inhibition of the renin-angiotensin system than ACE inhibitors, they do not affect the response to bradykinin, and are less likely to be associated with nonrenin-angiotensin effects (eg, cough and angioedema). Losartan increases urinary flow rate and in addition to being natriuretic and kaliuretic, increases excretion of chloride, magnesium, uric acid, calcium, and phosphate.

Pharmacodynamics/Kinetics

Onset of action: 6 hours

Distribution: V_d: Losartan: 34 L; E-3174: 12 L; does not cross blood brain barrier

Protein binding, plasma: High

Metabolism: Hepatic (14%) via CYP2C9 and 3A4 to active metabolite, E-3174 (40 times more potent than losartan); extensive first-pass effect

Bioavailability: 25% to 33%; AUC of E-3174 is four times greater than that of losartan

Half-life elimination: Losartan: 1.5-2 hours; E-3174: 6-9 hours

Time to peak, serum: Losartan: 1 hour; E-3174: 3-4 hours

Excretion: Urine (4% as unchanged drug, 6% as active metabolite)

Clearance: Plasma: Losartan: 600 mL/minute; Active metabolite: 50 mL/minute

Dosage

Geriatric & Adult

Hypertension: Oral: Usual starting dose: 50 mg once daily; can be administered once or twice daily with total daily doses ranging from 25-100 mg

Usual initial doses in patients receiving diuretics or those with intravascular volume depletion: 25 mg once daily

Nephropathy in patients with type 2 diabetes and hypertension: Oral: Initial: 50 mg once daily; can be increased to 100 mg once daily based on blood pressure response

Stroke reduction (HTN with LVH): Oral: 50 mg once daily (maximum daily dose: 100 mg); may be used in combination with a thiazide diuretic

Renal Impairment Adults: No adjustment necessary.

Hepatic Impairment Adults: Reduce the initial dose to 25 mg/day

Administration May be administered with or without food.

Monitoring Parameters Supine blood pressure, electrolytes, serum creatinine, BUN, urinalysis, symptomatic hypotension and tachycardia, CBC

Pharmacotherapy Pearls It is not uncommon to find hyperuricemia associated with hypertension. In those patients, losartan may offer an advantage due to its uricosuric action and may be of benefit in patients who have hyperuricemia and hypertension. Available in combination with hydrochlorothiazide as Hyzaar®.

Special Geriatric Considerations Serum concentrations of losartan and its metabolites are not significantly different and no initial dose adjustment is necessary even in low creatinine clearance states (<30 mL/minute). Many elderly may be volume depleted due to diuretic use and/or blunted thirst reflex resulting in inadequate fluid intake.

Dosage Forms Excipient information presented when available (limited, particularly for generics); consult specific product labeling.

Tablet, oral, as potassium: 25 mg, 50 mg, 100 mg

Cozaar®: 25 mg [contains potassium 2.12 mg (0.054 mEq)]

Cozaar®: 50 mg [contains potassium 4.24 mg (0.108 mEq)]

Cozaar®: 100 mg [contains potassium 8.48 mg (0.216 mEq)]

Extemporaneously Prepared To prepare losartan suspension, combine 10 mL of purified water and ten (10) losartan 50 mg tablets in an 8 ounce bottle. Shake well for ≥2 minutes. Allow concentrate to stand for 1 hour then shake for 1 minute. Separately, prepare 190 mL of a 50/50 mixture of Ora-Plus™ and Ora-Sweet SF™. Add to tablet and water mixture; shake for 1 minute. Resulting 200 mL suspension will contain losartan 2.5 mg/mL. Store under refrigeration for up to 4 weeks; shake well before use.

Selected References

Chobanian AV, Bakris GL, Black HR, et al, "The Seventh Report of the Joint National Committee on Prevention, Detection, Evaluation, and Treatment of High Blood Pressure: The JNC 7 Report," *JAMA*, 2003, 289(19):2560-71.

Cohn JN and Tognoni G, "Valsartan Heart Failure Trial Investigators. A Randomized Trial of the Angiotensin-Receptor Blocker Valsartan in Chronic Heart Failure," *N Engl J Med*, 2001, 345(23):1667-75.

Conlin P, Moore T, Swartz S, et al, "Effect of Indomethacin on Blood Pressure Lowering by Captopril and Losartan in Hypertensive Patients," *Hypertension*, 2000, 36(3):461-5.

Dahlof B, Devereux RB, Kjeldsen SE, et al, "Cardiovascular Morbidity and Mortality in the Losartan Intervention For Endpoint Reduction in Hypertension Study (LIFE): A Randomised Trial Against Atenolol," *Lancet*, 2002, 359 (9311):995-1003.

Dickstein K, Kjekshus J, et al, "Effects of Losartan and Captopril on Mortality and Morbidity in High-Risk Patients After Acute Myocardial Infarction: The OPTIMAAL Randomised Trial. Optimal Trial in Myocardial Infarction with Angiotensin II Antagonist Losartan," *Lancet*, 2002, 360(9335):752-60.

Epstein BJ and Gums JG, "Angiotensin Receptor Blockers Versus ACE Inhibitors: Prevention of Death and Myocardial Infarction in High-Risk Populations," *Ann Pharmacother*, 2005, 39(3):470-80.

Granger CB, McMurray JJ, Yusuf S, et al, "Effects of Candesartan in Patients With Chronic Heart Failure and Reduced Left-Ventricular Systolic Function Intolerant to Angiotensin-Converting-Enzyme Inhibitors: The CHARM-Alternative Trial," *Lancet*, 2003, 362(9386):772-6.

Hunt SA, Baker DW, Chin MH, et al, "ACC/AHA Guidelines for the Evaluation and Management of Chronic Heart Failure in the Adult: A Report of the American College of Cardiology/American Heart Association Task Force on Practice Guidelines (Committee to Revise the 1995 Guidelines for the Evaluation and Management of Heart Failure). 2001. American College of Cardiology Web site. Available at: http://www.acc.org/clinical/guidelines/failure/hf_index.-htm. Accessed June 9, 2003.

"K/DOQI Clinical Practice Guidelines for Chronic Kidney Disease: Evaluation, Classification, and Stratification. Kidney Disease Outcome Quality Initiative," *Am J Kidney Dis*, 2002, 39(2 Suppl 2):1-246. Available at: http://www.kidney.org/professionals/doqi/kdoqi/toc.htm. Accessed August 1, 2003.

McMurray JJ, Ostergren J, Swedberg K, et al, "Effects of Candesartan in Patients With Chronic Heart Failure and Reduced Left-Ventricular Systolic Function Taking Angiotensin-Converting-Enzyme Inhibitors: The CHARM-Added Trial," *Lancet*, 2003, 362(9386):767-71.

Pfeffer MA, McMurray JJ, Velazquez EJ, et al, "Valsartan, Captopril, or Both in Myocardial Infarction Complicated by Heart Failure, Left Ventricular Dysfunction, or Both," *N Engl J Med*, 2004, 350(2):203.

Pitt B, Poole-Wilson PA, Segal R, et al, "Effect of Losartan Compared With Captopril on Mortality in Patients With Symptomatic Heart Failure: Randomised Trial - The Losartan Heart Failure Survival Study ELITE II," *Lancet*, 2000, 355(9215):1582-7.

Losartan and Hydrochlorothiazide (loe SAR tan & hye droe klor oh THYE a zide)

Related Information

Hydrochlorothiazide *on page 876*

Losartan *on page 1092*

Medication Safety Issues

Sound-alike/look-alike issues:

Hyzaar® may be confused with Cozaar®

Brand Names: U.S. Hyzaar®

Brand Names: Canada Hyzaar®; Hyzaar® DS

Index Terms Hydrochlorothiazide and Losartan

Generic Availability (U.S.) Yes

Pharmacologic Category Angiotensin II Receptor Blocker; Diuretic, Thiazide

Use Treatment of hypertension; stroke risk reduction in patients with HTN and left ventricular hypertrophy (LVH)

Dosage

Geriatric Refer to dosing in individual monographs.

Adult Note: Dose is individualized (combination substituted for individual components); dose may be titrated after 2-4 weeks of therapy

Hypertension/stroke reduction in hypertension (with LVH): Usual recommended starting dose of losartan: 50 mg once daily when used as monotherapy in patients who are not volume depleted

Renal Impairment Cl_{cr} ≤30 mL/minute: Use of combination formulation is not recommended.

Hepatic Impairment Use is not recommended.

Special Geriatric Considerations Hydrochlorothiazide is not effective in patients with a Cl_{cr} <30 mL/minute; therefore, it may not be a useful agent in many elderly patients.

◀ **Dosage Forms** Excipient information presented when available (limited, particularly for generics); consult specific product labeling.

Tablet: 50/12.5: Losartan potassium 50 mg and hydrochlorothiazide 12.5 mg; 100/12.5: Losartan potassium 100 mg and hydrochlorothiazide 12.5 mg; 100/25: Losartan potassium 100 mg and hydrochlorothiazide 25 mg

Hyzaar® 50/12.5: Losartan potassium 50 mg and hydrochlorothiazide 12.5 mg [contains potassium 4.24 mg (0.108 mEq)]

Hyzaar® 100/12.5: Losartan potassium 100 mg and hydrochlorothiazide 12.5 mg [contains potassium 8.48 mg (0.216 mEq)]

Hyzaar® 100/25: Losartan potassium 100 mg and hydrochlorothiazide 25 mg [contains potassium 8.48 mg (0.216 mEq)]

- ♦ **Losartan Potassium** see Losartan on page 1092
- ♦ **Lotemax®** see Loteprednol on page 1096
- ♦ **Lotensin®** see Benazepril on page 188
- ♦ **Lotensin HCT®** see Benazepril and Hydrochlorothiazide on page 191

Loteprednol (loe te PRED nol)

Brand Names: U.S. Alrex®; Lotemax®
Brand Names: Canada Alrex®; Lotemax®
Index Terms Loteprednol Etabonate
Generic Availability (U.S.) No
Pharmacologic Category Corticosteroid, Ophthalmic
Use

Suspension, 0.2% (Alrex®): Temporary relief of signs and symptoms of seasonal allergic conjunctivitis

Suspension, 0.5% (Lotemax®): Inflammatory conditions (treatment of steroid-responsive inflammatory conditions of the palpebral and bulbar conjunctiva, cornea, and anterior segment of the globe such as allergic conjunctivitis, acne rosacea, superficial punctate keratitis, herpes zoster keratitis, iritis, cyclitis, selected infective conjunctivitis, when the inherent hazard of steroid use is accepted to obtain an advisable diminution in edema and inflammation) and treatment of postoperative inflammation following ocular surgery

Dosage

Geriatric & Adult

Seasonal allergic conjunctivitis: Ophthalmic: 0.2% suspension (Alrex®): Instill 1 drop into affected eye(s) 4 times/day.

Inflammatory conditions: Ophthalmic: 0.5% suspension (Lotemax®): Apply 1-2 drops into the conjunctival sac of the affected eye(s) 4 times/day. During the initial treatment within the first week, the dosing may be increased up to 1 drop every hour. Advise patients not to discontinue therapy prematurely. If signs and symptoms fail to improve after 2 days, re-evaluate the patient.

Postoperative inflammation: Ophthalmic: 0.5% suspension (Lotemax®): Apply 1-2 drops into the conjunctival sac of the operated eye(s) 4 times/day beginning 24 hours after surgery and continuing throughout the first 2 weeks of the postoperative period.

Special Geriatric Considerations Assess patient's ability to administer eye drops.
Product Availability

Lotemax® 0.5% ointment: FDA approved April 2011; expected availability undetermined

Lotemax® 0.5% ointment is a topical corticosteroid approved for the treatment of post-operative inflammation and pain following ocular surgery.

Dosage Forms Excipient information presented when available (limited, particularly for generics); consult specific product labeling.

Suspension, ophthalmic, as etabonate [drops]:

Alrex®: 0.2% (5 mL, 10 mL) [contains benzalkonium chloride]

Lotemax®: 0.5% (2.5 mL, 5 mL, 10 mL, 15 mL) [contains benzalkonium chloride]

Loteprednol and Tobramycin (loe te PRED nol & toe bra MYE sin)

Related Information

Loteprednol on page 1096

Brand Names: U.S. Zylet®
Index Terms Loteprednol Etabonate and Tobramycin; Tobramycin and Loteprednol Etabonate
Generic Availability (U.S.) No
Pharmacologic Category Antibiotic/Corticosteroid, Ophthalmic
Use Treatment of steroid-responsive ocular inflammatory conditions where either a superficial bacterial ocular infection or the risk of a superficial bacterial ocular infection exists

Dosage

Geriatric & Adult Ophthalmic: Instill 1-2 drops into the affected eye(s) every 4-6 hours; may increase frequency during the first 24-48 hours to every 1-2 hours. Interval should increase as signs and symptoms improve. Further evaluation should occur for use of greater than 20 mL.

Special Geriatric Considerations Evaluate the patient's or caregiver's ability to safely administer the correct dose of ophthalmic medication.

Dosage Forms Excipient information presented when available (limited, particularly for generics); consult specific product labeling.

Suspension, ophthalmic [drops]:

Zylet®: Loteprednol etabonate 0.5% and tobramycin 0.3% (2.5 mL, 5 mL, 10 mL) [contains benzalkonium chloride]

Lovastatin (LOE va sta tin)

Related Information
Hyperlipidemia Management on page 2021

Medication Safety Issues
Sound-alike/look-alike issues:
Lovastatin may be confused with atorvastatin, Leustatin®, Livostin®, Lotensin®, nystatin, pitavastatin
Mevacor® may be confused with Benicar®, Lipitor®, Mivacron®

International issues:
Lovacol [Chile and Finland] may be confused with Levatol brand name for penbutolol [U.S.]
Lovastin [Malaysia, Poland, and Singapore] may be confused with Livostin brand name for levocabastine [multiple international markets]

Brand Names: U.S. Altoprev®; Mevacor®

Brand Names: Canada Apo-Lovastatin®; CO Lovastatin; Dom-Lovastatin; Gen-Lovastatin; Mevacor®; Mylan-Lovastatin; Novo-Lovastatin; Nu-Lovastatin; PHL-Lovastatin; PMS-Lovastatin; PRO-Lovastatin; RAN™-Lovastatin; ratio-Lovastatin; Riva-Lovastatin; Sandoz-Lovastatin

Index Terms Mevinolin; Monacolin K

Generic Availability (U.S.) Yes: Exludes extended release tablet

Pharmacologic Category Antilipemic Agent, HMG-CoA Reductase Inhibitor

Use
Adjunct to dietary therapy to decrease elevated serum total and LDL-cholesterol concentrations in primary hypercholesterolemia
Primary prevention of coronary artery disease (patients without symptomatic disease with average to moderately elevated total and LDL-cholesterol and below average HDL-cholesterol); slow progression of coronary atherosclerosis in patients with coronary heart disease
Adjunct to dietary therapy in adolescent patients (10-17 years of age, females >1 year postmenarche) with heterozygous familial hypercholesterolemia having LDL >189 mg/dL, **or** LDL >160 mg/dL with positive family history of premature cardiovascular disease (CVD), **or** LDL >160 mg/dL with the presence of at least two other CVD risk factors

Contraindications Hypersensitivity to lovastatin or any component of the formulation; active liver disease; unexplained persistent elevations of serum transaminases

Warnings/Precautions Secondary causes of hyperlipidemia should be ruled out prior to therapy. Liver function must be monitored by periodic laboratory assessment. Rhabdomyolysis with or without acute renal failure has occurred. Risk is dose-related and is increased with concurrent use of lipid-lowering agents which may cause rhabdomyolysis (gemfibrozil, fibric acid derivatives, or niacin at doses ≥1 g/day) or during concurrent use with potent CYP3A4 inhibitors. Avoid concurrent use of azole antifungals, macrolide antibiotics, and protease inhibitors. Use caution/limit dose with amiodarone, cyclosporine, danazol, gemfibrozil (or other fibrates), lipid-lowering doses of niacin, or verapamil. Monitor closely if used with other drugs associated with myopathy (eg, colchicine). Patients should be instructed to report unexplained muscle pain or weakness; lovastatin should be discontinued if myopathy is suspected/confirmed. Temporarily discontinue in any patient experiencing an acute or serious condition predisposing to renal failure secondary to rhabdomyolysis. Based upon current evidence, HMG-CoA reductase inhibitor therapy should be continued in the perioperative period unless risk outweighs cardioprotective benefit. Use with caution in patients with advanced age, these patients are predisposed to myopathy. Use with caution in patients who consume large amounts of ethanol or have a history of liver disease.

Adverse Reactions (Reflective of adult population; not specific for elderly) Percentages as reported with immediate release tablets; similar adverse reactions seen with extended release tablets.

>10%: Neuromuscular & skeletal: CPK increased (>2x normal) (11%)

1% to 10%:

Central nervous system: Headache (2% to 3%), dizziness (≤1%)

Dermatologic: Rash (≤1%)

Gastrointestinal: Flatulence (4% to 5%), constipation (2% to 4%), abdominal pain (2% to 3%), diarrhea (2% to 3%), nausea (2% to 3%), dyspepsia (1% to 2%)

Neuromuscular & skeletal: Myalgia (2% to 3%), weakness (1% to 2%), muscle cramps (≤1%)

Ocular: Blurred vision (≤1%)

Additional class-related events or case reports (not necessarily reported with lovastatin therapy): Alkaline phosphatase increased, alteration in taste, anaphylaxis, angioedema, anorexia, anxiety, arthritis, cataracts, chills, cholestatic jaundice, cirrhosis, depression, dryness of skin/mucous membranes, dyspnea, eosinophilia, erectile dysfunction, erythema multiforme, ESR increased, facial paresis, fatty liver, fever, flushing, fulminant hepatic necrosis, GGT increased, gynecomastia, hemolytic anemia, hepatitis, hepatoma, hyperbilirubinemia, hypersensitivity reaction, impaired extraocular muscle movement, impotence, interstitial lung disease, leukopenia, libido decreased, malaise, memory loss, myopathy, nail changes, nodules, ophthalmoplegia, pancreatitis, peripheral nerve palsy, peripheral neuropathy, photosensitivity, polymyalgia rheumatica, positive ANA, psychic disturbance, purpura, renal failure (secondary to rhabdomyolysis), rhabdomyolysis, skin discoloration, Stevens-Johnson syndrome, systemic lupus erythematosus-like syndrome, thrombocytopenia, thyroid dysfunction, toxic epidermal necrolysis, transaminases increased, tremor, urticaria, vasculitis, vertigo

Drug Interactions

Metabolism/Transport Effects Substrate of CYP3A4 (major), P-glycoprotein; **Inhibits** CYP2C9 (weak), 2D6 (weak), 3A4 (weak)

Avoid Concomitant Use

Avoid concomitant use of Lovastatin with any of the following: Boceprevir; CYP3A4 Inhibitors (Strong); Erythromycin; Protease Inhibitors; Red Yeast Rice; Telaprevir

Increased Effect/Toxicity

Lovastatin may increase the levels/effects of: DAPTOmycin; Diltiazem; Trabectedin; Vitamin K Antagonists

The levels/effects of Lovastatin may be increased by: Amiodarone; Antifungal Agents (Azole Derivatives, Systemic); Boceprevir; Colchicine; CycloSPORINE; CycloSPORINE (Systemic); CYP3A4 Inhibitors (Moderate); CYP3A4 Inhibitors (Strong); Cyproterone; Danazol; Dasatinib; Diltiazem; Dronedarone; Erythromycin; Fenofibrate; Fenofibric Acid; Fluconazole; Gemfibrozil; Grapefruit Juice; Macrolide Antibiotics; Niacin; Niacinamide; P-Glycoprotein Inhibitors; Protease Inhibitors; QuiNINE; Red Yeast Rice; Rifamycin Derivatives; Sildenafil; Telaprevir; Ticagrelor; Verapamil

Decreased Effect

Lovastatin may decrease the levels/effects of: Lanthanum

The levels/effects of Lovastatin may be decreased by: Antacids; Bosentan; CYP3A4 Inducers (Strong); Deferasirox; Efavirenz; Etravirine; Fosphenytoin; P-Glycoprotein Inducers; Phenytoin; Rifamycin Derivatives; St Johns Wort; Tocilizumab

Ethanol/Nutrition/Herb Interactions

Ethanol: Avoid excessive ethanol consumption (due to potential hepatic effects).

Food: Food **decreases** the bioavailability of lovastatin extended release tablets and **increases** the bioavailability of lovastatin immediate release tablets. Lovastatin serum concentrations may be increased if taken with grapefruit juice; avoid concurrent intake of large quantities (>1 quart/day). Red yeast rice contains an estimated 2.4 mg lovastatin per 600 mg rice.

Herb/Nutraceutical: St John's wort may decrease lovastatin levels.

Stability

Tablet, immediate release: Store at 20°C to 25°C (68°F to 77°F). Protect from light

Tablet, extended release: Store between 20°C to 25°C (68°F to 77°F); excursions permitted between 15°C to 30°C (59°F to 86°F). Avoid excessive heat and humidity.

Mechanism of Action Lovastatin acts by competitively inhibiting 3-hydroxyl-3-methylglutaryl-coenzyme A (HMG-CoA) reductase, the enzyme that catalyzes the rate-limiting step in cholesterol biosynthesis

Pharmacodynamics/Kinetics

Onset of action: LDL-cholesterol reductions: 3 days

Absorption: 30%; increased with extended release tablets when taken in the fasting state

Protein binding: >95%

Metabolism: Hepatic; extensive first-pass effect; hydrolyzed to β-hydroxyacid (active)

Bioavailability: Increased with extended release tablets

Half-life elimination: 1.1-1.7 hours

Time to peak, serum: Immediate release: 2-4 hours; extended release: 12-14 hours

Excretion: Feces (~80% to 85%); urine (10%)

Dosage

Geriatric & Adult

Dyslipidemia and primary prevention of CAD: Oral: Initial: 20 mg with evening meal, then adjust at 4-week intervals; maximum: 80 mg/day immediate release tablet **or** 60 mg/day extended release tablet.

Note: Doses should be individualized according to the baseline LDL-cholesterol levels, the recommended goal of therapy, and patient response.

Dosage modification/limits based on concurrent therapy:

Cyclosporine or danazol: Initial dose: 10 mg/day with a maximum recommended dose of 20 mg/day

Concurrent therapy with fibrates and/or lipid-lowering doses of niacin (≥1 g/day): Maximum recommended dose: 20 mg/day. Concurrent use with fibrates should be avoided unless risk to benefit favors use.

Concurrent therapy with amiodarone or verapamil: Maximum recommended dose: 40 mg/day of immediate release or 20 mg/day with extended release.

Dosage adjustment in renal impairment: Cl_{cr} <30 mL/minute: Use doses >20 mg/day with caution.

Renal Impairment Cl_{cr} <30 mL/minute: Use with caution and carefully consider doses >20 mg/day.

Administration Administer immediate release tablets with meals. Administer extended-release tablet at bedtime; do not crush or chew.

Monitoring Parameters Obtain baseline LFTs and total cholesterol profile. LFTs should also be assessed prior to, at 6 and 12 weeks after initiation, and periodically thereafter; baseline CPK (recheck CPK in any patient with symptoms suggestive of myopathy).

Reference Range NCEP classification of pediatric patients with familial history of hyper-cholesterolemia or premature CVD: Acceptable total cholesterol: <170 mg/dL, LDL: <110 mg/dL

Test Interactions Altered thyroid function tests

Special Geriatric Considerations The definition of and, therefore, when to treat hyper-lipidemia in the elderly is a controversial issue. The National Cholesterol Education Program recommends that all adults maintain a plasma cholesterol <160 mg/dL. For elderly patients with one additional risk factor, goal LDL would be <130 mg/dL. It is the authors' belief that pharmacologic treatment be reserved for those who are unable to obtain a desirable plasma cholesterol concentration by diet alone and for whom the benefits of treatment are believed to outweigh the potential adverse effects, drug interactions, and cost of treatment. Age ≥65 years is a risk factor for myopathy.

Dosage Forms Excipient information presented when available (limited, particularly for generics); consult specific product labeling.

Tablet, oral: 10 mg, 20 mg, 40 mg

Mevacor®: 20 mg, 40 mg

Tablet, extended release, oral:

Altoprev®: 20 mg, 40 mg, 60 mg

Selected References

Fleisher LA, Beckman JA, Brown KA, et al, "ACC/AHA 2007 Guidelines on Perioperative Cardiovascular Evaluation and Care for Noncardiac Surgery: A Report of the American College of Cardiology/American Heart Association Task Force on Practice Guidelines (Writing Committee to Revise the 2002 Guidelines on Perioperative Cardiovascular Evaluation for Noncardiac Surgery) Developed in Collaboration With the American Society of Echocardiography, American Society of Nuclear Cardiology, Heart Rhythm Society, Society of Cardiovascular Anesthesiologists, Society for Cardiovascular Angiography and Interventions, Society for Vascular Medicine and Biology, and Society for Vascular Surgery," *J Am Coll Cardiol*, 2007, 50(17):e159-241.

Grundy SM, Cleeman JI, Merz CN, et al, "Implications of Recent Clinical Trials for the National Cholesterol Education Program Adult Treatment Panel III Guidelines," *J Am Coll Cardiol*, 2004, 44(3):720-32.

National Cholesterol Education Program (NCEP) Expert Panel on Detection, Evaluation, and Treatment of High Blood Cholesterol in Adults (Adult Treatment Panel III), "Third Report of the National Cholesterol Education Program (NCEP) Expert Panel on Detection, Evaluation, and Treatment of High Blood Cholesterol in Adults (Adult Treatment Panel III) Final Report," *Circulation*, 2002, 106(25):3143-421.

◆ **Lovastatin and Niacin** see Niacin and Lovastatin on page 1291
◆ **Lovaza®** see Omega-3-Acid Ethyl Esters on page 1338
◆ **Lovenox®** see Enoxaparin on page 598
◆ **Low-Molecular-Weight Iron Dextran (INFeD®)** see Iron Dextran Complex on page 977

Loxapine (LOKS a peen)

Related Information

Antipsychotic Agents *on page 1997*

Liquid Compatibility of Antidepressants, Antipsychotics, and Mood Stabilizers *on page 2111*

Medication Safety Issues

Sound-alike/look-alike issues:

Loxitane® may be confused with Lexapro®, Soriatane®

International issues:

Loxitane [U.S.] may be confused with Lexotan which is a brand name for bromazepam [multiple international markets]

Brand Names: U.S. Loxitane®

Brand Names: Canada Apo-Loxapine®; Dom-Loxapine; Loxapac® IM; Nu-Loxapine; PHL-Loxapine; Xylac

Index Terms Loxapine Succinate; Oxilapine Succinate

Generic Availability (U.S.) Yes

Pharmacologic Category Antipsychotic Agent, Typical

Use Management of psychotic disorders

Unlabeled/Investigational Use Psychosis/agitation related to Alzheimer's dementia

Contraindications Hypersensitivity to loxapine or any component of the formulation; severe CNS depression; coma

Warnings/Precautions [U.S. Boxed Warning]: Elderly patients with dementia-related psychosis treated with antipsychotics are at an increased risk of death compared to placebo. Most deaths appeared to be either cardiovascular (eg, heart failure, sudden death) or infectious (eg, pneumonia) in nature. Loxapine is not approved for the treatment of dementia-related psychosis.

May alter cardiac conduction; life-threatening arrhythmias have occurred with therapeutic doses of antipsychotics. Avoid use in patients with underlying QT prolongation, in those taking medicines that prolong the QT interval, or cause polymorphic ventricular tachycardia; monitor ECG closely for dose-related QT effects.

Leukopenia, neutropenia, and agranulocytosis (sometimes fatal) have been reported in clinical trials and postmarketing reports with antipsychotic use; presence of risk factors (eg, pre-existing low WBC or history of drug-induced leuko-/neutropenia) should prompt periodic blood count assessment. Discontinue therapy at first signs of blood dyscrasias or if absolute neutrophil count <1000/mm³.

Antipsychotic use has been associated with esophageal dysmotility and aspiration; use with caution in patients at risk of pneumonia (ie, Alzheimer's disease). May cause extrapyramidal symptoms (EPS), including pseudoparkinsonism, acute dystonic reactions, akathisia, and tardive dyskinesia. Risk of dystonia (and possibly other EPS) may be greater with increased doses, use of conventional antipsychotics, males, and younger patients. Increased incidence of EPS has been observed with I.M. administration compared to oral administration. Use may be associated with NMS; monitor for mental status changes, fever, muscle rigidity, and/or autonomic instability. May cause orthostatic hypotension; use with caution in patients at risk of this effect or in those who would not tolerate transient hypotensive episodes (cerebrovascular disease, cardiovascular disease, hypovolemia, or concurrent medication use which may predispose to hypotension/bradycardia). May be associated with pigmentary retinopathy. Impaired core body temperature regulation may occur; caution with strenuous exercise, heat exposure, dehydration, and concomitant medication possessing anticholinergic effects.

May be sedating, use with caution in disorders where CNS depression is a feature; patients must be cautioned about performing tasks which require mental alertness (eg, operating machinery or driving). Effects may be potentiated when used with other sedative drugs or ethanol. May cause anticholinergic effects (constipation, xerostomia, blurred vision, urinary retention); use with caution in patients with decreased gastrointestinal motility, paralytic ileus, urinary retention, BPH, xerostomia, or visual problems. Relative to other antipsychotics, loxapine has a low potency of cholinergic blockade. May mask toxicity of other drugs or conditions (eg, intestinal obstruction, Reye's syndrome, brain tumor) due to antiemetic effects. Use associated with increased prolactin levels; clinical significance of hyperprolactinemia in patients with breast cancer or other prolactin-dependent tumors is unknown. May cause pigmentary retinopathy, and lenticular and corneal deposits, particularly with prolonged therapy.

Use with caution in patients with severe cardiovascular disease, narrow-angle glaucoma, myasthenia gravis, Parkinson's disease, or seizure disorder. Use with caution in the elderly.

Adverse Reactions (Reflective of adult population; not specific for elderly) Frequency not defined.

Cardiovascular: Abnormal T waves with prolonged ventricular repolarization, arrhythmia, hyper-/hypotension, orthostatic hypotension, tachycardia, syncope

Central nervous system: Agitation, altered central temperature regulation, ataxia, confusion, dizziness, drowsiness, extrapyramidal reactions (akathisia, akinesia, dystonia, pseudoparkinsonism, tardive dyskinesia), faintness, headache, insomnia, lightheadedness, neuroleptic malignant syndrome (NMS), seizure, slurred speech, tension

Dermatologic: Alopecia, dermatitis, photosensitivity, pruritus, rash, seborrhea

Endocrine & metabolic: Amenorrhea, enlargement of breasts, galactorrhea, gynecomastia, menstrual irregularity

Gastrointestinal: Adynamic ileus, constipation, nausea, polydipsia, vomiting, weight gain/loss, xerostomia

Genitourinary: Sexual dysfunction, urinary retention

Hematologic: Agranulocytosis, leukopenia, thrombocytopenia

Neuromuscular & skeletal: Weakness

Ocular: Blurred vision

Respiratory: Nasal congestion

Drug Interactions

Avoid Concomitant Use

Avoid concomitant use of Loxapine with any of the following: Artemether; Dronedarone; Lumefantrine; Metoclopramide; Nilotinib; Pimozide; QUEtiapine; QuiNINE; Tetrabenazine; Thioridazine; Toremifene; Vandetanib; Vemurafenib; Ziprasidone

Increased Effect/Toxicity

Loxapine may increase the levels/effects of: Alcohol (Ethyl); Anticholinergics; Anti-Parkinson's Agents (Dopamine Agonist); CNS Depressants; Dronedarone; LORazepam; Methylphenidate; Pimozide; QTc-Prolonging Agents; QuiNINE; Selective Serotonin Reuptake Inhibitors; Tetrabenazine; Thioridazine; Toremifene; Vandetanib; Vemurafenib; Ziprasidone

The levels/effects of Loxapine may be increased by: Acetylcholinesterase Inhibitors (Central); Alfuzosin; Artemether; Chloroquine; Ciprofloxacin; Ciprofloxacin (Systemic); Gadobutrol; HydrOXYzine; Lithium formulations; Lumefantrine; Methylphenidate; Metoclopramide; Nilotinib; Pramlintide; QUEtiapine; QuiNINE; Tetrabenazine

Decreased Effect

Loxapine may decrease the levels/effects of: Amphetamines; Quinagolide

The levels/effects of Loxapine may be decreased by: Anti-Parkinson's Agents (Dopamine Agonist); Lithium formulations

Ethanol/Nutrition/Herb Interactions

Ethanol: May increase CNS depression; monitor for increased effects with coadministration. Caution patients about effects.

Herb/Nutraceutical: Avoid kava kava, gotu kola, valerian, St John's wort (may increase CNS depression).

Stability Protect from light. Dispense in amber or opaque vials.

Mechanism of Action Loxapine is a dibenzoxazepine antipsychotic which blocks postsynaptic mesolimbic D_1 and D_2 receptors in the brain, and also possesses serotonin 5-HT$_2$ blocking activity

Pharmacodynamics/Kinetics

Onset of action: Neuroleptic: Oral: 20-30 minutes

Peak effect: 1.5-3 hours

Duration: ~12 hours

Metabolism: Hepatic to glucuronide conjugates

Half-life elimination: Biphasic: Initial: 5 hours; Terminal: 12-19 hours

Excretion: Urine; feces (small amounts)

Dosage

Geriatric Oral: 20-60 mg/day

Adult Psychosis: Oral: 10 mg twice daily, increase dose until psychotic symptoms are controlled; usual dose range: 20-100 mg/day in divided doses 2-4 times/day; dosages >250 mg/day are not recommended.

Administration Dilute the oral concentrate with water or juice before administration; avoid skin contact with solution; may cause contact dermatitis.

Monitoring Parameters Vital signs, orthostatic blood pressures 3-5 days after initiation of therapy or a dose increase; lipid profile, fasting blood glucose/Hgb A$_{1c}$; BMI; mental status, abnormal involuntary movement scale (AIMS), extrapyramidal symptoms (EPS)

Test Interactions False-positives for phenylketonuria, amylase, uroporphyrins, urobilinogen

◀ **Special Geriatric Considerations** Many elderly patients receive antipsychotic medications for inappropriate nonpsychotic behavior. Before initiating antipsychotic medication, the clinician should investigate any possible reversible cause; any stress or stress from any disease can cause acute "confusion" or worsening of baseline nonpsychotic behavior. Most commonly acute changes in behavior are due to increases in drug dose or addition of new drug to regimen; fluid electrolyte loss; infections; and changes in environment.

Any changes in disease status in any organ system can result in behavior changes.

In the treatment of agitated, demented, elderly patients, authors of meta-analysis of controlled trials of the response to the traditional antipsychotics (phenothiazines, butyrophenones) in controlling agitation have concluded that the use of neuroleptics results in a response rate of 18%. Clearly neuroleptic therapy for behavior control should be limited with frequent attempts to withdraw the agent given for behavior control.

Dosage Forms Excipient information presented when available (limited, particularly for generics); consult specific product labeling.
Capsule, oral: 5 mg, 10 mg, 25 mg, 50 mg
  Loxitane®: 5 mg, 10 mg, 25 mg, 50 mg

Selected References

American Diabetes Association; American Psychiatric Association; American Association of Clinical Endocrinologists; North American Association for the Study of Obesity, "Consensus Development Conference on Antipsychotic Drugs and Obesity and Diabetes," *Diabetes Care*, 2004, 27(2):596-601.

Rabins PV, Blacker D, Rovner BW, et al, "Practice Guidelines for the Treatment of Patients With Alzheimer's Disease and Other Dementias," *Am J Psychiatry*, 2007, 164(12 Suppl):5-56. Available at http://www.psych.org/psych_pract/treatg/pg/prac_guide.cfm.

Schneider LS, Tariot PN, Dagerman KS, et al, "Effectiveness of Atypical Antipsychotic Drugs in Patients With Alzheimer's Disease," *N Engl J Med*, 2006, 355(15):1525-38.

Lubiprostone (loo bi PROS tone)

Related Information
  Laxatives, Classification and Properties on page 2012
Brand Names: U.S. Amitiza®
Index Terms RU 0211; SPI 0211
Generic Availability (U.S.) No
Pharmacologic Category Chloride Channel Activator; Gastrointestinal Agent, Miscellaneous
Use Treatment of chronic idiopathic constipation; treatment of irritable bowel syndrome with constipation in adult women
Contraindications Known or suspected mechanical bowel obstruction
Warnings/Precautions Symptoms of mechanical gastrointestinal obstruction should be evaluated before prescribing this medicine; use is contraindicated in patients with bowel obstruction. Avoid use in patients with severe diarrhea. Nausea may occur; administer with food to reduce symptoms. In long-term clinical studies for chronic idiopathic constipation, patients were allowed to reduce the dose to 24 mcg once daily if nausea was severe. Dyspnea, often described as chest tightness, has been observed with use, including postmarketing reports; generally occurs following the first dose with an acute onset (within 30-60 minutes) and resolves within a few hours; however, has been frequently reported with subsequent dosing. Dose adjustment is recommended in patients with moderate-to-severe hepatic impairment (Child Pugh class B or C). Not approved for use in males with irritable bowel syndrome with constipation.
Adverse Reactions (Reflective of adult population; not specific for elderly)
>10%:
  Central nervous system: Headache (3% to 11%)
  Gastrointestinal: Nausea (7% to 29%; severe: 4%; dose related), diarrhea (7% to 12%; severe 2%)

1% to 10%:
    Cardiovascular: Edema (3%), chest discomfort/pain (2%)
    Central nervous system: Dizziness (3%), fatigue (2%)
    Gastrointestinal: Abdominal pain (1% to 8%), abdominal distention (3% to 6%), flatulence (3% to 6%), vomiting (3%), loose stools (3%), dyspepsia (2%), xerostomia (1%)
    Respiratory: Dyspnea (2% to 3%)

Drug Interactions

Avoid Concomitant Use There are no known interactions where it is recommended to avoid concomitant use.

Increased Effect/Toxicity There are no known significant interactions involving an increase in effect.

Decreased Effect There are no known significant interactions involving a decrease in effect.

Stability Store at 25°C (77°F); excursions permitted to 15°C to 30°C (59°F to 86°F).

Mechanism of Action Bicyclic fatty acid that acts locally at the apical portion of the intestine as a chloride channel activator, increasing intestinal fluid secretion and intestinal motility. Does not alter serum sodium or potassium concentrations.

Pharmacodynamics/Kinetics
    Absorption: Systemic: Parent drug: Poor (below levels of detection); Active metabolite (M3): Low
    Distribution: Gastrointestinal tissue; minimal beyond gastrointestinal tissue
    Metabolism: Rapid and extensive within stomach and jejunum by carbonyl reductase to M3 (active metabolite) and others
    Bioavailability: Minimal
    Half-life elimination: M3: 0.9-1.4 hours
    Excretion: Parent drug and M3: Feces (trace amounts)

Dosage
    Geriatric & Adult
        Chronic idiopathic constipation: Adults: 24 mcg twice daily
        Irritable bowel syndrome with constipation: Females ≥18 years: 8 mcg twice daily
    Renal Impairment No dosage adjustment required.
    Hepatic Impairment
        Moderate hepatic impairment (Child-Pugh class B):
            Chronic idiopathic constipation: 16 mcg twice daily; may increase to 24 mcg twice daily if tolerated and an adequate response has not been obtained with lower dosage
            Irritable bowel syndrome with constipation: No dosage adjustment required
        Severe hepatic impairment (Child-Pugh class C):
            Chronic idiopathic constipation: 8 mcg twice daily; may increase to 16-24 mcg twice daily if tolerated and an adequate response has not been obtained with lower dosage
            Irritable bowel syndrome with constipation: 8 mcg once daily; may increase to 8 mcg twice daily if tolerated and an adequate response has not been obtained at lower dosage

Administration Administer with food and water. Swallow whole; do not break or chew.

Special Geriatric Considerations Elderly with chronic idiopathic constipation, when studied, demonstrated consistent efficacy to that seen in younger populations. Of note, the elderly experienced less nausea than younger subjects.

Dosage Forms Excipient information presented when available (limited, particularly for generics); consult specific product labeling.
    Capsule, softgel, oral:
        Amitiza®: 8 mcg, 24 mcg

Selected References
"Lubiprostone: RU 0211, SPI 0211," *Drugs R D*, 2005, 6(4):245-8.
Winpenny JP, "Lubiprostone," *IDrugs*, 2005, 8(5):416-22.

Lurasidone (loo RAS i done)

Related Information
Antipsychotic Agents *on page 1997*
Atypical Antipsychotics *on page 1999*
Medication Safety Issues
Sound-alike/look-alike issues:
Latuda® may be confused with Lantus®
Brand Names: U.S. Latuda®
Index Terms Lurasidone Hydrochloride; SM-13496
Generic Availability (U.S.) No
Pharmacologic Category Antipsychotic Agent, Atypical
Use Treatment of schizophrenia
Contraindications Hypersensitivity to lurasidone or any component of the formulation; concomitant use with potent CYP3A4 inhibitors (eg, ketoconazole) and inducers (eg, rifampin)
Warnings/Precautions [U.S. Boxed Warning]: Elderly patients with dementia-related psychosis treated with antipsychotics are at an increased risk of death compared to placebo. Most deaths appeared to be either cardiovascular (eg, heart failure, sudden death) or infectious (eg, pneumonia) in nature. Lurasidone is not approved for the treatment of dementia-related psychosis. An increased incidence of cerebrovascular effects (eg, transient ischemic attack, stroke), including fatalities, has been reported in placebo-controlled trials of antipsychotics for the unapproved use in elderly patients with dementia-related psychosis.

Leukopenia, neutropenia, and agranulocytosis (sometimes fatal) have been reported in clinical trials and postmarketing reports with antipsychotic use; presence of risk factors (eg, pre-existing low WBC or history of drug-induced leuko-/neutropenia) should prompt periodic blood count assessment. Discontinue therapy at first signs of blood dyscrasias or if absolute neutrophil count <1000/mm^3.

Low to moderately sedating, use with caution in disorders where CNS depression is a feature. Use with caution in Parkinson's disease. Caution in patients with predisposition to seizures. Use with caution in renal or hepatic dysfunction; dose reduction recommended in moderate-to-severe impairment. Esophageal dysmotility and aspiration have been associated with antipsychotic use; use with caution in patients at risk of aspiration pneumonia (ie, Alzheimer's disease). Use is associated with increased prolactin levels; clinical significance of hyper-prolactinemia in patients with breast cancer or other prolactin-dependent tumors is unknown. May alter temperature regulation.

Use with caution in patients with severe cardiac disease, hemodynamic instability, prior myocardial infarction or ischemic heart disease. May cause orthostatic hypotension; use with caution in patients at risk of this effect (eg, concurrent medication use which may predispose to hypotension/bradycardia or presence of hypovolemia) or in those who would not tolerate transient hypotensive episodes. Antipsychotics may alter cardiac conduction; life-threatening arrhythmias have occurred with therapeutic doses of antipsychotics. Relative to other antipsychotics, lurasidone has minimal effects on the QT$_c$ interval and therefore, risk for arrhythmias is low. Increases in total cholesterol and triglyceride concentrations have been observed with atypical antipsychotic use; during clinical trials of lurasidone, there were no significant changes in total cholesterol or triglycerides observed. Concurrent use with strong inhibitors/inducers of CYP3A4 is contraindicated; dosage adjustment is recommended with concurrent use of moderate CYP3A4 inhibitors (eg, diltiazem).

May cause extrapyramidal symptoms (EPS), including pseudoparkinsonism, acute dystonic reactions, akathisia, and tardive dyskinesia (potentially irreversible). Risk of tardive dyskinesia may be increased in elderly patients, particularly elderly women. Risk of dystonia (and probably other EPS) may be greater with increased doses, use of conventional antipsychotics, males, and younger patients. Use may be associated with neuroleptic malignant syndrome (NMS); monitor for mental status changes, fever, muscle rigidity and/or autonomic instability (risk may be increased in patients with Parkinson's disease or Lewy body dementia). May cause hyperglycemia; in some cases may be extreme and associated with ketoacidosis, hyperosmolar coma, or death. Use with caution in patients with diabetes or other disorders of glucose regulation; monitor for worsening of glucose control. Significant weight gain has been observed with antipsychotic therapy; incidence varies with product. Monitor waist circumference and BMI.

The possibility of a suicide attempt is inherent in psychotic illness or bipolar disorder; use caution in high-risk patients during initiation of therapy. Prescriptions should be written for the smallest quantity consistent with good patient care.

Adverse Reactions (Reflective of adult population; not specific for elderly)
10%:
Central nervous system: Somnolence (dose-related: 19% to 23%), akathisia (dose-related: 11% to 15%)
Endocrine & metabolic: Fasting glucose increased (10% to 14%)
Gastrointestinal: Nausea (12%)
Neuromuscular & skeletal: Extrapyramidal symptoms (24% to 26%), parkinsonism (11%)
1% to 10%:
Cardiovascular: Tachycardia
Central nervous system: Insomnia (8%), agitation (6%), anxiety (6%), dizziness (5%), dystonia (5%), fatigue (4%), restlessness (3%)
Dermatologic: Pruritus, rash
Endocrine & metabolic: Prolactin increased (≥5 x ULN: females: 8%; males: 2%)
Gastrointestinal: Dyspepsia (8%), vomiting (8%), weight gain (≥7% increase in baseline body weight: 6%), salivary hypersecretion (2%), abdominal pain, appetite decreased, diarrhea
Neuromuscular & skeletal: Back pain (4%), CPK increased
Ocular: Blurred vision
Renal: Creatinine increased (3%)

Drug Interactions

Metabolism/Transport Effects
Substrate of CYP3A4 (major); **Inhibits** CYP3A4 (weak)

Avoid Concomitant Use
Avoid concomitant use of Lurasidone with any of the following: CYP3A4 Inducers (Strong); CYP3A4 Inhibitors (Strong); DOPamine; EPINEPHrine; EPINEPHrine (Systemic, Oral Inhalation); Metoclopramide

Increased Effect/Toxicity
Lurasidone may increase the levels/effects of: Alcohol (Ethyl); CNS Depressants; Disopyramide; Methotrimeprazine; Methylphenidate; Procainamide; QuiNIDine; Selective Serotonin Reuptake Inhibitors

The levels/effects of Lurasidone may be increased by: Acetylcholinesterase Inhibitors (Central); CYP3A4 Inhibitors (Moderate); CYP3A4 Inhibitors (Strong); Dasatinib; DOPamine; Droperidol; EPINEPHrine; EPINEPHrine (Systemic, Oral Inhalation); HydrOXYzine; Lithium formulations; MAO Inhibitors; Methotrimeprazine; Methylphenidate; Metoclopramide; Tetrabenazine

Decreased Effect
Lurasidone may decrease the levels/effects of: Amphetamines; Anti-Parkinson's Agents (Dopamine Agonist); Quinagolide

The levels/effects of Lurasidone may be decreased by: CYP3A4 Inducers (Strong); Deferasirox; Herbs (CYP3A4 Inducers); Lithium formulations; Tocilizumab

Ethanol/Nutrition/Herb Interactions
Ethanol: May increase CNS depression; monitor for increased effects with coadministration. Caution patients about side effects.
Food: Administration with food (≥350 calories) increased C_{max} and AUC of lurasidone ~3 times and 2 times, respectively, compared to administration under fasting conditions. Lurasidone exposure was not affected by the fat content of the meal.

Stability Store at controlled room temperature of 25°C (77°F).

Mechanism of Action Lurasidone is a benzoisothiazol-derivative atypical antipsychotic with mixed serotonin-dopamine antagonist activity. It exhibits high affinity for D_2, $5-HT_{2A}$, and $5-HT_7$ receptors; moderate affinity for alpha$_{2C}$-adrenergic receptors; and is a partial agonist for $5-HT_{1A}$ receptors. Lurasidone has no significant affinity for muscarinic M_1 and histamine H_1 receptors. The addition of serotonin antagonism to dopamine antagonism (classic neuroleptic mechanism) is thought to improve negative symptoms of psychoses and reduce the incidence of extrapyramidal side effects as compared to typical antipsychotics.

Pharmacodynamics/Kinetics
Distribution: V_d: 6173 L
Protein binding: ~99%
Metabolism: Primarily via CYP3A4; two active metabolites (ID-14283 and ID-14326) and two major nonactive metabolites (ID-20219 and ID-20220) produced
Bioavailability: 9% to 19%
Half-life elimination: 18 hours; Main active metabolite, ID-14283 (exo-hydroxy metabolite), exhibits a half-life of 7.5-10 hours
Time to peak: 1-3 hours; steady state concentrations achieved within 7 days
Excretion: Urine (~9%); feces (~80%)

Dosage
  Geriatric & Adult Schizophrenia: Oral: Initial: 40 mg once daily; titration is not required; maximum recommended dose: 80 mg/day

  Concomitant CYP3A4 inhibitors/inducers:
    CYP3A4 inhibitors: If concomitant administration with a moderate CYP3A4 inhibitor (eg, diltiazem) is necessary, do not exceed 40 mg/day of lurasidone. Concomitant administration with a strong CYP3A4 inhibitor (eg, ketoconazole) is contraindicated.
    CYP3A4 inducers: Concomitant administration with a strong CYP3A4 inducer (eg, rifampin) is contraindicated.

  Renal Impairment Exposure is increased in renal impairment; use caution.
    Cl_{cr} ≥50 mL/minute: No dosage adjustment required.
    Cl_{cr} 10-49 mL/minute: Do not exceed 40 mg/day.

  Hepatic Impairment Exposure is increased in hepatic impairment; use caution.
    Mild hepatic impairment (Child-Pugh class A): No dosage adjustment required.
    Moderate-to-severe hepatic impairment (Child-Pugh class B or C): Do not exceed 40 mg/day.

Administration Administer with food (≥350 calories).

Monitoring Parameters Vital signs; fasting lipid profile and fasting blood glucose/Hgb A_{1c} (baseline and periodically); CBC frequently during first few months of therapy in patients with pre-existing low WBC or a history of drug-induced leukopenia/neutropenia; BMI, personal/ family history of obesity, waist circumference; blood pressure; mental status, abnormal involuntary movement scale (AIMS), extrapyramidal symptoms; orthostatic blood pressure changes for 3-5 days after starting or increasing dose. Weight should be assessed prior to treatment and regularly throughout therapy. Consider titrating to a different antipsychotic agent for a weight gain ≥5% of the initial weight.

Special Geriatric Considerations Clinical studies of schizophrenic patients did not include sufficient numbers of elderly to determine a difference in response compared to younger adults. Elderly with psychosis had similar serum concentrations to younger adults; therefore, no dosage adjustments are recommended for elderly patients with psychosis. This drug is not recommended/indicated for use in elderly patients with dementia-related psychosis. Such patients are at an increased risk of death compared to placebo. Most deaths were cardiovascular (eg, heart failure, sudden death) or infectious (eg, pneumonia) in nature.

Dosage Forms Excipient information presented when available (limited, particularly for generics); consult specific product labeling.
  Tablet, oral, as hydrochloride:
    Latuda®: 40 mg, 80 mg

Selected References
"Challenges and Solutions in Developing New Medications for Schizophrenia," *J Clin Psychiatry,* 2010, 71(10):1391-9.
Citrome L, "Lurasidone for Schizophrenia: A Brief Review of a New Second-Generation Antipsychotic," *Clin Schizophr Relat Psychoses,* 2011, 4(4):251-7.

Magaldrate and Simethicone (MAG al drate & sye METH i kone)

Related Information
Simethicone *on page 1679*
Medication Safety Issues
Sound-alike/look-alike issues:
Riopan Plus® may be confused with Repan®
Index Terms Riopan Plus; Simethicone and Magaldrate
Generic Availability (U.S.) Yes
Pharmacologic Category Antacid; Antiflatulent
Use Relief of hyperacidity associated with peptic ulcer, gastritis, peptic esophagitis, and hiatal hernia which are accompanied by symptoms of gas
Dosage
Geriatric & Adult Hyperacidity/gas: Oral: 5-10 mL (540-1080 mg magaldrate) between meals and at bedtime
Dosage Forms Excipient information presented when available (limited, particularly for generics); consult specific product labeling.
Suspension, oral: Magaldrate 540 mg and simethicone 20 mg per 5 mL (360 mL)

♦ **Mag-Al Ultimate [OTC]** *see* Aluminum Hydroxide and Magnesium Hydroxide *on page 81*
♦ **Magan®** *see* Salicylates (Various Salts) *on page 1647*
♦ **Mag Citrate** *see* Magnesium Citrate *on page 1107*
♦ **MagGel™ 600 [OTC]** *see* Magnesium Oxide *on page 1112*
♦ **Maginex™ [OTC]** *see* Magnesium L-aspartate Hydrochloride *on page 1111*
♦ **Maginex™ DS [OTC]** *see* Magnesium L-aspartate Hydrochloride *on page 1111*
♦ **Magnesia Magma** *see* Magnesium Hydroxide *on page 1109*
♦ **Magnesium L-lactate Dihydrate** *see* Magnesium L-lactate *on page 1112*
♦ **Magnesium Carbonate and Aluminum Hydroxide** *see* Aluminum Hydroxide and Magnesium Carbonate *on page 80*

Magnesium Citrate (mag NEE zhum SIT rate)

Related Information
Laxatives, Classification and Properties *on page 2012*
Brand Names: U.S. Citroma® [OTC]
Brand Names: Canada Citro-Mag®
Index Terms Citrate of Magnesia; Mag Citrate
Generic Availability (U.S.) Yes
Pharmacologic Category Laxative, Saline; Magnesium Salt
Use Evacuation of bowel prior to certain surgical and diagnostic procedures or overdose situations
Contraindications Renal failure, appendicitis, abdominal pain, intestinal impaction, obstruction or perforation, diabetes mellitus, complications in gastrointestinal tract, patients with colostomy or ileostomy, ulcerative colitis or diverticulitis
Warnings/Precautions Use with caution in patients with impaired renal function (accumulation of magnesium may lead to magnesium intoxication).

Constipation (self-medication, OTC use): For occasional use only; serious side effects may occur with prolonged use. For use only under the supervision of a healthcare provider in patients with kidney dysfunction, or with a sudden change in bowel habits which persist for >2 weeks. Do not use if abdominal pain, nausea, or vomiting are present.
Adverse Reactions (Reflective of adult population; not specific for elderly)
1% to 10%:
Cardiovascular: Hypotension
Endocrine & metabolic: Hypermagnesemia
Gastrointestinal: Abdominal cramps, diarrhea, gas formation
Respiratory: Respiratory depression
Drug Interactions
Avoid Concomitant Use
Avoid concomitant use of Magnesium Citrate with any of the following: Calcium Polystyrene Sulfonate; Sodium Polystyrene Sulfonate
Increased Effect/Toxicity
Magnesium Citrate may increase the levels/effects of: Aluminum Hydroxide; Calcium Channel Blockers; Calcium Polystyrene Sulfonate; Neuromuscular-Blocking Agents; Sodium Polystyrene Sulfonate

The levels/effects of Magnesium Citrate may be increased by: Alfacalcidol; Calcitriol; Calcium Channel Blockers

Decreased Effect

Magnesium Citrate may decrease the levels/effects of: Bisphosphonate Derivatives; Eltrombopag; Mycophenolate; Phosphate Supplements; Quinolone Antibiotics; Tetracycline Derivatives; Trientine

The levels/effects of Magnesium Citrate may be decreased by: Trientine

Mechanism of Action Promotes bowel evacuation by causing osmotic retention of fluid which distends the colon with increased peristaltic activity

Pharmacodynamics/Kinetics

Absorption: Oral: 15% to 30%

Excretion: Urine

Dosage

Geriatric & Adult Cathartic: Oral: 150-300 mL

Renal Impairment Patients in severe renal failure should not receive magnesium due to toxicity from accumulation. Patients with a Cl_{cr} <25 mL/minute should be monitored by serum magnesium levels.

Administration To increase palatability, chill the solution prior to administration.

Reference Range Serum magnesium: 1.5-2.5 mg/dL; slightly different ranges are reported by different laboratories

Test Interactions Increased magnesium; decreased protein, decreased calcium (S), decreased potassium (S)

Pharmacotherapy Pearls To increase palatability, manufacturer suggests chilling the solution prior to administration.

3.85-4.71 mEq of magnesium/5 mL

Special Geriatric Considerations Elderly, due to disease or drug therapy, may be predisposed to diarrhea. Diarrhea may result in electrolyte imbalance. Decreased renal function (Cl_{cr} <30 mL/minute) may result in toxicity; monitor for toxicity and Cl_{cr} <30 mL/minute.

Dosage Forms Excipient information presented when available (limited, particularly for generics); consult specific product labeling.

Solution, oral: 290 mg/5 mL (296 mL)

Citroma®: 290 mg/5 mL (340 mL) [contains benzoic acid, magnesium 48 mg/5 mL, sodium 0.5 mg/5 mL; grape flavor]

Citroma®: 290 mg/5 mL (296 mL) [contains magnesium 48 mg/5 mL, potassium 13 mg/5 mL; cherry flavor]

Citroma®: 290 mg/5 mL (296 mL) [contains magnesium 48 mg/5 mL, potassium 13 mg/5 mL; lemon flavor]

Citroma®: 290 mg/5 mL (296 mL) [contains magnesium 48 mg/5 mL, sodium 7.5 mg/5 mL; grape flavor]

Citroma®: 290 mg/5 mL (296 mL) [contains magnesium 48 mg/5 mL, sodium 7.5 mg/5 mL; lemon flavor]

Tablet, oral: Elemental magnesium 100 mg

◆ **Magnesium Gluceptate** see Magnesium Glucoheptonate *on page 1108*

Magnesium Glucoheptonate (mag NEE zhum gloo koh HEP toh nate)

Brand Names: Canada Magnesium Glucoheponate

Index Terms Magnesium Gluceptate

Pharmacologic Category Magnesium Salt

Use Dietary supplement

Dosage

Geriatric & Adult Note: Serum magnesium is poor reflection of repletional status as the majority of magnesium is intracellular; serum levels may be transiently normal for a few hours after a dose is given, therefore, aim for consistently high normal serum levels in patients with normal renal function for most efficient repletion.

RDA (elemental magnesium):

19-30 years:

Female: 310 mg/day

Male: 400 mg/day

≥31 years:

Female: 320 mg/day

Male: 420 mg/day

Hypomagnesemia: Oral: 1500-3000 mg (75-150 mg elemental magnesium) 1-3 times/day

Renal Impairment

Mild-to-moderate renal impairment: Use with caution; monitor serum magnesium levels carefully.

Severe renal impairment: Use is contraindicated.

Special Geriatric Considerations Elderly, due to disease or drug therapy, may be predisposed to diarrhea. Diarrhea may result in electrolyte imbalance. Decreased renal function (Cl_{cr} <30 mL/minute) may result in toxicity; monitor for toxicity and Cl_{cr} <30 mL/minute.

Product Availability Not available in U.S.

Dosage Forms: Canada Excipient information presented when available (limited, particularly for generics); consult specific product labeling.

Solution, oral: 100 mg/mL

Magnesium Hydroxide (mag NEE zhum hye DROKS ide)

Related Information

Laxatives, Classification and Properties *on page 2012*

Brand Names: U.S. Fleet® Pedia-Lax™ Chewable Tablet [OTC]; Little Phillips'® Milk of Magnesia [OTC]; Milk of Magnesia [OTC]; Phillips'® Milk of Magnesia [OTC]

Index Terms Magnesia Magma; Milk of Magnesia; MOM

Generic Availability (U.S.) Yes: Liquid

Pharmacologic Category Antacid; Laxative; Magnesium Salt

Use Short-term treatment of occasional constipation and symptoms of hyperacidity, laxative; dietary supplement

Contraindications Hypersensitivity to magnesium hydroxide or any component of the formulation

Warnings/Precautions Use magnesium with caution in patients with impaired renal function (accumulation of magnesium may lead to magnesium intoxication). Use with extreme caution in patients with myasthenia gravis or other neuromuscular disease.

For self-medication (OTC use): For occasional use only; serious side effects may occur with prolonged use. For use only under the supervision of a healthcare provider in patients with kidney dysfunction, or with a sudden change in bowel habits which persist for >2 weeks. Patients should notify healthcare provider of any sudden change in bowel habits which last >14 days, stomach pain, nausea, or vomiting or if use is needed for >1 week.

Drug Interactions

Avoid Concomitant Use

Avoid concomitant use of Magnesium Hydroxide with any of the following: Calcium Polystyrene Sulfonate; QuiNINE; Sodium Polystyrene Sulfonate

Increased Effect/Toxicity

Magnesium Hydroxide may increase the levels/effects of: Alpha-/Beta-Agonists; Amphetamines; Calcium Channel Blockers; Calcium Polystyrene Sulfonate; Dexmethylphenidate; Methylphenidate; Misoprostol; Neuromuscular-Blocking Agents; QuiNIDine; Sodium Polystyrene Sulfonate

The levels/effects of Magnesium Hydroxide may be increased by: Alfacalcidol; Calcitriol; Calcium Channel Blockers

Decreased Effect

Magnesium Hydroxide may decrease the levels/effects of: ACE Inhibitors; Allopurinol; Anticonvulsants (Hydantoin); Antipsychotic Agents (Phenothiazines); Atazanavir; Bisacodyl; Bisphosphonate Derivatives; Cefditoren; Cefpodoxime; Cefuroxime; Chloroquine; Corticosteroids (Oral); Dabigatran Etexilate; Dasatinib; Delavirdine; Eltrombopag; Erlotinib; Fexofenadine; Gabapentin; HMG-CoA Reductase Inhibitors; Iron Salts; Isoniazid; Itraconazole; Ketoconazole; Ketoconazole (Systemic); Mesalamine; Methenamine; Mycophenolate; Penicillamine; Phosphate Supplements; Protease Inhibitors; QuiNINE; Quinolone Antibiotics; Rilpivirine; Tetracycline Derivatives; Trientine

The levels/effects of Magnesium Hydroxide may be decreased by: Trientine

Mechanism of Action Promotes bowel evacuation by causing osmotic retention of fluid which distends the colon with increased peristaltic activity; reacts with hydrochloric acid in stomach to form magnesium chloride

Pharmacodynamics/Kinetics

Onset of action: Laxative: 30 minutes to 6 hours

Excretion: Urine (up to 30% as absorbed magnesium ions); feces (as unabsorbed drug)

◀ **Dosage**
Geriatric & Adult
Antacid: OTC labeling: Oral:
Liquid: Magnesium hydroxide 400 mg/5 mL: 5-15 mL as needed up to 4 times/day
Tablet: Magnesium hydroxide 311 mg/tablet: 2-4 tablets every 4 hours up to 4 times/day
Dietary supplement: OTC labeling (Phillips'® Chews): Oral: Magnesium 500 mg: 2-4 tablets/day once daily at bedtime or in divided doses
Laxative: OTC labeling: Oral:
Liquid:
Magnesium hydroxide 400 mg/5 mL: 30-60 mL/day once daily at bedtime or in divided doses
Magnesium hydroxide 800 mg/5 mL: 15-30 mL/day once daily at bedtime or in divided doses
Tablet: Magnesium hydroxide 311 mg/tablet: 8 tablets/day once daily at bedtime or in divided doses

Renal Impairment Patients in severe renal failure should not receive magnesium due to toxicity from accumulation. Patients with a Cl_{cr} <30 mL/minute should be monitored by serum magnesium levels.

Administration Liquid doses may be diluted with a small amount of water prior to administration. All doses should be followed by 8 ounces of water.

Reference Range Serum magnesium: 1.5-2.5 mg/dL; slightly different ranges are reported by different laboratories

Test Interactions Increased magnesium; decreased protein, calcium (S), decreased potassium (S)

Pharmacotherapy Pearls 1.05 g magnesium = ~87 mEq magnesium/30 mL

Special Geriatric Considerations Elderly, due to disease or drug therapy, may be predisposed to diarrhea. Diarrhea may result in electrolyte imbalance. Decreased renal function (Cl_{cr} <30 mL/minute) may result in toxicity; monitor for toxicity.

Dosage Forms Excipient information presented when available (limited, particularly for generics); consult specific product labeling.
Suspension, oral: 400 mg/5 mL (30 mL, 473 mL)
Milk of Magnesia: 400 mg/5 mL (360 mL, 480 mL)
Milk of Magnesia: 400 mg/5 mL (360 mL, 480 mL) [mint flavor]
Milk of Magnesia: 400 mg/5 mL (480 mL) [ethanol free, sugar free]
Phillips'® Milk of Magnesia: 400 mg/5 mL (120 mL, 360 mL, 780 mL) [contains magnesium 167 mg/5 mL; fresh mint flavor]
Phillips'® Milk of Magnesia: 400 mg/5 mL (120 mL, 360 mL, 780 mL) [contains magnesium 167 mg/5 mL; original flavor]
Phillips'® Milk of Magnesia: 400 mg/5 mL (120 mL, 240 mL, 360 mL, 780 mL) [contains magnesium 167 mg/5 mL, sodium 2 mg/5 mL; cherry flavor]
Suspension, oral [concentrate]: 2400 mg/10 mL (10 mL)
Little Phillips'® Milk of Magnesia: 800 mg/5 mL (120 mL) [contains magnesium 333 mg/5 mL, propylene glycol; strawberry flavor]
Milk of Magnesia: 800 mg/5 mL (100 mL, 400 mL) [contains sodium 20 mg/10 mL, sucrose 0.8 g/10 mL; lemon flavor]
Phillips'® Milk of Magnesia: 800 mg/5 mL (240 mL) [contains magnesium 333 mg/5 mL, propylene glycol; strawberry flavor]
Tablet, chewable, oral:
Fleet® Pedia-Lax™ Chewable Tablet: 400 mg [contains magnesium 170 mg/tablet; watermelon flavor]
Phillips'® Milk of Magnesia: 311 mg [mint flavor]
Phillips'® Milk of Magnesia: 311 mg [contains magnesium 130 mg/tablet; mint flavor]

◆ **Magnesium Hydroxide, Aluminum Hydroxide, and Simethicone** *see* Aluminum Hydroxide, Magnesium Hydroxide, and Simethicone *on page 84*
◆ **Magnesium Hydroxide and Aluminum Hydroxide** *see* Aluminum Hydroxide and Magnesium Hydroxide *on page 81*

Magnesium Hydroxide and Mineral Oil
(mag NEE zhum hye DROKS ide & MIN er al oyl)

Related Information
Magnesium Hydroxide *on page 1109*
Mineral Oil *on page 1217*
Brand Names: U.S. Phillips'® M-O [OTC]
Index Terms Haley's M-O; MOM/Mineral Oil Emulsion
Generic Availability (U.S.) No

Pharmacologic Category Laxative

Use Short-term treatment of occasional constipation

Contraindications Hypersensitivity magnesium hydroxide, mineral oil, or any component of the formulation

Warnings/Precautions Use magnesium with caution in patients with severe renal impairment (especially when doses are >50 mEq magnesium/day); hypermagnesemia and toxicity may occur due to decreased renal clearance of absorbed magnesium. Decreased renal function (Cl$_{cr}$ <30 mL/minute) may result in toxicity; monitor for toxicity.

For self-medication (OTC use): Patients should notify healthcare provider of any sudden change in bowel habits which last >14 days, stomach pain, nausea, vomiting, or if use is needed for >1 week. Not for OTC use in bedridden patients or patients with dysphagia. Avoid concomitant use with stool softener laxatives.

Drug Interactions

Avoid Concomitant Use

Avoid concomitant use of Magnesium Hydroxide and Mineral Oil with any of the following: Calcium Polystyrene Sulfonate; QuiNINE; Sodium Polystyrene Sulfonate

Increased Effect/Toxicity

Magnesium Hydroxide and Mineral Oil may increase the levels/effects of: Alpha-/Beta-Agonists; Amphetamines; Calcium Channel Blockers; Calcium Polystyrene Sulfonate; Dexmethylphenidate; Methylphenidate; Misoprostol; Neuromuscular-Blocking Agents; QuiNIDine; Sodium Polystyrene Sulfonate

The levels/effects of Magnesium Hydroxide and Mineral Oil may be increased by: Alfacalcidol; Calcitriol; Calcium Channel Blockers

Decreased Effect

Magnesium Hydroxide and Mineral Oil may decrease the levels/effects of: ACE Inhibitors; Allopurinol; Anticonvulsants (Hydantoin); Antipsychotic Agents (Phenothiazines); Atazanavir; Bisacodyl; Bisphosphonate Derivatives; Cefditoren; Cefpodoxime; Cefuroxime; Chloroquine; Corticosteroids (Oral); Dabigatran Etexilate; Dasatinib; Delavirdine; Eltrombopag; Erlotinib; Fexofenadine; Gabapentin; HMG-CoA Reductase Inhibitors; Iron Salts; Isoniazid; Itraconazole; Ketoconazole; Ketoconazole (Systemic); Mesalamine; Methenamine; Mycophenolate; Penicillamine; Phosphate Supplements; Phytonadione; Protease Inhibitors; QuiNINE; Quinolone Antibiotics; Rilpivirine; Tetracycline Derivatives; Trientine; Vitamin D Analogs

The levels/effects of Magnesium Hydroxide and Mineral Oil may be decreased by: Trientine

Pharmacodynamics/Kinetics

Onset of action: Laxative: 30 minutes to 6 hours hours

Excretion: Magnesium: Urine (up to 30% as absorbed magnesium ions); feces (as unabsorbed drug)

Dosage

Geriatric & Adult Laxative: OTC labeling: Oral: 45-60 mL at bedtime

Renal Impairment Patients in severe renal failure should not receive magnesium due to toxicity from accumulation. Patients with a Cl$_{cr}$ <30 mL/minute should be monitored by serum magnesium levels.

Administration Shake well; administer with full glass of water

Special Geriatric Considerations The use of mineral oil products may be hazardous in the elderly with conditions predisposing them to aspiration. Elderly, due to disease or drug therapy, may be predisposed to diarrhea. Diarrhea may result in electrolyte imbalance. Decreased renal function (Cl$_{cr}$ <30 mL/minute) may result in toxicity from magnesium absorption; monitor for toxicity.

Dosage Forms Excipient information presented when available (limited, particularly for generics); consult specific product labeling.

Suspension, oral:

Phillips'® M-O: Magnesium hydroxide 300 mg and mineral oil 1.25 mL per 5 mL (360 mL, 780 mL) [contains magnesium 125 mg and sodium 1.5 mg per 5 mL mint flavors]

◆ **Magnesium Hydroxide, Famotidine, and Calcium Carbonate** *see* Famotidine, Calcium Carbonate, and Magnesium Hydroxide *on page 696*

Magnesium L-aspartate Hydrochloride
(mag NEE zhum el as PAR tate hye droe KLOR ide)

Brand Names: U.S. Maginex™ DS [OTC]; Maginex™ [OTC]

Index Terms MAH

Generic Availability (U.S.) No

Pharmacologic Category Electrolyte Supplement, Oral; Magnesium Salt

Use Dietary supplement

Dosage

Geriatric & Adult

RDA (elemental magnesium):

19-30 years:

Female: 310 mg/day

Male: 400 mg/day

≥31 years:

Female: 320 mg/day

Male: 420 mg/day

Dietary supplement: Oral: Magnesium-L-aspartate 1230 mg (magnesium 122 mg) up to 3 times/day

Renal Impairment Cl$_{cr}$ <30 mL/minute: Use with caution; monitor for hypermagnesemia

Special Geriatric Considerations Elderly, due to disease or drug therapy, may be predisposed to diarrhea. Diarrhea may result in electrolyte imbalance. Decreased renal function (Cl$_{cr}$ <30 mL/minute) may result in toxicity; monitor for toxicity. Monitor for signs of confusion or worsening signs of dementia.

Dosage Forms Excipient information presented when available (limited, particularly for generics); consult specific product labeling.

Granules for solution, oral [preservative free]:

Maginex™ DS: 1230 mg/packet (30s) [sugar free; lemon flavor; equivalent to elemental magnesium 122 mg (10 mEq)]

Tablet, enteric coated, oral [preservative free]:

Maginex™: 615 mg [sugar free; equivalent to elemental magnesium 61 mg (5 mEq)]

Magnesium L-lactate (mag NEE zhum el LAK tate)

Brand Names: U.S. Mag-Tab® SR

Index Terms Magnesium L-lactate Dihydrate

Generic Availability (U.S.) No

Pharmacologic Category Electrolyte Supplement; Magnesium Salt

Use Dietary supplement

Dosage

Geriatric & Adult

Dietary supplement: Oral: 1-2 caplets every 12 hours

RDA (elemental magnesium):

19-30 years:

Female: 310 mg/day

Male: 400 mg/day

≥31 years:

Female: 320 mg/day

Male: 420 mg/day

Renal Impairment Cl$_{cr}$ <30 mL/minute: Use with caution; monitor for hypermagnesemia

Special Geriatric Considerations Elderly, due to disease or drug therapy, may be predisposed to diarrhea. Diarrhea may result in electrolyte imbalance. Decreased renal function (Cl$_{cr}$ <30 mL/minute) may result in toxicity; monitor for toxicity and Cl$_{cr}$ <30 mL/minute.

Dosage Forms Excipient information presented when available (limited, particularly for generics); consult specific product labeling.

Caplet, sustained release, oral:

Mag-Tab® SR: Elemental magnesium 84 mg [scored; 7 mEq]

Magnesium Oxide (mag NEE zhum OKS ide)

Brand Names: U.S. Mag-Ox® 400 [OTC]; MagGel™ 600 [OTC]; MAGnesium-Oxide™ [OTC]; Phillips'® Laxative Dietary Supplement Cramp-Free [OTC]; Uro-Mag® [OTC]

Index Terms Mag Oxide

Generic Availability (U.S.) Yes

Pharmacologic Category Electrolyte Supplement, Oral; Magnesium Salt

Use Electrolyte replacement

Contraindications Hypersensitivity to any component of the formulation

Warnings/Precautions Use magnesium with caution in patients with impaired renal function (accumulation of magnesium may lead to magnesium intoxication). Use with extreme caution in patients with myasthenia gravis or other neuromuscular disease.

Constipation (self-medication, OTC use): For occasional use only; serious side effects may occur with prolonged use. For use only under the supervision of a healthcare provider in patients with kidney dysfunction, or with a sudden change in bowel habits which persist for >2 weeks. Do not use if abdominal pain, nausea, or vomiting are present.

Adverse Reactions (Reflective of adult population; not specific for elderly) Frequency not defined: Gastrointestinal: Diarrhea (excessive oral doses)

Drug Interactions

Avoid Concomitant Use

Avoid concomitant use of Magnesium Oxide with any of the following: Calcium Polystyrene Sulfonate; Sodium Polystyrene Sulfonate

Increased Effect/Toxicity

Magnesium Oxide may increase the levels/effects of: Calcium Channel Blockers; Calcium Polystyrene Sulfonate; Neuromuscular-Blocking Agents; Sodium Polystyrene Sulfonate

The levels/effects of Magnesium Oxide may be increased by: Alfacalcidol; Calcitriol; Calcium Channel Blockers

Decreased Effect

Magnesium Oxide may decrease the levels/effects of: Bisphosphonate Derivatives; Eltrombopag; Mycophenolate; Phosphate Supplements; Quinolone Antibiotics; Tetracycline Derivatives; Trientine

The levels/effects of Magnesium Oxide may be decreased by: Trientine

Mechanism of Action Magnesium is important as a cofactor in many enzymatic reactions in the body involving protein synthesis and carbohydrate metabolism (at least 300 enzymatic reactions require magnesium). Actions on lipoprotein lipase have been found to be important in reducing serum cholesterol and on sodium/potassium ATPase in promoting polarization (eg, neuromuscular functioning).

Pharmacodynamics/Kinetics

Absorption: Oral: Inversely proportional to amount ingested; 40% to 60% under controlled dietary conditions; 15% to 36% at higher doses

Distribution: Bone (50% to 60%); extracellular fluid (1% to 2%)

Protein binding: 30%, to albumin

Excretion: Urine (as magnesium)

Dosage

Geriatric & Adult

RDA (elemental magnesium): Oral:

19-30 years:

Female: 310 mg/day

Male: 400 mg/day

≥31 years:

Female: 320 mg/day

Male: 420 mg/day

Dietary supplement: Oral:

Mag-Ox 400®: 2 tablets daily with food

Mag-Caps, Uro-Mag®: 4-5 capsules daily with food

Renal Impairment Cl_{cr} <30 mL/minute: Use with caution; monitor for hypermagnesemia

Reference Range Serum magnesium: 1.5-2.5 mg/dL; slightly different ranges are reported by different laboratories

Special Geriatric Considerations Elderly, due to disease or drug therapy, may be predisposed to diarrhea. Diarrhea may result in electrolyte imbalance. Decreased renal function (Cl_{cr} <30 mL/minute) may result in toxicity; monitor for toxicity.

Dosage Forms Excipient information presented when available (limited, particularly for generics); consult specific product labeling.

Caplet, oral: Elemental magnesium 250 mg

Phillips'® Laxative Dietary Supplement Cramp-Free: Elemental magnesium 500 mg

Capsule, oral:

Uro-Mag®: 140 mg [equivalent to elemental magnesium 84.5 mg (6.93 mEq)]

Capsule, softgel, oral:

MagGel™ 600: 600 mg [equivalent to elemental magnesium 348 mg (28.64 mEq)]

Tablet, oral: 400 mg [equivalent to elemental magnesium 240 mg (20 mEq)], 500 mg, Elemental magnesium 500 mg

Mag-Ox® 400: 400 mg [scored; equivalent to elemental magnesium 240 mg (20 mEq)]

MAGnesium-Oxide™: 400 mg [equivalent to elemental magnesium 240 mg (20 mEq)]

◆ **MAGnesium-Oxide™ [OTC]** *see* Magnesium Oxide *on page 1112*
◆ **Magnesium Salicylate** *see* Salicylates (Various Salts) *on page 1647*

Magnesium Salts (Various Salts) (mag NEE zhum salts)

Brand Names: U.S. Almora® [OTC]; Epsom Salt [OTC]; Magonate® [OTC]; Mg-plus® [OTC]; Slow-Mag® [OTC]

Generic Availability (U.S.) Yes

Stability Refrigeration of intact ampuls may result in precipitation or crystallization; stability of parenteral admixture at room temperature (25°C): 60 days

Mechanism of Action Promotes bowel evacuation by causing osmotic retention of fluid which distends the colon with increased peristaltic activity when taken orally; parenterally, decreases acetylcholine in motor nerve terminals and acts on myocardium by slowing rate of S-A node impulse formation and prolonging conduction time

Pharmacodynamics/Kinetics

Absorption: Absorbed magnesium is rapidly eliminated by the kidneys.

Elimination: Primarily excreted in feces

Test Interactions Increased magnesium; decreased protein, calcium (S), decreased potassium (S)

Pharmacotherapy Pearls 1 g magnesium = 8.3 mEq (41.1 mmol); see individual agents for magnesium content per dose

Special Geriatric Considerations Elderly, due to disease or drug therapy, may be predisposed to diarrhea. Diarrhea may result in electrolyte imbalance. Decreased renal function (Cl_{cr} <30 mL/minute) may result in toxicity; monitor for toxicity.

Dosage Forms

Granules, as sulfate: ~40 mEq magnesium/5 g (240 g)

Injection, as sulfate: 10% = 0.8 mEq/mL (2 mL, 10 mL, 20 mL, 30 mL, 50 mL); 20% = 1.97 mEq/mL (2 mL, 10 mL, 20 mL, 30 mL, 50 mL); 50% = 4 mEq/mL (2 mL, 10 mL, 20 mL, 30 mL, 50 mL)

Liquid, as sulfate: 54 mg/5 mL; gluconate: 54 mg/5 mL (gluconate has 27 mg magnesium)

Tablet, as various salts: 140 mg, 400 mg, 500 mg

◆ **Magnesium Trisilicate and Aluminum Hydroxide** see Aluminum Hydroxide and Magnesium Trisilicate on page 83

◆ **Magonate® [OTC]** see Magnesium Salts (Various Salts) on page 1114

◆ **Mag-Ox® 400 [OTC]** see Magnesium Oxide on page 1112

◆ **Mag Oxide** see Magnesium Oxide on page 1112

◆ **Mag-Tab® SR** see Magnesium L-lactate on page 1112

◆ **MAH** see Magnesium L-aspartate Hydrochloride on page 1111

◆ **Mallamint® [OTC]** see Calcium Salts (Oral) on page 256

Maltodextrin (mal toe DEK strin)

Brand Names: U.S. Carrington® Oral Wound Rinse [OTC]; Multidex® [OTC]

Generic Availability (U.S.) No

Pharmacologic Category Anti-inflammatory, Locally Applied

Use Topical: Treatment of infected or noninfected wounds

Dosage

Geriatric & Adult

Management of pain due to oral lesions: Carrington® Oral Wound Rinse: 1 tablespoonful, swish or gargle for ~1 minute, 4 times/day or more if needed

Wound dressing: Topical: Multidex®: After debridement and irrigation of wound, apply and cover with a nonadherent, nonocclusive dressing. Apply ¼" thick dressing over entire shallow wound. Completely fill in deep wounds with dressing. May be applied to moist or dry, infected or noninfected wounds. Change dressing once or twice daily.

Dosage Forms Excipient information presented when available (limited, particularly for generics); consult specific product labeling.

Gel, topical [preservative free]:

Multidex®: 7.1 mL (7.1 mL); 14.2 mL (14.2 mL); 85.2 mL (85.2 mL) [dye free]

Powder, topical [preservative free]:

Multidex®: 6 g (6 g); 12 g (12 g); 25 g (25 g); 45 g (45 g) [dye free]

Powder for suspension, oral:

Carrington® Oral Wound Rinse: 23 g [contains aloe, fructose, phenylalanine, sodium benzoate]

Solution, topical [spray, preservative free]:

Multidex®: 45 mL (45 mL) [dye free]

◆ **Mantoux** see Tuberculin Tests on page 1877

◆ **Mapap® [OTC]** see Acetaminophen on page 33

◆ **Mapap® Arthritis Pain [OTC]** see Acetaminophen on page 33

♦ **Mapap® Children's [OTC]** *see* Acetaminophen *on page 33*
♦ **Mapap® Extra Strength [OTC]** *see* Acetaminophen *on page 33*
♦ **Mapap® Infant's [OTC]** *see* Acetaminophen *on page 33*
♦ **Mapap® Junior Rapid Tabs [OTC]** *see* Acetaminophen *on page 33*
♦ **Mapap® Sinus Congestion and Pain Daytime [OTC]** *see* Acetaminophen and Phenylephrine *on page 38*

Maprotiline (ma PROE ti leen)

Related Information
  Antidepressant Agents *on page 1991*
Medication Safety Issues
  International issues
    Ludiomil [multiple international markets] may be confused with Lamictal brand name for lamotrigine [U.S., Canada, and multiple international markets]; lamotrigine [U.S., Canada, and multiple international markets]; Lomotil brand name for diphenoxylate [U.S, Canada, and multiple international markets] and brand name for loperamide [Mexico, Philippines]
Brand Names: Canada Novo-Maprotiline
Index Terms Ludiomil; Maprotiline Hydrochloride
Generic Availability (U.S.) Yes
Pharmacologic Category Antidepressant, Tetracyclic
Use Treatment of major depressive disorder (MDD) or of anxiety associated with depression
Unlabeled/Investigational Use Chronic pain; panic attacks
Medication Guide Available Yes
Dosage
  Geriatric Depression/anxiety: Oral: Initial: 25 mg/day for 2 weeks; Maintenance: Increase by 25 mg as tolerated; usual dose: 50-75 mg/day, higher doses may be necessary in nonresponders
  Adult
    Mild-to-moderate depression/anxiety: Oral: Initial: 75 mg/day for 2 weeks (lower doses may be considered in some patients); Maintenance: Increase by 25 mg as tolerated up to 150 mg/day; given in divided doses or in a single daily dose
  Severe depression: Oral: Initial: 100-150 mg/day for 2 weeks; Maintenance: Increase by 25 mg as tolerated up to 225 mg/day; given in divided doses or in a single daily dose
Special Geriatric Considerations Avoid in the elderly due to sedation and anticholinergic effects (eg, confusion, constipation, difficulty urinating, dry mouth).
Dosage Forms Excipient information presented when available (limited, particularly for generics); consult specific product labeling.
  Tablet, oral, as hydrochloride: 25 mg, 50 mg, 75 mg

♦ **Maprotiline Hydrochloride** *see* Maprotiline *on page 1115*
♦ **Mar-Cof® CG** *see* Guaifenesin and Codeine *on page 848*
♦ **Marezine® [OTC]** *see* Cyclizine *on page 426*
♦ **Margesic® H** *see* Hydrocodone and Acetaminophen *on page 880*
♦ **Marplan®** *see* Isocarboxazid *on page 982*
♦ **Matzim™ LA** *see* Diltiazem *on page 514*
♦ **Mavik®** *see* Trandolapril *on page 1843*
♦ **Maxair® Autohaler®** *see* Pirbuterol *on page 1468*
♦ **Maxalt®** *see* Rizatriptan *on page 1630*
♦ **Maxalt-MLT®** *see* Rizatriptan *on page 1630*
♦ **Maxaron® Forte** *see* Polysaccharide-Iron Complex, Vitamin B12, and Folic Acid *on page 1483*
♦ **Maxidex®** *see* Dexamethasone (Ophthalmic) *on page 487*
♦ **Maxidone®** *see* Hydrocodone and Acetaminophen *on page 880*
♦ **Maximum D3® [OTC]** *see* Cholecalciferol *on page 346*
♦ **Maxipime®** *see* Cefepime *on page 295*
♦ **Maxitrol®** *see* Neomycin, Polymyxin B, and Dexamethasone *on page 1280*
♦ **Maxzide®** *see* Hydrochlorothiazide and Triamterene *on page 879*
♦ **Maxzide®-25** *see* Hydrochlorothiazide and Triamterene *on page 879*
♦ **3M™ Cavilon™ Antifungal [OTC]** *see* Miconazole *on page 1206*
♦ **MCV** *see* Meningococcal (Groups A / C / Y and W-135) Diphtheria Conjugate Vaccine *on page 1137*
♦ **MCV4** *see* Meningococcal (Groups A / C / Y and W-135) Diphtheria Conjugate Vaccine *on page 1137*
♦ **MDL 73,147EF** *see* Dolasetron *on page 552*

Measles, Mumps, and Rubella Virus Vaccine
(MEE zels, mumpz & roo BEL a VYE rus vak SEEN)

Related Information
Immunization Administration Recommendations *on page 2037*
Immunization Recommendations *on page 2043*

Medication Safety Issues
Sound-alike/look-alike issues:
MMR (measles, mumps and rubella virus vaccine) may be confused with MMRV (measles, mumps, rubella, and varicella) vaccine

Brand Names: U.S. M-M-R® II

Brand Names: Canada M-M-R® II; Priorix™

Index Terms MMR; Mumps, Measles and Rubella Vaccines; Rubella, Measles and Mumps Vaccines

Generic Availability (U.S.) No

Pharmacologic Category Vaccine, Live (Viral)

Use Measles, mumps, and rubella prophylaxis
The Advisory Committee on Immunization Practices (ACIP) recommends routine vaccination for the following:
- All children (first dose given at 12-15 months of age)
- Adults born 1957 or later (without evidence of immunity or documentation of vaccination).
- Adults at higher risk for exposure to and transmission of measles mumps and rubella should receive special consideration for vaccination, unless an acceptable evidence of immunity exists. This includes international travelers, persons attending colleges and other post-high school education, persons working in healthcare facilities.

Contraindications Hypersensitivity to measles, mumps, and/or rubella vaccine or any component of the formulation; current febrile respiratory illness or other febrile infection; patients receiving immunosuppressive therapy (does not include corticosteroids as replacement therapy); primary and acquired immunodeficiency states; individuals with blood dyscrasias, leukemia, lymphomas, or other malignant neoplasms affecting the bone marrow or lymphatic systems; family history of congenital or hereditary immunodeficiency (until immune competence in the vaccine recipient is demonstrated)

Warnings/Precautions Use caution with history of cerebral injury, seizures, or other conditions where stress due to fever should be avoided. Immediate treatment for anaphylactic/anaphylactoid reaction should be available during vaccine use. Use caution in patients with thrombocytopenia and those who develop thrombocytopenia after first dose; thrombocytopenia may worsen. Consider delaying vaccination during acute moderate or severe febrile illness; per the ACIP, patients with minor illnesses with or without fever may receive vaccine. Use is contraindicated in severely immunocompromised patients. However, leukemia patients who are in remission and who have not received chemotherapy for at least 3 months may be vaccinated; patients with HIV infection, who are asymptomatic and not severely immunosuppressed may be vaccinated. In general, household and close contacts of persons with altered immunocompetence may receive all age appropriate vaccines. Recent administration of blood or blood products may interfere with immune response.

Therapy to treat tuberculosis should be started prior to administering vaccine to patients with active tuberculosis. Patients with untreated, active tuberculosis should not receive vaccine. Exposure to measles is not a contraindication to vaccine; use within 72 hours of exposure may provide some protection. Vaccine contains trace amounts of chick embryo antigen. Use caution in patients with history of immediate hypersensitivity/anaphylactic reactions following egg ingestion. Generally, the MMR vaccine can be safely administered to persons with an egg allergy (CDC, 2011). Manufactured with neomycin. Patients with history of anaphylaxis should not receive vaccine; contact dermatitis to neomycin is not a contraindication to the vaccine. Contains gelatin; contraindicated if known hypersensitivity to gelatin. In order to maximize vaccination rates, the ACIP recommends simultaneous administration of all age-appropriate vaccines (live or inactivated) for which a person is eligible at a single clinic visit, unless contraindications exist. The use of combination vaccines is generally preferred over separate injections, taking into consideration provider assessment, patient preference, and potential adverse events. Acceptable evidence of immunity is recommended healthcare workers prior to employment, students entering institutions of higher learning, and travelers to endemic areas.

Adverse Reactions (Reflective of adult population; not specific for elderly) All serious adverse reactions must be reported to the U.S. Department of Health and Human Services (DHHS) Vaccine Adverse Event Reporting System (VAERS) 1-800-822-7967 or online at https://vaers.hhs.gov/esub/index. In Canada, adverse reactions may be reported to local provincial/territorial health agencies or to the Vaccine Safety Section at Public Health Agency of Canada (1-866-844-0018).

Frequency not defined:

Cardiovascular: Syncope, vasculitis

Central nervous system: Ataxia, dizziness, febrile seizure, fever, encephalitis, encephalopathy, Guillain-Barré syndrome, headache, irritability, malaise, measles inclusion body encephalitis, polyneuritis, polyneuropathy, seizure, subacute sclerosing panencephalitis,

Dermatologic: Angioneurotic edema, erythema multiforme, measles-like rash, pruritus, purpura, rash, Stevens-Johnson syndrome, urticaria

Endocrine & metabolic: Diabetes mellitus, parotitis

Gastrointestinal: Diarrhea, nausea, pancreatitis, sore throat, vomiting

Genitourinary: Epididymitis, orchitis

Hematologic: Leukocytosis, thrombocytopenia

Local: Injection site reactions which include burning, induration, redness, stinging, swelling, tenderness, wheal and flare, vesiculation

Neuromuscular & skeletal: Arthralgia/arthritis (variable; highest rates in women, 12% to 26% versus children, up to 3%), myalgia, paresthesia

Ocular: Conjunctivitis, ocular palsies, optic neuritis, papillitis, retinitis, retrobulbar neuritis

Otic: Nerve deafness, otitis media

Renal: Conjunctivitis, retinitis, optic neuritis, papillitis, retrobulbar neuritis

Respiratory: Bronchospasm, cough, pneumonia, pneumonitis, rhinitis

Miscellaneous: Anaphylactoid reactions, anaphylaxis, atypical measles, panniculitis, regional lymphadenopathy

Drug Interactions

Avoid Concomitant Use

Avoid concomitant use of Measles, Mumps, and Rubella Virus Vaccine with any of the following: Belimumab; Fingolimod; Immunosuppressants

Increased Effect/Toxicity

The levels/effects of Measles, Mumps, and Rubella Virus Vaccine may be increased by: AzaTHIOprine; Belimumab; Corticosteroids (Systemic); Fingolimod; Hydroxychloroquine; Immunosuppressants; Leflunomide; Mercaptopurine; Methotrexate

Decreased Effect

Measles, Mumps, and Rubella Virus Vaccine may decrease the levels/effects of: Tuberculin Tests

The levels/effects of Measles, Mumps, and Rubella Virus Vaccine may be decreased by: Fingolimod; Immune Globulins; Immunosuppressants

Stability To maintain potency, the lyophilized vaccine must be stored between -50°C to 8°C (-58°F to 46°F). Temperatures below -50°C (-58°F) may occur if stored in dry ice. Prior to reconstitution, store the powder at 2°C to 8°C (36°F to 46°F). Protect from light. Diluent may be stored in refrigerator or at room temperature. Do not freeze diluent. Use entire contents of the provided diluent to reconstitute vaccine. Gently agitate to mix thoroughly. Discard if powder does not dissolve. Use as soon as possible following reconstitution (may be stored at 2°C to 8°C/36°F to 46°F; protect from light); discard if not used within 8 hours.

Mechanism of Action As a live, attenuated vaccine, MMR vaccine offers active immunity to disease caused by the measles, mumps, and rubella viruses.

Dosage

Adult

Immunization: SubQ: 0.5 mL

Birth year in or after 1957 without evidence of immunity: 1 or 2 doses (0.5 mL/dose); minimum interval between doses is 28 days

Adults born in or after 1957 without documentation of live vaccine on or after first birthday, or without physician-diagnosed measles or mumps, or without laboratory evidence of immunity, should be vaccinated with at least one dose; a second dose, separated by no less than 1 month, is indicated for those previously vaccinated with one dose of measles vaccine, students entering institutions of higher learning, recently exposed in an outbreak setting, healthcare workers at time of employment, and for travelers to endemic areas (CDC, 1998).

Persons vaccinated between 1963 and 1967 with a killed measles vaccine, followed by live vaccine within 3 months, or with a vaccine of unknown type should be revaccinated with live measles virus vaccine (CDC, 1998).

Healthcare personnel (unvaccinated) born prior to 1957 and who are without laboratory evidence of measles, mumps and/or rubella immunity or laboratory confirmation of disease: Consider 2 doses of MMR vaccine at the appropriate interval. Two doses of the MMR vaccine are needed for measles and mumps, one dose is needed for rubella (CDC, 2006).

◀ **Administration** Administer SubQ in outer aspect of the upper arm in patients ≥12 months. **Not for I.V. administration.**

Simultaneous administration of vaccines helps ensure the patients will be fully vaccinated by the appropriate age. Simultaneous administration of vaccines is defined as administering >1 vaccine on the same day at different anatomic sites. The use of licensed combination vaccines is generally preferred over separate injections of the equivalent components. Separate vaccines should not be combined in the same syringe unless indicated by product specific labeling. Separate needles and syringes should be used for each injection. The ACIP prefers each dose of a specific vaccine in a series come from the same manufacturer when possible. Adolescents and adults should be vaccinated while seated or lying down. In general, preterm infants should be vaccinated at the same chronological age as full-term infants (CDC, 2011).

Antipyretics have not been shown to prevent febrile seizures. Antipyretics may be used to treat fever or discomfort following vaccination (CDC, 2011). One study reported that routine prophylactic administration of acetaminophen to prevent fever prior to vaccination decreased the immune response of some vaccines; the clinical significance of this reduction in immune response has not been established (Prymula, 2009).

Monitoring Parameters Monitor for syncope for ≥15 minutes following vaccination.

Test Interactions Temporary suppression of TB skin test reactivity. Tuberculin test may be given simultaneously at separate sites on the same day as measles-containing vaccine or ≥4 weeks later.

Pharmacotherapy Pearls Federal law requires that the name of medication, date of administration, the vaccine manufacturer, lot number of vaccine, and the administering person's name, title, and address be entered into the patient's permanent medical record.

Acceptable presumptive evidence of immunity includes one of the following:
1. Documentation of adequate vaccination (for measles, mumps, and rubella). Adequate vaccination for mumps is defined as 1 dose of a live mumps virus vaccine for preschool children and adults not at high risk; 2 doses of a live mumps virus vaccine for school-aged children and high-risk adults. Healthcare workers, international travelers, and students in institutions of higher learning are considered high-risk adults.
2. Laboratory evidence of immunity (for measles, mumps, and rubella)
3. Birth prior to 1957 (measles and mumps); for women of childbearing potential, birth prior to 1957 is not acceptable evidence of immunity to rubella
4. Documentation of physician-diagnosed disease (for measles, mumps); exception, not acceptable evidence of immunity for healthcare workers

Special Geriatric Considerations Most adults and elderly are immune to measles (rubeola) and it is not necessary to vaccinate. If no history of measles exposure or patient is from an isolated community where measles is not endemic, vaccination may be required. Testing may be indicated; may need to test for rubella. Vaccinate those traveling into endemic areas with no evidence of immunity. No dose restriction necessary.

Dosage Forms Excipient information presented when available (limited, particularly for generics); consult specific product labeling.

Injection, powder for reconstitution [preservative free]:

M-M-R® II: Measles virus ≥1000 TCID$_{50}$, mumps virus ≥20,000 TCID$_{50}$, and rubella virus ≥1000 TCID$_{50}$ [contains albumin (human), bovine serum, chicken egg protein, gelatin, neomycin, sorbitol, and sucrose 1.9 mg/vial]

Selected References

Centers for Disease Control and Prevention (CDC), "Notice to Readers: Updated Recommendations of the Advisory Committee on Immunization Practices (ACIP) for the Control and Elimination of Mumps," *MMWR Recomm Rep*, 2006, 55(early release):1-2. Available at http://www.cdc.gov/mmwr/pdf/wk/mm55e601.pdf

Centers for Disease Control and Prevention (CDC), "Syncope After Vaccination – United States, January 2005-July 2007," *MMWR Morb Mortal Wkly Rep*, 2008, 57(17):457-60.

◆ **Mebaral® [DSC]** see Mephobarbital *on page 1143*

Meclizine (MEK li zeen)

Medication Safety Issues
Sound-alike/look-alike issues:
Antivert® may be confused with Anzemet®, Axert®

Brand Names: U.S. Antivert®; Bonine® [OTC]; Dramamine® Less Drowsy Formula [OTC]; Medi-Meclizine [OTC]; Trav-L-Tabs® [OTC]

Brand Names: Canada Bonamine™; Bonine®

Index Terms Meclizine Hydrochloride; Meclozine Hydrochloride

Generic Availability (U.S.) Yes

Pharmacologic Category Antiemetic; Histamine H₁ Antagonist; Histamine H₁ Antagonist, First Generation; Piperazine Derivative

Use Prevention and treatment of symptoms of motion sickness; management of vertigo with diseases affecting the vestibular system

Contraindications Hypersensitivity to meclizine or any component of the formulation

Warnings/Precautions Use with caution in patients with asthma, angle-closure glaucoma, prostatic hyperplasia, pyloric or duodenal obstruction, or bladder neck obstruction. Elderly may be at risk for anticholinergic side effects such as glaucoma, prostatic hyperplasia, constipation, GI obstructive disease. If vertigo does not respond in 1-2 weeks, it is advised to discontinue use. May be sedating, use with caution in disorders where CNS depression is a feature; patients must be cautioned about performing tasks which require mental alertness (eg, operating machinery or driving). Effects may be potentiated when used with other sedative drugs or ethanol.

Adverse Reactions (Reflective of adult population; not specific for elderly)
>10%:
  Central nervous system: Slight to moderate drowsiness
  Respiratory: Thickening of bronchial secretions
1% to 10%:
  Central nervous system: Headache, fatigue, nervousness, dizziness
  Gastrointestinal: Appetite increase, weight gain, nausea, diarrhea, abdominal pain, xerostomia
  Respiratory: Pharyngitis

Drug Interactions
  Avoid Concomitant Use There are no known interactions where it is recommended to avoid concomitant use.
  Increased Effect/Toxicity
  Meclizine may increase the levels/effects of: Alcohol (Ethyl); Anticholinergics; CNS Depressants; Selective Serotonin Reuptake Inhibitors

  The levels/effects of Meclizine may be increased by: Droperidol; HydrOXYzine; Pramlintide
  Decreased Effect
  Meclizine may decrease the levels/effects of: Acetylcholinesterase Inhibitors (Central); Benzylpenicilloyl Polylysine; Betahistine

  The levels/effects of Meclizine may be decreased by: Acetylcholinesterase Inhibitors (Central); Amphetamines

Ethanol/Nutrition/Herb Interactions Ethanol: May increase CNS depression; monitor for increased effects with coadministration. Caution patients about effects.

Mechanism of Action Has central anticholinergic action by blocking chemoreceptor trigger zone; decreases excitability of the middle ear labyrinth and blocks conduction in the middle ear vestibular-cerebellar pathways

Pharmacodynamics/Kinetics
  Onset of action: ~1 hour
  Duration: 8-24 hours
  Metabolism: Hepatic
  Half-life elimination: 6 hours
  Excretion: Urine (as metabolites); feces (as unchanged drug)

Dosage
  Geriatric & Adult
    Motion sickness: Oral: 12.5-25 mg 1 hour before travel, repeat dose every 12-24 hours if needed; doses up to 50 mg may be needed
    Vertigo: Oral: 25-100 mg/day in divided doses

Monitoring Parameters Monitor for CNS anticholinergic side effects in older adults, relief of symptoms

Special Geriatric Considerations Due to anticholinergic action, use lowest dose in divided doses to avoid side effects and their inconvenience. Limit use if possible. May cause confusion or aggravate symptoms of confusion in those with dementia. If vertigo does not respond in 1-2 weeks, discontinue use.

Dosage Forms Excipient information presented when available (limited, particularly for generics); consult specific product labeling.
  Caplet, oral, as hydrochloride: 12.5 mg
  Tablet, oral, as hydrochloride: 12.5 mg, 25 mg
    Antivert®: 12.5 mg, 25 mg, 50 mg
    Dramamine® Less Drowsy Formula: 25 mg
    Medi-Meclizine: 25 mg
    Trav-L-Tabs®: 25 mg
  Tablet, chewable, oral, as hydrochloride: 25 mg
    Bonine®: 25 mg [scored; raspberry flavor]

◆ **Meclizine Hydrochloride** *see* Meclizine *on page 1118*

Meclofenamate (me kloe fen AM ate)

Brand Names: Canada Meclomen®
Index Terms Meclofenamate Sodium
Generic Availability (U.S.) Yes
Pharmacologic Category Nonsteroidal Anti-inflammatory Drug (NSAID), Oral
Use Treatment of inflammatory disorders, arthritis, mild-to-moderate pain
Medication Guide Available Yes
Contraindications Hypersensitivity to meclofenamate, aspirin, other NSAIDs, or any component of the formulation; perioperative pain in the setting of coronary artery bypass graft (CABG) surgery
Warnings/Precautions NSAIDs are associated with an increased risk of adverse cardiovascular thrombotic events, including MI and stroke. Risk may be increased with duration of use or pre-existing cardiovascular risk factors or disease. Carefully evaluate individual cardiovascular risk profiles prior to prescribing. May cause new-onset hypertension or worsening of existing hypertension. Use caution with fluid retention. Avoid use in heart failure. Concurrent administration of ibuprofen, and potentially other nonselective NSAIDs, may interfere with aspirin's cardioprotective effect. Risk of MI and stroke may be increased with use following CABG surgery.

Platelet adhesion and aggregation may be decreased; may prolong bleeding time; patients with coagulation disorders or who are receiving anticoagulants should be monitored closely. Anemia may occur; patients on long-term NSAID therapy should be monitored for anemia. Rarely, NSAID use may cause severe blood dyscrasias (eg, agranulocytosis, aplastic anemia, thrombocytopenia).

NSAID use may compromise existing renal function; dose-dependent decreases in prostaglandin synthesis may result from NSAID use, reducing renal blood flow which may cause renal decompensation. NSAID use may increase the risk for hyperkalemia. Patients with impaired renal function, dehydration, heart failure, liver dysfunction, those taking diuretics, and ACE inhibitors, and the elderly are at greater risk of renal toxicity and hyperkalemia. Rehydrate patient before starting therapy; monitor renal function closely. Not recommended for use in patients with advanced renal disease. Long-term NSAID use may result in renal papillary necrosis.

NSAIDs may increase risk of gastrointestinal irritation, inflammation, ulceration, bleeding, and perforation. These events may occur at any time during therapy and without warning. Use caution with a history of GI disease (bleeding or ulcers), concurrent therapy with aspirin, anticoagulants and/or corticosteroids, smoking, use of alcohol, the elderly or debilitated patients. When used concomitantly with ≤325 mg of aspirin, a substantial increase in the risk of gastrointestinal complications (eg, ulcer) occurs; concomitant gastroprotective therapy (eg, proton pump inhibitors) is recommended (Bhatt, 2008).

Use the lowest effective dose for the shortest duration of time, consistent with individual patient goals, to reduce risk of cardiovascular or GI adverse events. Alternate therapies should be considered for patients at high risk.

NSAIDs may cause serious skin adverse events including exfoliative dermatitis, Stevens-Johnson syndrome (SJS) and toxic epidermal necrolysis (TEN); discontinue use at first sign of skin rash or hypersensitivity. Anaphylactoid reactions may occur, even without prior exposure; patients with "aspirin triad" (bronchial asthma, aspirin intolerance, rhinitis) may be at increased risk. Do not use in patients who experience bronchospasm, asthma, rhinitis, or urticaria with NSAID or aspirin therapy. Use caution in other forms of asthma.

Use with caution in patients with decreased hepatic function. Closely monitor patients with any abnormal LFT. Severe hepatic reactions (eg, fulminant hepatitis, liver failure) have occurred with NSAID use, rarely; discontinue if signs or symptoms of liver disease develop, or if systemic manifestations occur.

NSAIDS may cause drowsiness, dizziness, blurred vision and other neurologic effects which may impair physical or mental abilities; patients must be cautioned about performing tasks which require mental alertness (eg, operating machinery or driving). Discontinue use with blurred or diminished vision and perform ophthalmologic exam. Monitor vision with long-term therapy.

The elderly are at increased risk for adverse effects (especially peptic ulceration, CNS effects, renal toxicity) from NSAIDs even at low doses.

Withhold for at least 4-6 half-lives prior to surgical or dental procedures.

Adverse Reactions (Reflective of adult population; not specific for elderly)

>10%:

Central nervous system: Dizziness

Dermatologic: Rash

Gastrointestinal: Abdominal cramps, heartburn, indigestion, nausea

1% to 10%:

Central nervous system: Headache, nervousness

Dermatologic: Itching

Endocrine & metabolic: Fluid retention

Gastrointestinal: Vomiting

Otic: Tinnitus

Drug Interactions

Avoid Concomitant Use

Avoid concomitant use of Meclofenamate with any of the following: Floctafenine; Ketorolac; Ketorolac (Nasal); Ketorolac (Systemic)

Increased Effect/Toxicity

Meclofenamate may increase the levels/effects of: Aminoglycosides; Anticoagulants; Antiplatelet Agents; Bisphosphonate Derivatives; Collagenase (Systemic); CycloSPORINE; CycloSPORINE (Systemic); Deferasirox; Desmopressin; Digoxin; Drotrecogin Alfa; Eplerenone; Haloperidol; Ibritumomab; Lithium; Methotrexate; Nonsteroidal Anti-Inflammatory Agents; PEMEtrexed; Porfimer; Potassium-Sparing Diuretics; PRALAtrexate; Quinolone Antibiotics; Rivaroxaban; Salicylates; Thrombolytic Agents; Tositumomab and Iodine I 131 Tositumomab; Vancomycin; Vitamin K Antagonists

The levels/effects of Meclofenamate may be increased by: ACE Inhibitors; Angiotensin II Receptor Blockers; Antidepressants (Tricyclic, Tertiary Amine); Corticosteroids (Systemic); Dasatinib; Floctafenine; Glucosamine; Herbs (Anticoagulant/Antiplatelet Properties); Ketorolac; Ketorolac (Nasal); Ketorolac (Systemic); Nonsteroidal Anti-Inflammatory Agents; Omega-3-Acid Ethyl Esters; Pentosan Polysulfate Sodium; Pentoxifylline; Probenecid; Prostacyclin Analogues; Selective Serotonin Reuptake Inhibitors; Serotonin/Norepinephrine Reuptake Inhibitors; Sodium Phosphates; Treprostinil; Vitamin E

Decreased Effect

Meclofenamate may decrease the levels/effects of: ACE Inhibitors; Angiotensin II Receptor Blockers; Antiplatelet Agents; Beta-Blockers; Eplerenone; HydrALAZINE; Potassium-Sparing Diuretics; Salicylates; Selective Serotonin Reuptake Inhibitors; Thiazide Diuretics

The levels/effects of Meclofenamate may be decreased by: Bile Acid Sequestrants; Nonsteroidal Anti-Inflammatory Agents; Salicylates

Ethanol/Nutrition/Herb Interactions

Ethanol: Avoid ethanol (may enhance gastric mucosal irritation).

Herb/Nutraceutical: Avoid alfalfa, anise, bilberry, bladderwrack, bromelain, cat's claw, celery, chamomile, coleus, cordyceps, dong quai, evening primrose, fenugreek, feverfew, garlic, ginger, ginkgo biloba, ginseng (American, Panax, Siberian), grapeseed, green tea, guggul, horse chestnut seed, horseradish, licorice, prickly ash, red clover, reishi, SAMe (S-adenosylmethionine), sweet clover, turmeric, white willow (all have additional antiplatelet activity).

Mechanism of Action Reversibly inhibits cyclooxygenase-1 and 2 (COX-1 and 2) enzymes, which results in decreased formation of prostaglandin precursors; has antipyretic, analgesic, and anti-inflammatory properties.

Other proposed mechanisms not fully elucidated (and possibly contributing to the anti-inflammatory effect to varying degrees) include inhibiting chemotaxis, altering lymphocyte activity, inhibiting neutrophil aggregation/activation, and decreasing proinflammatory cytokine levels.

Pharmacodynamics/Kinetics

Duration: 2-4 hours

Distribution: Meclofenamate sodium: 9.1-43.2 L/kg

Protein binding: ≥99%

Metabolism: Metabolized to metabolite I (active) and ~6 other minor metabolites

Bioavailability: 100%

Half-life elimination: Meclofenamate sodium: 0.8-2.1 hours; metabolite I 15.3 hours

Time to peak, serum: Meclofenamate sodium 0.5-1.5 hours; metabolite I 0.5-4 hours

Excretion: Primarily urine (70%; primarily as metabolites); feces (30%)

◀ **Dosage**
Geriatric & Adult
Mild-to-moderate pain: Oral: 50 mg every 4-6 hours; increases to 100 mg may be required; maximum dose: 400 mg
Rheumatoid arthritis/osteoarthritis: Oral: 50 mg every 4-6 hours; increase, over weeks, to 200-400 mg/day in 3-4 divided doses; do not exceed 400 mg/day; maximal benefit for any dose may not be seen for 2-3 weeks

Monitoring Parameters Monitor response (pain, range of motion, grip strength, mobility, ADL function), inflammation; observe for weight gain, edema; monitor renal function; observe for bleeding, bruising; evaluate gastrointestinal effects (abdominal pain, bleeding, dyspepsia); mental confusion, disorientation, CBC, serum, creatinine, BUN, liver function tests

Test Interactions Increased chloride (S), increased sodium (S)

Pharmacotherapy Pearls There are no clinical guidelines to predict which NSAID will give response in a particular patient. Trials with each must be initiated until response determined. If diarrhea develops, reduce dose or discontinue use of meclofenamate for a short time (until diarrhea stops). Some patients are not able to tolerate further use. Consider dose, patient convenience, and cost.

Special Geriatric Considerations Elderly are a high-risk population for adverse effects from NSAIDs. As much as 60% of elderly can develop peptic ulceration and/or hemorrhage asymptomatically. The concomitant use of H_2 blockers and sucralfate is not effective as prophylaxis with the exception of NSAID-induced duodenal ulcers which may be prevented by the use of ranitidine. Misoprostol and proton pump inhibitors are the only agents proven to help prevent the development of NSAID-induced ulcers. Also, concomitant disease and drug use contribute to the risk for GI adverse effects. Use lowest effective dose for shortest period possible. Consider renal function decline with age. Use of NSAIDs can compromise existing renal function especially when Cl_{cr} is ≤30 mL/minute. Tinnitus may be a difficult and unreliable indication of toxicity due to age-related hearing loss or eighth cranial nerve damage. CNS adverse effects such as confusion, agitation, and hallucination are generally seen in overdose or high dose situations, but elderly may demonstrate these adverse effects at lower doses than younger adults.

Dosage Forms Excipient information presented when available (limited, particularly for generics); consult specific product labeling.
Capsule, oral, as sodium: 50 mg, 100 mg

♦ **Meclofenamate Sodium** see Meclofenamate on page 1120
♦ **Meclozine Hydrochloride** see Meclizine on page 1118
♦ **Medicone® Suppositories [OTC]** see Phenylephrine (Topical) on page 1443
♦ **Medi-First® Sinus Decongestant [OTC]** see Phenylephrine (Systemic) on page 1440
♦ **Medi-Meclizine [OTC]** see Meclizine on page 1118
♦ **Medi-Phenyl [OTC]** see Phenylephrine (Systemic) on page 1440
♦ **Mediproxen [OTC]** see Naproxen on page 1263
♦ **Medrol®** see MethylPREDNISolone on page 1183
♦ **Medrol Dose Pack** see MethylPREDNISolone on page 1183
♦ **Medrol® Dosepak™** see MethylPREDNISolone on page 1183

MedroxyPROGESTERone (me DROKS ee proe JES te rone)

Medication Safety Issues
Sound-alike/look-alike issues:
Depo-Provera® may be confused with depo-subQ provera 104™
depo-subQ provera 104™ may be confused with Depo-Provera®
MedroxyPROGESTERone may be confused with hydroxyprogesterone caproate, methyl-PREDNISolone, methylTESTOSTERone
Provera® may be confused with Covera®, Femara®, Parlodel®, Premarin®, Proscar®, PROzac®

Administration issues:
The injection dosage form is available in different formulations. Carefully review prescriptions to assure the correct formulation and route of administration.

Brand Names: U.S. Depo-Provera®; Depo-Provera® Contraceptive; depo-subQ provera 104®; Provera®

Brand Names: Canada Alti-MPA; Apo-Medroxy®; Depo-Prevera®; Depo-Provera®; Dom-Medroxyprogesterone; Gen-Medroxy; Medroxy; Medroxyprogesterone Acetate Injectable Suspension USP; Novo-Medrone; PMS-Medroxyprogesterone; Provera-Pak; Provera®; Teva-Medroxyprogesterone

Index Terms Acetoxymethylprogesterone; Medroxyprogesterone Acetate; Methylacetoxyprogesterone; MPA

Generic Availability (U.S.) Yes

Pharmacologic Category Contraceptive; Progestin

Use Secondary amenorrhea or abnormal uterine bleeding due to hormonal imbalance; reduction of endometrial hyperplasia in nonhysterectomized postmenopausal women receiving conjugated estrogens; management of endometriosis-associated pain; adjunctive therapy and palliative treatment of recurrent and metastatic endometrial carcinoma

Unlabeled/Investigational Use Treatment of low-grade endometrial stromal sarcoma

Contraindications Hypersensitivity to medroxyprogesterone or any component of the formulation; history of or current thrombophlebitis or venous thromboembolic disorders (including DVT, PE); cerebral vascular disease; severe hepatic dysfunction or disease; carcinoma of the breast or other estrogen- or progesterone-dependent neoplasia; undiagnosed vaginal bleeding

Warnings/Precautions [U.S. Boxed Warning]: Prolonged use of medroxyprogesterone contraceptive injection may result in a loss of bone mineral density (BMD). It is not known if use during adolescence or early adulthood will decrease peak bone mass accretion or increase the risk for osteoporotic fractures later in life. Loss is related to the duration of use, may not be completely reversible on discontinuation of the drug, and incidence is not significantly different between the SubQ and I.M. dosage forms. The impact on peak bone mass in adolescents should be weighed against the potential for unintended pregnancies in treatment decision. Consider alternative contraceptive methods in patients at risk for osteoporosis (eg, metabolic bone disease, family history of osteoporosis, chronic use of medications associated with osteoporosis such as corticosteroids). **[U.S. Boxed Warning]: Long-term use (ie, >2 years) should be limited to situations where other birth control methods are inadequate.** Consider other methods of birth control in women with (or at risk for) osteoporosis. **[U.S. Boxed Warning]: Inform patients that injectable contraceptives do not protect against HIV infection or other sexually-transmitted diseases.** When used for contraception, the possibility of ectopic pregnancy should be considered in patients with abdominal pain. Anaphylaxis or anaphylactoid reactions have been reported with use of the injection; medication for the treatment of hypersensitivity reactions should be available for immediate use.

[U.S. Boxed Warning]: Estrogens with or without progestin should not be used to prevent coronary heart disease. Use caution with cardiovascular disease or dysfunction. MPA used in combination with estrogen may increase the risks of hypertension, myocardial infarction (MI), stroke, pulmonary emboli (PE), and deep vein thrombosis; incidence of these effects was shown to be significantly increased in postmenopausal women using conjugated equine estrogens (CEE) in combination with MPA.

[U.S. Boxed Warning]: The risk of dementia may be increased in postmenopausal women; increased incidence was observed in women ≥65 years of age taking MPA in combination with CEE. An increased risk of invasive breast cancer was observed in postmenopausal women using MPA in combination with CEE. An increase in abnormal mammograms has also been reported with estrogen and progestin therapy. Use is contraindicated in patients with known or suspected breast cancer. Whenever possible, progestins in combination with estrogens should be discontinued at least 4-6 weeks prior to surgeries associated with an increased risk of thromboembolism or during periods of prolonged immobilization. If thrombosis develops with contraceptive treatment, discontinue treatment (unless no other acceptable contraceptive alternative). Progestins used in combination with estrogen should be used for shortest duration possible consistent with treatment goals. Conduct periodic risk:benefit assessments.

Discontinue pending examination in cases of sudden partial or complete vision loss, sudden onset of proptosis, diplopia, or migraine; discontinue permanently if papilledema or retinal vascular lesions are observed on examination. Use with caution in patients with diseases that may be exacerbated by fluid retention (including asthma, epilepsy, migraine, cardiac, or renal dysfunction). Contraceptive therapy with medroxyprogesterone commonly results in an average weight gain of ~2.5 kg after 1 year and ~3.7 kg after 2 years of treatment. Use caution with history of depression.

May have adverse effects on glucose tolerance; use caution in women with diabetes. MPA is extensively metabolized in the liver. Discontinue if jaundice develops or if acute or chronic hepatic disturbances occur. Use is contraindicated with severe hepatic disease. Unscheduled bleeding/spotting may occur. Presentation of irregular, unresolving vaginal bleeding following previously regular cycles warrants further evaluation including endometrial sampling, if indicated, to rule out malignancy. Not for use prior to menarche.

◄ **Adverse Reactions (Reflective of adult population; not specific for elderly)** Adverse effects as reported with any dosage form; percent ranges presented are noted with the MPA I.M. contraceptive injection:

>5%:

Central nervous system: Dizziness, headache, nervousness

Endocrine & metabolic: Libido decreased, menstrual irregularities (includes bleeding, amenorrhea, or both)

Gastrointestinal: Abdominal pain/discomfort, weight gain (>10 lbs at 24 months: 38%)

1% to 5%:

Cardiovascular: Edema

Central nervous system: Depression, fatigue, insomnia

Dermatologic: Acne, alopecia, rash

Endocrine & metabolic: Breast pain, hot flashes

Gastrointestinal: Bloating, nausea

Genitourinary: Dysmenorrhea, leukorrhea, vaginitis

Local: Injection site reaction (SubQ administration): Atrophy, induration, pain

Neuromuscular & skeletal: Arthralgia, backache, leg cramp, weakness

<1%, postmarketing, and/or case reports: Allergic reaction, anaphylaxis, anaphylactoid reactions, anemia, angioedema, anxiety, appetite changes, asthma, axillary swelling, blood dyscrasia, body odor, BMD loss, breast cancer, breast changes, cervical cancer, chest pain, chills, chloasma, cholestatic jaundice, deep vein thrombosis, diaphoresis, diarrhea, drowsiness, dry skin, dyspareunia, dyspnea, facial palsy, fainting, fever, galactorrhea, genitourinary infections, glucose tolerance decreased, hirsutism, hoarseness, jaundice, lack of return to fertility, lactation decreased, libido increased, melasma, nipple bleeding, oligomenorrhea, optic neuritis, osteoporosis, osteoporotic fractures, paralysis, paresthesia, pruritus, pulmonary embolus, rectal bleeding, retinal thrombosis, scleroderma, seizure, somnolence, syncope, tachycardia, thirst, thrombophlebitis, urticaria, uterine hyperplasia, vaginal cysts, varicose veins

In addition: Depo-Provera® aqueous suspension: Residual lump, sterile abscess, or skin discoloration at the injection

Drug Interactions

Metabolism/Transport Effects Substrate of CYP3A4 (major); **Induces** CYP3A4 (weak)

Avoid Concomitant Use

Avoid concomitant use of MedroxyPROGESTERone with any of the following: Griseofulvin

Increased Effect/Toxicity

MedroxyPROGESTERone may increase the levels/effects of: Benzodiazepines (metabolized by oxidation); Selegiline; Tranexamic Acid; Voriconazole

The levels/effects of MedroxyPROGESTERone may be increased by: Boceprevir; Conivaptan; Herbs (Progestogenic Properties); Voriconazole

Decreased Effect

MedroxyPROGESTERone may decrease the levels/effects of: Saxagliptin; Vitamin K Antagonists

The levels/effects of MedroxyPROGESTERone may be decreased by: Acitretin; Aminoglutethimide; Aprepitant; Artemether; Barbiturates; Bexarotene; Bexarotene (Systemic); Bile Acid Sequestrants; Bosentan; CarBAMazepine; CYP3A4 Inducers (Strong); Deferasirox; Felbamate; Fosaprepitant; Fosphenytoin; Griseofulvin; LamoTRIgine; Mycophenolate; OXcarbazepine; Phenytoin; Retinoic Acid Derivatives; Rifamycin Derivatives; St Johns Wort; Telaprevir; Tocilizumab; Topiramate

Ethanol/Nutrition/Herb Interactions

Ethanol: Avoid ethanol (may increase risk of osteoporosis).

Food: Bioavailability of the oral tablet is increased when taken with food; half-life is unchanged.

Herb/Nutraceutical: St John's wort may diminish the therapeutic effect of progestin contraceptives (contraceptive failure is possible).

Stability Store at controlled room temperature.

Mechanism of Action Inhibits secretion of pituitary gonadotropins, which prevents follicular maturation and ovulation; causes endometrial thinning

Pharmacodynamics/Kinetics

Absorption: Oral: Well absorbed; I.M.: Slow

Protein binding: 86% to 90% primarily to albumin; does not bind to sex hormone-binding globulin

Metabolism: Extensively hepatic via hydroxylation and conjugation; forms metabolites

Half-life elimination: Oral: 12-17 hours; I.M. (Depo-Provera® Contraceptive): ~50 days; SubQ: ~40 days

Time to peak: Oral: 2-4 hours; I.M. (Depo-Provera® Contraceptive): ~3 weeks; SubQ: ~1 week

Excretion: Urine

Dosage

Geriatric & Adult

Abnormal uterine bleeding: Oral: 5-10 mg for 5-10 days starting on day 16 or 21 of cycle

Endometriosis (depo-subQ provera 104™): SubQ: 104 mg every 3 months (every 12-14 weeks)

Endometrial carcinoma, recurrent or metastatic (adjunctive/palliative treatment) (Depo-Provera®): I.M.: 400-1000 mg/week

Accompanying cyclic estrogen therapy, postmenopausal: Oral: 5-10 mg for 12-14 consecutive days each month, starting on day 1 or day 16 of the cycle; lower doses may be used if given with estrogen continuously throughout the cycle

Hepatic Impairment Use is contraindicated with severe impairment. Discontinue with jaundice or if liver function disturbances occur. Consider lower dose or less frequent administration with mild-to-moderate impairment. Use of the contraceptive injection has not been studied in patients with hepatic impairment; consideration should be given to not readminister if jaundice develops

Administration

I.M.: Depo-Provera® Contraceptive: Administer first dose during the first 5 days of menstrual period, or within the first 5 days postpartum if not breast-feeding, or at the sixth week postpartum if breast-feeding exclusively. Shake vigorously prior to administration. Administer by deep I.M. injection in the gluteal or deltoid muscle.

When switching from combined hormonal contraceptives (estrogen plus progestin), the first injection should be on the day after the last active tablet or (at the latest) the day after the final inactive tablet. When switching from other contraceptive methods, ensure continuous contraceptive coverage.

SubQ: depo-subQ provera 104™: Administer first dose during the first 5 days of menstrual period, or at the sixth week postpartum if breast-feeding. Shake vigorously prior to administration. Administer by SubQ injection in the anterior thigh or abdomen; avoid boney areas and the umbilicus. Administer over 5-7 seconds. Do not rub the injection area. When switching from combined hormonal contraceptives (estrogen plus progestin), the first injection should be within 7 days after the last active pill, or removal of patch or ring. If switching from the I.M. to SubQ formulation, the next dose should be given within the prescribed dosing period for the I.M. injection to assure continuous coverage.

Monitoring Parameters Before starting therapy, a physical exam with reference to the breasts and pelvis are recommended, including a Papanicolaou smear. Monitor patient closely for loss of vision; sudden onset of proptosis, diplopia, or migraine; signs and symptoms of thromboembolic disorders; signs or symptoms of depression; glucose in patients with diabetes; or blood pressure. BMD with long-term use (per manufacturer).

Adequate diagnostic measures, including endometrial sampling, if indicated, should be performed to rule out malignancy in all cases of undiagnosed abnormal vaginal bleeding.

Test Interactions

The following tests may be decreased: Steroid levels (plasma and urinary), gonadotropin levels, SHBG concentration, T_3 uptake

The following tests may be increased: Protein-bound iodine, butanol extractable protein-bound iodine, Factors II, VII, VIII, IX, X

Pathologist should be advised of estrogen/progesterone therapy when specimens are submitted.

Dosage Forms Excipient information presented when available (limited, particularly for generics); consult specific product labeling.

Injection, suspension, as acetate: 150 mg/mL (1 mL)

Depo-Provera®: 400 mg/mL (2.5 mL)

Depo-Provera® Contraceptive: 150 mg/mL (1 mL) [contains polysorbate 80]

depo-subQ provera 104®: 104 mg/0.65 mL (0.65 mL) [contains polysorbate 80]

Tablet, oral, as acetate: 2.5 mg, 5 mg, 10 mg

Provera®: 2.5 mg, 5 mg, 10 mg [scored]

♦ **Medroxyprogesterone Acetate** *see* MedroxyPROGESTERone *on page 1122*

♦ **Medroxyprogesterone and Estrogens (Conjugated)** *see* Estrogens (Conjugated/Equine) and Medroxyprogesterone *on page 664*

Mefenamic Acid (me fe NAM ik AS id)

Medication Safety Issues
Sound-alike/look-alike issues:
Ponstel® may be confused with Pronestyl®

◀ **Brand Names: U.S.** Ponstel®

Brand Names: Canada Apo-Mefenamic®; Dom-Mefenamic Acid; Mefenamic-250; Nu-Mefenamic; PMS-Mefenamic Acid; Ponstan®

Generic Availability (U.S.) Yes

Pharmacologic Category Nonsteroidal Anti-inflammatory Drug (NSAID), Oral

Use Short-term relief of mild-to-moderate pain

Medication Guide Available Yes

Dosage

Geriatric & Adult Mild-moderate pain: Oral: Initial: 500 mg; then 250 mg every 4 hours as needed; maximum therapy: 1 week

Renal Impairment Not recommended for use

Special Geriatric Considerations Elderly are a high-risk population for adverse effects from NSAIDs. As much as 60% of elderly can develop peptic ulceration and/or hemorrhage asymptomatically. The concomitant use of H_2 blockers, omeprazole, and sucralfate is not effective as prophylaxis with the exception of NSAID-induced duodenal ulcers which may be prevented by the use of ranitidine. Misoprostol and proton pump inhibitors are the only agents proven to help prevent the development of NSAID-induced ulcers. Also, concomitant disease and drug use contribute to the risk for GI adverse effects. Use lowest effective dose for shortest period possible. Consider renal function decline with age. Use of NSAIDs can compromise existing renal function especially when Cl_{cr} is ≤30 mL/minute. Tinnitus may be a difficult and unreliable indication of toxicity due to age-related hearing loss or eighth cranial nerve damage. CNS adverse effects such as confusion, agitation, and hallucination are generally seen in overdose or high-dose situations, but elderly may demonstrate these adverse effects at lower doses than younger adults.

Dosage Forms Excipient information presented when available (limited, particularly for generics); consult specific product labeling.

Capsule, oral: 250 mg

Ponstel®: 250 mg

◆ **Mefoxin®** *see* CefOXitin *on page 303*
◆ **Megace®** *see* Megestrol *on page 1126*
◆ **Megace® ES** *see* Megestrol *on page 1126*
◆ **Megadophilus® [OTC]** *see* Lactobacillus *on page 1020*

Megestrol (me JES trole)

Medication Safety Issues

Sound-alike/look-alike issues:

Megace® may be confused with Reglan®

Megestrol may be confused with mesalamine

Brand Names: U.S. Megace®; Megace® ES

Brand Names: Canada Apo-Megestrol®; Megace®; Megace® OS; Nu-Megestrol

Index Terms 5071-1DL(6); Megestrol Acetate; NSC-71423

Generic Availability (U.S.) Yes: Excludes Megace® ES

Pharmacologic Category Antineoplastic Agent, Hormone; Appetite Stimulant; Progestin

Use Palliative treatment of breast and endometrial carcinoma; treatment of anorexia, cachexia, or unexplained significant weight loss in patients with AIDS

Unlabeled/Investigational Use Treatment of uterine bleeding

Contraindications Hypersensitivity to megestrol or any component of the formulation

Warnings/Precautions Hazardous agent - use appropriate precautions for handling and disposal. May suppress hypothalamic-pituitary-adrenal (HPA) axis during chronic administration; consider the possibility of adrenal suppression in any patient receiving or being withdrawn from chronic therapy when signs/symptoms suggestive of hypoadrenalism are noted (during stress or in unstressed state). Laboratory evaluation and replacement/stress doses of rapid-acting glucocorticoid should be considered. New-onset diabetes and exacerbation of pre-existing diabetes have been reported with long-term use. Use with caution in patients with a history of thromboembolic disease. Vaginal bleeding or discharge may occur in females. Megace® ES suspension is not equivalent to other formulations on a mg per mg basis; Megace® ES suspension 625 mg/5 mL is equivalent to megestrol acetate suspension 800 mg/20 mL.

Adverse Reactions (Reflective of adult population; not specific for elderly)

Frequency not always defined.

Cardiovascular: Hypertension (≤8%), cardiomyopathy (1% to 3%), chest pain (1% to 3%), edema (1% to 3%), palpitation (1% to 3%), peripheral edema (1% to 3%), heart failure

Central nervous system: Headache (≤10%), insomnia (≤6%), fever (1% to 6%), pain (≤6%, similar to placebo), abnormal thinking (1% to 3%), confusion (1% to 3%), depression (1% to 3%), hypoesthesia (1% to 3%), seizure (1% to 3%), mood changes, malaise, lethargy

Dermatologic: Rash (2% to 12%), alopecia (1% to 3%), pruritus (1% to 3%), vesiculobullous rash (1% to 3%)

Endocrine & metabolic: Hyperglycemia (≤6%), gynecomastia (1% to 3%), adrenal insufficiency, amenorrhea, breakthrough bleeding, cervical erosion and secretions (changes), breast tenderness increased, Cushing's syndrome, diabetes, glucose intolerance, HPA axis suppression, hot flashes, hypercalcemia, menstrual flow changes, spotting, vaginal bleeding pattern changes

Gastrointestinal: Diarrhea (6% to 15%, similar to placebo), flatulence (≤10%), vomiting (≤6%), nausea (≤5%), dyspepsia (≤4%), abdominal pain (1% to 3%), constipation (1% to 3%), salivation increased (1% to 3%), xerostomia (1% to 3%), weight gain (not attributed to edema or fluid retention)

Genitourinary: Impotence (4% to 14%), decreased libido (≤5%), urinary incontinence (1% to 3%), urinary tract infection (1% to 3%), urinary frequency (≤2%)

Hematologic: Anemia (≤5%), leukopenia (1% to 3%)

Hepatic: Hepatomegaly (1% to 3%), LDH increased (1% to 3%), cholestatic jaundice, hepatotoxicity

Neuromuscular & skeletal: Weakness (2% to 6%), neuropathy (1% to 3%), paresthesia (1% to 3%), carpal tunnel syndrome

Ocular: Amblyopia (1% to 3%)

Renal: Albuminuria (1% to 3%)

Respiratory: Dyspnea (1% to 3%), cough (1% to 3%), pharyngitis (1% to 3%), pneumonia (≤2%), hyperpnea

Miscellaneous: Diaphoresis (1% to 3%), herpes infection (1% to 3%), infection (1% to 3%), moniliasis (1% to 3%), tumor flare

Drug Interactions

Avoid Concomitant Use

Avoid concomitant use of Megestrol with any of the following: Dofetilide

Increased Effect/Toxicity

Megestrol may increase the levels/effects of: Dofetilide

The levels/effects of Megestrol may be increased by: Herbs (Progestogenic Properties)

Decreased Effect

The levels/effects of Megestrol may be decreased by: Aminoglutethimide

Ethanol/Nutrition/Herb Interactions Herb/Nutraceutical: Avoid herbs with progestogenic properties (eg, bloodroot, chasteberry, damiana, oregano, and yucca); may enhance the adverse/toxic effect of megestrol.

Stability

Suspension: Store at 15°C to 25°C (59°F to 77°F); protect from heat.

Tablet: Store at 25°C (77°F); excursions permitted to 15°C to 30°C (59°F to 86°F); protect from heat (temperatures >40°C [>104°F])

Mechanism of Action A synthetic progestin with antiestrogenic properties which disrupt the estrogen receptor cycle. Megestrol interferes with the normal estrogen cycle and results in a lower LH titer. May also have a direct effect on the endometrium. Megestrol is an antineoplastic progestin thought to act through an antileutenizing effect mediated via the pituitary. May stimulate appetite by antagonizing the metabolic effects of catabolic cytokines.

Pharmacodynamics/Kinetics

Absorption: Well absorbed orally

Metabolism: Hepatic (to free steroids and glucuronide conjugates)

Half-life elimination: 13-105 hours

Time to peak, serum: 1-3 hours

Excretion: Urine (57% to 78%; 5% to 8% as metabolites); feces (8% to 30%)

Dosage

Geriatric & Adult Note: Megace® ES suspension is not equivalent to other formulations on a mg-per-mg basis.

Breast carcinoma (females): Refer to individual protocols: Oral: Tablet: 40 mg 4 times/day

Endometrial carcinoma: Refer to individual protocols: Oral: Tablet: 40-320 mg/day in divided doses; use for 2 months to determine efficacy; maximum doses used have been up to 800 mg/day.

◄ **HIV-related cachexia (males/females):** Oral: Suspension:

Megace®: Initial dose: 800 mg/day; daily doses of 400 and 800 mg/day were found to be clinically effective

Megace® ES: 625 mg/day

Renal Impairment No data available; however, the urinary excretion of megestrol acetate administered in doses of 4-90 mg ranged from 57% to 78% within 10 days.

Administration Megestrol acetate (Megace®) oral suspension is compatible with water, orange juice, apple juice, or Sustacal H.C. for immediate consumption.

Monitoring Parameters Observe for signs of thromboembolic events; blood pressure, weight; serum glucose

Test Interactions Altered thyroid and liver function tests

Special Geriatric Considerations Elderly females may have vaginal bleeding or discharge and need to be forewarned of this side effect and inconvenience. No specific changes in dose are required for the elderly. Megestrol has been used in the treatment of the failure to thrive syndrome in cachectic elderly in addition to proper nutrition. Data does not support the use of megestrol for weight gain. The increase in weight tends to be mostly fat instead of lean body mass. Also, this agent is associated with DVTs.

Dosage Forms Excipient information presented when available (limited, particularly for generics); consult specific product labeling.

Suspension, oral, as acetate: 40 mg/mL (10 mL, 20 mL, 237 mL, 240 mL, 473 mL, 480 mL)

Megace®: 40 mg/mL (240 mL) [contains ethanol 0.06%, sodium benzoate; lemon-lime flavor]

Megace® ES: 125 mg/mL (150 mL) [contains ethanol 0.06%, sodium benzoate; lemon-lime flavor]

Tablet, oral, as acetate: 20 mg, 40 mg

Selected References

Farrar DJ, "Megestrol Acetate: Promises and Pitfalls," *AIDS Patient Care STDS*, 1999, 13(3):149-52.

◆ **Megestrol Acetate** see Megestrol *on page 1126*

Meloxicam (mel OKS i kam)

Brand Names: U.S. Mobic®

Brand Names: Canada Apo-Meloxicam®; CO Meloxicam; Dom-Meloxicam; Mobicox®; Mobic®; Mylan-Meloxicam; Novo-Meloxicam; PHL-Meloxicam; PMS-Meloxicam; ratio-Meloxicam; Teva-Meloxicam

Generic Availability (U.S.) Yes:

Pharmacologic Category Nonsteroidal Anti-inflammatory Drug (NSAID), Oral

Use Relief of signs and symptoms of osteoarthritis, rheumatoid arthritis, and juvenile idiopathic arthritis (JIA)

Medication Guide Available Yes

Contraindications Hypersensitivity (eg, asthma, urticaria, allergic-type reactions) to meloxicam, aspirin, other NSAIDs, or any component of the formulation; perioperative pain in the setting of coronary artery bypass graft (CABG) surgery

Warnings/Precautions [U.S. Boxed Warning]: NSAIDs are associated with an increased risk of adverse cardiovascular thrombotic events, including MI and stroke. Risk may be increased with duration of use or pre-existing cardiovascular risk factors or disease. Carefully evaluate individual cardiovascular risk profiles prior to prescribing. May cause new-onset hypertension or worsening of existing hypertension. Use caution with fluid retention. Avoid use in heart failure. Concurrent administration of ibuprofen, and potentially other nonselective NSAIDs, may interfere with aspirin's cardioprotective effect. **[U.S. Boxed Warning]: Use is contraindicated for treatment of perioperative pain in the setting of coronary artery bypass graft (CABG) surgery.** Risk of MI and stroke may be increased with use within the first 10-14 days following CABG surgery.

Platelet adhesion and aggregation may be decreased; may prolong bleeding time; patients with coagulation disorders or who are receiving anticoagulants should be monitored closely. Anemia may occur; patients on long-term NSAID therapy should be monitored for anemia. Rarely, NSAID use may cause severe blood dyscrasias (eg, agranulocytosis, aplastic anemia, thrombocytopenia).

NSAID use may compromise existing renal function; dose-dependent decreases in prostaglandin synthesis may result from NSAID use, reducing renal blood flow which may cause renal decompensation. NSAID use may increase the risk for hyperkalemia. Patients with impaired renal function, dehydration, heart failure, liver dysfunction, those taking diuretics, and ACE inhibitors, and the elderly are at greater risk of renal toxicity and hyperkalemia. Rehydrate patient before starting therapy; monitor renal function closely. Not recommended for use in patients with advanced renal disease. Long-term NSAID use may result in renal papillary necrosis.

[U.S. Boxed Warning]: NSAIDs may increase risk of gastrointestinal irritation, inflammation, ulceration, bleeding, and perforation. These events may occur at any time during therapy and without warning. Use caution with a history of GI disease (bleeding or ulcers), concurrent use with aspirin, anticoagulants and/or corticosteroids, smoking, use of alcohol, the elderly or debilitated patients. When used concomitantly with ≤325 mg of aspirin, a substantial increase in the risk of gastrointestinal complications (eg, ulcer) occurs; concomitant gastroprotective therapy (eg, proton pump inhibitors) is recommended (Bhatt, 2008).

Use the lowest effective dose for the shortest duration of time, consistent with individual patient goals, to reduce risk of cardiovascular or GI adverse events. Alternate therapies should be considered for patients at high risk.

NSAIDs may cause serious skin adverse events including exfoliative dermatitis, Stevens-Johnson syndrome (SJS) and toxic epidermal necrolysis (TEN); discontinue use at first sign of skin rash or hypersensitivity. Anaphylactoid reactions may occur, even without prior exposure; patients with "aspirin triad" (bronchial asthma, aspirin intolerance, rhinitis) may be at increased risk. Do not use in patients who experience bronchospasm, asthma, rhinitis, or urticaria with NSAID or aspirin therapy. Use caution in other forms of asthma.

Use with caution in patients with decreased hepatic function. Closely monitor patients with any abnormal LFT. Severe hepatic reactions (eg, fulminant hepatitis, liver failure) have occurred with NSAID use, rarely; discontinue if signs or symptoms of liver disease develop, or if systemic manifestations occur.

NSAIDS may cause drowsiness, dizziness, blurred vision and other neurologic effects which may impair physical or mental abilities; patients must be cautioned about performing tasks which require mental alertness (eg, operating machinery or driving). Discontinue use with blurred or diminished vision and perform ophthalmologic exam. Monitor vision with long-term therapy.

The elderly are at increased risk for adverse effects (especially peptic ulceration, CNS effects, renal toxicity) from NSAIDs even at low doses.

Oral suspension formulation may contain sorbitol. Concomitant use with sodium polystyrene sulfonate (Kayexalate®) may cause intestinal necrosis (including fatal cases); combined use should be avoided. Withhold for at least 4-6 half-lives prior to surgical or dental procedures.

Adverse Reactions (Reflective of adult population; not specific for elderly) Percentages reported in adult patients; abdominal pain, diarrhea, fever, headache, pyrexia, and vomiting were reported more commonly in pediatric patients
2% to 10%:
  Cardiovascular: Edema (≤5%)
  Central nervous system: Headache (2% to 8%), pain (1% to 5%), dizziness (≤4%), insomnia (≤4%)
  Dermatologic: Pruritus (≤2%), rash (≤3%)
  Gastrointestinal: Dyspepsia (4% to 10%), diarrhea (2% to 8%), nausea (2% to 7%), abdominal pain (2% to 5%), constipation (≤3%), flatulence (≤3%), vomiting (≤3%)
  Genitourinary: Urinary tract infection (≤7%), micturition (≤2%)
  Hematologic: Anemia (≤4%)
  Neuromuscular & skeletal: Arthralgia (≤5%), back pain (≤3%)
  Respiratory: Upper respiratory infection (≤8%), cough (≤2%), pharyngitis (≤3%)
  Miscellaneous: Flu-like syndrome (2% to 6%), falls (≤3%)
Drug Interactions
  Metabolism/Transport Effects Substrate (minor) of CYP2C9, 3A4; **Inhibits** CYP2C9 (weak)
  Avoid Concomitant Use
    Avoid concomitant use of Meloxicam with any of the following: Calcium Polystyrene Sulfonate; Floctafenine; Ketorolac; Ketorolac (Nasal); Ketorolac (Systemic); Sodium Polystyrene Sulfonate
  Increased Effect/Toxicity
    Meloxicam may increase the levels/effects of: Aminoglycosides; Anticoagulants; Antiplatelet Agents; Bisphosphonate Derivatives; Calcium Polystyrene Sulfonate; Collagenase (Systemic); CycloSPORINE; CycloSPORINE (Systemic); Deferasirox; Desmopressin; Digoxin; Drotrecogin Alfa; Eplerenone; Haloperidol; Ibritumomab; Lithium; Methotrexate; Nonsteroidal Anti-Inflammatory Agents; PEMEtrexed; Porfimer; Potassium-Sparing Diuretics; PRALAtrexate; Quinolone Antibiotics; Rivaroxaban; Salicylates; Sodium Polystyrene Sulfonate; Thrombolytic Agents; Tositumomab and Iodine I 131 Tositumomab; Vancomycin; Vitamin K Antagonists

The levels/effects of Meloxicam may be increased by: ACE Inhibitors; Angiotensin II Receptor Blockers; Antidepressants (Tricyclic, Tertiary Amine); Conivaptan; Corticosteroids (Systemic); Dasatinib; Floctafenine; Glucosamine; Herbs (Anticoagulant/Antiplatelet Properties); Ketorolac; Ketorolac (Nasal); Ketorolac (Systemic); Nonsteroidal Anti-Inflammatory Agents; Omega-3-Acid Ethyl Esters; Pentosan Polysulfate Sodium; Pentoxifylline; Probenecid; Prostacyclin Analogues; Selective Serotonin Reuptake Inhibitors; Serotonin/Norepinephrine Reuptake Inhibitors; Sodium Phosphates; Treprostinil; Vitamin E; Voriconazole

Decreased Effect

Meloxicam may decrease the levels/effects of: ACE Inhibitors; Angiotensin II Receptor Blockers; Antiplatelet Agents; Beta-Blockers; Eplerenone; HydrALAZINE; Potassium-Sparing Diuretics; Salicylates; Selective Serotonin Reuptake Inhibitors; Thiazide Diuretics

The levels/effects of Meloxicam may be decreased by: Bile Acid Sequestrants; Nonsteroidal Anti-Inflammatory Agents; Salicylates; Tocilizumab

Ethanol/Nutrition/Herb Interactions

Ethanol: Avoid ethanol (may enhance gastric mucosal irritation).

Herb/Nutraceutical: Avoid alfalfa, anise, bilberry, bladderwrack, bromelain, cat's claw, celery, chamomile, coleus, cordyceps, dong quai, evening primrose, fenugreek, feverfew, garlic, ginger, ginkgo biloba, ginseng (American, Panax, Siberian), grapeseed, green tea, guggul, horse chestnut seed, horseradish, licorice, prickly ash, red clover, reishi, SAMe (S-adenosylmethionine), sweet clover, turmeric, white willow (all have additional antiplatelet activity).

Stability Store at 25°C (77°F). Protect tablets from moisture.

Mechanism of Action Reversibly inhibits cyclooxygenase-1 and 2 (COX-1 and 2) enzymes, which results in decreased formation of prostaglandin precursors; has antipyretic, analgesic, and anti-inflammatory properties

Other proposed mechanisms not fully elucidated (and possibly contributing to the anti-inflammatory effect to varying degrees), include inhibiting chemotaxis, altering lymphocyte activity, inhibiting neutrophil aggregation/activation, and decreasing proinflammatory cytokine levels.

Pharmacodynamics/Kinetics

Distribution: 10 L

Protein binding: ~99%, primarily to albumin

Metabolism: Hepatic via CYP2C9 and CYP3A4 (minor); forms 4 metabolites (inactive)

Bioavailability: 89%

Half-life elimination: Adults: 15-20 hours

Time to peak: Initial: 4-5 hours; Secondary: 12-14 hours

Excretion: Urine and feces (as inactive metabolites)

Dosage

Geriatric & Adult Osteoarthritis, rheumatoid arthritis: Oral: Initial: 7.5 mg once daily; some patients may receive additional benefit from increasing dose to 15 mg once daily; maximum dose: 15 mg/day.

Renal Impairment

Mild-to-moderate impairment: No specific dosage recommendations

Significant impairment (Cl_{cr} ≤20 mL/minute): Patients with severe renal impairment have not been adequately studied; use not recommended.

Hemodialysis: Maximum dose: 7.5 mg/day

Hepatic Impairment

Mild (Child-Pugh class A) to moderate (Child-Pugh class B) hepatic dysfunction: No dosage adjustment is necessary

Severe hepatic impairment: Patients with severe hepatic impairment have not been adequately studied

Administration May be administered with or without meals; take with food or milk to minimize gastrointestinal irritation. Oral suspension: Shake gently prior to use.

Monitoring Parameters Periodic CBC, serum chemistries, liver function, renal function (serum BUN and creatinine) with long-term use; signs and symptoms of bleeding

Special Geriatric Considerations Men ≥65 years of age exhibited steady-state plasma concentrations and pharmacokinetics similar to younger men. Elderly women (≥65 years of age) had nearly a 50% greater AUC and 32% higher C_{max} compared to younger women.

Elderly are a high-risk population for adverse effects from NSAIDs. As much as 60% of elderly can develop peptic ulceration and/or hemorrhage asymptomatically. The concomitant use of H_2 blockers and sucralfate is not effective as prophylaxis with the exception of NSAID-induced duodenal ulcers which may be prevented by the use of ranitidine. Misoprostol and proton pump inhibitors are the only agents proven to help prevent the development of NSAID-induced ulcers. Also, concomitant disease and drug use contribute to the risk for GI adverse effects. Use lowest effective dose for shortest period possible. Consider renal function decline with age. Use of NSAIDs can compromise existing renal function especially when Cl$_{cr}$ is ≤30 mL/minute. Tinnitus may be a difficult and unreliable indication of toxicity due to age-related hearing loss or eighth cranial nerve damage. CNS adverse effects, such as confusion, agitation, and hallucination, are generally seen in overdose or high-dose situations, but the elderly may demonstrate these adverse effects at lower doses than younger adults.

Dosage Forms Excipient information presented when available (limited, particularly for generics); consult specific product labeling.

Suspension, oral: 7.5 mg/5 mL (100 mL)

Mobic®: 7.5 mg/5 mL (100 mL) [contains sodium benzoate; raspberry flavor]

Tablet, oral: 7.5 mg, 15 mg

Mobic®: 7.5 mg, 15 mg

Melphalan (MEL fa lan)

Medication Safety Issues

Sound-alike/look-alike issues:

Melphalan may be confused with Mephyton®, Myleran®

Alkeran® may be confused with Alferon®, Leukeran®, Myleran®

High alert medication:

This medication is in a class the Institute for Safe Medication Practices (ISMP) includes among its list of drug classes which have a heightened risk of causing significant patient harm when used in error.

Brand Names: U.S. Alkeran®

Brand Names: Canada Alkeran®

Index Terms L-PAM; L-Phenylalanine Mustard; L-Sarcolysin; Phenylalanine Mustard

Generic Availability (U.S.) Yes: Excludes tablet

Pharmacologic Category Antineoplastic Agent, Alkylating Agent

Use Palliative treatment of multiple myeloma and nonresectable epithelial ovarian carcinoma

Unlabeled/Investigational Use Treatment of Hodgkin's disease, amyloidosis; conditioning regimen for autologous hematopoietic stem cell transplantation in adults with hematologic disorders (eg, multiple myeloma) and autologous marrow or stem cell transplantation in pediatric neuroblastoma and Ewing's sarcoma

Contraindications Hypersensitivity to melphalan or any component of the formulation; patients whose disease was resistant to prior melphalan therapy

Warnings/Precautions [U.S. Boxed Warning]: Bone marrow suppression is common; may be severe and result in infection or bleeding; myelosuppression is dose-related. Monitor blood counts; may require treatment delay or dose modification for thrombocytopenia or neutropenia. Use with caution in patients with prior bone marrow suppression, impaired renal function (consider dose reduction), or who have received prior (or concurrent) chemotherapy or irradiation. Myelotoxicity is generally reversible, although irreversible bone marrow failure has been reported. In patients who are candidates for autologous transplantation, avoid melphalan-containing regimens prior to transplant (due to the effects on stem cell reserve). Myelosuppression has been demonstrated more with the I.V. formulation (compared to oral); may be dose-related. Signs of infection, such as fever and WBC rise, may not occur; lethargy and confusion may be more prominent signs of infection.

[U.S. Boxed Warning]: Hypersensitivity reactions have occurred in ~2% of patients receiving I.V. melphalan, usually after multiple treatment cycles. Discontinue infusion and treat symptomatically. Hypersensitivity may also occur (rarely) with oral melphalan. Do not readminister (oral or I.V.) in patients who experience hypersensitivity to melphalan.

Gastrointestinal toxicities, including nausea, vomiting, diarrhea and mucositis, are common. When administering high-dose melphalan in autologous transplantation, cryotherapy is recommended to prevent mucositis (Keefe, 2007). Abnormal liver function tests may occur; hepatitis and jaundice have also been reported; hepatic sinusoidal obstruction syndrome (SOS; formerly called veno-occlusive disease) has been reported with I.V. melphalan. Pulmonary fibrosis (some fatal) and interstitial pneumonitis have been observed with treatment. Dosage reduction is recommended with I.V. melphalan in patients with renal impairment; reduced initial doses may also be recommended with oral melphalan. Closely monitor patients with azotemia.

[U.S. Boxed Warning]: Produces chromosomal changes and is potentially mutagenic and leukemogenic; secondary malignancies (including acute myeloid leukemia, myeloproliferative disease, and carcinoma) have been reported reported (some patients were receiving combination chemotherapy or radiation therapy); the risk is increased with increased treatment duration and cumulative doses. Suppresses ovarian function and produces amenorrhea; may also cause testicular suppression.

◄ Extravasation may cause local tissue damage; administration by slow injection into a fast running I.V. solution into an injection port or via a central line is recommended; do not administer directly into a peripheral vein. **[U.S. Boxed Warning]: Should be administered under the supervision of an experienced cancer chemotherapy physician.** Avoid vaccination with live vaccines during treatment if immunocompromised. Toxicity may be increased in elderly; start with lowest recommended adult doses.

Adverse Reactions (Reflective of adult population; not specific for elderly)

>10%:

Gastrointestinal: Nausea/vomiting (oral low-dose: <10%; I.V.: 30% to 90%), oral ulceration

Hematologic: Myelosuppression, leukopenia (nadir: 14-21 days; recovery: 28-35 days), thrombocytopenia (nadir: 14-21 days; recovery: 28-35 days), anemia

Miscellaneous: Secondary malignancy (<2% to 20%; cumulative dose and duration dependent, includes acute myeloid leukemia, myeloproliferative syndrome, carcinoma)

1% to 10%: Miscellaneous: Hypersensitivity (I.V.: 2%; includes bronchospasm, dyspnea, edema, hypotension, pruritus, rash, tachycardia, urticaria)

Drug Interactions

Avoid Concomitant Use

Avoid concomitant use of Melphalan with any of the following: BCG; Nalidixic Acid; Natalizumab; Pimecrolimus; Tacrolimus (Topical); Vaccines (Live)

Increased Effect/Toxicity

Melphalan may increase the levels/effects of: Carmustine; CycloSPORINE; CycloSPORINE (Systemic); Leflunomide; Natalizumab; Vaccines (Live); Vitamin K Antagonists

The levels/effects of Melphalan may be increased by: Denosumab; Nalidixic Acid; Pimecrolimus; Roflumilast; Tacrolimus (Topical); Trastuzumab

Decreased Effect

Melphalan may decrease the levels/effects of: BCG; Cardiac Glycosides; Sipuleucel-T; Vaccines (Inactivated); Vaccines (Live); Vitamin K Antagonists

The levels/effects of Melphalan may be decreased by: Echinacea

Ethanol/Nutrition/Herb Interactions

Ethanol: Avoid ethanol (due to GI irritation).

Food: Food interferes with oral absorption.

Stability Use appropriate precautions for handling and disposal.

Tablet: Store in refrigerator at 2°C to 8°C (36°F to 46°F). Protect from light.

Injection: Store at room temperature of 15°C to 30°C (59°F to 86°F). Protect from light. Stability is limited; must be prepared fresh. **The time between reconstitution/dilution and administration of parenteral melphalan must be kept to a minimum (manufacturer recommends <60 minutes) because reconstituted and diluted solutions are unstable.** Dissolve powder initially with 10 mL of supplied diluent to a concentration of 5 mg/mL; shake immediately and vigorously to dissolve. This solution is chemically and physically stable for ≤90 minutes when stored at room temperature, although the manufacturer recommends administration be completed within 60 minutes of reconstitution. **Immediately** dilute dose in NS to a concentration of ≤0.45 mg/mL (manufacturer recommended concentration). Do not refrigerate solution; precipitation occurs.

Mechanism of Action Alkylating agent which is a derivative of mechlorethamine that inhibits DNA and RNA synthesis via formation of carbonium ions; cross-links strands of DNA; acts on both resting and rapidly dividing tumor cells.

Pharmacodynamics/Kinetics Note: Pharmacokinetics listed are for FDA-approved doses.

Absorption: Oral: Variable and incomplete

Distribution: V_d: 0.5-0.6 L/kg throughout total body water; low penetration into CSF

Protein binding: 60% to 90%; primarily to albumin, 20% to α_1-acid glycoprotein

Metabolism: Hepatic; chemical hydrolysis to monohydroxymelphalan and dihydroxymelphalan

Bioavailability: Unpredictable; 61% ± 26%, decreasing with repeated doses

Half-life elimination: Terminal: I.V.: 75 minutes; Oral: 1-2 hours

Time to peak, serum: ~1-2 hours

Excretion: Oral: Feces (20% to 50%); urine (~10% as unchanged drug)

Dosage

Geriatric Refer to adult dosing. Use caution and begin at the lower end of dosing range.

Adult Details regarding dosing in combination regimens should also be consulted. Adjust dose based on patient response and weekly blood counts.

Multiple myeloma (palliative treatment): Note: Response is gradual; may require repeated courses to realize benefit:

I.V.: 16 mg/m^2 administered at 2-week intervals for 4 doses, then administer at 4-week intervals after adequate hematologic recovery.

Oral: Usual dose (as described in the manufacturer's labeling):
6 mg once daily for 2-3 weeks initially, followed by up to 4 weeks rest, then a maintenance dose of 2 mg daily as hematologic recovery begins **or**
10 mg daily for 7-10 days; institute 2 mg daily maintenance dose after WBC >4000 cells/mm^3 and platelets >100,000 cells/mm^3 (~4-8 weeks); titrate maintenance dose to hematologic response **or**
0.15 mg/kg/day for 7 days, with a 2-6 week rest, followed by a maintenance dose of ≤0.05 mg/kg/day as hematologic recovery begins **or**
0.25 mg/kg/day for 4 days (or 0.2 mg/kg/day for 5 days); repeat at 4- to 6-week intervals as ANC and platelet counts return to normal
Other dosing regimens in combination therapy (unlabeled doses):
4 mg/m^2/day for 7 days every 4 weeks (Palumbo, 2006; Palumbo, 2008) **or**
6 mg/m^2/day for 7 days every 4 weeks (Palumbo, 2004) **or**
0.25 mg/kg/day for 4 days every 6 weeks (Facon, 2006; Facon, 2007) **or**
9 mg/m^2/day for 4 days every 6 weeks (Dimopoulos, 2009; San Miguel, 2008)
Ovarian carcinoma: Oral: 0.2 mg/kg/day for 5 days, repeat every 4-5 weeks **or**
Unlabeled dosing: 7 mg/m^2/day in 2 divided doses for 5 days, repeat every 28 days (Wadler, 1996)
Amyloidosis (unlabeled use): Oral: 0.22 mg/kg/day for 4 days every 28 days in combination with oral dexamethasone (Palladini, 2004)
Hodgkin's disease (unlabeled use): I.V.: 30 mg/m^2 on day 6 of combination chemotherapy (mini-BEAM) regimen (Colwill, 1995; Martin, 2001)
Conditioning regimen for autologous hematopoietic stem cell transplantation (unlabeled use): I.V.:
200 mg/m^2 alone 2 days prior to transplantation (Fermand, 2005; Moreau, 2002) **or**
140 mg/m^2 2 days prior to transplantation (combined with busulfan) (Fermand, 2005) **or**
140 mg/m^2 2 days prior to transplantation (combined with total body irradiation [TBI]) (Moreau, 2002) **or**
140 mg/m^2 5 days prior to transplantation (combined with TBI) (Barlogie, 2006)

Renal Impairment

The FDA-approved labeling contains the following adjustment recommendations (for approved dosing levels) based on route of administration:
Oral: Moderate-to-severe renal impairment: Consider a reduced dose initially.
I.V.: BUN ≥30 mg/dL: Reduce dose by up to 50%.

The following guidelines have been used by some clinicians:
Aronoff, 2007 (route of administration not specified): Adults (based on a 6 mg once-daily dose):
Cl_{cr} 10-50 mL/minute: Administer 75% of dose.
Cl_{cr} <10 mL/minute: Administer 50% of dose.
Hemodialysis: Administer dose after hemodialysis.
Continuous ambulatory peritoneal dialysis (CAPD): Administer 50% of dose.
Continuous renal replacement therapy (CRRT): Administer 75% of dose.
Badros, 2001: I.V.: Autologous stem cell transplant: Serum creatinine >2 mg/dL: Reduce dose from 200 mg/m^2 to 140 mg/m^2
Carlson, 2005: Oral (for melphalan-prednisone combination therapy; based on a study evaluating toxicity with melphalan dosed at 0.25 mg/kg/day for 4 days/cycle):
Cl_{cr} >10 to <30 mL/minute: Administer 75% of dose
Cl_{cr} ≤10 mL/minute: Data is insufficient for a recommendation
Kintzel, 1995:
Oral: Adjust dose in the presence of hematologic toxicity
I.V.:
Cl_{cr} 46-60 mL/minute: Administer 85% of normal dose.
Cl_{cr} 31-45 mL/minute: Administer 75% of normal dose.
Cl_{cr} <30 mL/minute: Administer 70% of normal dose.
Hepatic Impairment Melphalan is hepatically metabolized; however, dosage adjustment does not appear to be necessary (King, 2001).

Administration

Oral: Administer on an empty stomach (1 hour prior to or 2 hours after meals)
Parenteral: Due to limited stability, complete administration of I.V. dose should occur within 60 minutes of reconstitution
I.V.: Infuse over 15-30 minutes. Extravasation may cause local tissue damage; administration by slow injection into a fast running I.V. solution into an injection port or via a central line is recommended; do not administer by direct injection into a peripheral vein.
BMT only: Saline-based hydration preceding (2-4 hours), during, and following (6-12 hours) administration reduces risk of drug precipitation in renal tubules. Hydrolysis causes loss of 1% melphalan injection per 10 minutes.

◄ **Monitoring Parameters** CBC with differential and platelet count, serum electrolytes, serum uric acid

Test Interactions False-positive Coombs' test [direct]

Special Geriatric Considerations Toxicity to immunosuppressives is increased in the elderly. Start with lowest recommended adult doses. Signs of infection, such as fever and WBC rise, may not occur. Lethargy and confusion may be more prominent signs of infection.

Dosage Forms Excipient information presented when available (limited, particularly for generics); consult specific product labeling.

Injection, powder for reconstitution: 50 mg

Alkeran®: 50 mg [contains ethanol (in diluent), propylene glycol (in diluent)]

Tablet, oral:

Alkeran®: 2 mg

Selected References

Barlogie B, Kyle RA, Anderson KC, et al, "Standard Chemotherapy Compared With High-Dose Chemoradiotherapy for Multiple Myeloma: Final Results of Phase III US Intergroup Trial S9321," J Clin Oncol, 2006, 24(6):929-36.

Berthold F, Boos J, Burdach S, et al, "Myeloablative Megatherapy With Autologous Stem-Cell Rescue Versus Oral Maintenance Chemotherapy as Consolidation Treatment in Patients With High-Risk Neuroblastoma: A Randomised Controlled Trial," Lancet Oncol, 2005, 6(9):649-58.

Carlson K, Hjorth M, Knudsen LM, et al, "Toxicity in Standard Melphalan-Prednisone Therapy Among Myeloma Patients With Renal Failure - A Retrospective Analysis and Recommendations for Dose Adjustment," Br J Haematol, 2005, 128(5):631-5.

Dimopoulos MA, Richardson PG, Schlag R, et al, "VMP (Bortezomib, Melphalan, and Prednisone) is Active and Well Tolerated in Newly Diagnosed Patients With Multiple Myeloma With Moderately Impaired Renal Function, and Results in Reversal of Renal Impairment: Cohort Analysis of the Phase III VISTA Study," J Clin Oncol, 2009, 27 (36):6086-93.

Facon T, Mary JY, Hulin C, et al, "Melphalan and Prednisone Plus Thalidomide Versus Melphalan and Prednisone Alone or Reduced-Intensity Autologous Stem Cell Transplantation in Elderly Patients With Multiple Myeloma (IFM 99-06): A Randomised Trial," Lancet, 2007, 370(9594):1209-18.

Facon T, Mary JY, Pegourie B, et al, "Dexamethasone-Based Regimens Versus Melphalan-Prednisone for Elderly Multiple Myeloma Patients Ineligible for High-Dose Therapy," Blood, 2006, 107(4):1292-8.

Fermand JP, Katsahian S, Divine M, et al, "High-Dose Therapy and Autologous Blood Stem-Cell Transplantation Compared With Conventional Treatment in Myeloma Patients Aged 55 to 65 years: Long-Term Results of a Randomized Control Trial From the Group Myelome-Autogreffe," J Clin Oncol, 2005, 23(36):9227-33.

Keefe DM, Schubert MM, Elting LS, et al, "Updated Clinical Practice Guidelines for the Prevention and Treatment of Mucositis," Cancer, 2007, 109(5):820-31.

Nath CE, Shaw PJ, Montgomery K, et al, "Population Pharmacokinetics of Melphalan in Pediatric Blood or Marrow Transplant Recipients," Br J Clin Pharmacol, 2007, 64(2):151-64.

National Comprehensive Cancer Network® (NCCN), "Clinical Practice Guidelines in Oncology™: Hodgkin Disease/Lymphoma," Version 1.2010. Available at http://www.nccn.org/professionals/physician_gls/PDF/hodgkins.pdf

National Comprehensive Cancer Network® (NCCN), "Clinical Practice Guidelines in Oncology™: Multiple Myeloma," Version 3.2010. Available at http://www.nccn.org/professionals/physician_gls/PDF/myeloma.pdf.

National Comprehensive Cancer Network® (NCCN), "Clinical Practice Guidelines in Oncology™: Ovarian Cancer," Version 2.2010. Available at http://www.nccn.org/professionals/physician_gls/PDF/ovarian.pdf

Palumbo A, Bringhen S, Caravita T, et al, "Oral Melphalan and Prednisone Chemotherapy Plus Thalidomide Compared With Melphalan and Prednisone Alone in Elderly Patients With Multiple Myeloma: Randomised Controlled Trial," Lancet, 2006, 367(9513):825-31.

Palumbo A, Bringhen S, Liberati AM, et al, "Oral Melphalan, Prednisone, and Thalidomide in Elderly Patients With Multiple Myeloma: Updated Results of a Randomized Controlled Trial," Blood, 2008, 112(8):3107-14.

Pritchard J, Cotterill SJ, Germond SM, et al, "High Dose Melphalan in the Treatment of Advanced Neuroblastoma: Results of a Randomised Trial (ENSG-1) by the European Neuroblastoma Study Group," Pediatr Blood Cancer, 2005, 44(4):348-57.

San Miguel JF, Schlag R, Khuageva NK, et al, "Bortezomib Plus Melphalan and Prednisone for Initial Treatment of Multiple Myeloma," New Engl J Med, 2008, 359(9):906-17.

Seddon BM, Cassoni AM, Galloway MJ, et al, "Fatal Radiation Myelopathy After High-Dose Busulfan and Melphalan Chemotherapy and Radiotherapy for Ewing's Sarcoma: A Review of the Literature and Implications for Practice," Clin Oncol, 2005, 17(5):385-90.

Memantine (me MAN teen)

Medication Safety Issues

Sound-alike/look-alike issues:

Memantine may be confused with mesalamine

Brand Names: U.S. Namenda®

Brand Names: Canada CO Memantine; Ebixa®; PMS-Memantine; ratio-Memantine; Riva-Memantine; Sandoz-Memantine

Index Terms Memantine Hydrochloride; Namenda XR

Generic Availability (U.S.) No

Pharmacologic Category N-Methyl-D-Aspartate Receptor Antagonist

Use Treatment of moderate-to-severe dementia of the Alzheimer's type

Unlabeled/Investigational Use Treatment of mild-to-moderate vascular dementia

Contraindications Hypersensitivity to memantine or any component of the formulation

Warnings/Precautions Use with caution in patients with cardiovascular disease; an increased incidence of cardiac failure, angina, bradycardia, and hypertension (compared with placebo) was observed in clinical trials. Use caution with seizure disorders or severe hepatic impairment. Use with caution in moderate-to-severe renal impairment; dose adjustments may be required. Worsening of corneal condition has been observed in a clinical trial; periodic ophthalmic exams during use have been recommended (Canadian labeling). Clearance is significantly reduced by alkaline urine; use caution with medications, dietary changes, or patient conditions which may alter urine pH.

Adverse Reactions (Reflective of adult population; not specific for elderly)
1% to 10%:
Cardiovascular: Hypertension (4%), hypotension (2%), cardiac failure, cerebrovascular accident, syncope, transient ischemic attack
Central nervous system: Dizziness (5% to 7%), confusion (6%), headache (6%), anxiety (4%), depression (3%), hallucinations (3%), pain (3%), somnolence (3%), fatigue (2%), aggressive reaction (1% to 2%), ataxia, vertigo
Dermatologic: Rash
Gastrointestinal: Constipation (3% to 5%), diarrhea (5%), weight gain (3%), vomiting (2% to 3%), abdominal pain (2%), weight loss
Genitourinary: Urinary incontinence (2%), micturition
Hematologic: Anemia
Hepatic: Alkaline phosphatase increased
Neuromuscular & skeletal: Back pain (3%), hypokinesia
Ocular: Cataract, conjunctivitis
Respiratory: Cough (4%), dyspnea (2%), pneumonia
Miscellaneous: Influenza (4%)

Drug Interactions

Avoid Concomitant Use There are no known interactions where it is recommended to avoid concomitant use.

Increased Effect/Toxicity
Memantine may increase the levels/effects of: Trimethoprim

The levels/effects of Memantine may be increased by: Carbonic Anhydrase Inhibitors; Sodium Bicarbonate; Trimethoprim

Decreased Effect There are no known significant interactions involving a decrease in effect.

Stability Store at 25°C (77°F); excursions permitted to 15°C to 30°C (59°F to 86°F).

Mechanism of Action Glutamate, the primary excitatory amino acid in the CNS, may contribute to the pathogenesis of Alzheimer's disease (AD) by overstimulating various glutamate receptors leading to excitotoxicity and neuronal cell death. Memantine is an uncompetitive antagonist of the N-methyl-D-aspartate (NMDA) type of glutamate receptors, located ubiquitously throughout the brain. Under normal physiologic conditions, the (unstimulated) NMDA receptor ion channel is blocked by magnesium ions, which are displaced after agonist-induced depolarization. Pathologic or excessive receptor activation, as postulated to occur during AD, prevents magnesium from reentering and blocking the channel pore resulting in a chronically open state and excessive calcium influx. Memantine binds to the intra-pore magnesium site, but with longer dwell time, and thus functions as an effective receptor blocker only under conditions of excessive stimulation; memantine does not affect normal neurotransmission.

Pharmacodynamics/Kinetics
Distribution: 9-11 L/kg
Protein binding: 45%
Metabolism: Partially hepatic, primarily independent of the CYP enzyme system; forms 3 metabolites (minimal activity)
Half-life elimination: Terminal: ~60-80 hours; severe renal impairment (Cl_{cr} 5-29 mL/minute): 117-156 hours
Time to peak, serum: Immediate release: 3-7 hours; Extended release: 9-12 hours
Excretion: Urine (74%; ~48% of the total dose as unchanged drug; undergoes active tubular secretion moderated by pH-dependent tubular reabsorption; excretion reduced by alkaline urine pH)

Dosage

Geriatric & Adult

Alzheimer's disease: Oral:
Immediate release: Initial: 5 mg/day; increase dose by 5 mg/day to a target dose of 20 mg/day; wait ≥1 week between dosage changes. Doses >5 mg/day should be given in 2 divided doses.
Suggested titration: 5 mg/day for ≥1 week; 5 mg twice daily for ≥1 week; 15 mg/day given in 5 mg and 10 mg separated doses for ≥1 week; then 10 mg twice daily

◄ Extended release: Initial: 7 mg once daily, increase dose by 7 mg/day to a target maximum dose of 28 mg/day; wait ≥1 week between dosage changes

Note: When switching from the immediate release product to the extended release product, begin the extended release product the day after the last dose of the immediate release product. Patients on immediate release 10 mg twice daily should be switched to extended release 28 mg once daily.

Mild-to-moderate vascular dementia (unlabeled use): Oral: Immediate release: Initial: 5 mg/day, titrated by 5 mg/day weekly to a target dose of 10 mg twice daily (Orgogozo, 2002)

Renal Impairment

Mild impairment: No adjustment required.

Moderate impairment:

U.S. labeling: No adjustment required.

Canadian labeling: (Cl$_{cr}$ 30-49 mL/minute): Initial: 5 mg once daily; after at least 1 week of therapy and if tolerated, may titrate up to 5 mg twice daily; may further titrate dosage upward in weekly increments to 20 mg/day according to suggested titration schedule.

Severe impairment:

U.S. labeling: Cl$_{cr}$ 5-29 mL/minute: Immediate release: Initial: 5 mg once daily; after at least 1 week of therapy and if tolerated, may titrate up to 5 mg twice daily; Extended release: Target dose of 14 mg/day

Note: When switching from the immediate release product to the extended release product, begin the extended release product the day after the last dose of the immediate release product. Patients on immediate release 5 mg twice daily should be switched to extended release 14 mg once daily.

Canadian labeling: Cl$_{cr}$ 15-29 mL/minute: Initial: 5 mg once daily; after at least 1 week of therapy and if tolerated, may titrate up to 5 mg twice daily.

Hepatic Impairment

Mild-to-moderate impairment: No adjustment required.

Severe impairment: Use caution.

U.S. labeling: No specific dosing recommendations.

Canadian labeling: Avoid use.

Administration Administer without regard to meals. Extended release capsules may be swallowed whole or entire contents of capsule may be sprinkled on applesauce and swallowed immediately. Do not chew, crush, or divide.

Monitoring Parameters Periodic ophthalmic exam (Canadian labeling)

Special Geriatric Considerations In clinical trials, patients on memantine had less of a decline in cognitive function and activities of daily living (ADL) as compared to placebo. This was true for monotherapy with memantine, as well as combination therapy with donepezil, an acetylcholinesterase inhibitor.

Product Availability

Namenda XR™: FDA approved in June 2010; anticipated availability is currently undetermined

Namenda XR™ is an extended release capsule (once-daily administration) approved for the treatment of moderate-to-severe dementia associated with Alzheimer's disease

Dosage Forms Excipient information presented when available (limited, particularly for generics); consult specific product labeling.

Combination package, oral, as hydrochloride [titration pack contains two separate tablet formulations]:

Namenda®: Tablet: 5 mg (28s) and Tablet: 10 mg (21s)

Solution, oral, as hydrochloride:

Namenda®: 2 mg/mL (360 mL) [ethanol free, sugar free; contains propylene glycol; peppermint flavor]

Tablet, oral, as hydrochloride:

Namenda®: 5 mg, 10 mg

Selected References

Orgogozo JM, Rigaud AS, Stoffler A et al, "Efficacy and Safety of Memantine in Patients with Mild to Moderate Vascular Dementia: A Randomized, Placebo-Controlled Trial (MMM 300)," *Stroke,* 2002, 33:1834-39.

Reisberg B, Doody R, Stoffler A, et al, "Memantine in Moderate-to-Severe Alzheimer's Disease," *N Engl J Med,* 2003, 348(14):1333-41.

Tariot PN, Farlow MR, Grossberg GT, et al, "Memantine Treatment in Patients With Moderate to Severe Alzheimer Disease Already Receiving Donepezil: A Randomized Controlled Trial. The Memantine Study Group," *JAMA,* 2004, 291(3):317-24.

Wilcock G, Mobius HJ, Stoffler A et al, "A Double-Blind, Placebo-Controlled Multicentre Study of Memantine in Mild to Moderate Vascular Dementia (MMM 500)," *Int Clin Psychopharmacol,* 2002, 17(6):297-305.

◆ **Memantine Hydrochloride** *see* Memantine *on page 1134*

◆ **Menactra®** *see* Meningococcal (Groups A / C / Y and W-135) Diphtheria Conjugate Vaccine *on page 1137*

- ◆ **MenACWY-D (Menactra®)** *see* Meningococcal (Groups A / C / Y and W-135) Diphtheria Conjugate Vaccine *on page 1137*
- ◆ **MenACWY-CRM (Menveo®)** *see* Meningococcal (Groups A / C / Y and W-135) Diphtheria Conjugate Vaccine *on page 1137*
- ◆ **Menest® *see* Estrogens (Esterified) *on page 667*
- ◆ **Meningococcal Conjugate Vaccine** *see* Meningococcal (Groups A / C / Y and W-135) Diphtheria Conjugate Vaccine *on page 1137*

Meningococcal (Groups A / C / Y and W-135) Diphtheria Conjugate Vaccine
(me NIN joe kok al groops aye, see, why & dubl yoo won thur tee fyve dif THEER ee a KON joo gate vak SEEN)

Medication Safety Issues
Administration issue:
Menactra® (MCV4) should be administered by intramuscular (I.M.) injection only. Inadvertent subcutaneous (SubQ) administration has been reported; possibly due to confusion of this product with Menomume® (MPSV4), also a meningococcal polysaccharide vaccine, which is administered by the SubQ route.

Brand Names: U.S. Menactra®; Menveo®

Brand Names: Canada Menactra®; Menveo®

Index Terms MCV; MCV4; MenACWY-CRM (Menveo®); MenACWY-D (Menactra®); Meningococcal Conjugate Vaccine

Generic Availability (U.S.) No

Pharmacologic Category Vaccine, Inactivated (Bacterial)

Use Provide active immunization of children and adults against invasive meningococcal disease caused by *N. meningitidis* serogroups A, C, Y, and W-135.

The Advisory Committee on Immunization Practices (ACIP) recommends routine vaccination of all persons at age 11 or 12 years of age, followed by a booster at age 16 years of age (CDC, 60[3], 2011).

The ACIP also recommends vaccination for:
Children 9 through 23 months of age at increased risk for meningococcal disease (VFC Resolution No 6/11-1). Children at increased risk include:
- Children traveling to or who reside in countries where *N. meningitidisis* hyperendemic or epidemic, particularly if contact with local population will be prolonged
- Children with persistent complement component deficiencies (eg, C5-C9, properidin, factor H, or factor D)
- Children with HIV infection, if another indication for vaccination exists

Persons 2 through 55 years of age at increased risk for meningococcal disease (CDC, 60[3], 2011). Meningococcal conjugate vaccine (MCV4) is preferred for persons aged 2-55 years; meningococcal polysaccharide vaccine (MPSV4) is preferred in adults ≥56 years of age (CDC, 2005). Persons at increased risk include:
- Previously unvaccinated college freshmen living in dormitories
- Microbiologists routinely exposed to isolates of *N. meningitidis*
- Military recruits
- Persons traveling to or who reside in countries where *N. meningitidis* is hyperendemic or epidemic, particularly if contact with local population will be prolonged
- Persons with persistent complement component deficiencies (eg, C5-C9, properidin, factor H, or factor D)
- Persons with anatomic or functional asplenia
- Persons with HIV infection, if another indication for vaccination exists

Use is also recommended during meningococcal outbreaks caused by vaccine preventable serogroups (all recommended age groups) (CDC, 2005; VFC Resolution No. 6/11-1).

Dosage
Geriatric Safety and efficacy not established in patients >55 years.

Adult Immunization: I.M.:
Menactra®, Menveo®: Adults ≤55 years: 0.5 mL/dose given as single dose

ACIP recommendations:
Adults ≤55 years with persistent complement component deficiency; functional or anatomic asplenia; or with HIV infection and an indication for vaccination: Two doses, 2 months apart. A booster dose should be given every 5 years if still at risk for meningococcal disease. (CDC, 60[3], 2011).

Adults ≤55 years with prolonged increased risk of exposure: One dose. A booster dose should be given every 5 years if still at risk for meningococcal disease. (CDC, 60[3], 2011; VFC Resolution No. 6/11-1).

◀ College students: Persons ≤21 years of age should have documentation of vaccination ≤5 years prior to enrollment. If the primary dose was given at <16 years of age, a booster dose should be given anytime after the 16th birthday and prior to college enrollment. The minimum interval between doses is 8 weeks (CDC, 60[3], 2011).

Special Geriatric Considerations May be used though safety and efficacy have not been established in patients >55 years of age.

Dosage Forms Excipient information presented when available (limited, particularly for generics); consult specific product labeling.

Injection, solution [preservative free]:

Menactra®: 4 mcg each of polysaccharide antigen groups A, C, Y, and W-135 [bound to diphtheria toxoid 48 mcg] per 0.5 mL [MCV4 or MenACWY-D; contains natural rubber/natural latex in packaging]

Menveo®: MenA oligosaccharide 10 mcg, MenC oligosaccharide 5 mcg, MenY oligosaccharide 5 mcg, and MenW-135 oligosaccharide 5 mcg [bound to CRM$_{197}$ protein 32.7-64.1 mcg] per 0.5 mL (0.5 mL) [MenACWY-CRM; supplied in two vials, one containing MenA powder and one containing MenCYW-135 liquid]

♦ **Meningococcal Polysaccharide Vaccine** *see* Meningococcal Polysaccharide Vaccine (Groups A / C / Y and W-135) *on page* 1138

Meningococcal Polysaccharide Vaccine (Groups A / C / Y and W-135)

(me NIN joe kok al pol i SAK a ride vak SEEN groops aye, see, why & dubl yoo won thur tee fyve)

Related Information

Immunization Administration Recommendations *on page* 2037
Immunization Recommendations *on page* 2043

Medication Safety Issues

Administration issue:

Menomune® (MPSV4) should be administered by subcutaneous (SubQ) injection. Menactra® (MCV4), also a meningococcal polysaccharide vaccine, is to be administered by intramuscular (I.M.) injection only.

Brand Names: U.S. Menomune®-A/C/Y/W-135

Brand Names: Canada Menomune®-A/C/Y/W-135

Index Terms Meningococcal Polysaccharide Vaccine; MPSV; MPSV4

Generic Availability (U.S.) No

Pharmacologic Category Vaccine, Inactivated (Bacterial)

Use Provide active immunity to meningococcal serogroups contained in the vaccine

The Advisory Committee on Immunization Practices (ACIP) recommends routine vaccination for persons at increased risk for meningococcal disease. Meningococcal conjugate vaccine (MCV4) is preferred for persons aged 2-55 years; meningococcal polysaccharide vaccine (MPSV4) is preferred in adults ≥56 years of age (CDC, 2005).

Persons at increased risk include:

• Previously unvaccinated college freshmen living in dormitories
• Microbiologists routinely exposed to isolates of *N. meningitidis*
• Military recruits
• Persons traveling to or who reside in countries where *N. meningitidis* is hyperendemic or epidemic, particularly if contact with local population will be prolonged
• Persons with persistent complement component deficiencies (eg, C5-C9, properidin, factor H, or factor D)
• Persons with anatomic or functional asplenia
• Persons with HIV infection

Use is also recommended during meningococcal outbreaks caused by vaccine preventable serogroups.

Contraindications Hypersensitivity to any component of the formulation

Warnings/Precautions Immediate treatment (including epinephrine 1:1000) for anaphylactoid and/or hypersensitivity reactions should be available during vaccine use. Response may not be as great as desired in immunosuppressed patients. In general, household and close contacts of persons with altered immunocompetence may receive all age appropriate vaccines. Not to be used to treat meningococcal infections or to provide immunity against *N. meningitidis* serogroup B. May consider deferring administration in patients with moderate or severe acute illness (with or without fever); may administer to patients with mild acute illness (with or without fever). Use with caution in patients with latex sensitivity; the stopper to the vial contains dry, natural latex rubber. Some dosage forms contain thimerosal. In order to maximize vaccination rates, the ACIP recommends simultaneous administration of all age-appropriate vaccines (live or inactivated) for which a person is eligible at a single clinic visit, unless contraindications exist.

MENINGOCOCCAL POLYSACCHARIDE VACCINE (GROUPS A / C / Y AND W-135)

Adverse Reactions (Reflective of adult population; not specific for elderly) All serious adverse reactions must be reported to the U.S. Department of Health and Human Services (DHHS) Vaccine Adverse Event Reporting System (VAERS) 1-800-822-7967 or online at https://vaers.hhs.gov/esub/index. In Canada, adverse reactions may be reported to local provincial/territorial health agencies or to the Vaccine Safety Section at Public Health Agency of Canada (1-866-844-0018).

>10%:
  Central nervous system: Headache (29% to 42%), fatigue (25% to 32%), malaise (17% to 22%), irritability (12%), drowsiness (11%)
  Gastrointestinal: Diarrhea (10% to 14%)
  Local: Injection site: Pain (26% to 48%), redness (6% to 16%), induration (4% to 11%)
  Neuromuscular & skeletal: Arthralgia (5% to 16%)
1% to 10%:
  Central nervous system: Chills (4% to 6%), fever (≤5%)
  Dermatologic: Rash (≤3%)
  Gastrointestinal: Anorexia (8% to 10%), vomiting (1% to 3%)
  Local: Injection site: Swelling (3% to 8%)

Drug Interactions

Avoid Concomitant Use There are no known interactions where it is recommended to avoid concomitant use.

Increased Effect/Toxicity There are no known significant interactions involving an increase in effect.

Decreased Effect
The levels/effects of Meningococcal Polysaccharide Vaccine (Groups A / C / Y and W-135) may be decreased by: Belimumab; Fingolimod; Immunosuppressants

Stability Prior to and following reconstitution, store vaccine and diluent at 2°C to 8°C (35°F to 46°F); do not freeze. Reconstitute using provided diluent; shake well. Use single-dose vial within 30 minutes of reconstitution. Use single-dose vial immediately after reconstitution. Use multidose vial within 35 days of reconstitution.

Mechanism of Action Induces the formation of bactericidal antibodies to meningococcal antigens; the presence of these antibodies is strongly correlated with immunity to meningococcal disease caused by *Neisseria meningitidis* groups A, C, Y and W-135.

Pharmacodynamics/Kinetics
Onset of action: Antibody levels: 7-10 days
Duration: Antibodies against group A and C polysaccharides decline markedly (to prevaccination levels) over the first 3 years following a single dose of vaccine, especially in children <4 years of age

Dosage
Geriatric & Adult Immunization: SubQ: 0.5 mL/dose
ACIP recommendations:
  Adults ≤55 years: 0.5 mL/dose; however, use is not generally recommended; meningococcal conjugate vaccine (MCV4) is preferred (CDC, 2011); If MCV4 is unavailable, meningococcal polysaccharide vaccine (MPSV4) is an acceptable alternative (CDC, 2005). Persons at prolonged increased risk for meningococcal disease should be revaccinated with MCV4 (CDC, 2009).
  Adults >55 years: 0.5 mL/dose (MPSV4 preferred in this population) (CDC, 2005)

Administration Administer by SubQ injection to the deltoid region; do not administer intradermally, I.M., or I.V.

Simultaneous administration of vaccines helps ensure the patients will be fully vaccinated by the appropriate age. Simultaneous administration of vaccines is defined as administering ≥1 vaccine on the same day at different anatomic sites. Separate vaccines should not be combined in the same syringe unless indicated by product specific labeling. Separate needles and syringes should be used for each injection. The ACIP prefers each dose of a specific vaccine in a series come from the same manufacturer when possible. Adolescents and adults should be vaccinated while seated or lying down. In general, preterm infants should be vaccinated at the same chronological age as full-term infants (CDC, 2011).

Antipyretics have not been shown to prevent febrile seizures. Antipyretics may be used to treat fever or discomfort following vaccination (CDC, 2011). One study reported that routine prophylactic administration of acetaminophen to prevent fever prior to vaccination decreased the immune response of some vaccines; the clinical significance of this reduction in immune response has not been established (Prymula, 2009).

Monitoring Parameters Monitor for syncope for ≥15 minutes following vaccination.

Pharmacotherapy Pearls Federal law requires that the name of medication, date of administration, the vaccine manufacturer, lot number of vaccine, and the administering person's name, title and address be entered into the patient's permanent medical record.

Special Geriatric Considerations No specific data; only recommended when traveling to highly endemic areas.

Dosage Forms Excipient information presented when available (limited, particularly for generics); consult specific product labeling.

Injection, powder for reconstitution [MPSV4]:

Menomune®-A/C/Y/W-135: 50 mcg each of polysaccharide antigen groups A, C, Y, and W-135 per 0.5 mL dose [contains lactose 2.5-5 mg/0.5 mL, natural rubber/natural latex in packaging, thimerosal in diluent for multidose vial]

Selected References

Centers for Disease Control and Prevention (CDC), "Syncope After Vaccination - United States, January 2005-July 2007," *MMWR Morb Mortal Wkly Rep*, 2008, 57(17):457-60.

Centers for Disease Control, "Recommendations of the Advisory Committee on Immunization Practices (ACIP): General Recommendations on Immunization," *MMWR Recomm Rep*, 2006, 55(RR-15):1-48.

◆ **Menomune®-A/C/Y/W-135** *see* Meningococcal Polysaccharide Vaccine (Groups A / C / Y and W-135) *on page 1138*

◆ **Menostar®** *see* Estradiol (Systemic) *on page 641*

◆ **Menveo®** *see* Meningococcal (Groups A / C / Y and W-135) Diphtheria Conjugate Vaccine *on page 1137*

Meperidine (me PER i deen)

Related Information

Beers Criteria − Potentially Inappropriate Medications for Geriatrics *on page 2089*

Opioid Analgesics *on page 2013*

Patient Information for Disposal of Unused Medications *on page 2125*

Medication Safety Issues

Sound-alike/look-alike issues:

Meperidine may be confused with meprobamate

Demerol® may be confused with Demulen®, Desyrel, dicumarol, Dilaudid®, Dymelor®, Pamelor®

High alert medication:

The Institute for Safe Medication Practices (ISMP) includes this medication among its list of drug classes which have a heightened risk of causing significant patient harm when used in error.

BEERS Criteria medication:

This drug may be inappropriate for use in geriatric patients (high severity risk).

Other safety concerns:

Avoid the use of meperidine for pain control, especially in elderly and renally-compromised patients because of the risk of neurotoxicity (American Pain Society, 2008; Institute for Safe Medication Practices [ISMP], 2007)

Brand Names: U.S. Demerol®

Brand Names: Canada Demerol®

Index Terms Isonipecaine Hydrochloride; Meperidine Hydrochloride; Pethidine Hydrochloride

Generic Availability (U.S.) Yes

Pharmacologic Category Analgesic, Opioid

Use Management of moderate-to-severe pain; adjunct to anesthesia and preoperative sedation

Unlabeled/Investigational Use Reduce postoperative shivering; reduce rigors from amphotericin B (conventional)

Contraindications Hypersensitivity to meperidine or any component of the formulation; use with or within 14 days of MAO inhibitors

Warnings/Precautions Oral meperidine is not recommended for acute/chronic pain management. Meperidine should not be used for acute/cancer pain because of the risk of neurotoxicity. Normeperidine (an active metabolite and CNS stimulant) may accumulate and precipitate anxiety, tremors, or seizures; risk increases with CNS or renal dysfunction, prolonged use (>48 hours), and cumulative dose (>600 mg/24 hours). The Institute for Safe Medication Practice recommends avoiding the use of meperidine for pain control, especially in the elderly and renally-impaired (ISMP, 2007). In the elderly; meperidine is not an effective oral analgesic at commonly used doses; may cause confusion; other opioids are preferred in the elderly (Beers Criteria).

May cause CNS depression, which may impair physical or mental abilities; patients must be cautioned about performing tasks which require mental alertness (eg, operating machinery or driving). Effects may be potentiated when used with other sedative drugs or ethanol. Use only with extreme caution (if at all) in patients with head injury or increased intracranial pressure (ICP). Use caution with pulmonary, hepatic, or renal disorders, supraventricular tachycardias, acute abdominal conditions, hypothyroidism, toxic psychosis, kyphoscoliosis, morbid obesity, Addison's disease, BPH, or urethral stricture. Use with caution in patients with biliary tract dysfunction; acute pancreatitis may cause constriction of sphincter of Oddi. May cause hypotension; use with caution in patients with depleted blood volume or drugs which may exaggerate hypotensive effects (including phenothiazines or general anesthetics).

An opioid-containing analgesic regimen should be tailored to each patient's needs and based upon the type of pain being treated (acute versus chronic), the route of administration, degree of tolerance for opioids (naive versus chronic user), age, weight, and medical condition. The optimal analgesic dose varies widely among patients. Some preparations contain sulfites which may cause allergic reaction. Tolerance or drug dependence may result from extended use. Healthcare provider should be alert to problems of abuse, misuse, and diversion. Concurrent use of agonist/antagonist analgesics may precipitate withdrawal symptoms and/or reduced analgesic efficacy in patients following prolonged therapy with mu opioid agonists. Abrupt discontinuation following prolonged use may also lead to withdrawal symptoms. Avoid use in the elderly.

Adverse Reactions (Reflective of adult population; not specific for elderly) Frequency not defined.

Cardiovascular: Hypotension

Central nervous system: Fatigue, drowsiness, dizziness, nervousness, headache, restlessness, malaise, confusion, mental depression, hallucinations, paradoxical CNS stimulation, increased intracranial pressure, seizure (associated with metabolite accumulation), serotonin syndrome

Dermatologic: Rash, urticaria

Gastrointestinal: Nausea, vomiting, constipation, anorexia, stomach cramps, xerostomia, biliary spasm, paralytic ileus, sphincter of Oddi spasm

Genitourinary: Ureteral spasms, decreased urination

Local: Pain at injection site

Neuromuscular & skeletal: Weakness

Respiratory: Dyspnea

Miscellaneous: Anaphylaxis, histamine release, hypersensitivity reactions, physical and psychological dependence

Drug Interactions

Metabolism/Transport Effects Substrate (minor) of CYP2B6, 2C19, 3A4

Avoid Concomitant Use

Avoid concomitant use of Meperidine with any of the following: MAO Inhibitors; Sibutramine

Increased Effect/Toxicity

Meperidine may increase the levels/effects of: Alcohol (Ethyl); Alvimopan; CNS Depressants; Desmopressin; Selective Serotonin Reuptake Inhibitors; Serotonin Modulators; Thiazide Diuretics

The levels/effects of Meperidine may be increased by: Amphetamines; Antipsychotic Agents (Phenothiazines); Barbiturates; Droperidol; HydrOXYzine; MAO Inhibitors; Protease Inhibitors; Sibutramine; Succinylcholine

Decreased Effect

Meperidine may decrease the levels/effects of: Pegvisomant

The levels/effects of Meperidine may be decreased by: Ammonium Chloride; Fosphenytoin; Mixed Agonist / Antagonist Opioids; Phenytoin; Protease Inhibitors

Ethanol/Nutrition/Herb Interactions

Ethanol: May increase CNS depression; monitor for increased effects with coadministration. Caution patients about effects.

Herb/Nutraceutical: Avoid valerian, St John's wort, kava kava, gotu kola (may increase CNS depression).

Stability Meperidine injection should be stored at room temperature; do not freeze. Protect from light. Protect oral dosage forms from light.

Mechanism of Action Binds to opiate receptors in the CNS, causing inhibition of ascending pain pathways, altering the perception of and response to pain; produces generalized CNS depression

Pharmacodynamics/Kinetics

Onset of action: Analgesic: Oral, SubQ: 10-15 minutes; I.V.: ~5 minutes

Peak effect: SubQ.: ~1 hour; Oral: 2 hours

Duration: Oral, SubQ.: 2-4 hours

Absorption: I.M.: Erratic and highly variable

Protein binding: 65% to 75%

Metabolism: Hepatic; hydrolyzed to meperidinic acid (inactive) or undergoes N-demethylation to normeperidine (active; has 1/2 the analgesic effect and 2-3 times the CNS effects of meperidine)

Bioavailability: ~50% to 60%; increased with liver disease

Half-life elimination:
Parent drug: Terminal phase: Adults: 2.5-4 hours, Liver disease: 7-11 hours
Normeperidine (active metabolite): 15-30 hours; can accumulate with high doses (>600 mg/day) or with decreased renal function
Excretion: Urine (as metabolites)

Dosage
Geriatric Note: The American Pain Society (2008) and ISMP (2007) do not recommend meperidine's use as an analgesic.

Oral: 50 mg every 4 hours
I.M.: 25 mg every 4 hours

Adult Note: The American Pain Society (2008) and ISMP (2007) do not recommend meperidine's use as an analgesic. If use in acute pain (in patients without renal or CNS disease) cannot be avoided, treatment should be limited to ≤48 hours and doses should not exceed 600 mg/24 hours.

Pain (analgesic):
Oral: Initial: Opiate-naive: 50 mg every 3-4 hours as needed; usual dosage range: 50-150 mg every 2-4 hours as needed (manufacturers recommendation; oral route is not recommended for acute pain)
I.M., SubQ: Initial: Opiate-naive: 50-75 mg every 3-4 hours as needed; patients with prior opiate exposure may require higher initial doses.
Preoperatively: 50-100 mg given 30-90 minutes before the beginning of anesthesia
Slow I.V.: Initial: 5-10 mg every 5 minutes as needed
Postoperative shivering (unlabeled use): *I.V.:* 25-50 mg once (Crowley, 2008; Kranke, 2002; Mercandante, 1994; Wang, 1999)

Renal Impairment Avoid use in renal impairment.
Hepatic Impairment Increased narcotic effect in cirrhosis; reduction in dose is more important for oral than I.V. route.

Administration
Solution for injection: Meperidine may be administered I.M., SubQ, or I.V.; I.V. push should be administered slowly, use of a 10 mg/mL concentration has been recommended. For continuous I.V. infusions, a more dilute solution (eg, 1 mg/mL) should be used.
Oral solution: Administer solution in ½ glass of water; undiluted solution may exert topical anesthetic effect on mucous membranes

Monitoring Parameters Pain relief, respiratory and mental status, blood pressure; observe patient for excessive sedation, CNS depression, seizures, respiratory depression

Reference Range Therapeutic: 70-500 ng/mL (SI: 283-2020 nmol/L); Toxic: >1000 ng/mL (SI: >4043 nmol/L)

Test Interactions Increased amylase (S), increased BSP retention, increased CPK (I.M. injections)

Special Geriatric Considerations Meperidine is not recommended as a drug of first choice for the treatment of chronic pain in the elderly due to the accumulation of its metabolite, normeperidine, which leads to serious CNS side effects (eg, tremor, seizures). If used for acute pain, its use should be limited to 1-2 doses.

This medication is considered to be potentially inappropriate in this patient population (Beers Criteria severity: High).

Controlled Substance C-II
Dosage Forms Excipient information presented when available (limited, particularly for generics); consult specific product labeling.
Injection, solution, as hydrochloride: 25 mg/mL (1 mL); 50 mg/mL (1 mL); 100 mg/mL (1 mL)
Demerol®: 25 mg/mL (1 mL); 25 mg/0.5 mL (0.5 mL); 50 mg/mL (1 mL, 1.5 mL, 2 mL, 30 mL); 75 mg/mL (1 mL); 100 mg/mL (1 mL, 20 mL)
Injection, solution, as hydrochloride [for PCA pump]: 10 mg/mL (30 mL)
Solution, oral, as hydrochloride: 50 mg/5 mL (500 mL)
Tablet, oral, as hydrochloride: 50 mg, 100 mg
Demerol®: 50 mg [scored]
Demerol®: 100 mg

Selected References
American Geriatrics Society Panel on Pharmacological Management of Persistent Pain in Older Persons, "Pharmacological Management of Persistent Pain in Older Persons," *J Am Geriatr Soc*, 2009, 57(8):1331-46.
Institute for Safe Medication Practice, "High Alert Medication Feature: Reducing Patient Harm From Opiates," *ISMP Medication Safety Alert*, February 22, 2007. Available online at http://www.ismp.org/Newsletters/acutecare/articles/20070222.asp.
Latta KS, Ginsberg B, and Barkin RL, "Meperidine: A Critical Review," *Am J Ther*, 2002, 9(1):53-68.

◆ **Meperidine Hydrochloride** *see* Meperidine *on page 1140*

Mephobarbital (me foe BAR bi tal)

Medication Safety Issues
Sound-alike/look-alike issues:
Mephobarbital may be confused with methocarbamol
Mebaral® may be confused with Medrol®, Mellaril®, TEGretol®
BEERS Criteria medication:
This drug may be inappropriate for use in geriatric patients (high severity risk).
Brand Names: U.S. Mebaral® [DSC]
Brand Names: Canada Mebaral®
Index Terms Methylphenobarbital
Generic Availability (U.S.) No
Pharmacologic Category Barbiturate
Use Sedative; treatment of grand mal and petit mal epilepsy
Contraindications Hypersensitivity to mephobarbital, other barbiturates, or any component of the formulation; pre-existing CNS depression; respiratory depression; severe uncontrolled pain; history of porphyria
Warnings/Precautions Use with caution in patients with cardiovascular disease, depression or suicidal tendencies, myasthenia gravis, myxedema, respiratory disease, or in patients with acute or chronic pain or a history of substance abuse. Use caution in patients with hepatic or renal impairment; dosage adjustment recommended.

Use may cause CNS depression; use caution when performing tasks which require mental alertness. May cause paradoxical responses including agitation and hyperactivity. Effects may be potentiated when used concomitantly with sedatives or ethanol. Do not discontinue abruptly; therapy should be discontinued gradually to minimize the potential of increased seizure frequency.

May be inappropriate for use in the elderly due to increased risk for adverse effects and high addiction potential (Beers Criteria).

Adverse Reactions (Reflective of adult population; not specific for elderly)
>1%: Central nervous system: Somnolence

Drug Interactions
Metabolism/Transport Effects Substrate of CYP2B6 (minor), 2C9 (minor), 2C19 (major); **Inhibits** CYP2C19 (weak); **Induces** CYP2A6 (weak)

Avoid Concomitant Use
Avoid concomitant use of Mephobarbital with any of the following: Voriconazole

Increased Effect/Toxicity
Mephobarbital may increase the levels/effects of: Alcohol (Ethyl); CNS Depressants; Meperidine; QuiNIDine; Selective Serotonin Reuptake Inhibitors; Thiazide Diuretics

The levels/effects of Mephobarbital may be increased by: Chloramphenicol; CYP2C19 Inhibitors (Moderate); CYP2C19 Inhibitors (Strong); Divalproex; Droperidol; Felbamate; HydrOXYzine; Primidone; Valproic Acid

Decreased Effect
Mephobarbital may decrease the levels/effects of: Acetaminophen; Beta-Blockers; Calcium Channel Blockers; Chloramphenicol; Contraceptives (Estrogens); Contraceptives (Progestins); Corticosteroids (Systemic); CycloSPORINE; CycloSPORINE (Systemic); Disopyramide; Divalproex; Doxycycline; Etoposide; Etoposide Phosphate; Felbamate; Fosphenytoin; Griseofulvin; LamoTRIgine; Methadone; Phenytoin; Propafenone; QuiNIDine; Teniposide; Theophylline Derivatives; Tricyclic Antidepressants; Valproic Acid; Vitamin K Antagonists; Voriconazole

The levels/effects of Mephobarbital may be decreased by: CYP2C19 Inducers (Strong); Pyridoxine; Rifamycin Derivatives

Mechanism of Action Increases seizure threshold in the motor cortex; depresses monosynaptic and polysynaptic transmission in the CNS

Pharmacodynamics/Kinetics
Onset of action: 20-60 minutes
Duration: 6-8 hours
Absorption: ~50%
Half-life elimination, serum: 34 hours

Dosage
Geriatric Refer to adult dosing. Start at lowest recommended doses.
Adult
Epilepsy: Oral:
400-600 mg/day; **Note:** Initiate at low dose and gradually increase over 4-5 days. Taper other antiepileptics off as dose increases. When lowering or discontinuing dose, taper over 4-5 days.
Coadministration with phenobarbital: Average dose: 200-300 mg/day mephobarbital plus 50-100 mg/day of phenobarbital (doses should be approximately half the amount of those when used alone)
Coadministration with phenytoin: Use full dose of mephobarbital and reduce phenytoin dose (average dose: phenytoin 230 mg/day plus mephobarbital 600 mg/day)
Sedation: Oral: 32-100 mg 3-4 times/day
Renal Impairment Use with caution and reduce dose.
Hepatic Impairment Use with caution and reduce dose.
Administration Administer at bedtime if seizures occur at night and during the day if seizures are diurnal.
Pharmacotherapy Pearls May use in combination with phenobarbital or phenytoin. When using with phenobarbital, both agents should be started at $^1/_2$ dose. When mephobarbital is used with phenytoin, the dose of phenytoin must be reduced. Full doses of mephobarbital may be given.
Special Geriatric Considerations Using barbiturates in the elderly may induce paradoxical stimulation, cause or aggravate depression and confusion. Due to mephobarbital's long half-life and risk of dependence, it is not a drug of choice in the elderly as a sedative/hypnotic. Interpretive guidelines from Centers for Medicare and Medicaid Services (CMS) OBRA regulations discourage the use of barbiturates as sedative/hypnotics in nursing home patients.

This medication is considered to be potentially inappropriate in this patient population (Beers Criteria severity: High).
Controlled Substance C-IV
Dosage Forms Excipient information presented when available (limited, particularly for generics); consult specific product labeling. [DSC] = Discontinued product
Tablet, oral:
Mebaral®: 32 mg [DSC] [scored]
Mebaral®: 50 mg [DSC], 100 mg [DSC]

◆ **Mephyton®** *see* Phytonadione *on page 1450*

Meprobamate (me proe BA mate)

Related Information
Beers Criteria – Potentially Inappropriate Medications for Geriatrics *on page 2089*
Medication Safety Issues
Sound-alike/look-alike issues:
Meprobamate may be confused with Mepergan, meperidine
Equanil may be confused with Elavil®
BEERS Criteria medication:
This drug may be inappropriate for use in geriatric patients (high severity risk).
Brand Names: Canada Novo-Mepro
Index Terms Equanil
Generic Availability (U.S.) Yes
Pharmacologic Category Antianxiety Agent, Miscellaneous
Use Management of anxiety disorders
Unlabeled/Investigational Use Demonstrated value for muscle contraction, headache, external sphincter spasticity, muscle rigidity, opisthotonos-associated with tetanus
Contraindications Hypersensitivity to meprobamate, related compounds (including carisoprodol), or any component of the formulation; acute intermittent porphyria; pre-existing CNS depression; narrow-angle glaucoma; severe uncontrolled pain
Warnings/Precautions Physical and psychological dependence and abuse may occur; abrupt cessation may precipitate withdrawal. Use with caution in patients with depression or suicidal tendencies, or in patients with a history of drug abuse. May cause CNS depression, which may impair physical or mental abilities. Patients must be cautioned about performing tasks which require mental alertness (eg, operating machinery or driving). Effects with other sedative drugs or ethanol may be potentiated. Allergic reaction may occur in patients with history of dermatological condition (usually by fourth dose). Use with caution in patients with renal or hepatic impairment, or with a history of seizures. Use with caution in the elderly; may

cause confusion, cognitive impairment, excessive sedation, or addiction with prolonged use (Beers Criteria).

Adverse Reactions (Reflective of adult population; not specific for elderly) Frequency not defined.

Cardiovascular: Arrhythmia EEG abnormalities, hypotensive crisis, peripheral edema, palpitation, syncope, tachycardia

Central nervous system: Ataxia, chills, dizziness, drowsiness, euphoria, fever, headache, overstimulation, paradoxical excitement, slurred speech, vertigo

Dermatologic: Angioneurotic edema, bruising, dermatitis, erythema multiforme, petechiae, purpura, rash, Stevens-Johnson syndrome

Gastrointestinal: Diarrhea, nausea, proctitis, stomatitis, vomiting

Hematologic: Agranulocytosis, aplastic anemia, eosinophilia, leukopenia, porphyria exacerbation, thrombocytopenic purpura

Neuromuscular & skeletal: Paresthesia, weakness

Ocular: Impairment of accommodation

Renal: Anuria, oliguria

Respiratory: Bronchospasm

Miscellaneous: Anaphylaxis, hypersensitivity

Drug Interactions

Avoid Concomitant Use There are no known interactions where it is recommended to avoid concomitant use.

Increased Effect/Toxicity

Meprobamate may increase the levels/effects of: Alcohol (Ethyl); CNS Depressants; Methotrimeprazine; Selective Serotonin Reuptake Inhibitors

The levels/effects of Meprobamate may be increased by: Droperidol; HydrOXYzine; Methotrimeprazine

Decreased Effect

The levels/effects of Meprobamate may be decreased by: Yohimbine

Ethanol/Nutrition/Herb Interactions

Ethanol: May increase CNS depression; monitor for increased effects with coadministration. Caution patients about effects.

Herb/Nutraceutical: Avoid valerian, St John's wort, kava kava, gotu kola (may increase CNS depression).

Mechanism of Action Affects the thalamus and limbic system; also appears to inhibit multineuronal spinal reflexes

Pharmacodynamics/Kinetics

Onset of action: Sedation: ~1 hour

Metabolism: Hepatic

Half-life elimination: 10 hours

Excretion: Urine (8% to 20% as unchanged drug); feces (10% as metabolites)

Dosage

Adult Anxiety or muscle spasm (TMJ) pain (unlabeled use): Oral: 1200-1600 mg/day in 3-4 divided doses, up to 2400 mg/day

Renal Impairment

Cl_{cr} 10-50 mL/minute: Administer every 9-12 hours.

Cl_{cr} <10 mL/minute: Administer every 12-18 hours.

Moderately dialyzable (20% to 50%)

Hepatic Impairment Probably necessary in patients with liver disease; no specific recommendations.

Monitoring Parameters Mental status

Reference Range Therapeutic: 6-12 mcg/mL (SI: 28-55 μmol/L); Toxic: >60 mcg/mL (SI: >275 μmol/L)

Pharmacotherapy Pearls Withdrawal should be gradual over 1-2 weeks. Benzodiazepine and buspirone are better choices for treatment of anxiety disorders.

Special Geriatric Considerations Meprobamate is not considered a drug of choice in the elderly because of its potential to cause physical and psychological dependence. Interpretive guidelines from the Centers for Medicare and Medicaid Services (CMS) strongly discourage the use of meprobamate in residents of long-term care facilities.

This medication is considered to be potentially inappropriate in this patient population (Beers Criteria severity: High).

Controlled Substance C-IV

Dosage Forms Excipient information presented when available (limited, particularly for generics); consult specific product labeling.

Tablet, oral: 200 mg, 400 mg

Mercaptopurine (mer kap toe PYOOR een)

Medication Safety Issues
Sound-alike/look-alike issues:
Mercaptopurine may be confused with methotrexate
Purinethol® may be confused with propylthiouracil
High alert medication:
The Institute for Safe Medication Practices (ISMP) includes this medication among its list of drugs which have a heightened risk of causing significant patient harm when used in error.
Other safety concerns:
To avoid potentially serious dosage errors, the terms "6-mercaptopurine" or "6-MP" should be avoided; use of these terms has been associated with sixfold overdosages.
Azathioprine is metabolized to mercaptopurine; concurrent use of these commercially-available products has resulted in profound myelosuppression.

Brand Names: U.S. Purinethol®
Brand Names: Canada Purinethol®
Index Terms 6-Mercaptopurine (error-prone abbreviation); 6-MP (error-prone abbreviation); NSC-755
Generic Availability (U.S.) Yes
Pharmacologic Category Antineoplastic Agent, Antimetabolite; Antineoplastic Agent, Antimetabolite (Purine Analog); Immunosuppressant Agent
Use Treatment (maintenance and induction) of acute lymphoblastic leukemia (ALL)
Unlabeled/Investigational Use Steroid-sparing agent for corticosteroid-dependent Crohn's disease (CD) and ulcerative colitis (UC); maintenance of remission in CD; fistulizing Crohn's disease
Contraindications Hypersensitivity to mercaptopurine or any component of the formulation; patients whose disease showed prior resistance to mercaptopurine or thioguanine; severe liver disease, severe bone marrow suppression
Warnings/Precautions Hazardous agent - use appropriate precautions for handling and disposal. Consider adjusting dosage in patients with renal impairment or hepatic failure; use with caution in patients with prior bone marrow suppression. Toxicity to immunosuppressives is increased in elderly. Start with lowest recommended adult doses. Signs of infection, such as fever and WBC rise, may not occur. Lethargy and confusion may be more prominent signs of infection. Use caution with other hepatotoxic drugs or in dosages >2.5 mg/kg/day; hepatotoxicity may occur. Patients with genetic deficiency of thiopurine methyltransferase (TPMT) or concurrent therapy with drugs which may inhibit TPMT (eg, olsalazine) or xanthine oxidase (eg, allopurinol) may be sensitive to myelosuppressive effects. Azathioprine is metabolized to mercaptopurine; concomitant use may result in profound myelosuppression and should be avoided. Immune response to vaccines may be diminished.

To avoid potentially serious dosage errors, the terms "6-mercaptopurine" or "6-MP" should be avoided; use of these terms has been associated with sixfold overdosages.

Adverse Reactions (Reflective of adult population; not specific for elderly)
>10%:
Hematologic: Myelosuppression; leukopenia, thrombocytopenia, anemia
Onset: 7-10 days
Nadir: 14-16 days
Recovery: 21-28 days
Hepatic: Intrahepatic cholestasis and focal centralobular necrosis (40%), characterized by hyperbilirubinemia, increased alkaline phosphatase and AST, jaundice, ascites, encephalopathy; more common at doses >2.5 mg/kg/day. Usually occurs within 2 months of therapy but may occur within 1 week, or be delayed up to 8 years.
1% to 10%:
Central nervous system: Drug fever
Dermatologic: Hyperpigmentation, rash
Endocrine & metabolic: Hyperuricemia
Gastrointestinal: Anorexia, diarrhea, mucositis, nausea, pancreatitis, stomach pain, stomatitis, vomiting
Renal: Renal toxicity

Drug Interactions
Avoid Concomitant Use
Avoid concomitant use of Mercaptopurine with any of the following: AzaTHIOprine; BCG; Febuxostat; Natalizumab; Pimecrolimus; Tacrolimus (Topical)

Increased Effect/Toxicity

Mercaptopurine may increase the levels/effects of: Leflunomide; Natalizumab; Vaccines (Live); Vitamin K Antagonists

The levels/effects of Mercaptopurine may be increased by: 5-ASA Derivatives; Allopurinol; AzaTHIOprine; Denosumab; Febuxostat; Pimecrolimus; Roflumilast; Tacrolimus (Topical); Trastuzumab

Decreased Effect

Mercaptopurine may decrease the levels/effects of: BCG; Sipuleucel-T; Vaccines (Inactivated); Vitamin K Antagonists

The levels/effects of Mercaptopurine may be decreased by: Echinacea

Stability Store at room temperature of 15°C to 25°C (59°F to 77°F). Protect from moisture.

Mechanism of Action Purine antagonist which inhibits DNA and RNA synthesis; acts as false metabolite and is incorporated into DNA and RNA, eventually inhibiting their synthesis; specific for the S phase of the cell cycle

Pharmacodynamics/Kinetics

Absorption: Variable and incomplete (16% to 50%)

Distribution: V_d = total body water; CNS penetration is poor

Protein binding: 19%

Metabolism: Hepatic and in GI mucosa; hepatically via xanthine oxidase and methylation via TPMT to sulfate conjugates, 6-thiouric acid, and other inactive compounds; first-pass effect

Half-life elimination (age dependent): Adults: 47 minutes

Time to peak, serum: ~2 hours

Excretion: Urine (46% as mercaptopurine and metabolites)

Dosage

Geriatric Due to renal decline with age, start with lower recommended doses for adults.

Adult Refer to individual protocols.

ALL:

Induction: Oral: 2.5-5 mg/kg/day (100-200 mg)

Maintenance: Oral: 1.5-2.5 mg/kg/day **or** 80-100 mg/m²/day given once daily

Note: In ALL, administration in the evening (vs morning administration) may lower the risk of relapse.

Reduction of steroid use in CD or UC, maintenance of remission in CD or fistulizing disease (unlabeled uses): Oral: Initial: 50 mg/day; may increase by 25 mg/day every 1-2 weeks as tolerated to target dose of 1-1.5 mg/kg/day

Dosage adjustment with concurrent allopurinol: Reduce mercaptopurine dosage to ¼ to ⅓ the usual dose.

Dosage adjustment in TPMT-deficiency: Not established; substantial reductions are generally required only in homozygous deficiency.

Renal Impairment The FDA-approved labeling recommends starting with reduced doses in patients with renal impairment to avoid accumulation; however, specific guidelines are not available. The following guidelines have been used by some clinicians (Aronoff, 2007): Children:

Cl_{cr} <50 mL/minute: Administer every 48 hours

Hemodialysis: Administer every 48 hours

Continuous ambulatory peritoneal dialysis (CAPD): Administer every 48 hours

Continuous renal replacement therapy (CRRT): Administer every 48 hours

Hepatic Impairment The FDA-approved labeling recommends considering a reduced dose in patients with hepatic impairment; however, specific guidelines are not available.

Administration Preferably on an empty stomach (1 hour before or 2 hours after meals)

Monitoring Parameters CBC with differential and platelet count, liver function tests, uric acid, urinalysis; TPMT genotyping may identify individuals at risk for toxicity

For use as immunomodulatory therapy in CD or UC, monitor CBC with differential weekly for 1 month, then biweekly for 1 month, followed by monitoring every 1-2 months throughout the course of therapy. LFTs should be assessed every 3 months.

Special Geriatric Considerations Toxicity to immunosuppressives is increased in the elderly. Start with lowest recommended adult doses. Signs of infection, such as fever and WBC rise, may not occur. Lethargy and confusion may be more prominent signs of infection.

Dosage Forms Excipient information presented when available (limited, particularly for generics); consult specific product labeling.

Tablet, oral: 50 mg

Purinethol®: 50 mg [scored]

Selected References

Lichtenstein GR, Abreu MT, Cohen R, et al, "American Gastroenterological Association Institute Medical Position Statement on Corticosteroids, Immunomodulators, and Infliximab in Inflammatory Bowel Disease," *Gastroenterology*, 2006, 130(3):935-9.

◆ **6-Mercaptopurine (error-prone abbreviation)** *see* Mercaptopurine *on page 1146*

Meropenem (mer oh PEN em)

Medication Safety Issues
Sound-alike/look-alike issues:
Meropenem may be confused with ertapenem, imipenem, metronidazole.
Brand Names: U.S. Merrem® I.V.
Brand Names: Canada Merrem®
Generic Availability (U.S.) Yes
Pharmacologic Category Antibiotic, Carbapenem
Use
Treatment of intra-abdominal infections (complicated appendicitis and peritonitis); treatment of complicated skin and skin structure infections caused by susceptible organisms

Canadian labeling: Additional indications (not in U.S. labeling): Treatment of lower respiratory tract infections (community-acquired and nosocomial pneumonias), complicated urinary tract infections, gynecologic infections (excluding chlamydia), and septicemia; treatment of bacterial meningitis in adults caused by *S. pneumoniae*, *H. influenzae*, and *N. meningitidis* (use in adult meningitis based on pediatric data)

Unlabeled/Investigational Use *Burkholderia pseudomallei* (melioidosis), febrile neutropenia, liver abscess, otitis externa

Contraindications Hypersensitivity to meropenem, any component of the formulation, or other carbapenems (eg, doripenem, ertapenem, imipenem); patients who have experienced anaphylactic reactions to other beta-lactams

Warnings/Precautions Serious hypersensitivity reactions, including anaphylaxis, have been reported (some without a history of previous allergic reactions to beta-lactams). Carbapenems have been associated with CNS adverse effects, including confusional states and seizures (myoclonic); use caution with CNS disorders (eg, brain lesions and history of seizures) and adjust dose in renal impairment to avoid drug accumulation, which may increase seizure risk. Prolonged use may result in fungal or bacterial superinfection, including *C. difficile*-associated diarrhea (CDAD) and pseudomembranous colitis; CDAD has been observed >2 months postantibiotic treatment. Use with caution in patients with renal impairment; dosage adjustment required in patients with moderate-to-severe renal dysfunction. Thrombocytopenia has been reported in patients with renal dysfunction. Lower doses (based upon renal function) are often required in the elderly. May decrease divalproex sodium/valproic acid concentrations leading to breakthrough seizures; concomitant use not recommended. Alternative antimicrobial agents should be considered; if concurrent meropenem is necessary, consider additional antiseizure medication.

Adverse Reactions (Reflective of adult population; not specific for elderly)
1% to 10%:
Central nervous system: Headache (2% to 8%), pain (≤5%)
Dermatologic: Rash (2% to 3%, includes diaper-area moniliasis in pediatrics), pruritus (1%)
Endocrine & metabolic: Hypoglycemia
Gastrointestinal: Diarrhea (4% to 7%), nausea/vomiting (1% to 8%), constipation (1% to 7%), oral moniliasis (up to 2% in pediatric patients), glossitis (1%)
Hematologic: Anemia (≤6%)
Local: Inflammation at the injection site (2%), phlebitis/thrombophlebitis (1%), injection site reaction (1%)
Respiratory: Apnea (1%), pharyngitis, pneumonia
Miscellaneous: Sepsis (2%), shock (1%)
Drug Interactions
Avoid Concomitant Use
Avoid concomitant use of Meropenem with any of the following: BCG; Probenecid
Increased Effect/Toxicity
The levels/effects of Meropenem may be increased by: Probenecid
Decreased Effect
Meropenem may decrease the levels/effects of: BCG; Divalproex; Typhoid Vaccine; Valproic Acid

Stability Dry powder should be stored at controlled room temperature 20°C to 25°C (68°F to 77°F). Meropenem infusion vials may be reconstituted with SWFI or a compatible diluent (eg, NS). The 500 mg vials should be reconstituted with 10 mL, and 1 g vials with 20 mL. May be further diluted with compatible solutions for infusion. Consult detailed reference/product labeling for compatibility.
Injection reconstitution: Stability in vial when constituted (up to 50 mg/mL) with:
SWFI: Stable for up to 2 hours at controlled room temperature of 15°C to 25°C (59°F to 77°F) or for up to 12 hours under refrigeration.

Sodium chloride: Stable for up to 2 hours at controlled room temperature of 15°C to 25°C (59°F to 77°F) or for up to 18 hours under refrigeration.

Dextrose 5% injection: Stable for 1 hour at controlled room temperature of 15°C to 25°C (59°F to 77°F) or for 8 hours under refrigeration.

Infusion admixture (1-20 mg/mL): Solution stability when diluted in NS is 4 hours at controlled room temperature of 15°C to 25°C (59°F to 77°F) or 24 hours under refrigeration. Stability in D₅W is 1 hour at controlled room temperature of 15°C to 25°C (59°F to 77°F) or 4 hours under refrigeration. For other diluents, see prescribing information.

Mechanism of Action Inhibits bacterial cell wall synthesis by binding to several of the penicillin-binding proteins, which in turn inhibit the final transpeptidation step of peptidoglycan synthesis in bacterial cell walls, thus inhibiting cell wall biosynthesis; bacteria eventually lyse due to ongoing activity of cell wall autolytic enzymes (autolysins and murein hydrolases) while cell wall assembly is arrested

Pharmacodynamics/Kinetics

Distribution: V_d: ~0.3 L/kg; penetrates well into most body fluids and tissues; CSF concentrations approximate those of the plasma

Protein binding: ~2%

Metabolism: Hepatic; metabolized to open beta-lactam form (inactive)

Half-life elimination:

Normal renal function: 1-1.5 hours

Cl_{cr} 30-80 mL/minute: 1.9-3.3 hours

Cl_{cr} 2-30 mL/minute: 3.82-5.7 hours

Time to peak, tissue: 1 hour following infusion

Excretion: Urine (~70% as unchanged drug)

Dosage

Geriatric & Adult

Usual dosage range: I.V.: 1.5-6 g/day divided every 8 hours

Extended infusion method (unlabeled dosing): I.V.: 0.5-2 g over 3 hours every 8 hours (Crandon 2011; Dandekar, 2003). **Note:** Dosing used at some centers and is based on pharmacokinetic/pharmacodynamic modeling and not clinical efficacy data.

Indication-specific dosing:

***Burkholderia pseudomallei* (melioidosis) (unlabeled use), *Pseudomonas*:** I.V.: 1 g every 8 hours

Cholangitis, intra-abdominal infections, complicated: I.V.: 1 g every 8 hours. **Note:** 2010 IDSA guidelines recommend treatment duration of 4-7 days (provided source controlled). Not recommended for mild-to-moderate, community-acquired intra-abdominal infections due to risk of toxicity and the development of resistant organisms (Solomkin, 2010).

Febrile neutropenia, otitis externa, pneumonia (unlabeled uses): I.V.: 1 g every 8 hours

Gynecologic and pelvic inflammatory disease: *Canadian labeling (not in U.S. labeling):* I.V.: 500 mg every 8 hours

Liver abscess (unlabeled use): I.V.: 1 g every 8 hours for 2-3 weeks, then oral therapy for duration of 4-6 weeks

Meningitis: *Canadian labeling (not in U.S. labeling):* I.V.: 2 g every 8 hours

Mild-to-moderate infection, other severe infections (unlabeled use): I.V.: 1.5-3 g/day divided every 8 hours

Pneumonia (community-acquired): *Canadian labeling (not in U.S. labeling):* I.V.: 500 mg every 8 hours

Pneumonia (nosocomial): *Canadian labeling (not in U.S. labeling):* I.V.: 1 g every 8 hours

Septicemia: *Canadian labeling (not in U.S. labeling):* I.V.: 1 g every 8 hours

Skin and skin structure infections:

Complicated: I.V.: 500 mg every 8 hours; diabetic foot: 1 g every 8 hours

Uncomplicated: *Canadian labeling (not in U.S. labeling):* I.V.: 500 mg every 8 hours

Urinary tract infections (complicated): *Canadian labeling (not in U.S. labeling):* I.V.: 500 mg every 8 hours. **Note:** Up to 1 g every 8 hours may be administered (Pallett, 2010).

Renal Impairment

Adults:

Cl_{cr} 26-50 mL/minute: Administer recommended dose based on indication every 12 hours

Cl_{cr} 10-25 mL/minute: Administer one-half recommended dose based on indication every 12 hours

Cl_{cr} <10 mL/minute: Administer one-half recommended dose based on indication every 24 hours

Alternative dosing recommendations: (unlabeled dosing; Aronoff, 2007):

GFR 10-50 mL/minute: Administer recommended dose (based on indication) every 12 hours

GFR <10 mL/minute: Administer recommended dose (based on indication) every 24 hours

Intermittent hemodialysis (IHD) (administer after hemodialysis on dialysis days): Meropenem and its metabolite are readily dialyzable: 500 mg every 24 hours. **Note:** Dosing dependent on the assumption of 3 times/week, complete IHD sessions.

Peritoneal dialysis (unlabeled dose): Administer recommended dose (based on indication) every 24 hours (Aronoff, 2007).

Continuous renal replacement therapy (CRRT) (Heintz, 2009; Trotman, 2005): Drug clearance is highly dependent on the method of renal replacement, filter type, and flow rate. Appropriate dosing requires close monitoring of pharmacologic response, signs of adverse reactions due to drug accumulation, as well as drug concentrations in relation to target trough (if appropriate). The following are general recommendations only (based on dialysate flow/ultrafiltration rates of 1-2 L/hour and minimal residual renal function) and should not supersede clinical judgment:

CVVH: Loading dose of 1 g followed by either 0.5 g every 8 hours **or** 1 g every 12 hours
CVVHD/CVVHDF: Loading dose of 1 g followed by either 0.5 g every 6-8 hours **or** 1 g every 8-12 hours

Note: Consider giving patients receiving CVVHDF dosages of 750 mg every 8 hours **or** 1500 mg every 12 hours (Heintz, 2009). Substantial variability exists in various published recommendations, ranging from 1-3 g/day in 2-3 divided doses. One gram every 12 hours achieves a target trough of ~4 mg/L.

Administration Administer I.V. infusion over 15-30 minutes; I.V. bolus injection (5-20 mL) over 3-5 minutes

Extended infusion administration (unlabeled dosing): Administer over 3 hours (Crandon 2011; Dandekar, 2003). **Note:** Must consider meropenem's limited room temperature stability if using extended infusions

Monitoring Parameters Perform culture and sensitivity testing prior to initiating therapy. Monitor for signs of anaphylaxis during first dose. During prolonged therapy, monitor renal function, liver function, CBC.

Test Interactions Positive Coombs' [direct]

Special Geriatric Considerations Adjust dose based on renal function.

Dosage Forms Excipient information presented when available (limited, particularly for generics); consult specific product labeling.

Injection, powder for reconstitution: 500 mg, 1 g
Merrem® I.V.: 500 mg [contains sodium 45.1 mg as sodium carbonate (1.96 mEq)]
Merrem® I.V.: 1 g [contains sodium 90.2 mg as sodium carbonate (3.92 mEq)]

Selected References

Ljungberg B and Nilsson-Ehle I, "Pharmacokinetics of Meropenem an Its Metabolites in Young and Elderly Healthy Men," *Antimicrob Agents Chemother*, 1992, 36(7):1437-40.

Mandell LA, Wunderink RG, Anzueto A, et al, "Infectious Diseases Society of America/American Thoracic Society Consensus Guidelines on the Management of Community-Acquired Pneumonia in Adults," *Clin Infect Dis*, 2007, 44 Suppl 2:S27-72.

Wiseman LR, Wagstaff AJ, Brogden RN, et al, "Meropenem. A Review of Its Antibacterial Activity, Pharmacokinetic Properties and Clinical Efficacy," *Drugs*, 1995, 50(1):73-101.

◆ **Merrem® I.V.** *see* Meropenem *on page* 1148

Mesalamine (me SAL a meen)

Medication Safety Issues
Sound-alike/look-alike issues:
Mesalamine may be confused with mecamylamine, megestrol, memantine, metaxalone, methenamine
Apriso™ may be confused with Apri®
Asacol® may be confused with Ansaid®, Os-Cal®, Visicol®
Lialda® may be confused with Aldara®
Pentasa® may be confused with Pancrease®, Pangestyme™

Brand Names: U.S. Apriso™; Asacol®; Asacol® HD; Canasa®; Lialda®; Pentasa®; Rowasa®; sfRowasa™

Brand Names: Canada 5-ASA; Asacol®; Asacol® 800; Mesasal®; Mezavant®; Novo-5 ASA; Novo-5 ASA-ECT; Pentasa®; Salofalk®; Salofalk® 5-ASA

Index Terms 5-Aminosalicylic Acid; 5-ASA; Fisalamine; Mesalazine

Generic Availability (U.S.) Yes: Rectal suspension

Pharmacologic Category 5-Aminosalicylic Acid Derivative

Use

Oral:

Asacol®, Lialda®, Pentasa®: Treatment and maintenance of remission of mildly- to moderately-active ulcerative colitis

Apriso™: Maintenance of remission of ulcerative colitis

Asacol® HD: Treatment of moderately-active ulcerative colitis

Rectal: Treatment of active mild-to-moderate distal ulcerative colitis, proctosigmoiditis, or proctitis

Contraindications Hypersensitivity to mesalamine, aminosalicylates, salicylates, or any component of the formulation

Warnings/Precautions May cause an acute intolerance syndrome (cramping, acute abdominal pain, bloody diarrhea; sometimes fever, headache, rash); discontinue if this occurs. Use caution in patients with active peptic ulcers. Patients with pyloric stenosis may have prolonged gastric retention of tablets, delaying the release of mesalamine in the colon. Pericarditis or myocarditis should be considered in patients with chest pain; use with caution in patients predisposed to these conditions. Pancreatitis should be considered in patients with new abdominal discomfort. Symptomatic worsening of colitis/IBD may occur following initiation of therapy. Oligospermia (rare, reversible) has been reported in males. Use caution in patients with sulfasalazine hypersensitivity. Use caution in patients with impaired hepatic function; hepatic failure has been reported. Renal impairment (including minimal change nephropathy and acute/chronic interstitial nephritis) and rarely failure have been reported; use caution in patients with renal impairment. Use caution with other medications converted to mesalamine. Postmarketing reports suggest an increased incidence of blood dyscrasias in patients >65 years of age. In addition, elderly may have difficulty administering and retaining rectal suppositories or may have decreased renal function; use with caution and monitor.

Apriso™ contains phenylalanine. The Asacol® HD 800 mg tablet has not been shown to be bioequivalent to 2 Asacol® 400 mg tablets. Canasa® suppositories contain saturated vegetable fatty acid esters (contraindicated in patients with allergy to these components). Rowasa® enema contains potassium metabisulfite; may cause severe hypersensitivity reactions (ie, anaphylaxis) in patients with sulfite allergies.

Adverse Reactions (Reflective of adult population; not specific for elderly) Adverse effects vary depending upon dosage form. Incidence usually on lower end with enema and suppository dosage forms.

>10%:

Central nervous system: Headache (2% to 35%), pain (≤14%)

Gastrointestinal: Abdominal pain (1% to 18%), eructation (16%), nausea (3% to 13%)

Respiratory: Pharyngitis (11%)

1% to 10%:

Cardiovascular: Chest pain (3%), peripheral edema (3%), vasodilation (≥2%)

Central nervous system: Dizziness (2% to 8%), fever (1% to 6%), chills (3%), malaise (2% to 3%), fatigue (<3%), vertigo (<3%), anxiety (≥2%), migraine (≥2%), nervousness (≥2%), insomnia (2%),

Dermatologic: Rash (1% to 6%), pruritus (1% to 3%), alopecia (<3%), acne (1% to 2%)

Endocrine & metabolic: Triglyceride increased (<3%)

Gastrointestinal: Diarrhea (2% to 8%), dyspepsia (1% to 6%), flatulence (1% to 6%), constipation (5%), vomiting (1% to 5%), colitis exacerbation (1% to 3%), rectal bleeding (<3%), abdominal distention (≥2%), gastroenteritis (≥2%), gastrointestinal bleeding (≥2%), stool abnormalities (≥2%), tenesmus (≥2%), rectal pain (1% to 2%), hemorrhoids (1%)

Genitourinary: Polyuria (≥2%)

Hematologic: Hematocrit/hemoglobin decreased (<3%)

Hepatic: Cholestatic hepatitis (<3%), transaminases increased (<3%), ALT increased (1%)

Local: Pain on insertion of enema tip (1%)

Neuromuscular & skeletal: Back pain (1% to 7%), arthralgia (≤5%), hypertonia (5%), myalgia (3%), paresthesia (≥2%), weakness (≥2%), arthritis (2%), leg/joint pain (2%)

Ocular: Vision abnormalities (≥2%), conjunctivitis (2%)

Otic: Tinnitus (<3%), ear pain (≥2%)

Renal: Creatinine clearance decreased (<3%), hematuria (<3%)

Respiratory: Nasopharyngitis (1% to 4%), dyspnea (<3%), bronchitis (≥2%), sinusitis (≥2%), cough (≤2%)

Miscellaneous: Flu-like syndrome (1% to 5%), infection (≥2%), diaphoresis (3%), intolerance syndrome (3%)

Drug Interactions

Avoid Concomitant Use There are no known interactions where it is recommended to avoid concomitant use.

◀ **Increased Effect/Toxicity**

Mesalamine may increase the levels/effects of: Heparin; Heparin (Low Molecular Weight); Thiopurine Analogs; Varicella Virus-Containing Vaccines

Decreased Effect

Mesalamine may decrease the levels/effects of: Cardiac Glycosides

The levels/effects of Mesalamine may be decreased by: Antacids; H2-Antagonists; Proton Pump Inhibitors

Stability

Capsule:

Apriso™: Store at controlled room temperature of 20°C to 25°C (68°F to 77°F)

Pentasa®: Store at controlled room temperature of 15°C to 30°C (59°F to 86°F). Protect from light.

Enema: Store at controlled room temperature. Use promptly once foil wrap is removed. Contents may darken with time (do not use if dark brown).

Suppository: Store below 25°C (below 77°F). May store under refrigeration; do not freeze. Protect from direct heat, light, and humidity.

Tablet: Store at controlled room temperature:

Asacol®, Asacol® HD: 20°C to 25°C (68°F to 77°F)

Lialda®: 15°C to 30°C (59°F to 86°F)

Mezavant®: 15°C to 25°C (59°F to 77°F)

Mechanism of Action Mesalamine (5-aminosalicylic acid) is the active component of sulfasalazine; the specific mechanism of action of mesalamine is unknown; however, it is thought that it modulates local chemical mediators of the inflammatory response, especially leukotrienes, and is also postulated to be a free radical scavenger or an inhibitor of tumor necrosis factor (TNF); action appears topical rather than systemic

Pharmacodynamics/Kinetics

Absorption: Rectal: Variable and dependent upon retention time, underlying GI disease, and colonic pH; Oral: Tablet: ~20% to 28%, Capsule: ~20% to 40%

Distribution: ~18 L

Protein binding: 43%

Metabolism: Hepatic and via GI tract to acetyl-5-aminosalicylic acid

Half-life elimination: 5-ASA: 0.5-10 hours; N-acetyl-5-ASA: 2-15 hours

Time to peak, serum:

Capsule: Apriso™: ~4 hours; Pentasa®: 3 hours

Rectal: 4-7 hours

Tablet: Asacol®: 4-12 hours; Asacol® HD: 10-16 hours; Lialda™: 9-12 hours; Mezavant®: 8 hours

Excretion: Urine (primarily as metabolites, <8% as unchanged drug); feces (<2%)

Dosage

Geriatric & Adult

Treatment of ulcerative colitis: Oral: Usual course of therapy is 3-8 weeks:

Capsule (Pentasa®): 1 g 4 times/day; **Note:** Apriso™ capsules are approved for maintenance of remission only.

Tablet: Initial:

Asacol®: 800 mg 3 times/day for 6 weeks

Asacol® HD: 1.6 g 3 times/day for 6 weeks

Lialda®, Mezavant®: 2.4-4.8 g once daily for up to 8 weeks

Maintenance of remission of ulcerative colitis: Oral:

Capsule:

Apriso™: 1.5 g once daily in the morning

Pentasa®: 1 g 4 times/day

Tablet:

Asacol®: 1.6 g/day in divided doses

Lialda®: 2.4 g once daily

Note: Asacol® HD and Mezavant® tablets are approved for treatment only.

Active mild-to-moderate distal ulcerative colitis, proctosigmoiditis, or proctitis: Retention enema: 60 mL (4 g) at bedtime, retained overnight, approximately 8 hours

Active ulcerative proctitis: Rectal suppository (Canasa®): Insert one 1000 mg suppository in rectum daily at bedtime; retained for at least 1-3 hours to achieve maximum benefit

Note: Duration of rectal therapy is 3-6 weeks; some patients may require rectal and oral therapy concurrently.

Administration

Oral: Swallow capsules or tablets whole, do not break, chew, or crush.

Apriso™: Administer with or without food; do not administer with antacids

Asacol®: Do not break outer coating.

Asacol® HD: Do not break outer coating; administer with or without food.

Lialda™: Do not break outer coating; should be administered once daily with a meal

Mezavant®: Do not break outer coating; should be administered once daily with a meal

Rectal enema: Shake bottle well. Retain enemas for 8 hours or as long as practical.

Suppository: Remove foil wrapper; avoid excessive handling. Should be retained for at least 1-3 hours to achieve maximum benefit.

Monitoring Parameters Renal function (prior to and periodically during therapy); CBC (particularly in elderly patients)

Pharmacotherapy Pearls Patients hypersensitive to sulfasalazine may tolerate mesalamine rectally; however, use with caution.

Special Geriatric Considerations Use with caution. Elderly may have difficulty administering and retaining rectal suppositories. Given renal function decline with aging, monitor serum creatinine often during therapy.

Dosage Forms Excipient information presented when available (limited, particularly for generics); consult specific product labeling.

Capsule, controlled release, oral:

Pentasa®: 250 mg, 500 mg

Capsule, delayed and extended release, oral:

Apriso™: 0.375 g [contains phenylalanine 0.56 mg/capsule]

Suppository, rectal:

Canasa®: 1000 mg (30s, 42s) [contains saturated vegetable fatty esters]

Suspension, rectal: 4 g/60 mL (7s, 28s)

Rowasa®: 4 g/60 mL (7s) [contains potassium metabisulfite, sodium benzoate; packaged with wipes]

Rowasa®: 4 g/60 mL (28s) [contains potassium metabisulfite, sodium benzoate; packaged with wipes]

sfRowasa™: 4 g/60 mL (7s, 28s) [contains sodium benzoate]

Tablet, delayed release, enteric coated, oral:

Asacol®: 400 mg

Asacol® HD: 800 mg

Lialda®: 1.2 g

Dosage Forms: Canada Excipient information presented when available (limited, particularly for generics); consult specific product labeling.

Tablet, delayed and extended release:

Mezavant®: 1.2 g

Selected References

Kamm MA, Sandborn WJ, Gassull M, et al, "Once-Daily, High-Concentration MMX Mesalamine in Active Ulcerative Colitis," *Gastroenterology*, 2007, 132(1):66-75.

Metaprotenerol (met a proe TER e nol)

Related Information

Inhalant Agents *on page 2010*

Medication Safety Issues

Sound-alike/look-alike issues:

Metaproterenol may be confused with metipranolol, metoprolol

Alupent may be confused with Atrovent®

Brand Names: Canada Apo-Orciprenaline®; ratio-Orciprenaline®; Tanta-Orciprenaline®

Index Terms Alupent; Metaproterenol Sulfate; Orciprenaline Sulfate

Generic Availability (U.S.) Yes

Pharmacologic Category Beta$_2$-Adrenergic Agonist

Use Bronchodilator in reversible airway obstruction due to asthma or COPD

Contraindications Hypersensitivity to metaproterenol or any component of the formulation; pre-existing cardiac arrhythmias associated with tachycardia

Warnings/Precautions Use beta$_2$-agonists with caution in patients with cardiovascular disease (arrhythmia or hypertension or HF), convulsive disorders, diabetes, glaucoma, hyperthyroidism, or hypokalemia. Beta-agonists may cause elevation in blood pressure, heart rate, and result in CNS stimulation/excitation. Beta$_2$-agonists may increase risk of arrhythmia, increase serum glucose, or decrease serum potassium. Immediate hypersensitivity reactions (urticaria, angioedema, rash, bronchospasm) have been reported.

Asthma: Appropriate use: Metaproterenol (a less selective beta$_2$-agonist) is not recommended in the management of asthma due to potential for excessive cardiac stimulation. Oral systemic agents (eg, tablets, syrup) should be avoided due to increased risk of adverse effects (eg, excessive cardiac stimulation).

Chronic obstructive lung disease (COPD): Appropriate use: Inhaled bronchodilators are preferred therapy for COPD exacerbations; oral systemic agents (eg, tablets, syrup) should be avoided due to increased risk of adverse effects (eg, excessive cardiac stimulation).

Adverse Reactions (Reflective of adult population; not specific for elderly)
>10%:
Cardiovascular: Tachycardia (6% to 17%)
Central nervous system: Nervousness (5% to 20%), headache (1% to 7%)
Neuromuscular & skeletal: Tremor (2% to 17%)
1% to 10%:
Cardiovascular: Palpitation (4%)
Central nervous system: Dizziness (2%), insomnia (2%), fatigue (1%)
Gastrointestinal: Nausea (1% to 4%), diarrhea (1%)
Respiratory: Asthma exacerbation (2%)

Drug Interactions
Avoid Concomitant Use
Avoid concomitant use of Metaproterenol with any of the following: Iobenguane I 123
Increased Effect/Toxicity
Metaproterenol may increase the levels/effects of: Loop Diuretics; Sympathomimetics

The levels/effects of Metaproterenol may be increased by: Atomoxetine; Cannabinoids; MAO Inhibitors; Tricyclic Antidepressants
Decreased Effect
Metaproterenol may decrease the levels/effects of: Iobenguane I 123

The levels/effects of Metaproterenol may be decreased by: Alpha-/Beta-Blockers; Beta-Blockers (Beta1 Selective); Beta-Blockers (Nonselective); Betahistine

Stability Store at room temperature; protect from light. Protect tablets from moisture.

Mechanism of Action Stimulates beta$_2$-receptors which increases the conversion of adenosine triphosphate (ATP) to 3'-5'-cyclic adenosine monophosphate (cAMP), resulting in bronchial smooth muscle relaxation

Pharmacodynamics/Kinetics
Onset of action: Bronchodilation: Oral: ~30 minutes
Peak effect: Oral: ~1 hour
Duration: ~2-6 hours

Dosage
Geriatric & Adult Bronchoconstriction: Oral: 20 mg 3-4 times/day

Administration Administer orally without regards to food. May administer with food if GI upset occurs.

Monitoring Parameters Lung sounds, heart rate, and blood pressure; FEV$_1$, peak flow, and/or other pulmonary function tests; CNS stimulation; serum glucose, serum potassium (in selected patients)

Pharmacotherapy Pearls Use with caution perioperatively due to beta$_1$ effect of agent. Hypertension and tachycardia are increased with exogenous sympathomimetics.

Special Geriatric Considerations Oral systemic beta-agonists should be avoided due to the increased incidence of adverse effects compared to inhaled agents.

Dosage Forms Excipient information presented when available (limited, particularly for generics); consult specific product labeling.
Syrup, oral, as sulfate: 10 mg/5 mL (473 mL)
Tablet, oral, as sulfate: 10 mg, 20 mg

◆ **Metaproterenol Sulfate** *see* Metaproterenol *on page 1153*

MetFORMIN (met FOR min)

Related Information
Diabetes Mellitus Management, Adults *on page 2073*

Medication Safety Issues
Sound-alike/look-alike issues:
MetFORMIN may be confused with metroNIDAZOLE
Glucophage® may be confused with Glucotrol®, Glutofac®
International issues:
Dianben [Spain] may be confused with Diovan brand name for valsartan [U.S., Canada, and multiple international markets]

Brand Names: U.S. Fortamet®; Glucophage®; Glucophage® XR; Glumetza®; Riomet®

Brand Names: Canada Apo-Metformin®; CO Metformin; Dom-Metformin; Glucophage®; Glumetza®; Glycon; Med-Metformin; Mylan-Metformin; Novo-Metformin; Nu-Metformin; PHL-Metformin; PMS-Metformin; PRO-Metformin; RAN™-Metformin; ratio-Metformin; Riva-Metformin; Sandoz-Metformin FC

Index Terms Metformin Hydrochloride

Generic Availability (U.S.) Yes: Excludes solution

Pharmacologic Category Antidiabetic Agent, Biguanide

Use Management of type 2 diabetes mellitus (noninsulin dependent, NIDDM) when hyperglycemia cannot be managed with diet and exercise alone.

Unlabeled/Investigational Use Prevention of type 2 diabetes mellitus

Contraindications Hypersensitivity to metformin or any component of the formulation; renal disease or renal dysfunction (serum creatinine ≥1.5 mg/dL in males or ≥1.4 mg/dL in females) or abnormal creatinine clearance from any cause, including shock, acute myocardial infarction, or septicemia; acute or chronic metabolic acidosis with or without coma (including diabetic ketoacidosis)

Note: Temporarily discontinue in patients undergoing radiologic studies in which intravascular iodinated contrast media are utilized.

Warnings/Precautions [U.S. Boxed Warning]: Lactic acidosis is a rare, but potentially severe consequence of therapy with metformin. Lactic acidosis should be suspected in any patient with diabetes receiving metformin with evidence of acidosis but without evidence of ketoacidosis. Discontinue metformin in clinical situations predisposing to hypoxemia, including conditions such as cardiovascular collapse, respiratory failure, acute myocardial infarction, acute congestive heart failure, and septicemia. Use caution in patients with congestive heart failure requiring pharmacologic management, particularly in patients with unstable or acute CHF; risk of lactic acidosis may be increased secondary to hypoperfusion.

Metformin is substantially excreted by the kidney. The risk of accumulation and lactic acidosis increases with the degree of impairment of renal function. Patients with renal function below the limit of normal for their age should not receive metformin. In elderly patients, renal function should be monitored regularly; should not be initiated in patients ≥80 years of age unless normal renal function is confirmed. Use of concomitant medications that may affect renal function (ie, affect tubular secretion) may also affect metformin disposition. Metformin should be withheld in patients with dehydration and/or prerenal azotemia. Therapy should be suspended for any surgical procedures (resume only after normal oral intake resumed and normal renal function is verified). Therapy should be temporarily discontinued prior to or at the time of intravascular administration of iodinated contrast media (potential for acute alteration in renal function). Metformin should be withheld for 48 hours after the radiologic study and restarted only after renal function has been confirmed as normal. It may be necessary to discontinue metformin and administer insulin if the patient is exposed to stress (fever, trauma, infection, surgery).

Avoid use in patients with impaired liver function. Patient must be instructed to avoid excessive acute or chronic ethanol use; ethanol may potentiate metformin's effect on lactate metabolism. Administration of oral antidiabetic drugs has been reported to be associated with increased cardiovascular mortality; metformin does not appear to share this risk. Insoluble tablet shell of Glumetza® 1000 mg extended release tablet may remain intact and be visible in the stool. Other extended released tablets (Fortamet®, Glucophage® XR, Glumetza® 500 mg) may appear in the stool as a soft mass resembling the tablet.

Adverse Reactions (Reflective of adult population; not specific for elderly)
>10%:
Gastrointestinal: Diarrhea (10% to 53%), nausea/vomiting (7% to 26%), flatulence (12%)
Neuromuscular & skeletal: Weakness (9%)

◀ 1% to 10%:

Cardiovascular: Chest discomfort, flushing, palpitation

Central nervous system: Headache (6%), chills, dizziness, lightheadedness

Dermatologic: Rash

Endocrine & metabolic: Hypoglycemia

Gastrointestinal: Indigestion (7%), abdominal discomfort (6%), abdominal distention, abnormal stools, constipation, dyspepsia/ heartburn, taste disorder

Neuromuscular & skeletal: Myalgia

Respiratory: Dyspnea, upper respiratory tract infection

Miscellaneous: Decreased vitamin B_{12} levels (7%), increased diaphoresis, flu-like syndrome, nail disorder

Drug Interactions

Avoid Concomitant Use There are no known interactions where it is recommended to avoid concomitant use.

Increased Effect/Toxicity

MetFORMIN may increase the levels/effects of: Dofetilide

The levels/effects of MetFORMIN may be increased by: Cephalexin; Cimetidine; Glycopyrrolate; Iodinated Contrast Agents; Pegvisomant

Decreased Effect

The levels/effects of MetFORMIN may be decreased by: Corticosteroids (Orally Inhaled); Corticosteroids (Systemic); Luteinizing Hormone-Releasing Hormone Analogs; Somatropin; Thiazide Diuretics

Ethanol/Nutrition/Herb Interactions

Ethanol: Avoid or limit ethanol (incidence of lactic acidosis may be increased; may cause hypoglycemia).

Food: Food decreases the extent and slightly delays the absorption. May decrease absorption of vitamin B_{12} and/or folic acid.

Herb/Nutraceutical: Caution with chromium, garlic, gymnema (may cause hypoglycemia).

Stability

Oral solution: Store at 15°C to 30°C (59°F to 86°F).

Tablets: Store at 20°C to 25°C (68°F to 77°F); excursion permitted to 15°C to 30°C (59°F to 86°F). Protect from light and moisture.

Mechanism of Action Decreases hepatic glucose production, decreasing intestinal absorption of glucose and improves insulin sensitivity (increases peripheral glucose uptake and utilization).

Pharmacodynamics/Kinetics

Onset of action: Within days; maximum effects up to 2 weeks

Distribution: V_d: 654 ± 358 L; partitions into erythrocytes

Protein binding: Negligible

Metabolism: Not metabolized by the liver

Bioavailability: Absolute: Fasting: 50% to 60%

Half-life elimination: Plasma: 4-9 hours

Time to peak, serum: Immediate release: 2-3 hours; Extended release: 7 hours (range: 4-8 hours)

Excretion: Urine (90% as unchanged drug; active secretion)

Dosage

Geriatric The initial and maintenance dosing should be conservative, due to the potential for decreased renal function. Generally, elderly patients should **not** be titrated to the maximum dose of metformin. Do not use in patients ≥80 years of age unless normal renal function has been established.

Adult

Management of type 2 diabetes mellitus: Oral: **Note:** Allow 1-2 weeks between dose titrations: Generally, clinically significant responses are not seen at doses <1500 mg daily; however, a lower recommended starting dose and gradual increased dosage is recommended to minimize gastrointestinal symptoms.

Immediate release tablet or solution: Adults ≥17 years: Initial: 500 mg twice daily **or** 850 mg once daily; titrate in increments of 500 mg weekly or 850 mg every other week; may also titrate from 500 mg twice a day to 850 mg twice a day after 2 weeks

Doses of up to 2000 mg/day may be given twice daily. If a dose >2000 mg/day is required, it may be better tolerated in three divided doses. Maximum recommended dose 2550 mg/day.

Extended release tablet: **Note:** If glycemic control is not achieved at maximum dose, may divide dose and administer twice daily.

Fortamet®: Initial: 500-1000 mg once daily;dosage may be increased by 500 mg weekly; maximum dose: 2500 mg once daily

Glucophage® XR: Initial: 500 mg once daily; dosage may be increased by 500 mg weekly; maximum dose: 2000 mg once daily

Glumetza®: Initial: 1000 mg once daily; dosage may be increased by 500 mg weekly; maximum dose: 2000 mg once daily

Transfer from other antidiabetic agents: No transition period is generally necessary except when transferring from chlorpropamide. When transferring from chlorpropamide, care should be exercised during the first 2 weeks because of the prolonged retention of chlorpropamide in the body, leading to overlapping drug effects and possible hypoglycemia.

Concomitant metformin and oral sulfonylurea therapy: If patients have not responded to 4 weeks of the maximum dose of metformin monotherapy, consider a gradual addition of an oral sulfonylurea, even if prior primary or secondary failure to a sulfonylurea has occurred. Continue metformin at the maximum dose. If adequate response has not occurred following 3 months of metformin and sulfonylurea combination therapy, consider switching to insulin with or without metformin.

Failed sulfonylurea therapy: Patients with prior failure on glyburide may be treated by gradual addition of metformin. Initiate with glyburide 20 mg and metformin 500 mg daily. Metformin dosage may be increased by 500 mg/day at weekly intervals, up to a maximum metformin dose (dosage of glyburide maintained at 20 mg/day).

Concomitant metformin and insulin therapy: Initial: 500 mg metformin once daily, continue current insulin dose; increase by 500 mg metformin weekly until adequate glycemic control is achieved

Maximum daily dose: Immediate release and solution: 2550 mg metformin; Extended release: 2000-2500 mg (varies by product)

Decrease insulin dose 10% to 25% when FPG <120 mg/dL; monitor and make further adjustments as needed

Type 2 diabetes prevention (unlabeled use): *Immediate release tablet or solution:* Oral: Initial: 850 mg once daily; Target: 850 mg twice daily (Knowler, 2002)

Renal Impairment The plasma and blood half-life of metformin is prolonged and the renal clearance is decreased in proportion to the decrease in creatinine clearance. Per the manufacturer, metformin is contraindicated in the presence of renal dysfunction defined as a serum creatinine ≥1.5 mg/dL in males, or ≥1.4 mg/dL in females and in patients with abnormal clearance. The Canadian labeling recommends that metformin be avoided in patients with Cl_{cr} <60 mL/minute.

Hepatic Impairment Avoid metformin; liver disease is a risk factor for the development of lactic acidosis during metformin therapy.

Administration Administer with a meal (to decrease GI upset).

Extended release: Swallow whole; do not crush, break, or chew. Administer once daily doses with the evening meal. Fortamet® should also be administered with a full glass of water.

Monitoring Parameters Urine for glucose and ketones, fasting blood glucose, and hemoglobin A_{1c}. Initial and periodic monitoring of hematologic parameters (eg, hemoglobin/hematocrit and red blood cell indices) and renal function should be performed, at least annually. Check vitamin B_{12} and folate if anemia is present.

Reference Range Recommendations for glycemic control in adults with diabetes:

Hb A_{1c}: <7%

Preprandial capillary plasma glucose: 70-130 mg/dL

Peak postprandial capillary blood glucose: <180 mg/dL

Blood pressure: <130/80 mm Hg

Special Geriatric Considerations Limited data suggest that metformin's total body clearance may be decreased and AUC and half-life increased in elderly patients; presumably due to decreased renal clearance. Metformin has been well tolerated by the elderly but lower doses and frequent monitoring are recommended. In one study of elderly subjects, its effects could not be distinguished from tolbutamide, except for weight loss. The initial and maintenance dosing should be conservative, due to the potential for decreased renal function. Generally, elderly patients should not be titrated to the maximum dose of metformin. Do not use in patients ≥80 years of age unless normal renal function has been established. Intensive glucose control (HbA$_{1c}$ <6.5%) has been linked to increased all-cause and cardiovascular mortality, hypoglycemia requiring assistance, and weight gain in adult type 2 diabetes. How "tightly" to control a geriatric patient's blood glucose needs to be individualized. Such a decision should be based on several factors, including the patient's functional and cognitive status, how well he/she recognizes hypoglycemic or hyperglycemic symptoms, and how to respond to them and other disease states. An HbA$_{1c}$ <7.5% is an acceptable endpoint for a healthy older adult, while <8% is acceptable for frail elderly patients, those with a duration of illness >10 years, or those with comorbid conditions and requiring combination diabetes medications. Patients who are unable to accurately draw up their dose will need assistance, such as prefilled syringes. Initial doses may require considerations for renal function in the elderly with dosing adjusted subsequently based on blood glucose monitoring. For elderly patients with diabetes who are relatively healthy, attaining target goals for aspirin use, blood pressure, lipids, smoking cessation, and diet and exercise may be more important than normalized glycemic control.

Dosage Forms Excipient information presented when available (limited, particularly for generics); consult specific product labeling.

Solution, oral, as hydrochloride:

Riomet®: 100 mg/mL (118 mL, 473 mL) [dye free, ethanol free, sugar free; contains saccharin; cherry flavor]

Tablet, oral, as hydrochloride: 500 mg, 850 mg, 1000 mg

Glucophage®: 500 mg, 850 mg

Glucophage®: 1000 mg [scored]

Tablet, extended release, oral, as hydrochloride: 500 mg, 750 mg

Fortamet®: 500 mg, 1000 mg

Glucophage® XR: 500 mg, 750 mg

Glumetza®: 500 mg, 1000 mg

Selected References

Action to Control Cardiovascular Risk in Diabetes Study Group, Gerstein HC, Miller ME, et al, "Effects of Intensive Glucose Lowering in Type 2 Diabetes," *N Engl J Med*, 2008, 358(24):2545-59.

ADVANCE Collaborative Group, Patel A, MacMahon S, et al, "Intensive Blood Glucose Control and Vascular Outcomes in Patients With Type 2 Diabetes," *N Engl J Med*, 2008, 358(24):2560-72.

American Diabetes Association, "Standards of Medical Care in Diabetes – 2011," *Diabetes Care*, 2011, 34(Suppl 1):11-61.

Brown AF, Mangione CM, Saliba D, et al, "Guidelines for Improving the Care of the Older Person With Diabetes Mellitus," *J Am Geriatr Soc*, 2003, 51(5 Suppl Guidelines):265-80.

Josephkutty S and Potter JM, "Comparison of Tolbutamide and Metformin in Elderly Diabetic Patients," *Diabet Med*, 1990, 7(16):510-4.

Lalau JD, Vermersch A, Hary L, et al, "Type 2 Diabetes in the Elderly: An Assessment of Metformin," *Int J Clin Pharmacol Ther Toxicol*, 1990, 28(8):329-32.

"VA/DoD Clinical Practice Guideline for the Management of Diabetes Mellitus," 2010. Available at http://www.healthquality.va.gov/Diabetes_Mellitus.asp

◆ **Metformin and Glipizide** *see* Glipizide and Metformin *on page 826*

◆ **Metformin and Glyburide** *see* Glyburide and Metformin *on page 832*

◆ **Metformin and Repaglinide** *see* Repaglinide and Metformin *on page 1598*

◆ **Metformin and Rosiglitazone** *see* Rosiglitazone and Metformin *on page 1639*

◆ **Metformin and Saxagliptin** *see* Saxagliptin and Metformin *on page 1659*

◆ **Metformin and Sitagliptin** *see* Sitagliptin and Metformin *on page 1686*

◆ **Metformin Hydrochloride** *see* MetFORMIN *on page 1155*

◆ **Metformin Hydrochloride and Pioglitazone Hydrochloride** *see* Pioglitazone and Metformin *on page 1461*

◆ **Metformin Hydrochloride and Rosiglitazone Maleate** *see* Rosiglitazone and Metformin *on page 1639*

◆ **Metformin Hydrochloride and Saxagliptin** *see* Saxagliptin and Metformin *on page 1659*

Methadone (METH a done)

Related Information

Opioid Analgesics *on page 2013*

Patient Information for Disposal of Unused Medications *on page 2125*

Medication Safety Issues

Sound-alike/look-alike issues:

Methadone may be confused with dexmethylphenidate, Mephyton®, methylphenidate, Metadate® CD, Metadate® ER, morphine

High alert medication:

The Institute for Safe Medication Practices (ISMP) includes this medication among its list of drug classes which have a heightened risk of causing significant patient harm when used in error.

Brand Names: U.S. Dolophine®; Methadone Diskets®; Methadone Intensol™; Methadose®

Brand Names: Canada Metadol-D™; Metadol™

Index Terms Methadone Hydrochloride

Generic Availability (U.S.) Yes

Pharmacologic Category Analgesic, Opioid

Use Management of moderate-to-severe pain; detoxification and maintenance treatment of opioid addiction as part of an FDA-approved program

Prescribing and Access Restrictions When used for treatment of opioid addiction: May only be dispensed in accordance to guidelines established by the Substance Abuse and Mental Health Services Administration's (SAMHSA) Center for Substance Abuse Treatment (CSAT). Regulations regarding methadone use may vary by state and/or country. Obtain advice from appropriate regulatory agencies and/or consult with pain management/palliative care specialists.

Note: Regulatory Exceptions to the General Requirement to Provide Opioid Agonist Treatment (per manufacturer's labeling):

1. During inpatient care, when the patient was admitted for any condition other than concurrent opioid addiction, to facilitate the treatment of the primary admitting diagnosis.
2. During an emergency period of no longer than 3 days while definitive care for the addiction is being sought in an appropriately licensed facility.

Contraindications Hypersensitivity to methadone or any component of the formulation; respiratory depression (in the absence of resuscitative equipment or in an unmonitored setting); acute bronchial asthma or hypercarbia; paralytic ileus; concurrent use of selegiline

Warnings/Precautions An opioid-containing analgesic regimen should be tailored to each patient's needs and based upon the type of pain being treated (acute versus chronic), the route of administration, degree of tolerance for opioids (naive versus chronic user), age, weight, and medical condition. The optimal analgesic dose varies widely among patients. Doses should be titrated to pain relief/prevention. Patients maintained on stable doses of methadone may need higher and/or more frequent doses in case of acute pain (eg, postoperative pain, physical trauma). Methadone is ineffective for the relief of anxiety.

[U.S. Boxed Warning]: May prolong the QT_c interval and increase risk for torsade de pointes. Patients should be informed of the potential arrhythmia risk, evaluated for any history of structural heart disease, arrhythmia, syncope, and for existence of potential drug interactions including drugs that possess QT_c interval-prolonging properties, promote hypokalemia, hypomagnesemia, or hypocalcemia, or reduce elimination of methadone (eg, CYP3A4 inhibitors). Obtain baseline ECG for all patients and risk stratify according to QT_c interval (see Monitoring Parameters). Use with caution in patients at risk for QT_c prolongation, with medications known to prolong the QT_c interval, promote electrolyte depletion, or inhibit CYP3A4, or history of conduction abnormalities. QT_c interval prolongation and torsade de pointes may be associated with doses >100 mg/day, but have also been observed with lower doses. May cause severe hypotension; use caution with severe volume depletion or other conditions which may compromise maintenance of normal blood pressure. Use caution with cardiovascular disease or patients predisposed to dysrhythmias.

[U.S. Boxed Warning]: May cause respiratory depression. Use caution in patients with respiratory disease or pre-existing respiratory conditions (eg, severe obesity, asthma, COPD, sleep apnea, CNS depression). Because the respiratory effects last longer than the analgesic effects, slow titration is required. Use extreme caution during treatment initiation, dose titration and conversion from other opioid agonists. Incomplete cross tolerance may occur; patients tolerant to other mu opioid agonists may not be tolerant to methadone. Abrupt cessation may precipitate withdrawal symptoms.

May cause CNS depression, which may impair physical or mental abilities. Patients must be cautioned about performing tasks which require mental alertness (eg, operating machinery or driving). Effects with other sedative drugs or ethanol may be potentiated. Use with caution in patients with depression or suicidal tendencies, or in patients with a history of drug abuse. Tolerance or psychological and physical dependence may occur with prolonged use.

Use with caution in patients with head injury or increased intracranial pressure. May obscure diagnosis or clinical course of patients with acute abdominal conditions. Elderly may be more susceptible to adverse effects (eg, CNS, respiratory, gastrointestinal). Decrease initial dose and use caution in the elderly or debilitated; with hyper/hypothyroidism, morbid obesity, adrenal insufficiency, prostatic hyperplasia, or urethral stricture; or with severe renal or hepatic failure. Use with caution in patients with biliary tract dysfunction; acute pancreatitis may cause constriction of sphincter of Oddi. **[U.S. Boxed Warning]: For oral administration only; excipients to deter use by injection are contained in tablets.**

[U.S. Boxed Warning]: When used for treatment of narcotic addiction: May only be dispensed by opioid treatment programs certified by the Substance Abuse and Mental Health Services Administration (SAMHSA) and certified by the designated state authority. Exceptions include inpatient treatment of other conditions and emergency period (not >3 days) while definitive substance abuse treatment is being sought.

Adverse Reactions (Reflective of adult population; not specific for elderly) Frequency not defined. During prolonged administration, adverse effects may decrease over several weeks; however, constipation and sweating may persist.

Cardiovascular: Arrhythmia, bigeminal rhythms, bradycardia, cardiac arrest, cardiomyopathy, ECG changes, edema, extrasystoles, faintness, flushing, heart failure, hypotension, palpitation, peripheral vasodilation, phlebitis, orthostatic hypotension, QT interval prolonged, shock, syncope, tachycardia, torsade de pointes, T-wave inversion, ventricular fibrillation, ventricular tachycardia,

Central nervous system: Agitation, confusion, disorientation, dizziness, drowsiness, dysphoria, euphoria, hallucination, headache, insomnia, lightheadedness, sedation, seizure

Dermatologic: Hemorrhagic urticaria, pruritus, rash, urticaria

Endocrine & metabolic: Antidiuretic effect, amenorrhea, hypokalemia, hypomagnesemia, libido decreased

Gastrointestinal: Abdominal pain, anorexia, biliary tract spasm, constipation, glossitis, nausea, stomach cramps, vomiting, weight gain, xerostomia

Genitourinary: Impotence, urinary retention or hesitancy

Hematologic: Thrombocytopenia (reversible, reported in patients with chronic hepatitis)

Neuromuscular & skeletal: Weakness

Local: I.M./SubQ injection: Erythema, pain, swelling; I.V. injection: Hemorrhagic urticaria (rare), pruritus, urticaria, rash

Ocular: Miosis, visual disturbances

Respiratory: Pulmonary edema, respiratory depression, respiratory arrest

Miscellaneous: Death, diaphoresis, physical and psychological dependence

Drug Interactions

Metabolism/Transport Effects Substrate of CYP2B6 (major), 2C9 (minor), 2C19 (minor), 2D6 (minor), 3A4 (major); **Inhibits** CYP2D6 (moderate), 3A4 (weak)

Avoid Concomitant Use

Avoid concomitant use of Methadone with any of the following: Artemether; Conivaptan; Dronedarone; Lumefantrine; Nilotinib; Pimozide; QUEtiapine; QuiNINE; Tetrabenazine; Thioridazine; Toremifene; Vandetanib; Vemurafenib; Ziprasidone

Increased Effect/Toxicity

Methadone may increase the levels/effects of: Alcohol (Ethyl); Alvimopan; CNS Depressants; CYP2D6 Substrates; Desmopressin; Dronedarone; Fesoterodine; Nebivolol; Pimozide; QTc-Prolonging Agents; QuiNINE; Selective Serotonin Reuptake Inhibitors; Tamoxifen; Tetrabenazine; Thiazide Diuretics; Thioridazine; Toremifene; Vandetanib; Vemurafenib; Zidovudine; Ziprasidone

The levels/effects of Methadone may be increased by: Alfuzosin; Amphetamines; Antifungal Agents (Azole Derivatives, Systemic); Antipsychotic Agents (Phenothiazines); Artemether; Boceprevir; Chloroquine; Ciprofloxacin; Ciprofloxacin (Systemic); Conivaptan; CYP2B6 Inhibitors (Moderate); CYP2B6 Inhibitors (Strong); CYP3A4 Inhibitors (Moderate); CYP3A4 Inhibitors (Strong); Gadobutrol; HydrOXYzine; Interferons (Alfa); Lumefantrine; MAO Inhibitors; Nilotinib; Quazepam; QUEtiapine; QuiNINE; Selective Serotonin Reuptake Inhibitors; Succinylcholine

Decreased Effect

Methadone may decrease the levels/effects of: Codeine; Didanosine; Pegvisomant; TraMADol

The levels/effects of Methadone may be decreased by: Ammonium Chloride; Barbiturates; Boceprevir; CarBAMazepine; CYP2B6 Inducers (Strong); CYP3A4 Inducers (Strong); Deferasirox; Etravirine; Fosphenytoin; Herbs (CYP3A4 Inducers); Mixed Agonist / Antagonist Opioids; Phenytoin; Protease Inhibitors; Reverse Transcriptase Inhibitors (Non-Nucleoside); Rifamycin Derivatives; Telaprevir; Tocilizumab

Ethanol/Nutrition/Herb Interactions

Ethanol: May increase CNS depression; monitor for increased effects with coadministration. Caution patients about effects.

Herb/Nutraceutical: Avoid St John's wort (may decrease methadone levels; may increase CNS depression). Avoid valerian, kava kava, gotu kola (may increase CNS depression). Methadone is metabolized by CYP3A4 in the intestines; avoid concurrent use of grapefruit juice.

Stability

Injection: Store at controlled room temperature of 15°C to 30°C (59°F to 86°F). Protect from light.

Oral concentrate, oral solution, tablet: Store at controlled room temperature of 15°C to 30°C (59°F to 86°F).

Mechanism of Action Binds to opiate receptors in the CNS, causing inhibition of ascending pain pathways, altering the perception of and response to pain; produces generalized CNS depression

Pharmacodynamics/Kinetics

Onset of action: Oral: Analgesic: 0.5-1 hour; Parenteral: 10-20 minutes

Peak effect: Parenteral: 1-2 hours; Oral: Continuous dosing: 3-5 days

Duration of analgesia: Oral: 4-8 hours, increases to 22-48 hours with repeated doses

Distribution: V_{dss}: 1-8 L/kg

Protein binding: 85% to 90%

Metabolism: Hepatic; N-demethylation primarily via CYP3A4, CYP2B6, and CYP2C19 to inactive metabolites

Bioavailability: Oral: 36% to 100%
Half-life elimination: 8-59 hours; may be prolonged with alkaline pH
Time to peak, plasma: 1-7.5 hours
Excretion: Urine (<10% as unchanged drug); increased with urine pH <6

Dosage

Geriatric Oral, I.M.: 2.5 mg every 8-12 hours; refer to adult dosing.

Adult Regulations regarding methadone use may vary by state and/or country. Obtain advice from appropriate regulatory agencies and/or consult with pain management/palliative care specialists. **Note:** These are guidelines and do not represent the maximum doses that may be required in all patients. Methadone accumulates with repeated doses and dosage may need reduction after 3-5 days to prevent CNS depressant effects. Some patients may benefit from every 8-12 hour dosing interval for chronic pain management. Doses should be titrated to appropriate effects.

Acute pain (moderate-to-severe):
Opioid-naive: *Oral:* Initial: 2.5-10 mg every 8-12 hours; more frequent administration may be required during initiation to maintain adequate analgesia. Dosage interval may range from 4-12 hours, since duration of analgesia is relatively short during the first days of therapy, but increases substantially with continued administration.

Chronic pain (opioid-tolerant): Conversion from oral morphine to oral methadone:
Daily oral morphine dose <100 mg: Estimated daily oral methadone dose: 20% to 30% of total daily morphine dose
Daily oral morphine dose 100-300 mg: Estimated daily oral methadone dose: 10% to 20% of total daily morphine dose
Daily oral morphine dose 300-600 mg: Estimated daily oral methadone dose: 8% to 12% of total daily morphine dose
Daily oral morphine dose 600-1000 mg: Estimated daily oral methadone dose: 5% to 10% of total daily morphine dose.
Daily oral morphine dose >1000 mg: Estimated daily oral methadone dose: <5% of total daily morphine dose.
Note: The total daily methadone dose should then be divided to reflect the intended dosing schedule.

I.V.: Manufacturers labeling: Initial: 2.5-10 mg every 8-12 hours in opioid-naive patients; titrate slowly to effect; may also be administered by SubQ or I.M. injection

Conversion from oral to parenteral dose: Initial dose: Parenteral:Oral ratio: 1:2 (eg, 5 mg parenteral methadone equals 10 mg oral methadone)

Detoxification: *Oral:*
Initial: A single dose of 20-30 mg is usually sufficient to suppress symptoms. Should not exceed 30 mg; lower doses should be considered in patients with low tolerance at initiation (eg, absence of opioids ≥5 days); an additional 5-10 mg of methadone may be provided if withdrawal symptoms have not been suppressed or if symptoms reappear after 2-4 hours; total daily dose on the first day should not exceed 40 mg, unless the program physician documents in the patient's record that 40 mg did not control opiate abstinence symptoms.
Maintenance: Titrate to a dosage which prevents craving, attenuates euphoric effect of self-administered opiates, and tolerance to sedative effects of methadone. Usual range: 80-120 mg/day (titration should occur cautiously)
Withdrawal: Dose reductions should be <10% of the maintenance dose, every 10-14 days

Detoxification (short-term): *Oral:*
Initial: Titrate to ~40 mg/day in divided doses to achieve stabilization. May continue 40 mg dose for 2-3 days
Maintenance: Titrate to a dosage which prevents/attenuates euphoric effects of self-administered opioids, reduces drug craving, and withdrawal symptoms are prevented for 24 hours.
Withdrawal: Requires individualization. Decrease daily or every other day, keeping withdrawal symptoms tolerable; hospitalized patients may tolerate a 20% reduction/day; ambulatory patients may require a slower reduction

Renal Impairment Cl_{cr} <10 mL/minute: Administer 50% to 75% of normal dose.

Hepatic Impairment Avoid in severe liver disease.

Administration Oral dose for detoxification and maintenance may be administered in fruit juice or water. Dispersible tablet should not be chewed or swallowed; add to liquid and allow to dissolve before administering. May rinse if residual remains.

Monitoring Parameters Obtain baseline ECG (evaluate QT_c interval), within 30 days of initiation, and then annually for all patients receiving methadone. Increase ECG monitoring if patient receiving >100 mg/day or if unexplained syncope or seizure occurs while on methadone (Krantz, 2008).
If before or at anytime during therapy:
QT_c >450-499 msecs: Discuss potential risks and benefits; monitor QT_c more frequently

◀ QT$_c$ ≥500 msecs: Consider discontinuation or reducing methadone dose **or** eliminate factors promoting QT$_c$ prolongation (eg, potassium-wasting drugs) **or** use alternative therapy (eg, buprenorphine)

Pain relief, respiratory and mental status, blood pressure

Reference Range Prevention of opiate withdrawal: Therapeutic: 100-400 ng/mL (SI: 0.32-1.29 µmol/L); Toxic: >2 mcg/mL (SI: >6.46 µmol/L)

Test Interactions Some quinolones may produce a false-positive urine screening result for opiates using commercially-available immunoassay kits. This has been demonstrated most consistently for levofloxacin and ofloxacin, but other quinolones have shown cross-reactivity in certain assay kits. Confirmation of positive opiate screens by more specific methods should be considered.

Special Geriatric Considerations Because of its long half-life and risk of accumulation, methadone is difficult to titrate and is not considered a drug of first choice. It should be prescribed only by physicians who are experienced in using it. Elderly may be particularly susceptible to the CNS depressant and constipating effects of narcotics.

Controlled Substance C-II

Dosage Forms Excipient information presented when available (limited, particularly for generics); consult specific product labeling.

Injection, solution, as hydrochloride: 10 mg/mL (20 mL)

Solution, oral, as hydrochloride: 5 mg/5 mL (500 mL); 10 mg/5 mL (500 mL)

Solution, oral, as hydrochloride [concentrate]: 10 mg/mL (946 mL, 1000 mL, 1000s)

Methadone Intensol™: 10 mg/mL (30 mL) [dye free, sugar free; contains sodium benzoate; unflavored]

Methadose®: 10 mg/mL (1000 mL) [contains propylene glycol; cherry flavor]

Methadose®: 10 mg/mL (1000 mL) [dye free, sugar free; contains sodium benzoate; unflavored]

Tablet, oral, as hydrochloride: 5 mg, 10 mg

Dolophine®: 5 mg, 10 mg [scored]

Tablet, dispersible, oral, as hydrochloride: 40 mg

Methadone Diskets®: 40 mg [scored; orange-pineapple flavor]

Methadose®: 40 mg [scored]

Selected References

American Geriatrics Society Panel on Pharmacological Management of Persistent Pain in Older Persons, "Pharmacological Management of Persistent Pain in Older Persons," *J Am Geriatr Soc*, 2009, 57(8):1331-46.

Department of Health and Human Services: Substance Abuse and Mental Health Services Administration, "Opioid Drugs in Maintenance and Detoxification of Opiate Addiction; Final Rule," *Fed Regist*, 2001, 66(11): 4075-102.

Gazelle G and Fine PG, "Methadone for the Treatment of Pain #75," *J Palliat Med*, 2003, 6(4):620-1.

◆ **Methadone Diskets®** *see* Methadone *on page 1158*
◆ **Methadone Hydrochloride** *see* Methadone *on page 1158*
◆ **Methadone Intensol™** *see* Methadone *on page 1158*
◆ **Methadose®** *see* Methadone *on page 1158*
◆ **Methaminodiazepoxide Hydrochloride** *see* ChlordiazePOXIDE *on page 334*

Methazolamide (meth a ZOE la mide)

Related Information

Glaucoma Drug Therapy *on page 2008*

Medication Safety Issues

Sound-alike/look-alike issues:

Methazolamide may be confused with methenamine, metolazone

Neptazane™ may be confused with Nesacaine®

Brand Names: U.S. Neptazane™

Brand Names: Canada Apo-Methazolamide®

Generic Availability (U.S.) Yes

Pharmacologic Category Carbonic Anhydrase Inhibitor; Diuretic, Carbonic Anhydrase Inhibitor; Ophthalmic Agent, Antiglaucoma

Use Treatment of chronic open-angle or secondary glaucoma; short-term therapy of acute angle-closure glaucoma prior to surgery

Contraindications Marked kidney or liver dysfunction; adrenal gland failure; cirrhosis; hyperchloremic acidosis; hyponatremia; hypokalemia; long-term treatment of angle-closure glaucoma

Warnings/Precautions May impair mental alertness and/or physical coordination. Use with caution in patients with prediabetes or diabetes mellitus; may see a change in glucose control. Initially, potassium excretion may be increased; periodically monitor serum electrolytes and signs of hypokalemia in at risk patients. Use with caution in patients with respiratory disease such as emphysema or pulmonary obstruction; may precipitate or aggravate respiratory acidosis. Use with caution in patients with hepatic impairment; may precipitate hepatic encephalopathy. Use is contraindicated in patients with marked liver impairment or cirrhosis.

Chemical similarities are present among sulfonamides, sulfonylureas, carbonic anhydrase inhibitors, thiazides, and loop diuretics (except ethacrynic acid). Use in patients with sulfonylurea allergy is not specifically contraindicated in product labeling, however, a risk of cross-reaction exists in patients with allergy to any of these compounds; avoid use when previous reaction has been severe. Discontinue if signs of hypersensitivity are noted. Use with caution in patients taking high dose aspirin concurrently; may lead to severe adverse effects including death, coma, tachypnea, anorexia, and lethargy

Adverse Reactions (Reflective of adult population; not specific for elderly) Frequency not defined.

Central nervous system: Confusion, drowsiness, fatigue, fever, malaise, seizure

Dermatologic: Erythema multiforme, photosensitivity, rash, Stevens-Johnson syndrome, toxic epidermal necrolysis, urticaria

Endocrine & metabolic: Electrolyte imbalance, metabolic acidosis

Gastrointestinal: Appetite decreased, diarrhea, melena, nausea, taste alteration, vomiting

Genitourinary: Crystalluria, glycosuria, hematuria, polyuria, renal calculi

Hematologic: Agranulocytosis, aplastic anemia, bone marrow depression, hemolytic anemia, leukopenia, pancytopenia, thrombocytopenic purpura

Hepatic: Fulminant hepatic necrosis, hepatic insufficiency

Neuromuscular & skeletal: Flaccid paralysis, paresthesia

Ocular: Myopia

Otic: Hearing disturbance, tinnitus

Miscellaneous: Anaphylaxis, hypersensitivity

Drug Interactions

Avoid Concomitant Use

Avoid concomitant use of Methazolamide with any of the following: Carbonic Anhydrase Inhibitors

Increased Effect/Toxicity

Methazolamide may increase the levels/effects of: Alpha-/Beta-Agonists; Amifostine; Amphetamines; Anticonvulsants (Barbiturate); Anticonvulsants (Hydantoin); Antihypertensives; CarBAMazepine; Carbonic Anhydrase Inhibitors; Flecainide; Hypotensive Agents; Memantine; Primidone; QuiNIDine; RiTUXimab; Sodium Phosphates

The levels/effects of Methazolamide may be increased by: Alfuzosin; Diazoxide; Herbs (Hypotensive Properties); MAO Inhibitors; Pentoxifylline; Phosphodiesterase 5 Inhibitors; Prostacyclin Analogues; Salicylates

Decreased Effect

Methazolamide may decrease the levels/effects of: Lithium; Methenamine; Primidone; Trientine

The levels/effects of Methazolamide may be decreased by: Herbs (Hypertensive Properties); Methylphenidate; Yohimbine

Stability Store at 20°C to 25°C (68°F to 77°F).

Mechanism of Action Noncompetitive inhibition of the enzyme carbonic anhydrase; thought that carbonic anhydrase is located at the luminal border of cells of the proximal tubule. When the enzyme is inhibited, there is an increase in urine volume and a change to an alkaline pH with a subsequent increase in the excretion of titratable acid and ammonia.

Pharmacodynamics/Kinetics

Onset of action: Slow in comparison with acetazolamide (2-4 hours)

Peak effect: 6-8 hours

Duration: 10-18 hours

Absorption: Slow

Distribution: V_d: 17-23 L

Protein binding: ~55%

Metabolism: Slowly from GI tract

Half-life elimination: ~14 hours

Excretion: Urine (~25% as unchanged drug)

Dosage

Geriatric & Adult Glaucoma: Oral: 50-100 mg 2-3 times/day

Monitoring Parameters Intraocular pressure, serum potassium, serum bicarbonate, serum sodium

Special Geriatric Considerations Malaise and complaints of tiredness and myalgia are signs of excessive dosing and acidosis in the elderly.

◀ **Dosage Forms** Excipient information presented when available (limited, particularly for generics); consult specific product labeling.
Tablet, oral: 25 mg, 50 mg
  Neptazane™: 25 mg
  Neptazane™: 50 mg [scored]

Methenamine (meth EN a meen)

Medication Safety Issues
Sound-alike/look-alike issues:
  Hiprex® may be confused with Mirapex®
  Methenamine may be confused with mesalamine, methazolamide, methionine
  Urex may be confused with Eurax®, serax
International issues:
  Urex: Brand name for methenamine [U.S. (discontinued)], but also the brand name for furosemide [Australia, China, Turkey]
  Urex [U.S. (discontinued)] may be confused with Eurax brand name for crotamitin [U.S., Canada, and multiple international markets]
Brand Names: U.S. Hiprex®
Brand Names: Canada Dehydral®; Hiprex®; Mandelamine®; Urasal®
Index Terms Hexamethylenetetramine; Methenamine Hippurate; Methenamine Mandelate; Urex
Generic Availability (U.S.) Yes
Pharmacologic Category Antibiotic, Miscellaneous
Use Prophylaxis or suppression of recurrent urinary tract infections; urinary tract discomfort secondary to hypermotility
Contraindications Hypersensitivity to methenamine or any component of the formulation; severe dehydration, renal insufficiency, severe hepatic insufficiency; concurrent treatment with sulfonamides
Warnings/Precautions Methenamine should not be used to treat infections outside of the lower urinary tract. Use with caution in patients with hepatic disease (contraindicated with severe impairment), gout, and the elderly; doses of 8 g/day for 3-4 weeks may cause bladder irritation. Use care to maintain an acid pH of the urine, especially when treating infections due to urea splitting organisms (eg, *Proteus* and strains of *Pseudomonas*); reversible increases in LFTs have occurred during therapy especially in patients with hepatic dysfunction. Prolonged use may result in fungal or bacterial superinfection, including *C. difficile*-associated diarrhea (CDAD) and pseudomembranous colitis; CDAD has been observed >2 months postantibiotic treatment. Hiprex® contains tartrazine dye.
Adverse Reactions (Reflective of adult population; not specific for elderly)
<4%:
Dermatologic: Pruritus, rash
Gastrointestinal: Dyspepsia, nausea, vomiting
Hepatic: ALT increased (reversible; rare), AST increased (reversible; rare)
Note: Large doses (higher than recommended) have resulted in bladder irritation, frequent/painful micturition, albuminuria, and hematuria.
Drug Interactions
Avoid Concomitant Use
  Avoid concomitant use of Methenamine with any of the following: BCG; Sulfonamide Derivatives
Increased Effect/Toxicity
  Methenamine may increase the levels/effects of: Sulfonamide Derivatives
Decreased Effect
  Methenamine may decrease the levels/effects of: Amphetamines; BCG; Typhoid Vaccine
  The levels/effects of Methenamine may be decreased by: Antacids; Carbonic Anhydrase Inhibitors
Ethanol/Nutrition/Herb Interactions Food: Foods/diets which alkalinize urine (pH >5.5) decrease therapeutic effect of methenamine.
Stability Store at room temperature of 15°C to 30°C (59°F to 86°F). Protect from light.
Mechanism of Action Methenamine is hydrolyzed to formaldehyde and ammonia in acidic urine; formaldehyde has nonspecific bactericidal action. Other components, hippuric acid or mandelic acid, aid in maintaining urine acidity and may aid in suppressing bacteria.
Pharmacodynamics/Kinetics
Absorption: Readily
Metabolism: Gastric juices: Hydrolyze 10% to 30% unless protected via enteric coating; Hepatic: ~10% to 25%
Half-life elimination: 3-6 hours
Excretion: Urine (90% as unchanged drug) within 24 hours

Dosage
Geriatric & Adult Urinary tract infection: Oral:
Hippurate: 1 g twice daily
Mandelate: 1 g 4 times/day after meals and at bedtime
Renal Impairment Cl_{cr} <50 mL/minute: Avoid use.
Administration Administer around-the-clock to promote less variation in effect.
Monitoring Parameters Urinalysis, periodic liver function tests
Test Interactions Increased urinary catecholamines, 17-hydroxycorticosteroid and vanillyl-mandelic acid (VMA) levels; decreased urinary 5-hydroxyindoleacetic acid (5HIAA) and estriol levels

Pharmacotherapy Pearls Should not be used to treat infections outside of the lower urinary tract. Methenamine has little, if any, role in the treatment or prevention of infections in patients with indwelling urinary (Foley) catheters. Furthermore, in noncatheterized patients, more effective antibiotics are available for the prevention or treatment of urinary tract infections. The influence of decreased renal function on the pharmacologic effects of methenamine results are unknown.

Special Geriatric Considerations Methenamine has little, if any, role in the treatment or prevention of infections in patients with indwelling urinary (Foley) catheters. Furthermore, in noncatheterized patients, more effective antibiotics are available for the prevention or treatment of urinary tract infections. The influence of decreased renal function on the pharmacologic effects of methenamine results are unknown.

Dosage Forms Excipient information presented when available (limited, particularly for generics); consult specific product labeling.
Tablet, oral, as hippurate: 1 g
Hiprex®: 1 g [scored; contains tartrazine]
Tablet, oral, as mandelate: 500 mg, 1 g

Selected References
Vainrub B and Musher DM, "Lack of Effect of Methenamine in Suppression of, or Prophylaxis Against, Chronic Urinary Tract Infection," *Antimicrob Agents Chemother*, 1977, 12:625-9.

♦ **Methenamine Hippurate** *see* Methenamine *on page 1164*
♦ **Methenamine Mandelate** *see* Methenamine *on page 1164*

Methimazole (meth IM a zole)

Medication Safety Issues
Sound-alike/look-alike issues:
Methimazole may be confused with metolazone
Brand Names: U.S. Tapazole®
Brand Names: Canada Dom-Methimazole; PHL-Methimazole; Tapazole®
Index Terms Thiamazole
Generic Availability (U.S.) Yes
Pharmacologic Category Antithyroid Agent; Thioamide
Use Treatment of hyperthyroidism; improve hyperthyroidism prior to thyroidectomy or radio-active iodine therapy
Contraindications Hypersensitivity to methimazole or any component of the formulation
Warnings/Precautions Antithyroid agents have been associated (rarely) with significant bone marrow depression. The most severe manifestation is agranulocytosis. Aplastic anemia, thrombocytopenia, and leukopenia may also occur. Use with extreme caution in patients receiving other drugs known to cause myelosuppression (particularly agranulocytosis) and in patients >40 years of age; avoid doses ≥40 mg/day (increased myelosuppression). Monitor patients closely; discontinue if significant bone marrow suppression occurs, particularly agranulocytosis or aplastic anemia.

May cause hypoprothrombinemia and bleeding. Rare, severe hepatic reactions (hepatic necrosis, hepatitis, encephalopathy) may occur; possibly fatal. Symptoms suggestive of hepatic dysfunction should prompt evaluation. Discontinue in the presence of hepatitis (transaminase >3 times upper limit of normal). In addition, other rare hypersensitivity reactions to antithyroid agents have been reported, including the development of ANCA-positive vasculitis, drug fever, exfoliative dermatitis, glomerulonephritis, leukocytoclastic vasculitis, and a lupus-like syndrome; prompt discontinuation is warranted in patients who develop symptoms consistent with a form of autoimmunity or other hypersensitivity during therapy. Minor dermatologic reactions may not require discontinuation, depending on severity.
Adverse Reactions (Reflective of adult population; not specific for elderly) Frequency not defined.
Cardiovascular: ANCA-positive vasculitis, edema, leukocytoclastic vasculitis, periarteritis
Central nervous system: Drowsiness, fever, headache, neuritis, vertigo

◀ Dermatologic: Alopecia, exfoliative dermatitis, pruritus, skin pigmentation, skin rash, urticaria

Endocrine & metabolic: Goiter, hypoglycemic coma

Gastrointestinal: Constipation, epigastric distress, loss of taste perception, nausea, salivary gland swelling, vomiting, weight gain

Hematologic: Agranulocytosis, aplastic anemia, granulocytopenia, hypoprothrombinemia, leukopenia, thrombocytopenia

Hepatic: Hepatic necrosis, hepatitis, jaundice

Neuromuscular & skeletal: Arthralgia, myalgia, paresthesia

Renal: Nephritis

Miscellaneous: Insulin autoimmune syndrome, lymphadenopathy, SLE-like syndrome

Drug Interactions

Metabolism/Transport Effects Inhibits CYP1A2 (weak), 2A6 (weak), 2B6 (weak), 2C9 (weak), 2C19 (weak), 2D6 (moderate), 2E1 (weak), 3A4 (weak)

Avoid Concomitant Use

Avoid concomitant use of Methimazole with any of the following: Sodium Iodide I131

Increased Effect/Toxicity There are no known significant interactions involving an increase in effect.

Decreased Effect

Methimazole may decrease the levels/effects of: Sodium Iodide I131; Vitamin K Antagonists

Stability Store at 20°C to 25°C (68°F to 77°F); excursion permitted to 15°C to 30°C (59°F to 86°F). Protect from light.

Mechanism of Action Inhibits the synthesis of thyroid hormones by blocking the oxidation of iodine in the thyroid gland. As a result, methimazole inhibits the ability of iodine to combine with tyrosine to form thyroxine and triiodothyronine (T_3); does not inactivate circulating T_4 and T_3

Pharmacodynamics/Kinetics

Onset of action: Antithyroid: Oral: 12-18 hours

Duration: 36-72 hours

Distribution: Concentrated in thyroid gland

Protein binding, plasma: None

Metabolism: Hepatic

Bioavailability: ~93%

Half-life elimination: 4-6 hours

Time to peak, serum concentration: 1-2 hours

Excretion: Urine

Dosage

Geriatric & Adult

Hyperthyroidism: Oral: Initial: 15 mg/day in 3 divided doses (approximately every 8 hours) for mild hyperthyroidism; 30-40 mg/day in moderately severe hyperthyroidism; 60 mg/day in severe hyperthyroidism; maintenance: 5-15 mg/day (may be given as a single daily dose in many cases)

Adjust dosage as required to achieve and maintain serum T_3, T_4, and TSH levels in the normal range. An elevated T_3 may be the sole indicator of inadequate treatment. An elevated TSH indicates excessive antithyroid treatment.

Thyrotoxic crisis (unlabeled use): Note: Recommendations vary; use in combination with other specific agents. Dosages of 20-25 mg every 6 hours have been used; once stable, dosing frequency may be reduced to once or twice daily (Nayak, 2006). Rectal administration has been described (Nabil, 1982).

Administration Administer orally with meals. In thyrotoxic crisis, rectal administration has been described (Nabil, 1982).

Monitoring Parameters Monitor for signs of hypothyroidism, hyperthyroidism, T_4, T_3; CBC with differential, liver function (baseline and as needed), serum thyroxine, free thyroxine index; prothrombin time

Pharmacotherapy Pearls Periodic blood counts are recommended with chronic therapy. See Warnings/Precautions.

Special Geriatric Considerations The use of antithyroid thioamides is as effective in the elderly as they are in younger adults.

Dosage Forms Excipient information presented when available (limited, particularly for generics); consult specific product labeling.

Tablet, oral: 5 mg, 10 mg

Tapazole® 5 mg, 10 mg [scored]

Selected References

Nayak B and Burman K, "Thyrotoxicosis and Thyroid Storm," *Endocrinol Metab Clin North Am*, 2006, 35(4):663-86.

Ozaki N, Miura Y, Sakakibara A, et al, "A Case of Hypersensitivity Syndrome Induced by Methimazole for Graves' Disease," *Thyroid*, 2005, 15(12):1333-6.

◆ **Methitest™** *see* MethylTESTOSTERone *on page 1188*

Methocarbamol (meth oh KAR ba mole)

Related Information
Beers Criteria – Potentially Inappropriate Medications for Geriatrics *on page 2089*

Medication Safety Issues
Sound-alike/look-alike issues:
Methocarbamol may be confused with mephobarbital
Robaxin® may be confused with ribavirin, Rubex®, Skelaxin®
BEERS Criteria medication:
This drug may be inappropriate for use in geriatric patients (high severity risk).

Brand Names: U.S. Robaxin®; Robaxin®-750

Brand Names: Canada Robaxin®

Generic Availability (U.S.) Yes: Tablet

Pharmacologic Category Skeletal Muscle Relaxant

Use Adjunctive treatment of muscle spasm associated with acute painful musculoskeletal conditions (eg, tetanus)

Contraindications Hypersensitivity to methocarbamol or any component of the formulation; renal impairment (injection formulation)

Warnings/Precautions May cause CNS depression, which may impair physical or mental abilities; patients must be cautioned about performing tasks which require mental alertness (eg, operating machinery or driving). Effects may be potentiated when used with other sedative drugs or ethanol. Plasma protein binding and clearance are decreased and the half-life is increased in patients with hepatic impairment. This class of medication is poorly tolerated by the elderly due to anticholinergic effects, sedation, and weakness. Efficacy is questionable at dosages tolerated by elderly patients (Beers Criteria).

Injection: Contraindicated in renal impairment. Contains polyethylene glycol. Rate of injection should not exceed 3 mL/minute; solution is hypertonic; avoid extravasation. Use with caution in patients with a history of seizures. Use caution with hepatic impairment. Vial stopper contains latex. Recommended only for the treatment of tetanus in pediatric patients.

Adverse Reactions (Reflective of adult population; not specific for elderly) Frequency not defined.
Cardiovascular: Bradycardia, flushing, hypotension, syncope
Central nervous system: Amnesia, confusion, coordination impaired (mild), dizziness, drowsiness, fever, headache, insomnia, lightheadedness, sedation, seizures, vertigo
Dermatologic: Angioneurotic edema, pruritus, rash, urticaria
Gastrointestinal: Dyspepsia, metallic taste, nausea, vomiting
Hematologic: Leukopenia
Hepatic: Jaundice
Local: Pain at injection site, thrombophlebitis
Ocular: Blurred vision, conjunctivitis, diplopia, nystagmus
Respiratory: Nasal congestion
Miscellaneous: Hypersensitivity reactions including anaphylaxis

Drug Interactions
Avoid Concomitant Use There are no known interactions where it is recommended to avoid concomitant use.

Increased Effect/Toxicity
Methocarbamol may increase the levels/effects of: Alcohol (Ethyl); CNS Depressants; Methotrimeprazine; Selective Serotonin Reuptake Inhibitors

The levels/effects of Methocarbamol may be increased by: Droperidol; HydrOXYzine; Methotrimeprazine

Decreased Effect
Methocarbamol may decrease the levels/effects of: Pyridostigmine

Ethanol/Nutrition/Herb Interactions
Ethanol: May increase CNS depression; monitor for increased effects with coadministration. Caution patients about effects.
Herb/Nutraceutical: Avoid valerian, St John's wort, kava kava, gotu kola (may increase CNS depression).

Stability
Injection: Prior to dilution, store at controlled room temperature of 20°C to 25°C (68°F to 77°F); excursions permitted to 15°C to 30°C (59°F to 86°F).
Tablet: Store at controlled room temperature of 20°C to 25°C (68°F to 77°F).

Mechanism of Action Causes skeletal muscle relaxation by general CNS depression

Pharmacodynamics/Kinetics
Onset of action: Muscle relaxation: Oral: ~30 minutes
Protein binding: 46% to 50%
Metabolism: Hepatic via dealkylation and hydroxylation
Half-life elimination: 1-2 hours
Time to peak, serum: Oral: 1-2 hours
Excretion: Urine (primarily as metabolites)

Dosage

Adult

Muscle spasm:
Oral: 1.5 g 4 times/day for 2-3 days (up to 8 g/day may be given in severe conditions), then decrease to 4-4.5 g/day in 3-6 divided doses
I.M., I.V.: Initial: 1 g; may repeat every 8 hours if oral administration not possible; maximum dose: 3 g/day for no more than 3 consecutive days. If condition persists, may repeat course of therapy after a drug-free interval of 48 hours.
Tetanus: I.V.: Initial dose: 1-2 g by direct I.V. injection, which may be followed by an additional 1-2 g by infusion (maximum initial dose: 3 g total); may repeat initial dose every 6 hours until NG tube or oral therapy possible; total oral daily dose of up to 24 g may be needed; injection should not be used for more than 3 consecutive days

Renal Impairment Administration of the parenteral formulation is contraindicated in patients with renal dysfunction due to the presence of polyethylene glycol.

Hepatic Impairment Specific dosing guidelines are not available.

Administration
Injection:
I.M.: A maximum of 5 mL can be administered into each gluteal region.
I.V.: Maximum rate: 3 mL/minute; should not be used for more than 3 consecutive days; may be administered undiluted. Monitor closely for extravasation. Administer I.V. while in recumbent position. Maintain position 15-30 minutes following infusion.
Tablet: May be crushed and mixed with food or liquid if needed. Avoid alcohol.

Monitoring Parameters Relief of symptoms, mental status; blood pressure, pulse in I.V. administration

Test Interactions May cause color interference in certain screening tests for 5-HIAA using nitrosonaphthol reagent and in screening tests for urinary VMA using the Gitlow method.

Special Geriatric Considerations There is no specific information on the use of skeletal muscle relaxants in the elderly. Methocarbamol has a short half-life, so it may be considered one of the safer agents in this class.

This medication is considered to be potentially inappropriate in this patient population (Beers Criteria severity: High).

Dosage Forms Excipient information presented when available (limited, particularly for generics); consult specific product labeling.
Injection, solution:
Robaxin®: 100 mg/mL (10 mL) [contains natural rubber/natural latex in packaging, polyethylene glycol 300]
Tablet, oral: 500 mg, 750 mg
Robaxin®: 500 mg [scored]
Robaxin®-750: 750 mg

Methotrexate (meth oh TREKS ate)

Medication Safety Issues
Sound-alike/look-alike issues:
Methotrexate may be confused with mercaptopurine, methylPREDNISolone sodium succinate, metolazone, metroNIDAZOLE, mitoXANtrone, PRALAtrexate

High alert medication:
The Institute for Safe Medication Practices (ISMP) includes this medication among its list of drugs which have a heightened risk of causing significant patient harm when used in error.

Administration issues:
Errors have occurred (resulting in death) when methotrexate was administered as "daily" dose instead of the recommended "weekly" dose.

Intrathecal medication safety: The American Society of Clinical Oncology (ASCO)/Oncology Nursing Society (ONS) chemotherapy administration safety standards (Jacobson, 2009) encourage the following safety measures for intrathecal chemotherapy:
• Intrathecal medication should not be prepared during the preparation of any other agents
• After preparation, store in an isolated location or container clearly marked with a label identifying as "intrathecal" use only

- Delivery to the patient should only be with other medications intended for administration into the central nervous system

Other safety concerns:
MTX is an error-prone abbreviation (mistaken as mitoxantrone)

International issues:
Trexall [U.S.] may be confused with Trexol brand name for tamadol [Mexico]; Truxal brand name for chlorprothixene [multiple international markets]

Brand Names: U.S. Rheumatrex®; Trexall™

Brand Names: Canada Apo-Methotrexate®; ratio-Methotrexate

Index Terms Amethopterin; Methotrexate Sodium; Methotrexatum; MTX (error-prone abbreviation)

Generic Availability (U.S.) Yes

Pharmacologic Category Antineoplastic Agent, Antimetabolite (Antifolate); Antirheumatic, Disease Modifying; Immunosuppressant Agent

Use
Oncology-related uses: Treatment of trophoblastic neoplasms (gestational choriocarcinoma, chorioadenoma destruens and hydatidiform mole), acute lymphocytic leukemia (ALL), meningeal leukemia, breast cancer, head and neck cancer (epidermoid), cutaneous T-Cell lymphoma (advanced mycosis fungoides), lung cancer (squamous cell and small cell), advanced non-Hodgkin's lymphomas (NHL), osteosarcoma

Nononcology uses: Treatment of psoriasis (severe, recalcitrant, disabling) and severe rheumatoid arthritis (RA), including polyarticular-course juvenile idiopathic arthritis (JIA)

Unlabeled/Investigational Use Treatment and maintenance of remission in Crohn's disease; dermatomyositis; bladder cancer, central nervous system tumors (including nonleukemic meningeal cancers), acute promyelocytic leukemia (maintenance treatment), soft tissue sarcoma (desmoid tumors)

Contraindications Hypersensitivity to methotrexate or any component of the formulation

Additional contraindications for patients with psoriasis or rheumatoid arthritis: Alcoholism, alcoholic liver disease or other chronic liver disease, immunodeficiency syndrome (overt or laboratory evidence); pre-existing blood dyscrasias (eg, bone marrow hypoplasia, leukopenia, thrombocytopenia, significant anemia)

Warnings/Precautions Hazardous agent - use appropriate precautions for handling and disposal.

[U.S. Boxed Warning]: Methotrexate has been associated with acute (elevated transaminases) and potentially fatal chronic (fibrosis, cirrhosis) hepatotoxicity. Risk is related to cumulative dose and prolonged exposure. Monitor closely (with liver function tests, including serum albumin) for liver toxicities. Liver enzyme elevations may be noted, but may not be predictive of hepatic disease in long term treatment for psoriasis (but generally is predictive in rheumatoid arthritis [RA] treatment). With long-term use, liver biopsy may show histologic changes, fibrosis, or cirrhosis; periodic liver biopsy is recommended with long-term use for psoriasis patients with risk factors for hepatotoxicity and for persistent abnormal liver function tests in psoriasis patients without risk factors for hepatotoxicity and in RA patients; discontinue methotrexate with moderate-to-severe change in liver biopsy. Risk factors for hepatotoxicity include history of above moderate ethanol consumption, persistent abnormal liver chemistries, history of chronic liver disease (including hepatitis B or C), family history of inheritable liver disease, diabetes, obesity, hyperlipidemia, lack of folate supplementation during methotrexate therapy, and history of significant exposure to hepatotoxic drugs. Use caution with preexisting liver impairment; may require dosage reduction. Use caution when used with other hepatotoxic agents (azathioprine, retinoids, sulfasalazine). **[U.S. Boxed Warning]: Methotrexate elimination is reduced in patients with ascites;** may require dose reduction or discontinuation. Monitor closely for toxicity.

[U.S. Boxed Warning]: May cause renal damage leading to acute renal failure, especially with high-dose methotrexate; monitor renal function and methotrexate levels closely, maintain adequate hydration and urinary alkalinization. Use caution in osteosarcoma patients treated with high-dose methotrexate in combination with nephrotoxic chemotherapy (eg, cisplatin). **[U.S. Boxed Warning]: Methotrexate elimination is reduced in patients with renal impairment;** may require dose reduction or discontinuation; monitor closely for toxicity. **[U.S. Boxed Warning]: Tumor lysis syndrome may occur in patients with high tumor burden;** use appropriate prevention and treatment.

[U.S. Boxed Warning]: May cause potentially life-threatening pneumonitis (may occur at any time during therapy and at any dosage); monitor closely for pulmonary symptoms, particularly dry, nonproductive cough. Other potential symptoms include fever, dyspnea, hypoxemia, or pulmonary infiltrate. **[U.S. Boxed Warning]: Methotrexate elimination is reduced in patients with pleural effusions;** may require dose reduction or discontinuation. Monitor closely for toxicity.

METHOTREXATE

[U.S. Boxed Warning]: Bone marrow suppression may occur, resulting in anemia, aplastic anemia, pancytopenia, leukopenia, neutropenia, and/or thrombocytopenia. Use caution in patients with pre-existing bone marrow suppression. Discontinue therapy in RA or psoriasis if a significant decrease in hematologic components is noted. **[U.S. Boxed Warning]: Use of low dose methotrexate has been associated with the development of malignant lymphomas;** may regress upon discontinuation of therapy; treat lymphoma appropriately if regression is not induced by cessation of methotrexate.

[U.S. Boxed Warning]: Diarrhea and ulcerative stomatitis may require interruption of therapy; death from hemorrhagic enteritis or intestinal perforation has been reported. Use with caution in patients with peptic ulcer disease, ulcerative colitis.

May cause neurotoxicity including seizures (usually in pediatric ALL patients), leukoencephalopathy (usually with concurrent cranial irradiation) and stroke-like encephalopathy (usually with high-dose regimens). Chemical arachnoiditis (headache, back pain, nuchal rigidity, fever), myelopathy and chronic leukoencephalopathy may result from intrathecal administration.

[U.S. Boxed Warning]: Any dose level or route of administration may cause severe and potentially fatal dermatologic reactions, including toxic epidermal necrolysis, Stevens-Johnson syndrome, exfoliative dermatitis, skin necrosis, and erythema multiforme. Radiation dermatitis and sunburn may be precipitated by methotrexate administration. Psoriatic lesions may be worsened by concomitant exposure to ultraviolet radiation.

[U.S. Boxed Warning]: Concomitant administration with NSAIDs may cause severe bone marrow suppression, aplastic anemia, and GI toxicity. Do not administer NSAIDs prior to or during high dose methotrexate therapy; may increase and prolong serum methotrexate levels. Doses used for psoriasis may still lead to unexpected toxicities; use caution when administering NSAIDs or salicylates with lower doses of methotrexate for RA. Methotrexate may increase the levels and effects of mercaptopurine; may require dosage adjustments. Vitamins containing folate may decrease response to systemic methotrexate; folate deficiency may increase methotrexate toxicity. **[U.S. Boxed Warning]: Concomitant methotrexate administration with radiotherapy may increase the risk of soft tissue necrosis and osteonecrosis.**

[U.S. Boxed Warnings]: Should be administered under the supervision of a physician experienced in the use of antimetabolite therapy; serious and fatal toxicities have occurred at all dose levels. Immune suppression may lead to potentially fatal opportunistic infections. For rheumatoid arthritis and psoriasis, immunosuppressive therapy should only be used when disease is active and less toxic, traditional therapy is ineffective. Methotrexate formulations and/or diluents containing preservatives should not be used for intrathecal or high-dose therapy. May cause impairment of fertility, oligospermia, and menstrual dysfunction. Toxicity from methotrexate or any immunosuppressive is increased in the elderly.

When used for intrathecal administration, should not be prepared during the preparation of any other agents; after preparation, store intrathecal medications in an isolated location or container clearly marked with a label identifying as "intrathecal" use only; delivery of intrathecal medications to the patient should only be with other medications intended for administration into the central nervous system (Jacobson, 2009).

Adverse Reactions (Reflective of adult population; not specific for elderly) Note: Adverse reactions vary by route and dosage. Hematologic and/or gastrointestinal toxicities may be common at dosages used in chemotherapy; these reactions are much less frequent when used at typical dosages for rheumatic diseases.

>10%:
Central nervous system (with I.T. administration or very high-dose therapy):
Arachnoiditis: Acute reaction manifested as severe headache, nuchal rigidity, vomiting, and fever; may be alleviated by reducing the dose
Subacute toxicity: 10% of patients treated with 12-15 mg/m^2 of I.T. methotrexate may develop this in the second or third week of therapy; consists of motor paralysis of extremities, cranial nerve palsy, seizure, or coma. This has also been seen in pediatric cases receiving very high-dose I.V. methotrexate.
Demyelinating encephalopathy: Seen months or years after receiving methotrexate; usually in association with cranial irradiation or other systemic chemotherapy
Dermatologic: Reddening of skin
Endocrine & metabolic: Hyperuricemia, defective oogenesis or spermatogenesis
Gastrointestinal: Ulcerative stomatitis, glossitis, gingivitis, nausea, vomiting, diarrhea, anorexia, intestinal perforation, mucositis (dose dependent; appears in 3-7 days after therapy, resolving within 2 weeks)
Hematologic: Leukopenia, myelosuppression (nadir: 7-10 days), thrombocytopenia

Renal: Renal failure, azotemia, nephropathy
Respiratory: Pharyngitis

1% to 10%:
Cardiovascular: Vasculitis
Central nervous system: Dizziness, malaise, encephalopathy, seizure, fever, chills
Dermatologic: Alopecia, rash, photosensitivity, depigmentation or hyperpigmentation of skin
Endocrine & metabolic: Diabetes
Genitourinary: Cystitis
Hematologic: Hemorrhage
Hepatic: Cirrhosis and portal fibrosis have been associated with chronic methotrexate therapy; acute elevation of liver enzymes are common after high-dose methotrexate, and usually resolve within 10 days.
Neuromuscular & skeletal: Arthralgia
Ocular: Blurred vision
Renal: Renal dysfunction: Manifested by an abrupt rise in serum creatinine and BUN and a fall in urine output; more common with high-dose methotrexate, and may be due to precipitation of the drug.
Respiratory: Pneumonitis: Associated with fever, cough, and interstitial pulmonary infiltrates; treatment is to withhold methotrexate during the acute reaction; interstitial pneumonitis has been reported to occur with an incidence of 1% in patients with RA (dose 7.5-15 mg/week)

Drug Interactions

Metabolism/Transport Effects Substrate of P-glycoprotein, SLCO1B1

Avoid Concomitant Use

Avoid concomitant use of Methotrexate with any of the following: Acitretin; BCG; Natalizumab; Pimecrolimus; Tacrolimus (Topical)

Increased Effect/Toxicity

Methotrexate may increase the levels/effects of: CycloSPORINE; CycloSPORINE (Systemic); Leflunomide; Loop Diuretics; Natalizumab; Theophylline Derivatives; Vaccines (Live); Vitamin K Antagonists

The levels/effects of Methotrexate may be increased by: Acitretin; Ciprofloxacin; Ciprofloxacin (Systemic); CycloSPORINE; CycloSPORINE (Systemic); Denosumab; Eltrombopag; Loop Diuretics; Nonsteroidal Anti-Inflammatory Agents; Penicillins; P-Glycoprotein Inhibitors; Pimecrolimus; Probenecid; Proton Pump Inhibitors; Roflumilast; Salicylates; Sulfonamide Derivatives; Tacrolimus (Topical); Trastuzumab; Trimethoprim

Decreased Effect

Methotrexate may decrease the levels/effects of: BCG; Cardiac Glycosides; Loop Diuretics; Sapropterin; Sipuleucel-T; Vaccines (Inactivated); Vitamin K Antagonists

The levels/effects of Methotrexate may be decreased by: Bile Acid Sequestrants; Echinacea; P-Glycoprotein Inducers

Ethanol/Nutrition/Herb Interactions

Ethanol: Avoid ethanol (may be associated with increased liver injury).
Food: Methotrexate peak serum levels may be decreased if taken with food. Milk-rich foods may decrease methotrexate absorption. Folate may decrease drug response.
Herb/Nutraceutical: Avoid echinacea (has immunostimulant properties).

Stability Store tablets and intact vials at room temperature (15°C to 25°C). Use appropriate precautions for handling and disposal. Protect from light. **Use preservative-free preparations for intrathecal or high-dose methotrexate administration.**

I.M., I.V., SubQ: Dilute powder with D$_5$W or NS to a concentration of ≤25 mg/mL (20 mg and 50 mg vials) and 50 mg/mL (1 g vial). Further dilution in D$_5$W or NS is stable for 24 hours at room temperature (21°C to 25°C). Reconstituted solutions with a preservative may be stored under refrigeration for up to 3 months, and up to 4 weeks at room temperature.

Intrathecal: Prepare intrathecal solutions with preservative-free NS, lactated Ringer's, or Elliot's B solution to a final volume of up to 12 mL (volume generally based on institution or practitioner preference). Intrathecal methotrexate concentrations may be institution specific or based on practitioner preference, generally ranging from a final concentration of 1 mg/mL (per prescribing information; Grossman, 1993; Lin, 2008) up to ~2-4 mg/mL (de Lemos, 2009; Glantz, 1999). For triple intrathecal therapy (methotrexate 12 mg/hydrocortisone 24 mg/cytarabine 36 mg), preparation to final volume of 12 mL is reported (Lin, 2008). Intrathecal dilutions are preservative-free and should be used as soon as possible after preparation. Intrathecal medications should **NOT** be prepared during the preparation of any other agents. After preparation, store intrathecal medications (until use) in an isolated location or container clearly marked with a label identifying as "intrathecal" use only.

◀ **Mechanism of Action** Methotrexate is a folate antimetabolite that inhibits DNA synthesis. Methotrexate irreversibly binds to dihydrofolate reductase, inhibiting the formation of reduced folates, and thymidylate synthetase, resulting in inhibition of purine and thymidylic acid synthesis. Methotrexate is cell cycle specific for the S phase of the cycle.

The MOA in the treatment of rheumatoid arthritis is unknown, but may affect immune function. In psoriasis, methotrexate is thought to target rapidly proliferating epithelial cells in the skin.

In Crohn's disease, it may have immune modulator and anti-inflammatory activity.

Pharmacodynamics/Kinetics

Onset of action: Antirheumatic: 3-6 weeks; additional improvement may continue longer than 12 weeks

Absorption: Oral: Dose dependent; well absorbed at low doses (<30 mg/m^2), incomplete after higher doses; I.M. injection: Complete

Distribution: Penetrates slowly into 3rd space fluids (eg, pleural effusions, ascites), exits slowly from these compartments (slower than from plasma); sustained concentrations retained in kidney and liver

V_d: 0.18 L/kg (initial); 0.4-0.8 L/kg (steady state)

Protein binding: ~50%

Metabolism: <10%; degraded by intestinal flora to DAMPA by carboxypeptidase; hepatic aldehyde oxidase converts methotrexate to 7-OH methotrexate; polyglutamates are produced intracellularly and are just as potent as methotrexate; their production is dose- and duration-dependent and they are slowly eliminated by the cell once formed. Polyglutamated forms can be converted back to methotrexate.

Bioavailability: Dose dependent; ~60% at low doses

Half-life elimination: Low dose: 3-10 hours; High dose: 8-15 hours

Time to peak, serum: Oral: 1-2 hours; I.M.: 30-60 minutes

Excretion: Urine (44% to 100%); feces (small amounts)

Dosage

Geriatric Refer to individual protocols; adjust for renal impairment.

Meningeal leukemia: I.T.: Consider a dose reduction (CSF volume and turnover may decrease with age)

Rheumatoid arthritis/psoriasis: Oral: Initial: 5-7.5 mg/week, not to exceed 20 mg/week

Adult Details concerning dosing in combination regimens should also be consulted.

Note: Doses between 100-500 mg/m^2 **may require** leucovorin rescue. Doses >500 mg/m^2 **require** leucovorin rescue: I.V., I.M., Oral: Leucovorin 10-15 mg/m^2 every 6 hours for 8 or 10 doses, starting 24 hours after the start of methotrexate infusion. Continue until the methotrexate level is ≤0.1 micromolar (10^{-7} M). Some clinicians continue leucovorin until the methotrexate level is <0.05 micromolar (5 x 10^{-8} M) or 0.01 micromolar (10^{-8} M).

If the 48-hour methotrexate level is >1 micromolar (10^{-6} M) or the 72-hour methotrexate level is >0.2 micromolar (2 x 10^{-7} M): I.V., I.M, Oral: Leucovorin 100 mg/m^2 every 6 hours until the methotrexate level is ≤0.1 micromolar (10^{-7} M). Some clinicians continue leucovorin until the methotrexate level is <0.05 micromolar (5 x 10^{-8} M) or 0.01 micromolar (10^{-8} M).

Antineoplastic dosage range: I.V.: Range is wide from 30-40 mg/m^2/week to 100-12,000 mg/m^2 with leucovorin rescue

Trophoblastic neoplasms:
Oral, I.M.: 15-30 mg/day for 5 days; repeat in 7 days for 3-5 courses
I.V.: 11 mg/m^2 days 1 through 5 every 3 weeks

Head and neck cancer: Oral, I.M., I.V.: 25-50 mg/m^2 once weekly

Mycosis fungoides (cutaneous T-cell lymphoma): Oral, I.M.: Initial (early stages):
5-50 mg once weekly **or**
15-37.5 mg twice weekly

Breast cancer: I.V.: 30-60 mg/m^2 Day 1 and 8 every 3-4 weeks

Lymphoma, non-Hodgkin's: I.V.:
30 mg/m^2 days 3 and 10 every 3 weeks **or**
120 mg/m^2 day 8 and 15 every 3-4 weeks **or**
200 mg/m^2 day 8 and 15 every 3 weeks **or**
400 mg/m^2 every 4 weeks for 3 cycles **or**
1 g/m^2 every 3 weeks **or**
1.5 g/m^2 every 4 weeks

Meningeal leukemia: I.T.: Usual dose: 12 mg/dose

Osteosarcoma: I.V.: 8-12 g/m^2 weekly for 2-4 weeks

Rheumatoid arthritis: Some experts recommend concomitant folic acid at a dose of least 5 mg/week (except the day of methotrexate) to reduce hematologic, gastrointestinal, and hepatic adverse events related to methotrexate.

Oral (manufacturer labeling): 7.5 mg once weekly or 2.5 mg every 12 hours for 3 doses/ week (dosage exceeding 20 mg/week may cause a higher incidence and severity of adverse events); *alternatively,* 10-15 mg once weekly, increased by 5 mg every 2-4 weeks to a maximum of 20-30 mg once weekly has been recommended by some experts (Visser, 2009)

I.M., SubQ (unlabeled route): 15 mg once weekly (dosage varies, similar to oral) (Braun, 2008)

Psoriasis: Some experts recommend concomitant folic acid 1-5 mg/day (except the day of methotrexate) to reduce hematologic, gastrointestinal, and hepatic adverse events related to methotrexate.

Oral: 2.5-5 mg/dose every 12 hours for 3 doses given weekly **or**

Oral, I.M., SubQ: 10-25 mg/dose given once weekly; titrate to lowest effective dose

Note: An initial test dose of 2.5-5 mg is recommended in patients with risk factors for hematologic toxicity or renal impairment. (Kalb, 2009).

Bladder cancer (unlabeled use): I.V.:

30 mg/m^2 day 1 and 8 every 3 weeks **or**

30 mg/m^2 day 1, 15, and 22 every 4 weeks

Nonleukemic meningeal cancer (unlabeled uses): I.T.: 10-12 mg/dose twice weekly for 4 weeks, then weekly for 4 weeks, then monthly (NCCN CNS cancer guidelines v.2.2009) **or** 12 mg/dose twice weekly for 4 weeks, then weekly for 4 doses, then monthly for 4 doses (Glantz, 1998) **or** 10 mg twice weekly for 4 weeks, then weekly for 1 month, then every 2 weeks for 2 months (Glantz, 1999)

Active Crohn's disease (unlabeled use): Induction of remission: I.M., SubQ: 15-25 mg once weekly; remission maintenance: 15 mg once weekly

Note: Oral dosing has been reported as effective but oral absorption is highly variable. If patient relapses after a switch to oral, may consider returning to injectable.

Renal Impairment The FDA-approved labeling does not contain dosage adjustment guidelines.

The following guidelines have been used by some clinicians:

Cl_{cr} 61-80 mL/minute: Administer 75% of dose

Cl_{cr} 51-60 mL/minute: Administer 70% of dose

Cl_{cr} 10-50 mL/minute: Administer 30% to 50% of dose

Cl_{cr} <10 mL/minute: Avoid use

Hemodialysis: Not dialyzable (0% to 5%); supplemental dose is not necessary

Peritoneal dialysis effects: Supplemental dose is not necessary

CAVH effects: Unknown

Aronoff, 2007:

Adults:

Cl_{cr} 10-50 mL/minute: Administer 50% of dose

Cl_{cr} <10 mL/minute: Avoid use

Hemodialysis: Administer 50% of dose

Continuous renal replacement therapy (CRRT): Administer 50% of dose

Kintzel, 1995:

Cl_{cr} 46-60 mL/minute: Administer 65% of normal dose

Cl_{cr} 31-45 mL/minute: Administer 50% of normal dose

Cl_{cr} <30 mL/minute: Avoid use

Hepatic Impairment The FDA-approved labeling does not contain dosage adjustment guidelines. The following guidelines have been used by some clinicians (Floyd, 2006):

Bilirubin 3.1-5 mg/dL **or** transaminases >3 times ULN: Administer 75% of dose

Bilirubin >5 mg/dL: Avoid use

Administration Methotrexate may be administered I.M., I.V., or I.T.; I.V. administration may be as slow push, short bolus infusion, or 24- to 42-hour continuous infusion. Specific dosing schemes vary, but high dose should be followed by leucovorin calcium to prevent toxicity.

Monitoring Parameters

Laboratory tests should be performed on day 5 or day 6 of the weekly methotrexate cycle (eg, psoriasis, RA) to detect the leukopenia nadir and to avoid elevated LFTs 1-2 days after taking dose.

Patients with psoriasis:

CBC with differential and platelets (baseline, 7-14 days after initiating therapy or dosage increase, every 2-4 weeks for first few months, then every 1-3 months); BUN and serum creatinine (baseline and every 2-3 months); consider PPD for latent TB screening (baseline); LFTs (baseline, monthly for first 6 months, then every 1-2 months); chest x-ray (baseline if underlying lung disease)

Liver biopsy for patients with risk factors for hepatotoxicity: Baseline or after 2-6 months of therapy and with each 1-1.5 g cumulative dose interval

◀ Liver biopsy for patients **without** risk factors for hepatotoxicity: If persistent elevations in 5 of 9 AST levels during a 12-month period, or decline of serum albumin below the normal range with normal nutritional status. Consider biopsy after cumulative dose of 3.5-4 g and after each additional 1.5 g.

Patients with RA:
CBC with differential and platelets, serum creatinine and LFTs (baseline then every 2-4 weeks for initial 3 months of therapy, then every 8-12 weeks for 3-6 months of therapy and then every 12 weeks after 6 months of therapy); chest x-ray (baseline); pulmonary function test (if methotrexate-induced lung disease suspected); hepatitis B or C testing (baseline)

Liver biopsy: Baseline (if persistent abnormal baseline LFTs, history of alcoholism, or chronic hepatitis B or C) or during treatment if persistent LFT elevations (6 of 12 tests abnormal over 1 year or 5 of 9 results when LFTs performed at 6-week intervals)

Patients with cancer: Baseline and frequently during treatment: CBC with differential and platelets, serum creatinine, LFTs; chest x-ray (baseline); methotrexate levels and urine pH (with high-dose therapy); pulmonary function test (if methotrexate-induced lung disease suspected)

Reference Range Therapeutic levels: Variable; Toxic concentration: Variable; therapeutic range is dependent upon therapeutic approach.

High-dose regimens produce drug levels that are between 0.1-1 micromole/L 24-72 hours after drug infusion

Toxic: Low-dose therapy: >0.2 micromole/L; high-dose therapy: >1 micromole/L

Pharmacotherapy Pearls Oncology Comment: Methotrexate overexposure: The investigational rescue agent, glucarpidase, is an enzyme which rapidly hydrolyzes extracellular methotrexate into inactive metabolites, resulting in a rapid reduction of methotrexate concentrations. Glucarpidase is available for intrathecal (IT) use through an Emergency Use IND and for I.V. use under an Open-Label Treatment protocol.

Special Geriatric Considerations Toxicity to methotrexate or any immunosuppressive is increased in the elderly. Must monitor carefully. For rheumatoid arthritis and psoriasis, immunosuppressive therapy should only be used when disease is active and less toxic, traditional therapy is ineffective. Recommended doses should be reduced when initiating therapy in the elderly due to possible decreased metabolism, reduced renal function, and presence of interacting diseases and drugs. Adjust dose as needed for renal function (Cl_{cr}).

Dosage Forms Excipient information presented when available (limited, particularly for generics); consult specific product labeling.

Injection, powder for reconstitution: 1 g

Injection, solution: 25 mg/mL (2 mL, 10 mL)

Injection, solution [preservative free]: 25 mg/mL (2 mL, 4 mL, 8 mL, 10 mL, 40 mL)

Tablet, oral: 2.5 mg

Trexall™: 5 mg, 7.5 mg, 10 mg, 15 mg [scored]

Tablet, oral [dose-pack]:

Rheumatrex®: 2.5 mg [scored]

Selected References

Feagan BG, Fedorak RN, Irvine EJ, et al, "A Comparison of Methotrexate With Placebo for the Maintenance of Remission in Crohn's Disease. North American Crohn's Study Group Investigators." *N Engl J Med*, 2000, 342 (22):1627-32.

◆ **Methotrexate Sodium** *see* Methotrexate *on page 1168*

◆ **Methotrexatum** *see* Methotrexate *on page 1168*

Methsuximide (meth SUKS i mide)

Medication Safety Issues

Sound-alike/look-alike issues:

Methsuximide may be confused with ethosuximide

Brand Names: U.S. Celontin®

Brand Names: Canada Celontin®

Generic Availability (U.S.) No

Pharmacologic Category Anticonvulsant, Succinimide

Use Control of absence (petit mal) seizures that are refractory to other drugs

Unlabeled/Investigational Use Treatment of partial complex (psychomotor) seizures

Medication Guide Available Yes

Contraindications History of hypersensitivity to succinimides

Warnings/Precautions Antiepileptics are associated with an increased risk of suicidal behavior/thoughts with use (regardless of indication); patients should be monitored for signs/symptoms of depression, suicidal tendencies, and other unusual behavior changes during therapy and instructed to inform their healthcare provider immediately if symptoms occur. Use with caution in patients with hepatic or renal disease. Abrupt withdrawal of the drug may precipitate absence status. Methsuximide may increase tonic-clonic seizures when used alone in patients with mixed seizure disorders. Methsuximide must be used in combination with other anticonvulsants in patients with both absence and tonic-clonic seizures. May cause CNS depression, which may impair physical or mental abilities; patients must be cautioned about performing tasks which require mental alertness (eg, operating machinery or driving). Effects with other sedative drugs or ethanol may be potentiated. Consider evaluation of blood counts in patients with signs/symptoms of infection. Succinimides have been associated with severe blood dyscrasias and cases of systemic lupus erythematosus.

Adverse Reactions (Reflective of adult population; not specific for elderly) Frequency not defined.

Cardiovascular: Hyperemia

Central nervous system: Aggressiveness, ataxia, confusion, depression, dizziness, drowsiness, hallucinations (auditory), headache, hypochondriacal behavior, insomnia, irritability, mental instability, mental slowness, nervousness, psychosis, suicidal behavior

Dermatologic: Pruritus, rash, Stevens-Johnson syndrome, urticaria

Gastrointestinal: Abdominal pain, anorexia, constipation, diarrhea, epigastric pain, nausea, vomiting, weight loss

Genitourinary: Hematuria (microscopic), proteinuria

Hematologic: Eosinophilia, leukopenia, monocytosis, pancytopenia

Ocular: Blurred vision, periorbital edema, photophobia

Miscellaneous: Hiccups, systemic lupus erythematosus

Drug Interactions

Metabolism/Transport Effects Substrate of CYP2C19 (major); **Inhibits** CYP2C19 (weak)

Avoid Concomitant Use There are no known interactions where it is recommended to avoid concomitant use.

Increased Effect/Toxicity

Methsuximide may increase the levels/effects of: Alcohol (Ethyl); CNS Depressants; Methotrimeprazine; Selective Serotonin Reuptake Inhibitors

The levels/effects of Methsuximide may be increased by: CYP2C19 Inhibitors (Moderate); CYP2C19 Inhibitors (Strong); Droperidol; HydrOXYzine; Methotrimeprazine

Decreased Effect

The levels/effects of Methsuximide may be decreased by: CYP2C19 Inducers (Strong); Ketorolac; Ketorolac (Nasal); Ketorolac (Systemic); Mefloquine

Stability Store at 25°C (77°F); excursions permitted to 15°C to 30°C (59°F to 86°F); protect from excessive heat 40°C (104°F). Protect from light and moisture. **Note:** Methsuximide has a relatively low melting temperature (124°F); do not store in conditions that promote high temperatures (eg, in a closed vehicle).

Mechanism of Action Increases the seizure threshold and suppresses paroxysmal spike-and-wave pattern in absence seizures; depresses nerve transmission in the motor cortex

Pharmacodynamics/Kinetics

Metabolism: Hepatic; rapidly demethylated to N-desmethylmethsuximide (active metabolite)

Half-life elimination: 2-4 hours

Time to peak, serum: Within 1-3 hours

Excretion: Urine (<1% as unchanged drug)

Dosage

Geriatric & Adult Anticonvulsant: Oral: 300 mg/day for the first week; may increase by 300 mg/day at weekly intervals up to 1.2 g/day in 2-4 divided doses/day

Monitoring Parameters CBC, hepatic function tests, urinalysis; suicidality (eg, suicidal thoughts, depression, behavioral changes)

Reference Range Therapeutic: N-desmethylmethsuximide: 20-40 μg/m

Special Geriatric Considerations No specific data available for the elderly. This drug is rarely used in the elderly, however, if it is used for partial complex seizure control, monitor closely.

Dosage Forms Excipient information presented when available (limited, particularly for generics); consult specific product labeling.

Capsule, oral:

Celontin®: 150 mg, 300 mg

◆ **Methylacetoxyprogesterone** *see* MedroxyPROGESTERone *on page 1122*

◆ **Methylcobalamin, Acetylcysteine, and Methylfolate** *see* Methylfolate, Methylcobalamin, and Acetylcysteine *on page 1178*

Methyldopa (meth il DOE pa)

Related Information
  Beers Criteria – Potentially Inappropriate Medications for Geriatrics *on page 2089*
Medication Safety Issues
  Sound-alike/look-alike issues:
    Methyldopa may be confused with L-dopa, levodopa
  BEERS Criteria medication:
    This drug may be inappropriate for use in geriatric patients (high severity risk).
Brand Names: Canada Apo-Methyldopa®; Nu-Medopa
Index Terms Aldomet; Methyldopate Hydrochloride
Generic Availability (U.S.) Yes
Pharmacologic Category Alpha-Adrenergic Inhibitor; Alpha$_2$-Adrenergic Agonist
Use Management of moderate-to-severe hypertension
Contraindications Hypersensitivity to methyldopa or any component of the formulation; active hepatic disease; liver disorders previously associated with use of methyldopa; on MAO inhibitors; bisulfite allergy if using oral suspension or injectable
Warnings/Precautions May rarely produce hemolytic anemia and liver disorders; positive Coombs' test occurs in 10% to 20% of patients (perform periodic CBCs); sedation usually transient may occur during initial therapy or whenever the dose is increased. Use with caution in patients with previous liver disease or dysfunction, the active metabolites of methyldopa accumulate in uremia. Patients with impaired renal function may respond to smaller doses. Tolerance may occur usually between the second and third month of therapy. Adding a diuretic or increasing the dosage of methyldopa frequently restores blood pressure control. May be inappropriate in this age group due to a risk of bradycardia and depression (Beers Criteria). Use with caution in the elderly; may experience syncope (avoid by giving smaller doses); not considered a drug of choice in this age group. Do not use injectable if bisulfite allergy.
Adverse Reactions (Reflective of adult population; not specific for elderly)
  >10%: Cardiovascular: Peripheral edema
  1% to 10%:
    Central nervous system: Drug fever, mental depression, anxiety, nightmares, drowsiness, headache
    Gastrointestinal: Dry mouth
Drug Interactions
  Avoid Concomitant Use
    Avoid concomitant use of Methyldopa with any of the following: Iobenguane I 123; MAO Inhibitors
  Increased Effect/Toxicity
    Methyldopa may increase the levels/effects of: Lithium

    The levels/effects of Methyldopa may be increased by: COMT Inhibitors; MAO Inhibitors
  Decreased Effect
    Methyldopa may decrease the levels/effects of: Iobenguane I 123

    The levels/effects of Methyldopa may be decreased by: Iron Salts
Ethanol/Nutrition/Herb Interactions Herb/Nutraceutical: Avoid dong quai if using for hypertension (has estrogenic activity). Avoid ephedra, yohimbe, ginseng (may worsen hypertension). Avoid valerian, St John's wort, kava kava, gotu kola (may increase CNS depression). Avoid natural licorice (causes sodium and water retention and increases potassium loss). Avoid garlic (may have increased antihypertensive effect).
Stability Injectable dosage form is most stable at acid to neutral pH. Stability of parenteral admixture at room temperature (25°C) is 24 hours. Stability of parenteral admixture at refrigeration temperature (4°C) is 4 days. Standard diluent: 250-500 mg/100 mL D$_5$W.
Mechanism of Action Stimulation of central alpha-adrenergic receptors by a false transmitter that results in a decreased sympathetic outflow to the heart, kidneys, and peripheral vasculature
Pharmacodynamics/Kinetics
  Onset of action: Peak effect: Hypotensive: Oral/parenteral: 3-6 hours
  Duration: 12-24 hours
  Distribution: Crosses placenta
  Protein binding: <15%
  Metabolism: Intestinal and hepatic
  Half-life elimination: 75-80 minutes; End-stage renal disease: 6-16 hours
  Excretion: Urine (85% as metabolites) within 24 hours

Dosage
Geriatric Refer to adult dosing. Initiate at the lower end of the dosage range.
Adult Hypertension:
Oral: Initial: 250 mg 2-3 times/day; increase every 2 days as needed (maximum dose: 3 g/day); usual dose range (JNC 7): 250-1000 mg/day in 2 divided doses
I.V.: 250-1000 mg every 6-8 hours; maximum: 1 g every 6 hours
Renal Impairment
Cl_{cr} >50 mL/minute: Administer every 8 hours.
Cl_{cr} 10-50 mL/minute: Administer every 8-12 hours.
Cl_{cr} <10 mL/minute: Administer every 12-24 hours.
Slightly dialyzable (5% to 20%)
Administration Infuse over 30-60 minutes
Monitoring Parameters Blood pressure, standing and sitting/lying down, CBC, liver enzymes, Coombs' test (direct); blood pressure monitor required during I.V. administration
Test Interactions Methyldopa interferes with the following laboratory tests: urinary uric acid, serum creatinine (alkaline picrate method), AST (colorimetric method), and urinary catecholamines (falsely high levels)
Special Geriatric Considerations Because of its CNS effects, methyldopa is not considered a drug of first choice in the elderly. Adjust dose for renal function.

This medication is considered to be potentially inappropriate in this patient population (Beers Criteria severity: High).
Dosage Forms Excipient information presented when available (limited, particularly for generics); consult specific product labeling.
Injection, solution, as hydrochloride: 50 mg/mL (5 mL)
Tablet, oral: 250 mg, 500 mg

◆ **Methyldopate Hydrochloride** *see* Methyldopa *on page 1176*

Methylfolate (meth il FO late)

Brand Names: U.S. Deplin™
Index Terms 6(S)-5-methyltetrahydrofolate; 6(S)-5-MTHF; L-methylfolate
Generic Availability (U.S.) Yes
Pharmacologic Category Dietary Supplement
Use Medicinal food for management of patients with low plasma and/or low red blood cell folate
Contraindications Hypersensitivity to any component of the formulation
Warnings/Precautions Folate administration is not appropriate for monotherapy with pernicious or other megaloblastic anemias when anemia is present with vitamin B_{12} deficiency. Doses >0.1 mg/day may obscure pernicious anemia with continuing irreversible nerve damage progression. Product is a medicinal food for use only under the supervision of a healthcare provider.
Drug Interactions
Avoid Concomitant Use
Avoid concomitant use of Methylfolate with any of the following: Raltitrexed
Increased Effect/Toxicity There are no known significant interactions involving an increase in effect.
Decreased Effect
Methylfolate may decrease the levels/effects of: CarBAMazepine; Divalproex; Fosphenytoin; PHENobarbital; Phenytoin; Primidone; Pyrimethamine; Raltitrexed; Valproic Acid

The levels/effects of Methylfolate may be decreased by: Cholestyramine Resin; Colestipol; SulfaSALAzine
Stability Store at controlled room temperature of 15°C to 30°C (59°F to 86°F). Protect from light and moisture.
Mechanism of Action Methylfolate, or L-methylfolate, is the active form of folate in the body, which can be transported into peripheral tissues and across the blood brain barrier. Folate is necessary for formation of numerous coenzymes in many metabolic systems, particularly for purine, pyrimidine, and nucleoprotein synthesis, and maintenance in erythropoiesis; stimulates WBC and platelet production in folate deficiency anemia.
Dosage
Geriatric & Adult Medicinal food: Oral: One tablet (7.5 mg) daily
Pharmacotherapy Pearls Information in this monograph is currently limited to the fields presented. Consult product labeling for additional details.

The manufacturer of Deplin™ indicates a use of methylfolate in individuals who have a major depressive disorder that has not fully responded or may not fully respond to antidepressant therapy. Limited data exists of the investigational use of folate supplementation as an adjunct to the treatment of major depressive disorder. Adjunctive use in major depressive disorders requires further studies, but some studies (using various forms of folic acid) suggest a possible benefit of supplementation by augmentation of response to antidepressants, particularly in patients with low serum folate levels prior to supplementation.

Special Geriatric Considerations No special recommendations. Elderly frequently have combined nutritional deficiencies. Must rule out vitamin B_{12} deficiency before initiating folate therapy. Elderly, due to decreased nutrient intake, may benefit from daily intake of a multiple vitamin with minerals.

Dosage Forms Excipient information presented when available (limited, particularly for generics); consult specific product labeling.

Tablet, oral: 7.5 mg

Deplin™: L-methylfolate 7.5 mg [gluten free, sugar free]

Methylfolate, Methylcobalamin, and Acetylcysteine

(meth il FO late meth il koe BAL a min & a se teel SIS teen)

Related Information
Methylfolate on page 1177

Brand Names: U.S. Cerefolin® NAC

Index Terms Acetylcysteine, Methylcobalamin, and Methylfolate; Acetylcysteine, Methylfolate, and Methylcobalamin; L-methylfolate, Methylcobalamin, and N-acetylcysteine; Methylcobalamin, Acetylcysteine, and Methylfolate

Generic Availability (U.S.) No

Pharmacologic Category Dietary Supplement

Use Medicinal food for use in patients with neurovascular oxidative stress and/or hyperhomocysteinemia

Dosage
Adult Medicinal food: Oral: One caplet daily

Dosage Forms Excipient information presented when available (limited, particularly for generics); consult specific product labeling.

Caplet, oral:

Cerefolin® NAC: L-methylfolate 5.6 mg, methylcobalamin 2 mg, and N-acetylcysteine 600 mg [gluten free, sugar free]

◆ **Methylin®** see Methylphenidate on page 1179
◆ **Methylin® ER [DSC]** see Methylphenidate on page 1179
◆ **Methylmorphine** see Codeine on page 407

Methylnaltrexone (meth il nal TREKS one)

Medication Safety Issues
Sound-alike/look-alike issues:
Methylnaltrexone may be confused with naltrexone

Brand Names: U.S. Relistor®

Brand Names: Canada Relistor®

Index Terms Methylnaltrexone Bromide; N-methylnaltrexone Bromide

Generic Availability (U.S.) No

Pharmacologic Category Gastrointestinal Agent, Miscellaneous; Opioid Antagonist, Peripherally-Acting

Use Treatment of opioid-induced constipation in patients with advanced illness receiving palliative care with inadequate response to conventional laxative regimens

Dosage
Geriatric & Adult Opioid-induced constipation: SubQ: Dosing is according to body weight: Administer 1 dose every other day as needed; maximum: 1 dose/24 hours

<38 kg: 0.15 mg/kg (round dose up to nearest 0.1 mL of volume)

38 to <62 kg: 8 mg

62-114 kg: 12 mg

>114 kg: 0.15 mg/kg (round dose up to nearest 0.1 mL of volume)

Renal Impairment

Mild-to-moderate renal impairment: No adjustment required.

Severe renal impairment (Cl_{cr} <30 mL/minute): Administer 50% of normal dose.

End-stage renal impairment (dialysis-dependent): Has not been studied.

Hepatic Impairment

Mild-to-moderate hepatic impairment (Child-Pugh class A and B): No adjustment required.

Severe hepatic impairment: Has not been studied.

Special Geriatric Considerations In small studies (Phase 2 and 3), no differences in safety and efficacy were noted between elderly and young adults. No dose adjustment is required in elderly.

Dosage Forms Excipient information presented when available (limited, particularly for generics); consult specific product labeling.

Injection, solution:

Relistor®: 12 mg/0.6 mL (0.6 mL) [contains edetate calcium disodium]

◆ **Methylnaltrexone Bromide** see Methylnaltrexone on page 1178

Methylphenidate (meth il FEN i date)

Related Information

Beers Criteria – Potentially Inappropriate Medications for Geriatrics on page 2089
Patient Information for Disposal of Unused Medications on page 2125

Medication Safety Issues

Sound-alike/look-alike issues:

Metadate CD® may be confused with Metadate® ER
Metadate® ER may be confused with Metadate CD®, methadone
Methylphenidate may be confused with methadone
Ritalin® may be confused with Ismelin®, Rifadin®, ritodrine
Ritalin LA® may be confused with Ritalin-SR®
Ritalin-SR® may be confused with Ritalin LA®

Brand Names: U.S. Concerta®; Daytrana®; Metadate CD®; Metadate® ER; Methylin®; Methylin® ER [DSC]; Ritalin LA®; Ritalin-SR®; Ritalin®

Brand Names: Canada Apo-Methylphenidate®; Apo-Methylphenidate® SR; Biphentin®; Concerta®; Novo-Methylphenidate ER-C; PHL-Methylphenidate; PMS-Methylphenidate; ratio-Methylphenidate; Ritalin®; Ritalin® SR; Sandoz-Methylphenidate SR

Index Terms Methylphenidate Hydrochloride

Generic Availability (U.S.) Yes: Immediate release tablet, oral solution, sustained release tablet

Pharmacologic Category Central Nervous System Stimulant

Use Treatment of attention-deficit/hyperactivity disorder (ADHD); symptomatic management of narcolepsy

Unlabeled/Investigational Use Depression (especially elderly or medically ill)

Medication Guide Available Yes

Contraindications Hypersensitivity to methylphenidate, any component of the formulation, or idiosyncratic reactions to sympathomimetic amines; marked anxiety, tension, and agitation; glaucoma; use during or within 14 days following MAO inhibitor therapy; family history or diagnosis of Tourette's syndrome or tics

Metadate CD® and Metadate® ER: Additional contraindications: Severe hypertension, heart failure, arrhythmia, hyperthyroidism, recent MI or angina; concomitant use of halogenated anesthetics

Warnings/Precautions CNS stimulant use has been associated with serious cardiovascular events (eg, sudden death, stroke, and MI in adults) in patients with pre-existing structural cardiac abnormalities or other serious heart problems. These products should be avoided in patients with known serious structural cardiac abnormalities, cardiomyopathy, serious heart rhythm abnormalities, or other serious cardiac problems that could further increase their risk of sudden death. Patients should be carefully evaluated for cardiac disease prior to initiation of therapy. Use of stimulants can cause an increase in blood pressure (average 2-4 mm Hg) and increases in heart rate (average 3-6 bpm), although some patients may have larger than average increases. Use caution with hypertension, hyperthyroidism, or other cardiovascular conditions that might be exacerbated by increases in blood pressure or heart rate. Some products are contraindicated in patients with heart failure, arrhythmias, severe hypertension, hyperthyroidism, angina, or recent MI.

Has demonstrated value as part of a comprehensive treatment program for ADHD. Use with caution in patients with bipolar disorder (may induce mixed/manic episode). May exacerbate symptoms of behavior and thought disorder in psychotic patients; new-onset psychosis or mania may occur with stimulant use; observe for symptoms of aggression and/or hostility. Use caution with seizure disorders (may reduce seizure threshold). Use caution in patients with history of ethanol or drug abuse. May exacerbate symptoms of behavior and thought disorder in psychotic patients. **[U.S. Boxed Warning]: Potential for drug dependency exists - avoid abrupt discontinuation in patients who have received for prolonged periods.** Visual disturbances have been reported (rare).

◀ Concerta® should not be used in patients with esophageal motility disorders or pre-existing severe gastrointestinal narrowing (small bowel disease, short gut syndrome, history of peritonitis, cystic fibrosis, chronic intestinal pseudo-obstruction, Meckel's diverticulum). Metadate CD® and Metadate® ER contain sucrose and lactose, respectively; avoid administration in hereditary galactose intolerance, Lapp lactase deficiency, or glucose-galactose malabsorption. Concomitant use with halogenated anesthetics is contraindicated; may cause sudden elevations in blood pressure; if surgery is planned, do not administer Metadate CD® or Metadate® ER on the day of surgery. Transdermal system may cause allergic contact sensitization, characterized by intense local reactions (edema, papules) that may spread beyond the patch site; sensitization may subsequently manifest systemically with other routes of methylphenidate administration; monitor closely. Avoid exposure of application site to any direct external heat sources (eg, hair dryers, heating pads, electric blankets); may increase the rate and extent of absorption and risk of overdose. Efficacy of transdermal methylphenidate therapy for >7 weeks has not been established.

Adverse Reactions (Reflective of adult population; not specific for elderly)

Transdermal system: Frequency of adverse events as reported in trials of 7-week duration. Incidence of some events higher with extended use.

>10%:

Central nervous system: Headache (≤15%; long-term use in children: 28%), insomnia (6% to 13%; long-term use in children: 30%), irritability (7% to 11%)

Gastrointestinal: Appetite decreased (26%), nausea (10% to 12%)

Miscellaneous: Viral infection (long-term use in children: 28%)

1% to 10%:

Cardiovascular: Tachycardia (≤1%)

Central nervous system: Tic (7%), dizziness (adolescents 6%), emotional instability (6%)

Gastrointestinal: Vomiting (3% to 10%), weight loss (6% to 9%), abdominal pain (5% to 7%), anorexia (5%; long-term use in children: 46%)

Local: Application site reaction

Respiratory: Nasal congestion (6%) nasopharyngitis (5%)

Postmarketing and/or case reports (limited to important or life-threatening): Allergic contact dermatitis/sensitization, anaphylaxis, angioedema, hallucinations, seizures

All dosage forms: Frequency not defined:

Cardiovascular: Angina, cardiac arrhythmia, cerebral arteritis, cerebral hemorrhage, cerebral occlusion, cerebrovascular accidents, vasculitis, hyper-/hypotension, MI, murmur, palpitation, pulse increased/decreased, Raynaud's phenomenon, tachycardia

Central nervous system: Aggression, agitation, anger, anxiety, confusional state, depression, dizziness, drowsiness, fatigue, fever, headache, hypervigilance, insomnia, irritability, lethargy, mood alterations, nervousness, neuroleptic malignant syndrome (NMS) (rare), restlessness, stroke, tension, Tourette's syndrome (rare), toxic psychosis, tremor, vertigo

Dermatologic: Alopecia, erythema multiforme, exfoliative dermatitis, hyperhidrosis, rash, urticaria

Endocrine & metabolic: Dysmenorrhea, growth retardation, libido decreased

Gastrointestinal: Abdominal pain, anorexia, appetite decreased, bruxism, constipation, diarrhea, dyspepsia, nausea, vomiting, weight loss, xerostomia

Genitourinary: Erectile dysfunction

Hematologic: Anemia, leukopenia, pancytopenia, thrombocytopenic purpura, thrombocytopenia

Hepatic: Bilirubin increased, liver function tests abnormal, hepatic coma, transaminases increased

Neuromuscular & skeletal: Arthralgia, dyskinesia, muscle tightness, paresthesia

Ocular: Blurred vision, dry eyes, mydriasis, visual accommodation disturbance

Renal: Necrotizing vasculitis

Respiratory: Cough increased, dyspnea, pharyngitis, pharyngolaryngeal pain, rhinitis, sinusitis, upper respiratory tract infection

Miscellaneous: Accidental injury, hypersensitivity reactions

Drug Interactions

Metabolism/Transport Effects Inhibits CYP2D6 (weak)

Avoid Concomitant Use

Avoid concomitant use of Methylphenidate with any of the following: Inhalational Anesthetics; Iobenguane I 123; MAO Inhibitors

Increased Effect/Toxicity

Methylphenidate may increase the levels/effects of: Anti-Parkinson's Agents (Dopamine Agonist); Antipsychotics; CloNIDine; Fosphenytoin; Inhalational Anesthetics; PHENobarbital; Phenytoin; Primidone; Sympathomimetics; Tricyclic Antidepressants; Vitamin K Antagonists

The levels/effects of Methylphenidate may be increased by: Antacids; Antipsychotics; Atomoxetine; Cannabinoids; H2-Antagonists; MAO Inhibitors; Proton Pump Inhibitors

Decreased Effect

Methylphenidate may decrease the levels/effects of: Antihypertensives; Iobenguane I 123

Ethanol/Nutrition/Herb Interactions

Ethanol: Avoid ethanol (may cause CNS depression).

Food: Food may increase oral absorption; Concerta® formulation is not affected. Food delays early peak and high-fat meals increase C_{max} and AUC of Metadate CD® formulation.

Herb/Nutraceutical: Avoid ephedra (may cause hypertension or arrhythmias) and yohimbe (also has CNS stimulatory activity).

Stability

Capsule: *Extended release:* Store at 25°C (77°F); excursions permitted to 15°C to 30°C (59°F to 86°F). Protect from light.

Solution: Store at controlled room temperature of 20°C to 25°C (68°F to 77°F).

Tablet:

Chewable: Store at controlled room temperature of 20°C to 25°C (68°F to 77°F). Protect from light and moisture.

Extended and sustained release: Store at controlled room temperature of 20°C to 25°C (68°F to 77°F). Protect from light and moisture.

Immediate release: Store at controlled room temperature of 20°C to 25°C (68°F to 77°F). Protect from light and moisture.

Osmotic controlled release (Concerta®): Store at controlled room temperature of 25°C; excursions permitted to 15°C to 30°C (59°F to 86°F). Protect from humidity.

Transdermal system: Store at 25°C (77°F); excursions permitted to 15°C to 30°C (59°F to 86°F). Keep patches stored in protective pouch. Once tray is opened, use patches within 2 months; once an individual patch has been removed from the pouch and the protective liner removed, use immediately. Do not refrigerate or freeze.

Mechanism of Action Mild CNS stimulant; blocks the reuptake of norepinephrine and dopamine into presynaptic neurons; appears to stimulate the cerebral cortex and subcortical structures similar to amphetamines

Pharmacodynamics/Kinetics

Onset of action: Peak effect:

Immediate release tablet: Cerebral stimulation: ~2 hours

Extended release capsule (Metadate CD®, Ritalin LA®): Biphasic; initial peak similar to immediate release product, followed by second rising portion (corresponding to extended release portion)

Sustained release tablet: 4-7 hours

Osmotic release tablet (Concerta®): Initial: 1-2 hours

Transdermal: ~2 hours; may be expedited by the application of external heat

Duration: Immediate release tablet: 3-6 hours; Sustained release tablet: 8 hours; Extended release tablet: Methylin® ER, Metadate® ER: 8 hours, Concerta®: 12 hours

Absorption:

Oral: Readily absorbed

Transdermal: Absorption increased when applied to inflamed skin or exposed to heat. Absorption is continuous for 9 hours after application.

Distribution: V_d: *d*-methylphenidate: 2.65 ± 1.11 L/kg, *l*-methylphenidate: 1.80 ± 0.91 L/kg

Protein binding: 10% to 33%

Metabolism: Hepatic via carboxylesterase CES1A1 to minimally active metabolite

Half-life elimination: *d*-methylphenidate: 3-4 hours; *l*-methylphenidate: 1-3 hours

Time to peak: Concerta®: C_{max}: 6-8 hours; Daytrana™: 7.5-10.5 hours

Excretion: Urine (90% as metabolites and unchanged drug)

Dosage

Geriatric & Adult

ADHD: Oral:

Concerta®:

Patients not currently taking methylphenidate: Initial dose: 18-36 mg once daily in the morning

Patients currently taking methylphenidate: **Note:** Initial dose: Dosing based on current regimen and clinical judgment; suggested dosing listed below:

- Patients taking methylphenidate 5 mg 2-3 times/day: 18 mg once every morning
- Patients taking methylphenidate 10 mg 2-3 times/day: 36 mg once every morning
- Patients taking methylphenidate 15 mg 2-3 times/day: 54 mg once every morning
- Patients taking methylphenidate 20 mg 2-3 times/day: 72 mg once every morning

◄

Metadate® ER, Methylin® ER, Ritalin® SR: May be given in place of immediate release products, once the daily dose is titrated and the titrated 8-hour dosage corresponds to sustained or extended release tablet size; maximum: 60 mg/day

Metadate CD®, Ritalin LA®: Initial: 20 mg once daily; may be adjusted in 10-20 mg increments at weekly intervals; maximum: 60 mg/day

Narcolepsy: Oral: 10 mg 2-3 times/day, up to 60 mg/day

Depression (unlabeled use): Oral: Initial: 2.5 mg every morning before 9 AM; dosage may be increased by 2.5-5 mg every 2-3 days as tolerated to a maximum of 20 mg/day; may be divided (ie, 7 AM and 12 noon), but should not be given after noon; do not use sustained release product

Note: Discontinue periodically to re-evaluate or if no improvement occurs within 1 month.

Administration

Oral: Do not crush or allow patient to chew sustained or extended release dosage form. To effectively avoid insomnia, dosing should be completed by noon.

Concerta®: Administer dose once daily in the morning. May be taken with or without food, but must be taken with water, milk, or juice.

Metadate CD®, Ritalin LA®: Capsules may be opened and the contents sprinkled onto a small amount (equal to 1 tablespoon) of cold applesauce. Swallow applesauce without chewing. Do not crush or chew capsule contents.

Methylin® chewable tablet: Administer with at least 8 ounces of water or other fluid.

Topical: Transdermal (Daytrana™): Apply to clean, dry, non-oily, intact skin to the hip area, avoiding the waistline; do not premedicate the patch site with hydrocortisone or other solutions, creams, ointments, or emollients. Apply at the same time each day to alternating hips. Press firmly for 30 seconds to ensure proper adherence. Avoid exposure of application site to external heat source, which may increase the amount of drug absorbed. If difficulty is experienced when separating the patch from the liner or if any medication (sticky substance) remains on the liner after separation; discard that patch and apply a new patch. Do not use a patch that has been damaged or torn; do not cut patch. If patch should dislodge, may replace with new patch (to different site) but total wear time should not exceed 9 hours; do not reapply with dressings, tape, or common adhesives. Patch may be removed early if a shorter duration of effect is desired or if late day side effects occur. Wash hands with soap and water after handling. Avoid touching the sticky side of the patch. If patch removal is difficult, an oil-based product (eg, petroleum jelly, olive oil) may be applied to the patch edges to aid removal; never apply acetone-based products (eg, nail polish remover) to patch. Dispose of used patch by folding adhesive side onto itself, and discard in toilet or appropriate lidded container.

Monitoring Parameters Blood pressure, heart rate, signs and symptoms of depression, aggression, or hostility; CBC, differential and platelet counts, liver function tests; signs of central nervous system stimulation

Transdermal: Signs of worsening erythema, blistering or edema which does not improve within 48 hours of patch removal, or spreads beyond patch site.

When used for the treatment of ADHD, thoroughly evaluate for cardiovascular risk. Monitor heart rate, blood pressure, and consider obtaining ECG prior to initiation (Vetter, 2008).

Test Interactions May interfere with urine detection of amphetamines/methamphetamines (false-positive).

Pharmacotherapy Pearls Concerta® is an osmotic controlled release formulation (OROS®) of methylphenidate. The tablet has an immediate-release overcoat that provides an initial dose of methylphenidate within 1 hour. The overcoat covers a trilayer core. The trilayer core is composed of two layers containing the drug and excipients, and one layer of osmotic components. As water from the gastrointestinal tract enters the core, the osmotic components expand and methylphenidate is released.

Metadate CD® capsules contain a mixture of immediate release and extended release beads, designed to release 30% of the dose immediately and 70% over an extended period.

Ritalin LA® uses a combination of immediate release and enteric coated, delayed release beads.

Special Geriatric Considerations Methylphenidate is often useful in treating elderly patients who are discouraged, withdrawn, apathetic, or disinterested in their activities. In particular, it is useful in patients who are starting a rehabilitation program but have resigned themselves to fail; these patients may not have a major depressive disorder; will not improve memory or cognitive function; use with caution in patients with dementia who may have increased agitation and confusion.

Controlled Substance C-II

Dosage Forms Excipient information presented when available (limited, particularly for generics); consult specific product labeling. [DSC] = Discontinued product
Capsule, extended release, oral, as hydrochloride [bi-modal release]:
  Metadate CD®: 10 mg [contains sucrose; 3 mg immediate release, 7 mg extended release]
  Metadate CD®: 20 mg [contains sucrose; 6 mg immediate release, 14 mg extended release]
  Metadate CD®: 30 mg [contains sucrose; 9 mg immediate release, 21 mg extended release]
  Metadate CD®: 40 mg [contains sucrose; 12 mg immediate release, 28 mg extended release]
  Metadate CD®: 50 mg [contains sucrose; 15 mg immediate release, 35 mg extended release]
  Metadate CD®: 60 mg [contains sucrose; 18 mg immediate release, 42 mg extended release]
  Ritalin LA®: 10 mg [5 mg immediate release, 5 mg extended release]
  Ritalin LA®: 20 mg [10 mg immediate release, 10 mg extended release]
  Ritalin LA®: 30 mg [15 mg immediate release, 15 mg extended release]
  Ritalin LA®: 40 mg [20 mg immediate release, 20 mg extended release]
Patch, transdermal:
  Daytrana®: 10 mg/9 hours (30s) [12.5 cm^2, total methylphenidate 27.5 mg]
  Daytrana®: 15 mg/9 hours (30s) [18.75 cm^2, total methylphenidate 41.3 mg]
  Daytrana®: 20 mg/9 hours (30s) [25 cm^2, total methylphenidate 55 mg]
  Daytrana®: 30 mg/9 hours (30s) [37.5 cm^2, total methylphenidate 82.5 mg]
Solution, oral, as hydrochloride: 5 mg/5 mL (500 mL [DSC]); 10 mg/mL (500 mL [DSC])
  Methylin®: 5 mg/5 mL (500 mL); 10 mg/5 mL (500 mL) [grape flavor]
Tablet, oral, as hydrochloride: 5 mg, 10 mg, 20 mg
  Methylin®: 5 mg [DSC]
  Methylin®: 10 mg [DSC], 20 mg [DSC] [scored]
  Ritalin®: 5 mg
  Ritalin®: 10 mg, 20 mg [scored]
Tablet, chewable, oral, as hydrochloride:
  Methylin®: 2.5 mg [contains phenylalanine 0.42 mg/tablet; grape flavor]
  Methylin®: 5 mg [contains phenylalanine 0.84 mg/tablet; grape flavor]
  Methylin®: 10 mg [scored; contains phenylalanine 1.68 mg/tablet; grape flavor]
Tablet, extended release, oral, as hydrochloride: 10 mg, 20 mg, 36 mg
  Metadate® ER: 20 mg [contains lactose]
  Methylin® ER: 10 mg [DSC], 20 mg [DSC]
Tablet, extended release, oral, as hydrochloride [bi-modal release]: 18 mg, 27 mg, 54 mg
  Concerta®: 18 mg [4 mg immediate release, 14 mg extended release]
  Concerta®: 27 mg [6 mg immediate release, 21 mg extended release]
  Concerta®: 36 mg [8 mg immediate release, 28 mg extended release]
  Concerta®: 54 mg [12 mg immediate release, 42 mg extended release]
Tablet, sustained release, oral, as hydrochloride: 20 mg
  Ritalin-SR®: 20 mg [dye free]

Selected References
Emptage RE and Semla TP, "Depression in the Medically Ill Elderly: A Focus on Methylphenidate," *Ann Pharmacother*, 1996, 30(2):151-7.
Lazarus LW, Moberg PJ, Langsley PR, et al, "Methylphenidate and Nortriptyline in the Treatment of Poststroke Depression: A Retrospective Comparison," *Arch Phys Med Rehabil*, 1994, 75(4):403-6.
Nissen SE, "ADHD and Cardiovascular Risk," *New Eng J Med*, 2006, 354:1445-8.
Wallace AE, Kofoed LL and West AN, "Double-Blind, Placebo-Controlled Trial of Methylphenidate in Older, Depressed, Medically Ill Patients," *Am J Psychiatry*, 1995, 152(6):929-31.

◆ **Methylphenidate Hydrochloride** *see* Methylphenidate *on page 1179*
◆ **Methylphenobarbital** *see* Mephobarbital *on page 1143*
◆ **Methylphenyl Isoxazolyl Penicillin** *see* Oxacillin *on page 1356*
◆ **Methylphytyl Napthoquinone** *see* Phytonadione *on page 1450*

MethylPREDNISolone (meth il pred NIS oh lone)

Related Information
  Corticosteroids *on page 2005*
Medication Safety Issues
  Sound-alike/look-alike issues:
    MethylPREDNISolone may be confused with medroxyPROGESTERone, methotrexate, methylTESTOSTERone, predniSONE
    Depo-Medrol® may be confused with Solu-Medrol®

Medrol® may be confused with Mebaral®

Solu-MEDROL® may be confused with Depo-Medrol®, salmeterol, Solu-CORTEF®

International issues:

Medrol [U.S., Canada, and multiple international markets] may be confused with Medral brand name for omeprazole [Mexico]

Brand Names: U.S. A-Methapred®; Depo-Medrol®; Medrol®; Medrol® Dosepak™; Solu-MEDROL®

Brand Names: Canada Depo-Medrol®; Medrol®; Methylprednisolone Acetate; Solu-Medrol®

Index Terms 6-α-Methylprednisolone; A-Methapred; Medrol Dose Pack; Methylprednisolone Acetate; Methylprednisolone Sodium Succinate; Solumedrol

Generic Availability (U.S.) Yes: Excludes preservative free injection, suspension

Pharmacologic Category Corticosteroid, Systemic

Use Primarily as an anti-inflammatory or immunosuppressant agent in the treatment of a variety of diseases including those of hematologic, allergic, inflammatory, neoplastic, and autoimmune origin. Prevention and treatment of graft-versus-host disease following allogeneic bone marrow transplantation.

Unlabeled/Investigational Use Treatment of fibrosing-alveolitis phase of adult respiratory distress syndrome (ARDS)

Contraindications Hypersensitivity to methylprednisolone or any component of the formulation; systemic fungal infection (except intra-articular injection in localized joint conditions); administration of live virus vaccines. I.M. administration in idiopathic thrombocytopenia purpura; intrathecal administration

Warnings/Precautions Use with caution in patients with thyroid disease, hepatic impairment, renal impairment, cardiovascular disease, diabetes, glaucoma, cataracts, myasthenia gravis, patients at risk for osteoporosis, patients at risk for seizures, or GI diseases (diverticulitis, peptic ulcer, ulcerative colitis) due to perforation risk. Not recommended for the treatment of optic neuritis; may increase frequency of new episodes. Use caution following acute MI (corticosteroids have been associated with myocardial rupture). Cardiomegaly and congestive heart failure have been reported following concurrent use of amphotericin B and hydrocortisone for the management of fungal infections.

Because of the risk of adverse effects, systemic corticosteroids should be used cautiously in the elderly in the smallest possible effective dose for the shortest duration. Withdraw therapy with gradual tapering of dose.

May cause hypercorticism or suppression of hypothalamic-pituitary-adrenal (HPA) axis, particularly in patients receiving high doses for prolonged periods. HPA axis suppression may lead to adrenal crisis. Withdrawal and discontinuation of a corticosteroid should be done slowly and carefully. Particular care is required when patients are transferred from systemic corticosteroids to inhaled products due to possible adrenal insufficiency or withdrawal from steroids, including an increase in allergic symptoms. Patients receiving >20 mg per day of prednisone (or equivalent) may be most susceptible. Fatalities have occurred due to adrenal insufficiency in asthmatic patients during and after transfer from systemic corticosteroids to aerosol steroids; aerosol steroids do not provide the systemic steroid needed to treat patients having trauma, surgery, or infections.

Acute myopathy has been reported with high dose corticosteroids, usually in patients with neuromuscular transmission disorders; may involve ocular and/or respiratory muscles; monitor creatine kinase; recovery may be delayed. Corticosteroid use may cause psychiatric disturbances, including depression, euphoria, insomnia, mood swings, and personality changes. Pre-existing psychiatric conditions may be exacerbated by corticosteroid use. Prolonged use of corticosteroids may also increase the incidence of secondary infection, cause activation of latent infections, mask acute infection (including fungal infections), prolong or exacerbate viral or parasitic infections, or limit response to vaccines. Exposure to chickenpox or measles should be avoided; corticosteroids should not be used to treat ocular herpes simplex. Corticosteroids should not be used for cerebral malaria or viral hepatitis. Close observation is required in patients with latent tuberculosis and/or TB reactivity; restrict use in active TB (only in conjunction with antituberculosis treatment). Amebiasis should be ruled out in any patient with recent travel to tropic climates or unexplained diarrhea prior to initiation of corticosteroids. Prolonged treatment with corticosteroids has been associated with the development of Kaposi's sarcoma (case reports); discontinuation may result in clinical improvement.

High-dose corticosteroids should not be used to manage acute head injury. Rare cases of anaphylactoid reactions have been observed in patients receiving corticosteroids. Avoid injection or leakage into the dermis; dermal and/or subdermal skin depression may occur at the site of injection. Avoid deltoid muscle injection; subcutaneous atrophy may occur.

Adverse Reactions (Reflective of adult population; not specific for elderly) Frequency not defined.

Cardiovascular: Arrhythmias, bradycardia, cardiac arrest, cardiomegaly, circulatory collapse, congestive heart failure, edema, fat embolism, hypertension, hypertrophic cardiomyopathy in premature infants, myocardial rupture (post MI), syncope, tachycardia, thromboembolism, vasculitis

Central nervous system: Delirium, depression, emotional instability, euphoria, hallucinations, headache, intracranial pressure increased, insomnia, malaise, mood swings, nervousness, neuritis, personality changes, psychic disorders, pseudotumor cerebri (usually following discontinuation), seizure, vertigo

Dermatologic: Acne, allergic dermatitis, alopecia, dry scaly skin, ecchymoses, edema, erythema, hirsutism, hyper-/hypopigmentation, hypertrichosis, impaired wound healing, petechiae, rash, skin atrophy, sterile abscess, skin test reaction impaired, striae, urticaria

Endocrine & metabolic: Adrenal suppression, amenorrhea, carbohydrate intolerance increased, Cushing's syndrome, diabetes mellitus, fluid retention, glucose intolerance, growth suppression (children), hyperglycemia, hyperlipidemia, hypokalemia, hypokalemic alkalosis, menstrual irregularities, negative nitrogen balance, pituitary-adrenal axis suppression, protein catabolism, sodium and water retention

Gastrointestinal: Abdominal distention, appetite increased, bowel/bladder dysfunction (after intrathecal administration), gastrointestinal hemorrhage, gastrointestinal perforation, nausea, pancreatitis, peptic ulcer, perforation of the small and large intestine, ulcerative esophagitis, vomiting, weight gain

Hematologic: Leukocytosis (transient)

Hepatic: Hepatomegaly, transaminases increased

Local: Postinjection flare (intra-articular use), thrombophlebitis

Neuromuscular & skeletal: Arthralgia, arthropathy, aseptic necrosis (femoral and humoral heads), fractures, muscle mass loss, muscle weakness, myopathy (particularly in conjunction with neuromuscular disease or neuromuscular-blocking agents), neuropathy, osteoporosis, parasthesia, tendon rupture, vertebral compression fractures, weakness

Ocular: Cataracts, exophthalmoses, glaucoma, intraocular pressure increased

Renal: Glycosuria

Respiratory: Pulmonary edema

Miscellaneous: Abnormal fat disposition, anaphylactoid reaction, anaphylaxis, angioedema, avascular necrosis, diaphoresis, hiccups, hypersensitivity reactions, infections, secondary malignancy

Drug Interactions

Metabolism/Transport Effects Substrate of CYP3A4 (major); **Inhibits** CYP2C8 (weak), 3A4 (weak)

Avoid Concomitant Use

Avoid concomitant use of MethylPREDNISolone with any of the following: Aldesleukin; BCG; Natalizumab; Pimecrolimus; Tacrolimus (Topical)

Increased Effect/Toxicity

MethylPREDNISolone may increase the levels/effects of: Acetylcholinesterase Inhibitors; Amphotericin B; CycloSPORINE; CycloSPORINE (Systemic); Deferasirox; Leflunomide; Loop Diuretics; Natalizumab; NSAID (COX-2 Inhibitor); NSAID (Nonselective); Thiazide Diuretics; Vaccines (Live); Warfarin

The levels/effects of MethylPREDNISolone may be increased by: Antifungal Agents (Azole Derivatives, Systemic); Aprepitant; Calcium Channel Blockers (Nondihydropyridine); CycloSPORINE; CycloSPORINE (Systemic); CYP3A4 Inhibitors (Strong); Denosumab; Estrogen Derivatives; Fluconazole; Fosaprepitant; Macrolide Antibiotics; Neuromuscular-Blocking Agents (Nondepolarizing); Pimecrolimus; Quinolone Antibiotics; Roflumilast; Salicylates; Tacrolimus (Topical); Telaprevir; Trastuzumab

Decreased Effect

MethylPREDNISolone may decrease the levels/effects of: Aldesleukin; Antidiabetic Agents; BCG; Calcitriol; Corticorelin; CycloSPORINE; CycloSPORINE (Systemic); Isoniazid; Salicylates; Sipuleucel-T; Telaprevir; Vaccines (Inactivated)

The levels/effects of MethylPREDNISolone may be decreased by: Aminoglutethimide; Antacids; Barbiturates; Bile Acid Sequestrants; Echinacea; Mitotane; Primidone; Rifamycin Derivatives; Tocilizumab

Ethanol/Nutrition/Herb Interactions

Ethanol: Avoid ethanol (may increase gastric mucosal irritation).

Food: Methylprednisolone interferes with calcium absorption. Limit caffeine.

Herb/Nutraceutical: St John's wort may decrease methylprednisolone levels. Avoid cat's claw, echinacea (have immunostimulant properties).

◄ **Stability**
Intact vials of methylprednisolone sodium succinate should be stored at controlled room temperature of 20°C to 25°C (68°F to 77°F). Protect from light.
Reconstituted solutions of methylprednisolone sodium succinate should be stored at room temperature of 20°C to 25°C (68°F to 77°F), and used within 48 hours.
Stability of parenteral admixture at room temperature (25°C) and at refrigeration temperature (4°C) is 48 hours.
Standard diluent (Solu-Medrol®): 40 mg/50 mL D$_5$W; 125 mg/50 mL D$_5$W.
Minimum volume (Solu-Medrol®): 50 mL D$_5$W.

Mechanism of Action In a tissue-specific manner, corticosteroids regulate gene expression subsequent to binding specific intracellular receptors and translocation into the nucleus. Corticosteroids exert a wide array of physiologic effects including modulation of carbohydrate, protein, and lipid metabolism and maintenance of fluid and electrolyte homeostasis. Moreover cardiovascular, immunologic, musculoskeletal, endocrine, and neurologic physiology are influenced by corticosteroids. Decreases inflammation by suppression of migration of poly-morphonuclear leukocytes and reversal of increased capillary permeability.

Pharmacodynamics/Kinetics
Onset of action: Peak effect (route dependent): Oral: 1-2 hours; I.M.: 4-8 days; Intra-articular: 1 week; methylprednisolone sodium succinate is highly soluble and has a rapid effect by I.M. and I.V. routes
Duration (route dependent): Oral: 30-36 hours; I.M.: 1-4 weeks; Intra-articular: 1-5 weeks; methylprednisolone acetate has a low solubility and has a sustained I.M. effect
Distribution: V$_d$: 0.7-1.5 L/kg
Half-life elimination: 3-3.5 hours; reduced in obese
Excretion: Clearance: Reduced in obese

Dosage
Geriatric & Adult Only sodium succinate may be given I.V.; methylprednisolone sodium succinate is highly soluble and has a rapid effect by I.M. and I.V. routes. Methylprednisolone acetate has a low solubility and has a sustained I.M. effect.

Acute spinal cord injury (unlabeled use): I.V. (sodium succinate): 30 mg/kg over 15 minutes, followed in 45 minutes by a continuous infusion of 5.4 mg/kg/hour for 23 hours. **Note:** Due to insufficient evidence of clinical efficacy (ie, preserving or improving spinal cord function), the routine use of methylprednisolone in the treatment of acute spinal cord injury is no longer recommended. If used in this setting, methylprednisolone should not be initiated >8 hours after the injury; not effective in penetrating trauma (eg, gunshot) (Consortium for Spinal Cord Medicine, 2008).

Allergic conditions: Oral: Tapered-dosage schedule:
Day 1: 24 mg on day 1 administered as 8 mg before breakfast, 4 mg after lunch, 4 mg after supper, and 8 mg at bedtime **OR** 24 mg as a single dose or divided into 2 or 3 doses upon initiation (regardless of time of day)
Day 2: 20 mg on day 2 administered as 4 mg before breakfast, 4 mg after lunch, 4 mg after supper, and 8 mg at bedtime
Day 3: 16 mg on day 3 administered as 4 mg before breakfast, 4 mg after lunch, 4 mg after supper, and 4 mg at bedtime
Day 4: 12 mg on day 4 administered as 4 mg before breakfast, 4 mg after lunch, and 4 mg at bedtime
Day 5: 8 mg on day 5 administered as 4 mg before breakfast and 4 mg at bedtime
Day 6: 4 mg on day 6 administered as 4 mg before breakfast

Anti-inflammatory or immunosuppressive:
Oral: 2-60 mg/day in 1-4 divided doses to start, followed by gradual reduction in dosage to the lowest possible level consistent with maintaining an adequate clinical response.
I.M. (sodium succinate): 10-80 mg/day once daily
I.M. (acetate): 10-80 mg every 1-2 weeks
I.V. (sodium succinate): 10-40 mg over a period of several minutes and repeated I.V. or I.M. at intervals depending on clinical response; when high dosages are needed, give 30 mg/kg over a period ≥30 minutes and may be repeated every 4-6 hours for 48 hours.

Arthritis: Intra-articular (acetate): Administer every 1-5 weeks.
Large joints (eg, knee, ankle): 20-80 mg
Medium joints (eg, elbow, wrist): 10-40 mg
Small joints: 4-10 mg

Asthma exacerbations, including status asthmaticus (emergency medical care or hospital doses): Oral, I.V.: 40-80 mg/day in 1- 2 divided doses until peak expiratory flow is 70% of predicted or personal best (NIH Asthma Guidelines, NAEPP, 2007)

Asthma, severe persistent, long-term control: Oral: 7.5-60 mg/day (or on alternate days) (NIH Asthma Guidelines, NAEPP, 2007)

Dermatitis, acute severe: I.M. (acetate): 80-120 mg as a single dose
Dermatitis, chronic: I.M. (acetate): 40-120 mg every 5-10 days

Dermatologic conditions (eg, keloids, lichen planus): Intralesional (acetate): 20-60 mg

Dermatomyositis/polymyositis: I.V. (sodium succinate): 1 g/day for 3-5 days for severe muscle weakness, followed by conversion to oral prednisone (Drake, 1996)

Lupus nephritis: High-dose "pulse" therapy: I.V. (sodium succinate): 0.5-1 g/day for 3 days (Ponticelli, 2010)

***Pneumocystis* pneumonia in AIDS patients:** I.V.: 30 mg twice daily for 5 days, then 30 mg once daily for 5 days, then 15 mg once daily for 11 days

Renal Impairment

Hemodialysis effects: Slightly dialyzable (5% to 20%)

Administer dose posthemodialysis.

Administration Succinate: I.V. push over 1-15 minutes; intermittent infusion over 15-60 minutes; maximum concentration: IVP: 125 mg/mL

Monitoring Parameters Blood pressure, blood glucose, electrolytes

Test Interactions Interferes with skin tests

Pharmacotherapy Pearls Sodium content of 1 g sodium succinate injection: 2.01 mEq; 53 mg of sodium succinate salt is equivalent to 40 mg of methylprednisolone base

Methylprednisolone acetate: Depo-Medrol®; methylprednisolone sodium succinate: Solu-Medrol®

Withdrawal/tapering of therapy: Corticosteroid tapering following short-term use is limited primarily by the need to control the underlying disease state; tapering may be accomplished over a period of days. Following longer-term use, tapering over weeks to months may be necessary to avoid signs and symptoms of adrenal insufficiency and to allow recovery of the HPA axis. Testing of HPA axis responsiveness may be of value in selected patients. Subtle deficits in HPA response may persist for months after discontinuation of therapy, and may require supplemental dosing during periods of acute illness or surgical stress.

Special Geriatric Considerations Because of the risk of adverse effects, systemic corticosteroids should be used cautiously in the elderly, in the smallest possible dose, and for the shortest possible time.

Dosage Forms Excipient information presented when available (limited, particularly for generics); consult specific product labeling.

Injection, powder for reconstitution, as sodium succinate [strength expressed as base]: 40 mg, 125 mg, 500 mg, 1 g

A-Methapred®: 40 mg [contains benzyl alcohol (in diluent), lactose 25 mg/vial]

A-Methapred®: 40 mg [contains lactose 25 mg/vial]

A-Methapred®: 125 mg

A-Methapred®: 125 mg [contains benzyl alcohol (in diluent)]

Solu-MEDROL®: 500 mg, 1 g

Solu-MEDROL®: 2 g [contains benzyl alcohol (in diluent)]

Injection, powder for reconstitution, as sodium succinate [strength expressed as base, preservative free]:

Solu-MEDROL®: 40 mg [contains lactose 25 mg/vial; supplied with diluent]

Solu-MEDROL®: 125 mg, 500 mg, 1 g [supplied with diluent]

Injection, suspension, as acetate: 40 mg/mL (1 mL, 5 mL, 10 mL); 80 mg/mL (1 mL, 5 mL)

Depo-Medrol®: 20 mg/mL (5 mL); 40 mg/mL (5 mL, 10 mL); 80 mg/mL (5 mL) [contains benzyl alcohol, polysorbate 80]

Injection, suspension, as acetate [preservative free]:

Depo-Medrol®: 40 mg/mL (1 mL); 80 mg/mL (1 mL)

Tablet, oral: 4 mg, 8 mg, 16 mg, 32 mg

Medrol®: 2 mg, 4 mg, 8 mg, 16 mg, 32 mg [scored]

Tablet, oral [dose-pack]: 4 mg

Medrol® Dosepak™: 4 mg [scored]

Selected References

Tornatore KM, Logue G, Venuto RC, et al, "Pharmacokinetics of Methylprednisolone in Elderly and Young Healthy Males," *J Am Geriatr Soc*, 1994, 42(10):1118-22.

◆ **6-α-Methylprednisolone** see MethylPREDNISolone *on page 1183*

◆ **Methylprednisolone Acetate** see MethylPREDNISolone *on page 1183*

◆ **Methylprednisolone Sodium Succinate** see MethylPREDNISolone *on page 1183*

MethylTESTOSTERone (meth il tes TOS te rone)

Related Information
  Beers Criteria – Potentially Inappropriate Medications for Geriatrics *on page 2089*
Medication Safety Issues
  Sound-alike/look-alike issues:
    MethylTESTOSTERone may be confused with medroxyPROGESTERone, methylPREDNI-Solone
    Virilon® may be confused with Verelan®
  Beers Criteria medication:
    This drug may be inappropriate for use in geriatric patients (high severity risk).
Brand Names: U.S. Android®; Methitest™; Testred®
Generic Availability (U.S.) No
Pharmacologic Category Androgen
Use
  Male: Hypogonadism; impotence and climacteric symptoms
  Female: Palliative treatment of metastatic breast cancer
Unlabeled/Investigational Use Hypogonadism (male); delayed puberty (male)
Contraindications Hypersensitivity to methyltestosterone or any component of the formulation; in males, known or suspected carcinoma of the breast or the prostate
Warnings/Precautions Prolonged use and/or high doses may cause peliosis hepatis or liver cell tumors which may not be apparent until liver failure or intra-abdominal hemorrhage develops. Discontinue in case of cholestatic hepatitis with jaundice or abnormal liver function tests. Use with caution in patients with breast cancer; may cause hypercalcemia by stimulating osteolysis. Use with caution in patients with diabetes mellitus; monitor carefully. Use with caution in patients with conditions influenced by edema (eg, cardiovascular disease, migraine, seizure disorder, renal impairment); may cause fluid retention. Discontinue with evidence of mild virilization in women. Use with caution in hepatic impairment. May be inappropriate for use in the elderly due to increased risk of prostatic hypertrophy and cardiac problems (Beers Criteria). In addition, elderly patients may be at greater risk for fluid retention and transaminase elevations. Product may contain tartrazine.
Adverse Reactions (Reflective of adult population; not specific for elderly) Frequency not defined.
  Male: Gynecomastia, impotence, oligospermia (at high doses), priapism, prostatic carcinoma, prostatic hyperplasia, testicular atrophy, virilism
  Female: Atrophy, breast soreness, hirsutism, menstrual problems (amenorrhea), virilism
  Cardiovascular: Edema
  Central nervous system: Anxiety, depression, headache
  Dermatologic: Acne, "male pattern" baldness
  Endocrine & metabolic: Hypercalcemia, hypercholesterolemia, libido (changes in)
  Gastrointestinal: Nausea, vomiting
  Hematologic: Polycythemia, suppression of clotting factors
  Hepatic: Cholestatic hepatitis, hepatic dysfunction, hepatic necrosis, hepatocellular neoplasm (rare), jaundice, liver function tests (abnormal), peliosis hepatitis
  Neuromuscular & skeletal: Paresthesia
  Miscellaneous: Anaphylactoid reactions (rare)
Drug Interactions
  Avoid Concomitant Use There are no known interactions where it is recommended to avoid concomitant use.
  Increased Effect/Toxicity
    MethylTESTOSTERone may increase the levels/effects of: CycloSPORINE; CycloSPORINE (Systemic); Vitamin K Antagonists
  Decreased Effect There are no known significant interactions involving a decrease in effect.
Mechanism of Action Stimulates receptors in organs and tissues to promote growth and development of male sex organs and maintains secondary sex characteristics in androgen-deficient males
Pharmacodynamics/Kinetics
  Metabolism: Hepatic
  Excretion: Urine
Dosage
  Geriatric & Adult Note: Buccal absorption produces twice the androgenic activity of oral tablets.

  Hypogonadism; impotence and climacteric symptoms (Males):
    Oral: 10-40 mg/day
    Buccal: 5-25 mg/day

Breast pain/engorgement (Females):
Oral: 80 mg/day for 3-5 days
Buccal: 40 mg/day for 3-5 days
Breast cancer (Females):
Oral: 50-200 mg/day
Buccal: 25-100 mg/day
Monitoring Parameters Cholesterol, PSA, electrolyte changes
Special Geriatric Considerations Testosterone should be reserved for men with moderate to severe testosterone deficiency. Retention of sodium and water could be a problem in patients with CHF and hypertension.

This medication is considered to be potentially inappropriate in this patient population (Beers Criteria severity: High).
Controlled Substance C-III
Dosage Forms Excipient information presented when available (limited, particularly for generics); consult specific product labeling.
Capsule, oral:
Android®: 10 mg
Testred®: 10 mg
Tablet, oral:
Methitest™: 10 mg [scored]

Metipranolol (met i PRAN oh lol)

Related Information
Glaucoma Drug Therapy *on page 2008*
Medication Safety Issues
Sound-alike/look-alike issues:
Metipranolol may be confused with metaproterenol
International issues:
Betanol [Monaco] may be confused with Beta-Val brand name for betamethasone [U.S.]; Betimol brand name for timolol [U.S., Finland]; Patanol brand name for olopatadine [U.S., Canada, and multiple international markets]
Brand Names: U.S. OptiPranolol®
Brand Names: Canada OptiPranolol®
Index Terms Metipranolol Hydrochloride
Generic Availability (U.S.) Yes
Pharmacologic Category Beta-Adrenergic Blocker, Nonselective; Ophthalmic Agent, Anti-glaucoma
Use Treatment of chronic open-angle glaucoma or ocular hypertension
Contraindications Hypersensitivity to metipranolol or any component of the formulation; bronchial asthma, severe COPD, sinus bradycardia, second- and third-degree AV block, cardiac failure, cardiogenic shock
Warnings/Precautions Consider pre-existing conditions such as sick sinus syndrome before initiating. Use with caution in patients with bronchospastic disease, cardiac failure, diabetes mellitus, myasthenia gravis, peripheral vascular disease, or psychiatric disease. Systemic absorption and adverse effects may occur with ophthalmic use, including bradycardia and/or hypotension. Beta-blocker therapy should not be withdrawn abruptly (particularly in patients with CAD), but gradually tapered to avoid acute tachycardia, hypertension, and/or ischemia. Use caution with history of severe anaphylaxis to allergens; patients taking beta-blockers may become more sensitive to repeated challenges. Treatment of anaphylaxis (eg, epinephrine) in patients taking beta-blockers may be ineffective or promote undesirable effects. Some products may contain benzalkonium chloride which may be absorbed by soft contact lenses; do not administer while wearing soft contact lenses.
Adverse Reactions (Reflective of adult population; not specific for elderly) Frequency not defined.
Cardiovascular: Angina, atrial fibrillation, bradycardia, hypertension, MI, palpitation
Central nervous system: Anxiety, depression, dizziness, headache, nervousness, somnolence
Dermatologic: Rash
Gastrointestinal: Nausea
Neuromuscular & skeletal: Arthritis, myalgia, weakness
Ocular: Abnormal vision, blepharitis, blurred vision, browache, conjunctivitis, discomfort, edema, eyelid dermatitis, photophobia, tearing, uveitis
Respiratory: Bronchitis, cough, dyspnea, epistaxis, rhinitis
Miscellaneous: Allergic reaction

◀ **Drug Interactions**
Avoid Concomitant Use
Avoid concomitant use of Metipranolol with any of the following: Floctafenine; Methacholine
Increased Effect/Toxicity
Metipranolol may increase the levels/effects of: Alpha-/Beta-Agonists (Direct-Acting); Bupivacaine; Fingolimod; Hypotensive Agents; Lidocaine (Systemic); Lidocaine (Topical); Mepivacaine; Methacholine; Midodrine

The levels/effects of Metipranolol may be increased by: Anilidopiperidine Opioids; Dronedarone; Floctafenine; MAO Inhibitors; QuiNIDine; Reserpine
Decreased Effect
Metipranolol may decrease the levels/effects of: Beta2-Agonists; Theophylline Derivatives
Mechanism of Action Beta-adrenoceptor-blocking agent; lacks intrinsic sympathomimetic activity and membrane-stabilizing effects and possesses only slight local anesthetic activity; mechanism of action of metipranolol in reducing intraocular pressure appears to be via reduced production of aqueous humor. This effect may be related to a reduction in blood flow to the iris root-ciliary body. It remains unclear if the reduction in intraocular pressure observed with beta-blockers is actually secondary to beta-adrenoceptor blockade.
Pharmacodynamics/Kinetics
Onset of action: ≤30 minutes
Peak effect: Maximum: ~2 hours
Duration: Intraocular pressure reduction: Up to 24 hours
Metabolism: Rapid and complete to deacetyl metipranolol, an active metabolite
Half-life elimination: ~3 hours
Dosage
Geriatric & Adult Glaucoma: Ophthalmic: Instill 1 drop in the affected eye(s) twice daily
Administration Do not allow the dispenser tip to touch the eye. Remove contact lenses prior to administration and wait 15 minutes before reinserting.
Monitoring Parameters Intraocular pressure, funduscopic exam, visual field testing
Special Geriatric Considerations Because systemic absorption occurs with ophthalmic administration, elderly patients with other disease states or syndromes that may be affected by a beta-blocker (ie, CHF, COPD, etc) should be closely monitored. Evaluate the patient's or caregiver's ability to safely administer the correct dose of ophthalmic medication.
Dosage Forms Excipient information presented when available (limited, particularly for generics); consult specific product labeling.
Solution, ophthalmic [drops]: 0.3% (5 mL, 10 mL)
OptiPranolol®: 0.3% (5 mL, 10 mL) [contains benzalkonium chloride]

◆ **Metipranolol Hydrochloride** see Metipranolol on page 1189

Metoclopramide (met oh KLOE pra mide)

Related Information
Beers Criteria − Potentially Inappropriate Medications for Geriatrics on page 2089
Medication Safety Issues
Sound-alike/look-alike issues:
Metoclopramide may be confused with metolazone, metoprolol, metroNIDAZOLE
Reglan® may be confused with Megace®, Regonol®, Renagel®
Brand Names: U.S. Metozolv™ ODT; Reglan®
Brand Names: Canada Apo-Metoclop®; Metoclopramide Hydrochloride Injection; Metoclopramide Omega; Nu-Metoclopramide; PMS-Metoclopramide
Generic Availability (U.S.) Yes: Excludes oral-disintegrating tablet
Pharmacologic Category Antiemetic; Gastrointestinal Agent, Prokinetic
Use
Oral: Symptomatic treatment of diabetic gastroparesis; gastroesophageal reflux
I.V., I.M.: Symptomatic treatment of diabetic gastroparesis; postpyloric placement of enteral feeding tubes; prevention and/or treatment of nausea and vomiting associated with chemotherapy, or postsurgery; to stimulate gastric emptying and intestinal transit of barium during radiological examination of the stomach/small intestine
Medication Guide Available Yes
Contraindications Hypersensitivity to metoclopramide or any component of the formulation; GI obstruction, perforation or hemorrhage; pheochromocytoma; history of seizures or concomitant use of other agents likely to increase extrapyramidal reactions
Warnings/Precautions [U.S. Boxed Warning]: May cause tardive dyskinesia, which is often irreversible; duration of treatment and total cumulative dose are associated with an increased risk. Therapy durations >12 weeks should be avoided (except in rare cases following risk:benefit assessment). Risk appears to be increased in the elderly, women, and

diabetics; however, it is not possible to predict which patients will develop tardive dyskinesia. Therapy should be discontinued in any patient if signs/symptoms of tardive dyskinesia appear.

May cause extrapyramidal symptoms, generally manifested as acute dystonic reactions within the initial 24-48 hours of use. Risk of these reactions is increased at higher doses. Pseudoparkinsonism (eg, bradykinesia, tremor, rigidity) may also occur (usually within first 6 months of therapy) and is generally reversible following discontinuation. Use with caution or avoid in patients with Parkinson's disease. Use caution in the elderly; may have increased risk of tardive dyskinesia, particularly older women. Neuroleptic malignant syndrome (NMS) has been reported (rarely) with metoclopramide.

May cause transient increase in serum aldosterone; use caution in patients who are at risk of fluid overload (HF, cirrhosis). Use caution in patients with hypertension or following surgical anastomosis/closure. Use caution with a history of mental illness; has been associated with depression. Abrupt discontinuation may (rarely) result in withdrawal symptoms (dizziness, headache, nervousness). Use caution and adjust dose in renal impairment. Patients with NADH-cytochrome b5 reductase deficiency are at increased risk of methemoglobinemia and/ or sulfhemoglobinemia.

Adverse Reactions (Reflective of adult population; not specific for elderly) Frequency not always defined.

Cardiovascular: AV block, bradycardia, HF, fluid retention, flushing (following high I.V. doses), hyper-/hypotension, supraventricular tachycardia

Central nervous system: Drowsiness (~10% to 70%; dose related), acute dystonic reactions (<1% to 25%; dose and age related), fatigue (2% to 10%), lassitude (~10%), restlessness (~10%), headache (4% to 5%), dizziness (1% to 4%), somnolence (2% to 3%), akathisia, confusion, depression, hallucinations (rare), insomnia, neuroleptic malignant syndrome (rare), Parkinsonian-like symptoms, suicidal ideation, seizure, tardive dyskinesia

Dermatologic: Angioneurotic edema (rare), rash, urticaria

Endocrine & metabolic: Amenorrhea, galactorrhea, gynecomastia, hyperprolactinemia, impotence

Gastrointestinal: Nausea (4% to 6%), vomiting (1% to 2%), diarrhea

Hematologic: Agranulocytosis, leukopenia, neutropenia, porphyria

Hepatic: Hepatotoxicity (rare)

Ocular: Visual disturbance

Respiratory: Bronchospasm, laryngeal edema (rare), laryngospasm (rare)

Miscellaneous: Allergic reactions, methemoglobinemia, sulfhemoglobinemia

Drug Interactions

Metabolism/Transport Effects Substrate (minor) of CYP1A2, 2D6; **Inhibits** CYP2D6 (weak)

Avoid Concomitant Use

Avoid concomitant use of Metoclopramide with any of the following: Antipsychotics; Droperidol; Promethazine; Tetrabenazine

Increased Effect/Toxicity

Metoclopramide may increase the levels/effects of: Antipsychotics; CycloSPORINE; CycloSPORINE (Systemic); Promethazine; Selective Serotonin Reuptake Inhibitors; Tetrabenazine; Tricyclic Antidepressants; Venlafaxine

The levels/effects of Metoclopramide may be increased by: Droperidol

Decreased Effect

Metoclopramide may decrease the levels/effects of: Anti-Parkinson's Agents (Dopamine Agonist); Posaconazole; Quinagolide

The levels/effects of Metoclopramide may be decreased by: Cyproterone; Peginterferon Alfa-2b

Ethanol/Nutrition/Herb Interactions Ethanol: Avoid ethanol (may increase CNS depression).

Stability

Injection: Store intact vial at controlled room temperature. Injection is photosensitive and should be protected from light during storage. Parenteral admixtures in D_5W or NS are stable for at least 24 hours and do not require light protection if used within 24 hours.

Tablet: Store at controlled room temperature of 20°C to 25°C (68°F to 77°F).

Mechanism of Action Blocks dopamine receptors and (when given in higher doses) also blocks serotonin receptors in chemoreceptor trigger zone of the CNS; enhances the response to acetylcholine of tissue in upper GI tract causing enhanced motility and accelerated gastric emptying without stimulating gastric, biliary, or pancreatic secretions; increases lower esophageal sphincter tone

Pharmacodynamics/Kinetics
  Onset of action: Oral: 30-60 minutes; I.V.: 1-3 minutes; I.M.: 10-15 minutes
  Duration: Therapeutic: 1-2 hours, regardless of route
  Absorption: Oral: Rapid
  Distribution: V_d: ~3.5 L/kg
  Protein binding: ~30%
  Bioavailability: Oral: Range: 65% to 95%
  Half-life elimination: Normal renal function: Adults: 5-6 hours (may be dose dependent)
  Time to peak, serum: Oral: 1-2 hours
  Excretion: Urine (~85%)

Dosage
  Geriatric Initial: Dose at the lower end of the recommended range. Refer to adult dosing.
  Adult
    Gastroesophageal reflux: Oral: 10-15 mg/dose up to 4 times/day 30 minutes before meals or food and at bedtime; single doses of 20 mg are occasionally needed prior to provoking situations. Treatment >12 weeks is not recommended.
    Diabetic gastroparesis:
      Oral: 10 mg/dose up to 4 times/day 30 minutes before meals or food and at bedtime for 2-8 weeks
      I.M., I.V. (for severe symptoms): 10 mg over 1-2 minutes; 10 days of I.V. therapy may be necessary before symptoms are controlled to allow transition to oral administration
    Chemotherapy-induced emesis prophylaxis: I.V.: 1-2 mg/kg 30 minutes before chemotherapy and repeated every 2 hours for 2 doses, then every 3 hours for 3 doses (manufacturer labeling); pretreatment with diphenhydramine will decrease risk of extrapyramidal reactions
      Alternate dosing: **Note:** Metoclopramide is considered an antiemetic with a low therapeutic index; use is generally reserved for agents with low emetogenic potential or in patients intolerant/refractory to first line antiemetics.
        Low-risk chemotherapy (unlabeled): I.V., Oral: 10-40 mg prior to dose, then every 4-6 hours as needed (NCCN Antiemesis guidelines, v.4.2009)
        Breakthrough treatment (unlabeled): I.V., Oral: 10-40 mg every 4-6 hours (NCCN Antiemesis guidelines, v.4.2009)
        Delayed-emesis prophylaxis (unlabeled): Oral: 20-40 mg/dose (or 0.5 mg/kg/dose) 2-4 times/day for 3-4 days (in combination with dexamethasone [ASCO guidelines, 2006])
        Refractory or intolerant to antiemetics with a higher therapeutic index (unlabeled; Hesketh, 2008):
          I.V.: 1-2 mg/kg/dose before chemotherapy and repeat 2 hours after chemotherapy
          Oral: 0.5 mg/kg every 6 hours on days 2-4
    Postoperative nausea and vomiting prophylaxis: I.M., I.V. (unlabeled route): 10-20 mg near end of surgery. **Note:** Guidelines discourage use of 10 mg metoclopramide as being ineffective (Gan, 2007); comparative study indicates higher dose (20 mg) may be efficacious (Quaynor, 2002).
    Postpyloric feeding tube placement, radiological exam: I.V.: 10 mg as a single dose
  Renal Impairment
    Cl_{cr} <40 mL/minute: Administer 50% of normal dose.
    Not dialyzable (0% to 5%); supplemental dose is not necessary.

Administration
  Injection solution: May be given I.M., direct I.V. push, short infusion (15-30 minutes), or continuous infusion; lower doses (≤10 mg) of metoclopramide can be given I.V. push undiluted over 1-2 minutes; higher doses (>10 mg) to be diluted in 50 mL of compatible solution (preferably NS) and given IVPB over at least 15 minutes; continuous SubQ infusion and rectal administration have been reported. **Note:** Rapid I.V. administration may be associated with a transient (but intense) feeling of anxiety and restlessness, followed by drowsiness.
  Orally-disintegrating tablets: Administer on an empty stomach at least 30 minutes prior to food. Do not remove from packaging until time of administration. If tablet breaks or crumbles while handling, discard and remove new tablet. Using dry hands, place tablet on tongue and allow to dissolve. Swallow with saliva.

Monitoring Parameters Dystonic reactions; signs of hypoglycemia in patients using insulin and those being treated for gastroparesis; agitation, and confusion

Test Interactions Increased aminotransferase [ALT/AST] (S), increased amylase (S)

Special Geriatric Considerations Elderly are more likely to develop tardive dyskinesia syndrome (especially elderly females) reactions than younger adults. Use lowest recommended doses initially. Must consider renal function (estimate creatinine clearance). It is recommended to do involuntary movement assessments on elderly using this medication at high doses and for long-term therapy.

Dosage Forms Excipient information presented when available (limited, particularly for generics); consult specific product labeling.

Injection, solution [preservative free]: 5 mg/mL (2 mL)

  Reglan®: 5 mg/mL (2 mL, 10 mL, 30 mL)

Solution, oral: 5 mg/5 mL (10 mL, 473 mL)

Tablet, oral: 5 mg, 10 mg

  Reglan®: 5 mg

  Reglan®: 10 mg [scored]

Tablet, orally disintegrating, oral:

  Metozolv™ ODT: 5 mg, 10 mg [mint flavor]

Extemporaneously Prepared

Reglan® suppository: 5 pulverized tablets in polyethylene glycol; administer 1 suppository 30-60 minutes before meals and at bedtime; use ¹/₂ for older adults.

Metoclophen nausea suppository:

  Metoclopramide powder (USP) 40 mg

  Haloperidol powder (USP) 1 mg

  Dexamethasone powder (USP) 10 mg

  Diphenhydramine HCl (USP) 25 mg

  Benztropine mesylate (USP) 1 mg

  Silica gel powder 200 mg

  Fatty base (emulsifying type) qs 2.2 g

Metoclophen-modified nausea suppository:

  Metoclopramide powder (USP) 40 mg

  Haloperidol powder (USP) 1 mg

  Lorazepam (USP) 1 mg

  Benztropine mesylate (USP) 1 mg

  Fatty base (emulsifying type) qs 2.2 g

Grind all powders (and/or tablets) into a fine uniform powder. Melt the fatty base on low temperature, then add the powder. Stir the mixture until uniform. With continuous stirring, draw up part of the mixture and instill into calibrated suppository molds. Refrigerate.

Francom M, "Compounding Nausea Aid," Am Pharm, 1991, NS31(7):7.

Selected References

Hesketh PJ, "Chemotherapy-Induced Nausea and Vomiting," N Engl J Med, 2008, 358(23):2482-94.

Kris MG, Hesketh PJ, Somerfield MR, et al, "American Society of Clinical Oncology Guideline for Antiemetics in Oncology: Update 2006," J Clin Oncol, 2006, 24(18):2932-46.

Mary AM and Bhupalam L, "Metoclopramide-induced Methemoglobinemia in an Adult," J KY Med Assoc, 2000, 98 (6):245-7.

Multinational Association of Supportive Care in Cancer (MASCC), "Antiemetic Guidelines," Updated March 2008. Available at http://data.memberclicks.com/site/mascc/MASCC_Guidelines_Update.pdf

Metolazone (me TOLE a zone)

Medication Safety Issues

Sound-alike/look-alike issues:

Metolazone may be confused with metaxalone, methazolamide, methimazole, methotrexate, metoclopramide, metoprolol, minoxidil

Zaroxolyn® may be confused with Zarontin®

Brand Names: U.S. Zaroxolyn®

Brand Names: Canada Zaroxolyn®

Generic Availability (U.S.) Yes

Pharmacologic Category Diuretic, Thiazide-Related

Use Management of mild-to-moderate hypertension; treatment of edema in heart failure and nephrotic syndrome, impaired renal function

Contraindications Hypersensitivity to metolazone, any component of the formulation, other thiazides, and sulfonamide derivatives; anuria; hepatic coma

Warnings/Precautions Electrolyte disturbances (hypokalemia, hypochloremic alkalosis, hyponatremia) can occur. Large or prolonged fluid and electrolyte losses may occur with concomitant furosemide administration. Use with caution in severe hepatic dysfunction; hepatic encephalopathy can be caused by electrolyte disturbances. Gout can be precipitate in certain patients with a history of gout, a familial predisposition to gout, or chronic renal failure. Cautious use in patients with prediabetes or diabetes; may see a change in glucose control. Can cause SLE exacerbation or activation. Use caution in severe renal impairment. Use with caution in patients with moderate or high cholesterol concentrations. Photosensitization may occur.

Chemical similarities are present among sulfonamides, sulfonylureas, carbonic anhydrase inhibitors, thiazides, and loop diuretics (except ethacrynic acid). Use in patients with thiazide or sulfonamide allergy is specifically contraindicated in product labeling, however, a risk of cross-reaction exists in patients with allergy to any of these compounds; avoid use when previous reaction has been severe. Discontinue if signs of hypersensitivity are noted.

Adverse Reactions (Reflective of adult population; not specific for elderly) Frequency not defined.

Cardiovascular: Chest pain/discomfort, necrotizing angiitis, orthostatic hypotension, palpitation, syncope, venous thrombosis, vertigo, volume depletion

Central nervous system: Chills, depression, dizziness, drowsiness, fatigue, headache, lightheadedness, restlessness

Dermatologic: Petechiae, photosensitivity, pruritus, purpura, rash, skin necrosis, Stevens-Johnson syndrome, toxic epidermal necrolysis, urticaria

Endocrine & metabolic: Gout attacks, hypercalcemia, hyperglycemia, hyperuricemia, hypochloremia, hypochloremic alkalosis, hypokalemia, hypomagnesemia, hyponatremia, hypophosphatemia

Gastrointestinal: Abdominal bloating, abdominal pain, anorexia, constipation, diarrhea, epigastric distress, nausea, pancreatitis, vomiting, xerostomia

Genitourinary: Impotence

Hematologic: Agranulocytosis, aplastic/hypoplastic anemia, hemoconcentration, leukopenia, thrombocytopenia

Hepatic: Cholestatic jaundice, hepatitis

Neuromuscular & skeletal: Joint pain, muscle cramps/spasm, neuropathy, paresthesia, weakness

Ocular: Blurred vision (transient)

Renal: BUN increased, glucosuria

Drug Interactions

Avoid Concomitant Use

Avoid concomitant use of Metolazone with any of the following: Dofetilide

Increased Effect/Toxicity

Metolazone may increase the levels/effects of: ACE Inhibitors; Allopurinol; Amifostine; Antihypertensives; Calcium Salts; CarBAMazepine; Dofetilide; Hypotensive Agents; Lithium; OXcarbazepine; Porfimer; RiTUXimab; Sodium Phosphates; Topiramate; Toremifene; Vitamin D Analogs

The levels/effects of Metolazone may be increased by: Alcohol (Ethyl); Alfuzosin; Analgesics (Opioid); Barbiturates; Corticosteroids (Orally Inhaled); Corticosteroids (Systemic); Herbs (Hypotensive Properties); Licorice; MAO Inhibitors; Pentoxifylline; Phosphodiesterase 5 Inhibitors; Prostacyclin Analogues

Decreased Effect

Metolazone may decrease the levels/effects of: Antidiabetic Agents

The levels/effects of Metolazone may be decreased by: Bile Acid Sequestrants; Herbs (Hypertensive Properties); Methylphenidate; Nonsteroidal Anti-Inflammatory Agents; Yohimbine

Ethanol/Nutrition/Herb Interactions

Ethanol: May potentiate hypotensive effect of metazolone.

Herb/Nutraceutical: Avoid herbs with *hypertensive* properties (bayberry, blue cohosh, cayenne, ephedra, ginger, ginseng [American], kola, licorice); may diminish the antihypertensive effect of metolazone. Avoid herbs with *hypotensive* properties (black cohosh, California poppy, coleus, golden seal, hawthorn, mistletoe, periwinkle, quinine, shepherd's purse); may enhance the hypotensive effect of metolazone.

Mechanism of Action Inhibits sodium reabsorption in the distal tubules causing increased excretion of sodium and water, as well as, potassium and hydrogen ions

Pharmacodynamics/Kinetics

Onset of action: Diuresis: ~60 minutes

Duration: ≥24 hours

Absorption: Incomplete

Protein binding: 95%

Half-life elimination: 20 hours

Excretion: Urine (80%); bile (10%)

Dosage

Geriatric Oral: Initial: 2.5 mg/day or every other day

Adult

Edema: Oral: Initial: 2.5-10 mg once daily; may increase as necessary to 20 mg once daily (ACC/AHA 2009 Heart Failure Guidelines); **Note:** Dosing frequency may be adjusted based on patient-specific diuretic needs (eg, administration every other day or weekly) (Lindenfeld, 2010).

Hypertension: Oral: 2.5-5 mg/dose every 24 hours

Renal Impairment Not dialyzable (0% to 5%) via hemo- or peritoneal dialysis; supplemental dose is not necessary

Administration May be taken with food or milk. Take early in day to avoid nocturia. Take the last dose of multiple doses no later than 6 PM unless instructed otherwise.

Monitoring Parameters Serum electrolytes (potassium, sodium, chloride, bicarbonate), renal function, blood pressure (standing, sitting/supine)

Pharmacotherapy Pearls 5 mg is approximately equivalent to 50 mg of hydrochlorothiazide; may be effective in patients with glomerular filtration rate <20 mL/minute; metolazone is often used in combination with a loop diuretic in patients who are unresponsive to the loop diuretic alone

Special Geriatric Considerations When metolazone is used in combination with other diuretics, there is an increased risk of azotemia and electrolyte depletion, particularly in the elderly, monitor closely. May be effective in patients with glomerular filtration rate <20 mL/minute. Metolazone is often used in combination with a loop diuretic in patients who are unresponsive to the loop diuretic alone.

Dosage Forms Excipient information presented when available (limited, particularly for generics); consult specific product labeling.
Tablet, oral: 2.5 mg, 5 mg, 10 mg
Zaroxolyn®: 2.5 mg, 5 mg

Metoprolol (me toe PROE lole)

Related Information
Beta-Blockers *on page 2001*
Medication Safety Issues
  Sound-alike/look-alike issues:
    Lopressor® may be confused with Lyrica®
    Metoprolol may be confused with metaproterenol, metoclopramide, metolazone, misoprostol
    Metoprolol succinate may be confused with metoprolol tartrate
    Toprol-XL® may be confused with TEGretol®, TEGretol®-XR, Topamax®
  High alert medication:
    The Institute for Safe Medication Practices (ISMP) includes this medication among its list of drugs which have a heightened risk of causing significant patient harm when used in error.
  Administration issues:
    Significant differences exist between oral and I.V. dosing. Use caution when converting from one route of administration to another.
Brand Names: U.S. Lopressor®; Toprol-XL®
Brand Names: Canada Apo-Metoprolol (Type L®); Apo-Metoprolol SR®; Apo-Metoprolol®; Betaloc®; Dom-Metoprolol; JAMP-Metoprolol-L; Lopressor®; Metoprolol Tartrate Injection, USP; Metoprolol-25; Metoprolol-L; Mylan-Metoprolol (Type L); Nu-Metop; PHL-Metoprolol; PMS-Metoprolol; Riva-Metoprolol; Sandoz-Metoprolol (Type L); Sandoz-Metoprolol SR; Teva-Metoprolol
Index Terms Metoprolol Succinate; Metoprolol Tartrate
Generic Availability (U.S.) Yes
Pharmacologic Category Beta Blocker, Beta-1 Selective
Use Treatment of angina pectoris, hypertension, or hemodynamically-stable acute myocardial infarction
Extended release: Treatment of angina pectoris or hypertension; to reduce mortality/hospitalization in patients with heart failure (stable NYHA Class II or III) already receiving ACE inhibitors, diuretics, and/or digoxin
Unlabeled/Investigational Use Treatment of ventricular arrhythmias, atrial ectopy; migraine prophylaxis, essential tremor, aggressive behavior (not recommended for dementia-associated aggression); prevention of myocardial infarction, atrial fibrillation, and atrial flutter; symptomatic treatment of hypertrophic obstructive cardiomyopathy
Contraindications
Hypersensitivity to metoprolol, any component of the formulation, or other beta-blockers
  Note: Additional contraindications are formulation and/or indication specific.
  Immediate release tablets/injectable formulation:
    Hypertension and angina: Sinus bradycardia; second- and third-degree heart block; cardiogenic shock; overt heart failure; sick sinus syndrome (except in patients with a functioning artificial pacemaker); severe peripheral arterial disease; pheochromocytoma (without alpha blockade)
    Myocardial infarction: Severe sinus bradycardia (heart rate <45 beats/minute); significant first-degree heart block (P-R interval ≥0.24 seconds); second- and third-degree heart block; systolic blood pressure <100 mm Hg; moderate-to-severe cardiac failure

◀ **Extended release tablet:** Severe bradycardia, second- and third degree heart block; cardiogenic shock; decompensated heart failure; sick sinus syndrome (except in patients with a functioning artificial pacemaker)

Warnings/Precautions [U.S. Boxed Warning]: Beta-blocker therapy should not be withdrawn abruptly (particularly in patients with CAD), but gradually tapered over 1-2 weeks to avoid acute tachycardia, hypertension, and/or ischemia. Consider pre-existing conditions such as sick sinus syndrome before initiating. Metoprolol commonly produces mild first-degree heart block (P-R interval >0.2-0.24 sec). May also produce severe first- (P-R interval ≥0.26 sec), second-, or third-degree heart block. Patients with acute MI (especially right ventricular MI) have a high risk of developing heart block of varying degrees. If severe heart block occurs, metoprolol should be discontinued and measures to increase heart rate should be employed. Symptomatic hypotension may occur with use. May precipitate or aggravate symptoms of arterial insufficiency in patients with PVD and Raynaud's disease; use with caution and monitor for progression of arterial obstruction. Use caution with concurrent use of digoxin, verapamil, or diltiazem; bradycardia or heart block can occur; avoid concurrent I.V. use of both agents. Use with caution in patients receiving inhaled anesthetic agents known to depress myocardial contractility. Use with caution in patients receiving CYP2D6 inhibitors (eg, bupropion, chlorpromazine, cimetidine, diphenhydramine, hydroxychloroquine, fluoxetine, paroxetine, propafenone, propoxyphene, quinidine, ritonavir, terbinafine, thioridazine); concurrent use may increase metoprolol plasma concentrations.

In general, beta-blockers should be avoided in patients with bronchospastic disease. Metoprolol, with B$_1$ selectivity, should be used cautiously in bronchospastic disease with close monitoring. Use cautiously in patients with diabetes because it can mask prominent hypoglycemic symptoms. May mask signs of hyperthyroidism (eg, tachycardia); if hyperthyroidism is suspected, carefully manage and monitor; abrupt withdrawal may exacerbate symptoms of hyperthyroidism or precipitate thyroid storm. Alterations in thyroid function tests may be observed. Use caution with hepatic dysfunction. Use with caution in patients with myasthenia gravis or psychiatric disease (may cause CNS depression). Although perioperative beta-blocker therapy is recommended prior to elective surgery in selected patients, use of high-dose extended release metoprolol in patients naïve to beta-blocker therapy undergoing noncardiac surgery has been associated with bradycardia, hypotension, stroke, and death. Chronic beta-blocker therapy should not be routinely withdrawn prior to major surgery. Use of beta-blockers may unmask cardiac failure in patients without a history of dysfunction. Adequate alpha-blockade is required prior to use of any beta-blocker for patients with untreated pheochromocytoma. May induce or exacerbate psoriasis. Use caution with history of severe anaphylaxis to allergens; patients taking beta-blockers may become more sensitive to repeated allergen challenges. Treatment of anaphylaxis (eg, epinephrine) in patients taking beta-blockers may be ineffective or promote undesirable effects. Bradycardia may be observed more frequently in elderly patients (>65 years of age); dosage reductions may be necessary.

Extended release: Use with caution in patients with compensated heart failure; monitor for a worsening of heart failure.

Adverse Reactions (Reflective of adult population; not specific for elderly) Frequency may not be defined.

Cardiovascular: Hypotension (1% to 27%), bradycardia (2% to 16%), first-degree heart block (P-R interval ≥0.26 sec; 5%), arterial insufficiency (usually Raynaud type; 1%), chest pain (1%), CHF (1%), edema (peripheral; 1%), palpitation (1%), syncope (1%)

Central nervous system: Dizziness (2% to 10%), fatigue (1% to 10%), depression (5%), confusion, hallucinations, headache, insomnia, memory loss (short-term), nightmares, sleep disturbances, somnolence, vertigo

Dermatology: Pruritus (5%), rash (5%), photosensitivity, psoriasis exacerbated

Endocrine & metabolic: Libido decreased, Peyronie's disease (<1%), diabetes exacerbated

Gastrointestinal: Diarrhea (5%), constipation (1%), flatulence (1%), gastrointestinal pain (1%), heartburn (1%), nausea (1%), xerostomia (1%), vomiting

Hematologic: Claudication

Neuromuscular & skeletal: Musculoskeletal pain

Ocular: Blurred vision, visual disturbances

Otic: Tinnitus

Respiratory: Dyspnea (1% to 3%), bronchospasm (1%), wheezing (1%), rhinitis, shortness of breath

Miscellaneous: Cold extremities (1%)

Other events reported with beta-blockers: Catatonia, emotional lability, fever, hypersensitivity reactions, laryngospasm, nonthrombocytopenic purpura, respiratory distress, thrombocytopenic purpura

Drug Interactions
Metabolism/Transport Effects Substrate of CYP2C19 (minor), 2D6 (major); **Inhibits** CYP2D6 (weak)
Avoid Concomitant Use
Avoid concomitant use of Metoprolol with any of the following: Floctafenine; Methacholine
Increased Effect/Toxicity
Metoprolol may increase the levels/effects of: Alpha-/Beta-Agonists (Direct-Acting); Alpha1-Blockers; Alpha2-Agonists; Amifostine; Antihypertensives; Antipsychotic Agents (Phenothiazines); Bupivacaine; Cardiac Glycosides; Fingolimod; Hypotensive Agents; Insulin; Lidocaine; Lidocaine (Systemic); Lidocaine (Topical); Mepivacaine; Methacholine; Midodrine; RiTUXimab; Sulfonylureas

The levels/effects of Metoprolol may be increased by: Abiraterone Acetate; Acetylcholinesterase Inhibitors; Aminoquinolines (Antimalarial); Amiodarone; Anilidopiperidine Opioids; Antipsychotic Agents (Phenothiazines); Calcium Channel Blockers (Dihydropyridine); Calcium Channel Blockers (Nondihydropyridine); CYP2D6 Inhibitors (Moderate); CYP2D6 Inhibitors (Strong); Darunavir; Diazoxide; Dipyridamole; Disopyramide; Dronedarone; Floctafenine; Herbs (Hypotensive Properties); MAO Inhibitors; Pentoxifylline; Phosphodiesterase 5 Inhibitors; Propafenone; Propoxyphene; Prostacyclin Analogues; QuiNIDine; Reserpine; Selective Serotonin Reuptake Inhibitors
Decreased Effect
Metoprolol may decrease the levels/effects of: Beta2-Agonists; Theophylline Derivatives

The levels/effects of Metoprolol may be decreased by: Barbiturates; Herbs (Hypertensive Properties); Methylphenidate; Nonsteroidal Anti-Inflammatory Agents; Peginterferon Alfa-2b; Rifamycin Derivatives; Yohimbine
Ethanol/Nutrition/Herb Interactions
Food: Food increases absorption. Metoprolol serum levels may be increased if taken with food.
Herb/Nutraceutical: Avoid bayberry, blue cohosh, cayenne, ephedra, ginger, ginseng (American), gotu kola, licorice, (may worsen hypertension). Avoid black cohosh, California poppy, coleus, golden seal, hawthorn, mistletoe, periwinkle, quinine, shepherd's purse (may have increased antihypertensive effect).
Stability
Injection: Store at 25°C (77°F); excursions permitted to 15°C to 30°C (59°F to 86°F). Protect from light.
Tablet: Store at 25°C (77°F); excursions permitted to 15°C to 30°C (59°F to 86°F). Protect from moisture.
Mechanism of Action Selective inhibitor of beta$_1$-adrenergic receptors; competitively blocks beta$_1$-receptors, with little or no effect on beta$_2$-receptors at doses <100 mg; does not exhibit any membrane stabilizing or intrinsic sympathomimetic activity
Pharmacodynamics/Kinetics
Onset of action: Peak effect: Oral: 1.5-4 hours; I.V.: 20 minutes (when infused over 10 minutes)
Duration: Oral: Immediate release: 10-20 hours, Extended release: ~24 hours; I.V.: 5-8 hours
Absorption: 95%, rapid and complete
Distribution: V_d: 5.5 L/kg
Protein binding: 12% to albumin
Metabolism: Extensively hepatic via CYP2D6; significant first-pass effect (~50%)
Bioavailability: Oral: ~50%
Half-life elimination: 3-8 hours (dependent on rate of CYP2D6 metabolism)
Excretion: Urine (<5% to 10% as unchanged drug)
Dosage
Geriatric Refer to adult dosing. In the management of hypertension, consider lower initial doses and titrate to response (Aronow, 2011).
Adult
Angina: Oral:
Immediate release: Initial: 50 mg twice daily; usual dosage range: 50-200 mg twice daily; maximum: 400 mg/day; increase dose at weekly intervals to desired effect
Extended release: Initial: 100 mg/day (maximum: 400 mg/day)
Atrial fibrillation/flutter (ventricular rate control), supraventricular tachycardia (SVT) (acute treatment; unlabeled use; Antman, 2004; Fuster, 2006; Neumar, 2010): I.V.: 2.5-5 mg every 2-5 minutes (maximum total dose: 15 mg over a 10-15 minute period). **Note:** Initiate cautiously in patients with concomitant heart failure; avoid in patients with decompensated heart failure.
Maintenance: Oral (immediate release): 25-100 mg twice daily

◀ **Heart failure:** Oral: *Extended release:* Initial: 25 mg once daily (reduce to 12.5 mg once daily in NYHA class higher than class II); may double dosage every 2 weeks as tolerated (target dose: 200 mg/day)

Hypertension: Oral:
Immediate release: Initial: 50 mg twice daily; effective dosage range: 100-450 mg/day in 2-3 divided doses; increase dose at weekly intervals to desired effect; maximum: 450 mg/day; usual dosage range (JNC 7): 50-100 mg/day

Extended release: Initial: 25-100 mg once daily; increase doses at weekly (or longer) intervals to desired effect; maximum: 400 mg/day; usual dosage range (JNC 7): 50-100 mg/day

Hypertension/ventricular rate control: I.V. (in patients having nonfunctioning GI tract): Initial: 1.25-5 mg every 6-12 hours; titrate initial dose to response. Initially, low doses may be appropriate to establish response; however, although not routine, up to 15 mg administered as frequently as every 3 hours has been employed in patients with refractory tachycardia.

Myocardial infarction:
Acute: I.V.: 5 mg every 2 minutes for 3 doses in early treatment of myocardial infarction; thereafter, give 50 mg orally every 6 hours beginning 15 minutes after last I.V. dose and continue for 48 hours; then administer a maintenance dose of 100 mg twice daily. **Note:** Do not initiate this regimen in those with signs of heart failure, a low output state, increased risk of cardiogenic shock, or other contraindications (eg, second- or third-degree heart block). If initial I.V. dosing is not tolerated, may give 25-50 mg orally (depending on degree of intolerance) every 6 hours beginning 15 minutes after the last I.V. dose or as soon as clinical condition permits.

Secondary prevention (unlabeled use; Olsson, 1992): Oral: Immediate release: 25-100 mg twice daily; optimize dose based on heart rate and blood pressure; continue indefinitely.

Note: Switching dosage forms:
When switching from immediate release metoprolol to extended release, the same total daily dose of metoprolol should be used.
When switching between oral and intravenous dosage forms, equivalent beta-blocking effect is achieved when doses in a 2.5:1 (Oral:I.V.) ratio is used. For example, if the patient is receiving an oral dose of 25 mg twice daily (50 mg/day), this would translate to 5 mg I.V. every 6 hours; consider reducing initial I.V. dose to evaluate patient response.

Renal Impairment No adjustment required.

Hepatic Impairment Reduced dose may be necessary.

Administration
Oral: Extended release tablets: May be divided in half; do not crush or chew.

I.V.: When administered acutely for cardiac treatment, monitor ECG and blood pressure. May administer by rapid infusion (I.V. push) over 1 minute or by slow infusion (ie, 5-10 mg of metoprolol in 50 mL of fluid) over ~30 minutes. Necessary monitoring for surgical patients who are unable to take oral beta-blockers (prolonged ileus) has not been defined. Some institutions require monitoring of baseline and postinfusion heart rate and blood pressure when a patient's response to beta-blockade has not been characterized (ie, the patient's initial dose or following a change in dose). Consult individual institutional policies and procedures.

Monitoring Parameters Blood pressure, orthostatic hypotension, heart rate, CNS effects

Special Geriatric Considerations Due to alterations in the beta-adrenergic autonomic nervous system, beta-adrenergic blockade may result in less hemodynamic response than seen in younger adults. Studies indicate that despite decreased sensitivity to the chronotropic effects of beta-blockade with age, there appears to be an increased myocardial sensitivity to the negative inotropic effect during stress (ie, exercise). Controlled trials have shown the overall response rate for propranolol to be only 20% to 50% in the elderly populations. Therefore, all beta-adrenergic blocking drugs may result in a decreased response as compared to younger adults.

Dosage Forms Excipient information presented when available (limited, particularly for generics); consult specific product labeling.

Injection, solution, as tartrate: 1 mg/mL (5 mL)
Lopressor®: 1 mg/mL (5 mL)

Injection, solution, as tartrate [preservative free]: 1 mg/mL (5 mL)

Tablet, oral, as tartrate: 25 mg, 50 mg, 100 mg
Lopressor®: 50 mg, 100 mg [scored]

Tablet, extended release, oral, as succinate: 25 mg [expressed as mg equivalent to tartrate], 50 mg [expressed as mg equivalent to tartrate], 100 mg [expressed as mg equivalent to tartrate], 200 mg [expressed as mg equivalent to tartrate]
Toprol-XL®: 25 mg, 50 mg, 100 mg, 200 mg [scored; expressed as mg equivalent to tartrate]

Extemporaneously Prepared To prepare a metoprolol 10 mg/mL liquid, crush 12 metoprolol tartrate 100 mg tablets into a fine powder. Add ~20 mL of either Ora-Sweet® and Ora-Plus® (1:1 preparation), or Ora-Sweet® SF and Ora-Plus® (1:1 preparation), or cherry syrup. Mix to a uniform paste. Continue to add the vehicle to bring the final volume to 120 mL. The preparation is stable for 60 days; shake well before using and protect from light.

Allen LV and Erickson III MA, "Stability of Labetalol Hydrochloride, Metoprolol Tartrate, Verapamil Hydrochloride, and Spironolactone With Hydrochlorothiazide in Extemporaneously Compounded Oral Liquids," *Am J Health Syst Pharm*, 1996, 53:2304-9.

Selected References

Antman EM, Hand M, Armstrong PW, et al, "2007 Focused Update of the ACC/AHA 2004 Guidelines for the Management of Patients With ST-Elevation Myocardial Infarction. A Report of the American College of Cardiology/American Heart Association Task Force on Practice Guidelines," *J Am Coll Cardiol*, 2008, 51(2):210-49.

Fleisher LA, Beckman JA, Brown KA, et al, "ACC/AHA 2006 Guideline Update on Perioperative Cardiovascular Evaluation for Noncardiac Surgery: Focused Update on Perioperative Beta-Blocker Therapy. A Report of the American College of Cardiology/American Heart Association Task Force on Practice Guidelines (Writing Committee to Update the 2002 Guidelines on Perioperative Cardiovascular Evaluation for Noncardiac Surgery) Developed in Collaboration With the American Society of Echocardiography, American Society of Nuclear Cardiology, Heart Rhythm Society, Society of Cardiovascular Anesthesiologists, Society for Cardiovascular Angiography and Interventions, and Society for Vascular Medicine and Biology," *J Am Coll Cardiol*, 2006, 47(11):2343-55.

Fuster V, Ryden LE, Cannom DS, et al, "ACC/AHA/ESC 2006 Guidelines for the Management of Patients With Atrial Fibrillation-Executrive Summary. A Report of the American College of Cardiology/American Heart Association Task Force on Practice Guidelines and the European Society of Cardiology Committee for Practice Guidelines (Writing Committee to Revise the 2001 Guidelines for the Management of Patients With Atrial Fibrillation). Developed in Collaboration With the European Heart Rhythm Association and the Heart Rhythm Society)," *J Am Coll Cardiol*, 2006, 48(4):854-906.

Juul AB, Wetterslev J, Gluud C, et al, "Effect of Perioperative Beta Blockade in Patients With Diabetes Undergoing Major Non-Cardiac Surgery: Randomized Placebo Controlled, Blinded Multicentre Trial. DIPOM Trial Group," *BMJ*, 2006, 332(7556):1482.

Poole-Wilson PA, Swedberg K, Cleland JG, et al, "Comparison of Carvedilol and Metoprolol on Clinical Outcomes in Patients With Chronic Heart Failure in the Carvedilol or Metoprolol European Trial (COMET): Randomized Controlled Trial," *Lancet*, 2003, 362(9377):7-13.

Rabins PV, Blacker D, Rovner BW, et al, "Practice Guidelines for the Treatment of Patients With Alzheimer's Disease and Other Dementias," *Am J Psychiatry*, 2007, 164(12 Suppl):5-56. Available at http://www.psych.org/psych_pract/treatg/pg/prac_guide.cfm.

Metoprolol and Hydrochlorothiazide
(me toe PROE lole & hye droe klor oh THYE a zide)

Related Information
Hydrochlorothiazide *on page 876*
Metoprolol *on page 1195*

Brand Names: U.S. Lopressor HCT®

Index Terms Hydrochlorothiazide and Metoprolol; Hydrochlorothiazide and Metoprolol Tartrate; Metoprolol Tartrate and Hydrochlorothiazide

Generic Availability (U.S.) Yes

Pharmacologic Category Beta Blocker, Beta-1 Selective; Diuretic, Thiazide

Use Treatment of hypertension (not recommended for initial treatment)

Dosage
>   **Geriatric & Adult** Hypertension: Oral: Dosage should be determined by titration of the individual agents and the combination product substituted based upon the daily requirements.
>
>   Usual dose: Metoprolol 50-100 mg and hydrochlorothiazide 25-50 mg administered daily as single or divided doses (twice daily)
>
>   **Note:** Hydrochlorothiazide >50 mg/day is not recommended.
>
>   Concomitant therapy: It is recommended that if an additional antihypertensive agent is required, gradual titration should occur using 1/2 the usual starting dose of the other agent to avoid hypotension.

Special Geriatric Considerations See individual agents. Combination products are not recommended as first-line treatment. Use only if doses of individual agents correspond to the combination available.

Dosage Forms Excipient information presented when available (limited, particularly for generics); consult specific product labeling.

>   Tablet: 50/25: Metoprolol tartrate 50 mg and hydrochlorothiazide 25 mg; 100/25: Metoprolol tartrate 100 mg and hydrochlorothiazide 25 mg; 100/50: Metoprolol tartrate 100 mg and hydrochlorothiazide 50 mg
>
>   Lopressor HCT® 50/25: Metoprolol tartrate 50 mg and hydrochlorothiazide 25 mg
>
>   Lopressor HCT® 100/25: Metoprolol tartrate 100 mg and hydrochlorothiazide 25 mg

◆ **Metoprolol Succinate** *see* Metoprolol *on page 1195*

◆ **Metoprolol Tartrate** *see* Metoprolol *on page 1195*

◆ **Metoprolol Tartrate and Hydrochlorothiazide** *see* Metoprolol and Hydrochlorothiazide *on page 1199*

METRONIDAZOLE (SYSTEMIC)

- ◆ **Metozolv™ ODT** *see* Metoclopramide *on page 1190*
- ◆ **MetroCream®** *see* MetroNIDAZOLE (Topical) *on page 1203*
- ◆ **MetroGel®** *see* MetroNIDAZOLE (Topical) *on page 1203*
- ◆ **MetroGel® 1% Kit** *see* MetroNIDAZOLE (Topical) *on page 1203*
- ◆ **MetroGel-Vaginal®** *see* MetroNIDAZOLE (Topical) *on page 1203*
- ◆ **MetroLotion®** *see* MetroNIDAZOLE (Topical) *on page 1203*

MetroNIDAZOLE (Systemic) (met roe NYE da zole)

Related Information
Community-Acquired Pneumonia in Adults *on page 2059*
Helicobacter pylori Treatment in Adult Patients *on page 2009*

Medication Safety Issues
Sound-alike/look-alike issues:
MetroNIDAZOLE may be confused with mebendazole, meropenem, metFORMIN, methotrexate, metoclopramide, miconazole

Brand Names: U.S. Flagyl®; Flagyl® 375; Flagyl® ER

Brand Names: Canada Apo-Metronidazole®; Flagyl®; Florazole® ER

Index Terms Metronidazole Hydrochloride

Generic Availability (U.S.) Yes: Excludes extended release tablet

Pharmacologic Category Amebicide; Antibiotic, Miscellaneous; Antiprotozoal, Nitroimidazole

Use Treatment of susceptible anaerobic bacterial and protozoal infections in the following conditions: Amebiasis, symptomatic and asymptomatic trichomoniasis; skin and skin structure infections, bone and joint infections, CNS infections, endocarditis, gynecologic infections, intra-abdominal infections (as part of combination regimen); respiratory tract infections (lower), systemic anaerobic infections; treatment of antibiotic-associated pseudomembranous colitis (AAPC); as part of a multidrug regimen for *H. pylori* eradication to reduce the risk of duodenal ulcer recurrence; surgical prophylaxis (colorectal)

Unlabeled/Investigational Use Crohn's disease

Contraindications Hypersensitivity to metronidazole, nitroimidazole derivatives, or any component of the formulation

Warnings/Precautions Use with caution in patients with severe liver impairment due to potential accumulation, blood dyscrasias; history of seizures, CHF or other sodium-retaining states; reduce dosage in patients with severe liver impairment, CNS disease, and consider dosage reduction in longer-term therapy with severe renal failure (Cl_{cr} <10 mL/minute); if *H. pylori* is not eradicated in patients being treated with metronidazole in a regimen, it should be assumed that metronidazole-resistance has occurred and it should not again be used; aseptic meningitis, encephalopathy, seizures, and neuropathies have been reported especially with increased doses and chronic treatment; monitor and consider discontinuation of therapy if symptoms occur. **[U.S. Boxed Warning]: Possibly carcinogenic based on animal data.** Prolonged use may result in fungal or bacterial superinfection, including *C. difficile*-associated diarrhea (CDAD) and pseudomembranous colitis; CDAD has been observed >2 months postantibiotic treatment. The Infectious Disease Society of America (IDSA) recommends the use of oral metronidazole for initial treatment of mild-to-moderate *C. difficile* infection and the use of oral vancomycin for initial treatment of severe *C. difficile* infection with or without I.V. metronidazole depending on the presence of complications. May treat recurrent mild-to-moderate infection once with oral metronidazole; avoid use beyond first reoccurrence due to potential cumulative neurotoxicity (Cohen, 2010). Candidiasis infection (known or unknown) maybe more prominent during metronidazole treatment, antifungal treatment required. Disulfiram-like reactions to ethanol have been reported with oral metronidazole; avoid alcoholic beverages during therapy

Adverse Reactions (Reflective of adult population; not specific for elderly) Frequency not always defined.

Cardiovascular: Flattening of the T-wave, flushing, syncope

Central nervous system: Aseptic meningitis, ataxia, confusion, coordination impaired, depression, dizziness, encephalopathy, fever, headache, insomnia, irritability, seizure, vertigo

Dermatologic: Erythematous rash, pruritus, Stevens-Johnson syndrome, toxic epidermal necrolysis, urticaria

Endocrine & metabolic: Disulfiram-like reaction, dysmenorrhea

Gastrointestinal: Nausea (~12%), anorexia, abdominal cramping, constipation, diarrhea, epigastric distress, furry tongue, glossitis, pancreatitis (rare), proctitis, stomatitis, unusual/metallic taste, vomiting, xerostomia

Genitourinary: Cystitis, darkened urine (rare), dyspareunia, dysuria, incontinence, libido decreased, pelvic pressure, polyuria, vaginal dryness, vaginitis

Hematologic: Neutropenia (reversible), thrombocytopenia (reversible, rare)

Local: Thrombophlebitis

Neuromuscular & skeletal: Dysarthria, peripheral neuropathy, weakness

Ocular: Optic neuropathy

Respiratory: Nasal congestion, pharyngitis, rhinitis, sinusitis, pharyngitis

Miscellaneous: Flu-like syndrome, joint pains resembling serum sickness, moniliasis

Drug Interactions

Metabolism/Transport Effects Inhibits CYP2C9 (weak), 3A4 (moderate)

Avoid Concomitant Use

Avoid concomitant use of MetroNIDAZOLE (Systemic) with any of the following: BCG; Tolvaptan

Increased Effect/Toxicity

MetroNIDAZOLE (Systemic) may increase the levels/effects of: Alcohol (Ethyl); Budesonide (Systemic, Oral Inhalation); Busulfan; Calcineurin Inhibitors; Colchicine; CYP3A4 Substrates; Eplerenone; Everolimus; FentaNYL; Fosphenytoin; Halofantrine; Lurasidone; Phenytoin; Pimecrolimus; Ranolazine; Salmeterol; Saxagliptin; Tipranavir; Tolvaptan; Vilazodone; Vitamin K Antagonists

The levels/effects of MetroNIDAZOLE (Systemic) may be increased by: Disulfiram; Mebendazole

Decreased Effect

MetroNIDAZOLE (Systemic) may decrease the levels/effects of: BCG; Mycophenolate; Typhoid Vaccine

The levels/effects of MetroNIDAZOLE (Systemic) may be decreased by: Fosphenytoin; PHENobarbital; Phenytoin

Ethanol/Nutrition/Herb Interactions

Ethanol: The manufacturer recommends to avoid all ethanol or any ethanol-containing drugs (may cause disulfiram-like reaction characterized by flushing, headache, nausea, vomiting, sweating, or tachycardia).

Food: Peak antibiotic serum concentration lowered and delayed, but total drug absorbed not affected.

Stability

Injection: Store at controlled room temperature of 15°C to 30°C (59°F to 86°F). Protect from light. Keep in overwrap until ready to use. Product may be refrigerated but crystals may form. Crystals redissolve on warming to room temperature. Prolonged exposure to light will cause a darkening of the product. However, short-term exposure to normal room light does not adversely affect metronidazole stability. Direct sunlight should be avoided. Stability of parenteral admixture at room temperature (25°C); Out of overwrap stability: 30 days. Standard diluent: 500 mg/100 mL NS.

Tablets: Store at room temperature. Protect from light and moisture.

Mechanism of Action After diffusing into the organism, interacts with DNA to cause a loss of helical DNA structure and strand breakage resulting in inhibition of protein synthesis and cell death in susceptible organisms

Pharmacodynamics/Kinetics

Absorption: Oral: Well absorbed

Distribution: To saliva, bile, seminal fluid, bone, liver, and liver abscesses, lung and vaginal secretions; crosses blood-brain barrier

CSF:blood level ratio: Normal meninges: 16% to 43%; Inflamed meninges: 100%

Protein binding: <20%

Metabolism: Hepatic (30% to 60%)

Half-life elimination: 6-8 hours, prolonged with hepatic impairment; End-stage renal disease: 21 hours

Time to peak, serum: Oral: Immediate release: 1-2 hours

Excretion: Urine (60% to 80% as unchanged drug); feces (6% to 15%)

Dosage

Geriatric Refer to adult dosing. Use the lower end of the dosing recommendations for adults; do not administer as single dose as efficacy has not been established.

Adult

Anaerobic infections (diverticulitis, intra-abdominal, peritonitis, cholangitis, or abscess): Oral, I.V.: 500 mg every 6-8 hours, not to exceed 4 g/day; **Note:** Initial: 1 g I.V. loading dose may be administered

Amebiasis: Oral: 500-750 mg every 8 hours for 5-10 days

Antibiotic-associated pseudomembranous colitis: IDSA Guidelines (Cohen, 2010):
Mild-to-moderate infection: Oral: 500 mg 3 times/day for 10-14 days
Severe complicated infection: I.V.: 500 mg 3 times/day with oral vancomycin (recommended agent) for 10-14 days
Note: Due to the emergence of a new strain of *C. difficile*, some clinicians recommend converting to oral vancomycin therapy if the patient does not show a clear clinical response after 2 days of metronidazole therapy.
Giardiasis: 500 mg twice daily for 5-7 days
Intra-abdominal infection, complicated, community-acquired, mild-to-moderate (in combination with cephalosporin or fluoroquinolone): I.V.: 500 mg every 8-12 hours **or** 1.5 g every 24 hours for 4-7 days (provided source controlled)
Peptic ulcer disease: *Helicobacter pylori* eradication: Oral: 250-500 mg with meals and at bedtime for 14 days; requires combination therapy with at least one other antibiotic and an acid-suppressing agent (proton pump inhibitor or H_2 blocker)
Bacterial vaginosis or vaginitis due to *Gardnerella*, *Mobiluncus*: Oral: 500 mg twice daily (regular release) or 750 mg once daily (extended release tablet) for 7 days
Pelvic inflammatory disease (unlabeled use): Oral: 500 mg twice daily for 14 days (in combination with a cephalosporin and doxycycline) (CDC, 2010)
Trichomoniasis: Oral: 250 mg every 8 hours for 7 days **or** 375 mg twice daily for 7 days **or** 2 g as a single dose **or** 1 g twice daily for 2 doses (on same day)
Urethritis (unlabeled use): Oral: 2 g as a single dose with azithromycin (CDC, 2010)
Surgical prophylaxis (colorectal): I.V.: 15 mg/kg 1 hour prior to surgery; followed by 7.5 mg/kg 6 and 12 hours after initial dose
Renal Impairment Cl_{cr} <10 mL/minute (not on dialysis): Recommendations vary: To reduce possible accumulation in patients receiving multiple doses, consider reduction to 50% of dose or administer normal dose every 12 hours; **Note:** Dosage reduction is unnecessary in short courses of therapy. Some references do not recommend reduction at any level of renal impairment (Lamp, 1999).
Intermittent hemodialysis (IHD) (administer after hemodialysis on dialysis days): Dialyzable (50% to 100%): 500 mg every 8-12 hours. **Note:** Dosing regimen highly dependent on clinical indication (trichomoniasis vs *C. difficile* colitis) (Heintz, 2009). **Note:** Dosing dependent on the assumption of thrice weekly, complete IHD sessions.
Peritoneal dialysis (PD): Dose as for Cl_{cr} <10 mL/minute
Continuous renal replacement therapy (CRRT) (Heintz, 2009; Trotman, 2005): Drug clearance is highly dependent on the method of renal replacement, filter type, and flow rate. Appropriate dosing requires close monitoring of pharmacologic response, signs of adverse reactions due to drug accumulation, as well as drug concentrations in relation to target trough (if appropriate). The following are general recommendations only (based on dialysate flow/ultrafiltration rates of 1-2 L/hour and minimal residual renal function) and should not supersede clinical judgment:
CVVH/CVVHD/CVVHDF: 500 mg every 6-12 hours (or per clinical indication; dosage reduction generally not necessary)
Hepatic Impairment Unchanged in mild liver disease; reduce dosage in severe liver disease.

Administration
I.V.: Infuse intravenously over 30-60 minutes. Avoid contact of drug solution with equipment containing aluminum.
Oral: May be taken with food to minimize stomach upset. Extended release tablets should be taken on an empty stomach (1 hour before or 2 hours after meals).

Test Interactions May interfere with AST, ALT, triglycerides, glucose, and LDH testing
Special Geriatric Considerations Adjust dose based on renal function.
Dosage Forms Excipient information presented when available (limited, particularly for generics); consult specific product labeling.
Capsule, oral: 375 mg
Flagyl® 375: 375 mg
Infusion, premixed iso-osmotic sodium chloride solution: 500 mg (100 mL)
Tablet, oral: 250 mg, 500 mg
Flagyl®: 250 mg, 500 mg
Tablet, extended release, oral:
Flagyl® ER: 750 mg

Selected References
Lamp KC, Freeman CD, Klutman NE, et al, "Pharmacokinetics and Pharmacodynamics of the Nitroimidazole Antimicrobials," *Clin Pharmacokinet*, 1999, 36(5):353-73.
Ludwig E, Csiba A, Magyar T, et al, "Age-Associated Pharmacokinetic Changes of Metronidazole," *Int J Clin Pharmacol Ther Toxicol*, 1983, 21(2):87-91.

MetroNIDAZOLE (Topical) (met roe NYE da zole)

Brand Names: U.S. MetroCream®; MetroGel-Vaginal®; MetroGel®; MetroGel® 1% Kit; MetroLotion®; Noritate®; Vandazole®

Brand Names: Canada MetroCream®; Metrogel®; MetroLotion®; Nidagel™; Noritate®; Rosasol®

Index Terms Metronidazole Hydrochloride

Generic Availability (U.S.) Yes

Pharmacologic Category Antibiotic, Topical

Use
Topical: Treatment of inflammatory lesions and erythema of rosacea
Vaginal gel: Bacterial vaginosis

Dosage
Geriatric Use the lower end of the dosing recommendations for adults

Adult
Acne rosacea: Topical:
0.75%: Apply and rub a thin film twice daily, morning and evening, to entire affected areas after washing.
1%: Apply thin film to affected area once daily
Bacterial vaginosis or vaginitis due to *Gardnerella*, *Mobiluncus*: Vaginal: One applicatorful (~37.5 mg metronidazole) intravaginally once or twice daily for 5 days; apply once in morning and evening if using twice daily, if daily, use at bedtime

Dosage Forms Excipient information presented when available (limited, particularly for generics); consult specific product labeling.
Cream, topical: 0.75% (45 g)
  MetroCream®: 0.75% (45 g) [contains benzyl alcohol]
  Noritate®: 1% (60 g)
Gel, topical: 0.75% (45 g)
  MetroGel®: 1% (60 g)
  MetroGel® 1% Kit: 1% (60 g)
Gel, vaginal: 0.75% (70 g)
  MetroGel-Vaginal®: 0.75% (70 g)
  Vandazole®: 0.75% (70 g)
Lotion, topical: 0.75% (59 mL, 60 mL)
  MetroLotion®: 0.75% (59 mL) [contains benzyl alcohol]

◆ **Metronidazole Hydrochloride** *see* MetroNIDAZOLE (Systemic) *on page 1200*
◆ **Metronidazole Hydrochloride** *see* MetroNIDAZOLE (Topical) *on page 1203*
◆ **Mevacor®** *see* Lovastatin *on page 1097*
◆ **Mevinolin** *see* Lovastatin *on page 1097*

Mexiletine (meks IL e teen)

Brand Names: Canada Novo-Mexiletine

Generic Availability (U.S.) Yes

Pharmacologic Category Antiarrhythmic Agent, Class Ib

Use Management of serious ventricular arrhythmias; suppression of PVCs

Unlabeled/Investigational Use Treatment of diabetic neuropathy

Contraindications Hypersensitivity to mexiletine or any component of the formulation; cardiogenic shock; second- or third-degree AV block (except in patients with a functioning artificial pacemaker)

Warnings/Precautions [U.S. Boxed Warning]: In the Cardiac Arrhythmia Suppression Trial (CAST), recent (>6 days but <2 years ago) myocardial infarction patients with asymptomatic, non-life-threatening ventricular arrhythmias did not benefit and may have been harmed by attempts to suppress the arrhythmia with flecainide or encainide. An increased mortality or non-fatal cardiac arrest rate (7.7%) was seen in the active treatment group compared with patients in the placebo group (3%). The applicability of the CAST results to other populations is unknown. Antiarrhythmic agents should be reserved for patients with life-threatening ventricular arrhythmias. Can be proarrhythmic. Electrolyte disturbances alter response; should be corrected before initiating therapy. Use cautiously in patients with first-degree block, pre-existing sinus node dysfunction, intraventricular conduction delays, significant hepatic dysfunction, hypotension, or severe HF. Alterations in urinary pH may change urinary excretion. Rare hepatic toxicity may occur; may cause acute hepatic injury.

◄ **Adverse Reactions (Reflective of adult population; not specific for elderly)**
>10%:
Central nervous system: Lightheadedness (11% to 25%), dizziness (20% to 25%), nervousness (5% to 10%), incoordination (10%)
Gastrointestinal: GI distress (41%), nausea/vomiting (40%)
Neuromuscular & skeletal: Trembling, unsteady gait, tremor (13%), ataxia (10% to 20%)
1% to 10%:
Cardiovascular: Chest pain (3% to 8%), premature ventricular contractions (1% to 2%), palpitation (4% to 8%), angina (2%), proarrhythmia (10% to 15% in patients with malignant arrhythmia)
Central nervous system: Confusion, headache, insomnia (5% to 7%), depression (2%)
Dermatologic: Rash (4%)
Gastrointestinal: Constipation or diarrhea (4% to 5%), xerostomia (3%), abdominal pain (1%)
Neuromuscular & skeletal: Weakness (5%), numbness of fingers or toes (2% to 4%), paresthesia (2%), arthralgia (1%)
Ocular: Blurred vision (5% to 7%), nystagmus (6%)
Otic: Tinnitus (2% to 3%)
Respiratory: Dyspnea (3%)

Drug Interactions
Metabolism/Transport Effects Substrate (major) of CYP1A2, 2D6; **Inhibits** CYP1A2 (strong)
Avoid Concomitant Use There are no known interactions where it is recommended to avoid concomitant use.
Increased Effect/Toxicity
Mexiletine may increase the levels/effects of: Bendamustine; CYP1A2 Substrates; Theophylline Derivatives

The levels/effects of Mexiletine may be increased by: Abiraterone Acetate; CYP1A2 Inhibitors (Moderate); CYP1A2 Inhibitors (Strong); CYP2D6 Inhibitors (Moderate); CYP2D6 Inhibitors (Strong); Darunavir; Deferasirox; Selective Serotonin Reuptake Inhibitors
Decreased Effect
The levels/effects of Mexiletine may be decreased by: CYP1A2 Inducers (Strong); Cyproterone; Etravirine; Fosphenytoin; Peginterferon Alfa-2b; Phenytoin
Ethanol/Nutrition/Herb Interactions Food: Food may decrease the rate, but not the extent of oral absorption; diets which affect urine pH can increase or decrease excretion of mexiletine. Avoid dietary changes that alter urine pH.
Mechanism of Action Class IB antiarrhythmic, structurally related to lidocaine, which inhibits inward sodium current, decreases rate of rise of phase 0, increases effective refractory period/ action potential duration ratio
Pharmacodynamics/Kinetics
Absorption: Well absorbed; elderly have a slightly slower rate, but extent of absorption is the same as young adults
Distribution: V_d: 5-7 L/kg
Protein binding: 50% to 60%
Metabolism: Hepatic; low first-pass effect
Bioavailability: 80% to 95%
Half-life elimination: Adults: 10-14 hours (average: elderly: 14.4 hours, younger adults: 12 hours); prolonged with hepatic impairment or heart failure
Time to peak, serum: 2-3 hours
Excretion: Urine (10% to 15% as unchanged drug); urinary acidification increases excretion, alkalinization decreases excretion
Dosage
Geriatric & Adult Arrhythmias: Oral: Initial: 200 mg every 8 hours (may load with 400 mg if necessary); adjust dose every 2-3 days; usual dose: 200-300 mg every 8 hours; maximum: 1.2 g/day (some patients respond to every 12-hour dosing). When switching from another antiarrhythmic, initiate a 200 mg dose 6-12 hours after stopping former agents, 3-6 hours after stopping procainamide.
Hepatic Impairment Patients with hepatic impairment or CHF may require dose reduction; reduce dose to 25% to 30% of usual dose
Administration Administer with food, around-the-clock rather than 3 times/day to promote less variation in peak and trough serum levels.
Monitoring Parameters ECG, blood pressure, pulse, serum concentrations
Reference Range Therapeutic range: 0.5-2 mcg/mL; potentially toxic: >2 mcg/mL
Test Interactions Abnormal liver function test, positive ANA, thrombocytopenia
Special Geriatric Considerations No specific changes in dose are necessary.

Dosage Forms Excipient information presented when available (limited, particularly for generics); consult specific product labeling.
Capsule, oral, as hydrochloride: 150 mg, 200 mg, 250 mg

◆ **MG217® Sal-Acid [OTC]** *see* Salicylic Acid *on page 1648*
◆ **Mg-plus® [OTC]** *see* Magnesium Salts (Various Salts) *on page 1114*
◆ **Miacalcin®** *see* Calcitonin *on page 241*
◆ **Mi-Acid [OTC]** *see* Aluminum Hydroxide, Magnesium Hydroxide, and Simethicone *on page 84*
◆ **Mi-Acid Gas Relief [OTC]** *see* Simethicone *on page 1679*
◆ **Mi-Acid Maximum Strength [OTC] [DSC]** *see* Aluminum Hydroxide, Magnesium Hydroxide, and Simethicone *on page 84*
◆ **Micaderm® [OTC]** *see* Miconazole *on page 1206*

Micafungin (mi ka FUN gin)

Brand Names: U.S. Mycamine®
Brand Names: Canada Mycamine®
Index Terms Micafungin Sodium
Generic Availability (U.S.) No
Pharmacologic Category Antifungal Agent, Parenteral; Echinocandin
Use Treatment of esophageal candidiasis; *Candida* prophylaxis in patients undergoing hematopoietic stem cell transplant (HSCT); treatment of candidemia, acute disseminated candidiasis, and other *Candida* infections (peritonitis and abscesses)
Unlabeled/Investigational Use Treatment of infections due to *Aspergillus* spp; prophylaxis of HIV-related esophageal candidiasis
Contraindications Hypersensitivity to micafungin, other echinocandins, or any component of the formulation
Warnings/Precautions Anaphylactic reactions, including shock, have been reported. New onset or worsening hepatic failure has been reported; use caution in pre-existing mild-moderate hepatic impairment; safety in severe liver failure has not been evaluated. Hemolytic anemia and hemoglobinuria have been reported. Increased BUN, serum creatinine, renal dysfunction, and/or acute renal failure has been reported; use with caution in patients with pre-existing renal impairment and monitor closely.
Adverse Reactions (Reflective of adult population; not specific for elderly) Percentages reflect incidence across all approved indications (prophylaxis and treatment); however, in general, a higher frequency of adverse reactions was observed in studies with HSCT patients.

>10%:
  Central nervous system: Fever (7% to 20%), headache (2% to 16%)
  Endocrine & metabolic: Hypokalemia (14% to 18%), hypomagnesemia (6% to 13%)
  Gastrointestinal: Diarrhea (8% to 23%), nausea (7% to 22%), vomiting (7% to 22%), mucosal inflammation (14%), constipation (11%)
  Hematologic: Thrombocytopenia (4% to 15%), neutropenia (14%)
  Local: Phlebitis (5% to 19%)
1% to 10%:
  Cardiovascular: Hypotension (6% to 10%), tachycardia (3% to 8%), hypertension (3% to 5%), peripheral edema (7%), edema (5%), bradycardia (3% to 5%), atrial fibrillation (3% to 5%)
  Central nervous system: Insomnia (4% to 10%), anxiety (6%), fatigue (6%)
  Dermatologic: Rash (2% to 9%), pruritus (6%)
  Endocrine & metabolic: Hypocalcemia (7%), hypoglycemia (6% to 7%), hyperglycemia (6%), hypernatremia (4% to 6%), hyperkalemia (4% to 5%), fluid overload (5%)
  Gastrointestinal: Abdominal pain (2% to 10%), anorexia (6%), dyspepsia (6%)
  Hematologic: Anemia (3% to 10%), febrile neutropenia (6%)
  Hepatic: AST increased (6%), ALT increased (5%), serum alkaline phosphatase increased (6% to 8%)
  Neuromuscular & skeletal: Rigors (9%), back pain (5%)
  Respiratory: Cough (8%), dyspnea (6%), epistaxis (6%)
  Miscellaneous: Bacteremia (5% to 9%), sepsis (5% to 6%)
Drug Interactions
  Metabolism/Transport Effects Substrate of CYP3A4 (minor); **Inhibits** CYP3A4 (weak)
  Avoid Concomitant Use There are no known interactions where it is recommended to avoid concomitant use.
  Increased Effect/Toxicity
    The levels/effects of Micafungin may be increased by: Conivaptan

Decreased Effect
Micafungin may decrease the levels/effects of: Saccharomyces boulardii

The levels/effects of Micafungin may be decreased by: Tocilizumab

Stability Store at controlled room temperature of 25°C (77°F). Reconstituted and diluted solutions are stable for 24 hours at room temperature. Protect from light. Aseptically add 5 mL of NS (preservative-free) to each 50 or 100 mg vial. Swirl to dissolve; do not shake. Further dilute 50-150 mg in 100 mL NS. Protect from light. Alternatively, D_5W may be used for reconstitution and dilution.

Mechanism of Action Concentration-dependent inhibition of 1,3-beta-D-glucan synthase resulting in reduced formation of 1,3-beta-D-glucan, an essential polysaccharide comprising 30% to 60% of *Candida* cell walls (absent in mammalian cells); decreased glucan content leads to osmotic instability and cellular lysis

Pharmacodynamics/Kinetics
Distribution: 0.28-0.5 L/kg
Protein binding: >99%; primarily to albumin
Metabolism: Hepatic; forms M-1 (catechol) and M-2 (methoxy) metabolites (activity unknown)
Half-life elimination: 11-21 hours
Excretion: Primarily feces (71%); urine (<15%)

Dosage
Geriatric & Adult
Candidemia, acute disseminated candidiasis, and *Candida* peritonitis and abscesses: I.V.: 100 mg daily; mean duration of therapy (from clinical trials) was 15 days (range: 10-47 days)
Esophageal candidiasis: I.V.: 150 mg daily; mean duration of therapy (from clinical trials) was 15 days (range: 10-30 days)
Prophylaxis of *Candida* infection in hematopoietic stem cell transplantation: 50 mg daily

Renal Impairment No dosage adjustment required in renal impairment.
Poorly dialyzed; no supplemental dose or dosage adjustment necessary, including patients on intermittent hemodialysis, peritoneal dialysis, or continuous renal replacement therapy (eg, CVVHD).

Hepatic Impairment No dosage adjustment required for moderate hepatic impairment (Child-Pugh score 7-9). Patients with severe hepatic dysfunction have not been studied.

Administration For intravenous use only; infuse over 1 hour

Monitoring Parameters Liver function tests

Special Geriatric Considerations No specific data for the elderly; use does not require alteration in dose or dose intervals.

Dosage Forms Excipient information presented when available (limited, particularly for generics); consult specific product labeling.
Injection, powder for reconstitution, as sodium:
Mycamine®: 50 mg, 100 mg [contains lactose 200 mg]

◆ **Micafungin Sodium** *see* Micafungin *on page 1205*
◆ **Micardis®** *see* Telmisartan *on page 1747*
◆ **Micardis® HCT** *see* Telmisartan and Hydrochlorothiazide *on page 1750*
◆ **Micatin® [OTC]** *see* Miconazole *on page 1206*

Miconazole (mi KON a zole)

Medication Safety Issues
Sound-alike/look-alike issues:
Miconazole may be confused with metroNIDAZOLE, Micronase®, Micronor®
Lotrimin® may be confused with Lotrisone®, Otrivin®
Micatin® may be confused with Miacalcin®

Brand Names: U.S. 3M™ Cavilon™ Antifungal [OTC]; Aloe Vesta® Antifungal [OTC]; Baza® Antifungal [OTC]; Carrington® Antifungal [OTC]; Critic-Aid® Clear AF [OTC]; DermaFungal [OTC]; Dermagran® AF [OTC]; DiabetAid® Antifungal Foot Bath [OTC]; Fungoid® [OTC]; Lotrimin AF® [OTC]; Micaderm® [OTC]; Micatin® [OTC]; Micro-Guard® [OTC]; Miranel AF™ [OTC]; Mitrazol® [OTC]; Monistat® 1 Day or Night [OTC]; Monistat® 1 [OTC]; Monistat® 3 [OTC]; Monistat® 7 [OTC]; Neosporin® AF [OTC]; Podactin Cream [OTC]; Secura® Antifungal Extra Thick [OTC]; Secura® Antifungal Greaseless [OTC]; Ting® Spray Powder [OTC]; Zeasorb®-AF [OTC]

Brand Names: Canada Dermazole; Micatin®; Micozole; Monistat®; Monistat® 3

Index Terms Miconazole Nitrate

Generic Availability (U.S.) Yes: Combination package (topical/vaginal), cream (topical and vaginal), vaginal suppository

Pharmacologic Category Antifungal Agent, Topical; Antifungal Agent, Vaginal

Use Treatment of vulvovaginal candidiasis and a variety of skin and mucous membrane fungal infections

Contraindications Hypersensitivity to miconazole or any component of the formulation

Warnings/Precautions For topical use only; avoid contact with eyes. Discontinue if sensitivity or irritation develop. Petrolatum-based vaginal products may damage rubber or latex condoms or diaphragms. Separate use by 3 days. Consult with healthcare provider prior to self-medication (OTC use) of vaginal products if experiencing vaginal itching/discomfort, lower abdominal pain, back or shoulder pain, chills, nausea, vomiting, foul-smelling discharge, if this is the first vaginal yeast infection, or if exposed to HIV. Contact healthcare provider if symptoms do not begin to improve after 3 days or last longer than 7 days.

Fungoid® tincture: Patients with diabetes, circulatory problems, renal or hepatic dysfunction should contact healthcare provider prior to self-medication (OTC use).

Adverse Reactions (Reflective of adult population; not specific for elderly) Frequency not defined.

Topical: Allergic contact dermatitis, burning, maceration

Vaginal: Abdominal cramps, burning, irritation, itching

Drug Interactions

Metabolism/Transport Effects Substrate of CYP3A4 (major); **Inhibits** CYP1A2 (moderate), 2A6 (strong), 2B6 (strong), 2C9 (strong), 2C19 (strong), 2D6 (strong), 2E1 (moderate), 3A4 (strong)

Avoid Concomitant Use There are no known interactions where it is recommended to avoid concomitant use.

Increased Effect/Toxicity

Miconazole (Topical) may increase the levels/effects of: Vitamin K Antagonists

Decreased Effect There are no known significant interactions involving a decrease in effect.

Ethanol/Nutrition/Herb Interactions Herb/Nutraceutical: St John's wort may decrease miconazole levels.

Mechanism of Action Inhibits biosynthesis of ergosterol, damaging the fungal cell wall membrane, which increases permeability causing leaking of nutrients

Pharmacodynamics/Kinetics

Absorption: Topical: Negligible

Excretion: Feces; urine

Dosage

Geriatric & Adult

Tinea corporis: Topical: Apply twice daily for 4 weeks

Tinea pedis: Topical: Apply twice daily for 4 weeks

Effervescent tablet: Dissolve 1 tablet in ~1 gallon of water; soak feet for 15-30 minutes; pat dry

Tinea cruris: Topical: Apply twice daily for 2 weeks

Vulvovaginal candidiasis: Vaginal:

Cream, 2%: Insert 1 applicatorful at bedtime for 7 days

Cream, 4%: Insert 1 applicatorful at bedtime for 3 days

Suppository, 100 mg: Insert 1 suppository at bedtime for 7 days

Suppository, 200 mg: Insert 1 suppository at bedtime for 3 days

Suppository, 1200 mg: Insert 1 suppository (a one-time dose); may be used at bedtime or during the day

Note: Many products are available as a combination pack, with a suppository for vaginal instillation and cream to relieve external symptoms. External cream may be used twice daily, as needed, for up to 7 days.

Administration Administer I.V. dose over 2 hours; administer around-the-clock rather than 4 times/day, 3 times/day, etc (ie, 12-6-12-6, not 9-1-5-9) to promote less variation in peak and trough serum concentration

Monitoring Parameters Signs and symptoms of infection

Special Geriatric Considerations No specific data for the elderly; use does not require alteration in dose or dose intervals. Assess patient's ability to self administer, may be difficult in patients with arthritis or limited range of motion.

Dosage Forms Excipient information presented when available (limited, particularly for generics); consult specific product labeling. [DSC] = Discontinued product

Aerosol, topical, as nitrate:

Micatin®: 2% (90 g)

Micatin®: 2% (105 mL) [contains benzyl alcohol]

Neosporin® AF: 2% (105 mL)

◀ Aerosol, topical, as nitrate [powder]:
Lotrimin AF®: 2% (133 g)
Lotrimin AF®: 2% (133 g) [deodorant formulation]
Micatin®: 2% (90 g)
Neosporin® AF: 2% (85 g)
Ting® Spray Powder: 2% (128 g) [contains aloe, ethanol 10% w/w]
Combination package, topical/vaginal, as nitrate: Cream, topical: 2% (9 g) and Suppository,
vaginal: 200 mg (3s)
Monistat® 3: Cream, topical: 2% (9 g) and Insert, vaginal: 200 mg (3s)
Monistat® 7: Cream, topical: 2% (9 g) and Cream, vaginal: 2% (45 g), Cream, topical: 2%
(9 g) and Cream, vaginal: 2% (7 x 5 g) [contains benzoic acid]
Monistat® 3: Cream, topical: 2% (9 g) and Cream, vaginal: 4% (25 g), Cream, topical: 2%
(9 g) and Cream, vaginal: 4% (3 x 5 g) [contains benzoic acid; vaginal cream 200 mg/
applicator]
Monistat® 7: Cream, topical: 2% (9 g) and Suppository, vaginal: 100 mg (7s) [contains
benzoic acid (in cream)]
Monistat® 1: Cream, topical: 2% (9 g) and Insert, vaginal: 1200 mg (1) [contains benzoic
acid (in cream), soya lecithin (in insert)]
Monistat® 1 Day or Night: Cream, topical: 2% (9 g) and Insert, vaginal: 1200 mg (1)
[contains benzoic acid (in cream), mineral oil (in insert), soya lecithin (in insert)]
Cream, topical, as nitrate: 2% (15 g, 30 g, 45 g)
Baza® Antifungal: 2% (4 g, 57 g, 142 g) [zinc oxide based formula]
Carrington® Antifungal: 2% (150 g)
Micaderm®: 2% (30 g)
Micatin®: 2% (14 g) [contains benzoic acid]
Micro-Guard®: 2% (60 g)
Miranel AF™: 2% (28 g) [contains ethanol]
3M™ Cavilon™ Antifungal: 2% (56 g, 141 g) [contains castor oil]
Neosporin® AF: 2% (14 g, 15 g) [contains benzoic acid]
Podactin Cream: 2% (30 g)
Secura® Antifungal Extra Thick: 2% (97.5 g) [contains zinc oxide]
Secura® Antifungal Greaseless: 2% (60 g)
Cream, vaginal, as nitrate: 2% (45 g); 4% (25 g [DSC])
Monistat® 7: 2% (45 g) [contains benzoic acid; 100 mg/applicator]
Monistat® 3: 4% (15 g, 25 g) [contains benzoic acid; 200 mg/applicator]
Gel, topical, as nitrate:
Zeasorb®-AF: 2% (24 g)
Liquid, topical, as nitrate [spray]:
Lotrimin AF®: 2% (150 g)
Ointment, topical, as nitrate:
Aloe Vesta® Antifungal: 2% (60 g, 150 g) [contains aloe]
Critic-Aid® Clear AF: 2% (57 g, 142 g, 300s)
DermaFungal: 2% (120 g)
Dermagran® AF: 2% (120 g) [zinc oxide based formula]
Powder, topical, as nitrate:
Lotrimin AF®: 2% (90 g)
Micro-Guard®: 2% (90 g)
Mitrazol®: 2% (30 g)
Zeasorb®-AF: 2% (70 g)
Suppository, vaginal, as nitrate: 100 mg (7s); 200 mg (3s)
Tablet for solution, topical, as nitrate [effervescent]:
DiabetAid® Antifungal Foot Bath: 2% (10s)
Tincture, topical, as nitrate:
Fungoid®: 2% (7.39 mL, 30 mL) [contains isopropyl alcohol 30%]

Midazolam (MID aye zoe lam)

Related Information
Anxiolytic, Sedative / Hypnotic, and Miscellaneous Benzodiazepines *on page 2000*
Medication Safety Issues
Sound-alike/look-alike issues:
Versed may be confused with VePesid®, Vistaril®
High alert medication:
The Institute for Safe Medication Practices (ISMP) includes this medication among its list of drugs which have a heightened risk of causing significant patient harm when used in error.
Brand Names: Canada Apo-Midazolam®; Midazolam Injection
Index Terms Midazolam Hydrochloride; Versed
Generic Availability (U.S.) Yes
Pharmacologic Category Benzodiazepine
Use Preoperative sedation; moderate sedation prior to diagnostic or radiographic procedures; ICU sedation (continuous infusion); induction and maintenance of general anesthesia
Unlabeled/Investigational Use Treatment of anxiety, status epilepticus
Contraindications Hypersensitivity to midazolam or any component of the formulation, including benzyl alcohol (cross-sensitivity with other benzodiazepines may exist); parenteral form is not for intrathecal or epidural injection; narrow-angle glaucoma; concurrent use of potent inhibitors of CYP3A4 (amprenavir, atazanavir, or ritonavir)
Warnings/Precautions [U.S. Boxed Warning]: May cause severe respiratory depression, respiratory arrest, or apnea. Use with extreme caution, particularly in noncritical care settings. Appropriate resuscitative equipment and qualified personnel must be available for administration and monitoring. Initial dosing must be cautiously titrated and individualized, particularly in elderly or debilitated patients, patients with hepatic impairment (including alcoholics), or in renal impairment, particularly if other CNS depressants (including opiates) are used concurrently. **[U.S. Boxed Warning]: Initial doses in elderly or debilitated patients should be conservative; as little as 1 mg, but not to exceed 2.5 mg.** Use with caution in patients with respiratory disease or impaired gag reflex. Use during upper airway procedures may increase risk of hypoventilation. Prolonged responses have been noted following extended administration by continuous infusion (possibly due to metabolite accumulation) or in the presence of drugs which inhibit midazolam metabolism.

Causes CNS depression (dose-related) resulting in sedation, dizziness, confusion, or ataxia which may impair physical and mental capabilities. Patients must be cautioned about performing tasks which require mental alertness (eg, operating machinery or driving). A minimum of 1 day should elapse after midazolam administration before attempting these tasks. Use with caution in patients receiving other CNS depressants or psychoactive agents. Effects with other sedative drugs or ethanol may be potentiated. Benzodiazepines have been associated with falls and traumatic injury and should be used with extreme caution in patients who are at risk of these events (especially the elderly).

May cause hypotension - hemodynamic events are more common in patients with hemodynamic instability. Hypotension and/or respiratory depression may occur more frequently in patients who have received opioid analgesics. Use with caution in obese patients, chronic renal failure, and HF. Does not protect against increases in heart rate or blood pressure during intubation. Should not be used in shock, coma, or acute alcohol intoxication. **[U.S. Boxed Warning]: Parenteral form contains benzyl alcohol; avoid rapid injection in neonates or prolonged infusions.** Avoid intra-arterial administration or extravasation of parenteral formulation.

Midazolam causes anterograde amnesia. Paradoxical reactions, including hyperactive or aggressive behavior have been reported with benzodiazepines, particularly in psychiatric patients. Does not have analgesic, antidepressant, or antipsychotic properties.

Benzodiazepines have been associated with dependence and acute withdrawal symptoms on discontinuation or reduction in dose. Acute withdrawal, including seizures, may be precipitated after administration of flumazenil to patients receiving long-term benzodiazepine therapy.
Adverse Reactions (Reflective of adult population; not specific for elderly)
>10%: Respiratory: Decreased tidal volume and/or respiratory rate decrease, apnea
1% to 10%:
Cardiovascular: Hypotension
Central nervous system: Drowsiness (1%), oversedation, headache (1%), seizure-like activity
Gastrointestinal: Nausea (3%), vomiting (3%)

◄ Local: Pain and local reactions at injection site (4% I.M., 5% I.V.; severity less than diazepam)

Ocular: Nystagmus

Respiratory: Cough (1%)

Miscellaneous: Physical and psychological dependence with prolonged use, hiccups (4%), paradoxical reaction

Drug Interactions

Metabolism/Transport Effects Substrate of CYP2B6 (minor), 3A4 (major); **Inhibits** CYP2C8 (weak), 2C9 (weak), 3A4 (weak)

Avoid Concomitant Use

Avoid concomitant use of Midazolam with any of the following: Boceprevir; Conivaptan; Efavirenz; OLANZapine; Protease Inhibitors; Telaprevir

Increased Effect/Toxicity

Midazolam may increase the levels/effects of: Alcohol (Ethyl); CloZAPine; CNS Depressants; Fosphenytoin; Methotrimeprazine; Phenytoin; Propofol; Selective Serotonin Reuptake Inhibitors

The levels/effects of Midazolam may be increased by: Antifungal Agents (Azole Derivatives, Systemic); Aprepitant; Atorvastatin; Boceprevir; Calcium Channel Blockers (Nondihydropyridine); Cimetidine; Conivaptan; Contraceptives (Estrogens); Contraceptives (Progestins); CYP3A4 Inhibitors (Moderate); CYP3A4 Inhibitors (Strong); Dasatinib; Droperidol; Efavirenz; Fluconazole; Fosaprepitant; Grapefruit Juice; HydrOXYzine; Isoniazid; Macrolide Antibiotics; Methotrimeprazine; Nefazodone; OLANZapine; Propofol; Protease Inhibitors; Proton Pump Inhibitors; Selective Serotonin Reuptake Inhibitors; Telaprevir

Decreased Effect

The levels/effects of Midazolam may be decreased by: CarBAMazepine; CYP3A4 Inducers (Strong); Deferasirox; Ginkgo Biloba; Rifamycin Derivatives; St Johns Wort; Theophylline Derivatives; Tocilizumab; Yohimbine

Ethanol/Nutrition/Herb Interactions

Ethanol: May increase CNS depression; monitor for increased effects with coadministration. Caution patients about effects.

Food: Grapefruit juice may increase serum concentrations of midazolam; avoid concurrent use with oral form.

Herb/Nutraceutical: Avoid concurrent use with St John's wort (may decrease midazolam levels, may increase CNS depression). Avoid concurrent use with valerian, kava kava, gotu kola (may increase CNS depression).

Stability The manufacturer states that midazolam, at a final concentration of 0.5 mg/mL, is stable for up to 24 hours when diluted with D_5W or NS. A final concentration of 1 mg/mL in NS has been documented to be stable for up to 10 days (McMullen, 1995). Admixtures do not require protection from light for short-term storage.

Mechanism of Action Binds to stereospecific benzodiazepine receptors on the postsynaptic GABA neuron at several sites within the central nervous system, including the limbic system, reticular formation. Enhancement of the inhibitory effect of GABA on neuronal excitability results by increased neuronal membrane permeability to chloride ions. This shift in chloride ions results in hyperpolarization (a less excitable state) and stabilization.

Pharmacodynamics/Kinetics

Onset of action: I.M.: Sedation: ~15 minutes; I.V.: 3-5 minutes; Oral: 10-20 minutes

Peak effect: I.M.: 0.5-1 hour

Duration: I.M.: Up to 6 hours; Mean: 2 hours

Absorption: Oral: Rapid

Distribution: V_d: 1-3.1 L/kg; increased in females, elderly, and obesity

Protein binding: ~97%

Metabolism: Extensively hepatic via CYP3A4

Bioavailability: 36% (oral, children); >90% (I.M.)

Half-life elimination: 2-6 hours; prolonged in cirrhosis, congestive heart failure, obesity, and elderly

Excretion: Urine (as glucuronide conjugated metabolites); feces (~2% to 10%)

Dosage

Geriatric The dose of midazolam needs to be individualized based on the patient's age, underlying diseases, and concurrent medications. Consider reducing dose by 30% to 50% in elderly or debilitated patients and those receiving opioids or other CNS depressants.

I.V.: Conscious sedation: Initial: 0.5 mg slow I.V.; give no more than 1.5 mg in a 2-minute period. If additional titration is needed, give no more than 1 mg over 2 minutes, waiting another 2 or more minutes to evaluate sedative effect. A total dose >3.5 mg is rarely necessary.

Adult The dose of midazolam needs to be individualized based on the patient's age, underlying diseases, and concurrent medications. Consider reducing dose by 30% to 50% in elderly or debilitated patients and those receiving opioids or other CNS depressants.

Preoperative sedation:
I.M.: 0.07-0.08 mg/kg 30-60 minutes prior to surgery/procedure; usual dose: 5 mg
I.V.: 0.02-0.04 mg/kg; repeat every 5 minutes as needed to desired effect or up to 0.1-0.2 mg/kg
Intranasal (unlabeled route): 0.1 mg/kg; administer 10-20 minutes prior to surgery/proce-dure (Uygur-Bayramiçli, 2002). **Note:** Use 5 mg/mL injectable solution to deliver dose. Due to the low pH of the solution, burning upon administration is likely to occur.
Conscious sedation: I.V.: Initial: 0.5-2 mg slow I.V. over at least 2 minutes; slowly titrate to effect by repeating doses every 2-3 minutes if needed; usual total dose: 2.5-5 mg
Healthy adults <60 years:
Initial: Some patients respond to doses as low as 1 mg; no more than 2.5 mg should be administered over a period of 2 minutes. Additional doses of midazolam may be administered after a 2-minute waiting period and evaluation of sedation after each dose increment. A total dose >5 mg is generally not needed.
Maintenance: 25% of dose used to reach sedative effect
Adults ≥60 years, debilitated, or chronically ill: Refer to geriatric dosing.
Anesthesia: I.V.:
Induction:
Unpremedicated patients: 0.3-0.35 mg/kg (up to 0.6 mg/kg in resistant cases)
Premedicated patients: 0.15-0.35 mg/kg
Maintenance: 0.05-0.3 mg/kg as needed, or continuous infusion 0.25-1.5 mcg/kg/minute
Sedation in mechanically ventilated patients: Per the manufacturer: I.V.: Initial dose: 0.01-0.05 mg/kg (~0.5-4 mg); may repeat at 5- to 15-minute intervals until adequate sedation achieved; maintenance infusion: 0.02-0.1 mg/kg/hour. Titrate to reach desired level of sedation.
or
I.V.: Initial dose: 0.02-0.08 mg/kg (~1-5 mg in 70 kg adult); may repeat at 5- to 15-minute intervals until adequate sedation achieved; maintenance infusion: 0.04-0.2 mg/kg/hour. Titrate to reach desired level of sedation (Jacobi, 2002).
Refractory status epilepticus (unlabeled use): Note: Intubation required; adjust dose based on hemodynamics, seizure activity, and EEG. I.V.: 0.15-0.3 mg/kg (usual dose: 5-15 mg); may repeat every 10-15 minutes as needed **or** 0.2 mg/kg bolus followed by a continuous infusion of 0.05-0.6 mg/kg/hour (Lowenstein, 2005; Meierkord, 2010)

Renal Impairment There are no dosage adjustments provided in manufacturer's labeling; use with caution.
Hemodialysis: Supplemental dose is not necessary.
Peritoneal dialysis: Significant drug removal is unlikely based on physiochemical character-istics.

Hepatic Impairment Severe hepatic impairment: Reduce dose by 50%.

Administration See Dosage.

Monitoring Parameters Respiratory and cardiovascular status, blood pressure, blood pressure monitor required during I.V. administration

Pharmacotherapy Pearls Healthy adults <60 years of age: Some patients respond to doses as low as 1 mg; no more than 2.5 mg should be administered over a period of 2 minutes. Additional doses of midazolam may be administered after a 2-minute waiting period and evaluation of sedation after each dose increment. A total dose >5 mg is generally not needed. If narcotics or other CNS depressants are administered concomitantly, the midazolam dose should be reduced by 30%.

Special Geriatric Considerations In the elderly if concomitant CNS depressant medica-tions are used, the midazolam dose will be at least 50% less than doses used in healthy, young, unpremedicated patients.

Controlled Substance C-IV

Dosage Forms Excipient information presented when available (limited, particularly for generics); consult specific product labeling.
Injection, solution: 1 mg/mL (2 mL, 5 mL, 10 mL); 5 mg/mL (1 mL, 2 mL, 5 mL, 10 mL)
Injection, solution [preservative free]: 1 mg/mL (2 mL, 5 mL); 5 mg/mL (1 mL, 2 mL)
Syrup, oral: 2 mg/mL (118 mL)

Selected References
Kälviäinen R, "Status Epilepticus Treatment Guidelines," *Epilepsia*, 2007, 48(Suppl 8):99-102.
Kanto J, Aaltonen L, Himberg JJ, et al, "Midazolam as an Intravenous Induction Agent in the Elderly: A Clinical and Pharmacokinetic Study," *Anesth Analg*, 1986, 65(1):15-20.
Servin F, Enriquez I, Fournet M, et al, "Pharmacokinetics of Midazolam Used as an Intravenous Induction Agent for Patients Over 80 Years of Age," *Eur J Anaesthesiol*, 1987, 4(1):1-7.

◆ **Midazolam Hydrochloride** *see* Midazolam *on page 1209*

Midodrine (MI doe dreen)

Medication Safety Issues
Sound-alike/look-alike issues:
Midodrine may be confused with Midrin®, minoxidil
ProAmatine® may be confused with protamine

Brand Names: U.S. ProAmatine® [DSC]
Brand Names: Canada Amatine®; Apo-Midodrine®
Index Terms Midodrine Hydrochloride
Generic Availability (U.S.) Yes
Pharmacologic Category Alpha$_1$ Agonist
Use Orphan drug: Treatment of symptomatic orthostatic hypotension
Unlabeled/Investigational Use Investigational: Management of urinary incontinence
Contraindications Hypersensitivity to midodrine or any component of the formulation; severe organic heart disease; acute renal failure; urinary retention; pheochromocytoma; thyrotoxicosis; persistent and significant supine hypertension

Warnings/Precautions [U.S. Boxed Warning]: Indicated for patients for whom orthostatic hypotension significantly impairs their daily life despite standard clinical care. May cause hypertension. Use is not recommended with supine hypertension. May slow heart rate primarily due to vagal reflex. Use caution when administered concurrently with negative chronotropes (eg, digoxin, beta blockers). Use is not recommended with supine hypertension. Use cautiously in patients with renal impairment and initiate with a reduced dose; contraindicated in patients with acute renal failure. Caution should be exercised in patients with diabetes, visual problems (especially if receiving fludrocortisone), urinary retention (reduce initial dose), or hepatic dysfunction; monitor renal and hepatic function prior to and periodically during therapy.

Adverse Reactions (Reflective of adult population; not specific for elderly)
>10%:
Cardiovascular: Supine hypertension (7% to 13%)
Dermatologic: Piloerection (13%), pruritus (12%)
Genitourinary: Urinary urgency, retention, or polyuria, dysuria (up to 13%)
Neuromuscular & skeletal: Paresthesia (18%)
1% to 10%:
Central nervous system: Chills (5%), pain (5%)
Dermatologic: Rash (2%)
Gastrointestinal: Abdominal pain

Drug Interactions
Avoid Concomitant Use
Avoid concomitant use of Midodrine with any of the following: Iobenguane I 123; MAO Inhibitors

Increased Effect/Toxicity
Midodrine may increase the levels/effects of: Sympathomimetics

The levels/effects of Midodrine may be increased by: Atomoxetine; Beta-Blockers; Calcium Channel Blockers (Nondihydropyridine); Cannabinoids; Cardiac Glycosides; MAO Inhibitors; Tricyclic Antidepressants

Decreased Effect
Midodrine may decrease the levels/effects of: Benzylpenicilloyl Polylysine; Iobenguane I 123

Mechanism of Action Midodrine forms an active metabolite, desglymidodrine, which is an alpha$_1$-agonist. This agent increases arteriolar and venous tone resulting in a rise in standing, sitting, and supine systolic and diastolic blood pressure in patients with orthostatic hypotension.

Pharmacodynamics/Kinetics
Onset of action: ~1 hour
Duration: 2-3 hours
Absorption: Rapid
Distribution: V_d (desglymidodrine): <1.6 L/kg; poorly across membrane (eg, blood brain barrier)
Protein binding: Minimal
Metabolism: Hepatic and many other tissues; midodrine is a prodrug which undergoes rapid deglycination to desglymidodrine (active metabolite)
Bioavailability: Desglymidodrine: 93%
Half-life elimination: Desglymidodrine: ~3-4 hours; Midodrine: 25 minutes
Time to peak, serum: Desglymidodrine: 1-2 hours; Midodrine: 30 minutes
Excretion: Urine (Midodrine: Insignificant; Desglymidodrine: 80% by active renal secretion)

Dosage
Geriatric & Adult
Orthostatic hypotension: Oral: 10 mg 3 times/day during daytime hours (every 3-4 hours) when patient is upright (maximum: 40 mg/day)

Prevention of hemodialysis-induced hypotension (unlabeled use): Oral: 2.5-10 mg given 15-30 minutes prior to dialysis session (Cruz, 1998; KDOQI, 2005; Prakash, 2004)

Vasovagal syncope (unlabeled use): Oral: Initial: 5 mg 3 times/day during daytime hours (every 6 hours) increased up to 15 mg/dose if necessary (Perez-Lugones, 2001; Ward, 1998)

Renal Impairment Orthostatic hypotension: 2.5 mg 3 times/day; gradually increase as tolerated.

Hemodialysis: Dialyzable; dose after hemodialysis unless used for prevention of hemodialysis-induced hypotension.

Administration Doses may be given in approximately 3- to 4-hour intervals (eg, shortly before or upon rising in the morning, at midday, in the late afternoon not later than 6 PM). Avoid dosing after the evening meal or within 4 hours of bedtime. Continue therapy only in patients who appear to attain symptomatic improvement during initial treatment. Standing systolic blood pressure may be elevated 15-30 mm Hg at 1 hour after a 10 mg dose. Some effect may persist for 2-3 hours.

Monitoring Parameters Blood pressure (standing and sitting), renal and hepatic parameters, symptoms of orthostasis

Special Geriatric Considerations Adjust dosage for renal impairment.

Dosage Forms Excipient information presented when available (limited, particularly for generics); consult specific product labeling. [DSC] = Discontinued product

Tablet, oral, as hydrochloride: 2.5 mg, 5 mg, 10 mg

ProAmatine®: 2.5 mg [DSC], 5 mg [DSC], 10 mg [DSC] [scored]

◆ **Midodrine Hydrochloride** see Midodrine on page 1212
◆ **Midol® Cramps & Body Aches [OTC]** see Ibuprofen on page 908
◆ **Midol® Extended Relief [OTC]** see Naproxen on page 1263
◆ **Migergot®** see Ergotamine and Caffeine on page 623

Miglitol (MIG li tol)

Related Information
Diabetes Mellitus Management, Adults on page 2073

Medication Safety Issues
Sound-alike/look-alike issues:
Glyset® may be confused with Cycloset®

Brand Names: U.S. Glyset®

Brand Names: Canada Glyset®

Generic Availability (U.S.) No

Pharmacologic Category Antidiabetic Agent, Alpha-Glucosidase Inhibitor

Use Type 2 diabetes mellitus (noninsulin-dependent, NIDDM):

Monotherapy as an adjunct to diet to improve glycemic control in patients with type 2 diabetes mellitus (noninsulin-dependent, NIDDM) whose hyperglycemia cannot be managed with diet alone

Combination therapy with a sulfonylurea when diet plus either miglitol or a sulfonylurea alone do not result in adequate glycemic control. The effect of miglitol to enhance glycemic control is additive to that of sulfonylureas when used in combination.

Contraindications Hypersensitivity to miglitol or any of component of the formulation; diabetic ketoacidosis; inflammatory bowel disease; colonic ulceration; partial intestinal obstruction or predisposition to intestinal obstruction; chronic intestinal diseases associated with marked disorders of digestion or absorption or with conditions that may deteriorate as a result of increased gas formation in the intestine

Warnings/Precautions GI symptoms are the most common reactions. The incidence of abdominal pain and diarrhea tend to diminish considerably with continued treatment. Use with caution in patients with mild-to-moderate renal impairment; not recommended in severe impairment (serum creatinine >2 mg/dL); studies have not been conducted. In combination with a sulfonylurea will cause a further lowering of blood glucose and may increase the hypoglycemic potential of the sulfonylurea. It may be necessary to discontinue miglitol and administer insulin if the patient is exposed to stress (ie, fever, trauma, infection, surgery).

Adverse Reactions (Reflective of adult population; not specific for elderly)
>10%: Gastrointestinal: Flatulence (42%), diarrhea (29%), abdominal pain (12%)
1% to 10%: Dermatologic: Rash (4%)

Drug Interactions

Avoid Concomitant Use There are no known interactions where it is recommended to avoid concomitant use.

Increased Effect/Toxicity

Miglitol may increase the levels/effects of: Hypoglycemic Agents

The levels/effects of Miglitol may be increased by: Herbs (Hypoglycemic Properties); Pegvisomant

Decreased Effect

The levels/effects of Miglitol may be decreased by: Corticosteroids (Orally Inhaled); Corticosteroids (Systemic); Luteinizing Hormone-Releasing Hormone Analogs; Somatropin; Thiazide Diuretics

Stability Store at 25°C (77°F); excursions permitted to 15°C to 30°C (59°F to 86°F).

Mechanism of Action In contrast to sulfonylureas, miglitol does not enhance insulin secretion; the antihyperglycemic action of miglitol results from a reversible inhibition of membrane-bound intestinal alpha-glucosidases which hydrolyze oligosaccharides and disaccharides to glucose and other monosaccharides in the brush border of the small intestine. In patients with diabetes, this enzyme inhibition results in delayed glucose absorption and lowering of postprandial hyperglycemia.

Pharmacodynamics/Kinetics

Absorption: Saturable at high doses: 25 mg dose: Completely absorbed; 100 mg dose: 50% to 70% absorbed

Distribution: V_d: 0.18 L/kg

Protein binding: <4%

Metabolism: None

Half-life elimination: ~2 hours

Time to peak: 2-3 hours

Excretion: Urine (as unchanged drug)

Dosage

Geriatric & Adult Type 2 diabetes (noninsulin dependent, NIDDM): Oral: Initial: 25 mg 3 times/day with the first bite of food at each meal; the dose may be increased to 50 mg 3 times/day after 4-8 weeks; maximum recommended dose: 100 mg 3 times/day

Renal Impairment Miglitol is primarily excreted by the kidneys; no dosage adjustment recommended in mild-moderate impairment. Not recommended in patients with a S_{cr} >2 mg/dL; studies have not been conducted.

Hepatic Impairment No adjustment necessary.

Administration Should be taken orally at the start (with the first bite) of each main meal

Monitoring Parameters Monitor therapeutic response by periodic blood glucose tests; measurement of glycosylated hemoglobin is recommended for the monitoring of long-term glycemic control

Reference Range

Recommendations for glycemic control in adults with diabetes:

Hb A_{1c}: <7%

Preprandial capillary plasma glucose: 70-130 mg/dL

Peak postprandial capillary blood glucose: <180 mg/dL

Blood pressure: <130/80 mm Hg

Recommendations for glycemic control in older adults with diabetes:

Relatively healthy, cognitively intact, and with a ≥5-year life expectancy: See Adults

Frail, life expectancy <5-years or those for whom the risks of intensive glucose control outweigh the benefits:

Hb A_{1c}: <8% to 9%

Blood pressure: <140/80 mm Hg or <130/80 mm Hg if tolerated

Special Geriatric Considerations In a double-blind randomized, placebo-controlled trial, glyburide caused significantly greater reductions in hemoglobin A_{1c} compared to miglitol 25 mg or 50 mg three times per day, but was associated with more weight gain. Diarrhea, soft stools, and flatulence were more common with miglitol. Intensive glucose control (HbA$_{1c}$ <6.5%) has been linked to increased all-cause and cardiovascular mortality, hypoglycemia requiring assistance, and weight gain in adult type 2 diabetes. How "tightly" to control a geriatric patient's blood glucose needs to be individualized. Such a decision should be based on several factors, including the patient's functional and cognitive status, how well he/she recognizes hypoglycemic or hyperglycemic symptoms, and how to respond to them and other disease states. An HbA$_{1c}$ <7.5% is an acceptable endpoint for a healthy older adult, while <8% is acceptable for frail elderly patients, those with a duration of illness >10 years, or those with comorbid conditions and requiring combination diabetes medications. Patients who are unable to accurately draw up their dose will need assistance, such as prefilled syringes. Initial doses may require considerations for renal function in the elderly with dosing adjusted subsequently based on blood glucose monitoring. For elderly patients with diabetes who are relatively healthy, attaining target goals for aspirin use, blood pressure, lipids, smoking cessation, and diet and exercise may be more important than normalized glycemic control.

Dosage Forms Excipient information presented when available (limited, particularly for generics); consult specific product labeling.

Tablet, oral:

Glyset®: 25 mg, 50 mg, 100 mg

Selected References

Action to Control Cardiovascular Risk in Diabetes Study Group, Gerstein HC, Miller ME, et al, "Effects of Intensive Glucose Lowering in Type 2 Diabetes," *N Engl J Med*, 2008, 358(24):2545-59.

ADVANCE Collaborative Group, Patel A, MacMahon S, et al, "Intensive Blood Glucose Control and Vascular Outcomes in Patients With Type 2 Diabetes," *N Engl J Med*, 2008, 358(24):2560-72.

American Diabetes Association, "Standards of Medical Care in Diabetes – 2011," *Diabetes Care*, 2011, 34(Suppl 1):11-61.

Brown AF, Mangione CM, Saliba D, et al, "Guidelines for Improving the Care of the Older Person With Diabetes Mellitus," *J Am Geriatr Soc*, 2003, 51(5 Suppl Guidelines):265-80.

Johnston PS, Lebovitz HE, Coniff RF, et al, "Advantages of Alpha-Glucosidase Inhibition as Monotherapy in Elderly Type 2 Diabetic Patients," *J Clin Endocrinol Metab*, 1998, 83(5):1515-22.

"VA/DoD Clinical Practice Guideline for the Management of Diabetes Mellitus," 2010. Available at http://www.healthquality.va.gov/Diabetes_Mellitus.asp

◆ **Migranal®** *see* Dihydroergotamine *on page* 512
◆ **Mild-C® [OTC]** *see* Ascorbic Acid *on page* 149
◆ **Milkinol® [OTC]** *see* Mineral Oil *on page* 1217
◆ **Milk of Magnesia** *see* Magnesium Hydroxide *on page* 1109
◆ **Milk of Magnesia [OTC]** *see* Magnesium Hydroxide *on page* 1109
◆ **Millipred™** *see* PrednisoLONE (Systemic) *on page* 1507

Milnacipran (mil NAY ci pran)

Related Information
Antidepressant Agents *on page* 1991
Medication Safety Issues
Sound-alike/look-alike issues:
Savella® may be confused with cevimeline, sevelamer
Brand Names: U.S. Savella®
Generic Availability (U.S.) No
Pharmacologic Category Antidepressant, Serotonin/Norepinephrine Reuptake Inhibitor
Use Management of fibromyalgia
Medication Guide Available Yes
Contraindications Concomitant use or within 2 weeks of MAO inhibitors; uncontrolled narrow-angle glaucoma
Warnings/Precautions [U.S. Boxed Warning]: Milnacipran is a serotonin/norepinephrine reuptake inhibitor (SNRI) similar to SNRIs used to treat depression and other psychiatric disorders. **Antidepressants increase the risk of suicidal thinking and behavior in children, adolescents, and young adults (18-24 years of age) with major depressive disorder (MDD) and other psychiatric disorders**; consider risk prior to prescribing. Short-term studies did not show an increased risk in patients >24 years of age and showed a decreased risk in patients ≥65 years. Closely monitor for clinical worsening, suicidality, or unusual changes in behavior; the patient's family or caregiver should be instructed to closely observe the patient and communicate condition with healthcare provider. A medication guide should be dispensed with each prescription. **Milnacipran is not FDA approved for the treatment of major depressive disorder or for use in children.**

Suicide risks should be monitored in patients treated with SNRIs regardless of the indication. The possibility of a suicide attempt is inherent in major depression and may persist until remission occurs. Monitor for worsening of depression or suicidality, especially during initiation of therapy (generally first 1-2 months) or with dose increases or decreases. Use caution in high-risk patients. Worsening depression and severe abrupt suicidality that are not part of the presenting symptoms may require discontinuation or modification of drug therapy. The patient's family or caregiver should be alerted to monitor patients for the emergence of suicidality and associated behaviors (such as agitation, irritability, hostility, impulsivity, and hypomania) and call healthcare provider.

Patients with major depressive disorder were excluded from clinical trials evaluating milnacipran for fibromyalgia; however, mania has been reported in patients with mood disorders taking similar medications. May worsen psychosis in some patients or precipitate a shift to mania or hypomania in patients with bipolar disorder. Patients presenting with depressive symptoms should be screened for bipolar disorder. Monotherapy in patients with bipolar disorder should be avoided. **Milnacipran is not FDA approved for the treatment of bipolar depression.**

◀ Serotonin syndrome and neuroleptic malignant syndrome (NMS)-like reactions have occurred with serotonin/norepinephrine reuptake inhibitors (SNRIs) and selective serotonin reuptake inhibitors (SSRIs) when used alone, and particularly when used in combination with serotonergic agents (eg, triptans) or antidopaminergic agents (eg, antipsychotics). Concurrent use with MAO inhibitors is contraindicated. May cause sustained increase in blood pressure or heart rate. Control pre-existing hypertension and cardiovascular disease prior to initiation of milnacipran. Use caution in patients with renal impairment; dose reduction required in severe renal impairment. Use caution in patients with hepatic impairment. Avoid ethanol use. May cause hyponatremia/SIADH (elderly at increased risk); volume depletion (diuretics may increase risk). Use cautiously in patients with a history of seizures. May impair platelet aggregation, resulting in bleeding. May cause increased urinary resistance. Use caution in patients with controlled narrow-angle glaucoma; use is contraindicated with uncontrolled narrow-angle glaucoma.

Abrupt discontinuation or dosage reduction after extended therapy may lead to agitation, dysphoria, anxiety, and other symptoms. When discontinuing therapy, dosage should be tapered gradually. If intolerable symptoms occur following a decrease in dosage or upon discontinuation of therapy, then resuming the previous dose with a more gradual taper should be considered.

Adverse Reactions (Reflective of adult population; not specific for elderly)
>10%:
  Central nervous system: Headache (18%), insomnia (12%)
  Endocrine & metabolic: Hot flashes (12%)
  Gastrointestinal: Nausea (37%), constipation (16%)
1% to 10%:
  Cardiovascular: Palpitation (7%), heart rate increased (6%), hypertension (5%), flushing (3%), blood pressure increased (3%), tachycardia (2%), peripheral edema (≥1%)
  Central nervous system: Dizziness (10%), migraine (5%), chills (2%), tremor (2%), depression (≥1%), fatigue (≥1%), fever (≥1%), irritability (≥1%), somnolence (≥1%)
  Dermatologic: Hyperhidrosis (9%), rash (3%)
  Endocrine & metabolic: Hypercholesterolemia (≥1%)
  Gastrointestinal: Vomiting (7%), xerostomia (5%), abdominal pain (3%), appetite decreased (2%), abdominal distension (≥1%), abnormal taste (≥1%), diarrhea (≥1%), dyspepsia (≥1%), flatulence (≥1%), gastroesophageal reflux disease (≥1%), weight changes (≥1%)
  Genitourinary: Dysuria (≥2%), ejaculation disorder/failure (≥2%), erectile dysfunction (≥2%), libido decreased (≥2%), prostatitis (≥2%), scrotal pain (≥2%), testicular pain (≥2%), testicular swelling (≥2%), urethral pain (≥2%), urinary hesitation (≥2%), urinary retention (≥2%), urine flow decreased (≥2%), cystitis (≥1%), urinary tract infection (≥1%)
  Neuromuscular & skeletal: Falling (≥1%)
  Ocular: Blurred vision (2%)
  Respiratory: Dyspnea (2%)
  Miscellaneous: Night sweats (≥1%)
Drug Interactions
Avoid Concomitant Use
  Avoid concomitant use of Milnacipran with any of the following: Iobenguane I 123; MAO Inhibitors; Methylene Blue; Sibutramine
Increased Effect/Toxicity
  Milnacipran may increase the levels/effects of: Alpha-/Beta-Agonists; Aspirin; Digoxin; Methylene Blue; NSAID (Nonselective); Serotonin Modulators; Vitamin K Antagonists

  The levels/effects of Milnacipran may be increased by: Alcohol (Ethyl); ClomiPRAMINE; MAO Inhibitors; Sibutramine
Decreased Effect
  Milnacipran may decrease the levels/effects of: Alpha2-Agonists; Iobenguane I 123
Ethanol/Nutrition/Herb Interactions
  Ethanol: May increase CNS depression; monitor for increased effects with coadministration. Caution patients about effects.
  Herb/Nutraceutical: Avoid valerian, St John's wort, SAMe, kava kava, tryptophan (may increase risk of serotonin syndrome and/or excessive sedation).
Stability Store at 25°C (77°F); excursions permitted between 15°C to 30°C (59°F to 86°F).
Mechanism of Action Potent inhibitor of norepinephrine and serotonin reuptake (3:1). Milnacipran has no significant activity for serotonergic, alpha- and beta-adrenergic, muscarinic, histaminergic, dopaminergic, opiate, benzodiazepine, and GABA receptors. It does not possess MAO-inhibitory activity.
Pharmacodynamics/Kinetics
  Absorption: Well absorbed
  Distribution: I.V: V_d: ~400 L
  Protein binding: 13%

Metabolism: Hepatic to inactive metabolites
Bioavailability: 85% to 90%
Half-life elimination: 6-8 hours
Time to peak, plasma: Oral: 2-4 hours
Excretion: Urine (55% as unchanged drug)

Dosage

Geriatric & Adult Fibromyalgia: Oral: 50 mg twice daily (maximum dose: 200 mg/day).

Titration schedule: 12.5 mg once on day 1, then 12.5 mg twice daily on days 2-3, 25 mg twice daily on days 4-7, then 50 mg twice daily thereafter. Dose may be increased to 100 mg twice daily, based on individual response. Doses >200 mg/day have not been studied.

Discontinuation of therapy: Gradually taper dose. If intolerable symptoms occur following a dose reduction, consider resuming the previously prescribed dose and/or decrease dose at a more gradual rate.

Renal Impairment

Mild renal impairment: No dose adjustment is recommended.

Moderate renal impairment: Use with caution.

Severe renal impairment (Cl_{cr} ≤29 mL/minute): Reduce maintenance dose to 25 mg twice daily; dose may be increased to 50 mg twice daily, based on individual tolerance.

End-stage renal disease (ESRD): Use not recommended.

Hepatic Impairment

Mild-to-moderate hepatic impairment: No dose adjustment is recommended.

Severe hepatic impairment: Use with caution.

Administration May be administered with or without food; food may improve tolerability.

Monitoring Parameters Blood pressure and heart rate should be regularly monitored; renal function should be monitored for dosing purposes; mental status for suicidal ideation (especially at the beginning of therapy or when doses are increased or decreased); intraocular pressure should be monitored in those with baseline elevations or a history of glaucoma

Special Geriatric Considerations According to the manufacturer of milnacipran, 402 participants in the clinical trials were age 60 years and older; no difference in efficacy or safety were reported compared to younger participants. Milnacipran should be used cautiously in patients with moderate renal impairment and its dose reduced in patients with Cl_{cr} 5-29 mL/minute. The risk of hyponatremia may be greater in the elderly.

Dosage Forms Excipient information presented when available (limited, particularly for generics); consult specific product labeling.

Combination package, oral [titration pack contains three separate tablet formulations]:

Savella®: Tablet: 12.5 mg (5s), Tablet: 25 mg (8s), and Tablet: 50 mg (42s)

Tablet, oral:

Savella®: 12.5 mg, 25 mg, 50 mg, 100 mg

Mineral Oil (MIN er al oyl)

Related Information

Beers Criteria − Potentially Inappropriate Medications for Geriatrics on page 2089

Laxatives, Classification and Properties on page 2012

Medication Safety Issues

BEERS Criteria medication:

This drug may be inappropriate for use in geriatric patients (high severity risk).

Brand Names: U.S. Fleet® Mineral Oil Enema [OTC]; Kondremul® [OTC]; Milkinol® [OTC]; Neo-Cultol® [OTC]; Zymenol® [OTC]

Index Terms Heavy Mineral Oil; Liquid Paraffin; White Mineral Oil

Generic Availability (U.S.) Yes

Pharmacologic Category Laxative, Lubricant

Use Temporary relief of occasional constipation; relief of fecal impaction; removal of barium sulfate residues following barium administration

Contraindications Patients with colostomy or an ileostomy, appendicitis, ulcerative colitis, diverticulitis

Warnings/Precautions Lipid pneumonitis results from aspiration of mineral oil. Aspiration risk increased in patients in prolonged supine position or conditions which interfere with swallowing or epiglottal function (eg, stroke, Parkinson's disease, Alzheimer's disease, esophageal dysmotility). Due to potential for aspiration and other adverse effects, use in the elderly should be avoided (Beers Criteria).

When used for self-medication (OTC): Healthcare provider should be contacted in case of sudden changes in bowel habits which last over 2 weeks or if abdominal pain, nausea, vomiting, or rectal bleeding occur following use; do not use for >1 week, unless otherwise directed by healthcare provider.

Adverse Reactions (Reflective of adult population; not specific for elderly) Frequency not defined.

Gastrointestinal: Abdominal cramps, diarrhea, nausea, vomiting

Respiratory: Lipid pneumonitis with aspiration

Miscellaneous: Large doses may cause anal leakage causing anal itching, irritation, hemorrhoids, perianal discomfort, soiling of clothes

Drug Interactions

Avoid Concomitant Use There are no known interactions where it is recommended to avoid concomitant use.

Increased Effect/Toxicity There are no known significant interactions involving an increase in effect.

Decreased Effect

Mineral Oil may decrease the levels/effects of: Phytonadione; Vitamin D Analogs

Mechanism of Action Eases passage of stool by decreasing water absorption and lubricating the intestine; retards colonic absorption of water

Pharmacodynamics/Kinetics

Onset of action: Oral: 6-8 hours; Rectal: 2-15 minutes

Distribution: Site of action is the colon

Excretion: Feces

Dosage

Geriatric & Adult

Constipation:

Oral: 15-45 mL/day

Kondremul®: 30-75 mL/day

Liqui-Doss®: 15-45 mL at bedtime

Rectal (Fleet® Mineral Oil): 118 mL as a single dose

Fecal impaction or following barium studies: Rectal (Fleet® Mineral Oil): 118 mL as a single dose

Administration

Oral: Mineral oil may be more palatable if refrigerated. Administer on an empty stomach in an upright position.

Kondremul®: Shake well before use.

Liqui-Doss®: Shake well before use. Prior to use, mix with 120 mL of any beverage; administer only at bedtime.

Rectal (Fleet® Mineral Oil): Gently insert enema rectally with patient lying on left side and left knee slightly bent, right knee drawn to chest.

Monitoring Parameters Monitor for response (stool frequency, consistency). Avoid use in patients who may aspirate.

Pharmacotherapy Pearls Do not administer with food or meals because of the risk of aspiration; prolonged administration of mineral oil may decrease absorption of lipid-soluble vitamins A, D, E, and K. Light sterile mineral oils are not for injection.

Special Geriatric Considerations Other therapies should be attempted before using mineral oil to relieve constipation to avoid complications with mineral oil; doses, if used, should begin low and should be used as infrequently as possible.

This medication is considered to be potentially inappropriate in this patient population (Beers Criteria severity: High).

Dosage Forms

Emulsion: 1.4 g/5 mL (480 mL); 2.5 mL/5 mL (420 mL); 2.75 mL/5 mL (480 mL); 4.75 mL/5 mL (240 mL)

Jelly: 2.75 mL/5 mL (180 mL)

Liquid: 500 mL, 1000 mL, 4000 mL

Liquid, rectal: 133 mL

♦ **Minipress®** *see* Prazosin *on page 1505*
♦ **Minitran™** *see* Nitroglycerin *on page 1311*
♦ **Minocin®** *see* Minocycline *on page 1218*
♦ **Minocin® PAC** *see* Minocycline *on page 1218*

Minocycline (mi noe SYE kleen)

Medication Safety Issues

Sound-alike/look-alike issues:

Dynacin® may be confused with Dyazide®, Dynabac®, DynaCirc®, Dynapen®

Minocin® may be confused with Indocin®, Lincocin®, Minizide®, Mithracin®, niacin

Brand Names: U.S. Minocin®; Minocin® PAC; Solodyn®

Brand Names: Canada Apo-Minocycline®; Arestin Microspheres; Dom-Minocycline; Minocin®; Mylan-Minocycline; Novo-Minocycline; PHL-Minocycline; PMS-Minocycline; ratio-Minocycline; Riva-Minocycline; Sandoz-Minocycline

Index Terms Minocycline Hydrochloride

Generic Availability (U.S.) Yes: Excludes extended release tablet, injection, pellet-filled capsule

Pharmacologic Category Antibiotic, Tetracycline Derivative

Use Treatment of susceptible bacterial infections of both gram-negative and gram-positive organisms; treatment of anthrax (inhalational, cutaneous, and gastrointestinal); moderate-to-severe acne; meningococcal (asymptomatic) carrier state; Rickettsial diseases (including Rocky Mountain spotted fever, Q fever); nongonococcal urethritis, gonorrhea; acute intestinal amebiasis; respiratory tract infection; skin/soft tissue infections; chlamydial infections

Extended release (Solodyn®): Only indicated for treatment of inflammatory lesions of non-nodular moderate-to-severe acne

Unlabeled/Investigational Use Rheumatoid arthritis (patients with low disease activity of short duration); nocardiosis; alternative treatment for community-acquired MRSA infection

Contraindications Hypersensitivity to minocycline, other tetracyclines, or any component of the formulation

Warnings/Precautions May be associated with increases in BUN secondary to antianabolic effects; use caution in patients with renal impairment (Cl_{cr} <80 mL/minute). Hepatotoxicity has been reported; use caution in patients with hepatic insufficiency. Autoimmune syndromes (eg, lupus-like, hepatitis, and vasculitis) have been reported; discontinue if symptoms occur. CNS effects (lightheadedness, vertigo) may occur; patients must be cautioned about performing tasks which require mental alertness (eg, operating machinery or driving). Pseudotumor cerebri has been (rarely) reported with tetracycline use; usually resolves with discontinuation. May cause photosensitivity; discontinue if skin erythema occurs. Prolonged use may result in fungal or bacterial superinfection, including *C. difficile*-associated diarrhea (CDAD) and pseudomembranous colitis; CDAD has been observed >2 months postantibiotic treatment. Rash, along with eosinophilia, fever, and organ failure (Drug Rash with Eosinophilia and Systemic Symptoms [DRESS] syndrome) has been reported; discontinue treatment immediately if DRESS syndrome is suspected.

Adverse Reactions (Reflective of adult population; not specific for elderly) Frequency not defined.

Cardiovascular: Myocarditis, pericarditis, vasculitis

Central nervous system: Bulging fontanels, dizziness, fatigue, fever, headache, hypoesthesia, malaise, mood changes, paresthesia, pseudotumor cerebri, sedation, seizure, somnolence, vertigo

Dermatologic: Alopecia, angioedema, DRESS (Drug Rash with Eosinophilia and Systemic Symptoms) syndrome, erythema multiforme, erythema nodosum, erythematous rash, exfoliative dermatitis, hyperpigmentation of nails, maculopapular rash, photosensitivity, pigmentation of the skin and mucous membranes, pruritus, Stevens-Johnson syndrome, toxic epidermal necrolysis, urticaria

Endocrine & metabolic: Thyroid cancer, thyroid discoloration, thyroid dysfunction

Gastrointestinal: Anorexia, diarrhea, dyspepsia, dysphagia, enamel hypoplasia, enterocolitis, esophageal ulcerations, esophagitis, glossitis, inflammatory lesions (oral/anogenital), moniliasis, nausea, oral cavity discoloration, pancreatitis, pseudomembranous colitis, stomatitis, tooth discoloration, vomiting, xerostomia

Genitourinary: Balanitis, vulvovaginitis

Hematologic: Agranulocytosis, eosinophilia, hemolytic anemia, leukopenia, neutropenia, pancytopenia, thrombocytopenia

Hepatic: Autoimmune hepatitis, hepatic cholestasis, hepatic failure, hepatitis, hyperbilirubinemia, jaundice, liver enzyme increases

Local: Injection site reaction (I.V. administration)

Neuromuscular & skeletal: Arthralgia, arthritis, bone discoloration, joint stiffness, joint swelling, myalgia

Otic: Hearing loss, tinnitus

Renal: Acute renal failure, BUN increased, interstitial nephritis

Respiratory: Asthma, bronchospasm, cough, dyspnea, pneumonitis, pulmonary infiltrate (with eosinophilia)

Miscellaneous: Anaphylaxis, hypersensitivity, lupus erythematosus, lupus-like syndrome, serum sickness

Drug Interactions

Avoid Concomitant Use

Avoid concomitant use of Minocycline with any of the following: BCG; Retinoic Acid Derivatives

◀ **Increased Effect/Toxicity**
Minocycline may increase the levels/effects of: Neuromuscular-Blocking Agents; Porfimer; Retinoic Acid Derivatives; Vitamin K Antagonists

Decreased Effect
Minocycline may decrease the levels/effects of: Atazanavir; BCG; Penicillins; Typhoid Vaccine

The levels/effects of Minocycline may be decreased by: Antacids; Bile Acid Sequestrants; Bismuth; Bismuth Subsalicylate; Calcium Salts; Iron Salts; Lanthanum; Magnesium Salts; Quinapril; Sucralfate; Zinc Salts

Ethanol/Nutrition/Herb Interactions
Food: Minocycline serum concentrations are not significantly altered if taken with food or dairy products.
Herb/Nutraceutical: Avoid dong quai, St John's wort (may also cause photosensitization).

Stability
Capsule (including pellet-filled), tablet: Store at 20°C to 25°C (68°F to 77°F); protect from heat. Protect from light and moisture.
Extended release tablet: Store at 15°C to 30°C (59°F to 86°F); protect from heat. Protect from light and moisture.
Injection: Store vials at 20°C to 25°C (68°F to 77°F) prior to reconstitution. Reconstitute with 5 mL of sterile water for injection, and further dilute in 500-1000 mL of NS, D_5W, D_5NS, Ringer's injection, or LR. Reconstituted solution is stable at room temperature for 24 hours. Final dilutions should be administered immediately.

Mechanism of Action Inhibits bacterial protein synthesis by binding with the 30S and possibly the 50S ribosomal subunit(s) of susceptible bacteria; cell wall synthesis is not affected

Rheumatoid arthritis: The mechanism of action of minocycline in rheumatoid arthritis is not completely understood. It is thought to have antimicrobial, anti-inflammatory, immunomodulatory, and chondroprotective effects. More specifically, it is thought to be a potent inhibitor of metalloproteinases, which are active in rheumatoid arthritis joint destruction.

Pharmacodynamics/Kinetics
Absorption: Oral: Well absorbed
Protein binding: 70% to 75%
Metabolism: Hepatic to inactive metabolites
Half-life elimination: I.V.: 15-23 hours; Oral: 16 hours (range: 11-22 hours)
Time to peak: Capsule, pellet filled: 1-4 hours; Extended release tablet: 3.5-4 hours
Excretion: Urine, feces

Dosage
Geriatric & Adult
Usual dosage range:
I.V.: Initial: 200 mg, followed by 100 mg every 12 hours (maximum: 400 mg/day)
Oral: Initial: 200 mg, followed by 100 mg every 12 hours; more frequent dosing intervals may be used (100-200 mg initially, followed by 50 mg 4 times daily)

Acne: Oral: Capsule or immediate-release tablet: 50-100 mg twice daily
Inflammatory, non-nodular, moderate-to-severe acne (Solodyn®):
45-54 kg: 45 mg once daily
55-77 kg: 65 mg once daily
78-102 kg: 90 mg once daily
103-125 kg: 115 mg once daily
126-136 kg: 135 mg once daily
Note: Therapy should be continued for 12 weeks. Higher doses do not confer greater efficacy and may be associated with more acute vestibular side effects. Safety of use beyond 12 weeks has not been established.

Cellulitis (purulent) due to community-acquired MRSA (unlabeled use): Oral: Initial: 200 mg; Maintenance: 100 mg twice daily for 5-10 days (Liu, 2011)

Chlamydial or *Ureaplasma urealyticum* infection, uncomplicated: Oral, I.V.: Urethral, endocervical, or rectal: 100 mg every 12 hours for at least 7 days

Gonococcal infection, uncomplicated (males): Oral, I.V.:
Without urethritis or anorectal infection: Initial: 200 mg, followed by 100 mg every 12 hours for at least 4 days (cultures 2-3 days post-therapy)
Urethritis: 100 mg every 12 hours for 5 days

Meningococcal carrier state (manufacturer's labeling): Oral: 100 mg every 12 hours for 5 days. **Note:** CDC recommendations do not mention use of minocycline for eradicating nasopharyngeal carriage of meningococcal

Mycobacterium marinum: Oral: 100 mg every 12 hours for 6-8 weeks

Nocardiosis, cutaneous (non-CNS) (unlabeled use): Oral: 100-200 mg every 12 hours
Rheumatoid arthritis (unlabeled use): Oral: 100 mg twice daily (O'Dell, 2001)
Syphilis: Oral, I.V.: Initial: 200 mg, followed by 100 mg every 12 hours for 10-15 days
Renal Impairment Use with caution; monitor BUN and creatinine clearance. Consider decreasing dose or increasing dosing interval (extended release).
Cl$_{cr}$ <80 mL/minute: Do not exceed 200 mg/day

Administration

I.V.: Infuse slowly; avoid rapid administration. The manufacturer's labeling does not provide a recommended administration rate. The injectable route should be used only if the oral route is not feasible or adequate. Prolonged intravenous therapy may be associated with thrombophlebitis.

Oral: May be administered with or without food. Administer with adequate fluid to decrease the risk of esophageal irritation and ulceration. Swallow pellet-filled capsule and extended release tablet whole; do not chew, crush, or split.

Monitoring Parameters LFTs, BUN, renal function with long-term treatment; if symptomatic for autoimmune disorder, include ANA, CBC

Test Interactions May cause interference with fluorescence test for urinary catecholamines (false elevations)

Special Geriatric Considerations Minocycline has not been studied in the elderly but its CNS effects may limit its use. Dose reduction for renal function not necessary.

Dosage Forms Excipient information presented when available (limited, particularly for generics); consult specific product labeling.
Capsule, oral: 50 mg, 75 mg, 100 mg
Capsule, pellet filled, oral:
  Minocin®: 50 mg, 100 mg
  Minocin® PAC: 50 mg, 100 mg
Injection, powder for reconstitution:
  Minocin®: 100 mg
Tablet, oral: 50 mg, 75 mg, 100 mg
Tablet, extended release, oral:
  Solodyn®: 45 mg, 65 mg, 90 mg, 115 mg, 135 mg

◆ **Minocycline Hydrochloride** see Minocycline on page 1218

Minoxidil (Systemic) (mi NOKS i dil)

Medication Safety Issues
Sound-alike/look-alike issues:
Loniten® may be confused with Lipitor®
Minoxidil may be confused with metolazone, midodrine, Minipress®, Minocin®, Monopril®, Noxafil®

International issues:
Loniten [Canada and multiple international markets] may be confused with Linoten brand name for pamidronate [Spain]
Noxidil [Thailand] may be confused with Noxafil brand name for posaconazole [U.S. and multiple international markets]

Brand Names: Canada Loniten®
Generic Availability (U.S.) Yes
Pharmacologic Category Vasodilator, Direct-Acting
Use Management of severe hypertension (usually in combination with a diuretic and beta-blocker)
Contraindications Hypersensitivity to minoxidil or any component of the formulation; pheochromocytoma
Warnings/Precautions [U.S. Boxed Warning]: Minoxidil may cause pericarditis and pericardial effusion that may progress to tamponade; patients with renal impairment not on dialysis may be at higher risk. Observe patients closely. **[U.S. Boxed Warning]: May increase oxygen demand and exacerbate angina pectoris;** concomitant use with a beta-blocker (if no contraindication exists may help reduce the effect. Use with caution in patients with pulmonary hypertension, significant renal failure, or HF; use with caution in patients with coronary artery disease or recent myocardial infarction; renal failure or dialysis patients may require smaller doses; usually used with a beta-blocker (to treat minoxidil-induced tachycardia) and a diuretic (for treatment of water retention/edema). Compared to placebo minoxidil increased the frequency of clinical events, including increased need for diuretics, angina, ventricular arrhythmias, worsening heart failure and death (Franciosa, 1984). Use with caution in the elderly; initiate at the low end of the dosage range and monitor closely.

◀ **[U.S. Boxed Warning]: Maximum therapeutic doses of a diuretic and two antihypertensives should be used before this drug is ever added. Should be given with a diuretic to minimize fluid gain and a beta-blocker (if no contraindications) to prevent tachycardia. Anyone with malignant hypertension should be hospitalized with close medical supervision to ensure blood pressure is reducing and to prevent too rapid of a reduction in blood pressure.** Inform patients of excessive hair growth before initiating therapy; may take 1-6 months for hypertrichosis to reverse itself after discontinuation of the drug.

Adverse Reactions (Reflective of adult population; not specific for elderly) Frequency not always reported.

Cardiovascular: ECG changes (T-wave changes 60%), peripheral edema (7%), pericardial effusion with tamponade (3%), pericardial effusion without tamponade (3%), angina pectoris, heart failure, pericarditis, rebound hypertension (in children after a gradual withdrawal), sodium and water retention, tachycardia

Dermatologic: Hypertrichosis (common; 80%), bullous eruption (rare), rash, Stevens-Johnson syndrome (rare)

Endocrine & metabolic: Breast tenderness (rare; <1%)

Gastrointestinal: Nausea, vomiting, weight gain

Hematologic: Leukopenia (rare), thrombocytopenia (rare), transient decreased erythrocyte count (hemodilution), transient decreased hematocrit/hemoglobin (hemodilution)

Hepatic: Increased alkaline phosphatase

Renal: Transient increase in serum BUN and creatinine

Respiratory: Pulmonary edema

Drug Interactions

Avoid Concomitant Use There are no known interactions where it is recommended to avoid concomitant use.

Increased Effect/Toxicity

Minoxidil (Systemic) may increase the levels/effects of: Amifostine; Antihypertensives; Hypotensive Agents; RiTUXimab

The levels/effects of Minoxidil (Systemic) may be increased by: Alfuzosin; CycloSPORINE; CycloSPORINE (Systemic); Diazoxide; Herbs (Hypotensive Properties); MAO Inhibitors; Pentoxifylline; Phosphodiesterase 5 Inhibitors; Prostacyclin Analogues

Decreased Effect

The levels/effects of Minoxidil (Systemic) may be decreased by: Herbs (Hypertensive Properties); Methylphenidate; Yohimbine

Ethanol/Nutrition/Herb Interactions Herb/Nutraceutical: Bayberry, blue cohosh, cayenne, ephedra, ginger, ginseng (American), kola, licorice may diminish the antihypertensive effects of minoxidil. Black cohosh, California poppy, coleus, golden seal, hawthorn, mistletoe, periwinkle, quinine, shepherd's purse may enhance the hypotensive effects of minoxidil.

Stability Store at controlled room temperature of 15°C to 30°C (59°F to 86°F).

Mechanism of Action Produces vasodilation by directly relaxing arteriolar smooth muscle, with little effect on veins; effects may be mediated by cyclic AMP; stimulation of hair growth is secondary to vasodilation, increased cutaneous blood flow and stimulation of resting hair follicles

Pharmacodynamics/Kinetics

Onset of action: Hypotensive: ~30 minutes

  Peak effect: 2-8 hours

Duration: 2-5 days

Protein binding: None

Metabolism: 88%, primarily via glucuronidation

Bioavailability: 90%

Half-life elimination: Adults: 3.5-4.2 hours

Excretion: Urine (12% as unchanged drug)

Dosage

Geriatric Hypertension: Initial: 2.5 mg once daily; increase gradually.

Adult Hypertension: Oral: Initial: 5 mg once daily, increase gradually every 3 days (maximum: 100 mg/day); usual dosage range (JNC 7): 2.5-80 mg/day in 1-2 divided doses

  Note: Dosage adjustment is needed when added to concomitant therapy.

Renal Impairment Patient with renal failure and/or receiving dialysis may require dosage reduction.

  Supplemental dose is not necessary after hemo- or peritoneal dialysis.

Monitoring Parameters Blood pressure, standing and sitting/supine; fluid and electrolyte balance and body weight should be monitored. Any tests that are abnormal at the time of initiation (including, renal function tests, ECG, echocardiogram, chest x-ray) should be repeated initially every 1-3 months then every 6-12 months once stable.

Dosage Forms Excipient information presented when available (limited, particularly for generics); consult specific product labeling.
Tablet, oral: 2.5 mg, 10 mg

◆ **Mintab DM [DSC]** *see* Guaifenesin and Dextromethorphan *on page 848*
◆ **Mintox Plus [OTC]** *see* Aluminum Hydroxide, Magnesium Hydroxide, and Simethicone *on page 84*
◆ **Miochol®-E** *see* Acetylcholine *on page 41*
◆ **Miostat®** *see* Carbachol *on page 267*
◆ **MiraLAX® [OTC]** *see* Polyethylene Glycol 3350 *on page 1480*
◆ **Miranel AF™ [OTC]** *see* Miconazole *on page 1206*
◆ **Mirapex®** *see* Pramipexole *on page 1496*
◆ **Mirapex® ER®** *see* Pramipexole *on page 1496*

Mirtazapine (mir TAZ a peen)

Related Information
Antidepressant Agents *on page 1991*
Medication Safety Issues
Sound-alike/look-alike issues:
Remeron® may be confused with Premarin®, ramelteon, Rozerem®, Zemuron®
International issues:
Avanza [Australia] may be confused with Albenza brand name for albendazole [U.S.]; Avandia brand name for rosiglitazone [U.S., Canada, and multiple international markets]
Remeron [U.S., Canada, and multiple international markets] may be confused with Reneuron which is a brand name for fluoxetine [Spain]
Brand Names: U.S. Remeron SolTab®; Remeron®
Brand Names: Canada Apo-Mirtazapine®; CO Mirtazapine; Dom-Mirtazapine; Mylan-Mirtazapine; Novo-Mirtazapine; PHL-Mirtazapine; PMS-Mirtazapine; PRO-Mirtazapine; ratio-Mirtazapine; Remeron®; Remeron® RD; Riva-Mirtazapine; Sandoz-Mirtazapine; Sandoz-Mirtazapine FC; ZYM-Mirtazapine
Generic Availability (U.S.) Yes
Pharmacologic Category Antidepressant, Alpha-2 Antagonist
Use Treatment of depression
Unlabeled/Investigational Use Post-traumatic stress disorder (PTSD)
Medication Guide Available Yes
Contraindications Hypersensitivity to mirtazapine or any component of the formulation; use of MAO inhibitors within 14 days
Warnings/Precautions [U.S. Boxed Warning]: Antidepressants increase the risk of suicidal thinking and behavior in children, adolescents, and young adults (18-24 years of age) with major depressive disorder (MDD) and other psychiatric disorders; consider risk prior to prescribing. Short-term studies did not show an increased risk in patients >24 years of age and showed a decreased risk in patients ≥65 years. Closely monitor for clinical worsening, suicidality, or unusual changes in behavior; the patient's family or caregiver should be instructed to closely observe the patient and communicate condition with healthcare provider. A medication guide should be dispensed with each prescription. **Mirtazapine is not FDA approved for use in children.**

The possibility of a suicide attempt is inherent in major depression and may persist until remission occurs. Monitor for worsening of depression or suicidality, especially during initiation of therapy (generally first 1-2 months) or with dose increases or decreases. Use caution in high-risk patients. Worsening depression and severe abrupt suicidality that are not part of the presenting symptoms may require discontinuation or modification of drug therapy. The patient's family or caregiver should be alerted to monitor patients for the emergence of suicidality and associated behaviors (such as agitation, irritability, hostility, impulsivity, and hypomania) and call healthcare provider.

May worsen psychosis in some patients or precipitate a shift to mania or hypomania in patients with bipolar disorder. Patients presenting with depressive symptoms should be screened for bipolar disorder. Monotherapy in patients with bipolar disorder should be avoided. **Mirtazapine is not FDA approved for the treatment of bipolar depression.**

Patients should not discontinue treatment abruptly, unless significant life-threatening event, due to risk of withdrawal symptoms. A gradual reduction in the dose over several weeks is recommended.

Discontinue immediately if signs and symptoms of neutropenia/agranulocytosis occur. May cause sedation, resulting in impaired performance of tasks requiring alertness (eg, operating machinery or driving). Sedative effects may be additive with other CNS depressants and/or ▶

ethanol. The degree of sedation is moderate-high relative to other antidepressants. Conversely, may increase psychomotor restlessness within first few weeks of therapy. The risks of orthostatic hypotension or anticholinergic effects are low relative to other antidepressants. The incidence of sexual dysfunction with mirtazapine is generally lower than with SSRIs. Potential for severe reaction when used with MAO inhibitors; autonomic instability, coma, death, delirium, diaphoresis, hyperthermia, mental status changes/agitation, muscular rigidity, myoclonus, neuroleptic malignant syndrome features, and seizures may occur.

May increase appetite and stimulate weight gain. Weight gain of >7% of body weight reported in 7.5% of patients treated with mirtazapine compared to 0% for placebo; 8% of patients receiving mirtazapine discontinued treatment due to the weight gain. In an 8-week pediatric clinical trial, 49% of mirtazapine-treated patients had a weight gain of at least 7% (mean increase 4 kg) as compared to 5.7% of placebo-treated patients (mean increase 1 kg). May increase serum cholesterol and triglyceride levels.

Use caution in patients with a previous seizure disorder or condition predisposing to seizures such as brain damage, alcoholism, or concurrent therapy with other drugs which lower the seizure threshold. May cause hyponatremia.Use with caution in patients with hepatic or renal dysfunction and in elderly patients. Clinically significant transaminase elevations have been observed. SolTab® formulation contains phenylalanine.

Adverse Reactions (Reflective of adult population; not specific for elderly)
>10%:
  Central nervous system: Somnolence (54%)
  Endocrine & metabolic: Increased cholesterol
  Gastrointestinal: Constipation (13%), xerostomia (25%), increased appetite (17%), weight gain (12%; weight gain of >7% reported in 8% of adults, ≤49% of pediatric patients)
1% to 10%:
  Cardiovascular: Hypertension, vasodilatation, peripheral edema (2%), edema (1%)
  Central nervous system: Dizziness (7%), abnormal dreams (4%), abnormal thoughts (3%), confusion (2%), malaise
  Endocrine & metabolic: Increased triglycerides
  Gastrointestinal: Vomiting, anorexia, abdominal pain
  Genitourinary: Urinary frequency (2%)
  Hepatic: SGPT increased (≥3 times ULN: 2%)
  Neuromuscular & skeletal: Myalgia (2%), back pain (2%), arthralgia, tremor (2%), weakness (8%)
  Respiratory: Dyspnea (1%)
  Miscellaneous: Flu-like syndrome (5%), thirst

Drug Interactions
Metabolism/Transport Effects **Substrate** of CYP1A2 (major), 2C9 (minor), 2D6 (major), 3A4 (major); **Inhibits** CYP1A2 (weak), 3A4 (weak)

Avoid Concomitant Use
  Avoid concomitant use of Mirtazapine with any of the following: Conivaptan; MAO Inhibitors; Methylene Blue; Sibutramine

Increased Effect/Toxicity
  Mirtazapine may increase the levels/effects of: Alcohol (Ethyl); CNS Depressants; Methotrimeprazine; Methylene Blue; Serotonin Modulators; Warfarin

  The levels/effects of Mirtazapine may be increased by: Abiraterone Acetate; Conivaptan; CYP1A2 Inhibitors (Moderate); CYP1A2 Inhibitors (Strong); CYP2D6 Inhibitors (Moderate); CYP2D6 Inhibitors (Strong); CYP3A4 Inhibitors (Moderate); CYP3A4 Inhibitors (Strong); Darunavir; Dasatinib; Deferasirox; Droperidol; HydrOXYzine; MAO Inhibitors; Methotrimeprazine; Sibutramine

Decreased Effect
  Mirtazapine may decrease the levels/effects of: Alpha2-Agonists

  The levels/effects of Mirtazapine may be decreased by: CYP1A2 Inducers (Strong); CYP3A4 Inducers (Strong); Cyproterone; Deferasirox; Peginterferon Alfa-2b; Tocilizumab

Ethanol/Nutrition/Herb Interactions
  Ethanol: May increase CNS depression; monitor for increased effects with coadministration. Caution patients about effects.
  Herb/Nutraceutical: Avoid St John's wort (may decrease mirtazapine levels). Avoid valerian, St John's wort, SAMe, kava kava (may increase CNS depression).

Stability Store at controlled room temperature of 25°C (77°F); excursions permitted to 15°C to 30°C (59°F to 86°F). Protect from light and moisture.
  SolTab®: Protect from light and moisture. Use immediately upon opening tablet blister.

Mechanism of Action Mirtazapine is a tetracyclic antidepressant that works by its central presynaptic alpha$_2$-adrenergic antagonist effects, which results in increased release of norepinephrine and serotonin. It is also a potent antagonist of 5-HT$_2$ and 5-HT$_3$ serotonin receptors and H1 histamine receptors and a moderate peripheral alpha$_1$-adrenergic and muscarinic antagonist; it does not inhibit the reuptake of norepinephrine or serotonin.

Pharmacodynamics/Kinetics

Absorption: Rapid and complete

Distribution: 4.5 L/kg

Protein binding: 85%

Metabolism: Extensively hepatic via CYP1A2, 2C9, 2D6, 3A4 and via demethylation (forms demethylmirtazapine, an active metabolite) and hydroxylation (forms inactive metabolites)

Bioavailability: 50%

Half-life elimination: 20-40 hours; hampered with renal or hepatic impairment

Time to peak, serum: 2 hours

Excretion: Urine (75%) and feces (15%) as metabolites

Dosage

Geriatric Initial: 7.5 mg/day as a single bedtime dose; increase by 7.5-15 mg/day every 1-2 weeks; usual dose: 15-30 mg/day; maximum dose: 45 mg/day

Alzheimer's dementia-related depression: Initial: 7.5 mg at bedtime; may increase at 7.5-15 mg increments to 45-60 mg/day

Adult

Depression: Oral: Initial: 15 mg nightly, titrate up to 15-45 mg/day with dose increases made no more frequently than every 1-2 weeks. There is an inverse relationship between dose and sedation.

Post-traumatic stress disorder (PTSD) (unlabeled use): Oral: 30-60 mg/day

Renal Impairment

Cl$_{cr}$ 11-39 mL/minute: 30% decreased clearance

Cl$_{cr}$ <10 mL/minute: 50% decreased clearance

Hepatic Impairment Clearance is decreased by 30%.

Administration SolTab®: Open blister pack and place tablet on the tongue. Do not split tablet. Tablet is formulated to dissolve on the tongue without water.

Monitoring Parameters Patients should be monitored for signs of agranulocytosis or severe neutropenia such as sore throat, stomatitis or other signs of infection or a low WBC; mental status for depression, suicide ideation (especially at the beginning of therapy or when doses are increased or decreased), anxiety, social functioning, mania, panic attacks; lipid profile

Pharmacotherapy Pearls Note: At least 14 days should elapse between discontinuation of an MAO inhibitor and initiation of therapy with mirtazapine; at least 14 days should be allowed after discontinuing mirtazapine before starting an MAO inhibitor.

Special Geriatric Considerations Limited published data specifically in the elderly or addressing in vivo drug interactions.

Dosage Forms Excipient information presented when available (limited, particularly for generics); consult specific product labeling.

Tablet, oral: 7.5 mg, 15 mg, 30 mg, 45 mg

Remeron®: 15 mg, 30 mg [scored]

Remeron®: 45 mg

Tablet, orally disintegrating, oral: 15 mg, 30 mg, 45 mg

Remeron SolTab®: 15 mg [contains phenylalanine 2.6 mg/tablet; orange flavor]

Remeron SolTab®: 30 mg [contains phenylalanine 5.2 mg/tablet; orange flavor]

Remeron SolTab®: 45 mg [contains phenylalanine 7.8 mg/tablet; orange flavor]

Misoprostol (mye soe PROST ole)

Medication Safety Issues

Sound-alike/look-alike issues:

Cytotec® may be confused with Cytoxan, Sytobex®

Misoprostol may be confused with metoprolol, mifepristone

Brand Names: U.S. Cytotec®

Brand Names: Canada Apo-Misoprostol®; Novo-Misoprostol; PMS-Misoprostol

Generic Availability (U.S.) Yes

Pharmacologic Category Prostaglandin

Use Prevention of NSAID-induced gastric ulcers

Unlabeled/Investigational Use Fat malabsorption in cystic fibrosis

Contraindications Hypersensitivity to prostaglandins

Warnings/Precautions [U.S. Boxed Warning]: Due to the abortifacient property of this medication, patients must be warned not to give this drug to others. Use with caution in patients with renal impairment, cardiovascular disease and the elderly.

Adverse Reactions (Reflective of adult population; not specific for elderly)
>10%: Gastrointestinal: Diarrhea, abdominal pain
1% to 10%:
Central nervous system: Headache
Gastrointestinal: Constipation, dyspepsia, flatulence, nausea, vomiting

Drug Interactions

Avoid Concomitant Use
Avoid concomitant use of Misoprostol with any of the following: Carbetocin

Increased Effect/Toxicity
Misoprostol may increase the levels/effects of: Carbetocin; Oxytocin

The levels/effects of Misoprostol may be increased by: Antacids

Decreased Effect There are no known significant interactions involving a decrease in effect.

Ethanol/Nutrition/Herb Interactions Food: Misoprostol peak serum concentrations may be decreased if taken with food (not clinically significant).

Stability Store at or below 25°C (77°F).

Mechanism of Action Misoprostol is a synthetic prostaglandin E_1 analog that replaces the protective prostaglandins consumed with prostaglandin-inhibiting therapies (eg, NSAIDs); has been shown to induce uterine contractions

Pharmacodynamics/Kinetics
Absorption: Oral: Rapid
Half-life (parent and metabolite combined): 1.5 hours; metabolite: 20-40 minutes
Time to peak serum concentration (active metabolite): Within 15-30 minutes
Rapidly de-esterified to misoprostol acid
Elimination: In urine (64% to 73% in 24 hours) and feces (15% in 24 hours)
Since older adults have decreased clearance (increased AUC), it may be necessary to reduce dose to 100 mcg 4 times/day

Dosage
Geriatric Oral: 100-200 mcg 4 times/day with food; if 200 mcg 4 times/day not tolerated, reduce to 100 mcg 4 times/day. **Note:** To avoid the diarrhea potential, doses can be initiated at 100 mcg/day and increased 100 mcg/day at 3-day intervals until desired dose is achieved; also, recommend administering with food to decrease diarrhea incidence.

Adult Prevention of NSAID-induced ulcers: Oral: 200 mcg 4 times/day with food; if not tolerated, may decrease dose to 100 mcg 4 times/day with food. Last dose of the day should be taken at bedtime.

Renal Impairment Half-life, maximum plasma concentration, and bioavailability may be increased; however, a correlation has not been observed with degree of dysfunction. Decrease dose if recommended dose is not tolerated. It is not known if misoprostol is removed by dialysis.

Administration Incidence of diarrhea may be lessened by having patient take dose right after meals and avoiding magnesium-containing antacids.

Monitoring Parameters Adequate diagnostic measures in all cases of undiagnosed abnormal vaginal bleeding

Special Geriatric Considerations Elderly, due to extensive use of NSAIDs and the high percentage of asymptomatic hemorrhage and perforation from NSAIDs, are at risk for NSAID-induced ulcers and may be candidates for misoprostol use. However, routine use for prophylaxis is not justified. Patients must be selected upon demonstration that they are at risk for NSAID-induced lesions. Misoprostol should not be used as a first-line therapy for gastric or duodenal ulcers.

Dosage Forms Excipient information presented when available (limited, particularly for generics); consult specific product labeling.
Tablet, oral: 100 mcg, 200 mcg
Cytotec®: 100 mcg
Cytotec®: 200 mcg [scored]

◆ **Misoprostol and Diclofenac** see Diclofenac and Misoprostol on page 501
◆ **Mitrazol® [OTC]** see Miconazole on page 1206
◆ **MK-217** see Alendronate on page 53
◆ **MK383** see Tirofiban on page 1806
◆ **MK-0431** see SitaGLIPtin on page 1684
◆ **MK462** see Rizatriptan on page 1630
◆ **MK 0517** see Fosaprepitant on page 788
◆ **MK594** see Losartan on page 1092
◆ **MK0826** see Ertapenem on page 623
◆ **MK 869** see Aprepitant on page 139
◆ **MMR** see Measles, Mumps, and Rubella Virus Vaccine on page 1116
◆ **M-M-R® II** see Measles, Mumps, and Rubella Virus Vaccine on page 1116
◆ **Mobic®** see Meloxicam on page 1128

♦ **Mobidin®** see Salicylates (Various Salts) on page 1647

Modafinil (moe DAF i nil)

Brand Names: U.S. Provigil®
Brand Names: Canada Alertec®; Apo-Modafinil®
Generic Availability (U.S.) No
Pharmacologic Category Stimulant
Use Improve wakefulness in patients with excessive daytime sleepiness associated with narcolepsy and shift work sleep disorder (SWSD); adjunctive therapy for obstructive sleep apnea/hypopnea syndrome (OSAHS)
Unlabeled/Investigational Use Attention-deficit/hyperactivity disorder (ADHD); treatment of fatigue in MS and other disorders
Medication Guide Available Yes
Contraindications Hypersensitivity to modafinil, armodafinil, or any component of the formulation
Warnings/Precautions For use following complete evaluation of sleepiness and in conjunction with other standard treatments (eg, CPAP). The degree of sleepiness should be reassessed frequently; some patients may not return to a normal level of wakefulness. Use is not recommended with a history of angina, cardiac ischemia, recent history of myocardial infarction, left ventricular hypertrophy, or patients with mitral valve prolapse who have developed mitral valve prolapse syndrome with previous CNS stimulant use.

Serious and life-threatening rashes (including Stevens-Johnson syndrome and toxic epidermal necrolysis) have been reported with modafinil. Most cases have occurred within the first 5 weeks of therapy; however, rare cases have occurred after long-term use. No risk factors have been identified to predict occurrence or severity. Patients should be advised to discontinue at first sign of rash.

In addition, rare cases of multiorgan hypersensitivity reactions in association with modafinil use, and lone cases of angioedema and anaphylactoid reactions with armodafinil, have been reported. Signs and symptoms are diverse, reflecting the involvement of specific organs. Patients typically present with fever and rash associated with organ-system dysfunction. Patients should be advised to report any signs and symptoms related to these effects; discontinuation of therapy is recommended.

Caution should be exercised when modafinil is given to patients with a history of psychosis; may impair the ability to engage in potentially hazardous activities. Stimulants may unmask tics in individuals with coexisting Tourette's syndrome. Use caution with renal or hepatic impairment (dosage adjustment in hepatic dysfunction is recommended).

Adverse Reactions (Reflective of adult population; not specific for elderly)
>10%:
  Central nervous system: Headache (34%, dose related)
  Gastrointestinal: Nausea (11%)
1% to 10%:
  Cardiovascular: Chest pain (3%), hypertension (3%), palpitation (2%), tachycardia (2%), vasodilation (2%), edema (1%)
  Central nervous system: Nervousness (7%), dizziness (5%), anxiety (5%; dose related), insomnia (5%), depression (2%), somnolence (2%), chills (1%), agitation (1%), confusion (1%), emotional lability (1%), vertigo (1%)
  Dermatologic: Rash (1%; includes some severe cases requiring hospitalization)
  Gastrointestinal: Diarrhea (6%), dyspepsia (5%), xerostomia (4%), anorexia (4%), constipation (2%), flatulence (1%), mouth ulceration (1%), taste perversion (1%)
  Genitourinary: Abnormal urine (1%), hematuria (1%), pyuria (1%)
  Hematologic: Eosinophilia (1%)
  Hepatic: LFTs abnormal (2%)
  Neuromuscular & skeletal: Back pain (6%), paresthesia (2%), dyskinesia (1%), hyperkinesia (1%), hypertonia (1%), neck rigidity (1%), tremor (1%)
  Ocular: Amblyopia (1%), eye pain (1%), vision abnormal (1%)
  Respiratory: Rhinitis (7%), pharyngitis (4%), lung disorder (2%), asthma (1%), epistaxis (1%)
  Miscellaneous: Flu-like syndrome (4%), thirst (1%), diaphoresis (1%), herpes simplex infection (1%)
Drug Interactions
  Metabolism/Transport Effects Substrate of CYP3A4 (major); **Inhibits** CYP1A2 (weak), 2A6 (weak), 2C8/9 (weak), 2C19 (strong), 2E1 (weak), 3A4 (weak); **Induces** CYP1A2 (weak), 2B6 (weak), 3A4 (weak)

◀ **Avoid Concomitant Use**
Avoid concomitant use of Modafinil with any of the following: Clopidogrel; Conivaptan; Iobenguane I 123

Increased Effect/Toxicity Modafinil may increase the levels/effects of citalopram, diazepam, methsuximide, phenytoin, propranolol, sertraline, or other CYP2C19 substrates. Modafinil may increase levels of warfarin. In populations deficient in the CYP2D6 isoenzyme, where CYP2C19 acts as a secondary metabolic pathway, concentrations of tricyclic antidepressants and selective serotonin reuptake inhibitors may be increased during coadministration. The levels/effects of modafinil may be increased by azole antifungals, ciprofloxacin, clarithromycin, diclofenac, doxycycline, erythromycin, imatinib, isoniazid, nefazodone, nicardipine, propofol, protease inhibitors, quinidine, telithromycin, verapamil, or other CYP3A4 inhibitors.

Decreased Effect Modafinil may decrease serum concentrations of oral contraceptives, cyclosporine, and to a lesser degree, theophylline. The levels/effects of modafinil may be decreased by aminoglutethimide, carbamazepine, nafcillin, nevirapine, phenobarbital, phenytoin, rifamycins, and other CYP3A4 inducers. There is also evidence to suggest that modafinil may induce its own metabolism.

Ethanol/Nutrition/Herb Interactions
Ethanol: Avoid or limit ethanol.
Food: Delays absorption, but does not affect bioavailability.

Stability Store at 20°C to 25°C (68°F to 77°F).

Mechanism of Action The exact mechanism of action is unclear, it does not appear to alter the release of dopamine or norepinephrine, it may exert its stimulant effects by decreasing GABA-mediated neurotransmission, although this theory has not yet been fully evaluated; several studies also suggest that an intact central alpha-adrenergic system is required for modafinil's activity; the drug increases high-frequency alpha waves while decreasing both delta and theta wave activity, and these effects are consistent with generalized increases in mental alertness

Pharmacodynamics/Kinetics Modafinil is a racemic compound (10% *d*-isomer and 90% *l*-isomer at steady state) whose enantiomers have different pharmacokinetics

Distribution: V_d: 0.9 L/kg
Protein binding: ~60%, primarily to albumin
Metabolism: Hepatic; multiple pathways including CYP3A4
Half-life elimination: Effective half-life: 15 hours
Time to peak, serum: 2-4 hours
Excretion: Urine (as metabolites, <10% as unchanged drug)

Dosage
Geriatric Elimination of modafinil and its metabolites may be reduced as a consequence of aging and as a result, consider initiating at lower doses in this patient population.

Adult
ADHD (unlabeled use): Oral: 100-400 mg/day (Taylor, 2000)
Narcolepsy, obstructive sleep apnea/hypopnea syndrome (OSAHS): Oral: Initial: 200 mg as a single daily dose in the morning.
Shift work sleep disorder (SWSD): Oral: Initial: 200 mg as a single dose taken ~1 hour prior to start of work shift.
Note: Doses of 400 mg/day, given as a single dose, have been well tolerated, but there is no consistent evidence that this dose confers additional benefit.

Renal Impairment Safety and efficacy have not been established in severe renal impairment.

Hepatic Impairment Severe hepatic impairment: Dose should be reduced to one-half of that recommended for patients with normal liver function.

Administration For the treatment of narcolepsy and obstructive sleep apnea/hypopnea syndrome (OSAHS), administer dose in the morning. For the treatment of shift work sleep disorder (SWSD), administer dose ~1 hour prior to start of work shift.

Monitoring Parameters Levels of sleepiness; blood pressure in patients with hypertension

Special Geriatric Considerations Clearance of modafinil may be reduced in the elderly. Safety and effectiveness in persons >65 years of age have not been established. In the limited number of elderly patients studied, the incidence of adverse events was similar to younger patients.

Controlled Substance C-IV

Dosage Forms Excipient information presented when available (limited, particularly for generics); consult specific product labeling.
Tablet, oral:
Provigil®: 100 mg
Provigil®: 200 mg [scored]

◆ **Modified Shohl's Solution** *see* Sodium Citrate and Citric Acid *on page 1693*

Moexipril (mo EKS i pril)

Related Information
Angiotensin Agents *on page 1985*
Medication Safety Issues
  Sound-alike/look-alike issues:
    Moexipril may be confused with Monopril®
Brand Names: U.S. Univasc®
Index Terms Moexipril Hydrochloride
Generic Availability (U.S.) Yes
Pharmacologic Category Angiotensin-Converting Enzyme (ACE) Inhibitor
Use Treatment of hypertension, alone or in combination with thiazide diuretics
Contraindications Hypersensitivity to moexipril or any component of the formulation; angioedema related to previous treatment with an ACE inhibitor
Warnings/Precautions Anaphylactic reactions may occur rarely with ACE inhibitors. At any time during treatment (especially following first dose) angioedema may occur rarely with ACE inhibitors; it may involve the head and neck (potentially compromising airway) or the intestine (presenting with abdominal pain). African-Americans and patients with idiopathic or hereditary angioedema may be at an increased risk. Prolonged frequent monitoring may be required especially if tongue, glottis, or larynx are involved as they are associated with airway obstruction. Patients with a history of airway surgery may have a higher risk of airway obstruction. Aggressive early and appropriate management is critical. Use in patients with previous angioedema associated with ACE inhibitor therapy is contraindicated. Severe anaphylactoid reactions may be seen during hemodialysis (eg, CVVHD) with high-flux dialysis membranes (eg, AN69), and rarely, during low density lipoprotein apheresis with dextran sulfate cellulose. Rare cases of anaphylactoid reactions have been reported in patients undergoing sensitization treatment with hymenoptera (bee, wasp) venom while receiving ACE inhibitors.

Symptomatic hypotension with or without syncope can occur with ACE inhibitors (usually with the first several doses); effects are most often observed in volume depleted patients; correct volume depletion prior to initiation; close monitoring of patient is required especially with initial dosing and dosing increases; blood pressure must be lowered at a rate appropriate for the patient's clinical condition. Initiation of therapy in patients with ischemic heart disease or cerebrovascular disease warrants close observation due to the potential consequences posed by falling blood pressure (eg, MI, stroke). Use with caution in hypertrophic cardiomyopathy with outflow tract obstruction, severe aortic stenosis, or before, during, or immediately after major surgery.

Hyperkalemia may occur with ACE inhibitors; risk factors include renal dysfunction, diabetes mellitus, concomitant use of potassium-sparing diuretics, potassium supplements, and/or potassium-containing salts. Use cautiously, if at all, with these agents and monitor potassium closely. Cough may occur with ACE inhibitors. Other causes of cough should be considered (eg, pulmonary congestion in patients with heart failure) and excluded prior to discontinuation.

May be associated with deterioration of renal function and/or increases in serum creatinine, particularly in patients with low renal blood flow (eg, renal artery stenosis, heart failure) whose glomerular filtration rate (GFR) is dependent on efferent arteriolar vasoconstriction by angiotensin II; deterioration may result in oliguria, acute renal failure, and progressive azotemia. Small increases in serum creatinine may occur following initiation; consider discontinuation only in patients with progressive and/or significant deterioration in renal function. Use with caution in patients with unstented unilateral/bilateral renal artery stenosis. When unstented bilateral renal artery stenosis is present, use is generally avoided due to the elevated risk of deterioration in renal function unless possible benefits outweigh risks. Concurrent use of angiotensin receptor blockers may increase the risk of clinically-significant adverse events (eg, renal dysfunction, hyperkalemia).

Rare toxicities associated with ACE inhibitors include cholestatic jaundice (which may progress to fulminant hepatic necrosis), agranulocytosis, neutropenia, or leukopenia with myeloid hypoplasia. Patients with collagen vascular diseases (especially with concomitant renal impairment) or renal impairment alone may be at increased risk for hematologic toxicity; periodically monitor CBC with differential in these patients.
Adverse Reactions (Reflective of adult population; not specific for elderly)
1% to 10%:
Cardiovascular: Hypotension, peripheral edema
Central nervous system: Headache, dizziness, fatigue
Dermatologic: Flushing, rash
Endocrine & metabolic: Hyperkalemia, hyponatremia

◀ Gastrointestinal: Diarrhea, nausea, heartburn

Genitourinary: Polyuria

Neuromuscular & skeletal: Myalgia

Renal: Reversible increases in creatinine or BUN

Respiratory: Cough, pharyngitis, upper respiratory infection, sinusitis

Drug Interactions

Avoid Concomitant Use There are no known interactions where it is recommended to avoid concomitant use.

Increased Effect/Toxicity

Moexipril may increase the levels/effects of: Allopurinol; Amifostine; Antihypertensives; AzaTHIOprine; CycloSPORINE; CycloSPORINE (Systemic); Ferric Gluconate; Gold Sodium Thiomalate; Hypotensive Agents; Iron Dextran Complex; Lithium; Nonsteroidal Anti-Inflammatory Agents; RiTUXimab; Sodium Phosphates

The levels/effects of Moexipril may be increased by: Alfuzosin; Angiotensin II Receptor Blockers; Diazoxide; DPP-IV Inhibitors; Eplerenone; Everolimus; Herbs (Hypotensive Properties); Loop Diuretics; MAO Inhibitors; Pentoxifylline; Phosphodiesterase 5 Inhibitors; Potassium Salts; Potassium-Sparing Diuretics; Prostacyclin Analogues; Sirolimus; Temsirolimus; Thiazide Diuretics; TiZANidine; Tolvaptan; Trimethoprim

Decreased Effect

The levels/effects of Moexipril may be decreased by: Antacids; Aprotinin; Herbs (Hypertensive Properties); Icatibant; Lanthanum; Methylphenidate; Nonsteroidal Anti-Inflammatory Agents; Salicylates; Yohimbine

Ethanol/Nutrition/Herb Interactions

Food: Food may delay and reduce peak serum levels.

Herb/Nutraceutical: Avoid bayberry, blue cohosh, cayenne, ephedra, ginger, ginseng (American), kola, licorice (may worsen hypertension). Avoid black cohosh, California poppy, coleus, golden seal, hawthorn, mistletoe, periwinkle, quinine, shepherd's purse (may have increased antihypertensive effect).

Mechanism of Action Competitive inhibitor of angiotensin-converting enzyme (ACE); prevents conversion of angiotensin I to angiotensin II, a potent vasoconstrictor; results in lower levels of angiotensin II which causes an increase in plasma renin activity and a reduction in aldosterone secretion

Pharmacodynamics/Kinetics

Onset of action: Peak effect: 1-2 hours

Duration: >24 hours

Absorption: Incomplete

Distribution: V_d (moexiprilat): 180 L

Protein binding, plasma: Moexipril: 90%; Moexiprilat: 50% to 70%

Metabolism: Parent drug: Hepatic and via GI tract to moexiprilat, 1000 times more potent than parent

Bioavailability: Moexiprilat: 13%; reduced with food (AUC decreased by ~40%)

Half-life elimination: Moexipril: 1 hour; Moexiprilat: 2-9 hours

Time to peak: 1.5 hours

Excretion: Feces (50%)

Dosage

Geriatric Dose the same as adults; adjust for renal impairment. Tablet may be cut in half (3.75 mg) for starting therapy (see Dosage: Renal Impairment).

Adult Hypertension: Oral: Initial: 7.5 mg once daily (in patients **not** receiving diuretics), 1 hour prior to a meal **or** 3.75 mg once daily (when combined with thiazide diuretics); maintenance dose: 7.5-30 mg/day in 1 or 2 divided doses 1 hour before meals

Renal Impairment Cl_{cr} ≤40 mL/minute: Patients may be cautiously placed on 3.75 mg once daily, then upwardly titrated to a maximum of 15 mg/day.

Administration Administer on an empty stomach at least 1 hour before meals

Monitoring Parameters Blood pressure; serum creatinine and potassium; if patient has collagen vascular disease and/or renal impairment, periodically monitor CBC with differential

Test Interactions Increases BUN, creatinine, potassium, positive Coombs' [direct]; decreases cholesterol (S); may cause false-positive results in urine acetone determinations using sodium nitroprusside reagent

Pharmacotherapy Pearls The antihypertensive effect of moexipril may decrease towards the end of the dosing interval; blood pressure should be monitored prior to dosing. If blood pressure control is not adequate, an increased dose or divided dose may be attempted. Moexipril offers no therapeutic advantage over other ACE inhibitors. To reduce the risk of hypotension, discontinue therapy 2-3 days prior to starting moexipril if possible. If diuretics cannot be stopped for a short period, initiate dose at 3.75 mg/day.

Special Geriatric Considerations Due to frequent decreases in glomerular filtration (also creatinine clearance) with aging, elderly patients may have exaggerated responses to ACE inhibitors; differences in clinical response due to hepatic changes are not observed. ACE inhibitors may be preferred agents in elderly patients with congestive heart failure and diabetes mellitus. Diabetic proteinuria is reduced and insulin sensitivity is enhanced. In general, the side effect profile is favorable in the elderly and causes little or no CNS confusion; use lowest dose recommendations initially; adjust dose for renal function in the elderly. Many elderly may be volume depleted due to diuretic use and/or blunted thirst reflex resulting in inadequate fluid intake.

Dosage Forms Excipient information presented when available (limited, particularly for generics); consult specific product labeling.

Tablet, oral, as hydrochloride: 7.5 mg, 15 mg

    Univasc®: 7.5 mg, 15 mg [scored]

- ◆ **Moexipril Hydrochloride** see Moexipril on page 1229
- ◆ **Moi-Stir® [OTC]** see Saliva Substitute on page 1652
- ◆ **Moisture® Eyes [OTC]** see Artificial Tears on page 148
- ◆ **Moisture® Eyes PM [OTC]** see Artificial Tears on page 148
- ◆ **MOM** see Magnesium Hydroxide on page 1109

Mometasone (Oral Inhalation) (moe MET a sone)

Related Information

Asthma on page 2016
Corticosteroids on page 2005
Inhalant Agents on page 2010

Brand Names: U.S. Asmanex® Twisthaler®

Index Terms Mometasone Furoate

Generic Availability (U.S.) No

Pharmacologic Category Corticosteroid, Inhalant (Oral)

Use Maintenance treatment of asthma as prophylactic therapy

Contraindications Hypersensitivity to mometasone or any component of the formulation; hypersensitivity to milk proteins; primary treatment of status asthmaticus or acute bronchospasm

Warnings/Precautions May cause hypercorticism or suppression of hypothalamic-pituitary-adrenal (HPA) axis, particularly in patients receiving high doses for prolonged periods. HPA axis suppression may lead to adrenal crisis. Withdrawal and discontinuation of a corticosteroid should be done slowly and carefully. Particular care is required when patients are transferred from systemic corticosteroids to inhaled products due to possible adrenal insufficiency or withdrawal from steroids, including an increase in allergic symptoms. Patients receiving >20 mg per day of prednisone (or equivalent) may be most susceptible. Fatalities have occurred due to adrenal insufficiency in asthmatic patients during and after transfer from systemic corticosteroids to aerosol steroids; aerosol steroids do not provide the systemic steroid needed to treat patients having trauma, surgery, or infections. When transferring to oral inhaler, previously-suppressed allergic conditions (rhinitis, conjunctivitis, eczema) may be unmasked.

Bronchospasm may occur with wheezing after inhalation; if this occurs stop steroid and treat with a fast-acting bronchodilator. Supplemental steroids (oral or parenteral) may be needed during stress or severe asthma attacks. Not to be used in status asthmaticus or for the relief of acute bronchospasm. Corticosteroid use may cause psychiatric disturbances, including depression, euphoria, insomnia, mood swings, and personality changes. Pre-existing psychiatric conditions may be exacerbated by corticosteroid use. Prolonged use of corticosteroids may also increase the incidence of secondary infection, mask acute infection (including fungal infections), prolong or exacerbate viral infections, or limit response to vaccines. Exposure to chickenpox should be avoided; corticosteroids should not be used to treat ocular herpes simplex. Corticosteroids should not be used for cerebral malaria or viral hepatitis. Close observation is required in patients with latent tuberculosis and/or TB reactivity; restrict use in active TB (only in conjunction with antituberculosis treatment). Prolonged treatment with corticosteroids has been associated with the development of Kaposi's sarcoma (case reports); if noted, discontinuation of therapy should be considered.

Use with caution in patients with thyroid disease, hepatic impairment, renal impairment, cardiovascular disease, diabetes, cataracts, glaucoma, myasthenia gravis, patients with or who are at risk for osteoporosis, patients at risk for seizures, or GI diseases (diverticulitis, peptic ulcer, ulcerative colitis) due to perforation risk. Use caution following acute MI (corticosteroids have been associated with myocardial rupture). Because of the risk of adverse

◄ effects, systemic corticosteroids should be used cautiously in the elderly in the smallest possible effective dose for the shortest duration.

Adverse Reactions (Reflective of adult population; not specific for elderly)

>10%:

Central nervous system: Headache (17% to 22%), fatigue (1% to 13%), depression (11%)

Neuromuscular & skeletal: Musculoskeletal pain (4% to 22%), arthralgia (13%)

Respiratory: Sinusitis (5% to 22%), rhinitis (4% to 20%), upper respiratory infection (8% to 15%), pharyngitis (8% to 13%)

Miscellaneous: Oral candidiasis (4% to 22%)

1% to 10%:

Central nervous system: Fever (children 7%), pain (1% to <3%)

Dermatologic: Bruising (children 2%)

Gastrointestinal: Abdominal pain (2% to 6%), dyspepsia (3% to 5%), nausea (1% to 3%), vomiting (1% to ≤3%), anorexia (1% to <3%), dry throat (1% to <3%), gastroenteritis (1% to <3%)

Genitourinary: Dysmenorrhea (4% to 9%), urinary tract infection (children 2%)

Neuromuscular & skeletal: Back pain (3% to 6%), myalgia (2% to 3%)

Ocular: Ocular pressure increased (3%), cataracts (1%)

Otic: Earache (1% to <3%)

Respiratory: Sinus congestion (9%), dysphonia (1% to <3%), epistaxis (1% to <3%), nasal irritation (1% to <3%)

Miscellaneous: Flu-like syndrome (1% to <3%), infection (1% to <3%)

Drug Interactions

Metabolism/Transport Effects Substrate of CYP3A4 (major)

Avoid Concomitant Use

Avoid concomitant use of Mometasone (Oral Inhalation) with any of the following: Aldesleukin

Increased Effect/Toxicity

Mometasone (Oral Inhalation) may increase the levels/effects of: Amphotericin B; Deferasirox; Loop Diuretics; Thiazide Diuretics

The levels/effects of Mometasone (Oral Inhalation) may be increased by: CYP3A4 Inhibitors (Strong); Telaprevir

Decreased Effect

Mometasone (Oral Inhalation) may decrease the levels/effects of: Aldesleukin; Antidiabetic Agents; Corticorelin; Telaprevir

The levels/effects of Mometasone (Oral Inhalation) may be decreased by: Tocilizumab

Stability Store at 25°C (77°F); excursions permitted to 15°C to 30°C (59°F to 86°F). Discard when oral dose counter reads "00" (or 45 days after opening the foil pouch).

Mechanism of Action May depress the formation, release, and activity of endogenous chemical mediators of inflammation (kinins, histamine, liposomal enzymes, prostaglandins). Leukocytes and macrophages may have to be present for the initiation of responses mediated by the above substances. Inhibits the margination and subsequent cell migration to the area of injury, and also reverses the dilatation and increased vessel permeability in the area resulting in decreased access of cells to the sites of injury.

Pharmacodynamics/Kinetics

Absorption: <1%

Protein binding: 98% to 99%

Metabolism: Hepatic via CYP3A4; forms metabolite

Half-life elimination: 5 hours

Excretion: Feces, bile, urine

Dosage

Geriatric & Adult Asthma: Oral inhalation:

Bronchodilators or inhaled corticosteroids: Initial: 1 inhalation (220 mcg) daily (maximum: 2 inhalations or 440 mcg/day); may be given in the evening or in divided doses twice daily

Oral corticosteroids: Initial: 440 mcg twice daily (maximum: 880 mcg/day); prednisone should be reduced no faster than 2.5 mg/day on a weekly basis, beginning after at least 1 week of mometasone furoate use

NIH Asthma Guidelines (NIH, 2007):

"Low" dose: 220 mcg/day

"Medium" dose: 440 mcg/day

"High" dose: >440 mcg/day

Note: Maximum effects may not be evident for 1-2 weeks or longer; dose should be titrated to effect, using the lowest possible dose

Administration Exhale fully prior to bringing the Twisthaler® up to the mouth. Place between lips and inhale quickly and deeply. Do not breathe out through the inhaler. Remove inhaler and hold breath for 10 seconds if possible. Rinse mouth after use.

Monitoring Parameters HPA axis suppression
Asthma: FEV$_1$, peak flow, and/or other pulmonary function tests
Dosage Forms Excipient information presented when available (limited, particularly for generics); consult specific product labeling.
Powder, for oral inhalation, as furoate:
Asmanex® Twisthaler®: 110 mcg (30 units) [contains lactose; delivers 100 mcg/actuation]
Asmanex® Twisthaler®: 220 mcg (14 units, 30 units, 60 units, 120 units) [contains lactose; delivers 200 mcg/actuation]

Mometasone (Nasal) (moe MET a sone)

Related Information
Corticosteroids on page 2005
Brand Names: U.S. Nasonex®
Brand Names: Canada Nasonex®
Index Terms Mometasone Furoate
Generic Availability (U.S.) No
Pharmacologic Category Corticosteroid, Nasal
Use Treatment of nasal symptoms of seasonal and perennial allergic rhinitis; prevention of nasal symptoms associated with seasonal allergic rhinitis; treatment of nasal polyps in adults

Canadian labeling: Additional use (not in U.S. labeling): Treatment of mild-to-moderate uncomplicated rhinosinusitis or as adjunctive treatment (with antimicrobials) in acute rhinosinusitis
Dosage
Geriatric & Adult
Seasonal and perennial allergic rhinitis: Intranasal:
U.S. labeling:
Treatment: 2 sprays (100 mcg) in each nostril once daily
Prevention: 2 sprays (100 mcg) in each nostril once daily beginning 2-4 weeks prior to pollen season
Canadian labeling (not in U.S. labeling): Initial: 2 sprays (100 mcg) in each nostril once daily; upon symptom control, may consider dose reduction to 1 spray (50 mcg) in each nostril once daily as maintenance therapy. **Note:** If adequate symptom control is not achieved with initial dosing, may increase dose to 4 sprays (200 mcg) in each nostril once daily (total daily dose: 400 mcg). Dose reduction is recommended upon symptom control.
Treatment of nasal polyps: Intranasal: 2 sprays (100 mcg) in each nostril twice daily; 2 sprays (100 mcg) once daily may be effective in some patients
Rhinosinusitis, adjunctive treatment (acute): Intranasal: Canadian labeling (not in U.S. labeling): 2 sprays (100 mcg) in each nostril twice daily; if inadequate symptom control, may increase to 4 sprays (200 mcg) in each nostril twice daily (total daily dose: 800 mcg)
Rhinosinusitis treatment (acute, mild-to-moderate, uncomplicated): Intranasal: Canadian labeling (not in U.S. labeling): 2 sprays (100 mcg) in each nostril twice daily; use beyond 15 days has not been studied.
Dosage Forms Excipient information presented when available (limited, particularly for generics); consult specific product labeling.
Suspension, intranasal, as furoate [spray]:
Nasonex®: 50 mcg/spray (17 g) [contains benzalkonium chloride; delivers 120 sprays]
Dosage Forms: Canada Excipient information presented when available (limited, particularly for generics); consult specific product labeling.
Suspension, intranasal, as furoate [spray]:
Nasonex®: 50 mcg/spray [contains benzalkonium chloride; delivers 140 sprays]

Mometasone (Topical) (moe MET a sone)

Related Information
Corticosteroids on page 2005
Medication Safety Issues
Sound-alike/look-alike issues:
Elocon® lotion may be confused with ophthalmic solutions. Manufacturer's labeling emphasizes the product is **NOT** for use in the eyes.
Brand Names: U.S. Elocon®
Brand Names: Canada Elocom®; PMS-Mometasone; ratio-Mometasone; Taro-Mometasone
Index Terms Mometasone Furoate
Generic Availability (U.S.) Yes
Pharmacologic Category Corticosteroid, Topical

◀ **Use** Relief of the inflammatory and pruritic manifestations of corticosteroid-responsive dermatoses (medium potency topical corticosteroid)

Dosage

    Geriatric & Adult Treatment of corticosteroid-responsive dermatoses: Topical: Apply
sparingly, do not use occlusive dressings. Therapy should be discontinued when control is
achieved; if no improvement is seen in 2 weeks, reassessment of diagnosis may be
necessary.

    Cream, ointment: Apply a thin film to affected area once daily

    Lotion: Apply a few drops to affected area once daily

Special Geriatric Considerations Due to age-related changes in skin, limit use of topical
corticosteroids.

Dosage Forms Excipient information presented when available (limited, particularly for
generics); consult specific product labeling.

    Cream, topical, as furoate: 0.1% (15 g, 45 g)

      Elocon®: 0.1% (15 g, 45 g)

    Lotion, topical, as furoate: 0.1% (30 mL, 60 mL)

      Elocon®: 0.1% (30 mL, 60 mL) [contains isopropyl alcohol 40%]

    Ointment, topical, as furoate: 0.1% (15 g, 45 g)

      Elocon®: 0.1% (15 g, 45 g)

Mometasone and Formoterol (moe MET a sone & for MOH te rol)

Related Information

    Formoterol *on page 785*

    Mometasone (Oral Inhalation) *on page 1231*

Brand Names: U.S. Dulera®

Brand Names: Canada Zenhale™

Index Terms Formoterol and Mometasone; Formoterol and Mometasone Furoate; Formoterol
Fumarate Dihydrate and Mometasone

Generic Availability (U.S.) No

Pharmacologic Category Beta$_2$-Adrenergic Agonist; Beta$_2$-Adrenergic Agonist, Long-Acting; Corticosteroid, Inhalant (Oral)

Use Maintenance treatment of asthma where combination therapy is indicated

Medication Guide Available Yes

Contraindications Hypersensitivity to mometasone, formoterol, or any component of the
formulation; need for acute bronchodilation (including status asthmaticus)

**Warnings/Precautions [U.S. Boxed Warning]: Long-acting beta$_2$-agonists (LABAs),
such as formoterol, increase the risk of asthma-related deaths; mometasone and
formoterol should only be used in patients not adequately controlled on a long-term
asthma control medication (ie, inhaled corticosteroid) or whose disease severity
requires initiation of two maintenance therapies.** In a large, randomized, placebo-controlled U.S. clinical trial (SMART, 2006), salmeterol was associated with an increase in
asthma-related deaths (when added to usual asthma therapy); risk is considered a class
effect among all LABAs. Data are not available to determine if the addition of an inhaled
corticosteroid lessens this increased risk of death associated with LABA use. Assess patients
at regular intervals once asthma control is maintained on combination therapy to determine if
step-down therapy is appropriate (without loss of asthma control), and the patient can be
maintained on an inhaled corticosteroid only. LABAs are not appropriate in patients whose
asthma is adequately controlled on low- or medium-dose inhaled corticosteroids.

Do **not** use for acute bronchospasm. Short-acting beta$_2$-agonist (eg, albuterol) should be used
for acute symptoms and symptoms occurring between treatments. Do **not** initiate in patients
with significantly worsening or acutely deteriorating asthma. Patients must be instructed to
seek medical attention in cases where acute symptoms are not relieved by short-acting beta-
agonist (not formoterol) or a previous level of response is diminished. Medical evaluation must
not be delayed. Patients using inhaled, short-acting beta$_2$-agonists should be instructed to
discontinue routine use of these medications prior to beginning treatment with Dulera®; short-
acting agents should be reserved for symptomatic relief of acute symptoms. Patients should
not use additional long-acting beta2-adrenergic agonists.

Immediate hypersensitivity reactions (urticaria, angioedema, rash, bronchospasm) have been
reported. Do not exceed recommended dose; serious adverse events, including fatalities,
have been associated with excessive use of inhaled sympathomimetics. Rarely, paradoxical
bronchospasm may occur with use of inhaled bronchodilating agents; this should be
distinguished from inadequate response.

Use caution in patients with cardiovascular disease (arrhythmia or hypertension or HF), seizure disorders, diabetes, osteoporosis, ocular disease, thyroid disease, or hypokalemia. Beta agonists may cause elevation in blood pressure, heart rate, and result in CNS stimulation/excitation. Beta₂-agonists may increase risk of arrhythmia, increase serum glucose, or decrease serum potassium. Long-term use may affect bone mineral density in adults. Infections with *Candida albicans* in the mouth and throat (thrush) have been reported with use. Use with caution in patients taking strong CYP3A4 inhibitors (see Drug Interactions); consider alternative agents that avoid or lessen the potential for CYP-mediated interactions.

Mometasone may cause hypercorticism and/or suppression of hypothalamic-pituitary-adrenal (HPA) axis, particularly in patients receiving high doses for prolonged periods. Caution is required when patients are transferred from systemic corticosteroids to products with lower systemic bioavailability (ie, inhalation). May lead to possible adrenal insufficiency or withdrawal symptoms, including an increase in allergic symptoms. Patients receiving prolonged therapy ≥20 mg per day of prednisone (or equivalent) may be most susceptible. Aerosol steroids do not provide the systemic steroid needed to treat patients having trauma, surgery, or infections.

Prolonged use of corticosteroids may also increase the incidence of secondary infection, mask acute infection (including fungal infections), prolong or exacerbate viral infections, or limit response to vaccines. Exposure to chickenpox should be avoided; corticosteroids should not be used to treat ocular herpes simplex. Corticosteroids should not be used for cerebral malaria. Close observation is required in patients with latent tuberculosis and/or TB reactivity restrict use in active TB (only in conjunction with antituberculosis treatment).

Withdraw systemic therapy with gradual tapering of dose. There have been reports of systemic corticosteroid withdrawal symptoms (eg, joint/muscle pain, lassitude, depression) when withdrawing oral inhalation therapy.

Adverse Reactions (Reflective of adult population; not specific for elderly) Also see individual agents.

1% to 10%:
Central nervous system: Headache (up to 5%)
Respiratory: Nasopharyngitis (5%), dysphonia (4% to 5%), sinusitis (2% to 3%)

Drug Interactions

Metabolism/Transport Effects
Mometasone: **Substrate** (minor) of CYP3A4
Formoterol: **Substrate** (minor) of CYP2A6, 2C9, 2C19, 2D6

Avoid Concomitant Use
Avoid concomitant use of Mometasone and Formoterol with any of the following: Aldesleukin; BCG; Iobenguane I 123; Natalizumab; Pimecrolimus; Tacrolimus (Topical)

Increased Effect/Toxicity
Mometasone and Formoterol may increase the levels/effects of: Acetylcholinesterase Inhibitors; Amphotericin B; Deferasirox; Leflunomide; Loop Diuretics; Natalizumab; NSAID (COX-2 Inhibitor); NSAID (Nonselective); Sympathomimetics; Thiazide Diuretics; Vaccines (Live); Warfarin

The levels/effects of Mometasone and Formoterol may be increased by: Antifungal Agents (Azole Derivatives, Systemic); Aprepitant; Atomoxetine; Caffeine; Calcium Channel Blockers (Nondihydropyridine); Cannabinoids; CYP3A4 Inhibitors (Strong); Denosumab; Estrogen Derivatives; Fluconazole; Fosaprepitant; Macrolide Antibiotics; MAO Inhibitors; Neuromuscular-Blocking Agents (Nondepolarizing); Pimecrolimus; Quinolone Antibiotics; Roflumilast; Salicylates; Tacrolimus (Topical); Telaprevir; Theophylline Derivatives; Trastuzumab; Tricyclic Antidepressants

Decreased Effect
Mometasone and Formoterol may decrease the levels/effects of: Aldesleukin; Antidiabetic Agents; BCG; Calcitriol; Corticorelin; Iobenguane I 123; Isoniazid; Salicylates; Sipuleucel-T; Telaprevir; Vaccines (Inactivated)

The levels/effects of Mometasone and Formoterol may be decreased by: Alpha-/Beta-Blockers; Aminoglutethimide; Barbiturates; Beta-Blockers (Beta1 Selective); Beta-Blockers (Nonselective); Betahistine; Echinacea; Mitotane; Primidone; Rifamycin Derivatives; Tocilizumab

Stability Store at room temperature of 20°C to 25°C (68°F to 77°F). Do not puncture, incinerate, or store near heat or open flame. Discard inhaler after the labeled number of inhalations have been used.

◀ **Mechanism of Action** Formoterol relaxes bronchial smooth muscle by selective action on beta$_2$ receptors with little effect on heart rate. Formoterol has a long-acting effect. Mometasone is a corticosteroid which controls the rate of protein synthesis, depresses the migration of polymorphonuclear leukocytes/fibroblasts, and reverses capillary permeability and lysosomal stabilization at the cellular level to prevent or control inflammation.

Pharmacodynamics/Kinetics See individual agents.

Dosage

Geriatric & Adult Asthma: Oral inhalation:

Previous therapy included inhaled low-dose corticosteroids: Canadian labeling (not in U.S. labeling): Mometasone 50 mcg/formoterol 5 mcg: Two inhalations twice daily. Maximum daily dose: 4 inhalations

Previous therapy included inhaled medium-dose corticosteroids: Mometasone 100 mcg/ formoterol 5 mcg: Two inhalations twice daily. Consider the higher dose combination for patients not adequately controlled on the lower combination following 1-2 weeks of therapy. Maximum daily dose: 4 inhalations

Previous therapy included inhaled high-dose corticosteroids: Mometasone 200 mcg/formoterol 5 mcg: Two inhalations twice daily. Maximum daily dose: 4 inhalations

Hepatic Impairment Mometasone systemic exposure appears to increase with increasing extent of impairment; however, there is no dosage adjustment recommended in the manufacturer labeling.

Administration Prior to first use, inhaler must be primed by releasing 4 test sprays into the air; shake well before each spray. Inhaler must be reprimed if not used for >5 days. Shake well before each use. Discard inhaler after the labeled number of inhalations have been used.

Delivery of dose: Instruct patient to place mouthpiece gently between teeth, closing lips around inhaler. Instruct patient to inhale deeply and hold breath held for 5-10 seconds. The amount of drug delivered is small, and the individual will not sense the medication as it is inhaled. Remove mouthpiece from mouth prior to exhalation. Patient should not breathe out through the mouthpiece. After use of the inhaler, patient should rinse mouth/oropharynx with water and spit out rinse solution.

Monitoring Parameters FEV$_1$, peak flow meter, and/or other pulmonary function tests; monitor symptom relief, monitor for increased use if short-acting beta$_2$-adrenergic agonists (may be a sign of asthma deterioration).

Pharmacotherapy Pearls Effects of inhaled steroids on growth have been observed in the absence of laboratory evidence of HPA axis suppression, suggesting that growth velocity is a more sensitive indicator of systemic corticosteroid exposure in pediatric patients than some commonly used tests of HPA axis function. The long-term effects of this reduction in growth velocity associated with orally-inhaled corticosteroids, including the impact on final adult height, are unknown. The potential for "catch up" growth following discontinuation of treatment with inhaled corticosteroids has not been adequately studied.

Special Geriatric Considerations No significant difference in both safety and effectiveness was seen between elderly and young patients. Elderly patients should be specifically counseled about the proper use of metered-dose inhalers.

Dosage Forms Excipient information presented when available (limited, particularly for generics); consult specific product labeling.

Aerosol, for oral inhalation:

Dulera®: Mometasone furoate 100 mcg and formoterol fumarate dihydrate 5 mcg per inhalation (13 g) [120 metered actuations]

Dulera®: Mometasone furoate 200 mcg and formoterol fumarate dihydrate 5 mcg per inhalation (13 g) [120 metered actuations]

Dosage Forms: Canada Excipient information presented when available (limited, particularly for generics); consult specific product labeling.

Aerosol, for oral inhalation:

Zenhale™: Mometasone furoate 50 mcg and formoterol fumarate dihydrate 5 mcg per inhalation [120 metered actuations]

Selected References

National Asthma Education and Prevention Program, "Expert Panel Report 3 (EPR-3): Guidelines for the Diagnosis and Management of Asthma-Summary Report 2007," *J Allergy Clin Immunol*, 2007, 120(5 Suppl):94-138.

◆ **Monodox®** *see* Doxycycline *on page 570*
◆ **Monoket®** *see* Isosorbide Mononitrate *on page 990*
◆ **Monopril** *see* Fosinopril *on page 791*

Montelukast (mon te LOO kast)

Medication Safety Issues
Sound-alike/look-alike issues:
Singulair® may be confused with SINEquan®
Brand Names: U.S. Singulair®
Brand Names: Canada Singulair®
Index Terms Montelukast Sodium
Generic Availability (U.S.) No
Pharmacologic Category Leukotriene-Receptor Antagonist
Use Prophylaxis and chronic treatment of asthma; relief of symptoms of seasonal allergic rhinitis and perennial allergic rhinitis; prevention of exercise-induced bronchospasm
Unlabeled/Investigational Use Acute asthma
Contraindications Hypersensitivity to montelukast or any component of the formulation
Warnings/Precautions Montelukast is not FDA approved for use in the reversal of broncho-spasm in acute asthma attacks, including status asthmaticus; some clinicians, however, support its use as adjunctive therapy (Camargo, 2003; Cylly, 2003; Ferreira, 2001; Harmancik 2006). Appropriate rescue medication should be available. Appropriate clinical monitoring and caution are recommended when systemic corticosteroid reduction is considered in patients receiving montelukast. Patients should be instructed to notify prescriber if behavioral changes occur. Inform phenylketonuric patients that the chewable tablet contains phenylalanine.

In rare cases, patients on therapy with montelukast may present with systemic eosinophilia, sometimes presenting with clinical features of vasculitis consistent with Churg-Strauss syndrome, a condition which is often treated with systemic corticosteroid therapy. Healthcare providers should be alert to eosinophilia, vasculitic rash, worsening pulmonary symptoms, cardiac complications, and/or neuropathy presenting in their patients. A causal association between montelukast and these underlying conditions has not been established. Montelukast will not interrupt bronchoconstrictor response to aspirin or other NSAIDs; aspirin sensitive asthmatics should continue to avoid these agents. Postmarketing reports of behavior changes (agitation, aggression, depression, insomnia) have been noted in children and adults.
Adverse Reactions (Reflective of adult population; not specific for elderly)
1% to 10%:
Central nervous system: Dizziness (2%), fatigue (2%), fever (2%)
Dermatologic: Rash (2%)
Gastrointestinal: Abdominal pain (3%), dyspepsia (2%), dental pain (2%), gastroenteritis (2%)
Hepatic: AST increased (2%)
Neuromuscular & skeletal: Weakness (2%)
Respiratory: Cough (3%), nasal congestion (2%)
Drug Interactions
Metabolism/Transport Effects Substrate (major) of CYP2C9, 3A4; **Inhibits** CYP2C8 (weak), 2C9 (weak)
Avoid Concomitant Use There are no known interactions where it is recommended to avoid concomitant use.
Increased Effect/Toxicity
The levels/effects of Montelukast may be increased by: Conivaptan; CYP2C9 Inhibitors (Moderate); CYP2C9 Inhibitors (Strong)
Decreased Effect
The levels/effects of Montelukast may be decreased by: CYP2C9 Inducers (Highly Effective); CYP3A4 Inducers (Strong); Deferasirox; Herbs (CYP3A4 Inducers); Peginterferon Alfa-2b; Tocilizumab
Ethanol/Nutrition/Herb Interactions Herb/Nutraceutical: St John's wort may decrease montelukast levels.
Stability Store at room temperature of 25°C (77°F); excursions permitted to 15°C to 30°C (59°F to 86°F). Protect from moisture and light.
Granules: Store in original package; use within 15 minutes of opening packet.
Mechanism of Action Selective leukotriene receptor antagonist that inhibits the cysteinyl leukotriene receptor. Cysteinyl leukotrienes and leukotriene receptor occupation have been correlated with the pathophysiology of asthma, including airway edema, smooth muscle contraction, and altered cellular activity associated with the inflammatory process, which contribute to the signs and symptoms of asthma. Cysteinyl leukotrienes are also released from the nasal mucosa following allergen exposure leading to symptoms associated with allergic rhinitis.

Pharmacodynamics/Kinetics
Duration: >24 hours
Absorption: Rapid
Distribution: V_d: 8-11 L
Protein binding, plasma: >99%
Metabolism: Extensively hepatic via CYP3A4 and 2C9
Bioavailability: Tablet: 10 mg: Mean: 64%; 5 mg: 63% to 73%
Half-life elimination, plasma: Mean: 2.7-5.5 hours
Time to peak, serum: Tablet: 10 mg: 3-4 hours; 5 mg: 2-2.5 hours; 4 mg: 2 hours
Excretion: Feces (86%); urine (<0.2%)

Dosage

Geriatric & Adult

Asthma, allergic seasonal or perennial rhinitis: Oral: 10 mg once daily

Asthma, acute (unlabeled use): 10 mg as a single dose administered with first-line therapy (Camargo, 2003; Cylly, 2003)

Bronchoconstriction, exercise-induced (prevention): 10 mg at least 2 hours prior to exercise; additional doses should not be administered within 24 hours. Daily administration to prevent exercise-induced bronchoconstriction has not been evaluated.

Renal Impairment No adjustment is necessary.

Hepatic Impairment No adjustment necessary in mild-to-moderate hepatic disease. Patients with severe hepatic disease were **not** studied.

Administration When treating asthma, administer dose in the evening. Patients with allergic rhinitis may individualize administration time (morning or evening). Patients with both asthma and allergic rhinitis should take their dose in the evening. Granules may be administered directly in the mouth or mixed with a spoonful of applesauce, carrots, rice, ice cream, baby formula, or breast milk; do not add to any other liquids or foods. Administer within 15 minutes of opening packet. May administer without regard to meals.

Monitoring Parameters Mood or behavior changes, including suicidal thinking/behavior

Special Geriatric Considerations The pharmacokinetic profile in the elderly is similar to younger adults except the half-life is slightly longer in the elderly. Despite this difference, no adjustment in dose is necessary in the elderly. Elimination is mostly fecal and bile with insignificant amounts from renal elimination, which is an advantage for the elderly.

Dosage Forms Excipient information presented when available (limited, particularly for generics); consult specific product labeling.

Granules, oral:
  Singulair®: 4 mg/packet (30s)
Tablet, oral:
  Singulair®: 10 mg
Tablet, chewable, oral:
  Singulair®: 4 mg [contains phenylalanine 0.674 mg/tablet; cherry flavor]
  Singulair®: 5 mg [contains phenylalanine 0.842 mg/tablet; cherry flavor]

Selected References

Camargo CA Jr, Smithline HA, Malice MP, et al, "A Randomized Controlled Trial of Intravenous Montelukast in Acute Asthma," Am J Respir Crit Care Med, 2003, 167(4):528-33.

Cylly A, Kara A, Ozdemir T, et al, "Effects of Oral Montelukast on Airway Function in Acute Asthma," Respir Med, 2003, 97(5):533-6.

◆ **Montelukast Sodium** see Montelukast on page 1237
◆ **MoreDophilus® [OTC]** see Lactobacillus on page 1020

Morphine (Systemic) (MOR feen)

Related Information
Opioid Analgesics on page 2013
Patient Information for Disposal of Unused Medications on page 2125

Medication Safety Issues
Sound-alike/look-alike issues:
Morphine may be confused with HYDROmorphone, methadone
Morphine sulfate may be confused with magnesium sulfate
Kadian® may be confused with Kapidex [DSC]
MS Contin® may be confused with OxyCONTIN®

MSO$_4$ and MS are error-prone abbreviations (mistaken as magnesium sulfate)

AVINza® may be confused with Evista®, INVanz®

Roxanol may be confused with OxyFast®, Roxicet™, Roxicodone®

High alert medication:

The Institute for Safe Medication Practices (ISMP) includes this medication (I.V. formulation) among its list of drug classes which have a heightened risk of causing significant patient harm when used in error.

Other safety concerns:

Use care when prescribing and/or administering morphine solutions. These products are available in different concentrations. Always prescribe dosage in mg; **not** by volume (mL).

Use caution when selecting a morphine formulation for use in neurologic infusion pumps (eg, Medtronic delivery systems). The product should be appropriately labeled as "preservative-free" and suitable for intraspinal use via continuous infusion. In addition, the product should be formulated in a pH range that is compatible with the device operation specifications.

Significant differences exist between oral and I.V. dosing. Use caution when converting from one route of administration to another.

Brand Names: U.S. Astramorph®/PF; AVINza®; Duramorph; Infumorph 200; Infumorph 500; Kadian®; MS Contin®; Oramorph® SR

Brand Names: Canada Doloral; Kadian®; M-Eslon®; M.O.S.-SR®; M.O.S.-Sulfate®; M.O.S.® 10; M.O.S.® 20; M.O.S.® 30; Morphine Extra Forte Injection; Morphine Forte Injection; Morphine HP®; Morphine LP® Epidural; Morphine SR; Morphine-EPD; MS Contin SRT; MS Contin®; MS-IR®; Novo-Morphine SR; PMS-Morphine Sulfate SR; ratio-Morphine; ratio-Morphine SR; Sandoz-Morphine SR; Statex®

Index Terms MS (error-prone abbreviation and should not be used); MSO$_4$ (error-prone abbreviation and should not be used); Roxanol

Generic Availability (U.S.) Yes: Excludes capsule, sustained release tablet

Pharmacologic Category Analgesic, Opioid

Use Relief of moderate-to-severe acute and chronic pain; relief of pain of myocardial infarction; relief of dyspnea of acute left ventricular failure and pulmonary edema; preanesthetic medication

Infumorph®: Used in continuous microinfusion devices for intrathecal or epidural administration in treatment of intractable chronic pain

Controlled, extended, or sustained release products: Only intended/indicated for use when repeated doses for an extended period of time are required. The 100 mg and 200 mg tablets or capsules of Kadian®, MS Contin®, and morphine sulfate controlled-release tablets and the 60 mg, 90 mg, and 120 mg capsules of Avinza® should only be used in opioid-tolerant patients.

Medication Guide Available Yes

Contraindications Note: Some contraindications are product specific. For details, please see detailed product prescribing information.

Hypersensitivity to morphine sulfate or any component of the formulation; severe respiratory depression (without resuscitative equipment); acute or severe asthma; known or suspected paralytic ileus; sustained release products are not recommended with gastrointestinal obstruction or in acute/postoperative pain. Oral solutions contraindicated in patients with heart failure due to chronic lung disease, cardiac arrhythmias, head injuries, brain tumors, acute alcoholism, delirium tremens, seizure disorders, Injectable solution contraindicated during labor when a premature birth is anticipated. Some products contraindicated in patients with head injuries or increased intracranial pressure. MS Contin® and Kadian® contraindicated in patients with hypercarbia. Some immediate release formulations (tablets and solution) contraindicated in post biliary tract surgery, suspected surgical abdomen, surgical anastomosis, MAO inhibitor use (concurrent or within 14 days), general CNS depression.

Warnings/Precautions An opioid-containing analgesic regimen should be tailored to each patient's needs and based upon the type of pain being treated (acute versus chronic), the route of administration, degree of tolerance for opioids (naive versus chronic user), age, weight, and medical condition. The optimal analgesic dose varies widely among patients. Doses should be titrated to pain relief/prevention. When used as an epidural injection, monitor for delayed sedation. **[U.S. Boxed Warning]: Healthcare provider should be alert to problems of abuse, misuse, and diversion.**

May cause respiratory depression; use with caution in patients (particularly elderly or debilitated) with impaired respiratory function, morbid obesity, adrenal insufficiency, prostatic hyperplasia, urinary stricture, renal impairment, or severe hepatic dysfunction and in patients with hypersensitivity reactions to other phenanthrene derivative opioid agonists (codeine, hydrocodone, hydromorphone, levorphanol, oxycodone, oxymorphone). Use with caution in patients with biliary tract dysfunction; acute pancreatitis may cause constriction of sphincter of Oddi. Some preparations contain sulfites which may cause allergic reactions.

May cause CNS depression, which may impair physical or mental abilities; patients must be cautioned about performing tasks which require mental alertness (eg, operating machinery or driving). Effects may be potentiated when used with other sedative drugs or ethanol. May cause hypotension in patients with acute myocardial infarction, volume depletion, or concurrent drug therapy which may exaggerate vasodilation. Use with extreme caution in patients with head injury, intracranial lesions, or elevated intracranial pressure; exaggerated elevation of ICP may occur. May cause seizures if high doses are used; use with caution in patients with seizure disorders. Tolerance or drug dependence may result from extended use. Concurrent use of agonist/antagonist analgesics may precipitate withdrawal symptoms and/or reduced analgesic efficacy in patients following prolonged therapy with mu opioid agonists. Abrupt discontinuation following prolonged use may also lead to withdrawal symptoms. Elderly may be particularly susceptible to adverse effects of narcotics. May obscure diagnosis or clinical course of patients with acute abdominal conditions.

Extended or sustained-release formulations:

[U.S. Boxed Warning]: Extended or sustained release dosage forms should not be crushed or chewed. Controlled-, extended-, or sustained-release products are not intended for "as needed (PRN)" use. **MS Contin® 100 or 200 mg tablets and Kadian® 100 mg or 200 mg capsules are for use only in opioid-tolerant patients.** Avinza®, Kadian®, MS Contin®: **[U.S. Boxed Warning]: Indicated for the management of moderate-to-severe pain when around the clock pain control is needed for an extended time period.**

[U.S. Boxed Warning]: Avinza®: Do not administer with alcoholic beverages or ethanol-containing products, which may disrupt extended-release characteristic of product.

Highly concentrated oral solutions: [U.S. Boxed Warning]: Check doses carefully when using highly concentrated oral solutions.

Injections: Note: Products are designed for administration by specific routes (I.V., intrathecal, epidural). Use caution when prescribing, dispensing, or administering to use formulations only by intended route(s).

[U.S. Boxed Warning]: Duramorph®: Due to the risk of severe and/or sustained cardiopulmonary depressant effects of Duramorph® must be administered in a fully equipped and staffed environment. Naloxone injection should be immediately available. Patient should remain in this environment for at least 24 hours following the initial dose.

[U.S. Boxed Warning]: Intrathecal dosage is usually $^1/_{10}$ that of epidural dosage.

Infumorph® solutions are **for use in microinfusion devices only**; not for I.V., I.M., or SubQ administration, or for single-dose administration.

When used as an epidural injection, monitor for delayed sedation.

Adverse Reactions (Reflective of adult population; not specific for elderly) Note: Individual patient differences are unpredictable, and percentage may differ in acute pain (surgical) treatment. Reactions may be dose, formulation, and/or route dependent.

Frequency not defined:
Cardiovascular: Circulatory depression, flushing, shock
Central nervous system: Dysphonia, physical and psychological dependence, sedation
Endocrine & metabolic: Antidiuretic hormone release
>10%:
Cardiovascular: Bradycardia, hypotension
Central nervous system: Drowsiness (9% to 48%; tolerance usually develops to drowsiness with regular dosing for 1-2 weeks), dizziness (6% to 20%), fever (<3% to >10%), confusion, headache (following epidural or intrathecal use)
Dermatologic: Pruritus (may be dose related)
Gastrointestinal: Xerostomia (78%), constipation (9% to 40%; tolerance develops very slowly if at all), nausea (7% to 28%; tolerance usually develops to nausea and vomiting with chronic use), vomiting
Genitourinary: Urinary retention (16%; may be prolonged, up to 20 hours, following epidural or intrathecal use)
Hematologic: Anemia (following intrathecal use)
Local: Pain at injection site
Neuromuscular & skeletal: Weakness
Respiratory: Oxygen saturation decreased
Miscellaneous: Histamine release
1% to 10%:
Cardiovascular: Atrial fibrillation (<3%), chest pain (<3%), edema, hypertension, palpitation, peripheral edema, syncope, tachycardia, vasodilation

Central nervous system: Amnesia, agitation, anxiety, apathy, apprehension, ataxia, chills, coma, delirium, depression, dream abnormalities, euphoria, false sense of well being, hallucination, hypoesthesia, insomnia, lethargy, malaise, nervousness, restlessness, seizure, slurred speech, somnolence, vertigo

Dermatologic: Dry skin, rash, urticaria

Endocrine & metabolic: Gynecomastia (<3%), hypokalemia, hyponatremia, libido decreased

Gastrointestinal: Abdominal distension, abdominal pain, anorexia, biliary colic, diarrhea, dyspepsia, dysphagia, flatulence, gastroenteritis, GERD, GI irritation, paralytic ileus, rectal disorder, taste perversion, weight loss

Genitourinary: Bladder spasm, dysuria, ejaculation abnormal, impotence, urination decreased

Hematologic: Leukopenia (<3%), thrombocytopenia (<3%), hematocrit decreased

Hepatic: Liver function tests increased

Neuromuscular & skeletal: Arthralgia, back pain, bone pain, foot drop, gait abnormalities, paresthesia, rigors, skeletal muscle rigidity, tremor

Ocular: Amblyopia, conjunctivitis, eye pain, vision problems/disturbance

Renal: Oliguria

Respiratory: Asthma, atelectasis, dyspnea, hiccups, hypercapnia, hypoxia, pulmonary edema (noncardiogenic), respiratory depression, rhinitis

Miscellaneous: Diaphoresis, flu-like syndrome, infection, thirst, voice alteration, withdrawal syndrome

Drug Interactions

Metabolism/Transport Effects Substrate of CYP2D6 (minor)

Avoid Concomitant Use There are no known interactions where it is recommended to avoid concomitant use.

Increased Effect/Toxicity

Morphine (Systemic) may increase the levels/effects of: Alcohol (Ethyl); Alvimopan; CNS Depressants; Desmopressin; Selective Serotonin Reuptake Inhibitors; Thiazide Diuretics

The levels/effects of Morphine (Systemic) may be increased by: Amphetamines; Antipsychotic Agents (Phenothiazines); Droperidol; HydrOXYzine; Succinylcholine

Decreased Effect

Morphine (Systemic) may decrease the levels/effects of: Pegvisomant

The levels/effects of Morphine (Systemic) may be decreased by: Ammonium Chloride; Mixed Agonist / Antagonist Opioids; Peginterferon Alfa-2b; Rifamycin Derivatives

Ethanol/Nutrition/Herb Interactions

Ethanol: Alcoholic beverages or ethanol-containing products may disrupt extended-release formulation resulting in rapid release of entire morphine dose. Ethanol may also increase CNS depression; monitor for increased effects with coadministration. Caution patients about effects.

Food: Administration of oral morphine solution with food may increase bioavailability (ie, a report of 34% increase in morphine AUC when morphine oral solution followed a high-fat meal). The bioavailability of Avinza®, Oramorph SR®, or Kadian® does not appear to be affected by food.

Herb/Nutraceutical: Avoid valerian, St John's wort, kava kava, gotu kola (may increase CNS depression).

Stability

Capsule, sustained release (Avinza®, Kadian®): Store at 25°C (77°F); excursions permitted to 15°C to 30°C (59°F to 86°F). Protect from light and moisture.

Injection: Store at controlled room temperature of 20°C to 25°C (68°F to 77°F); do not freeze. Protect from light. Degradation depends on pH and presence of oxygen; relatively stable in pH ≤4; darkening of solutions indicate degradation. Usual concentration for continuous I.V. infusion: 0.1-1 mg/mL in D$_5$W.

Oral solution: Store at controlled room temperature of 25°C (68°F to 77°F); do not freeze.

Suppositories: Store at controlled room temperature 25°C (77°F). Protect from light.

Tablet, extended release: Store at controlled room temperature of 25°C (77°F).

Tablet, immediate release: Store at controlled room temperature of 25°C (77°F). Protect from moisture.

Mechanism of Action Binds to opiate receptors in the CNS, causing inhibition of ascending pain pathways, altering the perception of and response to pain; produces generalized CNS depression

Pharmacodynamics/Kinetics

Onset of action (patient dependent; dosing must be individualized): Oral (immediate release): ~30 minutes; I.V.: 5-10 minutes

Duration (patient dependent; dosing must be individualized): Pain relief:

Immediate release formulations: 4 hours

Extended release capsule and tablet: 8-24 hours (formulation dependent)

◀ Absorption: Variable

Distribution: V_d: 3-4 L/kg; binds to opioid receptors in the CNS and periphery (eg, GI tract)

Protein binding: 30% to 35%

Metabolism: Hepatic via conjugation with glucuronic acid primarily to morphine-6-glucuronide (active analgesic) morphine-3-glucuronide (inactive as analgesic); minor metabolites include morphine-3-6-diglucuronide; other minor metabolites include normorphine (active) and morphine 3-ethereal sulfate

Bioavailability: Oral: 17% to 33% (first-pass effect limits oral bioavailability; oral:parenteral effectiveness reportedly varies from 1:6 in opioid naive patients to 1:3 with chronic use)

Half-life elimination: Adults: 2-4 hours (immediate release forms)

Time to peak, plasma: Avinza®: 30 minutes (maintained for 24 hours); Kadian®: ~10 hours; Oramorph® SR: ~4 hours

Excretion: Urine (primarily as morphine-3-glucuronide, ~2% to 12% excreted unchanged); feces (~7% to 10%). It has been suggested that accumulation of morphine-6-glucuronide might cause toxicity with renal insufficiency. All of the metabolites (ie, morphine-3-glucuronide, morphine-6-glucuronide, and normorphine) have been suggested as possible causes of neurotoxicity (eg, myoclonus).

Dosage

Geriatric Refer to adult dosing. Use with caution; may require reduced dosage in the elderly and debilitated patients.

Adult These are guidelines and do not represent the doses that may be required in all patients. Doses and dosage intervals should be titrated to pain relief/prevention.

Acute pain (moderate-to-severe):

Oral (immediate release formulations: Opiate-naive: Initial: 10 mg every 4 hours as needed; patients with prior opiate exposure may require higher initial doses: usual dosage range: 10-30 mg every 4 hours as needed

I.M., SubQ: **Note:** Repeated SubQ administration causes local tissue irritation, pain, and induration.

Initial: Opiate-naive: 5-10 mg every 4 hours as needed; patients with prior opiate exposure may require higher initial doses; usual dosage range: 5-20 mg every 4 hours as needed

Rectal: 10-20 mg every 3-4 hours

I.V.: Initial: Opiate-naive: 2.5-5 mg every 3-4 hours; patients with prior opiate exposure may require higher initial doses. **Note:** Repeated doses (up to every 5 minutes if needed) in small increments (eg, 1-4 mg) may be preferred to larger and less frequent doses.

Acute myocardial infarction, analgesia (ACC/AHA 2004 Guidelines): Initial management: 2-4 mg, give 2-8 mg every 5-15 minutes as needed

Critically-ill patients (unlabeled dose): 0.7-10 mg (based on 70 kg patient) **or** 0.01-0.15 mg/kg every 1-2 hours as needed. **Note:** More frequent dosing may be needed (eg, mechanically-ventilated patients).

I.V., SubQ continuous infusion: 0.8-10 mg/hour; usual range: Up to 80 mg/hour

Continuous infusion: Usual dosage range: 5-35 mg/hour (based on 70 kg patient) **or** 0.07-0.5 mg/kg/hour

Patient-controlled analgesia (PCA): (Opiate-naive: Consider lower end of dosing range): Usual concentration: 1 mg/mL

Demand dose: Usual: 1 mg; range: 0.5-2.5 mg

Lockout interval: 5-10 minutes

Intrathecal (I.T.): **Note: Must be preservative-free.** Administer with extreme caution and in reduced dosage to geriatric or debilitated patients. I.T. dose is usually $^{1}/_{10}$ that of epidural dosage.

Opioid-naive: 0.2-1 mg/dose (may provide adequate relief for up to 24 hours); repeat doses are **not** recommended. **Note:** The American Pain Society recommends 0.1-0.3 mg/dose; adjust dose for age, injection site, and patient's medical condition and degree of opioid tolerance.

Continuous microinfusion (Infumorph®): Initial: 0.2-1 mg/day

Opioid-tolerant: 1-10 mg/day

Continuous microinfusion (Infumorph®): Initial: 1-10 mg/day, titrate to effect; usual maximum is ~20 mg/day

Epidural: Pain management **Note: Must be preservative-free.** Administer with extreme caution and in reduced dosage to geriatric or debilitated patients. Vigilant monitoring is particularly important in these patients.

Single-dose (Astromorph/PF™, Duramorph®): Initial: 5 mg, if pain relief not achieved in 1 hour, careful administration of 1-2 mg at intervals sufficient to assess effectiveness may be given; maximum: 10 mg/24 hours (single doses may provide adequate relief for up to 24 hours)

Infusion: Bolus dose: 1-6 mg; infusion rate: 0.1-0.2 mg/hour; maximum dose: 10 mg/24 hours.

Note: The American Pain Society recommends 1-6 mg/dose as a single dose or an infusion of 0.1-1 mg/hour; adjust dose for age, injection site, and patient's medical condition and degree of opioid tolerance.

Continuous microinfusion (Infumorph®):

Opioid-naive: Initial: 0.2-1 mg/day

Opioid-tolerant: Initial: 1-10 mg/day, titrate to effect; usual maximum is ~20 mg/day

Chronic pain: Note: Patients taking opioids chronically may become tolerant and require doses higher than the usual dosage range to maintain the desired effect. Tolerance can be managed by appropriate dose titration. There is no optimal or maximal dose for morphine in chronic pain. The appropriate dose is one that relieves pain throughout its dosing interval without causing unmanageable side effects.

Oral: Controlled-, extended-, or sustained-release formulations: A patient's morphine requirement should be established using prompt-release formulations. Conversion to long-acting products may be considered when chronic, continuous treatment is required. Higher dosages should be reserved for use only in opioid-tolerant patients.

Capsules, extended release (Avinza®): Daily dose administered once daily (for best results, administer at same time each day)

Capsules, sustained release (Kadian®): Daily dose administered once daily or in 2 divided doses daily (every 12 hours)

Tablets, controlled release (MS Contin®), sustained release (Oramorph SR®), or extended release: Daily dose divided and administered every 8 or every 12 hours

Renal Impairment

Cl_{cr} 10-50 mL/minute: Administer at 75% of normal dose

Cl_{cr} <10 mL/minute: Administer at 50% of normal dose

Intermittent HD: Adults: No dosage adjustment necessary

CRRT: Administer 75% of normal dose, titrate

Hepatic Impairment Unchanged in mild liver disease; substantial extrahepatic metabolism may occur. Excessive sedation may occur in cirrhosis.

Administration

Oral: Do not crush controlled release drug product, swallow whole. Kadian® and Avinza® can be opened and sprinkled on applesauce; do not crush or chew the beads. Contents of Kadian® capsules may be opened and sprinkled over 10 mL water and flushed through prewetted 16F gastrostomy tube; do not administer Kadian® through nasogastric tube.

I.V.: When giving morphine I.V. push, it is best to first dilute with sterile water or NS for a final concentration of 1-2 mg/mL and then administer slowly.

Epidural: Use preservative-free solutions for intrathecal or epidural use.

Monitoring Parameters Pain relief, respiratory and mental status, blood pressure

Astromorph/PF™, Duramorph®, Infumorph®: Patients should be observed in a fully-equipped and staffed environment for at least 24 hours following initiation, and as appropriate for the first several days after catheter implantation.

Test Interactions Some quinolones may produce a false-positive urine screening result for opiates using commercially-available immunoassay kits. This has been demonstrated most consistently for levofloxacin and ofloxacin, but other quinolones have shown cross-reactivity in certain assay kits. Confirmation of positive opiate screens by more specific methods should be considered.

Special Geriatric Considerations The elderly may be particularly susceptible to the CNS depressant and constipating effects of narcotics. For chronic administration of narcotic analgesics, morphine is preferable in the elderly due to its pharmacokinetics and side effect profile as compared to meperidine and methadone.

Controlled Substance C-II

Dosage Forms Excipient information presented when available (limited, particularly for generics); consult specific product labeling. [DSC] = Discontinued product

Capsule, extended release, oral, as sulfate:

AVINza®: 30 mg, 45 mg, 60 mg, 75 mg, 90 mg, 120 mg

Kadian®: 10 mg, 20 mg, 30 mg, 50 mg, 60 mg, 80 mg, 100 mg, 200 mg

Injection, solution, as sulfate: 1 mg/mL (10 mL); 2 mg/mL (1 mL); 4 mg/mL (1 mL); 5 mg/mL (1 mL); 8 mg/mL (1 mL); 10 mg/mL (1 mL, 10 mL); 10 mg/0.7 mL (0.7 mL); 15 mg/mL (1 mL, 20 mL); 25 mg/mL (4 mL, 10 mL); 50 mg/mL (20 mL, 50 mL)

Injection, solution, as sulfate [preservative free]: 0.5 mg/mL (10 mL); 1 mg/mL (10 mL); 25 mg/mL (10 mL)

Injection, solution, as sulfate [epidural or intrathecal infusion via microinfusion device, preservative free]:

Infumorph 200: 10 mg/mL (20 mL)

Infumorph 500: 25 mg/mL (20 mL)

Injection, solution, as sulfate [epidural, intrathecal, or I.V. infusion, preservative free]:

Astramorph®/PF: 0.5 mg/mL (2 mL, 10 mL); 1 mg/mL (2 mL, 10 mL)

Duramorph: 0.5 mg/mL (10 mL); 1 mg/mL (10 mL)

Injection, solution, as sulfate [for PCA pump]: 1 mg/mL (30 mL)
Injection, solution, as sulfate [for PCA pump, preservative free]: 0.5 mg/mL (30 mL [DSC]); 1 mg/mL (30 mL); 5 mg/mL (30 mL)
Solution, oral, as sulfate: 10 mg/5 mL (5 mL, 100 mL, 500 mL); 20 mg/5 mL (100 mL, 500 mL)
Solution, oral, as sulfate [concentrate]: 100 mg/5 mL (15 mL, 30 mL, 120 mL, 240 mL)
Suppository, rectal, as sulfate: 5 mg (12s); 10 mg (12s); 20 mg (12s); 30 mg (12s)
Tablet, oral, as sulfate: 15 mg, 30 mg
Tablet, controlled release, oral, as sulfate: 15 mg [DSC], 30 mg [DSC], 60 mg [DSC], 100 mg [DSC], 200 mg [DSC]
MS Contin®: 15 mg, 30 mg, 60 mg, 100 mg, 200 mg
Tablet, extended release, oral, as sulfate: 15 mg, 30 mg, 60 mg, 100 mg, 200 mg
Tablet, sustained release, oral, as sulfate:
Oramorph® SR: 15 mg, 30 mg, 60 mg, 100 mg
Dosage Forms: Canada Excipient information presented when available (limited, particularly for generics); consult specific product labeling.
Solution, oral, as sulfate:
Doloral: 1 mg/mL (10 mL, 250 mL, 500 mL); 5 mg/mL (10 mL, 250 mL, 500 mL)
Selected References
American Geriatrics Society Panel on Pharmacological Management of Persistent Pain in Older Persons, "Pharmacological Management of Persistent Pain in Older Persons," *J Am Geriatr Soc*, 2009, 57(8):1331-46.

Morphine (Liposomal) (MOR feen)

Related Information
Opioid Analgesics *on page 2013*
Medication Safety Issues
Sound-alike/look-alike issues:
Morphine may be confused with HYDROmorphone
Morphine sulfate may be confused with magnesium sulfate
MSO$_4$ and MS are error-prone abbreviations (mistaken as magnesium sulfate)
Brand Names: U.S. DepoDur®
Index Terms Extended Release Epidural Morphine; MS (error-prone abbreviation and should not be used); MSO$_4$ (error-prone abbreviation and should not be used)
Generic Availability (U.S.) No
Pharmacologic Category Analgesic, Opioid
Use Epidural (lumbar) single-dose management of surgical pain
Contraindications Hypersensitivity to morphine sulfate or any component of the formulation; severe respiratory depression (without resuscitative equipment); acute or severe asthma; known or suspected paralytic ileus; patients with head injuries or increased intracranial pressure; circulatory shock; upper airway obstruction.
Warnings/Precautions May cause respiratory depression. Risk increased in elderly patients, debilitated patients, and patients with conditions associated with hypoxia or hypercapnia. Prolonged, serious respiratory depression has been associated with nonapproved routes of administration (subarachnoid puncture and intrathecal). Although respiratory depression is reversible with naloxone, patients must be monitored for at least 48 hours due to the duration of action of the liposomal formulation and the potential for rebound sedation. Use with caution in patients with pre-existing respiratory compromise (hypoxia and/or hypercapnia), COPD or other obstructive pulmonary disease, and kyphoscoliosis or other skeletal disorder which may alter respiratory function.

May cause CNS depression and/or hypotension; use with caution in patients with hypovolemia, cardiovascular disease (including acute MI), circulatory shock, or drugs which may exaggerate hypotensive effects (including phenothiazines or general anesthetics). Use with caution in patients with CNS depression or coma. May cause orthostatic hypotension and syncope in ambulatory patients.

Use with caution in patients with hypersensitivity reactions to other phenanthrene derivative opioid agonists (codeine, hydrocodone, hydromorphone, levorphanol, oxycodone, oxymorphone). Use with caution in patients with biliary tract dysfunction and acute pancreatitis. Use may cause constriction of sphincter of Oddi diminishing biliary and pancreatic secretions. May obscure diagnosis or clinical course of patients with acute abdominal conditions. May worsen gastrointestinal ileus due to the effects on GI motility. Use with caution in patients with adrenal insufficiency, including Addison's disease. Use with caution in patients with severe hepatic impairment, renal impairment, prostatic hyperplasia, and/or urinary stricture. Use with caution in patients with seizure disorders or thyroid disease.

Use with caution in the elderly; may be more sensitive to adverse effects.

For lumbar administration only. Monitor for delayed sedation. Physician should evaluate patient for contraindications for epidural injection (eg, anticoagulant therapy, bleeding, diathesis). Intrathecal administration has resulted in prolonged respiratory depression. Freezing may adversely affect modified-release mechanism of drug; check freeze indicator within carton prior to administration. To minimize the pharmacokinetic interaction resulting in higher peak serum concentrations of morphine, administer the test dose of the local anesthetic at least 15 minutes prior to administration. Use of DepoDur® with epidural local anesthetics has not been studied. Other medications should not be administered into the epidural space for at least 48 hours after administration.

Adverse Reactions (Reflective of adult population; not specific for elderly)

>10%:
  Cardiovascular: Hypotension
  Central nervous system: Dizziness, fever, headache
  Dermatologic: Pruritus
  Gastrointestinal: Constipation, nausea, vomiting
  Genitourinary: Urinary retention (may be prolonged)
  Hematologic: Anemia
  Local: Pain at injection site
  Neuromuscular & skeletal: Weakness
  Respiratory: Oxygen saturation decreased

2% to 10%:
  Cardiovascular: Bradycardia, hypertension, tachycardia
  Central nervous system: Anxiety, insomnia, somnolence
  Gastrointestinal: Abdominal distension, dyspepsia, flatulence, paralytic ileus
  Genitourinary: Bladder spasm, oliguria
  Hematologic: Hematocrit decreased
  Neuromuscular & skeletal: Back pain, hypoesthesia, paresthesia, rigors
  Respiratory: Dyspnea, hypercapnea, hypoxia, respiratory depression
  Miscellaneous: Sweating increased

Drug Interactions

Metabolism/Transport Effects Substrate of CYP2D6 (minor)

Avoid Concomitant Use There are no known interactions where it is recommended to avoid concomitant use.

Increased Effect/Toxicity

Morphine (Liposomal) may increase the levels/effects of: Alcohol (Ethyl); Alvimopan; CNS Depressants; Desmopressin; Selective Serotonin Reuptake Inhibitors; Thiazide Diuretics

The levels/effects of Morphine (Liposomal) may be increased by: Amphetamines; Antipsychotic Agents (Phenothiazines); Droperidol; HydrOXYzine; Succinylcholine

Decreased Effect

Morphine (Liposomal) may decrease the levels/effects of: Pegvisomant

The levels/effects of Morphine (Liposomal) may be decreased by: Ammonium Chloride; Mixed Agonist / Antagonist Opioids; Peginterferon Alfa-2b

Stability DepoDur®: Store under refrigeration at 2°C to 8°C (36°F to 46°F); keep vials in carton during refrigeration; do not freeze. Check freeze indicator before administration; do not administer if bulb is pink or purple. May store at room temperature for up to 30 days in sealed, unopened vials. DepoDur® may be diluted in preservative-free NS to a volume of 5 mL. Gently invert to suspend particles prior to removal from vial. Once vial is opened, use within 4 hours.

Mechanism of Action Binds to opiate receptors in the CNS, causing inhibition of ascending pain pathways, altering the perception of and response to pain; produces generalized CNS depression

Pharmacodynamics/Kinetics

Duration (patient dependent; dosing must be individualized): >48 hours
Distribution: V_d: 3-4 L/kg; binds to opioid receptors in the CNS and periphery (eg, GI tract)
Protein binding: 30% to 35%
Metabolism: Hepatic via conjugation with glucuronic acid primarily to morphine-6-glucoronide (active analgesic) morphine-3-glucoronide (inactive as analgesic); minor metabolites include morphine-3-6-diglucoronide; other minor metabolites include normorphine (active) and morphine 3-ethereal sulfate
Excretion: Urine (primarily as morphine-3-glucoronide, ~2% to 12% excreted unchanged); feces (~7% to 10%). It has been suggested that accumulation of morphine-6-glucoronide might cause toxicity with renal insufficiency. All of the metabolites (ie, morphine-3-glucuronide, morphine-6-glucuronide, and normorphine) have been suggested as possible causes of neurotoxicity (eg, myoclonus).

◄ **Dosage**

Geriatric Refer to adult dosing. Use with caution; may require reduced dosage in the elderly and debilitated patients.

Adult Surgical anesthesia: Epidural: Single-dose (extended release, DepoDur®): Lumbar epidural only; not recommended in patients <18 years of age:

Cesarean section: 10 mg (after clamping umbilical cord)

Lower abdominal/pelvic surgery: 10-15 mg

Major orthopedic surgery of lower extremity: 15 mg; **Note:** Some patients may benefit from a 20 mg dose; however, the incidence of adverse effects may be increased.

To minimize the pharmacokinetic interaction resulting in higher peak serum concentrations of morphine, administer the test dose of the local anesthetic at least 15 minutes prior to administration. Use with epidural local anesthetics has not been studied. Other medications should not be administered into the epidural space for at least 48 hours after administration.

Renal Impairment Dosing adjustment is not required.

Hepatic Impairment Dosing adjustment is not required.

Administration Epidural: Intended for lumbar administration only. Thoracic administration has not been studied. May be administered undiluted or diluted up to 5 mL total volume in preservative-free NS. Do not use an in-line filter during administration. Not for I.V., I.M., or intrathecal administration.

Resedation may occur following epidural administration; this may be delayed ≥48 hours in patients receiving extended-release injections.

Administration of an epidural test dose (lidocaine 1.5% and epinephrine 1:200,000) may affect the release of morphine from the liposomal preparation. Delaying the dose for an interval of at least 15 minutes following the test dose minimizes this pharmacokinetic interaction. Except for a test dose, other epidural local anesthetics or medications should not be administered epidurally before or after this product for a minimum of 48 hours.

Monitoring Parameters Pain relief, respiratory and mental status, blood pressure; patient should be monitored for at least 48 hours following administration.

Controlled Substance C-II

Dosage Forms Excipient information presented when available (limited, particularly for generics); consult specific product labeling.

Injection, extended release liposomal suspension, as sulfate [lumbar epidural injection, preservative free]:

DepoDur®: 10 mg/mL (1 mL, 1.5 mL)

◆ **Mosco® Callus & Corn Remover [OTC]** *see* Salicylic Acid *on page 1648*
◆ **Mosco® One Step Corn Remover [OTC]** *see* Salicylic Acid *on page 1648*
◆ **Motrin® Children's [OTC]** *see* Ibuprofen *on page 908*
◆ **Motrin® IB [OTC]** *see* Ibuprofen *on page 908*
◆ **Motrin® Infants' [OTC]** *see* Ibuprofen *on page 908*
◆ **Motrin® Junior [OTC]** *see* Ibuprofen *on page 908*
◆ **Mouthkote® [OTC]** *see* Saliva Substitute *on page 1652*
◆ **Moxatag™** *see* Amoxicillin *on page 114*
◆ **Moxeza™** *see* Moxifloxacin (Ophthalmic) *on page 1249*

Moxifloxacin (Systemic) (moxs i FLOKS a sin)

Medication Safety Issues
Sound-alike/look-alike issues:
Avelox® may be confused with Avonex®

Brand Names: U.S. Avelox®; Avelox® ABC Pack; Avelox® I.V.

Brand Names: Canada Avelox®; Avelox® I.V.

Index Terms Moxifloxacin Hydrochloride

Generic Availability (U.S.) No

Pharmacologic Category Antibiotic, Quinolone; Respiratory Fluoroquinolone

Use Treatment of mild-to-moderate community-acquired pneumonia, including multidrug-resistant *Streptococcus pneumoniae* (MDRSP); acute bacterial exacerbation of chronic bronchitis; acute bacterial sinusitis; complicated and uncomplicated skin and skin structure infections; complicated intra-abdominal infections

Unlabeled/Investigational Use Treatment of *Legionella* pneumonia

Medication Guide Available Yes

Contraindications Hypersensitivity to moxifloxacin, other quinolone antibiotics, or any component of the formulation

Warnings/Precautions [U.S. Boxed Warning]: There have been reports of tendon inflammation and/or rupture with quinolone antibiotics; risk may be increased with concurrent corticosteroids, organ transplant recipients, and in patients >60 years of age. Rupture of the Achilles tendon sometimes requiring surgical repair has been reported most frequently; but other tendon sites (eg, rotator cuff, biceps) have also been reported. Strenuous physical activity, rheumatoid arthritis, and renal impairment may be an independent risk factor for tendonitis. Discontinue at first sign of tendon inflammation or pain. Tendon rupture may occur even after discontinuation of therapy. Use with caution in patients with rheumatoid arthritis or renal impairment; may increase risk of tendon rupture.

Use with caution in patients with significant bradycardia or acute myocardial ischemia. Moxifloxacin causes a concentration-dependent QT prolongation. Do not exceed recommended dose or infusion rate. Avoid use with uncorrected hypokalemia, with other drugs that prolong the QT interval or induce bradycardia, or with class Ia or III antiarrhythmic agents. Use with caution in individuals at risk of seizures (CNS disorders or concurrent therapy with medications which may lower seizure threshold). Potential for seizures, although very rare, may be increased with concomitant NSAID therapy. Discontinue in patients who experience significant CNS adverse effects (dizziness, hallucinations, suicidal ideation or actions). Use with caution in patients with mild, moderate, or severe hepatic impairment or liver cirrhosis; may increase the risk of QT prolongation. Fulminant hepatitis potentially leading to liver failure (including fatalities) has been reported with use. Use with caution in diabetes; glucose regulation may be altered.

Fluoroquinolones have been associated with the development of serious, and sometimes fatal, hypoglycemia, most often in elderly diabetics, but also in patients without diabetes. This occurred most frequently with gatifloxacin (no longer available systemically) but may occur at a lower frequency with other quinolones.

Severe hypersensitivity reactions, including anaphylaxis, have occurred with quinolone therapy. Reactions may present as typical allergic symptoms after a single dose, or may manifest as severe idiosyncratic dermatologic, vascular, pulmonary, renal, hepatic, and/or hematologic events, usually after multiple doses. Prompt discontinuation of drug should occur if skin rash or other symptoms arise. Avoid excessive sunlight and take precautions to limit exposure (eg, loose fitting clothing, sunscreen); may cause moderate-to-severe phototoxicity reactions. Discontinue use if photosensitivity occurs. Prolonged use may result in fungal or bacterial superinfection, including *C. difficile*-associated diarrhea (CDAD) and pseudomembranous colitis; CDAD has been observed >2 months postantibiotic treatment. **[U.S. Boxed Warning]: Quinolones may exacerbate myasthenia gravis; avoid use (rare, potentially life-threatening weakness of respiratory muscles may occur).** Peripheral neuropathy may rarely occur. Hemolytic reactions may (rarely) occur with quinolone use in patients with latent or actual G6PD deficiency. Adverse effects (eg, tendon rupture, QT changes) may be increased in the elderly. Some quinolones may exacerbate myasthenia gravis, use with caution (rare, potentially life-threatening weakness of respiratory muscles may occur).

Adverse Reactions (Reflective of adult population; not specific for elderly)
2% to 10%:
  Central nervous system: Dizziness (2%)
  Endocrine & metabolic: Serum chloride increased (≥2%), serum ionized calcium increased (≥2%), serum glucose decreased (≥2%)
  Gastrointestinal: Nausea (6%), diarrhea (5%), amylase decreased (≥2%)
  Hematologic: Decreased serum levels of the following (≥2%): Basophils, eosinophils, hemoglobin, RBC, neutrophils; increased serum levels of the following (≥2%): MCH, neutrophils, WBC
  Hepatic: Bilirubin decreased/increased (≥2%)
  Renal: Serum albumin increased (≥2%)
  Respiratory: PO_2 decreased (≥2%)
0.1% to <2%:
  Cardiovascular: Cardiac arrhythmias, palpitation, QT_c prolongation, tachycardia, vasodilation
  Central nervous system: Anxiety, headache, insomnia, malaise, nervousness, pain, somnolence, vertigo
  Dermatologic: Pruritus, rash (maculopapular, purpuric, pustular), urticaria
  Gastrointestinal: Abdominal pain, amylase increased, anorexia, constipation, dyspepsia, flatulence, glossitis, lactic dehydrogenase increased, stomatitis, taste perversion, vomiting, xerostomia
  Genitourinary: Vaginal moniliasis, vaginitis
  Hematologic: Eosinophilia, leukopenia, prothrombin time prolonged, increased INR, thrombocythemia
  Hepatic: GGTP increased, liver function test abnormal
  Local: Injection site reaction

Neuromuscular & skeletal: Arthralgia, myalgia, tremor, weakness

Respiratory: Pharyngitis, pneumonia, rhinitis, sinusitis

Miscellaneous: Allergic reaction, infection, diaphoresis, oral moniliasis

Drug Interactions

Avoid Concomitant Use

Avoid concomitant use of Moxifloxacin (Systemic) with any of the following: Artemether; BCG; Dronedarone; Lumefantrine; Nilotinib; Pimozide; QUEtiapine; QuiNINE; Tetrabenazine; Thioridazine; Toremifene; Vandetanib; Vemurafenib; Ziprasidone

Increased Effect/Toxicity

Moxifloxacin (Systemic) may increase the levels/effects of: Corticosteroids (Systemic); Dronedarone; Pimozide; Porfimer; QTc-Prolonging Agents; QuiNINE; Sulfonylureas; Tetrabenazine; Thioridazine; Toremifene; Vandetanib; Vemurafenib; Vitamin K Antagonists; Ziprasidone

The levels/effects of Moxifloxacin (Systemic) may be increased by: Alfuzosin; Artemether; Chloroquine; Ciprofloxacin; Ciprofloxacin (Systemic); Gadobutrol; Insulin; Lumefantrine; Nilotinib; Nonsteroidal Anti-Inflammatory Agents; Probenecid; QUEtiapine; QuiNINE

Decreased Effect

Moxifloxacin (Systemic) may decrease the levels/effects of: BCG; Mycophenolate; Sulfonylureas; Typhoid Vaccine

The levels/effects of Moxifloxacin (Systemic) may be decreased by: Antacids; Didanosine; Iron Salts; Lanthanum; Magnesium Salts; Quinapril; Sevelamer; Sucralfate; Zinc Salts

Ethanol/Nutrition/Herb Interactions Food: Absorption is not affected by administration with a high-fat meal or yogurt.

Stability Store at controlled room temperature of 25°C (77°F). Do not refrigerate infusion solution.

Mechanism of Action Moxifloxacin is a DNA gyrase inhibitor, and also inhibits topoisomerase IV. DNA gyrase (topoisomerase II) is an essential bacterial enzyme that maintains the superhelical structure of DNA. DNA gyrase is required for DNA replication and transcription, DNA repair, recombination, and transposition; inhibition is bactericidal.

Pharmacodynamics/Kinetics

Absorption: Well absorbed; not affected by high-fat meal or yogurt

Distribution: V_d: 1.7 to 2.7 L/kg; tissue concentrations often exceed plasma concentrations in respiratory tissues, alveolar macrophages, abdominal tissues/fluids, uterine tissue (endometrium, myometrium), and sinus tissues

Protein binding: ~30% to 50%

Metabolism: Hepatic (~52% of dose) via glucuronide (~14%) and sulfate (~38%) conjugation

Bioavailability: ~90%

Half-life elimination: Single dose: Oral: 12-16 hours; I.V.: 8-15 hours

Excretion: Urine (as unchanged drug [20%] and glucuronide conjugates); feces (as unchanged drug [25%] and sulfate conjugates)

Dosage

Geriatric & Adult

Acute bacterial sinusitis: Oral, I.V.: 400 mg every 24 hours for 10 days

Chronic bronchitis, acute bacterial exacerbation: Oral, I.V.: 400 mg every 24 hours for 5 days

Intra-abdominal infections, complicated: 400 mg every 24 hours for 5-14 days (initiate with I.V.); **Note:** 2010 IDSA guidelines recommend a treatment duration of 4-7 days (provided source controlled) for community-acquired, mild-to-moderate IAI

Pneumonia, community-acquired (including MDRSP): Oral, I.V.: 400 mg every 24 hours for 7-14 days

Skin and skin structure infections: Oral, I.V.:

Complicated: 400 mg every 24 hours for 7-21 days

Uncomplicated: 400 mg every 24 hours for 7 days

Renal Impairment No dosage adjustment required in renal impairment.

Poorly dialyzed; no supplemental dose or dosage adjustment necessary, including patients on intermittent hemodialysis, peritoneal dialysis, or continuous renal replacement therapy (eg, CVVHD).

Hepatic Impairment No dosage adjustment is required in mild, moderate, or severe hepatic insufficiency (Child-Pugh class A, B, or C); however, use with caution in this patient population secondary to the risk of QT prolongation.

Administration Administer without regard to meals.

I.V.: Infuse over 60 minutes; do not infuse by rapid or bolus intravenous infusion

Monitoring Parameters WBC, signs of infection

Test Interactions Some quinolones may produce a false-positive urine screening result for opiates using commercially-available immunoassay kits. This has been demonstrated most consistently for levofloxacin and ofloxacin, but other quinolones have shown cross-reactivity in certain assay kits. Confirmation of positive opiate screens by more specific methods should be considered.

Special Geriatric Considerations See Warnings/Precautions regarding tendon rupture in patients >60 years of age. No dosage adjustments are required based on age.

Dosage Forms Excipient information presented when available (limited, particularly for generics); consult specific product labeling.

Infusion, premixed in sodium chloride 0.8% [preservative free]:
Avelox® I.V.: 400 mg (250 mL) [contains sodium ~787 mg (34.2 mEq)/250 mL]

Tablet, oral:
Avelox®: 400 mg
Avelox® ABC Pack: 400 mg

Selected References
Khaliq Y and Zhanel GG, "Fluoroquinolone-Associated Tendinopathy: A Critical Review of the Literature," *Clin Infect Dis*, 2003, 36(11):1404-10.

Moxifloxacin (Ophthalmic) (moxs i FLOKS a sin)

Medication Safety Issues
International issues:
Vigamox [U.S., Canada, and multiple international markets] may be confused with Fisamox brand name for amoxicillin [Australia]

Brand Names: U.S. Moxeza™; Vigamox®

Brand Names: Canada Vigamox®

Index Terms Moxifloxacin Hydrochloride

Generic Availability (U.S.) No

Pharmacologic Category Antibiotic, Ophthalmic; Antibiotic, Quinolone

Use Treatment of bacterial conjunctivitis caused by susceptible organisms

Dosage
Geriatric & Adult Bacterial conjunctivitis: Ophthalmic:
Moxeza™: Instill 1 drop into affected eye(s) 2 times/day for 7 days
Vigamox®: Instill 1 drop into affected eye(s) 3 times/day for 7 days

Dosage Forms Excipient information presented when available (limited, particularly for generics); consult specific product labeling.

Solution, ophthalmic [drops]:
Moxeza™: 0.5% (3 mL)
Vigamox®: 0.5% (3 mL)

- **Mucinex® Kid's Cough [OTC]** *see* Guaifenesin and Dextromethorphan *on page 848*
- **Mucinex® Kid's Cough Mini-Melts™ [OTC]** *see* Guaifenesin and Dextromethorphan *on page 848*
- **Mucinex® Maximum Strength [OTC]** *see* GuaiFENesin *on page 846*

Mucosal Barrier Gel, Oral (myoo KOH sul BAR ee er GEL, OR al)

Brand Names: U.S. Gelclair®
Index Terms Mucosal Bioadherent Gel
Pharmacologic Category Gastrointestinal Agent, Miscellaneous
Use Management of oral mucosal pain caused by oral mucositis/stomatitis (resulting from chemotherapy or radiation therapy), irritation due to oral surgery, traumatic ulcers caused by braces/ill-fitting dentures or disease, diffuse aphthous ulcers (canker sores)
Dosage
  Geriatric & Adult Mucosal protection: Oral: Gargle and spit the mixture of 1 single-use packet (15 mL) and water 3 times daily, or as needed. May be used undiluted if water is unavailable.
Special Geriatric Considerations No specific data for elderly patients available. No dosage change necessary.
Dosage Forms Excipient information presented when available (limited, particularly for generics); consult specific product labeling.
  Gel, oral [concentrate]:
    Gelclair®: 15 mL/packet (15s) [contains benzalkonium chloride, castor oil, propylene glycol, sodium benzoate]

- **Mucosal Bioadherent Gel** *see* Mucosal Barrier Gel, Oral *on page 1250*
- **Mucus Relief [OTC]** *see* GuaiFENesin *on page 846*
- **Multaq®** *see* Dronedarone *on page 575*
- **Multidex® [OTC]** *see* Maltodextrin *on page 1114*
- **Mumps, Measles and Rubella Vaccines** *see* Measles, Mumps, and Rubella Virus Vaccine *on page 1116*

Mupirocin (myoo PEER oh sin)

Medication Safety Issues
  Sound-alike/look-alike issues:
    Bactroban® may be confused with bacitracin, baclofen, Bactrim™
Brand Names: U.S. Bactroban Cream®; Bactroban Nasal®; Bactroban®; Centany®; Centany® AT
Brand Names: Canada Bactroban®
Index Terms Mupirocin Calcium; Pseudomonic Acid A
Generic Availability (U.S.) Yes: Topical ointment
Pharmacologic Category Antibiotic, Topical
Use
  Intranasal: Eradication of nasal colonization with MRSA in adult patients and healthcare workers
  Topical: Treatment of impetigo or secondary infected traumatic skin lesions due to *S. aureus* and *S. pyogenes*
Unlabeled/Investigational Use Intranasal: Surgical prophylaxis to prevent wound infections
Contraindications Hypersensitivity to mupirocin or any component of the formulation
Warnings/Precautions Potentially toxic amounts of polyethylene glycol contained in some topical products may be absorbed percutaneously in patients with extensive burns or open wounds; use caution with renal impairment. Prolonged use may result in over growth of nonsusceptible organisms. For external use only; avoid contact with eyes. Not for treatment of pressure sores. If skin irritation occurs, discontinue use.
Adverse Reactions (Reflective of adult population; not specific for elderly) Frequency not defined.
  Central nervous system: Dizziness, headache
  Dermatologic: Cellulitis, dermatitis, dry skin, erythema, hives, pruritus, rash
  Gastrointestinal: Abdominal pain, diarrhea, nausea, taste perversion, ulcerative stomatitis, xerostomia
  Local: Burning, edema, pain, stinging, tenderness
  Ocular: Blepharitis
  Otic: Ear pain
  Respiratory: Cough, pharyngitis, rhinitis, upper respiratory tract congestion
  Miscellaneous: Secondary wound infection

Drug Interactions

Avoid Concomitant Use
Avoid concomitant use of Mupirocin with any of the following: BCG

Increased Effect/Toxicity There are no known significant interactions involving an increase in effect.

Decreased Effect
Mupirocin may decrease the levels/effects of: BCG; Typhoid Vaccine

Mechanism of Action Binds to bacterial isoleucyl transfer-RNA synthetase resulting in the inhibition of protein synthesis

Pharmacodynamics/Kinetics

Absorption: Topical: Penetrates outer layers of skin; systemic absorption minimal through intact skin

Metabolism: Skin: 3% to monic acid (inactive)

Excretion: Urine

Dosage

Geriatric & Adult

Impetigo: Topical: Ointment: Apply to affected area 3 times/day; re-evaluate after 3-5 days if no clinical response

Secondary skin infections: Topical: Cream: Apply to affected area 3 times/day for 10 days; re-evaluate after 3-5 days if no clinical response

Elimination of MRSA colonization: Intranasal: Approximately one-half of the ointment from the single-use tube should be applied into one nostril and the other half into the other nostril twice daily for 5 days

Administration

Intranasal ointment: After application into nostrils, press sides of nose together and gently massage to spread ointment throughout the insides of the nostrils; discard tube after use

Topical cream, ointment: For external use only; area may be covered with gauze if desired

Monitoring Parameters If no clinical response in 3-5 days, re-evaluate use

Pharmacotherapy Pearls Contains polyethylene glycol vehicle

Special Geriatric Considerations Not for treatment of pressure sores.

Dosage Forms Excipient information presented when available (limited, particularly for generics); consult specific product labeling.

Cream, topical, as calcium [strength expressed as base]:
Bactroban Cream®: 2% (15 g, 30 g) [contains benzyl alcohol]

Ointment, topical: 2% (22 g)
Bactroban®: 2% (22 g) [contains polyethylene glycol]
Centany®: 2% (30 g)
Centany® AT: 2% (1s) [kit includes Centany® ointment (30 g),12 gauze pads, and 24 cloth tape strips]

Ointment, intranasal, as calcium [strength expressed as base]:
Bactroban Nasal®: 2% (1 g)

◆ **Mysoline®** *see* Primidone *on page* 1517
◆ **Nabi-HB®** *see* Hepatitis B Immune Globulin (Human) *on page* 867

Nabumetone (na BYOO me tone)

Brand Names: Canada Apo-Nabumetone®; Gen-Nabumetone; Mylan-Nabumetone; Novo-Nabumetone; Relafen®; Rhoxal-nabumetone; Sandoz-Nabumetone
Index Terms Relafen
Generic Availability (U.S.) Yes
Pharmacologic Category Nonsteroidal Anti-inflammatory Drug (NSAID), Oral
Use Management of osteoarthritis and rheumatoid arthritis
Unlabeled/Investigational Use Treatment of sunburn, mild to moderate pain
Medication Guide Available Yes
Contraindications Hypersensitivity to nabumetone, aspirin, other NSAIDs, or any component of the formulation; perioperative pain in the setting of coronary artery bypass graft (CABG) surgery
Warnings/Precautions [U.S. Boxed Warning]: NSAIDs are associated with an increased risk of adverse cardiovascular thrombotic events, including MI and stroke. Risk may be increased with duration of use or pre-existing cardiovascular risk factors or disease. Carefully evaluate individual cardiovascular risk profiles prior to prescribing. May cause new-onset hypertension or worsening of existing hypertension. Use caution with fluid retention. Avoid use in heart failure. Concurrent administration of ibuprofen, and potentially other nonselective NSAIDs, may interfere with aspirin's cardioprotective effect. **[U.S. Boxed Warning]: Use is contraindicated for treatment of perioperative pain in the setting of coronary artery bypass graft (CABG) surgery.** Risk of MI and stroke may be increased with use following CABG surgery.

Platelet adhesion and aggregation may be decreased; may prolong bleeding time; patients with coagulation disorders or who are receiving anticoagulants should be monitored closely. Anemia may occur; patients on long-term NSAID therapy should be monitored for anemia. Rarely, NSAID use may cause severe blood dyscrasias (eg, agranulocytosis, aplastic anemia, thrombocytopenia).

NSAID use may compromise existing renal function; dose-dependent decreases in prostaglandin synthesis may result from NSAID use, reducing renal blood flow which may cause renal decompensation. NSAID use may increase the risk for hyperkalemia. Patients with impaired renal function, dehydration, heart failure, liver dysfunction, those taking diuretics, and ACE inhibitors, and the elderly are at greater risk of renal toxicity and hyperkalemia. Rehydrate patient before starting therapy; monitor renal function closely. Not recommended for use in patients with advanced renal disease. Long-term NSAID use may result in renal papillary necrosis.

[U.S. Boxed Warning]: NSAIDs may increase risk of gastrointestinal irritation, inflammation, ulceration, bleeding, and perforation. These events may occur at any time during therapy and without warning. Use caution with a history of GI disease (bleeding or ulcers), concurrent therapy with aspirin, anticoagulants and/or corticosteroids, smoking, use of alcohol, the elderly or debilitated patients. When used concomitantly with ≤325 mg of aspirin, a substantial increase in the risk of gastrointestinal complications (eg, ulcer) occurs; concomitant gastroprotective therapy (eg, proton pump inhibitors) is recommended (Bhatt, 2008).

Use the lowest effective dose for the shortest duration of time, consistent with individual patient goals, to reduce risk of cardiovascular or GI adverse events. Alternate therapies should be considered for patients at high risk.

NSAIDs may cause serious skin adverse events including exfoliative dermatitis, Stevens-Johnson syndrome (SJS) and toxic epidermal necrolysis (TEN); discontinue use at first sign of skin rash or hypersensitivity. Anaphylactoid reactions may occur, even without prior exposure; patients with "aspirin triad" (bronchial asthma, aspirin intolerance, rhinitis) may be at increased risk. Do not use in patients who experience bronchospasm, asthma, rhinitis, or urticaria with NSAID or aspirin therapy. Use caution in other forms of asthma.

Use with caution in patients with decreased hepatic function. Closely monitor patients with any abnormal LFT. Severe hepatic reactions (eg, fulminant hepatitis, liver failure) have occurred with NSAID use, rarely; discontinue if signs or symptoms of liver disease develop, or if systemic manifestations occur.

NSAIDS may cause drowsiness, dizziness, blurred vision and other neurologic effects which may impair physical or mental abilities; patients must be cautioned about performing tasks which require mental alertness (eg, operating machinery or driving). Discontinue use with blurred or diminished vision and perform ophthalmologic exam. Monitor vision with long-term therapy.

The elderly are at increased risk for adverse effects (especially peptic ulceration, CNS effects, renal toxicity) from NSAIDs even at low doses.

Withhold for at least 4-6 half-lives prior to surgical or dental procedures. May cause photosensitivity reactions.

Adverse Reactions (Reflective of adult population; not specific for elderly)

>10%: Gastrointestinal: Diarrhea (14%), dyspepsia (13%), abdominal pain (12%)

1% to 10%:

Cardiovascular: Edema (3% to 9%)

Central nervous system: Dizziness (3% to 9%), headache (3% to 9%), fatigue (1% to 3%), insomnia (1% to 3%), nervousness (1% to 3%), somnolence (1% to 3%)

Dermatologic: Pruritus (3% to 9%), rash (3% to 9%)

Gastrointestinal: Constipation (3% to 9%), flatulence (3% to 9%), guaiac positive (3% to 9%), nausea (3% to 9%), gastritis (1% to 3%), stomatitis (1% to 3%), vomiting (1% to 3%), xerostomia (1% to 3%)

Otic: Tinnitus

Miscellaneous: Diaphoresis (1% to 3%)

Drug Interactions

Avoid Concomitant Use

Avoid concomitant use of Nabumetone with any of the following: Floctafenine; Ketorolac; Ketorolac (Nasal); Ketorolac (Systemic)

Increased Effect/Toxicity

Nabumetone may increase the levels/effects of: Aminoglycosides; Anticoagulants; Antiplatelet Agents; Bisphosphonate Derivatives; Collagenase (Systemic); CycloSPORINE; CycloSPORINE (Systemic); Deferasirox; Desmopressin; Digoxin; Drotrecogin Alfa; Eplerenone; Haloperidol; Ibritumomab; Lithium; Methotrexate; Nonsteroidal Anti-Inflammatory Agents; PEMEtrexed; Porfimer; Potassium-Sparing Diuretics; PRALAtrexate; Quinolone Antibiotics; Rivaroxaban; Salicylates; Thrombolytic Agents; Tositumomab and Iodine I 131 Tositumomab; Vancomycin; Vitamin K Antagonists

The levels/effects of Nabumetone may be increased by: ACE Inhibitors; Angiotensin II Receptor Blockers; Antidepressants (Tricyclic, Tertiary Amine); Corticosteroids (Systemic); Dasatinib; Floctafenine; Glucosamine; Herbs (Anticoagulant/Antiplatelet Properties); Ketorolac; Ketorolac (Nasal); Ketorolac (Systemic); Nonsteroidal Anti-Inflammatory Agents; Omega-3-Acid Ethyl Esters; Pentosan Polysulfate Sodium; Pentoxifylline; Probenecid; Prostacyclin Analogues; Selective Serotonin Reuptake Inhibitors; Serotonin/Norepinephrine Reuptake Inhibitors; Sodium Phosphates; Treprostinil; Vitamin E

Decreased Effect

Nabumetone may decrease the levels/effects of: ACE Inhibitors; Angiotensin II Receptor Blockers; Antiplatelet Agents; Beta-Blockers; Eplerenone; HydrALAZINE; Potassium-Sparing Diuretics; Salicylates; Selective Serotonin Reuptake Inhibitors; Thiazide Diuretics

The levels/effects of Nabumetone may be decreased by: Bile Acid Sequestrants; Nonsteroidal Anti-Inflammatory Agents; Salicylates

Ethanol/Nutrition/Herb Interactions

Ethanol: Avoid ethanol (may enhance gastric mucosal irritation).

Food: Nabumetone peak serum concentrations may be increased if taken with food or dairy products.

Herb/Nutraceutical: Avoid alfalfa, anise, bilberry, bladderwrack, bromelain, cat's claw, celery, chamomile, coleus, cordyceps, dong quai, evening primrose, fenugreek, feverfew, garlic, ginger, ginkgo biloba, ginseng (American, Panax, Siberian), grapeseed, green tea, guggul, horse chestnut seed, horseradish, licorice, prickly ash, red clover, reishi, SAMe (S-adenosylmethionine), sweet clover, turmeric, white willow (all have additional antiplatelet activity).

Mechanism of Action Reversibly inhibits cyclooxygenase-1 and 2 (COX-1 and 2) enzymes, which results in decreased formation of prostaglandin precursors; has antipyretic, analgesic, and anti-inflammatory properties

Other proposed mechanisms not fully elucidated (and possibly contributing to the anti-inflammatory effect to varying degrees), include inhibiting chemotaxis, altering lymphocyte activity, inhibiting neutrophil aggregation/activation, and decreasing proinflammatory cytokine levels.

◀ **Pharmacodynamics/Kinetics**
Onset of action: Several days
Distribution: Diffusion occurs readily into synovial fluid
V_d: 6MNA: 29-82 L
Protein binding: 6MNA: >99%
Metabolism: Prodrug, rapidly metabolized in the liver to an active metabolite [6-methoxy-2-naphthylacetic acid (6MNA)] and inactive metabolites; extensive first-pass effect
Half-life elimination: 6MNA: ~24 hours
Time to peak, serum: 6MNA: Oral: 2.5-4 hours; Synovial fluid: 4-12 hours
Excretion: 6MNA: Urine (80%) and feces (9%)

Dosage
Geriatric Refer to adult dosing; do not exceed 2000 mg/day.
Adult Osteoarthritis, rheumatoid arthritis: Oral: 1000 mg/day; an additional 500-1000 mg may be needed in some patients to obtain more symptomatic relief; may be administered once or twice daily; maximum dose: 2000 mg/day
Note: Patients <50 kg are less likely to require doses >1000 mg/day.
Renal Impairment In general, NSAIDs are not recommended for use in patients with advanced renal disease, but the manufacturer of nabumetone does provide some guidelines for adjustment in renal dysfunction:
Moderate impairment (Cl_{cr} 30-49 mL/minute): Initial dose: 750 mg/day; maximum dose: 1500 mg/day
Severe impairment (Cl_{cr} <30 mL/minute): Initial dose: 500 mg/day; maximum dose: 1000 mg/day

Monitoring Parameters Monitor response (pain, range of motion, grip strength, mobility, ADL function), inflammation; observe for weight gain, edema; monitor renal function; observe for bleeding, bruising; evaluate gastrointestinal effects (abdominal pain, bleeding, dyspepsia); mental confusion, disorientation, CBC, serum, creatinine, BUN, liver function tests; perform baseline renal testing in patients with renal dysfunction and repeat in 1-2 weeks to determine if deterioration has occurred

Pharmacotherapy Pearls There are no clinical guidelines to predict which NSAID will give response in a particular patient. Trials with each must be initiated until response determined. Consider dose, patient convenience, and cost.

Special Geriatric Considerations In trials with nabumetone, no significant differences were noted between young and the elderly in regards to efficacy and safety. However, the elderly are a high-risk population for adverse effects from NSAIDs. As much as 60% of elderly can develop peptic ulceration and/or hemorrhage asymptomatically. The concomitant use of H_2 blockers and sucralfate is not effective as prophylaxis with the exception of NSAID-induced duodenal ulcers which may be prevented by the use of ranitidine. Misoprostol and proton pump inhibitors are the only agents proven to help prevent the development of NSAID-induced ulcers. Also, concomitant disease and drug use contribute to the risk for GI adverse effects. Use lowest effective dose for shortest period possible. Consider renal function decline with age. Use of NSAIDs can compromise existing renal function especially when Cl_{cr} is ≤30 mL/minute. Tinnitus may be a difficult and unreliable indication of toxicity due to age-related hearing loss or eighth cranial nerve damage. CNS adverse effects such as confusion, agitation, and hallucination are generally seen in overdose or high dose situations, but the elderly may demonstrate these adverse effects at lower doses than younger adults.

Dosage Forms Excipient information presented when available (limited, particularly for generics); consult specific product labeling.
Tablet, oral: 500 mg, 750 mg

♦ **N-Acetyl-P-Aminophenol** see Acetaminophen on page 33
♦ **NaCl** see Sodium Chloride on page 1690

Nadolol (NAY doe lol)

Related Information
Beta-Blockers on page 2001
Medication Safety Issues
Sound-alike/look-alike issues:
Nadolol may be confused with Mandol®
Corgard® may be confused with Cognex®, Coreg®
Brand Names: U.S. Corgard®
Brand Names: Canada Alti-Nadolol; Apo-Nadol®; Corgard®; Novo-Nadolol
Generic Availability (U.S.) Yes
Pharmacologic Category Beta-Adrenergic Blocker, Nonselective
Use Treatment of hypertension and angina pectoris; prophylaxis of migraine headaches
Unlabeled/Investigational Use Primary and secondary prophylaxis of variceal hemorrhage

Contraindications Hypersensitivity to nadolol or any component of the formulation; bronchial asthma; sinus bradycardia; sinus node dysfunction; heart block greater than first degree (except in patients with a functioning artificial pacemaker); cardiogenic shock; uncompensated cardiac failure

Warnings/Precautions Consider pre-existing conditions such as sick sinus syndrome before initiating. Administer only with extreme caution in patients with compensated heart failure, monitor for a worsening of the condition. Efficacy in heart failure has not been established for nadolol. **[U.S. Boxed Warning]: Beta-blocker therapy should not be withdrawn abruptly (particularly in patients with CAD), but gradually tapered to avoid acute tachycardia, hypertension, and/or ischemia.** Chronic beta-blocker therapy should not be routinely withdrawn prior to major surgery. Use with caution in patients on concurrent digoxin, verapamil or diltiazem; bradycardia or heart block can occur. Use with caution in patients receiving inhaled anesthetic agents known to depress myocardial contractility. In general, patients with bronchospastic disease should not receive beta-blockers. Nadolol, if used at all, should be used cautiously in bronchospastic disease with close monitoring. Use cautiously in diabetics because it can mask prominent hypoglycemic symptoms. May mask signs of hyperthyroidism (eg, tachycardia); if hyperthyroidism is suspected, carefully manage and monitor; abrupt withdrawal may exacerbate symptoms of hyperthyroidism or precipitate thyroid storm. Use cautiously in the renally impaired (dosage adjustments are required). Use with caution in patients with myasthenia gravis, peripheral vascular disease, or psychiatric disease (may cause CNS depression). Bradycardia may be observed more frequently in elderly patients (>65 years of age); dosage reductions may be necessary. Adequate alpha-blockade is required prior to use of any beta-blocker for patients with untreated pheochromocytoma. May induce or exacerbate psoriasis. Use caution with history of severe anaphylaxis to allergens; patients taking beta-blockers may become more sensitive to repeated challenges. Treatment of anaphylaxis (eg, epinephrine) in patients taking beta-blockers may be ineffective or promote undesirable effects.

Adverse Reactions (Reflective of adult population; not specific for elderly)
>10%:
  Central nervous system: Drowsiness, insomnia
  Endocrine & metabolic: Decreased sexual ability
1% to 10%:
  Cardiovascular: Bradycardia, palpitation, edema, CHF, reduced peripheral circulation
  Central nervous system: Mental depression
  Gastrointestinal: Diarrhea or constipation, nausea, vomiting, stomach discomfort
  Respiratory: Bronchospasm
  Miscellaneous: Cold extremities

Drug Interactions
  Metabolism/Transport Effects Substrate of P-glycoprotein
  Avoid Concomitant Use
    Avoid concomitant use of Nadolol with any of the following: Floctafenine; Methacholine
  Increased Effect/Toxicity
    Nadolol may increase the levels/effects of: Alpha-/Beta-Agonists (Direct-Acting); Alpha1-Blockers; Alpha2-Agonists; Amifostine; Antihypertensives; Bupivacaine; Cardiac Glycosides; Fingolimod; Hypotensive Agents; Insulin; Lidocaine; Lidocaine (Systemic); Lidocaine (Topical); Mepivacaine; Methacholine; Midodrine; RiTUXimab; Sulfonylureas

    The levels/effects of Nadolol may be increased by: Acetylcholinesterase Inhibitors; Amiodarone; Anilidopiperidine Opioids; Calcium Channel Blockers (Dihydropyridine); Calcium Channel Blockers (Nondihydropyridine); Diazoxide; Dipyridamole; Disopyramide; Dronedarone; Floctafenine; Herbs (Hypotensive Properties); MAO Inhibitors; Pentoxifylline; P-Glycoprotein Inhibitors; Phosphodiesterase 5 Inhibitors; Prostacyclin Analogues; Reserpine
  Decreased Effect
    Nadolol may decrease the levels/effects of: Beta2-Agonists; Theophylline Derivatives

    The levels/effects of Nadolol may be decreased by: Herbs (Hypertensive Properties); Methylphenidate; Nonsteroidal Anti-Inflammatory Agents; P-Glycoprotein Inducers; Yohimbine

Ethanol/Nutrition/Herb Interactions Herb/Nutraceutical: Avoid dong quai if using for hypertension (has estrogenic activity). Avoid ephedra, garlic, yohimbe, ginseng (may worsen hypertension). Avoid natural licorice (causes sodium and water retention and increases potassium loss).

Mechanism of Action Competitively blocks response to beta$_1$- and beta$_2$-adrenergic stimulation; does not exhibit any membrane stabilizing or intrinsic sympathomimetic activity. Nonselective beta-adrenergic blockers (propranolol, nadolol) reduce portal pressure by producing splanchnic vasoconstriction (beta$_2$ effect) thereby reducing portal blood flow.

◄ **Pharmacodynamics/Kinetics**
Duration: 17-24 hours
Absorption: 30% to 40%
Distribution: V_d: 1.9 L/kg
Protein binding: 30%
Metabolism: Not metabolized
Half-life elimination: Adults: 10-24 hours; prolonged with renal impairment; End-stage renal disease: 45 hours
Time to peak, serum: 2-4 hours
Excretion: Urine (as unchanged drug)

Dosage

Geriatric Refer to adult dosing. In the management of hypertension, consider lower initial doses (eg, 20 mg/day) and titrate to response (Aronow, 2011).

Adult

Hypertension, angina: Oral: Initial: 40-80 mg/day, increase dosage gradually by 40-80 mg increments at 3- to 7-day intervals until optimum clinical response is obtained with profound slowing of heart rate. Doses up to 160-240 mg/day in angina and 240-320 mg/day in hypertension may be necessary. Doses as high as 640 mg/day have been used.
Usual dosage range (JNC 7): 40-120 mg once daily

Variceal hemorrhage prophylaxis (unlabeled use) (Garcia-Tsao, 2007): Oral:
Primary prophylaxis: Initial: 40 mg once daily; adjust to maximal tolerated dose. **Note:** Risk factors for hemorrhage include Child-Pugh class B/C or variceal red wale markings on endoscopy.
Secondary prophylaxis: Initial: 40 mg once daily; adjust to maximal tolerated dose

Renal Impairment
Cl_{cr} 31-40 mL/minute: Administer every 24-36 hours or administer 50% of normal dose.
Cl_{cr} 10-30 mL/minute: Administer every 24-48 hours or administer 50% of normal dose.
Cl_{cr} <10 mL/minute: Administer every 40-60 hours or administer 25% of normal dose.
Hemodialysis effects: Moderately dialyzable (20% to 50%) via hemodialysis. Administer dose postdialysis or administer 40 mg supplemental dose. Supplemental dose is not necessary following peritoneal dialysis.

Hepatic Impairment Reduced dose is probably necessary.

Administration May be administered without regard to meals.

Special Geriatric Considerations Due to alterations in the beta-adrenergic autonomic nervous system, beta-adrenergic blockade may result in less hemodynamic response than seen in younger adults. Studies indicate that despite decreased sensitivity to the chronotropic effects of beta-blockade with age, there appears to be an increased myocardial sensitivity to the negative inotropic effect during stress (ie, exercise). Controlled trials have shown the overall response rate for propranolol to be only 20% to 50% in elderly populations. Therefore, all beta-adrenergic blocking drugs may result in a decreased response as compared to younger adults. Must adjust dose for renal function.

Dosage Forms Excipient information presented when available (limited, particularly for generics); consult specific product labeling.
Tablet, oral: 20 mg, 40 mg, 80 mg
Corgard®: 20 mg, 40 mg, 80 mg [scored]

Selected References
Chobanian AV, Bakris GL, Black HR, et al, "The Seventh Report of the Joint National Committee on Prevention, Detection, Evaluation, and Treatment of High Blood Pressure: The JNC 7 Report," *JAMA*, 2003, 289(19):2560-71.
Fleisher LA, Beckman JA, Brown KA, et al, "ACC/AHA 2006 Guideline Update on Perioperative Cardiovascular Evaluation for Noncardiac Surgery: Focused Update on Perioperative Beta-Blocker Therapy. A Report of the American College of Cardiology/American Heart Association Task Force on Practice Guidelines (Writing Committee to Update the 2002 Guidelines on Perioperative Cardiovascular Evaluation for Noncardiac Surgery) Developed in Collaboration With the American Society of Echocardiography, American Society of Nuclear Cardiology, Heart Rhythm Society, Society of Cardiovascular Anesthesiologists, Society for Cardiovascular Angiography and Interventions, and Society for Vascular Medicine and Biology," *J Am Coll Cardiol*, 2006, 47(11):2343-55.
Garcia-Tsao G, Sanyal AJ, Grace ND, et al, "Prevention and Management of Gastroesophageal Varices and Variceal Hemorrhage in Cirrhosis," *Hepatology*, 2007, 46(3):922-38.
Juul AB, Wetterslev J, Gluud C, et al, "Effect of Perioperative Beta Blockade in Patients With Diabetes Undergoing Major Non-Cardiac Surgery: Randomized Placebo Controlled, Blinded Multicentre Trial. DIPOM Trial Group," *BMJ*, 2006, 332(7556):1482.

Nafcillin (naf SIL in)

Related Information
Antibiotic Treatment of Adults With Infective Endocarditis *on page 2053*
Brand Names: Canada Nallpen®; Unipen®
Index Terms Ethoxynaphthamido Penicillin Sodium; Nafcillin Sodium; Nallpen; Sodium Nafcillin
Generic Availability (U.S.) Yes

Pharmacologic Category Antibiotic, Penicillin

Use Treatment of infections such as osteomyelitis, septicemia, endocarditis, and CNS infections caused by susceptible strains of staphylococci species

Contraindications Hypersensitivity to nafcillin, or any component of the formulation, or penicillins; premixed injection may contain corn-derived dextrose and its use is contraindicated in patients with allergy to corn-related products

Warnings/Precautions Serious and occasionally severe or fatal hypersensitivity (anaphylactoid) reactions have been reported in patients on penicillin therapy, especially with a history of beta-lactam hypersensitivity, history of sensitivity to multiple allergens, or previous IgE-mediated reactions (eg, anaphylaxis, angioedema, urticaria). Use with caution in asthmatic patients. Extravasation of I.V. infusions should be avoided. Modification of dosage is necessary in patients with both severe renal and hepatic impairment. Prolonged use may result in fungal or bacterial superinfection, including *C. difficile*-associated diarrhea (CDAD) and pseudomembranous colitis; CDAD has been observed >2 months postantibiotic treatment.

Adverse Reactions (Reflective of adult population; not specific for elderly) Frequency not defined.

Central nervous system: Neurotoxicity (high doses)

Gastrointestinal: Pseudomembranous colitis

Hematologic: Agranulocytosis, bone marrow depression, neutropenia

Local: Inflammation, pain, phlebitis, skin sloughing, swelling, and thrombophlebitis at the injection site; oxacillin (less likely to cause phlebitis) is often preferred in pediatric patients; tissue necrosis with sloughing (SubQ extravasation)

Renal: Interstitial nephritis (rare), renal tubular damage (rare)

Miscellaneous: Anaphylaxis, hypersensitivity reactions (immediate and delayed; general incidence of 1% to 10% for penicillins), serum sickness

Drug Interactions

Metabolism/Transport Effects Induces CYP3A4 (strong)

Avoid Concomitant Use

Avoid concomitant use of Nafcillin with any of the following: BCG; Crizotinib; Dienogest; Dronedarone; Everolimus; Lapatinib; Lurasidone; Nilotinib; Pazopanib; Praziquantel; Ranolazine; Roflumilast; RomiDEPsin; Ticagrelor; Tolvaptan; Vandetanib

Increased Effect/Toxicity

Nafcillin may increase the levels/effects of: Clarithromycin; Methotrexate

The levels/effects of Nafcillin may be increased by: Clarithromycin; Probenecid

Decreased Effect

Nafcillin may decrease the levels/effects of: BCG; Brentuximab Vedotin; Calcium Channel Blockers; Clarithromycin; Contraceptives (Estrogens); Crizotinib; CycloSPORINE; CycloSPORINE (Systemic); CYP3A4 Substrates; Dienogest; Dronedarone; Everolimus; Exemestane; Gefitinib; GuanFACINE; Imatinib; Ixabepilone; Lapatinib; Linagliptin; Lurasidone; Maraviroc; Mycophenolate; Nilotinib; Pazopanib; Praziquantel; Ranolazine; Rivaroxaban; Roflumilast; RomiDEPsin; Saxagliptin; SORAfenib; Tadalafil; Ticagrelor; Tolvaptan; Typhoid Vaccine; Ulipristal; Vandetanib; Vemurafenib; Vitamin K Antagonists

The levels/effects of Nafcillin may be decreased by: Fusidic Acid; Tetracycline Derivatives

Stability

Premixed infusions: Store in a freezer at -20°C (4°F). Thaw at room temperature or under refrigeration only. Thawed bags are stable for 21 days under refrigeration or 72 hours at room temperature. Do not refreeze.

Vials: Reconstituted parenteral solution is stable for 3 days at room temperature and 7 days when refrigerated or 12 weeks when frozen. For I.V. infusion in NS or D_5W, solution is stable for 24 hours at room temperature and 96 hours when refrigerated.

Mechanism of Action Interferes with bacterial cell wall synthesis during active multiplication, causing cell wall death and resultant bactericidal activity against susceptible bacteria

Pharmacodynamics/Kinetics

Distribution: Widely distributed; CSF penetration is poor but enhanced by meningeal inflammation

Protein binding: ~90%; primarily to albumin

Metabolism: Primarily hepatic; undergoes enterohepatic recirculation

Half-life elimination: Normal renal/hepatic function: 30-60 minutes

Time to peak, serum: I.M.: 30-60 minutes

Excretion: Primarily feces; urine (10% to 30% as unchanged drug)

Dosage

Geriatric & Adult

Susceptible infections:

I.M.: 500 mg every 4-6 hours

I.V.: 500-2000 mg every 4-6 hours

◀ **Endocarditis: MSSA:**
Native valve: I.V.: 12 g/24 hours in 4-6 divided doses for 6 weeks
Prosthetic valve: I.V.: 12 g/24 hours in 6 divided doses for ≥6 weeks (use with rifampin and gentamicin)
Joint:
Bursitis, septic: I.V.: 2 g every 4 hours
Prosthetic: I.V.: 2 g every 4-6 hours with rifampin for 6 weeks
***Staphylococcus aureus,* methicillin-susceptible infections, including brain abscess, empyema, erysipelas, mastitis, myositis, orbital cellulitis, osteomyelitis, pneumonia, splenic abscess, toxic shock, urinary tract (perinephric abscess):** I.V.: 2 g every 4 hours

Renal Impairment Not necessary unless renal impairment is in the setting of concomitant hepatic impairment.
Poorly dialyzed; no supplemental dose or dosage adjustment necessary, including patients on intermittent hemodialysis, peritoneal dialysis, or continuous renal replacement therapy (eg, CVVHD).

Hepatic Impairment In patients with both hepatic and renal impairment, modification of dosage may be necessary; no data available.

Administration Administer around-the-clock rather than 4 times/day, 3 times/day, etc (ie, 12-6-12-6, not 9-1-5-9) to promote less variation in peak and trough serum concentrations; burning on I.V. administration may be decreased by further diluting the preparation to 250 mL NS or D₅W

Monitoring Parameters Baseline and periodic CBC with differential; periodic urinalysis, BUN, serum creatinine, AST and ALT; observe for signs and symptoms of anaphylaxis during first dose

Test Interactions Positive Coombs' test (direct), false-positive urinary and serum proteins; may inactivate aminoglycosides *in vitro*

Pharmacotherapy Pearls Sodium content of 1 g: 66.7 mg (2.9 mEq)

Special Geriatric Considerations Nafcillin has not been studied exclusively in the elderly, however, given its route of elimination, dosage adjustments based upon age and renal function is not necessary

Dosage Forms Excipient information presented when available (limited, particularly for generics); consult specific product labeling.
Infusion, premixed iso-osmotic dextrose solution: 1 g (50 mL); 2 g (100 mL)
Injection, powder for reconstitution: 1 g, 2 g, 10 g

◆ **Nafcillin Sodium** *see* Nafcillin *on page 1256*

Naftifine (NAF ti feen)

Brand Names: U.S. Naftin®
Index Terms Naftifine Hydrochloride
Generic Availability (U.S.) No
Pharmacologic Category Antifungal Agent, Topical
Use Topical treatment of tinea cruris (jock itch), tinea corporis (ringworm), and tinea pedis (athlete's foot)
Contraindications Hypersensitivity to naftifine or any component of the formulation
Warnings/Precautions For topical use only; avoid contact with eyes, nose, mouth, or mucous membranes. Discontinue if sensitivity or irritation occurs.
Adverse Reactions (Reflective of adult population; not specific for elderly)
1% to 10%:
Dermatologic: Burning/stinging (5% to 6%), erythema (≤2%), pruritus (1% to 2%)
Local: Dryness (3%), irritation (2%)
Drug Interactions
Avoid Concomitant Use There are no known interactions where it is recommended to avoid concomitant use.
Increased Effect/Toxicity There are no known significant interactions involving an increase in effect.
Decreased Effect There are no known significant interactions involving a decrease in effect.
Mechanism of Action Synthetic, broad-spectrum antifungal agent in the allylamine class; appears to have both fungistatic and fungicidal activity. Exhibits antifungal activity by selectively inhibiting the enzyme squalene epoxidase in a dose-dependent manner which results in a reduced synthesis of ergosterol, the primary sterol within the fungal membrane.
Pharmacodynamics/Kinetics
Absorption: Systemic: Cream: 6%; Gel: ≤4%
Half-life elimination: 2-3 days
Excretion: Urine and feces (as unchanged drug and/or metabolites)

Dosage

Geriatric & Adult Tinea infection: Topical: Apply cream once daily and gel twice daily (morning and evening) for up to 4 weeks

Special Geriatric Considerations No specific recommendations for use in the elderly.

Dosage Forms Excipient information presented when available (limited, particularly for generics); consult specific product labeling.

Cream, topical, as hydrochloride:

Naftin®: 1% (30 g, 60 g, 90 g) [contains benzyl alcohol]

Gel, topical, as hydrochloride:

Naftin®: 1% (40 g, 60 g, 90 g) [contains ethanol 52%]

◆ **Naftifine Hydrochloride** see Naftifine on page 1258
◆ **Naftin®** see Naftifine on page 1258
◆ **NaHCO₃** see Sodium Bicarbonate on page 1688

Nalbuphine (NAL byoo feen)

Related Information

Opioid Analgesics on page 2013

Medication Safety Issues

Sound-alike/look-alike issues:

Nubain may be confused with Navane®, Nebcin®

High alert medication:

The Institute for Safe Medication Practices (ISMP) includes this medication among its list of drug classes which have a heightened risk of causing significant patient harm when used in error.

Index Terms Nalbuphine Hydrochloride; Nubain

Generic Availability (U.S.) Yes

Pharmacologic Category Analgesic, Opioid; Analgesic, Opioid Partial Agonist

Use Relief of moderate-to-severe pain; preoperative analgesia, postoperative and surgical anesthesia, and obstetrical analgesia during labor and delivery

Unlabeled/Investigational Use Opioid-induced pruritus

Contraindications Hypersensitivity to nalbuphine or any component of the formulation

Warnings/Precautions Use caution in CNS depression. Sedation and psychomotor impairment are likely, and are additive with other CNS depressants or ethanol. May cause respiratory depression. Ambulatory patients must be cautioned about performing tasks which require mental alertness (eg, operating machinery or driving). Effects may be potentiated when used with other sedative drugs or ethanol. Use with caution in patients with recent myocardial infarction, biliary tract impairment, morbid obesity, thyroid dysfunction, head trauma, or increased intracranial pressure. Use caution in patients with prostatic hyperplasia and/or urinary stricture, adrenal insufficiency, decreased hepatic or renal function. Use with caution in patients with pre-existing respiratory compromise (hypoxia and/or hypercapnia), COPD or other obstructive pulmonary disease; critical respiratory depression may occur, even at therapeutic dosages. May cause hypotension; use with caution in patients with hypovolemia, cardiovascular disease (including acute MI), or drugs which may exaggerate hypotensive effects (including phenothiazines or general anesthetics). May obscure diagnosis or clinical course of patients with acute abdominal conditions. May result in tolerance and/or drug dependence with chronic use; use with caution in patients with a history of drug dependence. Abrupt discontinuation following prolonged use may lead to withdrawal symptoms. May precipitate withdrawal symptoms in patients following prolonged therapy with mu opioid agonists. Use with caution in the elderly and debilitated patients; may be more sensitive to adverse effects.

Adverse Reactions (Reflective of adult population; not specific for elderly)

>10%: Central nervous system: Sedation (36%)

1% to 10%:

Central nervous system: Dizziness (5%), headache (3%)

Gastrointestinal: Nausea/vomiting (6%), xerostomia (4%)

Miscellaneous: Clamminess (9%)

Drug Interactions

Avoid Concomitant Use There are no known interactions where it is recommended to avoid concomitant use.

Increased Effect/Toxicity

Nalbuphine may increase the levels/effects of: Alcohol (Ethyl); Alvimopan; CNS Depressants; Desmopressin; Selective Serotonin Reuptake Inhibitors; Thiazide Diuretics

The levels/effects of Nalbuphine may be increased by: Amphetamines; Antipsychotic Agents (Phenothiazines); Droperidol; HydrOXYzine; Succinylcholine

◀ **Decreased Effect**
  Nalbuphine may decrease the levels/effects of: Analgesics (Opioid); Pegvisomant

  The levels/effects of Nalbuphine may be decreased by: Ammonium Chloride; Mixed Agonist/Antagonist Opioids

Ethanol/Nutrition/Herb Interactions
  Ethanol: May increase CNS depression; monitor for increased effects with coadministration. Caution patients about effects.
  Herb/Nutraceutical: Avoid valerian, St John's wort, kava kava, gotu kola (may increase CNS depression).

Stability Store at room temperature of 15°C to 30°C (59°F to 86°F). Protect from light.

Mechanism of Action Agonist of kappa opiate receptors and partial antagonist of mu opiate receptors in the CNS, causing inhibition of ascending pain pathways, altering the perception of and response to pain; produces generalized CNS depression

Pharmacodynamics/Kinetics
  Onset of action: Peak effect: SubQ, I.M.: <15 minutes; I.V.: 2-3 minutes
  Metabolism: Hepatic
  Half-life elimination: 5 hours
  Excretion: Feces; urine (~7% as metabolites)

Dosage
  Geriatric Refer to adult dosing; use with caution.
  Adult
    Pain management: I.M., I.V., SubQ: 10 mg/70 kg every 3-6 hours; maximum single dose in nonopioid-tolerant patients: 20 mg; maximum daily dose: 160 mg
    Surgical anesthesia supplement: I.V.: Induction: 0.3-3 mg/kg over 10-15 minutes; maintenance doses of 0.25-0.5 mg/kg may be given as required
    Opioid-induced pruritus (unlabeled use): I.V. 2.5-5 mg; may repeat dose
  Renal Impairment Use with caution and reduce dose. Monitor.
  Hepatic Impairment Use with caution and reduce dose.

Administration Administer I.M., SubQ, or I.V.

Monitoring Parameters Relief of pain, respiratory and mental status, blood pressure

Test Interactions May interfere with certain enzymatic methods used to detect opioids, depending on sensitivity and specificity of the test (refer to test manufacturer for details)

Special Geriatric Considerations The elderly may be particularly susceptible to CNS effects; monitor closely.

Dosage Forms Excipient information presented when available (limited, particularly for generics); consult specific product labeling.
  Injection, solution, as hydrochloride: 10 mg/mL (10 mL); 20 mg/mL (10 mL)
  Injection, solution, as hydrochloride [preservative free]: 10 mg/mL (1 mL); 20 mg/mL (1 mL)

Selected References
American Geriatrics Society Panel on Pharmacological Management of Persistent Pain in Older Persons, "Pharmacological Management of Persistent Pain in Older Persons," *J Am Geriatr Soc*, 2009, 57(8):1331-46.

◆ **Nalbuphine Hydrochloride** *see* Nalbuphine *on page* 1259
◆ **Nalfon®** *see* Fenoprofen *on page* 706
◆ **Nallpen** *see* Nafcillin *on page* 1256
◆ **N-allylnoroxymorphine Hydrochloride** *see* Naloxone *on page* 1260

Naloxone (nal OKS one)

Medication Safety Issues
  Sound-alike/look-alike issues:
    Naloxone may be confused with Lanoxin®, naltrexone
    Narcan® may be confused with Marcaine®, Norcuron®
  International issues:
    Narcan [multiple international markets] may be confused with Marcen brand name for ketazolam [Spain]

Brand Names: Canada Naloxone Hydrochloride Injection®

Index Terms N-allylnoroxymorphine Hydrochloride; Naloxone Hydrochloride; Narcan

Generic Availability (U.S.) Yes

Pharmacologic Category Antidote; Opioid Antagonist

Use Complete or partial reversal of opioid drug effects, including respiratory depression; management of known or suspected opioid overdose; diagnosis of suspected opioid dependence or acute opioid overdose

Unlabeled/Investigational Use Opioid-induced pruritus

Contraindications Hypersensitivity to naloxone or any component of the formulation

Warnings/Precautions Due to an association between naloxone and acute pulmonary edema, use with caution in patients with cardiovascular disease or in patients receiving medications with potential adverse cardiovascular effects (eg, hypotension, pulmonary edema, or arrhythmias). Administration of naloxone causes the release of catecholamines; may precipitate acute withdrawal or unmask pain in those who regularly take opioids. Excessive dosages should be avoided after use of opiates in surgery. Abrupt postoperative reversal may result in nausea, vomiting, sweating, tachycardia, hypertension, seizures, and other cardiovascular events (including pulmonary edema and arrhythmias). May precipitate withdrawal symptoms in patients addicted to opiates, including pain, hypertension, sweating, agitation, irritability; carefully titrate dose to reverse hypoventilation; do not fully awaken patient or reverse analgesic effect (postoperative patient). Use caution in patients with history of seizures; avoid use in treatment of meperidine-induced seizures. Recurrence of respiratory depression is possible if the opioid involved is long-acting; observe patients until there is no reasonable risk of recurrent respiratory depression.

Adverse Reactions (Reflective of adult population; not specific for elderly) Adverse reactions are related to reversing dependency and precipitating withdrawal. Withdrawal symptoms are the result of sympathetic excess. Adverse events occur secondarily to reversal (withdrawal) of narcotic analgesia and sedation.

Central nervous system: Narcotic withdrawal

Drug Interactions

Avoid Concomitant Use There are no known interactions where it is recommended to avoid concomitant use.

Increased Effect/Toxicity There are no known significant interactions involving an increase in effect.

Decreased Effect There are no known significant interactions involving a decrease in effect.

Stability Store at 25°C (77°F). Protect from light. Stable in 0.9% sodium chloride and D_5W at 4 mcg/mL for 24 hours.

Mechanism of Action Pure opioid antagonist that competes and displaces narcotics at opioid receptor sites

Pharmacodynamics/Kinetics

Onset of action: Endotracheal, I.M., SubQ: 2-5 minutes; I.V.: ~2 minutes

Duration: ~30-120 minutes depending on route of administration; I.V. has a shorter duration of action than I.M. administration; since naloxone's action is shorter than that of most opioids, repeated doses are usually needed

Metabolism: Primarily hepatic via glucuronidation

Half-life elimination: 0.5-1.5 hours

Excretion: Urine (as metabolites)

Dosage

Geriatric & Adult Note: I.M., I.V. (preferred), intranasal (adults only), and SubQ routes may be used. Endotracheal administration is the least desirable and is supported by only anecdotal evidence (case report) (ACLS, 2010):

Opioid overdose (with standard ACLS protocols):

I.V., I.M., SubQ: 2 mg; may need to repeat doses every 2-3 minutes; after reversal, may need to readminister dose(s) at a later interval (ie, 20-60 minutes) depending on type/duration of opioid. If no response is observed after 10 mg total, consider other causes of respiratory depression.

Continuous infusion (unlabeled dosing): I.V.: **Note:** For use with exposures to long-acting opioids (eg, methadone), sustained release product, and symptomatic body packers after initial naloxone response. Calculate dosage/hour based on effective intermittent dose used and duration of adequate response seen or use two-thirds (²/₃) of the initial effective naloxone bolus on an hourly basis (typically 0.25-6.25 mg/hour); one-half (¹/₂) of the initial bolus dose should be readministered 15 minutes after initiation of the continuous infusion to prevent a drop in naloxone levels; adjust infusion rate as needed to assure adequate ventilation and prevent withdrawal symptoms (Goldfrank, 1986).

Endotracheal (unlabeled route): 0.08-5 mg (dose is 2-2.5 times I.V. dose); may repeat (ACLS, 2010)

Intranasal administration (unlabeled route): 2 mg (1 mg per nostril); may repeat in 5 minutes if respiratory depression persists. **Note:** Onset of action is slightly delayed compared to I.M. or I.V. routes (ACLS, 2010; Kelly, 2005; Robertson, 2009).

Reversal of respiratory depression with therapeutic opioid doses: I.V., I.M., SubQ.: Initial: 0.04-0.4 mg; may repeat until desired response achieved. If desired response is not observed after 0.8 mg total, consider other causes of respiratory depression.

Continuous infusion (unlabeled dosing): I.V.: **Note:** For use with exposures to long-acting opioids (eg, methadone) or sustained release products. Calculate dosage/hour based on effective intermittent dose used and duration of adequate response seen or use two-thirds (²/₃) of the initial effective naloxone bolus on an hourly basis (typically 0.2-0.6 mg/hour); one-half (¹/₂) of the initial bolus dose should be readministered 15 minutes after initiation of the continuous infusion to prevent a drop in naloxone levels; adjust infusion rate as needed to assure adequate ventilation and prevent withdrawal symptoms (Goldfrank, 1986).

Opioid-dependent patients being treated for cancer pain (NCCN guidelines, v.2.2011): I.V.: 0.04-0.08 mg (40-80 mcg) slow I.V. push; administer every 30-60 seconds until improvement in symptoms; if no response is observed after total naloxone dose 1 mg, consider other causes of respiratory depression. **Note:** May dilute 0.4 mg/mL (1 mL) ampul into 9 mL of normal saline for a total volume of 10 mL to achieve a 0.04 mg/mL (40 mcg/mL) concentration.

Postoperative reversal: I.V.: 0.1-0.2 mg every 2-3 minutes until desired response (adequate ventilation and alertness without significant pain). **Note:** Repeat doses may be needed within 1-2 hour intervals depending on type, dose, and timing of the last dose of opioid administered.

Opioid-induced pruritus (unlabeled use): I.V. infusion: 0.25 mcg/kg/**hour**; **Note:** Monitor pain control; verify that the naloxone is not reversing analgesia (Gan, 1997)

Administration

Endotracheal: There is only anecdotal support for this route of administration. May require a slightly higher dose than used in other routes. Dilute to 1-2 mL with normal saline; flush with 5 cc of saline and then administer 5 ventilations

Intratracheal: Dilute to 1-2 mL with normal saline

I.V. push: Administer over 30 seconds as undiluted preparation **or** (unlabeled) administer as diluted preparation slow I.V. push by diluting 0.4 mg (1 mL) ampul with 9 mL of normal saline for a total volume of 10 mL to achieve a concentration of 0.04 mg/mL

I.V. continuous infusion: Dilute to 4 mcg/mL in D_5W or normal saline

Monitoring Parameters Respiratory rate, heart rate, blood pressure, temperature, level of consciousness, ABGs or pulse oximetry

Pharmacotherapy Pearls Too rapid a reversal of narcotic depression may result in nausea, vomiting, sweating, tachycardia, increased blood pressure, and tremulousness

Dosage Forms Excipient information presented when available (limited, particularly for generics); consult specific product labeling.

Injection, solution, as hydrochloride: 0.4 mg/mL (1 mL, 10 mL)

Injection, solution, as hydrochloride [preservative free]: 1 mg/mL (2 mL)

◆ **Naloxone Hydrochloride** *see* Naloxone *on page 1260*
◆ **Namenda**® *see* Memantine *on page 1134*
◆ **Namenda XR** *see* Memantine *on page 1134*

Naphazoline (Nasal) (naf AZ oh leen)

Brand Names: U.S. Privine® [OTC]
Index Terms Naphazoline Hydrochloride
Pharmacologic Category Alpha$_1$ Agonist
Use Temporary relief of nasal congestion associated with the common cold, upper respiratory allergies, or sinusitis

Dosage

Geriatric & Adult Nasal congestion (decongestant): Intranasal: 0.05%, instill 1-2 drops or sprays every 6 hours if needed; therapy should not exceed 3 days

Special Geriatric Considerations Evaluate patient's ability to self-administer; use cautiously in patients with cardiovascular disease.

Dosage Forms Excipient information presented when available (limited, particularly for generics); consult specific product labeling.

Solution, intranasal, as hydrochloride [drops]:
Privine®: 0.05% (25 mL) [contains benzalkonium chloride]
Solution, intranasal, as hydrochloride [spray]:
Privine®: 0.05% (20 mL) [contains benzalkonium chloride]

Naphazoline (Ophthalmic) (naf AZ oh leen)

Brand Names: U.S. AK-Con™; Clear eyes® for Dry Eyes Plus ACR Relief [OTC]; Clear eyes® for Dry Eyes plus Redness Relief [OTC]; Clear eyes® Redness Relief [OTC]; Clear eyes® Seasonal Relief [OTC]
Brand Names: Canada Naphcon Forte®; Vasocon®
Index Terms Naphazoline Hydrochloride
Generic Availability (U.S.) No
Pharmacologic Category Alpha$_1$ Agonist; Ophthalmic Agent, Vasoconstrictor
Use Topical ocular vasoconstrictor; relief of redness of the eye due to minor irritation

Dosage
  Geriatric & Adult Decrease in eye redness (vasoconstrictor): Ophthalmic:
    0.1% solution (prescription): 1-2 drops into conjuctival sac every 3-4 hours as needed
    0.012% or 0.025% solution (OTC): 1-2 drops into affected eye(s) up to 4 times a day; therapy
      should not exceed 3 days
Special Geriatric Considerations Evaluate the patient's or caregiver's ability to safely administer the correct dose of ophthalmic medication. Use cautiously in patients with cardiovascular disease.
Dosage Forms Excipient information presented when available (limited, particularly for generics); consult specific product labeling.
  Solution, ophthalmic, as hydrochloride [drops]:
    AK-Con™: 0.1% (15 mL) [contains benzalkonium chloride]
    Clear eyes® for Dry Eyes Plus ACR Relief: 0.025% (15 mL) [contains hypromellose, zinc
      sulfate]
    Clear eyes® for Dry Eyes plus Redness Relief: 0.012% (15 mL) [contains benzalkonium
      chloride, glycerin, hypromellose]
    Clear eyes® Redness Relief: 0.012% (6 mL, 15 mL, 30 mL) [contains benzalkonium
      chloride, glycerin]
    Clear eyes® Seasonal Relief: 0.012% (15 mL, 30 mL) [contains benzalkonium chloride,
      glycerin, zinc sulfate]

Naphazoline and Pheniramine (naf AZ oh leen & fen NIR a meen)

Related Information
  Naphazoline (Ophthalmic) on page 1262
Medication Safety Issues
  Sound-alike/look-alike issues:
    Visine® may be confused with Visken®
Brand Names: U.S. Naphcon-A® [OTC]; Opcon-A® [OTC]; Visine-A® [OTC]
Brand Names: Canada Naphcon-A®; Visine® Advanced Allergy
Index Terms Pheniramine and Naphazoline
Generic Availability (U.S.) No
Pharmacologic Category Alkylamine Derivative; Alpha$_1$ Agonist; Histamine H$_1$ Antagonist; Histamine H$_1$ Antagonist, First Generation; Imidazoline Derivative; Ophthalmic Agent, Vasoconstrictor
Use Treatment of ocular congestion, irritation, and itching
Dosage
  Geriatric & Adult Ophthalmic: 1-2 drops up to 4 times/day
Special Geriatric Considerations Evaluate the patient's or caregiver's ability to safely administer the correct dose of ophthalmic medication. Use cautiously in patients with cardiovascular disease.
Dosage Forms Excipient information presented when available (limited, particularly for generics); consult specific product labeling.
  Solution, ophthalmic:
    Naphcon-A®: Naphazoline hydrochloride 0.025% and pheniramine maleate 0.3% (5 mL)
      [contains benzalkonium chloride; 2 bottles/box], (15 mL) [contains benzalkonium chloride]
    Opcon-A®: Naphazoline hydrochloride 0.027% and pheniramine maleate 0.3% (15 mL)
      [contains benzalkonium chloride]
    Visine-A®: Naphazoline hydrochloride 0.025% and pheniramine maleate 0.3% (15 mL)
      [contains benzalkonium chloride]

◆ **Naphazoline Hydrochloride** see Naphazoline (Nasal) on page 1262
◆ **Naphazoline Hydrochloride** see Naphazoline (Ophthalmic) on page 1262
◆ **Naphcon-A® [OTC]** see Naphazoline and Pheniramine on page 1263
◆ **Naprelan®** see Naproxen on page 1263
◆ **Naprosyn®** see Naproxen on page 1263

Naproxen (na PROKS en)

Related Information
  Beers Criteria – Potentially Inappropriate Medications for Geriatrics on page 2089
Medication Safety Issues
  Sound-alike/look-alike issues:
    Naproxen may be confused with Natacyn®, Nebcin®
    Anaprox® may be confused with Anaspaz®, Avapro®
    Naprelan® may be confused with Naprosyn®

◀ Naprosyn® may be confused with Naprelan®, Natacyn®, Nebcin®

Beers Criteria medication:
This drug may be inappropriate for use in geriatric patients (high severity risk).

International issues:
Flogen [Mexico] may be confused with Flovent brand name for fluticasone [U.S., Canada]
Flogen [Mexico] may be confused with Floxin brand name for flunarizine [Thailand], norfloxacin [South Africa], ofloxacin [U.S., Canada], and perfloxacin [Philippines]

Brand Names: U.S. Aleve® [OTC]; Anaprox®; Anaprox® DS; EC-Naprosyn®; Mediproxen [OTC]; Midol® Extended Relief [OTC]; Naprelan®; Naprosyn®; Pamprin® Maximum Strength All Day Relief [OTC]

Brand Names: Canada Anaprox®; Anaprox® DS; Apo-Napro-Na DS®; Apo-Napro-Na®; Apo-Naproxen EC®; Apo-Naproxen SR®; Apo-Naproxen®; Mylan-Naproxen EC; Naprelan™; Naprosyn®; Naprosyn® E; Naprosyn® SR; Naproxen Sodium DS; Naproxen-NA; Naproxen-NA DF; PMS-Naproxen; PMS-Naproxen EC; PRO-Naproxen EC; Riva-Naproxen; Riva-Naproxen Sodium; Riva-Naproxen Sodium DS; Teva-Naproxen; Teva-Naproxen EC; Teva-Naproxen Sodium; Teva-Naproxen Sodium DS; Teva-Naproxen SR

Index Terms Naproxen Sodium

Generic Availability (U.S.) Yes: Caplet, suspension, tablet

Pharmacologic Category Nonsteroidal Anti-inflammatory Drug (NSAID), Oral

Use Management of ankylosing spondylitis, osteoarthritis, and rheumatoid disorders; acute gout; mild-to-moderate pain; tendonitis, bursitis; fever

Medication Guide Available Yes

Contraindications Hypersensitivity to naproxen, aspirin, other NSAIDs, or any component of the formulation; perioperative pain in the setting of coronary artery bypass graft (CABG) surgery

Warnings/Precautions [U.S. Boxed Warning]: NSAIDs are associated with an increased risk of adverse cardiovascular thrombotic events, including MI and stroke. Risk may be increased with duration of use or pre-existing cardiovascular risk factors or disease. Carefully evaluate individual cardiovascular risk profiles prior to prescribing. May cause new-onset hypertension or worsening of existing hypertension. Use caution with fluid retention. Avoid use in heart failure. Use the lowest effective dose for the shortest duration of time, consistent with individual patient goals, to reduce risk of cardiovascular or GI adverse events. Alternate therapies should be considered for patients at high risk. Concurrent administration of ibuprofen, and potentially other nonselective NSAIDs, may interfere with aspirin's cardioprotective effect. **[U.S. Boxed Warning]: Use is contraindicated for treatment of perioperative pain in the setting of coronary artery bypass graft (CABG) surgery.** Risk of MI and stroke may be increased with use following CABG surgery.

[U.S. Boxed Warning]: NSAIDs may increase risk of gastrointestinal irritation, inflammation, ulceration, bleeding, and perforation. These events may occur at any time during therapy and without warning. Use caution with a history of GI disease (bleeding or ulcers); concurrent therapy with aspirin, anticoagulants and/or corticosteroids, smoking, use of alcohol, the elderly or debilitated patients. When used concomitantly with ≤325 mg of aspirin, a substantial increase in the risk of gastrointestinal complications (eg, ulcer) occurs; concomitant gastroprotective therapy (eg, proton pump inhibitors) is recommended (Bhatt, 2008).

May increase the risk of aseptic meningitis, especially in patients with systemic lupus erythematosus (SLE) and mixed connective tissue disorders. Platelet adhesion and aggregation may be decreased; may prolong bleeding time; patients with coagulation disorders or who are receiving anticoagulants should be monitored closely. Anemia may occur; patients on long-term NSAID therapy should be monitored for anemia. Rarely, NSAID use may cause severe blood dyscrasias (eg, agranulocytosis, aplastic anemia, thrombocytopenia).

NSAID use may compromise existing renal function; dose-dependent decreases in prostaglandin synthesis may result from NSAID use, reducing renal blood flow which may cause renal decompensation. NSAID use may increase the risk for hyperkalemia. Patients with impaired renal function, dehydration, heart failure, liver dysfunction, those taking diuretics, and ACE inhibitors, and the elderly are at greater risk of renal toxicity and hyperkalemia. Rehydrate patient before starting therapy; monitor renal function closely. Not recommended for use in patients with advanced renal disease. Long-term NSAID use may result in renal papillary necrosis.

NSAIDs may cause serious skin adverse events including exfoliative dermatitis, Stevens-Johnson Syndrome (SJS) and toxic epidermal necrolysis (TEN); discontinue use at first sign of skin rash or hypersensitivity. Anaphylactoid reactions may occur, even without prior exposure; patients with "aspirin triad" (bronchial asthma, aspirin intolerance, rhinitis) may be at increased risk. Do not use in patients who experience bronchospasm, asthma, rhinitis, or urticaria with NSAID or aspirin therapy. Use caution in other forms of asthma.

Use with caution in patients with decreased hepatic function. Closely monitor patients with any abnormal LFT. Severe hepatic reactions (eg, fulminant hepatitis, liver failure) have occurred with NSAID use, rarely; discontinue if signs or symptoms of liver disease develop, or if systemic manifestations occur.

NSAIDS may cause drowsiness, dizziness, blurred vision and other neurologic effects which may impair physical or mental abilities; patients must be cautioned about performing tasks which require mental alertness (eg, operating machinery or driving). Discontinue use with blurred or diminished vision and perform ophthalmologic exam. Monitor vision with long-term therapy.

In the elderly, may be inappropriate for long-term use due to potential for GI bleeding, hypertension, heart failure, and renal failure (Beers Criteria).

Withhold for at least 4-6 half-lives prior to surgical or dental procedures.

OTC labeling: Prior to self-medication, patients should contact healthcare provider if they have had recurring stomach pain or upset, ulcers, bleeding problems, asthma, high blood pressure, heart or kidney disease, other serious medical problems, are currently taking a diuretic, anticoagulant, other NSAIDs, or are ≥60 years of age. Recommended dosages and duration should not be exceeded, due to an increased risk of GI bleeding, MI, and stroke. Patients should stop use and consult a healthcare provider if symptoms get worse, newly appear, or continue; if an allergic reaction occurs; if feeling faint, vomit blood or have bloody/ black stools; if having difficulty swallowing or heartburn, or if fever lasts for >3 days or pain >10 days. Consuming ≥3 alcoholic beverages/day or taking longer than recommended may increase the risk of GI bleeding.

Adverse Reactions (Reflective of adult population; not specific for elderly)

1% to 10%:

Cardiovascular: Edema (3% to 9%), palpitations (<3%)

Central nervous system: Dizziness (3% to 9%), drowsiness (3% to 9%), headache (3% to 9%), lightheadedness (<3%), vertigo (<3%)

Dermatologic: Pruritus (3% to 9%), skin eruption (3% to 9%), ecchymosis (3% to 9%), purpura (<3%), rash

Endocrine & metabolic: Fluid retention (3% to 9%)

Gastrointestinal: Abdominal pain (3% to 9%), constipation (3% to 9%), nausea (3% to 9%), heartburn (3% to 9%), diarrhea (<3%), dyspepsia (<3%), stomatitis (<3%), flatulence, gross bleeding/perforation, indigestion, ulcers, vomiting

Genitourinary: Abnormal renal function

Hematologic: Hemolysis (3% to 9%), ecchymosis (3% to 9%), anemia, bleeding time increased

Hepatic: LFTs increased

Ocular: Visual disturbances (<3%)

Otic: Tinnitus (3% to 9%), hearing disturbances (<3%)

Respiratory: Dyspnea (3% to 9%)

Miscellaneous: Diaphoresis (<3%), thirst (<3%)

Drug Interactions

Metabolism/Transport Effects Substrate (minor) of CYP1A2, 2C9

Avoid Concomitant Use

Avoid concomitant use of Naproxen with any of the following: Floctafenine; Ketorolac; Ketorolac (Nasal); Ketorolac (Systemic)

Increased Effect/Toxicity

Naproxen may increase the levels/effects of: Aminoglycosides; Anticoagulants; Antiplatelet Agents; Bisphosphonate Derivatives; Collagenase (Systemic); CycloSPORINE; Cyclo-SPORINE (Systemic); Deferasirox; Desmopressin; Digoxin; Drotrecogin Alfa; Eplerenone; Haloperidol; Ibritumomab; Lithium; Methotrexate; Nonsteroidal Anti-Inflammatory Agents; PEMEtrexed; Porfimer; Potassium-Sparing Diuretics; PRALAtrexate; Quinolone Antibiotics; Rivaroxaban; Salicylates; Thrombolytic Agents; Tositumomab and Iodine I 131 Tositumomab; Vancomycin; Vitamin K Antagonists

The levels/effects of Naproxen may be increased by: ACE Inhibitors; Angiotensin II Receptor Blockers; Antidepressants (Tricyclic, Tertiary Amine); Corticosteroids (Systemic); Dasatinib; Floctafenine; Glucosamine; Herbs (Anticoagulant/Antiplatelet Properties); Ketorolac; Ketorolac (Nasal); Ketorolac (Systemic); Nonsteroidal Anti-Inflammatory Agents; Omega-3-Acid Ethyl Esters; Pentosan Polysulfate Sodium; Pentoxifylline; Probenecid; Prostacyclin Analogues; Selective Serotonin Reuptake Inhibitors; Serotonin/Norepinephrine Reuptake Inhibitors; Sodium Phosphates; Treprostinil; Vitamin E

◀ **Decreased Effect**
Naproxen may decrease the levels/effects of: ACE Inhibitors; Angiotensin II Receptor Blockers; Antiplatelet Agents; Beta-Blockers; Eplerenone; HydrALAZINE; Potassium-Sparing Diuretics; Salicylates; Selective Serotonin Reuptake Inhibitors; Thiazide Diuretics

The levels/effects of Naproxen may be decreased by: Bile Acid Sequestrants; Cyproterone; Nonsteroidal Anti-Inflammatory Agents; Salicylates

Ethanol/Nutrition/Herb Interactions
Ethanol: Avoid ethanol (may enhance gastric mucosal irritation).
Food: Naproxen absorption rate/levels may be decreased if taken with food.
Herb/Nutraceutical: Avoid alfalfa, anise, bilberry, bladderwrack, bromelain, cat's claw, celery, chamomile, coleus, cordyceps, dong quai, evening primrose, fenugreek, feverfew, garlic, ginger, ginkgo biloba, ginseng (American, Panax, Siberian), grapeseed, green tea, guggul, horse chestnut seed, horseradish, licorice, prickly ash, red clover, reishi, SAMe (S-adenosylmethionine), sweet clover, turmeric, white willow (all have additional antiplatelet activity).

Stability Store oral suspension and tablet at 15°C to 30°C (59°F to 86°F).

Mechanism of Action Reversibly inhibits cyclooxygenase-1 and 2 (COX-1 and 2) enzymes, which results in decreased formation of prostaglandin precursors; has antipyretic, analgesic, and anti-inflammatory properties

Other proposed mechanisms not fully elucidated (and possibly contributing to the anti-inflammatory effect to varying degrees), include inhibiting chemotaxis, altering lymphocyte activity, inhibiting neutrophil aggregation/activation, and decreasing proinflammatory cytokine levels.

Pharmacodynamics/Kinetics
Onset of action: Analgesic: 1 hour; Anti-inflammatory: ~2 weeks
Peak effect: Anti-inflammatory: 2-4 weeks
Duration: Analgesic: ≤7 hours; Anti-inflammatory: ≤12 hours
Absorption: Almost 100%
Distribution: 0.16 L/kg
Protein binding: >99% to albumin; increased free fraction in elderly
Metabolism: Hepatic to metabolites
Bioavailability: 95%
Half-life elimination: Normal renal function: 12-17 hours; End-stage renal disease: No change
Time to peak, serum: 1-4 hours
Excretion: Urine (95%; primarily as metabolites); feces (≤3%)

Dosage
Geriatric & Adult Note: Dosage expressed as naproxen base; 200 mg naproxen base is equivalent to 220 mg naproxen sodium.
Gout, acute: Oral: Initial: 750 mg, followed by 250 mg every 8 hours until attack subsides. **Note:** EC-Naprosyn® is not recommended.
Migraine, acute (unlabeled use): Initial: 500-750 mg; an additional 250-500 mg may be given if needed (maximum: 1250 mg in 24 hours). **Note:** EC-Naprosyn® is not recommended.
Pain (mild-to-moderate), acute tendonitis, bursitis: Oral: Initial: 500 mg, then 250 mg every 6-8 hours; maximum: 1250 mg/day naproxen base
Rheumatoid arthritis, osteoarthritis, and ankylosing spondylitis: 500-1000 mg/day in 2 divided doses; may increase to 1.5 g/day of naproxen base for limited time period
OTC labeling: Pain/fever:
Adults ≤65 years: 200 mg naproxen base every 8-12 hours; if needed, may take 400 mg naproxen base for the initial dose; maximum: 600 mg naproxen base/24 hours
Adults >65 years: Refer to geriatric dosing
Renal Impairment Cl$_{cr}$ <30 mL/minute: use is not recommended.

Administration Administer with food, milk, or antacids to decrease GI adverse effects

Monitoring Parameters Monitor response (pain, range of motion, grip strength, mobility, ADL function), inflammation; observe for weight gain, edema; monitor renal function (serum creatinine, BUN); observe for bleeding, bruising; evaluate gastrointestinal effects (abdominal pain, bleeding, dyspepsia); mental confusion, disorientation, CBC, liver function tests; urine output

Test Interactions Naproxen may interfere with 5-HIAA urinary assays; due to an interaction with m-dinitrobenzene, naproxen should be discontinued 72 hours before adrenal function testing if the Porter-Silber test is used. May interfere with urine detection of cannabinoids and barbiturates (false-positives).

Special Geriatric Considerations Elderly are a high-risk population for adverse effects from NSAIDs. As much as 60% of the elderly can develop peptic ulceration and/or hemorrhage asymptomatically. The concomitant use of H$_2$ blockers and sucralfate is not effective as prophylaxis with the exception of NSAID-induced duodenal ulcers which may be prevented by the use of ranitidine. Misoprostol and proton pump inhibitors are the only agents proven to help prevent the development of NSAID-induced ulcers. Also, concomitant disease and drug use contribute to the risk for GI adverse effects. Use lowest effective dose for shortest period possible. Consider renal function decline with age. Use of NSAIDs can compromise existing renal function especially when Cl_{cr} is ≤30 mL/minute. Tinnitus may be a difficult and unreliable indication of toxicity due to age-related hearing loss or eighth cranial nerve damage. CNS adverse effects such as confusion, agitation, and hallucination are generally seen in overdose or high-dose situations, but elderly may demonstrate these adverse effects at lower doses than younger adults.

This medication is considered to be potentially inappropriate in this patient population (Beers Criteria severity: High).

Dosage Forms Excipient information presented when available (limited, particularly for generics); consult specific product labeling.
Caplet, oral, as sodium: 220 mg [equivalent to naproxen base 200 mg]
Aleve®: 220 mg [contains sodium 20 mg; equivalent to naproxen base 200 mg]
Midol® Extended Relief: 220 mg [contains sodium 20 mg; equivalent to naproxen base 200 mg]
Pamprin® Maximum Strength All Day Relief: 220 mg [contains sodium 20 mg; equivalent to naproxen base 200 mg]
Capsule, liquid gel, oral, as sodium:
Aleve®: 220 mg [contains sodium 20 mg; equivalent to naproxen base 200 mg]
Combination package, oral, as sodium [dose-pack/each package contains]:
Naprelan®: Day 1-3: Tablet, controlled release: 825 mg [equivalent to naproxen base 750 mg] (6s) [contains sodium 75 mg] and Day 4-10: Tablet, controlled release: 550 mg [equivalent to naproxen base 500 mg] (14s) [contains sodium 50 mg]
Gelcap, oral, as sodium:
Aleve®: 220 mg [contains sodium 20 mg; equivalent to naproxen base 200 mg]
Suspension, oral: 125 mg/5 mL (500 mL)
Naprosyn®: 125 mg/5 mL (473 mL) [contains sodium 39 mg (1.5 mEq)/5 mL; orange-pineapple flavor]
Tablet, oral: 250 mg, 375 mg, 500 mg
Naprosyn®: 250 mg [scored]
Naprosyn®: 375 mg
Naprosyn®: 500 mg [scored]
Tablet, oral, as sodium: 220 mg [equivalent to naproxen base 200 mg], 220 mg, 275 mg [equivalent to naproxen base 250 mg], 550 mg [equivalent to naproxen base 500 mg]
Aleve®: 220 mg [contains sodium 20 mg; equivalent to naproxen base 200 mg]
Anaprox®: 275 mg [contains sodium 25 mg; equivalent to naproxen base 250 mg]
Anaprox® DS: 550 mg [scored; contains sodium 50 mg; equivalent to naproxen base 500 mg]
Mediproxen: 220 mg [contains sodium 20 mg; equivalent to naproxen base 200 mg]
Tablet, controlled release, oral, as sodium:
Naprelan®: 412.5 mg [contains sodium 37.5 mg; equivalent to naproxen base 375 mg]
Naprelan®: 550 mg [contains sodium 50 mg; equivalent to naproxen base 500 mg]
Naprelan®: 825 mg [contains sodium 75 mg; equivalent to naproxen base 750 mg]
Tablet, delayed release, enteric coated, oral: 375 mg, 500 mg
EC-Naprosyn®: 375 mg, 500 mg

Naproxen and Esomeprazole (na PROKS en & es oh ME pray zol)

Related Information
Esomeprazole *on page 636*
Naproxen *on page 1263*
Medication Safety Issues
Sound-alike/look-alike issues:
Vimovo™ may be confused with Vimpat®
Brand Names: U.S. Vimovo™
Brand Names: Canada Vimovo™
Index Terms Esomeprazole and Naproxen
Generic Availability (U.S.) No
Pharmacologic Category Nonsteroidal Anti-inflammatory Drug (NSAID), Oral; Proton Pump Inhibitor; Substituted Benzimidazole
Use Reduction of the risk of NSAID-associated gastric ulcers in patients at risk of developing gastric ulcers who require an NSAID for the treatment of rheumatoid arthritis, osteoarthritis, and ankylosing spondylitis
Medication Guide Available Yes

◀ **Dosage**

Geriatric Naproxen: Dosing adjustment should be considered; use lowest effective dose. Refer to adult dosing.

Adult Reduce NSAID-associated gastric ulcers during treatment for arthritis: Oral: One tablet (375 mg naproxen/20 mg esomeprazole or 500 mg naproxen/20 mg esomeprazole) twice daily; maximum daily esomeprazole dose: 40 mg.

Note: If a daily dose of esomeprazole <40 mg/day is necessary, alternate treatment should be considered.

Renal Impairment Moderate-to-severe renal impairment (Cl_{cr} <30 mL/minute): Use is not recommended.

Hepatic Impairment Severe liver disease: Use of this combination product not recommended since esomeprazole dose will exceed 20 mg/day.

Special Geriatric Considerations An increased risk of fractures of the hip, spine, or wrist has been observed in epidemiologic studies with proton pump inhibitor (PPI) use, primarily in older adults ≥50 years of age. The greatest risk was seen in patients receiving high doses or on long-term therapy (≥1 year). Calcium and vitamin D supplementation and close monitoring are recommended to reduce the risk of fracture in high-risk patients.

Dosage Forms Excipient information presented when available (limited, particularly for generics); consult specific product labeling.

Tablet, variable release, oral:

Vimovo™: Naproxen [delayed release] 375 mg and esomeprazole [immediate release] 20 mg, Naproxen [delayed release] 500 mg and esomeprazole [immediate release] 20 mg

◆ **Naproxen and Sumatriptan** see Sumatriptan and Naproxen on page 1726
◆ **Naproxen Sodium** see Naproxen on page 1263
◆ **Naproxen Sodium and Sumatriptan** see Sumatriptan and Naproxen on page 1726
◆ **Naproxen Sodium and Sumatriptan Succinate** see Sumatriptan and Naproxen on page 1726

Naratriptan (NAR a trip tan)

Medication Safety Issues
Sound-alike/look-alike issues:
Amerge® may be confused with Altace®, Amaryl®

Brand Names: U.S. Amerge®

Brand Names: Canada Amerge®

Index Terms Naratriptan Hydrochloride

Generic Availability (U.S.) Yes

Pharmacologic Category Antimigraine Agent; Serotonin 5-HT$_{1B, 1D}$ Receptor Agonist

Use Treatment of acute migraine headache with or without aura

Contraindications Hypersensitivity to naratriptan or any component of the formulation; cerebrovascular, peripheral vascular disease (ischemic bowel disease), ischemic heart disease (angina pectoris, history of myocardial infarction, or proven silent ischemia); or in patients with symptoms consistent with ischemic heart disease, coronary artery vasospasm, or Prinzmetal's angina; uncontrolled hypertension or patients who have received within 24 hours another 5-HT agonist (sumatriptan, zolmitriptan) or ergotamine-containing product; patients with known risk factors associated with coronary artery disease; patients with severe hepatic (Child-Pugh grade C) or renal disease (Cl_{cr} <15 mL/minute); do not administer naratriptan to patients with hemiplegic or basilar migraine

Warnings/Precautions Use only if there is a clear diagnosis of migraine. Dosage reduction is required in mild-to-moderate hepatic impairment and moderate renal impairment; use is contraindicated in patients with severe hepatic or renal impairment. Do not give to patients with risk factors for CAD until a cardiovascular evaluation has been performed; if evaluation is satisfactory, the healthcare provider should administer the first dose (consider ECG monitoring) and cardiovascular status should be periodically re-evaluated. Cardiac events (coronary artery vasospasm, transient ischemia, myocardial infarction, ventricular tachycardia/fibrillation, cardiac arrest, and death), cerebral/subarachnoid hemorrhage, stroke, peripheral vascular ischemia, and colonic ischemia have been reported with 5-HT$_1$ agonist administration. Patients who experience sensations of chest pain/pressure/tightness or symptoms suggestive of angina following dosing should be evaluated for coronary artery disease or Prinzmetal's angina before receiving additional doses; if dosing is resumed and similar symptoms recur, monitor with ECG. Significant elevation in blood pressure, including hypertensive crisis, has also been reported on rare occasions in patients with and without a history of hypertension. Only indicated for the acute treatment of migraine; not indicated for migraine prophylaxis, or for the treatment of cluster headache, hemiplegic or basilar migraine. If a patient does not respond to the first dose, the diagnosis of migraine should be reconsidered;

rule out underlying neurologic disease in patients with atypical headache and in patients with no prior history of migraine.

Symptoms of agitation, confusion, hallucinations, hyper-reflexia, myoclonus, shivering, and tachycardia may occur with concomitant proserotonergic drugs (ie, SSRIs/SNRIs or triptans) or agents which reduce naratriptan's metabolism. Concurrent use of serotonin precursors (eg, tryptophan) is not recommended. If concomitant administration with SSRIs is warranted, monitor closely, especially at initiation and with dose increases.

Adverse Reactions (Reflective of adult population; not specific for elderly)

1% to 10%:

Central nervous system: Pain/pressure (2% to 4%), malaise/fatigue (2%), dizziness (1% to 2%), drowsiness (1% to 2%), vertigo (1%)

Gastrointestinal: Nausea (4% to 5%), hyposalivation (1%), vomiting (1%)

Neuromuscular & skeletal: Paresthesia (1% to 2%)

Ocular: Photophobia (1%)

Miscellaneous: Ear/nose/throat infection (1%), pressure/tightness/heaviness sensations (1%), warm/cold temperature sensations (1%)

Drug Interactions

Avoid Concomitant Use

Avoid concomitant use of Naratriptan with any of the following: Ergot Derivatives; Sibutramine

Increased Effect/Toxicity

Naratriptan may increase the levels/effects of: Ergot Derivatives; Serotonin Modulators

The levels/effects of Naratriptan may be increased by: Ergot Derivatives; Sibutramine

Decreased Effect There are no known significant interactions involving a decrease in effect.

Stability Store at 20°C to 25°C (68°F to 77°F).

Mechanism of Action Selective agonist for serotonin (5-HT$_{1B}$ and 5-HT$_{1D}$ receptors) in cranial arteries; causes vasoconstriction and reduces sterile inflammation associated with antidromic neuronal transmission correlating with relief of migraine

Pharmacodynamics/Kinetics

Onset of action: ~1-2 hours (Bomhof, 1999; Tfelt-Hansen, 2000)

Absorption: Well absorbed

Distribution: V$_{dss}$: 170 L

Protein binding, plasma: 28% to 31%

Metabolism: Hepatic via CYP

Bioavailability: ~70%

Half life, elimination: 6 hours; increased in renal impairment (moderate impairment; mean: 11 hours; range 7-20 hours); increased in hepatic impairment (moderate impairment: 8-16 hours)

Time to peak: 2-3 hours

Excretion: Urine (50% of total dose as unchanged drug; 30% of total dose as metabolites)

Dosage

Geriatric Not recommended for use in the elderly.

Adult Migraine: Oral: 1 mg to 2.5 mg at the onset of headache. It is recommended to use the lowest possible dose to minimize adverse effects. If headache returns or does not fully resolve, the dose may be repeated after 4 hours. Do not exceed 5 mg in 24 hours.

Renal Impairment

Mild-to-moderate renal impairment: Initial: 1 mg; do not exceed 2.5 mg in 24 hours.

Severe renal impairment (Cl$_{cr}$ <15 mL/minute): Use is contraindicated.

Hepatic Impairment

Mild-to-moderate hepatic impairment (Child-Pugh grade A or B): Initial: 1 mg; do not exceed 2.5 mg in 24 hours

Severe hepatic impairment (Child-Pugh grade C): Use is contraindicated.

Administration Do **not** crush or chew tablet; swallow whole with water.

Special Geriatric Considerations Naratriptan was not studied in patients >65 years of age. Use in elderly patients is not recommended because of the presence of risk factors associated with adverse effects. These include the presence of coronary artery disease, decreased liver or renal function, and the risk of pronounced blood pressure increases.

Dosage Forms Excipient information presented when available (limited, particularly for generics); consult specific product labeling.

Tablet, oral: 1 mg, 2.5 mg

Amerge®: 1 mg, 2.5 mg

♦ **Naratriptan Hydrochloride** see Naratriptan on page 1268
♦ **Narcan** see Naloxone on page 1260
♦ **Nardil®** see Phenelzine on page 1434
♦ **Nasacort® AQ** see Triamcinolone (Nasal) on page 1856

Natamycin (na ta MYE sin)

Medication Safety Issues

Sound-alike/look-alike issues:

Natacyn® may be confused with Naprosyn®

Brand Names: U.S. Natacyn®

Brand Names: Canada Natacyn®

Index Terms Pimaricin

Generic Availability (U.S.) No

Pharmacologic Category Antifungal Agent, Ophthalmic

Use Treatment of blepharitis, conjunctivitis, and keratitis caused by susceptible fungi (*Aspergillus*, *Candida*, *Cephalosporium*, *Fusarium*, and *Penicillium*)

Contraindications Hypersensitivity to natamycin or any component of the formulation

Warnings/Precautions For topical eye use only. Failure to improve (keratitis) after 7-10 days of administration suggests infection caused by a microorganism not susceptible to natamycin; efficacy as a single agent in fungal endophthalmitis has not been established. Suspension may adhere to epithelial ulcers; retention of the suspension in the fornices occurs regularly. Contains benzalkonium chloride which may be absorbed by contact lenses; remove contact lens prior to administration and wait 15 minutes before reinserting. Contact lens should not be worn if signs/symptoms of fungal blepharitis, conjunctivitis, and/or keratitis are present.

Adverse Reactions (Reflective of adult population; not specific for elderly) Postmarketing and/or case reports: Allergic reaction, chest pain, corneal opacity, dyspnea, eye discomfort, edema, hyperemia, irritation and/or pain, foreign body sensation, parasthesia, tearing, vision changes

Drug Interactions

Avoid Concomitant Use There are no known interactions where it is recommended to avoid concomitant use.

Increased Effect/Toxicity There are no known significant interactions involving an increase in effect.

Decreased Effect There are no known significant interactions involving a decrease in effect.

Stability Store at 2°C to 24°C (36°F to 75°F); do not freeze. Protect from excessive heat and light.

Mechanism of Action Increases cell membrane permeability in susceptible fungi

Pharmacodynamics/Kinetics

Absorption: Ophthalmic: Systemic, <2%; Gastrointestinal: Poor

Distribution: Adheres to cornea, retained in conjunctival fornices; does not produce effective intraocular fluid concentrations

Dosage

Geriatric & Adult

Fungal keratitis: Ophthalmic: Instill 1 drop in conjunctival sac every 1-2 hours, after 3-4 days reduce to one drop 6-8 times/day; usual course of therapy is 2-3 weeks or until resolution of active fungal keratitis (may be useful to gradually reduce dosage at 4-7 day intervals to assure elimination of organism)

Fungal blepharitis or conjunctivitis: Ophthalmic: Instill 1 drop in conjunctival sac every 4-6 hours

Administration Ophthalmic: Shake well before using, do not touch dropper to eye.

Monitoring Parameters Monitor tolerance to the drug at least twice weekly

Special Geriatric Considerations Assess patient's ability to self-administer ophthalmic drops.

Dosage Forms Excipient information presented when available (limited, particularly for generics); consult specific product labeling.

Suspension, ophthalmic [drops]:

Natacyn®: 5% (15 mL) [contains benzalkonium chloride]

Nateglinide (na te GLYE nide)

Related Information
Diabetes Mellitus Management, Adults *on page 2073*

Medication Safety Issues
High alert medication:
The Institute for Safe Medication Practices (ISMP) includes this medication among its list of drug classes which have a heightened risk of causing significant patient harm when used in error.

Brand Names: U.S. Starlix®
Brand Names: Canada Starlix®
Generic Availability (U.S.) Yes
Pharmacologic Category Antidiabetic Agent, Meglitinide Derivative

Use Management of type 2 diabetes mellitus (noninsulin dependent, NIDDM) as monotherapy when hyperglycemia cannot be managed by diet and exercise alone; in combination with metformin or a thiazolidinedione to lower blood glucose in patients whose hyperglycemia cannot be controlled by exercise, diet, or a single agent alone

Contraindications Hypersensitivity to nateglinide or any component of the formulation; diabetic ketoacidosis, with or without coma (treat with insulin); type 1 diabetes mellitus (insulin dependent, IDDM)

Warnings/Precautions Use with caution in patients with moderate-to-severe hepatic impairment. Use caution in severe renal dysfunction, elderly, malnourished, or patients with adrenal/pituitary dysfunction; may be more susceptible to glucose-lowering effects. All oral hypoglycemic agents are capable of producing hypoglycemia. Proper patient selection, dosage, and instructions to the patients are important to avoid hypoglycemic episodes. It may be necessary to discontinue nateglinide and administer insulin if the patient is exposed to stress (ie, fever, trauma, infection, surgery). Indicated for adjunctive therapy with metformin; not to be used as a substitute for metformin monotherapy. Combination treatment with sulfonylureas is not recommended (no additional benefit). Patients not adequately controlled on oral agents which stimulate insulin release (eg, glyburide) should not be switched to nateglinide or have nateglinide added to therapy.

Adverse Reactions (Reflective of adult population; not specific for elderly) As reported with nateglinide monotherapy: 1% to 10%:
Central nervous system: Dizziness (4%)
Endocrine & metabolic: Hypoglycemia (2%), increased uric acid
Gastrointestinal: Weight gain
Neuromuscular & skeletal: Arthropathy (3%)
Respiratory: Upper respiratory infection (10%)
Miscellaneous: Flu-like syndrome (4%)

Drug Interactions
Metabolism/Transport Effects Substrate (major) of CYP2C9, CYP3A4, SLCO1B1; **Inhibits** CYP2C9 (weak)

Avoid Concomitant Use
Avoid concomitant use of Nateglinide with any of the following: Conivaptan

Increased Effect/Toxicity
Nateglinide may increase the levels/effects of: Hypoglycemic Agents

The levels/effects of Nateglinide may be increased by: Conivaptan; CYP2C9 Inhibitors (Moderate); CYP2C9 Inhibitors (Strong); CYP3A4 Inhibitors (Moderate); CYP3A4 Inhibitors (Strong); Dasatinib; Eltrombopag; Herbs (Hypoglycemic Properties); Pegvisomant

Decreased Effect
The levels/effects of Nateglinide may be decreased by: Corticosteroids (Orally Inhaled); Corticosteroids (Systemic); CYP2C9 Inducers (Highly Effective); CYP3A4 Inducers (Strong); Deferasirox; Herbs (CYP3A4 Inducers); Luteinizing Hormone-Releasing Hormone Analogs; Peginterferon Alfa-2b; Somatropin; Thiazide Diuretics; Tocilizumab

Ethanol/Nutrition/Herb Interactions
Ethanol: Avoid ethanol (increased risk of hypoglycemia).
Food: Rate of absorption is decreased and time to T_{max} is delayed when taken with food. Food does not affect AUC. Multiple peak plasma concentrations may be observed if fasting. Not affected by composition of meal.
Herb/Nutraceutical: Avoid alfalfa, aloe, bilberry, bitter melon, burdock, celery, damiana, fenugreek, garcinia, garlic, ginger, ginseng (American), gymnema, marshmallow, and stinging nettle (may enhance the hypoglycemic effects of antidiabetic agents). St. John's wort may decrease the levels/effect of nateglinide.

Stability Store at 25°C (77°F).

◄ **Mechanism of Action** A phenylalanine derivative, nonsulfonylurea hypoglycemic agent used in the management of type 2 diabetes mellitus (noninsulin dependent, NIDDM); stimulates insulin release from the pancreatic beta cells to reduce postprandial hyperglycemia; amount of insulin release is dependent upon existing glucose levels

Pharmacodynamics/Kinetics

Onset of action: Insulin secretion: ~20 minutes
  Peak effect: 1 hour
Duration: 4 hours
Absorption: Rapid
Distribution: 10 L
Protein binding: 98%, primarily to albumin
Metabolism: Hepatic via hydroxylation followed by glucuronide conjugation via CYP2C9 (70%) and CYP3A4 (30%) to metabolites
Bioavailability: 73%
Half-life elimination: 1.5 hours
Time to peak: ≤1 hour
Excretion: Urine (83%, 16% as unchanged drug); feces (10%)

Dosage

Geriatric & Adult Management of type 2 diabetes mellitus: Oral: Initial and maintenance dose: 120 mg 3 times/day, 1-30 minutes before meals; may be given alone or in combination with metformin or a thiazolidinedione; patients close to Hb A_{1c} goal may be started at 60 mg 3 times/day

Renal Impairment No specific dosage adjustment is recommended for patients with mild-to-severe renal disease. Patients on dialysis showed reduced medication exposure and plasma protein binding. Patients with severe renal dysfunction are more susceptible to glucose-lowering effect; use with caution.

Hepatic Impairment Increased serum levels are seen with mild hepatic insufficiency; no dosage adjustment is needed. Has not been studied in patients with moderate-to-severe liver disease; use with caution.

Administration Patients who are anorexic or NPO will need to have their dose held to avoid hypoglycemia.

Monitoring Parameters Glucose and Hb A_{1c} levels, weight, lipid profile

Reference Range

Recommendations for glycemic control in adults with diabetes:
  Hb A_{1c}: <7%
  Preprandial capillary plasma glucose: 70-130 mg/dL
  Peak postprandial capillary blood glucose: <180 mg/dL
  Blood pressure: <130/80 mm Hg
Recommendations for glycemic control in older adults with diabetes:
  Relatively healthy, cognitively intact, and with a ≥5-year life expectancy: See Adults
  Frail, life expectancy <5-years or those for whom the risks of intensive glucose control outweigh the benefits:
  Hb A_{1c}: <8% to 9%
  Blood pressure: <140/80 mm Hg or <130/80 mm Hg if tolerated

Pharmacotherapy Pearls An increase in weight was seen in nateglinide monotherapy, which was not seen when used in combination with metformin.

Special Geriatric Considerations No changes in safety and efficacy were seen in patients ≥65 years; however, some older adults may show increased sensitivity to dosing. Intensive glucose control (HbA$_{1c}$ <6.5%) has been linked to increased all-cause and cardiovascular mortality, hypoglycemia requiring assistance, and weight gain in adult type 2 diabetes. How "tightly" to control a geriatric patient's blood glucose needs to be individualized. Such a decision should be based on several factors, including the patient's functional and cognitive status, how well he/she recognizes hypoglycemic or hyperglycemic symptoms, and how to respond to them and other disease states. An HbA$_{1c}$ <7.5% is an acceptable endpoint for a healthy older adult, while <8% is acceptable for frail elderly patients, those with a duration of illness >10 years, or those with comorbid conditions and requiring combination diabetes medications. Patients who are unable to accurately draw up their dose will need assistance, such as prefilled syringes. Initial doses may require considerations for renal function in the elderly with dosing adjusted subsequently based on blood glucose monitoring. For elderly patients with diabetes who are relatively healthy, attaining target goals for aspirin use, blood pressure, lipids, smoking cessation, and diet and exercise may be more important than normalized glycemic control.

Dosage Forms Excipient information presented when available (limited, particularly for generics); consult specific product labeling.
Tablet, oral: 60 mg, 120 mg
  Starlix®: 60 mg, 120 mg

Selected References

Action to Control Cardiovascular Risk in Diabetes Study Group, Gerstein HC, Miller ME, et al, "Effects of Intensive Glucose Lowering in Type 2 Diabetes," *N Engl J Med*, 2008, 358(24):2545-59.

ADVANCE Collaborative Group, Patel A, MacMahon S, et al, "Intensive Blood Glucose Control and Vascular Outcomes in Patients With Type 2 Diabetes," *N Engl J Med*, 2008, 358(24):2560-72.

American Diabetes Association, "Standards of Medical Care in Diabetes – 2011," *Diabetes Care*, 2011, 34(Suppl 1):11-61.

Brown AF, Mangione CM, Saliba D, et al, "Guidelines for Improving the Care of the Older Person With Diabetes Mellitus," *J Am Geriatr Soc*, 2003, 51(5 Suppl Guidelines):265-80.

"VA/DoD Clinical Practice Guideline for the Management of Diabetes Mellitus," 2010. Available at http://www.healthquality.va.gov/Diabetes_Mellitus.asp

Nebivolol (ne BIV oh lole)

Related Information
Beta-Blockers *on page 2001*
Brand Names: U.S. Bystolic®
Index Terms Nebivolol Hydrochloride
Generic Availability (U.S.) No
Pharmacologic Category Beta Blocker, Beta-1 Selective
Use Treatment of hypertension, alone or in combination with other agents
Unlabeled/Investigational Use Heart failure
Contraindications Hypersensitivity to nebivolol or any component of the formulation; severe bradycardia; heart block greater than first-degree (except in patients with a functioning artificial pacemaker); cardiogenic shock; decompensated cardiac failure; sick sinus syndrome (unless a permanent pacemaker is in place); severe hepatic impairment (Child-Pugh class C)
Warnings/Precautions Use caution in patients with heart failure (HF); use gradual and careful titration; monitor for symptoms of congestive heart failure. Patients should be stabilized on HF regimen prior to initiation of beta-blocker; adjustment of other medications (ACE inhibitors and/or diuretics) may be required. **Note:** Nebivolol has not been shown to reduce morbidity or mortality in the general HF population. Use with caution in patients with myasthenia gravis, psychiatric disease (may cause CNS depression), bronchospastic disease, undergoing anesthesia; and in those with impaired hepatic function. Bradycardia may be observed more frequently in elderly patients (>65 years of age); dosage reductions may be necessary. Nebivolol should not be withdrawn abruptly (particularly in patients with CAD), but gradually tapered over 1-2 weeks to avoid acute tachycardia, hypertension, and/or ischemia. Chronic beta-blocker therapy should not be routinely withdrawn prior to major surgery. Can precipitate or aggravate symptoms of arterial insufficiency in patients with PVD and Raynaud's disease. Use with caution and monitor for progression of arterial obstruction. Use caution with concurrent use of digoxin, verapamil, or diltiazem; bradycardia or heart block may occur. Use caution with concurrent use of CYP2D6 inhibitors. Use with caution in patients receiving inhaled anesthetic agents known to depress myocardial contractility.

Nebivolol, with beta$_1$-selectivity, may be used cautiously in bronchospastic disease with close monitoring. Use cautiously in patients with diabetes because it can mask prominent hypoglycemic symptoms. May mask signs of hyperthyroidism (eg, tachycardia); if hyperthyroidism is suspected, carefully manage and monitor; abrupt withdrawal may exacerbate symptoms of hyperthyroidism or precipitate thyroid storm. Dosage adjustment is required in patients with moderate hepatic or severe renal impairment. Adequate alpha-blockade is required prior to use of any beta-blocker for patients with untreated pheochromocytoma. May induce or exacerbate psoriasis. Use caution with history of severe anaphylaxis to allergens; patients taking beta-blockers may become more sensitive to repeated challenges. Treatment of anaphylaxis (eg, epinephrine) in patients taking beta-blockers may be ineffective or promote undesirable effects.

◀ **Adverse Reactions (Reflective of adult population; not specific for elderly)**
1% to 10%:
Cardiovascular: Peripheral edema (1%), bradycardia (≤1%), chest pain (≤1%)
Central nervous system: Headache (6% to 9%), fatigue (dose related; 2% to 5%), dizziness (2% to 4%), insomnia (1%)
Dermatologic: Rash (≤1%)
Endocrine & metabolic: HDL levels decreased, hypercholesterolemia, triglyceride levels increased, uric acid levels increased
Gastrointestinal: Diarrhea (dose related; 2% to 3%), nausea (1% to 3%), abdominal pain
Hematologic: Platelet count decreased
Neuromuscular & skeletal: Paresthesia, weakness
Renal: BUN increased
Respiratory: Dyspnea (≤1%)

Drug Interactions
Metabolism/Transport Effects Substrate of CYP2D6 (major)
Avoid Concomitant Use
Avoid concomitant use of Nebivolol with any of the following: Floctafenine; Methacholine
Increased Effect/Toxicity
Nebivolol may increase the levels/effects of: Alpha-/Beta-Agonists (Direct-Acting); Alpha1-Blockers; Alpha2-Agonists; Amifostine; Antihypertensives; Antipsychotic Agents (Phenothiazines); Bupivacaine; Cardiac Glycosides; Fingolimod; Hypotensive Agents; Insulin; Lidocaine; Lidocaine (Systemic); Lidocaine (Topical); Mepivacaine; Methacholine; Midodrine; RiTUXimab; Sulfonylureas

The levels/effects of Nebivolol may be increased by: Acetylcholinesterase Inhibitors; Aminoquinolines (Antimalarial); Amiodarone; Anilidopiperidine Opioids; Antpsychotic Agents (Phenothiazines); Calcium Channel Blockers (Dihydropyridine); Calcium Channel Blockers (Nondihydropyridine); CYP2D6 Inhibitors (Moderate); CYP2D6 Inhibitors (Strong); Diazoxide; Dipyridamole; Disopyramide; Dronedarone; Floctafenine; Herbs (Hypotensive Properties); MAO Inhibitors; Pentoxifylline; Phosphodiesterase 5 Inhibitors; Propafenone; Propoxyphene; Prostacyclin Analogues; QuiNIDine; Reserpine; Selective Serotonin Reuptake Inhibitors
Decreased Effect
Nebivolol may decrease the levels/effects of: Beta2-Agonists; Theophylline Derivatives

The levels/effects of Nebivolol may be decreased by: Barbiturates; Herbs (Hypertensive Properties); Methylphenidate; Nonsteroidal Anti-Inflammatory Agents; Peginterferon Alfa-2b; Rifamycin Derivatives; Yohimbine
Ethanol/Nutrition/Herb Interactions Herb/Nutraceutical: Avoid bayberry, blue cohosh, cayenne, ephedra, ginger, ginseng (American), kola, licorice (may worsen hypertension). Avoid black cohosh, California poppy, coleus, golden seal, hawthorn, mistletoe, periwinkle, quinine, shepherd's purse (may increase antihypertensive effect).
Stability Store at 20°C to 25°C (68°F to 77°F). Protect from light.
Mechanism of Action Highly-selective inhibitor of beta₁-adrenergic receptors; at doses ≤10 mg nebivolol preferentially blocks beta₁-receptors. Nebivolol, unlike other beta-blockers, also produces an endothelium-derived nitric oxide-dependent vasodilation resulting in a reduction of systemic vascular resistance.
Pharmacodynamics/Kinetics
Absorption: Rapid
Distribution: V_d: 8-12 L/kg
Protein binding: ~98%, primarily to albumin
Metabolism: Hepatic; via glucuronidation and CYP2D6; extensive first-pass metabolism to multiple active metabolites with variable activity
Bioavailability: ~12% (extensive metabolizers); 96% (poor metabolizers)
Half-life elimination: Terminal: 10-12 hours (extensive metabolizers); 19-32 hours in poor metabolizers
Time to peak, plasma: 1.5-4 hours
Excretion: Urine (extensive metabolizers: 38%; poor metabolizers: 67%; <0.5% of total dose as unchanged drug); feces (extensive metabolizers: 44%; poor metabolizers: 13%; <0.5% of total dose as unchanged drug)
Dosage
Geriatric & Adult
Hypertension: Oral: Initial: 5 mg once daily; if initial response is inadequate, may be increased at 2-week intervals to a maximum dose of 40 mg once daily
Heart failure (unlabeled use): Adults ≥70 years: Oral: Initial: 1.25 mg once daily; if tolerated, may increase by 2.5 mg at 1- to 2-week intervals to a maximum dose of 10 mg once daily (Flather, 2005). **Note:** Nebivolol has not been shown to reduce morbidity or mortality in the general HF population.

Renal Impairment Severe impairment (Cl$_{cr}$ <30 mL/minute): Initial: 2.5 mg/day; increase cautiously.

Hepatic Impairment Moderate impairment (Child-Pugh class B): Initial: 2.5 mg/day; increase cautiously.

Administration May be administered with or without food.

Monitoring Parameters Blood pressure, ECG; serum glucose (in diabetic patients)

Special Geriatric Considerations Due to alterations in the beta-adrenergic autonomic nervous system, beta-adrenergic blockade may result in less hemodynamic response than seen in younger adults. Studies indicate that despite decreased sensitivity to the chronotropic effects of beta-blockade with age, there appears to be an increased myocardial sensitivity to the negative inotropic effect during stress (eg, exercise). Controlled trials have shown the overall response rate for propranolol to be only 20% to 50% in elderly populations. Therefore, all beta-adrenergic blocking drugs may result in a decreased response as compared to younger adults.

Dosage Forms Excipient information presented when available (limited, particularly for generics); consult specific product labeling.

Tablet, oral:

Bystolic®: 2.5 mg, 5 mg, 10 mg, 20 mg

Selected References

Brixius K, Bundkirchen A, Bolck B, et al, "Nebivolol, Bucindolol, Metoprolol and Carvedilol are Devoid of Intrinsic Sympathomimetic Activity in Human Myocardium," *Br J Pharmacol*, 2001, 133(8):1330-8.

Chobanian AV, Bakris GL, Black HR, et al, "The Seventh Report of the Joint National Committee on Prevention, Detection, Evaluation, and Treatment of High Blood Pressure: The JNC 7 Report," *JAMA*, 2003, 289(19):2560-71.

Flather MD, Shibata MC, Coats AJ, et al, "Randomized Trial to Determine the Effect of Nebivolol on Mortality and Cardiovascular Hospital Admission in Elderly Patients With Heart Failure (SENIORS)," *Eur Heart J*, 2005, 26 (3):215-25.

Fleisher LA, Beckman JA, Brown KA, et al, "ACC/AHA 2007 Guidelines on Perioperative Cardiovascular Evaluation for Noncardiac Surgery: A Report of the American College of Cardiology/American Heart Association Task Force on Practice Guidelines (Writing Committee to Revise the 2002 Guidelines on Perioperative Cardiovascular Evaluation for Noncardiac Surgery) Developed in Collaboration With the American Society of Echocardiography, American Society of Nuclear Cardiology, Heart Rhythm Society, Society of Cardiovascular Anesthesiologists, Society for Cardiovascular Angiography and Interventions, Society for Vascular Medicine and Biology, and Society for Vascular Surgery," *J Am Coll Cardiol*, 2007, 50(17):e159-241.

Heart Failure Society of America, "HFSA 2006 Comprehensive Heart Failure Practice Guideline," *J Card Fail*, 2006, 12 (1):e1-119. Available at http://www.heartfailureguideline.org.

Juul AB, Wetterslev J, Gluud C, et al, "Effect of Perioperative Beta Blockade in Patients With Diabetes Undergoing Major Non-Cardiac Surgery: Randomized Placebo Controlled, Blinded Multicentre Trial. DIPOM Trial Group," *BMJ*, 2006, 332(7556):1482.

Lang DM, "Anaphylactoid and Anaphylactic Reactions. Hazards of Beta-Blockers," *Drug Saf*, 1995, 12(5):299-304.

Lindenauer PK, Pekow P, Wang K, et al, "Perioperative Beta-Blocker Therapy and Mortality After Noncardiac Surgery," *N Engl J Med*, 2005, 353(4):349-61.

Mokhlesi B, Leikin JB, Murray P, et al, "Adult Toxicology in Critical Care: Part II: Specific Poisonings," *Chest*, 2003, 123 (3):897-922.

Nuttall SL, Routledge HC, and Kendall MJ, "A Comparison of the Beta1-Selectivity of Three Beta1-Selective Beta-Blockers," *J Clin Pharm Ther*, 2003, 28(3):179-86.

Patrianakos AP, Parthenakis FI, Mavrakis HE, et al, "Comparative Efficacy of Nebivolol versus Carvedilol on Left Ventricular Function and Exercise Capacity in Patients With Non-Ischemic Cardiomyopathy. A 12-Month Study," *Am Heart J*, 2005, 150(5):985.

Prisant LM, "Nebivolol: Pharmacologic Profile of an Ultraselective, Vasodilatory [Beta]1-Blocker," *J Clin Pharm*, 2007 [epub ahead of print].

UK Prospective Diabetes Study Group, "Efficacy of Atenolol and Captopril in Reducing Risk of Macrovascular and Microvascular Complications in Type 2 Diabetes: UKPDS 39," *BMJ*, 1998, 317(7160):713-20.

Yang H, Raymer K, Butler R, et al, "The Effects of Perioperative Beta-Blockade: Results of the Metoprolol After Vascular Surgery (MaVS) Study, a Randomized Controlled Trial," *Am Hear J*, 2006, 152(5):983-90.

◆ **Nebivolol Hydrochloride** *see* Nebivolol *on page 1273*

Nedocromil (ne doe KROE mil)

Related Information

Asthma *on page 2016*

Inhalant Agents *on page 2010*

Brand Names: U.S. Alocril®

Brand Names: Canada Alocril®

Index Terms Nedocromil Sodium

Generic Availability (U.S.) No

Pharmacologic Category Mast Cell Stabilizer

Use Treatment of itching associated with allergic conjunctivitis

Contraindications Hypersensitivity to nedocromil or any component of the formulation

Warnings/Precautions Ophthalmic solution contains benzalkonium chloride, which may be absorbed by contact lenses; users of contact lenses should not wear them during periods of symptomatic allergic conjunctivitis.

◀ **Adverse Reactions (Reflective of adult population; not specific for elderly)**
>10%:
  Central nervous system: Headache (40%)
  Gastrointestinal: Unpleasant taste
  Ocular: Burning, irritation, stinging
  Respiratory: Nasal congestion
1% to 10%:
  Ocular: Conjunctivitis, eye redness, photophobia
  Respiratory: Asthma, rhinitis

Drug Interactions
  Avoid Concomitant Use There are no known interactions where it is recommended to avoid concomitant use.
  Increased Effect/Toxicity There are no known significant interactions involving an increase in effect.
  Decreased Effect There are no known significant interactions involving a decrease in effect.

Stability Store at 2°C to 25°C (36°F to 77°F).

Mechanism of Action Inhibits the activation of and mediator release from a variety of inflammatory cell types associated with hypersensitivity reactions including eosinophils, neutrophils, macrophages, mast cells, monocytes, and platelets; it inhibits the release of histamine, leukotrienes, and slow-reacting substance of anaphylaxis.

Pharmacodynamics/Kinetics
  Absorption: Low (<4%)
  Excretion: Urine 70% (as unchanged drug); feces 30% (as unchanged drug)

Dosage
  Geriatric & Adult Allergic conjunctivitis: Ophthalmic: 1-2 drops in each eye twice daily throughout the period of exposure to allergen

Administration If patient has aerosol (MDI) bronchodilators in their regimen, these should be used first, 5-10 minutes prior to use of nedocromil.

Monitoring Parameters Pulmonary function, spirometry

Pharmacotherapy Pearls Nedocromil has no known therapeutic systemic activity when delivered by inhalation.

Special Geriatric Considerations Evaluate the patient's or caregiver's ability to safely administer the correct dose of ophthalmic medication.

Dosage Forms Excipient information presented when available (limited, particularly for generics); consult specific product labeling.
  Solution, ophthalmic, as sodium [drops]:
    Alocril® 2% (5 mL) [contains benzalkonium chloride]

◆ **Nedocromil Sodium** see Nedocromil on page 1275

Nefazodone (nef AY zoe done)

Related Information
  Antidepressant Agents on page 1991
Medication Safety Issues
  Sound-alike/look-alike issues:
    Serzone® may be confused with selegiline, Serentil®, SEROquel®, sertraline
Index Terms Nefazodone Hydrochloride; Serzone
Generic Availability (U.S.) Yes
Pharmacologic Category Antidepressant, Serotonin Reuptake Inhibitor/Antagonist
Use Treatment of depression
Unlabeled/Investigational Use Treatment of post-traumatic stress disorder
Medication Guide Available Yes
Contraindications Hypersensitivity to nefazodone, related compounds (phenylpiperazines), or any component of the formulation; liver injury due to previous nefazodone treatment, active liver disease, or elevated serum transaminases; concurrent use or use of MAO inhibitors within previous 14 days; use in a patient during the acute recovery phase of MI; concurrent use with carbamazepine, cisapride, or pimozide; concurrent therapy with triazolam or alprazolam is generally contraindicated (dosage must be reduced by 75% for triazolam and 50% for alprazolam; such reductions may not be possible with available dosage forms).
Warnings/Precautions [U.S. Boxed Warning]: Antidepressants increase the risk of suicidal thinking and behavior in children, adolescents, and young adults (18-24 years of age) with major depressive disorder (MDD) and other psychiatric disorders; consider risk prior to prescribing. Short-term studies did not show an increased risk in patients >24 years of age and showed a decreased risk in patients ≥65 years. Closely monitor for clinical worsening, suicidality, or unusual changes in behavior; the patient's family or caregiver should

be instructed to closely observe the patient and communicate condition with healthcare provider. A medication guide should be dispensed with each prescription. **Nefazodone is not FDA approved for use in children.**

The possibility of a suicide attempt is inherent in major depression and may persist until remission occurs. Monitor for worsening of depression or suicidality, especially during initiation of therapy (generally first 1-2 months) or with dose increases or decreases. Use caution in high-risk patients. Worsening depression and severe abrupt suicidality that are not part of the presenting symptoms may require discontinuation or modification of drug therapy. The patient's family or caregiver should be alerted to monitor patients for the emergence of suicidality and associated behaviors (such as agitation, irritability, hostility, impulsivity, and hypomania) and call healthcare provider.

May worsen psychosis in some patients or precipitate a shift to mania or hypomania in patients with bipolar disorder. Patients presenting with depressive symptoms should be screened for bipolar disorder. Monotherapy in patients with bipolar disorder should be avoided. **Nefazodone is not FDA approved for the treatment of bipolar depression.**

Cases of life-threatening hepatic failure have been reported (risk should be considered when choosing an agent for the treatment of depression); discontinue if clinical signs or symptoms suggest liver failure. May cause sedation, resulting in impaired performance of tasks requiring alertness (eg, operating machinery or driving). May increase the risks associated with electroconvulsive therapy. Consider discontinuing, when possible, prior to elective surgery. Therapy should not be abruptly discontinued in patients receiving high doses for prolonged periods. Rare reports of priapism have occurred. The incidence of sexual dysfunction with nefazodone is generally lower than with SSRIs.

The risk of sedation, conduction disturbances, orthostatic hypotension, or anticholinergic effects are very low relative to other antidepressants. Use with caution in patients with a history of cardiovascular disease (including previous MI, stroke, tachycardia, or conduction abnormalities). Use with caution in patients with urinary retention, benign prostatic hyperplasia, narrow-angle glaucoma, xerostomia, visual problems, constipation, or history of bowel obstruction (due to anticholinergic effects).

Use caution in patients with a previous seizure disorder or condition predisposing to seizures such as brain damage, alcoholism, or concurrent therapy with other drugs which lower the seizure threshold. Use with caution in patients with renal dysfunction and in elderly patients.

Adverse Reactions (Reflective of adult population; not specific for elderly)
>10%:
Central nervous system: Headache, drowsiness, insomnia, agitation, dizziness
Gastrointestinal: Xerostomia, nausea, constipation
Neuromuscular & skeletal: Weakness
1% to 10%:
Cardiovascular: Bradycardia, hypotension, peripheral edema, postural hypotension, vasodilation
Central nervous system: Chills, fever, incoordination, lightheadedness, confusion, memory impairment, abnormal dreams, decreased concentration, ataxia, psychomotor retardation, tremor
Dermatologic: Pruritus, rash
Endocrine & metabolic: Breast pain, impotence, libido decreased
Gastrointestinal: Gastroenteritis, vomiting, dyspepsia, diarrhea, increased appetite, thirst, taste perversion
Genitourinary: Urinary frequency, urinary retention
Hematologic: Hematocrit decreased
Neuromuscular & skeletal: Arthralgia, hypertonia, paresthesia, neck rigidity, tremor
Ocular: Blurred vision (9%), abnormal vision (7%), eye pain, visual field defect
Otic: Tinnitus
Respiratory: Bronchitis, cough, dyspnea, pharyngitis
Miscellaneous: Flu syndrome, infection
Drug Interactions
Metabolism/Transport Effects Substrate (major) of CYP2D6, 3A4; **Inhibits** CYP1A2 (weak), 2B6 (weak), 2C8 (weak), 2D6 (weak), 3A4 (strong); **Induces** P-glycoprotein
Avoid Concomitant Use
Avoid concomitant use of Nefazodone with any of the following: Alfuzosin; CarBAMazepine; Cisapride; Conivaptan; Crizotinib; Dabigatran Etexilate; Dronedarone; Eplerenone; Everolimus; Fluticasone (Oral Inhalation); Halofantrine; Lapatinib; Lovastatin; Lurasidone; Methylene Blue; Nilotinib; Nisoldipine; Pimozide; Ranolazine; Rivaroxaban; RomiDEPsin; Salmeterol; Sibutramine; Silodosin; Simvastatin; Tamsulosin; Ticagrelor; Tolvaptan; Toremifene

Increased Effect/Toxicity

Nefazodone may increase the levels/effects of: Alfuzosin; Almotriptan; Alosetron; Benzo-diazepines (metabolized by oxidation); Bortezomib; Brentuximab Vedotin; Brinzolamide; Budesonide (Nasal); Budesonide (Systemic, Oral Inhalation); CarBAMazepine; Cardiac Glycosides; Ciclesonide; Cisapride; CloZAPine; Colchicine; Conivaptan; Corticosteroids (Orally Inhaled); Crizotinib; CYP3A4 Substrates; Dienogest; Dronedarone; Dutasteride; Eplerenone; Everolimus; FentaNYL; Fesoterodine; Fluticasone (Nasal); Fluticasone (Oral Inhalation); GuanFACINE; Halofantrine; Iloperidone; Ixabepilone; Lapatinib; Lovastatin; Lumefantrine; Lurasidone; Maraviroc; Methylene Blue; MethylPREDNISolone; Nilotinib; Nisoldipine; Paricalcitol; Pazopanib; Pimecrolimus; Pimozide; Ranolazine; Rivaroxaban; RomiDEPsin; Salmeterol; Saxagliptin; Serotonin Modulators; Sildenafil; Silodosin; Simvastatin; SORAfenib; Tacrolimus; Tacrolimus (Systemic); Tacrolimus (Topical); Tadalafil; Tamsulosin; Ticagrelor; Tolterodine; Tolvaptan; Toremifene; Vardenafil; Vemurafenib; Vilazodone

The levels/effects of Nefazodone may be increased by: Abiraterone Acetate; BusPIRone; CYP2D6 Inhibitors (Moderate); CYP2D6 Inhibitors (Strong); CYP3A4 Inhibitors (Moderate); CYP3A4 Inhibitors (Strong); Dasatinib; MAO Inhibitors; Protease Inhibitors; Selective Serotonin Reuptake Inhibitors; Sibutramine

Decreased Effect

Nefazodone may decrease the levels/effects of: Dabigatran Etexilate; Linagliptin; P-Glyco-protein Substrates; Prasugrel; Ticagrelor

The levels/effects of Nefazodone may be decreased by: CarBAMazepine; CYP3A4 Inducers (Strong); Deferasirox; Peginterferon Alfa-2b; Tocilizumab

Ethanol/Nutrition/Herb Interactions

Ethanol: May increase CNS depression; monitor for increased effects with coadministration. Caution patients about effects.

Food: Nefazodone absorption may be delayed and bioavailability may be decreased if taken with food.

Herb/Nutraceutical: Avoid valerian, St John's wort, SAMe, kava kava (may increase risk of serotonin syndrome and/or excessive sedation).

Stability Store at room temperature, below 40°C (104°F) in a tight container.

Mechanism of Action Inhibits neuronal reuptake of serotonin and norepinephrine; also blocks 5-HT$_2$ and alpha$_1$ receptors; has no significant affinity for alpha$_2$, beta-adrenergic, 5-HT$_{1A}$, cholinergic, dopaminergic, or benzodiazepine receptors

Pharmacodynamics/Kinetics

Onset of action: Therapeutic: Up to 6 weeks

Distribution: V$_d$: 0.22-0.87 L/kg

Protein binding: >99%

Metabolism: Hepatic to three active metabolites: Triazoledione, hydroxynefazodone, and m-chlorophenylpiperazine (mCPP)

Bioavailability: 20% (variable)

Half-life elimination: Parent drug: 2-4 hours; active metabolites persist longer

Time to peak, serum: 1 hour, prolonged in presence of food

Excretion: Primarily urine (as metabolites); feces

Dosage

Geriatric Oral: Initial: 50 mg twice daily; increase dose to 100 mg twice daily in 2 weeks; usual maintenance dose: 200-400 mg/day

Adult

Depression: Oral: 200 mg/day, administered in two divided doses initially, with a range of 300-600 mg/day in 2 divided doses thereafter.

Post-traumatic stress disorder (PTSD) (unlabeled use): Oral: Initial: 100 mg twice daily; target dose: 600 mg/day (average daily dose: 463 mg).

Administration Dosing after meals may decrease lightheadedness and postural hypotension, but may also decrease absorption and therefore effectiveness.

Monitoring Parameters If AST/ALT increase >3 times ULN, the drug should be discontinued and not reintroduced; mental status for depression, suicide ideation (especially at the beginning of therapy or when doses are increased or decreased), anxiety, social functioning, mania, panic attacks

Reference Range Therapeutic plasma levels have not yet been defined

Pharmacotherapy Pearls May cause less sexual dysfunction than other antidepressants. Women and elderly receiving single doses attain significant higher peak concentrations than male volunteers.

Special Geriatric Considerations Data on nefazodone in the elderly are limited, specifically regarding efficacy; clinical trials in adult patients have found it superior to placebo and similar to imipramine; nefazodone's C$_{max}$ and AUC have been reported to be increased twofold in the elderly and women after a single dose compared to younger patients, however, these differences were markedly reduced with multiple dosing with women having AUC values of nefazodone and its hydroxy metabolite remaining approximately 50% higher

Dosage Forms Excipient information presented when available (limited, particularly for generics); consult specific product labeling.

Tablet, oral, as hydrochloride: 50 mg, 100 mg, 150 mg, 200 mg, 250 mg

Selected References

Barbhaiya RH, Buch AB, and Greene DS, "A Study of the Effect of Age and Gender on the Pharmacokinetics of Nefazodone After Single and Multiple Doses," *J Clin Psychopharmacol*, 1996, 16(1):19-25.

Fontaine R, Ontiveros A, Elie R, et al, "A Double-Blind Comparison of Nefazodone, Imipramine, and Placebo in Major Depression," *J Clin Psychiatry*, 1994, 55(6):234-41.

Rickels K, Schweizer E, Clary C, et al, "Nefazodone and Imipramine in Major Depression: A Placebo-Controlled Trial," *Br J Psychiatry*, 1994, 164(6):802-5.

Shea JP, Shulka UA, Rittman KA, "Single Dose Pharmacokinetics of Nefazodone in Elderly Subjects, Renally Impaired Patients, and Patients With Hepatic Cirrhosis in Comparison to Healthy Volunteers," *Clin Pharmacol Ther*, 1988, 43:146.

♦ **Nefazodone Hydrochloride** see Nefazodone on page 1276
♦ **Neo-Calglucon® [OTC]** see Calcium Salts (Oral) on page 256
♦ **Neo-Cultol® [OTC]** see Mineral Oil on page 1217
♦ **Neofrin** see Phenylephrine (Ophthalmic) on page 1443

Neomycin and Polymyxin B (nee oh MYE sin & pol i MIKS in bee)

Brand Names: U.S. Neosporin® G.U. Irrigant
Brand Names: Canada Neosporin® Irrigating Solution
Index Terms Polymyxin B and Neomycin
Generic Availability (U.S.) Yes
Pharmacologic Category Antibiotic, Topical; Genitourinary Irrigant
Use Short-term as a continuous irrigant or rinse in the urinary bladder to prevent bacteriuria and gram-negative rod septicemia associated with the use of indwelling catheters
Contraindications Hypersensitivity to neomycin, polymyxin B, or any component of the formulation
Adverse Reactions (Reflective of adult population; not specific for elderly) Frequency not defined.

Dermatologic: Contact dermatitis, erythema, rash, urticaria
Genitourinary: Bladder irritation
Local: Burning
Neuromuscular & skeletal: Neuromuscular blockade
Otic: Ototoxicity
Renal: Nephrotoxicity

Drug Interactions

Avoid Concomitant Use
Avoid concomitant use of Neomycin and Polymyxin B with any of the following: BCG; Gallium Nitrate

Increased Effect/Toxicity
Neomycin and Polymyxin B may increase the levels/effects of: AbobotulinumtoxinA; Acarbose; Bisphosphonate Derivatives; CARBOplatin; Colistimethate; CycloSPORINE; CycloSPORINE (Systemic); Gallium Nitrate; Neuromuscular-Blocking Agents; OnabotulinumtoxinA; RimabotulinumtoxinB; Vitamin K Antagonists

The levels/effects of Neomycin and Polymyxin B may be increased by: Amphotericin B; Capreomycin; CISplatin; Loop Diuretics; Nonsteroidal Anti-Inflammatory Agents; Vancomycin

Decreased Effect
Neomycin and Polymyxin B may decrease the levels/effects of: BCG; Cardiac Glycosides; SORAfenib

The levels/effects of Neomycin and Polymyxin B may be decreased by: Penicillins

Stability Store irrigation solution in refrigerator. The following stability information has also been reported: May be stored at room temperature for up to 6 months if undiluted (Cohen, 2007). Aseptically prepared dilutions (1 mL/1 L) should be stored in the refrigerator and discarded after 48 hours.

Mechanism of Action
Neomycin: Interferes with bacterial protein synthesis by binding to 30S ribosomal subunits

Polymyxin B: Binds to phospholipids, alters permeability, and damages the bacterial cytoplasmic membrane permitting leakage of intracellular constituents

Pharmacodynamics/Kinetics Absorption: Topical: Clinically insignificant amounts of neomycin and polymyxin B are absorbed following irrigation of an intact urinary bladder. Systemic absorption may occur from a denuded bladder.

Dosage

Geriatric & Adult Bladder irrigation: **Not for I.V. injection**; add 1 mL irrigant to 1 L isotonic saline solution and connect container to the inflow of lumen of 3-way catheter. Continuous irrigant or rinse in the urinary bladder for up to a maximum of 10 days with administration rate adjusted to patient's urine output; usually no more than 1 L of irrigant is used per day.

Administration Bladder irrigant: Do not inject irrigant solution; concentrated irrigant solution must be diluted in 1 L normal saline before administration; connect irrigation container to the inflow lumen of a 3-way catheter to permit continuous irrigation of the urinary bladder

Dosage Forms Excipient information presented when available (limited, particularly for generics); consult specific product labeling.

Solution, irrigation: Neomycin 40 mg and polymyxin B sulfate 200,000 units per 1 mL (1 mL, 20 mL)

Neosporin® G.U. Irrigant: Neomycin 40 mg and polymyxin sulfate B 200,000 units per 1 mL (1 mL, 20 mL)

Neomycin, Colistin, Hydrocortisone, and Thonzonium

(nee oh MYE sin, koe LIS tin, hye droe KOR ti sone, & thon ZOE nee um)

Brand Names: U.S. Coly-Mycin® S; Cortisporin®-TC

Index Terms Colistin, Hydrocortisone, Neomycin, and Thonzonium; Hydrocortisone, Neomycin, Colistin, and Thonzonium; Thonzonium, Neomycin, Colistin, and Hydrocortisone

Generic Availability (U.S.) No

Pharmacologic Category Antibiotic, Otic; Antibiotic/Corticosteroid, Otic; Corticosteroid, Otic

Use Treatment of superficial and susceptible bacterial infections of the external auditory canal; for treatment of susceptible bacterial infections of mastoidectomy and fenestration cavities

Dosage

Geriatric & Adult Ear inflammation/infection: Otic:

Calibrated dropper: 5 drops in affected ear 3-4 times/day

Dropper bottle: 4 drops in affected ear 3-4 times/day

Note: Alternatively, a cotton wick may be inserted in the ear canal and saturated with suspension every 4 hours; wick should be replaced at least every 24 hours

Dosage Forms Excipient information presented when available (limited, particularly for generics); consult specific product labeling.

Suspension, otic [drops]:

Coly-Mycin® S: Neomycin 0.33%, colistin 0.3%, hydrocortisone acetate 1%, and thonzonium bromide 0.05% (5 mL) [contains thimerosal]

Cortisporin®-TC: Neomycin 0.33%, colistin 0.3%, hydrocortisone acetate 1%, and thonzonium bromide 0.05% (10 mL) [contains thimerosal]

Neomycin, Polymyxin B, and Dexamethasone

(nee oh MYE sin, pol i MIKS in bee, & deks a METH a sone)

Related Information

Dexamethasone (Ophthalmic) *on page 487*

Brand Names: U.S. Maxitrol®; Poly-Dex™ [DSC]

Brand Names: Canada Dioptrol®; Maxitrol®

Index Terms Dexamethasone, Neomycin, and Polymyxin B; Polymyxin B, Neomycin, and Dexamethasone

Generic Availability (U.S.) Yes

Pharmacologic Category Antibiotic/Corticosteroid, Ophthalmic

Use Steroid-responsive inflammatory ocular conditions in which a corticosteroid is indicated and where bacterial infection or a risk of bacterial infection exists

Contraindications Hypersensitivity to neomycin, polymyxin B, dexamethasone, or any component of the formulation; viral, fungal, or tuberculosis diseases of the eye

Warnings/Precautions For ophthalmic use only. Sensitivity to neomycin may develop; discontinue if sensitivity reaction occurs. Prolonged use of corticosteroids may result in glaucoma; damage to the optic nerve, defects in visual acuity and fields of vision, and posterior subcapsular cataract formation may occur. Prolonged use of corticosteroids may increase the incidence of secondary ocular infection or mask acute infection (including fungal infections); may prolong or exacerbate ocular viral infections; use following cataract surgery may delay healing or increase the incidence of bleb formation. A maximum of 8 g of ointment or 20 mL of suspension should be prescribed initially; patients should be evaluated prior to additional refills. Suspension contains benzalkonium chloride which may be adsorbed by contact lenses; contact lenses should not be worn during treatment of ophthalmic infections.

Adverse Reactions (Reflective of adult population; not specific for elderly) Frequency not defined: Ocular: Allergic sensitivity, cutaneous sensitization, eye pain, development of glaucoma, cataract, increased intraocular pressure, optic nerve damage, wound healing delayed

Drug Interactions

Avoid Concomitant Use

Avoid concomitant use of Neomycin, Polymyxin B, and Dexamethasone with any of the following: Aldesleukin; BCG; Conivaptan; Crizotinib; Dabigatran Etexilate; Dronedarone; Everolimus; Gallium Nitrate; Lapatinib; Lurasidone; Natalizumab; Nilotinib; Nisoldipine; Pazopanib; Pimecrolimus; Praziquantel; Ranolazine; Rilpivirine; RomiDEPsin; Tacrolimus (Topical); Ticagrelor; Tolvaptan; Vandetanib

Increased Effect/Toxicity

Neomycin, Polymyxin B, and Dexamethasone may increase the levels/effects of: AbobotulinumtoxinA; Acarbose; Acetylcholinesterase Inhibitors; Amphotericin B; Bisphosphonate Derivatives; CARBOplatin; Colistimethate; CycloSPORINE; CycloSPORINE (Systemic); Deferasirox; Gallium Nitrate; Leflunomide; Lenalidomide; Loop Diuretics; Natalizumab; Neuromuscular-Blocking Agents; NSAID (COX-2 Inhibitor); NSAID (Nonselective); OnabotulinumtoxinA; RimabotulinumtoxinB; Thalidomide; Thiazide Diuretics; Vaccines (Live); Vitamin K Antagonists; Warfarin

The levels/effects of Neomycin, Polymyxin B, and Dexamethasone may be increased by: Amphotericin B; Antifungal Agents (Azole Derivatives, Systemic); Aprepitant; Asparaginase; Calcium Channel Blockers (Nondihydropyridine); Capreomycin; CISplatin; Conivaptan; CycloSPORINE; CycloSPORINE (Systemic); CYP3A4 Inhibitors (Moderate); CYP3A4 Inhibitors (Strong); Dasatinib; Denosumab; Estrogen Derivatives; Fluconazole; Fosaprepitant; Loop Diuretics; Macrolide Antibiotics; Neuromuscular-Blocking Agents (Nondepolarizing); P-Glycoprotein Inhibitors; Pimecrolimus; Quinolone Antibiotics; Roflumilast; Salicylates; Tacrolimus (Topical); Telaprevir; Trastuzumab; Vancomycin

Decreased Effect

Neomycin, Polymyxin B, and Dexamethasone may decrease the levels/effects of: Aldesleukin; Antidiabetic Agents; BCG; Boceprevir; Brentuximab Vedotin; Calcitriol; Cardiac Glycosides; Caspofungin; Corticorelin; Crizotinib; CycloSPORINE; CycloSPORINE (Systemic); CYP3A4 Substrates; Dabigatran Etexilate; Dronedarone; Everolimus; Exemestane; Gefitinib; GuanFACINE; Imatinib; Isoniazid; Ixabepilone; Lapatinib; Lurasidone; Maraviroc; NIFEdipine; Nilotinib; Nisoldipine; Pazopanib; P-Glycoprotein Substrates; Praziquantel; Ranolazine; Rivaroxaban; RomiDEPsin; Salicylates; Sipuleucel-T; SORAfenib; Tadalafil; Telaprevir; Ticagrelor; Tolvaptan; Ulipristal; Vaccines (Inactivated); Vandetanib; Vemurafenib

The levels/effects of Neomycin, Polymyxin B, and Dexamethasone may be decreased by: Aminoglutethimide; Antacids; Barbiturates; Bile Acid Sequestrants; CYP3A4 Inducers (Strong); Echinacea; Herbs (CYP3A4 Inducers); Mitotane; Penicillins; P-Glycoprotein Inducers; Primidone; Rifamycin Derivatives; Rilpivirine; Tocilizumab

Mechanism of Action

Neomycin: Interferes with bacterial protein synthesis by binding to 30S ribosomal subunits

Polymyxin B: Binds to phospholipids, alters permeability, and damages the bacterial cytoplasmic membrane permitting leakage of intracellular constituents

Dexamethasone: Decreases inflammation by suppression of neutrophil migration, decreased production of inflammatory mediators, and reversal of increased capillary permeability; suppresses normal immune response. Dexamethasone's mechanism of antiemetic activity is unknown.

Pharmacodynamics/Kinetics See individual agents.

Dosage

Geriatric & Adult Ocular inflammation/infection: Ophthalmic:

Ointment: Place a small amount (~1/2") in the affected eye 3-4 times/day or apply at bedtime as an adjunct with drops

Suspension: Instill 1-2 drops into affected eye(s) every 3-4 hours; in severe disease, drops may be used hourly and tapered to discontinuation

Administration Shake well before using; tilt head back, place medication in conjunctival sac, and close eyes; apply finger pressure on lacrimal sac for 1 minute following instillation

Monitoring Parameters Monitor intraocular pressure with use longer than 10 days

Special Geriatric Considerations Evaluate the patient's or caregiver's ability to safely administer the correct dose of ophthalmic medication.

◀ **Dosage Forms** Excipient information presented when available (limited, particularly for generics); consult specific product labeling. [DSC] = Discontinued product

Ointment, ophthalmic: Neomycin 3.5 mg, polymyxin B sulfate 10,000 units, and dexamethasone 0.1% per g (3.5 g)

Maxitrol®: Neomycin 3.5 mg, polymyxin B sulfate 10,000 units, and dexamethasone 0.1% per g (3.5 g)

Poly-Dex™: Neomycin 3.5 mg, polymyxin B sulfate 10,000 units, and dexamethasone 0.1% per g (3.5 g) [DSC]

Suspension, ophthalmic [drops]: Neomycin 3.5 mg, polymyxin B sulfate 10,000 units, and dexamethasone 0.1% per 1 mL (5 mL)

Maxitrol®: Neomycin 3.5 mg, polymyxin B sulfate 10,000 units, and dexamethasone 0.1% per 1 mL (5 mL) [contains benzalkonium chloride]

Poly-Dex™: Neomycin 3.5 mg, polymyxin B sulfate 10,000 units, and dexamethasone 0.1% per 1 mL (5 mL) [contains benzalkonium chloride] [DSC]

Neomycin, Polymyxin B, and Gramicidin
(nee oh MYE sin, pol i MIKS in bee, & gram i SYE din)

Brand Names: U.S. Neosporin® Ophthalmic Solution

Brand Names: Canada Neosporin®; Optimyxin Plus®

Index Terms Gramicidin, Neomycin, and Polymyxin B; Polymyxin B, Neomycin, and Gramicidin

Generic Availability (U.S.) Yes

Pharmacologic Category Antibiotic, Ophthalmic

Use Treatment of superficial ocular infection

Contraindications Hypersensitivity to neomycin, polymyxin B, gramicidin or any component of the formulation

Warnings/Precautions Symptoms of neomycin sensitization include itching, reddening, edema, failure to heal; prolonged use may result in glaucoma, defects in visual acuity, posterior subcapsular cataract formation, and secondary ocular infections

Adverse Reactions (Reflective of adult population; not specific for elderly) Frequency not defined: Ocular: Transient irritation, burning, stinging, itching, inflammation, angioneurotic edema, urticaria, vesicular and maculopapular dermatitis

Drug Interactions

Avoid Concomitant Use

Avoid concomitant use of Neomycin, Polymyxin B, and Gramicidin with any of the following: BCG; Gallium Nitrate

Increased Effect/Toxicity

Neomycin, Polymyxin B, and Gramicidin may increase the levels/effects of: AbobotulinumtoxinA; Acarbose; Bisphosphonate Derivatives; CARBOplatin; Colistimethate; CycloSPORINE (Systemic); CycloSPORINE; Gallium Nitrate; Neuromuscular-Blocking Agents; OnabotulinumtoxinA; RimabotulinumtoxinB; Vitamin K Antagonists

The levels/effects of Neomycin, Polymyxin B, and Gramicidin may be increased by: Amphotericin B; Capreomycin; CISplatin; Loop Diuretics; Nonsteroidal Anti-Inflammatory Agents; Vancomycin

Decreased Effect

Neomycin, Polymyxin B, and Gramicidin may decrease the levels/effects of: BCG; Cardiac Glycosides; SORAfenib

The levels/effects of Neomycin, Polymyxin B, and Gramicidin may be decreased by: Penicillins

Mechanism of Action Interferes with bacterial protein synthesis by binding to 30S ribosomal subunits; binds to phospholipids, alters permeability, and damages the bacterial cytoplasmic membrane permitting leakage of intracellular constituents

Dosage

Geriatric & Adult Ophthalmic: Instill 1-2 drops 4-6 times/day or more frequently as required for severe infections

Special Geriatric Considerations Evaluate the patient's or caregiver's ability to safely administer the correct dose of ophthalmic medication.

Dosage Forms Excipient information presented when available (limited, particularly for generics); consult specific product labeling.

Solution, ophthalmic [drops]: Neomycin 1.75 mg, polymyxin B 10,000 units, and gramicidin 0.025 mg per 1 mL (10 mL)

Neosporin® Ophthalmic Solution: Neomycin 1.75 mg, polymyxin B 10,000 units, and gramicidin 0.025 mg per 1 mL (10 mL)

◆ **Neoral®** see CycloSPORINE (Systemic) *on page 432*

Neostigmine (nee oh STIG meen)

Medication Safety Issues
  Sound-alike/look-alike issues:
    Prostigmin® may be confused with physostigmine
Brand Names: U.S. Prostigmin®
Brand Names: Canada Prostigmin®
Index Terms Neostigmine Bromide; Neostigmine Methylsulfate
Generic Availability (U.S.) Yes: Injection
Pharmacologic Category Acetylcholinesterase Inhibitor
Use Reversal of the effects of nondepolarizing neuromuscular-blocking agents; treatment of myasthenia gravis; prevention and treatment of postoperative bladder distention and urinary retention
Contraindications Hypersensitivity to neostigmine, bromides, or any component of the formulation; GI or GU obstruction
Warnings/Precautions Does **not** antagonize and may prolong the Phase I block of depolarizing muscle relaxants (eg, succinylcholine). Use with caution in patients with epilepsy, asthma, bradycardia, hyperthyroidism, cardiac arrhythmias, or peptic ulcer; not generally recommended for use in patients with vagotonia. Adequate facilities should be available for cardiopulmonary resuscitation when testing and adjusting dose for myasthenia gravis. Have atropine and epinephrine ready to treat hypersensitivity reactions. Overdosage may result in cholinergic crisis, this must be distinguished from myasthenic crisis. Anticholinesterase insensitivity can develop for brief or prolonged periods.
Adverse Reactions (Reflective of adult population; not specific for elderly) Frequency not defined.
  Cardiovascular: Arrhythmias (especially bradycardia), AV block, cardiac arrest, flushing, hypotension, nodal rhythm, nonspecific ECG changes, syncope, tachycardia
  Central nervous system: Convulsions, dizziness, drowsiness, dysarthria, dysphonia, headache, loss of consciousness
  Dermatologic: Skin rash, thrombophlebitis (I.V.), urticaria
  Gastrointestinal: Diarrhea, dysphagia, flatulence, hyperperistalsis, nausea, salivation, stomach cramps, vomiting
  Genitourinary: Urinary urgency
  Neuromuscular & skeletal: Arthralgias, fasciculations, muscle cramps, spasms, weakness
  Ocular: Lacrimation, small pupils
  Respiratory: Bronchiolar constriction, bronchospasm, dyspnea, increased bronchial secretions, laryngospasm, respiratory arrest, respiratory depression, respiratory muscle paralysis
  Miscellaneous: Allergic reactions, anaphylaxis, diaphoresis increased
Drug Interactions
  Avoid Concomitant Use There are no known interactions where it is recommended to avoid concomitant use.
  Increased Effect/Toxicity
    Neostigmine may increase the levels/effects of: Beta-Blockers; Cholinergic Agonists; Succinylcholine

    The levels/effects of Neostigmine may be increased by: Corticosteroids (Systemic)
  Decreased Effect
    Neostigmine may decrease the levels/effects of: Neuromuscular-Blocking Agents (Nondepolarizing)
Mechanism of Action Inhibits destruction of acetylcholine by acetylcholinesterase which facilitates transmission of impulses across myoneural junction
Pharmacodynamics/Kinetics
  Onset of action: I.M.: 20-30 minutes; I.V.: 1-20 minutes
  Duration: I.M.: 2.5-4 hours; I.V.: 1-2 hours
  Absorption: Oral: Poor, <2%
  Metabolism: Hepatic
  Half-life elimination: Normal renal function: 0.5-2.1 hours; End-stage renal disease: Prolonged
  Excretion: Urine (50% as unchanged drug)

◄ **Dosage**

Geriatric & Adult

Myasthenia gravis, diagnosis: I.M.: 0.02 mg/kg as a single dose; **Note:** In the diagnosis of myasthenia gravis, all anticholinesterase medications should be discontinued for at least 8 hours before administering neostigmine.

Myasthenia gravis, treatment:

Oral: 15 mg/dose every 3-4 hours up to 375 mg/day maximum; interval between doses must be individualized to maximal response

I.M., I.V., SubQ: 0.5-2.5 mg every 1-3 hours up to 10 mg/24 hours maximum

Reversal of nondepolarizing neuromuscular blockade after surgery in conjunction with atropine: I.V.: 0.5-2.5 mg; total dose not to exceed 5 mg; must administer atropine several minutes prior to neostigmine

Bladder atony: I.M., SubQ:

Prevention: 0.25 mg every 4-6 hours for 2-3 days

Treatment: 0.5-1 mg every 3 hours for 5 doses after bladder has emptied

Renal Impairment

Cl_{cr} 10-50 mL/minute: Administer 50% of normal dose.

Cl_{cr} <10 mL/minute: Administer 25% of normal dose.

Administration May be administered undiluted by slow I.V. injection over several minutes

Monitoring Parameters Respiratory rate, pulse, blood pressure, signs of cholinergic crisis.

Pharmacotherapy Pearls In the diagnosis of myasthenia gravis, all anticholinesterase medications should be discontinued for at least 8 hours before administering neostigmine.

Special Geriatric Considerations Many elderly will have diseases which may influence the use of neostigmine. Also, many elderly will need doses reduced by 50% due to creatinine clearances in the 10-50 mL/minute range. Side effects or concomitant disease may warrant use of pyridostigmine.

Dosage Forms Excipient information presented when available (limited, particularly for generics); consult specific product labeling. [DSC] = Discontinued product

Injection, solution, as methylsulfate: 0.5 mg/mL (10 mL); 1 mg/mL (10 mL)

Prostigmin®: 0.5 mg/mL (1 mL [DSC], 10 mL [DSC]); 1 mg/mL (10 mL [DSC])

Tablet, oral, as bromide:

Prostigmin®: 15 mg [scored]

◆ **Neostigmine Bromide** *see* Neostigmine *on page 1283*

◆ **Neostigmine Methylsulfate** *see* Neostigmine *on page 1283*

◆ **Neo-Synephrine® Extra Strength [OTC]** *see* Phenylephrine (Nasal) *on page 1442*

◆ **Neo-Synephrine® Mild Formula [OTC]** *see* Phenylephrine (Nasal) *on page 1442*

◆ **Neo-Synephrine® Nighttime12-Hour [OTC]** *see* Oxymetazoline (Nasal) *on page 1374*

◆ **Neo-Synephrine® Regular Strength [OTC]** *see* Phenylephrine (Nasal) *on page 1442*

Nepafenac (ne pa FEN ak)

Brand Names: U.S. Nevanac®

Brand Names: Canada Nevanac®

Generic Availability (U.S.) No

Pharmacologic Category Nonsteroidal Anti-inflammatory Drug (NSAID), Ophthalmic

Use Treatment of pain and inflammation associated with cataract surgery

Contraindications Hypersensitivity to nepafenac, other NSAIDs, or any component of the formulation

Warnings/Precautions Use caution in patients with previous sensitivity to acetylsalicylic acid and phenylacetic acid derivatives, including patients who experience bronchospasm, asthma, rhinitis, or urticaria following NSAID or aspirin. May slow/delay healing or prolong bleeding time following surgery. Use caution in patients with a predisposition to bleeding (bleeding tendencies or medications which interfere with coagulation).

May cause keratitis; continued use of nepafenac in a patient with keratitis may cause severe corneal adverse reactions, potentially resulting in loss of vision. Immediately discontinue use in patients with evidence of corneal epithelial damage.

Use caution in patients with complicated ocular surgeries, corneal denervation, corneal epithelial defects, diabetes mellitus, ocular surface disease, rheumatoid arthritis, or repeat ocular surgeries (within a short timeframe); may be at risk of corneal adverse events, potentially resulting in loss of vision. Use more than 1 day prior to surgery or for 14 days beyond surgery may increase risk and severity of corneal adverse events. Patients using ophthalmic drops should not wear soft contact lenses.

Adverse Reactions (Reflective of adult population; not specific for elderly)
1% to 10%:
Cardiovascular: Hypertension (1% to 4%)
Central nervous system: Headache (1% to 4%)
Gastrointestinal: Nausea (1% to 4%), vomiting (1% to 4%)
Ocular: Capsular opacity (5% to 10%), foreign body sensation (5% to 10%), intraocular pressure increased (5% to 10%), sticky sensation (5% to 10%), visual acuity decreased (5% to 10%), conjunctival edema (1% to 5%), corneal edema (1% to 5%), dry eye (1% to 5%), lid margin crusting (1% to 5%), ocular discomfort (1% to 5%), ocular hyperemia (1% to 5%), ocular pain (1% to 5%), ocular pruritus (1% to 5%), photophobia (1% to 5%), tearing (1% to 5%), vitreous detachment (1% to 5%)
Respiratory: Sinusitis (1% to 4%)
Drug Interactions
Avoid Concomitant Use There are no known interactions where it is recommended to avoid concomitant use.
Increased Effect/Toxicity There are no known significant interactions involving an increase in effect.
Decreased Effect
Nepafenac may decrease the levels/effects of: Latanoprost
Stability Store at 2°C to 25°C (36°F to 77°F).
Mechanism of Action Nepafenac is a prodrug which once converted to amfenac inhibits prostaglandin synthesis by decreasing the activity of the enzyme, cyclooxygenase, which results in decreased formation of prostaglandin precursors.
Pharmacodynamics/Kinetics
Absorption: Low levels (0.2-0.5 ng/mL) of nepafenac and amfenac are detected in the plasma following ophthalmic administration
Metabolism: Hydrolyzed in ocular tissue to amfenac (active)
Dosage
Geriatric & Adult Pain, inflammation associated with cataract surgery: Ophthalmic: Instill 1 drop into affected eye(s) 3 times/day, beginning 1 day prior to surgery, the day of surgery, and through the first 2 weeks of the postoperative period
Administration Shake well prior to use.
Special Geriatric Considerations No differences in safety and efficacy noted between elderly and younger adults. No dosage adjustment necessary. Elderly may be taking other medications that will increase bleeding.
Dosage Forms Excipient information presented when available (limited, particularly for generics); consult specific product labeling.
Suspension, ophthalmic [drops]:
Nevanac®: 0.1% (3 mL) [contains benzalkonium chloride]

◆ **Nephro-Calci® [OTC]** *see* Calcium Salts (Oral) *on page* 256
◆ **Neptazane™** *see* Methazolamide *on page* 1162

Nesiritide (ni SIR i tide)

Medication Safety Issues
High alert medication:
The Institute for Safe Medication Practices (ISMP) includes this medication among its list of drugs which have a heightened risk of causing significant patient harm when used in error.
International issues:
Natrecor® may be confused with Nitrocor® which is a brand name for nitroglycerin in Chile and Italy
Brand Names: U.S. Natrecor®
Brand Names: Canada Natrecor®
Index Terms B-type Natriuretic Peptide (Human); hBNP; Natriuretic Peptide
Generic Availability (U.S.) No
Pharmacologic Category Natriuretic Peptide, B-Type, Human; Vasodilator
Use Treatment of acutely decompensated heart failure (HF) with dyspnea at rest or with minimal activity
Contraindications Hypersensitivity to natriuretic peptide or any component of the formulation; cardiogenic shock (when used as primary therapy); hypotension (systolic blood pressure <90 mm Hg)
Warnings/Precautions May cause hypotension; administer in clinical situations when blood pressure may be closely monitored. Use caution in patients systolic blood pressure <100 mm Hg (contraindicated if <90 mm Hg); more likely to experience hypotension. Effects may be additive with other agents capable of causing hypotension. Hypotensive effects may last for several hours.

Should not be used in patients with low cardiac filling pressures, or in patients with conditions which depend on venous return including significant valvular stenosis, restrictive or obstructive cardiomyopathy, constrictive pericarditis, and pericardial tamponade. May be associated with development of azotemia; use caution in patients with renal impairment or in patients where renal perfusion is dependent on renin-angiotensin-aldosterone system; avoid initiation at doses higher than recommended.

Monitor for allergic or anaphylactic reactions. Use caution with prolonged infusions; limited experience with infusions >48 hours.

Adverse Reactions (Reflective of adult population; not specific for elderly) Note: Frequencies cited below were recorded in VMAC trial at dosages similar to approved labeling. Higher frequencies have been observed in trials using higher dosages of nesiritide. The percentages marked with an asterisk (*) indicate frequency less than or equal to placebo or other standard therapy.

>10%:
  Cardiovascular: Hypotension (total: 11%; symptomatic: 4% at recommended dose, up to 17% at higher doses)
  Renal: Increased serum creatinine (28% with >0.5 mg/dL increase over baseline)
1% to 10%:
  Cardiovascular: Ventricular tachycardia (3%)*, ventricular extrasystoles (3%)*, angina (2%)*, bradycardia (1%), tachycardia, atrial fibrillation, AV node conduction abnormalities
  Central nervous system: Headache (8%)*, dizziness (3%), insomnia (2%)*, anxiety (3%), confusion, fever, paresthesia, somnolence, tremor
  Dermatologic: Pruritus, rash
  Gastrointestinal: Nausea (4%)*, abdominal pain (1%)*, vomiting (1%)*
  Hematologic: Anemia
  Local: Injection site reaction, catheter pain
  Neuromuscular & skeletal: Back pain (4%), leg cramps
  Ocular: Amblyopia
  Respiratory: Apnea, cough increased, hemoptysis
  Miscellaneous: Diaphoresis
Postmarketing and/or case reports: Hypersensitivity reactions (rare)

Drug Interactions
  Avoid Concomitant Use There are no known interactions where it is recommended to avoid concomitant use.
  Increased Effect/Toxicity
  Nesiritide may increase the levels/effects of: Hypotensive Agents
  Decreased Effect There are no known significant interactions involving a decrease in effect.

Ethanol/Nutrition/Herb Interactions Herb/Nutraceutical: Avoid bayberry, blue cohosh, cayenne, ephedra, ginger, ginseng (American), kola, and licorice (may increase blood pressure). Avoid black cohosh, California poppy, coleus, golden seal, hawthorn, mistletoe, periwinkle, quinine, and shepherd's purse (may enhance decreased blood pressure).

Stability Vials may be stored below 25°C (77°F); do not freeze. Protect from light. Following reconstitution, vials are stable at 2°C to 25°C (36°F to 77°F) for up to 24 hours. Use reconstituted solution within 24 hours.

Reconstitute 1.5 mg vial with 5 mL of diluent removed from a prefilled 250 mL plastic I.V. bag (compatible with D_5W, $D_5{}^1/_2NS$, $D_5{}^1/_4NS$, NS). Do not shake vial to dissolve (roll gently). Withdraw entire contents of vial and add to 250 mL I.V. bag. Invert several times to mix. Resultant concentration of solution is ~6 mcg/mL.

Mechanism of Action Binds to guanylate cyclase receptor on vascular smooth muscle and endothelial cells, increasing intracellular cyclic GMP, resulting in smooth muscle cell relaxation. Has been shown to produce dose-dependent reductions in pulmonary capillary wedge pressure (PCWP) and systemic arterial pressure.

Pharmacodynamics/Kinetics
Onset of action: 15 minutes (60% of 3-hour effect achieved)
Duration: >60 minutes (up to several hours) for systolic blood pressure; hemodynamic effects persist longer than serum half-life would predict
Distribution: V_{ss}: 0.19 L/kg
Metabolism: Proteolytic cleavage by vascular endopeptidases and proteolysis following binding to the membrane bound natriuretic peptide (NPR-C) and cellular internalization
Half-life elimination: Initial (distribution) 2 minutes; Terminal: 18 minutes
Time to peak: 1 hour
Excretion: Primarily eliminated by metabolism; also excreted in the urine

Dosage
Geriatric & Adult

Acute decompensated heart failure: I.V.: Initial: 2 mcg/kg (bolus optional); followed by continuous infusion at 0.01 mcg/kg/minute. **Note:** Should not be initiated at a dosage higher than initial recommended dose. There is limited experience with increasing the dose >0.01 mcg/kg/minute; in one trial, a limited number of patients received higher doses that were increased no faster than every 3 hours by 0.005 mcg/kg/minute (preceded by a bolus of 1 mcg/kg), up to a maximum of 0.03 mcg/kg/minute. Increases beyond the initial infusion rate should be limited to selected patients and accompanied by close hemodynamic and renal function monitoring.

Patients experiencing hypotension during the infusion: Infusion dose should be reduced or discontinued. Other measures to support blood pressure should be initiated (eg, I.V. fluids, Trendelenburg position). May attempt to restart at a lower dose (reduce previous infusion dose by 30% and omit bolus).

Maximum dosing weight: According to the manufacturer, the PRECEDENT Trial capped dosing weight at 160 kg and the VMAC Trial capped dosing weight at 175 kg. There are no specific guidelines on maximum dosing weight and clinical judgment should be used.

Renal Impairment No adjustment required but use cautiously in patients with renal impairment or those patients who rely on the renin-angiotensin-aldosterone system for renal perfusion. Monitor renal function closely.

Hepatic Impairment No dosage adjustment recommended.

Administration Do not administer through a heparin-coated catheter (concurrent administration of heparin via a separate catheter is acceptable, per manufacturer).

Prime I.V. tubing with 5 mL of infusion prior to connection with vascular access port and prior to administering bolus or starting the infusion. Withdraw bolus from the prepared infusion bag and administer over 60 seconds. Begin infusion immediately following administration of the bolus.

Monitoring Parameters Blood pressure, hemodynamic responses (PCWP, RAP, CI), BUN, creatinine; urine output

Pharmacotherapy Pearls The duration of symptomatic improvement with nesiritide following discontinuation of the infusion has been limited (generally lasting several days). Atrial natriuretic peptide, which is related to nesiritide, has been associated with increased vascular permeability. This has not been observed in clinical trials with nesiritide, but patients should be monitored for this effect.

Special Geriatric Considerations No specific data to date; elderly are liable to have hypotension, see Warnings/Precautions for blood pressure criteria. Elderly with reduced renal function should be monitored closely.

Dosage Forms Excipient information presented when available (limited, particularly for generics); consult specific product labeling.
Injection, powder for reconstitution:
Natrecor®: 1.5 mg

Selected References

Colucci WS, Elkayam U, Horton DP, et al, "Intravenous Nesiritide, A Natriuretic Peptide, in the Treatment of Decompensated Congestive Heart Failure. Nesiritide Study Group," *N Engl J Med*, 2000, 343(4):246-53.

Daniels LB and Maisel AS, "Natriuretic Peptides," *J Am Coll Cardiol*, 2007, 50(25):2357-68.

- ◆ **NESP** *see* Darbepoetin Alfa *on page 456*
- ◆ **Neulasta®** *see* Pegfilgrastim *on page 1402*
- ◆ **Neupogen®** *see* Filgrastim *on page 733*
- ◆ **Neurontin®** *see* Gabapentin *on page 803*
- ◆ **Neut®** *see* Sodium Bicarbonate *on page 1688*
- ◆ **NeutraCare®** *see* Fluoride *on page 751*
- ◆ **NeutraGard® Advanced** *see* Fluoride *on page 751*
- ◆ **Neutra-Phos** *see* Potassium Phosphate and Sodium Phosphate *on page 1494*
- ◆ **Neutra-Phos®-K [OTC] [DSC]** *see* Potassium Phosphate *on page 1492*
- ◆ **Neutrogena® Acne Stress Control [OTC]** *see* Salicylic Acid *on page 1648*
- ◆ **Neutrogena® Advanced Solutions™ [OTC]** *see* Salicylic Acid *on page 1648*
- ◆ **Neutrogena® Blackhead Eliminating™ 2-in-1 Foaming Pads [OTC]** *see* Salicylic Acid *on page 1648*
- ◆ **Neutrogena® Blackhead Eliminating™ Daily Scrub [OTC]** *see* Salicylic Acid *on page 1648*
- ◆ **Neutrogena® Blackhead Elinimating™ [OTC]** *see* Salicylic Acid *on page 1648*
- ◆ **Neutrogena® Body Clear® [OTC]** *see* Salicylic Acid *on page 1648*
- ◆ **Neutrogena® Clear Pore™ Oil-Controlling Astringent [OTC]** *see* Salicylic Acid *on page 1648*
- ◆ **Neutrogena® Maximum Strength T/Sal® [OTC]** *see* Salicylic Acid *on page 1648*
- ◆ **Neutrogena® Oil-Free Acne [OTC]** *see* Salicylic Acid *on page 1648*
- ◆ **Neutrogena® Oil-Free Acne Stress Control [OTC]** *see* Salicylic Acid *on page 1648*

- ◆ **Neutrogena® Oil-Free Acne Wash [OTC]** *see* Salicylic Acid *on page 1648*
- ◆ **Neutrogena® Oil-Free Acne Wash 60 Second Mask Scrub [OTC]** *see* Salicylic Acid *on page 1648*
- ◆ **Neutrogena® Oil-Free Acne Wash Cream Cleanser [OTC]** *see* Salicylic Acid *on page 1648*
- ◆ **Neutrogena® Oil-Free Acne Wash Foam Cleanser [OTC]** *see* Salicylic Acid *on page 1648*
- ◆ **Neutrogena® Oil-Free Anti-Acne [OTC]** *see* Salicylic Acid *on page 1648*
- ◆ **Neutrogena® Rapid Clear® [OTC]** *see* Salicylic Acid *on page 1648*
- ◆ **Neutrogena® Rapid Clear® Acne Defense [OTC]** *see* Salicylic Acid *on page 1648*
- ◆ **Neutrogena® Rapid Clear® Acne Eliminating [OTC]** *see* Salicylic Acid *on page 1648*
- ◆ **Nevanac®** *see* Nepafenac *on page 1284*
- ◆ **Nexiclon™ XR** *see* CloNIDine *on page 388*
- ◆ **NexIUM®** *see* Esomeprazole *on page 636*
- ◆ **NexIUM® I.V.** *see* Esomeprazole *on page 636*
- ◆ **Nexterone®** *see* Amiodarone *on page 97*
- ◆ **NGX-4010** *see* Capsaicin *on page 261*

Niacin (NYE a sin)

Related Information
Hyperlipidemia Management *on page 2021*
Medication Safety Issues
Sound-alike/look-alike issues:
Niacin may be confused with Minocin®, Niaspan®, Nispan®
Niaspan® may be confused with niacin
Nicobid® may be confused with Nitro-Bid®
Brand Names: U.S. Niacin-Time® [OTC]; Niacor®; Niaspan®; Slo-Niacin® [OTC]
Brand Names: Canada Niaspan®; Niaspan® FCT; Niodan
Index Terms Nicotinic Acid; Vitamin B_3
Generic Availability (U.S.) Yes
Pharmacologic Category Antilipemic Agent, Miscellaneous; Vitamin, Water Soluble
Use Treatment of dyslipidemias (Fredrickson types IIa and IIb or primary hypercholesterolemia) as mono- or adjunctive therapy; to lower the risk of recurrent MI in patients with a history of MI and hyperlipidemia; to slow progression or promote regression of coronary artery disease; treatment of hypertriglyceridemia in patients at risk of pancreatitis
Unlabeled/Investigational Use Treatment of pellagra; dietary supplement
Contraindications Hypersensitivity to niacin, niacinamide, or any component of the formulation; active hepatic disease or significant or unexplained persistent elevations in hepatic transaminases; active peptic ulcer; arterial hemorrhage
Warnings/Precautions Use with caution in patients with unstable angina or MI, diabetes (may interfere with glucose control), renal disease, active gallbladder disease (can exacerbate), gout, or with anticoagulants (may slightly increase prothrombin time). Use with caution in patients with a past history of hepatic impairment and/or who consume substantial amounts of ethanol; contraindicated with active liver disease or unexplained persistent transaminase elevation. Rare cases of rhabdomyolysis have occurred during concomitant use with HMG-CoA reductase inhibitors. With concurrent use or if symptoms suggestive of myopathy occur, monitor creatine phosphokinase (CPK) and potassium; use with caution in patients with renal impairment, inadequately treated hypothyroidism, patients with diabetes or the elderly; risk for myopathy and rhabdomyolysis may be increased.

Immediate and extended or sustained release products are not interchangeable. Cases of severe hepatotoxicity have occurred when immediate release (crystalline) niacin products have been substituted with sustained-release (modified release, timed-release) niacin products at equivalent doses. Patients should be initiated with low doses (eg, 500 mg at bedtime) with titration to achieve desired response. Flushing and pruritus, common adverse effects of niacin, may be attenuated with a gradual increase in dose, and/or by taking aspirin (adults: 325 mg) or an NSAID 30-60 minutes before dosing. Compliance is enhanced with twice-daily dosing (extended-release product excluded). Prior to initiation, secondary causes for hypercholesterolemia (eg, poorly controlled diabetes mellitus, hypothyroidism) should be excluded; management with diet and other nonpharmacologic measures (eg, exercise or weight reduction) should be attempted prior to initiation. Use has not been evaluated in Fredrickson type I or III dyslipidemias.

Adverse Reactions (Reflective of adult population; not specific for elderly) Frequency not defined.
Cardiovascular: Arrhythmias, atrial fibrillation, edema, flushing, hypotension, orthostasis, palpitation, syncope (rare), tachycardia
Central nervous system: Chills, dizziness, headache, insomnia, migraine, nervousness, pain

Dermatologic: Acanthosis nigricans, burning skin, dry skin, hyperpigmentation, maculopapular rash, pruritus, rash, skin discoloration, urticaria

Endocrine & metabolic: Glucose tolerance decreased, gout, phosphorous levels decreased, hyperuricemia

Gastrointestinal: Abdominal pain, amylase increased, diarrhea, dyspepsia, eructation, flatulence, nausea, peptic ulcers, vomiting

Hematologic: Platelet counts decreased

Hepatic: Hepatic necrosis (rare), hepatitis, jaundice, transaminases increased (dose-related), prothrombin time increased, total bilirubin increased

Neuromuscular & skeletal: CPK increased, leg cramps, myalgia, myasthenia, myopathy (with concurrent HMG-CoA reductase inhibitor), paresthesia, rhabdomyolysis (with concurrent HMG-CoA reductase inhibitor; rare), weakness

Ocular: Blurred vision, cystoid macular edema, toxic amblyopia

Respiratory: Cough, dyspnea

Miscellaneous: Diaphoresis, hypersensitivity reactions (rare; includes anaphylaxis, angioedema, laryngismus, vesiculobullous rash), LDH increased

Drug Interactions

Avoid Concomitant Use There are no known interactions where it is recommended to avoid concomitant use.

Increased Effect/Toxicity

Niacin may increase the levels/effects of: HMG-CoA Reductase Inhibitors

Decreased Effect

The levels/effects of Niacin may be decreased by: Bile Acid Sequestrants

Ethanol/Nutrition/Herb Interactions Ethanol: Avoid heavy use; avoid use around niacin dose.

Stability

Niaspan®: Store at room temperature of 20°C to 25°C (68°F to 77°F).

Niacor®: Store at controlled room temperature of 15°C to 30°C (59°F to 86°F).

Mechanism of Action Component of two coenzymes which is necessary for tissue respiration, lipid metabolism, and glycogenolysis; inhibits the synthesis of very low density lipoproteins (VLDL) and low density lipoproteins (LDL); may also increase the rate of chylomicron triglyceride removal from plasma.

Pharmacodynamics/Kinetics

Absorption: Rapid and extensive (60% to 76%)

Distribution: Mainly to hepatic, renal, and adipose tissue

Metabolism: Extensive first-pass effects; converted to nicotinamide adenine dinucleotide, nicotinuric acid, and other metabolites

Half-life elimination: 20-45 minutes

Time to peak, serum: Immediate release formulation: 30-60 minutes; extended release formulation: 4-5 hours

Excretion: Urine 60% to 88% (unchanged drug [up to 12% recovered after multiple dosing] and metabolites)

Dosage

Geriatric & Adult Note: Formulations of niacin (regular release versus extended release) are not interchangeable.

Recommended daily allowances (National Academy of Sciences, 1998): Oral:

≥19 years: Female: 14 mg/day; Male: 16 mg/day

Dietary supplement (OTC labeling): Oral: 50 mg twice daily or 100 mg once daily. **Note:** Many over-the-counter formulations exist.

Hyperlipidemia: Oral:

Regular release formulation (Niacor®): Initial: 250 mg once daily (with evening meal); increase frequency and/or dose every 4-7 days to desired response or first-level therapeutic dose (1.5-2 g/day in 2-3 divided doses); after 2 months, may increase at 2- to 4-week intervals to 3 g/day in 3 divided doses (maximum dose: 6 g/day [NCEP recommends 4.5 g/day] in 3 divided doses). Usual daily dose after titration (NCEP, 2002): 1.5-3 g/day. **Note:** Many over-the-counter formulations exist.

Sustained release (or controlled release) formulations: **Note:** Several over-the-counter formulations exist. Usual daily dose after titration (NCEP, 2002): 1-2 g/day

Extended release formulation (Niaspan®): Initial: 500 mg at bedtime for 4 weeks, then 1 g at bedtime for 4 weeks; adjust dose to response and tolerance; may increase dose every 4 weeks by 500 mg/day to a maximum of 2 g/day. Usual daily dose after titration (NCEP, 2002): 1-2 g once daily

If additional LDL-lowering is necessary with lovastatin or simvastatin: Recommended initial lovastatin or simvastatin dose: 20 mg/day (maximum lovastatin or simvastatin dose: 40 mg/day); **Note:** Lovastatin prescribing information recommends a maximum dose of 20 mg/day with concurrent use of niacin (>1 g/day).

◄ **Pellagra (unlabeled use):** Oral: 50-100 mg 3-4 times/day; maximum: 500 mg/day (some experts prefer niacinamide for treatment due to more favorable side effect profile)

Renal Impairment No dosage adjustment recommended; use with caution.

Hepatic Impairment Contraindicated in patients with significant or unexplained hepatic dysfunction, active liver disease or unexplained persistent transaminase elevations.

Administration Administer with food.

Niaspan®: Administer at bedtime. Tablet strengths are not interchangeable. When switching from immediate release tablet, initiate Niaspan® at lower dose and titrate. If therapy is interrupted for an extended period, dose should be retitrated. Long-acting forms should not be crushed, broken, or chewed. Do not substitute long-acting forms for immediate release ones.

Monitoring Parameters Blood glucose (in diabetic patients); CPK and serum potassium (if on concurrent HMG-CoA reductase inhibitor); liver function tests pretreatment, every 6-12 weeks for first year, then periodically (approximately every 6 months), monitor liver function more frequently if history of transaminase elevation with prior use; lipid profile; platelets; PT (if on anticoagulants); uric acid (if predisposed to gout); phosphorus (if predisposed to hypophosphatemia)

Test Interactions False elevations in some fluorometric determinations of plasma or urinary catecholamines; false-positive urine glucose (Benedict's reagent)

Pharmacotherapy Pearls If flushing is bothersome or persistent, 325 mg of aspirin 30 minutes before each dose or increasing the dose slowly with weekly increase may minimize this reaction; for explicit guidelines on the risk factors for CHD and when to treat high blood cholesterol. See Selected References. Due to liver function test abnormalities induced by sustained release niacin, these dosage forms are not currently recommended

Special Geriatric Considerations The definition of and, therefore, when to treat hyperlipidemia in the elderly is a controversial issue. The National Cholesterol Education Program recommends that all adults maintain a plasma cholesterol <160 mg/dL. Elderly with one additional risk factor, goal LDL would be <130 mg/dL. It is the authors' belief that pharmacologic treatment be reserved for those who are unable to obtain a desirable plasma cholesterol concentration by diet alone and for whom the benefits of treatment are believed to outweigh the potential adverse effects, drug interactions, and cost of treatment.

Dosage Forms Excipient information presented when available (limited, particularly for generics); consult specific product labeling.

Caplet, timed release, oral: 500 mg

Capsule, oral: 50 mg, 250 mg

Capsule, extended release, oral: 250 mg, 500 mg

Capsule, timed release, oral: 250 mg, 400 mg, 500 mg

Tablet, oral: 50 mg, 100 mg, 250 mg, 500 mg

Niacor®: 500 mg [scored]

Tablet, controlled release, oral:

Slo-Niacin®: 250 mg, 500 mg, 750 mg [scored]

Tablet, extended release, oral:

Niaspan®: 500 mg, 750 mg, 1000 mg

Tablet, timed release, oral: 250 mg, 500 mg, 750 mg, 1000 mg

Niacin-Time®: 500 mg

Selected References

National Cholesterol Education Program (NCEP) Expert Panel on Detection, Evaluation, and Treatment of High Blood Cholesterol in Adults (Adult Treatment Panel III), "Third Report of the National Cholesterol Education Program (NCEP) Expert Panel on Detection, Evaluation, and Treatment of High Blood Cholesterol in Adults (Adult Treatment Panel III) Final Report," *Circulation*, 2002, 106(25):3143-421.

"Third Report of The National Cholesterol Education Program (NCEP) Expert Panel on Detection, Evaluation, and Treatment of High Blood Cholesterol in Adults (Adult Treatment Panel III), Final Report," *Circulation*, 2002, 106 (25):3143-421.

Niacinamide (nye a SIN a mide)

Medication Safety Issues

Sound-alike/look-alike issues:

Niacinamide may be confused with niCARdipine

Brand Names: U.S. Nicomide-T™ [OTC]

Index Terms Nicotinamide; Nicotinic Acid Amide; Vitamin B₃

Generic Availability (U.S.) Yes: Tablet

Pharmacologic Category Vitamin, Water Soluble

Use

Oral: Prophylaxis and treatment of pellagra

Topical: Improve the appearance of acne and decrease visible inflammation and irritation caused by acne medications

Contraindications Hypersensitivity to niacin, niacinamide, or any component of the formulation; liver disease; active peptic ulcer

Warnings/Precautions Use caution in heavy ethanol users, unstable angina or CAD (risk of arrhythmias at high doses), diabetes (interferes with glucose control), renal disease, active gallbladder disease (can exacerbate), gout, or allergies. Avoid large pharmacological amounts in patients with a history of liver disease. Monitor liver function tests with high doses.

Adverse Reactions (Reflective of adult population; not specific for elderly) Frequency not defined.

Cardiovascular: Tachycardia
Dermatologic: Increased sebaceous gland activity, rash
Endocrine & metabolic: Hyperglycemia, hyperuricemia
Gastrointestinal: Bloating, flatulence, nausea
Neuromuscular & skeletal: Paresthesia in extremities
Ocular: Blurred vision
Respiratory: Wheezing

Drug Interactions

Avoid Concomitant Use There are no known interactions where it is recommended to avoid concomitant use.

Increased Effect/Toxicity
Niacinamide may increase the levels/effects of: HMG-CoA Reductase Inhibitors

Decreased Effect There are no known significant interactions involving a decrease in effect.

Mechanism of Action Used by the body as a source of niacin; is a component of two coenzymes which is necessary for tissue respiration, lipid metabolism, and glycogenolysis; does not have hypolipidemia or vasodilating effects. Niacinamide has anti-inflammatory properties which are believed to help decrease inflammatory acne lesions.

Pharmacodynamics/Kinetics
Absorption: Oral: Rapid; Topical: Absorbed systemically
Metabolism: Hepatic
Half-life elimination: 45 minutes
Time to peak, serum: 20-70 minutes
Excretion: Urine (as metabolites)

Dosage

Geriatric & Adult

Pellagra: Oral: 100 mg every 6 hours for several days (or until resolution of major signs and symptoms), followed by 50 mg every 8-12 hours until skin lesions heal (Hegyi, 2004)

Acne: Topical: Apply to affected area on face twice daily

Administration Topical: Prior to using cream or gel, wash face with mild cleanser. Apply thin layer to affected area. May apply under make-up or other acne medications. Re-evaluate after 8-12 weeks.

Test Interactions False elevations of urinary catecholamines in some fluorometric determinations

Special Geriatric Considerations Should not be confused with niacin.

Dosage Forms Excipient information presented when available (limited, particularly for generics); consult specific product labeling.

Cream, topical:
Nicomide-T™: 4% (30 g) [contains benzyl alcohol]
Gel, topical:
Nicomide-T™: 4% (30 g) [contains ethanol]
Tablet, oral: 100 mg, 250 mg, 500 mg

Niacin and Lovastatin (NYE a sin & LOE va sta tin)

Related Information
Hyperlipidemia Management *on page 2021*
Lovastatin *on page 1097*
Niacin *on page 1288*

Medication Safety Issues
Sound-alike/look-alike issues:
Advicor® may be confused with Adcirca®, Advair, Altocor™

Brand Names: U.S. Advicor®

Brand Names: Canada Advicor®

Index Terms Lovastatin and Niacin

Generic Availability (U.S.) No

Pharmacologic Category Antilipemic Agent, HMG-CoA Reductase Inhibitor; Antilipemic Agent, Miscellaneous

◀ **Use** For use when treatment with both extended-release niacin and lovastatin is appropriate in combination with a standard cholesterol-lowering diet:

Extended-release niacin: Adjunctive treatment of dyslipidemias (types IIa and IIb or primary hypercholesterolemia) to lower the risk of recurrent MI and/or slow progression of coronary artery disease, including combination therapy with other antidyslipidemic agents when additional triglyceride-lowering or HDL-increasing effects are desired; treatment of hyper-triglyceridemia in patients at risk of pancreatitis

Lovastatin: Treatment of primary hypercholesterolemia (Frederickson types IIa and IIb); primary and secondary prevention of cardiovascular disease

Dosage

Geriatric & Adult Dosage forms are a fixed combination of niacin and lovastatin.

Dyslipidemia: Oral: Lowest dose: Niacin 500 mg/lovastatin 20 mg; may increase by not more than 500 mg (niacin) at 4-week intervals (maximum dose: niacin 2000 mg/lovastatin 40 mg daily); should be taken at bedtime with a low-fat snack. **Note:** If therapy is interrupted for >7 days, reinstitution of therapy should begin with the lowest dose followed by retitration as needed.

Not for use as initial therapy of dyslipidemias. May be substituted for equivalent dose of Niaspan®, however, manufacturer does not recommend direct substitution with other niacin products.

Renal Impairment

Mild-to-moderate impairment: No dosage adjustment required

Cl_{cr} <30 mL/minute: Use doses of lovastatin >20 mg/day with caution

Hepatic Impairment Do not use in active liver disease or unexplained persistent elevations of serum transaminases.

Special Geriatric Considerations The definition of and, therefore, when to treat hyper-lipidemia in the elderly is a controversial issue. The National Cholesterol Education Program recommends that all adults maintain a plasma cholesterol <160 mg/dL. For elderly patients with one additional risk factor, the goal LDL would be <130 mg/dL. It is the authors' belief that pharmacologic treatment be reserved for those who are unable to obtain a desirable plasma cholesterol concentration by diet alone and for whom the benefits of treatment are believed to outweigh the potential adverse effects, drug interactions, and cost of treatment. Patients ≥65 years of age are at risk for myopathy.

Dosage Forms Excipient information presented when available (limited, particularly for generics); consult specific product labeling.

Tablet, variable release (Advicor®):

500/20: Niacin 500 mg [extended release] and lovastatin 20 mg [immediate release]

750/20: Niacin 750 mg [extended release] and lovastatin 20 mg [immediate release]

1000/20: Niacin 1000 mg [extended release] and lovastatin 20 mg [immediate release]

1000/40: Niacin 1000 mg [extended release] and lovastatin 40 mg [immediate release]

Niacin and Simvastatin (NYE a sin & sim va STAT in)

Related Information

Hyperlipidemia Management *on page 2021*

Niacin *on page 1288*

Simvastatin *on page 1681*

Medication Safety Issues

International issue:

Simcor® is also a brand name for simvastatin in Indonesia.

Brand Names: U.S. Simcor®

Index Terms Simvastatin and Niacin

Generic Availability (U.S.) No

Pharmacologic Category Antilipemic Agent, HMG-CoA Reductase Inhibitor; Antilipemic Agent, Miscellaneous

Use Reduce total cholesterol, LDL, Apo B, non-HDL, TG, and/or increase HDL in patients with primary hypercholesterolemia, mixed dyslipidemia, or hypertriglyceridemia in combination with standard cholesterol-lowering diet when simvastatin or niacin monotherapy is inadequate

Dosage

Adult Dosage forms are a fixed combination of niacin extended-release and simvastatin.

Dyslipidemia: Oral:

Initial dose:

Patients naïve to niacin therapy: Niacin 500 mg/simvastatin 20 mg once daily at bedtime; increase dose every 4 weeks as needed in increments of not more than 500 mg of niacin

Patients currently on immediate-release niacin products: Niacin 500 mg/simvastatin 20 mg once daily at bedtime; increase dose every 4 weeks as needed in increments of not more than 500 mg of niacin

Patients currently on simvastatin (20-40 mg/day): Niacin 500 mg/simvastatin 40 mg once daily at bedtime; increase dose every 4 weeks as needed in increments of not more than 500 mg of niacin

Maintenance dose: Niacin 1000-2000 mg/ simvastatin 20-40 mg once daily (maximum daily dose: niacin 2000 mg/simvastatin 40 mg)

Note: If therapy is interrupted for >7 days, reinstitution of therapy should begin with the lowest dose followed by retitration as tolerated. Not for use as initial therapy of dyslipidemias. May be substituted for equivalent dose of niacin extended-release, however, manufacturer does not recommend direct substitution with immediate-release preparations.

Dosage adjustment for simvastatin component with concomitant medications: *Amlodipine or ranolazine:* Dose should **not** exceed niacin 1000 mg/simvastatin 20 mg once daily

Renal Impairment

Mild-to-moderate impairment: No dosage adjustment required; use caution.

Severe renal impairment: Use with extreme caution or avoid unless patient already tolerating simvastatin doses ≥10 mg.

Hepatic Impairment Contraindicated in active liver disease or unexplained persistent elevations of serum transaminases.

Special Geriatric Considerations The definition of and, therefore, when to treat hyperlipidemia in the elderly is a controversial issue. The National Cholesterol Education Program recommends that all adults maintain a plasma cholesterol <160 mg/dL. For elderly patients with one additional risk factor, the goal LDL would be <130 mg/dL. It is the authors' belief that pharmacologic treatment be reserved for those who are unable to obtain a desirable plasma cholesterol concentration by diet alone and for whom the benefits of treatment are believed to outweigh the potential adverse effects, drug interactions, and cost of treatment. Patients ≥65 years of age are at risk for myopathy.

Dosage Forms Excipient information presented when available (limited, particularly for generics); consult specific product labeling.

Tablet, variable release, oral:

Simcor®:

500/20: Niacin 500 mg [extended release] and simvastatin 20 mg [immediate release]
500/40: Niacin 500 mg [extended release] and simvastatin 40 mg [immediate release]
750/20: Niacin 750 mg [extended release] and simvastatin 20 mg [immediate release]
1000/20: Niacin 1000 mg [extended release] and simvastatin 20 mg [immediate release]
1000/40: Niacin 1000 mg [extended release] and simvastatin 40 mg [immediate release]

◆ **Niacin-Time® [OTC]** *see* Niacin *on page 1288*
◆ **Niacor®** *see* Niacin *on page 1288*
◆ **Niaspan®** *see* Niacin *on page 1288*

NiCARdipine (nye KAR de peen)

Related Information

Calcium Channel Blockers *on page 2003*

Medication Safety Issues

Sound-alike/look-alike issues:

NiCARdipine may be confused with niacinamide, NIFEdipine, niMODipine

Cardene® may be confused with Cardizem®, Cardura®, codeine

Administration issues:

Significant differences exist between oral and I.V. dosing. Use caution when converting from one route of administration to another.

International issues:

Cardene [U.S., Great Britain, Netherlands] may be confused with Cardem brand name for celiprolol [Spain]; Cardin brand name for simvastatin [Poland]

Brand Names: U.S. Cardene® I.V.; Cardene® SR

Index Terms Nicardipine Hydrochloride

Generic Availability (U.S.) Yes: Capsule, injection

Pharmacologic Category Calcium Channel Blocker; Calcium Channel Blocker, Dihydropyridine

Use Chronic stable angina (immediate-release product only); management of hypertension (immediate and sustained release products); parenteral only for short-term use when oral treatment is not feasible

◀ **Unlabeled/Investigational Use** Congestive heart failure, control of blood pressure in acute ischemic stroke and spontaneous intracranial hemorrhage, postoperative hypertension associated with carotid endarterectomy, perioperative hypertension, prevention of migraine headaches, subarachnoid hemorrhage associated cerebral vasospasm

Contraindications Hypersensitivity to nicardipine or any component of the formulation; advanced aortic stenosis

Warnings/Precautions Symptomatic hypotension with or without syncope can rarely occur; blood pressure must be lowered at a rate appropriate for the patient's clinical condition. Close monitoring of blood pressure and heart rate is required. Reflex tachycardia may occur resulting in angina and/or MI in patients with obstructive coronary disease especially in the absence of concurrent beta blockade. The most common side effect is peripheral edema (dose-dependent); occurs within 2-3 weeks of starting therapy. Use with caution in CAD (can cause increase in angina), HF (can worsen heart failure symptoms), aortic stenosis (may reduce coronary perfusion resulting in ischemia; use is contraindicated in patients with advanced aortic stenosis), and hypertrophic cardiomyopathy with outflow tract obstruction. To minimize infusion site reactions, peripheral infusion sites (for I.V. therapy) should be changed every 12 hours; use of small peripheral veins should be avoided. Titrate I.V. dose cautiously in patients with HF, renal or hepatic dysfunction. Use the I.V. form cautiously in patients with portal hypertension (can cause increase in hepatic pressure gradient). Initiate at the low end of the dosage range in the elderly.

Adverse Reactions (Reflective of adult population; not specific for elderly)
1% to 10%:

Cardiovascular: Cardiovascular: Flushing (6% to 10%), peripheral edema (dose related; 6% to 8%), hypotension (I.V. 6%), increased angina (dose related; 6%), palpitation (3% to 4%), tachycardia (1% to 4%), vasodilation (I.V. to 5%), chest pain (I.V. 1%), ECG abnormal (I.V. 1%), extrasystoles (I.V. 1%), hemopericardium (I.V. 1%), hypertension (I.V. 1%), orthostasis (1%), supraventricular tachycardia (I.V. 1%), syncope (1%), ventricular extrasystoles (I.V. 1%), ventricular tachycardia (I.V. 1%)

Central nervous system: Headache (6% to 15%), dizziness (1% to 7%), hypoesthesia (1%), intracranial hemorrhage (1%) pain (1%), somnolence (1%)

Dermatologic: Rash (1%)

Endocrine & metabolic: Hypokalemia (I.V. 1%)

Gastrointestinal: Nausea (2% to 5%), vomiting (I.V. 5%), dyspepsia (oral 2%), abdominal pain (I.V. 1%), dry mouth (1%)

Genitourinary: Polyuria (1%)

Local: Injection site pain (I.V. 1%), injection site reaction (I.V. 1%)

Neuromuscular & skeletal: Weakness (1% to 6%), myalgia (1%), paresthesia (1%)

Renal: Hematuria (1%)

Respiratory: Dyspnea (1%)

Miscellaneous: Diaphoresis (1%)

Drug Interactions

Metabolism/Transport Effects Substrate of CYP1A2 (minor), CYP2C9 (minor), CYP2D6 (minor), CYP2E1 (minor), CYP3A4 (major), P-glycoprotein; **Inhibits** CYP2C9 (strong), CYP2C19 (moderate), CYP2D6 (moderate), CYP3A4 (strong), P-glycoprotein

Avoid Concomitant Use

Avoid concomitant use of NiCARdipine with any of the following: Alfuzosin; Conivaptan; Crizotinib; Dronedarone; Eplerenone; Everolimus; Fluticasone (Oral Inhalation); Halofantrine; Lapatinib; Lovastatin; Lurasidone; Nilotinib; Nisoldipine; Ranolazine; Rivaroxaban; RomiDEPsin; Salmeterol; Silodosin; Simvastatin; Tamsulosin; Thioridazine; Ticagrelor; Tolvaptan; Topotecan; Toremifene

Increased Effect/Toxicity

NiCARdipine may increase the levels/effects of: Alfuzosin; Almotriptan; Alosetron; Amifostine; Antihypertensives; Beta-Blockers; Bortezomib; Brentuximab Vedotin; Brinzolamide; Budesonide (Nasal); Budesonide (Systemic, Oral Inhalation); Calcium Channel Blockers (Nondihydropyridine); Ciclesonide; Colchicine; Conivaptan; Corticosteroids (Orally Inhaled); Crizotinib; CYP2C19 Substrates; CYP2C9 Substrates (High risk); CYP2D6 Substrates; CYP3A4 Substrates; Dabigatran Etexilate; Diclofenac; Dienogest; Dronedarone; Dutasteride; Eplerenone; Everolimus; FentaNYL; Fesoterodine; Fluticasone (Nasal); Fluticasone (Oral Inhalation); Fosphenytoin; GuanFACINE; Halofantrine; Hypotensive Agents; Iloperidone; Ixabepilone; Lapatinib; Lovastatin; Lumefantrine; Lurasidone; Magnesium Salts; Maraviroc; MethylPREDNISolone; Neuromuscular-Blocking Agents (Nondepolarizing); Nilotinib; Nisoldipine; Nitroprusside; Paricalcitol; Pazopanib; P-Glycoprotein Substrates; Phenytoin; Pimecrolimus; QuiNIDine; Ranolazine; RiTUXimab; Rivaroxaban; RomiDEPsin; Salmeterol; Saxagliptin; Sildenafil; Silodosin; Simvastatin; SORAfenib; Tacrolimus; Tacrolimus (Systemic); Tadalafil; Tamoxifen; Tamsulosin; Thioridazine; Ticagrelor; Tolterodine; Tolvaptan; Topotecan; Toremifene; Vardenafil; Vemurafenib; Vilazodone

The levels/effects of NiCARdipine may be increased by: Alpha1-Blockers; Antifungal Agents (Azole Derivatives, Systemic); Calcium Channel Blockers (Nondihydropyridine); Cyclo-SPORINE; CycloSPORINE (Systemic); CYP3A4 Inhibitors (Moderate); CYP3A4 Inhibitors (Strong); Dasatinib; Diazoxide; Fluconazole; Grapefruit Juice; Herbs (Hypotensive Properties); Macrolide Antibiotics; Magnesium Salts; MAO Inhibitors; Pentoxifylline; P-Glycoprotein Inhibitors; Prostacyclin Analogues; Protease Inhibitors; QuiNIDine

Decreased Effect

NiCARdipine may decrease the levels/effects of: Clopidogrel; Codeine; Prasugrel; QuiNI-Dine; Ticagrelor; TraMADol

The levels/effects of NiCARdipine may be decreased by: Barbiturates; Calcium Salts; CarBAMazepine; CYP3A4 Inducers (Strong); Cyproterone; Deferasirox; Herbs (CYP3A4 Inducers); Herbs (Hypertensive Properties); Methylphenidate; Nafcillin; Peginterferon Alfa-2b; Rifamycin Derivatives; Tocilizumab; Yohimbine

Ethanol/Nutrition/Herb Interactions

Ethanol: Avoid ethanol (may increase CNS depression).

Food: Nicardipine average peak concentrations may be decreased if taken with food. Serum concentrations/toxicity of nicardipine may be increased by grapefruit juice; avoid concurrent use.

Herb/Nutraceutical: St John's wort may decrease levels. Avoid bayberry, blue cohosh, cayenne, ephedra, ginger, ginseng (American), kola, licorice (may worsen hypertension). Avoid black cohosh, California poppy, coleus, golden seal, hawthorn, mistletoe, periwinkle, quinine, shepherd's purse (may have increased antihypertensive effect).

Stability

I.V.:

Premixed bags: Store at controlled room temperature of 20°C to 25°C (68°F to 77°F). Protect from light and excessive heat. Do not freeze.

Vials: Store at controlled room temperature of 20°C to 25°C (68°F to 77°F). Protect from light. Dilute 25 mg vial with 240 mL of compatible solution to provide a 250 mL total volume solution and a final concentration of 0.1 mg/mL. Diluted solution (0.1 mg/mL) is stable at room temperature for 24 hours in glass or PVC containers. Stability has also been demonstrated at room temperature at concentrations up to 0.5 mg/mL in PVC containers for 24 hours or in glass containers for up to 7 days (Baaske, 1996).

Oral (Cardene®, Cardene SR®): Store at 15°C to 30°C (59°F to 86°F). Protect from light. Freezing does not affect stability.

Mechanism of Action Inhibits calcium ion from entering the "slow channels" or select voltage-sensitive areas of vascular smooth muscle and myocardium during depolarization, producing a relaxation of coronary vascular smooth muscle and coronary vasodilation; increases myocardial oxygen delivery in patients with vasospastic angina

Pharmacodynamics/Kinetics

Onset of action: Oral: 0.5-2 hours; I.V.: 10 minutes; Hypotension: ~20 minutes

Duration:

I.V.: ≤8 hours

Oral: Immediate release capsules: ≤8 hours; Sustained release capsules: 8-12 hours

Absorption: Oral: ~100%

Protein binding: >95%

Metabolism: Hepatic; CYP3A4 substrate (major); extensive first-pass effect (saturable)

Bioavailability: 35%

Half-life elimination: 2-4 hours

Time to peak, serum: Oral: Immediate release: 30-120 minutes; Sustained release: 60-240 minutes

Excretion: Urine (49% to 60% as metabolites); feces (43% as metabolites)

Dosage

Geriatric Initiate at the low end of the dosage range. Specific guidelines for adjustment of nicardipine are not available, but careful monitoring is warranted and adjustment may be necessary.

Adult

Angina: Immediate release: Oral: 20 mg 3 times/day; usual range: 60-120 mg/day; increase dose at 3-day intervals

Hypertension: Oral:

Immediate release: Initial: 20 mg 3 times/day; usual: 20-40 mg 3 times/day (allow 3 days between dose increases)

Sustained release: Initial: 30 mg twice daily, titrate up to 60 mg twice daily

Note: The total daily dose of immediate-release product may not automatically be equivalent to the daily sustained-release dose; use caution in converting.

◀

Acute hypertension: I.V.: Initial: Initial: 5 mg/hour increased by 2.5 mg/hour every 5 minutes (for rapid titration) to every 15 minutes (for gradual titration) up to a maximum of 15 mg/hour; rapidly titrated patients, consider reduction to 3 mg/hour after response is achieved.

Arterial hypertension in acute ischemic stroke (unlabeled use [Adams, 2007; Jauch, 2010]): I.V.:

Patient otherwise eligible for reperfusion treatment (eg, alteplase): Blood pressure (BP): Systolic >185 mm Hg or diastolic >110 mm Hg: 5 mg/hour; titrate by 2.5 mg/hour at 5-15 minute intervals (maximum dose: 15 mg/hour). When goal BP obtained, reduce dose to 3 mg/hour. If BP does not decline and remains >185/110 mm Hg, alteplase should not be administered.

Management of BP during and after reperfusion treatment (eg, alteplase): BP: Systolic >230 mm Hg or diastolic >121-140 mm Hg: 5 mg/hour; titrate by 2.5 mg/hour at 5-minute intervals (maximum dose: 15 mg/hour). If hypertension is refractory, consider other I.V. antihypertensives (eg, nitroprusside).

Substitution for oral therapy (approximate equivalents):
20 mg every 8 hours oral, equivalent to 0.5 mg/hour I.V. infusion
30 mg every 8 hours oral, equivalent to 1.2 mg/hour I.V. infusion
40 mg every 8 hours oral, equivalent to 2.2 mg/hour I.V. infusion

Conversion to oral antihypertensive agent: Initiate oral antihypertensive at the same time that I.V. nicardipine is discontinued, if transitioning to oral nicardipine, start oral nicardipine 1 hour prior to I.V. discontinuation.

Renal Impairment

Oral: Per the manufacturer: Titrate dose beginning with 20 mg 3 times/day (immediate release) or 30 mg twice daily (sustained release capsule).

I.V.: Specific guidelines for adjustment of nicardipine are not available, but careful monitoring is warranted and adjustment may be necessary.

Hepatic Impairment

Oral: Per the manufacturer: Starting dose: 20 mg twice daily (immediate release) with titration. Refer to "**Note**" in adult dosing.

I.V.: Specific guidelines for adjustment of nicardipine are not available, but careful monitoring is warranted and adjustment may be necessary.

Administration

Oral: The total daily dose of immediate-release product may not automatically be equivalent to the daily sustained-release dose; use caution in converting. Do not chew or crush the sustained release formulation, swallow whole. Do not open or cut capsules.

I.V.:

Vials must be diluted before use. Administer as a slow continuous infusion at a concentration of 0.1 mg/mL or 0.2 mg/mL. Concentrations of 0.5 mg/mL may be administered via a central line only.

Premixed bags: No further dilution needed. For single use only, discard any unused portion. Use only if solution is clear; the manufacturer recommends not to admix or run in the same line as other medications.

Monitoring Parameters Blood pressure, heart rate

Special Geriatric Considerations Elderly may experience a greater hypotensive response. Constipation may be more of a problem in the elderly. Calcium channel blockers are no more effective in the elderly than other therapies; however, they do not cause significant CNS effects which is an advantage over some antihypertensive agents.

Dosage Forms Excipient information presented when available (limited, particularly for generics); consult specific product labeling.

Capsule, oral, as hydrochloride: 20 mg, 30 mg

Capsule, sustained release, oral, as hydrochloride:
Cardene® SR: 30 mg, 45 mg, 60 mg

Infusion, premixed iso-osmotic dextrose solution, as hydrochloride:
Cardene® I.V.: 20 mg (200 mL); 40 mg (200 mL)

Infusion, premixed iso-osmotic sodium chloride solution, as hydrochloride:
Cardene® I.V.: 20 mg (200 mL); 40 mg (200 mL)

Injection, solution, as hydrochloride: 2.5 mg/mL (10 mL)
Cardene® I.V.: 2.5 mg/mL (10 mL)

◆ **Nicardipine Hydrochloride** *see* NiCARdipine *on page* 1293
◆ **NicoDerm® CQ® [OTC]** *see* Nicotine *on page* 1297
◆ **Nicomide-T™ [OTC]** *see* Niacinamide *on page* 1290
◆ **Nicorelief [OTC]** *see* Nicotine *on page* 1297
◆ **Nicorette® [OTC]** *see* Nicotine *on page* 1297
◆ **Nicotinamide** *see* Niacinamide *on page* 1290

Nicotine (nik oh TEEN)

Medication Safety Issues
Sound-alike/look-alike issues:
NicoDerm® may be confused with Nitroderm
Nicorette® may be confused with Nordette®
Other safety concerns:
Transdermal patch may contain conducting metal (eg, aluminum); remove patch prior to MRI.

Brand Names: U.S. Commit® [OTC]; NicoDerm® CQ® [OTC]; Nicorelief [OTC]; Nicorette® [OTC]; Nicotrol® Inhaler; Nicotrol® NS; Thrive™ [OTC]

Brand Names: Canada Habitrol®; Nicoderm®; Nicorette®; Nicorette® Plus; Nicotrol®

Index Terms Habitrol; Nicotine Patch

Generic Availability (U.S.) Yes: Transdermal patch and gum

Pharmacologic Category Smoking Cessation Aid

Use Treatment to aid smoking cessation for the relief of nicotine withdrawal symptoms (including nicotine craving)

Unlabeled/Investigational Use Management of ulcerative colitis (transdermal)

Contraindications Hypersensitivity to nicotine or any component of the formulation; patients who are smoking during the postmyocardial infarction period; patients with life-threatening arrhythmias, or severe or worsening angina pectoris; active temporomandibular joint disease (gum); not for use in nonsmokers

Warnings/Precautions Hazardous agent - use appropriate precautions for handling and disposal. Use caution in patients with hyperthyroidism, pheochromocytoma, or insulin-dependent diabetes. Use with caution in oropharyngeal inflammation and in patients with history of esophagitis, peptic ulcer, coronary artery disease, recent MI, serious cardiac arrhythmias, vasospastic disease, angina, hypertension, hyperthyroidism, pheochromocy-toma, diabetes, severe renal dysfunction, and hepatic dysfunction. The oral inhaler and nasal spray should be used with caution in patients with bronchospastic disease (other forms of nicotine replacement may be preferred). Use of nasal product is not recommended with chronic nasal disorders (eg, allergy, rhinitis, nasal polyps, and sinusitis). Transdermal patch may contain conducting metal (eg, aluminum); remove patch prior to MRI. Cautious use of topical nicotine in patients with certain skin diseases. Hypersensitivity to the topical products can occur. Dental problems may be worsened by chewing the gum. Urge patients to stop smoking completely when initiating therapy.

Adverse Reactions (Reflective of adult population; not specific for elderly)
Nasal spray/inhaler:
>10%:
Central nervous system: Headache (18% to 26%)
Gastrointestinal: Inhaler: Mouth/throat irritation (66%), dyspepsia (18%)
Respiratory: Inhaler: Cough (32%), rhinitis (23%)
1% to 10%:
Dermatologic: Acne (3%)
Endocrine & metabolic: Dysmenorrhea (3%)
Gastrointestinal: Flatulence (4%), gum problems (4%), diarrhea, hiccup, nausea, taste disturbance, tooth abrasions
Neuromuscular & skeletal: Back pain (6%), arthralgia (5%), jaw/neck pain
Respiratory: Nasal burning (nasal spray), sinusitis
Miscellaneous: Withdrawal symptoms

Adverse events previously reported in prescription labeling for chewing gum, lozenge and/or transdermal systems. Frequency not defined; may be product or dose specific:
Central nervous system: Concentration impaired, depression, dizziness, headache, insomnia, nervousness, pain
Gastrointestinal: Aphthous stomatitis, constipation, cough, diarrhea, dyspepsia, flatulence, gingival bleeding, glossitis, hiccups, jaw pain, nausea, salivation increased, stomatitis, taste perversion, tooth abrasions, ulcerative stomatitis, xerostomia
Dermatologic: Rash
Local: Application site reaction, local edema, local erythema
Neuromuscular & skeletal: Arthralgia, myalgia, paresthesia
Respiratory: Cough, sinusitis
Miscellaneous: Allergic reaction, diaphoresis

Drug Interactions
Metabolism/Transport Effects Substrate (minor) of CYP1A2, 2A6, 2B6, 2C9, 2C19, 2D6, 2E1, 3A4; **Inhibits** CYP2A6 (weak), 2E1 (weak)

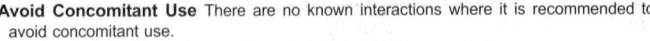

Avoid Concomitant Use There are no known interactions where it is recommended to avoid concomitant use.

Increased Effect/Toxicity

Nicotine may increase the levels/effects of: Adenosine

The levels/effects of Nicotine may be increased by: Cimetidine; Conivaptan

Decreased Effect

The levels/effects of Nicotine may be decreased by: Cyproterone; Peginterferon Alfa-2b; Tocilizumab

Ethanol/Nutrition/Herb Interactions Food: Lozenge: Acidic foods/beverages decrease absorption of nicotine.

Stability

Nicotrol®: Store inhaler cartridge at room temperature not to exceed 30°C (86°F). Protect cartridges from light.

Nicotrol® NS: Store at room temperature not to exceed 30°C (86°F).

Mechanism of Action Nicotine is one of two naturally-occurring alkaloids which exhibit their primary effects via autonomic ganglia stimulation. The other alkaloid is lobeline which has many actions similar to those of nicotine but is less potent. Nicotine is a potent ganglionic and central nervous system stimulant, the actions of which are mediated via nicotine-specific receptors. Biphasic actions are observed depending upon the dose administered. The main effect of nicotine in small doses is stimulation of all autonomic ganglia; with larger doses, initial stimulation is followed by blockade of transmission. Biphasic effects are also evident in the adrenal medulla; discharge of catecholamines occurs with small doses, whereas prevention of catecholamines release is seen with higher doses as a response to splanchnic nerve stimulation. Stimulation of the central nervous system (CNS) is characterized by tremors and respiratory excitation. However, convulsions may occur with higher doses, along with respiratory failure secondary to both central paralysis and peripheral blockade to respiratory muscles.

Pharmacodynamics/Kinetics

Onset of action: Intranasal: More closely approximate the time course of plasma nicotine levels observed after cigarette smoking than other dosage forms

Duration: Transdermal: 24 hours

Absorption: Transdermal: Slow

Metabolism: Hepatic, primarily to cotinine ($1/5$ as active)

Half-life elimination: 4 hours; Nasal spray: 1-2 hours

Time to peak, serum: Transdermal: 8-9 hours; Nasal spray: 10-20 minutes

Excretion: Urine

Clearance: Renal: pH dependent

Dosage

Geriatric & Adult

Tobacco cessation (patients should be advised to completely stop smoking upon initiation of therapy):

Gum: Chew 1 piece of gum when urge to smoke, up to 24 pieces/day. Patients who smoke <25 cigarettes/day should start with 2-mg strength; patients smoking ≥25 cigarettes/day should start with the 4-mg strength. Use according to the following 12-week dosing schedule:

Weeks 1-6: Chew 1 piece of gum every 1-2 hours; to increase chances of quitting, chew at least 9 pieces/day during the first 6 weeks

Weeks 7-9: Chew 1 piece of gum every 2-4 hours

Weeks 10-12: Chew 1 piece of gum every 4-8 hours

Inhaler: Oral: Usually 6-16 cartridges per day; best effect was achieved by frequent continuous puffing (20 minutes); recommended duration of treatment is 3 months, after which patients may be weaned from the inhaler by gradual reduction of the daily dose over 6-12 weeks

Lozenge: Oral: Patients who smoke their first cigarette within 30 minutes of waking should use the 4-mg strength; otherwise the 2-mg strength is recommended. Use according to the following 12-week dosing schedule:

Weeks 1-6: One lozenge every 1-2 hours

Weeks 7-9: One lozenge every 2-4 hours

Weeks 10-12: One lozenge every 4-8 hours

Note: Use at least 9 lozenges/day during first 6 weeks to improve chances of quitting; do not use more than one lozenge at a time (maximum: 5 lozenges every 6 hours, 20 lozenges/day)

Spray: Nasal: 1-2 sprays/hour; do not exceed more than 5 doses (10 sprays) per hour [maximum: 40 doses/day (80 sprays); each dose (2 sprays) contains 1 mg of nicotine]

Transdermal patch: Topical: Apply new patch every 24 hours to nonhairy, clean, dry skin on the upper body or upper outer arm; each patch should be applied to a different site. **Note:** Adjustment may be required during initial treatment (move to higher dose if experiencing withdrawal symptoms; lower dose if side effects are experienced).

NicoDerm CQ®:

Patients smoking >10 cigarettes/day: Begin with step 1 (21 mg/day) for 6 weeks, **followed by** step 2 (14 mg/day) for 2 weeks; **finish with** step 3 (7 mg/day) for 2 weeks

Patients smoking ≤10 cigarettes/day: Begin with step 2 (14 mg/day) for 6 weeks, **followed by** step 3 (7 mg/day) for 2 weeks

Note: Patients who are receiving >600 mg/day of cimetidine: Decrease to the next lower patch size

Benefits of use of nicotine transdermal patches beyond 3 months have not been demonstrated

Administration

Gum: Should be chewed slowly to avoid jaw ache and to maximize benefit. Chew slowly until it tingles, then park gum between cheek and gum until tingle is gone; repeat process until most of tingle is gone (~30 minutes).

Lozenge: Should not be chewed or swallowed; allow to dissolve slowly (~20-30 minutes)

Nasal spray: Prime pump prior to first use (pump 6-8 times until fine spray appears) or if it has not been used for 24 hours (pump 1-2 times). Blow nose prior to use. Tilt head back slightly and insert tip of bottle into nostril. Breathe through mouth and spray once in each nostril. Do not sniff, swallow, or inhale through the nose during administration. After administration, wait 2-3 minutes before blowing nose.

Oral Inhalant: Insert cartridge into inhaler and push hard until it pops into place. Replace mouthpiece and twist the top and bottom so that markings do not line up. Inhale deeply into the back of the throat or puff in short breaths. Nicotine in cartridge is used up after about 20 minutes of active puffing.

Transdermal patch: Do not cut patch; causes rapid evaporation, rendering the patch useless

Monitoring Parameters Heart rate and blood pressure periodically during therapy; discontinue therapy if signs of nicotine toxicity occur (eg, severe headache, dizziness, mental confusion, disturbed hearing and vision, abdominal pain; rapid, weak and irregular pulse; salivation, nausea, vomiting, diarrhea, cold sweat, weakness); therapy should be discontinued if rash develops; discontinuation may be considered if other adverse effects of patch occur such as myalgia, arthralgia, abnormal dreams, insomnia, nervousness, dry mouth, sweating

Pharmacotherapy Pearls A cigarette has 10-25 mg nicotine.

Special Geriatric Considerations Must evaluate benefit in the elderly who may have chronic diseases mentioned in Warning and Contraindications. The transdermal systems are as effective in the elderly as they are in younger adults; however, complaints of body aches, dizziness, and asthenia were reported more often in the elderly.

Dosage Forms Excipient information presented when available (limited, particularly for generics); consult specific product labeling.

Gum, chewing, oral, as polacrilex: 2 mg (20s, 40s, 50s, 100s, 110s); 4 mg (20s, 40s, 50s, 100s, 110s)

Nicorelief: 2 mg (50s, 110s)

Nicorelief: 2 mg (50s, 110s) [mint flavor]

Nicorelief: 4 mg (50s, 110s)

Nicorelief: 4 mg (50s, 110s) [mint flavor]

Nicorette®: 2 mg (40s, 100s) [fresh mint flavor]

Nicorette®: 2 mg (48s, 50s, 108s, 110s, 168s, 170s, 192s, 200s, 216s) [mint flavor]

Nicorette®: 2 mg (48s, 108s) [orange flavor]

Nicorette®: 2 mg (48s, 50s, 108s, 110s, 168s, 170s, 192s, 200s, 216s) [original flavor]

Nicorette®: 2 mg (40s, 100s) [contains calcium 94 mg/gum, sodium 11 mg/gum; fruit chill flavor]

Nicorette®: 4 mg (40s, 100s) [fresh mint flavor]

Nicorette®: 4 mg (48s, 108s, 110s, 168s, 170s, 192s, 200s, 216s) [mint flavor]

Nicorette®: 4 mg (48s, 108s, 110s) [orange flavor]

Nicorette®: 4 mg (48s, 50s, 108s, 110s, 168s, 170s, 192s, 200s, 216s) [original flavor]

Nicorette®: 4 mg (40s, 100s) [contains calcium 94 mg/gum, sodium 13 mg/gum; fruit chill flavor]

Thrive™: 2 mg (40s); 4 mg (40s) [gluten free, sucrose free; mint flavor]

Lozenge, oral, as polacrilex:

Commit®: 2 mg (48s, 72s); 4 mg (48s, 72s) [gluten free, sugar free; contains phenylalanine 3.4 mg/lozenge, sodium 18 mg/lozenge; mint flavor]

Nicorette®: 4 mg (50s) [mint flavor]

Oral inhalation system, for oral inhalation:

Nicotrol® Inhaler: 10 mg (10 mL) [contains menthol; delivering 4 mg nicotine]

Patch, transdermal: 7 mg/24 hours (7s, 14s); 14 mg/24 hours (7s, 14s); 21 mg/24 hours (7s, 14s)
NicoDerm® CQ®: 7 mg/24 hours (14s) [contains metal; step 3; clear patch]
NicoDerm® CQ®: 7 mg/24 hours (14s) [contains metal; step 3; tan patch]
NicoDerm® CQ®: 14 mg/24 hours (14s) [contains metal; step 2; clear patch]
NicoDerm® CQ®: 14 mg/24 hours (14s) [contains metal; step 2; tan patch]
NicoDerm® CQ®: 21 mg/24 hours (7s, 14s) [contains metal; step 1; clear patch]
NicoDerm® CQ®: 21 mg/24 hours (7s, 14s) [contains metal; step 1; tan patch]
Solution, intranasal [spray]:
Nicotrol® NS: 10 mg/mL (10 mL) [chlorofluorocarbon free; delivers ~0.5 mg/spray; ~200 sprays]

◆ **Nicotine Patch** see Nicotine on page 1297
◆ **Nicotinic Acid** see Niacin on page 1288
◆ **Nicotinic Acid Amide** see Niacinamide on page 1290
◆ **Nicotrol® Inhaler** see Nicotine on page 1297
◆ **Nicotrol® NS** see Nicotine on page 1297
◆ **Nifediac CC®** see NIFEdipine on page 1300
◆ **Nifedical XL®** see NIFEdipine on page 1300

NIFEdipine (nye FED i peen)

Related Information
Beers Criteria – Potentially Inappropriate Medications for Geriatrics on page 2089
Calcium Channel Blockers on page 2003
Medication Safety Issues
Sound-alike/look-alike issues:
NIFEdipine may be confused with niCARdipine, niMODipine, nisoldipine
Procardia XL® may be confused with Cartia XT®
Beers Criteria medication:
This drug may be inappropriate for use in geriatric patients (high severity risk).
International issues:
Depin [India] may be confused with Depen brand name for penicillamine [U.S.]; Depon brand name for acetaminophen [Greece]; Dipen brand name for diltiazem [Greece]
Nipin [Italy and Singapore] may be confused with Nipent brand name for pentostatin [U.S., Canada, and multiple international markets]
Brand Names: U.S. Adalat® CC; Afeditab® CR; Nifediac CC®; Nifedical XL®; Procardia XL®; Procardia®
Brand Names: Canada Adalat® XL®; Apo-Nifed PA®; Mylan-Nifedipine Extended Release; Nu-Nifed; Nu-Nifedipine-PA; PMS-Nifedipine
Generic Availability (U.S.) Yes
Pharmacologic Category Calcium Channel Blocker; Calcium Channel Blocker, Dihydropyridine
Use Management of chronic stable or vasospastic angina; treatment of hypertension (sustained release products only)
Unlabeled/Investigational Use Management of pulmonary hypertension, Raynaud's phenomenon
Contraindications Hypersensitivity to nifedipine or any component of the formulation; concomitant use with strong CYP3A4 inducers (eg, rifampin); cardiogenic shock; immediate release preparation for treatment of urgent or emergent hypertension (Chobanian, 2003); acute MI (Antman, 2004)
Warnings/Precautions Symptomatic hypotension with or without syncope can rarely occur; blood pressure must be lowered at a rate appropriate for the patient's clinical condition. **The use of immediate release nifedipine (sublingually or orally) in hypertensive emergencies and urgencies is neither safe nor effective.** Serious adverse events (eg, death, cerebrovascular ischemia, syncope, stroke, acute myocardial infarction, and fetal distress) have been reported. **Immediate release nifedipine should not be used for acute blood pressure reduction.**

Blood pressure lowering should be done at a rate appropriate for the patient's condition. Rapid drops in blood pressure can lead to arterial insufficiency. Increased angina and/or MI have occurred with initiation or dosage titration of dihydropyridine calcium channel blockers; use with caution in patients with obstructive coronary disease especially in the absence of concurrent beta-blockade. Use with caution before major surgery. Cardiopulmonary bypass, intraoperative blood loss or vasodilating anesthesia may result in severe hypotension and/or increased fluid requirements. Consider withdrawing nifedipine (>36 hours) before surgery if possible.

The most common side effect is peripheral edema; occurs within 2-3 weeks of starting therapy. Reflex tachycardia may occur with use. Use with caution in HF or severe aortic stenosis (especially with concomitant beta-adrenergic blocker), severe left ventricular dysfunction, renal impairment, hypertrophic cardiomyopathy (especially obstructive), concomitant therapy with beta-blockers or digoxin, and edema. Use caution in patients with severe hepatic impairment. Clearance of nifedipine is reduced in cirrhotic patients leading to increased systemic exposure; monitor closely for adverse effects/toxicity and consider dose adjustments. Mild and transient elevations in liver function enzymes may be apparent within 8 weeks of therapy initiation. Abrupt withdrawal may cause rebound angina in patients with CAD. Short-acting nifedipine may be inappropriate for use in the elderly due to potential to cause hypotension and constipation (Beers Criteria). Immediate release formulations should not be used to manage essential hypertension, adequate studies to evaluate outcomes have not been conducted. Avoid use of extended release tablets (Procardia XL®) in patients with known stricture/narrowing of the GI tract. Adalat® CC tablets contain lactose; do not use with galactose intolerance, Lapp lactase deficiency, or glucose-galactose malabsorption syndromes.

Use with caution in patients taking CYP3A4 inhibitors; may result in increased nifedipine concentrations; monitor for adverse effects/toxicity and consider dose adjustments. Use with strong CYP3A4 inducers (eg, rifampin, rifabutin, phenobarbital, phenytoin, carbamazepine, St John's wort) is contraindicated due to reduced bioavailability and efficacy.

Adverse Reactions (Reflective of adult population; not specific for elderly)
>10%:
  Cardiovascular: Flushing (10% to 25%; extended release products 3% to 4%), peripheral edema (dose related 7% to 30%)
  Central nervous system: Dizziness/lightheadedness/giddiness (10% to 27%), headache (10% to 23%)
  Gastrointestinal: Nausea/heartburn (10% to 11%)
≥1% to 10%:
  Cardiovascular: Palpitation (≤2% to 7%), transient hypotension (dose related 5%), CHF (2%)
  Central nervous system: Nervousness/mood changes (≤2% to 7%), fatigue (6%), shakiness (≤2%), jitteriness (≤2%), sleep disturbances (≤2%), difficulties in balance (≤2%), fever (≤2%), chills (≤2%)
  Dermatologic: Dermatitis (≤2%), pruritus (≤2%), urticaria (≤2%)
  Endocrine & metabolic: Sexual difficulties (≤2%)
  Gastrointestinal: Diarrhea (≤2%), constipation (≤2%), cramps (≤2%), flatulence (≤2%), gingival hyperplasia (≤10%)
  Neuromuscular & skeletal: Muscle cramps/tremor (≤2% to 8%), weakness (<3%), inflammation (≤2%), joint stiffness (≤2%)
  Ocular: Blurred vision (≤2%)
  Respiratory: Cough/wheezing (6%), nasal congestion/sore throat (≤2% to 6%), chest congestion (≤2%), dyspnea (≤2%)
  Miscellaneous: Diaphoresis (≤2%)
Drug Interactions
  Metabolism/Transport Effects Substrate of CYP2D6 (minor), 3A4 (major); **Inhibits** CYP1A2 (moderate), 2C9 (weak), 2D6 (weak), 3A4 (weak)
  Avoid Concomitant Use
    Avoid concomitant use of NIFEdipine with any of the following: Conivaptan; Grapefruit Juice
  Increased Effect/Toxicity
    NIFEdipine may increase the levels/effects of: Amifostine; Antihypertensives; Beta-Blockers; Calcium Channel Blockers (Nondihydropyridine); CYP1A2 Substrates; Digoxin; Fosphenytoin; Hypotensive Agents; Magnesium Salts; Neuromuscular-Blocking Agents (Nondepolarizing); Nitroprusside; Phenytoin; QuiNIDine; RiTUXimab; Tacrolimus; Tacrolimus (Systemic); VinCRIStine

    The levels/effects of NIFEdipine may be increased by: Alcohol (Ethyl); Alpha1-Blockers; Antifungal Agents (Azole Derivatives, Systemic); Calcium Channel Blockers (Nondihydropyridine); Cimetidine; Cisapride; Conivaptan; CycloSPORINE; CycloSPORINE (Systemic); CYP3A4 Inhibitors (Moderate); CYP3A4 Inhibitors (Strong); Dasatinib; Diazoxide; Fluconazole; FLUoxetine; Grapefruit Juice; Herbs (Hypotensive Properties); Macrolide Antibiotics; Magnesium Salts; MAO Inhibitors; Pentoxifylline; Phosphodiesterase 5 Inhibitors; Prostacyclin Analogues; Protease Inhibitors; QuiNIDine
  Decreased Effect
    NIFEdipine may decrease the levels/effects of: Clopidogrel; QuiNIDine

    The levels/effects of NIFEdipine may be decreased by: Barbiturates; Calcium Salts; CarBAMazepine; CYP3A4 Inducers (Strong); Deferasirox; Herbs (CYP3A4 Inducers); Herbs (Hypertensive Properties); Methylphenidate; Nafcillin; Peginterferon Alfa-2b; Rifamycin Derivatives; Tocilizumab; Yohimbine

Ethanol/Nutrition/Herb Interactions

Ethanol: Avoid ethanol (may increase CNS depression and may increase the effects of nifedipine). Monitor.

Food: Nifedipine serum levels may be decreased if taken with food. Food may decrease the rate but not the extent of absorption of Procardia XL®. Increased nifedipine concentrations resulting in therapeutic and vasodilator side effects, including severe hypotension and myocardial ischemia, may occur if nifedipine is taken by patients ingesting grapefruit.

Herb/Nutraceutical: St John's wort may decrease nifedipine levels (avoid use). Avoid use of bayberry, blue cohosh, cayenne, ephedra, ginger, ginseng (American), kola, licorice (may worsen hypertension). Avoid black cohosh, California poppy, coleus, golden seal, hawthorn, mistletoe, periwinkle, quinine, shepherd's purse (may have increased antihypertensive effect).

Mechanism of Action Inhibits calcium ion from entering the "slow channels" or select voltage-sensitive areas of vascular smooth muscle and myocardium during depolarization, producing a relaxation of coronary vascular smooth muscle and coronary vasodilation; increases myocardial oxygen delivery in patients with vasospastic angina; also reduces peripheral vascular resistance, producing a reduction in arterial blood pressure.

Pharmacodynamics/Kinetics

Onset of action: Immediate release: ~20 minutes

Protein binding (concentration dependent): 92% to 98%

Metabolism: Hepatic via CYP3A4 to inactive metabolites

Bioavailability: Capsule: 40% to 77%; Sustained release: 65% to 89% relative to immediate release capsules; bioavailability increased with significant hepatic disease

Half-life elimination: Adults: Healthy: 2-5 hours; Cirrhosis: 7 hours; Elderly: 7 hours (extended release tablet)

Excretion: Urine (60% to 80% as inactive metabolites); feces

Dosage

Geriatric Refer to adult dosing. In the management of hypertension, consider lower initial doses and titrate to response (Aronow, 2011).

Adult Dosage adjustments should occur at 7- to 14-day intervals, to allow for adequate assessment of new dose; when switching from immediate release to sustained release formulations, use same total daily dose.

Chronic stable or vasospastic angina: Oral:

Immediate release: Initial: 10 mg 3 times/day; usual dose: 10-20 mg 3 times/day; coronary artery spasm may require up to 20-30 mg 3-4 times/day; single doses >30 mg and total daily doses >120 mg are rarely needed; maximum: 180 mg/day; **Note:** Do not use for acute anginal episodes; may precipitate myocardial infarction

Extended release: Initial: 30 or 60 mg once daily; maximum: 120-180 mg/day

Hypertension: Oral: Extended release: Initial: 30 or 60 mg once daily; maximum: 90-120 mg/day

Pulmonary hypertension (unlabeled use; Galie, 2004): Oral: Extended release: Initial: 30 mg twice daily; may increase cautiously to 120-240 mg/day

Raynaud's phenomenon (unlabeled use; Wigley, 2002): Oral: Extended release: Dosage range: 30-120 mg once daily

Renal Impairment

Hemodialysis: Supplemental dose is not necessary.

Peritoneal dialysis effects: Supplemental dose is not necessary.

Hepatic Impairment Clearance of nifedipine is reduced in cirrhotic patients leading to increased systemic exposure; monitor closely for adverse effects/toxicity and consider dose adjustments.

Administration

Immediate release: In general, may be administered with or without food.

Extended release: Tablets should be swallowed whole; do not crush, split, or chew.

Adalat® CC, Afeditab® CR, Nifediac CC®: Administer on an empty stomach (per manufacturer). Other extended release products may not have this recommendation; consult product labeling.

Monitoring Parameters Heart rate, blood pressure, signs and symptoms of CHF, peripheral edema

Pharmacotherapy Pearls When measuring smaller doses from the liquid-filled capsules, consider the following concentrations (for Procardia®) 10 mg capsule = 10 mg/0.34 mL; 20 mg capsule = 20 mg/0.45 mL; may be used preoperative to treat hypertensive urgency.

Considerable attention has been directed to potential increases in mortality and morbidity when short-acting nifedipine is used in treating hypertension. The rapid reduction in blood pressure may precipitate adverse cardiovascular events.

Short-acting nifedipine should not be used for acute anginal episodes since this may precipitate myocardial infarction. Extended-release formulations are preferred for the management of chronic or vasospastic angina (Poole-Wilson, 2004).

Equivalency of extended release formulation (Adalat® CC): The manufacturer states that it is acceptable to interchange two 30 mg tablets with one 60 mg tablet to effectively deliver a 60 mg dose. However, it is not recommended to substitute one 90 mg tablet with three 30 mg tablets, since the resulting C_{max} is 29% higher compared to giving the single 90 mg tablet.

Special Geriatric Considerations Elderly may experience a greater hypotensive response. Theoretically, constipation may be more of a problem in elderly patients. The half-life of nifedipine is extended in elderly patients (6.7 hours) as compared to younger subjects (3.8 hours).

This medication is considered to be potentially inappropriate in this patient population (Beers Criteria severity: High).

Dosage Forms Excipient information presented when available (limited, particularly for generics); consult specific product labeling.

Capsule, softgel, oral: 10 mg, 20 mg
  Procardia®: 10 mg
Tablet, extended release, oral: 30 mg, 60 mg, 90 mg
  Adalat® CC: 30 mg, 60 mg, 90 mg
  Afeditab® CR: 30 mg, 60 mg
  Nifediac CC®: 30 mg, 60 mg
  Nifediac CC®: 90 mg [contains tartrazine]
  Nifedical XL®: 30 mg, 60 mg
  Procardia XL®: 30 mg, 60 mg, 90 mg

Selected References

Galie N, Torbicki A, Barst R, et al, "Guidelines on Diagnosis and Treatment of Pulmonary Arterial Hypertension. The Task Force on Diagnosis and Treatment of Pulmonary Arterial Hypertension of the European Society of Cardiology," Eur Heart J, 2004, 25(24):2243-78.

Gibbons RJ, Abrams J, Chatterjee K, et al, "ACC/AHA 2002 Guideline Update for the Management of Patients With Chronic Stable Angina: A Report of the American College of Cardiology/American Heart Association Task Force on Practice Guidelines (Committee to Update the 1999 Guidelines for the Management of Patients With Chronic Stable Angina)," 2002. Available at http://www.acc.org/qualityandscience/clinical/guidelines/stable/stable_clean.pdf.

Messerli FH, Kowey P, and Grodzicki T, "Sublingual Nifedipine for Hypertensive Emergencies," Lancet, 1991, 338 (8771):881.

Poole-Wilson PA, Lubsen J, Kirwan BA, et al, "Effect of Long-Acting Nifedipine on Mortality and Cardiovascular Morbidity in Patients with Stable Angina Requiring Treatment (Action Trial): Randomized Controlled Trial," Lancet, 2004, 364(9437):849-57.

Rosen WJ and Johnson CE, "Evaluation of Five Procedures for Measuring Nonstandard Doses of Nifedipine Liquid," Am J Hosp Pharm, 1989, 46(11):2313-7.

Silberschmidt AL, Kuhn-Velten WN, Juon AM, et al, "Nifedipine Concentration in Maternal and Umbilical Cord Blood After Nifedipine Gastrointestinal Therapeutic System for Tocolysis," BJOG, 2008, 115(4):480-85.

Sitbon O, Humbert M, Jais X, et al, "Long-Term Response to Calcium Channel Blockers in Idiopathic Pulmonary Arterial Hypertension," Circulation, 2005, 111(23):3105-11.

Wigley FM, "Clinical Practice. Raynaud's Phenomenon," N Engl J Med, 2002, 347(13):1001-8.

◆ **Niftolid** see Flutamide on page 766
◆ **Nilandron®** see Nilutamide on page 1303

Nilutamide (ni LOO ta mide)

Medication Safety Issues
  Sound-alike/look-alike issues:
    Nilutamide may be confused with nilotinib
Brand Names: U.S. Nilandron®
Brand Names: Canada Anandron®
Index Terms RU-23908
Generic Availability (U.S.) No
Pharmacologic Category Antiandrogen; Antineoplastic Agent, Antiandrogen
Use Treatment of metastatic prostate cancer (in combination with surgical castration)
Contraindications Hypersensitivity to nilutamide or any component of the formulation; severe hepatic impairment; severe respiratory insufficiency
Warnings/Precautions Hazardous agent - use appropriate precautions for handling and disposal. **[U.S. Boxed Warning]: Interstitial pneumonitis has been reported in 2% of patients exposed to nilutamide.** Symptoms typically include exertional dyspnea, cough, chest pain and fever; interstitial changes (including pulmonary fibrosis) leading to hospitalization and fatalities have been reported (rarely). The suggestive signs of pneumonitis most often occurred within the first 3 months of treatment. X-rays showed interstitial or alveolo-interstitial changes; pulmonary function tests revealed a restrictive pattern with decreased

◀ DLco. Consider baseline pulmonary function testing. Discontinue if signs and/or symptoms of interstitial pneumonitis are noted.

Hepatitis or marked increases in liver enzymes leading to drug discontinuation occurred in 1% of nilutamide patients; rare cases of hospitalization or deaths due to severe liver injury have been reported. Discontinue treatment for jaundice or ALT >2 times the upper limit of normal (ULN).

A delay in adaptation to dark has been reported; in clinical studies, this was reported by 13% to 57% of patients; the delay ranged from seconds to a few minutes after passing from a light to a dark area (this may not abate with continued treatment although may be alleviated by wearing tinted sunglasses); caution patients who experience adaptation delay about driving at night or through tunnels. Not indicated for use in women. Patients with disease progression while receiving antiandrogen therapy may experience clinical improvement with discontinuation of the antiandrogen.

Adverse Reactions (Reflective of adult population; not specific for elderly)
>10%:
Central nervous system: Insomnia (16%), headache (14%)
Endocrine & metabolic: Hot flashes (28% to 67%)
Gastrointestinal: Nausea (10% to 24%), constipation (7% to 20%), anorexia (11%), abdominal pain (10%)
Genitourinary: Testicular atrophy (16%), libido decreased (11%)
Hepatic: AST increased (8% to 13%), ALT increased (8% to 9%)
Ocular: Impaired dark adaptation (13% to 57%)
Respiratory: Dyspnea (6% to 11%)
1% to 10%:
Cardiovascular: Hypertension (5% to 9%), chest pain (7%), heart failure (3%), angina (2%), edema (2%), syncope (2%)
Central nervous system: Dizziness (7% to 10%), depression (9%), hypoesthesia (5%), malaise (2%), nervousness (2%)
Dermatologic: Alopecia (6%), dry skin (5%), rash (5%), pruritus (2%)
Endocrine & metabolic: Alcohol intolerance (5%), hyperglycemia (4%)
Gastrointestinal: Vomiting (6%), diarrhea (2%), GI hemorrhage (2%), melena (2%), weight loss (2%), xerostomia (2%), dyspepsia
Genitourinary: Nocturia (7%)
Hematologic: Anemia (7%), haptoglobin increased (2%), leukopenia (2%)
Hepatic: Alkaline phosphatase increased (3%)
Neuromuscular & skeletal: Bone pain (6%), arthritis (2%), paresthesia (2%)
Ocular: Chromatopsia (9%), impaired light adaptation (8%), abnormal vision (6% to 7%), cataract (2%), photophobia (2%)
Renal: Hematuria (8%), BUN increased (2%), creatinine increased (2%)
Respiratory: Pneumonia (5%), cough (2%), interstitial pneumonitis (2%), rhinitis (2%)
Miscellaneous: Flu-like syndrome (7%), diaphoresis (6%)
Drug Interactions
Metabolism/Transport Effects Substrate of CYP2C19 (major); **Inhibits** CYP2C19 (weak)
Avoid Concomitant Use There are no known interactions where it is recommended to avoid concomitant use.
Increased Effect/Toxicity
The levels/effects of Nilutamide may be increased by: CYP2C19 Inhibitors (Moderate); CYP2C19 Inhibitors (Strong)
Decreased Effect
The levels/effects of Nilutamide may be decreased by: CYP2C19 Inducers (Strong)
Ethanol/Nutrition/Herb Interactions Ethanol: Avoid ethanol (~5% of patients experience an intolerance [facial flushing, hypotension, malaise] when combined with nilutamide).
Stability Store at room temperature of 25°C (77°F); excursions permitted between 15°C to 30°C (59°F to 86°F). Protect from light.
Mechanism of Action Nonsteroidal antiandrogen which blocks testosterone effects at the androgen receptor level, preventing androgen response.
Pharmacodynamics/Kinetics
Absorption: Rapid and complete
Metabolism: Hepatic (extensive), forms active metabolites
Half-life elimination: Terminal: 38-59 hours; Metabolites: 59-126 hours
Excretion: Urine (62%; <2% as unchanged drug); feces (1% to 7%)
Dosage
Geriatric & Adult Prostate cancer, metastatic: Oral: 300 mg once daily (starting the same day or day after surgical castration) for 30 days, followed by 150 mg once daily

Hepatic Impairment
Prior to treatment initiation: Severe hepatic impairment: Use is contraindicated.
During treatment: ALT >2 times ULN or jaundice: Discontinue treatment.
Administration Administer without regard to meals.
Monitoring Parameters Hepatic enzymes (at baseline, regularly during the first 4 months of treatment, periodically thereafter); chest x-ray (at baseline); consider pulmonary function testing (at baseline)
Special Geriatric Considerations Eyes may be slow to adapt to darkness, tinted glasses may help; patients should be careful when driving at night.
Dosage Forms Excipient information presented when available (limited, particularly for generics); consult specific product labeling.
Tablet, oral:
Nilandron®: 150 mg

NiMODipine (nye MOE di peen)

Related Information
Calcium Channel Blockers *on page 2003*
Medication Safety Issues
Sound-alike/look-alike issues:
NiMODipine may be confused with niCARdipine, NIFEdipine, nisoldipine
Administration issues:
For oral administration only. For patients unable to swallow a capsule, the drug should be dispensed in an oral syringe (preferably amber in color) labeled **"WARNING: For ORAL use only"** or **"Not for I.V. use."** Nimodipine has inadvertently been administered I.V. when withdrawn from capsules into a syringe for subsequent nasogastric tube administration. Severe cardiovascular adverse events, including fatalities, have resulted. Employ precautions against such an event.
Brand Names: Canada Nimotop®
Generic Availability (U.S.) Yes
Pharmacologic Category Calcium Channel Blocker; Calcium Channel Blocker, Dihydropyridine
Use Vasospasm following subarachnoid hemorrhage from ruptured intracranial aneurysms
Unlabeled/Investigational Use Prevention of migraines (inconsistent data)
Contraindications Hypersensitivity to nimodipine or any component of the formulation
Warnings/Precautions Increased angina and/or MI has occurred with initiation or dosage titration of calcium channel blockers. The most common side effect is peripheral edema; occurs within 2-3 weeks of starting therapy. Reflex tachycardia may occur with use. Symptomatic hypotension with or without syncope can rarely occur; blood pressure must be lowered at a rate appropriate for the patient's clinical condition. Use caution in hepatic impairment. Intestinal pseudo-obstruction and ileus have been reported during the use of nimodipine. Use caution in patients with decreased GI motility of a history of bowel obstruction. Use caution when treating patients with hypertrophic cardiomyopathy.

[U.S. Boxed Warning]: Nimodipine has inadvertently been administered I.V. when withdrawn from capsules into a syringe for subsequent nasogastric administration. Severe cardiovascular adverse events, including fatalities, have resulted; precautions (eg, adequate labeling, use of oral syringes) should be employed against such an event.
Adverse Reactions (Reflective of adult population; not specific for elderly)
1% to 10%:
Cardiovascular: Reductions in systemic blood pressure (1% to 8%)
Central nervous system: Headache (1% to 4%)
Dermatologic: Rash (1% to 2%)
Gastrointestinal: Diarrhea (2% to 4%), abdominal discomfort (2%)
Drug Interactions
Metabolism/Transport Effects Substrate of CYP3A4 (major)
Avoid Concomitant Use
Avoid concomitant use of NiMODipine with any of the following: Conivaptan; Grapefruit Juice
Increased Effect/Toxicity
NiMODipine may increase the levels/effects of: Amifostine; Antihypertensives; Beta-Blockers; Calcium Channel Blockers (Nondihydropyridine); Fosphenytoin; Hypotensive Agents; Magnesium Salts; Neuromuscular-Blocking Agents (Nondepolarizing); Nitroprusside; Phenytoin; QuiNIDine; RiTUXimab; Tacrolimus; Tacrolimus (Systemic)

The levels/effects of NiMODipine may be increased by: Alpha1-Blockers; Antifungal Agents (Azole Derivatives, Systemic); Calcium Channel Blockers (Nondihydropyridine); Cimetidine; Conivaptan; CycloSPORINE; CycloSPORINE (Systemic); CYP3A4 Inhibitors (Moderate);

◄ CYP3A4 Inhibitors (Strong); Dasatinib; Diazoxide; Fluconazole; FLUoxetine; Grapefruit Juice; Herbs (Hypotensive Properties); Macrolide Antibiotics; Magnesium Salts; MAO Inhibitors; Pentoxifylline; Phosphodiesterase 5 Inhibitors; Prostacyclin Analogues; Protease Inhibitors; QuiNIDine

Decreased Effect

NiMODipine may decrease the levels/effects of: Clopidogrel; QuiNIDine

The levels/effects of NiMODipine may be decreased by: Barbiturates; Calcium Salts; CarBAMazepine; CYP3A4 Inducers (Strong); Deferasirox; Herbs (CYP3A4 Inducers); Herbs (Hypertensive Properties); Methylphenidate; Nafcillin; Rifamycin Derivatives; Tocilizumab; Yohimbine

Ethanol/Nutrition/Herb Interactions

Food: Nimodipine has shown a 1.5-fold increase in bioavailability when taken with grapefruit juice; avoid concurrent use.

Herb/Nutraceutical: St John's wort may decrease levels. Avoid dong quai if using for hypertension (has estrogenic activity). Avoid ephedra, yohimbe, ginseng (may worsen hypertension). Avoid garlic (may have increased antihypertensive effect).

Mechanism of Action Nimodipine shares the pharmacology of other calcium channel blockers; animal studies indicate that nimodipine has a greater effect on cerebral arterials than other arterials; this increased specificity may be due to the drug's increased lipophilicity and cerebral distribution as compared to nifedipine; inhibits calcium ion from entering the "slow channels" or select voltage sensitive areas of vascular smooth muscle and myocardium during depolarization

Pharmacodynamics/Kinetics

Protein binding: >95%

Metabolism: Extensively hepatic

Bioavailability: 13%

Half-life elimination: 1-2 hours; prolonged with renal impairment

Time to peak, serum: ~1 hour

Excretion: Urine (50%) and feces (32%) within 4 days

Dosage

Geriatric & Adult Note: Capsules and contents are for oral/NG tube administration **ONLY.**

Subarachnoid hemorrhage: Oral: 60 mg every 4 hours for 21 days, start therapy within 96 hours after subarachnoid hemorrhage.

Renal Impairment Not removed by hemo- or peritoneal dialysis; supplemental dose is not necessary.

Hepatic Impairment Reduce dosage to 30 mg every 4 hours in patients with liver failure.

Administration For oral administration ONLY. Life-threatening adverse events have occurred when administered parenterally. Administer on an empty stomach.

Nasogastric (NG) tube administration: If the capsules cannot be swallowed, the liquid may be removed by making a hole in each end of the capsule with an 18-gauge needle and extracting the contents into a syringe; transfer these contents into an oral syringe (amber-colored oral syringe preferred). It is strongly recommended that preparation be done in the pharmacy. Label oral syringe with **"WARNING: For ORAL use only"** or **"Not for I.V. use."** Follow with a flush of 30 mL NS.

Monitoring Parameters CNS response, heart rate, blood pressure, signs and symptoms of congestive heart failure

Special Geriatric Considerations Elderly may experience a greater hypotensive response. Constipation may be more of a problem in the elderly. Studies in the treatment of Alzheimer's disease have not demonstrated clear clinical effect.

Dosage Forms Excipient information presented when available (limited, particularly for generics); consult specific product labeling.

Capsule, liquid filled, oral: 30 mg

Capsule, softgel, oral: 30 mg

◆ Niravam™ *see ALPRAZolam on page 70*

Nisoldipine (nye SOL di peen)

Related Information

Calcium Channel Blockers *on page 2003*

Medication Safety Issues

Sound-alike/look-alike issues:

Nisoldipine may be confused with NIFEdipine, niMODipine

Brand Names: U.S. Sular®

Generic Availability (U.S.) Yes

Pharmacologic Category Calcium Channel Blocker; Calcium Channel Blocker, Dihydropyridine

Use Management of hypertension, alone or in combination with other antihypertensive agents

Contraindications Hypersensitivity to nisoldipine, any component of the formulation, or other dihydropyridine calcium channel blockers

Warnings/Precautions With initiation or dosage titration of dihydropyridine calcium channel blockers, reflex tachycardia may occur resulting in angina and/or MI in patients with obstructive coronary disease especially in the absence of concurrent beta-blockade. Use with caution in patients with severe aortic stenosis, HF, and hypertrophic cardiomyopathy with outflow tract obstruction. Use with caution in hepatic impairment; lower starting dose required. The most common side effect is peripheral edema; occurs within 2-3 weeks of starting therapy. Symptomatic hypotension with or without syncope can rarely occur; blood pressure must be lowered at a rate appropriate for the patient's clinical condition. Some dosage forms contain tartrazine, which may cause allergic reactions in certain individuals (eg, aspirin hypersensitivity). Use with caution in patients >65 years of age; lower starting dose recommended.

Adverse Reactions (Reflective of adult population; not specific for elderly)
>10%:
    Cardiovascular: Peripheral edema (dose related; 7% to 29%)
    Central nervous system: Headache (22%)
1% to 10%:
    Cardiovascular: Vasodilation (4%), palpitation (3%), angina exacerbation (2%), chest pain (2%)
    Central nervous system: Dizziness (3% to 10%)
    Dermatologic: Rash (2%)
    Gastrointestinal: Nausea (2%)
    Respiratory: Pharyngitis (5%), sinusitis (3%)

Drug Interactions
Metabolism/Transport Effects Substrate of CYP3A4 (major); **Inhibits** CYP1A2 (weak), 3A4 (weak)
Avoid Concomitant Use
Avoid concomitant use of Nisoldipine with any of the following: CYP3A4 Inducers (Strong); CYP3A4 Inhibitors (Strong); Grapefruit Juice
Increased Effect/Toxicity
Nisoldipine may increase the levels/effects of: Amifostine; Antihypertensives; Beta-Blockers; Calcium Channel Blockers (Nondihydropyridine); Fosphenytoin; Hypotensive Agents; Magnesium Salts; Neuromuscular-Blocking Agents (Nondepolarizing); Nitroprusside; Phenytoin; RiTUXimab; Tacrolimus; Tacrolimus (Systemic)

The levels/effects of Nisoldipine may be increased by: Alpha1-Blockers; Antifungal Agents (Azole Derivatives, Systemic); Calcium Channel Blockers (Nondihydropyridine); Cimetidine; CycloSPORINE; CycloSPORINE (Systemic); CYP3A4 Inhibitors (Moderate); CYP3A4 Inhibitors (Strong); Dasatinib; Diazoxide; Fluconazole; Grapefruit Juice; Herbs (Hypotensive Properties); Macrolide Antibiotics; Magnesium Salts; MAO Inhibitors; Pentoxifylline; Phosphodiesterase 5 Inhibitors; Prostacyclin Analogues; Protease Inhibitors
Decreased Effect
Nisoldipine may decrease the levels/effects of: Clopidogrel

The levels/effects of Nisoldipine may be decreased by: Barbiturates; Calcium Salts; CarBAMazepine; CYP3A4 Inducers (Strong); Deferasirox; Herbs (CYP3A4 Inducers); Herbs (Hypertensive Properties); Methylphenidate; Nafcillin; Rifamycin Derivatives; Tocilizumab; Yohimbine

Ethanol/Nutrition/Herb Interactions
Food: Peak concentrations of nisoldipine may be significantly increased if taken with high-lipid foods; however, total exposure (AUC) may be reduced. Grapefruit juice has been shown to significantly increase the bioavailability of nisoldipine; avoid grapefruit products before and after dosing.
Herb/Nutraceutical: Avoid St John's wort (may decrease nisoldipine levels). Avoid bayberry, blue cohosh, cayenne, ephedra, ginger, ginseng (American), kola, licorice (may worsen hypertension). Avoid black cohosh, California poppy, coleus, golden seal, hawthorn, mistletoe, periwinkle, quinine, shepherd's purse (may have increased antihypertensive effect).

Stability Store at controlled room temperature of 20°C to 25°C (68°F to 77°F). Protect from light; protect from moisture.

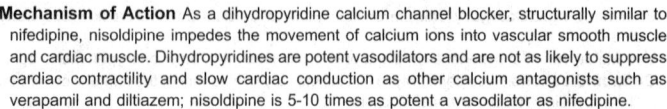

Mechanism of Action As a dihydropyridine calcium channel blocker, structurally similar to nifedipine, nisoldipine impedes the movement of calcium ions into vascular smooth muscle and cardiac muscle. Dihydropyridines are potent vasodilators and are not as likely to suppress cardiac contractility and slow cardiac conduction as other calcium antagonists such as verapamil and diltiazem; nisoldipine is 5-10 times as potent a vasodilator as nifedipine.

Pharmacodynamics/Kinetics

Duration: >24 hours

Absorption: Well absorbed. Peak concentrations significantly increased with high-lipid meals; however, AUC is reduced.

Protein binding: >99%

Metabolism: Extensively hepatic; 1 active metabolite (10% of activity of parent); first-pass effect

Bioavailability: ~5%

Half-life elimination: 9-18 hours

Time to peak: 4-14 hours

Excretion: Urine (60% to 80% as inactive metabolites); feces

Dosage

Geriatric Hypertension: Oral:

Sular® (Geomatrix® delivery system): Initial dose: 8.5 mg once daily; increase by 8.5 mg/week (or longer intervals) to attain adequate blood pressure control

Nisoldipine extended-release (original formulation): Initial dose: 10 mg once daily; increase by 10 mg/week (or longer intervals) to attain adequate blood pressure control.

Conversion from nisoldipine extended-release (original formulation) to Sular® Geomatrix® delivery system: Refer to adult dosing.

Adult Hypertension: Oral:

Sular® (Geomatrix® delivery system): Oral: Initial: 17 mg once daily, then increase by 8.5 mg/week (or longer intervals) to attain adequate control of blood pressure
Usual dose range: 17-34 mg once daily; doses >34 mg once daily are not recommended

Nisoldipine extended-release tablet (original formulation): Initial: 20 mg once daily, then increase by 10 mg/week (or longer intervals) to attain adequate control of blood pressure
Usual dose range (JNC 7): 10-40 mg once daily; doses >60 mg once daily are not recommended

Conversion from nisoldipine extended-release (original formulation) to Sular® Geomatrix® delivery system:

Nisoldipine Extended Release Dosing Equivalency

Original Extended Release Formulation	Sular® Extended Release (Geomatrix® delivery system)
10 mg	8.5 mg
20 mg	17 mg
30 mg	25.5 mg
40 mg	34 mg

Hepatic Impairment

Sular® (Geomatrix® delivery system): An initial dose exceeding 8.5 mg once daily is not recommended for patients with hepatic impairment.

Nisoldipine extended-release (original formulation): An initial dose exceeding 10 mg once daily is not recommended for patients with hepatic impairment.

Administration Administer at the same time each day to ensure minimal fluctuation of serum levels. Avoid high-fat diet. Administer on an empty stomach (1 hour before or 2 hours after a meal). Swallow whole; do not crush, break, split, or chew.

Monitoring Parameters Heart rate, blood pressure, signs and symptoms of CHF, peripheral edema

Special Geriatric Considerations Elderly have been found to have two- to threefold greater serum concentrations than younger adults. Therefore, begin therapy at lowest recommended doses. Elderly may experience a greater hypotensive response. Constipation may be more of a problem in the elderly. Calcium channel blockers are no more effective in the elderly than other therapies; however, they do not cause significant CNS effects which is an advantage over some antihypertensive agents.

Dosage Forms Excipient information presented when available (limited, particularly for generics); consult specific product labeling.
Tablet, extended release, oral: 8.5 mg, 17 mg, 25.5 mg, 34 mg
  Sular®: 8.5 mg
  Sular®: 17 mg [contains tartrazine]
  Sular®: 25.5 mg, 34 mg
Tablet, extended release, oral [original formula]: 20 mg, 30 mg, 40 mg

Selected References
Chobanian AV, Bakris GL, Black HR, et al, "The Seventh Report of the Joint National Committee on Prevention, Detection, Evaluation, and Treatment of High Blood Pressure: The JNC 7 Report," *JAMA*, 2003, 289(19):2560-71.

◆ **Nitalapram** see Citalopram on page 365
◆ **Nitro-Bid®** see Nitroglycerin on page 1311
◆ **Nitro-Dur®** see Nitroglycerin on page 1311

Nitrofurantoin (nye troe fyoor AN toyn)

Related Information
  Beers Criteria – Potentially Inappropriate Medications for Geriatrics on page 2089
Medication Safety Issues
  Sound alike/look alike issues:
    Macrobid® may be confused with microK®, Nitro-Bid®
    Nitrofurantoin may be confused with Neurontin®, nitroglycerin
  BEERS Criteria medication:
    This drug may be inappropriate for use in geriatric patients (high severity risk).
Brand Names: U.S. Furadantin®; Macrobid®; Macrodantin®
Brand Names: Canada Apo-Nitrofurantoin®; Macrobid®; Macrodantin®; Novo-Furantoin
Generic Availability (U.S.) Yes: Excludes suspension
Pharmacologic Category Antibiotic, Miscellaneous
Use Prevention and treatment of urinary tract infections caused by susceptible strains of *E. coli, S. aureus, Enterococcus, Klebsiella,* and *Enterobacter*
Contraindications Hypersensitivity to nitrofurantoin or any component of the formulation; significant renal impairment (anuria, oliguria, significantly elevated serum creatinine, or Cl_{cr} <60 mL/minute); use in patients with a history of cholestatic jaundice or hepatic impairment with previous nitrofurantoin therapy
Warnings/Precautions Use with caution in patients with G6PD deficiency (increased risk of hemolytic anemia). Therapeutic concentrations of nitrofurantoin are not attained in urine of patients with Cl_{cr} <60 mL/minute, therefore, use contraindicated in these patients. Use with caution if prolonged therapy is anticipated due to possible pulmonary toxicity. Acute, subacute, or chronic (usually after 6 months of therapy) pulmonary reactions (possibly fatal) have been observed in patients treated with nitrofurantoin; if these occur, discontinue therapy immediately; monitor closely for malaise, dyspnea, cough, fever, radiologic evidence of diffuse interstitial pneumonitis or fibrosis. Rare, but severe and sometimes fatal hepatic reactions (eg, cholestatic jaundice, hepatitis, hepatic necrosis) have been associated with nitrofurantoin (onset may be insidious); discontinue immediately if hepatitis occurs. Monitor liver function test periodically. Has been associated with peripheral neuropathy (rare); risk may be increased in patients with anemia, renal impairment, diabetes, vitamin B deficiency, debilitating disease, or electrolyte imbalance; use caution. Use in the elderly is not recommended due to potential for renal impairment; alternative agents preferred (Beers Criteria). Use in the elderly, particularly females receiving long-term prophylaxis for recurrent UTIs, has been associated with an increased risk of hepatic and pulmonary toxicity, and peripheral neuropathy. Avoid or use extreme caution when prescribing to elderly patients, particularly those with decreased renal function. Prolonged use may result in fungal or bacterial superinfection, including *C. difficile*-associated diarrhea (CDAD) and pseudomembranous colitis; CDAD has been observed >2 months postantibiotic treatment. Not indicated for the treatment of pyelonephritis or perinephric abscesses.
Adverse Reactions (Reflective of adult population; not specific for elderly) Frequency not defined.
  Cardiovascular: Cyanosis, ECG changes (nonspecific ST/T wave changes, bundle branch block)
  Central nervous system: Bulging fontanels (infants), chills, confusion, depression, dizziness, drowsiness, fever, headache, malaise, pseudotumor cerebri, psychotic reaction, vertigo
  Dermatologic: Alopecia, angioedema, erythema multiforme, exfoliative dermatitis, pruritus, rash (eczematous, erythematous, maculopapular), Stevens-Johnson syndrome, urticaria
  Endocrine & metabolic: Hyperphosphatemia
  Gastrointestinal: Abdominal pain, anorexia, *C. difficile* colitis, constipation, diarrhea, dyspepsia, flatulence, nausea, pancreatitis, pseudomembranous colitis, sialadenitis, vomiting

Genitourinary: Urine discoloration (brown)

Hematologic: Agranulocytosis, aplastic anemia, eosinophilia, glucose-6-phosphate dehydro-genase deficiency anemia, granulocytopenia, hemoglobin decreased, hemolytic anemia, leukopenia, megaloblastic anemia, thrombocytopenia

Hepatic: Hepatitis, hepatic necrosis, transaminases increased, jaundice (cholestatic)

Neuromuscular & skeletal: Arthralgia, myalgia, numbness, paresthesia, peripheral neuro-pathy, weakness

Ocular: Amblyopia, nystagmus, optic neuritis

Respiratory: Cough, dyspnea, pneumonitis, pulmonary fibrosis (with long-term use), pulmo-nary infiltration

Miscellaneous: Acute pulmonary reaction (symptoms include chills, chest pain, cough, dyspnea, fever, and eosinophilia), anaphylaxis, hypersensitivity (including acute pulmonary hypersensitivity), lupus-like syndrome, superinfections (eg, *Pseudomonas* or *Candida*)

Drug Interactions

Avoid Concomitant Use

Avoid concomitant use of Nitrofurantoin with any of the following: BCG; Magnesium Trisilicate; Norfloxacin

Increased Effect/Toxicity

The levels/effects of Nitrofurantoin may be increased by: Probenecid

Decreased Effect

Nitrofurantoin may decrease the levels/effects of: BCG; Norfloxacin; Typhoid Vaccine

The levels/effects of Nitrofurantoin may be decreased by: Magnesium Trisilicate

Ethanol/Nutrition/Herb Interactions

Ethanol: Avoid ethanol (may increase CNS depression).

Food: Nitrofurantoin serum concentrations may be increased if taken with food.

Stability Store at 20°C to 25°C (68°F to 77°F); excursions permitted to 15°C to 30°C (59°F to 86°F). Protect oral suspension from light.

Mechanism of Action Inhibits several bacterial enzyme systems including acetyl coenzyme A interfering with metabolism and possibly cell wall synthesis

Pharmacodynamics/Kinetics

Absorption: Well absorbed; macrocrystalline form absorbed more slowly due to slower dissolution (causes less GI distress)

Distribution: V_d: 0.8 L/kg

Protein binding: 60% to 90%

Metabolism: Body tissues (except plasma) metabolize 60% of drug to inactive metabolites

Bioavailability: Increased with food

Half-life elimination: 20-60 minutes; prolonged with renal impairment

Excretion:

Suspension: Urine (~40%) and feces (small amounts) as metabolites and unchanged drug

Macrocrystals: Urine (20% to 25% as unchanged drug)

Dosage

Geriatric Refer to adult dosing

Adult

UTI treatment:

Furadantin®, Macrodantin®: Oral: 50-100 mg/dose every 6 hours; administer for 7 days or at least 3 days after obtaining sterile urine

Macrobid®: Oral: 100 mg twice daily for 7 days

UTI prophylaxis (Furadantin®, Macrodantin®): Oral: 50-100 mg/dose at bedtime

Renal Impairment

Cl_{cr} <60 mL/minute: Contraindicated

Contraindicated in hemo- and peritoneal dialysis and continuous arteriovenous or venove-nous hemofiltration

Administration Administer with meals to improve absorption and decrease adverse effects; suspension may be mixed with water, milk, or fruit juice. Shake suspension well before use.

Monitoring Parameters Signs of pulmonary reaction; signs of numbness or tingling of the extremities; CBC, periodic liver function tests, periodic renal function tests with long-term use

Test Interactions False-positive urine glucose (Benedict's and Fehling's methods); no false positives with enzymatic tests

Special Geriatric Considerations Because of nitrofurantoin's decreased efficacy in patients with a Cl_{cr} <60 mL/minute and its side effect profile, it is not an antibiotic of choice for acute or prophylactic treatment of urinary tract infections in the elderly. An increased rate of severe hepatic toxicity has been suggested by postmarketing reports.

This medication is considered to be potentially inappropriate in this patient population (Beers Criteria severity: High).

Dosage Forms Excipient information presented when available (limited, particularly for generics); consult specific product labeling.

Capsule, oral [macrocrystal]: 50 mg, 100 mg

Macrodantin®: 25 mg, 50 mg, 100 mg

Capsule, oral [macrocrystal/monohydrate]: 100 mg

Macrobid®: 100 mg [nitrofurantoin macrocrystal 25% and nitrofurantoin monohydrate 75%]

Suspension, oral: 25 mg/5 mL (230 mL)

Furadantin®: 25 mg/5 mL (230 mL)

Nitroglycerin (nye troe GLI ser in)

Medication Safety Issues

Sound-alike/look-alike issues:

Nitroglycerin may be confused with nitrofurantoin, nitroprusse

Nitro-Bid® may be confused with Macrobid®, Nicobid®

Nitroderm may be confused with NicoDerm®

Nitrol® may be confused with Nizoral®

Nitrostat® may be confused with Nilstat®, nystatin

Other safety concerns:

Transdermal patch may contain conducting metal (eg, aluminum); remove patch prior to MRI.

International issues:

Nitrocor [Italy, Russia, and Venezuela] may be confused with Natrecor brand name for nesiritide [U.S., Canada, and multiple international markets] and Nutracort brand name for hydrocortisone in the [U.S. and multiple international markets]

Nitro-Dur [U.S., Canada, and multiple international markets] may be confused with Nitrocor [Italy, Russia, and Venezuela]

Brand Names: U.S. Minitran™; Nitro-Bid®; Nitro-Dur®; Nitro-Time®; Nitrolingual®; Nitro-Mist®; Nitrostat®

Brand Names: Canada Minitran™; Mylan-Nitro Sublingual Spray; Nitro-Dur®; Nitroglycerin Injection, USP; Nitrol®; Nitrostat®; Rho®-Nitro Pump Spray; Transderm-Nitro®; Trinipatch®

Index Terms Glyceryl Trinitrate; Nitroglycerol; NTG; Rectiv™; Tridil

Generic Availability (U.S.) Yes: Capsule, injection, patch, tablet

Pharmacologic Category Vasodilator

Use Treatment or prevention of angina pectoris

Intravenous (I.V.) administration: Treatment or prevention of angina pectoris; acute decompensated heart failure (especially when associated with acute myocardial infarction); perioperative hypertension (especially during cardiovascular surgery); induction of intraoperative hypotension

Unlabeled/Investigational Use Short-term management of pulmonary hypertension (I.V.); esophageal spastic disorders; uterine relaxation

Contraindications Hypersensitivity to organic nitrates or any component of the formulation (includes adhesives for transdermal product); concurrent use with phosphodiesterase-5 (PDE-5) inhibitors (sildenafil, tadalafil, or vardenafil); increased intracranial pressure; severe anemia

Additional contraindications for I.V. product: Inadequate cerebral circulation; constrictive pericarditis; pericardial tamponade; restrictive cardiomyopathy

Note: According to the 2010 American Heart Association guidelines for the treatment of acute coronary syndromes, nitrates are considered contraindicated in the following conditions: Hypotension (SBP <90 mm Hg or ≥30 mm Hg below baseline), extreme bradycardia (<50 bpm), tachycardia in the absence of heart failure (>100 bpm), and right ventricular infarction (O'Connor, 2010).

Warnings/Precautions Severe hypotension can occur. Use with caution in volume depletion, moderate hypotension, and extreme caution with inferior wall MI and suspected right ventricular involvement. Use considered contraindicated in patients with severe hypotension (SBP <90 mm Hg or ≥30 mm Hg below baseline), extreme bradycardia (<50 bpm), and right ventricular MI (O'Connor, 2010).

Paradoxical bradycardia and increased angina pectoris can accompany hypotension. Orthostatic hypotension can also occur. Ethanol can accentuate this. Tolerance does develop to nitrates and appropriate dosing is needed to minimize this (drug-free interval). Avoid use of long-acting agents in acute MI or acute HF; cannot easily reverse effects. Nitrates may aggravate angina caused by hypertrophic cardiomyopathy. Nitroglycerin may precipitate or aggravate increased intracranial pressure and subsequently may worsen clinical outcomes in patients with neurologic injury (eg, intracranial hemorrhage, traumatic brain injury). Nitroglycerin transdermal patches may contain conducting metal (eg, aluminum); remove patch

◀ prior to MRI. Avoid concurrent use with PDE-5 inhibitors. When nitrate administration becomes medically necessary, may administer nitrates only if 24 hours have elapsed after use of sildenafil or vardenafil (48 hours after tadalafil use) (Trujillo, 2007).

Adverse Reactions (Reflective of adult population; not specific for elderly) Frequency not defined.

Cardiovascular: Flushing, hypotension, peripheral edema, postural hypotension, syncope, tachycardia

Central nervous system: Headache (common), dizziness, lightheadedness

Gastrointestinal: Nausea, vomiting, xerostomia

Neuromuscular & skeletal: Paresthesia, weakness

Respiratory: Dyspnea, pharyngitis, rhinitis

Miscellaneous: Diaphoresis

Drug Interactions

Avoid Concomitant Use

Avoid concomitant use of Nitroglycerin with any of the following: Ergot Derivatives; Phosphodiesterase 5 Inhibitors

Increased Effect/Toxicity

Nitroglycerin may increase the levels/effects of: Ergot Derivatives; Hypotensive Agents; Rosiglitazone

The levels/effects of Nitroglycerin may be increased by: Alfuzosin; Phosphodiesterase 5 Inhibitors

Decreased Effect

Nitroglycerin may decrease the levels/effects of: Alteplase; Heparin

The levels/effects of Nitroglycerin may be decreased by: Ergot Derivatives

Ethanol/Nutrition/Herb Interactions

Ethanol: Avoid ethanol (may increase the hypotensive effects of nitroglycerin). Monitor.

Herb/Nutraceutical: Avoid bayberry, blue cohosh, cayenne, ephedra, ginger, ginseng (American), kola, licorice (may worsen hypertension). Avoid black cohosh, California poppy, coleus, golden seal, hawthorn, mistletoe, periwinkle, quinine, shepherd's purse (may cause hypotension).

Stability

I.V. solution: Doses should be made in glass bottles, EXCEL® or PAB® containers. Adsorption occurs to soft plastic (eg, PVC). Nitroglycerin diluted in D_5W or NS in glass containers is physically and chemically stable for 48 hours at room temperature and 7 days under refrigeration. In D_5W or NS in EXCEL®/PAB® containers it is physically and chemically stable for 24 hours at room temperature.

Premixed bottles are stable according to the manufacturer's expiration dating.

Standard diluent: 50 mg/250 mL D_5W; 50 mg/500 mL D_5W.

Minimum volume: 100 mg/250 mL D_5W; concentration should not exceed 400 mcg/mL.

Store sublingual tablets and ointment in tightly closed containers at 20°C to 25°C (68°F to 77°F); slow release capsules at 20°C to 25°C (68°F to 77°F); translingual spray and transdermal patch at 15°C to 30°C (59°F to 86°F).

Mechanism of Action Nitroglycerin forms free radical nitric oxide. In smooth muscle, nitric oxide activates guanylate cyclase which increases guanosine 3'5' monophosphate (cGMP) leading to dephosphorylation of myosin light chains and smooth muscle relaxation. Produces a vasodilator effect on the peripheral veins and arteries with more prominent effects on the veins. Primarily reduces cardiac oxygen demand by decreasing preload (left ventricular end-diastolic pressure); may modestly reduce afterload; dilates coronary arteries and improves collateral flow to ischemic regions

Pharmacodynamics/Kinetics

Onset of action: Sublingual tablet: 1-3 minutes; Translingual spray: Similar to sublingual tablet; Sustained release: ~60 minutes; Topical: 15-30 minutes; Transdermal: ~30 minutes; I.V.: Immediate

Peak effect: Sublingual tablet: 5 minutes; Translingual spray: 4-10 minutes; Sustained release: 2.5-4 hours; Topical: ~60 minutes; Transdermal: 120 minutes; I.V.: Immediate

Duration: Sublingual tablet: At least 25 minutes; Translingual spray: Similar to sublingual tablet; Sustained release: 4-8 hours; Topical: 7 hours; Transdermal: 10-12 hours; I.V.: 3-5 minutes

Distribution: V_d: ~3 L/kg

Protein binding: 60%

Metabolism: Extensive first-pass effect

Half-life elimination: 1-4 minutes

Excretion: Urine (as inactive metabolites)

Dosage

Geriatric & Adult Note: Hemodynamic and antianginal tolerance often develop within 24-48 hours of continuous nitrate administration. Nitrate-free interval (10-12 hours/day) is recommended to avoid tolerance development; gradually decrease dose in patients receiving NTG for prolonged period to avoid withdrawal reaction.

Angina/coronary artery disease:

Oral: 2.5-6.5 mg 3-4 times/day (maximum dose: 26 mg 4 times/day)

I.V.: 5 mcg/minute, increase by 5 mcg/minute every 3-5 minutes to 20 mcg/minute. If no response at 20 mcg/minute, may increase by 10-20 mcg/minute every 3-5 minutes (generally accepted maximum dose: 400 mcg/minute)

Topical ointment: 1/2" upon rising and 1/2" 6 hours later; if necessary, the dose may be doubled to 1" and subsequently doubled again to 2" if response is inadequate. Doses of 1/2" to 2" were used in clinical trials. Recommended maximum: 2 doses/day; include a nitrate free-interval ~10-12 hours/day.

Topical patch, transdermal: 0.2-0.4 mg/hour initially and titrate to doses of 0.4-0.8 mg/hour. Tolerance is minimized by using a patch-on period of 12-14 hours/day and patch-off period of 10-12 hours/day.

Sublingual: 0.3-0.6 mg every 5 minutes for maximum of 3 doses in 15 minutes; may also use prophylactically 5-10 minutes prior to activities which may provoke an attack.

Translingual: 1-2 sprays onto or under tongue every 3-5 minutes for maximum of 3 doses in 15 minutes, may also be used prophylactically 5-10 minutes prior to activities which may provoke an angina attack

Esophageal spastic disorders (unlabeled use): Sublingual: 0.3-0.6 mg (Swamy, 1977)

Uterine relaxation (unlabeled use): I.V. bolus: 100-200 mcg; may repeat dose every 2 minutes as necessary (Axemo, 1998; Chandraharan, 2005)

Administration

I.V.: Prepare in glass bottles, EXCEL® or PAB® containers. Adsorption occurs to soft plastic (eg, PVC); use administration sets intended for nitroglycerin

Oral (sustained release capsule): Swallow whole. Do not chew, break, or crush. Take with a full glass of water.

Sublingual: Do not crush sublingual product (tablet). Place under tongue and allow to dissolve.

Topical ointment: Wash hands prior to and after use. Application site should be clean, dry, and hair-free. Apply to chest or back with the applicator or dose-measuring paper. Spread in a thin layer over a 2.25 x 3.5 inch area. Do not rub into skin. Tape applicator into place.

Topical patch, transdermal: Application site should be clean, dry and hair-free. Remove patch after 12-14 hours. Rotate patch sites.

Translingual spray: Do not shake container. Prior to initial use, the pump must be primed by spraying 5 times (Nitrolingual®) or 10 times (Nitromist®) into the air. Priming sprays should be directed away from patient and others. Release spray onto or under tongue. Close mouth after administration. Do not rinse the mouth for at least 5-10 minutes. The end of the pump should be covered by the fluid in the bottle. If pump is unused for 6 weeks, a single priming spray (Nitrolingual®) or 2 priming sprays (Nitromist®) should be completed.

Monitoring Parameters Blood pressure, heart rate

Test Interactions I.V. formulation: Due to propylene glycol content, triglyceride assays dependent on glycerol oxidase may be falsely elevated.

Pharmacotherapy Pearls I.V. preparations contain alcohol and/or propylene glycol; may need to use nitrate-free interval (10-12 hours/day) to avoid tolerance development. Tolerance may possibly be reversed with acetylcysteine; gradually decrease dose in patients receiving NTG for prolonged period to avoid withdrawal reaction.

Concomitant use of sildenafil (Viagra®) or other phosphodiesterase-5 enzyme inhibitors (PDE-5) may precipitate acute hypotension, myocardial infarction, or death. Nitrates used in right ventricular infarction may induce acute hypotension. Nitrate use in severe pericardial effusion may reduce cardiac filling pressure and precipitate cardiac tamponade. In the management of heart failure, the combination of isosorbide dinitrate and hydralazine confers beneficial effects on disease progression and cardiac outcomes.

Special Geriatric Considerations Caution should be used when using nitrate therapy in the elderly due to hypotension. Hypotension is enhanced in the elderly due to decreased baroreceptor response, decreased venous tone, and often hypovolemia (dehydration) or other hypotensive drugs.

Product Availability

Rectiv™: FDA approved June 2011; availability expected during the first quarter of 2012

Rectiv™ (nitroglycerin 0.4% ointment) is approved for the treatment of moderate-to-severe pain associated with chronic anal fissure.

◄ **Dosage Forms** Excipient information presented when available (limited, particularly for generics); consult specific product labeling. [DSC] = Discontinued product

Aerosol, translingual [spray]:

NitroMist®: 0.4 mg/spray (8.5 g) [230 metered sprays]

Capsule, extended release, oral: 2.5 mg, 6.5 mg, 9 mg

Nitro-Time®: 2.5 mg, 6.5 mg, 9 mg

Capsule, sustained release, oral: 2.5 mg [DSC], 6.5 mg [DSC], 9 mg [DSC]

Infusion, premixed in D_5W: 25 mg (250 mL) [100 mcg/mL]; 50 mg (250 mL, 500 mL) [100 mcg/mL]; 50 mg (250 mL, 500 mL) [200 mcg/mL]; 100 mg (250 mL) [400 mcg/mL]

Injection, solution: 5 mg/mL (10 mL)

Ointment, topical:

Nitro-Bid®: 2% (1 g, 30 g, 60 g) [~15 mg/inch]

Patch, transdermal: 0.1 mg/hr (30s); 0.2 mg/hr (30s); 0.4 mg/hr (30s); 0.6 mg/hr (30s)

Minitran™: 0.1 mg/hr (30s); 0.2 mg/hr (30s); 0.4 mg/hr (30s); 0.6 mg/hr (30s)

Nitro-Dur®: 0.1 mg/hr (30s); 0.2 mg/hr (30s); 0.3 mg/hr (30s); 0.4 mg/hr (30s); 0.6 mg/hr (30s); 0.8 mg/hr (30s)

Solution, translingual [spray]: 0.4 mg/spray (4.9 g, 12 g)

Nitrolingual®: 0.4 mg/spray (12 g) [contains ethanol 20%; 200 metered sprays]

Nitrolingual®: 0.4 mg/spray (4.9 g) [contains ethanol 20%; 60 metered sprays]

Tablet, sublingual:

Nitrostat®: 0.3 mg, 0.4 mg, 0.6 mg

Selected References

Braunwald E, Antman EM, Beasley JW, et al, "ACC/AHA 2002 Guideline Update for the Management of Patients With Unstable Angina and Non-ST-Segment Elevation Myocardial Infarction - Summary Article: A Report of the American College of Cardiology/American Heart Association Task Force on Practice Guidelines (Committee on the Management of Patients With Unstable Angina)," J Am Coll Cardiol, 2002, 40(7):1366-74. Available at: http://www.acc.org/clinical/guidelines/unstable/incorporated/index.htm. Accessed May 20, 2003.

Gibbons RJ, Abrams J, Chatterjee K, et al, "ACC/AHA 2002 Guideline Update for the Management of Patients With Chronic Stable Angina - Summary Article: A Report of the American College of Cardiology/American Heart Association Task Force on Practice Guidelines (Committee on the Management of Patients With Chronic Stable Angina)," J Am Coll Cardiol, 2003, 41(1):159-68. Available at: http://http://www.acc.org/clinical/guidelines/stable/stable_clean.pdf. Accessed May 5, 2004.

◆ **Nitroglycerol** see Nitroglycerin on page 1311

◆ **Nitrolingual®** see Nitroglycerin on page 1311

◆ **NitroMist®** see Nitroglycerin on page 1311

◆ **Nitropress®** see Nitroprusside on page 1314

Nitroprusside (nye troe PRUS ide)

Medication Safety Issues

Sound-alike/look-alike issues:

Nitroprusside may be confused with nitroglycerin

High alert medication:

The Institute for Safe Medication Practices (ISMP) includes this medication among its list of drugs which have a heightened risk of causing significant patient harm when used in error.

Brand Names: U.S. Nitropress®

Brand Names: Canada Nipride®

Index Terms Nitroprusside Sodium; Sodium Nitroferricyanide; Sodium Nitroprusside

Generic Availability (U.S.) Yes

Pharmacologic Category Vasodilator

Use Management of hypertensive crises; acute decompensated heart failure (HF); used for controlled hypotension to reduce bleeding during surgery

Contraindications Hypersensitivity to nitroprusside or any component of the formulation; treatment of compensatory hypertension (aortic coarctation, arteriovenous shunting); high output failure; congenital optic atrophy or tobacco amblyopia

Warnings/Precautions [U.S. Boxed Warning]: Continuous blood pressure monitoring is needed. Except when used briefly or at low (<2 mcg/kg/minute) infusion rates, nitroprusside gives rise to large cyanide quantities. Do not use the maximum dose for more than 10 minutes; if blood pressure not controlled then discontinue infusion. Monitor for cyanide toxicity via acid-base balance and venous oxygen concentration. Use with extreme caution in patients with elevated intracranial pressure (head trauma, cerebral hemorrhage), severe renal impairment, hepatic failure, hypothyroidism. Use the lowest end of the dosage range with renal impairment. Cyanide toxicity may occur in patients with decreased liver function. Thiocyanate toxicity occurs in patients with renal impairment or those on prolonged infusions. **[U.S. Boxed Warning]: Should not be administered by direct injection; must be further diluted with 5% dextrose in water.**

Adverse Reactions (Reflective of adult population; not specific for elderly) Frequency not defined.

Cardiovascular: Excessive hypotensive response, palpitation, substernal distress

Central nervous system: Disorientation, psychosis, headache, restlessness

Endocrine & metabolic: Thyroid suppression (due to thiocyanate)

Gastrointestinal: Nausea, vomiting

Neuromuscular & skeletal: Hyper-reflexia (thiocyanate toxicity), muscle spasm, weakness

Ocular: Miosis (thiocyanate toxicity)

Otic: Tinnitus (thiocyanate toxicity)

Respiratory: Hypoxia

Miscellaneous: Diaphoresis

Drug Interactions

Avoid Concomitant Use There are no known interactions where it is recommended to avoid concomitant use.

Increased Effect/Toxicity

Nitroprusside may increase the levels/effects of: Amifostine; Antihypertensives; Hypotensive Agents; RiTUXimab

The levels/effects of Nitroprusside may be increased by: Alfuzosin; Calcium Channel Blockers; Diazoxide; Herbs (Hypotensive Properties); MAO Inhibitors; Pentoxifylline; Phosphodiesterase 5 Inhibitors; Prostacyclin Analogues

Decreased Effect

The levels/effects of Nitroprusside may be decreased by: Herbs (Hypertensive Properties); Methylphenidate; Yohimbine

Stability

Nitroprusside sodium should be reconstituted freshly by diluting 50 mg in 250-1000 mL of D_5W.

Use only clear solutions; solutions of nitroprusside exhibit a color described as brownish, brown, brownish-pink, light orange, and straw. Solutions are highly sensitive to light. Exposure to light causes decomposition, resulting in a highly colored solution of orange, dark brown or blue. **A blue color indicates almost complete degradation and breakdown to cyanide.**

Solutions should be wrapped with aluminum foil or other opaque material to protect from light (do as soon as possible).

Stability of parenteral admixture at room temperature (25°C) and at refrigeration temperature (4°C) is 24 hours.

Mechanism of Action Causes peripheral vasodilation by direct action on venous and arteriolar smooth muscle, thus reducing peripheral resistance; will increase cardiac output by decreasing afterload; reduces aortal and left ventricular impedance

Pharmacodynamics/Kinetics

Onset of action: BP reduction <2 minutes

Duration: 1-10 minutes

Metabolism: Nitroprusside is converted to cyanide ions in the bloodstream; decomposes to prussic acid which in the presence of sulfur donor is converted to thiocyanate (hepatic and renal rhodanase systems)

Half-life elimination: Parent drug: <10 minutes; Thiocyanate: 2.7-7 days

Excretion: Urine (as thiocyanate)

Dosage

Geriatric & Adult Acute hypertension: I.V.: Initial: 0.3-0.5 mcg/kg/minute; increase in increments of 0.5 mcg/kg/minute, titrating to the desired hemodynamic effect or the appearance of headache or nausea; usual dose: 3 mcg/kg/minute; rarely need >4 mcg/kg/minute; maximum: 10 mcg/kg/minute. When administered in doses >3 mcg/kg/minute for >72 hours, thiocyanate levels should be closely monitored.

Renal Impairment Limit use; accumulation of thiocyanate may occur.

Hepatic Impairment Limit use; risk of cyanide toxicity.

Administration I.V. infusion only, not for direct injection

Monitoring Parameters Blood pressure, heart rate; monitor for cyanide and thiocyanate toxicity; monitor acid-base status as acidosis can be the earliest sign of cyanide toxicity; monitor thiocyanate levels if requiring prolonged infusion (>3 days) or dose >3 mcg/kg/minute or patient has renal dysfunction; monitor cyanide blood levels in patients with decreased hepatic function; cardiac monitor and blood pressure monitor required

Reference Range Serum thiocyanate levels are not helpful in detecting toxicity. A level may be confirmatory if a patient is exhibiting signs and symptoms of thiocyanate toxicity. Initial signs of toxicity (eg, tinnitus) may be observed at levels >35 mcg/mL (manufacturer suggests 60 mcg/mL), but serious toxicity typically may not occur with levels <100 mcg/mL.

◀ **Pharmacotherapy Pearls** Nitroprusside is converted to cyanide ions in the bloodstream; decomposes to prussic acid which in the presence of sulfur donor is converted to thiocyanate (liver and kidney rhodanase systems); thiocyanate is then renally eliminated

Special Geriatric Considerations Elderly patients may have an increased sensitivity to nitroprusside possibly due to a decreased baroreceptor reflex, altered sensitivity to vaso-dilating effects or a resistance of cardiac adrenergic receptors to stimulation by catechol-amines.

Dosage Forms Excipient information presented when available (limited, particularly for generics); consult specific product labeling.

Injection, solution, as sodium:
Nitropress®: 25 mg/mL (2 mL)

◆ **Nitroprusside Sodium** see Nitroprusside on page 1314
◆ **Nitrostat®** see Nitroglycerin on page 1311
◆ **Nitro-Time®** see Nitroglycerin on page 1311
◆ **4'-Nitro-3'-Trifluoromethylisobutyrantide** see Flutamide on page 766
◆ **Nix® Complete Lice Treatment System [OTC]** see Permethrin on page 1429
◆ **Nix® Creme Rinse [OTC]** see Permethrin on page 1429
◆ **Nix® Creme Rinse Lice Treatment [OTC]** see Permethrin on page 1429
◆ **Nix® Lice Control Spray [OTC]** see Permethrin on page 1429

Nizatidine (ni ZA ti deen)

Medication Safety Issues
Sound-alike/look-alike issues:
Axid® may be confused with Ansaid®
International issues:
Tazac [Australia] may be confused with Tazact brand name for piperacillin/tazobactam [India]; Tiazac brand name for diltiazem [U.S., Canada]
Brand Names: U.S. Axid®
Brand Names: Canada Apo-Nizatidine®; Axid®; Gen-Nizatidine; Novo-Nizatidine; Nu-Niza-tidine; PMS-Nizatidine
Generic Availability (U.S.) Yes
Pharmacologic Category Histamine H_2 Antagonist
Use Treatment and maintenance of duodenal ulcer; treatment of benign gastric ulcer; treatment of gastroesophageal reflux disease (GERD)
Unlabeled/Investigational Use Part of a multidrug regimen for *H. pylori* eradication to reduce the risk of duodenal ulcer recurrence
Contraindications Hypersensitivity to nizatidine or any component of the formulation; hyper-sensitivity to other H_2 antagonists (cross-sensitivity has been observed)
Warnings/Precautions Relief of symptoms does not preclude the presence of a gastric malignancy. Use with caution in patients with liver and renal impairment. Dosage modification required in patients with renal impairment
Adverse Reactions (Reflective of adult population; not specific for elderly)
>10%: Central nervous system: Headache (16%)
1% to 10%:
Central nervous system: Anxiety, dizziness, fever (reported in children), insomnia, irritability (reported in children), somnolence, nervousness
Dermatologic: Pruritus, rash
Gastrointestinal: Abdominal pain, anorexia, constipation, diarrhea, dry mouth, flatulence, heartburn, nausea, vomiting
Respiratory: Reported in children: Cough, nasal congestion, nasopharyngitis
Drug Interactions
Metabolism/Transport Effects Inhibits 3A4 (weak)
Avoid Concomitant Use
Avoid concomitant use of Nizatidine with any of the following: Delavirdine
Increased Effect/Toxicity
Nizatidine may increase the levels/effects of: Dexmethylphenidate; Methylphenidate; Saqui-navir; Varenicline
Decreased Effect
Nizatidine may decrease the levels/effects of: Atazanavir; Cefditoren; Cefpodoxime; Cefur-oxime; Dasatinib; Delavirdine; Erlotinib; Fosamprenavir; Gefitinib; Indinavir; Iron Salts; Itraconazole; Ketoconazole; Ketoconazole (Systemic); Mesalamine; Nelfinavir; Posacona-zole; Rilpivirine
Ethanol/Nutrition/Herb Interactions
Ethanol: Avoid ethanol (may cause gastric mucosal irritation).
Food: Administration with apple juice may decrease absorption.

Mechanism of Action Competitive inhibition of histamine at H_2-receptors of the gastric parietal cells resulting in reduced gastric acid secretion, gastric volume and hydrogen ion concentration reduced. In healthy volunteers, nizatidine suppresses gastric acid secretion induced by pentagastrin infusion or food.

Pharmacodynamics/Kinetics

Distribution: V_d: 0.8-1.5 L/kg

Protein binding: 35% to α_1-acid glycoprotein

Metabolism: Partially hepatic; forms metabolites

Bioavailability: >70%

Half-life elimination: 1-2 hours; prolonged with renal impairment

Time to peak, plasma: 0.5-3.0 hours

Excretion: Urine (90%; ~60% as unchanged drug); feces (<6%)

Dosage

Geriatric & Adult

Duodenal ulcer: Oral:

Treatment of active ulcer: 300 mg at bedtime or 150 mg twice daily

Maintenance of healed ulcer: 150 mg/day at bedtime

Gastric ulcer: Oral: 150 mg twice daily or 300 mg at bedtime

GERD: Oral: 150 mg twice daily

Eradication of *Helicobacter pylori* (unlabeled use): Oral: 150 mg twice daily; requires combination therapy

Renal Impairment

Active treatment:

Cl_{cr} 20-50 mL/minute: 150 mg/day

Cl_{cr} <20 mL/minute: 150 mg every other day

Maintenance treatment:

Cl_{cr} 20-50 mL/minute: 150 mg every other day

Cl_{cr} <20 mL/minute: 150 mg every 3 days

Monitoring Parameters Signs and symptoms of peptic ulcer disease, occult blood with GI bleeding, gastric pH where necessary; monitor renal function to correct dose; monitor for side effects

Test Interactions False-positive urine protein using Multistix®, gastric acid secretion test, skin tests allergen extracts, serum creatinine and serum transaminase concentrations, urine protein test

Pharmacotherapy Pearls Giving a dose at 6 PM may more effectively suppress nocturnal acid secretion than giving a dose at 10 PM.

Special Geriatric Considerations H_2 blockers are the preferred drugs for treating peptic ulcer disorder (PUD) in the elderly due to cost and ease of administration. These agents are no less or more effective than any other therapy. The preferred agents (due to side effects and drug interaction profile and pharmacokinetics) are ranitidine, famotidine, and nizatidine. Treatment for PUD in the elderly is recommended for 12 weeks since their lesions are larger, and therefore, take longer to heal. Always adjust dose based upon creatinine clearance.

Dosage Forms Excipient information presented when available (limited, particularly for generics); consult specific product labeling.

Capsule, oral: 150 mg, 300 mg

Solution, oral: 15 mg/mL (473 mL)

Axid®: 15 mg/mL (480 mL) [bubblegum flavor]

◆ **Nizoral®** *see* Ketoconazole (Topical) *on page 1001*

◆ **Nizoral® A-D [OTC]** *see* Ketoconazole (Topical) *on page 1001*

◆ **N-methylnaltrexone Bromide** *see* Methylnaltrexone *on page 1178*

◆ **NN2211** *see* Liraglutide *on page 1077*

◆ **Nolvadex** *see* Tamoxifen *on page 1731*

◆ **Norco®** *see* Hydrocodone and Acetaminophen *on page 880*

◆ **Nordeoxyguanosine** *see* Ganciclovir (Ophthalmic) *on page 811*

◆ **Nordeoxyguanosine** *see* Ganciclovir (Systemic) *on page 809*

◆ **Norflex™** *see* Orphenadrine *on page 1351*

Norfloxacin (nor FLOKS a sin)

Medication Safety Issues

Sound-alike/look-alike issues:

Norfloxacin may be confused with Norflex™, Noroxin®

Noroxin® may be confused with Neurontin®, Norflex™, norfloxacin

Brand Names: U.S. Noroxin®

Brand Names: Canada Apo-Norflox®; CO Norfloxacin; Norfloxacine®; Novo-Norfloxacin; PMS-Norfloxacin; Riva-Norfloxacin

◀ **Generic Availability (U.S.)** No

Pharmacologic Category Antibiotic, Quinolone

Use Uncomplicated and complicated urinary tract infections caused by susceptible gram-negative and gram-positive bacteria; sexually-transmitted disease (eg, uncomplicated urethral and cervical gonorrhea) caused by *N. gonorrhoeae*; prostatitis due to *E. coli*

> **Note:** As of April 2007, the CDC no longer recommends the use of fluoroquinolones for the treatment of gonococcal disease.

Medication Guide Available Yes

Contraindications Hypersensitivity to norfloxacin, quinolones, or any component of the formulation; history of tendonitis or tendon rupture associated with quinolone use

Warnings/Precautions [U.S. Boxed Warning]: There have been reports of tendon inflammation and/or rupture with quinolone antibiotics; risk may be increased with concurrent corticosteroids, organ transplant recipients, and in patients >60 years of age. Rupture of the Achilles tendon sometimes requiring surgical repair has been reported most frequently; but other tendon sites (eg, rotator cuff, biceps) have also been reported. Strenuous physical activity, rheumatoid arthritis, and renal impairment may be an independent risk factor for tendonitis. Discontinue at first sign of tendon inflammation or pain. May occur even after discontinuation of therapy. Use with caution in patients with rheumatoid arthritis; may increase risk of tendon rupture. Use with caution in patients with known or suspected CNS disorders. CNS stimulation may occur which may lead to tremor, restlessness, confusion, and very rarely to hallucinations or convulsive seizures. Potential for seizures, although very rare, may be increased with concomitant NSAID therapy. Use with caution in individuals at risk of seizures. Use may be associated (rarely) with prolongation of QT_c interval; avoid concurrent use with class Ia and class III antiarrhythmics; use caution with other drugs may cause QT_c prolongation.

Fluoroquinolones have been associated with the development of serious, and sometimes fatal, hypoglycemia, most often in elderly diabetics, but also in patients without diabetes. This occurred most frequently with gatifloxacin (no longer available systemically) but may occur at a lower frequency with other quinolones.

Severe hypersensitivity reactions, including anaphylaxis, have occurred with quinolone therapy. Reactions may present as typical allergic symptoms after a single dose, or may manifest as severe idiosyncratic dermatologic, vascular, pulmonary, renal, hepatic, and/or hematologic events, usually after multiple doses. Prompt discontinuation of drug should occur if skin rash or other symptoms arise. Prolonged use may result in fungal or bacterial superinfection, including *C. difficile*-associated diarrhea (CDAD) and pseudomembranous colitis; CDAD has been observed >2 months postantibiotic treatment. Avoid excessive sunlight and take precautions to limit exposure (eg, loose fitting clothing, sunscreen); may cause moderate-to-severe phototoxicity reactions. Discontinue use if photosensitivity occurs. May be associated with the development of peripheral neuropathy and/or paresthesias; discontinue in patients who develop symptoms consistent with neuropathy. **[U.S. Boxed Warning]: Quinolones may exacerbate myasthenia gravis; avoid use (rare, potentially life-threatening weakness of respiratory muscles may occur).** Use caution with renal impairment. Since norfloxacin is ineffective in the treatment of syphilis and may mask symptoms, all patients should be tested for syphilis at the time of gonorrheal diagnosis and 3 months later. Hemolytic reactions may (rarely) occur with quinolone use in patients with latent or actual G6PD deficiency.

Adverse Reactions (Reflective of adult population; not specific for elderly)

>1% to 10%:
  Central nervous system: Headache (2% to 3%), dizziness (2% to 3%)
  Gastrointestinal: Nausea (3% to 4%), abdominal cramping (2%)
  Hematologic: Eosinophilia (1% to 2%)
  Hepatic: Liver enzymes increased (1% to 2%)

≥0.3% to 1%:
  Central nervous system: Fever, somnolence
  Dermatologic: Hyperhidrosis, pruritus, rash
  Gastrointestinal: Abdominal pain, anorectal pain, anorexia, constipation, diarrhea, dyspepsia, flatulence, loose stools, vomiting, xerostomia
  Hematologic: Hematocrit/hemoglobin decreased (1%), leukopenia (1%), thrombocytopenia (1%)
  Neuromuscular & skeletal: Back pain, paresthesia, weakness
  Renal: Proteinuria (1%)

Drug Interactions

Metabolism/Transport Effects Inhibits CYP1A2 (strong), 3A4 (moderate)

Avoid Concomitant Use

Avoid concomitant use of Norfloxacin with any of the following: Artemether; BCG; Dronedarone; Lumefantrine; Nilotinib; Nitrofurantoin; Pimozide; QUEtiapine; QuiNINE; Tetrabenazine; Thioridazine; Tolvaptan; Toremifene; Vandetanib; Vemurafenib; Ziprasidone

Increased Effect/Toxicity

Norfloxacin may increase the levels/effects of: Bendamustine; Caffeine; Colchicine; Corticosteroids (Systemic); CycloSPORINE; CycloSPORINE (Systemic); CYP1A2 Substrates; CYP3A4 Substrates; Dronedarone; Eplerenone; Everolimus; FentaNYL; Lurasidone; Pimecrolimus; Pimozide; Porfimer; QTc-Prolonging Agents; QuiNINE; Salmeterol; Saxagliptin; Sulfonylureas; Tetrabenazine; Theophylline Derivatives; Thioridazine; Tolvaptan; Toremifene; Vandetanib; Vemurafenib; Vilazodone; Vitamin K Antagonists; Ziprasidone

The levels/effects of Norfloxacin may be increased by: Alfuzosin; Artemether; Chloroquine; Ciprofloxacin; Ciprofloxacin (Systemic); Gadobutrol; Insulin; Lumefantrine; Nilotinib; Nonsteroidal Anti-Inflammatory Agents; Probenecid; QUEtiapine; QuiNINE

Decreased Effect

Norfloxacin may decrease the levels/effects of: BCG; Mycophenolate; Sulfonylureas; Typhoid Vaccine

The levels/effects of Norfloxacin may be decreased by: Antacids; Calcium Salts; Didanosine; Iron Salts; Lanthanum; Magnesium Salts; Nitrofurantoin; Quinapril; Sevelamer; Sucralfate; Zinc Salts

Ethanol/Nutrition/Herb Interactions

Food: Norfloxacin average peak serum concentrations may be decreased if taken with dairy products. Use caution with caffeine-containing beverages/foods; quinolones may increase blood levels of caffeine.

Herb/Nutraceutical: Avoid dong quai, St John's wort (may also cause photosensitization); avoid administration within 2 hours of multivitamins or other supplements containing iron, zinc, magnesium, or aluminum.

Stability Store at 25°C (77°F). Keep container tightly closed.

Mechanism of Action Norfloxacin is a DNA gyrase inhibitor. DNA gyrase is an essential bacterial enzyme that maintains the superhelical structure of DNA. DNA gyrase is required for DNA replication and transcription, DNA repair, recombination, and transposition; bactericidal

Pharmacodynamics/Kinetics

Absorption: Oral: Rapid, up to 40%

Protein binding: 10% to 15%

Metabolism: Hepatic

Half-life elimination: 3-4 hours; Renal impairment (Cl$_{cr}$ ≤30 mL/minute): 6.5 hours; Elderly: 4 hours

Time to peak, serum: 1-2 hours

Excretion: Urine (26% to 32% as unchanged drug; 5% to 8% as metabolites); feces (39%)

Dosage

Geriatric & Adult

Dysenteric enterocolitis *(Shigella* unlabeled use): Oral: 400 mg twice daily for 5 days

Prostatitis: Oral: 400 mg every 12 hours for 4-6 weeks

Traveler's diarrhea (unlabeled use): Oral: 400 mg twice daily for 3 days, single dose may also be effective

Uncomplicated gonorrhea: Oral: 800 mg as a single dose. **Note:** As of April 2007, the CDC no longer recommends the use of fluoroquinolones for the treatment of uncomplicated gonococcal disease.

Urinary tract infections: Oral:

Uncomplicated due to *E. coli, K. pneumoniae, P. mirabilis*: 400 mg twice daily for 3 days

Uncomplicated due to other organisms: 400 mg twice daily for 7-10 days

Complicated: 400 mg twice daily for 10-21 days

Renal Impairment Cl$_{cr}$ ≤30 mL/minute/1.73 m^2: Administer 400 mg every 24 hours

Administration Hold antacids, sucralfate, or multivitamins/supplements containing iron, zinc, magnesium, or aluminum for 2 hours after giving norfloxacin; do not administer together. Best taken on an empty stomach with water (1 hour before or 2 hours after meals, milk, or other dairy products).

Special Geriatric Considerations See Warnings/Precautions regarding tendon rupture in patients >60 years of age. Adjust dose for renal function.

Dosage Forms Excipient information presented when available (limited, particularly for generics); consult specific product labeling.

Tablet, oral:

Noroxin®: 400 mg

◀ **Selected References**

Khaliq Y and Zhanel GG, "Fluoroquinolone-Associated Tendinopathy: A Critical Review of the Literature," *Clin Infect Dis*, 2003, 36(11):1404-10.

Nilsson-Ehle I and Ljungberg B, "Quinolone Disposition in the Elderly: Practical Implications," *Drugs Aging*, 1991, 1 (4):279-88.

Nortriptyline (nor TRIP ti leen)

Related Information
Antidepressant Agents *on page 1991*

Medication Safety Issues
Sound-alike/look-alike issues:
Aventyl® HCl may be confused with Bentyl®
Nortriptyline may be confused with amitriptyline, desipramine, Norpramin®
Pamelor® may be confused with Demerol®, Dymelor®, Panlor®, Tambocor™

Brand Names: U.S. Pamelor®

Brand Names: Canada Alti-Nortriptyline; Apo-Nortriptyline®; Aventyl®; Gen-Nortriptyline; Norventyl; Novo-Nortriptyline; Nu-Nortriptyline; PMS-Nortriptyline

Index Terms Nortriptyline Hydrochloride

Generic Availability (U.S.) Yes

Pharmacologic Category Antidepressant, Tricyclic (Secondary Amine)

Use Treatment of symptoms of depression

Unlabeled/Investigational Use Treatment of chronic pain, anxiety disorders, enuresis, attention-deficit/hyperactivity disorder (ADHD); adjunctive therapy for smoking cessation

Medication Guide Available Yes

Contraindications Hypersensitivity to nortriptyline and similar chemical class, or any component of the formulation; use of MAO inhibitors within 14 days; use in a patient during the acute recovery phase of MI

Warnings/Precautions [U.S. Boxed Warning]: Antidepressants increase the risk of suicidal thinking and behavior in children, adolescents, and young adults (18-24 years of age) with major depressive disorder (MDD) and other psychiatric disorders; consider risk prior to prescribing. Short-term studies did not show an increased risk in patients >24 years of age and showed a decreased risk in patients ≥65 years. Closely monitor for clinical worsening, suicidality, or unusual changes in behavior; the patient's family or caregiver should be instructed to closely observe the patient and communicate condition with healthcare provider. A medication guide should be dispensed with each prescription. **Nortriptyline is not FDA approved for use in children.**

The possibility of a suicide attempt is inherent in major depression and may persist until remission occurs. Monitor for worsening of depression or suicidality, especially during initiation of therapy (generally first 1-2 months) or with dose increases or decreases. Use caution in high-risk patients. Worsening depression and severe abrupt suicidality that are not part of the presenting symptoms may require discontinuation or modification of drug therapy. The patient's family or caregiver should be alerted to monitor patients for the emergence of suicidality and associated behaviors (such as agitation, irritability, hostility, impulsivity, and hypomania) and call healthcare provider.

May worsen psychosis in some patients or precipitate a shift to mania or hypomania in patients with bipolar disorder. Patients presenting with depressive symptoms should be screened for bipolar disorder. Monotherapy in patients with bipolar disorder should be avoided. **Nortriptyline is not FDA approved for the treatment of bipolar depression.**

TCAs may rarely cause bone marrow suppression; monitor for any signs of infection and obtain CBC if symptoms (eg, fever, sore throat) evident. The risk of sedation and orthostatic effects are low relative to other antidepressants. However, nortriptyline may result in impaired performance of tasks requiring alertness (eg, operating machinery or driving). Sedative effects may be additive with other CNS depressants and/or ethanol. The degree of anticholinergic blockade produced by this agent is moderate relative to other cyclic antidepressants, however, caution should still be used in patients with urinary retention, benign prostatic hyperplasia, narrow-angle glaucoma, xerostomia, visual problems, constipation, or history of bowel obstruction. May cause orthostatic hypotension (risk is low relative to other antidepressants) or conduction disturbances. Use with caution in patients with a history of cardiovascular disease (including previous MI, stroke, tachycardia, or conduction abnormalities). The risk conduction abnormalities with this agent is moderate relative to other antidepressants.

Consider discontinuing, when possible, prior to elective surgery. Therapy should not be abruptly discontinued in patients receiving high doses for prolonged periods. May alter glucose regulation - use caution in patients with diabetes. Use caution in patients with a previous seizure disorder or condition predisposing to seizures such as brain damage, alcoholism, or concurrent therapy with other drugs which lower the seizure threshold. May increase the risks associated with electroconvulsive therapy. Use with caution in hyperthyroid patients or those receiving thyroid supplementation. Use with caution in patients with hepatic or renal dysfunction and in elderly patients.

Adverse Reactions (Reflective of adult population; not specific for elderly) Frequency not defined.

Cardiovascular: Arrhythmia, flushing, heart block, hypertension, MI, palpitation, postural hypotension, tachycardia

Central nervous system: Agitation, anxiety, ataxia, confusion, delirium, delusions, disorientation, dizziness, drowsiness, EEG changes, exacerbation of psychosis, extrapyramidal symptoms, fatigue, hallucinations, headache, hypomania, incoordination, insomnia, nightmares, panic, restlessness, seizure

Dermatologic: Alopecia, itching, petechiae, photosensitivity, rash, urticaria

Endocrine & metabolic: Blood sugar increased/decreased, breast enlargement, galactorrhea, gynecomastia, libido increased/decreased, sexual dysfunction, SIADH

Gastrointestinal: Abdominal cramps, anorexia, black tongue, constipation, diarrhea, epigastric distress, nausea, paralytic ileus, stomatitis, taste disturbance, vomiting, weight gain/loss, xerostomia

Genitourinary: Delayed micturition, impotence, nocturia, polyuria, testicular edema, urinary retention

Hematologic: Agranulocytosis (rare), eosinophilia, purpura, thrombocytopenia

Hepatic: Cholestatic jaundice, transaminases increased

Neuromuscular & skeletal: Numbness, paresthesia, peripheral neuropathy, tingling, tremor, weakness

Ocular: Blurred vision, disturbances in accommodation, eye pain, mydriasis

Otic: Tinnitus

Miscellaneous: Allergic reactions (eg, general edema or of the face/tongue), diaphoresis (excessive), withdrawal symptoms

Drug Interactions

Metabolism/Transport Effects Substrate of CYP1A2 (minor), 2C19 (minor), 2D6 (major), 3A4 (minor); **Inhibits** CYP2D6 (weak), 2E1 (weak)

Avoid Concomitant Use

Avoid concomitant use of Nortriptyline with any of the following: Artemether; Dronedarone; Iobenguane I 123; Lumefantrine; MAO Inhibitors; Methylene Blue; Nilotinib; Pimozide; QUEtiapine; QuiNINE; Sibutramine; Tetrabenazine; Thioridazine; Toremifene; Vandetanib; Vemurafenib; Ziprasidone

Increased Effect/Toxicity

Nortriptyline may increase the levels/effects of: Alpha-/Beta-Agonists (Direct-Acting); Alpha1-Agonists; Amphetamines; Anticholinergics; Beta2-Agonists; Desmopressin; Dronedarone; Methylene Blue; Pimozide; QTc-Prolonging Agents; QuiNIDine; QuiNINE; Serotonin Modulators; Sodium Phosphates; Sulfonylureas; Tetrabenazine; Thioridazine; Toremifene; TraMADol; Vandetanib; Vemurafenib; Vitamin K Antagonists; Yohimbine; Ziprasidone

The levels/effects of Nortriptyline may be increased by: Abiraterone Acetate; Alfuzosin; Altretamine; Artemether; BuPROPion; Chloroquine; Cimetidine; Cinacalcet; Ciprofloxacin; Ciprofloxacin (Systemic); Conivaptan; CYP2D6 Inhibitors (Moderate); CYP2D6 Inhibitors (Strong); Dexmethylphenidate; Divalproex; DULoxetine; Gadobutrol; Lithium; Lumefantrine; MAO Inhibitors; Methylphenidate; Metoclopramide; Nilotinib; Pramlintide; Propoxyphene; Protease Inhibitors; QUEtiapine; QuiNIDine; QuiNINE; Selective Serotonin Reuptake Inhibitors; Sibutramine; Terbinafine; Terbinafine (Systemic); Valproic Acid

Decreased Effect

Nortriptyline may decrease the levels/effects of: Acetylcholinesterase Inhibitors (Central); Alpha2-Agonists; Iobenguane I 123

The levels/effects of Nortriptyline may be decreased by: Acetylcholinesterase Inhibitors (Central); Barbiturates; CarBAMazepine; Cyproterone; Peginterferon Alfa-2b; St Johns Wort; Tocilizumab

◀ **Ethanol/Nutrition/Herb Interactions**

Ethanol: May increase CNS depression; monitor for increased effects with coadministration. Caution patients about effects.

Herb/Nutraceutical: Avoid valerian, St John's wort, SAMe, kava kava (may increase risk of serotonin syndrome and/or excessive sedation).

Stability Store at 20°C to 25°C (68°F to 77°F). Protect from light.

Mechanism of Action Traditionally believed to increase the synaptic concentration of serotonin and/or norepinephrine in the central nervous system by inhibition of their reuptake by the presynaptic neuronal membrane. However, additional receptor effects have been found including desensitization of adenyl cyclase, down regulation of beta-adrenergic receptors, and down regulation of serotonin receptors.

Pharmacodynamics/Kinetics

Onset of action: Therapeutic: 1-3 weeks

Distribution: V_d: 21 L/kg

Protein binding: 93% to 95%

Metabolism: Primarily hepatic; extensive first-pass effect

Half-life elimination: 28-31 hours

Geriatrics: Single-dose pharmacokinetic studies have found the mean half-life to range from 37-45 hours in older subjects; the mean metabolic clearance was significantly lower compared to younger subjects, 20 vs 54 L/hour

Time to peak, serum: 7-8.5 hours

Excretion: Urine (as metabolites and small amounts of unchanged drug); feces (small amounts)

Dosage

Geriatric Initial: 30-50 mg/day, given as a single daily dose or in divided doses. **Note:** Nortriptyline is one of the best tolerated TCAs in the elderly

Adult

Depression: Oral: 25 mg 3-4 times/day up to 150 mg/day; doses may be given once daily.

Chronic urticaria, angioedema, nocturnal pruritus (unlabeled use): Oral: 75 mg/day

Myofascial pain, neuralgia, burning mouth syndrome (unlabeled uses): Initial: 10-25 mg at bedtime; dosage may be increased by 25 mg/day weekly, if tolerated; usual maintenance dose: 75 mg as a single bedtime dose or 2 divided doses

Smoking cessation (unlabeled use; Fiore, 2008): Oral: Initial: 25 mg/day; titrate dose to 75-100 mg/day 10-28 days prior to selected "quit" date; continue therapy for ≥12 weeks after "quit" day

Hepatic Impairment Lower doses and slower titration are recommended dependent on individualization of dosage.

Monitoring Parameters Blood pressure and pulse rate (ECG, cardiac monitoring) prior to and during initial therapy in older adults; weight; blood levels are useful for therapeutic monitoring; suicide ideation (especially at the beginning of therapy or when doses are increased or decreased)

Reference Range

Plasma levels do not always correlate with clinical effectiveness

Therapeutic: 50-150 ng/mL (SI: 190-570 nmol/L)

Toxic: >500 ng/mL (SI: >1900 nmol/L)

Pharmacotherapy Pearls The maximum antidepressant effect of nortriptyline may not be seen for ≥2 weeks after initiation of therapy.

Special Geriatric Considerations Since nortriptyline is the least likely of the tricyclic antidepressants (TCAs) to cause orthostatic hypotension and one of the least anticholinergic and sedating TCAs, it is a preferred agent when a TCA is indicated.

Dosage Forms Excipient information presented when available (limited, particularly for generics); consult specific product labeling.

Capsule, oral: 10 mg, 25 mg, 50 mg, 75 mg

Pamelor®: 10 mg, 25 mg

Pamelor®: 50 mg [contains sodium bisulfite (may have trace amounts)]

Pamelor®: 75 mg

Solution, oral: 10 mg/5 mL (473 mL, 480 mL)

Pamelor®: 10 mg/5 mL (480 mL) [contains benzoic acid, ethanol 4%]

Selected References

Dawling S, Crome P, and Braithwaite R, "Pharmacokinetics of Single Oral Doses of Nortriptyline in Depressed Elderly Hospital Patients and Young Healthy Volunteers," *Clin Pharmacokinet*, 1980, 5(4):394-401.

Schneider LS, Cooper TB, Staples FR, et al, "Prediction of Individual Dosage of Nortriptyline in Depressed Elderly Outpatients," *J Clin Psychopharmacol*, 1987, 7(5):311-4.

Turbott J, Norman TR, Burrows GD, et al, "Pharmacokinetics of Nortriptyline in Elderly Volunteers," *Commun Psychopharmacol*, 1980, 4(3):225-31.

◆ **Nortriptyline Hydrochloride** *see* Nortriptyline *on page 1320*

◆ **Norvasc®** *see* AmLODIPine *on page 106*

◆ **Nostrilla® [OTC]** *see* Oxymetazoline (Nasal) *on page 1374*

Nystatin (Oral) (nye STAT in)

Medication Safety Issues
Sound-alike/look-alike issues:
Nystatin may be confused with HMG-CoA reductase inhibitors (also known as "statins"; eg, atorvastatin, fluvastatin, lovastatin, pitavastatin, pravastatin, rosuvastatin, simvastatin), Nitrostat®

Brand Names: U.S. Nystat-Rx [DSC]

Brand Names: Canada PMS-Nystatin

Generic Availability (U.S.) Yes

Pharmacologic Category Antifungal Agent, Oral Nonabsorbed

Use Treatment of susceptible cutaneous, mucocutaneous, and oral cavity fungal infections normally caused by the *Candida* species

Contraindications Hypersensitivity to nystatin or any component of the formulation

Adverse Reactions (Reflective of adult population; not specific for elderly)
1% to 10%: Gastrointestinal: Diarrhea, nausea, stomach pain, vomiting

Drug Interactions
Avoid Concomitant Use There are no known interactions where it is recommended to avoid concomitant use.

Increased Effect/Toxicity There are no known significant interactions involving an increase in effect.

Decreased Effect
Nystatin (Oral) may decrease the levels/effects of: Saccharomyces boulardii

Stability
Tablet and suspension: Store at controlled room temperature of 15°C to 25°C (59°F to 77°F).
Powder for suspension: Store under refrigeration at 2°C to 8°C (36°F to 46°F).

Mechanism of Action Binds to sterols in fungal cell membrane, changing the cell wall permeability allowing for leakage of cellular contents

Pharmacodynamics/Kinetics
Onset of action: Symptomatic relief from candidiasis: 24-72 hours
Absorption: Poorly absorbed
Excretion: Feces (as unchanged drug)

◀ **Dosage**

Geriatric & Adult

Oral candidiasis: Suspension (swish and swallow): 400,000-600,000 units 4 times/day; swish in the mouth and retain for as long as possible (several minutes) before swallowing

Intestinal infections: Oral tablets: 500,000-1,000,000 units every 8 hours

Note: Powder for compounding: 1/8 teaspoon (500,000 units) to equal approximately 1/2 cup of water; give 4 times/day

Administration Suspension: Shake well before using. Should be swished about the mouth and retained in the mouth for as long as possible (several minutes) before swallowing.

Special Geriatric Considerations For oral infections, patients who wear dentures must have them removed and cleaned in order to eliminate source of reinfection.

Dosage Forms Excipient information presented when available (limited, particularly for generics); consult specific product labeling. [DSC] = Discontinued product

Powder, for prescription compounding: 50 million units (10 g); 150 million units (30 g); 500 million units (100 g)

Nystat-Rx: 50 million units (10 g [DSC]); 150 million units (30 g [DSC]); 1 billion units (190 g [DSC]); 2 billion units (350 g [DSC])

Suspension, oral: 100,000 units/mL (5 mL, 60 mL, 473 mL, 480 mL [DSC])

Tablet, oral: 500,000 units

Nystatin (Topical) (nye STAT in)

Medication Safety Issues

Sound-alike/look-alike issues:

Nystatin may be confused with HMG-CoA reductase inhibitors (also known as "statins"; eg, atorvastatin, fluvastatin, lovastatin, pitavastatin, pravastatin, rosuvastatin, simvastatin), Nitrostat®

Brand Names: U.S. Nyamyc®; Nystop®; Pedi-Dri®; Pediaderm™ AF

Brand Names: Canada Candistatin®; Nyaderm

Generic Availability (U.S.) Yes

Pharmacologic Category Antifungal Agent, Topical; Antifungal Agent, Vaginal

Use Treatment of susceptible cutaneous and mucocutaneous fungal infections normally caused by the *Candida* species

Dosage

Geriatric & Adult

Mucocutaneous infections: Topical: Apply 2-3 times/day to affected areas; very moist topical lesions are treated best with powder.

Vaginal infections: Vaginal tablets: Insert 1 tablet/day at bedtime for 2 weeks. (May also be given orally.)

Dosage Forms Excipient information presented when available (limited, particularly for generics); consult specific product labeling.

Cream, topical: 100,000 units/g (15 g, 30 g)

Cream, topical [kit]:

Pediaderm™ AF: 100,000 units/g (30 g) [packaged with protective emollient]

Ointment, topical: 100,000 units/g (15 g, 30 g)

Powder, topical: 100,000 units/g (15 g, 30 g, 60 g)

Nyamyc®: 100,000 units/g (15 g, 30 g, 60 g) [contains talc]

Nystop®: 100,000 units/g (15 g, 30 g, 60 g) [contains talc]

Pedi-Dri®: 100,000 units/g (56.7 g) [contains talc]

Tablet, vaginal: 100,000 units

Nystatin and Triamcinolone (nye STAT in & trye am SIN oh lone)

Related Information

Nystatin (Topical) *on page 1324*

Triamcinolone (Topical) *on page 1857*

Index Terms Triamcinolone and Nystatin

Generic Availability (U.S.) Yes

Pharmacologic Category Antifungal Agent, Topical; Corticosteroid, Topical

Use Treatment of cutaneous candidiasis

Dosage

Geriatric & Adult Cutaneous *Candida*: Topical: Apply sparingly 2-4 times/day

Special Geriatric Considerations No specific dose adjustment or use consideration necessary in the elderly; for oral infections, patients who wear dentures must have them removed and cleaned in order to eliminate source of reinfection.

Dosage Forms Excipient information presented when available (limited, particularly for generics); consult specific product labeling.
Cream: Nystatin 100,000 units and triamcinolone acetonide 0.1% (15 g, 30 g, 60 g)
Ointment: Nystatin 100,000 units and triamcinolone acetonide 0.1% (15 g, 30 g, 60 g)

Ofloxacin (Systemic) (oh FLOKS a sin)

Brand Names: Canada Apo-Oflox®; Novo-Ofloxacin
Generic Availability (U.S.) Yes
Pharmacologic Category Antibiotic, Quinolone
Use Quinolone antibiotic for the treatment of acute exacerbations of chronic bronchitis, community-acquired pneumonia, skin and skin structure infections (uncomplicated), urethral and cervical gonorrhea (acute, uncomplicated), urethritis and cervicitis (nongonococcal), mixed infections of the urethra and cervix, pelvic inflammatory disease (acute), cystitis (uncomplicated), urinary tract infections (complicated), prostatitis
Note: As of April 2007, the CDC no longer recommends the use of fluoroquinolones for the treatment of gonococcal disease.
Unlabeled/Investigational Use Epididymitis (nongonococcal), leprosy, Traveler's diarrhea
Medication Guide Available Yes
Contraindications Hypersensitivity to ofloxacin or other members of the quinolone group, such as oxolinic acid, cinoxacin, norfloxacin, and ciprofloxacin; hypersensitivity to any component of the formulation
Warnings/Precautions [U.S. Boxed Warning]: There have been reports of tendon inflammation and/or rupture with quinolone antibiotics; risk may be increased with concurrent corticosteroids, organ transplant recipients, and in patients >60 years of age. Rupture of the Achilles tendon sometimes requiring surgical repair has been reported most frequently; but other tendon sites (eg, rotator cuff, biceps) have also been reported. Strenuous physical activity, rheumatoid arthritis, and renal impairment may be an independent risk factor for tendonitis. Discontinue at first sign of tendon inflammation or pain. May occur even after discontinuation of therapy. Use with caution in patients with rheumatoid arthritis; may increase risk of tendon rupture. Use with caution in patients with epilepsy or other CNS diseases which could predispose seizures; potential for seizures, although very rare, may be increased with concomitant NSAID therapy. Tremor, restlessness, confusion, and very rarely hallucinations or seizures may occur; use with caution in patients with known or suspected CNS disorder. Discontinue in patients who experience significant CNS adverse effects (eg, dizziness, hallucinations, suicidal ideations or actions). Use with caution in patients with renal or hepatic impairment. Peripheral neuropathies have been linked to ofloxacin use; discontinue if numbness, tingling, or weakness develops.

Fluoroquinolones have been associated with the development of serious, and sometimes fatal, hypoglycemia, most often in elderly diabetics, but also in patients without diabetes. This occurred most frequently with gatifloxacin (no longer available systemically) but may occur at a lower frequency with other quinolones.

Rare cases of torsade de pointes have been reported in patients receiving ofloxacin and other quinolones. Risk may be minimized by avoiding use in patients with known prolongation of the QT interval, bradycardia, hypokalemia, hypomagnesemia, cardiomyopathy, or in those receiving concurrent therapy with Class Ia or Class III antiarrhythmics.

Severe hypersensitivity reactions, including anaphylaxis, have occurred with quinolone therapy. Reactions may present as typical allergic symptoms after a single dose, or may manifest as severe idiosyncratic dermatologic, vascular, pulmonary, renal, hepatic, and/or hematologic events, usually after multiple doses. Prompt discontinuation of drug should occur if skin rash or other symptoms arise. Prolonged use may result in fungal or bacterial superinfection, including *C. difficile*-associated diarrhea (CDAD) and pseudomembranous colitis; CDAD has been observed >2 months postantibiotic treatment. **[U.S. Boxed Warning]: Quinolones may exacerbate myasthenia gravis; avoid use (rare, potentially life-threatening weakness of respiratory muscles may occur).** Avoid excessive sunlight and take precautions to limit exposure (eg, loose fitting clothing, sunscreen); may cause moderate-to-severe phototoxicity reactions. Discontinue use if photosensitivity occurs. Since ofloxacin is ineffective in the treatment of syphilis and may mask symptoms, all patients should be tested for syphilis at the time of gonorrheal diagnosis and 3 months later. Hemolytic reactions may (rarely) occur with quinolone use in patients with latent or actual G6PD deficiency.

Adverse Reactions (Reflective of adult population; not specific for elderly)
1% to 10%:
Cardiovascular: Chest pain (1% to 3%)
Central nervous system: Headache (1% to 9%), insomnia (3% to 7%), dizziness (1% to 5%), fatigue (1% to 3%), somnolence (1% to 3%), sleep disorders (1% to 3%), nervousness (1% to 3%), pyrexia (1% to 3%)
Dermatologic: Rash/pruritus (1% to 3%)
Gastrointestinal: Diarrhea (1% to 4%), vomiting (1% to 4%), GI distress (1% to 3%), abdominal cramps (1% to 3%), flatulence (1% to 3%), abnormal taste (1% to 3%), xerostomia (1% to 3%), appetite decreased (1% to 3%), nausea (3% to 10%), constipation (1% to 3%)
Genitourinary: Vaginitis (1% to 5%), external genital pruritus in women (1% to 3%)
Ocular: Visual disturbances (1% to 3%)
Respiratory: Pharyngitis (1% to 3%)
Miscellaneous: Trunk pain

Drug Interactions
  Metabolism/Transport Effects Inhibits CYP1A2 (strong)
  Avoid Concomitant Use
    Avoid concomitant use of Ofloxacin (Systemic) with any of the following: BCG
  Increased Effect/Toxicity
    Ofloxacin (Systemic) may increase the levels/effects of: Bendamustine; Corticosteroids (Systemic); CYP1A2 Substrates; Porfimer; Sulfonylureas; Theophylline Derivatives; Vitamin K Antagonists

    The levels/effects of Ofloxacin (Systemic) may be increased by: Insulin; Nonsteroidal Anti-Inflammatory Agents; Probenecid
  Decreased Effect
    Ofloxacin (Systemic) may decrease the levels/effects of: BCG; Mycophenolate; Sulfonylureas; Typhoid Vaccine

    The levels/effects of Ofloxacin (Systemic) may be decreased by: Antacids; Calcium Salts; Didanosine; Iron Salts; Lanthanum; Magnesium Salts; Quinapril; Sevelamer; Sucralfate; Zinc Salts

Ethanol/Nutrition/Herb Interactions
  Food: Ofloxacin average peak serum concentrations may be decreased by 20% if taken with food.
  Herb/Nutraceutical: Avoid dong quai, St John's wort (may also cause photosensitization).

Stability Store at 25°C (77°F); excursions permitted to 15°C to 30°C (59°F to 86°F).

Mechanism of Action Ofloxacin is a DNA gyrase inhibitor. DNA gyrase is an essential bacterial enzyme that maintains the superhelical structure of DNA. DNA gyrase is required for DNA replication and transcription, DNA repair, recombination, and transposition; bactericidal

Pharmacodynamics/Kinetics
  Absorption: Well absorbed; food causes only minor alterations
  Distribution: V_d: 2.4-3.5 L/kg
  Protein binding: 32%
  Bioavailability: 98%
  Half-life elimination: Biphasic: 4-5 hours and 20-25 hours (accounts for <5%); prolonged with renal impairment
  Excretion: Primarily urine (as unchanged drug)

Dosage
  Geriatric Oral: 200-400 mg every 12-24 hours (based on estimated renal function) for 7 days to 6 weeks depending on indication.

Adult

Cervicitis/urethritis (nongonococcal): Oral:
Nongonococcal: 300 mg every 12 hours for 7 days
Gonococcal (acute, uncomplicated): 400 mg as a single dose; **Note:** As of April 2007, the CDC no longer recommends the use of fluoroquinolones for the treatment of uncomplicated gonococcal disease.

Chronic bronchitis (acute exacerbation), community-acquired pneumonia, skin and skin structure infections (uncomplicated): Oral: 400 mg every 12 hours for 10 days

Epididymitis, nongonococcal (unlabeled use): Oral: 300 mg twice daily for 10 days

Leprosy (unlabeled use): Oral: 400 mg once daily

Pelvic inflammatory disease (acute): Oral: 400 mg every 12 hours for 10-14 days; **Note:** The CDC recommends use only if standard cephalosporin therapy is not feasible and community prevalence of quinolone-resistant gonococcal organisms is low. Culture sensitivity must be confirmed.

Prostatitis: Oral:
Acute: 400 mg for 1 dose, then 300 mg twice daily for 10 days
Chronic: 200 mg every 12 hours for 6 weeks

Traveler's diarrhea (unlabeled use): Oral: 300 mg twice daily for 3 days

UTI: Oral:
Uncomplicated: 200 mg every 12 hours for 3-7 days
Complicated: 200 mg every 12 hours for 10 days

Renal Impairment Adults: Oral: After a normal initial dose, adjust as follows:
Cl_{cr} 20-50 mL/minute: Administer usual dose every 24 hours
Cl_{cr} <20 mL/minute: Administer half the usual dose every 24 hours
Continuous arteriovenous or venovenous hemodiafiltration effects: Administer 300 mg every 24 hours

Hepatic Impairment Severe impairment: Maximum dose: 400 mg/day

Administration Do not take within 2 hours of food or any antacids which contain zinc, magnesium, or aluminum.

Test Interactions Some quinolones may produce a false-positive urine screening result for opiates using commercially-available immunoassay kits. This has been demonstrated most consistently for levofloxacin and ofloxacin, but other quinolones have shown cross-reactivity in certain assay kits. Confirmation of positive opiate screens by more specific methods should be considered.

Special Geriatric Considerations Dosage must be carefully adjusted to renal function. The half-life of ofloxacin may be prolonged and serum concentrations are elevated in elderly patients even in the absence of overt renal impairment. The risk of torsade de pointes and tendon inflammation and/or rupture associated with the concomitant use of corticosteroids and quinolones is increased in the elderly population. See Warnings/Precautions regarding tendon rupture in patients >60 years of age.

Dosage Forms Excipient information presented when available (limited, particularly for generics); consult specific product labeling.
Tablet, oral: 200 mg, 300 mg, 400 mg

Selected References
Khaliq Y and Zhanel GG, "Fluoroquinolone-Associated Tendinopathy: A Critical Review of the Literature," *Clin Infect Dis*, 2003, 36(11):1404-10.
Nilsson-Ehle I and Ljungberg B, "Quinolone Disposition in the Elderly: Practical Implications," *Drugs Aging*, 1991, 1 (4):279-88.

Ofloxacin (Ophthalmic) (oh FLOKS a sin)

Medication Safety Issues
Sound-alike/look-alike issues:
Ocuflox® may be confused with Occlusal®-HP, Ocufen®

Brand Names: U.S. Ocuflox®

Brand Names: Canada Ocuflox®

Generic Availability (U.S.) Yes

Pharmacologic Category Antibiotic, Ophthalmic; Antibiotic, Quinolone

Use Treatment of superficial ocular infections involving the conjunctiva or cornea due to strains of susceptible organisms

Dosage
Adult

Conjunctivitis: Ophthalmic: Instill 1-2 drops in affected eye(s) every 2-4 hours for the first 2 days, then use 4 times/day for an additional 5 days.

Corneal ulcer: Ophthalmic: Instill 1-2 drops every 30 minutes while awake and every 4-6 hours after retiring for the first 2 days; beginning on day 3, instill 1-2 drops every hour while awake for 4-6 additional days; thereafter, 1-2 drops 4 times/day until clinical cure.

◀ **Dosage Forms** Excipient information presented when available (limited, particularly for generics); consult specific product labeling.
Solution, ophthalmic [drops]: 0.3% (5 mL, 10 mL)
Ocuflox®: 0.3% (5 mL) [contains benzalkonium chloride]

Ofloxacin (Otic) (oh FLOKS a sin)

Medication Safety Issues
Sound-alike/look-alike issues:
Floxin® may be confused with Flexeril®
International issues:
Floxin: Brand name for ofloxacin [U.S., Canada], but also the brand name for flunarizine [Thailand], norfloxacin [South Africa], and perfloxacin [Philippines]
Floxin® [U.S., Canada] may be confused with Flexin brand name for diclofenac [Argentina], cyclobenzaprine [Chile], and orphenadrine [Israel]; Flogen brand name for naproxen [Mexico]; Fluoxin brand name for fluoxetine [Czech Republic]
Index Terms Floxin Otic Singles
Generic Availability (U.S.) Yes
Pharmacologic Category Antibiotic, Quinolone
Use Otitis externa, chronic suppurative otitis media, acute otitis media
Dosage
Adult
Otitis media, chronic suppurative with perforated tympanic membranes: Otic: Instill 10 drops (or the contents of 2 single-dose containers) into affected ear twice daily for 14 days
Otitis externa: Otic: Instill 10 drops (or the contents of 2 single-dose containers) into affected ear(s) once daily for 7 days
Dosage Forms Excipient information presented when available (limited, particularly for generics); consult specific product labeling.
Solution, otic [drops]: 0.3% (5 mL, 10 mL)

◆ **9-OH-risperidone** see Paliperidone on page 1378

OLANZapine (oh LAN za peen)

Related Information
Antipsychotic Agents on page 1997
Atypical Antipsychotics on page 1999
Beers Criteria – Potentially Inappropriate Medications for Geriatrics on page 2089
Medication Safety Issues
Sound-alike/look-alike issues:
OLANZapine may be confused with olsalazine, QUEtiapine
ZyPREXA® may be confused with CeleXA®, Reprexain™, Zestril®, ZyrTEC®
ZyPREXA® Zydis® may be confused with Zelapar®, zolpidem
ZyPREXA® Relprevv™ may be confused with ZyPREXA® IntraMuscular
Brand Names: U.S. ZyPREXA®; ZyPREXA® IntraMuscular; ZyPREXA® Relprevv™; ZyPREXA® Zydis®
Brand Names: Canada Apo-Olanzapine®; CO Olanzapine; CO Olanzapine ODT; Olanzapine ODT; PHL-Olanzapine; PHL-Olanzapine ODT; PMS-Olanzapine; PMS-Olanzapine ODT; Riva-Olanzapine; Riva-Olanzapine ODT; Sandoz-Olanzapine; Sandoz-Olanzapine ODT; Teva-Olanzapine; Teva-Olanzapine OD; Zyprex®; Zyprexa® Intramuscular; Zyprexa® Zydis®
Index Terms LY170053; Olanzapine Pamoate; Zyprexa Zydis
Generic Availability (U.S.) No
Pharmacologic Category Antimanic Agent; Antipsychotic Agent, Atypical
Use
Oral: Treatment of the manifestations of schizophrenia; treatment of acute or mixed mania episodes associated with bipolar I disorder (as monotherapy or in combination with lithium or valproate); maintenance treatment of bipolar disorder; in combination with fluoxetine for treatment-resistant or bipolar I depression
I.M., extended-release (Zyprexa® Relprevv™): Treatment of schizophrenia
I.M., short-acting (Zyprexa® IntraMuscular): Treatment of acute agitation associated with schizophrenia and bipolar I mania
Unlabeled/Investigational Use Chronic pain; prevention of chemotherapy-associated delayed nausea or vomiting; psychosis/agitation related to Alzheimer's dementia

Prescribing and Access Restrictions As a requirement of the REMS program, only prescribers, healthcare facilities, and pharmacies registered with the Zyprexa® Relprevv™ Patient Care Program are able to prescribe, distribute, or dispense Zyprexa® Relprevv™ for patients who are enrolled in and meet all conditions of the program. Zyprexa® Relprevv™ must be administered at a registered healthcare facility. Prescribers will need to be recertified every 3 years. Contact the Zyprexa® Relprevv™ Patient Care Program at 1-877-772-9390.

Medication Guide Available Yes

Contraindications There are no contraindications listed in the manufacturer's labeling.

Canadian labeling: Hypersensitivity to olanzapine or any component of the formulation

Warnings/Precautions [U.S. Boxed Warning]: Elderly patients with dementia-related psychosis treated with antipsychotics are at an increased risk of death compared to placebo. Most deaths appeared to be either cardiovascular (eg, heart failure, sudden death) or infectious (eg, pneumonia) in nature. In addition, an increased incidence of cerebrovascular effects (eg, transient ischemic attack, stroke) has been reported in studies of placebo-controlled trials of olanzapine in elderly patients with dementia-related psychosis. Olanzapine is not approved for the treatment of dementia-related psychosis.

Moderate to highly sedating, use with caution in disorders where CNS depression is a feature; patients must be cautioned about performing tasks which require mental alertness (eg, operating machinery or driving). Use caution in patients with cardiac disease. Use with caution in Parkinson's disease, predisposition to seizures, or severe hepatic or renal disease. Life-threatening arrhythmias have occurred with therapeutic doses of some neuroleptics. May induce orthostatic hypotension; use caution with history of cardiovascular disease, hemodynamic instability, prior myocardial infarction, or ischemic heart disease. Increases in cholesterol and triglycerides have been noted. Use with caution in patients with pre-existing abnormal lipid profile. Esophageal dysmotility and aspiration have been associated with antipsychotic use; use with caution in patients at risk of aspiration pneumonia. May increase prolactin levels; clinical significance of hyperprolactinemia in patients with breast cancer or other prolactin-dependent tumors is unknown. Significant weight gain (>7% of baseline weight) may occur; monitor waist circumference and BMI. Impaired core body temperature regulation may occur; caution with strenuous exercise, heat exposure, dehydration, and concomitant medication possessing anticholinergic effects.

Leukopenia, neutropenia, and agranulocytosis (sometimes fatal) have been reported in clinical trials and postmarketing reports with antipsychotic use; presence of risk factors (eg, pre-existing low WBC or history of drug-induced leuko-/neutropenia) should prompt periodic blood count assessment. Discontinue therapy at first signs of blood dyscrasias or if absolute neutrophil count <1000/mm^3.

May cause anticholinergic effects; use with caution in patients with decreased gastrointestinal motility, urinary retention, BPH, xerostomia, or narrow-angle glaucoma. Relative to other neuroleptics, olanzapine has a moderate potency of cholinergic blockade. May cause extrapyramidal symptoms (EPS), although risk of these reactions is lower relative to other neuroleptics. Risk of dystonia (and probably other EPS) may be greater with increased doses, use of conventional antipsychotics, males, and younger patients. May be associated with neuroleptic malignant syndrome (NMS). May cause extreme and life-threatening hyperglycemia; use with caution in patients with diabetes or other disorders of glucose regulation; monitor. Olanzapine levels may be lower in patients who smoke; the manufacturer does not require dosage adjustments, although dosage adjustments may be considered.

The possibility of a suicide attempt is inherent in psychotic illness or bipolar disorder; use caution in high-risk patients during initiation of therapy. Prescriptions should be written for the smallest quantity consistent with good patient care.

There are two Zyprexa® formulations for intramuscular injection: Zyprexa® Relprevv™ is an extended-release formulation and Zyprexa® Intramuscular is short-acting:

Extended-release I.M. injection (Zyprexa® Relprevv™): Monitor for post injection delirium/sedation syndrome; patients should be continuously watched (≥3 hours) for symptoms of olanzapine overdose. Only available through a restricted drug distribution program.

Short-acting I.M. injection (Zyprexa® IntraMuscular): Patients should remain recumbent if drowsy/dizzy until hypotension, bradycardia, and/or hypoventilation have been ruled out. Concurrent use of I.M./I.V. benzodiazepines is not recommended (fatalities have been reported, though causality not determined).

◄ **Adverse Reactions (Reflective of adult population; not specific for elderly)**

Oral: Unless otherwise noted, adverse events are reported for placebo-controlled trials in adult patients on monotherapy:

>10%:

Central nervous system: Somnolence (dose dependent; 20% to 39%; adolescents 39% to 48%), extrapyramidal symptoms (dose dependent; ≤32%), dizziness (11% to 18%), headache (adolescents 17%), fatigue (adolescents 3% to 14%), insomnia (12%)

Endocrine & metabolic: Prolactin increased (30%; adolescents 47%)

Gastrointestinal: Weight gain (5% to 6%, has been reported as high as 40%; adolescents 29% to 31%), appetite increased (3% to 6%; adolescents 17% to 29%), xerostomia (dose dependent; 3% to 22%), constipation (9% to 11%), dyspepsia (7% to 11%)

Hepatic: ALT increased ≥3 x ULN (adolescents 12%; adults 5%)

Neuromuscular & skeletal: Weakness (dose dependent; 8% to 20%)

Miscellaneous: Accidental injury (12%)

1% to 10%:

Cardiovascular: Chest pain, hypertension, peripheral edema, postural hypotension, tachycardia

Central nervous system: Fever, personality changes, restlessness (adolescents)

Dermatologic: Bruising

Endocrine & metabolic: Breast-related events ([adolescents] discharge, enlargement, galactorrhea, gynecomastia, lactation disorder); menstrual-related events (amenorrhea, hypomenorrhea, menstruation delayed, oligomenorrhea); sexual function-related events (anorgasmia, ejaculation delayed, erectile dysfunction, changes in libido, abnormal orgasm, sexual dysfunction)

Gastrointestinal: Abdominal pain (adolescents), diarrhea (adolescents), flatulence, nausea (dose dependent), vomiting

Genitourinary: Incontinence, UTI

Hepatic: Hepatic enzymes increased

Neuromuscular & skeletal: Abnormal gait, akathisia, articulation impairment, back pain, falling, hypertonia, joint/extremity pain, muscle stiffness (adolescents), tremor (dose dependent)

Ocular: Amblyopia

Respiratory: Cough, epistaxis (adolescents), pharyngitis, respiratory tract infection (adolescents), rhinitis, sinusitis (adolescents)

Injection: Unless otherwise noted, adverse events are reported for placebo-controlled trials in adult patients on extended-release I.M. injection (Zyprexa® Relprevv™). Also refer to adverse reactions noted with oral therapy.

>10%: Central nervous system: Headache (13% to 18%), sedation (8% to 13%)

1% to 10%:

Cardiovascular: Hypertension, hypotension (short-acting), postural hypotension (short-acting), QT prolongation

Central nervous system: Abnormal dreams, abnormal thinking, auditory hallucination, dizziness, dysarthria, extrapyramidal symptoms, fatigue, fever, pain, restlessness, somnolence

Dermatologic: Acne

Gastrointestinal: Abdominal pain, appetite increased, diarrhea, flatulence, nausea, vomiting, weight gain, xerostomia

Genitourinary: Vaginal discharge

Hepatic: Liver enzymes increased

Local: Injection site pain

Neuromuscular & skeletal: Arthralgia, back pain, muscle spasms, stiffness, tremor, weakness (short-acting)

Otic: Ear pain

Respiratory: Cough, nasal congestion, nasopharyngitis, pharyngolaryngeal pain, sneezing, upper respiratory tract infection

Miscellaneous: Toothache, tooth infection, viral infection

<1%, postmarketing, and/or case reports (limited to important or life-threatening): CPK increased, post-injection delirium/sedation syndrome, syncope (short-acting)

Drug Interactions

Metabolism/Transport Effects Substrate of CYP1A2 (major), 2D6 (minor); **Inhibits** CYP1A2 (weak), 2C9 (weak), 2C19 (weak), 2D6 (weak), 3A4 (weak)

Avoid Concomitant Use

Avoid concomitant use of OLANZapine with any of the following: Benzodiazepines; Metoclopramide

Increased Effect/Toxicity

OLANZapine may increase the levels/effects of: Alcohol (Ethyl); Anticholinergics; Benzodiazepines; CNS Depressants; Methotrimeprazine; Methylphenidate; Selective Serotonin Reuptake Inhibitors

The levels/effects of OLANZapine may be increased by: Abiraterone Acetate; Acetylcholinesterase Inhibitors (Central); CYP1A2 Inhibitors (Moderate); CYP1A2 Inhibitors (Strong); Deferasirox; Droperidol; FluvoxaMINE; HydrOXYzine; LamoTRIgine; Lithium formulations; Methotrimeprazine; Methylphenidate; Metoclopramide; Pramlintide; Tetrabenazine

Decreased Effect

OLANZapine may decrease the levels/effects of: Amphetamines; Anti-Parkinson's Agents (Dopamine Agonist); Quinagolide

The levels/effects of OLANZapine may be decreased by: CYP1A2 Inducers (Strong); Cyproterone; Lithium formulations; Peginterferon Alfa-2b

Ethanol/Nutrition/Herb Interactions

Ethanol: May increase CNS depression; monitor for increased effects with coadministration. Caution patients about effects.

Herb/Nutraceutical: Avoid dong quai, St John's wort (may also cause photosensitization). Avoid kava kava, gotu kola, valerian, St John's wort (may increase CNS depression).

Stability

Injection, extended-release: Store at 20°C to 25°C (68°F to 77°F); excursions permitted to 15°C to 30°C (59°F to 86°F). Dilute as directed to final concentration of 150 mg/mL. Shake vigorously to mix; will form yellow, opaque suspension. Following reconstitution, suspension may be stored at room temperature and used within 24 hours. Shake vigorously to resuspend prior to administration. Use immediately once suspension is in syringe. Suspension may be irritating to skin; wear gloves during reconstitution.

Injection, short-acting: Store at 20°C to 25°C (68°F to 77°F); excursions permitted to 15°C to 30°C (59°F to 86°F); do not freeze. Protect from light. Reconstitute 10 mg vial with 2.1 mL SWFI. Resulting solution is ~5 mg/mL. Use immediately (within 1 hour) following reconstitution. Discard any unused portion.

Tablet and orally-disintegrating tablet: Store at 20°C to 25°C (68°F to 77°F); excursions permitted to 15°C to 30°C (59°F to 86°F). Protect from light and moisture.

Mechanism of Action

Olanzapine is a second generation thienobenzodiazepine antipsychotic which displays potent antagonism of serotonin 5-HT_{2A} and 5-HT_{2C}, dopamine D_{1-4}, histamine H_1 and alpha$_1$-adrenergic receptors. Olanzapine shows moderate antagonism of 5-HT_3 and muscarinic M_{1-5} receptors, and weak binding to GABA-A, BZD, and beta-adrenergic receptors. Although the precise mechanism of action in schizophrenia and bipolar disorder is not known, the efficacy of olanzapine is thought to be mediated through combined antagonism of dopamine and serotonin type 2 receptor sites.

Pharmacodynamics/Kinetics

Absorption:

Oral: Well absorbed; not affected by food; tablets and orally-disintegrating tablets are bioequivalent

Short-acting injection: Rapidly absorbed

Distribution: V_d: Extensive, 1000 L

Protein binding, plasma: 93% bound to albumin and alpha$_1$-glycoprotein

Metabolism: Highly metabolized via direct glucuronidation and cytochrome P450 mediated oxidation (CYP1A2, CYP2D6); 40% removed via first pass metabolism

Half-life elimination: 21-54 hours; ~1.5 times greater in elderly; Extended-release injection: ~30 days

Time to peak, plasma: Maximum plasma concentrations after I.M. administration are 5 times higher than maximum plasma concentrations produced by an oral dose.

Extended-release injection: ~7 days

Short-acting injection: 15-45 minutes

Oral: ~6 hours

Excretion: Urine (57%, 7% as unchanged drug); feces (30%)

Clearance: 40% increase in olanzapine clearance in smokers; 30% decrease in females

Dosage

Geriatric & Adult

Schizophrenia:

Oral: Initial: 5-10 mg once daily (increase to 10 mg once daily within 5-7 days); thereafter, adjust by 5 mg/day at 1-week intervals, up to a recommended maximum of 20 mg/day. Maintenance: 10-20 mg once daily. Doses of 30-50 mg/day have been used; however, doses >10 mg/day have not demonstrated better efficacy, and safety and efficacy of doses >20 mg/day have not been evaluated.

◄ Extended-release I.M. injection: **Note:** Establish tolerance to oral olanzapine prior to changing to extended-release I.M. injection. Maximum dose: 300 mg/2 weeks or 405 mg/4 weeks

Patients established on oral olanzapine 10 mg/day: Initial dose: 210 mg every 2 weeks for 4 doses or 405 mg every 4 weeks for 2 doses; Maintenance dose: 150 mg every 2 weeks or 300 mg every 4 weeks

Patients established on oral olanzapine 15 mg/day: Initial dose: 300 mg every 2 weeks for 4 doses; Maintenance dose: 210 mg every 2 weeks or 405 mg every 4 weeks

Patients established on oral olanzapine 20 mg/day: Initial and maintenance dose: 300 mg every 2 weeks

Acute mania associated with bipolar disorder: Oral:

Monotherapy: Initial: 10-15 mg once daily; increase by 5 mg/day at intervals of not less than 24 hours. Maintenance: 5-20 mg/day; recommended maximum dose: 20 mg/day.

Combination therapy (with lithium or valproate): Initial: 10 mg once daily; dosing range: 5-20 mg/day

Agitation (acute, associated with bipolar disorder or schizophrenia): Short-acting I.M. injection: Initial dose: 10 mg (a lower dose of 5-7.5 mg may be considered when clinical factors warrant); additional doses (up to 10 mg) may be considered; however, 2-4 hours should be allowed between doses to evaluate response (maximum total daily dose: 30 mg, per manufacturer's recommendation)

Depression:

Depression associated with bipolar disorder (in combination with fluoxetine): Oral: Initial: 5 mg in the evening; adjust as tolerated to usual range of 5-12.5 mg/day. See **"Note."**

Treatment-resistant depression (in combination with fluoxetine): Oral: Initial: 5 mg in the evening; adjust as tolerated to range of 5-20 mg/day. See **"Note."**

Note: When using individual components of fluoxetine with olanzapine rather than fixed dose combination product (Symbyax®), approximate dosage correspondence is as follows:

Olanzapine 2.5 mg + fluoxetine 20 mg = Symbyax® 3/25

Olanzapine 5 mg + fluoxetine 20 mg = Symbyax® 6/25

Olanzapine 12.5 mg + fluoxetine 20 mg = Symbyax® 12/25

Olanzapine 5 mg + fluoxetine 50 mg = Symbyax® 6/50

Olanzapine 12.5 mg + fluoxetine 50 mg = Symbyax® 12/50

Delirium (unlabeled use): Oral: 5 mg once daily for up to 5 days (NICE, 2010)

Prevention of chemotherapy-associated delayed nausea or vomiting (unlabeled use; in combination with a corticosteroid and serotonin [$5HT_3$] antagonist): Oral: 10 mg once daily for 3-5 days, beginning on day 1 of chemotherapy **or** 5 mg once daily for 2 days before chemotherapy, followed by 10 mg once daily (beginning on the day of chemotherapy) for 3-8 days

Renal Impairment No dosage adjustment required. Not removed by dialysis.

Hepatic Impairment Dosage adjustment may be necessary; however, there are no specific recommendations. Monitor closely.

Administration

Short-acting I.M. injection: **For I.M. administration only**; do not administer injection intravenously or subcutaneously; inject slowly, deep into muscle. If dizziness and/or drowsiness are noted, patient should remain recumbent until examination indicates postural hypotension and/or bradycardia are not a problem.

Extended-release I.M. injection: **For I.M. gluteal injection only**; do not administer I.V. or subcutaneously. After needle insertion into muscle, aspirate to verify that no blood appears. Do not massage injection site. Use diluent, syringes, and needles provided in convenience kit; obtain a new kit if aspiration of blood occurs.

Tablet: May be administered without regard to meals.

Orally-disintegrating: Remove from foil blister by peeling back (do not push tablet through the foil); place tablet in mouth immediately upon removal; tablet dissolves rapidly in saliva and may be swallowed with or without liquid. May be administered with or without food/meals.

Monitoring Parameters Vital signs; fasting lipid profile and fasting blood glucose/Hgb A_{1c} (prior to treatment, at 3 months, then annually); periodic assessment of hepatic transaminases (in patients with hepatic disease); BMI, waist circumference; orthostatic blood pressure; mental status, abnormal involuntary movement scale (AIMS), extrapyramidal symptoms (EPS). Weight should be assessed prior to treatment, at 4 weeks, 8 weeks, 12 weeks, and then at quarterly intervals. Consider titrating to a different antipsychotic agent for a weight gain ≥5% of the initial weight.

Extended-release I.M. injection: Sedation/delirium for 3 hours after each dose

Special Geriatric Considerations Elderly patients have an increased risk of adverse response to side effects or adverse reactions to antipsychotics. A higher incidence of falls has been reported in elderly patients, particularly in debilitated patients. Olanzapine half-life that was 1.5 times that of younger (<65 years of age) adults; therefore, lower initial doses are recommended. Olanzapine is not indicated in dementia-related psychosis.

Studies with patients ≥65 years of age with schizophrenia showed no difference in tolerability compared to younger adults. Studies in the elderly with dementia-related psychosis suggested a different tolerability compared to younger patients with schizophrenia. In light of significant risks and adverse effects in the elderly population (compared with limited data demonstrating efficacy in the treatment of dementia-related psychosis, aggression, and agitation), an extensive risk:benefit analysis should be performed prior to use. Therefore, use with caution and at lower recommended doses.

Dosage Forms Excipient information presented when available (limited, particularly for generics); consult specific product labeling.

Injection, powder for reconstitution:
  ZyPREXA® IntraMuscular: 10 mg [contains lactose 50 mg]
Injection, powder for suspension, extended release:
  ZyPREXA® Relprevv™: 210 mg, 300 mg, 405 mg [contains polysorbate 80 (in diluent); supplied with diluent]
Tablet, oral:
  ZyPREXA®: 2.5 mg, 5 mg, 7.5 mg, 10 mg, 15 mg, 20 mg
Tablet, orally disintegrating, oral:
  ZyPREXA® Zydis®: 5 mg [contains phenylalanine 0.34 mg/tablet]
  ZyPREXA® Zydis®: 10 mg [contains phenylalanine 0.45 mg/tablet]
  ZyPREXA® Zydis®: 15 mg [contains phenylalanine 0.67 mg/tablet]
  ZyPREXA® Zydis®: 20 mg [contains phenylalanine 0.9 mg/tablet]

Selected References

American Diabetes Association; American Psychiatric Association; American Association of Clinical Endocrinologists; North American Association for the Study of Obesity, "Consensus Development Conference on Antipsychotic Drugs and Obesity and Diabetes," *Diabetes Care*, 2004, 27(2):596-601.

Farwell WR, Stump TE, Wang J, et al, "Weight Gain and New Onset Diabetes Associated With Olanzapine and Risperidone," *J Gen Intern Med*, 2004, 19(12):1200-5.

Rabins PV, Blacker D, Rovner BW, et al, "Practice Guidelines for the Treatment of Patients With Alzheimer's Disease and Other Dementias," *Am J Psychiatry*, 2007, 164(12 Suppl):5-56. Available at http://www.psych.org/psych_pract/treatg/pg/prac_guide.cfm.

Schneider LS, Tariot PN, Dagerman KS, et al, "Effectiveness of Atypical Antipsychotic Drugs in Patients With Alzheimer's Disease," *N Engl J Med*, 2006, 355(15):1525-38.

Sorsaburu S, Hornbuckle K, Blake D, et al, "The First 21 Months of Safety Experience with Post-Marketing Use of Olanzapine's Intramuscular Formulation," College of Psychiatric and Neurologic Pharmacists, April, 2006, Baltimore, MD.

◆ **Olanzapine Pamoate** *see* OLANZapine *on page 1328*
◆ **Oleptro™** *see* TraZODone *on page 1850*
◆ **Oleum Ricini** *see* Castor Oil *on page 287*

Olmesartan (ole me SAR tan)

Related Information
  Angiotensin Agents *on page 1985*
Medication Safety Issues
  Sound-alike/look-alike issues:
    Benicar® may be confused with Mevacor®
Brand Names: U.S. Benicar®
Brand Names: Canada Olmetec®
Index Terms Olmesartan Medoxomil
Generic Availability (U.S.) No
Pharmacologic Category Angiotensin II Receptor Blocker
Use Treatment of hypertension with or without concurrent use of other antihypertensive agents
Contraindications There are no contraindications listed in the manufacturer's labeling.
Warnings/Precautions May cause hyperkalemia; avoid potassium supplementation unless specifically required by healthcare provider. Avoid use or use a smaller dose in patients who are volume depleted; correct depletion first. May be associated with deterioration of renal function and/or increases in serum creatinine, particularly in patients with low renal blood flow (eg, renal artery stenosis, heart failure) whose glomerular filtration rate (GFR) is dependent on efferent arteriolar vasoconstriction by angiotensin II. Use with caution in unstented unilateral/bilateral renal artery stenosis. When unstented bilateral renal artery stenosis is present, use is generally avoided due to the elevated risk of deterioration in renal function unless possible benefits outweigh risks. Use with caution with pre-existing renal insufficiency; significant aortic/mitral stenosis. Concurrent use of ACE inhibitors may increase the risk of clinically-significant adverse events (eg, renal dysfunction, hyperkalemia).

◄ **Adverse Reactions (Reflective of adult population; not specific for elderly)**
1% to 10%:
Central nervous system: Dizziness (3%), headache
Endocrine & metabolic: Hyperglycemia, hypertriglyceridemia
Gastrointestinal: Diarrhea
Neuromuscular & skeletal: Back pain, CPK increased
Renal: Hematuria
Respiratory: Bronchitis, pharyngitis, rhinitis, sinusitis
Miscellaneous: Flu-like syndrome

Drug Interactions
Metabolism/Transport Effects Substrate of SLCO1B1
Avoid Concomitant Use There are no known interactions where it is recommended to avoid concomitant use.
Increased Effect/Toxicity
Olmesartan may increase the levels/effects of: ACE Inhibitors; Amifostine; Antihypertensives; Hypotensive Agents; Lithium; Nonsteroidal Anti-Inflammatory Agents; Potassium-Sparing Diuretics; RiTUXimab; Sodium Phosphates

The levels/effects of Olmesartan may be increased by: Alfuzosin; Diazoxide; Eltrombopag; Eplerenone; Herbs (Hypotensive Properties); MAO Inhibitors; Pentoxifylline; Phosphodiesterase 5 Inhibitors; Potassium Salts; Prostacyclin Analogues; Tolvaptan; Trimethoprim

Decreased Effect
The levels/effects of Olmesartan may be decreased by: Herbs (Hypertensive Properties); Methylphenidate; Nonsteroidal Anti-Inflammatory Agents; Yohimbine

Ethanol/Nutrition/Herb Interactions
Food: Does not affect olmesartan bioavailability.
Herb/Nutraceutical: Avoid bayberry, blue cohosh, cayenne, ephedra, ginger, ginseng (American), kola, licorice (may worsen hypertension). Avoid black cohosh, California poppy, coleus, golden seal, hawthorn, mistletoe, periwinkle, quinine, shepherd's purse (may have increased antihypertensive effect).

Stability Store at 20°C to 25°C (68°F to 77°F).

Mechanism of Action As a selective and competitive, nonpeptide angiotensin II receptor antagonist, olmesartan blocks the vasoconstrictor and aldosterone-secreting effects of angiotensin II; olmesartan interacts reversibly at the AT1 and AT2 receptors of many tissues and has slow dissociation kinetics; its affinity for the AT1 receptor is 12,500 times greater than the AT2 receptor. Angiotensin II receptor antagonists may induce a more complete inhibition of the renin-angiotensin system than ACE inhibitors, they do not affect the response to bradykinin, and are less likely to be associated with nonrenin-angiotensin effects (eg, cough and angioedema). Olmesartan increases urinary flow rate and, in addition to being natriuretic and kaliuretic, increases excretion of chloride, magnesium, uric acid, calcium, and phosphate.

Pharmacodynamics/Kinetics
Distribution: 17 L; does not cross the blood-brain barrier (animal studies)
Protein binding: 99%
Metabolism: Olmesartan medoxomil is hydrolyzed in the GI tract to active olmesartan. No further metabolism occurs.
Bioavailability: 26%
Half-life elimination: Terminal: 13 hours
Time to peak: 1-2 hours
Excretion: All as unchanged drug: Feces (50% to 65%); urine (35% to 50%)

Dosage
Geriatric No initial dosage adjustment necessary per labeling; however, may consider starting at 5-10 mg/day (due to concomitant disease or age changes).
Adult Hypertension: Oral: Initial: Usual starting dose is 20 mg once daily; if initial response is inadequate, may be increased to 40 mg once daily after 2 weeks. May administer with other antihypertensive agents if blood pressure inadequately controlled with olmesartan. Consider lower starting dose in patients with possible depletion of intravascular volume (eg, patients receiving diuretics).
Renal Impairment No specific guidelines for dosage adjustment; patients undergoing hemodialysis have not been studied.
Hepatic Impairment No initial dosage adjustment necessary.
Administration May be administered with or without food.
Monitoring Parameters Blood pressure, serum potassium
Special Geriatric Considerations No dosage adjustment is necessary when initiating angiotensin II receptor antagonists in the elderly. In clinical studies, no differences between younger adults and the elderly were demonstrated.

For age alone, consider hydration status to avoid hypotension; many elderly are volume depleted due to age-related blunting of the thirst reflex and diuretic use. May consider starting this medication at 5-10 mg once daily.

Dosage Forms Excipient information presented when available (limited, particularly for generics); consult specific product labeling.

Tablet, oral, as medoxomil:

Benicar®: 5 mg, 20 mg, 40 mg

Olmesartan, Amlodipine, and Hydrochlorothiazide
(ole me SAR tan, am LOE di peen, & hye droe klor oh THYE a zide)

Related Information

AmLODIPine *on page 106*

Hydrochlorothiazide *on page 876*

Olmesartan *on page 1333*

Brand Names: U.S. Tribenzor™

Index Terms Amlodipine Besylate, Olmesartan Medoxomil, and Hydrochlorothiazide; Amlodipine, Hydrochlorothiazide, and Olmesartan; Hydrochlorothiazide, Olmesartan, and Amlodipine; Olmesartan, Hydrochlorothiazide, and Amlodipine

Generic Availability (U.S.) No

Pharmacologic Category Angiotensin II Receptor Blocker; Calcium Channel Blocker; Calcium Channel Blocker, Dihydropyridine; Diuretic, Thiazide

Use Treatment of hypertension (not for initial therapy)

Dosage

Geriatric Patients ≥75 years of age should start amlodipine at 2.5 mg (combination product dosage form not available in this strength).

Adult Note: Not for initial therapy. Dose is individualized; combination product may be substituted for individual components in patients currently maintained on all 3 agents separately or in patients not adequately controlled with any 2 of the following antihypertensive classes: Calcium channel blockers, angiotensin II receptor blockers, and diuretics.

Hypertension: Oral: Add-on/switch/replacement therapy: Amlodipine 5-10 mg, olmesartan 20-40 mg, and hydrochlorothiazide 12.5-25 mg once daily; dose may be titrated after 2 weeks of therapy. Maximum recommended daily dose: Amlodipine 10 mg/olmesartan 40 mg/hydrochlorothiazide 25 mg

Renal Impairment

Cl_{cr} >30 mL/minute: No adjustment needed.

Cl_{cr} ≤30 mL/minute: Use of combination not recommended; contraindicated in patients with anuria

Hepatic Impairment

Mild-to-moderate hepatic impairment: Use with caution; specific dosing recommendations are not provided in manufacturer's labeling.

Severe hepatic impairment: Patients with severe hepatic impairment should start amlodipine at 2.5 mg (combination product dosage form not available).

Special Geriatric Considerations Consider hydration status to avoid hypotension; many elderly are volume depleted due to age-related blunting of the thirst reflex and diuretic use. Elderly may experience a greater hypotensive response to amlodipine. Constipation due to amlodipine may be more of a problem in the elderly. See individual agents.

Dosage Forms Excipient information presented when available (limited, particularly for generics); consult specific product labeling.

Tablet, oral:

Tribenzor™:Olmesartan medoxomil 20 mg, amlodipine 5 mg, and hydrochlorothiazide 12.5 mg

Tribenzor™: Olmesartan medoxomil 40 mg, amlodipine 5 mg, and hydrochlorothiazide 12.5 mg

Tribenzor™: Olmesartan medoxomil 40 mg, amlodipine 5 mg, and hydrochlorothiazide 25 mg

Tribenzor™: Olmesartan medoxomil 40 mg, amlodipine 10 mg, and hydrochlorothiazide 12.5 mg

Tribenzor™: Olmesartan medoxomil 40 mg, amlodipine 10 mg, and hydrochlorothiazide 25 mg

◆ **Olmesartan and Amlodipine** *see* Amlodipine and Olmesartan *on page 108*

Olmesartan and Hydrochlorothiazide
(ole me SAR tan & hye droe klor oh THYE a zide)

Related Information
Hydrochlorothiazide *on page 876*
Olmesartan *on page 1333*
Brand Names: U.S. Benicar HCT®
Brand Names: Canada Olmetec Plus®
Index Terms Hydrochlorothiazide and Olmesartan Medoxomil; Olmesartan Medoxomil and Hydrochlorothiazide
Generic Availability (U.S.) No
Pharmacologic Category Angiotensin II Receptor Blocker; Diuretic, Thiazide
Use Treatment of hypertension (not recommended for initial treatment)
Dosage
Geriatric & Adult
Hypertension: Oral: Dosage must be individualized; may be titrated at 2- to 4-week intervals.
Replacement therapy: May be substituted for titrated components.
Patients not controlled with single-agent therapy: Initiate by adding the lowest available dose of the alternative component (hydrochlorothiazide 12.5 mg or olmesartan 20 mg). Titrate to effect (maximum hydrochlorothiazide dose: 25 mg, maximum olmesartan dose: 40 mg).
Renal Impairment Not recommended in patients with Cl$_{cr}$ <30 mL/minute.
Special Geriatric Considerations Combination products are not recommended as first-line treatment. Use only if doses of individual agents correspond to the combination available.
Dosage Forms Excipient information presented when available (limited, particularly for generics); consult specific product labeling.
Tablet:
20/12.5: Olmesartan medoxomil 20 mg and hydrochlorothiazide 12.5 mg
40/12.5: Olmesartan medoxomil 40 mg and hydrochlorothiazide 12.5 mg
40/25: Olmesartan medoxomil 40 mg and hydrochlorothiazide 25 mg

- ◆ **Olmesartan, Hydrochlorothiazide, and Amlodipine** *see* Olmesartan, Amlodipine, and Hydrochlorothiazide *on page 1335*
- ◆ **Olmesartan Medoxomil** *see* Olmesartan *on page 1333*
- ◆ **Olmesartan Medoxomil and Hydrochlorothiazide** *see* Olmesartan and Hydrochlorothiazide *on page 1336*

Olopatadine (Nasal) (oh la PAT a deen)

Brand Names: U.S. Patanase®
Index Terms Olopatadine Hydrochloride
Generic Availability (U.S.) No
Pharmacologic Category Histamine H$_1$ Antagonist; Histamine H$_1$ Antagonist, Second Generation; Piperidine Derivative
Use Treatment of the symptoms of seasonal allergic rhinitis
Dosage
Geriatric & Adult Seasonal allergic rhinitis: Intranasal: 2 sprays into each nostril twice daily
Special Geriatric Considerations No specific information in the elderly.
Dosage Forms Excipient information presented when available (limited, particularly for generics); consult specific product labeling.
Solution, intranasal [spray]:
Patanase®: 0.6% (30.5 g) [contains benzalkonium chloride; equivalent to olopatadine hydrochloride 665 mcg/100 microliters; 240 metered sprays]

Olopatadine (Ophthalmic) (oh la PAT a deen)

Medication Safety Issues
Sound-alike/look-alike issues:
Patanol® may be confused with Platinol®
International issues:
Patanol [U.S., Canada, and multiple international markets] may be confused with Bétanol brand name for metipranolol [Monaco]
Brand Names: U.S. Pataday™; Patanol®

Brand Names: Canada Pataday™; Patanol®
Index Terms Olopatadine Hydrochloride
Generic Availability (U.S.) No
Pharmacologic Category Histamine H$_1$ Antagonist; Histamine H$_1$ Antagonist, Second Generation; Piperidine Derivative
Use Treatment of the signs and symptoms of allergic conjunctivitis
Dosage
 Geriatric & Adult Allergic conjunctivitis: Ophthalmic:
  Patanol®: Instill 1drop into affected eye(s) twice daily (allowing 6-8 hours between doses); results from an environmental study demonstrated that olopatadine was effective when dosed twice daily for up to 6 weeks
  Pataday™: Instill 1 drop into affected eye(s) once daily
Special Geriatric Considerations No specific information in the elderly.
Dosage Forms Excipient information presented when available (limited, particularly for generics); consult specific product labeling.
 Solution, ophthalmic [drops]:
  Pataday™: 0.2% (2.5 mL) [contains benzalkonium chloride]
  Patanol®: 0.1% (5 mL) [contains benzalkonium chloride]

◆ **Olopatadine Hydrochloride** see Olopatadine (Nasal) on page 1336
◆ **Olopatadine Hydrochloride** see Olopatadine (Ophthalmic) on page 1336

Olsalazine (ole SAL a zeen)

Medication Safety Issues
 Sound-alike/look-alike issues:
  Olsalazine may be confused with OLANZapine
  Dipentum® may be confused with Dilantin®
Brand Names: U.S. Dipentum®
Brand Names: Canada Dipentum®
Index Terms Olsalazine Sodium
Generic Availability (U.S.) No
Pharmacologic Category 5-Aminosalicylic Acid Derivative
Use Maintenance of remission of ulcerative colitis in patients intolerant to sulfasalazine
Contraindications Hypersensitivity to olsalazine, salicylates, or any component of the formulation
Warnings/Precautions Diarrhea is a common adverse effect of olsalazine. May exacerbate symptoms of colitis. Use with caution in patients with renal or hepatic impairment. Use with caution in elderly patients. Use with caution in patients with severe allergies or asthma.
Adverse Reactions (Reflective of adult population; not specific for elderly)
 >10%: Gastrointestinal: Diarrhea (11% to 17%; dose related)
 1% to 10%:
  Central nervous system: Depression (2%), dizziness/vertigo (1%)
  Dermatologic: Rash (2%), pruritus (1%)
  Gastrointestinal: Abdominal pain/cramps (10%), nausea (5%), bloating (2%), stomatitis (1%), vomiting (1%)
  Neuromuscular & skeletal: Arthralgia (4%)
  Respiratory: Upper respiratory infection (2%)
Drug Interactions
 Avoid Concomitant Use There are no known interactions where it is recommended to avoid concomitant use.
 Increased Effect/Toxicity
  Olsalazine may increase the levels/effects of: Heparin; Heparin (Low Molecular Weight); Thiopurine Analogs; Varicella Virus-Containing Vaccines
 Decreased Effect
  Olsalazine may decrease the levels/effects of: Cardiac Glycosides
Stability Store at 20°C to 25°C (77°F); excursions permitted to 15°C to 30°C (59°F to 86°F).
Mechanism of Action Mesalamine (5-aminosalicylic acid) is the active component of olsalazine; the specific mechanism of action of mesalamine is unknown; however, it is thought that it modulates local chemical mediators of the inflammatory response, especially leukotrienes, and is also postulated to be a free radical scavenger or an inhibitor of tumor necrosis factor (TNF); action appears topical rather than systemic.
Pharmacodynamics/Kinetics
 Absorption: <3%; very little intact olsalazine is systemically absorbed
 Protein binding, plasma: >99%
 Metabolism: Primarily via colonic bacteria to active drug, 5-aminosalicylic acid (5-ASA)

OLSALAZINE

Half-life elimination: 54 minutes
Time to peak: ~1 hour
Excretion: Primarily feces; urine (<1%)
Dosage
Geriatric & Adult Ulcerative colitis: Oral: 1 g/day in 2 divided doses
Administration Take with food in evenly divided doses.
Monitoring Parameters CBC, hepatic function, renal function; stool frequency
Special Geriatric Considerations No specific data is available on elderly to suggest the drug needs alterations in dose. Since so little is absorbed, dosing should not be changed for reasons of age. Diarrhea may pose a serious problem for elderly in that it may cause dehydration, electrolyte imbalance, hypotension, and confusion.
Dosage Forms Excipient information presented when available (limited, particularly for generics); consult specific product labeling.
Capsule, oral, as sodium:
Dipentum®: 250 mg

♦ **Olsalazine Sodium** *see* Olsalazine *on page 1337*
♦ **Olux®** *see* Clobetasol *on page 380*
♦ **Olux-E™** *see* Clobetasol *on page 380*
♦ **Olux®/Olux-E™ CP [DSC]** *see* Clobetasol *on page 380*
♦ **Omega 3** *see* Omega-3-Acid Ethyl Esters *on page 1338*

Omega-3-Acid Ethyl Esters (oh MEG a three AS id ETH il ES ters)

Medication Safety Issues
Sound-alike/look-alike issues:
Lovaza® may be confused with LORazepam
Omacor® may be confused with Amicar®
Other safety concerns:
The Institute for Safe Medication Practices (ISMP) reported a case of a foam plastic cup dissolving after contact with the liquid contents from a Lovaza® capsule. ISMP is requesting the manufacturer to add warnings to its labeling and that healthcare providers add Lovaza® to their list of medications to not crush.
Brand Names: U.S. Lovaza®
Index Terms Ethyl Esters of Omega-3 Fatty Acids; Fish Oil; Omega 3; P-OM3
Pharmacologic Category Antilipemic Agent, Miscellaneous
Use Lovaza®: Adjunct to diet therapy in the treatment of hypertriglyceridemia (≥500 mg/dL)
Note: A number of OTC formulations containing omega-3 fatty acids are marketed as nutritional supplements; these do not have FDA-approved indications and may not contain the same amounts of the active ingredient.
Unlabeled/Investigational Use Omacor®: Treatment of IgA nephropathy
Contraindications Hypersensitivity to omega-3-acid ethyl esters or any component of the formulation
Warnings/Precautions Use with caution in patients with known allergy or sensitivity to fish. Should be used as an adjunct to diet therapy and exercise and only in those with very high triglyceride levels (≥500 mg/dL). Treatment of primary metabolic disorders (eg, diabetes, thyroid disease) and/or evaluation of the patient's medication regimen for possible etiologic agents should be completed prior to a decision to initiate therapy. Secondary causes of hyperlipidemia should be ruled out prior to therapy. If triglyceride levels do not adequately respond after 2 months of treatment with omega-3-acid ethyl esters, discontinue treatment. ALT may be increased without ALT increasing. May increase LDL levels; periodically monitor LDL levels. Prolongation of bleeding time has been observed in some clinical studies; use with caution in patients with coagulopathy or in those receiving therapeutic anticoagulation; monitor INR.
Adverse Reactions (Reflective of adult population; not specific for elderly)
Cardiovascular: Angina (1%)
Central nervous system: Pain (2%)
Dermatologic: Rash (2%)
Gastrointestinal: Eructation (5%), dyspepsia (3%), taste perversion (3%)
Neuromuscular & skeletal: Back pain (2%)
Miscellaneous: Flu-like syndrome (4%), infection (4%)
Drug Interactions
Avoid Concomitant Use There are no known interactions where it is recommended to avoid concomitant use.
Increased Effect/Toxicity
Omega-3-Acid Ethyl Esters may increase the levels/effects of: Antiplatelet Agents; Warfarin
Decreased Effect There are no known significant interactions involving a decrease in effect.

Ethanol/Nutrition/Herb Interactions Ethanol: Monitor ethanol use (alcohol use may increase triglycerides).

Stability Store at controlled room temperature of 25°C (77°F); do not freeze.

Mechanism of Action Mechanism has not been completely defined. Possible mechanisms include inhibition of acyl CoA:1,2 diacylglycerol acyltransferase, increased hepatic beta-oxidation, a reduction in the hepatic synthesis of triglycerides, or an increase in plasma lipoprotein lipase activity.

Dosage

Geriatric & Adult

Hypertriglyceridemia: Oral: 4 g/day as a single daily dose or in 2 divided doses.

Treatment of IgA nephropathy (unlabeled use): Oral: 4 g/day

Renal Impairment No dosage adjustment required.

Administration May be administered with meals.

Monitoring Parameters Triglycerides and other lipids (LDL-C) should be monitored at baseline and periodically. Hepatic transaminase levels, particularly ALT, should be monitored periodically.

Pharmacotherapy Pearls Due to reports of prescribing errors associated with the similarity between Omacor® and Amicar,® (aminocaproic acid) the name Omacor® has been changed to Lovaza®. The size, strength, ingredients, and dose all remain the same

Special Geriatric Considerations Specific information about the safety and efficacy of omega-3-acid ethyl esters is limited. The manufacturer states there were no apparent differences between persons <60 and >60 years of age.

Dosage Forms Excipient information presented when available (limited, particularly for generics); consult specific product labeling.

Capsule, liquid gel, oral:

Lovaza®: 1 g [contains DHA ~375 mg/capsule, EPA ~465 mg/capsule, soybean oil]

Selected References

Donadio JV and Grande JP, "The Role of Fish Oil/Omega-3 Fatty Acids in the Treatment of IgA Nephropathy," *Semin Nephrol*, 2004, 24(3):225-43.

Grundy SM, Cleeman JI, Merz CN, et al, "Implications of Recent Clinical Trials for the National Cholesterol Education Program Adult Treatment Panel III Guidelines," *J Am Coll Cardiol*, 2004, 44(3):720-32.

National Cholesterol Education Program (NCEP) Expert Panel on Detection, Evaluation, and Treatment of High Blood Cholesterol in Adults (Adult Treatment Panel III), "Third Report of the National Cholesterol Education Program (NCEP) Expert Panel on Detection, Evaluation, and Treatment of High Blood Cholesterol in Adults (Adult Treatment Panel III) Final Report," *Circulation*, 2002, 106(25):3143-421.

Omeprazole (oh MEP ra zole)

Related Information

Helicobacter pylori Treatment in Adult Patients *on page 2009*

Medication Safety Issues

Sound-alike/look-alike issues:

Omeprazole may be confused with aripiprazole, fomepizole

PriLOSEC® may be confused with Plendil®, Prevacid®, predniSONE, prilocaine, Prinivil®, Proventil®, PROzac®

International issues:

Losec [multiple international markets] may be confused with Lasix, a brand name for furosemide [U.S., Canada, and multiple international markets]

Medral [Mexico] may be confused with Medrol brand name for methylprednisolone [U.S., Canada, and multiple international markets]

Norpramin: Brand name for omeprazole [Spain], but also the brand name for desipramine [U.S., Canada] and enalapril/hydrochlorothiazide [Portugal]

Brand Names: U.S. PriLOSEC OTC® [OTC]; PriLOSEC®

Brand Names: Canada Apo-Omeprazole®; Losec®; Mylan-Omeprazole; PMS-Omeprazole; PMS-Omeprazole DR; ratio-Omeprazole; Sandoz-Omeprazole

Index Terms Omeprazole Magnesium

Generic Availability (U.S.) Yes: Excludes granules for suspension

Pharmacologic Category Proton Pump Inhibitor; Substituted Benzimidazole

Use Short-term (4-8 weeks) treatment of active duodenal ulcer disease or active benign gastric ulcer; treatment of heartburn and other symptoms associated with gastroesophageal reflux disease (GERD); short-term (4-8 weeks) treatment of endoscopically-diagnosed erosive esophagitis; maintenance healing of erosive esophagitis; long-term treatment of pathological hypersecretory conditions; as part of a multidrug regimen for *H. pylori* eradication to reduce the risk of duodenal ulcer recurrence

OTC labeling: Short-term treatment of frequent, uncomplicated heartburn occurring ≥2 days/week

◀ **Unlabeled/Investigational Use** Healing NSAID-induced ulcers; prevention of NSAID-induced ulcer; stress-ulcer prophylaxis in the critically-ill

Contraindications Hypersensitivity to omeprazole, substituted benzimidazoles (eg, esomeprazole, lansoprazole), or any component of the formulation

Warnings/Precautions Use of proton pump inhibitors may increase the risk of gastrointestinal infections (eg, *Salmonella, Campylobacter*). Relief of symptoms does not preclude the presence of a gastric malignancy. Atrophic gastritis (by biopsy) has been noted with long-term omeprazole therapy. In long-term (2-year) studies in rats, omeprazole produced a dose-related increase in gastric carcinoid tumors. While available endoscopic evaluations and histologic examinations of biopsy specimens from human stomachs have not detected a risk from short-term exposure to omeprazole, further human data on the effect of sustained hypochlorhydria and hypergastrinemia are needed to rule out the possibility of an increased risk for the development of tumors in humans receiving long-term therapy. Proton pump inhibitors may diminish the therapeutic effect of clopidogrel thought to be due to reduced formation of the active metabolite of clopidogrel; an increase in the risk of cardiovascular events may occur. The manufacturer of clopidogrel recommends avoidance of concomitant administration of omeprazole even when scheduled 12 hours apart.

Increased incidence of osteoporosis-related bone fractures of the hip, spine, or wrist may occur with proton pump inhibitor therapy. Patients on high-dose (multiple daily doses)or long-term (≥1 year) therapy should be monitored. Use the lowest effective dose for the shortest duration of time, use vitamin D and calcium supplementation, and follow appropriate guidelines to reduce risk of fractures in patients at risk.

Hypomagnesemia, reported rarely, usually with prolonged PPI use of >3 months (most cases >1 year of therapy); may be symptomatic or asymptomatic; severe cases may cause tetany, seizures, and cardiac arrhythmias. Consider obtaining serum magnesium concentrations prior to beginning long-term therapy, especially if taking concomitant digoxin, diuretics, or other drugs known to cause hypomagnesemia; and periodically thereafter. Hypomagnesemia may be corrected by magnesium supplementation, although discontinuation of omeprazole may be necessary; magnesium levels typically return to normal within 1 week of stopping.

Decreased *H. pylori* eradication rates have been observed with short-term (≤7 days) combination therapy. The American College of Gastroenterology recommends 10-14 days of therapy (triple or quadruple) for eradication of *H. pylori* (Chey, 2007). Bioavailability may be increased in Asian populations and patients with hepatic dysfunction; consider dosage reductions, especially for maintenance healing of erosive esophagitis. Bioavailability may be increased in the elderly. When used for self-medication (OTC), do not use for >14 days.

Adverse Reactions (Reflective of adult population; not specific for elderly)

1% to 10%:

Central nervous system: Headache (7%), dizziness (2%)

Dermatologic: Rash (2%)

Gastrointestinal: Abdominal pain (5%), diarrhea (4%), nausea (4%), vomiting (3%), flatulence (3%), acid regurgitation (2%), constipation (2%)

Neuromuscular & skeletal: Back pain (1%), weakness (1%)

Respiratory: Upper respiratory infection (2%), cough (1%)

Drug Interactions

Metabolism/Transport Effects Substrate of CYP2A6 (minor), 2C9 (minor), 2C19 (major), 2D6 (minor), 3A4 (major); **Inhibits** CYP1A2 (weak), 2C9 (moderate), 2C19 (moderate), 2D6 (weak), 3A4 (weak); **Induces** CYP1A2 (weak)

Avoid Concomitant Use

Avoid concomitant use of Omeprazole with any of the following: Clopidogrel; Delavirdine; Erlotinib; Nelfinavir; Posaconazole; Rifampin; Rilpivirine; St Johns Wort

Increased Effect/Toxicity

Omeprazole may increase the levels/effects of: Amphetamines; Benzodiazepines (metabolized by oxidation); Carvedilol; Cilostazol; CloZAPine; CycloSPORINE; CycloSPORINE (Systemic); CYP2C19 Substrates; CYP2C9 Substrates (High risk); Dexmethylphenidate; Fosphenytoin; Methotrexate; Methylphenidate; Phenytoin; Raltegravir; Saquinavir; Tacrolimus; Tacrolimus (Systemic); Vitamin K Antagonists; Voriconazole

The levels/effects of Omeprazole may be increased by: Conivaptan; Fluconazole; Ketoconazole; Ketoconazole (Systemic)

Decreased Effect

Omeprazole may decrease the levels/effects of: Atazanavir; Bisphosphonate Derivatives; Cefditoren; Clopidogrel; CloZAPine; Dabigatran Etexilate; Dasatinib; Delavirdine; Erlotinib; Gefitinib; Indinavir; Iron Salts; Itraconazole; Ketoconazole; Ketoconazole (Systemic); Mesalamine; Mycophenolate; Nelfinavir; Posaconazole; Rilpivirine

The levels/effects of Omeprazole may be decreased by: CYP2C19 Inducers (Strong); Peginterferon Alfa-2b; Rifampin; St Johns Wort; Tipranavir; Tocilizumab

Ethanol/Nutrition/Herb Interactions

Ethanol: Avoid ethanol (may cause gastric mucosal irritation).

Food: Food delays absorption.

Stability

Capsules, tablets: Store at 15°C to 30°C (59°F to 86°F). Protect from light and moisture.

Granules for oral suspension: Store at 25°C (77°F); excursions permitted to 15°C to 30°C (59°F to 86°F). For oral administration, empty the contents of the 2.5 mg packet into 5 mL of water (10 mg packet into 15 mL of water); stir. For NG administration, add 5 mL of water into a catheter-tipped syringe, and then add the contents of a 2.5 mg packet (15 mL water for the 10 mg packet); shake. **Note:** Regardless of the route of administration, the suspension should be left to thicken for 2-3 minutes prior to administration.

Mechanism of Action
Proton pump inhibitor; suppresses gastric basal and stimulated acid secretion by inhibiting the parietal cell H+/K+ ATP pump

Pharmacodynamics/Kinetics

Onset of action: Antisecretory: ~1 hour

Peak effect: Within 2 hours

Duration: Up to 72 hours; 50% of maximum effect at 24 hours; after stopping treatment, secretory activity gradually returns over 3-5 days

Absorption: Rapid

Protein binding: ~95%

Metabolism: Hepatic via CYP2C19 primarily and (to a lesser extent) via 3A4 to hydroxy, desmethyl, and sulfone metabolites (all inactive); saturable first-pass effect

Bioavailability: Oral: ~30% to 40%; increased in Asian patients, elderly patients, and patients with hepatic dysfunction

Half-life elimination: 0.5-1 hour; hepatic impairment: ~3 hours

Time to peak, plasma: 0.5-3.5 hours

Excretion: Urine (~77% as metabolites, very small amount as unchanged drug); feces

Dosage

Geriatric & Adult

Active duodenal ulcer: Oral: 20 mg once daily for 4-8 weeks

Gastric ulcers: Oral: 40 mg once daily for 4-8 weeks

Symptomatic GERD (without esophageal lesions): Oral: 20 mg once daily for up to 4 weeks

Erosive esophagitis: Oral: 20 mg once daily for 4-8 weeks; maintenance of healing: 20 mg once daily for up to 12 months total therapy (including treatment period of 4-8 weeks)

Helicobacter pylori eradication: Oral: Dose varies with regimen:

Manufacturer labeling: 40 mg once daily administered with clarithromycin 500 mg 3 times/day for 14 days **or** 20 mg twice daily administered with amoxicillin 1000 mg *and* clarithromycin 500 mg twice daily for 10 days. **Note:** Presence of ulcer at time of therapy initiation may necessitate an additional 14-18 days of omeprazole 20 mg/day (mono-therapy) after completion of combination therapy.

American College of Gastroenterology guidelines (Chey, 2007):

Nonpenicillin allergy: 20 mg twice daily administered with amoxicillin 1000 mg *and* clarithromycin 500 mg twice daily for 10-14 days

Penicillin allergy: 20 mg twice daily administered with clarithromycin 500 mg *and* metronidazole 500 mg twice daily for 10-14 days **or** 20 mg once or twice daily administered with bismuth subsalicylate 525 mg *and* metronidazole 250 mg *plus* tetracycline 500 mg 4 times/day for 10-14 days

Pathological hypersecretory conditions: Oral: Initial: 60 mg once daily; doses up to 120 mg 3 times/day have been administered; administer daily doses >80 mg in divided doses

Stress-ulcer prophylaxis (ICU patients; unlabeled use): Oral: 40 mg once daily; periodically evaluate patient for continued need (Levy, 1997)

Frequent heartburn (OTC labeling): Oral: 20 mg once daily for 14 days; treatment may be repeated after 4 months if needed

Renal Impairment No adjustment is necessary.

Hepatic Impairment Bioavailability is increased with chronic liver disease. Consider dosage adjustment, especially for maintenance of erosive esophagitis. Specific guidelines are not available.

Administration

Oral: Best if administered before breakfast.

Capsule: Should be swallowed whole; do not chew or crush. Delayed release capsule may be opened and contents added to 1 tablespoon of applesauce (use immediately after adding to applesauce); mixture should not be chewed or warmed.

Oral suspension: Following reconstitution, the suspension should be left to thicken for 2-3 minutes and administered within 30 minutes. If any material remains after administration, add more water, stir, and administer immediately.

Tablet: Should be swallowed whole; do not crush or chew.

Nasogastric/orogastric (NG/OG) tube administration:

Capsule: When using capsules to extemporaneously prepare a solution for NG administration, the manufacturers of Prilosec® recommend the use of an acidic juice for preparation and administration. Alternative methods have been described as follows:

NG/OG tube administration for the prevention of stress-related mucosal damage in ventilated, critically-ill patients:

Study 1 (Phillips, 1996): Pour the contents of one or two 20 mg omeprazole delayed release capsules (depending on the dose) into a syringe (after removing plunger); withdraw 10-20 mL of an 8.4% sodium bicarbonate solution into the syringe; allow 30 minutes for the enteric-coated omeprazole granules to break down. Shake the resulting milky substance prior to administration. Flush the NG tube with 5-10 mL of water and clamp for at least 1 hour.

Study 2 (Balaban, 1997): Open the omeprazole delayed release capsule (20 mg or 40 mg), then pour the intact granules into a container holding 30 mL of water. Pour one-third to one-half of the granules into a 30 mL syringe (with the plunger removed) attached to a nasogastric tube (NG). Replace the plunger with 1 cm of air between the granules and the plunger top while the plunger is depressed. Repeat this process until all the granules are flushed, then flush a final 15 mL of water through the tube.

Oral suspension: Following reconstitution in a catheter-tipped syringe, shake the suspension well and leave to thicken for 2-3 minutes. Administer within 30 minutes of reconstitution. Use an NG tube or gastric tube that is a size 6 French or larger; flush the syringe and tube with water.

Monitoring Parameters Monitor symptoms, occult blood; use of gastroscopy is preferred; INR for patients on warfarin

Special Geriatric Considerations In clinical trials, the incidence of side effects in the elderly is no different than that of younger adults (≤65 years) despite slight decrease in elimination and increase in bioavailability. Bioavailability may be increased in the elderly (≥65 years of age), however, dosage adjustments are not necessary.

An increased risk of fractures of the hip, spine, or wrist has been observed in epidemiologic studies with proton pump inhibitor (PPI) use, primarily in older adults ≥50 years of age. The greatest risk was seen in patients receiving high doses or on long-term therapy (≥1 year). Calcium and vitamin D supplementation and close monitoring are recommended to reduce the risk of fracture in high-risk patients.

Dosage Forms Excipient information presented when available (limited, particularly for generics); consult specific product labeling.

Capsule, delayed release, oral: 10 mg, 20 mg, 40 mg

PriLOSEC®: 10 mg, 20 mg, 40 mg

Capsule, delayed release, oral [strength expressed as base]: 40 mg

Granules for suspension, delayed release, oral:

PriLOSEC®: 2.5 mg/packet (30s); 10 mg/packet (30s)

Tablet, delayed release, oral: 20 mg

PriLOSEC OTC®: 20 mg

Selected References

Anderson T, Hasan-Alin M, Hasselgren G, et al, "Drug Interactions Studies With Esomeprazole, the (S)-Isomer of Omeprazole," *Clin Pharmacokinet*, 2001, 40(7):523-37.

Blume H, Donath F, Warnke A, et al, "Pharmacokinetic Drug Interaction Profiles of Proton Pump Inhibitors," *Drug Saf*, 2006, 29(9): 769-84.

Chey WD, Wong BC, et al, "American College of Gastroenterology Guideline on the Management of *Helicobacter pylori* Infection," *Am J Gastroent*, 2007, 102(8):1808-25.

Natsch S, Vinks MH, Voogt AK, et al, "Anaphylactic Reactions to Proton-Pump Inhibitors," *Ann Pharmacother*, 2000, 34(4):474-6.

Paoluzi P, Iacopini F, Crispino P, et al, "2-Week Triple Therapy for *Helicobacter pylori* Infection is Better Than 1-Week in Clinical Practice: a Large Prospective Single-Center Randomized Study," *Helicobacter*, 2006, 11(6):562-8.

Omeprazole and Sodium Bicarbonate

(oh MEP ra zole & SOW dee um bye KAR bun ate)

Related Information

Omeprazole *on page 1339*

Sodium Bicarbonate *on page 1688*

Medication Safety Issues

Sound-alike/look-alike issues:

Zegerid® may be confused with Zestril®

Brand Names: U.S. Zegerid OTC™ [OTC]; Zegerid®

Index Terms Sodium Bicarbonate and Omeprazole

Generic Availability (U.S.) Yes: Capsule

Pharmacologic Category Proton Pump Inhibitor; Substituted Benzimidazole

Use Short-term (4-8 weeks) treatment of active duodenal ulcer or active benign gastric ulcer; treatment of heartburn and other symptoms associated with gastroesophageal reflux disease (GERD); short-term (4-8 weeks) treatment of endoscopically-diagnosed erosive esophagitis; maintenance healing of erosive esophagitis; reduction of risk of upper gastrointestinal bleeding in critically-ill patients

OTC labeling: Short-term (2 weeks) treatment of frequent (2 days/week), uncomplicated heartburn

Contraindications Hypersensitivity to omeprazole, sodium bicarbonate, or any component of the formulation

Warnings/Precautions Use of proton pump inhibitors may increase the risk of gastrointestinal infections (eg, *Salmonella, Campylobacter*). Relief of symptoms does not preclude the presence of a gastric malignancy. Atrophic gastritis (observed on biopsy) has been reported with long-term use. In long-term (2-year) studies in rats, omeprazole produced a dose-related increase in gastric carcinoid tumors. While available endoscopic evaluations and histologic examinations of biopsy specimens from human stomachs have not detected a risk from short-term exposure to omeprazole, further human data on the effect of sustained hypochlorhydria and hypergastrinemia are needed to rule out the possibility of an increased risk for the development of tumors in humans receiving long-term therapy. Bioavailability may be increased in the elderly, Asian population, and with hepatic dysfunction. Use with caution in patients with Bartter's syndrome, hypocalcemia, hypokalemia, sodium-restricted diets, and respiratory alkalosis (contains sodium bicarbonate). Proton pump inhibitors may diminish the therapeutic effect of clopidogrel, thought to be due to reduced formation of the active metabolite of clopidogrel; an increase in the risk of cardiovascular events may occur. The manufacturer of clopidogrel recommends avoidance of concomitant administration of omeprazole even when scheduled 12 hours apart.

Increased incidence of osteoporosis-related bone fractures of the hip, spine, or wrist may occur with proton pump inhibitor therapy. Patients on high-dose or long-term therapy should be monitored. Use the lowest effective dose for the shortest duration of time, use vitamin D and calcium supplementation, and follow appropriate guidelines to reduce risk of fractures in patients at risk.

Hypomagnesemia, reported rarely, usually with prolonged PPI use of >3 months (most cases >1 year of therapy); may be symptomatic or asymptomatic; severe cases may cause tetany, seizures, and cardiac arrhythmias. Consider obtaining serum magnesium concentrations prior to beginning long-term therapy, especially if taking concomitant digoxin, diuretics, or other drugs known to cause hypomagnesemia; and periodically thereafter. Hypomagnesemia may be corrected by magnesium supplementation, although discontinuation of omeprazole may be necessary; magnesium levels typically return to normal within 1 week of stopping.

When used for self-medication (OTC), patients should be instructed not to use if they have difficulty swallowing, are vomiting blood, or have bloody or black stools. Prior to use, patients should contact healthcare provider if they have heartburn for >3 months, heartburn with dizziness, lightheadedness, or sweating, MI symptoms, frequent chest pain, frequent wheezing (especially with heartburn), unexplained weight loss, nausea/vomiting, stomach pain, on a sodium-restricted diet, or are taking antifungals, HIV antivirals, diazepam, digoxin, tacrolimus, warfarin or other prescription medications. Patients should stop use and consult a healthcare provider if heartburn continues or worsens, or if they need to take for >14 days or more often than every 4 months. Patients should be informed that it may take 1-4 days for full effect to be seen.

Adverse Reactions (Reflective of adult population; not specific for elderly)

Percentages of adverse events reported from a controlled clinical trial of 359 critically-ill patients receiving the oral powder for suspension

>10%:

Central nervous system: Pyrexia (20%)

Endocrine & metabolic: Hypokalemia (12%), hyperglycemia (11%)

Respiratory: Nosocomial pneumonia (11%)

1% to 10%:

Cardiovascular: Hypotension (10%), hypertension (8%), atrial fibrillation (6%), ventricular tachycardia (5%), bradycardia (4%), tachycardia (3%), supraventricular tachycardia (3%), edema (3%)

Central nervous system: Hyperpyrexia (5%), agitation (3%)

Dermatological: Rash (6%), decubitus ulcer (3%)

◄

Endocrine & metabolic: Hypomagnesemia (10%), hypocalcemia (6%), hypophosphatemia (6%), fluid overload (5%), hypoglycemia (3%), hyponatremia (4%), hypernatremia (2%), hyperkalemia (2%)

Gastrointestinal: Constipation (5%), diarrhea (4%), hypomotility (2%)

Genitourinary: Urinary tract infection (2%)

Hematological: Thrombocytopenia (10%), anemia (8%), anemia increased (2%)

Hepatic: LFTs increased (2%)

Respiratory: ARDS (3%), respiratory failure (2%), pneumothorax (1%)

Miscellaneous: Sepsis (5%), oral candidiasis (4%), candidal infection (2%)

Drug Interactions

Metabolism/Transport Effects Substrate of CYP2A6 (minor), 2C9 (minor), 2C19 (major), 2D6 (minor), 3A4 (minor); **Inhibits** CYP1A2 (weak), 2C9 (moderate), 2C19 (strong), 2D6 (weak), 3A4 (weak); **Induces** CYP1A2 (weak)

Avoid Concomitant Use

Avoid concomitant use of Omeprazole and Sodium Bicarbonate with any of the following: Clopidogrel; Delavirdine; Erlotinib; Nelfinavir; Posaconazole; Rifampin; Rilpivirine; St Johns Wort

Increased Effect/Toxicity

Omeprazole and Sodium Bicarbonate may increase the levels/effects of: Alpha-/Beta-Agonists; Amphetamines; Benzodiazepines (metabolized by oxidation); Calcium Polystyrene Sulfonate; Cilostazol; CloZAPine; CycloSPORINE; CycloSPORINE (Systemic); CYP2C19 Substrates; CYP2C9 Substrates (High risk); Dexmethylphenidate; Flecainide; Fosphenytoin; Memantine; Methotrexate; Methylphenidate; Phenytoin; QuiNIDine; QuiNINE; Raltegravir; Saquinavir; Tacrolimus; Tacrolimus (Systemic); Vitamin K Antagonists; Voriconazole

The levels/effects of Omeprazole and Sodium Bicarbonate may be increased by: Conivaptan; Fluconazole; Ketoconazole; Ketoconazole (Systemic)

Decreased Effect

Omeprazole and Sodium Bicarbonate may decrease the levels/effects of: ACE Inhibitors; Anticonvulsants (Hydantoin); Antipsychotic Agents (Phenothiazines); Atazanavir; Bisacodyl; Bisphosphonate Derivatives; Cefditoren; Cefpodoxime; Cefuroxime; Chloroquine; Clopidogrel; CloZAPine; Corticosteroids (Oral); Dabigatran Etexilate; Dasatinib; Delavirdine; Erlotinib; Flecainide; Gabapentin; Gefitinib; HMG-CoA Reductase Inhibitors; Indinavir; Iron Salts; Isoniazid; Itraconazole; Ketoconazole; Ketoconazole (Systemic); Lithium; Mesalamine; Methenamine; Mycophenolate; Nelfinavir; Penicillamine; Phosphate Supplements; Posaconazole; Protease Inhibitors; Rilpivirine; Tetracycline Derivatives; Trientine

The levels/effects of Omeprazole and Sodium Bicarbonate may be decreased by: CYP2C19 Inducers (Strong); Peginterferon Alfa-2b; Rifampin; St Johns Wort; Tipranavir; Tocilizumab

Ethanol/Nutrition/Herb Interactions

Ethanol: Avoid ethanol (may cause gastric mucosal irritation).

Food: Food delays absorption. When given 1 hour after a meal, absorption is reduced.

Herb/Nutraceutical: St John's wort may decrease omeprazole levels.

Stability

Capsules, powder for oral suspension: Store at 25°C (77°F); excursions permitted to 15°C to 30°C (59°F to 86°F). Protect from light.

OTC capsules: Store at 20°C to 25°C (68°F to 77°F).

Mechanism of Action Suppresses gastric basal and stimulated acid secretion by inhibiting the parietal cell H+/K+ ATP pump

Pharmacodynamics/Kinetics

Onset of action: Antisecretory: ~1 hour; Peak antisecretory effect: 2 hours; Full therapeutic effect: 1-4 days

Duration: 72 hours

Absorption: Rapid

Protein binding: ~95%

Metabolism: Extensively hepatic to inactive metabolites

Bioavailability: Oral: ~30% to 40%; increased in Asian patients and patients with hepatic dysfunction

Half-life elimination: ~1 hour (range: 0.4-3.2 hours)

Time to peak, serum: ~30 minutes

Excretion: Urine (77% as metabolites, very small amount as unchanged drug); feces

Dosage

Geriatric & Adult Note: Both strengths of Zegerid® capsule and powder for oral suspension have identical sodium bicarbonate content, respectively. Do not substitute two 20 mg capsules/packets for one 40 mg dose.

Active duodenal ulcer: Oral: 20 mg/day for 4-8 weeks

Gastric ulcers: Oral: 40 mg/day for 4-8 weeks

Heartburn (OTC labeling): Oral: 20 mg once daily for 14 days. Do not take for >14 days or more often than every 4 months, unless instructed by healthcare provider.

Symptomatic GERD: Oral: 20 mg/day for up to 4 weeks

Erosive esophagitis: Oral: 20 mg/day for 4-8 weeks; maintenance of healing: 20 mg/day for up to 12 months total therapy (including treatment period of 4-8 weeks)

Risk reduction of upper GI bleeding in critically-ill patients (Zegerid® powder for oral suspension): Oral:

Loading dose: Day 1: 40 mg every 6-8 hours for two doses

Maintenance dose: 40 mg/day for up to 14 days; therapy >14 days has not been evaluated

Renal Impairment No adjustment is necessary.

Hepatic Impairment Bioavailability is increased with chronic liver disease. Consider dosage adjustment, especially for maintenance of healing of erosive esophagitis. Specific guidelines are not available.

Administration Note: Both strengths of Zegerid® capsule and powder for oral suspension have identical sodium bicarbonate content, respectively. Do not substitute two 20 mg capsules/packets for one 40 mg dose.

Capsule: Should be swallowed whole with water (do not use other liquids); do not chew or crush. Capsules should **not** be opened, sprinkled on food, or administered via NG. Best if taken at least 1 hour before breakfast.

Powder for oral suspension:

Oral: Administer 1 hour before a meal. Mix with 1-2 tablespoons of water; stir well and drink immediately. Rinse cup with water and drink. Do not use other liquids or sprinkle on food.

Nasogastric/orogastric tube: Mix well with 20 mL of water (do not use other liquids) and administer immediately; flush tube with an additional 20 mL of water. Suspend enteral feeding for 3 hours before and 1 hour after administering.

Special Geriatric Considerations The incidence of side effects in the elderly is no different than that of younger adults (≤65 years of age) despite slight decrease in elimination and increase in bioavailability. Dosage adjustments are not necessary. Use cautiously in patients requiring sodium restriction, hypertension, or congestive heart failure.

An increased risk of fractures of the hip, spine, or wrist has been observed in epidemiologic studies with proton pump inhibitor (PPI) use, primarily in older adults ≥50 years of age. The greatest risk was seen in patients receiving high doses or on long-term therapy (≥1 year). Calcium and vitamin D supplementation and close monitoring are recommended to reduce the risk of fracture in high-risk patients.

Dosage Forms Excipient information presented when available (limited, particularly for generics); consult specific product labeling.

Capsule, oral: Omeprazole 20 mg [immediate release] and sodium bicarbonate 1100 mg; omeprazole 40 mg [immediate release] and sodium bicarbonate 1100 mg

Zegerid®: Omeprazole 20 mg [immediate release] and sodium bicarbonate 1100 mg [contains sodium 304 mg (13 mEq) per capsule]

Zegerid®: Omeprazole 40 mg [immediate release] and sodium bicarbonate 1100 mg [contains sodium 304 mg (13 mEq) per capsule]

Zegerid OTC™: Omeprazole 20 mg [immediate release] and sodium bicarbonate 1100 mg [contains sodium 303 mg (13 mEq) per capsule]

Powder for oral suspension:

Zegerid®: Omeprazole 20 mg and sodium bicarbonate 1680 mg per packet (30s) [contains sodium 460 mg (20 mEq) per packet]

Zegerid®: Omeprazole 40 mg and sodium bicarbonate 1680 mg per packet (30s) [contains sodium 460 mg (20 mEq) per packet]

◆ **Omeprazole Magnesium** see Omeprazole on page 1339
◆ **Omnaris™** see Ciclesonide (Nasal) on page 353
◆ **Omnicef®** see Cefdinir on page 292
◆ **Omni Gel™ [OTC]** see Fluoride on page 751
◆ **Omnipred™** see PrednisoLONE (Ophthalmic) on page 1510

OnabotulinumtoxinA (oh nuh BOT yoo lin num TOKS in aye)

Medication Safety Issues

Other safety concerns:

Botulinum products are not interchangeable; potency differences may exist between the products.

Brand Names: U.S. Botox®; Botox® Cosmetic

Brand Names: Canada Botox®; Botox® Cosmetic

Index Terms Botulinum Toxin Type A; BTX-A

Generic Availability (U.S.) No

Pharmacologic Category Neuromuscular Blocker Agent, Toxin; Ophthalmic Agent, Toxin

◀ **Use** Treatment of strabismus and blepharospasm associated with dystonia (including benign essential blepharospasm or VII nerve disorders) in patients ≥12 years of age; treatment of cervical dystonia (spasmodic torticollis) in patients ≥16 years of age; temporary improvement in the appearance of lines/wrinkles of the face (moderate-to-severe glabellar lines associated with corrugator and/or procerus muscle activity) in adult patients ≤65 years of age; treatment of severe primary axillary hyperhidrosis in adults not adequately controlled with topical treatments; treatment of focal spasticity (specifically upper limb spasticity) in adults; prophylaxis of chronic migraine headache (≥15 days/month with ≥4 hours/day headache duration) in adults

Canadian labeling: Additional use (not in U.S. labeling): Treatment of forehead, lateral canthus, and glabellar lines in adults >65 years of age

Unlabeled/Investigational Use Treatment of oromandibular dystonia, spasmodic dysphonia (laryngeal dystonia) and other dystonias (ie, writer's cramp, focal task-specific dystonias)

Medication Guide Available Yes

Dosage

Geriatric Initiate therapy at lowest recommended dose. Refer to adult dosing.

Adult Note: In adults treated for more than one indication, the maximum cumulative dose should be ≤360 units/3 months. Canadian labeling recommends a maximum cumulative dose of 6 units/kg (up to 360 units) over 3 months in adult patients receiving additional treatment for noncosmetic indications.

Blepharospasm: I.M.:
Botox®: Initial dose: 1.25-2.5 units injected into the medial and lateral pretarsal orbicularis oculi of the upper lid and lateral pretarsal orbicularis oculi of lower lid
Dose may be increased up to twice the previous dose if the response from the initial dose lasted ≤2 months; maximum dose per site: 5 units. Tolerance may occur if treatments are given more often than every 3 months, but the effect is not usually permanent. Cumulative dose:
U.S. labeling: ≤200 units in 30-day period
Canadian labeling (not in U.S. labeling): Botox®: ≤200 units in 2-month period

Cervical dystonia: I.M.: For dosing guidance, the mean dose is 236 units (25th to 75th percentile range 198-300 units) divided among the affected muscles in patients previously treated with botulinum toxin (maximum: ≤50 units/site). Initial dose in previously untreated patients should be lower. Sequential dosing should be based on the patient's head and neck position, localization of pain, muscle hypertrophy, patient response, and previous adverse reactions. The total dose injected into the sternocleidomastoid muscles should be ≤100 units to decrease the occurrence of dysphagia.
Canadian labeling (not in U.S. labeling): I.M.: Botox®: Effective range of 200-360 units has been used in clinical practice; administer no more frequently than every 2 months

Chronic migraine: I.M.: Administer 5 units/0.1 mL per site. Recommended total dose is 155 units once every 12 weeks. Each 155 unit dose should be equally divided and administered bilaterally, into 31 total sites as described below (refer to prescribing information for specific diagrams of recommended injection sites):
Corrugator: 5 units to each side (2 sites)
Procerus: 5 units (1 site only)
Frontalis: 10 units to each side (divided into 2 sites/side)
Temporalis: 20 units to each side (divided into 4 sites/side)
Occipitalis: 15 units to each side (divided into 3 sites/side)
Cervical paraspinal: 10 units to each side (divided into 2 sites/side)
Trapezius: 15 units to each side (divided into 3 sites/side)

Spasticity (focal): I.M.: Individualize dose based on patient size, extent, and location of muscle involvement, degree of spasticity, local muscle weakness, and response to prior treatment. In clinical trials, total doses up to 360 units (Botox®) were administered as separate injections typically divided among selected muscles; may repeat therapy at ≥3 months with appropriate dosage based upon the clinical condition of patient at time of retreatment.
Suggested guidelines for the treatment of upper limb spasticity. The lowest recommended starting dose should be used and ≤50 units/site should be administered. **Note:** Dose listed is total dose administered as individual or separate intramuscular injection(s):
Biceps brachii: 100-200 units (divided into 4 sites)
Flexor digitorum profundus: 30-50 units (1 site)
Flexor digitorum sublimes: 30-50 units (1 site)
Flexor carpi radialis: 12.5-50 units (1 site)
Flexor carpi ulnaris: 12.5-50 units (1 site)

Suggested guidelines for the treatment of stroke-related upper limb spasticity: *Canadian labeling:* **Note:** Dose listed is total dose administered as individual or separate intramuscular injection(s):

Biceps brachii: 100-200 units (up to 4 sites)
Flexor digitorum profundus: 15-50 units (1-2 sites)
Flexor digitorum sublimes: 15-50 units (1-2 sites)
Flexor carpi radialis: 15-60 units (1-2 sites)
Flexor carpi ulnaris: 10-50 units (1-2 sites)
Adductor pollicis: 20 units (1-2 sites)
Flexor pollicis longus: 20 units (1-2 sites)

Strabismus: I.M.: **Note:** Several minutes prior to injection, administration of local anesthetic and ocular decongestant drops are recommended.

Initial dose:

Vertical muscles and for horizontal strabismus <20 prism diopters: 1.25-2.5 units in any one muscle

Horizontal strabismus of 20-50 prism diopters: 2.5-5 units in any one muscle

Persistent VI nerve palsy ≥1 month: 1.25-2.5 units in the medial rectus muscle

Re-examine patients 7-14 days after each injection to assess the effect of that dose. Subsequent doses for patients experiencing incomplete paralysis of the target may be increased up to twice the previous administered dose. The maximum recommended dose as a single injection for any one muscle is 25 units. Do not administer subsequent injections until the effects of the previous dose are gone.

Primary axillary hyperhidrosis: Intradermal: 50 units/axilla. Injection area should be defined by standard staining techniques. Injections should be evenly distributed into multiple sites (10-15), administered in 0.1-0.2 mL aliquots, ~1-2 cm apart. May repeat when clinical effect diminishes.

Cosmetic uses:

Reduction of glabellar lines: Adults ≤65 years: I.M.: An effective dose is determined by gross observation of the patient's ability to activate the superficial muscles injected. The location, size and use of muscles may vary markedly among individuals. Inject 0.1 mL (4 units) dose into each of five sites, two in each corrugator muscle and one in the procerus muscle for a total dose 0.5 mL (20 units) administered no more frequently than every 3-4 months. **Note:** Treatment of adults >65 years is approved in the Canadian labeling.

Reduction of forehead lines *(Canadian labeling; not in U.S. labeling):* I.M.: Inject 2-6 units into each of four sites in the frontalis muscle every 1-2 cm along either side of forehead crease and 2-3 cm above eyebrows for total dose of 24 units.

Reduction of lateral canthus lines; *(Canadian labeling; not in U.S. labeling):* I.M.: Inject 2-6 units into each of 1-3 injection sites, lateral to the lateral orbital rim.

Special Geriatric Considerations No specific dosing adjustment recommended.

Dosage Forms Excipient information presented when available (limited, particularly for generics); consult specific product labeling. [DSC] = Discontinued product

Injection, powder for reconstitution [preservative free]:

Botox®: *Clostridium botulinum* type A neurotoxin complex 100 units, *Clostridium botulinum* type A neurotoxin complex 200 units [contains albumin (human)]

Botox® Cosmetic: *Clostridium botulinum* type A neurotoxin complex 50 units [DSC], *Clostridium botulinum* type A neurotoxin complex 100 units [contains albumin (human)]

Powder for reconstitution, for injection [preservative free]:

Botox® Cosmetic: *Clostridium botulinum* type A neurotoxin complex 50 units [contains albumin (human)]

Dosage Forms: Canada Excipient information presented when available (limited, particularly for generics); consult specific product labeling.

Injection, powder for reconstitution [preservative free]:

Botox®: Botulinum toxin A 50 units [contains albumin (human)], 100 units [contains albumin (human)], 200 units [contains albumin (human)]

Botox Cosmetic®: Botulinum toxin A 50 units [contains albumin (human)], 100 units [contains albumin (human)], 200 units [contains albumin (human)]

Ondansetron (on DAN se tron)

Medication Safety Issues

Sound-alike/look-alike issues:

Ondansetron may be confused with dolasetron, granisetron, palonosetron

Zofran® may be confused with Zantac®, Zosyn®

Brand Names: U.S. Zofran®; Zofran® ODT; Zuplenz®

ONDANSETRON

Brand Names: Canada Apo-Ondansetron®; CO Ondansetron; Dom-Ondansetron; JAMP-Ondansetron; Mint-Ondansetron; Mylan-Ondansetron; Ondansetron Injection; Ondansetron Injection USP; Ondansetron-Odan; Ondansetron-Omega; PHL-Ondansetron; PMS-Ondansetron; RAN™-Ondansetron; ratio-Ondansetron; Sandoz-Ondansetron; Teva-Ondansetron; Zofran®; Zofran® ODT; ZYM-Ondansetron

Index Terms GR38032R; Ondansetron Hydrochloride; Zuplenz®

Generic Availability (U.S.) Yes: Excludes oral soluble film

Pharmacologic Category Antiemetic; Selective 5-HT$_3$ Receptor Antagonist

Use Prevention of nausea and vomiting associated with moderately- to highly-emetogenic cancer chemotherapy; radiotherapy; prevention of postoperative nausea and vomiting (PONV); treatment of PONV if no prophylactic dose of ondansetron received

Unlabeled/Investigational Use Hyperemesis gravidarum; breakthrough treatment of nausea and vomiting associated with chemotherapy

Contraindications Hypersensitivity to ondansetron, other selective 5-HT$_3$ antagonists, or any component of the formulation; concomitant use of apomorphine

Warnings/Precautions Ondansetron should be used on a scheduled basis, not on an **"as needed" (PRN) basis,** since data support the use of this drug only in the prevention of nausea and vomiting (due to antineoplastic therapy) and not in the rescue of nausea and vomiting. Ondansetron should only be used in the first 24-48 hours of chemotherapy. Data do not support any increased efficacy of ondansetron in delayed nausea and vomiting. Does not stimulate gastric or intestinal peristalsis; may mask progressive ileus and/or gastric distension. Use with caution in patients allergic to other 5-HT$_3$ receptor antagonists; cross-reactivity has been reported.

Use with caution in patients with congenital long QT syndrome or other risk factors for QT prolongation (eg, medications known to prolong QT interval, electrolyte abnormalities, and cumulative high-dose anthracycline therapy). 5-HT$_3$ antagonists have been associated with a number of dose-dependent increases in ECG intervals (eg, PR, QRS duration, QT/QT$_c$, JT), usually occurring 1-2 hours after I.V. administration. In general, these changes are not clinically relevant, however, when used in conjunction with other agents that prolong these intervals, arrhythmia may occur. When used with agents that prolong the QT interval (eg, Class I and III antiarrhythmics), clinically relevant QT interval prolongation may occur resulting in torsade de pointes. I.V. formulations of 5-HT$_3$ antagonists have more association with ECG interval changes, compared to oral formulations. Dose recommendations provided for patients with severe hepatic impairment (Child-Pugh class C); use with caution in mild-moderate hepatic impairment; clearance is decreased and half-life increased in hepatic impairment.

Orally-disintegrating tablets contain phenylalanine.

Adverse Reactions (Reflective of adult population; not specific for elderly) Note: Percentages reported in adult patients.

>10%:
  Central nervous system: Headache (9% to 27%), malaise/fatigue (9% to 13%)
  Gastrointestinal: Constipation (6% to 11%)

1% to 10%:
  Central nervous system: Drowsiness (8%), fever (2% to 8%), dizziness (4% to 7%), anxiety (6%), cold sensation (2%)
  Dermatologic: Pruritus (2% to 5%), rash (1%)
  Gastrointestinal: Diarrhea (2% to 7%)
  Genitourinary: Gynecological disorder (7%), urinary retention (5%)
  Hepatic: ALT increased (1% to 5%), AST increased (1% to 5%)
  Local: Injection site reaction (4%; pain, redness, burning)
  Neuromuscular & skeletal: Paresthesia (2%)
  Respiratory: Hypoxia (9%)

Drug Interactions

Metabolism/Transport Effects Substrate of CYP1A2 (minor), CYP2C9 (minor), CYP2D6 (minor), CYP2E1 (minor), CYP3A4 (major), P-glycoprotein; **Inhibits** CYP1A2 (weak), 2C9 (weak), 2D6 (weak)

Avoid Concomitant Use

Avoid concomitant use of Ondansetron with any of the following: Apomorphine; Artemether; Dronedarone; Lumefantrine; Nilotinib; Pimozide; QUEtiapine; QuiNINE; Tetrabenazine; Thioridazine; Toremifene; Vandetanib; Vemurafenib; Ziprasidone

Increased Effect/Toxicity

Ondansetron may increase the levels/effects of: Apomorphine; Dronedarone; Pimozide; QTc-Prolonging Agents; QuiNINE; Tetrabenazine; Thioridazine; Toremifene; Vandetanib; Vemurafenib; Ziprasidone

The levels/effects of Ondansetron may be increased by: Alfuzosin; Artemether; Chloroquine; Ciprofloxacin; Ciprofloxacin (Systemic); Conivaptan; Gadobutrol; Lumefantrine; Nilotinib; P-Glycoprotein Inhibitors; QUEtiapine; QuiNINE

Decreased Effect

The levels/effects of Ondansetron may be decreased by: CYP3A4 Inducers (Strong); Cyproterone; Deferasirox; Herbs (CYP3A4 Inducers); Peginterferon Alfa-2b; P-Glycoprotein Inducers; Rifamycin Derivatives; Tocilizumab

Ethanol/Nutrition/Herb Interactions

Food: Tablet: Food slightly increases the extent of absorption.

Herb/Nutraceutical: St John's wort may decrease ondansetron levels.

Stability

Oral soluble film: Store between 20°C and 25°C (68°F and 77°F). Store pouches in cartons; keep film in individual pouch until ready to use.

Oral solution: Store between 15°C and 30°C (59°F and 86°F). Protect from light.

Premixed bag: Store between 2°C and 30°C (36°F and 86°F). Protect from light.

Tablet: Store between 2°C and 30°C (36°F and 86°F).

Vial: Store between 2°C and 30°C (36°F and 86°F). Protect from light. Prior to I.V. infusion, dilute in 50 mL D_5W or NS. Solution is stable for 48 hours at room temperature.

Mechanism of Action Selective 5-HT_3-receptor antagonist, blocking serotonin, both peripherally on vagal nerve terminals and centrally in the chemoreceptor trigger zone

Pharmacodynamics/Kinetics

Onset of action: ~30 minutes

Absorption: Oral: Well absorbed from GI tract

Distribution: V_d: Adults: 2.2-2.5 L/kg

Protein binding, plasma: 70% to 76%

Metabolism: Extensively hepatic via hydroxylation, followed by glucuronide or sulfate conjugation; CYP1A2, CYP2D6, and CYP3A4 substrate; some demethylation occurs

Bioavailability: Oral: 56% to 71% (some first pass metabolism); Rectal: 58% to 74%

Half-life elimination: Adults: 3-6 hours

Mild-to-moderate hepatic impairment (Child-Pugh classes A and B): Adults: 12 hours

Severe hepatic impairment (Child-Pugh class C): Adults: 20 hours

Time to peak: Oral: ~2 hours; Oral soluble film: ~1 hour

Excretion: Urine (44% to 60% as metabolites, ~5% as unchanged drug); feces (~25%)

Dosage

Geriatric & Adult

Prevention of chemotherapy-induced emesis:

I.V.:

0.15 mg/kg 3 times/day beginning 30 minutes prior to chemotherapy **or**

0.45 mg/kg once daily **or**

8-10 mg 1-2 times/day **or**

24 mg or 32 mg once daily

Highly-emetogenic agents/single-day therapy: Oral: 24 mg given 30 minutes prior to the start of therapy

Moderately-emetogenic agents: Oral: 8 mg beginning 30 minutes before chemotherapy; repeat dose 8 hours after initial dose, then 8 mg every 12 hours for 1-2 days after chemotherapy completed

Radiation-induced emesis prophylaxis:

Total body irradiation: Oral: 8 mg 1-2 hours before each daily fraction of radiotherapy

Single high-dose fraction radiotherapy to abdomen: Oral: 8 mg 1-2 hours before irradiation, then 8 mg every 8 hours after first dose for 1-2 days after completion of radiotherapy

Daily fractionated radiotherapy to abdomen: Oral: 8 mg 1-2 hours before irradiation, then 8 mg 8 hours after first dose for each day of radiotherapy

Postoperative nausea and vomiting (PONV):

Oral: 16 mg given 1 hour prior to induction of anesthesia

I.M., I.V.: 4 mg as a single dose approximately 30 minutes before the end of anesthesia (see Note below) or as treatment if vomiting occurs after surgery (Gan, 2007).

Note: The manufacturer recommends administration immediately before induction of anesthesia; however, this has been shown not to be as effective as administration at the end of surgery (Sun, 1997). Repeat doses given in response to inadequate control of nausea/vomiting from preoperative doses are generally ineffective.

Treatment of hyperemesis gravidum (unlabeled use):

Oral: 8 mg every 12 hours

I.V.: 8 mg administered over 15 minutes every 12 hours or 1 mg/hour infused continuously for up to 24 hours

Renal Impairment No adjustment is necessary.

Hepatic Impairment Severe liver disease (Child-Pugh C): Maximum daily dose: 8 mg

◀ **Administration**

Oral: Oral dosage forms should be administered 30 minutes prior to chemotherapy; 1-2 hours before radiotherapy; 1 hour prior to the induction of anesthesia.

Orally-disintegrating tablets: Do not remove from blister until needed. Peel backing off the blister, do not push tablet through. Using dry hands, place tablet on tongue and allow to dissolve. Swallow with saliva.

Oral soluble film: Do not remove from pouch until immediately before use. Using dry hands, place film on top of tongue and allow to dissolve (4-20 seconds). Swallow with or without liquid. If using more than one film, each film should be allowed to dissolve completely before administering the next film.

I.M.: Should be administered undiluted.

I.V.:

IVPB: Dilute in 50 mL D_5W or NS. Infuse over 15-30 minutes; 24-hour continuous infusions have been reported, but are rarely used.

Chemotherapy-induced nausea and vomiting: Give first dose 30 minutes prior to beginning chemotherapy.

I.V. push: Prevention of postoperative nausea and vomiting: Single doses may be administered I.V. injection over 2-5 minutes as undiluted solution.

Monitoring Parameters Emetic episodes, diarrhea, headache

Special Geriatric Considerations Elderly have a slightly decreased hepatic clearance rate. This does not, however, require a dose adjustment.

Dosage Forms Excipient information presented when available (limited, particularly for generics); consult specific product labeling. [DSC] = Discontinued product

Film, soluble, oral:
Zuplenz®: 4 mg (10s); 8 mg (10s) [peppermint flavor]
Infusion, premixed in D_5W [preservative free]: 32 mg (50 mL)
Zofran®: 32 mg (50 mL)
Infusion, premixed in NS [preservative free]: 32 mg (50 mL)
Injection, solution: 2 mg/mL (2 mL, 20 mL)
Zofran®: 2 mg/mL (2 mL [DSC], 20 mL)
Injection, solution [preservative free]: 2 mg/mL (2 mL)
Solution, oral: 4 mg/5 mL (5 mL, 50 mL)
Zofran®: 4 mg/5 mL (50 mL) [contains sodium benzoate; strawberry flavor]
Tablet, oral: 4 mg, 8 mg, 24 mg [DSC]
Zofran®: 4 mg, 8 mg
Tablet, orally disintegrating, oral: 4 mg, 8 mg
Zofran® ODT: 4 mg, 8 mg [contains phenylalanine <0.03 mg/tablet; strawberry flavor]

Extemporaneously Prepared A 0.8 mg/mL syrup may be made by crushing ten 8 mg tablets; flaking of the tablet coating occurs. Mix thoroughly with 50 mL of the suspending vehicle, Ora-Plus® (Paddock), in 5 mL increments. Add sufficient volume of any of the following syrups: Cherry syrup USP, Syrpalta® (Humco), Ora-Sweet® (Paddock), or Ora-Sweet® Sugar-Free (Paddock) to make a final volume of 100 mL. Stability is 42 days refrigerated.

Trissel LA, "Trissel's Stability of Compounded Formulations," American Pharmaceutical Association, 1996.

Rectal suppositories: Calibrate a suppository mold for the base being used. Determine the displacement factor (DF) for ondansetron for the base being used (Fattibase® = 1.1; Polybase® = 0.6). Weigh the ondansetron tablet. Divide the tablet weight by the DF. Subtract the weight of base displaced from the calculated weight of base required for each suppository. Grind the ondansetron tablets to a fine powder in a mortar. Weigh out the appropriate weight of suppository base. Melt the base over a water bath (<55°C). Add the ondansetron powder to the suppository base and mix well. Pour the mixture into the suppository mold and cool. Stable for at least 30 days under refrigeration.

Allen LV, "Ondansetron Suppositories," *US Pharm*, 20(7):84-6.

◆ **Ondansetron Hydrochloride** *see* Ondansetron *on page 1347*
◆ **One Gram C [OTC]** *see* Ascorbic Acid *on page 149*
◆ **Onglyza™** *see* Saxagliptin *on page 1658*
◆ **Onsolis™** *see* FentaNYL *on page 709*
◆ **Opana®** *see* Oxymorphone *on page 1375*
◆ **Opana® ER** *see* Oxymorphone *on page 1375*
◆ **OPC-13013** *see* Cilostazol *on page 355*
◆ **OPC-14597** *see* ARIPiprazole *on page 143*
◆ **OPC-41061** *see* Tolvaptan *on page 1830*
◆ **Opcon-A® [OTC]** *see* Naphazoline and Pheniramine *on page 1263*
◆ **OPT-80** *see* Fidaxomicin (Systemic) *on page 732*
◆ **Optase™** *see* Trypsin, Balsam Peru, and Castor Oil *on page 1876*
◆ **Opti-Clear [OTC]** *see* Tetrahydrozoline (Ophthalmic) *on page 1774*

◆ **OptiPranolol®** *see* Metipranolol *on page 1189*
◆ **Optivar®** *see* Azelastine (Ophthalmic) *on page 172*
◆ **Oracea®** *see* Doxycycline *on page 570*
◆ **Oracit®** *see* Sodium Citrate and Citric Acid *on page 1693*
◆ **Orajel® Dry Mouth [OTC]** *see* Glycerin *on page 833*
◆ **Oral Balance® [OTC]** *see* Saliva Substitute *on page 1652*
◆ **Oralone®** *see* Triamcinolone (Topical) *on page 1857*
◆ **Oramorph® SR** *see* Morphine (Systemic) *on page 1238*
◆ **Oranyl [OTC]** *see* Pseudoephedrine *on page 1545*
◆ **Orap®** *see* Pimozide *on page 1453*
◆ **Orapred®** *see* PrednisoLONE (Systemic) *on page 1507*
◆ **Orapred ODT®** *see* PrednisoLONE (Systemic) *on page 1507*
◆ **Oraxyl™** *see* Doxycycline *on page 570*
◆ **Orazinc® 110 [OTC]** *see* Zinc Sulfate *on page 1947*
◆ **Orazinc® 220 [OTC]** *see* Zinc Sulfate *on page 1947*
◆ **Orciprenaline Sulfate** *see* Metaproterenol *on page 1153*
◆ **Orencia®** *see* Abatacept *on page 22*
◆ **Organidin® NR [OTC] [DSC]** *see* GuaiFENesin *on page 846*
◆ **Original Doan's® [OTC]** *see* Salicylates (Various Salts) *on page 1647*
◆ **Orinase** *see* TOLBUTamide *on page 1820*

Orlistat (OR li stat)

Medication Safety Issues
Sound-alike/look-alike issues:
Xenical® may be confused with Xeloda®
Brand Names: U.S. Alli® [OTC]; Xenical®
Brand Names: Canada Xenical®
Generic Availability (U.S.) No
Pharmacologic Category Lipase Inhibitor
Use Management of obesity, including weight loss and weight management, when used in conjunction with a reduced-calorie and low-fat diet; reduce the risk of weight regain after prior weight loss; indicated for obese patients with an initial body mass index (BMI) ≥30 kg/m^2 or ≥27 kg/m^2 in the presence of other risk factors (eg, diabetes, dyslipidemia, hypertension)
Dosage
Geriatric & Adult Obesity: Oral:
Xenical®: 120 mg 3 times/day with each main meal containing fat (during or up to 1 hour after the meal); omit dose if meal is occasionally missed or contains no fat.
Alli™: OTC labeling: 60 mg 3 times/day with each main meal containing fat
Dosage Forms Excipient information presented when available (limited, particularly for generics); consult specific product labeling.
Capsule, oral:
Alli®: 60 mg
Xenical®: 120 mg

Orphenadrine (or FEN a dreen)

Related Information
Beers Criteria – Potentially Inappropriate Medications for Geriatrics *on page 2089*
Medication Safety Issues
Sound-alike/look-alike issues:
Norflex™ may be confused with norfloxacin, Noroxin®
BEERS Criteria medication:
This drug may be inappropriate for use in geriatric patients (high severity risk).
International issues:
Flexin: Brand name for orphenadrine [Israel] but is also the brand name for cyclobenzaprine [Chile] and diclofenac [Argentina]
Flexin [Israel] may be confused with Floxin which is a brand name for flunarizine [Thailand], norfloxacin [South Africa], ofloxacin [U.S., Canada], and perfloxacin [Philippines]; Fluoxin brand name for fluoxetine [Czech Republic]
Brand Names: U.S. Norflex™
Brand Names: Canada Norflex™; Orphenace®; Rhoxal-orphendrine
Index Terms Orphenadrine Citrate
Generic Availability (U.S.) Yes
Pharmacologic Category Skeletal Muscle Relaxant
Use Treatment of muscle spasm associated with acute painful musculoskeletal conditions

◄ **Contraindications** Hypersensitivity to orphenadrine or any component of the formulation; glaucoma; GI obstruction, stenosing peptic ulcer; prostatic hypertrophy, bladder neck obstruction; cardiospasm; myasthenia gravis

Warnings/Precautions Use with caution in patients with HF, cardiac decompensation, coronary insufficiency, tachycardia or cardiac arrhythmias. May cause CNS depression, which may impair physical or mental abilities. May be inappropriate for use in the elderly due to excessive sedation and anticholinergic effects; alternative agents preferred (Beers Criteria). Potential for abuse; use with caution in patients with history of drug abuse. Solution for injection contains sodium bisulfite which may cause allergic reaction in some individuals. Has not been evaluated for continuous long-term use; monitor closely.

Adverse Reactions (Reflective of adult population; not specific for elderly) Frequency not defined.

Cardiovascular: Palpitation, tachycardia

Central nervous system: Agitation, dizziness, drowsiness, euphoria, hallucination, headache, mental confusion

Dermatologic: Pruritus, urticaria

Gastrointestinal: Constipation, gastric irritation, nausea, vomiting, xerostomia

Genitourinary: Urination hesitancy, urinary retention

Hematologic: Aplastic anemia (rare)

Neuromuscular & skeletal: Tremor, weakness

Ocular: Blurred vision, intraocular pressure increased, nystagmus, pupil dilation

Respiratory: Nasal congestion

Miscellaneous: Anaphylactic reaction (injection, rare), hypersensitivity

Drug Interactions

Metabolism/Transport Effects Substrate (minor) of CYP1A2, 2B6, 2D6, 3A4; **Inhibits** CYP1A2 (weak), 2A6 (weak), 2B6 (weak), 2C9 (weak), 2C19 (weak), 2D6 (weak), 2E1 (weak), 3A4 (weak)

Avoid Concomitant Use There are no known interactions where it is recommended to avoid concomitant use.

Increased Effect/Toxicity

Orphenadrine may increase the levels/effects of: AbobotulinumtoxinA; Alcohol (Ethyl); Anticholinergics; Cannabinoids; CNS Depressants; Methotrimeprazine; OnabotulinumtoxininA; Potassium Chloride; RimabotulinumtoxinB; Selective Serotonin Reuptake Inhibitors

The levels/effects of Orphenadrine may be increased by: Conivaptan; Droperidol; HydrOXYzine; Methotrimeprazine; Pramlintide

Decreased Effect

Orphenadrine may decrease the levels/effects of: Acetylcholinesterase Inhibitors (Central); Secretin

The levels/effects of Orphenadrine may be decreased by: Acetylcholinesterase Inhibitors (Central); Cyproterone; Peginterferon Alfa-2b; Tocilizumab

Ethanol/Nutrition/Herb Interactions

Ethanol: Avoid ethanol (may increase CNS depression).

Herb/Nutraceutical: Avoid valerian, St John's wort, kava kava, gotu kola (may increase CNS depression).

Stability Store at 15°C to 30°C (59°F to 86°F). Protect injection solution from light.

Mechanism of Action Indirect skeletal muscle relaxant thought to work by central atropine-like effects; has some euphorigenic and analgesic properties

Pharmacodynamics/Kinetics

Onset of effect: Peak effect: Oral: 2-4 hours

Duration: 4-6 hours

Protein binding: 20%

Metabolism: Extensively hepatic

Half-life elimination: 14-16 hours

Excretion: Primarily urine (8% as unchanged drug)

Dosage

Geriatric Use caution; generally not recommended for use in the elderly.

Adult Muscle spasms:

Oral: 100 mg twice daily

I.M., I.V.: 60 mg every 12 hours

Administration Do not crush sustained release drug product.

Monitoring Parameters Relief of symptoms, mental status, anticholinergic effects

Special Geriatric Considerations Because of its anticholinergic side effects (eg, constipation, urinary retention, confusion), orphenadrine is not a drug of choice in the elderly.

This medication is considered to be potentially inappropriate in this patient population (Beers Criteria severity: High).

Dosage Forms Excipient information presented when available (limited, particularly for generics); consult specific product labeling.

Injection, solution, as citrate: 30 mg/mL (2 mL)

Norflex™: 30 mg/mL (2 mL) [contains sodium bisulfite]

Tablet, extended release, oral, as citrate: 100 mg

Selected References

Olanow CW, Watts RL, and Koller WC, "An Algorithm (Decision Tree) for the Management of Parkinson's Disease (2001): Treatment Guidelines," *Neurology,* 2001, 56(11 Suppl 5):S1-S88.

◆ **Orphenadrine Citrate** *see* Orphenadrine *on page 1351*
◆ **Ortho Prefest** *see* Estradiol and Norgestimate *on page 649*
◆ **OrthoWash™** *see* Fluoride *on page 751*
◆ **Os-Cal® 500 [OTC]** *see* Calcium Salts (Oral) *on page 256*
◆ **Os-Cal® 500+D [OTC]** *see* Calcium and Vitamin D *on page 248*

Oseltamivir (oh sel TAM i vir)

Related Information

Community-Acquired Pneumonia in Adults *on page 2059*

Medication Safety Issues

Sound-alike/look-alike issues:

Tamiflu® may be confused with Thera-Flu®

Tamiflu® may be confused with Tambocor™

Other safety concerns:

Oseltamivir (Tamiflu®) oral suspension is packaged with an oral syringe. When dispensing commercially prepared oseltamivir oral suspension, verify the intended concentration to be dispensed and the correct dose, dosing instructions, and oral dosing device provided for the patient. Oseltamivir oral suspension is available in a 6 mg/mL concentration. The previous concentration (12 mg/mL) has been discontinued, but may be still be on the market until product expires. The 6 mg/mL concentration is packaged with an oral syringe calibrated in **milliliters** up to a total of 10 mL. The previous, discontinued concentration (12 mg/mL) was packaged with an oral syringe calibrated in mg (30 mg, 45 mg, and 60 mg graduations). **When the oral syringe is dispensed, instructions to the patient should be provided based on these units of measure (ie, mL or mg). Do NOT dispense an oral syringe with units of measure in milligrams when providing oseltamivir suspension for children <1 year of age** instead supply an oral syringe capable of measuring mL doses. Patients should always be provided with a measuring device calibrated the same way as their labeled instructions.

When commercially-prepared oseltamivir oral suspension is not available, an extemporaneously prepared suspension may be compounded to provide a 6 mg/mL concentration (to match the preferred, currently manufactured commercially available oral suspension concentration).

Brand Names: U.S. Tamiflu®

Brand Names: Canada Tamiflu®

Generic Availability (U.S.) No

Pharmacologic Category Antiviral Agent; Neuraminidase Inhibitor

Use Treatment of uncomplicated acute illness due to influenza (A or B) infection who have been symptomatic for no more than 2 days; prophylaxis against influenza (A or B) infection

The Advisory Committee on Immunization Practices (ACIP) recommends that **treatment** be considered for the following:

• Persons with severe, complicated or progressive illness
• Hospitalized persons
• Persons at higher risk for influenza complications:
  - Adults ≥65 years of age
  - Persons with chronic disorders of the pulmonary (including asthma) or cardiovascular systems (except hypertension)
  - Persons with chronic metabolic diseases (including diabetes mellitus), hepatic disease, renal dysfunction, hematologic disorders (including sickle cell disease), or immunosuppression (including immunosuppression caused by medications or HIV)
  - Persons with neurologic/neuromuscular conditions (including conditions such as spinal cord injuries, seizure disorders, cerebral palsy, stroke, mental retardation, moderate to severe developmental delay, or muscular dystrophy) which may compromise respiratory function, the handling of respiratory secretions, or that can increase the risk of aspiration
  - American Indians and Alaskan Natives
  - Persons who are morbidly obese (BMI ≥40)
  - Residents of nursing homes or other chronic care facilities

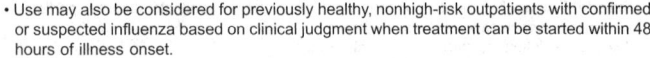

• Use may also be considered for previously healthy, nonhigh-risk outpatients with confirmed or suspected influenza based on clinical judgment when treatment can be started within 48 hours of illness onset.

The ACIP recommends that **prophylaxis** be considered for the following:
• Postexposure prophylaxis may be considered for family or close contacts of suspected or confirmed cases, who are at higher risk of influenza complications, and who have not been vaccinated against the circulating strain at the time of the exposure.
• Postexposure prophylaxis may be considered for unvaccinated healthcare workers who had occupational exposure without protective equipment.
• Pre-exposure prophylaxis should only be used for persons at very high risk of influenza complications who cannot be otherwise protected at times of high risk for exposure.
• Prophylaxis should also be administered to all eligible residents of institutions that house patients at high risk when needed to control outbreaks.

Contraindications Hypersensitivity to oseltamivir or any component of the formulation

Warnings/Precautions Oseltamivir is not a substitute for the influenza virus vaccine. It has not been shown to prevent primary or concomitant bacterial infections that may occur with influenza virus. Use caution with renal impairment; dosage adjustment is required for creatinine clearance <30 mL/minute. Safety and efficacy for use in patients with chronic cardiac and/or kidney disease, severe hepatic impairment, or for treatment or prophylaxis in immunocompromised patients have not been established. Rare but severe hypersensitivity reactions (anaphylaxis, severe dermatologic reactions) have been associated with use. Rare occurrences of neuropsychiatric events (including confusion, delirium, hallucinations, and/or self-injury) have been reported from postmarketing surveillance (primarily in pediatric patients); direct causation is difficult to establish (influenza infection may also be associated with behavioral and neurologic changes). Monitor closely for signs of any unusual behavior.

Antiviral treatment should begin within 48 hours of symptom onset. However, the CDC recommends that treatment may still be beneficial and should be started in hospitalized patients with severe, complicated or progressive illness if >48 hours. Nonhospitalized persons who are not at high risk for developing severe or complicated illness and who have a mild disease are not likely to benefit if treatment is started >48 hours after symptom onset. Nonhospitalized persons who are already beginning to recover do not need treatment.

Adverse Reactions (Reflective of adult population; not specific for elderly)
>10%: Gastrointestinal: Vomiting (2% to 15%)
1% to 10%:
Gastrointestinal: Nausea (4% to 10%), abdominal pain (2% to 5%), diarrhea (1% to 3%)
Ocular: Conjunctivitis (1%)
Respiratory: Epistaxis (1%)

Drug Interactions
Avoid Concomitant Use There are no known interactions where it is recommended to avoid concomitant use.
Increased Effect/Toxicity
The levels/effects of Oseltamivir may be increased by: Probenecid
Decreased Effect
Oseltamivir may decrease the levels/effects of: Influenza Virus Vaccine (Live/Attenuated)

Stability
Capsules: Store at 25°C (77°F); excursions permitted to 15°C to 30°C (59°F to 86°F).
Oral suspension: Store powder for suspension at 25°C (77°F); excursions permitted to 15°C to 30°C (59°F to 86°F). Once reconstituted, store suspension under refrigeration at 2°C to 8°C (36°F to 46°F); do not freeze. Use within 10 days of preparation if stored at room temperature or within 17 days of preparation if stored under refrigeration.
New concentration (6 mg/mL): Reconstitute with 55 mL of water to a final concentration of 6 mg/mL (to make 60 mL total suspension).
Discontinued concentration (12 mg/mL): Reconstitute with 23 mL of water to a final concentration of 12 mg/mL (to make 25 mL total suspension).

Mechanism of Action Oseltamivir, a prodrug, is hydrolyzed to the active form, oseltamivir carboxylate (OC). OC inhibits influenza virus neuraminidase, an enzyme known to cleave the budding viral progeny from its cellular envelope attachment point (neuraminic acid) just prior to release.

Pharmacodynamics/Kinetics
Absorption: Well absorbed
Distribution: V_d: 23-26 L (oseltamivir carboxylate)
Protein binding, plasma: Oseltamivir carboxylate: 3%; Oseltamivir: 42%
Metabolism: Hepatic (90%) to oseltamivir carboxylate; neither the parent drug nor active metabolite has any effect on the cytochrome P450 system
Bioavailability: 75% as oseltamivir carboxylate

Half-life elimination: Oseltamivir: 1-3 hours; Oseltamivir carboxylate: 6-10 hours
Excretion: Urine (>90% as oseltamivir carboxylate); feces

Dosage

Geriatric & Adult

Influenza prophylaxis: Oral: 75 mg once daily; initiate prophylaxis within 48 hours of contact with an infected individual; duration of prophylaxis: 10 days. During community outbreaks, duration of protection lasts for length of dosing period; safety and efficacy have been demonstrated for use up to 6 weeks in immunocompetent patients and safety has been demonstrated for use up to 12 weeks in patients who are immunocompromised.

Prophylaxis (institutional outbreak, CDC 2011 recommendations): Continue for ≥2 weeks and until ~10 days after identification of illness onset in the last patient

Influenza treatment:

Treatment of influenza: Oral: 75 mg twice daily initiated within 48 hours of onset of symptoms; duration of treatment: 5 days

Note: Hospitalized patients with severe influenza infection may require longer (eg, ≥10 days) treatment courses. Some experts also recommend empirically doubling the treatment dose. Initiate as early as possible in any hospitalized patient with suspected/confirmed influenza (CDC, 2011); may be administered via naso- or orogastric tube in mechanically-ventilated patients (Taylor, 2008).

Renal Impairment

Cl_{cr} 10-30 mL/minute: Adults:

Treatment: Reduce dose to 75 mg once daily for 5 days

High-dose treatment (unlabeled [eg, severely-ill hospitalized patients with 2009 H1N1 influenza]): Currently no data are available; consider 150 mg once daily

Prophylaxis: Administer 75 mg every other day or 30 mg once daily.

CAPD (unlabeled dose): Adults: 30 mg once weekly (Robson, 2006)

Hemodialysis: Adults (unlabeled dose; Robson, 2006): 30 mg after every other session

Hepatic Impairment

Mild-to-moderate impairment: No adjustment necessary

Severe impairment: Pharmacokinetics and safety have not been evaluated

Administration May be administered without regard to meals; take with food to improve tolerance.

Capsules may be opened and mixed with sweetened liquid (eg, chocolate syrup).

Mechanically-ventilated critically-ill patients: May administer via naso- or orogastric (NG/OG) tube. For a 150 mg dose, dissolve powder from two 75 mg capsules in 20 mL of sterile water and inject down the NG/OG tube; follow with a 10 mL sterile water flush (Taylor, 2008).

Monitoring Parameters Signs or symptoms of unusual behavior, including attempts at self-injury, confusion, and/or delirium

Critically-ill patients: Repeat rRT-PCR or viral culture may help to determine on-going viral replication

Pharmacotherapy Pearls In clinical studies of the influenza virus, 1.3% of post-treatment isolates in adults and adolescents had decreased neuraminidase susceptibility *in vitro* to oseltamivir carboxylate.

The absence of symptoms does not rule out viral influenza infection and clinical judgment should guide the decision for therapy. Treatment should not be delayed while waiting for the results of diagnostic tests. Treatment should be considered for high-risk patients with symptoms despite a negative rapid influenza test when the illness cannot be contributed to another cause. Use of oseltamivir is not a substitute for vaccination (when available); susceptibility to influenza infection returns once therapy is discontinued.

Special Geriatric Considerations Preferred influenza antiviral because of its ease of use compared to zanamivir and resistance associated with amantadine and rimantadine.

Dosage Forms Excipient information presented when available (limited, particularly for generics); consult specific product labeling. [DSC] = Discontinued product

Capsule, oral, as phosphate:

Tamiflu®: 30 mg, 45 mg, 75 mg

Powder for suspension, oral:

Tamiflu®: 6 mg/mL (60 mL); 12 mg/mL (25 mL [DSC]) [contains sodium benzoate; tutti frutti flavor]

Extemporaneously Prepared

If the commercially prepared oral suspension is not available, the manufacturer provides the following compounding information to prepare a **15 mg/mL** suspension in emergency situations. **Note:** The strength and dosing instructions differ from that of the commercially prepared product (see chart on next page).

1. Calculate the total volume needed by patient weight (refer to chart on next page).
2. Calculate the number of capsules and required volume of vehicle (refer to chart on next page). **Note:** Acceptable vehicles are cherry syrup or Ora-Sweet® SF.

3. Transfer contents of capsules into mortar and triturate granules into a fine powder.
4. Add ~1/3 of vehicle and triturate into a uniform suspension.
5. Add another 1/3 of vehicle and triturate, transfer to amber prescription bottle.
6. Add remaining vehicle to prescription bottle; shake well.

Suspension is stable for 35 days under refrigeration at 2°C to 8°C (36°F to 46°F) or 5 days at room temperature of 25°C (77°F). Shake gently prior to use. Do **not** dispense with dosing device provided with commercially-available product.

Preparation of Oseltamivir 15 mg/mL Suspension

Body Weight	Total Volume per Patient[1]	# of 75 mg Capsules[2]	Required Volume of Vehicle[2,3]	Treatment Dose (wt based)[4]	Prophylactic Dose (wt based)[4]
24-40 kg	50 mL	10	48 mL	4 mL (60 mg) twice daily for 5 days	4 mL (60 mg) once daily for 10 days
≥41 kg	60 mL	12	57 mL	5 mL (75 mg) twice daily for 5 days	5 mL (75 mg) once daily for 10 days

[1]Entire course of therapy.

[2]Based on total volume per patient.

[3]Acceptable vehicles are cherry syrup or Ora-Sweet® SF.

[4]Using 15 mg/mL suspension.

Selected References

Centers for Disease Control and Prevention, "2010-2011 Influenza Antiviral Medications: Summary for Clinicians," 2011. Available at http://www.cdc.gov/flu/professionals/antivirals/summary-clinicians.htm

He G, Massarella J, and Ward P, "Clinical Pharmacokinetics of the Prodrug Oseltamivir and Its Active Metabolite Ro 64-0802," *Clin Pharmacokinet*, 1999, 37(6):471-84.

◆ **OsmoPrep®** *see* Sodium Phosphates *on page 1694*
◆ **OTFC (Oral Transmucosal Fentanyl Citrate)** *see* FentaNYL *on page 709*
◆ **Otix® [OTC]** *see* Carbamide Peroxide *on page 272*
◆ **Ovace®** *see* Sulfacetamide (Topical) *on page 1713*
◆ **Ovace® Plus** *see* Sulfacetamide (Topical) *on page 1713*

Oxacillin (oks a SIL in)

Related Information
Antibiotic Treatment of Adults With Infective Endocarditis *on page 2053*
Index Terms Methylphenyl Isoxazolyl Penicillin; Oxacillin Sodium
Generic Availability (U.S.) Yes
Pharmacologic Category Antibiotic, Penicillin
Use Treatment of infections such as osteomyelitis, septicemia, endocarditis, and CNS infections caused by susceptible strains of *Staphylococcus*
Contraindications Hypersensitivity to oxacillin or other penicillins or any component of the formulation
Warnings/Precautions Modify dosage in patients with renal impairment and in the elderly. Serious and occasionally severe or fatal hypersensitivity (anaphylactoid) reactions have been reported in patients on penicillin therapy, especially with a history of beta-lactam hypersensitivity, history of sensitivity to multiple allergens, or previous IgE-mediated reactions (eg, anaphylaxis, angioedema, urticaria). Use with caution in asthmatic patients. Prolonged use may result in fungal or bacterial superinfection, including *C. difficile*-associated diarrhea (CDAD) and pseudomembranous colitis; CDAD has been observed >2 months postantibiotic treatment.
Adverse Reactions (Reflective of adult population; not specific for elderly) Frequency not defined.
Central nervous system: Fever
Dermatologic: Rash
Gastrointestinal: Nausea, diarrhea, vomiting
Hematologic: Eosinophilia, leukopenia, neutropenia, thrombocytopenia, agranulocytosis
Hepatic: Hepatotoxicity, AST increased
Renal: Acute interstitial nephritis, hematuria
Miscellaneous: Serum sickness-like reactions
Drug Interactions
Avoid Concomitant Use
Avoid concomitant use of Oxacillin with any of the following: BCG

Increased Effect/Toxicity
  Oxacillin may increase the levels/effects of: Methotrexate

  The levels/effects of Oxacillin may be increased by: Probenecid
Decreased Effect
  Oxacillin may decrease the levels/effects of: BCG; Mycophenolate; Typhoid Vaccine

  The levels/effects of Oxacillin may be decreased by: Fusidic Acid; Tetracycline Derivatives
Stability Reconstituted parenteral solution is stable for 3 days at room temperature and 7 days when refrigerated. For I.V. infusion in NS or D_5W, solution is stable for 24 hours at room temperature.
Mechanism of Action Inhibits bacterial cell wall synthesis by binding to one or more of the penicillin-binding proteins (PBPs); which in turn inhibits the final transpeptidation step of peptidoglycan synthesis in bacterial cell walls, thus inhibiting cell wall biosynthesis. Bacteria eventually lyse due to ongoing activity of cell wall autolytic enzymes (autolysins and murein hydrolases) while cell wall assembly is arrested.
Pharmacodynamics/Kinetics
  Distribution: Into bile, synovial and pleural fluids, bronchial secretions; also distributes to peritoneal and pericardial fluids; penetrates the blood-brain barrier only when meninges are inflamed
  Protein binding: ~94%
  Metabolism: Hepatic to active metabolites
  Half-life elimination: Adults: 23-60 minutes; prolonged with renal impairment
  Time to peak, serum: I.M.: 30-60 minutes
  Excretion: Urine and feces (small amounts as unchanged drug and metabolites)
Dosage
  Geriatric & Adult
    Endocarditis: I.V.: 2 g every 4 hours with gentamicin
    Mild-to-moderate infections: I.M., I.V.: 250-500 mg every 4-6 hours
    Prosthetic joint infection: I.V.: 2 g every 4 hours with rifampin
    Severe infections: I.M., I.V.: 1-2 g every 4-6 hours
    ***Staphylococcus aureus,* methicillin-susceptible infections, including brain abscess, bursitis, erysipelas, mastitis, mastoiditis, osteomyelitis, perinephric abscess, pneumonia, pyomyositis, scalded skin syndrome, toxic shock syndrome:** I.V.: 2 g every 4 hours
  Renal Impairment
    Cl_{cr} <10 mL/minute: Clinical practice varies; some clinicians recommend adjustment to the lower range of the usual dosage as based on severity of infection.
    Not dialyzable (0% to 5%)
Administration Administer around-the-clock to promote less variation in peak and trough serum concentrations. Administer IVP over 10 minutes. Administer IVPB over 30 minutes.
Monitoring Parameters Observe for signs and symptoms of anaphylaxis during first dose; monitor periodic CBC, urinalysis, BUN, serum creatinine, AST and ALT
Test Interactions May interfere with urinary glucose tests using cupric sulfate (Benedict's solution, Clinitest®); may inactivate aminoglycosides *in vitro*; false-positive urinary and serum proteins
Pharmacotherapy Pearls Sodium content of 1 g: 2.5 mEq
Special Geriatric Considerations Oxacillin has not been studied in the elderly. Dosing adjustments are not necessary except in renal failure (eg, Cl_{cr} <10 mL/minute). Consider sodium content in patients who may be sensitive to volume expansion (ie, CHF).
Dosage Forms Excipient information presented when available (limited, particularly for generics); consult specific product labeling.
  Infusion, premixed iso-osmotic solution: 1 g (50 mL); 2 g (50 mL)
  Injection, powder for reconstitution: 1 g, 2 g, 10 g
Selected References
  Yoshikawa TT, "Antimicrobial Therapy for the Elderly Patient," *J Am Geriatr Soc,* 1990, 38(12):1353-72.

◆ **Oxacillin Sodium** *see* Oxacillin *on page 1356*

Oxaprozin (oks a PROE zin)

Related Information
  Beers Criteria – Potentially Inappropriate Medications for Geriatrics *on page 2089*
Medication Safety Issues
  Sound-alike/look-alike issues:
    Daypro® may be confused with Diupres®

▶

◀ Oxaprozin may be confused with oxazepam

BEERS Criteria medication:
This drug may be inappropriate for use in geriatric patients (high severity risk).

Brand Names: U.S. Daypro®

Brand Names: Canada Apo-Oxaprozin®; Daypro®

Generic Availability (U.S.) Yes

Pharmacologic Category Nonsteroidal Anti-inflammatory Drug (NSAID), Oral

Use Acute and long-term use in the management of signs and symptoms of osteoarthritis and rheumatoid arthritis; juvenile idiopathic arthritis (JIA)

Medication Guide Available Yes

Contraindications Hypersensitivity to oxaprozin, aspirin, other NSAIDs, or any component of the formulation; perioperative pain in the setting of coronary artery bypass graft (CABG) surgery

Warnings/Precautions [U.S. Boxed Warning]: NSAIDs are associated with an increased risk of adverse cardiovascular thrombotic events, including MI and stroke. Risk may be increased with duration of use or pre-existing cardiovascular risk factors or disease. Carefully evaluate individual cardiovascular risk profiles prior to prescribing. May cause new onset hypertension or worsening of existing hypertension. Use caution with fluid retention. Avoid use in heart failure. Concurrent administration of ibuprofen, and potentially other nonselective NSAIDs, may interfere with aspirin's cardioprotective effect. **[U.S. Boxed Warning]: Use is contraindicated for treatment of perioperative pain in the setting of coronary artery bypass graft (CABG) surgery.** Risk of MI and stroke may be increased with use following CABG surgery.

Platelet adhesion and aggregation may be decreased; may prolong bleeding time; patients with coagulation disorders or who are receiving anticoagulants should be monitored closely. Anemia may occur; patients on long-term NSAID therapy should be monitored for anemia. Rarely, NSAID use may cause severe blood dyscrasias (eg, agranulocytosis, aplastic anemia, thrombocytopenia).

NSAID use may compromise existing renal function; dose-dependent decreases in prosta-glandin synthesis may result from NSAID use, reducing renal blood flow which may cause renal decompensation. NSAID use may increase the risk for hyperkalemia. Patients with impaired renal function, dehydration, heart failure, liver dysfunction, those taking diuretics, and ACE inhibitors, and the elderly are at greater risk of renal toxicity and hyperkalemia. In the elderly, may be inappropriate for long-term use due to potential for GI bleeding, hypertension, heart failure, and renal failure (Beers Criteria). Rehydrate patient before starting therapy; monitor renal function closely. Not recommended for use in patients with advanced renal disease. Long-term NSAID use may result in renal papillary necrosis.

[U.S. Boxed Warning]: NSAIDs may increase risk of gastrointestinal irritation, inflam-mation, ulceration, bleeding, and perforation. These events may occur at any time during therapy and without warning. Use caution with a history of GI disease (bleeding or ulcers); concurrent therapy with aspirin, anticoagulants, and/or corticosteroids; smoking; use of alcohol; and the elderly or debilitated patients. When used concomitantly with ≤325 mg of aspirin, a substantial increase in the risk of gastrointestinal complications (eg, ulcer) occurs; concomitant gastroprotective therapy (eg, proton pump inhibitors) is recommended (Bhatt, 2008).

Use the lowest effective dose for the shortest duration of time, consistent with individual patient goals, to reduce risk of cardiovascular or GI adverse events. Alternate therapies should be considered for patients at high risk.

NSAIDs may cause serious skin adverse events including exfoliative dermatitis, Stevens-Johnson syndrome (SJS), and toxic epidermal necrolysis (TEN); discontinue use at first sign of skin rash or hypersensitivity. Anaphylactoid reactions may occur, even without prior exposure; patients with "aspirin triad" (bronchial asthma, aspirin intolerance, rhinitis) may be at increased risk. Do not use in patients who experience bronchospasm, asthma, rhinitis, or urticaria with NSAID or aspirin therapy. Use caution in other forms of asthma.

Use with caution in patients with decreased hepatic function. Closely monitor patients with any abnormal LFT. Severe hepatic reactions (eg, fulminant hepatitis, liver failure) have occurred with NSAID use, rarely; discontinue if signs or symptoms of liver disease develop, or if systemic manifestations occur.

NSAIDS may cause drowsiness, dizziness, blurred vision and other neurologic effects which may impair physical or mental abilities; patients must be cautioned about performing tasks which require mental alertness (eg, operating machinery or driving). Discontinue use with blurred or diminished vision and perform ophthalmologic exam. Monitor vision with long-term therapy.

The elderly are at increased risk for adverse effects (especially peptic ulceration, CNS effects, renal toxicity) from NSAIDs even at low doses.

Withhold for at least 4-6 half-lives prior to surgical or dental procedures. May cause mild photosensitivity reactions.

Adverse Reactions (Reflective of adult population; not specific for elderly)

1% to 10%:

Cardiovascular: Edema

Central nervous system: Confusion, depression, dizziness, headache, sedation, sleep disturbance, somnolence

Dermatologic: Pruritus, rash

Gastrointestinal: Abdominal distress, abdominal pain, anorexia, constipation, diarrhea, flatulence, gastrointestinal ulcer, gross bleeding with perforation, heartburn, nausea, vomiting

Hematologic: Anemia, bleeding time increased

Hepatic: Liver enzyme elevation

Otic: Tinnitus

Renal: Dysuria, renal function abnormal, urinary frequency

Drug Interactions

Avoid Concomitant Use

Avoid concomitant use of Oxaprozin with any of the following: Floctafenine; Ketorolac; Ketorolac (Nasal); Ketorolac (Systemic)

Increased Effect/Toxicity

Oxaprozin may increase the levels/effects of: Aminoglycosides; Anticoagulants; Antiplatelet Agents; Bisphosphonate Derivatives; Collagenase (Systemic); CycloSPORINE; CycloSPORINE (Systemic); Deferasirox; Desmopressin; Digoxin; Drotrecogin Alfa; Eplerenone; Haloperidol; Ibritumomab; Lithium; Methotrexate; Nonsteroidal Anti-Inflammatory Agents; PEMEtrexed; Porfimer; Potassium-Sparing Diuretics; PRALAtrexate; Quinolone Antibiotics; Rivaroxaban; Salicylates; Thrombolytic Agents; Tositumomab and Iodine I 131 Tositumomab; Vancomycin; Vitamin K Antagonists

The levels/effects of Oxaprozin may be increased by: ACE Inhibitors; Angiotensin II Receptor Blockers; Antidepressants (Tricyclic, Tertiary Amine); Corticosteroids (Systemic); Dasatinib; Floctafenine; Glucosamine; Herbs (Anticoagulant/Antiplatelet Properties); Ketorolac; Ketorolac (Nasal); Ketorolac (Systemic); Nonsteroidal Anti-Inflammatory Agents; Omega-3-Acid Ethyl Esters; Pentosan Polysulfate Sodium; Pentoxifylline; Probenecid; Prostacyclin Analogues; Selective Serotonin Reuptake Inhibitors; Serotonin/Norepinephrine Reuptake Inhibitors; Sodium Phosphates; Treprostinil; Vitamin E

Decreased Effect

Oxaprozin may decrease the levels/effects of: ACE Inhibitors; Angiotensin II Receptor Blockers; Antiplatelet Agents; Beta-Blockers; Eplerenone; HydrALAZINE; Potassium-Sparing Diuretics; Salicylates; Selective Serotonin Reuptake Inhibitors; Thiazide Diuretics

The levels/effects of Oxaprozin may be decreased by: Bile Acid Sequestrants; Nonsteroidal Anti-Inflammatory Agents; Salicylates

Ethanol/Nutrition/Herb Interactions

Ethanol: Avoid ethanol (may enhance gastric mucosal irritation).

Herb/Nutraceutical: Avoid alfalfa, anise, bilberry, bladderwrack, bromelain, cat's claw, celery, chamomile, coleus, cordyceps, dong quai, evening primrose, fenugreek, feverfew, garlic, ginger, ginkgo biloba, ginseng (American, Panax, Siberian), grapeseed, green tea, guggul, horse chestnut seed, horseradish, licorice, prickly ash, red clover, reishi, SAMe (S-adenosylmethionine), sweet clover, turmeric, white willow (all have additional antiplatelet activity).

Stability Store at 25°C (77°F). Protect from light; keep bottle tightly closed.

Mechanism of Action Reversibly inhibits cyclooxygenase-1 and 2 (COX-1 and 2) enzymes, which results in decreased formation of prostaglandin precursors; has antipyretic, analgesic, and anti-inflammatory properties.

Other proposed mechanisms not fully elucidated (and possibly contributing to the anti-inflammatory effect to varying degrees) include inhibiting chemotaxis, altering lymphocyte activity, inhibiting neutrophil aggregation/activation, and decreasing proinflammatory cytokine levels.

Pharmacodynamics/Kinetics

Absorption: Oral: 95%

Distribution: V_d: 11-17 L/70 kg

Protein binding: >99% primarily to albumin

Metabolism: Hepatic via oxidation and glucuronidation; no active metabolites

Half-life elimination: 40-50 hours

Time to peak: 2-4 hours

Excretion: Urine (5% unchanged, 65% as metabolites); feces (35% as metabolites)

Dosage

Geriatric & Adult

Osteoarthritis: Oral: 600-1200 mg once daily; patients should be titrated to lowest dose possible; patients with low body weight should start with 600 mg daily

Rheumatoid arthritis: Oral: 1200 mg once daily; a one-time loading dose of up to 1800 mg/day or 26 mg/kg (whichever is lower) may be given

Maximum doses:

Patient <50 kg: Maximum: 1200 mg/day

Patient >50 kg with normal renal/hepatic function and low risk of peptic ulcer: Maximum: 1800 mg or 26 mg/kg (whichever is lower) in divided doses

Renal Impairment In general, NSAIDs are not recommended for use in patients with advanced renal disease but the manufacturer of oxaprozin does provide some guidelines for adjustment in renal dysfunction.

Severe renal impairment or on dialysis: 600 mg once daily; may increase cautiously to 1200 mg/day with close monitoring.

Hepatic Impairment Use caution in patients with severe dysfunction.

Monitoring Parameters Monitor response (pain, range of motion, grip strength, mobility, ADL function), inflammation; observe for weight gain, edema; monitor renal function; observe for bleeding, bruising; evaluate gastrointestinal effects (abdominal pain, bleeding, dyspepsia); mental confusion, disorientation, CBC, serum, creatinine, BUN, liver function tests

Test Interactions False-positive urine immunoassay screening tests for benzodiazepines have been reported and may occur several days after discontinuing oxaprozin.

Pharmacotherapy Pearls There are no clinical guidelines to predict which NSAID will give response in a particular patient; trials with each must be initiated until response determined; consider dose, patient convenience, and cost

Special Geriatric Considerations Elderly are a high-risk population for adverse effects from NSAIDs. As much as 60% of the elderly can develop peptic ulceration and/or hemorrhage asymptomatically. The concomitant use of H_2 blockers and sucralfate is not generally effective as prophylaxis with the exception of NSAID-induced duodenal ulcers which may be prevented by the use of ranitidine. Misoprostol and proton pump inhibitors are the only agents proven to help prevent the development of NSAID-induced ulcers. Also, concomitant disease and drug use contribute to the risk for GI adverse effects. Use lowest effective dose for shortest period possible. Consider renal function decline with age. Use of NSAIDs can compromise existing renal function especially when Cl_{cr} is ≤30 mL/minute. Tinnitus may be a difficult and unreliable indication of toxicity due to age-related hearing loss or eighth cranial nerve damage. CNS adverse effects, such as confusion, agitation, and hallucination, are generally seen in overdose or high dose situations, but the elderly may demonstrate these adverse effects at lower doses than younger adults.

This medication is considered to be potentially inappropriate in this patient population (Beers Criteria severity: High).

Dosage Forms Excipient information presented when available (limited, particularly for generics); consult specific product labeling.

Caplet, oral:

Daypro®: 600 mg [scored]

Tablet, oral: 600 mg

Selected References

Morgan TO, Anderson A, and Bertram D, "Effect of Indomethacin on Blood Pressure in Elderly People With Essential Hypertension Well Controlled on Amlodipine or Enalapril," *Am J Hypertens*, 2000, 13:1161-7.

Page J and Henry D, "Consumption of NSAIDs and the Development of Congestive Heart Failure in Elderly Patients: An Underrecognized Public Health Problem," *Arch Intern Med*, 2000, 160(6):777-84.

Oxazepam (oks A ze pam)

Related Information

Anxiolytic, Sedative / Hypnotic, and Miscellaneous Benzodiazepines *on page 2000*

Beers Criteria – Potentially Inappropriate Medications for Geriatrics *on page 2089*

Medication Safety Issues

Sound-alike/look-alike issues:

Oxazepam may be confused with oxaprozin, quazepam

Serax may be confused with Eurax®, Urex, ZyrTEC®

BEERS Criteria medication:

This drug may be inappropriate for use in geriatric patients (high severity risk).

International issues:

Murelax [Australia] may be confused with MiraLax brand name for polyethylene glycol 3350 [U.S.]

Brand Names: Canada Apo-Oxazepam®; Bio-Oxazepam; Novoxapram®; Oxpam®; Oxpram®; PMS-Oxazepam; Riva-Oxazepam

Index Terms Serax

Generic Availability (U.S.) Yes

Pharmacologic Category Benzodiazepine

Use Treatment of anxiety; management of ethanol withdrawal

Unlabeled/Investigational Use Anticonvulsant in management of simple partial seizures; hypnotic

Contraindications Hypersensitivity to oxazepam or any component of the formulation (cross-sensitivity with other benzodiazepines may exist); narrow-angle glaucoma (not in product labeling, however, benzodiazepines are contraindicated); not indicated for use in the treatment of psychosis

Warnings/Precautions May cause hypotension (rare) - use with caution in patients with cardiovascular or cerebrovascular disease, or in patients who would not tolerate transient decreases in blood pressure. Serax® 15 contains tartrazine.

Use with caution in elderly or debilitated patients, patients with hepatic disease (including alcoholics), or renal impairment. Due to increased sensitivity in the elderly, smaller doses of benzodiazepines may be safer and as effective; in this age group, avoid using doses >60 mg daily of oxazepam (Beers Criteria). Use with caution in patients with respiratory disease or impaired gag reflex. Avoid use in patients with sleep apnea.

Causes CNS depression (dose-related) resulting in sedation, dizziness, confusion, or ataxia which may impair physical and mental capabilities. Patients must be cautioned about performing tasks which require mental alertness (eg, operating machinery or driving). Use with caution in patients receiving other CNS depressants or psychoactive agents. Benzodiazepines have been associated with falls and traumatic injury and should be used with extreme caution in patients who are at risk of these events (especially the elderly).

Use caution in patients with depression, particularly if suicidal risk may be present. Use with caution in patients with a history of drug dependence. Benzodiazepines have been associated with dependence and acute withdrawal symptoms on discontinuation or reduction in dose. Acute withdrawal, including seizures, may be precipitated after administration of flumazenil to patients receiving long-term benzodiazepine therapy.

Benzodiazepines have been associated with anterograde amnesia. Paradoxical reactions, including hyperactive or aggressive behavior have been reported with benzodiazepines, particularly in psychiatric patients. Does not have analgesic, antidepressant, or antipsychotic properties.

Adverse Reactions (Reflective of adult population; not specific for elderly) Frequency not defined.

Cardiovascular: Syncope (rare), edema

Central nervous system: Drowsiness, ataxia, dizziness, vertigo, memory impairment, headache, paradoxical reactions (excitement, stimulation of effect), lethargy, amnesia, euphoria

Dermatologic: Rash

Endocrine & metabolic: Decreased libido, menstrual irregularities

Genitourinary: Incontinence

Hematologic: Leukopenia, blood dyscrasias

Hepatic: Jaundice

Neuromuscular & skeletal: Dysarthria, tremor, reflex slowing

Ocular: Blurred vision, diplopia

Miscellaneous: Drug dependence

Drug Interactions

Avoid Concomitant Use

Avoid concomitant use of Oxazepam with any of the following: OLANZapine

Increased Effect/Toxicity

Oxazepam may increase the levels/effects of: Alcohol (Ethyl); CloZAPine; CNS Depressants; Fosphenytoin; Methotrimeprazine; Phenytoin; Selective Serotonin Reuptake Inhibitors

The levels/effects of Oxazepam may be increased by: Droperidol; HydrOXYzine; Methotrimeprazine; OLANZapine

Decreased Effect

The levels/effects of Oxazepam may be decreased by: Theophylline Derivatives; Yohimbine

Ethanol/Nutrition/Herb Interactions

Ethanol: May increase CNS depression; monitor for increased effects with coadministration. Caution patients about effects.

Herb/Nutraceutical: Avoid valerian, St John's wort, kava kava, gotu kola (may increase CNS depression).

Mechanism of Action Binds to stereospecific benzodiazepine receptors on the postsynaptic GABA neuron at several sites within the central nervous system, including the limbic system, reticular formation. Enhancement of the inhibitory effect of GABA on neuronal excitability results by increased neuronal membrane permeability to chloride ions. This shift in chloride ions results in hyperpolarization (a less excitable state) and stabilization.

Pharmacodynamics/Kinetics

Absorption: Almost complete

Protein binding: 86% to 99%

Metabolism: Hepatic to inactive compounds (primarily as glucuronides)

Half-life elimination: 2.8-5.7 hours

Time to peak, serum: 2-4 hours

Excretion: Urine (as unchanged drug [50%] and metabolites)

Dosage

Geriatric Oral: Anxiety: 10 mg 2-3 times/day; increase gradually as needed to a total of 30-45 mg/day. Dose titration should be slow to evaluate sensitivity.

Adult

Anxiety: Oral: 10-30 mg 3-4 times/day

Ethanol withdrawal: Oral: 15-30 mg 3-4 times/day

Hypnotic: Oral: 15-30 mg

Renal Impairment Not dialyzable (0% to 5%)

Administration Administer orally in divided doses.

Monitoring Parameters Respiratory and cardiovascular status

Reference Range Therapeutic: 0.2-1.4 mcg/mL (SI: 0.7-4.9 µmol/L)

Pharmacotherapy Pearls Not intended for management of anxieties and minor distresses associated with everyday life. Treatment longer than 4 months should be re-evaluated to determine the patient's need for the drug. Abrupt discontinuation after sustained use (generally >10 days) may cause withdrawal symptoms.

Special Geriatric Considerations Because of its relatively short half-life and its lack of active metabolites, oxazepam could be considered for use in the elderly when a benzodiazepine is indicated.

This medication is considered to be potentially inappropriate in this patient population (Beers Criteria severity: High).

Controlled Substance C-IV

Dosage Forms Excipient information presented when available (limited, particularly for generics); consult specific product labeling.

Capsule, oral: 10 mg, 15 mg, 30 mg

Selected References

Hicks R, Dysken MW, Davis JM, et al, "The Pharmacokinetics of Psychotropic Medication in the Elderly: A Review," *J Clin Psychiatry*, 1981, 42(10)374-85.

OXcarbazepine (ox car BAZ e peen)

Medication Safety Issues

Sound-alike/look-alike issues:

OXcarbazepine may be confused with carBAMazepine

Trileptal® may be confused with TriLipix™

Brand Names: U.S. Trileptal®

Brand Names: Canada Apo-Oxcarbazepine®; Trileptal®

Index Terms GP 47680; OCBZ

Generic Availability (U.S.) Yes

Pharmacologic Category Anticonvulsant, Miscellaneous

Use Monotherapy or adjunctive therapy in the treatment of partial seizures

Unlabeled/Investigational Use Bipolar disorder; treatment of neuropathic pain

Medication Guide Available Yes

Contraindications Hypersensitivity to oxcarbazepine or any component of the formulation

Warnings/Precautions Antiepileptics are associated with an increased risk of suicidal behavior/thoughts with use (regardless of indication); patients should be monitored for signs/symptoms of depression, suicidal tendencies, and other unusual behavior changes during therapy and instructed to inform their healthcare provider immediately if symptoms occur.

Clinically-significant hyponatremia (serum sodium <125 mmol/L) may develop during oxcarbazepine use. Rare cases of anaphylaxis and angioedema have been reported, even after initial dosing; permanently discontinue should symptoms occur. Use caution in patients with previous hypersensitivity to carbamazepine (cross-sensitivity occurs in 25% to 30%). Potentially serious, sometimes fatal, dermatologic reactions (eg, Stevens-Johnson, toxic epidermal necrolysis) and multiorgan hypersensitivity reactions have been reported in adults and children; monitor for signs and symptoms of skin reactions and possible disparate manifestations associated with lymphatic, hepatic, renal, and/or hematologic organ systems; discontinuation and conversion to alternate therapy may be required. As with all antiepileptic drugs, oxcarbazepine should be withdrawn gradually to minimize the potential of increased seizure frequency. Use of oxcarbazepine has been associated with CNS-related adverse events, most significant of these were cognitive symptoms including psychomotor slowing, difficulty with concentration, speech or language problems, somnolence or fatigue, and coordination abnormalities, including ataxia and gait disturbances. Effects with other sedative drugs or ethanol may be potentiated. Single-dose studies show that half-life of the primary active metabolite is prolonged 3-4 fold and AUC is doubled in patients with Cl_{cr} <30 mL/minute; dose adjustment required in these patients. May reduce the efficacy of oral contraceptives (nonhormonal contraceptive measures are recommended). Agranulocytosis, leukopenia, and pancytopenia have been reported with use (rare). Discontinuation and conversion to alternate therapy may be required.

Adverse Reactions (Reflective of adult population; not specific for elderly) As reported in adults with doses of up to 2400 mg/day (includes patients on monotherapy, adjunctive therapy, and those not previously on AEDs); incidence in children was similar.

>10%:
  Central nervous system: Dizziness (22% to 49%), somnolence (20% to 36%), headache (13% to 32%), ataxia (5% to 31%), fatigue (12% to 15%), vertigo (6% to 15%)
  Gastrointestinal: Vomiting (7% to 36%), nausea (15% to 29%), abdominal pain (10% to 13%)
  Neuromuscular & skeletal: Abnormal gait (5% to 17%), tremor (3% to 16%)
  Ocular: Diplopia (14% to 40%), nystagmus (7% to 26%), abnormal vision (4% to 14%)
1% to 10%:
  Cardiovascular: Hypotension (≤2%), leg edema (1% to 2%)
  Central nervous system: Nervousness (2% to 5%), amnesia (4%), abnormal thinking (≤4%), insomnia (2% to 4%), fever (3%), speech disorder (1% to 3%), abnormal feelings (≤2%), EEG abnormalities (≤2%), agitation (1% to 2%), confusion (1% to 2%)
  Dermatologic: Rash (4%), acne (1% to 2%)
  Endocrine & metabolic: Hyponatremia (1% to 3%)
  Gastrointestinal: Diarrhea (5% to 7%), dyspepsia (5% to 6%), constipation (2% to 6%), taste perversion (5%), xerostomia (3%), gastritis (1% to 2%), weight gain (1% to 2%)
  Genitourinary: Micturition (2%)
  Neuromuscular & skeletal: Weakness (3% to 6%), back pain (4%), falling down (4%), abnormal coordination (1% to 4%), dysmetria (1% to 3%), sprains/strains (≤2%), muscle weakness (1% to 2%)
  Ocular: Abnormal accommodation (≤2%)
  Respiratory: Upper respiratory tract infection (7%), rhinitis (2% to 5%), chest infection (4%), epistaxis (4%), sinusitis (4%)

Drug Interactions

Metabolism/Transport Effects Inhibits CYP2C19 (weak); **Induces** CYP3A4 (strong)

Avoid Concomitant Use

Avoid concomitant use of OXcarbazepine with any of the following: Crizotinib; Dronedarone; Everolimus; Lapatinib; Lurasidone; Nilotinib; Nisoldipine; Pazopanib; Praziquantel; Ranolazine; Rilpivirine; Roflumilast; RomiDEPsin; Selegiline; Ticagrelor; Tolvaptan; Vandetanib

Increased Effect/Toxicity

OXcarbazepine may increase the levels/effects of: Clarithromycin; Phenytoin; Selegiline

The levels/effects of OXcarbazepine may be increased by: Clarithromycin; Thiazide Diuretics

Decreased Effect

OXcarbazepine may decrease the levels/effects of: Brentuximab Vedotin; Clarithromycin; Contraceptives (Estrogens); Contraceptives (Progestins); Crizotinib; CYP3A4 Substrates; Dronedarone; Everolimus; Exemestane; Gefitinib; GuanFACINE; Imatinib; Ixabepilone; Lapatinib; Linagliptin; Lurasidone; Maraviroc; NIFEdipine; Nilotinib; Nisoldipine; Pazopanib; Praziquantel; Ranolazine; Rilpivirine; Rivaroxaban; Roflumilast; RomiDEPsin; Saxagliptin; SORAfenib; Tadalafil; Ticagrelor; Tolvaptan; Uliprital; Vandetanib; Vemurafenib

The levels/effects of OXcarbazepine may be decreased by: Divalproex; PHENobarbital; Phenytoin; Valproic Acid

Ethanol/Nutrition/Herb Interactions

Ethanol: Avoid ethanol (may increase CNS depression).
Herb/Nutraceutical: St John's wort may decrease oxcarbazepine levels. Avoid evening primrose (seizure threshold decreased). Avoid valerian, St John's wort, kava kava, gotu kola.

Stability Store tablets and suspension at 25°C (77°F). Use suspension within 7 weeks of first opening container.

◀ **Mechanism of Action** Pharmacological activity results from both oxcarbazepine and its monohydroxy metabolite (MHD). Precise mechanism of anticonvulsant effect has not been defined. Oxcarbazepine and MHD block voltage-sensitive sodium channels, stabilizing hyper-excited neuronal membranes, inhibiting repetitive firing, and decreasing the propagation of synaptic impulses. These actions are believed to prevent the spread of seizures. Oxcarba-zepine and MHD also increase potassium conductance and modulate the activity of high-voltage activated calcium channels.

Pharmacodynamics/Kinetics

Absorption: Complete; food has no affect on rate or extent

Distribution: MHD: V_d: 49 L

Protein binding, serum: MHD: 40% primarily to albumin

Metabolism: Hepatic to 10-monohydroxy metabolite (MHD; active); MHD is further glucur-onidated or oxidized to a 10,11-dihydroxy metabolite (DHD; inactive)

Bioavailability: Increased in elderly >60 years

Half-life elimination: Parent drug: 2 hours; MHD: 9 hours; renal impairment (Cl$_{cr}$ 30 mL/minute): MHD: 19 hours

Time to peak, serum (median): Tablets: 4.5 hours; oral suspension: 6 hours

Excretion: Urine (95%, <1% as unchanged oxcarbazepine, 27% as unchanged MHD, 49% as MHD glucuronides); feces (<4%)

Dosage

Geriatric & Adult

Adjunctive therapy, partial seizures (epilepsy): Oral: Initial: 600 mg/day in 2 divided doses; dosage may be increased by 600 mg/day at approximate weekly intervals. Recommended daily dose is 1200 mg/day in 2 divided doses. Although daily doses >1200 mg/day were somewhat more efficacious, most patients were unable to tolerate 2400 mg/day (due to CNS effects).

Conversion to monotherapy, partial seizures (epilepsy): Oral: Patients receiving con-comitant antiepileptic drugs (AEDs): Initial: 600 mg/day in 2 divided doses while simulta-neously reducing the dose of concomitant AEDs. Withdraw concomitant AEDs completely over 3-6 weeks, while increasing the oxcarbazine dose in increments of 600 mg/day at weekly intervals, reaching the maximum oxcarbazine dose (2400 mg/day) in about 2-4 weeks (lower doses have been effective in patients in whom monotherapy has been initiated).

Initiation of monotherapy, partial seizures (epilepsy): Oral: Patients not receiving prior AEDs: Initial: 600 mg/day in 2 divided doses. Increase dose by 300 mg/day every third day to a dose of 1200 mg/day. Higher dosages (2400 mg/day) have been shown to be effective in patients converted to monotherapy from other AEDs.

Renal Impairment Cl$_{cr}$ <30 mL/minute: Therapy should be initiated at one-half the usual starting dose (300 mg/day in adults) and increased slowly to achieve the desired clinical response

Hepatic Impairment Adjustment not needed for mild-to-moderate impairment. No data in patients with severe impairment.

Administration Suspension: Prior to using for the first time, firmly insert the plastic adapter provided with the bottle. Cover adapter with child-resistant cap when not in use. Shake bottle for at least 10 seconds, remove child-resistant cap and insert the oral dosing syringe provided to withdraw appropriate dose. Dose may be taken directly from oral syringe or may be mixed in a small glass of water immediately prior to swallowing. Rinse syringe with warm water after use and allow to dry thoroughly. Discard any unused portion after 7 weeks of first opening bottle.

Monitoring Parameters Seizure frequency, serum sodium as deemed necessary (particu-larly during first 3 months of therapy), symptoms of CNS depression (dizziness, headache, somnolence). Additional serum sodium monitoring recommended during maintenance treat-ment in patients receiving other medications known to decrease sodium levels, in patients with signs/symptoms of hyponatremia, and in patients with an increase in seizure frequency or severity. Monitor for suicidality (eg, suicidal thoughts, depression, behavioral changes). Serum levels of concomitant antiepileptic drugs during titration as necessary.

Test Interactions Thyroid function tests; may depress serum T_4 without affecting T_3 levels or TSH

Special Geriatric Considerations Studies in elderly volunteers (60-82 years of age) with both single dose (300 mg) and multiple doses (600 mg/day) reported maximum plasma concentrations and AUC as being 30% to 60% higher than younger volunteers (18-32 years of age). These results were due to differences in creatinine clearance between the two groups. Since elderly may have Cl$_{cr}$ <30 mL/minute, dose reductions may be needed.

Dosage Forms Excipient information presented when available (limited, particularly for generics); consult specific product labeling.
Suspension, oral: 300 mg/5 mL (250 mL)
  Trileptal®: 300 mg/5 mL (250 mL) [contains ethanol, propylene glycol]
Tablet, oral: 150 mg, 300 mg, 600 mg
  Trileptal®: 150 mg, 300 mg, 600 mg [scored]

Selected References
Carrazana E and Mikoshiba I, "Rationale and Evidence for the Use of Oxcarbazepine in Neuropathic Pain," *J Pain Symptom Manage*, 2003, 25(5 Suppl):S31-5.
Irving GA, "Contemporary Assessment and Management of Neuropathic Pain," *Neurology*, 2005, 64(12 Suppl 3): S21-7.

◆ **Oxecta™** see OxyCODONE on page 1368
◆ **Oxilapine Succinate** see Loxapine on page 1100
◆ **Oxpentifylline** see Pentoxifylline on page 1425
◆ **OXY® [OTC]** see Salicylic Acid on page 1648
◆ **OXY® Body Wash [OTC]** see Salicylic Acid on page 1648

Oxybutynin (oks i BYOO ti nin)

Related Information
Beers Criteria – Potentially Inappropriate Medications for Geriatrics on page 2089
Pharmacotherapy of Urinary Incontinence on page 2032

Medication Safety Issues
Sound-alike/look-alike issues:
Oxybutynin may be confused with OxyCONTIN®
Ditropan may be confused with Detrol®, diazepam, Diprivan®, dithranol
Beers Criteria medication:
This drug may be inappropriate for use in geriatric patients (high severity risk).
Other safety concerns:
Transdermal patch may contain conducting metal (eg, aluminum); remove patch prior to MRI.

Brand Names: U.S. Ditropan XL®; Gelnique®; Oxytrol®
Brand Names: Canada Apo-Oxybutynin®; Ditropan XL®; Dom-Oxybutynin; Mylan-Oxybutynin; Novo-Oxybutynin; Nu-Oxybutyn; Oxybutyn; Oxybutynine; Oxytrol®; PHL-Oxybutynin; PMS-Oxybutynin; Riva-Oxybutynin; Uromax®
Index Terms Ditropan; Oxybutynin Chloride
Generic Availability (U.S.) Yes: Excludes gel, transdermal patch
Pharmacologic Category Antispasmodic Agent, Urinary
Use Antispasmodic for neurogenic bladder (urgency, frequency, leakage, urge incontinence, dysuria); extended release formulation also indicated for treatment of symptoms associated with detrusor overactivity due to a neurological condition (eg, spina bifida)
Contraindications Hypersensitivity to oxybutynin or any component of the formulation; patients with or at risk for uncontrolled narrow-angle glaucoma, urinary retention, gastric retention or conditions with severely decreased GI motility
Warnings/Precautions Cases of angioedema have been reported with oral oxybutynin; some cases have occurred after a single dose. Discontinue immediately if develops. Use with caution in patients with bladder outflow obstruction, angle-closure glaucoma (treated), hyperthyroidism, reflux esophagitis (including concurrent therapy with oral bisphosphonates or drugs which may increase the risk of esophagitis), heart disease, hepatic or renal disease, prostatic hyperplasia, autonomic neuropathy, ulcerative colitis (may cause ileus and toxic megacolon), hypertension, hiatal hernia, myasthenia gravis, dementia, ulcerative colitis, or intestinal atony. May increase the risk of heat prostration. May cause anticholinergic effects (agitation, confusion, hallucinations, somnolence) which may require dose reduction or discontinuation of therapy. May cause CNS depression, which may impair physical or mental abilities; patients must be cautioned about performing tasks which require mental alertness (eg, operating machinery or driving).

This class of medication is poorly tolerated by the elderly due to anticholinergic effects, sedation, and weakness. Efficacy is questionable at dosages tolerated by elderly patients. Oxybutynin extended-release is considered an exception. (Beers Criteria).

The extended release formulation consists of drug within a nondeformable matrix; following drug release/absorption, the matrix/shell is expelled in the stool. The use of nondeformable products in patients with known stricture/narrowing of the GI tract has been associated with symptoms of obstruction. Transdermal patch may contain conducting metal (eg, aluminum); remove patch prior to MRI. When using the topical gel, cover treatment area with clothing after gel has dried to minimize transferring medication to others. Discontinue gel if skin irritation occurs. Gel contains ethanol; do not expose to open flame or smoking until gel has dried.

◀ **Adverse Reactions (Reflective of adult population; not specific for elderly)**
Oral:
>10%:
Central nervous system: Dizziness (4% to 17%), somnolence (2% to 14%)
Gastrointestinal: Xerostomia (29% to 71%; dose related), constipation (7% to 15%), nausea (2% to 12%)
5% to 10%:
Central nervous system: Headache (6% to 10%), pain (1% to 7%), nervousness (1% to 7%), insomnia (1% to 6%)
Gastrointestinal: Diarrhea (1% to 9%), dyspepsia (5% to 7%)
Genitourinary: Urinary hesitation (9%), urinary tract infection (5% to 7%), urinary retention (6%)
Neuromuscular & skeletal: Weakness (3% to 7%)
Ocular: Blurred vision (1% to 10%), dry eyes (3% to 6%)
Respiratory: Rhinitis (2% to 6%)

Topical gel:
1% to 10%:
Central nervous system: Dizziness (2% to 3%), fatigue (2%), headache (2%)
Dermatologic: Pruritus (1%)
Gastrointestinal: Xerostomia (7% to 8%), gastroenteritis (2%), constipation (1%)
Genitourinary: Urinary tract infection (7%)
Local: Application site reaction (5%; includes anesthesia, dermatitis, erythema, irritation, pain, papules, pruritus)
Respiratory: Nasopharyngitis (3%)

Transdermal:
>10%: Local: Application site reaction (17%), pruritus (14%)
1% to 10%:
Gastrointestinal: Xerostomia (4% to 10%), diarrhea (3%), constipation (3%)
Genitourinary: Dysuria (2%)
Local: Erythema (6% to 8%), vesicles (3%), rash (3%)
Ocular: Vision changes (3%)

Drug Interactions
Metabolism/Transport Effects Substrate of CYP3A4 (minor); **Inhibits** CYP2C8 (weak), 2D6 (weak), 3A4 (weak)
Avoid Concomitant Use There are no known interactions where it is recommended to avoid concomitant use.
Increased Effect/Toxicity
Oxybutynin may increase the levels/effects of: AbobotulinumtoxinA; Anticholinergics; Cannabinoids; OnabotulinumtoxinA; Potassium Chloride; RimabotulinumtoxinB

The levels/effects of Oxybutynin may be increased by: Conivaptan; Pramlintide
Decreased Effect
Oxybutynin may decrease the levels/effects of: Acetylcholinesterase Inhibitors (Central); Secretin

The levels/effects of Oxybutynin may be decreased by: Acetylcholinesterase Inhibitors (Central); Tocilizumab
Ethanol/Nutrition/Herb Interactions Ethanol: Use ethanol with caution (may increase CNS depression and toxicity). Watch for sedation.
Stability
Immediate release: Store at controlled room temperature of 15°C to 30°C (59°F to 86°F). Protect syrup from light.
Extended release: Store at 25°C (77°F); excursions permitted to 15°C to 30°C (59°F to 86°F). Protect from moisture and humidity.
Gel sachet, transdermal patch: Store at 25°C (77°F); excursions permitted to 15°C to 30°C (59°F to 86°F). Protect from moisture and humidity. Keel gel away from open flame. Keep patch in sealed pouch. Throw away used sachets or patches where children and pets cannot reach.
Mechanism of Action Direct antispasmodic effect on smooth muscle, also inhibits the action of acetylcholine on smooth muscle (exhibits $1/5$ the anticholinergic activity of atropine, but is 4-10 times the antispasmodic activity); does not block effects at skeletal muscle or at autonomic ganglia; increases bladder capacity, decreases uninhibited contractions, and delays desire to void, therefore, decreases urgency and frequency
Pharmacodynamics/Kinetics
Onset of action: Oral: 30-60 minutes
Peak effect: 3-6 hours
Duration: 6-10 hours (up to 24 hours for extended release oral formulation)

Absorption: Oral: Rapid and well absorbed; Transdermal: High

Distribution: I.V.: V_d: 193 L

Metabolism: Hepatic via CYP3A4; Oral: High first-pass metabolism; forms active and inactive metabolites

Bioavailability: Oral: ~6%

Half-life elimination: I.V.: ~2 hours (parent drug), 7-8 hours (metabolites); Oral: ~2-3 hours

Time to peak, serum: Oral: Immediate release: ~60 minutes; Extended release: 4-6 hours; Transdermal: 24-48 hours

Excretion: Urine, as metabolites and unchanged drug (<0.1%)

Dosage

Geriatric

Oral: Regular release: Initial dose: 2.5 mg 2-3 times/day; increase as needed to 5 mg 2-3 times/day

Topical gel, transdermal patch: Refer to adult dosing. **Note:** Should be discontinued periodically to determine whether the patient can manage without the drug and to minimize resistance to the drug.

Adult

Bladder spasms:

Oral:

Regular release: 5 mg 2-3 times/day up to maximum of 5 mg 4 times/day

Extended release: Initial: 5-10 mg once daily, adjust dose in 5 mg increments at weekly intervals; maximum: 30 mg daily

Topical gel: Apply contents of 1 sachet (100 mg/g) once daily

Transdermal: Apply one 3.9 mg/day patch twice weekly (every 3-4 days)

Note: Should be discontinued periodically to determine whether the patient can manage without the drug and to minimize resistance to the drug.

Administration

Oral: Immediate release tablets and solution should be administered on an empty stomach with water. Extended release tablets may be taken with or without food and must be swallowed whole; do not crush, divide, or chew.

Topical gel: For topical use only. Apply to clean, dry, intact skin on abdomen, thighs, or upper arms/shoulders. Rotate site; do not apply to same site on consecutive days. Wash hands after use. Cover treated area with clothing after gel has dried to prevent transfer of medication to others. Do not bathe, shower, or swim until 1 hour after gel applied. Use of sunscreens, before or after, does not affect absorption.

Transdermal: Apply to clean, dry skin on abdomen, hip, or buttock. Select a new site for each new system (avoid reapplication to same site within 7 days).

Monitoring Parameters Incontinence episodes, postvoid residual (PVR)

Test Interactions May suppress the wheal and flare reactions to skin test antigens.

Special Geriatric Considerations Caution should be used in the elderly due to anticholinergic activity (eg, confusion, constipation, blurred vision, and tachycardia). Start with lower doses. Transdermal dosage form may have less potential for these effects. Oxybutynin may cause memory problems in the elderly. A study of 12 healthy volunteers with an average age of 69 showed cognitive decline while taking the drug (*J Am Geriatr Soc*, 1998, L46:8-13). Studies using transdermal dosage form did not reveal any differences in safety or efficacy between elderly and younger adults.

This medication is considered to be potentially inappropriate in this patient population (Beers Criteria severity: High).

Dosage Forms Excipient information presented when available (limited, particularly for generics); consult specific product labeling.

Gel, topical, as chloride:

Gelnique®: 10% (1 g) [contains ethanol]

Patch, transdermal:

Oxytrol®: 3.9 mg/24 hours (8s) [39 cm²; total oxybutynin 36 mg]

Syrup, oral, as chloride: 5 mg/5 mL (5 mL, 473 mL)

Tablet, oral, as chloride: 5 mg

Tablet, extended release, oral, as chloride: 5 mg, 10 mg, 15 mg

Ditropan XL®: 5 mg, 10 mg, 15 mg

♦ **Oxybutynin Chloride** *see* Oxybutynin *on page 1365*

♦ **OXY® Chill Factor® [OTC]** *see* Salicylic Acid *on page 1648*

OxyCODONE (oks i KOE done)

Related Information
Opioid Analgesics *on page 2013*
Patient Information for Disposal of Unused Medications *on page 2125*
Medication Safety Issues
Sound-alike/look-alike issues:
OxyCODONE may be confused with HYDROcodone, OxyCONTIN®, oxymorphone
OxyCONTIN® may be confused with MS Contin®, oxybutynin, oxyCODONE
OxyFast® may be confused with Roxanol
Roxicodone® may be confused with Roxanol
High alert medication:
The Institute for Safe Medication Practices (ISMP) includes this medication among its list of drug classes which have a heightened risk of causing significant patient harm when used in error.
International issues:
Supeudol® [Canada] may be confused with Supadol Mono which is a brand name for acetaminophen in Luxembourg
Brand Names: U.S. OxyCONTIN®; Roxicodone®
Brand Names: Canada Oxy.IR®; OxyContin®; PMS-Oxycodone; Supeudol®
Index Terms Dihydrohydroxycodeinone; Oxecta™; Oxycodone Hydrochloride
Generic Availability (U.S.) Yes: Excludes liquid, controlled release tablet
Pharmacologic Category Analgesic, Opioid
Use Management of moderate-to-severe pain, normally used in combination with nonopioid analgesics

OxyContin® is indicated for around-the-clock management of moderate-to-severe pain when an analgesic is needed for an extended period of time.
Prescribing and Access Restrictions As a requirement of the REMS program, healthcare providers who prescribe OxyContin® need to receive training on the proper use and potential risks of OxyContin®. For training, please refer to http://www.oxycontinrems.com. Prescribers will need retraining every 2 years or following any significant changes to the OxyContin® REMS program.
Medication Guide Available Yes
Contraindications Hypersensitivity to oxycodone or any component of the formulation; significant respiratory depression; hypercarbia; acute or severe bronchial asthma; paralytic ileus (known or suspected)
Warnings/Precautions May cause CNS depression, which may impair physical or mental abilities; patients must be cautioned about performing tasks which require mental alertness (eg, operating machinery or driving). Effects may be potentiated when used with other sedative drugs or ethanol. Use with caution in patients with hypersensitivity reactions to other phenanthrene derivative opioid agonists (morphine, hydrocodone, hydromorphone, levorphanol, oxymorphone), respiratory diseases including asthma, emphysema, or COPD. Use with caution in pancreatitis or biliary tract disease, acute alcoholism (including delirium tremens), morbid obesity, adrenocortical insufficiency, history of seizure disorders, CNS depression/coma, kyphoscoliosis (or other skeletal disorder which may alter respiratory function), hypothyroidism (including myxedema), prostatic hyperplasia, urethral stricture, and toxic psychosis. May obscure diagnosis or clinical course of patients with acute abdominal conditions.

Use with caution in the elderly, debilitated, and hepatic or renal function. Hemodynamic effects (hypotension, orthostasis) may be exaggerated in patients with hypovolemia, concurrent vasodilating drugs, or in patients with head injury. Respiratory depressant effects and capacity to elevate CSF pressure may be exaggerated in presence of head injury, other intracranial lesion, or pre-existing intracranial pressure.

[U.S. Boxed Warning]: Concomitant use with CYP3A4 inhibitors may result in increased effects and potentially fatal respiratory depression. Concurrent use of agonist/antagonist analgesics may precipitate withdrawal symptoms and/or reduced analgesic efficacy in patients following prolonged therapy with mu opioid agonists. Abrupt discontinuation following prolonged use may also lead to withdrawal symptoms. **[U.S. Boxed Warning]: Healthcare provider should be alert to problems of abuse, misuse, and diversion.** Tolerance or drug dependence may result from extended use. Patients should be assessed for risk of abuse or addition prior to therapy and all patients should be monitored for signs of misuse, abuse, and addiction.

Controlled-release formulations: [U.S. Boxed Warning]: OxyContin® is not intended for use as an "as needed" analgesic or for immediately-postoperative pain management (should be used postoperatively only if the patient has received it prior to surgery or if severe, persistent pain is anticipated). **[U.S. Boxed Warning]: Do NOT crush, break, or chew controlled-release tablets**; 60 mg and 80 mg strengths, a single dose >40 mg, or a total dose of >80 mg/day are for use only in opioid-tolerant patients.

Adverse Reactions (Reflective of adult population; not specific for elderly) Note: Percentages as reported with OxyContin®

>10%:

Central nervous system: Somnolence (23%), dizziness (13%)

Dermatologic: Pruritus (13%)

Gastrointestinal: Constipation (23%), nausea (23%), vomiting (12%)

1% to 10%:

Cardiovascular: Postural hypotension (1% to 5%)

Central nervous system: Headache (7%), abnormal dreams (1% to 5%), anxiety (1% to 5%), chills (1% to 5%), confusion (1% to 5%), dysphoria (1% to 5%), euphoria (1% to 5%), fever (1% to 5%), insomnia (1% to 5%), nervousness (1% to 5%), thought abnormalities (1% to 5%)

Dermatologic: Rash (1% to 5%)

Gastrointestinal: Xerostomia (6%), abdominal pain (1% to 5%), anorexia (1% to 5%), diarrhea (1% to 5%), dyspepsia (1% to 5%), gastritis (1% to 5%)

Neuromuscular & skeletal: Weakness (6%), twitching (1% to 5%)

Respiratory: Dyspnea (1% to 5%), hiccups (1% to 5%)

Miscellaneous: Diaphoresis (5%)

Drug Interactions

Metabolism/Transport Effects Substrate of CYP2D6 (minor), 3A4 (major)

Avoid Concomitant Use

Avoid concomitant use of OxyCODONE with any of the following: Conivaptan

Increased Effect/Toxicity

OxyCODONE may increase the levels/effects of: Alcohol (Ethyl); Alvimopan; CNS Depressants; Desmopressin; Selective Serotonin Reuptake Inhibitors; Thiazide Diuretics

The levels/effects of OxyCODONE may be increased by: Amphetamines; Antipsychotic Agents (Phenothiazines); Conivaptan; CYP3A4 Inhibitors (Moderate); CYP3A4 Inhibitors (Strong); Dasatinib; Droperidol; HydrOXYzine; Succinylcholine; Voriconazole

Decreased Effect

OxyCODONE may decrease the levels/effects of: Pegvisomant

The levels/effects of OxyCODONE may be decreased by: Ammonium Chloride; CYP3A4 Inducers (Strong); Deferasirox; Mixed Agonist / Antagonist Opioids; Rifampin; St Johns Wort; Tocilizumab

Ethanol/Nutrition/Herb Interactions

Ethanol: May increase CNS depression; monitor for increased effects with coadministration. Caution patients about effects.

Herb/Nutraceutical: Avoid valerian, St John's wort, kava kava, gotu kola (may increase CNS depression).

Stability Store at 25°C (77°F); excursions permitted between 15°C to 30°C (59°F to 86°F). Protect from light.

Mechanism of Action Binds to opiate receptors in the CNS, causing inhibition of ascending pain pathways, altering the perception of and response to pain; produces generalized CNS depression

Pharmacodynamics/Kinetics

Onset of action: Pain relief: Immediate release: 10-15 minutes

Peak effect: Immediate release: 0.5-1 hour

Duration: Immediate release: 3-6 hours; Controlled release: ≤12 hours

Distribution: V_d: 2.6 L/kg; distributed to skeletal muscle, liver, intestinal tract, lungs, spleen, and brain

Protein binding: ~45%

Metabolism: Hepatically via CYP3A4 to noroxycodone (has weak analgesic), noroxymorphone, and alpha- and beta-noroxycodol. CYP2D6 mediated metabolism produces oxymorphone (has analgesic activity; low plasma concentrations), alpha- and beta-oxymorphol.

Bioavailability: Controlled release, immediate release: 60% to 87%

Half-life elimination: Immediate release: 2-3 hours; controlled release: ~5 hours

Time to peak, plasma: Immediate release: 1.4-1.9 hours; Controlled release: 4-5 hours

Excretion: Urine (~19% as parent; >64% as metabolites)

Dosage

Geriatric & Adult Management of pain: Oral:

Regular or immediate release formulations: Initial: 5-15 mg every 4-6 hours as needed; dosing range: 5-20 mg/dose (APS 6th edition). For severe chronic pain, administer on a regularly scheduled basis, every 4-6 hours, at the lowest dose that will achieve adequate analgesia.

OXYCODONE

Controlled release:

Opioid-naïve: 10 mg every 12 hours

Concurrent CNS depressants: Reduce usual dose by ⅓ to ½

Conversion from transdermal fentanyl: For each 25 mcg/hour transdermal dose, substitute 10 mg controlled release oxycodone every 12 hours; should be initiated 18 hours after the removal of the transdermal fentanyl patch

Currently on opioids: Use standard conversion chart to convert daily dose to oxycodone equivalent. Divide daily dose in 2 (for twice-daily dosing, usually every 12 hours) and round down to nearest dosage form.

Dose adjustment: Doses may be adjusted by changing the total daily dose (not by changing the dosing interval). Doses may be adjusted every 1-2 days and may be increased by 25% to 50%. Dose should be gradually tapered when no longer required in order to prevent withdrawal.

Note: 60 mg and 80 mg strengths, a single dose >40 mg, or a total dose of >80 mg/day are for use only in opioid-tolerant patients.

Multiplication factors for converting the daily dose of current oral opioid to the daily dose of oral oxycodone:

Current opioid mg/day dose x factor = Oxycodone mg/day dose

Codeine mg/day oral dose **x** 0.15 = Oxycodone mg/day dose

Hydrocodone mg/day oral dose **x** 0.9 = Oxycodone mg/day dose

Hydromorphone mg/day oral dose **x** 4 = Oxycodone mg/day dose

Levorphanol mg/day oral dose **x** 7.5 = Oxycodone mg/day dose

Meperidine mg/day oral dose **x** 0.1 = Oxycodone mg/day dose

Methadone mg/day oral dose **x** 1.5 = Oxycodone mg/day dose

Morphine mg/day oral dose **x** 0.5 = Oxycodone mg/day dose

Note: Divide the oxycodone mg/day dose into the appropriate dosing interval for the specific form being used.

Renal Impairment Serum concentrations are increased ~50% in patients with Cl_{cr} <60 mL/minute; adjust dose based on clinical situation.

Hepatic Impairment Reduce dosage in patients with liver disease. Decrease the dose of controlled release tablets to ⅓ to ½ the usual starting dose; titrate carefully.

Administration Do not crush, break, or chew controlled release tablets. Controlled release tablets are not indicated for rectal administration; increased risk of adverse events due to better rectal absorption. Controlled release tablets should be administered one at a time and each followed with water immediately after placing in the mouth.

Appropriate laxatives should be administered to avoid the constipating side effects associated with use. Antiemetics may be needed for persistent nausea.

Monitoring Parameters Pain relief, respiratory and mental status, blood pressure; signs of misuse, abuse, and addiction

Reference Range Blood level of 5 mg/L associated with fatality

Test Interactions Some quinolones may produce a false-positive urine screening result for opiates using commercially-available immunoassay kits. This has been demonstrated most consistently for levofloxacin and ofloxacin, but other quinolones have shown cross-reactivity in certain assay kits. Confirmation of positive opiate screens by more specific methods should be considered.

Special Geriatric Considerations The elderly may be particularly susceptible to the CNS depressant and constipating effects of narcotics. Prophylactic use of a laxative should be considered. Serum concentrations at a given dose may also be increased relative to concentrations in younger patients.

Product Availability

Oxecta™: FDA approved June 2011; availability expected late third quarter 2011 or early fourth quarter 2011.

Oxecta™ is an immediate release tablet formulation of oxycodone that uses technology designed to discourage common methods of tampering that may help decrease opioid abuse and misuse.

Controlled Substance C-II

Dosage Forms Excipient information presented when available (limited, particularly for generics); consult specific product labeling. [DSC] = Discontinued product

Capsule, oral, as hydrochloride: 5 mg

Liquid, oral, as hydrochloride [concentrate]:

Roxicodone®: 20 mg/mL (30 mL [DSC]) [contains sodium benzoate]

Solution, oral, as hydrochloride: 5 mg/5 mL (100 mL [DSC], 500 mL [DSC])

Roxicodone®: 5 mg/5 mL (5 mL [DSC], 500 mL [DSC]) [contains ethanol]

Solution, oral, as hydrochloride [concentrate]: 20 mg/mL (30 mL)

Tablet, oral, as hydrochloride: 5 mg, 10 mg, 15 mg, 20 mg, 30 mg
  Roxicodone®: 5 mg, 15 mg, 30 mg [scored]
Tablet, controlled release, oral, as hydrochloride:
  OxyCONTIN®: 10 mg, 15 mg, 20 mg, 30 mg, 40 mg, 60 mg, 80 mg

Selected References

American Geriatrics Society Panel on Pharmacological Management of Persistent Pain in Older Persons, "Pharmacological Management of Persistent Pain in Older Persons," *J Am Geriatr Soc*, 2009, 57(8):1331-46.

Oxycodone and Acetaminophen (oks i KOE done & a seet a MIN oh fen)

Related Information

Acetaminophen *on page 33*
Opioid Analgesics *on page 2013*
OxyCODONE *on page 1368*
Patient Information for Disposal of Unused Medications *on page 2125*

Medication Safety Issues

Sound-alike/look-alike issues:
  Endocet® may be confused with Indocid®
  Percocet® may be confused with Darvocet®, Fioricet®, Percodan®
  Roxicet™ may be confused with Roxanol
  Tylox® may be confused with Trimox®, Tylenol®, Wymox®, Xanax®

High alert medication:
  The Institute for Safe Medication Practices (ISMP) includes this medication among its list of drug classes which have a heightened risk of causing significant patient harm when used in error.

Other safety concerns:
  Duplicate therapy issues: This product contains acetaminophen, which may be a component of other combination products. Do not exceed the maximum recommended daily dose of acetaminophen.

Brand Names: U.S. Endocet®; Percocet®; Primlev™; Roxicet™; Roxicet™ 5/500; Tylox®

Brand Names: Canada Endocet®; Novo-Oxycodone Acet; Oxycocet®; Percocet®; Percocet®-Demi; PMS-Oxycodone-Acetaminophen

Index Terms Acetaminophen and Oxycodone

Generic Availability (U.S.) Yes: Excludes caplet and solution

Pharmacologic Category Analgesic, Opioid

Use Management of moderate-to-severe pain

Contraindications Hypersensitivity to oxycodone, acetaminophen, or any component of the formulation; severe respiratory depression (in absence of resuscitative equipment or ventilatory support)

Warnings/Precautions Use with caution in patients with hypersensitivity reactions to other phenanthrene-derivative opioid agonists (morphine, codeine, hydrocodone, hydromorphone, levorphanol, oxymorphone); respiratory diseases including asthma, emphysema, COPD; severe liver or renal insufficiency; hypothyroidism; Addison's disease; seizure disorder; toxic psychosis; morbid obesity; CNS depression/coma; biliary tract impairment; prostatic hyperplasia; or urethral stricture. May obscure diagnosis or clinical course of patients with acute abdominal conditions. Some preparations contain sulfites which may cause allergic reactions. May be habit-forming. Causes sedation; caution must be used in performing tasks which require alertness (eg, operating machinery or driving). Effects may be potentiated when used with other sedative drugs or ethanol. May cause hypotension. Concurrent use of agonist/antagonist analgesics may precipitate withdrawal symptoms and/or reduced analgesic efficacy in patients following prolonged therapy with mu opioid agonists. Abrupt discontinuation following prolonged use may also lead to withdrawal symptoms.

Use with caution in patients with head injury and increased intracranial pressure (respiratory depressant effects increased and may also elevate CSF pressure).

Enhanced analgesia has been seen in elderly and debilitated patients on therapeutic doses of narcotics. Duration of action may be increased in the elderly. The elderly may be particularly susceptible to the CNS depressant and constipating effects of narcotics.

[U.S. Boxed Warning]: Acetaminophen may cause severe hepatotoxicity, potentially requiring liver transplant or resulting in death; hepatotoxicity is usually associated with excessive acetaminophen intake (>4 g/day). Risk is increased with alcohol use, preexisting liver disease, and intake of more than one source of acetaminophen-containing medications. Chronic daily dosing in adults has also resulted in liver damage in some patients. Hypersensitivity and anaphylactic reactions have been reported with acetaminophen use; discontinue immediately if symptoms of allergic or hypersensitivity reactions occur. Use with caution in patients with known G6PD deficiency.

◀ **Adverse Reactions (Reflective of adult population; not specific for elderly)** Frequency not defined (also see individual agents): Allergic reaction, constipation, dizziness, dysphoria, euphoria, lightheadedness, nausea, pruritus, respiratory depression, sedation, skin rash, vomiting

Drug Interactions

Metabolism/Transport Effects

Oxycodone: **Substrate** of CYP2D6 (minor), 3A4 (major)

Acetaminophen: **Substrate** (minor) of CYP1A2, 2A6, 2C9, 2D6, 2E1, 3A4

Avoid Concomitant Use

Avoid concomitant use of Oxycodone and Acetaminophen with any of the following: Conivaptan

Increased Effect/Toxicity

Oxycodone and Acetaminophen may increase the levels/effects of: Alcohol (Ethyl); Alvimopan; CNS Depressants; Dasatinib; Desmopressin; Imatinib; Selective Serotonin Reuptake Inhibitors; SORAfenib; Thiazide Diuretics; Vitamin K Antagonists

The levels/effects of Oxycodone and Acetaminophen may be increased by: Amphetamines; Antipsychotic Agents (Phenothiazines); Conivaptan; CYP3A4 Inhibitors (Moderate); CYP3A4 Inhibitors (Strong); Dasatinib; Droperidol; HydrOXYzine; Imatinib; Isoniazid; Metyrapone; Probenecid; SORAfenib; Succinylcholine; Voriconazole

Decreased Effect

Oxycodone and Acetaminophen may decrease the levels/effects of: Pegvisomant

The levels/effects of Oxycodone and Acetaminophen may be decreased by: Ammonium Chloride; Anticonvulsants (Hydantoin); Barbiturates; CarBAMazepine; Cholestyramine Resin; CYP3A4 Inducers (Strong); Cyproterone; Deferasirox; Mixed Agonist / Antagonist Opioids; Peginterferon Alfa-2b; Rifampin; St Johns Wort; Tocilizumab

Ethanol/Nutrition/Herb Interactions Ethanol: Excessive intake of ethanol may increase the risk of acetaminophen-induced hepatotoxicity. Avoid ethanol or limit to <3 drinks/day. Ethanol may also increase CNS depression; monitor for increased effects with co-administration. Caution patients about effects.

Stability Store at controlled room temperature of 20°C to 25°C (68°F to 77°F). Protect from moisture.

Mechanism of Action

Oxycodone, as with other narcotic (opiate) analgesics, blocks pain perception in the cerebral cortex by binding to specific receptor molecules (opiate receptors) within the neuronal membranes of synapses. This binding results in a decreased synaptic chemical transmission throughout the CNS thus inhibiting the flow of pain sensations into the higher centers. Mu and kappa are the two subtypes of the opiate receptor to which oxycodone binds to cause analgesia.

Acetaminophen inhibits the synthesis of prostaglandins in the CNS and peripherally blocks pain impulse generation; produces antipyresis from inhibition of hypothalamic heat-regulating center.

Pharmacodynamics/Kinetics See individual agents.

Dosage

Geriatric Doses should be titrated to appropriate analgesic effects: Oral: Initial dose, **based on oxycodone content:** 2.5-5 mg every 6 hours. Do not exceed 4 g/day of acetaminophen.

Adult

Note: Initial dose is based on the **oxycodone** content; however, the maximum daily dose is based on the **acetaminophen** content.

Management of pain: Doses should be given every 4-6 hours as needed and titrated to appropriate analgesic effects.

Maximum daily dose, based on acetaminophen content: Oral: 4 g/day.

Mild-to-moderate pain: Oral: Initial dose, **based on oxycodone content:** 2.5-5 mg

Severe pain: Oral: Initial dose, **based on oxycodone content:** 10-30 mg

Hepatic Impairment Dose should be reduced in patients with severe liver disease.

Monitoring Parameters Monitor for pain relief, respiratory and mental status, blood pressure, constipation

Special Geriatric Considerations The elderly may be particularly susceptible to the CNS depressant and constipating effects of narcotics. Prophylactic use of a laxative should be considered.

Controlled Substance C-II

Dosage Forms Excipient information presented when available (limited, particularly for generics); consult specific product labeling.

Caplet:

Roxicet™ 5/500: Oxycodone hydrochloride 5 mg and acetaminophen 500 mg

Capsule: 5/500: Oxycodone hydrochloride 5 mg and acetaminophen 500 mg
  Tylox®: 5/500: Oxycodone hydrochloride 5 mg and acetaminophen 500 mg [contains sodium benzoate and sodium metabisulfite]
Solution, oral:
  Roxicet™: Oxycodone hydrochloride 5 mg and acetaminophen 325 mg per 5 mL (5 mL, 500 mL) [contains ethanol <0.5%; mint flavor]
Tablet: 2.5/325: Oxycodone hydrochloride 2.5 mg and acetaminophen 325 mg; 5/325: Oxycodone hydrochloride 5 mg and acetaminophen 325 mg; 7.5/325: Oxycodone hydrochloride 7.5 mg and acetaminophen 325 mg; 7.5/500: Oxycodone hydrochloride 7.5 mg and acetaminophen 500 mg; 10/325: Oxycodone hydrochloride 10 mg and acetaminophen 325 mg; 10/650: Oxycodone hydrochloride 10 mg and acetaminophen 650 mg
  Endocet® 5/325 [scored]: Oxycodone hydrochloride 5 mg and acetaminophen 325 mg
  Endocet® 7.5/325: Oxycodone hydrochloride 7.5 mg and acetaminophen 325 mg
  Endocet® 7.5/500: Oxycodone hydrochloride 7.5 mg and acetaminophen 500 mg
  Endocet® 10/325: Oxycodone hydrochloride 10 mg and acetaminophen 325 mg
  Endocet® 10/650: Oxycodone hydrochloride 10 mg and acetaminophen 650 mg
  Percocet® 2.5/325: Oxycodone hydrochloride 2.5 mg and acetaminophen 325 mg
  Percocet® 5/325 [scored]: Oxycodone hydrochloride 5 mg and acetaminophen 325 mg
  Percocet® 7.5/325: Oxycodone hydrochloride 7.5 mg and acetaminophen 325 mg
  Percocet® 7.5/500: Oxycodone hydrochloride 7.5 mg and acetaminophen 500 mg
  Percocet® 10/325: Oxycodone hydrochloride 10 mg and acetaminophen 325 mg
  Percocet® 10/650: Oxycodone hydrochloride 10 mg and acetaminophen 650 mg
  Primlev™ 5/300: Oxycodone hydrochloride 5 mg and acetaminophen 300 mg
  Primlev™ 7.5/300: Oxycodone hydrochloride 7.5 mg and acetaminophen 300 mg
  Primlev™ 10/300: Oxycodone hydrochloride 10 mg and acetaminophen 300 mg
  Roxicet™ [scored]: Oxycodone hydrochloride 5 mg and acetaminophen 325 mg

Selected References
American Geriatrics Society Panel on Pharmacological Management of Persistent Pain in Older Persons, "Pharmacological Management of Persistent Pain in Older Persons," *J Am Geriatr Soc*, 2009, 57(8):1331-46.

Oxycodone and Aspirin (oks i KOE done & AS pir in)

Related Information
Aspirin *on page 153*
Opioid Analgesics *on page 2013*
OxyCODONE *on page 1368*
Patient Information for Disposal of Unused Medications *on page 2125*

Medication Safety Issues
Sound-alike/look-alike issues:
  Percodan® may be confused with Decadron®, Percocet®, Percogesic®, Periactin®
High alert medication:
  The Institute for Safe Medication Practices (ISMP) includes this medication among its list of drug classes which have a heightened risk of causing significant patient harm when used in error.

Brand Names: U.S. Endodan®; Percodan®
Brand Names: Canada Endodan®; Oxycodan®; Percodan®
Index Terms Aspirin and Oxycodone
Generic Availability (U.S.) Yes
Pharmacologic Category Analgesic, Opioid
Use Management of moderate- to moderately-severe pain
Dosage
  Geriatric & Adult Analgesic: Oral: One tablet every 6 hours as needed for pain; maximum aspirin dose should not exceed 4 g/day.
  Renal Impairment Use with caution. Avoid use of aspirin in patients with Cl_{cr} <10 mL/minute.
  Hepatic Impairment Use with caution. Avoid use of aspirin-containing products in severe impairment.
Special Geriatric Considerations Enhanced analgesia has been seen in the elderly patients on therapeutic doses of narcotics; duration of action may be increased. Elderly may be particularly susceptible to the CNS depressant and constipating effects of narcotics.
Controlled Substance C-II
Dosage Forms Excipient information presented when available (limited, particularly for generics); consult specific product labeling.
  Tablet: Oxycodone hydrochloride 4.5 mg, oxycodone terephthalate 0.38 mg, and aspirin 325 mg
  Endodan®, Percodan®: Oxycodone hydrochloride 4.8355 mg and aspirin 325 mg

♦ **Oxycodone Hydrochloride** *see* OxyCODONE *on page 1368*
♦ **OxyCONTIN®** *see* OxyCODONE *on page 1368*
♦ **OXY® Daily [OTC]** *see* Salicylic Acid *on page 1648*
♦ **OXY® Daily Cleansing [OTC]** *see* Salicylic Acid *on page 1648*
♦ **OXY® Face Wash [OTC]** *see* Salicylic Acid *on page 1648*
♦ **OXY® Maximum [OTC]** *see* Salicylic Acid *on page 1648*
♦ **OXY® Maximum Daily Cleansing [OTC]** *see* Salicylic Acid *on page 1648*

Oxymetazoline (Nasal) (oks i met AZ oh leen)

Medication Safety Issues
Sound-alike/look-alike issues:
Oxymetazoline may be confused with oxymetholone
Afrin® may be confused with aspirin
Afrin® (oxymetazoline) may be confused with Afrin® (saline)
Neo-Synephrine® (oxymetazoline) may be confused with Neo-Synephrine® (phenylephrine, nasal)

Brand Names: U.S. 12 Hour Nasal Relief [OTC]; 4-Way® 12 Hour [OTC]; Afrin® Extra Moisturizing [OTC]; Afrin® Original [OTC]; Afrin® Severe Congestion [OTC]; Afrin® Sinus [OTC]; Dristan® [OTC]; Duramist Plus [OTC]; Neo-Synephrine® Nighttime12-Hour [OTC]; Nostrilla® [OTC]; NRS® [OTC]; Sudafed OM® Sinus Congestion [DSC]; Vicks® Sinex® VapoSpray 12-Hour; Vicks® Sinex® VapoSpray 12-Hour UltraFine Mist [OTC]; Vicks® Sinex® VapoSpray Moisturizing 12-Hour UltraFine Mist [OTC]

Brand Names: Canada Claritin® Allergic Decongestant; Dristan® Long Lasting Nasal; Drixoral® Nasal

Index Terms Oxymetazoline Hydrochloride

Generic Availability (U.S.) Yes: Intranasal solution (spray)

Pharmacologic Category Adrenergic Agonist Agent; Imidazoline Derivative

Use Adjunctive therapy for nasal congestion, associated with acute or chronic rhinitis, the common cold, sinusitis, hay fever, or other allergies

Dosage
Geriatric & Adult Nasal congestion: Intranasal: Instill 2-3 sprays into each nostril twice daily for ≤3 days

Special Geriatric Considerations Evaluate the patient's or caregiver's ability to safely administer the correct dose. Use with caution in patients with cardiovascular disease.

Dosage Forms Excipient information presented when available (limited, particularly for generics); consult specific product labeling. [DSC] = Discontinued product
Solution, intranasal, as hydrochloride [mist]:
Afrin® Original: 0.05% (15 mL) [contains benzalkonium chloride]
Vicks® Sinex® VapoSpray 12-Hour UltraFine Mist: 0.05% (15 mL) [contains benzalkonium chloride, menthol]
Vicks® Sinex® VapoSpray Moisturizing 12-Hour UltraFine Mist: 0.05% (15 mL) [contains aloe, benzalkonium chloride]
Solution, intranasal, as hydrochloride [mist/no drip formula]:
Afrin® Extra Moisturizing: 0.05% (15 mL) [contains benzyl alcohol, glycerin]
Afrin® Original: 0.05% (15 mL) [contains benzalkonium chloride, benzyl alcohol]
Afrin® Severe Congestion: 0.05% (15 mL) [contains benzalkonium chloride, benzyl alcohol, camphor, menthol]
Afrin® Sinus: 0.05% (15 mL) [contains benzalkonium chloride, benzyl alcohol, camphor, menthol]
Solution, intranasal, as hydrochloride [spray]: 0.05% (15 mL, 30 mL)
12 Hour Nasal Relief: 0.05% (15 mL, 30 mL)
4-Way® 12 Hour: 0.05% (15 mL) [contains benzalkonium chloride]
Afrin® Extra Moisturizing: 0.05% (15 mL) [contains benzalkonium chloride, glycerin]
Afrin® Original: 0.05% (15 mL, 30 mL) [contains benzalkonium chloride]
Afrin® Severe Congestion: 0.05% (15 mL) [contains benzalkonium chloride, benzyl alcohol, camphor, menthol]
Afrin® Sinus: 0.05% (15 mL) [contains benzalkonium chloride, benzyl alcohol, camphor, menthol]
Dristan®: 0.05% (15 mL) [contains benzalkonium chloride, benzyl alcohol]
Duramist Plus: 0.05% (15 mL) [contains benzalkonium chloride]
Neo-Synephrine® Nighttime12-Hour: 0.05% (15 mL) [contains benzalkonium chloride, glycerin]
Nostrilla®: 0.05% (15 mL) [contains benzalkonium chloride]
NRS®: 0.05% (15 mL, 30 mL) [contains benzalkonium chloride]

Sudafed OM® Sinus Congestion: 0.05% (15 mL [DSC]) [contains benzalkonium chloride, glycerin]

Vicks® Sinex® VapoSpray 12-Hour: 0.05% (15 mL) [contains benzalkonium chloride]

Oxymetazoline (Ophthalmic) (oks i met AZ oh leen)

Medication Safety Issues
Sound-alike/look-alike issues:
Oxymetazoline may be confused with oxymetholone
Visine® may be confused with Visken®

Brand Names: U.S. Visine® L.R.® [OTC]

Index Terms Oxymetazoline Hydrochloride

Pharmacologic Category Vasoconstrictor

Use Relief of redness of eye due to minor eye irritations

Dosage
Geriatric & Adult Relief of eye redness: Ophthalmic: Instill 1-2 drops in affected eye(s) every 6 hours as needed or as directed by healthcare provider for ≤72 hours

Special Geriatric Considerations Evaluate the patient's or caregiver's ability to safely administer the correct dose of ophthalmic medication.

Dosage Forms Excipient information presented when available (limited, particularly for generics); consult specific product labeling.
Solution, ophthalmic, as hydrochloride [drops]:
Visine® L.R.®: 0.025% (15 mL, 30 mL) [contains benzalkonium chloride]

◆ **Oxymetazoline Hydrochloride** see Oxymetazoline (Nasal) on page 1374
◆ **Oxymetazoline Hydrochloride** see Oxymetazoline (Ophthalmic) on page 1375

Oxymorphone (oks i MOR fone)

Related Information
Opioid Analgesics on page 2013
Patient Information for Disposal of Unused Medications on page 2125

Medication Safety Issues
Sound-alike/look-alike issues:
Oxymorphone may be confused with oxycodone, oxymetholone

High alert medication:
The Institute for Safe Medication Practices (ISMP) includes this medication among its list of drug classes which have a heightened risk of causing significant patient harm when used in error.

Brand Names: U.S. Opana®; Opana® ER

Index Terms Oxymorphone Hydrochloride

Generic Availability (U.S.) Yes: Excludes injection solution

Pharmacologic Category Analgesic, Opioid

Use
Parenteral: Management of moderate-to-severe acute pain; relief of anxiety in patients with dyspnea associated with pulmonary edema secondary to acute left ventricular failure
Oral, regular release: Management of moderate-to-severe acute pain
Oral, extended release: Management of moderate-to-severe pain in patients requiring around-the-clock opioid treatment for an extended period of time

Contraindications Hypersensitivity to oxymorphone, other morphine analogs (phenanthrene derivatives), or any component of the formulation; paralytic ileus (known or suspected); moderate-to-severe hepatic impairment; severe respiratory depression (unless in monitored setting with resuscitative equipment); acute/severe bronchial asthma; hypercarbia

Note: Injection formulation is also contraindicated in the treatment of upper airway obstruction and pulmonary edema due to a chemical respiratory irritant.

Warnings/Precautions An opioid-containing analgesic regimen should be tailored to each patient's needs and based upon the type of pain being treated (acute versus chronic), the route of administration, degree of tolerance for opioids (naive versus chronic user), age, weight, and medical condition. The optimal analgesic dose varies widely among patients. Doses should be titrated to pain relief/prevention.

May cause CNS depression, which may impair physical or mental abilities; patients must be cautioned about performing tasks which require mental alertness (eg, operating machinery or driving). Effects may be potentiated when used with other sedative drugs or ethanol. Use not recommended within 14 days of MAO inhibitors. Use with caution in patients with hypersensitivity reactions to other phenanthrene-derivative opioid agonists (codeine, hydrocodone, hydromorphone, levorphanol, oxycodone). May cause respiratory depression. Use extreme

◀ caution in patients with COPD or other chronic respiratory conditions characterized by hypoxia, hypercapnia, or diminished respiratory reserve (myxedema, cor pulmonale, kyphoscoliosis, obstructive sleep apnea, severe obesity. Use with caution in patients (particularly elderly or debilitated) with impaired respiratory function, adrenal disease, morbid obesity, seizure disorders, toxic psychosis, thyroid dysfunction, prostatic hyperplasia, or renal impairment. Use caution in mild hepatic dysfunction; use is contraindicated in moderate-to-severe hepatic impairment. Use only with extreme caution (if at all) in patients with head injury or increased intracranial pressure (ICP); potential to elevate ICP and/or blunt papillary response may be greatly exaggerated in these patients. Use with caution in biliary tract disease or acute pancreatitis (may cause constriction of sphincter of Oddi). May obscure diagnosis or clinical course of patients with acute abdominal conditions.

Oxymorphone shares the toxic potential of opiate agonists and usual precautions of opiate agonist therapy should be observed; may cause hypotension in patients with acute myocardial infarction, volume depletion, or concurrent drug therapy which may exaggerate vasodilation. The elderly may be particularly susceptible to adverse effects of narcotics.

[U.S. Boxed Warning]: Healthcare provider should be alert to problems of abuse, misuse, and diversion. Tolerance or drug dependence may result from extended use. Use caution in patients with a history of drug dependence or abuse. Abrupt discontinuation may precipitate withdrawal syndrome.

Extended release formulation:

[U.S. Boxed Warnings]: Opana® ER is an extended release oral formulation of oxymorphone and is not suitable for use as an "as needed" analgesic. Tablets should not be broken, chewed, dissolved, or crushed; tablets should be swallowed whole. Opana® ER is intended for use in long-term, continuous management of moderate-to-severe chronic pain. It is not indicated for use in the immediate postoperative period (12-24 hours). **[U.S. Boxed Warning]: The coingestion of ethanol or ethanol-containing medications with Opana® ER may result in accelerated release of drug from the dosage form, abruptly increasing plasma levels, which may have fatal consequences.**

Adverse Reactions (Reflective of adult population; not specific for elderly) Incidence usually on higher end with extended release tablet.
>10%:
  Central nervous system: Somnolence (9% to 19%), dizziness (7% to 18%), fever (1% to 14%), headache (7% to 12%)
  Dermatologic: Pruritus (8% to 15%)
  Gastrointestinal: Nausea (19% to 33%), constipation (4% to 28%), vomiting (9% to 16%)
1% to 10%:
  Cardiovascular: Hypotension (<10%), tachycardia (<10%), edema (<10%), flushing (<10%), hypertension (<10%)
  Central nervous system: Anxiety (1% to <10%), sedation (1% to <10%), depression (<10%), disorientation (<10%), lethargy (<10%), nervousness (<10%), restlessness (<10%), fatigue (≤4%), insomnia (≤4%), confusion (3%)
  Endocrine & metabolic: Dehydration (<10%)
  Gastrointestinal: Abdominal distension (<10%), flatulence (1% to <10%), xerostomia (1% to <10%), dyspepsia (<10%), weight loss (<10%), diarrhea (≤4%), abdominal pain (≤3%), appetite decreased (≤3%)
  Neuromuscular & skeletal: Weakness (<10%)
  Ocular: Blurred vision (<10%)
  Respiratory: Hypoxia (<10%), dyspnea (<10%)
  Miscellaneous: Diaphoresis (1% to <10%)
Drug Interactions
  Avoid Concomitant Use
    Avoid concomitant use of Oxymorphone with any of the following: MAO Inhibitors
  Increased Effect/Toxicity
    Oxymorphone may increase the levels/effects of: Alcohol (Ethyl); Alvimopan; CNS Depressants; Desmopressin; MAO Inhibitors; Selective Serotonin Reuptake Inhibitors; Thiazide Diuretics

    The levels/effects of Oxymorphone may be increased by: Amphetamines; Antipsychotic Agents (Phenothiazines); Droperidol; HydrOXYzine; Succinylcholine
  Decreased Effect
    Oxymorphone may decrease the levels/effects of: Pegvisomant

    The levels/effects of Oxymorphone may be decreased by: Ammonium Chloride; Mixed Agonist / Antagonist Opioids

Ethanol/Nutrition/Herb Interactions

Ethanol: Ethanol ingestion with extended-release tablets is specifically contraindicated due to possible accelerated release and potentially fatal overdose. Ethanol may also increase CNS depression; monitor for increased effects with coadministration. Caution patients about effects.

Food: When taken orally with a high-fat meal, peak concentration is 38% to 50% greater. Both immediate-release and extended-release tablets should be taken 1 hour before or 2 hours after eating.

Herb/Nutraceutical: Avoid valerian, St John's wort, kava kava, gotu kola (may increase CNS depression).

Stability Injection solution, tablet: Store at 25°C (77°F); excursions permitted to 15°C to 30°C (59°F to 86°F). Protect injection from light.

Mechanism of Action Oxymorphone hydrochloride is a potent narcotic analgesic with uses similar to those of morphine. The drug is a semisynthetic derivative of morphine (phenanthrene derivative) and is closely related to hydromorphone chemically (Dilaudid®).

Pharmacodynamics/Kinetics

Onset of action: Parenteral: 5-10 minutes

Duration: Analgesic: Parenteral: 3-6 hours

Distribution: V_d: I.V.: 1.94-4.22 L/kg

Protein binding: 10% to 12%

Metabolism: Hepatic via glucuronidation to active and inactive metabolites

Bioavailability: Oral: ~10%

Half-life elimination: Oral: Immediate release: 7-9 hours; Extended release: 9-11 hours

Excretion: Urine (<1% as unchanged drug); feces

Dosage

Geriatric Refer to adult dosing. **Note:** Initiate dosing at the lower end of the dosage range.

Adult Analgesia: **Note:** Dosage must be individualized.

I.M., SubQ: Initial: 1-1.5 mg; may repeat every 4-6 hours as needed

I.V.: Initial: 0.5 mg

Oral:

Immediate release:

Opioid-naive: 10-20 mg every 4-6 hours as needed. Initial dosages as low as 5 mg may be considered in selected patients and/or patients with renal impairment. Dosage adjustment should be based on level of analgesia, side effects, and pain intensity. Initiation of therapy with initial dose >20 mg is **not** recommended.

Currently on stable dose of parenteral oxymorphone: ~10 times the daily parenteral requirement. The calculated amount should be divided and given in 4-6 equal doses.

Currently on other opioids: Use standard conversion chart to convert daily dose to oxymorphone equivalent. Generally start with 1/2 the calculated daily oxymorphone dosage and administered in divided doses every 4-6 hours.

Extended release (Opana® ER):

Opioid-naive: Initial: 5 mg every 12 hours. Supplemental doses of immediate-release oxymorphone may be used as "rescue" medication as dosage is titrated.

Note: Continued requirement for supplemental dosing may be used to titrate the dose of extended-release continuous therapy. Adjust therapy incrementally, by 5-10 mg every 12 hours at intervals of every 3-7 days. Ideally, basal dosage may be titrated to generally mild pain or no pain with the regular use of fewer than 2 supplemental doses per 24 hours.

Currently on stable dose of parenteral oxymorphone: Approximately 10 times the daily parenteral requirement. The calculated amount should be given in 2 divided doses (every 12 hours).

Currently on opioids: Use conversion chart (see Note below) to convert daily dose to oxymorphone equivalent. Generally start with 1/2 the calculated daily oxymorphone dosage. Divide daily dose in 2 (for every 12-hour dosing) and round down to nearest dosage form. **Note:** Per manufacturer, the following approximate oral dosages are equivalent to oxymorphone 10 mg:

Hydrocodone 20 mg

Oxycodone 20 mg

Methadone 20 mg

Morphine 30 mg

Conversion of stable dose of immediate-release oxymorphone to extended-release oxymorphone: Administer 1/2 of the daily dose of immediate-release oxymorphone (Opana®) as the extended-release formulation (Opana® ER) every 12 hours

Renal Impairment Cl_{cr} <50 mL/minute: Reduce initial dosage of oral formulations (bioavailability increased 57% to 65%). Begin therapy at lowest dose and titrate carefully.

Hepatic Impairment Generally, contraindicated for use in patients with moderate-to-severe liver disease. Initiate with lowest possible dose and titrate slowly in mild impairment.

◀ **Administration** Administer immediate release and extended release tablets 1 hour before or 2 hours after eating. Opana® ER tablet should be swallowed; do not break, crush, or chew.

Monitoring Parameters Respiratory rate, heart rate, blood pressure, CNS activity

Test Interactions Some quinolones may produce a false-positive urine screening result for opiates using commercially-available immunoassay kits. This has been demonstrated most consistently for levofloxacin and ofloxacin, but other quinolones have shown cross-reactivity in certain assay kits. Confirmation of positive opiate screens by more specific methods should be considered. May cause elevation in amylase (due to constriction of the sphincter of Oddi).

Special Geriatric Considerations Elderly may be particularly susceptible to the CNS depressant and constipating effects of narcotics. Plasma levels of oxymorphone were about 40% higher in elderly patients as compared to younger patients.

Controlled Substance C-II

Dosage Forms Excipient information presented when available (limited, particularly for generics); consult specific product labeling. [DSC] = Discontinued product

Injection, solution, as hydrochloride:
Opana®: 1 mg/mL (1 mL)
Tablet, oral, as hydrochloride: 5 mg, 10 mg
Opana®: 5 mg, 10 mg
Tablet, extended release, oral, as hydrochloride: 7.5 mg, 15 mg
Opana® ER: 5 mg, 7.5 mg [DSC], 10 mg, 15 mg [DSC], 20 mg, 30 mg, 40 mg

Selected References

American Geriatrics Society Panel on Pharmacological Management of Persistent Pain in Older Persons, "Pharmacological Management of Persistent Pain in Older Persons," *J Am Geriatr Soc*, 2009, 57(8):1331-46.

◆ **Oxymorphone Hydrochloride** *see* Oxymorphone *on page 1375*
◆ **OXY® Post-Shave [OTC]** *see* Salicylic Acid *on page 1648*
◆ **OXY® Spot Treatment [OTC]** *see* Salicylic Acid *on page 1648*
◆ **Oxytrol®** *see* Oxybutynin *on page 1365*
◆ **Oysco D [OTC]** *see* Calcium and Vitamin D *on page 248*
◆ **Oysco 500+D [OTC]** *see* Calcium and Vitamin D *on page 248*
◆ **Oyst-Cal-D [OTC]** *see* Calcium and Vitamin D *on page 248*
◆ **Oyst-Cal 500 [OTC]** *see* Calcium Salts (Oral) *on page 256*
◆ **Oyst-Cal-D 500 [OTC]** *see* Calcium and Vitamin D *on page 248*
◆ **Oystercal® 500** *see* Calcium Salts (Oral) *on page 256*
◆ **Ozurdex®** *see* Dexamethasone (Ophthalmic) *on page 487*
◆ **P-071** *see* Cetirizine *on page 327*
◆ **Pacerone®** *see* Amiodarone *on page 97*
◆ **Pain Eze [OTC]** *see* Acetaminophen *on page 33*
◆ **Pain & Fever Children's [OTC]** *see* Acetaminophen *on page 33*

Paliperidone (pal ee PER i done)

Related Information
Antipsychotic Agents *on page 1997*
Atypical Antipsychotics *on page 1999*

Brand Names: U.S. Invega®; Invega® Sustenna®

Brand Names: Canada Invega®; Invega® Sustenna®

Index Terms 9-hydroxy-risperidone; 9-OH-risperidone; Paliperidone Palmitate

Generic Availability (U.S.) No

Pharmacologic Category Antipsychotic Agent, Atypical

Use
Oral: Acute and maintenance treatment of schizophrenia; acute treatment of schizoaffective disorder (monotherapy or adjunctive therapy to mood stabilizers and/or antidepressants)
Injection: Acute and maintenance treatment of schizophrenia

Unlabeled/Investigational Use Psychosis/agitation related to Alzheimer's dementia

Contraindications Hypersensitivity to paliperidone, risperidone, or any component of the formulation

Warnings/Precautions [U.S. Boxed Warning]: Elderly patients with dementia-related psychosis treated with antipsychotics are at an increased risk of death compared to placebo. Most deaths appeared to be either cardiovascular (eg, heart failure, sudden death) or infectious (eg, pneumonia) in nature. In addition, an increased incidence of cerebrovascular adverse effects (eg, transient ischemic attack, cerebrovascular accidents) has been reported in studies of placebo-controlled trials of risperidone (paliperidone is the primary active metabolite of risperidone) in elderly patients with dementia-related psychosis. Paliperidone is not approved for the treatment of dementia-related psychosis.

Compared with risperidone, paliperidone is low to moderately sedating; use with caution in disorders where CNS depression is a feature. Use caution in patients with predisposition to seizures. Use with caution in renal dysfunction; dose reduction recommended. Esophageal dysmotility and aspiration have been associated with antipsychotic use; use with caution in patients at risk of aspiration pneumonia (eg, Alzheimer's disease).

Leukopenia, neutropenia, and agranulocytosis (sometimes fatal) have been reported in clinical trials and postmarketing reports with antipsychotic use; presence of risk factors (eg, pre-existing low WBC or history of drug-induced leuko-/neutropenia) should prompt periodic blood count assessment. Discontinue therapy at first signs of blood dyscrasias or if absolute neutrophil count <1000/mm^3.

Paliperidone is associated with increased prolactin levels; clinical significance of hyper-prolactinemia in patients with breast cancer or other prolactin-dependent tumors is unknown. May alter temperature regulation. May mask toxicity of other drugs or conditions (eg intestinal obstruction, Reyes syndrome, brain tumor) due to antiemetic effects. Priapism has been reported rarely with use.

May cause orthostasis and syncope. Use with caution in patients with cardiovascular diseases (eg, heart failure, history of myocardial infarction or ischemia, cerebrovascular disease, conduction abnormalities). Use caution in patients receiving medications for hypertension (orthostatic effects may be exacerbated) or in patients with hypovolemia or dehydration. May alter cardiac conduction; life-threatening arrhythmias have occurred with therapeutic doses of neuroleptics. Avoid use in combination with QT$_c$-prolonging drugs. Avoid use in patients with congenital long QT syndrome and in patients with history of cardiac arrhythmia.

May cause extrapyramidal symptoms (EPS), including pseudoparkinsonism, acute dystonic reactions, akathisia, and tardive dyskinesia (risk of these reactions is low relative to other neuroleptics, and is dose dependent). Risk of dystonia (and probably other EPS) may be greater with increased doses, use of conventional antipsychotics, males, and younger patients. Risk of neuroleptic malignant syndrome (NMS) may be increased in patients with Parkinson's disease or Lewy body dementia; monitor for symptoms of confusion, obtundation, postural instability and extrapyramidal symptoms. May cause hyperglycemia; in some cases may be extreme and associated with ketoacidosis, hyperosmolar coma, or death. Use with caution in patients with diabetes (or risk factors) or other disorders of glucose regulation; monitor for worsening of glucose control. Significant weight gain has been observed with antipsychotic therapy; incidence varies with product. Monitor waist circumference and BMI. May cause lipid abnormalities (LDL and triglycerides increased; HDL decreased).

The possibility of a suicide attempt is inherent in psychotic illness or bipolar disorder; use caution in high-risk patients during initiation of therapy. Prescriptions should be written for the smallest quantity consistent with good patient care.

The tablet formulation consists of drug within a nonabsorbable shell that is expelled and may be visible in the stool. Use is not recommended in patients with pre-existing severe gastrointestinal narrowing disorders. Patients with upper GI tract alterations in transit time may have increased or decreased bioavailability of paliperidone. Do not use in patients unable to swallow the tablet whole.

Adverse Reactions (Reflective of adult population; not specific for elderly) Unless otherwise noted, frequency of adverse effects is reported for the oral/I.M. formulation in adults.

>10%:
Cardiovascular: Tachycardia (1% to 14%)
Central nervous system: EPS (≤26%; dose dependent), insomnia (10% to 15%), headache (6% to 15%), parkinsonism (3% to 14%; dose dependent), somnolence (adolescents 9% to 26%; adults 1% to 12%; dose dependent)
Neuromuscular & skeletal: Tremor (2% to 12%)
3% to 10%:
Cardiovascular: Orthostatic hypotension (1% to 4%; dose dependent), bundle branch block (≤3%)
Central nervous system: Agitation (4% to 10%), akathisia (adolescents 4% to 17%; adults 1% to 10%; dose dependent), anxiety (adolescents ≤9%; adults 3% to 8%), dizziness (1% to 6%), dystonia (1% to 5%; dose dependent), dysarthria (1% to 4%; dose dependent), fatigue (adolescents ≤4%), sleep disorder (≤3%), lethargy (adolescents ≤3%)
Endocrine & metabolic: Amenorrhea (adolescents ≤6%), galactorrhea (adolescents ≤4%), gynecomastia (adolescents ≤3%)

◄ Gastrointestinal: Weight gain (1% to 9%; dose dependent), nausea (2% to 8%), dyspepsia (5% to 6%), vomiting (adolescents ≤11%; adults 2% to 5%), constipation (1% to 5%), salivation increased (adolescents ≤6%; adults ≤4%; dose dependent), appetite increased (2% to 3%), toothache (1% to 3%), abdominal pain (≤3%), diarrhea (≤3%), xerostomia (≤3%); tongue swelling (adolescents ≤3%), tongue paralysis (adolescents ≤3%)

Local: I.M. formulation: Injection site reaction (≤10%)

Neuromuscular & skeletal: Hyperkinesia (2% to 10% dose dependent), dyskinesia (1% to 9%), weakness (≤4%), myalgia (≤4% dose dependent), back pain (1% to 3%), extremity pain (≤3%)

Ocular: Blurred vision (adolescents ≤3%)

Respiratory: Nasopharyngitis (≤5%; dose dependent), upper respiratory tract infection (1% to 4%), cough (≤3%; dose dependent), rhinitis (1% to 3%; dose dependent)

Drug Interactions

Metabolism/Transport Effects Substrate of P-glycoprotein

Avoid Concomitant Use

Avoid concomitant use of Paliperidone with any of the following: Metoclopramide

Increased Effect/Toxicity

Paliperidone may increase the levels/effects of: Alcohol (Ethyl); CNS Depressants; Methotrimeprazine; Methylphenidate; Selective Serotonin Reuptake Inhibitors

The levels/effects of Paliperidone may be increased by: Acetylcholinesterase Inhibitors (Central); Divalproex; Droperidol; HydrOXYzine; Itraconazole; Lithium formulations; Methotrimeprazine; Methylphenidate; Metoclopramide; P-Glycoprotein Inhibitors; RisperiDONE; Tetrabenazine; Valproic Acid

Decreased Effect

Paliperidone may decrease the levels/effects of: Amphetamines; Anti-Parkinson's Agents (Dopamine Agonist); Quinagolide

The levels/effects of Paliperidone may be decreased by: CarBAMazepine; Lithium formulations; P-Glycoprotein Inducers

Ethanol/Nutrition/Herb Interactions

Ethanol: May increase CNS depression; monitor for increased effects with coadministration. Caution patients about effects.

Herb/Nutraceutical: Avoid kava kava, gotu kola, valerian, St John's wort (may increase CNS depression).

Stability Store at controlled room temperature of ≤25°C (77°F); excursions permitted to 15°C to 30°C (59°F to 86°F). Protect tablets from moisture.

Mechanism of Action Paliperidone is considered a benzisoxazole atypical antipsychotic as it is the primary active metabolite of risperidone. As with other atypical antipsychotics, its therapeutic efficacy is believed to result from mixed central serotonergic and dopaminergic antagonism. The addition of serotonin antagonism to dopamine antagonism (classic neuroleptic mechanism) is thought to improve negative symptoms of psychoses and reduce the incidence of extrapyramidal side effects. Similar to risperidone, paliperidone demonstrates high affinity to α_1, D_2, H_1, and 5-HT_{2C} receptors, and low affinity for muscarinic and 5-HT_{1A} receptors. In contrast to risperidone, paliperidone displays nearly 10-fold lower affinity for α_2 and 5-HT_{2A} receptors, and nearly three- to fivefold less affinity for 5-HT_{1A} and 5-HT_{1D}, respectively.

Pharmacodynamics/Kinetics

Absorption: I.M.: Slow release (begins on day 1 and continues up to 126 days)

Distribution: V_d: 391-487 L

Protein binding: 74%

Metabolism: Hepatic via CYP2D6 and 3A4 (limited role in elimination); minor metabolism (<10% each) via dealkylation, hydroxylation, dehydrogenation, and benzisoxazole scission

Bioavailability: 28%

Half-life elimination:

Oral: 23 hours; 24-51 hours with renal impairment (Cl_{cr} <80 mL/minute)

I.M. (following a single-dose administration): Range: 25-49 days

Time to peak, plasma: Oral: ~24 hours; I.M.: 13 days

Excretion: Urine (80%); feces (11%)

Dosage

Geriatric Refer to adult dosing. Additional monitoring of renal function and orthostatic blood pressure may be warranted.

Adult

U.S. labeling:

Schizoaffective disorder, schizophrenia: Oral: Usual: 6 mg once daily in the morning; titration not required, though some may benefit from higher or lower doses. If exceeding 6 mg/day, increases of 3 mg/day are recommended no more frequently than every 4 days in schizoaffective disorder or every 5 days in schizophrenia, up to a maximum of 12 mg/day. Some patients may require only 3 mg/day.

Schizophrenia: I.M.: **Note:** Prior to initiation of I.M therapy, tolerability should be established with oral paliperidone or oral risperidone. Previous oral antipsychotics can be discontinued at the time of initiation of I.M. therapy. **Dosing based on paliperidone palmitate.**

Initiation of therapy:

Initial: 234 mg on treatment day 1 followed by 156 mg 1 week later. The second dose may be administered 2 days before or after the weekly timepoint.

Maintenance: Following the 1-week initiation regimen, begin a maintenance dose of 117 mg every month. Some patients may benefit from higher or lower monthly maintenance doses (monthly maintenance dosage range: 39-234 mg). The monthly maintenance dose may be administered 7 days before or after the monthly timepoint.

Conversion from oral paliperidone to I.M paliperidone: Initiate I.M. therapy as described using the 1-week initiation regimen. Patients previously stabilized on oral doses can expect similar steady state exposure during maintenance treatment with I.M. therapy using the following conversion:

Oral extended release dose of 12 mg, then I.M. maintenance dose of 234 mg

Oral extended release dose of 6 mg, then I.M. maintenance dose of 117 mg

Oral extended release dose of 3 mg, then I.M. maintenance dose of 39-78 mg

Switching from other long-acting injectable antipsychotics to I.M. paliperidone: Initiate I.M. paliperidone in the place of the next scheduled injection and continue at monthly intervals. The 1-week initiation regimen is not required in these patients.

Dosage adjustments: Adjustments may be made monthly (full effect from adjustments may not be seen for several months)

Missed doses:

If <6 weeks has elapsed since the last monthly injection: Administer the missed dose as soon as possible and continue therapy at monthly intervals.

If >6 weeks and ≤6 months has elapsed since the last monthly injection: Therapy may be resumed at same dose the patient was previously stabilized on, if the maintenance dose was <234 mg. If the dose was 234 mg, then administer a 156 mg dose as soon as possible, followed by a second dose of 156 mg 1 week later, then resume monthly maintenance dosing.

If >6 months has elapsed since last monthly maintenance injection: Therapy must be reinitiated following dosing recommendations for initiation of therapy.

Canadian labeling:

Schizophrenia: Oral: Usual: 6 mg once daily in the morning; titration not required, though some may benefit from higher or lower doses. If exceeding 6 mg/day, increases of 3 mg/day are recommended no more frequently than every 5 days in schizophrenia, up to a maximum of 12 mg/day. Some patients may require only 3 mg/day.

Schizophrenia: I.M.: **Note:** Prior to initiation of I.M therapy, tolerability should be established with oral paliperidone or oral risperidone. Previous oral antipsychotics can be discontinued at the time of initiation of I.M. therapy. **Dosing based on paliperidone.**

Initiation of therapy:

Initial: 150 mg on treatment day 1 followed by 100 mg 1 week later (day 8). The second dose may be administered 2 days before or after the weekly timepoint.

Maintenance: Following the 1-week initiation regimen, begin a maintenance dose of 75 mg every month. Some patients may benefit from higher or lower monthly maintenance doses (monthly maintenance dosage range: 25-150 mg). The monthly maintenance dose may be administered 7 days before or after the monthly timepoint.

Conversion from oral paliperidone to I.M paliperidone: Initiate I.M. therapy as described using the 1-week initiation regimen. Patients previously stabilized on oral doses can expect similar steady state exposure during maintenance treatment with I.M. therapy using the following conversion:

Oral extended release dose of 12 mg, then I.M. maintenance dose of 150 mg

Oral extended release dose of 6 mg, then I.M. maintenance dose of 75 mg

Oral extended release dose of 3 mg, then I.M. maintenance dose of 25-50 mg

Switching from injectable risperidone (Risperdal® Consta®) to I.M. paliperidone:

Risperdal® Consta® dose of 25 mg every 2 weeks, then I.M. paliperidone maintenance dose of 50 mg

Risperdal® Consta® dose of 37.5 mg every 2 weeks, then I.M. paliperidone maintenance dose of 75 mg

Risperdal® Consta® dose of 50 mg every 2 weeks, then I.M. paliperidone maintenance dose of 100 mg

Switching from other long-acting injectable antipsychotics to I.M. paliperidone: Initiate I.M. paliperidone in the place of the next scheduled injection and continue at monthly intervals. The 1-week initiation regimen is not required in these patients.

Dosage adjustments: Adjustments may be made monthly (full effect from adjustments may not be seen for several months)

Missed doses:

If <6 weeks has elapsed since the last monthly injection: Administer the missed dose as soon as possible and continue therapy at monthly intervals.

If >6 weeks and ≤6 months has elapsed since the last monthly injection: Therapy may be resumed at same dose (25-100 mg) the patient was previously stabilized on and then repeated 1 week later (day 8). Resume usual monthly maintenance dosing cycle thereafter. If the dose was 150 mg, administer a 100 mg dose as soon as possible and repeat 1 week later (day 8), then resume usual monthly maintenance dosing cycle 25-150 mg.

If >6 months has elapsed since last monthly maintenance injection: Therapy must be reinitiated following dosing recommendations for initiation of therapy.

Renal Impairment Clearance is decreased in renal impairment; adjust dose according to renal function:

Oral:

Mild impairment (Cl_{cr} 50-79 mL/minute): Initial dose: 3 mg once daily; maximum dose: 6 mg once daily

Moderate-to-severe impairment (Cl_{cr} 10-49 mL/minute): Initial dose: 1.5 mg once daily; maximum dose: 3 mg once daily

Severe impairment (Cl_{cr} <10 mL/minute): Use not recommended; not studied in this population

I.M., U.S. labeling:

Mild impairment (Cl_{cr} 50-79 mL/minute): Initiation of therapy: 156 mg on treatment day 1, followed by 117 mg 1 week later, followed by a maintenance dose of 78 mg every month

Moderate-to-severe impairment (Cl_{cr} <50 mL/minute): Use not recommended

I.M., Canadian labeling:

Mild impairment (Cl_{cr} 50-79 mL/minute): Initiation of therapy: 100 mg on treatment day 1, followed by 75 mg 1 week later followed by a maintenance dose of 50 mg every month

Moderate-to-severe impairment (Cl_{cr} <50 mL/minute): Use not recommended

Hepatic Impairment Oral, I.M.: No adjustment necessary for mild-to-moderate (Child-Pugh class A and B) impairment. Not studied in severe impairment.

Administration

Oral: Administer in the morning without regard to meals. Extended release tablets should be swallowed whole with liquids; do not crush, chew, or divide.

Injection: Invega® Sustenna™ should be administered by I.M. route only as a single injection (do not divide); do not administer I.V. or subcutaneously. Avoid inadvertent injection into vasculature. Prior to injection, shake syringe for at least 10 seconds to ensure a homogenous suspension. The 2 initial injections should be administered in the deltoid muscle using a 1½ inch, 22-gauge needle for patients ≥90 kg, and a 1 inch, 23-gauge needle for patients <90 kg. The 2 initial deltoid intramuscular injections help attain therapeutic concentrations rapidly. Alternate deltoid injections (right and left deltoid muscle). The second dose may be administered 2 days before or after the weekly timepoint. Monthly maintenance doses can be administered in either the deltoid or gluteal muscle. Administer injections in the gluteal muscle using a 1½ inch, 22-gauge needle in the upper-outer quadrant of the gluteal area. Alternate gluteal injections (right and left gluteal muscle). The monthly maintenance dose may be administered 7 days before or after the monthly timepoint.

Monitoring Parameters Vital signs; fasting lipid profile and fasting blood glucose/Hgb A_{1c} (prior to treatment, at 3 months, then annually); prolactin levels, CBC frequently during first few months of therapy in patients with pre-existing low WBC or a history of drug-induced leukopenia/neutropenia; BMI, personal/family history of obesity, diabetes, waist circumference; blood pressure; mental status, abnormal involuntary movement scale (AIMS), extrapyramidal symptoms; orthostatic blood pressure changes for 3-5 days after starting or increasing dose. Weight should be assessed prior to treatment, at 4 weeks, 8 weeks, 12 weeks, and then at quarterly intervals. Consider titrating to a different antipsychotic agent for a weight gain ≥5% of the initial weight.

Pharmacotherapy Pearls Invega® is an extended release tablet based on the OROS® osmotic delivery system. Water from the GI tract enters through a semipermeable membrane coating the tablet, solubilizing the drug into a gelatinous form which, through hydrophilic expansion, is then expelled through laser-drilled holes in the coating.

Special Geriatric Considerations Any changes in disease status in any organ system can result in behavior changes. Extrapyramidal syndrome symptoms occur less with this agent when total daily dose remains ≤6 mg as compared with phenothiazines and butyrophenone classes of antipsychotics.

In the treatment of agitated, demented, elderly patients, authors of meta-analysis of controlled trials of the response to the traditional antipsychotics (phenothiazines, butyrophenones) in controlling agitation have concluded that the use of neuroleptics results in a response rate of 18%. Clearly neuroleptic therapy for behavior control should be limited with frequent attempts to withdraw the agent given for behavior control. In light of significant risks and adverse effects in elderly population compared with limited data demonstrating efficacy in the treatment of dementia related psychosis, aggression, and agitation, an extensive risk:benefit analysis should be performed prior to use.

Dosage Forms Excipient information presented when available (limited, particularly for generics); consult specific product labeling.

Injection, suspension, extended release, as palmitate:

Invega® Sustenna®: 39 mg/0.25 mL (0.25 mL); 78 mg/0.5 mL (0.5 mL); 117 mg/0.75 mL (0.75 mL); 156 mg/mL (1 mL); 234 mg/1.5 mL (1.5 mL)

Tablet, extended release, oral:

Invega®: 1.5 mg, 3 mg, 6 mg, 9 mg [osmotic controlled release]

Dosage Forms: Canada Excipient information presented when available (limited, particularly for generics); consult specific product labeling.

Injection, suspension, extended release:

Invega® Sustenna™: 25 mg/0.25 mL (0.25 mL), 50 mg/0.5 mL (0.5 mL), 75 mg/0.75 mL (0.75 mL), 100 mg/1 mL (1 mL), 150 mg/1.5 mL (1.5 mL)

Selected References

Jung SM, Kim K-A, Cho H-K, et al, "Cytochrome P450 3A Inhibitor Itraconazole Affects Plasma Concentrations of Risperidone and 9-Hydroxyrisperidone in Schizophrenic Patients," Clin Pharmacol Ther, 2005, 78(5):520-8.

Rabins PV, Blacker D, Rovner BW, et al, "Practice Guidelines for the Treatment of Patients With Alzheimer's Disease and Other Dementias," Am J Psychiatry, 2007, 164(12 Suppl):5-56. Available at http://www.psych.org/psych_pract/treatg/pg/prac_guide.cfm.

Richelson E and Souder T, "Binding of Antipsychotic Drugs to Human Brain Receptors. Focus on Newer Generation Compounds," Life Sci, 2000, 68(1):29-39.

Schneider LS, Tariot PN, Dagerman KS, et al, "Effectiveness of Atypical Antipsychotic Drugs in Patients With Alzheimer's Disease," N Engl J Med, 2006, 355(15):1525-38.

Spina E, Avenoso A, Facciola G, et al, "Plasma Concentrations of Risperidone and 9-Hydroxyrisperidone: Effect of Comedication with Carbamazepine or Valproate," Ther Drug Monit, 2000, 22:481-5.

◆ **Paliperidone Palmitate** see Paliperidone on page 1378

◆ **Palmer's® Skin Success Acne Cleanser [OTC]** see Salicylic Acid on page 1648

◆ **Pamelor®** see Nortriptyline on page 1320

Pamidronate (pa mi DROE nate)

Medication Safety Issues

Sound-alike/look-alike issues:

Aredia® may be confused with Adriamycin, Meridia®

Pamidronate may be confused with papaverine

International issues:

Linoten [Spain] may be confused with Loniten brand name for minoxidil [Canada and multiple international markets]

Brand Names: U.S. Aredia®

Brand Names: Canada Aredia®; Pamidronate Disodium Omega; Pamidronate Disodium®; PMS-Pamidronate; Rhoxal-pamidronate

Index Terms Pamidronate Disodium

Generic Availability (U.S.) Yes

Pharmacologic Category Antidote; Bisphosphonate Derivative

Use Treatment of moderate or severe hypercalcemia associated with malignancy (in conjunction with adequate hydration) with or without bone metastases; treatment of osteolytic bone lesions associated with multiple myeloma or metastatic breast cancer; moderate-to-severe Paget's disease of bone

Unlabeled/Investigational Use Treatment of osteogenesis imperfecta; treatment of symptomatic bone metastases of thyroid cancer; prevention of bone loss associated with androgen deprivation treatment in prostate cancer

Contraindications Hypersensitivity to pamidronate, other bisphosphonates, or any component of the formulation

Warnings/Precautions Osteonecrosis of the jaw (ONJ) has been reported in patients receiving bisphosphonates. Risk factors include invasive dental procedures (eg, tooth extraction, dental implants, boney surgery); a diagnosis of cancer, with concomitant chemotherapy, radiotherapy, or corticosteroids; poor oral hygiene, ill-fitting dentures; and comorbid disorders (anemia, coagulopathy, infection, pre-existing dental disease). Most reported cases occurred after I.V. bisphosphonate therapy; however, cases have been reported following oral therapy. A dental exam and preventative dentistry should be performed prior to placing patients with risk factors on chronic bisphosphonate therapy. The manufacturer's labeling states that discontinuing bisphosphonates in patients requiring invasive dental procedures reduces the risk of ONJ. However, other experts suggest that there is no evidence that discontinuing therapy reduces the risk of developing ONJ (Assael, 2009). The benefit/risk must be assessed by the treating physician and/or dentist/surgeon prior to any invasive dental procedure. Patients developing ONJ while on bisphosphonates should receive care by an oral surgeon.

Infrequently, severe (and occasionally debilitating) musculoskeletal (bone, joint, and/or muscle) pain have been reported during bisphosphonate treatment. The onset of pain ranged from a single day to several months. Consider discontinuing therapy in patients who experience severe symptoms; symptoms usually resolve upon discontinuation. Some patients experienced recurrence when rechallenged with same drug or another bisphosphonate; avoid use in patients with a history of these symptoms in association with bisphosphonate therapy.

Initial or single doses have been associated with renal deterioration, progressing to renal failure and dialysis. Withhold pamidronate treatment (until renal function returns to baseline) in patients with evidence of renal deterioration. Glomerulosclerosis (focal segmental) with or without nephrotic syndrome has also been reported. Longer infusion times (>2 hours) may reduce the risk for renal toxicity, especially in patients with pre-existing renal insufficiency. Single pamidronate doses should not exceed 90 mg. Patients with serum creatinine >3 mg/dL were not studied in clinical trials; limited data are available in patients with Cl_{cr} <30 mL/minute. Evaluate serum creatinine prior to each treatment. For the treatment of bone metastases, use is not recommended in patients with severe renal impairment; for renal impairment in indications other than bone metastases, use clinical judgment to determine if benefits outweigh potential risks.

Use has been associated with asymptomatic electrolyte abnormalities (including hypophosphatemia, hypokalemia, hypomagnesemia, and hypocalcemia). Rare cases of symptomatic hypocalcemia, including tetany have been reported. Patients with a history of thyroid surgery may have relative hypoparathyroidism; predisposing them to pamidronate-related hypocalcemia. Patients with pre-existing anemia, leukopenia, or thrombocytopenia should be closely monitored during the first 2 weeks of treatment.

According to the American Society of Clinical Oncology (ASCO) guidelines for bisphosphonates in multiple myeloma, treatment with pamidronate is not recommended for asymptomatic (smoldering) or indolent myeloma or with solitary plasmacytoma (Kyle, 2007). The National Comprehensive Cancer Network® (NCCN) multiple myeloma guidelines (v.1.2011) also do not recommend pamidronate use in stage 1 or smoldering disease, unless part of a clinical trial.

Adequate hydration is required during treatment (urine output ~2 L/day); avoid overhydration, especially in patients with heart failure. Vein irritation and thrombophlebitis may occur with infusions.

Adverse Reactions (Reflective of adult population; not specific for elderly) Note: Actual percentages may vary by indication; treatment for multiple myeloma is associated with higher percentage.

>10%:
  Central nervous system: Fever (18% to 39%; transient), fatigue (≤37%), headache (≤26%), insomnia (≤22%)
  Endocrine & metabolic: Hypophosphatemia (≤18%), hypokalemia (4% to 18%), hypomagnesemia (4% to 12%), hypocalcemia (≤12%)
  Gastrointestinal: Nausea (≤54%), vomiting (≤36%), anorexia (≤26%), abdominal pain (≤23%), dyspepsia (≤23%)
  Genitourinary: Urinary tract infection (≤19%)
  Hematologic: Anemia (≤43%), granulocytopenia (≤20%)
  Local: Infusion site reaction (≤18%; includes induration, pain, redness and swelling)
  Neuromuscular & skeletal: Myalgia (≤26%), weakness (≤22%), arthralgia (≤14%), osteonecrosis of the jaw (cancer patients: 1% to 11%)
  Renal: Serum creatinine increased (≤19%)
  Respiratory: Dyspnea (≤30%), cough (≤26%), upper respiratory tract infection (≤24%), sinusitis (≤16%), pleural effusion (≤11%)
1% to 10%:
  Cardiovascular: Atrial fibrillation (≤6%), hypertension (≤6%), syncope (≤6%), tachycardia (≤6%), atrial flutter (≤1%), cardiac failure (≤1%), edema (≤1%)
  Central nervous system: Somnolence (≤6%), psychosis (≤4%), seizure (≤2%)
  Endocrine & metabolic: Hypothyroidism (≤6%)
  Gastrointestinal: Constipation (≤6%), gastrointestinal hemorrhage (≤6%), diarrhea (≤1%), stomatitis (≤1%)
  Hematologic: Leukopenia (≤4%), neutropenia (≤1%), thrombocytopenia (≤1%)
  Neuromuscular & skeletal: Back pain, bone pain

Renal: Uremia (≤4%)
Respiratory: Rales (≤6%), rhinitis (≤6%)
Miscellaneous: Moniliasis (≤6%)

Drug Interactions

Avoid Concomitant Use There are no known interactions where it is recommended to avoid concomitant use.

Increased Effect/Toxicity

Pamidronate may increase the levels/effects of: Deferasirox; Phosphate Supplements

The levels/effects of Pamidronate may be increased by: Aminoglycosides; Nonsteroidal Anti-Inflammatory Agents; Thalidomide

Decreased Effect

The levels/effects of Pamidronate may be decreased by: Proton Pump Inhibitors

Stability

Powder for injection: Store below 30°C (86°F). Reconstitute by adding 10 mL of SWFI to each vial of lyophilized pamidronate disodium powder; the resulting solution will be 30 mg/10 mL or 90 mg/10 mL. The reconstituted solution is stable for 24 hours stored under refrigeration at 2°C to 8°C (36°F to 46°F).

Solution for injection: Store at 20°C to 25°C (68°F to 77°F).

Pamidronate may be further diluted in 250-1000 mL of 0.45% or 0.9% sodium chloride or 5% dextrose. (The manufacturer recommends dilution in 1000 mL for hypercalcemia of malignancy, 500 mL for Paget's disease and bone metastases of myeloma, and 250 mL for bone metastases of breast cancer.) Pamidronate solution for infusion is stable at room temperature for up to 24 hours.

Mechanism of Action A bisphosphonate which inhibits bone resorption via actions on osteoclasts and/or on osteoclast precursors. Does not appear to produce any significant effects on renal tubular calcium handling and is poorly absorbed following oral administration (high oral doses have been reported effective); therefore, I.V. therapy is preferred.

Pharmacodynamics/Kinetics

Onset of action: 24-48 hours
  Peak effect: Maximum: 5-7 days
Absorption: Poor; pharmacokinetic studies lacking
Metabolism: Not metabolized
Half-life elimination: 21-35 hours
Excretion: Biphasic; urine (30% to 62% as unchanged drug; lower in patients with renal dysfunction) within 120 hours

Dosage

Geriatric Refer to adult dosing. Begin at lower end of adult dosing range.

Adult Note: Single doses should not exceed 90 mg.

Hypercalcemia of malignancy: I.V.:
Moderate cancer-related hypercalcemia (corrected serum calcium: 12-13.5 mg/dL): 60-90 mg, as a single dose over 2-24 hours
Severe cancer-related hypercalcemia (corrected serum calcium: >13.5 mg/dL): 90 mg, as a single dose over 2-24 hours
Retreatment in patients who show an initial complete or partial response (allow at least 7 days to elapse prior to retreatment): May retreat at the same dose if serum calcium does not return to normal or does not remain normal after initial treatment.

Multiple myeloma, osteolytic bone lesions: I.V.: 90 mg over 4 hours monthly
Lytic disease: American Society of Clinical Oncology (ASCO) guidelines: 90 mg over at least 2 hours every 3-4 weeks for 2 years; discontinue after 2 years in patients with responsive and/or stable disease; resume therapy with new-onset skeletal-related events (Kyle, 2007)
Newly-diagnosed, symptomatic (unlabeled dose): 30 mg over 2.5 hours monthly for at least 3 years (Gimsing, 2010)

Breast cancer, osteolytic bone metastases: I.V.: 90 mg over 2 hours every 3-4 weeks

Paget's disease (moderate-to-severe): I.V.: 30 mg over 4 hours daily for 3 consecutive days (total dose = 90 mg); may retreat at initial dose if clinically indicated

Prevention of androgen deprivation-induced osteoporosis (unlabeled use): I.V.: 60 mg over 2 hours every 3 months (Smith, 2001) **or** 90 mg as a single dose over 3-4 hours (Diamond, 2001)

Renal Impairment Patients with serum creatinine >3 mg/dL were excluded from clinical trials; there are only limited pharmacokinetic data in patients with Cl$_{cr}$ <30 mL/minute.
Manufacturer recommends the following guidelines:
Treatment of bone metastases: Use is not recommended in patients with severe renal impairment.
Renal impairment in indications other than bone metastases: Use clinical judgment to determine if benefits outweigh potential risks.

Multiple myeloma: American Society of Clinical Oncology (ASCO) guidelines (Kyle, 2007):
Severe renal impairment (serum creatinine >3 mg/dL **or** Cl_{cr} <30 mL/minute) and extensive bone disease: 90 mg over 4-6 hours. However, a reduced initial dose should be considered if renal impairment was pre-existing.

Albuminuria >500 mg/24 hours (unexplained): Withhold dose until returns to baseline, then recheck every 3-4 weeks; consider reinitiating at a dose not to exceed 90 mg every 4 weeks and with a longer infusion time of at least 4 hours

Dosing adjustment in renal toxicity: In patients with bone metastases, treatment should be withheld for deterioration in renal function (increase of serum creatinine ≥0.5 mg/dL in patients with normal baseline or ≥1.0 mg/dL in patients with abnormal baseline). Resumption of therapy may be considered when serum creatinine returns to within 10% of baseline.

Hepatic Impairment No adjustment required in patients with mild-to-moderate hepatic impairment; not studied in patients with severe hepatic impairment.

Administration I.V.: Infusion rate varies by indication. Longer infusion times (>2 hours) may reduce the risk for renal toxicity, especially in patients with pre-existing renal insufficiency. The manufacturer recommends infusing over 2-24 hours for hypercalcemia of malignancy; over 2 hours for osteolytic bone lesions with metastatic breast cancer; and over 4 hours for Paget's disease and for osteolytic bone lesions with multiple myeloma. The ASCO guidelines for bisphosphonate use in multiple myeloma recommend infusing pamidronate over at least 2 hours; if therapy is withheld due to renal toxicity, infuse over at least 4 hours upon reintroduction of treatment after renal recovery.

Monitoring Parameters Serum creatinine (prior to each treatment); serum electrolytes, including calcium, phosphate, magnesium, and potassium; CBC with differential; monitor for hypocalcemia for at least 2 weeks after therapy; dental exam and preventative dentistry prior to therapy for patients at risk of osteonecrosis, including all cancer patients; patients with pre-existing anemia, leukopenia, or thrombocytopenia should be closely monitored during the first 2 weeks of treatment; in addition, monitor urine albumin every 3-6 months in multiple myeloma patients

Reference Range Calcium (total): Adults: 9.0-11.0 mg/dL (SI: 2.05-2.54 mmol/L), may slightly decrease with aging; Phosphorus: 2.5-4.5 mg/dL (SI: 0.81-1.45 mmol/L)

Test Interactions Bisphosphonates may interfere with diagnostic imaging agents such as technetium-99m-diphosphonate in bone scans.

Pharmacotherapy Pearls

Oncology Comment:

Metastatic breast cancer: The American Society of Clinical Oncology (ASCO) updated guidelines on the role of bone-modifying agents (BMAs) in the prevention and treatment of skeletal-related events for metastatic breast cancer patients (Van Poznak, 2011). The guidelines recommend initiating a BMA (denosumab, pamidronate, zoledronic acid) in patients with metastatic breast cancer to the bone. There is currently no literature indicating the superiority of one particular BMA. Optimal duration is not defined; however, the guidelines recommend continuing therapy until substantial decline in patient's performance status. In patients with normal Cl_{cr} (>60 mL/minute), no dosage/interval/infusion rate changes for pamidronate or zoledronic acid are necessary. For patients with Cl_{cr} <30 mL/minute, pamidronate and zoledronic acid are not recommended. While no renal dose adjustments are recommended for denosumab, close monitoring is advised for risk of hypocalcemia in patients with Cl_{cr} <30 mL/minute or on dialysis. The ASCO guidelines are in alignment with package insert guidelines for dosing, renal dose adjustments, infusion times, prevention and management of osteonecrosis of the jaw, and monitoring of laboratory parameter recommendations. BMAs are not the first-line therapy for pain. BMAs are to be used as adjunctive therapy for cancer-related bone pain associated with bone metastasis, demonstrating a modest pain control benefit. BMAs should be used in conjunction with agents such as NSAIDs, opioid and nonopioid analgesics, corticosteroids, radiation/surgery, and interventional procedures.

Multiple myeloma: The American Society of Clinical Oncology (ASCO) has also published guidelines on the use of bisphosphonates for prevention and treatment of bone disease in multiple myeloma (Kyle, 2007). Pamidronate or zoledronic acid use is recommended in multiple myeloma patients with lytic bone destruction or compression spine fracture from osteopenia. Clodronate (not available in the U.S.; available in Canada), administered orally or I.V., is an alternative treatment. The use of the bisphosphonates pamidronate and zoledronic acid may be considered in patients with pain secondary to osteolytic disease, adjunct therapy to stabilize fractures or impending fractures, and I.V. bisphosphonates for multiple myeloma patients with osteopenia but no radiographic evidence of lytic bone disease. Bisphosphonates are not recommended in patients with solitary plasmacytoma, smoldering (asymptomatic) or indolent myeloma, or monoclonal gammopathy of undetermined significance. The guidelines recommend monthly treatment for a period of 2 years. At that time, physicians need to consider discontinuing in responsive and stable patients, and reinitiate if a new-onset skeletal-related event occurs. The ASCO guidelines are in alignment with package insert guidelines for dosing, renal dose adjustments, infusion times, prevention and management of osteonecrosis of the jaw, and monitoring of laboratory parameter recommendations. The guidelines also recommend in patients with extensive bone disease with existing severe renal disease (a serum creatinine >3 mg/dL or Cl$_{cr}$ <30 mL/minute) pamidronate at a dose of 90 mg over 4-6 hours (unless pre-existing renal disease in which a reduced initial dose should be considered). ASCO also recommends monitoring for albuminuria every 3-6 months. In patients with unexplained albuminuria >500 mg/24 hours, withhold the dose until level returns to baseline, then recheck every 3-4 weeks. Pamidronate may be reinitiated at a dose not to exceed 90 mg every 4 weeks with a longer infusion time of at least 4 hours. Also consider increasing the infusion time of zoledronic acid to at least 30 minutes; although one study demonstrated that extending the infusion to 30 minutes did not change the safety profile (Berenson, 2011).

Special Geriatric Considerations The elderly are frequently treated long-term for osteoporosis. Elderly patients should be advised to report any lower extremity, jaw (osteonecrosis), or muscle pain that cannot be explained or lasts longer than 2 weeks. Additionally, elderly often receive concomitant diuretic therapy and therefore their electrolyte status (eg, calcium, phosphate) should be periodically evaluated.

Dosage Forms Excipient information presented when available (limited, particularly for generics); consult specific product labeling. [DSC] = Discontinued product

Injection, powder for reconstitution, as disodium: 30 mg, 90 mg

Aredia®: 30 mg, 90 mg [DSC]

Injection, solution, as disodium: 3 mg/mL (10 mL); 6 mg/mL (10 mL); 9 mg/mL (10 mL)

Injection, solution, as disodium [preservative free]: 3 mg/mL (10 mL); 9 mg/mL (10 mL)

Selected References

Bamias A, Kastritis E, Bamia C, et al, "Osteonecrosis of the Jaw in Cancer After Treatment With Bisphosphonates: Incidence and Risk Factors," *J Clin Oncol*, 2005, 23(34):8580-7.

Diamond TH, Winters J, Smith A, et al, "The Antiosteoporotic Efficacy of Intravenous Pamidronate in Men With Prostate Carcinoma Receiving Combined Androgen Blockade: A Double Blind, Randomized, Placebo-Controlled Crossover Study," *Cancer*, 2001, 92(6):1444-50.

Hillner BE, Ingel JN, Chlebowski RT, et al, "American Society of Clinical Oncology 2003 Update on the Role of Bisphosphonates and Bone Health Issues in Women With Breast Cancer," *J Clin Oncol*, 2003, 21(21):4042-57.

Kyle RA, Yee GC, Somerfield MR, et al, "American Society of Clinical Oncology 2007 Clinical Practice Guideline Update on the Role of Bisphosphonates in Multiple Myeloma," *J Clin Oncol*, 2007, 25(17):2464-72.

National Comprehensive Cancer Network® (NCCN), "Clinical Practice Guidelines in Oncology™: Multiple Myeloma," Version 2, 2009. Available at http://www.nccn.org/professionals/physician_gls/PDF/myeloma.pdf.

National Comprehensive Cancer Network® (NCCN), "Clinical Practice Guidelines in Oncology™: Thyroid Carcinoma," Version 1, 2008. Available at http://www.nccn.org/professionals/physicians_gls/PDF/thyroid.pdf

Smith MR, McGovern FJ, Zietman AL, et al, "Pamidronate to Prevent Bone Loss During Androgen-Deprivation Therapy For Prostate Cancer," *N Engl J Med*, 2001, 345(13):948-55.

Pancrelipase (pan kre LYE pase)

Medication Safety Issues

Sound-alike/look-alike issues:

Pancrelipase may be confused with pancreatin

Brand Names: U.S. Creon®; Pancreaze™; Pancrelipase™; Zenpep™

Brand Names: Canada Cotazym®; Creon®; Pancrease® MT; Ultrase®; Ultrase® MT; Viokase®

Index Terms Amylase, Lipase, and Protease; Lipancreatin; Lipase, Protease, and Amylase; Pancreatic Enzymes; Protease, Lipase, and Amylase

Generic Availability (U.S.) Yes

Pharmacologic Category Enzyme

Use Treatment of exocrine pancreatic insufficiency (EPI) due to conditions such as cystic fibrosis (Creon®, Pancreaze™, Zenpep™); chronic pancreatitis (Creon®); or pancreatectomy (Creon®)

Medication Guide Available Yes

Contraindications There are no contraindications listed in the manufacturer's labeling.

Warnings/Precautions Fibrosing colonopathy advancing to colonic strictures have been reported with doses of lipase >6000 units/kg/meal over long periods of time in children <12 years of age. Patients taking doses of lipase >6000 units/kg/meal should be examined and the dose decreased. Doses of lipase >2500 units/kg/meal (or lipase >10,000 units/kg/day) should be used with caution and only with documentation of 3-day fecal fat measures. Crushing or chewing the contents of the capsules, or mixing the contents with foods outside of product labeling, may cause early release of the enzymes, causing irritation of the oral mucosa and/or loss of enzyme activity. When mixing the contents of capsules with food, the mixture should be swallowed immediately and followed with water or juice to ensure complete ingestion. Use caution in patients with gout, hyperuricemia, or renal impairment; products contain purines which may increase uric acid concentrations. Products are derived from porcine pancreatic glands. Severe, allergic reactions (rare) have been observed; use with caution in patients hypersensitive to pork proteins. Transmission of porcine viruses is theoretically a risk; however, testing and/or inactivation or removal of certain viruses, reduces the risk. There have been no cases of transmission of an infectious illness reported. Available brand products are **not** interchangeable.

Adverse Reactions (Reflective of adult population; not specific for elderly) The following adverse reactions were reported in a short-term safety studies; actual frequency varies with different products; adverse events, particularly gastrointestinal events, were often greater with placebo:

10%:

Central nervous system: Headache (6% to 15%)

Gastrointestinal: Abdominal pain (4% to 18%)

1% to 10%:

Central nervous system: Dizziness (4% to 6%)

Endocrine & metabolic: Diabetes mellitus exacerbation (4%), hyperglycemia (4% to 8%), hypoglycemia (4%)

Gastrointestinal: Flatulence (4% to 9%), early satiety (6%), weight loss (3% to 6%), vomiting (6%), upper abdominal pain (≤5%), diarrhea (≤4%), feces abnormal (≤4%)

Respiratory: Cough (4% to 6%), nasopharyngitis (4%)

Drug Interactions

Avoid Concomitant Use There are no known interactions where it is recommended to avoid concomitant use.

Increased Effect/Toxicity There are no known significant interactions involving an increase in effect.

Decreased Effect

Pancrelipase may decrease the levels/effects of: Iron Salts

Ethanol/Nutrition/Herb Interactions Food: Avoid placing contents of opened capsules on alkaline food; pancrelipase may impair absorption of oral iron.

Stability

Creon®: Store at room temperature of 25°C (77°F); excursions permitted between 25°C to 40°C (77°F to 104°F) for ≤30 days. Protect from moisture, and discard if moisture conditions are >70%. Keep bottle tightly closed.

Pancreaze™: Store at ≤25°C (77°F). Protect from moisture; keep bottle tightly closed.

Zenpep™: Store at room temperature 20°C to 25°C (68°F to 77°F). Protect from moisture; keep bottle tightly closed after opening.

Mechanism of Action Pancrelipase is a natural product harvested from the porcine pancreatic glands. It contains a combination of lipase, amylase, and protease. Products are formulated to dissolve in the more basic pH of the duodenum so that they may act locally to break down fats, protein, and starch.

Pharmacodynamics/Kinetics

Absorption: None; acts locally in GI tract

Excretion: Feces

Dosage

Geriatric Refer to adult dosing.

Adult Note: Adjust dose based on body weight, clinical symptoms, and stool fat content. Allow several days between dose adjustments. Total daily dose reflects ~3 meals/day and 2-3 snacks/day, with half the mealtime dose given with a snack. Doses of lipase >2500 units/kg/meal (or lipase > 10,000 units/kg/day) should be used with caution and only with documentation of 3-day fecal fat measures. Doses of lipase >6000 units/kg/meal are associated with colonic stricture and should be decreased.

Pancreatic insufficiency: Oral: Initial: Lipase 500 units/kg/meal. Dosage range: Lipase 500-2500 units/kg/meal. Maximum dose: Lipase 10,000 units/kg/day **or** lipase 4000 units/g of fat per day

Pancreatic insufficiency due to chronic pancreatitis or pancreatectomy (Creon®): Oral: Lipase 72,000 units/meal while consuming ≥100 g of fat per day; alternatively, lower initial doses of lipase 500 units/kg/meal with individualized dosage titrations have also been used

Administration Oral: Administer with meals or snacks and swallow whole with a generous amount of liquid. Do not crush or chew; retention in the mouth before swallowing may cause mucosal irritation and stomatitis. If necessary, capsules may also be opened and contents added to a small amount of an acidic food (pH ≤4.5), such as applesauce. The food should be at room temperature and swallowed immediately after mixing. The contents of the capsule should not be crushed or chewed. Follow with water or juice to ensure complete ingestion and that no medication remains in the mouth.

Creon®: Capsules contain enteric coated spheres which are 0.71-1.6 mm in diameter
Pancreaze™: Capsules contain enteric coated microtablets which are ~2 mm in diameter
Zenpep™: Capsules contain enteric coated beads which are 1.8-2.5 mm in diameter

Monitoring Parameters Abdominal symptoms, nutritional intake, weight, stool character, fecal fat

Pharmacotherapy Pearls Unapproved PEPs are no longer allowed to be distributed in the U.S. There are three PEPs with FDA approval commercially available in the U.S.: Creon®, Pancreaze™, and Zenpep™. PEPs are **not** interchangeable, and patients will require new prescriptions when changing from one product to another. However, Pancrelipase™ lipase 5000 units strength (manufactured by Eurand Pharmaceuticals and distributed by X-Gen Pharmaceuticals) is an authorized generic which may be used interchangeably with the Zenpep™ lipase 5000 units product (manufactured by Eurand Pharmaceuticals).

Special Geriatric Considerations No special considerations are necessary since drug is dosed to response; however, drug-induced diarrhea can result in unwanted side effects (eg, confusion, hypotension, lethargy, fluid and electrolyte loss).

Dosage Forms Excipient information presented when available (limited, particularly for generics); consult specific product labeling.

Capsule, delayed release, enteric coated beads [porcine derived]:
Pancrelipase™: Lipase 5000 units, protease 17,000 units, amylase 27,000 units
Zenpep™: Lipase 3000 units, protease 10,000 units, amylase 16,000 units
Zenpep™: Lipase 5000 units, protease 17,000 units, amylase 27,000 units
Zenpep™: Lipase 10,000 units, protease 34,000 units, amylase 55,000 units
Zenpep™: Lipase 15,000 units, protease 51,000 units, amylase 82,000 units
Zenpep™: Lipase 20,000 units, protease 68,000 units, amylase 109,000 units
Capsule, delayed release, enteric coated microspheres [new formulation; porcine derived]:
Creon®: Lipase 3000 units, protease 9500 units, and amylase 15,000 units
Creon®: Lipase 6000 units, protease 19,000 units, and amylase 30,000 units
Creon®: Lipase 12000 units, protease 38,000 units, and amylase 60,000 units
Creon®: Lipase 24,000 units, protease 76,000 units, and amylase 120,000 units
Capsule, delayed release, enteric coated microtablets [porcine derived]:
Pancreaze™: Lipase 4200 units, protease 10,000 units, and amylase 17,500 units
Pancreaze™: Lipase 10,500 units, protease 25,000 units, and amylase 43,750 units
Pancreaze™: Lipase 16,800 units, protease 40,000 units, and amylase 70,000 units
Pancreaze™: Lipase 21,000 units, protease 37,000 units, and amylase 61,000 units

Selected References
Baker SS, "Delayed Release Pancrelipase for the Treatment of Pancreatic Exocrine Insufficiency Associated With Cystic Fibrosis," *Ther Clin Risk Manag*, 2008, 4(5):1079-84.
Marcuard SP and Stegall KS, "Unclogging Feeding Tubes With Pancreatic Enzyme," *JPEN J Parenter Enteral Nutr*, 1990, 14(2):198-200.

♦ **Pancrelipase™** *see* Pancrelipase *on page 1387*
♦ **Pandel®** *see* Hydrocortisone (Topical) *on page 886*
♦ **Panglobulin** *see* Immune Globulin *on page 922*

Pantoprazole (pan TOE pra zole)

Medication Safety Issues
Sound-alike/look-alike issues:
Pantoprazole may be confused with ARIPiprazole
Protonix® may be confused with Lotronex®, Lovenox®, protamine
Administration issues:
Vials containing Protonix® I.V. for injection are not recommended for use with spiked I.V. system adaptors. Nurses and pharmacists have reported breakage of the glass vials during attempts to connect spiked I.V. system adaptors, which may potentially result in injury to healthcare professionals.
International issues:
Protonix [U.S., Canada] may be confused with Pretanix brand name for indapamide [Hungary]

Brand Names: U.S. Protonix®; Protonix® I.V.

Brand Names: Canada Apo-Pantoprazole®; CO Pantoprazole; Mylan-Pantoprazole; Pantoloc®; Pantoprazole for Injection; Panto™ I.V.; PMS-Pantoprazole; RAN™-Pantoprazole; ratio-Pantoprazole; Riva-Pantoprazole; Sandoz-Pantoprazole; Tecta™; Teva-Pantoprazole

Generic Availability (U.S.) Yes: Delayed release tablet

Pharmacologic Category Proton Pump Inhibitor; Substituted Benzimidazole

◀ **Use**

Oral: Treatment and maintenance of healing of erosive esophagitis associated with GERD; reduction in relapse rates of daytime and nighttime heartburn symptoms in GERD; hypersecretory disorders associated with Zollinger-Ellison syndrome or other GI hypersecretory disorders

I.V.: Short-term treatment (7-10 days) of patients with gastroesophageal reflux disease (GERD) and a history of erosive esophagitis; hypersecretory disorders associated with Zollinger-Ellison syndrome or other neoplastic disorders

Unlabeled/Investigational Use Peptic ulcer disease, active ulcer bleeding (parenteral formulation); adjunct treatment with antibiotics for *Helicobacter pylori* eradication; stress-ulcer prophylaxis in the critically-ill

Contraindications Hypersensitivity to pantoprazole, substituted benzamidazoles (eg, esomeprazole, lansoprazole, omeprazole, rabeprazole), or any component of the formulation

Canadian labeling: Additional contraindication (not in U.S. labeling): Concomitant use with atazanavir

Warnings/Precautions Use of proton pump inhibitors may increase the risk of gastrointestinal infections (eg, *Salmonella, Campylobacter*). Relief of symptoms does not preclude the presence of a gastric malignancy. Long-term pantoprazole therapy (especially in patients who were *H. pylori* positive) has caused biopsy-proven atrophic gastritis. No reports of enterochromaffin-like (ECL) cell carcinoids, dysplasia, or neoplasia such as those seen in rodent studies have occurred in humans. Not indicated for maintenance therapy; safety and efficacy for use beyond 16 weeks have not been established. Prolonged treatment (typically >3 years) may lead to vitamin B_{12} malabsorption and subsequent deficiency. Intravenous preparation contains edetate sodium (EDTA); use caution in patients who are at risk for zinc deficiency if other EDTA-containing solutions are coadministered. Decreased *H. pylori* eradication rates have been observed with short-term (≤7 days) combination therapy. The American College of Gastroenterology recommends 10-14 days of therapy (triple or quadruple) for eradication of *H. pylori* (Chey, 2007). Proton pump inhibitors may diminish the therapeutic effect of clopidogrel, thought to be due to reduced formation of the active metabolite of clopidogrel; an increase in the risk of cardiovascular events may occur. Of the PPIs, pantoprazole has the lowest degree of CYP2C19 inhibition and is preferred if concomitant use of a PPI is necessary.

Increased incidence of osteoporosis-related bone fractures of the hip, spine, or wrist may occur with proton pump inhibitor therapy. Patients on high-dose or long-term therapy should be monitored. Use the lowest effective dose for the shortest duration of time, use vitamin D and calcium supplementation, and follow appropriate guidelines to reduce risk of fractures in patients at risk.

Hypomagnesemia, reported rarely, usually with prolonged PPI use of >3 months (most cases >1 year of therapy); may be symptomatic or asymptomatic; severe cases may cause tetany, seizures, and cardiac arrhythmias. Consider obtaining serum magnesium concentrations prior to beginning long-term therapy, especially if taking concomitant digoxin, diuretics, or other drugs known to cause hypomagnesemia; and periodically thereafter. Hypomagnesemia may be corrected by magnesium supplementation, although discontinuation of pantoprazole may be necessary; magnesium levels typically return to normal within 1 week of stopping.

Adverse Reactions (Reflective of adult population; not specific for elderly)

≥1%:

Cardiovascular: Chest pain

Central nervous system: Headache (2% to 9%), insomnia (≤1%), anxiety, dizziness, migraine, pain

Dermatologic: Rash (≤2%)

Endocrine & metabolic: Hyperglycemia (≤1%), hyperlipidemia

Gastrointestinal: Diarrhea (2% to 6%), flatulence (2% to 4%), abdominal pain (1% to 4%), nausea (≤2%), vomiting (≤2%), eructation (≤1%), constipation, dyspepsia, gastroenteritis, rectal disorder

Genitourinary: Urinary frequency, UTI

Hepatic: Liver function tests abnormal (≤2%)

Local: Injection site reaction (includes thrombophlebitis and abscess)

Neuromuscular & skeletal: Arthralgia, back pain, hypertonia, neck pain, weakness

Respiratory: Bronchitis, cough, dyspnea, pharyngitis, rhinitis, sinusitis, upper respiratory tract infection

Miscellaneous: Flu syndrome, infection

Drug Interactions

Metabolism/Transport Effects Substrate of CYP2C9 (minor), 2C19 (major), 2D6 (minor), 3A4 (minor); **Inhibits** CYP2C9 (weak), 2C19 (moderate), ABCG2; **Induces** CYP1A2 (weak), 3A4 (weak)

Avoid Concomitant Use

Avoid concomitant use of Pantoprazole with any of the following: Delavirdine; Erlotinib; Nelfinavir; Posaconazole; Rilpivirine

Increased Effect/Toxicity

Pantoprazole may increase the levels/effects of: Amphetamines; CYP2C19 Substrates; Dexmethylphenidate; Methotrexate; Methylphenidate; Raltegravir; Saquinavir; Topotecan; Voriconazole

The levels/effects of Pantoprazole may be increased by: Conivaptan; Fluconazole; Ketoconazole; Ketoconazole (Systemic)

Decreased Effect

Pantoprazole may decrease the levels/effects of: Atazanavir; Bisphosphonate Derivatives; Cefditoren; Clopidogrel; Dabigatran Etexilate; Dasatinib; Delavirdine; Erlotinib; Gefitinib; Indinavir; Iron Salts; Itraconazole; Ketoconazole; Ketoconazole (Systemic); Mesalamine; Mycophenolate; Nelfinavir; Posaconazole; Rilpivirine

The levels/effects of Pantoprazole may be decreased by: CYP2C19 Inducers (Strong); Peginterferon Alfa-2b; Tipranavir; Tocilizumab

Ethanol/Nutrition/Herb Interactions

Ethanol: Avoid ethanol (may cause gastric mucosal irritation).

Herb/Nutraceutical: Prolonged treatment (typically >3 years) may lead to vitamin B_{12} malabsorption and subsequent deficiency.

Stability

Oral: Store tablet and oral suspension at controlled room temperature of 20°C to 25°C (68°F to 77°F).

I.V.: Prior to reconstitution, store at controlled room temperature of 20°C to 25°C (68°F to 77°F). Protect from light. Reconstitute with 10 mL NS (final concentration 4 mg/mL). Reconstituted solution may be given intravenously (over 2 minutes) or may be added to 100 mL D_5W, NS, or LR (for 15-minute infusion). When reconstituted, solution is stable up to 96 hours at room temperature (Johnson, 2005). The preparation should be stored at 3°C to 5°C (37°F to 41°F) if it is stored beyond 48 hours to minimize discoloration. If further diluting in 100 mL of D_5W, LR, or NS, dilute within 6 hours of reconstitution. Diluted solution is stable at room temperature for up to 24 hours from the time of initial reconstitution; protection from light is not required.

Mechanism of Action Suppresses gastric acid secretion by inhibiting the parietal cell H^+/K^+ ATP pump

Pharmacodynamics/Kinetics

Absorption: Rapid, well absorbed

Distribution: V_d: 11-24 L

Protein binding: 98%, primarily to albumin

Metabolism: Extensively hepatic; CYP2C19 (demethylation), CYP3A4; no evidence that metabolites have pharmacologic activity

Bioavailability: 77%

Half-life elimination: 1 hour; increased to 3.5-10 hours with CYP2C19 deficiency

Time to peak: Oral: 2.5 hours

Excretion: Urine (71%); feces (18%)

Dosage

Geriatric & Adult

Erosive esophagitis associated with GERD:

Oral:

Treatment: 40 mg once daily for up to 8 weeks; an additional 8 weeks may be used in patients who have not healed after an 8-week course

Maintenance of healing: 40 mg once daily

Note: Lower doses (20 mg once daily) have been used successfully in mild GERD treatment and maintenance of healing

I.V.: 40 mg once daily for 7-10 days

Hypersecretory disorders (including Zollinger-Ellison):

Oral: Initial: 40 mg twice daily; adjust dose based on patient needs; doses up to 240 mg/day have been administered

I.V.: 80 mg twice daily; adjust dose based on acid output measurements; 160-240 mg/day in divided doses has been used for a limited period (up to 7 days)

Prevention of rebleeding in peptic ulcer bleed (unlabeled use): I.V.: 80 mg, followed by 8 mg/hour infusion for 72 hours. **Note:** A daily infusion of 40 mg does not raise gastric pH sufficiently to enhance coagulation in active GI bleeds.

◄

Helicobacter pylori eradication (unlabeled use): *Oral:* American College of Gastro-enterology guidelines (Chey, 2007):

Nonpenicillin allergy: 40 mg twice daily administered with amoxicillin 1000 mg *and* clarithromycin 500 mg twice daily for 10-14 days

Penicillin allergy: 40 mg twice daily administered with clarithromycin 500 mg *and* metronidazole 500 mg twice daily for 10-14 days **or** 40 mg once or twice daily administered with bismuth subsalicylate 525 mg *and* metronidazole 250 mg *plus* tetracycline 500 mg 4 times/day for 10-14 days

Renal Impairment No adjustment is required. Pantoprazole is not removed by hemodialysis.

Hepatic Impairment No adjustment is required.

Administration

I.V.: Flush I.V. line before and after administration. In-line filter not required.

2-minute infusion: The volume of reconstituted solution (4 mg/mL) to be injected may be administered intravenously over at least 2 minutes.

15-minute infusion: Infuse over 15 minutes at a rate not to exceed 7 mL/minute (3 mg/minute).

Oral:

Tablet: Should be swallowed whole, do not crush or chew. Best if taken before breakfast.

Delayed-release oral suspension: Should only be administered in apple juice or applesauce and taken ~30 minutes before a meal. Do not administer with any other liquid (eg, water) or foods.

Oral administration in **applesauce**: Sprinkle intact granules on 1 tablespoon of applesauce and swallow within 10 minutes of preparation.

Oral administration in **apple juice**: Empty intact granules into 5 mL of apple juice (~1 teaspoonful), stir for 5 seconds, and swallow immediately after preparation. Rinse container once or twice with apple juice and swallow immediately.

Nasogastric tube administration: Separate the plunger from the barrel of a 60 mL catheter tip syringe and connect to a ≥16 French nasogastric tube. Holding the syringe attached to the tubing as high as possible, empty the contents of the packet into barrel of the syringe, add 10 mL of apple juice and gently tap/shake the barrel of the syringe to help empty the syringe. Add an additional 10 mL of apple juice and gently tap/shake the barrel to help rinse. Repeat rinse with at least 2-10 mL aliquots of apple juice. No granules should remain in the syringe.

Monitoring Parameters Hypersecretory disorders: Acid output measurements, target level <10 mEq/hour (<5 mEq/hour if prior gastric acid-reducing surgery)

Test Interactions False-positive urine screening tests for tetrahydrocannabinol (THC) have been noted in patients receiving proton pump inhibitors, including pantoprazole.

Special Geriatric Considerations Dosage adjustment not required.

Dosage Forms Excipient information presented when available (limited, particularly for generics); consult specific product labeling.

Granules for suspension, delayed release, enteric coated, oral:

Protonix®: 40 mg/packet (30s)

Injection, powder for reconstitution:

Protonix® I.V.: 40 mg [contains edetate disodium]

Tablet, delayed release, oral: 20 mg, 40 mg

Protonix®: 20 mg, 40 mg

Dosage Forms: Canada Excipient information presented when available (limited, particularly for generics); consult specific product labeling.

Note: Strength expressed as base

Tablet, enteric coated, as magnesium:

Pantoloc®: 40 mg

Selected References

Chey WD, Wong BC, et al, "American College of Gastroenterology Guideline on the Management of *Helicobacter pylori* Infection," *Am J Gastroent*, 2007, 102(8):1808-25.

Johnson CE, "Stability of Pantoprazole in 0.9% Sodium Chloride Injection in Polypropylene Syringes," *Am J Health Syst Pharm*, 2005, 62(22):2410-2.

Paoluzi P, Iacopini F, Crispino P, et al, "2-Week Triple Therapy for *Helicobacter pylori* Infection is Better Than 1-Week in Clinical Practice: a Large Prospective Single-Center Randomized Study," *Helicobacter*, 2006, 11(6):562-8.

Papaverine (pa PAV er een)

Medication Safety Issues

Sound-alike/look-alike issues:

Papaverine may be confused with pamidronate

Index Terms Papaverine Hydrochloride; Pavabid [DSC]

Generic Availability (U.S.) Yes

Pharmacologic Category Vasodilator

Use Oral: Relief of peripheral and cerebral ischemia associated with arterial spasm and myocardial ischemia complicated by arrhythmias

Unlabeled/Investigational Use Investigational: Parenteral: Various vascular spasms associated with muscle spasms as in myocardial infarction, angina, peripheral and pulmonary embolism, peripheral vascular disease, angiospastic states, and visceral spasm (ureteral, biliary, and GI colic); testing for impotence

Papaverine has been used for many conditions where vasodilatation is felt to be of some benefit; however, to date, insufficient scientific evidence exists for any therapeutic value to its use except in testing for impotence.

Dosage

Geriatric & Adult Arterial spasm:

Oral, sustained release: 150-300 mg every 12 hours; in difficult cases: 150 mg every 8 hours

I.M., I.V.: 30-65 mg (rarely up to 120 mg); may repeat every 3 hours

Special Geriatric Considerations Vasodilators have been used to treat dementia upon the premise that dementia is secondary to a cerebral blood flow insufficiency. The hypothesis is that if blood flow could be increased, cognitive function would be increased. This hypothesis is no longer valid. The use of vasodilators for cognitive dysfunction is not recommended or proven by appropriate scientific study.

Dosage Forms Excipient information presented when available (limited, particularly for generics); consult specific product labeling. [DSC] = Discontinued product

Capsule, sustained release, oral, as hydrochloride: 150 mg [DSC]

Injection, solution, as hydrochloride: 30 mg/mL (2 mL, 10 mL)

- ◆ **Papaverine Hydrochloride** see Papaverine on page 1392
- ◆ **PAR-101** see Fidaxomicin (Systemic) on page 732
- ◆ **Para-Aminosalicylate Sodium** see Aminosalicylic Acid on page 97
- ◆ **Paracetamol** see Acetaminophen on page 33
- ◆ **Parafon Forte® DSC** see Chlorzoxazone on page 345
- ◆ **Parathyroid Hormone (1-34)** see Teriparatide on page 1760
- ◆ **Parcopa®** see Carbidopa and Levodopa on page 274

Paricalcitol (pah ri KAL si tole)

Medication Safety Issues

Sound alike/look alike issues:

Paricalcitol may be confused with calcitriol

Zemplar® may be confused with zaleplon, Zelapar®, zolpidem, ZyPREXA® Zydis®

Brand Names: U.S. Zemplar®

Brand Names: Canada Zemplar®

Generic Availability (U.S.) No

Pharmacologic Category Vitamin D Analog

Use

I.V.: Prevention and treatment of secondary hyperparathyroidism associated with stage 5 chronic kidney disease (CKD)

Oral: Prevention and treatment of secondary hyperparathyroidism associated with stage 3 and 4 CKD and stage 5 CKD patients on hemodialysis or peritoneal dialysis

Contraindications Hypersensitivity to paricalcitol or any component of the formulation; patients with evidence of vitamin D toxicity; hypercalcemia

Warnings/Precautions Excessive administration may lead to over suppression of PTH, hypercalcemia, hypercalciuria, hyperphosphatemia and adynamic bone disease. Acute hypercalcemia may increase risk of cardiac arrhythmias and seizures; use caution with cardiac glycosides as digitalis toxicity may be increased. Chronic hypercalcemia may lead to generalized vascular and other soft-tissue calcification. Phosphate and vitamin D (and its derivatives) should be withheld during therapy to avoid hypercalcemia. Risk of hypercalcemia may be increased by concomitant use of calcium-containing supplements and/or medications that increase serum calcium (eg, thiazide diuretics). Avoid regular administration to prevent aluminum overload and toxicity. Dialysate concentration of aluminum should be maintained at <10 mcg/L.

Adverse Reactions (Reflective of adult population; not specific for elderly)

>10%:

Gastrointestinal: Nausea (5% to 13%), diarrhea (7% to 12%)

Miscellaneous: Infection (bacterial, fungal, viral: 3% to 15%)

2% to 10%:

Cardiovascular: Edema (7%), hypertension (7%), hypervolemia (5%), hypotension (5%), palpitation (3%), chest pain (3%), peripheral edema (3%), syncope (3%)

Central nervous system: Pain (8%), dizziness (5% to 7%), chills (5%), insomnia (5%), lightheadedness (5%), vertigo (5%), fever (3% to 5%), headache (3% to 5%), anxiety (3%), depression (3%)

Dermatologic: Rash (6%), bruising (3%), skin ulcer (3%)

Endocrine & metabolic: Dehydration (3%), hypoglycemia (3%)

Gastrointestinal: Vomiting (5% to 8%), GI bleeding (5%), constipation (4% to 5%), abdominal pain (4%), dyspepsia (3%), xerostomia (3%)

Genitourinary: Urinary tract infection (3%)

Neuromuscular & skeletal: Arthritis (5%), weakness (3% to 5%), back pain (4%), leg cramps (3%)

Renal: Uremia (3%)

Respiratory: Pneumonia (5%), rhinitis (5%), oropharyngeal pain (4%), bronchitis (3%), cough (3%), sinusitis (3%)

Miscellaneous: Allergic reaction (6%), flu-like syndrome (5%), peritonitis (5%), sepsis (5%)

Drug Interactions

Metabolism/Transport Effects
Substrate of CYP3A4 (major)

Avoid Concomitant Use
Avoid concomitant use of Paricalcitol with any of the following: Aluminum Hydroxide; Sucralfate; Vitamin D Analogs

Increased Effect/Toxicity
Paricalcitol may increase the levels/effects of: Aluminum Hydroxide; Cardiac Glycosides; Digoxin; Sucralfate; Vitamin D Analogs

The levels/effects of Paricalcitol may be increased by: Calcium Salts; CYP3A4 Inhibitors (Strong); Thiazide Diuretics

Decreased Effect
The levels/effects of Paricalcitol may be decreased by: Bile Acid Sequestrants; Mineral Oil; Orlistat; Tocilizumab

Stability Store at 25°C (77°F); excursions permitted between 15°C to 30°C (59°F to 86°F).

Mechanism of Action Decreased renal conversion of vitamin D to its primary active metabolite (1,25-hydroxyvitamin D) in chronic renal failure leads to reduced activation of vitamin D receptor (VDR), which subsequently removes inhibitory suppression of parathyroid hormone (PTH) release; increased serum PTH (secondary hyperparathyroidism) reduces calcium excretion and enhances bone resorption. Paricalcitol is a synthetic vitamin D analog which binds to and activates the VDR in kidney, parathyroid gland, intestine and bone, thus reducing PTH levels and improving calcium and phosphate homeostasis.

Pharmacodynamics/Kinetics

Distribution: V_d:
  Healthy subjects: Oral: 34 L; I.V.: 24 L
  Stage 3 and 4 CKD: Oral: 44-46 L
  Stage 5 CKD: Oral: 38-49 L; I.V.: 31-35 L

Protein binding: >99%

Metabolism: Hydroxylation and glucuronidation via hepatic and nonhepatic enzymes, including CYP24, CYP3A4, UGT1A4; forms metabolites (at least one active)

Bioavailability: Oral: 72% to 86% in healthy subjects

Half-life elimination:
  Healthy subjects: Oral: 4-6 hours; I.V.: 5-7 hours
  Stage 3 and 4 CKD: Oral: 14-20 hours
  Stage 5 CKD: Oral: 14-20 hours; I.V.: 14-15 hours

Time to peak, plasma: 3 hours: Delayed by food

Excretion: Healthy subjects: Feces (oral: 70%; I.V.: 63%); urine (oral: 18%, I.V.: 19%)

Dosage

Geriatric & Adult Note: In stage 3 -5 CKD maintain Ca x P <55 mg^2/dL^2, reduce or interrupt dosing if recommended calcium phosphorus product (Ca x P) is exceeded or hypercalcemia is observed (K/DOQI Clinical Practice Guidelines, 2003).

Secondary hyperparathyroidism associated with chronic renal failure (stage 5 CKD):
  I.V.: 0.04-0.1 mcg/kg (2.8-7 mcg) given as a bolus dose no more frequently than every other day at any time during dialysis; dose may be increased by 2-4 mcg every 2-4 weeks; doses as high as 0.24 mcg/kg (16.8 mcg) have been administered safely; the dose of paricalcitol should be adjusted based on serum intact PTH (iPTH) levels, as follows:
    Same or increasing iPTH level: Increase paricalcitol dose
    iPTH level decreased by <30%: Increase paricalcitol dose
    iPTH level decreased by >30% and <60%: Maintain paricalcitol dose
    iPTH level decrease by >60%: Decrease paricalcitol dose
    iPTH level 1.5-3 times upper limit of normal: Maintain paricalcitol dose

Oral: Initial dose, in mcg, based on baseline iPTH level divided by 80. Administered 3 times weekly, no more frequently than every other day. **Note:** To reduce the risk of hypercalcemia initiate only after baseline serum calcium has been adjusted to ≤9.5 mg/dL.
Dose titration:
Titration dose (mcg) = Most recent iPTH level (pg/mL) divided by 80
Note: In situations where monitoring of iPTH, calcium, and phosphorus occurs less frequently than once per week, a more modest initial and dose titration rate may be warranted:
Modest titration dose (mcg) = Most recent iPTH level (pg/mL) divided by 100
Dosage adjustment for hypercalcemia or elevated Ca x P: Decrease calculated dose by 2-4 mcg. If further adjustment is required, dose should be reduced or interrupted until these parameters are normalized. If applicable, phosphate binder dosing may also be adjusted or withheld, or switch to a noncalcium-based phosphate binder

Secondary hyperparathyroidism associated with stage 3 and 4 CKD: Adults: Oral: Initial dose based on baseline serum iPTH:
iPTH ≤500 pg/mL: 1 mcg/day or 2 mcg 3 times/week
iPTH >500 pg/mL: 2 mcg/day or 4 mcg 3 times/week

Dosage adjustment based on iPTH level relative to baseline, adjust dose at 2-4 week intervals:
iPTH same or increased: Increase paricalcitol dose by 1 mcg/day or 2 mcg 3 times/week
iPTH decreased by <30%: Increase paricalcitol dose by 1 mcg/day or 2 mcg 3 times/week
iPTH decreased by ≥30% and ≤60%: Maintain paricalcitol dose
iPTH decreased by >60%: Decrease paricalcitol dose by 1 mcg/day* or 2 mcg 3 times/week
iPTH <60 pg/mL: Decrease paricalcitol dose by 1 mcg/day* or 2 mcg 3 times/week
*If patient is taking the lowest dose on a once-daily regimen, but further dose reduction is needed, decrease dose to 1 mcg 3 times/week. If further dose reduction is required, withhold drug as needed and restart at a lower dose. If applicable, calcium-phosphate binder dosing may also be adjusted or withheld, or switch to noncalcium-based binder.
Renal Impairment Refer to Dosage: Geriatric & Adult.
Hepatic Impairment
Mild-to-moderate hepatic impairment: No dosage adjustment required.
Severe hepatic impairment: Use has not been evaluated.
Administration
Oral: May be administered with or without food. With the 3 times/week dosing schedule, doses should not be given more frequently than every other day.
I.V.: Administered as a bolus dose at anytime during dialysis. Doses should not be administered more often than every other day.
Monitoring Parameters
Signs and symptoms of vitamin D intoxication
Serum calcium and phosphorus (closely monitor levels during dosage titration and after initiation of a strong CYP3A4 inhibitor):
I.V.: Twice weekly during initial phase, then at least monthly once dose established
Oral: At least every 2 weeks for 3 months or following dose adjustment, then monthly for 3 months, then every 3 months
Serum or plasma intact PTH (iPTH):
I.V.: Every 3 months
Oral: At least every 2 weeks for 3 months or following dose adjustment, then monthly for 3 months, then every 3 months
Reference Range
Corrected total serum calcium (K/DOQI, 2003): CKD stages 3 and 4: 8.4-10.2 mg/dL (2.1-2.6 mmol/L); CKD stage 5: 8.4-9.5 mg/dL (2.1-2.37 mmol/L); KDIGO guidelines recommend maintaining normal ranges for all stages of CKD (3-5D) (KDIGO, 2009)
Phosphorus (K/DOQI, 2003):
CKD stages 3 and 4: 2.7-4.6 mg/dL (0.87-1.48 mmol/L) (adults); maintain within age-appropriate limits (children)
CKD stage 5 (including those treated with dialysis): 3.5-5.5 mg/dL (1.13-1.78 mmol/L) (children > 12 years and adults); 4-6 mg/dL (1.29-1.94 mmol/L) (children 1-12 years)
KDIGO guidelines recommend maintaining normal ranges for CKD stages 3-5 and lowering elevated phosphorus levels toward the normal range for CKD stage 5D (KDIGO, 2009)
Serum calcium-phosphorus product (K/DOQI, 2003): CKD stage 3-5: <55 mg^2/dL^2 (children >12 years and adults); <65 mg^2/dL^2 (children ≤12 years)
PTH: Whole molecule, immunochemiluminometric assay (ICMA): 1.0-5.2 pmol/L; whole molecule, radioimmunoassay (RIA): 10.0-65.0 pg/mL; whole molecule, immunoradiometric, double antibody (IRMA): 1.0-6.0 pmol/L

Target ranges by stage of chronic kidney disease (KDIGO, 2009): CKD stage 3-5: Optimal iPTH is unknown; maintain normal range (assay-dependent); CKD stage 5D: Maintain iPTH within 2-9 times the upper limit of normal for the assay used

Special Geriatric Considerations No specific dose changes necessary. Monitor closely. It may be advised to obtain baseline electrolytes, calcium, phosphorous, and digoxin serum concentrations, if applicable.

Dosage Forms Excipient information presented when available (limited, particularly for generics); consult specific product labeling.

Capsule, soft gelatin, oral:
Zemplar®: 1 mcg, 2 mcg, 4 mcg [contains coconut oil (may have trace amounts), ethanol, palm kernel oil (may have trace amounts)]

Injection, solution:
Zemplar®: 2 mcg/mL (1 mL); 5 mcg/mL (1 mL, 2 mL) [contains ethanol 20%, propylene glycol 30%]

Selected References

"K/DOQI Clinical Practice Guidelines for Bone Metabolism and Disease in Chronic Kidney Disease. Guideline 1. Evaluation of Calcium and Phosphorus Metabolism," *Am J Kidney Dis*, 2003, 42(4 Suppl 3):52-7.

"K/DOQI Clinical Practice Guidelines for Bone Metabolism and Disease in Chronic Kidney Disease. Guideline 3. Evaluation of Serum Phosphorus Levels," *Am J Kidney Dis*, 2003, 42(4 Suppl 3):62-3.

"K/DOQI Clinical Practice Guidelines for Chronic Kidney Disease: Evaluation, Classification, and Stratification, Part 4. Definition and Classification of Stages of Chronic Kidney Disease," *Am J Kidney Dis*, 2002, 39(2 Suppl 1):46-75.

◆ **Pariprazole** see RABEprazole on page 1571
◆ **Parlodel®** see Bromocriptine on page 214
◆ **Parlodel® SnapTabs®** see Bromocriptine on page 214
◆ **Parnate®** see Tranylcypromine on page 1846

PARoxetine (pa ROKS e teen)

Related Information
Antidepressant Agents on page 1991
Beers Criteria – Potentially Inappropriate Medications for Geriatrics on page 2089
Liquid Compatibility of Antidepressants, Antipsychotics, and Mood Stabilizers on page 2111

Medication Safety Issues
Sound-alike/look-alike issues:
PARoxetine may be confused with FLUoxetine, PACLitaxel, piroxicam, pyridoxine
Paxil® may be confused with Doxil®, paclitaxel, Plavix®, PROzac®, Taxol®

Brand Names: U.S. Paxil CR®; Paxil®; Pexeva®

Brand Names: Canada Apo-Paroxetine®; CO Paroxetine; Dom-Paroxetine; Mylan-Paroxetine; Novo-Paroxetine; Paxil CR®; Paxil®; PHL-Paroxetine; PMS-Paroxetine; ratio-Paroxetine; Riva-paroxetine; Sandoz-Paroxetine; Teva-Paroxetine

Index Terms Paroxetine Hydrochloride; Paroxetine Mesylate

Generic Availability (U.S.) Yes: Excludes suspension, tablet (mesylate)

Pharmacologic Category Antidepressant, Selective Serotonin Reuptake Inhibitor

Use Treatment of major depressive disorder (MDD); treatment of panic disorder with or without agoraphobia; obsessive-compulsive disorder (OCD); social anxiety disorder (social phobia); generalized anxiety disorder (GAD); post-traumatic stress disorder (PTSD)

Unlabeled/Investigational Use May be useful in eating disorders, impulse control disorders, self-injurious behavior; vasomotor symptoms of menopause; treatment of depression and obsessive-compulsive disorder (OCD); treatment of mild dementia-associated agitation in nonpsychotic patients

Medication Guide Available Yes

Contraindications Hypersensitivity to paroxetine or any component of the formulation; use with or within 14 days of MAO inhibitors; concurrent use with thioridazine or pimozide

Warnings/Precautions [U.S. Boxed Warning]: Antidepressants increase the risk of suicidal thinking and behavior in children, adolescents, and young adults (18-24 years of age) with major depressive disorder (MDD) and other psychiatric disorders; consider risk prior to prescribing. Short-term studies did not show an increased risk in patients >24 years of age and showed a decreased risk in patients ≥65 years. Closely monitor patients for clinical worsening, suicidality, or unusual changes in behavior, particularly during the initial 1-2 months of therapy or during periods of dosage adjustments (increases or decreases); the patient's family or caregiver should be instructed to closely observe the patient and communicate condition with healthcare provider. A medication guide concerning the use of antidepressants should be dispensed with each prescription. **Paroxetine is not FDA approved for use in children.**

The possibility of a suicide attempt is inherent in major depression and may persist until remission occurs. Patients treated with antidepressants (for any indication) should be observed for clinical worsening and suicidality, especially during the initial few months of a course of drug therapy, or at times of dose changes, either increases or decreases. Use caution in high-risk patients. Worsening depression and severe abrupt suicidality that are not part of the presenting symptoms may require discontinuation or modification of drug therapy. The patient's family or caregiver should be alerted to monitor patients for the emergence of suicidality and associated behaviors (such as agitation, irritability, hostility, impulsivity, and hypomania) and call healthcare provider.

May worsen psychosis in some patients or precipitate a shift to mania or hypomania in patients with bipolar disorder. Patients presenting with depressive symptoms should be screened for bipolar disorder. Monotherapy in patients with bipolar disorder should be avoided. **Paroxetine is not FDA approved for the treatment of bipolar depression.**

Serotonin syndrome and neuroleptic malignant syndrome (NMS)-like reactions have occurred with serotonin/norepinephrine reuptake inhibitors (SNRIs) and selective serotonin reuptake inhibitors (SSRIs) when used alone, and particularly when used in combination with serotonergic agents (eg, triptans) or antidopaminergic agents (eg, antipsychotics). Concurrent use with MAO inhibitors is contraindicated. May increase the risks associated with electro-convulsive therapy. Has a low potential to impair cognitive or motor performance - caution operating hazardous machinery or driving. Symptoms of agitation and/or restlessness may occur during initial few weeks of therapy. Low potential for sedation or anticholinergic effects relative to cyclic antidepressants.

Use caution in patients with a previous seizure disorder or condition predisposing to seizures such as brain damage, alcoholism, or concurrent therapy with other drugs which lower the seizure threshold. Use with caution in patients with hepatic dysfunction and in elderly patients. May cause hyponatremia/SIADH (elderly at increased risk); volume depletion (diuretics may increase risk). Use with concomitant use of NSAIDs, ASA, or other drugs that affect coagulation; the risk of bleeding may be potentiated. Use with caution in patients with renal insufficiency or other concurrent illness (due to limited experience); dose reduction recommended with severe renal impairment. May cause or exacerbate sexual dysfunction. Use caution in patients with narrow-angle glaucoma.

Upon discontinuation of paroxetine therapy, gradually taper dose and monitor for discontinuation symptoms (eg, dizziness, dysphoric mood, irritability, agitation, confusion, paresthesias). If intolerable symptoms occur following a decrease in dosage or upon discontinuation of therapy, then resuming the previous dose with a more gradual taper should be considered.

Adverse Reactions (Reflective of adult population; not specific for elderly) Frequency varies by dose and indication. Adverse reactions reported as a composite of all indications.

>10%:
Central nervous system: Somnolence (15% to 24%), insomnia (11% to 24%), headache (17% to 18%), dizziness (6% to 14%)
Endocrine & metabolic: Libido decreased (3% to 15%)
Gastrointestinal: Nausea (19% to 26%), xerostomia (9% to 18%), constipation (5% to 16%), diarrhea (9% to 12%)
Genitourinary: Ejaculatory disturbances (13% to 28%)
Neuromuscular & skeletal: Weakness (12% to 22%), tremor (4% to 11%)
Miscellaneous: Diaphoresis (5% to 14%)
1% to 10%:
Cardiovascular: Vasodilation (2% to 4%), chest pain (3%), palpitation (2% to 3%), hypertension (≥1%), tachycardia (≥1%)
Central nervous system: Nervousness (4% to 9%), anxiety (5%), agitation (3% to 5%), abnormal dreams (3% to 4%), concentration impaired (3% to 4%), yawning (2% to 4%), depersonalization (up to 3%), amnesia (2%), chills (2%), emotional lability (≥1%), vertigo (≥1%), confusion (1%)
Dermatologic: Rash (2% to 3%), pruritus (≥1%)
Endocrine & metabolic: Orgasmic disturbance (2% to 9%), dysmenorrhea (5%)
Gastrointestinal: Appetite decreased (5% to 9%), dyspepsia (2% to 5%), flatulence (4%), abdominal pain (4%), appetite increased (2% to 4%), vomiting (2% to 3%), taste perversion (2%), weight gain (≥1%)
Genitourinary: Genital disorder (male 10%; female 2% to 9%), impotence (2% to 9%), urinary frequency (2% to 3%), urinary tract infection (2%)
Neuromuscular & skeletal: Paresthesia (4%), myalgia (2% to 4%), back pain (3%), myoclonus (2% to 3%), myopathy (2%), myasthenia (1%), arthralgia (≥1%)
Ocular: Blurred vision (4%), abnormal vision (2% to 4%)
Otic: Tinnitus (≥1%)

◀ Respiratory: Respiratory disorder (up to 7%), pharyngitis (4%), sinusitis (up to 4%), rhinitis (3%)

Miscellaneous: Infection (5% to 6%)

Drug Interactions

Metabolism/Transport Effects Substrate of CYP2D6 (major); **Inhibits** CYP1A2 (weak), 2B6 (moderate), 2C9 (weak), 2C19 (weak), 2D6 (strong), 3A4 (weak)

Avoid Concomitant Use

Avoid concomitant use of PARoxetine with any of the following: Iobenguane I 123; MAO Inhibitors; Methylene Blue; Pimozide; Sibutramine; Tamoxifen; Thioridazine; Tryptophan

Increased Effect/Toxicity

PARoxetine may increase the levels/effects of: Alpha-/Beta-Blockers; Anticoagulants; Antidepressants (Serotonin Reuptake Inhibitor/Antagonist); Antiplatelet Agents; Aspirin; Atomoxetine; Beta-Blockers; BusPIRone; CarBAMazepine; CloZAPine; Collagenase (Systemic); CYP2B6 Substrates; CYP2D6 Substrates; Desmopressin; Dextromethorphan; Drotrecogin Alfa; DULoxetine; Fesoterodine; Galantamine; Haloperidol; Ibritumomab; Iloperidone; Lithium; Methadone; Methylene Blue; Mexiletine; NSAID (COX-2 Inhibitor); NSAID (Nonselective); Pimozide; Propafenone; RisperiDONE; Rivaroxaban; Salicylates; Serotonin Modulators; Tamoxifen; Tetrabenazine; Thioridazine; Thrombolytic Agents; Tositumomab and Iodine I 131 Tositumomab; TraMADol; Tricyclic Antidepressants; Vitamin K Antagonists

The levels/effects of PARoxetine may be increased by: Abiraterone Acetate; Alcohol (Ethyl); Analgesics (Opioid); Asenapine; BusPIRone; Cimetidine; CNS Depressants; CYP2D6 Inhibitors (Moderate); CYP2D6 Inhibitors (Strong); Dasatinib; Glucosamine; Herbs (Anticoagulant/Antiplatelet Properties); MAO Inhibitors; Metoclopramide; Omega-3-Acid Ethyl Esters; Pentosan Polysulfate Sodium; Pentoxifylline; Pravastatin; Prostacyclin Analogues; Sibutramine; TraMADol; Tryptophan; Vitamin E

Decreased Effect

PARoxetine may decrease the levels/effects of: Aprepitant; Fosaprepitant; Iloperidone; Iobenguane I 123

The levels/effects of PARoxetine may be decreased by: Aprepitant; CarBAMazepine; Cyproheptadine; Darunavir; Fosamprenavir; Fosaprepitant; NSAID (Nonselective); Peginterferon Alfa-2b

Ethanol/Nutrition/Herb Interactions

Ethanol: May increase CNS depression; monitor for increased effects with coadministration. Caution patients about effects.

Food: Peak concentration is increased, but bioavailability is not significantly altered by food.

Herb/Nutraceutical: Avoid valerian, St John's wort, SAMe, kava kava.

Stability

Suspension: Store at ≤25°C (≤77°F).

Tablet: Store at 15°C to 30°C (59°F to 86°F).

Mechanism of Action Paroxetine is a selective serotonin reuptake inhibitor, chemically unrelated to tricyclic, tetracyclic, or other antidepressants; presumably, the inhibition of serotonin reuptake from brain synapse stimulated serotonic activity in the brain

Pharmacodynamics/Kinetics

Onset of action: Depression: The onset of action is within a week; however, individual response varies greatly and full response may not be seen until 8-12 weeks after initiation of treatment.

Absorption: Completely absorbed following oral administration

Distribution: V_d: 8.7 L/kg (3-28 L/kg)

Protein binding: 93% to 95%

Metabolism: Extensively hepatic via CYP2D6 enzymes; primary metabolites are formed via oxidation and methylation of parent drug, with subsequent glucuronide/sulfate conjugation; nonlinear pharmacokinetics (via 2D6 saturation) may be seen with higher doses and longer duration of therapy. Metabolites exhibit ~2% potency of parent compound. C_{min} concentrations are 70% to 80% greater in the elderly compared to nonelderly patients; clearance is also decreased.

Half-life elimination: 21 hours (3-65 hours)

Time to peak: Immediate release: 5.2 hours; controlled release: 6-10 hours

Excretion: Urine (64%, 2% as unchanged drug); feces (36% primarily via bile, <1% as unchanged drug)

Dosage

Geriatric

Major depressive disorder, obsessive compulsive disorder, panic attack, social anxiety disorder:

Paxil®, Pexeva®: Oral: Initial: 10 mg/day; increase if needed by 10 mg/day increments at intervals of at least 1 week; maximum dose: 40 mg/day

Paxil CR®: Initial: 12.5 mg/day; increase if needed by 12.5 mg/day increments at intervals of at least 1 week; maximum dose: 50 mg/day

Note: Upon discontinuation of paroxetine therapy, gradually taper dose:
Paxil®, Pexeva®: 10 mg/day at weekly intervals; when 20 mg/day dose is reached, continue for 1 week before treatment is discontinued. Some patients may need to be titrated to 10 mg/day for 1 week before discontinuation.
Paxil CR®: Patients receiving 37.5 mg/day in clinical trials had their dose decreased by 12.5 mg/day to a dose of 25 mg/day and remained at a dose of 25 mg/day for 1 week before treatment was discontinued.

Adult
MDD: Oral:
Paxil®, Pexeva®: Initial: 20 mg once daily, preferably in the morning; increase if needed by 10 mg/day increments at intervals of at least 1 week; maximum dose: 50 mg/day
Paxil CR®: Initial: 25 mg once daily; increase if needed by 12.5 mg/day increments at intervals of at least 1 week; maximum dose: 62.5 mg/day
GAD (Paxil®, Pexeva®): Oral: Initial: 20 mg once daily, preferably in the morning (if dose is increased, adjust in increments of 10 mg/day at 1-week intervals); doses of 20-50 mg/day were used in clinical trials, however, no greater benefit was seen with doses >20 mg.
OCD (Paxil®, Pexeva®): Oral: Initial: 20 mg once daily, preferably in the morning; increase if needed by 10 mg/day increments at intervals of at least 1 week; recommended dose: 40 mg/day; range: 20-60 mg/day; maximum dose: 60 mg/day
Panic disorder: Oral:
Paxil®, Pexeva®: Initial: 10 mg once daily, preferably in the morning; increase if needed by 10 mg/day increments at intervals of at least 1 week; recommended dose: 40 mg/day; range: 10-60 mg/day; maximum dose: 60 mg/day
Paxil CR®: Initial: 12.5 mg once daily; increase if needed by 12.5 mg/day at intervals of at least 1 week; maximum dose: 75 mg/day
PTSD (Paxil®): Oral: Initial: 20 mg once daily, preferably in the morning; increase if needed by 10 mg/day increments at intervals of at least 1 week; range: 20-50 mg. Limited data suggest doses of 40 mg/day were not more efficacious than 20 mg/day.
Social anxiety disorder: Oral:
Paxil®: Initial: 20 mg once daily, preferably in the morning; recommended dose: 20 mg/day; range: 20-60 mg/day; doses >20 mg may not have additional benefit
Paxil CR®: Initial: 12.5 mg once daily, preferably in the morning; may be increased by 12.5 mg/day at intervals of at least 1 week; maximum dose: 37.5 mg/day
Menopause-associated vasomotor symptoms (unlabeled use, Paxil CR®): Oral: 12.5-25 mg/day

Note: Upon discontinuation of paroxetine therapy, gradually taper dose:
Paxil®, Pexeva®: 10 mg/day at weekly intervals; when 20 mg/day dose is reached, continue for 1 week before treatment is discontinued. Some patients may need to be titrated to 10 mg/day for 1 week before discontinuation.
Paxil CR®: Patients receiving 37.5 mg/day in clinical trials had their dose decreased by 12.5 mg/day to a dose of 25 mg/day and remained at a dose of 25 mg/day for 1 week before treatment was discontinued.

Renal Impairment
Cl_{cr} <30 mL/minute: Mean plasma concentrations ~4 times that seen in normal function.
Cl_{cr} 30-60 mL/minute: Plasma concentrations 2 times that seen in normal function.
Paxil®, Pexeva®: Adults: Initial: 10 mg/day; increase if needed by 10 mg/day increments at intervals of at least 1 week; maximum dose: 40 mg/day
Paxil CR®: Initial: 12.5 mg/day; increase if needed by 12.5 mg/day increments at intervals of at least 1 week; maximum dose: 50 mg/day
Hepatic Impairment In hepatic dysfunction, plasma concentration is 2 times that seen in normal function.
Paxil®, Pexeva®: Initial: 10 mg/day; increase if needed by 10 mg/day increments at intervals of at least 1 week; maximum dose: 40 mg/day
Paxil CR®: Initial: 12.5 mg/day; increase if needed by 12.5 mg/day increments at intervals of at least 1 week; maximum dose: 50 mg/day
Administration Best given in the morning unless too sedating; then administer as divided dose or at bedtime
Monitoring Parameters Mental status for depression, suicide ideation (especially at the beginning of therapy or when doses are increased or decreased), anxiety, social functioning, mania, panic attacks; akathisia
Pharmacotherapy Pearls Paxil CR™ incorporates a degradable polymeric matrix (Geo-matrix™) to control dissolution rate over a period of 4-5 hours. An enteric coating delays the start of drug release until tablets have left the stomach.

◀ **Special Geriatric Considerations** Paroxetine is the most sedating and anticholinergic of the selective serotonin reuptake inhibitors. The elderly are more prone to SSRI/SNRI-induced hyponatremia.

Dosage Forms Excipient information presented when available (limited, particularly for generics); consult specific product labeling.

Suspension, oral, as hydrochloride [strength expressed as base]:

Paxil®: 10 mg/5 mL (250 mL) [contains propylene glycol; orange flavor]

Tablet, oral, as hydrochloride [strength expressed as base]: 10 mg, 20 mg, 30 mg, 40 mg

Paxil®: 10 mg, 20 mg [scored]

Paxil®: 30 mg, 40 mg

Tablet, oral, as mesylate [strength expressed as base]:

Pexeva®: 10 mg

Pexeva®: 20 mg [scored]

Pexeva®: 30 mg, 40 mg

Tablet, controlled release, oral, as hydrochloride [strength expressed as base]:

Paxil CR®: 12.5 mg, 25 mg, 37.5 mg

Tablet, controlled release, enteric coated, oral, as hydrochloride [strength expressed as base]: 12.5 mg, 25 mg, 37.5 mg

Tablet, extended release, enteric coated, oral, as hydrochloride [strength expressed as base]: 12.5 mg, 25 mg

Selected References

Hebenstreit GF, Fellerer K, Zochling R, et al, "A Pharmacokinetic Dose Titration Study in Adult and Elderly Depressed Patients," *Acta Psychiatr Scand Suppl*, 1989, 350:81-4.

Lundmark J, Scheel Thomsen I, Fjord-Larsen T, et al, "Paroxetine: Pharmacokinetic and Antidepressant Effect in the Elderly," *Acta Psychiatr Scand Suppl*, 1989, 350:76-80.

Schone W and Ludwig M, "A Double-Blind Study of Paroxetine Compared With Fluoxetine in Geriatric Patients With Major Depression," *J Clin Psychopharmacol*, 1993, 13(6 Suppl 2):34S-9S.

◆ **Paroxetine Hydrochloride** see PARoxetine on page 1396
◆ **Paroxetine Mesylate** see PARoxetine on page 1396
◆ **PAS** see Aminosalicylic Acid on page 97
◆ **Paser®** see Aminosalicylic Acid on page 97
◆ **Pataday™** see Olopatadine (Ophthalmic) on page 1336
◆ **Patanase®** see Olopatadine (Nasal) on page 1336
◆ **Patanol®** see Olopatadine (Ophthalmic) on page 1336
◆ **Pavabid [DSC]** see Papaverine on page 1392
◆ **Paxil®** see PARoxetine on page 1396
◆ **Paxil CR®** see PARoxetine on page 1396
◆ **PCA (error-prone abbreviation)** see Procainamide on page 1521
◆ **PCE®** see Erythromycin (Systemic) on page 625
◆ **PCEC** see Rabies Vaccine on page 1575
◆ **PediaCare® Children's Allergy [OTC]** see DiphenhydrAMINE (Systemic) on page 520
◆ **PediaCare® Children's Decongestant [OTC]** see Phenylephrine (Systemic) on page 1440
◆ **PediaCare® Children's Long-Acting Cough [OTC]** see Dextromethorphan on page 490
◆ **PediaCare® Children's NightTime Cough [OTC]** see DiphenhydrAMINE (Systemic) on page 520
◆ **Pediaderm™ AF** see Nystatin (Topical) on page 1324
◆ **Pediaderm™ HC** see Hydrocortisone (Topical) on page 886
◆ **Pediaderm™ TA** see Triamcinolone (Topical) on page 1857
◆ **Pediapred®** see PrednisoLONE (Systemic) on page 1507
◆ **Pediatex® TD** see Triprolidine and Pseudoephedrine on page 1872
◆ **Pedi-Boro® [OTC]** see Aluminum Sulfate and Calcium Acetate on page 85
◆ **Pedi-Dri®** see Nystatin (Topical) on page 1324
◆ **PEG** see Polyethylene Glycol 3350 on page 1480

Pegaptanib (peg AP ta nib)

Brand Names: U.S. Macugen®
Brand Names: Canada Macugen®
Index Terms EYE001; Pegaptanib Sodium
Generic Availability (U.S.) No
Pharmacologic Category Ophthalmic Agent; Vascular Endothelial Growth Factor (VEGF) Inhibitor
Use Treatment of neovascular (wet) age-related macular degeneration (AMD)
Contraindications Hypersensitivity to pegaptanib or any component of the formulation; ocular or periocular infection

Warnings/Precautions Intravitreous injections may be associated with endophthalmitis; patients should be instructed to report any signs of infection immediately. Intraocular pressure may increase following injection. Safety and efficacy for administration into both eyes concurrently have not been studied. Safety and efficacy have not been established with hepatic impairment, or in patients requiring hemodialysis. Rare hypersensitivity reactions (including anaphylaxis) have been associated with pegaptanib, occurring within several hours of use; monitor closely. Equipment and appropriate personnel should be available for monitoring and treatment of anaphylaxis.

Adverse Reactions (Reflective of adult population; not specific for elderly)

10% to 40%:

Cardiovascular: Hypertension

Ocular: Anterior chamber inflammation, blurred vision, cataract, conjunctival hemorrhage, corneal edema, eye discharge, eye irritation, eye pain, intraocular pressure increased, ocular discomfort, punctate keratitis, visual acuity decreased, visual disturbance, vitreous floaters, vitreous opacities

1% to 10%:

Cardiovascular: Carotid artery occlusion (1% to 5%), cerebrovascular accident (1% to 5%), chest pain (1% to 5%), transient ischemic attack (1% to 5%)

Central nervous system: Dizziness (6% to 10%), headache (6% to 10%), vertigo (1% to 5%)

Dermatologic: Contact dermatitis (1% to 5%)

Endocrine & metabolic: Diabetes mellitus (1% to 5%)

Gastrointestinal: Diarrhea (6% to 10%), nausea (6% to 10%), dyspepsia (1% to 5%), vomiting (1% to 5%)

Genitourinary: Urinary retention (1% to 5%)

Neuromuscular & skeletal: Arthritis (1% to 5%), bone spur (1% to 5%)

Ocular: Blepharitis (6% to 10%), conjunctivitis (6% to 10%), photopsia (6% to 10%), vitreous disorder (6% to 10%), allergic conjunctivitis (1% to 5%), conjunctival edema (1% to 5%), corneal abrasion (1% to 5%), corneal deposits (1% to 5%), corneal epithelium disorder (1% to 5%), endophthalmitis (1% to 5%), eye inflammation (1% to 5%), eye swelling (1% to 5%), eyelid irritation (1% to 5%), meibomianitis (1% to 5%), mydriasis (1% to 5%), periorbital hematoma (1% to 5%), retinal edema (1% to 5%), vitreous hemorrhage (1% to 5%)

Otic: Hearing loss (1% to 5%)

Renal: Urinary tract infection (6% to 10%)

Respiratory: Bronchitis (6% to 10%), pleural effusion (1% to 5%)

Miscellaneous: Contusion (1% to 5%)

Drug Interactions

Avoid Concomitant Use There are no known interactions where it is recommended to avoid concomitant use.

Increased Effect/Toxicity There are no known significant interactions involving an increase in effect.

Decreased Effect

The levels/effects of Pegaptanib may be decreased by: Pegloticase

Stability Store under refrigeration at 2°C to 8°C (36°F to 46°F); do not freeze. Do not shake vigorously.

Mechanism of Action Pegaptanib is an apatamer, an oligonucleotide covalently bound to polyethylene glycol, which can adopt a three-dimensional shape and bind to vascular endothelial growth factor (VEGF). Pegaptanib binds to extracellular VEGF, inhibiting VEGF from binding to its receptors and thereby suppressing neovascularization and slowing vision loss.

Pharmacodynamics/Kinetics

Absorption: Slow systemic absorption following intravitreous injection

Metabolism: Metabolized by endo- and exonucleases

Half-life elimination: Plasma: 6-14 days

Dosage

Geriatric & Adult AMD: Intravitreous injection: 0.3 mg into affected eye every 6 weeks

Renal Impairment Adjustment not required with renal impairment; information not available for patients requiring hemodialysis.

Administration For intravitreous injection only; adequate anesthesia and a broad spectrum antibiotic should be administered prior to injection

pH: 6-7

Monitoring Parameters Intraocular pressure (within 30 minutes and 2-7 days after injection); endophthalmitis

Special Geriatric Considerations In studies, 94% of patients treated with pegaptanib were ≥65 years of age. No difference in efficacy was seen as compared to younger adults.

Dosage Forms Excipient information presented when available (limited, particularly for generics); consult specific product labeling.
Injection, solution [preservative free]:
  Macugen®: 0.3 mg/0.09 mL (0.09 mL)

Selected References
Gragoudas ES, Adamis AP, Cunningham ET, et al, "Pegaptanib for Neovascular Age-Related Macular Degeneration," *N Engl J Med*, 2004, 351(27):2805-16.

◆ **Pegaptanib Sodium** *see* Pegaptanib *on page 1400*

Pegfilgrastim (peg fil GRA stim)

Medication Safety Issues
  Sound-alike/look-alike issues:
    Neulasta® may be confused with Neumega®, Neupogen®, and Lunesta®
Brand Names: U.S. Neulasta®
Brand Names: Canada Neulasta®
Index Terms G-CSF (PEG Conjugate); Granulocyte Colony Stimulating Factor (PEG Conjugate); NSC-725961; Pegylated G-CSF; SD/01
Generic Availability (U.S.) No
Pharmacologic Category Colony Stimulating Factor
Use To decrease the incidence of infection, by stimulation of granulocyte production, in patients with nonmyeloid malignancies receiving myelosuppressive therapy associated with a significant risk of febrile neutropenia
Contraindications Hypersensitivity to pegfilgrastim, filgrastim, or any component of the formulation
Warnings/Precautions Do not use pegfilgrastim in the period 14 days before to 24 hours after administration of cytotoxic chemotherapy because of the potential sensitivity of rapidly dividing myeloid cells to cytotoxic chemotherapy. Benefit has not been demonstrated with regimens under a two-week duration. Administration on the same day as chemotherapy is not recommended (NCCN Myeloid Growth Factor Guidelines, v.1.2009). Pegfilgrastim can potentially act as a growth factor for any tumor type, particularly myeloid malignancies. Caution should be exercised in the usage of pegfilgrastim in any malignancy with myeloid characteristics. Tumors of nonhematopoietic origin may have surface receptors for pegfilgrastim. Pegfilgrastim has not been evaluated with patients receiving radiation therapy, or with chemotherapy associated with delayed myelosuppression (nitrosoureas, mitomycin C). Safety and efficacy have not been evaluated for peripheral blood progenitor cell (PBPC) mobilization.

Allergic-type reactions (anaphylaxis, angioedema, erythema, skin rash, urticaria) have occurred primarily with the initial dose and may recur (possibly delayed) after discontinuation; close follow up for several days and permanent discontinuation are recommended for severe reactions. Rare cases of splenic rupture have been reported; patients must be instructed to report left upper quadrant pain or shoulder tip pain. Acute respiratory distress syndrome (ARDS) has been associated with use; evaluate patients with pulmonary symptoms such as fever, lung infiltrates, or respiratory distress; discontinue or withhold pegfilgrastim if ARDS occurs. May precipitate sickle cell crises in patients with sickle cell disease; carefully evaluate potential risks and benefits. The packaging (needle cover) contains latex.

Adverse Reactions (Reflective of adult population; not specific for elderly)
  >10%:
    Cardiovascular: Peripheral edema (12%)
    Central nervous system: Headache (16%)
    Gastrointestinal: Vomiting (13%)
    Neuromuscular & skeletal: Bone pain (31% to 57%), myalgia (21%), arthralgia (16%), weakness (13%)
  1% to 10%:
    Gastrointestinal: Constipation (10%)
    Miscellaneous: Antibody formation (1% to 6%)

Drug Interactions
  Avoid Concomitant Use There are no known interactions where it is recommended to avoid concomitant use.
  Increased Effect/Toxicity There are no known significant interactions involving an increase in effect.
  Decreased Effect
    The levels/effects of Pegfilgrastim may be decreased by: Pegloticase

Stability Store under refrigeration 2°C to 8°C (36°F to 46°F); do not freeze. If inadvertently frozen, allow to thaw in refrigerator; discard if frozen more than one time. Protect from light. Do not shake. Allow to reach room temperature prior to injection. May be kept at room temperature for up to 48 hours.

Mechanism of Action Stimulates the production, maturation, and activation of neutrophils, pegfilgrastim activates neutrophils to increase both their migration and cytotoxicity. Pegfil-grastim has a prolonged duration of effect relative to filgrastim and a reduced renal clearance.

Pharmacodynamics/Kinetics Half-life elimination: SubQ: Adults: 15-80 hours

Dosage

Geriatric & Adult Do not administer in the period between 14 days before and 24 hours after administration of cytotoxic chemotherapy. According to the NCCN guidelines, efficacy has been demonstrated with every-2-week chemotherapy regimens, however, benefit has not been demonstrated with regimens under a two-week duration (NCCN Myeloid Growth Factor Guidelines, v.1.2009)

Prevention of chemotherapy-induced neutropenia: SubQ: 6 mg once per chemotherapy cycle, beginning 24-72 hours after completion of chemotherapy

Renal Impairment No adjustment necessary.

Administration Administer subcutaneously. Engage/activate needle guard following use to prevent accidental needlesticks.

Monitoring Parameters Complete blood count (with differential) and platelet count should be obtained prior to chemotherapy. Leukocytosis (white blood cell counts 100,000/mm^3) has been observed in <1% of patients receiving pegfilgrastim. Monitor platelets and hematocrit regularly. Evaluate fever, pulmonary infiltrates, and respiratory distress; evaluate for left upper abdominal pain, shoulder tip pain, or splenomegaly. Monitor for sickle cell crisis (in patients with sickle cell anemia).

Test Interactions May interfere with bone imaging studies; increased hematopoietic activity of the bone marrow may appear as transient positive bone imaging changes

Special Geriatric Considerations Not for patients <45 kg.

Dosage Forms Excipient information presented when available (limited, particularly for generics); consult specific product labeling.

Injection, solution [preservative free]:

Neulasta®: 6 mg/0.6 mL (0.6 mL) [contains natural rubber/natural latex in packaging]

Selected References

Smith TJ, Khatcheressian J, Lyman GH, et al, "2006 Update of Recommendations for the Use of White Blood Cell Growth Factors: An Evidence-Based Clinical Practice Guideline," *J Clin Oncol*, 2006, 24(19):3187-205.

◆ **PEG-IFN Alfa-2b** *see* Peginterferon Alfa-2b *on page 1403*

Peginterferon Alfa-2b (peg in ter FEER on AL fa too bee)

Medication Safety Issues

Sound-alike/look-alike issues:

Peginterferon alfa-2b may be confused with interferon alfa-2a, interferon alfa-2b, interferon alfa-n3, peginterferon alfa-2a

PegIntron® may be confused with Intron® A

International issues:

Peginterferon alfa-2b may be confused with interferon alpha multi-subtype which is available in international markets

Brand Names: U.S. PegIntron®; PegIntron™ Redipen®; Sylatron™

Brand Names: Canada PegIntron®

Index Terms Interferon Alfa-2b (PEG Conjugate); PEG-IFN Alfa-2b; Pegylated Interferon Alfa-2b; Polyethylene Glycol Interferon Alfa-2b; Sylatron™

Generic Availability (U.S.) No

Pharmacologic Category Interferon

Use

PegIntron®: Treatment of chronic hepatitis C (CHC; in combination with ribavirin) in patients who have compensated liver disease; treatment of chronic hepatitis C (as monotherapy) in adult patients with compensated liver disease who have never received alfa interferons

Sylatron™: Adjuvant treatment of melanoma (with microscopic or gross nodal involvement within 84 days of definitive surgical resection, including lymphadenectomy)

Medication Guide Available Yes

Contraindications Hypersensitivity (including urticaria, angioedema, bronchoconstriction, anaphylaxis, Stevens Johnson syndrome and toxic epidermal necrolysis) to peginterferon alfa-2b, interferon alfa-2b, other alfa interferons, or any component of the formulation; autoimmune hepatitis; decompensated liver disease (Child-Pugh score >6, classes B and C)

Combination therapy with peginterferon alfa-2b and ribavirin is also contraindicated in males with pregnant partners; hemoglobinopathies (eg, thalassemia major, sickle-cell anemia); renal dysfunction (Cl$_{cr}$ <50 mL/minute)

◀ **Warnings/Precautions** Hazardous agent - use appropriate precautions for handling and disposal.

[U.S. Boxed Warnings]: May cause or aggravate severe depression or other neuro-psychiatric adverse events (including suicide and suicidal ideation) in patients with and without a history of psychiatric disorder; may be irreversible; discontinue treatment permanently with worsening or persistently severe signs/symptoms of neuropsychi-atric disorders (eg, depression, encephalopathy, psychosis). May cause or aggravate fatal or life-threatening autoimmune disorders, infectious disorders, ischemic disorders, and/or hemorrhagic cerebrovascular events; discontinue treatment for persistent severe or worsening symptoms.

Neuropsychiatric disorders: Neuropsychiatric effects may occur in patients with and without a history of psychiatric disorder; addiction relapse, aggression, depression, homicidal ideation and suicidal behavior/ideation have been observed with peginterferon alfa-2b; bipolar dis-order, encephalopathy, hallucinations, mania, and psychosis have been observed with other alfa interferons. Onset may be delayed (up to 6 months after discontinuation). Higher doses may be associated with the development of encephalopathy (higher risk in elderly patients). Use with extreme caution in patients with a history of psychiatric disorders, including depression. Monitor all patients for evidence of depression; patients being treated for melanoma should be monitored for depression and psychiatric symptoms every 3 weeks during the first eight weeks of treatment and every 6 months thereafter; discontinue treatment if psychiatric symptoms persist, worsen or if suicidal behavior develops. All patients should continue to be monitored for 6 months after completion of therapy.

Bone marrow suppression: Causes bone marrow suppression, including potentially severe cytopenias; alfa interferons may (rarely) cause aplastic anemia. Use with caution in patients who are chronically immunosuppressed, with low peripheral blood counts or myelosuppres-sion, including concurrent use of myelosuppressive therapy. Use with caution in patients with an increased risk for severe anemia (eg, spherocytosis, history of GI bleeding). Dosage modification may be necessary for hematologic toxicity. Combination therapy with ribavirin may potentiate the neutropenic effects of alfa interferons. When used in combination with ribavirin, an increased incidence of anemia was observed when using ribavirin weight-based dosing, as compared to flat-dose ribavirin.

Hepatic disease: Use is contraindicated in patients with hepatic decompensation. Discontinue treatment immediately with hepatic decompensation (Child Pugh score >6). Patients with chronic hepatitis C (CHC) with cirrhosis receiving peginterferon alfa-2b are at risk for hepatic decompensation. CHC patients coinfected with human immunodeficiency virus (HIV) are at increased risk for hepatic decompensation when receiving highly active antiretroviral therapy (HAART); monitor closely. A transient increase in ALT (2-5 times above baseline) which is not associated with deterioration of liver function may occur with peginterferon alfa-2b use (for the treatment of chronic hepatitis C); therapy generally may continue with monitoring.

Gastrointestinal disorders: Pancreatitis has been observed with alfa interferon therapy; discontinue therapy if known or suspected pancreatitis develops. Ulcerative or hemorrha-gic/ischemic colitis has been observed with alfa interferons; withhold treatment for suspected pancreatitis; discontinue therapy for known pancreatitis. Ulcerative or hemorrhagic/ischemic colitis has been observed with alfa interferons; discontinue therapy if signs of colitis (abdominal pain, bloody diarrhea, fever) develop; symptoms typically resolve within 1-3 weeks.

Autoimmune disorders: Thyroiditis, thrombotic thrombocytopenic purpura, idiopathic thrombo-cytopenic purpura, rheumatoid arthritis, interstitial nephritis, systemic lupus erythematosus, and psoriasis have been reported with therapy; use with caution in patients with autoimmune disorders.

Cardiovascular disease: Use with caution in patients with cardiovascular disease or a history of cardiovascular disease; hypotension, arrhythmia, bundle branch block, tachycardia, car-diomyopathy, angina pectoris and MI have been observed with treatment. Patients with pre-existing cardiac abnormalities should have baseline ECGs prior to combination treatment with ribavirin; closely monitor patients with a history of MI or arrhythmia. Patients with a history of significant or unstable cardiac disease should not receive combination treatment with ribavirin. Discontinue treatment (permanently) for new-onset ventricular arrhythmia or cardiovascular decompensation.

Endocrine disorders: Diabetes mellitus (including new-onset type I diabetes), hyperglycemia, and thyroid disorders have been reported; discontinue peginterferon alfa-2b if cannot be effectively managed with medication. Use caution in patients with a history of diabetes mellitus, particularly if prone to DKA. Use with caution in patients with thyroid disorders; may cause or aggravate hyper- or hypothyroidism.

Pulmonary disease: May cause or aggravate dyspnea, pulmonary infiltrates, pneumonia, bronchiolitis obliterans, interstitial pneumonitis, pulmonary hypertension, and sarcoidosis which may result in respiratory failure; may recur upon rechallenge with treatment; monitor closely. Use with caution in patients with existing pulmonary disease (eg, chronic obstructive pulmonary disease). Withhold combination therapy with ribavirin for development of pulmonary infiltrate or pulmonary function impairment.

Ophthalmic disorders: Ophthalmologic disorders (including decreased visual acuity, blindness, macular edema, retinal hemorrhages, optic neuritis, papilledema, cotton wool spots, retinal detachment [serous], and retinal artery or vein thrombosis) have occurred with peginterferon alfa-2b and/or with other alfa interferons. Prior to start of therapy, ophthalmic exams are recommended for all patients; patients with diabetic or hypertensive retinopathy should have periodic ophthalmic exams during treatment; a complete eye exam should be done promptly in patients who develop ocular symptoms. Permanently discontinue treatment with new or worsening ophthalmic disorder.

[U.S. Boxed Warning]: Combination treatment with ribavirin may cause birth defects and/or fetal mortality (avoid pregnancy in females and female partners of male patients); hemolytic anemia (which may worsen cardiac disease), genotoxicity, mutagenicity, and may possibly be carcinogenic. Interferon therapy is commonly associated with flu-like symptoms, including fever; rule out other causes/infection with persistent or high fever. Acute hypersensitivity reactions and cutaneous reactions (eg, Stevens-Johnson syndrome, toxic epidermal necrolysis) have been reported (rarely) with alfa interferons; prompt discontinuation is recommended; transient rashes do not require interruption of therapy. Hypertriglyceridemia has been reported with use; discontinue if persistent and severe (triglycerides >1000 mg/dL), particularly if combined with symptoms of pancreatitis. Use with caution in patients with renal impairment (Cl_{cr} <50 mL/minute); monitor closely. For the treatment of chronic hepatitis C, dosage adjustments are recommended with monotherapy in patients with moderate-to-severe impairment; do not use combination therapy with ribavirin in adult patients renal dysfunction (Cl_{cr} <50 mL/minute); discontinue if serum creatinine >2 mg/dL in children. Has not been studied in melanoma patients with renal impairment. Serum creatinine increases have been reported in patients with renal insufficiency. Use with caution in the elderly; the potential adverse effects may be more pronounced in the elderly. Elderly patients generally do not respond to interferon treatment as well as younger patients. Dental/periodontal disorders have been reported with combination therapy; dry mouth may affect teeth and mucous membranes; instruct patients to brush teeth twice daily; encourage regular dental exams.

Combination therapy with ribavirin is preferred over monotherapy for the treatment of chronic hepatitis C (combination therapy provides a better response). Safety and efficacy have not been established in patients who have received organ transplants, are coinfected with HIV or hepatitis B, or received treatment for >1 year. Patients with significant bridging fibrosis or cirrhosis, genotype 1 infection or who have not responded to prior therapy, including previous pegylated interferon treatment are less likely to benefit from combination therapy with peginterferon alfa-2b and ribavirin. Due to differences in dosage, patients should not change brands of interferon.

Adverse Reactions (Reflective of adult population; not specific for elderly) Note:
Percentages reported for adults receiving monotherapy unless noted:
>10%:
  Central nervous system: Fatigue (52% to 94%), fever (22% to 75%), headache (56% to 70%), chills (≤63%), depression (29% to 59%; may be severe), dizziness (12% to 35%), anxiety/emotional liability/irritability (28%), insomnia (23%), olfactory nerve disorder (≤23%)
  Dermatologic: Rash (6% to 36%), alopecia (22% to 34%), pruritus (12%), dry skin (11%)
  Gastrointestinal: Anorexia (20% to 69%), nausea (26% to 64%), taste perversion (≤38%), diarrhea (18% to 37%), vomiting (7% to 26%), abdominal pain (15%), weight loss (11%)
  Hematologic: Neutropenia (6% to 70%; grade 4: 1%), thrombocytopenia (7% to 20%; grades 3/4: <4%), anemia (6%; in combination with ribavirin: 12% to 47%)
  Hepatic: Transaminases increased (10% to 77%), alkaline phosphatase increased (≤23%)
  Local: Injection site inflammation/reaction (23% to 62%)
  Neuromuscular & skeletal: Myalgia (54% to 68%), weakness (52%), arthralgia (23% to 51%), musculoskeletal pain (28%), rigors (23%), paresthesia (21%)
  Miscellaneous: Viral infection (11%)
>1% to 10%:
  Cardiovascular: Chest pain (6%), flushing (6%)
  Central nervous system: Concentration impaired (10%), malaise (7%), nervousness (4%), agitation (2%), suicidal behavior (ideation/attempt/suicide ≤2%)
  Endocrine & metabolic: Hypothyroidism (5%), menstrual disorder (4%), hyperthyroidism (3%)

◀

Gastrointestinal: Dyspepsia (6%), xerostomia (6%), constipation (1%)
Hepatic: GGT increased (8%), hepatomegaly (6%)
Local: Injection site pain (2% to 3%)
Ocular: Conjunctivitis (4%), blurred vision (2%)
Renal: Proteinuria (≤7%)
Respiratory: Pharyngitis (10%), cough (5% to 8%), sinusitis (7%), dyspnea (4% to 6%), rhinitis (2%)
Miscellaneous: Diaphoresis (6%), neutralizing antibodies (2%)

Drug Interactions

Metabolism/Transport Effects Inhibits CYP1A2 (weak)

Avoid Concomitant Use

Avoid concomitant use of Peginterferon Alfa-2b with any of the following: Telbivudine

Increased Effect/Toxicity

Peginterferon Alfa-2b may increase the levels/effects of: Aldesleukin; Methadone; Ribavirin; Telbivudine; Theophylline Derivatives; Zidovudine

Decreased Effect

Peginterferon Alfa-2b may decrease the levels/effects of: CYP2C9 Substrates (High risk); CYP2D6 Substrates; FLUoxetine

The levels/effects of Peginterferon Alfa-2b may be decreased by: Pegloticase

Ethanol/Nutrition/Herb Interactions Ethanol: Avoid use in patients with hepatitis C virus.

Stability Prior to reconstitution, store Redipen® at 2°C to 8°C (36°F to 46°F). Store intact vials at 25°C (77°F); excursions permitted to 15°C to 30°C (59°F to 86°F). Do not freeze.

Redipen®: Hold cartridge upright and press the two halves together until there is a "click". Gently invert to mix; do not shake. Single-use pen.

Pegintron® (vial): Add 0.7 mL sterile water for injection, USP (supplied single-use diluent) to the vial. Gently swirl. Do not re-enter vial after dose removed.

Sylatron™ (vial): Add 0.7 mL sterile water for injection and swirl gently, resulting in the following concentrations:
296 mcg vial: 40 mcg/0.1 mL
444 mcg vial: 60 mcg/0.1 mL
888 mcg vial: 120 mcg/0.1 mL

Once reconstituted each product should be used immediately or may be stored for ≤24 hours at 2°C to 8°C (36°F to 46°F); do not freeze. Do not shake. Products do not contain preservative.

Mechanism of Action Alpha interferons are a family of proteins, produced by nucleated cells, that have antiviral, antiproliferative, and immune-regulating activity. There are 16 known subtypes of alpha interferons. Interferons interact with cells through high affinity cell surface receptors. Following attachment, multiple effects can be detected including induction of gene transcription. Inhibits cellular growth, alters the state of cellular differentiation, interferes with oncogene expression, alters cell surface antigen expression, increases phagocytic activity of macrophages, and augments cytotoxicity of lymphocytes for target cells.

Pharmacodynamics/Kinetics

Bioavailability: Increases with chronic dosing
Half-life elimination: CHC: ~40 hours (range: 22-60 hours); Melanoma: ~43-51 hours
Time to peak: CHC: 15-44 hours
Excretion: Urine (~30%)

Dosage

Geriatric May require dosage reduction based upon renal dysfunction; however, no established guidelines are available.

Adult

Melanoma: SubQ: 6 mcg/kg/week for 8 doses, followed by 3 mcg/kg/week for up to 5 years. **Note:** Premedicate with acetaminophen (500-1000 mg orally) 30 minutes prior to the first dose and as needed thereafter.

Chronic hepatitis C (CHC): SubQ: Administer dose once weekly; **Note:** Treatment duration is 48 weeks for genotype 1, 24 weeks for genotypes 2 and 3, or 48 weeks for patients who previously failed therapy (regardless of genotype). Discontinue after 12 weeks in patients with HCV (genotype 1) if HCV RNA decreases <2 log (compared to pretreatment) or if detectable HCV RNA at 24.

Monotherapy: Initial (based on average weekly dose of 1 mcg/kg):
≤45 kg: 40 mcg once weekly
46-56 kg: 50 mcg once weekly
57-72 kg: 64 mcg once weekly
73-88 kg: 80 mcg once weekly
89-106 kg: 96 mcg once weekly
107-136 kg: 120 mcg once weekly
137-160 kg: 150 mcg once weekly

Combination therapy with ribavirin: Initial (based on average weekly dose of 1.5 mcg/kg):
<40 kg: 50 mcg once weekly (with ribavirin 800 mg/day)
40-50 kg: 64 mcg once weekly (with ribavirin 800 mg/day)
51-60 kg: 80 mcg once weekly (with ribavirin 800 mg/day)
61-65 kg: 96 mcg once weekly (with ribavirin 800 mg/day)
66-75 kg: 96 mcg once weekly (with ribavirin 1000 mg/day)
76-80 kg: 120 mcg once weekly (with ribavirin 1000 mg/day)
81-85 kg: 120 mcg once weekly (with ribavirin 1200 mg/day)
86-105 kg: 150 mcg once weekly (with ribavirin 1200 mg/day)
>105 kg: 1.5 mcg/kg once weekly (with ribavirin 1400 mg/day)

Note: *American Association for the Study of Liver Diseases (AASLD) guidelines recommendation:* Adults with chronic HCV infection: Treatment of choice: Ribavirin plus **peginterferon**; clinical condition and ability of patient to tolerate therapy should be evaluated to determine length and/or likely benefit of therapy. Recommended treatment duration (AASLD guidelines; Ghany, 2009): Genotypes 1,4: 48 weeks; Genotypes 2,3: 24 weeks; Coinfection with HIV: 48 weeks.

Renal Impairment Chronic hepatitis C:
Peginterferon alfa-2b monotherapy:
Cl_{cr} 30-50 mL/minute: Reduce dose by 25%
Cl_{cr} 10-29 mL/minute: Reduce dose by 50%
Hemodialysis: Reduce dose by 50%
Discontinue use if renal function declines during treatment.
Peginterferon alfa-2b combination with ribavirin: Cl_{cr} <50 mL/minute: Combination therapy with ribavirin is not recommended.

Hepatic Impairment Contraindicated in decompensated liver disease

Administration For SubQ administration; rotate injection site; thigh, outer surface of upper arm, and abdomen are preferred injection sites; do not inject near navel or waistline; patients who are thin should only use thigh or upper arm. Do not inject into bruised, infected, irritated, red, or scarred skin. The weekly dose may be administered at bedtime to reduce flu-like symptoms.

Monitoring Parameters Baseline and periodic TSH (for patients being treated for melanoma, obtain baseline within 4 weeks prior to treatment initiation, and then at 3 and 6 months, and every 6 months thereafter during treatment); hematology (including hemoglobin, CBC with differential, platelets); chemistry (including LFTs) testing, renal function, triglycerides. Clinical studies (for combination therapy) tested as follows: CBC (including hemoglobin, WBC, and platelets) and chemistries (including liver function tests and uric acid) measured at weeks 2, 4, 8, and 12, and then every 6 weeks; TSH measured every 12 weeks during treatment.

Serum HCV RNA levels (pretreatment, 12 and 24 weeks after therapy initiation, 24 weeks after completion of therapy). **Note:** Discontinuation of therapy may be considered after 12 weeks in patients with HCV (genotype 1) who fail to achieve an early virologic response (EVR) (defined as ≥2-log decrease in HCV RNA compared to pretreatment) or after 24 weeks with detectable HCV RNA. Treat patients with HCV (genotypes 2,3) for 24 weeks (if tolerated) and then evaluate HCV RNA levels (Ghany, 2009).

Evaluate for depression and other psychiatric symptoms before and after initiation of therapy; patients being treated for melanoma should be monitored for depression and psychiatric symptoms every 3 weeks during the first eight weeks of treatment and every 6 months thereafter; baseline ophthalmic eye examination; periodic ophthalmic exam in patients with diabetic or hypertensive retinopathy; baseline ECG in patients with cardiac disease; serum glucose or Hb A_{1c} (for patients with diabetes mellitus). In combination therapy with ribavirin, pregnancy tests (for women of childbearing age who are receiving treatment or who have male partners who are receiving treatment), continue monthly up to 6 months after discontinuation of therapy.

Reference Range Chronic hepatitis C:
Early viral response (EVR): ≥2 log decrease in HCV RNA after 12 weeks of treatment
End of treatment response (ETR): Absence of detectable HCV RNA at end of the recommended treatment period
Sustained treatment response (STR): Absence of HCV RNA in the serum 6 months following completion of full treatment course

Special Geriatric Considerations May require dosage reduction based upon renal dysfunction, but no established guidelines are available. Geriatric patients often have Cl_{cr} <50 mL/minute, as well as, many diseases that put them at risk for adverse effects with this agent. Calculation and measuring creatinine clearance must be done prior to initiating this drug.

◀ **Dosage Forms** Excipient information presented when available (limited, particularly for generics); consult specific product labeling.

Injection, powder for reconstitution:

Sylatron™: 296 mcg [contains polysorbate 80, sucrose 59.2 mg; supplied with diluent]

Sylatron™: 444 mcg [contains polysorbate 80, sucrose 59.2 mg; supplied with diluent]

Sylatron™: 888 mcg [contains polysorbate 80, sucrose 59.2 mg; supplied with diluent]

Injection, powder for reconstitution [preservative free]:

PegIntron®: 50 mcg, 80 mcg, 120 mcg, 150 mcg [contains polysorbate 80, sucrose 59.2 mg; supplied with diluent]

PegIntron™ Redipen®: 50 mcg, 80 mcg, 120 mcg, 150 mcg [contains polysorbate 80, sucrose 54 mg; supplied with diluent]

Selected References

Bottomley A, Coens C, Suciu S, et al, "Adjuvant Therapy With Pegylated Interferon Alfa-2b Versus Observation in Resected Stage III Melanoma: A Phase III Randomized Controlled Trial of Health-Related Quality of Life and Symptoms by the European Organisation for Research and Treatment of Cancer Melanoma Group," *J Clin Oncol*, 2009 [epub ahead of print].

Eggermont AM, Suciu S, Santinami M, et al, "Adjuvant Therapy With Pegylated Interferon Alfa-2b Versus Observation Alone in Resected Stage III Melanoma: Final Results of EORTC 18991, A Randomised Phase III Trial," *Lancet*, 2008, 372(9633):117-26.

Heathcote EJ, Shiffman ML, Cooksley GE, et al, "Peginterferon Alfa-2a in Patients With Chronic Hepatitis C and Cirrhosis," *N Engl J Med*, 2000, 343(23):1673-80.

McHutchison JG, Lawitz EJ, Shiffman ML, et al, "Peginterferon Alfa-2b or Alfa-2a With Ribavirin for Treatment of Hepatitis C Infection," *N Engl J Med*, 2009, 361(6):580-93.

Poynard T, Colombo M, Bruix J, et al, "Peginterferon Alfa-2b and Ribavirin: Effective in Patients With Hepatitis C Who Failed Interferon Alfa/Ribavirin Therapy," *Gastroenterology*, 2009, 136(5):1618-28.

Zeuzem S, Feinman V, Rasenack J, et al, "Peginterferon Alfa-2a in Patients With Chronic Hepatitis C," *N Engl J Med*, 2000, 343(23):1666-72.

◆ **PegIntron®** *see* Peginterferon Alfa-2b *on page 1403*
◆ **PegIntron™ Redipen®** *see* Peginterferon Alfa-2b *on page 1403*

Pegloticase (peg LOE ti kase)

Brand Names: U.S. Krystexxa™
Index Terms PEG-Uricase; Pegylated Urate Oxidase; Polyethylene Glycol-Conjugated Uricase; Recombinant Urate Oxidase, Pegylated; Urate Oxidase, Pegylated
Generic Availability (U.S.) No
Pharmacologic Category Enzyme; Enzyme, Urate-Oxidase (Recombinant)
Use Treatment of chronic gout refractory to conventional therapy
Medication Guide Available Yes
Contraindications Glucose-6-phosphate dehydrogenase (G6PD) deficiency
Warnings/Precautions [U.S. Boxed Warning]: Anaphylaxis and infusion reactions have been reported during and after administration; patients should be closely monitored during infusion and for an appropriate period of time after the infusion. Therapy should be administered in a healthcare facility by skilled medical personnel prepared for the immediate treatment of anaphylaxis. All patients should be premedicated with antihistamines and corticosteroids. Anaphylaxis may occur at any time during treatment (including the initial dose). **Reactions generally occur within 2 hours of administration; however, delayed hypersensitivity reactions have also been reported.** Infusion reactions are varied; symptoms range from chest pain, pruritus/urticaria, or dyspnea to a clinical presentation of anaphylaxis (eg, hemodynamic instability, perioral or lingual edema). If a less severe (non-anaphylactic) infusion reaction occurs, the infusion may be slowed, or stopped and restarted at a slower rate, at the physician's discretion. **Risk of an infusion reaction is increased in patients whose uric acid is >6 mg/dL; therefore, monitor serum uric acid concentrations prior to infusion and consider discontinuing treatment if concentrations exceed 6 mg/dL, particularly in the event of 2 consecutive concentrations >6 mg/dL.**

Therapy with antihyperuricemic agents commonly results in gout flare, particularly upon initiation due to rapid lowering of urate concentrations; gout flare-ups during treatment do not warrant discontinuation of therapy. Gout flare prophylaxis is recommended, using non-steroidal anti-inflammatory agents (NSAID) or colchicines, unless contraindicated, beginning ≥1 week before initiation of pegloticase and continuing for at least 6 months. Exacerbation of heart failure has been observed in clinical trials; use caution in patients with pre-existing heart failure. Due to the risk for hemolysis and methemoglobinemia, pegloticase is contraindicated in patients with G6PD deficiency. Patients at higher risk for G6PD deficiency (eg, African, Mediterranean) should be screened prior to therapy. Therapy is not appropriate for the treatment of asymptomatic hyperuricemia. Potential for immunogenicity exists with the use of therapeutic proteins. Antipegloticase antibodies and antiPEG antibodies commonly occurred during clinical trials in pegloticase-treated patients. High antipegloticase antibody titers were associated with failure to maintain uric acid normalization and were also associated with a higher incidence of infusion reactions. Due to potential for immunogenicity, closely monitor patients who reinitiate therapy after discontinuing treatment for >4 weeks; patients may be at increased risk for anaphylaxis and infusion reactions.

Adverse Reactions (Reflective of adult population; not specific for elderly)

>10%:

Dermatologic: Bruising (11%), urticaria (11%)

Gastrointestinal: Nausea (12%)

Miscellaneous: Antibody formation (antipegloticase antibodies: 92%; antiPEG antibodies: 42%), gout flare (74% within the first 3 months), infusion reactions (26%)

1% to 10%:

Cardiovascular: Chest pain (6% to 10%)

Dermatologic: Erythema (10%), pruritus (10%)

Gastrointestinal: Constipation (6%), vomiting (5%)

Respiratory: Dyspnea (7%), nasopharyngitis (7%)

Miscellaneous: Anaphylaxis (≤7%)

Frequency not defined: Anemia, diarrhea, headache, muscle spasms, nephrolithiasis

Drug Interactions

Avoid Concomitant Use There are no known interactions where it is recommended to avoid concomitant use.

Increased Effect/Toxicity There are no known significant interactions involving an increase in effect.

Decreased Effect

Pegloticase may decrease the levels/effects of: Certolizumab Pegol; Pegademase Bovine; Pegaptanib; Pegaspargase; Pegfilgrastim; Peginterferon Alfa-2a; Peginterferon Alfa-2b; Pegvisomant

Stability Prior to use, vials must be stored in the carton to protect from light and kept under refrigeration between 2°C to 8°C (36° to 46°F) at all times. Do **not** shake or freeze.

To prepare solution for administration, withdraw 1 mL (8 mg) and add to a 250 mL bag of NS or ½NS; invert bag several times to mix thoroughly (do **not** shake). Do not use vial if particulate matter is present or if solution is discolored (solution should be a clear and colorless). After withdrawal, discard any unused portion of the product remaining in the vial. Diluted solution may be stored up to 4 hours at 2°C to 8°C (36°F to 46°F). Diluted solution is also stable for 4 hours at room temperature of 20°C to 25°C (68°F to 77°F); however, refrigeration is preferred. The diluted solution should be protected from light, not frozen, and used within 4 hours of dilution. Prior to administration, allow the diluted solution to reach room temperature; do not warm to room temperature using any form of artificial heating such as a microwave or warm water bath.

Mechanism of Action Pegloticase is a pegylated recombinant form of urate-oxidase enzyme, also known as uricase (an enzyme normally absent in humans and high primates), which converts uric acid to allantoin (an inactive and water soluble metabolite of uric acid); it does not inhibit the formation of uric acid.

Pharmacodynamics/Kinetics

Onset of action: ~24 hours following the first dose, serum uric acid concentrations decreased

Duration: >300 hours (12.5 days)

Half-life elimination: Median: ~14 days

Dosage

Geriatric & Adult Refractory gout: I.V.: 8 mg every 2 weeks

Note: Premedicate with antihistamines and corticosteroids. Gout flare prophylaxis with either NSAIDs or colchicine is also recommended, beginning at least 1 week prior to initiation and continuing for at least 6 months.

Renal Impairment Creatinine clearance did not alter the pharmacokinetics; dosage adjustments are not needed.

Administration Administer diluted solution by I.V. infusion over ≥120 minutes via gravity feed or an infusion pump or syringe-type pump. Do **not** administer by I.V. push or bolus. Administer in a healthcare setting by healthcare providers prepared to manage potential anaphylaxis. Monitor closely for infusion reactions during infusion and for an appropriate period of time after the infusion (anaphylaxis has been reported within 2 hours of the infusion). In the event or a less severe infusion reaction, infusion may be slowed, or stopped and restarted at a slower rate, based on the discretion of the physician.

Reference Range

Uric acid, serum: An increase occurs during childhood

Adults:

Male: 3.4-7 mg/dL or slightly more

Female: 2.4-6 mg/dL or slightly more

Values >7 mg/dL are sometimes arbitrarily regarded as hyperuricemia, but there is no sharp line between normals on the one hand, and the serum uric acid of those with clinical gout. Normal ranges cannot be adjusted for purine ingestion, but high purine diet increases uric acid. Uric acid may be increased with body size, exercise, and stress.

Dosage Forms Excipient information presented when available (limited, particularly for generics); consult specific product labeling.

Injection, solution:

Krystexxa™: Uricase protein 8 mg/mL (2 mL)

Selected References

Dalbeth N and So A, "Hyperuricaemia and Gout: State of the Art and Future Perspectives," *Ann Rheum Dis*, 2010, 69 (10):1738-43.

Sundy JS, Becker MA, Baraf HS, et al, "Reduction of Plasma Urate Levels following Treatment With Multiple Doses of Pegloticase (Polyethylene Glycol-Conjugated Uricase) in Patients With Treatment-Failure Gout: Results of a Phase II Randomized Study," *Arthritis Rheum*, 2008, 58(9):2882-91.

Whelton A, "Current and Future Therapeutic Options for the Management of Gout," *Am J Ther*, 2010, 17(4):402-17.

Yue CS, Huang W, Alton M, et al, "Population Pharmacokinetic and Pharmacodynamic Analysis of Pegloticase in Subjects With Hyperuricemia and Treatment-Failure Gout," *J Clin Pharmacol*, 2008, 48(6):708-18.

◆ **PEG-Uricase** *see* Pegloticase *on page 1408*
◆ **Pegylated G-CSF** *see* Pegfilgrastim *on page 1402*
◆ **Pegylated Interferon Alfa-2b** *see* Peginterferon Alfa-2b *on page 1403*
◆ **Pegylated Urate Oxidase** *see* Pegloticase *on page 1408*

Penbutolol (pen BYOO toe lole)

Related Information
Beta-Blockers *on page 2001*

Medication Safety Issues
Sound-alike/look-alike issues:
Levatol® may be confused with Lipitor®
International issues:
Levatol [U.S.] may be confused with Lovacol brand name for lovastatin [Chile and Finland]

Brand Names: U.S. Levatol®

Brand Names: Canada Levatol®

Index Terms Penbutolol Sulfate

Generic Availability (U.S.) No

Pharmacologic Category Beta Blocker With Intrinsic Sympathomimetic Activity

Use Treatment of mild-to-moderate arterial hypertension

Contraindications Hypersensitivity to penbutolol or any component of the formulation; uncompensated congestive heart failure; cardiogenic shock; bradycardia or heart block (except in patients with a functioning artificial pacemaker); sinus node dysfunction; asthma; bronchospastic disease; COPD; pulmonary edema

Warnings/Precautions Consider pre-existing conditions such as sick sinus syndrome before initiating. Beta-blocker therapy should not be withdrawn abruptly (particularly in patients with CAD), but gradually tapered to avoid acute tachycardia, hypertension, and/or ischemia. Chronic beta-blocker therapy should not be routinely withdrawn prior to major surgery. In general, patients with bronchospastic disease should not receive beta-blockers; if used at all, should be used cautiously with close monitoring. Bradycardia may be observed more frequently in elderly patients (>65 years of age); dosage reductions may be necessary. Use caution with concurrent use of digoxin, verapamil, or diltiazem; bradycardia or heart block can occur. Use with caution in patients receiving inhaled anesthetic agents known to depress myocardial contractility. Can precipitate or aggravate symptoms of arterial insufficiency in patients with PVD and Raynaud's disease. Use with caution and monitor for progression of arterial obstruction.

Use with caution in patients with psychiatric disease (may cause CNS depression) or myasthenia gravis. Use cautiously in patients with diabetes because it can mask prominent hypoglycemic symptoms. May mask signs of hyperthyroidism (eg, tachycardia); if hyperthyroidism is suspected, carefully manage and monitor; abrupt withdrawal may exacerbate symptoms of hyperthyroidism or precipitate thyroid storm. Beta-blockers with intrinsic sympathomimetic activity (including penbutolol) do not appear to be of benefit in HF. Adequate alpha-blockade is required prior to use of any beta-blocker for patients with untreated pheochromocytoma. Use caution with history of severe anaphylaxis to allergens; patients taking beta-blockers may become more sensitive to repeated challenges. Treatment of anaphylaxis (eg, epinephrine) in patients taking beta-blockers may be ineffective or promote undesirable effects.

Adverse Reactions (Reflective of adult population; not specific for elderly)
1% to 10%:
Cardiovascular: CHF, arrhythmia
Central nervous system: Mental depression, headache, dizziness, fatigue
Gastrointestinal: Nausea, diarrhea, dyspepsia
Neuromuscular & skeletal: Arthralgia

Drug Interactions

Avoid Concomitant Use

Avoid concomitant use of Penbutolol with any of the following: Floctafenine; Methacholine

Increased Effect/Toxicity

Penbutolol may increase the levels/effects of: Alpha-/Beta-Agonists (Direct-Acting); Alpha1-Blockers; Alpha2-Agonists; Amifostine; Antihypertensives; Antipsychotic Agents (Phenothiazines); Bupivacaine; Cardiac Glycosides; Fingolimod; Hypotensive Agents; Insulin; Lidocaine; Lidocaine (Systemic); Lidocaine (Topical); Mepivacaine; Methacholine; Midodrine; RiTUXimab; Sulfonylureas

The levels/effects of Penbutolol may be increased by: Acetylcholinesterase Inhibitors; Aminoquinolines (Antimalarial); Amiodarone; Anilidopiperidine Opioids; Antipsychotic Agents (Phenothiazines); Calcium Channel Blockers (Dihydropyridine); Calcium Channel Blockers (Nondihydropyridine); Diazoxide; Dipyridamole; Disopyramide; Dronedarone; Floctafenine; Herbs (Hypotensive Properties); MAO Inhibitors; Pentoxifylline; Phosphodiesterase 5 Inhibitors; Propafenone; Propoxyphene; Prostacyclin Analogues; QuiNIDine; Reserpine

Decreased Effect

Penbutolol may decrease the levels/effects of: Beta2-Agonists; Theophylline Derivatives

The levels/effects of Penbutolol may be decreased by: Barbiturates; Herbs (Hypertensive Properties); Methylphenidate; Nonsteroidal Anti-Inflammatory Agents; Rifamycin Derivatives; Yohimbine

Mechanism of Action Blocks both $beta_1$- and $beta_2$-receptors and has mild intrinsic sympathomimetic activity; has negative inotropic and chronotropic effects and can significantly slow AV nodal conduction

Pharmacodynamics/Kinetics
Onset of action: Peak effect: 1.3-3 hours
Duration: >20 hours
Absorption: ~100%
Protein binding: 80% to 98%
Metabolism: Extensively hepatic (oxidation and conjugation)
Bioavailability: ~100%
Half-life elimination: Penbutolol: 5 hours; Conjugated metabolite: ~20 hours with normal renal function, 100 hours with end-stage renal disease
Time to peak, plasma: 2-3 hours
Excretion: Urine

Dosage

Geriatric & Adult Hypertension: Oral: Initial: 20 mg once daily, full effect of a 20 or 40 mg dose is seen by the end of a 2-week period, doses of 40-80 mg have been tolerated but have shown little additional antihypertensive effects; usual dose range (JNC 7): 10-40 mg once daily

Monitoring Parameters Blood pressure, orthostatic hypotension, heart rate, CNS effects

Special Geriatric Considerations Due to alterations in the beta-adrenergic autonomic nervous system, beta-adrenergic blockade may result in less hemodynamic response than seen in younger adults. Studies indicate that despite decreased sensitivity to the chronotropic effects of beta-blockade with age, there appears to be an increased myocardial sensitivity to the negative inotropic effect during stress (ie, exercise). Controlled trials have shown the overall response rate for propranolol to be only 20% to 50% in elderly populations. Therefore, all beta-adrenergic blocking drugs may result in a decreased response as compared to younger adults.

Dosage Forms Excipient information presented when available (limited, particularly for generics); consult specific product labeling.
Tablet, oral, as sulfate:
  Levatol®: 20 mg [scored]

Selected References
Chobanian AV, Bakris GL, Black HR, et al, "The Seventh Report of the Joint National Committee on Prevention, Detection, Evaluation, and Treatment of High Blood Pressure: The JNC 7 Report," *JAMA*, 2003, 289(19):2560-71.

◆ **Penbutolol Sulfate** *see* Penbutolol *on page 1410*

Penicillamine (pen i SIL a meen)

Medication Safety Issues
Sound-alike/look-alike issues:
Penicillamine may be confused with penicillin
International issues:
Depen [U.S.] may be confused with Depin brand name for nifedipine [India]; Depon brand name for acetaminophen [Greece]; Dipen brand name for diltiazem [Greece]
Pemine [Italy] may be confused with Pamine brand name for methscopolamine [U.S., Canada]

Brand Names: U.S. Cuprimine®; Depen®
Brand Names: Canada Cuprimine®; Depen®
Index Terms D-3-Mercaptovaline; D-Penicillamine; β,β-Dimethylcysteine
Generic Availability (U.S.) No
Pharmacologic Category Chelating Agent
Use Treatment of Wilson's disease, cystinuria; adjunctive treatment of rheumatoid arthritis
Unlabeled/Investigational Use Chelation therapy for the treatment of lead poisoning (third-line agent)
Contraindications Hypersensitivity to penicillamine or any component of the formulation; renal insufficiency (in patients with rheumatoid arthritis); patients with previous penicillamine-related aplastic anemia or agranulocytosis
Warnings/Precautions Patients with a penicillin allergy may theoretically have cross-sensitivity to penicillamine; however, the possibility has been eliminated now that penicillamine is produced synthetically and no longer contains trace amounts of penicillin. Once instituted for Wilson's disease or cystinuria, continue treatment on a daily basis; interruptions of even a few days have been followed by hypersensitivity with reinstitution of therapy. Penicillamine has been associated with fatalities due to agranulocytosis, aplastic anemia, thrombocytopenia, Goodpasture's syndrome, and myasthenia gravis. **[U.S. Boxed Warning]: Patients should be warned to report promptly any symptoms suggesting toxicity (fever, sore throat, chills, bruising, or bleeding);** approximately 33% of patients will experience an allergic reaction; toxicity may be dose related, use caution in the elderly. Use caution with other hematopoietic-depressant drugs (eg, gold, immunosuppressants, antimalarials, phenylbutazone); hematologic and renal adverse reactions are similar. Proteinuria or hematuria may develop; monitor for membranous glomerulopathy which can lead to nephrotic syndrome. In rheumatoid arthritis patients, discontinue if gross hematuria or persistent microscopic hematuria develop. Monitor liver function tests periodically due to rare reports of intrahepatic cholestasis or toxic hepatitis. **[U.S. Boxed Warning]: Should be administered under the close supervision of a physician familiar with the toxicity and dosage considerations.**

Lead poisoning: Investigate, identify, and remove sources of lead exposure prior to treatment. Penicillamine should only be used when unacceptable reactions have occurred with edetate CALCIUM disodium and succimer. Primary care providers should consult experts in chemotherapy of lead toxicity before using chelation drug therapy.

Adverse Reactions (Reflective of adult population; not specific for elderly) Frequency not defined, may vary by indication. Adverse effects requiring discontinuation of treatment have been reported in 20% to 30% of patients with Wilson's disease.
Cardiovascular: Vasculitis
Central nervous system: Anxiety, agitation, fever, hyperpyrexia, psychiatric disturbances; worsening neurologic symptoms (10% to 50% patients with Wilson's disease)
Dermatologic: Alopecia, cheilosis, dermatomyositis, exfoliative dermatitis, lichen planus, rash (early and late 5%), pemphigus, pruritus, skin friability increased, toxic epidermal necrolysis, urticaria, wrinkling (excessive), yellow nail syndrome
Endocrine & metabolic: Hypoglycemia, thyroiditis
Gastrointestinal: Anorexia, diarrhea (17%), epigastric pain, gingivostomatitis, glossitis, nausea, oral ulcerations, pancreatitis, peptic ulcer reactivation, taste alteration (12%), vomiting
Hematologic: Eosinophilia, hemolytic anemia, leukocytosis, leukopenia (2% to 5%), monocytosis, red cell aplasia, thrombocytopenia (4% to 5%), thrombotic thrombocytopenia purpura, thrombocytosis
Hepatic: Alkaline phosphatase increased, hepatic failure, intrahepatic cholestasis, toxic hepatitis
Local: Thrombophlebitis, white papules at venipuncture and surgical sites
Neuromuscular & skeletal: Arthralgia, dystonia, myasthenia gravis, muscle weakness, neuropathies, polyarthralgia (migratory, often with objective synovitis), polymyositis
Ocular: Diplopia, extraocular muscle weakness, optic neuritis, ptosis, visual disturbances
Otic: Tinnitus
Renal: Goodpasture's syndrome, hematuria, nephrotic syndrome, proteinuria (6%), renal failure, renal vasculitis

Respiratory: Asthma, interstitial pneumonitis, pulmonary fibrosis, obliterative bronchiolitis

Miscellaneous: Allergic alveolitis, anetoderma, elastosis perforans serpiginosa, lupus-like syndrome, lactic dehydrogenase increased, lymphadenopathy, mammary hyperplasia, positive ANA test

Drug Interactions

Avoid Concomitant Use There are no known interactions where it is recommended to avoid concomitant use.

Increased Effect/Toxicity There are no known significant interactions involving an increase in effect.

Decreased Effect

Penicillamine may decrease the levels/effects of: Digoxin

The levels/effects of Penicillamine may be decreased by: Antacids; Iron Salts

Ethanol/Nutrition/Herb Interactions

Ethanol: Avoid or limit ethanol.

Food: Penicillamine serum levels may be decreased if taken with food. Do not administer with milk.

Stability Store in tight, well-closed containers.

Mechanism of Action Chelates with lead, copper, mercury and other heavy metals to form stable, soluble complexes that are excreted in urine; depresses circulating IgM rheumatoid factor, depresses T-cell but not B-cell activity; combines with cystine to form a compound which is more soluble, thus cystine calculi are prevented

Pharmacodynamics/Kinetics

Onset of action: Rheumatoid arthritis: 2-3 months; Wilson's disease: 1-3 months

Absorption: 40% to 70%

Protein binding: 80% to albumin and ceruloplasmin

Metabolism: Hepatic (small amounts metabolized to s-methyl-d-penicillamine)

Half-life elimination: 1.7-7 hours

Time to peak, serum: 1-3 hours

Excretion: Urine (>80% as unchanged drug)

Dosage

Geriatric & Adult

Rheumatoid arthritis: Oral: 125-250 mg/day, may increase dose at 1- to 3-month intervals up to 1-1.5 g/day (maximum in older adults: 750 mg/day)

Wilson's disease: Note: Decrease dose for surgery

Oral: 750-1500 mg/day in divided doses (dose that results in an initial 24-hour urinary copper excretion >2 mg/day should be continued for ~3 months; maintenance dose defined by amount resulting in <10 mcg serum free copper/dL); maximum dose: 2000 mg/day. **Note:** Therapy in elderly patients should be initiated at low end of dosing range and titrated upward cautiously.

AASLD guidelines recommend to increase tolerability, therapy may be initiated at 250-500 mg/day then titrated upward 250 mg every 4-7 days; usual maintenance dose: 750–1000 mg/day in 2 divided doses; maximum: 1000-1500 mg/day in 2-4 divided doses (Roberts, 2008)

Cystinuria: Note: Adjust dose to limit cystine excretion to 100-200 mg/day (<100 mg/day with history of stone formation): Oral: 1-4 g/day in 4 divided doses; usual dose: 2 g/day

Renal Impairment Cl_{cr} <50 mL/minute: Avoid use.

Hemodialysis: Dialyzable; a dosing decrease from 250 mg/day to 250 mg 3 times/week after dialysis has been suggested in the treatment of rheumatoid arthritis.

Administration For patients who cannot swallow, contents of capsules may be administered in 15-30 mL of chilled puréed fruit or fruit juice. Give on an empty stomach (1 hour before meals and at bedtime).

Cystinuria: If administering 4 equal doses is not feasible, administer the larger dose at bedtime.

Rheumatoid arthritis: Doses ≤500 mg/day may be given as a single dose; >500 mg administer in divided doses

Monitoring Parameters Urinalysis, CBC with differential, platelet count, skin, lymph nodes, and body temperature twice weekly during the first month of therapy, then every 2 weeks for 5 months, then monthly; LFTs every 6 months

Cystinuria: Urinary cystine, annual X-ray for renal stones

Lead poisoning: Serum lead concentration (baseline and 7-21 days after completing chelation therapy); hemoglobin or hematocrit, iron status, free erythrocyte protoporphyrin or zinc protoporphyrin; neurodevelopmental changes

Wilson's disease: Serum non-ceruloplasmin bound copper, 24-hour urinary copper excretion, LFTs every 3 months during the first year of treatment; periodic ophthalmic exam

CBC: WBC <3500/mm^3 indicate need to stop therapy immediately; platelet counts <100,000/mm^3 indicate need to stop therapy until numbers of platelets increase

Urinalysis: Monitor for proteinuria and hematuria. A quantitative 24-hour urine protein at 1- to 2-week intervals initially (first 2-3 months) is recommended if proteinuria develops; in patients with rheumatoid arthritis, discontinue or decrease dose with proteinuria >1 g/24 hours, progressively increasing proteinuria or hematuria.

Reference Range Wilson's disease: 24-hour urinary copper excretion: 200-500 mcg (3-8 micromoles)/day

Special Geriatric Considerations Close monitoring of elderly is necessary; since steady-state serum/tissue concentrations rise slowly, "go slow" with dose increase intervals; steady-state concentrations decline slowly after discontinuation suggesting extensive tissue distribution. Skin rashes and taste abnormalities occur more frequently in the elderly than in young adults; leukopenia, thrombocytopenia, and proteinuria occur with equal frequency in both younger adults and elderly. Since toxicity may be dose related, it is recommended not to exceed 750 mg/day in the elderly.

Dosage Forms Excipient information presented when available (limited, particularly for generics); consult specific product labeling.

Capsule, oral:
　Cuprimine®: 250 mg
Tablet, oral:
　Depen®: 250 mg [scored]

Selected References

Kosnett MJ, Wedeen RP, Rothenberg SJ, et al, "Recommendations for Medical Management of Adult Lead Exposure," *Environ Health Perspect*, 2007, 115(3):463-71.

Roberts EA and Schilsky ML, "Diagnosis and Treatment of Wilson Disease: An Update. American Association for Study of Liver Diseases (AASLD)," *Hepatology*, 2008, 47(6):2089-111.

Swarup A, Sachdeva N, and Schumacher Jr HP, "Dosing of Antirheumatic Drugs in Renal Disease and Dialysis," *J Clin Rheumatol*, 2004, 10(4):190-204.

Penicillin G Benzathine (pen i SIL in jee BENZ a theen)

Medication Safety Issues
Sound-alike/look-alike issues:
Penicillin may be confused with penicillamine
Bicillin® may be confused with Wycillin®

Administration issues:
Penicillin G benzathine may only be administered by deep intramuscular injection; intravenous administration of penicillin G benzathine has been associated with cardiopulmonary arrest and death.

Other safety concerns:
Bicillin® C-R (penicillin G benzathine and penicillin G procaine) may be confused with Bicillin® L-A (penicillin G benzathine). Penicillin G benzathine is the only product currently approved for the treatment of syphilis. Administration of penicillin G benzathine and penicillin G procaine combination instead of Bicillin® L-A may result in inadequate treatment response.

Brand Names: U.S. Bicillin® L-A

Brand Names: Canada Bicillin® L-A

Index Terms Benzathine Benzylpenicillin; Benzathine Penicillin G; Benzylpenicillin Benzathine

Generic Availability (U.S.) No

Pharmacologic Category Antibiotic, Penicillin

Use Active against some gram-positive organisms, few gram-negative organisms such as *Neisseria gonorrhoeae*, and some anaerobes and spirochetes; used in the treatment of syphilis; used only for the treatment of mild to moderately-severe upper respiratory tract infections caused by organisms susceptible to low concentrations of penicillin G or for prophylaxis of infections caused by these organisms; primary and secondary prevention of rheumatic fever

Contraindications Hypersensitivity to penicillin(s) or any component of the formulation

Warnings/Precautions Use with caution in patients with impaired renal function, seizure disorder, or history of hypersensitivity to other beta-lactams; CDC and AAP do not currently recommend the use of penicillin G benzathine to treat congenital syphilis or neurosyphilis due to reported treatment failures and lack of published clinical data on its efficacy. Prolonged use may result in fungal or bacterial superinfection, including *C. difficile*-associated diarrhea (CDAD) and pseudomembranous colitis; CDAD has been observed >2 months postantibiotic treatment. **[U.S. Boxed Warning]: Not for intravenous use; cardiopulmonary arrest and death have occurred from inadvertent I.V. administration;** administer by deep I.M. injection only; injection into or near an artery or nerve could result in severe neurovascular damage or permanent neurological damage. Extended duration of therapy or use associated with high serum concentrations may be associated with an increased risk for some adverse reactions.

Adverse Reactions (Reflective of adult population; not specific for elderly) Frequency not defined.

Cardiovascular: Cardiac arrest, cerebral vascular accident, cyanosis, gangrene, hypotension, pallor, palpitations, syncope, tachycardia, vasodilation, vasospasm, vasovagal reaction

Central nervous system: Anxiety, coma, confusion, dizziness, euphoria, fatigue, headache, nervousness, pain, seizure, somnolence

In addition, a syndrome of CNS symptoms has been reported which includes: Severe agitation with confusion, hallucinations (auditory and visual), and fear of death (Hoigne's syndrome); other symptoms include cyanosis, dizziness, palpitations, psychosis, seizures, tachycardia, taste disturbance, tinnitus

Gastrointestinal: Bloody stool, intestinal necrosis, nausea, vomiting

Genitourinary: Impotence, priapism

Hepatic: AST increased

Local: Injection site reactions: Abscess, atrophy, bruising, cellulitis, edema, hemorrhage, inflammation, lump, necrosis, pain, skin ulcer

Neuromuscular & skeletal: Arthritis exacerbation, joint disorder, neurovascular damage, numbness, periostitis, rhabdomyolysis, transverse myelitis, tremor, weakness

Ocular: Blindness, blurred vision

Renal: BUN increased, creatinine increased, hematuria, myoglobinuria, neurogenic bladder, proteinuria, renal failure

Miscellaneous: Diaphoresis, hypersensitivity reactions, Jarisch-Herxheimer reaction, lymphadenopathy, mottling, warmth

Drug Interactions

Avoid Concomitant Use

Avoid concomitant use of Penicillin G Benzathine with any of the following: BCG

Increased Effect/Toxicity

Penicillin G Benzathine may increase the levels/effects of: Methotrexate

The levels/effects of Penicillin G Benzathine may be increased by: Probenecid

Decreased Effect

Penicillin G Benzathine may decrease the levels/effects of: BCG; Mycophenolate; Typhoid Vaccine

The levels/effects of Penicillin G Benzathine may be decreased by: Fusidic Acid; Tetracycline Derivatives

Stability Refrigerate at 2°C to 8°C (36°F to 46°F); do not freeze. The following stability information has also been reported: May be stored at 25°C (77°F) for 7 days (Cohen, 2007).

Mechanism of Action Interferes with bacterial cell wall synthesis during active multiplication, causing cell wall death and resultant bactericidal activity against susceptible bacteria

Pharmacodynamics/Kinetics

Duration: 1-4 weeks (dose dependent); larger doses result in more sustained levels

Distribution: Highest levels in the kidney; lesser amounts in liver, skin, intestines

Protein Binding: ~60%

Absorption: I.M.: Slow

Time to peak, serum: 12-24 hours

Dosage

Geriatric & Adult

Usual dosage range: I.M.: 1.2-2.4 million units as a single dose

Group A streptococcal upper respiratory infection: 1.2 million units as a single dose

Secondary prevention of glomerulonephritis: 1.2 million units every 4 weeks or 600,000 units twice monthly

Secondary prevention of rheumatic fever: 1.2 million units every 3-4 weeks or 600,000 units twice monthly

Syphilis (CDC, 2010):

Primary, Secondary, Early Latent (<1 year duration): 2.4 million units as a single dose in 2 injection sites

Late Latent, Latent with unknown duration: 2.4 million units in 2 injection sites once weekly for 3 doses

Neurosyphilis: Not indicated as single-drug therapy, but may be given once weekly for 3 weeks following I.V. treatment; refer to Penicillin G (Parenteral/Aqueous) monograph for dosing

Administration I.M. Administer undiluted injection by deep injection in the upper outer quadrant of the buttock do **not** administer I.V., intra-arterially, or SubQ

Monitoring Parameters Observe for signs and symptoms of anaphylaxis during first dose

Test Interactions Positive Coombs' [direct], false-positive urinary and/or serum proteins; false-positive or negative urinary glucose using Clinitest®

◀ **Special Geriatric Considerations** Not indicated as single drug therapy for neurosyphilis, but may be given 1 time/week for 3 weeks following I.V. treatment with Penicillin G (Parenteral/ Aqueous). No adjustment for renal function or age is necessary.

Dosage Forms Excipient information presented when available (limited, particularly for generics); consult specific product labeling.

Injection, suspension:

Bicillin® L-A: 600,000 units/mL (1 mL, 2 mL, 4 mL)

Selected References

Collart P, Poitevin M, Milovanovic A, et al, "Kinetic Study of Serum Penicillin Concentrations After Single Doses of Benzathine and Benethamine Penicillins in Young and Old People," *Br J Vener Dis*, 1980, 56(6):355-62.

WHO Study Group, "Rheumatic Fever and Rheumatic Heart Disease," *World Health Organ Tech Rep Ser*, 1988, 764:1-58.

Penicillin G Benzathine and Penicillin G Procaine
(pen i SIL in jee BENZ a theen & pen i SIL in jee PROE kane)

Related Information
Penicillin G Benzathine *on page 1414*
Penicillin G Procaine *on page 1420*

Medication Safety Issues
Sound-alike/look-alike issues:
Penicillin may be confused with penicillamine
Bicillin® may be confused with Wycillin®

Administration issues:
Penicillin G benzathine may only be administered by deep intramuscular injection; intravenous administration of penicillin G benzathine has been associated with cardiopulmonary arrest and death.

Other safety concerns:
Bicillin® C-R (penicillin G benzathine and penicillin G procaine) may be confused with Bicillin® L-A (penicillin G benzathine). Penicillin G benzathine is the only product currently approved for the treatment of syphilis. Administration of penicillin G benzathine and penicillin G procaine combination instead of Bicillin® L-A may result in inadequate treatment response.

Brand Names: U.S. Bicillin® C-R; Bicillin® C-R 900/300

Index Terms Penicillin G Procaine and Benzathine Combined

Generic Availability (U.S.) No

Pharmacologic Category Antibiotic, Penicillin

Use May be used in specific situations in the treatment of streptococcal infections; primary prevention of rheumatic fever

Contraindications Hypersensitivity to penicillin(s), procaine, or any component of the formulation

Warnings/Precautions Use with caution in patients with impaired renal function. Serious and occasionally severe or fatal hypersensitivity (anaphylactoid) reactions have been reported in patients on penicillin therapy, especially with a history of beta-lactam hypersensitivity, history of sensitivity to multiple allergens, or previous IgE-mediated reactions (eg, anaphylaxis, angioedema, urticaria). Use with caution in asthmatic patients. Prolonged use may result in fungal or bacterial superinfection, including *C. difficile*-associated diarrhea (CDAD) and pseudomembranous colitis; CDAD has been observed >2 months postantibiotic treatment. **[U.S. Boxed Warning]: Not for intravenous use; cardiopulmonary arrest and death have occurred from inadvertent I.V. administration;** administer by deep I.M. injection only; injection into or near an artery or nerve could result in severe neurovascular damage or permanent neurological damage. Extended duration of therapy or use associated with high serum concentrations may be associated with an increased risk for some adverse reactions.

Adverse Reactions (Reflective of adult population; not specific for elderly) See individual agents.

Drug Interactions
Avoid Concomitant Use
Avoid concomitant use of Penicillin G Benzathine and Penicillin G Procaine with any of the following: BCG

Increased Effect/Toxicity
Penicillin G Benzathine and Penicillin G Procaine may increase the levels/effects of: Methotrexate

The levels/effects of Penicillin G Benzathine and Penicillin G Procaine may be increased by: Probenecid

Decreased Effect

Penicillin G Benzathine and Penicillin G Procaine may decrease the levels/effects of: BCG; Mycophenolate; Typhoid Vaccine

The levels/effects of Penicillin G Benzathine and Penicillin G Procaine may be decreased by: Fusidic Acid; Tetracycline Derivatives

Stability Refrigerate at 2°C to 8°C (36°F to 46°F); do not freeze. The following stability information has also been reported: May be stored at 25°C (77°F) for 7 days (Cohen, 2007).

Mechanism of Action Inhibits bacterial cell wall synthesis by binding to one or more of the penicillin-binding proteins (PBPs); which in turn inhibits the final transpeptidation step of peptidoglycan synthesis in bacterial cell walls, thus inhibiting cell wall biosynthesis. Bacteria eventually lyse due to ongoing activity of cell wall autolytic enzymes (autolysins and murein hydrolases) while cell wall assembly is arrested.

Pharmacodynamics/Kinetics

Absorption: I.M.: Released slowly

Distribution: Highest levels in the kidney; lesser amounts in liver, skin, intestines

Protein binding: ~60%

Time to peak, serum: I.M.: Within 3 hours

Dosage

Geriatric & Adult Streptococcal infections: I.M.: 2.4 million units in a single dose

Administration Administer by deep I.M. injection in the upper outer quadrant of the buttock do **not** administer I.V., intravascularly, or intra-arterially

Monitoring Parameters Observe for signs and symptoms of anaphylaxis during first dose

Test Interactions May interfere with urinary glucose tests using cupric sulfate (Benedict's solution, Clinitest®); may inactivate aminoglycosides *in vitro*; positive Coombs' [direct], increased protein

Special Geriatric Considerations No adjustment for renal function or age is necessary.

Dosage Forms Excipient information presented when available (limited, particularly for generics); consult specific product labeling. [DSC] = Discontinued product

Injection, suspension [prefilled syringe]:

Bicillin® C-R:

600,000 units: Penicillin G benzathine 300,000 units and penicillin G procaine 300,000 units per 1 mL (1 mL) [DSC]

1,200,000 units: Penicillin G benzathine 600,000 units and penicillin G procaine 600,000 units per 2 mL (2 mL)

2,400,000 units: Penicillin G benzathine 1,200,000 units and penicillin G procaine 1,200,000 units per 4 mL (4 mL) [DSC]

Bicillin® C-R 900/300: 1,200,000 units: Penicillin G benzathine 900,000 units and penicillin G procaine 300,000 units per 2 mL (2 mL)

Penicillin G (Parenteral/Aqueous) (pen i SIL in jee, pa REN ter al, AYE kwee us)

Related Information

Antibiotic Treatment of Adults With Infective Endocarditis *on page 2053*

Medication Safety Issues

Sound-alike/look-alike issues:

Penicillin may be confused with penicillamine

Brand Names: U.S. Pfizerpen®

Brand Names: Canada Crystapen®

Index Terms Benzylpenicillin Potassium; Benzylpenicillin Sodium; Crystalline Penicillin; Penicillin G Potassium; Penicillin G Sodium

Generic Availability (U.S.) Yes

Pharmacologic Category Antibiotic, Penicillin

Use Treatment of infections (including sepsis, pneumonia, pericarditis, endocarditis, meningitis, anthrax) caused by susceptible organisms; active against some gram-positive organisms, generally not *Staphylococcus aureus*; some gram-negative organisms such as *Neisseria gonorrhoeae*, and some anaerobes and spirochetes

Contraindications Hypersensitivity to penicillin or any component of the formulation

Warnings/Precautions Avoid intra-arterial administration or injection into or near major peripheral nerves or blood vessels since such injections may cause severe and/or permanent neurovascular damage; use with caution in patients with renal impairment (dosage reduction required), concomitant renal and hepatic impairment (further dosage adjustment may be required), pre-existing seizure disorders, or with a history of hypersensitivity to cephalosporins. Prolonged use may result in fungal or bacterial superinfection, including *C. difficile*-associated diarrhea (CDAD) and pseudomembranous colitis; CDAD has been observed >2 months postantibiotic treatment. Serious and occasionally severe or fatal hypersensitivity (anaphylactoid) reactions have been reported in patients on penicillin therapy, especially with a history of beta-lactam hypersensitivity, history of sensitivity to multiple allergens, or previous IgE-mediated reactions (eg, anaphylaxis, angioedema, urticaria). Use with caution in asthmatic patients. Extended duration of therapy or use associated with high serum concentrations may be associated with an increased risk for some adverse reactions. Product contains sodium and potassium; high doses of I.V. therapy may alter serum levels.

Adverse Reactions (Reflective of adult population; not specific for elderly) Frequency not defined.

Central nervous system: Coma (high doses), hyper-reflexia (high doses), seizures (high doses)

Dermatologic: Contact dermatitis, rash

Endocrine & metabolic: Electrolyte imbalance (high doses)

Gastrointestinal: Pseudomembranous colitis

Hematologic: Neutropenia, positive Coombs' hemolytic anemia (rare, high doses)

Local: Injection site reaction, phlebitis, thrombophlebitis

Neuromuscular & skeletal: Myoclonus (high doses)

Renal: Acute interstitial nephritis (high doses), renal tubular damage (high doses)

Miscellaneous: Anaphylaxis, hypersensitivity reactions (immediate and delayed), Jarisch-Herxheimer reaction, serum sickness

Drug Interactions

Avoid Concomitant Use

Avoid concomitant use of Penicillin G (Parenteral/Aqueous) with any of the following: BCG

Increased Effect/Toxicity

Penicillin G (Parenteral/Aqueous) may increase the levels/effects of: Methotrexate

The levels/effects of Penicillin G (Parenteral/Aqueous) may be increased by: Probenecid

Decreased Effect

Penicillin G (Parenteral/Aqueous) may decrease the levels/effects of: BCG; Mycophenolate; Typhoid Vaccine

The levels/effects of Penicillin G (Parenteral/Aqueous) may be decreased by: Fusidic Acid; Tetracycline Derivatives

Stability

Penicillin G potassium powder for injection should be stored below 86°F (30°C). Following reconstitution, solution may be stored for up to 7 days under refrigeration. Premixed bags for infusion should be stored in the freezer (-20°C to -4°F); frozen bags may be thawed at room temperature or in refrigerator. Once thawed, solution is stable for 14 days if stored in refrigerator or for 24 hours when stored at room temperature. Do not refreeze once thawed.

Penicillin G sodium powder for injection should be stored at controlled room temperature. Reconstituted solution may be stored under refrigeration for up to 3 days.

Reconstitution:

Intermittent I.V.: 5 million unit vial: Add 8.2 mL for a final concentration of 500,000 units/mL; add 3.2 mL for a final concentration of 1,000,000 units/mL. Dilute further to 50,000-145,000 units/mL prior to infusion.

Continuous I.V. infusion: 20 million unit vial: Add 11.5 mL for a final concentration of 1,000,000 units/mL. Dilute further in 1-2 L of infusion solution and administer over a 24-hour period.

Mechanism of Action Interferes with bacterial cell wall synthesis during active multiplication, causing cell wall death and resultant bactericidal activity against susceptible bacteria

Pharmacodynamics/Kinetics

Distribution: Poor penetration across blood-brain barrier, despite inflamed meninges

Relative diffusion from blood into CSF: Poor unless meninges inflamed (exceeds usual MICs)

CSF:blood level ratio: Normal meninges: <1%; Inflamed meninges: 2% to 6%

Protein binding: 65%

Metabolism: Hepatic (30%) to penicilloic acid

Half-life elimination:

Normal renal function: 30-50 minutes

End-stage renal disease: 3.3-5.1 hours

Time to peak, serum: I.M.: ~30 minutes; I.V.: ~1 hour

Excretion: Urine (58% to 85% as unchanged drug)

Dosage

Geriatric & Adult

Actinomyces species: I.V.: 10-20 million units/day divided every 4-6 hours for 4-6 weeks

Clostridium perfringens: I.V.: 24 million units/day divided every 4-6 hours with clindamycin

Corynebacterium diptheriae: I.V.: 2-3 million units/day in divided doses every 4-6 hours for 10-12 days

Erysipelas: I.V.: 1-2 million units every 4-6 hours
Erysipelothrix: I.V.: 2-4 million units every 4 hours
Fascial space infections: I.V.: 2-4 million units every 4-6 hours with metronidazole
Leptospirosis: I.V.: 1.5 million units every 6 hours for 7 days
Listeria: I.V.: 15-20 million units/day in divided doses every 4-6 hours for 2 weeks (meningitis) or 4 weeks (endocarditis)
Lyme disease (meningitis): I.V.: 20 million units/day in divided doses
Neurosyphilis: I.V.: 18-24 million units/day in divided doses every 4 hours (or by continuous infusion) for 10-14 days
Streptococcus:
  Brain abscess: I.V.: 18-24 million units/day in divided doses every 4 hours with metronidazole
  Endocarditis or osteomyelitis: I.V.: 3-4 million units every 4 hours for at least 4 weeks
  Skin and soft tissue: I.V.: 3-4 million units every 4 hours for 10 days
  Toxic shock: I.V.: 24 million units/day in divided doses with clindamycin
Streptococcal pneumonia: I.V.: 2-3 million units every 4 hours
Whipple's disease: I.V.: 2 million units every 4 hours for 2 weeks, followed by oral trimethoprim/sulfamethoxazole or doxycycline for 1 year
  Relapse or CNS involvement: 4 million units every 4 hours for 4 weeks

Renal Impairment
Uremic patients with Cl_{cr} >10 mL/minute/1.73 m^2: Administer full loading dose followed by $1/2$ of the loading dose given every 4-5 hours
Cl_{cr} <10 mL/minute/1.73 m^2: Administer full loading dose followed by $1/2$ of the loading dose given every 8-10 hours
Intermittent hemodialysis (IHD) (administer after hemodialysis on dialysis days): Administer normal loading dose followed by either 25% to 50% of normal dose every 4-6 hours **or** 50% to 100% of normal dose every 8-12 hours. For mild-to-moderate infections, administer 0.5-1 million units every 4-6 hours **or** 1-2 million units every 8-12 hours. For neurosyphilis, endocarditis, or serious infections, administer up to 2 million units every 4-6 hours; administer after dialysis on dialysis days **or** supplement with 500,000 units after dialysis (Heintz, 2009). **Note:** Dosing dependent on the assumption of 3 times/week, complete IHD sessions.
Continuous renal replacement therapy (CRRT) (Heintz, 2009; Trotman, 2005): Drug clearance is highly dependent on the method of renal replacement, filter type, and flow rate. Appropriate dosing requires close monitoring of pharmacologic response, signs of adverse reactions due to drug accumulation, as well as drug concentrations in relation to target trough (if appropriate). The following are general recommendations only (based on dialysate flow/ultrafiltration rates of 1-2 L/hour and minimal residual renal function) and should not supersede clinical judgment:
  CVVH: Loading dose of 4 million units, followed by 2 million units every 4-6 hours
  CVVHD: Loading dose of 4 million units, followed by 2-3 million units every 4-6 hours
  CVVHDF: Loading dose of 4 million units, followed by 2-4 million units every 4-6 hours

Administration
I.M.; Administer I.M. by deep injection in the upper outer quadrant of the buttock
I.V.: **Note:** The 20 million unit dosage form may be administered by continuous I.V. infusion only.
  Intermittent I.V.: May be dissolved in small amounts of SWFI, NS, D_5W and administered peripherally as a 50,000-100,000 unit/mL solution. In fluid-restricted patients, 146,000 units/mL in SW results in a maximum recommended osmolality for peripheral infusion. Infuse over 15-30 minutes.
  Continuous I.V. infusion: Determine the volume of fluid and rate of its administration required by the patient in a 24-hour period. Add the appropriate daily dosage of penicillin to this fluid. For example, if the daily dose is 10 million units and 2 L of fluid/day is required, add 5 million units to 1 L and adjust the rate of flow so the liter will be infused over 12 hours (83 mL/hour). Repeat steps (5 million units/L at 83 mL/hour) for the remaining 12 hours.

Monitoring Parameters Periodic electrolyte, hepatic, renal, cardiac and hematologic function tests during prolonged/high-dose therapy; observe for signs and symptoms of anaphylaxis during first dose

Test Interactions False-positive or negative urinary glucose determination using Clinitest®; positive Coombs' [direct]; false-positive urinary and/or serum proteins

Pharmacotherapy Pearls 1 million units is approximately equal to 625 mg.

Special Geriatric Considerations Despite a reported prolonged half-life, it is usually not necessary to adjust the dose of penicillin G or VK in elderly to account for renal function changes with age, however, it is advised to calculate an estimated creatinine clearance and adjust dose accordingly.

PENICILLIN G (PARENTERAL/AQUEOUS)

◄ **Dosage Forms** Excipient information presented when available (limited, particularly for generics); consult specific product labeling.

Infusion, premixed iso-osmotic dextrose solution, as potassium: 1 million units (50 mL); 2 million units (50 mL); 3 million units (50 mL)

Injection, powder for reconstitution, as potassium: 5 million units, 20 million units

Pfizerpen®: 5 million units, 20 million units [contains potassium 65.6 mg (1.68 mEq) per 1 million units, sodium 6.8 mg (0.3 mEq) per 1 million units]

Injection, powder for reconstitution, as sodium: 5 million units

Selected References

Hansen JM, Kampmann J, and Laursen H, "Renal Excretion of Drugs in the Elderly," *Lancet*, 1970, 1(657):1170.
Leikola E and Vartia KO, "On Penicillin Levels in Young and Geriatric Subjects," *J Gerontol*, 1957, 12:48-52.
Yoshikawa TT, "Antimicrobial Therapy for the Elderly Patient," *J Am Geriatr Soc*, 1990, 38(12):1353-72.

◆ **Penicillin G Potassium** see Penicillin G (Parenteral/Aqueous) *on page 1417*

Penicillin G Procaine (pen i SIL in jee PROE kane)

Medication Safety Issues
Sound-alike/look-alike issues:
Penicillin G procaine may be confused with penicillin V potassium
Wycillin® may be confused with Bicillin®

Brand Names: Canada Pfizerpen-AS®; Wycillin®

Index Terms APPG; Aqueous Procaine Penicillin G; Procaine Benzylpenicillin; Procaine Penicillin G; Wycillin [DSC]

Generic Availability (U.S.) Yes

Pharmacologic Category Antibiotic, Penicillin

Use Treatment of moderately-severe infections due to *Treponema pallidum* and other penicillin G-sensitive microorganisms that are susceptible to low, but prolonged serum penicillin concentrations; anthrax due to *Bacillus anthracis* (postexposure) to reduce the incidence or progression of disease following exposure to aerolized *Bacillus anthracis*

Contraindications Hypersensitivity to penicillin, procaine, or any component of the formulation

Warnings/Precautions May need to modify dosage in patients with severe renal impairment or seizure disorders; avoid I.V., intravascular, or intra-arterial administration of penicillin G procaine since severe and/or permanent neurovascular damage may occur. Serious and occasionally severe or fatal hypersensitivity (anaphylactoid) reactions have been reported in patients on penicillin therapy, especially with a history of beta-lactam hypersensitivity, history of sensitivity to multiple allergens, or previous IgE-mediated reactions (eg, anaphylaxis, angioedema, urticaria). Use with caution in asthmatic patients. Extended duration of therapy or use associated with high serum concentrations may be associated with an increased risk for some adverse reactions. Prolonged use may result in fungal or bacterial superinfection, including *C. difficile*-associated diarrhea (CDAD) and pseudomembranous colitis; CDAD has been observed >2 months postantibiotic treatment.

Adverse Reactions (Reflective of adult population; not specific for elderly) Frequency not defined.
Cardiovascular: Conduction disturbances, myocardial depression, vasodilation
Central nervous system: CNS stimulation, confusion, drowsiness, myoclonus, seizure
Hematologic: Hemolytic anemia, neutropenia, positive Coombs' reaction
Local: Pain at injection site, sterile abscess at injection site, thrombophlebitis
Renal: Interstitial nephritis
Miscellaneous: Hypersensitivity reactions, Jarisch-Herxheimer reaction, pseudoanaphylactic reactions, serum sickness

Drug Interactions
Avoid Concomitant Use
Avoid concomitant use of Penicillin G Procaine with any of the following: BCG

Increased Effect/Toxicity
Penicillin G Procaine may increase the levels/effects of: Methotrexate

The levels/effects of Penicillin G Procaine may be increased by: Probenecid

Decreased Effect
Penicillin G Procaine may decrease the levels/effects of: BCG; Mycophenolate; Typhoid Vaccine

The levels/effects of Penicillin G Procaine may be decreased by: Fusidic Acid; Tetracycline Derivatives

Stability Refrigerate

Mechanism of Action Inhibits bacterial cell wall synthesis by binding to one or more of the penicillin-binding proteins (PBPs); which in turn inhibits the final transpeptidation step of peptidoglycan synthesis in bacterial cell walls, thus inhibiting cell wall biosynthesis. Bacteria eventually lyse due to ongoing activity of cell wall autolytic enzymes (autolysins and murein hydrolases) while cell wall assembly is arrested.

Pharmacodynamics/Kinetics
Absorption: I.M.: Slow
Distribution: Penetration across the blood-brain barrier is poor, despite inflamed meninges
Protein binding: 65%
Half-life: 20-50 minutes
Time to peak serum concentration: Within 1-4 hours and can persist within the therapeutic range for 15-24 hours
Elimination: 60% to 90% of drug is excreted unchanged via renal tubular excretion; ~30% of dose inactivated in the liver
Renal clearance is delayed in patients with impaired renal function

Dosage
Geriatric & Adult
Anthrax:
Inhalational (postexposure prophylaxis): I.M.: 1,200,000 units every 12 hours
Note: Overall treatment duration should be 60 days. Available safety data suggest continued administration of penicillin G procaine for longer than 2 weeks may incur additional risk of adverse reactions. Clinicians may consider switching to effective alternative treatment for completion of therapy beyond 2 weeks.
Cutaneous (treatment): I.M.: 600,000-1,200,000 units/day; alternative therapy is recommended in severe cutaneous or other forms of anthrax infection
Endocarditis caused by susceptible viridans *Streptococcus* (when used in conjunction with an aminoglycoside): I.M.: 1.2 million units every 6 hours for 2-4 weeks
Gonorrhea (uncomplicated): 4.8 million units as a single dose divided in 2 sites given 30 minutes after probenecid 1 g orally
Neurosyphilis: I.M.: 2.4 million units/day with 500 mg probenecid by mouth 4 times/day for 10-14 days; **Note: penicillin G aqueous I.V. is the preferred agent**
Whipple's disease: I.M.: 1.2 million units/day (with streptomycin) for 10-14 days, followed by oral trimethoprim/sulfamethoxazole or doxycycline for 1 year

Renal Impairment
Cl_{cr} 10-30 mL/minute: Administer every 8-12 hours.
Cl_{cr} <10 mL/minute: Administer every 12-18 hours.
Moderately dialyzable (20% to 50%)

Administration Procaine suspension for deep I.M. injection only; administer around-the-clock rather than 4 times/day, etc (ie, 12-6-12-6, not 9-1-5-9) to promote less variation in peak and trough serum concentrations; when doses are repeated, rotate the injection site; avoid I.V., intravascular, or intra-arterial administration of penicillin G procaine since severe and/or permanent neurovascular damage may occur; renal and hematologic systems should be evaluated periodically during prolonged therapy

Monitoring Parameters Periodic renal and hematologic function tests with prolonged therapy; fever, mental status, WBC count

Test Interactions Positive Coombs' [direct], false-positive urinary and/or serum proteins

Special Geriatric Considerations Dosage does not usually need to be adjusted in the elderly, however, if multiple doses are to be given, adjust dose for renal function.

Dosage Forms Excipient information presented when available (limited, particularly for generics); consult specific product labeling.
Injection, suspension: 600,000 units/mL (1 mL, 2 mL)

Selected References
Yoshikawa TT, "Antimicrobial Therapy for the Elderly Patient," *J Am Geriatr Soc*, 1990, 38(12):1353-72.

◆ **Penicillin G Procaine and Benzathine Combined** *see* Penicillin G Benzathine and Penicillin G Procaine *on page 1416*
◆ **Penicillin G Sodium** *see* Penicillin G (Parenteral/Aqueous) *on page 1417*

Penicillin V Potassium (pen i SIL in vee poe TASS ee um)

Medication Safety Issues
Sound-alike/look-alike issues:
Penicillin V procaine may be confused with penicillin G potassium
Brand Names: Canada Apo-Pen VK®; Novo-Pen-VK; Nu-Pen-VK
Index Terms Pen VK; Phenoxymethyl Penicillin
Generic Availability (U.S.) Yes
Pharmacologic Category Antibiotic, Penicillin

PENICILLIN V POTASSIUM

Use Treatment of infections caused by susceptible organisms involving the respiratory tract, otitis media, sinusitis, skin, and urinary tract; prophylaxis in rheumatic fever

Contraindications Hypersensitivity to penicillin or any component of the formulation

Warnings/Precautions Use with caution in patients with severe renal impairment (modify dosage) or history of seizures. Serious and occasionally severe or fatal hypersensitivity (anaphylactoid) reactions have been reported in patients on penicillin therapy, especially with a history of beta-lactam hypersensitivity, history of sensitivity to multiple allergens, or previous IgE-mediated reactions (eg, anaphylaxis, angioedema, urticaria). Use with caution in asthmatic patients. Extended duration of therapy or use associated with high serum concentrations may be associated with an increased risk for some adverse reactions. Prolonged use may result in fungal or bacterial superinfection, including *C. difficile*-associated diarrhea (CDAD) and pseudomembranous colitis; CDAD has been observed >2 months postantibiotic treatment.

Adverse Reactions (Reflective of adult population; not specific for elderly)
>10%: Gastrointestinal: Mild diarrhea, vomiting, nausea, oral candidiasis

Drug Interactions

Avoid Concomitant Use
Avoid concomitant use of Penicillin V Potassium with any of the following: BCG

Increased Effect/Toxicity
Penicillin V Potassium may increase the levels/effects of: Methotrexate

The levels/effects of Penicillin V Potassium may be increased by: Probenecid

Decreased Effect
Penicillin V Potassium may decrease the levels/effects of: BCG; Mycophenolate; Typhoid Vaccine

The levels/effects of Penicillin V Potassium may be decreased by: Fusidic Acid; Tetracycline Derivatives

Ethanol/Nutrition/Herb Interactions Food: Decreases drug absorption rate; decreases drug serum concentration.

Stability Refrigerate suspension after reconstitution; discard after 14 days

Mechanism of Action Inhibits bacterial cell wall synthesis by binding to one or more of the penicillin-binding proteins (PBPs); which in turn inhibits the final transpeptidation step of peptidoglycan synthesis in bacterial cell walls, thus inhibiting cell wall biosynthesis. Bacteria eventually lyse due to ongoing activity of cell wall autolytic enzymes (autolysins and murein hydrolases) while cell wall assembly is arrested.

Pharmacodynamics/Kinetics
Absorption: 60% to 73%
Distribution: Widely distributed to kidneys, liver, skin, tonsils, and into synovial, pleural, and pericardial fluids
Protein binding, plasma: 80%
Half-life elimination: 30 minutes; prolonged with renal impairment
Time to peak, serum: 0.5-1 hour
Excretion: Urine (as unchanged drug and metabolites)

Dosage

Geriatric & Adult

Actinomycosis:
Mild: 2-4 g/day in 4 divided doses for 8 weeks
Surgical: 2-4 g/day in 4 divided doses for 6-12 months (after I.V. penicillin G therapy of 4-6 weeks)

Erysipelas: 500 mg 4 times/day

Pharyngitis (streptococcal): 500 mg 3-4 times/day for 10 days

Prophylaxis of pneumococcal or recurrent rheumatic fever infections: 250 mg twice daily

Renal Impairment
Cl$_{cr}$ 10-50 mL/minute: Administer every 8-12 hours.
Cl$_{cr}$ <10 mL/minute: Administer every 12-16 hours.

Administration Administer on an empty stomach (ie, 1 hour prior to, or 2 hours after meals) to increase total absorption; administer around-the-clock rather than 4 times/day, 3 times/day, etc (ie, 12-6-12-6, not 9-1-5-9) to promote less variation in peak and trough serum concentrations

Monitoring Parameters Periodic renal and hematologic function tests during prolonged therapy; monitor for signs of anaphylaxis during first dose

Test Interactions False-positive or negative urinary glucose determination using Clinitest®; positive Coombs' [direct]; false-positive urinary and/or serum proteins

Pharmacotherapy Pearls 0.7 mEq of potassium per 250 mg penicillin V; 250 mg equals 400,000 units of penicillin

Special Geriatric Considerations Dosage adjustment in the elderly is usually not necessary.

Dosage Forms Excipient information presented when available (limited, particularly for generics); consult specific product labeling.

Powder for solution, oral: 125 mg/5 mL (100 mL, 200 mL); 250 mg/5 mL (100 mL, 200 mL)

Tablet, oral: 250 mg, 500 mg

◆ **Penlac®** see Ciclopirox on page 354
◆ **Pennsaid®** see Diclofenac (Topical) on page 500
◆ **Pentasa®** see Mesalamine on page 1150

Pentazocine (pen TAZ oh seen)

Related Information

Beers Criteria − Potentially Inappropriate Medications for Geriatrics on page 2089
Opioid Analgesics on page 2013

Medication Safety Issues

High alert medication:

The Institute for Safe Medication Practices (ISMP) includes this medication among its list of drug classes which have a heightened risk of causing significant patient harm when used in error.

BEERS Criteria medication:

This drug may be inappropriate for use in geriatric patients (high severity risk).

Brand Names: U.S. Talwin®

Brand Names: Canada Talwin®

Index Terms Pentazocine Lactate

Generic Availability (U.S.) No

Pharmacologic Category Analgesic, Opioid; Analgesic, Opioid Partial Agonist

Use Relief of moderate-to-severe pain; has also been used as a sedative prior to surgery and as a supplement to surgical anesthesia

Contraindications Hypersensitivity to pentazocine or any component of the formulation

Warnings/Precautions May increase systemic and pulmonary arterial pressure and systemic vascular resistance; use with caution in patients who may not tolerate these alterations in hemodynamics (eg, heart failure). May cause CNS depression, which may impair physical or mental abilities; patients must be cautioned about performing tasks which require mental alertness (eg, operating machinery or driving). Effects may be potentiated when used with other sedative drugs or ethanol. Use with caution in seizure-prone patients, acute myocardial infarction, patients undergoing biliary tract impairment, thyroid dysfunction, prostatic hyperplasia/urinary stricture, patients with respiratory, adrenal insufficiency, morbid obesity, renal and hepatic dysfunction, head trauma, increased intracranial pressure, and patients with a history of prior opioid dependence or abuse; pentazocine may precipitate opiate withdrawal symptoms in patients who have been receiving opiates regularly; injection contains sulfites which may cause allergic reaction; tolerance or drug dependence may result from extended use. May cause hypotension; use with caution in patients with hypovolemia, cardiovascular disease (including acute MI), or drugs which may exaggerate hypotensive effects (including phenothiazines or general anesthetics). May obscure diagnosis or clinical course of patients with acute abdominal conditions. Abrupt discontinuation may result in withdrawal symptoms; taper dose to decrease risk of withdrawal symptoms. Severe sclerosis has occurred at the injection-site following multiple injections; rotate sites of injection. Use with caution in the elderly and debilitated patients; may be more sensitive to adverse effects. May be inappropriate for use in the elderly due to increased risk of CNS effects (confusion and hallucinations), in addition to its activity as a mixed opioid agonist and antagonist (Beers Criteria). If used in the elderly, use lower initial doses.

Adverse Reactions (Reflective of adult population; not specific for elderly) Frequency not defined.

Cardiovascular: Circulatory depression, facial edema, flushing, hyper-/hypotension, shock, syncope, systemic vascular resistance increased, tachycardia

Central nervous system: Chills, CNS depression, confusion, disorientation, dizziness, drowsiness, euphoria, excitement, hallucinations, headache, insomnia, irritability, lightheadedness, malaise, nightmares, sedation

Dermatologic: Dermatitis, erythema multiforme, pruritus, rash, Stevens-Johnson syndrome, toxic epidermal necrolysis, urticaria

Gastrointestinal: Abdominal distress, anorexia, constipation, diarrhea, nausea, taste alteration, vomiting, xerostomia

Genitourinary: Urinary retention

Hematologic: Agranulocytosis (rare), eosinophilia, WBCs decreased

Local: Injection site reaction (tissue damage and irritation)

◄ Neuromuscular & skeletal: Paresthesia, tremor, weakness
Ocular: Blurred vision, diplopia, miosis, nystagmus
Otic: Tinnitus
Respiratory: Dyspnea, respiratory depression (rare)
Miscellaneous: Anaphylaxis, diaphoresis, physical and psychological dependence

Drug Interactions

Avoid Concomitant Use There are no known interactions where it is recommended to avoid concomitant use.

Increased Effect/Toxicity

Pentazocine may increase the levels/effects of: Alcohol (Ethyl); Alvimopan; CNS Depressants; Desmopressin; Selective Serotonin Reuptake Inhibitors; Thiazide Diuretics

The levels/effects of Pentazocine may be increased by: Amphetamines; Antipsychotic Agents (Phenothiazines); Droperidol; HydrOXYzine; Succinylcholine

Decreased Effect

Pentazocine may decrease the levels/effects of: Analgesics (Opioid); Pegvisomant

The levels/effects of Pentazocine may be decreased by: Ammonium Chloride

Stability Store at 20°C to 25°C (68°F to 77°F).

Mechanism of Action Agonist of kappa opiate receptors and partial agonist of mu opiate receptors in the CNS, causing inhibition of ascending pain pathways, altering the perception of and response to pain; produces analgesia, respiratory depression and sedation similar to opioids

Pharmacodynamics/Kinetics

Onset of action: I.M., SubQ: 15-20 minutes; I.V.: 2-3 minutes
Duration: 2-3 hours
Protein binding: 60%
Metabolism: Hepatic via oxidative and glucuronide conjugation pathways; extensive first-pass effect
Half-life elimination: 2-3 hours; prolonged with hepatic impairment
Excretion: Urine (small amounts as unchanged drug)

Dosage

Geriatric Use with caution; may be more sensitive to analgesic and sedative effects; decrease initial dose and monitor closely

Adult

Analgesic:

I.M., SubQ: 30-60 mg every 3-4 hours; do **not** exceed 60 mg/dose (maximum: 360 mg/day)

I.V.: 30 mg every 3-4 hours; do **not** exceed 30 mg/dose (maximum: 360 mg/day)

Renal Impairment

Cl$_{cr}$ 10-50 mL/minute: Administer 75% of normal dose.
Cl$_{cr}$ <10 mL/minute: Administer 50% of normal dose.

Hepatic Impairment Reduce dose or avoid use in patients with liver disease.

Administration Rotate injection site for I.M.; avoid intra-arterial injection; avoid SubQ use unless absolutely necessary (may cause tissue damage)

Monitoring Parameters Relief of pain, respiratory and mental status, blood pressure

Special Geriatric Considerations Pentazocine is not recommended for use in the elderly because of its propensity to cause delirium and agitation. If pentazocine must be used, be sure to adjust dose for renal function.

This medication is considered to be potentially inappropriate in this patient population (Beers Criteria severity: High).

Controlled Substance C-IV

Dosage Forms Excipient information presented when available (limited, particularly for generics); consult specific product labeling.

Injection, solution:
Talwin®: 30 mg/mL (1 mL)
Talwin®: 30 mg/mL (10 mL) [contains sodium bisulfite]

Selected References

American Geriatrics Society Panel on Pharmacological Management of Persistent Pain in Older Persons, "Pharmacological Management of Persistent Pain in Older Persons," *J Am Geriatr Soc*, 2009, 57(8):1331-46.

◆ **Pentazocine Lactate** see Pentazocine on page 1423

Pentoxifylline (pen toks IF i lin)

Medication Safety Issues
Sound-alike/look-alike issues:
Pentoxifylline may be confused with tamoxifen
TRENtal® may be confused with Bentyl®, TEGretol®, Trandate®

Brand Names: U.S. TRENtal®

Brand Names: Canada Albert® Pentoxifylline; Apo-Pentoxifylline SR®; Nu-Pentoxifylline SR; ratio-Pentoxifylline; Trental®

Index Terms Oxpentifylline

Generic Availability (U.S.) Yes

Pharmacologic Category Blood Viscosity Reducer Agent

Use Treatment of intermittent claudication on the basis of chronic occlusive arterial disease of the limbs; may improve function and symptoms, but not intended to replace more definitive therapy

Unlabeled/Investigational Use Venous leg ulcers (Jull, 2007)

Contraindications Hypersensitivity to pentoxifylline, xanthines (eg, caffeine, theophylline), or any component of the formulation; recent cerebral and/or retinal hemorrhage

Warnings/Precautions Use with caution in renal impairment; active metabolite may accumulate in renal impairment leading to increased risk of adverse effects. Use caution in the elderly and assess renal function before initiating.

Adverse Reactions (Reflective of adult population; not specific for elderly)
1% to 10%: Gastrointestinal: Nausea (2%), vomiting (1%)

Drug Interactions

Metabolism/Transport Effects Inhibits CYP1A2 (weak)

Avoid Concomitant Use
Avoid concomitant use of Pentoxifylline with any of the following: Ketorolac; Ketorolac (Nasal); Ketorolac (Systemic)

Increased Effect/Toxicity
Pentoxifylline may increase the levels/effects of: Antihypertensives; Antiplatelet Agents; Heparin; Heparin (Low Molecular Weight); Theophylline Derivatives; Vitamin K Antagonists

The levels/effects of Pentoxifylline may be increased by: Cimetidine; Ciprofloxacin; Ciprofloxacin (Systemic); Ketorolac; Ketorolac (Nasal); Ketorolac (Systemic)

Decreased Effect There are no known significant interactions involving a decrease in effect.

Ethanol/Nutrition/Herb Interactions Food: Food may decrease rate but not extent of absorption. Pentoxifylline peak serum levels may be decreased if taken with food.

Stability Store between 15°C to 30°C (59°F to 86°F).

Mechanism of Action Reduces blood viscosity via increased leukocyte and erythrocyte deformability and decreased neutrophil adhesion/activation; improves peripheral tissue oxygenation presumably through enhanced blood flow.

Pharmacodynamics/Kinetics
Absorption: Well absorbed
Metabolism: Hepatic to 3-carboxybutyl (M-IV, inactive) and 3-carboxypropyl (M-V, active) and via erythrocytes to 5-hydroxyhexyl (M-I, active); extensive first-pass effect; M-I is further metabolized in the liver
Half-life elimination: Parent drug: 24-48 minutes; Metabolites: 60-96 minutes
Time to peak, serum: 2-4 hours
Excretion: Primarily urine (50% to 80% as M-V, 20% as other metabolites); feces (<4%)

Dosage
Geriatric Refer to adult dosing. Dosage adjustment based on creatinine clearance can be considered (see Dosage: Renal Impairment).
Adult Peripheral vascular disease: Oral: 400 mg 3 times/day with meals; maximal therapeutic benefit may take 2-4 weeks to develop; recommended to maintain therapy for at least 8 weeks. May reduce to 400 mg twice daily if GI or CNS side effects occur.
Renal Impairment Dosage adjustments are not required by manufacturer; however, consider dosing adjustments based on degree of renal impairment (Paap, 1996):
Moderate renal impairment (Cl_{cr} ~60 mL/minute): 400 mg twice daily
Severe renal impairment (Cl_{cr} ~20 mL/minute): 400 mg once daily; further reduction may be required; Paap suggests 200 mg once daily, but with current products (extended or controlled release; unscored) may require adaptation to 400 mg once every other day

Administration Tablets should be swallowed whole; do not chew, break, or crush. May be administered with food.

Monitoring Parameters PT, PTT if used in conjunction with other agents that may affect coagulation or platelet aggregation, clotting time

Test Interactions Decreased calcium (S), magnesium (S); false-positive theophylline levels ▶

◀ **Special Geriatric Considerations** Pentoxifylline's value in the treatment of intermittent claudication is controversial. Walking distance improved statistically in some clinical trials, but the actual distance was minimal when applied to improving physical activity. Dose adjustment in moderate and severe kidney impairment has been recommended based on accumulation of two active metabolites. However, these doses have not been studied for clinical or safety outcomes.

Dosage Forms Excipient information presented when available (limited, particularly for generics); consult specific product labeling.

Tablet, controlled release, oral:
TRENtal®: 400 mg
Tablet, extended release, oral: 400 mg

Selected References
Jull A, Arroll B, Paraq V, et al, "Pentoxifylline for Treating Venous Leg Ulcers," *Cochrane Database Syst Rev*, 2007, (3): CD001733.

♦ **Pen VK** *see* Penicillin V Potassium *on page* 1421
♦ **Pepcid®** *see* Famotidine *on page* 693
♦ **Pepcid® AC [OTC]** *see* Famotidine *on page* 693
♦ **Pepcid® AC Maximum Strength [OTC]** *see* Famotidine *on page* 693
♦ **Pepcid® Complete® [OTC]** *see* Famotidine, Calcium Carbonate, and Magnesium Hydroxide *on page* 696
♦ **Peptic Relief [OTC]** *see* Bismuth *on page* 207
♦ **Pepto-Bismol® [OTC]** *see* Bismuth *on page* 207
♦ **Pepto-Bismol® Maximum Strength [OTC]** *see* Bismuth *on page* 207
♦ **Pepto Relief [OTC]** *see* Bismuth *on page* 207
♦ **Percocet®** *see* Oxycodone and Acetaminophen *on page* 1371
♦ **Percodan®** *see* Oxycodone and Aspirin *on page* 1373
♦ **Perdiem® Overnight Relief [OTC]** *see* Senna *on page* 1667
♦ **Performist®** *see* Formoterol *on page* 785
♦ **Periactin** *see* Cyproheptadine *on page* 438
♦ **Peri-Colace® [OTC]** *see* Docusate and Senna *on page* 548

Perindopril Erbumine (per IN doe pril er BYOO meen)

Related Information
Angiotensin Agents *on page* 1985
Brand Names: U.S. Aceon®
Brand Names: Canada Apo-Perindopril®; Coversyl®
Generic Availability (U.S.) Yes
Pharmacologic Category Angiotensin-Converting Enzyme (ACE) Inhibitor
Use Treatment of hypertension; reduction of cardiovascular mortality or nonfatal myocardial infarction in patients with stable coronary artery disease

Canadian labeling: Additional use (unlabeled use in U.S.): Treatment of mild-moderate (NYHA I-III) heart failure

Unlabeled/Investigational Use To delay the progression of nephropathy and reduce risks of cardiovascular events in hypertensive patients with type 1 or 2 diabetes mellitus

Contraindications Hypersensitivity to perindopril, any other ACE inhibitor, or any component of the formulation; angioedema related to previous treatment with an ACE inhibitor

Canadian labeling: Additional contraindications (not in U.S. labeling): History of hereditary/idiopathic angioedema

Warnings/Precautions Anaphylactic reactions may occur rarely with ACE inhibitors. At any time during treatment (especially following first dose), angioedema may occur rarely with ACE inhibitors; it may involve the head and neck (potentially compromising airway) or the intestine (presenting with abdominal pain). African-Americans and patients with idiopathic or hereditary angioedema may be at an increased risk. Prolonged frequent monitoring may be required especially if tongue, glottis, or larynx are involved as they are associated with airway obstruction. Patients with a history of airway surgery may have a higher risk of airway obstruction. Aggressive early and appropriate management is critical. Use in patients with previous angioedema associated with ACE inhibitor therapy is contraindicated. Severe anaphylactoid reactions may be seen during hemodialysis (eg, CVVHD) with high-flux dialysis membranes (eg, AN69), and rarely, during low density lipoprotein apheresis with dextran sulfate cellulose. Rare cases of anaphylactoid reactions have been reported in patients undergoing sensitization treatment with hymenoptera (bee, wasp) venom while receiving ACE inhibitors.

Symptomatic hypotension with or without syncope can occur with ACE inhibitors (usually with the first several doses); effects are most often observed in volume-depleted patients; correct volume depletion prior to initiation; close monitoring of patient is required especially with initial dosing and dosing increases; blood pressure must be lowered at a rate appropriate for the patient's clinical condition. Initiation of therapy in patients with ischemic heart disease or cerebrovascular disease warrants close observation due to the potential consequences posed by falling blood pressure (eg, MI, stroke). Use with caution in hypertrophic cardiomyopathy with outflow tract obstruction, severe aortic stenosis, or before, during, or immediately after major surgery.

Hyperkalemia may occur with ACE inhibitors; risk factors include renal dysfunction, diabetes mellitus, concomitant use of potassium-sparing diuretics, potassium supplements, and/or potassium-containing salts. Use cautiously, if at all, with these agents and monitor potassium closely. Cough may occur with ACE inhibitors. Other causes of cough should be considered (eg, pulmonary congestion in patients with heart failure) and excluded prior to discontinuation.

May be associated with deterioration of renal function and/or increases in serum creatinine, particularly in patients with low renal blood flow (eg, renal artery stenosis, heart failure) whose glomerular filtration rate (GFR) is dependent on efferent arteriolar vasoconstriction by angiotensin II; deterioration may result in oliguria, acute renal failure, and progressive azotemia. Small increases in serum creatinine may occur following initiation; consider discontinuation only in patients with progressive and/or significant deterioration in renal function. Use with caution in patients with unstented unilateral/bilateral renal artery stenosis. When unstented bilateral renal artery stenosis is present, use is generally avoided due to the elevated risk of deterioration in renal function unless possible benefits outweigh risks. Concurrent use of angiotensin receptor blockers may increase the risk of clinically-significant adverse events (eg, renal dysfunction, hyperkalemia).

Rare toxicities associated with ACE inhibitors include cholestatic jaundice (which may progress to fulminant hepatic necrosis), agranulocytosis, neutropenia or leukopenia with myeloid hypoplasia. Patients with collagen vascular diseases (especially with concomitant renal impairment) or renal impairment alone may be at increased risk for hematologic toxicity; periodically monitor CBC with differential in these patients.

Adverse Reactions (Reflective of adult population; not specific for elderly)
>10%:
  Central nervous system: Headache (24%)
  Respiratory: Cough (incidence is higher in women, 3:1) (12%)
1% to 10%:
  Cardiovascular: Edema (4%), chest pain (2%), ECG abnormal (2%), palpitation (1%)
  Central nervous system: Dizziness (8%, less than placebo), sleep disorders (3%), depression (2%), fever (2%), nervousness (1%), somnolence (1%)
  Dermatologic: Rash (2%)
  Endocrine & metabolic: Hyperkalemia (1%, less than placebo), triglycerides increased (1%), menstrual disorder (1%)
  Gastrointestinal: Diarrhea (4%), abdominal pain (3%), nausea (2%), vomiting (2%), dyspepsia (2%), flatulence (1%)
  Genitourinary: Urinary tract infection (3%), sexual dysfunction (male 1%)
  Hepatic: ALT increased (2%)
  Neuromuscular & skeletal: Weakness (8%), back pain (6%), lower extremity pain (5%), upper extremity pain (3%), hypertonia (3%), paresthesia (2%), joint pain (1%), myalgia (1%), arthritis (1%), neck pain (1%)
  Renal: Proteinuria (2%)
  Respiratory: Upper respiratory tract infection (9%), sinusitis (5%), rhinitis (5%), pharyngitis (3%)
  Otic: Tinnitus (2%), ear infection (1%)
  Miscellaneous: Viral infection (3%), seasonal allergy (2%)
  Note: Some reactions occurred at an incidence >1% but ≤ placebo.

Additional adverse effects that have been reported with **ACE inhibitors** include agranulocytosis (especially in patients with renal impairment or collagen vascular disease), neutropenia, anemia, bullous pemphigoid, cardiac arrest, eosinophilic pneumonitis, exfoliative dermatitis, falls, hepatic failure, hyponatremia, jaundice, pancreatitis (acute), pancytopenia, pemphigus, psoriasis, thrombocytopenia; decreases in creatinine clearance in some elderly hypertensive patients or those with chronic renal failure, and worsening of renal function in patients with bilateral renal artery stenosis or hypovolemic patients (diuretic therapy). In addition, a syndrome which may include fever, myalgia, arthralgia, interstitial nephritis, vasculitis, rash, eosinophilia and positive ANA, and elevated ESR has been reported with ACE inhibitors.

Drug Interactions
  Avoid Concomitant Use There are no known interactions where it is recommended to avoid concomitant use.

PERINDOPRIL ERBUMINE

Increased Effect/Toxicity

Perindopril Erbumine may increase the levels/effects of: Allopurinol; Amifostine; Antihypertensives; AzaTHIOprine; CycloSPORINE; CycloSPORINE (Systemic); Ferric Gluconate; Gold Sodium Thiomalate; Hypotensive Agents; Iron Dextran Complex; Lithium; Nonsteroidal Anti-Inflammatory Agents; RiTUXimab; Sodium Phosphates

The levels/effects of Perindopril Erbumine may be increased by: Alfuzosin; Angiotensin II Receptor Blockers; Diazoxide; DPP-IV Inhibitors; Eplerenone; Everolimus; Herbs (Hypotensive Properties); Loop Diuretics; MAO Inhibitors; Pentoxifylline; Phosphodiesterase 5 Inhibitors; Potassium Salts; Potassium-Sparing Diuretics; Prostacyclin Analogues; Sirolimus; Temsirolimus; Thiazide Diuretics; TiZANidine; Tolvaptan; Trimethoprim

Decreased Effect

The levels/effects of Perindopril Erbumine may be decreased by: Antacids; Aprotinin; Herbs (Hypertensive Properties); Icatibant; Lanthanum; Methylphenidate; Nonsteroidal Anti-Inflammatory Agents; Salicylates; Yohimbine

Ethanol/Nutrition/Herb Interactions

Food: Perindopril active metabolite concentrations may be lowered if taken with food.

Herb/Nutraceutical: Avoid bayberry, blue cohosh, cayenne, ephedra, ginger, ginseng (American), kola, licorice (may worsen hypertension). Avoid black cohosh, California poppy, coleus, golden seal, hawthorn, mistletoe, periwinkle, quinine, shepherd's purse (may have increased antihypertensive effect).

Stability Store at room temperature of 20°C to 25°C (68°F to 77°F). Protect from moisture.

Mechanism of Action Perindopril is a prodrug for perindoprilat, which acts as a competitive inhibitor of angiotensin-converting enzyme (ACE); prevents conversion of angiotensin I to angiotensin II, a potent vasoconstrictor; results in lower levels of angiotensin II which, in turn, causes an increase in plasma renin activity and a reduction in aldosterone secretion

Pharmacodynamics/Kinetics

Onset of action: Peak effect: 1-2 hours

Protein binding: Perindopril: 60%; Perindoprilat: 10% to 20%

Metabolism: Hepatically hydrolyzed to active metabolite, perindoprilat (~17% to 20% of a dose) and other inactive metabolites

Bioavailability: Perindopril: 75%; Perindoprilat ~25% (~16% with food)

Half-life elimination: Parent drug: 1.5-3 hours; Metabolite: Effective: 3-10 hours, Terminal: 30-120 hours

Time to peak: Chronic therapy: Perindopril: 1 hour; Perindoprilat: 3-7 hours (maximum perindoprilat serum levels are 2-3 times higher and T_{max} is shorter following chronic therapy); CHF: Perindoprilat: 6 hours

Excretion: Urine (75%, 4% to 12% as unchanged drug)

Dosage

Geriatric

Hypertension: >65 years: Oral:

U.S. labeling: Initial: 4 mg/day; maintenance: 8 mg/day; experience with doses >8 mg/day is limited; may be given in 1-2 divided doses

Canadian labeling: Initial: 2 mg/day; if necessary may increase dose after 4 weeks to 4 mg/day; then to 8 mg/day (based on renal function); may be given in 1 or 2 divided doses.

ACCF/AHA Expert Consensus recommendations: Consider lower initial doses and titrating to response (Aronow, 2011)

Stable coronary artery disease: >70 years: Oral: Initial: 2 mg/day for 1 week; then increase as tolerated to 4 mg/day for 1 week; then increase as tolerated to 8 mg/day.

Adult

Heart failure (Canadian labeling; unlabeled use in U.S.): Initial: 2 mg once daily; if necessary, may titrate over 2-4 weeks to 4 mg once daily. The American College of Cardiology/ American Heart Association (ACC/AHA) 2009 Heart Failure Guidelines recommend an initial dose of 2 mg once daily with dose titration at 1- to 2- week intervals to a target dose of 8-16 mg once daily.

Hypertension: Oral: Initial: 4 mg/day but may be titrated to response; usual range: 4-8 mg/day (may be given in 2 divided doses); increase at 1- to 2-week intervals (maximum: 16 mg/day). **Note:** The Canadian labeling recommended maximum dose is 8 mg/day.

Concomitant therapy with diuretics: To reduce the risk of hypotension, discontinue diuretic, if possible, 2-3 days prior to initiating perindopril. If unable to stop diuretic, initiate perindopril at 2-4 mg/day (given in 1-2 divided doses) and monitor blood pressure closely for the first 2 weeks of therapy, and after any dose adjustment of perindopril or diuretic.

Stable coronary artery disease: Oral: Initial: 4 mg once daily for 2 weeks; then increase as tolerated to 8 mg once daily.

Renal Impairment
U.S. labeling:
Cl_{cr} >30 mL/minute: Initial: 2 mg/day; maintenance dosing not to exceed 8 mg/day
Cl_{cr} <30 mL/minute: Safety and efficacy not established.
Hemodialysis: Perindopril and its metabolites are dialyzable
Canadian labeling:
Cl_{cr} ≥60 mL/minute: Initial: 4 mg/day; maintenance dosing not to exceed 8 mg/day
Cl_{cr} 30-60 mL/minute: 2 mg/day
Cl_{cr} 15-30 mL/minute: 2 mg every other day
Hemodialysis (Cl_{cr} <15 mL/minute): 2 mg on dialysis days (given after dialysis)
Hepatic Impairment No adjustment necessary.
Administration Administer prior to a meal.
Monitoring Parameters Blood pressure; serum creatinine and potassium; if patient has collagen vascular disease and/or renal impairment, periodically monitor CBC with differential
Special Geriatric Considerations Due to frequent decreases in glomerular filtration (also creatinine clearance) with aging, elderly patients may have exaggerated responses to ACE inhibitors; differences in clinical response due to hepatic changes are not observed. ACE inhibitors may be preferred agents in elderly patients with congestive heart failure and diabetes mellitus. Diabetic proteinuria is reduced and insulin sensitivity is enhanced. In general, the side effect profile is favorable in elderly and causes little or no CNS confusion; use lowest dose recommendations initially. Many elderly may be volume depleted due to diuretic use and/or blunted thirst reflex resulting in inadequate fluid intake.
Dosage Forms Excipient information presented when available (limited, particularly for generics); consult specific product labeling.
Tablet, oral: 2 mg, 4 mg, 8 mg
Aceon®: 2 mg, 4 mg, 8 mg [scored]

Selected References
American Diabetes Association, "Standards of Medical Care in Diabetes Mellitus – 2009," *Diabetes Care*, 2009, 32 (Suppl 1):13-61.
Braunwald E, Antman EM, Beasley JW, et al, "ACC/AHA Guidelines for the Management of Patients With Unstable Angina and Non-ST-Segment Elevation Myocardial Infarction. A Report of the American College of Cardiology/American Heart Association Task Force on Practice Guidelines (Committee on the Management of Patients With Unstable Angina)," *J Am Coll Cardiol*, 2000, 36(3):970-1062.
Conlin P, Moore T, Swartz S, et al, "Effect of Indomethacin on Blood Pressure Lowering by Captopril and Losartan in Hypertensive Patients," *Hypertension*, 2000, 36:461-5.
Fox KM and EURopean Trial on Reduction of Cardiac Events With Perindopril in Stable Coronary Artery Disease Investigators, "Efficacy of Perindopril in Reduction of Cardiovascular Events Among Patients With Stable Coronary Artery Disease: Randomised, Double-Blind, Placebo-Controlled, Multicentre Trial (The EUROPA Study)," *Lancet*, 2003, 362(9386):782-8.
Hunt SA, Abraham WT, Chin MH, et al, "ACC/AHA 2005 Guideline Update for the Diagnosis and Management of Chronic Heart Failure in the Adult-Summary Article A Report of the American College of Cardiology/American Heart Association Task Force on Practice Guidelines (Writing Committee to Update the 2001 Guidelines for the Evaluation and Management of Heart Failure)," *J Am Coll Cardiol*, 2005, 46(6):1116-43.
"K/DOQI Clinical Practice Guidelines for Chronic Kidney Disease: Evaluation, Classification, and Stratification. Kidney Disease Outcome Quality Initiative," *Am J Kidney Dis*, 2002, 39(2 Suppl 2):1-246. Available at: http://www.kidney.org/professionals/doqi/kdoqi/toc.htm. Accessed August 1, 2003.

◆ **PerioMed™** *see* Fluoride *on page* 751
◆ **Periostat®** *see* Doxycycline *on page* 570

***

Permethrin (per METH rin)

Brand Names: U.S. A200® Lice [OTC]; Acticin® [DSC]; Nix® Complete Lice Treatment System [OTC]; Nix® Creme Rinse Lice Treatment [OTC]; Nix® Creme Rinse [OTC]; Nix® Lice Control Spray [OTC]; Rid® [OTC]
Brand Names: Canada Kwellada-P™; Nix®
Index Terms Elimite
Generic Availability (U.S.) Yes: Excludes liquid spray
Pharmacologic Category Antiparasitic Agent, Topical; Pediculocide; Scabicidal Agent
Use Single-application treatment of infestation with *Pediculus humanus capitis* (head louse) and its nits or *Sarcoptes scabiei* (scabies); indicated for prophylactic use during epidemics of lice
Contraindications Hypersensitivity to pyrethroid, pyrethrin, chrysanthemums, or any component of the formulation
Warnings/Precautions Treatment may temporarily exacerbate the symptoms of itching, redness, swelling; for external use only.
Adverse Reactions (Reflective of adult population; not specific for elderly)
1% to 10%:
Dermatologic: Pruritus, erythema, rash of the scalp
Local: Burning, stinging, tingling, numbness or scalp discomfort, edema

1429

◀ **Drug Interactions**
Avoid Concomitant Use There are no known interactions where it is recommended to avoid concomitant use.
Increased Effect/Toxicity There are no known significant interactions involving an increase in effect.
Decreased Effect There are no known significant interactions involving a decrease in effect.
Mechanism of Action Inhibits sodium ion influx through nerve cell membrane channels in parasites resulting in delayed repolarization and thus paralysis and death of the pest
Pharmacodynamics/Kinetics
Absorption: <2%
Metabolism: Hepatic via ester hydrolysis to inactive metabolites
Excretion: Urine
Dosage
Geriatric & Adult
Head lice: Topical: After hair has been washed with shampoo, rinsed with water and towel dried, apply a sufficient volume of creme rinse to saturate the hair and scalp; also apply behind the ears and at the base of the neck; leave on hair for 10 minutes before rinsing off with water; remove remaining nits. May repeat in 1 week if lice or nits still present; in areas of head lice resistance to 1% permethrin, 5% permethrin has been applied to clean, dry hair and left on overnight (8-14 hours) under a shower cap.
Scabies: Topical: Apply cream from head to toe; leave on for 8-14 hours before washing off with water; may reapply in 1 week if live mites appear. Time of application was limited to 6 hours before rinsing with soap and water.
Administration Because scabies and lice are so contagious, use caution to avoid spreading or infecting oneself; wear gloves when applying. See Dosage.
Special Geriatric Considerations Because of its minimal absorption, permethrin is a drug of choice and is preferred over lindane.
Dosage Forms Excipient information presented when available (limited, particularly for generics); consult specific product labeling. [DSC] = Discontinued product
Cream, topical: 5% (60 g)
Acticin®: 5% (60 g [DSC]) [contains coconut oil]
Liquid, topical [creme rinse formulation]:
Nix® Complete Lice Treatment System: 1% (1s) [contains isopropyl alcohol 20%]
Nix® Creme Rinse: 1% (60 mL) [contains isopropyl alcohol 20%]
Nix® Creme Rinse Lice Treatment: 1% (60 mL) [contains isopropyl alcohol 20%]
Liquid, topical [for bedding, furniture and garments/spray]:
Nix® Lice Control Spray: 0.25% (150 mL)
Lotion, topical: 1% (60 mL)
Solution, topical [for bedding, furniture and garments/spray]:
A200® Lice: 0.5% (170.1 g)
Rid®: 0.5% (150 mL)

Perphenazine (per FEN a zeen)

Related Information
Antipsychotic Agents on page 1997
Medication Safety Issues
Sound-alike/look-alike issues:
Trilafon® may be confused with Tri-Levlen®
Brand Names: Canada Apo-Perphenazine®
Generic Availability (U.S.) Yes
Pharmacologic Category Antiemetic; Antipsychotic Agent, Typical, Phenothiazine
Use Treatment of schizophrenia; severe nausea and vomiting
Unlabeled/Investigational Use Ethanol withdrawal; behavioral symptoms associated with dementia (elderly); Tourette's syndrome; Huntington's chorea; spasmodic torticollis; Reye's syndrome; psychosis; psychosis/agitation related to Alzheimer's dementia
Contraindications Hypersensitivity to perphenazine or any component of the formulation (cross-reactivity between phenothiazines may occur); severe CNS depression (comatose or patients receiving large doses of CNS depressants); subcortical brain damage; bone marrow suppression; blood dyscrasias; liver damage
Warnings/Precautions [U.S. Boxed Warning]: Elderly patients with dementia-related psychosis treated with antipsychotics are at an increased risk of death compared to placebo. Most deaths appeared to be either cardiovascular (eg, heart failure, sudden death) or infectious (eg, pneumonia) in nature. Perphenazine is not approved for the treatment of dementia-related psychosis.

Leukopenia, neutropenia, and agranulocytosis (sometimes fatal) have been reported in clinical trials and postmarketing reports with antipsychotic use; presence of risk factors (eg, pre-existing low WBC or history of drug-induced leuko-/neutropenia) should prompt periodic blood count assessment. Discontinue therapy at first signs of blood dyscrasias or if absolute neutrophil count <1000/mm³.

May cause hypotension. May be sedating, use with caution in disorders where CNS depression is a feature. Use with caution in depressed patients. Use with caution in Parkinson's disease. Caution in patients with hemodynamic instability; predisposition to seizures; severe cardiac, hepatic, renal, or respiratory disease. Esophageal dysmotility and aspiration have been associated with antipsychotic use; use with caution in patients at risk of pneumonia (eg, Alzheimer's disease). Use associated with increased prolactin levels; clinical significance of hyperprolactinemia in patients with breast cancer or other prolactin-dependent tumors is unknown. May alter temperature regulation or mask toxicity of other drugs due to antiemetic effects. May alter cardiac conduction; life-threatening arrhythmias have occurred with therapeutic doses of phenothiazines. May cause orthostatic hypotension; use with caution in patients at risk of this effect or those who would tolerate transient hypotensive episodes (cerebrovascular disease, cardiovascular disease, or other medications which may predispose).

Phenothiazines may cause anticholinergic effects (confusion, agitation, constipation, xerostomia, blurred vision, urinary retention); therefore, they should be used with caution in patients with decreased gastrointestinal motility, urinary retention, BPH, xerostomia, or visual problems. Conditions which also may be exacerbated by cholinergic blockade include narrow-angle glaucoma and worsening of myasthenia gravis. Relative to other neuroleptics, perphenazine has a low incidence of cholinergic blockade. Use with caution in patients with reduced functional alleles of CYP2D6. Poor metabolizers may have higher plasma concentrations at usual doses, increasing risk for adverse reactions.

May cause extrapyramidal reactions (EPS), including pseudoparkinsonism, acute dystonic reactions, akathisia, and tardive dyskinesia. Risk of dystonia (and possibly other EPS) may be greater with increased doses, use of conventional antipsychotics, males, and younger patients.May be associated with neuroleptic malignant syndrome (NMS). May cause pigmentary retinopathy, and lenticular and corneal deposits, particularly with prolonged therapy. May cause photosensitization. Use with caution in the elderly.

Adverse Reactions (Reflective of adult population; not specific for elderly) Frequency not defined.

Cardiovascular: Bradycardia, cardiac arrest, ECG changes, hyper-/hypotension, orthostatic hypotension, pallor, peripheral edema, sudden death, tachycardia

Central nervous system: Bizarre dreams, catatonic-like states, cerebral edema, dizziness, drowsiness, extrapyramidal symptoms (pseudoparkinsonism, akathisia, dystonias, tardive dyskinesia), faintness, headache, hyperactivity, hyperpyrexia, impairment of temperature regulation, insomnia, lethargy, neuroleptic malignant syndrome (NMS), nocturnal confusion, paradoxical excitement, paranoid reactions, restlessness, seizure

Dermatologic: Discoloration of skin (blue-gray), photosensitivity, rash

Endocrine & metabolic: Amenorrhea, breast enlargement, hyper-/hypoglycemia, galactorrhea, lactation, libido changes, gynecomastia, menstrual irregularity, parotid swelling (rare), SIADH

Gastrointestinal: Adynamic ileus, anorexia, appetite increased, constipation, diarrhea, fecal impaction, obstipation, nausea, salivation, stomach pain, vomiting, weight gain, xerostomia

Genitourinary: Bladder paralysis, ejaculatory disturbances, incontinence, polyuria, priapism, urinary retention

Hematologic: Agranulocytosis, eosinophilia, hemolytic anemia, leukopenia, pancytopenia, thrombocytopenic purpura

Hepatic: Hepatotoxicity, jaundice

Neuromuscular & skeletal: Muscle weakness, tremor

Ocular: Blurred vision, cornea and lens changes, epithelial keratopathies, glaucoma, mydriasis, myosis, pigmentary photophobia, retinopathy

Renal: Glycosuria

Respiratory: Nasal congestion

Miscellaneous: Allergic reactions, diaphoresis, systemic lupus erythematosus-like syndrome

Drug Interactions

Metabolism/Transport Effects Substrate of CYP1A2 (minor), 2C9 (minor), 2C19 (minor), 2D6 (major), 3A4 (minor); **Inhibits** CYP1A2 (weak), 2D6 (weak)

Avoid Concomitant Use

Avoid concomitant use of Perphenazine with any of the following: Metoclopramide

◄ **Increased Effect/Toxicity**
Perphenazine may increase the levels/effects of: Alcohol (Ethyl); Analgesics (Opioid); Anticholinergics; Anti-Parkinson's Agents (Dopamine Agonist); Beta-Blockers; CNS Depressants; Methotrimeprazine; Methylphenidate; Porfimer; Selective Serotonin Reuptake Inhibitors

The levels/effects of Perphenazine may be increased by: Abiraterone Acetate; Acetylcholinesterase Inhibitors (Central); Antimalarial Agents; Beta-Blockers; Conivaptan; CYP2D6 Inhibitors (Moderate); CYP2D6 Inhibitors (Strong); Darunavir; Droperidol; Lithium formulations; Methotrimeprazine; Methylphenidate; Metoclopramide; Pramlintide; Tetrabenazine

Decreased Effect
Perphenazine may decrease the levels/effects of: Amphetamines; Quinagolide

The levels/effects of Perphenazine may be decreased by: Antacids; Anti-Parkinson's Agents (Dopamine Agonist); Cyproterone; Lithium formulations; Peginterferon Alfa-2b; Tocilizumab

Ethanol/Nutrition/Herb Interactions
Ethanol: May increase CNS depression; monitor for increased effects with coadministration. Caution patients about effects.
Herb/Nutraceutical: Avoid kava kava, gotu kola, valerian, St John's wort (may increase CNS depression).

Stability Store at controlled room temperature of 20°C to 25°C (68°F to 77°F). Protect from light.

Mechanism of Action Perphenazine is a piperazine phenothiazine antipsychotic which blocks postsynaptic mesolimbic dopaminergic receptors in the brain; exhibits alpha-adrenergic blocking effect and depresses the release of hypothalamic and hypophyseal hormones

Pharmacodynamics/Kinetics
Absorption: Oral: Well absorbed; absorption may be affected by the inherent anticholinergic action on the gastrointestinal tissue causing variable absorption. Absorption from tablets is erratic with less variation seen with solutions. These agents are widely distributed in tissues with CNS concentrations exceeding that of plasma due to their lipophilic characteristics.
Protein binding: Antipsychotic agents are bound 90% to 99% to plasma or proteins; highly bound to brain and lung tissue and other tissues with a high blood perfusion
Metabolism: Extensively hepatic to metabolites via sulfoxidation, hydroxylation, dealkylation, and glucuronidation
Time to peak: Peak serum concentrations occur within 4-8 hours; peak concentrations between 2-4 hours
Elimination: Excreted in urine and bile; excretion occurs through hepatic metabolism (oxidation) where numerous active metabolites are produced; active metabolites excreted in urine; elimination half-lives of antipsychotics ranges from 20-40 hours which may be extended in older adults due to decline in oxidative hepatic reactions (phase I) with age.
The biologic effect of a single dose persists for 24 hours. When the patient has accommodated to initial side effects (sedation), once daily dosing is possible due to the long half-life of antipsychotics.
Steady-state plasma concentrations are achieved in 4-7 days; therefore, if possible, do not make dose adjustments more than once in a 7-day period. Due to the long half-lives of antipsychotics, as needed (prn) use is ineffective since repeated doses are necessary to achieve therapeutic tissue concentrations in the CNS.

Dosage
Geriatric Behavioral symptoms associated with dementia (unlabeled use): Oral: Initial: 2-4 mg 1-2 times/day; increase at 4- to 7-day intervals by 2-4 mg/day. Increase dose intervals (bid, tid, etc) as necessary to control behavior response or side effects. Maximum daily dose: 32 mg; gradual increase (titration) and bedtime administration may prevent some side effects or decrease their severity.
Adult
Schizophrenia/psychoses:
Nonhospitalized: Initial: 4-8 mg 3 times/day; reduce dose as soon as possible to minimum effective dosage (maximum: 64 mg/day)
Hospitalized: 8-16 mg 2-4 times/day (maximum: 64 mg/day)
Nausea/vomiting: Oral: 8-16 mg/day in divided doses up to 24 mg/day (maximum: 24 mg/day)
Renal Impairment Not dialyzable (0% to 5%)
Hepatic Impairment Dosage reductions should be considered in patients with liver disease although no specific guidelines are available.
Monitoring Parameters Orthostatic blood pressures; tremors, gait changes, abnormal movement in trunk, neck, buccal area, or extremities; monitor target behaviors for which the agent is given
Reference Range 2-6 nmol/L

Special Geriatric Considerations Any changes in disease status in any organ system can result in behavior changes.

Many elderly patients receive antipsychotic medications for inappropriate nonpsychotic behavior. Before initiating antipsychotic medication, the clinician should investigate any possible reversible cause; any stress or stress from any disease can cause acute "confusion" or worsening of baseline nonpsychotic behavior. Most commonly acute changes in behavior are due to increases in drug dose or addition of new drug to regimen; fluid electrolyte loss; infections; and changes in environment.

In the treatment of agitated, demented, elderly patients, authors of meta-analysis of controlled trials of the response to the traditional antipsychotics (phenothiazines, butyrophenones) in controlling agitation have concluded that the use of neuroleptics results in a response rate of 18%. Clearly neuroleptic therapy for behavior control should be limited with frequent attempts to withdraw the agent given for behavior control.

Dosage Forms Excipient information presented when available (limited, particularly for generics); consult specific product labeling.

Tablet, oral: 2 mg, 4 mg, 8 mg, 16 mg

Selected References

Rabins PV, Blacker D, Rovner BW, et al, "Practice Guidelines for the Treatment of Patients With Alzheimer's Disease and Other Dementias," *Am J Psychiatry*, 2007, 164(12 Suppl):5-56. Available at http://www.psych.org/psych_pract/treatg/pg/prac_guide.cfm.

Schneider LS, Tariot PN, Dagerman KS, et al, "Effectiveness of Atypical Antipsychotic Drugs in Patients With Alzheimer's Disease," *N Engl J Med*, 2006, 355(15):1525-38.

- ◆ **Persantine®** *see* Dipyridamole *on page* 537
- ◆ **Pethidine Hydrochloride** *see* Meperidine *on page* 1140
- ◆ **Pexeva®** *see* PARoxetine *on page* 1396
- ◆ **Pfizerpen®** *see* Penicillin G (Parenteral/Aqueous) *on page* 1417
- ◆ **PGE₁** *see* Alprostadil *on page* 73
- ◆ **Phazyme® Ultra Strength [OTC]** *see* Simethicone *on page* 1679
- ◆ **Phenadoz®** *see* Promethazine *on page* 1530

Phenazopyridine (fen az oh PEER i deen)

Medication Safety Issues

Sound-alike/look-alike issues:

Phenazopyridine may be confused with phenoxybenzamine

Pyridium® may be confused with Dyrenium®, Perdiem®, pyridoxine, pyrithione

Brand Names: U.S. AZO Standard® Maximum Strength [OTC]; AZO Standard® [OTC]; Azo-Gesic™ [OTC]; Baridium [OTC]; Pyridium®; ReAzo [OTC]; UTI Relief® [OTC]

Brand Names: Canada Phenazo™

Index Terms Phenazopyridine Hydrochloride; Phenylazo Diamino Pyridine Hydrochloride

Generic Availability (U.S.) Yes

Pharmacologic Category Analgesic, Urinary

Use Symptomatic relief of urinary burning, itching, frequency, and urgency in association with urinary tract infection or following urologic procedures

Contraindications Hypersensitivity to phenazopyridine or any component of the formulation; kidney or liver disease; patients with a Cl_{cr} <50 mL/minute

Warnings/Precautions Does not treat urinary infection, acts only as an analgesic; drug should be discontinued if skin or sclera develop a yellow color; use with caution in patients with renal impairment. Use of this agent in the elderly is limited since accumulation of phenazopyridine can occur in patients with renal insufficiency. Use is contraindicated in patients with a Cl_{cr} <50 mL/minute.

Adverse Reactions (Reflective of adult population; not specific for elderly)

1% to 10%:

Central nervous system: Headache, dizziness

Gastrointestinal: Stomach cramps

Drug Interactions

Avoid Concomitant Use There are no known interactions where it is recommended to avoid concomitant use.

Increased Effect/Toxicity There are no known significant interactions involving an increase in effect.

Decreased Effect There are no known significant interactions involving a decrease in effect.

Mechanism of Action An azo dye which exerts local anesthetic or analgesic action on urinary tract mucosa through an unknown mechanism

◄ **Pharmacodynamics/Kinetics**
Metabolism: Hepatic and via other tissues
Excretion: Urine (65% as unchanged drug)
Dosage
Geriatric & Adult Urinary analgesic: Oral: 100-200 mg 3 times/day after meals for 2 days when used concomitantly with an antibacterial agent
Renal Impairment
Cl_{cr} 50-80 mL/minute: Administer every 8-16 hours.
Cl_{cr} <50 mL/minute: Avoid use.
Administration Administer after meals.
Monitoring Parameters Relief of urinary discomfort
Test Interactions Phenazopyridine may cause delayed reactions with glucose oxidase reagents (Clinistix®, Tes-Tape®); occasional false-positive tests occur with Tes-Tape®; cupric sulfate tests (Clinitest®) are not affected; interference may also occur with urine ketone tests (Acetest®, Ketostix®) and urinary protein tests; tests for urinary steroids and porphyrins may also occur
Special Geriatric Considerations Use of this agent in older adults is limited since accumulation of phenazopyridine can occur in patients with renal insufficiency.
Dosage Forms Excipient information presented when available (limited, particularly for generics); consult specific product labeling.
Tablet, oral, as hydrochloride: 100 mg, 200 mg
AZO Standard®: 95 mg [gluten free]
AZO Standard® Maximum Strength: 97.5 mg
AZO Standard® Maximum Strength: 97.5 mg [gluten free]
Azo-Gesic™: 95 mg
Baridium: 97.2 mg
Pyridium®: 100 mg, 200 mg
ReAzo: 95 mg
UTI Relief®: 97.2 mg

♦ **Phenazopyridine Hydrochloride** see Phenazopyridine on page 1433

Phenelzine (FEN el zeen)

Related Information
Antidepressant Agents on page 1991
Medication Safety Issues
Sound-alike/look-alike issues:
Phenelzine may be confused with phenytoin
Nardil® may be confused with Norinyl®
Brand Names: U.S. Nardil®
Brand Names: Canada Nardil®
Index Terms Phenelzine Sulfate
Generic Availability (U.S.) Yes
Pharmacologic Category Antidepressant, Monoamine Oxidase Inhibitor
Use Symptomatic treatment of atypical, nonendogenous, or neurotic depression
Unlabeled/Investigational Use Treatment of selective mutism
Medication Guide Available Yes
Contraindications Hypersensitivity to phenelzine or any component of the formulation; congestive heart failure; pheochromocytoma; abnormal liver function tests or history of hepatic disease; renal impairment or severe renal disease/impairment
Concurrent use of sympathomimetics (including amphetamines, cocaine, dopamine, epinephrine, methylphenidate, norepinephrine, or phenylephrine) and related compounds (methyldopa, levodopa, phenylalanine, tryptophan, or tyrosine), ophthalmic alpha$_2$-agonists (apraclonidine, brimonidine), CNS depressants, cyclobenzaprine, dextromethorphan, ethanol, meperidine, bupropion, or buspirone
At least 2 weeks should elapse between the discontinuation of serotoninergic agents (including SNRIs, SSRIs, and tricyclics) and other MAO inhibitors and the initiation of phenelzine. At least 5 weeks should elapse between the discontinuation of fluoxetine and the initiation of phenelzine. In all cases, a sufficient amount of time must be allowed for the clearance of the serotoninergic agent and any active metabolites prior to the initiation of phenelzine.
At least 2 weeks should elapse between the discontinuation of phenelzine and the initiation of the following agents: Serotoninergic agents (including SNRIs, SSRIs, fluoxetine, and tricyclics), bupropion, buspirone, and other antidepressants.

General anesthesia, spinal anesthesia (hypotension may be exaggerated). Use caution with local anesthetics containing sympathomimetic agents. Phenelzine should be discontinued ≥10 days prior to elective surgery.

Foods high in tyramine or dopamine content; foods and/or supplements containing tyrosine, phenylalanine, tryptophan, or caffeine

Warnings/Precautions [U.S. Boxed Warning]: Antidepressants increase the risk of suicidal thinking and behavior in children, adolescents, and young adults (18-24 years of age) with major depressive disorder (MDD) and other psychiatric disorders; consider risk prior to prescribing. Short-term studies did not show an increased risk in patients >24 years of age and showed a decreased risk in patients ≥65 years. Closely monitor for clinical worsening, suicidality, or unusual changes in behavior; the patient's family or caregiver should be instructed to closely observe the patient and communicate condition with healthcare provider. Such observation would generally include at least weekly face-to-face contact with patients or their family members or caregivers during the first 4 weeks of treatment, then every other week visits for the next 4 weeks, then at 12 weeks, and as clinically indicated beyond 12 weeks. Additional contact by telephone may be appropriate between face-to-face visits. Adults treated with antidepressants should be observed similarly for clinical worsening and suicidality, especially during the initial few months of a course of drug therapy, or at times of dose changes, either increases or decreases. A medication guide should be dispensed with each prescription. Phenelzine is not generally considered a first-line agent for the treatment of depression; phenelzine is typically used in patients who have failed to respond to other treatments. **Phenelzine is not FDA approved for the treatment of depression in children ≤16 years of age.**

The possibility of a suicide attempt is inherent in major depression and may persist until remission occurs. Monitor for worsening of depression or suicidality, especially during initiation of therapy (generally first 1-2 months) or with dose increases or decreases. Worsening depression and severe abrupt suicidality that are not part of the presenting symptoms may require discontinuation or modification of drug therapy. Use caution in high-risk patients during initiation of therapy. Prescriptions should be written for the smallest quantity consistent with good patient care. The patient's family or caregiver should be alerted to monitor patients for the emergence of suicidality and associated behaviors such as anxiety, agitation, panic attacks, insomnia, irritability, hostility, impulsivity, akathisia, hypomania, and mania; patients should be instructed to notify their healthcare provider if any of these symptoms or worsening depression occur.

May worsen psychosis in some patients or precipitate a shift to mania or hypomania in patients with bipolar disorder. Monotherapy in patients with bipolar disorder should be avoided. Patients presenting with depressive symptoms should be screened for bipolar disorder. Phenelzine is not FDA approved for the treatment of bipolar depression.

Sensitization to the effects of insulin may occur; monitor blood glucose closely in patients with diabetes. Use with caution in patients who have glaucoma, or hyperthyroidism. Cases of hypertensive crisis (sometimes fatal) have occurred; symptoms include: severe headache, nausea/vomiting, neck stiffness/soreness, photophobia, and sweating. Monitor blood pressure closely in all patients. Hypertensive crisis may occur with tyramine-, tryptophan-, or dopamine-containing foods. Phentolamine is recommended for the treatment of hypertensive crisis. Do not use with other MAO inhibitors or antidepressants. Do not use within 5 weeks of fluoxetine discontinuation or 2 weeks of other antidepressant discontinuation. Avoid products containing sympathomimetic stimulants or dextromethorphan. Concurrent use with antihypertensive agents may lead to exaggeration of hypotensive effects. May cause orthostatic hypotension; use with caution in patients with hypotension or patients who would not tolerate transient hypotensive episodes (cardiovascular or cerebrovascular disease); effects may be additive with other agents which cause orthostasis. Use with caution in patients at risk of seizures, or in patients receiving other drugs which may lower seizure threshold. Discontinue at least 48 hours prior to myelography. May increase the risks associated with electroconvulsive therapy. Consider discontinuing, when possible, prior to elective surgery. Pyridoxine deficiency has occurred; symptoms include numbness and edema of hands; may respond to supplementation.

Adverse Reactions (Reflective of adult population; not specific for elderly) Frequency not defined.

Cardiovascular: Edema, orthostatic hypotension

Central nervous system: Anxiety (acute), ataxia, coma, delirium, dizziness, drowsiness, euphoria, fatigue, fever, headache, hyper-reflexia, hypersomnia, insomnia, mania, schizophrenia, seizure, twitching

Dermatologic: Pruritus, rash

Endocrine & metabolic: Decreased sexual ability (anorgasmia, ejaculatory disturbances, impotence), hypermetabolic syndrome, hypernatremia

Gastrointestinal: Constipation, weight gain, xerostomia

◀ Genitourinary: Urinary retention

Hematologic: Leukopenia

Hepatic: Jaundice, necrotizing hepatocellular necrosis (rare), transaminases increased

Neuromuscular & skeletal: Myoclonia, paresthesia, tremor, weakness

Ocular: Blurred vision, glaucoma, nystagmus

Respiratory: Edema (glottis)

Miscellaneous: Diaphoresis, Lupus-like syndrome, transient cardiac or respiratory depression (following ECT), withdrawal syndrome (nausea, vomiting, malaise)

Drug Interactions

Avoid Concomitant Use

Avoid concomitant use of Phenelzine with any of the following: Alpha-/Beta-Agonists (Indirect-Acting); Alpha1-Agonists; Alpha2-Agonists (Ophthalmic); Amphetamines; Anilidopiperidine Opioids; Atomoxetine; Bezafibrate; Buprenorphine; BuPROPion; BusPIRone; CarBAMazepine; Cyclobenzaprine; Dexmethylphenidate; Dextromethorphan; Diethylpropion; HYDROmorphone; Linezolid; Maprotiline; Meperidine; Methyldopa; Methylene Blue; Methylphenidate; Mirtazapine; Oxymorphone; Pizotifen; Propoxyphene; Selective Serotonin Reuptake Inhibitors; Serotonin 5-HT1D Receptor Agonists; Serotonin/Norepinephrine Reuptake Inhibitors; Sibutramine; Tapentadol; Tetrabenazine; Tetrahydrozoline; Tetrahydrozoline (Nasal); Tricyclic Antidepressants; Tryptophan

Increased Effect/Toxicity

Phenelzine may increase the levels/effects of: Alpha-/Beta-Agonists (Direct-Acting); Alpha-/Beta-Agonists (Indirect-Acting); Alpha1-Agonists; Alpha2-Agonists (Ophthalmic); Amphetamines; Anticholinergics; Antihypertensives; Atomoxetine; Beta2-Agonists; Bezafibrate; BuPROPion; Dexmethylphenidate; Dextromethorphan; Diethylpropion; Doxapram; HYDROmorphone; Linezolid; Lithium; Meperidine; Methadone; Methyldopa; Methylene Blue; Methylphenidate; Mirtazapine; Orthostatic Hypotension Producing Agents; Pizotifen; Reserpine; Selective Serotonin Reuptake Inhibitors; Serotonin 5-HT1D Receptor Agonists; Serotonin Modulators; Serotonin/Norepinephrine Reuptake Inhibitors; Succinylcholine; Tetrahydrozoline; Tetrahydrozoline (Nasal); Tricyclic Antidepressants

The levels/effects of Phenelzine may be increased by: Altretamine; Anilidopiperidine Opioids; Buprenorphine; BusPIRone; CarBAMazepine; COMT Inhibitors; Cyclobenzaprine; Levodopa; MAO Inhibitors; Maprotiline; Oxymorphone; Pramlintide; Propoxyphene; Sibutramine; Tapentadol; Tetrabenazine; TraMADol; Tryptophan

Decreased Effect

Phenelzine may decrease the levels/effects of: Acetylcholinesterase Inhibitors (Central)

The levels/effects of Phenelzine may be decreased by: Acetylcholinesterase Inhibitors (Central)

Ethanol/Nutrition/Herb Interactions

Ethanol: May increase CNS depression; monitor for increased effects with coadministration. Caution patients about effects. Avoid beverages containing tyramine (hearty red wine and beer).

Food: Concurrent ingestion of foods rich in tyramine may cause sudden and severe high blood pressure (hypertensive crisis). Avoid tyramine-containing foods with MAOIs.

Herb/Nutraceutical: Avoid valerian, St John's wort, SAMe, kava kava (may increase risk of serotonin syndrome and/or excessive sedation); Avoid supplements containing caffeine, tyrosine, tryptophan, or phenylalanine. Ingestion of large quantities may increase the risk of severe side effects (eg, hypertensive reactions, serotonin syndrome).

Stability Store at 20°C to 25°C (68°F to 77°F). Protect from heat and light.

Mechanism of Action Thought to act by increasing endogenous concentrations of norepinephrine, dopamine, and serotonin through inhibition of the enzyme (monoamine oxidase) responsible for the breakdown of these neurotransmitters

Pharmacodynamics/Kinetics

Onset of action: Therapeutic: 2-4 weeks; geriatric patients receiving an average of 55 mg/day developed a mean platelet MAO activity inhibition of about 85%.

Duration: May continue to have a therapeutic effect and interactions 2 weeks after discontinuing therapy

Absorption: Well absorbed

Metabolism: Oxidized via monoamine oxidase (primary pathway) and acetylation (minor pathway)

Half-life elimination: 12 hours

Excretion: Urine (73% as metabolites)

Dosage

Geriatric Oral: Initial: 7.5 mg/day; increase by 7.5-15 mg/day every 3-4 days as tolerated; usual therapeutic dose: 15-60 mg/day in 3-4 divided doses.

Adult Depression: Oral: Initial: 15 mg 3 times/day

Early phase: Increase rapidly, based on patient tolerance, to 60-90 mg/day (may take 4 weeks of 60 mg/day therapy before clinical response)

Maintenance: After maximum benefit is obtained, slowly reduce dose over several weeks; dose may be as low as 15 mg/day to 15 mg every other day

Monitoring Parameters Blood pressure, heart rate; diet, weight; mood (if depressive symptoms), suicide ideation (especially during the initial months of therapy or when doses are increased or decreased)

Special Geriatric Considerations The MAO inhibitors are effective and generally well tolerated by elderly patients. It is their potential interactions with tyramine or tryptophan-containing food and other drugs and their effects on blood pressure that have limited their use. The MAO inhibitors are usually reserved for patients who do not tolerate or respond to the traditional "cyclic" or "second generation" antidepressants. Phenelzine is less stimulating than tranylcypromine.

Dosage Forms Excipient information presented when available (limited, particularly for generics); consult specific product labeling.

Tablet, oral: 15 mg

Nardil®: 15 mg

Selected References

Georgotas A, Friedman E, McCarthy M, et al, "Resistant Geriatric Depression and Therapeutic Response to Monoamine-Oxidase Inhibitors," *Biol Psychiatry,* 1983, 18:195-205.

Goff DC and Jenike MA, "Treatment-Resistant Depression in the Elderly," *J Am Geriatr Soc,* 1986, 34(1):63-70.

♦ **Phenelzine Sulfate** *see* Phenelzine *on page 1434*

♦ **Phenergan®** *see* Promethazine *on page 1530*

♦ **Pheniramine and Naphazoline** *see* Naphazoline and Pheniramine *on page 1263*

PHENobarbital (fee noe BAR bi tal)

Medication Safety Issues

Sound-alike/look-alike issues:

PHENobarbital may be confused with PENTobarbital, Phenergan®, phenytoin

Luminal® may be confused with Tuinal®

Brand Names: Canada PMS-Phenobarbital

Index Terms Luminal Sodium; Phenobarbital Sodium; Phenobarbitone; Phenylethylmalonylurea

Generic Availability (U.S.) Yes

Pharmacologic Category Anticonvulsant, Barbiturate; Barbiturate

Use Management of generalized tonic-clonic (grand mal), status epilepticus, and partial seizures; sedative/hypnotic

Note: Use to treat insomnia is not recommended (Schutte-Rodin, 2008)

Unlabeled/Investigational Use Management of sedative/hypnotic withdrawal

Contraindications Hypersensitivity to barbiturates or any component of the formulation; marked hepatic impairment; dyspnea or airway obstruction; porphyria (manifest and latent); intra-arterial administration, subcutaneous administration (not recommended); use in patients with a history of sedative/hypnotic addiction is not recommended; nephritic patients (large doses)

Warnings/Precautions Potential for drug dependency exists, abrupt cessation may precipitate withdrawal, including status epilepticus in epileptic patients. Do not administer to patients in acute pain. Use caution in elderly, debilitated, and renal or hepatic dysfunction. May cause paradoxical responses, including agitation and hyperactivity, particularly in acute pain patients. Use with caution in patients with depression or suicidal tendencies, or in patients with a history of drug abuse. Tolerance, psychological and physical dependence may occur with prolonged use. May cause CNS depression, which may impair physical or mental abilities. Effects with other sedative drugs or ethanol may be potentiated. May cause respiratory depression or hypotension, particularly when administered intravenously. Use with caution in hemodynamically unstable patients (hypovolemic shock, CHF) or patients with respiratory disease. Due to its long half-life and risk of dependence, phenobarbital is not recommended as a sedative in the elderly. Use with caution in patients with hypoadrenalism. Intra-arterial administration may cause reactions ranging from transient pain to gangrene and is contraindicated. Subcutaneous administration may cause tissue irritation (eg, redness, tenderness, necrosis) and is not recommended.

Adverse Reactions (Reflective of adult population; not specific for elderly) Frequency not defined.

Cardiovascular: Bradycardia, hypotension, syncope

Central nervous system: Agitation, anxiety, ataxia, CNS excitation or depression, confusion, dizziness drowsiness, hallucinations, "hangover" effect, headache, hyperkinesia, impaired judgment, insomnia, lethargy, nervousness, nightmares, somnolence

◄ Dermatologic: Exfoliative dermatitis, rash, Stevens-Johnson syndrome
Gastrointestinal: Nausea, vomiting, constipation
Hematologic: Agranulocytosis, thrombocytopenia, megaloblastic anemia
Local: Pain at injection site, thrombophlebitis with I.V. use
Renal: Oliguria
Respiratory: Laryngospasm, respiratory depression, apnea (especially with rapid I.V. use), hypoventilation
Miscellaneous: Gangrene with inadvertent intra-arterial injection

Drug Interactions

Metabolism/Transport Effects Substrate of CYP2C9 (minor), 2C19 (major), 2E1 (minor); **Induces** CYP1A2 (strong), 2A6 (strong), 2B6 (strong), 2C8 (strong), 2C9 (strong), 3A4 (strong)

Avoid Concomitant Use

Avoid concomitant use of PHENobarbital with any of the following: Boceprevir; Crizotinib; Darunavir; Dronedarone; Etravirine; Everolimus; Lapatinib; Lurasidone; Nilotinib; Pazopanib; Praziquantel; Ranolazine; Rilpivirine; Roflumilast; RomiDEPsin; Telaprevir; Ticagrelor; Tolvaptan; Vandetanib; Voriconazole

Increased Effect/Toxicity

PHENobarbital may increase the levels/effects of: Alcohol (Ethyl); Clarithromycin; CNS Depressants; Meperidine; QuiNIDine; Selective Serotonin Reuptake Inhibitors; Thiazide Diuretics

The levels/effects of PHENobarbital may be increased by: Carbonic Anhydrase Inhibitors; Chloramphenicol; Clarithromycin; CYP2C19 Inhibitors (Moderate); CYP2C19 Inhibitors (Strong); Dexmethylphenidate; Divalproex; Droperidol; Felbamate; HydrOXYzine; Methylphenidate; Primidone; QuiNINE; Rufinamide; Telaprevir; Valproic Acid

Decreased Effect

PHENobarbital may decrease the levels/effects of: Acetaminophen; Bendamustine; Beta-Blockers; Boceprevir; Brentuximab Vedotin; Calcium Channel Blockers; Chloramphenicol; Clarithromycin; Contraceptives (Estrogens); Contraceptives (Progestins); Corticosteroids (Systemic); Crizotinib; CycloSPORINE; CycloSPORINE (Systemic); CYP1A2 Substrates; CYP2A6 Substrates; CYP2B6 Substrates; CYP2C8 Substrates (High risk); CYP2C9 Substrates (High risk); CYP3A4 Substrates; Darunavir; Deferasirox; Diclofenac; Disopyramide; Divalproex; Doxycycline; Dronedarone; Etoposide; Etoposide Phosphate; Etravirine; Everolimus; Exemestane; Felbamate; Fosphenytoin; Gefitinib; Griseofulvin; GuanFACINE; Imatinib; Irinotecan; Ixabepilone; Lacosamide; LamoTRIgine; Lapatinib; Linagliptin; Lopinavir; Lurasidone; Maraviroc; Methadone; MetroNIDAZOLE; MetroNIDAZOLE (Systemic); Nilotinib; OXcarbazepine; Pazopanib; Phenytoin; Praziquantel; Propafenone; QuiNIDine; QuiNINE; Ranolazine; Rilpivirine; Rivaroxaban; Roflumilast; RomiDEPsin; Rufinamide; Saxagliptin; SORAfenib; Tadalafil; Telaprevir; Teniposide; Theophylline Derivatives; Ticagrelor; Tipranavir; Tolvaptan; Treprostinil; Tricyclic Antidepressants; Ulipristal; Valproic Acid; Vandetanib; Vemurafenib; Vitamin K Antagonists; Voriconazole; Zonisamide

The levels/effects of PHENobarbital may be decreased by: Amphetamines; Cholestyramine Resin; CYP2C19 Inducers (Strong); Cyproterone; Folic Acid; Ketorolac; Ketorolac (Nasal); Ketorolac (Systemic); Leucovorin Calcium-Levoleucovorin; Levomefolate; Mefloquine; Methylfolate; Pyridoxine; Rifamycin Derivatives; Telaprevir; Tipranavir

Ethanol/Nutrition/Herb Interactions

Ethanol: May increase CNS depression; monitor for increased effects with coadministration. Caution patients about effects.
Food: May cause decrease in vitamin D and calcium.
Herb/Nutraceutical: Avoid evening primrose (seizure threshold decreased). Avoid valerian, St John's wort, kava kava, gotu kola (may increase CNS depression).

Stability Protect elixir from light. Not stable in aqueous solutions; use only clear solutions. Do not add to acidic solutions; precipitation may occur.

Mechanism of Action Long-acting barbiturate with sedative, hypnotic, and anticonvulsant properties. Barbiturates depress the sensory cortex, decrease motor activity, alter cerebellar function, and produce drowsiness, sedation, and hypnosis. In high doses, barbiturates exhibit anticonvulsant activity; barbiturates produce dose-dependent respiratory depression.

Pharmacodynamics/Kinetics

Onset of action: Oral: Hypnosis: 20-60 minutes; I.V.: ~5 minutes
  Peak effect: I.V.: ~30 minutes
Duration: Oral: 6-10 hours; I.V.: 4-10 hours
Absorption: Oral: 70% to 90%
Protein binding: 20% to 45%
Metabolism: Hepatic via hydroxylation and glucuronide conjugation
Half-life elimination: 53-140 hours

Time to peak, serum: Oral: 1-6 hours

Excretion: Urine (20% to 50% as unchanged drug)

Dosage

Geriatric Geriatric patients should be started at the lowest recommended dose. Refer to adult dosing.

Adult

Sedation: Oral, I.M.: 30-120 mg/day in 2-3 divided doses

Preoperative sedation: I.M.: 100-200 mg 1-1.5 hours before procedure

Anticonvulsant/status epilepticus:

Loading dose: I.V.: 10-20 mg/kg (maximum rate ≤60 mg/minute in patients ≥60 kg); may repeat dose in 20-minute intervals as needed (maximum total dose: 30 mg/kg)

Maintenance dose: Oral, I.V.: 1-3 mg/kg/day in divided doses or 50-100 mg 2-3 times/day

Sedative/hypnotic withdrawal (unlabeled use): Initial daily requirement is determined by substituting phenobarbital 30 mg for every 100 mg pentobarbital used during tolerance testing; then daily requirement is decreased by 10% of initial dose.

Renal Impairment

Cl_{cr} <10 mL/minute: Administer every 12-16 hours.

Moderately dialyzable (20% to 50%)

Hepatic Impairment Reduce dose in patients with hepatic impairment.

Administration May be administered I.V., I.M. or orally. Avoid rapid I.V. administration >60 mg/minute; intra-arterial injection is contraindicated; avoid subcutaneous administration; parenteral solutions are highly alkaline; avoid extravasation. For I.M. administration, inject deep into muscle. Do not exceed 5 mL per injection site due to potential for tissue irritation

Monitoring Parameters Phenobarbital serum concentrations, mental status, CBC, LFTs, seizure activity

Reference Range

Therapeutic: Adults: 20-40 mcg/mL (SI: 86-172 µmol/L)

Toxic: >40 mcg/mL (SI: >172 µmol/L)

Toxic concentration: Slowness, ataxia, nystagmus: 35-80 mcg/mL (SI: 150-344 µmol/L)

Coma with reflexes: 65-117 mcg/mL (SI: 279-502 µmol/L)

Coma without reflexes: >100 mcg/mL (SI: >430 µmol/L)

Test Interactions Assay interference of LDH

Pharmacotherapy Pearls Injectable solutions contain propylene glycol.

Phenobarbital tablets are also available from some generic manufacturers in strengths that are exactly equivalent to fractional grain strengths: 16.2 mg (1/4 grain), 32.4 mg (1/2 grain), 64.8 mg (1 grain). To avoid medication errors, do not prescribe phenobarbital in grains.

Special Geriatric Considerations Using barbiturates in elderly may induce paradoxical stimulation, cause or aggravate depression and confusion. Due to its long half-life and risk of dependence, phenobarbital is not recommended as a sedative or hypnotic in the elderly. Interpretive guidelines from the Centers for Medicare and Medicaid Services (CMS) discourage the use of this agent as a sedative/hypnotic in long-term care residents.

Controlled Substance C-IV

Dosage Forms Excipient information presented when available (limited, particularly for generics); consult specific product labeling.

Elixir, oral: 20 mg/5 mL (5 mL, 7.5 mL, 15 mL, 473 mL)

Injection, solution, as sodium: 65 mg/mL (1 mL); 130 mg/mL (1 mL)

Tablet, oral: 15 mg, 30 mg, 60 mg, 100 mg

Extemporaneously Prepared An alcohol-free phenobarbital 10 mg/mL suspension can be prepared as follows: Levigate ten phenobarbital 60 mg tablets in a glass mortar into a fine powder. Mix 30 mL of Ora-Plus® and 30 mL of either Ora-Sweet® or Ora-Sweet® SF; stir vigorously. Add 15 mL of the Ora-Plus®/Ora-Sweet® (or Ora-Sweet® SF) mixture to the powder; triturate well. Transfer to a 2 ounce amber plastic bottle; qs to a final volume of 60 mL. Stable for up to 115 days at room temperature. Shake well prior to use.

May mix dose with chocolate syrup (1:1 volume) immediately before administration to mask the bitter aftertaste.

Cober M and Johnson CE, "Stability of an Extemporaneously Prepared Alcohol-Free Phenobarbital Suspension," *Am J Health Syst Pharm*, 2007, 64(6):644-6.

◆ **Phenobarbital, Hyoscyamine, Atropine, and Scopolamine** see Hyoscyamine, Atropine, Scopolamine, and Phenobarbital on page 905

◆ **Phenobarbital Sodium** see PHENobarbital on page 1437

◆ **Phenobarbitone** see PHENobarbital on page 1437

Phenoxybenzamine (fen oks ee BEN za meen)

Medication Safety Issues
Sound-alike/look-alike issues:
Phenoxybenzamine may be confused with phenazopyridine
Brand Names: U.S. Dibenzyline®
Index Terms Phenoxybenzamine Hydrochloride
Generic Availability (U.S.) No
Pharmacologic Category Alpha₁ Blocker; Antidote
Use Symptomatic management of pheochromocytoma
Unlabeled/Investigational Use Micturition problems associated with neurogenic bladder, functional outlet obstruction, and partial prostate obstruction; treatment of hypertensive crisis caused by sympathomimetic amines
Dosage
Geriatric & Adult
Pheochromocytoma, hypertension: Oral: Initial: 10 mg twice daily, increase by 10 mg every other day until optimal blood pressure response is achieved; usual range: 20-40 mg 2-3 times/day. Doses up to 240 mg/day have been reported (Kinney, 2000).
Micturition disorders (unlabeled use): Oral: 10-20 mg 1-2 times/day
Special Geriatric Considerations Because of the risk of adverse effects, avoid the use of this medication in the elderly if possible.
Dosage Forms Excipient information presented when available (limited, particularly for generics); consult specific product labeling.
Capsule, oral, as hydrochloride:
Dibenzyline®: 10 mg

◆ **Phenoxybenzamine Hydrochloride** see Phenoxybenzamine on page 1440
◆ **Phenoxymethyl Penicillin** see Penicillin V Potassium on page 1421
◆ **Phenylalanine Mustard** see Melphalan on page 1131
◆ **Phenylazo Diamino Pyridine Hydrochloride** see Phenazopyridine on page 1433

Phenylephrine (Systemic) (fen il EF rin)

Medication Safety Issues
Sound-alike/look-alike issues:
Sudafed PE™ may be confused with Sudafed®
High alert medication:
The Institute for Safe Medication Practices (ISMP) includes this medication among its list of drugs which have a heightened risk of causing significant patient harm when used in error.
Brand Names: U.S. LuSonal™ [DSC]; Medi-First® Sinus Decongestant [OTC]; Medi-Phenyl [OTC]; PediaCare® Children's Decongestant [OTC]; Sudafed PE® Children's [OTC]; Sudafed PE® Congestion [OTC]; Sudafed PE™ Nasal Decongestant [OTC]; Sudogest™ PE [OTC]; Triaminic Thin Strips® Children's Cold with Stuffy Nose [OTC]
Index Terms Phenylephrine Hydrochloride
Generic Availability (U.S.) Yes: Excludes liquid, strips
Pharmacologic Category Alpha-Adrenergic Agonist
Use Treatment of hypotension, vascular failure in shock; as a vasoconstrictor in regional analgesia; supraventricular tachycardia (**Note:** Not for routine use in treatment of supraventricular tachycardias); as a decongestant [OTC]
Contraindications Hypersensitivity to phenylephrine or any component of the formulation; hypertension; ventricular tachycardia
Oral: Use with or within 14 days of MAO inhibitor therapy
Warnings/Precautions Some products contain sulfites which may cause allergic reactions in susceptible individuals. Use with extreme caution in patients taking MAO inhibitors.

Intravenous: Use with caution in the elderly, patients with hyperthyroidism, bradycardia, partial heart block, myocardial disease, or severe CAD. Avoid or use with extreme caution in patients with heart failure or cardiogenic shock; increased systemic vascular resistance may significantly reduce cardiac output. Assure adequate circulatory volume to minimize need for vasoconstrictors. Avoid hypertension; monitor blood pressure closely and adjust infusion rate. Avoid extravasation; infuse into a large vein if possible. Avoid infusion into leg veins. Watch I.V. site closely. If extravasation occurs, infiltrate the area subcutaneously with diluted phentolamine (5-10 mg in 10 mL of saline) with a fine hypodermic needle. **Phentolamine should be administered as soon as possible after extravasation is noted. [U.S. Boxed Warning]: Should be administered by adequately trained individuals familiar with its use.**

Oral: Use caution with asthma, bowel obstruction/narrowing, hyperthyroidism, diabetes mellitus, cardiovascular disease, ischemic heart disease, increased intraocular pressure, prostatic hyperplasia or in the elderly. Notify healthcare provider if symptoms do not improve within 7 days or are accompanied by fever. Discontinue and contact healthcare provider if nervousness, dizziness, or sleeplessness occur.

Adverse Reactions (Reflective of adult population; not specific for elderly) Frequency not defined.

Injection:

Cardiovascular: Arrhythmia (rare), decreased cardiac output, hypertension, pallor, precordial pain or discomfort, reflex bradycardia, severe peripheral and visceral vasoconstriction

Central nervous system: Anxiety, dizziness, excitability, giddiness, headache, insomnia, nervousness, restlessness

Endocrine & metabolic: Metabolic acidosis

Gastrointestinal: Gastric irritation, nausea

Local: I.V.: Extravasation which may lead to necrosis and sloughing of surrounding tissue, blanching of skin

Neuromuscular & skeletal: Paresthesia, pilomotor response, tremor, weakness

Renal: Decreased renal perfusion, reduced urine output

Respiratory: Respiratory distress

Miscellaneous: Hypersensitivity reactions (including rash, urticaria, leukopenia, agranulocytosis, thrombocytopenia)

Oral: Central nervous system: Anxiety, dizziness, excitability, giddiness, headache, insomnia, nervousness, restlessness

Drug Interactions

Avoid Concomitant Use

Avoid concomitant use of Phenylephrine (Systemic) with any of the following: Iobenguane I 123; MAO Inhibitors

Increased Effect/Toxicity

Phenylephrine (Systemic) may increase the levels/effects of: Sympathomimetics

The levels/effects of Phenylephrine (Systemic) may be increased by: Atomoxetine; Cannabinoids; MAO Inhibitors; Tricyclic Antidepressants

Decreased Effect

Phenylephrine (Systemic) may decrease the levels/effects of: Benzylpenicilloyl Polylysine; Iobenguane I 123

Ethanol/Nutrition/Herb Interactions Herb/Nutraceutical: Avoid ephedra, yohimbe (may cause CNS stimulation).

Stability

Solution for injection: Store vials at controlled room temperature of 15°C to 30°C (59°F to 86°F). Protect from light. Do not use solution if brown or contains a precipitate.

I.V. infusion: Usual concentration: 10 mg in 500 mL NS or D_5W. May also dilute 50 mg in 500 mL NS or 100 mg in 500 mL NS; both concentrations are stable for at least 14 days at room temperature of 25°C (77°F) (Gupta, 2004). Dilution of 1250 mg in 500 mL NS retained potency for at least 24 hours at 22°C (Weber, 1970).

I.V. injection: May dilute with SWFI to a concentration of 1 mg/mL.

Stability in syringes (Kiser, 2007): Concentration of 0.1 mg/mL in NS (polypropylene syringes) is stable for at least 30 days at -20°C (-4°F), 3°C to 5°C (37°F to 41°F), or 23°C to 25°C (73.4°F to 77°F).

Oral: Store at controlled room temperature of 15°C to 25°C (59°F to 77°F). Protect from light.

Mechanism of Action Potent, direct-acting alpha-adrenergic agonist with virtually no beta-adrenergic activity; produces systemic arterial vasoconstriction. Such increases in systemic vascular resistance result in dose dependent increases in systolic and diastolic blood pressure and reductions in heart rate and cardiac output especially in patients with heart failure.

Pharmacodynamics/Kinetics

Onset of action:

Blood pressure increase/vasoconstriction: I.M., SubQ: 10-15 minutes; I.V.: Immediate

Nasal decongestant: Oral: 15-30 minutes (Kollar, 2007)

Duration:

Blood pressure increase/vasoconstriction: I.M.: 1-2 hours; I.V.: ~15-20 minutes; SubQ: 50 minutes

Nasal decongestant: Oral: ≤4 hours (Kollar, 2007)

Absorption: Oral: Rapid and complete (Kanfer, 1993)

Distribution: V_d: Initial: 26-61 L; V_{dss}: 184-543 L (mean: 340 L) (Hengstmann 1982)

Metabolism: Hepatic via oxidative deamination (Oral: 24%; I.V.: 50%); Undergoes sulfation (Oral [mostly within gut wall]: 46%; I.V.: 8%) and some glucuronidation; forms inactive metabolites (Kanfer 1993)

Bioavailability: Oral: ≤38% (Hengstmann, 1982; Kanfer, 1993)

Half-life elimination: Alpha phase: ~5 minutes; Terminal phase: 2-3 hours (Hengstmann, 1982; Kanfer, 1993)

Time to peak: Oral: 0.75-2 hours (Kanfer, 1993)

Excretion: Urine (mostly as inactive metabolites)

Dosage

Geriatric & Adult

Hypotension/shock:

I.V. bolus: 100-500 mcg/dose every 10-15 minutes as needed (initial dose should not exceed 500 mcg)

I.V. infusion: Initial dose: 100-180 mcg/minute, **or alternatively,** 0.5 mcg/kg/minute; titrate to desired response. Dosing ranges between 0.4-9.1 mcg/kg/minute have been reported when treating septic shock (Gregory, 1991).

Nasal congestion: Oral: 10-20 mg every 4 hours as needed for ≤7 days

Paroxysmal supraventricular tachycardia (Note: Not recommended for routine use in treatment of supraventricular tachycardias): *I.V.:* 250-500 mcg/dose over 20-30 seconds

Administration I.V.: May cause necrosis or sloughing tissue if extravasation occurs during I.V. administration or SubQ administration.

Extravasation management: Use phentolamine as antidote; mix 5-10 mg with 10 mL of NS. Inject a small amount of this dilution subcutaneously into extravasated area. Blanching should reverse immediately. Monitor site. If blanching should recur, additional injections of phentolamine may be needed.

Monitoring Parameters Blood pressure (or mean arterial pressure), heart rate; cardiac output (as appropriate), intravascular volume status, pulmonary capillary wedge pressure (as appropriate); monitor infusion site closely

Special Geriatric Considerations Elderly are more predisposed to the adverse effects of sympathomimetics since they frequently have cardiovascular disease and diabetes mellitus and are on multiple medications. Elderly patients should be counseled about their proper use of OTC products and in what disease states they should be avoided.

Dosage Forms Excipient information presented when available (limited, particularly for generics); consult specific product labeling. [DSC] = Discontinued product

Injection, solution, as hydrochloride: 1% [10 mg/mL] (1 mL, 2 mL [DSC], 5 mL, 10 mL)

Liquid, oral, as hydrochloride:

LuSonal™: 7.5 mg/5 mL (473 mL [DSC]) [contains phenylalanine; strawberry flavor]

PediaCare® Children's Decongestant: 2.5 mg/5 mL (118 mL) [contains sodium 14 mg/5 mL, sodium benzoate; raspberry flavor]

Sudafed PE® Children's: 2.5 mg/5 mL (118 mL) [ethanol free, sugar free; contains sodium 14 mg/5 mL, sodium benzoate; raspberry flavor]

Strip, orally disintegrating, oral, as hydrochloride:

Triaminic Thin Strips® Children's Cold with Stuffy Nose: 2.5 mg (14s) [raspberry flavor]

Tablet, oral, as hydrochloride:

Medi-First® Sinus Decongestant: 10 mg

Medi-Phenyl: 5 mg

Sudafed PE® Congestion: 10 mg

Sudafed PE™ Nasal Decongestant: 10 mg

Sudogest™ PE: 10 mg

Selected References

Kollar C, Schneider H, Waksman J, et al, "Meta-Analysis of the Efficacy of Single Dose of Phenylephrine 10 Mg Compared With Placebo in Adults With Acute Nasal Congestion Due to the Common Cold," *Clin Ther,* 2007, 29 (6):1057-70.

Phenylephrine (Nasal) (fen il EF rin)

Medication Safety Issues

Sound-alike/look-alike issues:

Neo-Synephrine® (phenylephrine, nasal) may be confused with Neo-Synephrine® (oxy-metazoline)

Brand Names: U.S. 4 Way® Fast Acting [OTC]; 4 Way® Menthol [OTC]; Little Noses® Decongestant [OTC]; Neo-Synephrine® Extra Strength [OTC]; Neo-Synephrine® Mild Formula [OTC]; Neo-Synephrine® Regular Strength [OTC]; Rhinall® [OTC]; Vicks® Sinex® VapoSpray™ 4 Hour Decongestant [OTC]

Brand Names: Canada Neo-Synephrine®

Index Terms Phenylephrine Hydrochloride

Pharmacologic Category Alpha-Adrenergic Agonist

Use For OTC use as symptomatic relief of nasal and nasopharyngeal mucosal congestion

Dosage
Geriatric & Adult Nasal congestion: Intranasal: 0.25% to 1% solution: Instill 2-3 sprays or 2-3 drops in each nostril every 4 hours as needed for ≤3 days

Dosage Forms Excipient information presented when available (limited, particularly for generics); consult specific product labeling.

Solution, intranasal, as hydrochloride [drops]:
Little Noses® Decongestant: 0.125% (15 mL) [ethanol free; contains benzalkonium chloride]
Rhinall®: 0.25% (30 mL) [contains benzalkonium chloride, sodium bisulfite]
Solution, intranasal, as hydrochloride [spray]:
4 Way® Fast Acting: 1% (15 mL, 30 mL, 37 mL) [contains benzalkonium chloride]
4 Way® Menthol: 1% (15 mL, 30 mL) [contains benzalkonium chloride, menthol]
Neo-Synephrine® Extra Strength: 1% (15 mL) [contains benzalkonium chloride]
Neo-Synephrine® Mild Formula: 0.25% (15 mL) [contains benzalkonium chloride]
Neo-Synephrine® Regular Strength: 0.5% (15 mL) [contains benzalkonium chloride]
Rhinall®: 0.25% (40 mL) [contains benzalkonium chloride, sodium bisulfite]
Vicks® Sinex® VapoSpray™ 4 Hour Decongestant: 0.5% (15 mL) [contains benzalkonium chloride, menthol]

Phenylephrine (Ophthalmic) (fen il EF rin)

Medication Safety Issues
Sound-alike/look-alike issues:
Mydfrin® may be confused with Midrin®
Brand Names: U.S. AK-Dilate™; Altafrin; Mydfrin®; Neofrin; OcuNefrin™ [OTC] [DSC]
Brand Names: Canada Dionephrine®; Mydfrin®
Index Terms Phenylephrine Hydrochloride
Generic Availability (U.S.) Yes
Pharmacologic Category Alpha-Adrenergic Agonist; Ophthalmic Agent, Antiglaucoma; Ophthalmic Agent, Mydriatic
Use Used as a mydriatic in ophthalmic procedures and treatment of wide-angle glaucoma; OTC use as symptomatic relief of redness of the eye due to irritation

Dosage
Geriatric
Ophthalmic preparations for pupil dilation: Instill 1 drop of 2.5% solution; may repeat in 1 hour if necessary
Other indications: Refer to adult dosing.
Adult
Ocular procedures: Ophthalmic: Instill 1 drop of 2.5% or 10% solution; may repeat in 10-60 minutes as needed
Ophthalmic irritation (OTC formulation): Ophthalmic: Instill 1-2 drops 0.12% solution into affected eye up to 4 times/day; do not use for >72 hours

Dosage Forms Excipient information presented when available (limited, particularly for generics); consult specific product labeling. [DSC] = Discontinued product

Solution, ophthalmic, as hydrochloride [drops]: 2.5% (2 mL, 3 mL, 5 mL, 15 mL)
AK-Dilate™: 2.5% (2 mL, 15 mL); 10% (5 mL) [contains benzalkonium chloride]
Altafrin: 2.5% (15 mL); 10% (5 mL) [contains benzalkonium chloride]
Mydfrin®: 2.5% (3 mL, 5 mL) [contains benzalkonium chloride, sodium bisulfite]
Neofrin: 2.5% (15 mL); 10% (5 mL)
OcuNefrin™: 0.12% (15 mL [DSC])

Phenylephrine (Topical) (fen il EF rin)

Brand Names: U.S. Anu-Med [OTC]; Formulation R™ [OTC]; Medicone® Suppositories [OTC]; Preparation H® [OTC]; Rectacaine [OTC]; Tronolane® Suppository [OTC]
Index Terms Phenylephrine Hydrochloride
Pharmacologic Category Alpha-Adrenergic Agonist
Use For OTC use as treatment of hemorrhoids
Dosage
Geriatric & Adult Hemorrhoids: Rectal:
Ointment: Apply to clean, dry area up to 4 times/day
Suppository: Insert 1 suppository rectally up to 4 times/day
Special Geriatric Considerations Since topical phenylephrine products can be obtained OTC, elderly patients should be counseled about their proper use and in what disease states they should be avoided.

◄ **Dosage Forms** Excipient information presented when available (limited, particularly for generics); consult specific product labeling. [DSC] = Discontinued product

Ointment, rectal, as hydrochloride:
  Formulation R™: 0.25% (30 g, 60 g) [contains benzoic acid]
  Preparation H®: 0.25% (30 g, 60 g) [contains benzoic acid]
  Rectacaine: 0.25% (60 g [DSC])
Suppository, rectal, as hydrochloride: 0.25% (12s)
  Anu-Med: 0.25% (12s)
  Medicone® Suppositories: 0.25% (12s, 24s)
  Preparation H®: 0.25% (12s, 24s, 48s)
  Rectacaine: 0.25% (12s)
  Tronolane® Suppository: 0.25% (12s, 24s)

♦ **Phenylephrine Hydrochloride** *see* Phenylephrine (Nasal) *on page 1442*
♦ **Phenylephrine Hydrochloride** *see* Phenylephrine (Ophthalmic) *on page 1443*
♦ **Phenylephrine Hydrochloride** *see* Phenylephrine (Systemic) *on page 1440*
♦ **Phenylephrine Hydrochloride** *see* Phenylephrine (Topical) *on page 1443*
♦ **Phenylephrine Hydrochloride and Acetaminophen** *see* Acetaminophen and Phenylephrine *on page 38*
♦ **Phenylethylmalonylurea** *see* PHENobarbital *on page 1437*
♦ **Phenytek®** *see* Phenytoin *on page 1444*

Phenytoin (FEN i toyn)

Medication Safety Issues
  Sound-alike/look-alike issues:
    Phenytoin may be confused with phenelzine, phentermine, PHENobarbital
    Dilantin® may be confused with Dilaudid®, diltiazem, Dipentum®
  High alert medication:
    The Institute for Safe Medication Practices (ISMP) includes this medication (I.V. formulation) among its list of drug classes which have a heightened risk of causing significant patient harm when used in error.
  International issues:
    Dilantin [U.S., Canada, and multiple international markets] may be confused with Dolantine brand name for pethidine [Belgium]

Brand Names: U.S. Dilantin-125®; Dilantin®; Phenytek®

Brand Names: Canada Dilantin®

Index Terms Diphenylhydantoin; DPH; Phenytoin Sodium; Phenytoin Sodium, Extended; Phenytoin Sodium, Prompt

Generic Availability (U.S.) Yes: Excludes chewable tablet

Pharmacologic Category Anticonvulsant, Hydantoin

Use Management of generalized tonic-clonic (grand mal), complex partial seizures; prevention of seizures following head trauma/neurosurgery

Medication Guide Available Yes

Contraindications Hypersensitivity to phenytoin, other hydantoins, or any component of the formulation

Warnings/Precautions Antiepileptics are associated with an increased risk of suicidal behavior/thoughts with use (regardless of indication); patients should be monitored for signs/symptoms of depression, suicidal tendencies, and other unusual behavior changes during therapy and instructed to inform their healthcare provider immediately if symptoms occur.

[U.S. Boxed Warning]: Phenytoin must be administered slowly. Intravenous administration should not exceed 50 mg/minute in adult patients. In neonates, intravenous administration rate should not exceed 1-3 mg/kg/minute (most clinicians use a lower maximum rate of infusion in neonates of 0.5-1 mg/kg/minute). Hypotension may occur with rapid administration. I.V. form may cause skin necrosis at I.V. site; avoid I.V. administration in small veins; may increase frequency of petit mal seizures; use with caution in patients with porphyria; discontinue if rash or lymphadenopathy occurs; a spectrum of hematologic effects have been reported with use (eg, neutropenia, leukopenia, thrombocytopenia, pancytopenia, and anemias); use with caution in patients with hepatic dysfunction, sinus bradycardia, S-A block, or AV block; use with caution in elderly or debilitated patients, or in any condition associated with low serum albumin levels, which will increase the free fraction of phenytoin in the serum and, therefore, the pharmacologic response. Sedation, confusional states, or cerebellar dysfunction (loss of motor coordination) may occur at higher total serum concentrations, or at lower total serum concentrations when the free fraction of phenytoin is increased. Effects with other sedative drugs or ethanol may be potentiated. Abrupt withdrawal may precipitate status epilepticus. Severe reactions, including toxic epidermal necrolysis and

Stevens-Johnson syndromes, although rarely reported, have resulted in fatalities; drug should be discontinued if there are any signs of rash. Patients of Asian descent with the variant *HLA-B*1502* may be at an increased risk of developing Stevens-Johnson syndrome and/or toxic epidermal necrolysis.

Adverse Reactions (Reflective of adult population; not specific for elderly) I.V. effects: Hypotension, bradycardia, cardiac arrhythmia, cardiovascular collapse (especially with rapid I.V. use), venous irritation and pain, thrombophlebitis

Effects not related to plasma phenytoin concentrations: Hypertrichosis, gingival hypertrophy, thickening of facial features, carbohydrate intolerance, folic acid deficiency, peripheral neuropathy, vitamin D deficiency, osteomalacia, systemic lupus erythematosus

Concentration-related effects: Nystagmus, blurred vision, diplopia, ataxia, slurred speech, dizziness, drowsiness, lethargy, coma, rash, fever, nausea, vomiting, gum tenderness, confusion, mood changes, folic acid depletion, osteomalacia, hyperglycemia

Related to elevated concentrations:
>20 mcg/mL: Far lateral nystagmus
>30 mcg/mL: 45° lateral gaze nystagmus and ataxia
>40 mcg/mL: Decreased mentation
>100 mcg/mL: Death

Cardiovascular: Hypotension, bradycardia, cardiac arrhythmia, cardiovascular collapse
Central nervous system: Psychiatric changes, slurred speech, dizziness, drowsiness, headache, insomnia
Dermatologic: Rash
Gastrointestinal: Constipation, nausea, vomiting, gingival hyperplasia, enlargement of lips
Hematologic: Leukopenia, thrombocytopenia, agranulocytosis
Hepatic: Hepatitis
Local: Thrombophlebitis
Neuromuscular & skeletal: Tremor, peripheral neuropathy, paresthesia
Ocular: Diplopia, nystagmus, blurred vision
Rarely seen effects: Blood dyscrasias, coarsening of facial features, dyskinesias, hepatitis, hypertrichosis, lymphadenopathy, lymphoma, pseudolymphoma, SLE-like syndrome, Stevens-Johnson syndrome, toxic epidermal necrolysis, venous irritation and pain

Drug Interactions
Metabolism/Transport Effects Substrate of CYP2C9 (major), 2C19 (major), 3A4 (minor); **Induces** CYP2B6 (strong), 2C8 (strong), 2C9 (strong), 2C19 (strong), 3A4 (strong)
Avoid Concomitant Use
Avoid concomitant use of Phenytoin with any of the following: Boceprevir; Crizotinib; Darunavir; Dronedarone; Etravirine; Everolimus; Lapatinib; Lurasidone; Nilotinib; Pazopanib; Praziquantel; Ranolazine; Rilpivirine; Roflumilast; RomiDEPsin; Telaprevir; Ticagrelor; Tolvaptan; Vandetanib
Increased Effect/Toxicity
Phenytoin may increase the levels/effects of: Alcohol (Ethyl); Clarithromycin; CNS Depressants; Fosamprenavir; Lithium; Methotrimeprazine; Selective Serotonin Reuptake Inhibitors; Vecuronium; Vitamin K Antagonists

The levels/effects of Phenytoin may be increased by: Allopurinol; Amiodarone; Antifungal Agents (Azole Derivatives, Systemic); Benzodiazepines; Calcium Channel Blockers; Capecitabine; CarBAMazepine; Carbonic Anhydrase Inhibitors; CeFAZolin; Chloramphenicol; Cimetidine; Clarithromycin; Conivaptan; CYP2C19 Inhibitors (Moderate); CYP2C19 Inhibitors (Strong); CYP2C9 Inhibitors (Moderate); CYP2C9 Inhibitors (Strong); Dexmethylphenidate; Disulfiram; Droperidol; Efavirenz; Felbamate; Floxuridine; Fluconazole; Fluorouracil; Fluorouracil (Systemic); Fluorouracil (Topical); FLUoxetine; FluvoxaMINE; HydrOXYzine; Isoniazid; Methotrimeprazine; Methylphenidate; MetroNIDAZOLE; MetroNIDAZOLE (Systemic); OXcarbazepine; Proton Pump Inhibitors; Rufinamide; Sertraline; Sulfonamide Derivatives; Tacrolimus; Tacrolimus (Systemic); Telaprevir; Ticlopidine; Topiramate; Trimethoprim; Vitamin K Antagonists
Decreased Effect
Phenytoin may decrease the levels/effects of: Acetaminophen; Amiodarone; Antifungal Agents (Azole Derivatives, Systemic); Boceprevir; Brentuximab Vedotin; CarBAMazepine; Caspofungin; Chloramphenicol; Clarithromycin; CloZAPine; Contraceptives (Estrogens); Contraceptives (Progestins); Crizotinib; CycloSPORINE; CycloSPORINE (Systemic); CYP2B6 Substrates; CYP2C19 Substrates; CYP2C8 Substrates (High risk); CYP2C9 Substrates (High risk); CYP3A4 Substrates; Darunavir; Deferasirox; Diclofenac; Disopyramide; Divalproex; Doxycycline; Dronedarone; Efavirenz; Etoposide; Etoposide Phosphate; Etravirine; Everolimus; Exemestane; Felbamate; Flunarizine; Gefitinib; GuanFACINE; HMG-CoA Reductase Inhibitors; Imatinib; Irinotecan; Ixabepilone; Lacosamide; LamoTRIgine; Lapatinib; Levodopa; Linagliptin; Loop Diuretics; Lopinavir; Lurasidone; Maraviroc; Mebendazole; Meperidine; Methadone; MetroNIDAZOLE; MetroNIDAZOLE (Systemic);

1445

Metyrapone; Mexiletine; Nilotinib; OXcarbazepine; Pazopanib; Praziquantel; Primidone; QUEtiapine; QuiNIDine; QuiNINE; Ranolazine; Rilpivirine; Ritonavir; Rivaroxaban; Roflumilast; RomiDEPsin; Rufinamide; Saxagliptin; Sertraline; Sirolimus; SORAfenib; Tacrolimus; Tacrolimus (Systemic); Tadalafil; Telaprevir; Temsirolimus; Teniposide; Theophylline Derivatives; Thyroid Products; Ticagrelor; Tipranavir; Tolvaptan; Topiramate; Treprostinil; Ulipristal; Valproic Acid; Vandetanib; Vecuronium; Vemurafenib; Zonisamide

The levels/effects of Phenytoin may be decreased by: Amphetamines; Antacids; Barbiturates; CarBAMazepine; Ciprofloxacin; Ciprofloxacin (Systemic); CISplatin; Colesevelam; CYP2C19 Inducers (Strong); CYP2C9 Inducers (Highly Effective); Diazoxide; Divalproex; Folic Acid; Fosamprenavir; Ketorolac; Ketorolac (Nasal); Ketorolac (Systemic); Leucovorin Calcium-Levoleucovorin; Levomefolate; Lopinavir; Mefloquine; Methylfolate; Peginterferon Alfa-2b; Pyridoxine; Rifamycin Derivatives; Ritonavir; Telaprevir; Theophylline Derivatives; Tipranavir; Tocilizumab; Valproic Acid; Vigabatrin

Ethanol/Nutrition/Herb Interactions
Ethanol:
Acute use: Avoid or limit ethanol (inhibits metabolism of phenytoin). Ethanol may also increase CNS depression; monitor for increased effects with coadministration. Caution patients about effects.
Chronic use: Avoid or limit ethanol (stimulates metabolism of phenytoin).
Food: Phenytoin serum concentrations may be altered if taken with food. If taken with enteral nutrition, phenytoin serum concentrations may be decreased. Tube feedings decrease bioavailability; hold tube feedings 1-2 hours before and 1-2 hours after phenytoin administration. May decrease calcium, folic acid, and vitamin D levels.
Herb/Nutraceutical: Avoid evening primrose (seizure threshold decreased). Avoid valerian, St John's wort, kava kava, gotu kola (may increase CNS depression).

Stability
Capsule, tablet: Store at controlled room temperature. Protect from light and moisture.
Oral suspension: Store at room temperature of 20°C to 25°C (68°F to 77°F); do not freeze. Protect from light.
Solution for injection: Store at room temperature of 15°C to 30°C (59°F to 86°F). Use only clear solutions free of precipitate and haziness; slightly yellow solutions may be used. Precipitation may occur if solution is refrigerated and may dissolve at room temperature.
Further dilution of the solution for I.V. infusion is controversial and no consensus exists as to the optimal concentration and length of stability. Stability is concentration and pH dependent. Based on limited clinical consensus, NS or LR are recommended diluents. Dilutions of 1-10 mg/mL have been used and should be administered as soon as possible after preparation (some recommend to discard if not used within 4 hours). Do not refrigerate.

Mechanism of Action Stabilizes neuronal membranes and decreases seizure activity by increasing efflux or decreasing influx of sodium ions across cell membranes in the motor cortex during generation of nerve impulses; prolongs effective refractory period and suppresses ventricular pacemaker automaticity, shortens action potential in the heart

Pharmacodynamics/Kinetics
Onset of action: I.V.: ~0.5-1 hour
Absorption: Oral: Slow
Distribution: V_d: 0.6-0.7 L/kg
Protein binding:
Adults: 90% to 95%
Others: Decreased protein binding
Disease states resulting in a decrease in serum albumin concentration: Burns, hepatic cirrhosis, nephrotic syndrome, cystic fibrosis
Disease states resulting in an apparent decrease in affinity of phenytoin for serum albumin: Renal failure, jaundice (severe), other drugs (displacers), hyperbilirubinemia (total bilirubin >15 mg/dL), Cl_{cr} <25 mL/minute (unbound fraction is increased two- to threefold in uremia)
Metabolism: Follows dose-dependent capacity-limited (Michaelis-Menten) pharmacokinetics with increased V_{max} in infants >6 months of age and children versus adults; major metabolite (via oxidation), HPPA, undergoes enterohepatic recirculation
Bioavailability: Form dependent
Half-life elimination: Oral: 22 hours (range: 7-42 hours)
Time to peak, serum (form dependent): Oral: Extended-release capsule: 4-12 hours; Immediate release preparation: 2-3 hours
Excretion: Urine (<5% as unchanged drug); as glucuronides
Clearance: Highly variable, dependent upon intrinsic hepatic function and dose administered; increased clearance and decreased serum concentrations with febrile illness

Dosage

Geriatric & Adult Note: Phenytoin base (eg, oral suspension, chewable tablets) contains ~8% more drug than phenytoin sodium (~92 mg base is equivalent to 100 mg phenytoin sodium). Dosage adjustments and closer serum monitoring may be necessary when switching dosage forms.

Status epilepticus: I.V.: Loading dose: Manufacturer recommends 10-15 mg/kg, however, 15-20 mg/kg is generally recommended; maximum rate: 50 mg/minute; initial maintenance dose: I.V. or Oral: 100 mg every 6-8 hours

Anticonvulsant: Oral: Loading dose: 15-20 mg/kg; consider prior phenytoin serum concentrations and/or recent dosing history if available; administer oral loading dose in 3 divided doses given every 2-4 hours to decrease GI adverse effects and to ensure complete oral absorption; initial maintenance dose: 300 mg/day in 3 divided doses; may also administer in 1-2 divided doses using extended release formulation; adjust dosage based on individual requirements; usual maintenance dose range: 300-600 mg/day

Dosage adjustment in obesity: Loading dose: Use adjusted body weight (ABW) correction based on a pharmacokinetic study of phenytoin loading doses in obese patients (Abernethy, 1985). The larger correction factor (ie, 1.33) is due to a doubling of V_d estimated in these obese patients.

ABW = [(Actual body weight – IBW) x 1.33] + IBW

Maximum loading dose: I.V.: 2000 mg (Erstad, 2004)

Maintenance doses should be based on ideal body weight, conventional daily doses with adjustments based upon therapeutic drug monitoring and clinical effectiveness. (Abernethy, 1985; Erstad, 2002; Erstad, 2004)

Neurosurgery (prophylactic): I.V.: 100-200 mg at ~4-hour intervals during surgery and the immediate postoperative period. **Note:** While the manufacturer recommends I.M. administration, this route should be **avoided** due to severe risk of local tissue destruction and necrosis; use **fos**phenytoin if I.M. administration necessary (Boucher, 1996; Meek, 1999).

Renal Impairment Phenytoin level in serum may be difficult to interpret in renal failure. Monitoring of free (unbound) concentrations or adjustment to allow interpretation is recommended.

Hepatic Impairment Safe in usual doses in mild liver disease; clearance may be substantially reduced in cirrhosis and plasma level monitoring with dose adjustment advisable. Free phenytoin levels should be monitored closely.

Administration

Oral: Suspension: Shake well prior to use. Absorption is impaired when phenytoin suspension is given concurrently to patients who are receiving continuous nasogastric feedings. A method to resolve this interaction is to divide the daily dose of phenytoin and withhold the administration of nutritional supplements for 1-2 hours before and after each phenytoin dose.

I.M.: **Avoid** this route (manufacturer recommends I.M. administration) due to severe risk of local tissue destruction and necrosis; use **fos**phenytoin if I.M. administration necessary (Boucher, 1996; Meek, 1999).

I.V.: Vesicant. Fosphenytoin may be considered for loading in patients who are in status epilepticus, hemodynamically unstable, or develop hypotension/bradycardia with I.V. administration of phenytoin. Phenytoin may be administered by IVP or IVPB administration. The maximum rate of I.V. administration is 50 mg/minute in adults. In neonates, the manufacturer recommends a maximum rate of 1-3 mg/kg/minute; however, a lower maximum rate of 0.5-1 mg/kg/minute is used clinically (Sankar, 2010; Shields, 1989). Highly sensitive patients (eg, elderly, patients with pre-existing cardiovascular conditions) should receive phenytoin more slowly (eg, 20 mg/minute). An in-line 0.22-5 micron filter is recommended for IVPB solutions due to the high potential for precipitation of the solution. Avoid extravasation. Following I.V. administration, NS should be injected through the same needle or I.V. catheter to prevent irritation.

pH: 10.0-12.3

SubQ: SubQ administration is not recommended because of the possibility of local tissue damage (due to high pH).

Monitoring Parameters Blood pressure, vital signs (with I.V. use); plasma phenytoin level, CBC, liver function. **Note:** If available, free phenytoin concentrations should be obtained in patients with renal impairment and/or hypoalbuminemia. If free phenytoin levels are unavailable, the adjusted total level is based upon equations in adult patients. Monitor for suicidality (eg, suicidal thoughts, depression, behavioral changes).

Reference Range Timing of serum samples: Because it is slowly absorbed, peak blood levels may occur 4-8 hours after ingestion of an oral dose. The serum half-life varies with the dosage and the drug follows Michaelis-Menten kinetics. The average adult half-life is about 24 hours. Steady-state concentrations are reached in 5-10 days.

Adults: Toxicity is measured clinically, and some patients require levels outside the suggested therapeutic range

Therapeutic range:

Total phenytoin: 10-20 mcg/mL

Concentrations of 5-10 mcg/mL may be therapeutic for some patients but concentrations <5 mcg/mL are not likely to be effective

50% of patients show decreased frequency of seizures at concentrations >10 mcg/mL

86% of patients show decreased frequency of seizures at concentrations >15 mcg/mL

Add another anticonvulsant if satisfactory therapeutic response is not achieved with a phenytoin concentration of 20 mcg/mL

Free phenytoin: 1-2.5 mcg/mL

Toxic: >30 mcg/mL (SI: <120-200 μmol/L)

Lethal: >100 mcg/mL (SI: >400 μmol/L)

When to draw levels: This is dependent on the disease state being treated and the clinical condition of the patient

Key points:

Slow absorption of extended capsules and prolonged half-life minimize fluctuations between peak and trough concentrations, timing of sampling not crucial

Trough concentrations are generally recommended for routine monitoring. Daily levels are not necessary and may result in incorrect dosage adjustments. If it is determined essential to monitor free phenytoin concentrations, concomitant monitoring of total phenytoin concentrations is not necessary and expensive.

After a loading dose: Draw level within 48-96 hours

Rapid achievement: Draw within 2-3 days of therapy initiation to ensure that the patient's metabolism is not remarkably different from that which would be predicted by average literature-derived pharmacokinetic parameters; early levels should be used cautiously in design of new dosing regimens

Second concentration: Draw within 6-7 days with subsequent doses of phenytoin adjusted accordingly

If plasma concentrations have not changed over a 3- to 5-day period, monitoring interval may be increased to once weekly in the acute clinical setting

In stable patients requiring long-term therapy, generally monitor levels at 3- to 12-month intervals

Adjustment of serum concentration: See tables.

Adjustment of Serum Concentration in Patients With Low Serum Albumin

Measured Total Phenytoin Concentration (mcg/mL)	Patient's Serum Albumin (g/dL)			
	3.5	3	2.5	2
	Adjusted Total Phenytoin Concentration (mcg/mL)[1]			
5	6	7	8	10
10	13	14	17	20
15	19	21	25	30

[1]Adjusted concentration = measured total concentration divided by [(0.2 x albumin) + 0.1].

Adjustment of Serum Concentration in Patients With Renal Failure (Cl$_{cr}$ ≤10 mL/min)

Measured Total Phenytoin Concentration (mcg/mL)	Patient's Serum Albumin (g/dL)				
	4	3.5	3	2.5	2
	Adjusted Total Phenytoin Concentration (mcg/mL)[1]				
5	10	11	13	14	17
10	20	22	25	29	33
15	30	33	38	43	50

[1]Adjusted concentration = measured total concentration divided by [(0.1 x albumin) + 0.1].

Special Geriatric Considerations Elderly may have reduced hepatic clearance due to age decline in phase I metabolism. Elderly may have low albumin which will increase free fraction and, therefore, pharmacologic response. Monitor closely in those who are hypoalbuminemic. Free fraction measurements advised, also elderly may display a higher incidence of adverse effects (cardiovascular) when using the I.V. loading regimen; therefore, recommended to decrease loading I.V. dose to 25 mg/minute.

Dosage Forms Excipient information presented when available (limited, particularly for generics); consult specific product labeling.

Capsule, extended release, oral, as sodium: 100 mg, 200 mg, 300 mg

Dilantin®: 30 mg, 100 mg

Phenytek®: 200 mg, 300 mg

Injection, solution, as sodium: 50 mg/mL (2 mL, 5 mL)

Suspension, oral: 100 mg/4 mL (4 mL); 125 mg/5 mL (120 mL, 237 mL, 240 mL)

Dilantin-125®: 125 mg/5 mL (240 mL) [contains ethanol ≤0.6%, sodium benzoate; orange-vanilla flavor]

Tablet, chewable, oral:

Dilantin®: 50 mg [scored]

Selected References

Kälviäinen R, "Status Epilepticus Treatment Guidelines," *Epilepsia*, 2007, 48(Suppl 8):99-102.

Lowenstein DH, "Treatment Options for Status Epilepticus," *Curr Opin Pharmacol*, 2005, 5(3):334-9.

◆ **Phenytoin Sodium** *see* Phenytoin *on page 1444*

◆ **Phenytoin Sodium, Extended** *see* Phenytoin *on page 1444*

◆ **Phenytoin Sodium, Prompt** *see* Phenytoin *on page 1444*

◆ **Phillips'® M-O [OTC]** *see* Magnesium Hydroxide and Mineral Oil *on page 1110*

◆ **Phillips'® Laxative Dietary Supplement Cramp-Free [OTC]** *see* Magnesium Oxide *on page 1112*

◆ **Phillips'® Liquid-Gels® [OTC]** *see* Docusate *on page 547*

◆ **Phillips'® Milk of Magnesia [OTC]** *see* Magnesium Hydroxide *on page 1109*

◆ **Phillips'® Stool Softener Laxative [OTC]** *see* Docusate *on page 547*

◆ **Phos-Flur® [OTC]** *see* Fluoride *on page 751*

◆ **Phos-Flur® Rinse [OTC]** *see* Fluoride *on page 751*

◆ **PhosLo®** *see* Calcium Acetate *on page 247*

◆ **Phoslyra™** *see* Calcium Acetate *on page 247*

◆ **Phos-NaK** *see* Potassium Phosphate and Sodium Phosphate *on page 1494*

◆ **Phospha 250™ Neutral** *see* Potassium Phosphate and Sodium Phosphate *on page 1494*

◆ **Phosphate, Potassium** *see* Potassium Phosphate *on page 1492*

◆ **Phosphates, Sodium** *see* Sodium Phosphates *on page 1694*

◆ **Phospholine Iodide®** *see* Echothiophate Iodide *on page 589*

◆ *p*-Hydroxyampicillin *see* Amoxicillin *on page 114*

◆ **Phylloquinone** *see* Phytonadione *on page 1450*

Physostigmine (fye zoe STIG meen)

Related Information

Glaucoma Drug Therapy *on page 2008*

Medication Safety Issues

Sound-alike/look-alike issues:

Physostigmine may be confused with Prostigmin®, pyridostigmine

Index Terms Eserine Salicylate; Physostigmine Salicylate; Physostigmine Sulfate

Generic Availability (U.S.) Yes

Pharmacologic Category Acetylcholinesterase Inhibitor

Use Reverse toxic, life-threatening delirium caused by atropine, diphenhydramine, dimenhydrinate, *Atropa belladonna* (deadly nightshade), or jimson weed (*Datura* spp)

Contraindications Hypersensitivity to physostigmine or any component of the formulation; GI or GU obstruction; asthma; gangrene; diabetes, cardiovascular disease; any vagotonic state; coadministration of choline esters and depolarizing neuromuscular-blocking agents

Warnings/Precautions Hazardous agent - use appropriate precautions for handling and disposal. Patient must have a normal QRS interval, as measured by ECG, in order to receive; use caution in poisoning with agents known to prolong intraventricular conduction. Concomitant administration of choline esters or depolarizing neuromuscular-blocking agents (ie, succinylcholine) are contraindicated. Use with caution in patients with epilepsy, asthma, diabetes, gangrene, cardiovascular disease, bradycardia. Discontinue if excessive salivation or emesis, frequent urination or diarrhea occur. Reduce dosage if excessive sweating or nausea occurs. Administer slowly over 5 minutes to prevent respiratory distress and seizures. Continuous infusions should never be used. Due to the possibility of hypersensitivity or overdose/cholinergic crisis, atropine should be readily available; not intended as a first-line agent for anticholinergic toxicity or Parkinson's disease. Asystole and seizures have been reported when physostigmine was administered to TCA poisoned patients. Physostigmine is not recommended in patients with known or suspected TCA intoxication. Products may contain benzyl alcohol. Products may contain sodium bisulfate.

◀ **Adverse Reactions (Reflective of adult population; not specific for elderly)** Frequency not defined.
Cardiovascular: Asystole, bradycardia, palpitation
Central nervous system: Hallucinations, nervousness, restlessness, seizure
Gastrointestinal: Diarrhea, nausea, salivation, stomach pain
Genitourinary: Urinary frequency
Neuromuscular & skeletal: Twitching
Ocular: Lacrimation, miosis
Respiratory: Bronchospasm, dyspnea, pulmonary edema, respiratory paralysis
Miscellaneous: Diaphoresis

Drug Interactions

Avoid Concomitant Use There are no known interactions where it is recommended to avoid concomitant use.

Increased Effect/Toxicity
Physostigmine may increase the levels/effects of: Beta-Blockers; Cholinergic Agonists; Succinylcholine

The levels/effects of Physostigmine may be increased by: Corticosteroids (Systemic)

Decreased Effect
Physostigmine may decrease the levels/effects of: Neuromuscular-Blocking Agents (Non-depolarizing)

Ethanol/Nutrition/Herb Interactions Herb/Nutraceutical: Ginkgo biloba may enhance the adverse/toxic effect of physostigmine; monitor.

Stability Do not use solution if cloudy or dark brown.

Mechanism of Action Inhibits destruction of acetylcholine by acetylcholinesterase which facilitates transmission of impulses across myoneural junction and prolongs the central and peripheral effects of acetylcholine

Pharmacodynamics/Kinetics
Onset of action: ~5 minutes
Duration: 1-2 hours
Absorption: I.M.: Readily absorbed
Distribution: Crosses blood-brain barrier readily and reverses both central and peripheral anticholinergic effects
Metabolism: Hepatic and via hydrolysis by cholinesterases
Half-life elimination: 15-40 minutes

Dosage

Geriatric & Adult Reversal of toxic anticholinergic effects: Note: Administer slowly over 5 minutes to prevent respiratory distress and seizures. Continuous infusions of physostigmine should never be used.
I.M., I.V.: 0.5-2 mg to start; repeat every 20 minutes until response occurs or adverse effect occurs; repeat 1-4 mg every 30-60 minutes as life-threatening symptoms recur

Administration Injection: Infuse slowly I.V. over 5 minutes. Too rapid administration can cause bradycardia and hypersalivation leading to respiratory distress and seizures.

Monitoring Parameters ECG, vital signs

Test Interactions Increased aminotransferase [ALT/AST] (S), increased amylase (S)

Special Geriatric Considerations See Warnings/Precautions.

Dosage Forms Excipient information presented when available (limited, particularly for generics); consult specific product labeling.
Injection, solution, as salicylate: 1 mg/mL (2 mL)

Selected References
Jenike MA, Albert MS, Heller H, et al, "Oral Physostigmine Treatment for Patients With Presenile and Senile Dementia of the Alzheimer's Type: A Double-Blind Placebo-Controlled Trial," *J Clin Psychiatry*, 1990, 51(1):3-7.

◆ **Physostigmine Salicylate** *see Physostigmine on page 1449*
◆ **Physostigmine Sulfate** *see Physostigmine on page 1449*
◆ **Phytomenadione** *see Phytonadione on page 1450*

Phytonadione (fye toe na DYE one)

Medication Safety Issues
Sound-alike/look-alike issues:
Mephyton® may be confused with melphalan, methadone
Brand Names: U.S. Mephyton®
Brand Names: Canada AquaMEPHYTON®; Konakion; Mephyton®
Index Terms Methylphytyl Napthoquinone; Phylloquinone; Phytomenadione; Vitamin K_1
Generic Availability (U.S.) Yes
Pharmacologic Category Vitamin, Fat Soluble

Use Prevention and treatment of hypoprothrombinemia caused by coumarin derivative-induced or other drug-induced vitamin K deficiency, hypoprothrombinemia caused by malabsorption or inability to synthesize vitamin K

Unlabeled/Investigational Use Treatment of hypoprothrombinemia caused by anticoagulant rodenticides

Contraindications Hypersensitivity to phytonadione or any component of the formulation

Warnings/Precautions [U.S. Boxed Warning]: Severe reactions resembling hypersensitivity (eg, anaphylaxis) reactions have occurred rarely during or immediately after I.V. administration. Allergic reactions have also occurred with I.M. and SubQ injections; oral administration is the safest. In obstructive jaundice or with biliary fistulas concurrent administration of bile salts is necessary. Manufacturers recommend the SubQ route over other parenteral routes. SubQ is less predictable when compared to the oral route. The American College of Chest Physicians recommends the I.V. route in patients with serious or life-threatening bleeding secondary to warfarin. The I.V. route should be restricted to emergency situations where oral phytonadione cannot be used. Efficacy is delayed regardless of route of administration; patient management may require other treatments in the interim. Administer a dose that will quickly lower the INR into a safe range without causing resistance to warfarin. High phytonadione doses may lead to warfarin resistance for at least one week. In liver disease, if initial doses do not reverse coagulopathy then higher doses are unlikely to have any effect. Ineffective in hereditary hypoprothrombinemia. Use caution with renal dysfunction. Injectable products may contain aluminum; may result in toxic levels following prolonged administration. Product may contain polysorbate 80.

Adverse Reactions (Reflective of adult population; not specific for elderly) Parenteral administration: Frequency not defined.
Cardiovascular: Cyanosis, flushing, hypotension
Central nervous system: Dizziness
Dermatologic: Scleroderma-like lesions
Endocrine & metabolic: Hyperbilirubinemia (newborn; greater than recommended doses)
Gastrointestinal: Abnormal taste
Local: Injection site reactions
Respiratory: Dyspnea
Miscellaneous: Anaphylactoid reactions, diaphoresis, hypersensitivity reactions

Drug Interactions

Avoid Concomitant Use There are no known interactions where it is recommended to avoid concomitant use.

Increased Effect/Toxicity There are no known significant interactions involving an increase in effect.

Decreased Effect
Phytonadione may decrease the levels/effects of: Vitamin K Antagonists

The levels/effects of Phytonadione may be decreased by: Mineral Oil; Orlistat

Stability
Injection: Store at 15°C to 30°C (59°F to 86°F). Dilute in preservative-free NS, D_5W, or D_5NS.
Note: Store Hospira product at 20°C to 25°C (68°F to 77°F).
Oral: Store tablets at 15°C to 30°C (59°F to 86°F). Protect from light.

Mechanism of Action Promotes liver synthesis of clotting factors (II, VII, IX, X); however, the exact mechanism as to this stimulation is unknown. Menadiol is a water soluble form of vitamin K; phytonadione has a more rapid and prolonged effect than menadione; menadiol sodium diphosphate (K_4) is half as potent as menadione (K_3).

Pharmacodynamics/Kinetics
Onset of action: Increased coagulation factors: Oral: 6-10 hours; I.V.: 1-2 hours
Peak effect: INR values return to normal: Oral: 24-48 hours; I.V.: 12-14 hours
Absorption: Oral: From intestines in presence of bile; SubQ: Variable
Metabolism: Rapidly hepatic
Excretion: Urine and feces

Dosage
Geriatric & Adult Note: According to the manufacturer, SubQ is the preferred parenteral route; I.M. route should be avoided due to the risk of hematoma formation; I.V. route should be restricted to emergency use only. The American College of Chest Physicians recommends the I.V. route in patients with serious or life-threatening bleeding secondary to use of vitamin K antagonists.
Adequate intake: Males: 120 mcg/day; Females: 90 mcg/day
Hypoprothrombinemia due to drugs (other than coumarin derivatives) or factors limiting absorption or synthesis: Oral, SubQ, I.M., I.V.: Initial: 2.5-25 mg (rarely up to 50 mg)

◄ **Vitamin K deficiency (supratherapeutic INR) secondary to coumarin derivative** (Ansell, 2008):

If INR above therapeutic range to <5 (no significant bleeding and rapid reversal unnecessary): Lower or hold next dose and monitor frequently; when INR approaches desired range, resume dosing with a lower dose.

If INR ≥5 and <9 (no significant bleeding): If no risk factors for bleeding exist, omit next 1 or 2 doses, monitor INR more frequently, and resume with an appropriately adjusted dose when INR in desired range.

Alternatively, if other risk factors for bleeding exist, omit next dose and administer vitamin K orally 1-2.5 mg; resume with an appropriately adjusted dose when INR in desired range.

If INR ≥5 and <9 (no significant bleeding and rapid reversal required for surgery): Administer vitamin K orally ≤5 mg and hold warfarin. Expect INR to be reduced within 24 hours; if INR still elevated, another 1-2 mg of vitamin K orally may be given.

If INR ≥9 (no significant bleeding): Hold warfarin, administer vitamin K orally 2.5-5 mg, expect INR to be reduced within 24-48 hours, monitor INR more frequently and give additional vitamin K at an appropriate dose if necessary. Resume warfarin at an appropriately adjusted dose when INR is in desired range.

If serious bleeding at any INR elevation: Hold warfarin, administer vitamin K 10 mg by slow I.V. infusion and supplement with FFP, PCC, or rFVIIa depending on the urgency of the situation; I.V. vitamin K may be repeated every 12 hours.

If life-threatening bleeding: Hold warfarin, give FFP, PCC, or rFVIIa supplemented with vitamin K 10 mg slow I.V. infusion; repeat if necessary, depending on INR.

Notes:

If mild-moderate INR elevation without major bleeding occurs, administer vitamin K orally instead of subcutaneously.

Use of high doses of vitamin K (eg, 10-15 mg) may cause warfarin resistance for ≥1 week. During this period of resistance, heparin or low molecular weight heparin may be given until INR responds.

FFP=fresh frozen plasma; PCC=prothrombin complex concentrate; rFVIIa=recombinant factor VIIa

Administration I.V. administration: Infuse slowly; rate of infusion should not exceed 1 mg/minute. The injectable route should be used only if the oral route is not feasible or there is a greater urgency to reverse anticoagulation.

Monitoring Parameters PT, INR

Dosage Forms Excipient information presented when available (limited, particularly for generics); consult specific product labeling.

Injection, aqueous colloidal: 1 mg/0.5 mL (0.5 mL) [contains benzyl alcohol]; 10 mg/mL (1 mL) [contains benzyl alcohol]

Injection, aqueous colloidal [preservative free]: 1 mg/0.5 mL (0.5 mL) [contains polysorbate 80, propylene glycol 10.4 mg/0.5 mL]

Tablet, oral: 100 mcg

Mephyton®: 5 mg [scored]

Selected References

Ansell J, Hirsh J, Poller L, et al, "The Pharmacology and Management of the Vitamin K Antagonists: The Seventh ACCP Conference on Antithrombotic and Thrombolytic Therapy," *Chest,* 2004, 126(3 Suppl):204-33.

Crowther MA, Douketis JD, Schnurr T, et al, "Oral Vitamin K Lowers the International Normalized Ratio More Rapidly Than Subcutaneous Vitamin K in the Treatment of Warfarin-Associated Coagulopathy. A Randomized, Controlled Trial," *Ann Intern Med,* 2002, 137(4):251-4.

"Dietary Reference Intakes for Vitamin A, Vitamin K, Arsenic, Boron, Chromium, Copper, Iodine, Iron, Manganese, Molybdenum, Nickel, Silicon, Vanadium, and Zinc," Food and Nutrition Board, Institute of Medicine. National Academy of Sciences, Washington, DC: National Academy Press, 2001, 162-84.

Fiore LD, Scola MA, Cantillon CE, et al, "Anaphylactoid Reactions to Vitamin K," *J Thromb Thrombolysis,* 2001, 11 (2):175-83.

Pilocarpine (Ophthalmic) (pye loe KAR peen)

Related Information

Glaucoma Drug Therapy *on page 2008*

Medication Safety Issues

Sound-alike/look-alike issues:

Isopto® Carpine may be confused with Isopto® Carbachol

Brand Names: U.S. Isopto® Carpine; Pilopine HS®

Brand Names: Canada Diocarpine; Isopto® Carpine; Pilopine HS®

Index Terms Pilocarpine Hydrochloride

Generic Availability (U.S.) Yes: Excludes gel

Pharmacologic Category Ophthalmic Agent, Antiglaucoma; Ophthalmic Agent, Miotic

Use Management of chronic simple glaucoma, chronic and acute angle-closure glaucoma

Unlabeled/Investigational Use Counter effects of cycloplegics

Dosage

Geriatric & Adult

Glaucoma: Ophthalmic:

Solution: Instill 1-2 drops up to 6 times/day; adjust the concentration and frequency as required to control elevated intraocular pressure.

Gel: Instill 0.5" ribbon into lower conjunctival sac once daily at bedtime.

To counteract the mydriatic effects of sympathomimetic agents (unlabeled use): Ophthalmic: *Solution:* Instill 1 drop of a 1% solution in the affected eye.

Special Geriatric Considerations Evaluate the patient's or caregiver's ability to safely administer the correct dose of ophthalmic medication.

Dosage Forms Excipient information presented when available (limited, particularly for generics); consult specific product labeling.

Gel, ophthalmic, as hydrochloride:

Pilopine HS®: 4% (4 g) [contains benzalkonium chloride]

Solution, ophthalmic, as hydrochloride [drops]: 1% (15 mL); 2% (15 mL); 4% (15 mL)

Isopto® Carpine: 1% (15 mL); 2% (15 mL); 4% (15 mL) [contains benzalkonium chloride]

- ◆ **Pilocarpine Hydrochloride** see Pilocarpine (Ophthalmic) *on page 1452*
- ◆ **Pilopine HS®** see Pilocarpine (Ophthalmic) *on page 1452*
- ◆ **Pimaricin** see Natamycin *on page 1270*

Pimozide (PI moe zide)

Related Information

Antipsychotic Agents *on page 1997*

Brand Names: U.S. Orap®

Brand Names: Canada Apo-Pimozide®; Orap®; PMS-Pimozide

Generic Availability (U.S.) No

Pharmacologic Category Antipsychotic Agent, Typical

Use Suppression of severe motor and phonic tics in patients with Tourette's disorder who have failed to respond satisfactorily to standard treatment

Unlabeled/Investigational Use Psychosis; reported use in individuals with delusions focused on physical symptoms (ie, preoccupation with parasitic infestation); Huntington's chorea

Contraindications Hypersensitivity to pimozide or any component of the formulation; severe toxic CNS depression; coma; history of cardiac arrhythmias; congenital long QT syndrome; concurrent use with QT_c-prolonging agents; hypokalemia or hypomagnesemia; concurrent use of drugs that are inhibitors of CYP3A4, including concurrent use of the azole antifungals itraconazole and ketoconazole, macrolide antibiotics (eg, clarithromycin or erythromycin [Note: The manufacturer lists azithromycin and dirithromycin in its list of contraindicated macrolides; however, these drugs do not inhibit CYP3A4 and are not expected to interact with pimozide]), protease inhibitors (ie, atazanavir, indinavir, nelfinavir, ritonavir, saquinavir), citalopram, escitalopram, nefazodone, sertraline, and other less potent inhibitors of CYP3A4 (eg, fluvoxamine, zileuton); concurrent use with medications that may cause motor or phonic tics (eg, amphetamines, methylphenidate, pemoline) until it is determined if medications or Tourette's is causing tics; simple tics or tics other than Tourette's

Warnings/Precautions [U.S. Boxed Warning]: Elderly patients with dementia-related psychosis treated with antipsychotics are at an increased risk of death compared to placebo. Most deaths appeared to be either cardiovascular (eg, heart failure, sudden death) or infectious (eg, pneumonia) in nature. Pimozide is not approved for the treatment of dementia-related psychosis.

May alter cardiac conduction; life-threatening arrhythmias have occurred with therapeutic doses of antipsychotics. Contraindicated in patients with underlying QT prolongation, in those taking medicines that prolong the QT interval, or cause polymorphic ventricular tachycardia; monitor ECG closely for dose-related QT effects. Sudden unexplained deaths have occurred in patients taking high doses (>10 mg).

Leukopenia, neutropenia, and agranulocytosis (sometimes fatal) have been reported in clinical trials and postmarketing reports with antipsychotic use; presence of risk factors (eg, pre-existing low WBC or history of drug-induced leuko-/neutropenia) should prompt periodic blood count assessment. Discontinue therapy at first signs of blood dyscrasias or if absolute neutrophil count <1000/mm^3

Antipsychotic use has been associated with esophageal dysmotility and aspiration; use with caution in patients at risk of pneumonia (ie, Alzheimer's disease). May cause extrapyramidal symptoms (EPS), including pseudoparkinsonism, acute dystonic reactions, akathisia, and

◀ tardive dyskinesia. Risk of dystonia (and possibly other EPS) may be greater with increased doses, use of conventional antipsychotics, males, and younger patients. The risk for tardive dyskinesia (may be irreversible) increases with long-term treatment and higher cumulative doses. Use may be associated with NMS; monitor for mental status changes, fever, muscle rigidity, and/or autonomic instability; may also be associated with increased CPK, myoglobiuria, and acute renal failure. Discontinue use; may recur upon rechallenge. May cause orthostatic hypotension; use with caution in patients at risk of this effect or in those who would not tolerate transient hypotensive episodes (cerebrovascular disease, cardiovascular disease, hypovolemia, or concurrent medication use which may predispose to hypotension/bradycardia). May be associated with pigmentary retinopathy. Impaired core body temperature regulation may occur; caution with strenuous exercise, heat exposure, dehydration, and concomitant medication possessing anticholinergic effects.

May be sedating, use with caution in disorders where CNS depression is a feature; patients must be cautioned about performing tasks which require mental alertness (eg, operating machinery or driving). Effects may be potentiated when used with other sedative drugs or ethanol. May cause anticholinergic effects (constipation, xerostomia, blurred vision, urinary retention); use with caution in patients with decreased gastrointestinal motility, paralytic ileus, urinary retention, BPH, xerostomia, or visual problems. Relative to neuroleptics, pimozide has a moderate potency of cholinergic blockade. May mask toxicity of other drugs or conditions (eg, intestinal obstruction, Reye's syndrome, brain tumor) due to antiemetic effects. Antipsychotics are associated with increased prolactin levels; clinical significance of hyperprolactinemia in patients with breast cancer or other prolactin-dependent tumors is unknown.

Use with caution in patients with severe cardiovascular disease, narrow-angle glaucoma, hepatic impairment, myasthenia gravis, Parkinson's disease, renal impairment, or seizure disorder. Use with caution in the elderly.

Adverse Reactions (Reflective of adult population; not specific for elderly)

Frequencies >1% reported in adults (limited data) with Tourette's disorder:

Cardiovascular: Abnormal ECG (3%)

Central nervous system: Somnolence, sedation (14%), akathisia (8%), drowsiness (7%), hyperkinesias (6%), insomnia (2%), depression (2%), headache (1%), nervousness (1% to 8%)

Dermatologic: Rash (8%)

Gastrointestinal: Xerostomia (25%), constipation (20%), increased salivation (14%), diarrhea (5%), thirst (5%), appetite increased (5%), taste disturbance (5%), dysphagia (3%)

Genitourinary: Impotence (15%)

Neuromuscular & skeletal: Weakness (22%), muscle tightness (15%), rigidity (10%), myalgia (3%), torticollis (3%), tremor (1%)

Ocular: Visual disturbance (6% to 20%), accommodation decreased (20%)

Miscellaneous: Speech disorder (10%)

Frequency not established (reported in disorders other than Tourette's disorder): Blood dyscrasias, breast edema, chest pain, dizziness, extrapyramidal symptoms (akathisia, akinesia, dystonia, pseudoparkinsonism, tardive dyskinesia); facial edema, gingival hyperplasia (case report), hyper-/hypotension, hyponatremia, jaundice, libido decreased, neuroleptic malignant syndrome, orthostatic hypotension, palpitation, periorbital edema, postural hypotension, QT_c prolongation, seizure, tachycardia, ventricular arrhythmia, vomiting, weight gain/loss

Drug Interactions

Metabolism/Transport Effects Substrate (major) of CYP1A2, 3A4; **Inhibits** CYP2C19 (weak), 2D6 (weak), 2E1 (weak), 3A4 (weak)

Avoid Concomitant Use

Avoid concomitant use of Pimozide with any of the following: Antifungal Agents (Azole Derivatives, Systemic); Aprepitant; Artemether; Boceprevir; Conivaptan; Crizotinib; Dronedarone; Efavirenz; Fosaprepitant; Lumefantrine; Macrolide Antibiotics; Metoclopramide; Nefazodone; Nilotinib; Protease Inhibitors; QTc-Prolonging Agents; QUEtiapine; QuiNINE; Selective Serotonin Reuptake Inhibitors; Telaprevir; Tetrabenazine; Thioridazine; Toremifene; Vandetanib; Vemurafenib; Ziprasidone

Increased Effect/Toxicity

Pimozide may increase the levels/effects of: Alcohol (Ethyl); Anticholinergics; Anti-Parkinson's Agents (Dopamine Agonist); CNS Depressants; Dronedarone; Methylphenidate; QTc-Prolonging Agents; QuiNINE; Tetrabenazine; Thioridazine; Toremifene; Vandetanib; Vemurafenib; Ziprasidone

The levels/effects of Pimozide may be increased by: Abiraterone Acetate; Acetylcholinesterase Inhibitors (Central); Alfuzosin; Antifungal Agents (Azole Derivatives, Systemic); Aprepitant; Artemether; Boceprevir; Chloroquine; Ciprofloxacin; Ciprofloxacin (Systemic); Conivaptan; Crizotinib; CYP1A2 Inhibitors (Moderate); CYP1A2 Inhibitors (Strong); CYP3A4 Inhibitors (Moderate); CYP3A4 Inhibitors (Strong); Deferasirox; Efavirenz; Fosaprepitant;

Gadobutrol; HydrOXYzine; Lithium formulations; Lumefantrine; Macrolide Antibiotics; Methylphenidate; Metoclopramide; Nefazodone; Nilotinib; Pramlintide; Protease Inhibitors; QTc-Prolonging Agents; QUEtiapine; QuiNINE; Selective Serotonin Reuptake Inhibitors; Telaprevir; Tetrabenazine

Decreased Effect

Pimozide may decrease the levels/effects of: Amphetamines; Quinagolide

The levels/effects of Pimozide may be decreased by: Anti-Parkinson's Agents (Dopamine Agonist); CYP1A2 Inducers (Strong); CYP3A4 Inducers (Strong); Cyproterone; Deferasirox; Herbs (CYP3A4 Inducers); Lithium formulations; Tocilizumab

Ethanol/Nutrition/Herb Interactions

Ethanol: May increase CNS depression; monitor for increased effects with coadministration. Caution patients about effects.

Food: Pimozide serum concentration may be increased when taken with grapefruit juice; avoid concurrent use.

Herb/Nutraceutical: St John's wort may decrease pimozide levels. Avoid kava kava, gotu kola, valerian, St John's wort (may increase CNS depression).

Stability Store at 25°C (77°F); excursion permitted to 15°C to 30°C (59°F to 86°F).

Mechanism of Action Pimozide, a diphenylbutylperidine conventional antipsychotic, is a potent centrally-acting dopamine-receptor antagonist resulting in its characteristic neuroleptic effects

Pharmacodynamics/Kinetics

Absorption: ≥50%

Protein binding: 99%

Metabolism: Hepatic via N-dealkylation; significant first-pass effect

Half-life elimination: ~55 hours

Time to peak, serum: 6-8 hours (range: 4-12 hours)

Excretion: Urine

Dosage

Geriatric Recommend initial dose of 1 mg/day; periodically attempt gradual reduction of dose to determine if tic persists; follow up for 1-2 weeks before concluding the tic is a persistent disease phenomenon and not a manifestation of drug withdrawal. **Note:** An ECG should be performed baseline and periodically thereafter, especially during dosage adjustment.

Adult

Tourette's disorder: Oral: Initial: 1-2 mg/day, then increase dosage as needed every other day; range is usually 7-10 mg/day; maximum: 10 mg/day or 0.2 mg/kg/day (whichever is less)

Note: An ECG should be performed baseline and periodically thereafter, especially during dosage adjustment.

Monitoring Parameters ECG should be performed baseline and periodically thereafter, especially during dosage adjustment; vital signs; electrolytes, lipid profile, fasting blood glucose/Hgb A_{1c}; BMI; mental status, abnormal involuntary movement scale (AIMS), extrapyramidal symptoms (EPS)

Pharmacotherapy Pearls Causes less sedation, but is more likely to cause acute extrapyramidal symptoms than chlorpromazine.

Special Geriatric Considerations No specific clinical studies in the use of this drug in elderly; use with extreme caution in elderly due to cardiovascular effects. Consider cardiovascular effects of drugs an elderly patient may be receiving.

In the treatment of agitated, demented, older adult patients, authors of meta-analysis of controlled trials of the response to the traditional antipsychotics (phenothiazines, butyrophenones) in controlling agitation have concluded that the use of neuroleptics results in a response rate of 18%. Clearly neuroleptic therapy for behavior control should be limited with frequent attempts to withdraw the agent given for behavior control.

Dosage Forms Excipient information presented when available (limited, particularly for generics); consult specific product labeling.

Tablet, oral:

Orap®: 1 mg, 2 mg [scored]

Selected References

Rabins PV, Blacker D, Rovner BW, et al, "Practice Guidelines for the Treatment of Patients With Alzheimer's Disease and Other Dementias," *Am J Psychiatry*, 2007, 164(12 Suppl):5-56. Available at http://www.psych.org/psych_pract/treatg/pg/prac_guide.cfm.

Schneider LS, Tariot PN, Dagerman KS, et al, "Effectiveness of Atypical Antipsychotic Drugs in Patients With Alzheimer's Disease," *N Engl J Med*, 2006, 355(15):1525-38.

Pindolol (PIN doe lole)

Related Information
Beta-Blockers *on page 2001*
Medication Safety Issues
Sound-alike/look-alike issues:
Pindolol may be confused with Parlodel®, Plendil®
Visken® may be confused with Visine®, Viskazide®
Brand Names: Canada Apo-Pindol®; Dom-Pindolol; Mylan-Pindolol; Novo-Pindol; Nu-Pindol; PMS-Pindolol; Sandoz-Pindolol; Visken®
Generic Availability (U.S.) Yes
Pharmacologic Category Beta Blocker With Intrinsic Sympathomimetic Activity
Use Treatment of hypertension, alone or in combination with other agents
Unlabeled/Investigational Use Potential augmenting agent for antidepressants; treatment of ventricular arrhythmias/tachycardia, antipsychotic-induced akathisia, situational anxiety, aggressive behavior associated with dementia
Contraindications Bronchial asthma; cardiogenic shock; heart block (2nd or 3rd degree) except in patients with a functioning artificial pacemaker; overt cardiac failure; severe bradycardia
Warnings/Precautions Consider pre-existing conditions such as sick sinus syndrome before initiating. Use with caution in patients with inadequate myocardial function, bronchospastic disease, myasthenia gravis, peripheral vascular disease, renal impairment, psychiatric disease (may cause CNS depression) or impaired hepatic function. Use with caution in patients with diabetes mellitus; may potentiate hypoglycemia and/or mask signs and symptoms. May mask signs of hyperthyroidism (eg, tachycardia); if hyperthyroidism is suspected, carefully manage and monitor; abrupt withdrawal may exacerbate symptoms of hyperthyroidism or precipitate thyroid storm. Bradycardia may be observed more frequently in elderly patients (>65 years of age); dosage reductions may be necessary. Beta-blockers with intrinsic sympathomimetic activity (including pindolol) do not appear to be of benefit in HF. If use is warranted with compensated HF, use with caution and monitor for a worsening of the condition. If condition worsens, consider temporary discontinuation or dosage reduction of pindolol. Beta-blocker therapy should not be withdrawn abruptly (particularly in patients with CAD), but gradually tapered to avoid acute tachycardia, hypertension, and/or ischemia. Chronic beta-blocker therapy should not be routinely withdrawn prior to major surgery. Adequate alpha-blockade is required prior to use of any beta-blocker for patients with untreated pheochromocytoma. Use caution with history of severe anaphylaxis to allergens; patients taking beta-blockers may become more sensitive to repeated challenges. Treatment of anaphylaxis (eg, epinephrine) in patients taking beta-blockers may be ineffective or promote undesirable effects. Use with caution in patients on concurrent digoxin, verapamil, or diltiazem; bradycardia or heart block may occur. Use with caution in patients receiving inhaled anesthetic agents known to depress myocardial contractility.
Adverse Reactions (Reflective of adult population; not specific for elderly)
1% to 10%:
Cardiovascular: Edema (6%), chest pain (3%), bradycardia (≤2%), heart block (≤2%), hypotension (≤2%), syncope (≤2%), tachycardia (≤2%), palpitation (≤1%)
Central nervous system: Insomnia (10%), dizziness (9%), fatigue (8%), nervousness (7%), nightmares/vivid dreams (5%), anxiety (≤2%), lethargy (≤2%)
Dermatologic: Hyperhidrosis (≤2%), pruritus (1%)
Gastrointestinal: Nausea (5%), diarrhea (≤2%), vomiting (≤2%), weight gain (≤2%)
Genitourinary: Impotence (≤2%)
Hematologic: Claudication (≤2%)
Hepatic: ALT increased (7%), AST increased (7%)
Neuromuscular & skeletal: Muscle pain (10%), arthralgia (7%), weakness (4%), paresthesia (3%), muscle cramps (3%)
Ocular: Burning eyes (≤2%), visual disturbances (≤2%), eye discomfort (≤2%)
Renal: Polyuria (≤2%)
Respiratory: Dyspnea (5%), wheezing (≤2%)
Miscellaneous: Cold extremities (≤2%)
Other adverse reactions (noted with other beta-adrenergic-blocking agents that should be considered potential adverse events with pindolol): Agranulocytosis, alopecia, catatonia, clouded sensorium, disorientation, emotional lability, fever, intensification of pre-existing AV block, ischemic colitis, laryngospasm, mental depression, mesenteric artery thrombosis, nonthrombocytopenic purpura, Peyronie's disease, rash (erythematous), respiratory distress, short-term memory loss, thrombocytopenic purpura
Drug Interactions
Metabolism/Transport Effects Substrate of CYP2D6 (major); **Inhibits** CYP2D6 (weak)

Avoid Concomitant Use
Avoid concomitant use of Pindolol with any of the following: Floctafenine; Methacholine
Increased Effect/Toxicity
Pindolol may increase the levels/effects of: Alpha-/Beta-Agonists (Direct-Acting); Alpha1-Blockers; Alpha2-Agonists; Amifostine; Antihypertensives; Antipsychotic Agents (Phenothiazines); Bupivacaine; Cardiac Glycosides; Fingolimod; Hypotensive Agents; Insulin; Lidocaine; Lidocaine (Systemic); Lidocaine (Topical); Mepivacaine; Methacholine; Midodrine; RiTUXimab; Sulfonylureas

The levels/effects of Pindolol may be increased by: Acetylcholinesterase Inhibitors; Aminoquinolines (Antimalarial); Amiodarone; Anilidopiperidine Opioids; Antipsychotic Agents (Phenothiazines); Calcium Channel Blockers (Dihydropyridine); Calcium Channel Blockers (Nondihydropyridine); Diazoxide; Dipyridamole; Disopyramide; Dronedarone; Floctafenine; Herbs (Hypotensive Properties); MAO Inhibitors; Pentoxifylline; Phosphodiesterase 5 Inhibitors; Propafenone; Propoxyphene; Prostacyclin Analogues; QuiNIDine; Reserpine; Selective Serotonin Reuptake Inhibitors
Decreased Effect
Pindolol may decrease the levels/effects of: Beta2-Agonists; Theophylline Derivatives

The levels/effects of Pindolol may be decreased by: Barbiturates; Herbs (Hypertensive Properties); Methylphenidate; Nonsteroidal Anti-Inflammatory Agents; Peginterferon Alfa-2b; Rifamycin Derivatives; Yohimbine
Ethanol/Nutrition/Herb Interactions Herb/Nutraceutical: Avoid bayberry, blue cohosh, cayenne, ephedra, ginger, ginseng (American), kola, and licorice (may worsen hypertension). Avoid black cohosh, california poppy, coleus, golden seal, hawthorn, mistletoe, periwinkle, quinine, and shepherd's purse (may increase antihypertensive effect).
Stability Store below 30°C (86°F). Protect from light.
Mechanism of Action Blocks both beta$_1$- and beta$_2$-receptors and has mild intrinsic sympathomimetic activity; pindolol has negative inotropic and chronotropic effects and can significantly slow AV nodal conduction. Augmentive action of antidepressants thought to be mediated via a serotonin 1A autoreceptor antagonism.
Pharmacodynamics/Kinetics
Absorption: Rapid, 50% to 95%
Distribution: V$_d$: ~2 L/kg
Protein binding: 40%
Metabolism: Hepatic (60% to 65%) to conjugates
Half-life elimination: 3-4 hours; prolonged with advanced age, and cirrhosis (range: 2.5-30 hours)
Time to peak, serum: ~1 hour
Excretion: Urine (35% to 40% as unchanged drug); feces (6% to 9%)
Dosage
Geriatric Oral: Initial: 5 mg once daily; increase as necessary by 5 mg/day every 3-4 weeks.
Adult
Hypertension: Oral: Initial: 5 mg twice daily, increase as necessary by 10 mg/day every 3-4 weeks (maximum daily dose: 60 mg); usual dose range (JNC 7): 10-40 mg twice daily.
Antidepressant augmentation (unlabeled use): Oral: 2.5 mg 3 times/day
Renal Impairment Use with caution. Clearance significantly decreased in uremic patients. Dosage reduction may be necessary.
Hepatic Impairment Use with caution. Elimination half-life in cirrhotic patients may be 10 times as long compared to normal patients. Dosage reduction is necessary in severely impaired.
Administration May be administered without regard to meals.
Monitoring Parameters Blood pressure, heart rate, respiratory function
Special Geriatric Considerations Due to alterations in the beta-adrenergic autonomic nervous system, beta-adrenergic blockade may result in less hemodynamic response than seen in younger adults. Studies indicate that despite decreased sensitivity to the chronotropic effects of beta-blockade with age, there appears to be an increased myocardial sensitivity to the negative inotropic effect during stress (eg, exercise). Controlled trials have shown the overall response rate for propranolol to be only 20% to 50% in elderly populations. Therefore, all beta-adrenergic blocking drugs may result in a decreased response as compared to younger adults.
Dosage Forms Excipient information presented when available (limited, particularly for generics); consult specific product labeling.
Tablet, oral: 5 mg, 10 mg
♦ **Pink Bismuth** see Bismuth on page 207

Pioglitazone (pye oh GLI ta zone)

Related Information
Diabetes Mellitus Management, Adults on page 2073

Medication Safety Issues
Sound-alike/look-alike issues:
Actos® may be confused with Actidose®, Actonel®
International issues:
Tiazac: Brand name for piogitazone [Chile], but also the brand name for diltiazem [U.S, Canada]

Brand Names: U.S. Actos®

Brand Names: Canada Accel-Pioglitazone; Actos®; Apo-Pioglitazone®; CO Pioglitazone; Dom-Pioglitazone; JAMP-Pioglitazone; Mint-Pioglitazone; Mylan-Pioglitazone; Novo-Pioglitazone; PHL-Pioglitazone; PMS-Pioglitazone; PRO-Pioglitazone; ratio-Pioglitazone; Sandoz-Pioglitazone; Teva-Pioglitazone; ZYM-Pioglitazone

Generic Availability (U.S.) No

Pharmacologic Category Antidiabetic Agent, Thiazolidinedione

Use
Type 2 diabetes mellitus (noninsulin dependent, NIDDM), monotherapy: Adjunct to diet and exercise, to improve glycemic control
Type 2 diabetes mellitus (noninsulin dependent, NIDDM), combination therapy with sulfonylurea, metformin, or insulin: When diet, exercise, and a single agent alone does not result in adequate glycemic control

Medication Guide Available Yes

Contraindications Hypersensitivity to pioglitazone or any component of the formulation; NYHA Class III/IV heart failure (initiation of therapy)

Canadian labeling: Additional contraindications (not in U.S. labeling): Any stage of heart failure (eg, NYHA Class I, II, III, IV); serious hepatic impairment

Warnings/Precautions [U.S. Boxed Warning]: Thiazolidinediones, including pioglitazone, may cause or exacerbate heart failure; closely monitor for signs and symptoms of heart failure (eg, rapid weight gain, dyspnea, edema), particularly after initiation or dose increases. Not recommended for use in any patient with symptomatic heart failure. In the U.S., initiation of therapy is contraindicated in patients with NYHA class III or IV heart failure. If used in patients with NYHA class II (systolic heart failure), initiate at lowest dosage and monitor closely. In Canada, use in any stage of heart failure (NYHA I, II, III, IV) is contraindicated. Use with caution in patients with edema; may increase plasma volume and/or cause fluid retention. Dose reduction or discontinuation is recommended if heart failure suspected. Dose-related weight gain observed with use; mechanism unknown but likely associated with fluid retention and fat accumulation.

Should not be used in diabetic ketoacidosis. Mechanism requires the presence of insulin; therefore use in type 1 diabetes is not recommended. Use with caution in patients with anemia (may reduce hemoglobin and hematocrit). Increased incidence of bone fractures in females treated with pioglitazone; majority of fractures occurred in the lower limb and distal upper limb.

Use with caution in patients with elevated transaminases (AST or ALT); do not initiate in patients with active liver disease of ALT >2.5 times the upper limit of normal at baseline. During therapy, if ALT >3 times the upper limit of normal, re-evaluate levels promptly and discontinue if elevation persists or if jaundice occurs at any time during use. Idiosyncratic hepatotoxicity has been reported with another thiazolidinedione agent (troglitazone); avoid use in patients who previously experienced jaundice during troglitazone therapy. Monitoring should include periodic determinations of liver function. Use caution with pre-existing macular edema or diabetic retinopathy. Postmarketing reports of new-onset or worsening diabetic macular edema with decreased visual acuity has been reported.

Canadian labeling (not in U.S. labeling) states use with insulin **or** as part of triple therapy (pioglitazone in combination with a sulfonylurea and metformin) is not indicated.

Adverse Reactions (Reflective of adult population; not specific for elderly)
>10%:
Cardiovascular: Edema (5%; in combination trials with sulfonlyureas or insulin, the incidence of edema was as high as 15%)
Respiratory: Upper respiratory tract infection (13%)
1% to 10%:
Cardiovascular: Heart failure (requiring hospitalization; up to 6% in patients with prior macrovascular disease)
Central nervous system: Headache (9%), fatigue (4%)
Hematologic: Anemia (≤2%)

Neuromuscular & skeletal: Myalgia (5%)
Respiratory: Sinusitis (6%), pharyngitis (5%)
Frequency not defined: HDL-cholesterol increased, hematocrit/hemoglobin decreased, hypoglycemia (in combination trials with sulfonylureas or insulin), serum triglycerides decreased, weight gain/loss

Drug Interactions

Metabolism/Transport Effects Substrate of CYP2C8 (major), 3A4 (minor); **Inhibits** CYP2C8 (moderate), 2C9 (weak), 2C19 (weak) **Induces** CYP3A4 (weak)

Avoid Concomitant Use There are no known interactions where it is recommended to avoid concomitant use.

Increased Effect/Toxicity

Pioglitazone may increase the levels/effects of: CYP2C8 Substrates (High risk); Hypoglycemic Agents

The levels/effects of Pioglitazone may be increased by: Conivaptan; CYP2C8 Inhibitors (Moderate); CYP2C8 Inhibitors (Strong); Deferasirox; Gemfibrozil; Herbs (Hypoglycemic Properties); Insulin; Pegvisomant; Pregabalin; Trimethoprim

Decreased Effect

Pioglitazone may decrease the levels/effects of: Saxagliptin

The levels/effects of Pioglitazone may be decreased by: Bile Acid Sequestrants; Corticosteroids (Orally Inhaled); Corticosteroids (Systemic); CYP2C8 Inducers (Highly Effective); Luteinizing Hormone-Releasing Hormone Analogs; Rifampin; Somatropin; Thiazide Diuretics; Tocilizumab

Ethanol/Nutrition/Herb Interactions

Ethanol: Caution with ethanol (may cause hypoglycemia).
Food: Peak concentrations are delayed when administered with food, but the extent of absorption is not affected. Pioglitazone may be taken without regard to meals.
Herb/Nutraceutical: Caution with alfalfa, aloe, bilberry, bitter melon, burdock, celery, damiana, fenugreek, garcinia, garlic, ginger, ginseng (American), gymnema, marshmallow, and stinging nettle (may cause hypoglycemia).

Mechanism of Action Thiazolidinedione antidiabetic agent that lowers blood glucose by improving target cell response to insulin, without increasing pancreatic insulin secretion. It has a mechanism of action that is dependent on the presence of insulin for activity. Pioglitazone is a potent and selective agonist for peroxisome proliferator-activated receptor-gamma (PPAR-gamma). Activation of nuclear PPARgamma receptors influences the production of a number of gene products involved in glucose and lipid metabolism. PPARgamma is abundant in the cells within the renal collecting tubules; fluid retention results from stimulation by thiazolidinediones which increases sodium reabsorption.

Pharmacodynamics/Kinetics

Onset of action: Delayed
  Peak effect: Glucose control: Several weeks
Distribution: V_{ss} (apparent): 0.63 L/kg
Protein binding: Pioglitazone >99% and active metabolites >98%; primarily to albumin
Metabolism: Hepatic (99%) via CYP2C8 and 3A4 to both active and inactive metabolites
Half-life elimination: Parent drug: 3-7 hours; Total: 16-24 hours
Time to peak: ~2 hours; delayed with food
Excretion: Urine (15% to 30%) and feces as metabolites

Dosage

Geriatric & Adult Type 2 diabetes: Oral:

Monotherapy: Initial: 15-30 mg once daily; if response is inadequate, the dosage may be increased in increments up to 45 mg once daily; maximum recommended dose: 45 mg once daily

Combination therapy:

Note: Maximum recommended dose: 45 mg/day

With sulfonylureas: Initial: 15-30 mg once daily; dose of sulfonylurea should be reduced if the patient reports hypoglycemia

With metformin: Initial: 15-30 mg once daily; it is unlikely that the dose of metformin will need to be reduced due to hypoglycemia

With insulin: Initial: 15-30 mg once daily; dose of insulin should be reduced by 10% to 25% if the patient reports hypoglycemia or if the plasma glucose falls to below 100 mg/dL.

Dosage adjustment in patients with CHF (NYHA Class II) in mono- or combination therapy: Oral: Initial: 15 mg once daily; may be increased after several months of treatment, with close attention to heart failure symptoms

Renal Impairment No adjustment is necessary.

◄ **Hepatic Impairment** Clearance is significantly lower in hepatic impairment (Child-Pugh Grade B/C). Therapy should not be initiated if the patient exhibits active liver disease or increased transaminases (>2.5 times ULN) at baseline. During treatment if ALT levels elevate >3 times ULN, the test should be repeated as soon as possible. If ALT levels remain >3 times ULN or if the patient is jaundiced, therapy should be discontinued.

Administration May be administered without regard to meals

Monitoring Parameters Hemoglobin A$_{1c}$, serum glucose; signs and symptoms of heart failure; liver enzymes prior to initiation and periodically during treatment (per clinician judgment). If the ALT is increased to >2.5 times the upper limit of normal, liver function testing should be performed more frequently until the levels return to normal or pretreatment values. Patients with an elevation in ALT >3 times the upper limit of normal should be rechecked as soon as possible. If the ALT levels remain >3 times the upper limit of normal, therapy with pioglitazone should be discontinued. Routine ophthalmic exams are recommended; patients reporting visual deterioration should have a prompt referral to an ophthalmologist and consideration should be given to discontinuing pioglitazone.

Reference Range Recommendations for glycemic control in adults with diabetes:
Hb A$_{1c}$: <7%
Preprandial capillary plasma glucose: 70-130 mg/dL
Peak postprandial capillary blood glucose: <180 mg/dL

Special Geriatric Considerations Intensive glucose control (HbA$_{1c}$ <6.5%) has been linked to increased all-cause and cardiovascular mortality, hypoglycemia requiring assistance, and weight gain in adult type 2 diabetes. How "tightly" to control a geriatric patient's blood glucose needs to be individualized. Such a decision should be based on several factors, including the patient's functional and cognitive status, how well he/she recognizes hypoglycemic or hyperglycemic symptoms, and how to respond to them and other disease states. An HbA$_{1c}$ <7.5% is an acceptable endpoint for a healthy older adult, while <8% is acceptable for frail elderly patients, those with a duration of illness >10 years, or those with comorbid conditions and requiring combination diabetes medications. Patients who are unable to accurately draw up their dose will need assistance, such as prefilled syringes. Initial doses may require considerations for renal function in the elderly with dosing adjusted subsequently based on blood glucose monitoring. For elderly patients with diabetes who are relatively healthy, attaining target goals for aspirin use, blood pressure, lipids, smoking cessation, and diet and exercise may be more important than normalized glycemic control.

Dosage Forms Excipient information presented when available (limited, particularly for generics); consult specific product labeling.
Tablet, oral:
Actos®: 15 mg, 30 mg, 45 mg

Selected References

Action to Control Cardiovascular Risk in Diabetes Study Group, Gerstein HC, Miller ME, et al, "Effects of Intensive Glucose Lowering in Type 2 Diabetes," *N Engl J Med*, 2008, 358(24):2545-59.

ADVANCE Collaborative Group, Patel A, MacMahon S, et al, "Intensive Blood Glucose Control and Vascular Outcomes in Patients With Type 2 Diabetes," *N Engl J Med*, 2008, 358(24):2560-72.

American Diabetes Association, "Standards of Medical Care in Diabetes – 2011," *Diabetes Care*, 2011, 34(Suppl 1):11-61.

Brown AF, Mangione CM, Saliba D, et al, "Guidelines for Improving the Care of the Older Person With Diabetes Mellitus," *J Am Geriatr Soc*, 2003, 51(5 Suppl Guidelines):265-80.

Lago RM, Singh PP, and Nesto RW, "Congestive Heart Failure and Cardiovascular Death in Patients with Prediabetes and Type 2 Diabetes Given Thiazolidinediones: A Meta-Analysis of Randomised Clinical Trials," *Lancet*, 2007, 370 (9593):1129-36.

Lincoff AM, Wolski K, Nicholls SJ, et al, "Pioglitazone an Risk of Cardiovascular Events in Patients With Type 2 Diabetes Mellitus," *JAMA*, 2007, 298(10):1180-8.

Schwartz AV, Sellmeyer DE, Vittinghoff E, et al, "Thiazolidinedione Use and Bone Loss in Older Diabetic Adults," *J Clin Endocrin Metab*, 2006, 91(9):3349-54.

"VA/DoD Clinical Practice Guideline for the Management of Diabetes Mellitus," 2010. Available at http://www.healthquality.va.gov/Diabetes_Mellitus.asp

Yaturu S, Bryant B, Jain SK, "Thiazolidinedione Treatment Decreases Bone Mineral Density in Type 2 Diabetic Men," *Diabetes Care*, 2007, 30(6):1574-76.

Pioglitazone and Glimepiride (pye oh GLI ta zone & GLYE me pye ride)

Related Information
Glimepiride *on page 820*
Pioglitazone *on page 1458*

Medication Safety Issues
High alert medication:
The Institute for Safe Medication Practices (ISMP) includes this medication among its list of drugs which have a heightened risk of causing significant patient harm when used in error.

Brand Names: U.S. Duetact™

Index Terms Glimepiride and Pioglitazone; Glimepiride and Pioglitazone Hydrochloride

Generic Availability (U.S.) No

Pharmacologic Category Antidiabetic Agent, Sulfonylurea; Antidiabetic Agent, Thiazolidinedione; Hypoglycemic Agent, Oral

Use Management of type 2 diabetes mellitus (noninsulin dependent, NIDDM) as an adjunct to diet and exercise

Medication Guide Available Yes

Dosage

Geriatric Initial: Glimepiride 1 mg/day prior to initiating Duetact™; dose titration and maintenance dosing should be conservative to avoid hypoglycemia. Refer to adult dosing.

Adult Type 2 diabetes mellitus: Oral: Initial dose should be based on current dose of pioglitazone and/or sulfonylurea.

Patients inadequately controlled on **glimepiride** alone: Initial dose: 30 mg/2 mg or 30 mg/4 mg once daily

Patients inadequately controlled on **pioglitazone** alone: Initial dose: 30 mg/2 mg once daily

Patients with systolic dysfunction (eg, NYHA Class I and II): Initiate only after patient has been safely titrated to 30 mg of pioglitazone. Initial dose: 30 mg/2 mg or 30 mg/4 mg once daily.

Note: No exact dosing relationship exists between glimepiride and other sulfonlyureas. Dosing should be limited to less than or equal to the maximum initial dose of glimepiride (2 mg). When converting patients from other sulfonylureas with longer half-lives (eg, chlorpropamide) to glimepiride, observe patient carefully for 1-2 weeks due to overlapping hypoglycemic effects.

Dosing adjustment: Dosage may be increased up to max dose and formulation strengths available; tablet should not be given more than once daily; see individual agents for frequency of adjustments. Dosage adjustments in patients with systolic dysfunction should be done carefully and patient monitored for symptoms of worsening heart failure.

Maximum dose: Pioglitazone 45 mg/glimepiride 8 mg daily

Renal Impairment Cl_{cr} <22 mL/minute: Initial dose should be 1 mg of glimepiride and dosage increments should be based on fasting blood glucose levels.

Hepatic Impairment Do not initiate treatment with active liver disease or ALT >2.5 times ULN. During treatment, if ALT levels elevate >3 times ULN, the test should be repeated as soon as possible. If ALT levels remain >3 times ULN or if the patient is jaundiced, Duetact™ should be discontinued.

Special Geriatric Considerations Rapid and prolonged hypoglycemia (>12 hours) despite hypertonic glucose injections have been reported with glimepiride. Age, hepatic impairment, and renal impairment are independent risk factors for hypoglycemia; dosage titration should be made at weekly intervals. Intensive glucose control (HbA_{1c} <6.5%) has been linked to increased all-cause and cardiovascular mortality, hypoglycemia requiring assistance, and weight gain in adult type 2 diabetes. How "tightly" to control a geriatric patient's blood glucose needs to be individualized. Such a decision should be based on several factors, including the patient's functional and cognitive status, how well he/she recognizes hypoglycemic or hyperglycemic symptoms, and how to respond to them and other disease states. An HbA_{1c} <7.5% is an acceptable endpoint for a healthy older adult, while <8% is acceptable for frail elderly patients, those with a duration of illness >10 years, or those with comorbid conditions and requiring combination diabetes medications. Patients who are unable to accurately draw up their dose will need assistance, such as prefilled syringes. Initial doses may require considerations for renal function in the elderly with dosing adjusted subsequently based on blood glucose monitoring. For elderly patients with diabetes who are relatively healthy, attaining target goals for aspirin use, blood pressure, lipids, smoking cessation, and diet and exercise may be more important than normalized glycemic control.

Dosage Forms Excipient information presented when available (limited, particularly for generics); consult specific product labeling.

Tablet:

Duetact™:

30 mg/2 mg: Pioglitazone 30 mg and glimepiride 2 mg

30 mg/4 mg: Pioglitazone 30 mg and glimepiride 4 mg

Pioglitazone and Metformin (pye oh GLI ta zone & met FOR min)

Related Information

MetFORMIN *on page 1155*

Pioglitazone *on page 1458*

Brand Names: U.S. Actoplus Met®; Actoplus Met® XR

Index Terms Metformin Hydrochloride and Pioglitazone Hydrochloride

Generic Availability (U.S.) No

Pharmacologic Category Antidiabetic Agent, Biguanide; Antidiabetic Agent, Thiazolidinedione

◀ **Use** Management of type 2 diabetes mellitus (noninsulin dependent, NIDDM)

Medication Guide Available Yes

Dosage

Geriatric Refer to adult dosing. The initial and maintenance dosing should be conservative, due to the potential for decreased renal function (monitor). Generally, elderly patients should not be titrated to the maximum; do not use in patients ≥80 years of age unless normal renal function has been established.

Adult Type 2 diabetes mellitus: Oral: Initial dose should be based on current dose of pioglitazone and/or metformin; metformin dose may be titrated every 1-2 weeks and pioglitazone dose may be titrated every 2-3 months as necessary to achieve goals

Immediate release tablet: **Note:** Daily doses higher than pioglitazone 15 mg plus metformin 850 mg should be divided. Initial: Pioglitazone 15 mg plus metformin 500 mg **or** pioglitazone 15 mg plus metformin 850 mg tablets once or twice daily. Maximum daily dose: Pioglitazone 45 mg/metformin 2550 mg

Variable release tablet: Pioglitazone 15 mg plus metformin 1000 mg tablet **or** pioglitazone 30 mg plus metformin 1000 mg tablet once daily with evening meal. Maximum daily dose: Pioglitazone 45 mg/metformin 2000 mg

Renal Impairment Do not use with renal disease or renal dysfunction (serum creatinine ≥1.5 mg/dL in males or ≥1.4 mg/dL in females or abnormal clearance).

Hepatic Impairment Do not initiate treatment with active liver disease or ALT >2.5 times ULN. During treatment, if ALT concentrations increase >3 times ULN, the test should be repeated as soon as possible. If ALT concentrations remain >3 times ULN or if the patient is jaundiced, therapy should be discontinued.

Special Geriatric Considerations Metformin should not be used in patients ≥80 years of age unless renal function is verified as normal. **Do not titrate to maximum dose.** Intensive glucose control (HbA$_{1c}$ <6.5%) has been linked to increased all-cause and cardiovascular mortality, hypoglycemia requiring assistance, and weight gain in adult type 2 diabetes. How "tightly" to control a geriatric patient's blood glucose needs to be individualized. Such a decision should be based on several factors, including the patient's functional and cognitive status, how well he/she recognizes hypoglycemic or hyperglycemic symptoms, and how to respond to them and other disease states. An HbA$_{1c}$ <7.5% is an acceptable endpoint for a healthy older adult, while <8% is acceptable for frail elderly patients, those with a duration of illness >10 years, or those with comorbid conditions and requiring combination diabetes medications. Patients who are unable to accurately draw up their dose will need assistance, such as prefilled syringes. Initial doses may require considerations for renal function in the elderly with dosing adjusted subsequently based on blood glucose monitoring. For elderly patients with diabetes who are relatively healthy, attaining target goals for aspirin use, blood pressure, lipids, smoking cessation, and diet and exercise may be more important than normalized glycemic control.

Dosage Forms Excipient information presented when available (limited, particularly for generics); consult specific product labeling.

Tablet, oral:

Actoplus Met®:

15/500: Pioglitazone 15 mg and metformin hydrochloride 500 mg

15/850: Pioglitazone 15 mg and metformin hydrochloride 850 mg

Tablet, variable release, oral:

Actoplus Met® XR:

15/1000: Pioglitazone 15 mg [immediate release] and metformin hydrochloride 1000 mg [extended release]

30/1000: Pioglitazone 30 mg [immediate release] and metformin hydrochloride 1000 mg [extended release]

Piperacillin (pi PER a sil in)

Brand Names: Canada Piperacillin for Injection, USP

Index Terms Piperacillin Sodium

Generic Availability (U.S.) Yes

Pharmacologic Category Antibiotic, Penicillin

Use Treatment of susceptible infections such as septicemia, acute and chronic respiratory tract infections, skin and soft tissue infections, and urinary tract infections due to susceptible strains of *Pseudomonas*, *Proteus*, and *Escherichia coli* and *Enterobacter*; active against some streptococci and some anaerobic bacteria; febrile neutropenia (as part of combination regimen)

Contraindications Hypersensitivity to piperacillin, other beta-lactam antibiotics (penicillins or cephalosporins), or any component of the formulation

Warnings/Precautions Serious and occasionally severe or fatal hypersensitivity (anaphylactoid) reactions have been reported in patients on penicillin therapy, especially with a history of beta-lactam hypersensitivity, history of sensitivity to multiple allergens, or previous IgE-mediated reactions (eg, anaphylaxis, angioedema, urticaria). Use with caution in asthmatic patients. Bleeding disorders have been observed, particularly in patients with renal impairment; discontinue if thrombocytopenia or bleeding occurs. Due to sodium load and adverse effects (anemia, neuropsychological changes), use with caution and modify dosage in patients with renal impairment. Use caution in patients with history of seizure activity. Leukopenia and neutropenia have been reported (during prolonged therapy). An increased frequency of fever and rash has been reported in patients with cystic fibrosis. Prolonged use may result in fungal or bacterial superinfection, including *C. difficile*-associated diarrhea (CDAD) and pseudomembranous colitis; CDAD has been observed >2 months postantibiotic treatment.

Adverse Reactions (Reflective of adult population; not specific for elderly) Frequency not defined.

Central nervous system: Confusion, convulsions, drowsiness, fever, Jarisch-Herxheimer reaction

Dermatologic: Rash, toxic epidermal necrolysis, urticaria

Endocrine & metabolic: Electrolyte imbalance, hypokalemia

Hematologic: Abnormal platelet aggregation and prolonged PT (high doses), agranulocytosis, Coombs' reaction (positive), hemolytic anemia, pancytopenia

Local: Thrombophlebitis

Neuromuscular & skeletal: Myoclonus

Renal: Acute interstitial nephritis, acute renal failure

Miscellaneous: Anaphylaxis, hypersensitivity reactions

Drug Interactions

Avoid Concomitant Use

Avoid concomitant use of Piperacillin with any of the following: BCG

Increased Effect/Toxicity

Piperacillin may increase the levels/effects of: Methotrexate

The levels/effects of Piperacillin may be increased by: Probenecid

Decreased Effect

Piperacillin may decrease the levels/effects of: Aminoglycosides; BCG; Mycophenolate; Typhoid Vaccine

The levels/effects of Piperacillin may be decreased by: Fusidic Acid; Tetracycline Derivatives

Stability Reconstituted solution is stable (I.V. infusion) in NS or D_5W for 24 hours at room temperature, 7 days when refrigerated, or 4 weeks when frozen. After freezing, thawed solution is stable for 24 hours at room temperature or 48 hours when refrigerated. 40 g bulk vial should **not** be frozen after reconstitution.

Mechanism of Action Inhibits bacterial cell wall synthesis by binding to one or more of the penicillin-binding proteins (PBPs); which in turn inhibits the final transpeptidation step of peptidoglycan synthesis in bacterial cell walls, thus inhibiting cell wall biosynthesis. Bacteria eventually lyse due to ongoing activity of cell wall autolytic enzymes (autolysins and murein hydrolases) while cell wall assembly is arrested.

Pharmacodynamics/Kinetics

Absorption: I.M.: 70% to 80%

Protein binding: ~16%

Bioavailability: Not well absorbed when given orally

Half-life elimination (dose dependent; prolonged with moderately severe renal or hepatic impairment): 36-80 minutes

Time to peak, serum: I.M.: 30-50 minutes

Excretion: Primarily urine; partially feces

Dosage

Geriatric Adjust dose for renal impairment:

I.M.: 1-2 g every 8-12 hours

I.V.: 2-4 g every 6-8 hours

Adult

Usual dosage range:

I.M.: 2-3 g/dose every 6-12 hours; maximum: 24 g/24 hours

I.V.: 3-4 g/dose every 4-6 hours; maximum: 24 g/24 hours

Burn wound sepsis: I.V.: 4 g every 4 hours with vancomycin and amikacin

Cholangitis, acute: I.V.: 4 g every 6 hours

Keratitis *(Pseudomonas):* Ophthalmic: 6-12 mg/mL every 15-60 minutes around the clock for 24-72 hours, then slow reduction

Malignant otitis externa: I.V.: 4-6 g every 4-6 hours with tobramycin

Moderate infections: I.M., I.V.: 2-3 g/dose every 6-12 hours (maximum: 2 g I.M./site)

◄ **Prosthetic joint *(Pseudomonas):*** I.V.: 3 g every 6 hours with aminoglycoside
Pseudomonas infections: I.V.: 4 g every 4 hours
Severe infections: I.M., I.V.: 3-4 g/dose every 4-6 hours (maximum: 24 g/24 hours)
Urinary tract infections: I.V.: 2-3 g/dose every 6-12 hours
Uncomplicated gonorrhea: I.M.: 2 g in a single dose accompanied by 1 g probenecid 30 minutes prior to injection

Renal Impairment
Cl_{cr} 10-50 mL/minute: Administer every 6-8 hours.
Cl_{cr} <10 mL/minute: Administer every 8 hours.
Moderately dialyzable (20% to 50%)
Continuous arteriovenous or venovenous hemofiltration: Dose as for Cl_{cr} 10-50 mL/minute.

Administration Administer around-the-clock to promote less variation in peak and trough serum levels. Give at least 1 hour apart from aminoglycosides. Rapid administration can lead to seizures. Administer direct I.V. over 3-5 minutes. Intermittently infusion over 30 minutes. Do not administer more than 2 g per I.M. injection site.

Some penicillins (eg, carbenicillin, ticarcillin and piperacillin) have been shown to inactivate aminoglycosides *in vitro*. This has been observed to a greater extent with tobramycin and gentamicin, while amikacin has shown greater stability against inactivation. Concurrent use of these agents may pose a risk of reduced antibacterial efficacy *in vivo*, particularly in the setting of profound renal impairment. However, definitive clinical evidence is lacking. If combination penicillin/aminoglycoside therapy is desired in a patient with renal dysfunction, separation of doses (if feasible), and routine monitoring of aminoglycoside levels, CBC, and clinical response should be considered.

Monitoring Parameters Observe for signs and symptoms of anaphylaxis during first dose

Test Interactions May interfere with urinary glucose tests using cupric sulfate (Benedict's solution, Clinitest®); false-positive urinary and serum proteins, positive Coombs' test [direct]. False-positive Platelia® *Aspergillus* EIA test (Bio-Rad Laboratories) have been reported.

Some penicillin derivatives may accelerate the degradation of aminoglycosides *in vitro*, leading to a potential underestimation of aminoglycoside serum concentration.

Pharmacotherapy Pearls Sodium content of 1 g: 1.85 mEq. Administer 1 hour apart from aminoglycosides.

Special Geriatric Considerations Because of piperacillin's lower sodium content, it is preferred over ticarcillin in patients with a history of heart failure and/or renal or hepatic disease. Adjust dose for renal function.

Dosage Forms Excipient information presented when available (limited, particularly for generics); consult specific product labeling. [DSC] = Discontinued product
Injection, powder for reconstitution: 2 g [DSC], 3 g [DSC], 4 g [DSC], 40 g [DSC]

Selected References
Yoshikawa TT, "Antimicrobial Therapy for the Elderly Patient," *J Am Geriatr Soc,* 1990, 38(12):1353-72.

Piperacillin and Tazobactam Sodium
(pi PER a sil in & ta zoe BAK tam SOW dee um)

Related Information
Piperacillin *on page 1462*

Medication Safety Issues
Sound-alike/look-alike issues:
Zosyn® may be confused with Zofran®, Zyvox®
International issues:
Tazact [India] may be confused with Tazac brand name for nizatidine [Australia]; Tiazac brand name for diltiazem [U.S., Canada]

Brand Names: U.S. Zosyn®

Brand Names: Canada Piperacillin and Tazobactam for Injection; Tazocin®

Index Terms Piperacillin Sodium and Tazobactam Sodium; Tazobactam and Piperacillin

Generic Availability (U.S.) Yes: Excludes infusion

Pharmacologic Category Antibiotic, Penicillin

Use Treatment of moderate-to-severe infections caused by susceptible organisms, including infections of the lower respiratory tract (community-acquired pneumonia, nosocomial pneumonia); urinary tract; uncomplicated and complicated skin and skin structures; gynecologic (endometritis, pelvic inflammatory disease); bone and joint infections; intra-abdominal infections (appendicitis with rupture/abscess, peritonitis); and septicemia. Tazobactam expands activity of piperacillin to include beta-lactamase producing strains of *S. aureus, H. influenzae, Bacteroides,* and other gram-negative bacteria.

Contraindications Hypersensitivity to penicillins, beta-lactamase inhibitors, or any component of the formulation

Warnings/Precautions Bleeding disorders have been observed, particularly in patients with renal impairment; discontinue if thrombocytopenia or bleeding occurs. Due to sodium load and to the adverse effects of high serum concentrations of penicillins, dosage modification is required in patients with impaired or underdeveloped renal function; use with caution in patients with seizures or in patients with history of beta-lactam allergy; associated with an increased incidence of rash and fever in cystic fibrosis patients. Prolonged use may result in fungal or bacterial superinfection, including *C. difficile*-associated diarrhea (CDAD) and pseudomembranous colitis; CDAD has been observed >2 months postantibiotic treatment.

Adverse Reactions (Reflective of adult population; not specific for elderly)

>10%: Gastrointestinal: Diarrhea (7% to 11%)

>1% to 10%:

Cardiovascular: Hypertension (2%)

Central nervous system: Insomnia (7%), headache (8%), fever (2% to 5%), agitation (2%), pain (2%)

Dermatologic: Rash (4%), pruritus (3%)

Gastrointestinal: Constipation (1% to 8%), nausea (7%), vomiting (3% to 4%), dyspepsia (3%), stool changes (2%), abdominal pain (1% to 2%)

Hepatic: Transaminases increased

Local: Local reaction (3%), abscess (2%)

Respiratory: Pharyngitis (2%)

Miscellaneous: Moniliasis (2%), sepsis (2%), infection (2%)

Drug Interactions

Avoid Concomitant Use

Avoid concomitant use of Piperacillin and Tazobactam Sodium with any of the following: BCG

Increased Effect/Toxicity

Piperacillin and Tazobactam Sodium may increase the levels/effects of: Methotrexate

The levels/effects of Piperacillin and Tazobactam Sodium may be increased by: Probenecid

Decreased Effect

Piperacillin and Tazobactam Sodium may decrease the levels/effects of: Aminoglycosides; BCG; Mycophenolate; Typhoid Vaccine

The levels/effects of Piperacillin and Tazobactam Sodium may be decreased by: Fusidic Acid; Tetracycline Derivatives

Stability

Vials: Store at controlled room temperature of 20°C to 25°C (68°F to 77°F). Use single-dose vials immediately after reconstitution (discard unused portions after 24 hours at room temperature and 48 hours if refrigerated). Reconstitute with 5 mL of diluent per 1 g of piperacillin and then further dilute. After reconstitution, vials or solution are stable in NS or D_5W for 24 hours at room temperature and 48 hours (vials) or 7 days (solution) when refrigerated.

Premixed solution: Store frozen at -20°C (-4°F). Thawed solution is stable for 24 hours at room temperature or 14 days under refrigeration; do not refreeze.

Mechanism of Action Inhibits bacterial cell wall synthesis by binding to one or more of the penicillin-binding proteins (PBPs); which in turn inhibits the final transpeptidation step of peptidoglycan synthesis in bacterial cell walls, thus inhibiting cell wall biosynthesis. Bacteria eventually lyse due to ongoing activity of cell wall autolytic enzymes (autolysins and murein hydrolases) while cell wall assembly is arrested. Tazobactam inhibits many beta-lactamases, including staphylococcal penicillinase and Richmond and Sykes types II, III, IV, and V, including extended spectrum enzymes; it has only limited activity against class I beta-lactamases other than class Ic types.

Pharmacodynamics/Kinetics Both AUC and peak concentrations are dose proportional; hepatic impairment does not affect kinetics

Distribution: Well into lungs, intestinal mucosa, skin, muscle, uterus, ovary, prostate, gall-bladder, and bile; penetration into CSF is low in subject with noninflamed meninges

Protein binding: Piperacillin and tazobactam: ~30%

Metabolism:

Piperacillin: 6% to 9% to desethyl metabolite (weak activity)

Tazobactam: ~26% to inactive metabolite

Bioavailability:

Piperacillin: I.M.: 71%

Tazobactam: I.M.: 84%

Half-life elimination: Piperacillin and tazobactam: 0.7-1.2 hours

Time to peak, plasma: Immediately following infusion of 30 minutes

Excretion: Clearance of both piperacillin and tazobactam are directly proportional to renal function

Piperacillin: Urine (68% as unchanged drug); feces (10% to 20%)

Tazobactam: Urine (80% as unchanged drug; remainder as inactive metabolite)

Dosage

Geriatric & Adult

Usual dosage range: I.V.: 3.375 g every 6 hours **or** 4.5 g every 6-8 hours; maximum: 18 g/day

Extended infusion method (unlabeled dosing): 3.375-4.5 g I.V. over 4 hours every 8 hours (Kim, 2007; Shea, 2009); an alternative regimen of 4.5 g I.V. over 3 hours every 6 hours has also been described (Kim, 2007)

Indication-specific dosing: I.V.: **Note:** Dosing based on piperacillin component:

Diverticulitis, intra-abdominal abscess, peritonitis: I.V.: 3.375 g every 6 hours; **Note:** Some clinicians use 4.5 g every 8 hours for empiric coverage since the %time>MIC is similar between the regimens for most pathogens; however, this regimen is NOT recommended for nosocomial pneumonia or *Pseudomonas* coverage.

Intra-abdominal infection, severe: I.V.: 3.375 g every 6 hours for 4-7 days (provided source controlled). **Note:** Increase to 3.375 g every 4 hours or 4.5 g every 6 hours if *P. aeruginosa* suspected. Not recommended for mild-to-moderate, community-acquired intra-abdominal infections due to risk of toxicity and the development of resistant organisms (Solomkin, 2010).

Pneumonia (nosocomial): I.V.: 4.5 g every 6 hours for 7-14 days (when used empirically, combination with an aminoglycoside or antipseudomonal fluoroquinolone is recommended; consider discontinuation of additional agent if *P. aeruginosa* is not isolated)

Severe infections: I.V.: 3.375 g every 6 hours for 7-10 days; **Note:** Some clinicians use 4.5 g every 8 hours for empiric coverage since the %time>MIC is similar between the regimens for most pathogens; however, this regimen is NOT recommended for nosocomial pneumonia or *Pseudomonas* coverage.

Renal Impairment

Cl$_{cr}$ >40 mL/minute: No dosage adjustment required.

Cl$_{cr}$ 20-40 mL/minute: Administer 2.25 g every 6 hours (3.375 g every 6 hours for nosocomial pneumonia)

Cl$_{cr}$ <20 mL/minute: Administer 2.25 g every 8 hours (2.25 g every 6 hours for nosocomial pneumonia)

Intermittent hemodialysis (IHD)/peritoneal dialysis (PD): 2.25 g every 12 hours (2.25 g every 8 hours for nosocomial pneumonia). **Note:** Dosing dependent on the assumption of 3 times/week, complete IHD sessions. Administer scheduled doses after hemodialysis on dialysis days; if next regularly scheduled dose is not due right after dialysis session, administer an additional dose of 0.75 g after the dialysis session.

Continuous renal replacement therapy (CRRT) (Heintz, 2009; Trotman, 2005): Drug clearance is highly dependent on the method of renal replacement, filter type, and flow rate. Appropriate dosing requires close monitoring of pharmacologic response, signs of adverse reactions due to drug accumulation, as well as drug concentrations in relation to target trough (if appropriate). The following are general recommendations only (based on dialysate flow/ultrafiltration rates of 1-2 L/hour and minimal residual renal function) and should not supersede clinical judgment (Trotman, 2005):

CVVH: 2.25-3.375 g every 6-8 hours

CVVHD: 2.25-3.375 g every 6 hours

CVVHDF: 3.375 g every 6 hours

Note: Higher dose of 3.375 g should be considered when treating resistant pathogens (especially *Pseudomonas* spp); alternative recommendations suggest dosing of 4.5 g every 8 hours (Valtonen, 2001); regardless of regimen, there is some concern of tazobactam (TAZ) accumulation, given its lower clearance relative to piperacillin (PIP). Some clinicians advocate dosing with PIP to alternate with PIP/TAZ, particularly in CVVH-dependent patients, to lessen this concern.

Hepatic Impairment Hepatic impairment does not affect the kinetics of piperacillin or tazobactam significantly.

Administration Administer by I.V. infusion over 30 minutes

Some penicillins (eg, carbenicillin, ticarcillin and piperacillin) have been shown to inactivate aminoglycosides *in vitro*. This has been observed to a greater extent with tobramycin and gentamicin, while amikacin has shown greater stability against inactivation. Concurrent use of these agents may pose a risk of reduced antibacterial efficacy *in vivo*, particularly in the setting of profound renal impairment. However, definitive clinical evidence is lacking. If combination penicillin/aminoglycoside therapy is desired in a patient with renal dysfunction, separation of doses (if feasible), and routine monitoring of aminoglycoside levels, CBC, and clinical response should be considered. **Note:** Reformulated Zosyn® containing EDTA has been shown to be compatible *in vitro* for Y-site infusion with amikacin and gentamicin, but not compatible with tobramycin.

Monitoring Parameters Creatinine, BUN, CBC with differential, PT, PTT; signs of bleeding; monitor for signs of anaphylaxis during first dose

Test Interactions Positive Coombs' [direct] test; false positive reaction for urine glucose using copper-reduction method (Clinitest®); may result in false positive results with the Platelia® *Aspergillus* enzyme immunoassay (EIA)

Some penicillin derivatives may accelerate the degradation of aminoglycosides *in vitro*, leading to a potential underestimation of aminoglycoside serum concentration. **Note:** Reformulated Zosyn® containing EDTA has been shown to be compatible *in vitro* for Y-site infusion with amikacin and gentamicin, but not compatible with tobramycin.

Pharmacotherapy Pearls Administer 1 hour apart from aminoglycosides.

Special Geriatric Considerations Has not been studied exclusively in the elderly.

Dosage Forms Excipient information presented when available (limited, particularly for generics); consult specific product labeling.

Note: 8:1 ratio of piperacillin sodium/tazobactam sodium

Infusion [premixed iso-osmotic solution]:

Zosyn®: 2.25 g: Piperacillin 2 g and tazobactam 0.25 g (50 mL) [contains edetate disodium, sodium 128 mg (5.58 mEq)]

Zosyn®: 3.375 g: Piperacillin 3 g and tazobactam 0.375 g (50 mL) [contains edetate disodium, sodium 192 mg (8.38 mEq)]

Zosyn®: 4.5 g: Piperacillin 4 g and tazobactam 0.5 g (100 mL) [contains edetate disodium, sodium 256 mg (11.17 mEq)]

Injection, powder for reconstitution: 2.25 g: Piperacillin 2 g and tazobactam 0.25 g; 3.375 g: Piperacillin 3 g and tazobactam 0.375 g; 4.5 g: Piperacillin 4 g and tazobactam 0.5 g; 40.5 g: Piperacillin 36 g and tazobactam 4.5 g

Zosyn®: 2.25 g: Piperacillin 2 g and tazobactam 0.25 g [contains edetate disodium, sodium 128 mg (5.58 mEq)]

Zosyn®: 3.375 g: Piperacillin 3 g and tazobactam 0.375 g [contains edetate disodium, sodium 192 mg (8.38 mEq)]

Zosyn®: 4.5 g: Piperacillin 4 g and tazobactam 0.5 g [contains edetate disodium, sodium 256 mg (11.17 mEq)]

Zosyn®: 40.5 g: Piperacillin 36 g and tazobactam 4.5 g [contains edetate disodium, sodium 2304 mg (100.4 mEq); bulk pharmacy vial]

Selected References

Mandell LA, Wunderink RG, Anzueto A, et al, "Infectious Diseases Society of America/American Thoracic Society Consensus Guidelines on the Management of Community-Acquired Pneumonia in Adults," *Clin Infect Dis*, 2007, 44 Suppl 2:S27-72.

◆ **Piperacillin Sodium** *see* Piperacillin *on page 1462*
◆ **Piperacillin Sodium and Tazobactam Sodium** *see* Piperacillin and Tazobactam Sodium *on page 1464*

Piperazine (PI per a zeen)

Brand Names: Canada Entacyl®
Index Terms Piperazine Citrate
Generic Availability (U.S.) Yes
Pharmacologic Category Anthelmintic
Use Treatment of pinworm and roundworm infections (used as an alternative to first-line agents, mebendazole, or pyrantel pamoate)
Contraindications Hypersensitivity to piperazine or any component of the formulation; seizure disorders; liver or kidney impairment
Warnings/Precautions Use with caution in patients with anemia or malnutrition.
Drug Interactions
Avoid Concomitant Use There are no known interactions where it is recommended to avoid concomitant use.
Increased Effect/Toxicity There are no known significant interactions involving an increase in effect.
Decreased Effect
The levels/effects of Piperazine may be decreased by: Aminoquinolines (Antimalarial)
Mechanism of Action Causes muscle paralysis of the roundworm by blocking the effects of acetylcholine at the neuromuscular junction
Pharmacodynamics/Kinetics
Absorption: Well absorbed
Time to peak, serum: 1 hour
Excretion: Urine (as unchanged drug and metabolites)

◀ **Dosage**
Geriatric & Adult
Pinworm eradication: Oral: 65 mg/kg/day (not to exceed 2.5 g/day) as a single daily dose for 7 days; in severe infections, repeat course after a 1-week interval
Roundworm eradication: Oral: 3.5 g/day for 2 days (in severe infections, repeat course, after a 1-week interval)
Monitoring Parameters Stool exam for worms and ova
Special Geriatric Considerations Not a drug of choice. Monitor closely in the elderly.
Dosage Forms Excipient information presented when available (limited, particularly for generics); consult specific product labeling.
Piperazine citrate is available from Panorama Pharmacy (1-800-247-9767).

◆ **Piperazine Citrate** *see* Piperazine *on page 1467*

Pirbuterol (peer BYOO ter ole)

Related Information
Inhalant Agents *on page 2010*
Brand Names: U.S. Maxair® Autohaler®
Index Terms Pirbuterol Acetate
Generic Availability (U.S.) No
Pharmacologic Category Beta$_2$-Adrenergic Agonist
Use Prevention and treatment of reversible bronchospasm including asthma
Contraindications Hypersensitivity to pirbuterol, albuterol, or any component of the formulation

Warnings/Precautions Optimize anti-inflammatory treatment before initiating maintenance treatment with pirbuterol. Do not use as a component of chronic therapy without an anti-inflammatory agent. Only the mildest form of asthma (Step 1 and/or exercise-induced) would not require concurrent use based upon asthma guidelines. Patient must be instructed to seek medical attention in cases where acute symptoms are not relieved or a previous level of response is diminished. The need to increase frequency of use may indicate deterioration of asthma, and treatment must not be delayed.

Use caution in patients with cardiovascular disease (arrhythmia or hypertension or CHF), convulsive disorders, diabetes, glaucoma, hyperthyroidism, or hypokalemia. Beta-agonists may cause elevation in blood pressure, heart rate, and result in CNS stimulation/excitation. Beta$_2$-agonists may increase risk of arrhythmia, increase serum glucose, or decrease serum potassium.

Do not exceed recommended dose; serious adverse events including fatalities, have been associated with excessive use of inhaled sympathomimetics. Rarely, paradoxical bronchospasm may occur with use of inhaled bronchodilating agents; this should be distinguished from inadequate response. All patients should utilize a spacer device when using a metered-dose inhaler.

Adverse Reactions (Reflective of adult population; not specific for elderly)
>10%:
Central nervous system: Nervousness (7%)
Endocrine & metabolic: Serum glucose increased, serum potassium decreased
Neuromuscular & skeletal: Trembling (6%)
1% to 10%:
Cardiovascular: Palpitation (2%), tachycardia (1%)
Central nervous system: Headache (2%), dizziness (1%)
Gastrointestinal: Nausea (2%)
Respiratory: Cough (1%)
Drug Interactions
Avoid Concomitant Use
Avoid concomitant use of Pirbuterol with any of the following: Iobenguane I 123
Increased Effect/Toxicity
Pirbuterol may increase the levels/effects of: Loop Diuretics; Sympathomimetics

The levels/effects of Pirbuterol may be increased by: Atomoxetine; Cannabinoids; MAO Inhibitors; Tricyclic Antidepressants
Decreased Effect
Pirbuterol may decrease the levels/effects of: Iobenguane I 123

The levels/effects of Pirbuterol may be decreased by: Alpha-/Beta-Blockers; Beta-Blockers (Beta1 Selective); Beta-Blockers (Nonselective); Betahistine
Stability Store between 15°C and 30°C (59°F and 86°F).

Mechanism of Action Pirbuterol is a beta$_2$-adrenergic agonist with a similar structure to albuterol, specifically a pyridine ring has been substituted for the benzene ring in albuterol. The increased beta$_2$ selectivity of pirbuterol results from the substitution of a tertiary butyl group on the nitrogen of the side chain, which additionally imparts resistance of pirbuterol to degradation by monoamine oxidase and provides a lengthened duration of action in comparison to the less selective previous beta-agonist agents.

Pharmacodynamics/Kinetics
Onset of action: Peak effect: Therapeutic: Oral: 2-3 hours with peak serum concentration of 6.2-9.8 mcg/L; Inhalation: 0.5-1 hour
Half-life elimination: 2-3 hours
Metabolism: Hepatic
Excretion: Urine (10% as unchanged drug)

Dosage
Geriatric & Adult Bronchospasm: Inhalation: 2 inhalations every 4-6 hours for prevention; 2 inhalations at an interval of at least 1-3 minutes, followed by a third inhalation in treatment of bronchospasm, not to exceed 12 inhalations/day

Administration Inhalation: Shake inhaler well before use.

Monitoring Parameters Respiratory rate; FEV$_1$, peak flow, and/or other pulmonary function tests; blood pressure, heart rate; CNS stimulation; serum glucose, serum potassium

Special Geriatric Considerations Elderly patients may find it beneficial to utilize a spacer device when using a metered dose inhaler. Difficulty in using the inhaler often limits its effectiveness. The Maxair™ Autohaler™ may be easier for the elderly to use.

Dosage Forms Excipient information presented when available (limited, particularly for generics); consult specific product labeling.
Aerosol, for oral inhalation, as acetate:
Maxair® Autohaler®: 200 mcg/actuation (14 g) [contains chlorofluorocarbon; 400 actuations]

◆ **Pirbuterol Acetate** see Pirbuterol on page 1468

Piroxicam (peer OKS i kam)

Related Information
Beers Criteria – Potentially Inappropriate Medications for Geriatrics on page 2089

Medication Safety Issues
Sound-alike/look-alike issues:
Feldene® may be confused with FLUoxetine
Piroxicam may be confused with PARoxetine
BEERS Criteria medication:
This drug may be inappropriate for use in geriatric patients (high severity risk).
International issues:
Flogene [Brazil] may be confused with Florone brand name for diflorasone [Germany, Greece]

Brand Names: U.S. Feldene®

Brand Names: Canada Apo-Piroxicam®; Dom-Piroxicam; Gen-Piroxicam; Novo-Pirocam; Nu-Pirox; PMS-Piroxicam; PRO-Piroxicam

Generic Availability (U.S.) Yes

Pharmacologic Category Nonsteroidal Anti-inflammatory Drug (NSAID), Oral

Use Symptomatic treatment of acute and chronic rheumatoid arthritis and osteoarthritis

Unlabeled/Investigational Use Ankylosing spondylitis

Medication Guide Available Yes

Contraindications Hypersensitivity to piroxicam, aspirin, other NSAIDs or any component of the formulation; perioperative pain in the setting of coronary artery bypass graft (CABG) surgery

Warnings/Precautions [U.S. Boxed Warning]: NSAIDs are associated with an increased risk of adverse cardiovascular thrombotic events, including MI and stroke. Risk may be increased with duration of use or pre-existing cardiovascular risk factors or disease. Carefully evaluate individual cardiovascular risk profiles prior to prescribing. May cause new-onset hypertension or worsening of existing hypertension. Use caution with fluid retention. Avoid use in heart failure. Concurrent administration of ibuprofen, and potentially other nonselective NSAIDs, may interfere with aspirin's cardioprotective effect. **[U.S. Boxed Warning]: Use is contraindicated for treatment of perioperative pain in the setting of coronary artery bypass graft (CABG) surgery.** Risk of MI and stroke may be increased with use following CABG surgery.

Platelet adhesion and aggregation may be decreased; may prolong bleeding time; patients with coagulation disorders or who are receiving anticoagulants should be monitored closely.

◀ Anemia may occur; patients on long-term NSAID therapy should be monitored for anemia. Rarely, NSAID use may cause severe blood dyscrasias (eg, agranulocytosis, aplastic anemia, thrombocytopenia).

NSAID use may compromise existing renal function; dose-dependent decreases in prostaglandin synthesis may result from NSAID use, reducing renal blood flow which may cause renal decompensation. NSAID use may increase the risk for hyperkalemia. Patients with impaired renal function, dehydration, heart failure, liver dysfunction, those taking diuretics, and ACE inhibitors, and the elderly are at greater risk of renal toxicity and hyperkalemia. Rehydrate patient before starting therapy; monitor renal function closely. Not recommended for use in patients with advanced renal disease. Long-term NSAID use may result in renal papillary necrosis.

[U.S. Boxed Warning]: NSAIDs may increase risk of gastrointestinal irritation, inflammation, ulceration, bleeding, and perforation. These events may occur at any time during therapy and without warning. Use caution with a history of GI disease (bleeding or ulcers), concurrent therapy with aspirin, anticoagulants and/or corticosteroids, smoking, use of alcohol, the elderly or debilitated patients. When used concomitantly with ≤325 mg of aspirin, a substantial increase in the risk of gastrointestinal complications (eg, ulcer) occurs; concomitant gastroprotective therapy (eg, proton pump inhibitors) is recommended (Bhatt, 2008).

Use the lowest effective dose for the shortest duration of time, consistent with individual patient goals, to reduce risk of cardiovascular or GI adverse events. Alternate therapies should be considered for patients at high risk.

NSAIDs may cause serious skin adverse events including exfoliative dermatitis, Stevens-Johnson syndrome (SJS) and toxic epidermal necrolysis (TEN); discontinue use at first sign of skin rash or hypersensitivity. Anaphylactoid reactions may occur, even without prior exposure; patients with "aspirin triad" (bronchial asthma, aspirin intolerance, rhinitis) may be at increased risk. Do not use in patients who experience bronchospasm, asthma, rhinitis, or urticaria with NSAID or aspirin therapy. Use caution with other forms of asthma. A serum sickness-like reaction can rarely occur; watch for arthralgias, pruritus, fever, fatigue, and rash.

Use with caution in patients with decreased hepatic function. Closely monitor patients with any abnormal LFT. Severe hepatic reactions (eg, fulminant hepatitis, liver failure) have occurred with NSAID use, rarely; discontinue if signs or symptoms of liver disease develop, or if systemic manifestations occur.

NSAIDS may cause drowsiness, dizziness, blurred vision and other neurologic effects which may impair physical or mental abilities; patients must be cautioned about performing tasks which require mental alertness (eg, operating machinery or driving). Discontinue use with blurred or diminished vision and perform ophthalmologic exam. Monitor vision with long-term therapy.

In the elderly, may be inappropriate for long-term use due to potential for GI bleeding, hypertension, heart failure, and renal failure (Beers Criteria).

Withhold for at least 4-6 half-lives prior to surgical or dental procedures.

Adverse Reactions (Reflective of adult population; not specific for elderly)
>10%:
Central nervous system: Dizziness
Dermatologic: Rash
Gastrointestinal: Abdominal cramps, heartburn, indigestion, nausea
1% to 10%:
Central nervous system: Headache, nervousness
Dermatologic: Itching
Endocrine & metabolic: Fluid retention
Gastrointestinal: Vomiting
Otic: Tinnitus

Drug Interactions
Metabolism/Transport Effects Substrate of CYP2C9 (minor); **Inhibits** CYP2C9 (strong)
Avoid Concomitant Use
Avoid concomitant use of Piroxicam with any of the following: Floctafenine; Ketorolac; Ketorolac (Nasal); Ketorolac (Systemic)
Increased Effect/Toxicity
Piroxicam may increase the levels/effects of: Aminoglycosides; Anticoagulants; Antiplatelet Agents; Bisphosphonate Derivatives; Collagenase (Systemic); CycloSPORINE; CycloSPORINE (Systemic); Deferasirox; Desmopressin; Digoxin; Drotrecogin Alfa; Eplerenone; Haloperidol; Ibritumomab; Lithium; Methotrexate; Nonsteroidal Anti-Inflammatory Agents; PEMEtrexed; Porfimer; Potassium-Sparing Diuretics; PRALAtrexate; Quinolone Antibiotics;

Rivaroxaban; Salicylates; Thrombolytic Agents; Tositumomab and Iodine I 131 Tositumomab; Vancomycin; Vitamin K Antagonists

The levels/effects of Piroxicam may be increased by: ACE Inhibitors; Angiotensin II Receptor Blockers; Antidepressants (Tricyclic, Tertiary Amine); Corticosteroids (Systemic); Dasatinib; Floctafenine; Glucosamine; Herbs (Anticoagulant/Antiplatelet Properties); Ketorolac; Ketorolac (Nasal); Ketorolac (Systemic); Nonsteroidal Anti-Inflammatory Agents; Omega-3-Acid Ethyl Esters; Pentosan Polysulfate Sodium; Pentoxifylline; Prostacyclin Analogues; Selective Serotonin Reuptake Inhibitors; Serotonin/Norepinephrine Reuptake Inhibitors; Sodium Phosphates; Treprostinil; Vitamin E

Decreased Effect

Piroxicam may decrease the levels/effects of: ACE Inhibitors; Angiotensin II Receptor Blockers; Antiplatelet Agents; Beta-Blockers; Eplerenone; HydrALAZINE; Potassium-Sparing Diuretics; Salicylates; Selective Serotonin Reuptake Inhibitors; Thiazide Diuretics

The levels/effects of Piroxicam may be decreased by: Bile Acid Sequestrants; Nonsteroidal Anti-Inflammatory Agents; Salicylates

Ethanol/Nutrition/Herb Interactions

Ethanol: Avoid ethanol (may enhance gastric mucosal irritation).

Food: Onset of effect may be delayed if piroxicam is taken with food.

Herb/Nutraceutical: Avoid alfalfa, anise, bilberry, bladderwrack, bromelain, cat's claw, celery, chamomile, coleus, cordyceps, dong quai, evening primrose, fenugreek, feverfew, garlic, ginger, ginkgo biloba, ginseng (American, Panax, Siberian), grapeseed, green tea, guggul, horse chestnut seed, horseradish, licorice, prickly ash, red clover, reishi, SAMe (S-adenosylmethionine), sweet clover, turmeric, white willow (all have additional antiplatelet activity).

Mechanism of Action Reversibly inhibits cyclooxygenase-1 and 2 (COX-1 and 2) enzymes, which results in decreased formation of prostaglandin precursors; has antipyretic, analgesic, and anti-inflammatory properties

Other proposed mechanisms not fully elucidated (and possibly contributing to the anti-inflammatory effect to varying degrees), include inhibiting chemotaxis, altering lymphocyte activity, inhibiting neutrophil aggregation/activation, and decreasing proinflammatory cytokine levels.

Pharmacodynamics/Kinetics

Onset of action: Analgesic: ~1 hour

Distribution: V_d: 0.14 L/kg

Protein binding: 99%

Metabolism: Hepatic

Half-life elimination: 50 hours

Time to peak: 3-5 hours

Excretion: Primarily urine and feces (small amounts) as unchanged drug (5%) and metabolites

Dosage

Geriatric Refer to adult dosing. **Note:** Some clinicians have used 10 mg every other day to initiate therapy in the elderly to avoid side effects and produce therapeutic effect at minimal dose. Maximum dose: 20 mg/day.

Adult Inflammation, rheumatoid arthritis: Oral: 10-20 mg/day once daily; although associated with increase in GI adverse effects, doses >20 mg/day have been used (ie, 30-40 mg/day); maximum dose: 20 mg/day

Renal Impairment Not recommended in patients with advanced renal disease.

Hepatic Impairment Reduced dose is necessary.

Monitoring Parameters Occult blood loss, hemoglobin, hematocrit, and periodic renal and hepatic function tests; periodic ophthalmologic exams with chronic use

Test Interactions Increased chloride (S), increased sodium (S), increased bleeding time

Pharmacotherapy Pearls Because of its long half-life, may be dosed once daily. There are no clinical guidelines to predict which NSAID will give response in a particular patient. Trials with each must be initiated until response determined. Consider dose, patient convenience, and cost.

Special Geriatric Considerations Elderly are a high-risk population for adverse effects from NSAIDs. As much as 60% of elderly can develop peptic ulceration and/or hemorrhage asymptomatically. The concomitant use of H_2 blockers and sucralfate is not generally effective as prophylaxis with the exception of NSAID-induced duodenal ulcers which may be prevented by the use of ranitidine. Misoprostol and proton pump inhibitors are the only agents proven to help prevent the development of NSAID-induced ulcers. Also, concomitant disease and drug use contribute to the risk for GI adverse effects. Use lowest effective dose for shortest period possible. Consider renal function decline with age. Use of NSAIDs can compromise existing renal function especially when Cl_{cr} is ≤30 mL/minute. Tinnitus may be a difficult and unreliable indication of toxicity due to age-related hearing loss or eighth cranial nerve damage. CNS adverse effects such as confusion, agitation, and hallucination are generally seen in overdose or high dose situations, but elderly may demonstrate these adverse effects at lower doses than younger adults.

This medication is considered to be potentially inappropriate in this patient population (Beers Criteria severity: High).

Dosage Forms Excipient information presented when available (limited, particularly for generics); consult specific product labeling.
Capsule, oral: 10 mg, 20 mg
Feldene®: 10 mg, 20 mg

◆ *p*-Isobutylhydratropic Acid *see* Ibuprofen *on page 908*

Pitavastatin (pi TA va sta tin)

Related Information
Hyperlipidemia Management *on page 2021*
Medication Safety Issues
Sound-alike/look-alike issues:
Pitavastatin may be confused with atorvastatin, fluvastatin, lovastatin, nystatin, pravastatin, rosuvastatin, simvastatin
Brand Names: U.S. Livalo®
Index Terms Pitavastatin Calcium
Generic Availability (U.S.) No
Pharmacologic Category Antilipemic Agent, HMG-CoA Reductase Inhibitor
Use Adjunct to dietary therapy to reduce elevations in total cholesterol (TC), LDL-C, apolipoprotein B (Apo B), and triglycerides (TG), and to increase low HDL-C in patients with primary hyperlipidemia and mixed dyslipidemia
Contraindications Hypersensitivity to pitavastatin or any component of the formulation; active liver disease including unexplained persistent elevations of hepatic transaminases; concurrent use with cyclosporine
Warnings/Precautions Secondary causes of hyperlipidemia should be ruled out prior to therapy. Pitavastatin has not been studied when the primary lipid abnormality is chylomicron elevation (Fredrickson types I and V) or in familial dysbetalipoproteinemia (Fredrickson type III). May cause hepatic dysfunction; in all patients, liver function must be monitored by periodic laboratory assessment. Use with caution in patients who consume large amounts of ethanol or have a history of liver disease; use is contraindicated in patients with active liver disease or unexplained persistent elevations of serum transaminases.

Myopathy and rhabdomyolysis with acute renal failure have occurred with use. Risk is dose related and is increased with concurrent use of lipid-lowering agents which may cause rhabdomyolysis (fibric acid derivatives or niacin at doses ≥1 g/day) or during concurrent use with erythromycin or protease inhibitors. Use caution in patients with renal impairment, inadequately treated hypothyroidism, and those taking other drugs associated with myopathy (eg, colchicine); these patients are predisposed to myopathy. Monitor closely if used with other drugs associated with myopathy. Weigh the risk versus benefit when combining any of these drugs with pitavastatin. The manufacturer recommends temporary discontinuation for elective major surgery, acute medical or surgical conditions, or in any patient experiencing an acute or serious condition predisposing to renal failure (eg, sepsis, hypotension, trauma, uncontrolled seizures). However, based upon current evidence, HMG-CoA reductase inhibitor therapy should be continued in the perioperative period unless risk outweighs cardioprotective benefit. Patients should be instructed to report unexplained muscle pain, tenderness, weakness, or brown urine. Concurrent use with cyclosporine is contraindicated. Ensure patient is on the lowest effective pitavastatin dose. Use with caution in elderly patients, as these patients are predisposed to myopathy.

Adverse Reactions (Reflective of adult population; not specific for elderly)
2% to 10%:
Gastrointestinal: Constipation (2% to 4%), diarrhea (2% to 3%)
Neuromuscular & skeletal: Back pain (1% to 4%), myalgia (2% to 3%), pain in extremities (1% to 2%)
Additional class-related events or case reports (not necessarily reported with pitavastatin therapy): Cataracts, cirrhosis, dermatomyositis, eosinophilia, extraocular muscle movement impaired, fulminant hepatic necrosis, gynecomastia, hypersensitivity syndrome (symptoms may include anaphylaxis, angioedema, arthralgia, erythema multiforme, eosinophilia, hemolytic anemia, interstitial lung disease, lupus syndrome, photosensitivity, polymyalgia rheumatica, positive ANA, purpura, Stevens-Johnson syndrome, toxic epidermal necrolysis,

urticaria, vasculitis), ophthalmoplegia, peripheral nerve palsy, rhabdomyolysis, renal failure (secondary to rhabdomyolysis), thyroid dysfunction, tremor, vertigo

Drug Interactions

Metabolism/Transport Effects Substrate of OATP1B1; (major) of UGT1A3 and UGT2B7; (minor) of CYP2C9, 2C8

Avoid Concomitant Use

Avoid concomitant use of Pitavastatin with any of the following: CycloSPORINE; Cyclo-SPORINE (Systemic); Red Yeast Rice

Increased Effect/Toxicity

Pitavastatin may increase the levels/effects of: DAPTOmycin; Trabectedin; Vitamin K Antagonists

The levels/effects of Pitavastatin may be increased by: Atazanavir; Colchicine; Cyclo-SPORINE; CycloSPORINE (Systemic); Danazol; Eltrombopag; Fenofibrate; Fenofibric Acid; Gemfibrozil; Macrolide Antibiotics; Niacin; Niacinamide; Protease Inhibitors; Red Yeast Rice; Rifamycin Derivatives; Sildenafil

Decreased Effect

Pitavastatin may decrease the levels/effects of: Lanthanum

The levels/effects of Pitavastatin may be decreased by: Antacids; Bosentan; Rifamycin Derivatives; St Johns Wort

Ethanol/Nutrition/Herb Interactions

Ethanol: Avoid excessive ethanol consumption (due to potential hepatic effects).

Food: Red yeast rice contains an estimated 2.4 mg lovastatin per 600 mg rice.

Stability Store at controlled room temperature of 15°C to 30°C (59°F to 86°F). Protect from light.

Mechanism of Action Inhibitor of 3-hydroxy-3-methylglutaryl coenzyme A (HMG-CoA) reductase, the rate-limiting enzyme in cholesterol synthesis (reduces the production of mevalonic acid from HMG-CoA); this then results in a compensatory increase in the expression of LDL receptors on hepatocyte membranes and a stimulation of LDL catabolism

Pharmacodynamics/Kinetics

Distribution: V_d: ~148 L

Protein binding: >99%

Metabolism: Hepatic, via UGT1A3 and UGT 2B7; minimal metabolism via CYP2C9 and CYP2C8

Bioavailability: 51%

Half-life elimination: ~12 hours

Time to peak, plasma: ~1 hour

Excretion: Feces (79%); urine (15%)

Dosage

Geriatric & Adult

Primary hyperlipidemia and mixed dyslipidemia: Oral: Initial: 2 mg once daily; may be increased to maximum 4 mg once daily

Note: Doses should be individualized according to the baseline LDL-cholesterol levels, the recommended goal of therapy, and patient response; adjustments should be made at intervals of 4 weeks.

Dosage adjustment with concomitant medications:

Erythromycin: Pitavastatin dose should not exceed 1 mg once daily

Rifampin: Pitavastatin dose should not exceed 2 mg once daily

Renal Impairment Cl_{cr} <60 mL/minute/1.73 m^2 including hemodialysis: Initial: 1 mg once daily; maximum: 2 mg once daily

Hepatic Impairment Contraindicated in active liver disease or in patients with unexplained persistent elevations of serum transaminases.

Administration May be administered with or without food; may take without regard to time of day.

Monitoring Parameters Total cholesterol, LDL, and HDL cholesterol within 4 weeks of treatment initiation or dose change; LFTs; CPK

It is recommended that liver function tests (LFTs) be performed prior to and at 12 weeks following both the initiation of therapy and any elevation in dose, and periodically (eg, semiannually) thereafter.

Special Geriatric Considerations The definition of and, therefore, when to treat hyperlipidemia in the elderly is a controversial issue. The National Cholesterol Education Program recommends that all adults maintain a plasma cholesterol <160 mg/dL. For elderly patients with one additional risk factor, goal LDL would be <130 mg/dL. It is the authors' belief that pharmacologic treatment be reserved for those who are unable to obtain a desirable plasma cholesterol concentration by diet alone and for whom the benefits of treatment are believed to outweigh the potential adverse effects, drug interactions, and cost of treatment. Age ≥65 years is a risk factor for myopathy.

◀ **Dosage Forms** Excipient information presented when available (limited, particularly for generics); consult specific product labeling.
Tablet, oral:
Livalo®: 1 mg, 2 mg, 4 mg

Selected References

"Executive Summary of The Third Report of The National Cholesterol Education Program (NCEP) Expert Panel on Detection, Evaluation, and Treatment of High Blood Cholesterol in Adults (Adult Treatment Panel III)," *JAMA*, 2001, 285(19):2486-97.

Fleisher LA, Beckman JA, Brown KA, et al, "ACC/AHA 2007 Guidelines on Perioperative Cardiovascular Evaluation and Care for Noncardiac Surgery: A Report of the American College of Cardiology/American Heart Association Task Force on Practice Guidelines (Writing Committee to Revise the 2002 Guidelines on Perioperative Cardiovascular Evaluation for Noncardiac Surgery) Developed in Collaboration With the American Society of Echocardiography, American Society of Nuclear Cardiology, Heart Rhythm Society, Society of Cardiovascular Anesthesiologists, Society for Cardiovascular Angiography and Interventions, Society for Vascular Medicine and Biology, and Society for Vascular Surgery," *J Am Coll Cardiol*, 2007, 50(17):e159-241.

Grundy SM, Cleeman JI, Merz CN, et al, "Implications of Recent Clinical Trials for the National Cholesterol Education Program Adult Treatment Panel III Guidelines," *J Am Coll Cardiol*, 2004, 44(3):720-32.

Smith SC Jr, Allen J, Blair SN, et al, "AHA/ACC Guidelines for Secondary Prevention for Patients With Coronary and Other Atherosclerotic Vascular Disease: 2006 Update: Endorsed by the National Heart, Lung, and Blood Institute," *J Am Coll Cardiol*, 2006, 47(10):2130-9.

Pneumococcal Polysaccharide Vaccine (Polyvalent)
(noo moe KOK al pol i SAK a ride vak SEEN, pol i VAY lent)

Related Information

Immunization Administration Recommendations *on page 2037*
Immunization Recommendations *on page 2043*

Medication Safety Issues

Sound-alike/look-alike issues:
Pneumococcal 23-Valent Polysaccharide Vaccine (Pneumovax® 23) may be confused with Pneumococcal 7-Valent Conjugate Vaccine (Prevnar®) or with Pneumococcal 13-Valent Conjugate Vaccine (Prevnar 13™)

Brand Names: U.S. Pneumovax® 23

Brand Names: Canada Pneumo 23™; Pneumovax® 23

Index Terms 23-Valent Pneumococcal Polysaccharide Vaccine; 23PS; PPSV; PPSV23; PPV23

Generic Availability (U.S.) No

Pharmacologic Category Vaccine, Inactivated (Bacterial)

Use Immunization against pneumococcal disease caused by serotypes included in the vaccine. Routine vaccination is recommended for persons ≥50 years of age and persons ≥2 years in certain situations.

The Advisory Committee on Immunization Practices (ACIP) recommends routine vaccination for the following:

All immunocompetent patients ≥65 years of age

Patients 2-18 years of age with certain high-risk condition(s):
- Chronic heart disease (particularly cyanotic congenital heart disease and cardiac failure)
- Chronic lung disease (including asthma if treated with high-dose oral corticosteroids)

Patients 2-64 years of age with certain high-risk condition(s):
- Diabetes mellitus
- Cochlear implants
- Cerebrospinal fluid leaks
- Functional or anatomic asplenia (including sickle cell disease and other hemoglobino-pathies, splenic dysfunction, or splenectomy)
- Immunocompromising conditions including congenital immunodeficiency (includes B- or T-lymphocyte deficiency, complement deficiencies, and phagocytic disorders [excluding chronic granulomatous disease]); HIV infection; leukemia, lymphoma, Hodgkin's disease, multiple myeloma, generalized malignancy; chronic renal failure, nephrotic syndrome; patients requiring treatment with immunosuppressive therapy, including chemotherapy, long-term systemic corticosteroids, or radiation therapy; patients who have received a solid organ transplant

Patients 19-64 years of age with certain high-risk condition(s):
- Chronic heart disease (including heart failure and cardiomyopathy, and excluding hypertension)
- Chronic lung disease (including COPD, emphysema, and asthma)
- Persons who smoke cigarettes
- Alcoholism
- Chronic liver disease (including cirrhosis)

Routine vaccination is not recommended for Alaska Natives or American Indian persons unless they have underlying conditions which are indications for vaccination; in special situations, vaccination may be recommended when living in an area at increased risk of invasive pneumococcal disease.

Contraindications Hypersensitivity to pneumococcal vaccine or any component of the formulation

Warnings/Precautions Use caution in patients with severely compromised cardiovascular function or pulmonary disease where a systemic reaction may pose a significant risk. May cause relapse in patients with stable idiopathic thrombocytopenia purpura. Epinephrine injection (1:1000) must be immediately available in the case of anaphylaxis.

Patients who will be receiving immunosuppressive therapy (including Hodgkin's disease, cancer chemotherapy, or transplantation) should be vaccinated at least 2 weeks prior to the initiation of therapy. Immune responses may be impaired for several months following intensive immunosuppressive therapy (up to 2 years in Hodgkin's disease patients). Patients who will undergo splenectomy should also be vaccinated 2 weeks prior to surgery, if possible. In general, household and close contacts of persons with altered immunocompetence may receive all age appropriate vaccines. Patients with HIV should be vaccinated as soon as possible (following confirmation of the diagnosis). The decision to administer or delay vaccination because of current or recent febrile illness depends on the severity of symptoms and the etiology of the disease. Immunization should be delayed during the course of an acute febrile illness or other active infection. In order to maximize vaccination rates, the ACIP recommends simultaneous administration of all age-appropriate vaccines (live or inactivated) for which a person is eligible at a single clinic visit, unless contraindications exist. If a person has not received any pneumococcal vaccine or if pneumococcal vaccination status is unknown, PPSV23 should be administered as indicated. Postmarketing reports of adverse effects in the elderly, especially those with comorbidities, have been significant enough to require hospitalization.

Adverse Reactions (Reflective of adult population; not specific for elderly) All serious adverse reactions must be reported to the U.S. Department of Health and Human Services (DHHS) Vaccine Adverse Event Reporting System (VAERS) 1-800-822-7967 or online at https://vaers.hhs.gov/esub/index.

Frequency not defined.

Central nervous system: Chills, Guillain-Barré syndrome, fever ≤102°F*, fever >102°F, headache, malaise, pain, radiculoneuropathy, seizure (febrile)

Dermatologic: Angioneurotic edema, cellulitis, rash, urticaria

Gastrointestinal: Nausea, vomiting

Hematologic: Hemolytic anemia (in patients with other hematologic disorders), leukocytosis, thrombocytopenia (in patients with stabilized ITP)

Local: Injection site reaction* (erythema, induration, swelling, soreness, warmth); peripheral edema in injected extremity

Neuromuscular & skeletal: Arthralgia, arthritis, limb mobility decreased, myalgia, paresthesia, weakness

Miscellaneous: Anaphylactoid reaction, C-reactive protein increased, lymphadenitis, lymphadenopathy, serum sickness

*Reactions most commonly reported in clinical trials.

Drug Interactions

Avoid Concomitant Use There are no known interactions where it is recommended to avoid concomitant use.

Increased Effect/Toxicity There are no known significant interactions involving an increase in effect.

Decreased Effect

Pneumococcal Polysaccharide Vaccine (Polyvalent) may decrease the levels/effects of: Zoster Vaccine

The levels/effects of Pneumococcal Polysaccharide Vaccine (Polyvalent) may be decreased by: Belimumab; Fingolimod; Immunosuppressants

Stability Store under refrigeration at 2°C to 8°C (36°F to 46°F).

PNEUMOCOCCAL POLYSACCHARIDE VACCINE (POLYVALENT)

Mechanism of Action Although there are more than 80 known pneumococcal capsular types, pneumococcal disease is mainly caused by only a few types of pneumococci. Pneumococcal vaccine contains capsular polysaccharides of 23 pneumococcal types of *Streptococcal pneumoniae* which represent at least 85% to 90% of pneumococcal disease isolates in the United States. The 23 capsular pneumococcal vaccine contains purified capsular polysaccharides of pneumococcal types 1, 2, 3, 4, 5, 6B, 7F, 8, 9N, 9V, 10A, 11A, 12F, 14, 15B, 17F, 18C, 19F, 19A, 20, 22F, 23F, and 33F.

Dosage

Geriatric

Primary immunization: I.M., SubQ: Refer to adult dosing.

Revaccination: I.M., SubQ: ≥65 years: One revaccination if ≥5 years after first dose of PPSV23 and if <65 years of age at the time of the initial vaccination (CDC, September 3, 2010).

Adult Immunization: I.M., SubQ: 0.5 mL

Revaccination: I.M., SubQ:

Immunocompetent individuals: Revaccination generally not recommended

Adults at highest risk for pneumococcal disease: One revaccination ≥5 years after first dose of PPSV23. Patients at highest risk for infection include those with asplenia or immunocompromising conditions (eg, sickle cell anemia, HIV infection, leukemia, lymphoma, Hodgkin's disease, multiple myeloma, generalized malignancy, chronic renal failure, nephrotic syndrome, solid organ transplant, and patients on immunosuppressive therapy [including corticosteroids]) (CDC, September 3, 2010; CDC, December 10, 2010).

Administration Do not inject I.V.; avoid intradermal administration (may cause severe local reactions); administer SubQ or I.M. (deltoid muscle or lateral midthigh)

For patients at risk of hemorrhage following intramuscular injection, the ACIP recommends "it should be administered intramuscularly if, in the opinion of the physician familiar with the patients bleeding risk, the vaccine can be administered by this route with reasonable safety. If the patient receives antihemophilia or other similar therapy, intramuscular vaccination can be scheduled shortly after such therapy is administered. A fine needle (23 gauge or smaller) can be used for the vaccination and firm pressure applied to the site (without rubbing) for at least 2 minutes. The patient should be instructed concerning the risk of hematoma from the injection." Patients on anticoagulant therapy should be considered to have the same bleeding risks and treated as those with clotting factor disorders (CDC, 2011).

Antipyretics have not been shown to prevent febrile seizures. Antipyretics may be used to treat fever or discomfort following vaccination (CDC, 2011). One study reported that routine prophylactic administration of acetaminophen to prevent fever prior to vaccination decreased the immune response of some vaccines; the clinical significance of this reduction in immune response has not been established (Prymula, 2009).

Simultaneous administration of vaccines helps ensure the patients will be fully vaccinated by the appropriate age. Simultaneous administration of vaccines is defined as administering >1 vaccine on the same day at different anatomic sites. Separate vaccines should not be combined in the same syringe unless indicated by product specific labeling. Separate needles and syringes should be used for each injection. The ACIP prefers each dose of a specific vaccine in a series come from the same manufacturer when possible. Adolescents and adults should be vaccinated while seated or lying down. In general, preterm infants should be vaccinated at the same chronological age as full-term infants (CDC, 2011).

Monitoring Parameters Monitor for syncope for ≥15 minutes following vaccination.

Pharmacotherapy Pearls Federal law requires that the name of medication, date of administration, the vaccine manufacturer, lot number of vaccine, and the administering person's name, title, and address be entered into the patient's permanent medical record.

Special Geriatric Considerations Elderly have ~3 times the incidence of pneumococcal pneumonia than younger adults and 30% of all pneumococcal meningitis occurs in persons >50 years of age with a 20% mortality. Limited data on the elderly; however, elderly, compared to young adults, develop slightly lower antibody titers; provides 60% to 70% protection for bacterial pneumonia. 90% protection for pneumococcal pneumonia strains; 20% of the elderly with pneumococcal pneumonia have an associated bacteremia with a 17% to 40% fatality. All persons ≥65 years of age should receive the pneumococcal vaccine including previously unvaccinated persons and persons who have not been vaccinated within 5 years. All persons of unknown vaccination status should receive one dose of vaccine. Postmarketing reports of adverse effects in the elderly, especially those with comorbidities, have been significant enough to require hospitalization.

Dosage Forms Excipient information presented when available (limited, particularly for generics); consult specific product labeling.

Injection, solution:

Pneumovax® 23: 25 mcg each of 23 capsular polysaccharide isolates/0.5 mL (0.5 mL, 2.5 mL)

Selected References

ACIP Provisional Recommendations for Use of Pneumococcal Vaccines, available at http://www.cdc.gov/vaccines/recs/provisional/downloads/pneumo-oct-2008-508.pdf.

Centers for Disease Control and Prevention (CDC), "Syncope After Vaccination – United States, January 2005-July 2007," *MMWR Morb Mortal Wkly Rep*, 2008, 57(17):457-60.

Centers for Disease Control, "Recommendations of the Advisory Committee on Immunization Practices (ACIP): General Recommendations on Immunization," *MMWR Recomm Rep*, 2006, 55(RR-15):1-48.

♦ **Pneumovax® 23** *see* Pneumococcal Polysaccharide Vaccine (Polyvalent) *on page 1474*
♦ **Podactin Cream [OTC]** *see* Miconazole *on page 1206*
♦ **Podactin Powder [OTC]** *see* Tolnaftate *on page 1827*
♦ **Polio Vaccine** *see* Poliovirus Vaccine (Inactivated) *on page 1477*
♦ **Poliovirus, Inactivated (IPV)** *see* Diphtheria and Tetanus Toxoids, Acellular Pertussis, and Poliovirus Vaccine *on page 528*

Poliovirus Vaccine (Inactivated) (POE lee oh VYE rus vak SEEN, in ak ti VAY ted)

Related Information

Immunization Administration Recommendations *on page 2037*
Immunization Recommendations *on page 2043*

Medication Safety Issues

Administration issues:

Poliovirus vaccine (inactivated) may be confused with tuberculin products. Medication errors have occurred when poliovirus vaccine (IPV) has been inadvertently administered instead of ttuberculin skin tests (PPD). These products are refrigerated and often stored in close proximity to each other.

Brand Names: U.S. IPOL®
Brand Names: Canada Imovax® Polio
Index Terms Enhanced-Potency Inactivated Poliovirus Vaccine; IPV; Polio Vaccine; Salk Vaccine
Generic Availability (U.S.) No
Pharmacologic Category Vaccine, Inactivated (Viral)
Use Active immunization against poliomyelitis caused by poliovirus types 1, 2 and 3. **Note:** Combination products containing polio vaccine are also available and may be preferred in certain age groups if recipients are likely to be susceptible to the agents contained within each vaccine.

The Advisory Committee on Immunization Practices (ACIP) recommends routine vaccination for the following:

• All children (first dose given at 2 months of age)

Routine immunization of adults in the United States is generally not recommended. Adults with previous wild poliovirus disease, who have never been immunized, or those who are incompletely immunized may receive inactivated poliovirus vaccine if they fall into one of the following categories:

• Travelers to regions or countries where poliomyelitis is endemic or epidemic
• Healthcare workers in close contact with patients who may be excreting poliovirus
• Laboratory workers handling specimens that may contain poliovirus
• Members of communities or specific population groups with diseases caused by wild poliovirus
• Incompletely vaccinated or unvaccinated adults in a household or with other close contact with children receiving oral poliovirus (may be at increased risk of vaccine associated paralytic poliomyelitis)

Contraindications Hypersensitivity to any component of the vaccine
Warnings/Precautions Patients with prior clinical poliomyelitis, incomplete immunization with oral poliovirus vaccine (OPV), HIV infection, severe combined immunodeficiency, hypogammaglobulinemia, agammaglobulinemia, or altered immunity (due to corticosteroids, alkylating agents, antimetabolites or radiation) may receive inactivated poliovirus vaccine (IPV). In general, household and close contacts of persons with altered immunocompetence may receive all age appropriate vaccines. Immune response may be decreased in patients receiving immune globulin. Vaccination may be deferred with an acute febrile illness; minor illnesses with or without a low-grade fever are not reasons to postpone vaccination. Immediate treatment for anaphylactic/anaphylactoid reaction should be available during vaccine use. In order to maximize vaccination rates, the ACIP recommends simultaneous

◀ administration of all age-appropriate vaccines (live or inactivated) for which a person is eligible at a single clinic visit, unless contraindications exist. The use of combination vaccines is generally preferred over separate injections, taking into consideration provider assessment, patient preference, and adverse events.

The injection contains 2-phenoxyethanol, calf serum protein, formaldehyde, neomycin, streptomycin, and polymyxin B; the packaging contains natural latex rubber. Use of the minimum age and minimum intervals during the first 6 months of life should only be done when the vaccine recipient is at risk for imminent exposure to circulating poliovirus (shorter intervals and earlier start dates may lead to lower seroconversion).

Adverse Reactions (Reflective of adult population; not specific for elderly) All serious adverse reactions must be reported to the U.S. Department of Health and Human Services (DHHS) Vaccine Adverse Event Reporting System (VAERS) 1-800-822-7967 or online at https://vaers.hhs.gov/esub/index. In Canada, adverse reactions may be reported to local provincial/territorial health agencies or to the Vaccine Safety Section at Public Health Agency of Canada (1-866-844-0018).

Percentages noted with concomitant administration of DTP or DTaP vaccine and observed within 48 hours of injection.

>10%:
  Central nervous system: Irritability (7% to 65%), tiredness (4% to 61%), fever ≥39°C (≤38%)
  Gastrointestinal: Anorexia (1% to 17%)
  Local: Injection Site: Tenderness (≤29%), swelling (≤11%)
1% to 10%:
  Central nervous system: Fever >39°C (≤4%)
  Gastrointestinal: Vomiting (1% to 3%)
  Local: Injection site: Erythema (≤3%)
  Miscellaneous: Persistent crying (up to 1% reported within 72 hours)

Drug Interactions

Avoid Concomitant Use There are no known interactions where it is recommended to avoid concomitant use.

Increased Effect/Toxicity There are no known significant interactions involving an increase in effect.

Decreased Effect
  The levels/effects of Poliovirus Vaccine (Inactivated) may be decreased by: Belimumab; Fingolimod; Immunosuppressants

Stability Store under refrigeration 2°C to 8°C (35°F to 46°F); do not freeze.

Dosage

Geriatric & Adult Immunization: I.M., SubQ:
  Previously unvaccinated: Two 0.5 mL doses administered at 1- to 2-month intervals, followed by a third dose 6-12 months later. If <3 months, but at least 2 months are available before protection is needed, 3 doses may be administered at least 1 month apart. If administration must be completed within 1-2 months, give 2 doses at least 1 month apart. If <1 month is available, give 1 dose.
  Incompletely vaccinated: Adults with at least 1 previous dose of OPV, <3 doses of IPV, or a combination of OPV and IPV equaling <3 doses, administer at least one 0.5 mL dose of IPV. Additional doses to complete the series may be given if time permits.
  Completely vaccinated and at increased risk of exposure: One 0.5 mL dose

Administration Do not administer I.V.; for I.M. or SubQ administration. Administer in the deltoid area to adults.

Simultaneous administration of vaccines helps ensure the patients will be fully vaccinated by the appropriate age. Simultaneous administration of vaccines is defined as administering >1 vaccine on the same day at different anatomic sites. The use of licensed combination vaccines is generally preferred over separate injections of the equivalent components. Separate vaccines should not be combined in the same syringe unless indicated by product specific labeling. Separate needles and syringes should be used for each injection. The ACIP prefers each dose of a specific vaccine in a series come from the same manufacturer when possible. Adolescents and adults should be vaccinated while seated or lying down. In general, preterm infants should be vaccinated at the same chronological age as full-term infants (CDC, 2011).

Antipyretics have not been shown to prevent febrile seizures. Antipyretics may be used to treat fever or discomfort following vaccination (CDC, 2011). One study reported that routine prophylactic administration of acetaminophen to prevent fever prior to vaccination decreased the immune response of some vaccines; the clinical significance of this reduction in immune response has not been established (Prymula, 2009).

Monitoring Parameters Monitor for syncope for ≥15 minutes following vaccination.

Test Interactions May temporarily suppress tuberculin skin test sensitivity (4-6 weeks)

Pharmacotherapy Pearls Federal law requires that the name of medication, date of administration, the vaccine manufacturer, lot number of vaccine, and the administering person's name, title, and address be entered into the patient's permanent medical record.

Currently, the primary risk for paralytic polio in U.S. residents is through travel to countries where polio remains endemic or where polio outbreaks are occurring. Unvaccinated persons traveling to countries that use OPV should be aware of the risk caused by OPV and should consider polio vaccination prior to travel.

Special Geriatric Considerations For the elderly who cannot document a primary immunization series or at risk due to contact or travel, administer the initial series. Boosters may be necessary for travel since antibody titers may diminish with age.

Dosage Forms Excipient information presented when available (limited, particularly for generics); consult specific product labeling.

Injection, suspension:

IPOL®: Type 1 poliovirus 40 D-antigen units, type 2 poliovirus 8 D-antigen units, and type 3 poliovirus 32 D-antigen units per 0.5 mL (0.5 mL, 5 mL) [contains 2-phenoxyethanol, formaldehyde, calf serum protein, neomycin (may have trace amounts), streptomycin (may have trace amounts), and polymyxin B (may have trace amounts)]

Selected References

Centers for Disease Control and Prevention, "Imported Vaccine-Associated Paralytic Poliomyelitis – United States," *MMWR Recomm Rep*, 2005, 55(RR 4):97-9.

Centers for Disease Control and Prevention, "Poliomyelitis Prevention in the United States: Updated Recommendations of the Advisory Committee on Immunization Practices (ACIP)," *MMWR Recomm Rep*, 2000, 49(RR-5):14.

Centers for Disease Control and Prevention (CDC),"Syncope After Vaccination – United States, January 2005-July 2007," *MMWR Morb Mortal Wkly Rep*, 2008, 57(17):457-60.

Polycarbophil (pol i KAR boe fil)

Brand Names: U.S. Equalactin® [OTC]; Fiber-Lax [OTC]; Fiber-Tabs™ [OTC]; FiberCon® [OTC]; Konsyl® Fiber [OTC]

Generic Availability (U.S.) Yes

Pharmacologic Category Antidiarrheal; Fiber Supplement; Laxative, Bulk-Producing

Use Treatment of constipation or diarrhea

Warnings/Precautions Use caution in patients who have difficulty swallowing; taking products without adequate fluid may cause it to swell and block throat or esophagus.

Adverse Reactions (Reflective of adult population; not specific for elderly) Frequency not defined: Gastrointestinal: Abdominal fullness

Drug Interactions

Avoid Concomitant Use

Avoid concomitant use of Polycarbophil with any of the following: Calcium Acetate

Increased Effect/Toxicity

Polycarbophil may increase the levels/effects of: Calcium Acetate; Vitamin D Analogs

The levels/effects of Polycarbophil may be increased by: Thiazide Diuretics

Decreased Effect

Polycarbophil may decrease the levels/effects of: Bisphosphonate Derivatives; Calcium Channel Blockers; DOBUTamine; Eltrombopag; Estramustine; Phosphate Supplements; Quinolone Antibiotics; Tetracycline Derivatives; Thyroid Products; Trientine

The levels/effects of Polycarbophil may be decreased by: Trientine

Mechanism of Action Restoring a more normal moisture level and providing bulk in the patient's intestinal tract

Dosage

Geriatric & Adult Constipation or diarrhea: General dosing guidelines (OTC labeling): Oral: 1250 mg calcium polycarbophil 1-4 times/day

Administration Patient should drink adequate fluids (8 oz of water or other fluids) with each dose.

Monitoring Parameters Monitor for diarrhea, abdominal pain, bowel obstruction, or impaction

Pharmacotherapy Pearls Each calcium polycarbophil tablet contains ~100 mg of absorbable elemental calcium; chewable tablets are available

Special Geriatric Considerations Elderly may have insufficient fluid intake which may predispose them to fecal impaction and bowel obstruction. Bloating and flatulence may be a problem when used short-term. Use cautiously in patients with a history of bowel impaction/obstruction.

◄ **Dosage Forms** Excipient information presented when available (limited, particularly for generics); consult specific product labeling. [DSC] = Discontinued product
Caplet, oral: Calcium polycarbophil 625 mg [equivalent to polycarbophil 500 mg]
FiberCon®: Calcium polycarbophil 625 mg [scored; contains calcium 140 mg/caplet, magnesium 10 mg/caplet; equivalent to polycarbophil 500 mg]
Konsyl® Fiber: Calcium polycarbophil 625 mg [sugar free; contains calcium 125 mg/caplet; equivalent to polycarbophil 500 mg]
Captab, oral:
Fiber-Lax: Calcium polycarbophil 625 mg [contains calcium 170 mg/caplet; equivalent to polycarbophil 500 mg]
Tablet, oral: Calcium polycarbophil 625 mg [DSC] [equivalent to polycarbophil 500 mg]
Fiber-Tabs™: Calcium polycarbophil 625 mg [scored; equivalent to polycarbophil 500 mg]
Tablet, chewable, oral:
Equalactin®: Calcium polycarbophil 625 mg [citrus flavor; equivalent to polycarbophil 500 mg]

◆ **Polycitra** see Citric Acid, Sodium Citrate, and Potassium Citrate on page 368
◆ **Poly-Dex™ [DSC]** see Neomycin, Polymyxin B, and Dexamethasone on page 1280

Polyethylene Glycol 3350 (pol i ETH i leen GLY kol 3350)

Related Information
Laxatives, Classification and Properties on page 2012
Medication Safety Issues
Sound-alike/look-alike issues:
MiraLax™ may be confused with Mirapex®
Polyethylene glycol 3350 may be confused with polyethylene glycol electrolyte solution
International issues:
MiraLax may be confused with Murelax brand name for oxazepam [Australia]
Brand Names: U.S. Dulcolax Balance® [OTC]; MiraLAX® [OTC]
Index Terms PEG
Generic Availability (U.S.) Yes
Pharmacologic Category Laxative, Osmotic
Use Treatment of occasional constipation in adults
Unlabeled/Investigational Use Bowel preparation before colonoscopy
Contraindications Hypersensitivity to polyethylene glycol or any component of the formulation
Warnings/Precautions Evaluate patients with symptoms of bowel obstruction (nausea, vomiting, abdominal pain, or distension) prior to use; avoid use in patients with known or suspected bowel obstruction. Use with caution in patients with renal impairment. Do not use for longer than 1 week; 2-4 days may be required to produce bowel movement. Prolonged, frequent, or excessive use may lead to electrolyte imbalance. When using for self medication, patients should consult healthcare provider prior to use if they have nausea, vomiting, or abdominal pain, irritable bowel syndrome, kidney disease, or a sudden change in bowel habits for >2 weeks. Patients should be instructed to discontinue use and consult healthcare provider if they have diarrhea, rectal bleeding, if abdominal pain, bloating, cramping, or nausea gets worse, or if need to use for >1 week.
Adverse Reactions (Reflective of adult population; not specific for elderly) Frequency not defined.
Dermatologic: Urticaria
Gastrointestinal: Abdominal bloating, cramping, diarrhea, flatulence, nausea
Drug Interactions
Avoid Concomitant Use There are no known interactions where it is recommended to avoid concomitant use.
Increased Effect/Toxicity There are no known significant interactions involving an increase in effect.
Decreased Effect There are no known significant interactions involving a decrease in effect.
Stability Store at room temperature before reconstitution. Dissolve powder in 4-8 ounces of water, juice, cola, or tea.
Mechanism of Action An osmotic agent, polyethylene glycol 3350 causes water retention in the stool; increases stool frequency.
Pharmacodynamics/Kinetics
Onset of action: Oral: 24-96 hours
Absorption: Minimal
Bioavailability: 0.2%
Excretion: Feces (93%); urine (0.2%)

Dosage

Geriatric & Adult

Occasional constipation: Oral: 17 g of powder (~1 heaping tablespoon) dissolved in 4-8 ounces of beverage, once daily; do not use for >1 week unless directed by healthcare provider

Bowel preparation before colonoscopy (unlabeled use): Oral: Mix 17 g of powder (~1 heaping tablespoon) in 8 ounces of clear liquid and administer the entire mixture every 10 minutes until 2 L are consumed (start within 6 hours after administering 20 mg bisacodyl delayed-release tablets) (Wexner, 2006).

Administration

Occasional constipation: Stir powder in 4-8 ounces of water, juice, soda, coffee or tea until dissolved and drink.

Bowel preparation for colonoscopy: Stir powder in 8 ounces of clear liquid until dissolved and drink.

Special Geriatric Considerations Elderly are more likely to show CNS signs of dehydration and electrolyte loss than younger adults. Therefore, monitor closely for fluid and electrolyte loss with chronic use.

Dosage Forms Excipient information presented when available (limited, particularly for generics); consult specific product labeling.

Powder for solution, oral: 17 g/dose (119 g, 238 g, 255 g, 510 g, 527 g); 17 g/packet (14s, 30s)

Dulcolax Balance®: 17 g/dose (119 g, 238 g, 510 g)

MiraLAX®: 17 g/dose (119 g, 238 g, 510 g); 17 g/packet (10s)

Selected References

Pelham RW, Nix LC, Chavira RE, et al, "Clinical Trial: Single- and Multiple-Dose Pharmacokinetics of Polyethylene Glycol (PEG-3350) in Healthy Young and Elderly Subjects," *Aliment Pharmaco Ther*, 2008, 28(2):256-65.

Wexner SD, Beck DE, Baron TH, et al, "A Consensus Document on Bowel Preparation Before Colonoscopy: Prepared by a Task Force from The American Society of Colon and Rectal Surgeons (ASCRS), The American Society for Gastrointestinal and Endoscopy (ASGE) and The Society of American Gastrointestinal and Endoscopic Surgeons (SAGES)," *Dis Colon Rectum*, 2006, 49(6):792-809.

◆ **Polyethylene Glycol-Conjugated Uricase** *see* Pegloticase *on page 1408*

Polyethylene Glycol-Electrolyte Solution and Bisacodyl
(pol i ETH i leen GLY kol ee LEK troe lite soe LOO shun & bis a KOE dil)

Related Information

Bisacodyl *on page 205*

Brand Names: U.S. HalfLytely® and Bisacodyl

Index Terms Bisacodyl and Polyethylene Glycol-Electrolyte Solution; Electrolyte Lavage Solution

Generic Availability (U.S.) No

Pharmacologic Category Laxative, Bowel Evacuant; Laxative, Stimulant

Use Bowel cleansing prior to colonoscopy

Medication Guide Available Yes

Contraindications Gastrointestinal obstruction; bowel perforation; toxic colitis; toxic mega-colon; gastric retention; ileus

Warnings/Precautions Serious arrhythmias have been reported (rarely) with the use of ionic osmotic laxative products. Use with caution in patients who may be at risk of cardiac arrhythmias (e.g. patients with a history of prolonged QT, uncontrolled arrhythmias, recent MI, unstable angina, CHF, or cardiomyopathy). Consider pre-dose and post-colonoscopy ECGs in these patients. Evaluate patients with symptoms of bowel obstruction or perforation prior to use. Correct electrolyte abnormalities in patients prior to use. Fluid and electrolyte disturbances can lead to arrhythmias, seizures, and renal impairment. Advise patients to maintain adequate hydration before, during, and after treatment. If patient becomes dehydrated or experiences significant vomiting after treatment, consider post-colonoscopy lab tests (electrolytes, creatinine, and BUN).

No additional ingredients or flavors (other than the flavor packs provided) should be added to the polyethylene glycol-electrolyte solution. Use with caution in patients with severe ulcerative colitis, or renal impairment. Observe unconscious or semiconscious patients with impaired gag reflex or those who are prone to regurgitation or aspiration during administration. Closely monitor patients with impaired renal function who develop nausea and vomiting. Generalized tonic-clonic seizures have occurred in patients without a prior history of seizures (4 L solution); use caution in patients taking medications which increase the risk for electrolyte abnormalities (eg, diuretics) and/or patients with pre-existing electrolyte abnormalities. Evaluation of electrolytes pre- and post-colonoscopy is warranted in this population. Rare cases of ischemic colitis have been reported; development of severe abdominal pain or rectal bleeding should prompt further evaluation.

Adverse Reactions (Reflective of adult population; not specific for elderly)
>10%:
Gastrointestinal: Fullness (40%), cramping (38%), nausea (34%)
Miscellaneous: Overall discomfort (57%)
1% to 10%: Gastrointestinal: Vomiting (10%)

Drug Interactions
Avoid Concomitant Use There are no known interactions where it is recommended to avoid concomitant use.
Increased Effect/Toxicity There are no known significant interactions involving an increase in effect.
Decreased Effect
The levels/effects of Polyethylene Glycol-Electrolyte Solution and Bisacodyl may be decreased by: Antacids

Ethanol/Nutrition/Herb Interactions Food: Take clear liquid diet the day of and during the bowel preparation; after consuming the solution, avoid drinking large quantities of clear liquids until colonoscopy.

Stability Store at 20°C to 25°C (68°F to 77°F); excursions permitted to 15°C to 30°C (59°F to 86°F). Fill the container with water to the fill mark; may add flavor packet provided in kit to the solution; no other ingredients should be added to the solution. Shake well. When polyethylene glycol-electrolyte solution is reconstituted, may refrigerate. Use within 48 hours.

Mechanism of Action Bisacodyl acts on the colonic mucosa to increase peristalsis throughout the large intestine. Polyethylene glycol-electrolyte solution induces catharsis through strong electrolyte and osmotic effects.

Pharmacodynamics/Kinetics See individual agents.

Dosage
Geriatric & Adult Bowel cleansing: Oral:
Bisacodyl: 5 mg as a single dose. After bowel movement or 6 hours (whichever occurs first), initiate polyethylene glycol-electrolyte solution
Polyethylene glycol-electrolyte solution: 8 ounces every 10 minutes until 2 L are consumed

Administration Administer bisacodyl tablet with water; do not chew or crush tablet. Do not take antacids within 1 hour of taking bisacodyl. Rapidly drinking the polyethylene glycol-electrolyte solution is preferred to drinking small amount continuously. If severe bloating, distention, or abdominal pain occurs, administration should be slowed or temporarily discontinued until symptoms resolve.

Monitoring Parameters Bowel movements; electrolytes, renal function

Special Geriatric Considerations Studies of this combination preparation drug included 28% of patients >65 years of age with 7% being >75 years. Rates of success appear to be lower in patients >65 years. No adjustments in dose are necessary.

Dosage Forms Excipient information presented when available (limited, particularly for generics); consult specific product labeling. [DSC]] = Discontinued product
Kit [each kit contains]:
HalfLytely® and Bisacodyl [DSC]:
Powder for solution, oral (HalfLytely®): PEG 3350 210 g, sodium bicarbonate 2.86 g, sodium chloride 5.6 g, potassium chloride 0.74 g (2000 mL) [sulfate-free; cherry, lemon-lime, orange flavor] [DSC]
Tablet, delayed release (Bisacodyl): 5 mg (2s) [DSC]
HalfLytely® and Bisacodyl:
Powder for solution, oral (HalfLytely®): PEG 3350 210 g, sodium bicarbonate 2.86 g, sodium chloride 5.6 g, potassium chloride 0.74 g (2000 mL) [contains 4 flavor packs (each 1 g) cherry, lemon-lime, orange, pineapple flavors]
Tablet, delayed release (Bisacodyl): 5 mg (1s)

Selected References
DiPalma JA, McGowan J, and Cleveland M, "Clinical Trial: An Efficacy Evaluation of Reduced Bisacodyl Given as Part of a Polyethylene Glycol Electrolyte Solution Preparation Prior to Colonoscopy," *Aliment Pharmacol Ther*, 2007, 26 (8):113-9.
DiPalma JA, Wolff BG, Meagher A, et al, "Comparison of Reduced Volume Versus Four Liters Sulfate-Free Electrolyte Lavage Solutions for Colonoscopy Colon Cleansing," *Am J Gastroenterol*, 2003, 98(10):2187-91.

◆ **Polyethylene Glycol Interferon Alfa-2b** *see* Peginterferon Alfa-2b *on page 1403*
◆ **Poly-Iron 150 Forte** *see* Polysaccharide-Iron Complex, Vitamin B12, and Folic Acid *on page 1483*
◆ **Polymyxin B and Neomycin** *see* Neomycin and Polymyxin B *on page 1279*
◆ **Polymyxin B, Neomycin, and Dexamethasone** *see* Neomycin, Polymyxin B, and Dexamethasone *on page 1280*
◆ **Polymyxin B, Neomycin, and Gramicidin** *see* Neomycin, Polymyxin B, and Gramicidin *on page 1282*

♦ **Polysaccharide Iron 150 Forte** *see* Polysaccharide-Iron Complex, Vitamin B12, and Folic Acid *on page 1483*

Polysaccharide-Iron Complex, Vitamin B12, and Folic Acid
(pol i SAK a ride-EYE ern KOM pleks, VYE ta min bee twelve & FOE lik AS id)

Related Information
Folic Acid *on page 781*
Brand Names: U.S. Ferrex™ 150 Forte; Ferrex™ 150 Forte Plus; Maxaron® Forte; Poly-Iron 150 Forte; Polysaccharide Iron 150 Forte
Index Terms Iron-Polysaccharide Complex, Vitamin B12, and Folic Acid
Generic Availability (U.S.) No
Pharmacologic Category Iron Salt
Use Prevention and treatment of iron-deficiency anemias and/or nutritional megaloblastic anemias
Warnings/Precautions [U.S. Boxed Warning]: Accidental overdose of iron-containing products is a leading cause of fatal poisoning in children under 6 years of age. Keep this product out of the reach of children. In case of accidental overdose call the poison control center immediately. Not appropriate for use with pernicious, aplastic, or normocytic anemias when anemia is present with vitamin B_{12} deficiency. Folate doses >0.1 mg/day may obscure pernicious anemia.
Adverse Reactions (Reflective of adult population; not specific for elderly) Frequency not defined.
Gastrointestinal: Abdominal pain, constipation, dark stools, diarrhea, epigastric pain, GI irritation, nausea, stomach cramping, vomiting
Genitourinary: Discolored urine
Miscellaneous: Hypersensitivity reaction
Drug Interactions
Avoid Concomitant Use
Avoid concomitant use of Polysaccharide-Iron Complex, Vitamin B12, and Folic Acid with any of the following: Dimercaprol; Raltitrexed
Increased Effect/Toxicity
The levels/effects of Polysaccharide-Iron Complex, Vitamin B12, and Folic Acid may be increased by: Dimercaprol
Decreased Effect
Polysaccharide-Iron Complex, Vitamin B12, and Folic Acid may decrease the levels/effects of: Bisphosphonate Derivatives; Cefdinir; Eltrombopag; Fosphenytoin; Levodopa; Levothyroxine; Methyldopa; Penicillamine; PHENobarbital; Phenytoin; Phosphate Supplements; Primidone; Quinolone Antibiotics; Raltitrexed; Tetracycline Derivatives; Trientine

The levels/effects of Polysaccharide-Iron Complex, Vitamin B12, and Folic Acid may be decreased by: Antacids; Green Tea; H2-Antagonists; Pancrelipase; Proton Pump Inhibitors; Trientine
Stability Store at 25°C (77°F); excursions permitted to 15°C to 30°C (59°F to 86°F).
Poly-Iron 150 Forte: Store at 15°C to 30°C (59°F to 86°F).
Dosage
Geriatric & Adult Iron deficiency (prevention/treatment): Oral: 1-2 capsules daily
Dosage Forms Excipient information presented when available (limited, particularly for generics); consult specific product labeling.
Capsule, oral:
Ferrex™ 150 Forte: Elemental iron 150 mg, cyanocobalamin 25 mcg, and folic acid 1 mg
Ferrex™ 150 Forte Plus: Elemental iron 150 mg (50 mg as ferrous asparto glycinate), cyanocobalamin 25 mcg, and folic acid 1 mg [contains ascorbic acid 60 mg and succinic acid 50 mg]
Maxaron® Forte: Elemental iron 150 mg (80 mg as ferrous bisglycinate), cyanocobalamin 25 mcg, and folic acid 1 mg [contains ascorbic acid 60 mg]
Poly-Iron 150 Forte: Elemental iron 150 mg, cyanocobalamin 25 mcg, and folic acid 1 mg
Polysaccharide Iron 150 Forte: Elemental iron 150 mg, cyanocobalamin 25 mcg, and folic acid 1 mg
Selected References
"Dietary Reference Intakes for Vitamin A, Vitamin K, Arsenic, Boron, Chromium, Copper, Iodine, Iron, Manganese, Molybdenum, Nickel, Silicon, Vanadium, and Zinc." Standing Committee on the Scientific Evaluation of Dietary Reference Intakes, Food and Nutrition Board, Institute of Medicine, National Academy of Sciences, Washington, DC: National Academy Press, 2000. Available at http://www.nap.edu.

♦ **Polyvinyl Alcohol** *see* Artificial Tears *on page 148*
♦ **P-OM3** *see* Omega-3-Acid Ethyl Esters *on page 1338*
♦ **Ponstel®** *see* Mefenamic Acid *on page 1125*

Posaconazole (poe sa KON a zole)

Medication Safety Issues
Sound-alike/look-alike issues:
Noxafil® may be confused with minoxidil
International issues:
Noxafil [U.S. and multiple international markets] may be confused with Noxidil brand name for minoxidil [Thailand]

Brand Names: U.S. Noxafil®

Brand Names: Canada Posanol™

Index Terms SCH 56592

Generic Availability (U.S.) No

Pharmacologic Category Antifungal Agent, Oral

Use Prophylaxis of invasive *Aspergillus* and *Candida* infections in severely-immunocompromised patients [eg, hematopoietic stem cell transplant (HSCT) recipients with graft-versus-host disease (GVHD) or those with prolonged neutropenia secondary to chemotherapy for hematologic malignancies]; treatment of oropharyngeal candidiasis (including patients refractory to itraconazole and/or fluconazole)

Unlabeled/Investigational Use Salvage therapy of refractory or relapsed invasive fungal infections; mucormycosis; pulmonary infection (nonimmunosuppressed)

Contraindications Hypersensitivity to posaconazole, other azole antifungals, or any component of the formulation; coadministration of cisapride, ergot alkaloids, pimozide, quinidine, simvastatin, or sirolimus

Warnings/Precautions Hepatic dysfunction has occurred, ranging from reversible mild/moderate increases of ALT, AST, alkaline phosphatase, total bilirubin, and/or clinical hepatitis to severe reactions (cholestasis, hepatic failure including death). Consider discontinuation of therapy in patients who develop clinical evidence of liver disease that may be secondary to posaconazole. Use caution in patients with an increased risk of arrhythmia (long QT syndrome, concurrent QT_c-prolonging drugs, hypokalemia). Correct electrolyte abnormalities (eg, potassium, magnesium, and calcium) before initiating therapy. Concurrent use with cyclosporine or tacrolimus may significantly increase cyclosporine/tacrolimus concentrations and may result in rare serious adverse events (eg, nephrotoxicity, leukoencephalopathy, and death); dose reduction and close monitoring are recommended with initiation of posaconazole therapy. Concurrent use with midazolam may increase midazolam concentrations and potentiate midazolam-related adverse effects.

Use caution in hypersensitivity with other azole antifungal agents; cross-reaction may occur, but has not been established. Consider alternative therapy or closely monitor for breakthrough fungal infections in patients receiving drugs that decrease absorption or increase the metabolism of posaconazole or in any patient unable to eat or tolerate an oral liquid nutritional supplement. Use caution in severe renal impairment or GI disturbances; monitor for breakthrough fungal infections.

Adverse Reactions (Reflective of adult population; not specific for elderly) Note: Percentages reflect data from use in comparator trials with multiple concomitant conditions and medications; some adverse reactions may be due to underlying condition(s).
>10%:
Cardiovascular: Hypertension (18%), edema (9% to 15%), hypotension (14%), tachycardia (12%)
Central nervous system: Fever (6% to 45%), headache (8% to 28%), fatigue (3% to 17%), insomnia (1% to 17%), dizziness (11%), pain (1% to 11%)
Endocrine & metabolic: Hypokalemia (≤30%), hypomagnesemia (18%), dehydration (1% to 11%), hyperglycemia (11%)
Gastrointestinal: Diarrhea (10% to 42%), nausea (9% to 38%), vomiting (7% to 29%), abdominal pain (5% to 27%), constipation (21%), anorexia (2% to 19%), mucositis (17%), weight loss (1% to 14%), oral candidiasis (1% to 12%)
Hematologic: Thrombocytopenia (29%), anemia (2% to 25%), neutropenia (4% to 23%), neutropenic fever (20%)
Hepatic: ALT increased (6% to 17%)
Neuromuscular & skeletal: Rigors (≤20%), musculoskeletal pain (16%), weakness (2% to 13%), arthralgia (11%)
Respiratory: Cough (3% to 25%), dyspnea (1% to 20%), epistaxis (14%), pharyngitis (12%)
Miscellaneous: Bacteremia (18%), herpes simplex (3% to 15%), CMV infection (14%)
1% to 10%:
Central nervous system: Anxiety (9%)
Endocrine & metabolic: Hypocalcemia (9%)
Gastrointestinal: Dyspepsia (10%)
Genitourinary: Vaginal hemorrhage (10%)

Hepatic: Hyperbilirubinemia (7% to 10%), AST increased (3% to 4%), alkaline phosphatase increased (1% to 3%)

Neuromuscular & skeletal: Back pain (10%)

Respiratory: Pneumonia (3% to 10%), upper respiratory infection (7%)

Miscellaneous: Diaphoresis (2% to 10%)

Drug Interactions

Metabolism/Transport Effects Inhibits CYP3A4 (strong)

Avoid Concomitant Use

Avoid concomitant use of Posaconazole with any of the following: Alfuzosin; Cisapride; Conivaptan; Crizotinib; Dofetilide; Dronedarone; Efavirenz; Eplerenone; Ergot Derivatives; Everolimus; Fluticasone (Oral Inhalation); Halofantrine; Lapatinib; Lovastatin; Lurasidone; Nilotinib; Nisoldipine; Pimozide; Proton Pump Inhibitors; QuiNIDine; Ranolazine; Rivaroxaban; RomiDEPsin; Salmeterol; Silodosin; Simvastatin; Sirolimus; Tamsulosin; Ticagrelor; Tolvaptan; Toremifene

Increased Effect/Toxicity

Posaconazole may increase the levels/effects of: Alfentanil; Alfuzosin; Almotriptan; Alosetron; Antineoplastic Agents (Vinca Alkaloids); Aprepitant; Benzodiazepines (metabolized by oxidation); Boceprevir; Bortezomib; Bosentan; Brentuximab Vedotin; Brinzolamide; Budesonide (Nasal); Budesonide (Systemic, Oral Inhalation); BusPIRone; Busulfan; Calcium Channel Blockers; CarBAMazepine; Cardiac Glycosides; Ciclesonide; Cilostazol; Cinacalcet; Cisapride; Colchicine; Conivaptan; Corticosteroids (Orally Inhaled); Corticosteroids (Systemic); Crizotinib; CycloSPORINE; CycloSPORINE (Systemic); CYP3A4 Substrates; Dienogest; DOCEtaxel; Dofetilide; Dronedarone; Dutasteride; Eletriptan; Eplerenone; Ergot Derivatives; Erlotinib; Eszopiclone; Etravirine; Everolimus; FentaNYL; Fesoterodine; Fluticasone (Nasal); Fluticasone (Oral Inhalation); Fosamprenavir; Fosaprepitant; Fosphenytoin; Gefitinib; GlipiZIDE; GuanFACINE; Halofantrine; HMG-CoA Reductase Inhibitors; Iloperidone; Imatinib; Irinotecan; Ixabepilone; Lapatinib; Losartan; Lovastatin; Lumefantrine; Lurasidone; Macrolide Antibiotics; Maraviroc; Methadone; MethylPREDNISolone; Nilotinib; Nisoldipine; Paricalcitol; Pazopanib; Phenytoin; Phosphodiesterase 5 Inhibitors; Pimecrolimus; Pimozide; Protease Inhibitors; QuiNIDine; Ramelteon; Ranolazine; Repaglinide; Rifamycin Derivatives; Rivaroxaban; RomiDEPsin; Salmeterol; Saxagliptin; Sildenafil; Silodosin; Simvastatin; Sirolimus; Solifenacin; SORAfenib; SUNItinib; Tacrolimus; Tacrolimus (Systemic); Tacrolimus (Topical); Tadalafil; Tamsulosin; Telaprevir; Temsirolimus; Ticagrelor; Tolterodine; Tolvaptan; Toremifene; Vardenafil; Vemurafenib; Vilazodone; Vitamin K Antagonists; Ziprasidone; Zolpidem

The levels/effects of Posaconazole may be increased by: Boceprevir; Etravirine; Grapefruit Juice; Macrolide Antibiotics; Protease Inhibitors; Tacrolimus; Telaprevir

Decreased Effect

Posaconazole may decrease the levels/effects of: Amphotericin B; Prasugrel; Saccharomyces boulardii; Ticagrelor

The levels/effects of Posaconazole may be decreased by: Didanosine; Efavirenz; Etravirine; Fosamprenavir; Fosphenytoin; H2-Antagonists; Metoclopramide; Phenytoin; Proton Pump Inhibitors; Rifamycin Derivatives; Sucralfate

Ethanol/Nutrition/Herb Interactions Food: Bioavailability increased ~3 times when posaconazole is administered with a nonfat meal or an oral liquid nutritional supplement; increased ~4 times when administered with a high-fat meal. Grapefruit juice may decrease the levels/effects of posaconazole; concurrent use should be avoided.

Stability Store at 25°C (77°F); excursions permitted to 15°C to 30°C (59°F to 86°F). Do not freeze.

Mechanism of Action Interferes with fungal cytochrome P450 (latosterol-14α-demethylase) activity, decreasing ergosterol synthesis (principal sterol in fungal cell membrane) and inhibiting fungal cell membrane formation.

Pharmacodynamics/Kinetics

Absorption: Coadministration with food, liquid nutritional supplements, and/or acidic carbonated beverages (eg, ginger ale) increases absorption; fasting states do not provide sufficient absorption to ensure adequate plasma concentrations.

Distribution: V_d: 465-1774 L

Protein binding: >98%; predominantly bound to albumin

Metabolism: Not significantly metabolized; ~15% to 17% undergoes non-CYP-mediated metabolism, primarily via hepatic glucuronidation into metabolites

Half-life elimination: 35 hours (range: 20-66 hours)

Time to peak, plasma: ~3-5 hours

Excretion: Feces 71% to 77% (~66% of the total dose as unchanged drug); urine 13% to 14% (<0.2% of the total dose as unchanged drug)

◀ **Dosage**
Geriatric & Adult
Aspergillosis, invasive: Oral:
Prophylaxis: 200 mg 3 times/day; duration of therapy is based on based on recovery from neutropenia or immunosuppression
Salvage treatment of refractory infection (unlabeled use): 200 mg 4 times/day initially; after disease stabilization may decrease frequency to 400 mg 2 times/day (Walsh, 2007). **Note:** Duration of therapy should be a minimum of 6-12 weeks or throughout period of immunosuppression (Walsh, 2008).

Candidal infections: Oral:
Prophylaxis: 200 mg 3 times/day; duration of therapy is based on recovery from neutropenia or immunosuppression
Treatment of oropharyngeal infection: Initial: 100 mg 2 times/day for 1 day; maintenance: 100 mg once daily for 13 days
Treatment of refractory oropharyngeal infection: 400 mg 2 times/day; duration of therapy is based on underlying disease and clinical response

Mucormycosis (unlabeled use): Oral: 800 mg/day in 2 or 4 divided doses; duration of therapy is based on response and risk of relapse due to immunosuppression (Greenburg, 2006)

Cryptococcal infections: Oral:
Pulmonary, nonimmunosuppressed (unlabeled use): 400 mg 2 times/day. **Note:** Fluconazole is considered first-line treatment (Perfect, 2010).
Salvage treatment of relapsed infection (unlabeled use): 400 mg 2 times/day (or 200 mg 4 times/day) for 10-12 weeks. **Note:** Salvage treatment should only be started after an appropriate course of an induction regimen (Perfect, 2010).

Renal Impairment
Mild-to-moderate renal insufficiency (Cl$_{cr}$ 20-80 mL/minute/1.73 m^2): No adjustment necessary
Severe renal insufficiency (Cl$_{cr}$ <20 mL/minute/1.73 m^2): No adjustment necessary; however, monitor for breakthrough fungal infections due to variability in posaconazole exposure.

Hepatic Impairment
Mild-to-severe hepatic insufficiency (Child-Pugh classes A, B, and C): No adjustment necessary.
Clinical signs and symptoms of liver disease due to posaconazole: Consider discontinuing therapy.

Administration Oral: Shake well before use. Must be administered during or within 20 minutes following a full meal or an oral liquid nutritional supplement; alternatively, posaconazole may be administered with an acidic carbonated beverage (eg, ginger ale). In patients able to swallow, administer oral suspension using dosing spoon provided by the manufacturer; spoon should be rinsed clean with water after each use and before storage.

Monitoring Parameters Hepatic function (eg, AST/ALT, alkaline phosphatase and bilirubin) prior to initiation and during treatment; renal function; electrolyte disturbances (eg, calcium, magnesium, potassium); CBC

Special Geriatric Considerations Dosage adjustment not necessary.

Dosage Forms Excipient information presented when available (limited, particularly for generics); consult specific product labeling.
Suspension, oral:
Noxafil®: 40 mg/mL (123 mL) [contains sodium benzoate; cherry flavor; delivers 105 mL of suspension]

Selected References
Walsh TJ, Anaissie EJ, Denning DW, et al, "Treatment of Aspergillosis: Clinical Practice Guidelines of the Infectious Diseases Society of America," *Clin Infect Dis*, 2008, 46(3):327-60.

◆ **Posture® [OTC]** *see* Calcium Salts (Oral) *on page 256*

Potassium Acid Phosphate (poe TASS ee um AS id FOS fate)

Brand Names: U.S. K-Phos® Original
Generic Availability (U.S.) No
Pharmacologic Category Urinary Acidifying Agent
Use Acidifies urine and lowers urinary calcium concentration; reduces odor and rash caused by ammoniacal urine; increases the antibacterial activity of methenamine
Contraindications Severe renal impairment; hyperkalemia, hyperphosphatemia; infected magnesium ammonium phosphate stones

Warnings/Precautions Use with caution in patients receiving concomitant medications or therapies that increase potassium (eg, ACEI, potassium-sparing diuretics, potassium containing salt substitutes). Use caution in patients with renal insufficiency or severe tissue breakdown (eg, chemotherapy or hemodialysis). May cause GI upset (eg, nausea, vomiting, diarrhea, abdominal pain, discomfort) and lead to GI ulceration, bleeding, perforation and/or obstruction. Close monitoring of serum potassium concentrations is needed to avoid hyperkalemia.

Adverse Reactions (Reflective of adult population; not specific for elderly)
>10%: Gastrointestinal: Diarrhea, nausea, stomach pain, flatulence, vomiting
1% to 10%:
Cardiovascular: Bradycardia
Endocrine & metabolic: Hyperkalemia
Local: Local tissue necrosis with extravasation
Neuromuscular & skeletal: Weakness
Respiratory: Dyspnea

Drug Interactions
Avoid Concomitant Use There are no known interactions where it is recommended to avoid concomitant use.
Increased Effect/Toxicity
Potassium Acid Phosphate may increase the levels/effects of: ACE Inhibitors; Angiotensin II Receptor Blockers; Potassium-Sparing Diuretics

The levels/effects of Potassium Acid Phosphate may be increased by: Eplerenone
Decreased Effect There are no known significant interactions involving a decrease in effect.

Mechanism of Action The principal intracellular cation; involved in transmission of nerve impulses, muscle contractions, enzyme activity, and glucose utilization

Pharmacodynamics/Kinetics
Absorption: Well absorbed from upper GI tract
Distribution: Enters cells via active transport from extracellular fluid
Excretion: Primarily urine; skin and feces (small amounts); most intestinal potassium reabsorbed

Dosage
Geriatric & Adult Urine acidification: Oral: 1000 mg dissolved in 6-8 oz of water 4 times/day with meals and at bedtime; for best results, soak tablets in water for 2-5 minutes, then stir and swallow

Monitoring Parameters Serum potassium, sodium, phosphate, calcium; serum salicylates (if taking salicylates); signs of muscle weakness, cramps

Reference Range Note: Reference ranges may vary depending on the laboratory
Serum phosphorus: Both low and high ends of the normal range are higher in children than in adults.
Infants: 4.5-7.5 mg/dL (1.45-2.42 mmol/L)
Children: ~4-6 mg/dL (1.29-1.94 mmol/L)
Adults: 2.5-4.5 mg/dL (0.81-1.45 mmol/L)
Urinary pH: 4.6-8.0

Test Interactions Decreased ammonia (B)

Special Geriatric Considerations A complete drug history should be taken to rule out potential drug interactions since the elderly frequently may be taking potassium and potassium-sparing diuretics, salicylates, or antacids. Use with caution in renal impairment (low Cl$_{cr}$).

Dosage Forms Excipient information presented when available (limited, particularly for generics); consult specific product labeling.
Tablet, oral:
K-Phos® Original: 500 mg [scored; phosphorus 114 mg and potassium 144 mg (3.7 mEq) per tablet]

Potassium Chloride (poe TASS ee um KLOR ide)

Medication Safety Issues
Sound-alike/look-alike issues:
Kaon-Cl-10® may be confused with kaolin
KCl may be confused with HCl
Klor-Con® may be confused with Klaron®

◀ microK® may be confused with Macrobid®, Micronase®

High alert medication:
The Institute for Safe Medication Practices (ISMP) includes this medication (I.V. formulation) among its list of drugs which have a heightened risk of causing significant patient harm when used in error.

Other safety concerns:
Per JCAHO recommendations, concentrated electrolyte solutions should not be available in patient care areas.

Consider special storage requirements for intravenous potassium salts; I.V. potassium salts have been administered IVP in error, leading to fatal outcomes.

Brand Names: U.S. Epiklor™; Epiklor™/25; K-Tab®; Kaon-CL® 10; Klor-Con®; Klor-Con® 10; Klor-Con® 8; Klor-Con® M10; Klor-Con® M15; Klor-Con® M20; Klor-Con®/25; microK®; microK® 10

Brand Names: Canada Apo-K®; K-10®; K-Dur®; Micro-K Extencaps®; Roychlor®; Slo-Pot; Slow-K®

Index Terms KCl; Kdur

Generic Availability (U.S.) Yes: Excludes powder for solution

Pharmacologic Category Electrolyte Supplement, Oral; Electrolyte Supplement, Parenteral

Use Treatment or prevention of hypokalemia

Contraindications Hypersensitivity to any component of the formulation; hyperkalemia. In addition, solid oral dosage forms are contraindicated in patients in whom there is a structural, pathological, and/or pharmacologic cause for delay or arrest in passage through the GI tract.

Warnings/Precautions Close monitoring of serum potassium concentrations is needed to avoid hyperkalemia. Use with caution in patients with renal impairment, cardiac disease, acid/base disorders, or potassium-altering conditions/disorders. Use with caution in digitalized patients or patients receiving concomitant medications or therapies that increase potassium (eg, ACEI, potassium-sparing diuretics, potassium containing salt substitutes). Do **NOT** administer undiluted or I.V. push; inappropriate parenteral administration may be fatal. Always administer potassium further diluted; refer to appropriate dilution and administration rate recommendations. Pain and phlebitis may occur during parenteral infusion requiring a decrease in infusion rate or potassium concentration. Avoid administering potassium diluted in dextrose solutions during initial therapy; potential for transient decreases in serum potassium due to intracellular shift of potassium from dextrose-stimulated insulin release. May cause GI upset (eg, nausea, vomiting, diarrhea, abdominal pain, discomfort) and lead to GI ulceration, bleeding, perforation, and/or obstruction. Oral liquid preparations (not solid) should be used in patients with esophageal compression or delayed gastric emptying.

Adverse Reactions (Reflective of adult population; not specific for elderly) Frequency not defined.

Dermatologic: Rash

Endocrine & metabolic: Hyperkalemia

Gastrointestinal: Abdominal pain/discomfort, diarrhea, flatulence, GI bleeding (oral), GI obstruction (oral), GI perforation (oral), nausea, vomiting

Drug Interactions

Avoid Concomitant Use
Avoid concomitant use of Potassium Chloride with any of the following: Glycopyrrolate

Increased Effect/Toxicity
Potassium Chloride may increase the levels/effects of: ACE Inhibitors; Angiotensin II Receptor Blockers; Potassium-Sparing Diuretics

The levels/effects of Potassium Chloride may be increased by: Anticholinergic Agents; Eplerenone; Glycopyrrolate

Decreased Effect There are no known significant interactions involving a decrease in effect.

Stability
Capsule: MicroK®: Store between 20°C to 25°C (68°F to 77°F).

Powder for oral solution: Klor-Con®: Store at room temperature of 15°C to 30°C (59°F to 86°F).

Solution for injection: Store at room temperature; do not freeze. Use only clear solutions. Use admixtures within 24 hours.

Tablet: K-Tab®: Store below 30°C (86°F).

Mechanism of Action Potassium is the major cation of intracellular fluid and is essential for the conduction of nerve impulses in heart, brain, and skeletal muscle; contraction of cardiac, skeletal and smooth muscles; maintenance of normal renal function, acid-base balance, carbohydrate metabolism, and gastric secretion

Pharmacodynamics/Kinetics

Absorption: Well absorbed from upper GI tract

Distribution: Enters cells via active transport from extracellular fluid

Excretion: Primarily urine; skin and feces (small amounts); most intestinal potassium reabsorbed

Dosage

Geriatric & Adult I.V. doses should be incorporated into the patient's maintenance I.V. fluids; intermittent I.V. potassium administration should be reserved for severe depletion situations in patients undergoing ECG monitoring. Doses expressed as mEq of potassium.

Normal daily requirements: *Oral, I.V.:* 40-80 mEq/day

Prevention of hypokalemia: *Oral:* 20-40 mEq/day in 1-2 divided doses

Treatment of hypokalemia:

Oral:

Asymptomatic, mild hypokalemia: Usual dosage range: 40-100 mEq/day divided in 2-5 doses; generally recommended to limit doses to 20-25 mEq/dose to avoid GI discomfort.

Mild-to-moderate hypokalemia: Some clinicians may administer up to 120-240 mEq/day divided in 3-4 doses; generally recommended to limit doses to 40-60 mEq/dose. If deficits are severe or ongoing losses are great, I.V. route should be considered.

I.V. intermittent infusion: Peripheral or central line: ≤10 mEq/hour; repeat as needed based on frequently obtained lab values; central line infusion and continuous ECG monitoring highly recommended for infusions >10 mEq/hour.

Potassium dosage/rate of infusion general guidelines (per product labeling): **Note:** High variability exists in dosing/infusion rate recommendations; therapy guided by patient condition and specific institutional guidelines.

Serum potassium >2.5 mEq/L: Maximum infusion rate: 10 mEq/hour; maximum concentration: 40 mEq/L; maximum 24-hour dose: 200 mEq

Serum potassium <2 mEq/L and symptomatic (excluding emergency treatment of cardiac arrest): Maximum infusion rate (central line only): 40 mEq/hour in presence of continuous ECG monitoring and frequent lab monitoring; In selected situations, patients may require up to 400 mEq/24 hours.

Administration

Parenteral: Potassium must be diluted prior to parenteral administration. Do not administer I.V. push. In general, the dose, concentration of infusion and rate of administration may be dependant on patient condition and specific institution policy. Some clinicians recommend that the maximum concentration for peripheral infusion is 10 mEq/100 mL and maximum rate of administration for peripheral infusion is 10 mEq/hour. ECG monitoring is recommended for peripheral or central infusions >10 mEq/hour in adults. Concentrations and rates of infusion may be greater with central line administration. Some clinicians recommend that the maximum concentration for central infusion is 20-40 mEq/100 mL and maximum rate of administration for central infusion is 40 mEq/hour.

Oral: Oral dosage forms should be taken with meals and a full glass of water or other liquid.

Capsule: MicroK®: Swallow whole, do not chew. Capsules may also be opened and contents sprinkled on a spoonful of applesauce or pudding and should be swallowed immediately without chewing. No more than 20 mEq should be given as a single dose.

Powder: Klor-Con®: Dissolve in 4-5 ounces of water or other beverage prior to administration.

Tablet:

K-Tab®, Kaon-Cl®, Klor-Con®: Swallow tablets whole; do not crush, chew or suck on tablet. No more than 20 mEq should be given as a single dose.

Klor-Con® M: Tablet may also be broken in half and each half swallowed separately; the whole tablet may be dissolved in ~4 ounces of water (allow ~2 minutes to dissolve, stir well and drink immediately)

Monitoring Parameters Serum potassium, glucose, chloride, pH, urine output (if indicated), cardiac monitor (if intermittent infusion or potassium infusion rates >10 mEq/hour in adults)

Reference Range Note: Reference ranges may vary depending on the laboratory

Serum potassium: 3.5-5.2 mEq/L

Special Geriatric Considerations Elderly may require less potassium than younger adults due to decreased renal function. For the elderly who do not respond to replacement therapy, check serum magnesium. Long-term use of diuretics may result in hypomagnesemic.

Dosage Forms Excipient information presented when available (limited, particularly for generics); consult specific product labeling. [DSC] = Discontinued product

Capsule, extended release, microencapsulated, oral: 8 mEq, 10 mEq

microK®: 8 mEq [600 mg]

microK® 10: 10 mEq [750 mg]

Infusion, premixed in 1/2 NS: 20 mEq (1000 mL)

Infusion, premixed in D_{10} 1/4 NS: 5 mEq (250 mL)

◀ Infusion, premixed in D_5 1/2 NS: 10 mEq (500 mL, 1000 mL); 20 mEq (1000 mL); 30 mEq (1000 mL); 40 mEq (1000 mL)

Infusion, premixed in D_5 1/3 NS: 10 mEq (500 mL [DSC]); 20 mEq (1000 mL)

Infusion, premixed in D_5 1/4 NS: 5 mEq (250 mL); 10 mEq (500 mL, 1000 mL); 20 mEq (1000 mL); 30 mEq (1000 mL); 40 mEq (1000 mL)

Infusion, premixed in D_5LR: 20 mEq (1000 mL); 40 mEq (1000 mL [DSC])

Infusion, premixed in D_5NS: 20 mEq (1000 mL); 40 mEq (1000 mL)

Infusion, premixed in D_5W: 20 mEq (1000 mL); 30 mEq (1000 mL [DSC]); 40 mEq (1000 mL)

Infusion, premixed in NS: 20 mEq (1000 mL); 40 mEq (1000 mL)

Infusion, premixed in water for injection [highly concentrated]: 10 mEq (50 mL, 100 mL); 20 mEq (50 mL, 100 mL); 30 mEq (100 mL); 40 mEq (100 mL)

Injection, solution [concentrate]: 2 mEq/mL (5 mL, 10 mL, 15 mL, 20 mL, 30 mL, 250 mL, 500 mL)

Injection, solution [concentrate, preservative free]: 2 mEq/mL (5 mL, 10 mL, 15 mL, 20 mL)

Powder for solution, oral:

    Epiklor™: 20 mEq/packet (30s, 100s) [sugar free; orange flavor]

    Epiklor™/25: 25 mEq/packet (30s, 100s) [sugar free; orange flavor]

    Klor-Con®: 20 mEq/packet (30s, 100s) [sugar free; fruit flavor]

    Klor-Con®/25: 25 mEq/packet (30s, 100s) [sugar free; fruit flavor]

Solution, oral: 20 mEq/15 mL (15 mL, 30 mL, 473 mL); 40 mEq/15 mL (15 mL, 473 mL)

Tablet, extended release, microencapsulated, oral: 8 mEq, 10 mEq, 20 mEq

    Klor-Con® M10: 10 mEq [750 mg]

    Klor-Con® M15: 15 mEq [scored; 1125 mg]

    Klor-Con® M20: 20 mEq [scored; 1500 mg]

Tablet, extended release, wax matrix, oral: 8 mEq, 10 mEq

    K-Tab®: 10 mEq [750 mg]

    Kaon-CL® 10: 10 mEq [750 mg]

    Klor-Con® 8: 8 mEq [600 mg]

    Klor-Con® 10: 10 mEq [750 mg]

Selected References

Alfonzo AV, Isles C, Geddes C, et al, "Potassium Disorders – Clinical Spectrum and Emergency Management," *Resuscitation*, 2006, 70(1):10-25.

ASPEN Board of Directors and the Clinical Guidelines Task Force, "Guidelines for the Use of Parenteral and Enteral Nutrition in Adult and Pediatric Patients," *JPEN J Parenter Enteral Nutr*, 2002, 26(1 Suppl):22-4.

ASPEN Board of Directors and the Clinical Guidelines Task Force, "Guidelines for the Use of Parenteral and Enteral Nutrition in Adult and Pediatric Patients," *JPEN J Parenter Enteral Nutr*, 2002, 26(1 Suppl):25-32.

"Dietary Reference Intakes for Water, Potassium, Sodium, Chloride, and Sulfate. Standing Committee on the Scientific Evaluation of Dietary Reference Intakes, Food and Nutrition Board, Institute of Medicine," National Academy of Sciences, Washington, DC: National Academy Press, 2004. Available at http://www.nap.edu.

Joint Commission on Accreditation of Healthcare Organizations, "2005 National Patient Safety Goals," available at http://www.jcaho.org/accredited+organizations/patient+safety/05_npsg_guidelines Last accessed October 15, 2004.

Weiss-Guillet EM, Takala J, and Jakob SM, "Diagnosis and Management of Electrolyte Emergencies," *Best Pract Res Clin Endocrinol Metab*, 2003, 17(4):623-51.

◆ **Potassium Citrate, Citric Acid, and Sodium Citrate** *see* Citric Acid, Sodium Citrate, and Potassium Citrate *on page 368*

Potassium Gluconate (poe TASS ee um GLOO coe nate)

Generic Availability (U.S.) Yes

Pharmacologic Category Electrolyte Supplement, Oral

Use Treatment or prevention of hypokalemia

Contraindications Severe renal impairment, untreated Addison's disease, heat cramps, hyperkalemia, severe tissue trauma; solid oral dosage forms are contraindicated in patients in whom there is a structural, pathological, and/or pharmacologic cause for delay or arrest in passage through the GI tract

Warnings/Precautions Use caution in patients with acid/base disorders, cardiovascular disease, potassium-altering conditions/disorders, or renal impairment. Use with caution in patients receiving concomitant medications or therapies that increase potassium (eg, ACEI, potassium-sparing diuretics, potassium containing salt substitutes). Close monitoring of serum potassium concentrations is needed to avoid hyperkalemia. May cause GI upset (eg, nausea, vomiting, diarrhea, abdominal pain, discomfort) and lead to GI ulceration, bleeding, perforation and/or obstruction. Oral liquid preparations (not solid) should be used in patients with esophageal compression or delayed gastric emptying.

Adverse Reactions (Reflective of adult population; not specific for elderly)

>10%: Gastrointestinal: Diarrhea, nausea, stomach pain, flatulence, vomiting (oral)

1% to 10%:

    Cardiovascular: Bradycardia

    Endocrine & metabolic: Hyperkalemia

Neuromuscular & skeletal: Weakness
Respiratory: Dyspnea

Drug Interactions

Avoid Concomitant Use There are no known interactions where it is recommended to avoid concomitant use.

Increased Effect/Toxicity

Potassium Gluconate may increase the levels/effects of: ACE Inhibitors; Angiotensin II Receptor Blockers; Potassium-Sparing Diuretics

The levels/effects of Potassium Gluconate may be increased by: Eplerenone

Decreased Effect There are no known significant interactions involving a decrease in effect.

Stability Store at room temperature.

Mechanism of Action Potassium is the major cation of intracellular fluid and is essential for the conduction of nerve impulses in heart, brain, and skeletal muscle; contraction of cardiac, skeletal and smooth muscles; maintenance of normal renal function, acid-base balance, carbohydrate metabolism, and gastric secretion

Pharmacodynamics/Kinetics

Absorption: Well absorbed from upper GI tract

Distribution: Enters cells via active transport from extracellular fluid

Excretion: Primarily urine; skin and feces (small amounts); most intestinal potassium reabsorbed

Dosage

Geriatric & Adult Note: Doses listed as mEq of potassium (approximately 4.3 mEq potassium/g potassium gluconate, and 1 mEq potassium is equivalent to 39 mg elemental potassium):

Normal daily requirement: Oral: 40-80 mEq/day

Prevention of hypokalemia during diuretic therapy: Oral: 16-24 mEq/day in 1-2 divided doses

Treatment of hypokalemia: Oral: 40-100 mEq/day in 2-4 divided doses

Monitoring Parameters Serum potassium, blood pressure, pulse, ECG (as needed), signs of muscle weakness, cramps; serum magnesium for failure to respond to replacement

Reference Range Note: Reference ranges may vary depending on the laboratory

Serum potassium: 3.5-5.2 mEq/L

Test Interactions Decreased ammonia (B)

Pharmacotherapy Pearls 9.4 g potassium gluconate is approximately equal to 40 mEq potassium (4.3 mEq potassium/g salt)

Special Geriatric Considerations Elderly may require less potassium than younger adults due to decreased renal function. For the elderly who do not respond to replacement therapy, check serum magnesium. Long-term use of diuretics may result in hypomagnesemia.

Dosage Forms Excipient information presented when available (limited, particularly for generics); consult specific product labeling.

Caplet, oral: 595 mg [equivalent to potassium 99 mg]

Capsule, oral [strength expressed as base]: 99 mg

Tablet, oral: 550 mg [equivalent to potassium 90 mg], 595 mg [equivalent to potassium 99 mg]

Tablet, oral [strength expressed as base]: 99 mg

Tablet, timed release, oral [strength expressed as base]: 95 mg

Potassium Iodide and Iodine (poe TASS ee um EYE oh dide & EYE oh dine)

Medication Safety Issues

Sound-alike/look-alike issues:

Potassium iodide and iodine (Strong Iodide Solution or Lugol's solution) may be confused with potassium iodide products, including saturated solution of potassium iodide (SSKI®)

Index Terms Iodine and Potassium Iodide; Lugol's Solution; Strong Iodine Solution

Generic Availability (U.S.) Yes

Pharmacologic Category Antithyroid Agent

Use Reduce thyroid vascularity prior to thyroidectomy and management of thyrotoxic crisis; block thyroidal uptake of radioactive isotopes of iodine in a radiation emergency or after therapeutic/diagnostic use of radioactive iodine; topical antiseptic

Dosage

Geriatric & Adult RDA: 150 mcg (iodine)

Preoperative thyroidectomy: Oral: 0.1-0.3 mL (3-5 drops) 3 times/day; administer for 10 days before surgery

Thyrotoxic crisis: Oral: 4-8 drops every 6-8 hours; begin administration ≥1 hour following the initial dose of either propylthiouracil or methimazole (Nayak, 2006)

◀ **Thyroid gland protection during radiopharmaceutical use:** Oral: 1 drop/kg/day; (maximum: 40 drops/day or 20 drops twice daily) (Giammarile, 2008); alternatively, 20 drops 3 times/day has also been used (Bexxar® prescribing information, 2005)

    Note: Initiate 1-48 hours prior to radiopharmaceutical exposure and continue after radiopharmaceutical administration until risk of exposure has diminished (treatment initiation time and duration is dependent on the radiopharmaceutical agent used, consult specific protocol or labeling).

Special Geriatric Considerations Elderly may have reduced renal function and require close monitoring of serum potassium. May be also recommended to check serum magnesium.

Dosage Forms Excipient information presented when available (limited, particularly for generics); consult specific product labeling.

Solution, oral: Potassium iodide 100 mg/mL and iodine 50 mg/mL (480 mL)

Solution, topical: Potassium iodide 100 mg/mL and iodine 50 mg/mL (8 mL)

Potassium Phosphate (poe TASS ee um FOS fate)

Medication Safety Issues
High alert medication:

The Institute for Safe Medication Practices (ISMP) includes this medication (I.V. formulation) among its list of drugs which have a heightened risk of causing significant patient harm when used in error.

Other safety concerns:

Per JCAHO recommendations, concentrated electrolyte solutions should not be available in patient care areas.

Consider special storage requirements for intravenous potassium salts; I.V. potassium salts have been administered IVP in error, leading to fatal outcomes.

Safe Prescribing: Because inorganic phosphate exists as monobasic and dibasic anions, with the mixture of valences dependent on pH, ordering by mEq amounts is unreliable and may lead to large dosing errors. In addition, I.V. phosphate is available in the sodium and potassium salt; therefore, the content of these cations must be considered when ordering phosphate. The most reliable method of ordering I.V. phosphate is by millimoles, then specifying the potassium or sodium salt. For example, an order for 15 mmol of phosphate as potassium phosphate in one liter of normal saline.

Brand Names: U.S. Neutra-Phos®-K [OTC] [DSC]

Index Terms Phosphate, Potassium

Generic Availability (U.S.) Yes: Injection

Pharmacologic Category Electrolyte Supplement, Parenteral

Use Treatment and prevention of hypophosphatemia; **Note:** The concomitant amount of potassium must be calculated into the total electrolyte content. For each 1 mmol of phosphate, ~1.5 mEq of potassium will be administered. Therefore, if ordering 30 mmol of potassium phosphate, the patient will receive ~45 mEq of potassium.

Contraindications Hyperphosphatemia, hyperkalemia, hypocalcemia, hypomagnesemia, renal failure (oral product)

Warnings/Precautions Close monitoring of serum potassium concentrations is needed to avoid hyperkalemia. Use with caution in patients with renal insufficiency, cardiac disease, metabolic alkalosis. Use with caution in digitalized patients and patients receiving concomitant potassium-altering therapies. Parenteral potassium may cause pain and phlebitis, requiring a decrease in infusion rate or potassium concentration. Solutions for injection may contain aluminum; toxic levels may occur following prolonged administration in patients with renal impairment.

Adverse Reactions (Reflective of adult population; not specific for elderly) Frequency not defined.

Cardiovascular: Arrhythmia, bradycardia, chest pain, ECG changes, edema, heart block, hypotension

Central nervous system: Listlessness, mental confusion, tetany (with large doses of phosphate)

Endocrine & metabolic: Hyperkalemia

Gastrointestinal: Diarrhea, nausea, stomach pain, vomiting

Genitourinary: Urine output decreased

Local: Phlebitis

Neuromuscular & skeletal: Paralysis, paresthesia, weakness

Renal: Acute renal failure

Respiratory: Dyspnea

Drug Interactions

Avoid Concomitant Use There are no known interactions where it is recommended to avoid concomitant use.

Increased Effect/Toxicity
Potassium Phosphate may increase the levels/effects of: ACE Inhibitors; Angiotensin II Receptor Blockers; Potassium-Sparing Diuretics

The levels/effects of Potassium Phosphate may be increased by: Bisphosphonate Derivatives; Eplerenone

Decreased Effect There are no known significant interactions involving a decrease in effect.

Ethanol/Nutrition/Herb Interactions Food: Avoid administering with oxalate (berries, nuts, chocolate, beans, celery, tomato) or phytate-containing foods (bran, whole wheat).

Stability Store at room temperature; do not freeze. Use only clear solutions. Up to 10-15 mEq of calcium may be added per liter before precipitate may occur.

Stability of parenteral admixture at room temperature (25°C) is 24 hours.

Phosphate salts may precipitate when mixed with calcium salts. Solubility is improved in amino acid parenteral nutrition solutions. Check with a pharmacist to determine compatibility.

Dosage

Geriatric & Adult Caution: The concomitant amount of potassium must be calculated into the total electrolyte content. For each 1 mmol of phosphate, ~1.5 mEq of potassium will be administered. Therefore, if ordering 30 mmol of potassium phosphate, the patient will receive ~45 mEq of potassium. With orders for I.V. phosphate, there is considerable confusion associated with the use of millimoles (mmol) versus milliequivalents (mEq) to express the phosphate requirement. The most reliable method of ordering I.V. phosphate is by millimoles, then specifying the potassium or sodium salt. Doses listed as mmol of phosphate.

Acute treatment of hypophosphatemia: Repletion of severe hypophosphatemia should be done I.V. because large doses of oral phosphate may cause diarrhea and intestinal absorption may be unreliable. Reserve intermittent I.V. infusion for severe depletion situations; may require continuous cardiac monitoring depending on potassium administration rate. Guidelines differ based on degree of illness, need/use of parenteral nutrition, and severity of hypophosphatemia. If potassium >4.0 mEq/L consider phosphate replacement strategy without potassium (eg, sodium phosphates). Patients with severe renal impairment were excluded from phosphate supplement trials. **Note:** 1 mmol phosphate = 31 mg phosphorus; 1 mg phosphorus = 0.032 mmol phosphate.

General replacement guidelines (Lentz, 1978):
Low dose, if serum phosphate losses are recent and uncomplicated: 0.08 mmol/kg over 6 hours
Intermediate dose, if serum phosphorus level 0.5-1 mg/dL (0.16-0.32 mmol/L): 0.16-0.24 mmol/kg over 4-6 hours
Note: The initial dose may be increased by 25% to 50% if the patient is symptomatic secondary to hypophosphatemia and lowered by 25% to 50% if the patient is hypercalcemic.

Critically-ill adult patients receiving concurrent enteral/parenteral nutrition (Brown, 2006; Clark, 2006): Note: Round doses to the nearest 7.5 mmol for ease of preparation. If administering with phosphate-containing parenteral nutrition, do not exceed 15 mmol/L within parenteral nutrition. May use adjusted body weight for patients weighing >130% of ideal body weight (and BMI<40 kg/m^2) by using [IBW + 0.25 (ABW-IBW)]:
Low dose, serum phosphorus level 2.3-3 mg/dL (0.74-0.96 mmol/L): 0.16-0.32 mmol/kg over 4-6 hours
Intermediate dose, serum phosphorus level 1.6-2.2 mg/dL (0.51-0.71 mmol/L): 0.32-0.64 mmol/kg over 4-6 hours
High dose, serum phosphorus <1.5 mg/dL (<0.5 mmol/L): 0.64-1 mmol/kg over 8-12 hours

Parenteral nutrition: I.V.: 10-15 mmol/1000 kcal (Hicks, 2001) **or** 20-40 mmol/24 hours (Mirtallo, 2004 [ASPEN guidelines])

Administration Injection must be diluted in appropriate I.V. solution and volume prior to administration. In general, the dose, concentration of infusion, and rate of administration may be dependent on patient condition and specific institution policy. Must consider administration precautions for phosphate and potassium when prescribing.

For adult patients with severe symptomatic hypophosphatemia (ie, <1.5 mg/dL), may administer at rates up to 15 mmol phosphate/hour (this rate will deliver potassium at 22.5 mEq/hour) (Rosen, 1995, Charron, 2003). Potassium infusion rates >10 mEq/hour should be administered via central line (minimizes burning and phlebitis). ECG monitoring is recommended for potassium infusions >10 mEq/hour in adults. In patients with renal dysfunction and/or less severe hypophosphatemia, slower administration rates (eg, over 4-6 hours) or oral repletion is recommended.

Intermittent infusion doses of potassium phosphate are typically prepared in 100-250 mL of NS or D_5W (usual phosphate concentration range: 0.15 - 0.6 mmol/mL) (Rosen, 1995, Charron, 2003). Suggested maximum concentrations:

Peripheral line administration: 6.7 mmoL potassium phosphate/100 mL (10 mEq potassium/100 mL)

Central line administration: 26.8 mmoL potassium phosphate/100 mL (40 mEq potassium/100 mL)

Monitoring Parameters Serum potassium, calcium, phosphorus, magnesium (to facilitate potassium repletion); cardiac monitor (if intermittent infusion or potassium infusion rates 0.5 mEq/kg/hour in children or >10 mEq/hour in adults); to assess adequate replacement, repeat serum potassium and phosphorus levels 2-4 hours after dose

Reference Range Note: Reference ranges may vary depending on the laboratory

Serum calcium: 8.4-10.2 mg/dL

Serum phosphorus: Both low and high ends of the normal range are higher in children than in adults.

Infants: 4.5-7.5 mg/dL (1.45-2.42 mmol/L)

Children: ~4-6 mg/dL (1.29-1.94 mmol/L)

Adults: 2.5-4.5 mg/dL (0.81-1.45 mmol/L)

Serum potassium: 3.5-5.2 mEq/L

Special Geriatric Considerations Elderly may require less potassium than younger adults due to decreased renal function. Elderly who do not respond to replacement therapy, check serum magnesium. Long-term use of diuretics may result in hypomagnesemia. Monitor closely in elderly with Cl_{cr} <30 mL/minute.

Dosage Forms Excipient information presented when available (limited, particularly for generics); consult specific product labeling. [DSC] = Discontinued product

Injection, solution: Potassium 4.4 mEq and phosphorus 3 mmol per mL (5 mL, 15 mL, 50 mL) [equivalent to potassium 170 mg and elemental phosphorus 93 mg per mL]

Selected References

Brown KA, Dickerson RN, Morgan LM, et al, "A New Graduated Dosing Regimen for Phosphorus Replacement in Patients Receiving Nutrition Support," *JPEN J Parenter Enteral Nutr*, 2006, 30(3):209-14.

Potassium Phosphate and Sodium Phosphate
(poe TASS ee um FOS fate & SOW dee um FOS fate)

Related Information

Potassium Phosphate *on page 1492*

Sodium Phosphates *on page 1694*

Medication Safety Issues

Sound-alike/look-alike issues:

K-Phos® Neutral may be confused with Neutra-Phos-K®

Brand Names: U.S. K-Phos® MF; K-Phos® Neutral; K-Phos® No. 2; Phos-NaK; Phospha 250™ Neutral

Index Terms Neutra-Phos; Sodium Phosphate and Potassium Phosphate

Generic Availability (U.S.) Yes

Pharmacologic Category Electrolyte Supplement, Oral

Use Treatment of conditions associated with excessive renal phosphate loss or inadequate GI absorption of phosphate; to acidify the urine to lower calcium concentrations; to increase the antibacterial activity of methenamine; reduce odor and rash caused by ammonia in urine

Contraindications Addison's disease, hyperkalemia, hyperphosphatemia, infected urolithiasis or struvite stone formation, patients with severely impaired renal function

Warnings/Precautions Use with caution in patients with renal disease, cardiac disease, metabolic alkalosis, acute dehydration, hepatic impairment, hypernatremia, and hypotension.

Adverse Reactions (Reflective of adult population; not specific for elderly) Frequency not defined.

Cardiovascular: Bradycardia, arrhythmia, chest pain, edema, tachycardia

Central nervous system: Mental confusion, tetany (with large doses of phosphate), headache, dizziness, seizure

Endocrine & metabolic: Hyperkalemia, alkalosis

Gastrointestinal: Diarrhea, nausea, stomach pain, flatulence, vomiting, throat pain, weight gain

Genitourinary: Urine output decreased

Local: Phlebitis

Neuromuscular & skeletal: Weakness, arthralgia, bone pain, paralysis, paresthesia, pain/weakness of extremities, muscle cramps

Renal: Acute renal failure

Respiratory: Dyspnea

Miscellaneous: Thirst

Drug Interactions

Avoid Concomitant Use There are no known interactions where it is recommended to avoid concomitant use.

Increased Effect/Toxicity

Potassium Phosphate and Sodium Phosphate may increase the levels/effects of: ACE Inhibitors; Angiotensin II Receptor Blockers; Potassium-Sparing Diuretics

The levels/effects of Potassium Phosphate and Sodium Phosphate may be increased by: Bisphosphonate Derivatives; Eplerenone

Decreased Effect There are no known significant interactions involving a decrease in effect.

Pharmacodynamics/Kinetics Excretion: Urine

Dosage

Geriatric & Adult Phosphate supplement: Oral: Elemental phosphorus 250-500 mg 4 times/day after meals and at bedtime

Administration

Powder: Following dilution of powder, solution may be chilled to increase palatability.

Tablet: Should be taken with a full glass of water.

Monitoring Parameters Serum potassium, sodium, magnesium (failure to respond to replacement), calcium, phosphate, ECG; signs of muscle weakness, cramps

Reference Range Note: Reference ranges may vary depending on the laboratory

Serum potassium: 3.5-5.2 mEq/L

Serum phosphorus: Both low and high ends of the normal range are higher in children than in adults.

Infants: 4.5-7.5 mg/dL (1.45-2.42 mmol/L)

Children: ~4.0-6.0 mg/dL (1.29-1.94 mmol/L)

Adults: 2.5-4.5 mg/dL (0.81-1.45 mmol/L)

Pharmacotherapy Pearls Each mmol of phosphate contains 31 mg elemental phosphorus

Additional terminology for the potassium and sodium salts:

Sodium phosphate monobasic = Sodium acid phosphate

Sodium phosphate dibasic = Disodium phosphate

Potassium phosphate monobasic = Potassium acid phosphate

Potassium phosphate dibasic = Dipotassium phosphate

Special Geriatric Considerations A complete drug history should be taken to rule out potential drug interactions since elderly frequently may be taking potassium and potassium-sparing diuretics or salicylates as antacids. Elderly may require less potassium than younger adults due to decreased renal function. Elderly who do not respond to replacement therapy, check serum magnesium. Long-term use of diuretics may result in hypomagnesemia.

Dosage Forms Excipient information presented when available (limited, particularly for generics); consult specific product labeling.

Powder, for oral solution:

Phos-NaK: Dibasic potassium phosphate, monobasic potassium phosphate, dibasic sodium phosphate, and monobasic sodium phosphate per packet (100s) [sugar free; equivalent to elemental phosphorus 250 mg (8 mmol), sodium 160 mg (6.9 mEq), and potassium 280 mg (7.1 mEq) per packet; fruit flavor]

Tablet:

K-Phos® MF: Potassium acid phosphate 155 mg and sodium acid phosphate 350 mg [equivalent to elemental phosphorus 125.6 mg (4 mmol), sodium 67 mg (2.9 mEq), and potassium 44.5 mg (1.1 mEq)]

K-Phos® Neutral: Monobasic potassium phosphate 155 mg, dibasic sodium phosphate 852 mg, and monobasic sodium phosphate 130 mg [equivalent to elemental phosphorus 250 mg (8 mmol), sodium 298 mg (13 mEq), and potassium 45 mg (1.1 mEq)]

K-Phos® No. 2: Potassium acid phosphate 305 mg and sodium acid phosphate 700 mg [equivalent to elemental phosphorus 250 mg (8 mmol), sodium 134 mg (5.8 mEq), and potassium 88 mg (2.3 mEq)]

Phospha 250™ Neutral: Monobasic potassium phosphate 155 mg, dibasic sodium phosphate 852 mg, and monobasic sodium phosphate 130 mg [equivalent to elemental phosphorus 250 mg (8 mmol), sodium 298 mg (13 mEq), and potassium 45 mg (1.1 mEq)]

◆ **PPD** *see* Tuberculin Tests *on page 1877*

◆ **PPI-0903** *see* Ceftaroline Fosamil *on page 307*

◆ **PPI-0903M** *see* Ceftaroline Fosamil *on page 307*

◆ **PPSV** *see* Pneumococcal Polysaccharide Vaccine (Polyvalent) *on page 1474*

◆ **PPSV23** *see* Pneumococcal Polysaccharide Vaccine (Polyvalent) *on page 1474*

◆ **PPV23** *see* Pneumococcal Polysaccharide Vaccine (Polyvalent) *on page 1474*

◆ **Pradaxa®** *see* Dabigatran Etexilate *on page 440*

Pramipexole (pra mi PEKS ole)

Related Information
Antiparkinsonian Agents *on page 1995*

Medication Safety Issues
Sound-alike/look-alike issues:
Mirapex® may be confused with Hiprex®, Mifeprex®, MiraLax™

Brand Names: U.S. Mirapex®; Mirapex® ER®

Brand Names: Canada Apo-Pramipexole®; CO Pramipexole; Mirapex®; Novo-Pramipexole; PHL-Pramipexole; PMS-Pramipexole; Sandoz-Pramipexole

Index Terms Pramipexole Dihydrochloride Monohydrate

Generic Availability (U.S.) Yes: Excludes extended release tablet

Pharmacologic Category Anti-Parkinson's Agent, Dopamine Agonist

Use
Immediate release: Treatment of the signs and symptoms of idiopathic Parkinson's disease; treatment of moderate-to-severe primary Restless Legs Syndrome (RLS)

Extended release: Treatment of the signs and symptoms of idiopathic Parkinson's disease

Unlabeled/Investigational Use Treatment of depression; treatment of fibromyalgia

Contraindications Hypersensitivity to pramipexole or any component of the formulation

Warnings/Precautions Caution should be taken in patients with renal insufficiency; dose adjustment necessary. May cause or exacerbate dyskinesias; use caution in patients with pre-existing dyskinesias. May cause orthostatic hypotension; Parkinson's disease patients appear to have an impaired capacity to respond to a postural challenge. Use with caution in patients at risk of hypotension or where transient hypotensive episodes would be poorly tolerated. Parkinson's patients being treated with dopaminergic agonists ordinarily require careful monitoring for signs and symptoms of postural hypotension, especially during dose escalation. May cause hallucinations.

Dopamine agonists have been associated with compulsive behaviors and/or loss of impulse control, which has manifested as pathological gambling, libido increases (hypersexuality), and/or binge eating. Causality has not been established, and controversy exists as to whether this phenomenon is related to the underlying disease, prior behaviors/addictions and/or drug therapy. Dose reduction or discontinuation of therapy has been reported to reverse these behaviors in some, but not all cases. Risk for melanoma development is increased in Parkinson's disease patients; drug causation or factors contributing to risk have not been established. Patients should be monitored closely and periodic skin examinations should be performed.

Taper gradually over a period of 1 week when discontinuing therapy; dopaminergic agents have been associated with a syndrome resembling neuroleptic malignant syndrome on abrupt withdrawal or significant dosage reduction after long-term use. Ergot-derived dopamine agonists have been associated with fibrotic complications (eg, retroperitoneal fibrosis, pleural thickening, and pulmonary infiltrates). Although pramipexole is not an ergot, there have been postmarketing reports of possible fibrotic complications with pramipexole; monitor closely for signs and symptoms of fibrosis.

Pramipexole has been associated with somnolence, particularly at higher dosages (>1.5 mg/day). In addition, patients have been reported to fall asleep during activities of daily living, including driving, while taking this medication. Whether these patients exhibited somnolence prior to these events is not clear. Patients should be advised of this issue and factors which may increase risk (sleep disorders, other sedating medications, or concomitant medications which increase pramipexole concentrations) and instructed to report daytime somnolence or sleepiness to the prescriber. Patients should use caution in performing activities which require alertness (driving or operating machinery), and to avoid other medications which may cause CNS depression, including ethanol. Use caution in the elderly as they may be more sensitive to these adverse drug reactions.

Pathologic degenerative changes were observed in the retinas of albino rats during studies with this agent, but were not observed in the retinas of albino mice or in other species. The significance of these data for humans remains uncertain. Augmentation (earlier onset of symptoms in the evening/afternoon, increase and/or spread of symptoms to other extremities) or rebound (shifting of symptoms to early morning hours) may occur in some RLS patients.

Adverse Reactions (Reflective of adult population; not specific for elderly)

Parkinson's disease: Actual frequency may be dependent on dose and/or formulation:

>10%:

Cardiovascular: Postural hypotension (dose related; ≤53%)

Central nervous system: Somnolence (dose related; 9% to 36%), extrapyramidal syndrome (28%), insomnia (4% to 27%), dizziness (2% to 26%), hallucinations (5% to 17%), abnormal dreams (11%), headache (4% to 7%)

Gastrointestinal: Nausea (dose related; 11% to 28%), constipation (dose related; 6% to 14%)

Neuromuscular & skeletal: Dyskinesia (17% to 47%), weakness (1% to 14%)

1% to 10%:

Cardiovascular: Edema (2% to 8%), chest pain (3%)

Central nervous system: Confusion (4% to 10%), dystonia (2% to 8%), fatigue (6%), amnesia (dose related; 4% to 6%), sudden onset of sleep (3% to 6%), vertigo (2% to 4%), hypesthesia (3%), abnormal thinking (2% to 3%), akathisia (2% to 3%), malaise (2% to 3%), paranoia (2%), sleep disorder (1% to 3%), depression (≤2%), delusions (1%), fever (1%), myoclonus (1%)

Endocrine & metabolic: Libido decreased (1%)

Gastrointestinal: Xerostomia (4% to 7%), anorexia (1% to 5%), vomiting (4%), abdominal discomfort/pain (1% to 4%), dyspepsia (3%), appetite increased (2% to 3%), dysphagia (2%), weight loss (2%), salivary hypersecretion (≤2%), diarrhea (1% to 2%)

Genitourinary: Urinary frequency (6%), urinary tract infection (4%), impotence (2%), urinary incontinence (2%)

Neuromuscular & skeletal: Gait abnormalities (7%), hypertonia (7%), muscle spasm (3% to 5%), falls (4%), arthritis (3%), tremor (3%), back pain (2% to 3%), bursitis (2%), muscle twitching (2%), balance abnormalities (≤2%), CPK increased (1%), myasthenia (1%)

Ocular: Accommodation abnormalities (4%), vision abnormalities (3%), diplopia (1%)

Respiratory: Dyspnea (4%), cough (3%), rhinitis (3%), pneumonia (2%)

Restless legs syndrome: Actual frequency may be dependent on dose:

>10%:

Central nervous system: Headache (16%), insomnia (9% to 13%), abnormal dreams (1% to 8%), somnolence (6%)

Gastrointestinal: Nausea (11% to 27%), constipation (4%)

1% to 10%:

Central nervous system: Fatigue (3% to 9%)

Gastrointestinal: Diarrhea (1% to 7%), xerostomia (3%)

Neuromuscular & skeletal: Extremity pain (3% to 7%)

Respiratory: Nasal congestion (≤6%)

Miscellaneous: Influenza (1% to 7%)

Drug Interactions

Avoid Concomitant Use There are no known interactions where it is recommended to avoid concomitant use.

Increased Effect/Toxicity

Pramipexole may increase the levels/effects of: Alcohol (Ethyl); CNS Depressants; Selective Serotonin Reuptake Inhibitors

The levels/effects of Pramipexole may be increased by: Antipsychotics (Typical); Cimetidine; HydrOXYzine; MAO Inhibitors; Methylphenidate

Decreased Effect

Pramipexole may decrease the levels/effects of: Antipsychotics (Typical)

The levels/effects of Pramipexole may be decreased by: Antipsychotics (Atypical); Metoclopramide

Ethanol/Nutrition/Herb Interactions

Ethanol: May increase CNS depression; monitor for increased effects with coadministration. Caution patients about effects.

Food: Food intake does not affect the extent of drug absorption although the time to maximal plasma concentration is delayed when taken with a meal.

Herb/Nutraceutical: Avoid valerian, St John's wort, SAMe, kava kava (may increase risk of serotonin syndrome and/or excessive sedation).

Stability Store at 25°C (77°F); excursions permitted to 15°C to 30°C (59°F to 86°F). Protect from light and high humidity.

Mechanism of Action Pramipexole is a nonergot dopamine agonist with specificity for the D_2 subfamily dopamine receptor, and has also been shown to bind to D_3 and D_4 receptors. By binding to these receptors, it is thought that pramipexole can stimulate dopamine activity on the nerves of the striatum and substantia nigra.

Pharmacodynamics/Kinetics
Absorption: Rapid
Distribution: V_d: 500 L
Metabolism: Minimal
Bioavailability: >90%
Half-life: Adults: 8 hours; older adults: 12 hours
Elimination: 90% eliminated unchanged in the urine
  Clearance is decreased in older adults, likely due to decreased renal function. Clearance in Parkinson's patients was 30% less than healthy older adult volunteers. Clearance is decreased 60% when creatinine clearance is 40 mL/minute; 75% when clearance is 20 mL/minute.

Dosage
Geriatric & Adult
Parkinson's disease: Oral:
  Immediate release formulation: Initial: 0.375 mg/day given in 3 divided doses; increase gradually every 5-7 days; range: 1.5-4.5 mg/day.
  Extended release formulation (Mirapex® ER™): Initial: 0.375 mg once daily; increase gradually to 0.75 mg once daily. If necessary, may increase by 0.75 mg/dose not more frequently than every 5-7 days; maximum recommended dose 4.5 mg/day
  Note: Converting from immediate release to extended release: May initiate extended release preparation the morning after the last immediate release evening tablet is taken. The total daily dose should remain the same.
Restless legs syndrome: Oral: Initial: 0.125 mg once daily 2-3 hours before bedtime. Dose may be doubled every 4-7 days up to 0.5 mg/day. Maximum dose: 0.5 mg/day (manufacturer's recommendation).
  Note: Most patients require <0.5 mg/day, but higher doses have been used (2 mg/day). If augmentation occurs, dose earlier in the day.
Depression (unlabeled use): Initial: 0.25-0.375 mg/day given in 2-3 divided doses with a gradual titration; mean dose: 1.6-1.7 mg/day (Aiken, 2007; Goldberg, 2004)
Fibromyalgia (unlabeled use): Initial: 0.25 mg once daily at bedtime; may be increased weekly by 0.25 mg/day increments up to 4.5 mg/day (Holman, 2005)
Renal Impairment Use caution; renally-eliminated
Parkinson's disease: Immediate release formulation:
  Cl_{cr} 35-59 mL/minute: Initial: 0.125 mg twice daily (maximum dose: 1.5 mg twice daily)
  Cl_{cr} 15-34 mL/minute: Initial: 0.125 mg once daily (maximum dose: 1.5 mg once daily)
  Cl_{cr} <15 mL/minute: Not adequately studied
  Hemodialysis: Not adequately studied; a negligible amount of pramipexole is removed by dialysis
Parkinson's disease: Extended release formulation:
  Cl_{cr} >50 mL/minute: Dosing adjustment not necessary
  Cl_{cr} 30-50 mL/minute: Initial: 0.375 mg every other day; may increase to 0.375 mg once daily no sooner than 1 week after initiation. If necessary, may increase by 0.375 mg/dose not more frequently than every 7 days; maximum recommended dose: 2.25 mg/day
  Cl_{cr} <30 mL/minute: Not recommended
  Hemodialysis: Not recommended; a negligible amount of pramipexole is removed by dialysis
Restless legs syndrome: Immediate release formulation:
  Cl_{cr} 20-60 mL/minute: Duration between titration should be increased to 14 days
  Cl_{cr} <20 mL/minute: Not adequately studied
Administration Doses should be titrated gradually in all patients to avoid the onset of intolerable side effects. The dosage should be increased to achieve a maximum therapeutic effect, balanced against the side effects of dyskinesia, hallucinations, somnolence, and dry mouth. May be administered with or without food; may be administered with food to decrease nausea. Extended release tablets should be swallowed whole and not chewed, crushed, or divided.
Monitoring Parameters Blood pressure, heart rate; body weight changes; CNS depression, fall risk
Special Geriatric Considerations Since the dose is titrated to clinical response, no specific dosage adjustment is necessary in the elderly.
Dosage Forms Excipient information presented when available (limited, particularly for generics); consult specific product labeling.
  Tablet, oral, as dihydrochloride monohydrate: 0.125 mg, 0.25 mg, 0.5 mg, 0.75 mg, 1 mg, 1.5 mg
  Mirapex®: 0.125 mg
  Mirapex®: 0.25 mg, 0.5 mg [scored]
  Mirapex®: 0.75 mg
  Mirapex®: 1 mg, 1.5 mg [scored]

Tablet, extended release, oral, as dihydrochloride monohydrate:
Mirapex® ER®: 0.375 mg, 0.75 mg, 1.5 mg, 2.25 mg, 3 mg, 3.75 mg, 4.5 mg

Selected References

Aiken CB, "Pramipexole In Psychiatry: A Systematic Review Of The Literature," *J Clin Psychiatry*, 2007, 68(8):1230-6.

Carville SF, Arendt-Nielsen S, Bliddal H, et la, "EULAR Evidence-Based Recommendations for the Management of Fibromyalgia Syndrome," *Ann Rheum Dis*, 2008, 67(4):536-41.

Factor SA, "Current Status of Symptomatic Medical Therapy in Parkinson's Disease," *Neurotherapeutics*, 2008, 5 (2):164-80.

Olanow CW, Watts RL, and Koller WC, "An Algorithm (Decision Tree) for the Management of Parkinson's Disease (2001): Treatment Guidelines," *Neurology*, 2001, 56(11 Suppl 5):S1-S88.

"RLS Medical Bulletin," Restless Legs Syndrome Foundation, 2005, 1-34. Available at www.rls.org. Last accessed December 13, 2006.

Weintraub D, Siderowf AD, Potenza MN, et al, "Association of Dopamine Agonist Use With Impulse Control Disorders in Parkinson Disease," *Arch Neurol*, 2006, 63(7):969-73.

◆ **Pramipexole Dihydrochloride Monohydrate** *see* Pramipexole *on page 1496*

Pramlintide (PRAM lin tide)

Related Information
Diabetes Mellitus Management, Adults *on page 2073*

Medication Safety Issues
High alert medication:
The Institute for Safe Medication Practices (ISMP) includes this medication among its list of drug classes which have a heightened risk of causing significant patient harm when used in error.

Administration issues:
Use caution when drawing up doses from the vial (concentration 600 micrograms (mcg)/mL). Manufacturer recommended dosing ranges from 15 mcg to 120 mcg, which corresponds to injectable volumes of 0.025 mL to 0.2 mL. Patients and healthcare providers should exercise caution when administering this product to avoid inadvertent calculation of the dose based on "units," which could result in a sixfold overdose.

Brand Names: U.S. SymlinPen®; Symlin® [DSC]

Index Terms Pramlintide Acetate

Generic Availability (U.S.) No

Pharmacologic Category Amylinomimetic; Antidiabetic Agent

Use
Adjunctive treatment with mealtime insulin in type 1 diabetes mellitus (insulin dependent, IDDM) patients who have failed to achieve desired glucose control despite optimal insulin therapy

Adjunctive treatment with mealtime insulin in type 2 diabetes mellitus (noninsulin dependent, NIDDM) patients who have failed to achieve desired glucose control despite optimal insulin therapy, with or without concurrent sulfonylurea and/or metformin

Medication Guide Available Yes

Contraindications Hypersensitivity to pramlintide or any component of the formulation; confirmed diagnosis of gastroparesis; hypoglycemia unawareness

Warnings/Precautions [U.S. Boxed Warning]: Coadministration with insulin may induce severe hypoglycemia (usually within 3 hours following administration); coadministration with insulin therapy is an approved indication but does require an initial dosage reduction of insulin and frequent pre and post blood glucose monitoring to reduce risk of severe hypoglycemia. Concurrent use of other glucose-lowering agents may increase risk of hypoglycemia. Avoid use in patients with poor compliance with their insulin regimen and/or blood glucose monitoring. Do not use in patients with Hb A$_{1c}$ levels >9% or recent, recurrent episodes of hypoglycemia; obtain detailed history of glucose control (eg, Hb A$_{1c}$, incidence of hypoglycemia, glucose monitoring, and medication compliance) and body weight before initiating therapy. Use caution in patients with visual or dexterity impairment. Use caution when driving or operating heavy machinery until effects on blood sugar are known. Use caution with certain antihypertensive agents (eg, beta-adrenergic blockers) or neuropathic conditions which may mask signs/symptoms of hypoglycemia. Use caution in patients with history of nausea; avoid use in patients with conditions or concurrent medications likely to impair gastric motility (eg, anticholinergics); do not use in patients requiring medication(s) to stimulate gastric emptying.

Adverse Reactions (Reflective of adult population; not specific for elderly)
>10%:
Central nervous system: Headache (5% to 13%)
Gastrointestinal: Nausea (28% to 48%), vomiting (7% to 11%), anorexia (≤17%)
Endocrine & metabolic: Severe hypoglycemia (type 1 diabetes ≤17%)
Miscellaneous: Inflicted injury (8% to 14%)

1% to 10%:
 Central nervous system: Fatigue (3% to 7%), dizziness (2% to 6%)
 Endocrine & metabolic: Severe hypoglycemia (type 2 diabetes ≤8%)
 Gastrointestinal: Abdominal pain (2% to 8%)
 Respiratory: Pharyngitis (3% to 5%), cough (2% to 6%)
 Neuromuscular & skeletal: Arthralgia (2% to 7%)
 Miscellaneous: Allergic reaction (≤6%)

Drug Interactions

Avoid Concomitant Use There are no known interactions where it is recommended to avoid concomitant use.

Increased Effect/Toxicity
 Pramlintide may increase the levels/effects of: Anticholinergics

Decreased Effect There are no known significant interactions involving a decrease in effect.

Ethanol/Nutrition/Herb Interactions
 Ethanol: Use caution with ethanol (may increase hypoglycemia).
 Herb/Nutraceutical: Use caution with garlic, chromium, gymnema (may increase hypoglycemia).

Stability Store unopened vials at 2°C to 8°C (36°F to 46°F); do not freeze. Opened vials may be kept refrigerated or at room temperature ≤30°C (≤86°F). Discard opened vial after 30 days. Protect from light.

Mechanism of Action Synthetic analog of human amylin cosecreted with insulin by pancreatic beta cells; reduces postprandial glucose increases via the following mechanisms: 1) prolongation of gastric emptying time, 2) reduction of postprandial glucagon secretion, and 3) reduction of caloric intake through centrally-mediated appetite suppression

Pharmacodynamics/Kinetics Note: Pharmacokinetic studies have not been conducted in the elderly.
 Protein binding: 60%
 Metabolism: Primarily renal to des-lys^1 pramlintide (active metabolite)
 Bioavailability: 30% to 40%
 Half-life elimination: 48 minutes
 Time to peak, plasma: 20 minutes
 Excretion: Primarily urine

Dosage

Geriatric & Adult Note: When initiating pramlintide, reduce current insulin dose (including rapidly- and mixed-acting preparations) by 50% to avoid hypoglycemia. If pramlintide is discontinued for any reason, restart therapy with same initial titration protocol.

 Type 1 diabetes mellitus (insulin dependent, IDDM): SubQ: Initial: 15 mcg immediately prior to meals; titrate in 15 mcg increments every 3 days (if no significant nausea occurs) to target dose of 30-60 mcg (consider discontinuation if intolerant of 30 mcg dose)

 Type 2 diabetes mellitus (noninsulin dependent, NIDDM): SubQ: Initial: 60 mcg immediately prior to meals; after 3-7 days, increase to 120 mcg prior to meals if no significant nausea occurs (if nausea occurs at 120 mcg dose, reduce to 60 mcg)

Renal Impairment No dosage adjustment required; not evaluated in dialysis patients

Administration Do not mix with insulins; administer subcutaneously into abdominal or thigh areas at sites distinct from concomitant insulin injections (do not administer into arm due to variable absorption); rotate injection sites frequently. For oral medications in which a rapid onset of action is desired, administer 1 hour before, or 2 hours after pramlintide, if possible.

Monitoring Parameters Prior to initiating therapy: Hb A$_{1c}$, hypoglycemic history, body weight. During therapy: urine sugar and acetone, pre- and postprandial and bedtime serum glucose, electrolytes, Hb A$_{1c}$, lipid profile

Special Geriatric Considerations Patients must be able to adhere to their insulin regimen and self-monitor their blood glucose. In premarketing studies, the change in the Hb A$_{1c}$ values and hypoglycemia frequencies did not differ by age. Monitor regimen closely. Intensive glucose control (HbA$_{1c}$ <6.5%) has been linked to increased all-cause and cardiovascular mortality, hypoglycemia requiring assistance, and weight gain in adult type 2 diabetes. How "tightly" to control a geriatric patient's blood glucose needs to be individualized. Such a decision should be based on several factors, including the patient's functional and cognitive status, how well he/she recognizes hypoglycemic or hyperglycemic symptoms, and how to respond to them and other disease states. An HbA$_{1c}$ <7.5% is an acceptable endpoint for a healthy older adult, while <8% is acceptable for frail elderly patients, those with a duration of illness >10 years, or those with comorbid conditions and requiring combination diabetes medications. Patients who are unable to accurately draw up their dose will need assistance, such as prefilled syringes. Initial doses may require considerations for renal function in the elderly with dosing adjusted subsequently based on blood glucose monitoring. For elderly patients with diabetes who are relatively healthy, attaining target goals for aspirin use, blood pressure, lipids, smoking cessation, and diet and exercise may be more important than normalized glycemic control.

Dosage Forms Excipient information presented when available (limited, particularly for generics); consult specific product labeling. [DSC] = Discontinued product

Injection, solution, as acetate:

SymlinPen®: 1000 mcg/mL (2.7 mL) [120 pen-injector]

SymlinPen®: 1000 mcg/mL (1.5 mL) [60 pen-injector]

Symlin®: 600 mcg/mL (5 mL [DSC])

Selected References

Action to Control Cardiovascular Risk in Diabetes Study Group, Gerstein HC, Miller ME, et al, "Effects of Intensive Glucose Lowering in Type 2 Diabetes," N Engl J Med, 2008, 358(24):2545-59.

ADVANCE Collaborative Group, Patel A, MacMahon S, et al, "Intensive Blood Glucose Control and Vascular Outcomes in Patients With Type 2 Diabetes," N Engl J Med, 2008, 358(24):2560-72.

American Diabetes Association, "Standards of Medical Care in Diabetes – 2011," Diabetes Care, 2011, 34(Suppl 1):11-61.

Brown AF, Mangione CM, Saliba D, et al, "Guidelines for Improving the Care of the Older Person With Diabetes Mellitus," J Am Geriatr Soc, 2003, 51(5 Suppl Guidelines):265-80.

"VA/DoD Clinical Practice Guideline for the Management of Diabetes Mellitus," 2010. Available at http://www.healthquality.va.gov/Diabetes_Mellitus.asp

◆ **Pramlintide Acetate** see Pramlintide on page 1499
◆ **PrandiMet®** see Repaglinide and Metformin on page 1598
◆ **Prandin®** see Repaglinide on page 1596

Prasugrel (PRA soo grel)

Medication Safety Issues

Sound-alike/look-alike issues:

Prasugrel may be confused with pravastatin, propranolol

Brand Names: U.S. Effient®

Index Terms CS-747; LY-640315; Prasugrel Hydrochloride

Generic Availability (U.S.) No

Pharmacologic Category Antiplatelet Agent; Antiplatelet Agent, Thienopyridine

Use Reduces rate of thrombotic cardiovascular events (eg, stent thrombosis) in patients with unstable angina, non-ST-segment elevation MI, or ST-elevation MI (STEMI) managed with percutaneous coronary intervention (PCI)

Medication Guide Available Yes

Contraindications Active pathological bleeding such as peptic ulcer disease (PUD) or intracranial hemorrhage; history of transient ischemic attack (TIA) or stroke

Warnings/Precautions [U.S. Boxed Warning]: May cause significant or fatal bleeding. Use is contraindicated in patients with active pathological bleeding or history of TIA or stroke. Use with caution in patients who may be at risk of increased bleeding, including patients with active PUD, recent or recurrent GI bleeding, severe hepatic impairment, trauma, or surgery. Additional risk factors include body weight <60 kg, CABG or other surgical procedure, concomitant use of medications that increase risk of bleeding.

[U.S. Boxed Warning]: In patients ≥75 years of age, use is not recommended due to increased risk of fatal and intracranial bleeding and uncertain benefit; use may be considered in high-risk situations (eg, patients with diabetes or history of MI). **[U.S. Boxed Warning]: Discontinue ≥7 days before CABG;** increased risk of bleeding; do not initiate therapy in patients likely to undergo CABG.

If necessary, discontinue therapy for active bleeding, elective surgery, stroke, or TIA; reinitiate therapy as soon as possible unless patient suffers stroke or TIA where subsequent use is contraindicated. If possible, manage bleeding without discontinuing prasugrel. Use caution in concurrent treatment with oral anticoagulants (eg, warfarin), NSAIDs, or fibrinolytic agents; bleeding risk is increased. Use with caution in patients with severe liver impairment or end-stage renal disease (experience is limited). Cases of thrombotic thrombocytopenic purpura (usually occurring within the first 2 weeks of therapy), resulting in some fatalities, have been reported with other thienopyridines; urgent plasmapheresis is required. In patients <60 kg, risk of bleeding increased; consider lower maintenance dose.

Adverse Reactions (Reflective of adult population; not specific for elderly) As with all drugs which may affect hemostasis, bleeding is associated with prasugrel. Hemorrhage may occur at virtually any site. Risk is dependent on multiple variables, including patient susceptibility and concurrent use of multiple agents which alter hemostasis.

2% to 10%:

Cardiovascular: Hypertension (8%), hypotension (4%), atrial fibrillation (3%), bradycardia (3%), noncardiac chest pain (3%), peripheral edema (3%)

Central nervous system: Headache (6%), dizziness (4%), fatigue (4%), fever (3%), extremity pain (3%)

Dermatologic: Rash (3%)

Endocrine & metabolic: Hypercholesterolemia/hyperlipidemia (7%)

◀ Gastrointestinal: Nausea (5%), diarrhea (2%), gastrointestinal hemorrhage (2%)
Hematologic: Leukopenia (3%), anemia (2%)
Neuromuscular & skeletal: Back pain (5%)
Respiratory: Epistaxis (6%), dyspnea (5%), cough (4%)

Drug Interactions

Avoid Concomitant Use There are no known interactions where it is recommended to avoid concomitant use.

Increased Effect/Toxicity

Prasugrel may increase the levels/effects of: Anticoagulants; Antiplatelet Agents; Collagenase (Systemic); Drotrecogin Alfa; Ibritumomab; Rivaroxaban; Salicylates; Thrombolytic Agents; Tositumomab and Iodine I 131 Tositumomab

The levels/effects of Prasugrel may be increased by: Dasatinib; Glucosamine; Herbs (Anticoagulant/Antiplatelet Properties); Nonsteroidal Anti-Inflammatory Agents; Omega-3-Acid Ethyl Esters; Pentosan Polysulfate Sodium; Pentoxifylline; Prostacyclin Analogues; Vitamin E

Decreased Effect

The levels/effects of Prasugrel may be decreased by: CYP3A4 Inhibitors (Strong); Nonsteroidal Anti-Inflammatory Agents; Ranitidine; Rifampin; Tocilizumab

Stability Store at 25°C (77°F); excursions permitted to 15°C to 30°C (59°F to 86°F).

Mechanism of Action Prasugrel is a prodrug that is metabolized to both active (R-138727) and inactive metabolites. The active metabolite irreversibly blocks the P2Y$_{12}$ component of ADP receptors on the platelet, which prevents activation of the GPIIb/IIIa receptor complex, thereby reducing platelet activation and aggregation. Platelet aggregation returns to baseline within 5-9 days of discontinuation.

Pharmacodynamics/Kinetics

Onset of action: Inhibition of platelet aggregation (IPA): Dose dependent: 60 mg loading dose: <30 minutes; median time to reach 20% IPA: 30 minutes (Brandt, 2007)

Peak effect: Time to maximal IPA: Dose-dependent: **Note:** Degree of IPA based on adenosine diphosphate (ADP) concentration used during light aggregometry: 60 mg loading dose: Occurs 4 hours post administration; mean IPA (ADP 5 µmol/L): 78.8%: mean IPA (ADP 20 µmol/L): 84.1%

Duration of effect: >3 days; platelet aggregation gradually returns to baseline values over 5-9 days after discontinuation; reflective of new platelet production

Absorption: Rapid; ≥79%

Distribution: V$_d$: 44-68 L

Protein binding: Active metabolite: ~98%

Metabolism: Rapid intestinal and serum metabolism via esterase-mediated hydrolysis to a thiolactone (inactive), which is then converted, via CYP450-mediated (primarily CYP3A4 and CYP2B6) oxidation, to an active metabolite (R-138727)

Half-life elimination: Active metabolite: ~7 hours (range 2-15 hours)

Time to peak, plasma: Active metabolite: ~30 minutes (peak plasma levels begin to decrease at ~24 hours); with high-fat/high-calorie meal: 1.5 hours

Excretion: Urine (~68% inactive metabolites); feces (27% inactive metabolites)

Dosage

Geriatric Refer to adult dosing. Patients ≥75 years: Use not recommended; may be considered in high-risk situations (eg, patients with diabetes or history of MI).

Adult Acute coronary syndrome managed with PCI: Oral: Loading dose: 60 mg administered promptly (as soon as coronary anatomy is known or before if risk for bleeding is low and need for CABG considered unlikely) and no later than 1 hour after PCI; Maintenance dose: 10 mg once daily (in combination with aspirin 81-325 mg/day). **Note:** In patients weighing <60 kg, the manufacturer suggests to consider decreasing maintenance dose to 5 mg once daily; however, prospective clinical trial data does not exist to support this recommendation and may place some patients at risk of thrombotic complications (eg, stent thrombosis); consider use of full dose while monitoring closely for bleeding complications or administration of an alternative agent (eg, clopidogrel).

Duration of prasugrel (in combination with aspirin) after stent placement: **Premature interruption of therapy may result in stent thrombosis with subsequent fatal and nonfatal MI.** With STEMI, prasugrel for at least 12 months regardless of stent type (ie, either bare metal or drug eluting stent) is recommended (Kushner, 2009). With UA/NSTEMI, at least 12 months of prasugrel regardless of stent type is recommended and for up to 15 months unless the risk of bleeding outweighs the benefits (Wright, 2011). In either setting, a duration >15 months may be considered in patients with DES placement (Kushner, 2009; Wright 2011).

Renal Impairment No dosage adjustment necessary.

Hepatic Impairment No dosage adjustment necessary for mild-to-moderate hepatic impairment; use in severe hepatic impairment has not been evaluated.

Administration Administer without regard to meals.

Monitoring Parameters Hemoglobin and hematocrit periodically. Consider platelet function testing to determine platelet inhibitory response if results of testing may alter management (Wright, 2011).

Special Geriatric Considerations See Warnings/Precautions. Not recommended for use in elderly ≥75 years due to risk of fatal intracranial bleeding and lack of certain benefit in this age group. Exceptions may be high-risk patients (eg, diabetics or patients with a history of myocardial infarction). In the TRITON-TIMI 38 study, the AUC of the active metabolite was 19% higher in those ≥75 years of age compared to those participants <75 years.

Dosage Forms Excipient information presented when available (limited, particularly for generics); consult specific product labeling.

Tablet, oral:
　Effient®: 5 mg, 10 mg

Selected References

Brandt JT, Payne CD, Wiviott SD, et al, "A Comparison of Prasugrel and Clopidogrel Loading Doses on Platelet Function: Magnitude of Platelet Inhibition is Related to Active Metabolite Formation," *Am Heart J*, 2007, 153(1):66. e9-16.

Kushner FG, Hand M, Smith SC, et al, "2009 Focused Updates: ACC/AHA Guidelines for the Management of Patients With ST-Elevation Myocardial Infarction (Updating the 2004 Guideline and 2007 Focused Update) and ACC/AHA/SCAI Guidelines on Percutaneous Coronary Intervention (Updating the 2005 Guideline and 2007 Focused Update): A Report of the American College of Cardiology Foundation/American Heart Association Task Force on Practice Guidelines," *J Am Coll Cardiol*, 2009, 54(23):2205-41.

Smith SC, Feldman TE, Hirshfeld JW, et al, "ACC/AHA/SCAI 2005 Guidelines of Percutaneous Coronary Intervention. A Report of the American College of Cardiology/American Heart Association Task Force on Practice Guidelines (ACC/AHA/SCAI Writing Committee to Update the 2001 Guidelines for Percutaneous Coronary Intervention)." Available online at http://www.acc.org/clinical/guidelines/percutaneous/update/index_rev.pdf. Last accessed December 21, 2005.

◆ **Prasugrel Hydrochloride** *see* Prasugrel *on page 1501*
◆ **Pravachol®** *see* Pravastatin *on page 1503*

Pravastatin (prav a STAT in)

Related Information
Hyperlipidemia Management *on page 2021*

Medication Safety Issues
Sound-alike/look-alike issues:
Pravachol® may be confused with atorvastatin, Prevacid®, Prinivil®, propranolol
Pravastatin may be confused with nystatin, pitavastatin, prasugrel

Brand Names: U.S. Pravachol®

Brand Names: Canada Apo-Pravastatin®; CO Pravastatin; Dom-Pravastatin; Mylan-Pravastatin; Novo-Pravastatin; Nu-Pravastatin; PHL-Pravastatin; PMS-Pravastatin; Pravachol®; RAN™-Pravastatin; ratio-Pravastatin; Riva-Pravastatin; Sandoz-Pravastatin; ZYM-Pravastatin

Index Terms Pravastatin Sodium

Generic Availability (U.S.) Yes

Pharmacologic Category Antilipemic Agent, HMG-CoA Reductase Inhibitor

Use Use with dietary therapy for the following:

Primary prevention of coronary events: In hypercholesterolemic patients without established coronary heart disease to reduce cardiovascular morbidity (myocardial infarction, coronary revascularization procedures) and mortality.

Secondary prevention of cardiovascular events in patients with established coronary heart disease: To slow the progression of coronary atherosclerosis; to reduce cardiovascular morbidity (myocardial infarction, coronary vascular procedures) and to reduce mortality; to reduce the risk of stroke and transient ischemic attacks

Hyperlipidemia: Reduce elevations in total cholesterol, LDL-C, apolipoprotein B, and triglycerides (elevations of 1 or more components are present in Fredrickson type IIa, IIb, III, and IV hyperlipidemias)

Contraindications Hypersensitivity to pravastatin or any component of the formulation; active liver disease; unexplained persistent elevations of serum transaminases

Warnings/Precautions Secondary causes of hyperlipidemia should be ruled out prior to therapy. Liver function must be monitored by periodic laboratory assessment. Rhabdomyolysis with acute renal failure has occurred. Risk may be increased with concurrent use of other drugs which may cause rhabdomyolysis (including colchicine, gemfibrozil, fibric acid derivatives, or niacin at doses ≥1 g/day). Temporarily discontinue in any patient experiencing an acute or serious condition predisposing to renal failure secondary to rhabdomyolysis. Based upon current evidence, HMG-CoA reductase inhibitor therapy should be continued in the perioperative period unless risk outweighs cardioprotective benefit. Use with caution in patients with advanced age, these patients are predisposed to myopathy. Use caution in patients with previous liver disease or heavy ethanol use.

Adverse Reactions (Reflective of adult population; not specific for elderly) As reported in short-term trials; safety and tolerability with long-term use were similar to placebo 1% to 10%:

Cardiovascular: Chest pain (4%)

Central nervous system: Headache (2% to 6%), fatigue (4%), dizziness (1% to 3%)

Dermatologic: Rash (4%)

Gastrointestinal: Nausea/vomiting (7%), diarrhea (6%), heartburn (3%)

Hepatic: Transaminases increased (>3x normal on two occasions - 1%)

Neuromuscular & skeletal: Myalgia (2%)

Respiratory: Cough (3%)

Miscellaneous: Influenza (2%)

Additional class-related events or case reports (not necessarily reported with pravastatin therapy): Angioedema, cataracts, depression, dyspnea, eosinophilia, erectile dysfunction, facial paresis, hypersensitivity reaction, impaired extraocular muscle movement, impotence, interstitial lung disease, leukopenia, malaise, memory loss, ophthalmoplegia, paresthesia, peripheral neuropathy, photosensitivity, psychic disturbance, skin discoloration, thrombocytopenia, thyroid dysfunction, toxic epidermal necrolysis, transaminases increased, vomiting

Drug Interactions

Metabolism/Transport Effects Substrate of CYP3A4 (minor), P-glycoprotein, SLCO1B1; **Inhibits** CYP2C9 (weak), 2D6 (weak), 3A4 (weak)

Avoid Concomitant Use

Avoid concomitant use of Pravastatin with any of the following: Red Yeast Rice

Increased Effect/Toxicity

Pravastatin may increase the levels/effects of: DAPTOmycin; PARoxetine; Trabectedin; Vitamin K Antagonists

The levels/effects of Pravastatin may be increased by: Antifungal Agents (Azole Derivatives, Systemic); Colchicine; Conivaptan; CycloSPORINE; CycloSPORINE (Systemic); Eltrombopag; Fenofibrate; Fenofibric Acid; Gemfibrozil; Niacin; Niacinamide; P-Glycoprotein Inhibitors; Protease Inhibitors; Red Yeast Rice; Rifamycin Derivatives

Decreased Effect

Pravastatin may decrease the levels/effects of: Lanthanum

The levels/effects of Pravastatin may be decreased by: Antacids; Bile Acid Sequestrants; Efavirenz; Fosphenytoin; P-Glycoprotein Inducers; Phenytoin; Rifamycin Derivatives; Tocilizumab

Ethanol/Nutrition/Herb Interactions

Ethanol: Consumption of large amounts of ethanol may increase the risk of liver damage with HMG-CoA reductase inhibitors.

Food: Red yeast rice contains an estimated 2.4 mg lovastatin per 600 mg rice.

Herb/Nutraceutical: St John's wort may decrease pravastatin levels.

Stability Store at 25°C (77°F); excursions permitted to 15°C to 30°C (59°F to 86°F). Protect from moisture and light.

Mechanism of Action Pravastatin is a competitive inhibitor of 3-hydroxy-3-methylglutaryl coenzyme A (HMG-CoA) reductase, which is the rate-limiting enzyme involved in *de novo* cholesterol synthesis.

Pharmacodynamics/Kinetics

Onset of action: Several days

Peak effect: 4 weeks

Absorption: Rapidly absorbed; average absorption 34%

Protein binding: 50%

Metabolism: Hepatic multiple metabolites; primary metabolite is 3α-hydroxy-iso-pravastatin (2.5% to 10% activity of parent drug)

Bioavailability: 17%

Half-life elimination: 77 hours (including all metabolites); pravastatin: ~2-3 hours (Pan, 1990); 3α-hydroxy-iso-pravastatin: ~1.5 hours (Gustavson, 2005)

Time to peak, serum: 1-1.5 hours

Excretion: Feces (70%); urine (≤20%, 8% as unchanged drug)

Dosage

Geriatric & Adult

Hyperlipidemias, primary prevention of coronary events, secondary prevention of cardiovascular events: Oral: Initial: 40 mg once daily; titrate dosage to response (usual range: 10-80 mg) (maximum dose: 80 mg once daily)

Dosage adjustment based on concomitant cyclosporine: Oral: Initial: 10 mg/day, titrate with caution (maximum dose: 20 mg/day)

Note: Doses should be individualized according to the baseline LDL-cholesterol levels, the recommended goal of therapy, and patient response; adjustments should be made at intervals of 4 weeks or more; doses may need adjusted based on concomitant medications

Renal Impairment Initial: 10 mg/day

Hepatic Impairment Initial: 10 mg/day

Administration May be administered without regard to meals.

Monitoring Parameters Obtain baseline LFTs and total cholesterol profile; creatine phosphokinase due to possibility of myopathy. Repeat LFTs prior to elevation of dose. May be measured when clinically indicated and/or periodically thereafter; baseline CPK (recheck CPK in any patient with symptoms suggestive of myopathy). Monitor LDL-C at intervals no less than 4 weeks.

Special Geriatric Considerations Effective and well tolerated in the elderly. No specific dosage recommendations. Clearance is reduced in the elderly, resulting in an increase in AUC between 25% to 50%; however, substantial accumulation is not expected.

The definition of and, therefore, when to treat hyperlipidemia in elderly is a controversial issue. The National Cholesterol Education Program recommends that all adults maintain a plasma cholesterol <160 mg/dL. For the elderly with one additional risk factor, goal LDL would be <130 mg/dL. It is the authors' belief that pharmacologic treatment be reserved for those who are unable to obtain a desirable plasma cholesterol concentration by diet alone and for whom the benefits of treatment are believed to outweigh the potential adverse effects, drug interactions, and cost of treatment. Age ≥65 years is a risk factor for myopathy.

Dosage Forms Excipient information presented when available (limited, particularly for generics); consult specific product labeling.

Tablet, oral, as sodium: 10 mg, 20 mg, 40 mg, 80 mg

Pravachol®: 10 mg, 20 mg, 40 mg, 80 mg

Selected References

Fleisher LA, Beckman JA, Brown KA, et al, "ACC/AHA 2007 Guidelines on Perioperative Cardiovascular Evaluation and Care for Noncardiac Surgery: A Report of the American College of Cardiology/American Heart Association Task Force on Practice Guidelines (Writing Committee to Revise the 2002 Guidelines on Perioperative Cardiovascular Evaluation for Noncardiac Surgery) Developed in Collaboration With the American Society of Echocardiography, American Society of Nuclear Cardiology, Heart Rhythm Society, Society of Cardiovascular Anesthesiologists, Society for Cardiovascular Angiography and Interventions, Society for Vascular Medicine and Biology, and Society for Vascular Surgery," *J Am Coll Cardiol*, 2007, 50(17):e159-241.

Grundy SM, Cleeman JI, Merz CN, et al, "Implications of Recent Clinical Trials for the National Cholesterol Education Program Adult Treatment Panel III Guidelines," *J Am Coll Cardiol*, 2004, 44(3):720-32.

National Cholesterol Education Program (NCEP) Expert Panel on Detection, Evaluation, and Treatment of High Blood Cholesterol in Adults (Adult Treatment Panel III), "Third Report of the National Cholesterol Education Program (NCEP) Expert Panel on Detection, Evaluation, and Treatment of High Blood Cholesterol in Adults (Adult Treatment Panel III) Final Report," *Circulation*, 2002, 106(25):3143-421.

◆ **Pravastatin Sodium** see Pravastatin on page 1503

Prazosin (PRAZ oh sin)

Related Information

Beers Criteria – Potentially Inappropriate Medications for Geriatrics on page 2089

Medication Safety Issues

Sound-alike/look-alike issues:

Prazosin may be confused with predniSONE

International issues:

Prazepam [multiple international markets] may be confused with prazosin

Brand Names: U.S. Minipress®

Brand Names: Canada Apo-Prazo®; Minipress®; Novo-Prazin; Nu-Prazo

Index Terms Furazosin; Prazosin Hydrochloride

Generic Availability (U.S.) Yes

Pharmacologic Category Alpha$_1$ Blocker

Use Treatment of hypertension

Unlabeled/Investigational Use Post-traumatic stress disorder (PTSD) related nightmares and sleep disruption; benign prostatic hyperplasia; Raynaud's syndrome

Contraindications Hypersensitivity to prazosin, quinazolines (eg, doxazosin, terazosin) or any component of the formulation

Warnings/Precautions May cause significant orthostatic hypotension and syncope, especially with first dose; anticipate a similar effect if therapy is interrupted for a few days, if dosage is rapidly increased, or if another antihypertensive drug (particularly vasodilators) or a PDE-5 inhibitor is introduced. Intraoperative floppy iris syndrome (IFIS) has been observed during cataract surgery in some patients treated with alpha$_1$-blockers. Patients should be cautioned about performing hazardous tasks when starting new therapy or adjusting dosage upward. Discontinue if symptoms of angina occur or worsen. Should rule out prostatic carcinoma before beginning therapy.

Adverse Reactions (Reflective of adult population; not specific for elderly)

>4%:
  Cardiovascular: Palpitation (5%)
  Central nervous system: Dizziness (10%), headache (8%), drowsiness (8%)
  Endocrine & metabolic: Decreased energy (7%)
  Gastrointestinal: Nausea (5%)
  Neuromuscular & skeletal: Weakness (7%)

1% to 4%:
  Cardiovascular: Edema, orthostatic hypotension, syncope
  Central nervous system: Depression, nervousness, vertigo
  Dermatologic: Rash
  Gastrointestinal: Constipation, diarrhea, vomiting, xerostomia
  Genitourinary: Urinary frequency
  Ocular: Blurred vision, reddened sclera
  Respiratory: Dyspnea, epistaxis, nasal congestion

Drug Interactions

Metabolism/Transport Effects Induces P-glycoprotein

Avoid Concomitant Use

Avoid concomitant use of Prazosin with any of the following: Alpha1-Blockers; Dabigatran Etexilate

Increased Effect/Toxicity

Prazosin may increase the levels/effects of: Alpha1-Blockers; Amifostine; Antihypertensives; Calcium Channel Blockers; Hypotensive Agents; RiTUXimab

The levels/effects of Prazosin may be increased by: Beta-Blockers; Diazoxide; Herbs (Hypotensive Properties); MAO Inhibitors; Pentoxifylline; Phosphodiesterase 5 Inhibitors; Prostacyclin Analogues

Decreased Effect

Prazosin may decrease the levels/effects of: Dabigatran Etexilate; Linagliptin; P-Glycoprotein Substrates

The levels/effects of Prazosin may be decreased by: Herbs (Hypertensive Properties); Methylphenidate; Yohimbine

Ethanol/Nutrition/Herb Interactions

Ethanol: Avoid ethanol (may increase vasodilation).
Food: Food has variable effects on absorption.
Herb/Nutraceutical: Avoid dong quai if using for hypertension (has estrogenic activity). Avoid ephedra, yohimbe, ginseng (may worsen hypertension). Avoid saw palmetto (due to limited experience with this combination). Avoid garlic (may have increased antihypertensive effect).

Stability Store in airtight container. Protect from light.

Mechanism of Action Competitively inhibits postsynaptic alpha-adrenergic receptors which results in vasodilation of veins and arterioles and a decrease in total peripheral resistance and blood pressure

Pharmacodynamics/Kinetics

Onset of action: Anithypertensive: ~2 hours
  Peak effect: Antihypertensive: 2-4 hours
Duration: 10-24 hours
Distribution: Hypertensive adults: V_d: 0.5 L/kg
Protein binding: 92% to 97%
Metabolism: Extensively hepatic
Bioavailability: 43% to 82%
Time to peak, plasma: ~3 hours
Half-life elimination: 2-3 hours; prolonged with congestive heart failure
Excretion: Feces, urine (6% to 10% as unchanged drug)

Dosage

Geriatric Refer to adult dosing. In the management of hypertension, consider lower initial doses and titrate to response (Aronow, 2011).

Adult

Hypertension: Oral: Initial: 1 mg/dose 2-3 times/day; usual maintenance dose: 2-20 mg/day in divided doses 2-3 times/day (JNC 7); maximum daily dose: 20 mg

PTSD-related nightmares and sleep disruption (unlabeled use): Oral: Initial: 1 mg at bedtime (Raskind, 2002; Raskind, 2007); titrate as tolerated to 2-15 mg at bedtime (Benedek, 2009)

Raynaud's (unlabeled use): Oral: Dosage range: 1-5 mg twice daily (Bakst, 2008)

Benign prostatic hyperplasia (unlabeled use): Oral: Initial: 0.5 mg twice daily; titrate as tolerated to 2 mg twice daily (Moran, 2001)

Monitoring Parameters Blood pressure, standing and sitting/supine

Test Interactions Increased urinary VMA 17%, norepinephrine metabolite 42%; therefore, false positives may occur in screening for pheochromocytoma. If elevated VMA is found, discontinue prazosin and retest after one month.

Special Geriatric Considerations Adverse effects such as orthostatic hypotension, dry mouth, and urinary problems can be particularly bothersome in the elderly.

Dosage Forms Excipient information presented when available (limited, particularly for generics); consult specific product labeling.

Capsule, oral, as hydrochloride: 1 mg, 2 mg, 5 mg

Minipress®: 1 mg, 2 mg, 5 mg

Selected References

Chobanian AV, Bakris GL, Black HR, et al, "The Seventh Report of the Joint National Committee on Prevention, Detection, Evaluation, and Treatment of High Blood Pressure: The JNC 7 Report," *JAMA*, 2003, 289(19):2560-71.

Rubin PC, Scott PJ, and Reid JL, "Prazosin Disposition in Young and Elderly Subjects," *Br J Clin Pharmacol*, 1981, 12 (3):401-4.

♦ **Prazosin Hydrochloride** *see* Prazosin *on page 1505*
♦ **Precose®** *see* Acarbose *on page 28*
♦ **Pred Forte®** *see* PrednisoLONE (Ophthalmic) *on page 1510*
♦ **Pred-G®** *see* Prednisolone and Gentamicin *on page 1510*
♦ **Pred Mild®** *see* PrednisoLONE (Ophthalmic) *on page 1510*

Prednicarbate (pred ni KAR bate)

Related Information
Corticosteroids *on page 2005*

Medication Safety Issues
Sound-alike/look-alike issues:
Dermatop® may be confused with Dimetapp®

Brand Names: U.S. Dermatop®

Brand Names: Canada Dermatop®

Generic Availability (U.S.) Yes

Pharmacologic Category Corticosteroid, Topical

Use Relief of the inflammatory and pruritic manifestations of corticosteroid-responsive dermatoses (medium potency topical corticosteroid)

Dosage

Geriatric & Adult Steroid-responsive dermatoses: Topical: Cream, ointment: Apply a thin film to affected area twice daily. Therapy should be discontinued when control is achieved; if no improvement is seen within 2 weeks, reassessment of diagnosis may be necessary.

Special Geriatric Considerations Due to age-related changes in skin, limit use of topical corticosteroids.

Dosage Forms Excipient information presented when available (limited, particularly for generics); consult specific product labeling.

Cream, topical: 0.1% (15 g, 60 g)
Dermatop®: 0.1% (60 g)
Ointment, topical: 0.1% (15 g, 60 g)
Dermatop®: 0.1% (60 g)

PrednisoLONE (Systemic) (pred NISS oh lone)

Related Information
Corticosteroids *on page 2005*

Medication Safety Issues
Sound-alike/look-alike issues:
PrednisoLONE may be confused with predniSONE
Pediapred® may be confused with Pediazole®
Prelone® may be confused with Prozac®

Brand Names: U.S. Flo-Pred™; Millipred™; Orapred ODT®; Orapred®; Pediapred®; Prelone®; Veripred™ 20

Brand Names: Canada Hydeltra T.B.A.®; Novo-Prednisolone; Pediapred®

Index Terms Prednisolone Sodium Phosphate

Generic Availability (U.S.) Yes: Excludes orally disintegrating tablet, oral suspension

Pharmacologic Category Corticosteroid, Systemic

PREDNISOLONE (SYSTEMIC)

Use Treatment of endocrine disorders, rheumatic disorders, collagen diseases, allergic states, respiratory diseases, hematologic disorders, neoplastic diseases, edematous states, and gastrointestinal diseases; resolution of acute exacerbations of multiple sclerosis; management of fulminating or disseminated tuberculosis and trichinosis; acute or chronic solid organ rejection

Contraindications Hypersensitivity to prednisolone or any component of the formulation; acute superficial herpes simplex keratitis; live or attenuated virus vaccines (with immunosuppressive doses of corticosteroids); systemic fungal infections; varicella

Warnings/Precautions May cause hypercorticism or suppression of hypothalamic-pituitary-adrenal (HPA) axis, particularly in patients receiving high doses for prolonged periods. HPA axis suppression may lead to adrenal crisis. Withdrawal and discontinuation of a corticosteroid should be done slowly and carefully. Particular care is required when patients are transferred from systemic corticosteroids to inhaled products due to possible adrenal insufficiency or withdrawal from steroids, including an increase in allergic symptoms. Patients receiving >20 mg per day of prednisone (or equivalent) may be most susceptible. Fatalities have occurred due to adrenal insufficiency in asthmatic patients during and after transfer from systemic corticosteroids to aerosol steroids; aerosol steroids do **not** provide the systemic steroid needed to treat patients having trauma, surgery, or infections.

Acute myopathy has been reported with high dose corticosteroids, usually in patients with neuromuscular transmission disorders; may involve ocular and/or respiratory muscles; monitor creatine kinase; recovery may be delayed. Corticosteroid use may cause psychiatric disturbances, including depression, euphoria, insomnia, mood swings, and personality changes. Pre-existing psychiatric conditions may be exacerbated by corticosteroid use. Prolonged use of corticosteroids may also increase the incidence of secondary infection, mask acute infection (including fungal infections), prolong or exacerbate viral infections, or limit response to vaccines. Exposure to chickenpox should be avoided; corticosteroids should not be used to treat ocular herpes simplex. Corticosteroids should not be used for cerebral malaria or viral hepatitis. Close observation is required in patients with latent tuberculosis and/or TB reactivity; restrict use in active TB (only in conjunction with antituberculosis treatment). Prolonged use of corticosteroids may result in glaucoma; cataract formation may occur. Prolonged treatment with corticosteroids has been associated with the development of Kaposi's sarcoma (case reports); if noted, discontinuation of therapy should be considered.

Use with caution in patients with thyroid disease, hepatic impairment, renal impairment, cardiovascular disease, diabetes, glaucoma, cataracts, myasthenia gravis, patients at risk for osteoporosis, patients at risk for seizures, or GI diseases (diverticulitis, peptic ulcer, ulcerative colitis) due to perforation risk. Use caution following acute MI (corticosteroids have been associated with myocardial rupture). Because of the risk of adverse effects, systemic corticosteroids should be used cautiously in the elderly in the smallest possible effective dose for the shortest duration.

Adverse Reactions (Reflective of adult population; not specific for elderly) Frequency not defined.

Cardiovascular: Cardiomyopathy, CHF, edema, facial edema, hypertension

Central nervous system: Headache, insomnia, malaise, nervousness, pseudotumor cerebri, psychic disorders, seizure, vertigo

Dermatologic: Bruising, facial erythema, hirsutism, petechiae, skin test reaction suppression, thin fragile skin, urticaria

Endocrine & metabolic: Carbohydrate tolerance decreased, Cushing's syndrome, diabetes mellitus, growth suppression, hyperglycemia, hypernatremia, hypokalemia, hypokalemic alkalosis, menstrual irregularities, negative nitrogen balance, pituitary adrenal axis suppression

Gastrointestinal: Abdominal distention, increased appetite, indigestion, nausea, pancreatitis, peptic ulcer, ulcerative esophagitis, weight gain

Hepatic: LFTs increased (usually reversible)

Neuromuscular & skeletal: Arthralgia, aseptic necrosis (humeral/femoral heads), fractures, muscle mass decreased, muscle weakness, osteoporosis, steroid myopathy, tendon rupture, weakness

Ocular: Cataracts, exophthalmus, eyelid edema, glaucoma, intraocular pressure increased, irritation

Respiratory: Epistaxis

Miscellaneous: Diaphoresis increased, impaired wound healing

Drug Interactions

Metabolism/Transport Effects Substrate of CYP3A4 (minor); **Inhibits** CYP3A4 (weak)

Avoid Concomitant Use

Avoid concomitant use of PrednisoLONE (Systemic) with any of the following: Aldesleukin; BCG; Natalizumab; Pimecrolimus; Tacrolimus (Topical)

Increased Effect/Toxicity

PrednisoLONE (Systemic) may increase the levels/effects of: Acetylcholinesterase Inhibitors; Amphotericin B; CycloSPORINE; CycloSPORINE (Systemic); Deferasirox; Leflunomide; Loop Diuretics; Natalizumab; NSAID (COX-2 Inhibitor); NSAID (Nonselective); Thiazide Diuretics; Vaccines (Live); Warfarin

The levels/effects of PrednisoLONE (Systemic) may be increased by: Antifungal Agents (Azole Derivatives, Systemic); Aprepitant; Calcium Channel Blockers (Nondihydropyridine); Conivaptan; CycloSPORINE; CycloSPORINE (Systemic); Denosumab; Estrogen Derivatives; Fluconazole; Fosaprepitant; Macrolide Antibiotics; Neuromuscular-Blocking Agents (Nondepolarizing); Pimecrolimus; Quinolone Antibiotics; Roflumilast; Salicylates; Tacrolimus (Topical); Telaprevir; Trastuzumab

Decreased Effect

PrednisoLONE (Systemic) may decrease the levels/effects of: Aldesleukin; Antidiabetic Agents; BCG; Calcitriol; Corticorelin; CycloSPORINE; CycloSPORINE (Systemic); Isoniazid; Salicylates; Sipuleucel-T; Telaprevir; Vaccines (Inactivated)

The levels/effects of PrednisoLONE (Systemic) may be decreased by: Aminoglutethimide; Antacids; Barbiturates; Bile Acid Sequestrants; Echinacea; Mitotane; Primidone; Rifamycin Derivatives; Tocilizumab

Ethanol/Nutrition/Herb Interactions

Ethanol: Avoid ethanol (may increase gastric mucosal irritation).

Food: Prednisolone interferes with calcium absorption. Limit caffeine.

Herb/Nutraceutical: St John's wort may decrease prednisolone levels. Avoid cat's claw, echinacea (have immunostimulant properties).

Stability

Flo-Pred™: Store at 20°C to 25°C (68°F to 77°F). Flo-Pred™ should be dispensed in the original container (to avoid loss of formulation during transfer).

Millipred™: Store at 20°C to 25°C (68°F to 77°F).

Orapred ODT®: Store at 20°C to 25°C (68°F to 77°F) in blister pack. Protect from moisture.

Orapred®, Veripred™ 20: 2°C to 8°C (36°F to 46°F).

Pediapred®: 4°C to 25°C (39°F to 77°F); may be refrigerated.

Prelone®: 15°C to 30°C (59°F to 86°F).

Mechanism of Action

Decreases inflammation by suppression of migration of polymorphonuclear leukocytes and reversal of increased capillary permeability; suppresses the immune system by reducing activity and volume of the lymphatic system

Pharmacodynamics/Kinetics

Duration: 18-36 hours

Protein binding (concentration dependent): 65% to 91%; decreased in elderly

Metabolism: Primarily hepatic, but also metabolized in most tissues, to inactive compounds

Half-life elimination: 3.6 hours; End-stage renal disease: 3-5 hours

Excretion: Primarily urine (as glucuronides, sulfates, and unconjugated metabolites)

Dosage

Geriatric Use lowest effective adult dose. Dose depends upon condition being treated and response of patient; alternate day dosing may be attempted in some disease states.

Adult Dose depends upon condition being treated and response of patient. Oral dosage expressed in terms of prednisolone base. Consider alternate day therapy for long-term therapy. Discontinuation of long-term therapy requires gradual withdrawal by tapering the dose. Patients undergoing unusual stress while receiving corticosteroids, should receive increased doses prior to, during, and after the stressful situation.

Usual dose (range): Oral: 5-60 mg/day

Rheumatoid arthritis: Oral: Initial: 5-7.5 mg/day, adjust dose as necessary

Multiple sclerosis: Oral: 200 mg/day for 1 week followed by 80 mg every other day for 1 month

Dosing adjustment in hyperthyroidism: Prednisolone dose may need to be increased to achieve adequate therapeutic effects.

Renal Impairment

Hemodialysis: Slightly dialyzable (5% to 20%); administer dose posthemodialysis

Peritoneal dialysis: Supplemental dose is not necessary

Administration Administer oral formulation with food or milk to decrease GI effects.

Flo-Pred™: Administer using the provided calibrated syringe (supplied by manufacturer) to accurately measure the dose. Syringe should be washed prior to next use.

Orapred ODT®: Do not break or use partial tablet. Remove tablet from blister pack just prior to use. May swallow whole or allow to dissolve on tongue.

Monitoring Parameters Blood pressure; blood glucose, electrolytes; intraocular pressure (use >6 weeks); bone mineral density

Test Interactions Response to skin tests

◀ **Pharmacotherapy Pearls Withdrawal/tapering of therapy:** Corticosteroid tapering following short-term use is limited primarily by the need to control the underlying disease state; tapering may be accomplished over a period of days. Following longer-term use, tapering over weeks to months may be necessary to avoid signs and symptoms of adrenal insufficiency and to allow recovery of the HPA axis. Testing of HPA axis responsiveness may be of value in selected patients. Subtle deficits in HPA response may persist for months after discontinuation of therapy, and may require supplemental dosing during periods of acute illness or surgical stress.

Special Geriatric Considerations Useful in patients with inability to activate prednisone (liver disease). Because of the risk of adverse effects, systemic corticosteroids should be used cautiously in the elderly, in the smallest possible dose, and for the shortest possible time. For long-term use, monitor bone mineral density and institute fracture prevention strategies.

Dosage Forms Excipient information presented when available (limited, particularly for generics); consult specific product labeling.

Solution, oral, as base: 15 mg/5 mL (240 mL, 480 mL)

Solution, oral, as sodium phosphate [strength expressed as base]: 5 mg/5 mL (120 mL); 15 mg/5 mL (237 mL, 473 mL)

Millipred™: 10 mg/5 mL (237 mL) [dye free; grape flavor]

Orapred®: 15 mg/5 mL (20 mL, 237 mL) [dye free; contains ethanol 2%, sodium benzoate; grape flavor]

Pediapred®: 5 mg/5 mL (120 mL) [dye free; raspberry flavor]

Veripred™ 20: 20 mg/5 mL (237 mL) [dye free, ethanol free; grape flavor]

Suspension, oral:

Flo-Pred™: 15 mg/5 mL (52 mL) [contains propylene glycol; cherry flavor]

Syrup, oral, as base: 15 mg/5 mL (240 mL, 480 mL)

Prelone®: 15 mg/5 mL (240 mL, 480 mL) [contains benzoic acid, ethanol 5%, propylene glycol; wild cherry flavor]

Tablet, orally disintegrating, oral, as sodium phosphate [strength expressed as base]:

Orapred ODT®: 10 mg, 15 mg, 30 mg [grape flavor]

PrednisoLONE (Ophthalmic) (pred NISS oh lone)

Medication Safety Issues

Sound-alike/look-alike issues:

PrednisoLONE may be confused with predniSONE

Brand Names: U.S. Omnipred™; Pred Forte®; Pred Mild®

Brand Names: Canada Diopred®; Ophtho-Tate®; Pred Forte®; Pred Mild®

Index Terms Econopred; Prednisolone Acetate, Ophthalmic; Prednisolone Sodium Phosphate, Ophthalmic

Generic Availability (U.S.) Yes

Pharmacologic Category Corticosteroid, Ophthalmic

Use Treatment of palpebral and bulbar conjunctivitis; corneal injury from chemical, radiation, thermal burns, or foreign body penetration; steroid-responsive inflammatory ophthalmic diseases

Dosage

Geriatric & Adult Conjunctivitis: Ophthalmic (suspension/solution): Instill 1-2 drops in the eye 2-4 times daily

Dosage Forms Excipient information presented when available (limited, particularly for generics); consult specific product labeling.

Solution, ophthalmic, as sodium phosphate [drops]: 1% (5 mL, 10 mL, 15 mL)

Suspension, ophthalmic, as acetate [drops]: 1% (5 mL, 10 mL, 15 mL)

Omnipred™: 1% (5 mL, 10 mL) [contains benzalkonium chloride]

Pred Forte®: 1% (1 mL, 5 mL, 10 mL, 15 mL) [contains benzalkonium chloride, sodium bisulfite]

Pred Mild®: 0.12% (5 mL, 10 mL) [contains benzalkonium chloride, sodium bisulfite]

◆ **Prednisolone Acetate, Ophthalmic** see PrednisoLONE (Ophthalmic) on page 1510

Prednisolone and Gentamicin (pred NIS oh lone & jen ta MYE sin)

Related Information

Gentamicin (Ophthalmic) on page 820

PrednisoLONE (Ophthalmic) on page 1510

Brand Names: U.S. Pred-G®

Index Terms Gentamicin and Prednisolone

Generic Availability (U.S.) No

Pharmacologic Category Antibiotic/Corticosteroid, Ophthalmic
Use Treatment of steroid responsive inflammatory conditions and superficial ocular infections due to microorganisms susceptible to gentamicin
Dosage
  Geriatric & Adult Inflammatory conditions and superficial ocular infections: Ophthalmic:
    Ointment: Apply ½ inch ribbon in the conjunctival sac 1-3 times/day
    Suspension: 1 drop 2-4 times/day; during the initial 24-48 hours, the dosing frequency may be increased if necessary up to 1 drop every hour
Special Geriatric Considerations Evaluate the patient's or caregiver's ability to safely administer the correct dose of ophthalmic medication.
Dosage Forms Excipient information presented when available (limited, particularly for generics); consult specific product labeling. [DSC] = Discontinued product
  Ointment, ophthalmic:
    Pred-G®: Prednisolone acetate 0.6% and gentamicin sulfate 0.3% (3.5 g)
  Suspension, ophthalmic:
    Pred-G®: Prednisolone acetate 1% and gentamicin sulfate 0.3% (5 mL, 10 mL) [contains benzalkonium chloride] [DSC]

◆ **Prednisolone and Sulfacetamide** see Sulfacetamide and Prednisolone on page 1714
◆ **Prednisolone Sodium Phosphate** see PredniSOLONE (Systemic) on page 1507
◆ **Prednisolone Sodium Phosphate, Ophthalmic** see PredniSOLONE (Ophthalmic) on page 1510

PredniSONE (PRED ni sone)

Related Information
  Corticosteroids on page 2005
Medication Safety Issues
  Sound-alike/look-alike issues:
    PredniSONE may be confused with methylPREDNISolone, Pramosone®, prazosin, predniSOLONE, PriLOSEC®, primidone, promethazine
Brand Names: U.S. PredniSONE Intensol™
Brand Names: Canada Apo-Prednisone®; Novo-Prednisone; Winpred™
Index Terms Deltacortisone; Deltadehydrocortisone
Generic Availability (U.S.) Yes
Pharmacologic Category Corticosteroid, Systemic
Use Treatment of a variety of diseases, including:
  Allergic states (including adjunctive treatment of anaphylaxis)
  Autoimmune disorders (including systemic lupus erythematosus [SLE])
  Collagen diseases
  Dermatologic conditions/diseases
  Edematous states (including nephrotic syndrome)
  Endocrine disorders
  Gastrointestinal diseases
  Hematologic disorders (including idiopathic thrombocytopenia purpura [ITP])
  Multiple sclerosis exacerbations
  Neoplastic diseases
  Ophthalmic diseases
  Respiratory diseases (including acute asthma exacerbation)
  Rheumatic disorders (including rheumatoid arthritis)
  Trichinosis with neurologic or myocardial involvement
  Tuberculous meningitis
Unlabeled/Investigational Use Adjunctive therapy for Pneumocystis jiroveci (formerly carinii) pneumonia (PCP); autoimmune hepatitis; adjunctive therapy for pain management in immunocompetent patients with herpes zoster; tuberculosis (severe, paradoxical reactions)
Contraindications Hypersensitivity to any component of the formulation; systemic fungal infections; administration of live or live attenuated vaccines with immunosuppressive doses of prednisone
Warnings/Precautions May cause hypercorticism or suppression of hypothalamic-pituitary-adrenal (HPA) axis, particularly in patients receiving high doses for prolonged periods. HPA axis suppression may lead to adrenal crisis. Withdrawal and discontinuation of a corticosteroid should be done slowly and carefully. Particular care is required when patients are transferred from systemic corticosteroids to inhaled products due to possible adrenal insufficiency or withdrawal from steroids, including an increase in allergic symptoms. Patients receiving >20 mg per day of prednisone (or equivalent) may be most susceptible. Fatalities have occurred due to adrenal insufficiency in asthmatic patients during and after transfer from ▶

◄ systemic corticosteroids to aerosol steroids; aerosol steroids do **not** provide the systemic steroid needed to treat patients having trauma, surgery, or infections.

Acute myopathy has been reported with high dose corticosteroids, usually in patients with neuromuscular transmission disorders; may involve ocular and/or respiratory muscles; monitor creatine kinase; recovery may be delayed. Prolonged use of corticosteroids may increase the incidence of secondary infection, mask acute infection (including fungal infections), prolong or exacerbate viral infections, or limit response to vaccines. Exposure to chickenpox should be avoided. Corticosteroids should not be used to treat ocular herpes simplex or cerebral malaria. Close observation is required in patients with latent tuberculosis and/or TB reactivity; restrict use in active TB (only in conjunction with antituberculosis treatment). Prolonged treatment with corticosteroids has been associated with the development of Kaposi's sarcoma (case reports); if noted, discontinuation of therapy should be considered. Prolonged use may cause posterior subcapsular cataracts, glaucoma (with possible nerve damage) and may increase the risk for ocular infections. Corticosteroid use may cause psychiatric disturbances, including depression, euphoria, insomnia, mood swings, and personality changes. Pre-existing psychiatric conditions may be exacerbated by corticosteroid use.

Use with caution in patients with HF, diabetes, GI diseases (diverticulitis, peptic ulcer, ulcerative colitis; due to risk of perforation), hepatic impairment, myasthenia gravis, MI, patients with or who are at risk for osteoporosis, seizure disorders or thyroid disease.

Prior to use, the dose and duration of treatment should be based on the risk versus benefit for each individual patient. In general, use the smallest effective dose for the shortest duration of time to minimize adverse events. A gradual tapering of dose may be required prior to discontinuing therapy.

Adverse Reactions (Reflective of adult population; not specific for elderly) Frequency not defined.

Cardiovascular: Congestive heart failure (in susceptible patients), hypertension

Central nervous system: Emotional instability, headache, intracranial pressure increased (with papilledema), psychic derangements (including euphoria, insomnia, mood swings, personality changes, severe depression), seizure, vertigo

Dermatologic: Bruising, facial erythema, petechiae, thin fragile skin, urticaria, wound healing impaired

Endocrine & metabolic: Adrenocortical and pituitary unresponsiveness (in times of stress), carbohydrate intolerance, Cushing's syndrome, diabetes mellitus, fluid retention, growth suppression (in children), hypokalemic alkalosis, hypothyroidism enhanced, menstrual irregularities, negative nitrogen balance due to protein catabolism, potassium loss, sodium retention

Gastrointestinal: Abdominal distension, pancreatitis, peptic ulcer (with possible perforation and hemorrhage), ulcerative esophagitis

Hepatic: ALT increased, AST increased, alkaline phosphatase increased

Neuromuscular & skeletal: Aseptic necrosis of femoral and humeral heads, muscle mass loss, muscle weakness, osteoporosis, pathologic fracture of long bones, steroid myopathy, tendon rupture (particularly Achilles tendon), vertebral compression fractures

Ocular: Exophthalmos, glaucoma, intraocular pressure increased, posterior subcapsular cataracts

Miscellaneous: Allergic reactions, anaphylactic reactions, diaphoresis, hypersensitivity reactions, infections, Kaposi's sarcoma

Drug Interactions

Metabolism/Transport Effects Substrate of CYP3A4 (minor); **Induces** CYP2C19 (weak), 3A4 (weak)

Avoid Concomitant Use

Avoid concomitant use of PredniSONE with any of the following: Aldesleukin; BCG; Natalizumab; Pimecrolimus; Tacrolimus (Topical)

Increased Effect/Toxicity

PredniSONE may increase the levels/effects of: Acetylcholinesterase Inhibitors; Amphotericin B; CycloSPORINE; CycloSPORINE (Systemic); Deferasirox; Leflunomide; Loop Diuretics; Natalizumab; NSAID (COX-2 Inhibitor); NSAID (Nonselective); Thiazide Diuretics; Vaccines (Live); Warfarin

The levels/effects of PredniSONE may be increased by: Antifungal Agents (Azole Derivatives, Systemic); Aprepitant; Calcium Channel Blockers (Nondihydropyridine); Conivaptan; CycloSPORINE; CycloSPORINE (Systemic); Denosumab; Estrogen Derivatives; Fluconazole; Fosaprepitant; Macrolide Antibiotics; Neuromuscular-Blocking Agents (Nondepolarizing); Pimecrolimus; Quinolone Antibiotics; Ritonavir; Roflumilast; Salicylates; Tacrolimus (Topical); Telaprevir; Trastuzumab

Decreased Effect

PredniSONE may decrease the levels/effects of: Aldesleukin; Antidiabetic Agents; BCG; Calcitriol; Corticorelin; CycloSPORINE; CycloSPORINE (Systemic); Isoniazid; Salicylates; Sipuleucel-T; Telaprevir; Vaccines (Inactivated)

The levels/effects of PredniSONE may be decreased by: Aminoglutethimide; Antacids; Barbiturates; Bile Acid Sequestrants; Echinacea; Mitotane; Primidone; Rifamycin Derivatives; Somatropin; Tesamorelin; Tocilizumab

Ethanol/Nutrition/Herb Interactions

Ethanol: Avoid ethanol (may increase gastric mucosal irritation)

Food: Prednisone interferes with calcium absorption. Limit caffeine.

Herb/Nutraceutical: St John's wort may decrease prednisone levels. Avoid cat's claw, echinacea (have immunostimulant properties).

Mechanism of Action

Decreases inflammation by suppression of migration of polymorpho-nuclear leukocytes and reversal of increased capillary permeability; suppresses the immune system by reducing activity and volume of the lymphatic system; suppresses adrenal function at high doses. Antitumor effects may be related to inhibition of glucose transport, phosphorylation, or induction of cell death in immature lymphocytes. Antiemetic effects are thought to occur due to blockade of cerebral innervation of the emetic center via inhibition of prostaglandin synthesis.

Pharmacodynamics/Kinetics

Absorption: 50% to 90% (may be altered in IBS or hyperthyroidism)

Protein binding (concentration dependent): 65% to 91%

Metabolism: Hepatically converted from prednisone (inactive) to prednisolone (active); may be impaired with hepatic dysfunction

Half-life elimination: Normal renal function: ~3.5 hours

Excretion: Urine (small portion)

Dosage

Geriatric Refer to adult dosing; use the lowest effective dose. Oral dose depends upon condition being treated and response of patient. Alternate day dosing may be attempted.

Adult General dosing range: Oral: Initial: 5-60 mg/day: **Note:** Dose depends upon condition being treated and response of patient. Consider alternate day therapy for long-term therapy. Discontinuation of long-term therapy requires gradual withdrawal by tapering the dose.

Prednisone taper (other regimens also available):

Day 1: 30 mg divided as 10 mg before breakfast, 5 mg at lunch, 5 mg at dinner, 10 mg at bedtime

Day 2: 5 mg at breakfast, 5 mg at lunch, 5 mg at dinner, 10 mg at bedtime

Day 3: 5 mg 4 times/day (with meals and at bedtime)

Day 4: 5 mg 3 times/day (breakfast, lunch, bedtime)

Day 5: 5 mg 2 times/day (breakfast, bedtime)

Day 6: 5 mg before breakfast

Indication-specific dosing:

Acute asthma (NIH guidelines, 2007): Oral: 40-60 mg per day for 3-10 days; administer as single or 2divided doses

Anaphylaxis, adjunctive treatment (Lieberman 2005): Oral: 0.5 mg/kg

Antineoplastic: Oral: Usual range: 10 mg/day to 100 mg/m² /day (depending on indication). **Note:** Details concerning dosing in combination regimens should also be consulted.

Autoimmune hepatitis (unlabeled use; Czaja 2002): Oral: Initial treatment: 60 mg/day for 1 week, *followed by* 40 mg/day for 1 week, *then* 30 mg/day for 2 weeks, *then* 20 mg/day. Half this dose should be given when used in combination with azathioprine

Herpes zoster (unlabeled use; Dworkin 2007): Oral: 60 mg/day for 7 days, *followed by* 30 mg/day for 7 days, *then* 15 mg/day for 7 days

Idiopathic thrombocytopenia purpura (American Society of Hematology 1997): Oral: 1-2 mg/kg/day

PCP pneumonia (AIDSinfo guidelines, 2008): Note: Begin within 72 hours of PCP therapy: 40 mg twice daily for 5 days, *followed by* 40 mg once daily for 5 days, *followed by* 20 mg once daily for 11 days or until antimicrobial regimen is completed

Rheumatoid arthritis (American College of Rheumatology 2002): Oral: ≤10 mg/day

Systemic lupus erythematosus (American College of Rheumatology 1999): Oral: Mild SLE: ≤10 mg/day

Refractory or severe organ-threatening disease: 20-60 mg/day

Thyrotoxicosis (type II amiodarone induced; unlabeled use): Oral: 30-40 mg/day for 7-14 days, gradually taper over 3 months

Tuberculosis, severe, paradoxical reactions (unlabeled use, AIDS info guidelines 2008): Oral: 1 mg/kg/day, gradually reduce after 1-2 weeks

Renal Impairment Hemodialysis effects: Supplemental dose is not necessary.

Administration Administer with food to decrease gastrointestinal upset

◀ **Monitoring Parameters** Blood pressure, blood glucose, electrolytes

Following prolonged use: Bone mass density, signs and symptoms of infection, cataract formation

Test Interactions Decreased response to skin tests

Pharmacotherapy Pearls Tapering of corticosteroids after a short course of therapy (<7-10 days) is generally not required unless the disease/inflammatory process is slow to respond. Tapering after prolonged exposure is dependent upon the individual patient, duration of corticosteroid treatments, and size of steroid dose. Recovery of the HPA axis may require several months. Subtle but important HPA axis suppression may be present for as long as several months after a course of as few as 10-14 days duration. Testing of HPA axis (cosyntropin) may be required, and signs/symptoms of adrenal insufficiency should be monitored in patients with a history of use.

Special Geriatric Considerations Because of the risk of adverse effects, systemic corticosteroids should be used cautiously in the elderly, in the smallest possible dose, and for the shortest possible time. For long-term use, monitor bone mineral density and institute fracture prevention strategies.

Dosage Forms Excipient information presented when available (limited, particularly for generics); consult specific product labeling.

Solution, oral: 1 mg/mL (5 mL, 120 mL, 500 mL)

Solution, oral [concentrate]:

PredniSONE Intensol™: 5 mg/mL (30 mL) [dye free, sugar free; contains ethanol 30%, propylene glycol]

Tablet, oral: 1 mg, 2.5 mg, 5 mg, 10 mg, 20 mg, 50 mg

◆ **PredniSONE Intensol™** *see* PredniSONE *on page 1511*

◆ **Prefest™** *see* Estradiol and Norgestimate *on page 649*

Pregabalin (pre GAB a lin)

Medication Safety Issues

Sound-alike/look-alike issues:

Lyrica® may be confused with Lopressor®

Brand Names: U.S. Lyrica®

Brand Names: Canada Lyrica®

Index Terms CI-1008; S-(+)-3-isobutylgaba

Generic Availability (U.S.) No

Pharmacologic Category Analgesic, Miscellaneous; Anticonvulsant, Miscellaneous

Use Management of pain associated with diabetic peripheral neuropathy; management of postherpetic neuralgia; adjunctive therapy for partial-onset seizure disorder in adults; management of fibromyalgia

Medication Guide Available Yes

Contraindications Hypersensitivity to pregabalin or any component of the formulation

Warnings/Precautions Antiepileptics are associated with an increased risk of suicidal behavior/thoughts with use (regardless of indication); patients should be monitored for signs/symptoms of depression, suicidal tendencies, and other unusual behavior changes during therapy and instructed to inform their healthcare provider immediately if symptoms occur.

Angioedema has been reported; may be life threatening; use with caution in patients with a history of angioedema episodes. Concurrent use with other drugs known to cause angioedema (eg, ACE inhibitors) may increase risk. Hypersensitivity reactions, including skin redness, blistering, hives, rash, dyspnea and wheezing have been reported; discontinue treatment of hypersensitivity occurs. May cause CNS depression and/or dizziness, which may impair physical or mental abilities. Patients must be cautioned about performing tasks which require mental alertness (eg, operating machinery or driving). Effects with other sedative drugs or ethanol may be potentiated. Visual disturbances (blurred vision, decreased acuity and visual field changes) have been associated with pregabalin therapy; patients should be instructed to notify their physician if these effects are noted.

Pregabalin has been associated with increases in CPK and rare cases of rhabdomyolysis. Patients should be instructed to notify their prescriber if unexplained muscle pain, tenderness, or weakness, particularly if fever and/or malaise are associated with these symptoms. Use may be associated with weight gain and peripheral edema; use caution in patients with congestive heart failure, hypertension, or diabetes. Effect on weight gain/edema may be additive to thiazolidinedione antidiabetic agent; particularly in patients with prior cardiovascular disease. May decrease platelet count or prolong PR interval.

Has been noted to be tumorigenic (increased incidence of hemangiosarcoma) in animal studies; significance of these findings in humans is unknown. Pregabalin has been associated with discontinuation symptoms following abrupt cessation, and increases in seizure frequency (when used as an antiepileptic) may occur. Should not be discontinued abruptly; dosage tapering over at least 1 week is recommended. Use caution in renal impairment; dosage adjustment required.

Adverse Reactions (Reflective of adult population; not specific for elderly) Note: Frequency of adverse effects may be influenced by dose or concurrent therapy. In add-on trials in epilepsy, frequency of CNS and visual adverse effects were higher than those reported in pain management trials. Range noted below is inclusive of all trials.

>10%:

Cardiovascular: Peripheral edema (up to 16%)

Central nervous system: Dizziness (8% to 45%), somnolence (4% to 28%), ataxia (up to 20%), headache (up to 14%)

Gastrointestinal: Weight gain (up to 16%), xerostomia (1% to 15%)

Neuromuscular & skeletal: Tremor (up to 11%)

Ocular: Blurred vision (1% to 12%), diplopia (up to 12%)

Miscellaneous: Infection (up to 14%), accidental injury (2% to 11%)

1% to 10%:

Cardiovascular: Chest pain (up to 4%), edema (up to 6%)

Central nervous system: Neuropathy (up to 9%), thinking abnormal (up to 9%), fatigue (up to 8%), confusion (up to 7%), euphoria (up to 7%), speech disorder (up to 7%), attention disturbance (up to 6%), incoordination (up to 6%), amnesia (up to 6%), pain (up to 5%), memory impaired (up to 4%), vertigo (up to 4%), feeling abnormal (up to 3%), hypoesthesia (up to 3%), anxiety (up to 2%), depression (up to 2%), disorientation (up to 2%), lethargy (up to 2%), depersonalization (≥1%), hypertonia (≥1%), stupor (≥1%), nervousness (up to 1%)

Dermatologic: Facial edema (up to 3%), bruising (≥1%), pruritus (≥1%)

Endocrine & metabolic: Fluid retention (up to 3%), hypoglycemia (up to 3%), libido decreased (≥1%)

Gastrointestinal: Constipation (up to 10%), appetite increased (up to 7%), flatulence (up to 3%), vomiting (up to 3%), abdominal distension (up to 2%), abdominal pain (≥1%), gastroenteritis (≥1%)

Genitourinary: Incontinence (up to 2%), anorgasmia (≥1%), impotence (≥1%), urinary frequency (≥1%)

Hematologic: Thrombocytopenia (3%)

Neuromuscular & skeletal: Balance disorder (up to 9%), abnormal gait (up to 8%), weakness (up to 7%), arthralgia (up to 6%), twitching (up to 5%), back pain (up to 4%), muscle spasm (up to 4%), myoclonus (up to 4%), paresthesia (>2%), CPK increased (2%), leg cramps (≥1%), myalgia (≥1%), myasthenia (up to 1%)

Ocular: Visual abnormalities (up to 5%), visual field defect (≥2%), eye disorder (up to 2%), nystagmus (>2%), conjunctivitis (≥1%)

Otic: Otitis media (≥1%), tinnitus (≥1%)

Respiratory: Sinusitis (up to 7%), dyspnea (up to 3%), bronchitis (up to 3%), pharyngolaryngeal pain (up to 3%)

Miscellaneous: Flu-like syndrome (up to 2%), allergic reaction (≥1%)

Drug Interactions

Avoid Concomitant Use There are no known interactions where it is recommended to avoid concomitant use.

Increased Effect/Toxicity

Pregabalin may increase the levels/effects of: Alcohol (Ethyl); Antidiabetic Agents (Thiazolidinedione); CNS Depressants; Methotrimeprazine; Selective Serotonin Reuptake Inhibitors

The levels/effects of Pregabalin may be increased by: Droperidol; HydrOXYzine; Methotrimeprazine

Decreased Effect

The levels/effects of Pregabalin may be decreased by: Ketorolac; Ketorolac (Nasal); Ketorolac (Systemic); Mefloquine

Ethanol/Nutrition/Herb Interactions

Ethanol: May increase CNS depression; monitor for increased effects with coadministration. Caution patients about effects.

Herb/Nutraceutical: Avoid valerian, St John's wort, kava kava, gotu kola (may increase CNS depression).

Stability Store at 15°C to 30°C (59°F to 86°F).

Mechanism of Action Binds to alpha$_2$-delta subunit of voltage-gated calcium channels within the CNS, inhibiting excitatory neurotransmitter release. Although structurally related to GABA, it does not bind to GABA or benzodiazepine receptors. Exerts antinociceptive and anticonvulsant activity. Decreases symptoms of painful peripheral neuropathies and, as adjunctive therapy in partial seizures, decreases the frequency of seizures.

Pharmacodynamics/Kinetics

Onset of action: Pain management: Effects may be noted as early as the first week of therapy.

Distribution: V_d: 0.5 L/kg

Protein binding: 0%

Metabolism: Negligible

Bioavailability: >90%

Half-life elimination: 6.3 hours

Time to peak, plasma: 1.5 hours (3 hours with food)

Excretion: Urine (90% as unchanged drug; minor metabolites)

Dosage

Geriatric & Adult

Fibromyalgia: Oral: Initial: 150 mg/day in divided doses (75 mg 2 times/day); may be increased to 300 mg/day (150 mg 2 times/day) within 1 week based on tolerability and effect; may be further increased to 450 mg/day (225 mg 2 times/day). Maximum dose: 450 mg/day (dosages up to 600 mg/day were evaluated with no significant additional benefit and an increase in adverse effects)

Neuropathic pain (diabetes-associated): Oral: Initial: 150 mg/day in divided doses (50 mg 3 times/day); may be increased within 1 week based on tolerability and effect; maximum dose: 300 mg/day (dosages up to 600 mg/day were evaluated with no significant additional benefit and an increase in adverse effects)

Postherpetic neuralgia: Oral: Initial: 150 mg/day in divided doses (75 mg 2 times/day or 50 mg 3 times/day); may be increased to 300 mg/day within 1 week based on tolerability and effect; further titration (to 600 mg/day) after 2-4 weeks may be considered in patients who do not experience sufficient relief of pain provided they are able to tolerate pregabalin. Maximum dose: 600 mg/day

Partial onset seizures (adjunctive therapy): Oral: Initial: 150 mg per day in divided doses (75 mg 2 times/day or 50 mg 3 times/day); may be increased based on tolerability and effect (optimal titration schedule has not been defined). Maximum dose: 600 mg/day

Note: Discontinuing therapy: Pregabalin should not be abruptly discontinued; taper dosage over at least 1 week

Renal Impairment Renal function may be estimated using the Cockcroft-Gault formula. Then determine recommended dosage regimen based on the indication-specific total daily dose for normal renal function ($Cl_{cr} \geq 60$ mL/minute). For example, if the indication-specific daily dose is 450 mg/day for normal renal function, the daily dose should be reduced to 225 mg/day (in 2-3 divided doses) for a creatinine clearance of 30-60 mL/minute (see table).

Pregabalin Renal Impairment Dosing

Cl_{cr} (mL/minute)	Total Pregabalin Daily Dose (mg/day)				Dosing Frequency
≥60 (normal renal function)	150	300	450	600	2-3 divided doses
30-60	75	150	225	300	2-3 divided doses
15-30	25-50	75	100-150	150	1-2 divided doses
<15	25	25-50	50-75	75	Single daily dose

Posthemodialysis supplementary dosage (as a single additional dose):
25 mg/day schedule: Single supplementary dose of 25 mg **or** 50 mg
25-50 mg/day schedule: Single supplementary dose of 50 mg **or** 75 mg
50-75 mg/day schedule: Single supplementary dose of 75 mg **or** 100 mg
75 mg/day schedule: Single supplementary dose of 100 mg **or** 150 mg

Administration May be administered with or without food.

Monitoring Parameters Measures of efficacy (pain intensity/seizure frequency); degree of sedation; symptoms of myopathy or ocular disturbance; weight gain/edema; CPK; skin integrity (in patients with diabetes); suicidality (eg, suicidal thoughts, depression, behavioral changes)

Special Geriatric Considerations In clinical studies, no differences in safety and efficacy were noted between elderly. Since pregabalin is primarily excreted renally, dosage adjustment, based on Cl_{cr} is necessary.

Product Availability Lyrica® oral solution: FDA approved December 2009; anticipated availability is currently undetermined

Controlled Substance C-V

Dosage Forms Excipient information presented when available (limited, particularly for generics); consult specific product labeling.
Capsule, oral:
  Lyrica®: 25 mg, 50 mg, 75 mg, 100 mg, 150 mg, 200 mg, 225 mg, 300 mg
Selected References
Hill CM, Balkenohl M, Thomas DW, et al, "Pregabalin in Patients With Postoperative Dental Pain," *Eur J Pain*, 2001, 5 (2):119-24.

◆ **Pregnenedione** *see* Progesterone *on page 1528*
◆ **Prelone®** *see* PrednisoLONE (Systemic) *on page 1507*
◆ **Premarin®** *see* Estrogens (Conjugated/Equine, Systemic) *on page 658*
◆ **Premarin®** *see* Estrogens (Conjugated/Equine, Topical) *on page 661*
◆ **Premjact®** *see* Lidocaine (Topical) *on page 1064*
◆ **Premphase®** *see* Estrogens (Conjugated/Equine) and Medroxyprogesterone *on page 664*
◆ **Prempro®** *see* Estrogens (Conjugated/Equine) and Medroxyprogesterone *on page 664*
◆ **Preparation H® [OTC]** *see* Phenylephrine (Topical) *on page 1443*
◆ **Preparation H® Hydrocortisone [OTC]** *see* Hydrocortisone (Topical) *on page 886*
◆ **Pretz® [OTC]** *see* Sodium Chloride *on page 1690*
◆ **Prevacid®** *see* Lansoprazole *on page 1029*
◆ **Prevacid® 24 HR [OTC]** *see* Lansoprazole *on page 1029*
◆ **Prevacid® SoluTab™** *see* Lansoprazole *on page 1029*
◆ **Prevalite®** *see* Cholestyramine Resin *on page 348*
◆ **PreviDent®** *see* Fluoride *on page 751*
◆ **PreviDent® 5000 Booster** *see* Fluoride *on page 751*
◆ **PreviDent® 5000 Dry Mouth** *see* Fluoride *on page 751*
◆ **PreviDent® 5000 Plus®** *see* Fluoride *on page 751*
◆ **PreviDent® 5000 Sensitive** *see* Fluoride *on page 751*
◆ **Prialt®** *see* Ziconotide *on page 1944*
◆ **Priftin®** *see* Rifapentine *on page 1612*
◆ **PriLOSEC®** *see* Omeprazole *on page 1339*
◆ **PriLOSEC OTC® [OTC]** *see* Omeprazole *on page 1339*
◆ **Primaclone** *see* Primidone *on page 1517*
◆ **Primatene® Mist [OTC]** *see* EPINEPHrine (Systemic, Oral Inhalation) *on page 606*
◆ **Primaxin® I.M. [DSC]** *see* Imipenem and Cilastatin *on page 916*
◆ **Primaxin® I.V.** *see* Imipenem and Cilastatin *on page 916*

Primidone (PRI mi done)

Medication Safety Issues
  Sound-alike/look-alike issues:
    Primidone may be confused with predniSONE, primaquine, pyridoxine
Brand Names: U.S. Mysoline®
Brand Names: Canada Apo-Primidone®
Index Terms Desoxyphenobarbital; Primaclone
Generic Availability (U.S.) Yes
Pharmacologic Category Anticonvulsant, Miscellaneous; Barbiturate
Use Management of grand mal, psychomotor, and focal seizures
Unlabeled/Investigational Use Benign familial tremor (essential tremor)
Medication Guide Available Yes
Contraindications Hypersensitivity to phenobarbital; porphyria
Warnings/Precautions Antiepileptics are associated with an increased risk of suicidal behavior/thoughts with use (regardless of indication); patients should be monitored for signs/symptoms of depression, suicidal tendencies, and other unusual behavior changes during therapy and instructed to inform their healthcare provider immediately if symptoms occur.

Use with caution in patients with renal or hepatic impairment, pulmonary insufficiency; abrupt withdrawal may precipitate status epilepticus. Potential for drug dependency exists. Do not administer to patients in acute pain. Use caution in elderly or debilitated patients - may cause paradoxical responses. May cause CNS depression, which may impair physical or mental abilities. Patients must cautioned about performing tasks which require mental alertness (eg, operating machinery or driving). Effects with other sedative drugs or ethanol may be potentiated. Use with caution in patients with depression or suicidal tendencies, or in patients with a history of drug abuse. Tolerance or psychological and physical dependence may occur with prolonged use. Use with caution in patients with hypoadrenalism.

◀ **Adverse Reactions (Reflective of adult population; not specific for elderly)** Frequency not defined.

Central nervous system: Ataxia, drowsiness, emotional disturbances, fatigue, hyperirritability, suicidal ideation, vertigo

Dermatologic: Morbilliform skin eruptions

Gastrointestinal: Anorexia, nausea, vomiting

Genitourinary: Impotence

Hematologic: Agranulocytosis, granulocytopenia, megaloblastic anemia (idiosyncratic), red cell aplasia/hypoplasia

Ocular: Diplopia, nystagmus

Drug Interactions

Metabolism/Transport Effects Metabolized to phenobarbital; **Induces** CYP1A2 (strong), 2B6 (strong), 2C8 (strong), 2C9 (strong), 3A4 (strong)

Avoid Concomitant Use

Avoid concomitant use of Primidone with any of the following: Boceprevir; Crizotinib; Dienogest; Dronedarone; Everolimus; Lapatinib; Lurasidone; Nilotinib; Nisoldipine; Pazopanib; Praziquantel; Ranolazine; Rilpivirine; Roflumilast; RomiDEPsin; Ticagrelor; Tolvaptan; Vandetanib

Increased Effect/Toxicity

Primidone may increase the levels/effects of: Alcohol (Ethyl); Barbiturates; Clarithromycin; CNS Depressants; Methotrimeprazine; Selective Serotonin Reuptake Inhibitors

The levels/effects of Primidone may be increased by: Carbonic Anhydrase Inhibitors; Clarithromycin; Dexmethylphenidate; Divalproex; Droperidol; Felbamate; HydrOXYzine; Methotrimeprazine; Methylphenidate; Valproic Acid

Decreased Effect

Primidone may decrease the levels/effects of: Bendamustine; Boceprevir; Brentuximab Vedotin; Clarithromycin; Corticosteroids (Systemic); Crizotinib; CYP1A2 Substrates; CYP2B6 Substrates; CYP2C8 Substrates (High risk); CYP2C9 Substrates (High risk); CYP3A4 Substrates; Diclofenac; Dienogest; Divalproex; Dronedarone; Everolimus; Exemestane; Felbamate; Gefitinib; GuanFACINE; Imatinib; Ixabepilone; LamoTRIgine; Lapatinib; Linagliptin; Lurasidone; Maraviroc; NIFEdipine; Nilotinib; Nisoldipine; Pazopanib; Praziquantel; QuiNIDine; Ranolazine; Rilpivirine; Rivaroxaban; Roflumilast; RomiDEPsin; Rufinamide; Saxagliptin; SORAfenib; Tadalafil; Ticagrelor; Tolvaptan; Treprostinil; Ulipristal; Valproic Acid; Vandetanib; Vemurafenib

The levels/effects of Primidone may be decreased by: Carbonic Anhydrase Inhibitors; Folic Acid; Fosphenytoin; Ketorolac; Ketorolac (Nasal); Ketorolac (Systemic); Leucovorin Calcium-Levoleucovorin; Levomefolate; Mefloquine; Methylfolate; Phenytoin

Ethanol/Nutrition/Herb Interactions

Ethanol: May increase CNS depression; monitor for increased effects with coadministration. Caution patients about effects.

Food: Protein-deficient diets increase duration of action of primidone.

Herb/Nutraceutical: Avoid valerian, St John's wort, kava kava, gotu kola (may increase CNS depression).

Stability Store at 20°C to 25°C (68°F to 77°F).

Mechanism of Action Decreases neuron excitability, raises seizure threshold similar to phenobarbital; primidone has two active metabolites, phenobarbital and phenylethylmalonamide (PEMA); PEMA may enhance the activity of phenobarbital

Pharmacodynamics/Kinetics

Absorption: 60% to 80%

Distribution: Adults: V_d: 0.6 L/kg

Protein binding: 30%

Metabolism: Hepatic to phenobarbital (active) by oxidation and to phenylethylmalonamide (PEMA; active) by scission of the heterocyclic ring

Half-life elimination (age dependent): Primidone: Mean: 5-15 hours (variable); PEMA: 16 hours (variable)

Time to peak, serum: ~3 hours (variable)

Excretion: Urine (40% as unchanged drug; the remainder is unconjugated PEMA, phenobarbital and its metabolites)

Dosage

Geriatric & Adult

Seizure disorders (grand mal, psychomotor, and focal): Oral: Days 1-3: 100-125 mg/day at bedtime; days 4-6: 100-125 twice daily; days 7-9: 100-125 mg 3 times daily; usual dose: 750-1500 mg/day in divided doses 3-4 times/day with maximum dosage of 2 g/day

Patients already receiving other anticonvulsants: Initial: 100-125 mg at bedtime; gradually increase to maintenance dose as other drug is gradually decreased, continue until desired level obtained or other drug completely withdrawn. If goal is monotherapy, conversion should be completed over ≥2 weeks.

Essential tremor (unlabeled use): Oral: Initial 12.5-25 mg/day at bedtime; titrate up to 250 mg/day in 1-2 divided doses; doses up to 750 mg/day may be beneficial

Renal Impairment

Adults (Aronoff, 2007): **Note:** Avoid in renal failure if possible; due to active metabolites with long half-lives and complex kinetics:

Cl_{cr} ≥50 mL/minute: Administer every 12 hours

Cl_{cr} 10-50 mL/minute: Administer every 12-24 hours

Cl_{cr} <10 mL/minute: Administer every 24 hours

Hemodialysis: Administer dose postdialysis

Hepatic Impairment Increased side effects may occur in severe liver disease. Monitor plasma levels and adjust dose accordingly.

Monitoring Parameters Serum primidone and phenobarbital concentration, neurological status. Due to CNS effects, monitor closely when initiating drug in elderly. Monitor CBC and sequential multiple analysis-12 (SMA-12) at 6-month intervals to compare with baseline obtained at start of therapy. Monitor for suicidality (eg, suicidal thoughts, depression, behavioral changes). Since elderly metabolize phenobarbital at a slower rate than younger adults, it is suggested to measure both primidone and phenobarbital levels together.

Reference Range Therapeutic: Adults: 5-12 mcg/mL (SI: 23-55 µmol/L); toxic effects rarely present with levels <10 mcg/mL (SI: 46 µmol/L) if phenobarbital concentrations are low. Dosage of primidone is adjusted with reference mostly to the phenobarbital level; Toxic: >15 mcg/mL (SI: >69 µmol/L)

Pharmacotherapy Pearls Bioequivalence problems have been noted with primidone from one manufacturer to another, therefore, brand interchange is not recommended

Special Geriatric Considerations Due to CNS effects, monitor closely when initiating drug in elderly. Monitor CBC at 6-month intervals to compare with baseline obtained at start of therapy. Since elderly metabolize phenobarbital at a slower rate than younger adults, it is suggested to measure both primidone and phenobarbital serum concentrations together. Adjust dose for renal function in elderly when initiating or changing dose.

Dosage Forms Excipient information presented when available (limited, particularly for generics); consult specific product labeling.

Tablet, oral: 50 mg, 250 mg

Mysoline®: 50 mg, 250 mg [scored]

Dosage Forms: Canada Excipient information presented when available (limited, particularly for generics); consult specific product labeling.

Tablet, oral:

Apo-Primidone®: 125 mg, 250 mg

Selected References

Chen JJ and Swope DM, "Essential Tremor: Diagnosis and Treatment," *Pharmacotherapy*, 2003, 23(9):1105-22.

Louis ED, "Clinical Practice. Essential Tremor," *N Engl J Med*, 2001, 345(12):887-91.

McNamara JO, "Drugs Effective in the Therapy of the Epilepsies," Gardman JG, Limbird LE, eds, *Goodman and Gilman's The Pharmacological Basis of Therapeutics*, 10th ed, New York, NY: McGraw-Hill, 2001:532.

Pahwa R and Lyons KE, "Essential Tremor: Differential Diagnosis and Current Therapy," *Am J Med*, 2003, 115 (2):134-42.

Probenecid (proe BEN e sid)

Medication Safety Issues

Sound-alike/look-alike issues:

Probenecid may be confused with Procanbid®

Brand Names: Canada Benuryl™

Index Terms Benemid [DSC]

Generic Availability (U.S.) Yes

Pharmacologic Category Uricosuric Agent

Use Treatment of hyperuricemia associated with gout or gouty arthritis; prolongation and elevation of beta-lactam plasma levels (eg, uncomplicated gonococcal infection)

◀ **Unlabeled/Investigational Use** Prolongation and elevation of beta-lactam plasma levels (eg, neurosyphilis, pelvic inflammatory disease)

Contraindications Hypersensitivity to probenecid or any component of the formulation; small- or large-dose aspirin therapy; blood dyscrasias; uric acid kidney stones; initiation during an acute gout attack

Warnings/Precautions Use with caution in patients with peptic ulcer. Salicylates may diminish the therapeutic effect of probenecid. This effect may be more pronounced with high, chronic doses, however, the manufacturer recommends the use of an alternative analgesic even in place of small doses of aspirin. Use of probenecid with penicillin in patients with renal insufficiency is not recommended. Probenecid monotherapy may not be effective in patients with a creatinine clearance <30 mL/minute. Probenecid may increase the serum concentration of methotrexate. Avoid concomitant use of probenecid and methotrexate if possible. If used together, consider lower methotrexate doses and monitor for methotrexate toxicity. May cause exacerbation of acute gouty attack. If hypersensitivity reaction or anaphylaxis occurs, discontinue medication. Use caution in patients with G6PD deficiency; may increase risk for hemolytic anemia.

Adverse Reactions (Reflective of adult population; not specific for elderly) Frequency not defined.

Cardiovascular: Flushing

Central nervous system: Dizziness, fever, headache

Dermatologic: Alopecia, dermatitis, pruritus, rash

Gastrointestinal: Anorexia, dyspepsia, gastroesophageal reflux, nausea, sore gums, vomiting

Genitourinary: Hematuria, polyuria

Hematologic: Anemia, aplastic anemia, hemolytic anemia (in G6PD deficiency), leukopenia

Hepatic: Hepatic necrosis

Neuromuscular & skeletal: Costovertebral pain, gouty arthritis (acute)

Renal: Nephrotic syndrome, renal colic

Miscellaneous: Anaphylaxis, hypersensitivity

Drug Interactions

Metabolism/Transport Effects Inhibits CYP2C19 (weak)

Avoid Concomitant Use

Avoid concomitant use of Probenecid with any of the following: Doripenem; Ketorolac; Ketorolac (Nasal); Ketorolac (Systemic); Meropenem

Increased Effect/Toxicity

Probenecid may increase the levels/effects of: Acetaminophen; Cephalosporins; Dapsone; Dapsone (Systemic); Doripenem; Ganciclovir-Valganciclovir; Gemifloxacin; Imipenem; Ketoprofen; Ketorolac; Ketorolac (Nasal); Ketorolac (Systemic); Loop Diuretics; LORazepam; Meropenem; Methotrexate; Mycophenolate; Nitrofurantoin; Nonsteroidal Anti-Inflammatory Agents; Oseltamivir; Penicillins; PRALAtrexate; Quinolone Antibiotics; Sodium Benzoate; Sodium Phenylacetate; Theophylline Derivatives; Zidovudine

Decreased Effect

Probenecid may decrease the levels/effects of: Loop Diuretics

The levels/effects of Probenecid may be decreased by: Salicylates

Stability Store at 20°C to 25°C (68°F to 77°F). Protect from light.

Mechanism of Action Competitively inhibits the reabsorption of uric acid at the proximal convoluted tubule, thereby promoting its excretion and reducing serum uric acid levels; increases plasma levels of weak organic acids (penicillins, cephalosporins, or other beta-lactam antibiotics) by competitively inhibiting their renal tubular secretion

Pharmacodynamics/Kinetics

Onset of action: Effect on penicillin levels: 2 hours

Absorption: Rapid and complete

Metabolism: Hepatic

Half-life elimination (dose dependent): Normal renal function: 6-12 hours

Time to peak, serum: 2-4 hours

Excretion: Urine

Dosage

Geriatric & Adult

Hyperuricemia with gout: Oral: 250 mg twice daily for 1 week; may increase to 500 mg twice daily; if needed, may increase to a maximum of 2 g/day (increase dosage in 500 mg increments every 4 weeks). If serum uric acid levels are within normal limits and gout attacks have been absent for 6 months, daily dosage may be reduced by 500 mg every 6 months.

Prolong penicillin serum levels: Oral: 500 mg 4 times/day. **Note:** Dosing per manufacturer, see indication-specific dosing.

Gonorrhea, uncomplicated infections of cervix, urethra, and rectum: Oral: 1 g once with cefoxitin 2 g I.M. (CDC, 2010)

Pelvic inflammatory disease (unlabeled use): Oral: 1 g once with cefoxitin 2 g I.M. plus doxycycline (CDC, 2010)

Neurosyphilis (unlabeled use): Oral: 500 mg 4 times/day with procaine penicillin 2.4 million units/day I.M for 10-14 days (CDC, 2010). **Note:** Penicillin G aqueous I.V. is the preferred agent.

Renal Impairment Cl_{cr} <30 mL/minute: Avoid use.

Administration Administer with food or antacids to minimize GI effects.

Monitoring Parameters Uric acid, renal function, CBC

Reference Range

Uric acid, serum: An increase occurs during childhood

Adults:

Male: 3.4-7 mg/dL or slightly more

Female: 2.4-6 mg/dL or slightly more

Target: <6 mg/dL

Values >7 mg/dL are sometimes arbitrarily regarded as hyperuricemia, but there is no sharp line between normals and the serum uric acid of those with clinical gout. Normal ranges cannot be adjusted for purine ingestion, but high-purine diet increases uric acid. Uric acid may be increased with body size, exercise, and stress.

Test Interactions False-positive glucosuria with Clinitest®, a falsely high determination of theophylline has occurred and the renal excretion of phenolsulfonphthalein 17-ketosteroids and bromsulfophthalein (BSP) may be inhibited

Pharmacotherapy Pearls Avoid fluctuation in uric acid (increase or decrease); may precipitate gout attack. The manufacturer recommends the use of sodium bicarbonate (3-7.5 g daily) or potassium citrate (7.5 g daily) is suggested until serum uric acid normalizes and tophaceous deposits disappear.

Special Geriatric Considerations Since probenecid loses its effectiveness when the Cl_{cr} is <30 mL/minute, its usefulness in the elderly is limited.

Dosage Forms Excipient information presented when available (limited, particularly for generics); consult specific product labeling.

Tablet, oral: 500 mg

◆ **Probenecid and Colchicine** see Colchicine and Probenecid on page 412

Procainamide (pro KANE a mide)

Medication Safety Issues

Sound-alike/look-alike issues:

Procanbid may be confused with probenecid, Procan SR®

Procan SR® may be confused with procanbid

Pronestyl may be confused with Ponstel®

High alert medication:

The Institute for Safe Medication Practices (ISMP) includes this medication among its list of drugs which have a heightened risk of causing significant patient harm when used in error.

Administration issues:

Procainamide hydrochloride is available in 10 mL vials of 100 mg/mL and in 2 mL vials with 500 mg/mL. Note that **BOTH** vials contain 1 gram of drug; confusing the strengths can lead to massive overdoses or underdoses.

Other safety concerns:

PCA is an error-prone abbreviation (mistaken as patient controlled analgesia)

Brand Names: Canada Apo-Procainamide®; Procainamide Hydrochloride Injection, USP; Procan SR®

Index Terms PCA (error-prone abbreviation); Procainamide Hydrochloride; Procaine Amide Hydrochloride; Procanbid; Pronestyl

Generic Availability (U.S.) Yes

Pharmacologic Category Antiarrhythmic Agent, Class Ia

Use

Intravenous: Treatment of life-threatening ventricular arrhythmias

Oral (Canadian labeling; not available in U.S.): Treatment of supraventricular arrhythmias. **Note:** In the treatment of atrial fibrillation, use only when preferred treatment is ineffective or cannot be used. Use in paroxysmal atrial tachycardia when reflex stimulation or other measures are ineffective.

PROCAINAMIDE

Unlabeled/Investigational Use

Paroxysmal supraventricular tachycardia (PSVT); prevent recurrence of ventricular tachycardia; symptomatic premature ventricular contractions

ACLS guidelines: I.V.: Treatment of the following arrhythmias in patients with preserved left ventricular function: Stable monomorphic VT; atrial fibrillation or atrial flutter, including preexcitation syndrome; AV re-entrant narrow complex tachycardias (eg, re-entrant SVT), uncontrolled by adenosine and vagal maneuvers; and stable wide complex regular tachycardia (likely VT)

PALS guidelines: I.V.: Tachycardia with pulses and poor perfusion (probable SVT [unresponsive to vagal maneuvers and adenosine or synchronized cardioversion]; probable VT [unresponsive to synchronized cardioversion or adenosine])

Contraindications Hypersensitivity to procainamide, procaine, other ester-type local anesthetics, or any component of the formulation; complete heart block; second-degree AV block or various types of hemiblock (without a functional artificial pacemaker); SLE; torsade de pointes

Warnings/Precautions Monitor and adjust dose to prevent QT_c prolongation. Watch for proarrhythmic effects. Avoid use in patients with QT prolongation (ACLS, 2010). May precipitate or exacerbate HF due to negative inotropic actions; use with caution or avoid (ACLS, 2010) in patients with HF. Correct electrolyte disturbances, especially hypokalemia or hypomagnesemia, prior to use and throughout therapy. Reduce dosage in renal impairment. May increase ventricular response rate in patients with atrial fibrillation or flutter; control AV conduction before initiating. Correct hypokalemia before initiating therapy; hypokalemia may worsen toxicity. Reduce dose if first-degree heart block occurs. Use caution with concurrent use of other antiarrhythmics; may exacerbate or increase the risk of conduction disturbances. Avoid concurrent use with other drugs known to prolong QT_c interval. Avoid use in myasthenia gravis (may worsen condition). Use caution and dose cautiously; renal clearance of procainamide/NAPA declines in patients ≥50 years of age (independent of creatinine clearance reductions) and in the presence of concomitant renal impairment. This product contains sodium metabisulfite which may cause allergic-type reactions, including anaphylactic symptoms and life-threatening asthmatic episodes in susceptible people; this is seen more frequently in asthmatics.

[U.S. Boxed Warning]: Potentially fatal blood dyscrasias (eg, agranulocytosis) have occurred with therapeutic doses; weekly monitoring is recommended during the first 3 months of therapy and periodically thereafter. Discontinue procainamide if this occurs.

[U.S. Boxed Warning]: Long-term administration leads to the development of a positive antinuclear antibody (ANA) test in 50% of patients which may result in a drug-induced lupus erythematosus-like syndrome (in 20% to 30% of patients); discontinue procainamide with rising ANA titers or with SLE symptoms and choose an alternative agent.

[U.S. Boxed Warning]: In the Cardiac Arrhythmia Suppression Trial (CAST), recent (>6 days but <2 years ago) myocardial infarction patients with asymptomatic, non-life-threatening ventricular arrhythmias did not benefit and may have been harmed by attempts to suppress the arrhythmia with flecainide or encainide. An increased mortality or nonfatal cardiac arrest rate (7.7%) was seen in the active treatment group compared with patients in the placebo group (3%). The applicability of the CAST results to other populations is unknown. Procainamide should be reserved for patients with life-threatening ventricular arrhythmias.

Adverse Reactions (Reflective of adult population; not specific for elderly)

>1%:

Cardiovascular: Hypotension (I.V. up to 5%)

Dermatologic: Rash

Gastrointestinal: Diarrhea (oral: 3% to 4%), nausea (oral: 3% to 4%), taste disorder (oral: 3% to 4%), vomiting (oral: 3% to 4%)

Miscellaneous: Positive ANA (≤50%), SLE-like syndrome (≤30%, increased incidence with long-term therapy or slow acetylators; syndrome may include abdominal pain, arthralgia, arthritis, chills, fever, hepatomegaly, myalgia, pericarditis, pleural effusion, pulmonary infiltrates, rash)

Drug Interactions

Metabolism/Transport Effects Substrate of CYP2D6 (major)

Avoid Concomitant Use

Avoid concomitant use of Procainamide with any of the following: Artemether; Dronedarone; Lumefantrine; Nilotinib; Pimozide; QUEtiapine; QuiNINE; Tetrabenazine; Thioridazine; Toremifene; Vandetanib; Vemurafenib; Ziprasidone

Increased Effect/Toxicity

Procainamide may increase the levels/effects of: Dronedarone; Neuromuscular-Blocking Agents; Pimozide; QTc-Prolonging Agents; QuiNINE; Tetrabenazine; Thioridazine; Toremifene; Vandetanib; Vemurafenib; Ziprasidone

The levels/effects of Procainamide may be increased by: Abiraterone Acetate; Alfuzosin; Amiodarone; Artemether; Chloroquine; Cimetidine; Ciprofloxacin; Ciprofloxacin (Systemic); CYP2D6 Inhibitors (Moderate); CYP2D6 Inhibitors (Strong); Darunavir; Eribulin; Fingolimod; Gadobutrol; Lumefantrine; Lurasidone; Nilotinib; QUEtiapine; QuiNINE; Ranitidine; Trimethoprim

Decreased Effect

The levels/effects of Procainamide may be decreased by: Peginterferon Alfa-2b

Ethanol/Nutrition/Herb Interactions

Ethanol: Avoid ethanol (acute ethanol administration reduces procainamide serum concentrations).

Herb/Nutraceutical: Avoid ephedra (may worsen arrhythmia).

Stability Store undiluted vials at room temperature of 15°C to 30°C (59°F to 86°F). The solution is initially colorless but may turn slightly yellow on standing. Injection of air into the vial causes solution to darken. Discard solutions darker than light amber. Color formation may occur upon refrigeration.

Maximum concentration (loading dose only): 20 mg/mL

Maximum admixture concentration: 8 mg/mL

Usual admixture concentration: 1 g/250 mL NS/D$_5$W or 1 g/500 mL NS/D$_5$W

When admixed in NS or D$_5$W to a final concentration of 2-4 mg/mL, solution is stable at room temperature for 24 hours and for 7 days under refrigeration.

Some information indicates that procainamide may be subject to greater decomposition in D$_5$W unless the admixture is refrigerated or the pH is adjusted. Procainamide is believed to form an association complex with dextrose - the bioavailability of procainamide in this complex is not known and the complex formation is reversible (Raymond, 1988).

Mechanism of Action Decreases myocardial excitability and conduction velocity and may depress myocardial contractility, by increasing the electrical stimulation threshold of ventricle, His-Purkinje system and through direct cardiac effects

Pharmacodynamics/Kinetics

Onset of action: I.M. 10-30 minutes

Distribution: V$_d$: 2 L/kg; decreased with congestive heart failure or shock

Protein binding: 15% to 20%

Metabolism: Hepatic via acetylation to produce N-acetyl procainamide (NAPA) (active metabolite)

Half-life elimination:

Procainamide (hepatic acetylator, phenotype, cardiac and renal function dependent): 2.5-4.7 hours; Anephric: 11 hours

NAPA (dependent upon renal function): 6-8 hours; Anephric: 42 hours

Time to peak, serum: I.M.: 15-60 minutes

Excretion: Urine (30% to 60% unchanged procainamide; 6% to 52% as NAPA); feces (<5% unchanged procainamide. **Note:** >80% of formed NAPA is renally eliminated in contrast to procainamide which is ~50% renally eliminated (Gibson, 1977).

Dosage

Geriatric Refer to adult dosing. Initiate doses at lower end of dosage range.

Adult Dose must be titrated to patient's response.

Antiarrhythmic:

I.M.: 50 mg/kg/day divided every 3-6 hours **or** 0.5-1 g every 4-8 hours (Koch-Weser, 1971)

I.V.:

Loading dose: 15-18 mg/kg administered as slow infusion over 25-30 minutes **or** 100 mg/dose at a rate not to exceed 50 mg/minute repeated every 5 minutes as needed to a total dose of 1 g.

Hemodynamically stable monomorphic VT or pre-excited atrial fibrillation (ACLS, 2010): Loading dose: Infuse 20-50 mg/minute **or** 100 mg every 5 minutes until arrhythmia controlled, hypotension occurs, QRS complex widens by 50% of its original width, or total of 17 mg/kg is given. Follow with a continuous infusion of 1-4 mg/minute. **Note:** Not recommended for use in ongoing ventricular fibrillation (VF) or pulseless ventricular tachycardia (VT) due to prolonged administration time and uncertain efficacy.

Maintenance dose: 1-4 mg/minute by continuous infusion. Maintenance infusions should be reduced by one-third in patients with moderate renal or cardiac impairment and by two-thirds in patients with severe renal or cardiac impairment.

Oral (not available in the U.S.; Canadian labeling): Sustained release formulation (Procan SR®): Maintenance: 50 mg/kg/24 hours given in divided doses every 6 hours

Suggested Procan SR® maintenance dose:

<55 kg: 500 mg every 6 hours

55-91 kg: 750 mg every 6 hours

>91 kg: 1000 mg every 6 hours

Renal Impairment
Oral:
Cl_{cr} 10-50 mL/minute: Administer every 6-12 hours.
Cl_{cr} <10 mL/minute: Administer every 8-24 hours.
I.V.:
Loading dose: Reduce dose to 12 mg/kg in severe renal impairment.
Maintenance infusion: Reduce dose by one-third in patients with mild renal impairment. Reduce dose by two-thirds in patients with severe renal impairment.
Dialysis:
Procainamide: Moderately hemodialyzable (20% to 50%): Monitor procainamide/N-acetyl-procainamide (NAPA) concentrations; supplementation may be necessary.
NAPA: Not dialyzable (0% to 5%)
Procainamide/NAPA: Not peritoneal dialyzable (0% to 5%)
Procainamide/NAPA: Replace according to blood concentration monitoring during continuous arteriovenous or venovenous hemofiltration.

Hepatic Impairment
Reduce dose by 50%.

Administration
Oral: Do **not** crush or chew sustained release drug products (not available in the U.S.).
I.V.: Must dilute prior to I.V. administration. Loading dose: Maximum rate: 50 mg/minute

Monitoring Parameters
ECG, blood pressure, renal function; with prolonged use monitor CBC with differential, platelet count; procainamide and NAPA blood concentrations in patients with hepatic impairment, renal impairment, or receiving constant infusion >3 mg/minute for longer than 24 hours; ANA titers

Reference Range
Timing of serum samples: Draw 6-12 hours after I.V. infusion has started; half-life is 2.5-5 hours
Therapeutic concentrations: Procainamide: 4-10 mcg/mL; NAPA 15-25 mcg/mL; Combined: 10-30 mcg/mL
Toxic concentration: Procainamide: >10-12 mcg/mL

Test Interactions
In the presence of propranolol or suprapharmacologic concentrations of lidocaine or meprobamate, tests which depend on fluorescence to measure procainamide/NAPA concentrations may be affected.

Special Geriatric Considerations
Monitor closely since clearance is reduced in those >60 years of age. If clinically possible, start doses at lowest recommended dose. Also, elderly frequently have drug therapy which may interfere with the use of procainamide. Adjust dose for renal function in the elderly.

Dosage Forms
Excipient information presented when available (limited, particularly for generics); consult specific product labeling.
Injection, solution, as hydrochloride: 100 mg/mL (10 mL); 500 mg/mL (2 mL)

Dosage Forms: Canada
Excipient information presented when available (limited, particularly for generics); consult specific product labeling.
Tablet, sustained release, oral, as hydrochloride:
Procan SR®: 250 mg, 500 mg, 750 mg

Selected References
"2005 American Heart Association Guidelines for Cardiopulmonary Resuscitation and Emergency Cardiovascular Care," *Circulation*, 2005, 112(24 Suppl):1-211.

♦ **Procainamide Hydrochloride** *see* Procainamide *on page 1521*
♦ **Procaine Amide Hydrochloride** *see* Procainamide *on page 1521*
♦ **Procaine Benzylpenicillin** *see* Penicillin G Procaine *on page 1420*
♦ **Procaine Penicillin G** *see* Penicillin G Procaine *on page 1420*
♦ **Procanbid** *see* Procainamide *on page 1521*
♦ **Procardia®** *see* NIFEdipine *on page 1300*
♦ **Procardia XL®** *see* NIFEdipine *on page 1300*
♦ **Procetofene** *see* Fenofibrate *on page 701*
♦ **Prochieve® [DSC]** *see* Progesterone *on page 1528*

Prochlorperazine (proe klor PER a zeen)

Medication Safety Issues
Sound-alike/look-alike issues:
Prochlorperazine may be confused with chlorproMAZINE
Compazine® may be confused with Copaxone®, Coumadin®
Other safety concerns:
CPZ (occasional abbreviation for Compazine®) is an error-prone abbreviation (mistaken as chlorpromazine)

Brand Names: U.S.
Compro®

Brand Names: Canada Apo-Prochlorperazine®; Nu-Prochlor; Stemetil®

Index Terms Chlormeprazine; Compazine; Prochlorperazine Edisylate; Prochlorperazine Maleate

Generic Availability (U.S.) Yes

Pharmacologic Category Antiemetic; Antipsychotic Agent, Typical, Phenothiazine

Use Management of nausea and vomiting; psychotic disorders, including schizophrenia and anxiety

Unlabeled/Investigational Use Treatment of behavioral syndromes in dementia

Contraindications Hypersensitivity to prochlorperazine or any component of the formulation (cross-reactivity between phenothiazines may occur); severe CNS depression; coma

Warnings/Precautions [U.S. Boxed Warning]: Elderly patients with dementia-related psychosis treated with antipsychotics are at an increased risk of death compared to placebo. Most deaths appeared to be either cardiovascular (eg, heart failure, sudden death) or infectious (eg, pneumonia) in nature. Prochlorperazine is not approved for the treatment of dementia-related psychosis.

Leukopenia, neutropenia, and agranulocytosis (sometimes fatal) have been reported in clinical trials and postmarketing reports with antipsychotic use; presence of risk factors (eg, pre-existing low WBC or history of drug-induced leuko-/neutropenia) should prompt periodic blood count assessment. Discontinue therapy at first signs of blood dyscrasias or if absolute neutrophil count <1000/mm^3.

May be sedating; use with caution in disorders where CNS depression is a feature. May obscure intestinal obstruction or brain tumor. May impair physical or mental abilities. Effects with other sedative drugs or ethanol may be potentiated. Use with caution in Parkinson's disease; hemodynamic instability; predisposition to seizures; subcortical brain damage; and in severe cardiac, hepatic, or renal disease. May alter temperature regulation or mask toxicity of other drugs. Use caution with exposure to heat. May alter cardiac conduction. May cause orthostatic hypotension. Hypotension may occur following administration, particularly when parenteral form is used or in high dosages. Antipsychotic use has been associated with esophageal dysmotility and aspiration; use with caution in patients at risk of pneumonia (ie, Alzheimer's disease).

May cause pigmentary retinopathy, and lenticular and corneal deposits, particularly with prolonged therapy. Use associated with increased prolactin levels; clinical significance of hyperprolactinemia in patients with breast cancer or other prolactin-dependent tumors is unknown.

Phenothiazines may cause anticholinergic effects; therefore, they should be used with caution in patients with decreased gastrointestinal motility, urinary retention, BPH, xerostomia, or visual problems. Conditions which also may be exacerbated by cholinergic blockade include narrow-angle glaucoma and worsening of myasthenia gravis. May cause extrapyramidal symptoms (EPS), including pseudoparkinsonism, acute dystonic reactions, akathisia, and tardive dyskinesia (risk of these reactions is high relative to other neuroleptics). Risk of dystonia (and possibly other EPS) may be greater with increased doses, use of conventional antipsychotics, males. Use caution in the elderly. May be associated with neuroleptic malignant syndrome (NMS).

Adverse Reactions (Reflective of adult population; not specific for elderly) Reported with prochlorperazine or other phenothiazines. Frequency not defined.

Cardiovascular: Cardiac arrest, hypotension, peripheral edema, Q-wave distortions, T-wave distortions

Central nervous system: Agitation, catatonia, cerebral edema, cough reflex suppressed, dizziness, drowsiness, fever (mild - I.M.), headache, hyperactivity, hyperpyrexia, impairment of temperature regulation, insomnia, neuroleptic malignant syndrome (NMS), paradoxical excitement, restlessness, seizure

Dermatologic: Angioedema, contact dermatitis, discoloration of skin (blue-gray), epithelial keratopathy, erythema, eczema, exfoliative dermatitis (injectable), itching, photosensitivity, rash, skin pigmentation, urticaria

Endocrine & metabolic: Amenorrhea, breast enlargement, galactorrhea, gynecomastia, glucosuria, hyper-/hypoglycemia, lactation, libido (changes in), menstrual irregularity, SIADH

Gastrointestinal: Appetite increased, atonic colon, constipation, ileus, nausea, weight gain, xerostomia

Genitourinary: Ejaculating dysfunction, ejaculatory disturbances, impotence, incontinence, polyuria, priapism, urinary retention, urination difficulty

Hematologic: Agranulocytosis, aplastic anemia, eosinophilia, hemolytic anemia, leukopenia, pancytopenia, thrombocytopenic purpura

Hepatic: Biliary stasis, cholestatic jaundice, hepatotoxicity

Neuromuscular & skeletal: Dystonias (torticollis, opisthotonos, carpopedal spasm, trismus, oculogyric crisis, protrusion of tongue); extrapyramidal symptoms (pseudoparkinsonism, akathisia, dystonias, tardive dyskinesia); SLE-like syndrome; tremor

Ocular: blurred vision, cornea and lens changes, lenticular/corneal deposits, miosis, mydriasis, pigmentary retinopathy

Respiratory: Asthma, laryngeal edema, nasal congestion

Miscellaneous: Allergic reactions, diaphoresis

Drug Interactions

Avoid Concomitant Use

Avoid concomitant use of Prochlorperazine with any of the following: Dofetilide; Metoclopramide

Increased Effect/Toxicity

Prochlorperazine may increase the levels/effects of: Alcohol (Ethyl); Analgesics (Opioid); Anticholinergics; Anti-Parkinson's Agents (Dopamine Agonist); Beta-Blockers; CNS Depressants; Dofetilide; Methotrimeprazine; Methylphenidate; Porfimer; Selective Serotonin Reuptake Inhibitors

The levels/effects of Prochlorperazine may be increased by: Acetylcholinesterase Inhibitors (Central); Antimalarial Agents; Beta-Blockers; Deferoxamine; Droperidol; Lithium formulations; Methotrimeprazine; Methylphenidate; Metoclopramide; Pramlintide; Tetrabenazine

Decreased Effect

Prochlorperazine may decrease the levels/effects of: Amphetamines; Quinagolide

The levels/effects of Prochlorperazine may be decreased by: Antacids; Anti-Parkinson's Agents (Dopamine Agonist); Lithium formulations

Ethanol/Nutrition/Herb Interactions

Ethanol: May increase CNS depression; monitor for increased effects with coadministration. Caution patients about effects.

Food: Limit caffeine.

Herb/Nutraceutical: Avoid dong quai, St John's wort (may also cause photosensitization). Avoid kava kava, gotu kola, valerian, St John's wort (may increase CNS depression).

Stability

Injection: Store at <30°C (<86°F); do not freeze. Protect from light. Clear or slightly yellow solutions may be used.

I.V. infusion: Injection may be diluted in 50-100 mL NS or D_5W.

Suppository, tablet: Store at 15°C to 30°C (59°F to 86°F). Protect from light.

Mechanism of Action
Prochlorperazine is a piperazine phenothiazine antipsychotic which blocks postsynaptic mesolimbic dopaminergic D_1 and D_2 receptors in the brain, including the chemoreceptor trigger zone; exhibits a strong alpha-adrenergic and anticholinergic blocking effect and depresses the release of hypothalamic and hypophyseal hormones; believed to depress the reticular activating system, thus affecting basal metabolism, body temperature, wakefulness, vasomotor tone and emesis

Pharmacodynamics/Kinetics

Onset of action: Oral: 30-40 minutes; I.M.: 10-20 minutes; Rectal: ~60 minutes

Peak antiemetic effect: I.V.: 30-60 minutes

Duration: Rectal: 12 hours; Oral: 3-4 hours; I.M., I.V.: Adults: 4-6 hours

Distribution: V_d: 1400-1548 L

Metabolism: Primarily hepatic; N-desmethyl prochlorperazine (major active metabolite)

Bioavailability: Oral: 12.5%

Half-life elimination: Oral: 6-10 hours (single dose), 14-22 hours (repeated dosing); I.V.: 6-10 hours

Dosage

Geriatric Dementia behavior (nonpsychotic, unlabeled use): Initial: 2.5-5 mg 1-2 times/day; increase dose at 4- to 7-day intervals by 2.5-5 mg/day. Increase dosing intervals (twice daily, 3 times/day, etc) as necessary to control response or side effects. Maximum daily dose should probably not exceed 75 mg in the elderly. Gradual increases (titration) may prevent some side effects or decrease their severity.

Adult

Antiemetic:

Oral (tablet): 5-10 mg 3-4 times/day; usual maximum: 40 mg/day; larger doses may rarely be required

I.M. (deep): 5-10 mg every 3-4 hours; usual maximum: 40 mg/day

I.V.: 2.5-10 mg; maximum: 10 mg/dose or 40 mg/day; may repeat dose every 3-4 hours as needed

Rectal: 25 mg twice daily

Surgical nausea/vomiting: Note: Should not exceed 40 mg/day
  I.M.: 5-10 mg 1-2 hours before induction or to control symptoms during or after surgery; may repeat once if necessary
  I.V. (administer slow IVP <5 mg/minute): 5-10 mg 15-30 minutes before induction or to control symptoms during or after surgery; may repeat once if necessary
  Rectal (unlabeled use): 25 mg
Antipsychotic:
  Oral: 5-10 mg 3-4 times/day; titrate dose slowly every 2-3 days; doses up to 150 mg/day may be required in some patients for treatment of severe disturbances
  I.M.: Initial: 10-20 mg; if necessary repeat initial dose every 1-4 hours to gain control; more than 3-4 doses are rarely needed. If parenteral administration is still required; give 10-20 mg every 4-6 hours; change to oral as soon as possible.
Nonpsychotic anxiety: Oral *(tablet):* Usual dose: 15-20 mg/day in divided doses; do not give doses >20 mg/day or for longer than 12 weeks
Administration May be administered orally, I.M., or I.V.
I.M.: Inject by deep IM into outer quadrant of buttocks.
I.V.: Administer slow I.V. at a rate not exceeding 5 mg/minute. To reduce the risk of hypotension, patients receiving I.V. prochlorperazine must remain lying down and be observed for at least 30 minutes following administration.
Monitoring Parameters Orthostatic blood pressures; tremors, gait changes, abnormal movement in trunk, neck, buccal area, or extremities; monitor target behaviors for which the agent is given; CBC with differential and periodic ophthalmic exams (if chronically used); baseline and periodic hepatic and renal function tests; monitor orthostatic blood pressures 3-5 days after initiation of therapy or a dose increase
Test Interactions False-positives for phenylketonuria, urinary amylase, uroporphyrins, urobilinogen
Pharmacotherapy Pearls Not recommended as an antipsychotic due to inferior efficacy compared to other phenothiazines.
Special Geriatric Considerations Due to side effect profile (dystonias, EPS) this is not a preferred drug in the elderly for antiemetic therapy.

Many elderly patients receive antipsychotic medications for inappropriate nonpsychotic behavior. Before initiating antipsychotic medication, the clinician should investigate any possible reversible cause; any stress or stress from any disease can cause acute "confusion" or worsening of baseline nonpsychotic behavior. Most commonly acute changes in behavior are due to increases in drug dose or addition of new drug to regimen, fluid electrolyte loss, infections, and changes in environment.

Any changes in disease status in any organ system can result in behavior changes.

In the treatment of agitated, demented, older adult patients, authors of meta-analysis of controlled trials of the response to the traditional antipsychotics (phenothiazines, butyrophenones) in controlling agitation have concluded that the use of neuroleptics results in a response rate of 18%. Clearly neuroleptic therapy for behavior control should be limited with frequent attempts to withdraw the agent given for behavior control.
Dosage Forms Excipient information presented when available (limited, particularly for generics); consult specific product labeling.
Injection, solution, as edisylate [strength expressed as base]: 5 mg/mL (2 mL, 10 mL)
Suppository, rectal: 25 mg (12s)
  Compro®: 25 mg (12s) [contains coconut oil, palm oil]
Tablet, oral, as maleate [strength expressed as base]: 5 mg, 10 mg
Selected References
Ernst AA, Weiss SJ, Park S, et al, "Prochlorperazine Versus Promethazine for Uncomplicated Nausea and Vomiting in the Emergency Department: A Randomized, Double-Blind Clinical Trial," *Ann Emerg Med*, 2000, 36 (2):89-94.
Golembiewski J, Chernin E, and Chopra T, "Prevention and Treatment of Postoperative Nausea and Vomiting," *Am J Health-Syst Pharm*, 2005, 62:1247-60.
Rabins PV, Blacker D, Rovner BW, et al, "Practice Guidelines for the Treatment of Patients With Alzheimer's Disease and Other Dementias," *Am J Psychiatry*, 2007, 164(12 Suppl):5-56. Available at http://www.psych.org/psych_pract/treatg/pg/prac_guide.cfm.
Schneider LS, Tariot PN, Dagerman KS, et al, "Effectiveness of Atypical Antipsychotic Drugs in Patients With Alzheimer's Disease," *N Engl J Med*, 2006, 355(15):1525-38.

Progesterone (proe JES ter one)

Brand Names: U.S. Crinone®; Endometrin®; First™-Progesterone VGS 100; First™-Progesterone VGS 200; First™-Progesterone VGS 25; First™-Progesterone VGS 400; First™-Progesterone VGS 50; Prochieve® [DSC]; Prometrium®

Brand Names: Canada Crinone®; Prometrium®

Index Terms Pregnenedione; Progestin

Generic Availability (U.S.) Yes: Injection, powder

Pharmacologic Category Progestin

Use

Oral: Prevention of endometrial hyperplasia in nonhysterectomized, postmenopausal women who are receiving conjugated estrogen tablets

I.M.: Abnormal uterine bleeding due to hormonal imbalance

Contraindications Hypersensitivity to progesterone or any component of the formulation; undiagnosed abnormal vaginal bleeding; history of or current thrombophlebitis or venous thromboembolic disorders (including DVT, PE); history of, active or recent (within 1 year) arterial thromboembolic disease (eg, stroke, MI); history of or known or suspected carcinoma of the breast or genital organs; hepatic dysfunction or disease

Warnings/Precautions [U.S. Boxed Warning]: Progestins used in combination with estrogen should not be used to prevent cardiovascular disease. Use caution with cardiovascular disease or dysfunction. Progestins used in combination with estrogen may increase the risks of hypertension, myocardial infarction (MI), stroke, pulmonary emboli (PE), and deep vein thrombosis; incidence of these effects was shown to be significantly increased in postmenopausal women using CEE in combination with MPA. Similar risk should be assumed with other progestins.

[U.S. Boxed Warning]: The risk of dementia may be increased in postmenopausal women; progestins used in combination with estrogen should not be used to prevent dementia. Increased incidence was observed in women ≥65 years of age taking CEE alone or in combination with MPA.

[U.S. Boxed Warning]: An increased risk of invasive breast cancer was observed in postmenopausal women using conjugated equine estrogens (CEE) in combination with medroxyprogesterone acetate (MPA). An increase in abnormal mammograms has also been reported with estrogen and progestin therapy

Unopposed estrogens may increase the risk of endometrial carcinoma in postmenopausal women with an intact uterus. Risk appears to be associated with long-term use. The use of a progestin should be considered when administering estrogens to postmenopausal women with an intact uterus. Adequate diagnostic measures, including endometrial sampling (if indicated), should be performed to rule out malignancy in all cases of undiagnosed abnormal vaginal bleeding. Postmenopausal estrogen therapy and combined estrogen/progesterone therapy may increase the risk of ovarian cancer; however, the absolute risk to an individual woman is small. Although results from various studies are not consistent, risk does not appear to be significantly associated with the duration, route, or dose of therapy. In one study, the risk decreased after 2 years following discontinuation of therapy.

Discontinue pending examination in cases of sudden partial or complete vision loss, sudden onset of proptosis, diplopia, or migraine; discontinue permanently if papilledema or retinal vascular lesions are observed on examination. Use with caution in patients with diseases that may be exacerbated by fluid retention, including asthma, epilepsy, migraine, diabetes or renal dysfunction. Use caution with history of depression. Patients should be warned that progesterone might cause transient dizziness or drowsiness during initial therapy. Whenever possible, progestins in combination with estrogens should be discontinued at least 4-6 weeks prior to surgeries associated with an increased risk of thromboembolism or during periods of prolonged immobilization. Progestins used in combination with estrogen should be used for shortest duration possible consistent with treatment goals. Conduct periodic risk:benefit assessments.

Products may contain palm oil, peanut oil, sesame oil, or benzyl alcohol. Not for use prior to menarche.

Adverse Reactions (Reflective of adult population; not specific for elderly)

Injection (I.M.):

Cardiovascular: Cerebral edema, cerebral thrombosis, edema

Central nervous system: Depression, fever, insomnia, somnolence

Dermatologic: Acne, allergic rash (rare), alopecia, hirsutism, pruritus, rash, urticaria

Endocrine & metabolic: Amenorrhea, breakthrough bleeding, breast tenderness, galactorrhea, menstrual flow changes, spotting

PROGESTERONE

Gastrointestinal: Nausea, weight gain/loss
Genitourinary: Cervical erosion changes, cervical secretion changes
Hepatic: Cholestatic jaundice
Local: Injection site: Irritation, pain, redness
Ocular: Optic neuritis, retinal thrombosis
Respiratory: Pulmonary embolism
Miscellaneous: Anaphylactoid reactions

Oral capsule (percentages reported when used in combination with or cycled with conjugated estrogens):
>10%:
Central nervous system: Headache (16% to 31%), dizziness (15% to 24%), depression (19%)
Endocrine & metabolic: Breast tenderness (27%), breast pain (6% to 16%)
Gastrointestinal: Abdominal pain (10% to 20%), abdominal bloating (8% to 12%)
Genitourinary: Urinary problems (11%)
Neuromuscular & skeletal: Joint pain (20%), musculoskeletal pain (12%)
Miscellaneous: Viral infection (12%)
5% to 10%:
Cardiovascular: Chest pain (7%)
Central nervous system: Fatigue (8%), irritability (8%), worry (8%)
Gastrointestinal: Nausea/vomiting (8%), diarrhea (7% to 8%)
Genitourinary: Vaginal discharge (10%)
Respiratory: Cough (8%)
<5%: Breast biopsy, breast cancer, cholecystectomy, constipation
Drug Interactions
Metabolism/Transport Effects Substrate of CYP1A2 (minor), 2A6 (minor), 2C9 (minor), 2C19 (major), 2D6 (minor), 3A4 (major); **Inhibits** CYP2C9 (weak), CYP2C19 (weak), CYP3A4 (weak), P-glycoprotein
Avoid Concomitant Use
Avoid concomitant use of Progesterone with any of the following: Silodosin; Topotecan
Increased Effect/Toxicity
Progesterone may increase the levels/effects of: Colchicine; Dabigatran Etexilate; Everolimus; P-Glycoprotein Substrates; Rivaroxaban; Silodosin; Topotecan

The levels/effects of Progesterone may be increased by: Conivaptan; Herbs (Progestogenic Properties)
Decreased Effect
The levels/effects of Progesterone may be decreased by: Aminoglutethimide; CYP2C19 Inducers (Strong); CYP3A4 Inducers (Strong); Cyproterone; Deferasirox; Herbs (CYP3A4 Inducers); Peginterferon Alfa-2b; Tocilizumab
Ethanol/Nutrition/Herb Interactions
Food: Food increases oral bioavailability.
Herb/Nutraceutical: St John's wort may decrease progesterone levels. Herbs with progestogenic properties may enhance the adverse/toxic effects of progestin; example herbs include bloodroot, chasteberry, damiana, oregano, yucca.
Stability Store at controlled room temperature. Protect capsules from excessive moisture.
Mechanism of Action Natural steroid hormone that induces secretory changes in the endometrium, promotes mammary gland development, relaxes uterine smooth muscle
Pharmacodynamics/Kinetics
Absorption: Vaginal gel: Prolonged
Absorption half-life: 25-50 hours
Protein binding: Albumin (50% to 54%) and cortisol-binding protein (43% to 48%)
Metabolism: Hepatic to metabolites
Half-life elimination: Vaginal gel: 5-20 minutes
Time to peak: Oral: Within 3 hours; I.M.: ~8 hours; Vaginal tablet: ~17-24 hours
Excretion: Urine, bile, feces
Dosage
Geriatric & Adult Females:
Endometrial hyperplasia prevention (in postmenopausal women with a uterus who are receiving daily conjugated estrogen tablets): Oral: 200 mg as a single daily dose every evening for 12 days sequentially per 28-day cycle
Functional uterine bleeding: I.M.: 5-10 mg/day for 6 doses
Administration
I.M.: Administer deep I.M. only
Oral capsule: For patients who experience difficulty swallowing the capsules, taking with a full glass of water in the standing position may be beneficial.

◀ **Monitoring Parameters** Routine physical examination that includes blood pressure and Papanicolaou smear, breast exam, mammogram. Adequate diagnostic measures, including endometrial sampling, if indicated, should be performed to rule out malignancy in all cases of undiagnosed abnormal vaginal bleeding. Signs and symptoms of thromboembolic disorders, vision changes

Test Interactions Thyroid function, metyrapone, liver function, coagulation tests, endocrine function tests

Special Geriatric Considerations Not a progestin of choice in the elderly for hormonal cycling.

Dosage Forms Excipient information presented when available (limited, particularly for generics); consult specific product labeling.
Capsule:
Prometrium®: 100 mg, 200 mg [contains peanut oil]
Injection, oil: 50 mg/mL (10 mL) [contains benzyl alcohol 10%, sesame oil]

Selected References

Mørch LS, Løkkegaard E, Andreasen AH, et al, "Hormone Therapy and Ovarian Cancer," *JAMA*, 2009, 302 (3):298-305.

◆ **Progestin** *see* Progesterone *on page 1528*
◆ **Prolia™** *see* Denosumab *on page 468*

Promethazine (proe METH a zeen)

Related Information
Beers Criteria – Potentially Inappropriate Medications for Geriatrics *on page 2089*

Medication Safety Issues
Sound-alike/look-alike issues:
Promethazine may be confused with chlorproMAZINE, predniSONE, promazine
Phenergan® may be confused with Phenaphen®, PHENobarbital, Phrenilin®, Theragran®

High alert medication:
The Institute for Safe Medication Practices (ISMP) includes this medication (I.V. formulation) among its list of drugs which have a heightened risk of causing significant patient harm when used in error.

Beers Criteria medication:
This drug may be inappropriate for use in geriatric patients (high severity risk).

Administration issues:
To prevent or minimize tissue damage during I.V. administration, the Institute for Safe Medication Practices (ISMP) has the following recommendations:
- Limit concentration available to the 25 mg/mL product
- Consider limiting initial doses to 6.25-12.5 mg
- Further dilute the 25 mg/mL strength into 10-20 mL NS
- Administer through a large bore vein (not hand or wrist)
- Administer via running I.V. line at port farthest from patient's vein
- Consider administering over 10-15 minutes
- Instruct patients to report immediately signs of pain or burning

International issues:
Sominex: Brand name for promethazine in Great Britain, but also is a brand name for diphenhydrAMINE in the U.S.

Brand Names: U.S. Phenadoz®; Phenergan®; Promethegan™
Brand Names: Canada Bioniche Promethazine; Histantil; Phenergan®; PMS-Promethazine
Index Terms Promethazine Hydrochloride
Generic Availability (U.S.) Yes
Pharmacologic Category Antiemetic; Histamine H_1 Antagonist; Histamine H_1 Antagonist, First Generation; Phenothiazine Derivative
Use Symptomatic treatment of various allergic conditions; antiemetic; motion sickness; sedative; adjunct to postoperative analgesia and anesthesia
Contraindications Hypersensitivity to promethazine or any component of the formulation (cross-reactivity between phenothiazines may occur); coma; treatment of lower respiratory tract symptoms, including asthma; intra-arterial or subcutaneous administration
Warnings/Precautions [U.S. Boxed Warning]: Promethazine injection can cause severe tissue injury (including gangrene) regardless of the route of administration. Tissue irritation and damage may result from perivascular extravasation, unintentional intra-arterial administration, and intraneuronal or perineuronal infiltration. In addition to gangrene, adverse events reported include tissue necrosis, abscesses, burning, pain, erythema, edema, paralysis, severe spasm of distal vessels, phlebitis, thrombophlebitis, venous thrombosis, sensory loss, paralysis, and palsies. Surgical intervention including fasciotomy, skin graft, and/or amputation have been necessary in some

cases. **The preferred route of administration is by deep intramuscular (I.M.) injection. Subcutaneous administration is contraindicated. Discontinue intravenous injection immediately with onset of pain and evaluate for arterial injection or perivascular extravasation. Although there is no proven successful management of unintentional intra-arterial injection or perivascular extravasation, sympathetic block and heparinization have been used in the acute management of unintentional intra-arterial injection based on results from animal studies.**

May be sedating; use with caution in disorders where CNS depression is a feature. May impair physical or mental abilities; patients must be cautioned about performing tasks which require mental alertness. Use with caution in hemodynamic instability; bone marrow suppression; subcortical brain damage; and in severe cardiac, hepatic or respiratory disease. Avoid use in Reye's syndrome. May lower seizure threshold; use caution in persons with seizure disorders or in persons using narcotics or local anesthetics which may also affect seizure threshold. May alter temperature regulation or mask toxicity of other drugs due to antiemetic effects. May alter cardiac conduction (life-threatening arrhythmias have occurred with therapeutic doses of phenothiazines). May cause orthostatic hypotension; use with caution in patients at risk of hypotension or where transient hypotensive episodes would be poorly tolerated (cardiovascular disease or cerebrovascular disease).

Phenothiazines may cause anticholinergic effects; therefore, they should be used with caution in patients with decreased gastrointestinal motility, GI or GU obstruction, urinary retention, BPH, xerostomia, or visual problems. Conditions which also may be exacerbated by cholinergic blockade include narrow-angle glaucoma (screening is recommended) and worsening of myasthenia gravis. Use with caution in Parkinson's disease. May cause extrapyramidal symptoms, including pseudoparkinsonism, acute dystonic reactions, akathisia, and tardive dyskinesia. May be associated with neuroleptic malignant syndrome (NMS). May cause photosensitivity. May be inappropriate for use in the elderly due to potent anticholinergic effects (Beers Criteria). Injection may contain sodium metabisulfite.

Adverse Reactions (Reflective of adult population; not specific for elderly) Frequency not defined.

Cardiovascular: Bradycardia, hyper-/hypotension, nonspecific QT changes, postural hypotension, tachycardia.

Central nervous system: Agitation akathisia, catatonic states, confusion, delirium, disorientation, dizziness, drowsiness, dystonias, euphoria, excitation, extrapyramidal symptoms, faintness, fatigue, hallucinations, hysteria, insomnia, lassitude, pseudoparkinsonism, tardive dyskinesia, nervousness, neuroleptic malignant syndrome, nightmares, sedation, seizure, somnolence

Dermatologic: Angioneurotic edema, dermatitis, photosensitivity, skin pigmentation (slate gray), urticaria

Endocrine & metabolic: Amenorrhea, breast engorgement, gynecomastia, hyperglycemia, lactation

Gastrointestinal: Constipation, nausea, vomiting, xerostomia

Genitourinary: Ejaculatory disorder, impotence, urinary retention

Hematologic: Agranulocytosis, leukopenia, thrombocytopenia, thrombocytopenic purpura

Hepatic: Jaundice

Local: Abscess, distal vessel spasm, gangrene, injection site reactions (burning, edema, erythema, pain), palsies, paralysis, phlebitis, sensory loss, thrombophlebitis, tissue necrosis, venous thrombosis

Neuromuscular & skeletal: Incoordination, tremor

Ocular: Blurred vision, corneal and lenticular changes, diplopia, epithelial keratopathy, pigmentary retinopathy

Otic: Tinnitus

Respiratory: Apnea, asthma, nasal congestion, respiratory depression

Drug Interactions

Metabolism/Transport Effects Substrate (major) of CYP2B6, 2D6; **Inhibits** CYP2D6 (weak)

Avoid Concomitant Use

Avoid concomitant use of Promethazine with any of the following: Metoclopramide; Sibutramine

Increased Effect/Toxicity

Promethazine may increase the levels/effects of: Anticholinergics; Serotonin Modulators

The levels/effects of Promethazine may be increased by: Abiraterone Acetate; CYP2B6 Inhibitors (Moderate); CYP2B6 Inhibitors (Strong); CYP2D6 Inhibitors (Moderate); CYP2D6 Inhibitors (Strong); Darunavir; MAO Inhibitors; Metoclopramide; Pramlintide; Quazepam; Sibutramine

◀ **Decreased Effect**
Promethazine may decrease the levels/effects of: Acetylcholinesterase Inhibitors (Central)

The levels/effects of Promethazine may be decreased by: Acetylcholinesterase Inhibitors (Central); CYP2B6 Inducers (Strong); Peginterferon Alfa-2b

Ethanol/Nutrition/Herb Interactions
Ethanol: Avoid ethanol (may increase CNS depression).
Herb/Nutraceutical: Avoid valerian, St John's wort, kava kava, gotu kola (may increase CNS depression).

Stability
Injection: Prior to dilution, store at 20°C to 25°C (68°F to 77°F). Protect from light. Solutions in NS or D_5W are stable for 24 hours at room temperature.
Oral solution: Store at 15°C to 25°C (59°F to 77°F). Protect from light.
Suppositories: Store refrigerated at 2°C to 8°C (36°F to 46°F).
Tablets: Store at 20°C to 25°C (68°F to 77°F). Protect from light.

Mechanism of Action Phenothiazine derivative; blocks postsynaptic mesolimbic dopaminergic receptors in the brain; exhibits a strong alpha-adrenergic blocking effect and depresses the release of hypothalamic and hypophyseal hormones; competes with histamine for the H_1-receptor; muscarinic-blocking effect may be responsible for antiemetic activity; reduces stimuli to the brainstem reticular system

Pharmacodynamics/Kinetics
Onset of action: Oral, I.M.: ~20 minutes; I.V.: ~5 minutes
Peak effect: C_{max}: ~9 ng/mL (suppository); ~19 ng/mL (syrup)
Duration: Usually 4-6 hours (up to 12 hours)
Absorption:
    I.M.: Bioavailability may be greater than with oral or rectal administration
    Oral: Rapid and complete; large first pass effect limits systemic bioavailability
Distribution: V_d: 970 L
Protein binding: 93%
Metabolism: Hepatic; primarily oxidation; forms metabolites
Half-life elimination: 9-16 hours
Time to maximum serum concentration: ~4.5 hours (syrup); ~7-9 hours (suppositories)
Excretion: Primarily urine and feces (as inactive metabolites)

Dosage
Geriatric & Adult
Allergic conditions (including allergic reactions to blood or plasma):
    Oral, rectal: 25 mg at bedtime **or** 12.5 mg before meals and at bedtime (range: 6.25-12.5 mg 3 times/day)
    I.M., I.V.: 25 mg, may repeat in 2 hours when necessary; switch to oral route as soon as feasible
Antiemetic: Oral, I.M., I.V., rectal: 12.5-25 mg every 4-6 hours as needed
Motion sickness: Oral, rectal: 25 mg 30-60 minutes before departure, then every 12 hours as needed
Obstetrics (labor) analgesia adjunct: I.M., I.V.: Early labor: 50 mg; Established labor: 25-75 mg in combination with analgesic at reduced dosage; may repeat every 4 hours for up to 2 additional doses (maximum: 100 mg/day while in labor)
Pre-/postoperative analgesia/hypnotic adjunct: I.M., I.V.: 25-50 mg in combination with analgesic or hypnotic (at reduced dosage)
Sedation: Oral, I.M., I.V., rectal: 12.5-50 mg/dose

Administration Formulations available for oral, rectal, I.M./I.V.; not for SubQ or intra-arterial administration. Administer I.M. into deep muscle (preferred route of administration). I.V. administration is **not** the preferred route; severe tissue damage may occur. Solution for injection should be administered in a maximum concentration of 25 mg/mL (more dilute solutions are recommended). Administer via running I.V. line at port farthest from patient's vein, or through a large bore vein (not hand or wrist). Consider administering over 10-15 minutes (maximum: 25 mg/minute). Discontinue immediately if burning or pain occurs with administration.

Monitoring Parameters Relief of symptoms, mental status; signs and symptoms of tissue injury (burning or pain at injection site, phlebitis, edema) with I.V. administration

Test Interactions Alters the flare response in intradermal allergen tests; increased serum glucose may be seen with glucose tolerance tests

Special Geriatric Considerations Because promethazine is a phenothiazine (and can, therefore, cause side effects such as extrapyramidal symptoms), it is not considered an antihistamine of choice in the elderly.

This medication is considered to be potentially inappropriate in this patient population (Beers Criteria severity: High).

Dosage Forms Excipient information presented when available (limited, particularly for generics); consult specific product labeling.

Injection, solution, as hydrochloride: 25 mg/mL (1 mL); 50 mg/mL (1 mL)

Phenergan®: 25 mg/mL (1 mL); 50 mg/mL (1 mL) [contains edetate disodium, sodium metabisulfite]

Suppository, rectal, as hydrochloride: 12.5 mg (12s); 25 mg (12s)

Phenadoz®: 12.5 mg (12s); 25 mg (12s)

Promethegan™: 12.5 mg (12s); 25 mg (12s); 50 mg (12s)

Syrup, oral, as hydrochloride: 6.25 mg/5 mL (118 mL, 473 mL)

Tablet, oral, as hydrochloride: 12.5 mg, 25 mg, 50 mg

◆ **Promethazine Hydrochloride** see Promethazine on page 1530

◆ **Promethegan™** see Promethazine on page 1530

◆ **Prometrium®** see Progesterone on page 1528

◆ **Pronestyl** see Procainamide on page 1521

Propafenone (pro PAF en one)

Brand Names: U.S. Rythmol®; Rythmol® SR

Brand Names: Canada Apo-Propafenone®; Mylan-Propafenone; PMS-Propafenone; Rythmol® Gen-Propafenone

Index Terms Propafenone Hydrochloride

Generic Availability (U.S.) Yes

Pharmacologic Category Antiarrhythmic Agent, Class Ic

Use Treatment of life-threatening ventricular arrhythmias

Rythmol® SR: Maintenance of normal sinus rhythm in patients with symptomatic atrial fibrillation

Unlabeled/Investigational Use Treatment of supraventricular tachycardias, including those patients with Wolff-Parkinson-White syndrome

Contraindications Hypersensitivity to propafenone or any component of the formulation; sinoatrial, AV, and intraventricular disorders of impulse generation and/or conduction (except in patients with a functioning artificial pacemaker); sinus bradycardia; cardiogenic shock; uncompensated cardiac failure; hypotension; bronchospastic disorders; uncorrected electrolyte abnormalities; concurrent use of ritonavir (see Drug Interactions)

Warnings/Precautions Monitor for proarrhythmic events. May prolong QT_c interval; use caution with other QT_c-prolonging drugs. **[U.S. Boxed Warning]: In the Cardiac Arrhythmia Suppression Trial (CAST), recent (>6 days but <2 years ago) myocardial infarction patients with asymptomatic, non-life-threatening ventricular arrhythmias did not benefit and may have been harmed by attempts to suppress the arrhythmia with flecainide or encainide. An increased mortality or nonfatal cardiac arrest rate (7.7%) was seen in the active treatment group compared with patients in the placebo group (3%). The applicability of the CAST results to other populations is unknown. Antiarrhythmic agents should be reserved for patients with life-threatening ventricular arrhythmias.** Can cause or unmask a variety of conduction disturbances. May alter pacing and sensing thresholds of artificial pacemakers. Patients with bronchospastic disease should generally not receive this drug. Monitor for worsening HF if patient has underlying condition. Correct electrolyte disturbances, especially hypokalemia or hypomagnesemia, prior to use and throughout therapy. Administer cautiously in significant hepatic dysfunction. Use with caution in patients with myasthenia gravis; may exacerbate condition.

Adverse Reactions (Reflective of adult population; not specific for elderly)

1% to 10%:

Cardiovascular: New or worsened arrhythmia (proarrhythmic effect) (2% to 10%), angina (2% to 5%), CHF (1% to 4%), ventricular tachycardia (1% to 3%), palpitation (1% to 3%), AV block (first-degree) (1% to 3%), syncope (1% to 2%), increased QRS interval (1% to 2%), chest pain (1% to 2%), PVCs (1% to 2%), bradycardia (1% to 2%), edema (0% to 1%), bundle branch block (0% to 1%), atrial fibrillation (1%), hypotension (0% to 1%), intraventricular conduction delay (0% to 1%)

Central nervous system: Dizziness (4% to 15%), fatigue (2% to 6%), headache (2% to 5%), ataxia (0% to 2%), insomnia (0% to 2%), anxiety (1% to 2%), drowsiness (1%)

Dermatologic: Rash (1% to 3%)

Gastrointestinal: Nausea/vomiting (2% to 11%), unusual taste (3% to 23%), constipation (2% to 7%), dyspepsia (1% to 3%), diarrhea (1% to 3%), xerostomia (1% to 2%), anorexia (1% to 2%), abdominal pain (1% to 2%), flatulence (0% to 1%)

Neuromuscular & skeletal: Tremor (0% to 1%), arthralgia (0% to 1%), weakness (1% to 2%)

Ocular: Blurred vision (1% to 6%)

Respiratory: Dyspnea (2% to 5%)

Miscellaneous: Diaphoresis (1%)

Drug Interactions

Metabolism/Transport Effects Substrate of CYP1A2 (minor), 2D6 (major), 3A4 (minor); **Inhibits** CYP1A2 (weak), 2D6 (weak)

Avoid Concomitant Use

Avoid concomitant use of Propafenone with any of the following: Artemether; Dronedarone; Lumefantrine; Nilotinib; Pimozide; QUEtiapine; QuiNINE; Ritonavir; Saquinavir; Tetrabenazine; Thioridazine; Tipranavir; Toremifene; Vandetanib; Vemurafenib; Ziprasidone

Increased Effect/Toxicity

Propafenone may increase the levels/effects of: Beta-Blockers; Cardiac Glycosides; Dronedarone; Pimozide; Propranolol; QTc-Prolonging Agents; QuiNINE; Tetrabenazine; Theophylline Derivatives; Thioridazine; Toremifene; Vandetanib; Vemurafenib; Venlafaxine; Vitamin K Antagonists; Ziprasidone

The levels/effects of Propafenone may be increased by: Abiraterone Acetate; Alfuzosin; Artemether; Boceprevir; Chloroquine; Cimetidine; Ciprofloxacin; Ciprofloxacin (Systemic); Conivaptan; CYP2D6 Inhibitors (Moderate); CYP2D6 Inhibitors (Strong); Darunavir; FLUoxetine; FluvoxaMINE; Gadobutrol; Lumefantrine; Nilotinib; PARoxetine; QUEtiapine; QuiNINE; Ritonavir; Saquinavir; Telaprevir; Tipranavir

Decreased Effect

The levels/effects of Propafenone may be decreased by: Barbiturates; Cyproterone; Etravirine; Peginterferon Alfa-2b; Rifamycin Derivatives; Tocilizumab

Ethanol/Nutrition/Herb Interactions

Food: Propafenone serum concentrations may be increased if taken with food.

Herb/Nutraceutical: St John's wort may decrease propafenone levels. Avoid ephedra (may worsen arrhythmia).

Stability Store at 25°C (77°F); excursions permitted to 15°C to 30°C (59°F to 86°F).

Mechanism of Action Propafenone is a class 1c antiarrhythmic agent which possesses local anesthetic properties, blocks the fast inward sodium current, and slows the rate of increase of the action potential. Prolongs conduction and refractoriness in all areas of the myocardium, with a slightly more pronounced effect on intraventricular conduction; it prolongs effective refractory period, reduces spontaneous automaticity and exhibits some beta-blockade activity.

Pharmacodynamics/Kinetics

Absorption: Well absorbed

Distribution: V_d: Adults: 2-5 L/kg

Protein binding: 85% to 95%

Metabolism: Hepatic; two genetically determined metabolism groups exist (extensive and poor metabolizers); 10% of Caucasians are poor metabolizers. Exhibits nonlinear pharmacokinetics; when dose is increased from 300-900 mg/day, serum concentrations increase tenfold; this nonlinearity is thought to be due to saturable first-pass effect.

Bioavailability: 150 mg: 3.4%; 300 mg: 10.6%

Half-life elimination: Extensive metabolizers: 2-10 hours; Poor metabolizers: 10-32 hours

Time to peak, serum: 3.5 hours

Dosage

Geriatric & Adult Note: Patients who exhibit significant widening of QRS complex or second- or third-degree AV block may need dose reduction.

Ventricular arrhythmias: Oral:

Immediate release tablet: Initial: 150 mg every 8 hours, increase at 3- to 4-day intervals up to 300 mg every 8 hours.

Extended release capsule: Initial: 225 mg every 12 hours; dosage increase may be made at a minimum of 5-day intervals; may increase to 325 mg every 12 hours; if further increase is necessary, may increase to 425 mg every 12 hours

Paroxysmal atrial fibrillation (unlabeled dose): Oral: *Immediate release:* Outpatient: "Pill-in-the-pocket" dose: 450 mg (weight <70 kg); 600 mg (weight ≥70 kg). May not repeat in ≤24 hours. **Note:** An initial inpatient conversion trial should have been successful before sending patient home on this approach. Patient must be taking an AV nodal-blocking agent (eg, beta-blocker, nondihydropyridine calcium channel blocker) prior to initiation of antiarrhythmic.

Hepatic Impairment Reduction is necessary; however, specific guidelines are not available.

Administration Capsules should be swallowed whole; do not crush or chew; may be taken without regard to meals.

Monitoring Parameters ECG, blood pressure, pulse (particularly at initiation of therapy)

Pharmacotherapy Pearls An oral sodium channel blocker similar to flecainide; in clinical trials was used effectively to treat atrial flutter, atrial fibrillation, and other arrhythmias, but are not labeled indications; can worsen or even cause new ventricular arrhythmias (proarrhythmic effect)

Special Geriatric Considerations Elderly may have age-related decreases in hepatic Phase I metabolism. Propafenone is dependent upon liver metabolism, therefore, monitor closely in the elderly and adjust dose more gradually during initial treatment. No differences in clearance noted with impaired renal function and, therefore, no adjustment for renal function in the elderly is necessary.

Dosage Forms Excipient information presented when available (limited, particularly for generics); consult specific product labeling. [DSC] = Discontinued product
Capsule, extended release, oral, as hydrochloride: 225 mg, 325 mg, 425 mg
Rythmol® SR: 225 mg, 325 mg, 425 mg [contains soy lecithin]
Tablet, oral, as hydrochloride: 150 mg, 225 mg, 300 mg
Rythmol®: 150 mg, 225 mg, 300 mg [DSC] [scored]

◆ **Propafenone Hydrochloride** see Propafenone on page 1533

Propantheline (proe PAN the leen)

Related Information
Beers Criteria – Potentially Inappropriate Medications for Geriatrics on page 2089
Pharmacotherapy of Urinary Incontinence on page 2032

Medication Safety Issues
BEERS Criteria medication:
This drug may be inappropriate for use in geriatric patients (high severity risk).

Index Terms Propantheline Bromide

Generic Availability (U.S.) Yes

Pharmacologic Category Anticholinergic Agent

Use Adjunctive treatment of peptic ulcer

Unlabeled/Investigational Use Decreased salivation and drooling

Contraindications Severe ulcerative colitis, toxic megacolon, obstructive disease of the GI or urinary tract; glaucoma; myasthenia gravis; unstable cardiovascular adjustment in acute hemorrhage; intestinal atony of elderly or debilitated patients

Warnings/Precautions May cause drowsiness and/or blurred vision, which may impair physical or mental abilities; patients must be cautioned about performing tasks which require mental alertness (eg, operating machinery or driving). Use with caution in patients with hyperthyroidism, hiatal hernia with reflux esophagitis, autonomic neuropathy, hepatic, cardiac, or renal disease, hypertension, GI infections, or other endocrine diseases. In the elderly, avoid long-term use due to anticholinergic adverse effects and uncertain effectiveness (Beers Criteria). Heat prostration may occur in the presence of increased environmental temperature; use caution in hot weather and/or exercise. Diarrhea may be a sign of incomplete intestinal obstruction, treatment should be discontinued if this occurs.

Adverse Reactions (Reflective of adult population; not specific for elderly) Frequency not defined.
Cardiovascular: Palpitation, tachycardia
Central nervous system: Confusion, dizziness, drowsiness, headache, insomnia, nervousness
Endocrine & metabolic: Suppression of lactation
Gastrointestinal: Bloated feeling, constipation, loss of taste, nausea, vomiting, xerostomia
Genitourinary: Impotence, urinary hesitancy, urinary retention
Neuromuscular & skeletal: Weakness
Ocular: Blurred vision, cycloplegia, mydriasis, ocular tension increased
Miscellaneous: Allergic reactions, anaphylaxis, diaphoresis decreased

Drug Interactions
Avoid Concomitant Use There are no known interactions where it is recommended to avoid concomitant use.
Increased Effect/Toxicity
Propantheline may increase the levels/effects of: AbobotulinumtoxinA; Anticholinergics; Cannabinoids; OnabotulinumtoxinA; Potassium Chloride; RimabotulinumtoxinB

The levels/effects of Propantheline may be increased by: MAO Inhibitors; Pramlintide
Decreased Effect
Propantheline may decrease the levels/effects of: Acetylcholinesterase Inhibitors (Central); Secretin

The levels/effects of Propantheline may be decreased by: Acetylcholinesterase Inhibitors (Central)

Stability Store at 20°C to 25°C (68°F to 77°F).

Mechanism of Action Competitively blocks the action of acetylcholine at postganglionic parasympathetic receptor sites

Pharmacodynamics/Kinetics
Onset of action: 30-45 minutes
Duration: 4-6 hours
Half-life elimination, serum: Average: 1.6 hours

Dosage
Geriatric Antisecretory (unlabeled use): 7.5 mg 3 times/day before meals and at bedtime; increase as necessary to a maximum of 30 mg 3 times/day
Adult Antisecretory (unlabeled use), antispasmodic: Oral: 15 mg 3 times/day before meals or food and 30 mg at bedtime

Administration Administer 30 minutes before meals and at bedtime.

Monitoring Parameters Anticholinergic effects, blood pressure, pulse, urinary output, postvoid residual, GI symptoms

Pharmacotherapy Pearls Because propantheline is a quaternary ammonium compound, it does not cross the blood-brain barrier and is less likely to cause CNS effects as compared to atropine

Special Geriatric Considerations The primary use of propantheline in the geriatric population was for treatment of urinary incontinence due to detrusor instability. It is rarely used presently since newer agents, with fewer side effects, have been introduced. Even though it does not cross the blood-brain barrier, CNS effects have been reported. Orthostatic hypotension may also occur.

This medication is considered to be potentially inappropriate in this patient population (Beers Criteria severity: High).

Dosage Forms Excipient information presented when available (limited, particularly for generics); consult specific product labeling.
Tablet, oral, as bromide: 15 mg

◆ **Propantheline Bromide** see Propantheline on page 1535
◆ **Propecia®** see Finasteride on page 736

Propranolol (proe PRAN oh lole)

Related Information
Beers Criteria – Potentially Inappropriate Medications for Geriatrics on page 2089
Beta-Blockers on page 2001

Medication Safety Issues
Sound-alike/look-alike issues:
Propranolol may be confused with prasugrel, Pravachol®, Propulsid®
Inderal® may be confused with Adderall®, Enduron®, Enduronyl®, Imdur®, Imuran®, Inderide®, Isordil®, Toradol®
Inderal® 40 may be confused with Endurony® Forte
High alert medication:
The Institute for Safe Medication Practices (ISMP) includes this medication among its list of drugs which have a heightened risk of causing significant patient harm when used in error.
Administration issues:
Significant differences exist between oral and I.V. dosing. Use caution when converting from one route of administration to another.
International issues:
Inderal [Canada and multiple international markets] and Inderal LA [U.S.] may be confused with Indiaral brand name for loperamide [France]

Brand Names: U.S. Inderal® LA; InnoPran XL®

Brand Names: Canada Apo-Propranolol®; Dom-Propranolol; Inderal®; Inderal® LA; Novo-Pranol; Nu-Propranolol; PMS-Propranolol; Propranolol Hydrochloride Injection, USP

Index Terms Propranolol Hydrochloride

Generic Availability (U.S.) Yes

Pharmacologic Category Antiarrhythmic Agent, Class II; Beta-Adrenergic Blocker, Nonselective

Use Management of hypertension; angina pectoris; pheochromocytoma; essential tremor; supraventricular arrhythmias (such as atrial fibrillation and flutter, AV nodal re-entrant tachycardias), ventricular tachycardias (catecholamine-induced arrhythmias, digoxin toxicity); prevention of myocardial infarction; migraine headache prophylaxis; symptomatic treatment of hypertrophic subaortic stenosis (hypertrophic obstructive cardiomyopathy)

Unlabeled/Investigational Use Tremor due to Parkinson's disease; ethanol withdrawal; aggressive behavior (not recommended for dementia-associated aggression), anxiety, schizophrenia; antipsychotic-induced akathisia; primary and secondary prophylaxis of variceal hemorrhage; acute panic; thyrotoxicosis; tetralogy of Fallot (TOF) hypercyanotic spells

Contraindications Hypersensitivity to propranolol, beta-blockers, or any component of the formulation; uncompensated congestive heart failure (unless the failure is due to tachyarrhythmias being treated with propranolol), cardiogenic shock, severe sinus bradycardia or heart block greater than first-degree (except in patients with a functioning artificial pacemaker), severe hyperactive airway disease (asthma or COPD)

Warnings/Precautions Consider pre-existing conditions such as sick sinus syndrome before initiating. Administer cautiously in compensated heart failure and monitor for a worsening of the condition (efficacy of propranolol in HF has not been demonstrated). **[U.S. Boxed Warning]: Beta-blocker therapy should not be withdrawn abruptly (particularly in patients with CAD), but gradually tapered to avoid acute tachycardia, hypertension, and/or ischemia.** Chronic beta-blocker therapy should not be routinely withdrawn prior to major surgery. May precipitate or aggravate symptoms of arterial insufficiency in patients with PVD and Raynaud's disease; use with caution and monitor for progression of arterial obstruction. Bradycardia may be observed more frequently in elderly patients (>65 years of age); dosage reductions may be necessary. Use caution with concurrent use of digoxin, verapamil, or diltiazem; bradycardia or heart block can occur. Avoid concurrent I.V. use of both agents. Use with caution in patients receiving inhaled anesthetic agents known to depress myocardial contractility.

Use cautiously in patients with diabetes because it can mask prominent hypoglycemic symptoms. May mask signs of hyperthyroidism (eg, tachycardia); if hyperthyroidism is suspected, carefully manage and monitor; abrupt withdrawal may exacerbate symptoms of hyperthyroidism or precipitate thyroid storm. May alter thyroid-function tests. Use with caution in myasthenia gravis or psychiatric disease (may cause CNS depression). Use cautiously in renal and hepatic dysfunction; dosage adjustment required in hepatic impairment. In general, patients with bronchospastic disease should not receive beta-blockers; if used at all, should be used cautiously with close monitoring. Adequate alpha-blockade is required prior to use of any beta-blocker for patients with untreated pheochromocytoma. May induce or exacerbate psoriasis. Use caution with history of severe anaphylaxis to allergens; patients taking beta-blockers may become more sensitive to repeated challenges. Treatment of anaphylaxis (eg, epinephrine) in patients taking beta-blockers may be ineffective or promote undesirable effects.

Adverse Reactions (Reflective of adult population; not specific for elderly) Frequency not defined.

Cardiovascular: Angina, arterial insufficiency, AV conduction disturbance increased, bradycardia, cardiogenic shock, CHF, hypotension, impaired myocardial contractility, mesenteric arterial thrombosis (rare), Raynaud's syndrome, syncope

Central nervous system: Amnesia, catatonia, cognitive dysfunction, confusion, depression, dizziness, emotional lability, fatigue, hallucinations, hypersomnolence, insomnia, lethargy, lightheadedness, psychosis, vertigo, vivid dreams

Dermatologic: Alopecia, contact dermatitis, cutaneous ulcers, eczematous eruptions, erythema multiforme, exfoliative dermatitis, hyperkeratosis, nail changes, oculomucocutaneous reactions, pruritus, psoriasiform eruptions, rash, Stevens-Johnson syndrome, toxic epidermal necrolysis, ulcers, ulcerative lichenoid, urticaria

Endocrine & metabolic: Hyper-/hypoglycemia, hyperkalemia, hyperlipidemia

Gastrointestinal: Anorexia, cramping, constipation, diarrhea, ischemic colitis, nausea, stomach discomfort, vomiting

Genitourinary: Impotence, interstitial nephritis (rare), oliguria (rare), Peyronie's disease, proteinuria (rare)

Hematologic: Agranulocytosis, nonthrombocytopenic purpura, thrombocytopenia, thrombocytopenic purpura

Hepatic: Alkaline phosphatase increased, transaminases increased

Neuromuscular & skeletal: Arthropathy, carpal tunnel syndrome (rare), myotonus, paresthesia, polyarthritis, weakness

Ocular: Hyperemia of the conjunctiva, mydriasis, visual acuity decreased, visual disturbances, xerophthalmia

Renal: BUN increased

Respiratory: Bronchospasm, dyspnea, laryngospasm, pharyngitis, pulmonary edema, respiratory distress, wheezing

Miscellaneous: Anaphylactic/anaphylactoid allergic reaction, cold extremities, lupus-like syndrome (rare)

Drug Interactions

Metabolism/Transport Effects Substrate of CYP1A2 (major), 2C19 (minor), 2D6 (major), 3A4 (minor); **Inhibits** CYP1A2 (weak), CYP2D6 (weak), P-glycoprotein

Avoid Concomitant Use

Avoid concomitant use of Propranolol with any of the following: Floctafenine; Methacholine; Topotecan

◀ **Increased Effect/Toxicity**

Propranolol may increase the levels/effects of: Alpha-/Beta-Agonists (Direct-Acting); Alpha1-Blockers; Alpha2-Agonists; Amifostine; Antihypertensives; Antipsychotic Agents (Phenothiazines); Bupivacaine; Cardiac Glycosides; Colchicine; Dabigatran Etexilate; Everolimus; Fingolimod; Hypotensive Agents; Insulin; Lidocaine; Lidocaine (Systemic); Lidocaine (Topical); Mepivacaine; Methacholine; Midodrine; P-Glycoprotein Substrates; RiTUXimab; Rivaroxaban; Rizatriptan; Sulfonylureas; Topotecan; ZOLMitriptan

The levels/effects of Propranolol may be increased by: Abiraterone Acetate; Acetylcholinesterase Inhibitors; Alcohol (Ethyl); Aminoquinolines (Antimalarial); Amiodarone; Anilidopiperidine Opioids; Antipsychotic Agents (Phenothiazines); Calcium Channel Blockers (Dihydropyridine); Calcium Channel Blockers (Nondihydropyridine); Conivaptan; CYP1A2 Inhibitors (Moderate); CYP1A2 Inhibitors (Strong); CYP2D6 Inhibitors (Moderate); CYP2D6 Inhibitors (Strong); Darunavir; Deferasirox; Diazoxide; Dipyridamole; Disopyramide; Dronedarone; Floctafenine; FluvoxaMINE; Herbs (Hypotensive Properties); Lacidipine; MAO Inhibitors; Pentoxifylline; Phosphodiesterase 5 Inhibitors; Propafenone; Propoxyphene; Prostacyclin Analogues; QuiNIDine; Reserpine; Selective Serotonin Reuptake Inhibitors; Zileuton

Decreased Effect

Propranolol may decrease the levels/effects of: Beta2-Agonists; Lacidipine; Theophylline Derivatives

The levels/effects of Propranolol may be decreased by: Alcohol (Ethyl); Barbiturates; Bile Acid Sequestrants; CYP1A2 Inducers (Strong); Cyproterone; Herbs (Hypertensive Properties); Methylphenidate; Nonsteroidal Anti-Inflammatory Agents; Peginterferon Alfa-2b; Rifamycin Derivatives; Tocilizumab; Yohimbine

Ethanol/Nutrition/Herb Interactions

Ethanol: Ethanol may increase or decrease plasma levels of propranolol. Reports are variable and have shown both enhanced as well as inhibited hepatic metabolism (of propranolol). Caution advised with consumption of alcohol and monitor for heart rate and/or blood pressure changes.

Food: Propranolol serum levels may be increased if taken with food. Protein-rich foods may increase bioavailability; a change in diet from high carbohydrate/low protein to low carbohydrate/high protein may result in increased oral clearance.

Cigarette: Smoking may decrease plasma levels of propranolol by increasing metabolism.

Herb/Nutraceutical: Avoid dong quai if using for hypertension (has estrogenic activity). Avoid bayberry, blue cohosh, cayenne, ephedra, ginger, ginseng (American), gotu kola, licorice, yohimbe (may worsen hypertension). Avoid black cohosh, california poppy, coleus, garlic, golden seal, hawthorn, mistletoe, periwinkle, quinine, shepherd's purse (have antihypertensive activity, may cause hypotension).

Stability

Injection: Store at 20°C to 25°C (68°F to 77°F); protect from freezing or excessive heat. Once diluted, propranolol is stable for 24 hours at room temperature in D_5W or NS. Protect from light. Solution has a maximum stability at pH of 3 and decomposes rapidly in alkaline pH.

Capsule, tablet: Store at 20°C to 25°C (68°F to 77°F); protect from freezing or excessive heat. Protect from light and moisture.

Mechanism of Action Nonselective beta-adrenergic blocker (class II antiarrhythmic); competitively blocks response to beta$_1$- and beta$_2$-adrenergic stimulation which results in decreases in heart rate, myocardial contractility, blood pressure, and myocardial oxygen demand. Nonselective beta-adrenergic blockers (propranolol, nadolol) reduce portal pressure by producing splanchnic vasoconstriction (beta$_2$ effect) thereby reducing portal blood flow.

Pharmacodynamics/Kinetics

Onset of action: Beta-blockade: Oral: 1-2 hours

Duration: Immediate release: 6-12 hours; Extended-release formulations: ~24-27 hours

Absorption: Oral: Rapid and complete

Distribution: V_d: 4 L/kg in adults

Protein binding: ~90% (S-isomer primarily to alpha$_1$-acid glycoprotein; R-isomer primarily to albumin)

Metabolism: Hepatic via CYP2D6, and CYP1A2 to 4-hydroxypropranolol (active) and inactive compounds; extensive first-pass effect

Bioavailability: ~25% reaches systemic circulation due to high first-pass metabolism; protein-rich foods increase bioavailability by ~50%

Half-life elimination: Immediate release formulation: 3-6 hours; Extended-release formulations: 8-10 hours

Time to peak: Immediate release: 1-4 hours; Extended-release formulations: ~6-14 hours

Excretion: Metabolites are excreted primarily in urine (96% to 99%); <1% excreted in urine as unchanged drug

Dosage

Geriatric

I.V.: Use caution; initiate at lower end of the dosing range.

Oral:

Hypertension: Consider lower initial doses and titrate to response (Aronow, 2011)

Tachyarrhythmias: Initial: 10 mg twice daily; increase dosage every 3-7 days; usual dose range: 10-320 mg/day given in 1-2 divided doses.

Refer to adult dosing for additional uses.

Adult

Akathisia (unlabeled use): Oral: 30-120 mg/day in 2-3 divided doses

Essential tremor: Oral: 40 mg twice daily initially; maintenance doses: Usually 120-320 mg/day

Hypertension: Initial: Oral: 40 mg twice daily; increase dosage every 3-7 days; usual dose: 120-240 mg divided in 2-3 doses/day; maximum daily dose: 640 mg; usual dosage range (JNC 7): 40-160 mg/day in 2 divided doses

Extended release formulations:

Inderal® LA: Initial: 80 mg once daily; usual maintenance: 120-160 mg once daily; maximum daily dose: 640 mg; usual dosage range (JNC 7): 60-180 mg/day once daily

InnoPran XL®: Initial: 80 mg once daily at bedtime; if initial response is inadequate, may be increased at 2-3 week intervals to a maximum dose of 120 mg

Hypertrophic subaortic stenosis: Oral: 20-40 mg 3-4 times/day

Inderal® LA: 80-160 mg once daily

Migraine headache prophylaxis: Oral: Initial: 80 mg/day divided every 6-8 hours; increase by 20-40 mg/dose every 3-4 weeks to a maximum of 160-240 mg/day given in divided doses every 6-8 hours; if satisfactory response not achieved within 6 weeks of starting therapy, drug should be withdrawn gradually over several weeks

Inderal® LA: Initial: 80 mg once daily; effective dose range: 160-240 mg once daily

Pheochromocytoma: Oral: 30-60 mg/day in divided doses

Post-MI mortality reduction: Oral: 180-240 mg/day in 3-4 divided doses

Stable angina: Oral: 80-320 mg/day in doses divided 2-4 times/day

Inderal® LA: Initial: 80 mg once daily; maximum dose: 320 mg once daily

Tachyarrhythmias:

Oral: 10-30 mg/dose every 6-8 hours

I.V.: 1-3 mg/dose slow IVP; repeat every 2-5 minutes up to a total of 5 mg; titrate initial dose to desired response

or

0.5-1 mg over 1 minute; may repeat, if necessary, up to a total maximum dose of 0.1 mg/kg (ACLS guidelines, 2010)

Note: Once response achieved or maximum dose administered, additional doses should not be given for at least 4 hours.

Thyrotoxicosis (unlabeled use):

Oral: 10-40 mg/dose every 6 hours

I.V.: 1-3 mg/dose slow IVP as a single dose

Variceal hemorrhage prophylaxis (unlabeled use) (Garcia-Tsao, 2007): Oral:

Primary prophylaxis: Initial: 20 mg twice daily; adjust to maximal tolerated dose. **Note:** Risk factors for hemorrhage include Child-Pugh class B/C or variceal red wale markings on endoscopy.

Secondary prophylaxis: Initial: 20 mg twice daily; adjust to maximal tolerated dose

Renal Impairment

Not dialyzable (0% to 5%); supplemental dose is not necessary.

Peritoneal dialysis effects: Supplemental dose is not necessary.

Hepatic Impairment Marked slowing of heart rate may occur in chronic liver disease with conventional doses; low initial dose and regular heart rate monitoring.

Administration I.V. administration should not exceed 1 mg/minute; I.V. dose much smaller than oral dose; monitor ECG and CV

Monitoring Parameters Blood pressure, orthostatic hypotension, heart rate, CNS effects

Reference Range Therapeutic: 50-100 ng/mL (SI: 190-390 nmol/L) at end of dose interval

Special Geriatric Considerations Since bioavailability increased in about twofold in elderly patients, geriatrics may require lower maintenance doses. Also, as serum and tissue concentrations increase beta$_1$ selectivity diminishes. Beta-adrenergic blockade may result in less hemodynamic response than seen in younger adults due to alterations in the beta-adrenergic autonomic system. Studies indicate that despite decreased sensitivity to the chronotropic effects of beta-blockade with age, there appears to be an increased myocardial sensitivity to the negative inotropic effect during stress (ie, exercise). Controlled trials have shown the overall response rate for propranolol to be only 20% to 50% in elderly populations. Therefore, all beta-adrenergic blocking drugs may result in a decreased response as compared to younger adults. Due to propranolol's CNS penetration and nonselective action, it may not be the beta-blocker of choice for use in elderly.

Dosage Forms Excipient information presented when available (limited, particularly for generics); consult specific product labeling.

Capsule, extended release, oral, as hydrochloride: 60 mg, 80 mg, 120 mg, 160 mg
InnoPran XL®: 80 mg, 120 mg

Capsule, sustained release, oral, as hydrochloride:
Inderal® LA: 60 mg, 80 mg, 120 mg, 160 mg

Injection, solution, as hydrochloride: 1 mg/mL (1 mL)

Injection, solution, as hydrochloride [preservative free]: 1 mg/mL (1 mL)

Solution, oral, as hydrochloride: 4 mg/mL (500 mL); 8 mg/mL (500 mL)

Tablet, oral, as hydrochloride: 10 mg, 20 mg, 40 mg, 60 mg, 80 mg

Selected References

Chobanian AV, Bakris GL, Black HR, et al, "The Seventh Report of the Joint National Committee on Prevention, Detection, Evaluation, and Treatment of High Blood Pressure: The JNC 7 Report," *JAMA*, 2003, 289(19):2560-71.

Fleisher LA, Beckman JA, Brown KA, et al, "ACC/AHA 2006 Guideline Update on Perioperative Cardiovascular Evaluation for Noncardiac Surgery: Focused Update on Perioperative Beta-Blocker Therapy. A Report of the American College of Cardiology/American Heart Association Task Force on Practice Guidelines (Writing Committee to Update the 2002 Guidelines on Perioperative Cardiovascular Evaluation for Noncardiac Surgery) Developed in Collaboration With the American Society of Echocardiography, American Society of Nuclear Cardiology, Heart Rhythm Society, Society of Cardiovascular Anesthesiologists, Society for Cardiovascular Angiography and Interventions, and Society for Vascular Medicine and Biology," *J Am Coll Cardiol*, 2006, 47(11):2343-55.

Garcia-Tsao G, Sanyal AJ, Grace ND, et al, "Prevention and Management of Gastroesophageal Varices and Variceal Hemorrhage in Cirrhosis," *Hepatology*, 2007, 46(3):922-38.

Juul AB, Wetterslev J, Gluud C, et al, "Effect of Perioperative Beta Blockade in Patients With Diabetes Undergoing Major Non-Cardiac Surgery: Randomized Placebo Controlled, Blinded Multicentre Trial. DIPOM Trial Group," *BMJ*, 2006, 332(7556):1482.

Propranolol and Hydrochlorothiazide
(proe PRAN oh lole & hye droe klor oh THYE a zide)

Related Information
Hydrochlorothiazide *on page 876*
Propranolol *on page 1536*

Medication Safety Issues
Sound-alike/look-alike issues:
Inderide® may be confused with Inderal®

Index Terms Hydrochlorothiazide and Propranolol; Inderide

Generic Availability (U.S.) Yes

Pharmacologic Category Beta Blocker, Nonselective; Diuretic, Thiazide

Use Management of hypertension

Dosage
Geriatric & Adult
Hypertension: Oral: Dose is individualized; typical dosages of **hydrochlorothiazide**: 12.5-50 mg/day; initial dose of **propranolol** 80 mg/day

Note: Daily dose of tablet form should be divided into 2 daily doses; may be used to maximum dosage of up to 160 mg of propranolol; higher dosages would result in higher than optimal thiazide dosages.

Special Geriatric Considerations Divided doses of diuretics may increase the incidence of nocturia in the elderly. Hydrochlorothiazide is not effective in patients with a Cl_{cr} <30 mL/minute; therefore, it may not be a useful agent in many elderly patients.

Dosage Forms Excipient information presented when available (limited, particularly for generics); consult specific product labeling.

Tablet: Propranolol hydrochloride 40 mg and hydrochlorothiazide 25 mg; propranolol hydrochloride 80 mg and hydrochlorothiazide 25 mg

◆ **Propranolol Hydrochloride** *see* Propranolol *on page 1536*
◆ **Proprinal® [OTC]** *see* Ibuprofen *on page 908*
◆ **2-Propylpentanoic Acid** *see* Valproic Acid *on page 1888*

Propylthiouracil (proe pil thye oh YOOR a sil)

Medication Safety Issues
Sound-alike/look-alike issues:
Propylthiouracil may be confused with Purinethol®
PTU is an error-prone abbreviation (mistaken as mercaptopurine [Purinethol®; 6-MP])

Brand Names: Canada Propyl-Thyracil®

Index Terms PTU (error-prone abbreviation)

Generic Availability (U.S.) Yes

Pharmacologic Category Antithyroid Agent; Thioamide

Use Adjunctive therapy in patients intolerant of methimazole to ameliorate hyperthyroidism symptoms in preparation for surgical treatment or radioactive iodine therapy; treatment of hyperthyroidism in patients intolerant of methimazole and not candidates for surgical/radiotherapy

Unlabeled/Investigational Use Management of thyrotoxic crisis

Medication Guide Available Yes

Contraindications Hypersensitivity to propylthiouracil or any component of the formulation

Warnings/Precautions [U.S. Boxed Warning]: Severe liver injury (some fatal) and acute liver failure (some cases requiring transplantation) have been reported. Patients should be counseled to recognize and report symptoms suggestive of hepatic dysfunction (especially in first 6 months of treatment), which should prompt immediate discontinuation. Routine liver function test monitoring may not reduce risk due to unpredictable and rapid onset.

Has been associated with significant bone marrow depression. The most severe manifestation is agranulocytosis (commonly within first 3 months of therapy). Aplastic anemia, thrombocytopenia, and leukopenia may also occur. Use with caution in patients receiving other drugs known to cause myelosuppression particularly agranulocytosis. Discontinue if significant bone marrow suppression occurs, particularly agranulocytosis or aplastic anemia.

Rare hypersensitivity reactions have been reported, including the development of ANCA-positive vasculitis, drug fever, interstitial pneumonitis, exfoliative dermatitis, glomerulonephritis, leukocytoclastic vasculitis, and a lupus-like syndrome; prompt discontinuation is warranted in patients who develop symptoms consistent with a form of autoimmunity or other hypersensitivity during therapy. May cause hypoprothrombinemia and bleeding.

Adverse Reactions (Reflective of adult population; not specific for elderly) Frequency not defined.

Cardiovascular: Periarteritis, vasculitis (ANCA-positive, cutaneous, leukocytoclastic)

Central nervous system: Drowsiness, drug fever, fever, headache, neuritis, vertigo

Dermatologic: Alopecia, erythema nodosum, exfoliative dermatitis, pruritus, skin pigmentation, skin rash, skin ulcers, urticaria

Endocrine & metabolic: Goiter, weight gain

Gastrointestinal: Constipation, loss of taste, nausea, sialoadenopathy, splenomegaly, stomach pain, taste perversion, vomiting

Hematologic: Agranulocytosis, aplastic anemia, bleeding, granulopenia, hypoprothrombinemia, leukopenia, thrombocytopenia

Hepatic: Acute liver failure, cholestatic jaundice, hepatitis

Neuromuscular & skeletal: Arthralgia, myalgia, paresthesia

Renal: Acute renal failure, glomerulonephritis, nephritis

Respiratory: Alveolar hemorrhage, interstitial pneumonitis

Miscellaneous: Lymphadenopathy, SLE-like syndrome

Drug Interactions

Avoid Concomitant Use

Avoid concomitant use of Propylthiouracil with any of the following: Sodium Iodide I131

Increased Effect/Toxicity There are no known significant interactions involving an increase in effect.

Decreased Effect

Propylthiouracil may decrease the levels/effects of: Sodium Iodide I131; Vitamin K Antagonists

Ethanol/Nutrition/Herb Interactions Food: Propylthiouracil serum levels may be altered if taken with food.

Stability Store at 25°C (77°F); excursions permitted to 15°C to 30°C (59°F to 86°F).

Mechanism of Action Inhibits the synthesis of thyroid hormones by blocking the oxidation of iodine in the thyroid gland; blocks synthesis of thyroxine and triiodothyronine

Pharmacodynamics/Kinetics

Onset of action: Therapeutic: 24-36 hours

Peak effect: Remission: 4 months of continued therapy

Duration: 2-3 hours

Distribution: Concentrated in the thyroid gland

Protein binding: 75% to 80%

Metabolism: Hepatic

Bioavailability: 80% to 95%

Half-life elimination: 1.5-5 hours; End-stage renal disease: 8.5 hours

Time to peak, serum: ~1 hour

Excretion: Urine (35%)

Dosage
Adult
Hyperthyroidism: Oral: Initial: 300 mg/day in 3 divided doses; 400 mg/day in patients with severe hyperthyroidism and/or very large goiters; an occasional patient will require 600-900 mg/day; usual maintenance: 100-150 mg/day

Thyrotoxic crisis/thyroid storm (unlabeled use): **Note:** Recommendations vary widely and have not been evaluated in comparative trials. Typical dosing is 800-1200 mg/day given as 200-300 mg every 4-6 hours; some clinicians advocate an initial loading dose of 600-1000 mg. After initial response, dose may be reduced gradually to a maintenance dosage (100-600 mg/day in divided doses) (Goldberg, 2003; Nayak, 2006).

Duration of therapy: Clinical improvement generally occurs in 1-3 months, after which dosage reduction may be employed (to prevent hypothyroidism), with discontinuation considered after 12-18 months of therapy. Thyroid function should be monitored every 2 months thereafter for 6 months until remission is confirmed, followed by annual evaluations (Cooper, 2005).
Renal Impairment Adjustment is not necessary.
Administration Administer at the same time in relation to meals each day, either always with meals or always between meals.
Monitoring Parameters CBC with differential, prothrombin time, liver function tests (bilirubin, alkaline phosphatase, transaminases), and thyroid function tests (TSH, T_3, T_4) every 4-6 weeks until euthyroid; periodic blood counts are recommended for chronic therapy
Reference Range Normal laboratory values:
Total T_4: 5-12 mcg/dL
Serum T_3: 90-185 ng/dL
Free thyroxine index (FT$_4$ I): 6-10.5
TSH: 0.5-4.0 microunits/mL
Pharmacotherapy Pearls Preferred over methimazole in thyroid storm due to inhibition of peripheral conversion as well as synthesis of thyroid hormone.

Graves' hyperthyroidism: Elevated T_3 may be the sole indicator of inadequate treatment. Elevated TSH indicates excessive antithyroid treatment. Monitoring of TSH is a poor indicator of treatment effectiveness, as levels may remain suppressed for months, despite euthyroid state (Cooper, 2005).
Special Geriatric Considerations The use of antithyroid thioamides is as effective in the elderly as they are in younger adults.
Dosage Forms Excipient information presented when available (limited, particularly for generics); consult specific product labeling.
Tablet, oral: 50 mg

- ◆ **2-Propylvaleric Acid** see Valproic Acid on page 1888
- ◆ **Proscar®** see Finasteride on page 736
- ◆ **ProSom** see Estazolam on page 639
- ◆ **Prostaglandin E$_1$** see Alprostadil on page 73
- ◆ **Prostate Cancer Vaccine, Cell-Based** see Sipuleucel-T on page 1684
- ◆ **Prostigmin®** see Neostigmine on page 1283
- ◆ **Protease, Lipase, and Amylase** see Pancrelipase on page 1387
- ◆ **Protonix®** see Pantoprazole on page 1389
- ◆ **Protonix® I.V.** see Pantoprazole on page 1389

Protriptyline (proe TRIP ti leen)

Related Information
Antidepressant Agents on page 1991
Medication Safety Issues
Sound-alike/look-alike issues:
Vivactil® may be confused with Vyvanse™
Brand Names: U.S. Vivactil®
Index Terms Protriptyline Hydrochloride
Generic Availability (U.S.) Yes
Pharmacologic Category Antidepressant, Tricyclic (Secondary Amine)
Use Treatment of depression
Medication Guide Available Yes
Contraindications Hypersensitivity to protriptyline (cross-reactivity to other cyclic antidepressants may occur) or any component of the formulation; use of MAO inhibitors within 14 days; use of cisapride; use in a patient during the acute recovery phase of MI

Warnings/Precautions [U.S. Boxed Warning]: Antidepressants increase the risk of suicidal thinking and behavior in children, adolescents, and young adults (18-24 years of age) with major depressive disorder (MDD) and other psychiatric disorders; consider risk prior to prescribing. Short-term studies did not show an increased risk in patients >24 years of age and showed a decreased risk in patients ≥65 years. Closely monitor for clinical worsening, suicidality, or unusual changes in behavior; the patient's family or caregiver should be instructed to closely observe the patient and communicate condition with healthcare provider. A medication guide should be dispensed with each prescription. **Protriptyline is FDA approved for the treatment of depression in adolescents.**

The possibility of a suicide attempt is inherent in major depression and may persist until remission occurs. Monitor for worsening of depression or suicidality, especially during initiation of therapy (generally first 1-2 months) or with dose increases or decreases. Use caution in high-risk patients. Worsening depression and severe abrupt suicidality that are not part of the presenting symptoms may require discontinuation or modification of drug therapy. The patient's family or caregiver should be alerted to monitor patients for the emergence of suicidality and associated behaviors (such as agitation, irritability, hostility, impulsivity, and hypomania) and call healthcare provider.

May worsen psychosis in some patients or precipitate a shift to mania or hypomania in patients with bipolar disorder. Patients presenting with depressive symptoms should be screened for bipolar disorder. Monotherapy in patients with bipolar disorder should be avoided. **Protriptyline is not FDA approved for the treatment of bipolar depression.**

TCAs may rarely cause bone marrow suppression; monitor for any signs of infection and obtain CBC if symptoms (eg, fever, sore throat) evident. Although the degree of sedation is low relative to other antidepressant agents, protriptyline may cause sedation, resulting in impaired performance of tasks requiring alertness (eg, operating machinery or driving). Sedative effects may be additive with other CNS depressants and/or ethanol. Protriptyline may aggravate aggressive behavior. Consider discontinuing, when possible, prior to elective surgery. Therapy should not be abruptly discontinued in patients receiving high doses for prolonged periods. May alter glucose regulation - use with caution in patients with diabetes.

May cause orthostatic hypotension or conduction abnormalities (risks are moderate relative to other antidepressants). Use with caution in patients with a history of cardiovascular disease (including previous MI, stroke, tachycardia, or conduction abnormalities). The degree of anticholinergic blockade produced by this agent is moderate relative to other cyclic antidepressants; however, caution should still be used in patients with urinary retention, benign prostatic hyperplasia, narrow-angle glaucoma, xerostomia, visual problems, constipation, or history of bowel obstruction.

Hyperpyrexia has been observed with TCAs in combination with anticholinergics and/or neuroleptics, particularly during hot weather. Use caution in patients with a previous seizure disorder or condition predisposing to seizures such as brain damage, alcoholism, or concurrent therapy with other drugs which lower the seizure threshold. May increase the risks associated with electroconvulsive therapy. Use with caution in hyperthyroid patients or those receiving thyroid supplementation. Use with caution in patients with hepatic or renal dysfunction and in elderly patients.

Adverse Reactions (Reflective of adult population; not specific for elderly) Frequency not defined.

Cardiovascular: Arrhythmias, heart block, hyper-/hypotension, MI, palpitation, stroke, tachycardia

Central nervous system: Agitation, anxiety, ataxia, confusion, delirium, delusions, dizziness, drowsiness, EPS, exacerbation of psychosis, fatigue, hallucinations, headache, hypomania, incoordination, insomnia, nightmares, panic, restlessness, seizure

Dermatologic: Alopecia, itching, petechiae, photosensitivity, rash, urticaria

Endocrine & metabolic: Breast enlargement, galactorrhea, gynecomastia, increased or decreased libido, syndrome of inappropriate ADH secretion (SIADH)

Gastrointestinal: Anorexia, constipation, decreased lower esophageal sphincter tone may cause GE reflux, diarrhea, heartburn, increased appetite, nausea, trouble with gums, unpleasant taste, vomiting, weight gain/loss, xerostomia

Genitourinary: Difficult urination, impotence, testicular edema

Hematologic: Agranulocytosis, eosinophilia, leukopenia, purpura, thrombocytopenia

Hepatic: Cholestatic jaundice, increased liver enzymes

Neuromuscular & skeletal: Fine muscle tremor, numbness, tingling, tremor, weakness

Ocular: Blurred vision, eye pain, increased intraocular pressure

Otic: Tinnitus

Miscellaneous: Allergic reactions, excessive diaphoresis

Drug Interactions

Metabolism/Transport Effects Substrate of CYP2D6 (major)

◄ **Avoid Concomitant Use**

Avoid concomitant use of Protriptyline with any of the following: Artemether; Cisapride; Dronedarone; Iobenguane I 123; Lumefantrine; MAO Inhibitors; Methylene Blue; Nilotinib; Pimozide; QUEtiapine; QuiNINE; Sibutramine; Tetrabenazine; Thioridazine; Toremifene; Vandetanib; Vemurafenib; Ziprasidone

Increased Effect/Toxicity

Protriptyline may increase the levels/effects of: Alpha-/Beta-Agonists (Direct-Acting); Alpha1-Agonists; Amphetamines; Anticholinergics; Beta2-Agonists; Cisapride; Desmopressin; Dronedarone; Methylene Blue; Pimozide; QTc-Prolonging Agents; QuiNIDine; QuiNINE; Serotonin Modulators; Sodium Phosphates; Sulfonylureas; Tetrabenazine; Thioridazine; Toremifene; TraMADol; Vandetanib; Vemurafenib; Vitamin K Antagonists; Yohimbine; Ziprasidone

The levels/effects of Protriptyline may be increased by: Abiraterone Acetate; Alfuzosin; Altretamine; Artemether; Chloroquine; Cimetidine; Cinacalcet; Ciprofloxacin; Ciprofloxacin (Systemic); CYP2D6 Inhibitors (Moderate); CYP2D6 Inhibitors (Strong); Dexmethylphenidate; Divalproex; DULoxetine; Gadobutrol; Lithium; Lumefantrine; MAO Inhibitors; Methylphenidate; Metoclopramide; Nilotinib; Pramlintide; Propoxyphene; Protease Inhibitors; QUEtiapine; QuiNIDine; QuiNINE; Selective Serotonin Reuptake Inhibitors; Sibutramine; Terbinafine; Terbinafine (Systemic); Valproic Acid

Decreased Effect

Protriptyline may decrease the levels/effects of: Acetylcholinesterase Inhibitors (Central); Alpha2-Agonists; Iobenguane I 123

The levels/effects of Protriptyline may be decreased by: Acetylcholinesterase Inhibitors (Central); Barbiturates; CarBAMazepine; Peginterferon Alfa-2b; St Johns Wort

Ethanol/Nutrition/Herb Interactions

Ethanol: May increase CNS depression; monitor for increased effects with coadministration. Caution patients about effects.

Food: Grapefruit juice may inhibit the metabolism of some TCAs and clinical toxicity may result.

Herb/Nutraceutical: Avoid valerian, St John's wort, SAMe, kava kava (may increase risk of serotonin syndrome and/or excessive sedation).

Mechanism of Action Increases the synaptic concentration of serotonin and/or norepinephrine in the central nervous system by inhibition of their reuptake by the presynaptic neuronal membrane

Pharmacodynamics/Kinetics

Protein binding: 92%

Metabolism: Undergoes first-pass metabolism (10% to 25%); extensively metabolized in the liver by N-oxidation, hydroxylation and glucuronidation

Half-life: 54-92 hours, averaging 74 hours

Time to peak serum concentration: Oral: Within 24-30 hours

Elimination: In urine

Dosage

Geriatric Oral: Initial: 5-10 mg/day; increase every 3-7 days by 5-10 mg; usual dose: 15-20 mg/day

Adult Depression: Oral: 15-60 mg/day in 3-4 divided doses

Administration Make any dosage increase in the morning dose

Monitoring Parameters Monitor for cardiac abnormalities in elderly patients receiving doses >20 mg; suicide ideation (especially at the beginning of therapy or when doses are increased or decreased)

Reference Range Therapeutic: 70-250 ng/mL (SI: 266-950 nmol/L); Toxic: >500 ng/mL (SI: >1900 nmol/L)

Special Geriatric Considerations Little data on its use in the elderly. Strong anticholinergic properties which may limit its use; more often stimulating rather than sedating.

Dosage Forms Excipient information presented when available (limited, particularly for generics); consult specific product labeling.

Tablet, oral, as hydrochloride: 5 mg, 10 mg

Vivactil®: 5 mg, 10 mg

◆ **Protriptyline Hydrochloride** *see* Protriptyline *on page 1542*
◆ **Provenge®** *see* Sipuleucel-T *on page 1684*
◆ **Proventil® HFA** *see* Albuterol *on page 50*
◆ **Provera®** *see* MedroxyPROGESTERone *on page 1122*
◆ **Provigil®** *see* Modafinil *on page 1227*
◆ **PROzac®** *see* FLUoxetine *on page 753*
◆ **PROzac® Weekly™** *see* FLUoxetine *on page 753*
◆ **Prudoxin™** *see* Doxepin (Topical) *on page 567*

◆ **P&S® [OTC]** *see* Salicylic Acid *on page 1648*
◆ **23PS** *see* Pneumococcal Polysaccharide Vaccine (Polyvalent) *on page 1474*

Pseudoephedrine (soo doe e FED rin)

Related Information
Beers Criteria – Potentially Inappropriate Medications for Geriatrics *on page 2089*
Medication Safety Issues
Sound-alike/look-alike issues:
Sudafed® may be confused with sotalol, Sudafed PE™, Sufenta®
Brand Names: U.S. Children's Nasal Decongestant [OTC]; Genaphed™ [OTC] [DSC]; Oranyl [OTC]; Silfedrine Children's [OTC]; Sudafed® 12 Hour [OTC]; Sudafed® 24 Hour [OTC]; Sudafed® Children's [OTC]; Sudafed® Maximum Strength Nasal Decongestant [OTC]; Sudo-Tab® [OTC]; SudoGest 12 Hour [OTC]; SudoGest Children's [OTC]; SudoGest [OTC]
Brand Names: Canada Balminil Decongestant; Benylin® D for Infants; Contac® Cold 12 Hour Relief Non Drowsy; Drixoral® ND; Eltor®; PMS-Pseudoephedrine; Pseudofrin; Robi-drine®; Sudafed® Decongestant
Index Terms *d*-Isoephedrine Hydrochloride; Pseudoephedrine Hydrochloride; Pseudoephedrine Sulfate; Sudafed
Generic Availability (U.S.) Yes: Excludes extended release products
Pharmacologic Category Alpha/Beta Agonist
Use Temporary symptomatic relief of nasal congestion due to common cold, upper respiratory allergies, and sinusitis; also promotes nasal or sinus drainage
Contraindications Hypersensitivity to pseudoephedrine or any component of the formulation; with or within 14 days of MAO inhibitor therapy
Warnings/Precautions Use with caution in the elderly; may be more sensitive to adverse effects; administer with caution to patients with hypertension, hyperthyroidism, diabetes mellitus, cardiovascular disease, ischemic heart disease, increased intraocular pressure, prostatic hyperplasia, seizure disorders, or renal impairment. When used for self-medication (OTC), notify healthcare provider if symptoms do not improve within 7 days or are accompanied by fever. Discontinue and contact healthcare provider if nervousness, dizziness, or sleeplessness occur. Some products may contain sodium.
Adverse Reactions (Reflective of adult population; not specific for elderly) Frequency not defined.
Cardiovascular: Arrhythmia, cardiovascular collapse with hypotension, hypertension, palpitation, tachycardia
Central nervous system: Chills, confusion, coordination impaired, dizziness, drowsiness, excitability, fatigue, hallucination, headache, insomnia, nervousness, neuritis, restlessness, seizure, transient stimulation, vertigo
Dermatologic: Photosensitivity, rash, urticaria
Gastrointestinal: Anorexia, constipation, diarrhea, dry throat, ischemic colitis, nausea, vomiting, xerostomia
Genitourinary: Difficult urination, dysuria, polyuria, urinary retention
Hematologic: Agranulocytosis, hemolytic anemia, thrombocytopenia
Neuromuscular & skeletal: Tremor, weakness
Ocular: Blurred vision, diplopia
Otic: Tinnitus
Respiratory: Chest/throat tightness, dry nose, dyspnea, nasal congestion, thickening of bronchial secretions, wheezing
Miscellaneous: Anaphylaxis, diaphoresis
Drug Interactions
Avoid Concomitant Use
Avoid concomitant use of Pseudoephedrine with any of the following: Iobenguane I 123; MAO Inhibitors
Increased Effect/Toxicity
Pseudoephedrine may increase the levels/effects of: Bromocriptine; Sympathomimetics

The levels/effects of Pseudoephedrine may be increased by: Antacids; Atomoxetine; Cannabinoids; Carbonic Anhydrase Inhibitors; MAO Inhibitors; Serotonin/Norepinephrine Reuptake Inhibitors
Decreased Effect
Pseudoephedrine may decrease the levels/effects of: Benzylpenicilloyl Polylysine; Iobenguane I 123

The levels/effects of Pseudoephedrine may be decreased by: Spironolactone

▶

◀ **Ethanol/Nutrition/Herb Interactions**
Food: Onset of effect may be delayed if pseudoephedrine is taken with food.
Herb/Nutraceutical: Avoid ephedra, yohimbe (may cause hypertension).

Mechanism of Action Directly stimulates alpha-adrenergic receptors of respiratory mucosa causing vasoconstriction; directly stimulates beta-adrenergic receptors causing bronchial relaxation, increased heart rate and contractility

Pharmacodynamics/Kinetics
Onset of action: Decongestant: Oral: 30 minutes (Chua, 1989)
    Peak effect: Decongestant: Oral: ~1-2 hours (Chua, 1989)
Duration: Immediate release tablet: 3-8 hours (Chua, 1989)
Absorption: Rapid (Simons, 1996)
Distribution: Adults: 2.64-3.51 L/kg (Kanfer, 1993)
Metabolism: Undergoes n-demethylation to norpseudoephedrine (active) (Chua, 1989; Kanfer, 1993); Hepatic (<1%) (Kanfer, 1993)
Half-life elimination: Varies by urine pH and flow rate; alkaline urine decreases renal elimination of pseudoephedrine (Kanfer, 1993)
Adults: 9-16 hours (pH 8); 3-6 hours (pH 5) (Chua, 1989)
Time to peak: Adults (immediate release): 1-3 hours (dose dependent) (Kanfer, 1993)
Excretion: Urine (43% to 96% as unchanged drug, 1% to 6% as active norpseudoephedrine); dependent on urine pH and flow rate; alkaline urine decreases renal elimination of pseudoephedrine (Kanfer, 1993)

Dosage
Geriatric Nasal congestion: Use caution in this population; initiate using immediate release formulation: 30-60 mg every 6 hours as needed
Adult Nasal congestion: General dosing guidelines: Oral: Immediate release: 60 mg every 4-6 hours; Extended release: 120 mg every 12 hours **or** 240 mg every 24 hours; maximum: 240 mg/24 hours
Renal Impairment Consider reducing dose.

Administration Do not crush extended release drug product, swallow whole. May administer with or without food. Sudafed® 24 Hour tablet may not completely dissolve and appear in stool

Monitoring Parameters Blood pressure, pulse, relief of symptoms, urinary output, episodes of incontinence

Test Interactions Interferes with urine detection of amphetamine (false-positive)

Special Geriatric Considerations Elderly patients should be counseled about the proper use of over-the-counter cough and cold preparations. Elderly are more predisposed to adverse effects of sympathomimetics since they frequently have cardiovascular diseases and diabetes mellitus as well as multiple drug therapies. It may be advisable to treat with a short-acting/immediate-release formulation before initiating sustained-release/long-acting formulations.

Dosage Forms Excipient information presented when available (limited, particularly for generics); consult specific product labeling. [DSC] = Discontinued product
Caplet, extended release, oral, as hydrochloride:
    Sudafed® 12 Hour: 120 mg
Liquid, oral, as hydrochloride: 30 mg/5 mL (473 mL)
    Children's Nasal Decongestant: 30 mg/5 mL (118 mL) [contains sodium benzoate; raspberry flavor]
    Silfedrine Children's: 15 mg/5 mL (118 mL, 237 mL) [ethanol free, sugar free; grape flavor]
    Sudafed® Children's: 15 mg/5 mL (118 mL) [ethanol free, sugar free; contains menthol, sodium 5 mg/5 mL, sodium benzoate; grape flavor]
Syrup, oral, as hydrochloride: 30 mg/5 mL (118 mL)
    SudoGest Children's: 15 mg/5 mL (118 mL) [ethanol free, sugar free; contains sodium 5 mg/5 mL, sodium benzoate; grape flavor]
Tablet, oral, as hydrochloride: 30 mg
    Genaphed™: 30 mg [DSC]
    Oranyl: 30 mg [sugar free]
    Sudafed® Maximum Strength Nasal Decongestant: 30 mg [contains sodium benzoate]
    Sudo-Tab®: 30 mg [contains sodium benzoate]
    SudoGest: 30 mg
    SudoGest: 60 mg [scored]
Tablet, extended release, oral, as hydrochloride:
    Sudafed® 24 Hour: 240 mg
    SudoGest 12 Hour: 120 mg

Selected References
Chua SS, Benrimoj SI, and Triggs EJ, "Pharmacokinetics of Non-Prescription Sympathomimetic Agents," *Biopharm Drug Dispos*, 1989, 10(1):1-14.
Kanfer I, Dowse R, and Vuma V, "Pharmacokinetics of Oral Decongestants," *Pharmacotherapy*, 1993, 13(6 Pt 2):116-28; discussion 143-6.

♦ **Pseudoephedrine and Triprolidine** *see* Triprolidine and Pseudoephedrine *on page 1872*
♦ **Pseudoephedrine Hydrochloride** *see* Pseudoephedrine *on page 1545*
♦ **Pseudoephedrine Sulfate** *see* Pseudoephedrine *on page 1545*
♦ **Pseudomonic Acid A** *see* Mupirocin *on page 1250*

Psyllium (SIL i yum)

Related Information
Laxatives, Classification and Properties *on page 2012*
Medication Safety Issues
Sound-alike/look-alike issues:
Fiberall® may be confused with Feverall®
Hydrocil® may be confused with Hydrocet®
Brand Names: U.S. Bulk-K [OTC]; Fiberall® [OTC]; Fibro-Lax [OTC]; Fibro-XL [OTC]; Genfiber™ [OTC] [DSC]; Hydrocil® Instant [OTC]; Konsyl-D™ [OTC]; Konsyl® Easy Mix™ [OTC]; Konsyl® Orange [OTC]; Konsyl® Original [OTC]; Konsyl® [OTC]; Metamucil® Plus Calcium [OTC]; Metamucil® Smooth Texture [OTC]; Metamucil® [OTC]; Natural Fiber Therapy Smooth Texture [OTC]; Natural Fiber Therapy [OTC]; Reguloid [OTC]
Brand Names: Canada Metamucil®
Index Terms Plantago Seed; Plantain Seed; Psyllium Husk; Psyllium Hydrophilic Mucilloid
Generic Availability (U.S.) Yes: Excludes wafers
Pharmacologic Category Antidiarrheal; Fiber Supplement; Laxative, Bulk-Producing
Use OTC labeling: Dietary fiber supplement; treatment of occasional constipation; reduce risk of coronary heart disease (CHD)
Unlabeled/Investigational Use Treatment of diarrhea, chronic constipation, irritable bowel syndrome, inflammatory bowel disease, colon cancer, or diabetes
Contraindications Hypersensitivity to psyllium or any component of the formulation; fecal impaction; GI obstruction
Warnings/Precautions Use with caution in patients with esophageal strictures, ulcers, stenosis, intestinal adhesions, or difficulty swallowing. Use with caution in the elderly; may have insufficient fluid intake which may predispose them to fecal impaction and bowel obstruction. Products must be taken with at least 8 ounces of fluid in order to prevent choking. To reduce the risk of CHD, the soluble fiber from psyllium should be used in conjunction with a diet low in saturated fat and cholesterol. Some products may contain calcium, potassium, sodium, soy lecithin, or phenylalanine.

When used for self-medication (OTC), do not use in the presence of abdominal pain, nausea, or vomiting. Notify healthcare provider in case of sudden changes of bowel habits which last >2 weeks or in case of rectal bleeding. Not for self-treatment of constipation lasting >1 week
Adverse Reactions (Reflective of adult population; not specific for elderly) Frequency not defined.
Gastrointestinal: Abdominal cramps, constipation, diarrhea, esophageal or bowel obstruction
Respiratory: Bronchospasm
Miscellaneous: Anaphylaxis upon inhalation in susceptible individuals, rhinoconjunctivitis
Drug Interactions
Avoid Concomitant Use There are no known interactions where it is recommended to avoid concomitant use.
Increased Effect/Toxicity There are no known significant interactions involving an increase in effect.
Decreased Effect There are no known significant interactions involving a decrease in effect.
Mechanism of Action Psyllium is a soluble fiber. It absorbs water in the intestine to form a viscous liquid which promotes peristalsis and reduces transit time.
Pharmacodynamics/Kinetics
Onset of action: Relief of constipation: 12-72 hours
Absorption: None; small amounts of grain extracts present in the preparation have been reportedly absorbed following colonic hydrolysis
Dosage
Geriatric & Adult General dosing guidelines; consult specific product labeling.
Adequate intake for total fiber: Oral: **Note:** The definition of "fiber" varies, however, the soluble fiber in psyllium is only one type of fiber which makes up the daily recommended intake of total fiber.
Adults ≥51 years: Male: 30 g/day; Female: 21 g/day
Constipation: Oral: Psyllium: 2.5-30 g per day in divided doses
Reduce risk of CHD: Oral: Soluble fiber ≥7 g (psyllium seed husk ≥10.2 g) per day

◀ **Administration** Inhalation of psyllium dust may cause sensitivity to psyllium (eg, runny nose, watery eyes, wheezing). Drink at least 8 ounces of liquid with each dose. Powder must be mixed in a glass of water or juice. Capsules should be swallowed one at a time. When more than one dose is required, they should be divided throughout the day. Separate dose by at least 2 hours from other drug therapies.

Monitoring Parameters Monitor for diarrhea, abdominal pain, bowel obstruction, or impaction

Pharmacotherapy Pearls 3.4 g psyllium hydrophilic mucilloid per 7 g powder is equivalent to a rounded teaspoonful or one packet; fiber therapy results in increased frequency of defecation. Diabetic patients may need or prefer sugar-free products; psyllium using aspartame is available for diabetic patients. Bloating and flatulence are mostly a problem in first 4 weeks of therapy.

Special Geriatric Considerations Elderly may have insufficient fluid intake which may predispose them to fecal impaction and bowel obstruction. Patients should have a 1 month trial, with at least 14 g/day, before effects in bowel function are determined. Bloating and flatulence are mostly a problem in first 4 weeks of therapy. See Warnings/Precautions.

Dosage Forms Excipient information presented when available (limited, particularly for generics); consult specific product labeling. [DSC] = Discontinued product

Capsule, oral: 500 mg

Fibro-XL: 0.675 g [sugar free; provides dietary fiber 3.8 g and soluble fiber 3 g per 7 capsules]

Genfiber™: 0.52 g [DSC] [provides dietary fiber 3 g and soluble fiber 2 g per 6 capsules]

Konsyl®: 0.52 g [sugar free; contains calcium 8 mg/capsule, potassium <11 mg/capsule, sodium 1 mg/capsule; provides dietary fiber 3 g and soluble fiber 2 g per 5 capsules]

Metamucil®: 0.52 g [contains potassium 5 mg/capsule; provides dietary fiber 3 g and soluble fiber 2.1 g per 6 capsules]

Metamucil® Plus Calcium: 0.52 g [contains calcium 60 mg/capsule, potassium 6 mg/capsule; provides dietary fiber 3 g and soluble fiber 2.1 g per 5 capsules]

Reguloid: 0.52 g [provides dietary fiber 3 g and soluble fiber 2 g per 6 capsules]

Powder, oral: (454 g)

Bulk-K: (392 g)

Fiberall®: (454 g) [sugar free; contains phenylalanine; orange flavor; psyllium is in combination with other fiber sources; also contains vitamins and minerals]

Fibro-Lax: (140 g, 392 g)

Genfiber™: (397 g [DSC]) [contains sodium; natural flavor]

Genfiber™: (397 g [DSC]) [contains sodium; orange flavor]

Hydrocil® Instant: (300 g) [sugar free]

Hydrocil® Instant: 3.5 g/packet (30s, 500s) [sugar free; provides dietary fiber 3 g and soluble fiber 2.4 g per packet]

Konsyl-D™: (325 g, 397 g, 500 g) [contains calcium, dextrose, potassium, sodium]

Konsyl-D™: 3.4 g/packet (100s, 500s) [contains calcium 6 mg/packet, dextrose 3.1 g/packet, potassium 31 mg/packet, sodium 3 mg/packet; provides dietary fiber 3 g and soluble fiber 2 g per packet]

Konsyl® Easy Mix™: (250 g) [sugar free; contains calcium, potassium, sodium]

Konsyl® Easy Mix™: 6 g/packet (500s) [sugar free; contains calcium 10 mg/packet, potassium 55 mg/packet, sodium 5 mg/packet; provides dietary fiber 5 g and soluble fiber 3 g per packet]

Konsyl® Orange: (538 g) [contains calcium, potassium, sodium, sucrose; orange flavor]

Konsyl® Orange: 3.4 g/packet (30s) [contains calcium 6 mg/packet, potassium 31 mg/packet, sodium 3 mg/packet, sucrose 8 g/packet; orange flavor; provides dietary fiber 3 g and soluble fiber 2 g per packet]

Konsyl® Orange: (425 g) [sugar free; contains calcium, phenylalanine, potassium, sodium; orange flavor]

Konsyl® Original: (300 g, 450 g) [sugar free; contains calcium, potassium, sodium]

Konsyl® Original: 6 g/packet (30s, 100s, 500s) [sugar free; contains calcium 10 mg/packet, potassium 55 mg/packet, sodium 5 mg/packet; provides dietary fiber 5 g and soluble fiber 3 g per packet]

Metamucil®: (390 g, 570 g, 870 g) [contains potassium, sodium; unflavored]

Metamucil®: (570 g, 870 g, 1254 g) [contains potassium, sodium; orange flavor]

Metamucil® Smooth Texture: (609 g, 912 g, 1368 g) [contains potassium, sodium; orange flavor]

Metamucil® Smooth Texture: 3.4 g/packet (30s) [contains potassium 30 mg/packet, sodium 5 mg/packet; orange flavor; provides dietary fiber 3 g and soluble fiber ~2 g per packet]

Metamucil® Smooth Texture: (283 g, 425 g, 660 g) [sugar free; contains phenylalanine, potassium, sodium; berry burst flavor]

Metamucil® Smooth Texture: (173 g, 300 g, 450 g, 660 g, 1020 g) [sugar free; contains phenylalanine, potassium, sodium; orange flavor]

Metamucil® Smooth Texture: (288 g, 432 g, 684 g) [sugar free; contains phenylalanine, potassium, sodium; pink lemonade flavor]

Metamucil® Smooth Texture: (300 g, 450 g, 690 g) [sugar free; contains potassium, sodium; unflavored]

Metamucil® Smooth Texture: 3.4 g/packet (30s) [sugar free; contains phenylalanine 16 mg/packet, potassium 30 mg/packet, sodium 5 mg/packet; berry burst flavor; provides dietary fiber 3 g and soluble fiber ~2 g per packet]

Metamucil® Smooth Texture: 3.4 g/packet (30s) [sugar free; contains phenylalanine 25 mg/packet, potassium 30 mg/packet, sodium 5 mg/packet; orange flavor; provides dietary fiber 3 g and soluble fiber ~2 g per packet]

Natural Fiber Therapy: (390 g, 539 g) [natural flavor]

Natural Fiber Therapy: (390 g, 539 g) [contains sodium; orange flavor]

Natural Fiber Therapy Smooth Texture: (300 g) [sugar free; orange flavor]

Reguloid: (369 g, 540 g) [contains sodium; orange flavor]

Reguloid: (369 g, 540 g) [contains sodium; regular flavor]

Reguloid: (284 g, 426 g) [sugar free; contains phenylalanine, sodium; orange flavor]

Reguloid: (284 g, 426 g) [sugar free; contains phenylalanine, sodium; regular flavor]

Wafer, oral:

Metamucil®: 3.4 g/2 wafers (24s) [contains potassium 60 mg/2 wafers, sodium 20 mg/2 wafers, soya lecithin; apple flavor; provides dietary fiber 6 g and soluble fiber 3 g per 2 wafers]

Metamucil®: 3.4 g/2 wafers (24s) [contains potassium 60 mg/2 wafers, sodium 20 mg/2 wafers, soya lecithin; cinnamon-spice flavor; provides dietary fiber 6 g and soluble fiber 3 g per 2 wafers]

Selected References

"Dietary Reference Intakes for Energy, Carbohydrate, Fiber, Fat, Fatty Acids, Cholesterol, Protein and Amino Acids," Standing Committee on the Scientific Evaluation of Dietary Reference Intakes, Food and Nutrition Board, Institute of Medicine, National Academy of Sciences, Washington, DC: National Academy Press, 2005. Available at http://www.nap.edu.

James SL, Muir JG, Curtis SL, et al, "Dietary Fibre: A Roughage Guide," *Intern Med J*, 2003, 33(7):291-6.

Singh B, "Psyllium as Therapeutic and Drug Delivery Agent," *Int J Pharm*, 2007, 334(1-2):1-14.

- ◆ **Psyllium Husk** *see* Psyllium *on page 1547*
- ◆ **Psyllium Hydrophilic Mucilloid** *see* Psyllium *on page 1547*
- ◆ **P-Tann [DSC]** *see* Chlorpheniramine *on page 337*
- ◆ **Pteroylglutamic Acid** *see* Folic Acid *on page 781*
- ◆ **PTU (error-prone abbreviation)** *see* Propylthiouracil *on page 1540*
- ◆ **Pulmicort Flexhaler®** *see* Budesonide (Systemic, Oral Inhalation) *on page 219*
- ◆ **Pulmicort Respules®** *see* Budesonide (Systemic, Oral Inhalation) *on page 219*
- ◆ **Purified Chick Embryo Cell** *see* Rabies Vaccine *on page 1575*
- ◆ **Purinethol®** *see* Mercaptopurine *on page 1146*

Pyrazinamide (peer a ZIN a mide)

Brand Names: Canada Tebrazid™

Index Terms Pyrazinoic Acid Amide

Generic Availability (U.S.) Yes

Pharmacologic Category Antitubercular Agent

Use Adjunctive treatment of tuberculosis in combination with other antituberculosis agents

Contraindications Hypersensitivity to pyrazinamide or any component of the formulation; acute gout; severe hepatic damage

Warnings/Precautions Use with caution in patients with a history of alcoholism, renal failure, chronic gout, diabetes mellitus, or porphyria. Dose-related hepatotoxicity ranging from transient ALT/AST elevations to jaundice, hepatitis and/or liver atrophy (rare) has occurred. Use with caution in patients receiving concurrent medications associated with hepatotoxicity (particularly with rifampin).

Adverse Reactions (Reflective of adult population; not specific for elderly)

1% to 10%:

Central nervous system: Malaise

Gastrointestinal: Anorexia, nausea, vomiting

Neuromuscular & skeletal: Arthralgia, myalgia

Drug Interactions

Avoid Concomitant Use There are no known interactions where it is recommended to avoid concomitant use.

Increased Effect/Toxicity

Pyrazinamide may increase the levels/effects of: CycloSPORINE (Systemic); Rifampin

Decreased Effect

Pyrazinamide may decrease the levels/effects of: CycloSPORINE

◀ **Stability** Store at controlled room temperature of 15°C to 30°C (59°F to 86°F).

Mechanism of Action Converted to pyrazinoic acid in susceptible strains of *Mycobacterium* which lowers the pH of the environment; exact mechanism of action has not been elucidated

Pharmacodynamics/Kinetics Bacteriostatic or bactericidal depending on drug's concentration at infection site

Absorption: Well absorbed

Distribution: Widely into body tissues and fluids including liver, lung, and CSF

Relative diffusion from blood into CSF: Adequate with or without inflammation (exceeds usual MICs)

CSF:blood level ratio: Inflamed meninges: 100%

Protein binding: 50%

Metabolism: Hepatic

Half-life elimination: 9-10 hours

Time to peak, serum: Within 2 hours

Excretion: Urine (4% as unchanged drug)

Dosage

Adult Tuberculosis treatment: Oral: **Note:** Used as part of a multidrug regimen. Treatment regimens consist of an initial 2-month phase, followed by a continuation phase of 4 or 7 additional months; pyrazinamide is administered in the initial phase of treatment.

Suggested dosing based on lean body weight (Blumberg, 2003; CDC, 2003):

Daily therapy:

40-55 kg: 1000 mg

56-75 kg: 1500 mg

76-90 kg: 2000 mg (maximum dose regardless of weight)

Twice weekly directly observed therapy (DOT):

40-55 kg: 2000 mg

56-75 kg: 3000 mg

76-90 kg: 4000 mg (maximum dose regardless of weight)

Three times/week DOT:

40-55 kg: 1500 mg

56-75 kg: 2500 mg

76-90 kg: 3000 mg (maximum dose regardless of weight)

Renal Impairment Adults: Cl_{cr} <30 mL/minute or receiving hemodialysis: Treatment of TB: 25-35 mg/kg/dose 3 times per week administered after dialysis (Blumberg, 2003; CDC, 2003)

Monitoring Parameters Periodic liver function tests, serum uric acid, sputum culture, chest x-ray 2-3 months into treatment and at completion

Test Interactions Reacts with Acetest® and Ketostix® to produce pinkish-brown color

Special Geriatric Considerations Pyrazinamide is used in the 2-month intensive treatment phase of a 6-month treatment plan. Most elderly acquired their *Mycobacterium tuberculosis* infection before effective chemotherapy was available; however, older persons with new infections (not reactivation), or who are from areas where drug-resistant *M. tuberculosis* is endemic, or who are HIV-infected should receive 3-4 drug therapies including pyrazinamide.

Dosage Forms Excipient information presented when available (limited, particularly for generics); consult specific product labeling.

Tablet, oral: 500 mg

Selected References

American Thoracic Society, "Treatment of Tuberculosis," *MMWR Recomm Rep*, 2003, 52(RR-11):1-77. Available at http://www.cdc.gov/mmwr/preview/mmwrhtml/rr5211a1.htm

Yoshikawa TT, "Tuberculosis in Aging Adults," *J Am Geriatr Soc*, 1992, 40(2):178-87.

◆ **Pyrazinoic Acid Amide** *see* Pyrazinamide *on page 1549*

◆ **Pyri-500 [OTC]** *see* Pyridoxine *on page 1552*

◆ **Pyridium®** *see* Phenazopyridine *on page 1433*

Pyridostigmine (peer id oh STIG meen)

Medication Safety Issues

Sound-alike/look-alike issues:

Pyridostigmine may be confused with physostigmine

Mestinon® may be confused with Metatensin®

Regonol® may be confused with Reglan®, Renagel®

Brand Names: U.S. Mestinon®; Mestinon® Timespan®; Regonol®

Brand Names: Canada Mestinon®; Mestinon®-SR

Index Terms Pyridostigmine Bromide

Generic Availability (U.S.) Yes: Tablet

Pharmacologic Category Acetylcholinesterase Inhibitor

Use Symptomatic treatment of myasthenia gravis; antagonism of nondepolarizing neuro-muscular blockers
Military use: Pretreatment for Soman nerve gas exposure

Contraindications Hypersensitivity to pyridostigmine, bromides, or any component of the formulation; GI or GU obstruction

Warnings/Precautions Use with caution in patients with epilepsy, bradycardia, hyperthyroid-ism, cardiac arrhythmias, or peptic ulcer; use with extreme caution in patients with asthma or bronchospastic disease; adequate facilities should be available for cardiopulmonary resusci-tation when testing and adjusting dose for myasthenia gravis; have atropine and epinephrine ready to treat hypersensitivity reactions; overdosage may result in cholinergic crisis, this must be distinguished from myasthenic crisis; anticholinesterase insensitivity can develop for brief or prolonged periods. Regonol® injection contains 1% benzyl alcohol as the preservative.
[U.S. Boxed Warning]: Regonol® injection must be administered by trained personnel.

Adverse Reactions (Reflective of adult population; not specific for elderly) Fre-quency not defined.
Cardiovascular: Arrhythmias (especially bradycardia), AV block, cardiac arrest, decreased carbon monoxide, flushing, hypotension, nodal rhythm, nonspecific ECG changes, syncope, tachycardia
Central nervous system: Convulsions, dizziness, drowsiness, dysphonia, headache, loss of consciousness
Dermatologic: Skin rash, thrombophlebitis (I.V.), urticaria
Gastrointestinal: Abdominal pain, diarrhea, dysphagia, flatulence, hyperperistalsis, nausea, salivation, stomach cramps, vomiting
Genitourinary: Urinary urgency
Neuromuscular & skeletal: Arthralgia, dysarthria, fasciculations, muscle cramps, myalgia, spasms, weakness
Ocular: Amblyopia, lacrimation, small pupils
Respiratory: Bronchial secretions increased, bronchiolar constriction, bronchospasm, dysp-nea, laryngospasm, respiratory arrest, respiratory depression, respiratory muscle paralysis
Miscellaneous: Allergic reactions, anaphylaxis, diaphoresis increased

Drug Interactions

Avoid Concomitant Use There are no known interactions where it is recommended to avoid concomitant use.

Increased Effect/Toxicity
Pyridostigmine may increase the levels/effects of: Beta-Blockers; Cholinergic Agonists; Succinylcholine

The levels/effects of Pyridostigmine may be increased by: Corticosteroids (Systemic)

Decreased Effect
Pyridostigmine may decrease the levels/effects of: Neuromuscular-Blocking Agents (Non-depolarizing)

The levels/effects of Pyridostigmine may be decreased by: Methocarbamol

Stability
Injection: Protect from light.
Tablet:
30 mg: Store under refrigeration at 2°C to 8°C (36°F to 46°F). Protect from light. Stable at room temperature for up to 3 months.
Mestinon®: Store at 25°C (77°F). Protect from moisture.

Mechanism of Action Inhibits destruction of acetylcholine by acetylcholinesterase which facilitates transmission of impulses across myoneural junction

Pharmacodynamics/Kinetics
Onset of action: Oral, I.M.: 15-30 minutes; I.V. injection: 2-5 minutes
Duration: Oral: Up to 6-8 hours (due to slow absorption); I.V.: 2-3 hours
Absorption: Oral: Very poor
Distribution: 19 ± 12 L
Metabolism: Hepatic
Bioavailability: 10% to 20%
Half-life elimination: 1-2 hours; Renal failure: ≤6 hours
Excretion: Urine (80% to 90% as unchanged drug)

Dosage
Geriatric & Adult
Myasthenia gravis:
Oral: Highly individualized dosing ranges: 60-1500 mg/day, usually 600 mg/day divided into 5-6 doses, spaced to provide maximum relief
Sustained release formulation: Highly individualized dosing ranges: 180-540 mg once or twice daily (doses separated by at least 6 hours); **Note:** Most clinicians reserve sustained release dosage form for bedtime dose only.

◀ *I.M. or slow I.V. Push:* To supplement oral dosage pre- and postoperatively, during myasthenic crisis, or when oral therapy is impractical): ~1/30th of oral dose; observe patient closely for cholinergic reactions

I.V. infusion: To supplement oral dosage pre- and postoperatively, during myasthenic crisis, or when oral therapy is impractical): Initial: 2 mg/hour with gradual titration in increments of 0.5-1 mg/hour, up to a maximum rate of 4 mg/hour

Pretreatment for Soman nerve gas exposure (military use): Oral: 30 mg every 8 hours beginning several hours prior to exposure; discontinue at first sign of nerve agent exposure, then begin atropine and pralidoxime

Reversal of nondepolarizing muscle relaxants: I.V.: 0.1-0.25 mg/kg/dose; 10-20 mg is usually sufficient (full recovery usually occurs ≤15 minutes, but ≥30 minutes may be required).

Note: Atropine sulfate (0.6-1.2 mg) I.V. immediately prior to pyridostigmine to minimize side effects:

Renal Impairment Lower dosages may be required due to prolonged elimination; no specific recommendations have been published.

Administration When giving for reversal of neuromuscular blockade, keep patient well ventilated until recovered

Monitoring Parameters Observe for cholinergic reactions, particularly when administered I.V.

Test Interactions Increased aminotransferase [ALT/AST] (S), increased amylase (S)

Pharmacotherapy Pearls Myasthenia gravis: Not a cure; patient may develop resistance to the drug; normally, sustained release dosage form is used at bedtime for patients who complain of morning weakness

Special Geriatric Considerations Many elderly may have pulmonary or cardiovascular diseases which will require cautious use of pyridostigmine.

Dosage Forms Excipient information presented when available (limited, particularly for generics); consult specific product labeling.

Injection, solution, as bromide:
Regonol®: 5 mg/mL (2 mL) [contains benzyl alcohol]
Syrup, oral, as bromide:
Mestinon®: 60 mg/5 mL (480 mL) [contains ethanol 5%, sodium benzoate; raspberry flavor]
Tablet, oral, as bromide: 60 mg
Mestinon®: 60 mg [scored]
Tablet, sustained release, oral, as bromide:
Mestinon® Timespan®: 180 mg [scored]

◆ **Pyridostigmine Bromide** *see* Pyridostigmine *on page 1550*

Pyridoxine (peer i DOKS een)

Medication Safety Issues
Sound-alike/look-alike issues:
Pyridoxine may be confused with paroxetine, pralidoxime, Pyridium®
International issues:
Doxal® [Brazil] may be confused with Doxil® which is a brand name for doxorubicin in the U.S.
Doxal® [Brazil]: Brand name for doxycycline in Austria; brand name for pyridoxine/thiamine combination in Brazil; brand name for doxepin in Finland
Brand Names: U.S. Aminoxin® [OTC]; Pyri-500 [OTC]
Index Terms B6; B_6; Pyridoxine Hydrochloride; Vitamin B_6
Generic Availability (U.S.) Yes
Pharmacologic Category Vitamin, Water Soluble
Use Prevention and treatment of vitamin B_6 deficiency
Unlabeled/Investigational Use Treatment and prophylaxis of neurological toxicities (ie, seizures, coma) associated with isoniazid, hydrazine, and Gyromitrin-containing mushroom (false morel) overdose/toxicity
Contraindications Hypersensitivity to pyridoxine or any component of the formulation
Warnings/Precautions Severe, permanent peripheral neuropathies have been reported; neurotoxicity is more common with long-term administration of large doses (>2 g/day). Dependence and withdrawal may occur with doses >200 mg/day. Single vitamin deficiency is rare; evaluate for other deficiencies. Some parenteral products contain aluminum; use caution in patients with impaired renal function. Guidelines suggest that at least 8-24 g be stocked. This is enough to treat 1 patient weighing 100 kg for an initial 8- to 24-hour period. In areas where tuberculosis is common, hospitals should consider stocking 24 g. This is enough to treat 1 patient for 24 hours (Dart, 2009).

Adverse Reactions (Reflective of adult population; not specific for elderly) Frequency not defined.

Central nervous system: Headache, seizure (following very large I.V. doses), somnolence

Endocrine & metabolic: Acidosis, folic acid decreased

Gastrointestinal: Nausea

Hepatic: AST increased

Neuromuscular & skeletal: Neuropathy, paresthesia

Miscellaneous: Allergic reactions

Drug Interactions

Avoid Concomitant Use There are no known interactions where it is recommended to avoid concomitant use.

Increased Effect/Toxicity There are no known significant interactions involving an increase in effect.

Decreased Effect

Pyridoxine may decrease the levels/effects of: Altretamine; Barbiturates; Fosphenytoin; Levodopa; Phenytoin

Stability Store at 20°C to 25°C (68°F to 77°F). Protect from light.

Mechanism of Action Precursor to pyridoxal, which functions in the metabolism of proteins, carbohydrates, and fats; pyridoxal also aids in the release of liver and muscle-stored glycogen and in the synthesis of GABA (within the central nervous system) and heme

Pharmacodynamics/Kinetics

Absorption: Enteral, parenteral: Well absorbed

Metabolism: Hepatic to 4-pyridoxic acid (active form) and other metabolites

Half-life elimination: Biologic: 15-20 days

Excretion: Urine

Dosage

Geriatric & Adult

Recommended daily allowance (RDA):

Male: 1.7-2 mg

Female: 1.4-1.6 mg

Dietary deficiency: Oral: 10-20 mg/day for 3 weeks

Drug-induced neuritis (eg, isoniazid, hydralazine, penicillamine, cycloserine): Oral:

Treatment: 100-200 mg/24 hours

Prophylaxis: 25-100 mg/24 hours

Treatment of isoniazid-induced seizures and/or coma (unlabeled use): I.V.:

Acute ingestion of known amount: Initial: A total dose of pyridoxine equal to the amount of isoniazid ingested (maximum dose: 5 g); administer at a rate of 0.5-1 g/minute until seizures stop or the maximum initial dose has been administered; may repeat every 5-10 minutes as needed to control persistent seizure activity and/or CNS toxicity. If seizures stop prior to the administration of the calculated initial dose, infuse the remaining pyridoxine over 4-6 hours (Howland, 2006; Morrow, 2006).

Acute ingestion of unknown amount: Initial: 5 g; administer at a rate of 0.5-1 g/minute; may repeat every 5-10 minutes as needed to control persistent seizure activity and/or CNS toxicity (Howland, 2006; Morrow, 2006)

Prevention of isoniazid-induced seizures and/or coma (unlabeled use): I.V.: Asymptomatic patients who present within 2 hours of ingesting a potentially toxic amount of isoniazid should receive a prophylactic dose of pyridoxine (Boyer, 2006). Dosing recommendations are the same as for the treatment of symptomatic patients.

Treatment of acute hydrazine toxicity (unlabeled use): I.V.: A total dose of 25 mg/kg should be given over 15-30 minutes

Treatment of seizures from acute Gyromitrin-containing mushroom toxicity (unlabeled use; Diaz, 2005): I.V.: 25 mg/kg over 15-30 minutes; repeat dose as needed to control seizures

Administration Administer slow I.V. Burning may occur at the injection site after I.M. or SubQ administration; seizures have occurred following I.V. administration of very large doses

Monitoring Parameters For treatment of isoniazid, hydrazine, or Gyromitrin-containing mushroom toxicity: Anion gap, arterial blood gases, electrolytes, neurological exam, seizure activity

Reference Range Over 50 ng/mL (SI: 243 nmol/L) (varies considerably with method). A broad range is ~25-80 ng/mL (SI: 122-389 nmol/L). HPLC method for pyridoxal phosphate has normal range of 3.5-18 ng/mL (SI: 17-88 nmol/L).

Test Interactions False positive urobilinogen spot test using Ehrlich's reagent

Special Geriatric Considerations Use with caution in patients with Parkinson's disease treated with levodopa.

◀ **Dosage Forms** Excipient information presented when available (limited, particularly for generics); consult specific product labeling.

Capsule, oral, as hydrochloride: 50 mg, 250 mg
Aminoxin®: 20 mg
Injection, solution, as hydrochloride: 100 mg/mL (1 mL)
Liquid, oral, as hydrochloride: 200 mg/5 mL (120 mL)
Tablet, oral, as hydrochloride: 25 mg, 50 mg, 100 mg, 250 mg, 500 mg
Tablet, sustained release, oral, as hydrochloride:
Pyri-500: 500 mg

Selected References

Schnyder G, Roffi M, Flammer Y, et al, "Effect of Homocysteine-Lowering Therapy With Folic Acid, Vitamin B12, and Vitamin B6 on Clinical Outcome After Percutaneous Coronary Intervention: The Swiss Heart Study: A Randomized Controlled Trial," *JAMA*, 2002, 288(8):973-9.

◆ **Pyridoxine Hydrochloride** *see* Pyridoxine *on page 1552*
◆ **Qualaquin®** *see* QuiNINE *on page 1567*

Quazepam (KWAZ e pam)

Related Information

Anxiolytic, Sedative / Hypnotic, and Miscellaneous Benzodiazepines *on page 2000*
Beers Criteria − Potentially Inappropriate Medications for Geriatrics *on page 2089*

Medication Safety Issues

Sound-alike/look-alike issues:
Quazepam may be confused with oxazepam

Beers Criteria medication:
This drug may be inappropriate for use in geriatric patients (high severity risk).

Brand Names: U.S. Doral®
Brand Names: Canada Doral®
Generic Availability (U.S.) No
Pharmacologic Category Benzodiazepine
Use Treatment of insomnia
Medication Guide Available Yes
Contraindications Hypersensitivity to quazepam, other benzodiazepines, or any component of the formulation; sleep apnea

Note: Product labeling does not include narrow-angle glaucoma; however, use in narrow-angle glaucoma is contraindicated with other benzodiazepines.

Warnings/Precautions Should be used only after evaluation of potential causes of sleep disturbance. Failure of sleep disturbance to resolve after 7-10 days may indicate psychiatric or medical illness. A worsening of insomnia or the emergence of new abnormalities of thought or behavior may represent unrecognized psychiatric or medical illness and requires immediate and careful evaluation. Use with caution in elderly or debilitated patients, patients with hepatic disease (including alcoholics), or renal impairment. Use with caution in patients with respiratory disease or impaired gag reflex. Avoid use in patients with sleep apnea.

Causes CNS depression (dose related) resulting in sedation, dizziness, confusion, or ataxia which may impair physical and mental capabilities. Patients must be cautioned about performing tasks which require mental alertness (operating machinery or driving). Use with caution in patients receiving other CNS depressants or psychoactive agents. Postmarketing studies have indicated that the use of hypnotic/sedative agents for sleep has been associated with hypersensitivity reactions including anaphylaxis as well as angioedema. An increased risk for hazardous sleep-related activities such as sleep-driving; cooking and eating food, and making phone calls while asleep have also been noted. Effects with other sedative drugs or ethanol may be potentiated. Benzodiazepines have been associated with falls and traumatic injury and should be used with extreme caution in patients who are at risk of these events (especially the elderly). Benzodiazepines with long half-lives may produce prolonged sedation and increase the risk of falls and fracture. Short- or intermediate-acting benzodiazepines are preferred in elderly patients (Beers Criteria).

Use caution in patients with depression, particularly if suicidal risk may be present. Use with caution in patients with a history of drug dependence. Benzodiazepines have been associated with dependence and acute withdrawal symptoms on discontinuation or reduction in dose. Acute withdrawal, including seizures, may be precipitated after administration of flumazenil to patients receiving long-term benzodiazepine therapy.

Benzodiazepines have been associated with anterograde amnesia. Paradoxical reactions, including hyperactive or aggressive behavior have been reported with benzodiazepines, particularly in psychiatric patients. Does not have analgesic, antidepressant, or antipsychotic properties. Use lowest effective dose.

Adverse Reactions (Reflective of adult population; not specific for elderly)
>10%: Central nervous system: Daytime drowsiness (12%)
<10%:
    Central nervous system: Headache (5%), dizziness (2%), fatigue (2%)
    Gastrointestinal: Xerostomia (2%), dyspepsia (1%)

Frequency not defined. **Note:** Asterisked (*) reactions are those reported with benzodiazepines.
    Cardiovascular: Palpitation
    Central nervous system: Abnormal thinking, agitation, amnesia, anxiety, apathy, ataxia, confusion, depression, dystonia*, euphoria, hallucinations*, hyper-/hypokinesia, incoordination, irritability*, malaise, nervousness, nightmare, paranoid reaction, sleep disturbances*, slurred speech*, speech disorder, stimulation*
    Dermatologic: Pruritus, rash
    Endocrine & metabolic: Libido decreased, menstrual irregularities*
    Gastrointestinal: Abdominal pain, abnormal taste perception, anorexia, constipation, diarrhea, nausea
    Genitourinary: Impotence, incontinence, urinary retention*
    Hepatic: Jaundice*
    Neuromuscular & skeletal: Dysarthria*, muscle spasticity*, tremor, weakness
    Ocular: Abnormal vision, cataract
    Miscellaneous: Drug dependence, withdrawal*

Drug Interactions
    Metabolism/Transport Effects Substrate of CYP2C19 (minor), 3A4 (major)
    Avoid Concomitant Use
        Avoid concomitant use of Quazepam with any of the following: OLANZapine
    Increased Effect/Toxicity
        Quazepam may increase the levels/effects of: Alcohol (Ethyl); CloZAPine; CNS Depressants; CYP2B6 Substrates; Fosphenytoin; Methotrimeprazine; Phenytoin; Selective Serotonin Reuptake Inhibitors

        The levels/effects of Quazepam may be increased by: Aprepitant; Calcium Channel Blockers (Nondihydropyridine); Cimetidine; Conivaptan; Contraceptives (Estrogens); Contraceptives (Progestins); Droperidol; Fluconazole; Fosaprepitant; Grapefruit Juice; HydrOXYzine; Isoniazid; Macrolide Antibiotics; Methotrimeprazine; Nefazodone; OLANZapine; Proton Pump Inhibitors; Selective Serotonin Reuptake Inhibitors
    Decreased Effect
        The levels/effects of Quazepam may be decreased by: CarBAMazepine; Rifamycin Derivatives; St Johns Wort; Theophylline Derivatives; Tocilizumab; Yohimbine

Ethanol/Nutrition/Herb Interactions
    Ethanol: May increase CNS depression; monitor for increased effects with coadministration. Caution patients about effects.
    Food: Grapefruit juice may decrease the metabolism of quazepam.
    Herb/Nutraceutical: Avoid St John's wort (may increase the metabolism of quazepam).

Stability Store at controlled room temperature of 20°C to 25°C (68°F to 77°F).

Mechanism of Action Binds to stereospecific benzodiazepine receptors on the postsynaptic GABA neuron at several sites within the central nervous system, including the limbic system, reticular formation. Enhancement of the inhibitory effect of GABA on neuronal excitability results by increased neuronal membrane permeability to chloride ions. This shift in chloride ions results in hyperpolarization (a less excitable state) and stabilization.

Pharmacodynamics/Kinetics
    Absorption: Rapid
    Protein binding: >95%
    Metabolism: Hepatic; forms metabolites (active)- 2-oxoquasepam and N-desalkyl-2-oxoquazepam
    Half-life elimination, serum: Quazepam, 2-oxoquasepam: 39 hours; N-desalkyl-2-oxoquazepam: 73 hours
    Time to peak, plasma: ~2 hours
    Excretion: Urine (31%, only trace amounts as unchanged drug); feces (23%)

Dosage
    Geriatric Dosing should be cautious; begin at lower end of dosing range (ie, 7.5 mg)
    Adult Hypnotic: Oral: Initial: 15 mg at bedtime; in some patients, the dose may be reduced to 7.5 mg after a few nights

Renal Impairment Use caution; monitor for signs of excessive sedation or impaired coordination.

Hepatic Impairment Use caution; monitor for signs of excessive sedation or impaired coordination.

Monitoring Parameters Respiratory status; mental status

Pharmacotherapy Pearls More likely than short-acting benzodiazepine to cause daytime sedation and fatigue. Classified as a long-acting benzodiazepine hypnotic (eg, flurazepam), this long duration of action may prevent withdrawal symptoms when therapy is discontinued. Abrupt discontinuation after sustained use (generally >10 days) may cause withdrawal symptoms.

Special Geriatric Considerations Because of the long half-life of one of its active metabolites, quazepam is not a drug of choice in the elderly. Long-acting benzodiazepines have been associated with falls in the elderly and are not recommended for use in older patients.

This medication is considered to be potentially inappropriate in this patient population (Beers Criteria severity: High).

Controlled Substance C-IV

Dosage Forms Excipient information presented when available (limited, particularly for generics); consult specific product labeling.

Tablet, oral:

Doral®: 15 mg

♦ **Questran®** see Cholestyramine Resin on page 348
♦ **Questran® Light** see Cholestyramine Resin on page 348

QUEtiapine (kwe TYE a peen)

Related Information

Antipsychotic Agents on page 1997
Atypical Antipsychotics on page 1999

Medication Safety Issues

Sound-alike/look-alike issues:

QUEtiapine may be confused with OLANZapine
SEROquel® may be confused with Serentil®, Serzone®, SINEquan®

Brand Names: U.S. SEROquel XR®; SEROquel®

Brand Names: Canada Apo-Quetiapine®; CO Quetiapine; Dom-Quetiapine; JAMP-Quetiapine; Mylan-Quetiapine; PHL-Quetiapine; PMS-Quetiapine; PRO-Quetiapine; ratio-Quetiapine; Riva-Quetiapine; Sandoz-Quetiapine; Seroquel XR®; Seroquel®; Teva-Quetiapine

Index Terms Quetiapine Fumarate

Generic Availability (U.S.) No

Pharmacologic Category Antipsychotic Agent, Atypical

Use Treatment of schizophrenia; treatment of acute manic or mixed episodes associated with bipolar I disorder (as monotherapy or in combination with lithium or divalproex); maintenance treatment of bipolar I disorder (in combination with lithium or divalproex); treatment of acute depressive episodes associated with bipolar disorder; adjunctive treatment of major depressive disorder

Unlabeled/Investigational Use Autism; delirium in the critically-ill patient; psychosis/agitation related to Alzheimer's dementia

Medication Guide Available Yes

Contraindications There are no contraindications listed in manufacturers labeling.

Canadian labeling: Hypersensitivity to quetiapine or any component of the formulation

Warnings/Precautions [U.S. Boxed Warning]: Antidepressants increase the risk of suicidal thinking and behavior in children, adolescents, and young adults (18-24 years of age) with major depressive disorder (MDD) and other psychiatric disorders; consider risk prior to prescribing. Short-term studies did not show an increased risk in patients >24 years of age and showed a decreased risk in patients ≥65 years. Closely monitor all patients for clinical worsening, suicidality, or unusual changes in behavior; particularly during the initial 1-2 months of therapy or during periods of dosage adjustments (increased or decreases); the patient's family or caregiver should be instructed to closely observe the patient and communicate condition with healthcare provider. A medication guide concerning the use of antidepressants should be dispensed with each prescription.

[U.S. Boxed Warning]: Elderly patients with dementia-related psychosis treated with antipsychotics are at an increased risk of death compared to placebo. Most deaths appeared to be either cardiovascular (eg, heart failure, sudden death) or infectious (eg, pneumonia) in nature. Quetiapine is not approved for the treatment of dementia-related psychosis.

Leukopenia, neutropenia, and agranulocytosis (sometimes fatal) have been reported in clinical trials and postmarketing reports with antipsychotic use; presence of risk factors (eg, pre-existing low WBC or history of drug-induced leuko-/neutropenia) should prompt periodic blood count assessment. Discontinue therapy at first signs of blood dyscrasias or if absolute neutrophil count <1000/mm^3.

May be sedating, use with caution in disorders where CNS depression is a feature. Use with caution in Parkinson's disease. May induce orthostatic hypotension associated with dizziness, tachycardia, and, in some cases, syncope, especially during the initial dose titration period. Should be used with particular caution in patients with known cardiovascular disease (history of MI or ischemic heart disease, heart failure, or conduction abnormalities), cerebrovascular disease, or conditions that predispose to hypotension. Use has been associated with QT prolongation; postmarketing reports have occurred in patients with concomitant illness, quetiapine overdose, or who were receiving concomitant therapy known to affect QT interval or cause electrolyte imbalance. Esophageal dysmotility and aspiration have been associated with antipsychotic use; use with caution in patients at risk of aspiration pneumonia (eg, Alzheimer's disease). May cause dose-related decreases in thyroid levels, including cases requiring thyroid replacement therapy. Development of cataracts has been observed in animal studies; lens changes have been observed in humans during long-term treatment. Lens examination on initiation of therapy and every 6 months thereafter is recommended.

Due to anticholinergic effects, use with caution in patients with decreased gastrointestinal motility, urinary retention, BPH, xerostomia, visual problems, and narrow-angle glaucoma. Relative to other antipsychotics, quetiapine has a moderate potency of cholinergic blockade. May cause extrapyramidal symptoms (EPS), pseudoparkinsonism, and/or tardive dyskinesia. Risk of dystonia (and probably other EPS) may be greater with increased doses, use of conventional antipsychotics, males, and younger patients. Impaired core body temperature regulation may occur; caution with strenuous exercise, heat exposure, dehydration, and concomitant medication possessing anticholinergic effects. Neuroleptic malignant syndrome (NMS) is a potentially fatal symptom complex that has been reported in association with administration of antipsychotic drugs. Clinical manifestations of NMS are hyperpyrexia, muscle rigidity, altered mental status, and evidence of autonomic instability (irregular pulse or blood pressure, tachycardia, diaphoresis, and cardiac dysrhythmia). Management of NMS should include immediate discontinuation of antipsychotic drugs and other drugs not essential to concurrent therapy, intensive symptomatic treatment and medication monitoring, and treatment of any concomitant medical problems for which specific treatment are available.

Use caution in patients with a history of seizures. May cause decreases in total free thyroxine, elevations of liver enzymes, cholesterol levels, and/or triglyceride increases. Rare cases of priapism have been reported. May increase prolactin levels; clinical significance of hyperprolactinemia in patients with breast cancer or other prolactin-dependent tumors is unknown.

May cause hyperglycemia; in some cases may be extreme and associated with ketoacidosis, hyperosmolar coma, or death. Use with caution in patients with diabetes or other disorders of glucose regulation; monitor for worsening of glucose control. Significant weight gain has been observed with antipsychotic therapy; incidence varies with product. Monitor waist circumference and BMI. Patients using immediate release tablets may be switched to extended release tablets at the same total daily dose taken once daily. Dosage adjustments may be necessary based on response and tolerability. May cause withdrawal symptoms (rare) with abrupt cessation; gradually taper dose during discontinuation.

Adverse Reactions (Reflective of adult population; not specific for elderly) Actual frequency may be dependent upon dose and/or indication. Unless otherwise noted, frequency of adverse effects is reported for adult patients; spectrum and incidence of adverse effects similar in children (with significant exceptions noted).

>10%:

Cardiovascular: Diastolic blood pressure increased (children and adolescents, 41%), systolic blood pressure increased (children and adolescents, 15%)

Central nervous system: Somnolence (18% to 57%), headache (7% to 21%), agitation (5% to 20%), dizziness (1% to 18%), fatigue (3% to 14%), extrapyramidal symptoms (1% to 13%)

Endocrine & metabolic: Triglycerides increased (≥200 mg/dL, 8% to 22%), HDL cholesterol decreased (≤40 mg/dL, 6% to 19%), total cholesterol increased (≥240 mg/dL, 7% to 18%), LDL cholesterol increased (≥160 mg/dL, 4% to 17%), hyperglycemia (≥200 mg/dL post glucose challenge or fasting glucose ≥126 mg/dL, 2% to 12%)

◀ Gastrointestinal: Xerostomia (9% to 44%), weight gain (dose related; 3% to 23%), appetite increased (2% to 12%), constipation (6% to 11%)

1% to 10%:

Cardiovascular: Orthostatic hypotension (2% to 7%; children and adolescents <1%), tachycardia (1% to 6%), syncope (<5%), palpitation (4%), peripheral edema (4%), hypotension (3%), hypertension (1% to 2%)

Central nervous system: Insomnia (9%), akathisia (≤8%), pain (1% to 7%), dystonia (≤6%), lethargy (1% to 5%), tardive dyskinesia (<5%), anxiety (2% to 4%), irritability (1% to 4%), parkinsonism (≤4%), abnormal dreams (2% to 3%), depression (1% to 3%), hypersomnia (1% to 3%), abnormal thinking (2%), ataxia (2%), attention disturbance (2%), coordination impaired (2%), disorientation (2%), hypoesthesia (2%), mental impairment (2%), migraine (2%), sluggishness (2%), vertigo (2%), confusion (1% to 2%), restlessness (1% to 2%), fever (1% to 2%), chills (1%)

Dermatologic: Rash (4%), hyperhidrosis (2%)

Endocrine & metabolic: Hyperprolactinemia (4%), libido decreased (≤2%), hypothyroidism (≤2%), female lactation (1%)

Gastrointestinal: Nausea (7% to 8%), abdominal pain (dose related; 4% to 7%), dyspepsia (dose related; 2% to 7%), vomiting (1% to 6%), drooling (<5%), gastroenteritis (2% to 4%), toothache (2% to 3%), appetite decreased (2%), dysphagia (2%), flatulence (2%), GERD (2%), anorexia (≥1%), abnormal taste (1%), abdominal distension (≤1%)

Genitourinary: Pollakiuria (2%), urinary tract infection (2%), impotence (1%)

Hematologic: Neutropenia (≤2%), leukopenia (≥1%), hemorrhage (1%)

Hepatic: Transaminases increased (1% to 6%), GGT increased (1%)

Neuromuscular & skeletal: Weakness (2% to 10%), tremor (2% to 8%), back pain (3% to 5%), dysarthria (1% to 5%), hypertonia (4%), twitching (4%), dyskinesia (≤4%), arthralgia (1% to 4%), paresthesia (3%), muscle spasm (1% to 3%), limb pain (2%), myalgia (2%), neck pain (2%), neck rigidity (1%)

Ocular: Blurred vision (1% to 4%), amblyopia (2% to 3%)

Otic: Ear pain (1% to 2%)

Respiratory: Pharyngitis (4% to 6%), nasal congestion (5%), rhinitis (3% to 4%), upper respiratory tract infection (2% to 3%), sinus congestion (2%), sinus headache (2%), sinusitis (2%), cough (3%), dyspnea (≥1%), dry throat (1%)

Miscellaneous: Diaphoresis (2%), restless legs syndrome (2%), flu-like syndrome (1% to 2%), lymphadenopathy (1%)

Drug Interactions

Metabolism/Transport Effects Substrate of CYP2D6 (minor), 3A4 (major)

Avoid Concomitant Use

Avoid concomitant use of QUEtiapine with any of the following: Artemether; Conivaptan; Dronedarone; Lumefantrine; Metoclopramide; Nilotinib; Pimozide; QTc-Prolonging Agents; QuiNINE; Tetrabenazine; Thioridazine; Toremifene; Vandetanib; Vemurafenib; Ziprasidone

Increased Effect/Toxicity

QUEtiapine may increase the levels/effects of: Alcohol (Ethyl); Anticholinergics; CNS Depressants; Dronedarone; Methylphenidate; Pimozide; QTc-Prolonging Agents; QuiNINE; Selective Serotonin Reuptake Inhibitors; Tetrabenazine; Thioridazine; Toremifene; Vandetanib; Vemurafenib; Ziprasidone

The levels/effects of QUEtiapine may be increased by: Acetylcholinesterase Inhibitors (Central); Alfuzosin; Artemether; Chloroquine; Ciprofloxacin; Ciprofloxacin (Systemic); Conivaptan; CYP3A4 Inhibitors (Moderate); CYP3A4 Inhibitors (Strong); Gadobutrol; HydrOX-Yzine; Lithium formulations; Lumefantrine; Methylphenidate; Metoclopramide; Nilotinib; Pramlintide; QuiNINE; Tetrabenazine

Decreased Effect

QUEtiapine may decrease the levels/effects of: Amphetamines; Anti-Parkinson's Agents (Dopamine Agonist); Quinagolide

The levels/effects of QUEtiapine may be decreased by: CYP3A4 Inducers (Strong); Deferasirox; Fosphenytoin; Herbs (CYP3A4 Inducers); Lithium formulations; Peginterferon Alfa-2b; Phenytoin; Tocilizumab

Ethanol/Nutrition/Herb Interactions

Ethanol: May increase CNS depression; monitor for increased effects with coadministration. Caution patients about effects.

Food: In healthy volunteers, administration of quetiapine (immediate release) with food resulted in an increase in the peak serum concentration and AUC by 25% and 15%, respectively, compared to the fasting state. Administration of the extended release formulation with a high-fat meal (~800-1000 calories) resulted in an increase in peak serum concentration by 44% to 52% and AUC by 20% to 22% for the 50 mg and 300 mg tablets; administration with a light meal (≤300 calories) had no significant effect on the C_{max} or AUC.

Herb/Nutraceutical: St John's wort may decrease quetiapine levels. Avoid valerian, St John's wort, kava kava, gotu kola (may increase CNS depression).

Stability Store at controlled room temperature of 25°C (77°F); excursions permitted to 15°C to 30°C (59°F to 86°F).

Mechanism of Action Quetiapine is a dibenzothiazepine atypical antipsychotic. It has been proposed that this drug's antipsychotic activity is mediated through a combination of dopamine type 2 (D_2) and serotonin type 2 (5-HT_2) antagonism. It is an antagonist at multiple neurotransmitter receptors in the brain: Serotonin 5-HT_{1A} and 5-HT_2, dopamine D_1 and D_2, histamine H_1, and adrenergic alpha$_1$- and alpha$_2$- receptors; but appears to have no appreciable affinity at cholinergic muscarinic and benzodiazepine receptors. Norquetiapine, an active metabolite, differs from its parent molecule by exhibiting high affinity for muscarinic M1 receptors.

Antagonism at receptors other than dopamine and 5-HT_2 with similar receptor affinities may explain some of the other effects of quetiapine. The drug's antagonism of histamine H_1-receptors may explain the somnolence observed. The drug's antagonism of adrenergic alpha$_1$-receptors may explain the orthostatic hypotension observed.

Pharmacodynamics/Kinetics

Absorption: Rapidly absorbed following oral administration

Distribution: V_d: 6-14 L/kg

Protein binding, plasma: 83%

Metabolism: Primarily hepatic; via CYP3A4; forms the metabolite N-desalkyl quetiapine (active) and two inactive metabolites

Bioavailability: 100% (relative to oral solution)

Half-life elimination:
  Mean: Terminal: Quetiapine: ~6 hours; Extended release: ~7 hours
  Metabolite: N-desalkyl quetiapine: 9-12 hours

Time to peak, plasma: Immediate release: 1.5 hours; Extended release: 6 hours

Excretion: Urine (73% as metabolites, <1% of total dose as unchanged drug); feces (20%)

Dosage

Geriatric Adults >65 years: 40% lower mean oral clearance of quetiapine in adults >65 years of age; higher plasma levels expected and, therefore, dosage adjustment may be needed; elderly patients usually require 50-200 mg/day of immediate release tablets or 50 mg/day of extended release tablets with a slower titration schedule. Increase immediate release dose by 25-50 mg/day or extended release dose by 50 mg/day to effective dose, based on clinical response and tolerability. If initiated with immediate release tablets, patient may transition to extended release formulation (at equivalent total daily dose) when effective dose has been reached. See "Note" in adult dosing.

Psychosis/agitation related to Alzheimer's dementia (unlabeled use): Initial: 12.5-50 mg/day; if necessary, gradually increase as tolerated not to exceed 200-300 mg/day (Rabins, 2007)

Adult

Bipolar disorder: Oral:

Depression:

Immediate release tablet: Initial: 50 mg once daily the first day; increase to 100 mg once daily on day 2, further increasing by 100 mg/day each day until a target dose of 300 mg once daily is reached by day 4. Further increases up to 600 mg once daily by day 8 have been evaluated in clinical trials, but no additional antidepressant efficacy was noted.

Extended release tablet: Initial: 50 mg/day the first day; increase to 100 mg on day 2, further increasing by 100 mg/day each day until a target dose of 300 mg/day is reached by day 4.

Mania:

Immediate release tablet: Initial: 50 mg twice daily on day 1, increase dose in increments of 100 mg/day to 200 mg twice daily on day 4; may increase to a target dose of 800 mg/day by day 6 at increments ≤200 mg/day. Usual dosage range: 400-800 mg/day.

Extended release tablet: Initial: 300 mg on day 1; increase to 600 mg on day 2 and adjust dose to 400-800 mg once daily on day 3, depending on response and tolerance.

Maintenance therapy: Immediate release tablet: 200-400 mg twice daily with lithium or divalproex; **Note:** Average time of stabilization was 15 weeks in clinical trials.

Major depressive disorder (adjunct to antidepressants): Oral: Extended release tablet: Initial: 50 mg once daily; may be increased to 150 mg on day 3. Usual dosage range: 150-300 mg/day

QUETIAPINE

Schizophrenia/psychoses: Oral:

Immediate release tablet: Initial: 25 mg twice daily; followed by increases in the total daily dose on the second and third day in increments of 25-50 mg divided 2-3 times/day, if tolerated, to a target dose of 300-400 mg/day in 2-3 divided doses by day 4. Make further adjustments as needed at intervals of at least 2 days in adjustments of 25-50 mg divided twice daily. Usual maintenance range: 300-800 mg/day.

Extended-release tablet: Initial: 300 mg once daily; increase in increments of up to 300 mg/day (in intervals of ≥1 day). Usual maintenance range: 400-800 mg/day.

Note: Dose reductions should be attempted periodically to establish lowest effective dose in patients with psychosis. Patients being restarted after 1 week of no drug need to be titrated as above.

ICU delirium: Oral: Initial: 50 mg twice daily; may increase as necessary on a daily basis in increments of 50 mg twice daily to a maximum dose of 400 mg/day (Devlin, 2010)

Renal Impairment No dosage adjustment required: 25% lower mean oral clearance of quetiapine than normal subjects; however, plasma concentrations similar to normal subjects receiving the same dose.

Hepatic Impairment Lower clearance in hepatic impairment (30%), may result in higher concentrations. Dosage adjustment may be required.

Immediate release tablet: Oral: Initial: 25 mg/day, increase dose by 25-50 mg/day to effective dose, based on clinical response and tolerability to patient. If initiated with immediate-release formulation, patient may transition to extended-release formulation (at equivalent total daily dose) when effective dose has been reached.

Extended release tablet Oral: Initial: 50 mg/day; increase dose by 50 mg/day to effective dose, based on clinical response and tolerability to patient.

Administration

Oral:

Immediate release tablet: May be administered with or without food.

Extended release tablet: Administer without food or with a light meal (≤300 calories), preferably in the evening. Swallow tablet whole; do not break, crush, or chew.

Nasogastric/enteral tube (unlabeled route): Hold tube feeds for 30 minutes before administration; flush with 25 mL of sterile water. Crush dose using immediate-release formulation, mix in 10 mL water and administer via NG/enteral tube; follow with a 50 mL flush of sterile water (Devlin, 2010).

Monitoring Parameters Vital signs; fasting lipid profile and fasting blood glucose/Hgb A_{1c} (prior to treatment, at 3 months, then annually); CBC frequently during first few months of therapy in patients with pre-existing low WBC or a history of drug-induced leukopenia/neutropenia; BMI, personal/family history of obesity, waist circumference; mental status, abnormal involuntary movement scale (AIMS). Weight should be assessed prior to treatment, at 4 weeks, 8 weeks, 12 weeks, and then at quarterly intervals. Consider titrating to a different antipsychotic agent for a weight gain ≥5% of the initial weight. Patients should have eyes checked for cataracts every 6 months while on this medication. Observe for new or worsening depression, anxiety, irritability, aggression, or other symptoms of unusual behavior, mood, or suicide ideation (especially at the beginning of therapy or when doses are increased or decreased).

Test Interactions May interfere with urine detection of methadone (false-positives); may cause false-positive serum TCA screen

Special Geriatric Considerations Any changes in disease status in any organ system can result in behavior changes.

Extrapyramidal syndrome symptoms occur less often than with traditional antipsychotics from the phenothiazine and butyrophenone classes. Many elderly patients receive antipsychotic medications for inappropriate nonpsychotic behavior. Before initiating antipsychotic medication, the clinician should investigate any possible reversible cause; any stress or stress from any disease can cause acute "confusion" or worsening of baseline nonpsychotic behavior. Most commonly acute changes in behavior are due to increases in drug dose or addition of new drug to regimen; fluid electrolyte loss; infections; and changes in environment.

In the treatment of agitated, demented elderly patients, authors of meta-analyses of controlled trials of the response to the traditional antipsychotics (eg, phenothiazines, butyrophenones) in controlling agitation, have concluded that the use of neuroleptics results in a response rate of 18%. Clearly neuroleptic therapy for behavior control should be limited with frequent attempts to withdraw the agent given for behavior control. In light of significant risks and adverse effects in elderly population compared with limited data demonstrating efficacy in the treatment of dementia related psychosis, aggression, and agitation, an extensive risk:benefit analysis should be performed prior to use.

Dosage Forms Excipient information presented when available (limited, particularly for generics); consult specific product labeling.
Tablet, oral:
SEROquel®: 25 mg, 50 mg, 100 mg, 200 mg, 300 mg, 400 mg
Tablet, extended release, oral:
SEROquel XR®: 50 mg, 150 mg, 200 mg, 300 mg, 400 mg
Dosage Forms: Canada Excipient information presented when available (limited, particularly for generics); consult specific product labeling.
Tablet:
Seroquel®: 25 mg, 50 mg, 100 mg, 200 mg, 300 mg, 400 mg
Tablet, extended release:
Seroquel XR®: 50 mg, 150 mg, 200 mg, 300 mg, 400 mg

Selected References

American Diabetes Association; American Psychiatric Association; American Association of Clinical Endocrinologists; North American Association for the Study of Obesity, "Consensus Development Conference on Antipsychotic Drugs and Obesity and Diabetes," *Diabetes Care*, 2004, 27(2):596-601.

Bauer M, Pretorius HW, Constant EL, et al, "Extended-Release Quetiapine as Adjunct to an Antidepressant in Patients with Major Depressive Disorder: Results of a Randomized, Placebo-Controlled, Double-Blind Study," *J Clin Psychiatry*, 2009, 70(4):540-9.

Devlin JW, Roberts RJ, Fong JJ, et al, "Efficacy and Safety of Quetiapine in Critically Ill Patients With Delirium: A Prospective, Multicenter, Randomized, Double-Blind, Placebo-Controlled Pilot Study," *Crit Care Med*, 2010, 38 (2):419-27.

Rabins PV, Blacker D, Rovner BW, et al, "Practice Guidelines for the Treatment of Patients With Alzheimer's Disease and Other Dementias," *Am J Psychiatry*, 2007, 164(12 Suppl):5-56. Available at http://www.psych.org/psych_pract/treatg/pg/prac_guide.cfm.

Schneider LS, Tariot PN, Dagerman KS, et al, "Effectiveness of Atypical Antipsychotic Drugs in Patients With Alzheimer's Disease," *N Engl J Med*, 2006, 355(15):1525-38.

♦ **Quetiapine Fumarate** *see* QUEtiapine *on page 1556*

Quinapril (KWIN a pril)

Related Information
Angiotensin Agents *on page 1985*
Medication Safety Issues
Sound-alike/look-alike issues:
Accupril® may be confused with Accolate®, Accutane®, AcipHex®, Monopril®
International issues:
Accupril [U.S., Canada] may be confused with Acepril which is a brand name for captopril [Great Britain]; enalapril [Hungary, Switzerland]; lisinopril [Malaysia]
Brand Names: U.S. Accupril®
Brand Names: Canada Accupril®
Index Terms Quinapril Hydrochloride
Generic Availability (U.S.) Yes
Pharmacologic Category Angiotensin-Converting Enzyme (ACE) Inhibitor
Use Treatment of hypertension; treatment of heart failure
Unlabeled/Investigational Use Treatment of left ventricular dysfunction after myocardial infarction; to delay the progression of nephropathy and reduce risks of cardiovascular events in hypertensive patients with type 1 or 2 diabetes mellitus
Contraindications Hypersensitivity to quinapril or any component of the formulation; angioedema related to previous treatment with an ACE inhibitor
Warnings/Precautions Anaphylactic reactions may occur rarely with ACE inhibitors. At any time during treatment (especially following first dose) angioedema may occur rarely with ACE inhibitors; it may involve the head and neck (potentially compromising airway) or the intestine (presenting with abdominal pain). African-Americans and patients with idiopathic or hereditary angioedema may be at an increased risk. Prolonged frequent monitoring may be required especially if tongue, glottis, or larynx are involved as they are associated with airway obstruction. Patients with a history of airway surgery may have a higher risk of airway obstruction. Aggressive early and appropriate management is critical. Use in patients with previous angioedema associated with ACE inhibitor therapy is contraindicated. Severe anaphylactoid reactions may be seen during hemodialysis (eg, CVVHD) with high-flux dialysis membranes (eg, AN69), and rarely, during low density lipoprotein apheresis with dextran sulfate cellulose. Rare cases of anaphylactoid reactions have been reported in patients undergoing sensitization treatment with hymenoptera (bee, wasp) venom while receiving ACE inhibitors.

Symptomatic hypotension with or without syncope can occur with ACE inhibitors (usually with the first several doses); effects are most often observed in volume-depleted patients; close monitoring of patient is required especially with initial dosing and dosing increases; blood pressure must be lowered at a rate appropriate for the patient's clinical condition. Initiation of therapy in patients with ischemic heart disease or cerebrovascular disease warrants close observation due to the potential consequences posed by falling blood pressure (eg, MI, stroke). Use with caution in hypertrophic cardiomyopathy with outflow tract obstruction, severe aortic stenosis, or before, during, or immediately after major surgery.

Hyperkalemia may occur with ACE inhibitors; risk factors include renal dysfunction, diabetes mellitus, concomitant use of potassium-sparing diuretics, potassium supplements, and/or potassium-containing salts. Use cautiously, if at all, with these agents and monitor potassium closely. Cough may occur with ACE inhibitors. Other causes of cough should be considered (eg, pulmonary congestion in patients with heart failure) and excluded prior to discontinuation.

May be associated with deterioration of renal function and/or increases in serum creatinine, particularly in patients with low renal blood flow (eg, renal artery stenosis, heart failure) whose glomerular filtration rate (GFR) is dependent on efferent arteriolar vasoconstriction by angiotensin II; deterioration may result in oliguria, acute renal failure, and progressive azotemia. Small increases in serum creatinine may occur following initiation; consider discontinuation only in patients with progressive and/or significant deterioration in renal function. Use with caution in patients with unstented unilateral/bilateral renal artery stenosis. When unstented bilateral renal artery stenosis is present, use is generally avoided due to the elevated risk of deterioration in renal function unless possible benefits outweigh risks. Concurrent use of angiotensin receptor blockers may increase the risk of clinically-significant adverse events (eg, renal dysfunction, hyperkalemia).

Rare toxicities associated with ACE inhibitors include cholestatic jaundice (which may progress to fulminant hepatic necrosis), agranulocytosis, neutropenia, or leukopenia with myeloid hypoplasia. Patients with collagen vascular diseases (especially with concomitant renal impairment) or renal impairment alone may be at increased risk for hematologic toxicity; periodically monitor CBC with differential in these patients.

Adverse Reactions (Reflective of adult population; not specific for elderly) Note: Frequency ranges include data from hypertension and heart failure trials. Higher rates of adverse reactions have generally been noted in patients with CHF. However, the frequency of adverse effects associated with placebo is also increased in this population.

1% to 10%:
Cardiovascular: Hypotension (3%), chest pain (2%), first-dose hypotension (up to 3%)
Central nervous system: Dizziness (4% to 8%), headache (2% to 6%), fatigue (3%)
Dermatologic: Rash (1%)
Endocrine & metabolic: Hyperkalemia (2%)
Gastrointestinal: Vomiting/nausea (1% to 2%), diarrhea (2%)
Neuromuscular & skeletal: Myalgias (2% to 5%), back pain (1%)
Renal: BUN/serum creatinine increased (2%, transient elevations may occur with a higher frequency), worsening of renal function (in patients with bilateral renal artery stenosis or hypovolemia)
Respiratory: Upper respiratory symptoms, cough (2% to 4%; up to 13% in some studies), dyspnea (2%)

Drug Interactions
Avoid Concomitant Use There are no known interactions where it is recommended to avoid concomitant use.
Increased Effect/Toxicity
Quinapril may increase the levels/effects of: Allopurinol; Amifostine; Antihypertensives; AzaTHIOprine; CycloSPORINE; CycloSPORINE (Systemic); Ferric Gluconate; Gold Sodium Thiomalate; Hypotensive Agents; Iron Dextran Complex; Lithium; Nonsteroidal Anti-Inflammatory Agents; RiTUXimab; Sodium Phosphates

The levels/effects of Quinapril may be increased by: Alfuzosin; Angiotensin II Receptor Blockers; Diazoxide; DPP-IV Inhibitors; Eplerenone; Everolimus; Herbs (Hypotensive Properties); Loop Diuretics; MAO Inhibitors; Pentoxifylline; Phosphodiesterase 5 Inhibitors; Potassium Salts; Potassium-Sparing Diuretics; Prostacyclin Analogues; Sirolimus; Temsirolimus; Thiazide Diuretics; TiZANidine; Tolvaptan; Trimethoprim

Decreased Effect
Quinapril may decrease the levels/effects of: Quinolone Antibiotics; Tetracycline Derivatives

The levels/effects of Quinapril may be decreased by: Antacids; Aprotinin; Herbs (Hypertensive Properties); Icatibant; Lanthanum; Methylphenidate; Nonsteroidal Anti-Inflammatory Agents; Salicylates; Yohimbine

Ethanol/Nutrition/Herb Interactions Herb/Nutraceutical: Avoid bayberry, blue cohosh, cayenne, ephedra, ginger, ginseng (American), kola, licorice (may worsen hypertension). Avoid black cohosh, California poppy, coleus, golden seal, hawthorn, mistletoe, periwinkle, quinine, shepherd's purse (may have increased antihypertensive effect).

Stability Store at room temperature. To prepare solution for oral administration, mix prior to administration and use within 10 minutes.

Mechanism of Action Competitive inhibitor of angiotensin-converting enzyme (ACE); prevents conversion of angiotensin I to angiotensin II, a potent vasoconstrictor; results in lower levels of angiotensin II which causes an increase in plasma renin activity and a reduction in aldosterone secretion; a CNS mechanism may also be involved in hypotensive effect as angiotensin II increases adrenergic outflow from CNS; vasoactive kallikreins may be decreased in conversion to active hormones by ACE inhibitors, thus reducing blood pressure

Pharmacodynamics/Kinetics

Onset of action: 1 hour

Duration: 24 hours

Absorption: Quinapril: ≥60%

Protein binding: Quinapril: 97%; Quinaprilat: 97%

Metabolism: Rapidly hydrolyzed to quinaprilat, the active metabolite

Half-life elimination: Quinapril: 0.8 hour; Quinaprilat: 3 hours; increases as Cl_{cr} decreases

Time to peak, serum: Quinapril: 1 hour; Quinaprilat: ~2 hours

Excretion: Urine (50% to 60% primarily as quinaprilat)

Dosage

Geriatric Oral: Initial: 2.5-5 mg/day; increase dosage at increments of 2.5-5 mg at 1- to 2-week intervals; adjust for renal impairment.

Adult

Heart failure: Oral: Initial: 5 mg once or twice daily, titrated at weekly intervals to 20-40 mg daily in 2 divided doses; target dose (heart failure): 20 mg twice daily (ACC/AHA 2009 Heart Failure Guidelines)

Hypertension: Oral: Initial: 10-20 mg once daily, adjust according to blood pressure response at peak and trough blood levels; initial dose may be reduced to 5 mg in patients receiving diuretic therapy if the diuretic is continued.

Usual dose range (JNC 7): 10-40 mg once daily

Renal Impairment Lower initial doses should be used; after initial dose (if tolerated), administer initial dose twice daily; may be increased at weekly intervals to optimal response:

Heart failure: Oral: Initial:

Cl_{cr} >30 mL/minute: Administer 5 mg/day

Cl_{cr} 10-30 mL/minute: Administer 2.5 mg/day

Hypertension: Oral: Initial:

Cl_{cr} >60 mL/minute: Administer 10 mg/day

Cl_{cr} 30-60 mL/minute: Administer 5 mg/day

Cl_{cr} 10-30 mL/minute: Administer 2.5 mg/day

Hepatic Impairment In patients with alcoholic cirrhosis, hydrolysis of quinapril to quinaprilat is impaired; however, the subsequent elimination of quinaprilat is unaltered.

Monitoring Parameters Blood pressure; serum creatinine and potassium; if patient has collagen vascular disease and/or renal impairment, periodically monitor CBC with differential

Pharmacotherapy Pearls Patients taking diuretics are at risk for developing hypotension on initial dosing; to prevent this, discontinue diuretics 2-3 days prior to initiating quinapril; may restart diuretics if blood pressure is not controlled by quinapril alone

Special Geriatric Considerations Due to frequent decreases in glomerular filtration (also creatinine clearance) with aging, elderly patients may have exaggerated responses to ACE inhibitors; differences in clinical response due to hepatic changes are not observed. ACE inhibitors may be preferred agents in elderly patients with CHF and diabetes mellitus. Diabetic proteinuria is reduced and insulin sensitivity is enhanced. In general, the side effect profile is favorable in elderly and causes little or no CNS confusion; use lowest dose recommendations initially. Adjust for renal function. Many elderly may be volume depleted due to diuretic use and/or blunted thirst reflex resulting in inadequate fluid intake.

Dosage Forms Excipient information presented when available (limited, particularly for generics); consult specific product labeling.

Tablet, oral: 5 mg, 10 mg, 20 mg, 40 mg

Accupril®: 5 mg, 10 mg, 20 mg [scored]

Accupril®: 40 mg

Selected References

American Diabetes Association, "Standards of Medical Care in Diabetes Mellitus – 2009," *Diabetes Care*, 2009, 32 (Suppl 1):13-61.

Chobanian AV, Bakris GL, Black HR, et al, "The Seventh Report of the Joint National Committee on Prevention, Detection, Evaluation, and Treatment of High Blood Pressure: The JNC 7 Report," *JAMA*, 2003, 289(19):2560-71.

Quinapril and Hydrochlorothiazide (KWIN a pril & hye droe klor oh THYE a zide)

Related Information
Hydrochlorothiazide on page 876
Quinapril on page 1561

Brand Names: U.S. Accuretic®
Brand Names: Canada Accuretic®
Index Terms Hydrochlorothiazide and Quinapril; Quinaretic
Generic Availability (U.S.) Yes
Pharmacologic Category Angiotensin-Converting Enzyme (ACE) Inhibitor; Diuretic, Thiazide
Use Treatment of hypertension (not for initial therapy)

Dosage

Geriatric If previous response to individual components is unknown, initial dose selection should be cautious, at the low end of adult dosage range; titration should occur at 1- to 2-week intervals.

Adult

Hypertension: Oral:

Patients with inadequate response to quinapril monotherapy: Quinapril 10 mg/hydrochlorothiazide 12.5 mg **or** quinapril 20 mg/hydrochlorothiazide 12.5 mg once daily

Patients with adequate blood pressure control on hydrochlorothiazide 25 mg/day, but significant potassium loss: Quinapril 10 mg/hydrochlorothiazide 12.5 mg **or** quinapril 20 mg/hydrochlorothiazide 12.5 mg once daily

Note: Clinical trials of quinapril/hydrochlorothiazide combinations used quinapril doses of 2.5-40 mg/day and hydrochlorothiazide doses of 6.25-25 mg/day.

Renal Impairment Cl_{cr} <30 mL/minute/1.73 m^2 or serum creatinine ≥3 mg/dL: Use is not recommended.

Special Geriatric Considerations Hydrochlorothiazide is not effective in patients with a Cl_{cr} <30 mL/minute; therefore, it may not be a useful agent in many elderly patients.

Dosage Forms Excipient information presented when available (limited, particularly for generics); consult specific product labeling.

Tablet:
10/12.5: Quinapril 10 mg and hydrochlorothiazide 12.5 mg
20/12.5: Quinapril 20 mg and hydrochlorothiazide 12.5 mg
20/25: Quinapril 20 mg and hydrochlorothiazide 25 mg
Accuretic® 10/12.5: Quinapril 10 mg and hydrochlorothiazide 12.5 mg
Accuretic® 20/12.5: Quinapril 20 mg and hydrochlorothiazide 12.5 mg
Accuretic® 20/25: Quinapril 20 mg and hydrochlorothiazide 25 mg

◆ **Quinapril Hydrochloride** see Quinapril on page 1561
◆ **Quinaretic** see Quinapril and Hydrochlorothiazide on page 1564

QuiNIDine (KWIN i deen)

Medication Safety Issues

Sound-alike/look-alike issues:
QuiNIDine may be confused with cloNIDine, quiNINE, Quinora®

High alert medication:
The Institute for Safe Medication Practices (ISMP) includes this medication (I.V. formulation) among its list of drug classes which have a heightened risk of causing significant patient harm when used in error.

Brand Names: Canada Apo-Quinidine®; BioQuin® Durules™; Novo-Quinidin; Quinate®
Index Terms Quinidine Gluconate; Quinidine Polygalacturonate; Quinidine Sulfate
Generic Availability (U.S.) Yes
Pharmacologic Category Antiarrhythmic Agent, Class Ia

Use

Quinidine gluconate and sulfate salts: Conversion and prevention of relapse into atrial fibrillation and/or flutter; suppression of ventricular arrhythmias. **Note:** Due to proarrhythmic effects, use should be reserved for life-threatening arrhythmias. Moreover, the use of quinidine has largely been replaced by more effective/safer antiarrhythmic agents and/or nonpharmacologic therapies (eg, radiofrequency ablation).

Quinidine gluconate (I.V. formulation): Conversion of atrial fibrillation/flutter and ventricular tachycardia. **Note:** The use of I.V. quinidine gluconate for these indications has been replaced by more effective/safer antiarrhythmic agents (eg, amiodarone and procainamide).

Quinidine gluconate (I.V. formulation) and quinidine sulfate: Treatment of malaria (*Plasmodium falciparum*)

Unlabeled/Investigational Use Paroxysmal supraventricular tachycardia, paroxysmal AV junctional rhythm, and symptomatic atrial or ventricular premature contractions; short QT syndrome; Brugada syndrome

Contraindications Hypersensitivity to quinidine or any component of the formulation; thrombocytopenia; thrombocytopenic purpura; myasthenia gravis; heart block greater than first degree; idioventricular conduction delays (except in patients with a functioning artificial pacemaker); those adversely affected by anticholinergic activity; concurrent use of quinolone antibiotics which prolong QT interval, cisapride, amprenavir, or ritonavir

Warnings/Precautions Watch for proarrhythmic effects; may cause QT prolongation and subsequent torsade de pointes. Monitor and adjust dose to prevent QT_c prolongation. Avoid use in patients with diagnosed or suspected congenital long QT syndrome. Correct hypokalemia before initiating therapy. Hypokalemia may worsen toxicity. **[U.S. Boxed Warning]: Antiarrhythmic drugs have not been shown to enhance survival in non-life-threatening ventricular arrhythmias and may increase mortality; the risk is greatest with structural heart disease. Quinidine may increase mortality in treatment of atrial fibrillation/flutter.** May precipitate or exacerbate HF. Reduce dosage in hepatic impairment. Use may cause digoxin-induced toxicity (adjust digoxin's dose). Use caution with concurrent use of other antiarrhythmics. Hypersensitivity reactions can occur. Can unmask sick sinus syndrome (causes bradycardia); use with caution in patients with heart block. Has been associated with severe hepatotoxic reactions, including granulomatous hepatitis. Hemolysis may occur in patients with G6PD (glucose-6-phosphate dehydrogenase) deficiency. Different salt products are not interchangeable.

Adverse Reactions (Reflective of adult population; not specific for elderly)

Frequency not defined: Hypotension, syncope

>10%:
Cardiovascular: QT_c prolongation (modest prolongation is common, however, excessive prolongation is rare and indicates toxicity)
Central nervous system: Lightheadedness (15%)
Gastrointestinal: Diarrhea (35%), upper GI distress, bitter taste, diarrhea, anorexia, nausea, vomiting, stomach cramping (22%)

1% to 10%:
Cardiovascular: Angina (6%), palpitation (7%), new or worsened arrhythmia (proarrhythmic effect)
Central nervous system: Syncope (1% to 8%), headache (7%), fatigue (7%), sleep disturbance (3%), tremor (2%), nervousness (2%), incoordination (1%)
Dermatologic: Rash (5%)
Neuromuscular & skeletal: Weakness (5%)
Ocular: Blurred vision
Otic: Tinnitus
Respiratory: Wheezing

Note: Cinchonism, a syndrome which may include tinnitus, high-frequency hearing loss, deafness, vertigo, blurred vision, diplopia, photophobia, headache, confusion, and delirium has been associated with quinidine use. Usually associated with chronic toxicity, this syndrome has also been described after brief exposure to a moderate dose in sensitive patients. Vomiting and diarrhea may also occur as isolated reactions to therapeutic quinidine levels.

Drug Interactions

Metabolism/Transport Effects Substrate of CYP2C9 (minor), CYP2E1 (minor), CYP3A4 (major), P-glycoprotein; **Inhibits** CYP2C9 (weak), CYP2D6 (strong), CYP3A4 (strong), P-glycoprotein

Avoid Concomitant Use

Avoid concomitant use of QuiNIDine with any of the following: Alfuzosin; Antifungal Agents (Azole Derivatives, Systemic); Artemether; Conivaptan; Crizotinib; Dronedarone; Eplerenone; Everolimus; Fluticasone (Oral Inhalation); Halofantrine; Lapatinib; Lovastatin; Lumefantrine; Lurasidone; Mefloquine; Nilotinib; Nisoldipine; Pimozide; Protease Inhibitors; QUEtiapine; QuiNINE; Ranolazine; Rivaroxaban; RomiDEPsin; Salmeterol; Silodosin; Simvastatin; Tamoxifen; Tamsulosin; Tetrabenazine; Thioridazine; Ticagrelor; Tolvaptan; Topotecan; Toremifene; Vandetanib; Vemurafenib; Ziprasidone

Increased Effect/Toxicity

QuiNIDine may increase the levels/effects of: Alfuzosin; Almotriptan; Alosetron; Atomoxetine; Beta-Blockers; Bortezomib; Brentuximab Vedotin; Brinzolamide; Budesonide (Nasal); Budesonide (Systemic, Oral Inhalation); Calcium Channel Blockers (Dihydropyridine); Cardiac Glycosides; Ciclesonide; Colchicine; Conivaptan; Corticosteroids (Orally Inhaled); Crizotinib; CYP2D6 Substrates; CYP3A4 Substrates; Dabigatran Etexilate; Dextromethorphan; Dienogest; Dronedarone; Dutasteride; Eplerenone; Everolimus; FentaNYL; Fesoterodine; Fluticasone (Nasal); Fluticasone (Oral Inhalation); GuanFACINE; Halofantrine; Haloperidol; Iloperidone; Ixabepilone; Lapatinib; Lovastatin; Lumefantrine; Lurasidone;

Maraviroc; Mefloquine; MethylPREDNISolone; Neuromuscular-Blocking Agents; Nilotinib; Nisoldipine; Paricalcitol; Pazopanib; P-Glycoprotein Substrates; Pimecrolimus; Pimozide; QTc-Prolonging Agents; QuiNINE; Ranolazine; Rivaroxaban; RomiDEPsin; Salmeterol; Saxagliptin; Sildenafil; Silodosin; Simvastatin; SORAfenib; Tadalafil; Tamoxifen; Tamsulosin; Tetrabenazine; Thioridazine; Ticagrelor; Tolterodine; Tolvaptan; Topotecan; Toremifene; Tricyclic Antidepressants; Vandetanib; Vardenafil; Vemurafenib; Verapamil; Vilazodone; Vitamin K Antagonists; Ziprasidone

The levels/effects of QuiNIDine may be increased by: Alfuzosin; Amiodarone; Antacids; Antifungal Agents (Azole Derivatives, Systemic); Artemether; Barbiturates; Boceprevir; Calcium Channel Blockers (Dihydropyridine); Carbonic Anhydrase Inhibitors; Chloroquine; Cimetidine; Ciprofloxacin; Ciprofloxacin (Systemic); CYP3A4 Inhibitors (Moderate); CYP3A4 Inhibitors (Strong); Diltiazem; Eribulin; Fingolimod; Fluconazole; Gadobutrol; Haloperidol; Lumefantrine; Lurasidone; Macrolide Antibiotics; Nilotinib; P-Glycoprotein Inhibitors; Protease Inhibitors; QUEtiapine; QuiNINE; Reserpine; Selective Serotonin Reuptake Inhibitors; Telaprevir; Tricyclic Antidepressants; Verapamil

Decreased Effect

QuiNIDine may decrease the levels/effects of: Codeine; Dihydrocodeine; Hydrocodone; Prasugrel; Ticagrelor; TraMADol

The levels/effects of QuiNIDine may be decreased by: Barbiturates; Calcium Channel Blockers (Dihydropyridine); CYP3A4 Inducers (Strong); Cyproterone; Deferasirox; Etravirine; Fosphenytoin; Herbs (CYP3A4 Inducers); Kaolin; P-Glycoprotein Inducers; Phenytoin; Potassium-Sparing Diuretics; Primidone; Rifamycin Derivatives; Sucralfate; Tocilizumab

Ethanol/Nutrition/Herb Interactions

Food: Dietary salt intake may alter the rate and extent of quinidine absorption. A decrease in dietary salt may lead to an increase in quinidine serum concentrations. Avoid changes in dietary salt intake. Quinidine serum levels may be increased if taken with food. Food has a variable effect on absorption of sustained release formulation. The rate of absorption of quinidine may be decreased following the ingestion of grapefruit juice. In addition, CYP3A4 metabolism of quinidine may be reduced by grapefruit juice. Grapefruit juice should be avoided. Excessive intake of fruit juices or vitamin C may decrease urine pH and result in increased clearance of quinidine with decreased serum concentration. Alkaline foods may result in increased quinidine serum concentrations.

Herb/Nutraceutical: St John's wort may decrease quinidine levels. Avoid ephedra (may worsen arrhythmia).

Stability

Solution for injection: Store at room temperature of 25°C (77°F).

Tablets: Store at controlled room temperature of 20°C to 25°C (68°F to 77°F). Protect from light.

Mechanism of Action Class Ia antiarrhythmic agent; depresses phase O of the action potential; decreases myocardial excitability and conduction velocity, and myocardial contractility by decreasing sodium influx during depolarization and potassium efflux in repolarization; also reduces calcium transport across cell membrane

Pharmacodynamics/Kinetics

Distribution: V_d: Adults: 2-3 L/kg, decreased with congestive heart failure, malaria; increased with cirrhosis

Protein binding: 80% to 90%

Metabolism: Extensively hepatic (50% to 90%) to inactive compounds

Bioavailability: Sulfate: 80%; Gluconate: 70%

Half-life elimination, plasma: 6-8 hours; prolonged with elderly, cirrhosis, and congestive heart failure

Time to peak, serum: Sulfate: 2 hours; Gluconate: 3-5 hours

Excretion: Urine (15% to 25% as unchanged drug)

Dosage

Geriatric & Adult

Note: Dosage expressed in terms of the salt: 267 mg of quinidine gluconate = 200 mg of quinidine sulfate.

Antiarrhythmic: Oral:

Immediate release formulations: Quinidine sulfate: Initial: 200-400 mg/dose every 6 hours the dose may be increased cautiously to desired effect

Extended release formulations:

Quinidine sulfate: Initial: 300 mg every 8-12 hours; the dose may be increased cautiously to desired effect

Quinidine gluconate: Initial: 324 mg every 8-12 hours; the dose may be increased cautiously to desired effect

Severe malaria, treatment: I.V. (quinidine gluconate): 10 mg/kg infused over 60-120 minutes followed by 0.02 mg/kg/minute continuous infusion for ≥24 hours; alternatively, may administer 24 mg/kg loading dose over 4 hours, followed by 12 mg/kg over 4 hours every 8 hours (beginning 8 hours after initiation of the loading dose); complete treatment with oral quinine once parasite density <1% and patient can receive oral medication; total duration of treatment (quinidine/quinine): 3 days (Africa or South America) or 7 days (Southeast Asia); use in combination with doxycycline, tetracycline or clindamycin (CDC malaria guidelines, 2009). **Note:** Close monitoring, including telemetry, required.

Renal Impairment The FDA-approved labeling recommends that caution should be used in patients with renal impairment; however, no specific dosage adjustment guidelines are available. The following guidelines have been used by some clinicians (Aronoff, 2007): Oral: Cl_{cr} ≥10 mL/minute: No adjustment required.

Cl_{cr} <10 mL/minute: Administer 75% of normal dose.

Hemodialysis: Dose following hemodialysis.

Peritoneal dialysis: Supplemental dose is not necessary.

CRRT: No dosage adjustment required; monitor serum concentrations.

Hepatic Impairment Use caution; hepatic impairment decreases clearance; dosage adjustments are not provided in the manufacturers' labeling although toxicity may occur if the dose is not appropriately adjusted.

Administration Administer around-the-clock to promote less variation in peak and trough serum levels

Oral: Do not crush, chew, or break sustained release dosage forms.

Parenteral: When injecting I.M., aspirate carefully to avoid injection into a vessel; maximum I.V. infusion rate: 10 mg/minute

Monitoring Parameters Cardiac monitor required during I.V. administration; CBC, liver and renal function tests, should be routinely performed during long-term administration

Reference Range Therapeutic: 2-5 mcg/mL (SI: 6.2-15.4 µmol/L). Patient-dependent therapeutic response occurs at levels of 3-6 mcg/mL (SI: 9.2-18.5 µmol/L). Optimal therapeutic level is method dependent; >6 mcg/mL (SI: >18 µmol/L).

Special Geriatric Considerations Clearance may be decreased with a resultant increased half-life. Must individualize dose. Bioavailability and half-life are increased in the elderly due to decreases in both renal and hepatic function with age.

Dosage Forms Excipient information presented when available (limited, particularly for generics); consult specific product labeling.

Injection, solution, as gluconate: 80 mg/mL (10 mL) [equivalent to quinidine base 50 mg/mL]

Tablet, oral, as sulfate: 200 mg, 300 mg

Tablet, extended release, oral, as gluconate: 324 mg [equivalent to quinidine base 202 mg]

Tablet, extended release, oral, as sulfate: 300 mg [equivalent to quinidine base 249 mg]

◆ **Quinidine Gluconate** see QuiNIDine on page 1564
◆ **Quinidine Polygalacturonate** see QuiNIDine on page 1564
◆ **Quinidine Sulfate** see QuiNIDine on page 1564

QuiNINE (KWYE nine)

Medication Safety Issues

Sound-alike/look-alike issues:

QuiNINE may be confused with quiNIDine

Brand Names: U.S. Qualaquin®

Brand Names: Canada Apo-Quinine®; Novo-Quinine; Quinine-Odan

Index Terms Quinine Sulfate

Generic Availability (U.S.) No

Pharmacologic Category Antimalarial Agent

Use In conjunction with other antimalarial agents, treatment of uncomplicated chloroquine-resistant *P. falciparum* malaria

Unlabeled/Investigational Use Treatment of *Babesia microti* infection in conjunction with clindamycin; treatment of uncomplicated chloroquine-resistant *P. vivax* malaria (in conjunction with other antimalarial agents)

Medication Guide Available Yes

Contraindications Hypersensitivity to quinine or any component of the formulation; hypersensitivity to mefloquine or quinidine (cross sensitivity reported); history of potential hypersensitivity reactions (including black water fever, thrombotic thrombocytopenia purpura [TTP], hemolytic uremic syndrome [HUS], or thrombocytopenia) associated with prior quinine use; prolonged QT interval; myasthenia gravis; optic neuritis; G6PD deficiency

◄ **Warnings/Precautions [U.S. Boxed Warning]:** Quinine is not recommended for the prevention/treatment of nocturnal leg cramps due to the potential for severe and/or life-threatening side effects (eg, cardiac arrhythmias, thrombocytopenia, HUS/TTP, severe hypersensitivity reactions). These risks, as well as the absence of clinical effectiveness, do not justify its use in the unapproved/unlabeled prevention and/or treatment of leg cramps.

Quinine may cause QT interval prolongation, with maximum increase corresponding to maximum plasma concentration. Use caution with medications or clinical conditions which may further prolong the QT interval or cause cardiac arrhythmias. Use caution with atrial fibrillation or flutter, renal or hepatic impairment. Quinine interacts with many medications due to its hepatic metabolism; use caution with other medications metabolized via the CYP3A4 isoenzyme system. Severe hypersensitivity reactions (eg, Stevens-Johnson syndrome, anaphylactic shock) have occurred; discontinue following any signs of sensitivity. Other events (including acute interstitial nephritis, neutropenia, and granulomatous hepatitis) may also be attributed to hypersensitivity reactions. Immune-mediated thrombocytopenia, including life-threatening cases and hemolytic uremic syndrome/thrombotic thrombocytopenic purpura (HUS/TTP), has occurred with use. Chronic renal failure associated with TTP has also been reported. Thrombocytopenia generally resolves within a week upon discontinuation. Re-exposure may result in increased severity of thrombocytopenia and faster onset.

Use may cause significant hypoglycemia due to quinine-induced insulin release. Use with caution in patients with hepatic impairment. Use with caution in patients with renal impairment; dosage adjustment recommended. Quinine should not be used for the prevention of malaria or in the treatment of complicated or severe *P. falciparum* malaria (oral antimalarial agents are not appropriate for initial therapy of severe malaria).

Adverse Reactions (Reflective of adult population; not specific for elderly)
Frequency not defined.

Cardiovascular: Atrial fibrillation, atrioventricular block, bradycardia, cardiac arrest, chest pain, hypotension, irregular rhythm, nodal escape beats, palpitation, postural hypotension, QT prolongation, syncope, tachycardia, torsade de pointes, unifocal premature ventricular contractions, U waves, vasodilation, ventricular fibrillation, ventricular tachycardia

Central nervous system: Aphasia, ataxia, chills, coma, confusion, disorientation, dizziness, dystonic reaction, fever, flushing, headache, mental status altered, restlessness, seizure, suicide, vertigo

Dermatologic: Acral necrosis, allergic contact dermatitis, bullous dermatitis, bruising, cutaneous rash (urticaria, papular, scarlatinal), cutaneous vasculitis, exfoliative dermatitis, erythema multiforme, petechiae, photosensitivity, pruritus, Stevens-Johnson syndrome, toxic epidermal necrolysis

Endocrine & metabolic: Hypoglycemia

Gastrointestinal: Abdominal pain, anorexia, diarrhea, esophagitis, gastric irritation, nausea, vomiting

Hematologic: Agranulocytosis, aplastic anemia, coagulopathy, disseminated intravascular coagulation, hemolytic anemia, hemolytic uremic syndrome, hemorrhage, hypoprothrombinemia, idiopathic thrombocytopenic purpura, leukopenia, neutropenia, pancytopenia, thrombocytopenia, thrombotic thrombocytopenic purpura

Hepatic: Granulomatous hepatitis, hepatitis, jaundice, liver function test abnormalities

Neuromuscular & skeletal: Myalgia, tremor, weakness

Ocular: Blindness, blurred vision (with or without scotomata), color vision disturbance, diminished visual fields, diplopia, night blindness, optic neuritis, photophobia, pupillary dilation, vision loss (sudden)

Otic: Deafness, hearing impaired, tinnitus

Renal: Acute interstitial nephritis, hemoglobinuria, renal failure, renal impairment

Respiratory: Asthma, dyspnea, pulmonary edema

Miscellaneous: Black water fever, diaphoresis, hypersensitivity reaction, lupus anticoagulant, lupus-like syndrome

Drug Interactions

Metabolism/Transport Effects Substrate of CYP1A2 (minor), 2C19 (minor), 3A4 (major); **Inhibits** CYP2C8 (moderate), 2C9 (moderate), 2D6 (moderate), 3A4 (weak)

Avoid Concomitant Use

Avoid concomitant use of QuiNINE with any of the following: Antacids; Artemether; Conivaptan; Halofantrine; Lumefantrine; Macrolide Antibiotics; Mefloquine; Neuromuscular-Blocking Agents; QTc-Prolonging Agents; Rifampin; Ritonavir; Silodosin; Topotecan

Increased Effect/Toxicity

QuiNINE may increase the levels/effects of: Antihypertensives; Antipsychotic Agents (Phenothiazines); CarBAMazepine; Cardiac Glycosides; Carvedilol; Colchicine; CYP2C8 Substrates (High risk); CYP2C9 Substrates (High risk); CYP2D6 Substrates; Dabigatran Etexilate; Dapsone; Dapsone (Systemic); Dapsone (Topical); Everolimus; Fesoterodine;

Halofantrine; Herbs (Hypotensive Properties); HMG-CoA Reductase Inhibitors; Lumefantrine; Mefloquine; Nebivolol; Neuromuscular-Blocking Agents; P-Glycoprotein Substrates; PHENobarbital; QTc-Prolonging Agents; Ritonavir; Rivaroxaban; Silodosin; Tamoxifen; Theophylline Derivatives; Topotecan; Vitamin K Antagonists

The levels/effects of QuiNINE may be increased by: Alkalinizing Agents; Artemether; Cimetidine; Conivaptan; CYP3A4 Inhibitors (Moderate); CYP3A4 Inhibitors (Strong); Dapsone; Dapsone (Systemic); Macrolide Antibiotics; Mefloquine; P-Glycoprotein Inhibitors; QTc-Prolonging Agents; Ritonavir

Decreased Effect

QuiNINE may decrease the levels/effects of: Codeine; TraMADol

The levels/effects of QuiNINE may be decreased by: Antacids; CarBAMazepine; CYP3A4 Inducers (Strong); Cyproterone; Deferasirox; Fosphenytoin; Herbs (CYP3A4 Inducers); P-Glycoprotein Inducers; PHENobarbital; Phenytoin; Rifampin; Tocilizumab

Ethanol/Nutrition/Herb Interactions Herb/Nutraceutical: St John's wort may decrease quinine levels. Black cohosh, California poppy, coleus, golden seal, hawthorn, mistletoe, periwinkle, and shepherd's purse may cause excessive decreases in blood pressure.

Stability Store at 20°C to 25°C (68°F to 77°F).

Mechanism of Action Depresses oxygen uptake and carbohydrate metabolism; intercalates into DNA, disrupting the parasite's replication and transcription; cardiovascular effects similar to quinidine

Pharmacodynamics/Kinetics

Absorption: Readily, mainly from upper small intestine

Distribution: Adults: 2.5-7.1 L/kg (varies with severity of infection)
Intraerythrocytic levels are ~30% to 50% of the plasma concentration; distributes poorly to the CSF (~2% to 7% of plasma concentration)

Protein binding: 69% to 92% in healthy subjects; 78% to 95% with malaria

Metabolism: Hepatic via CYP450 enzymes, primarily CYP3A4; forms metabolites; major metabolite, 3-hydroxyquinine, is less active than parent

Bioavailability: 76% to 88% in healthy subjects; increased with malaria

Half-life elimination:
Healthy adults: 10-13 hours
Healthy elderly subjects: 18 hours

Time to peak, serum: Adults: 2-4 hours in healthy subjects; 1-11 hours with malaria

Excretion: Urine (<20% as unchanged drug)

Dosage

Geriatric & Adult Note: Actual duration of quinine treatment for malaria may be dependent upon the geographic region or pathogen. Dosage expressed in terms of the salt; 1 capsule Qualaquin® = 324 mg of quinine sulfate = 269 mg of base.

Treatment of uncomplicated chloroquine-resistant *P. falciparum* malaria (CDC guidelines): 648 mg every 8 hours for 3-7 days. Tetracycline, doxycycline, or clindamycin should also be given.

Treatment of uncomplicated chloroquine-resistant *P. vivax* malaria (unlabeled use; CDC guidelines): 648 mg every 8 hours for 3-7 days. Tetracycline or doxycycline plus primaquine should also be given.

Babesiosis (unlabeled use): 650 mg every 8 hours for 7-10 days with clindamycin

Renal Impairment

Cl_{cr} 10-50 mL/minute: Administer every 8-12 hours

Cl_{cr} <10 mL/minute: Administer every 24 hours

Severe chronic renal failure not on dialysis: Initial dose: 648 mg followed by 324 mg every 12 hours

Dialysis: Administer dose after dialysis. **Note:** Clearance of ~6.5% achieved with 1 hour of hemodialysis.

Not removed by hemo- or peritoneal dialysis; dose as for Cl_{cr} <10 mL/minute.

Continuous arteriovenous or hemodialysis: Dose as for Cl_{cr} 10-50 mL/minute.

Hepatic Impairment

Mild-to-moderate impairment: No dosing adjustment required; monitor closely.

Severe impairment (Child-Pugh class C): Data not available.

Administration Avoid use of aluminum- or magnesium-containing antacids because of drug absorption problems. Swallow dose whole to avoid bitter taste. May be administered with food.

Monitoring Parameters Monitor CBC with platelet count, liver function tests, blood glucose, ophthalmologic examination

Test Interactions May interfere with urine detection of opioids (false-positive); positive Coombs' [direct]; false elevation of urinary steroids (when assayed by Zimmerman method) and catecholamines

◀ **Special Geriatric Considerations** Quinine's efficacy as a treatment for nocturnal leg cramps is not well supported in the medical and pharmacy literature. The FDA's decision to remove all quinine products (except one that is indicated for the treatment of malaria) indicates that quinine's benefits for nocturnal leg cramps do not outweigh its risks.

Dosage Forms Excipient information presented when available (limited, particularly for generics); consult specific product labeling.

Capsule, oral, as sulfate:

Qualaquin®: 324 mg

Selected References

Centers for Disease Control and Prevention (CDC), "Treatment of Malaria (Guidelines for Clinicians)." Available at http://www.cdc.gov/malaria/pdf/clinicalguidance.pdf

Centers for Disease Control and Prevention (CDC), "Guidelines for Treatment of Malaria in the United States," Treatment Table Update, May 18, 2009. Available at http://www.cdc.gov/malaria/pdf/treatmenttable.pdf

◆ **Quinine Sulfate** *see* QuiNINE *on page 1567*

Quinupristin and Dalfopristin (kwi NYOO pris tin & dal FOE pris tin)

Related Information

Antibiotic Treatment of Adults With Infective Endocarditis *on page 2053*

Brand Names: U.S. Synercid®

Brand Names: Canada Synercid®

Index Terms Dalfopristin and Quinupristin; Pristinamycin; RP-59500

Generic Availability (U.S.) No

Pharmacologic Category Antibiotic, Streptogramin

Use Treatment of complicated skin and skin structure infections caused by methicillin-susceptible *Staphylococcus aureus* or *Streptococcus pyogenes*

Contraindications Hypersensitivity to quinupristin, dalfopristin, pristinamycin, or virginiamycin, or any component of the formulation

Warnings/Precautions Use with caution in patients with hepatic or renal dysfunction. May cause pain and phlebitis when infused through a peripheral line (not relieved by hydrocortisone or diphenhydramine). Prolonged use may result in fungal or bacterial superinfection, including *C. difficile*-associated diarrhea (CDAD) and pseudomembranous colitis; CDAD has been observed >2 months postantibiotic treatment. May cause arthralgias, myalgias, and hyperbilirubinemia. May inhibit the metabolism of many drugs metabolized by CYP3A4. Concurrent therapy with cisapride (which may prolong QT_c interval and lead to arrhythmias) should be avoided.

Adverse Reactions (Reflective of adult population; not specific for elderly)

>10%:

Hepatic: Hyperbilirubinemia (3% to 35%)

Local: Local pain (40% to 44%), inflammation at infusion site (38% to 42%), local edema (17% to 18%), infusion site reaction (12% to 13%)

Neuromuscular & skeletal: Arthralgia (up to 47%), myalgia (up to 47%)

1% to 10%:

Central nervous system: Pain (2% to 3%), headache (2%)

Dermatologic: Rash (3%), pruritus (2%)

Endocrine & metabolic: Hyperglycemia (1%)

Gastrointestinal: Nausea (3% to 5%), vomiting (3% to 4%), diarrhea (3%)

Hematologic: Anemia (3%)

Hepatic: GGT increased (2%), LDH increased (3%)

Local: Thrombophlebitis (2%)

Neuromuscular & skeletal: CPK increased (2%)

Drug Interactions

Metabolism/Transport Effects Quinupristin: **Inhibits** CYP3A4 (weak)

Avoid Concomitant Use There are no known interactions where it is recommended to avoid concomitant use.

Increased Effect/Toxicity

Quinupristin and Dalfopristin may increase the levels/effects of: CycloSPORINE; CycloSPORINE (Systemic)

Decreased Effect There are no known significant interactions involving a decrease in effect.

Stability Store unopened vials under refrigeration at 2°C to 8°C (36°F to 46°F). The following stability information has also been reported: May be stored at room temperature for up to 7 days (Cohen, 2007).

Reconstitute single dose vial with 5 mL of 5% dextrose in water or sterile water for injection. Swirl gently to dissolve; do not shake (to limit foam formation). The reconstituted solution should be diluted within 30 minutes. Stability of the diluted solution prior to the infusion is established as 5 hours at room temperature or 54 hours if refrigerated at 2°C to 8°C (36°F to 46°F). Reconstituted solution should be added to at least 250 mL of 5% dextrose in water for peripheral administration (increase to 500 mL or 750 mL if necessary to limit venous irritation). An infusion volume of 100 mL may be used for central line infusions. Do not freeze solution.

Mechanism of Action Quinupristin/dalfopristin inhibits bacterial protein synthesis by binding to different sites on the 50S bacterial ribosomal subunit thereby inhibiting protein synthesis

Pharmacodynamics/Kinetics

Distribution: Quinupristin: 0.45 L/kg; Dalfopristin: 0.24 L/kg

Metabolism: To active metabolites via nonenzymatic reactions

Half-life elimination: Quinupristin: 0.85 hour; Dalfopristin: 0.7 hour (mean elimination half-lives, including metabolites: 3 and 1 hours, respectively)

Excretion: Feces (75% to 77% as unchanged drug and metabolites); urine (15% to 19%)

Dosage

Geriatric & Adult Complicated skin and skin structure infection: I.V.: 7.5 mg/kg every 12 hours for at least 7 days

Renal Impairment No adjustment is necessary in renal failure, hemodialysis, or peritoneal dialysis.

Hepatic Impairment Pharmacokinetic data suggest dosage adjustment may be necessary; however, specific recommendations have not been proposed.

Administration Line should be flushed with 5% dextrose in water prior to and following administration. Infusion should be completed over 60 minutes (toxicity may be increased with shorter infusion). If severe venous irritation occurs following peripheral administration of quinupristin/dalfopristin diluted in 250 mL 5% dextrose in water, consideration should be given to increasing the infusion volume to 500 mL or 750 mL, changing the infusion site, or infusing by a peripherally-inserted central catheter (PICC) or a central venous catheter.

Special Geriatric Considerations No pharmacokinetic changes in the elderly in one study. No dose adjustment necessary.

Dosage Forms Excipient information presented when available (limited, particularly for generics); consult specific product labeling.

Injection, powder for reconstitution:
Synercid®: 500 mg: Quinupristin 150 mg and dalfopristin 350 mg

Selected References
Bryson HM and Spencer CM, "Quinupristin/Dalfopristin," *Drugs*, 1996, 52(3):406-15.

Chant C and Rybak MH, "Quinupristin/Dalfopristin (RP 59500): A New Streptogramin Antibiotic," *Ann Pharmacother*, 1995, 29(10):1022-7.

Griswold MW, Lomaestro BM, and Briceland LL, "Quinupristin-Dalfopristin (RP 59500): An Injectable Streptogramin Combination," *Am J Health Syst Pharm*, 1996, 53(17):2045-53.

◆ **Quixin®** see Levofloxacin (Ophthalmic) *on page 1055*
◆ **Qutenza™** see Capsaicin *on page 261*
◆ **QVAR®** see Beclomethasone (Oral Inhalation) *on page 184*
◆ **R-1569** see Tocilizumab *on page 1816*
◆ **RabAvert®** see Rabies Vaccine *on page 1575*

RABEprazole (ra BEP ra zole)

Related Information
Helicobacter pylori Treatment in Adult Patients *on page 2009*

Medication Safety Issues
Sound-alike/look-alike issues:
AcipHex® may be confused with Acephen®, Accupril®, Aricept®, pHisoHex®
RABEprazole may be confused with ARIPiprazole, donepezil, lansoprazole, omeprazole, raloxifene

Brand Names: U.S. AcipHex®

Brand Names: Canada Pariet®; PMS-Rabeprazole EC; PRO-Rabeprazole; Rabeprazole EC; RAN™-Rabeprazole; Riva-Rabeprazole EC; Sandoz-Rabeprazole; Teva-Rabeprazole EC

Index Terms Pariprazole

Generic Availability (U.S.) No

Pharmacologic Category Proton Pump Inhibitor; Substituted Benzimidazole

Use Short-term (4-8 weeks) treatment and maintenance of erosive or ulcerative gastro-esophageal reflux disease (GERD); symptomatic GERD; short-term (up to 4 weeks) treatment of duodenal ulcers; long-term treatment of pathological hypersecretory conditions, including Zollinger-Ellison syndrome; *H. pylori* eradication (in combination therapy)

Canadian labeling: Additional uses (not in U.S. labeling): Treatment of nonerosive reflux disease (NERD); treatment of gastric ulcers

Unlabeled/Investigational Use Maintenance of duodenal ulcer

◄ **Contraindications** Hypersensitivity to rabeprazole, substituted benzimidazoles (ie, esome-prazole, lansoprazole, omeprazole, pantoprazole), or any component of the formulation

Warnings/Precautions Use of proton pump inhibitors may increase the risk of gastro-intestinal infections (eg, *Salmonella, Campylobacter*). Use caution in severe hepatic impairment. Relief of symptoms with rabeprazole does not preclude the presence of a gastric malignancy. Decreased *H. pylori* eradication rates have been observed with short-term (≤7 days) combination therapy. The American College of Gastroenterology recommends 10-14 days of therapy (triple or quadruple) for eradication of *H. pylori* (Chey, 2007). Proton pump inhibitors may diminish the therapeutic effect of clopidogrel, thought to be due to reduced formation of the active metabolite of clopidogrel; an increase in the risk of cardiovascular events may occur. The manufacturer of clopidogrel recommends avoidance of concomitant administration of another PPI (ie, omeprazole); given the potency of CYP2C19 inhibitory activity, similar recommendations with rabeprazole would appear prudent. Increased incidence of osteoporosis-related bone fractures of the hip, spine, or wrist may occur with proton pump inhibitor therapy. Patients on high-dose (multiple daily doses) or long-term therapy (≥1 year) should be monitored. Use the lowest effective dose for the shortest duration of time, use vitamin D and calcium supplementation, and follow appropriate guidelines to reduce risk of fractures in patients at risk.

Hypomagnesemia, reported rarely, usually with prolonged PPI use of >3 months (most cases >1 year of therapy); may be symptomatic or asymptomatic; severe cases may cause tetany, seizures, and cardiac arrhythmias. Consider obtaining serum magnesium concentrations prior to beginning long-term therapy, especially if taking concomitant digoxin, diuretics, or other drugs known to cause hypomagnesemia; and periodically thereafter. Hypomagnesemia may be corrected by magnesium supplementation, although discontinuation of rabeprazole may be necessary; magnesium levels typically return to normal within 1 week of stopping.

Adverse Reactions (Reflective of adult population; not specific for elderly)
1% to 10%:
Central nervous system: Pain (3%), headache (2% to 5%)
Gastrointestinal: Diarrhea (3%), flatulence (3%), constipation (2%), nausea (2%)
Respiratory: Pharyngitis (3%)
Miscellaneous: Infection (2%)

Drug Interactions
Metabolism/Transport Effects Substrate (major) of CYP2C19, 3A4; **Inhibits** CYP2C8 (moderate), 2C19 (moderate), 2D6 (weak), 3A4 (weak)

Avoid Concomitant Use
Avoid concomitant use of RABEprazole with any of the following: Delavirdine; Erlotinib; Nelfinavir; Posaconazole; Rilpivirine

Increased Effect/Toxicity
RABEprazole may increase the levels/effects of: Amphetamines; CYP2C19 Substrates; CYP2C8 Substrates (High risk); Dexmethylphenidate; Methotrexate; Methylphenidate; Raltegravir; Saquinavir; Tacrolimus; Tacrolimus (Systemic); Voriconazole

The levels/effects of RABEprazole may be increased by: Conivaptan; Fluconazole; Keto-conazole; Ketoconazole (Systemic)

Decreased Effect
RABEprazole may decrease the levels/effects of: Atazanavir; Bisphosphonate Derivatives; Cefditoren; Clopidogrel; Dabigatran Etexilate; Dasatinib; Delavirdine; Erlotinib; Gefitinib; Indinavir; Iron Salts; Itraconazole; Ketoconazole; Ketoconazole (Systemic); Mesalamine; Mycophenolate; Nelfinavir; Posaconazole; Rilpivirine

The levels/effects of RABEprazole may be decreased by: CYP2C19 Inducers (Strong); CYP3A4 Inducers (Strong); Deferasirox; Herbs (CYP3A4 Inducers); Tipranavir; Tocilizumab

Ethanol/Nutrition/Herb Interactions
Ethanol: Avoid ethanol (may cause gastric mucosal irritation).
Food: High-fat meals may delay absorption, but C_{max} and AUC are not altered.
Herb/Nutraceutical: St John's wort may increase the metabolism and thus decrease the levels/ effects of rabeprazole.

Stability Store at 25°C (77°F). Protect from moisture.

Mechanism of Action Potent proton pump inhibitor; suppresses gastric acid secretion by inhibiting the parietal cell H+/K+ ATP pump

Pharmacodynamics/Kinetics
Onset of action: Within 1 hour
Duration: 24 hours
Absorption: Oral: Well absorbed within 1 hour
Protein binding, serum: ~96%
Metabolism: Hepatic via CYP3A and 2C19 to inactive metabolites
Bioavailability: Oral: ~52%

Half-life elimination (dose dependent): 1-2 hours
Time to peak, plasma: 2-5 hours
Excretion: Urine (90% primarily as thioether carboxylic acid metabolites); remainder in feces

Dosage

Geriatric & Adult

GERD, erosive/ulcerative: Oral: Treatment: 20 mg once daily for 4-8 weeks; if inadequate response, may repeat up to an additional 8 weeks; maintenance: 20 mg once daily
Canadian labeling: Oral: 20 mg once daily for 4 weeks; if inadequate response, may repeat for an additional 4 weeks (lack of symptom control after 4 weeks warrants further evaluation); maintenance: 10 mg once daily (maximum: 20 mg once daily)

GERD, symptomatic: Oral: Treatment: 20 mg once daily for 4 weeks; if inadequate response, may repeat for an additional 4 weeks
Canadian labeling: 10 mg once daily (maximum: 20 mg once daily) for 4 weeks; lack of symptom control after 4 weeks warrants further evaluation

Duodenal ulcer: Oral: 20 mg/day before breakfast for 4 weeks; additional therapy may be required for some patients

Gastric ulcers (*Canadian labeling*): Oral: 20 mg once daily up to 6 weeks; additional therapy may be required for some patients

Helicobacter pylori **eradication:** Oral:
Manufacturer labeling: 20 mg twice daily administered with amoxicillin 1000 mg *and* clarithromycin 500 mg twice daily for 7 days
American College of Gastroenterology guidelines (Chey, 2007):
Nonpenicillin allergy: 20 mg twice daily administered with amoxicillin 1000 mg *and* clarithromycin 500 mg twice daily for 10-14 days
Penicillin allergy: 20 mg twice daily administered with clarithromycin 500 mg *and* metronidazole 500 mg twice daily for 10-14 days **or** 20 mg once or twice daily administered with bismuth subsalicylate 525 mg *and* metronidazole 250 mg *plus* tetracycline 500 mg 4 times/day for 10-14 days

Hypersecretory conditions: Oral: 60 mg once daily; dose may need to be adjusted as necessary. Doses as high as 100 mg once daily and 60 mg twice daily have been used, and continued as long as necessary (up to 1 year in some patients).

NERD (*Canadian labeling*): Oral: Treatment: 10 mg (maximum: 20 mg once daily) for 4 weeks; lack of symptom control after 4 weeks warrants further evaluation

Renal Impairment No dosage adjustment required.

Hepatic Impairment
Mild-to-moderate: Elimination decreased; no dosage adjustment required.
Severe: Use caution.

Administration May be administered without regard to meals; best if taken before breakfast. Do not crush, split, or chew tablet. May be administered with an antacid.

Special Geriatric Considerations No difference in efficacy or safety was noted in elderly subjects as compared to younger subjects. No dosage adjustment is necessary in the elderly.

An increased risk of fractures of the hip, spine, or wrist has been observed in epidemiologic studies with proton pump inhibitor (PPI) use, primarily in older adults ≥50 years of age. The greatest risk was seen in patients receiving high doses or on long-term therapy (≥1 year). Calcium and vitamin D supplementation and close monitoring are recommended to reduce the risk of fracture in high-risk patients.

Dosage Forms Excipient information presented when available (limited, particularly for generics); consult specific product labeling.
Tablet, delayed release, enteric coated, oral, as sodium:
AcipHex®: 20 mg

Dosage Forms: Canada Excipient information presented when available (limited, particularly for generics); consult specific product labeling.
Tablet, delayed release, enteric coated, as sodium:
Pariet®: 10 mg, 20 mg

Selected References
Chey WD, Wong BC, et al, "American College of Gastroenterology Guideline on the Management of *Helicobacter pylori* Infection," *Am J Gastroent*, 2007, 102(8):1808-25.
Paoluzi P, Iacopini F, Crispino P, et al, "2-Week Triple Therapy for *Helicobacter pylori* Infection is Better Than 1-Week in Clinical Practice: a Large Prospective Single-Center Randomized Study," *Helicobacter*, 2006, 11(6):562-8.

Rabies Immune Globulin (Human) (RAY beez i MYUN GLOB yoo lin, HYU man)

Related Information
Immunization Administration Recommendations *on page 2037*
Immunization Recommendations *on page 2043*
Brand Names: U.S. HyperRAB™ S/D; Imogam® Rabies-HT
Brand Names: Canada HyperRAB™ S/D; Imogam® Rabies Pasteurized

Index Terms HRIG; RIG

Generic Availability (U.S.) No

Pharmacologic Category Blood Product Derivative; Immune Globulin

Use Part of postexposure prophylaxis of persons with rabies exposure. Provides passive immunity until active immunity with rabies vaccine is established. Not for use in persons with a history of pre-exposure vaccination, history of postexposure prophylaxis, or previous vaccination with rabies vaccine and documentation of antibody response.

Contraindications There are no contraindications listed within the FDA-approved manufacturer's labeling.

Warnings/Precautions Hypersensitivity and anaphylactic reactions can occur; immediate treatment (including epinephrine 1:1000) should be available. Use with caution in patients with isolated immunoglobulin A deficiency or a history of systemic hypersensitivity to human immunoglobulins. Use with caution in patients with thrombocytopenia or coagulation disorders; I.M. injections may be contraindicated. Product of human plasma; may potentially contain infectious agents which could transmit disease. Screening of donors, as well as testing and/or inactivation or removal of certain viruses, reduces the risk. Infections thought to be transmitted by this product should be reported to the manufacturer. Not for intravenous administration.

Adverse Reactions (Reflective of adult population; not specific for elderly) Frequency not defined.

Central nervous system: Fever (mild), headache, malaise

Dermatologic: Angioneurotic edema, rash

Local: Injection site: Pain, stiffness, soreness, tenderness

Renal: Nephrotic syndrome

Miscellaneous: Anaphylaxis

Drug Interactions

Avoid Concomitant Use There are no known interactions where it is recommended to avoid concomitant use.

Increased Effect/Toxicity There are no known significant interactions involving an increase in effect.

Decreased Effect

Rabies Immune Globulin (Human) may decrease the levels/effects of: Vaccines (Live)

Stability Store between 2°C to 8°C (36°F to 46°F); do not freeze. Discard product exposed to freezing. The following stability information has also been reported for HyperRAB™ S/D: May be exposed to room temperature for a cumulative 7 days (Cohen, 2007).

Mechanism of Action Rabies immune globulin is a solution of globulins dried from the plasma or serum of selected adult human donors who have been immunized with rabies vaccine and have developed high titers of rabies antibody. It generally contains 10% to 18% of protein of which not less than 80% is monomeric immunoglobulin G.

Dosage

Geriatric & Adult Postexposure prophylaxis: Local wound infiltration: 20 units/kg in a single dose, RIG should always be administered as part of rabies vaccine regimen. If anatomically feasible, the full rabies immune globulin dose should be infiltrated around and into the wound(s); remaining volume should be administered I.M. at a site distant from the vaccine administration site. If rabies vaccine was initiated without rabies immune globulin, rabies immune globulin may be administered through the seventh day after the administration of the first dose of the vaccine. Administration of RIG is not recommended after the seventh day post vaccine since an antibody response to the vaccine is expected during this time period.

Note: Not for use in persons with a history of pre-exposure vaccination, history of postexposure prophylaxis, or previous vaccination with rabies vaccine and documentation of antibody response.

Administration Do not administer I.V.

Postexposure wound infiltration: If anatomically feasible, the full rabies immune globulin dose should be infiltrated around and into the wound(s); remaining volume should be administered I.M. in the deltoid muscle of the upper arm or lateral thigh muscle. The gluteal area should be avoided to reduce the risk of sciatic nerve damage. Do not administer rabies vaccine in the same syringe or at the same administration site as RIG.

Monitoring Parameters Monitor for adverse effects

Special Geriatric Considerations No special considerations are needed for initiating therapy. No specific data relevant to the elderly to date.

Dosage Forms Excipient information presented when available (limited, particularly for generics); consult specific product labeling.

Injection, solution [preservative free]:

HyperRAB™ S/D: 150 int. units/mL (2 mL, 10 mL) [solvent/detergent treated]

Imogam® Rabies-HT: 150 int. units/mL (2 mL, 10 mL) [heat treated]

Selected References
Centers for Disease Control, "Recommendations of the Advisory Committee on Immunization Practices (ACIP): General Recommendations on Immunization," *MMWR Recomm Rep*, 2002, 51(RR-2):1-36.
Centers for Disease Control and Prevention, "Human Rabies Prevention - United States, 2008 Recommendations of the Advisory Committee on Immunization Practices (ACIP)," *MMWR Recomm Rep*, 2008, 57(RR-3):1-28.

Rabies Vaccine (RAY beez vak SEEN)

Related Information
Immunization Administration Recommendations *on page 2037*
Immunization Recommendations *on page 2043*
Brand Names: U.S. Imovax® Rabies; RabAvert®
Brand Names: Canada Imovax® Rabies; RabAvert®
Index Terms HDCV; Human Diploid Cell Cultures Rabies Vaccine; PCEC; Purified Chick Embryo Cell
Generic Availability (U.S.) No
Pharmacologic Category Vaccine, Inactivated (Viral)
Use Pre-exposure and postexposure vaccination against rabies

The Advisory Committee on Immunization Practices (ACIP) recommends a primary course of prophylactic immunization (pre-exposure vaccination) for the following:
• Persons with continuous risk of infection, including rabies research laboratory and biologics production workers
• Persons with frequent risk of infection in areas where rabies is enzootic, including rabies diagnostic laboratory workers, cavers, veterinarians and their staff, and animal control and wildlife workers; persons who frequently handle bats
• Persons with infrequent risk of infection, including veterinarians and animal control staff with terrestrial animals in areas where rabies infection is rare, veterinary students, and travelers visiting areas where rabies is enzootic and immediate access to medical care and biologicals is limited

The ACIP recommends the use of postexposure vaccination for a particular person be assessed by the severity and likelihood versus the actual risk of acquiring rabies. Consideration should include the type of exposure, epidemiology of rabies in the area, species of the animal, circumstances of the incident, and the availability of the exposing animal for observation or rabies testing. Postexposure vaccination is used in both previously vaccinated and previously unvaccinated individuals.

Contraindications
Pre-exposure prophylaxis: Hypersensitivity to rabies vaccine or any component of the formulation
Postexposure prophylaxis: There are no contraindications listed within the FDA-approved manufacturer's labeling.

Warnings/Precautions Rabies vaccine should not be used in persons with a confirmed diagnosis of rabies; use after the onset of symptoms may be detrimental. Postexposure vaccination may begin regardless of the length of time from documented or likely exposure, as long as clinical signs of rabies are not present. Immediate treatment (including epinephrine 1:1000) for anaphylactoid and/or hypersensitivity reactions should be available during vaccine use. Once postexposure prophylaxis has begun, administration should generally not be interrupted or discontinued due to local or mild adverse events. Continuation of vaccination following severe systemic reactions should consider the persons risk of developing rabies. Report serious reactions to the State Health Department or the manufacturer/distributor. An immune complex reaction is possible 2-21 days following booster doses of HDCV. Symptoms may include arthralgia, arthritis, angioedema, fever, generalized urticaria, malaise, nausea, and vomiting. Use with caution in severely immunocompromised patients (eg, patients receiving chemo/radiation therapy or other immunosuppressive therapy [including high-dose corticosteroids]); may have a reduced response to vaccination. Withhold nonessential immunosuppressive agents during postexposure prophylaxis; if possible postpone pre-exposure prophylaxis until the immunocompromising condition is resolved. Persons with altered immunocompetence should receive the five-dose postexposure vaccine regimen. In general, household and close contacts of persons with altered immunocompetence may receive all age appropriate vaccines. Imovax® Rabies contains albumin and neomycin. RabAvert® contains amphotericin B, bovine gelatin, chicken protein, chlortetracycline, and neomycin. For I. M. administration only.

Adverse Reactions (Reflective of adult population; not specific for elderly) All serious adverse reactions must be reported to the U.S. Department of Health and Human Services (DHHS) Vaccine Adverse Event Reporting System (VAERS) 1-800-822-7967 or online at https://vaers.hhs.gov/esub/index. In Canada, adverse reactions may be reported to local provincial/territorial health agencies or to the Vaccine Safety Section at Public Health Agency of Canada (1-866-844-0018).

>10%:
Central nervous system: Dizziness, headache, malaise
Gastrointestinal: Abdominal pain, nausea
Local: Erythema, itching, pain, swelling
Neuromuscular & skeletal: Myalgia
Miscellaneous: Lymphadenopathy
Uncommon, frequency not defined, postmarketing, and/or case reports:
Cardiovascular: Circulatory reactions, edema, palpitation
Central nervous system: Chills, fatigue, fever >38°C (100°F), Guillain-Barré syndrome, encephalitis, meningitis, multiple sclerosis, myelitis, neuroparalysis, vertigo
Dermatologic: Pruritus, urticaria, urticaria pigmentosa
Endocrine & metabolic: Hot flashes
Local: Limb swelling (extensive)
Neuromuscular & skeletal: Limb pain, monoarthritis, paralysis (transient), paresthesias (transient)
Ocular: Retrobulbar neuritis, visual disturbances
Respiratory: Bronchospasm
Miscellaneous: Allergic reactions, anaphylaxis, hypersensitivity reactions, swollen lymph nodes

Drug Interactions

Avoid Concomitant Use There are no known interactions where it is recommended to avoid concomitant use.

Increased Effect/Toxicity There are no known significant interactions involving an increase in effect.

Decreased Effect
The levels/effects of Rabies Vaccine may be decreased by: Belimumab; Chloroquine; Fingolimod; Immunosuppressants

Stability Prior to reconstitution, store under refrigeration at 2°C to 8°C (36°F to 46°F); do not freeze. Protect from light. Reconstitute with provided diluent; gently swirl to dissolve. Use immediately after reconstitution.
Imovax®: Suspension will appear pink to red
RabAvert®: Suspension will appear clear to slightly opaque

Mechanism of Action Rabies vaccine is an inactivated virus vaccine which promotes immunity by inducing an active immune response. The production of specific antibodies requires about 7-10 days to develop. Rabies immune globulin or antirabies serum, equine (ARS) is given in conjunction with rabies vaccine to provide immune protection until an antibody response can occur.

Pharmacodynamics/Kinetics
Onset of action: I.M.: Rabies antibody: ~7-10 days
Peak effect: ~30-60 days
Duration: ≥1 year

Dosage

Geriatric & Adult

Pre-exposure vaccination: I.M.: A total of 3 doses, 1 mL each, on days 0, 7, and 21-28.
Note: Prolonging the interval between doses does not interfere with immunity achieved after the concluding dose of the basic series.

Postexposure vaccination: All postexposure treatment should begin with immediate cleansing of the wound with soap and water
Persons not previously immunized as above: I.M.: 5 doses (1 mL each) on days 0, 3, 7, 14, 28. In addition, patients should receive rabies immune globulin with the first dose (day 0).
Note: A regimen of 4 doses (1 mL each) on days 0, 3, 7, 14 may be used in persons who are not immunosuppressed (ACIP recommendations, 2010).

Persons who have previously received postexposure prophylaxis with rabies vaccine, received a recommended I.M. pre-exposure series of rabies vaccine or have a previously documented rabies antibody titer considered adequate: I.M.: Two doses (1 mL each) on days 0 and 3; do not administer rabies immune globulin

Booster (for persons with continuous or frequent risk of infection): I.M.: 1 mL based on antibody titers

Administration For I.M. administration only; this rabies vaccine product must not be administered intradermally; in adults, administer I.M. injections in the deltoid muscle, not the gluteal. Postexposure prophylaxis should begin with immediate cleansing of wounds with soap and water; if available, a virucidal agent (eg povidone-iodine solution) should be used to irrigate the wounds.

For patients at risk of hemorrhage following intramuscular injection, the ACIP recommends "it should be administered intramuscularly if, in the opinion of the physician familiar with the patients bleeding risk, the vaccine can be administered by this route with reasonable safety. If the patient receives antihemophilia or other similar therapy, intramuscular vaccination can be scheduled shortly after such therapy is administered. A fine needle (23 gauge or smaller) can be used for the vaccination and firm pressure applied to the site (without rubbing) for at least 2 minutes. The patient should be instructed concerning the risk of hematoma from the injection." Patients on anticoagulant therapy should be considered to have the same bleeding risks and treated as those with clotting factor disorders (CDC, 2011).

Simultaneous administration of vaccines helps ensure the patients will be fully vaccinated by the appropriate age. Simultaneous administration of vaccines is defined as administering >1 vaccine on the same day at different anatomic sites. The use of licensed combination vaccines is generally preferred over separate injections of the equivalent components. Separate vaccines should not be combined in the same syringe unless indicated by product specific labeling. Separate needles and syringes should be used for each injection. The ACIP prefers each dose of a specific vaccine in a series come from the same manufacturer when possible. Adolescents and adults should be vaccinated while seated or lying down. In general, preterm infants should be vaccinated at the same chronological age as full-term infants (CDC, 2011).

Antipyretics have not been shown to prevent febrile seizures. Antipyretics may be used to treat fever or discomfort following vaccination (CDC, 2011). One study reported that routine prophylactic administration of acetaminophen to prevent fever prior to vaccination decreased the immune response of some vaccines; the clinical significance of this reduction in immune response has not been established (Prymula, 2009).

Monitoring Parameters Monitor for syncope for ≥15 minutes following vaccination.

Antibody response to vaccination is not recommended for otherwise healthy persons who complete the pre-exposure or postexposure regimen. Serologic testing to determine if the antibody titer is at an acceptable level is required for the following persons (booster vaccination recommended if titer is below the acceptable level):

Persons with continuous risk of infection: Serologic testing every 6 months

Persons with frequent risk of infection: Serologic testing every 2 years

Persons who are immunocompromised: Serologic testing after completion of pre-exposure or postexposure prophylaxis series

Monitoring of antibody response to vaccination is not recommended for otherwise healthy persons who complete the pre-exposure or postexposure regimen.

Reference Range Adequate adaptive immune response: antibody titers of 0.5 int. units/mL [WHO] or complete virus neutralization at a 1:5 serum dilution by the rapid fluorescent focus inhibition test (RFFIT) [ACIP]

Pharmacotherapy Pearls Federal law requires that the name of medication, date of administration, the vaccine manufacturer, lot number of vaccine, and the administering person's name, title, and address be entered into the patient's permanent medical record.

Special Geriatric Considerations No specific data for use in the elderly. Use as recommended in elderly patients for whom this vaccine would be indicated.

Dosage Forms Excipient information presented when available (limited, particularly for generics); consult specific product labeling.

Injection, powder for reconstitution [preservative free]:

Imovax® Rabies: ≥ 2.5 int. units [contains albumin (human), neomycin (may have trace amounts); HDCV; grown in human diploid cell culture]

RabAvert®: ≥ 2.5 int. units [contains albumin (human), amphotericin B (may have trace amounts), bovine gelatin, chicken egg protein, chlortetracycline (may have trace amounts), neomycin (may have trace amounts); PCEC; grown in chicken fibroblast culture]

Selected References

Centers for Disease Control and Prevention, "ACIP Provisional Recommendations for the Prevention of Human Rabies," available at http://www.cdc.gov/vaccines/recs/provisional/downloads/rabies-July2009-508.pdf

Centers for Disease Control, "Recommendations of the Advisory Committee on Immunization Practices (ACIP): General Recommendations on Immunization," *MMWR Recomm Rep*, 2006, 55(RR-15):1-48.

Centers for Disease Control and Prevention, "Human Rabies Prevention - United States, 2008 Recommendations of the Advisory Committee on Immunization Practices (ACIP)," *MMWR Recomm Rep*, 2008, 57(RR-3):1-28.

Dreesen DW and Hanlon CA, "Current Recommendations for the Prophylaxis and Treatment of Rabies," *Drugs*, 1998, 56(5):801-9.

◆ **Racemic Epinephrine** *see* EPINEPHrine (Systemic, Oral Inhalation) *on page 606*

◆ **Racepinephrine** *see* EPINEPHrine (Systemic, Oral Inhalation) *on page 606*

◆ **R-albuterol** *see* Levalbuterol *on page 1043*

Raloxifene (ral OKS i feen)

Related Information
Osteoporosis Management *on page 2027*

Medication Safety Issues
Sound-alike/look-alike issues:
Evista® may be confused with Avinza™, Eovist®

Brand Names: U.S. Evista®

Brand Names: Canada Apo-Raloxifene®; Evista®; Novo-Raloxifene

Index Terms Keoxifene Hydrochloride; Raloxifene Hydrochloride

Generic Availability (U.S.) No

Pharmacologic Category Selective Estrogen Receptor Modulator (SERM)

Use Prevention and treatment of osteoporosis in postmenopausal women; risk reduction for invasive breast cancer in postmenopausal women with osteoporosis and in postmenopausal women with high risk for invasive breast cancer

Medication Guide Available Yes

Contraindications History of or current venous thromboembolic disorders (including DVT, PE, and retinal vein thrombosis)

Warnings/Precautions Hazardous agent - use appropriate precautions for handling and disposal. **[U.S. Boxed Warning]: May increase the risk for DVT or PE; use contra-indicated in patients with history of or current venous thromboembolic disorders.** Use with caution in patients at high risk for venous thromboembolism; the risk for DVT and PE are higher in the first 4 months of treatment. Discontinue at least 72 hours prior to and during prolonged immobilization (postoperative recovery or prolonged bedrest). **[U.S. Boxed Warning]: The risk of death due to stroke may be increased in women with coronary heart disease or in women at risk for coronary events;** use with caution in patients with cardiovascular disease. Not be used for the prevention of cardiovascular disease. Use caution with moderate-to-severe renal dysfunction, hepatic impairment, unexplained uterine bleeding, and in women with a history of elevated triglycerides in response to treatment with oral estrogens (or estrogen/progestin). Safety with concomitant estrogen therapy has not been established. Safety and efficacy in premenopausal women or men have not been established. Not indicated for treatment of invasive breast cancer, to reduce the risk of recurrence of invasive breast cancer or to reduce the risk of noninvasive breast cancer. The efficacy (for breast cancer risk reduction) in women with inherited BRCA1 and BRCA1 mutations has not been established.

Adverse Reactions (Reflective of adult population; not specific for elderly) Note: Raloxifene has been associated with increased risk of thromboembolism (DVT, PE) and superficial thrombophlebitis; risk is similar to reported risk of HRT
>10%:
Cardiovascular: Peripheral edema (3% to 14%)
Endocrine & metabolic: Hot flashes (8% to 29%)
Neuromuscular & skeletal: Arthralgia (11% to 16%), leg cramps/muscle spasm (6% to 12%)
Miscellaneous: Flu syndrome (14% to 15%), infection (11%)
1% to 10%:
Cardiovascular: Chest pain (3%), venous thromboembolism (1% to 2%)
Central nervous system: Insomnia (6%)
Dermatologic: Rash (6%)
Endocrine & metabolic: Breast pain (4%)
Gastrointestinal: Weight gain (9%), abdominal pain (7%), vomiting (5%), flatulence (2% to 3%), cholelithiasis (≤3%), gastroenteritis (≤3%)
Genitourinary: Vaginal bleeding (6%), leukorrhea (3%), urinary tract disorder (3%), uterine disorder (3%), vaginal hemorrhage (3%), endometrial disorder (≤3%)
Neuromuscular & skeletal: Myalgia (8%), tendon disorder (4%)
Respiratory: Bronchitis (10%), sinusitis (10%), pharyngitis (8%), pneumonia (3%), laryngitis (≤2%)
Miscellaneous: Diaphoresis (3%)

Drug Interactions
Avoid Concomitant Use There are no known interactions where it is recommended to avoid concomitant use.
Increased Effect/Toxicity There are no known significant interactions involving an increase in effect.
Decreased Effect
Raloxifene may decrease the levels/effects of: Levothyroxine

The levels/effects of Raloxifene may be decreased by: Bile Acid Sequestrants

Ethanol/Nutrition/Herb Interactions Ethanol: Avoid ethanol (may increase risk of osteoporosis).

Stability Store at controlled room temperature of 20°C to 25°C (68°F to 77°F); excursions permitted to 15°C to 30°C (59°F to 86°F).

Mechanism of Action A selective estrogen receptor modulator (SERM), meaning that it affects some of the same receptors that estrogen does, but not all, and in some instances, it antagonizes or blocks estrogen; it acts like estrogen to prevent bone loss and has the potential to block some estrogen effects in the breast and uterine tissues. Raloxifene decreases bone resorption, increasing bone mineral density and decreasing fracture incidence.

Pharmacodynamics/Kinetics
Onset of action: 8 weeks
Absorption: Rapid; ~60%
Distribution: 2348 L/kg
Protein binding: >95% to albumin and α-glycoprotein; does not bind to sex-hormone-binding globulin
Metabolism: Hepatic, extensive first-pass effect; metabolized to glucuronide conjugates
Bioavailability: ~2%
Half-life elimination: 28-33 hours
Excretion: Primarily feces; urine (<0.2% as unchanged drug; <6% as glucuronide conjugates)

Dosage
Geriatric & Adult
Osteoporosis: Females: Oral: 60 mg once daily
Invasive breast cancer risk reduction: Female: Oral: 60 mg once daily for 5 years per ASCO guidelines (Visvanathan, 2009)
Renal Impairment Moderate-to-severe impairment: Use caution; safety and efficacy have not been established.
Hepatic Impairment Mild impairment (Child-Pugh class A): Plasma concentrations were higher and correlated with total bilirubin. Safety and efficacy in hepatic insufficiency have not been established.

Administration May be administered any time of the day without regard to meals.

Monitoring Parameters Bone mineral density (BMD), lipid profile; adequate diagnostic measures, including endometrial sampling, if indicated, should be performed to rule out malignancy in all cases of undiagnosed abnormal vaginal bleeding

Pharmacotherapy Pearls The decrease in estrogen-related adverse effects with the selective estrogen-receptor modulators in general and raloxifene in particular should improve compliance and decrease the incidence of cardiovascular events and fractures while not increasing breast cancer.

Oncology Comment: The American Society of Clinical Oncology (ASCO) guidelines for breast cancer risk reduction (Visvanathan, 2009) recommend raloxifene (for 5 years) as an option to reduce the risk of ER-positive invasive breast cancer in postmenopausal women with a 5-year projected risk (based on NCI trial model) of ≥1.66%, or with lobular carcinoma *in situ*. Raloxifene should not be used in premenopausal women. Women with osteoporosis may use raloxifene beyond 5 years of treatment. According to the NCCN breast cancer risk reduction guidelines (v.2.2009), raloxifene is only recommended for postmenopausal women (≥35 years of age), and is equivalent to tamoxifen although, raloxifene has a better adverse event profile; however, tamoxifen is superior in reducing the risk on noninvasive breast cancer.

Special Geriatric Considerations Raloxifene has only been shown to prevent vertebral fractures. Women may experience hot flushes, leg cramps, and peripheral edema. Avoid in bedbound patients due to increased risk of thromboembolism. The U.S. Preventive Services Task Force (USPSTF) recommends against routine use of raloxifene (or tamoxifen) for the primary prevention of breast cancer in women at low or average risk.

Dosage Forms Excipient information presented when available (limited, particularly for generics); consult specific product labeling.
Tablet, oral, as hydrochloride:
Evista®: 60 mg

Selected References
Delmas PD, Bjarnason NH, Mitlak BH, et al, "Effects of Raloxifene on Bone Mineral Density, Serum Cholesterol Concentrations, and Uterine Endometrium in Postmenopausal Women," N Engl J Med, 1997, 337(23):1641-7.
Land SR, Wickerham DL, Costantino JP, et al, "Patient-Reported Symptoms and Quality of Life During Treatment With Tamoxifen or Raloxifene for Breast Cancer Prevention: The NSABP Study of Tamoxifen and Raloxifene (STAR) P-2 Trial," JAMA, 2006, 295(23):2742-51.
NCCN (National Comprehensive Cancer Network), "Practice Guidelines in Oncology: Breast Cancer Risk Reduction Version 1.2007," available at http://www.nccn.org/professionals/physician_gls/PDF/breast_risk.pdf
Vogel VG, Costantino JP, Wickerham DL, "Effects of Tamoxifen vs Raloxifene on the Risk of Developing Invasive Breast Cancer and Other Disease Outcomes: The NSABP Study of Tamoxifen and Raloxifene (STAR) P-2 Trial," JAMA, 2006, 295(23):2727-41.

◆ **Raloxifene Hydrochloride** see Raloxifene on page 1578

Ramelteon (ra MEL tee on)

Medication Safety Issues
Sound-alike/look-alike issues:
Ramelteon may be confused with Remeron®
Rozerem® may be confused with Razadyne®, Remeron®

Brand Names: U.S. Rozerem™
Index Terms TAK-375
Generic Availability (U.S.) No
Pharmacologic Category Hypnotic, Nonbenzodiazepine
Use Treatment of insomnia characterized by difficulty with sleep onset
Medication Guide Available Yes
Contraindications History of angioedema with previous ramelteon therapy (do not rechallenge); concurrent use with fluvoxamine
Warnings/Precautions Symptomatic treatment of insomnia should be initiated only after careful evaluation of potential causes of sleep disturbance. Failure of sleep disturbance to resolve after a reasonable period of treatment may indicate psychiatric and/or medical illness. Because of the rapid onset of action, administer immediately prior to bedtime or after the patient has gone to bed and is having difficulty falling asleep. Hypnotics/sedatives have been associated with abnormal thinking and behavior changes including decreased inhibition, aggression, bizarre behavior, agitation, hallucinations, and depersonalization. These changes may occur unpredictably and may indicate previously unrecognized psychiatric disorders; evaluate appropriately. Postmarketing studies have indicated that the use of hypnotic/sedative agents (including ramelteon) for sleep has been associated with hypersensitivity reactions including anaphylaxis as well as angioedema. Do not rechallenge patients who have developed angioedema with ramelteon therapy. An increased risk for hazardous sleep-related activities such as sleep-driving; cooking and eating food, and making phone calls while asleep have also been noted. Use caution with pre-existing depression or other psychiatric conditions. Caution when using with other CNS depressants; avoid engaging in hazardous activities or activities requiring mental alertness. Not recommended for use in patients with severe sleep apnea or COPD. Use caution with moderate hepatic impairment; not recommended in patients with severe impairment. May cause disturbances of hormonal regulation. Use caution when administered concomitantly with strong CYP1A2 inhibitors.

Adverse Reactions (Reflective of adult population; not specific for elderly)
1% to 10%:
Central nervous system: Dizziness (4% to 5%), somnolence (3% to 5%), fatigue (3% to 4%), insomnia worsened (3%), depression (2%)
Endocrine & metabolic: Serum cortisol decreased (1%)
Gastrointestinal: Nausea (3%), taste perversion (2%)
Neuromuscular & skeletal: Myalgia (2%), arthralgia (2%)
Respiratory: Upper respiratory infection (3%)
Miscellaneous: Influenza (1%)

Drug Interactions
Metabolism/Transport Effects Substrate of CYP1A2 (major), CYP3A4 (minor), CYP2C family (minor)
Avoid Concomitant Use
Avoid concomitant use of Ramelteon with any of the following: FluvoxaMINE
Increased Effect/Toxicity
Ramelteon may increase the levels/effects of: Alcohol (Ethyl); CNS Depressants; Methotrimeprazine; Selective Serotonin Reuptake Inhibitors

The levels/effects of Ramelteon may be increased by: Abiraterone Acetate; Antifungal Agents (Azole Derivatives, Systemic); Conivaptan; CYP1A2 Inhibitors (Moderate); CYP1A2 Inhibitors (Strong); Deferasirox; Droperidol; Fluconazole; FluvoxaMINE; HydrOXYzine; Methotrimeprazine
Decreased Effect
The levels/effects of Ramelteon may be decreased by: Cyproterone; Rifamycin Derivatives; Tocilizumab

Ethanol/Nutrition/Herb Interactions
Ethanol: May increase CNS depression; monitor for increased effects with coadministration. Caution patients about effects.
Food: Taking with high-fat meal delays T_{max} and increases AUC (~31%).
Herb/Nutraceutical: Avoid valerian, St John's wort, kava kava, gotu kola (may increase CNS depression).

Stability Store at 25°C (77°F); excursions permitted to 15°C to 30°C (59°F to 86°F). Protect from moisture.

Mechanism of Action Potent, selective agonist of melatonin receptors MT_1 and MT_2 (with little affinity for MT_3) within the suprachiasmic nucleus of the hypothalamus, an area responsible for determination of circadian rhythms and synchronization of the sleep-wake cycle. Agonism of MT_1 is thought to preferentially induce sleepiness, while MT_2 receptor activation preferentially influences regulation of circadian rhythms. Ramelteon is eightfold more selective for MT_1 than MT_2 and exhibits nearly sixfold higher affinity for MT_1 than melatonin, presumably allowing for enhanced effects on sleep induction.

Pharmacodynamics/Kinetics
Onset of action: 30 minutes
Absorption: Rapid; high-fat meal delays T_{max} and increases AUC (~31%)
Distribution: 74 L
Protein binding: ~82%
Metabolism: Extensive first-pass effect; oxidative metabolism primarily through CYP1A2 and to a lesser extent through CYP2C and CYP3A4; forms active metabolite (M-II)
Bioavailability: Absolute: 1.8%
Half-life elimination: Ramelteon: 1-2.6 hours; M-II: 2-5 hours
Time to peak, plasma: Median: 0.5-1.5 hours
Excretion: Primarily as metabolites: Urine (84%); feces (4%)

Dosage
Geriatric & Adult Insomnia: Oral: One 8 mg tablet within 30 minutes of bedtime
Renal Impairment No dosage adjustment required
Hepatic Impairment No adjustment required for mild-to-moderate impairment; use caution. Not recommended with severe impairment.

Administration Do not administer with a high-fat meal. Swallow tablet whole; do not break.

Monitoring Parameters Mental status

Special Geriatric Considerations Although the C_{max} and AUC of ramelteon were increased in elderly patients, in clinical trials there were no significant differences in safety or efficacy between elderly and younger adult subjects.

Dosage Forms Excipient information presented when available (limited, particularly for generics); consult specific product labeling.
Tablet, oral:
Rozerem™: 8 mg

Ramipril (RA mi pril)

Related Information
Angiotensin Agents *on page 1985*

Medication Safety Issues
Sound-alike/look-alike issues:
Ramipril may be confused with enalapril, Monopril®
Altace® may be confused with alteplase, Amaryl®, Amerge®, Artane®
International issues:
Altace [Canada] may be confused with Altace HCT brand name for ramipril/hydrochlorothiazide [Canada]

Brand Names: U.S. Altace®

Brand Names: Canada Altace®; Apo-Ramipril®; CO Ramipril; Dom-Ramipril; JAMP-Ramipril; Mylan-Ramipril; PHL-Ramipril; PMS-Ramipril; RAN™-Ramipril; ratio-Ramipril; Sandoz-Ramipril; Teva-Ramipril

Generic Availability (U.S.) Yes: Capsule

Pharmacologic Category Angiotensin-Converting Enzyme (ACE) Inhibitor

Use Treatment of hypertension, alone or in combination with thiazide diuretics; treatment of left ventricular dysfunction after MI; to reduce risk of MI, stroke, and death in patients at increased risk for these events

Unlabeled/Investigational Use Treatment of heart failure; to delay the progression of nephropathy and reduce risks of cardiovascular events in hypertensive patients with type 1 or 2 diabetes mellitus

Contraindications Hypersensitivity to ramipril or any component of the formulation; prior hypersensitivity (including angioedema) to ACE inhibitors

Warnings/Precautions Anaphylactic reactions may occur rarely with ACE inhibitors. At any time during treatment (especially following first dose) angioedema may occur rarely with ACE inhibitors; it may involve the head and neck (potentially compromising airway) or the intestine (presenting with abdominal pain). African-Americans and patients with idiopathic or hereditary angioedema may be at an increased risk. Prolonged frequent monitoring may be required especially if tongue, glottis, or larynx are involved as they are associated with airway obstruction. Patients with a history of airway surgery may have a higher risk of airway obstruction. Aggressive early and appropriate management is critical. Use in patients with previous angioedema associated with ACE inhibitor therapy is contraindicated. Severe anaphylactoid reactions may be seen during hemodialysis (eg, CVVHD) with high-flux dialysis membranes (eg, AN69), and rarely, during low density lipoprotein apheresis with dextran sulfate cellulose. Rare cases of anaphylactoid reactions have been reported in patients undergoing sensitization treatment with hymenoptera (bee, wasp) venom while receiving ACE inhibitors.

Symptomatic hypotension with or without syncope can occur with ACE inhibitors (usually with the first several doses); effects are most often observed in volume-depleted patients; close monitoring of patient is required especially with initial dosing and dosing increases; blood pressure must be lowered at a rate appropriate for the patient's clinical condition. Initiation of therapy in patients with ischemic heart disease or cerebrovascular disease warrants close observation due to the potential consequences posed by falling blood pressure (eg, MI, stroke). Use with caution in hypertrophic cardiomyopathy with outflow tract obstruction, severe aortic stenosis, or before, during, or immediately after major surgery.

Hyperkalemia may occur with ACE inhibitors; risk factors include renal dysfunction, diabetes mellitus, concomitant use of potassium-sparing diuretics, potassium supplements, and/or potassium containing salts. Use cautiously, if at all, with these agents and monitor potassium closely. Cough may occur with ACE inhibitors. Other causes of cough should be considered (eg, pulmonary congestion in patients with heart failure) and excluded prior to discontinuation.

May be associated with deterioration of renal function and/or increases in serum creatinine, particularly in patients with low renal blood flow (eg, renal artery stenosis, heart failure) whose glomerular filtration rate (GFR) is dependent on efferent arteriolar vasoconstriction by angiotensin II; deterioration may result in oliguria, acute renal failure, and progressive azotemia. Small increases in serum creatinine may occur following initiation; consider discontinuation only in patients with progressive and/or significant deterioration in renal function. Use with caution in patients with unstented unilateral/bilateral renal artery stenosis. When unstented bilateral renal artery stenosis is present, use is generally avoided due to the elevated risk of deterioration in renal function unless possible benefits outweigh risks. Concurrent use of angiotensin receptor blockers may increase the risk of clinically-significant adverse events (eg, renal dysfunction, hyperkalemia). Concurrent use with telmisartan is not recommended.

Rare toxicities associated with ACE inhibitors include cholestatic jaundice (which may progress to fulminant hepatic necrosis), agranulocytosis, neutropenia, or leukopenia with myeloid hypoplasia. Patients with collagen vascular diseases (especially with concomitant renal impairment) or renal impairment alone may be at increased risk for hematologic toxicity; periodically monitor CBC with differential in these patients.

Adverse Reactions (Reflective of adult population; not specific for elderly) Note: Frequency ranges include data from hypertension and heart failure trials. Higher rates of adverse reactions have generally been noted in patients with CHF. However, the frequency of adverse effects associated with placebo is also increased in this population.

>10%: Respiratory: Cough increased (7% to 12%)

1% to 10%:
Cardiovascular: Hypotension (11%), angina (up to 3%), postural hypotension (2%), syncope (up to 2%)
Central nervous system: Headache (1% to 5%), dizziness (2% to 4%), fatigue (2%), vertigo (up to 2%)
Endocrine & metabolic: Hyperkalemia (1% to 10%)
Gastrointestinal: Nausea/vomiting (1% to 2%)
Neuromuscular & skeletal: Chest pain (noncardiac) (1%)
Renal: Renal dysfunction (1%), serum creatinine increased (1% to 2%), BUN increased (<1% to 3%); transient increases of creatinine and/or BUN may occur more frequently
Respiratory: Cough (estimated 1% to 10%)

Worsening of renal function may occur in patients with bilateral renal artery stenosis or in hypovolemia. In addition, a syndrome which may include fever, myalgia, arthralgia, interstitial nephritis, vasculitis, rash, eosinophilia and positive ANA, and elevated ESR has been reported with ACE inhibitors. Risk of pancreatitis and agranulocytosis may be increased in patients with collagen vascular disease or renal impairment.

Drug Interactions

Avoid Concomitant Use There are no known interactions where it is recommended to avoid concomitant use.

Increased Effect/Toxicity
Ramipril may increase the levels/effects of: Allopurinol; Amifostine; Antihypertensives; AzaTHIOprine; CycloSPORINE; CycloSPORINE (Systemic); Ferric Gluconate; Gold Sodium Thiomalate; Hypotensive Agents; Iron Dextran Complex; Lithium; Nonsteroidal Anti-Inflammatory Agents; RiTUXimab; Sodium Phosphates

The levels/effects of Ramipril may be increased by: Alfuzosin; Angiotensin II Receptor Blockers; Diazoxide; DPP-IV Inhibitors; Eplerenone; Everolimus; Herbs (Hypotensive Properties); Loop Diuretics; MAO Inhibitors; Pentoxifylline; Phosphodiesterase 5 Inhibitors; Potassium Salts; Potassium-Sparing Diuretics; Prostacyclin Analogues; Sirolimus; Telmisartan; Temsirolimus; Thiazide Diuretics; TiZANidine; Tolvaptan; Trimethoprim

Decreased Effect

The levels/effects of Ramipril may be decreased by: Aprotinin; Herbs (Hypertensive Properties); Icatibant; Lanthanum; Methylphenidate; Nonsteroidal Anti-Inflammatory Agents; Salicylates; Yohimbine

Ethanol/Nutrition/Herb Interactions Herb/Nutraceutical: Avoid bayberry, blue cohosh, cayenne, ephedra, ginger, ginseng (American), kola, licorice (may worsen hypertension). Avoid black cohosh, California poppy, coleus, golden seal, hawthorn, mistletoe, periwinkle, quinine, shepherd's purse (may have increased antihypertensive effect).

Stability Store at controlled room temperature.

Mechanism of Action Ramipril is an ACE inhibitor which prevents the formation of angiotensin II from angiotensin I and exhibits pharmacologic effects that are similar to captopril. Ramipril must undergo enzymatic saponification by esterases in the liver to its biologically active metabolite, ramiprilat. The pharmacodynamic effects of ramipril result from the high-affinity, competitive, reversible binding of ramiprilat to angiotensin-converting enzyme, thus preventing the formation of the potent vasoconstrictor angiotensin II. This isomerized enzyme-inhibitor complex has a slow rate of dissociation, which results in high potency and a long duration of action; a CNS mechanism may also be involved in the hypotensive effect as angiotensin II increases adrenergic outflow from CNS; vasoactive kallikreins may be decreased in conversion to active hormones by ACE inhibitors, thus reducing blood pressure

Pharmacodynamics/Kinetics

Onset of action: 1-2 hours

Duration: 24 hours

Absorption: Well absorbed (50% to 60%)

Distribution: Plasma levels decline in a triphasic fashion; rapid decline is a distribution phase to peripheral compartment, plasma protein and tissue ACE (half-life: 2-4 hours); second phase is an apparent elimination phase representing the clearance of free ramiprilat (half-life: 9-18 hours); and final phase is the terminal elimination phase representing the equilibrium phase between tissue binding and dissociation

Protein binding: Ramipril: 73%; Ramiprilat: 56%

Metabolism: Hepatic to the active form, ramiprilat

Bioavailability: Ramipril: 28%; Ramiprilat: 44%

Half-life elimination: Ramiprilat: Effective: 13-17 hours; Terminal: >50 hours

Time to peak, serum: Ramipril: ~1 hour; Ramiprilat: 2-4 hours

Excretion: Urine (60%) and feces (40%) as parent drug and metabolites

Dosage

Geriatric Refer to adult dosing. Adjust for renal function for elderly since glomerular filtration rates are decreased; may see exaggerated hypotensive effects if renal clearance is not considered.

In the management of hypertension, consider lower initial doses and titrate to response (Aronow, 2011).

Adult

Heart failure (unlabeled use): Initial: 1.25-2.5 mg once daily; target dose: 10 mg once daily (ACC/AHA 2009 Heart Failure Guidelines)

Hypertension: Oral: 2.5-5 mg once daily, maximum: 20 mg/day

LV dysfunction postmyocardial infarction: Oral: Initial: 2.5 mg twice daily titrated upward, if possible, to 5 mg twice daily

To reduce the risk of MI, stroke, and death from cardiovascular causes: Oral: Initial: 2.5 mg once daily for 1 week, then 5 mg once daily for the next 3 weeks, then increase as tolerated to 10 mg once daily (may be given as divided dose)

Note: The dose of any concomitant diuretic should be reduced. If the diuretic cannot be discontinued, initiate therapy with 1.25 mg. After the initial dose, the patient should be monitored carefully until blood pressure has stabilized.

Renal Impairment

Cl_{cr} <40 mL/minute: Administer 25% of normal dose.

Renal failure and heart failure: Administer 1.25 mg once daily, increasing to 1.25 mg twice daily up to 2.5 mg twice daily as tolerated.

Renal failure and hypertension: Administer 1.25 mg once daily, titrated upward as possible; maximum daily dose 5 mg.

Administration Capsule is usually swallowed whole, but may be may be mixed in water, apple juice, or applesauce.

◀ **Monitoring Parameters** Blood pressure; serum creatinine and potassium; if patient has collagen vascular disease and/or renal impairment, periodically monitor CBC with differential

Test Interactions Positive Coombs' [direct]; may cause false-positive results in urine acetone determinations using sodium nitroprusside reagent

Pharmacotherapy Pearls Some patients may have a decreased hypotensive effect between 12 and 16 hours; consider dividing total daily dose into 2 doses 12 hours apart. If patient is receiving a diuretic, a potential for first-dose hypotension is increased. To decrease this potential, stop diuretic for 2-3 days prior to initiating ramipril. If diuretic cannot be stopped temporarily, then initiate therapy with 1.25 mg daily. Continue diuretic if needed to control blood pressure. Capsules should be swallowed whole; if this cannot be done, capsule contents may be mixed with applesauce; also, contents may be mixed with apple juice or water. Mixtures in juice and water are stable for 24 hours at room temperature or 48 hours with refrigeration.

Special Geriatric Considerations Due to frequent decreases in glomerular filtration (also creatinine clearance) with aging, elderly patients may have exaggerated responses to ACE inhibitors; differences in clinical response due to hepatic changes are not observed. ACE inhibitors may be preferred agents in elderly patients with CHF and diabetes mellitus. Diabetic proteinuria is reduced and insulin sensitivity is enhanced. In general, the side effect profile is favorable in the elderly and causes little or no CNS confusion; use lowest dose recommendations initially. Many elderly may be volume depleted due to diuretic use and/or blunted thirst reflex resulting in inadequate fluid intake.

Dosage Forms Excipient information presented when available (limited, particularly for generics); consult specific product labeling. [DSC] = Discontinued product

Capsule, oral: 1.25 mg, 2.5 mg, 5 mg, 10 mg
  Altace®: 1.25 mg, 2.5 mg, 5 mg, 10 mg

Tablet, oral:
  Altace®: 1.25 mg [DSC], 2.5 mg [DSC], 5 mg [DSC], 10 mg [DSC]

Selected References

American Diabetes Association, "Standards of Medical Care in Diabetes Mellitus – 2009," *Diabetes Care*, 2009, 32 (Suppl 1):13-61.

Yusuf S, Sleight P, Pogue J, et al, "Effects of an Angiotensin-Converting-Enzyme Inhibitor, Ramipril, on Cardiovascular Events in High-Risk Patients. The Heart Outcomes Prevention Evaluation Study Investigators," *N Engl J Med*, 2000, 342(3):145-53.

Ramipril and Hydrochlorothiazide (RA mi pril & hye droe klor oh THYE a zide)

Related Information
  Hydrochlorothiazide *on page 876*
  Ramipril *on page 1581*

Medication Safety Issues
  Sound-alike/look-alike issues:
    Altace® HCT may be confused with alteplase, Artane®, Altace®

Brand Names: Canada Altace® HCT; PMS-Ramipril HCTZ

Index Terms Hydrochlorothiazide and Ramipril

Pharmacologic Category Angiotensin-Converting Enzyme (ACE) Inhibitor; Diuretic, Thiazide

Use Treatment of essential hypertension (not for initial therapy)

Dosage
  Geriatric & Adult Hypertension: Oral: **Note:** Not for initial therapy; titration of individual agents to an appropriate clinical response is required before patient is converted over to an equivalent dose of the combination product.
    Usual dosage: Ramipril 2.5 mg/hydrochlorothiazide 12.5 mg once daily; titrate to maximum ramipril 10 mg/hydrochlorothiazide 50 mg once daily
  Renal Impairment
    Cl_{cr} 30-60 mL/minute: Use caution; maximum dose: Ramipril 5 mg/hydrochlorothiazide 25 mg once daily
    Cl_{cr} <30 mL/minute: Hydrochlorothiazide is usually ineffective
  Hepatic Impairment No specific dosing available.

Special Geriatric Considerations See individual agents. Hydrochlorothiazide is not effective in patients with a Cl_{cr} <30 mL/minute; therefore, it may not be a useful agent in many elderly patients.

Product Availability Not available in U.S.

Dosage Forms: Canada Excipient information presented when available (limited, particularly for generics); consult specific product labeling.
  Tablet, oral:
    Altace® HCT 2.5/12.5: Ramipril 2.5 mg and hydrochlorothiazide 12.5 mg
    Altace® HCT 5/12.5: Ramipril 5 mg and hydrochlorothiazide 12.5 mg

Altace® HCT 5/25: Ramipril 5 mg and hydrochlorothiazide 25 mg
Altace® HCT 10/12.5: Ramipril 10 mg and hydrochlorothiazide 12.5 mg
Altace® HCT 10/25: Ramipril 10 mg and hydrochlorothiazide 25 mg

♦ **Ranexa®** *see* Ranolazine *on page 1589*

Ranibizumab (ra ni BIZ oo mab)

Brand Names: U.S. Lucentis®
Brand Names: Canada Lucentis®
Index Terms rhuFabV2
Generic Availability (U.S.) No
Pharmacologic Category Monoclonal Antibody; Ophthalmic Agent; Vascular Endothelial Growth Factor (VEGF) Inhibitor
Use Treatment of neovascular (wet) age-related macular degeneration (AMD); treatment of macular edema following retinal vein occlusion (RVO)
Contraindications Hypersensitivity to ranibizumab or any component of the formulation; ocular or periocular infection

Canadian labeling: Additional contraindications (not in U.S.labeling): Active intraocular inflammation

Warnings/Precautions Intravitreous injections may be associated with endophthalmitis and retinal detachments. Proper aseptic injection techniques should be used and patients should be instructed to report any signs of infection immediately. Intraocular pressure may increase following injection. Intravitreal injections of ranibizumab may induce temporary visual disturbances that impair the ability to drive or operate machinery. Affected patients should be advised to abstain from driving or using machinery until resolution of disturbances. Use for >24 months has not been evaluated.

Risk of thromboembolic events, particularly stroke, may be increased following intravitreal administration of VEGF inhibitors. Rare hypersensitivity reactions (including anaphylaxis) have been associated with another VEGF inhibitor, pegaptanib, occurring within several hours of use; monitor closely. Equipment and appropriate personnel should be available for monitoring and treatment of anaphylaxis.

Adverse Reactions (Reflective of adult population; not specific for elderly) **Note:** Rates of ocular adverse reactions reported for control group when percentages overlapped with treatment group.
>10%:
  Central nervous system: Headache (3% to 12%)
  Neuromuscular & skeletal: Arthralgia (2% to 11%)
  Ocular: Conjunctival hemorrhage (48% to 74%; control: 37% to 60%), eye pain (17% to 35%; control 12% to 30%), vitreous floaters (7% to 27%), intraocular pressure increased (7% to 24%), blurred vision/visual disturbance (5% to 18%), intraocular inflammation (1% to 18%; control 3% to 8%), blepharitis (≤12%), maculopathy (6% to 11%; control 6% to 9%), ocular hyperemia (5% to 11%; control 3% to 8%)
    Note: Cataract, dry eye, eye irritation, foreign body sensation, lacrimation increased, pruritus, and vitreous detachment occurred in >10% of patients, but also occurred in similar percentages to the control; visual acuity blurred/decreased occurred more often in the control.
  Respiratory: Nasopharyngitis (5% to 16%), bronchitis (≤11%)
1% to 10%:
  Cardiovascular: Atrial fibrillation (1% to 5%), arterial thromboembolic events (4%; stroke ≤3%)
  Gastrointestinal: Nausea (1% to 9%), viral gastroenteritis (1% to 4%)
  Hematologic: Anemia (1% to 8%; control up to 7%)
  Ocular: Retinal disorder (2% to 10%), retinal degeneration (1% to 8%), posterior capsule opacification (≤7%), injection site hemorrhage (≤5%)
    Note: Conjunctival hyperemia and ocular discomfort occurred in 1% to 10% of patients, but also occurred in similar percentages to the control; retinal exudates occurred more often in the control.
  Respiratory: Cough (2% to 9%), upper respiratory tract infection (≤9%), sinusitis (3% to 8%), chronic obstructive pulmonary disease (COPD) (≤6%), dyspnea (≤4%)
  Miscellaneous: Ranibizumab antibodies (1% to 8%), influenza (3% to 7%)
Drug Interactions
  Avoid Concomitant Use There are no known interactions where it is recommended to avoid concomitant use.
  Increased Effect/Toxicity There are no known significant interactions involving an increase in effect.

Decreased Effect There are no known significant interactions involving a decrease in effect.

Stability Store in original carton under refrigeration at 2°C to 8°C (36°F to 46°F); protect from light. Do not freeze.

Mechanism of Action Ranibizumab is a recombinant humanized monoclonal antibody fragment which binds to and inhibits human vascular endothelial growth factor A (VEGF-A). Ranibizumab inhibits VEGF from binding to its receptors and thereby suppressing neovascularization and slowing vision loss.

Pharmacodynamics/Kinetics
Absorption: Low levels are detected in the serum following intravitreal injection
Half-life elimination: Vitreous: ~9 days

Dosage

Geriatric & Adult

Age-related macular degeneration (AMD): Intravitreal injection: 0.5 mg (0.05 mL) once a month. **Note:** Frequency may be reduced after the first 4 injections to once every 3 months if monthly injections are not feasible; however, this regimen has reportedly resulted in an ~5 letter (1 line) loss of visual acuity over 9 months, as compared to monthly dosing.

Canadian labeling: Intravitreal injection: 0.5 mg (0.05 mL) once a month. Frequency may be reduced after the first 3 injections to once every 3 months if monthly injections are not feasible.

Macular edema following retinal vein occlusion (RVO): Intravitreal injection: 0.5 mg (0.05 mL) once a month

Renal Impairment Dose adjustment not expected.

Hepatic Impairment Dose adjustment not expected.

Administration For ophthalmic intravitreal injection only. Remove contents from vial using a 5 micron 19-gauge filter needle attached to a tuberculin syringe. Discard filter needle and replace with a sterile 30 gauge ¹/₂ inch needle for injection. Adequate anesthesia and a broad-spectrum antimicrobial agent should be administered prior to the procedure.

Monitoring Parameters Intraocular pressure (within 30 minutes and between 2-7 days following administration); retinal perfusion, endophthalmitis

Special Geriatric Considerations In clinical trials, ~94% of the patients were >65 years and 68% were >75 years of age. No differences were seen in efficacy with increasing age. After correcting for creatinine clearance, age did not affect systemic exposure of ranibizumab.

Dosage Forms Excipient information presented when available (limited, particularly for generics); consult specific product labeling.
Injection, solution [preservative free]:
Lucentis®: 10 mg/mL (0.2 mL)

Dosage Forms: Canada Excipient information presented when available (limited, particularly for generics); consult specific product labeling.
Injection, solution [preservative free]:
Lucentis®: 10 mg/mL (0.3 mL)

Selected References
Rosenfeld PJ, Brown DM, Heier JS, et al, "Ranibizumab for Neovascular Age-Related Macular Degeneration," *N Engl J Med*, 2006, 355(14):1419-31.

Ranitidine (ra NI ti deen)

Medication Safety Issues
Sound-alike/look-alike issues:
Ranitidine may be confused with amantadine, rimantadine
Zantac® may be confused with Xanax®, Zarontin®, Zofran®, ZyrTEC®
International issues:
Antagon®: Brand name for astemizole in Mexico; brand name for ganirelix in the U.S.

Brand Names: U.S. Zantac 150® [OTC]; Zantac 75® [OTC]; Zantac®; Zantac® EFFER-dose®

Brand Names: Canada Acid Reducer; Apo-Ranitidine®; CO Ranitidine; Dom-Ranitidine; Myl-Ranitidine; Mylan-Ranitidine; Nu-Ranit; PHL-Ranitidine; PMS-Ranitidine; Ranitidine Injection, USP; RAN™-Ranitidine; ratio-Ranitidine; Riva-Ranitidine; Sandoz-Ranitidine; Schein-Pharm Ranitidine; Teva-Ranitidine; Zantac 75®; Zantac Maximum Strength Non-Prescription; Zantac®

Index Terms Ranitidine Hydrochloride

Generic Availability (U.S.) Yes: Excludes effervescent tablet, premixed infusion

Pharmacologic Category Histamine H_2 Antagonist

Use

Zantac®: Short-term and maintenance therapy of duodenal ulcer, gastric ulcer, gastro-esophageal reflux disease (GERD), active benign ulcer, erosive esophagitis, and pathological hypersecretory conditions; as part of a multidrug regimen for *H. pylori* eradication to reduce the risk of duodenal ulcer recurrence

Zantac 75® [OTC]: Relief of heartburn, acid indigestion, and sour stomach

Unlabeled/Investigational Use Treatment of recurrent postoperative ulcer, upper GI bleeding; prevention of acid-aspiration pneumonitis during surgery, stress-induced ulcers

Contraindications Hypersensitivity to ranitidine or any component of the formulation

Warnings/Precautions Ranitidine has been associated with confusional states (rare). Use with caution in patients with hepatic impairment; use with caution in renal impairment, dosage modification required. Avoid use in patients with history of acute porphyria (may precipitate attacks); long-term therapy may be associated with vitamin B_{12} deficiency. Symptoms of GI distress may be associated with a variety of conditions; symptomatic response to H_2 antagonists does not rule out the potential for significant pathology (eg, malignancy). EFFERdose® formulation contains phenylalanine.

Adverse Reactions (Reflective of adult population; not specific for elderly) Frequency not defined.

Cardiovascular: Asystole, atrioventricular block, bradycardia (with rapid I.V. administration), premature ventricular beats, tachycardia, vasculitis

Central nervous system: Agitation, dizziness, depression, hallucinations, headache, insomnia, malaise, mental confusion, somnolence, vertigo

Dermatologic: Alopecia, erythema multiforme, rash

Endocrine & metabolic: Prolactin levels increased

Gastrointestinal: Abdominal discomfort/pain, constipation, diarrhea, nausea, pancreatitis, vomiting

Hematologic: Acquired immune hemolytic anemia, acute porphyritic attack, agranulocytosis, aplastic anemia, granulocytopenia, leukopenia, pancytopenia, thrombocytopenia

Hepatic: Cholestatic hepatitis, hepatic failure, hepatitis, jaundice

Local: Transient pain, burning or itching at the injection site

Neuromuscular & skeletal: Arthralgia, involuntary motor disturbance, myalgia

Ocular: Blurred vision

Renal: Acute interstitial nephritis, serum creatinine increased

Respiratory: Pneumonia (causal relationship not established)

Miscellaneous: Anaphylaxis, angioneurotic edema, hypersensitivity reactions (eg, bronchospasm, fever, eosinophilia)

Drug Interactions

Metabolism/Transport Effects Substrate of CYP1A2 (minor), CYP2C19 (minor), CYP2D6 (minor), P-glycoprotein; **Inhibits** CYP1A2 (weak), 2D6 (weak)

Avoid Concomitant Use

Avoid concomitant use of Ranitidine with any of the following: Delavirdine

Increased Effect/Toxicity

Ranitidine may increase the levels/effects of: Dexmethylphenidate; Methylphenidate; Procainamide; Saquinavir; Sulfonylureas; Varenicline; Warfarin

The levels/effects of Ranitidine may be increased by: P-Glycoprotein Inhibitors

Decreased Effect

Ranitidine may decrease the levels/effects of: Atazanavir; Cefditoren; Cefpodoxime; Cefuroxime; Dasatinib; Delavirdine; Erlotinib; Fosamprenavir; Gefitinib; Indinavir; Iron Salts; Itraconazole; Ketoconazole; Ketoconazole (Systemic); Mesalamine; Nelfinavir; Posaconazole; Prasugrel; Rilpivirine

The levels/effects of Ranitidine may be decreased by: Cyproterone; Peginterferon Alfa-2b; P-Glycoprotein Inducers

Ethanol/Nutrition/Herb Interactions

Ethanol: Avoid ethanol (may cause gastric mucosal irritation).

Food: Does not interfere with absorption of ranitidine.

Stability

Injection: Vials: Store between 4°C to 25°C (39°F to 77°F); excursion permitted to 30°C (86°F). Protect from light. Solution is a clear, colorless to yellow solution; slight darkening does not affect potency.

Premixed bag: Store between 2°C to 25°C (36°F to 77°F). Protect from light.

EFFERdose® formulations: Store between 2°C to 30°C (36°F to 86°F).

Syrup: Store between 4°C to 25°C (39°F to 77°F). Protect from light.

Tablet: Store in dry place, between 15°C to 30°C (59°F to 86°F). Protect from light.

◀ Vials can be mixed with NS or D_5W; solutions are stable for 48 hours at room temperature.
Intermittent bolus injection, continuous infusion: Dilute to maximum of 2.5 mg/mL.
Intermittent infusion: Dilute to maximum of 0.5 mg/mL.

Mechanism of Action Competitive inhibition of histamine at H_2-receptors of the gastric parietal cells, which inhibits gastric acid secretion, gastric volume, and hydrogen ion concentration are reduced. Does not affect pepsin secretion, pentagastrin-stimulated intrinsic factor secretion, or serum gastrin.

Pharmacodynamics/Kinetics

Absorption: Oral: 50%

Distribution: Normal renal function: V_d: ~1.4 L/kg; Cl_{cr} 25-35 mL/minute: 1.76 L/kg minimally penetrates the blood-brain barrier

Protein binding: 15%

Metabolism: Hepatic to N-oxide, S-oxide, and N-desmethyl metabolites

Bioavailability: Oral: 48% to 50%; I.M.: 90% to 100%

Half-life elimination:

Oral: Normal renal function: 2.5-3 hours; Cl_{cr} 25-35 mL/minute: 4.8 hours

I.V.: Normal renal function: 2-2.5 hours

Time to peak, serum: Oral: 2-3 hours; I.M.: ≤15 minutes

Excretion: Urine: Oral: 30%, I.V.: 70% (as unchanged drug); feces (as metabolites)

Dosage

Geriatric & Adult

Duodenal ulcer: Oral: Treatment: 150 mg twice daily, or 300 mg once daily after the evening meal or at bedtime; maintenance: 150 mg once daily at bedtime

Eradication of *Helicobacter pylori*: Oral: 150 mg twice daily; requires combination therapy

Pathological hypersecretory conditions:

Oral: 150 mg twice daily; adjust dose or frequency as clinically indicated; doses of up to 6 g/day have been used

I.V.: Continuous infusion for Zollinger-Ellison: Initial: 1 mg/kg/hour; measure gastric acid output at 4 hours, if >10 mEq or if patient is symptomatic, increase dose in increments of 0.5 mg/kg/hour; doses of up to 2.5 mg/kg/hour (or 220 mg/hour) have been used

Gastric ulcer, benign: *Oral:* 150 mg twice daily; maintenance: 150 mg once daily at bedtime

GERD: *Oral:* 150 mg twice daily

Erosive esophagitis: *Oral:* Treatment: 150 mg 4 times/day; maintenance: 150 mg twice daily

Prevention of heartburn: *Oral:* Zantac 75® [OTC]: 75 mg 30-60 minutes before eating food or drinking beverages which cause heartburn; maximum: 150 mg in 24 hours; do not use for more than 14 days

Patients not able to take oral medication:

I.M.: 50 mg every 6-8 hours

I.V.: Intermittent bolus or infusion: 50 mg every 6-8 hours

Continuous I.V. infusion: 6.25 mg/hour

Renal Impairment Adults: Cl_{cr} <50 mL/minute:

Oral: 150 mg every 24 hours; adjust dose cautiously if needed

I.V.: 50 mg every 18-24 hours; adjust dose cautiously if needed

Hemodialysis: Adjust dosing schedule so that dose coincides with the end of hemodialysis.

Hepatic Impairment Patients with hepatic impairment may have minor changes in ranitidine half-life, distribution, clearance, and bioavailability; dosing adjustments are not necessary; monitor patient.

Administration

Ranitidine injection may be administered I.M. or I.V.:

I.M.: Injection is administered undiluted

I.V.: Must be diluted; may be administered I.V. push, intermittent I.V. infusion, or continuous I.V. infusion

I.V. push: Ranitidine (usually 50 mg) should be diluted to a total of 20 mL (or a concentration not exceeding 2.5 mg/mL) with NS or D_5W and administered over at least 5 minutes or a maximum rate of 10 mg/minute

Intermittent I.V. infusion: Dilute to a maximum concentration of 0.5 mg/mL; administer over 15-20 minutes

Continuous I.V. infusion: Dilute to a maximum concentration of 2.5 mg/mL. Titrate dosage based on gastric pH.

EFFERdose®: Should not be chewed; swallowed whole, or dissolved on tongue: 25 mg tablet: Dissolve in at least 5 mL (1 teaspoonful) of water; wait until completely dissolved before administering

Monitoring Parameters AST, ALT, serum creatinine; when used to prevent stress-related GI bleeding, measure the intragastric pH and try to maintain pH >4; signs and symptoms of peptic ulcer disease, occult blood with GI bleeding, monitor renal function to correct dose

Test Interactions False-positive urine protein using Multistix®; gastric acid secretion test; skin test allergen extracts. May also interfere with urine detection of amphetamine/methamphetamine (false-positive).

Pharmacotherapy Pearls Giving dose at 6 PM may be better than 10 PM bedtime, the highest acid production usually starts at approximately 7 PM, thus giving at 6 PM controls acid secretion better; administer I.V. administration over a 30 minute period to avoid bradycardia; causes fewer adverse reactions and interactions than cimetidine; most patient's ulcers have healed within 4 weeks, however, older adults require 12 weeks of therapy; long-term therapy may cause vitamin B_{12} deficiency

Special Geriatric Considerations Ulcer healing rates and incidence of adverse effects are similar in the elderly, when compared to younger patients; dosing adjustments not necessary based on age alone. Always adjust dose based upon creatinine clearance. Serum half-life is increased to 3-4 hours in elderly patients. H_2 blockers are the preferred drugs for treating PUD in the elderly due to cost and ease of administration. These agents are no less or more effective than any other therapy. The preferred agents, due to side effects and drug interaction profile and pharmacokinetics are ranitidine, famotidine, and nizatidine. Treatment for PUD in the elderly is recommended for 12 weeks since their lesions are larger; therefore, take longer to heal. This drug is substantially cleared renally, and elderly, having decreased renal function in general, should be monitored closely for adverse effects, especially CNS.

Dosage Forms Excipient information presented when available (limited, particularly for generics); consult specific product labeling.
Capsule, oral: 150 mg, 300 mg
Infusion, premixed in 1/2 NS [preservative free]:
  Zantac®: 50 mg (50 mL)
Injection, solution: 25 mg/mL (2 mL, 6 mL, 40 mL)
  Zantac®: 25 mg/mL (2 mL, 6 mL, 40 mL)
Syrup, oral: 15 mg/mL (5 mL, 10 mL, 120 mL, 473 mL, 480 mL)
  Zantac®: 15 mg/mL (480 mL) [contains ethanol 7.5%; peppermint flavor]
Tablet, oral: 75 mg, 150 mg, 300 mg
  Zantac 150®: 150 mg
  Zantac 150®: 150 mg [cool mint flavor]
  Zantac 75®: 75 mg
  Zantac 75®: 75 mg [sugar free]
  Zantac®: 150 mg, 300 mg
Tablet for solution, oral [effervescent]:
  Zantac® EFFERdose®: 25 mg [contains phenylalanine 2.81 mg/tablet, sodium 1.33 mEq/tablet, sodium benzoate]

◆ **Ranitidine Hydrochloride** see Ranitidine on page 1586

Ranolazine (ra NOE la zeen)

Medication Safety Issues
  Sound-alike/look-alike issues:
    Ranexa® may be confused with Celexa®
  Brand Names: U.S. Ranexa®
  Generic Availability (U.S.) No
  Pharmacologic Category Cardiovascular Agent, Miscellaneous
  Use Treatment of chronic angina
  Contraindications Clinically significant hepatic impairment; concurrent strong CYP3A inhibitors; concurrent inducers of CYP3A
  Warnings/Precautions Ranolazine does not relieve acute angina attacks. Has been shown to prolong QT interval in a dose/plasma concentration-related manner. Hepatically-impaired patients may have a more significant increase in QT interval. Use with caution in patients with mild (Child-Pugh class A) or moderate (Child-Pugh class B) hepatic impairment; use is contraindicated with clinically significant hepatic impairment. Use caution in patients ≥75 years of age; they may experience more adverse events. Use caution and monitor blood pressure in patients with renal dysfunction; has not been evaluated in patients requiring dialysis.

  Ranolazine is a substrate for and a moderate inhibitor of P-glycoprotein. Inhibitors of P-glycoprotein may increase serum concentrations of ranolazine. Ranolazine may increase serum concentrations of substrates for P-glycoprotein (eg, digoxin). Ranolazine is primarily metabolized by CYP3A; use is contraindicated with inducers and strong inhibitors of CYP3A. Ranolazine has potential to prolong the QT-interval; use caution when administered concomitantly with QT-prolonging drugs. Use caution when administering ranolazine to patients with a history of malignant neoplasms or adenomatous polyps.

Adverse Reactions (Reflective of adult population; not specific for elderly)
>10%:
Central nervous system: Dizziness (5% to 13%; dose related)
Gastrointestinal: Constipation (5% to 8%; 19% in the elderly)
>0.5% to 10%:
Cardiovascular: Syncope (≤3%), bradycardia (≤2%), hypotension (≤2%), orthostatic hypotension (≤2%), palpitation (≤2%), peripheral edema (≤2%), QT_c prolongation (>500 msec: ≤1%)
Central nervous system: Headache (3% to 6%), vertigo (≤2%)
Gastrointestinal: Nausea (4% to 9%), abdominal pain (≤2%), vomiting (≤2%), xerostomia (≤2%)
Hematologic: Hematocrit decreased (1%)
Otic: Tinnitus (≤2%)
Respiratory: Dyspnea (≤2%)

Drug Interactions
Metabolism/Transport Effects Substrate of CYP3A4 (major), CYP2D6 (minor), P-glycoprotein; **Inhibits** CYP3A4 (weak), CYP2D6 (moderate), P-glycoprotein
Avoid Concomitant Use
Avoid concomitant use of Ranolazine with any of the following: Antifungal Agents (Azole Derivatives, Systemic); Artemether; CYP3A4 Inducers (Strong); CYP3A4 Inhibitors (Strong); Dronedarone; Lumefantrine; Nilotinib; Pimozide; QUEtiapine; QuiNINE; Rifampin; Silodosin; Tetrabenazine; Thioridazine; Topotecan; Toremifene; Vandetanib; Vemurafenib; Ziprasidone
Increased Effect/Toxicity
Ranolazine may increase the levels/effects of: Colchicine; CYP2D6 Substrates; Dabigatran Etexilate; Digoxin; Dronedarone; Everolimus; Fesoterodine; Nebivolol; P-Glycoprotein Substrates; Pimozide; QTc-Prolonging Agents; QuiNINE; Rivaroxaban; Silodosin; Simvastatin; Tacrolimus; Tacrolimus (Systemic); Tamoxifen; Tetrabenazine; Thioridazine; Topotecan; Toremifene; Vandetanib; Vemurafenib; Ziprasidone

The levels/effects of Ranolazine may be increased by: Alfuzosin; Antifungal Agents (Azole Derivatives, Systemic); Artemether; Calcium Channel Blockers (Nondihydropyridine); Chloroquine; Ciprofloxacin; Ciprofloxacin (Systemic); CYP3A4 Inhibitors (Moderate); CYP3A4 Inhibitors (Strong); Gadobutrol; Lumefantrine; Nilotinib; P-Glycoprotein Inhibitors; QUEtiapine; QuiNINE
Decreased Effect
Ranolazine may decrease the levels/effects of: Codeine; TraMADol

The levels/effects of Ranolazine may be decreased by: CYP3A4 Inducers (Strong); Deferasirox; Herbs (CYP3A4 Inducers); Peginterferon Alfa-2b; P-Glycoprotein Inducers; Rifampin; Tocilizumab
Ethanol/Nutrition/Herb Interactions Food: Limit the use of grapefruit, grapefruit juice, or grapefruit-containing products; if use is significant and consistent, the dose of ranolazine should be limited to 500 mg twice daily.
Stability Store at 25°C (77°F); excursions permitted to 15°C to 30°C (59°F to 86°F).
Mechanism of Action Ranolazine exerts antianginal and anti-ischemic effects without changing hemodynamic parameters (heart rate or blood pressure). At therapeutic levels, ranolazine inhibits the late phase of the inward sodium channel (late I_{Na}) in ischemic cardiac myocytes during cardiac repolarization reducing intracellular sodium concentrations and thereby reducing calcium influx via Na^+-Ca^{2+} exchange. Decreased intracellular calcium reduces ventricular tension and myocardial oxygen consumption. It is thought that ranolazine produces myocardial relaxation and reduces anginal symptoms through this mechanism although this is uncertain. At higher concentrations, ranolazine inhibits the rapid delayed rectifier potassium current (I_{Kr}) thus prolonging the ventricular action potential duration and subsequent prolongation of the QT interval.
Pharmacodynamics/Kinetics
Absorption: Highly variable; ranolazine is a substrate of P-glycoprotein; concurrent use of P-glycoprotein inhibitors may increase absorption
Protein binding: ~62%
Metabolism: Hepatic via CYP3A (major) and 2D6 (minor); gut
Bioavailability: 35% to 55%
Half-life elimination: Terminal: 7 hours
Time to peak, plasma: 2-5 hours
Excretion: Primarily urine (75% mostly as metabolites); feces (25% mostly as metabolites); in feces and urine, <5% to 7% excreted unchanged
Dosage
Geriatric Refer to adult dosing. Select dose cautiously, starting at the lower end of the dosing range.

Adult

Chronic angina: Oral: Initial: 500 mg twice daily; maximum recommended dose: 1000 mg twice daily

Dosage adjustment for ranolazine with concomitant medications:

Diltiazem, verapamil, and other moderate CYP3A inhibitors: Dose should not exceed 500 mg twice daily

P-glycoprotein inhibitors (eg, cyclosporine): Down-titrate ranolazine based on clinical response

Renal Impairment Dosage adjustment recommendations have not been established. However, plasma ranolazine levels increased ~50% in patients with varying degrees of renal dysfunction. Patients with severe renal dysfunction had an increase in mean diastolic blood pressure of 10-15 mm Hg. Monitor blood pressure closely in these patients. Ranolazine has not been evaluated in patients requiring dialysis.

Hepatic Impairment Use with caution in patients with mild (Child-Pugh class A) and moderate (Child-Pugh class B) hepatic impairment. Use is contraindicated with clinically significant hepatic impairment.

Administration May be taken with or without meals. Swallow tablet whole; do not crush, break, or chew.

Monitoring Parameters Baseline and follow up ECG to evaluate QT interval; blood pressure in patients with renal dysfunction; correct and maintain serum potassium in normal limits

Special Geriatric Considerations Elderly comprised 48% of study group participants. For those elderly, no overall difference in efficacy was observed between younger and older adults. There was, however, a higher incidence of adverse effects for those ≥75 years of age, resulting in drug discontinuations. The most common adverse effects were constipation (19%), nausea (6%), and dizziness (6%). Therefore, start dosing at lower end of dosing range recommended.

Dosage Forms Excipient information presented when available (limited, particularly for generics); consult specific product labeling.

Tablet, extended release, oral:

Ranexa®: 500 mg, 1000 mg

Selected References

Abdallah H and Jerling M, "Effect of Hepatic Impairment on the Multiple-Dose Pharmacokinetics of Ranolazine Sustained Release Tablets," *J Clin Pharmacol,* 2005, 45(7):802-9.

Chaitman BR, Pepine CJ, Parker JO, et al, "Effects of Ranolazine With Atenolol, Amlodipine, or Diltiazem on Exercise Tolerance and Angina Frequency in Patients With Severe Chronic Angina. A Randomized Controlled Trial," *JAMA,* 2004, 291(3):309-16.

Chaitman BR, Skettino SL, Parker JO, et al, "Anti-ischemic Effects and Long-term Survival During Ranolazine Monotherapy in Patients With Chronic Severe Angina," *J Am Coll Cardiol,* 2004, 43(8):1375-82.

Dobesh PP and Trujillo TC, "Ranolazine: A New Option in the Management of Chronic Stable Angina," *Pharmaco-therapy,* 2007, 27(12):1659-76.

Jerling M and Abdallah H, "Effect of Renal Impairment on Multiple-Dose Pharmacokinetics of Extended Release Ranolazine," *Clin Pharmacol Ther,* 2005, 78(3):288-97.

◆ **Rapaflo®** see Silodosin on page *1677*

Rasagiline (ra SA ji leen)

Related Information

Antiparkinsonian Agents on page *1995*

Medication Safety Issues

Sound-alike/look-alike issues:

Azilect® may be confused with Aricept®

Brand Names: U.S. Azilect®

Index Terms AGN 1135; Rasagiline Mesylate; TVP-1012

Generic Availability (U.S.) No

Pharmacologic Category Anti-Parkinson's Agent, MAO Type B Inhibitor

Use Treatment of idiopathic Parkinson's disease (initial monotherapy or as adjunct to levodopa)

Contraindications Concomitant use of cyclobenzaprine, dextromethorphan, methadone, propoxyphene, St John's wort, or tramadol; concomitant use of meperidine or an MAO inhibitor (including selective MAO-B inhibitors) within 14 days of rasagiline

Warnings/Precautions Hazardous agent - use appropriate precautions for handling and disposal.

Cardiovascular system: May cause orthostatic hypotension, particularly in combination with levodopa; use with caution in patients with hypotension or patients who would not tolerate transient hypotensive episodes (cardiovascular or cerebrovascular disease); orthostasis is usually most problematic during first 2 months of therapy and tends to abate thereafter. Due to the potential for hemodynamic instability, patients should not undergo elective surgery requiring general anesthesia and should avoid local anesthesia containing sympathomimetic vasoconstrictors within 14 days of discontinuing rasagiline. If surgery is required, benzodiazepines, mivacurium, fentanyl, morphine or codeine may be used cautiously. In patients taking recommended doses of rasagiline, dietary restriction of most tyramine-containing products is not necessary; however, certain foods (eg, aged cheeses) may contain high amounts (>150 mg) of tyramine and could lead to hypertensive crisis. Avoid concomitant use with foods high in tyramine.

Central nervous system: Serotonin syndrome (SS)/neuroleptic malignant syndrome (NMS)-like reactions may occur rarely, particularly when used at doses exceeding recommendations or when used in combination with an antidepressant (eg, SSRI, SNRI, TCA). May cause hallucinations; signs of severe CNS toxicity (some fatal), including hyperpyrexia, hyperthermia, rigidity, altered mental status, seizure and coma have been reported with selective and nonselective MAO inhibitor use in combination with antidepressants. Do not use within 5 weeks of fluoxetine discontinuation; do not initiate tricyclic, SSRI, or SNRI therapy within 2 weeks of discontinuing rasagiline. Addition to levodopa therapy may result in exacerbation of dyskinesias, requiring a reduction in levodopa dosage.

Dermatologic: Risk of melanoma may be increased with rasagiline, although increased risk has been associated with Parkinson's disease itself; patients should have regular and frequent skin examinations.

Organ dysfunction: Use caution in mild hepatic impairment; dose reduction recommended. Do not use with moderate-to-severe hepatic impairment.

Adverse Reactions (Reflective of adult population; not specific for elderly) Unless otherwise noted, the following adverse reactions are as reported for monotherapy. Spectrum of adverse events was generally similar with adjunctive (levodopa) therapy, though the incidence tended to be higher.

>10%:

    Cardiovascular: Postural hypotension (6% to 13% adjunct therapy, dose dependent)

    Central nervous system: Dyskinesia (18% adjunct therapy), headache (14%)

    Gastrointestinal: Nausea (10% to 12% adjunct therapy)

1% to 10%:

    Cardiovascular: Angina, bundle branch block, chest pain, syncope

    Central nervous system: Depression (5%), hallucinations (4% to 5% adjunct therapy), fever (3%), malaise (2%), vertigo (2%), anxiety, dizziness

    Dermatologic: Bruising (2%), alopecia, skin carcinoma, vesiculobullous rash

    Endocrine & metabolic: Impotence, libido decreased

    Gastrointestinal: Constipation (4% to 9% adjunct therapy), weight loss (2% to 9% adjunct therapy; dose dependent), dyspepsia (7%), xerostomia (2% to 6% adjunct therapy; dose dependent), gastroenteritis (3%), anorexia, diarrhea, gastrointestinal hemorrhage, vomiting

    Genitourinary: Hematuria, urinary incontinence

    Hematologic: Leukopenia

    Hepatic: Liver function tests increased

    Neuromuscular & skeletal: Arthralgia (7%), neck pain (2%), arthritis (2%), paresthesia (2%), abnormal gait, hyperkinesias, hypertonia, neuropathy, tremor, weakness

    Ocular: Conjunctivitis (3%)

    Renal: Albuminuria

    Respiratory: Rhinitis (3%), asthma, cough increased

    Miscellaneous: Fall (5%), flu-like syndrome (5%), allergic reaction

Drug Interactions

Metabolism/Transport Effects Substrate of CYP1A2 (major)

Avoid Concomitant Use

Avoid concomitant use of Rasagiline with any of the following: Alpha-/Beta-Agonists (Indirect-Acting); Alpha1-Agonists; Alpha2-Agonists (Ophthalmic); Amphetamines; Anilidopiperidine Opioids; Atomoxetine; Bezafibrate; Buprenorphine; BuPROPion; BusPIRone; CarBAMazepine; Cyclobenzaprine; Dexmethylphenidate; Dextromethorphan; Diethylpropion; HYDROmorphone; Linezolid; Maprotiline; Meperidine; Methyldopa; Methylene Blue; Methylphenidate; Mirtazapine; Oxymorphone; Pizotifen; Propoxyphene; Selective Serotonin Reuptake Inhibitors; Serotonin 5-HT1D Receptor Agonists; Serotonin/Norepinephrine Reuptake Inhibitors; Sibutramine; Tapentadol; Tetrabenazine; Tetrahydrozoline; Tetrahydrozoline (Nasal); Tricyclic Antidepressants; Tryptophan

Increased Effect/Toxicity

Rasagiline may increase the levels/effects of: Alpha-/Beta-Agonists (Direct-Acting); Alpha-/Beta-Agonists (Indirect-Acting); Alpha1-Agonists; Alpha2-Agonists (Ophthalmic); Amphetamines; Antihypertensives; Atomoxetine; Beta2-Agonists; Bezafibrate; BuPROPion; Dexmethylphenidate; Dextromethorphan; Diethylpropion; Doxapram; HYDROmorphone; Linezolid; Lithium; Meperidine; Methadone; Methyldopa; Methylene Blue; Methylphenidate; Mirtazapine; Orthostatic Hypotension Producing Agents; Pizotifen; Reserpine; Selective

Serotonin Reuptake Inhibitors; Serotonin 5-HT1D Receptor Agonists; Serotonin Modulators; Serotonin/Norepinephrine Reuptake Inhibitors; Tetrahydrozoline; Tetrahydrozoline (Nasal); Tricyclic Antidepressants

The levels/effects of Rasagiline may be increased by: Abiraterone Acetate; Altretamine; Anilidopiperidine Opioids; Buprenorphine; BusPIRone; CarBAMazepine; COMT Inhibitors; Cyclobenzaprine; CYP1A2 Inhibitors (Moderate); CYP1A2 Inhibitors (Strong); Deferasirox; Levodopa; MAO Inhibitors; Maprotiline; Oxymorphone; Propoxyphene; Sibutramine; Tapentadol; Tetrabenazine; TraMADol; Tryptophan

Decreased Effect

The levels/effects of Rasagiline may be decreased by: CYP1A2 Inducers (Strong); Cyproterone

Ethanol/Nutrition/Herb Interactions

Ethanol: Avoid ethanol.

Food: Concurrent ingestion of foods rich in tyramine may cause sudden and severe high blood pressure (hypertensive crisis). Avoid foods (such as aged cheeses) containing high amounts (>150 mg) of tyramine.

Herb/Nutraceutical: Avoid valerian, St John's wort, SAMe, kava kava (may increase risk of serotonin syndrome and/or excessive sedation); Avoid supplements containing caffeine, tyrosine, tryptophan, or phenylalanine. Ingestion of large quantities may increase the risk of severe side effects (eg, hypertensive reactions, serotonin syndrome).

Stability Store at 25°C (77°F); excursions permitted to 15°C to 30°C (59°F to 86°F).

Mechanism of Action Potent, irreversible and selective inhibitor of brain monoamine oxidase (MAO) type B, which plays a major role in the catabolism of dopamine. Inhibition of dopamine depletion in the striatal region of the brain reduces the symptomatic motor deficits of Parkinson's disease. There is also experimental evidence of rasagiline conferring neuroprotective effects (antioxidant, antiapoptotic), which may delay onset of symptoms and progression of neuronal deterioration.

Pharmacodynamics/Kinetics

Onset of action: Therapeutic: Within 1 hour

Duration: ~1 week (irreversible inhibition); may require ~14-40 days for complete restoration of (brain) MAO-B activity

Absorption: Rapid

Protein binding: 88% to 94%, primarily to albumin

Metabolism: Hepatic N-dealkylation and/or hydroxylation via CYP1A2 to multiple inactive metabolites (nonamphetamine derivatives)

Distribution: V_{dss}: 87 L

Bioavailability: ~36%

Half-life elimination: ~1.3-3 hours (no correlation with biologic effect due to irreversible inhibition)

Time to peak, plasma: ~1 hour

Excretion: Urine (62%, <1% of total dose as unchanged drug); feces (7%)

Dosage

Geriatric & Adult Parkinson's disease: Oral:

Monotherapy: 1 mg once daily

Adjunctive therapy with levodopa: Initial: 0.5 mg once daily; may increase to 1 mg once daily based on response and tolerability

Note: When added to existing levodopa therapy, a dose reduction of levodopa may be required to avoid exacerbation of dyskinesias; typical dose reductions of ~9% to 13% were employed in clinical trials.

Dose reduction with concomitant ciprofloxacin or other CYP1A2 inhibitors: 0.5 mg once daily

Renal Impairment

Mild-to-moderate impairment: No adjustment necessary.

Severe impairment: Not studied.

Hepatic Impairment

Mild impairment (Child-Pugh ≤6): 0.5 mg once daily

Moderate-to-severe impairment: Not recommended.

Administration Administer without regard to meals.

Monitoring Parameters Blood pressure; symptoms of parkinsonism; general mood and behavior (increased anxiety, or presence of mania or agitation); skin examination for presence of melanoma (higher incidence in Parkinson's patients- drug causation not established)

Pharmacotherapy Pearls When adding rasagiline to levodopa/carbidopa, the dose of the latter can usually be decreased. Studies are investigating the use of rasagiline in early Parkinson's disease to slow the progression of the disease.

Special Geriatric Considerations In clinical trials, no significant differences in the safety profile were seen between elderly and younger adults.

Dosage Forms Excipient information presented when available (limited, particularly for generics); consult specific product labeling.

Tablet, oral:

Azilect®: 0.5 mg, 1 mg

Selected References

Chen JJ and Ly A-V, "Rasagiline: A Second-Generation Monoamine Oxidase Type-B Inhibitor for the Treatment of Parkinson's Disease," *Am J Health-Syst Pharm*, 2006, 63(10):915-28.

Parkinson Study Group, "A Randomized Placebo-Controlled Trial of Rasagiline in Levodopa-Treated Patients with Parkinson Disease and Motor Fluctuations. The PRESTO Study," *Arch Neurol*, 2005 62(2):241-8.

Parkinson Study Group, "A Controlled, Randomized, Delayed-Start Study of Rasagiline in Early Parkinson Disease," *Arch Neurol*, 2004, 61(4):561-66.

Parkinson Study Group, "A Controlled Trial of Rasagiline in Early Parkinson Disease: the TEMPO Study," *Arch Neurol*, 2002, 59(12):1937-43.

Rascol O, Brooks DJ, Melamed E et al, "Rasagiline as an Adjunct to Levodopa in Patients with Parkinson's Disease and Motor Fluctuations (LARGO, Lasting effect in Adjunct therapy With Rasagiline Given Once Daily, Study): A Randomized, Double-Blind, Parallel-Group Trial," *Lancet*, 2005, 365(9463):947-54.

Regadenoson (re ga DEN of son)

Brand Names: U.S. Lexiscan®

Index Terms CVT-3146

Generic Availability (U.S.) No

Pharmacologic Category Diagnostic Agent

Use Radionuclide myocardial perfusion imaging (MPI) in patients unable to undergo adequate exercise stress testing

Contraindications Second- or third-degree heart block or sinus node dysfunction in patients without a functioning artificial pacemaker

Warnings/Precautions Pharmacological stress agents may produce myocardial ischemia resulting in life threatening ventricular arrhythmias, MI, and fatal cardiac arrest. Regadenoson decreases conduction through the AV node and may produce first-, second-, or third-degree heart block, or sinus bradycardia. Third-degree heart block and asystole within minutes of administration have been observed. Use caution in patients with first-degree AV block or bundle branch block. Functional pacemaker must be in place to use in patients with second- or third-degree AV block or sinus node dysfunction. May produce profound vasodilation with subsequent hypotension. Syncope and transient ischemic attacks have been reported. Use with caution in patients with autonomic dysfunction, carotid stenosis (with cerebrovascular insufficiency), uncorrected hypovolemia, left main coronary artery stenosis, pericarditis, pericardial effusion and/or stenotic valvular heart disease. May produce hypertension; typically within 10-15 minutes of administration, although some patients may not experience until 45 minutes after administration. Use with caution in patients with underlying hypertension, especially when low-level exercise is used during MPI. May cause bronchoconstriction in patients with asthma; should be used cautiously in patients with obstructive lung disease not associated with bronchoconstriction (eg, COPD/emphysema, bronchitis). When possible, dipyridamole should be withheld for at least 2 days prior to regadenoson administration. Patients should avoid consumption of any products containing theophylline derivatives (eg, aminophylline, caffeine) for at least 12 hours prior to regadenoson administration.

Adverse Reactions (Reflective of adult population; not specific for elderly)

>10%:

Cardiovascular: Tachycardia (22%), flushing (16%), premature ventricular contractions (14%), chest discomfort (13%), angina or ST segment depression (12%)

Central nervous system: Headache (26%)

Respiratory: Dyspnea (28% to 61%; incidence increased in patients with respiratory disease), bronchoconstriction (COPD patients: 12%)

1% to 10%:

Cardiovascular: Chest pain (7%), premature atrial contractions (7%), systolic blood pressure decreased >35 mm Hg (7%), systolic blood pressure increased ≥180 mm Hg and ≥20 mm Hg from baseline (5%), ventricular conduction abnormalities (6%) diastolic blood pressure decreased >25 mm Hg (4%), first-degree AV block (PR prolongation >220 msec; 3%), diastolic blood pressure increased ≥30 mm Hg (1%)

Central nervous system: Dizziness (8%)

Gastrointestinal: Nausea (6%), abdominal discomfort (5%), abnormal taste (5%)

Miscellaneous: Feeling hot (5%)

Drug Interactions

Avoid Concomitant Use There are no known interactions where it is recommended to avoid concomitant use.

Increased Effect/Toxicity

The levels/effects of Regadenoson may be increased by: Dipyridamole

Decreased Effect

The levels/effects of Regadenoson may be decreased by: Aminophylline; Caffeine; Theophylline

Ethanol/Nutrition/Herb Interactions Food: Avoid food or drugs with caffeine. Regadenoson's diagnostic effect may be decreased if used concurrently with caffeine. Avoid dietary caffeine for at least 12 hours prior to pharmacologic stress testing.

Stability Store at controlled room temperature of 25°C (77°F); excursions permitted to 15°C to 30°C (59°F to 86°F).

Mechanism of Action Regadenoson, a low affinity agonist of the A_{2A} adenosine receptor, increases coronary blood flow (CBF) and mimics the increase in CBF caused by exercise. Myocardial uptake of the radiopharmaceutical is proportional to CBF creating the contrast required to identify stenotic coronary arteries.

Pharmacodynamics/Kinetics

Distribution: 11.5 L

Metabolism: Unknown

Half-life elimination: Intermediate phase: 30 minutes; Terminal phase: 2 hours

Time to peak, plasma: 1-4 minutes

Excretion: Urine (57% as unchanged drug)

Dosage

Geriatric & Adult Myocardial perfusion imaging: I.V.: 0.4 mg (5 mL) over ~10 seconds, followed immediately by a 5 mL saline flush. Wait 10-20 seconds, then administer the radionuclide myocardial perfusion imaging agent.

Administration Administer over approximately 10 seconds into a peripheral vein using a ≥22-gauge catheter or needle, followed immediately by a 5 mL saline flush. Wait 10-20 seconds, then administer the radionuclide myocardial perfusion imaging agent. The radionuclide may be injected directly into the same catheter as regadenoson.

Monitoring Parameters Heart rate, blood pressure, continuous cardiac monitoring, oxygen saturation

Special Geriatric Considerations In initial studies, elderly had a higher incidence of hypotension (2% vs <1%).

Dosage Forms Excipient information presented when available (limited, particularly for generics); consult specific product labeling.

Injection, solution [preservative free]:

Lexiscan®: 0.08 mg/mL (5 mL) [contains edetate disodium, propylene glycol 150 mg/mL]

Selected References

American Society of Nuclear Cardiology, "Imaging Guidelines for Nuclear Cardiology Procedures: A Report of The American Society of Nuclear Cardiology Quality Assurance Committee," *J Nucl Cardiol*, 2006, 13(6):e21-171.

Gordi T, Frohna P, Sun HL, et al, "A Population Pharmacokinetic/Pharmacodynamic Analysis of Regadenoson, an Adenosine A2A-Receptor Agonist, in Healthy Male Volunteers," *Clin Pharmacokinet*, 2006, 45(12):1201-12.

Iskandrian AE, Bateman TM, Belardinelli L, et al, "Adenosine Versus Regadenoson Comparative Evaluation in Myocardial Perfusion Imaging: Results of the ADVANCE Phase 3 Multicenter International Trial," *J Nucl Cardiol*, 2007, 14(5):645-58.

◆ **Regenecare®** *see* Lidocaine (Topical) *on page 1064*

◆ **Regenecare® HA [OTC]** *see* Lidocaine (Topical) *on page 1064*

◆ **Reglan®** *see* Metoclopramide *on page 1190*

◆ **Regonol®** *see* Pyridostigmine *on page 1550*

◆ **Regranex®** *see* Becaplermin *on page 183*

- **Regular Insulin** *see* Insulin Regular *on page 963*
- **Reguloid [OTC]** *see* Psyllium *on page 1547*
- **Relafen** *see* Nabumetone *on page 1252*
- **Relenza®** *see* Zanamivir *on page 1941*
- **Relistor®** *see* Methylnaltrexone *on page 1178*
- **Relpax®** *see* Eletriptan *on page 592*
- **Remeron®** *see* Mirtazapine *on page 1223*
- **Remeron SolTab®** *see* Mirtazapine *on page 1223*
- **Renagel®** *see* Sevelamer *on page 1672*
- **Renvela®** *see* Sevelamer *on page 1672*

Repaglinide (re PAG li nide)

Related Information
Diabetes Mellitus Management, Adults *on page 2073*

Medication Safety Issues
Sound-alike/look-alike issues:
Prandin® may be confused with Avandia®
High alert medication:
The Institute for Safe Medication Practices (ISMP) includes this medication among its list of drug classes which have a heightened risk of causing significant patient harm when used in error.

Brand Names: U.S. Prandin®
Brand Names: Canada GlucoNorm®; Prandin®
Generic Availability (U.S.) No
Pharmacologic Category Antidiabetic Agent, Meglitinide Derivative
Use Management of type 2 diabetes mellitus (noninsulin dependent, NIDDM) as an adjunct to diet and exercise; may be used in combination with metformin or thiazolidinediones
Contraindications Hypersensitivity to repaglinide or any component of the formulation; diabetic ketoacidosis, with or without coma; type 1 diabetes (insulin dependent, IDDM); concurrent gemfibrozil therapy
Warnings/Precautions Use with caution in patients with hepatic impairment. Use caution in severe renal dysfunction, elderly, malnourished, or patients with adrenal/pituitary dysfunction; may be more susceptible to glucose-lowering effects. May cause hypoglycemia; appropriate patient selection, dosage, and patient education are important to avoid hypoglycemic episodes. It may be necessary to discontinue repaglinide and administer insulin if the patient is exposed to stress (fever, trauma, infection, surgery). Theoretically, repaglinide may increase cardiovascular events as observed in some studies using sulfonylureas, but there are no long-term studies assessing this concern. Not indicated for use in combination with NPH insulin as there have been case reports of myocardial ischemia; further evaluation required to assess the safety of this combination.

Adverse Reactions (Reflective of adult population; not specific for elderly)
>10%:
  Central nervous system: Headache (9% to 11%)
  Endocrine & metabolic: Hypoglycemia (16% to 31%)
  Respiratory: Upper respiratory tract infection (10% to 16%)
1% to 10%:
  Cardiovascular: Ischemia (4%), chest pain (2% to 3%)
  Gastrointestinal: Diarrhea (4% to 5%), constipation (2% to 3%)
  Genitourinary: Urinary tract infection (2% to 3%)
  Neuromuscular & skeletal: Back pain (5% to 6%), arthralgia (3% to 6%)
  Respiratory: Sinusitis (3% to 6%), bronchitis (2% to 6%)
  Miscellaneous: Allergy (1% to 2%)

Drug Interactions
Metabolism/Transport Effects Substrate of CYP2C8 (major), CYP3A4 (major), SLCO1B1
Avoid Concomitant Use
Avoid concomitant use of Repaglinide with any of the following: Conivaptan; Gemfibrozil
Increased Effect/Toxicity
Repaglinide may increase the levels/effects of: Hypoglycemic Agents

The levels/effects of Repaglinide may be increased by: Antifungal Agents (Azole Derivatives, Systemic); Conivaptan; CycloSPORINE; CycloSPORINE (Systemic); CYP2C8 Inhibitors (Moderate); CYP2C8 Inhibitors (Strong); CYP3A4 Inhibitors (Moderate); CYP3A4 Inhibitors (Strong); Dasatinib; Deferasirox; Eltrombopag; Gemfibrozil; Herbs (Hypoglycemic Properties); Macrolide Antibiotics; Pegvisomant; Trimethoprim

Decreased Effect

The levels/effects of Repaglinide may be decreased by: Corticosteroids (Orally Inhaled); Corticosteroids (Systemic); CYP2C8 Inducers (Highly Effective); CYP3A4 Inducers (Strong); Deferasirox; Herbs (CYP3A4 Inducers); Luteinizing Hormone-Releasing Hormone Analogs; Rifamycin Derivatives; Somatropin; Thiazide Diuretics; Tocilizumab

Ethanol/Nutrition/Herb Interactions

Ethanol: Avoid ethanol; may increase risk of hypoglycemia.

Food: When given with food, the AUC of repaglinide is decreased.

Herb/Nutraceutical: Avoid alfalfa, aloe, bilberry, bitter melon, burdock, celery, damiana, fenugreek, garcinia, garlic, ginger, ginseng (American), gymnema, marshmallow, and stinging nettle (may enhance the hypoglycemic effects of antidiabetic agents). St John's wort may decrease the levels/effect of repaglinide.

Stability Do not store above 25°C (77°F). Protect from moisture.

Mechanism of Action Nonsulfonylurea hypoglycemic agent which blocks ATP-dependent potassium channels, depolarizing the membrane and facilitating calcium entry through calcium channels. Increased intracellular calcium stimulates insulin release from the pancreatic beta cells. Repaglinide-induced insulin release is glucose-dependent.

Pharmacodynamics/Kinetics

Onset of action: Single dose: Increased insulin levels: ~15-60 minutes

Duration: 4-6 hours

Absorption: Rapid and complete

Distribution: V_d: 31 L

Protein binding, plasma: >98% to albumin

Metabolism: Hepatic via CYP3A4 and CYP2C8 isoenzymes and glucuronidation to inactive metabolites

Bioavailability: ~56%

Half-life elimination: ~1 hour

Time to peak, plasma: ~1 hour

Excretion: Feces (~90%, <2% as unchanged drug); Urine (~8%, 0.1% as unchanged drug)

Dosage

Geriatric & Adult

Type 2 diabetes: Oral:

Patients not previously treated or whose Hb A_{1c} is <8%: Initial: 0.5 mg before each meal

Patients previously treated with blood glucose-lowering agents whose Hb A_{1c} is ≥8%: Initial: 1 or 2 mg before each meal.

Dose adjustment: Determine dosing adjustments by blood glucose response, usually fasting blood glucose. Double the preprandial dose up to 4 mg until satisfactory blood glucose response is achieved. At least 1 week should elapse to assess response after each dose adjustment.

Dose range: 0.5-4 mg taken with meals. Repaglinide may be dosed preprandially 2, 3, or 4 times/day in response to changes in the patient's meal pattern. Maximum recommended daily dose: 16 mg.

Patients receiving other oral hypoglycemic agents: When repaglinide is used to replace therapy with other oral hypoglycemic agents, it may be started the day after the final dose is given. Observe patients carefully for hypoglycemia because of potential overlapping of drug effects. When transferred from longer half-life sulfonylureas (eg, chlorpropamide), close monitoring may be indicated for up to ≥1 week.

Note: Combination therapy: If repaglinide monotherapy does not result in adequate glycemic control, metformin or a thiazolidinedione may be added. Or, if metformin or thiazolidinedione therapy does not provide adequate control, repaglinide may be added. The starting dose and dose adjustments for combination therapy are the same as repaglinide monotherapy. Carefully adjust the dose of each drug to determine the minimal dose required to achieve the desired pharmacologic effect. Failure to do so could result in an increase in the incidence of hypoglycemic episodes. Use appropriate monitoring of FPG and Hb A_{1c} measurements to ensure that the patient is not subjected to excessive drug exposure or increased probability of secondary drug failure. If glucose is not achieved after a suitable trial of combination therapy, consider discontinuing these drugs and using insulin.

Renal Impairment

Cl_{cr} 40-80 mL/minute (mild-to-moderate renal dysfunction): Initial dosage adjustment does not appear to be necessary.

Cl_{cr} 20-40 mL/minute (severe renal impairment): Initial: 0.5 mg with meals; titrate carefully.

Cl_{cr} <20 mL/minute: Not studied.

Hemodialysis: Not studied

Hepatic Impairment Use conservative initial and maintenance doses. Use longer intervals between dosage adjustments.

◀ **Administration** Administer 15 minutes before meals; however, time may vary from immediately preceding a meal to as long as 30 minutes before a meal. If the patient misses a meal or is unable to take anything by mouth, repaglinide should not be administered to avoid hypoglycemia. Patients consuming extra meals should be instructed to add a dose for the extra meal.

Monitoring Parameters Monitor fasting blood glucose (periodically) and glycosylated hemoglobin (Hb A_{1c}) levels (every 3 months) with a goal of decreasing these levels towards the normal range. During dose adjustment, fasting glucose can be used to determine response.

Reference Range
Recommendations for glycemic control in adults with diabetes:
Hb A_{1c}: <7%
Preprandial capillary plasma glucose: 70-130 mg/dL
Peak postprandial capillary blood glucose: <180 mg/dL
Blood pressure: <130/80 mm Hg
Recommendations for glycemic control in older adults with diabetes:
Relatively healthy, cognitively intact, and with a ≥5-year life expectancy: See Adults
Frail, life expectancy <5-years or those for whom the risks of intensive glucose control outweigh the benefits:
Hb A_{1c}: <8% to 9%
Blood pressure: <140/80 mm Hg or <130/80 mm Hg if tolerated

Special Geriatric Considerations Repaglinide has not been studied exclusively in the elderly; information from the manufacturer states that no differences in its effectiveness or adverse effects had been identified between persons younger than and older than 65 years of age. Intensive glucose control (HbA_{1c} <6.5%) has been linked to increased all-cause and cardiovascular mortality, hypoglycemia requiring assistance, and weight gain in adult type 2 diabetes. How "tightly" to control a geriatric patient's blood glucose needs to be individualized. Such a decision should be based on several factors, including the patient's functional and cognitive status, how well he/she recognizes hypoglycemic or hyperglycemic symptoms, and how to respond to them and other disease states. An HbA_{1c} <7.5% is an acceptable endpoint for a healthy older adult, while <8% is acceptable for frail elderly patients, those with a duration of illness >10 years, or those with comorbid conditions and requiring combination diabetes medications. Patients who are unable to accurately draw up their dose will need assistance, such as prefilled syringes. Initial doses may require considerations for renal function in the elderly with dosing adjusted subsequently based on blood glucose monitoring. For elderly patients with diabetes who are relatively healthy, attaining target goals for aspirin use, blood pressure, lipids, smoking cessation, and diet and exercise may be more important than normalized glycemic control.

Dosage Forms Excipient information presented when available (limited, particularly for generics); consult specific product labeling.
Tablet, oral:
Prandin®: 0.5 mg, 1 mg, 2 mg

Selected References
Action to Control Cardiovascular Risk in Diabetes Study Group, Gerstein HC, Miller ME, et al, "Effects of Intensive Glucose Lowering in Type 2 Diabetes," *N Engl J Med*, 2008, 358(24):2545-59.
ADVANCE Collaborative Group, Patel A, MacMahon S, et al, "Intensive Blood Glucose Control and Vascular Outcomes in Patients With Type 2 Diabetes," *N Engl J Med*, 2008, 358(24):2560-72.
American Diabetes Association, "Standards of Medical Care in Diabetes – 2011," *Diabetes Care*, 2011, 34(Suppl 1):11-61.
Brown AF, Mangione CM, Saliba D, et al, "Guidelines for Improving the Care of the Older Person With Diabetes Mellitus," *J Am Geriatr Soc*, 2003, 51(5 Suppl Guidelines):265-80.
"VA/DoD Clinical Practice Guideline for the Management of Diabetes Mellitus," 2010. Available at http://www.healthquality.va.gov/Diabetes_Mellitus.asp

Repaglinide and Metformin (re PAG li nide & met FOR min)

Related Information
Diabetes Mellitus Management, Adults *on page 2073*
MetFORMIN *on page 1155*
Repaglinide *on page 1596*

Medication Safety Issues
Sound-alike/look-alike issues:
PrandiMet® may be confused with Avandamet®, Prandin®
High alert medication:
The Institute for Safe Medication Practices (ISMP) includes this medication among its list of drug classes which have a heightened risk of causing significant patient harm when used in error.

Brand Names: U.S. PrandiMet®

Index Terms Metformin and Repaglinide; Repaglinide and Metformin Hydrochloride
Generic Availability (U.S.) No
Pharmacologic Category Antidiabetic Agent, Biguanide; Antidiabetic Agent, Meglitinide Derivative; Hypoglycemic Agent, Oral
Use Management of type 2 diabetes mellitus (noninsulin dependent, NIDDM), as an adjunct to diet and exercise, in patients currently receiving or not adequately controlled on metformin and/or a meglitinide
Dosage

Geriatric & Adult Type 2 diabetes mellitus: Oral: **Note:** Daily doses should be divided and given 2-3 times daily with meals (maximum single dose: 4 mg/dose [repaglinide], 1000 mg/dose [metformin]; maximum daily dose: 10 mg/day [repaglinide], 2500 mg/day [metformin])
Patients currently taking repaglinide and metformin: Initial doses should be based on (but not exceeding) the patient's current doses of repaglinide and metformin; titrate as needed to the maximum daily dose to achieve targeted glycemic control
Patients inadequately controlled on metformin alone: Initial dose: repaglinide 1 mg/ metformin 500 mg twice daily with meals. Titrate slowly to reduce the risk of repaglinide-induced hypoglycemia.
Patients inadequately controlled on a meglitinide alone: Initial dose: metformin 500 mg twice daily plus repaglinide at a dose similar to (but not exceeding) the patient's current dose. Titrate slowly to reduce the risk of metformin-induced gastrointestinal adverse effects.

Renal Impairment Do not use in renal impairment; metformin use is contraindicated in patients with renal impairment (serum creatinine ≥1.5 mg/dL in males or ≥1.4 mg/dL in females).

Hepatic Impairment Avoid use in patients with impaired liver function.

Special Geriatric Considerations Metformin should not be used in patients ≥80 years of age unless renal function is verified as normal. **Do not titrate to maximum dose.** Intensive glucose control (HbA$_{1c}$ <6.5%) has been linked to increased all-cause and cardiovascular mortality, hypoglycemia requiring assistance, and weight gain in adult type 2 diabetes. How "tightly" to control a geriatric patient's blood glucose needs to be individualized. Such a decision should be based on several factors, including the patient's functional and cognitive status, how well he/she recognizes hypoglycemic or hyperglycemic symptoms, and how to respond to them and other disease states. An HbA$_{1c}$ <7.5% is an acceptable endpoint for a healthy older adult, while <8% is acceptable for frail elderly patients, those with a duration of illness >10 years, or those with comorbid conditions and requiring combination diabetes medications. Patients who are unable to accurately draw up their dose will need assistance, such as prefilled syringes. Initial doses may require considerations for renal function in the elderly with dosing adjusted subsequently based on blood glucose monitoring. For elderly patients with diabetes who are relatively healthy, attaining target goals for aspirin use, blood pressure, lipids, smoking cessation, and diet and exercise may be more important than normalized glycemic control.

Dosage Forms Excipient information presented when available (limited, particularly for generics); consult specific product labeling.
Tablet:
PrandiMet®:
1/500: Repaglinide 1 mg and metformin hydrochloride 500 mg
2/500: Repaglinide 2 mg and metformin hydrochloride 500 mg

◆ **Repaglinide and Metformin Hydrochloride** see Repaglinide and Metformin *on page 1598*
◆ **Requip®** see ROPINIRole *on page 1632*
◆ **Requip® XL™** see ROPINIRole *on page 1632*

Reserpine (re SER peen)

Related Information
Beers Criteria − Potentially Inappropriate Medications for Geriatrics *on page 2089*
Medication Safety Issues
Sound-alike/look-alike issues:
Reserpine may be confused with RisperDAL®, risperiDONE
BEERS Criteria medication:
This drug may be inappropriate for use in geriatric patients (low severity risk).
Generic Availability (U.S.) Yes
Pharmacologic Category Central Monoamine-Depleting Agent; Rauwolfia Alkaloid
Use Management of mild-to-moderate hypertension; treatment of agitated psychotic states (schizophrenia)
Unlabeled/Investigational Use Management of tardive dyskinesia

Dosage

Geriatric Oral: Initial: 0.05 mg once daily increasing by 0.05 mg every week as necessary; full antihypertensive effects may take as long as 3 weeks (Beers Criteria: Avoid doses >0.25 mg daily)

Adult

Hypertension:

Manufacturer's labeling: Initial: 0.5 mg/day for 1-2 weeks; maintenance: 0.1-0.25 mg/day

Note: Clinically, the need for a "loading" period (as recommended by the manufacturer) is not well supported, and alternative dosing is preferred.

Alternative dosing (unlabeled): Initial: 0.1 mg once daily; adjust as necessary based on response.

Usual dose range (JNC 7): 0.05-0.25 mg once daily; 0.1 mg every other day may be given to achieve 0.05 mg once daily

Schizophrenia (labeled use) or tardive dyskinesia (unlabeled use): Dosing recommendations vary; initial dose recommendations generally range from 0.05-0.25 mg (although manufacturer recommends 0.5 mg once daily initially in schizophrenia). May be increased in increments of 0.1-0.25 mg; maximum dose in tardive dyskinesia: 5 mg/day.

Renal Impairment

Cl_{cr} <10 mL/minute: Avoid use.

Not removed by hemo- or peritoneal dialysis; supplemental dose is not necessary.

Special Geriatric Considerations Some older studies advocated the use of reserpine because of its low cost, long half-life, and efficacy, but it is generally not considered a first-line drug.

This medication is considered to be potentially inappropriate in this patient population (Beers Criteria severity: Low).

Dosage Forms Excipient information presented when available (limited, particularly for generics); consult specific product labeling.

Tablet, oral: 0.1 mg, 0.25 mg

- ◆ **Resistant Dextrin** *see* Wheat Dextrin *on page 1933*
- ◆ **Resistant Maltodextrin** *see* Wheat Dextrin *on page 1933*
- ◆ **Respa®-BR [DSC]** *see* Brompheniramine *on page 217*
- ◆ **Restasis®** *see* CycloSPORINE (Ophthalmic) *on page 438*
- ◆ **Restoril™** *see* Temazepam *on page 1751*

Retapamulin (re te PAM ue lin)

Brand Names: U.S. Altabax™

Generic Availability (U.S.) No

Pharmacologic Category Antibiotic, Pleuromutilin; Antibiotic, Topical

Use Treatment of impetigo caused by susceptible strains of *S. pyogenes* or methicillin-susceptible *S. aureus*

Contraindications Hypersensitivity to retapamulin or any component of the formulation

Warnings/Precautions For treatment of impetigo covering up to 100 cm² total area in adults. For external use only; not for intranasal, intravaginal, ophthalmic, oral, or mucosal application. May cause superinfection. Concomitant use with other topical products to the same treatment area has not been evaluated. If skin irritation occurs, discontinue use.

Adverse Reactions (Reflective of adult population; not specific for elderly)

1% to 10%:

Central nervous system: Headache (1% to 2%), pyrexia (1%)

Dermatologic: Pruritus (2%), eczema (1%)

Gastrointestinal: Diarrhea (1% to 2%), nausea (1%)

Local: Application site irritation (2%), application site pruritus (2%)

Respiratory: Nasopharyngitis (1% to 2%)

Drug Interactions

Avoid Concomitant Use There are no known interactions where it is recommended to avoid concomitant use.

Increased Effect/Toxicity There are no known significant interactions involving an increase in effect.

Decreased Effect There are no known significant interactions involving a decrease in effect.

Stability Store at room temperature of 15°C to 30°C (59°F to 86°F).

Mechanism of Action Primarily bacteriostatic. Inhibits normal bacterial protein biosynthesis by binding at a unique site (protein L3) on the ribosomal 50S subunit; prevents formation of active 50S ribosomal subunits by inhibiting peptidyl transfer and blocking P-site interactions at this site

Pharmacodynamics/Kinetics

Absorption: Topical: Low; increased when applied to abraded skin

Protein binding: 94%

Metabolism: Hepatic via CYP 3A4; extensively metabolized by mono-oxygenation and di-oxygenation to multiple metabolites

Dosage

Adult Impetigo: Topical: Apply to affected area twice daily for 5 days. Total treatment area should not exceed 100 cm^2 total body surface area.

Administration Topical: May cover treatment area with sterile bandage or gauze dressing if needed. Concomitant use with other topical products to the same treatment area has not been evaluated.

Special Geriatric Considerations Evaluate the patient's or caregiver's ability to safely administer the correct dose of ophthalmic medication.

Dosage Forms Excipient information presented when available (limited, particularly for generics); consult specific product labeling. [DSC] = Discontinued product

Ointment, topical:

Altabax™: 1% (5 g [DSC], 10 g [DSC], 15 g)

Selected References

Parish LC, Jorizzo JL, Breton JJ, et al, "Topical Retapamulin Ointment (1%, wt/wt) Twice Daily for 5 Days Versus Oral Cephalexin Twice Daily for 10 Days in the Treatment of Secondarily Infected Dermatitis: Results of a Randomized Controlled Trial," *J Am Acad Dermatol*, 2006, 55(6):1003-13.

◆ **Retavase®** see Reteplase *on page 1601*

Reteplase (RE ta plase)

Medication Safety Issues

High alert medication:

The Institute for Safe Medication Practices (ISMP) includes this medication (I.V.) among its list of drugs which have a heightened risk of causing significant patient harm when used in error.

Brand Names: U.S. Retavase®

Brand Names: Canada Retavase®

Index Terms r-PA; Recombinant Plasminogen Activator

Generic Availability (U.S.) No

Pharmacologic Category Thrombolytic Agent

Use Management of ST-elevation myocardial infarction (STEMI); improvement of ventricular function; reduction of the incidence of CHF and the reduction of mortality following AMI

Recommended criteria for treatment: STEMI: Chest pain ≥20 minutes duration, onset of chest pain within 12 hours of treatment (or within prior 12-24 hours in patients with continuing ischemic symptoms), and ST-segment elevation >0.1 mV in at least two contiguous precordial leads or two adjacent limb leads on ECG or new or presumably new left bundle branch block (LBBB)

Contraindications Hypersensitivity to reteplase or any component of the formulation; active internal bleeding; history of cerebrovascular accident; recent intracranial or intraspinal surgery or trauma; intracranial neoplasm, arteriovenous malformations, or aneurysm; known bleeding diathesis; severe uncontrolled hypertension

Warnings/Precautions Concurrent heparin anticoagulation can contribute to bleeding; careful attention to all potential bleeding sites. I.M. injections and nonessential handling of the patient should be avoided. Venipunctures should be performed carefully and only when necessary. If arterial puncture is necessary, use an upper extremity vessel that can be manually compressed. If serious bleeding occurs then the infusion of anistreplase and heparin should be stopped.

For the following conditions the risk of bleeding is higher with use of reteplase and should be weighed against the benefits of therapy: recent major surgery (eg, CABG, obstetrical delivery, organ biopsy, previous puncture of noncompressible vessels), cerebrovascular disease, recent gastrointestinal or genitourinary bleeding, recent trauma including CPR, hypertension (systolic BP >180 mm Hg and/or diastolic BP >110 mm Hg), high likelihood of left heart thrombus (eg, mitral stenosis with atrial fibrillation), acute pericarditis, subacute bacterial endocarditis, hemostatic defects including ones caused by severe renal or hepatic dysfunction, significant hepatic dysfunction, diabetic hemorrhagic retinopathy or other hemorrhagic ophthalmic conditions, septic thrombophlebitis or occluded AV cannula at seriously infected site, advanced age (eg, >75 years), patients receiving oral anticoagulants, any other condition in which bleeding constitutes a significant hazard or would be particularly difficult to manage because of location.

◄ Coronary thrombolysis may result in reperfusion arrhythmias. Follow standard MI management. Rare anaphylactic reactions can occur.

Adverse Reactions (Reflective of adult population; not specific for elderly) Bleeding is the most frequent adverse effect associated with reteplase. Heparin and aspirin have been administered concurrently with reteplase in clinical trials. The incidence of adverse events is a reflection of these combined therapies, and are comparable with comparison thrombolytics.

>10%: Local: Injection site bleeding (4.6% to 48.6%)
1% to 10%:
  Gastrointestinal: Bleeding (1.8% to 9.0%)
  Genitourinary: Bleeding (0.9% to 9.5%)
  Hematologic: Anemia (0.9% to 2.6%)
Other adverse effects noted are frequently associated with MI (and therefore may or may not be attributable to Retavase®) and include arrhythmia, hypotension, cardiogenic shock, pulmonary edema, cardiac arrest, reinfarction, pericarditis, tamponade, thrombosis, and embolism.

Drug Interactions

Avoid Concomitant Use There are no known interactions where it is recommended to avoid concomitant use.

Increased Effect/Toxicity
Reteplase may increase the levels/effects of: Anticoagulants; Drotrecogin Alfa

The levels/effects of Reteplase may be increased by: Antiplatelet Agents; Herbs (Anticoagulant/Antiplatelet Properties); Nonsteroidal Anti-Inflammatory Agents; Salicylates

Decreased Effect
The levels/effects of Reteplase may be decreased by: Aprotinin

Stability Dosage kits should be stored at 2°C to 25°C (36°F to 77°F) and remain sealed until use in order to protect from light. Reteplase should be reconstituted using the diluent, syringe, needle, and dispensing pin provided with each kit.

Mechanism of Action Reteplase is a nonglycosylated form of tPA produced by recombinant DNA technology using *E. coli*; it initiates local fibrinolysis by binding to fibrin in a thrombus (clot) and converts entrapped plasminogen to plasmin

Pharmacodynamics/Kinetics
Onset of action: Thrombolysis: 30-90 minutes
Half-life elimination: 13-16 minutes
Excretion: Feces and urine
  Clearance: Plasma: 250-450 mL/minute

Dosage
Geriatric & Adult
STEMI: I.V.: 10 units I.V. over 2 minutes, followed by a second dose 30 minutes later of 10 units I.V. over 2 minutes; withhold second dose if serious bleeding or anaphylaxis occurs.
Note: All patients should receive 162-325 mg of chewable nonenteric coated aspirin as soon as possible and then daily. Administer concurrently with heparin 60 units/kg bolus (maximum: 4000 units) followed by continuous infusion of 12 units/kg/hour (maximum: 1000 units/hour) and adjust to aPTT target of 50-70 seconds (or 1.5-2 times the upper limit of control).

Administration Reteplase should be reconstituted using the diluent, syringe, needle and dispensing pin provided with each kit and the each reconstituted dose should be administered I.V. over 2 minutes; no other medication should be added to the injection solution

Monitoring Parameters Monitor for signs of bleeding (hematuria, GI bleeding, gingival bleeding)

Pharmacotherapy Pearls The dosage of reteplase in clinical trials was expressed in terms of million unit (MU); however, reteplase is being marketed in units (U) with 1 unit equivalent to 1 million units, reteplase units are expressed using a reference standard specific for reteplase and are not comparable with units used for other thrombolytic agents, 10 units is equivalent to 17.4 mg

Special Geriatric Considerations No specific changes in use in the elderly are necessary.

Dosage Forms Excipient information presented when available (limited, particularly for generics); consult specific product labeling.
Injection, powder for reconstitution [preservative free]:
  Retavase®: 10.4 units [contains polysorbate 80, sucrose 364 mg/vial; equivalent to reteplase 18.1 mg; supplied with diluent]

◆ **Retisert**® *see* Fluocinolone (Ophthalmic) *on page 748*
◆ **Revatio**® *see* Sildenafil *on page 1674*
◆ **Revonto**™ *see* Dantrolene *on page 452*
◆ **Rexolate**® *see* Salicylates (Various Salts) *on page 1647*
◆ **Rheumatrex**® *see* Methotrexate *on page 1168*

◆ **Rhinall® [OTC]** *see* Phenylephrine (Nasal) *on page 1442*
◆ **Rhinaris® [OTC]** *see* Sodium Chloride *on page 1690*
◆ **Rhinocort Aqua®** *see* Budesonide (Nasal) *on page 222*
◆ **r-Hirudin** *see* Desirudin *on page 474*
◆ **rhPTH(1-34)** *see* Teriparatide *on page 1760*
◆ **rHuEPO** *see* Epoetin Alfa *on page 611*
◆ **rhuFabV2** *see* Ranibizumab *on page 1585*
◆ **Ribasphere®** *see* Ribavirin *on page 1603*
◆ **Ribasphere® RibaPak®** *see* Ribavirin *on page 1603*

Ribavirin (rye ba VYE rin)

Medication Safety Issues
  Sound-alike/look-alike issues:
    Ribavirin may be confused with riboflavin, rifampin, Robaxin®
Brand Names: U.S. Copegus®; Rebetol®; Ribasphere®; Ribasphere® RibaPak®; Virazole®
Brand Names: Canada Virazole®
Index Terms RTCA; Tribavirin
Generic Availability (U.S.) Yes: Capsule, tablet
Pharmacologic Category Antiviral Agent
Use
  Inhalation: Treatment of hospitalized infants and young children with respiratory syncytial virus
    (RSV) infections; specially indicated for treatment of severe lower respiratory tract RSV
    infections in patients with an underlying compromising condition (prematurity, cardiopulmo-
    nary disease, or immunosuppression)
  Oral capsule:
    In combination with interferon alfa-2b (Intron® A) injection for the treatment of chronic
      hepatitis C in patients with compensated liver disease who have relapsed after alpha
      interferon therapy or were previously untreated with alpha interferons
    In combination with peginterferon alfa-2b (PEG-Intron®) injection for the treatment of chronic
      hepatitis C in patients with compensated liver disease who were previously untreated with
      alpha interferons
  Oral solution: In combination with interferon alfa 2b (Intron® A) injection for the treatment of
    chronic hepatitis C in patients with compensated liver disease who were previously
    untreated with alpha interferons or patients who have relapsed after alpha interferon therapy
  Oral tablet: In combination with peginterferon alfa-2a (Pegasys®) injection for the treatment of
    chronic hepatitis C in patients with compensated liver disease who were previously
    untreated with alpha interferons (includes patients with histological evidence of cirrhosis
    [Child-Pugh class A] and patients with clinically-stable HIV disease)
Unlabeled/Investigational Use
  Inhalation: Treatment for RSV in adult hematopoietic stem cell or heart/lung transplant
    recipients
  Used in other viral infections including influenza A and B and adenovirus
Medication Guide Available Yes
Contraindications Hypersensitivity to ribavirin or any component of the formulation

  Additional contraindications for oral formulation: Male partners of pregnant women; hemoglo-
    binopathies (eg, thalassemia major, sickle cell anemia); patients with autoimmune hepatitis;
    ribavirin tablets are contraindicated in patients with hepatic decompensation (Child-Pugh
    class B and C); concomitant use of didanosine
Warnings/Precautions Oral: **[U.S. Boxed Warning]: Significant teratogenic effects have
  been observed in all animal studies.** A negative pregnancy test is required before initiation
  and monthly thereafter. Avoid pregnancy in female patients and female partners of male
  patients, during therapy, and for at least 6 months after treatment; two forms of contraception
  should be used. Safety and efficacy have not been established in patients who have failed
  other alfa interferon therapy, received organ transplants, or been coinfected with hepatitis B or
  HIV (Copegus® may be used in HIV coinfected patients unless CD4+ cell count is <100 cells/
  microL). Oral products should not be used for HIV infection, adenovirus, RSV, or influenza
  infections.

  [U.S. Boxed Warning]: Monotherapy not effective for chronic hepatitis C infection.
  Severe psychiatric events have occurred including depression and suicidal behavior during
  combination therapy. Avoid use in patients with a psychiatric history; discontinue if severe
  psychiatric symptoms occur. Acute hypersensitivity reactions (eg, anaphylaxis, angioedema,
  bronchoconstriction, and urticaria) have been observed (rarely) with ribavirin and alfa
  interferon combination therapy. Severe cutaneous reactions, including Stevens-Johnson
  syndrome and exfoliative dermatitis have been reported (rarely) with ribavirin and alfa

interferon combination therapy; discontinue with signs or symptoms of severe skin reactions. Use with caution in patients with renal impairment; avoid use in patients with Cl_{cr} <50 mL/minute. Elderly patients are more susceptible to adverse effects; use caution.

[U.S. Boxed Warning]: Hemolytic anemia is the primary toxicity of oral therapy; usually occurring within 1-2 weeks of therapy initiation; observed in ~10% to 13% of patients when alfa interferons were combined with ribavirin. Assess cardiac disease before initiation. Anemia may worsen underlying cardiac disease; avoid use in patients with significant/unstable cardiac disease. If deterioration in cardiovascular status occurs, discontinue therapy. Patients with renal dysfunction and/or those >50 years of age should be carefully assessed for development of anemia. Pancytopenia and bone marrow suppression have been reported with the combination of ribavirin, interferon, and azathioprine. Use caution in pulmonary disease; pulmonary symptoms have been associated with administration. Discontinue therapy if evidence of hepatic decompensation (Child-Pugh score ≥6) is observed. Use caution in patients with sarcoidosis (exacerbation reported). Dental and periodontal disorders have been reported with ribavirin and interferon therapy; patients should be instructed to brush teeth twice daily and have regular dental exams. Serious ophthalmologic disorders have occurred with combination therapy. All patients require an eye exam at baseline; those with pre-existing ophthalmologic disorders (eg, diabetic or hypertensive retinopathy) require periodic follow up.

Inhalation: **[U.S. Boxed Warning]: Use with caution in patients requiring assisted ventilation because precipitation of the drug in the respiratory equipment may interfere with safe and effective patient ventilation; sudden deterioration of respiratory function has been observed;** monitor carefully in patients with COPD and asthma for deterioration of respiratory function. Ribavirin is potentially mutagenic, tumor-promoting, and gonadotoxic. Although anemia has not been reported with inhalation therapy, consider monitoring for anemia 1-2 weeks post-treatment. Pregnant healthcare workers may consider unnecessary occupational exposure; ribavirin has been detected in healthcare workers' urine. Healthcare professionals or family members who are pregnant (or may become pregnant) should be counseled about potential risks of exposure and counseled about risk reduction strategies. Hazardous agent - use appropriate precautions for handling and disposal.

Adverse Reactions (Reflective of adult population; not specific for elderly)

Inhalation:

1% to 10%:
  Central nervous system: Fatigue, headache, insomnia
  Gastrointestinal: Nausea, anorexia
  Hematologic: Anemia

<1%: Hypotension, cardiac arrest, digitalis toxicity, conjunctivitis, mild bronchospasm, worsening of respiratory function, apnea

Note: Incidence of adverse effects (approximate) in healthcare workers: Headache (51%); conjunctivitis (32%); rhinitis, nausea, rash, dizziness, pharyngitis, and lacrimation (10% to 20%); bronchospasm and/or chest pain (case reports in individuals with underlying airway disease)

Oral (all adverse reactions are documented while receiving combination therapy with alfa interferons; percentages as reported in adults); asterisked (*) percentages are those similar to interferon therapy alone:

>10%:
  Central nervous system: Fatigue (60% to 70%)*, headache (43% to 66%)*, fever (32% to 55%)*, insomnia (26% to 41%), depression (20% to 36%)*, irritability (23% to 33%), dizziness (14% to 26%), impaired concentration (10% to 21%)*, emotional lability (7% to 12%)*
  Dermatologic: Alopecia (27% to 36%), pruritus (13% to 29%), rash (5% to 28%), dry skin (10% to 24%), dermatitis (≤16%)
  Endocrine and metabolic: Hyperuricemia (33% to 38%)
  Gastrointestinal: Nausea (25% to 47%), anorexia (21% to 32%), weight decrease (10% to 29%), vomiting (9% to 25%)*, diarrhea (10% to 22%), dyspepsia (6% to 16%), abdominal pain (8% to 13%), xerostomia (≤12%), RUQ pain (≤12%)
  Hematologic: Leukopenia (6% to 45%), neutropenia (8% to 42%; grade 4: 2% to 11%; 40% with HIV coinfection), hemoglobin decreased (11% to 35%), anemia (11% to 17%), thrombocytopenia (<1% to 15%), lymphopenia (12% to 14%), hemolytic anemia (10% to 13%)
  Hepatic: Bilirubin increase (10% to 32%)
  Neuromuscular & skeletal: Myalgia (40% to 64%)*, rigors (25% to 48%), arthralgia (22% to 34%)*, musculoskeletal pain (19% to 28%)
  Respiratory: Dyspnea (13% to 26%), cough (7% to 23%), pharyngitis (≤13%), sinusitis (≤12%)*
  Miscellaneous: Flu-like syndrome (13% to 18%)*, viral infection (≤12%), diaphoresis (≤11%)

1% to 10%:

Cardiovascular: Chest pain (5% to 9%)*, flushing (≤4%)

Central nervous system: Pain (≤10%), mood alteration (≤6%; 9% with HIV coinfection), agitation (5% to 8%), nervousness (6%)*, memory impairment (≤6%), malaise (≤6%), suicidal ideation (adolescents: 2%; adults: 1%)

Dermatologic: Eczema (4% to 5%)

Endocrine & metabolic: Menstrual disorder (≤7%), hypothyroidism (≤5%)

Gastrointestinal: Taste perversion (4% to 9%), constipation (5%)

Hepatic: Hepatomegaly (4%), transaminases increased (1% to 3%), hepatic decompensation (2% with HIV coinfection)

Neuromuscular & skeletal: Weakness (9% to 10%), back pain (5%)

Ocular: Blurred vision (≤6%), conjunctivitis (≤5%)

Respiratory: Rhinitis (≤8%), exertional dyspnea (≤7%)

Miscellaneous: Fungal infection (≤6%), bacterial infection (3% to 5%)

Note: Incidence of anorexia, headache, fever, suicidal ideation, and vomiting are higher in children.

Drug Interactions

Avoid Concomitant Use

Avoid concomitant use of Ribavirin with any of the following: Didanosine

Increased Effect/Toxicity

Ribavirin may increase the levels/effects of: AzaTHIOprine; Didanosine; Reverse Transcriptase Inhibitors (Nucleoside)

The levels/effects of Ribavirin may be increased by: Interferons (Alfa); Zidovudine

Decreased Effect

Ribavirin may decrease the levels/effects of: Influenza Virus Vaccine (Live/Attenuated)

Ethanol/Nutrition/Herb Interactions Food: Oral: High-fat meal increases the AUC and C_{max}.

Stability

Inhalation: Store vials in a dry place at 15°C to 30°C (59°F to 86°F). Do not use any water containing an antimicrobial agent to reconstitute drug. Reconstituted solution is stable for 24 hours at room temperature. Should not be mixed with other aerosolized medication.

Oral: Store at controlled room temperature of 25°C (77°F). Solution may also be refrigerated at 2°C to 8°C (36°F to 46°F).

Mechanism of Action Inhibits replication of RNA and DNA viruses; inhibits influenza virus RNA polymerase activity and inhibits the initiation and elongation of RNA fragments resulting in inhibition of viral protein synthesis

Pharmacodynamics/Kinetics

Absorption: Inhalation: Systemic; dependent upon respiratory factors and method of drug delivery; maximal absorption occurs with the use of aerosol generator via endotracheal tube; highest concentrations in respiratory tract and erythrocytes

Distribution: Oral capsule: Single dose: V_d: 2825 L; distribution significantly prolonged in the erythrocyte (16-40 days), which can be used as a marker for intracellular metabolism

Protein binding: Oral: None

Metabolism: Hepatically and intracellularly (forms active metabolites); may be necessary for drug action

Bioavailability: Oral: 64%

Half-life elimination, plasma:

Adults: Oral:

Capsule, single dose (Rebetol®, Ribasphere®): 24 hours in healthy adults, 44 hours with chronic hepatitis C infection (increases to ~298 hours at steady state)

Tablet, single dose (Copegus®): ~120-170 hours

Time to peak, serum: Inhalation: At end of inhalation period; Oral capsule: Multiple doses: 3 hours; Tablet: 2 hours

Excretion: Inhalation: Urine (40% as unchanged drug and metabolites); Oral capsule: Urine (61%), feces (12%)

Dosage

Geriatric & Adult

Chronic hepatitis C (in combination with peginterferon alfa-2a): Oral: Tablet (Copegus®):

Monoinfection, genotype 1,4:

<75 kg: 1000 mg/day, in 2 divided doses for 48 weeks

≥75 kg: 1200 mg/day, in 2 divided doses for 48 weeks

Monoinfection, genotype 2,3: 800 mg/day, in 2 divided doses for 24 weeks

Coinfection with HIV: 800 mg/day in 2 divided doses for 48 weeks (regardless of genotype)

◀

Chronic hepatitis C (in combination with interferon alfa-2b): Oral: Capsule (Rebetol®, Ribasphere®):

≤75 kg: 400 mg in the morning, then 600 mg in the evening

>75 kg: 600 mg in the morning, then 600 mg in the evening

Chronic hepatitis C (in combination with peginterferon alfa-2b): Oral: Capsule (Rebetol®, Ribasphere®): 400 mg twice daily

Note: *American Association for the Study of Liver Diseases (AASLD) guidelines recommendation:* Adults with chronic HCV infection (Ghany, 2009): Treatment of choice: Ribavirin plus **peginterferon**; clinical condition and ability of patient to tolerate therapy should be evaluated to determine length and/or likely benefit of therapy. Recommended treatment duration (AASLD guidelines): Genotypes 1,4: 48 weeks; Genotypes 2,3: 24 weeks; Coinfection with HIV: 48 weeks.

RSV Infection in hematopoietic cell or heart/lung transplant recipients (unlabeled use): Aerosol inhalation: 2 g (over 2 hours) every 8 hours

Note: Heart/lung transplant recipients also received IVIG, methylprednisolone and palivizumab. Dosage and protocol may be institution specific. (Boeckh, 2007; Chemaly, 2006; Liu, 2010).

Renal Impairment Cl_{cr} <50 mL/minute: Oral route is not recommended.

Hepatic Impairment Hepatic decompensation (Child-Pugh class B and C): Use of ribavirin tablets is contraindicated.

Administration

Inhalation: Ribavirin should be administered in well-ventilated rooms (at least 6 air changes/hour). In mechanically-ventilated patients, ribavirin can potentially be deposited in the ventilator delivery system depending on temperature, humidity, and electrostatic forces; this deposition can lead to malfunction or obstruction of the expiratory valve, resulting in inadvertently high positive end-expiratory pressures. The use of one-way valves in the inspiratory lines, a breathing circuit filter in the expiratory line, and frequent monitoring and filter replacement have been effective in preventing these problems. Solutions in SPAG-2 unit should be discarded at least every 24 hours and when the liquid level is low before adding newly reconstituted solution. Should not be mixed with other aerosolized medication.

Oral: Administer concurrently with interferon alfa injection. Capsule should not be opened, crushed, chewed, or broken. Use oral solution for those who cannot swallow capsules.

Capsule, in combination with interferon alfa-2b: May be administered with or without food, but always in a consistent manner in regard to food intake.

Capsule, in combination with peginterferon alfa-2b: Administer with food.

Solution, in combination with interferon alfa-2b: May be administered with or without food, but always in a consistent manner in regard to food intake.

Tablet: Should be administered with food.

Monitoring Parameters

Inhalation: Respiratory function, hemoglobin, reticulocyte count, CBC with differential, I & O

Oral: Clinical studies tested as follows: CBC (including hemoglobin, WBC, and platelets) and chemistries (including liver function tests and uric acid) measured at weeks 1, 2, 4, 6, and 8, and then every 4 weeks; TSH measured every 12 weeks

Baseline values used in clinical trials:

Platelet count ≥90,000/mm^3 (75,000/mm^3 for cirrhosis or 70,000/mm^3 for coinfection with HIV)

ANC ≥1500/mm^3

Hemoglobin ≥12 g/dL for women and ≥13 g/dL for men (11 g/dL for HIV coinfected women and 12 g/dL for HIV coinfected men)

TSH and T_4 within normal limits or adequately controlled

CD4$^+$ cell count ≥200 cells/microL or CD4$^+$ cell count 100-200 cells/microL and HIV-1 RNA <5000 copies/mL for coinfection with HIV

Serum HCV RNA (pretreatment, week 12 and week 24, and 24 weeks after completion of therapy). **Note:** Discontinuation of therapy may be considered after 12 weeks in patients with HCV (genotypes 1,4) who fail to achieve an early virologic response (EVR) (defined as ≥2-log decrease in HCV RNA compared to pretreatment) or after 24 weeks with detectable HCV RNA. Treat patients with HCV (genotypes 2,3) for 24 weeks (if tolerated) and then evaluate HCV RNA levels (Ghany, 2009).

Pretreatment ECG in patients with pre-existing cardiac disease; dental exams; ophthalmic exam pretreatment (all patients) and periodically for those with pre-existing ophthalmologic disorders.

Reference Range

Rapid virological response (RVR): Absence of detectable HCV RNA after 4 weeks of treatment

Early viral response (EVR): ≥2-log decrease in HCV RNA after 12 weeks of treatment

End of treatment response (ETR): Absence of detectable HCV RNA at end of the recommended treatment period

Sustained treatment response (STR): Absence of HCV RNA in the serum 6 months following completion of full treatment course

Special Geriatric Considerations No specific recommendations are necessary in the elderly; however, in patients with creatinine clearance <50 mL/minute, the oral route not recommended. Many elderly will fall into this category.

Dosage Forms Excipient information presented when available (limited, particularly for generics); consult specific product labeling.

Capsule, oral: 200 mg
  Rebetol®: 200 mg
  Ribasphere®: 200 mg
Combination package, oral [dose-pack/each package contains]:
  Ribasphere® RibaPak®: Tablet: 400 mg (7s) [medium blue tablets] and Tablet: 600 mg (7s) [dark blue tablets] (14s, 56s)
Powder for solution, for nebulization:
  Virazole®: 6 g [reconstituted product contains ribavirin 20 mg/mL]
Solution, oral:
  Rebetol®: 40 mg/mL (100 mL) [contains propylene glycol, sodium benzoate; bubblegum flavor]
Tablet, oral: 200 mg
  Copegus®: 200 mg
  Ribasphere®: 200 mg, 400 mg, 600 mg
Tablet, oral [dose-pack]:
  Ribasphere® RibaPak®: 400 mg, 600 mg

Selected References

Ghany MG, Strader DB, Thomas DL, et al, "Diagnosis, Management And Treatment Of Hepatitis C: An Update," Hepatology, 2009, 49(4):1335-74.

◆ **Rid® [OTC]** see Permethrin on page 1429
◆ **Ridaura®** see Auranofin on page 168

Rifabutin (rif a BYOO tin)

Medication Safety Issues
  Sound-alike/look-alike issues:
    Rifabutin may be confused with rifampin

Brand Names: U.S. Mycobutin®

Brand Names: Canada Mycobutin®

Index Terms Ansamycin

Generic Availability (U.S.) No

Pharmacologic Category Antibiotic, Miscellaneous; Antitubercular Agent

Use Prevention of disseminated *Mycobacterium avium* complex (MAC) in patients with advanced HIV infection

Unlabeled/Investigational Use Utilized in multidrug regimens for treatment of MAC; alternative to rifampin as prophylaxis for latent tuberculosis infection (LTBI) or part of multidrug regimen for treatment active tuberculosis infection

Contraindications Hypersensitivity to rifabutin, any other rifamycins, or any component of the formulation

Warnings/Precautions Rifabutin must not be administered for MAC prophylaxis to patients with active tuberculosis since its use may lead to the development of tuberculosis that is resistant to both rifabutin and rifampin. May be associated with neutropenia and/or thrombocytopenia (rarely). Dosage reduction recommended in severe impairment (Cl$_{cr}$ <30 mL/minute). Prolonged use may result in fungal or bacterial superinfection, including *C. difficile*-associated diarrhea (CDAD) and pseudomembranous colitis; CDAD has been observed >2 months postantibiotic treatment. May cause brown/orange discoloration of urine, feces, saliva, sweat, tears, and skin. Remove soft contact lenses during therapy since permanent staining may occur.

Adverse Reactions (Reflective of adult population; not specific for elderly)
>10%:
  Dermatologic: Rash (11%)
  Genitourinary: Discoloration of urine (30%)
  Hematologic: Neutropenia (25%), leukopenia (17%)
1% to 10%:
  Central nervous system: Headache (3%), fever (2%)
  Gastrointestinal: Nausea (3% to 6%), abdominal pain (4%), dyspepsia (3%), eructation (3%), taste perversion (3%), vomiting (3%), flatulence (2%)

Hematologic: Thrombocytopenia (5%)

Hepatic: ALT increased (7% to 9%; incidence less than placebo), AST increased (7% to 9%; incidence less than placebo)

Neuromuscular & skeletal: Myalgia (2%)

Drug Interactions

Metabolism/Transport Effects Substrate of CYP3A4 (major); **Induces** CYP3A4 (strong)

Avoid Concomitant Use

Avoid concomitant use of Rifabutin with any of the following: BCG; Boceprevir; Crizotinib; Dronedarone; Everolimus; Lapatinib; Lurasidone; Mycophenolate; Nilotinib; Pazopanib; Praziquantel; Ranolazine; Rilpivirine; Roflumilast; RomiDEPsin; Telaprevir; Ticagrelor; Tolvaptan; Vandetanib; Voriconazole

Increased Effect/Toxicity

Rifabutin may increase the levels/effects of: Clopidogrel; Darunavir; Fosamprenavir; HMG-CoA Reductase Inhibitors; Isoniazid; Lopinavir

The levels/effects of Rifabutin may be increased by: Antifungal Agents (Azole Derivatives, Systemic); Atazanavir; Boceprevir; Conivaptan; Darunavir; Delavirdine; Fluconazole; Fosamprenavir; Indinavir; Lopinavir; Macrolide Antibiotics; Nelfinavir; Nevirapine; Ritonavir; Saquinavir; Telaprevir; Tipranavir; Voriconazole

Decreased Effect

Rifabutin may decrease the levels/effects of: Alfentanil; Amiodarone; Angiotensin II Receptor Blockers; Antiemetics (5HT3 Antagonists); Antifungal Agents (Azole Derivatives, Systemic); Aprepitant; Atovaquone; Barbiturates; BCG; Benzodiazepines (metabolized by oxidation); Boceprevir; Brentuximab Vedotin; BusPIRone; Calcium Channel Blockers; Contraceptives (Estrogens); Contraceptives (Progestins); Corticosteroids (Systemic); Crizotinib; CycloSPORINE; CycloSPORINE (Systemic); CYP3A4 Substrates; Dapsone; Dapsone (Systemic); Delavirdine; Disopyramide; Dronedarone; Efavirenz; Etravirine; Everolimus; Exemestane; FentaNYL; Fluconazole; Fosphenytoin; Gefitinib; GuanFACINE; HMG-CoA Reductase Inhibitors; Imatinib; Indinavir; Ixabepilone; Lapatinib; Linagliptin; Lurasidone; Maraviroc; Morphine (Systemic); Morphine Sulfate; Mycophenolate; Nelfinavir; Nevirapine; Nilotinib; Pazopanib; Phenytoin; Praziquantel; Propafenone; QuiNIDine; Rameltenon; Ranolazine; Repaglinide; Rilpivirine; Rivaroxaban; Roflumilast; RomiDEPsin; Saxagliptin; SORAfenib; SUNItinib; Tacrolimus; Tacrolimus (Systemic); Tadalafil; Tamoxifen; Telaprevir; Temsirolimus; Terbinafine (Systemic); Ticagrelor; Tolvaptan; Typhoid Vaccine; Ulipristal; Vandetanib; Vemurafenib; Vitamin K Antagonists; Voriconazole; Zaleplon; Zolpidem

The levels/effects of Rifabutin may be decreased by: CYP3A4 Inducers (Strong); Cyproterone; Deferasirox; Efavirenz; Herbs (CYP3A4 Inducers); Nevirapine; Tocilizumab

Ethanol/Nutrition/Herb Interactions Food: High-fat meal may decrease the rate but not the extent of absorption.

Stability Store at 25°C (77°F); excursions permitted to 15°C to 30°C (59°F to 86°F).

Mechanism of Action Inhibits DNA-dependent RNA polymerase at the beta subunit which prevents chain initiation

Pharmacodynamics/Kinetics

Absorption: Readily, 53%

Distribution: V_d: 9.32 L/kg; distributes to body tissues including the lungs, liver, spleen, eyes, and kidneys

Protein binding: 85%

Metabolism: To 5 metabolites; predominantly 25-O-desacetyl-rifabutin (antimicrobial activity equivalent to parent drug; serum AUC 10% of parent drug) and 31-hydroxy-rifabutin (serum AUC 7% of parent drug)

Bioavailability: Absolute: HIV: 20%

Half-life elimination: Terminal: 45 hours (range: 16-69 hours)

Time to peak, serum: 2-4 hours

Excretion: Urine (53% as metabolites); feces (30%)

Dosage

Geriatric & Adult

Disseminated MAC in advanced HIV infection: Oral:

Prophylaxis: 300 mg once daily or 150 mg twice daily to reduce gastrointestinal upset

Treatment (unlabeled use; AIDSinfo guidelines): 300 mg once daily as an optional add-on to primary therapy of clarithromycin and ethambutol

Tuberculosis (unlabeled use as alternative to rifampin; AIDS *info* guidelines): Oral:

Prophylaxis of LTBI: 300 mg once daily for 4 months

Treatment of active TB: 300 mg once daily or intermittently 2-3 times weekly as part of multidrug regimen

Dosage adjustment for concurrent nelfinavir, amprenavir, indinavir: Reduce rifabutin dose to 150 mg/day; no change in dose if administered twice weekly

Dosage adjustment for concurrent efavirenz (no concomitant protease inhibitor): Increase rifabutin dose to 450-600 mg daily, or 600 mg 3 times/week

Renal Impairment Cl$_{cr}$ <30 mL/minute: Reduce dose by 50%

Administration May be mixed with food (ie, applesauce)

Monitoring Parameters Periodic liver function tests, CBC with differential, platelet count

Special Geriatric Considerations No specific recommendations for the elderly.

Dosage Forms Excipient information presented when available (limited, particularly for generics); consult specific product labeling.

Capsule, oral:

Mycobutin®: 150 mg

♦ **Rifadin®** see Rifampin on page 1609
♦ **Rifampicin** see Rifampin on page 1609

Rifampin (rif AM pin)

Related Information

Antibiotic Treatment of Adults With Infective Endocarditis on page 2053

Medication Safety Issues

Sound-alike/look-alike issues:

Rifadin® may be confused with Rifater®, Ritalin®

Rifampin may be confused with ribavirin, rifabutin, Rifamate®, rifapentine, rifaximin

Brand Names: U.S. Rifadin®

Brand Names: Canada Rifadin®; Rofact™

Index Terms Rifampicin

Generic Availability (U.S.) Yes

Pharmacologic Category Antibiotic, Miscellaneous; Antitubercular Agent

Use Management of active tuberculosis in combination with other agents; elimination of meningococci from the nasopharynx in asymptomatic carriers

Unlabeled/Investigational Use Prophylaxis of *Haemophilus influenzae* type b infection; *Legionella* pneumonia; used in combination with other anti-infectives in the treatment of staphylococcal infections; treatment of *M. leprae* infections

Contraindications Hypersensitivity to rifampin, any rifamycins, or any component of the formulation; concurrent use of amprenavir, saquinavir/ritonavir (possibly other protease inhibitors)

Warnings/Precautions Use with caution and modify dosage in patients with liver impairment; observe for hyperbilirubinemia; discontinue therapy if this in conjunction with clinical symptoms or any signs of significant hepatocellular damage develop. Use with caution in patients receiving concurrent medications associated with hepatotoxicity. Use with caution in patients with a history of alcoholism (even if ethanol consumption is discontinued during therapy). Since rifampin since rifampin has enzyme-inducing properties, porphyria exacerbation is possible; use with caution in patients with porphyria; do not use for meningococcal disease, only for short-term treatment of asymptomatic carrier states

Regimens of >600 mg once or twice weekly have been associated with a high incidence of adverse reactions including a flu-like syndrome, hypersensitivity, thrombocytopenia, leukopenia, and anemia. Urine, feces, saliva, sweat, tears, and CSF may be discolored to red/orange; remove soft contact lenses during therapy since permanent staining may occur. Do not administer I.V. form via I.M. or SubQ routes; restart infusion at another site if extravasation occurs. Prolonged use may result in fungal or bacterial superinfection, including *C. difficile*-associated diarrhea (CDAD) and pseudomembranous colitis; CDAD has been observed >2 months postantibiotic treatment. Monitor for compliance in patients on intermittent therapy.

Adverse Reactions (Reflective of adult population; not specific for elderly)

1% to 10%:

Dermatologic: Rash (1% to 5%)

Gastrointestinal (1% to 2%): Anorexia, cramps, diarrhea, epigastric distress, flatulence, heartburn, nausea, pseudomembranous colitis, pancreatitis, vomiting

Hepatic: LFTs increased (up to 14%)

Frequency not defined:

Cardiovascular: Edema, flushing

Central nervous system: Ataxia, behavioral changes, concentration impaired, confusion, dizziness, drowsiness, fatigue, fever, headache, numbness, psychosis

Dermatologic: Pemphigoid reaction, pruritus, urticaria

Endocrine & metabolic: Adrenal insufficiency, menstrual disorders

Hematologic: Agranulocytosis (rare), DIC, eosinophilia, hemoglobin decreased, hemolysis, hemolytic anemia, leukopenia, thrombocytopenia (especially with high-dose therapy)

Hepatic: Hepatitis (rare), jaundice

Neuromuscular & skeletal: Myalgia, osteomalacia, weakness

Ocular: Exudative conjunctivitis, visual changes

Renal: Acute renal failure, BUN increased, hemoglobinuria, hematuria, interstitial nephritis, uric acid increased

Miscellaneous: Flu-like syndrome

Drug Interactions

Metabolism/Transport Effects Substrate of P-glycoprotein, SLCO1B1; **Induces** CYP1A2 (strong), CYP2A6 (strong), CYP2B6 (strong), CYP2C8 (strong), CYP2C9 (strong), CYP2C19 (strong), CYP3A4 (strong), P-glycoprotein

Avoid Concomitant Use

Avoid concomitant use of Rifampin with any of the following: Atazanavir; BCG; Boceprevir; Crizotinib; Dabigatran Etexilate; Darunavir; Dronedarone; Esomeprazole; Etravirine; Everolimus; Fosamprenavir; Indinavir; Lapatinib; Lopinavir; Lurasidone; Mycophenolate; Nelfinavir; Nilotinib; Omeprazole; Pazopanib; Praziquantel; QuiNINE; Ranolazine; Rilpivirine; Ritonavir; Roflumilast; RomiDEPsin; Saquinavir; Telaprevir; Ticagrelor; Tipranavir; Tolvaptan; Vandetanib; Voriconazole

Increased Effect/Toxicity

Rifampin may increase the levels/effects of: Clopidogrel; Gadoxetate; HMG-CoA Reductase Inhibitors; Isoniazid; Leflunomide; Lopinavir; Saquinavir

The levels/effects of Rifampin may be increased by: Antifungal Agents (Azole Derivatives, Systemic); Delavirdine; Eltrombopag; Fluconazole; Macrolide Antibiotics; P-Glycoprotein Inhibitors; Pyrazinamide; Voriconazole

Decreased Effect

Rifampin may decrease the levels/effects of: Alfentanil; Amiodarone; Angiotensin II Receptor Blockers; Antidiabetic Agents (Thiazolidinedione); Antiemetics (5HT3 Antagonists); Antifungal Agents (Azole Derivatives, Systemic); Aprepitant; Atazanavir; Atovaquone; Barbiturates; BCG; Bendamustine; Benzodiazepines (metabolized by oxidation); Beta-Blockers; Boceprevir; Brentuximab Vedotin; BusPIRone; Calcium Channel Blockers; Caspofungin; Chloramphenicol; Contraceptives (Estrogens); Contraceptives (Progestins); Corticosteroids (Systemic); Crizotinib; CycloSPORINE; CycloSPORINE (Systemic); CYP1A2 Substrates; CYP2A6 Substrates; CYP2B6 Substrates; CYP2C19 Substrates; CYP2C8 Substrates (High risk); CYP2C9 Substrates (High risk); CYP3A4 Substrates; Dabigatran Etexilate; Dapsone; Dapsone (Systemic); Darunavir; Deferasirox; Delavirdine; Diclofenac; Disopyramide; Divalproex; Dronedarone; Efavirenz; Erlotinib; Esomeprazole; Etravirine; Everolimus; Exemestane; FentaNYL; Fexofenadine; Fluconazole; Fosamprenavir; Fosaprepitant; Fosphenytoin; Gefitinib; GuanFACINE; HMG-CoA Reductase Inhibitors; Imatinib; Indinavir; Ixabepilone; LamoTRIgine; Lapatinib; Linagliptin; Lopinavir; Lurasidone; Maraviroc; Methadone; Morphine (Systemic); Morphine Sulfate; Mycophenolate; Nelfinavir; Nevirapine; Nilotinib; Omeprazole; OxyCODONE; Pazopanib; P-Glycoprotein Substrates; Phenytoin; Prasugrel; Praziquantel; Propafenone; QuiNIDine; QuiNINE; Raltegravir; Ramelteon; Ranolazine; Repaglinide; Rilpivirine; Ritonavir; Rivaroxaban; Roflumilast; RomiDEPsin; Saquinavir; Saxagliptin; Sirolimus; SORAfenib; Sulfonylureas; SUNItinib; Tacrolimus; Tacrolimus (Systemic); Tadalafil; Tamoxifen; Telaprevir; Temsirolimus; Terbinafine; Terbinafine (Systemic); Thyroid Products; Ticagrelor; Tipranavir; Tolvaptan; Treprostinil; Typhoid Vaccine; Ulipristal; Valproic Acid; Vandetanib; Vemurafenib; Vitamin K Antagonists; Voriconazole; Zaleplon; Zidovudine; Zolpidem

The levels/effects of Rifampin may be decreased by: P-Glycoprotein Inducers

Ethanol/Nutrition/Herb Interactions

Ethanol: Avoid ethanol (may increase risk of hepatotoxicity).

Food: Food decreases the extent of absorption; rifampin concentrations may be decreased if taken with food.

Herb/Nutraceutical: St John's wort may decrease rifampin levels.

Stability Rifampin powder is reddish brown. Intact vials should be stored at room temperature and protected from excessive heat and light. Reconstitute powder for injection with SWFI. Prior to injection, dilute in appropriate volume of compatible diluent (eg, 100 mL D_5W). Reconstituted vials are stable for 24 hours at room temperature.

Stability of parenteral admixture at room temperature (25°C) is 4 hours for D_5W and 24 hours for NS.

Mechanism of Action Inhibits bacterial RNA synthesis by binding to the beta subunit of DNA-dependent RNA polymerase, blocking RNA transcription

Pharmacodynamics/Kinetics

Duration: ≤24 hours

Absorption: Oral: Well absorbed; food may delay or slightly reduce peak

Distribution: Highly lipophilic; crosses blood-brain barrier well

Relative diffusion from blood into CSF: Adequate with or without inflammation (exceeds usual MICs)

CSF:blood level ratio: Inflamed meninges: 25%

Protein binding: 80%

Metabolism: Hepatic; undergoes enterohepatic recirculation

Half-life elimination: 3-4 hours; prolonged with hepatic impairment; End-stage renal disease: 1.8-11 hours

Time to peak, serum: Oral: 2-4 hours

Excretion: Feces (60% to 65%) and urine (~30%) as unchanged drug

Dosage

Geriatric & Adult

Tuberculosis, active: Oral, I.V.: **Note:** A four-drug regimen (isoniazid, rifampin, pyrazinamide, and ethambutol) is preferred for the initial, empiric treatment of TB. When the drug susceptibility results are available, the regimen should be altered as appropriate.

Daily therapy: 10 mg/kg/day (maximum: 600 mg/day)

Twice weekly directly observed therapy (DOT): 10 mg/kg (maximum: 600 mg); 3 times/ week: 10 mg/kg (maximum: 600 mg)

Tuberculosis, latent infection (LTBI): As an alternative to isoniazid: Oral, I.V.: 10 mg/kg/ day (maximum: 600 mg/day) for 4 months. **Note:** Combination with pyrazinamide should not generally be offered (*MMWR*, Aug 8, 2003).

Endocarditis, prosthetic valve due to MRSA (unlabeled use): Oral, I.V.: 300 mg every 8 hours for at least 6 weeks (combine with vancomycin for the entire duration of therapy and gentamicin for the first 2 weeks) (Liu, 2011).

***H. influenzae* prophylaxis (unlabeled use):** Oral, I.V.: 600 mg every 24 hours for 4 days

Leprosy (unlabeled use): Oral, I.V.:

Multibacillary: 600 mg once monthly for 24 months in combination with ofloxacin and minocycline

Paucibacillary: 600 mg once monthly for 6 months in combination with dapsone

Single lesion: 600 mg as a single dose in combination with ofloxacin 400 mg and minocycline 100 mg

Meningococcal meningitis prophylaxis (unlabeled use): Oral, I.V.: 600 mg every 12 hours for 2 days

Meningitis *(Pneumococcus* or *Staphylococcus)* (unlabeled use): Oral, I.V.: 600 mg once daily

Nasal carriers of *Staphylococcus aureus* (unlabeled use): Oral, I.V.: 600 mg/day for 5-10 days; **Note: Must be used in combination with at least one other systemic antistaphylococcal antibiotic.** Not recommended as first-line drug for decolonization; evidence is weak for use in patients with recurrent infections (Liu, 2011).

Nontuberculous mycobacterium *(M. kansasii)* (unlabeled use): Oral, I.V.: 10 mg/kg/day (maximum: 600 mg/day) for duration to include 12 months of culture-negative sputum; typically used in combination with ethambutol and isoniazid

***Staphylococcus aureus* infections, adjunctive therapy (unlabeled use):** Oral, I.V.: 600 mg once daily or 300-450 mg every 12 hours with other antibiotics. **Note:** Must be used in combination with another antistaphylococcal antibiotic to avoid rapid development of resistance (Liu, 2011).

Renal Impairment No dosage adjustment required in renal impairment.

Poorly dialyzed; no supplemental dose or dosage adjustment necessary, including patients on intermittent hemodialysis, peritoneal dialysis, or continuous renal replacement therapy (eg, CVVHD).

Hepatic Impairment Dose reductions are necessary to reduce hepatotoxicity.

Administration

I.V.: Administer I.V. preparation by slow I.V. infusion over 30 minutes to 3 hours at a final concentration not to exceed 6 mg/mL.

Oral: Administer on an empty stomach (ie, 1 hour prior to, or 2 hours after meals or antacids) to increase total absorption. The compounded oral suspension must be shaken well before using. May mix contents of capsule with applesauce or jelly.

Monitoring Parameters Periodic (baseline and every 2-4 weeks during therapy) monitoring of liver function (AST, ALT, bilirubin), CBC, mental status, sputum culture, chest x-ray 2-3 months into treatment

Test Interactions May interfere with urine detection of opiates (false-positive); positive Coombs' reaction [direct], rifampin inhibits standard assay's ability to measure serum folate and B$_{12}$; transient increase in LFTs and decreased biliary excretion of contrast media

Special Geriatric Considerations Rifampin, in combination with isoniazid, is the foundation of tuberculosis treatment. Since most older patients acquired their *Mycobacterium tuberculosis* infection before effective chemotherapy was available, either a 9-month regimen of isoniazid and rifampin or a 6-month regimen of isoniazid and rifampin with pyrazinamide (the first 2 months) should be effective.

◀ **Dosage Forms** Excipient information presented when available (limited, particularly for generics); consult specific product labeling.
Capsule, oral: 150 mg, 300 mg
  Rifadin®: 150 mg, 300 mg
Injection, powder for reconstitution: 600 mg
  Rifadin®: 600 mg

Selected References

Advenier C, Gobert C, Houin G, et al, "Pharmacokinetic Studies of Rifampicin in the Elderly," *Ther Drug Monit*, 1983, 5 (1):61-5.
American Thoracic Society, "Treatment of Tuberculosis," *MMWR Recomm Rep*, 2003, 52(RR-11):1-77. Available at http://www.cdc.gov/mmwr/preview/mmwrhtml/rr5211a1.htm
Yoshikawa TT, "Tuberculosis in Aging Adults," *J Am Geriatr Soc*, 1992, 40(2):178-87.

Rifapentine (rif a PEN teen)

Medication Safety Issues
  Sound-alike/look-alike issues:
    Rifapentine may be confused with rifampin
Brand Names: U.S. Priftin®
Brand Names: Canada Priftin®
Generic Availability (U.S.) No
Pharmacologic Category Antitubercular Agent

Use Treatment of pulmonary tuberculosis; rifapentine must always be used in conjunction with at least one other antituberculosis drug to which the isolate is susceptible; it may also be necessary to add a third agent (either streptomycin or ethambutol) until susceptibility is known.

Contraindications Hypersensitivity to rifapentine, rifampin, rifabutin, any rifamycin analog, or any component of the formulation

Warnings/Precautions Patients with abnormal liver tests and/or liver disease should only be given rifapentine when absolutely necessary and under strict medical supervision. Monitoring of liver function tests should be carried out prior to therapy and then every 2-4 weeks during therapy if signs of liver disease occur or worsen, rifapentine should be discontinued. All patients treated with rifapentine should have baseline measurements of liver function tests and enzymes, bilirubin, and a complete blood count. Patients should be seen monthly and specifically questioned regarding symptoms associated with adverse reactions. Routine laboratory monitoring in people with normal baseline measurements is generally not necessary. Use with caution in patients with porphyria; exacerbation is possible.

Rifapentine may produce a red-orange discoloration of body tissues/fluids including skin, teeth, tongue, urine, feces, saliva, sputum, tears, sweat, and cerebral spinal fluid. Contact lenses may become permanently stained. Prolonged use may result in fungal or bacterial superinfection, including *C. difficile*-associated diarrhea (CDAD) and pseudomembranous colitis; CDAD has been observed >2 months postantibiotic treatment. Experience in treating TB in HIV-infected patients is limited. Compliance with dosing regimen is absolutely necessary for successful drug therapy.

Adverse Reactions (Reflective of adult population; not specific for elderly)
>10%: Endocrine & metabolic: Hyperuricemia (most likely due to pyrazinamide from initiation phase combination therapy)
1% to 10%:
  Cardiovascular: Hypertension
  Central nervous system: Headache, dizziness
  Dermatologic: Rash, pruritus, acne
  Gastrointestinal: Anorexia, nausea, vomiting, dyspepsia, diarrhea
  Hematologic: Neutropenia, lymphopenia, anemia, leukopenia, thrombocytosis
  Hepatic: ALT increased, AST increased
  Neuromuscular & skeletal: Arthralgia, pain
  Renal: Pyuria, proteinuria, hematuria, urinary casts
  Respiratory: Hemoptysis

Drug Interactions
  Metabolism/Transport Effects Induces CYP2C8 (strong), 2C9 (strong), 3A4 (strong)
  Avoid Concomitant Use
    Avoid concomitant use of Rifapentine with any of the following: Crizotinib; Dronedarone; Etravirine; Everolimus; Lapatinib; Lurasidone; Mycophenolate; Nilotinib; Pazopanib; Praziquantel; Ranolazine; Rilpivirine; Roflumilast; RomiDEPsin; Ticagrelor; Tolvaptan; Vandetanib; Voriconazole
  Increased Effect/Toxicity
    Rifapentine may increase the levels/effects of: Clarithromycin; Clopidogrel; HMG-CoA Reductase Inhibitors; Isoniazid

The levels/effects of Rifapentine may be increased by: Antifungal Agents (Azole Derivatives, Systemic); Clarithromycin; Delavirdine; Fluconazole; Voriconazole

Decreased Effect

Rifapentine may decrease the levels/effects of: Alfentanil; Amiodarone; Angiotensin II Receptor Blockers; Antiemetics (5HT3 Antagonists); Antifungal Agents (Azole Derivatives, Systemic); Aprepitant; Atovaquone; Barbiturates; Benzodiazepines (metabolized by oxidation); Beta-Blockers; Brentuximab Vedotin; BusPIRone; Calcium Channel Blockers; Clarithromycin; Contraceptives (Estrogens); Contraceptives (Progestins); Corticosteroids (Systemic); Crizotinib; CycloSPORINE; CycloSPORINE (Systemic); CYP2C8 Substrates (High risk); CYP2C9 Substrates (High risk); CYP3A4 Substrates (High risk); Dapsone; Dapsone (Systemic); Delavirdine; Diclofenac; Disopyramide; Dronedarone; Etravirine; Everolimus; Exemestane; FentaNYL; Fluconazole; Fosphenytoin; Gefitinib; GuanFACINE; HMG-CoA Reductase Inhibitors; Imatinib; Ixabepilone; Lapatinib; Linagliptin; Lurasidone; Maraviroc; Methadone; Morphine (Systemic); Morphine Sulfate; Mycophenolate; Nilotinib; Pazopanib; Phenytoin; Praziquantel; Propafenone; QuiNIDine; Ramelteon; Ranolazine; Repaglinide; Rilpivirine; Rivaroxaban; Roflumilast; RomiDEPsin; Saxagliptin; SORAfenib; SUNItinib; Tacrolimus; Tacrolimus (Systemic); Tadalafil; Tamoxifen; Temsirolimus; Terbinafine (Systemic); Ticagrelor; Tolvaptan; Treprostinil; Ulipristal; Vandetanib; Vemurafenib; Vitamin K Antagonists; Voriconazole; Zaleplon; Zidovudine; Zolpidem

Ethanol/Nutrition/Herb Interactions Food: Food increases AUC and maximum serum concentration by 43% and 44% respectively as compared to fasting conditions.

Stability Store at room temperature (15°C to 30°C; 59°F to 86°F). Protect from excessive heat and humidity.

Mechanism of Action Inhibits DNA-dependent RNA polymerase in susceptible strains of *Mycobacterium tuberculosis* (but not in mammalian cells). Rifapentine is bactericidal against both intracellular and extracellular MTB organisms. MTB resistant to other rifamycins including rifampin are likely to be resistant to rifapentine. Cross-resistance does not appear between rifapentine and other nonrifamycin antimycobacterial agents.

Pharmacodynamics/Kinetics

Absorption: Food increases AUC and C_{max} by 43% and 44% respectively.

Distribution: V_d: ~70.2 L; rifapentine and metabolite accumulate in human monocyte-derived macrophages with intracellular/extracellular ratios of 24:1 and 7:1 respectively

Protein binding: Rifapentine and 25-desacetyl metabolite: 97.7% and 93.2%, primarily to albumin

Metabolism: Hepatic; hydrolyzed by an esterase and esterase enzyme to form the active metabolite 25-desacetyl rifapentine

Bioavailability: ~70%

Half-life elimination: Rifapentine: 14-17 hours; 25-desacetyl rifapentine: 13 hours

Time to peak, serum: 5-6 hours

Excretion: Urine (17% primarily as metabolites)

Dosage

Geriatric & Adult Note: Rifapentine should not be used alone; initial phase should include a 3- to 4-drug regimen.

Tuberculosis, intensive phase (initial 2 months) of short-term therapy: 600 mg (four 150 mg tablets) given twice weekly (with an interval of not less than 72 hours between doses); following the intensive phase, treatment should continue with rifapentine 600 mg once weekly for 4 months in combination with INH or appropriate agent for susceptible organisms.

Monitoring Parameters Patients with pre-existing hepatic problems should have liver function tests monitored every 2-4 weeks during therapy

Test Interactions Rifampin has been shown to inhibit standard microbiological assays for serum folate and vitamin B_{12}; this should be considered for rifapentine; therefore, alternative assay methods should be considered.

Pharmacotherapy Pearls Rifapentine has only been studied in patients with tuberculosis receiving a 6-month short-course intensive regimen approval; outcomes have been based on 6-month follow-up treatment observed in clinical trial 008 as a surrogate for the 2-year follow-up generally accepted as evidence for efficacy in the treatment of pulmonary tuberculosis

Dosage Forms Excipient information presented when available (limited, particularly for generics); consult specific product labeling.

Tablet, oral:

Priftin®: 150 mg

Selected References

American Thoracic Society, "Treatment of Tuberculosis," *MMWR Recomm Rep*, 2003, 52(RR-11):1-77. Available at http://www.cdc.gov/mmwr/preview/mmwrhtml/rr5211a1.htm

Rifaximin (rif AX i min)

Medication Safety Issues
Sound-alike/look-alike issues:
Rifaximin may be confused with rifampin
Brand Names: U.S. Xifaxan®
Generic Availability (U.S.) No
Pharmacologic Category Antibiotic, Miscellaneous
Use Treatment of travelers' diarrhea caused by noninvasive strains of *E. coli*; reduction in the risk of overt hepatic encephalopathy (HE) recurrence
Unlabeled/Investigational Use Treatment of hepatic encephalopathy; alternative treatment for *Clostridium difficile*-associated diarrhea (CDAD)

Dosage
Geriatric & Adult
Hepatic encephalopathy: Oral:
Reduction of overt hepatic encephalopathy recurrence: 550 mg 2 times/day. **Note:** Supporting clinical trial evaluated efficacy over 6-month treatment period.
Treatment of hepatic encephalopathy (unlabeled use): 400 mg every 8 hours for 5-10 days (Mas, 2003)
Travelers' diarrhea: Oral: 200 mg 3 times/day for 3 days
***Clostridium difficile* -associated diarrhea (unlabeled use):** Oral: 200-400 mg 2-3 times/day for 14 days (Johnson, 2007)
Renal Impairment Not studied; no dosing recommendation available.
Hepatic Impairment No adjustment necessary, but use with caution in severe impairment (Child-Pugh class C) as systemic absorption does occur and pharmacokinetic parameters are highly variable.
Special Geriatric Considerations In one clinical trial, ~20% of subjects assigned to rifaximin (n=27) or placebo (n=31) were ≥65 years. The risk of a breakthrough episode of hepatitis encephalopathy over 6 months was reduced with rifaximin, similar to younger subjects. Adverse drug events were not stratified by age.
Dosage Forms Excipient information presented when available (limited, particularly for generics); consult specific product labeling.
Tablet, oral:
Xifaxan®: 200 mg, 550 mg

◆ **rIFN beta-1b** see Interferon Beta-1b *on page 970*
◆ **RIG** see Rabies Immune Globulin (Human) *on page 1573*

Rilpivirine (ril pi VIR een)

Brand Names: U.S. Edurant™
Index Terms TMC278
Generic Availability (U.S.) No
Pharmacologic Category Antiretroviral Agent, Reverse Transcriptase Inhibitor (Non-nucleoside)
Use Treatment of HIV-1 infections in combination with at least two other antiretroviral agents

Dosage
Adult Treatment of HIV-1 infection: Oral: 25 mg once daily
Renal Impairment
Mild-to-moderate renal impairment: No dosage adjustment recommended.
Severe or end-stage renal impairment: Use with caution; monitor for adverse events.
Hemodialysis/peritoneal dialysis: Due to extensive protein binding, significant removal by hemodialysis or peritoneal dialysis is unlikely.
Hepatic Impairment
Mild-to-moderate impairment (Child-Pugh class A, B): No dosage adjustment recommended.
Severe impairment (Child-Pugh class C): Has not been studied.
Special Geriatric Considerations In clinical studies of rilpivirine, there were not sufficient numbers of elderly ≥65 years of age to demonstrate a difference in response between elderly and younger adults. It is generally recommended to use caution when using this agent in the elderly due to age-related declines in renal and hepatic function, and/or other concomitant drug therapy.
Dosage Forms Excipient information presented when available (limited, particularly for generics); consult specific product labeling.
Tablet, oral:
Edurant™: 25 mg

◆ **Rilutek®** *see* Riluzole *on page 1615*

Riluzole (RIL yoo zole)

Brand Names: U.S. Rilutek®
Brand Names: Canada Rilutek®
Index Terms 2-Amino-6-Trifluoromethoxy-benzothiazole; RP-54274
Generic Availability (U.S.) No
Pharmacologic Category Glutamate Inhibitor
Use Treatment of amyotrophic lateral sclerosis (ALS); riluzole can extend survival or time to tracheostomy
Contraindications Severe hypersensitivity reactions to riluzole or any component of the formulation
Warnings/Precautions Among 4000 patients given riluzole for ALS, there were 3 cases of marked neutropenia (ANC <500/mm³), all seen within the first 2 months of treatment. Interstitial lung disease (primarily hypersensitivity pneumonitis) has occurred, requires prompt evaluation and possible discontinuation. Use with caution in patients with concomitant renal insufficiency. Use with caution in patients with current evidence or history of abnormal liver function; do not administer if baseline liver function tests are elevated. May cause elevations in transaminases (usually transient). May cause elevations in transaminases (usually transient) within first 3 months of therapy; discontinue if ALT levels are ≥5 times upper limit of normal or if jaundice develops. The elderly or female patients may have decreased clearance of riluzole; use with caution. May cause dizziness or somnolence; caution should be used performing tasks which require alertness (operating machinery or driving).
Adverse Reactions (Reflective of adult population; not specific for elderly)
>10%:
  Gastrointestinal: Nausea (16%)
  Neuromuscular & skeletal: Weakness (19%)
1% to 10%:
  Cardiovascular: Hypertension (5%), peripheral edema (3%), tachycardia (3%)
  Central nervous system: Dizziness (4%), somnolence (2%), vertigo (2%), malaise (1%)
  Dermatologic: Pruritus (4%), eczema (2%), exfoliative dermatitis (1%)
  Gastrointestinal: Abdominal pain (5%), vomiting (4%), flatulence (3%), oral moniliasis (1%), stomatitis (1%), tooth caries (1%)
  Genitourinary: Urinary tract infection (3%), dysuria (1%)
  Hepatic: Liver function tests increased (8% >3 x ULN; 2% >5 x ULN)
  Neuromuscular & skeletal: Arthralgia (4%), paresthesia (circumoral; 2%), tremor (1%)
  Respiratory: Lung function decreased (10%), cough increased (3%)
Drug Interactions
  Metabolism/Transport Effects Substrate of CYP1A2 (major)
  Avoid Concomitant Use There are no known interactions where it is recommended to avoid concomitant use.
  Increased Effect/Toxicity There are no known significant interactions involving an increase in effect.
  Decreased Effect
    The levels/effects of Riluzole may be decreased by: CYP1A2 Inducers (Strong); Cyproterone
Ethanol/Nutrition/Herb Interactions
  Ethanol: Avoid ethanol (due to CNS depression and possible risk of liver toxicity).
  Food: A high-fat meal decreases absorption of riluzole (decreasing AUC by 20% and peak blood levels by 45%). Charbroiled food may increase riluzole elimination.
Stability Store at 20°C to 25°C (68°F to 77°F). Protect from bright light.
Mechanism of Action Mechanism of action is not known. Pharmacologic properties include inhibitory effect on glutamate release, inactivation of voltage-dependent sodium channels; and ability to interfere with intracellular events that follow transmitter binding at excitatory amino acid receptors
Pharmacodynamics/Kinetics
  Absorption: ~90%; high-fat meal decreases AUC by 20% and peak blood levels by 45%
  Protein binding, plasma: 96%, primarily to albumin and lipoproteins
  Metabolism: Extensively hepatic to six major and a number of minor metabolites via CYP1A2 dependent hydroxylation and glucuronidation
  Bioavailability: Oral: Absolute: ~60%
  Half-life elimination: 12 hours
  Excretion: Urine (90%; 85% as metabolites, 2% as unchanged drug) and feces (5%) within 7 days

◀ **Dosage**
Geriatric & Adult
ALS treatment: Oral: 50 mg every 12 hours; no increased benefit can be expected from higher daily doses, but adverse events are increased.
Dosage adjustment in smoking: Cigarette smoking is known to induce CYP1A2; patients who smoke cigarettes would be expected to eliminate riluzole faster. There is no information, however, on the effect of, or need for, dosage adjustment in these patients.
Renal Impairment No specific dosage adjustments recommended by manufacturer; use caution.
Hepatic Impairment No specific dosage adjustments recommended by manufacturer; use caution.
Administration Administer at the same time each day, 1 hour before or 2 hours after a meal.
Monitoring Parameters Monitor serum aminotransferases including ALT levels before and during therapy. Evaluate serum ALT levels every month during the first 3 months of therapy, every 3 months during the remainder of the first year and periodically thereafter. Evaluate ALT levels more frequently in patients who develop elevations. Maximum increases in serum ALT usually occurred within 3 months after the start of therapy and were usually transient when <5 times ULN (upper limits of normal). Discontinue therapy if ALT levels are ≥5 times upper limit of normal or if jaundice develops.

In trials, if ALT levels were <5 times ULN, treatment continued and ALT levels usually returned to below 2 times ULN within 2-6 months. There is no experience with continued treatment of ALS patients once ALT values exceed 5 times ULN.
Special Geriatric Considerations In clinical trials, no difference was demonstrated between elderly and younger adults. However, renal and hepatic changes with age can be expected to result in higher serum concentrations of the parent drug and its metabolites.
Dosage Forms Excipient information presented when available (limited, particularly for generics); consult specific product labeling.
Tablet, oral:
Rilutek®: 50 mg

RimabotulinumtoxinB (rime uh BOT yoo lin num TOKS in bee)

Medication Safety Issues
Other safety concerns:
Botulinum products are not interchangeable; potency differences may exist between the products.
Brand Names: U.S. Myobloc®
Index Terms Botulinum Toxin Type B
Generic Availability (U.S.) No
Pharmacologic Category Neuromuscular Blocker Agent, Toxin
Use Treatment of cervical dystonia (spasmodic torticollis)
Unlabeled/Investigational Use Treatment of cervical dystonia in patients who have developed resistance to botulinum toxin type A
Medication Guide Available Yes
Dosage
Geriatric & Adult Cervical dystonia: I.M.: Initial: 2500-5000 units divided among the affected muscles in patients **previously treated** with botulinum toxin; initial dose in **previously untreated** patients should be lower. Subsequent dosing should be optimized according to patient's response.
Renal Impairment No adjustment is recommended.
Hepatic Impairment No adjustment necessary.
Special Geriatric Considerations No dosage adjustments required, but limited experience in patients ≥75 years of age.
Dosage Forms Excipient information presented when available (limited, particularly for generics); consult specific product labeling.
Injection, solution [preservative free]:
Myobloc®: 5000 units/mL (0.5 mL, 1 mL, 2 mL) [contains albumin (human)]

Rimantadine (ri MAN ta deen)

Medication Safety Issues
Sound-alike/look-alike issues:
Rimantadine may be confused with amantadine, ranitidine, Rimactane®
Flumadine® may be confused with fludarabine, flunisolide, flutamide
Brand Names: U.S. Flumadine®

Brand Names: Canada Flumadine®
Index Terms Rimantadine Hydrochloride
Generic Availability (U.S.) Yes
Pharmacologic Category Antiviral Agent; Antiviral Agent, Adamantane
Use Prophylaxis and treatment of influenza A viral infection (per manufacturer labeling; also refer to current ACIP guidelines for recommendations during current flu season)

Note: In certain circumstances, the ACIP recommends use of rimantadine in combination with oseltamivir for the treatment or prophylaxis of influenza A infection when resistance to oseltamivir is suspected.

Contraindications Hypersensitivity to drugs of the adamantine class, including rimantadine and amantadine, or any component of the formulation

Warnings/Precautions Use with caution in patients with renal and hepatic dysfunction; avoid use, if possible, in patients with uncontrolled psychosis or severe psychoneurosis. An increase in seizure incidence may occur in patients with seizure disorders; discontinue drug if seizures occur; resistance may develop during treatment; viruses exhibit cross-resistance between amantadine and rimantadine. Due to increased resistance, the ACIP has recommended that rimantadine and amantadine no longer be used for the treatment or prophylaxis of influenza A in the United States until susceptibility has been re-established; consult current guidelines. Rimantadine is not effective in the prevention or treatment of influenza B virus infections. The elderly are at higher risk for CNS (eg, dizziness, headache, weakness) and gastrointestinal (eg, nausea/vomiting, abdominal pain) adverse events; dosage adjustment is recommended in elderly patients >65 years of age.

Adverse Reactions (Reflective of adult population; not specific for elderly)
1% to 10%:
Central nervous system: Insomnia (2% to 3%), concentration impaired (≤2%), dizziness (1% to 2%), nervousness (1% to 2%), fatigue (1%), headache (1%)
Gastrointestinal: Nausea (3%), anorexia (2%), vomiting (2%), xerostomia (2%), abdominal pain (1%)
Neuromuscular & skeletal: Weakness (1%)

Drug Interactions

Avoid Concomitant Use There are no known interactions where it is recommended to avoid concomitant use.

Increased Effect/Toxicity
The levels/effects of Rimantadine may be increased by: MAO Inhibitors

Decreased Effect
Rimantadine may decrease the levels/effects of: Influenza Virus Vaccine (Live/Attenuated)

Ethanol/Nutrition/Herb Interactions Food: Food does not affect rate or extent of absorption

Stability Store at 25°C (77°F); excursions permitted to 15°C to 30°C (59°F to 86°F).

Mechanism of Action Exerts its inhibitory effect on three antigenic subtypes of influenza A virus (H1N1, H2N2, H3N2) early in the viral replicative cycle, possibly inhibiting the uncoating process; it has no activity against influenza B virus and is two- to eightfold more active than amantadine

Pharmacodynamics/Kinetics
Onset of action: Antiviral activity: No data exist establishing a correlation between plasma concentration and antiviral effect
Protein Binding: ~40%, primarily to albumin
Metabolism: Extensively hepatic
Half-life elimination: 25.4 hours; prolonged in elderly, severe liver and severe renal impairment
Time to peak: 6 hours
Excretion: Urine (<25% as unchanged drug)
Clearance: Hemodialysis does not contribute to clearance

Dosage
Geriatric Prophylaxis or treatment of influenza A: Oral: 100 mg daily in the elderly (≥65 years), including elderly nursing home patients.
Adult
Prophylaxis of influenza A: Oral: 100 mg twice daily
Note: Prophylaxis (institutional outbreak): In order to control outbreaks in institutions, if influenza A virus subtyping is unavailable and oseltamivir resistant viruses are circulating, rimantadine may be used in combination with oseltamivir if zanamivir cannot be used. Treatment should continue for ≥2 weeks and until ~10 days after illness onset in the last patient (CDC, 2011; Harper 2009).
Treatment of influenza A: Oral: 100 mg twice daily
Renal Impairment
Cl$_{cr}$ ≥30 mL/minute: Dose adjustment not required.
Cl$_{cr}$ <30 mL/minute: 100 mg daily

◀ **Hepatic Impairment** Severe dysfunction: 100 mg daily

Administration Initiation of rimantadine within 48 hours of the onset of influenza A illness halves the duration of illness and significantly reduces the duration of viral shedding and increased peripheral airways resistance; continue therapy for 5-7 days after symptoms begin; discontinue as soon as clinically warranted to reduce the emergence of antiviral drug resistant viruses

Monitoring Parameters Monitor for CNS or GI effects in elderly or patients with renal or hepatic impairment

Special Geriatric Considerations No longer recommended for the treatment or prevention of influenza in the United States because of concerns about resistance and CNS adverse effects. Refer to current CDC guidelines. Monitor GI effects in the elderly or patients with renal or hepatic impairment. Dosing must be individualized (100 mg 1-2 times/day). It is recommended that nursing home patients receive 100 mg/day.

Dosage Forms Excipient information presented when available (limited, particularly for generics); consult specific product labeling.

Tablet, oral: 100 mg

Tablet, oral, as hydrochloride: 100 mg

Flumadine®: 100 mg

◆ **Rimantadine Hydrochloride** see Rimantadine on page 1616

Rimexolone (ri MEKS oh lone)

Medication Safety Issues

Sound-alike/look-alike issues:

Vexol® may be confused with VoSol®

Brand Names: U.S. Vexol®

Brand Names: Canada Vexol®

Generic Availability (U.S.) No

Pharmacologic Category Corticosteroid, Ophthalmic

Use Treatment of inflammation after ocular surgery and the treatment of anterior uveitis

Contraindications Hypersensitivity to rimexolone or any component of the formulation; fungal, mycobacterial, viral (including dendritic keratitis, vaccinia, varicella), or untreated pus-forming bacterial ocular infections

Warnings/Precautions Prolonged use has been associated with the development of corneal or scleral perforation and posterior subcapsular cataracts; may delay healing after cataract surgery; Intraocular pressure should be monitored if this product is used >10 days. Prolonged use of corticosteroids may increase the incidence of secondary infection, mask acute infection (including fungal infections), or prolong or exacerbate viral infections. Corticosteroids should not be used to treat ocular herpes simplex. Fungal infection should be suspected in any patient with persistent corneal ulceration who has received corticosteroids.

Adverse Reactions (Reflective of adult population; not specific for elderly)

1% to 5%: Ocular: Blurred vision, discharge, discomfort, pain, increased intraocular pressure, foreign body sensation, hyperemia, pruritus

<2%:

Cardiovascular: Hypotension

Central nervous system: Headache

Gastrointestinal: Taste perversion

Respiratory: Pharyngitis, rhinitis

Frequency not defined: Cataracts, damage to the optic nerve, defects in visual activity, perforation of globe, secondary ocular infection

Drug Interactions

Avoid Concomitant Use

Avoid concomitant use of Rimexolone with any of the following: Aldesleukin

Increased Effect/Toxicity

Rimexolone may increase the levels/effects of: Deferasirox

The levels/effects of Rimexolone may be increased by: Telaprevir

Decreased Effect

Rimexolone may decrease the levels/effects of: Aldesleukin; Corticorelin; Telaprevir

Mechanism of Action Decreases inflammation by suppression of migration of polymorpho-nuclear leukocytes and reversal of increased capillary permeability

Pharmacodynamics/Kinetics

Absorption: Through aqueous humor

Metabolism: Hepatic for any amount of drug absorbed

Excretion: Urine and feces

Dosage
  Geriatric & Adult
    Anti-inflammatory: Ophthalmic: Instill 1-2 drops in conjunctival sac of affected eye 4 times/day beginning 24 hours after surgery and continuing through the first 2 weeks of the postoperative period
    Anterior uveitis: Ophthalmic: Instill 1-2 drops in conjunctival sac of affected eye every hour during waking hours for the first week, then 1 drop every 2 hours during waking hours of the second week, and then taper until uveitis is resolved

Monitoring Parameters Intraocular pressure and periodic examination of lens (with prolonged use)

Special Geriatric Considerations No special considerations; must limit the time steroids are used to prevent adverse effects.

Dosage Forms Excipient information presented when available (limited, particularly for generics); consult specific product labeling.
  Suspension, ophthalmic [drops]:
    Vexol®: 1% (5 mL, 10 mL) [contains benzalkonium chloride]

◆ **Riomet®** see MetFORMIN on page 1155
◆ **Riopan Plus** see Magaldrate and Simethicone on page 1107
◆ **RisaQuad™ [OTC]** see Lactobacillus on page 1020
◆ **RisaQuad®-2 [OTC]** see Lactobacillus on page 1020

Risedronate (ris ED roe nate)

Related Information
  Osteoporosis Management on page 2027
Medication Safety Issues
  Sound-alike/look-alike issues:
    Actonel® may be confused with Actos®
    Risedronate may be confused with alendronate
Brand Names: U.S. Actonel®; Atelvia™
Brand Names: Canada Actonel®; Actonel® DR; Apo-Risedronate®; Dom-Risedronate; Novo-Risedronate; PMS-Risedronate; ratio-Risedronate; Riva-Risedronate; Sandoz-Risedronate; Teva-Risedronate
Index Terms Risedronate Sodium
Generic Availability (U.S.) No
Pharmacologic Category Bisphosphonate Derivative
Use
  Actonel®: Treatment of Paget's disease of the bone; treatment and prevention of glucocorticoid-induced osteoporosis; treatment and prevention of osteoporosis in postmenopausal women; treatment of osteoporosis in men
  Atelvia™: Treatment of osteoporosis in postmenopausal women
Medication Guide Available Yes
Contraindications Hypersensitivity to risedronate, bisphosphonates, or any component of the formulation; hypocalcemia; inability to stand or sit upright for at least 30 minutes; abnormalities of the esophagus which delay esophageal emptying, such as stricture or achalasia
Warnings/Precautions Bisphosphonates may cause upper gastrointestinal disorders such as dysphagia, esophagitis, esophageal ulcer, and gastric ulcer; risk increases in patients unable to comply with dosing instructions. Use with caution in patients with dysphagia, esophageal disease, gastritis, duodenitis, or ulcers (may worsen underlying condition). Discontinue if new or worsening symptoms occur. Use caution in patients with renal impairment (not recommended in patients with a Cl$_{cr}$ <30 mL/minute). Hypocalcemia must be corrected before therapy initiation with risedronate. Ensure adequate calcium and vitamin D intake, especially for patients with Paget's disease in whom the pretreatment rate of bone turnover may be greatly elevated.

Bisphosphonate therapy has been associated with osteonecrosis, primarily of the jaw. Risk factors for osteonecrosis of the jaw (ONJ) include invasive dental procedures (eg, tooth extraction, dental implants, boney surgery); a diagnosis of cancer, with concomitant chemotherapy or corticosteroids; poor oral hygiene, ill-fitting dentures; and comorbid disorders (anemia, coagulopathy, infection, pre-existing dental disease). Most reported cases occurred after I.V. bisphosphonate therapy; however, cases have been reported following oral therapy. A dental exam and preventative dentistry should be performed prior to placing patients with risk factors on chronic bisphosphonate therapy. The manufacturer's labeling states that discontinuing bisphosphonates in patients requiring invasive dental procedures may reduce the risk of ONJ. However, other experts suggest that there is no evidence that discontinuing therapy reduces the risk of developing ONJ (Assael, 2009). The benefit/risk must be assessed by the treating physician and/or dentist/surgeon prior to any invasive dental procedure. Patients developing ONJ while on bisphosphonates should receive care by an oral surgeon.

Infrequently, severe (and occasionally debilitating) bone, joint, and/or muscle pain have been reported during bisphosphonate treatment. The onset of pain ranged from a single day to several months. Consider discontinuing therapy in patients who experience severe symptoms; symptoms usually resolve upon discontinuation. Some patients experienced recurrence when rechallenged with same drug or another bisphosphonate; avoid use in patients with a history of these symptoms in association with bisphosphonate therapy.

When using for glucocorticoid-induced osteoporosis, evaluate sex steroid hormonal status prior to treatment initiation; consider appropriate hormone replacement if necessary.

Adverse Reactions (Reflective of adult population; not specific for elderly) Frequency may vary with product, dose, and indication.

>10%:
 Cardiovascular: Hypertension (11%)
 Central nervous system: Headache (3% to 18%)
 Dermatologic: Rash (8% to 12%)
 Endocrine & metabolic: Serum PTH levels increased (transient; <30%)
 Gastrointestinal: Diarrhea (5% to 20%), nausea (4% to 13%), constipation (3% to 13%), abdominal pain (2% to 12%), dyspepsia (4% to 11%)
 Genitourinary: Urinary tract infection (11%)
 Neuromuscular & skeletal: Arthralgia (7% to 33%), back pain (6% to 28%)
 Miscellaneous: Infection (≤31%)
1% to 10%:
 Cardiovascular: Peripheral edema (8%), chest pain (5% to 7%), arrhythmia (2%)
 Central nervous system: Depression (7%), dizziness (3% to 7%)
 Endocrine & metabolic: Hypocalcemia (≤5%), hypophosphatemia (<3%)
 Gastrointestinal: Vomiting (2% to 5%), gastritis (3%), duodenitis (≤1%), glossitis (≤1%)
 Genitourinary: Prostatic hyperplasia (5%; benign), nephrolithiasis (3%)
 Neuromuscular & skeletal: Joint disorder (7%), myalgia (2% to 7%), neck pain (5%), muscle spasm (1% to 2%)
 Ocular: Cataract (7%)
 Respiratory: Bronchitis (3% to 10%), pharyngitis (6%), rhinitis (6%), dyspnea (4%)
 Miscellaneous: Flu-like syndrome (10%), acute phase reaction (≤8%; includes fever, influenza-like illness)

Drug Interactions

Avoid Concomitant Use There are no known interactions where it is recommended to avoid concomitant use.

Increased Effect/Toxicity

Risedronate may increase the levels/effects of: Deferasirox; Phosphate Supplements

The levels/effects of Risedronate may be increased by: Aminoglycosides; Nonsteroidal Anti-Inflammatory Agents

Decreased Effect

The levels/effects of Risedronate may be decreased by: Antacids; Calcium Salts; Iron Salts; Magnesium Salts; Proton Pump Inhibitors

Ethanol/Nutrition/Herb Interactions

Ethanol: Avoid ethanol (may increase risk of osteoporosis).
Food: Food reduces absorption (similar to other bisphosphonates); mean oral bioavailability is decreased when given with food.

Stability Store at room temperature of 20°C to 25°C (68°F to 77°F).

Mechanism of Action A bisphosphonate which inhibits bone resorption via actions on osteoclasts or on osteoclast precursors; decreases the rate of bone resorption, leading to an indirect increase in bone mineral density. In Paget's disease, characterized by disordered resorption and formation of bone, inhibition of resorption leads to an indirect decrease in bone formation; but the newly-formed bone has a more normal architecture.

Pharmacodynamics/Kinetics

Onset of action: May require weeks
Absorption: Rapid
Distribution: V_d: 13.8 L/kg
Protein binding: ~24%
Metabolism: None
Bioavailability: Poor, ~0.54% to 0.75%
Half-life elimination: Initial: 1.5 hours; Terminal: 480-561 hours
Time to peak, serum: 1-3 hours
Excretion: Urine (up to 85%); feces (as unabsorbed drug)

Dosage

Geriatric & Adult Note: Patients should receive supplemental calcium and vitamin D if dietary intake is inadequate.

Paget's disease of bone: Oral: *Immediate release tablet:* 30 mg once daily for 2 months
Note: Retreatment may be considered (following post-treatment observation of at least 2 months) if relapse occurs, or if treatment fails to normalize serum alkaline phosphatase. For retreatment, the dose and duration of therapy are the same as for initial treatment. No data are available on more than one course of retreatment.

Osteoporosis (postmenopausal): Oral:
Immediate release tablet: Prevention and treatment: 5 mg once daily **or** 35 mg once weekly **or** 150 mg once a month
Delayed release tablet: Treatment: 35 mg once weekly

Osteoporosis (male) treatment: Oral: *Immediate release tablet:* 35 mg once weekly

Osteoporosis (glucocorticoid-induced) prevention and treatment: Oral: *Immediate release tablet:* 5 mg once daily

Renal Impairment

Cl_{cr} ≥30 mL/minute: No adjustment required
Cl_{cr} <30 mL/minute: Use is not recommended

Hepatic Impairment No studies performed in hepatic impairment; no dosage adjustment necessary due to lack of hepatic metabolism.

Administration Note: Avoid administration of oral calcium supplements, antacids, magnesium supplements/laxatives, and iron preparations within 30 minutes of risedronate administration.

Immediate release tablet: Risedronate immediate release tablets must be taken on an empty stomach with a full glass (6-8 oz) of **plain water** (not mineral water) at least 30 minutes before any food, drink, or other medications orally to avoid interference with absorption. Patient must remain sitting upright or standing for at least 30 minutes after taking (to reduce esophageal irritation). Tablet should be swallowed whole; do not crush or chew.

Delayed release tablet: Risedronate delayed release tablets must be taken with at least 4 oz of **plain water** (not mineral water) immediately after breakfast. Patient must remain sitting upright or standing for at least 30 minutes after taking (to reduce esophageal irritation). Tablet should be swallowed whole; do not cut, split, crush, or chew.

Monitoring Parameters

Osteoporosis: Bone mineral density as measured by central dual-energy x-ray absorptiometry (DXA) of the hip or spine prior to initiation of therapy and at least every 2 years thereafter (6-12 months post-baseline if combined glucocorticoid and risedronate treatment, then every 2 years thereafter); annual measurements of height and weight, assessment of chronic back pain; serum calcium and 25(OH)D; consider measuring biochemical markers of bone turnover

Paget's disease: Alkaline phosphatase; pain; serum calcium and 25(OH)D

Test Interactions Bisphosphonates may interfere with diagnostic imaging agents such as technetium-99m-diphosphonate in bone scans.

Pharmacotherapy Pearls Esophageal irritation and gastric pain have been reported frequently. Proper administration may prevent or decrease this common adverse effect. Patients need to take supplemental calcium while treated with risedronate appropriate for age and hormonal status; vitamin D supplements suggested if patient is deficient in this vitamin.

Special Geriatric Considerations The elderly are frequently treated long-term for osteoporosis. Elderly patients should be advised to report any lower extremity, jaw (osteonecrosis), or muscle pain that cannot be explained or lasts longer than 2 weeks. Additionally, elderly often receive concomitant diuretic therapy and therefore their electrolyte status (eg, calcium, phosphate) should be periodically evaluated.

Dosage Forms Excipient information presented when available (limited, particularly for generics); consult specific product labeling.

Tablet, oral, as sodium:
Actonel®: 5 mg, 30 mg, 35 mg, 150 mg
Tablet, delayed release, oral, as sodium:
Atelvia™: 35 mg

Selected References

Hillner BE, Ingle JN, Chlebowski RT, et al, "American Society of Clinical Oncology 2003 Update on the Role of Bisphosphonates and Bone Health Issues in Women With Breast Cancer," *J Clin Oncol*, 2003, 21(21):4042-57.

Risedronate and Calcium (ris ED roe nate & KAL see um)

Medication Safety Issues

Sound-alike/look-alike issues:
Actonel® may be confused with Actos®

◄ **Brand Names: U.S.** Actonel® and Calcium
Brand Names: Canada Actonel Plus Calcium
Index Terms Calcium and Risedronate; Risedronate Sodium and Calcium Carbonate
Generic Availability (U.S.) No
Pharmacologic Category Bisphosphonate Derivative; Calcium Salt
Use Treatment and prevention of osteoporosis in postmenopausal women
Medication Guide Available Yes
Dosage
  Geriatric & Adult Osteoporosis in postmenopausal females: Oral:
    Risedronate: 35 mg once weekly on day 1 of 7-day treatment cycle
    Calcium carbonate: 1250 mg (elemental calcium 500 mg) once daily on days 2 through 7 of
      7-day treatment cycle
  Renal Impairment Cl_{cr} <30 mL/minute: Not recommended for use.
Special Geriatric Considerations See individual agents. The elderly are frequently treated long-term for osteoporosis and patients should be advised to report any lower extremity pain that cannot be explained or lasts for more than a week. Combination products are not recommended as first-line treatment. Use only if doses of individual agents correspond to the combination available.
Dosage Forms Excipient information presented when available (limited, particularly for generics); consult specific product labeling.
  Combination package [each package contains]:
    Tablet (Actonel®): Risedronate 35 mg (4s)
    Tablet: Calcium carbonate 1250 mg (24s) [equivalent to elemental calcium 500 mg]

◆ **Risedronate Sodium** see Risedronate on page 1619
◆ **Risedronate Sodium and Calcium Carbonate** see Risedronate and Calcium on page 1621
◆ **RisperDAL®** see RisperiDONE on page 1622
◆ **Risperdal M-Tab** see RisperiDONE on page 1622
◆ **RisperDAL® M-Tab®** see RisperiDONE on page 1622
◆ **RisperDAL® Consta®** see RisperiDONE on page 1622

RisperiDONE (ris PER i done)

Related Information
  Antipsychotic Agents on page 1997
  Atypical Antipsychotics on page 1999
  Liquid Compatibility of Antidepressants, Antipsychotics, and Mood Stabilizers on page 2111
Medication Safety Issues
  Sound-alike/look-alike issues:
    RisperiDONE may be confused with reserpine, rOPINIRole
    RisperDAL® may be confused with lisinopril, reserpine, Restoril™
Brand Names: U.S. RisperDAL®; RisperDAL® Consta®; RisperDAL® M-Tab®
Brand Names: Canada Apo-Risperidone®; CO Risperidone; Dom-Risperidone; JAMP-Risperidone; Mint-Risperidon; Mylan-Risperidone; Novo-Risperidone; PHL-Risperidone; PMS-Risperidone; PMS-Risperidone ODT; PRO-Risperidone; RAN™-Risperidone; ratio-Risperidone; RBX-Risperidone; Risperdal®; Risperdal® Consta®; Risperdal® M-Tab®; Riva-Risperidone; Sandoz-Risperidone
Index Terms Risperdal M-Tab
Generic Availability (U.S.) Yes: Excludes injection
Pharmacologic Category Antimanic Agent; Antipsychotic Agent, Atypical
Use
  Oral: Treatment of schizophrenia; treatment of acute mania or mixed episodes associated with bipolar I disorder (as monotherapy or in combination with lithium or valproate); treatment of irritability/aggression associated with autistic disorder
  Injection: Treatment of schizophrenia; maintenance treatment of bipolar I disorder in adults as monotherapy or in combination with lithium and valproate
Unlabeled/Investigational Use Treatment of Tourette's syndrome; treatment of pervasive developmental disorder; psychosis/agitation related to Alzheimer's dementia; post-traumatic stress disorder (PTSD)
Contraindications Hypersensitivity to risperidone or any component of the formulation
Warnings/Precautions Hazardous agent - use appropriate precautions for handling and disposal. **[U.S. Boxed Warning]: Elderly patients with dementia-related psychosis treated with antipsychotics are at an increased risk of death compared to placebo.** Most deaths appeared to be either cardiovascular (eg, heart failure, sudden death) or infectious (eg, pneumonia) in nature. In addition, an increased incidence of cerebrovascular effects (eg, transient ischemic attack, cerebrovascular accidents) has been reported in studies

of placebo-controlled trials of risperidone in elderly patients with dementia-related psychosis. Risperidone is not approved for the treatment of dementia-related psychosis.

Leukopenia, neutropenia, and agranulocytosis (sometimes fatal) have been reported in clinical trials and postmarketing reports with antipsychotic use; presence of risk factors (eg, pre-existing low WBC or history of drug-induced leuko-/neutropenia) should prompt periodic blood count assessment. Discontinue therapy at first signs of blood dyscrasias or if absolute neutrophil count <1000/mm^3.

Low to moderately sedating, use with caution in disorders where CNS depression is a feature. Use with caution in Parkinson's disease. Caution in patients with predisposition to seizures. Use with caution in renal or hepatic dysfunction; dose reduction recommended. Esophageal dysmotility and aspiration have been associated with antipsychotic use; use with caution in patients at risk of aspiration pneumonia (ie, Alzheimer's disease). Use is associated with increased prolactin levels; clinical significance of hyperprolactinemia in patients with breast cancer or other prolactin-dependent tumors is unknown. May alter temperature regulation. May mask toxicity of other drugs or conditions (eg intestinal obstruction, Reyes syndrome, brain tumor) due to antiemetic effects. Neutropenia has been reported with antipsychotic use, including fatal cases of agranulocytosis. Pre-existing myelosuppression (disease or drug-induced) increases risk and these patients should have frequent CBC monitoring; decreased blood counts in absence of other causative factors should prompt discontinuation of therapy.

Use with caution in patients with cardiovascular diseases (eg, heart failure, history of myocardial infarction or ischemia, cerebrovascular disease, conduction abnormalities). May cause orthostatic hypotension; use with caution in patients at risk of this effect (eg, concurrent medication use which may predispose to hypotension/bradycardia or presence of hypovolemia) or in those who would not tolerate transient hypotensive episodes. May alter cardiac conduction (low risk relative to other neuroleptics); life-threatening arrhythmias have occurred with therapeutic doses of neuroleptics.

May cause anticholinergic effects (confusion, agitation, constipation, xerostomia, blurred vision, urinary retention); therefore, they should be used with caution in patients with decreased gastrointestinal motility, urinary retention, BPH, xerostomia, or visual problems (including narrow-angle glaucoma). Relative to other neuroleptics, risperidone has a low potency of cholinergic blockade.

May cause extrapyramidal symptoms (EPS), including pseudoparkinsonism, acute dystonic reactions, akathisia, and tardive dyskinesia (risk of these reactions is low relative to other neuroleptics, and is dose dependent). Risk of dystonia (and probably other EPS) may be greater with increased doses, use of conventional antipsychotics, males, and younger patients. Risk of neuroleptic malignant syndrome (NMS) may be increased in patients with Parkinson's disease or Lewy body dementia; monitor for symptoms of confusion, obtundation, postural instability and extrapyramidal symptoms. May cause hyperglycemia; in some cases may be extreme and associated with ketoacidosis, hyperosmolar coma, or death. Use with caution in patients with diabetes or other disorders of glucose regulation; monitor for worsening of glucose control. Significant weight gain has been observed with antipsychotic therapy; incidence varies with product. Monitor waist circumference and BMI. Rare cases of priapism have been reported.

The possibility of a suicide attempt is inherent in psychotic illness or bipolar disorder; use caution in high-risk patients during initiation of therapy. Prescriptions should be written for the smallest quantity consistent with good patient care. Long-term effects on growth or sexual maturation have not been evaluated. Vehicle used in injectable (polylactide-co-glycolide microspheres) has rarely been associated with retinal artery occlusion in patients with abnormal arteriovenous anastomosis.

Adverse Reactions (Reflective of adult population; not specific for elderly) The frequency of adverse effects is reported as absolute percentages and is not based upon net frequencies as compared to placebo. Actual frequency may be dependent upon dose and/or indication. Events are reported from placebo-controlled studies and not with combination therapy. Unless otherwise noted, frequency of adverse effects is reported for the oral formulation in adults.

>10%:

Central nervous system: Somnolence (children 12% to 67%; adults 5% to 14%; I.M. injection 5% to 6%), fatigue (children 18% to 42%; adults 1% to 3%), headache (I.M. injection 15% to 21%), fever (children 20%; adults 1% to 2%), dystonia (children 9% to 18%; adults 5% to 11%), anxiety (children ≤16%; adults 2% to 16%), dizziness (children 7% to 16%; adults 4% to 10%), Parkinsonism (children 2% to 16%; adults 12% to 20%)

Dermatologic: Rash (children ≤11%; adults 2% to 4%)

Gastrointestinal: Appetite increased (children 4% to 49%), vomiting (children 10% to 25%), salivation increased (children ≤22%; adults 1% to 3%), constipation (children 21%; adults 8% to 9%), abdominal pain (children 15% to 18%; adults 3% to 4%), nausea (children 8% to 16%; adults 4% to 9%), dyspepsia (children 5% to 16%; adults 4% to 10%), xerostomia (children 13%; adults ≤4%)

Genitourinary: Urinary incontinence (children 5% to 22%; adults <2%)

Neuromuscular & skeletal: Tremor (adults 6%; children 10% to 12%)

Respiratory: Rhinitis (children 13% to 36%; adults 7% to 11%), upper respiratory infection (children 34%; adults 2% to 3%), cough (children 34%; adults 3%)

1% to 10%:

Cardiovascular: Tachycardia (children ≤7%; adults 1% to 5%), hypertension (I.M. injection 3%), chest pain (1% to 3%), creatine phosphokinase increased (≤2%), postural hypotension (≤2%), arrhythmia (≤1%), edema (≤1%), hypotension (≤1%), syncope (≤1%)

Central nervous system: Akathisia (children ≤10%; adults 5% to 9%), automatism (children 7%), confusion (children 5%)

Dermatologic: Seborrhea (up to 2%), acne (1%)

Endocrine & metabolic: Lactation nonpuerperal (children 2% to 5%; adults 1%), ejaculation failure (≤1%)

Gastrointestinal: Diarrhea (children 7% to 8%; adults ≤3%), anorexia (children 8%; adults ≤2%;), weight gain (children 5%; adults ≤1%), toothache (I.M. injection 1% to 3%)

Genitourinary: Urinary tract infection (≤3%)

Hematologic: Neutropenia (I.M. injection <2%), anemia (I.M. injection <2%; oral ≤1%)

Hepatic: Transaminases increased (I.M. injection ≥1%; oral 1%)

Neuromuscular & skeletal: Dyskinesia (children 7%; adults 1%), arthralgia (2% to 3%), back pain (2% to 3%), myalgia (≤2%), weakness (1%)

Ocular: Abnormal vision (children 4% to 7%; adults 1% to 3%), blurred vision (I.M. injection 2% to 3%)

Otic: Earache (1%)

Respiratory: Dyspnea (children 2% to 5%; adults 2%), epistaxis (≤2%)

Drug Interactions

Metabolism/Transport Effects Substrate of CYP2D6 (major), 3A4 (minor); **Inhibits** CYP2D6 (weak), 3A4 (weak)

Avoid Concomitant Use

Avoid concomitant use of RisperiDONE with any of the following: Artemether; Dronedarone; Lumefantrine; Metoclopramide; Nilotinib; Pimozide; QUEtiapine; QuiNINE; Tetrabenazine; Thioridazine; Toremifene; Vandetanib; Vemurafenib; Ziprasidone

Increased Effect/Toxicity

RisperiDONE may increase the levels/effects of: Alcohol (Ethyl); Anticholinergics; CNS Depressants; Dronedarone; Methylphenidate; Paliperidone; Pimozide; QTc-Prolonging Agents; QuiNINE; Selective Serotonin Reuptake Inhibitors; Tetrabenazine; Thioridazine; Toremifene; Vandetanib; Vemurafenib; Ziprasidone

The levels/effects of RisperiDONE may be increased by: Abiraterone Acetate; Acetylcholinesterase Inhibitors (Central); Alfuzosin; Artemether; Chloroquine; Ciprofloxacin; Ciprofloxacin (Systemic); Conivaptan; CYP2D6 Inhibitors (Moderate); CYP2D6 Inhibitors (Strong); Darunavir; Divalproex; Gadobutrol; HydrOXYzine; Lithium formulations; Loop Diuretics; Lumefantrine; Methylphenidate; Metoclopramide; Nilotinib; Pramlintide; QUEtiapine; QuiNINE; Selective Serotonin Reuptake Inhibitors; Tetrabenazine; Valproic Acid; Verapamil

Decreased Effect

RisperiDONE may decrease the levels/effects of: Amphetamines; Anti-Parkinson's Agents (Dopamine Agonist); Quinagolide

The levels/effects of RisperiDONE may be decreased by: CarBAMazepine; Lithium formulations; Peginterferon Alfa-2b; Tocilizumab

Ethanol/Nutrition/Herb Interactions

Ethanol: May increase CNS depression; monitor for increased effects with coadministration. Caution patients about effects.

Herb/Nutraceutical: Avoid kava kava, gotu kola, valerian, St John's wort (may increase CNS depression).

Stability

Injection: Risperdal® Consta®: Store in refrigerator at 2°C to 8°C (36°F to 46°F) and protect from light. May be stored at room temperature of 25°C (77°F) for up to 7 days prior to administration. Bring to room temperature prior to reconstitution. Reconstitute with provided diluent only. Shake vigorously to mix; will form thick, milky suspension. Following reconstitution, store at room temperature and use within 6 hours. Suspension settles in ~2 minutes; shake vigorously to resuspend prior to administration.

Oral solution, tablet: Store at 15°C to 25°C (59°F to 77°F). Protect from light and moisture. Keep orally-disintegrating tablets sealed in foil pouch until ready to use. Do not freeze solution.

Mechanism of Action Risperidone is a benzisoxazole atypical antipsychotic with mixed serotonin-dopamine antagonist activity that binds to $5-HT_2$-receptors in the CNS and in the periphery with a very high affinity; binds to dopamine-D_2 receptors with less affinity. The binding affinity to the dopamine-D_2 receptor is 20 times lower than the $5-HT_2$ affinity. The addition of serotonin antagonism to dopamine antagonism (classic neuroleptic mechanism) is thought to improve negative symptoms of psychoses and reduce the incidence of extrapyramidal side effects. Alpha$_1$, alpha$_2$ adrenergic, and histaminergic receptors are also antagonized with high affinity. Risperidone has low to moderate affinity for $5-HT_{1C}$, $5-HT_{1D}$, and $5-HT_{1A}$ receptors, weak affinity for D_1 and no affinity for muscarinics or beta$_1$ and beta$_2$ receptors

Pharmacodynamics/Kinetics
Absorption:
Oral: Rapid and well absorbed; food does not affect rate or extent
Injection: <1% absorbed initially; main release occurs at ~3 weeks and is maintained from 4-6 weeks
Distribution: V_d: 1-2 L/kg
Protein binding, plasma: Risperidone 90%; 9-hydroxyrisperidone: 77%
Metabolism: Extensively hepatic via CYP2D6 to 9-hydroxyrisperidone (similar pharmacological activity as risperidone); *N*-dealkylation is a second minor pathway
Bioavailability: Oral: 70%; Tablet (relative to solution): 94%; orally-disintegrating tablets and oral solution are bioequivalent to tablets
Half-life elimination: Active moiety (risperidone and its active metabolite 9-hydroxyrisperidone)
Oral: 20 hours (mean)
Extensive metabolizers: Risperidone: 3 hours; 9-hydroxyrisperidone: 21 hours
Poor metabolizers: Risperidone: 20 hours; 9-hydroxyrisperidone: 30 hours
Injection: 3-6 days; related to microsphere erosion and subsequent absorption of risperidone
Time to peak, plasma: Oral: Risperidone: Within 1 hour; 9-hydroxyrisperidone: Extensive metabolizers: 3 hours; Poor metabolizers: 17 hours
Excretion: Urine (70%); feces (14%)

Dosage
Geriatric
Oral: Initial: 0.5 mg twice daily; titration should progress slowly in increments of no more than 0.5 mg twice daily; increases to dosages >1.5 mg twice daily should occur at intervals of ≥1 week.
Note: Additional monitoring of renal function and orthostatic blood pressure may be warranted. If once-a-day dosing in the elderly or debilitated patient is considered, a twice daily regimen should be used to titrate to the target dose, and this dose should be maintained for 2-3 days prior to attempts to switch to a once-daily regimen.
Psychosis/agitation related to Alzheimer's dementia (unlabeled use): Initial: 0.25-1 mg/day; if necessary, gradually increase as tolerated not to exceed 1.5-2 mg/day; doses >1 mg/day are associated with higher rates of extrapyramidal symptoms (Rabins, 2007)
I.M. (Risperdal® Consta®): 25 mg every 2 weeks; a lower initial dose of 12.5 mg may be appropriate in some patients.
Note: Oral risperidone (or other antipsychotic) should be administered with the initial injection of Risperdal® Consta® and continued for 3 weeks (then discontinued) to maintain adequate therapeutic plasma concentrations prior to main release phase of risperidone from injection site. When switching from depot administration to a short-acting formulation, administer short-acting agent in place of the next regularly-scheduled depot injection.
Adult Note: When reinitiating treatment after discontinuation, the initial titration schedule should be followed.
Bipolar mania: *Oral:* Recommended starting dose: 2-3 mg once daily; if needed, adjust dose by 1 mg/day in intervals ≥24 hours; dosing range: 1-6 mg/day.
Maintenance: No dosing recommendation available for treatment >3 weeks duration
Bipolar I maintenance: *I.M. (Risperdal® Consta®):* 25 mg every 2 weeks; if unresponsive, some may benefit from larger doses (37.5-50 mg); maximum dose: 50 mg every 2 weeks. Dosage adjustments should not be made more frequently than every 4 weeks. A lower initial dose of 12.5 mg may be appropriate in some patients (eg, demonstrated poor tolerability to other psychotropic medications).
Note: Oral risperidone (or other antipsychotic) should be administered with the initial injection of Risperdal® Consta® and continued for 3 weeks (then discontinued) to maintain adequate therapeutic plasma concentrations prior to main release phase of risperidone from injection site. When switching from depot administration to a short-acting

formulation, administer short-acting agent in place of the next regularly-scheduled depot injection.

Schizophrenia:

Oral: Initial: 2 mg/day in 1-2 divided doses; may be increased by 1-2 mg/day at intervals ≥24 hours to a recommended dosage range of 4-8 mg/day; may be given as a single daily dose once maintenance dose is achieved; daily dosages >6 mg do not appear to confer any additional benefit, and the incidence of extrapyramidal symptoms is higher than with lower doses. Further dose adjustments should be made in increments/decrements of 1-2 mg/day on a weekly basis. Dose range studied in clinical trials: 4-16 mg/day. Maintenance: Recommended dosage range: 2-8 mg/day

I.M. (Risperdal® Consta®): Initial: 25 mg every 2 weeks; if unresponsive, some may benefit from larger doses (37.5-50 mg); maximum dose: 50 mg every 2 weeks. Dosage adjustments should not be made more frequently than every 4 weeks. A lower initial dose of 12.5 mg may be appropriate in some patients (eg, demonstrated poor tolerability to other psychotropic medications).

Note: Oral risperidone (or other antipsychotic) should be administered with the initial injection of Risperdal® Consta® and continued for 3 weeks (then discontinued) to maintain adequate therapeutic plasma concentrations prior to main release phase of risperidone from injection site. When switching from depot administration to a short-acting formulation, administer short-acting agent in place of the next regularly-scheduled depot injection.

Post-traumatic stress disorder (PTSD) (unlabeled use): *Oral:* 0.5-8 mg/day (Bandelow, 2008; Benedek, 2009)

Tourette's syndrome (unlabeled use): *Oral:* Initial: 0.25 mg once daily for 2 days, then 0.25 mg twice daily for 3 days, then 0.5 mg twice daily for 2 days; titrate slowly thereafter in increments/decrements ≤0.5 mg twice daily and at intervals ≥3 days; maximum dose: 6 mg/day (Dion, 2002)

Renal Impairment

Oral: Starting dose of 0.5 mg twice daily; titration should progress slowly in increments of no more than 0.5 mg twice daily; increases to dosages >1.5 mg twice daily should occur at intervals of ≥1 week. Clearance of the active moiety is decreased by 60% in patients with moderate-to-severe renal disease compared to healthy subjects.

I.M.: Initiate with **oral** dosing (0.5 mg twice daily for 1 week then 2 mg/day for 1 week); if tolerated, begin 25 mg **I.M.** every 2 weeks; continue oral dosing for 3 weeks after the first I.M. injection. An initial I.M. dose of 12.5 mg may also be considered.

Hepatic Impairment

Oral: Starting dose of 0.5 mg twice daily; titration should progress slowly in increments of no more than 0.5 mg twice daily; increases to dosages >1.5 mg twice daily should occur at intervals of ≥1 week. The mean free fraction of risperidone in plasma was increased by 35% in patients with hepatic impairment compared to healthy subjects.

I.M.: Initiate with **oral** dosing (0.5 mg twice daily for 1 week then 2 mg/day for 1 week); if tolerated, begin 25 mg **I.M.** every 2 weeks; continue oral dosing for 3 weeks after the first I.M. injection. An initial I.M. dose of 12.5 mg may also be considered.

Administration

Oral: May be administered without regard to meals.

Oral solution can be administered directly from the provided pipette or may be mixed with water, coffee, orange juice, or low-fat milk, but is **not compatible** with cola or tea.

Risperdal® M-Tab® should not be removed from blister pack until administered. Using dry hands, place immediately on tongue. Tablet will dissolve within seconds, and may be swallowed with or without liquid. Do not split or chew.

I.M.: Risperdal® Consta® should be administered into either the deltoid muscle or the upper outer quadrant of the gluteal area. Avoid inadvertent injection into vasculature. Injection should alternate between the two arms or buttocks. Do not combine two different dosage strengths into one single administration. Do not substitute any components of the dose-pack; administer with needle provided (1-inch needle for deltoid administration or 2-inch needle for gluteal administration).

Monitoring Parameters Vital signs; fasting lipid profile and fasting blood glucose/Hgb A$_{1c}$ (prior to treatment, at 3 months, then annually); CBC; BMI, personal/family history of obesity, waist circumference; blood pressure; mental status, abnormal involuntary movement scale (AIMS), extrapyramidal symptoms; orthostatic blood pressure changes for 3-5 days after starting or increasing dose. Weight should be assessed prior to treatment, at 4 weeks, 8 weeks, 12 weeks, and then at quarterly intervals. Consider titrating to a different antipsychotic agent for a weight gain ≥5% of the initial weight.

Pharmacotherapy Pearls Risperdal® Consta® is an injectable formulation of risperidone using the extended release Medisorb® drug-delivery system; small polymeric microspheres degrade slowly, releasing the medication at a controlled rate.

Special Geriatric Considerations Acute changes in mental status and/or behavior from baseline are often caused by changes in fluid/electrolytes, infections, addition or increases in CNS active medications, changes in the environment (eg, moving, remodeling, new room-mate, etc.), and changes in disease status of any organ system. These changes in behavior need to be assessed before initiating or increasing antipsychotic therapy.

Extrapyramidal syndrome symptoms occur less with this agent when total daily dose remains <6 mg as compared with phenothiazines and butyrophenone classes of antipsychotics. Many elderly patients receive antipsychotic medications for inappropriate nonpsychotic behavior. Before initiating antipsychotic medication, the clinician should investigate any possible reversible cause; any stress or stress from any disease can cause acute "confusion" or worsening of baseline nonpsychotic behavior. Most commonly acute changes in behavior are due to increases in drug dose or addition of new drug to regimen, fluid electrolyte loss, infections, and changes in environment.

In the treatment of agitated, demented, elderly patients, authors of meta-analysis of controlled trials of the response to the traditional antipsychotics (phenothiazines, butyrophenones) in controlling agitation have concluded that the use of neuroleptics results in a response rate of 18%. Clearly, neuroleptic therapy for behavior control should be limited with frequent attempts to withdraw the agent given for behavior control. In light of significant risks and adverse effects in elderly population compared with limited data demonstrating efficacy in the treatment of dementia-related psychosis, aggression, and agitation, an extensive risk:benefit analysis should be performed prior to use.

Dosage Forms Excipient information presented when available (limited, particularly for generics); consult specific product labeling.

Injection, microspheres for reconstitution, extended release:
RisperDAL® Consta®: 12.5 mg, 25 mg, 37.5 mg, 50 mg [contains polylactide-co-glycolide; supplied in a dose-pack containing vial with active ingredient in microsphere formulation, prefilled syringe with diluent, needle-free vial access device, and 2 safety needles (a 21 G UTW 1-inch and a 20 G TW 2-inch)]

Solution, oral: 1 mg/mL (30 mL)
RisperDAL®: 1 mg/mL (30 mL) [contains benzoic acid]

Tablet, oral: 0.25 mg, 0.5 mg, 1 mg, 2 mg, 3 mg, 4 mg
RisperDAL®: 0.25 mg, 0.5 mg
RisperDAL®: 1 mg [scored]
RisperDAL®: 2 mg, 3 mg, 4 mg

Tablet, orally disintegrating, oral: 0.25 mg, 0.5 mg, 1 mg, 2 mg, 3 mg, 4 mg
RisperDAL® M-Tab®: 0.5 mg [contains phenylalanine 0.14 mg/tablet]
RisperDAL® M-Tab®: 1 mg [contains phenylalanine 0.28 mg/tablet]
RisperDAL® M-Tab®: 2 mg [contains phenylalanine 0.42 mg/tablet]
RisperDAL® M-Tab®: 3 mg [contains phenylalanine 0.63 mg/tablet]
RisperDAL® M-Tab®: 4 mg [contains phenylalanine 0.84 mg/tablet]

Selected References

Rabins PV, Blacker D, Rovner BW, et al, "Practice Guidelines for the Treatment of Patients With Alzheimer's Disease and Other Dementias," *Am J Psychiatry*, 2007, 164(12 Suppl):5-56. Available at http://www.psych.org/psych_pract/treatg/pg/prac_guide.cfm.

Schneider LS, Tariot PN, Dagerman KS, et al, "Effectiveness of Atypical Antipsychotic Drugs in Patients With Alzheimer's Disease," *N Engl J Med*, 2006, 355(15):1525-38.

◆ **Ritalin®** *see* Methylphenidate *on page 1179*
◆ **Ritalin LA®** *see* Methylphenidate *on page 1179*
◆ **Ritalin-SR®** *see* Methylphenidate *on page 1179*

Rivastigmine (ri va STIG meen)

Brand Names: U.S. Exelon®
Brand Names: Canada Exelon®; Mylan-Rivastigmine; Novo-Rivastigmine; PMS-Rivastigmine; ratio-Rivastigmine; Sandoz-Rivastigmine
Index Terms ENA 713; Rivastigmine Tartrate; SDZ ENA 713
Generic Availability (U.S.) Yes: Capsule
Pharmacologic Category Acetylcholinesterase Inhibitor (Central)
Use Treatment of mild-to-moderate dementia associated with Alzheimer's disease or Parkinson's disease
Unlabeled/Investigational Use Severe dementia associated with Alzheimer's disease; Lewy body dementia
Contraindications Hypersensitivity to rivastigmine, other carbamate derivatives (eg, neostigmine, pyridostigmine, physostigmine), or any component of the formulation

◀ **Warnings/Precautions** Significant nausea, vomiting, anorexia, and weight loss are associated with use; occurs more frequently in women and during the titration phase. Nausea and/or vomiting may be severe, particularly at doses higher than recommended. Monitor weight during therapy. Therapy should be initiated at lowest dose and titrated; if treatment is interrupted for more than several days, reinstate at the lowest daily dose. Cholinesterase inhibitors may have vagotonic effects which may cause bradycardia and/or heart block with or without a history of cardiac disease. Alzheimer's treatment guidelines consider bradycardia to be a relative contraindication for use of centrally-active cholinesterase inhibitors. Post-market cases of overdose (including a few fatalities) have been reported in association with medication errors/improper use of rivastigmine transdermal patches. No more than 1 patch should be applied daily and existing patch must be removed prior to applying new patch.

Use caution in patients with a history of peptic ulcer disease or concurrent NSAID use. Use caution in patients undergoing anesthesia who will receive succinylcholine-type muscle relaxation, patients with sick-sinus syndrome, bradycardia or supraventricular conduction conditions, urinary obstruction, seizure disorders, or pulmonary conditions such as asthma or COPD. Use caution in patients with low body weight (<50 kg) due to increased risk of adverse reactions.

Adverse Reactions (Reflective of adult population; not specific for elderly) Note: Many concentration-related effects are reported at a lower frequency by transdermal route.
>10%:
Central nervous system: Dizziness (2% to 21%), headache (3% to 17%)
Gastrointestinal: Nausea (7% to 47%), vomiting (6% to 31%), diarrhea (5% to 19%), anorexia (3% to 17%), abdominal pain (1% to 13%)
1% to 10%:
Cardiovascular: Syncope (3%), hypertension (3%)
Central nervous system: Fatigue (2% to 9%), insomnia (1% to 9%), confusion (8%), depression (4% to 6%), anxiety (2% to 5%), malaise (5%), somnolence (4% to 5%), hallucinations (4%), aggressiveness (3%), parkinsonism symptoms worsening (2% to 3%), vertigo (≤2%)
Gastrointestinal: Dyspepsia (9%), constipation (5%), flatulence (4%), weight loss (3% to 8%), eructation (2%), dehydration (2%)
Genitourinary: Urinary tract infection (1% to 7%)
Neuromuscular & skeletal: Weakness (2% to 6%), tremor (1%; up to 10% in Parkinson's patients)
Respiratory: Rhinitis (4%)
Miscellaneous: Diaphoresis (4%), flu-like syndrome (3%)

Drug Interactions
Avoid Concomitant Use There are no known interactions where it is recommended to avoid concomitant use.
Increased Effect/Toxicity
Rivastigmine may increase the levels/effects of: Antipsychotics; Beta-Blockers; Cholinergic Agonists; Succinylcholine

The levels/effects of Rivastigmine may be increased by: Corticosteroids (Systemic)
Decreased Effect
Rivastigmine may decrease the levels/effects of: Anticholinergics; Neuromuscular-Blocking Agents (Nondepolarizing)

The levels/effects of Rivastigmine may be decreased by: Anticholinergics
Ethanol/Nutrition/Herb Interactions
Smoking: Nicotine increases the clearance of rivastigmine by 23%.
Ethanol: Avoid ethanol (due to risk of sedation; may increase GI irritation).
Food: Food delays absorption by 90 minutes, lowers C_{max} by 30% and increases AUC by 30%.
Herb/Nutraceutical: Avoid ginkgo biloba (may increase cholinergic effects).
Stability
Oral: Store at 15°C to 30°C (59°F to 86°F); do not freeze. Store solution in an upright position.
Transdermal patch: Store at 15°C to 30°C (59°F to 86°F). Patches should be kept in sealed pouch until use.
Mechanism of Action A deficiency of cortical acetylcholine is thought to account for some of the symptoms of Alzheimer's disease and the dementia of Parkinson's disease; rivastigmine increases acetylcholine in the central nervous system through reversible inhibition of its hydrolysis by cholinesterase

Pharmacodynamics/Kinetics

Duration: Anticholinesterase activity (CSF): ~10 hours (6 mg oral dose)

Absorption: Oral: Fasting: Rapid and complete within 1 hour

Distribution: V_d: 1.8-2.7 L/kg; penetrates blood-brain barrier (CSF levels are ~40% of plasma levels following oral administration)

Protein binding: 40%

Metabolism: Extensively via cholinesterase-mediated hydrolysis in the brain; metabolite undergoes N-demethylation and/or sulfate conjugation hepatically; CYP minimally involved; linear kinetics at 3 mg twice daily, but nonlinear at higher doses

Bioavailability: Oral: 36% to 40%

Half-life elimination: Oral: 1.5 hours; Transdermal patch: 3 hours (after removal)

Time to peak: Oral: 1 hour; Transdermal patch: 10-16 hours following first dose

Excretion: Urine (97% as metabolites); feces (0.4%)

Dosage

Geriatric Following oral administration, clearance is significantly lower in patients >60 years of age, but dosage adjustments are not recommended. Age was not associated with exposure in patients treated transdermally. Titrate dose to individual's tolerance. Refer to adult dosing.

Adult Note: Exelon® oral solution and capsules are bioequivalent.

Mild-to-moderate Alzheimer's dementia:

Oral: Initial: 1.5 mg twice daily; may increase by 3 mg/day (1.5 mg/dose) every 2 weeks based on tolerability (maximum recommended dose: 6 mg twice daily)

Note: If GI adverse events occur, discontinue treatment for several doses then restart at the same or next lower dosage level; antiemetics have been used to control GI symptoms. If treatment is interrupted for longer than several days, restart the treatment at the lowest dose and titrate as previously described.

Transdermal patch: Initial: 4.6 mg/24 hours; if well tolerated, may be increased (after at least 4 weeks) to 9.5 mg/24 hours (recommended effective dose). Maintenance: 9.5 mg/24 hours (maximum dose: 9.5 mg/24 hours).

Note: If intolerance is noted (nausea, vomiting), patch should be removed and treatment interrupted for several days and restarted at the same or lower dosage. If interrupted for more than several days, reinitiate at lowest dosage and increase to maintenance dose after 4 weeks.

Conversion from oral therapy: If oral daily dose <6 mg, switch to 4.6 mg/24 hours patch; if oral daily dose 6-12 mg, switch to 9.5 mg/24 hours patch. Apply patch on the next day following last oral dose.

Mild-to-moderate Parkinson's-related dementia:

Oral: Initial: 1.5 mg twice daily; may increase by 3 mg/day (1.5 mg/dose) every 4 weeks based on tolerability (maximum recommended dose: 6 mg twice daily)

Transdermal patch: See transdermal dosing for Alzheimer's dementia.

Renal Impairment Dosage adjustments are not recommended; however, titrate the dose to the individual's tolerance.

Hepatic Impairment Clearance is significantly reduced in mild to moderately impaired patients. Although dosage adjustments are not recommended, use lowest possible dose and titrate according to individual's tolerance. Consider intervals of >2 weeks between dosage adjustments.

Administration

Oral: Should be administered with meals (breakfast or dinner). Capsule should be swallowed whole. Liquid form is available for patients who cannot swallow capsules (can be swallowed directly from syringe or mixed with water, soda, or cold fruit juice). Stir well and drink within 4 hours of mixing.

Topical: Apply transdermal patch to upper or lower back (alternatively, may apply to upper arm or chest). Avoid reapplication to same spot of skin for 14 days (may rotate sections of back, for example). Do not apply to red, irritated, or broken skin. Avoid areas of recent application of lotion or powder. After removal, fold patch to press adhesive surfaces together, and discard. Avoid eye contact; wash hands after handling patch. Replace patch every 24 hours. Avoid exposing the patch to external sources of heat (eg, sauna, excessive light) for prolonged periods of time. No more than 1 patch should be applied daily and existing patch must be removed prior to applying new patch.

Monitoring Parameters Cognitive function at periodic intervals, symptoms of GI intolerance, weight

Special Geriatric Considerations Titrate dose to tolerance.

Dosage Forms Excipient information presented when available (limited, particularly for generics); consult specific product labeling.

Capsule, oral: 1.5 mg, 3 mg, 4.5 mg, 6 mg

Exelon®: 1.5 mg, 3 mg, 4.5 mg, 6 mg

Patch, transdermal:
Exelon®: 4.6 mg/24 hours (30s) [5 cm^2; contains rivastigmine 9 mg]
Exelon®: 9.5 mg/24 hours (30s) [10 cm^2; contains rivastigmine 18 mg]
Solution, oral:
Exelon®: 2 mg/mL (120 mL) [contains sodium benzoate]

Selected References
Rabins PV, Blacker D, Rovner BW, et al, "Practice Guidelines for the Treatment of Patients With Alzheimer's Disease and Other Dementias," *Am J Psychiatry*, 2007, 164(12 Suppl):5-56. Available at http://www.psych.org/psych_pract/treatg/pg/prac_guide.cfm.

♦ **Rivastigmine Tartrate** *see* Rivastigmine *on page* 1627

Rizatriptan (rye za TRIP tan)

Brand Names: U.S. Maxalt-MLT®; Maxalt®
Brand Names: Canada Maxalt RPD™; Maxalt™
Index Terms MK462
Generic Availability (U.S.) No
Pharmacologic Category Antimigraine Agent; Serotonin 5-HT$_{1B, 1D}$ Receptor Agonist
Use Acute treatment of migraine with or without aura
Contraindications Hypersensitivity to rizatriptan or any component of the formulation; documented ischemic heart disease or Prinzmetal's angina; uncontrolled hypertension; basilar or hemiplegic migraine; during or within 2 weeks of MAO inhibitors; during or within 24 hours of treatment with another 5-HT$_1$ agonist, or an ergot-containing or ergot-type medication (eg, methysergide, dihydroergotamine)
Warnings/Precautions Only indicated for treatment of acute migraine; if a patient does not respond to the first dose, the diagnosis of migraine should be reconsidered. Coronary artery vasospasm, transient ischemia, myocardial infarction, ventricular tachycardia/fibrillation, cardiac arrest, and death have been reported with 5-HT$_1$ agonist administration. Patients who experience sensations of chest pain/pressure/tightness or symptoms suggestive of angina following dosing should be evaluated for coronary artery disease or Prinzmetal's angina before receiving additional doses; if dosing is resumed and similar symptoms recur, monitor with ECG. Should not be given to patients who have risk factors for CAD (eg, hypertension, hypercholesterolemia, smoker, obesity, diabetes, strong family history of CAD, menopause, male >40 years of age) without adequate cardiac evaluation. Patients with suspected CAD should have cardiovascular evaluation to rule out CAD before considering use; if cardiovascular evaluation is "satisfactory," first dose should be given in the healthcare provider's office (consider ECG monitoring). Periodic evaluation of cardiovascular status should be done in all patients. Significant elevation in blood pressure, including hypertensive crisis, has also been reported on rare occasions in patients with and without a history of hypertension. Cerebral/subarachnoid hemorrhage, stroke, peripheral vascular ischemia, and colonic ischemia have been reported with 5-HT$_1$ agonist administration.

Use with caution in elderly or patients with hepatic or renal impairment (including dialysis patients). Symptoms of agitation, confusion, hallucinations, hyper-reflexia, myoclonus, shivering, and tachycardia may occur with concomitant proserotonergic drugs (eg, SSRIs/SNRIs or triptans) or agents which reduce rizatriptan's metabolism. Concurrent use of serotonin precursors (eg, tryptophan) is not recommended. If concomitant administration with SSRIs is warranted, monitor closely, especially at initiation and with dose increases. Maxalt-MLT® tablets contain phenylalanine.

Adverse Reactions (Reflective of adult population; not specific for elderly)
1% to 10%:
Cardiovascular: Systolic/diastolic blood pressure increases (5-10 mm Hg), chest pain (5%), palpitation
Central nervous system: Dizziness, drowsiness, fatigue (13% to 30%, dose related)
Dermatologic: Skin flushing
Endocrine & metabolic: Mild increase in growth hormone, hot flashes
Gastrointestinal: Abdominal pain, dry mouth (<5%), nausea
Respiratory: Dyspnea

Drug Interactions
Avoid Concomitant Use
Avoid concomitant use of Rizatriptan with any of the following: Ergot Derivatives; MAO Inhibitors; Sibutramine
Increased Effect/Toxicity
Rizatriptan may increase the levels/effects of: Ergot Derivatives; Serotonin Modulators

The levels/effects of Rizatriptan may be increased by: Ergot Derivatives; MAO Inhibitors; Propranolol; Sibutramine

Decreased Effect There are no known significant interactions involving a decrease in effect.
Ethanol/Nutrition/Herb Interactions Food: Food delays absorption.
Stability Store in blister pack until administration.
Mechanism of Action Selective agonist for serotonin (5-HT$_{1B}$ and 5-HT$_{1D}$receptors) in cranial arteries; causes vasoconstriction and reduces sterile inflammation associated with antidromic neuronal transmission correlating with relief of migraine
Pharmacodynamics/Kinetics
  Onset of action: ~30 minutes
  Duration: 14-16 hours
  Protein binding: 14%
  Metabolism: Via monoamine oxidase-A; first-pass effect
  Bioavailability: 40% to 50%
  Half-life elimination: 2-3 hours
  Time to peak: 1-1.5 hours
  Excretion: Urine (82%, 8% to 16% as unchanged drug); feces (12%)
Dosage
  Geriatric & Adult Note: In patients with risk factors for coronary artery disease, following adequate evaluation to establish the absence of coronary artery disease, the initial dose should be administered in a setting where response may be evaluated (physician's office or similarly staffed setting). ECG monitoring may be considered.

  Migraine: Oral: 5-10 mg, repeat after 2 hours if significant relief is not attained; maximum: 30 mg in a 24-hour period (use 5 mg dose in patients receiving propranolol with a maximum of 15 mg in 24 hours)
  Note: For orally-disintegrating tablets (Maxalt-MLT®): Patient should be instructed to place tablet on tongue and allow to dissolve. Dissolved tablet will be swallowed with saliva.
Monitoring Parameters Headache severity, signs/symptoms suggestive of angina; consider monitoring blood pressure, heart rate, and/or ECG with first dose in patients with likelihood of unrecognized coronary disease, such as patients with significant hypertension, hypercholesterolemia, obese patients, patients with diabetes, smokers with other risk factors or strong family history of coronary artery disease
Special Geriatric Considerations Since the elderly often have cardiovascular disease, careful evaluation of the use of 5-HT agonists is needed to avoid complications with the use of these agents. The pharmacokinetic disposition of these agents is similar to that seen in younger adults.
Dosage Forms Excipient information presented when available (limited, particularly for generics); consult specific product labeling.
  Tablet, oral:
    Maxalt®: 5 mg, 10 mg
  Tablet, orally disintegrating, oral:
    Maxalt-MLT®: 5 mg [contains phenylalanine 1.05 mg/tablet; peppermint flavor]
    Maxalt-MLT®: 10 mg [contains phenylalanine 2.1 mg/tablet; peppermint flavor]

◆ **R-modafinil** *see* Armodafinil *on page 146*
◆ **RoActemra®** *see* Tocilizumab *on page 1816*
◆ **Robafen [OTC]** *see* GuaiFENesin *on page 846*
◆ **Robafen AC** *see* Guaifenesin and Codeine *on page 848*
◆ **Robafen Cough [OTC]** *see* Dextromethorphan *on page 490*
◆ **Robafen DM [OTC]** *see* Guaifenesin and Dextromethorphan *on page 848*
◆ **Robafen DM Clear [OTC]** *see* Guaifenesin and Dextromethorphan *on page 848*
◆ **Robaxin®** *see* Methocarbamol *on page 1167*
◆ **Robaxin®-750** *see* Methocarbamol *on page 1167*
◆ **Robinul®** *see* Glycopyrrolate *on page 834*
◆ **Robinul® Forte** *see* Glycopyrrolate *on page 834*
◆ **Robitussin AC** *see* Guaifenesin and Codeine *on page 848*
◆ **Robitussin® Children's Cough Long-Acting [OTC]** *see* Dextromethorphan *on page 490*
◆ **Robitussin® Cough & Chest Congestion DM [OTC]** *see* Guaifenesin and Dextromethorphan *on page 848*
◆ **Robitussin® Cough & Chest Congestion DM Max [OTC]** *see* Guaifenesin and Dextromethorphan *on page 848*
◆ **Robitussin® Cough & Chest Congestion Sugar-Free DM [OTC]** *see* Guaifenesin and Dextromethorphan *on page 848*
◆ **Robitussin® CoughGels™ Long-Acting [OTC]** *see* Dextromethorphan *on page 490*
◆ **Robitussin® Cough Long Acting [OTC]** *see* Dextromethorphan *on page 490*
◆ **Rocaltrol®** *see* Calcitriol *on page 243*
◆ **Rocephin®** *see* CefTRIAXone *on page 313*
◆ **Rolaids® Calcium Rich [OTC]** *see* Calcium Salts (Oral) *on page 256*

ROPINIRole (roe PIN i role)

Related Information
Antiparkinsonian Agents *on page 1995*

Medication Safety Issues
Sound-alike/look-alike issues:
Requip® may be confused with Reglan®
ROPINIRole may be confused with RisperDAL®, risperiDONE, ropivacaine

Brand Names: U.S. Requip®; Requip® XL™
Brand Names: Canada CO Ropinirole; JAMP-Ropinirole; PMS-Ropinirole; RAN™-Ropinirole; Requip®
Index Terms Ropinirole Hydrochloride
Generic Availability (U.S.) Yes: Excludes combination package, extended-release tablets
Pharmacologic Category Anti-Parkinson's Agent, Dopamine Agonist
Use Treatment of idiopathic Parkinson's disease; in patients with early Parkinson's disease who were not receiving concomitant levodopa therapy as well as in patients with advanced disease on concomitant levodopa; treatment of moderate-to-severe primary Restless Legs Syndrome (RLS)
Contraindications Hypersensitivity to ropinirole or any component of the formulation
Warnings/Precautions Syncope, sometimes associated with bradycardia, was observed in association with ropinirole in both early Parkinson's disease (without levodopa) patients and advanced Parkinson's disease (with levodopa) patients. Dopamine agonists appear to impair the systemic regulation of blood pressure resulting in postural hypotension, especially during dose escalation. Parkinson's disease patients appear to have an impaired capacity to respond to a postural challenge; use with caution in patients at risk of hypotension (ie, those receiving antihypertensive or antiarrhythmic drugs) or where transient hypotensive episodes would be poorly tolerated (cardiovascular disease or cerebrovascular disease). Parkinson's patients being treated with dopaminergic agonists ordinarily require careful monitoring for signs and symptoms of postural hypotension, especially during dose escalation, and should be informed of this risk.

May cause hallucinations (dose dependent); risk may be increased in the elderly. Use with caution in patients with pre-existing dyskinesia, hepatic or severe renal dysfunction (use in patients with severe renal impairment and who are not undergoing regular hemodialysis is not recommended in the Canadian labeling). Avoid use in patients with a major psychotic disorder; may exacerbate psychosis.

Patients treated with ropinirole have reported falling asleep while engaging in activities of daily living; this has been reported to occur without significant warning signs. Monitor for daytime somnolence or pre-existing sleep disorder; caution with concomitant sedating medication; discontinue if significant daytime sleepiness or episodes of falling asleep occur. Patients must be cautioned about performing tasks which require mental alertness (eg, operating machinery or driving). Use with caution in patients receiving other CNS depressants or psychoactive agents. Effects with other sedative drugs or ethanol may be potentiated.

Dopamine agonists have been associated with compulsive behaviors and/or loss of impulse control, which has manifested as pathological gambling, libido increases (hypersexuality), and/or binge eating. Causality has not been established, and controversy exists as to whether this phenomenon is related to the underlying disease, prior behaviors/addictions and/or drug therapy. Dose reduction or discontinuation of therapy has been reported to reverse these behaviors in some, but not all cases. Risk for melanoma development is increased in Parkinson's disease patients; drug causation or factors contributing to risk have not been established. Patients should be monitored closely and periodic skin examinations should be performed.

Some patients treated for RLS may experience worsening of symptoms in the early morning hours (rebound) or an increase and/or spread of daytime symptoms (augmentation); clinical management of these phenomena has not been evaluated in controlled clinical trials. Pathologic degenerative changes were observed in the retinas of albino rats during studies with this agent, but were not observed in the retinas of albino mice or in other species. The significance of these data for humans remains uncertain.

Other dopaminergic agents have been associated with a syndrome resembling neuroleptic malignant syndrome on withdrawal or significant dosage reduction after long-term use. Risk of fibrotic complications (eg, pleural effusion/fibrosis, interstitial lung disease) and melanoma has been reported in patients receiving ropinirole; drug causation has not been established.

Adverse Reactions (Reflective of adult population; not specific for elderly)

Data inclusive of trials in early Parkinson's disease (without levodopa) and Restless Legs Syndrome:

>10%:

Cardiovascular: Syncope (1% to 12%)

Central nervous system: Somnolence (11% to 40%), dizziness (6% to 40%), fatigue (8% to 11%)

Gastrointestinal: Nausea (immediate release: 40% to 60%; extended release: 19%), vomiting (11% to 12%)

Miscellaneous: Viral infection (11%)

1% to 10%:

Cardiovascular: Dependent/leg edema (2% to 7%), orthostasis (1% to 6%), hypertension (5%), chest pain (4%), flushing (3%), palpitation (3%), peripheral ischemia (2% to 3%), atrial fibrillation (2%), extrasystoles (2%), hypotension (2%), tachycardia (2%)

Central nervous system: Pain (3% to 8%), headache (extended release: 6%), confusion (5%), hallucinations (up to 5%; dose related), hypoesthesia (4%), amnesia (3%), malaise (3%), yawning (3%), concentration impaired (2%), vertigo (2%)

Dermatologic: Hyperhidrosis (3%)

Gastrointestinal: Dyspepsia (4% to 10%), abdominal pain (3% to 7%), constipation (≥5%), xerostomia (3% to 5%), diarrhea (5%), anorexia (4%), flatulence (3%)

Genitourinary: Urinary tract infection (5%), impotence (3%)

Hepatic: Alkaline phosphatase increased (3%)

Neuromuscular & skeletal: Weakness (6%), arthralgia (4%), muscle cramps (3%), paresthesia (3%), hyperkinesia (2%)

Ocular: Abnormal vision (6%), xerophthalmia (2%)

Respiratory: Pharyngitis (6% to 9%), rhinitis (4%), sinusitis (4%), bronchitis (3%), dyspnea (3%), influenza (3%), cough (3%), nasal congestion (2%)

Miscellaneous: Diaphoresis increased (3% to 6%)

Advanced Parkinson's disease (with levodopa):

>10%:

Central nervous system: Dizziness (immediate release: 26%; extended-release: 8%), somnolence (immediate release: 20%, extended release: 7%), headache (17%)

Gastrointestinal: Nausea (immediate release: 30%; extended-release: 11%)

Neuromuscular & skeletal: Dyskinesias (immediate release: 34%; extended-release: 13%; dose related)

1% to 10%:

Cardiovascular: Hypotension (2% to 5%; including orthostatic), peripheral edema (4%), syncope (3%), hypertension (3%; dose related)

Central nervous system: Hallucinations (7% to 10%; dose related), confusion (9%), anxiety (2% to 6%), amnesia (5%), nervousness (5%), pain (5%), vertigo (4%), abnormal dreaming (3%), paresis (3%), aggravated parkinsonism, insomnia

Gastrointestinal: Abdominal pain (6% to 9%), vomiting (7%), constipation (4% to 6%), diarrhea (3% to 5%), xerostomia (2% to 5%), dysphagia (2%), flatulence (2%), salivation increased (2%), weight loss (2%)

Genitourinary: Urinary tract infection (6%), pyuria (2%), urinary incontinence (2%)

Hematologic: Anemia (2%)

Neuromuscular & skeletal: Falls (2% to 10%; dose related), arthralgia (7%), tremor (6%), hypokinesia (5%), paresthesia (5%), arthritis (3%), back pain (3%)

Ocular: Diplopia (2%)

Respiratory: Upper respiratory tract infection (9%), dyspnea (3%)

Miscellaneous: Injury, diaphoresis increased (7%), viral infection, increased drug level (7%)

Other adverse effects (all phase 2/3 trials for Parkinson's disease and Restless Leg Syndrome): ≥1%: Asthma, BUN increased, depression, gastroenteritis, gastrointestinal reflux, irritability, migraine, muscle spasm, myalgia, neck pain, neuralgia, osteoarthritis, pharyngolaryngeal pain, rash, rigors, sleep disorder, tendonitis

Drug Interactions

Metabolism/Transport Effects Substrate of CYP1A2 (major), 3A4 (minor); **Inhibits** CYP1A2 (weak)

Avoid Concomitant Use There are no known interactions where it is recommended to avoid concomitant use.

Increased Effect/Toxicity

The levels/effects of ROPINIRole may be increased by: Abiraterone Acetate; Antipsychotics (Typical); Ciprofloxacin; Ciprofloxacin (Systemic); Conivaptan; CYP1A2 Inhibitors (Moderate); CYP1A2 Inhibitors (Strong); Deferasirox; Estrogen Derivatives; MAO Inhibitors; Methylphenidate

Decreased Effect
ROPINIRole may decrease the levels/effects of: Antipsychotics (Typical)

The levels/effects of ROPINIRole may be decreased by: Antipsychotics (Atypical); CYP1A2 Inducers (Strong); Cyproterone; Metoclopramide; Tocilizumab

Ethanol/Nutrition/Herb Interactions
Ethanol: Avoid ethanol (may increase CNS depression).
Herb/Nutraceutical: Avoid kava kava, gotu kola, valerian, St John's wort (may increase CNS depression).

Stability Store at controlled room temperature of 20°C to 25°C (68°F to 77°F). Protect from light.

Mechanism of Action Ropinirole has a high relative *in vitro* specificity and full intrinsic activity at the D_2 and D_3 dopamine receptor subtypes, binding with higher affinity to D_3 than to D_2 or D_4 receptor subtypes; relevance of D_3 receptor binding in Parkinson's disease is unknown. Ropinirole has moderate *in vitro* affinity for opioid receptors. Ropinirole and its metabolites have negligible *in vitro* affinity for dopamine D_1, 5-HT$_1$, 5-HT$_2$, benzodiazepine, GABA, muscarinic, alpha$_1$-, alpha$_2$-, and beta-adrenoreceptors. Although precise mechanism of action of ropinirole is unknown, it is believed to be due to stimulation of postsynaptic dopamine D_2-type receptors within the caudate putamen in the brain. Ropinirole caused decreases in systolic and diastolic blood pressure at doses >0.25 mg. The mechanism of ropinirole-induced postural hypotension is believed to be due to D_2-mediated blunting of the noradrenergic response to standing and subsequent decrease in peripheral vascular resistance.

Pharmacodynamics/Kinetics
Absorption: Not affected by food
Distribution: V_d: 525 L
Protein binding: 40%
Metabolism: Extensively hepatic via CYP1A2 to inactive metabolites; first-pass effect
Bioavailability: Absolute: 45% to 55%
Half-life elimination: ~6 hours
Time to peak: Immediate release: ~1-2 hours; Extended release: 6-10 hours; T_{max} increased by 2.5-3 hours when drug taken with food
Excretion: Urine (<10% as unchanged drug, 60% as metabolites)
Clearance: Reduced by 15% to 30% in patients >65 years of age

Dosage
Geriatric Clearance is reduced; however, no dosage adjustment necessary. Titrate dose to clinical response. Refer to adult dosing.

Adult
Parkinson's disease: Oral:
Immediate release tablet: The dosage should be increased to achieve a maximum therapeutic effect, balanced against the principal side effects of nausea, dizziness, somnolence and dyskinesia. Recommended starting dose is 0.25 mg 3 times/day; based on individual patient response, the dosage should be titrated with weekly increments as described below:
- Week 1: 0.25 mg 3 times/day; total daily dose: 0.75 mg
- Week 2: 0.5 mg 3 times/day; total daily dose: 1.5 mg
- Week 3: 0.75 mg 3 times/day; total daily dose: 2.25 mg
- Week 4: 1 mg 3 times/day; total daily dose: 3 mg
  Note: After week 4, if necessary, daily dosage may be increased by 1.5 mg/day on a weekly basis up to a dose of 9 mg/day, and then by up to 3 mg/day weekly to a total of 24 mg/day
Parkinson's disease discontinuation taper: Ropinirole should be gradually tapered over 7 days as follows: reduce frequency of administration from 3 times daily to twice daily for 4 days, then reduce to once daily for remaining 3 days.
Extended release tablet: Initial: 2 mg once daily for 1-2 weeks, followed by increases of 2 mg/day at weekly or longer intervals based on therapeutic response and tolerability (maximum: 24 mg/day); **Note:** When discontinuing gradually taper over 7 days.

Restless legs syndrome: Oral: Immediate release tablets: Initial: 0.25 mg once daily 1-3 hours before bedtime. Dose may be increased after 2 days to 0.5 mg daily, and after 7 days to 1 mg daily. Dose may be further titrated upward in 0.5 mg increments every week until reaching a daily dose of 3 mg during week 6. If symptoms persist or reappear, the daily dose may be increased to a maximum of 4 mg beginning week 7.
Note: Doses up to 4 mg per day may be discontinued without tapering.

Converting from ropinirole immediate release tablets to ropinirole extended-release tablets: Choose a once daily extended-release dose that most closely matches current immediate-release daily dose.

Renal Impairment

Moderate renal impairment (Cl_{cr} 30-50 mL/minute): No adjustment needed

Severe renal impairment (Cl_{cr} <30 mL/minute): Use with caution; has not been studied in this patient population. **Note:** The Canadian labeling recommends to avoid use in patients with severe renal impairment and who are not undergoing regular hemodialysis.

Hemodialysis: Canadian labeling (not in U.S. labeling): Initial: 0.25 mg 3 times daily; may titrate dose upward based on tolerability and efficacy (maximum dose: 18 mg/day); postdialysis supplemental doses are not required

Hepatic Impairment Titrate with caution; has not been studied.

Administration May be administered with or without food; taking with food may reduce nausea. Swallow extended-release tablet whole; do not crush, split, or chew.

Monitoring Parameters Blood pressure (orthostatic); daytime alertness

Pharmacotherapy Pearls If therapy with a drug known to be a potent inhibitor of CYP1A2 is stopped or started during treatment with ropinirole, adjustment of ropinirole dose may be required. Ropinirole binds to melanin-containing tissues (ie, eyes, skin) in pigmented rats. After a single dose, long-term retention of drug was demonstrated, with a half-life in the eye of 20 days; not known if ropinirole accumulates in these tissues over time.

Special Geriatric Considerations Since the dose is titrated to clinical response, no specific dosage adjustment is necessary in the elderly.

Dosage Forms Excipient information presented when available (limited, particularly for generics); consult specific product labeling.

Tablet, oral: 0.25 mg, 0.5 mg, 1 mg, 2 mg, 3 mg, 4 mg, 5 mg

Requip®: 0.25 mg, 0.5 mg, 1 mg, 2 mg, 3 mg, 4 mg, 5 mg

Tablet, extended release, oral:

Requip® XL™: 2 mg, 4 mg, 6 mg, 8 mg, 12 mg

Selected References

Factor SA, "Current Status of Symptomatic Medical Therapy in Parkinson's Disease," *Neurotherapeutics*, 2008, 5 (2):164-80.

Olanow CW, Watts RL, and Koller WC, "An Algorithm (Decision Tree) for the Management of Parkinson's Disease (2001): Treatment Guidelines," *Neurology*, 2001, 56(11 Suppl 5):S1-S88.

Weintraub D, Siderowf AD, Potenza MN, et al, "Association of Dopamine Agonist Use With Impulse Control Disorders in Parkinson Disease," *Arch Neurol*, 2006, 63(7):969-73.

◆ **Ropinirole Hydrochloride** *see* ROPINIRole *on page 1632*

Rosiglitazone (roh si GLI ta zone)

Related Information

Diabetes Mellitus Management, Adults *on page 2073*

Medication Safety Issues

Sound-alike/look-alike issues:

Avandia® may be confused with Avalide®, Coumadin®, Prandin®

International issues:

Avandia [U.S., Canada, and multiple international markets] may be confused with Avanza brand name for mirtazapine [Australia]

Brand Names: U.S. Avandia®

Brand Names: Canada Avandia®

Generic Availability (U.S.) No

Pharmacologic Category Antidiabetic Agent, Thiazolidinedione

Use Type 2 diabetes mellitus (noninsulin dependent, NIDDM):

Monotherapy: Improve glycemic control as an adjunct to diet and exercise

Note: Canadian labeling approves use as monotherapy only when metformin is contra-indicated or not tolerated.

Combination therapy: **Note:** Use when diet, exercise, and a single agent do not result in adequate glycemic control.

U.S. labeling: In combination with a sulfonylurea, metformin, or sulfonylurea plus metformin

Canadian labeling: In combination with metformin; in combination with a sulfonylurea only when metformin use is contraindicated or not tolerated

Prescribing and Access Restrictions Health Canada requires written informed consent for new and current patients receiving rosiglitazone.

Medication Guide Available Yes

Contraindications

U.S. labeling: NYHA Class III/IV heart failure (initiation of therapy)

Canadian labeling: Hypersensitivity to rosiglitazone or any component of the formulation; any stage of heart failure (eg, NYHA Class I, II, III, IV); serious hepatic impairment

◄ **Warnings/Precautions [U.S. Boxed Warning]: Thiazolidinediones, including rosiglitazone, may cause or exacerbate congestive heart failure; closely monitor for signs/symptoms of congestive heart failure** (eg, rapid weight gain, dyspnea, edema), particularly after initiation or dose increases. Not recommended for use in any patient with symptomatic heart failure. In the U.S., initiation of therapy is contraindicated in patients with NYHA class III or IV heart failure; in Canada use is contraindicated in patients with any stage of heart failure (NYHA Class I, II, III, IV). Use with caution in patients with edema; may increase plasma volume and/or cause fluid retention, leading to heart failure. Dose-related weight gain observed with use; mechanism unknown but likely associated with fluid retention and fat accumulation. Use may also be associated with an increased risk of angina and MI. Use caution in patients at risk for cardiovascular events and monitor closely. Discontinue if any deterioration in cardiac status occurs.

Should not be used in diabetic ketoacidosis. Mechanism requires the presence of insulin; therefore, use in type 1 diabetes (insulin dependent, IDDM) is not recommended. Combination therapy with other hypoglycemic agents may increase risk for hypoglycemic events; dose reduction with the concomitant agent may be warranted. Concomitant use with nitrates is not recommended due to increased risk of myocardial ischemia. Avoid use with insulin due to an increased risk of edema, congestive heart failure, and myocardial ischemic events.

Use with caution in patients with elevated transaminases (AST or ALT); do not initiate in patients with active liver disease or ALT >2.5 times ULN at baseline; evaluate patients with ALT ≤2.5 times ULN at baseline or during therapy for cause of enzyme elevation; during therapy, if ALT >3 times ULN, reevaluate levels promptly and discontinue if elevation persists or if jaundice occurs at any time during use. Idiosyncratic hepatotoxicity has been reported with another thiazolidinedione agent (troglitazone); avoid use in patients who previously experienced jaundice during troglitazone therapy. Monitoring should include periodic determinations of liver function. Increased incidence of bone fractures in females treated with rosiglitazone observed during analysis of long-term trial; majority of fractures occurred in the upper arm, hand, and foot (differing from the hip or spine fractures usually associated with postmenopausal osteoporosis). May decrease hemoglobin/hematocrit and/or WBC count (slight); effects may be related to increased plasma volume and/or dose related; use with caution in patients with anemia.

Rosiglitazone has been associated with new onset and/or worsening of macular edema in patients with diabetes. Rosiglitazone should be used with caution in patients with a preexisting macular edema or diabetic retinopathy. Discontinuation of rosiglitazone should be considered in any patient who reports visual deterioration. In addition, ophthalmological consultation should be initiated in these patients.

Additional Canadian warnings (not included in U.S. labeling): If glycemic control is inadequate, rosiglitazone may be added to metformin or a sulfonylurea (if metformin use is contraindicated or not tolerated); use of triple therapy (rosiglitazone in combination with both metformin and a sulfonylurea) is not recommended due to increased risks of heart failure and fluid retention.

Adverse Reactions (Reflective of adult population; not specific for elderly) Note: The rate of certain adverse reactions (eg, anemia, edema, hypoglycemia) may be higher with some combination therapies.

>10%: Endocrine & metabolic: HDL-cholesterol increased, LDL-cholesterol increased, total cholesterol increased, weight gain

1% to 10%:
Cardiovascular: Edema (5%), hypertension (4%); heart failure/CHF (up to 2% to 3% in patients receiving insulin; incidence likely higher in patients with pre-existing HF; myocardial ischemia (3%; incidence likely higher in patients with preexisting CAD)
Central nervous system: Headache (6%)
Endocrine & metabolic: Hypoglycemia (1% to 3%; combination therapy with insulin: 12% to 14%)
Gastrointestinal: Diarrhea (3%)
Hematologic: Anemia (2%)
Neuromuscular & skeletal: Fractures (up to 9%; incidence greater in females; usually upper arm, hand, or foot), arthralgia (5%), back pain (4% to 5%)
Respiratory: Upper respiratory tract infection (4% to 10%), nasopharyngitis (6%)
Miscellaneous: Injury (8%)

Drug Interactions
Metabolism/Transport Effects Substrate of CYP2C8 (major), 2C9 (minor); **Inhibits** CYP2C8 (moderate), 2C9 (weak), 2C19 (weak)
Avoid Concomitant Use There are no known interactions where it is recommended to avoid concomitant use.

Increased Effect/Toxicity

Rosiglitazone may increase the levels/effects of: CYP2C8 Substrates (High risk); Hypoglycemic Agents

The levels/effects of Rosiglitazone may be increased by: CYP2C8 Inhibitors (Moderate); CYP2C8 Inhibitors (Strong); Deferasirox; Gemfibrozil; Herbs (Hypoglycemic Properties); Insulin; Pegvisomant; Pregabalin; Trimethoprim; Vasodilators (Organic Nitrates)

Decreased Effect

The levels/effects of Rosiglitazone may be decreased by: Bile Acid Sequestrants; Corticosteroids (Orally Inhaled); Corticosteroids (Systemic); CYP2C8 Inducers (Highly Effective); Luteinizing Hormone-Releasing Hormone Analogs; Rifampin; Somatropin; Thiazide Diuretics

Ethanol/Nutrition/Herb Interactions

Ethanol: Avoid ethanol (may cause hypoglycemia).

Food: Peak concentrations are lower by 28% and delayed when administered with food, but these effects are not believed to be clinically significant.

Herb/Nutraceutical: Avoid alfalfa, aloe, bilberry, bitter melon, burdock, celery, damiana, fenugreek, garcinia, garlic, ginger, ginseng (American), gymnema, marshmallow, stinging nettle (may cause hypoglycemia).

Stability
Store at 15°C to 30°C (59°F to 86°F). Protect from light.

Mechanism of Action
Thiazolidinedione antidiabetic agent that lowers blood glucose by improving target cell response to insulin, without increasing pancreatic insulin secretion. It has a mechanism of action that is dependent on the presence of insulin for activity. Rosiglitazone is an agonist for peroxisome proliferator-activated receptor-gamma (PPARgamma). Activation of nuclear PPARgamma receptors influences the production of a number of gene products involved in glucose and lipid metabolism. PPARgamma is abundant in the cells within the renal collecting tubules; fluid retention results from stimulation by thiazolidinediones which increases sodium reabsorption.

Pharmacodynamics/Kinetics

Onset of action: Delayed; Maximum effect: Up to 12 weeks

Distribution: V_{dss} (apparent): 17.6 L

Protein binding: 99.8%; primarily albumin

Metabolism: Hepatic (99%) via CYP2C8; minor metabolism via CYP2C9

Bioavailability: 99%

Half-life elimination: 3-4 hours

Time to peak, plasma: 1 hour; delayed with food

Excretion: Urine (~64%) and feces (~23%) as metabolites

Dosage

Geriatric & Adult Type 2 diabetes: Oral: **Note:** All patients should be initiated at the lowest recommended dose.

Monotherapy: Initial: 4 mg daily as a single daily dose or in divided doses twice daily. If response is inadequate after 8-12 weeks of treatment, the dosage may be increased to 8 mg daily as a single daily dose or in divided doses twice daily. In clinical trials, the 4 mg twice-daily regimen resulted in the greatest reduction in fasting plasma glucose and Hb A_{1c}.

Combination therapy: When adding rosiglitazone to existing therapy, continue current dose(s) of previous agents:

U.S. labeling: With sulfonylureas or metformin (or sulfonylurea plus metformin): Initial: 4 mg daily as a single daily dose or in divided doses twice daily. If response is inadequate after 8-12 weeks of treatment, the dosage may be increased to 8 mg daily as a single daily dose or in divided doses twice daily. Reduce dose of sulfonylurea if hypoglycemia occurs. It is unlikely that the dose of metformin will need to be reduced due to hypoglycemia.

Canadian labeling:

With metformin: Initial: 4 mg daily as a single daily dose or in divided doses twice daily. If response is inadequate after 8-12 weeks of treatment, the dosage may be increased to 8 mg daily as a single daily dose or in divided doses twice daily.

With a sulfonylurea: 4 mg daily as a single daily dose or in divided doses twice daily. Dose should not exceed 4 mg daily when using in combination with a sulfonylurea. Reduce dose of sulfonylurea if hypoglycemia occurs.

Renal Impairment No adjustment is necessary.

Hepatic Impairment Clearance is significantly lower in hepatic impairment. Therapy should not be initiated if the patient exhibits active liver disease or increased transaminases (ALT >2.5 times the upper limit of normal) at baseline.

Administration May be administered without regard to meals.

Monitoring Parameters Hemoglobin A$_{1c}$, fasting serum glucose; signs and symptoms of fluid retention or heart failure; liver enzymes (prior to initiation of therapy, then periodically thereafter); ophthalmic exams. Evaluate patients with ALT ≤2.5 times ULN at baseline or during therapy for cause of enzyme elevation. Patients with an elevation in ALT >3 times ULN should be rechecked as soon as possible. If the ALT levels remain >3 times ULN, therapy with rosiglitazone should be discontinued.

Reference Range Recommendations for glycemic control in adults with diabetes:

Hb A$_{1c}$: <7%

Preprandial capillary plasma glucose: 70-130 mg/dL

Peak postprandial capillary blood glucose: <180 mg/dL

Special Geriatric Considerations Intensive glucose control (HbA$_{1c}$ <6.5%) has been linked to increased all-cause and cardiovascular mortality, hypoglycemia requiring assistance, and weight gain in adult type 2 diabetes. How "tightly" to control a geriatric patient's blood glucose needs to be individualized. Such a decision should be based on several factors, including the patient's functional and cognitive status, how well he/she recognizes hypoglycemic or hyperglycemic symptoms, and how to respond to them and other disease states. An HbA$_{1c}$ <7.5% is an acceptable endpoint for a healthy older adult, while <8% is acceptable for frail elderly patients, those with a duration of illness >10 years, or those with comorbid conditions and requiring combination diabetes medications. Patients who are unable to accurately draw up their dose will need assistance, such as prefilled syringes. Initial doses may require considerations for renal function in the elderly with dosing adjusted subsequently based on blood glucose monitoring. For elderly patients with diabetes who are relatively healthy, attaining target goals for aspirin use, blood pressure, lipids, smoking cessation, and diet and exercise may be more important than normalized glycemic control.

Dosage Forms Excipient information presented when available (limited, particularly for generics); consult specific product labeling.

Tablet, oral:

Avandia®: 2 mg, 4 mg, 8 mg

Selected References

Action to Control Cardiovascular Risk in Diabetes Study Group, Gerstein HC, Miller ME, et al, "Effects of Intensive Glucose Lowering in Type 2 Diabetes," *N Engl J Med*, 2008, 358(24):2545-59.

ADVANCE Collaborative Group, Patel A, MacMahon S, et al, "Intensive Blood Glucose Control and Vascular Outcomes in Patients With Type 2 Diabetes," *N Engl J Med*, 2008, 358(24):2560-72.

American Diabetes Association, "Standards of Medical Care in Diabetes – 2011," *Diabetes Care*, 2011, 34(Suppl 1):11-61.

Brown AF, Mangione CM, Saliba D, et al, "Guidelines for Improving the Care of the Older Person With Diabetes Mellitus," *J Am Geriatr Soc*, 2003, 51(5 Suppl Guidelines):265-80.

Home PD, Pocock SJ, Beck-Nielsen H, et al, "Rosiglitazone Evaluated for Cardiovascular Outcomes - An Interim Analysis," *N Engl J Med*, 2007, 357(1):28-38.

Lago RM, Singh PP, and Nesto RW, "Congestive Heart Failure and Cardiovascular Death in Patients With Prediabetes and Type 2 Diabetes Given Thiazolidinediones: A Meta-Analysis of Randomized Clinical Trials," *Lancet*, 2007, 370 (9593):1129-36.

Schwartz AV, Sellmeyer DE, Vittinghoff E, et al, "Thiazolidinedione Use and Bone Loss in Older Diabetic Adults," *J Clin Endocrin Metab*, 2006, 91(9):3349-54.

Singh S, Loke YK, and Furberg CD, "Long-Term Risk of Cardiovascular Events With Rosiglitazone," *JAMA*, 2007, 298 (10):1189-95.

"VA/DoD Clinical Practice Guideline for the Management of Diabetes Mellitus," 2010. Available at http://www.healthquality.va.gov/Diabetes_Mellitus.asp

Yaturu S, Bryant B, Jain SK, "Thiazolidinedione Treatment Decreases Bone Mineral Density in Type 2 Diabetic Men," *Diabetes Care*, 2007, 30(6):1574-76.

Rosiglitazone and Glimepiride (roh si GLI ta zone & GLYE me pye ride)

Related Information

Glimepiride *on page 820*

Rosiglitazone *on page 1635*

Medication Safety Issues

High alert medication:

The Institute for Safe Medication Practices (ISMP) includes this medication among its list of drugs which have a heightened risk of causing significant patient harm when used in error.

Brand Names: U.S. Avandaryl®

Brand Names: Canada Avandaryl®

Index Terms Glimepiride and Rosiglitazone Maleate

Generic Availability (U.S.) No

Pharmacologic Category Antidiabetic Agent, Sulfonylurea; Antidiabetic Agent, Thiazolidinedione

Use Management of type 2 diabetes mellitus (noninsulin dependent, NIDDM) as an adjunct to diet and exercise

Prescribing and Access Restrictions Health Canada requires written informed consent for new and current patients receiving rosiglitazone

Medication Guide Available Yes

Dosage

Geriatric Rosiglitazone 4 mg and glimepiride 1 mg once daily. Carefully titrate dose.

Adult Type 2 diabetes mellitus: Oral: Initial: Rosiglitazone 4 mg and glimepiride 1 mg once daily **or** rosiglitazone 4 mg and glimepiride 2 mg once daily (for patients previously treated with sulfonylurea or thiazolidinedione monotherapy)

Patients switching from combination rosiglitazone and glimepiride as separate tablets: Use current dose.

Titration:

Dose adjustment in patients previously on sulfonylurea monotherapy: May take 2 weeks to observe decreased blood glucose and 2-3 months to see full effects of rosiglitazone component. If not adequately controlled after 8-12 weeks, increase daily dose of rosiglitazone component.

Dose adjustment in patients previously on thiazolidinedione monotherapy: If not adequately controlled after 1-2 weeks, increase daily dose of glimepiride component in ≤2 mg increments in 1-2 week intervals.

Maximum dose:

U.S. labeling: Rosiglitazone 8 mg and glimepiride 4 mg once daily

Canadian labeling: Rosiglitazone 4 mg and glimepiride 4 mg once daily

Renal Impairment Rosiglitazone 4 mg and glimepiride 1 mg once daily. Carefully titrate dose.

Hepatic Impairment Rosiglitazone 4 mg and glimepiride 1 mg once daily. Carefully titrate dose.

ALT ≤2.5 times ULN: Use with caution.

ALT >2.5 times ULN: Do not initiate therapy.

ALT >3 times ULN or jaundice: Discontinue.

Special Geriatric Considerations Rapid and prolonged hypoglycemia (>12 hours) despite hypertonic glucose injections have been reported; age, hepatic, and renal impairment are independent risk factors for hypoglycemia; dosage titration should be made at weekly intervals. Intensive glucose control (HbA$_{1c}$ <6.5%) has been linked to increased all-cause and cardiovascular mortality, hypoglycemia requiring assistance, and weight gain in adult type 2 diabetes. How "tightly" to control a geriatric patient's blood glucose needs to be individualized. Such a decision should be based on several factors, including the patient's functional and cognitive status, how well he/she recognizes hypoglycemic or hyperglycemic symptoms, and how to respond to them and other disease states. An HbA$_{1c}$ <7.5% is an acceptable endpoint for a healthy older adult, while <8% is acceptable for frail elderly patients, those with a duration of illness >10 years, or those with comorbid conditions and requiring combination diabetes medications. Patients who are unable to accurately draw up their dose will need assistance, such as prefilled syringes. Initial doses may require considerations for renal function in the elderly with dosing adjusted subsequently based on blood glucose monitoring. For elderly patients with diabetes who are relatively healthy, attaining target goals for aspirin use, blood pressure, lipids, smoking cessation, and diet and exercise may be more important than normalized glycemic control.

Dosage Forms Excipient information presented when available (limited, particularly for generics); consult specific product labeling.

Tablet:

Avandaryl® 4 mg/1 mg: Rosiglitazone maleate 4 mg and glimepiride 1 mg

Avandaryl® 4 mg/2 mg: Rosiglitazone maleate 4 mg and glimepiride 2 mg

Avandaryl® 4 mg/4 mg: Rosiglitazone maleate 4 mg and glimepiride 4 mg

Avandaryl® 8 mg/2 mg: Rosiglitazone maleate 8 mg and glimepiride 2 mg

Avandaryl® 8 mg/4 mg: Rosiglitazone maleate 8 mg and glimepiride 4 mg

---

Rosiglitazone and Metformin (roh si GLI ta zone & met FOR min)

Related Information

MetFORMIN *on page 1155*
Rosiglitazone *on page 1635*

Medication Safety Issues

Sound-alike/look-alike issues:

Avandamet® may be confused with Anzemet®

Brand Names: U.S. Avandamet®

Brand Names: Canada Avandamet®

Index Terms Metformin and Rosiglitazone; Metformin Hydrochloride and Rosiglitazone Maleate; Rosiglitazone Maleate and Metformin Hydrochloride

Generic Availability (U.S.) No

◄ **Pharmacologic Category** Antidiabetic Agent, Biguanide; Antidiabetic Agent, Thiazolidine-dione

Use Management of type 2 diabetes mellitus (noninsulin dependent, NIDDM) as an adjunct to diet and exercise in patients where dual rosiglitazone and metformin therapy is appropriate

Prescribing and Access Restrictions Health Canada requires written informed consent for new and current patients receiving rosiglitazone.

Medication Guide Available Yes

Dosage

Geriatric The initial and maintenance dosing should be conservative, due to the potential for decreased renal function (monitor). Generally, elderly patients should not be titrated to the maximum. Do not use in patients ≥80 years unless normal renal function has been established.

Adult Type 2 diabetes mellitus: Oral:

First-line therapy (drug-naive patients): Initial: Rosiglitazone 2 mg and metformin 500 mg once or twice daily; may increase by 2 mg/500 mg per day after 4 weeks to a maximum of 8 mg/2000 mg per day.

Second-line therapy:

Patients inadequately controlled on metformin alone: Initial dose: Rosiglitazone 4 mg/day plus current dose of metformin

Patients inadequately controlled on rosiglitazone alone: Initial dose: Metformin 1000 mg/day plus current dose of rosiglitazone

Note: When switching from combination rosiglitazone and metformin as separate tablets: Use current dose

Dose adjustment: Doses may be increased as increments of rosiglitazone 4 mg and/or metformin 500 mg, up to the maximum dose; doses should be titrated gradually.

After a change in the metformin dosage, titration can be done after 1-2 weeks

After a change in the rosiglitazone dosage, titration can be done after 8-12 weeks

Maximum dose: Rosiglitazone 8 mg/metformin 2000 mg daily

Renal Impairment Do not use with renal disease or renal dysfunction (serum creatinine ≥1.5 mg/dL in males or ≥1.4 mg/dL in females or abnormal clearance).

Hepatic Impairment Do not initiate therapy with active liver disease or ALT >2.5 times the upper limit of normal.

Special Geriatric Considerations Metformin should not be used in patients ≥80 years of age unless renal function is verified as normal. **Do not titrate to maximum dose.** Intensive glucose control (HbA$_{1c}$ <6.5%) has been linked to increased all-cause and cardiovascular mortality, hypoglycemia requiring assistance, and weight gain in adult type 2 diabetes. How "tightly" to control a geriatric patient's blood glucose needs to be individualized. Such a decision should be based on several factors, including the patient's functional and cognitive status, how well he/she recognizes hypoglycemic or hyperglycemic symptoms, and how to respond to them and other disease states. An HbA$_{1c}$ <7.5% is an acceptable endpoint for a healthy older adult, while <8% is acceptable for frail elderly patients, those with a duration of illness >10 years, or those with comorbid conditions and requiring combination diabetes medications. Patients who are unable to accurately draw up their dose will need assistance, such as prefilled syringes. Initial doses may require considerations for renal function in the elderly with dosing adjusted subsequently based on blood glucose monitoring. For elderly patients with diabetes who are relatively healthy, attaining target goals for aspirin use, blood pressure, lipids, smoking cessation, and diet and exercise may be more important than normalized glycemic control.

Dosage Forms Excipient information presented when available (limited, particularly for generics); consult specific product labeling.

Tablet:

Avandamet®: 2/500: Rosiglitazone 2 mg and metformin hydrochloride 500 mg

Avandamet®: 4/500: Rosiglitazone 4 mg and metformin hydrochloride 500 mg

Avandamet®: 2/1000: Rosiglitazone 2 mg and metformin hydrochloride 1000 mg

Avandamet®: 4/1000: Rosiglitazone 4 mg and metformin hydrochloride 1000 mg

◆ **Rosiglitazone Maleate and Metformin Hydrochloride** *see* Rosiglitazone and Metformin *on page 1639*

◆ **Rosula® NS** *see* Sulfacetamide (Topical) *on page 1713*

Rosuvastatin (roe soo va STAT in)

Related Information

Hyperlipidemia Management *on page 2021*

Medication Safety Issues

Sound-alike/look-alike issues:

Rosuvastatin may be confused with atorvastatin, nystatin, pitavastatin

Brand Names: U.S. Crestor®
Brand Names: Canada Crestor®
Index Terms Rosuvastatin Calcium
Generic Availability (U.S.) No
Pharmacologic Category Antilipemic Agent, HMG-CoA Reductase Inhibitor
Use

Treatment of dyslipidemias:

Used with dietary therapy for hyperlipidemias to reduce elevations in total cholesterol (TC), LDL-C, apolipoprotein B, nonHDL-C, and triglycerides (TG) in patients with primary hypercholesterolemia (elevations of 1 or more components are present in Fredrickson type IIa, IIb, and IV hyperlipidemias); increase HDL-C; treatment of primary dysbetalipoproteinemia (Fredrickson type III hyperlipidemia); treatment of homozygous familial hypercholesterolemia (FH); to slow progression of atherosclerosis as an adjunct to diet to lower TC and LDL-C

Heterozygous familial hypercholesterolemia (HeFH): In adolescent patients (10-17 years of age, females >1 year postmenarche) with HeFH having LDL-C >190 mg/dL or LDL >160 mg/dL with positive family history of premature cardiovascular disease (CVD), or ≥2 other CVD risk factors.

Primary prevention of cardiovascular disease: To reduce the risk of stroke, myocardial infarction, or arterial revascularization procedures in patients without clinically evident coronary heart disease or lipid abnormalities but with all of the following: 1) an increased risk of cardiovascular disease based on age ≥50 years old in men and ≥60 years old in women, 2) hsCRP ≥2 mg/L, and 3) the presence of at least one additional cardiovascular disease risk factor such as hypertension, low HDL-C, smoking, or a family history of premature coronary heart disease.

Secondary prevention of cardiovascular disease: To slow progression of atherosclerosis

Contraindications Hypersensitivity to rosuvastatin or any component of the formulation; active liver disease; unexplained persistent elevations of serum transaminases (>3 times ULN)

Canadian labeling: Additional contraindications (not in U.S. labeling): Concomitant administration of cyclosporine; use of 40 mg dose in Asian patients, patients with predisposing risk factors for myopathy/rhabdomyolysis (eg, hereditary muscle disorders, history of myotoxicity with other HMC-CoA reductase inhibitors, concomitant use with fibrates or niacin, severe hepatic impairment, severe renal impairment [Cl$_{cr}$ <30 mL/minute/1.73 m^2], hypothyroidism, alcohol abuse)

Warnings/Precautions Secondary causes of hyperlipidemia should be ruled out prior to therapy. Rosuvastatin has not been studied when the primary lipid abnormality is chylomicron elevation (Fredrickson types I and V). Liver function must be monitored by periodic laboratory assessment. Use with caution in patients who consume large amounts of ethanol or have a history of liver disease. Use is contraindicated with active liver disease or unexplained transaminase elevations; may cause hepatic dysfunction. Rhabdomyolysis with acute renal failure has occurred. Hematuria (microscopic) and proteinuria have been observed; more commonly reported in patients receiving rosuvastatin 40 mg daily. Typically, transient and not associated with a decrease in renal function. Consider dosage reduction if unexplained hematuria and proteinuria persists. Discontinue in any patient in which CPK levels are markedly elevated (>10 times ULN) or if myopathy is suspected/diagnosed. An increased incidence of rosuvastatin-associated myopathy has been reported during concomitant therapy with fibric acid derivatives, niacin, cyclosporine, and lopinavir/ritonavir, and in certain subgroups of the Asian population; dosage adjustment should be considered for patients of Asian descent. The Canadian labeling contraindicates concomitant use of rosuvastatin with cyclosporine and the use of rosuvastatin 40 mg/day in Asian patients and/or patients receiving fibrates or niacin. Use with caution with concurrent protease inhibitor/ritonavir combinations. Atazanavir/ritonavir and lopinavir/ritonavir significantly increase rosuvastatin serum concentration; limit dose of rosuvastatin to 10 mg/day. Monitor closely if used with other drugs associated with myopathy (eg, colchicine). Risk is also elevated at higher dosages of rosuvastatin. Patients should be instructed to report unexplained muscle pain, tenderness, or weakness, particularly if associated with fever and/or malaise. Use caution in patients predisposed to myopathy (eg, renal failure, advanced age, inadequately treated hypothyroidism). The manufacturer recommends temporary discontinuation for elective major surgery, acute medical or surgical conditions, or in any patient experiencing an acute or serious condition predisposing to renal failure (eg, sepsis, hypotension, trauma, uncontrolled seizures). However, based upon current evidence, HMG-CoA reductase inhibitor therapy should be continued in the perioperative period unless risk outweighs cardioprotective benefit. In the JUPITER study, small increases in hemoglobin (Hb) A1c (mean HbA1c increased by ~0.1%) and physician-reported diabetes was significantly higher in the rosuvastatin group compared to placebo (Ridker, 2008). Overall, evidence supporting an association with diabetes risk is lacking. Because the clear benefits on cardiovascular disease risk outweigh any potential detrimental effects on glucose metabolism, the use of HMG-CoA reductase inhibitors in patients with diabetes continues to be recommended (ADA, 2011).

Adverse Reactions (Reflective of adult population; not specific for elderly)
>10%: Neuromuscular & skeletal: Myalgia (3% to 13%)
2% to 10%:
  Central nervous system: Headache (6%), dizziness (4%)
  Gastrointestinal: Nausea (3%), abdominal pain (2%), constipation (2%)
  Hepatic: ALT increased (2%; >3 times ULN)
  Neuromuscular & skeletal: Arthralgia (4% to 10%), CPK increased (3%; >10 x ULN: Children 3%), weakness (3%)
Adverse reactions reported with other HMG-CoA reductase inhibitors (not necessarily reported with rosuvastatin therapy) include a hypersensitivity syndrome (symptoms may include anaphylaxis, angioedema, arthralgia, erythema multiforme, eosinophilia, hemolytic anemia, interstitial lung disease, lupus syndrome, photosensitivity, polymyalgia rheumatica, positive ANA, purpura, Stevens-Johnson syndrome, toxic epidermal necrolysis, urticaria, vasculitis)

Drug Interactions
  Metabolism/Transport Effects Substrate (minor) of CYP2C9, CYP3A4, SLCO1B1
  Avoid Concomitant Use
    Avoid concomitant use of Rosuvastatin with any of the following: Red Yeast Rice
  Increased Effect/Toxicity
    Rosuvastatin may increase the levels/effects of: DAPTOmycin; Trabectedin; Vitamin K Antagonists

    The levels/effects of Rosuvastatin may be increased by: Amiodarone; Colchicine; Conivaptan; CycloSPORINE; CycloSPORINE (Systemic); Eltrombopag; Fenofibrate; Fenofibric Acid; Gemfibrozil; Niacin; Niacinamide; Protease Inhibitors; Red Yeast Rice
  Decreased Effect
    Rosuvastatin may decrease the levels/effects of: Lanthanum

    The levels/effects of Rosuvastatin may be decreased by: Antacids; Tocilizumab
Ethanol/Nutrition/Herb Interactions
  Ethanol: Avoid excessive ethanol consumption (due to potential hepatic effects).
  Food: Red yeast rice contains an estimated 2.4 mg lovastatin per 600 mg rice.
Stability Store between 20°C and 25°C (68°F to 77°F). Protect from moisture.
Mechanism of Action Inhibitor of 3-hydroxy-3-methylglutaryl coenzyme A (HMG-CoA) reductase, the rate-limiting enzyme in cholesterol synthesis (reduces the production of mevalonic acid from HMG-CoA); this then results in a compensatory increase in the expression of LDL receptors on hepatocyte membranes and a stimulation of LDL catabolism
Pharmacodynamics/Kinetics
  Onset of action: Within 1 week; maximal at 4 weeks
  Distribution: V_d: 134 L
  Protein binding: 88%
  Metabolism: Hepatic (10%), via CYP2C9 (1 active metabolite identified: N-desmethyl rosuvastatin, one-sixth to one-half the HMG-CoA reductase activity of the parent compound)
  Bioavailability: 20% (high first-pass extraction by liver)
    Asian patients have been noted to have increased bioavailability.
  Half-life elimination: 19 hours
  Time to peak, plasma: 3-5 hours
  Excretion: Feces (90%), primarily as unchanged drug
Dosage
  Geriatric & Adult Note: Doses should be individualized according to the baseline LDL-cholesterol levels, the recommended goal of therapy, and patient response; adjustments should be made at intervals of 4 weeks or more.
    Hyperlipidemia, mixed dyslipidemia, hypertriglyceridemia, primary dysbetalipoproteinemia, slowing progression of atherosclerosis: Oral:
      Initial dose:
        General dosing: 10 mg once daily; 20 mg once daily may be used in patients with severe hyperlipidemia (LDL >190 mg/dL) and aggressive lipid targets
        Conservative dosing: Patients requiring less aggressive treatment or predisposed to myopathy (including patients of Asian descent): 5 mg once daily
      Titration: After 2 weeks, may be increased by 5-10 mg once daily; dosing range: 5-40 mg/day (maximum dose: 40 mg once daily)
      Note: The 40 mg dose should be reserved for patients who have not achieved goal cholesterol levels on a dose of 20 mg/day, including patients switched from another HMG-CoA reductase inhibitor.
    Homozygous familial hypercholesterolemia (FH): Oral: Initial: 20 mg once daily (maximum dose: 40 mg/day)

Dosage adjustment with concomitant medications: Oral:

U.S. labeling:

Cyclosporine: Rosuvastatin dose should not exceed 5 mg/day

Gemfibrozil: Avoid concurrent use; if unable to avoid concurrent use, rosuvastatin dose should not exceed 10 mg/day

Atazanavir/ritonavir or lopinavir/ritonavir: Rosuvastatin dose should not exceed 10 mg/day

Canadian labeling:

Cyclosporine: Concomitant use is contraindicated

Gemfibrozil: Rosuvastatin dose should not exceed 20 mg/day

Dosage adjustment for hematuria and/or persistent, unexplained proteinuria while on 40 mg/day: Reduce dose and evaluate causes.

Renal Impairment

Mild-to-moderate impairment: No dosage adjustment required.

Cl_{cr} <30 mL/minute/1.73 m^2: Initial: 5 mg/day; do not exceed 10 mg once daily

Hepatic Impairment

U.S. labeling: Active hepatic disease, including unexplained persistent transaminase elevations: Use is contraindicated.

Canadian labeling:

Active hepatic disease or unexplained persistent transaminase >3 x ULN: Use is contraindicated.

Mild-to-moderate impairment: No dosage adjustment required.

Severe impairment: Initial: 5 mg/day; do not exceed 20 mg once daily.

Administration May be administered with or without food. May be taken at any time of the day.

Monitoring Parameters Total cholesterol, LDL, and HDL cholesterol within 2-4 weeks of treatment initiation or dose change; liver function tests to be determined at baseline (prior to initiation), 3 months following initiation, 3 months after any increase in dose, and periodically thereafter (eg, semiannually); baseline CPK (recheck CPK in any patient with symptoms suggestive of myopathy). Monitor LDL-C at intervals no less than 4 weeks.

Special Geriatric Considerations Effective and well tolerated in the elderly. The definition of and, therefore, when to treat hyperlipidemia in geriatrics is a controversial issue. The National Cholesterol Education Program recommends that all adults maintain a plasma cholesterol <160 mg/dL. For elderly patients with one additional risk factor, goal LDL would be <130 mg/dL. It is the authors' belief that pharmacologic treatment be reserved for those who are unable to obtain a desirable plasma cholesterol concentration by diet alone and for whom the benefits of treatment are believed to outweigh the potential adverse effects, drug interactions, and cost of treatment. Age ≥65 years is a risk factor for myopathy.

Dosage Forms Excipient information presented when available (limited, particularly for generics); consult specific product labeling.

Tablet, oral:

Crestor®: 5 mg, 10 mg, 20 mg, 40 mg

Selected References

Anderson JL, Adams CD, Antman EM, et al, "ACC/AHA 2007 Guidelines for the Management of Patients With Unstable Angina/Non ST-Elevation Myocardial Infarction: Executive Summary. A Report of the American College of Cardiology/American Heart Association Task Force on Practice Guidelines (Writing Committee to Revise the 2002 Guidelines for the Management of Patients with Unstable Angina/Non ST-Elevation Myocardial Infarction) Developed in Collaboration With the American College of Emergency Physicians, The Society of Cardiovascular Angiography and Interventions, and the Society of Thoracic Surgeons," *J Am Coll Cardiol*, 2007, 50(7):1-157.

Fleisher LA, Beckman JA, Brown KA, et al, "ACC/AHA 2007 Guidelines on Perioperative Cardiovascular Evaluation and Care for Noncardiac Surgery: A Report of the American College of Cardiology/American Heart Association Task Force on Practice Guidelines (Writing Committee to Revise the 2002 Guidelines on Perioperative Cardiovascular Evaluation for Noncardiac Surgery) Developed in Collaboration With the American Society of Echocardiography, American Society of Nuclear Cardiology, Heart Rhythm Society, Society of Cardiovascular Anesthesiologists, Society for Cardiovascular Angiography and Interventions, Society for Vascular Medicine and Biology, and Society for Vascular Surgery," *J Am Coll Cardiol*, 2007, 50(17):e159-241.

Grundy SM, Cleeman JI, Merz CN, et al, "Implications of Recent Clinical Trials for the National Cholesterol Education Program Adult Treatment Panel III Guidelines," *J Am Coll Cardiol*, 2004, 44(3):720-32.

National Cholesterol Education Program (NCEP) Expert Panel on Detection, Evaluation, and Treatment of High Blood Cholesterol in Adults (Adult Treatment Panel III), "Third Report of the National Cholesterol Education Program (NCEP) Expert Panel on Detection, Evaluation, and Treatment of High Blood Cholesterol in Adults (Adult Treatment Panel III) Final Report," *Circulation*, 2002, 106(25):3143-421.

Rufinamide (roo FIN a mide)

Brand Names: U.S. Banzel®
Index Terms CGP 33101; E 2080; RUF 331; Xilep
Generic Availability (U.S.) No
Pharmacologic Category Anticonvulsant, Triazole Derivative
Use Adjunctive therapy in the treatment of generalized seizures of Lennox-Gastaut syndrome
Medication Guide Available Yes
Contraindications Patients with familial short QT syndrome
Warnings/Precautions Has been associated with shortening of the QT interval. Use caution in patients receiving concurrent medications that shorten the QT interval. Contraindicated in patients with familial short-QT syndrome. Use has been associated with CNS-related adverse events, most significant of these were cognitive symptoms (including somnolence and fatigue) and coordination abnormalities (including ataxia, dizziness, and gait disturbances). Caution patients about performing tasks which require mental alertness (eg, operating machinery or driving). Effects with other sedative drugs or ethanol may be potentiated. Potentially serious, sometimes fatal, multiorgan hypersensitivity reactions have been reported with some anti-epileptic drugs, including rufinamide; monitor for signs and symptoms of possible disparate manifestations associated with lymphatic, hepatic, renal, and/or hematologic organ systems; gradual discontinuation and conversion to alternate therapy may be required. Closely monitor any patient who develops a rash; instruct patients to report any rash associated with fever.

Antiepileptics are associated with an increased risk of suicidal behavior/thoughts with use (regardless of indication); patients should be monitored for signs/symptoms of depression, suicidal tendencies, and other unusual behavior changes during therapy and instructed to inform their healthcare provider immediately if symptoms occur. Use with caution in patients with mild-to-moderate hepatic impairment; use in not recommended in patients with severe hepatic impairment. Concurrent use with hormonal contraceptives may lead to contraceptive failure. Anticonvulsants should not be discontinued abruptly because of the possibility of increasing seizure frequency; therapy should be withdrawn gradually to minimize the potential of increased seizure frequency, unless safety concerns require a more rapid withdrawal. Reducing dose by ~25% every two days was effective in trials.
Adverse Reactions (Reflective of adult population; not specific for elderly)
>10%:
  Cardiovascular: QT shortening (46% to 65%; dose related)
  Central nervous system: Headache (16% to 27%), somnolence (11% to 24%), dizziness (3% to 19%), fatigue (9% to 16%)
  Gastrointestinal: Vomiting (5% to 17%), nausea (7% to 12%)
1% to 10%:
  Central nervous system: Ataxia (4% to 5%), seizure (children 5%), status epilepticus (≤4%), aggression (children 3%), anxiety (adults 3%), attention disturbance (children 3%), hyperactivity (children 3%), vertigo (adults 3%)
  Dermatologic: Rash (children 4%), pruritus (children 3%)
  Gastrointestinal: Appetite decreased (≥1% to 5%), abdominal pain (3%), constipation (adults 3%), dyspepsia (adults 3%), appetite increased (≥1%)
  Hematologic: Leukopenia (≤4%), anemia (≥1%)
  Neuromuscular & skeletal: Tremor (adults 6%), back pain (adults 3%), gait disturbance (1% to 3%)
  Ocular: Diplopia (4% to 9%), blurred vision (adults 6%), nystagmus (adults 6%)
  Otic: Otitis media (children 3%)
  Renal: Pollakiuria (≥1%)
  Respiratory: Nasopharyngitis (children 5%), bronchitis (children 3%), sinusitis (children 3%)
  Miscellaneous: Influenza (children 5%)
Drug Interactions
  Avoid Concomitant Use There are no known interactions where it is recommended to avoid concomitant use.

Increased Effect/Toxicity

Rufinamide may increase the levels/effects of: PHENobarbital; Phenytoin

The levels/effects of Rufinamide may be increased by: Divalproex; Valproic Acid

Decreased Effect

Rufinamide may decrease the levels/effects of: CarBAMazepine; Ethinyl Estradiol; Norethindrone; Saxagliptin

The levels/effects of Rufinamide may be decreased by: CarBAMazepine; PHENobarbital; Phenytoin; Primidone

Ethanol/Nutrition/Herb Interactions

Ethanol: Avoid ethanol (may increase CNS depression).

Food: Food increases the absorption of rufinamide.

Herb/Nutraceutical: Avoid evening primrose (seizure threshold decreased).

Stability Store at 25°C (77°F); excursions permitted to 15°C to 30°C (59°F to 86°F). Protect tablets from moisture. The cap to the oral suspension bottle fits over the adapter.

Mechanism of Action A triazole-derivative antiepileptic whose exact mechanism is unknown. *In vitro*, it prolongs the inactive state of the sodium channels, thereby limiting repetitive firing of sodium-dependent action potentials mediating anticonvulsant effects.

Pharmacodynamics/Kinetics

Absorption: Slow; extensive ≥85%; increased with food

Distribution: V_d: ~50 L

Protein binding: 34%, primarily to albumin

Metabolism: Extensively via carboxylesterase-mediated hydrolysis of the carboxylamide group to CGP 47292 (inactive metabolite); weak inhibitor of CYP2E1 and weak inducer of CYP3A4

Bioavailability: Extent decreased with increased dose; oral tablets and oral suspension are bioequivalent

Half-life elimination: ~6-10 hours

Time to peak, plasma: 4-6 hours

Excretion: Urine (85%, ~66% as CGP 47292, <2% as unchanged drug)

Dosage

Geriatric & Adult Lennox-Gastaut (adjunctive): Oral: Initial: 400-800 mg/day in 2 equally divided doses; increase dose by 400-800 mg/day every other day to a maximum dose of 3200 mg/day in 2 equally divided doses

Dosage adjustment for concomitant medications: Valproate: Initial rufinamide dose should be <400 mg/day

Renal Impairment

Cl_{cr} <30 mL/minute: No dosage adjustment needed.

Hemodialysis: No specific guidelines available; consider dosage adjustment for loss of drug.

Hepatic Impairment

Mild-to-moderate impairment: Use caution.

Severe impairment: Use in severe impairment has not been studied and is not recommended.

Administration Administer with food. Tablets may be swallowed whole, split in half, or crushed. Oral suspension should be administered using the provided adapter and oral syringe; shake well before every administration.

Monitoring Parameters Seizure (frequency and duration); serum levels of concurrent anticonvulsants; suicidality (eg, suicidal thoughts, depression, behavioral changes)

Special Geriatric Considerations Limited study in the elderly; however, to date, no data to demonstrate differences in pharmacokinetic between elderly and young adults. No dosage adjustment necessary.

Dosage Forms Excipient information presented when available (limited, particularly for generics); consult specific product labeling.

Suspension, oral:

Banzel®: 40 mg/mL (460 mL) [dye free, gluten free, lactose free; contains propylene glycol; orange flavor]

Tablet, oral:

Banzel®: 200 mg, 400 mg [scored]

Selected References

Deeks ED and Scott LJ, "Rufinamide," *CNS Drugs*, 2006, 20(9):751-60.

Glauser T, Kluger G, Sachdeo R, et al, "Rufinamide for Generalized Seizures Associated With Lennox-Gastaut Syndrome," *Neurology*, 2008, 70(21):1950-8.

Perucca E, Cloyd J, Critchley D, et al, "Rufinamide: Clinical Pharmacokinetics and Concentration-Response Relationships in Patients With Epilepsy," *Epilepsia*, 2008, 49(7):1123-41.

◆ **Rulox [OTC]** *see* Aluminum Hydroxide, Magnesium Hydroxide, and Simethicone *on page 84*

◆ **Rybix™ ODT** *see* TraMADol *on page 1839*

◆ **Rythmol®** *see* Propafenone *on page 1533*

- **Rythmol® SR** *see* Propafenone *on page 1533*
- **Ryzolt™** *see* TraMADol *on page 1839*
- **S2® [OTC]** *see* EPINEPHrine (Systemic, Oral Inhalation) *on page 606*
- **S-(+)-3-isobutylgaba** *see* Pregabalin *on page 1514*
- **6(S)-5-methyltetrahydrofolate** *see* Methylfolate *on page 1177*
- **6(S)-5-MTHF** *see* Methylfolate *on page 1177*
- **S-4661** *see* Doripenem *on page 558*
- **Sabril®** *see* Vigabatrin *on page 1916*

Saccharomyces boulardii (sak roe MYE sees boo LAR dee)

Medication Safety Issues
International issues:
Codex: Brand name for *saccharomyces boulardii* [Italy], but also the brand name for acetaminophen/codeine [Brazil]

Codex [Italy] may be confused with Cedax brand name for ceftibuten [U.S. and multiple international markets]; Clobex® brand name for clobetasol [U.S., Canada, and multiple international markets]

Precosa [Finland, Sweden] may be confused with Precose brand name for acarbose [U.S., Malaysia]

Brand Names: U.S. Florastor® Kids [OTC]; Florastor® [OTC]

Index Terms *S. boulardii*; *Saccharomyces boulardii lyo*

Generic Availability (U.S.) No

Pharmacologic Category Dietary Supplement; Probiotic

Use Promote maintenance of normal microflora in the gastrointestinal tract; used in management of bloating, gas, and diarrhea, particularly to decrease the incidence of diarrhea associated with antibiotic use

Contraindications Hypersensitivity to *Saccharomyces boulardii* or any component of the formulation

Warnings/Precautions *S. boulardii*, a nonpathogenic yeast, has been associated with case reports of invasive fungemias in immunocompromised, debilitated, or critically ill patients; use caution or avoid use in these patients, particularly those with a central venous catheter and/or previous or current antibiotic therapy. Use caution in patients allergic to yeast; *S. boulardii* is a live yeast preparation and a subtype of the species, *S. cervasiae*, which is also referred to as "baker's yeast" or "brewer's yeast." Avoid use in patients on systemic antifungal therapy; *S. boulardii* may be susceptible. Probiotic products are classified as dietary supplements; therefore, there are no safety reviews or approved therapeutic indications by the FDA. There is no conclusive evidence to support widespread use in the treatment of diarrhea. Significant differences may exist from one preparation of *S. boulardii* compared to another with respect to biologic activity and composition. Some products may contain lactose.

Adverse Reactions (Reflective of adult population; not specific for elderly) Frequency not defined.
Gastrointestinal: Constipation, flatulence
Miscellaneous: Thirst

Drug Interactions
Avoid Concomitant Use There are no known interactions where it is recommended to avoid concomitant use.

Increased Effect/Toxicity There are no known significant interactions involving an increase in effect.

Decreased Effect
The levels/effects of Saccharomyces boulardii may be decreased by: Antifungal Agents

Stability Some preparations may need to be refrigerated or stored in freezer; consult individual product labeling.
Florastor®, Florastor® Kids: Store at ≤25°C (≤77°F); refrigeration not necessary.

Mechanism of Action *S. boulardii*, a nonpathogenic live yeast probiotic, acts as temporary flora to help re-establish the normal gastrointestinal microflora. May also modulate the immune system by inducing cytokines and suppress pathogenic bacteria growth.

Pharmacodynamics/Kinetics
Onset of action: Yeast cell release from capsules/powder: 30 minutes
Duration: Yeast cells cleared in 5-7 days

Dosage
Geriatric Refer to adult dosing. Use caution in debilitated patients.

Adult Dietary supplement: Oral: Dosing varies by manufacturer; consult product labeling.
Florastor®: 250 mg twice daily

Administration
Florastor®: Swallow capsule whole or capsules may be opened and emptied on tongue (wash down with water or juice) or sprinkled on semi-solid food (eg, applesauce, sour cream, yogurt) or added to a drink (eg, water, apple or orange juice, milk or formula); may be administered with or without food.
Florastor® Kids: Add powder to a drink or sprinkle on semi-solid food; may be administered with or without food.

Special Geriatric Considerations Use caution in debilitated patients.

Dosage Forms Excipient information presented when available (limited, particularly for generics); consult specific product labeling.
Capsule, oral:
Florastor®: S. boulardii lyo 250 mg [contains lactose 32.5 mg/capsule, magnesium 2.85 mg/capsule; provides 5 billion live cells]
Powder, oral:
Florastor® Kids: S. boulardii lyo 250 mg/packet (10s) [contains lactose 32.5 mg/packet, magnesium 2.85 mg/packet; tutti frutti flavor; provides 5 billion live cells]

Selected References
Enache-Angoulvant A and Hennequin C, "Invasive Saccharomyces Infection: A Comprehensive Review," *Clin Infect Dis*, 2005, 41(11):1559-68.

◆ **Saccharomyces boulardii lyo** *see* Saccharomyces boulardii *on page 1646*
◆ **Safe Tussin® DM [OTC]** *see* Guaifenesin and Dextromethorphan *on page 848*
◆ **Salactic® [OTC]** *see* Salicylic Acid *on page 1648*
◆ **Salbutamol** *see* Albuterol *on page 50*
◆ **Salbutamol and Ipratropium** *see* Ipratropium and Albuterol *on page 975*
◆ **Salbutamol Sulphate** *see* Albuterol *on page 50*
◆ **Salex®** *see* Salicylic Acid *on page 1648*

Salicylates (Various Salts) (sa LIS i lates)

Brand Names: U.S. Arthropan®; Asproject®; Extra Strength Doan's® [OTC]; Magan®; Mobidin®; Original Doan's® [OTC]; Rexolate®; Tusal®

Index Terms Choline Salicylate; Magnesium Salicylate; Sodium Salicylate; Sodium Thiosalicylate

Generic Availability (U.S.) Yes

Pharmacologic Category Analgesic, Nonopioid; Anti-inflammatory Agent; Antiplatelet Agent; Antipyretic; Nonsteroidal Anti-inflammatory Drug (NSAID), Oral; Salicylate

Use Treatment of mild to moderate pain, inflammation and fever; may be used as a prophylaxis of myocardial infarction and transient ischemic attacks (TIA)

Contraindications Bleeding disorders, hypersensitivity to salicylates or other nonsteroidal anti-inflammatory drugs (NSAIDs)

Stability Keep suppositories in refrigerator, do not freeze; hydrolysis of aspirin occurs upon exposure to water or moist air, resulting in salicylate and acetate, which possess a vinegar-like odor; do not use if a strong odor is present

Mechanism of Action Inhibits prostaglandin synthesis, acts on the hypothalamus heat-regulating center to reduce fever, blocks prostaglandin synthetase action which prevents formation of the platelet-aggregating substance thromboxane A_2; inhibits both vitamin K-dependent and independent clotting factors

Pharmacodynamics/Kinetics
Absorption: From the stomach and small intestine
Distribution: Readily into most body fluids and tissues
Aspirin is hydrolyzed to salicylate (active) by esterases in the GI mucosa, red blood cells, synovial fluid and blood
Metabolism: Metabolism of salicylate occurs primarily by hepatic microsomal enzymes
Half-life, aspirin: 15-20 minutes; metabolic pathways are saturable such that salicylate half-life is dose-dependent ranging from 3 hours at lower doses (300-600 mg), 5-6 hours (after 1 g) and 15-30 hours with higher doses; in therapeutic anti-inflammatory doses, half-lives generally range from 6-12 hours
Time to peak plasma concentration: ~1-2 hours

Monitoring Parameters Serum concentrations, renal function; hearing changes or tinnitus; monitor for response (ie, pain, inflammation, range of motion, grip strength); observe for abnormal bleeding, bruising, weight gain

Reference Range
Sample size: 1.5-2 mL blood (lavender top (EDTA) tube)

Timing of serum samples: Peak levels usually occur 2 hours after ingestion; half-life increases with dosage (eg, the half-life after 300 mg is 3 hours, and after 1 g is 5-6 hours, and after 8-10 g is 10 hours)

SALICYLATES (VARIOUS SALTS)

Salicylate serum concentrations correlate with the pharmacological actions and adverse effects observed.

Test Interactions False-negative results for glucose oxidase urinary glucose tests (Clinistix®); false-positives using the cupric sulfate method (Clinitest®); also, interferes with Gerhardt test (urinary ketone analysis), VMA determination; 5-HIAA, xylose tolerance test, and T_3 and T_4; increased PBI; increased uric acid

Pharmacotherapy Pearls Liquid dosage form may be useful for those who have difficulty swallowing tablets or caplets. These agents do not appear to inhibit platelet aggregation. Nonacetylated salicylates have less GI toxicity and renal effects than aspirin and other NSAIDs. They also do not cause reactions in aspirin sensitive patients.

Choline salicylate: Arthropan®

Sodium thiosalicylate: Asproject®; Rexolate®; Tusal®

Magnesium salicylate: Extra Strength Doan's® [OTC]; Magan®; Mobidin®; Original Doan's® [OTC]

Special Geriatric Considerations Elderly are a high-risk population for adverse effects from NSAIDs. As much as 60% of elderly can develop peptic ulceration and/or hemorrhage asymptomatically. The concomitant use of H_2 blockers, omeprazole, and sucralfate is not effective as prophylaxis with the exception of NSAID-induced duodenal ulcers which may be prevented by the use of ranitidine. Misoprostol and proton pump inhibitors are the only agents proven to help prevent the development of NSAID-induced ulcers. Also, concomitant disease and drug use contribute to the risk for GI adverse effects. Use lowest effective dose for shortest period possible. Consider renal function decline with age. Use of NSAIDs can compromise existing renal function especially when Cl_{cr} is ≤30 mL/minute. Tinnitus may be a difficult and unreliable indication of toxicity due to age-related hearing loss or eighth cranial nerve damage. CNS adverse effects such as confusion, agitation, and hallucination are generally seen in overdose or high dose situations, but elderly may demonstrate these adverse effects at lower doses than younger adults.

Dosage Forms

Injection: 50 mg/mL

Liquid: 870 mg/mL (choline salicylate)

Tablet, enteric coated: 325 mg, 545 mg, 600 mg, 650 mg

Selected References

AGS Panel on Persistent Pain in Older Persons, "The Management of Persistent Pain in Older Persons," *J Am Geriatr Soc*, 2002, 50(6 Suppl):S205-24.

◆ **Salicylazosulfapyridine** *see* SulfaSALAzine *on page 1719*

Salicylic Acid (sal i SIL ik AS id)

Medication Safety Issues

Sound-alike/look-alike issues:

Occlusal®-HP may be confused with Ocuflox®

Other safety concerns:

Transdermal patch may contain conducting metal (eg, aluminum); remove patch prior to MRI.

Brand Names: U.S. Aliclen™; Beta Sal® [OTC]; Clean & Clear® Advantage® Acne Cleanser [OTC]; Clean & Clear® Advantage® Acne Spot Treatment [OTC]; Clean & Clear® Advantage® Invisible Acne Patch [OTC]; Clean & Clear® Advantage® Oil-Free Acne [OTC]; Clean & Clear® Blackhead Clearing Daily Cleansing [OTC]; Clean & Clear® Blackhead Clearing Scrub [OTC]; Clean & Clear® Continuous Control® Acne Wash [OTC]; Clean & Clear® Deep Cleaning [OTC]; Clean & Clear® Dual Action Moisturizer [OTC]; Clean & Clear® Invisible Blemish Treatment [OTC]; Compound W® One Step Invisible Strip [OTC]; Compound W® One Step Wart Remover for Feet [OTC]; Compound W® One-Step Wart Remover for Kids [OTC]; Compound W® One-Step Wart Remover [OTC]; Compound W® [OTC]; Curad® Mediplast® [OTC]; Denorex® Extra Strength Protection 2-in-1 [OTC]; Denorex® Extra Strength Protection [OTC]; Dermarest® Psoriasis Medicated Moisturizer [OTC]; Dermarest® Psoriasis Medicated Scalp Treatment [OTC]; Dermarest® Psoriasis Medicated Shampoo/ Conditioner [OTC]; Dermarest® Psoriasis Medicated Skin Treatment [OTC]; Dermarest® Psoriasis Overnight Treatment [OTC]; DHS™ Sal [OTC]; Dr. Scholl's® Callus Removers [OTC]; Dr. Scholl's® Clear Away® One Step Wart Remover [OTC]; Dr. Scholl's® Clear Away® Plantar Wart Remover For Feet [OTC]; Dr. Scholl's® Clear Away® Wart Remover Fast-Acting [OTC]; Dr. Scholl's® Clear Away® Wart Remover Invisible Strips [OTC]; Dr. Scholl's® Clear Away® Wart Remover [OTC]; Dr. Scholl's® Corn Removers [OTC]; Dr. Scholl's® Corn/Callus Remover [OTC]; Dr. Scholl's® Extra Thick Corn Removers [OTC]; Dr. Scholl's® Extra-Thick Callus Removers [OTC]; Dr. Scholl's® For Her Corn Removers [OTC]; Dr. Scholl's® OneStep Callus Removers [OTC]; Dr. Scholl's® OneStep Corn Removers [OTC]; Dr. Scholl's® Small Corn Removers [OTC]; Dr. Scholl's® Ultra-Thin Corn Removers [OTC]; DuoFilm® [OTC]; Durasal™; Freezone® [OTC]; Fung-O® [OTC]; Gets-It® [OTC]; Gordofilm [OTC]; Hydrisalic®

[OTC]; Ionil Plus® [OTC]; Ionil® [OTC]; Keralyt®; Keralyt® [OTC]; LupiCare® Dandruff [OTC]; LupiCare® Psoriasis [OTC]; MG217® Sal-Acid [OTC]; Mosco® Callus & Corn Remover [OTC]; Mosco® One Step Corn Remover [OTC]; Neutrogena® Acne Stress Control [OTC]; Neutrogena® Advanced Solutions™ [OTC]; Neutrogena® Blackhead Eliminating™ 2-in-1 Foaming Pads [OTC]; Neutrogena® Blackhead Eliminating™ Daily Scrub [OTC]; Neutrogena® Blackhead Elinimating™ [OTC]; Neutrogena® Body Clear® [OTC]; Neutrogena® Clear Pore™ Oil-Controlling Astringent [OTC]; Neutrogena® Maximum Strength T/Sal® [OTC]; Neutrogena® Oil-Free Acne Stress Control [OTC]; Neutrogena® Oil-Free Acne Wash 60 Second Mask Scrub [OTC]; Neutrogena® Oil-Free Acne Wash Cream Cleanser [OTC]; Neutrogena® Oil-Free Acne Wash Foam Cleanser [OTC]; Neutrogena® Oil-Free Acne Wash [OTC]; Neutrogena® Oil-Free Acne [OTC]; Neutrogena® Oil-Free Anti-Acne [OTC]; Neutrogena® Rapid Clear® Acne Defense [OTC]; Neutrogena® Rapid Clear® Acne Eliminating [OTC]; Neutrogena® Rapid Clear® [OTC]; OXY® Body Wash [OTC]; OXY® Chill Factor® [OTC]; OXY® Daily Cleansing [OTC]; OXY® Daily [OTC]; OXY® Face Wash [OTC]; OXY® Maximum Daily Cleansing [OTC]; OXY® Maximum [OTC]; OXY® Post-Shave [OTC]; OXY® Spot Treatment [OTC]; OXY® [OTC]; P&S® [OTC]; Palmer's® Skin Success Acne Cleanser [OTC]; Sal-Plant® [OTC]; Salactic® [OTC]; Salex®; Salitop™; Salvax; Scalpicin® Anti-Itch [OTC]; Stridex® Essential Care® [OTC]; Stridex® Facewipes To Go® [OTC]; Stridex® Maximum Strength [OTC]; Stridex® Sensitive Skin [OTC]; Thera-Sal [OTC]; Tinamed® Corn and Callus Remover [OTC]; Tinamed® Wart Remover [OTC]; Trans-Ver-Sal® [OTC]; Wart-Off® Maximum Strength [OTC]; Zapzyt® Acne Wash [OTC]; Zapzyt® Pore Treatment [OTC]

Brand Names: Canada Duofilm®; Duoforte® 27; Occlusal™-HP; Sebcur®; Soluver®; Soluver® Plus; Trans-Plantar®; Trans-Ver-Sal®

Generic Availability (U.S.) Yes: Aerosol, Bar, Cream, gel, lotion, shampoo, soap

Pharmacologic Category Acne Products; Keratolytic Agent; Topical Skin Product, Acne

Use Topically for its keratolytic effect in controlling seborrheic dermatitis or psoriasis of body and scalp, dandruff, and other scaling dermatoses; also used to remove warts, corns, and calluses; acne

Contraindications Hypersensitivity to salicylic acid or any component of the formulation

Warnings/Precautions Prior to OTC use, consult with healthcare provider if you have diabetes or poor circulation. Not for application to areas that are irritated, infected, reddened, birthmarks, genital or facial warts, or mucous membranes. Avoid contact with eyes.

Adverse Reactions (Reflective of adult population; not specific for elderly) Frequency not defined.

Central nervous system: Dizziness, headache, mental confusion

Local: Burning and irritation at site of exposure on normal tissue, peeling, scaling

Otic: Tinnitus

Respiratory: Hyperventilation

Drug Interactions

Avoid Concomitant Use There are no known interactions where it is recommended to avoid concomitant use.

Increased Effect/Toxicity There are no known significant interactions involving an increase in effect.

Decreased Effect There are no known significant interactions involving a decrease in effect.

Mechanism of Action Produces desquamation of hyperkeratotic epithelium via dissolution of the intercellular cement which causes the cornified tissue to swell, soften, macerate, and desquamate. Salicylic acid is keratolytic at concentrations of 3% to 6%; it becomes destructive to tissue at concentrations >6%. Concentrations of 6% to 60% are used to remove corns and warts and in the treatment of psoriasis and other hyperkeratotic disorders.

Pharmacodynamics/Kinetics

Absorption: Absorbed percutaneously, but systemic toxicity is unlikely with normal use

Time to peak serum concentration: Topical: Within 5 hours of application with occlusion

Elimination: Salicyluric acid (52%), salicylate glucuronides (42%), and salicylic acid (6%) are major metabolites identified in urine after percutaneous absorption

Dosage

Geriatric & Adult

Acne: Topical:

Cream, cloth, foam, or liquid cleansers (2%): Use to cleanse skin once or twice daily. Massage gently into skin, work into lather and rinse thoroughly. Cloths should be wet with water prior to using and disposed of (not flushed) after use.

Gel (0.5% or 2%): Apply small amount to face in the morning or evening; if peeling occurs, may be used every other day. Some products may be labeled for OTC use up to 3 or 4 times per day. Apply to clean, dry skin

Pads (0.5% or 2%): Use pad to cover affected area with thin layer of salicylic acid 1-3 times/day. Apply to clean, dry skin. Do not leave pad on skin.

◀

Patch (2%): At bedtime, after washing face, allow skin to dry at least 5 minutes. Apply patch directly over pimple being treated. Remove in the morning.

Shower/bath gels or soap (2%): Use once daily in shower or bath to massage over skin prone to acne. Rinse well.

Callus, corns, or warts: Topical:

Foam: Apply to affected area twice daily; rub into skin until completely absorbed.

Gel or liquid (17%): Apply to each wart and allow to dry. May repeat once or twice daily, up to 12 weeks. Apply to clean dry area.

Gel (6%): Apply to affected area once daily, generally used at night and rinsed off in the morning.

Transdermal patch (15%): Apply directly over affected area at bedtime, leave in place overnight and remove in the morning. Patch should be trimmed to cover affected area. May repeat daily for up to 12 weeks.

Transdermal patch (40%): Apply directly over affected area, leave in place for 48 hours. Some products may be cut to fit area or secured with adhesive strips. May repeat procedure for up to 12 weeks. Apply to clean, dry skin

Dandruff, psoriasis, or seborrheic dermatitis: Topical:

Cream (2.5%): Apply to affected area 3-4 times daily. Apply to clean, dry skin. Some products may be left in place overnight.

Foam: Apply to affected area twice daily; rub into skin until completely absorbed.

Ointment (3%): Apply to scales or plaques on skin up to 4 times per day (not for scalp or face)

Shampoo (1.8% to 3%): Massage into wet hair or affected area; leave in place for several minutes; rinse thoroughly. Labeled for OTC use 2-3 times a week, or as directed by healthcare provider. Some products may be left in place overnight.

Administration For warts: Before applying product, soak area in warm water for 5 minutes; dry area thoroughly, then apply medication

Special Geriatric Considerations No specific considerations are needed if used according to recommended doses and duration of use. Many elderly may have diabetes or impaired circulation and avoidance of topical salicylic acid would be advised.

Dosage Forms Excipient information presented when available (limited, particularly for generics); consult specific product labeling.

Aerosol, topical [foam]: 6% (70 g)
  Salvax: 6% (70 g, 200 g) [ethanol free]
Bar, topical [soap]: 2% (113 g)
  OXY®: 0.5% (119 g)
Cloth, topical:
  Neutrogena® Oil-Free Acne Wash: 2% (30s)
Cream, topical: 6% (400 g)
  Clean & Clear® Advantage® Acne Cleanser: 2% (148 mL)
  Clean & Clear® Advantage® Acne Spot Treatment: 2% (22 g) [contains benzalkonium chloride, ethanol 14%]
  Clean & Clear® Blackhead Clearing Scrub: 2% (141 g, 226 g) [contains ethanol]
  Clean & Clear® Dual Action Moisturizer: 0.5% (120 mL) [contains ethanol]
  LupiCare® Psoriasis: 2% (227 g)
  Neutrogena® Acne Stress Control: 2% (125 g) [with microbeads]
  Neutrogena® Oil-Free Acne: 2% (125 mL) [contains ethanol, tartrazine; with microbeads]
  Neutrogena® Oil-Free Acne Wash Cream Cleanser: 2% (200 mL) [contains ethanol]
  Neutrogena® Oil-Free Anti-Acne: 0.5% (50 g) [contains aloe]
  Salex®: 6% (454 g)
  Salitop™: 6% (400 g) [contains ethanol]
Cream, topical [wash]:
  Neutrogena® Oil-Free Acne Stress Control: 2% (172 g)
Gel, topical:
  Clean & Clear® Advantage® Invisible Acne Patch: 2% (1.9 mL) [contains ethanol]
  Clean & Clear® Invisible Blemish Treatment: 2% (22 mL) [contains ethanol 28%]
  Compound W®: 17.6% (7 g) [contains ethanol 67.5%]
  Dermarest® Psoriasis Medicated Scalp Treatment: 3% (118 mL)
  Dermarest® Psoriasis Medicated Skin Treatment: 3% (118 mL)
  Dermarest® Psoriasis Overnight Treatment: 3% (56.7 g)
  Hydrisalic®: 6% (28 g) [contains ethanol]
  Keralyt®: 3% (30 g); 6% (40 g, 100 g) [contains ethanol 21%]
  Neutrogena® Oil-Free Acne Wash: 2% (177 mL, 296 mL) [contains tartrazine]
  Neutrogena® Rapid Clear® Acne Eliminating: 2% (15 mL) [contains ethanol 38%]
  OXY®: 2% (355 mL) [contains aloe]
  OXY® Body Wash: 2% (355 mL)
  OXY® Body Wash: 2% (355 mL) [contains aloe]
  OXY® Chill Factor®: 2% (142 g)

OXY® Face Wash: 2% (177 mL) [contains aloe]
OXY® Maximum: 2% (142 g)
OXY® Spot Treatment: 1% (14.7 g) [contains aloe]
Sal-Plant®: 17% (14 g) [contains isopropyl alcohol]
Zapzyt® Acne Wash: 2% (188.5 g) [ethanol free]
Zapzyt® Pore Treatment: 2% (22 mL) [ethanol free]
Gel, topical [peel]:
Neutrogena® Advanced Solutions™: 2% (40 g)
Liquid, topical:
Clean & Clear® Advantage® Oil-Free Acne: 0.5% (120 mL) [contains benzalkonium chloride]
Clean & Clear® Deep Cleaning: 2% (240 mL) [contains benzoic acid, ethanol]
Compound W®: 17.6% (9 mL) [contains ethanol 21.2%]
Dr. Scholl's® Clear Away® Wart Remover Fast-Acting: 17% (9.8 mL) [contains ethanol 18% w/w; includes 20 cover-up discs]
Dr. Scholl's® Corn/Callus Remover: 12.6% (9.8 mL)
Dr. Scholl's® Corn/Callus Remover: 12.6% (9.8 mL) [contains ethanol 18% w/w]
DuoFilm®: 17% (9.8 mL) [contains ethanol]
Durasal™: 26% (10 mL) [contains isopropyl alcohol]
Freezone®: 17.6% (9.3 mL) [contains ethanol]
Fung-O®: 17% (15 mL) [contains ethanol 2%]
Gets-It®: 13.9% (15 mL)
Gordofilm: 16.7% (15 mL)
Mosco® Callus & Corn Remover: 17.6% (9 mL) [contains ethanol 27%]
Neutrogena® Blackhead Eliminating™ Daily Scrub: 2% (125 mL)
Neutrogena® Clear Pore™ Oil-Controlling Astringent: 2% (236 mL) [contains ethanol 45%]
Neutrogena® Oil-Free Acne Stress Control: 2% (50 mL)
Palmer's® Skin Success Acne Cleanser: 0.5% (240 mL) [contains aloe, vitamin E]
Salactic®: 17% (15 mL) [contains isopropyl alcohol]
Scalpicin® Anti-Itch: 3% (44 mL, 74 mL) [contains aloe]
Tinamed® Corn and Callus Remover: 17% (15 mL)
Tinamed® Wart Remover: 17% (15 mL)
Wart-Off® Maximum Strength: 17.5% (14.8 mL) [contains ethanol]
Liquid, topical [body scrub with microbeads]:
Neutrogena® Body Clear®: 2% (250 mL) [contains tartrazine]
Liquid, topical [body wash]:
Neutrogena® Body Clear®: 2% (250 mL) [contains tartrazine]
Liquid, topical [foam]:
Neutrogena® Oil-Free Acne Wash Foam Cleanser: 2% (150 mL)
Liquid, topical [foam/wash]:
Clean & Clear® Continuous Control® Acne Wash: 2% (177 mL)
Neutrogena® Oil-Free Acne Stress Control: 0.5% (177 mL)
Liquid, topical [mask/wash]:
Neutrogena® Oil-Free Acne Wash 60 Second Mask Scrub: 1% (170 g) [ethanol free]
Lotion, topical: 6% (414 mL)
Dermarest® Psoriasis Medicated Moisturizer: 2% (118 mL)
Neutrogena® Rapid Clear® Acne Defense: 2% (50 mL) [contains ethanol]
OXY® Post-Shave: 0.5% (50 g) [contains aloe]
Salex®: 6% (237 mL)
Salitop™: 6% (414 mL) [contains ethanol]
Ointment, topical:
MG217® Sal-Acid: 3% (57 g) [contains vitamin E]
Pad, topical:
Clean & Clear® Blackhead Clearing Daily Cleansing: 1% (70s) [contains ethanol 39%]
Curad® Mediplast®: 40% (25s)
Neutrogena® Blackhead Eliminating™ 2-in-1 Foaming Pads: 0.5% (28s)
Neutrogena® Blackhead Elinimating™: 0.5% (28s)
Neutrogena® Rapid Clear®: 2% (60s) [contains benzalkonium chloride, ethanol 35%]
OXY® Chill Factor®: 2% (90s) [contains ethanol 46% v/v]
OXY® Daily: 0.2% (90s) [contains ethanol 46% v/v]
OXY® Daily Cleansing: 0.5% (90s) [contains ethanol 34% v/v]
OXY® Maximum Daily Cleansing: 2% (55s, 90s) [contains ethanol 46% v/v]
Stridex® Essential Care®: 1% (55s) [ethanol free; contains vitamin A, vitamin E]
Stridex® Facewipes To Go®: 0.5% (32s) [contains aloe, ethanol 28%]
Stridex® Maximum Strength: 2% (55s, 90s) [ethanol free]
Stridex® Sensitive Skin: 0.5% (55s, 90s) [ethanol free]

Patch, topical:
  Compound W® One Step Invisible Strip: 14% (14s)
  Compound W® One Step Wart Remover for Feet: 40% (20s)
  Compound W® One-Step Wart Remover: 40% (14s)
  Compound W® One-Step Wart Remover for Kids: 40% (12s)
  Dr. Scholl's® Callus Removers: 40% (4s)
  Dr. Scholl's® Callus Removers: 40% (4s) [includes 6 cushions]
  Dr. Scholl's® Clear Away® One Step Wart Remover: 40% (14s)
  Dr. Scholl's® Clear Away® Plantar Wart Remover For Feet: 40% (24s)
  Dr. Scholl's® Clear Away® Wart Remover: 40% (18s)
  Dr. Scholl's® Clear Away® Wart Remover Invisible Strips: 40% (18s)
  Dr. Scholl's® Corn Removers: 40% (9s)
  Dr. Scholl's® Corn Removers: 40% (9s) [includes 9 cushions]
  Dr. Scholl's® Extra Thick Corn Removers: 40% (9s)
  Dr. Scholl's® Extra-Thick Callus Removers: 40% (4s)
  Dr. Scholl's® Extra-Thick Callus Removers: 40% (4s) [includes 4 cushions]
  Dr. Scholl's® For Her Corn Removers: 40% (6s) [includes 6 cushions]
  Dr. Scholl's® OneStep Callus Removers: 40% (4s)
  Dr. Scholl's® OneStep Corn Removers: 40% (6s)
  Dr. Scholl's® Small Corn Removers: 40% (9s)
  Dr. Scholl's® Ultra-Thin Corn Removers: 40% (9s) [includes 9 covers]
  Mosco® One Step Corn Remover: 40% (8s)
  Trans-Ver-Sal®: 15% (10s, 25s) [20 mm PlantarPatch]
  Trans-Ver-Sal®: 15% (15s, 40s) [contains propylene glycol]
  Trans-Ver-Sal®: 15% (12s, 40s) [contains propylene glycol; 12 mm AdultPatch]
Shampoo, topical: 6% (177 mL)
  Aliclen™: 6% (177 mL)
  Beta Sal®: 3% (480 mL)
  Denorex® Extra Strength Protection: 3% (118 mL, 355 mL)
  DHS™ Sal: 3% (120 mL)
  Ionil Plus®: 2% (240 mL) [conditioning shampoo]
  Ionil®: 2% (120 mL)
  LupiCare® Dandruff: 2% (237 mL)
  LupiCare® Psoriasis: 2% (237 mL)
  Neutrogena® Maximum Strength T/Sal®: 3% (135 mL)
  P&S®: 2% (118 mL, 236 mL)
  Salex®: 6% (177 mL)
  Thera-Sal: 3% (180 mL)
Shampoo/Conditioner, topical:
  Denorex® Extra Strength Protection 2-in-1: 3% (118 mL, 355 mL)
  Dermarest® Psoriasis Medicated Shampoo/Conditioner: 3% (236 mL)

- ◆ **Salicylsalicylic Acid** *see* Salsalate *on page 1656*
- ◆ **Saline** *see* Sodium Chloride *on page 1690*
- ◆ **Saline Mist [OTC]** *see* Sodium Chloride *on page 1690*
- ◆ **Salitop™** *see* Salicylic Acid *on page 1648*

Saliva Substitute (sa LYE va SUB stee tute)

Brand Names: U.S. Aquoral™; Caphosol®; Entertainer's Secret® [OTC]; Moi-Stir® [OTC]; Mouthkote® [OTC]; Numoisyn™; Oasis®; Oral Balance® [OTC]; SalivaSure™ [OTC]
Index Terms Artificial Saliva
Generic Availability (U.S.) No
Pharmacologic Category Gastrointestinal Agent, Miscellaneous
Use Relief of dry mouth and throat in xerostomia or hyposalivation; adjunct to standard oral care in relief of symptoms associated with chemotherapy or radiation therapy-induced mucositis
Dosage
  Geriatric & Adult
    Mucositis (due to high-dose chemotherapy or radiation therapy): Caphosol®: Swish and spit 4-10 doses per day beginning at onset of chemo- or radiation therapy
    Xerostomia: Oral: Use as needed, or product-specific dosing:
      Caphosol®: Swish and spit 2-10 doses per day
      Numoisyn™ liquid: Use 2 mL as needed
      Numoisyn™ lozenges: Dissolve 1 lozenge in mouth as needed; maximum 16 lozenges/day
      Oasis® mouthwash: Rinse mouth with ~30 mL twice daily or as needed; do not swallow

Oasis® spray: 1-2 sprays as needed; maximum 60 sprays/day

Oral Balance®: Use after meals, at bedtime, and as needed

Special Geriatric Considerations Saliva production has not been shown to change with aging, however, many drugs used by elderly can cause dry mouth. These patients may benefit from a saliva substitute.

Dosage Forms Excipient information presented when available (limited, particularly for generics); consult specific product labeling.

Liquid:

Numoisyn™: Water, sorbitol, linseed extract, *Chondrus crispus*, methylparaben, sodium benzoate, potassium sorbate, dipotassium phosphate, propylparaben (300 mL)

Oral Balance®: Water, starch, sunflower oil, propylene glycol, xylitol, glycerine, purified milk extract (45 mL) [sugar-free]

Lozenge:

Numoisyn™: Sorbitol 0.3 g/lozenge, polyethylene glycol, malic acid, sodium citrate, calcium phosphate dibasic, hydrogenated cottonseed oil, citric acid, magnesium stearate, silicon dioxide (100s)

SalivaSure™: Xylitol, citric acid, apple acid, sodium citrate dihydrate, sodium carboxyme-thylcellulose, dibasic calcium phosphate, silica colloidal, magnesium stearate, stearic acid (90s)

Solution, oral:

Caphosol®: Dibasic sodium phosphate 0.032%, monobasic sodium phosphate 0.009%, calcium chloride 0.052%, sodium chloride 0.569%, purified water (30 mL) [packaged in two 15 mL ampuls when mixed together provide one 30 mL dose]

Entertainer's Secret®: Sodium carboxymethylcellulose, aloe vera gel, glycerin (60 mL) [ethanol free; honey-apple flavor]

Solution, oral [mouthwash/gargle]:

Oasis®: Water, glycerin, sorbitol, poloxamer 338, PEG-60, hydrogenated castor oil, copo-vidone, sodium benzoate, carboxymethycellulose (473 mL) [ethanol free, sugar free; mild mint flavor]

Solution, oral [spray]:

Aquoral™: Oxidized glycerol triesters and silicon dioxide (40 mL) [contains aspartame; delivers 400 sprays, citrus flavor]

Moi-Stir®: Water, sorbitol, sodium carboxymethylcellulose, methylparaben, propylparaben, potassium chloride, dibasic sodium phosphate, calcium chloride, magnesium chloride, sodium chloride (120 mL)

Mouthkote®: Water, xylitol, sorbitol, yerba santa, citric acid, ascorbic acid, sodium saccharin, sodium benzoate (5 mL, 60 mL, 240 mL) [ethanol free, sugar free; lemon-lime flavor]

Oasis®: Glycerin, cetylpyridinium, copovidone (30 mL) [ethanol free, sugar free; contains sodium benzoate; delivers ~150 sprays, mild mint flavor]

◆ SalivaSure™ [OTC] *see* Saliva Substitute *on page 1652*
◆ Salk Vaccine *see* Poliovirus Vaccine (Inactivated) *on page 1477*

Salmeterol (sal ME te role)

Related Information

Inhalant Agents *on page 2010*

Medication Safety Issues

Sound-alike/look-alike issues:

Salmeterol may be confused with Salbutamol, Solu-Medrol®

Serevent® may be confused with Atrovent®, Combivent®, Serentil®, sertraline, Sinemet®, Spiriva®, Zoloft®

Brand Names: U.S. Serevent® Diskus®

Brand Names: Canada Serevent® Diskhaler® Disk; Serevent® Diskus®

Index Terms Salmeterol Xinafoate

Generic Availability (U.S.) No

Pharmacologic Category Beta$_2$-Adrenergic Agonist; Beta$_2$-Adrenergic Agonist, Long-Acting

Use Maintenance treatment of asthma and prevention of bronchospasm (as concomitant therapy) in patients with reversible obstructive airway disease, including patients with symptoms of nocturnal asthma; prevention of exercise-induced bronchospasm (monotherapy may be indicated in patients without persistent asthma); maintenance treatment of broncho-spasm associated with COPD

Medication Guide Available Yes

Contraindications Hypersensitivity to salmeterol or any component of the formulation (milk proteins); monotherapy in the treatment of asthma (ie, use without a concomitant long-term asthma control medication, such as an inhaled corticosteroid); status asthmaticus or other acute episodes of asthma or COPD

◀ **Warnings/Precautions**

Asthma treatment: [U.S. Boxed Warning]: **Long-acting beta₂-agonists (LABAs) increase the risk of asthma-related deaths. Salmeterol should only be used in asthma patients as adjuvant therapy in patients who are currently receiving but are not adequately controlled on a long-term asthma control medication (ie, an inhaled corticosteroid).** Monotherapy with an LABA is contraindicated in the treatment of asthma. In a large, randomized, placebo-controlled U.S. clinical trial (SMART, 2006), salmeterol was associated with an increase in asthma-related deaths (when added to usual asthma therapy); risk is considered a class effect among all LABAs. Data are not available to determine if the addition of an inhaled corticosteroid lessens this increased risk of death associated with LABA use. Assess patients at regular intervals once asthma control is maintained on combination therapy to determine if step-down therapy is appropriate and the LABA can be discontinued (without loss of asthma control), and the patient can be maintained on an inhaled corticosteroid. LABAs are not appropriate in patients whose asthma is adequately controlled on low- or medium-dose inhaled corticosteroids. Do **not** use for acute bronchospasm. Short-acting beta₂-agonist (eg, albuterol) should be used for acute symptoms and symptoms occurring between treatments. Do **not** initiate in patients with significantly worsening or acutely deteriorating asthma; reports of severe (sometimes fatal) respiratory events have been reported when salmeterol has been initiated in this situation. Corticosteroids should not be stopped or reduced when salmeterol is initiated. During initiation, watch for signs of worsening asthma. Patients must be instructed to use short-acting beta₂-agonists (eg, albuterol) for acute asthmatic or COPD symptoms and to seek medical attention in cases where acute symptoms are not relieved or a previous level of response is diminished. The need to increase frequency of use of short-acting beta₂-agonist may indicate deterioration of asthma, and treatment must not be delayed. Because LABAs may disguise poorly controlled persistent asthma, frequent or chronic use of LABAs for exercise-induced bronchospasm is discouraged by the NIH Asthma Guidelines (NIH, 2007). Salmeterol should not be used more than twice daily; do not use with other long-acting beta₂-agonists.

COPD treatment: Appropriate use: Do **not** use for acute episodes of COPD. Do **not** initiate in patients with significantly worsening or acutely deteriorating COPD. Data are not available to determine if LABA use increases the risk of death in patients with COPD.

Concurrent diseases: Use caution in patients with cardiovascular disease (eg, arrhythmia, hypertension, or HF), seizure disorders, diabetes, hyperthyroidism, hepatic impairment, or hypokalemia. Beta-agonists may cause elevation in blood pressure, heart rate, CNS stimulation/excitation, increased risk of arrhythmia, increase serum glucose, or decrease serum potassium.

Adverse events: Immediate hypersensitivity reactions (urticaria, angioedema, rash, bronchospasm) have been reported. There have been reports of laryngeal spasm, irritation, swelling (stridor, choking) with use. Salmeterol should not be used more than twice daily; do not exceed recommended dose; do not use with other long-acting beta₂-agonists; serious adverse events have been associated with excessive use of inhaled sympathomimetics. Rarely, paradoxical bronchospasm may occur with use of inhaled bronchodilating agents; this should be distinguished from inadequate response. Use with strong CYP3A4 inhibitors (see Drug Interactions) is not recommended due to potential for an increased risk of cardiovascular events. Powder for oral inhalation contains lactose; very rare anaphylactic reactions have been reported in patients with severe milk protein allergy.

Adverse Reactions (Reflective of adult population; not specific for elderly)

>10%:
  Central nervous system: Headache (13% to 17%)
  Neuromuscular & skeletal: Pain (1% to 12%)
1% to 10%:
  Cardiovascular: Hypertension (4%), edema (1% to 3%), pallor
  Central nervous system: Dizziness (4%), sleep disturbance (1% to 3%), fever (1% to 3%), anxiety (1% to 3%), migraine (1% to 3%)
  Dermatologic: Rash (1% to 4%), contact dermatitis (1% to 3%), eczema (1% to 3%), urticaria (3%), photodermatitis (1% to 2%)
  Endocrine & metabolic: Hyperglycemia (1% to 3%)
  Gastrointestinal: Throat irritation (7%), nausea (1% to 3%), dyspepsia (1% to 3%), dental pain (1% to 3%), gastrointestinal infection (1% to 3%), oropharyngeal candidiasis (1% to 3%), xerostomia (1% to 3%)
  Hepatic: Liver enzymes increased
  Neuromuscular & skeletal: Muscular cramps/spasm (3%), articular rheumatism (1% to 3%), arthralgia (1% to 3%), joint pain (1% to 3%), muscular stiffness (1% to 3%), paresthesia (1% to 3%), rigidity (1% to 3%)

Ocular: Keratitis/conjunctivitis (1% to 3%)

Respiratory: Nasal congestion (4% to 9%), tracheitis/bronchitis (7%), pharyngitis (≤6%), cough (5%), influenza (5%), viral respiratory tract infection (5%), sinusitis (4% to 5%), rhinitis (4% to 5%), asthma (3% to 4%)

Drug Interactions

Metabolism/Transport Effects Substrate of CYP3A4 (major)

Avoid Concomitant Use

Avoid concomitant use of Salmeterol with any of the following: CYP3A4 Inhibitors (Strong); Iobenguane I 123; Telaprevir

Increased Effect/Toxicity

Salmeterol may increase the levels/effects of: Loop Diuretics; Sympathomimetics

The levels/effects of Salmeterol may be increased by: Atomoxetine; Cannabinoids; CYP3A4 Inhibitors (Moderate); CYP3A4 Inhibitors (Strong); MAO Inhibitors; Telaprevir; Tricyclic Antidepressants

Decreased Effect

Salmeterol may decrease the levels/effects of: Iobenguane I 123

The levels/effects of Salmeterol may be decreased by: Alpha-/Beta-Blockers; Beta-Blockers (Beta1 Selective); Beta-Blockers (Nonselective); Betahistine

Stability Inhalation powder: Store at controlled room temperature 20°C to 25°C (68°F to 77°F) in a dry place away from direct heat or sunlight. Stable for 6 weeks after removal from foil pouch.

Mechanism of Action Relaxes bronchial smooth muscle by selective action on beta$_2$-receptors with little effect on heart rate; salmeterol acts locally in the lung.

Pharmacodynamics/Kinetics

Onset of action: Asthma: 30-48 minutes, COPD: 2 hours

Peak effect: Asthma: 3 hours, COPD: 2-5 hours

Duration: 12 hours

Absorption: Systemic: Inhalation: Undetectable to poor

Protein binding: 96%

Metabolism: Hepatic; hydroxylated via CYP3A4

Half-life elimination: 5.5 hours

Time to peak, serum: ~20 minutes

Excretion: Feces (60%); urine (25%)

Dosage

Geriatric & Adult

Asthma, maintenance and prevention: Inhalation, powder (50 mcg/inhalation): One inhalation twice daily (~12 hours apart); maximum: 1 inhalation twice daily. **Note:** For asthma control, long acting beta$_2$-agonists (LABAs) should be used in combination with inhaled corticosteroids and not as monotherapy.

Exercise-induced asthma, prevention: Inhalation, powder (50 mcg/inhalation): One inhalation at least 30 minutes prior to exercise; additional doses should not be used for 12 hours; should not be used in individuals already receiving salmeterol twice daily. **Note:** Because LABAs may disguise poorly controlled persistent asthma, frequent or chronic use of LABAs for exercise-induced bronchospasm is discouraged by the NIH Asthma Guidelines (NIH, 2007).

COPD maintenance: Inhalation, powder (50 mcg/inhalation): One inhalation twice daily (~12 hours apart); maximum: 1 inhalation twice daily

Hepatic Impairment No dosage adjustment required; manufacturer suggests close monitoring of patients with hepatic impairment.

Administration Inhalation: **Not** to be used for the relief of acute attacks. Not for use with a spacer device. Administer with Diskus® in a level, horizontal position. Do not wash mouthpiece; Diskus® should be kept dry. Discard device 6 weeks after removal from foil pouch or when the dose counter reads "0" (whichever comes first).

Monitoring Parameters FEV$_1$, peak flow, and/or other pulmonary function tests; blood pressure, heart rate; CNS stimulation. Monitor for increased use of short-acting beta$_2$-agonist inhalers; may be marker of a deteriorating asthma condition.

Special Geriatric Considerations Geriatric patients were included in four clinical studies of salmeterol; no apparent differences in efficacy and safety were noted in geriatric patients compared to younger adults. Because salmeterol is only to be used for prevention of bronchospasm, patients also need a short-acting beta-agonist to treat acute attacks. Elderly patients should be carefully counseled about which inhaler to use and the proper scheduling of doses.

Dosage Forms Excipient information presented when available (limited, particularly for generics); consult specific product labeling.

Powder, for oral inhalation:

Serevent® Diskus®: 50 mcg (28s, 60s) [contains lactose]

◀ **Dosage Forms: Canada** Excipient information presented when available (limited, particularly for generics); consult specific product labeling.
Powder for oral inhalation:
Serevent® Diskhaler® Disk: Salmeterol xinafoate 50 mcg (60s) [delivers 50 mcg/inhalation; contains lactose]

Selected References
National Asthma Education and Prevention Program, "Expert Panel Report 3 (EPR-3): Guidelines for the Diagnosis and Management of Asthma-Summary Report 2007," *J Allergy Clin Immunol*, 2007, 120(5 Suppl):94-138.
Nelson HS, Weiss ST, Bleecker ER, et al, "The Salmeterol Multicenter Asthma Research Trial: A Comparison of Usual Pharmacotherapy for Asthma or Usual Pharmacotherapy Plus Salmeterol," *Chest*, 2006, 129(1):15-26.

◆ **Salmeterol and Fluticasone** *see* Fluticasone and Salmeterol *on page* 772
◆ **Salmeterol Xinafoate** *see* Salmeterol *on page* 1653
◆ **Salonpas® Hot [OTC]** *see* Capsaicin *on page* 261
◆ **Sal-Plant® [OTC]** *see* Salicylic Acid *on page* 1648

Salsalate (SAL sa late)

Medication Safety Issues
Sound-alike/look-alike issues:
Salsalate may be confused with sucralfate, sulfaSALAzine
Brand Names: Canada Amigesic®; Salflex®
Index Terms Disalicylic Acid; Salicylsalicylic Acid
Generic Availability (U.S.) Yes
Pharmacologic Category Salicylate
Use Treatment of rheumatoid arthritis, osteoarthritis, and related rheumatic disorders
Contraindications Hypersensitivity to salsalate or any component of the formulation; GI ulcer or bleeding
Warnings/Precautions Use with caution in patients with platelet and bleeding disorders, dehydration, renal dysfunction, erosive gastritis, or peptic ulcer disease; patients with sensitivity to tartrazine dyes, nasal polyps, and asthma may have an increased risk of salicylate sensitivity, previous nonreaction does not guarantee future safe taking of medication.
Adverse Reactions (Reflective of adult population; not specific for elderly) Frequency not defined.
Cardiovascular: Hypotension
Central nervous system: Vertigo
Dermatologic: Angioedema, rash, Stevens-Johnson syndrome, toxic epidermal necrolysis, urticaria
Gastrointestinal: Abdominal pain, diarrhea, GI bleeding, GI perforation, GI ulceration, nausea
Hematologic: Anemia
Hepatic: Hepatitis, liver function abnormal
Otic: Hearing impairment, tinnitus
Renal: Creatinine clearance decreased, nephritis
Respiratory: Bronchospasm
Miscellaneous: Anaphylactic shock

Drug Interactions
Avoid Concomitant Use
Avoid concomitant use of Salsalate with any of the following: Influenza Virus Vaccine (Live/Attenuated)
Increased Effect/Toxicity
Salsalate may increase the levels/effects of: Anticoagulants; Carbonic Anhydrase Inhibitors; Corticosteroids (Systemic); Divalproex; Drotrecogin Alfa; Methotrexate; PRALAtrexate; Salicylates; Sulfonylureas; Thrombolytic Agents; Valproic Acid; Varicella Virus-Containing Vaccines

The levels/effects of Salsalate may be increased by: Antiplatelet Agents; Calcium Channel Blockers (Nondihydropyridine); Ginkgo Biloba; Herbs (Anticoagulant/Antiplatelet Properties); Influenza Virus Vaccine (Live/Attenuated); Loop Diuretics; NSAID (Nonselective); Treprostinil
Decreased Effect
Salsalate may decrease the levels/effects of: ACE Inhibitors; Loop Diuretics; NSAID (Nonselective); Probenecid

The levels/effects of Salsalate may be decreased by: Corticosteroids (Systemic); NSAID (Nonselective)

Ethanol/Nutrition/Herb Interactions

Ethanol: Avoid ethanol (may enhance gastric mucosal irritation).

Food: Salsalate peak serum levels may be delayed if taken with food.

Herb/Nutraceutical: Avoid cat's claw, dong quai, evening primrose, feverfew, garlic, ginger, ginkgo, red clover, horse chestnut, green tea, ginseng (all have additional antiplatelet activity).

Mechanism of Action Weakly inhibits cyclooxygenase enzymes, which results in decreased formation of prostaglandin precursors; has antipyretic, analgesic, and anti-inflammatory properties

Other proposed mechanisms not fully elucidated (and possibly contributing to the anti-inflammatory effect to varying degrees) include inhibiting chemotaxis, altering lymphocyte activity, inhibiting neutrophil aggregation/activation, and decreasing proinflammatory cytokine levels.

Pharmacodynamics/Kinetics

Onset of action: Therapeutic: 3-4 days of continuous dosing

Absorption: Complete from small intestine

Metabolism: Hepatically hydrolyzed to two moles of salicylic acid (active)

Half-life elimination: 7-8 hours

Excretion: Primarily urine

Dosage

Geriatric Refer to adult dosing. May require lower dosage.

Adult Pain, inflammation (arthritis): Oral: 3 g/day in 2-3 divided doses

Administration May be administered with food to decrease GI distress.

Monitoring Parameters Serum concentrations, renal function; hearing changes or tinnitus; monitor for response (ie, pain, inflammation, range of motion, grip strength); observe for abnormal bleeding, bruising, weight gain

Test Interactions False-negative results for glucose oxidase urinary glucose tests (Clinistix®); false-positives using the cupric sulfate method (Clinitest®); also, interferes with Gerhardt test, VMA determination; 5-HIAA, xylose tolerance test and T_3 and T_4

Pharmacotherapy Pearls Does not appear to inhibit platelet aggregation; salsalate causes less GI and renal toxicity than aspirin and other NSAIDs

Special Geriatric Considerations Elderly are a high-risk population for adverse effects from NSAIDs. As much as 60% of the elderly can develop peptic ulceration and/or hemorrhage asymptomatically. The concomitant use of H_2 blockers and sucralfate is not effective as prophylaxis with the exception of NSAID-induced duodenal ulcers which may be prevented by the use of ranitidine. Misoprostol and proton pump inhibitors are the only agents proven to help prevent the development of NSAID-induced ulcers. Also, concomitant disease and drug use contribute to the risk for GI adverse effects. Use lowest effective dose for shortest period possible. Consider renal function decline with age. Use of NSAIDs can compromise existing renal function especially when Cl_{cr} is ≤30 mL/minute. Tinnitus may be a difficult and unreliable indication of toxicity due to age-related hearing loss or eighth cranial nerve damage. CNS adverse effects such as confusion, agitation, and hallucinations are generally seen in overdose or high dose situations, but elderly may demonstrate these adverse effects at lower doses than younger adults.

Dosage Forms Excipient information presented when available (limited, particularly for generics); consult specific product labeling.

Tablet, oral: 500 mg, 750 mg

Saxagliptin (sax a GLIP tin)

Related Information
Diabetes Mellitus Management, Adults *on page 2073*

Medication Safety Issues
Sound-alike/look-alike issues:
Saxagliptin may be confused with sitaGLIPtin, SUMAtriptan

Brand Names: U.S. Onglyza™

Brand Names: Canada Onglyza™

Index Terms BMS-477118

Generic Availability (U.S.) No

Pharmacologic Category Antidiabetic Agent, Dipeptidyl Peptidase IV (DPP-IV) Inhibitor

Use Treatment of type 2 diabetes mellitus (noninsulin dependent, NIDDM) as an adjunct to diet and exercise as monotherapy or in combination therapy with other antidiabetic agents to improve glycemic control

Contraindications There are no contraindications listed within the manufacturer's labeling.

Warnings/Precautions Use with caution in patients with moderate-to-severe renal dysfunction, end-stage renal disease (ESRD) requiring hemodialysis, and in patients taking strong CYP3A4/5 inhibitors (eg, atazanavir, clarithromycin, indinavir, itraconazole, nefazodone, nelfinavir, ritonavir, saquinavir, telithromycin [also see Drug Interactions]); dosing adjustment required. Use caution when used in conjunction with insulin secretagogues (eg, sulfonylureas); risk of hypoglycemia is increased. Monitor blood glucose closely; dosage adjustments of the insulin secretagogue may be necessary.

Adverse Reactions (Reflective of adult population; not specific for elderly) Note:
Frequencies and adverse reactions reported with monotherapy unless otherwise noted.
1% to 10%:
Cardiovascular: Peripheral edema (≤4%; incidence increased in conjunction with thiazolidinediones: ≤8%)
Central nervous system: Headache (7%)
Endocrine & metabolic: Hypoglycemia (≤6%; incidence increased in conjunction with insulin secretagogues: ≤15%)
Gastrointestinal: Abdominal pain (2%), gastroenteritis (2%), vomiting (2%)
Genitourinary: Urinary tract infection (7%)
Hematologic: Lymphopenia (≤2%; dose related)
Respiratory: Sinusitis (3%)
Miscellaneous: Hypersensitivity reactions (2%; including urticaria and facial edema)

Drug Interactions

Metabolism/Transport Effects Substrate of CYP3A4 (major), P-glycoprotein

Avoid Concomitant Use There are no known interactions where it is recommended to avoid concomitant use.

Increased Effect/Toxicity
Saxagliptin may increase the levels/effects of: ACE Inhibitors; Hypoglycemic Agents

The levels/effects of Saxagliptin may be increased by: CYP3A4 Inhibitors (Moderate); CYP3A4 Inhibitors (Strong); Dasatinib; Herbs (Hypoglycemic Properties); Pegvisomant; P-Glycoprotein Inhibitors

Decreased Effect
The levels/effects of Saxagliptin may be decreased by: Corticosteroids (Orally Inhaled); Corticosteroids (Systemic); CYP3A4 Inducers; Luteinizing Hormone-Releasing Hormone Analogs; P-Glycoprotein Inducers; Somatropin; Thiazide Diuretics; Tocilizumab

Stability Store at 20°C to 25°C (68°F to 77°F); excursions permitted between 15°C to 30°C (59°F to 86°F).

Mechanism of Action Saxagliptin inhibits dipeptidyl peptidase IV (DPP-IV) enzyme resulting in prolonged active incretin levels. Incretin hormones (eg, glucagon-like peptide-1 [GLP-1] and glucose-dependent insulinotropic polypeptide [GIP]) regulate glucose homeostasis by increasing insulin synthesis and release from pancreatic beta cells and decreasing glucagon secretion from pancreatic alpha cells. Decreased glucagon secretion results in decreased hepatic glucose production. Under normal physiologic circumstances, incretin hormones are released by the intestine throughout the day and levels are increased in response to a meal; incretin hormones are rapidly inactivated by the DPP-IV enzyme.

Pharmacodynamics/Kinetics
Duration: 24 hours
Protein binding: Negligible
Metabolism: Hepatic via CYP3A4/5 to 5-hydroxy saxagliptin (active; ~50% potency of the parent compound)
Half-life elimination: Saxagliptin: 2.5 hours; 5-hydroxy saxagliptin: 3.1 hours

Time to peak, plasma: Saxagliptin: 2 hours; 5-hydroxy saxagliptin: 4 hours

Excretion: Urine (75%, 24% of the total dose as saxagliptin, 36% of the total dose as 5-hydroxy saxagliptin); feces (22%)

Dosage

Geriatric & Adult Type 2 diabetes: Oral: 2.5-5 mg once daily

Concomitant use with strong CYP3A4/5 inhibitors: 2.5 mg once daily

Concomitant use with insulin secretagogues: Reduced dose of the insulin secretagogue (eg, sulfonylurea) may be needed

Renal Impairment Note: Renal function may be estimated using the Cockcroft-Gault formula or the MDRD formula for dosage adjustment purposes.

Cl_{cr} >50 mL/minute: No adjustment required.

Cl_{cr} ≤50 mL/minute: 2.5 mg once daily.

ESRD requiring hemodialysis: 2.5 mg once daily; administer postdialysis.

Peritoneal dialysis: Not studied.

Hepatic Impairment No dosage adjustment required.

Administration May be administered without regard to meals.

Monitoring Parameters Plasma glucose, Hb A_{1c}, renal function

Reference Range

Recommendations for glycemic control in adults with diabetes mellitus (ADA, 2009):

Hb A_{1c}: <7%

Preprandial capillary plasma glucose: 70-130 mg/dL

Peak postprandial capillary blood glucose: <180 mg/dL

Recommendations for glycemic control in older adults with diabetes:

Relatively healthy, cognitively intact, and with a ≥5-year life expectancy: See Adults

Frail, life expectancy <5-years or those for whom the risks of intensive glucose control outweigh the benefits:

Hb A_{1c}: <8% to 9%

Blood pressure: <140/80 mm Hg or <130/80 mm Hg if tolerated

Special Geriatric Considerations Persons up to age 77 years were eligible for clinical trials with saxagliptin; ~15% of subjects were 65 years and older. Intensive glucose control (HbA$_{1c}$ <6.5%) has been linked to increased all-cause and cardiovascular mortality, hypoglycemia requiring assistance, and weight gain in adult type 2 diabetes. How "tightly" to control a geriatric patient's blood glucose needs to be individualized. Such a decision should be based on several factors, including the patient's functional and cognitive status, how well he/she recognizes hypoglycemic or hyperglycemic symptoms, and how to respond to them and other disease states. An HbA$_{1c}$ <7.5% is an acceptable endpoint for a healthy older adult, while <8% is acceptable for frail elderly patients, those with a duration of illness >10 years, or those with comorbid conditions and requiring combination diabetes medications. Patients who are unable to accurately draw up their dose will need assistance, such as prefilled syringes. Initial doses may require considerations for renal function in the elderly with dosing adjusted subsequently based on blood glucose monitoring. For elderly patients with diabetes who are relatively healthy, attaining target goals for aspirin use, blood pressure, lipids, smoking cessation, and diet and exercise may be more important than normalized glycemic control.

Dosage Forms Excipient information presented when available (limited, particularly for generics); consult specific product labeling.

Tablet, oral:

Onglyza™: 2.5 mg, 5 mg

Selected References

Action to Control Cardiovascular Risk in Diabetes Study Group, Gerstein HC, Miller ME, et al, "Effects of Intensive Glucose Lowering in Type 2 Diabetes," *N Engl J Med*, 2008, 358(24):2545-59.

ADVANCE Collaborative Group, Patel A, MacMahon S, et al, "Intensive Blood Glucose Control and Vascular Outcomes in Patients With Type 2 Diabetes," *N Engl J Med*, 2008, 358(24):2560-72.

American Diabetes Association, "Standards of Medical Care in Diabetes – 2011," *Diabetes Care*, 2011, 34(Suppl 1):11-61.

Brown AF, Mangione CM, Saliba D, et al, "Guidelines for Improving the Care of the Older Person With Diabetes Mellitus," *J Am Geriatr Soc*, 2003, 51(5 Suppl Guidelines):265-80.

"VA/DoD Clinical Practice Guideline for the Management of Diabetes Mellitus," 2010. Available at http://www.healthquality.va.gov/Diabetes_Mellitus.asp

Saxagliptin and Metformin (sax a GLIP tin & met FOR min)

Related Information

Diabetes Mellitus Management, Adults *on page 2073*

MetFORMIN *on page 1155*

Saxagliptin *on page 1658*

Medication Safety Issues

Sound-alike/look-alike issues:

Saxagliptin and Metformin may be confused with sitaGLIPtin and Metformin

SAXAGLIPTIN AND METFORMIN

Brand Names: U.S. Kombiglyze™ XR

Index Terms Metformin and Saxagliptin; Metformin Hydrochloride and Saxagliptin; Saxagliptin and Metformin Hydrochloride

Pharmacologic Category Antidiabetic Agent, Biguanide; Antidiabetic Agent, Dipeptidyl Peptidase IV (DPP-IV) Inhibitor

Use Management of type 2 diabetes mellitus (noninsulin dependent, NIDDM) as an adjunct to diet and exercise when treatment with both saxagliptin and metformin is appropriate

Dosage

Geriatric Refer to adult dosing. The initial and maintenance dosing should be conservative, due to the potential for decreased renal function (monitor). Do not use in patients ≥80 years of age unless normal renal function has been established.

Adult Note: Patients receiving concomitant insulin secretagogues (eg, sulfonylureas) may require dosage adjustments of these agents.

Type 2 diabetes mellitus: Oral: Initial doses should be based on current dose of saxagliptin and metformin; daily doses should be given once daily with the evening meal. Maximum: Saxagliptin 5 mg/metformin 2000 mg daily

Patients inadequately controlled on metformin alone: Initial dose: Saxagliptin 2.5-5 mg/day plus current dose of metformin. **Note:** Patients who require saxagliptin 2.5 mg (eg, dose adjusted for concomitant use of strong CYP3A4/5 inhibitors) and metformin >1000 mg should not be switched to the combination product.

Patients inadequately controlled on saxagliptin alone: Initial dose: Metformin 500 mg/day plus saxagliptin 5 mg/day. **Note:** Metformin-naïve patients currently receiving saxagliptin 2.5 mg daily (eg, dose adjusted for concomitant use of strong CYP3A4/5 inhibitors) should not be switched to the combination product.

Concomitant use with strong CYP3A4/5 inhibitors: Maximum: Saxagliptin 2.5 mg/metformin 1000 mg daily

Renal Impairment Do not use in patients with renal disease or renal dysfunction (serum creatinine ≥1.5 mg/dL [≥136 µmol/L] in males or ≥1.4 mg/dL [≥124 µmol/L] in females or abnormal clearance).

Hepatic Impairment Avoid metformin; liver disease is a risk factor for the development of lactic acidosis during metformin therapy.

Special Geriatric Considerations Metformin should not be used in patients ≥80 years of age unless renal function is verified as normal. **Do not titrate to maximum dose.** Intensive glucose control (HbA$_{1c}$ <6.5%) has been linked to increased all-cause and cardiovascular mortality, hypoglycemia requiring assistance, and weight gain in adult type 2 diabetes. How "tightly" to control a geriatric patient's blood glucose needs to be individualized. Such a decision should be based on several factors, including the patient's functional and cognitive status, how well he/she recognizes hypoglycemic or hyperglycemic symptoms, and how to respond to them and other disease states. An HbA$_{1c}$ <7.5% is an acceptable endpoint for a healthy older adult, while <8% is acceptable for frail elderly patients, those with a duration of illness >10 years, or those with comorbid conditions and requiring combination diabetes medications. Patients who are unable to accurately draw up their dose will need assistance, such as prefilled syringes. Initial doses may require considerations for renal function in the elderly with dosing adjusted subsequently based on blood glucose monitoring. For elderly patients with diabetes who are relatively healthy, attaining target goals for aspirin use, blood pressure, lipids, smoking cessation, and diet and exercise may be more important than normalized glycemic control.

Dosage Forms Excipient information presented when available (limited, particularly for generics); consult specific product labeling.

Tablet, variable release, oral:

Kombiglyze™ XR 2.5/1000: Saxagliptin 2.5 mg [immediate release] and metformin hydrochloride 1000 mg [extended release]

Kombiglyze™ XR 5/500: Saxagliptin 5 mg [immediate release] and metformin hydrochloride 500 mg [extended release]

Kombiglyze™ XR 5/1000: Saxagliptin 5 mg [immediate release] and metformin hydrochloride 1000 mg [extended release]

♦ **Saxagliptin and Metformin Hydrochloride** see Saxagliptin and Metformin *on page 1659*

♦ **SB-265805** *see* Gemifloxacin *on page 814*

♦ **SB659746-A** *see* Vilazodone *on page 1919*

♦ ***S. boulardii*** *see Saccharomyces boulardii on page 1646*

♦ **Scalpana [OTC]** *see* Hydrocortisone (Topical) *on page 886*

♦ **Scalpicin® Anti-Itch [OTC]** *see* Salicylic Acid *on page 1648*

♦ **SCH 13521** *see* Flutamide *on page 766*

♦ **SCH 56592** *see* Posaconazole *on page 1484*

♦ **SCIG** *see* Immune Globulin *on page 922*

♦ **S-Citalopram** *see* Escitalopram *on page 630*

♦ **Scopace™ [DSC]** *see* Scopolamine (Systemic) *on page 1661*

Scopolamine (Systemic) (skoe POL a mee)

Medication Safety Issues
Other safety concerns:
Transdermal patch may contain conducting metal (eg, aluminum); remove patch prior to MRI.

Brand Names: U.S. Scopace™ [DSC]; Transderm Scōp®
Brand Names: Canada Buscopan®; Transderm-V®
Index Terms Hyoscine Butylbromide; Scopolamine Base; Scopolamine Butylbromide; Scopolamine Hydrobromide
Generic Availability (U.S.) Yes: Injection
Pharmacologic Category Anticholinergic Agent
Use
Scopolamine base: Transdermal: Prevention of nausea/vomiting associated with motion sickness and recovery from anesthesia and surgery
Scopolamine hydrobromide:
Injection: Preoperative medication to produce amnesia, sedation, tranquilization, antiemetic effects, and decrease salivary and respiratory secretions
Oral: Symptomatic treatment of postencephalitic parkinsonism and paralysis agitans; in spastic states; inhibits excessive motility and hypertonus of the gastrointestinal tract in such conditions as the irritable colon syndrome, mild dysentery, diverticulitis, pylorospasm, and cardiospasm
Scopolamine butylbromide [not available in the U.S.]: Oral/injection: Treatment of smooth muscle spasm of the genitourinary or gastrointestinal tract; injection may also be used to prior to radiological/diagnostic procedures to prevent spasm
Unlabeled/Investigational Use Scopolamine base: Transdermal: Breakthrough treatment of nausea and vomiting associated with chemotherapy
Contraindications Hypersensitivity to scopolamine, other belladonna alkaloids, or any component of the formulation; narrow-angle glaucoma; acute hemorrhage; paralytic ileus; tachycardia secondary to cardiac insufficiency; myasthenia gravis
Tablet formulations are also contraindicated in patients with prostatic hyperplasia, pyloric obstruction, or patients with an idiosyncrasy to anticholinergic drugs.
Injectable formulations are also contraindicated in patients with chronic lung disease (repeated administration).
Warnings/Precautions Use with caution in patients with coronary artery disease, tachyarrhythmias, heart failure, or hypertension; evaluate tachycardia prior to administration. Use with caution with hepatic or renal impairment; adverse CNS effects occur more often in these patients. Use injectable and transdermal products with caution in patients with prostatic hyperplasia (nonobstructive) or urinary retention; oral products are contraindicated. Discontinue if patient reports unusual visual disturbances or pain within the eye. Use caution in hiatal hernia, reflux esophagitis, and ulcerative colitis. Use with caution in patients with a history of seizure or psychosis; may exacerbate these conditions. Patients with idiosyncratic reaction to anticholinergics, including scopolamine, may experience disorientation, delirium and/or marked somnolence; may be accompanied by dilated pupils, rapid pulse and xerostomia. May cause CNS depression, which may impair physical or mental abilities; patients must be cautioned about performing tasks which require mental alertness (eg, operating machinery or driving).

Transdermal patch may contain conducting metal (eg, aluminum); remove patch prior to MRI.
Scopolamine (hyoscine) hydrobromide should not be interchanged with scopolamine butylbromide formulations; dosages are not equivalent.
Adverse Reactions (Reflective of adult population; not specific for elderly) Frequency not defined.
Cardiovascular: Orthostatic hypotension, ventricular fibrillation, tachycardia, palpitation
Central nervous system: Confusion, drowsiness, headache, loss of memory, ataxia, fatigue
Dermatologic: Dry skin, photosensitivity increased, rash
Endocrine & metabolic: Decreased flow of breast milk
Gastrointestinal: Constipation, xerostomia, dry throat, dysphagia, bloated feeling, nausea, vomiting
Genitourinary: Dysuria
Local: Irritation at injection site
Neuromuscular & skeletal: Weakness
Ocular: Increased intraocular pain, blurred vision
Respiratory: Dry nose
Miscellaneous: Diaphoresis decreased

◀ **Drug Interactions**

Avoid Concomitant Use There are no known interactions where it is recommended to avoid concomitant use.

Increased Effect/Toxicity

Scopolamine (Systemic) may increase the levels/effects of: AbobotulinumtoxinA; Alcohol (Ethyl); Anticholinergics; Cannabinoids; CNS Depressants; Methotrimeprazine; Onabotulinumtoxin A; Potassium Chloride; RimabotulinumtoxinB; Selective Serotonin Reuptake Inhibitors

The levels/effects of Scopolamine (Systemic) may be increased by: Droperidol; HydrOX-Yzine; Methotrimeprazine; Pramlintide

Decreased Effect

Scopolamine (Systemic) may decrease the levels/effects of: Acetylcholinesterase Inhibitors (Central); Secretin

The levels/effects of Scopolamine (Systemic) may be decreased by: Acetylcholinesterase Inhibitors (Central)

Ethanol/Nutrition/Herb Interactions Ethanol: May increase CNS depression; monitor for increased effects with coadministration. Caution patients about effects.

Stability

Injection: Store at room temperature of 15°C to 30°C (58°F to 86°F). Protect from light. Hydrobromide injection: Avoid acid solutions, hydrolysis occurs at pH <3. Butylbromide injection: Stable in D_5W, NS, $D_{10}W$, and LR for up to 8 hours. Tablet: Store at room temperature of 15°C to 30°C (58°F to 86°F). Transdermal system: Store at 20°C to 25°C (68°F to 77°F).

Mechanism of Action Blocks the action of acetylcholine at parasympathetic sites in smooth muscle, secretory glands and the CNS; increases cardiac output, dries secretions, antagonizes histamine and serotonin

Pharmacodynamics/Kinetics

Onset of action: Oral, I.M.: 0.5-1 hour; I.V.: 10 minutes

Peak effect: 20-60 minutes; may take 3-7 days for full recovery; transdermal: 24 hours

Duration: Oral, I.M.: 4-6 hours; I.V.: 2 hours

Absorption: Tertiary salts (hydrobromide) are well absorbed; quaternary salts (butylbromide) are poorly absorbed (local concentrations in the GI tract following oral dosing may be high)

Metabolism: Hepatic

Half-life elimination: Hyoscine-N-butylbromide: 4.8 hours; Scopolamine: 9.5 hours

Excretion: Urine (<10%, as parent drug and metabolites)

Dosage

Geriatric & Adult Note: Scopolamine (hyoscine) hydrobromide should not be interchanged with scopolamine butylbromide formulations. Dosages are not equivalent.

Scopolamine base:

Preoperative: Transdermal patch: Apply 1 patch to hairless area behind ear the night before surgery; remove 24 hours after surgery

Motion sickness: Transdermal patch: Apply 1 patch behind the ear at least 4 hours prior to exposure and every 3 days as needed; effective if applied as soon as 2-3 hours before anticipated need, best if 12 hours before

Scopolamine hydrobromide:

Antiemetic: SubQ: 0.6-1 mg

Preoperative: I.M., I.V., SubQ: 0.3-0.65 mg

Sedation, tranquilization: I.M., I.V., SubQ: 0.6 mg 3-4 times/day

Parkinsonism, spasticity, motion sickness: Oral: 0.4-0.8 mg. May repeat every 8-12 hours as needed; the dosage may be cautiously increased in parkinsonism and spastic states. For motion sickness, administration at least 1 hour before exposure is recommended.

Scopolamine butylbromide: *Gastrointestinal/genitourinary spasm* (Buscopan® [CAN]; not available in the U.S.):

Oral: 10-20 mg daily (1-2 tablets); maximum: 6 tablets/day

I.M., I.V., SubQ: 10-20 mg; maximum: 100 mg/day. Intramuscular injections should be administered 10-15 minutes prior to radiological/diagnostic procedures

Administration

I.M.: **Butylbromide:** Intramuscular injections should be administered 10-15 minutes prior to radiological/diagnostic procedures.

I.V.:

Hydrobromide: Dilute with an equal volume of sterile water and administer by direct I.V.; inject over 2-3 minutes

Butylbromide: No dilution is necessary prior to injection; inject at a rate of 1 mL/minute

Transdermal: Topical patch is programmed to deliver 1 mg over 3 days. Once applied, do not remove the patch for 3 full days. Apply to hairless area of skin behind the ear. Wash hands before and after applying the disc to avoid drug contact with eyes.

Monitoring Parameters Body temperature, heart rate, urinary output, intraocular pressure

Test Interactions Interferes with gastric secretion test

Special Geriatric Considerations Anticholinergic agents are not well tolerated in the elderly and their use should be avoided when possible.

Dosage Forms Excipient information presented when available (limited, particularly for generics); consult specific product labeling. [DSC] = Discontinued product

Injection, solution, as hydrobromide: 0.4 mg/mL (1 mL)

Patch, transdermal:

Transderm Scōp®: 1.5 mg (4s, 10s, 24s) [contains metal; releases ~1 mg over 72 hours]

Tablet, soluble, oral, as hydrobromide:

Scopace™: 0.4 mg [DSC]

Dosage Forms: Canada Excipient information presented when available (limited, particularly for generics); consult specific product labeling.

Injection, solution, as hyoscine-N-butylbromide:

Buscopan®: 20 mg/mL [not available in U.S.]

Tablet, as hyoscine-N-butylbromide:

Buscopan®: 10 mg

Selected References

Feinberg M, "The Problems of Anticholinergic Adverse Effects in Older Patients," *Drugs Aging*, 1993, 3(4):335-48.

Scopolamine (Ophthalmic) (skoe POL a meen)

Brand Names: U.S. Isopto® Hyoscine

Index Terms Hyoscine Hydrobromide; Scopolamine Hydrobromide

Generic Availability (U.S.) No

Pharmacologic Category Anticholinergic Agent; Anticholinergic Agent, Ophthalmic; Ophthalmic Agent, Mydriatic

Use Scopolamine hydrobromide: Produce cycloplegia and mydriasis; treatment of iridocyclitis

Dosage

Geriatric & Adult Scopolamine hydrobromide:

Refraction: Ophthalmic: Instill 1-2 drops of 0.25% to eye(s) 1 hour before procedure

Iridocyclitis: Ophthalmic: Instill 1-2 drops of 0.25% to eye(s) up to 4 times/day

Special Geriatric Considerations Because of its long duration of action as a mydriatic agent, it should be avoided in elderly patients.

Dosage Forms Excipient information presented when available (limited, particularly for generics); consult specific product labeling.

Solution, ophthalmic, as hydrobromide [drops]:

Isopto® Hyoscine: 0.25% (5 mL) [contains benzalkonium chloride]

Selegiline (se LE ji leen)

Related Information

Antidepressant Agents *on page 1991*

Antiparkinsonian Agents *on page 1995*

Medication Safety Issues

Sound-alike/look-alike issues:

Selegiline may be confused with Salagen®, Serentil®, sertraline, Serzone®, Stelazine®

Eldepryl® may be confused with Elavil®, enalapril

Zelapar® may be confused with zaleplon, Zemplar®, zolpidem, ZyPREXA® Zydis®

SELEGILINE

Brand Names: U.S. Eldepryl®; Emsam®; Zelapar®
Brand Names: Canada Apo-Selegiline®; Gen-Selegiline; Mylan-Selegiline; Novo-Selegiline; Nu-Selegiline
Index Terms Deprenyl; L-Deprenyl; Selegiline Hydrochloride
Generic Availability (U.S.) Yes: Capsule, tablet
Pharmacologic Category Anti-Parkinson's Agent, MAO Type B Inhibitor; Antidepressant, Monoamine Oxidase Inhibitor
Use Adjunct in the management of parkinsonian patients in which levodopa/carbidopa therapy is deteriorating (oral products); treatment of major depressive disorder (transdermal product)
Unlabeled/Investigational Use Early Parkinson's disease; attention-deficit/hyperactivity disorder (ADHD)
Medication Guide Available Yes
Contraindications Hypersensitivity to selegiline or any component of the formulation; concomitant use of meperidine

Orally disintegrating tablet: Additional contraindications: Concomitant use of dextromethorphan, methadone, propoxyphene, tramadol, oral selegiline, other MAO inhibitors

Transdermal: Additional contraindications: Pheochromocytoma; concomitant use of bupropion, selective or dual serotonin reuptake inhibitors (including SSRIs and SNRIs), tricyclic antidepressants, tramadol, propoxyphene, methadone, dextromethorphan, St. John's wort, mirtazapine, cyclobenzaprine, oral selegiline and other MAO inhibitors; carbamazepine, and oxcarbazepine; elective surgery requiring general anesthesia, local anesthesia containing sympathomimetic vasoconstrictors; sympathomimetics (and related compounds); foods high in tyramine content; supplements containing tyrosine, phenylalanine, tryptophan, or caffeine

Warnings/Precautions

Oral: MAO-B selective inhibition should not pose a problem with tyramine-containing products as long as the typical oral doses are employed, however, rare reactions have been reported. Increased risk of nonselective MAO inhibition occurs with oral capsule/tablet doses >10 mg/day or orally disintegrating tablet doses >2.5 mg/day. Use of oral selegiline with tricyclic antidepressants and SSRIs has also been associated with rare reactions and should generally be avoided. Addition to levodopa therapy may result in exacerbation of levodopa adverse effects, requiring a reduction in levodopa dosage. Dopaminergic agents used for Parkinson's disease or restless legs syndrome have been associated with compulsive behaviors and/or loss of impulse control, which has manifested as pathological gambling, libido increases (hypersexuality), and/or binge eating. Causality has not been established, and controversy exists as to whether this phenomenon is related to the underlying disease, prior behaviors/addictions and/or drug therapy. Dose reduction or discontinuation of therapy has been reported to reverse these behaviors in some, but not all cases. Use caution in patients with hepatic or renal impairment. Incidence of orthostatic hypotension may be increased in older adults and when titrating to the 2.5 mg dosage in patients taking the orally disintegrating tablet. Risk for melanoma development is increased in Parkinson's disease patients; drug causation or factors contributing to risk have not been established. Patients should be monitored closely and periodic skin examinations should be performed. Orally disintegrating tablet may cause oral mucosa edema, irritation, pain, ulceration and/or swallowing pain. Do not use orally disintegrating tablet concurrently with other selegiline products; wait at least 14 days from discontinuation before initiating treatment with another selegiline dosage form. Some products may contain phenylalanine.

Transdermal: Nonselective MAO inhibition occurs with transdermal delivery and is necessary for antidepressant efficacy. Hypertensive crisis as a result of ingesting tyramine-rich foods is always a concern with nonselective MAO inhibition. Although transdermal delivery minimizes inhibition of MAO-A in the gut, there is limited data with higher transdermal doses; dietary modifications are recommended with doses >6 mg/24 hours.

Transdermal patch: May cause orthostatic hypotension; use with caution in patients at risk of this effect or in those who would not tolerate transient hypotensive episodes (cerebrovascular disease, cardiovascular disease, hypovolemia, or concurrent medication use which may predispose to hypotension/bradycardia). Discontinue transdermal product at least 10 days prior to elective surgery. May contain conducting metal (eg, aluminum); remove patch prior to MRI. Avoid exposure of application site and surrounding area to direct external heat sources.

Transdermal: **[U.S. Boxed Warning]: Antidepressants increase the risk of suicidal thinking and behavior in children, adolescents, and young adults (18-24 years of age) with major depressive disorder (MDD) and other psychiatric disorders;** consider risk prior to prescribing. Short-term studies did not show an increased risk in patients >24 years of age and showed a decreased risk in patients ≥65 years. Closely monitor patients for worsening of depression, suicidality and/or associated behaviors, particularly during the initial 1-2 months of therapy or during periods of dosage adjustments (increases or decreases); the patient's family or caregiver should be instructed to closely observe the patient and communicate condition with healthcare provider. A medication guide concerning the use of antidepressants should be dispensed with each prescription.

Transdermal: The possibility of a suicide attempt is inherit in major depression and may persist until remission occurs. Patients treated with antidepressants (for any indication) should be observed for clinical worsening and suicidality, especially during the initial few months of a course of drug therapy, or at times of dose changes, either increases or decreases. Use caution in high-risk patients. Worsening depression and severe abrupt suicidality that are not part of the presenting symptoms may require discontinuation or modification of drug therapy. Use caution in high-risk patients during initiation of therapy. The patient's family or caregiver should be alerted to monitor patients for the emergence of suicidality and associated behaviors (such as agitation, irritability, hostility, and hypomania) and call healthcare provider.

Transdermal selegiline may worsen psychosis in some patients or precipitate a shift to mania or hypomania in patients with bipolar disorder. Monotherapy in patients with bipolar disorder should be avoided. Patients presenting with depressive symptoms should be screened for bipolar disorder. **Selegiline is not FDA approved for the treatment of bipolar depression.**

Adverse Reactions (Reflective of adult population; not specific for elderly) Unless otherwise noted, the percentage of adverse events is reported for the transdermal patch (**Note:** ODT = orally disintegrating tablet, Oral = capsule/tablet)

>10%:
  Central nervous system: Headache (18%; ODT 7%; oral 4%), insomnia (12%; ODT 7%), dizziness (oral 14%; ODT 11%)
  Gastrointestinal: Nausea (oral 20%; ODT 11%)
  Local: Application site reaction (24%)

1% to 10%:
  Cardiovascular: Hypotension (including postural 3% to 10%), palpitation (oral 2%), chest pain (≥1%; ODT 2%), hypertension (≥1%; ODT 3%), peripheral edema (≥1%)
  Central nervous system: Pain (ODT 8%; oral 2%), hallucinations (oral 6%; ODT 4%), confusion (oral 6%; ODT 4%), vivid dreams (oral 4%), ataxia (ODT 3%), somnolence (ODT 3%), lethargy (oral 2%), agitation (≥1%), amnesia (≥1%), paresthesia (≥1%), thinking abnormal (≥1%), depression (<1%; ODT 2%)
  Dermatologic: Rash (4%), bruising (≥1%; ODT 2%), pruritus (≥1%), acne (≥1%)
  Endocrine & metabolic: Weight loss (5%; oral 2%), hypokalemia (ODT 2%), sexual side effects (≤1%)
  Gastrointestinal: Diarrhea (9%; ODT 2%; oral 2%), xerostomia (8%; oral 6%; ODT 4%), stomatitis (ODT 5%), abdominal pain (oral 8%), dyspepsia (4%; ODT 5%), dysphagia (ODT 2%), dental caries (ODT 2%), constipation (≥1%; ODT 4%), flatulence (≥1%; ODT 2%), anorexia (≥1%), gastroenteritis (≥1%), taste perversion (≥1%; ODT 2%), vomiting (≥1%; ODT 3%)
  Genitourinary: Urinary retention (oral 2%), dysmenorrhea (≥1%), metrorrhagia (≥1%), UTI (≥1%), urinary frequency (≥1%)
  Neuromuscular & skeletal: Dyskinesia (ODT 6%), back pain (ODT 5%; oral 2%), ataxia (<1%; ODT 3%), leg cramps (ODT 3%; oral 2%), myalgia (≥1%; ODT 3%), neck pain (≥1%), tremor (<1%; ODT 3%)
  Otic: Tinnitus (≥1%)
  Respiratory: Rhinitis (ODT 7%), pharyngitis (3%; ODT 4%), sinusitis (3%), cough (≥1%; ODT 3%), bronchitis (≥1%), dyspnea (<1%; ODT 3%)
  Miscellaneous: Diaphoresis (≥1%)

Drug Interactions

Metabolism/Transport Effects Substrate of CYP1A2 (minor), 2A6 (minor), 2B6 (major), 2C8 (minor), 2C19 (minor), 2D6 (minor), 3A4 (minor); **Inhibits** CYP1A2 (weak), 2A6 (weak), 2C9 (weak), 2C19 (weak), 2D6 (weak), 2E1 (weak), 3A4 (weak)

Avoid Concomitant Use

Avoid concomitant use of Selegiline with any of the following: Alpha-/Beta-Agonists (Indirect-Acting); Alpha1-Agonists; Alpha2-Agonists (Ophthalmic); Amphetamines; Anilidopiperidine Opioids; Atomoxetine; Bezafibrate; Buprenorphine; BuPROPion; BusPIRone; CarBAMazepine; Cyclobenzaprine; Dexmethylphenidate; Dextromethorphan; Diethylpropion; HYDROmorphone; Linezolid; Maprotiline; Meperidine; Methyldopa; Methylene Blue; Methylphenidate; Mirtazapine; OXcarbazepine; Oxymorphone; Pizotifen; Propoxyphene; Selective Serotonin Reuptake Inhibitors; Serotonin 5-HT1D Receptor Agonists; Serotonin/Norepinephrine Reuptake Inhibitors; Sibutramine; Tapentadol; Tetrabenazine; Tetrahydrozoline; Tetrahydrozoline (Nasal); Tricyclic Antidepressants; Tryptophan

Increased Effect/Toxicity

Selegiline may increase the levels/effects of: Alpha-/Beta-Agonists (Direct-Acting); Alpha-/Beta-Agonists (Indirect-Acting); Alpha1-Agonists; Alpha2-Agonists (Ophthalmic); Amphetamines; Antihypertensives; Atomoxetine; Beta2-Agonists; Bezafibrate; BuPROPion; Dexmethylphenidate; Dextromethorphan; Diethylpropion; Doxapram; HYDROmorphone;

◄

Linezolid; Lithium; Meperidine; Methadone; Methyldopa; Methylene Blue; Methylphenidate; Mirtazapine; Orthostatic Hypotension Producing Agents; Pizotifen; Reserpine; Selective Serotonin Reuptake Inhibitors; Serotonin 5-HT1D Receptor Agonists; Serotonin Modulators; Serotonin/Norepinephrine Reuptake Inhibitors; Tetrahydrozoline; Tetrahydrozoline (Nasal); Tricyclic Antidepressants

The levels/effects of Selegiline may be increased by: Altretamine; Anilidopiperidine Opioids; Buprenorphine; BusPIRone; CarBAMazepine; COMT Inhibitors; Conivaptan; Contraceptives (Estrogens); Contraceptives (Progestins); Cyclobenzaprine; CYP2B6 Inhibitors (Moderate); CYP2B6 Inhibitors (Strong); Levodopa; MAO Inhibitors; Maprotiline; OXcarbazepine; Oxymorphone; Propoxyphene; Quazepam; Sibutramine; Tapentadol; Tetrabenazine; TraMADol; Tryptophan

Decreased Effect

The levels/effects of Selegiline may be decreased by: CYP2B6 Inducers (Strong); Cyproterone; Peginterferon Alfa-2b; Tocilizumab

Ethanol/Nutrition/Herb Interactions

Ethanol: Avoid ethanol (based on CNS depressant effects and potential tyramine content)

Food: Concurrent ingestion of foods rich in tyramine may cause sudden and severe high blood pressure (hypertensive crisis). Avoid or limit tyramine-containing foods with MAO-Is (product and/or dose-dependent).

Herb/Nutraceuticals: Avoid valerian, St John's wort, SAMe, kava kava. Avoid supplements containing caffeine, tryptophan, or phenylalanine. Ingestion of large quantities may increase the risk of severe side effects (eg, hypertensive reactions, serotonin syndrome).

Stability

Capsule, tablet, transdermal: Store at 20°C to 25°C (68°F to 77°F). Store patch in sealed pouch and apply immediately after removal.

Orally disintegrating tablet: Store at controlled room temperature 25°C (77°F); excursions permitted to 15°C to 30°C (59°F to 86°F). Use within 3 months of opening pouch and immediately after opening individual blister.

Mechanism of Action Potent, irreversible inhibitor of monoamine oxidase (MAO). Plasma concentrations achieved via administration of oral dosage forms in recommended doses confer selective inhibition of MAO type B, which plays a major role in the metabolism of dopamine; selegiline may also increase dopaminergic activity by interfering with dopamine reuptake at the synapse. When administered transdermally in recommended doses, selegiline achieves higher blood levels and effectively inhibits both MAO-A and MAO-B, which blocks catabolism of other centrally-active biogenic amine neurotransmitters.

Pharmacodynamics/Kinetics

Onset of action: Therapeutic: Oral: Within 1 hour

Duration: Oral: 24-72 hours

Absorption:

Orally disintegrating tablet: Rapid; greater bioavailability than capsule/tablet

Transdermal: 25% to 30% (of total selegiline content) over 24 hours

Protein binding: ~90%

Metabolism: Hepatic, primarily via CYP2B6 to active (N-desmethylselegiline, amphetamine, methamphetamine) and inactive metabolites

Half-life elimination: Oral: 10 hours; Transdermal: 18-25 hours

Excretion: Urine (primarily metabolites); feces

Dosage

Geriatric

Parkinson's disease:

Capsule/tablet: ≤5 mg/day (when combined with levodopa) is recommended by some clinicians to decrease the enhanced dopaminergic side effects (Olanow, 2001)

Orally disintegrating tablet (Zelapar®): Refer to adult dosing

Depression: Transdermal (Emsam®): 6 mg/24 hours

Adult

Parkinson's disease:

Capsule/tablet: 5 mg twice daily with breakfast and lunch

Orally disintegrating tablet (Zelapar®): Initial 1.25 mg daily for at least 6 weeks; may increase to 2.5 mg daily based on clinical response (maximum: 2.5 mg daily)

Depression: Transdermal (Emsam®): Initial: 6 mg/24 hours once daily; may titrate based on clinical response in increments of 3 mg/day every 2 weeks up to a maximum of 12 mg/24 hours

Renal Impairment

Oral: Use caution, has not been studied.

Transdermal: No adjustment required in patients with mild-to-moderate impairment.

Hepatic Impairment

Oral: Use caution, has not been studied.

Transdermal: No adjustment required in patients with mild-to-moderate impairment.

Administration

Oral: Orally disintegrating tablet (Zelapar®): Take in morning before breakfast; place on top of tongue and allow to dissolve. Avoid food or liquid 5 minutes before and after administration.

Topical: Transdermal (Emsam®): Apply to clean, dry, intact skin to the upper torso (below the neck and above the waist), upper thigh, or outer surface of the upper arm. Avoid exposure of application site to external heat source, which may increase the amount of drug absorbed. Apply at the same time each day and rotate application sites. Wash hands with soap and water after handling. Avoid touching the sticky side of the patch.

Monitoring Parameters Blood pressure; symptoms of parkinsonism; general mood and behavior (increased anxiety, presence of mania or agitation); suicidal ideation (especially at the beginning of therapy or when doses are increased or decreased)

Test Interactions May interfere with urine detection of amphetamine/methamphetamine (false-positive).

Pharmacotherapy Pearls When adding selegiline to levodopa/carbidopa, the dose of the latter can usually be decreased.

Special Geriatric Considerations Do not use capsule/tablet at doses >10 mg/day or orally disintegrating tablet at doses >2.5 mg/day because of the risks associated with nonselective inhibition of MAO.

Orally-disintegrating tablets: In clinical trials, adverse effects were seen more frequently in the elderly compared to younger adults. This is particularly of concern for hypertension, orthostatic hypotension, dizziness, and somnolence. If using the orally disintegrating tablets, administer at the lowest dose and monitor for side effects.

Dosage Forms Excipient information presented when available (limited, particularly for generics); consult specific product labeling.

Capsule, oral, as hydrochloride: 5 mg

Eldepryl®: 5 mg

Patch, transdermal:

Emsam®: 6 mg/24 hours (30s) [20 cm², total selegiline 20 mg]

Emsam®: 9 mg/24 hours (30s) [30 cm², total selegiline 30 mg]

Emsam®: 12 mg/24 hours (30s) [40 cm², total selegiline 40 mg]

Tablet, oral, as hydrochloride: 5 mg

Tablet, orally disintegrating, oral:

Zelapar®: 1.25 mg [contains phenylalanine 1.25 mg/tablet; grapefruit flavor]

Selected References

Lawlor BA, Aisen PS, and Green C, "Selegiline in the Treatment of Behavioural Disturbances in Alzheimer's Disease," *Int J Geriatr Psychiatry*, 1997, 12(3):319-22.

Olanow CW, Watts RL, and Koller WC, "An Algorithm (Decision Tree) for the Management of Parkinson's Disease (2001): Treatment Guidelines," *Neurology*, 2001, 56(11 Suppl 5):S1-S88.

Sano M, Ernesto C, Thomas RG, et al, "A Controlled Trial of Selegiline, Alpha-Tocopherol, or Both as Treatment for Alzheimer's Disease," *N Engl J Med*, 1997, 336(17):1216-22.

The Parkinson Study Group, "Effects of Tocopherol and Deprenyl on the Progression of Disability in Early Parkinson's Disease," *N Engl J Med*, 1993, 328(3):176-83.

◆ **Selegiline Hydrochloride** *see* Selegiline *on page 1663*

◆ **Selfemra® [DSC]** *see* FLUoxetine *on page 753*

◆ **Senexon [OTC]** *see* Senna *on page 1667*

◆ **Senexon-S [OTC]** *see* Docusate and Senna *on page 548*

Senna (SEN na)

Related Information

Laxatives, Classification and Properties *on page 2012*

Treatment Options for Constipation *on page 2035*

Medication Safety Issues

Sound-alike/look-alike issues:

Perdiem® may be confused with Pyridium®

Senexon® may be confused with Cenestin®

Senokot® may be confused with Depakote®

Brand Names: U.S. Black Draught® [OTC]; Evac-U-Gen® [OTC]; ex-lax® Maximum Strength [OTC]; ex-lax® [OTC]; Fleet® Pedia-Lax™ Quick Dissolve [OTC]; Fletcher's® [OTC]; Little Tummys® Laxative [OTC]; Perdiem® Overnight Relief [OTC]; Senexon [OTC]; SennaGen [OTC]; Senokot® [OTC]

Index Terms Sennosides

Generic Availability (U.S.) Yes

Pharmacologic Category Laxative, Stimulant

◀ **Use** Short-term treatment of constipation; evacuate the colon for bowel or rectal examinations

Contraindications Per Commission E: Intestinal obstruction, acute intestinal inflammation (eg, Crohn's disease), colitis ulcerosa, appendicitis, abdominal pain of unknown origin

Warnings/Precautions Not recommended for over-the-counter (OTC) use in patients experiencing stomach pain, nausea, vomiting, or a sudden change in bowel movements which lasts >2 weeks.

Adverse Reactions (Reflective of adult population; not specific for elderly) Frequency not defined: Gastrointestinal: Abdominal cramps, diarrhea, nausea, vomiting

Drug Interactions

  Avoid Concomitant Use There are no known interactions where it is recommended to avoid concomitant use.

  Increased Effect/Toxicity There are no known significant interactions involving an increase in effect.

  Decreased Effect There are no known significant interactions involving a decrease in effect.

Pharmacodynamics/Kinetics

  Metabolism: In the liver

  Elimination: In feces (via bile) and urine

Dosage

  Geriatric & Adult

    Bowel evacuation: Oral: OTC labeling: Usual dose: Sennosides 130 mg between 2-4 PM the afternoon of the day prior to procedure

    Constipation: Oral: OTC ranges: Sennosides 15 mg once daily (maximum: 70-100 mg/day, divided twice daily)

Administration Oral: Once daily doses should be taken at bedtime. Granules may be eaten plain, sprinkled on food, or mixed in liquids

Monitoring Parameters Monitor stools daily for consistency, occult or gross blood; also with chronic use, monitor serum electrolytes; monitor for dehydration and hypotension

Pharmacotherapy Pearls Some products that may have previously been labeled as standardized senna concentrate are now labeled as sennosides. For example, Senokot® tablets, previously labeled as standardized senna concentrate 187 mg, are now labeled as sennosides 8.6 mg. The actual content of senna in this product did not change. Individual product labeling should be consulted prior to dosing.

Special Geriatric Considerations Elderly are often predisposed to constipation due to disease, immobility, drugs, and a decreased "thirst reflex" with age enhancing the possibility of dehydration. Avoid stimulant cathartic use on a chronic basis if possible. Use osmotic, lubricant, stool softeners, and bulk agents as prophylaxis. Patients should be instructed for proper dietary fiber and fluid intake as well as regular exercise. Monitor closely for fluid/electrolyte imbalance, CNS signs of fluid/electrolyte loss, and hypotension.

Dosage Forms Excipient information presented when available (limited, particularly for generics); consult specific product labeling.

  Liquid, oral:

    Senexon: Sennosides 8.8 mg/5 mL (237 mL) [contains propylene glycol]

  Liquid, oral [concentrate]:

    Fletcher's®: Senna concentrate 33.3 mg/mL (75 mL) [ethanol free; contains sodium benzoate; rootbeer flavor]

  Liquid, oral [concentrate/drops]:

    Little Tummys® Laxative: Sennosides 8.8 mg/mL (30 mL) [dye free, ethanol free; contains propylene glycol, soya lecithin; chocolate flavor]

  Strip, orally disintegrating, oral:

    Fleet® Pedia-Lax™ Quick Dissolve: Sennosides 8.6 mg (12s) [grape flavor]

  Syrup, oral: Sennosides 8.8 mg/5 mL (237 mL, 240 mL)

  Tablet, oral: Sennosides 8.6 mg

    ex-lax®: Sennosides USP 15 mg

    ex-lax® Maximum Strength: Sennosides USP 25 mg

    Perdiem® Overnight Relief: Sennosides USP 15 mg

    Senexon: Sennosides 8.6 mg

    SennaGen: Sennosides 8.6 mg

    Senokot®: Sennosides 8.6 mg

  Tablet, chewable, oral:

    Black Draught®: Sennosides 10 mg

    Evac-U-Gen®: Sennosides 10 mg

    ex-lax®: Sennosides USP 15 mg [chocolate flavor]

◆ **Senna and Docusate** *see* Docusate and Senna *on page 548*
◆ **SennaGen [OTC]** *see* Senna *on page 1667*
◆ **Senna-S** *see* Docusate and Senna *on page 548*
◆ **Sennosides** *see* Senna *on page 1667*

◆ **Senokot® [OTC]** *see* Senna *on page 1667*
◆ **Senokot-S® [OTC]** *see* Docusate and Senna *on page 548*
◆ **SenoSol™-SS [OTC]** *see* Docusate and Senna *on page 548*
◆ **Septra® [DSC]** *see* Sulfamethoxazole and Trimethoprim *on page 1714*
◆ **Septra® DS** *see* Sulfamethoxazole and Trimethoprim *on page 1714*
◆ **Serax** *see* Oxazepam *on page 1360*
◆ **Serevent® Diskus®** *see* Salmeterol *on page 1653*
◆ **Seromycin®** *see* CycloSERINE *on page 431*
◆ **SEROquel®** *see* QUEtiapine *on page 1556*
◆ **SEROquel XR®** *see* QUEtiapine *on page 1556*

Sertraline (SER tra leen)

Related Information
Antidepressant Agents *on page 1991*
Beers Criteria – Potentially Inappropriate Medications for Geriatrics *on page 2089*
Liquid Compatibility of Antidepressants, Antipsychotics, and Mood Stabilizers *on page 2111*
Medication Safety Issues
Sound-alike/look-alike issues:
Sertraline may be confused with selegiline, Serentil®, Serevent®, Soriatane®
Zoloft® may be confused with Zocor®
Brand Names: U.S. Zoloft®
Brand Names: Canada Apo-Sertraline®; CO Sertraline; Dom-Sertraline; GD-Sertraline; Mylan-Sertraline; Nu-Sertraline; PHL-Sertraline; PMS-Sertraline; ratio-Sertraline; Riva-Sertraline; Sandoz-Sertraline; Teva-Sertraline; Zoloft®
Index Terms Sertraline Hydrochloride
Generic Availability (U.S.) Yes
Pharmacologic Category Antidepressant, Selective Serotonin Reuptake Inhibitor
Use Treatment of major depression; obsessive-compulsive disorder (OCD); panic disorder; post-traumatic stress disorder (PTSD); social anxiety disorder
Unlabeled/Investigational Use Eating disorders; generalized anxiety disorder (GAD); impulse control disorders; treatment of mild dementia-associated agitation in nonpsychotic patients
Medication Guide Available Yes
Contraindications Hypersensitivity to sertraline or any component of the formulation; use of MAO inhibitors within 14 days; concurrent use of pimozide; concurrent use of sertraline oral concentrate with disulfiram
Warnings/Precautions [U.S. Boxed Warning]: Antidepressants increase the risk of suicidal thinking and behavior in children, adolescents, and young adults (18-24 years of age) with major depressive disorder (MDD) and other psychiatric disorders; consider risk prior to prescribing. Short-term studies did not show an increased risk in patients >24 years of age and showed a decreased risk in patients ≥65 years. Closely monitor patients for clinical worsening, suicidality, or unusual changes in behavior, particularly during the initial 1-2 months of therapy or during periods of dosage adjustments (increases or decreases); the patient's family or caregiver should be instructed to closely observe the patient and communicate condition with healthcare provider. A medication guide concerning the use of antidepressants should be dispensed with each prescription. **Sertraline is not FDA approved for use in children with major depressive disorder (MDD). However, it is approved for the treatment of obsessive-compulsive disorder (OCD) in children ≥6 years of age.**

The possibility of a suicide attempt is inherent in major depression and may persist until remission occurs. Use caution in high-risk patients. Worsening depression and severe abrupt suicidality that are not part of the presenting symptoms may require discontinuation or modification of drug therapy. The patient's family or caregiver should be alerted to monitor patients for the emergence of suicidality and associated behaviors (such as agitation, irritability, hostility, impulsivity, and hypomania) and call healthcare provider.

May worsen psychosis in some patients or precipitate a shift to mania or hypomania in patients with bipolar disorder. Patients presenting with depressive symptoms should be screened for bipolar disorder. Monotherapy in patients with bipolar disorder should be avoided. **Sertraline is not FDA approved for the treatment of bipolar depression.**

Serotonin syndrome and neuroleptic malignant syndrome (NMS)-like reactions have occurred with serotonin/norepinephrine reuptake inhibitors (SNRIs) and selective serotonin reuptake inhibitors (SSRIs) when used alone, and particularly when used in combination with serotonergic agents (eg, triptans) or antidopaminergic agents (eg, antipsychotics). Concurrent use with MAO inhibitors is contraindicated. Has a very low potential to impair cognitive or motor performance. However, caution patients regarding activities requiring alertness until response to sertraline is known. Does not appear to potentiate the effects of alcohol, however, ethanol use is not advised.

Use caution in patients with a previous seizure disorder or condition predisposing to seizures such as brain damage, alcoholism, or concurrent therapy with other drugs which lower the seizure threshold. May increase the risks associated with electroconvulsive therapy. Use with caution in patients with hepatic or renal dysfunction and in elderly patients. May cause hyponatremia/SIADH (elderly at increased risk); volume depletion (diuretics may increase risk). Use with caution in patients with renal insufficiency or other concurrent illness (due to limited experience). Sertraline acts as a mild uricosuric; use with caution in patients at risk of uric acid nephropathy. Use caution with concomitant use of NSAIDs, ASA, or other drugs that affect coagulation; the risk of bleeding may be potentiated. Use with caution in patients where weight loss is undesirable. May cause or exacerbate sexual dysfunction.

Use oral concentrate formulation with caution in patients with latex sensitivity; dropper dispenser contains dry natural rubber. Discontinuation symptoms (eg, dysphoric mood, irritability, agitation, confusion, anxiety, insomnia, hypomania) may occur upon abrupt discontinuation. Taper dose when discontinuing therapy.

Adverse Reactions (Reflective of adult population; not specific for elderly)
>10%:
Central nervous system: Dizziness, fatigue, headache, insomnia, somnolence
Endocrine & metabolic: Libido decreased
Gastrointestinal: Anorexia, diarrhea, nausea, xerostomia
Genitourinary: Ejaculatory disturbances
Neuromuscular & skeletal: Tremors
Miscellaneous: Diaphoresis
1% to 10%:
Cardiovascular: Chest pain, palpitation
Central nervous system: Agitation, anxiety, hypoesthesia, malaise, nervousness, pain
Dermatologic: Rash
Endocrine & metabolic: Impotence
Gastrointestinal: Appetite increased, constipation, dyspepsia, flatulence, vomiting, weight gain
Neuromuscular & skeletal: Back pain, hypertonia, myalgia, paresthesia, weakness
Ocular: Visual difficulty, abnormal vision
Otic: Tinnitus
Respiratory: Rhinitis
Miscellaneous: Yawning

Additional adverse reactions reported in pediatric patients (frequency >2%): Aggressiveness, epistaxis, hyperkinesia, purpura, sinusitis, urinary incontinence

Drug Interactions
Metabolism/Transport Effects Substrate of CYP2B6 (minor), 2C9 (minor), 2C19 (major), 2D6 (major), 3A4 (minor); **Inhibits** CYP1A2 (weak), 2B6 (moderate), 2C8 (weak), 2C9 (weak), 2C19 (moderate), 2D6 (moderate), 3A4 (moderate)

Avoid Concomitant Use
Avoid concomitant use of Sertraline with any of the following: Clopidogrel; Disulfiram; Iobenguane I 123; MAO Inhibitors; Methylene Blue; Pimozide; Sibutramine; Thioridazine; Tolvaptan; Tryptophan

Increased Effect/Toxicity
Sertraline may increase the levels/effects of: Alpha-/Beta-Blockers; Anticoagulants; Antidepressants (Serotonin Reuptake Inhibitor/Antagonist); Antiplatelet Agents; Aspirin; Beta-Blockers; Budesonide (Systemic, Oral Inhalation); BusPIRone; CarBAMazepine; CloZAPine; Colchicine; Collagenase (Systemic); CYP2B6 Substrates; CYP2C19 Substrates; CYP2D6 Substrates; CYP3A4 Substrates; Desmopressin; Dextromethorphan; Drotrecogin Alfa; Eplerenone; Everolimus; Fesoterodine; Fosphenytoin; Galantamine; Halofantrine; Haloperidol; Ibritumomab; Lithium; Lurasidone; Methadone; Methylene Blue; NSAID (COX-2 Inhibitor); NSAID (Nonselective); Phenytoin; Pimecrolimus; Pimozide; Ranolazine; RisperiDONE; Rivaroxaban; Salicylates; Salmeterol; Saxagliptin; Serotonin Modulators; Tamoxifen; Thioridazine; Thrombolytic Agents; Tolvaptan; Tositumomab and Iodine I 131 Tositumomab; TraMADol; Tricyclic Antidepressants; Vitamin K Antagonists

The levels/effects of Sertraline may be increased by: Abiraterone Acetate; Alcohol (Ethyl); Analgesics (Opioid); BusPIRone; Cimetidine; CNS Depressants; Conivaptan; CYP2D6 Inhibitors (Moderate); CYP2D6 Inhibitors (Strong); Dasatinib; Disulfiram; Glucosamine; Herbs (Anticoagulant/Antiplatelet Properties); Macrolide Antibiotics; MAO Inhibitors; Metoclopramide; Omega-3-Acid Ethyl Esters; Pentosan Polysulfate Sodium; Pentoxifylline; Prostacyclin Analogues; Sibutramine; TraMADol; Tryptophan; Vitamin E

Decreased Effect

Sertraline may decrease the levels/effects of: Clopidogrel; Iobenguane I 123

The levels/effects of Sertraline may be decreased by: CarBAMazepine; Cyproheptadine; Darunavir; Efavirenz; Fosphenytoin; NSAID (Nonselective); Peginterferon Alfa-2b; Phenytoin; Tocilizumab

Ethanol/Nutrition/Herb Interactions

Ethanol: May increase CNS depression; monitor for increased effects with coadministration. Caution patients about effects.

Food: Sertraline average peak serum levels may be increased if taken with food.

Herb/Nutraceutical: Avoid valerian, St John's wort, kava kava, gotu kola (may increase CNS depression).

Stability Tablets and oral solution should be stored at controlled room temperature of 15°C to 30°C (59°F to 86°F).

Mechanism of Action Antidepressant with selective inhibitory effects on presynaptic serotonin (5-HT) reuptake and only very weak effects on norepinephrine and dopamine neuronal uptake. *In vitro* studies demonstrate no significant affinity for adrenergic, cholinergic, GABA, dopaminergic, histaminergic, serotonergic, or benzodiazepine receptors.

Pharmacodynamics/Kinetics

Onset of action: Depression: The onset of action is within a week, however, individual response varies greatly and full response may not be seen until 8-12 weeks after initiation of treatment.

Absorption: Slow

Protein binding: 98%

Metabolism: Hepatic; may involve CYP2C19 and CYP2D6; extensive first pass metabolism; forms metabolite N-desmethylsertraline

Bioavailability: Bioavailability of tablets and solution are equivalent

Half-life elimination: Sertraline: 26 hours; N-desmethylsertraline: 66 hours (range: 62-104 hours)

Time to peak, plasma: Sertraline: 4.5-8.4 hours

Excretion: Urine and feces

Sertraline's clearance has been found to be reduced by 40% in older adults

Dosage

Geriatric Oral: Initial: 25 mg/day in the morning; increase by 25 mg/day increments every 2-3 days if tolerated to 50-100 mg/day; additional increases may be necessary; maximum: 200 mg/day. **Note:** Patients with Alzheimer's dementia-related depression may require a lower starting dosage of 12.5 mg/day, with titration intervals of 1-2 weeks, up to 150-200 mg/day maximum.

Adult

Depression/OCD: Oral: Initial: 50 mg/day

Note: May increase daily dose, at intervals of not less than 1 week, to a maximum of 200 mg/day. If somnolence is noted, give at bedtime.

Panic disorder, PTSD, social anxiety disorder: Oral: Initial: 25 mg once daily; increased after 1 week to 50 mg once daily (see "Note" above)

Renal Impairment Multiple-dose pharmacokinetics are unaffected by renal impairment. Hemodialysis effect: Not removed by hemodialysis

Hepatic Impairment Sertraline is extensively metabolized by the liver. Caution should be used in patients with hepatic impairment. A lower dose or less frequent dosing should be used.

Administration Oral concentrate: Must be diluted before use. Immediately before administration, use the dropper provided to measure the required amount of concentrate; mix with 4 ounces (1/2 cup) of water, ginger ale, lemon/lime soda, lemonade, or orange juice **only**. Do not mix with any other liquids than these. The dose should be taken immediately after mixing; do not mix in advance. A slight haze may appear after mixing; this is normal. **Note:** Use with caution in patients with latex sensitivity; dropper dispenser contains dry natural rubber.

Monitoring Parameters Monitor nutritional intake and weight; mental status for depression, suicidal ideation, anxiety, social functioning, mania, panic attacks; akathisia

Test Interactions Increased (minor) serum triglycerides, LFTs; decreased serum uric acid; may interfere with urine detection of benzodiazepines (false-positive)

Pharmacotherapy Pearls Buspirone (15-60 mg/day) may be useful in treatment of sexual dysfunction during treatment with a selective serotonin reuptake inhibitor. May exacerbate tics in Tourette's syndrome.

Special Geriatric Considerations Sertraline's favorable side effect profile makes it a preferred SSRI in older adults. It has the shortest half-life of the currently marketed serotonin-reuptake inhibitors. The elderly are more prone to SSRI/SNRI-induced hyponatremia.

◀ **Dosage Forms** Excipient information presented when available (limited, particularly for generics); consult specific product labeling.

Solution, oral [concentrate]: 20 mg/mL (60 mL)

Zoloft®: 20 mg/mL (60 mL) [contains ethanol 12%, natural rubber/natural latex in packaging]

Tablet, oral: 25 mg, 50 mg, 100 mg

Zoloft®: 25 mg, 50 mg, 100 mg [scored]

Selected References

Cohn CK, Shrivastava R, Mendels J, et al, "Double-Blind, Multicenter Comparison of Sertraline and Amitriptyline in Elderly Depressed Patients," *J Clin Psychiatry*, 1990, 51(Suppl B):28-33.

♦ **Sertraline Hydrochloride** *see* Sertraline *on page 1669*

♦ **Serzone** *see* Nefazodone *on page 1276*

Sevelamer (se VEL a mer)

Medication Safety Issues

Sound-alike/look-alike issues:

Renagel® may be confused with Reglan®, Regonol®, Renal Caps, Renvela®

Renvela® may be confused with Reglan®, Regonol®, Renagel®, Renal Caps

Sevelamer may be confused with Savella®

International issues:

Renagel [U.S., Canada, and multiple international markets] may be confused with Remegel brand name for aluminium hydroxide and magnesium carbonate [Netherlands] and for calcium carbonate [Hungary, Great Britain and Ireland] and with Remegel Wind Relief brand name for calcium carbonate and simethicone [Great Britain]

Brand Names: U.S. Renagel®; Renvela®

Brand Names: Canada Renagel®

Index Terms Sevelamer Carbonate; Sevelamer Hydrochloride

Generic Availability (U.S.) No

Pharmacologic Category Phosphate Binder

Use Reduction or control of serum phosphorous in patients with chronic kidney disease on hemodialysis

Contraindications Bowel obstruction

Warnings/Precautions Use with caution in patients with gastrointestinal disorders including dysphagia, swallowing disorders, severe gastrointestinal motility disorders (including constipation), or major gastrointestinal surgery. May cause reductions in vitamin D, E, K, or folic acid absorption. May bind to some drugs in the gastrointestinal tract and decrease their absorption; when changes in absorption of oral medications may have significant clinical consequences (such as antiarrhythmic and antiseizure medications), these medications should be taken at least 1 hour before or 3 hours after a dose of sevelamer. Tablets should not be taken apart or chewed; broken or crushed tablets will rapidly expand in water/saliva and may be a choking hazard.

Adverse Reactions (Reflective of adult population; not specific for elderly)

>10%: Gastrointestinal: Vomiting (22%), nausea (20%), diarrhea (19%), dyspepsia (16%)

1% to 10%:

Endocrine & metabolic: Hypercalcemia (5% to 7%)

Gastrointestinal: Abdominal pain (9%), flatulence (8%), constipation (8%)

Miscellaneous: Peritonitis (peritoneal dialysis): 8%)

Drug Interactions

Avoid Concomitant Use There are no known interactions where it is recommended to avoid concomitant use.

Increased Effect/Toxicity There are no known significant interactions involving an increase in effect.

Decreased Effect

Sevelamer may decrease the levels/effects of: Calcitriol; Levothyroxine; Mycophenolate; Quinolone Antibiotics

Stability Store at controlled room temperature of 25°C (77°F); excursions permitted to 15°C to 30°C (59°F to 86°F). Protect from moisture.

Mechanism of Action Sevelamer (a polymeric compound) binds phosphate within the intestinal lumen, limiting absorption and decreasing serum phosphate concentrations without altering calcium, aluminum, or bicarbonate concentrations.

Pharmacodynamics/Kinetics

Absorption: Not systemically absorbed

Excretion: Feces

Dosage

Geriatric & Adult Note: The dosing of sevelamer carbonate and sevelamer hydrochloride are similar; when switching from one product to another, the same dose (on a mg per mg basis) should be utilized.

Control of serum phosphorous: Oral:

Patients not taking a phosphate binder: 800-1600 mg 3 times/day with meals; the initial dose may be based on serum phosphorous levels:

>5.5 mg/dL to <7.5 mg/dL: 800 mg 3 times/day

≥7.5 mg/dL to <9.0 mg/dL: 1200-1600 mg 3 times/day

≥9.0 mg/dL: 1600 mg 3 times/day

Maintenance dose adjustment based on serum phosphorous concentration (goal range of 3.5-5.5 mg/dL; maximum dose studied was equivalent to 13 g/day [sevelamer hydrochloride] or 14 g/day [sevelamer carbonate]):

>5.5 mg/dL: Increase by 400-800 mg per meal at 2-week intervals

3.5-5.5 mg/dL: Maintain current dose

<3.5 mg/dL: Decrease by 400-800 mg per meal

Dosage adjustment when switching between phosphate-binder products: 667 mg of calcium acetate is equivalent to ~800 mg sevelamer (carbonate or hydrochloride)

Conversion based on dose per meal:

Calcium acetate 667 mg: Convert to 800 mg Renagel® / Renvela®

Calcium acetate 1334 mg: Convert to 1600 mg Renagel® 800 mg/ Renvela® **or** 1200 mg Renagel® 400 mg

Calcium acetate 2001 mg: Convert to 2400 mg Renagel® 800 mg / Renvela® **or** 2000 mg Renagel® 400 mg

Administration Must be administered with meals. Tablets should be swallowed whole; do not crush, chew, or break.

Monitoring Parameters

Serum chemistries, including bicarbonate and chloride

Serum calcium and phosphorus: Frequency of measurement may be dependent upon the presence and magnitude of abnormalities, the rate of progression of CKD, and the use of treatments for CKD-mineral and bone disorders (KDIGO, 2009):

CKD stage 3: Every 6-12 months

CKD stage 4: Every 3-6 months

CKD stage 5 and 5D: Every 1-3 months

Periodic 24-hour urinary calcium and phosphorus; magnesium; alkaline phosphatase every 12 months or more frequently in the presence of elevated PTH; creatinine, BUN, albumin; intact parathyroid hormone (iPTH) every 3-12 months depending on CKD severity

Reference Range

Corrected total serum calcium (K/DOQI, 2003): CKD stages 3 and 4: 8.4-10.2 mg/dL (2.1-2.6 mmol/L); CKD stage 5: 8.4-9.5 mg/dL (2.1-2.37 mmol/L); KDIGO guidelines recommend maintaining normal ranges for all stages of CKD (3-5D) (KDIGO, 2009)

Phosphorus (K/DOQI, 2003):

CKD stages 3 and 4: 2.7-4.6 mg/dL (0.87-1.48 mmol/L) (adults); maintain within age-appropriate limits (children)

CKD stage 5 (including those treated with dialysis): 3.5-5.5 mg/dL (1.13-1.78 mmol/L) (children >12 years and adults); 4-6 mg/dL (1.29-1.94 mmol/L) (children 1-12 years)

KDIGO guidelines recommend maintaining normal ranges for CKD stages 3-5 and lowering elevated phosphorus levels toward the normal range for CKD stage 5D (KDIGO, 2009)

Serum calcium-phosphorus product (K/DOQI, 2003): CKD stage 3-5: <55 mg^2/dL^2 (children >12 years and adults); <65 mg2/dL2 (children ≤12 years)

PTH: Whole molecule, immunochemiluminometric assay (ICMA): 1.0-5.2 pmol/L; whole molecule, radioimmunoassay (RIA): 10.0-65.0 pg/mL; whole molecule, immunoradiometric, double antibody (IRMA): 1.0-6.0 pmol/L

Target ranges by stage of chronic kidney disease (KDIGO, 2009): CKD stage 3-5: Optimal iPTH is unknown; maintain normal range (assay-dependent); CKD stage 5D: Maintain iPTH within 2-9 times the upper limit of normal for the assay used

Pharmacotherapy Pearls Switching patients from calcium acetate to sevelamer: 667 mg of calcium acetate is equivalent to 800 mg sevelamer

Special Geriatric Considerations No specific dose changes needed for the elderly. Since electrolyte changes (ie, phosphorus, calcium) can have dramatic effects in the elderly, monitor closely.

Dosage Forms Excipient information presented when available (limited, particularly for generics); consult specific product labeling.

Powder for suspension, oral, as carbonate:

Renvela®: 0.8 g/packet (90s); 2.4 g/packet (90s) [contains propylene glycol; citrus-cream flavor]

◀ Tablet, oral, as carbonate:
Renvela®: 800 mg
Tablet, oral, as hydrochloride:
Renagel®: 400 mg, 800 mg

Selected References
Delmez J, Block G, Robertson J, et al, "A Randomized, Double-Blind, Crossover Design Study of Sevelamer Hydrochloride and Sevelamer Carbonate in Patients on Hemodialysis," *Clin Nephrol*, 2007, 68(6):386-91.

Sildenafil (sil DEN a fil)

Medication Safety Issues
Sound-alike/look-alike issues:
Revatio® may be confused with ReVia®, Revonto™
Sildenafil may be confused with silodosin, tadalafil, vardenafil
Viagra® may be confused with Allegra®, Vaniqa®

Brand Names: U.S. Revatio®; Viagra®
Brand Names: Canada ratio-Sildenafil R; Revatio®; Viagra®
Index Terms Sildenafil Citrate; UK92480
Generic Availability (U.S.) No
Pharmacologic Category Phosphodiesterase-5 Enzyme Inhibitor
Use
Revatio®: Treatment of pulmonary arterial hypertension (PAH) (WHO Group I) to improve exercise ability and delay clinical worsening
Viagra®: Treatment of erectile dysfunction (ED)

Unlabeled/Investigational Use No geriatric-specific information.

Contraindications Hypersensitivity to sildenafil or any component of the formulation; concurrent use (regularly/intermittently) of organic nitrates in any form (eg, nitroglycerin, isosorbide dinitrate); concurrent use with a protease inhibitor regimen when sildenafil used for pulmonary artery hypertension (eg, Revatio®)

Warnings/Precautions Decreases in blood pressure may occur due to vasodilator effects; use with caution in patients with left ventricular outflow obstruction (aortic stenosis or hypertrophic obstructive cardiomyopathy); may be more sensitive to hypotensive actions. Concurrent use with alpha-adrenergic antagonist therapy or substantial ethanol consumption may cause symptomatic hypotension; patients should be hemodynamically stable prior to initiating therapy at the lowest possible dose. Use with caution in patients with hypotension (<90/50 mm Hg); uncontrolled hypertension (>170/110 mm Hg); life-threatening arrhythmias, stroke or MI within the last 6 months; cardiac failure or coronary artery disease causing unstable angina; safety and efficacy have not been studied in these patients. There is a degree of cardiac risk associated with sexual activity; therefore, physicians should consider the cardiovascular status of their patients prior to initiating any treatment for erectile dysfunction. If pulmonary edema occurs when treating pulmonary arterial hypertension (PAH), consider the possibility of pulmonary veno-occlusive disease (PVOD); continued use is not recommended in patient with PVOD.

Sildenafil should be used with caution in patients with anatomical deformation of the penis (angulation, cavernosal fibrosis, or Peyronie's disease) and in patients who have conditions which may predispose them to priapism (sickle cell anemia, multiple myeloma, leukemia). All patients should be instructed to seek medical attention if erection persists >4 hours.

Vision loss may occur rarely and be a sign of nonarteritic anterior ischemic optic neuropathy (NAION). Risk may be increased with history of vision loss. Other risk factors for NAION include low cup-to-disc ratio ("crowded disc"), coronary artery disease, diabetes, hypertension, hyperlipidemia, smoking, and age >50 years. May cause dose-related impairment of color discrimination. Use caution in patients with retinitis pigmentosa; a minority have genetic disorders of retinal phosphodiesterases (no safety information available). Sudden decrease or loss of hearing has been reported rarely; hearing changes may be accompanied

SILDENAFIL

by tinnitus and dizziness. A direct relationship between therapy and vision or hearing loss has not been determined.

The potential underlying causes of erectile dysfunction should be evaluated prior to treatment. The safety and efficacy of sildenafil with other treatments for erectile dysfunction have not been established; use is not recommended. Efficacy with concurrent bosentan therapy has not been evaluated; use with caution. Use with caution in patients taking strong CYP3A4 inhibitors or alpha-blockers. Concomitant use with all forms of nitrates is contraindicated. If nitrate administration is medically necessary, it is not known when nitrates can be safely administered following the use of sildenafil (per manufacturer); the ACC/AHA 2007 guidelines supports administration of nitrates only if 24 hours have elapsed.

Avoid abrupt discontinuation, especially if used as monotherapy in PAH as exacerbation may occur. Use caution in patients with bleeding disorders or with active peptic ulcer disease; safety and efficacy have not been established. Efficacy has not been established for treatment of pulmonary hypertension associated with sickle cell disease. Use with caution in the elderly, or patients with renal or hepatic dysfunction; dose adjustment may be needed.

Adverse Reactions (Reflective of adult population; not specific for elderly) Based upon normal doses for either indication or route. (Adverse effects such as flushing, diarrhea, myalgia, and visual disturbances may be increased with doses >100 mg/24 hours.)

>10%:
Central nervous system: Headache (16% to 46%)
Gastrointestinal: Dyspepsia (7% to 17%; dose related)

2% to 10%:
Cardiovascular: Flushing (10%)
Central nervous system: Insomnia (≤7%), pyrexia (6%), dizziness (2%)
Dermatologic: Erythema (6%), rash (2%)
Gastrointestinal: Diarrhea (3% to 9%), gastritis (≤3%)
Genitourinary: Urinary tract infection (3%)
Hepatic: LFTs increased
Neuromuscular & skeletal: Myalgia (≤7%), paresthesia (≤3%)
Ocular: Abnormal vision (color changes, blurred vision, or increased sensitivity to light 3% to 11%; dose related)
Respiratory: Epistaxis (9% to 13%), dyspnea exacerbated (≤7%), nasal congestion (4%), rhinitis (4%), sinusitis (3%)

Drug Interactions
Metabolism/Transport Effects Substrate of CYP2C9 (minor), 3A4 (major); **Inhibits** CYP1A2 (weak), 2C9 (weak), 2C19 (weak), 2D6 (weak), 2E1 (weak), 3A4 (weak)

Avoid Concomitant Use
Avoid concomitant use of Sildenafil with any of the following: Amyl Nitrite; Boceprevir; Phosphodiesterase 5 Inhibitors; Telaprevir; Vasodilators (Organic Nitrates)

Increased Effect/Toxicity
Sildenafil may increase the levels/effects of: Alpha1-Blockers; Amyl Nitrite; Antihypertensives; Bosentan; HMG-CoA Reductase Inhibitors; Phosphodiesterase 5 Inhibitors; Vasodilators (Organic Nitrates)

The levels/effects of Sildenafil may be increased by: Antifungal Agents (Azole Derivatives, Systemic); Boceprevir; CYP3A4 Inhibitors (Moderate); CYP3A4 Inhibitors (Strong); Dasatinib; Erythromycin; Protease Inhibitors; Sapropterin; Telaprevir

Decreased Effect
The levels/effects of Sildenafil may be decreased by: Bosentan; CYP3A4 Inducers (Strong); Cyproterone; Deferasirox; Etravirine; Herbs (CYP3A4 Inducers); Peginterferon Alfa-2b; Tocilizumab

Ethanol/Nutrition/Herb Interactions
Food: Amount and rate of absorption of sildenafil is reduced when taken with a high-fat meal. Serum concentrations/toxicity may be increased with grapefruit juice; avoid concurrent use.
Herb/Nutraceutical: St John's wort may decrease sildenafil levels.

Stability Store at controlled room temperature of 25°C (77°F); excursions permitted to 15°C to 30°C (59°F to 86°F).

Mechanism of Action
Erectile dysfunction: Does not directly cause penile erections, but affects the response to sexual stimulation. The physiologic mechanism of erection of the penis involves release of nitric oxide (NO) in the corpus cavernosum during sexual stimulation. NO then activates the enzyme guanylate cyclase, which results in increased levels of cyclic guanosine monophosphate (cGMP), producing smooth muscle relaxation and inflow of blood to the corpus cavernosum. Sildenafil enhances the effect of NO by inhibiting phosphodiesterase type 5 (PDE-5), which is responsible for degradation of cGMP in the corpus cavernosum; when sexual stimulation causes local release of NO, inhibition of PDE-5 by sildenafil causes

1675

increased levels of cGMP in the corpus cavernosum, resulting in smooth muscle relaxation and inflow of blood to the corpus cavernosum; at recommended doses, it has no effect in the absence of sexual stimulation.

Pulmonary arterial hypertension (PAH): Inhibits phosphodiesterase type 5 (PDE-5) in smooth muscle of pulmonary vasculature where PDE-5 is responsible for the degradation of cyclic guanosine monophosphate (cGMP). Increased cGMP concentration results in pulmonary vasculature relaxation; vasodilation in the pulmonary bed and the systemic circulation (to a lesser degree) may occur.

Pharmacodynamics/Kinetics

Onset of action: ~60 minutes

Duration: 2-4 hours

Absorption: Rapid; slower with a high-fat meal

Distribution: V_{dss}: 105 L

Protein binding, plasma: ~96%

Metabolism: Hepatic via CYP3A4 (major) and CYP2C9 (minor route); forms N-desmethyl metabolite (active)

Bioavailability: 40% (25% to 63%)

Half-life elimination: ~4 hours; the elderly and those with severe renal impairment have reduced clearance of sildenafil and its active N-desmethyl metabolite

Time to peak: 30-120 minutes; delayed by 60 minutes with a high-fat meal

Excretion: Feces (~80%); urine (~13%)

Dosage

Geriatric Elderly >65 years: Use with caution.

Revatio®: Refer to adult dosing.

Viagra®: Starting dose of 25 mg should be considered.

Adult

Erectile dysfunction (Viagra®): Oral: Usual dose: 50 mg once daily 1 hour (range: 30 minutes to 4 hours) before sexual activity; dosing range: 25-100 mg once daily.

Pulmonary arterial hypertension (PAH) (Revatio®):

I.V.: 10 mg 3 times/day

Oral: 20 mg 3 times/day, taken 4-6 hours apart. **Note:** A delay in clinical worsening was observed in a short-term trial in which most patients achieved a target dose of 80 mg 3 times daily (unlabeled dose). The patients had an incremental dosage escalation while on a stable epoprostenol regimen (Simonneau, 2008).

Dosage considerations for patients stable on alpha-blockers: Viagra®: Initial: 25 mg

Dosage adjustment for concomitant use of potent CYP34A inhibitors:

Revatio®:

Erythromycin: No dosage adjustment

Itraconazole, ketoconazole: Not recommended

Viagra®:

Erythromycin, itraconazole, ketoconazole: Starting dose of 25 mg should be considered

Protease inhibitors: Maximum sildenafil dose: 25 mg every 48 hours

Renal Impairment

Revatio®: Dose adjustment not necessary

Viagra®: Cl_{cr} <30 mL/minute: Starting dose of 25 mg should be considered.

Hepatic Impairment

Revatio®: Child-Pugh class A and B: Dose adjustment not necessary; not studied in severe impairment (Child-Pugh class C).

Viagra®: Child-Pugh class A and B: Starting dose of 25 mg should be considered; not studied in severe impairment (Child-Pugh class C).

Administration

Revatio®: Administer tablets without regard to meals at least 4-6 hours apart. Administer injection as an I.V. bolus.

Viagra®: Administer orally 30 minutes to 4 hours before sexual activity

Pharmacotherapy Pearls Sildenafil is ~10 times more selective for PDE-5 as compared to PDE6. This enzyme is found in the retina and is involved in phototransduction. At higher plasma levels, interference with PDE6 is believed to be the basis for changes in color vision noted in some patients.

Special Geriatric Considerations Since the elderly often have concomitant diseases, many of which may contraindicate the use of sildenafil, a thorough knowledge of diseases and medications used must be assessed. Adjust dose for renal/hepatic function.

Dosage Forms Excipient information presented when available (limited, particularly for generics); consult specific product labeling.

Injection, solution:

Revatio®: 0.8 mg/mL (12.5 mL)

Tablet, oral:
Revatio®: 20 mg
Viagra®: 25 mg, 50 mg, 100 mg

Selected References

Galie N, Ghofrani HA, Torbicki A, et al, "Sildenafil Citrate Therapy for Pulmonary Arterial Hypertension," *N Engl J Med*, 2005, 353(20):2148-57.

Geelen P, Drolet B, Rail J, et al, "Sildenafil (Viagra) Prolongs Cardiac Repolarization by Blocking the Rapid Component of the Delayed Rectifier Potassium Current," *Circulation*, 2000, 102(3):275-7.

Ishikura F, Beppu S, Hamada T, et al, "Effects of Sildenafil Citrate (Viagra) Combined With Nitrate on the Heart," *Circulation*, 2000, 102(20):2516-21.

Phillips BG, Kato M, Pesek CA, et al, "Sympathetic Activation by Sildenafil," *Circulation*, 2000, 102(25):3068-73.

Traverse JH, Chen YJ, Du R, et al, "Cyclic Nucleotide Phosphodiesterase Type 5 Activity Limits Blood Flow to Hypoperfused Myocardium During Exercise," *Circulation*, 2000, 102(24):2997-3002.

◆ **Sildenafil Citrate** *see* Sildenafil *on page 1674*
◆ **Silenor®** *see* Doxepin (Systemic) *on page 564*
◆ **Silexin [OTC]** *see* Guaifenesin and Dextromethorphan *on page 848*
◆ **Silfedrine Children's [OTC]** *see* Pseudoephedrine *on page 1545*

Silodosin (SI lo doe sin)

Related Information

Pharmacotherapy of Urinary Incontinence *on page 2032*

Medication Safety Issues

Sound-alike/look-alike issues:
Rapaflo™ may be confused with Rapamune®, Raptiva®
Silodosin may be confused with sildenafil

Brand Names: U.S. Rapaflo®

Index Terms KMD 3213

Generic Availability (U.S.) No

Pharmacologic Category Alpha$_1$ Blocker

Use Treatment of signs and symptoms of benign prostatic hyperplasia (BPH)

Contraindications Concurrent use with strong CYP3A4 inhibitors (eg, clarithromycin, itraconazole, ketoconazole, ritonavir); severe renal impairment (Cl$_{cr}$ <30 mL/minute); severe hepatic impairment (Child-Pugh class C)

Warnings/Precautions Not intended for use as an antihypertensive drug. May cause significant orthostatic hypotension and syncope, especially with first dose; anticipate a similar effect if therapy is interrupted for a few days, if dosage is rapidly increased, or if another antihypertensive drug (particularly vasodilators) or a PDE-5 inhibitor (eg, sildenafil, tadalafil, vardenafil) is introduced. "First-dose" orthostatic hypotension may occur 4-8 hours after dosing; may be dose related. Patients should be cautioned about performing hazardous tasks when starting new therapy or adjusting dosage upward. Rule out prostatic carcinoma before beginning therapy with silodosin. Intraoperative floppy iris syndrome has been observed in cataract surgery patients who were on or were previously treated with alpha$_1$-blockers; causality has not been established and there appears to be no benefit in discontinuing alpha-blocker therapy prior to surgery. Use with caution in patients with mild-to-moderate hepatic impairment; contraindicated with severe impairment; not studied. Use with caution in patients with moderate renal impairment; dosage adjustment recommended. Contraindicated in patients with severe impairment (Cl$_{cr}$ <30 mL/minute). Not indicated for use in women.

Adverse Reactions (Reflective of adult population; not specific for elderly)

>10%: Miscellaneous: Retrograde ejaculation (28%)

1% to 10%:
Cardiovascular: Orthostatic hypotension (3%)
Central nervous system: Dizziness (3%), headache (2%), insomnia (1% to 2%)
Gastrointestinal: Diarrhea (3%), abdominal pain (1% to 2%)
Genitourinary: PSA increased (1% to 2%)
Neuromuscular & skeletal: Weakness (1% to 2%)
Respiratory: Nasal congestion (2%), nasopharyngitis (2%), rhinorrhea (1% to 2%), sinusitis (1% to 2%)

Drug Interactions

Metabolism/Transport Effects Substrate of CYP3A4, UGT2B7, P-glycoprotein

Avoid Concomitant Use
Avoid concomitant use of Silodosin with any of the following: Alpha1-Blockers; CYP3A4 Inhibitors (Strong); P-Glycoprotein Inhibitors

◀

Increased Effect/Toxicity
Silodosin may increase the levels/effects of: Alpha1-Blockers; Calcium Channel Blockers

The levels/effects of Silodosin may be increased by: Beta-Blockers; CYP3A4 Inhibitors (Moderate); CYP3A4 Inhibitors (Strong); Dasatinib; MAO Inhibitors; P-Glycoprotein Inhibitors; Phosphodiesterase 5 Inhibitors

Decreased Effect
The levels/effects of Silodosin may be decreased by: CYP3A4 Inducers (Strong); Deferasirox; Herbs (CYP3A4 Inducers); P-Glycoprotein Inducers; Tocilizumab

Ethanol/Nutrition/Herb Interactions
Food: AUC decrease by 4% to 49% and C_{max} decreased by ~18% to 43% with moderate calorie/fat meal.
Herb/Nutraceutical: Avoid St. John's wort (may decrease the levels/effects of silodosin). Avoid herbs with hypotensive properties (black cohosh, California poppy, coleus, golden seal, hawthorn, mistletoe, periwinkle, quinine, Shepherd's purse); may enhance the hypotensive effect of silodosin. Avoid saw palmetto (due to limited experience with this combination).

Stability Store at room temperature of 25°C (77°F); excursions permitted to 15°C to 30°C (59°F to 86°F). Protect from light. Protect from moisture.

Mechanism of Action Silodosin is a selective antagonist of alpha$_{1A}$-adrenoreceptors in the prostate and bladder. Smooth muscle tone in the prostate is mediated by alpha$_{1A}$-adrenoreceptors; blocking them leads to relaxation of smooth muscle in the bladder neck and prostate causing an improvement of urine flow and decreased symptoms of BPH. Approximately 75% of the alpha1-receptors in the prostate are of the alpha$_{1A}$ subtype.

Pharmacodynamics/Kinetics
Distribution: V_d: 49.5 L
Protein binding: ~97%
Metabolism: Extensive, via CYP3A4, glucuronidation, and alcohol and aldehyde dehydrogenase pathways; KMD-3213G (active *in vitro*) and KMD-3293 (not significant) metabolites formed
Bioavailability: ~32%
Half-life elimination: Healthy volunteers: Silodosin: 5-21 hours; KMD-3213G: ~24 hours
Time to peak, plasma: ~3 hours
Excretion: Feces (55%); urine (34%)

Dosage
Geriatric & Adult BPH: Oral: 8 mg once daily with a meal
Renal Impairment
Cl$_{cr}$ >50 mL/minute: No adjustment needed.
Cl$_{cr}$ 30-50 mL/minute: 4 mg once daily.
Cl$_{cr}$ <30 mL/minute: Use is contraindicated.
Hepatic Impairment
Mild-to-moderate impairment (Child-Pugh classes A and B): No adjustment needed.
Severe impairment (Child-Pugh class C): Use is contraindicated.

Administration Administer once daily with a meal.

Monitoring Parameters Blood pressure; urinary symptoms

Special Geriatric Considerations See Dosage: Renal Impairment. In clinical studies, older men had a higher incidence of orthostatic hypotension when using silodosin.

Dosage Forms Excipient information presented when available (limited, particularly for generics); consult specific product labeling.
Capsule, oral:
Rapaflo®: 4 mg, 8 mg

Selected References
Chang DF and Campbell JR, "Intraoperative Floppy Iris Syndrome Associated With Tamsulosin," *J Cataract Refract Surg,* 2005, 31(4):664-73.

◆ **Silphen [OTC]** *see* DiphenhydrAMINE (Systemic) *on page 520*
◆ **Silphen-DM [OTC]** *see* Dextromethorphan *on page 490*
◆ **Siltussin DAS [OTC] [DSC]** *see* GuaiFENesin *on page 846*
◆ **Siltussin DM [OTC]** *see* Guaifenesin and Dextromethorphan *on page 848*
◆ **Siltussin DM DAS [OTC]** *see* Guaifenesin and Dextromethorphan *on page 848*
◆ **Siltussin SA [OTC]** *see* GuaiFENesin *on page 846*
◆ **Silvadene®** *see* Silver Sulfadiazine *on page 1678*

Silver Sulfadiazine (SIL ver sul fa DYE a zeen)

Brand Names: U.S. Silvadene®; SSD AF®; SSD®; Thermazene®
Brand Names: Canada Flamazine®
Generic Availability (U.S.) Yes

Pharmacologic Category Antibiotic, Topical

Use Prevention and treatment of infection in second and third degree burns

Contraindications Hypersensitivity to silver sulfadiazine or any component of the formulation

Warnings/Precautions Use with caution in patients with G6PD deficiency, renal impairment, or history of allergy to other sulfonamides; sulfadiazine may accumulate in patients with impaired hepatic or renal function. Prolonged use may result in fungal or bacterial super-infection, including *C. difficile*-associated diarrhea (CDAD) and pseudomembranous colitis; CDAD has been observed >2 months postantibiotic treatment. Use of analgesic might be needed before application; systemic absorption may be significant and adverse reactions may occur

Adverse Reactions (Reflective of adult population; not specific for elderly) Frequency not defined.

Dermatologic: Discoloration of skin, erythema multiforme, itching, photosensitivity, rash

Hematologic: Agranulocytosis, aplastic anemia, hemolytic anemia, leukopenia

Hepatic: Hepatitis

Renal: Interstitial nephritis

Miscellaneous: Allergic reactions may be related to sulfa component

Drug Interactions

Avoid Concomitant Use

Avoid concomitant use of Silver Sulfadiazine with any of the following: BCG

Increased Effect/Toxicity There are no known significant interactions involving an increase in effect.

Decreased Effect

Silver Sulfadiazine may decrease the levels/effects of: BCG

Stability Silvadene® cream will occasionally darken either in the jar or after application to the skin. This color change results from a light catalyzed reaction which is a common characteristic of all silver salts. A similar analogy is the oxidation of silverware. The product of this color change reaction is silver oxide which ranges in color from gray to black. Silver oxide has rarely been associated with permanent skin discoloration. Additionally, the antimicrobial activity of the product is not substantially diminished because the color change reaction involves such a small amount of the active drug and is largely a surface phenomenon.

Mechanism of Action Acts upon the bacterial cell wall and cell membrane. Bactericidal for many gram-negative and gram-positive bacteria and is effective against yeast. Active against *Pseudomonas aeruginosa*, *Pseudomonas maltophilia*, *Enterobacter* species, *Klebsiella* species, *Serratia* species, *Escherichia coli*, *Proteus mirabilis*, *Morganella morganii*, *Providencia rettgeri*, *Proteus vulgaris*, *Providencia* species, *Citrobacter* species, *Acinetobacter calcoaceticus*, *Staphylococcus aureus*, *Staphylococcus epidermidis*, *Enterococcus* species, *Candida albicans*, *Corynebacterium diphtheriae*, and *Clostridium perfringens*

Pharmacodynamics/Kinetics

Absorption: Significant percutaneous absorption of silver sulfadiazine can occur especially when applied to extensive burns

Half-life elimination: 10 hours; prolonged with renal impairment

Time to peak, serum: 3-11 days of continuous therapy

Excretion: Urine (~50% as unchanged drug)

Dosage

Geriatric & Adult Antiseptic, burns: Topical: Apply once or twice daily

Administration Apply with a sterile-gloved hand. Apply to a thickness 1/16". Burned area should be covered with cream at all times.

Monitoring Parameters Serum electrolytes, urinalysis, renal function tests, CBC in patients with extensive burns on long-term treatment

Pharmacotherapy Pearls Contains methylparaben and propylene glycol

Special Geriatric Considerations No specific recommendations for use in the elderly.

Dosage Forms Excipient information presented when available (limited, particularly for generics); consult specific product labeling.

Cream, topical: 1% (20 g, 25 g, 50 g, 85 g, 400 g)

Silvadene®: 1% (20 g, 50 g, 85 g, 400 g, 1000 g)

SSD AF®: 1% (50 g, 400 g)

SSD®: 1% (25 g, 50 g, 85 g, 400 g)

Thermazene®: 1% (20 g, 50 g, 85 g, 400 g, 1000 g)

◆ **Simcor®** see Niacin and Simvastatin on page 1292

Simethicone (sye METH i kone)

Medication Safety Issues

Sound-alike/look-alike issues:

Simethicone may be confused with cimetidine

Mylanta® may be confused with Mynatal®
Mylicon® may be confused with Modicon®, Myleran®
Phazyme® may be confused with Pherazine®

Brand Names: U.S. Equalizer Gas Relief [OTC]; Gas Free Extra Strength [OTC]; Gas Relief Ultra Strength [OTC]; Gas-X® Children's Tongue Twisters™ [OTC]; Gas-X® Extra Strength [OTC]; Gas-X® Maximum Strength [OTC]; Gas-X® Thin Strips™ [OTC]; Gas-X® [OTC]; Gax-X® Infant [OTC]; Infantaire Gas [OTC]; Infants Gas Relief Drops [OTC]; Little Tummys® Gas Relief [OTC]; Mi-Acid Gas Relief [OTC]; Mylanta® Gas Maximum Strength [OTC]; Mylicon® Infants' [OTC]; Phazyme® Ultra Strength [OTC]

Brand Names: Canada Ovol®; Phazyme™

Index Terms Activated Dimethicone; Activated Methylpolysiloxane

Generic Availability (U.S.) Yes

Pharmacologic Category Antiflatulent

Use Postoperative gas pain or for use in endoscopic examination; relief of bloating, pressure, and discomfort of gas

Contraindications Hypersensitivity to simethicone or any component of the formulation

Adverse Reactions (Reflective of adult population; not specific for elderly) No data reported

Drug Interactions

    Avoid Concomitant Use There are no known interactions where it is recommended to avoid concomitant use.

    Increased Effect/Toxicity There are no known significant interactions involving an increase in effect.

    Decreased Effect There are no known significant interactions involving a decrease in effect.

Ethanol/Nutrition/Herb Interactions Food: Avoid carbonated beverages and gas-forming foods.

Stability Store at room temperature. Avoid high humidity and excessive heat.

Mechanism of Action Decreases the surface tension of gas bubbles thereby disperses and prevents gas pockets in the GI system

Pharmacodynamics/Kinetics Elimination: In feces

Dosage

    Geriatric & Adult Flatulence/bloating: Oral: 40-360 mg after meals and at bedtime, as needed

Administration Shake oral suspension (drops) before using; mix with water or other liquids.

Monitoring Parameters Monitor for feelings of relief, decreased pain, bloating

Special Geriatric Considerations Before treating excess gas or pain due to gas accumulation, a thorough evaluation must be made to determine cause since many bowel diseases may present with flatulence and bloating.

Dosage Forms Excipient information presented when available (limited, particularly for generics); consult specific product labeling.

Capsule, softgel, oral:
    Gas Free Extra Strength: 125 mg
    Gas Relief Ultra Strength: 180 mg
    Gas-X® Extra Strength: 125 mg
    Gas-X® Maximum Strength: 166 mg
    Mylanta® Gas Maximum Strength: 125 mg
    Phazyme® Ultra Strength: 180 mg

Strip, orally disintegrating, oral:
    Gas-X® Children's Tongue Twisters™: 40 mg (16s) [cinnamon flavor]
    Gas-X® Thin Strips™: 62.5 mg (18s) [cinnamon flavor]
    Gas-X® Thin Strips™: 62.5 mg (18s, 32s) [peppermint flavor]

Suspension, oral [drops]: 40 mg/0.6 mL (30 mL)
    Equalizer Gas Relief: 40 mg/0.6 mL (30 mL) [contains sodium 0.15 mg/0.6 mL]
    Gax-X® Infant: 40 mg/0.6 mL (30 mL) [ethanol free; contains sodium benzoate]
    Infantaire Gas: 40 mg/0.6 mL (30 mL)
    Infants Gas Relief Drops: 40 mg/0.6 mL (30 mL) [vanilla flavor]
    Little Tummys® Gas Relief: 40 mg/0.6 mL (30 mL, 45 mL) [dye free, ethanol free; contains sodium benzoate; strawberry flavor]
    Mylicon® Infants': 40 mg/0.6 mL (15 mL, 30 mL) [dye free, ethanol free; contains sodium benzoate; non-staining formula]
    Mylicon® Infants': 40 mg/0.6 mL (15 mL, 30 mL) [ethanol free; contains sodium benzoate]

Tablet, chewable, oral: 80 mg, 125 mg
    Gas-X®: 80 mg [scored; contains calcium 30 mg/tablet; cherry crème flavor]
    Gas-X®: 80 mg [contains calcium 30 mg/tablet; peppermint crème flavor]
    Gas-X® Extra Strength: 125 mg [contains calcium 45 mg/tablet; cherry crème flavor]
    Gas-X® Extra Strength: 125 mg [contains calcium 45 mg/tablet; peppermint crème flavor]

Mi-Acid Gas Relief: 80 mg
Mylanta® Gas Maximum Strength: 125 mg [scored; cherry flavor]
Mylanta® Gas Maximum Strength: 125 mg [mint flavor]

♦ **Simethicone, Aluminum Hydroxide, and Magnesium Hydroxide** *see* Aluminum Hydroxide, Magnesium Hydroxide, and Simethicone *on page 84*
♦ **Simethicone and Loperamide Hydrochloride** *see* Loperamide and Simethicone *on page 1087*
♦ **Simethicone and Magaldrate** *see* Magaldrate and Simethicone *on page 1107*
♦ **Simply Saline® [OTC]** *see* Sodium Chloride *on page 1690*
♦ **Simply Saline® Baby [OTC]** *see* Sodium Chloride *on page 1690*
♦ **Simply Saline® Nasal Moist® [OTC]** *see* Sodium Chloride *on page 1690*
♦ **Simply Sleep® [OTC]** *see* DiphenhydrAMINE (Systemic) *on page 520*
♦ **Simponi®** *see* Golimumab *on page 837*
♦ **Simuc-DM [DSC]** *see* Guaifenesin and Dextromethorphan *on page 848*

Simvastatin (sim va STAT in)

Related Information
Hyperlipidemia Management *on page 2021*
Medication Safety Issues
Sound-alike/look-alike issues:
Simvastatin may be confused with atorvastatin, nystatin, pitavastatin
Zocor® may be confused with Cozaar®, Lipitor®, Yocon®, Zoloft®, ZyrTEC®
International issues:
Cardin [Poland] may be confused with Cardem brand name for celiprolol [Spain]; Cardene brand name for nicardipine [U.S., Great Britain, Netherlands]
Brand Names: U.S. Zocor®
Brand Names: Canada Apo-Simvastatin®; CO Simvastatin; Dom-Simvastatin; JAMP-Simvastatin; Mylan-Simvastatin; Nu-Simvastatin; PHL-Simvastatin; PMS-Simvastatin; RAN™-Simvastatin; ratio-Simvastatin; Riva-Simvastatin; Sandoz-Simvastatin; Taro-Simvastatin; Teva-Simvastatin; Zocor®; ZYM-Simvastatin
Generic Availability (U.S.) Yes
Pharmacologic Category Antilipemic Agent, HMG-CoA Reductase Inhibitor
Use Used with dietary therapy for the following:
Secondary prevention of cardiovascular events in hypercholesterolemic patients with established coronary heart disease (CHD) or at high risk for CHD: To reduce cardiovascular morbidity (myocardial infarction, coronary/noncoronary revascularization procedures) and mortality; to reduce the risk of stroke
Hyperlipidemias: To reduce elevations in total cholesterol (total-C), LDL-C, apolipoprotein B, triglycerides, and VLDL-C, and to increase HDL-C in patients with primary hypercholesterolemia (elevations of 1 or more components are present in Fredrickson type IIa, IIb, III, and IV hyperlipidemias); treatment of homozygous familial hypercholesterolemia
Heterozygous familial hypercholesterolemia (HeFH): In adolescent patients (10-17 years of age, females >1 year postmenarche) with HeFH having LDL-C ≥190 mg/dL **or** LDL-C ≥160 mg/dL with positive family history of premature cardiovascular disease (CVD), or 2 or more CVD risk factors in the adolescent patient
Contraindications Hypersensitivity to simvastatin or any component of the formulation; active liver disease; unexplained persistent elevations of serum transaminases; concomitant use of strong CYP3A4 inhibitors (eg, clarithromycin, erythromycin, HIV protease inhibitors, itraconazole, ketoconazole, nefazodone, posaconazole, telithromycin), cyclosporine, danazol, and gemfibrozil
Warnings/Precautions Secondary causes of hyperlipidemia should be ruled out prior to therapy. Liver function must be monitored by laboratory assessment. Rhabdomyolysis with acute renal failure has occurred. Risk is dose-related and is increased with high doses (80 mg), concurrent use of lipid-lowering agents which may cause rhabdomyolysis (gemfibrozil, other fibric acid derivatives, or niacin at doses ≥1 g/day) or moderate-to-strong CYP3A4 inhibitors (including amiodarone, cyclosporine, grapefruit juice in large quantities, or verapamil), age >65, female gender, uncontrolled hypothyroidism, and renal dysfunction. If concurrent use of a contraindicated interacting medication is unavoidable, treatment with simvastatin should be suspended during use or consider the use of an alternative HMG-CoA reductase inhibitor void of CYP3A4 metabolism. Monitor closely if used with other drugs associated with myopathy (eg, colchicine). Weigh the risk versus benefit when combining any of these drugs with simvastatin. The manufacturer recommends temporary discontinuation for elective major surgery, acute medical or surgical conditions, or in any patient experiencing an acute or serious condition predisposing to renal failure (eg, sepsis, hypotension, trauma, uncontrolled seizures). However, based upon current evidence, HMG-CoA reductase inhibitor

therapy should be continued in the perioperative period unless risk outweighs cardioprotective benefit. Use with caution in patients who consume large amounts of ethanol or have a history of liver disease. Use is contraindicated with active liver disease and with unexplained transaminase elevations. Concomitant use of high-dose simvastatin (80 mg) and niacin ≥1 g/day may increase risk of myopathy in Chinese patients.

Adverse Reactions (Reflective of adult population; not specific for elderly)

1% to 10%:

Cardiovascular: Atrial fibrillation (6%; placebo 5%), edema (3%; placebo 2%)

Central nervous system: Headache (3% to 7%), vertigo (5%)

Dermatologic: Eczema (5%)

Gastrointestinal: Abdominal pain (7%), constipation (2% to 7%), gastritis (5%), nausea (5%)

Hepatic: Transaminases increased (>3 x ULN; 1%)

Neuromuscular & skeletal: CPK increased (>3 x normal; 5%), myalgia (4%)

Respiratory: Upper respiratory infections (9%), bronchitis (7%)

Additional class-related events or case reports (not necessarily reported with simvastatin therapy): Alteration in taste, anorexia, anxiety, bilirubin increased, cataracts, cholestatic jaundice, cirrhosis, decreased libido, depression, erectile dysfunction/impotence, facial paresis, fatty liver, fulminant hepatic necrosis, gynecomastia, hepatoma, hyperbilirubinemia, impaired extraocular muscle movement, increased CPK (>10 x normal), interstitial lung disease, ophthalmoplegia, peripheral nerve palsy, psychic disturbance, renal failure (secondary to rhabdomyolysis), thyroid dysfunction, tremor, vertigo

Drug Interactions

Metabolism/Transport Effects Substrate of CYP3A4 (major), SLCO1B1; **Inhibits** CYP2C8 (weak), 2C9 (weak), 2D6 (weak)

Avoid Concomitant Use

Avoid concomitant use of Simvastatin with any of the following: Boceprevir; CYP3A4 Inhibitors (Strong); Erythromycin; Gemfibrozil; Protease Inhibitors; Red Yeast Rice; Telaprevir

Increased Effect/Toxicity

Simvastatin may increase the levels/effects of: DAPTOmycin; Diltiazem; Trabectedin; Vitamin K Antagonists

The levels/effects of Simvastatin may be increased by: Amiodarone; AmLODIPine; Antifungal Agents (Azole Derivatives, Systemic); Boceprevir; Colchicine; CycloSPORINE; CycloSPORINE (Systemic); CYP3A4 Inhibitors (Moderate); CYP3A4 Inhibitors (Strong); Cyproterone; Danazol; Dasatinib; Diltiazem; Dronedarone; Eltrombopag; Erythromycin; Fenofibrate; Fenofibric Acid; Fluconazole; Fusidic Acid; Gemfibrozil; Grapefruit Juice; Green Tea; Imatinib; Macrolide Antibiotics; Niacin; Niacinamide; Protease Inhibitors; QuiNINE; Ranolazine; Red Yeast Rice; Rifamycin Derivatives; Sildenafil; Telaprevir; Ticagrelor; Verapamil

Decreased Effect

Simvastatin may decrease the levels/effects of: Lanthanum

The levels/effects of Simvastatin may be decreased by: Antacids; Bosentan; CYP3A4 Inducers (Strong); Deferasirox; Efavirenz; Etravirine; Fosphenytoin; Phenytoin; Rifamycin Derivatives; St Johns Wort; Tocilizumab

Ethanol/Nutrition/Herb Interactions

Ethanol: Avoid excessive ethanol consumption (due to potential hepatic effects).

Food: Simvastatin serum concentration may be increased when taken with grapefruit juice; avoid concurrent intake of large quantities (>1 quart/day). Red yeast rice contains an estimated 2.4 mg lovastatin per 600 mg rice.

Herb/Nutraceutical: St John's wort may decrease simvastatin levels.

Stability Tablets should be stored in tightly-closed containers at temperatures between 5°C to 30°C (41°F to 86°F).

Mechanism of Action Simvastatin is a methylated derivative of lovastatin that acts by competitively inhibiting 3-hydroxy-3-methylglutaryl-coenzyme A (HMG-CoA) reductase, the enzyme that catalyzes the rate-limiting step in cholesterol biosynthesis

Pharmacodynamics/Kinetics

Onset of action: >3 days

Peak effect: 2 weeks

Absorption: 85%

Protein binding: ~95%

Metabolism: Hepatic via CYP3A4; extensive first-pass effect

Bioavailability: <5%

Half-life elimination: Unknown

Time to peak: 1.3-2.4 hours

Excretion: Feces (60%); urine (13%)

Dosage

Geriatric Oral: Initial: Maximum reductions in LDL-cholesterol may be achieved with daily dose ≤20 mg.

Adult Note: Doses should be individualized according to the baseline LDL-cholesterol levels, the recommended goal of therapy, and the patient's response; adjustments should be made at intervals of 4 weeks or more; doses may need adjusted based on concomitant medications

Note: Dosing limitation: Simvastatin 80 mg is limited to patients that have been taking this dose for >12 consecutive months without evidence of myopathy and are not currently taking or beginning to take a simvastatin dose-limiting or contraindicated interacting medication.

Homozygous familial hypercholesterolemia: Oral: 40 mg once daily in the evening

Prevention of cardiovascular events, hyperlipidemias: Oral: 20-40 mg once daily in the evening; range: 5-40 mg/day

Patients requiring only moderate reduction of LDL-cholesterol: May be started at 10 mg once daily in the evening

Patients requiring reduction of >45% in low-density lipoprotein (LDL) cholesterol: May be started at 40 mg once daily in the evening

Patients with CHD or at high risk for CHD: Dosing should be started at 40 mg once daily in the evening; simvastatin should be started simultaneously with diet therapy.

Dosage adjustment for simvastatin with concomitant medications:

Amiodarone, diltiazem or verapamil: Simvastatin dose should **not** exceed 10 mg/day

Amlodipine or ranolazine: Simvastatin dose should **not** exceed 20 mg/day

Dosage adjustment in Chinese patients on niacin doses ≥1 g/day: Use caution with simvastatin doses exceeding 20 mg/day; because of an increased risk of myopathy, do not administer simvastatin 80 mg concurrently.

Renal Impairment Because simvastatin does not undergo significant renal excretion, modification of dose should not be necessary in patients with mild-to-moderate renal insufficiency.

Severe renal impairment: Cl_{cr} <10 mL/minute: Initial: 5 mg/day with close monitoring.

Administration May be administered without regard to meals. Administer in the evening for maximal efficacy.

Monitoring Parameters Serum cholesterol (total and fractionated); baseline CPK (recheck CPK in any patient with symptoms suggestive of myopathy)

Obtain liver function tests prior to initiation and thereafter when clinically indicated. Patients with elevated transaminase levels should have a second (confirmatory) test and frequent monitoring until values normalize. Discontinue if increase in ALT/AST is persistently >3 times ULN. Monitor LDL-C at intervals no less than 4 weeks.

Special Geriatric Considerations Effective and well tolerated in the elderly. The definition of and, therefore, when to treat hyperlipidemia in the elderly is a controversial issue. The National Cholesterol Education Program recommends that all adults maintain a plasma cholesterol <160 mg/dL. In elderly patients with one additional risk factor, goal LDL would be <130 mg/dL. It is the authors' belief that pharmacologic treatment be reserved for those who are unable to obtain a desirable plasma cholesterol concentration by diet alone and for whom the benefits of treatment are believed to outweigh the potential adverse effects, drug interactions, and cost of treatment. Age ≥65 years is a risk factor for myopathy.

Dosage Forms Excipient information presented when available (limited, particularly for generics); consult specific product labeling.

Tablet, oral: 5 mg, 10 mg, 20 mg, 40 mg, 80 mg

Zocor®: 5 mg, 10 mg, 20 mg, 40 mg, 80 mg

Selected References

Bach LA, Cooper ME, O'Brien RC, et al, "The Use of Simvastatin, an HMG-CoA Reductase Inhibitor, in Older Patients With Hypercholesterolemia and Atherosclerosis," *J Am Geriatr Soc*, 1990, 38(1):10-4.

Fleisher LA, Beckman JA, Brown KA, et al, "ACC/AHA 2007 Guidelines on Perioperative Cardiovascular Evaluation and Care for Noncardiac Surgery: A Report of the American College of Cardiology/American Heart Association Task Force on Practice Guidelines (Writing Committee to Revise the 2002 Guidelines on Perioperative Cardiovascular Evaluation for Noncardiac Surgery) Developed in Collaboration With the American Society of Echocardiography, American Society of Nuclear Cardiology, Heart Rhythm Society, Society of Cardiovascular Anesthesiologists, Society for Cardiovascular Angiography and Interventions, Society for Vascular Medicine and Biology, and Society for Vascular Surgery," *J Am Coll Cardiol*, 2007, 50(17):e159-241.

Grundy SM, Cleeman JI, Merz CN, et al, "Implications of Recent Clinical Trials for the National Cholesterol Education Program Adult Treatment Panel III Guidelines," *J Am Coll Cardiol*, 2004, 44(3):720-32.

National Cholesterol Education Program (NCEP) Expert Panel on Detection, Evaluation, and Treatment of High Blood Cholesterol in Adults (Adult Treatment Panel III), "Third Report of the National Cholesterol Education Program (NCEP) Expert Panel on Detection, Evaluation, and Treatment of High Blood Cholesterol in Adults (Adult Treatment Panel III) Final Report," *Circulation*, 2002, 106(25):3143-421.

◆ **Simvastatin and Ezetimibe** see Ezetimibe and Simvastatin *on page 691*
◆ **Simvastatin and Niacin** see Niacin and Simvastatin *on page 1292*

- ◆ **Sinemet®** *see* Carbidopa and Levodopa *on page 274*
- ◆ **Sinemet® CR** *see* Carbidopa and Levodopa *on page 274*
- ◆ **Singulair®** *see* Montelukast *on page 1237*
- ◆ **Sinus Pain & Pressure [OTC]** *see* Acetaminophen and Phenylephrine *on page 38*
- ◆ **Sinutab® Sinus [OTC]** *see* Acetaminophen and Phenylephrine *on page 38*

Sipuleucel-T (si pu LOO sel tee)

Medication Safety Issues
Other safety concerns:
For autologous use only; patient identity must be matched to the patient identifiers on the infusion bag and on the "Cell Product Disposition Form" prior to infusion. Healthcare providers should apply universal precautions when handling both the initial leukapheresis product and the activated product.

Brand Names: U.S. Provenge®
Index Terms APC8015; Prostate Cancer Vaccine, Cell-Based
Generic Availability (U.S.) No
Pharmacologic Category Cellular Immunotherapy, Autologous
Use Treatment of metastatic hormone-refractory prostate cancer in patients who are asymptomatic or minimally symptomatic
Prescribing and Access Restrictions Patients may currently receive Sipuleucel-T at one of the ~50 sites that participated in the clinical trials until the program is expanded to additional sites. Physicians must go through an inservice and register to prescribe the treatment; patients must also complete an enrollment form. Information on registration and enrollment is available at 1-877-336-3736.

Dosage
Geriatric & Adult Note: Premedicate with oral acetaminophen 650 mg and an antihistamine (eg, diphenhydramine 50 mg) ~30 minutes prior to infusion. For autologous use only.
Prostate cancer, metastatic: I.V.: Each dose contains ≥50 million autologous CD54+ cells (obtained through leukapheresis) activated with PAP-GM-CSF; administer doses at ~2 week intervals for a total of 3 doses
Dosage Forms Excipient information presented when available (limited, particularly for generics); consult specific product labeling.
Infusion, premixed in LR [preservative free]:
Provenge®: ≥50 million autologous CD54$^+$ cells activated with PAP-GM-CSF (250 mL)

- ◆ **Sirdalud®** *see* TiZANidine *on page 1808*

SitaGLIPtin (sit a GLIP tin)

Related Information
Diabetes Mellitus Management, Adults *on page 2073*
Medication Safety Issues
Sound-alike/look-alike issues:
Januvia® may be confused with Enjuvia™, Janumet®, Jantoven™
SitaGLIPtin may be confused with saxagliptin, SUMAtriptan

Brand Names: U.S. Januvia®
Brand Names: Canada Januvia®
Index Terms MK-0431; Sitagliptin Phosphate
Generic Availability (U.S.) No
Pharmacologic Category Antidiabetic Agent, Dipeptidyl Peptidase IV (DPP-IV) Inhibitor
Use Management of type 2 diabetes mellitus (noninsulin dependent, NIDDM) as an adjunct to diet and exercise as monotherapy or in combination therapy with other antidiabetic agents
Medication Guide Available Yes
Contraindications Serious hypersensitivity (eg, anaphylaxis, angioedema) to sitagliptin or any component of the formulation
Warnings/Precautions Avoid use in type 1 diabetes mellitus (insulin dependent, IDDM) and diabetic ketoacidosis (DKA) due to lack of efficacy in these populations. Use caution when used in conjunction with insulin or insulin secretagogues; risk of hypoglycemia is increased. Monitor blood glucose closely; dosage adjustments of insulin or insulin secretagogues may be necessary. Use with caution in patients with moderate-to-severe renal dysfunction and end-stage renal disease (ESRD) requiring hemodialysis or peritoneal dialysis; dosing adjustment required. Safety and efficacy have not been established in severe hepatic dysfunction.

Rare hypersensitivity reactions, including anaphylaxis, angioedema, and/or severe dermatologic reactions (such as Stevens-Johnson syndrome), have been reported in postmarketing surveillance; discontinue if signs/symptoms of hypersensitivity reactions occur. Cases of acute pancreatitis (including hemorrhagic and necrotizing with some fatalities) have been reported with use; monitor for signs/symptoms of pancreatitis. Discontinue use immediately if pancreatitis is suspected and initiate appropriate management. Use with caution in patients with a history of pancreatitis (not known if this population is at greater risk).

Clinical trials included only a limited number of patients with heart failure (HF). No specific recommendations regarding this population are provided in the approved U.S. labeling (Canadian labeling recommends against use in this population). Diabetes self-management education (DSME) is essential to maximize the effectiveness of therapy.

Adverse Reactions (Reflective of adult population; not specific for elderly) As reported with monotherapy: 1% to 10%:

Cardiovascular: Peripheral edema (2%)

Endocrine & metabolic: Hypoglycemia (1%)

Gastrointestinal: Diarrhea (4%), constipation (3%), nausea (2%)

Neuromuscular & skeletal: Osteoarthritis (1%)

Respiratory: Nasopharyngitis (5%), pharyngitis (1%), upper respiratory tract infection (viral; 1%)

Drug Interactions

Metabolism/Transport Effects Substrate of CYP2C8 (minor), CYP3A4 (minor), P-glycoprotein

Avoid Concomitant Use There are no known interactions where it is recommended to avoid concomitant use.

Increased Effect/Toxicity

SitaGLIPtin may increase the levels/effects of: ACE Inhibitors; Digoxin; Hypoglycemic Agents

The levels/effects of SitaGLIPtin may be increased by: Herbs (Hypoglycemic Properties); Pegvisomant; P-Glycoprotein Inhibitors

Decreased Effect

The levels/effects of SitaGLIPtin may be decreased by: Corticosteroids (Orally Inhaled); Corticosteroids (Systemic); Luteinizing Hormone-Releasing Hormone Analogs; P-Glycoprotein Inducers; Somatropin; Thiazide Diuretics

Stability Store at 20°C to 25°C (68°F to 77°F); excursions permitted to 15°C to 30°C (59°F to 86°F).

Mechanism of Action Sitagliptin inhibits dipeptidyl peptidase IV (DPP-IV) enzyme resulting in prolonged active incretin levels. Incretin hormones (eg, glucagon-like peptide-1 [GLP-1] and glucose-dependent insulinotropic polypeptide [GIP]) regulate glucose homeostasis by increasing insulin synthesis and release from pancreatic beta cells and decreasing glucagon secretion from pancreatic alpha cells. Decreased glucagon secretion results in decreased hepatic glucose production. Under normal physiologic circumstances, incretin hormones are released by the intestine throughout the day and levels are increased in response to a meal; incretin hormones are rapidly inactivated by the DPP-IV enzyme.

Pharmacodynamics/Kinetics

Absorption: Rapid

Distribution: ~198 L

Protein binding: 38%

Metabolism: Not extensively metabolized; minor metabolism via CYP3A4 and 2C8 to metabolites (inactive) suggested by *in vitro* studies

Bioavailability: ~87%

Half-life elimination: 12 hours

Time to peak, plasma: 1-4 hours

Excretion: Urine 87% (79% as unchanged drug, 16% as metabolites); feces 13%

Dosage

Adult Type 2 diabetes: Oral: 100 mg once daily

Concomitant use with insulin and/or insulin secretagogues (eg, sulfonylureas): Reduced dose of insulin and/or insulin secretagogues may be needed.

Renal Impairment

Cl_{cr} ≥50 mL/minute: No adjustment required

Cl_{cr} ≥30 to <50 mL/minute: 50 mg once daily

S_{cr}: Males: >1.7 to ≤3.0 mg/dL; Females: >1.5 to ≤2.5 mg/dL: 50 mg once daily

Cl_{cr}<30 mL/minute: 25 mg once daily

S_{cr}: Males: >3.0 mg/dL; Females: >2.5 mg/dL: 25 mg once daily

ESRD requiring hemodialysis or peritoneal dialysis: 25 mg once daily; administered without regard to timing of hemodialysis

Hepatic Impairment

Mild-to-moderate impairment (Child-Pugh score 7-9): No dosage adjustment required

Severe impairment (Child-Pugh score >9): Not studied

◀ **Administration** May be administered with or without food.

Monitoring Parameters Hb A$_{1c}$, serum glucose; renal function prior to initiation and periodically during treatment

Reference Range

Recommendations for glycemic control in adults with diabetes:

Hb A$_{1c}$: <7%

Preprandial capillary plasma glucose: 70-130 mg/dL

Peak postprandial capillary blood glucose: <180 mg/dL

Blood pressure: <130/80 mm Hg

Recommendations for glycemic control in older adults with diabetes:

Relatively healthy, cognitively intact, and with a ≥5-year life expectancy: See Adults

Frail, life expectancy <5-years or those for whom the risks of intensive glucose control outweigh the benefits:

Hb A$_{1c}$: <8% to 9%

Blood pressure: <140/80 mm Hg or <130/80 mm Hg if tolerated

Special Geriatric Considerations Sitagliptin has not been studied exclusively in the elderly. The manufacturer reports that 725 out of 3884 patients in clinical trials were >65 years (only 61 were age 75 years and older), with no difference in safety or efficacy compared to younger patients. Intensive glucose control (HbA$_{1c}$ <6.5%) has been linked to increased all-cause and cardiovascular mortality, hypoglycemia requiring assistance, and weight gain in adult type 2 diabetes. How "tightly" to control a geriatric patient's blood glucose needs to be individualized. Such a decision should be based on several factors, including the patient's functional and cognitive status, how well he/she recognizes hypoglycemic or hyperglycemic symptoms, and how to respond to them and other disease states. An HbA$_{1c}$ <7.5% is an acceptable endpoint for a healthy older adult, while <8% is acceptable for frail elderly patients, those with a duration of illness >10 years, or those with comorbid conditions and requiring combination diabetes medications. Patients who are unable to accurately draw up their dose will need assistance, such as prefilled syringes. Initial doses may require considerations for renal function in the elderly with dosing adjusted subsequently based on blood glucose monitoring. For elderly patients with diabetes who are relatively healthy, attaining target goals for aspirin use, blood pressure, lipids, smoking cessation, and diet and exercise may be more important than normalized glycemic control.

Dosage Forms Excipient information presented when available (limited, particularly for generics); consult specific product labeling.

Tablet, oral:

Januvia®: 25 mg, 50 mg, 100 mg

Selected References

Action to Control Cardiovascular Risk in Diabetes Study Group, Gerstein HC, Miller ME, et al, "Effects of Intensive Glucose Lowering in Type 2 Diabetes," *N Engl J Med*, 2008, 358(24):2545-59.

ADVANCE Collaborative Group, Patel A, MacMahon S, et al, "Intensive Blood Glucose Control and Vascular Outcomes in Patients With Type 2 Diabetes," *N Engl J Med*, 2008, 358(24):2560-72.

American Diabetes Association, "Standards of Medical Care in Diabetes – 2011," *Diabetes Care*, 2011, 34(Suppl 1):11-61.

Brown AF, Mangione CM, Saliba D, et al, "Guidelines for Improving the Care of the Older Person With Diabetes Mellitus," *J Am Geriatr Soc*, 2003, 51(5 Suppl Guidelines):265-80.

"VA/DoD Clinical Practice Guideline for the Management of Diabetes Mellitus," 2010. Available at http://www.-healthquality.va.gov/Diabetes_Mellitus.asp

Sitagliptin and Metformin (sit a GLIP tin & met FOR min)

Related Information

MetFORMIN *on page 1155*

SitaGLIPtin *on page 1684*

Medication Safety Issues

Sound-alike/look-alike issues:

Janumet® may be confused with Jantoven™, Januvia®

Brand Names: U.S. Janumet®

Brand Names: Canada Janumet®

Index Terms Metformin and Sitagliptin; Sitagliptin Phosphate and Metformin Hydrochloride

Generic Availability (U.S.) No

Pharmacologic Category Antidiabetic Agent, Biguanide; Antidiabetic Agent, Dipeptidyl Peptidase IV (DPP-IV) Inhibitor; Hypoglycemic Agent, Oral

Use Management of type 2 diabetes mellitus (noninsulin dependent, NIDDM) as an adjunct to diet and exercise in patients not adequately controlled on metformin or sitagliptin monotherapy

Medication Guide Available Yes

Dosage

Geriatric Refer to adult dosing. The initial and maintenance dosing should be conservative, due to the potential for decreased renal function (monitor). Do not use in patients ≥80 years of age unless normal renal function has been established.

Adult Note: Patients receiving concomitant insulin and/or insulin secretagogues (eg, sulfonylureas) may require dosage adjustments of these agents.

Type 2 diabetes mellitus: Oral: Initial doses should be based on current dose of sitagliptin and metformin; daily doses should be divided and given twice daily with meals. Maximum: Sitagliptin 100 mg/metformin 2000 mg daily

  Patients inadequately controlled on metformin alone: Initial dose: Sitagliptin 100 mg/day plus current dose of metformin. **Note:** The U.S. labeling recommends that patients currently receiving metformin 850 mg twice daily receive an initial dose of sitagliptin 50 mg and metformin 1000 mg twice daily

  Patients inadequately controlled on sitagliptin alone: Initial dose: Metformin 1000 mg/day plus sitagliptin 100 mg/day. **Note:** Patients currently receiving a renally adjusted dose of sitagliptin should not be switched to combination product.

Dosing adjustment: Metformin component may be gradually increased up to the maximum dose. Maximum dose: Sitagliptin 100 mg/metformin 2000 mg daily

Renal Impairment Do not use with renal disease or renal dysfunction (serum creatinine ≥1.5 mg/dL [≥136 μmol/L] in males or ≥1.4 mg/dL [≥124 μmol/L] in females or abnormal clearance).

Hepatic Impairment Avoid metformin; liver disease is a risk factor for the development of lactic acidosis during metformin therapy.

Special Geriatric Considerations Sitagliptin has not been studied exclusively in the elderly. The manufacturer reports that 725 out of 3884 patients in clinical trials were >65 years of age (only 61 were ≥75 years), with no difference in safety or efficacy compared to younger patients. Limited data suggest that metformin's total body clearance may be decreased and AUC and half-life increased in elderly patients, presumably due to decreased renal clearance. Metformin should not be used in patients ≥80 years of age unless renal function is verified as normal. **Do not titrate to maximum dose.** Intensive glucose control (HbA$_{1c}$ <6.5%) has been linked to increased all-cause and cardiovascular mortality, hypoglycemia requiring assistance, and weight gain in adult type 2 diabetes. How "tightly" to control a geriatric patient's blood glucose needs to be individualized. Such a decision should be based on several factors, including the patient's functional and cognitive status, how well he/she recognizes hypoglycemic or hyperglycemic symptoms, and how to respond to them and other disease states. An HbA$_{1c}$ <7.5% is an acceptable endpoint for a healthy older adult, while <8% is acceptable for frail elderly patients, those with a duration of illness >10 years, or those with comorbid conditions and requiring combination diabetes medications. Patients who are unable to accurately draw up their dose will need assistance, such as prefilled syringes. Initial doses may require considerations for renal function in the elderly with dosing adjusted subsequently based on blood glucose monitoring. For elderly patients with diabetes who are relatively healthy, attaining target goals for aspirin use, blood pressure, lipids, smoking cessation, and diet and exercise may be more important than normalized glycemic control.

Dosage Forms Excipient information presented when available (limited, particularly for generics); consult specific product labeling.

Tablet, oral:

  Janumet® 50/500: Sitagliptin 50 mg and metformin hydrochloride 500 mg
  Janumet® 50/1000: Sitagliptin 50 mg and metformin hydrochloride 1000 mg

Dosage Forms: Canada Excipient information presented when available (limited, particularly for generics); consult specific product labeling.

Tablet, oral:

  Janumet® 50/850: Sitagliptin 50 mg and metformin hydrochloride 850 mg

◆ **(+)-(S)-N-Methyl-γ-(1-naphthyloxy)-2-thiophenepropylamine Hydrochloride** *see* DULoxetine *on page 583*
◆ **Sodium L-Triiodothyronine** *see* Liothyronine *on page 1072*
◆ **Sodium Acid Carbonate** *see* Sodium Bicarbonate *on page 1688*
◆ **Sodium Aurothiomalate** *see* Gold Sodium Thiomalate *on page 836*

Sodium Bicarbonate (SOW dee um bye KAR bun ate)

Brand Names: U.S. Brioschi® [OTC]; Neut®
Index Terms Baking Soda; $NaHCO_3$; Sodium Acid Carbonate; Sodium Hydrogen Carbonate
Generic Availability (U.S.) Yes: Excludes granules
Pharmacologic Category Alkalinizing Agent; Antacid; Electrolyte Supplement, Oral; Electrolyte Supplement, Parenteral
Use Management of metabolic acidosis; gastric hyperacidity; as an alkalinization agent for the urine; treatment of hyperkalemia; management of overdose of certain drugs, including tricyclic antidepressants and aspirin
Unlabeled/Investigational Use Prevention of contrast-induced nephropathy (CIN)
Contraindications Alkalosis, hypernatremia, severe pulmonary edema, hypocalcemia, unknown abdominal pain
Warnings/Precautions Use of I.V. $NaHCO_3$ should be reserved for documented metabolic acidosis and for hyperkalemia-induced cardiac arrest. Routine use in cardiac arrest is not recommended. Avoid extravasation, tissue necrosis can occur due to the hypertonicity of $NaHCO_3$. May cause sodium retention especially if renal function is impaired; not to be used in treatment of peptic ulcer; use with caution in patients with HF, edema, cirrhosis, or renal failure. Not the antacid of choice for the elderly because of sodium content and potential for systemic alkalosis.
Adverse Reactions (Reflective of adult population; not specific for elderly) Frequency not defined.
Cardiovascular: Cerebral hemorrhage, CHF (aggravated), edema
Central nervous system: Tetany
Gastrointestinal: Belching, flatulence (with oral), gastric distension
Endocrine & metabolic: Hypernatremia, hyperosmolality, hypocalcemia, hypokalemia, increased affinity of hemoglobin for oxygen-reduced pH in myocardial tissue necrosis when extravasated, intracranial acidosis, metabolic alkalosis, milk-alkali syndrome (especially with renal dysfunction)
Respiratory: Pulmonary edema
Drug Interactions
Avoid Concomitant Use There are no known interactions where it is recommended to avoid concomitant use.
Increased Effect/Toxicity
Sodium Bicarbonate may increase the levels/effects of: Alpha-/Beta-Agonists; Amphetamines; Calcium Polystyrene Sulfonate; Dexmethylphenidate; Flecainide; Memantine; Methylphenidate; QuiNIDine; QuiNINE
Decreased Effect
Sodium Bicarbonate may decrease the levels/effects of: ACE Inhibitors; Anticonvulsants (Hydantoin); Antipsychotic Agents (Phenothiazines); Atazanavir; Bisacodyl; Cefditoren; Cefpodoxime; Cefuroxime; Chloroquine; Corticosteroids (Oral); Dabigatran Etexilate; Dasatinib; Delavirdine; Erlotinib; Flecainide; Gabapentin; HMG-CoA Reductase Inhibitors; Iron Salts; Isoniazid; Itraconazole; Ketoconazole; Ketoconazole (Systemic); Lithium; Mesalamine; Methenamine; Penicillamine; Phosphate Supplements; Protease Inhibitors; Rilpivirine; Tetracycline Derivatives; Trientine
Ethanol/Nutrition/Herb Interactions Herb/Nutraceutical: Concurrent doses with iron may decrease iron absorption.
Stability Store injection at room temperature; do not freeze. Protect from heat. Use only clear solutions.
Prevention of contrast-induced nephropathy (unlabeled use): Remove 154 mL from 1000 mL bag of D_5W; replace with 154 mL of 8.4% sodium bicarbonate; resultant concentration is 154 mEq/L (Merten, 2004); more practically, institutions may remove 150 mL from 1000 mL bag of D_5W and replace with 150 mL of 8.4% sodium bicarbonate; resultant concentration is 150 mEq/L
Mechanism of Action Dissociates to provide bicarbonate ion which neutralizes hydrogen ion concentration and raises blood and urinary pH
Pharmacodynamics/Kinetics
Onset of action: Oral: Rapid; I.V.: 15 minutes
Duration: Oral: 8-10 minutes; I.V.: 1-2 hours

Absorption: Oral: Well absorbed

Excretion: Urine (<1%)

Dosage

Geriatric & Adult

Cardiac arrest (ACLS, 2010): I.V.: Initial: 1 mEq/kg/dose; repeat doses should be guided by arterial blood gases

Routine use of NaHCO₃ is not recommended. May be considered in the setting of prolonged cardiac arrest only after adequate alveolar ventilation has been established and effective cardiac compressions. **Note:** In some cardiac arrest situations (eg, metabolic acidosis, hyperkalemia, or tricyclic antidepressant overdose), sodium bicarbonate may be beneficial.

Metabolic acidosis: I.V.: Dosage should be based on the following formula if blood gases and pH measurements are available:

$HCO_3^-(mEq) = 0.5 \times$ weight (kg) $\times$ [24 - serum $HCO_3^-(mEq/L)$] **or** $HCO_3^-(mEq) = 0.5 \times$ weight (kg) x [desired increase in serum $HCO_3^-(mEq/L)$]

Administer ½ dose initially, then remaining ½ dose over the next 24 hours; monitor pH, serum HCO_3^-, and clinical status. **Note:** These equations provide an estimated replacement dose. The underlying cause and degree of acidosis may result in the need for larger or smaller replacement doses. In most cases, the initial goal of therapy is to target a pH of ~7.2 and a plasma bicarbonate level of ~10 mEq/L to prevent overalkalinization.

Note: If acid-base status is not available: 2-5 mEq/kg I.V. infusion over 4-8 hours; subsequent doses should be based on patient's acid-base status

Hyperkalemia (ACLS, 2010): I.V.: 50 mEq over 5 minutes (as appropriate, consider methods of enhancing potassium removal/excretion)

Chronic renal failure: Oral: Initiate when plasma HCO_3^- <15 mEq/L Start with 20-36 mEq/ day in divided doses, titrate to bicarbonate level of 18-20 mEq/L

Renal tubular acidosis: Oral:

Distal: 0.5-2 mEq/kg/day in 4-5 divided doses

Proximal: Initial: 5-10 mEq/kg/day; maintenance: Increase as required to maintain serum bicarbonate in the normal range

Urine alkalinization: Oral: Initial: 48 mEq (4 g), then 12-24 mEq (1-2 g) every 4 hours; dose should be titrated to desired urinary pH; doses up to 16 g/day (200 mEq) in patients <60 years and 8 g (100 mEq) in patients >60 years

Antacid: Oral: 325 mg to 2 g 1-4 times/day

Prevention of contrast-induced nephropathy (unlabeled use): I.V. infusion: 154 mEq/L sodium bicarbonate in D₅W solution: 3 mL/kg/hour for 1 hour immediately before contrast injection, then 1mL/kg/hour during contrast exposure and for 6 hours after procedure

To prepare solution, remove 154 mL from 1000 mL bag of D₅W; replace with 154 mL of 8.4% sodium bicarbonate; resultant concentration is 154 mEq/L (Merten, 2004); more practically, institutions may remove 150 mL from 1000 mL bag of D₅W and replace with 150 mL of 8.4% sodium bicarbonate; resultant concentration is 150 mEq/L

Administration Observe for extravasation when giving I.V. Oral product should be administered 1-3 hours after meals.

Special Geriatric Considerations Not the antacid of choice for the elderly because of sodium content and potential for systemic alkalosis (see maximum daily dose under Dosage).

Dosage Forms Excipient information presented when available (limited, particularly for generics); consult specific product labeling. [DSC] = Discontinued product

Granules for solution, oral [effervescent]:

Brioschi®: 2.69 g/capful (120 g, 240 g) [contains sodium 770 mg/capful; lemon flavor]

Brioschi®: 2.69 g/packet (12s) [contains sodium 770 mg/packet; lemon flavor]

Infusion, premixed in water for injection: 5% (500 mL [DSC]) [5.95 mEq/10 mL]

Injection, solution: 4.2% (10 mL) [5 mEq/10 mL]; 7.5% (50 mL [DSC]) [8.92 mEq/10 mL]; 8.4% (50 mL, 250 mL, 500 mL) [10 mEq/10 mL]

Neut®: 4% (5 mL) [contains edetate disodium; 2.4 mEq/5 mL]

Injection, solution [preservative free]: 4.2% (5 mL) [5 mEq/10 mL]; 7.5% (50 mL) [8.92 mEq/10 mL]; 8.4% (10 mL, 50 mL) [10 mEq/10 mL]

Powder, oral: USP: 100% (120 g, 480 g)

Tablet, oral: 325 mg [3.8 mEq], 650 mg [7.6 mEq]

Selected References

Dellinger RP, Levy MM, Carlet JM, et al, "Surviving Sepsis Campaign: International Guidelines for Management of Severe Sepsis and Septic Shock: 2008," *Intensive Care Med*, 2007 [epub ahead of print].

◆ **Sodium Bicarbonate and Omeprazole** see Omeprazole and Sodium Bicarbonate on page 1342

Sodium Chloride (SOW dee um KLOR ide)

Medication Safety Issues
High alert medication:
The Institute for Safe Medication Practices (ISMP) includes this medication (I.V. formulation >0.9% concentration) among its list of drugs which have a heightened risk of causing significant patient harm when used in error.

Other safety concerns:
Per The Joint Commission (TJC) recommendations, concentrated electrolyte solutions (eg, NaCl >0.9%) should not be available in patient care areas.

Inappropriate use of low sodium or sodium-free intravenous fluids (eg, D_5W, hypotonic saline) in pediatric patients can lead to significant morbidity and mortality due to hyponatremia (ISMP, 2009).

Brand Names: U.S. 4-Way® Saline Moisturizing Mist [OTC]; Altachlore [OTC]; Altamist [OTC]; Ayr® Allergy Sinus [OTC]; Ayr® Baby Saline [OTC]; Ayr® Saline No-Drip [OTC]; Ayr® Saline [OTC]; Breathe Free® [OTC]; Deep Sea [OTC]; Entsol® [OTC]; HuMist® for Kids [OTC]; HuMist® [OTC]; Hyper-Sal™; Little Noses® Saline [OTC]; Little Noses® Stuffy Nose Kit [OTC]; Muro 128® [OTC]; Na-Zone® [OTC]; Nasal Moist® Saline [OTC]; Nasal Spray [OTC] [DSC]; NāSal™ [OTC]; Ocean® for Kids [OTC]; Ocean® [OTC]; Pretz® [OTC]; Rhinaris® [OTC]; Saline Mist [OTC]; Simply Saline® Baby [OTC]; Simply Saline® Nasal Moist® [OTC]; Simply Saline® [OTC]; Syrex; Wound Wash Saline™ [OTC]

Index Terms Hypertonic Saline; NaCl; Normal Saline; Saline; Salt

Generic Availability (U.S.) Yes

Pharmacologic Category Electrolyte Supplement, Parenteral; Genitourinary Irrigant; Irrigant; Lubricant, Ocular; Sodium Salt

Use
Parenteral: Restores sodium ion in patients with restricted oral intake (especially hyponatremia states or low salt syndrome).
Concentrated sodium chloride: Additive for parenteral fluid therapy
Hypertonic sodium chloride: For severe hyponatremia and hypochloremia
Hypotonic sodium chloride: Hydrating solution
Normal saline: Restores water/sodium losses
Ophthalmic: Reduces corneal edema
Inhalation: Restores moisture to pulmonary system; loosens and thins congestion caused by colds or allergies; diluent for bronchodilator solutions that require dilution before inhalation
Intranasal: Restores moisture to nasal membranes
Irrigation: Wound cleansing, irrigation, and flushing

Unlabeled/Investigational Use Traumatic brain injury (hypertonic sodium chloride)

Dosage
Geriatric & Adult
Refractory elevated ICP due to various etiologies (eg, subarachnoid hemorrhage, trauma, neoplasm), transtentorial herniation syndromes (unlabeled use): I.V.: Hypertonic saline: 23.4% (30-60 mL) given over 2-20 minutes administered via central venous access only (Koenig, 2008; Suarez, 1998; Ware, 2005)

Subarachnoid hemorrhage with hyponatremia (ie, ≤135 mEq/L) to enhance cerebral perfusion (unlabeled use): I.V.: Hypertonic saline: 3% sodium chloride/acetate (50:50 mixture) 100-200 mL/hour administered via central venous catheter; titrate to clinical response up to a maximum serum sodium between 150-160 mEq/L (achieved at a rate of 0.5-1 mEq/L/hour) (Suarez, 1999)

Traumatic brain injury with elevated ICP (unlabeled use): I.V.: Hypertonic saline: **Note:** Optimal dose has not been established; due to insufficient evidence, the Brain Trauma Foundation guidelines (Bratton, 2007) do not make specific recommendations on the use of hypertonic saline for the treatment of traumatic intracranial hypertension. Clinical trials are small; few are prospective. **Some concentrations may not be commercially available; administer via central venous catheter;** protocols include:
3%: 300 mL administered over 20 minutes when ICP values exceed 20 mm Hg (Huang, 2006)
7.2%: 1.5 mL/kg administered over 15 minutes when ICP values exceed 15 mm Hg (Munar, 2000)
7.5%: 2 mL/kg administered over 20 minutes when ICP values exceed 25 mm Hg (Vialet, 2003)
23.4%: 30 mL administered over 2 minutes (Ware, 2005) **or** over >30 minutes when ICP values exceed 20 mm Hg (Kerwin, 2009)

GU irrigant: Irrigation: 1-3 L/day by intermittent irrigation

Replacement: I.V.: Determined by laboratory determinations mEq

Hyponatremia: Sodium deficiency (mEq/kg) = [% dehydration (L/kg)/100 x 70 (mEq/L)] + [0.6 (L/kg) x (140 - serum sodium) (mEq/L)]

To correct acute, serious hyponatremia: mEq sodium = [desired sodium (mEq/L) - actual sodium (mEq/L)] x [0.6 x wt (kg)]; for acute correction use 125 mEq/L as the desired serum sodium; acutely correct serum sodium in 5 mEq/L/dose increments; more gradual correction in increments of 10 mEq/L/day is indicated in the asymptomatic patient

Approximate Deficits of Water and Electrolytes in Moderately Severe Dehydration[1]

Condition	Water (mL/kg)	Sodium (mEq/kg)
Fasting and thirsting	100-120	5-7
Diarrhea		
isonatremic	100-120	8-10
hypernatremic	100-120	2-4
hyponatremic	100-120	10-12
Pyloric stenosis	100-120	8-10
Diabetic acidosis	100-120	9-10

[1]A **negative** deficit indicates total body **excess** prior to treatment.

Adapted from Behrman RE, Kleigman RM, Nelson WE, et al, eds, *Nelson Textbook of Pediatrics*, 14th ed, WB Saunders Co, 1992.

Ophthalmic:
Ointment: Apply once daily or more often
Solution: Instill 1-2 drops into affected eye(s) every 3-4 hours
Bronchodilator diluent: Inhalation: 1-3 sprays (1-3 mL) to dilute bronchodilator solution in nebulizer before administration
Nasal congestion: Intranasal: 2-3 sprays in each nostril as needed
Irrigation: Spray affected area

Dosage Forms Excipient information presented when available (limited, particularly for generics); consult specific product labeling. [DSC] = Discontinued product
Aerosol, intranasal [spray, preservative free]:
Entsol®: 3% (100 mL) [chlorofluorocarbon free]
Gel, intranasal:
Ayr® Saline: < 0.5% (14 g) [contains aloe, soybean oil]
Entsol®: 3% (20 g) [contains aloe, benzalkonium chloride, vitamin E]
Rhinaris®: 0.2% (28.4 g) [contains benzalkonium chloride]
Simply Saline® Nasal Moist®: 0.65% (30 g) [contains aloe]
Gel, intranasal [spray]:
Ayr® Saline No-Drip: < 0.5% (22 mL) [contains benzalkonium chloride, benzyl alcohol, soybean oil]
Injection, solution: 0.45% (25 mL [DSC], 50 mL, 100 mL, 250 mL, 500 mL, 1000 mL); 0.9% (25 mL, 50 mL, 100 mL, 150 mL, 250 mL, 500 mL, 1000 mL); 3% (500 mL); 5% (500 mL)
Injection, solution [preservative free]: 0.9% (2 mL, 3 mL, 5 mL, 10 mL, 20 mL, 50 mL, 100 mL)
Injection, solution [I.V. flush]: 0.9% (10 mL)
Injection, solution [I.V. flush, preservative free]: 0.9% (1 mL, 2 mL, 2.5 mL, 3 mL, 5 mL, 10 mL, 50 mL, 125 mL)
Syrex: 0.9% (2.5 mL, 3 mL, 5 mL, 10 mL)
Injection, solution [bacteriostatic]: 0.9% (10 mL, 20 mL, 30 mL)
Injection, solution [concentrate]: 14.6% (20 mL, 40 mL, 250 mL [DSC]); 23.4% (100 mL, 250 mL)
Injection, solution [concentrate, preservative free]: 14.6% (20 mL, 40 mL); 23.4% (30 mL, 100 mL, 200 mL)
Ointment, ophthalmic: 5% (3.5 g)
Altachlore: 5% (3.5 g)
Ointment, ophthalmic [preservative free]:
Muro 128®: 5% (3.5 g)
Powder for solution, intranasal [preservative free]:
Entsol®: 3% (10s)
Powder for solution, intranasal [concentrate, preservative free]:
Pretz®: 1 teaspoon/dose (360 g) [with yerba santa]
Solution, for blood processing [not for injection]: 0.9% (3000 mL)
Solution, for inhalation [preservative free]: 0.9% (3 mL, 5 mL, 15 mL); 3% (15 mL); 10% (15 mL)

◀ Solution, for irrigation: 0.45% (2000 mL [DSC]); 0.9% (250 mL, 500 mL, 1000 mL, 1500 mL, 2000 mL, 3000 mL, 4000 mL, 5000 mL)

Solution, for irrigation [preservative free]: 0.9% (250 mL, 500 mL, 1000 mL, 1500 mL, 2000 mL, 3000 mL)

Solution, for irrigation [slush solution]: 0.9% (1000 mL)

Solution, for nebulization [preservative free]:
  Hyper-Sal™: 7% (4 mL)

Solution, intranasal [preservative free]:
  Simply Saline®: 3% (44 mL)

Solution, intranasal [buffered/spray, preservative free]:
  Pretz®: 0.75% (20 mL) [chlorofluorocarbon free; with yerba santa]

Solution, intranasal [drops]:
  Ayr® Saline: 0.65% (50 mL) [ethanol free; contains benzalkonium chloride]

Solution, intranasal [drops/mist/spray]:
  HuMist®: 0.65% (45 mL) [ethanol free]
  HuMist® for Kids: 0.65% (30 mL) [ethanol free; bubblegum flavor]
  Ocean®: 0.65% (45 mL, 473 mL) [gluten free; contains benzalkonium chloride, benzyl alcohol]
  Ocean® for Kids: 0.65% (37.5 mL) [ethanol free; contains benzalkonium chloride]

Solution, intranasal [drops/spray]:
  Ayr® Baby Saline: 0.65% (30 mL) [ethanol free; contains benzalkonium chloride]
  Little Noses® Saline: 0.65% (30 mL) [contains benzalkonium chloride]
  Little Noses® Stuffy Nose Kit: 0.65% (15 mL) [contains benzalkonium chloride]

Solution, intranasal [irrigation]:
  Pretz®: 0.75% (237 mL [DSC], 960 mL) [contains benzalkonium chloride, sodium benzoate; with yerba santa]

Solution, intranasal [isotonic, buffered/spray]:
  Pretz®: 0.75% (50 mL) [contains benzalkonium chloride, sodium benzoate; with yerba santa]

Solution, intranasal [mist]:
  4-Way® Saline Moisturizing Mist: 0.74% (29.6 mL) [ethanol free; contains benzalkonium chloride, menthol]
  Ayr® Allergy Sinus: 2.65% (50 mL)
  Ayr® Saline: 0.65% (50 mL) [ethanol free; contains benzalkonium chloride]
  Entsol®: 3% (30 mL) [contains benzalkonium chloride]
  Rhinaris®: 0.2% (30 mL) [contains benzalkonium chloride]
  Saline Mist: 0.65% (45 mL) [contains benzalkonium chloride]

Solution, intranasal [mist, preservative free]:
  Simply Saline®: 0.9% (44 mL, 90 mL)
  Simply Saline® Baby: 0.9% (45 mL)

Solution, intranasal [nasal wash, preservative free]:
  Entsol®: 3% (240 mL)

Solution, intranasal [spray]:
  Altamist: 0.65% (60 mL) [contains benzalkonium chloride]
  Breathe Free®: 0.65% (44.3 mL) [contains benzalkonium chloride]
  Deep Sea: 0.65% (45 mL) [contains benzalkonium chloride, benzyl alcohol]
  Na-Zone®: 0.65% (60 mL) [contains benzalkonium chloride]
  Nasal Moist® Saline: 0.65% (45 mL)
  Nasal Spray: 0.65% (45 mL [DSC]) [contains benzalkonium chloride, benzyl alcohol]
  NāSal™: 0.65% (30 mL) [ethanol free; contains benzalkonium chloride, thimerosal]

Solution, intranasal [spray, isotonic, buffered]:
  Pretz®: 0.75% (50 mL [DSC]) [contains benzalkonium chloride, sodium benzoate; with yerba santa]

Solution, ophthalmic [drops]: 5% (15 mL)
  Altachlore: 5% (15 mL, 30 mL)
  Muro 128®: 2% (15 mL); 5% (15 mL, 30 mL)

Solution, topical [preservative free]:
  Wound Wash Saline™: 0.9% (90 mL, 210 mL)

Swab, intranasal:
  Ayr® Saline: < 0.5% (20s) [contains aloe, soybean oil]

Tablet, oral: 1 g

Tablet for solution, topical: 1000 mg

Sodium Citrate and Citric Acid (SOW dee um SIT rate & SI trik AS id)

Medication Safety Issues
Sound-alike/look-alike issues:
Bicitra may be confused with Polycitra®

Brand Names: U.S. Cytra-2; Oracit®; Shohl's Solution (Modified)
Brand Names: Canada PMS-Dicitrate
Index Terms Bicitra; Citric Acid and Sodium Citrate; Modified Shohl's Solution
Generic Availability (U.S.) Yes
Pharmacologic Category Alkalinizing Agent, Oral
Use Treatment of metabolic acidosis; alkalinizing agent in conditions where long-term maintenance of an alkaline urine is desirable
Contraindications Hypersensitivity to sodium citrate, citric acid, or any component of the formulation; severe renal insufficiency; sodium-restricted diet
Warnings/Precautions Conversion to bicarbonate may be impaired in patients with hepatic failure, in shock, or who are severely ill. Use caution with cardiac failure, hypertension, impaired renal function, and peripheral or pulmonary edema; contains sodium.
Adverse Reactions (Reflective of adult population; not specific for elderly) Frequency not defined. Generally well tolerated with normal renal function.
Central nervous system: Tetany
Endocrine & metabolic: Metabolic alkalosis, hyperkalemia
Gastrointestinal: Diarrhea, nausea, vomiting
Drug Interactions
Avoid Concomitant Use There are no known interactions where it is recommended to avoid concomitant use.
Increased Effect/Toxicity
Sodium Citrate and Citric Acid may increase the levels/effects of: Aluminum Hydroxide
Decreased Effect There are no known significant interactions involving a decrease in effect.
Stability Store at controlled room temperature of 15°C to 30°C (59°F to 86°F); do not freeze. Protect from excessive heat.
Pharmacodynamics/Kinetics
Metabolism: Oxidized to sodium bicarbonate
Excretion: Urine (<5% as sodium citrate)
Dosage
Geriatric & Adult Systemic alkalization: Oral: 10-30 mL with water after meals and at bedtime
Administration Administer after meals. Dilute with 30-90 mL of water to enhance taste. Chilling solution prior to dosing helps to enhance palatability.
Monitoring Parameters Blood gas for pH and bicarbonate; serum bicarbonate
Pharmacotherapy Pearls 1 mL of solution contains 1 mEq of sodium and is metabolized to form the equivalent of 1 mEq of bicarbonate/mL
Dosage Forms Excipient information presented when available (limited, particularly for generics); consult specific product labeling. **Note:** Contains sodium 1 mEq/mL and is equivalent to bicarbonate 1 mEq/mL
Solution, oral: Sodium citrate 500 mg and citric acid 334 mg per 5 mL (480 mL)
Cytra-2: Sodium citrate 500 mg and citric acid 334 mg per 5 mL (480 mL) [alcohol free, dye free, sugar free; contains propylene glycol and sodium benzoate; grape flavor]
Oracit®: Sodium citrate 490 mg and citric acid 640 mg per 5 mL (15 mL, 30 mL, 500 mL, 3840 mL)
Shohl's Solution (Modified): Sodium citrate 500 mg and citric acid 300 mg per 5 mL (480 mL) [contains alcohol]

Sodium Phosphates (SOW dee um FOS fates)

Related Information

Laxatives, Classification and Properties *on page 2012*

Treatment Options for Constipation *on page 2035*

Medication Safety Issues

Sound-alike/look-alike issues:

Visicol® may be confused with Asacol®, VESIcare®

Administration issues:

Enemas and oral solution are available in pediatric and adult sizes; prescribe by "volume" not by "bottle."

Because inorganic phosphate exists as monobasic and dibasic anions, with the mixture of valences dependent on pH, ordering by mEq amounts is unreliable and may lead to large dosing errors. In addition, I.V. phosphate is available in the sodium and potassium salt; therefore, the content of these cations must be considered when ordering phosphate. The most reliable method of ordering I.V. phosphate is by millimoles, then specifying the potassium or sodium salt.

Brand Names: U.S. Fleet® Enema Extra® [OTC]; Fleet® Enema [OTC]; Fleet® Pedia-Lax™ Enema [OTC]; Fleet® Phospho-soda® EZ-Prep™ [OTC] [DSC]; Fleet® Phospho-soda® [OTC] [DSC]; LaCrosse Complete [OTC]; OsmoPrep®; Visicol®

Brand Names: Canada Fleet Enema®

Index Terms Phosphates, Sodium

Generic Availability (U.S.) Yes: Enema, injection, oral solution

Pharmacologic Category Cathartic; Electrolyte Supplement, Parenteral; Laxative, Bowel Evacuant

Use

Oral, rectal: Short-term treatment of constipation and to evacuate the colon for rectal and bowel exams

I.V.: Source of phosphate in large volume I.V. fluids and parenteral nutrition; treatment and prevention of hypophosphatemia

Medication Guide Available Yes

Contraindications Hypersensitivity to sodium phosphate salts or any component of the formulation; additional contraindications vary by product:

Enema: Ascites, clinically significant renal impairment, heart failure, imperforate anus, known or suspected GI obstruction, megacolon (congenital or acquired)

Intravenous preparation: Diseases with hyperphosphatemia, hypocalcemia, or hypernatremia

Oral preparation: Acute phosphate nephropathy (biopsy proven), bowel obstruction, congenital megacolon, toxic megacolon

Warnings/Precautions [U.S. Boxed Warning]: Acute phosphate nephropathy has been reported (rarely) with use of oral products as a colon cleanser prior to colonoscopy. Some cases have resulted in permanent renal impairment (some requiring dialysis). Risk factors for acute phosphate nephropathy may include increased age (>55 years of age), pre-existing renal dysfunction, bowel obstruction, active colitis, or dehydration, and the use of medicines that affect renal perfusion or function (eg, ACE inhibitors, angiotensin receptor blockers, diuretics, and possibly NSAIDs), although some cases have been reported in patients without apparent risk factors. Other preventive measures may include avoid exceeding maximum recommended doses and concurrent use of other laxatives containing sodium phosphate; encourage patients to adequately hydrate before, during, and after use; obtain baseline and postprocedure labs in patients at risk; consider hospitalization and intravenous hydration during bowel cleansing for patients unable to hydrate themselves (eg, frail patients).

Use with caution in patients with impaired renal dysfunction, pre-existing electrolyte imbalances, risk of electrolyte disturbance (hypocalcemia, hyperphosphatemia, hypernatremia), or dehydration. If using as a bowel evacuant, correct electrolyte abnormalities before administration. Use caution in patients with unstable angina, history of myocardial infarction arrhythmia, cardiomyopathy; use caution in patients with or at risk for arrhythmias (eg, cardiomyopathy, prolonged QT interval, history of uncontrolled arrhythmias, recent MI) or with concurrent use of other QT-prolonging medications; pre-/postdose ECGs should be considered in high-risk patients.

Use caution in inflammatory bowel disease; may induce colonic aphthous ulceration. Use caution in patients with any of the following: Bowel obstruction (including pseudo) or perforation, gastric retention or hypomotility, ileus, severe, chronic constipation, colitis, gastric bypass or bariatric surgery.

Use with caution in patients with a history of seizures and those at higher risk of seizures. Inadequate fluid intake may lead to dehydration. Use with caution in debilitated patients; consider each patient's ability to hydrate properly. Use with caution in geriatric patients. Laxatives and purgatives have the potential for abuse by bulimia nervosa patients. Other oral medications may not be well absorbed when given during bowel evacuation because of rapid intestinal peristalsis. Solutions for injection may contain aluminum; toxic levels may occur following prolonged administration in patients with renal impairment. Enemas and oral solution are available in pediatric and adult sizes; prescribe by "volume" not by "bottle."

Visicol®: Use caution with history of swallowing difficulties or esophageal narrowing. Tablet particles may be seen in the stool.

Adverse Reactions (Reflective of adult population; not specific for elderly) Frequency not defined.

Cardiovascular: Edema, hypotension

Central nervous system: Dizziness, headache

Endocrine & metabolic: Hypocalcemia, hypernatremia, hyperphosphatemia, calcium phosphate precipitation

Gastrointestinal: Nausea, vomiting, diarrhea, abdominal bloating, abdominal pain, mucosal bleeding, superficial mucosal ulcerations

Renal: Acute renal failure

Postmarketing and/or case reports: Acute phosphate nephropathy, anaphylaxis, arrhythmia, atrial fibrillation (following severe vomiting [tablet formulation]), BUN increased, creatinine increased, nephrocalcinosis (oral solution), pruritus, rash, renal tubular necrosis, swelling (face, lips, tongue), urticaria, seizure

Drug Interactions

Avoid Concomitant Use There are no known interactions where it is recommended to avoid concomitant use.

Increased Effect/Toxicity

Sodium Phosphates may increase the levels/effects of: Nonsteroidal Anti-Inflammatory Agents

The levels/effects of Sodium Phosphates may be increased by: ACE Inhibitors; Angiotensin II Receptor Blockers; Bisphosphonate Derivatives; Diuretics; Tricyclic Antidepressants

Decreased Effect

The levels/effects of Sodium Phosphates may be decreased by: Antacids; Calcium Salts; Iron Salts; Magnesium Salts; Sucralfate

Stability Store at 15°C to 30°C (59°F to 86°F).

Mechanism of Action As a laxative, exerts osmotic effect in the small intestine by drawing water into the lumen of the gut, producing distention and promoting peristalsis and evacuation of the bowel; phosphorous participates in bone deposition, calcium metabolism, utilization of B complex vitamins, and as a buffer in acid-base equilibrium

Pharmacodynamics/Kinetics

Onset of action: Cathartic: 3-6 hours; Rectal: 2-5 minutes

Absorption: Oral: ~1% to 20%

Excretion: Urine

Dosage

Geriatric & Adult Caution: With orders for I.V. phosphate, there is considerable confusion associated with the use of millimoles (mmol) versus milliequivalents (mEq) to express the phosphate requirement. The most reliable method of ordering I.V. phosphate is by millimoles, then specifying the potassium or sodium salt. Intravenous doses listed as mmol of phosphate.

Acute treatment of hypophosphatemia: I.V.: It is difficult to provide concrete guidelines for the treatment of severe hypophosphatemia because the extent of total body deficits and response to therapy are difficult to predict. Aggressive doses of phosphate may result in a transient serum elevation followed by redistribution into intracellular compartments or bone tissue. It is recommended that repletion of severe hypophosphatemia be done I.V. because large doses of oral phosphate may cause diarrhea and intestinal absorption may be unreliable. Intermittent I.V. infusion should be reserved for severe depletion situations; requires continuous cardiac monitoring. Guidelines differ based on degree of illness, need/ use of TPN, and severity of hypophosphatemia. If hypokalemia exists (some clinicians recommend threshold of <4 mmol/L), consider phosphate replacement strategy with potassium (eg, potassium phosphates). Obese patients and/or severe renal impairment were excluded from phosphate supplement trials. **Note:** 1 mmol phosphate = 31 mg phosphorus; 1 mg phosphorus = 0.032 mmol phosphate.

General replacement guidelines (Lentz, 1978):

Low dose, serum phosphorus losses are recent and uncomplicated: 0.08 mmol/kg over 6 hours

Intermediate dose, serum phosphorus level 0.5-1 mg/dL (0.16-0.32 mmol/L): 0.16-0.24 mmol/kg over 6 hours

Note: The initial dose may be increased by 25% to 50% if the patient is symptomatic secondary to hypophosphatemia and lowered by 25% to 50% if the patient is hypercalcemic.

Critically-ill adult patients receiving concurrent enteral/parenteral nutrition (Brown, 2006; Clark, 1995): **Note:** Round doses to the nearest 7.5 mmol for ease of preparation. If administering with phosphate-containing parenteral nutrition, do not exceed 15 mmol/L within parenteral nutrition. May use adjusted body weight for patients weighing >130% of ideal body weight (and BMI <40 kg/m^2) by using [IBW + 0.25 (ABW-IBW)]:

Low dose, serum phosphorus level 2.3-3 mg/dL (0.74-0.96 mmol/L): 0.16-0.32 mmol/kg over 4-6 hours

Intermediate dose, serum phosphorus level 1.6-2.2 mg/dL (0.51-0.71 mmol/L): 0.32-0.64 mmol/kg over 4-6 hours

High dose, serum phosphorus <1.5 mg/dL (<0.5 mmol/L): 0.64-1 mmol/kg over 8-12 hours

Parenteral nutrition: I.V.: 10-15 mmol/1000 kcal (Hicks, 2001) **or** 20-40 mmol/24 hours (Mirtallo, 2004 [ASPEN guidelines])

Laxative (Fleet®): Rectal: Contents of one 4.5-ounce enema as a single dose, may repeat

Laxative (Fleet® Phospho-soda®): Oral: Take on an empty stomach; dilute dose with 8 ounces cool water, then follow dose with 8 ounces water; **do not repeat dose within 24 hours:** 15 mL as a single dose; maximum daily dose: 45 mL

Bowel cleansing prior to colonoscopy: Oral: **Note:** Each dose should be taken with a minimum of 8 ounces of clear liquids. Do not repeat treatment within 7 days. Do not use additional agents, especially sodium phosphate products.

Fleet® Phospho-Soda® (as component of Fleet® Prep Kit 3): Prior to procedure (timing of doses determined by prescriber): Mix 15 mL with 240 mL clear liquid; drink, then follow with 240 mL clear liquid; repeat every 10 minutes for a total of 45 mL

Visicol®: A total of 40 tablets divided as follows:

Evening before colonoscopy: 3 tablets every 15 minutes for 6 doses, then 2 additional tablets in 15 minutes (total of 20 tablets)

3-5 hours prior to colonoscopy: 3 tablets every 15 minutes for 6 doses, then 2 additional tablets in 15 minutes (total of 20 tablets)

OsmoPrep®: A total of 32 tablets divided as follows:

Evening before colonoscopy: 4 tablets every 15 minutes for 5 doses (total of 20 tablets)

3-5 hours prior to colonoscopy: 4 tablets every 15 minutes for 3 doses (total of 12 tablets)

Renal Impairment Use with caution; ionized inorganic phosphate is excreted by the kidneys. Oral solution is contraindicated in patients with kidney disease.

Administration

Intermittent I.V. infusion; do **not** administer I.V. push. Must be diluted prior to parenteral administration. In general, the dose, concentration of infusion, and rate of administration may be dependent on patient condition and specific institution policy. Intermittent infusion doses are typically prepared in 100-250 mL of NS or D$_5$W (usual concentration range: 0.15-0.6 mmol/mL). For adult patients with severe symptomatic hypophosphatemia (ie, <1.5 mg/dL), may administer at rates up to 15 mmol/hour (Rosen, 1995; Charron, 2003). In patients with renal dysfunction and/or less severe hypophosphatemia, slower administration rates (eg, over 4-6 hours) or oral repletion is recommended.

Bowel cleansing: Have patient drink ~8 ounces of water with each dose of sodium phosphate (total of 2 quarts/64 ounces); have patient rehydrate before and after colonoscopy

Monitoring Parameters

I.V.: Serum calcium, sodium and phosphorus levels; renal function; after I.V. phosphate repletion, repeat serum phosphorus level should be checked 2-4 hours later

Oral: Bowel cleansing: Baseline and postprocedure labs (electrolytes, calcium, phosphorus, BUN, creatinine) in patients at risk for acute renal nephropathy, seizure, or who have a history of electrolyte abnormality; ECG in patients with risks for prolonged QT or arrhythmias. Ensure euvolemia before initiating bowel preparation.

Reference Range Note: Reference ranges may vary depending on the laboratory

Serum calcium: 8.4-10.2 mg/dL

Serum phosphorus: Both low and high ends of the normal range are higher in children than in adults.

Infants: 4.5-7.5 mg/dL (1.45-2.42 mmol/L)

Children: ~4.0-6.0 mg/dL (1.29-1.94 mmol/L)

Adults: 2.5-4.5 mg/dL (0.81-1.45 mmol/L)

Pharmacotherapy Pearls Phosphate salts may precipitate when mixed with calcium salts; solubility is improved in amino acid parenteral nutrition solutions; check with a pharmacist to determine compatibility.

Special Geriatric Considerations The use of laxatives should be limited in the elderly since abuse could lead to fluid/electrolyte deficiencies. Since elderly often have reduced renal function, or disease that could predispose them to adverse effects, caution must be used with parenteral sodium phosphate.

Dosage Forms Excipient information presented when available (limited, particularly for generics); consult specific product labeling. [DSC] = Discontinued product

Kit [packaged as a two-dose kit which contains]:

Fleet® Phospho-soda® EZ-Prep™ [DSC]:

Solution, oral: Monobasic sodium phosphate monohydrate 2.4 g and dibasic sodium phosphate heptahydrate 0.9 g per 5 mL (30 mL) [sugar-free; contains sodium 556 mg/5 mL and phosphate 62.25 mEq/5 mL; packaged with lemonade flavor packets which contain phenylalanine]

Solution, oral: Monobasic sodium phosphate monohydrate 2.4 g and dibasic sodium phosphate heptahydrate 0.9 g per 5 mL (45 mL) [sugar-free; contains sodium 556 mg/5 mL and phosphate 62.25 mEq/5 mL; packaged with lemonade flavor packets which contain phenylalanine]

Injection, solution [concentrate; preservative free]: Phosphorus 3 mmol and sodium 4 mEq per 1 mL (5 mL, 15 mL, 50 mL) [equivalent to phosphorus 93 mg and sodium 92 mg per 1 mL; source of electrolytes; monobasic and dibasic sodium phosphate]

Solution, oral: Monobasic sodium phosphate monohydrate 2.4 g and dibasic sodium phosphate heptahydrate 0.9 g per 5 mL (45 mL)

Fleet® Phospho-soda®: Monobasic sodium phosphate monohydrate 2.4 g and dibasic sodium phosphate heptahydrate 0.9 g per 5 mL (45 mL) [sugar free; contains sodium 556 mg/5 mL, sodium benzoate, and phosphate 62.25 mEq/5 mL; unflavored or ginger-lemon flavor] [DSC]

Solution, rectal [enema]: Monobasic sodium phosphate monohydrate 19 g and dibasic sodium phosphate heptahydrate 7 g per 118 mL delivered dose (133 mL)

Fleet® Enema: Monobasic sodium phosphate monohydrate 19 g and dibasic sodium phosphate heptahydrate 7 g per 118 mL delivered dose (133 mL) [contains sodium 4.4 g/118 mL]

Fleet® Enema Extra®: Monobasic sodium phosphate monohydrate 19 g and dibasic sodium phosphate heptahydrate 7 g per 197 mL delivered dose (230 mL) [contains sodium 4.4 g/197 mL]

Fleet® Pedia-Lax™ Enema: Monobasic sodium phosphate monohydrate 9.5 g and dibasic sodium phosphate heptahydrate 3.5 g per 59 mL delivered dose (66 mL) [contains sodium 2.2 g/59 mL]

LaCrosse Complete: Monobasic sodium phosphate monohydrate 19 g and dibasic sodium phosphate heptahydrate 7 g per 118 mL delivered dose (133 mL) [contains sodium 4.4 g/118 mL]

Tablet, oral [scored]:

OsmoPrep®, Visicol®: Monobasic sodium phosphate monohydrate 1.102 g and dibasic sodium phosphate anhydrous 0.398 g [sodium phosphate 1.5 g per tablet; gluten free]

Selected References

Khurana A, McLean L, Atkinson S, et al, "The Effect of Oral Sodium Phosphate Drug Products on Renal Function in Adults Undergoing Bowel Endoscopy," Arch Intern Med, 2008, 168(6):593-7.

Roy HK and Bianchi LK, "Purging the Colon While Preserving the Kidneys," Arch Intern Med, 2008, 168(6): 565-7.

Sodium Polystyrene Sulfonate (SOW dee um pol ee STYE reen SUL fon ate)

Medication Safety Issues

Sound-alike/look-alike issues:

Kayexalate® may be confused with Kaopectate®

Sodium polystyrene sulfonate may be confused with calcium polystyrene sulfonate

Administration issues:

Always prescribe either one-time doses or as a specific number of doses (eg, 15 g q6h x 2 doses). Scheduled doses with no dosage limit could be given for days leading to dangerous hypokalemia.

International issues:

Kionex [U.S.] may be confused with Kinex brand name for biperiden [Mexico]

Brand Names: U.S. Kalexate; Kayexalate®; Kionex®; SPS®

Brand Names: Canada Kayexalate®; PMS-Sodium Polystyrene Sulfonate

Generic Availability (U.S.) No

SODIUM POLYSTYRENE SULFONATE

Pharmacologic Category Antidote

Use Treatment of hyperkalemia

Contraindications Hypersensitivity to sodium polystyrene sulfonate or any component of the formulation; hypokalemia; obstructive bowel disease

Additional contraindications: Sodium polystyrene sulfonate suspension (**with** sorbitol): Any postoperative patient until normal bowel function resumes

Warnings/Precautions Intestinal necrosis (including fatalities) and other serious gastrointestinal events (eg, bleeding, ischemic colitis, perforation) have been reported, especially when administered with sorbitol. Increased risk may be associated with a history of intestinal disease or surgery, hypovolemia, and renal insufficiency or failure; use with sorbitol is not recommended. Avoid use in any postoperative patient until normal bowel function resumes or in patients at risk for constipation or impaction; discontinue use if constipation occurs. Use with caution in patients with severe HF, hypertension, or edema; sodium load may exacerbate condition. Effective lowering of serum potassium from sodium polystyrene sulfonate may take hours to days after administration; consider alternative measures (eg, dialysis) or concomitant therapy (eg, I.V. sodium bicarbonate) in situations where rapid correction of severe hyperkalemia is required. Severe hypokalemia may occur; frequent monitoring of serum potassium is recommended within each 24-hour period; ECG monitoring may be appropriate in select patients. In addition to serum potassium-lowering effects, cation-exchange resins may also affect other cation concentrations possibly resulting in decreased serum magnesium and calcium. Large oral doses may cause fecal impaction (especially in elderly).

Concomitant administration of oral sodium polystyrene sulfonate with nonabsorbable cation-donating antacids or laxatives (eg, magnesium hydroxide) may result in systemic alkalosis and may diminish ability to reduce serum potassium concentrations; use with such agents is not recommended. In addition, intestinal obstruction has been reported with concomitant administration of aluminum hydroxide due to concretion formation. Enema will reduce the serum potassium faster than oral administration, but the oral route will result in a greater reduction over several hours.

Adverse Reactions (Reflective of adult population; not specific for elderly) Frequency not defined.

Endocrine & metabolic: Hypernatremia, hypocalcemia, hypokalemia, hypomagnesemia, sodium retention

Gastrointestinal: Anorexia, constipation, diarrhea, fecal impaction, intestinal necrosis (rare), intestinal obstruction (due to concretions in association with aluminum hydroxide), nausea, vomiting

Drug Interactions

Avoid Concomitant Use

Avoid concomitant use of Sodium Polystyrene Sulfonate with any of the following: Laxatives; Meloxicam; Sorbitol

Increased Effect/Toxicity

Sodium Polystyrene Sulfonate may increase the levels/effects of: Aluminum Hydroxide; Digoxin

The levels/effects of Sodium Polystyrene Sulfonate may be increased by: Antacids; Laxatives; Meloxicam; Sorbitol

Decreased Effect

Sodium Polystyrene Sulfonate may decrease the levels/effects of: Lithium; Thyroid Products

Stability Store at 25°C (77°F); excursions permitted to 15°C to 30°C (59°F to 86°F). Store repackaged product in refrigerator and use within 14 days. Freshly prepared suspensions should be used within 24 hours. Do not heat resin suspension.

Mechanism of Action Removes potassium by exchanging sodium ions for potassium ions in the intestine (especially the large intestine) before the resin is passed from the body; exchange capacity is 1 mEq/g in vivo, and in vitro capacity is 3.1 mEq/g, therefore, a wide range of exchange capacity exists such that close monitoring of serum electrolytes is necessary

Pharmacodynamics/Kinetics

Onset of action: 2-24 hours

Absorption: None

Excretion: Completely feces (primarily as potassium polystyrene sulfonate)

Dosage

Geriatric & Adult Hyperkalemia:

Oral: 15 g 1-4 times/day

Rectal: 30-50 g every 6 hours

Administration

Oral: Shake suspension well prior to administration. Administer orally (or via NG tube) as a suspension. **Do not mix in orange juice.** Chilling the oral mixture will increase palatability. Powder for suspension: For each 1 g of the powdered resin, add 3-4 mL of water or syrup (amount of fluid usually ranges from 20-100 mL)

Rectal: Enema route is less effective than oral administration. Administer cleansing enema first. Each dose of the powder for suspension should be suspended in 100 mL of aqueous vehicle and administered as a warm emulsion (body temperature). The commercially available suspension should also be warmed to body temperature. During administration, the solution should be agitated gently. Retain enema in colon for at least 30-60 minutes and for several hours, if possible. Once retention time is complete, irrigate colon with a non-sodium-containing solution to remove resin.

Monitoring Parameters Serum electrolytes (potassium, sodium, calcium, magnesium); ECG in select patients

Reference Range Serum potassium: Adults: 3.5-5.2 mEq/L

Pharmacotherapy Pearls 1 g of resin binds approximately 1 mEq of potassium

Historically, sorbitol was often recommended as a cathartic agent to be administered with sodium polystyrene sulfonate (SPS) to prevent SPS-induced fecal impaction. However, SPS, particularly when used with sorbitol, has been associated with cases of intestinal necrosis and other serious GI adverse events. Due to the concern that sorbitol may increase the risk of intestinal necrosis, concomitant use of sorbitol is no longer recommended.

Sodium polystyrene sulfonate is commercially available in a liquid suspension containing 33% sorbitol (~20 grams sorbitol per 60 mL suspension).

Special Geriatric Considerations Large doses in the elderly may cause fecal impaction and intestinal obstruction.

Dosage Forms Excipient information presented when available (limited, particularly for generics); consult specific product labeling.

Powder for suspension, oral/rectal: (454 g)

Kalexate: (454 g) [contains sodium 100 mg (4.1 mEq)/g]

Kayexalate®: (454 g) [contains sodium 100 mg (4.1 mEq)/g]

Kionex®: (454 g) [contains sodium 100 mg (4.1 mEq)/g]

Suspension, oral/rectal:

Kionex®: 15 g/60 mL (60 mL, 480 mL) [contains ethanol 0.2%, propylene glycol, sodium 1500 mg (65 mEq)/60 mL, sorbitol; raspberry flavor]

SPS®: 15 g/60 mL (60 mL, 120 mL, 473 mL) [contains ethanol 0.3%, propylene glycol, sodium 1500 mg (65 mEq)/60 mL, sorbitol; cherry flavor]

Selected References

McGowan CE, Saha S, Chu G, et al, "Intestinal Necrosis Due to Sodium Polystyrene Sulfonate (Kayexalate) in Sorbitol," *South Med J,* 2009, 102(5):493-7.

◆ **Sodium Salicylate** *see* Salicylates (Various Salts) *on page 1647*

◆ **Sodium Sulfacetamide** *see* Sulfacetamide (Ophthalmic) *on page 1713*

◆ **Sodium Sulfacetamide** *see* Sulfacetamide (Topical) *on page 1713*

◆ **Sodium Thiosalicylate** *see* Salicylates (Various Salts) *on page 1647*

◆ **Solaraze®** *see* Diclofenac (Topical) *on page 500*

◆ **Solarcaine® cool aloe Burn Relief [OTC]** *see* Lidocaine (Topical) *on page 1064*

Solifenacin (sol i FEN a sin)

Related Information

Pharmacotherapy of Urinary Incontinence *on page 2032*

Medication Safety Issues

Sound-alike/look-alike issues:

VESIcare® may be confused with Vesinoid®, Visicol®

Brand Names: U.S. VESIcare®

Index Terms Solifenacin Succinate; YM905

Generic Availability (U.S.) No

Pharmacologic Category Anticholinergic Agent

Use Treatment of overactive bladder with symptoms of urinary frequency, urgency, or urge incontinence

Contraindications Hypersensitivity to solifenacin or any component of the formulation; urinary retention; gastric retention; uncontrolled narrow-angle glaucoma.

◄ **Warnings/Precautions** Cases of angioedema involving the face, lips, tongue, and/or larynx have been reported. Immediately discontinue if tongue, hypopharynx, or larynx are involved. May cause drowsiness and/or blurred vision, which may impair physical or mental abilities; patients must be cautioned about performing tasks which require mental alertness (eg, operating machinery or driving). Heat prostration may occur in the presence of increased environmental temperature; use caution in hot weather and/or exercise. Use with caution in patients with bladder outflow obstruction, gastrointestinal obstructive disorders, and decreased gastrointestinal motility. Use with caution in patients with a known history of QT prolongation or other risk factors for QT prolongation (eg, concomitant use of medications known to prolong QT interval and/or electrolyte abnormalities); the risk for QT prolongation is dose-related. Use with caution in patients with controlled (treated) narrow-angle glaucoma; use is contraindicated with uncontrolled narrow-angle glaucoma. Dosage adjustment is required for patients with severe renal impairment (Cl_{cr} <30 mL/minute) or moderate (Child-Pugh class B) hepatic impairment; use is not recommended with severe hepatic impairment (Child-Pugh class C). Patients on potent CYP3A4 inhibitors require the lower dose of solifenacin.

Adverse Reactions (Reflective of adult population; not specific for elderly)
>10%: Gastrointestinal: Xerostomia (11% to 28%; dose-related), constipation (5% to 13%; dose-related)
1% to 10%:
Cardiovascular: Edema (≤1%), hypertension (≤1%)
Central nervous system: Headache (3% to 6%), fatigue (1% to 2%), depression (≤1%)
Gastrointestinal: Dyspepsia (1% to 4%), nausea (2% to 3%), upper abdominal pain (1% to 2%)
Genitourinary: Urinary tract infection (3% to 5%), urinary retention (≤1%)
Ocular: Blurred vision (4% to 5%), dry eyes (≤2%)
Respiratory: Cough (≤1%)
Miscellaneous: Influenza (≤2%)

Drug Interactions
Metabolism/Transport Effects Substrate of CYP3A4 (major)
Avoid Concomitant Use
Avoid concomitant use of Solifenacin with any of the following: Conivaptan
Increased Effect/Toxicity
Solifenacin may increase the levels/effects of: AbobotulinumtoxinA; Anticholinergics; Cannabinoids; OnabotulinumtoxinA; Potassium Chloride; RimabotulinumtoxinB

The levels/effects of Solifenacin may be increased by: Antifungal Agents (Azole Derivatives, Systemic); Conivaptan; CYP3A4 Inhibitors (Moderate); CYP3A4 Inhibitors (Strong); Dasatinib; Pramlintide
Decreased Effect
Solifenacin may decrease the levels/effects of: Acetylcholinesterase Inhibitors (Central); Secretin

The levels/effects of Solifenacin may be decreased by: Acetylcholinesterase Inhibitors (Central); CYP3A4 Inducers (Strong); Deferasirox; Herbs (CYP3A4 Inducers); Tocilizumab
Ethanol/Nutrition/Herb Interactions
Food: Grapefruit juice may increase the serum level effects of solifenacin.
Herb/Nutraceutical: St John's wort (*Hypericum*) may decrease the levels/effects of solifenacin.
Stability Store at controlled room temperature of 25°C (77°F); excursions permitted to 15°C to 30°C (59°F to 86°F).
Mechanism of Action Inhibits muscarinic receptors resulting in decreased urinary bladder contraction, increased residual urine volume, and decreased detrusor muscle pressure.
Pharmacodynamics/Kinetics
Distribution: V_d: 600 L
Protein binding: ~98% bound primarily to alpha$_1$-acid glycoprotein
Metabolism: Extensively hepatic; via N-oxidation and 4 R-hydroxylation, forms 1 active and 3 inactive metabolites; primary pathway for elimination is via CYP3A4
Bioavailability: ~90%
Half-life elimination: 45-68 hours following chronic dosing; prolonged in severe renal (Cl_{cr} <30 mL/minute) or moderate hepatic (Child-Pugh class B) impairment
Time to peak, plasma: 3-8 hours
Excretion: Urine 69% (<15% as unchanged drug); feces 23%
Dosage
Geriatric Base dosing on renal/hepatic function.
Adult Overactive bladder: Oral: 5 mg once daily; if tolerated, may increase to 10 mg once daily
Dosage adjustment with concomitant CYP3A4 inhibitors: Maximum solifenacin dose: 5 mg/day

Renal Impairment Use with caution in reduced renal function; Cl_{cr} <30 mL/minute: Maximum dose: 5 mg/day

Hepatic Impairment Use with caution in reduced hepatic function:
Moderate (Child-Pugh class B): Maximum dose: 5 mg/day
Severe (Child-Pugh class C): Use is not recommended

Administration Swallow tablet whole; administer with liquids; may be administered without regard to meals.

Monitoring Parameters Anticholinergic effects (eg, fixed and dilated pupils, blurred vision, tremors, or dry skin); creatinine clearance (prior to treatment for dosing adjustment); liver function

Special Geriatric Considerations In patients with Cl_{cr} <30 mL/minute, doses >5 mg/day are not recommended. Similar safety and effectiveness were observed in elderly and younger patients.

Dosage Forms Excipient information presented when available (limited, particularly for generics); consult specific product labeling.
Tablet, oral, as succinate:
VESIcare®: 5 mg, 10 mg

◆ **Solifenacin Succinate** see Solifenacin on page 1699
◆ **Solodyn®** see Minocycline on page 1218
◆ **Solu-CORTEF®** see Hydrocortisone (Systemic) on page 883
◆ **Solumedrol** see MethylPREDNISolone on page 1183
◆ **Solu-MEDROL®** see MethylPREDNISolone on page 1183
◆ **Solzira** see Gabapentin Enacarbil on page 805
◆ **Soma®** see Carisoprodol on page 279
◆ **Sominex® [OTC]** see DiphenhydrAMINE (Systemic) on page 520
◆ **Sominex® Maximum Strength [OTC]** see DiphenhydrAMINE (Systemic) on page 520
◆ **Somnote®** see Chloral Hydrate on page 330
◆ **Sonata®** see Zaleplon on page 1939
◆ **Soothe® [OTC]** see Artificial Tears on page 148

Sorbitol (SOR bi tole)

Related Information
Laxatives, Classification and Properties on page 2012
Treatment Options for Constipation on page 2035

Generic Availability (U.S.) Yes

Pharmacologic Category Genitourinary Irrigant; Laxative, Osmotic

Use Genitourinary irrigant in transurethral prostatic resection or other transurethral resection or other transurethral surgical procedures; diuretic; humectant; sweetening agent; hyperosmotic laxative; facilitate the passage of sodium polystyrene sulfonate through the intestinal tract

Contraindications Anuria

Warnings/Precautions Use with caution in patients with severe cardiopulmonary or renal impairment and in patients unable to metabolize sorbitol; large volumes may result in fluid overload and/or electrolyte changes.

Adverse Reactions (Reflective of adult population; not specific for elderly) Frequency not defined.
Cardiovascular: Edema
Endocrine & metabolic: Fluid and electrolyte losses, hyperglycemia, lactic acidosis
Gastrointestinal: Abdominal discomfort, diarrhea, dry mouth, nausea, vomiting, xerostomia

Drug Interactions

Avoid Concomitant Use
Avoid concomitant use of Sorbitol with any of the following: Calcium Polystyrene Sulfonate; Sodium Polystyrene Sulfonate

Increased Effect/Toxicity
Sorbitol may increase the levels/effects of: Calcium Polystyrene Sulfonate; Sodium Polystyrene Sulfonate

Decreased Effect There are no known significant interactions involving a decrease in effect.

Stability Avoid storage in temperatures >150°F; do not freeze.

Mechanism of Action A polyalcoholic sugar with osmotic cathartic actions

Pharmacodynamics/Kinetics
Onset of action: 0.25-1 hour
Absorption: Oral, rectal: Poor
Metabolism: Primarily hepatic to fructose

◀ **Dosage**
Geriatric & Adult
Hyperosmotic laxative (as single dose, at infrequent intervals):
Oral: 30-150 mL (as 70% solution)
Rectal enema: 120 mL as 25% to 30% solution
Adjunct to sodium polystyrene sulfonate: 15 mL as 70% solution orally until diarrhea occurs (10-20 mL/2 hours) or 20-100 mL as an oral vehicle for the sodium polystyrene sulfonate resin
When administered with charcoal:
Oral: 4.3 mL/kg of 70% sorbitol with 1 g/kg of activated charcoal every 4 hours until first stool containing charcoal is passed
Transurethral surgical procedures: Irrigation: Topical: 3% to 3.3% as transurethral surgical procedure irrigation

Monitoring Parameters Monitor for fluid overload and/or electrolyte disturbances following large volumes; changes may be delayed due to slow absorption

Special Geriatric Considerations Causes for constipation must be evaluated prior to initiating treatment. Nonpharmacological dietary treatment should be initiated before laxative use. Sorbitol is as effective as lactulose but is much less expensive.

Dosage Forms Excipient information presented when available (limited, particularly for generics); consult specific product labeling. [DSC] = Discontinued product
Solution, genitourinary irrigation [preservative free]: 3% (3000 mL, 5000 mL [DSC]); 3.3% (2000 mL, 4000 mL)
Solution, oral: 70% (30 mL, 473 mL, 480 mL, 3840 mL)

◆ **Sorine®** see Sotalol on page 1702

Sotalol (SOE ta lole)

Related Information
Beta-Blockers on page 2001
Medication Safety Issues
Sound-alike/look-alike issues:
Sotalol may be confused with Stadol®, Sudafed®
Betapace® may be confused with Betapace AF®
Betapace AF® may be confused with Betapace®
Brand Names: U.S. Betapace AF®; Betapace®; Sorine®
Brand Names: Canada Apo-Sotalol®; CO Sotalol; Dom-Sotalol; Med-Sotalol; Mylan-Sotalol; Novo-Sotalol; Nu-Sotalol; PHL-Sotalol; PMS-Sotalol; PRO-Sotalol; ratio-Sotalol; Rhoxal-sotalol; Riva-Sotalol; Rylosol; Sandoz-Sotalol; ZYM-Sotalol
Index Terms Sotalol Hydrochloride
Generic Availability (U.S.) Yes
Pharmacologic Category Antiarrhythmic Agent, Class II; Antiarrhythmic Agent, Class III; Beta-Adrenergic Blocker, Nonselective
Use Treatment of documented ventricular arrhythmias (ie, sustained ventricular tachycardia), that in the judgment of the physician are life-threatening; maintenance of normal sinus rhythm in patients with symptomatic atrial fibrillation and atrial flutter who are currently in sinus rhythm. Manufacturer states substitutions should not be made for Betapace AF® since Betapace AF® is distributed with a patient package insert specific for atrial fibrillation/flutter.

Injection: Substitution for oral sotalol in those who are unable to take sotalol orally
Unlabeled/Investigational Use Fetal tachycardia
Injection: Hemodynamically stable monomorphic ventricular tachycardia (ACLS, 2010)
Contraindications Hypersensitivity to sotalol or any component of the formulation; bronchial asthma; sinus bradycardia; second- or third-degree AV block (unless a functioning pacemaker is present); congenital or acquired long QT syndromes; cardiogenic shock; uncontrolled heart failure

Additional contraindications: Betapace AF® and the injectable formulation: Baseline QT_c interval >450 msec; bronchospastic conditions; Cl_{cr} <40 mL/minute; serum potassium <4 mEq/L; sick sinus syndrome

Warnings/Precautions [U.S. Boxed Warning] Manufacturer recommends initiation (or reinitiation) and doses increased in a hospital setting with continuous monitoring and staff familiar with the recognition and treatment of life-threatening arrhythmias. Some experts will initiate therapy on an outpatient basis in a patient without heart disease or bradycardia, who has a baseline uncorrected QT interval <450 msec, and normal serum potassium and magnesium levels; close ECG monitoring during this time is necessary. ACC/AHA guidelines for management of atrial fibrillation also recommend that for outpatient initiation the patient not have risk factors predisposing to drug-induced ventricular proarrhythmia (Fuster, 2006). Dosage should be adjusted gradually with 3 days between dosing increments to achieve steady-state concentrations, and to allow time to monitor QT intervals. **[U.S. Boxed Warning]: Adjust dosing interval based on creatinine clearance to decrease risk of proarrhythmia; QT interval prolongation is directly related to sotalol concentration.** Creatinine clearance must be calculated with dose initiation and dose increases. Use cautiously in the renally-impaired (dosage adjustment required). Betapace AF® and the injectable formulation are contraindicated in patients with Cl$_{cr}$ <40 mL/minute.

[U.S. Boxed Warning]: Sotalol injection: Sotalol can cause life-threatening ventricular tachycardia associated with QT-interval prolongation (ie, torsade de pointes). Do not initiate if baseline QTc interval is >450 msec. If QT$_c$ exceeds 500 msec during therapy, reduce the dose, prolong the infusion duration, or discontinue use. If while on oral sotalol therapy baseline QT$_c$ interval is >500 msec, use I.V. sotalol with particular caution; serious consideration should be given to reducing the dose or discontinuing I.V. sotalol when QT$_c$ exceeds 520 msec. QT$_c$ prolongation is directly related to the concentration of sotalol; reduced creatinine clearance, female gender, and large doses increase the risk of QT$_c$ prolongation and subsequent torsade de pointes. Monitor and adjust dose to prevent QT$_c$ prolongation. Concurrent use with other QT$_c$-prolonging drugs (including Class I and Class III antiarrhythmics) and use within 3 months of discontinuing amiodarone is generally not recommended. To reduce the chance of excessive QT$_c$-prolongation, withhold QT$_c$-prolonging drugs for at least 3 half-lives (or 3 months for amiodarone) before initiating sotalol.

Correct electrolyte imbalances before initiating (especially hypokalemia and hypomagnesemia). Consider pre-existing conditions such as sick sinus syndrome before initiating. Conduction abnormalities can occur particularly sinus bradycardia. Use cautiously within the first 2 weeks post-MI especially in patients with markedly impaired ventricular function (experience limited). Administer cautiously in compensated heart failure and monitor for a worsening of the condition. May precipitate or aggravate symptoms of arterial insufficiency in patients with PVD and Raynaud's disease; use with caution and monitor for progression of arterial obstruction. Bradycardia may be observed more frequently in elderly patients (>65 years of age); dosage reductions may be necessary. Beta-blocker therapy should not be withdrawn abruptly (particularly in patients with CAD), but gradually tapered to avoid acute tachycardia, hypertension, and/or ischemia. Chronic beta-blocker therapy should not be routinely withdrawn prior to major surgery. Use caution with concurrent use of digoxin, verapamil, or diltiazem; bradycardia or heart block can occur. Use with caution in patients receiving inhaled anesthetic agents known to depress myocardial contractility. Use cautiously in diabetics because it can mask prominent hypoglycemic symptoms. Use with caution in patients with bronchospastic disease, myasthenia gravis or psychiatric disease. Adequate alpha-blockade is required prior to use of any beta-blocker for patients with untreated pheochromocytoma. May mask signs of hyperthyroidism (eg, tachycardia); if hyperthyroidism is suspected, carefully manage and monitor; abrupt withdrawal may exacerbate symptoms of hyperthyroidism or precipitate thyroid storm. Use caution with history of severe anaphylaxis to allergens; patients taking beta-blockers may become more sensitive to repeated challenges. Treatment of anaphylaxis (eg, epinephrine) in patients taking beta-blockers may be ineffective or promote undesirable effects.

[U.S. Boxed Warning]: Betapace® should not be substituted for Betapace® AF; Betapace® AF is distributed with an educational insert specifically for patients with atrial fibrillation/flutter.

Adverse Reactions (Reflective of adult population; not specific for elderly) Note: No clinical experience with I.V. sotalol; however, since exposure is similar between I.V. and oral sotalol, adverse reactions are expected to be similar.

>10%:
  Cardiovascular: Bradycardia (13% to 16%), chest pain (3% to 16%), palpitation (14%)
  Central nervous system: Fatigue (20%), dizziness (20%), lightheadedness (12%)
  Neuromuscular & skeletal: Weakness (13%)
  Respiratory: Dyspnea (21%)
1% to 10%:
  Cardiovascular: Edema (8%), abnormal ECG (7%), hypotension (6%), proarrhythmia (5%), syncope (5%), CHF (5%), torsade de pointes (dose related; 1% to 4%), peripheral vascular disorders (3%), ventricular tachycardia worsened (1%), QT$_c$ interval prolongation (dose related)
  Central nervous system: Headache (8%), sleep problems (8%), mental confusion (6%), anxiety (4%), depression (4%)
  Dermatologic: Itching/rash (5%)
  Endocrine & metabolic: Sexual ability decreased (3%)
  Gastrointestinal: Nausea/vomiting (10%), diarrhea (7%), stomach discomfort (3% to 6%), flatulence (2%)
  Genitourinary: Impotence (2%)

◄ Hematologic: Bleeding (2%)
Neuromuscular & skeletal: Extremity pain (7%), paresthesia (4%), back pain (3%)
Ocular: Visual problems (5%)
Respiratory: Upper respiratory problems (5% to 8%), asthma (2%)

Drug Interactions

Avoid Concomitant Use

Avoid concomitant use of Sotalol with any of the following: Artemether; Dronedarone; Floctafenine; Lumefantrine; Methacholine; Nilotinib; Pimozide; QUEtiapine; QuiNINE; Tetrabenazine; Thioridazine; Toremifene; Vandetanib; Vemurafenib; Ziprasidone

Increased Effect/Toxicity

Sotalol may increase the levels/effects of: Alpha-/Beta-Agonists (Direct-Acting); Alpha1-Blockers; Alpha2-Agonists; Amifostine; Antihypertensives; Antipsychotic Agents (Phenothiazines); Bupivacaine; Cardiac Glycosides; Dronedarone; Fingolimod; Hypotensive Agents; Insulin; Lidocaine; Lidocaine (Systemic); Lidocaine (Topical); Mepivacaine; Methacholine; Midodrine; Pimozide; QTc-Prolonging Agents; QuiNINE; RiTUXimab; Sulfonylureas; Tetrabenazine; Thioridazine; Toremifene; Vandetanib; Vemurafenib; Ziprasidone

The levels/effects of Sotalol may be increased by: Acetylcholinesterase Inhibitors; Alfuzosin; Aminoquinolines (Antimalarial); Amiodarone; Anilidopiperidine Opioids; Antipsychotic Agents (Phenothiazines); Artemether; Calcium Channel Blockers (Dihydropyridine); Calcium Channel Blockers (Nondihydropyridine); Chloroquine; Ciprofloxacin; Ciprofloxacin (Systemic); Diazoxide; Dipyridamole; Disopyramide; Dronedarone; Eribulin; Fingolimod; Floctafenine; Gadobutrol; Herbs (Hypotensive Properties); Lumefantrine; MAO Inhibitors; Nilotinib; Pentoxifylline; Phosphodiesterase 5 Inhibitors; Propafenone; Propoxyphene; Prostacyclin Analogues; QUEtiapine; QuiNIDine; QuiNINE; Reserpine

Decreased Effect

Sotalol may decrease the levels/effects of: Beta2-Agonists; Theophylline Derivatives

The levels/effects of Sotalol may be decreased by: Barbiturates; Herbs (Hypertensive Properties); Methylphenidate; Nonsteroidal Anti-Inflammatory Agents; Rifamycin Derivatives; Yohimbine

Ethanol/Nutrition/Herb Interactions

Food: Sotalol peak serum concentrations may be decreased if taken with food.
Herb/Nutraceutical: Avoid ephedra (may worsen arrhythmia).

Stability Store at 25°C (77°F); excursions permitted to 15°C to 30°C (59°F to 86°F). To prepare sotalol infusion, see manufacturer's prescribing information.

Mechanism of Action

Beta-blocker which contains both beta-adrenoreceptor-blocking (Vaughan Williams Class II) and cardiac action potential duration prolongation (Vaughan Williams Class III) properties
Class II effects: Increased sinus cycle length, slowed heart rate, decreased AV nodal conduction, and increased AV nodal refractoriness
Class III effects: Prolongation of the atrial and ventricular monophasic action potentials, and effective refractory prolongation of atrial muscle, ventricular muscle, and atrioventricular accessory pathways in both the antegrade and retrograde directions
Sotalol is a racemic mixture of *d*- and *l*-sotalol; both isomers have similar Class III antiarrhythmic effects while the *l*-isomer is responsible for virtually all of the beta-blocking activity
Sotalol has both beta$_1$- and beta$_2$-receptor blocking activity. The beta-blocking effect of sotalol is a noncardioselective [half maximal at about 80 mg/day and maximal at doses of 320-640 mg/day]. Significant beta-blockade occurs at oral doses as low as 25 mg/day.
The Class III effects are seen only at oral doses ≥160 mg/day

Pharmacodynamics/Kinetics

Onset of action: Rapid, 1-2 hours
Duration: 8-16 hours
Absorption: Oral: Decreased 20% to 30% by meals compared to fasting
Distribution: V_d: 1.2-2.4 L/kg
Protein binding: None
Metabolism: None
Bioavailability: Oral: 90% to 100%
Half-life elimination: 12 hours; increases with renal dysfunction
Time to peak, serum: 2.5-4 hours
Excretion: Urine (as unchanged drug)

Dosage

Geriatric & Adult Baseline QT_c interval and creatinine clearance must be determined prior to initiation. Sotalol should be initiated and doses increased in a hospital with facilities for cardiac rhythm monitoring and assessment. Proarrhythmic events can occur after initiation of therapy and with each upward dosage adjustment.

Conversion from oral sotalol to I.V. sotalol:
  80 mg oral equivalent to 75 mg I.V.
  120 mg oral equivalent to 112.5 mg I.V.
  160 mg oral equivalent to 150 mg I.V.

Ventricular arrhythmias:
I.V.: **Note:** The effects of the initial I.V. dose must be monitored and the dose titrated either upward or downward, if needed, based on clinical effect, QT_c interval, or adverse reactions.
  Substitution for oral sotalol: Initial dose: 75 mg infused over 5 hours twice daily
    Dose adjustment: If the frequency of relapse does not reduce and excessive QT_c prolongation does not occur, may increase to 112.5 mg twice daily. For ventricular arrhythmias, may increase dose every 3 days in increments of 75 mg/day.
    Dose range: Usual therapeutic dose: 75-150 mg twice daily; maximum dose: 300 mg twice daily.
  Hemodynamically stable monomorphic VT, ongoing (unlabeled use): 1.5 mg/kg over 5 minutes (ACLS, 2010); **Note:** Clinical trial employed standard dose of 100 mg (Ho, 1994).
Oral (Betapace®, Sorine®):
  Initial: 80 mg twice daily; dose may be increased gradually to 240-320 mg/day; allow 3 days between dosing increments (to attain steady-state plasma concentrations and to allow monitoring of QT_c intervals).
  Usual range: Most patients respond to 160-320 mg/day in 2-3 divided doses.
  Maximum: Some patients, with life-threatening refractory ventricular arrhythmias, may require doses as high as 480-640 mg/day; prescribed ONLY when the potential benefit outweighs the increased of adverse events.

Atrial fibrillation or atrial flutter:
I.V.: **Note:** The effects of the initial I.V. dose must be monitored and the dose titrated either upward or downward, if needed, based on clinical effect, QT_c interval, or adverse reactions.
  Substitution for oral sotalol: Initial dose: 75 mg infused over 5 hours twice daily
    Dose adjustment: If the frequency of relapse does not reduce and excessive QT_c prolongation does not occur, may increase to 112.5 mg twice daily. For ventricular arrhythmias, may increase dose every 3 days in increments of 75 mg/day.
    Dose range: Usual therapeutic dose: 112.5 mg twice daily; maximum dose: 150 mg twice daily
Oral (Betapace AF®): Initial: 80 mg twice daily. If the frequency of relapse does not reduce and excessive QT_c prolongation does not occur after 3 days, the dose may be increased to 120 mg twice daily; may further increase to 160 mg twice daily if response is inadequate and QT_c prolongation is not excessive.

Renal Impairment Adults: Impaired renal function can increase the terminal half-life, resulting in increased drug accumulation. Sotalol (Betapace AF®, injectable formulation) is contraindicated per the manufacturers for treatment of atrial fibrillation/flutter in patients with a Cl_{cr} <40 mL/minute.
Ventricular arrhythmias (Betapace®, Sorine®):
  Cl_{cr} >60 mL/minute: Administer every 12 hours.
  Cl_{cr} 30-60 mL/minute: Administer every 24 hours.
  Cl_{cr} 10-29 mL/minute: Administer every 36-48 hours.
  Cl_{cr} <10 mL/minute: Individualize dose.
Atrial fibrillation/flutter (Betapace AF®):
  Cl_{cr} >60 mL/minute: Administer every 12 hours.
  Cl_{cr} 40-60 mL/minute: Administer every 24 hours.
  Cl_{cr} <40 mL/minute: Use is contraindicated.
Note: The manufacturer of the injectable formulation recommends adjustment similar to that used for Betapace AF®. However, the injectable formulation may be used for either indication.

Dialysis: Hemodialysis would be expected to reduce sotalol plasma concentrations because sotalol is not bound to plasma proteins and does not undergo extensive metabolism. Administer dose postdialysis or administer supplemental 80 mg dose. Peritoneal dialysis does not remove sotalol; supplemental dose is not necessary.

Administration
Oral: Administer without regard to meals.
I.V.:
  Substitution for oral: Administer over 5 hours.
  Hemodynamically stable monomorphic VT: Administer I.V. push over 5 minutes; use with caution due to increased risk of adverse events (eg, bradycardia, hypotension, torsade de pointes) (ACLS, 2010)

Monitoring Parameters Serum creatinine, magnesium, potassium; heart rate, blood pressure; ECG (eg, QT_c interval, PR interval). If baseline QT_c >450 msec (or JT interval >330 msec if QRS over 100 msec), sotalol is contraindicated.

For oral use (Betapace AF®) during initiation period, monitor QT_c interval 2-4 hours after each dose. If QT_c interval ≥500 msec, discontinue use; if QT_c interval <500 msec after 3 days (after fifth or sixth dose if patient receiving once-daily dosing), patient may be discharged on current regimen. Monitor QT_c interval periodically thereafter.

For I.V. use, measure QT_c interval after completion of each infusion.

Test Interactions May falsely increase urinary metanephrine values when fluorimetric or photometric methods are used; does not interact with HPLC assay with solid phase extraction for determination of urinary catecholamines

Pharmacotherapy Pearls If patients are receiving another antiarrhythmic, it is best to withdraw the agent, with careful monitoring, for at least 2-3 half-lives of the agent if clinical condition allows before initiating sotalol; treatment with sotalol has been initiated in some with patients receiving I.V. lidocaine without problems; if patients are receiving amiodarone, **do not** start sotalol until QT interval is normal

Special Geriatric Considerations Since elderly frequently have Cl_{cr} <60 mL/minute, attention to dose, creatinine clearance, and monitoring is important. Make dosage adjustments at 3-day intervals or after 5-6 doses at any dosage.

Dosage Forms Excipient information presented when available (limited, particularly for generics); consult specific product labeling.

Injection, solution, as hydrochloride [preservative free]: 15 mg/mL (10 mL)

Tablet, oral, as hydrochloride: 80 mg [atrial fibrillation], 80 mg, 120 mg [atrial fibrillation], 120 mg, 160 mg [atrial fibrillation], 160 mg, 240 mg

Betapace AF®: 80 mg, 120 mg, 160 mg [scored; atrial fibrillation]

Betapace®: 80 mg, 120 mg, 160 mg, 240 mg [scored]

Sorine®: 80 mg, 120 mg, 160 mg, 240 mg [scored]

Extemporaneously Prepared To make a 5 mg/mL oral solution, using a 6-ounce amber plastic prescription bottle, add five sotalol 120 mg tablets to 120 mL of simple syrup containing 0.1% sodium benzoate (tablets do not need to be crushed). Shake well. Allow tablets to hydrate for ~2 hours; shake intermittently until tablets completely disintegrate. Store at room temperature; shake well before use. Stable for 3 months. (Refer to manufacturer's current labeling.)

Selected References

Fuster V, Ryden LE, Cannom DS, et al, "ACC/AHA/ESC 2006 Guidelines for the Management of Patients With Atrial Fibrillation-Excutrive Summary. A Report of the American College of Cardiology/American Heart Association Task Force on Practice Guidelines and the European Society of Cardiology Committee for Practice Guidelines (Writing Committee to Revise the 2001 Guidelines for the Management of Patients With Atrial Fibrillation). Developed in Collaboration With the European Heart Rhythm Association and the Heart Rhythm Society," *J Am Coll Cardiol*, 2006, 48(4):854-906.

◆ **Sotalol Hydrochloride** see Sotalol on page 1702
◆ **SPD417** see CarBAMazepine on page 268
◆ **Spectracef®** see Cefditoren on page 294
◆ **SPI 0211** see Lubiprostone on page 1102

Spinosad (SPIN oh sad)

Brand Names: U.S. Natroba™
Index Terms NatrOVA
Pharmacologic Category Antiparasitic Agent, Topical; Pediculocide
Use Topical treatment of head lice (*Pediculosis capitis*) infestation in adults and children ≥4 years of age
Unlabeled/Investigational Use Topical treatment of head lice (*Pediculosis capitis*) infestation in children ≥6 months and <4 years of age
Contraindications There are no contraindications listed in the manufacturer's labeling
Warnings/Precautions For topical use on scalp and scalp hair only; avoid contact with eyes. Wash hands after application. The suspension contains benzyl alcohol.
Adverse Reactions (Reflective of adult population; not specific for elderly)
1% to 10%:
Dermatologic: Application site erythema (3%), application site irritation (1%), skin irritation
Ocular: Erythema (2%), hyperemia (2%), irritation
Drug Interactions
Avoid Concomitant Use There are no known interactions where it is recommended to avoid concomitant use.
Increased Effect/Toxicity There are no known significant interactions involving an increase in effect.

Decreased Effect There are no known significant interactions involving a decrease in effect.

Stability Store at 25°C (77°F); excursions permitted between 15°C to 30°C (59°F to 86°F).

Mechanism of Action Insect paralysis and death is caused by central nervous system excitation and involuntary muscle contractions. Spinosad is thought to be both pediculocidal and ovicidal (Stough, 2009).

Pharmacodynamics/Kinetics Absorption: Not absorbed topically (not detectable in a pediatric patient plasma sampling study); absorption of the benzyl alcohol was not analyzed in this study.

Dosage

Geriatric Refer to adult dosing.

Adult Head lice: Topical: Apply sufficient amount to cover dry scalp and completely cover dry hair; 120 mL may be necessary depending on the length of hair. If live lice are seen 7 days after first treatment, repeat with second application.

Administration Topical suspension. For external use only. Shake bottle well. Apply to dry scalp and rub gently until the scalp is thoroughly moistened, then apply to dry hair; completely covering scalp and hair. Leave on for 10 minutes (start timing treatment after the scalp and hair have been completely covered). The hair should then be rinsed thoroughly with warm water. Shampoo may be used immediately after the product is completely rinsed off. If live lice are seen 7 days after the first treatment, repeat with second application. Avoid contact with the eyes. Nit combing is not required, although a fine-tooth comb may be used to remove treated lice and nits.

Spinosad should be a portion of a whole lice removal program, which should include washing or dry cleaning all clothing, hats, bedding and towels recently worn or used by the patient and washing combs, brushes and hair accessories in hot water.

Monitoring Parameters Monitor scalp for lice

Special Geriatric Considerations Specific information on the safety and efficacy of spinosad in persons ≥65 years of age is not available as this age group was not sufficiently represented in clinical trials.

Dosage Forms Excipient information presented when available (limited, particularly for generics); consult specific product labeling.

Suspension, topical:
  Natroba™: 0.9% (120 mL) [contains benzyl alcohol, isopropyl alcohol]

Selected References
Frankowski BL and Bocchini JA Jr, "Head Lice," *Pediatrics*, 2010, 126(2):392-403.
Stough D, Shellabarger S, Quiring J, et al, "Efficacy and Safety of Spinosad and PermethrinCreme Rinses for PediculosisCapitis (Head Lice)," *Pediatrics*, 2009, 124(3):e389-95.

◆ **Spiriva® HandiHaler®** see Tiotropium on page 1804

Spironolactone (speer on oh LAK tone)

Medication Safety Issues
Sound-alike/look-alike issues:
  Aldactone® may be confused with Aldactazide®
International issues:
  Aldactone: Brand name for spironolactone [U.S., Canada], but also the brand name for potassium canrenoate [Austria, Czech Republic, Germany, Hungary, Poland]

Brand Names: U.S. Aldactone®
Brand Names: Canada Aldactone®; Novo-Spiroton; Teva-Spironolactone
Generic Availability (U.S.) Yes
Pharmacologic Category Diuretic, Potassium-Sparing; Selective Aldosterone Blocker
Use Management of edema associated with excessive aldosterone excretion; hypertension; primary hyperaldosteronism; hypokalemia; cirrhosis of liver accompanied by edema or ascites; nephrotic syndrome; severe heart failure (NYHA class III-IV) to increase survival and reduce hospitalization when added to standard therapy
Unlabeled/Investigational Use Female acne (adjunctive therapy); hirsutism
Contraindications Hypersensitivity to spironolactone or any component of the formulation; anuria; acute renal insufficiency; significant impairment of renal excretory function; hyperkalemia
Warnings/Precautions Monitor serum potassium closely in patients being treated for heart failure. Avoid potassium supplements, potassium-containing salt substitutes, a diet rich in potassium, or other drugs that can cause hyperkalemia. Excess amounts can lead to profound diuresis with fluid and electrolyte loss; close medical supervision and dose evaluation are required. Watch for and correct electrolyte disturbances; adjust dose to avoid dehydration. In cirrhosis, avoid electrolyte and acid/base imbalances that might lead to hepatic encephalopathy. Gynecomastia is related to dose and duration of therapy. Discontinue use prior to adrenal vein catheterization. When evaluating a heart failure patient for spironolactone

◀ treatment, creatinine should be ≤2.5 mg/dL in men or ≤2 mg/dL in women and potassium <5 mEq/L. Discontinue or interrupt therapy if serum potassium >5 mEq/L or serum creatinine >4 mg/dL. **[U.S. Boxed Warning]: Shown to be a tumorigen in chronic toxicity animal studies. Avoid unnecessary use.**

Adverse Reactions (Reflective of adult population; not specific for elderly) Frequency not defined.

Cardiovascular: Vasculitis

Central nervous system: Ataxia, confusion, drowsiness, fever, headache, lethargy

Dermatologic: Maculopapular or erythematous cutaneous eruptions, urticaria

Endocrine & metabolic: Gynecomastia, hyperkalemia, impotence, irregular menses, amenorrhea, postmenopausal bleeding

Gastrointestinal: Cramps, diarrhea, gastritis, gastric bleeding, nausea, ulceration, vomiting

Hematologic: Agranulocytosis

Hepatic: Cholestatic/hepatocellular toxicity

Renal: BUN increased, renal dysfunction, renal failure

Miscellaneous: Anaphylactic reaction, breast cancer

Drug Interactions

Avoid Concomitant Use

Avoid concomitant use of Spironolactone with any of the following: Tacrolimus

Increased Effect/Toxicity

Spironolactone may increase the levels/effects of: ACE Inhibitors; Amifostine; Ammonium Chloride; Antihypertensives; Cardiac Glycosides; Digoxin; Hypotensive Agents; Neuromuscular-Blocking Agents (Nondepolarizing); RiTUXimab; Sodium Phosphates; Tacrolimus

The levels/effects of Spironolactone may be increased by: Alfuzosin; Angiotensin II Receptor Blockers; Diazoxide; Drospirenone; Eplerenone; Herbs (Hypotensive Properties); MAO Inhibitors; Nonsteroidal Anti-Inflammatory Agents; Pentoxifylline; Phosphodiesterase 5 Inhibitors; Potassium Salts; Prostacyclin Analogues; Tolvaptan

Decreased Effect

Spironolactone may decrease the levels/effects of: Alpha-/Beta-Agonists; Cardiac Glycosides; Mitotane; QuiNIDine

The levels/effects of Spironolactone may be decreased by: Herbs (Hypertensive Properties); Methylphenidate; Nonsteroidal Anti-Inflammatory Agents; Yohimbine

Ethanol/Nutrition/Herb Interactions

Ethanol: Increases risk of orthostasis.

Food: Food increases absorption.

Herb/Nutraceutical: Avoid natural licorice (due to mineralocorticoid activity)

Stability Store below 25°C (77°F).

Mechanism of Action Competes with aldosterone for receptor sites in the distal renal tubules, increasing sodium chloride and water excretion while conserving potassium and hydrogen ions; may block the effect of aldosterone on arteriolar smooth muscle as well

Pharmacodynamics/Kinetics

Duration: 2-3 days

Protein binding: 91% to 98%

Metabolism: Hepatic to multiple metabolites, including active metabolites canrenone and 7-alpha-spirolactone

Half-life elimination: Spironolactone: 78-84 minutes; Canrenone: 10-23 hours; 7-alpha-spirolactone: 7-20 hours

Time to peak, serum: 3-4 hours (primarily as the active metabolite)

Excretion: Urine and feces

Dosage

Geriatric Oral: Indication specific: Initial: 25-50 mg/day in 1-2 divided doses; increase by 25-50 mg every 5 days as needed. Adjust for renal impairment.

Adult To reduce delay in onset of effect, a loading dose of 2 or 3 times the daily dose may be administered on the first day of therapy.

Edema: Oral: 25-200 mg/day in 1-2 divided doses

Hypokalemia: Oral: 25-100 mg daily

Hypertension (JNC 7): Oral: 25-50 mg/day in 1-2 divided doses

Diagnosis of primary aldosteronism: Oral: Long test: 400 mg daily for 3-4 weeks; short test: 400 mg daily for 4 days; maintenance until surgical correction: 100-400 mg/day in 1-2 divided doses

Heart failure, severe (NYHA class III-IV; with ACE inhibitor and a loop diuretic ± digoxin): 12.5-25 mg/day; maximum daily dose: 50 mg. If 25 mg once daily not tolerated, reduce to 25 mg every other day was the lowest maintenance dose possible.

Note: If potassium >5 mEq/L or serum creatinine >4 mg/dL, discontinue or interrupt therapy.

Acne in women (unlabeled use): Oral: 25-200 mg once daily

Hirsutism in women (unlabeled use): Oral: 50-200 mg/day in 1-2 divided doses (Koulouri, 2008; Martin, 2008)

Renal Impairment Heart failure:

Cl_{cr} 31-50 mL/minute: Decrease initial dose to 12.5 mg once daily.

Cl_{cr} <30 mL/minute: Not recommended.

Monitoring Parameters Blood pressure, serum electrolytes (potassium, sodium), renal function, I & O ratios and daily weight throughout therapy

HF: Potassium levels and renal function should be checked in 3 days and 1 week after initiation or increase in dose, then every 2-4 weeks for 3 months, then quarterly for a year, then every 6 months thereafter.

Test Interactions May cause false elevation in serum digoxin concentrations measured by RIA

Pharmacotherapy Pearls Maximum diuretic effect may be delayed 2-3 days and maximum hypertensive effects may be delayed 2-3 weeks.

Special Geriatric Considerations When used in combination with ACE inhibitors, monitor patient for hyperkalemia.

Dosage Forms Excipient information presented when available (limited, particularly for generics); consult specific product labeling.

Tablet, oral: 25 mg, 50 mg, 100 mg

Aldactone®: 25 mg

Aldactone®: 50 mg, 100 mg [scored]

Selected References

Bozkurt B, Agoston I, and Knowlton AA, "Complications of Inappropriate Use of Spironolactone in Heart Failure: When an Old Medicine Spirals Out of New Guidelines," *J Am Coll Cardiol*, 2003, 41(2):211-4.

Hunt SA, Abraham WT, Chin MH, et al, "2009 Focused Update Incorporated Into the ACC/AHA 2005 Guidelines for the Diagnosis and Management of Heart Failure in Adults A Report of the American College of Cardiology Foundation/American Heart Association Task Force on Practice Guidelines Developed in Collaboration With the International Society for Heart and Lung Transplantation," *J Am Coll Cardiol*, 2009, 53(15):e1-e90.

Juurlink DN, Mamdani MM, Lee DS, et al, "Rates of Hyperkalemia After Publication of the Randomized Aldactone Evaluation Study," *N Engl J Med*, 2004, 351(6):543-51.

Pitt B, Zannad F, Remme WJ, et al, "The Effect of Spironolactone on Morbidity and Mortality in Patients With Severe Heart Failure," *N Engl J Med*, 1999, 341(10):709-17.

Streptomycin (strep toe MYE sin)

Medication Safety Issues

Sound-alike/look-alike issues:

Streptomycin may be confused with streptozocin

Index Terms Streptomycin Sulfate

Generic Availability (U.S.) Yes

Pharmacologic Category Antibiotic, Aminoglycoside; Antitubercular Agent

Use Part of combination therapy of active tuberculosis; used in combination with other agents for treatment of streptococcal or enterococcal endocarditis, mycobacterial infections, plague, tularemia, and brucellosis

Contraindications Hypersensitivity to streptomycin or any component of the formulation

Warnings/Precautions [U.S. Boxed Warning]: May cause neurotoxicity, nephrotoxicity, and/or neuromuscular blockade and respiratory paralysis; usual risk factors include pre-existing renal impairment, concomitant neuro-/nephrotoxic medications, advanced age and dehydration. The drug's neurotoxicity can result in respiratory paralysis from neuromuscular blockade, especially when the drug is given soon after anesthesia or muscle relaxants. Use with caution in patients with pre-existing vertigo, tinnitus, hearing loss, neuromuscular disorders, or renal impairment; modify dosage in patients with renal impairment; ototoxicity is directly proportional to the amount of drug given and the duration of treatment; tinnitus or vertigo are indications of vestibular injury and impending bilateral irreversible damage; renal damage is usually reversible. **[U.S. Boxed Warning]: Parenteral form should be used only where appropriate audiometric and laboratory testing facilities are available.** Prolonged use may result in fungal or bacterial superinfection, including *C. difficile*-associated diarrhea (CDAD) and pseudomembranous colitis; CDAD has been observed >2 months postantibiotic treatment.

Adverse Reactions (Reflective of adult population; not specific for elderly) Frequency not defined.

Cardiovascular: Hypotension

Central nervous system: Neurotoxicity, drowsiness, headache, drug fever, paresthesia

Dermatologic: Skin rash

Gastrointestinal: Nausea, vomiting

Hematologic: Eosinophilia, anemia

Neuromuscular & skeletal: Arthralgia, weakness, tremor

Otic: Ototoxicity (auditory), ototoxicity (vestibular)

Renal: Nephrotoxicity

Respiratory: Difficulty in breathing

Drug Interactions

Avoid Concomitant Use

Avoid concomitant use of Streptomycin with any of the following: BCG; Gallium Nitrate

Increased Effect/Toxicity

Streptomycin may increase the levels/effects of: AbobotulinumtoxinA; Bisphosphonate Derivatives; CARBOplatin; Colistimethate; CycloSPORINE; CycloSPORINE (Systemic); Gallium Nitrate; Neuromuscular-Blocking Agents; OnabotulinumtoxinA; Rimabotulinumtoxin B

The levels/effects of Streptomycin may be increased by: Amphotericin B; Capreomycin; CISplatin; Loop Diuretics; Nonsteroidal Anti-Inflammatory Agents; Vancomycin

Decreased Effect

Streptomycin may decrease the levels/effects of: BCG; Typhoid Vaccine

The levels/effects of Streptomycin may be decreased by: Penicillins

Stability Depending upon manufacturer, reconstituted solution remains stable for 2-4 weeks when refrigerated. Exposure to light causes darkening of solution without apparent loss of potency.

Mechanism of Action Inhibits bacterial protein synthesis by binding directly to the 30S ribosomal subunits causing faulty peptide sequence to form in the protein chain

Pharmacodynamics/Kinetics

Absorption: Oral: Poorly absorbed; I.M.: Well absorbed

Distribution: To extracellular fluid including serum, abscesses, ascitic, pericardial, pleural, synovial, lymphatic, and peritoneal fluids; poorly distributed into CSF

Protein binding: 34%

Half-life elimination: Newborns: 4-10 hours; Adults: 2-4.7 hours, prolonged with renal impairment

Time to peak: I.M.: Within 1 hour

Excretion: Urine (90% as unchanged drug); feces, saliva, sweat, and tears (<1%)

Dosage

Geriatric I.M.: 10 mg/kg/day, not to exceed 750 mg/day; dosing interval should be adjusted for renal function. Some authors suggest not to give more than 5 days/week or give as 20-25 mg/kg/dose twice weekly.

Adult

Brucellosis: I.M.: 1 g/day for 14-21 days (with doxycycline, 100 mg twice daily for 6 weeks)

Endocarditis: I.M.:

Enterococcal: 1 g every 12 hours for 2 weeks, 500 mg every 12 hours for 4 weeks in combination with penicillin

Streptococcal: 1 g every 12 hours for 1 week

Mycobacterium avium **complex:** I.M.: Adjunct therapy (with macrolide, rifamycin, and ethambutol): 15 mg/kg 3 times/week for first 2-3 months for severe disease

Plague: I.M.: 15 mg/kg (or 1 g) every 12 hours until the patient is afebrile for at least 3 days

Tuberculosis: I.M.:
  Daily therapy: 15 mg/kg/day (maximum: 1 g)
  Directly observed therapy (DOT), twice weekly: 25-30 mg/kg (maximum: 1.5 g)
  Directly observed therapy (DOT), 3 times/week: 25-30 mg/kg (maximum: 1.5 g)
Tularemia: I.M.: 10-15 mg/kg every 12 hours (maximum: 2 g/day) for 7-10 days or until patient is afebrile for 5-7 days

Renal Impairment
  Cl_{cr} 10-50 mL/minute: Administer every 24-72 hours.
  Cl_{cr} <10 mL/minute: Administer every 72-96 hours.
  Removed by hemo- and peritoneal dialysis: Administer dose postdialysis.

Administration Inject deep I.M. into large muscle mass; I.V. administration is not recommended

Monitoring Parameters Hearing (audiogram), BUN, creatinine; serum concentration of the drug should be monitored in all patients; eighth cranial nerve damage is usually preceded by high-pitched tinnitus, roaring noises, sense of fullness in ears, or impaired hearing and may persist for weeks after drug is discontinued

Reference Range Therapeutic: Peak: 20-30 mcg/mL; Trough: <5 mcg/mL; Toxic: Peak: >50 mcg/mL; Trough: >10 mcg/mL

Test Interactions False-positive urine glucose with Benedict's solution or Clinitest®; penicillin may decrease aminoglycoside serum concentrations *in vitro*

Pharmacotherapy Pearls Eighth cranial nerve damage is usually preceded by high-pitched tinnitus, roaring noises, sense of fullness in ears, or impaired hearing and may persist for weeks after drug is discontinued.

Special Geriatric Considerations Streptomycin is indicated for persons from endemic areas of drug-resistant *Mycobacterium tuberculosis* or who are HIV infected. Since most older patients acquired the *M. tuberculosis* infection prior to the availability of effective chemotherapy, isoniazid and rifampin are usually effective unless resistant organisms are suspected or the patient is HIV infected. Adjust dose interval for renal function.

Dosage Forms Excipient information presented when available (limited, particularly for generics); consult specific product labeling.
  Injection, powder for reconstitution: 1 g

Selected References
Stead WW and Dutt AK, "Tuberculosis: A Special Problem in the Elderly," *Principles of Geriatric Medicine and Gerontology,* 2nd ed, 1990, 522.
Yoshikawa TT, "Tuberculosis in Aging Adults," *J Am Geriatr Soc,* 1992, 40(2):178-87.

- ◆ **Streptomycin Sulfate** *see* Streptomycin *on page 1709*
- ◆ **Striant®** *see* Testosterone *on page 1761*
- ◆ **Stridex® Essential Care® [OTC]** *see* Salicylic Acid *on page 1648*
- ◆ **Stridex® Facewipes To Go® [OTC]** *see* Salicylic Acid *on page 1648*
- ◆ **Stridex® Maximum Strength [OTC]** *see* Salicylic Acid *on page 1648*
- ◆ **Stridex® Sensitive Skin [OTC]** *see* Salicylic Acid *on page 1648*
- ◆ **Strong Iodine Solution** *see* Potassium Iodide and Iodine *on page 1491*
- ◆ **Subutex®** *see* Buprenorphine *on page 225*

Sucralfate (soo KRAL fate)

Medication Safety Issues
  Sound-alike/look-alike issues:
    Sucralfate may be confused with salsalate
    Carafate® may be confused with Cafergot®

Brand Names: U.S. Carafate®

Brand Names: Canada Apo-Sucralfate; Dom-Sucralfate; Novo-Sucralate; Nu-Sucralate; PMS-Sucralate; Sucralfate-1; Sulcrate®; Sulcrate® Suspension Plus; Teva-Sucralfate

Index Terms Aluminum Sucrose Sulfate, Basic

Generic Availability (U.S.) Yes

Pharmacologic Category Gastrointestinal Agent, Miscellaneous

Use Short-term (≤8 weeks) management of duodenal ulcers; maintenance therapy for duodenal ulcers

Unlabeled/Investigational Use Treatment of gastric ulcers, stomatitis due to cancer chemotherapy and other causes of esophageal and gastric erosions (suspension), GERD, esophagitis, NSAID mucosal damage; prevention of stress ulcers; postsclerotherapy for esophageal variceal bleeding

Contraindications Hypersensitivity to sucralfate or any component of the formulation

Warnings/Precautions Because sucralfate acts locally at the ulcer site, successful therapy with sucralfate should not be expected to alter the posthealing frequency of recurrence or the severity of duodenal ulceration. Use with caution in patients with chronic renal failure; sucralfate is an aluminum complex, small amounts of aluminum are absorbed following oral administration. Excretion of aluminum may be decreased in patients with chronic renal failure. Because of the potential for sucralfate to alter the absorption of some drugs, separate administration (take other medication 2 hours before sucralfate) should be considered when alterations in bioavailability are believed to be critical.

Adverse Reactions (Reflective of adult population; not specific for elderly)
1% to 10%: Gastrointestinal: Constipation (2%)

Drug Interactions

Avoid Concomitant Use
Avoid concomitant use of Sucralfate with any of the following: Vitamin D Analogs

Increased Effect/Toxicity
The levels/effects of Sucralfate may be increased by: Vitamin D Analogs

Decreased Effect
Sucralfate may decrease the levels/effects of: Antifungal Agents (Azole Derivatives, Systemic); Digoxin; Eltrombopag; Furosemide; Levothyroxine; Phosphate Supplements; QuiNIDine; Quinolone Antibiotics; Tetracycline Derivatives; Vitamin K Antagonists

Ethanol/Nutrition/Herb Interactions Food: Sucralfate may interfere with absorption of vitamin A, vitamin D, vitamin E, and vitamin K.

Stability Suspension: Shake well. Store at 20°C to 25°C (68°F to 77°F); do **not** freeze.

Mechanism of Action Forms a complex by binding with positively charged proteins in exudates, forming a viscous paste-like, adhesive substance. This selectively forms a protective coating that acts locally to protect the gastric lining against peptic acid, pepsin, and bile salts.

Pharmacodynamics/Kinetics
Onset of action: Paste formation and ulcer adhesion: 1-2 hours
Duration: Up to 6 hours
Absorption: Oral: <5%
Distribution: Acts locally at ulcer sites; unbound in GI tract to aluminum and sucrose octasulfate
Metabolism: None
Excretion: Urine (small amounts as unchanged compounds)

Dosage

Geriatric & Adult
Stress ulcer prophylaxis (unlabeled use): Oral: 1 g 4 times/day
Stress ulcer treatment (unlabeled use): Oral: 1 g every 4 hours
Treatment of duodenal ulcer: Oral:
Initial treatment: 1 g 4 times/day, 1 hour before meals or food and at bedtime for 4-8 weeks, or alternatively 2 g twice daily; treatment is recommended for 4-8 weeks in adults
Maintenance/prophylaxis of duodenal ulcer: 1 g twice daily
Stomatitis (unlabeled use): Oral: 10 mL (1 g/10 mL suspension); swish and spit or swish and swallow 4 times/day.

Renal Impairment Aluminum salt is minimally absorbed (<5%), however, may accumulate in renal failure.

Administration Tablet may be broken or dissolved in water before ingestion. Administer with water on an empty stomach.

Monitoring Parameters Monitor signs and symptoms of disease process and adverse effects; evaluate by endoscopic examination or x-ray

Pharmacotherapy Pearls May decrease gastric emptying; many trials have demonstrated sucralfate is equivalent in efficacy to antacids and H$_2$ blockers; equivalence of sucralfate suspension to sucralfate tablets has not been established in studies

Special Geriatric Considerations Caution should be used in the elderly due to reduced renal function. Patients with Cl$_{cr}$ <30 mL/minute may be at risk for aluminum intoxication. Due to low side effect profile, this may be an agent of choice in the elderly with PUD.

Dosage Forms Excipient information presented when available (limited, particularly for generics); consult specific product labeling.
Suspension, oral: 1 g/10 mL (10 mL)
  Carafate®: 1 g/10 mL (420 mL)
Tablet, oral: 1 g
  Carafate®: 1 g [scored]

◆ **Sudafed** *see* Pseudoephedrine *on page 1545*
◆ **Sudafed® 12 Hour [OTC]** *see* Pseudoephedrine *on page 1545*
◆ **Sudafed® 24 Hour [OTC]** *see* Pseudoephedrine *on page 1545*
◆ **Sudafed® Children's [OTC]** *see* Pseudoephedrine *on page 1545*

♦ **Sudafed® Maximum Strength Nasal Decongestant [OTC]** *see* Pseudoephedrine *on page 1545*
♦ **Sudafed OM® Sinus Congestion [OTC] [DSC]** *see* Oxymetazoline (Nasal) *on page 1374*
♦ **Sudafed PE® Children's [OTC]** *see* Phenylephrine (Systemic) *on page 1440*
♦ **Sudafed PE® Congestion [OTC]** *see* Phenylephrine (Systemic) *on page 1440*
♦ **Sudafed PE™ Nasal Decongestant [OTC]** *see* Phenylephrine (Systemic) *on page 1440*
♦ **Sudafed PE® Pressure + Pain [OTC]** *see* Acetaminophen and Phenylephrine *on page 38*
♦ **SudoGest [OTC]** *see* Pseudoephedrine *on page 1545*
♦ **SudoGest 12 Hour [OTC]** *see* Pseudoephedrine *on page 1545*
♦ **SudoGest Children's [OTC]** *see* Pseudoephedrine *on page 1545*
♦ **Sudogest™ PE [OTC]** *see* Phenylephrine (Systemic) *on page 1440*
♦ **Sudo-Tab® [OTC]** *see* Pseudoephedrine *on page 1545*
♦ **Sulamyd** *see* Sulfacetamide (Ophthalmic) *on page 1713*
♦ **Sulamyd** *see* Sulfacetamide (Topical) *on page 1713*
♦ **Sular®** *see* Nisoldipine *on page 1306*
♦ **Sulbactam and Ampicillin** *see* Ampicillin and Sulbactam *on page 130*

Sulfacetamide (Ophthalmic) (sul fa SEE ta mide)

Medication Safety Issues
  Sound-alike/look-alike issues:
    Bleph®-10 may be confused with Blephamide®
Brand Names: U.S. Bleph®-10; Sulfamide
Brand Names: Canada AK Sulf Liq; Bleph 10 DPS; Diosulf™; PMS-Sulfacetamide; Sodium Sulamyd
Index Terms Sodium Sulfacetamide; Sulamyd
Generic Availability (U.S.) Yes
Pharmacologic Category Antibiotic, Ophthalmic
Use Treatment and prophylaxis of conjunctivitis due to susceptible organisms; corneal ulcers; adjunctive treatment with systemic sulfonamides for therapy of trachoma
Dosage
  Geriatric & Adult Conjunctivitis: Ophthalmic: Solution: Instill 1-2 drops several times daily up to every 2-3 hours in lower conjunctival sac during waking hours and less frequently at night; increase dosing interval as condition responds. Usual duration of treatment: 7-10 days
    Trachoma: Instill 2 drops into the conjunctival sac every 2 hours; must be used in conjunction with systemic therapy
Special Geriatric Considerations Evaluate the patient's or caregiver's ability to safely administer the correct dose of ophthalmic medication.
Dosage Forms Excipient information presented when available (limited, particularly for generics); consult specific product labeling.
  Solution, ophthalmic, as sodium [drops]: 10% (15 mL)
    Bleph®-10: 10% (5 mL) [contains benzalkonium chloride]
    Sulfamide: 10% (15 mL)

Sulfacetamide (Topical) (sul fa SEE ta mide)

Medication Safety Issues
  Sound-alike/look-alike issues:
    Klaron® may be confused with Klor-Con®
Brand Names: U.S. Carmol® Scalp Treatment; Klaron®; Ovace®; Ovace® Plus; Rosula® NS; Seb-Prev™
Brand Names: Canada Sulfacet-R
Index Terms Sodium Sulfacetamide; Sulamyd; Sulfacetamide Sodium
Generic Availability (U.S.) Yes: Lotion, suspension
Pharmacologic Category Acne Products; Antibiotic, Sulfonamide Derivative; Topical Skin Product, Acne
Use Scaling dermatosis (seborrheic); bacterial infections of the skin; acne vulgaris
Dosage
  Geriatric & Adult
    Acne: Topical: Apply thin film to affected area twice daily
    Seborrheic dermatitis: Topical: Apply at bedtime and allow to remain overnight; in severe cases, may apply twice daily. Duration of therapy is usually 8-10 applications; dosing interval may be increased as eruption subsides. Applications once or twice weekly, or every other week may be used to prevent eruptions.
    Secondary cutaneous bacterial infections: Topical: Apply 2-4 times/day until infection clears

◀ **Special Geriatric Considerations** Assess whether patient can adequately use topically.
Dosage Forms Excipient information presented when available (limited, particularly for generics); consult specific product labeling. [DSC] = Discontinued product
Aerosol, topical, as sodium [foam]:
Ovace®: 10% (70 g)
Cream, topical, as sodium:
Seb-Prev™: 10% (30 g [DSC], 60 g [DSC]) [contains benzyl alcohol]
Gel, topical, as sodium:
Seb-Prev™: 10% (30 g [DSC], 60 g [DSC])
Lotion, topical, as sodium: 10% (118 mL)
Carmol® Scalp Treatment: 10% (85 g) [contains urea 10%]
Klaron®: 10% (118 mL) [contains sodium metabisulfite]
Lotion, topical, as sodium [emulsion-based/wash]:
Ovace® Plus: 10% (480 mL)
Lotion, topical, as sodium [wash]:
Ovace®: 10% (180 mL, 360 mL)
Pad, topical, as sodium: 10% (30s)
Rosula® NS: 10% (30s) [contains urea 10%]
Soap, topical, as sodium [wash]:
Seb-Prev™: 10% (170 mL, 340 mL)
Suspension, topical, as sodium: 10% (118 mL)

Sulfacetamide and Prednisolone (sul fa SEE ta mide & pred NIS oh lone)

Related Information
PrednisoLONE (Ophthalmic) on page 1510
Sulfacetamide (Ophthalmic) on page 1713
Medication Safety Issues
Sound-alike/look-alike issues:
Blephamide® may be confused with Bleph®-10
Brand Names: U.S. Blephamide®
Brand Names: Canada AK Cide Oph; Blephamide®; Dioptimyd®
Index Terms Prednisolone and Sulfacetamide
Generic Availability (U.S.) Yes: Solution
Pharmacologic Category Antibiotic/Corticosteroid, Ophthalmic
Use Steroid-responsive inflammatory ocular conditions in which a corticosteroid is indicated and where infection is present or there is a risk of infection
Dosage
Geriatric & Adult Conjunctivitis: Ophthalmic:
Ointment: Apply ~1/2 inch ribbon to lower conjunctival sac 3-4 times/day and 1-2 times at night
Solution: Instill 2 drops every 4 hours
Suspension: Instill 2 drops every 4 hours during the day and at bedtime
Special Geriatric Considerations Evaluate the patient's or caregiver's ability to safely administer the correct dose of ophthalmic medication.
Dosage Forms Excipient information presented when available (limited, particularly for generics); consult specific product labeling.
Ointment, ophthalmic:
Blephamide®: Sulfacetamide sodium 10% and prednisolone acetate 0.2% (3.5 g)
Solution, ophthalmic [drops]: Sulfacetamide sodium 10% and prednisolone sodium phosphate 0.25% (5 mL, 10 mL)
Suspension, ophthalmic [drops]:
Blephamide®: Sulfacetamide sodium 10% and prednisolone acetate 0.2% (5 mL, 10 mL) [contains benzalkonium chloride]

◆ **Sulfacetamide Sodium** see Sulfacetamide (Topical) on page 1713

Sulfamethoxazole and Trimethoprim
(sul fa meth OKS a zole & trye METH oh prim)

Related Information
Trimethoprim on page 1868
Medication Safety Issues
Sound-alike/look-alike issues:
Bactrim™ may be confused with bacitracin, Bactine®, Bactroban®
Co-trimoxazole may be confused with clotrimazole

Septra® may be confused with Ceptaz®, Sectral®

Septra® DS may be confused with Semprex®-D

Brand Names: U.S. Bactrim™; Bactrim™ DS; Septra® DS; Septra® [DSC]

Brand Names: Canada Apo-Sulfatrim®; Apo-Sulfatrim® DS; Apo-Sulfatrim® Pediatric; Novo-Trimel; Novo-Trimel D.S.; Nu-Cotrimox; Septra® Injection

Index Terms Co-Trimoxazole; SMX-TMP; SMZ-TMP; Sulfatrim; TMP-SMX; TMP-SMZ; Trimethoprim and Sulfamethoxazole

Generic Availability (U.S.) Yes

Pharmacologic Category Antibiotic, Miscellaneous; Antibiotic, Sulfonamide Derivative

Use

Oral treatment of urinary tract infections due to *E. coli, Klebsiella* and *Enterobacter* sp, *M. morganii, P. mirabilis* and *P. vulgaris*; acute exacerbations of chronic bronchitis in adults due to susceptible strains of *H. influenzae* or *S. pneumoniae*; treatment and prophylaxis of *Pneumocystis jirovecii* pneumonia (PCP); traveler's diarrhea due to enterotoxigenic *E. coli*; treatment of enteritis caused by *Shigella flexneri* or *Shigella sonnei*

I.V. treatment of severe or complicated infections when oral therapy is not feasible, for documented PCP, empiric treatment of PCP in immune compromised patients; treatment of documented or suspected shigellosis, typhoid fever, *Nocardia asteroides* infection, or other infections caused by susceptible bacteria

Unlabeled/Investigational Use Cholera and *Salmonella*-type infections and nocardiosis; chronic prostatitis; as prophylaxis in neutropenic patients with *P. jirovecii* infections, in leukemia patients, and in patients following renal transplantation, to decrease incidence of PCP; treatment of *Cyclospora* infection, typhoid fever, *Nocardia asteroides* infection; prophylaxis against urinary tract infection; alternative treatment for MRSA infections

Contraindications Hypersensitivity to any sulfa drug, trimethoprim, or any component of the formulation; megaloblastic anemia due to folate deficiency; marked hepatic damage or severe renal disease (if patient not monitored)

Warnings/Precautions Use with caution in patients with G6PD deficiency, impaired renal or hepatic function or potential folate deficiency (malnourished, chronic anticonvulsant therapy, or elderly); maintain adequate hydration to prevent crystalluria; adjust dosage in patients with renal impairment. Injection vehicle contains benzyl alcohol and sodium metabisulfite.

Chemical similarities are present among sulfonamides, sulfonylureas, carbonic anhydrase inhibitors, thiazides, and loop diuretics (except ethacrynic acid). Use in patients with sulfonamide allergy is specifically contraindicated in product labeling, however, a risk of cross-reaction exists in patients with allergy to any of these compounds; avoid use when previous reaction has been severe.

Fatalities associated with severe reactions including Stevens-Johnson syndrome, toxic epidermal necrolysis, hepatic necrosis, agranulocytosis, aplastic anemia, and other blood dyscrasias; discontinue use at first sign of rash or serious adverse reactions. Elderly patients appear at greater risk for more severe adverse reactions. May cause hypoglycemia, particularly in malnourished, or patients with renal or hepatic impairment. Use with caution in patients with porphyria or thyroid dysfunction. Slow acetylators may be more prone to adverse reactions. Caution in patients with allergies or asthma. May cause hyperkalemia (associated with high doses of trimethoprim). Incidence of adverse effects appears to be increased in patients with AIDS. Prolonged use may result in fungal or bacterial super-infection, including *C. difficile*-associated diarrhea (CDAD) and pseudomembranous colitis; CDAD has been observed >2 months postantibiotic treatment.

Adverse Reactions (Reflective of adult population; not specific for elderly) The most common adverse reactions include gastrointestinal upset (nausea, vomiting, anorexia) and dermatologic reactions (rash or urticaria). Rare, life-threatening reactions have been associated with co-trimoxazole, including severe dermatologic reactions, blood dyscrasias, and hepatotoxic reactions. Most other reactions listed are rare, however, frequency cannot be accurately estimated.

Cardiovascular: Allergic myocarditis

Central nervous system: Apathy, aseptic meningitis, ataxia, chills, depression, fatigue, fever, hallucinations, headache, insomnia, kernicterus (in neonates), nervousness, peripheral neuritis, seizure, vertigo

Dermatologic: Photosensitivity, pruritus, rash, skin eruptions, urticaria; rare reactions include erythema multiforme, exfoliative dermatitis, Henoch-Schönlein purpura, Stevens-Johnson syndrome, and toxic epidermal necrolysis

Endocrine & metabolic: Hyperkalemia (generally at high dosages), hypoglycemia (rare), hyponatremia

Gastrointestinal: Abdominal pain, anorexia, diarrhea, glottitis, nausea, pancreatitis, pseudomembranous colitis, stomatitis, vomiting

Hematologic: Agranulocytosis, aplastic anemia, eosinophilia, hemolysis (with G6PD deficiency), hemolytic anemia, hypoprothrombinemia, leukopenia, megaloblastic anemia, methemoglobinemia, neutropenia, thrombocytopenia

Hepatic: Hepatotoxicity (including hepatitis, cholestasis, and hepatic necrosis), hyperbilirubinemia, transaminases increased

Neuromuscular & skeletal: Arthralgia, myalgia, rhabdomyolysis, weakness

Otic: Tinnitus

Renal: BUN increased, crystalluria, diuresis (rare), interstitial nephritis, nephrotoxicity (in association with cyclosporine), renal failure, serum creatinine increased, toxic nephrosis (with anuria and oliguria)

Respiratory: Cough, dyspnea, pulmonary infiltrates

Miscellaneous: Allergic reaction, anaphylaxis, angioedema, periarteritis nodosa (rare), serum sickness, systemic lupus erythematosus (rare)

Drug Interactions

Metabolism/Transport Effects

Sulfamethoxazole: **Substrate** of CYP2C9 (major), 3A4 (minor); **Inhibits** CYP2C9 (moderate)

Trimethoprim: **Substrate** (major) of CYP2C9, 3A4; **Inhibits** CYP2C8 (moderate), 2C9 (moderate)

Avoid Concomitant Use

Avoid concomitant use of Sulfamethoxazole and Trimethoprim with any of the following: BCG; Dofetilide; Methenamine; Potassium P-Aminobenzoate; Procaine

Increased Effect/Toxicity

Sulfamethoxazole and Trimethoprim may increase the levels/effects of: ACE Inhibitors; Amantadine; Angiotensin II Receptor Blockers; Antidiabetic Agents (Thiazolidinedione); AzaTHIOprine; Carvedilol; CycloSPORINE; CycloSPORINE (Systemic); CYP2C8 Substrates (High risk); CYP2C9 Substrates (High risk); Dapsone; Dapsone (Systemic); Dapsone (Topical); Dofetilide; Fosphenytoin; LamiVUDine; Memantine; Methotrexate; Phenytoin; Porfimer; PRALAtrexate; Procainamide; Repaglinide; Sulfonylureas; Varenicline; Vitamin K Antagonists

The levels/effects of Sulfamethoxazole and Trimethoprim may be increased by: Amantadine; Conivaptan; CYP2C9 Inhibitors (Moderate); CYP2C9 Inhibitors (Strong); Dapsone; Dapsone (Systemic); Memantine; Methenamine

Decreased Effect

Sulfamethoxazole and Trimethoprim may decrease the levels/effects of: BCG; CycloSPORINE; CycloSPORINE (Systemic); Typhoid Vaccine

The levels/effects of Sulfamethoxazole and Trimethoprim may be decreased by: CYP2C9 Inducers (Highly Effective); CYP3A4 Inducers (Strong); Deferasirox; Herbs (CYP3A4 Inducers); Leucovorin Calcium-Levoleucovorin; Peginterferon Alfa-2b; Potassium P-Aminobenzoate; Procaine; Tocilizumab

Ethanol/Nutrition/Herb Interactions Herb/Nutraceutical: Avoid dong quai; St John's wort (may diminish effects and also cause photosensitization).

Stability

Injection: Store at room temperature; do not refrigerate. Less soluble in more alkaline pH. Protect from light. Solution must be diluted prior to administration. Following dilution, store at room temperature; do not refrigerate. Manufacturer recommended dilutions and stability of parenteral admixture at room temperature (25°C):

5 mL/125 mL D_5W; stable for 6 hours.

5 mL/100 mL D_5W; stable for 4 hours.

5 mL/75 mL D_5W; stable for 2 hours.

Studies have also confirmed limited stability in NS; detailed references should be consulted.

Suspension, tablet: Store at controlled room temperature of 15°C to 25°C (59°F to 77°F). Protect from light.

Mechanism of Action Sulfamethoxazole interferes with bacterial folic acid synthesis and growth via inhibition of dihydrofolic acid formation from para-aminobenzoic acid; trimethoprim inhibits dihydrofolic acid reduction to tetrahydrofolate resulting in sequential inhibition of enzymes of the folic acid pathway

Pharmacodynamics/Kinetics

Absorption: Oral: Almost completely, 90% to 100%

Protein binding: SMX: 68%, TMP: 45%

Metabolism: SMX: N-acetylated and glucuronidated; TMP: Metabolized to oxide and hydroxylated metabolites

Half-life elimination: SMX: 9 hours, TMP: 6-17 hours; both are prolonged in renal failure

Time to peak, serum: Within 1-4 hours

Excretion: Both are excreted in urine as metabolites and unchanged drug

Effects of aging on the pharmacokinetics of both agents has been variable; increase in half-life and decreases in clearance have been associated with reduced creatinine clearance

Dosage

Geriatric & Adult Dosage recommendations are based on the trimethoprim component. double-strength tablets are equivalent to sulfamethoxazole 800 mg and trimethoprim 160 mg.

General dosing guidelines:

Oral: 1-2 double-strength tablets (sulfamethoxazole 800 mg; trimethoprim 160 mg) every 12-24 hours

I.V.: 8-20 mg TMP/kg/day divided every 6-12 hours

Chronic bronchitis (acute): Oral: One double-strength tablet every 12 hours for 10-14 days

Cyclosporiasis (unlabeled use): Oral, I.V.: 160 mg TMP twice daily for 7-10 days. **Note:** AIDS patients: Oral: One double-strength tablet 2-4 times/day for 10 days, then 1 double-strength tablet 3 times/week for 10 weeks (Pape, 1994; Verdier, 2000).

Granuloma inguinale (donovanosis) (unlabeled use): Oral: One double-strength tablet every 12 hours for at least 3 weeks and until lesions have healed (CDC, 2010)

Meningitis (bacterial): I.V.: 10-20 mg TMP/kg/day in divided doses every 6-12 hours

Nocardia (unlabeled use): Oral, I.V.:

Cutaneous infections: 5-10 mg TMP/kg/day in 2-4 divided doses

Severe infections (pulmonary/cerebral): 15 mg TMP/kg/day in 2-4 divided doses for 3-4 weeks, then 10 mg TMP/kg/day in 2-4 divided doses. Treatment duration is controversial; an average of 7 months has been reported.

Note: Therapy for severe infection may be initiated I.V. and converted to oral therapy (frequently converted to approximate dosages of oral solid dosage forms: 2 DS tablets every 8-12 hours). Although not widely available, sulfonamide levels should be considered in patients with questionable absorption, at risk for dose-related toxicity, or those with poor therapeutic response.

Osteomyelitis due to MRSA (unlabeled use): Oral, I.V.: 3.5-4 mg TMP/kg/dose every 8-12 hours for a minimum of 8 weeks with rifampin 600 mg once daily (Liu, 2011)

Pneumocystis jirovecii:

Prophylaxis: Oral: One double-strength tablet daily or 3 times/week

Treatment: Oral, I.V.: 15-20 mg TMP/kg/day in 3-4 divided doses

Sepsis: I.V.: 20 TMP/kg/day divided every 6 hours

Septic arthritis due to MRSA (unlabeled use): Oral, I.V.: 3.5-4 mg TMP/kg/dose every 8-12 hours for 3-4 weeks (some experts combine with rifampin) (Liu, 2011)

Shigellosis:

Oral: One double-strength tablet every 12 hours for 5 days

I.V.: 8-10 mg TMP/kg/day in divided doses every 6, 8, or 12 hours for up to 5 days

Skin/soft tissue infection due to community-acquired MRSA (unlabeled use): Oral: 1-2 double-strength tablets every 12 hours for 5-10 days (Liu, 2011); **Note:** If beta-hemolytic *Streptococcus* spp are also suspected, a beta-lactam antibiotic should be added to the regimen (Liu, 2011)

Stenotrophomonas maltophilia (ventilator-associated pneumonia): I.V.: Most clinicians have utilized 12-15 mg TMP/kg/day for the treatment of VAP caused by *Stenotrophomonas maltophilia*. Higher doses (up to 20 mg TMP/kg/day) have been mentioned for treatment of severe infection in patients with normal renal function (Vartivarian, 1989; Looney, 2009; Wood, 2010)

Travelers' diarrhea: Oral: One double-strength tablet every 12 hours for 5 days

Urinary tract infection:

Oral: One double-strength tablet every 12 hours

Duration of therapy: Uncomplicated: 3-5 days; Complicated: 7-10 days

Pyelonephritis: 14 days

Prostatitis: Acute: 2 weeks; Chronic: 2-3 months

I.V.: 8-10 mg TMP/kg/day in divided doses every 6, 8, or 12 hours for up to 14 days with severe infections

Renal Impairment Oral, I.V.:

Manufacturer's recommendation: Adults:

Cl_{cr} 15-30 mL/minute: Administer 50% of recommended dose

Cl_{cr} <15 mL/minute: Use is not recommended

Alternate recommendations:

Cl_{cr} 15-30 mL/minute:

Treatment: Administer full daily dose (divided every 12 hours) for 24-48 hours, then decrease daily dose by 50% and administer every 24 hours (**Note:** For serious infections including *Pneumocystis jirovecii* pneumonia (PCP), full daily dose is given in divided doses every 6-8 hours for 2 days, followed by reduction to 50% daily dose divided every 12 hours) (Nahata, 1995).

PCP prophylaxis: One-half single-strength tablet (40 mg trimethoprim) daily **or** 1 single-strength tablet (80 mg trimethoprim) daily or 3 times weekly (Masur, 2002).

Cl_{cr} <15 mL/minute:

Treatment: Administer full daily dose every 48 hours (Nahata, 1995)

PCP prophylaxis: One-half single-strength tablet (40 mg trimethoprim) daily **or** 1 single-strength tablet (80 mg trimethoprim) 3 times weekly (Masur, 2002). While the guidelines do acknowledge the alternative of giving 1 single-strength tablet daily, this may be inadvisable in the uremic/ESRD patient.

Intermittent Hemodialysis (IHD) (administer after hemodialysis on dialysis days):

Treatment: Full daily dose before dialysis and 50% dose after dialysis (Nahata, 1995)

PCP prophylaxis: One single-strength tablet (80 mg trimethoprim) after each dialysis session (Masur, 2002)

Note: Dosing dependent on the assumption of 3 times/week, complete IHD sessions.

Peritoneal dialysis (PD):

Use Cl_{cr} <15 mL/minute dosing recommendations. Not significantly removed by PD; supplemental dosing is not required (Aronoff, 2007):

Exit-site and tunnel infections: Oral: One single-strength tablet daily (Li, 2010)

Peritonitis: Oral: One double-strength tablet twice daily (Li, 2010)

Continuous renal replacement therapy (CRRT) (Heintz, 2009; Trotman, 2005): Drug clearance is highly dependent on the method of renal replacement, filter type, and flow rate. Appropriate dosing requires close monitoring of pharmacologic response, signs of adverse reactions due to drug accumulation, as well as drug concentrations in relation to target trough (if appropriate). The following are general recommendations only (based on dialysate flow/ultrafiltration rates of 1-2 L/hour and minimal residual renal function) and should not supersede clinical judgment:

CVVH/CVVHD/CVVHDF: 2.5-7.5 mg/kg of TMP every 12 hours. **Note:** Dosing regimen dependent on clinical indication. Critically-ill patients with *P. jirovecii* pneumonia receiving CVVHDF may require up to 10 mg/kg every 12 hours (Heintz, 2009).

Administration

I.V.: Infuse over 60-90 minutes, must dilute well before giving (ie, 1:15 to 1:25, which equates to 5 mL of drug solution diluted in 75-125 mL base solution); not for I.M. injection

Oral: Administer without regard to meals. Administer with at least 8 ounces of water.

Monitoring Parameters Perform culture and sensitivity testing prior to initiating therapy; CBC, serum potassium, creatinine, BUN

Test Interactions Increased creatinine (Jaffé alkaline picrate reaction); increased serum methotrexate by dihydrofolate reductase method

Special Geriatric Considerations Elderly patients appear at greater risk for more severe adverse reactions.

Dosage Forms Excipient information presented when available (limited, particularly for generics); consult specific product labeling. **Note:** The 5:1 ratio (SMX:TMP) remains constant in all dosage forms. [DSC] = Discontinued products

Injection, solution: Sulfamethoxazole 80 mg and trimethoprim 16 mg per mL (5 mL, 10 mL, 30 mL) [contains benzyl alcohol, ethanol 12.2%, propylene glycol 400 mg/mL, sodium metabisulfite]

Suspension, oral: Sulfamethoxazole 200 mg and trimethoprim 40 mg per 5 mL (480 mL)

Tablet: Sulfamethoxazole 400 mg and trimethoprim 80 mg

Bactrim™: Sulfamethoxazole 400 mg and trimethoprim 80 mg

Septra®: Sulfamethoxazole 400 mg and trimethoprim 80 mg [DSC]

Tablet, double-strength: Sulfamethoxazole 800 mg and trimethoprim 160 mg

Bactrim™ DS: Sulfamethoxazole 800 mg and trimethoprim 160 mg

Septra® DS: Sulfamethoxazole 800 mg and trimethoprim 160 mg

Selected References

Naber K, Vergin H, and Weigand W, "Pharmacokinetics of Co-trimoxazole and Co-tetroxazine in Geriatric Patients," Infection, 1981, 9(5):239-43.

Varoquaux O, Lajoie D, Gobert C, et al, "Pharmacokinetics of the Trimethoprim-Sulfamethoxazole Combination in the Elderly," Br J Clin Pharmacol, 1985, 20(6):575-81.

◆ **Sulfamide** *see* Sulfacetamide (Ophthalmic) *on page 1713*

Sulfanilamide (sul fa NIL a mide)

Brand Names: U.S. AVC™

Index Terms p-amino-benzenesulfonamide

Pharmacologic Category Antifungal Agent, Vaginal

Use Treatment of vulvovaginitis caused by *Candida albicans*

Dosage

Adult Vulvovaginitis due to *Candida albicans*: Intravaginal: Insert one applicatorful intravaginally once or twice daily; treatment should continue for a period of 30 days

Special Geriatric Considerations Localized fungal infections frequently follow broad-spectrum antimicrobial therapy, specifically, oral and vaginal infections due to *Candida*.

Dosage Forms Excipient information presented when available (limited, particularly for generics); consult specific product labeling.

Cream, vaginal:

AVC™: 15% (120 g) [~6 g/applicator]

SulfaSALAzine (sul fa SAL a zeen)

Medication Safety Issues

Sound-alike/look-alike issues:

SulfaSALAzine may be confused with salsalate, sulfADIAZINE, sulfiSOXAZOLE

Azulfidine® may be confused with Augmentin®, azaTHIOprine

Brand Names: U.S. Azulfidine EN-tabs®; Azulfidine®

Brand Names: Canada Alti-Sulfasalazine; Salazopyrin En-Tabs®; Salazopyrin®

Index Terms Salicylazosulfapyridine

Generic Availability (U.S.) Yes

Pharmacologic Category 5-Aminosalicylic Acid Derivative

Use Treatment of mild-to-moderate ulcerative colitis or as adjunctive therapy in severe ulcerative colitis; enteric coated tablets are also used for rheumatoid arthritis (including juvenile idiopathic arthritis [JIA]) in patients who inadequately respond to analgesics and NSAIDs

Unlabeled/Investigational Use Ankylosing spondylitis, Crohn's disease, psoriasis, psoriatic arthritis

Contraindications Hypersensitivity to sulfasalazine, sulfa drugs, salicylates, or any component of the formulation; porphyria; GI or GU obstruction

Warnings/Precautions Use with extreme caution in patients with renal impairment, impaired hepatic function or blood dyscrasias. Use caution in patients with severe allergies or asthma, or G6PD deficiency; may cause folate deficiency (consider providing 1 mg/day folate supplement). Deaths from irreversible neuromuscular or central nervous system changes, fibrosing alveolitis, agranulocytosis, aplastic anemia, and other blood dyscrasias have been reported. In males, oligospermia (rare) has been reported. Chemical similarities are present among sulfonamides, sulfonylureas, carbonic anhydrase inhibitors, thiazides, and loop diuretics (except ethacrynic acid). Nausea, vomiting, and abdominal discomfort commonly occur; titration of dose and/or using the enteric coated formulation may decrease GI adverse effects. Use in patients with sulfonamide allergy is specifically contraindicated in product labeling, however, a risk of cross-reaction exists in patients with allergy to any of these compounds; avoid use when previous reaction has been severe. Slow acetylators may be more prone to adverse reactions.

Adverse Reactions (Reflective of adult population; not specific for elderly)

>10%:

Central nervous system: Headache

Dermatologic: Rash

Gastrointestinal: Anorexia, dyspepsia, gastric distress, nausea, vomiting

Genitourinary: Oligospermia (reversible)

1% to 10%:

Cardiovascular: Cyanosis

Central nervous system: Dizziness, fever

Dermatologic: Pruritus, urticaria

Gastrointestinal: Abdominal pain, stomatitis

Hematologic: Heinz body anemia, hemolytic anemia, leukopenia, thrombocytopenia

Hepatic: Liver function tests abnormal

Drug Interactions

Avoid Concomitant Use There are no known interactions where it is recommended to avoid concomitant use.

Increased Effect/Toxicity

SulfaSALAzine may increase the levels/effects of: Heparin; Heparin (Low Molecular Weight); Thiopurine Analogs; Varicella Virus-Containing Vaccines

Decreased Effect

SulfaSALAzine may decrease the levels/effects of: Cardiac Glycosides; Methylfolate

Ethanol/Nutrition/Herb Interactions

Food: May impair folate absorption.

Herb/Nutraceutical: Avoid dong quai, St John's wort (may also cause photosensitization)

Stability Store at 25°C (77°F); excursions permitted to 15°C to 30°C (59°F to 86°F).

Mechanism of Action Acts locally in the colon to decrease the inflammatory response and systemically interferes with secretion by inhibiting prostaglandin synthesis

◀ **Pharmacodynamics/Kinetics**
Absorption: ≤15% as unchanged drug from small intestine
Metabolism: Via colonic intestinal flora to sulfapyridine and 5-aminosalicylic acid (5-ASA). Following absorption, sulfapyridine undergoes acetylation to form AcSP and ring hydroxylation while 5-ASA undergoes N-acetylation (non-acetylation phenotype dependent process); rate of metabolism via acetylation dependent on acetylation phenotype
Bioavailability: Sulfasalazine: <15%; sulfapyridine: ~60%; 5-aminosalicylic acid: ~10% to 30%
Half-life elimination: 5.7-10 hours (prolonged in elderly); sulfapyridine half-life prolonged in slow acetylators (14.8 hours)
Time to peak: Sulfasalazine: 3-12 hours (mean: 6 hours); metabolites: ~10 hours
Excretion: Primarily urine (as unchanged drug, components, and acetylated metabolites)

Dosage

Geriatric & Adult

Ulcerative colitis: Oral:
Initial: 3-4 g/day in evenly divided doses at ≤8-hour intervals. **Note:** American College of Gastroenterology guideline recommendations: Titrate to 4-6 g/day in 4 divided doses (Kornbluth, 2010).
Maintenance dose: 2 g/day in evenly divided doses at ≤8-hour intervals; may initiate therapy with 1-2 g/day to reduce GI intolerance

Rheumatoid arthritis: Oral (enteric coated tablet): Initial: 0.5-1 g/day; increase weekly to maintenance dose of 2 g/day in 2 divided doses; maximum: 3 g/day (if response to 2 g/day is inadequate after 12 weeks of treatment)

Renal Impairment Use not recommended; weigh risk vs benefit.

Hepatic Impairment Use not recommended; weigh risk vs benefit.

Administration GI intolerance is common during the first few days of therapy (administer with meals). Do not crush enteric coated tablets.

Monitoring Parameters CBC with differential and liver function tests (prior to therapy, then every other week for first 3 months of therapy, followed by every month for the second 3 months, then once every 3 months thereafter); periodic urinalysis and renal function tests; stool frequency; signs of infection

Pharmacotherapy Pearls This drug should be administered after food to reduce GI irritation. Sulfasalazine can be used as a disease-modifying agent (DMARD) in the treatment of progressive rheumatoid arthritis that has not responded adequately to anti-inflammatory agents.

Special Geriatric Considerations Adjust dose for renal function.

Dosage Forms Excipient information presented when available (limited, particularly for generics); consult specific product labeling.
Tablet, oral: 500 mg
Azulfidine®: 500 mg [scored]
Tablet, delayed release, enteric coated, oral: 500 mg
Azulfidine EN-tabs®: 500 mg

◆ **Sulfatrim** see Sulfamethoxazole and Trimethoprim on page 1714
◆ **Sulfisoxazole and Erythromycin** see Erythromycin and Sulfisoxazole on page 629

Sulindac (SUL in dak)

Medication Safety Issues
Sound-alike/look-alike issues:
Clinoril® may be confused with Cleocin®, Clozaril®
Brand Names: U.S. Clinoril®
Brand Names: Canada Apo-Sulin®; Novo-Sundac; Nu-Sulindac; Nu-Sundac; Teva-Sulindac
Generic Availability (U.S.) Yes
Pharmacologic Category Nonsteroidal Anti-inflammatory Drug (NSAID), Oral
Use Management of inflammatory diseases including osteoarthritis, rheumatoid arthritis, acute gouty arthritis, ankylosing spondylitis, acute painful shoulder (bursitis/tendonitis)
Unlabeled/Investigational Use Management of preterm labor
Medication Guide Available Yes
Contraindications Hypersensitivity or allergic-type reactions to sulindac, aspirin, other NSAIDs, or any component of the formulation; perioperative pain in the setting of coronary artery bypass graft (CABG) surgery
Warnings/Precautions [U.S. Boxed Warning]: NSAIDs are associated with an increased risk of adverse cardiovascular thrombotic events, including MI and stroke. Use caution with fluid retention. Avoid use in heart failure. Concurrent administration of ibuprofen, and potentially other nonselective NSAIDs, may interfere with aspirin's cardioprotective effect. May cause new-onset hypertension or worsening of existing hypertension. NSAID use may compromise existing renal function; dose-dependent decreases in prostaglandin synthesis

may result from NSAID use, reducing renal blood flow which may cause renal decompensation. NSAID use may increase the risk for hyperkalemia. Patients with impaired renal function, dehydration, heart failure, liver dysfunction, those taking diuretics, and ACE inhibitors, and the elderly are at greater risk of renal toxicity and hyperkalemia. Rehydrate patient before starting therapy; monitor renal function closely. Not recommended for use in patients with advanced renal disease. Long-term NSAID use may result in renal papillary necrosis. Use caution in patients with renal lithiasis; sulindac metabolites have been reported as components of renal stones. Maintain adequate hydration in patients with a history of renal stones. Use with caution in patients with decreased hepatic function. May require dosage adjustment in hepatic dysfunction; sulfide and sulfone metabolites may accumulate. The elderly are at increased risk for adverse effects. **[U.S. Boxed Warning]: Use is contraindicated for treatment of perioperative pain in the setting of coronary artery bypass graft (CABG) surgery.** Risk of MI and stroke may be increased with use following CABG surgery.

[U.S. Boxed Warning]: NSAIDs may increase risk of gastrointestinal irritation, inflammation, ulceration, bleeding, and perforation. Use the lowest effective dose for the shortest duration of time, consistent with individual patient goals, to reduce risk of cardiovascular or GI adverse events. When used concomitantly with ≤325 mg of aspirin, a substantial increase in the risk of gastrointestinal complications (eg, ulcer) occurs; concomitant gastroprotective therapy (eg, proton pump inhibitors) is recommended (Bhatt, 2008). Pancreatitis has been reported; discontinue with suspected pancreatitis.

NSAIDS may cause drowsiness, dizziness, blurred vision and other neurologic effects which may impair physical or mental abilities; patients must be cautioned about performing tasks which require mental alertness (eg, operating machinery or driving). Discontinue use with blurred or diminished vision and perform ophthalmologic exam. Monitor vision with long-term therapy.

Platelet adhesion and aggregation may be decreased, may prolong bleeding time; patients with coagulation disorders or who are receiving anticoagulants should be monitored closely. Anemia may occur; patients on long-term NSAID therapy should be monitored for anemia. Rarely, NSAID use may cause severe blood dyscrasias (eg, agranulocytosis, aplastic anemia, thrombocytopenia). NSAIDs may cause serious skin adverse events including exfoliative dermatitis, Stevens-Johnson syndrome (SJS) and toxic epidermal necrolysis (TEN); discontinue use at first sign of skin rash or hypersensitivity. Anaphylactoid reactions may occur. Do not use in patients who experience bronchospasm, asthma, rhinitis, or urticaria with NSAID or aspirin therapy. Use caution in other forms of asthma. May increase the risk of aseptic meningitis, especially in patients with systemic lupus erythematosus (SLE) and mixed connective tissue disorders.

Withhold for at least 4-6 half-lives prior to surgical or dental procedures.

Adverse Reactions (Reflective of adult population; not specific for elderly)

1% to 10%:

Cardiovascular: Edema (1% to 3%)

Central nervous system: Dizziness (3% to 9%), headache (3% to 9%), nervousness (1% to 3%)

Dermatologic: Rash (3% to 9%), pruritus (1% to 3%)

Gastrointestinal: GI pain (10%), constipation (3% to 9%), diarrhea (3% to 9%), dyspepsia (3% to 9%), nausea (3% to 9%), abdominal cramps (1% to 3%), anorexia (1% to 3%), flatulence (1% to 3%), vomiting (1% to 3%)

Otic: Tinnitus (1% to 3%)

Drug Interactions

Avoid Concomitant Use

Avoid concomitant use of Sulindac with any of the following: Floctafenine; Ketorolac; Ketorolac (Nasal); Ketorolac (Systemic)

Increased Effect/Toxicity

Sulindac may increase the levels/effects of: Aminoglycosides; Anticoagulants; Antiplatelet Agents; Bisphosphonate Derivatives; Collagenase (Systemic); CycloSPORINE; CycloSPORINE (Systemic); Deferasirox; Desmopressin; Digoxin; Drotrecogin Alfa; Eplerenone; Haloperidol; Ibritumomab; Methotrexate; Nonsteroidal Anti-Inflammatory Agents; PEMEtrexed; Porfimer; Potassium-Sparing Diuretics; PRALAtrexate; Quinolone Antibiotics; Rivaroxaban; Salicylates; Thrombolytic Agents; Tositumomab and Iodine I 131 Tositumomab; Vancomycin; Vitamin K Antagonists

The levels/effects of Sulindac may be increased by: ACE Inhibitors; Angiotensin II Receptor Blockers; Antidepressants (Tricyclic, Tertiary Amine); Corticosteroids (Systemic); Dasatinib; Dimethyl Sulfoxide; Floctafenine; Glucosamine; Herbs (Anticoagulant/Antiplatelet Properties); Ketorolac; Ketorolac (Nasal); Ketorolac (Systemic); Nonsteroidal Anti-Inflammatory Agents; Omega-3-Acid Ethyl Esters; Pentosan Polysulfate Sodium; Pentoxifylline;

Probenecid; Prostacyclin Analogues; Selective Serotonin Reuptake Inhibitors; Serotonin/ Norepinephrine Reuptake Inhibitors; Sodium Phosphates; Treprostinil; Vitamin E

Decreased Effect

Sulindac may decrease the levels/effects of: ACE Inhibitors; Angiotensin II Receptor Blockers; Antiplatelet Agents; Beta-Blockers; Eplerenone; HydrALAZINE; Potassium-Sparing Diuretics; Salicylates; Selective Serotonin Reuptake Inhibitors; Thiazide Diuretics

The levels/effects of Sulindac may be decreased by: Bile Acid Sequestrants; Nonsteroidal Anti-Inflammatory Agents; Salicylates

Ethanol/Nutrition/Herb Interactions

Ethanol: Avoid ethanol (may enhance gastric mucosal irritation).

Herb/Nutraceutical: Avoid alfalfa, anise, bilberry, bladderwrack, bromelain, cat's claw, celery, chamomile, coleus, cordyceps, dong quai, evening primrose, fenugreek, feverfew, garlic, ginger, ginkgo biloba, ginseng (American, Panax, Siberian), grapeseed, green tea, guggul, horse chestnut seed, horseradish, licorice, prickly ash, red clover, reishi, SAMe (S-adenosylmethionine), sweet clover, turmeric, white willow (all have additional antiplatelet activity).

Stability Store at room temperature of 15°C to 30°C (59°F to 86°F).

Mechanism of Action Reversibly inhibits cyclooxygenase-1 and 2 (COX-1 and 2) enzymes, which results in decreased formation of prostaglandin precursors; has antipyretic, analgesic, and anti-inflammatory properties

Other proposed mechanisms not fully elucidated (and possibly contributing to the anti-inflammatory effect to varying degrees), include inhibiting chemotaxis, altering lymphocyte activity, inhibiting neutrophil aggregation/activation, and decreasing proinflammatory cytokine levels.

Pharmacodynamics/Kinetics

Absorption: 90%

Distribution: Crosses blood-brain barrier (brain concentrations <4% of plasma concentrations)

Protein binding: Sulindac: 93%, sulfone metabolite: 95%, sulfide metabolite: 98%; primarily to albumin

Metabolism: Hepatic; prodrug metabolized to sulfide metabolite (active) for therapeutic effects and to sulfone metabolites (inactive); parent and inactive sulfone metabolite undergo extensive enterohepatic recirculation

Half-life elimination: Sulindac: ~8 hours; Sulfide metabolite: ~16 hours

Time to peak: Sulindac: 3-4 hours; Sulfide and sulfone metabolites: 5-6 hours

Excretion: Urine (~50%, primarily as inactive metabolites, <1% as active metabolite); feces (~25%, primarily as metabolites)

Dosage

Geriatric & Adult Note: Maximum daily dose: 400 mg

Osteoarthritis, rheumatoid arthritis, ankylosing spondylitis: 150 mg twice daily

Acute painful shoulder (bursitis/tendonitis): 200 mg twice daily; usual treatment: 7-14 days

Acute gouty arthritis: 200 mg twice daily; usual treatment: 7 days

Renal Impairment Not recommended with advanced renal impairment; if required, decrease dose and monitor closely.

Hepatic Impairment Dose reduction is necessary; discontinue if abnormal liver function tests occur.

Administration Should be administered with food or milk.

Monitoring Parameters Liver enzymes, BUN, serum creatinine, CBC, blood pressure; signs and symptoms of GI bleeding; ophthalmic exam (if ocular complaints develop during treatment)

Test Interactions Increased chloride (S), increased sodium (S), increased bleeding time

Pharmacotherapy Pearls Structurally similar to indomethacin but acts like aspirin; associated with the highest (one study) incidence of upper GI bleeds among NSAIDs; safest NSAID for use in mild renal impairment; maximum therapeutic response may not be realized for up to 3 weeks. There are no clinical guidelines to predict which NSAID will give which response in a particular patient. Trials with each must be initiated until response determined. Consider dose, patient convenience, and cost.

Special Geriatric Considerations Elderly are a high-risk population for adverse effects from NSAIDs. As much as 60% of the elderly who develop GI complications can develop peptic ulceration and/or hemorrhage asymptomatically. The concomitant use of H_2 blockers and sucralfate is not effective as prophylaxis with the exception of NSAID-induced duodenal ulcers which may be prevented by the use of ranitidine. Misoprostol and proton pump inhibitors are the only agents proven to help prevent the development of NSAID-induced ulcers. Also, concomitant disease and drug use contribute to the risk for GI adverse effects. Use lowest effective dose for shortest period possible. Consider renal function decline with age. Use of NSAIDs can compromise existing renal function especially when Cl_{cr} is ≤30 mL/minute.

Tinnitus may be a difficult and unreliable indication of toxicity due to age-related hearing loss or eighth cranial nerve damage. CNS adverse effects such as confusion, agitation, and hallucination are generally seen in overdose or high-dose situations, but the elderly may demonstrate these adverse effects at lower doses than younger adults.

Dosage Forms Excipient information presented when available (limited, particularly for generics); consult specific product labeling.

Tablet, oral: 150 mg, 200 mg

Clinoril®: 200 mg [scored]

SUMAtriptan (soo ma TRIP tan)

Medication Safety Issues

Sound-alike/look-alike issues:

SUMAtriptan may be confused with saxagliptin, sitaGLIPtin, somatropin, ZOLMitriptan

Brand Names: U.S. Alsuma™; Imitrex®; Sumavel™ DosePro™

Brand Names: Canada Apo-Sumatriptan®; CO Sumatriptan; Dom-Sumatriptan; Gen-Suma-triptan; Imitrex®; Imitrex® DF; Imitrex® Injection; Imitrex® Nasal Spray; Mylan-Sumatriptan; Novo-Sumatriptan; PHL-Sumatriptan; PMS-Sumatriptan; ratio-Sumatriptan; Rhoxal-sumatriptan; Riva-Sumatriptan; Sandoz-Sumatriptan; Sumatriptan Injection; Sumatriptan Sun Injection; Sumatryx; Teva-Sumatriptan; Teva-Sumatriptan DF

Index Terms Sumatriptan Succinate

Generic Availability (U.S.) Yes

Pharmacologic Category Antimigraine Agent; Serotonin 5-HT$_{1B, 1D}$ Receptor Agonist

Use

Intranasal, Oral, SubQ: Acute treatment of migraine with or without aura

SubQ: Acute treatment of cluster headache episodes

Contraindications Hypersensitivity to sumatriptan or any component of the formulation; patients with ischemic heart disease or signs or symptoms of ischemic heart disease (including Prinzmetal's angina, angina pectoris, myocardial infarction, silent myocardial ischemia); cerebrovascular syndromes (including strokes, transient ischemic attacks); peripheral vascular disease (including ischemic bowel disease); uncontrolled hypertension; use within 24 hours of ergotamine derivatives; use within 24 hours of another 5-HT$_1$ agonist; concurrent administration or within 2 weeks of discontinuing an MAO type A inhibitors (oral and nasal sumatriptan only; see Warnings/Precautions); management of hemiplegic or basilar migraine; severe hepatic impairment (oral and nasal sumatriptan, and injectable Imitrex® only); not for I.V. administration

Warnings/Precautions Sumatriptan is only indicated for the acute treatment of migraine or cluster headache (product dependent); not indicated for migraine prophylaxis, or for the treatment of hemiplegic or basilar migraine. If a patient does not respond to the first dose, the diagnosis of migraine or cluster headache should be reconsidered; rule out underlying neurologic disease in patients with atypical headache and in patients with no prior history of migraine or cluster headache. Cardiac events (coronary artery vasospasm, transient ischemia, myocardial infarction, ventricular tachycardia/fibrillation, cardiac arrest and death), cerebral/subarachnoid hemorrhage, and stroke have been reported with 5-HT$_1$ agonist administration. Patients who experience sensations of chest pain/pressure/tightness or symptoms suggestive of angina following dosing should be evaluated for coronary artery disease or Prinzmetal's angina before receiving additional doses; if dosing is resumed and similar symptoms recur, monitor with ECG. Do not give to patients with risk factors for CAD until a cardiovascular evaluation has been performed; if evaluation is satisfactory, the healthcare provider should administer the first dose (consider ECG monitoring) and cardiovascular status should be periodically evaluated.

Significant elevation in blood pressure, including hypertensive crisis, has also been reported on rare occasions in patients with and without a history of hypertension; use is contraindicated in patients with uncontrolled hypertension. Vasospasm-related reactions have been reported other than coronary artery vasospasm. Peripheral vascular ischemia and colonic ischemia with abdominal pain and bloody diarrhea have occurred. Transient and permanent blindness and significant partial vision loss have been very rarely reported. Use with caution in patients with a history of seizure disorder or in patients with a lowered seizure threshold. Use the oral formulation with caution (and with dosage limitations) in patients with hepatic impairment where treatment is necessary and advisable. Presystemic clearance of orally administered sumatriptan is reduced in hepatic impairment, leading to increased plasma concentrations; dosage reduction of the oral product is recommended. Non-oral routes of administration (nasal, subcutaneous formulations) do not undergo similar hepatic first-pass metabolism and are not expected to result in significantly altered pharmacokinetics in patients with hepatic impairment. Use of the oral, nasal, or Imitrex® injectable is contraindicated in severe hepatic impairment.

◀ Symptoms of agitation, confusion, hallucinations, hyper-reflexia, myoclonus, shivering, and tachycardia (serotonin syndrome) may occur with concomitant proserotonergic drugs (ie, SSRIs/SNRIs or triptans) or agents which reduce sumatriptan's metabolism. Concurrent use of serotonin precursors (eg, tryptophan) is not recommended. If concomitant administration with SSRIs is warranted, monitor closely, especially at initiation and with dose increases. Concurrent use with an MAO inhibitor may result in increased sumatriptan concentrations and increased risk for dose-related adverse effects (eg, serotonin syndrome); use with oral or nasal sumatriptan is contraindicated. Although generally not recommended, if concomitant use of MAO inhibitors with injectable sumatriptan is deemed necessary, careful monitoring and appropriate dosage adjustments are required. I.V. administration is contraindicated due to the potential to cause coronary vasospasm. Not recommended for use in elderly patients; older adults are at a higher risk for coronary artery disease and may be more likely to have reduced hepatic function.

Adverse Reactions (Reflective of adult population; not specific for elderly)
Injection:
>10%:
Central nervous system: Dizziness (12%), warm/hot sensation (11%)
Local: Injection site reaction (≤86%; includes bleeding, bruising, edema, and erythema)
Neuromuscular & skeletal: Paresthesia (5% to 14%)
1% to 10%:
Cardiovascular: Chest discomfort/tightness/pressure (2% to 5%)
Central nervous system: Burning sensation (7%), feeling of heaviness (7%), flushing (7%), pressure sensation (7%), feeling of tightness (5%), drowsiness (3%), feeling strange (2%), headache (2%), tight feeling in head (2%), anxiety (1%), cold sensation (1%), malaise/fatigue (1%)
Gastrointestinal: Nausea/vomiting (4%), abdominal discomfort (1%), dysphagia (1%)
Neuromuscular & skeletal: Neck pain/stiffness (5%), numbness (5%), weakness (5%), jaw discomfort (2%), myalgia (2%), muscle cramps (1%)
Ocular: Vision alterations (1%)
Respiratory: Throat discomfort (3%), nasal disorder/discomfort (2%), bronchospasm (1%)
Miscellaneous: Diaphoresis (2%)

Nasal spray:
>10%: Gastrointestinal: Bad taste (13% to 24%), nausea (11% to 13%), vomiting (11% to 13%)
1% to 10%:
Central nervous system: Dizziness (1% to 2%)
Respiratory: Nasal disorder/discomfort (2% to 4%), throat discomfort (1% to 2%)

Tablet:
1% to 10%:
Cardiovascular: Chest pain/tightness/heaviness/pressure (1% to 2%), palpitation (1%), syncope (1%)
Central nervous system: Burning (1%), dizziness (>1%), drowsiness (>1%), malaise/fatigue (2% to 3%), headache (>1%), nonspecified pain (1% to 2%, placebo 1%), vertigo (<1% to 2%), migraine (>1%), sleepiness (>1%)
Gastrointestinal: Diarrhea (1%), nausea (>1%), vomiting (>1%), hyposalivation (>1%)
Hematologic: Hemolytic anemia (1%)
Neuromuscular & skeletal: Neck, throat, and jaw pain/tightness/pressure (2% to 3%), paresthesia (3% to 5%), myalgia (1%), numbness (1%)
Otic: Ear hemorrhage (1%), hearing loss (1%), sensitivity to noise (1%), tinnitus (1%)
Renal: Hematuria (1%)
Respiratory: Allergic rhinitis (1%), dyspnea (1%), nasal inflammation (1%), nose/throat hemorrhage (1%), sinusitis (1%), upper respiratory inflammation (1%)
Miscellaneous: Hypersensitivity reactions (1%), nonspecified pressure/tightness/heaviness (1% to 3%, placebo 2%); warm/cold sensation (2% to 3%, placebo 2%)

Drug Interactions
Avoid Concomitant Use
Avoid concomitant use of SUMAtriptan with any of the following: Ergot Derivatives; MAO Inhibitors; Sibutramine
Increased Effect/Toxicity
SUMAtriptan may increase the levels/effects of: Ergot Derivatives; Serotonin Modulators

The levels/effects of SUMAtriptan may be increased by: Ergot Derivatives; MAO Inhibitors; Sibutramine
Decreased Effect There are no known significant interactions involving a decrease in effect.

Stability

Alsuma™: Store at 25°C (77°F); excursions permitted between 15°C and 30°C (59°F and 86°F); do not refrigerate. Protect from light.

Imitrex® injectable, tablet, nasal spray: Store at 2°C to 30°C (36°F to 86°F). Protect from light.

Sumavel™ DosePro™: Store at 20°C to 25°C (68°F to 77°F); excursions permitted between 15°C and 30°C (59°F and 86°F); do not freeze.

Mechanism of Action Selective agonist for serotonin (5-HT$_{1B}$ and 5-HT$_{1D}$receptors) in cranial arteries; causes vasoconstriction and reduces neurogenic inflammation associated with antidromic neuronal transmission correlating with relief of migraine

Pharmacodynamics/Kinetics

Onset of action: Oral: ~30 minutes; Nasal: ~15-30 minutes; SubQ: ~10 minutes

Distribution: V_d: 2.4 L/kg

Protein binding: 14% to 21%

Metabolism: Hepatic, primarily via MAO-A isoenzyme; extensive first-pass metabolism following oral administration

Bioavailability: Nasal: 17% (compared to SubQ); Oral: 15%; SubQ: 97% ± 16%

Half-life elimination: ~2-2.5 hours

Time to peak, serum: Oral: 2-2.5 hours; SubQ: 12 minutes (range: 4-20 minutes)

Excretion:

Nasal spray: Urine (42% of total dose as indole acetic acid metabolite; 3% of total dose as unchanged drug)

Oral: Urine (~60% of total dose, mostly as indole acetic acid metabolite; 3% of total dose as unchanged drug); feces (~40%)

SubQ: Urine (38% of total dose as indole acetic acid metabolite; 22% of total dose as unchanged drug)

Dosage

Geriatric Use is not recommended (due to increased potential for adverse effects).

Adult

Migraine:

Oral: A single dose of 25 mg, 50 mg, or 100 mg (taken with fluids). If a satisfactory response has not been obtained at 2 hours, a second dose may be administered. Results from clinical trials show that initial doses of 50 mg and 100 mg are more effective than doses of 25 mg, and that 100 mg doses do not provide a greater effect than 50 mg and may have increased incidence of side effects. Although doses of up to 300 mg/day have been studied, the total daily dose should not exceed 200 mg. The safety of treating an average of >4 headaches in a 30-day period have not been established.

Intranasal: A single dose of 5 mg, 10 mg, or 20 mg administered in one nostril. A 10 mg dose may be achieved by administering a single 5 mg dose in each nostril. If headache returns, the dose may be repeated once after 2 hours, not to exceed a total daily dose of 40 mg. In clinical trials, a greater number of patients responded to initial doses of 20 mg versus 5 or 10 mg. The safety of treating an average of >4 headaches in a 30-day period has not been established.

SubQ: Initial: Up to 6 mg; may repeat if needed ≥1 hour after initial dose (maximum: Two 6 mg injections per 24-hour period). However, controlled clinical trials have failed to document a benefit with administration of a second 6 mg dose in nonresponders.

Cluster headache: SubQ: Initial: Up to 6 mg; may repeat if needed ≥1 hour after initial dose (maximum: Two 6 mg injections per 24-hour period)

Renal Impairment No dosage adjustments are recommended.

Hepatic Impairment

Mild-to-moderate hepatic impairment:

Oral: Bioavailability of oral sumatriptan is increased with liver disease. If treatment is needed, do not exceed single doses of 50 mg.

Nasal spray: Has not been studied in patients with hepatic impairment, however, because the spray does not undergo first-pass metabolism, levels would not be expected to be altered.

Subcutaneous: Has been studied and pharmacokinetics were not altered in patients with hepatic impairment compared to healthy patients.

Severe hepatic impairment: Oral, nasal, and subcutaneous (limited to Imitrex® injection, per prescribing information) formulations are contraindicated with severe hepatic impairment.

Administration

Should be administered as soon as symptoms appear.

Intranasal: Each nasal spray unit is preloaded with 1 dose; **do not** test the spray unit before use; remove unit from plastic pack when ready to use; while sitting down, gently blow nose to clear nasal passages; keep head upright and close one nostril gently with index finger; hold container with other hand, with thumb supporting bottom and index and middle fingers on either side of nozzle; insert nozzle into nostril about ¹/₂ inch; close mouth; take a breath through nose while releasing spray into nostril by pressing firmly on blue plunger; remove nozzle from nostril; keep head level for 10-20 seconds and gently breathe in through nose and out through mouth; **do not breathe deeply**

SubQ: Not for I.M. or I.V. use. Needle penetrates ¼ inch of skin; use in areas of the body with adequate skin and subcutaneous thickness. Alsuma™ is a prefilled single-use autoinjector device.

Needleless administration (Sumavel™ DosePro™): Administer to the abdomen (>2 inches from the navel) or thigh; not for I.M. or I.V. administration. Do not administer to other areas of the body (eg, arm). Device is for single use only, discard after use; do not use if the tip of the device is tilted or broken.

Special Geriatric Considerations Use is not recommended in the elderly, particularly since many elderly have cardiovascular disease which would put them at risk for cardiovascular adverse effects. Safety and efficacy in the elderly (>65 years) have not been established. Pharmacokinetic disposition is, however, similar to that in young adults.

Dosage Forms Excipient information presented when available (limited, particularly for generics); consult specific product labeling.

Injection, solution, as succinate [strength expressed as base]: 4 mg/0.5 mL (0.5 mL); 6 mg/0.5 mL (0.5 mL)

Alsuma™: 6 mg/0.5 mL (0.5 mL) [autoinjector]

Imitrex®: 4 mg/0.5 mL (0.5 mL); 6 mg/0.5 mL (0.5 mL) [cartridge]

Imitrex®: 6 mg/0.5 mL (0.5 mL) [vial]

Sumavel™ DosePro™: 6 mg/0.5 mL (0.5 mL) [needleless autoinjector]

Injection, solution, as succinate [strength expressed as base, preservative free]: 6 mg/0.5 mL (0.5 mL)

Solution, intranasal [spray]: 5 mg/0.1 mL (6s); 20 mg/0.1 mL (6s)

Imitrex®: 5 mg/0.1 mL (6s); 20 mg/0.1 mL (6s)

Tablet, oral, as succinate [strength expressed as base]: 25 mg, 50 mg, 100 mg

Imitrex®: 25 mg, 50 mg, 100 mg

Sumatriptan and Naproxen (soo ma TRIP tan & na PROKS en)

Related Information
Naproxen on page 1263
SUMAtriptan on page 1723

Medication Safety Issues
Sound-alike/look-alike issues:
Naproxen may be confused with Natacyn®, Nebcin®, neomycin, niacin
SUMAtriptan may be confused with somatropin, ZOLMitriptan
Treximet™ may be confused with Trexall™

Brand Names: U.S. Treximet™

Index Terms Naproxen and Sumatriptan; Naproxen Sodium and Sumatriptan; Naproxen Sodium and Sumatriptan Succinate; Sumatriptan Succinate and Naproxen; Sumatriptan Succinate and Naproxen Sodium

Generic Availability (U.S.) No

Pharmacologic Category Antimigraine Agent; Nonsteroidal Anti-inflammatory Drug (NSAID), Oral; Serotonin 5-HT$_{1B, 1D}$ Receptor Agonist

Use Acute treatment of migraine with or without aura

Medication Guide Available Yes

Dosage
Geriatric & Adult Migraine: Oral: 1 tablet (sumatriptan 85 mg and naproxen 500 mg). If a satisfactory response has not been obtained at 2 hours, a second dose may be administered (maximum: 2 tablets/24 hours). **Note:** The safety of treating an average of >5 migraine headaches in a 30-day period has not been established.

Renal Impairment
Cl$_{cr}$ ≥30 mL/minute Dosage adjustment not necessary.
Cl$_{cr}$ <30 mL/minute: Use not recommended.

Hepatic Impairment Mild-to-severe impairment: Use is contraindicated by the manufacturer.

Special Geriatric Considerations See individual agents.

Dosage Forms Excipient information presented when available (limited, particularly for generics); consult specific product labeling.

Tablet:
Treximet™ 85/500: Sumatriptan 85 mg and naproxen sodium 500 mg [contains sodium 61.2 mg/tablet (~2.7 mEq/tablet)]

◆ **Sumatriptan Succinate** see SUMAtriptan on page 1723
◆ **Sumatriptan Succinate and Naproxen** see Sumatriptan and Naproxen on page 1726

Tadalafil (tah DA la fil)

Medication Safety Issues
Sound-alike/look-alike issues:
Tadalafil may be confused with sildenafil, vardenafil
Adcirca® may be confused with Advair® Diskus®, Advair® HFA, Advicor®

Brand Names: U.S. Adcirca®; Cialis®
Brand Names: Canada Adcirca®; Cialis®
Index Terms GF196960
Generic Availability (U.S.) No
Pharmacologic Category Phosphodiesterase-5 Enzyme Inhibitor
Use

Adcirca®: Treatment of pulmonary arterial hypertension (PAH) (WHO Group I) to improve exercise ability
Cialis®: Treatment of erectile dysfunction (ED)

Contraindications Known serious hypersensitivity to tadalafil; concurrent use (regularly/intermittently) of organic nitrates in any form (eg, nitroglycerin, isosorbide dinitrate)

Warnings/Precautions There is a degree of cardiac risk associated with sexual activity; therefore, physicians should consider the cardiovascular status of their patients prior to initiation. Use for erectile dysfunction is not recommended in patients with hypotension (<90/50 mm Hg), uncontrolled hypertension (>170/100 mm Hg), NYHA class II-IV heart failure within the last 6 months, uncontrolled arrhythmias, stroke within the last 6 months, MI within the last 3 months, unstable angina or angina during sexual intercourse; safety and efficacy have not been evaluated in these patients. Safety and efficacy in PAH have not been evaluated in patients with clinically significant aortic and/or mitral valve disease, life-threatening arrhythmias, hypotension (<90/50 mm Hg), uncontrolled hypertension, significant left ventricular dysfunction, pericardial constriction, restrictive or congestive cardiomyopathy, symptomatic coronary artery disease. Use caution in patients with left ventricular outflow obstruction (eg, aortic stenosis, hypertrophic obstructive cardiomyopathy); may be more sensitive to vasodilator effects.

Patients experiencing anginal chest pain after tadalafil administration should seek immediate medical attention. Concomitant use (regularly/intermittently) with all forms of nitrates is contraindicated. When used for either erectile dysfunction or PAH and nitrate administration is medically necessary following use, at least 48 hours should elapse after the tadalafil dose and nitrate administration. When used for PAH, per the manufacturer, nitrate may be administered within 48 hours of tadalafil. For both situations, administration of nitrates should only be done under close medical supervision with hemodynamic monitoring.

Concurrent use with alpha-adrenergic antagonist therapy or substantial alcohol consumption may cause symptomatic hypotension; patients should be hemodynamically stable prior to initiating tadalafil therapy at the lowest possible dose. When used for erectile dysfunction, use caution in patients receiving strong CYP3A4 inhibitors. When used for PAH, avoid use in patients taking strong CYP3A4 inducers/inhibitors. Use in patients receiving or about to receive ritonavir requires dosage adjustment or interruption of therapy, respectively. Pulmonary vasodilators may exacerbate the cardiovascular status in patients with pulmonary veno-occlusive disease (PVOD); use is not recommended. In patients with unrecognized PVOD, signs of pulmonary edema should prompt investigation into this diagnosis. Use with caution in patients with mild-to-moderate hepatic impairment; dosage adjustment/limitation is needed. Use is not recommended in patients with severe hepatic impairment or cirrhosis. Use with caution in patients with renal impairment; dosage adjustment/limitation is needed. Safety and efficacy with other tadalafil brands or other PDE-5 inhibitors (ie, sildenafil and vardenafil) have not been established. Patients should be informed not to take with other tadalafil brands or other PDE-5 inhibitors. Use caution in patients with bleeding disorders or peptic ulcer disease due to effect on platelets (bleeding).

When used to treat erectile dysfunction, potential underlying causes of erectile dysfunction should be evaluated prior to treatment. Use with caution in patients with anatomical deformation of the penis (angulation, cavernosal fibrosis, or Peyronie's disease), or who have conditions which may predispose them to priapism (sickle cell anemia, multiple myeloma, leukemia). Instruct patients to seek immediate medical attention if erection persists >4 hours. Safety and efficacy with other tadalafil brands or other PDE-5 inhibitors (ie, sildenafil and vardenafil) have not been established. Patients should be informed not to take with other tadalafil brands or other PDE-5 inhibitors. The safety and efficacy of tadalafil with other treatments for erectile dysfunction have not been studied and are, therefore, not recommended as combination therapy.

Rare cases of nonarteritic anterior ischemic optic neuropathy (NAION) have been reported; risk may be increased with history of vision loss or NAION in one eye. Other risk factors for NAION include heart disease, diabetes, hypertension, smoking, age >50 years, or history of certain eye problems. Sudden decrease or loss of hearing has been reported rarely; hearing changes may be accompanied by tinnitus and dizziness. A direct relationship between therapy and vision or hearing loss has not been determined. Instruct patients to seek medical assistance for sudden loss of vision in one or both eyes, sudden decrease in hearing, or sudden loss of hearing.

Patients with genetic retinal disorders (eg, retinitis pigmentosa) were not evaluated in clinical trials; use is not recommended. Use with caution in the elderly.

Adverse Reactions (Reflective of adult population; not specific for elderly) Based upon usual doses for either indication. For erectile dysfunction, similar adverse events are reported with once-daily versus intermittent dosing, but are generally lower than with doses used intermittently.

>10%:
Cardiovascular: Flushing (1% to 13%; dose related)
Central nervous system: Headache (3% to 42%; dose related)
Gastrointestinal: Dyspepsia (1% to 13%), nausea (10% to 11%)
Neuromuscular & skeletal: Myalgia (1% to 14%; dose related), back pain (2% to 12%), extremity pain (1% to 11%)
Respiratory: Respiratory tract infection (3% to 13%), nasopharyngitis (2% to 13%)
2% to 10%:
Cardiovascular: Hypertension (1% to 3%)
Gastrointestinal: Gastroenteritis (viral; 3% to 5%), GERD (1% to 3%), abdominal pain (1% to 2%), diarrhea (1% to 2%)
Genitourinary: Urinary tract infection (≤2%)
Respiratory: Nasal congestion (≤9%), cough (2% to 4%), bronchitis (≤2%)
Miscellaneous: Flu-like syndrome (2% to 5%)

Drug Interactions
Metabolism/Transport Effects Substrate of CYP3A4 (major)
Avoid Concomitant Use
Avoid concomitant use of Tadalafil with any of the following: Amyl Nitrite; Boceprevir; Phosphodiesterase 5 Inhibitors; Telaprevir; Vasodilators (Organic Nitrates)
Increased Effect/Toxicity
Tadalafil may increase the levels/effects of: Alpha1-Blockers; Amyl Nitrite; Antihypertensives; Bosentan; Phosphodiesterase 5 Inhibitors; Vasodilators (Organic Nitrates)

The levels/effects of Tadalafil may be increased by: Antifungal Agents (Azole Derivatives, Systemic); Boceprevir; CYP3A4 Inhibitors (Moderate); CYP3A4 Inhibitors (Strong); Dasatinib; Ritonavir; Sapropterin; Telaprevir

Decreased Effect

The levels/effects of Tadalafil may be decreased by: Bosentan; CYP3A4 Inducers (Strong); Etravirine; Tocilizumab

Ethanol/Nutrition/Herb Interactions

Ethanol: Substantial consumption of ethanol may increase the risk of hypotension and orthostasis. Lower ethanol consumption has not been associated with significant changes in blood pressure or increase in orthostatic symptoms.

Food: Rate and extent of absorption are not affected by food. Grapefruit juice may increase serum levels/toxicity of tadalafil. Use tadalafil with caution in patients who regularly consume grapefruit juice. In general, use of grapefruit juice should be limited or avoided; the manufacturer does not give specific recommendations.

Herb/Nutraceutical: St John's wort: Use caution with concomitant use.

Stability Store at 25°C (77°F); excursions permitted to 15°C to 30°C (59°F to 86°F).

Mechanism of Action

Erectile dysfunction: Does not directly cause penile erections, but affects the response to sexual stimulation. The physiologic mechanism of erection of the penis involves release of nitric oxide (NO) in the corpus cavernosum during sexual stimulation. NO then activates the enzyme guanylate cyclase, which results in increased levels of cyclic guanosine mono-phosphate (cGMP), producing smooth muscle relaxation and inflow of blood to the corpus cavernosum. Tadalafil enhances the effect of NO by inhibiting phosphodiesterase type 5 (PDE-5), which is responsible for degradation of cGMP in the corpus cavernosum; when sexual stimulation causes local release of NO, inhibition of PDE-5 by tadalafil causes increased levels of cGMP in the corpus cavernosum, resulting in smooth muscle relaxation and inflow of blood to the corpus cavernosum. At recommended doses, it has no effect in the absence of sexual stimulation.

PAH: Inhibits phosphodiesterase type 5 (PDE-5) in smooth muscle of pulmonary vasculature where PDE-5 is responsible for the degradation of cyclic guanosine monophosphate (cGMP). Increased cGMP concentration results in pulmonary vasculature relaxation; vaso-dilation in the pulmonary bed and the systemic circulation (to a lesser degree) may occur.

Pharmacodynamics/Kinetics

Onset of action: Within 1 hour

Peak effect (pulmonary artery vasodilation): 75-90 minutes (Ghofrani, 2004)

Duration: Erectile dysfunction: Up to 36 hours

Distribution: V_d: 63-77 L

Protein binding: 94%

Metabolism: Hepatic, via CYP3A4 to metabolites (inactive)

Half-life elimination: 15-17.5 hours; Pulmonary hypertension (not receiving bosentan): 35 hours

Time to peak, plasma: ~2-4 hours (range: 30 minutes to 8 hours)

Excretion: Feces (~61%, predominantly as metabolites); urine (~36%, predominantly as metabolites)

Dosage

Geriatric Refer to adult dosing. No dose adjustment for patients >65 years of age in the absence of renal or hepatic impairment.

Adult

Erectile dysfunction (Cialis®): Oral:

As-needed dosing: 10 mg at least 30 minutes prior to anticipated sexual activity (dosing range: 5-20 mg); to be given as one single dose and not given more than once daily. **Note:** Erectile function may be improved for up to 36 hours following a single dose; adjust dose.

Once-daily dosing: 2.5 mg once daily (dosing range: 2.5-5 mg/day) to be given at approximately the same time daily without regard to timing of sexual activity

Dosing adjustment with concomitant medications:

Alpha₁-blockers: If stabilized on either alpha-blockers or tadalafil therapy, initiate new therapy with the other agent at the lowest possible dose.

Protease inhibitors: Maximum tadalafil dose: 10 mg in a 72-hour period

Other CYP3A4 inhibitors: Dose reduction of tadalafil is recommended with strong CYP3A4 inhibitors. When used on an as-needed basis, the dose of tadalafil should not exceed 10 mg, and tadalafil should not be taken more frequently than once every 72 hours. When used on a once-daily basis, the dose of tadalafil should not exceed 2.5 mg. Examples of such inhibitors include clarithromycin, conivaptan, delavirdine, diclofenac, imatinib, isoniazid, itraconazole, ketoconazole, miconazole, nefazodone, nicardipine, propofol, quinidine, and telithromycin.

Pulmonary arterial hypertension (Adcirca®): Oral: 40 mg once daily

◀ **Dosing adjustment with concomitant medications:**

Coadministration with protease inhibitor regimen:

Concurrent use with atazanavir/ritonavir, darunavir/ritonavir, fosamprenavir, ritonavir, saquinavir/ritonavir, tipranavir/ritonavir:

Coadministration of tadalafil in patients currently receiving one of these protease inhibitor regimens for at least 1 week: Initiate tadalafil at 20 mg once daily; increase to 40 mg once daily based on individual tolerability.

Coadministration of one of these protease inhibitor regimens in patients currently receiving tadalafil: Discontinue tadalafil at least 24 hours prior to the initiation of the protease inhibitor regimen. After at least 1 week of the protease inhibitor regimen, resume tadalafil at 20 mg once daily; increase to 40 mg once daily based on individual tolerability.

Concurrent use with indinavir or nelfinavir:

Patient receiving indinavir/nelfinavir when initiating tadalafil: Initiate tadalafil at 20 mg once daily; increase to 40 mg once daily based on individual tolerability

Patient receiving tadalafil when initiating indinavir/nelfinavir: Adjust tadalafil to 20 mg once daily; increase to 40 mg once daily based on individual tolerability

Other potent CYP3A4 inhibitors: Avoid concurrent use when tadalafil used for PAH. Examples of such inhibitors include clarithromycin, conivaptan, delavirdine, diclofenac, imatinib, isoniazid, itraconazole, ketoconazole, miconazole, nefazodone, nicardipine, propofol, quinidine, and telithromycin.

Potent CYP3A4 inducers (eg, rifampin): Avoid concurrent use when tadalafil used for PAH.

Renal Impairment

Erectile dysfunction (Cialis®):

As-needed use:

Cl_{cr} ≥51 mL/minute: Dosage adjustment not required.

Cl_{cr} 31-50 mL/minute: Initial: 5 mg once daily; maximum: 10 mg (not to be given more frequently than every 48 hours).

Cl_{cr} <30 mL/minute and on hemodialysis: Maximum: 5 mg (not to be given more frequently than every 72 hours).

Once-daily use:

Cl_{cr} ≥31 mL/minute: Dose adjustment not required.

Cl_{cr} <30 mL/minute and on hemodialysis: Use not recommended.

Pulmonary arterial hypertension (Adcirca®):

Cl_{cr} 31-80 mL/minute: Initial: 20 mg once daily; increase to 40 mg once daily based on individual tolerability.

Cl_{cr} <30 mL/minute and on hemodialysis: Avoid use due to increased tadalafil exposure, limited clinical experience, and lack of ability to influence clearance by dialysis.

Hepatic Impairment

Erectile dysfunction (Cialis®):

As-needed use:

Mild-to-moderate hepatic impairment (Child-Pugh class A or B): Use with caution; dose should not exceed 10 mg once daily.

Severe hepatic impairment (Child-Pugh class C): Use is not recommended.

Once-daily use:

Mild-to-moderate hepatic impairment (Child-Pugh class A or B): Use with caution.

Severe hepatic impairment (Child-Pugh class C): Use is not recommended.

Pulmonary arterial hypertension (Adcirca®):

Mild-to-moderate hepatic impairment (Child-Pugh class A or B): Use with caution; consider initial dose of 20 mg once daily.

Severe hepatic impairment (Child-Pugh class C): Avoid use; has not been studied in patients with severe hepatic cirrhosis.

Administration May be administered with or without food.

Adcirca®: Administer daily dose all at once; dividing doses throughout the day is not advised.

Cialis®: When used on an as-needed basis, should be taken at least 30 minutes prior to sexual activity. When used on a once-daily basis, should be taken at the same time each day, without regard to timing of sexual activity.

Monitoring Parameters Blood pressure; response and adverse effects

Special Geriatric Considerations No significant differences in pharmacokinetics were seen in elderly men versus younger men. Dosing should be adjusted for renal function. Since older adults often have concomitant diseases, many of which may be contraindicated with the use of tadalafil, prescriber should complete a thorough review of diseases and medications prior to prescribing tadalafil.

Dosage Forms Excipient information presented when available (limited, particularly for generics); consult specific product labeling.

Tablet, oral:

Adcirca®: 20 mg

Cialis®: 2.5 mg, 5 mg, 10 mg, 20 mg

Selected References

Anderson JL, Adams CD, Antman EM, et al, "ACC/AHA 2007 Guidelines for the Management of Patients With Unstable Angina/Non ST-Elevation Myocardial Infarction: Executive Summary. A Report of the American College of Cardiology/American Heart Association Task Force on Practice Guidelines (Writing Committee to Revise the 2002 Guidelines for the Management of Patients with Unstable Angina/Non ST-Elevation Myocardial Infarction) Developed in Collaboration With the American College of Emergency Physicians, The Society of Cardiovascular Angiography and Interventions, and the Society of Thoracic Surgeons," *J Am Coll Cardiol*, 2007, 50(7):1-157. Available at http://content.onlinejacc.org/cgi/reprint/50/7/e1

Antman EM, Anbe DT, Armstrong PW, et al, "ACC/AHA Guidelines for the Management of Patients With ST-Elevation Myocardial Infarction: A Report of the American College of Cardiology/American Heart Association Task Force on Practice Guidelines (Committee to Revise the 1999 Guidelines for the Management of Patients with Acute Myocardial Infarction)," *Circulation*, 2004, 110(9):e82-292.

Curran M and Keating G, "Tadalafil," *Drugs*, 2003, 63(20):2203-12; discussion 2213-4.

Galie N, Brundage BH, Ghofrani HA, et al, "Tadalafil Therapy for Pulmonary Arterial Hypertenstion," *Circulation*, 2009, 119 [epub ahead of print]

Ghofrani HA, Voswinckel R, Reichenberger F, et al, "Differences in Hemodynamic and Oxygenation Responses to Three Different Phosphodiesterase-5 Inhibitors in Patients with Pulmonary Arterial Hypertension," *J Am Coll Cardiol*, 2004, 44(7):1488-96.

Jackson G, Rosen RC, Kloner RA, et al, "The Second Princeton Consensus on Sexual Dysfunction and Cardiac Risk: New Guidelines for Sexual Medicine," *J Sex Med*, 2006, 3(1):28-36.

◆ **Tagamet HB 200® [OTC]** *see* Cimetidine *on page 357*
◆ **TAK-375** *see* Ramelteon *on page 1580*
◆ **TAK-390MR** *see* Dexlansoprazole *on page 489*
◆ **TAK-599** *see* Ceftaroline Fosamil *on page 307*
◆ **Talwin®** *see* Pentazocine *on page 1423*
◆ **Tambocor™** *see* Flecainide *on page 739*
◆ **Tamiflu®** *see* Oseltamivir *on page 1353*

Tamoxifen (ta MOKS i fen)

Medication Safety Issues

Sound-alike/look-alike issues:

Tamoxifen may be confused with pentoxifylline, Tambocor™, tamsulosin, temazepam

Brand Names: Canada Apo-Tamox®; Mylan-Tamoxifen; Nolvadex®-D; PMS-Tamoxifen; Teva-Tamoxifen

Index Terms ICI-46474; Nolvadex; Tamoxifen Citras; Tamoxifen Citrate

Generic Availability (U.S.) Yes

Pharmacologic Category Antineoplastic Agent, Estrogen Receptor Antagonist; Selective Estrogen Receptor Modulator (SERM)

Use Treatment of metastatic (female and male) breast cancer; adjuvant treatment of breast cancer after primary treatment with surgery and radiation; reduce risk of invasive breast cancer in women with ductal carcinoma *in situ* (DCIS) after surgery and radiation; reduce the incidence of breast cancer in women at high risk

Unlabeled/Investigational Use Treatment of mastalgia, gynecomastia, ovarian cancer, endometrial cancer, uterine sarcoma, and desmoid tumors; risk reduction in women with Paget's disease of the breast (with DCIS or without associated cancer)

Medication Guide Available Yes

Contraindications Hypersensitivity to tamoxifen or any component of the formulation; concurrent warfarin therapy or history of deep vein thrombosis or pulmonary embolism (when tamoxifen is used for cancer risk reduction in women at high-risk for breast cancer and in women with DCIS)

Warnings/Precautions Hazardous agent - use appropriate precautions for handling and disposal. **[U.S. Boxed Warning]: Serious and life-threatening events (including stroke, pulmonary emboli, and uterine malignancy) have occurred at an incidence greater than placebo during use for breast cancer risk reduction in women at high-risk for breast cancer and in women with DCIS;** these events are rare, but require consideration in risk: benefit evaluation. An increased incidence of thromboembolic events, including DVT and pulmonary embolism, has been associated with use for breast cancer; risk is increased with concomitant chemotherapy; use with caution in individuals with a history of thromboembolic events. Thrombocytopenia and/or leukopenia may occur; neutropenia and pancytopenia have been reported rarely. Although the relationship to tamoxifen therapy is uncertain, rare hemorrhagic episodes have occurred in patients with significant thrombocytopenia. Use with caution in patients with hyperlipidemias; infrequent postmarketing cases of hyperlipidemias have been reported. Decreased visual acuity, retinal vein thrombosis, retinopathy, corneal changes, color perception changes, and increased incidence of cataracts (and the need for

◄ cataract surgery), have been reported. Hypercalcemia has occurred in patients with bone metastasis, usually within a few weeks of therapy initiation; institute appropriate hypercalcemia management; discontinue if severe. Local disease flare and increased bone and tumor pain may occur in patients with metastatic breast cancer; may be associated with (good) tumor response.

Tamoxifen is associated with a high potential for drug interactions, including CYP- and Pgp-mediated interactions. Decreased efficacy and an increased risk of breast cancer recurrence has been reported with concurrent moderate or strong CYP2D6 inhibitors (Aubert, 2009; Dezentje, 2009). Concomitant use with select SSRIs may result in decreased tamoxifen efficacy. Strong CYP2D6 inhibitors (eg, fluoxetine, paroxetine) and moderate CYP2D6 inhibitors (eg, sertraline) are reported to interfere with transformation to the active metabolite endoxifen. Weak CYP2D6 inhibitors (eg, venlafaxine, citalopram) have minimal effect on the conversion to endoxifen (Jin, 2005; NCCN Breast Cancer Risk Reduction Guidelines v.2.2010); escitalopram is also a weak CYP2D6 inhibitor. Lower plasma concentrations of endoxifen (active metabolite) have been observed in patients associated with reduced CYP2D6 activity (Jin, 2005) and may be associated with reduced efficacy. In a retrospective analysis of breast cancer patients taking tamoxifen and SSRIs, concomitant use of paroxetine and tamoxifen was associated with an increased risk of death due to breast cancer (Kelly, 2010).

Tamoxifen use may be associated with changes in bone mineral density (BMD) and the effects may be dependent upon menstrual status. In postmenopausal women, tamoxifen use is associated with a protective effect on bone mineral density (BMD), preventing loss of BMD which lasts over the 5-year treatment period. In premenopausal women, a decline (from baseline) in BMD mineral density has been observed in women who continued to menstruate; may be associated with an increased risk of fractures. Liver abnormalities such as cholestasis, fatty liver, hepatitis, and hepatic necrosis have occurred. Hepatocellular carcinomas have been reported in some studies; relationship to treatment is unclear. Tamoxifen is associated with an increased incidence of uterine or endometrial cancers. Endometrial hyperplasia, polyps, endometriosis, uterine fibroids, and ovarian cysts have occurred. Monitor and promptly evaluate any report of abnormal vaginal bleeding. Amenorrhea and menstrual irregularities have been reported with tamoxifen use.

Adverse Reactions (Reflective of adult population; not specific for elderly)

>10%:
  Cardiovascular: Vasodilation (41%), flushing (33%), hypertension (11%), peripheral edema (11%)
  Central nervous system: Mood changes (12% to 18%), pain (3% to 16%), depression (2% to 12%)
  Dermatologic: Skin changes (6% to 19%), rash (13%)
  Endocrine & metabolic: Hot flashes (3% to 80%), fluid retention (32%), altered menses (13% to 25%), amenorrhea (16%)
  Gastrointestinal: Nausea (5% to 26%), weight loss (23%), vomiting (12%)
  Genitourinary: Vaginal discharge (13% to 55%), vaginal bleeding (2% to 23%)
  Neuromuscular & skeletal: Weakness (18%), arthritis (14%), arthralgia (11%)
  Respiratory: Pharyngitis (14%)
  Miscellaneous: Lymphedema (11%)

1% to 10%:
  Cardiovascular: Chest pain (5%), venous thrombotic events (5%), edema (4%), cardiovascular ischemia (3%), angina (2%), deep venous thrombus (≤2%), MI (1%)
  Central nervous system: Insomnia (9%), dizziness (8%), headache (8%), anxiety (6%), fatigue (4%)
  Dermatologic: Alopecia (≤5%)
  Endocrine & metabolic: Oligomenorrhea (9%), breast pain (6%), menstrual disorder (6%), breast neoplasm (5%), hypercholesterolemia (4%)
  Gastrointestinal: Abdominal pain (9%), weight gain (9%), constipation (4% to 8%), diarrhea (7%), dyspepsia (6%), throat irritation (oral solution 5%), abdominal cramps (1%), anorexia (1%)
  Genitourinary: Urinary tract infection (10%), leukorrhea (9%), vaginal hemorrhage (6%), vaginitis (5%), vulvovaginitis (5%), ovarian cyst (3%)
  Hematologic: Thrombocytopenia (≤10%), anemia (5%)
  Hepatic: AST increased (5%), serum bilirubin increased (2%)
  Neuromuscular & skeletal: Back pain (10%), bone pain (6% to 10%), osteoporosis (7%), fracture (7%), arthrosis (5%), joint disorder (5%), myalgia (5%), paresthesia (5%), musculoskeletal pain (3%)
  Ocular: Cataract (7%)
  Renal: Serum creatinine increased (≤2%)

Respiratory: Cough (4% to 9%), dyspnea (8%), bronchitis (5%), sinusitis (5%)

Miscellaneous: Infection/sepsis (≤9%), diaphoresis (6%), flu-like syndrome (6%), cyst (5%), neoplasm (5%), allergic reaction (3%)

Drug Interactions

Metabolism/Transport Effects Substrate of CYP2A6 (minor), 2B6 (minor), 2C9 (major), 2D6 (major), 2E1 (minor), 3A4 (major); **Inhibits** CYP2B6 (weak), 2C8 (moderate), 2C9 (weak), 3A4 (weak), p-glycoprotein

Avoid Concomitant Use

Avoid concomitant use of Tamoxifen with any of the following: Conivaptan; CYP2D6 Inhibitors (Strong); Silodosin; Topotecan; Vitamin K Antagonists

Increased Effect/Toxicity

Tamoxifen may increase the levels/effects of: Colchicine; CYP2C8 Substrates (High risk); Dabigatran Etexilate; Everolimus; P-Glycoprotein Substrates; Rivaroxaban; Silodosin; Topotecan; Vitamin K Antagonists

The levels/effects of Tamoxifen may be increased by: Abiraterone Acetate; Conivaptan; CYP2C9 Inhibitors (Moderate); CYP2C9 Inhibitors (Strong); CYP2D6 Inhibitors (Moderate); CYP2D6 Inhibitors (Strong); CYP3A4 Inhibitors (Moderate); CYP3A4 Inhibitors (Strong); Darunavir; Dasatinib

Decreased Effect

Tamoxifen may decrease the levels/effects of: Anastrozole; Letrozole

The levels/effects of Tamoxifen may be decreased by: Aminoglutethimide; CYP2C9 Inducers (Highly Effective); CYP3A4 Inducers (Strong); Cyproterone; Deferasirox; Herbs (CYP3A4 Inducers); Peginterferon Alfa-2b; Rifamycin Derivatives; Tocilizumab

Ethanol/Nutrition/Herb Interactions

Food: Avoid grapefruit juice (may decrease the metabolism of tamoxifen).

Herb/Nutraceutical: Avoid black cohosh, dong quai in estrogen-dependent tumors. Avoid St John's wort (may decrease levels/effects of tamoxifen).

Stability Store at room temperature of 20°C to 25°C (68°F to 77°F). Protect from light.

Mechanism of Action Competitively binds to estrogen receptors on tumors and other tissue targets, producing a nuclear complex that decreases DNA synthesis and inhibits estrogen effects; nonsteroidal agent with potent antiestrogenic properties which compete with estrogen for binding sites in breast and other tissues; cells accumulate in the G_0 and G_1 phases; therefore, tamoxifen is cytostatic rather than cytocidal.

Pharmacodynamics/Kinetics

Absorption: Well absorbed

Distribution: High concentrations found in uterus, endometrial and breast tissue

Protein binding: 99%

Metabolism: Hepatic; via CYP2D6 to 4-hydroxytamoxifen and via CYP3A4/5 to N-desmethyl-tamoxifen. Each is then further metabolized into endoxifen (4-hydroxy-tamoxifen via CYP3A4/5 and N-desmethyl-tamoxifen via CYP2D6); both 4-hydroxy-tamoxifen and endoxifen are 30- to 100-fold more potent than tamoxifen

Half-life elimination: Tamoxifen: ~5-7 days; N-desmethyl tamoxifen: ~14 days

Time to peak, serum: ~5 hours

Excretion: Feces (26% to 51%); urine (9% to 13%)

Dosage

Geriatric & Adult Note: For the treatment of breast cancer, patients receiving both tamoxifen and chemotherapy, should receive treatment sequentially, with tamoxifen following completion of chemotherapy.

Breast cancer treatment:

Adjuvant therapy (females): 20 mg once daily for 5 years

Metastatic (males and females): 20-40 mg/day (doses >20 mg should be given in 2 divided doses). **Note:** Although the FDA-approved labeling recommends dosing up to 40 mg/day, clinical benefit has not been demonstrated with doses above 20 mg/day (Bratherton, 1984).

Premenopausal women: Duration of treatment is 5 years (NCCN Breast Cancer guidelines v.1.2011)

Postmenopausal women: Duration of tamoxifen treatment is 2-3 years followed by an aromatase inhibitor (AI) to complete 5 years; if contraindications or intolerant to AI, may take tamoxifen for the full 5 years **or** extended therapy: 4.5-6 years of tamoxifen followed by 5 years of an AI (NCCN Breast Cancer guidelines v.1.2011)

DCIS (females), to reduce the risk for invasive breast cancer: 20 mg once daily for 5 years

Breast cancer risk reduction (pre- and postmenopausal high-risk females): 20 mg once daily for 5 years

Paget's disease of the breast (risk reduction; with DCIS or without associated cancer): 20 mg once daily for 5 years (NCCN Breast Cancer Guidelines, v.1.2011)

◄ **Dosage adjustment for DVT, pulmonary embolism, cerebrovascular accident, or prolonged immobilization:** Discontinue tamoxifen (NCCN Breast Cancer Risk Reduction Guidelines, v.2.2010)

Administration Administer orally with or without food.

Monitoring Parameters CBC with platelets, serum calcium, LFTs; triglycerides and cholesterol (in patients with pre-existing hyperlipidemias); INR and PT (in patients on vitamin K antagonists); abnormal vaginal bleeding; breast and gynecologic exams (baseline and routine), mammogram (baseline and routine); signs/symptoms of DVT (leg swelling, tenderness) or PE (shortness of breath); ophthalmic exam (if vision problem or cataracts); bone mineral density (premenopausal women)

Test Interactions T_4 elevations (which may be explained by increases in thyroid-binding globulin) have been reported; not accompanied by clinical hyperthyroidism

Pharmacotherapy Pearls Estrogen receptor status may predict if adjuvant treatment with tamoxifen is of benefit. In metastatic breast cancer, patients with estrogen receptor positive tumors are more likely to benefit from tamoxifen treatment. With tamoxifen use to reduce the incidence of breast cancer in high risk-women, high risk is defined as women ≥35 years of age with a 5 year NCI Gail model predicted risk of breast cancer ≥1.67%.

Oncology Comment: The American Society of Clinical Oncology (ASCO) guidelines for adjuvant endocrine therapy in postmenopausal women with HR-positive breast cancer (Burstein, 2010) recommend considering aromatase inhibitor (AI) therapy at some point in the treatment course (primary, sequentially, or extended). Optimal duration at this time is not known; however, treatment with an AI should not exceed 5 years in primary and extended therapies, and 2-3 years if followed by tamoxifen in sequential therapy (total of 5 years). If initial therapy with AI has been discontinued before the 5 years, consideration should be taken to receive tamoxifen for a total of 5 years. The optimal time to switch to an AI is also not known; but data supports switching after 2-3 years of tamoxifen (sequential) or after 5 years of tamoxifen (extended). If patient becomes intolerant or has poor adherence, consideration should be made to switch to another AI or initiate tamoxifen.

The adjuvant endocrine therapy of choice is tamoxifen for men with breast cancer and for pre- or perimenopausal women at diagnosis. CYP2D6 genotyping is not recommended, however, due to the potential for drug-drug interactions use caution and consider avoiding concomitant therapy with tamoxifen and known CYP2D6 inhibitors.

Special Geriatric Considerations Studies have shown tamoxifen to be effective in the treatment of primary breast cancer in elderly women. Comparative studies with other antineoplastic agents in elderly women with breast cancer had more favorable survival rates with tamoxifen. Initiation of hormone therapy rather than chemotherapy is justified for elderly patients with metastatic breast cancer who are responsive. Reduction of mortality and recurrence was greater in those studies that used tamoxifen for ≥2 years than those that use it for <2 years.

Dosage Forms Excipient information presented when available (limited, particularly for generics); consult specific product labeling.
Tablet, oral: 10 mg, 20 mg

Selected References

Eastell R, Adams JE, Coleman RE, et al, "Effect of Anastrozole on Bone Mineral Density: 5-Year Results From the Anastrozole, Tamoxifen, Alone or in Combination Trial 18233230," *J Clin Oncol*, 2008, 26(7):1051-7.

National Comprehensive Cancer Network® (NCCN), "Clinical Practice Guidelines in Oncology™: Breast Cancer," Version 1.2009. Available at http://www.nccn.org/professionals/physician_gls/PDF/breast.pdf.

National Comprehensive Cancer Network® (NCCN), "Clinical Practice Guidelines in Oncology™: Breast Cancer Risk Reduction, Version 1.2009." Accessible at http://www.nccn.org/professionals/physician_gls/PDF/breast_risk.pdf

Visvanathan K, Chlebowski RT, Hurley P, et al, "American Society of Clinical Oncology Clinical Practice Guideline Update on the Use of Pharmacologic Interventions Including Tamoxifen, Raloxifene, and Aromatase Inhibition for Breast Cancer Risk Reduction," *J Clin Oncol*, 2009, 27(19):3235-58.

Winer EP, Hudis C, Burstein HJ, et al, "American Society of Clinical Oncology Technology Assessment on the Use of Aromatase Inhibitors as Adjuvant Therapy for Postmenopausal Women With Hormone Receptor-Positive Breast Cancer: Status Report 2004," *J Clin Oncol*, 2005, 23(3):619-29.

◆ **Tamoxifen Citras** see Tamoxifen on page 1731
◆ **Tamoxifen Citrate** see Tamoxifen on page 1731

Tamsulosin (tam SOO loe sin)

Related Information
Pharmacotherapy of Urinary Incontinence on page 2032

Medication Safety Issues
Sound-alike/look-alike issues:
Flomax® may be confused with Flonase®, Flovent®, Foltx®, Fosamax®

Tamsulosin may be confused with tacrolimus, tamoxifen, terazosin

International issues:

Flomax [U.S., Canada, and multiple international markets] may be confused with Flomox brand name for cefcapene [Japan] and Volmax brand name for salbutamol [multiple international markets]

Flomax: Brand name for tamsulosin [U.S., Canada, and multiple international markets], but also the brand name for morniflumate [Italy]

Brand Names: U.S. Flomax®

Brand Names: Canada Flomax® CR; JAMP-Tamsulosin; Mylan-Tamsulosin; RAN™-Tamsulosin; ratio-Tamsulosin; Sandoz-Tamsulosin; Sandoz-Tamsulosin CR; Teva-Tamsulosin

Index Terms Tamsulosin Hydrochloride

Generic Availability (U.S.) Yes

Pharmacologic Category Alpha₁ Blocker

Use Treatment of signs and symptoms of benign prostatic hyperplasia (BPH)

Unlabeled/Investigational Use Symptomatic treatment of bladder outlet obstruction or dysfunction

Contraindications Hypersensitivity to tamsulosin or any component of the formulation

Warnings/Precautions Not intended for use as an antihypertensive drug. May cause significant orthostatic hypotension and syncope, especially with first dose; anticipate a similar effect if therapy is interrupted for a few days, if dosage is rapidly increased, or if another antihypertensive drug (particularly vasodilators) or a PDE-5 inhibitor (eg, sildenafil, tadalafil, vardenafil) is introduced. "First-dose" orthostatic hypotension may occur 4-8 hours after dosing; may be dose related. Patients should be cautioned about performing hazardous tasks when starting new therapy or adjusting dosage upward. Discontinue if symptoms of angina occur or worsen. Rule out prostatic carcinoma before beginning therapy with tamsulosin. Intraoperative floppy iris syndrome has been observed in cataract surgery patients who were on or were previously treated with alpha₁-blockers; causality has not been established and there appears to be no benefit in discontinuing alpha-blocker therapy prior to surgery; instruct patients to inform ophthalmologist of tamsulosin use when considering eye surgery. Priapism has been associated with use (rarely). Rarely, patients with a sulfa allergy have also developed an allergic reaction to tamsulosin; avoid use when previous reaction has been severe.

Adverse Reactions (Reflective of adult population; not specific for elderly)

>10%:

Cardiovascular: Orthostatic hypotension (6 % to 19%)

Central nervous system: Headache (19% to 21%), dizziness (15% to 17%)

Genitourinary: Abnormal ejaculation (8% to 18%)

Respiratory: Rhinitis (13% to 18%)

Miscellaneous: Infection (9% to 11%)

1% to 10%:

Cardiovascular: Chest pain (4%)

Central nervous system: Somnolence (3% to 4%), insomnia (1% to 2%), vertigo (≤1%)

Endocrine & metabolic: Libido decreased (1% to 2%)

Gastrointestinal: Diarrhea (4% to 6%), nausea (3% to 4%), gum pain, toothache

Neuromuscular & skeletal: Weakness (8% to 9%), back pain (7% to 8%)

Ocular: Blurred vision (≤2%)

Respiratory: Pharyngitis (5% to 6%), cough (3% to 5%), sinusitis (2% to 4%)

Drug Interactions

Metabolism/Transport Effects Substrate (major) of CYP2D6, 3A4

Avoid Concomitant Use

Avoid concomitant use of Tamsulosin with any of the following: Alpha1-Blockers; CYP3A4 Inhibitors (Strong)

Increased Effect/Toxicity

Tamsulosin may increase the levels/effects of: Alpha1-Blockers; Calcium Channel Blockers

The levels/effects of Tamsulosin may be increased by: Abiraterone Acetate; Beta-Blockers; CYP2D6 Inhibitors (Moderate); CYP2D6 Inhibitors (Strong); CYP3A4 Inhibitors (Moderate); CYP3A4 Inhibitors (Strong); Dasatinib; MAO Inhibitors; Phosphodiesterase 5 Inhibitors

Decreased Effect

The levels/effects of Tamsulosin may be decreased by: CYP3A4 Inducers (Strong); Deferasirox; Herbs (CYP3A4 Inducers); Peginterferon Alfa-2b; Tocilizumab

Ethanol/Nutrition/Herb Interactions

Food: Fasting increases bioavailability by 30% and peak concentration 40% to 70%.

Herb/Nutraceutical: St John's wort: May decrease the levels/effects of tamsulosin. Avoid herbs with hypotensive properties (black cohosh, California poppy, coleus, golden seal, hawthorn, mistletoe, periwinkle, quinine, Shepherd's purse); may enhance the hypotensive effect of tamsulosin. Avoid saw palmetto (due to limited experience with this combination).

◄ **Stability** Store at room temperature of 25°C (77°F); excursions permitted to 15°C to 30°C (59°F to 86°F).

Mechanism of Action Tamsulosin is an antagonist of alpha$_{1A}$-adrenoreceptors in the prostate. Smooth muscle tone in the prostate is mediated by alpha$_{1A}$-adrenoreceptors; blocking them leads to relaxation of smooth muscle in the bladder neck and prostate causing an improvement of urine flow and decreased symptoms of BPH. Approximately 75% of the alpha$_1$-receptors in the prostate are of the alpha$_{1A}$ subtype.

Pharmacodynamics/Kinetics

Absorption: >90% under fasting conditions

Protein binding: 94% to 99% to alpha$_1$-glycoprotein

Metabolism: Hepatic via CYP3A4 and 2D6; metabolites undergo extensive conjugation to glucuronide or sulfate

Bioavailability: Fasting: 30% increase

Half-life:

Healthy volunteers: 9-13 hours

Target population: 14-15 hours

Geriatrics: Slightly prolonged and AUC is increased by 40%

Elimination: 76% in urine as metabolites

Dosage

Geriatric & Adult

Benign prostatic hyperplasia (BPH): Oral: 0.4 mg once daily ~30 minutes after the same meal each day; dose may be increased after 2-4 weeks to 0.8 mg once daily in patients who fail to respond. If therapy is interrupted for several days, restart with 0.4 mg once daily.

Bladder outlet obstruction symptoms (unlabeled use): Oral: 0.4 mg once daily (Rossi, 2001)

Ureteral stones, expulsion (unlabeled use): Oral: 0.4 mg once daily, discontinue after successful expulsion (average time to expulsion was 1-2 weeks) (Agrawal, 2009; Ahmed, 2010). **Note:** Patients with stones >10 mm were excluded from studies.

Renal Impairment

Cl$_{cr}$ ≥10 mL/minute: No adjustment needed.

Cl$_{cr}$ <10 mL/minute: Not studied.

Hepatic Impairment

Mild-to-moderate impairment: No adjustment needed

Severe impairment: Not studied

Administration Administer 30 minutes after the same meal each day. Capsules should be swallowed whole; do not crush, chew, or open.

Monitoring Parameters Relief of symptoms, blood pressure

Special Geriatric Considerations Metabolism of tamsulosin may be slower, and older patients may be more sensitive to the orthostatic hypotension caused by this medication. A 40% higher exposure (AUC) is anticipated in patients between 55 and 75 years of age as compared to younger subjects (20-32 years).

Dosage Forms Excipient information presented when available (limited, particularly for generics); consult specific product labeling.

Capsule, oral, as hydrochloride: 0.4 mg

Flomax®: 0.4 mg

Tablet, oral, as hydrochloride: 0.4 mg

Selected References

Goldman HB and Zimmern PE, "The Treatment of Female Bladder Outlet Obstruction," *BJU Int*, 2006, 98(Suppl 1):17-23.

Pischedda A, Pirozzi Farina F, Madonia M, et al, "Use of Alpha$_1$-Blockers in Female Functional Bladder Neck Obstruction," *Urol Int*, 2005, 74(3):256-61.

◆ **Tamsulosin and Dutasteride** see Dutasteride and Tamsulosin *on page 588*

◆ **Tamsulosin Hydrochloride** see Tamsulosin *on page 1734*

◆ **Tamsulosin Hydrochloride and Dutasteride** see Dutasteride and Tamsulosin *on page 588*

◆ **TanaCof-XR [DSC]** see Brompheniramine *on page 217*

◆ **TAP-144** see Leuprolide *on page 1039*

◆ **Tapazole®** see Methimazole *on page 1165*

Tapentadol (ta PEN ta dol)

Medication Safety Issues

Sound-alike/look-alike issues:

Tapentadol may be confused with traMADol

Brand Names: U.S. Nucynta®; Nucynta® ER

Brand Names: Canada Nucynta™ CR

Index Terms CG5503; Tapentadol Hydrochloride

Generic Availability (U.S.) No

Pharmacologic Category Analgesic, Opioid

Use

Immediate release formulation: Relief of moderate-to-severe acute pain

Long acting formulations: Relief of moderate-to-severe chronic pain when continuous, around-the-clock analgesia is necessary for an extended period of time

Medication Guide Available Yes

Contraindications Impaired pulmonary function (severe respiratory depression, acute or severe asthma or hypercapnia) in unmonitored settings or in absence of resuscitative equipment or ventilatory support; paralytic ileus; use of MAO inhibitors within 14 days

Canadian labeling: Additional contraindications (not in U.S. labeling): Hypersensitivity to tapentadol, opioids, or any component of the formulation or container; any disease/condition that affects bowel transit (eg, ileus of any type, strictures); severe renal impairment (Cl$_{cr}$ <30 mL/minute); severe hepatic impairment (Child-Pugh class C); mild, intermittent, or short-duration pain that can be managed with alternative pain medication; management of perioperative pain; acute alcoholism, delirium tremens, and seizure disorders; severe CNS depression, increased cerebrospinal or intracranial pressure or head injury

Warnings/Precautions Extended release tablets: **[U.S. Boxed Warning]: Use of alcohol or alcohol-containing medications should be avoided;** concomitant use with alcohol may increase tapentadol systemic exposure which may lead to possible fatal overdose. **[U.S. Boxed warning]: NOT intended for use as an as-needed analgesic; NOT intended for the management of acute or postoperative pain;** approved for the treatment of chronic pain only (not as an as-needed basis). **[U.S. Boxed Warning]: Extended-release tablets must be swallowed whole and should NOT be split, crushed, broken, chewed or dissolved. [U.S. Boxed Warning]: Healthcare provider should be alert to problems of abuse, misuse, and diversion.** May cause severe hypotension; use with caution in patients with risk factors (eg. hypovolemia, concomitant use of other hypotensive agents).

Use with caution in patients with respiratory disease or respiratory compromise (eg, asthma, chronic obstructive pulmonary disease [COPD], cor pulmonale, sleep apnea, severe obesity, kyphoscoliosis, hypoxia, hypercapnia); critical respiratory depression may occur, even at therapeutic dosages. May cause CNS depression, which may impair physical or mental abilities; patients must be cautioned about performing tasks which require mental alertness (eg, operating machinery or driving). Use with caution in patients with CNS depression or coma. Effects may be potentiated when used with other sedative drugs or ethanol. Use with caution in patients with adrenal insufficiency, hypothyroidism or prostatic hyperplasia/urinary stricture.

Serotonin syndrome (SS) may occur with serotonin/norepinephrine reuptake inhibitors (SNRIs), including tapentadol. Signs of SS may include agitation, tachycardia, hyperthermia, nausea, and vomiting. Avoid use with serotonergic agents such as TCAs, triptans, venlafaxine, trazodone, lithium, sibutramine, meperidine, dextromethorphan, St John's wort, SNRIs, and SSRIs; concomitant use has been associated with the development of serotonin syndrome. Contraindicated with MAO inhibitor use within 14 days.

Use caution in patients with biliary tract dysfunction or acute pancreatitis; opioids may cause spasm of the sphincter of Oddi. Opioid use may obscure diagnosis or clinical course of patients with acute abdominal conditions. Use with extreme caution in patients with head injury, intracranial lesions, or elevated intracranial pressure (ICP); exaggerated elevation of ICP may occur. Serum concentrations are increased in hepatic impairment; use with caution in patients with moderate hepatic impairment (dosage adjustment required). Not recommended for use in severe hepatic impairment (not studied). Use with caution in patients with mild-to-moderate renal impairment (no dosage adjustment recommended). Not recommended for use in severe renal impairment (not studied). Use caution in patients with a history of seizures or conditions predisposing patients to seizures; patients with a history of seizures were excluded in clinical trials of tapentadol. Tramadol, an analgesic with similar pharmacologic properties to tapentadol, has been associated with seizures, particularly in patients with predisposing factors.

Prolonged use increases risk of abuse, addiction, and withdrawal symptoms. An opioid-containing regimen should be tailored to each patient's needs with respect to degree of tolerance for opioids (naïve versus chronic user), age, weight, and medical condition. Healthcare provider should be alert to problems of abuse, misuse, and diversion. Abrupt discontinuation may lead to withdrawal symptoms. Symptoms may be decreased by tapering prior to discontinuation. Use opioids with caution in elderly; consider decreasing initial dose. Use caution in debilitated patients; there is a greater potential for critical respiratory depression, even at therapeutic dosages.

◀ During dosage adjustments, the Canadian labeling recommends that immediate release tramadol may be used as rescue medication (maximum dose: 400 mg/day) and that fentanyl should not be used as rescue medication.

Adverse Reactions (Reflective of adult population; not specific for elderly)

Immediate release;

>10%:

Central nervous system: Dizziness (24%), somnolence (15%)

Gastrointestinal: Nausea (30%), vomiting (18%), constipation (8%)

≤1% to 10%:

Central nervous system: Fatigue (3%), insomnia (2%), anxiety (1%), confusion (1%), dreams abnormal (1%), lethargy (1%), attention disturbances (<1%), headache (<1%)

Dermatologic: Pruritus (3% to 5%), hyperhidrosis (3%), rash (1%)

Endocrine & metabolic: Hot flushes (1%)

Gastrointestinal: Xerostomia (4%), appetite decreased (2%), dyspepsia (2%)

Genitourinary: Urinary tract infection (1%)

Neuromuscular & skeletal: Arthralgia (1%), tremor (1%)

Respiratory: Nasopharyngitis (1%), upper respiratory tract infection (1%), dyspnea (<1%)

Extended release:

>10%:

Central nervous system: Dizziness (17%), headache (15%), somnolence (12%)

Gastrointestinal: Nausea (21%), constipation (17%), vomiting (8%)

1% to 10%:

Central nervous system: Fatigue (9%), insomnia (4%), anxiety (2%), lethargy (2%), vertigo (2%), attention disturbances (1%), chills (1%), depression/depressed mood (1%)

Dermatologic: Hyperhidrosis (5%), pruritus (5%), rash (1%)

Endocrine & metabolic: Hot flushes (2%)

Gastrointestinal: Xerostomia (7%), dyspepsia (3%), appetite decreased (2%)

Genitourinary: Erectile dysfunction (1%)

Neuromuscular & skeletal: Weakness (2%), tremor (1%)

Ocular: Vision blurred (1%)

Respiratory: Dyspnea (1%)

Drug Interactions

Avoid Concomitant Use

Avoid concomitant use of Tapentadol with any of the following: MAO Inhibitors; Sibutramine

Increased Effect/Toxicity

Tapentadol may increase the levels/effects of: Alcohol (Ethyl); Alvimopan; CNS Depressants; Desmopressin; MAO Inhibitors; Selective Serotonin Reuptake Inhibitors; Serotonin Modulators; Thiazide Diuretics

The levels/effects of Tapentadol may be increased by: Amphetamines; Antipsychotic Agents (Phenothiazines); Droperidol; HydrOXYzine; Sibutramine; Succinylcholine

Decreased Effect

Tapentadol may decrease the levels/effects of: Pegvisomant

The levels/effects of Tapentadol may be decreased by: Ammonium Chloride; Mixed Agonist / Antagonist Opioids; Peginterferon Alfa-2b

Ethanol/Nutrition/Herb Interactions

Ethanol: May increase CNS depression; monitor for increased effects with coadministration. Caution patients about effects. Bioavailability of extended release tablets may be increased by alcohol; combined use should be avoided.

Food: When administered after a high fat/calorie meal, the AUC and C_{max} increased by 25% and 16%, respectively; may administer without regard to meals.

Herb/Nutraceutical: Avoid St John's wort (may increase CNS depression and risk of serotonin syndrome).

Stability Store at room temperature up to 25°C (77°F); excursions permitted to 15°C to 30°C (59°F to 86°F). Protect from moisture.

Mechanism of Action Binds to μ-opiate receptors in the CNS causing inhibition of ascending pain pathways, altering the perception of and response to pain; also inhibits the reuptake of norepinephrine, which also modifies the ascending pain pathway

Pharmacodynamics/Kinetics

Absorption: Rapid and complete

Distribution: V_d: I.V.: 442-638 L

Protein binding: ~20%

Metabolism: Extensive metabolism, including first pass metabolism; metabolized primarily via phase 2 glucuronidation to glucuronides (major metabolite: tapentadol-O-glucuronide); minimal phase 1 oxidative metabolism; also metabolized to a lesser degree by CYP2C9, CYP2C19, and CYP2D6; all metabolites pharmacologically inactive

Bioavailability: ~32%

Half-life elimination: Immediate release: ~4 hours; Long acting formulations: ~5-6 hours

Time to peak, plasma: Immediate release: 1.25 hours; Long acting formulations: 3-6 hours

Excretion: Urine (99%: 70% conjugated metabolites; 3% unchanged drug)

Dosage

Geriatric Initial: Consider initiating at lower range of dosing. Refer to adult dosing.

Adult Dose and dosage intervals should be individualized according to pain severity with respect to patient's previous experience with similar opioid analgesics. To reduce the risk of withdrawal symptoms, it is recommended to taper the dose when discontinuing therapy.

Acute moderate-severe pain: Oral: *U.S. labeling (immediate release):* Day 1: 50-100 mg every 4-6 hours as needed; may administer a second dose ≥1 hour after the initial dose (maximum dose on first day: 700 mg/day); Day 2 and subsequent dosing: 50-100 mg every 4-6 hours as needed (maximum: 600 mg/day)

Chronic moderate-severe pain: Oral:

U.S. labeling (extended release):

Opioid naive: Initial: 50 mg twice daily (recommended interval: ~12 hours); titrate in increments of 50 mg no more frequently than twice daily every 3 days to effective dose (therapeutic range: 100-250 mg twice daily) (maximum dose: 500 mg/day)

Opioid experienced: Initial: 50 mg titrated to an effective dose; titrate in increments of 50 mg no more frequently than twice daily every 3 days (therapeutic range: 100-250 mg twice daily) (maximum dose: 500 mg/day). **Note:** No adequate data on converting patients from other opioids to tapentadol extended release.

Conversion from Nucynta® immediate release to extended release: Convert using same total daily dose but divide into two equal doses and administer twice daily (recommended interval: ~12 hours) (maximum dose: 500 mg/day).

Canadian labeling (controlled release):

Opioid naive: Initial: 50 mg twice daily (recommended interval: ~12 hours); titrate to effective dose (therapeutic range: 100-250 mg twice daily)

Opioid experienced (**Note:** Decrease initial dose by 50% when switching from other opioid analgesics): Titrate in increments of 50 mg twice daily every 3 days to recommended dosing range of 100-250 mg twice daily (maximum dose should not exceed 500 mg/day)

Renal Impairment

Mild-moderate renal impairment: No adjustment necessary.

Severe renal impairment: Not recommended (not studied); use is contraindicated in the Canadian labeling.

Hepatic Impairment

Mild hepatic impairment: No adjustment necessary.

Moderate hepatic impairment:

U.S. labeling:

Immediate release: Initial: 50 mg every 8 hours or longer (maximum: 3 doses/24 hours). Further treatment for maintenance of analgesia may be achieved by either shortening or lengthening the dosing interval.

Extended release: Initial: 50 mg every 24 hours; maximum: 100 mg once daily

Canadian labeling (controlled release): Initial: 50 mg every 24 hours; titrate dose cautiously; manufacturer labeling does not provide specific recommendations.

Severe hepatic impairment: Not recommended (not studied); use is contraindicated in the Canadian labeling.

Administration Administer orally with or without food. Long acting formulations must be swallowed whole and should **not** be split, crushed, broken, chewed, or dissolved.

Special Geriatric Considerations In clinical studies, patients ≥65 years had a higher incidence of constipation as compared to younger patients. See Dosage: Geriatric.

Controlled Substance C-II

Dosage Forms Excipient information presented when available (limited, particularly for generics); consult specific product labeling.

Tablet, oral:

Nucynta®: 50 mg, 75 mg, 100 mg

Tablet, extended release, oral:

Nucynta® ER: 50 mg, 100 mg, 150 mg, 200 mg, 250 mg

Dosage Forms: Canada Excipient information presented when available (limited, particularly for generics); consult specific product labeling.

Tablet, controlled release, oral, as hydrochloride:

Nucynta™ CR: 50 mg, 100 mg, 150 mg, 200 mg, 250 mg

Selected References

Hartrick C, Van Hove I, Stegmann JU, et al, "Efficacy and Tolerability of Tapentadol Immediate Release and Oxycodone HCl Immediate Release in Patients Awaiting Primary Joint Replacement Surgery for End-Stage Joint Disease: A 10-Day, Phase III, Randomized, Double-Blind, Active- and Placebo-Controlled Study," *Clin Ther*, 2009, 31(2):260-71.

Kleinert R, Lange C, Steup A, et al, "Single Dose Analgesic Efficacy of Tapentadol in Postsurgical Dental Pain: The Results of a Randomized, Double-Blind, Placebo-Controlled Study," *Anesth Analg*, 2008, 107(6):2048-55.

Tegaserod (teg a SER od)

Brand Names: U.S. Zelnorm®
Brand Names: Canada Zelnorm® [DSC]
Index Terms HTF919; Tegaserod Maleate
Generic Availability (U.S.) No
Pharmacologic Category Serotonin 5-HT$_4$ Receptor Agonist
Use Emergency treatment of irritable bowel syndrome with constipation (IBS-C) and chronic idiopathic constipation (CIC) in women (<55 years of age) in which no alternative therapy exists
Prescribing and Access Restrictions Available in U.S. under an emergency investigational new drug (IND) process. Emergency situations are defined as immediately life-threatening or requiring hospitalization. Physicians with patients who may qualify can contact the FDA's Division of Drug Information via email (druginfo@fda.hhs.gov). The FDA may either deny the request or authorize shipment of Zelnorm® by Novartis. Additional information can be found at http://www.fda.gov/Drugs/DrugSafety/PostmarketDrugSafetyInformationforPatientsandProviders/ucm103223.htm.
Contraindications Per product labeling: Hypersensitivity to tegaserod or any component of the formulation; severe renal impairment; moderate or severe hepatic impairment; history of bowel obstruction, symptomatic gallbladder disease, suspected sphincter of Oddi dysfunction, or abdominal adhesions. Treatment should not be started in patients with diarrhea or in those who experience diarrhea frequently.

Exclusion criteria under the emergency-IND process: Unstable angina, history of MI or stroke, hypertension, hyperlipidemia, diabetes, age ≥55 years, smoking, obesity, depression, anxiety, or suicidal ideation.
Warnings/Precautions Serious cardiovascular events (eg, MI, stroke, unstable angina) may occur; patients should seek emergency care following any sign and symptom suggestive of a serious cardiac event. Use under the emergency IND process will not be permitted in patients with unstable angina, a history of MI or stroke, cigarette smoking, hypertension, hyperlipidemia, obesity, or diabetes. In addition, use will not be permitted in patients with depression, anxiety, or with any signs of suicidal ideation or behavior. Use has been associated with rare intestinal ischemic events. Discontinue immediately with new or sudden worsening abdominal pain or rectal bleeding. Diarrhea may occur after the start of treatment, most cases reported as a single episode within the first week of therapy, and may resolve with continued dosing. However, serious consequences of diarrhea (hypovolemia, syncope) have been reported. Patients should be warned to contact healthcare provider immediately if they develop severe diarrhea, or diarrhea with severe cramping, abdominal pain, or dizziness. Use caution with mild hepatic impairment; not recommended with moderate or severe impairment.

Potential benefits should be weighed against potential risks in patients eligible for emergency-IND use. Safety and efficacy have not been established in males with IBS. Use in elderly women (≥55 years of age) is contraindicated.

Adverse Reactions (Reflective of adult population; not specific for elderly)
>10%:
  Central nervous system: Headache (15%)
  Gastrointestinal: Abdominal pain (12%)
1% to 10%:
  Central nervous system: Dizziness (4%), migraine (2%)
  Gastrointestinal: Diarrhea (9%; severe <1%), nausea (8%), flatulence (6%)
  Neuromuscular & skeletal: Back pain (5%), arthropathy (2%), leg pain (1%)

Drug Interactions
  Avoid Concomitant Use There are no known interactions where it is recommended to avoid concomitant use.
  Increased Effect/Toxicity There are no known significant interactions involving an increase in effect.
  Decreased Effect There are no known significant interactions involving a decrease in effect.

Ethanol/Nutrition/Herb Interactions Food: Bioavailability is decreased by 40% to 65% and C_{max} is decreased by 20% to 40% when taken with food. T_{max} is prolonged from 1 hour up to 2 hours when taken following a meal, but decreased to 0.7 hours when taken 30 minutes before a meal.

Stability Store at controlled room temperature of 15°C to 30°C (59°F to 86°F). Protect from moisture.

Mechanism of Action Tegaserod is a partial neuronal 5-HT$_4$ receptor agonist. Its action at the receptor site leads to stimulation of the peristaltic reflex and intestinal secretion, and moderation of visceral sensitivity.

Pharmacodynamics/Kinetics
  Distribution: V_d: 368 ± 223 L
  Protein binding: 98% primarily to α_1-acid glycoprotein
  Metabolism: GI: Hydrolysis in the stomach; Hepatic: Oxidation, conjugation, and glucuronidation; metabolite (negligible activity); significant first-pass effect
  Bioavailability: Fasting: 10%
  Half-life elimination: I.V.: 11 ± 5 hours
  Time to peak: 1 hour
  Excretion: Feces (~66% as unchanged drug); urine (~33% as metabolites)

Dosage
  Geriatric Use in elderly women (≥55 years of age) is contraindicated.
  Adult
    IBS with constipation: Females <55 years of age: Oral: 6 mg twice daily, before meals, for 4-6 weeks; may consider continuing treatment for an additional 4-6 weeks in patients who respond initially
    Chronic idiopathic constipation: Females <55 years of age: Oral: 6 mg twice daily, before meals; the need for continued therapy should be reassessed periodically
  Renal Impairment C_{max} and AUC of the inactive metabolite are increased with renal impairment.
    Mild-to-moderate impairment: No dosage adjustment recommended
    Severe impairment: Use is contraindicated
  Hepatic Impairment C_{max} and AUC of tegaserod are increased with hepatic impairment.
    Mild impairment: No dosage adjustment recommended; however, use caution
    Moderate-to-severe impairment: Use is contraindicated

Administration Administer 30 minutes before meals.

Special Geriatric Considerations Use in elderly women (≥55 years of age) is contraindicated.

Dosage Forms Excipient information presented when available (limited, particularly for generics); consult specific product labeling.
  Tablet, oral:
    Zelnorm®: 2 mg, 6 mg

Telavancin (tel a VAN sin)

Medication Safety Issues
Sound-alike/look-alike issues:
Telavancin may be confused with telithromycin
Vibativ™ may be confused with Viactiv®, Vibramycin®, vigabatrin
Brand Names: U.S. Vibativ™
Index Terms TD-6424; Telavancin Hydrochloride
Generic Availability (U.S.) No
Pharmacologic Category Glycopeptide
Use Treatment of complicated skin and skin structure infections caused by susceptible gram-positive organisms including methicillin-susceptible or -resistant *Staphylococcus aureus*, vancomycin-susceptible *Enterococcus faecalis*, and *Streptococcus pyogenes*, *Streptococcus agalactiae*, or *Streptococcus anginosus* group
Medication Guide Available Yes
Contraindications There are no contraindications listed within the manufacturers labeling.
Warnings/Precautions May prolong QT$_c$ interval; avoid use in patients with a history of QT$_c$ prolongation, uncompensated heart failure, severe left ventricular hypertrophy, or concurrent administration of other medications known to prolong the QT interval (including Class Ia and Class III antiarrhythmics, cisapride, erythromycin, antipsychotics, and tricyclic antidepressants). Clinical studies indicate mean maximal QT$_c$ prolongation of 12-15 msec at the end of 10 mg/kg infusion. Use with caution in patients with renal impairment or those receiving other nephrotoxic drugs; dosage modification required and efficacy may be reduced in patients with Cl$_{cr}$ ≤50 mL/minute. May cause nephrotoxicity; usual risk factors include pre-existing renal impairment, concomitant nephrotoxic medications, advanced age, and dehydration. Monitor renal function prior to, during, and following therapy. Contains solubilizer cyclodextrin (hydroxypropyl-beta-cyclodextrin) which may accumulate in patients with renal dysfunction. Prolonged use may result in fungal or bacterial superinfection, including *C. difficile*-associated diarrhea (CDAD) and pseudomembranous colitis; CDAD has been observed >2 months postantibiotic treatment.

May interfere with tests used to monitor coagulation (eg, prothrombin time, INR, activated partial thromboplastin time, activated clotting time, coagulation based factor Xa tests) when samples drawn ≤18 hours after drug administration. Blood samples should be collected as close to the next dose of telavancin as possible. Rapid I.V. administration may result in flushing, rash, urticaria, and/or pruritus; slowing or stopping the infusion may alleviate these symptoms. In the elderly, lower doses are often required secondary to age-related decreases in renal function.

Adverse Reactions (Reflective of adult population; not specific for elderly)
>10%:
Central nervous system: Insomnia (13%), psychiatric disorder (12%), headache (11%)
Gastrointestinal: Metallic/soapy taste (33%), nausea (27%), vomiting (14%)
Genitourinary: Foamy urine (13%)
1% to 10%:
Central nervous system: Dizziness (6%)
Dermatologic: Pruritus (3% to 6%), rash (4%)
Endocrine & metabolic: Hypokalemia (7%)
Gastrointestinal: Diarrhea (7%), appetite decreased (3%), abdominal pain (2%)
Hematologic: Thrombocytopenia (7%)
Local: Infusion site pain (4%), infusion site erythema (3%)
Neuromuscular & skeletal: Paresthesia (5%), rigors (4%)
Renal: Serum creatinine increased (8%), microalbuminuria (7%)
Respiratory: Dyspnea (8%)

Drug Interactions
Avoid Concomitant Use
Avoid concomitant use of Telavancin with any of the following: Artemether; BCG; Dronedarone; Lumefantrine; Nilotinib; Pimozide; QUEtiapine; QuiNINE; Tetrabenazine; Thioridazine; Toremifene; Vandetanib; Vemurafenib; Ziprasidone

Increased Effect/Toxicity
Telavancin may increase the levels/effects of: Dronedarone; Pimozide; QTc-Prolonging Agents; QuiNINE; Tetrabenazine; Thioridazine; Toremifene; Vandetanib; Vemurafenib; Ziprasidone

The levels/effects of Telavancin may be increased by: Alfuzosin; Artemether; Chloroquine; Ciprofloxacin; Ciprofloxacin (Systemic); Gadobutrol; Lumefantrine; Nilotinib; QUEtiapine; QuiNINE

Decreased Effect
Telavancin may decrease the levels/effects of: BCG; Typhoid Vaccine

Stability Store at 2°C to 8°C (35°F to 46°F); excursions permitted up to 25°C (77°F); avoid excess heat. **Note:** Vials contain no bacteriostatic agent.
Reconstitute 250 mg vial with 15 mL of D_5W, NS, or SWFI to yield 15 mg/mL (total volume of ~17 mL). Reconstitute 750 mg vial with 45 mL of of D_5W, NS, or SWFI to yield 15 mg/mL (total volume of ~50 mL). Reconstitution may take 2-20 minutes. Discard vial if vacuum did not pull the diluent into the vial. Prior to administration, dilute dose in 100-250 mL D_5W, LR, or NS to a final concentration of 0.6-8 mg/mL.
Reconstituted solution in the vial or admixed in either D_5W, NS, or SWFI are stable at room temperature for 4 hours or under refrigeration for 72 hours. Total time in vial **plus** time in infusion bag should not exceed 4 hours at room temperature or 72 hours if refrigerated at 2°C to 8°C (35°F to 46°F).

Mechanism of Action Exerts concentration-dependent bactericidal activity; inhibits bacterial cell wall synthesis by blocking polymerization and cross-linking of peptidoglycan by binding to D-Ala-D-Ala portion of cell wall. Unlike vancomycin, additional mechanism involves disruption of membrane potential and changes cell permeability due to presence of lipophilic side chain moiety.

Pharmacodynamics/Kinetics
Distribution: V_{ss}: 0.13 L/kg
Protein binding: ~90%; primarily to albumin
Half-life elimination: 6.6-9.6 hours
Excretion: Urine (~76%); feces (<1%)

Dosage

Geriatric & Adult Complicated skin and skin structure Infection: I.V.: 10 mg/kg every 24 hours for 1-2 weeks

Renal Impairment *Note: Renal function may be estimated using the Cockcroft-Gault formula for dosage adjustment purposes.*
Cl_{cr} 30-50 mL/minute: 7.5 mg/kg every 24 hours.
Cl_{cr} 10 to <30 mL/minute: 10 mg/kg every 48 hours.
Cl_{cr} <10 mL/minute and hemodialysis patients: Dosage adjustment recommendations are not available; use caution or avoid.

Hepatic Impairment
Mild-to-moderate hepatic impairment: no dosage adjustment necessary.
Severe hepatic impairment: Has not been evaluated.

Administration Administer I.V. over 60 minutes. Other medications should not be infused simultaneously through the same I.V. line. When the same intravenous line is used for sequential infusion of other medications, flush line with D_5W, LR, or NS before and after infusing telavancin.
Red-man syndrome may occur if the infusion is too rapid. It is not an allergic reaction, but may be characterized by hypotension and/or a maculopapular rash appearing on the face, neck, trunk, and/or upper extremities. If this should occur, discontinuing or slowing the infusion rate may eliminate these reactions.

Monitoring Parameters Renal function

Test Interactions Interferes with the following coagulation assessments (causes artificially increased clotting times): PT, INR, aPTT, ACT, Xa; interferes with urine protein via qualitative dipstick and quantitative dye methods

Special Geriatric Considerations Of the more than 900 patients treated with telavancin in clinical trials to treat complicated skin and skin-structure infections, 18.7% were ≥65 years of age and 9.4% were ≥75 years of age. The results of subgroup, post-hoc analyses found lower cure rates with telavancin in patients ≥65 years compared to those <65 years of age, 72.1% vs 86.6%, respectively. Lower cure rates were also noted in patients with a Cl_{cr} ≤50 mL/minute. The frequency of adverse events in patients ≥65 years of age was 75% compared to 83% in patients >65 years of age. Renal adverse events were reported in 8.6% of patients ≥65 years and 1.9% of patients <65 years. Common comorbidities in these patients include pre-existing kidney disease, diabetes mellitus, heart failure or hypertension. Concomitant medications that affect kidney function were commonly used, such as NSAIDs, ACE inhibitors, and loop diuretics.

Dosage Forms Excipient information presented when available (limited, particularly for generics); consult specific product labeling.
Injection, powder for reconstitution:
Vibativ™: 250 mg, 750 mg [contains cyclodextrin]

Selected References
Stryjewski ME, Chu VH, O'Riordan WD, et al, "Telavancin Versus Standard Therapy for Treatment of Complicated Skin and Skin-Structure Infections Caused by Gram-Positive Bacteria: Fast 2 Study," *Antimicrob Agents Chemother*, 2006, 50(3):862-7.
Stryjewski ME, Graham DR, Wilson SE, et al, "Telavancin Versus Vancomycin for the Treatment of Complicated Skin and Skin-Structure Infections Caused by Gram-Positive Organisms," *Clin Infect Dis*, 2008, 46(11):1683-93.

TELAVANCIN

Stryjewski ME, O'Riordan WD, Lau WK, et al, "Telavancin Versus Standard Therapy for Treatment of Complicated Skin and Soft-Tissue Infections Due to Gram-Positive Bacteria," *Clin Infect Dis*, 2005, 40(11):1601-7.

Wilson SE, O'Riordan W, Hopkins A, et al, "Telavancin Versus Vancomycin for the Treatment of Complicated Skin and Skin-Structure Infections Associated With Surgical Procedures," *Am J Surg*, 2009, 197(6):791-6.

◆ **Telavancin Hydrochloride** *see* Telavancin *on page 1742*

Telbivudine (tel BI vyoo deen)

Brand Names: U.S. Tyzeka®
Brand Names: Canada Sebivo®
Index Terms L-Deoxythymidine; LdT
Generic Availability (U.S.) No
Pharmacologic Category Antiretroviral Agent, Reverse Transcriptase Inhibitor (Nucleoside)
Use Treatment of chronic hepatitis B with evidence of viral replication and either persistent transaminase elevations or histologically-active disease
Medication Guide Available Yes
Contraindications There are no contraindications in the manufacturers labeling.
Warnings/Precautions [U.S. Boxed Warnings]: Cases of lactic acidosis and severe hepatomegaly with steatosis, some fatal, have been reported with the use of nucleoside analogues. Severe, acute exacerbation of hepatitis B may occur upon discontinuation. Monitor liver function several months after stopping treatment; reinitiation of antihepatitis B therapy may be required. Myopathy (eg, unexplained muscle aches and/or muscle weakness in conjunction with increases serum creatine kinase) has been reported with telbivudine initiation after several weeks to months; therapy should be interrupted if myopathy suspected and discontinued if diagnosed. Patients taking concomitant medications associated with myopathy should be monitored closely. Concomitant use with peginterferon alfa-2a has been associated with an increased risk of peripheral neuropathy; interrupt therapy for suspected peripheral neuropathy and discontinue if confirmed. Use caution in patients with renal impairment or patients receiving concomitant therapy which may reduce renal function; dosage adjustment required (Cl$_{cr}$ <50 mL/minute). Monitor renal function before and during treatment in liver transplant patients receiving concurrent therapy of cyclosporine or tacrolimus; telbivudine may need to be adjusted. Safety and efficacy in liver transplant patients have not been established.

Not recommended as first-line therapy of chronic HBV due to high rate of resistance; use may be appropriate in short-term treatment of acute HBV (Lok, 2009). Cross-resistance among other antivirals for hepatitis B may occur; use caution in patients failing previous therapy with lamivudine. Telbivudine does not exhibit any clinically-relevant activity against human immunodeficiency virus (HIV type 1). Safety and efficacy have not been studied in patients coinfected with HIV, hepatitis C virus (HCV), or hepatitis D virus (HDV).

Adverse Reactions (Reflective of adult population; not specific for elderly)
>10%:
  Central nervous system: Fatigue (13%), headache (10%)
  Neuromuscular & skeletal: CPK increased (79%; grades 3/4: 13%)
1% to 10%:
  Central nervous system: Dizziness (4%), fever (4%), insomnia (3%)
  Dermatologic: Rash (4%), pruritus (2%)
  Endocrine & metabolic: Lipase increased (grades 3/4: 2%)
  Gastrointestinal: Abdominal pain (3% to 6%), diarrhea (6%), nausea (5%), abdominal distension (3%), dyspepsia (3%)
  Hematologic: Neutropenia (grades 3/4: 2%)
  Hepatic: ALT increased (grades 3/4: 5% to 7%), AST increased (grades 3/4: 6%)
  Neuromuscular & skeletal: Arthralgia (4%), back pain (4%), myalgia (3%)
  Respiratory: Cough (6%), pharyngolaryngeal pain (5%)
Drug Interactions
  Avoid Concomitant Use
    Avoid concomitant use of Telbivudine with any of the following: Interferon Alfa-2b; Peginterferon Alfa-2a; Peginterferon Alfa-2b
  Increased Effect/Toxicity
    The levels/effects of Telbivudine may be increased by: Interferon Alfa-2b; Peginterferon Alfa-2a; Peginterferon Alfa-2b
  Decreased Effect There are no known significant interactions involving a decrease in effect.
Ethanol/Nutrition/Herb Interactions
  Ethanol: Should be avoided in hepatitis B infection due to potential hepatic toxicity.
  Food: Does not have a significant effect on telbivudine absorption.
Stability Store at 25°C (77°F); excursions permitted to 15°C to 30°C (59°F to 86°F).

Mechanism of Action Telbivudine, a synthetic thymidine nucleoside analogue (L-enantiomer of thymidine), is intracellularly phosphorylated to the active triphosphate form, which competes with the natural substrate, thymidine 5'-triphosphate, to inhibit hepatitis B viral DNA polymerase; enzyme inhibition blocks reverse transcriptase activity thereby reducing viral DNA replication.

Pharmacodynamics/Kinetics

Distribution: V_d: > total body water

Protein binding: ~3%

Metabolism: No metabolites detected

Half-life elimination: Terminal: 40-49 hours

Time to peak, plasma: 1-4 hours

Excretion: Urine (as unchanged drug)

Dosage

Adult Chronic hepatitis B: Oral: 600 mg once daily.

Treatment duration (AASLD practice guidelines):

Hepatitis Be antigen (HBeAg) positive chronic hepatitis: Treat ≥1 year until HBeAg seroconversion and undetectable serum HBV DNA; continue therapy for ≥6 months after HBeAg seroconversion.

HBeAg negative chronic hepatitis: Treat >1 year until hepatitis B surface antigen (HBsAg) clearance.

Note: Patients achieving <2 log decrease in serum HBV DNA after at least 6 months of therapy should either receive additional treatment or be switched to an alternative therapy (Lok, 2009).

Renal Impairment

Cl_{cr} 30-49 mL/minute: 600 mg every 48 hours

Cl_{cr} <30 mL/minute (not requiring dialysis): 600 mg every 72 hours

End-stage renal disease: 600 mg every 96 hours

Hemodialysis: Administer after dialysis session

Hepatic Impairment No adjustment necessary.

Administration May be administered without regard to food.

Monitoring Parameters LFTs (eg, AST and ALT) periodically during therapy and for several months following discontinuation of therapy; renal function prior to initiation and periodically during treatment; signs and symptoms of peripheral neuropathy (eg, weakness, paresthesia, leg pain) or myopathy (eg, unexplained muscle pain, tenderness or weakness); serum creatine kinase; HBV DNA (every 3-6 months during therapy); HBeAg and anti-HBe signs/symptoms of HBV relapse/exacerbation after discontinuation of therapy.

Pharmacotherapy Pearls Telbivudine is the L-enantiomer of thymidine

Special Geriatric Considerations Insufficient clinical data in elderly to determine differences between aged patients and younger patients. Since elderly often have Cl_{cr} <50 mL/minute, dosage should be determined accordingly.

Product Availability Tyzeka® oral solution: FDA approved April 2009; anticipated availability is currently undetermined

Dosage Forms Excipient information presented when available (limited, particularly for generics); consult specific product labeling.

Tablet, oral:

Tyzeka®: 600 mg

Selected References

Lok AS and McMahon BJ, "Chronic Hepatitis B: Update 2009," *Hepatology*, 2009, 50(3):661-2.

◆ **Teldrin® HBP [OTC]** *see* Chlorpheniramine *on page 337*

Telithromycin (tel ith roe MYE sin)

Medication Safety Issues

Sound-alike/look-alike issues:

Telithromycin may be confused with telavancin

Brand Names: U.S. Ketek®

Brand Names: Canada Ketek®

Index Terms HMR 3647

Generic Availability (U.S.) No

Pharmacologic Category Antibiotic, Ketolide

Use Treatment of community-acquired pneumonia (mild-to-moderate) caused by susceptible strains of *Streptococcus pneumoniae* (including multidrug-resistant isolates), *Haemophilus influenzae*, *Chlamydophila pneumoniae*, *Moraxella catarrhalis*, and *Mycoplasma pneumoniae*

Medication Guide Available Yes

◀ **Contraindications** Hypersensitivity to telithromycin, macrolide antibiotics, or any component of the formulation; myasthenia gravis; history of hepatitis and/or jaundice associated with telithromycin or other macrolide antibiotic use; concurrent use of cisapride or pimozide

Warnings/Precautions Acute hepatic failure and severe liver injury, including hepatitis and hepatic necrosis (leading to some fatalities) have been reported, in some cases after only a few doses; if signs/symptoms of hepatitis or liver damage occur, discontinue therapy and initiate liver function tests. **[U.S. Boxed Warning]: Life-threatening (including fatal) respiratory failure has occurred in patients with myasthenia gravis;** use in these patients is contraindicated. May prolong QT_c interval, leading to a risk of ventricular arrhythmias; closely-related antibiotics have been associated with malignant ventricular arrhythmias and torsade de pointes. Avoid in patients with prolongation of QTc interval due to congenital causes, history of long QT syndrome, uncorrected electrolyte disturbances (hypokalemia or hypomagnesemia), significant bradycardia (<50 bpm), or concurrent therapy with QT_c-prolonging drugs (eg, class Ia and class III antiarrhythmics). Avoid use in patients with a prior history of confirmed cardiogenic syncope or ventricular arrhythmias while receiving macrolide antibiotics or other QT_c-prolonging drugs. May cause severe visual disturbances (eg, changes in accommodation ability, diplopia, blurred vision). May cause loss of consciousness (possibly vagal-related); caution patients that these events may interfere with ability to operate machinery or drive, and to use caution until effects are known. Use caution in renal impairment; severe impairment (Cl_{cr} <30 mL/minute) requires dosage adjustment. Pseudomembranous colitis has been reported.

Adverse Reactions (Reflective of adult population; not specific for elderly)

>10%: Gastrointestinal: Diarrhea (10% to 11%)

2% to 10%:

Central nervous system: Headache (2% to 6%), dizziness (3% to 4%)

Gastrointestinal: Nausea (7% to 8%), vomiting (2% to 3%), loose stools (2%), dysgeusia (2%)

≥0.2% to <2%:

Central nervous system: Fatigue, insomnia, somnolence, vertigo

Dermatologic: Rash

Gastrointestinal: Abdominal distension, abdominal pain, anorexia, constipation, dyspepsia, flatulence, gastritis, gastroenteritis, GI upset, glossitis, stomatitis, watery stools, xerostomia

Genitourinary: Vaginal candidiasis

Hematologic: Platelets increased

Hepatic: Transaminases increased

Ocular: Blurred vision, accommodation delayed, diplopia

Miscellaneous: Candidiasis, diaphoresis increased

Drug Interactions

Metabolism/Transport Effects Substrate of CYP1A2 (minor), 3A4 (major); **Inhibits** CYP2D6 (weak), 3A4 (strong)

Avoid Concomitant Use

Avoid concomitant use of Telithromycin with any of the following: Alfuzosin; Artemether; BCG; Cisapride; Conivaptan; Crizotinib; Disopyramide; Dronedarone; Eplerenone; Everolimus; Fluticasone (Oral Inhalation); Halofantrine; Lapatinib; Lovastatin; Lumefantrine; Lurasidone; Nilotinib; Nisoldipine; Pimozide; QUEtiapine; QuiNINE; Ranolazine; Rivaroxaban; RomiDEPsin; Salmeterol; Silodosin; Simvastatin; Tamsulosin; Terfenadine; Tetrabenazine; Thioridazine; Ticagrelor; Tolvaptan; Toremifene; Vandetanib; Vemurafenib; Ziprasidone

Increased Effect/Toxicity

Telithromycin may increase the levels/effects of: Alfentanil; Alfuzosin; Almotriptan; Alosetron; Antifungal Agents (Azole Derivatives, Systemic); Antineoplastic Agents (Vinca Alkaloids); Benzodiazepines (metabolized by oxidation); Bortezomib; Brentuximab Vedotin; Brinzolamide; Budesonide (Nasal); Budesonide (Systemic, Oral Inhalation); BusPIRone; Calcium Channel Blockers; CarBAMazepine; Cardiac Glycosides; Ciclesonide; Cilostazol; Cisapride; CloZAPine; Colchicine; Conivaptan; Corticosteroids (Orally Inhaled); Corticosteroids (Systemic); Crizotinib; CycloSPORINE; CycloSPORINE (Systemic); CYP3A4 Substrates; Dienogest; Disopyramide; Dronedarone; Dutasteride; Eletriptan; Eplerenone; Ergot Derivatives; Everolimus; FentaNYL; Fesoterodine; Fluticasone (Nasal); Fluticasone (Oral Inhalation); GuanFACINE; Halofantrine; HMG-CoA Reductase Inhibitors; Iloperidone; Ixabepilone; Lapatinib; Lovastatin; Lumefantrine; Lurasidone; Maraviroc; MethylPREDNISolone; Nilotinib; Nisoldipine; Paricalcitol; Pazopanib; Pimecrolimus; Pimozide; QTc-Prolonging Agents; QuiNIDine; QuiNINE; Ranolazine; Repaglinide; Rifamycin Derivatives; Rivaroxaban; RomiDEPsin; Salmeterol; Saxagliptin; Selective Serotonin Reuptake Inhibitors; Sildenafil; Silodosin; Simvastatin; Sirolimus; SORAfenib; Tacrolimus; Tacrolimus (Systemic); Tacrolimus (Topical); Tadalafil; Tamsulosin; Telaprevir; Temsirolimus; Terfenadine; Tetrabenazine; Thioridazine; Ticagrelor; Tolterodine; Tolvaptan; Toremifene; Vandetanib; Vardenafil; Vemurafenib; Verapamil; Vilazodone; Vitamin K Antagonists; Ziprasidone; Zopiclone

The levels/effects of Telithromycin may be increased by: Alfuzosin; Antifungal Agents (Azole Derivatives, Systemic); Artemether; Chloroquine; Ciprofloxacin; Ciprofloxacin (Systemic); CYP3A4 Inhibitors (Moderate); CYP3A4 Inhibitors (Strong); Gadobutrol; Lumefantrine; Nilotinib; QUEtiapine; QuiNINE; Telaprevir

Decreased Effect

Telithromycin may decrease the levels/effects of: BCG; Clopidogrel; Prasugrel; Ticagrelor; Typhoid Vaccine

The levels/effects of Telithromycin may be decreased by: CYP3A4 Inducers (Strong); Cyproterone; Deferasirox; Etravirine; Herbs (CYP3A4 Inducers); Tocilizumab

Ethanol/Nutrition/Herb Interactions Herb/nutraceutical: St John's wort: May decrease the levels/effects of telithromycin.

Stability Store at 15°C to 30°C (59°F to 86°F).

Mechanism of Action Inhibits bacterial protein synthesis by binding to two sites on the 50S ribosomal subunit. Telithromycin has also been demonstrated to alter secretion of IL-1alpha and TNF-alpha; the clinical significance of this immunomodulatory effect has not been evaluated.

Pharmacodynamics/Kinetics

Absorption: Rapid

Distribution: 2.9 L/kg

Protein binding: 60% to 70%; primarily to albumin

Metabolism: Hepatic, via CYP3A4 (50%) and non-CYP-mediated pathways

Bioavailability: 57% (significant first-pass metabolism)

Half-life elimination: 10 hours

Time to peak, plasma: 1 hour

Excretion: Urine (13% unchanged drug, remainder as metabolites); feces (7%)

Dosage

Geriatric & Adult

Community-acquired pneumonia: Oral: 800 mg once daily for 7-10 days

Renal Impairment

Cl_{cr} <30 mL/minute, including dialysis:

U.S. product labeling: 600 mg once daily; when renal impairment is accompanied by hepatic impairment, reduce dosage to 400 mg once daily

Canadian product labeling: Reduce dose to 400 mg once daily

Hemodialysis: Administer following dialysis

Hepatic Impairment No adjustment recommended, unless concurrent severe renal impairment is present.

Administration May be administered with or without food.

Monitoring Parameters Liver function tests; signs/symptoms of liver failure (eg, jaundice, fatigue, malaise, anorexia, nausea, bilirubinemia, acholic stools, liver tenderness, hepatomegaly); visual acuity

Special Geriatric Considerations Bioavailability (57%) equivalent in persons ≥65 years compared to younger adults; although a 1.4- to 2-fold increase in AUC found in older adults. No dosage adjustment required.

Dosage Forms Excipient information presented when available (limited, particularly for generics); consult specific product labeling.

Tablet, oral:

Ketek®: 300 mg, 400 mg

Dosage Forms: Canada Excipient information presented when available (limited, particularly for generics); consult specific product labeling.

Tablet:

Ketek®: 400 mg

Selected References

Perret C, Lenfant B, Weinling E, et al, "Pharmacokinetics and Absolute Oral Bioavailability of an 800-mg Oral Dose of Telithromycin in Healthy Young and Elderly Volunteers," *Chemotherapy*, 2002, 48(5):217-23.

Telmisartan (tel mi SAR tan)

Related Information

Angiotensin Agents *on page 1985*

Brand Names: U.S. Micardis®

Brand Names: Canada Micardis®

Generic Availability (U.S.) No

Pharmacologic Category Angiotensin II Receptor Blocker

Use Treatment of hypertension (may be used alone or in combination with other antihypertensive agents); cardiovascular risk reduction in patients ≥55 years of age unable to take ACE inhibitors and who are at high risk of major cardiovascular events (eg, MI, stroke, death)

◄ **Contraindications** There are no contraindications listed in manufacturer's labeling.

Canadian labeling: Hypersensitivity to telmisartan or any component of the formulation; fructose intolerance

Warnings/Precautions May cause hyperkalemia; avoid potassium supplementation unless specifically required by healthcare provider. Avoid use or use a smaller dose in patients who are volume depleted; correct depletion first. May be associated with deterioration of renal function and/or increases in serum creatinine, particularly in patients with low renal blood flow (eg, renal artery stenosis, heart failure) whose glomerular filtration rate (GFR) is dependent on efferent arteriolar vasoconstriction by angiotensin II. Use with caution in unstented unilateral/ bilateral renal artery stenosis. When unstented bilateral renal artery stenosis is present, use is generally avoided due to the elevated risk of deterioration in renal function unless possible benefits outweigh risks. Use with caution with pre-existing renal insufficiency; significant aortic/mitral stenosis. Concurrent use of ACE inhibitors may increase the risk of clinically-significant adverse events (eg, renal dysfunction, hyperkalemia). Concurrent use with ramipril is not recommended. Use with caution in patients who have biliary obstructive disorders or hepatic dysfunction. Product contains sorbitol. The Canadian labeling (not in U.S. labeling) contraindicates use in fructose intolerant patients.

Adverse Reactions (Reflective of adult population; not specific for elderly) May be associated with worsening of renal function in patients dependent on renin-angiotensin-aldosterone system.

1% to 10%:
Cardiovascular: Intermittent claudication (7%; placebo 6%), chest pain (≥1%), hypertension (≥1%), peripheral edema (≥1%)
Central nervous system: Dizziness (≥1%), fatigue (≥1%), headache (≥1%), pain (≥1%)
Dermatologic: Skin ulcer (3%; placebo 2%)
Gastrointestinal: Diarrhea (3%), abdominal pain (≥1%), dyspepsia (≥1%), nausea (≥1%)
Genitourinary: Urinary tract infection (≥1%)
Neuromuscular & skeletal: Back pain (3%), myalgia (≥1%)
Respiratory: Upper respiratory infection (7%), sinusitis (3%), cough (≥1%), pharyngitis (1%)

Drug Interactions

Metabolism/Transport Effects Inhibits CYP2C19 (weak)

Avoid Concomitant Use There are no known interactions where it is recommended to avoid concomitant use.

Increased Effect/Toxicity
Telmisartan may increase the levels/effects of: ACE Inhibitors; Amifostine; Antihypertensives; Cardiac Glycosides; Hypotensive Agents; Lithium; Nonsteroidal Anti-Inflammatory Agents; Potassium-Sparing Diuretics; Ramipril; RiTUXimab; Sodium Phosphates

The levels/effects of Telmisartan may be increased by: Alfuzosin; Diazoxide; Eplerenone; Herbs (Hypotensive Properties); MAO Inhibitors; Pentoxifylline; Phosphodiesterase 5 Inhibitors; Potassium Salts; Prostacyclin Analogues; Tolvaptan; Trimethoprim

Decreased Effect
The levels/effects of Telmisartan may be decreased by: Herbs (Hypertensive Properties); Methylphenidate; Nonsteroidal Anti-Inflammatory Agents; Yohimbine

Ethanol/Nutrition/Herb Interactions Herb/Nutraceutical: Avoid herbs with hypertensive properties (bayberry, blue cohosh, cayenne, ephedra, ginger, ginseng [American], kola, licorice); may diminish the antihypertensive effect of telmisartan. Avoid herbs with hypotensive properties (black cohosh, California poppy, coleus, golden seal, hawthorn, mistletoe, periwinkle, quinine, shepherd's purse); may enhance the hypotensive effect of telmisartan.

Stability Store at 25°C (77°F); excursions between 15°C to 30°C (59°F to 86°F) permitted. Protect from moisture and do not remove from blister pack until immediately before use.

Mechanism of Action Angiotensin II acts as a vasoconstrictor. In addition to causing direct vasoconstriction, angiotensin II also stimulates the release of aldosterone. Once aldosterone is released, sodium as well as water are reabsorbed. The end result is an elevation in blood pressure. Telmisartan is a nonpeptide AT1 angiotensin II receptor antagonist. This binding prevents angiotensin II from binding to the receptor thereby blocking the vasoconstriction and the aldosterone secreting effects of angiotensin II.

Pharmacodynamics/Kinetics Orally active, not a prodrug
Onset of action: 1-2 hours
Duration: Up to 24 hours
Distribution: V_d: 500 L
Protein binding: >99.5%; primarily to albumin and alpha$_1$-acid glycoprotein
Metabolism: Hepatic via conjugation to inactive metabolites; not metabolized via CYP
Bioavailability (dose dependent): 42% to 58%; Hepatic impairment: Approaches 100%
Half-life elimination: Terminal: 24 hours
Time to peak, plasma: 0.5-1 hours

Excretion: Feces (97%)
Clearance: Total body: 800 mL/minute
Dosage
Geriatric
Hypertension: Oral: Initial: 20 mg/day; usual maintenance dose range: 20-80 mg/day
Cardiovascular risk reduction: Oral: Initial 80 mg once daily
Adult
Hypertension: Oral: Initial: 40 mg once daily; usual maintenance dose range: 20-80 mg/day. Patients with volume depletion should be initiated on the lower dosage with close supervision.
Cardiovascular risk reduction: Oral: Initial: 80 mg once daily. **Note:** It is unknown whether doses <80 mg/day are associated with a reduction in risk of cardiovascular morbidity or mortality.
Renal Impairment No adjustment required; hemodialysis patients are more susceptible to orthostatic hypotension
Hepatic Impairment Initiate therapy with low dose; titrate slowly and monitor closely.
Canadian labeling: Recommended initial dose: 40 mg/day
Administration May be administered without regard to meals.
Monitoring Parameters Blood pressure; electrolytes, serum creatinine, BUN
Special Geriatric Considerations No initial dose adjustment is required. There appear to be no significant differences in response between the elderly and younger adults (limited data available). Monitor closely during initiation phase. Many elderly may be volume depleted due to diuretics and/or blunted thirst reflex resulting in inadequate fluid intake.
Dosage Forms Excipient information presented when available (limited, particularly for generics); consult specific product labeling.
Tablet, oral:
Micardis®: 20 mg
Micardis®: 40 mg, 80 mg [scored]
Selected References
The Telmisartan Randomised Assessment Study in ACE Intolerant Subjects with Cardiovascular Disease (TRAN-SCEND) Investigators, "Effects of the Angiotensin-Receptor Blocker Telmisartan on Cardiovascular Events in High-risk Patients Intolerant to Angiotensin-Converting Enzyme Inhibitors: A Randomized Controlled Trial," *Lancet*, 2008, 372(9644):1174-83.

Telmisartan and Amlodipine (tel mi SAR tan & am LOE di peen)

Related Information
AmLODIPine on page 106
Telmisartan on page 1747
Brand Names: U.S. Twynsta®
Index Terms Amlodipine and Telmisartan; Amlodipine Besylate and Telmisartan
Generic Availability (U.S.) No
Pharmacologic Category Angiotensin II Receptor Blocker; Calcium Channel Blocker; Calcium Channel Blocker, Dihydropyridine
Use Treatment of hypertension, including initial treatment in patients who will require multiple antihypertensives for adequate control
Dosage
Geriatric Initial therapy is not recommended in patients ≥75 years. Amlodipine therapy should be initiated at 2.5 mg once daily and slowly titrated up. The appropriate combination form is not available.
Adult Dose is individualized; combination product may be substituted for individual components in patients currently maintained on both agents separately or in patients not adequately controlled with monotherapy (using one of the agents or an agent within the same antihypertensive class). May also be used as initial therapy in patients who are likely to need >1 antihypertensive to control blood pressure.
Hypertension: Oral:
Initial therapy (antihypertensive naive): Telmisartan 40 mg/amlodipine 5 mg once daily; dose may be increased after 2 weeks of therapy. Patients requiring larger blood pressure reductions may be started on telmisartan 80 mg/amlodipine 5 mg once daily. Maximum recommended dose: Telmisartan 80 mg/day, amlodipine 10 mg/day
Add-on/replacement therapy: Telmisartan 40-80 mg and amlodipine 5-10 mg once daily depending upon previous doses, current control, and goals of therapy; dose may be titrated after 2 weeks of therapy. Maximum recommended dose: Telmisartan 80 mg/day; amlodipine 10 mg/day
Renal Impairment
Mild-to-moderate impairment: No adjustment necessary.
Severe impairment: Titrate slowly.

◀ **Hepatic Impairment** Initial therapy is not recommended. Initiate amlodipine therapy at 2.5 mg once daily and titrate slowly. The appropriate combination form is not available.

Special Geriatric Considerations See individual agents. Combination products are not recommended as first-line treatment. Use only if doses of individual agents correspond to the combination available.

Dosage Forms Excipient information presented when available (limited, particularly for generics); consult specific product labeling.

Tablet, oral:

Twynsta® 40/5: Telmisartan 40 mg and amlodipine 5 mg

Twynsta® 40/10: Telmisartan 40 mg and amlodipine 10 mg

Twynsta® 80/5: Telmisartan 80 mg and amlodipine 5 mg

Twynsta® 80/10: Telmisartan 80 mg and amlodipine 10 mg

Telmisartan and Hydrochlorothiazide
(tel mi SAR tan & hye droe klor oh THYE a zide)

Related Information
Hydrochlorothiazide on page 876

Telmisartan on page 1747

Brand Names: U.S. Micardis® HCT

Brand Names: Canada Micardis® Plus

Index Terms Hydrochlorothiazide and Telmisartan

Generic Availability (U.S.) No

Pharmacologic Category Angiotensin II Receptor Blocker; Diuretic, Thiazide

Use Treatment of hypertension; combination product should not be used for initial therapy

Dosage

Geriatric Refer to adult dosing. Monitor renal function.

Adult Hypertension: Oral: Replacement therapy: Combination product can be substituted for individual titrated agents. Initiation of combination therapy when monotherapy has failed to achieve desired effects:

Patients currently on telmisartan: Initial dose if blood pressure is not currently controlled on monotherapy of 80 mg telmisartan: Telmisartan 80 mg/hydrochlorothiazide 12.5 mg once daily; may titrate up to telmisartan 160 mg/hydrochlorothiazide 25 mg if needed.

Patients currently on hydrochlorothiazide: Initial dose if blood pressure is not currently controlled on monotherapy of 25 mg once daily: Telmisartan 80 mg/hydrochlorothiazide 12.5 mg once daily or telmisartan 80 mg/hydrochlorothiazide 25 mg once daily; may titrate up to telmisartan 160 mg/hydrochlorothiazide 25 mg if blood pressure remains uncontrolled after 2-4 weeks of therapy. Patients who develop hypokalemia while on hydrochlorothiazide 25 mg may be switched to telmisartan 80 mg/hydrochlorothiazide 12.5 mg.

Renal Impairment

Cl_{cr} >30 mL/minute: No dosage adjustment necessary.

Cl_{cr} ≤30 mL/minute: Not recommended.

Hepatic Impairment

Mild-to-moderate hepatic impairment or biliary obstructive disorders: Initial: Telmisartan 40 mg/hydrochlorothiazide 12.5 mg.

Severe hepatic impairment: Not recommended.

Special Geriatric Considerations No dosing adjustment is needed based on age. Monitor renal function. Combination products are not recommended as first-line treatment. Use only if doses of individual agents correspond to the combination available.

Dosage Forms Excipient information presented when available (limited, particularly for generics); consult specific product labeling.

Tablet, oral:

Micardis® HCT:

40/12.5: Telmisartan 40 mg and hydrochlorothiazide 12.5 mg

80/12.5: Telmisartan 80 mg and hydrochlorothiazide 12.5 mg

80/25: Telmisartan 80 mg and hydrochlorothiazide 25 mg

Dosage Forms: Canada Excipient information presented when available (limited, particularly for generics); consult specific product labeling.

Tablet, oral:

Micardis® Plus: 80/25: Telmisartan 80 mg and hydrochlorothiazide 25 mg

Temazepam (te MAZ e pam)

Related Information

Anxiolytic, Sedative / Hypnotic, and Miscellaneous Benzodiazepines *on page 2000*
Beers Criteria – Potentially Inappropriate Medications for Geriatrics *on page 2089*

Medication Safety Issues

Sound-alike/look-alike issues:

Temazepam may be confused with flurazepam, LORazepam, tamoxifen

Restoril™ may be confused with, RisperDAL®, Vistaril®, Zestril®

BEERS Criteria medication:

This drug may be inappropriate for use in geriatric patients (high severity risk).

Brand Names: U.S. Restoril™

Brand Names: Canada Apo-Temazepam®; CO Temazepam; Dom-Temazepam; Gen-Temazepam; Novo-Temazepam; Nu-Temazepam; PHL-Temazepam; PMS-Temazepam; ratio-Temazepam; Restoril™

Generic Availability (U.S.) Yes

Pharmacologic Category Hypnotic, Benzodiazepine

Use Short-term treatment of insomnia

Unlabeled/Investigational Use Treatment of anxiety

Medication Guide Available Yes

Contraindications Hypersensitivity to temazepam or any component of the formulation (cross-sensitivity with other benzodiazepines may exist); narrow-angle glaucoma (not in product labeling, however, benzodiazepines are contraindicated)

Warnings/Precautions As a hypnotic, should be used only after evaluation of potential causes of sleep disturbance. Failure of sleep disturbance to resolve after 7-10 days may indicate psychiatric or medical illness. A worsening of insomnia or the emergence of new abnormalities of thought or behavior may represent unrecognized psychiatric or medical illness and requires immediate and careful evaluation.

Use with caution in elderly or debilitated patients, patients with hepatic disease (including alcoholics), or renal impairment. Due to increased sensitivity in the elderly, smaller doses of benzodiazepines may be safer and as effective. Avoid using doses >15 mg daily of temazepam (Beers Criteria). Use with caution in patients with respiratory disease, or impaired gag reflex. Avoid use inpatients with sleep apnea.

Causes CNS depression (dose-related) resulting in sedation, dizziness, confusion, or ataxia which may impair physical and mental capabilities. Patients must be cautioned about performing tasks which require mental alertness (eg, operating machinery or driving). Use with caution in patients receiving other CNS depressants or psychoactive agents. Postmarketing studies have indicated that the use of hypnotic/sedative agents for sleep has been associated with hypersensitivity reactions including anaphylaxis as well as angioedema. An increased risk for hazardous sleep-related activities such as sleep-driving; cooking and eating food, and making phone calls while asleep have also been noted. Effects with other sedative drugs or ethanol may be potentiated. Benzodiazepines have been associated with falls and traumatic injury and should be used with extreme caution in patients who are at risk of these events (especially the elderly).

Use caution in patients with suicidal risk. Use with caution in patients with a history of drug dependence. Benzodiazepines have been associated with dependence and acute withdrawal symptoms on discontinuation or reduction in dose (may occur after as little as 10 days). Acute withdrawal, including seizures, may be precipitated after administration of flumazenil to patients receiving long-term benzodiazepine therapy.

Benzodiazepines have been associated with anterograde amnesia. Paradoxical reactions, including hyperactive or aggressive behavior, have been reported with benzodiazepines, particularly in psychiatric patients. Does not have analgesic, antidepressant, or antipsychotic properties.

Adverse Reactions (Reflective of adult population; not specific for elderly)

1% to 10%:

Central nervous system: Anxiety, confusion, dizziness, drowsiness, euphoria, fatigue, hangover, headache, lethargy, vertigo

Dermatologic: Rash

Endocrine & metabolic: Libido decreased

Gastrointestinal: Diarrhea

Neuromuscular & skeletal: Dysarthria, weakness

Ocular: Blurred vision

Miscellaneous: Diaphoresis

Drug Interactions

Metabolism/Transport Effects Substrate (minor) of CYP2B6, 2C9, 2C19, 3A4

Avoid Concomitant Use

Avoid concomitant use of Temazepam with any of the following: OLANZapine

Increased Effect/Toxicity

Temazepam may increase the levels/effects of: Alcohol (Ethyl); CloZAPine; CNS Depressants; Fosphenytoin; Methotrimeprazine; Phenytoin; Selective Serotonin Reuptake Inhibitors

The levels/effects of Temazepam may be increased by: Conivaptan; Droperidol; HydrOXYzine; Methotrimeprazine; OLANZapine

Decreased Effect

The levels/effects of Temazepam may be decreased by: Theophylline Derivatives; Tocilizumab; Yohimbine

Ethanol/Nutrition/Herb Interactions

Ethanol: May increase CNS depression; monitor for increased effects with coadministration. Caution patients about effects.

Food: Serum levels may be increased by grapefruit juice.

Herb/Nutraceutical: St John's wort may decrease temazepam levels. Avoid valerian, St John's wort, kava kava, gotu kola (may increase CNS depression).

Mechanism of Action Binds to stereospecific benzodiazepine receptors on the postsynaptic GABA neuron at several sites within the central nervous system, including the limbic system, reticular formation. Enhancement of the inhibitory effect of GABA on neuronal excitability results by increased neuronal membrane permeability to chloride ions. This shift in chloride ions results in hyperpolarization (a less excitable state) and stabilization.

Pharmacodynamics/Kinetics

Distribution: V_d: 1.4 L/kg

Protein binding: 96%

Metabolism: Hepatic

Half-life elimination: 9.5-12.4 hours

Time to peak, serum: 2-3 hours

Excretion: Urine (80% to 90% as inactive metabolites)

Dosage

Geriatric Initial: 7.5 mg in elderly or debilitated patients at bedtime

Adult Insomnia: Oral: Usual dose: 15-30 mg at bedtime; some patients may respond to 7.5 mg in transient insomnia

Monitoring Parameters Respiratory and cardiovascular status

Reference Range Therapeutic: 26 ng/mL after 24 hours

Pharmacotherapy Pearls Abrupt discontinuation after sustained use (generally >10 days) may cause withdrawal symptoms.

Special Geriatric Considerations Because of its lack of active metabolites, temazepam could be considered in the elderly when a benzodiazepine hypnotic is indicated. Hypnotic use should be limited to 10-14 days. If insomnia persists, the patient should be evaluated for etiology.

This medication is considered to be potentially inappropriate in this patient population (Beers Criteria severity: High).

Controlled Substance C-IV

Dosage Forms Excipient information presented when available (limited, particularly for generics); consult specific product labeling.

Capsule, oral: 7.5 mg, 15 mg, 22.5 mg, 30 mg

Restoril™: 7.5 mg, 15 mg, 22.5 mg, 30 mg

Selected References

Divoll M, Greenblatt DJ, Harmatz JS, et al, "Effect of Age and Gender on Disposition of Temazepam," *J Pharm Sci*, 1981, 70(10):1104-7.

Scharf MB, Berkowitz DV, and Brannen DE, "Effectiveness of Low-Dose Temazepam on Sleep Patterns in Geriatric Insomniac Subjects," *Consult Pharm*, 1993, 8(12):1367-73.

◆ **Temovate®** *see* Clobetasol *on page 380*

◆ **Temovate E®** *see* Clobetasol *on page 380*

◆ **Tenex®** *see* GuanFACINE *on page 851*

◆ **Tenormin®** *see* Atenolol *on page 160*

◆ **Terazol® 3** *see* Terconazole *on page 1759*

◆ **Terazol® 7** *see* Terconazole *on page 1759*

Terazosin (ter AY zoe sin)

Related Information

Beers Criteria – Potentially Inappropriate Medications for Geriatrics *on page 2089*

Pharmacotherapy of Urinary Incontinence *on page 2032*

Brand Names: Canada Apo-Terazosin®; Dom-Terazosin; Hytrin®; Nu-Terazosin; PHL-Terazosin; PMS-Terazosin; ratio-Terazosin; Teva-Terazosin

Index Terms Hytrin

Generic Availability (U.S.) Yes

Pharmacologic Category Alpha₁ Blocker

Use Management of mild-to-moderate hypertension; alone or in combination with other agents such as diuretics or beta-blockers; benign prostate hyperplasia (BPH)

Contraindications Hypersensitivity to terazosin or any component of the formulation

Warnings/Precautions Can cause significant orthostatic hypotension and syncope, especially with first dose; anticipate a similar effect if therapy is interrupted for a few days, if dosage is rapidly increased, or if another antihypertensive drug (particularly vasodilators) or a PDE-5 inhibitor is introduced. Discontinue if symptoms of angina occur or worsen. Patients should be cautioned about performing hazardous tasks when starting new therapy or adjusting dosage upward. Prostate cancer should be ruled out before starting for BPH. Intraoperative floppy iris syndrome has been observed in cataract surgery patients who were on or were previously treated with alpha₁-blockers. Causality has not been established and there appears to be no benefit in discontinuing alpha-blocker therapy prior to surgery. Priapism has been associated with use (rarely).

Adverse Reactions (Reflective of adult population; not specific for elderly)

>10%:

Central nervous system: Dizziness (9% to 19%)

Neuromuscular & skeletal: Muscle weakness (7% to 11%)

1% to 10%:

Cardiovascular: Peripheral edema (1% to 6%), orthostatic hypotension (1% to 4%), palpitation (≤4%), tachycardia (≤2%), syncope (≤1%)

Central nervous system: Somnolence (4% to 5%), vertigo (1%)

Gastrointestinal: Nausea (2% to 4%)

Genitourinary: Impotence (≤2%), libido decreased (≤1%)

Neuromuscular & skeletal: Extremity pain (≤4%), paresthesia (≤3%), back pain (≤2%)

Ocular: Blurred vision (≤2%)

Respiratory: Nasal congestion (2% to 6%), dyspnea (2% to 3%), sinusitis (≤3%)

Drug Interactions

Avoid Concomitant Use

Avoid concomitant use of Terazosin with any of the following: Alpha1-Blockers

Increased Effect/Toxicity

Terazosin may increase the levels/effects of: Alpha1-Blockers; Amifostine; Antihypertensives; Calcium Channel Blockers; Hypotensive Agents; RiTUXimab

The levels/effects of Terazosin may be increased by: Beta-Blockers; Diazoxide; Herbs (Hypotensive Properties); MAO Inhibitors; Pentoxifylline; Phosphodiesterase 5 Inhibitors; Prostacyclin Analogues

Decreased Effect

The levels/effects of Terazosin may be decreased by: Herbs (Hypertensive Properties); Methylphenidate; Yohimbine

Ethanol/Nutrition/Herb Interactions Herb/Nutraceutical: Avoid dong quai if using for hypertension (has estrogenic activity). Avoid ephedra, yohimbe, ginseng (may worsen hypertension). Avoid saw palmetto. Avoid garlic (may have increased antihypertensive effect).

Stability Store below 30°C (86°F).

Mechanism of Action Alpha₁-specific blocking agent with minimal alpha₂ effects; this allows peripheral postsynaptic blockade, with the resultant decrease in arterial tone, while preserving the negative feedback loop which is mediated by the peripheral presynaptic alpha₂-receptors; terazosin relaxes the smooth muscle of the bladder neck, thus reducing bladder outlet obstruction

Pharmacodynamics/Kinetics

Onset of action: 1-2 hours

Absorption: Rapid and complete

Protein binding: 90% to 95%

Metabolism: Hepatic; minimal first-pass

Half-life elimination: ~12 hours; half-life is not significantly prolonged in older adults

Time to peak, serum: ~1 hour

Excretion: Feces (~60%, ~20% as unchanged drug); urine (~40%, ~10% as unchanged drug)

◀ **Dosage**

Geriatric Refer to adult dosing. In the management of hypertension, consider lower initial doses (eg, immediate release: 0.5 mg once daily) and titrate to response (Aronow, 2011).

Adult Note: If drug is discontinued for greater than several days, consider beginning with initial dose and retitrate as needed.

Hypertension: Oral: Initial: 1 mg at bedtime; slowly increase dose to achieve desired blood pressure, up to 20 mg/day; usual dose range (JNC 7): 1-20 mg once daily. **Note:** Dosage may be given on a twice daily regimen if response is diminished at 24 hours and hypotension is observed at 2-4 hours following a dose.

Benign prostatic hyperplasia: Oral: Initial: 1 mg at bedtime; thereafter, titrate upwards, if needed, over several weeks, balancing therapeutic benefit with terazosin-induced postural hypotension; most patients require 10 mg day; if no response after 4-6 weeks of 10 mg/day, may increase to 20 mg/day

Dosage adjustment with concurrent medication:

Concurrent use with a diuretic or other antihypertensive agent (especially verapamil): Dosage reduction may be needed when adding

Concurrent use with PDE-5 inhibitors: Initiate PDE-5 inhibitor therapy at the lowest dose due to additive orthostatic and blood pressure lowering effects

Administration Administer without regard to meals at the same time each day.

Monitoring Parameters Standing and sitting/supine blood pressure, especially following the initial dose at 2-4 hours following the dose and thereafter at the trough point to ensure adequate control throughout the dosing interval; urinary symptoms

Pharmacotherapy Pearls Syncope may occur usually within 90 minutes of the initial dose; administer initial dose at bedtime.

Special Geriatric Considerations Adverse reactions such as orthostatic hypotension, dry mouth, and urinary problems can be particularly bothersome in the elderly.

Dosage Forms Excipient information presented when available (limited, particularly for generics); consult specific product labeling.

Capsule, oral: 1 mg, 2 mg, 5 mg, 10 mg

Terbinafine (Systemic) (TER bin a feen)

Medication Safety Issues

Sound-alike/look-alike issues:

Terbinafine may be confused with terbutaline

LamISIL® may be confused with LaMICtal®, Lomotil®

Brand Names: U.S. LamISIL®; Terbinex™

Brand Names: Canada Apo-Terbinafine®; Auro-Terbinafine; CO Terbinafine; Dom-Terbinafine; JAMP-Terbinafine; Lamisil®; Mylan-Terbinafine; Nu-Terbinafine; PHL-Terbinafine; PMS-Terbinafine; Riva-Terbinafine; Sandoz-Terbinafine; Teva-Terbinafine

Index Terms Terbinafine Hydrochloride

Generic Availability (U.S.) Yes: Tablet

Pharmacologic Category Antifungal Agent, Oral

Use Active against most strains of *Trichophyton mentagrophytes*, *Trichophyton rubrum*; may be effective for infections of *Microsporum gypseum* and *M. nanum*, *Trichophyton verrucosum*, *Epidermophyton floccosum*, *Candida albicans*, and *Scopulariopsis brevicaulis*

Onychomycosis of the toenail or fingernail due to susceptible dermatophytes; treatment of tinea capitis

Contraindications Hypersensitivity to terbinafine or any component of the formulation

Warnings/Precautions While rare, the following complications have been reported and may require discontinuation of therapy: Changes in the ocular lens and retina, pancytopenia, neutropenia, Stevens-Johnson syndrome, toxic epidermal necrolysis. Precipitation or exacerbation of cutaneous or systemic lupus erythematosus has been observed; discontinue if signs and/or symptoms develop. Rare cases of hepatic failure, including fatal cases, have been reported following treatment of onychomycosis. Not recommended for use in patients with active or chronic liver disease. Discontinue if symptoms or signs of hepatobiliary dysfunction or cholestatic hepatitis develop. Products are not recommended for use with pre-existing liver or renal disease (Cl_{cr} ≤50 mL/minute). Use caution in patients sensitive to allylamine antifungals (eg, naftifine, butenafine); cross sensitivity to terbinafine may exist.

Adverse Reactions (Reflective of adult population; not specific for elderly) Adverse events listed for tablets unless otherwise specified. Granules were studied in patients 4-12 years of age.

>10%: Central nervous system: Headache (13%; granules 7%)

1% to 10%:

Central nervous system: Fever (granules 7%)

Dermatologic: Rash (6%; granules 2%), pruritus (3%; granules 1%), urticaria (1%)

Gastrointestinal: Diarrhea (6%; granules 3%), vomiting (granules 5%), dyspepsia (4%), nausea (3%; granules 2%), taste disturbance (3%), abdominal pain (2%; granules 2% to 4%), toothache (granules 1%)

Hepatic: Liver enzyme abnormalities (3%)

Respiratory: Nasopharyngitis (granules 10%), cough (granules 6%), nasal congestion (granules 2%), pharyngeal pain (granules 2%), rhinorrhea (granules 2%)

Drug Interactions

Metabolism/Transport Effects Substrate (minor) of 1A2, 2C9, 2C19, 3A4; **Inhibits** CYP2D6 (strong); **Induces** CYP3A4 (weak)

Avoid Concomitant Use

Avoid concomitant use of Terbinafine (Systemic) with any of the following: Tamoxifen; Thioridazine

Increased Effect/Toxicity

Terbinafine (Systemic) may increase the levels/effects of: Atomoxetine; CYP2D6 Substrates; Fesoterodine; Iloperidone; Nebivolol; Tamoxifen; Tetrabenazine; Thioridazine; Tricyclic Antidepressants

The levels/effects of Terbinafine (Systemic) may be increased by: Conivaptan

Decreased Effect

Terbinafine (Systemic) may decrease the levels/effects of: Codeine; CycloSPORINE; Iloperidone; Saccharomyces boulardii; Saxagliptin; TraMADol

The levels/effects of Terbinafine (Systemic) may be decreased by: Cyproterone; Rifamycin Derivatives; Tocilizumab

Stability

Granules: Store at controlled room temperature of 15°C to 30°C (59°F to 86°F).

Tablet: Store below 25°C (77°F). Protect from light.

Mechanism of Action Synthetic allylamine derivative which inhibits squalene epoxidase, a key enzyme in sterol biosynthesis in fungi. This results in a deficiency in ergosterol within the fungal cell wall and results in fungal cell death.

Pharmacodynamics/Kinetics

Absorption: >70%

Distribution: V_d: 1000 L; distributed to sebum and skin predominantly

Protein binding: Plasma: >99%

Metabolism: Hepatic; no active metabolites; first-pass effect; little effect on CYP

Bioavailability: 40%

Half-life elimination: Terminal half-life: 200-400 hours; very slow release of drug from skin and adipose tissues occurs; effective half-life: ~36 hours

Time to peak, plasma: 1-2 hours

Excretion: Urine (70% to 75%)

Dosage

Geriatric & Adult

Superficial mycoses (onychomycosis): Oral:

Fingernail: 250 mg daily for up to 6 weeks; may be given in 2 divided doses

Toenail: 250 mg daily for 12 weeks; may be given in 2 divided doses

Systemic mycosis (unlabeled use): Oral: 250-500 mg/day for up to 16 months

Renal Impairment Cl_{cr} <50 mL/minute: Oral administration is not recommended; clearance is decreased by ~50%.

Hepatic Impairment Hepatic cirrhosis: Oral administration is not recommended; clearance is decreased by ~50%.

Administration Tablets may be administered without regard to meals. Granules should be sprinkled on a spoonful of nonacidic food (eg, mashed potatoes); swallow granules without chewing.

Monitoring Parameters AST/ALT prior to initiation, repeat if used >6 weeks; CBC

Pharmacotherapy Pearls Due to potential toxicity, the manufacturer recommends confirmation of diagnosis testing of nail specimens prior to treatment of onychomycosis. Patients should not be considered therapeutic failures until they have been symptom-free for 2-4 weeks off following a course of treatment; GI complaints usually subside with continued administration.

A meta-analysis of efficacy studies for toenail infections revealed that weighted average mycological cure rates for continuous therapy were 36.7% (griseofulvin), 54.7% (itraconazole), and 77% (terbinafine). Cure rate for 4-month pulse therapy for itraconazole and terbinafine were 73.3% and 80%. Additionally, the final outcome measure of final costs per cured infections for continuous therapy was significantly lower for terbinafine.

◀ **Special Geriatric Considerations** No specific information on use in the elderly is available; however, since many elderly will have creatinine clearances <50 mL/minute, this drug is not a drug of choice for elderly with onychomycosis.

Dosage Forms Excipient information presented when available (limited, particularly for generics); consult specific product labeling.

Granules, oral:
LamISIL®: 125 mg/packet (14s, 42s); 187.5 mg/packet (14s, 42s)
Tablet, oral: 250 mg
LamISIL®: 250 mg
Terbinex™: 250 mg [kit includes Terbinex™ tablets (42s) and Eco-Formula™ nail enhancer]

Selected References

Abdel-Rahman SM, Herron J, Fallon-Friedlander S, et al, "Pharmacokinetics of Terbinafine in Young Children Treated for Tinea Capitis," *Pediatr Infect Dis J*, 2005, 24(10):886-91.

Gupta AK, Sibbald RG, Knowles SR, et al, "Terbinafine Therapy May Be Associated With the Development of Psoriasis De Novo or Its Exacerbation: Four Case Reports and a Review of Drug Induced Psoriasis," *J Am Acad Dermatol*, 1997, 36(5 Part 2):858-62.

Terbinafine (Topical) (TER bin a feen)

Medication Safety Issues
Sound-alike/look-alike issues:
Terbinafine may be confused with terbutaline
Brand Names: U.S. LamISIL AT® [OTC]
Brand Names: Canada Lamisil®
Index Terms Terbinafine Hydrochloride
Generic Availability (U.S.) Yes: Cream
Pharmacologic Category Antifungal Agent, Topical
Use Antifungal for the treatment of tinea pedis (athlete's foot), tinea cruris (jock itch), and tinea corporis (ringworm) [OTC/prescription formulations]; tinea versicolor [prescription formulations]

Dosage
Geriatric & Adult
Athlete's foot (tinea pedis): Topical:
Cream: Apply to affected area once daily for at least 1 week, not to exceed 4 weeks [OTC/Canadian/prescription formulations]
Gel: Apply to affected area once daily for at least 1 week, not to exceed 4 weeks [OTC/Canadian/prescription formulations]
Solution: Apply to affected area once daily for at least 1 week, not to exceed 4 weeks [OTC/Canadian/prescription formulations]
Cutaneous candidiasis: Topical:
Cream: Apply to affected area once or twice daily for 7-14 days
Gel: Apply to affected area once or twice daily for 7-14 days
Solution: Apply to affected area once or twice daily for 7-14 days
Ringworm and jock itch (tinea corporis/tinea versicolor, tinea cruris): Topical:
Cream: Apply to affected area once daily for at least 1 week, not to exceed 4 weeks [OTC formulations]; apply to affected area once or twice daily for 2 weeks in tinea versicolor [Canadian/prescription formulation]
Gel: Apply to affected area once daily for 7 days [OTC formulations]
Solution: Apply to affected area once daily for 7 days in tinea corporis and tinea cruris [OTC formulations]; apply to affected area once or twice daily for 2 weeks in tinea versicolor [Canadian/prescription formulation]

Dosage Forms Excipient information presented when available (limited, particularly for generics); consult specific product labeling. [DSC] = Discontinued product
Cream, topical, as hydrochloride: 1% (12 g [DSC], 15 g, 24 g [DSC], 30 g)
LamISIL AT®: 1% (12 g, 15 g, 24 g, 30 g, 36 g) [contains benzyl alcohol]
Gel, topical:
LamISIL AT®: 1% (6 g, 12 g) [contains benzyl alcohol]
Solution, topical, as hydrochloride [spray]:
LamISIL AT®: 1% (30 mL) [contains ethanol]
Dosage Forms: Canada Excipient information presented when available (limited, particularly for generics); consult specific product labeling.
Cream, topical, as hydrochloride: 1% (12 g, 24 g)
Lamisil®: 1% (15 g, 30 g)
Solution, topical, as hydrochloride [spray]:
Lamisil®: 1% (30 mL)

◆ **Terbinafine Hydrochloride** *see* Terbinafine (Systemic) *on page 1754*
◆ **Terbinafine Hydrochloride** *see* Terbinafine (Topical) *on page 1756*

◆ **Terbinex™** *see* Terbinafine (Systemic) *on page 1754*

Terbutaline (ter BYOO ta leen)

Related Information
Inhalant Agents *on page 2010*

Medication Safety Issues
Sound-alike/look-alike issues:
Brethine may be confused with Methergine®
Terbutaline may be confused with terbinafine, TOLBUTamide
Terbutaline and methylergonovine parenteral dosage forms look similar. Due to their contrasting indications, use care when administering these agents.

Brand Names: Canada Bricanyl®

Index Terms Brethaire [DSC]; Brethine; Bricanyl [DSC]

Generic Availability (U.S.) Yes

Pharmacologic Category Beta₂-Adrenergic Agonist

Use Bronchodilator in reversible airway obstruction and bronchial asthma

Unlabeled/Investigational Use Injection: Tocolytic agent (short-term [≤72 hours] prevention or management of preterm labor

Contraindications Hypersensitivity to terbutaline or any component of the formulation; cardiac arrhythmias associated with tachycardia; tachycardia caused by digitalis intoxication

Injection: Additional contraindications: Prolonged (>72 hours) prevention or management of preterm labor

Oral: Additional contraindications: Prevention or treatment of preterm labor

Warnings/Precautions Use caution in patients with cardiovascular disease (arrhythmia or hypertension or HF), convulsive disorders, diabetes, glaucoma, hyperthyroidism, or hypokalemia. Beta-agonists may cause elevation in blood pressure, heart rate, and result in CNS stimulation/excitation. Beta₂-agonists may increase risk of arrhythmia, increase serum glucose, or decrease serum potassium.

When used as a bronchodilator, optimize anti-inflammatory treatment before initiating maintenance treatment with terbutaline. Do not use as a component of chronic therapy without an anti-inflammatory agent. Only the mildest form of asthma (Step 1 and/or exercise-induced) would not require concurrent use based upon asthma guidelines. Patient must be instructed to seek medical attention in cases where acute symptoms are not relieved or a previous level of response is diminished. The need to increase frequency of use may indicate deterioration of asthma, and treatment must not be delayed.

Immediate hypersensitivity reactions (urticaria, angioedema, rash, bronchospasm) have been reported. Do not exceed recommended dose; serious adverse events including fatalities, have been associated with excessive use of inhaled sympathomimetics. Rarely, paradoxical bronchospasm may occur with use of inhaled bronchodilating agents; this should be distinguished from inadequate response.

Adverse Reactions (Reflective of adult population; not specific for elderly)
>10%:
Central nervous system: Nervousness, restlessness
Endocrine & metabolic: Serum glucose increased, serum potassium decreased
Neuromuscular & skeletal: Trembling
1% to 10%:
Cardiovascular: Tachycardia, hypertension
Central nervous system: Dizziness, drowsiness, headache, insomnia
Gastrointestinal: Xerostomia, nausea, vomiting, bad taste in mouth
Neuromuscular & skeletal: Muscle cramps, weakness
Miscellaneous: Diaphoresis

Drug Interactions
Avoid Concomitant Use
Avoid concomitant use of Terbutaline with any of the following: Iobenguane I 123

Increased Effect/Toxicity
Terbutaline may increase the levels/effects of: Loop Diuretics; Sympathomimetics

The levels/effects of Terbutaline may be increased by: Atomoxetine; Cannabinoids; MAO Inhibitors; Tricyclic Antidepressants

Decreased Effect

Terbutaline may decrease the levels/effects of: Iobenguane I 123

The levels/effects of Terbutaline may be decreased by: Alpha-/Beta-Blockers; Beta-Blockers (Beta1 Selective); Beta-Blockers (Nonselective); Betahistine

Ethanol/Nutrition/Herb Interactions Herb/Nutraceutical: Avoid ephedra, yohimbe (may cause CNS stimulation).

Stability Store injection at room temperature; do not freeze. Protect from heat and light. Use only clear solutions. Store powder for inhalation (Bricanyl® Turbuhaler [CAN]) at room temperature between 15°C and 30°C (58°F and 86°F).

Mechanism of Action Relaxes bronchial and uterine smooth muscle by action on beta$_2$-receptors with less effect on heart rate

Pharmacodynamics/Kinetics

Onset of action: Oral: 30-45 minutes; SubQ: 6-15 minutes

Protein binding: 25%

Metabolism: Hepatic to inactive sulfate conjugates

Bioavailability: SubQ doses are more bioavailable than oral

Half-life elimination: 11-16 hours

Excretion: Urine

Dosage

Geriatric & Adult

Asthma or bronchoconstriction:

Oral: 5 mg/dose every 6 hours 3 times/day; if side effects occur, reduce dose to 2.5 mg every 6 hours; not to exceed 15 mg in 24 hours.

SubQ:

Manufacturer's labeling: 0.25 mg/dose; may repeat in 15-30 minutes (maximum: 0.5 mg/4-hour period)

Unlabeled dose: 0.25 mg/dose; may repeat every 20 minutes for 3 doses (maximum: 0.75 mg/1-hour period) (NIH Guidelines, 2007)

Bronchospasm (acute): *Inhalation* (Bricanyl® [CAN] MDI: 500 mcg/puff, *not labeled for use in the U.S.*): One puff as needed; may repeat with 1 inhalation (after 5 minutes); more than 6 inhalations should not be necessary in any 24 hour period. **Note:** If a previously effective dosage regimen fails to provide the usual relief, or the effects of a dose last for >3 hours, medical advice should be sought immediately; this is a sign of seriously worsening asthma that requires reassessment of therapy.

Premature labor (acute; short-term [≤72 hours] tocolysis; unlabeled use):

I.V.: 2.5-5 mcg/minute; increased gradually every 20-30 minutes by 2.5-5 mcg/minute; effective maximum dosages from 17.5-30 mcg/minute have been used with caution. Duration of infusion is at least 12 hours (Travis, 1993).

SubQ: 0.25 mg every 20 minutes to 3 hours; hold for pulse >120 beats per minute. Terbutaline has not been approved for and should not be used for prolonged tocolysis (beyond 48-72 hours) (ACOG, 2003)

Renal Impairment

Cl$_{cr}$ 10-50 mL/minute: Administer 50% of normal dose.

Cl$_{cr}$ <10 mL/minute: Avoid use.

Administration

I.V.: Use infusion pump.

Oral: Administer around-the-clock to promote less variation in peak and trough serum levels

Monitoring Parameters Serum potassium, glucose; intake/output; heart rate, blood pressure, respiratory rate; chest pain, shortness of breath; monitor for signs and symptoms of pulmonary edema (when used as a tocolytic); monitor FEV$_1$, peak flow, and/or other pulmonary function tests (when used as bronchodilator)

Special Geriatric Considerations Oral terbutaline should be avoided in the elderly due to the increased incidence of adverse effects as compared to the inhaled form.

Dosage Forms Excipient information presented when available (limited, particularly for generics); consult specific product labeling.

Injection, solution, as sulfate: 1 mg/mL (1 mL)

Tablet, oral, as sulfate: 2.5 mg, 5 mg

Dosage Forms: Canada Excipient information presented when available (limited, particularly for generics); consult specific product labeling.

Powder for oral inhalation:

Bricanyl® Turbuhaler: 500 mcg/actuation [50 or 200 metered actuations]

Terconazole (ter KONE a zole)

Medication Safety Issues
Sound-alike/look-alike issues:
Terconazole may be confused with tioconazole
International issues:
Terazol [U.S., Canada] may be confused with Theradol brand name for tramadol [Netherlands]

Brand Names: U.S. Terazol® 3; Terazol® 7; Zazole™ [DSC]

Brand Names: Canada Terazol®

Index Terms Triaconazole

Generic Availability (U.S.) Yes

Pharmacologic Category Antifungal Agent, Vaginal

Use Local treatment of vulvovaginal candidiasis

Contraindications Hypersensitivity to terconazole or any component of the formulation

Warnings/Precautions Should be discontinued if sensitization or irritation occurs. Microbiological studies (KOH smear and/or cultures) should be repeated in patients not responding to terconazole in order to confirm the diagnosis and rule out other pathogens. Petrolatum-based vaginal products may damage rubber or latex condoms or diaphragms; separate use by 3 days.

Adverse Reactions (Reflective of adult population; not specific for elderly)
>10%: Central nervous system: Headache
1% to 10%:
Central nervous system: Chills, fever, pain
Gastrointestinal: Abdominal pain
Genitourinary: Dysmenorrhea; vulvar/vaginal burning, irritation, or itching

Drug Interactions
Avoid Concomitant Use There are no known interactions where it is recommended to avoid concomitant use.

Increased Effect/Toxicity There are no known significant interactions involving an increase in effect.

Decreased Effect There are no known significant interactions involving a decrease in effect.

Stability Store at room temperature of 15°C to 30°C (59°F to 86°F).

Mechanism of Action Triazole ketal antifungal agent; involves inhibition of fungal cytochrome P450. Specifically, terconazole inhibits cytochrome P450-dependent 14-alpha-demethylase which results in accumulation of membrane disturbing 14-alpha-demethylsterols and ergosterol depletion.

Pharmacodynamics/Kinetics Absorption: Extent of systemic absorption after vaginal administration may be dependent on presence of a uterus; 5% to 8% in women who had a hysterectomy versus 12% to 16% in nonhysterectomy women

Dosage
Geriatric & Adult Vulvovaginal candidiasis: Intravaginal:
Terazol® 3, Zazole™ (0.8%) vaginal cream: Insert 1 applicatorful intravaginally at bedtime for 3 consecutive days.
Terazol® 7, Zazole™ (0.4%) vaginal cream: Insert 1 applicatorful intravaginally at bedtime for 7 consecutive days.
Terazol® 3 vaginal suppository: Insert 1 suppository intravaginally at bedtime for 3 consecutive days.

Administration
Vaginal cream: Use applicator provided by manufacturer. Insertion should be as far as possible into the vagina without causing discomfort. Wash applicator after each use; allow to dry thoroughly before putting back together.
Vaginal suppository: Remove foil package prior to use. Insertion should be as far as possible into the vagina without causing discomfort. If the provided applicator is used for insertion, wash and dry thoroughly prior to additional use.

Monitoring Parameters Response to treatment

Pharmacotherapy Pearls Watch for local irritation; assist patient in administration, if necessary; assess patient's ability to self-administer, may be difficult in patients with arthritis or limited range of motion

Special Geriatric Considerations Assess patient's ability to self-administer; may be difficult in patients with arthritis or limited range of motion.

◀ **Dosage Forms** Excipient information presented when available (limited, particularly for generics); consult specific product labeling. [DSC] = Discontinued product

Cream, vaginal: 0.4% (45 g); 0.8% (20 g)
Terazol® 7: 0.4% (45 g)
Terazol® 3: 0.8% (20 g)
Zazole™: 0.4% (45 g [DSC]); 0.8% (20 g [DSC])

Suppository, vaginal: 80 mg (3s)
Terazol® 3: 80 mg (3s) [contains coconut oil (may have trace amounts), palm kernel oil (may have trace amounts)]

Teriparatide (ter i PAR a tide)

Related Information
Osteoporosis Management *on page 2027*

Brand Names: U.S. Forteo®

Brand Names: Canada Forteo®

Index Terms Parathyroid Hormone (1-34); Recombinant Human Parathyroid Hormone (1-34); rhPTH(1-34)

Generic Availability (U.S.) No

Pharmacologic Category Parathyroid Hormone Analog

Use Treatment of osteoporosis in postmenopausal women at high risk of fracture; treatment of primary or hypogonadal osteoporosis in men at high risk of fracture; treatment of glucocorticoid-induced osteoporosis in men and women at high risk for fracture

Medication Guide Available Yes

Contraindications Hypersensitivity to teriparatide or any component of the formulation

Canadian labeling: Additional contraindications (not in U.S. labeling): Pre-existing hypercalcemia; severe renal impairment; metabolic bone diseases other than primary osteoporosis (including hyperparathyroidism and Paget's disease of the bone); unexplained elevations of alkaline phosphatase; prior external beam or implant radiation therapy involving the skeleton; bone metastases or history of skeletal malignancies

Warnings/Precautions [U.S. Boxed Warning]: In animal studies, teriparatide has been associated with an increase in osteosarcoma; risk was dependent on both dose and duration. Avoid use in patients with an increased risk of osteosarcoma (including Paget's disease, prior radiation, unexplained elevation of alkaline phosphatase, or in patients with open epiphyses). Do not use in patients with a history of skeletal metastases, hyperparathyroidism, or pre-existing hypercalcemia. Not for use in patients with metabolic bone disease other than osteoporosis. Use caution in patients with active or recent urolithiasis. Use caution in patients at risk of orthostasis (including concurrent antihypertensive therapy), or in patients who may not tolerate transient hypotension (cardiovascular or cerebrovascular disease). Use caution in patients with cardiac, renal or hepatic impairment (limited data available concerning safety and efficacy). Use of teriparatide for longer than 2 years is not recommended.

Adverse Reactions (Reflective of adult population; not specific for elderly)

>10%: Endocrine & metabolic: Hypercalcemia (transient increases noted 4-6 hours postdose [women 11%; men 6%])

1% to 10%:
Cardiovascular: Orthostatic hypotension (5%; transient), chest pain (3%), syncope (3%)
Central nervous system: Dizziness (8%), insomnia (4% to 5%), anxiety (≤4%), depression (4%), vertigo (4%)
Dermatologic: Rash (5%)
Endocrine & metabolic: Hyperuricemia (3%)
Gastrointestinal: Nausea (9% to 14%), gastritis (≤7%), dyspepsia (5%), vomiting (3%)
Neuromuscular & skeletal: Arthralgia (10%), weakness (9%), leg cramps (3%)
Respiratory: Rhinitis (10%), pharyngitis (6%), dyspnea (4% to 6%), pneumonia (4% to 6%)
Miscellaneous: Antibodies to teriparatide (3% of women in long-term treatment; hypersensitivity reactions or decreased efficacy were not associated in preclinical trials), herpes zoster (≤3%)

Drug Interactions

Avoid Concomitant Use There are no known interactions where it is recommended to avoid concomitant use.

Increased Effect/Toxicity There are no known significant interactions involving an increase in effect.

Decreased Effect There are no known significant interactions involving a decrease in effect.

Ethanol/Nutrition/Herb Interactions
Ethanol: Excessive intake may increase risk of osteoporosis.
Herb/Nutraceutical: Ensure adequate calcium and vitamin D intake.

Stability Store at 2°C to 8°C (36°F to 46°F); do not freeze. Protect from light. Discard pen 28 days after first injection. Do not use if solution is cloudy, colored or contains solid particles.

Mechanism of Action Teriparatide is a recombinant formulation of endogenous parathyroid hormone (PTH), containing a 34-amino-acid sequence which is identical to the N-terminal portion of this hormone. The pharmacologic activity of teriparatide, which is similar to the physiologic activity of PTH, includes stimulating osteoblast function, increasing gastrointestinal calcium absorption, and increasing renal tubular reabsorption of calcium. Treatment with teriparatide results in increased bone mineral density, bone mass, and strength. In postmenopausal women, teriparatide has been shown to decrease osteoporosis-related fractures.

Pharmacodynamics/Kinetics
Distribution: V_d: ~0.12 L/kg
Metabolism: Hepatic (nonspecific proteolysis)
Bioavailability: 95%
Half-life elimination: I.V.: 5 minutes; SubQ: ~1 hour
Time to peak, serum: ~30 minutes
Excretion: Urine (as metabolites)

Dosage
  Geriatric & Adult Osteoporosis: SubQ: 20 mcg once daily; **Note:** Initial administration should occur under circumstances in which the patient may sit or lie down, in the event of orthostasis.

  Renal Impairment No dosage adjustment required. Bioavailability and half-life increase with Cl_{cr} <30 mL/minute. Use in severe renal impairment is contraindicated in the Canadian labeling.

Administration Administer by subcutaneous injection into the thigh or abdominal wall. Initial administration should occur under circumstances in which the patient may sit or lie down, in the event of orthostasis. **Note:** The 3 mL prefilled pen (Canadian availability; not available in U.S.) must be primed prior to each dose.

Monitoring Parameters Serum calcium, serum phosphorus, uric acid; blood pressure; bone mineral density

Test Interactions Transiently increases serum calcium; maximal effect 4-6 hours postdose; generally returns to baseline ~16 hours postdose

Pharmacotherapy Pearls Teriparatide was formerly marketed as a diagnostic agent (Perithar™); that agent was withdrawn from the market in 1997. Teriparatide (Forteo®) is manufactured through recombinant DNA technology using a strain of *E. coli.*

Patients are encouraged to enroll in the Forteo® Patient Registry which is designed to monitor the potential risk of osteosarcoma and teriparatide treatment. Enrollment information may be found at www.forteoregistry.rti.org or by calling 1-866-382-6813.

Special Geriatric Considerations No age-related differences in pharmacokinetics have been seen. In studies, no significant difference was seen in either efficacy or adverse effects between older patients and younger patients. Teriparatide should be considered an alternative in patients who cannot tolerate or have not responded to other treatments for osteoporosis.

Dosage Forms Excipient information presented when available (limited, particularly for generics); consult specific product labeling.
Injection, solution:
  Forteo®: 250 mcg/mL (2.4 mL) [delivers teriparatide 20 mcg/dose]

Dosage Forms: Canada Excipient information presented when available (limited, particularly for generics); consult specific product labeling.
Injection, solution:
  Forteo®: 250 mcg/mL (3 mL) [delivers teriparatide 20 mcg/dose]

Selected References
Body JJ, Gaich GA, Scheele WH, et al, "A Randomized Double-blind Trial to Compare the Efficacy of Teriparatide [Recombinant Human Parathyroid Hormone (1-34)] With Alendronate in Postmenopausal Women With Osteoporosis," *J Clin Endocrinol Metab*, 2002, 87(10):4528-35.
Neer RM, Arnaud CD, Zanchetta JR, et al, "Effect of Parathyroid Hormone (1-34) on Fractures and Bone Mineral Density in Postmenopausal Women With Osteoporosis," *N Engl J Med*, 2001, 344(19):1434-41.

◆ **Tessalon®** *see* Benzonatate *on page 191*
◆ **Tessalon Perles** *see* Benzonatate *on page 191*
◆ **Testim®** *see* Testosterone *on page 1761*
◆ **Testopel®** *see* Testosterone *on page 1761*

Testosterone (tes TOS ter one)

Medication Safety Issues
  Sound-alike/look-alike issues:
    Testosterone may be confused with testolactone
    Testoderm® may be confused with Estraderm®

◀ AndroGel® 1% may be confused with AndroGel® 1.62%

Other safety concerns:

Transdermal patch may contain conducting metal (eg, aluminum); remove patch prior to MRI.

Brand Names: U.S. Androderm®; AndroGel®; Axiron®; Delatestryl®; Depo®-Testosterone; First®-Testosterone; First®-Testosterone MC; Fortesta™; Striant®; Testim®; Testopel®

Brand Names: Canada Andriol®; Androderm®; AndroGel®; Andropository®; Delatestryl®; Depotest® 100; Everone® 200; PMS-Testosterone; Testim®

Index Terms Axiron®; Testosterone Cypionate; Testosterone Enanthate

Generic Availability (U.S.) Yes: Injection, powder

Pharmacologic Category Androgen

Use

Injection: Male hypogonadism (primary or hypogonadotropic); inoperable metastatic female breast cancer (enanthate only)

Pellet: Male hypogonadism (primary or hypogonadotropic)

Buccal system, topical gel, topical solution, transdermal system: Male hypogonadism (primary or hypogonadotropic)

Capsule (not available in U.S.): Conditions associated with a deficiency or absence of endogenous testosterone

Unlabeled/Investigational Use Androgen deficiency in men with AIDS wasting; postmenopausal women (short-term use in select cases)

Medication Guide Available Yes

Contraindications Hypersensitivity to testosterone or any component of the formulation; males with known or suspected carcinoma of the breast or prostate; specific products are contraindicated in women

Depo®-Testosterone: Also contraindicated in serious hepatic, renal, or cardiac disease

Warnings/Precautions When used to treat delayed male puberty, perform radiographic examination of the hand and wrist every 6 months to determine the rate of bone maturation. May cause hypercalcemia in patients with prolonged immobilization or cancer. May accelerate bone maturation without producing compensating gain in linear growth. Has both androgenic and anabolic activity, the anabolic action may enhance hypoglycemia. May alter serum cholesterol; use caution with history of MI or coronary artery disease. Use caution in elderly patients or patients with other demographic factors which may increase the risk of prostatic carcinoma; careful monitoring is required. Urethral obstruction may develop in patients with BPH; treatment should be discontinued if this should occur (use lower dose if restarted). Withhold treatment pending urological evaluation in patients with palpable prostate nodule or induration, PSA >4 ng/mL, or PSA >3 ng/mL in men at high risk of prostate cancer (Bhasin, 2010). Use with caution in patients with conditions influenced by edema (eg, cardiovascular disease, migraine, seizure disorder, renal or hepatic impairment) or medications that enhance edema formation (eg, corticosteroids); testosterone may cause fluid retention. May cause gynecomastia. Large doses may suppress spermatogenesis. During treatment for metastatic breast cancer, women should be monitored for signs of virilization; discontinue if mild virilization is present to prevent irreversible symptoms.

Prolonged use of high doses of androgens has been associated with serious hepatic effects (peliosis hepatis, hepatic neoplasms, cholestatic hepatitis, jaundice). May potentiate sleep apnea in some male patients (obesity or chronic lung disease). May increase hematocrit requiring dose adjustment or discontinuation; monitor.

[U.S. Boxed Warning]: Virilization in children has been reported following contact with unwashed or unclothed application sites of men using topical testosterone. Patients should strictly adhere to instructions for use in order to prevent secondary exposure. Virilization of female sexual partners has also been reported with male use of topical testosterone. Symptoms of virilization generally regress following removal of exposure; however, in some children, enlarged genitalia and bone age did not fully return to age appropriate normal. Signs of inappropriate virilization in women or children following secondary exposure to topical testosterone should be brought to the attention of a healthcare provider. Axiron® and Fortesta™ are not interchangeable with other topical testosterone products. Transdermal patch may contain conducting metal (eg, aluminum); remove patch prior to MRI. Some testosterone products may be chemically synthesized from soy. Some products may contain benzyl alcohol. Use of Axiron® in males with BMI >35 kg/m^2 has not been established.

Adverse Reactions (Reflective of adult population; not specific for elderly) Frequency not always defined.

Cardiovascular: Deep venous thrombosis, edema, hypertension, vasodilation

Central nervous system: Abnormal dreams, aggressive behavior, anger, amnesia, anxiety, blood pressure decreased, depression, dizziness, emotional lability, excitation, headache, hostility, insomnia, malaise, memory loss, mood swings, nervousness, seizure, sleep apnea, sleeplessness

Dermatologic: Acne, alopecia, contact dermatitis, dry skin, folliculitis, hair discoloration, hirsutism (increase in pubic hair growth), pruritus, rash, seborrhea

Endocrine & metabolic: Breast pain/soreness, gonadotropin secretion decreased, growth acceleration, gynecomastia, hot flashes, hypercalcemia, hyperchloremia, hypercholesterolemia, hyper-/hypoglycemia, hyper-/hypokalemia, hyperlipidemia, hypernatremia, inorganic phosphate retention, libido changes, menstrual problems (including amenorrhea), virilism, water retention

Gastrointestinal: Appetite increased, diarrhea, GI bleeding, GI irritation, nausea, taste disorder, vomiting, weight gain

Following buccal administration (most common): Bitter taste, gum edema, gum or mouth irritation, gum pain, gum tenderness, taste perversion

Genitourinary: Bladder irritability, impotence, oligospermia, penile erections (spontaneous), priapism, prostatic carcinoma, prostatic hyperplasia, PSA increased, testicular atrophy, urination impaired

Hepatic: Bilirubin increased, cholestatic hepatitis, cholestatic jaundice, hepatic dysfunction, hepatic necrosis, hepatocellular neoplasms, liver function test changes, peliosis hepatis

Hematologic: Anemia, bleeding, hematocrit/hemoglobin increased, leukopenia, polycythemia, suppression of clotting factors

Local: Application site reaction (gel, solution), injection site inflammation/pain

Transdermal system: Pruritus at application site (37%), burn-like blisters under system (12%), erythema at application site (7%), vesicles at application site (6%), allergic contact dermatitis to system (4%), burning at application site (3%), induration at application site (3%)

Neuromuscular & skeletal: Hyperkinesias, paresthesia, weakness

Ocular: Lacrimation increased

Renal: Creatinine increased

Respiratory: Dyspnea, nasopharyngitis

Miscellaneous: Anaphylactoid reactions, diaphoresis, hypersensitivity reactions, smell disorder

Drug Interactions

Metabolism/Transport Effects Substrate (minor) of CYP2B6, 2C9, 2C19, 3A4; **Inhibits** CYP3A4 (weak)

Avoid Concomitant Use There are no known interactions where it is recommended to avoid concomitant use.

Increased Effect/Toxicity

Testosterone may increase the levels/effects of: CycloSPORINE; CycloSPORINE (Systemic); Vitamin K Antagonists

The levels/effects of Testosterone may be increased by: Conivaptan

Decreased Effect

The levels/effects of Testosterone may be decreased by: Tocilizumab

Ethanol/Nutrition/Herb Interactions Herb/Nutraceutical: St John's wort may decrease testosterone levels.

Stability

Androderm®: Store at room temperature. Do not store outside of pouch. Excessive heat may cause system to burst.

AndroGel® 1%, AndroGel® 1.62%, Axiron®, Delatestryl®, Striant®, Testim®: Store at room temperature.

Depo® Testosterone: Store at room temperature. Protect from light.

Fortesta™: Store at room temperature; do not freeze

Testopel®: Store in a cool location.

Mechanism of Action Principal endogenous androgen responsible for promoting the growth and development of the male sex organs and maintaining secondary sex characteristics in androgen-deficient males

Pharmacodynamics/Kinetics

Duration (route and ester dependent): I.M.: Cypionate and enanthate esters have longest duration, ≤2-4 weeks; gel: 24-48 hours

Absorption: Transdermal gel: ~10% of applied dose

Protein binding: 98%; bound to sex hormone-binding globulin (40%) and albumin

Metabolism: Hepatic; forms metabolites, including dihydrotestosterone (DHT) and estradiol (both active)

◀ Half-life elimination: Variable: 10-100 minutes
Excretion: Urine (90%); feces (6%)

Dosage

Geriatric & Adult

Conditions associated with a deficiency or absence of endogenous testosterone: *Oral capsule (Andriol®; not available in U.S.):* Initial: 120-160 mg/day in 2 divided doses for 2-3 weeks; adjust according to individual response; usual maintenance dose: 40-120 mg/day (in divided doses)

Inoperable metastatic breast cancer (females): *I.M. (testosterone enanthate):* 200-400 mg every 2-4 weeks

Hypogonadism or hypogonadotropic hypogonadism (males):

I.M. (testosterone enanthate or testosterone cipionate): 50-400 mg every 2-4 weeks (FDA-approved dosing range); 75-100 mg/week or 150-200 mg every 2 weeks (Bhasin, 2010)

Pellet (for subcutaneous implantation): 150-450 mg every 3-6 months

Topical:

Buccal: 30 mg twice daily (every 12 hours) applied to the gum region above the incisor tooth

Transdermal system: Androderm®: Primary hypogonadism or hypogonadotropic hypogonadism: Initial: Apply 5 mg/day once nightly; dosing range: 2.5-7.5 mg/day; in non-virilized patients, dose may be initiated at 2.5 mg/day. Apply to clean, dry, intact skin. **Do not apply to the scrotum.**

Gel: Apply to clean, dry, intact skin. **Do not apply testosterone gel to the genitals.**

AndroGel®, Testim®: 5 g (to deliver 50 mg of testosterone with 5 mg systemically absorbed) applied once daily (preferably in the morning) to clean, dry, intact skin of the shoulder and upper arms. AndroGel® may also be applied to the abdomen. Dosage may be increased to a maximum of 10 g (100 mg).

Dose adjustment based on testosterone levels:

Less than normal range: Increase dose from 5 g to 7.5 g to 10 g

Greater than normal range: Decrease dose. Discontinue if consistently above normal at 5 g/day

Fortesta™: 40 mg once daily in the morning. Apply to the thighs. Dosing range: 10-70 mg/day

Dose adjustment based on serum testosterone levels:

≥2500 ng/dL: Decrease dose by 20 mg/day

≥1250 to <2500 ng/dL: Decrease dose by 10 mg/day

≥500 and <1250 ng/dL: Maintain current dose

<500 ng/dL: Increase by 10 mg/day

Solution (Axiron®): 60 mg once daily. (Dosage range 30-120 mg/day). Apply to the axilla at the same time each morning; do not apply to other parts of the body. Apply to clean, dry, intact skin. **Do not apply testosterone solution to the genitals.**

Dose adjustment based on serum testosterone levels:

>1050 ng/dL: Decrease 60 mg/day dose to 30 mg/day; if levels >1050 ng/dL persist after dose reduction discontinue therapy

<300 ng/dL: Increase 60 mg/day dose to 90 mg/day, or increase 90 mg/day dose to 120 mg/day

Renal Impairment Use with caution; may enhance edema formation.

Hepatic Impairment Use with caution; may enhance edema formation.

Administration

I.M.: Warm to room temperature; shaking vial will help redissolve crystals that have formed after storage. Administer by deep I.M. injection into the upper outer quadrant of the gluteus maximus.

Oral, buccal application (Striant®): One mucoadhesive for buccal application (buccal system) should be applied to a comfortable area above the incisor tooth. Apply flat side of system to gum. Rotate to alternate sides of mouth with each application. Hold buccal system firmly in place for 30 seconds to ensure adhesion. The buccal system should adhere to gum for 12 hours. If the buccal system falls out, replace with a new system. If the system falls out within 4 hours of next dose, the new buccal system should remain in place until the time of the following scheduled dose. System will soften and mold to shape of gum as it absorbs moisture from mouth. Do not chew or swallow the buccal system. The buccal system will not dissolve; gently remove by sliding downwards from gum; avoid scratching gum.

Oral, capsule (Andriol®; not available in the U.S.): Should be administered with meals. Should be swallowed whole; do not crush or chew.

Transdermal patch (Androderm®): Apply patch to clean, dry area of skin on the back, abdomen, upper arms, or thigh. Do not apply to bony areas or parts of the body that are subject to prolonged pressure while sleeping or sitting. **Do not apply to the scrotum.** Following patch removal, mild skin irritation may be treated with OTC hydrocortisone cream. A small amount of triamcinolone acetonide 0.1% cream may be applied under the system to decrease irritation; do not use ointment. Patch should be applied nightly. Rotate administration sites, allowing 7 days between applying to the same site.

Topical gel and solution: Apply to clean, dry, intact skin. Application sites should be allowed to dry for a few minutes prior to dressing. Hands should be washed with soap and water after application. **Do not apply testosterone gel or solution to the genitals.** Alcohol-based gels and solutions are flammable; avoid fire or smoking until dry. Testosterone may be transferred to another person following skin-to-skin contact with the application site. Strict adherence to application instructions is needed in order to decrease secondary exposure. Thoroughly wash hands after application and cover application site with clothing (ie, shirt) once gel or solution has dried, or clean application site thoroughly with soap and water prior to contact in order to minimize transfer. In addition to skin-to-skin contact, secondary exposure has also been reported following exposure to secondary items (eg, towel, shirt, sheets). If secondary exposure occurs, the other person should thoroughly wash the skin with soap and water as soon as possible.

AndroGel® 1%, AndroGel® 1.62%, Testim®: Apply (preferably in the morning) to clean, dry, intact skin of the shoulder and upper arms. AndroGel® 1% may also be applied to the abdomen; do not apply AndroGel® 1.62% or Testim® to the abdomen. Area of application should be limited to what will be covered by a short sleeve t-shirt. Apply at the same time each day. Upon opening the packet(s), the entire contents should be squeezed into the palm of the hand and immediately applied to the application site(s). Alternatively, a portion may be squeezed onto palm of hand and applied, repeating the process until entire packet has been applied. Application site should not be washed for ≥2 hours following application of AndroGel® 1.62% or Testim®, or >5 hours for AndroGel® 1%.

AndroGel® 1% multidose pump: Prime pump 3 times (and discard this portion of product) prior to initial use. Each actuation delivers 1.25 g of gel (4 actuations = 5 g; 6 actuations = 7.5 g; 8 actuations = 10 g); each actuation may be applied individually or all at the same time.

AndroGel® 1.62% multidose pump: Prime pump 3 times (and discard this portion of product) prior to initial use. Each actuation delivers 20.25 mg of gel (2 actuations = 40.5 mg; 3 actuations = 60.75 mg; 4 actuations = 81 mg); each actuation may be applied individually or all at the same time.

Axiron®: Apply using the applicator to the axilla at the same time each morning. Do not apply to other parts of the body (eg, abdomen, genitals, shoulders, upper arms). Avoid washing the site or swimming for 2 hours after application. Prior to first use, prime the applicator pump by depressing it 3 times (discard this portion of the product). After priming, position the nozzle over the applicator cup and depress pump fully one time; ensure liquid enters cup. Each pump actuation delivers testosterone 30 mg. No more than 30 mg (one pump) should be added to the cup at one time. The total dose should be divided between axilla (example, 30 mg/day: apply to one axilla only; 60 mg/day: apply 30 mg to each axilla; 90 mg/day: apply 30 mg to each axilla, allow to dry, then apply an additional 30 mg to one axilla; etc). To apply dose, keep applicator upright and wipe into the axilla; if solution runs or drips, use cup to wipe. Do not rub into skin with fingers or hand. If more than one 30 mg dose is needed, repeat process. Apply roll-on or stick antiperspirants or deodorants prior to testosterone. Once application site is dry, cover with clothing. After use, rinse applicator under running water and pat dry with a tissue. The application site and dose of this product are not interchangeable with other topical testosterone products.

Fortesta™: Apply to skin of front and inner thighs. Do not apply to other parts of the body. Use one finger to rub gel evenly onto skin of each thigh. Avoid showering, washing the site, or swimming for 2 hours after application. Prior to first dose, prime the pump by holding canister upright and fully depressing the pump 8 times (discard this portion of the product). Each pump actuation delivers testosterone 10 mg. The total dose should be divided between thighs (example, 10 mg/day: apply 10 mg to one thigh only; 20 mg/day: apply 10 mg to each thigh; 30 mg/day: apply 20 mg to one thigh and 10 mg to the other thigh; etc). Once application site is dry, cover with clothing. The application site and dose of this product are not interchangeable with other topical testosterone products.

Monitoring Parameters Periodic liver function tests, cholesterol, hemoglobin and hematocrit (prior to therapy, at 3-6 months, then annually). Withhold initial treatment with hematocrit >54%, hyperviscosity, untreated obstructive sleep apnea, or uncontrolled severe heart failure. Monitor urine and serum calcium and signs of virilization in women treated for breast cancer. Serum glucose (may be decreased by testosterone, monitor patients with diabetes). Evaluate males for response to treatment and adverse events 3-6 months after initiation and then annually.

Bone mineral density: Monitor after 1-2 years of therapy in hypogonadal men with osteoporosis or low trauma fracture (Bhasin, 2010)

PSA: In men >40 years of age with baseline PSA >0.6 ng/mL, PSA and prostate exam (prior to therapy, at 3-6 months, then as based on current guidelines). Withhold treatment pending urological evaluation in patients with palpable prostate nodule or induration or PSA >4 ng/mL or if PSA >3 ng/mL in men at high risk of prostate cancer (Bhasin, 2010).

TESTOSTERONE

◀ Do not treat with severe untreated BPH with IPSS symptom score >19.

Serum testosterone: Monitor 3-6 months after initiating treatment, then annually.

Injection: Measure midway between injections. Adjust dose or frequency if testosterone concentration is <400 ng/dL or >700 ng/dL (Bhasin, 2010).

AndroGel® 1%, Testim®: Morning serum testosterone levels ~14 days after start of therapy

AndroGel® 1.62%: Morning serum testosterone levels after 14 and 28 days of starting therapy or dose adjustments and periodically thereafter

Androderm®: Morning serum testosterone levels following application the previous evening

Axiron®: Serum testosterone levels can be measured 2-8 hours after application and after 14 days of starting therapy or dose adjustments

Fortesta™: Serum testosterone levels can be measured 2 hours after application and after 14 and 35 days of starting therapy or dose adjustments

Striant®: Application area of gums; total serum testosterone 4-12 weeks after initiating treatment, prior to morning dose

Testopel®: Measure at the end of the dosing interval (Bhasin, 2010)

Reference Range

Total testosterone, male:

12-13 years: <800 ng/dL

14 years: <1200 ng/dL

15-16 years: 100-1200ng/dL

17-18 years: 300-1200 ng/dL

19-40 years: 300-950 ng/dL

>40 years: 240-950 ng/dL

Free testosterone, male: 9-30 ng/dL

Test Interactions Testosterone may decrease thyroxine-binding globulin, resulting in decreased total T_4; free thyroid hormone levels are not changed.

Special Geriatric Considerations Elderly males treated with androgens may be at increased risk of developing prostatic hyperplasia and prostatic carcinoma. Increase in libido may occur.

Controlled Substance C-III

Dosage Forms Excipient information presented when available (limited, particularly for generics); consult specific product labeling.

Cream, topical [compounding kit]:

First®-Testosterone MC: 2% (60 g) [contains benzyl alcohol, sesame oil]

Gel, topical:

AndroGel®: 1% [5 g gel/packet] (30s); 1% [2.5 g gel/packet] (30s); 1% [1.25 g gel/actuation] (75 g) [contains ethanol 67%; may be chemically synthesized from soy]

AndroGel®: 1.62% [1.25 g gel/actuation] (75 g) [contains ethanol]

Fortesta™: 10 mg/actuation (60 g) [contains ethanol; 0.5 g gel/actuation; 120 metered actuations]

Testim®: 1% [5 g gel/tube] (30s) [contains ethanol 74%; may be chemically synthesized from soy]

Implant, subcutaneous:

Testopel®: 75 mg (10s, 24s, 100s)

Injection, oil, as cypionate: 100 mg/mL (10 mL); 200 mg/mL (1 mL, 10 mL)

Depo®-Testosterone: 100 mg/mL (10 mL); 200 mg/mL (1 mL, 10 mL) [contains benzyl alcohol, benzyl benzoate, cottonseed oil]

Injection, oil, as enanthate: 200 mg/mL (5 mL)

Delatestryl®: 200 mg/mL (5 mL) [contains chlorobutanol, sesame oil]

Mucoadhesive, for buccal application [buccal system]:

Striant®: 30 mg (60s) [may be chemically synthesized from soy]

Ointment, topical [compounding kit]:

First®-Testosterone: 2% (60 g) [contains benzyl alcohol, sesame oil]

Patch, transdermal:

Androderm®: 2.5 mg/24 hours (60s); 5 mg/24 hours (30s) [contains ethanol, metal]

Powder, for prescription compounding [micronized]: USP: 100% (5 g, 25 g)

Powder, for prescription compounding, as propionate: USP: 100% (5 g, 25 g)

Solution, topical:

Axiron®: 30 mg/actuation (110 mL) [contains ethanol, isopropyl alcohol; 60 metered actuations]

Dosage Forms: Canada Excipient information presented when available (limited, particularly for generics); consult specific product labeling.

Capsule, gelatin, as undecanoate:

Andriol™: 40 mg (10s)

Selected References

Bhasin S, Cunningham GR, Hayes FJ, et al, "Testosterone Therapy in Adult Men With Androgen Deficiency Syndromes: An Endocrine Society Clinical Practice Guideline," *J Clin Endocrinol Metab*, 2006, 91(6):1995-2010.

NAMS Board of Trustees, "The Role of Testosterone Therapy in Postmenopausal Women: Position Statement of The North American Menopause Society," *Menopause*, 2005, 12(5):497-511.

◆ **Testosterone Cypionate** *see* Testosterone *on page 1761*
◆ **Testosterone Enanthate** *see* Testosterone *on page 1761*
◆ **Testred®** *see* MethylTESTOSTERone *on page 1188*
◆ **Tetanus and Diphtheria Toxoid** *see* Diphtheria and Tetanus Toxoids *on page 525*

Tetanus Immune Globulin (Human) (TET a nus i MYUN GLOB yoo lin HYU man)

Related Information

Immunization Administration Recommendations *on page 2037*
Immunization Recommendations *on page 2043*
Brand Names: U.S. HyperTET™ S/D
Brand Names: Canada HyperTET™ S/D
Index Terms TIG
Generic Availability (U.S.) No
Pharmacologic Category Immune Globulin
Use Prophylaxis against tetanus following injury in patients where immunization status is not known or uncertain

The Advisory Committee on Immunization Practices (ACIP) recommends passive immunization with TIG for the following:
- Persons with a wound that is not clean or minor and in whom contraindications to a tetanus-toxoid containing vaccine exist and they have not completed a primary series of tetanus toxoid immunization.
- Persons who are wounded in bombings or similar mass casualty events who have penetrating injuries or nonintact skin exposure and who cannot confirm receipt of a tetanus booster within the previous 5 years. In case of shortage, use should be reserved for persons ≥60 years of age.

Warnings/Precautions Hypersensitivity and anaphylactic reactions can occur; immediate treatment (including epinephrine 1:1000) should be available. Use caution in patients with isolated immunoglobulin A deficiency or a history of systemic hypersensitivity to human immunoglobulins. Use with caution in patients with thrombocytopenia or coagulation disorders; I.M. injections may be contraindicated. Product of human plasma; may potentially contain infectious agents which could transmit disease. Screening of donors, as well as testing and/or inactivation or removal of certain viruses, reduces the risk. Infections thought to be transmitted by this product should be reported to the manufacturer. Skin testing should not be performed as local irritation can occur and be misinterpreted as a positive reaction. Not for intravenous administration.

Adverse Reactions (Reflective of adult population; not specific for elderly) Frequency not defined.

Central nervous system: Temperature increased
Dermatologic: Angioneurotic edema (rare)
Local: Injection site: Pain, soreness, tenderness
Renal: Nephritic syndrome (rare)
Miscellaneous: Anaphylactic shock (rare)

Drug Interactions

Avoid Concomitant Use There are no known interactions where it is recommended to avoid concomitant use.

Increased Effect/Toxicity There are no known significant interactions involving an increase in effect.

Decreased Effect
Tetanus Immune Globulin (Human) may decrease the levels/effects of: Vaccines (Live)

Stability Store at 2°C to 8°C (26°F to 46°F). Do not use if frozen. The following stability information has also been reported for HyperTET™ S/D: May be exposed to room temperature for a cumulative 7 days (Cohen, 2007).

Mechanism of Action Passive immunity toward tetanus

Pharmacodynamics/Kinetics Absorption: Well absorbed

Dosage

Geriatric & Adult
Prophylaxis of tetanus: I.M.: 250 units
Tetanus prophylaxis in wound management: I.M.: Tetanus prophylaxis in patients with wounds should consider if the wound is clean or contaminated, the immunization status of the patient, proper use of tetanus toxoid and/or tetanus immune globulin (TIG), wound

cleaning, and (if required) surgical debridement and the proper use of antibiotics. Patients with an uncertain or incomplete tetanus immunization status should have additional follow up to ensure a series is completed. Patients with a history of Arthus reaction following a previous dose of a tetanus toxoid-containing vaccine should not receive a tetanus toxoid-containing vaccine until >10 years after the most recent dose even if they have a wound that is neither clean nor minor. See table.

Tetanus Prophylaxis in Wound Management

History of Tetanus Immunization Doses	Clean, Minor Wounds		All Other Wounds[1]	
	Tetanus Toxoid[2]	TIG	Tetanus Toxoid[2]	TIG
Uncertain or <3 doses	Yes	No	Yes	Yes
3 or more doses	No[3]	No	No[4]	No

[1]Such as, but not limited to, wounds contaminated with dirt, feces, soil, and saliva; puncture wounds; wounds from crushing, tears, burns, and frostbite.

[2]Tetanus toxoid in this chart refers to a tetanus toxoid-containing vaccine. For children <7 years of age, DTaP (DT, if pertussis vaccine contraindicated) is preferred to tetanus toxoid alone. For children ≥7 years and Adults, Td preferred to tetanus toxoid alone; Tdap may be preferred if the patient has not previously been vaccinated with Tdap.

[3]Yes, if ≥10 years since last dose.

[4]Yes, if ≥5 years since last dose.

Adapted from CDC "Yellow Book" (*Health Information for International Travel 2010*), "Routine Vaccine-Preventable Diseases, Tetanus" (available at http://www.cdc.gov/yellowbook) and *MMWR* 2006, 55(RR-17).

Abbreviations: **DT** = Diphtheria and Tetanus Toxoids (formulation for age ≤6 years); **DTaP** = Diphtheria and Tetanus Toxoids, and Acellular Pertussis (formulation for age ≤6 years; Daptacel®, Infanrix®, Tripedia®); **Td** = Diphtheria and Tetanus Toxoids (formulation for age ≥7 years; Decavac®); **TT**= Tetanus toxoid (adsorbed [formulation for age ≥7 years]); **Tdap** = Diphtheria and Tetanus Toxoids, and Acellular Pertussis (Adacel® or Boostrix® [formulations for age ≥7 years]); **TIG** = Tetanus Immune Globulin

Treatment of tetanus: I.M.: 500-6000 units. Infiltration of part of the dose around the wound is recommended.

Administration Do not administer I.V.; I.M. use only

Monitoring Parameters Monitor for hypersensitivity reactions

Pharmacotherapy Pearls Tetanus immune globulin (TIG) must not contain <50 units/mL. Protein makes up 10% to 18% of TIG preparations. The great majority of this (≥90%) is IgG. TIG has almost no color or odor and it is a sterile, nonpyrogenic, concentrated preparation of immunoglobulins that has been derived from the plasma of adults hyperimmunized with tetanus toxoid. The pooled material from which the immunoglobulin is derived may be from fewer than 1000 donors. This plasma has been shown to be free of hepatitis B surface antigen.

Special Geriatric Considerations Tetanus is a rare disease in the U.S. with <50 cases annually; 40% of cases occurred in persons ≥60 years of age; protective tetanus and diphtheria antibodies decline with age; it is estimated that <50% of the elderly are protected.

Elderly are at risk because:
Many lack proper immunization maintenance
Higher case fatality ratio
Immunizations are not available from childhood
Indications for vaccination:
Primary series with combined tetanus-diphtheria (Td) should be given to all elderly lacking a clear history of vaccination
Boosters with Td (may substitute a single dose of Tdap for a single dose of Td as a one-time replacement) should be given at 10-year intervals (earlier for wounds)
Elderly are more likely to require tetanus immune globulin with infection of tetanus due to lower antibody titer.

Dosage Forms Excipient information presented when available (limited, particularly for generics); consult specific product labeling.
Injection, solution [preservative free]:
HyperTET™ S/D: 250 units/mL (~1 mL)

Selected References

Centers for Disease Control and Prevention (CDC), "Preventing Tetanus, Diphtheria, and Pertussis Among Adults: Use of Tetanus Toxoid, Reduced Diphtheria Toxoid and Acellular Pertussis Vaccine, Recommendations of the Advisory Committee on Immunization Practices (ACIP) and Recommendation of ACIP, Supported by the Healthcare Infection Control Practices Advisory Committee (HICPAC), for Use of Tdap Among Health-Care Personnel," *MMWR Recomm Rep*, 2006, 55(RR-17):1-37.

Centers for Disease Control and Prevention (CDC), "Updated Recommendations for Use of Tetanus Toxoid, Reduced Diphtheria Toxoid and Acellular Pertussis (Tdap) Vaccine From the Advisory Committee on Immunization Practices, 2010," *MMWR Morb Mortal Wkly Rep*, 2011, 60(1):13-5.

McQuillan GM, Kruszon-Moran D, Deforest A, et al, "Serologic Immunity to Diphtheria and Tetanus in the United States," *Ann Intern Med*, 2002, 136(9):660-6.

Tetanus Toxoid (Adsorbed) (TET a nus TOKS oyd, ad SORBED)

Related Information
Immunization Administration Recommendations *on page 2037*
Immunization Recommendations *on page 2043*

Medication Safety Issues
Sound-alike/look-alike issues:
Tetanus toxoid products may be confused with influenza virus vaccine and tuberculin products. Medication errors have occurred when tetanus toxoid products have been inadvertently administered instead of tuberculin skin tests (PPD) and influenza virus vaccine. These products are refrigerated and often stored in close proximity to each other.

Index Terms TT

Generic Availability (U.S.) No

Pharmacologic Category Vaccine, Inactivated (Bacterial)

Use Active immunization against tetanus when combination antigen preparations are not indicated; tetanus prophylaxis in wound management. **Note:** Tetanus and diphtheria toxoids for adult use (Td) is the preferred immunizing agent for most adults and for children after their seventh birthday. Young children should receive trivalent DTaP (diphtheria/tetanus/acellular pertussis) as part of their childhood immunization program, unless pertussis is contra-indicated, then DT is warranted.

Contraindications Hypersensitivity to tetanus toxoid or any component of the formulation

Warnings/Precautions Avoid injection into a blood vessel; allergic reactions may occur; epinephrine 1:1000 must be available. Patients who are immunocompromised may have reduced response; may be used in patients with HIV infection. May defer elective immunization during febrile illness or acute infection; defer elective immunization during outbreaks of poliomyelitis. In patients with a history of severe local reaction (Arthus-type) or temperature of >39.4°C (>103°F) following previous dose, do not give further routine or emergency doses of tetanus and diphtheria toxoids for 10 years. Use caution in patients on anticoagulants, with thrombocytopenia, or bleeding disorders (bleeding may occur following intramuscular injection). Use with caution if Guillain-Barré syndrome occurred within 6 weeks of prior tetanus toxoid. Contains thimerosal; vial stopper may contain natural latex rubber. In order to maximize vaccination rates, the ACIP recommends simultaneous administration of all age-appropriate vaccines (live or inactivated) for which a person is eligible at a single clinic visit, unless contraindications exist. The use of combination vaccines is generally preferred over separate injections, taking into consideration provider assessment, patient preference, and adverse events.

Adverse Reactions (Reflective of adult population; not specific for elderly) All serious adverse reactions must be reported to the U.S. Department of Health and Human Services (DHHS) Vaccine Adverse Event Reporting System (VAERS) 1-800-822-7967 or online at https://vaers.hhs.gov/esub/index.
Frequency not defined.
Cardiovascular: Hypotension
Central nervous system: Brachial neuritis, fever, malaise, pain
Gastrointestinal: Nausea
Local: Edema, induration (with or without tenderness), rash, redness, urticaria, warmth
Neuromuscular: Arthralgia, Guillain-Barré syndrome
Miscellaneous: Anaphylactic reaction, Arthus-type hypersensitivity reaction

Drug Interactions
Avoid Concomitant Use There are no known interactions where it is recommended to avoid concomitant use.

Increased Effect/Toxicity There are no known significant interactions involving an increase in effect.

Decreased Effect
The levels/effects of Tetanus Toxoid (Adsorbed) may be decreased by: Belimumab; Fingolimod; Immunosuppressants

Stability Store at 2°C to 8°C (26°F to 46°F); do not freeze.

Mechanism of Action Tetanus toxoid preparations contain the toxin produced by virulent tetanus bacilli (detoxified growth products of *Clostridium tetani*). The toxin has been modified by treatment with formaldehyde so that it has lost toxicity but still retains ability to act as antigen and produce active immunity; the aluminum salt, a mineral adjuvant, delays the rate of absorption and prolongs and enhances its properties; duration ~10 years.

Pharmacodynamics/Kinetics Duration: Primary immunization: ~10 years

TETANUS TOXOID (ADSORBED)

◄ **Dosage**

Geriatric & Adult Note: In most patients, Td is the recommended product for primary immunization, booster doses, and tetanus immunization in wound management (refer to Diphtheria and Tetanus Toxoids monograph).

Primary immunization: I.M.: 0.5 mL; repeat 0.5 mL at 4-8 weeks after first dose and at 6-12 months after second dose

Routine booster dose: Recommended every 10 years

Tetanus prophylaxis in wound management: Tetanus prophylaxis in patients with wounds should consider if the wound is clean or contaminated, the immunization status of the patient, proper use of tetanus toxoid and/or tetanus immune globulin (TIG), wound cleaning, and (if required) surgical debridement and the proper use of antibiotics. Patients with an uncertain or incomplete tetanus immunization status should have additional follow up to ensure a series is completed. Patients with a history of Arthus reaction following a previous dose of a tetanus toxoid-containing vaccine should not receive a tetanus toxoid-containing vaccine until >10 years after the most recent dose even if they have a wound that is neither clean nor minor. See table.

Tetanus Prophylaxis in Wound Management

History of Tetanus Immunization Doses	Clean, Minor Wounds		All Other Wounds[1]	
	Tetanus Toxoid[2]	TIG	Tetanus Toxoid[2]	TIG
Uncertain or <3 doses	Yes	No	Yes	Yes
3 or more doses	No[3]	No	No[4]	No

[1]Such as, but not limited to, wounds contaminated with dirt, feces, soil, and saliva; puncture wounds; wounds from crushing, tears, burns, and frostbite.

[2]Tetanus toxoid in this chart refers to a tetanus toxoid-containing vaccine. For children <7 years of age, DTaP (DT, if pertussis vaccine contraindicated) is preferred to tetanus toxoid alone. For children ≥7 years and Adults, Td preferred to tetanus toxoid alone; Tdap may be preferred if the patient has not previously been vaccinated with Tdap.

[3]Yes, if ≥10 years since last dose.

[4]Yes, if ≥5 years since last dose.

Adapted from CDC "Yellow Book" (*Health Information for International Travel 2010*), "Routine Vaccine-Preventable Diseases, Tetanus" (available at http://www.cdc.gov/yellowbook) and *MMWR* 2006, 55(RR-17).

Abbreviations: **DT** = Diphtheria and Tetanus Toxoids (formulation for age ≤6 years); **DTaP** = Diphtheria and Tetanus Toxoids, and Acellular Pertussis (formulation for age ≤6 years; Daptacel®, Infanrix®, Tripedia®); **Td** = Diphtheria and Tetanus Toxoids (formulation for age ≥7 years; Decavac®); **TT**= Tetanus toxoid (adsorbed [formulation for age ≥7 years]); **Tdap** = Diphtheria and Tetanus Toxoids, and Acellular Pertussis (Adacel® or Boostrix® [formulations for age ≥7 years]); **TIG** = Tetanus Immune Globulin

Administration Inject intramuscularly in the area of the vastus lateralis (midthigh laterally) or deltoid. Do not inject into gluteal area. Shake well prior to withdrawing dose; do not use if product does not form a suspension.

For patients at risk of hemorrhage following intramuscular injection, the ACIP recommends "it should be administered intramuscularly if, in the opinion of the physician familiar with the patients bleeding risk, the vaccine can be administered by this route with reasonable safety. If the patient receives antihemophilia or other similar therapy, intramuscular vaccination can be scheduled shortly after such therapy is administered. A fine needle (23 gauge or smaller) can be used for the vaccination and firm pressure applied to the site (without rubbing) for at least 2 minutes. The patient should be instructed concerning the risk of hematoma from the injection." Patients on anticoagulant therapy should be considered to have the same bleeding risks and treated as those with clotting factor disorders (CDC, 2011).

Simultaneous administration of vaccines helps ensure the patients will be fully vaccinated by the appropriate age. Simultaneous administration of vaccines is defined as administering >1 vaccine on the same day at different anatomic sites. The use of licensed combination vaccines is generally preferred over separate injections of the equivalent components. Separate vaccines should not be combined in the same syringe unless indicated by product specific labeling. Separate needles and syringes should be used for each injection. The ACIP prefers each dose of a specific vaccine in a series come from the same manufacturer when possible. Adolescents and adults should be vaccinated while seated or lying down. In general, preterm infants should be vaccinated at the same chronological age as full-term infants (CDC, 2011).

Antipyretics have not been shown to prevent febrile seizures. Antipyretics may be used to treat fever or discomfort following vaccination (CDC, 2011). One study reported that routine prophylactic administration of acetaminophen to prevent fever prior to vaccination decreased the immune response of some vaccines; the clinical significance of this reduction in immune response has not been established (Prymula, 2009).

Pharmacotherapy Pearls Federal law requires that the name of medication, date of administration, the vaccine manufacturer, lot number of vaccine, and the administering person's name, title and address be entered into the patient's permanent medical record.

Special Geriatric Considerations Tetanus is a rare disease in the U.S. with <50 cases annually; 40% of cases occurred in persons ≥60 years of age; protective tetanus and diphtheria antibodies decline with age; it is estimated that <50% of the elderly are protected.

Elderly are at risk because:
  Many lack proper immunization maintenance
  Higher case fatality ratio
  Immunizations are not available from childhood
Indications for vaccination:
  Primary series with combined tetanus-diphtheria (Td) should be given to all elderly lacking a clean history of vaccination
  Boosters with Td (may substitute a single dose of Tdap for a single dose of Td as a one-time replacement) should be given at 10-year intervals (earlier for wounds)
  Elderly are more likely to require tetanus immune globulin with infection of tetanus due to lower antibody titer.

Dosage Forms Excipient information presented when available (limited, particularly for generics); consult specific product labeling.

Injection, suspension: 5 Lf units/0.5 mL (0.5 mL) [contains aluminum and thimerosal (may have trace amounts]

Selected References

Centers for Disease Control and Prevention (CDC), "Preventing Tetanus, Diphtheria, and Pertussis Among Adults: Use of Tetanus Toxoid, Reduced Diphtheria Toxoid and Acellular Pertussis Vaccine, Recommendations of the Advisory Committee on Immunization Practices (ACIP) and Recommendation of ACIP, Supported by the Healthcare Infection Control Practices Advisory Committee (HICPAC), for Use of Tdap Among Health-Care Personnel,"*MMWR Recomm Rep*, 2006, 55(RR-17):1-37.

Centers for Disease Control and Prevention (CDC), "Updated Recommendations for Use of Tetanus Toxoid, Reduced Diphtheria Toxoid and Acellular Pertussis (Tdap) Vaccine From the Advisory Committee on Immunization Practices, 2010," *MMWR Morb Mortal Wkly Rep*, 2011, 60(1):13-5.

McQuillan GM, Kruszon-Moran D, Deforest A, et al, "Serologic Immunity to Diphtheria and Tetanus in the United States," *Ann Intern Med*, 2002, 136(9):660-6.

◆ **Tetanus Toxoid, Reduced Diphtheria Toxoid, and Acellular Pertussis, Adsorbed** *see* Diphtheria and Tetanus Toxoids, and Acellular Pertussis Vaccine *on page* 531

Tetrabenazine (tet ra BEN a zeen)

Brand Names: U.S. Xenazine®
Brand Names: Canada Nitoman™
Pharmacologic Category Central Monoamine-Depleting Agent
Use Treatment of chorea associated with Huntington's disease

Canadian labeling: Treatment of hyperkinetic movement disorders, including Huntington's chorea, hemiballismus, senile chorea, Tourette syndrome, and tardive dyskinesia

Prescribing and Access Restrictions Xenazine® is available only through specialty pharmacies. For more information regarding the procurement of Xenazine®, healthcare providers, patients, and caregivers may contact the Xenazine® Information Center (XIC) at 1-888-882-6013 or at:
  Healthcare providers: http://www.xenazineusa.com/HCP/PrescribingXenazine/Default.aspx
  Patients and caregivers: http://www.xenazineusa.com/AboutXenazine/Getting-Your-Prescription.aspx

Medication Guide Available Yes

Dosage
  Geriatric Canadian labeling: Elderly and/or debilitated patients: Consider initiation at lower doses; must be titrated slowly to individualize dosage.
  Adult Dose should be individualized; titrate slowly
    Chorea associated with Huntington's disease: Oral:
      Initial: 12.5 mg once daily, may increase to 12.5 mg twice daily after 1 week
      Maintenance: May be increased by 12.5 mg/day at weekly intervals; doses >37.5 mg/day should be divided into 3 doses (maximum single dose: 25 mg)
      Patients requiring doses >50 mg/day: Genotype for CYP2D6:
        Extensive/intermediate metabolizers: Maximum: 100 mg/day; 37.5 mg/dose
        Poor metabolizers: Maximum: 50 mg/day; 25 mg/dose

◄ *Concomitant use with strong CYP2D6 inhibitors (eg, fluoxetine, paroxetine, quinidine):* Dose of tetrabenazine should be reduced by 50% in patients receiving strong CYP2D6 inhibitors, follow dosing for poor CYP2D6 metabolizers. Use caution when adding a CYP2D6 inhibitor to patients already taking tetrabenazine.

Note: If treatment is interrupted for >5 days, retitration is recommended. If treatment is interrupted for <5 days resume at previous maintenance dose.

Canadian labeling: Hyperkinetic movement disorders: Initial: 12.5 mg twice daily (may be given 3 times/day); may be increased by 12.5 mg/day every 3-5 days; should be titrated slowly to maximal tolerated and effective dose (dose is individualized)

Usual maximum tolerated dosage: 25 mg 3 times/day; maximum recommended dose: 200 mg/day

Note: If there is no improvement at the maximum tolerated dose after 7 days, improvement is unlikely; discontinuation should be considered.

Hepatic Impairment Use is contraindicated.

Special Geriatric Considerations No specific geriatric information is available.

Dosage Forms Excipient information presented when available (limited, particularly for generics); consult specific product labeling.

Tablet, oral:
Xenazine®: 12.5 mg
Xenazine®: 25 mg [scored]

Dosage Forms: Canada Excipient information presented when available (limited, particularly for generics); consult specific product labeling.

Tablet:
Nitoman™: 25 mg

◆ **Tetracaine and Lidocaine** see Lidocaine and Tetracaine on page 1066

Tetracycline (tet ra SYE kleen)

Related Information
Helicobacter pylori Treatment in Adult Patients on page 2009

Medication Safety Issues
Sound-alike/look-alike issues:
Tetracycline may be confused with tetradecyl sulfate
Achromycin may be confused with actinomycin, Adriamycin PFS®

Brand Names: Canada Apo-Tetra®; Nu-Tetra

Index Terms Achromycin; TCN; Tetracycline Hydrochloride

Generic Availability (U.S.) Yes: Capsule

Pharmacologic Category Antibiotic, Tetracycline Derivative

Use Treatment of susceptible bacterial infections of both gram-positive and gram-negative organisms; also infections due to *Mycoplasma*, *Chlamydia*, and *Rickettsia*; indicated for acne, exacerbations of chronic bronchitis, and treatment of gonorrhea and syphilis in patients who are allergic to penicillin; as part of a multidrug regimen for *H. pylori* eradication to reduce the risk of duodenal ulcer recurrence

Unlabeled/Investigational Use Treatment of periodontitis associated with presence of *Actinobacillus actinomycetemcomitans* (AA)

Contraindications Hypersensitivity to tetracycline or any component of the formulation

Warnings/Precautions Use with caution in patients with renal or hepatic impairment (eg, elderly); dosage modification required in patients with renal impairment since it may increase BUN as an antianabolic agent. Hepatotoxicity has been reported rarely; risk may be increased in patients with pre-existing hepatic or renal impairment. Pseudotumor cerebri has been reported with tetracycline use (usually resolves with discontinuation); outdated drug can cause nephropathy; use protective measure to avoid photosensitivity. Prolonged use may result in fungal or bacterial superinfection, including *C. difficile*-associated diarrhea (CDAD) and pseudomembranous colitis; CDAD has been observed >2 months postantibiotic treatment.

Adverse Reactions (Reflective of adult population; not specific for elderly) Frequency not defined.
Cardiovascular: Pericarditis
Central nervous system: Bulging fontanels in infants, increased intracranial pressure, paresthesia, pseudotumor cerebri
Dermatologic: Exfoliative dermatitis, photosensitivity, pigmentation of nails, pruritus
Endocrine & metabolic: Diabetes insipidus syndrome
Gastrointestinal: Abdominal cramps, anorexia, antibiotic-associated pseudomembranous colitis, diarrhea, discoloration of teeth and enamel hypoplasia (young children), esophagitis, nausea, pancreatitis, staphylococcal enterocolitis, vomiting

Hematologic: Thrombophlebitis

Hepatic: Hepatotoxicity

Renal: Acute renal failure, azotemia, renal damage

Miscellaneous: Anaphylaxis, candidal superinfection, hypersensitivity reactions, superinfection

Drug Interactions

Metabolism/Transport Effects Substrate of CYP3A4 (major); **Inhibits** CYP3A4 (moderate)

Avoid Concomitant Use

Avoid concomitant use of Tetracycline with any of the following: BCG; Retinoic Acid Derivatives; Tolvaptan

Increased Effect/Toxicity

Tetracycline may increase the levels/effects of: Budesonide (Systemic, Oral Inhalation); Colchicine; CYP3A4 Substrates; Eplerenone; Everolimus; FentaNYL; Halofantrine; Lurasidone; Neuromuscular-Blocking Agents; Pimecrolimus; Porfimer; Ranolazine; Retinoic Acid Derivatives; Salmeterol; Saxagliptin; Tolvaptan; Vilazodone; Vitamin K Antagonists

The levels/effects of Tetracycline may be increased by: Conivaptan

Decreased Effect

Tetracycline may decrease the levels/effects of: Atovaquone; BCG; Penicillins; Typhoid Vaccine

The levels/effects of Tetracycline may be decreased by: Antacids; Bile Acid Sequestrants; Bismuth; Bismuth Subsalicylate; Calcium Salts; CYP3A4 Inducers (Strong); Deferasirox; Herbs (CYP3A4 Inducers); Iron Salts; Lanthanum; Magnesium Salts; Quinapril; Sucralfate; Tocilizumab; Zinc Salts

Ethanol/Nutrition/Herb Interactions

Food: Serum concentrations may be decreased if taken with dairy products.

Herb/Nutraceutical: Avoid dong quai, St John's wort (may also cause photosensitization)

Stability Outdated tetracyclines have caused a Fanconi-like syndrome. Protect oral dosage forms from light.

Mechanism of Action Inhibits bacterial protein synthesis by binding with the 30S and possibly the 50S ribosomal subunit(s) of susceptible bacteria; may also cause alterations in the cytoplasmic membrane

Pharmacodynamics/Kinetics

Absorption: Oral: 75%

Distribution: Small amount appears in bile

Relative diffusion from blood into CSF: Good only with inflammation (exceeds usual MICs)

CSF:blood level ratio: Inflamed meninges: 25%

Protein binding: ~65%

Half-life elimination: Normal renal function: 8-11 hours; End-stage renal disease: 57-108 hours

Time to peak, serum: Oral: 2-4 hours

Excretion: Urine (60% as unchanged drug); feces (as active form)

Dosage

Geriatric & Adult

Usual dosage range: Oral: 250-500 mg every 6 hours

Acne: Oral: 250-500 twice daily

Chronic bronchitis, acute exacerbation: Oral: 500 mg 4 times/day

Erlichiosis: Oral: 500 mg 4 times/day for 7-14 days

Peptic ulcer disease: Eradication of *Helicobacter pylori*: Oral: 500 mg 2-4 times/day depending on regimen; requires combination therapy with at least one other antibiotic and an acid-suppressing agent (proton pump inhibitor or H_2 blocker)

Periodontitis (unlabeled use): Oral: 250 mg every 6 hours until improvement (usually 10 days)

Vibrio cholerae: Oral: 500 mg 4 times/day for 3 days

Renal Impairment

Cl_{cr} 50-80 mL/minute: Administer every 8-12 hours.

Cl_{cr} 10-50 mL/minute: Administer every 12-24 hours.

Cl_{cr} <10 mL/minute: Administer every 24 hours.

Slightly dialyzable (5% to 20%) via hemo- and peritoneal dialysis or via continuous arteriovenous or venovenous hemofiltration; supplemental dose is not necessary.

Hepatic Impairment Use caution; no dosing adjustment required

Administration Should be administered on an empty stomach (ie, 1 hour prior to, or 2 hours after meals) to increase total absorption. Administer at least 1-2 hours prior to, or 4 hours after antacid because aluminum and magnesium cations may chelate with tetracycline and reduce its total absorption.

Monitoring Parameters Renal, hepatic, and hematologic function test, temperature, WBC, cultures and sensitivity, appetite, mental status

◄ **Test Interactions** False-negative urine glucose with Clinistix®

Pharmacotherapy Pearls Use of tetracycline in animal feed has caused emergence of resistant organisms

Tetracycline: Achromycin® V oral suspension, Sumycin® syrup, Tetralan® syrup

Tetracycline hydrochloride: Achromycin® injection, Achromycin® V capsule, Nor-tet® capsule, Panmycin® capsule, Robitet® capsule, Sumycin® capsule and tablet, Teline® capsule, Tetracyn® capsule, Tetralan® capsule

Special Geriatric Considerations The role of tetracycline has decreased because of the emergence of resistant organisms. Doxycycline is the tetracycline of choice when one is indicated because of its better GI absorption, less interactions with divalent cations, longer half-life, and the fact that the majority is cleared by nonrenal mechanisms.

Dosage Forms Excipient information presented when available (limited, particularly for generics); consult specific product labeling.

Capsule, oral, as hydrochloride: 250 mg, 500 mg

Selected References

Yoshikawa TT, "Antimicrobial Therapy for the Elderly Patient," *J Am Geriatr Soc*, 1990, 38(12):1353-72.

◆ **Tetracycline Hydrochloride** see Tetracycline on page 1772
◆ **Tetrahydrocannabinol** see Dronabinol on page 574

Tetrahydrozoline (Nasal) (tet ra hye DROZ a leen)

Brand Names: U.S. Tyzine®; Tyzine® Pediatric
Index Terms Tetrahydrozoline Hydrochloride; Tetryzoline
Generic Availability (U.S.) No
Pharmacologic Category Adrenergic Agonist Agent; Decongestant; Imidazoline Derivative
Use Symptomatic relief of nasal congestion
Dosage
Geriatric & Adult Nasal congestion: Intranasal: Instill 2-4 drops or 3-4 sprays of 0.1% solution into each nostril every 3-4 hours as needed, no more frequently than every 3 hours
Special Geriatric Considerations Evaluate the patient's or caregiver's ability to safely administer the correct dose. Use with caution in patients with cardiovascular disease.
Dosage Forms Excipient information presented when available (limited, particularly for generics); consult specific product labeling.
Solution, intranasal, as hydrochloride [drops]:
Tyzine®: 0.1% (30 mL) [contains benzalkonium chloride]
Tyzine® Pediatric: 0.05% (15 mL) [contains benzalkonium chloride]
Solution, intranasal, as hydrochloride [spray]:
Tyzine®: 0.1% (15 mL) [contains benzalkonium chloride]

Tetrahydrozoline (Ophthalmic) (tet ra hye DROZ a leen)

Medication Safety Issues
Sound-alike/look-alike issues:
Visine® may be confused with Visken®
Brand Names: U.S. Murine® Tears Plus [OTC]; Opti-Clear [OTC]; Visine® Advanced Relief [OTC]; Visine® Original [OTC]
Index Terms Tetrahydrozoline Hydrochloride; Tetryzoline
Pharmacologic Category Adrenergic Agonist Agent; Imidazoline Derivative; Ophthalmic Agent, Vasoconstrictor
Use Symptomatic relief of conjunctival congestion
Contraindications Hypersensitivity to tetrahydrozoline or any component of the formulation.
Warnings/Precautions For ophthalmic use only. Stop use if vision changes, condition worsens, or symptoms persist >72 hours. Use with caution in patients with cardiovascular disease, including hypertension and coronary artery disease. Use with caution in patients with endocrine disorders, including diabetes and hyperthyroidism.
Adverse Reactions (Reflective of adult population; not specific for elderly) Frequency not established
Cardiovascular: Hypertension, palpitation, tachycardia
Central nervous system: Headache
Local: Transient stinging
Neuromuscular & skeletal: Tremor
Ocular: Blurred vision
Drug Interactions
Avoid Concomitant Use There are no known interactions where it is recommended to avoid concomitant use.

Increased Effect/Toxicity There are no known significant interactions involving an increase in effect.

Decreased Effect There are no known significant interactions involving a decrease in effect.

Stability Do not use if solution changes color or becomes cloudy.

Mechanism of Action Stimulates alpha-adrenergic receptors in the arterioles of the conjunctiva to produce vasoconstriction

Pharmacodynamics/Kinetics Duration: Vasoconstriction: 2-3 hours

Dosage

  Geriatric & Adult Conjunctival congestion: Ophthalmic: Instill 1-2 drops in each eye 2-4 times/day

Monitoring Parameters Blood pressure, heart rate

Special Geriatric Considerations Use with caution in patients with cardiovascular disease. Evaluate the patient's or caregiver's ability to safely administer the correct dose of ophthalmic medication.

Dosage Forms Excipient information presented when available (limited, particularly for generics); consult specific product labeling.

  Solution, ophthalmic, as hydrochloride [drops]: 0.05% (15 mL)

    Murine® Tears Plus: 0.05% (15 mL) [contains benzalkonium chloride]

    Opti-Clear: 0.05% (15 mL)

    Visine® Advanced Relief: 0.05% (15 mL, 30 mL) [contains benzalkonium chloride; contains polyethylene glycol]

    Visine® Original: 0.05% (15 mL, 30 mL) [contains benzalkonium chloride]

Theophylline (thee OFF i lin)

Related Information

  Asthma on page 2016

  Beers Criteria – Potentially Inappropriate Medications for Geriatrics on page 2089

Brand Names: U.S. Elixophyllin® Elixir; Theo-24®

Brand Names: Canada Apo-Theo LA®; Novo-Theophyl SR; PMS-Theophylline; Pulmophylline; ratio-Theo-Bronc; Teva-Theophylline SR; Theo ER; Theochron® SR; Theolair; Uniphyl

Index Terms Theophylline Anhydrous

Generic Availability (U.S.) Yes: Extended release tablet, infusion, solution

Pharmacologic Category Theophylline Derivative

Use Treatment of symptoms and reversible airway obstruction due to chronic asthma, or other chronic lung diseases

  Note: The National Heart, Lung, and Blood Institute Guidelines (2007) do not recommend oral theophylline as a long-term control medication for asthma in children ≤4years of age; use may be considered as an alternative (but not preferred) agent in older children and adults. The guidelines do not recommend theophylline I.V. for the treatment of exacerbations of asthma.

Contraindications Hypersensitivity to theophylline or any component of the formulation; premixed injection may contain corn-derived dextrose and its use is contraindicated in patients with allergy to corn-related products

Warnings/Precautions If a patient develops signs and symptoms of theophylline toxicity (eg, persistent, repetitive vomiting), a serum theophylline level should be measured and subsequent doses held. Due to potential saturation of theophylline clearance at serum levels in or (in some patients) less than the therapeutic range, dosage adjustment should be made in small increments (maximum: 25%). Due to wider interpatient variability, theophylline serum level measurements must be used to optimize therapy and prevent serious toxicity. Use with caution in patients with peptic ulcer, hyperthyroidism, seizure disorders, and patients with tachyarrhythmias (eg, sinus tachycardia, atrial fibrillation); use may exacerbate these conditions. Theophylline clearance may be decreased in patients with acute pulmonary edema, congestive heart failure, cor-pulmonale, fever, hepatic disease, acute hepatitis, cirrhosis, hypothyroidism, sepsis with multiorgan failure, and shock; clearance may also be decreased in the elderly >60 years of age and patients following cessation of smoking.

Adverse Reactions (Reflective of adult population; not specific for elderly) Frequency not defined. Adverse events observed at therapeutic serum levels:

Cardiovascular: Flutter, tachycardia

Central nervous system: Headache, hyperactivity (children), insomnia, restlessness, seizures

Endocrine & metabolic: Hypercalcemia (with concomitant hyperthyroid disease)

Gastrointestinal: Nausea, reflux or ulcer aggravation, vomiting

Genitourinary: Difficulty urinating (elderly males with prostatism)

Neuromuscular & skeletal: Tremor

Renal: Diuresis (transient)

Drug Interactions

Metabolism/Transport Effects Substrate of CYP1A2 (major), 2C9 (minor), 2D6 (minor), 2E1 (major), 3A4 (major); **Inhibits** CYP1A2 (weak)

Avoid Concomitant Use

Avoid concomitant use of Theophylline with any of the following: Conivaptan; Deferasirox; Iobenguane I 123

Increased Effect/Toxicity

Theophylline may increase the levels/effects of: Formoterol; Pancuronium; Sympathomimetics

The levels/effects of Theophylline may be increased by: Abiraterone Acetate; Allopurinol; Atomoxetine; Cannabinoids; Cimetidine; Conivaptan; Contraceptives (Estrogens); CYP1A2 Inhibitors (Moderate); CYP1A2 Inhibitors (Strong); CYP3A4 Inhibitors (Moderate); CYP3A4 Inhibitors (Strong); Dasatinib; Deferasirox; Disulfiram; Febuxostat; FluvoxaMINE; Interferons; Isoniazid; Macrolide Antibiotics; Methotrexate; Mexiletine; Pentoxifylline; Propafenone; QuiNINE; Quinolone Antibiotics; Thiabendazole; Ticlopidine; Zafirlukast; Zileuton

Decreased Effect

Theophylline may decrease the levels/effects of: Adenosine; Benzodiazepines; CarBAMazepine; Fosphenytoin; Iobenguane I 123; Lithium; Pancuronium; Phenytoin; Regadenoson; Zafirlukast

The levels/effects of Theophylline may be decreased by: Aminoglutethimide; Barbiturates; Beta-Blockers (Beta1 Selective); Beta-Blockers (Nonselective); CarBAMazepine; CYP1A2 Inducers (Strong); CYP3A4 Inducers (Strong); Cyproterone; Fosphenytoin; Herbs (CYP3A4 Inducers); Isoproterenol; Phenytoin; Protease Inhibitors; Thyroid Products; Tocilizumab

Ethanol/Nutrition/Herb Interactions Food: Food does not appreciably affect the absorption of liquid, fast-release products, and most sustained release products; however, food may induce a sudden release (dose-dumping) of once-daily sustained release products resulting in an increase in serum drug levels and potential toxicity. Avoid excessive amounts of caffeine. Avoid extremes of dietary protein and carbohydrate intake. Changes in diet may affect the elimination of theophylline; charbroiled foods may increase elimination, reducing half-life by 50%.

Stability Tablet, premixed infusion, solution: Store at controlled room temperature of 25°C (77°F).

Mechanism of Action Causes bronchodilatation, diuresis, CNS and cardiac stimulation, and gastric acid secretion by blocking phosphodiesterase which increases tissue concentrations of cyclic adenine monophosphate (cAMP) which in turn promotes catecholamine stimulation of lipolysis, glycogenolysis, and gluconeogenesis and induces release of epinephrine from adrenal medulla cells

Pharmacodynamics/Kinetics

Absorption: Oral: Up to 100%, depending upon the formulation used

Distribution: 0.45 L/kg (range: 0.3-0.7 L/kg) based on ideal body weight; distributes poorly into body fat; V_d may increase in patients with hepatic cirrhosis, acidemia (uncorrected), the elderly

Metabolism: In the liver by demethylation

Protein binding: 40%, primarily to albumin

Half-life elimination: Highly variable and dependent upon age, liver function, cardiac function, lung disease, and smoking history

Adults 16-60 years with asthma, nonsmoking, otherwise healthy: 8.7 hours (range: 6.1-12.8 hours)

Time to peak plasma concentration: 1-2 hours, 4 hours for sustained release

Excretion: Urine (~10% as unchanged theophylline)

Dosage

Geriatric

Acute symptoms: Adults >60 years:

Loading dose: Oral, I.V.: Refer to adult dosing.

Maintenance dose: I.V.: 0.3 mg/kg/hour; maximum 400 mg/day unless serum levels indicate need for larger dose

Chronic conditions: Oral: Adults >60 years: Do not exceed a dose of 400 mg/day

Cardiac decompensation, cor pulmonale, hepatic dysfunction, sepsis with multiorgan failure, shock: Refer to adult dosing.

Adult Note: Doses should be individualized based on peak serum concentrations and should be based on ideal body weight.

Acute symptoms: Loading dose: Oral, I.V.:

If no theophylline received within the previous 24 hours: 4.6 mg/kg loading dose (~5.8 mg/kg hydrous aminophylline) I.V. or 5 mg/kg orally. Loading dose intended to achieve a serum level of approximately 10 mcg/mL; loading doses should be given intravenously (preferred) or with a rapidly absorbed oral product (not an extended-release product). **Note:** On the average, for every 1 mg/kg theophylline given, blood levels will rise 2 mcg/mL.

If theophylline has been administered in the previous 24 hours: A loading dose is not recommended without obtaining a serum theophylline concentration. The loading dose should be calculated as follows:

Dose = (desired serum theophylline concentration - measured serum theophylline concentration) (V_d)

Acute symptoms: Maintenance dose: I.V.: **Note:** To achieve a target concentration of 10 mcg/mL unless otherwise noted. Lower initial doses may be required in patients with reduced theophylline clearance. Dosage should be adjusted according to serum level measurements during the first 12- to 24-hour period.

Adults 16-60 years (otherwise healthy, nonsmokers): 0.4 mg/kg/hour; maximum 900 mg/day unless serum levels indicate need for larger dose

Adults >60 years: 0.3 mg/kg/hour; maximum 400 mg/day unless serum levels indicate need for larger dose

Cardiac decompensation, cor pulmonale, hepatic dysfunction, sepsis with multiorgan failure, shock: 0.2 mg/kg/hour; maximum 400 mg/day unless serum levels indicate need for larger dose

Treatment of chronic conditions: Oral:

Adults 16-60 years **without** risk factors for impaired theophylline clearance: 300 mg/day in divided doses every 6-8 hours for 3 days, then increase to 400 mg/day in divided doses every 6-8 hours for 3 days; maintenance dose: 600 mg/day in divided doses every 6-8 hours

Increase dose only if tolerated. Consider lowering dose or using a slower titration if caffeine-like adverse events occur. Smaller doses given more frequently may be used in patients with a more rapid metabolism to prevent breakthrough symptoms which could occur due to low trough concentration prior to the next dose. Reliably absorbed slow release formulations can be used to decrease serum fluctuations and permit longer dosing intervals.

Dose adjustment in patients **with** risk factors for impaired theophylline clearance and patients in whom monitoring serum theophylline levels is not feasible: Do not exceed a dose of 400 mg/day

Dosage adjustment after serum theophylline measurement:

Within normal limits: 10-19.9 mcg/mL: Maintain dosage if tolerated. Recheck serum theophylline concentration at 24-hour intervals (for acute I.V. dosing) or at 6- to 12-month intervals (for oral dosing). Finer adjustments in dosage may be needed for some patients. If levels ≥15 mcg/mL, consider 10% dose reduction to improve safety margin.

Too high:

20-24.9 mcg/mL: Decrease doses by about 25%. Recheck serum theophylline concentrations (see "Note").

25-30 mcg/mL: Skip next dose (oral) or stop infusion for 24 hours and decrease subsequent doses by about 25%. Recheck serum theophylline concentrations (see "Note").

>30 mcg/mL: Stop dosing and treat overdose; if resumed, decrease subsequent doses by 50%. Recheck serum theophylline concentrations (see "Note").

Too low: <9.9 mcg/mL: If tolerated, but symptoms remain, increase dose by about 25%. Recheck serum theophylline concentrations (see "Note").

Note: Recheck serum theophylline levels after 3 days when using oral dosing, or after 24 hours when dosing intravenously. Patients maintained with oral therapy may be reassessed at 6- to 12-month intervals.

◀ **Administration** Oral: Long-acting preparations should be taken with a full glass of water, swallowed whole, or cut in half if scored. Do **not** crush. Extended release capsule forms may be opened and the contents sprinkled on soft foods; do **not** chew beads.

Monitoring Parameters Monitor heart rate, CNS effects (insomnia, irritability); respiratory rate (COPD patients often have resting controlled respiratory rates in low 20s); arterial or capillary blood gases (if applicable)

Theophylline levels: Serum theophylline levels should be monitored prior to making dose increases; in the presence of signs or symptoms of toxicity; or when a new illness, worsening of a present illness, or medication changes occur that may change theophylline clearance

I.V. loading dose: Measure serum concentrations 30 minutes after the end of an I.V. loading dose

I.V. infusion: Measure serum concentrations one half-life after starting a continuous infusion, then every 12-24 hours

Reference Range Therapeutic levels: Asthma:

Children: 5-10 mcg/mL

Adults: 5-15 mcg/mL

Test Interactions Plasma glucose, uric acid, free fatty acids, total cholesterol, HDL, HDL/LDL ratio, and urinary free cortisol excretion may be increased by theophylline. Theophylline may decrease triiodothyronine.

Pharmacotherapy Pearls Saliva levels are approximately equal to 60% of plasma concentrations. Charcoal-broiled foods may increase elimination, reducing half-life by 50%; cigarette smoking may require an increase of dosage by 50% to 100%. Because different salts of theophylline have different theophylline content, various salts are equivalent. The following are percent content of theophylline for various salts:

Theophylline anhydrous: 100%

Theophylline monohydrate: 91%

Aminophylline anhydrous: 86%

Oxtriphylline: 64%

Most preparations are now labeled with actual milligram content delivered by the particular product.

Theophylline immediate release tablet/capsule: Bronkodyl®, Elixophyllin®, Quibron®-T, Slo-Phyllin®, Somophyllin®-T, Theolair™

Theophylline liquid: Accurbron®, Aerolate®, Aquaphyllin®, Asmalix®, Elixicon®, Elixophyllin®, Lixolin®, Theon®

Theophylline timed release capsule: Aerolate III®, Aerolate JR®, Aerolate SR®, Elixophyllin® SR, Lodrane®, Slo-bid™ Gyrocaps®, Slo-Phyllin® Gyrocaps®, Somophyllin®-CRT, Theobid®, Theoclear® L.A., Theophyl-SR®, Theospan®-SR, Theospan®-SR

Theophylline timed release tablet: Constant-T®, Duraphyl™, LaBID®, Quibron®-T/S, Respbid®, Sustaire®, Theochron®, Theo-Dur®, Theolair™-SR, Theo-Time®, Uniphyl®

Special Geriatric Considerations Although there is a great intersubject variability for half-lives of methylxanthines (2-10 hours), elderly as a group have slower hepatic clearance. Therefore, use lower initial doses and monitor closely for response and adverse reactions. Additionally, elderly are at greater risk for toxicity due to concomitant disease (eg, CHF, arrhythmias), and drug use (eg, cimetidine, ciprofloxacin).

Dosage Forms Excipient information presented when available (limited, particularly for generics); consult specific product labeling. [DSC] = Discontinued product

Capsule, extended release, oral:

Theo-24®: 100 mg, 200 mg, 300 mg, 400 mg [24 hours]

Infusion, premixed in D₅W: 400 mg (250 mL [DSC], 500 mL); 800 mg (250 mL [DSC], 500 mL)

Solution, oral: 80 mg/15 mL (15 mL)

Elixophyllin® Elixir: 80 mg/15 mL (473 mL) [contains ethanol 20%; mixed fruit flavor]

Tablet, extended release, oral: 100 mg, 200 mg, 300 mg, 400 mg, 450 mg, 600 mg

Selected References

Expert Panel Report 3, "Guidelines for the Diagnosis and Management of Asthma," Clinical Practice Guidelines, National Institutes of Health, National Heart, Lung, and Blood Institute, NIH Publication No. 08-4051, prepublication 2007. Available at http://www.nhlbi.nih.gov/guidelines/asthma/asthgdln.htm

◆ **Theophylline Anhydrous** see Theophylline on page 1775

◆ **Theophylline Ethylenediamine** see Aminophylline on page 94

◆ **Theraflu® Thin Strips® Multi Symptom [OTC]** see DiphenhydrAMINE (Systemic) on page 520

◆ **Thera-Sal [OTC]** see Salicylic Acid on page 1648

◆ **Thermazene®** see Silver Sulfadiazine on page 1678

◆ **Thiamazole** see Methimazole on page 1165

◆ **Thiamin** see Thiamine on page 1779

Thiamine (THYE a min)

Medication Safety Issues
Sound-alike/look-alike issues:
Thiamine may be confused with Tenormin®, Thalomid®, Thorazine®
International issues:
Doxal® [Brazil] may be confused with Doxil® which is a brand name for doxorubicin in the U.S.
Doxal® [Brazil]: Brand name for doxycycline in Austria; brand name for pyridoxine/thiamine combination in Brazil; brand name for doxepin in Finland

Brand Names: Canada Betaxin®

Index Terms Aneurine Hydrochloride; Thiamin; Thiamine Hydrochloride; Thiaminium Chloride Hydrochloride; Vitamin B_1

Generic Availability (U.S.) Yes

Pharmacologic Category Vitamin, Water Soluble

Use Treatment of thiamine deficiency including beriberi, Wernicke's encephalopathy, Korsakoff's syndrome, or in alcoholic patients; dietary supplement

Contraindications Hypersensitivity to thiamine or any component of the formulation

Warnings/Precautions Use with caution with parenteral route (especially I.V.) of administration. Hypersensitivity reactions have been reported following repeated parenteral doses; consider skin test in individuals with history of allergic reactions. Single vitamin deficiency is rare; evaluate for other deficiencies. Dextrose administration may precipitate acute symptoms of thiamine deficiency; use caution when thiamine status is marginal or suspect. Some parenteral products contain aluminum; use caution in patients with impaired renal function.

Adverse Reactions (Reflective of adult population; not specific for elderly) Adverse reactions reported with injection. Frequency not defined.
Cardiovascular: Cyanosis
Central nervous system: Restlessness
Dermatologic: Angioneurotic edema, pruritus, urticaria
Gastrointestinal: Hemorrhage into GI tract, nausea, tightness of the throat
Local: Induration and/or tenderness at the injection site (following I.M. administration)
Neuromuscular & skeletal: Weakness
Respiratory: Pulmonary edema
Miscellaneous: Anaphylactic/hypersensitivity reactions (following I.V. administration), diaphoresis, warmth

Drug Interactions
Avoid Concomitant Use There are no known interactions where it is recommended to avoid concomitant use.
Increased Effect/Toxicity There are no known significant interactions involving an increase in effect.
Decreased Effect There are no known significant interactions involving a decrease in effect.

Ethanol/Nutrition/Herb Interactions
Ethanol: May decrease thiamine absorption.
Food: High carbohydrate diets may increase thiamine requirement.

Stability Injection: Store at 15°C to 30°C (59°F to 86°F). Protect from light

Mechanism of Action An essential coenzyme in carbohydrate metabolism by combining with adenosine triphosphate to form thiamine pyrophosphate

Pharmacodynamics/Kinetics
Absorption: Oral: Adequate; I.M.: Rapid and complete
Distribution: Highest concentrations found in brain, heart, kidney, liver; crosses the placenta, enters breast milk
Excretion: Urine (as unchanged drug and as pyrimidine after body storage sites become saturated)

Dosage
Geriatric & Adult
Recommended daily intake: Female: 1.1 mg; Male: 1.2 mg
Parenteral nutrition supplementation: 6 mg/day; may be increased to 25-50 mg/day with history of alcohol abuse
Thiamine deficiency (beriberi): 5-30 mg/dose I.M. or I.V. 3 times/day (if critically ill); then orally 5-30 mg/day in single or divided doses 3 times/day for 1 month
Alcohol withdrawal syndrome: 100 mg/day I.M. or I.V. for several days, followed by 50-100 mg/day orally

◄   **Wernicke's encephalopathy:** Treatment (manufacturer labeling): Initial: 100 mg I.V., then 50-100 mg/day I.M. or I.V. until consuming a regular, balanced diet. However, larger doses may be required based on failure of lower doses to produce clinical improvement in some patients.

    Alternate dosage: The Royal College of Physicians (U.K.) has recommended the use of higher doses of thiamine (in combination with other B vitamins, ascorbic acid, potassium, phosphate, and magnesium) for the management of Wernicke's encephalopathy (Thomson, 2002):

    Prophylaxis: 250 mg I.V. once daily for 3-5 days

    Treatment: Initial: 500 mg I.V. 3 times/day for 3 days. If response to thiamine after 3 days, continue with 250 mg I.M. or I.V. once daily for an additional 5 days or until clinical improvement.

Administration Parenteral form may be administered by I.M. or I.V. injection. Various rates of administration have been reported. Local injection reactions may be minimized by slow administration (~30 minutes) into larger, more proximal veins. Thiamine should be administered prior to parenteral glucose solutions to prevent precipitation of acute symptoms of thiamine deficiency in the poorly nourished.

Reference Range Normal, serum: 1.1-1.6 mg/dL

Test Interactions False-positive for uric acid using the phosphotungstate method and for urobilinogen using the Ehrlich's reagent; large doses may interfere with the spectrophotometric determination of serum theophylline concentration

Pharmacotherapy Pearls Thiamine (vitamin B_1) is unstable in alkaline or neutral solutions, therefore, do not mix with carbonates, citrates, barbiturates. Also, any solution containing sulfites is incompatible with thiamine. Recommended thiamine intake is 0.5 mg/1000 Kcal.

Special Geriatric Considerations No special recommendations are necessary. Elderly are treated the same as younger adults.

Dosage Forms Excipient information presented when available (limited, particularly for generics); consult specific product labeling.

Injection, solution, as hydrochloride: 100 mg/mL (2 mL)

Tablet, oral, as hydrochloride: 50 mg, 100 mg, 250 mg, 500 mg

Selected References

Bayard M, McIntyre J, Hill K, et al, "Alcohol Withdrawal Syndrome," *Am Fam Physician*, 2004, 69(6):1443-50.

Mirtallo J, Canada T, Johnson D, et al, "Safe Practices for Parenteral Nutrition. Task Force for the Revision of Safe Practices for Parenteral Nutrition,"*JPEN J Parenter Enteral Nutr*, 2004, 28(6):39-70.

Sechi G and Serra A, "Wernicke's Encephalopathy: New Clinical Settings and Recent Advances in Diagnosis and Management," *Lancet Neurol*, 2007, 6(5):442-55.

Thomson AD, Cook CC, Touquet R, et al, "The Royal College of Physicians Report on Alcohol: Guidelines for Managing Wernicke's Encephalopathy in the Accident and Emergency Department," *Alcohol Alcohol*, 2002, 37 (6):513-21.

◆ **Thiamine Hydrochloride** *see* Thiamine *on page 1779*
◆ **Thiaminium Chloride Hydrochloride** *see* Thiamine *on page 1779*

Thioridazine (thye oh RID a zeen)

Related Information

Antipsychotic Agents *on page 1997*

Beers Criteria – Potentially Inappropriate Medications for Geriatrics *on page 2089*

Liquid Compatibility of Antidepressants, Antipsychotics, and Mood Stabilizers *on page 2111*

Medication Safety Issues

Sound-alike/look-alike issues:

Thioridazine may be confused with thiothixene, Thorazine®

Mellaril® may be confused with Elavil®, Mebaral®

BEERS Criteria medication:

This drug may be inappropriate for use in geriatric patients (high severity risk).

Index Terms Thioridazine Hydrochloride

Generic Availability (U.S.) Yes

Pharmacologic Category Antipsychotic Agent, Typical, Phenothiazine

Use Management of schizophrenic patients who fail to respond adequately to treatment with other antipsychotic drugs, either because of insufficient effectiveness or the inability to achieve an effective dose due to intolerable adverse effects from those medications

Unlabeled/Investigational Use Behavioral symptoms associated with dementia (elderly); psychosis/agitation related to Alzheimer's dementia

Contraindications Severe CNS depression; severe hyper-/hypotensive heart disease; coma; in combination with other drugs that are known to prolong the QT_c interval and/or CYP2D6 inhibitors; in patients with congenital long QT syndrome or a history of cardiac arrhythmias; concurrent use with medications that inhibit the metabolism of thioridazine (fluoxetine, paroxetine, fluvoxamine, propranolol, pindolol); patients known to have genetic defect leading to reduced levels of activity of CYP2D6

Warnings/Precautions [U.S. Boxed Warning]: Thioridazine has dose-related effects on ventricular repolarization leading to QT_c prolongation, a potentially life-threatening effect. Therefore, it should be reserved for patients with schizophrenia who have failed to respond to adequate levels of other antipsychotic drugs. Due to potential for QT_c prolongation; use contraindicated with concomitant CYP2D6 inhibitors and/or concomitant use with other agents that prolong the QT_c interval. May cause orthostatic hypotension; use with caution in patients at risk of this effect or those who would tolerate transient hypotensive episodes (cerebrovascular disease, cardiovascular disease, or other medications which may predispose). **[U.S. Boxed Warning]: Elderly patients with dementia-related psychosis treated with antipsychotics are at an increased risk of death compared to placebo.** Most deaths appeared to be either cardiovascular (eg, heart failure, sudden death) or infectious (eg, pneumonia) in nature. Thioridazine is not approved for the treatment of dementia-related psychosis.

Leukopenia, neutropenia, and agranulocytosis (sometimes fatal) have been reported in clinical trials and postmarketing reports with antipsychotic use; presence of risk factors (eg, pre-existing low WBC or history of drug-induced leuko-/neutropenia) should prompt periodic blood count assessment. Discontinue therapy at first signs of blood dyscrasias or if absolute neutrophil count <1000/mm^3.

Highly sedating, use with caution in disorders where CNS depression is a feature. Use with caution in Parkinson's disease. Use caution in patients with hemodynamic instability; predisposition to seizures; subcortical brain damage; severe cardiac, hepatic, or renal disease. Esophageal dysmotility and aspiration have been associated with antipsychotic use; use with caution in patients at risk of pneumonia (ie, Alzheimer's disease). Use associated with increased prolactin levels; clinical significance of hyperprolactinemia in patients with breast cancer or other prolactin-dependent tumors is unknown. May alter temperature regulation or mask toxicity of other drugs due to antiemetic effects.

Phenothiazines may cause anticholinergic effects (confusion, agitation, constipation, xerostomia, blurred vision, urinary retention); therefore, they should be used with caution in patients with decreased gastrointestinal motility, urinary retention, BPH, xerostomia, or visual problems. Conditions which also may be exacerbated by cholinergic blockade include narrow-angle glaucoma and worsening of myasthenia gravis. Relative to other neuroleptics, thioridazine has a high potency of cholinergic blockade.

May cause extrapyramidal symptoms (EPS), including pseudoparkinsonism, acute dystonic reactions, akathisia, and tardive dyskinesia. Risk of dystonia (and possibly other EPS) may be greater with increased doses, use of conventional antipsychotics, males, and younger patients. May be inappropriate for use in the elderly due to risk of CNS and EPS adverse effects (Beers Criteria). May be associated with neuroleptic malignant syndrome (NMS). May cause pigmentary retinopathy, and lenticular and corneal deposits, particularly with prolonged therapy.

Adverse Reactions (Reflective of adult population; not specific for elderly) Frequency not defined.

Cardiovascular: Hypotension, orthostatic hypotension, peripheral edema, ECG changes

Central nervous system: EPS (pseudoparkinsonism, akathisia, dystonias, tardive dyskinesia), dizziness, drowsiness, neuroleptic malignant syndrome (NMS), impairment of temperature regulation, lowering of seizure threshold, seizure

Dermatologic: Increased sensitivity to sun, rash, discoloration of skin (blue-gray)

Endocrine & metabolic: Changes in menstrual cycle, libido (changes in), breast pain, galactorrhea, amenorrhea

Gastrointestinal: Constipation, weight gain, nausea, vomiting, stomach pain, xerostomia, nausea, vomiting, diarrhea

Genitourinary: Difficulty in urination, ejaculatory disturbances, urinary retention, priapism

Hematologic: Agranulocytosis, leukopenia

Hepatic: Cholestatic jaundice, hepatotoxicity

Neuromuscular & skeletal: Tremor

Ocular: Pigmentary retinopathy, blurred vision, cornea and lens changes

Respiratory: Nasal congestion

Drug Interactions

Metabolism/Transport Effects Substrate of CYP2C19 (minor), 2D6 (major); **Inhibits** CYP1A2 (weak), 2C9 (weak), 2D6 (moderate), 2E1 (weak)

THIORIDAZINE

◄ **Avoid Concomitant Use**

Avoid concomitant use of Thioridazine with any of the following: Artemether; CYP2D6 Inhibitors; Dronedarone; FluvoxaMINE; Lumefantrine; Metoclopramide; Moclobemide; Nilotinib; Pimozide; QTc-Prolonging Agents; QUEtiapine; QuiNINE; Tamoxifen; Tetrabenazine; Toremifene; Vandetanib; Vemurafenib; Ziprasidone

Increased Effect/Toxicity

Thioridazine may increase the levels/effects of: Alcohol (Ethyl); Analgesics (Opioid); Anticholinergics; Anti-Parkinson's Agents (Dopamine Agonist); Atomoxetine; Beta-Blockers; CNS Depressants; CYP2D6 Substrates; Dronedarone; Fesoterodine; Methylphenidate; Pimozide; Porfimer; QTc-Prolonging Agents; QuiNINE; Selective Serotonin Reuptake Inhibitors; Tamoxifen; Tetrabenazine; Toremifene; Vandetanib; Vemurafenib; Ziprasidone

The levels/effects of Thioridazine may be increased by: Abiraterone Acetate; Acetylcholinesterase Inhibitors (Central); Alfuzosin; Antimalarial Agents; Artemether; Beta-Blockers; Chloroquine; Ciprofloxacin; Ciprofloxacin (Systemic); CYP2D6 Inhibitors; Darunavir; FluvoxaMINE; Gadobutrol; Lithium formulations; Lumefantrine; Methylphenidate; Metoclopramide; Moclobemide; Nilotinib; Pramlintide; QTc-Prolonging Agents; QUEtiapine; QuiNINE; Tetrabenazine

Decreased Effect

Thioridazine may decrease the levels/effects of: Amphetamines; Quinagolide

The levels/effects of Thioridazine may be decreased by: Antacids; Anti-Parkinson's Agents (Dopamine Agonist); Lithium formulations; Peginterferon Alfa-2b

Ethanol/Nutrition/Herb Interactions

Ethanol: May increase CNS depression; monitor for increased effects with coadministration. Caution patients about effects.

Herb/Nutraceutical: Avoid kava kava, valerian, St John's wort, gotu kola (may increase CNS depression). Avoid dong quai, St John's wort (may also cause photosensitization).

Stability Protect from light.

Mechanism of Action Thioridazine is a piperidine phenothiazine which blocks postsynaptic mesolimbic dopaminergic receptors in the brain; exhibits a strong alpha-adrenergic blocking effect and depresses the release of hypothalamic and hypophyseal hormones

Pharmacodynamics/Kinetics

Absorption: May be affected by the inherent anticholinergic action on the gastrointestinal tissue causing variable absorption. Absorption from tablets is erratic with less variation seen with solutions. These agents are widely distributed in tissues with CNS concentrations exceeding that of plasma due to their lipophilic characteristics.

Protein binding: Antipsychotic agents are bound 90% to 99% to plasma proteins; highly bound to brain and lung tissue and other tissues with a high blood perfusion.

Metabolism: Hepatic

Time to peak concentration: Oral: 2-4 hours

Elimination: Occurs through hepatic metabolism (oxidation) where numerous active metabolites are produced; active metabolites excreted in urine; elimination half-lives of antipsychotics ranges from 20-40 hours which may be extended in older adults due to decline in oxidative hepatic reactions (phase I) with age.

The biologic effect of a single dose persists for 24 hours. When the patient has accommodated to initial side effects (sedation), once daily dosing is possible due to the long half-life of antipsychotics.

Steady-state plasma concentrations are achieved in 4-7 days; therefore, if possible, do not make dose adjustments more than once in a 7-day period. Due to the long half-lives of antipsychotics, as needed (prn) use is ineffective since repeated doses are necessary to achieve therapeutic tissue concentrations in the CNS.

Dosage

Geriatric Behavioral symptoms associated with dementia (unlabeled use): Oral: Initial: 10-25 mg 1-2 times/day; increase at 4- to 7-day intervals by 10-25 mg/day; increase dose intervals (once daily, twice daily, etc) as necessary to control response or side effects. Maximum daily dose: 400 mg; gradual increases (titration) may prevent some side effects or decrease their severity.

Adult

Schizophrenia/psychosis: Oral: Initial: 50-100 mg 3 times/day with gradual increments as needed and tolerated; maximum: 800 mg/day in 2-4 divided doses

Depressive disorders, dementia (unlabeled use): Oral: Initial: 25 mg 3 times/day; maintenance dose: 20-200 mg/day

Renal Impairment Not dialyzable (0% to 5%)

Administration Oral concentrate must be diluted in 2-4 oz of liquid (eg, water, fruit juice, carbonated drinks, milk, or pudding) before administration. Do not take antacid within 2 hours of taking drug. Thioridazine concentrate is not compatible with carbamazepine suspension; schedule dosing at least 1-2 hours apart from each other. **Note:** Avoid skin contact with oral suspension or solution; may cause contact dermatitis.

Monitoring Parameters Orthostatic blood pressures; tremors, gait changes, abnormal movement in trunk, neck, buccal area, or extremities; monitor target behaviors for which the agent is given. Baseline and periodic ECG and serum potassium; periodic eye exam, CBC with differential, blood pressure, liver enzyme tests; do not initiate if QT_c >450 msec

Reference Range Toxic: >1 mg/mL; lethal: 2-8 mg/dL

Test Interactions False-positives for phenylketonuria, urinary amylase, uroporphyrins, urobilinogen; may interfere with urine detection of methadone and PCP (false-positives)

Pharmacotherapy Pearls May cause stomach upset; may cause thermoregulatory changes.

Special Geriatric Considerations Any changes in disease status in any organ system can result in behavior changes.

Many elderly patients receive antipsychotic medications for inappropriate nonpsychotic behavior. Before initiating antipsychotic medication, the clinician should investigate any possible reversible cause; any stress or stress from any disease can cause acute "confusion" or worsening of baseline nonpsychotic behavior. Most commonly acute changes in behavior are due to increases in drug dose or addition of new drug to regimen; fluid electrolyte loss; infections; and changes in environment.

In the treatment of agitated, demented, older adult patients, authors of meta-analysis of controlled trials of the response to the traditional antipsychotics (phenothiazines, butyrophenones) in controlling agitation have concluded that the use of neuroleptics results in a response rate of 18%. Clearly neuroleptic therapy for behavior control should be limited with frequent attempts to withdraw the agent given for behavior control.

This medication is considered to be potentially inappropriate in this patient population (Beers Criteria severity: High).

Dosage Forms Excipient information presented when available (limited, particularly for generics); consult specific product labeling.

Tablet, oral, as hydrochloride: 10 mg, 25 mg, 50 mg, 100 mg

Selected References

Appell RA, Shield DE, and McGuire EJ, "Thioridazine-Induced Priapism," *Br J Urol*, 1977, 49(2):160.

Rabins PV, Blacker D, Rovner BW, et al, "Practice Guidelines for the Treatment of Patients With Alzheimer's Disease and Other Dementias," *Am J Psychiatry*, 2007, 164(12 Suppl):5-56. Available at http://www.psych.org/psych_pract/treatg/pg/prac_guide.cfm.

Schneider LS, Tariot PN, Dagerman KS, et al, "Effectiveness of Atypical Antipsychotic Drugs in Patients With Alzheimer's Disease," *N Engl J Med*, 2006, 355(15):1525-38.

◆ **Thioridazine Hydrochloride** *see* Thioridazine *on page 1780*

Thiothixene (thye oh THIKS een)

Related Information

Antipsychotic Agents *on page 1997*

Beers Criteria – Potentially Inappropriate Medications for Geriatrics *on page 2089*

Liquid Compatibility of Antidepressants, Antipsychotics, and Mood Stabilizers *on page 2111*

Medication Safety Issues

Sound-alike/look-alike issues:

Thiothixene may be confused with FLUoxetine, thioridazine

Navane® may be confused with Norvasc®, Nubain®

Brand Names: U.S. Navane®

Brand Names: Canada Navane®

Index Terms Tiotixene

Generic Availability (U.S.) Yes

Pharmacologic Category Antipsychotic Agent, Typical

Use Management of schizophrenia

Unlabeled/Investigational Use Nonpsychotic patient, dementia behavior (elderly); psychosis/agitation related to Alzheimer's dementia

Contraindications Hypersensitivity to thiothixene or any component of the formulation; severe CNS depression; circulatory collapse; blood dyscrasias; coma

Warnings/Precautions [U.S. Boxed Warning]: Elderly patients with dementia-related psychosis treated with antipsychotics are at an increased risk of death compared to placebo. Most deaths appeared to be either cardiovascular (eg, heart failure, sudden death) or infectious (eg, pneumonia) in nature. Thiothixene is not approved for the treatment of dementia-related psychosis.

◄ May alter cardiac conduction; life-threatening arrhythmias have occurred with therapeutic doses of antipsychotics. Avoid use in patients with underlying QT prolongation, in those taking medicines that prolong the QT interval, or cause polymorphic ventricular tachycardia; monitor ECG closely for dose-related QT effects.

Leukopenia, neutropenia, and agranulocytosis (sometimes fatal) have been reported in clinical trials and postmarketing reports with antipsychotic use; presence of risk factors (eg, pre-existing low WBC or history of drug-induced leuko-/neutropenia) should prompt periodic blood count assessment. Discontinue therapy at first signs of blood dyscrasias or if absolute neutrophil count <1000/mm^3.

Antipsychotic use has been associated with esophageal dysmotility and aspiration; use with caution in patients at risk of pneumonia (ie, Alzheimer's disease). May cause extrapyramidal symptoms (EPS), including pseudoparkinsonism, acute dystonic reactions, akathisia, and tardive dyskinesia. Risk of dystonia (and possibly other EPS) may be greater with increased doses, use of conventional antipsychotics, males, and younger patients. Use may be associated with NMS; monitor for mental status changes, fever, muscle rigidity, and/or autonomic instability. May cause orthostatic hypotension; use with caution in patients at risk of this effect or in those who would not tolerate transient hypotensive episodes (cerebrovascular disease, cardiovascular disease, hypovolemia, or concurrent medication use which may predispose to hypotension/bradycardia). May rarely cause pigmentary retinopathy and lenticular pigmentation. Impaired core body temperature regulation may occur; caution with strenuous exercise, heat exposure, dehydration, and concomitant medication possessing anticholinergic effects.

May be sedating, use with caution in disorders where CNS depression is a feature; patients must be cautioned about performing tasks which require mental alertness (eg, operating machinery or driving). Effects may be potentiated when used with other sedative drugs or ethanol. May cause anticholinergic effects (constipation, xerostomia, blurred vision, urinary retention); use with caution in patients with decreased gastrointestinal motility, paralytic ileus, urinary retention, BPH, xerostomia, or visual problems. Relative to other neuroleptics, thiothixene has a low potency of cholinergic blockade. May mask toxicity of other drugs or conditions (eg, intestinal obstruction, Reye's syndrome, brain tumor) due to antiemetic effects. Use is associated with increased prolactin levels; clinical significance of hyperprolactinemia in patients with breast cancer or other prolactin-dependent tumors is unknown.

Use with caution in patients with severe cardiovascular disease, narrow-angle glaucoma, hepatic impairment, myasthenia gravis, Parkinson's disease, renal impairment, or seizure disorder. Use with caution in the elderly.

Adverse Reactions (Reflective of adult population; not specific for elderly) Frequency not defined.

Cardiovascular: Hypotension, nonspecific ECG changes, syncope, tachycardia

Central nervous system: Agitation, dizziness, drowsiness, extrapyramidal symptoms (akathisia, dystonias, lightheadedness, pseudoparkinsonism, tardive dyskinesia), insomnia restlessness

Dermatologic: Discoloration of skin (blue-gray), photosensitivity, pruritus, rash, urticaria

Endocrine & metabolic: Amenorrhea, breast pain, libido (changes in), changes in menstrual cycle, galactorrhea, gynecomastia, hyper-/hypoglycemia, hyperprolactinemia, lactation

Gastrointestinal: Constipation, nausea, salivation increased, stomach pain, vomiting, weight gain, xerostomia

Genitourinary: Difficulty in urination, ejaculatory disturbances, impotence

Hematologic: Leukocytes, leukopenia

Neuromuscular & skeletal: Tremors

Ocular: Blurred vision, pigmentary retinopathy

Respiratory: Nasal congestion

Miscellaneous: Diaphoresis

Drug Interactions

Metabolism/Transport Effects Substrate of CYP1A2 (major); **Inhibits** CYP2D6 (weak)

Avoid Concomitant Use

Avoid concomitant use of Thiothixene with any of the following: Artemether; Dronedarone; Lumefantrine; Metoclopramide; Nilotinib; Pimozide; QUEtiapine; QuiNINE; Tetrabenazine; Thioridazine; Toremifene; Vandetanib; Vemurafenib; Ziprasidone

Increased Effect/Toxicity

Thiothixene may increase the levels/effects of: Alcohol (Ethyl); Anticholinergics; Anti-Parkinson's Agents (Dopamine Agonist); CNS Depressants; Dronedarone; Methylphenidate; Pimozide; QTc-Prolonging Agents; QuiNINE; Selective Serotonin Reuptake Inhibitors; Tetrabenazine; Thioridazine; Toremifene; Vandetanib; Vemurafenib; Ziprasidone

The levels/effects of Thiothixene may be increased by: Abiraterone Acetate; Acetylcholinesterase Inhibitors (Central); Alfuzosin; Artemether; Chloroquine; Ciprofloxacin; Ciprofloxacin (Systemic); CYP1A2 Inhibitors (Moderate); CYP1A2 Inhibitors (Strong); Deferasirox; Gadobutrol; HydrOXYzine; Lithium formulations; Lumefantrine; Methylphenidate; Metoclopramide; Nilotinib; Pramlintide; QUEtiapine; QuiNINE; Tetrabenazine

Decreased Effect

Thiothixene may decrease the levels/effects of: Amphetamines; Quinagolide

The levels/effects of Thiothixene may be decreased by: Anti-Parkinson's Agents (Dopamine Agonist); CYP1A2 Inducers (Strong); Cyproterone; Lithium formulations

Ethanol/Nutrition/Herb Interactions

Ethanol: May increase CNS depression; monitor for increased effects with coadministration. Caution patients about effects.

Herb/Nutraceutical: Avoid kava kava, valerian, St John's wort, gotu kola (may increase CNS depression).

Mechanism of Action Thiothixene is a thioxanthene antipsychotic which elicits antipsychotic activity by postsynaptic blockade of CNS dopamine receptors resulting in inhibition of dopamine-mediated effects; also has alpha-adrenergic blocking activity

Pharmacodynamics/Kinetics

Absorption: May be affected by the inherent anticholinergic action on the gastrointestinal tissue causing variable absorption. Absorption from tablets is erratic with less variation seen with solutions. These agents are widely distributed in tissues with CNS concentrations exceeding that of plasma due to their lipophilic characteristics.

Protein binding: Antipsychotic agents are bound 90% to 99% to plasma proteins; highly bound to brain and lung tissue and other tissues with a high blood perfusion.

Metabolism: Extensive in the liver

Half-life: >24 hours with chronic use

Time to peak serum concentration: Oral: 2-4 hours

Elimination: Occurs through hepatic metabolism (oxidation) where numerous active metabolites are produced; active metabolites excreted in urine; elimination half-lives of antipsychotics ranges from 20-40 hours which may be extended in older adults due to decline in oxidative hepatic reactions (phase I) with age.

The biologic effect of a single dose persists for 24 hours. When the patient has accommodated to initial side effects (sedation), once daily dosing is possible due to the long half-life of antipsychotics.

Steady-state plasma concentrations are achieved in 4-7 days; therefore, if possible, do not make dose adjustments more than once in a 7-day period. Due to the long half-lives of antipsychotics, as needed (prn) use is ineffective since repeated doses are necessary to achieve therapeutic tissue concentrations in the CNS.

Dosage

Geriatric Nonpsychotic patient, dementia behavior (unlabeled use): Initial: 1-2 mg 1-2 times/day; increase dose at 4- to 7-day intervals by 1-2 mg/day. Increase dosing intervals (bid, tid, etc) as necessary to control response or side effects; maximum daily dose: 30 mg. Gradual increases in dose may prevent some side effects or decrease their severity.

Adult

Mild-to-moderate psychosis: Oral: 2 mg 3 times/day, up to 20-30 mg/day; more severe psychosis: Initial: 5 mg 2 times/day, may increase gradually, if necessary; maximum: 60 mg/day

Rapid tranquilization of the agitated patient (administered every 30-60 minutes): Oral: 5-10 mg; average total dose for tranquilization: 15-30 mg

Renal Impairment Not dialyzable (0% to 5%)

Administration Oral (concentrate) solution: Dilute immediately before administration with water, fruit juice, milk, etc. **Note:** Avoid skin contact with oral medication; may cause contact dermatitis.

Monitoring Parameters Orthostatic blood pressures; tremors; gait changes, abnormal movement in trunk, neck, buccal area, or extremities; monitor target behaviors for which the agent is given. Monitor orthostatic blood pressures 3-5 days after initiation of therapy or a dose increase.

Special Geriatric Considerations Any changes in disease status in any organ system can result in behavior changes.

Many elderly patients receive antipsychotic medications for inappropriate nonpsychotic behavior. Before initiating antipsychotic medication, the clinician should investigate any possible reversible cause; any stress or stress from any disease can cause acute "confusion" or worsening of baseline nonpsychotic behavior. Most commonly acute changes in behavior are due to increases in drug dose or addition of new drug to regimen; fluid electrolyte loss; infections; and changes in environment.

In the treatment of agitated, demented, elderly patients, authors of meta-analysis of controlled trials of the response to the traditional antipsychotics (phenothiazines, butyrophenones) in controlling agitation have concluded that the use of neuroleptics results in a response rate of 18%. Clearly neuroleptic therapy for behavior control should be limited with frequent attempts to withdraw the agent given for behavior control.

Dosage Forms Excipient information presented when available (limited, particularly for generics); consult specific product labeling. [DSC] = Discontinued product

Capsule, oral: 1 mg, 2 mg, 5 mg, 10 mg

Navane®: 2 mg, 5 mg [DSC], 10 mg, 20 mg

Selected References

Rabins PV, Blacker D, Rovner BW, et al, "Practice Guidelines for the Treatment of Patients With Alzheimer's Disease and Other Dementias," *Am J Psychiatry*, 2007, 164(12 Suppl):5-56. Available at http://www.psych.org/psych_pract/treatg/pg/prac_guide.cfm.

Schneider LS, Tariot PN, Dagerman KS, et al, "Effectiveness of Atypical Antipsychotic Drugs in Patients With Alzheimer's Disease," *N Engl J Med*, 2006, 355(15):1525-38.

◆ **Thonzonium, Neomycin, Colistin, and Hydrocortisone** *see* Neomycin, Colistin, Hydrocortisone, and Thonzonium *on page 1280*

◆ **Thorazine** *see* ChlorproMAZINE *on page 339*

◆ **Thrive™ [OTC]** *see* Nicotine *on page 1297*

Thyroid, Desiccated (THYE roid DES i kay tid)

Related Information

Beers Criteria – Potentially Inappropriate Medications for Geriatrics *on page 2089*

Medication Safety Issues

BEERS Criteria medication:

This drug may be inappropriate for use in geriatric patients (high severity risk).

Brand Names: U.S. Armour® Thyroid; Nature-Throid™; Westhroid™

Index Terms Desiccated Thyroid; Levothyroxine and Liothyronine; Tetraiodothyronine and Triiodothyronine; Thyroid Extract; Thyroid USP

Generic Availability (U.S.) Yes

Pharmacologic Category Thyroid Product

Use Replacement or supplemental therapy in hypothyroidism; pituitary TSH suppressants (thyroid nodules, thyroiditis, multinodular goiter, thyroid cancer)

Contraindications Hypersensitivity to beef or pork or any component of the formulation; untreated thyrotoxicosis; uncorrected adrenal insufficiency

Warnings/Precautions [U.S. Boxed Warning]: In euthyroid patients, thyroid supplements are ineffective and potentially toxic for weight reduction. High doses may produce serious or even life-threatening toxic effects particularly when used with some anorectic drugs. Thyroid supplements are not recommended for the treatment of female or male infertility, unless associated with hypothyroidism. Use with caution and reduce dosage in patients with angina pectoris or other cardiovascular disease and elderly since they may be more likely to have compromised cardiovascular function (Beers Criteria); chronic hypothyroidism predisposes patients to coronary artery disease. Use with caution in patients with adrenal insufficiency (contraindicated with uncorrected adrenal insufficiency), diabetes mellitus or insipidus, and myxedema; symptoms may be exaggerated or aggravated; initial dosage reduction is recommended in patients with long-standing myxedema. Desiccated thyroid contains variable amounts of T_3, T_4, and other triiodothyronine compounds which are more likely to cause cardiac signs or symptoms due to fluctuating levels. Should avoid use in the elderly for this reason. Many clinicians consider levothyroxine to be the drug of choice for thyroid replacement.

Drug Interactions

Avoid Concomitant Use

Avoid concomitant use of Thyroid, Desiccated with any of the following: Sodium Iodide I131

Increased Effect/Toxicity

Thyroid, Desiccated may increase the levels/effects of: Vitamin K Antagonists

Decreased Effect

Thyroid, Desiccated may decrease the levels/effects of: Sodium Iodide I131; Theophylline Derivatives

The levels/effects of Thyroid, Desiccated may be decreased by: Bile Acid Sequestrants; Calcium Polystyrene Sulfonate; Calcium Salts; CarBAMazepine; Estrogen Derivatives; Fosphenytoin; Lanthanum; Phenytoin; Rifampin; Sodium Polystyrene Sulfonate

Mechanism of Action The primary active compound is T_3 (triiodothyronine), which may be converted from T_4 (thyroxine) and then circulates throughout the body to influence growth and maturation of various tissues; exact mechanism of action is unknown; however, it is believed the thyroid hormone exerts its many metabolic effects through control of DNA transcription and protein synthesis; involved in normal metabolism, growth, and development; promotes gluconeogenesis, increases utilization and mobilization of glycogen stores and stimulates protein synthesis, increases basal metabolic rate

Pharmacodynamics/Kinetics
Onset of action: Liothyronine (T_3): ~3 hours
Absorption: Thyroxine (T_4): 40% to 80%; T_3: 95%; desiccated thyroid contains T_4, T_3, and iodine (primarily bound)
Protein binding: T_4: >99% bound to plasma proteins including thyroxine-binding globulin, thyroxine-binding prealbumin, and albumin
Metabolism: Hepatic to triiodothyronine (active); ~80% T_4 deiodinated in kidney and periphery; glucuronidation/conjugation also occurs; undergoes enterohepatic recirculation
Half-life elimination, serum:
T_4: Euthyroid: 6-7 days; Hyperthyroid: 3-4 days; Hypothyroid: 9-10 days
T_3: 2.5 days
Time to peak: Serum: T_4: 2-4 hours; T_3: 2-3 days
Excretion: Urine (major route of elimination); partially feces

Dosage
Geriatric Not recommended for use in the elderly.
Adult Note: The American Association of Clinical Endocrinologists does not recommend the use of desiccated thyroid for thyroid replacement therapy for hypothyroidism (Baskin, 2002).
Hypothyroidism: Oral: Initial: 15-30 mg; increase with 15 mg increments every 2-3 weeks; use 15 mg in patients with cardiovascular disease or long-standing myxedema. Maintenance dose: Usually 60-120 mg/day; monitor TSH and clinical symptoms.
Administration Administer on an empty stomach. Take in the morning before breakfast.
Monitoring Parameters T_4, TSH, heart rate, blood pressure, clinical signs of hypo- and hyperthyroidism; TSH is the most reliable guide for evaluating adequacy of thyroid replacement dosage. TSH may be elevated during the first few months of thyroid replacement despite patients being clinically euthyroid. In cases where T_4 remains low and TSH is within normal limits, an evaluation of "free" (unbound) T_4 is needed to evaluate further increase in dosage.
Pharmacotherapy Pearls Equivalent doses: The following statement on relative potency of thyroid products is included in a joint statement by American Thyroid Association (ATA), American Association of Clinical Endocrinologists (AACE) and The Endocrine Society (TES): For purposes of conversion, levothyroxine sodium (T_4) 100 mcg is usually considered equivalent to desiccated thyroid 60 mg, thyroglobulin 60 mg, or liothyronine sodium (T_3) 25 mcg. However, these are rough guidelines only and do not obviate the careful re-evaluation of a patient when switching thyroid hormone preparations, including a change from one brand of levothyroxine to another. Joint position statement is available at http://www.thyroid.org/professionals/advocacy/04_12_08_thyroxine.html.
Special Geriatric Considerations Desiccated thyroid contains variable amounts of T_3, T_4, and other triiodothyronine compounds which are more likely to cause cardiac signs or symptoms due to fluctuating levels. Should avoid use in the elderly for this reason. Many clinicians consider levothyroxine to be the drug of choice. (Beers Criteria severity: High)
Dosage Forms Excipient information presented when available (limited, particularly for generics); consult specific product labeling. [DSC] = Discontinued product
Tablet, oral: 30 mg [DSC], 60 mg [DSC], 120 mg [DSC]
Armour® Thyroid: 15 mg, 30 mg, 60 mg, 90 mg, 120 mg
Armour® Thyroid: 180 mg [scored]
Armour® Thyroid: 240 mg
Armour® Thyroid: 300 mg [scored]
Nature-Throid™: 16.25 mg, 32.5 mg, 65 mg, 130 mg, 195 mg
Westhroid™: 32.5 mg, 65 mg, 130 mg

◆ **Thyroid Extract** see Thyroid, Desiccated on page 1786
◆ **Thyroid USP** see Thyroid, Desiccated on page 1786
◆ **Thyrolar®** see Liotrix on page 1074
◆ **Tiacumicin B** see Fidaxomicin (Systemic) on page 732

TiaGABine (tye AG a been)

Medication Safety Issues
Sound-alike/look-alike issues:
TiaGABine may be confused with tiZANidine
Brand Names: U.S. Gabitril®
Brand Names: Canada Gabitril®
Index Terms Tiagabine Hydrochloride
Generic Availability (U.S.) No
Pharmacologic Category Anticonvulsant, Miscellaneous

◀ **Use** Adjunctive therapy in the treatment of partial seizures

Medication Guide Available Yes

Contraindications Hypersensitivity to tiagabine or any component of the formulation

Warnings/Precautions Antiepileptics are associated with an increased risk of suicidal behavior/thoughts with use (regardless of indication); patients should be monitored for signs/symptoms of depression, suicidal tendencies, and other unusual behavior changes during therapy and instructed to inform their healthcare provider immediately if symptoms occur. New-onset seizures and status epilepticus have been associated with tiagabine use when taken for unlabeled indications. Often these seizures have occurred shortly after the initiation of treatment or shortly after a dosage increase. Seizures have also occurred with very low doses or after several months of therapy. In most cases, patients were using concomitant medications (eg, antidepressants, antipsychotics, stimulants, narcotics). In these instances, the discontinuation of tiagabine, followed by an evaluation for an underlying seizure disorder, is suggested. Use for unapproved indications, however, has not been proven to be safe or effective and is not recommended. When tiagabine is used as an adjunct in partial seizures (an FDA-approved indication), it should not be abruptly discontinued because of the possibility of increasing seizure frequency, unless safety concerns require a more rapid withdrawal. Rarely, nonconvulsive status epilepticus has been reported following abrupt discontinuation or dosage reduction.

Use with caution in patients with hepatic impairment. Experience in patients not receiving enzyme-inducing drugs has been limited; caution should be used in treating any patient who is not receiving one of these medications (decreased dose and slower titration may be required). Weakness, sedation, and confusion may occur with tiagabine use. Patients must be cautioned about performing tasks which require mental alertness (eg, operating machinery or driving). Effects with other sedative drugs or ethanol may be potentiated. May cause serious rash, including Stevens-Johnson syndrome.

Adverse Reactions (Reflective of adult population; not specific for elderly)

>10%:

Central nervous system: Concentration decreased, dizziness, nervousness, somnolence

Gastrointestinal: Nausea

Neuromuscular & skeletal: Weakness, tremor

1% to 10%:

Cardiovascular: Chest pain, edema, hypertension, palpitation, peripheral edema, syncope, tachycardia, vasodilation

Central nervous system: Agitation, ataxia, chills, confusion, difficulty with memory, confusion, depersonalization, depression, euphoria, hallucination, hostility, insomnia, malaise, migraine, paranoid reaction, personality disorder, speech disorder

Dermatologic: Alopecia, bruising, dry skin, pruritus, rash

Gastrointestinal: Abdominal pain, diarrhea, gingivitis, increased appetite, mouth ulceration, stomatitis, vomiting, weight gain/loss

Neuromuscular & skeletal: Abnormal gait, arthralgia, dysarthria, hyper-/hypokinesia, hyper-/hypotonia, myasthenia, myalgia, myoclonus, neck pain, paresthesia, reflexes decreased, stupor, twitching, vertigo

Ocular: Abnormal vision, amblyopia, nystagmus

Otic: Ear pain, hearing impairment, otitis media, tinnitus

Respiratory: Bronchitis, cough, dyspnea, epistaxis, pneumonia

Miscellaneous: Allergic reaction, cyst, diaphoresis, flu-like syndrome, lymphadenopathy

Drug Interactions

Metabolism/Transport Effects Substrate of 3A4 (major)

Avoid Concomitant Use

Avoid concomitant use of TiaGABine with any of the following: Conivaptan

Increased Effect/Toxicity

TiaGABine may increase the levels/effects of: Alcohol (Ethyl); CNS Depressants; Methotrimeprazine; Selective Serotonin Reuptake Inhibitors

The levels/effects of TiaGABine may be increased by: Conivaptan; CYP3A4 Inhibitors (Moderate); CYP3A4 Inhibitors (Strong); Dasatinib; Droperidol; HydrOXYzine; Methotrimeprazine

Decreased Effect

The levels/effects of TiaGABine may be decreased by: CYP3A4 Inducers (Strong); Deferasirox; Herbs (CYP3A4 Inducers); Ketorolac; Ketorolac (Nasal); Ketorolac (Systemic); Mefloquine; Tocilizumab

Ethanol/Nutrition/Herb Interactions

Ethanol: May increase CNS depression; monitor for increased effects with coadministration. Caution patients about effects.

Food: Food reduces the rate but not the extent of absorption.

Herb/Nutraceutical: St John's wort may decrease tiagabine levels. Avoid valerian, St John's wort, kava kava, gotu kola (may increase CNS depression).

Mechanism of Action The exact mechanism by which tiagabine exerts antiseizure activity is not definitively known; however, *in vitro* experiments demonstrate that it enhances the activity of gamma aminobutyric acid (GABA), the major neuroinhibitory transmitter in the nervous system; it is thought that binding to the GABA uptake carrier inhibits the uptake of GABA into presynaptic neurons, allowing an increased amount of GABA to be available to postsynaptic neurons; based on *in vitro* studies, tiagabine does not inhibit the uptake of dopamine, norepinephrine, serotonin, glutamate, or choline

Pharmacodynamics/Kinetics

Absorption: Rapid (45 minutes); prolonged with food

Protein binding: 96%, primarily to albumin and α_1-acid glycoprotein

Metabolism: Hepatic via CYP (primarily 3A4)

Bioavailability: Oral: Absolute: 90%

Half-life elimination: 2-5 hours when administered with enzyme inducers; 7-9 hours when administered without enzyme inducers

Time to peak, plasma: 45 minutes

Excretion: Feces (63%); urine (25%); 2% as unchanged drug; primarily as metabolites

Dosage

Geriatric & Adult Partial seizures (adjunct): Oral:

Patients receiving enzyme-inducing AED regimens: 4 mg once daily for 1 week; may increase by 4-8 mg weekly to response or up to 56 mg daily in 2-4 divided doses; usual maintenance: 32-56 mg/day

Patients **not** receiving enzyme-inducing AED regimens: The estimated plasma concentrations of tiagabine in patients not taking enzyme-inducing medications is twice that of patients receiving enzyme-inducing AEDs. Lower doses are required; slower titration may be necessary.

Monitoring Parameters A reduction in seizure frequency is indicative of therapeutic response to tiagabine in patients with partial seizures; complete blood counts, renal function tests, liver function tests, and routine blood chemistry should be monitored periodically during therapy; suicidality (eg, suicidal thoughts, depression, behavioral changes)

Reference Range Maximal plasma level after a 24 mg/dose: 552 ng/mL

Pharmacotherapy Pearls Animal studies suggest that tiagabine may bind to retina and uvea; however, no treatment-related ophthalmoscopic changes were seen long-term; periodic monitoring may be considered.

Special Geriatric Considerations No special recommendations are made for the elderly; dose according to response.

Dosage Forms Excipient information presented when available (limited, particularly for generics); consult specific product labeling.

Tablet, oral, as hydrochloride:

Gabitril®: 2 mg, 4 mg, 12 mg, 16 mg

Selected References

Patsalos PN and Sander JW, "Newer Antiepileptic Drugs: Towards an Improved Risk-Benefit Ratio," *Drug Saf*, 1994, 11(1):37-67.

◆ **Tiagabine Hydrochloride** see TiaGABine *on page 1787*

◆ **Tiazac®** see Diltiazem *on page 514*

Ticarcillin and Clavulanate Potassium

(tye kar SIL in & klav yoo LAN ate poe TASS ee um)

Brand Names: U.S. Timentin®

Brand Names: Canada Timentin®

Index Terms Ticarcillin and Clavulanic Acid

Generic Availability (U.S.) No

Pharmacologic Category Antibiotic, Penicillin

Use Treatment of lower respiratory tract, urinary tract, skin and skin structures, bone and joint, gynecologic (endometritis) and intra-abdominal (peritonitis) infections, and septicemia caused by susceptible organisms. Clavulanate expands activity of ticarcillin to include beta-lactamase producing strains of *S. aureus*, *H. influenzae*, *Bacteroides* species, and some other gram-negative bacilli

Contraindications Hypersensitivity to ticarcillin, clavulanate, any penicillin, or any component of the formulation

Warnings/Precautions Use with caution and modify dosage in patients with renal impairment; serious and occasionally severe or fatal hypersensitivity (anaphylactoid) reactions have been reported in patients on penicillin therapy (especially with a history of beta-lactam hypersensitivity and/or a history of sensitivity to multiple allergens); use with caution in

◄ patients with seizures and in patients with HF due to high sodium load. Particularly in patients with renal impairment, bleeding disorders have been observed; discontinue if thrombocytopenia or bleeding occurs. Prolonged use may result in fungal or bacterial superinfection, including *C. difficile*-associated diarrhea (CDAD) and pseudomembranous colitis; CDAD has been observed >2 months postantibiotic treatment.

Adverse Reactions (Reflective of adult population; not specific for elderly) Frequency not defined.

Central nervous system: Confusion, drowsiness, fever, headache, Jarisch-Herxheimer reaction, seizure

Dermatologic: Erythema multiforme, pruritus, rash, Stevens-Johnson syndrome, toxic epidermal necrolysis, urticaria

Endocrine & metabolic: Electrolyte imbalance

Gastrointestinal: *Clostridium difficile* colitis, diarrhea, nausea, vomiting

Hematologic: Bleeding, eosinophilia, hemolytic anemia, leukopenia, neutropenia, positive Coombs' reaction, prothrombin time prolonged, thrombocytopenia

Hepatic: Hepatotoxicity, jaundice

Local: Injection site reaction (pain, burning, induration); thrombophlebitis

Neuromuscular & skeletal: Myoclonus

Renal: BUN increased, interstitial nephritis (acute), serum creatinine increased

Miscellaneous: Anaphylaxis, hypersensitivity reactions

Drug Interactions

Avoid Concomitant Use

Avoid concomitant use of Ticarcillin and Clavulanate Potassium with any of the following: BCG

Increased Effect/Toxicity

Ticarcillin and Clavulanate Potassium may increase the levels/effects of: Methotrexate

The levels/effects of Ticarcillin and Clavulanate Potassium may be increased by: Probenecid

Decreased Effect

Ticarcillin and Clavulanate Potassium may decrease the levels/effects of: Aminoglycosides; BCG; Mycophenolate; Typhoid Vaccine

The levels/effects of Ticarcillin and Clavulanate Potassium may be decreased by: Fusidic Acid; Tetracycline Derivatives

Stability

Vials: Store intact vials at <24°C (<75°F). Reconstituted solution is stable for 6 hours at room temperature and 72 hours when refrigerated. I.V. infusion in NS or LR is stable for 24 hours at room temperature, 7 days when refrigerated, or 30 days when frozen. I.V. infusion in D_5W solution is stable for 24 hours at room temperature, 3 days when refrigerated, or 7 days when frozen. After freezing, thawed solution is stable for 8 hours at room temperature. Darkening of drug indicates loss of potency of clavulanate potassium.

Premixed solution: Store frozen at ≤-20°C (-4°F). Thawed solution is stable for 24 hours at room temperature or 7 days under refrigeration; do not refreeze.

Mechanism of Action Inhibits bacterial cell wall synthesis by binding to one or more of the penicillin-binding proteins (PBPs); which in turn inhibits the final transpeptidation step of peptidoglycan synthesis in bacterial cell walls, thus inhibiting cell wall biosynthesis. Bacteria eventually lyse due to ongoing activity of cell wall autolytic enzymes (autolysins and murein hydrolases) while cell wall assembly is arrested.

Pharmacodynamics/Kinetics

Absorption: Ticarcillin: Not absorbed orally

Protein binding: Ticarcillin: ~45%; Clavulanic acid: ~25%

Metabolism: Clavulanic acid: Hepatic

Half-life elimination: Ticarcillin: 1.1 hours; Clavulanic acid: 1.1 hours

Excretion: Ticarcillin: Urine (60% to 70%); Clavulanic acid: Urine (35% to 45% as unchanged drug)

Clearance: Clavulanic acid does not affect clearance of ticarcillin

Dosage

Geriatric I.V.: 3.1 g every 4-6 hours; adjust for renal function.

Adult Note: Timentin® (ticarcillin/clavulanate) is a combination product; each 3.1 g dosage form contains 3 g ticarcillin disodium and 0.1 g clavulanic acid.

Systemic infections: I.V.: 3.1 g (ticarcillin 3 g plus clavulanic acid 0.1 g) every 4-6 hours (maximum: 24 g of ticarcillin component/day)

Amnionitis, cholangitis, diverticulitis, endometritis, epididymo-orchitis, mastoiditis, orbital cellulitis, peritonitis, pneumonia (aspiration): I.V.: 3.1 g every 6 hours

Intra-abdominal infection, complicated, community-acquired, mild-to-moderate: I.V.: 3.1 g every 6 hours for 4-7 days (provided source controlled)

Liver abscess, parafascial space infections, septic thrombophlebitis: I.V.: 3.1 g every 4 hours

Pseudomonas **infections:** I.V.: 3.1 g every 4 hours

Urinary tract infections: I.V.: 3.1 g every 6-8 hours

Renal Impairment

Loading dose: I.V.: 3.1 g one dose, followed by maintenance dose based on creatinine clearance:

Cl_{cr} 30-60 mL/minute: Administer 2 g of ticarcillin component every 4 hours or 3.1 g every 8 hours

Cl_{cr} 10-30 mL/minute: Administer 2 g of ticarcillin component every 8 hours or 3.1 g every 12 hours

Cl_{cr} <10 mL/minute: Administer 2 g of ticarcillin component every 12 hours

Cl_{cr} <10 mL/minute with concomitant hepatic dysfunction: 2 g of ticarcillin component every 24 hours

Intermittent hemodialysis (IHD) (administer after hemodialysis on dialysis days): Dialyzable (20% to 50%): 2 g of ticarcillin component every 12 hours; supplemented with 3.1 g (ticarcillin/clavulanate) after each dialysis session. Alternatively, administer 2 g every 8 hours without a supplemental dose for deep-seated infections (Heintz, 2009). **Note:** Dosing dependent on the assumption of 3 times/week, complete IHD sessions.

Peritoneal dialysis (PD): 3.1 g every 12 hours

Continuous renal replacement therapy (CRRT) (Heintz, 2009; Trotman, 2005): Drug clearance is highly dependent on the method of renal replacement, filter type, and flow rate. Appropriate dosing requires close monitoring of pharmacologic response, signs of adverse reactions due to drug accumulation, as well as drug concentrations in relation to target trough (if appropriate). The following are general recommendations only (based on dialysate flow/ultrafiltration rates of 1-2 L/hour and minimal residual renal function) and should not supersede clinical judgment:

CVVH: Loading dose of 3.1g followed by 2 g every 6-8 hours

CVVHD: Loading dose of 3.1 g followed by 3.1 g every 6-8 hours

CVVHDF: Loading dose of 3.1 g followed by 3.1 g every 6 hours

Note: Do not administer in intervals exceeding every 8 hours. Clavulanate component is hepatically eliminated; extending the dosing interval beyond 8 hours may result in loss of beta-lactamase inhibition.

Hepatic Impairment With concomitant renal dysfunction (Cl_{cr} <10 mL/minute): 2 g of ticarcillin component every 24 hours.

Administration Infuse over 30 minutes. Administer 1 hour apart from aminoglycosides. Give around-the-clock. Rapid administration may lead to seizures.

Monitoring Parameters Observe for signs and symptoms of anaphylaxis during first dose.

Test Interactions Positive Coombs' test, false-positive urinary proteins

Some penicillin derivatives may accelerate the degradation of aminoglycosides *in vitro*, leading to a potential underestimation of aminoglycoside serum concentration.

Special Geriatric Considerations When used as empiric therapy or for a documented pseudomonal pneumonia, it is best to combine with an aminoglycoside such as gentamicin or tobramycin. High sodium content may limit use in patients with congestive heart failure. Adjust dose for renal function.

Dosage Forms Excipient information presented when available (limited, particularly for generics); consult specific product labeling.

Infusion [premixed, frozen]: Ticarcillin 3 g and clavulanic acid 0.1 g (100 mL) [contains sodium 4.51 mEq and potassium 0.15 mEq per g]

Injection, powder for reconstitution: Ticarcillin 3 g and clavulanic acid 0.1 g (3.1 g, 31 g) [contains sodium 4.51 mEq and potassium 0.15 mEq per g]

◆ **Ticarcillin and Clavulanic Acid** see Ticarcillin and Clavulanate Potassium *on page 1789*

Ticlopidine (tye KLOE pi deen)

Related Information

Beers Criteria – Potentially Inappropriate Medications for Geriatrics *on page 2089*

Medication Safety Issues

BEERS Criteria medication:

This drug may be inappropriate for use in geriatric patients (high severity risk).

Brand Names: Canada Apo-Ticlopidine®; Dom-Ticlopidine; Gen-Ticlopidine; Mylan-Ticlopidine; Novo-Ticlopidine; Nu-Ticlopidine; PMS-Ticlopidine; Sandoz-Ticlopidine; Teva-Ticlopidine

Index Terms Ticlopidine Hydrochloride

Generic Availability (U.S.) Yes

Pharmacologic Category Antiplatelet Agent; Antiplatelet Agent, Thienopyridine

TICLOPIDINE

◄ **Use** Platelet aggregation inhibitor that reduces the risk of thrombotic stroke in patients who have had a stroke or stroke precursors. **Note:** Due to its association with life-threatening hematologic disorders, ticlopidine should be reserved for patients who are intolerant to aspirin, or who have failed aspirin therapy. Adjunctive therapy (with aspirin) following successful coronary stent implantation to reduce the incidence of subacute stent thrombosis.

Unlabeled/Investigational Use Protection of aortocoronary bypass grafts, diabetic microangiopathy, ischemic heart disease, prevention of postoperative DVT, reduction of graft loss following renal transplant

Contraindications Hypersensitivity to ticlopidine or any component of the formulation; active pathological bleeding such as peptic ulcer disease (PUD) or intracranial hemorrhage; severe liver dysfunction; hematopoietic disorders (neutropenia, thrombocytopenia, a past history of TTP or aplastic anemia)

Warnings/Precautions Use with caution in patients who may be at risk of increased bleeding (eg, PUD, trauma, or surgery). Consider discontinuing 10-14 days before elective surgery (except in patients with cardiac stents that have not completed their full course of dual antiplatelet therapy; patient-specific situations need to be discussed with cardiologist; AHA/ACC/SCAI/ACS/ADA Science Advisory provides recommendations). Use caution in concurrent treatment with anticoagulants (eg, heparin, warfarin) or other antiplatelet drugs; bleeding risk is increased. Use with caution in patients with mild-to-moderate hepatic impairment; use is contraindicated with severe hepatic impairment. Use with caution in patients with moderate-to-severe renal impairment (experience is limited); bleeding times may be significantly prolonged and the risk of hematologic adverse effects (eg, neutropenia) may be increased. **[U.S. Boxed Warning]: May cause life-threatening hematologic reactions, including neutropenia, agranulocytosis, thrombotic thrombocytopenia purpura (TTP), and aplastic anemia.** Routine monitoring is required (see Monitoring Parameters). Monitor for signs and symptoms of neutropenia including WBC count. Discontinue if the absolute neutrophil count falls to <1200/mm^3 or if the platelet count falls to <80,000/mm^3. Not recommended for use in the elderly as this medication has been shown to be no better than aspirin as an antiplatet agent and may have more significant adverse effects (Beers Criteria).

Adverse Reactions (Reflective of adult population; not specific for elderly) As with all drugs which may affect hemostasis, bleeding is associated with ticlopidine. Hemorrhage may occur at virtually any site. Risk is dependent on multiple variables, including the use of multiple agents which alter hemostasis and patient susceptibility.

>10%:
  Endocrine & metabolic: Total cholesterol increased (increases of ~8% to 10% within 1 month of therapy), triglycerides increased
  Gastrointestinal: Diarrhea (13%)
1% to 10%:
  Central nervous system: Dizziness (1%)
  Dermatologic: Rash (5%), purpura (2%), pruritus (1%)
  Gastrointestinal: Nausea (7%), dyspepsia (7%), gastrointestinal pain (4%), vomiting (2%), flatulence (2%), anorexia (1%)
  Hematologic: Neutropenia (2%)
  Hepatic: Alkaline phosphatase increased (>2 x upper limit of normal; 8%), abnormal liver function test (1%)

Drug Interactions

Metabolism/Transport Effects Substrate of CYP3A4 (major); **Inhibits** CYP1A2 (weak), 2B6 (moderate), 2C9 (weak), 2C19 (strong), 2D6 (moderate), 2E1 (weak), 3A4 (weak)

Avoid Concomitant Use

Avoid concomitant use of Ticlopidine with any of the following: Clopidogrel; Thioridazine

Increased Effect/Toxicity

Ticlopidine may increase the levels/effects of: Anticoagulants; Antiplatelet Agents; Collagenase (Systemic); CYP2B6 Substrates; CYP2C19 Substrates; CYP2D6 Substrates; Drotrecogin Alfa; Fesoterodine; Fosphenytoin; Ibritumomab; Nebivolol; Phenytoin; Rivaroxaban; Salicylates; Tamoxifen; Theophylline Derivatives; Thioridazine; Thrombolytic Agents; Tositumomab and Iodine I 131 Tositumomab

The levels/effects of Ticlopidine may be increased by: Conivaptan; Dasatinib; Glucosamine; Herbs (Anticoagulant/Antiplatelet Properties); Nonsteroidal Anti-Inflammatory Agents; Omega-3-Acid Ethyl Esters; Pentosan Polysulfate Sodium; Pentoxifylline; Prostacyclin Analogues; Vitamin E

Decreased Effect

Ticlopidine may decrease the levels/effects of: Clopidogrel; Codeine; TraMADol

The levels/effects of Ticlopidine may be decreased by: CYP3A4 Inducers (Strong); Deferasirox; Herbs (CYP3A4 Inducers); Nonsteroidal Anti-Inflammatory Agents; Tocilizumab

Ethanol/Nutrition/Herb Interactions

Food: Ticlopidine bioavailability may be increased (20%) if taken with food. High-fat meals increase absorption, antacids decrease absorption.

Herb/Nutraceutical: Avoid alfalfa, anise, bilberry, bladderwrack, bromelain, cat's claw, chamomile, coleus, cordyceps, dong quai, evening primrose oil, fenugreek, feverfew, garlic, ginger, ginkgo biloba, ginseng (American), ginseng (Panax), ginseng (Siberian), grape seed, green tea, guggul, horse chestnut seed, horseradish, licorice, prickly ash, red clover, reishi, SAMe (S-adenosylmethionine), sweet clover, turmeric, white willow (all have additional antiplatelet activity).

Mechanism of Action Ticlopidine requires *in vivo* biotransformation to an unidentified active metabolite. This active metabolite irreversibly blocks the P2Y12 component of ADP receptors, which prevents activation of the GPIIb/IIIa receptor complex, thereby reducing platelet aggregation. Platelets blocked by ticlopidine are affected for the remainder of their lifespan.

Pharmacodynamics/Kinetics

Onset of action: ~6 hours

Peak effect: 3-5 days; serum levels do not correlate with clinical antiplatelet activity

Absorption: Well absorbed

Protein binding: Parent drug: 98%; <15% bound to alpha$_1$-acid glycoprotein

Metabolism: Extensively hepatic; has at least 1 active metabolite

Half-life elimination: 13 hours

Time to peak, serum: ~2 hours

Excretion: Urine (60%); feces (23%)

Dosage

Geriatric 250 mg twice daily with food; dosage in older patients has not been determined; however, in two large clinical trials, the average age of subjects was 63 and 66 years. A dosage decrease may be necessary if bleeding develops.

Adult

Stroke prevention: Oral: 250 mg twice daily

Coronary artery stenting (initiate after successful implantation): Oral: 250 mg twice daily (in combination with antiplatelet doses of aspirin) for up to 30 days

Unstable angina, non-ST-segment elevation myocardial infarction (UA/NSTEMI) undergoing percutaneous coronary intervention (PCI) in patients unable to receive clopidogrel (unlabeled dosing): Initial: 500 mg loading dose given at least 6 hours prior to PCI, followed by 250 mg twice daily (in combination with aspirin 75-325 mg once daily). Duration of therapy dependent upon type of stent implanted during PCI.

Note: *Coronary artery stents:* Duration of ticlopidine (clopidogrel preferred) in combination with aspirin: According to the ACC/AHA/SCAI guidelines, ideally 12 months following drug-eluting stent (DES) placement in patients not at high risk for bleeding; at a minimum, 1, 3, and 6 months for bare metal (BMS), sirolimus-eluting, and paclitaxel-eluting stents, respectively, for uninterrupted therapy (Smith, 2005). The 2008 *Chest* guidelines recommend for patients who undergo PCI and receive a BMS (with ongoing ACS) or a DES (with or without ongoing ACS) that ticlopidine (clopidogrel preferred) be continued for at least 12 months. In patients receiving a BMS without ongoing ACS, ticlopidine (or clopidogrel) may be continued for at least 1 month. In patients receiving a DES, therapy with ticlopidine (or clopidogrel) beyond 12 months may be considered in patients without bleeding or tolerability issues (Becker, 2008). Premature interruption of therapy may result in stent thrombosis with subsequent fatal and nonfatal myocardial infarction.

Renal Impairment No adjustment is necessary.

Hepatic Impairment No specific guidelines for patients with hepatic impairment; use with caution. Use is contraindicated with severe renal impairment.

Administration Oral: Administer with food.

Monitoring Parameters Signs of bleeding; CBC with differential every 2 weeks starting the second week through the third month of treatment; more frequent monitoring is recommended for patients whose absolute neutrophil counts have been consistently declining or are 30% less than baseline values. The peak incidence of TTP occurs between 3-4 weeks, the peak incidence of neutropenia occurs at approximately 4-6 weeks, and the incidence of aplastic anemia peaks after 4-8 weeks of therapy. Few cases have been reported after 3 months of treatment. Liver function tests (alkaline phosphatase and transaminases) should be performed in the first 4 months of therapy if liver dysfunction is suspected.

Special Geriatric Considerations Because of the risk of neutropenia and its relative expense as compared with aspirin, ticlopidine should only be used in patients with a documented intolerance to aspirin.

This medication is considered to be potentially inappropriate in this patient population (Beers Criteria severity: High).

◀ **Dosage Forms** Excipient information presented when available (limited, particularly for generics); consult specific product labeling.
Tablet, oral, as hydrochloride: 250 mg

♦ **Ticlopidine Hydrochloride** *see* Ticlopidine *on page 1791*
♦ **TIG** *see* Tetanus Immune Globulin (Human) *on page 1767*
♦ **Tigan®** *see* Trimethobenzamide *on page 1866*

Tigecycline (tye ge SYE kleen)

Brand Names: U.S. Tygacil®
Brand Names: Canada Tygacil®
Index Terms GAR-936
Generic Availability (U.S.) No
Pharmacologic Category Antibiotic, Glycylcycline
Use Treatment of complicated skin and skin structure infections caused by susceptible organisms, including methicillin-resistant *Staphylococcus aureus* and vancomycin-sensitive *Enterococcus faecalis*; complicated intra-abdominal infections (cIAI); community-acquired pneumonia
Contraindications Hypersensitivity to tigecycline or any component of the formulation
Warnings/Precautions In Phase 3 and 4 clinical trials, an increase in all-cause mortality was observed in patients treated with tigecycline compared to those treated with comparator antibiotics; cause has not been established. In general, deaths were the result of worsening infection, complications of infection, or underlying comorbidity. May cause life-threatening anaphylaxis/anaphylactoid reactions. Due to structural similarity with tetracyclines, use caution in patients with prior hypersensitivity and/or severe adverse reactions associated with tetracycline use. Due to structural similarities with tetracyclines, may be associated with photosensitivity, pseudotumor cerebri, pancreatitis, and antianabolic effects (including increased BUN, azotemia, acidosis, and hyperphosphatemia) observed with this class. Acute pancreatitis (including fatalities) has been reported, including patients without known risk factors; discontinue use when suspected.

Use caution in hepatic impairment; dosage adjustment recommended in severe hepatic impairment. Abnormal liver function tests (increased total bilirubin, prothrombin time, transaminases) have been reported. Isolated cases of significant hepatic dysfunction and hepatic failure have occurred. Closely monitor for worsening hepatic function in patients that develop abnormal liver function tests during therapy. Adverse hepatic effects may occur after drug discontinuation.

Prolonged use may result in fungal or bacterial superinfection, including *C. difficile*-associated diarrhea (CDAD) and pseudomembranous colitis; CDAD has been observed >2 months postantibiotic treatment. Use with caution if using as monotherapy for patients with intestinal perforation (in the small sample of available cases, septic shock occurred more frequently than patients treated with imipenem/cilastatin comparator). Demonstrated inferior efficacy (versus comparator antibiotic), including lower cure rates and increased mortality in the subgroup of patients with VAP (particularly those with VAP and concurrent bacteremia at baseline).
Adverse Reactions (Reflective of adult population; not specific for elderly) Note: Frequencies relative to placebo are not available; some frequencies are lower than those experienced with comparator drugs.
>10%: Gastrointestinal: Nausea (26%; severe: 1%), vomiting (18%; severe: 1%), diarrhea (12%)
2% to 10%:
Central nervous system: Headache (6%), dizziness (3%)
Dermatologic: Rash (3%)
Endocrine & metabolic: Hypoproteinemia (5%)
Gastrointestinal: Abdominal pain (6%), dyspepsia (2%)
Hematologic: Anemia (4%)
Hepatic: ALT increased (5%), AST increased (4%), alkaline phosphatase increased (4%), amylase increased (3%), bilirubin increased (2%)
Local: Phlebitis (3%)
Neuromuscular & skeletal: Weakness (3%)
Renal: BUN increased (3%)
Miscellaneous: Infection (8%), abnormal healing (4%), abscess (3%)
Drug Interactions
Avoid Concomitant Use There are no known interactions where it is recommended to avoid concomitant use.

Increased Effect/Toxicity
Tigecycline may increase the levels/effects of: Warfarin

Decreased Effect There are no known significant interactions involving a decrease in effect.

Stability Prior to reconstitution, store at 20°C to 25°C (68°F to 77°F); excursions permitted to 15°C to 30°C (59°F to 86°F). Add 5.3 mL NS, D_5W, or LR to each 50 mg vial. Swirl gently to dissolve. Resulting solution is 10 mg/mL. Reconstituted solution must be further diluted to allow I.V. administration. Transfer to 100 mL I.V. bag for infusion (final concentration should not exceed 1 mg/mL). Reconstituted solution may be stored at room temperature for up to 6 hours or up to 24 hours if further diluted in a compatible I.V. solution. Alternatively, may be stored refrigerated at 2°C to 8°C (36°F to 46°F) for up to 48 hours following immediate transfer of the reconstituted solution into NS or D_5W. Reconstituted solution should be yellow-orange; discard if not this color.

Mechanism of Action A glycylcycline antibiotic that binds to the 30S ribosomal subunit of susceptible bacteria, thereby, inhibiting protein synthesis. Generally considered bacteriostatic; however, bactericidal activity has been demonstrated against isolates of *S. pneumoniae* and *L. pneumophila*. Tigecycline is a derivative of minocycline (9-t-butylglycylamido minocycline), and while not classified as a tetracycline, it may share some class-associated adverse effects. Tigecycline has demonstrated activity against a variety of gram-positive and -negative bacterial pathogens including methicillin-resistant staphylococci.

Pharmacodynamics/Kinetics Note: Systemic clearance is reduced by 55% and half-life increased by 43% in severe hepatic impairment.

Distribution: V_d: 7-9 L/kg; extensive tissue distribution

Protein binding: 71% to 89%

Metabolism: Hepatic, via glucuronidation, N-acetylation, and epimerization to several metabolites, each <10% of the dose

Half-life elimination: Single dose: 27 hours; following multiple doses: 42 hours

Excretion: Feces (59%, primarily as unchanged drug); urine (33%, with 22% of the total dose as unchanged drug)

Dosage

Geriatric & Adult Note: Duration of therapy dependent on severity/site of infection and clinical status and response to therapy.

Pneumonia, community-acquired: I.V.: Initial: 100 mg as a single dose; Maintenance dose: 50 mg every 12 hours for 7-14 days

Intra-abdominal infections, complicated (cIAI): I.V.: Initial: 100 mg as a single dose; Maintenance dose: 50 mg every 12 hours for 5-14 days; **Note:** 2010 IDSA guidelines recommend a treatment duration of 4-7 days (provided source controlled) for community-acquired, mild-to-moderate IAI

Skin/skin structure infections, complicated: I.V.: Initial: 100 mg as a single dose; Maintenance dose: 50 mg every 12 hours for 5-14 days

Renal Impairment No dosage adjustment required in renal impairment.

Poorly dialyzed; no supplemental dose or dosage adjustment necessary, including patients on intermittent hemodialysis, peritoneal dialysis, or continuous renal replacement therapy (eg, CVVHD).

Hepatic Impairment

Mild-to-moderate hepatic impairment (Child-Pugh classes A and B): No dosage adjustment required.

Severe hepatic impairment (Child-Pugh class C): Initial: 100 mg single dose; Maintenance: 25 mg every 12 hours.

Administration Infuse over 30-60 minutes through dedicated line or via Y-site

Special Geriatric Considerations The manufacturer reports no significant differences in tigecycline's pharmacokinetics in small numbers of healthy older adults 65-75 years of age and >75 years compared to younger adults following a single 100 mg dose. No dosage adjustment is recommended.

Dosage Forms Excipient information presented when available (limited, particularly for generics); consult specific product labeling.

Injection, powder for reconstitution:

Tygacil®: 50 mg [contains lactose 100 mg]

Selected References
Conte JE Jr, Golden JA, Kelly MG, et al, "Steady-State Serum and Intrapulmonary Pharmacokinetics and Pharmacodynamics of Tigecycline," *Int J Antimicrob Agents*, 2005, 25(6):523-9.

◆ Tikosyn® *see* Dofetilide *on page 549*

Tiludronate (tye LOO droe nate)

Brand Names: U.S. Skelid®
Index Terms Tiludronate Disodium

TILUDRONATE

Generic Availability (U.S.) No

Pharmacologic Category Bisphosphonate Derivative

Use Treatment of Paget's disease of the bone (osteitis deformans) in patients who have a level of serum alkaline phosphatase (SAP) at least twice the upper limit of normal, or who are symptomatic, or who are at risk for future complications of their disease

Contraindications Hypersensitivity to tiludronate, bisphosphonates, or any component of the formulation; inability to stand or sit upright for at least 30 minutes

Warnings/Precautions Not recommended in patients with severe renal impairment (Cl$_{cr}$ <30 mL/minute). Use with caution in patients with active upper GI problems (eg, dysphagia, symptomatic esophageal diseases, gastritis, duodenitis, ulcers); discontinue use if new or worsening symptoms develop.

Osteonecrosis of the jaw (ONJ) has been reported in patients receiving bisphosphonates. Risk factors include invasive dental procedures (eg, tooth extraction, dental implants, boney surgery); a diagnosis of cancer, with concomitant chemotherapy or corticosteroids; poor oral hygiene, ill-fitting dentures; and comorbid disorders (anemia, coagulopathy, infection, pre-existing dental disease). Most reported cases occurred after I.V. bisphosphonate therapy; however, cases have been reported following oral therapy. A dental exam and preventative dentistry should be performed prior to placing patients with risk factors on chronic bisphosphonate therapy. The manufacturer's labeling states that discontinuing bisphosphonates in patients requiring invasive dental procedures may reduce the risk of ONJ. However, other experts suggest that there is no evidence that discontinuing therapy reduces the risk of developing ONJ (Assael, 2009). The benefit/risk must be assessed by the treating physician and/or dentist/surgeon prior to any invasive dental procedure. Patients developing ONJ while on bisphosphonates should receive care by an oral surgeon.

Infrequently, severe (and occasionally debilitating) bone, joint, and/or muscle pain have been reported during bisphosphonate treatment. The onset of pain ranged from a single day to several months. Consider discontinuing therapy in patients who experience severe symptoms; symptoms usually resolve upon discontinuation. Some patients experienced recurrence when rechallenged with same drug or another bisphosphonate; avoid use in patients with a history of these symptoms in association with bisphosphonate therapy.

Adverse Reactions (Reflective of adult population; not specific for elderly)

1% to 10%:

Cardiovascular: Chest pain (3%), edema (3%), peripheral edema (3%), flushing, hypertension, syncope

Central nervous system: Anxiety, fatigue, insomnia, nervousness, somnolence, vertigo

Dermatologic: Rash (3%), skin disorder (3%), pruritus

Endocrine & metabolic: Hyperparathyroidism (3%)

Gastrointestinal: Nausea (9%), diarrhea (9%), dyspepsia (5%), vomiting (4%), flatulence (3%), abdominal pain, anorexia, constipation, gastritis, xerostomia

Genitourinary: Urinary tract infection

Neuromuscular & skeletal: Paresthesia (4%), arthrosis (3%), fractures, muscle spasm, weakness

Ocular: Cataract (3%), conjunctivitis (3%), glaucoma (3%)

Respiratory: Rhinitis (5%), sinusitis (5%), pharyngitis (3%), bronchitis

Miscellaneous: Accidental injury (4%), infection (3%), diaphoresis

Drug Interactions

Avoid Concomitant Use There are no known interactions where it is recommended to avoid concomitant use.

Increased Effect/Toxicity

Tiludronate may increase the levels/effects of: Deferasirox; Phosphate Supplements

The levels/effects of Tiludronate may be increased by: Aminoglycosides; Indomethacin; Nonsteroidal Anti-Inflammatory Agents

Decreased Effect

The levels/effects of Tiludronate may be decreased by: Antacids; Aspirin; Calcium Salts; Iron Salts; Magnesium Salts; Proton Pump Inhibitors

Ethanol/Nutrition/Herb Interactions Food: In single-dose studies, the bioavailability of tiludronate was reduced by 90% when an oral dose was administered with, or 2 hours after, a standard breakfast compared to the same dose administered after an overnight fast and 4 hours before a standard breakfast.

Stability Store at 25°C (77°F); excursions permitted to 15°C to 30°C (59°F to 86°F). Do not remove tablets from foil strips until they are to be used.

Mechanism of Action Inhibition of normal and abnormal bone resorption. Inhibits osteoclasts through at least two mechanisms: disruption of the cytoskeletal ring structure, possibly by inhibition of protein-tyrosine-phosphatase, thus leading to the detachment of osteoclasts from the bone surface area and the inhibition of the osteoclast proton pump.

Pharmacodynamics/Kinetics
Onset of action: Delayed, may require several weeks
Absorption: Rapid
Distribution: Widely to bone and soft tissue
Protein binding: ~90%, primarily to albumin
Metabolism: Little, if any
Bioavailability: ~6% (range: 2% to 11%); reduced by 90% when given with food
Half-life elimination: Healthy volunteers: Single dose: 50 hours; Cl_{cr} 11-18 mL/minute: 205 hours; Pagetic patients: Repeated dosing: 150 hours
Time to peak, plasma: Within 2 hours
Excretion: Urine (~60%, as tiludronic acid within 13 days)

Dosage
Geriatric & Adult Paget's disease: Oral: 400 mg (2 tablets of tiludronic acid) daily for a period of 3 months
Renal Impairment Tiludronate is excreted renally. It is not recommended for use in patients with severe renal impairment (Cl_{cr} <30 mL/minute) and is not removed by dialysis.

Administration Administer as a single oral dose, take with 6-8 oz of plain water. Should not be taken with beverages containing minerals (eg, mineral water), food, or with other medications (may reduce absorption). Do not take within 2 hours of food. Take calcium or mineral supplements at least 2 hours before or after tiludronate. Take aluminum- or magnesium-containing antacids at least 2 hours after taking tiludronate. Do not take tiludronate within 2 hours of indomethacin.

Monitoring Parameters Alkaline phosphatase; pain; serum calcium and 25(OH)D

Test Interactions Bisphosphonates may interfere with diagnostic imaging agents such as technetium-99m-diphosphonate in bone scans.

Pharmacotherapy Pearls Three months of treatment is recommended; because of bioavailability problems, tiludronate should not be taken with beverages other than water or within 2 hours of food, calcium or mineral supplements, aspirin, or indomethacin; aluminum- or magnesium-containing antacids should be taken at least 2 hours after tiludronate

Special Geriatric Considerations The elderly are frequently treated long-term for osteoporosis. Elderly patients should be advised to report any lower extremity, jaw (osteonecrosis), or muscle pain that cannot be explained or lasts longer than 2 weeks. Additionally, elderly often receive concomitant diuretic therapy and therefore their electrolyte status (eg, calcium, phosphate) should be periodically evaluated.

Dosage Forms Excipient information presented when available (limited, particularly for generics); consult specific product labeling.
Tablet, oral, as tiludronic acid:
Skelid® 200 mg [equivalent tiludronate disodium 240 mg]

Selected References
Hillner BE, Ingle JN, Chlebowski RT, et al, "American Society of Clinical Oncology 2003 Update on the Role of Bisphosphonates and Bone Health Issues in Women With Breast Cancer," *J Clin Oncol*, 2003, 21(21):4042-57.

◆ **Tiludronate Disodium** *see* Tiludronate *on page 1795*
◆ **Time-C® [OTC]** *see* Ascorbic Acid *on page 149*
◆ **Timentin®** *see* Ticarcillin and Clavulanate Potassium *on page 1789*

Timolol (Systemic) (TIM oh lol)

Related Information
Beta-Blockers *on page 2001*
Medication Safety Issues
Sound-alike/look-alike issues:
Timolol may be confused with atenolol, Tylenol®
Brand Names: Canada Apo-Timol®; Nu-Timolol; Teva-Timolol
Index Terms Timolol Maleate
Generic Availability (U.S.) Yes
Pharmacologic Category Beta-Adrenergic Blocker, Nonselective
Use Treatment of hypertension and angina; to reduce mortality following myocardial infarction; prophylaxis of migraine
Contraindications Hypersensitivity to timolol or any component of the formulation; sinus bradycardia; sinus node dysfunction; heart block greater than first degree (except in patients with a functioning artificial pacemaker); cardiogenic shock; uncompensated cardiac failure; bronchospastic disease
Warnings/Precautions Consider pre-existing conditions, such as sick sinus syndrome before initiating. Administer cautiously in compensated heart failure and monitor for a worsening of the condition. **[U.S. Boxed Warning]: Beta-blocker therapy should not be withdrawn abruptly (particularly in patients with CAD), but gradually tapered to avoid acute**

◄ **tachycardia, hypertension, and/or ischemia.** Chronic beta-blocker therapy should not be routinely withdrawn prior to major surgery. Use caution with concurrent use of digoxin, verapamil or diltiazem; bradycardia or heart block can occur. Use with caution in patients receiving inhaled anesthetic agents known to depress myocardial contractility. May precipitate or aggravate symptoms of arterial insufficiency in patients with PVD and Raynaud's disease; use with caution and monitor for progression of arterial obstruction. Patients with broncho-spastic disease should generally not receive beta-blockers - monitor closely if used in patients with potential risk of bronchospasm. Use cautiously in patients with diabetes because it can mask prominent hypoglycemic symptoms.

May mask signs of hyperthyroidism (eg, tachycardia); if hyperthyroidism is suspected, carefully manage and monitor; abrupt withdrawal may exacerbate symptoms of hyperthyroid-ism or precipitate thyroid storm. Bradycardia may be observed more frequently in elderly patients (>65 years of age); dosage reductions may be necessary. Use cautiously in severe renal impairment: marked hypotension can occur in patients maintained on hemodialysis. Can worsen myasthenia gravis. Use with caution in patients with a history of psychiatric illness; may cause or exacerbate CNS depression. Adequate alpha-blockade is required prior to use of any beta-blocker for patients with untreated pheochromocytoma. May induce or exacerbate psoriasis. Use caution with history of severe anaphylaxis to allergens; patients taking beta-blockers may become more sensitive to repeated challenges. Treatment of anaphylaxis (eg, epinephrine) in patients taking beta-blockers may be ineffective or promote undesirable effects.

Adverse Reactions (Reflective of adult population; not specific for elderly)
1% to 10%:
Cardiovascular: Bradycardia
Central nervous system: Fatigue, dizziness
Respiratory: Dyspnea

Frequency not defined:
Cardiovascular: Angina pectoris, arrhythmia, cardiac failure, cardiac arrest, cerebral vas-cular accident, cerebral ischemia, edema, hypotension, heart block, palpitation, Raynaud's phenomenon
Central nervous system: Anxiety, confusion, depression, disorientation, hallucinations, insomnia, memory loss, nervousness, nightmares, somnolence
Dermatologic: Alopecia, angioedema, pseudopemphigoid, psoriasiform rash, psoriasis exacerbation, rash, urticaria
Endocrine & metabolic: Hypoglycemia masked, libido decreased
Gastrointestinal: Anorexia, diarrhea, dyspepsia, nausea, xerostomia
Genitourinary: Impotence, retoperitoneal fibrosis
Hematologic: Claudication
Neuromuscular & skeletal: Myasthenia gravis exacerbation, paresthesia
Ocular: Blepharitis, conjunctivitis, corneal sensitivity decreased, cystoid macular edema, diplopia, dry eyes, foreign body sensation, keratitis, ocular discharge, ocular pain, ptosis, refractive changes, tearing, visual disturbances
Otic: Tinnitus
Respiratory: Bronchospasm, cough, nasal congestion, pulmonary edema, respiratory failure
Miscellaneous: Allergic reactions, cold hands/feet, Peyronie's disease, systemic lupus erythematosus

Drug Interactions
Metabolism/Transport Effects Substrate of CYP2D6 (major); **Inhibits** CYP2D6 (weak)
Avoid Concomitant Use
Avoid concomitant use of Timolol (Systemic) with any of the following: Floctafenine; Methacholine

Increased Effect/Toxicity
Timolol (Systemic) may increase the levels/effects of: Alpha-/Beta-Agonists (Direct-Acting); Alpha1-Blockers; Alpha2-Agonists; Amifostine; Antihypertensives; Antipsychotic Agents (Phenothiazines); Bupivacaine; Cardiac Glycosides; Fingolimod; Hypotensive Agents; Insu-lin; Lidocaine; Lidocaine (Systemic); Lidocaine (Topical); Mepivacaine; Methacholine; Mido-drine; RiTUXimab; Sulfonylureas

The levels/effects of Timolol (Systemic) may be increased by: Abiraterone Acetate; Acetylcholinesterase Inhibitors; Aminoquinolines (Antimalarial); Amiodarone; Anilidopiper-idine Opioids; Antipsychotic Agents (Phenothiazines); Calcium Channel Blockers (Dihydro-pyridine); Calcium Channel Blockers (Nondihydropyridine); CYP2D6 Inhibitors (Moderate); CYP2D6 Inhibitors (Strong); Darunavir; Diazoxide; Dipyridamole; Disopyramide; Dronedar-one; Floctafenine; Herbs (Hypotensive Properties); MAO Inhibitors; Pentoxifylline; Phos-phodiesterase 5 Inhibitors; Propafenone; Propoxyphene; Prostacyclin Analogues; QuiNIDine; Reserpine; Selective Serotonin Reuptake Inhibitors

Decreased Effect

Timolol (Systemic) may decrease the levels/effects of: Beta2-Agonists; Theophylline Derivatives

The levels/effects of Timolol (Systemic) may be decreased by: Barbiturates; Herbs (Hypertensive Properties); Methylphenidate; Nonsteroidal Anti-Inflammatory Agents; Peginterferon Alfa-2b; Rifamycin Derivatives; Yohimbine

Mechanism of Action Blocks both beta$_1$- and beta$_2$-adrenergic receptors; reduces blood pressure by blocking adrenergic receptors and decreasing sympathetic outflow, produces a negative chronotropic and inotropic activity through an unknown mechanism

Pharmacodynamics/Kinetics

Onset of action: Hypotensive: 15-45 minutes

Peak effect: 0.5-2.5 hours

Duration: ~4 hours

Absorption: Rapid and complete (~90%)

Distribution: V_d: 1.7 L/kg

Protein binding: 60%

Metabolism: Extensively hepatic via CYP2D6; extensive first-pass effect

Bioavailability: 50%

Half-life elimination: 2-2.7 hours; prolonged with renal impairment

Time to peak, plasma: 1-2 hours

Excretion: Urine (15% to 20% as unchanged drug)

Dosage

Geriatric & Adult

Hypertension: Oral: Initial: 10 mg twice daily, increase gradually every 7 days, usual dosage: 20-40 mg/day in 2 divided doses; maximum: 60 mg/day.

Prevention of myocardial infarction: Oral: 10 mg twice daily initiated within 1-4 weeks after infarction.

Migraine prophylaxis: Oral: Initial: 10 mg twice daily, increase to maximum of 30 mg/day.

Monitoring Parameters Blood pressure, apical and radial pulses, fluid I & O, daily weight, respirations, mental status, and circulation in extremities before and during therapy; monitor for systemic effect of beta-blockade

Special Geriatric Considerations Since bioavailability increased in about twofold in elderly patients, geriatrics may require lower maintenance doses. Also, as serum and tissue concentrations increase beta$_1$ selectivity diminishes. Beta-adrenergic blockade may result in less hemodynamic response than seen in younger adults due to alterations in the beta-adrenergic autonomic system. Studies indicate that despite decreased sensitivity to the chronotropic effects of beta-blockade with age, there appears to be an increased myocardial sensitivity to the negative inotropic effect during stress (ie, exercise). Controlled trials have shown the overall response rate for propranolol to be only 20% to 50% in elderly populations. Therefore, all beta-adrenergic blocking drugs may result in a decreased response as compared to younger adults. Due to propranolol's CNS penetration and nonselective action, it may not be the beta-blocker of choice for use in elderly.

Dosage Forms Excipient information presented when available (limited, particularly for generics); consult specific product labeling.

Tablet, oral, as maleate: 5 mg, 10 mg, 20 mg

Selected References

Fleisher LA, Beckman JA, Brown KA, "2009 ACCF/AHA Focused Update on Perioperative Beta Blockade Incorporated Into the ACC/AHA 2007 Guidelines on Perioperative Cardiovascular Evaluation and Care for Noncardiac Surgery. A Report of the American College of Cardiology Foundation/American Heart Association Task Force on Practice Guidelines," *J Am Coll Cardiol*, 2009, 54(22):e13-118.

Juul AB, Wetterslev J, Gluud C, et al, "Effect of Perioperative Beta Blockade in Patients With Diabetes Undergoing Major Non-Cardiac Surgery: Randomized Placebo Controlled, Blinded Multicentre Trial. DIPOM Trial Group," *BMJ*, 2006, 332(7556):1482.

Kligman EW and Higbee MD, "Drug Therapy for Hypertension in the Elderly," *J Fam Pract*, 1989, 28(1):81-7.

Levison SP, "Treating Hypertension in the Elderly," *Clin Geriatr Med*, 1988, 4(1):1-12.

Timolol (Ophthalmic) (TIM oh lol)

Related Information

Glaucoma Drug Therapy *on page 2008*

Medication Safety Issues

Sound-alike/look-alike issues:

Timolol may be confused with atenolol, Tylenol®

◀ Timoptic® may be confused with Betoptic® S, Talacen, Viroptic®

Other safety concerns:

Bottle cap color change: Timoptic®: Both the 0.25% and 0.5% strengths are now packaged in bottles with yellow caps; previously, the color of the cap on the product corresponded to different strengths.

International issues:

Betimol [U.S., Finland] may be confused with Betanol brand name for metipranolol [Monaco]

Brand Names: U.S. Betimol®; Istalol®; Timolol GFS; Timoptic-XE®; Timoptic®; Timoptic® in OcuDose®

Brand Names: Canada Apo-Timop®; Dom-Timolol; Mylan-Timolol; Novo-Timol; PMS-Timolol; Sandoz-Timolol; Tim-AK; Timolol Maleate-EX; Timoptic-XE®; Timoptic®

Index Terms Timolol Hemihydrate; Timolol Maleate

Generic Availability (U.S.) Yes: Excludes solution as maleate (preservative free), solution as hemihydrate

Pharmacologic Category Beta-Adrenergic Blocker, Nonselective; Ophthalmic Agent, Antiglaucoma

Use Treatment of elevated intraocular pressure such as glaucoma or ocular hypertension

Dosage

Geriatric & Adult Glaucoma: Ophthalmic:

Solution: Initial: 0.25% solution, instill 1 drop twice daily into affected eye(s); increase to 0.5% solution if response not adequate; decrease to 1 drop/day if controlled; do not exceed 1 drop twice daily of 0.5% solution.

Istalol®: Instill 1 drop (0.5% solution) once daily in the morning.

Gel-forming solution (Timolol GFS, Timoptic-XE®): Instill 1 drop (either 0.25% or 0.5%) once daily

Special Geriatric Considerations Evaluate the patient's or caregiver's ability to safely administer the correct dose of ophthalmic medication.

Dosage Forms Excipient information presented when available (limited, particularly for generics); consult specific product labeling.

Gel forming solution, ophthalmic, as maleate [strength expressed as base, drops]: 0.25% (5 mL); 0.5% (5 mL)

Timolol GFS: 0.25% (5 mL); 0.5% (5 mL)

Timoptic-XE®: 0.25% (5 mL); 0.5% (5 mL)

Solution, ophthalmic, as hemihydrate [strength expressed as base, drops]:

Betimol®: 0.25% (5 mL); 0.5% (5 mL, 10 mL, 15 mL) [contains benzalkonium chloride]

Solution, ophthalmic, as maleate [strength expressed as base, drops]: 0.25% (5 mL, 10 mL, 15 mL); 0.5% (5 mL, 10 mL, 15 mL)

Istalol®: 0.5% (2.5 mL, 5 mL) [contains benzalkonium chloride]

Timoptic®: 0.25% (5 mL); 0.5% (5 mL, 10 mL) [contains benzalkonium chloride]

Solution, ophthalmic, as maleate [strength expressed as base, drops, preservative free]:

Timoptic® in OcuDose®: 0.25% (0.2 mL); 0.5% (0.2 mL)

Tinzaparin (tin ZA pa rin)

Related Information

Anticoagulants, Injectable *on page 1989*

Medication Safety Issues

High alert medication:

The Institute for Safe Medication Practices (ISMP) includes this medication among its list of drug classes which have a heightened risk of causing significant patient harm when used in error.

2009 National Patient Safety Goals:

The Joint Commission (TJC) requires healthcare organizations that provide anticoagulant therapy to have a process in place to reduce the risk of anticoagulant-associated patient harm. Patients receiving anticoagulants should receive individualized care through a defined process that includes standardized ordering, dispensing, administration, monitoring and education. This does not apply to routine short-term use of anticoagulants for prevention of venous thromboembolism when the expectation is that the patient's laboratory values will remain within or close to normal values (NPSG.03.05.01).

Brand Names: U.S. Innohep® [DSC]

Brand Names: Canada Innohep®

Index Terms Tinzaparin Sodium

Generic Availability (U.S.) No

Pharmacologic Category Low Molecular Weight Heparin

Use Treatment of acute symptomatic deep vein thrombosis, with or without pulmonary embolism, in conjunction with warfarin sodium

Unlabeled/Investigational Use Prophylaxis of deep vein thrombosis following hip or knee replacement surgery, and general surgery

Contraindications Hypersensitivity to tinzaparin sodium, heparin, or any component of the formulation; active major bleeding; heparin-induced thrombocytopenia (current or history of)

Warnings/Precautions [U.S. Boxed Warning]: Spinal or epidural hematomas, including subsequent paralysis, may occur with recent or anticipated neuraxial anesthesia (epidural or spinal) or spinal puncture in patients anticoagulated with LMWH or heparinoids. Consider risk versus benefit prior to spinal procedures; risk is increased by the use of concomitant agents which may alter hemostasis, the use of indwelling epidural catheters for analgesia, a history of spinal deformity or spinal surgery, as well as traumatic or repeated epidural or spinal punctures. Patient should be observed closely for signs and symptoms of neurological impairment. Not to be used interchangeably (unit for unit) with heparin or any other low molecular weight heparins.

Monitor patient closely for signs or symptoms of bleeding. Certain patients are at increased risk of bleeding. Risk factors include bacterial endocarditis; congenital or acquired bleeding disorders; active ulcerative or angiodysplastic GI diseases; severe uncontrolled hypertension; history of hemorrhagic stroke; use shortly after brain, spinal, or ophthalmologic surgery; patients treated concomitantly with platelet inhibitors; recent GI bleeding; thrombocytopenia or platelet defects; severe liver disease; hypertensive or diabetic retinopathy; or in patients undergoing invasive procedures. Monitor platelet count closely. Rare cases of thrombocytopenia have occurred. Manufacturer recommends discontinuation of therapy if platelets are <100,000/mm^3. Rare cases of thrombocytopenia with thrombosis have occurred.

Reduced tinzaparin clearance was observed in patients with moderate-to-severe renal impairment; use with caution or avoid use in patients with renal insufficiency. The 2008 *Chest* guidelines recommend that patients with Cl$_{cr}$ <30 mL/minute be treated with unfractionated heparin instead of LMWH (Hirsh, 2008). Use with caution in the elderly (delayed elimination may occur). Use in patients ≥70 years of age with renal insufficiency (Cl$_{cr}$ ≤30 mL/minute or ≥75 years of age and Cl$_{cr}$ ≤60 mL/minute) has been associated with an increased risk of death compared to use of unfractionated heparin; consider alternative treatments in these patients.

Heparin can cause hyperkalemia by suppressing aldosterone production; similar reactions could occur with LMWHs. Monitor for hyperkalemia which most commonly occurs in patients with risk factors for the development of hyperkalemia (eg, renal dysfunction, concomitant use of potassium-sparing diuretics or potassium supplements, hematoma in body tissues). For subcutaneous use only; do not administer intramuscularly or intravenously. Clinical experience is limited in patients with BMI >40 kg/m^2. Derived from porcine intestinal mucosa. Contains benzyl alcohol and sodium metabisulfite.

Adverse Reactions (Reflective of adult population; not specific for elderly) As with all anticoagulants, bleeding is the major adverse effect of tinzaparin. Hemorrhage may occur at virtually any site. Risk is dependent on multiple variables.

>10%:
  Hepatic: ALT increased (13%)
  Local: Injection site hematoma (16%)
1% to 10%:
  Cardiovascular: Angina pectoris, chest pain (2%), hyper-/hypotension, tachycardia
  Central nervous system: Confusion, dizziness, fever (2%), headache (2%), insomnia, pain (2%)
  Dermatologic: Bullous eruption, pruritus, rash (1%), skin disorder
  Gastrointestinal: Constipation (1%), dyspepsia, flatulence, nausea (2%), nonspecified gastrointestinal disorder, vomiting (1%)
  Genitourinary: Dysuria, urinary retention, urinary tract infection (4%)
  Hematologic: Anemia, hematoma, hemorrhage (2%), thrombocytopenia (1%)
  Hepatic: AST increased (9%)
  Local: Thrombophlebitis (deep)
  Neuromuscular & skeletal: Back pain (2%)
  Renal: Hematuria (1%)
  Respiratory: Dyspnea (1%), epistaxis (2%), pneumonia, pulmonary embolism (2%), respiratory disorder
  Miscellaneous: Impaired healing, infection, unclassified reactions

Drug Interactions
Avoid Concomitant Use
  Avoid concomitant use of Tinzaparin with any of the following: Rivaroxaban
Increased Effect/Toxicity
  Tinzaparin may increase the levels/effects of: Anticoagulants; Collagenase (Systemic); Deferasirox; Drotrecogin Alfa; Ibritumomab; Rivaroxaban; Tositumomab and Iodine I 131 Tositumomab

  The levels/effects of Tinzaparin may be increased by: 5-ASA Derivatives; Antiplatelet Agents; Dasatinib; Herbs (Anticoagulant/Antiplatelet Properties); Nonsteroidal Anti-Inflammatory Agents; Pentosan Polysulfate Sodium; Pentoxifylline; Prostacyclin Analogues; Salicylates; Thrombolytic Agents

Decreased Effect There are no known significant interactions involving a decrease in effect.
Stability Store at 15°C to 30°C (59°F to 86°F).
Mechanism of Action Standard heparin consists of components with molecular weights ranging from 4000-30,000 daltons with a mean of 16,000 daltons. Heparin acts as an anticoagulant by enhancing the inhibition rate of clotting proteases by antithrombin III, impairing normal hemostasis and inhibition of factor Xa. Low molecular weight heparins have a small effect on the activated partial thromboplastin time and strongly inhibit factor Xa. The primary inhibitory activity of tinzaparin is through antithrombin. Tinzaparin is derived from porcine heparin that undergoes controlled enzymatic depolymerization. The average molecular weight of tinzaparin ranges between 5500 and 7500 daltons which is distributed as <2000 daltons (<10%), 2000-8000 daltons (60% to 72%), and >8000 daltons (22% to 36%). The anti-Xa activity is approximately 100 int. units/mg.

Pharmacodynamics/Kinetics
Onset of action: 2-3 hours
Distribution: 3-5 L
Half-life elimination: 3-4 hours
Metabolism: Partially metabolized by desulphation and depolymerization
Bioavailability: 87%
Time to peak: 4-5 hours
Excretion: Urine

Dosage
  Geriatric Refer to adult dosing. Increased sensitivity to tinzaparin in elderly patients may be possible due to a decline in renal function. Increased all-cause mortality noted in patients ≥70 years of age with Cl_{cr} ≤30 mL/minute or ≥75 years of age and Cl_{cr} ≤60 mL/minute; consider alternative treatments in these patients.
  Adult Note: Each 100 int. units of anti-Xa activity is equal to 1 mg of tinzaparin.
  Note: A pharmacokinetic study confirmed that weight-based dosing (single doses of 75 or 175 units/kg) using actual body weight in heavy/obese patients between 100 and 165 kg led to achievement of similar anti-Xa activity levels compared to normal-weight patients (Hainer, 2002). However, there is limited clinical experience in patients with a BMI >40 kg/m^2.

DVT (with or without PE) treatment: SubQ: 175 anti-Xa int. units/kg once daily. The 2008 *Chest* guidelines recommend starting warfarin on the first treatment day and continuing tinzaparin until INR is between 2 and 3 (usually 5-7 days). Administer tinzaparin for at least 5 days and until INR ≥2 for at least 24 hours (Hirsh, 2008).

DVT prophylaxis (unlabeled use): SubQ:

Hip replacement surgery: 75 anti-Xa int. units/kg once daily, with initial dose given 18-24 hours after surgery for up to 14 days **or** 4500 anti-Xa int. units once daily, with initial dose given 12 hours prior to surgery and continued for up to 15 days (Hull, 1993; Planes, 1999)

Knee replacement surgery: 75 anti-Xa int. units/kg once daily, with initial dose given 18-24 hours after surgery and continued for up to 14 days (Hull, 1993)

General surgery: 3500 anti-Xa int. units once daily, with initial dose given 2 hours prior to surgery and continued for 7-10 days (Leizorovicz, 1991)

Renal Impairment

Cl$_{cr}$ ≤50 mL/minute: Use with caution; clearance is decreased.

Cl$_{cr}$ <30 mL/minute: Per manufacturer's labeling, use with caution. The 2008 *Chest* guidelines recommend avoiding use (in patients requiring therapeutic anticoagulation); if used, consider monitoring anti-Xa levels (Hirsh, 2008).

Hepatic Impairment No adjustment necessary.

Administration Patient should be lying down or sitting. Administer by deep SubQ injection, alternating between the left and right anterolateral and left and right posterolateral abdominal wall. Vary site daily. The entire needle should be introduced into the skin fold formed by the thumb and forefinger. Hold the skin fold until injection is complete. To minimize bruising, do not rub the injection site.

Monitoring Parameters CBC including platelet count and hematocrit or hemoglobin, and stool for occult blood; the monitoring of PT and/or aPTT is not of clinical value. Patients receiving both warfarin and tinzaparin should have their INR drawn just prior to the next scheduled dose of tinzaparin.

According to 2008 *Chest* guidelines, routine monitoring of anti-Xa levels is generally not recommended; however, anti-Xa levels may be beneficial in certain patients (eg, obese patients, patients with severe renal insufficiency receiving therapeutic doses, and possibly pregnant women receiving therapeutic doses; Hirsh, 2008)

Special Geriatric Considerations No significant differences in safety or response were seen when used in patients ≥65 years of age. However, increased sensitivity to tinzaparin in elderly patients may be possible due to a decline in renal function. Results from the Innohep in Renal Insufficiency Study (IRIS) study showed an increase in all-cause mortality in elderly patients receiving tinzaparin compared to unfractionated heparin for treatment of DVT and/or PE. The at-risk population has defined as patients ≥70 years of age with Cl$_{cr}$ ≤30 mL/minute or ≥75 years of age and Cl$_{cr}$ ≤60 mL/minute.

Dosage Forms Excipient information presented when available (limited, particularly for generics); consult specific product labeling. [DSC] = Discontinued product

Injection, solution, as sodium:

Innohep®: 20,000 anti-Xa int. units/mL (2 mL [DSC]) [contains benzyl alcohol, sodium metabisulfite]

Selected References

Hainer JW, Barrett JS, Assaid CA, et al, "Dosing in Heavy-weight/Obese Patients With the LMWH, Tinzaparin: A Pharmacodynamic Study," *Thromb Haemost*, 2002, 87(5):817-23.

Hirsh J, Bauer KA, Donati MB, et al, "Parenteral Anticoagulants: American College of Chest Physicians Evidence-Based Clinical Practice Guidelines (8th Edition)," *Chest*, 2008, 133(6 Suppl):141-59.

Kearon C, Kahn SR, Agnelli G, et al, "Antithrombotic Therapy for Venous Thromboembolic Disease: American College of Chest Physicians Evidence-Based Clinical Practice Guidelines (8th Edition)," *Chest*, 2008, 33(6 Suppl):454-545.

♦ Tinzaparin Sodium *see* Tinzaparin *on page 1801*

Tioconazole (tye oh KONE a zole)

Medication Safety Issues

Sound-alike/look-alike issues:

Tioconazole may be confused with terconazole

Brand Names: U.S. 1-Day™ [OTC]; Vagistat®-1 [OTC]

Generic Availability (U.S.) No

Pharmacologic Category Antifungal Agent, Vaginal

Use Local treatment of vulvovaginal candidiasis

Contraindications Hypersensitivity to tioconazole or any component of the formulation

Warnings/Precautions If irritation or sensitization occurs, discontinue use. Petrolatum-based vaginal products may damage rubber or latex condoms or diaphragms. Separate use by 3 days.

Adverse Reactions (Reflective of adult population; not specific for elderly) Frequency not defined.
Central nervous system: Headache
Gastrointestinal: Abdominal pain
Dermatologic: Burning, desquamation
Genitourinary: Discharge, dyspareunia, dysuria, irritation, itching, nocturia, vaginal pain, vaginitis, vulvar swelling

Drug Interactions
Metabolism/Transport Effects Inhibits CYP1A2 (weak), 2A6 (weak), 2C9 (weak), 2C19 (weak), 2D6 (weak), 2E1 (weak)
Avoid Concomitant Use There are no known interactions where it is recommended to avoid concomitant use.
Increased Effect/Toxicity There are no known significant interactions involving an increase in effect.
Decreased Effect There are no known significant interactions involving a decrease in effect.

Stability Store at room temperature.
Mechanism of Action A 1-substituted imidazole derivative with a broad antifungal spectrum against a wide variety of dermatophytes and yeasts, including *Trichophyton mentagrophytes*, *T. rubrum*, *T. erinacei*, *T. tonsurans*, *Microsporum canis*, *Microsporum gypseum*, and *Candida albicans*. Both agents appear to be similarly effective against *Epidermophyton floccosum*.

Pharmacodynamics/Kinetics
Onset of action: Some improvement: Within 24 hours; Complete relief: Within 7 days
Absorption: Intravaginal: Systemic (small amounts)
Distribution: Vaginal fluid: 24-72 hours
Excretion: Urine and feces

Dosage
Geriatric & Adult Vulvovaginal candidiasis: Vaginal: Insert 1 applicatorful in vagina, just prior to bedtime, as a single dose
Administration Insert high into vagina
Special Geriatric Considerations Assess patient's ability to self-administer; may be difficult in patients with arthritis or limited range of motion.
Dosage Forms Excipient information presented when available (limited, particularly for generics); consult specific product labeling.
Ointment, vaginal:
1-Day™: 6.5% (4.6 g)
Vagistat®-1: 6.5% (4.6 g) [applicator delivers approximately 300 mg of tioconazole]

◆ **Tiotixene** see Thiothixene on page 1783

Tiotropium (ty oh TRO pee um)

Related Information
Inhalant Agents on page 2010
Medication Safety Issues
Sound-alike/look-alike issues:
Spiriva® may be confused with Inspra™, Serevent®
Tiotropium may be confused with ipratropium
Administration issues:
Spiriva® capsules for inhalation are for administration via HandiHaler® device and are **not** for oral use

Brand Names: U.S. Spiriva® HandiHaler®
Brand Names: Canada Spiriva®
Index Terms Tiotropium Bromide Monohydrate
Generic Availability (U.S.) No
Pharmacologic Category Anticholinergic Agent
Use Maintenance treatment of bronchospasm associated with COPD (including bronchitis and emphysema); reduction of COPD exacerbations
Contraindications Hypersensitivity to tiotropium or ipratropium, or any component of the formulation (contains lactose)
Warnings/Precautions Rarely, paradoxical bronchospasm may occur with use of inhaled bronchodilating agents; discontinue use and consider other therapy if bronchospasm occurs.

Not indicated for the initial (rescue) treatment of acute episodes of bronchospasm. Use with caution in patients with myasthenia gravis, narrow-angle glaucoma, prostatic hyperplasia, moderate-severe renal impairment (Cl_{cr} ≤50 mL/minute), or bladder neck obstruction; avoid inadvertent instillation of powder into the eyes. Immediate hypersensitivity reactions may occur; discontinue immediately if signs/symptoms occur. Use with caution in patients with a history of hypersensitivity to atropine.

The contents of Spiriva® capsules are for inhalation only via the HandiHaler® device. There have been reports of incorrect administration (swallowing of the capsules). Capsule for oral inhalation contains lactose; use with caution in patients with severe milk protein allergy.

Adverse Reactions (Reflective of adult population; not specific for elderly)

>10%:

Gastrointestinal: Xerostomia (5% to 16%)

Respiratory: Upper respiratory tract infection (41%), pharyngitis (9% to 13%), sinusitis (7% to 11%)

1% to 10%:

Cardiovascular: Chest pain (1% to 7%), edema (dependent, 5%)

Central nervous system: Headache (6%), insomnia (4%), depression (1% to 4%), dysphonia (1% to 3%)

Dermatologic: Rash (4%)

Endocrine & metabolic: Hypercholesterolemia (1% to 3%), hyperglycemia (1% to 3%)

Gastrointestinal: Dyspepsia (6%), abdominal pain (5%), constipation (4% to 5%), vomiting (4%), gastroesophageal reflux (1% to 3%), stomatitis (including ulcerative; 1% to 3%)

Genitourinary: Urinary tract infection (7%)

Neuromuscular & skeletal: Arthralgia (4%), myalgia (4%), arthritis (≥3%), leg pain (1% to 3%), paresthesia (1% to 3%), skeletal pain (1% to 3%)

Ocular: Cataract (1% to 3%)

Respiratory: Rhinitis (6%), epistaxis (4%), cough (≥3%), laryngitis (1% to 3%)

Miscellaneous: Infection (4%), moniliasis (4%), flu-like syndrome (≥3%), allergic reaction (1% to 3%), herpes zoster (1% to 3%)

Drug Interactions

Metabolism/Transport Effects Substrate (minor) of CYP2D6, 3A4

Avoid Concomitant Use There are no known interactions where it is recommended to avoid concomitant use.

Increased Effect/Toxicity

Tiotropium may increase the levels/effects of: AbobotulinumtoxinA; Anticholinergics; Cannabinoids; OnabotulinumtoxinA; Potassium Chloride; RimabotulinumtoxinB

The levels/effects of Tiotropium may be increased by: Conivaptan; Pramlintide

Decreased Effect

Tiotropium may decrease the levels/effects of: Acetylcholinesterase Inhibitors (Central); Secretin

The levels/effects of Tiotropium may be decreased by: Acetylcholinesterase Inhibitors (Central); Peginterferon Alfa-2b; Tocilizumab

Stability Store at 25°C (77°F); excursions permitted to 15°C to 30°C (59°F to 86°F). Avoid excessive temperatures and moisture. Do not store capsules in HandiHaler® device. Capsules should be stored in the blister pack and only removed immediately before use. Once protective foil is peeled back and/or removed the capsule should be used immediately; if capsule is not used immediately it should be discarded.

Mechanism of Action Competitively and reversibly inhibits the action of acetylcholine at type 3 muscarinic (M_3) receptors in bronchial smooth muscle causing bronchodilation

Pharmacodynamics/Kinetics

Absorption: Poorly absorbed from GI tract, systemic absorption may occur from lung

Distribution: V_d: 32 L/kg

Protein binding: 72%

Metabolism: Hepatic (minimal), via CYP2D6 and CYP3A4

Bioavailability: Following inhalation, 19.5%; oral solution: 2% to 3%

Half-life elimination: 5-6 days

Time to peak, plasma: 5 minutes (following inhalation)

Excretion: Urine (14% of an inhaled dose); feces (primarily nonabsorbed drug)

Dosage

Geriatric & Adult COPD: Oral inhalation: Contents of 1 capsule (18 mcg) inhaled once daily using HandiHaler® device. **Note:** To ensure drug delivery the contents of each capsule should be inhaled twice.

Renal Impairment Plasma concentrations may increase in renal impairment. Use caution in moderate-to-severe impairment (Cl_{cr} ≤50 mL/minute); although no dosage adjustment is required, monitor closely.

Administration Administer once daily at the same time each day. Remove capsule from foil blister immediately before use. Place capsule in the capsule-chamber in the base of the HandiHaler® Inhaler. Must only use the HandiHaler® Inhaler. Close mouthpiece until a click is heard, leaving dustcap open. Exhale fully. Do not exhale into inhaler. Tilt head slightly back and inhale (rapidly, steadily and deeply); the capsule vibration may be heard within the device. Hold breath as long as possible. If any powder remains in capsule, exhale and inhale again. Repeat until capsule is empty. Throw away empty capsule; do not leave in inhaler. Do not use a spacer with the HandiHaler® Inhaler. Always keep capsules and inhaler dry.

Delivery of dose: Instruct patient to place mouthpiece gently between teeth, closing lips around inhaler. Instruct patient to inhale deeply and hold breath held for 5-10 seconds. The amount of drug delivered is small, and the individual will not sense the medication as it is inhaled. Remove mouthpiece prior to exhalation. Patient should not breathe out through the mouthpiece.

Monitoring Parameters FEV_1, peak flow (or other pulmonary function studies)

Special Geriatric Considerations Assess patient's ability to use the HandiHaler®. In elderly patients, renal clearance of tiotropium was decreased and plasma concentrations were increased, due to decreased renal function. In clinical trials, the incidence of constipation, UTIs and xerostomia increased with age. No dosage adjustments are recommended due to age or renal function. However, the manufacturer recommends monitoring patients with moderate-to-severe renal impairment.

Dosage Forms Excipient information presented when available (limited, particularly for generics); consult specific product labeling.

Powder, for oral inhalation [capsule]:

Spiriva® HandiHaler®: 18 mcg/capsule (5s, 30s, 90s) [contains lactose]

Selected References

Expert Panel Report 3, "Guidelines for the Diagnosis and Management of Asthma," *Clinical Practice Guidelines*, National Institutes of Health, National Heart, Lung, and Blood Institute, NIH Publication No. 08-4051, prepublication 2007. Available at http://www.nhlbi.nih.gov/guidelines/asthma/asthgdln.htm

♦ **Tiotropium Bromide Monohydrate** see Tiotropium on page 1804

Tirofiban (tye roe FYE ban)

Medication Safety Issues

Sound-alike/look-alike issues:

Aggrastat® may be confused with Aggrenox®, argatroban

High alert medication:

The Institute for Safe Medication Practices (ISMP) includes this medication among its list of drugs which have a heightened risk of causing significant patient harm when used in error.

Brand Names: U.S. Aggrastat®

Brand Names: Canada Aggrastat®

Index Terms MK383; Tirofiban Hydrochloride

Generic Availability (U.S.) No

Pharmacologic Category Antiplatelet Agent, Glycoprotein IIb/IIIa Inhibitor

Use Treatment of acute coronary syndrome (ie, unstable angina/non-ST-elevation myocardial infarction [UA/NSTEMI]) in combination with heparin

Unlabeled/Investigational Use To support PCI during ST-elevation myocardial infarction (STEMI) (administered at the time of primary PCI)

Contraindications Hypersensitivity to tirofiban or any component of the formulation; active internal bleeding or a history of bleeding diathesis within the previous 30 days; history of intracranial hemorrhage, intracranial neoplasm, arteriovenous malformation, or aneurysm; history of thrombocytopenia following prior exposure; history of CVA within 30 days or any history of hemorrhagic stroke; major surgical procedure or severe physical trauma within the previous month; history, symptoms, or findings suggestive of aortic dissection; severe hypertension (systolic BP >180 mm Hg and/or diastolic BP >110 mm Hg); concomitant use of another parenteral GP IIb/IIIa inhibitor; acute pericarditis

Warnings/Precautions Bleeding is the most common complication encountered during this therapy; most major bleeding occurs at the arterial access site for cardiac catheterization. Caution in patients with platelets <150,000/mm^3; patients with hemorrhagic retinopathy; chronic dialysis patients; when used in combination with other drugs impacting on coagulation. Prior to pulling the sheath, heparin should be discontinued for 3-4 hours and ACT <180 seconds or aPTT <45 seconds. Use standard compression techniques after sheath removal. Watch the site closely afterwards for further bleeding. Sheath hemostasis should be achieved at least 4 hours before hospital discharge. Other trauma and vascular punctures should be minimized. Avoid obtaining vascular access through a noncompressible site (eg, subclavian or jugular vein). Patients with severe renal insufficiency require dosage reduction.

Adverse Reactions (Reflective of adult population; not specific for elderly) Bleeding is the major drug-related adverse effect. Patients received background treatment with aspirin and heparin. Major bleeding was reported in 1.4% to 2.2%; minor bleeding in 10.5% to 12%; transfusion was required in 4% to 4.3%.

>1% (nonbleeding adverse events):

Cardiovascular: Coronary artery dissection (5%), bradycardia (4%), edema (2%)

Central nervous system: Dizziness (3%), vasovagal reaction (2%), fever (>1%), headache (>1%)

Gastrointestinal: Nausea (>1%)

Genitourinary: Pelvic pain (6%)

Hematologic: Thrombocytopenia: <90,000/mm^3 (1.5%), <50,000/mm^3 (0.3%)

Neuromuscular & skeletal: Leg pain (3%)

Miscellaneous: Diaphoresis (2%)

Drug Interactions

Avoid Concomitant Use There are no known interactions where it is recommended to avoid concomitant use.

Increased Effect/Toxicity

Tirofiban may increase the levels/effects of: Anticoagulants; Antiplatelet Agents; Collagenase (Systemic); Drotrecogin Alfa; Ibritumomab; Rivaroxaban; Salicylates; Thrombolytic Agents; Tositumomab and Iodine I 131 Tositumomab

The levels/effects of Tirofiban may be increased by: Dasatinib; Glucosamine; Herbs (Anticoagulant/Antiplatelet Properties); Nonsteroidal Anti-Inflammatory Agents; Omega-3-Acid Ethyl Esters; Pentosan Polysulfate Sodium; Pentoxifylline; Prostacyclin Analogues; Vitamin E

Decreased Effect

The levels/effects of Tirofiban may be decreased by: Nonsteroidal Anti-Inflammatory Agents

Stability Store at 25°C (77°F); do not freeze. Protect from light during storage.

Mechanism of Action A reversible antagonist of fibrinogen binding to the GP IIb/IIIa receptor, the major platelet surface receptor involved in platelet aggregation. When administered intravenously, it inhibits *ex vivo* platelet aggregation in a dose- and concentration-dependent manner. When given according to the recommended regimen, >90% inhibition is attained by the end of the 30-minute infusion. Platelet aggregation inhibition is reversible following cessation of the infusion.

Pharmacodynamics/Kinetics

Distribution: 35% unbound

Metabolism: Minimally hepatic

Half-life elimination: 2 hours

Excretion: Urine (65%) and feces (25%) primarily as unchanged drug

Clearance: Elderly: Reduced by 19% to 26%

Dosage

Geriatric & Adult

Unstable angina/non-ST-elevation myocardial infarction (UA/NSTEMI): I.V.: Initial rate of 0.4 mcg/kg/minute for 30 minutes and then continued at 0.1 mcg/kg/minute. Dosing should be continued through angiography and for 12-24 hours after angioplasty or atherectomy.

ST-elevation myocardial infarction (STEMI) undergoing percutaneous coronary intervention (PCI) (unlabeled use): Loading dose: 25 mcg/kg over 3 minutes at the time of PCI; Maintenance infusion: 0.15 mcg/kg/minute continued for up to 18 hours (Kushner, 2009)

Renal Impairment Cl$_{cr}$ <30 mL/minute: Reduce dose to 50% of normal rate.

Administration Intended for intravenous delivery using sterile equipment and technique. Do not add other drugs or remove solution directly from the bag with a syringe. Do not use plastic containers in series connections; such use can result in air embolism by drawing air from the first container if it is empty of solution. Discard unused solution 24 hours following the start of infusion. May be administered through the same catheter as heparin. Tirofiban injection must be diluted to a concentration of 50 mcg/mL (premixed solution does not require dilution). For unstable angina/non-ST-elevation MI (UA/NSTEMI), infuse loading dose over 30 minutes, followed by continuous infusion. When used during percutaneous coronary intervention (PCI), may administer loading dose over 3 minutes, followed by continuous infusion.

Monitoring Parameters Platelet count. Hemoglobin and hematocrit should be monitored prior to treatment, within 6 hours following loading infusion, and at least daily thereafter during therapy. Platelet count may need to be monitored earlier in patients who received prior glycoprotein IIb/IIIa antagonists. Persistent reductions of platelet counts <90,000/mm^3 may require interruption or discontinuation of infusion. Because tirofiban requires concurrent heparin therapy, aPTT levels should also be followed. Monitor vital signs and laboratory results prior to, during, and after therapy. Assess infusion insertion site during and after therapy (every 15 minutes or as institutional policy). Observe and teach patient bleeding precautions (avoid invasive procedures and activities that could result in injury). Monitor closely for signs of unusual or excessive bleeding (eg, CNS changes, blood in urine, stool, or vomitus, unusual bruising or bleeding).

Special Geriatric Considerations Elderly patients receiving tirofiban with heparin or heparin alone had a higher incidence of bleeding in clinical trials. Caution must be used when using other drugs affecting hemostasis, which are commonly used in elderly.

Dosage Forms Excipient information presented when available (limited, particularly for generics); consult specific product labeling. [DSC] = Discontinued product

Infusion, premixed in NS [preservative free]:
Aggrastat®: 50 mcg/mL (100 mL [DSC], 250 mL)

Selected References

Braunwald E, Antman EM, Beasley JW, et al, "ACC/AHA Guidelines for the Management of Patients With Unstable Angina and Non-ST-Segment Elevation Myocardial Infarction. A Report of the American College of Cardiology/American Heart Association Task Force on Practice Guidelines (Committee on the Management of Patients With Unstable Angina)," J Am Coll Cardiol, 2000, 36(3):970-1062.

Goodman SG, Menon V, Cannon CP, et al, "Acute ST-Segment Elevation Myocardial Infarction: American College of Chest Physicians Evidence-Based Clinical Practice Guidelines (8th Edition)," Chest, 2008, 133(6 Suppl):708-75.

Kushner FG, Hand M, Smith SC, et al, "2009 Focused Updates: ACC/AHA Guidelines for the Management of Patients With ST-Elevation Myocardial Infarction (Updating the 2004 Guideline and 2007 Focused Update) and ACC/AHA/SCAI Guidelines on Percutaneous Coronary Intervention (Updating the 2005 Guideline and 2007 Focused Update): A Report of the American College of Cardiology Foundation/American Heart Association Task Force on Practice Guidelines," J Am Coll Cardiol, 2009, 54(23):2205-41.

◆ **Tirofiban Hydrochloride** see Tirofiban on page 1806
◆ **Tirosint®** see Levothyroxine on page 1058
◆ **Titralac® Plus Liquid [OTC]** see Calcium Salts (Oral) on page 256
◆ **TIV** see Influenza Virus Vaccine (Inactivated) on page 936

TiZANidine (tye ZAN i deen)

Medication Safety Issues
Sound-alike/look-alike issues:
TiZANidine may be confused with tiaGABine
Zanaflex® may be confused with Xiaflex™

Other safety concerns:
Zanaflex® capsules and Zanaflex® tablets (or generic tizanidine tablets) are not interchangeable

Brand Names: U.S. Zanaflex Capsules®; Zanaflex®
Brand Names: Canada Apo-Tizanidine®; Gen-Tizanidine; Mylan-Tizanidine; Zanaflex®
Index Terms Sirdalud®
Generic Availability (U.S.) Yes: Tablet
Pharmacologic Category Alpha$_2$-Adrenergic Agonist
Use Skeletal muscle relaxant used for treatment of muscle spasticity
Unlabeled/Investigational Use Treatment of tension headaches, low back pain, trigeminal neuralgia
Contraindications Hypersensitivity to tizanidine or any component of the formulation; concomitant therapy with ciprofloxacin or fluvoxamine (potent CYP1A2 inhibitors)
Warnings/Precautions Significant hypotension (possibly with bradycardia or orthostatic hypotension) and sedation may occur; use caution in patients with cardiac disease or those at risk for severe hypotensive or sedative effects. Should not be used with other alpha$_2$-adrenergic agonists. Avoid concomitant administration with CYP1A2 inhibitors; increased tizanidine levels/effects (severe hypotension and sedation) may occur. These effects may also be increased with concomitant administration with other CNS depressants and/or antihypertensives; use caution. Elderly patients are at risk due to decreased clearance, particulary in elderly patients with renal insufficiency (Cl$_{cr}$ <25 mL/minute) compared to healthy elderly subjects; this may lead to an increased risk of adverse effects and/or a longer duration of effects. Use caution in any patient with renal impairment; reduced initial doses recommended in patient with Cl$_{cr}$ <25 mL/minute. Use with extreme caution or avoid in hepatic impairment due to extensive hepatic metabolism and potential hepatotoxicity; AST/ALT elevations (≥2 times baseline) and rarely hepatic failure have occurred; monitoring recommended.

Use has been associated with visual hallucinations or delusions, generally in first 6 weeks of therapy; use caution in patients with psychiatric disorders. Withdrawal resulting in rebound hypertension, tachycardia, and hypertonia may occur upon discontinuation; doses should be decreased slowly, particularly in patients receiving high doses for prolonged periods. Pharmacokinetics and bioequivalence between capsules and tablets altered by nonfasting vs fasting conditions. Limited data exists for chronic use of single doses >8 mg and multiple doses >24 mg/day.

Adverse Reactions (Reflective of adult population; not specific for elderly) Frequency percentages below reported during multiple-dose studies, unless specified otherwise.
>10%:
    Cardiovascular: Hypotension (single-dose study with doses ≥8 mg: 16% to 33%)
    Central nervous system: Somnolence (48%), dizziness (16%)
    Gastrointestinal: Xerostomia (49%)
    Neuromuscular & skeletal: Weakness (41%)
1% to 10%:
    Cardiovascular: Bradycardia (single-dose study with doses ≥8 mg: 2% to 10%)
    Central nervous system: Nervousness (3%), speech disorder (3%), visual hallucinations/delusions (3%; generally occurring in first 6 weeks of therapy), anxiety (1%), depression (1%), fever (1%)
    Dermatologic: Rash (1%), skin ulcer (1%)
    Gastrointestinal: Constipation (4%), vomiting (3%), abdominal pain (1%), diarrhea (1%), dyspepsia (1%)
    Genitourinary: UTI (10%), urinary frequency (3%)
    Hepatic: Liver enzymes increased (3% to 5%)
    Neuromuscular & skeletal: Dyskinesia (3%), back pain (1%), myasthenia (1%), paresthesia (1%)
    Ocular: Blurred vision (3%)
    Respiratory: Pharyngitis (3%), rhinitis (3%)
    Miscellaneous: Infection (6%), flu-like syndrome (3%), diaphoresis (1%)
Drug Interactions
  Metabolism/Transport Effects Substrate of CYP1A2 (major)
  Avoid Concomitant Use
    Avoid concomitant use of TiZANidine with any of the following: Ciprofloxacin; Ciprofloxacin (Systemic); FluvoxaMINE; Iobenguane I 123
  Increased Effect/Toxicity
    TiZANidine may increase the levels/effects of: ACE Inhibitors; Alcohol (Ethyl); CNS Depressants; Hypotensive Agents; Lisinopril; Methotrimeprazine; Selective Serotonin Reuptake Inhibitors

    The levels/effects of TiZANidine may be increased by: Abiraterone Acetate; Beta-Blockers; Ciprofloxacin; Ciprofloxacin (Systemic); Contraceptives (Estrogens); CYP1A2 Inhibitors (Moderate); CYP1A2 Inhibitors (Strong); Deferasirox; Droperidol; FluvoxaMINE; HydrOXYzine; MAO Inhibitors; Methotrimeprazine
  Decreased Effect
    TiZANidine may decrease the levels/effects of: Iobenguane I 123

    The levels/effects of TiZANidine may be decreased by: Antidepressants (Alpha2-Antagonist); Cyproterone; Serotonin/Norepinephrine Reuptake Inhibitors; Tricyclic Antidepressants
Ethanol/Nutrition/Herb Interactions
  Ethanol: May increase CNS depression; monitor for increased effects with coadministration. Caution patients about effects.
  Food: The tablet and capsule dosage forms are not bioequivalent when administered with food. Food increases both the time to peak concentration and the extent of absorption for both the tablet and capsule. However, maximal concentrations of tizanidine achieved when administered with food were increased by 30% for the tablet, but decreased by 20% for the capsule. Under fed conditions, the capsule is approximately 80% bioavailable relative to the tablet.
  Herb/Nutraceutical: Avoid valerian, St John's wort, kava kava, gotu kola (may increase CNS depression). Avoid black cohosh, California poppy, coleus, golden seal, hawthorn, mistletoe, periwinkle, quinine, shepherd's purse (may increase hypotensive effects).
Stability Store at 25°C (77°F); excursions permitted to 15°C to 30°C (59°F to 86°F).
Mechanism of Action An alpha$_2$-adrenergic agonist agent which decreases excitatory input to alpha motor neurons; an imidazole derivative chemically-related to clonidine, which acts as a centrally acting muscle relaxant with alpha$_2$-adrenergic agonist properties; acts on the level of the spinal cord
Pharmacodynamics/Kinetics
  Absorption: Tablets and capsules are bioequivalent under fasting conditions, but not under nonfasting conditions.
    Tablets administered with food: Peak plasma concentration is increased by ~30%; time to peak increased by 25 minutes; extent of absorption increased by ~30%.
    Capsules administered with food: Peak plasma concentration decreased by 20%; time to peak increased by 2-3 hours; extent of absorption increased by ~10%.
    Capsules opened and sprinkled on applesauce are not bioequivalent to administration of intact capsules under fasting conditions. Peak plasma concentration and AUC are increased by 15% to 20%.

Distribution: V_d: 204 L/kg
Protein binding: ~30%
Metabolism: Extensively hepatic
Bioavailability: ~40% (extensive first-pass metabolism)
Half-life elimination: 2 hours
Time to peak serum:
  Fasting state: Capsule, tablet: 1 hour
  Fed state: Capsule: 3-4 hours, Tablet: 1.5 hours
Excretion: Urine (60%); feces (20%)

Dosage

Geriatric No specific dosing guidelines exist; clearance is decreased; dose cautiously.

Adult Spasticity: Usual initial dose: 4 mg, may increase by 2-4 mg as needed for satisfactory reduction of muscle tone every 6-8 hours to a maximum of 3 doses in any 24 hour period
Range: 2-4 mg 3 times/day
Maximum: 36 mg/day

Renal Impairment Cl_{cr} <25 mL/minute: Use with caution; clearance reduced >50%. During initial dose titration, use reduced doses. If higher doses necessary, increase dose instead of increasing dosing frequency.

Hepatic Impairment Avoid use in hepatic impairment; if used, lowest possible dose should be used initially with close monitoring for adverse effects (eg, hypotension).

Administration Capsules may be opened and contents sprinkled on food; however, extent of absorption is increased up to 20% relative to administration of the capsule under fasted conditions.

Monitoring Parameters Monitor liver function (aminotransferases) at baseline, 1, 3, 6 months and periodically thereafter; blood pressure; renal function

Pharmacotherapy Pearls Single doses of 8 mg reduce muscle tone for a period of several hours; the effect peaks in 1-2 hours and lasts 3-6 hours; effects are dose-related, however, it is prudent to start at lower doses as above.

Special Geriatric Considerations Since elderly commonly have renal function of Cl_{cr} <30 mL/minute, creatinine clearance should be estimated before dosing this medication. Low doses should be started initially because of the possibility of CNS effects.

Dosage Forms Excipient information presented when available (limited, particularly for generics); consult specific product labeling.
Capsule, oral:
  Zanaflex Capsules®: 2 mg, 4 mg, 6 mg
Tablet, oral: 2 mg, 4 mg
  Zanaflex®: 4 mg [scored]

◆ **TMC278** see Rilpivirine on page 1614
◆ **TMP** see Trimethoprim on page 1868
◆ **TMP-SMX** see Sulfamethoxazole and Trimethoprim on page 1714
◆ **TMP-SMZ** see Sulfamethoxazole and Trimethoprim on page 1714
◆ **TMX-67** see Febuxostat on page 696
◆ **TOBI®** see Tobramycin (Systemic, Oral Inhalation) on page 1810
◆ **TobraDex®** see Tobramycin and Dexamethasone on page 1815
◆ **TobraDex® ST** see Tobramycin and Dexamethasone on page 1815

Tobramycin (Systemic, Oral Inhalation) (toe bra MYE sin)

Related Information
Aminoglycoside Dosing and Monitoring on page 2050

Medication Safety Issues
Sound-alike/look-alike issues:
Tobramycin may be confused with Trobicin®, vancomycin
Nebcin® may be confused with Inapsine®, Naprosyn®, Nubain®
High alert medication:
The Institute for Safe Medication Practices (ISMP) includes this medication (intrathecal administration) among its list of drug classes which have a heightened risk of causing significant patient harm when used in error.

Brand Names: U.S. TOBI®
Brand Names: Canada TOBI®; TOBI® Podhaler®; Tobramycin Injection, USP
Index Terms Tobramycin Sulfate
Generic Availability (U.S.) Yes: Excludes solution for nebulization
Pharmacologic Category Antibiotic, Aminoglycoside
Use Treatment of documented or suspected infections caused by susceptible gram-negative bacilli, including *Pseudomonas aeruginosa*.

Contraindications Hypersensitivity to tobramycin, other aminoglycosides, or any component of the formulation

Warnings/Precautions [U.S. Boxed Warning]: Aminoglycosides may cause neurotoxicity and/or nephrotoxicity; usual risk factors include pre-existing renal impairment, concomitant neuro-/nephrotoxic medications, advanced age, and dehydration. Ototoxicity may be directly proportional to the amount of drug given and the duration of treatment; tinnitus or vertigo are indications of vestibular injury and impending hearing loss; renal damage is usually reversible. May cause neuromuscular blockade and respiratory paralysis, especially when given soon after anesthesia or muscle relaxants.

Not intended for long-term therapy due to toxic hazards associated with extended administration; use caution in pre-existing renal insufficiency, vestibular or cochlear impairment, myasthenia gravis, hypocalcemia, and conditions which depress neuromuscular transmission. Dosage modification required in patients with impaired renal function. Prolonged use may result in fungal or bacterial superinfection, including *C. difficile*-associated diarrhea (CDAD) and pseudomembranous colitis; CDAD has been observed >2 months postantibiotic treatment. Solution may contain sodium metabisulfate; use caution in patients with sulfite allergy.

Adverse Reactions (Reflective of adult population; not specific for elderly)
Injection: Frequency not defined:
Central nervous system: Confusion, disorientation, dizziness, fever, headache, lethargy, vertigo
Dermatologic: Exfoliative dermatitis, itching, rash, urticaria
Endocrine & metabolic: Serum calcium, magnesium, potassium, and/or sodium decreased
Gastrointestinal: Diarrhea, nausea, vomiting
Hematologic: Anemia, eosinophilia, granulocytopenia, leukocytosis, leukopenia, thrombocytopenia
Hepatic: ALT increased, AST increased, bilirubin increased, LDH increased
Local: Pain at the injection site
Otic: Hearing loss, tinnitus, ototoxicity (auditory), ototoxicity (vestibular), roaring in the ears
Renal: BUN increased, cylindruria, serum creatinine increased, oliguria, proteinuria

Inhalation (as reported for solution for inhalation unless otherwise noted):
>10%:
Gastrointestinal: Sputum discoloration (21%)
Respiratory: Cough (22% [powder for inhalation]), voice alteration (13%)
1% to 10%:
Cardiovascular: Chest discomfort (3% [powder for inhalation])
Central nervous system: Malaise (6%), pyrexia (1% [powder for inhalation])
Gastrointestinal: Abnormal taste (5% [powder for inhalation]), xerostomia (2% [powder for inhalation])
Otic: Tinnitus (3%)
Respiratory: Dyspnea (4% [powder for inhalation]), oropharyngeal pain (4% [powder for inhalation]), throat irritation (3% [powder for inhalation]), FEV decreased (2% [powder for inhalation]), pulmonary function decreased (2% [powder for inhalation]), bronchospasm (1% [powder for inhalation]), upper respiratory tract infection (1% [powder for inhalation])

Drug Interactions
Avoid Concomitant Use
Avoid concomitant use of Tobramycin (Systemic, Oral Inhalation) with any of the following:
BCG; Gallium Nitrate
Increased Effect/Toxicity
Tobramycin (Systemic, Oral Inhalation) may increase the levels/effects of: AbobotulinumtoxinA; Bisphosphonate Derivatives; CARBOplatin; Colistimethate; CycloSPORINE; CycloSPORINE (Systemic); Gallium Nitrate; Neuromuscular-Blocking Agents; OnabotulinumtoxinA; RimabotulinumtoxinB

The levels/effects of Tobramycin (Systemic, Oral Inhalation) may be increased by: Amphotericin B; Capreomycin; CISplatin; Loop Diuretics; Nonsteroidal Anti-Inflammatory Agents; Vancomycin
Decreased Effect
Tobramycin (Systemic, Oral Inhalation) may decrease the levels/effects of: BCG; Typhoid Vaccine

The levels/effects of Tobramycin (Systemic, Oral Inhalation) may be decreased by: Penicillins
Stability
Injection: Stable at room temperature both as the clear, colorless solution and as the dry powder. Reconstituted solutions remain stable for 24 hours at room temperature and 96 hours when refrigerated. Dilute in 50-100 mL NS, D_5W for I.V. infusion.

Powder, for inhalation (TOBI® Podhaler®) [Canadian availability; not available in the U.S.]): Store in original package at 15°C to 30°C (59°F to 86°F). Protect from moisture.

Solution, for inhalation (TOBI®): Store under refrigeration at 2°C to 8°C (36°F to 46°F). May be stored in foil pouch at room temperature of 25°C (77°F) for up to 28 days. Avoid intense light. Solution may darken over time; however, do not use if cloudy or contains particles.

Mechanism of Action Interferes with bacterial protein synthesis by binding to 30S and 50S ribosomal subunits, resulting in a defective bacterial cell membrane

Pharmacodynamics/Kinetics

Absorption:

Oral: Poorly absorbed

I.M.: Rapid and complete

Inhalation: Peak serum concentrations are ~1 mcg/mL following a 300 mg dose

Distribution: V_d: 0.2-0.3 L/kg; to extracellular fluid, including serum, abscesses, ascitic, pericardial, pleural, synovial, lymphatic, and peritoneal fluids; poor penetration into CSF, eye, bone, prostate

Inhalation: Tobramycin remains concentrated primarily in the airways

Protein binding: <30%

Half-life elimination:

Adults: 2-3 hours; directly dependent upon glomerular filtration rate

Adults with impaired renal function: 5-70 hours

Time to peak, serum: I.M.: 30-60 minutes; I.V.: ~30 minutes

Excretion: Normal renal function: Urine (~90% to 95%) within 24 hours

Dosage

Geriatric Dosage should be based on an estimate of ideal body weight.

I.M., I.V.: 1.5-5 mg/kg/day in 1-2 divided doses

I.V.: Once daily or extended interval: 5-7 mg/kg/dose given every 24, 36, or 48 hours based on creatinine clearance

Adult Note: Individualization is **critical** because of the low therapeutic index.

Use of ideal body weight (IBW) for determining the mg/kg/dose appears to be more accurate than dosing on the basis of total body weight (TBW). In morbid obesity, dosage requirement may best be estimated using a dosing weight of IBW + 0.4 (TBW - IBW).

Initial and periodic plasma drug levels (eg, peak and trough with conventional dosing) should be determined, particularly in critically-ill patients with serious infections or in disease states known to significantly alter aminoglycoside pharmacokinetics (eg, cystic fibrosis, burns, or major surgery).

Severe life-threatening infections: I.M., I.V.:

Conventional: 1-2.5 mg/kg/dose every 8-12 hours; to ensure adequate peak concentrations early in therapy, higher initial dosage may be considered in selected patients when extracellular water is increased (edema, septic shock, postsurgical, and/or trauma)

Once-daily: 4-7 mg/kg/dose once daily; some clinicians recommend this approach for all patients with normal renal function; this dose is at least as efficacious with similar, if not less, toxicity than conventional dosing.

Brucellosis: I.M., I.V.: 240 mg (I.M.) daily or 5 mg/kg (I.V.) daily for 7 days; either regimen recommended in combination with doxycycline

Cholangitis: I.M., I.V.: 4-6 mg/kg once daily with ampicillin

CNS shunt infection: Intrathecal (unlabeled route): 5-20 mg/day (Tunkel, 2004)

Diverticulitis, complicated: I.M., I.V.: 1.5-2 mg/kg every 8 hours (with ampicillin and metronidazole)

Infective endocarditis or synergy (for gram-positive infections): I.M., I.V.: 1 mg/kg every 8 hours (with ampicillin)

Meningitis (Enterococcus or Pseudomonas aeruginosa): I.V.: 5 mg/kg/day in divided doses every 8 hours (administered with another bacteriocidal drug)

Pelvic inflammatory disease: I.M., I.V.: Loading dose: 2 mg/kg, then 1.5 mg/kg every 8 hours **or** 4.5 mg/kg once daily

Plague (Yersinia pestis): I.M., I.V.: Treatment: 5 mg/kg/day, followed by postexposure prophylaxis with doxycycline

Pneumonia, hospital- or ventilator-associated: I.M., I.V.: 7 mg/kg/day (with antipseudomonal beta-lactam or carbapenem)

Prophylaxis against endocarditis (dental, oral, upper respiratory procedures, GI/GU procedures): I.M., I.V.: 1.5 mg/kg with ampicillin (50 mg/kg) 30 minutes prior to procedure. **Note:** AHA guidelines now recommend prophylaxis only in patients undergoing invasive procedures and in whom underlying cardiac conditions may predispose to a higher risk of adverse outcomes should infection occur. As of April 2007, routine prophylaxis no longer recommended by the AHA.

Tularemia: I.M., I.V.: 5 mg/kg/day divided every 8 hours for 1-2 weeks

Urinary tract infection: I.M., I.V.: 1.5 mg/kg/dose every 8 hours

Renal Impairment I.M., I.V.:

Conventional dosing:

Cl_{cr} ≥60 mL/minute: Administer every 8 hours.

Cl_{cr} 40-60 mL/minute: Administer every 12 hours.

Cl_{cr} 20-40 mL/minute: Administer every 24 hours.

Cl_{cr} 10-20 mL/minute: Administer every 48 hours.

Cl_{cr} <10 mL/minute: Administer every 72 hours.

High-dose therapy: Interval may be extended (eg, every 48 hours) in patients with moderate renal impairment (Cl_{cr} 30-59 mL/minute) and/or adjusted based on serum level determinations.

Intermittent hemodialysis (IHD) (administer after hemodialysis on dialysis days) (Heintz, 2009): Dialyzable (25% to 70%; variable; dependent on filter, duration, and type of HD): I.V.:

Loading dose of 2-3 mg/kg, followed by:

Mild UTI or synergy: I.V.: 1 mg/kg every 48-72 hours; consider redosing for pre-HD or post-HD concentrations <1mg/L

Moderate-to-severe UTI: I.V. 1-1.5 mg/kg every 48-72 hours; consider redosing for pre-HD concentrations <1.5-2 mg/L or post-HD concentrations <1 mg/L

Systemic gram-negative infection: I.V.: 1.5-2 mg/kg every 48-72 hours; consider redosing for pre-HD concentrations <3-5 mg/L or post-HD concentrations <2 mg/L

Note: Dosing dependent on the assumption of 3 times/week, complete IHD sessions.

Peritoneal dialysis (PD):

Administration via peritoneal dialysis (PD) fluid:

Gram-negative infection: 4-8 mg/L (4-8 mcg/mL) of PD fluid

Gram-positive infection (ie, synergy): 3-4 mg/L (3-4 mcg/mL) of PD fluid

Administration IVPB/I.M.: Dose as for Cl_{cr} <10 mL/minute and follow levels

Continuous renal replacement therapy (CRRT) (Heintz, 2009; Trotman, 2005): Drug clearance is highly dependent on the method of renal replacement, filter type, and flow rate. Appropriate dosing requires close monitoring of pharmacologic response, signs of adverse reactions due to drug accumulation, as well as drug concentrations in relation to target trough (if appropriate). The following are general recommendations only (based on dialysate flow/ultrafiltration rates of 1-2 L/hour and minimal residual renal function) and should not supersede clinical judgment:

CVVH/CVVHD/CVVHDF: I.V.: Loading dose of 2-3 mg/kg, followed by:

Mild UTI or synergy: I.V. 1 mg/kg every 24-36 hours (redose when concentration <1 mg/L)

Moderate-severe UTI: I.V.: 1-1.5 mg/kg every 24-36 hours (redose when concentration <1.5-2 mg/L)

Systemic gram-negative infection: I.V.: 1.5-2.5 mg/kg every 24-48 hours (redose when concentration <3-5 mg/L)

Hepatic Impairment No dosage adjustment necessary in hepatic impairment; monitor plasma concentrations as appropriate.

Administration

I.V.: Infuse over 30-60 minutes. Flush with saline before and after administration.

Inhalation:

TOBI®: To be inhaled over ~15 minutes using a handheld nebulizer (PARI-LC PLUS™). If multiple different nebulizer treatments are required, administer bronchodilator first, followed by chest physiotherapy, any other nebulized medications, and then TOBI® last. Do not mix with other nebulizer medications.

TOBI® Podhaler® (Canadian availability; not available in the U.S.): Capsules should be administered by oral inhalation via Podhaler® device following manufacturer recommendations for use and handling. Capsules should not be swallowed. Patients requiring bronchodilator therapy should administer the bronchodilator 15-90 minutes prior to TOBI® Podhaler®. The sequence of chest physiotherapy and additional inhaled therapies is at the discretion of the healthcare provider however TOBI® Podhaler® should always be administered last.

Some penicillins (eg, carbenicillin, ticarcillin, and piperacillin) have been shown to inactivate aminoglycosides *in vitro*. This has been observed to a greater extent with tobramycin and gentamicin, while amikacin has shown greater stability against inactivation. Concurrent use of these agents may pose a risk of reduced antibacterial efficacy *in vivo*, particularly in the setting of profound renal impairment. However, definitive clinical evidence is lacking. If combination penicillin/aminoglycoside therapy is desired in a patient with renal dysfunction, separation of doses (if feasible), and routine monitoring of aminoglycoside levels, CBC, and clinical response should be considered.

Monitoring Parameters Urinalysis, urine output, BUN, serum creatinine, peak and trough plasma tobramycin levels; be alert to ototoxicity; hearing should be tested before and during treatment

◀ Some penicillin derivatives may accelerate the degradation of aminoglycosides *in vitro*. This may be clinically-significant for certain penicillin (ticarcillin, piperacillin, carbenicillin) and aminoglycoside (gentamicin, tobramycin) combination therapy in patients with significant renal impairment. Close monitoring of aminoglycoside levels is warranted.

Reference Range

Timing of serum samples: Draw peak 30 minutes after 30-minute infusion has been completed or 1 hour following I.M. injection or beginning of infusion; draw trough immediately before next dose

Therapeutic levels:

Peak:

Serious infections: 6-8 mcg/mL (SI: 12-17 µmol/L)

Life-threatening infections: 8-10 mcg/mL (SI: 17-21 µmol/L)

Urinary tract infections: 4-6 mcg/mL (SI: 7-12 µmol/L)

Synergy against gram-positive organisms: 3-5 mcg/mL

Trough:

Serious infections: 0.5-1 mcg/mL

Life-threatening infections: 1-2 mcg/mL

The American Thoracic Society (ATS) recommends trough levels of <1 mcg/mL for patients with hospital-acquired pneumonia.

Monitor serum creatinine and urine output; obtain drug levels after the third dose unless otherwise directed

Inhalation: Serum levels are ~1 mcg/mL one hour following a 300 mg dose in patients with normal renal function.

Test Interactions Some penicillin derivatives may accelerate the degradation of aminoglycosides *in vitro*, leading to a potential underestimation of aminoglycoside serum concentration.

Pharmacotherapy Pearls Once-daily dosing: Higher peak serum drug concentration to MIC ratios, demonstrated aminoglycoside postantibiotic effect, decreased renal cortex drug uptake, and improved cost-time efficiency are supportive reasons for the use of once daily dosing regimens for aminoglycosides. Current research indicates these regimens to be as effective for nonlife-threatening infections, with no higher incidence of nephrotoxicity, as those requiring multiple daily doses. Doses are determined by calculating the entire day's dose via usual multiple dose calculation techniques and administering this quantity as a single dose. Doses are then adjusted to maintain mean serum concentrations above the MIC(s) of the causative organism(s). (Example: 2.5-5 mg/kg as a single dose; expected Cp_{max}: 10-20 mcg/mL and Cp_{min}: <1 mcg/mL). Further research is needed for universal recommendation in all patient populations and gram-negative disease; exceptions may include those with known high clearance (eg, patients with burns who may require shorter dosage intervals) and patients with renal function impairment for whom longer than conventional dosage intervals are usually required.

Special Geriatric Considerations The aminoglycosides are an important therapeutic intervention for susceptible organisms and as empiric therapy in seriously ill patients. Their use is not without risk of toxicity; however, these risks can be minimized if initial dosing is adjusted for estimated renal function and appropriate monitoring is performed. High dose, once daily aminoglycosides have been advocated as an alternative to traditional dosing regimens. Once daily or extended interval dosing is as effective and may be safer than traditional dosing. Interval must be adjusted for renal function.

Dosage Forms Excipient information presented when available (limited, particularly for generics); consult specific product labeling. [DSC] = Discontinued product

Infusion, premixed in NS: 60 mg (50 mL [DSC]); 80 mg (100 mL)

Injection, powder for reconstitution: 1.2 g

Injection, solution: 10 mg/mL (2 mL); 40 mg/mL (2 mL, 30 mL, 50 mL)

Solution, for nebulization [preservative free]:

TOBI®: 300 mg/5 mL (56s)

Dosage Forms: Canada Excipient information presented when available (limited, particularly for generics); consult specific product labeling.

Powder, for oral inhalation [capsule]:

TOBI® Podhaler®: 28 mg/capsule (224s)

Selected References

Bauer LA and Blouin RA, "Influence of Age on Tobramycin. Pharmacokinetics in Patients With Normal Renal Function," *Antimicrob Agents Chemother*, 1981, 20:587-9.

Matzke GR, Jameson JJ, and Halstenson CE, "Gentamicin Disposition in Young and Elderly Patients With Various Degrees of Renal Function," *J Clin Pharmacol*, 1987, 27(3):216-20.

Mayer PR, Brown CH, Carter RA, et al, "Intramuscular Tobramycin Pharmacokinetics in Geriatric Patients," *Drug Intell Clin Pharm*, 1986, 20:611-5.

Nicolau DP, Freeman CD, Belliveau PP, et al, "Experience With a Once-Daily Aminoglycoside Program Administered to 2184 Adult Patients," *Antimicrob Agents Chemother*, 1995, 39(3):650-5.

Preston SL and Briceland LL, "Single Daily Dosing of Aminoglycosides," *Pharmacotherapy*, 1995, 15(3):297-316.

Zaske DE, Irvine P, Strand LM, et al, "Wide Interpatient Variations in Gentamicin Dose Requirements for Geriatric Patients," *JAMA*, 1982, 248(23):3122-6.

Tobramycin (Ophthalmic) (toe bra MYE sin)

Medication Safety Issues
Sound-alike/look-alike issues:
Tobramycin may be confused with Trobicin®, vancomycin
AKTob® may be confused with AK-Trol®
Tobrex® may be confused with TobraDex®
Brand Names: U.S. AK-Tob™; Tobrex®
Brand Names: Canada PMS-Tobramycin; Sandoz-Tobramycin; Tobrex®
Index Terms Tobramycin Sulfate
Generic Availability (U.S.) Yes: Solution
Pharmacologic Category Antibiotic, Aminoglycoside; Antibiotic, Ophthalmic
Use Treatment of superficial ophthalmic infections caused by susceptible bacteria
Dosage
Adult Ocular infections: Ophthalmic:
Ointment: Instill ½" (1.25 cm) 2-3 times/day; for severe infections, apply every 3-4 hours
Solution: Instill 1-2 drops every 2-4 hours; for severe infections, instill up to 2 drops every hour until improved, then reduce to less frequent intervals
Dosage Forms Excipient information presented when available (limited, particularly for generics); consult specific product labeling.
Ointment, ophthalmic:
Tobrex®: 0.3% (3.5 g) [contains chlorobutanol]
Solution, ophthalmic [drops]: 0.3% (5 mL)
AK-Tob™: 0.3% (5 mL) [contains benzalkonium chloride]
Tobrex®: 0.3% (5 mL) [contains benzalkonium chloride]

Tobramycin and Dexamethasone (toe bra MYE sin & deks a METH a sone)

Related Information
Dexamethasone (Ophthalmic) on page 487
Tobramycin (Ophthalmic) on page 1815
Medication Safety Issues
Sound-alike/look-alike issues:
TobraDex® may be confused with Tobrex®
Brand Names: U.S. TobraDex®; TobraDex® ST
Brand Names: Canada Tobradex®
Index Terms Dexamethasone and Tobramycin
Generic Availability (U.S.) Yes: Suspension
Pharmacologic Category Antibiotic/Corticosteroid, Ophthalmic
Use Treatment of external ocular infection caused by susceptible gram-negative bacteria and steroid responsive inflammatory conditions of the palpebral and bulbar conjunctiva, cornea, and anterior segment of the globe
Dosage
Geriatric & Adult Ocular infection/inflammation: Ophthalmic:
Ointment: Apply a small amount (~½-inch ribbon of ointment) up to 3-4 times/day
Suspension: Instill 1-2 drops every 4-6 hours; may be increased to 1-2 drops every 2 hours for the first 24-48 hours, then reduce to less frequent intervals
Special Geriatric Considerations Evaluate the patient's or caregiver's ability to safely administer the correct dose of ophthalmic medication.
Dosage Forms Excipient information presented when available (limited, particularly for generics); consult specific product labeling.
Ointment, ophthalmic:
TobraDex®: Tobramycin 0.3% and dexamethasone 0.1% (3.5 g) [contains chlorobutanol]
Suspension, ophthalmic: Tobramycin 0.3% and dexamethasone 0.1% (2.5 mL, 5 mL, 10 mL)
TobraDex®: Tobramycin 0.3% and dexamethasone 0.1% (2.5 mL, 5 mL, 10 mL) [contains benzalkonium chloride]
TobraDex® ST: Tobramycin 0.3% and dexamethasone 0.05% (5 mL) [contains benzalkonium chloride]

♦ **Tobramycin and Loteprednol Etabonate** see Loteprednol and Tobramycin on page 1096
♦ **Tobramycin Sulfate** see Tobramycin (Ophthalmic) on page 1815
♦ **Tobramycin Sulfate** see Tobramycin (Systemic, Oral Inhalation) on page 1810
♦ **Tobrex®** see Tobramycin (Ophthalmic) on page 1815

Tocilizumab (toe si LIZ oo mab)

Brand Names: U.S. Actemra®
Brand Names: Canada Actemra®
Index Terms Atlizumab; MRA; R-1569; RoActemra®
Generic Availability (U.S.) No
Pharmacologic Category Antirheumatic, Disease Modifying; Interleukin-6 Receptor Antagonist
Use Treatment of moderately- to severely-active rheumatoid arthritis in adult patients who have had an inadequate response to one or more TNF antagonists (as monotherapy or in combination with nonbiological disease modifying antirheumatic drugs [DMARDs]); treatment of active systemic juvenile idiopathic arthritis (SJIA) (as monotherapy or in combination with methotrexate)
Medication Guide Available Yes
Contraindications Hypersensitivity to tocilizumab or any component of the formulation
Warnings/Precautions [U.S. Boxed Warning]: Serious and potentially fatal infections (including tuberculosis, invasive fungal, bacterial, viral, protozoal, and other opportunistic infections) have been reported in patients receiving tocilizumab. Most of the serious infections have occurred in patients on concomitant immunosuppressive therapy. Do not administer tocilizumab to a patient with an active infection, including localized infection. Caution should be exercised when considering use in patients with chronic or recurrent infections, previous exposure to tuberculosis, previous residence or travel in an area of endemic tuberculosis or mycoses, or predisposition to infection. Patients should be closely monitored for signs and symptoms of infection during and after treatment. If a patient develops a serious infection, therapy should be discontinued. **[U.S. Boxed Warning]: Tuberculosis (disseminated or extrapulmonary) has been reported in patients receiving tocilizumab; both reactivation of latent infection and new infections have been reported.** Patients should be evaluated for latent tuberculosis infection with a tuberculin skin test prior to starting therapy. Treatment of latent tuberculosis should be initiated before therapy is used. Some patients who test negative prior to therapy may develop active infection; monitor for signs and symptoms of tuberculosis in all patients. Rare reactivation of herpes zoster has been reported. Patients should be brought up to date with all immunizations before initiating therapy. Live vaccines should not be given concurrently; there is no data available concerning secondary transmission of infection from live vaccines in patients receiving therapy.

Impact on the development and course of malignancies is not fully defined, however, malignancies were observed in clinical trials. Use with caution in patients with pre-existing or recent onset CNS demyelinating disorders; rare cases of CNS demyelinating disorders (eg, multiple sclerosis) have occurred. All patients should be monitored for signs and symptoms of demyelinating disorders. May cause hypersensitivity, anaphylaxis, or anaphylactoid reactions; permanently discontinue treatment in patients who develop a hypersensitivity reaction to tocilizumab. Medications for the treatment of hypersensitivity reactions should be available for immediate use. Use is not recommended in patients with active hepatic disease or hepatic impairment; use with caution in patients at increased risk for gastrointestinal perforation.

Use may cause increases in total cholesterol, triglycerides, LDL and HDL cholesterol; hyperlipidemia should be managed according to current guidelines. Therapy should not be initiated in patients with an ANC <2000/mm^3, platelet count <100,000/mm^3, or ALT/AST >1.5 times the upper limit of normal (ULN); discontinue treatment in patients who develop an ANC <500/mm^3, platelet count <50,000/mm^3, or ALT/AST >5 x ULN.

Due to higher incidence of serious infections, concomitant use with other biological DMARDs (eg, TNF blockers, IL-1 receptor blockers, anti-CD20 monoclonal antibodies, selective costimulation modulators) should be avoided. Cautious use is recommended in elderly patients due to an increased incidence of serious infections.
Adverse Reactions (Reflective of adult population; not specific for elderly) Incidence as reported for monotherapy, except where noted. Combination therapy refers to use in rheumatoid arthritis with nonbiological DMARDs or use in SJIA in trials where most patients (~70%) were taking methotrexate at baseline.
>10%: Hepatic: ALT increased (≤36%; grades 3/4: <1%), AST increased (≤22%; grades 3/4: <1%)
1% to 10%:
  Cardiovascular: Hypertension (1% to 6%), peripheral edema (<2%)
  Central nervous system: Headache (1% to 7%), dizziness (3%)
  Dermatologic: Rash (2%), skin reaction (combination therapy; 1% [includes pruritus, urticaria])

Endocrine & metabolic: LDL cholesterol increased (>1.5-2 x ULN; combination therapy; children 2%), total cholesterol increased (>1.5-2 x ULN; combination therapy; children 2%), hypothyroidism (<2%)

Gastrointestinal: Diarrhea (children ≤5%), abdominal pain (2%), mouth ulceration (2%), gastric ulcer (<2%), stomatitis (<2%), weight gain (<2%), gastritis (1%)

Hematologic: Neutropenia (combination therapy; grade 3: 2% to 7%; grade 4: <1%), thrombocytopenia (combination therapy; 1% to 2%), leukopenia (<2%)

Hepatic: Bilirubin increased (<2%)

Local: Infusion-related reactions (combination therapy; 4% to 16%)

Ocular: Conjunctivitis (<2%)

Renal: Nephrolithiasis (<2%)

Respiratory: Upper respiratory tract infection (7%), nasopharyngitis (7%), bronchitis (3%), cough (<2%), dyspnea (<2%)

Miscellaneous: Anti-tocilizumab antibody formation (2%), herpes simplex (<2%)

Drug Interactions

Avoid Concomitant Use

Avoid concomitant use of Tocilizumab with any of the following: BCG; Belimumab; Natalizumab; Pimecrolimus; Tacrolimus (Topical); Vaccines (Live)

Increased Effect/Toxicity

Tocilizumab may increase the levels/effects of: Belimumab; Leflunomide; Natalizumab; Vaccines (Live)

The levels/effects of Tocilizumab may be increased by: Abciximab; Denosumab; Pimecrolimus; Roflumilast; Tacrolimus (Topical); Trastuzumab

Decreased Effect

Tocilizumab may decrease the levels/effects of: BCG; CYP3A4 Substrates; Sipuleucel-T; Vaccines (Inactivated); Vaccines (Live)

The levels/effects of Tocilizumab may be decreased by: Echinacea

Stability Store unopened vials at 2°C to 8°C (36°F to 46°F); do not freeze. Protect from light. Prior to administration, dilute to 50 mL (children <30 kg) or 100 mL (children ≥30 kg and adults) using 0.9% sodium chloride. Diluted solutions may be stored under refrigeration or at room temperature for up to 24 hours and are compatible with polypropylene, polyethylene (PE), polyvinyl chloride (PVC), and glass infusion containers.

Mechanism of Action Antagonist of the interleukin-6 (IL-6) receptor. Endogenous IL-6 is induced by inflammatory stimuli and mediates a variety of immunological responses. Inhibition of IL-6 receptors by tocilizumab leads to a reduction in cytokine and acute phase reactant production.

Pharmacodynamics/Kinetics

Distribution: V_{dss}: Adults: 6.4 L

Half life elimination: Terminal, single dose: 6.3 days (concentration-dependent; may be increased up to 13 days [adults] at steady state)

Dosage

Adult Rheumatoid arthritis: I.V.: Initial: 4 mg/kg every 4 weeks; may be increased to 8 mg/kg based on clinical response (maximum: 800 mg per infusion).

Renal Impairment

Mild renal impairment: No dosage adjustment required.

Moderate-to-severe renal impairment: Limited experience; no specific dosage adjustment recommended by the manufacturer.

Hepatic Impairment Not recommended for use in patients with active hepatic disease or hepatic impairment.

Administration I.V.: Allow diluted solution to reach room temperature prior to administration; infuse over 60 minutes using a dedicated I.V. line. Do not infuse other agents through same I.V. line. Do not administer I.V. push or I.V. bolus. Do not use if opaque particles or discoloration is visible.

Monitoring Parameters Signs and symptoms of infection (prior to and during therapy); latent TB screening prior to therapy initiation; CBC with differential (prior to and every 2-4 weeks [SJIA] or 4-8 weeks [RA] during therapy); ALT/AST (prior to and every 2-4 weeks [SJIA] or 4-8 weeks [RA] during therapy); additional liver function tests (eg, bilirubin) as clinically indicated; lipid panel (prior to, at 4-8 weeks following initiation, and every ~6 months during therapy); signs and symptoms of CNS demyelinating disorders

Special Geriatric Considerations Due to higher infection rate in elderly, this medication should be used cautiously and patients should be monitored closely for infection. In clinical studies, patients over the age of 65 had a higher infection rate than those younger than 65 years of age.

◄ **Dosage Forms** Excipient information presented when available (limited, particularly for generics); consult specific product labeling.

Injection, solution [preservative free]:

Actemra®: 20 mg/mL (4 mL, 10 mL, 20 mL) [contains polysorbate 80, sucrose 50 mg/mL]

Selected References

Emery P, Keystone E, Tony HP, et al, "IL-6 Receptor Inhibition With Tocilizumab Improves Treatment Outcomes in Patients With Rheumatoid Arthritis Refractory to Anti-Tumour Necrosis Factor Biologicals: Results from a 24-Week Multicentre Randomised Placebo-Controlled Trial," *Ann Rheum Dis*, 2008, 67(11):1516-23.

Genovese MC, McKay JD, Nasonov EL, et al, "Interleukin-6 Receptor Inhibition With Tocilizumab Reduces Disease Activity in Rheumatoid Arthritis With Inadequate Response to Disease-Modifying Antirheumatic Drugs: The Tocilizumab in Combination With Traditional Disease-Modifying Antirheumatic Drug Therapy Study," *Arthritis Rheum*, 2008, 58(10):2968-80.

Maini RN, Taylor PC, Szechinski J, et al, "Double-Blind Randomized Controlled Clinical Trial of the Interleukin-6 Receptor Antagonist, Tocilizumab, in European Patients With Rheumatoid Arthritis Who had an Incomplete Response to Methotrexate," *Arthritis Rheum*, 2006, 54(9):2817-29.

Nishimoto N, Hashimoto J, Miyasaka N, et al, "Study of Active Controlled Monotherapy Used for Rheumatoid Arthritis, and IL-6 Inhibitor (SAMURAI): Evidence of Clinical and Radiographic Benefit from an X-Ray Reader-Blinded Randomised Controlled Trial of Tocilizumab," *Ann Rheum Dis*, 2007, 66(9):1162-7.

Nishimoto N, Miyasaka N, Yamamoto K, et al, "Long-Term Safety and Efficacy of Tocilizumab, an Anti-IL-6 Receptor Monoclonal Antibody, in Monotherapy, in Patients With Rheumatoid Arthritis (the STREAM study): Evidence of Safety and Efficacy in a 5-Year Extension Study," *Ann Rheum Dis*, 2009, 68(10):1580-4.

Nishimoto N, Miyasaka N, Yamamoto K, et al, "Study of Active Controlled Tocilizumab Monotherapy for Rheumatoid Arthritis Patients With an Inadequate Response to Methotrexate (SATORI): Significant Reduction in Disease Activity and Serum Vascular Endothelial Growth Factor by IL-6 Receptor Inhibition Therapy," *Mod Rheum*, 2009, 19(1):12-9.

Oldfield V, Dhillon S, and Plosker GL, "Tocilizumab: A Review of its Use in the Management of Rheumatoid Arthritis," *Drugs*, 2009, 69(5):609-32.

Plushner SL, "Tocilizumab: An Interleukin-6 Receptor Inhibitor for the Treatment of Rheumatoid Arthritis," *Ann Pharmacother*, 2008, 429(11):1660-8.

Smolen JS, Beaulieu A, Rubbert-Roth A, et al, "Effect of Interleukin-6 Receptor Inhibition With Tocilizumab in Patients With Rheumatoid Arthritis (OPTION study): A Double-Blind, Placebo-Controlled, Randomised Trial," *Lancet*, 2008, 371(9617):987-97.

◆ **Tofranil®** see Imipramine *on page 919*
◆ **Tofranil-PM®** see Imipramine *on page 919*

TOLAZamide (tole AZ a mide)

Related Information

Diabetes Mellitus Management, Adults *on page 2073*

Medication Safety Issues

Sound-alike/look-alike issues:

TOLAZamide may be confused with tolazoline, TOLBUTamide

Tolinase® may be confused with Orinase®

High alert medication:

The Institute for Safe Medication Practices (ISMP) includes this medication among its list of drugs which have a heightened risk of causing significant patient harm when used in error.

Brand Names: Canada Tolinase®

Generic Availability (U.S.) Yes

Pharmacologic Category Antidiabetic Agent, Sulfonylurea

Use Adjunct to diet for the management of mild-to-moderately severe, stable, type 2 diabetes mellitus (noninsulin dependent, NIDDM)

Contraindications Hypersensitivity to tolazamide, sulfonylureas, or any component of the formulation; type 1 diabetes mellitus (insulin dependent, IDDM) therapy; diabetic ketoacidosis

Warnings/Precautions All sulfonylurea drugs are capable of producing severe hypoglycemia. Hypoglycemia is more likely to occur when caloric intake is deficient, after severe or prolonged exercise, when ethanol is ingested, or when more than one glucose-lowering drug is used. It is also more likely in elderly patients, malnourished patients and in patients with impaired renal or hepatic function; use with caution.

Loss of efficacy may be observed following prolonged use as a result of the progression of type 2 diabetes mellitus which results in continued beta cell destruction. In patients who were previously responding to sulfonylurea therapy, consider additional factors which may be contributing to decreased efficacy (eg, inappropriate dose, nonadherence to diet and exercise regimen). If no contributing factors can be identified, consider discontinuing use of the sulfonylurea due to secondary failure of treatment. Additional antidiabetic therapy (eg, insulin) will be required. It may be necessary to discontinue therapy and administer insulin if the patient is exposed to stress (fever, trauma, infection, surgery).

Chemical similarities are present among sulfonamides, sulfonylureas, carbonic anhydrase inhibitors, thiazides, and loop diuretics (except ethacrynic acid). Use in patients with sulfonylurea allergy is specifically contraindicated in product labeling, however, a risk of cross-reaction exists in patients with allergy to any of these compounds; avoid use when previous reaction has been severe. Patients with G6PD deficiency may be at an increased risk of sulfonylurea-induced hemolytic anemia; however, cases have also been described in patients without G6PD deficiency during postmarketing surveillance. Use with caution and consider a nonsulfonylurea alternative in patients with G6PD deficiency.

Product labeling states oral hypoglycemic drugs may be associated with an increased cardiovascular mortality as compared to treatment with diet alone or diet plus insulin. Data to support this association are limited, and several studies, including a large prospective trial (UKPDS) have not supported an association.

Adverse Reactions (Reflective of adult population; not specific for elderly) Frequency not defined.

Central nervous system: Dizziness, fatigue, headache, malaise, vertigo

Dermatologic: Maculopapular eruptions, morbilliform eruptions, photosensitivity, pruritus, rash, urticaria

Endocrine & metabolic: Disulfiram-like reaction, hypoglycemia, hyponatremia, SIADH

Gastrointestinal: Anorexia, constipation, diarrhea, epigastric fullness, heartburn, nausea, vomiting

Hematologic: Agranulocytosis, aplastic anemia, hemolytic anemia, leukopenia, pancytopenia, porphyria cutanea tarda, thrombocytopenia

Hepatic: Cholestatic jaundice, hepatic porphyria

Neuromuscular & skeletal: Weakness

Renal: Diuretic effect

Drug Interactions

Avoid Concomitant Use There are no known interactions where it is recommended to avoid concomitant use.

Increased Effect/Toxicity

TOLAZamide may increase the levels/effects of: Alcohol (Ethyl); Hypoglycemic Agents; Porfimer

The levels/effects of TOLAZamide may be increased by: Beta-Blockers; Chloramphenicol; Cimetidine; Cyclic Antidepressants; Fibric Acid Derivatives; Fluconazole; GLP-1 Agonists; Herbs (Hypoglycemic Properties); Pegvisomant; Quinolone Antibiotics; Ranitidine; Salicylates; Sulfonamide Derivatives; Voriconazole

Decreased Effect

The levels/effects of TOLAZamide may be decreased by: Corticosteroids (Orally Inhaled); Corticosteroids (Systemic); Luteinizing Hormone-Releasing Hormone Analogs; Quinolone Antibiotics; Rifampin; Somatropin; Thiazide Diuretics

Ethanol/Nutrition/Herb Interactions

Ethanol: Avoid ethanol (possible disulfiram-like reaction).

Herb/Nutraceutical: Herbs with hypoglycemic properties may enhance the hypoglycemic effect of tolazamide. This includes alfalfa, aloe, bilberry, bitter melon, burdock, celery, damiana, fenugreek, garcinia, garlic, ginger, ginseng (American), gymnema, marshmallow, stinging nettle.

Mechanism of Action Stimulates insulin release from the pancreatic beta cells; reduces glucose output from the liver; insulin sensitivity is increased at peripheral target sites

Pharmacodynamics/Kinetics

Onset of hypoglycemic effect: 20 minutes

Peak hypoglycemic effect: 4-6 hours

Duration: 10-24 hours

Absorption: Rapid

Protein binding: 94%

Metabolism: Extensively hepatic to 5 metabolites (activity 0% to 70%)

Half-life elimination: 7 hours

Time to peak, serum: 3-4 hours

Excretion: Urine (85%); feces (7%)

Dosage

Geriatric & Adult

Type 2 diabetes: Oral (doses >500 mg/day should be given in 2 divided doses):

Initial: 100-250 mg/day with breakfast or the first main meal of the day

Fasting blood sugar <200 mg/dL: 100 mg/day

Fasting blood sugar >200 mg/dL: 250 mg/day

Patient is malnourished, underweight, elderly, or not eating properly: 100 mg/day

Adjustment/titration: Increase in increments of 100-250 mg/day at weekly intervals to response; maximum daily dose: 1 g (doses >1 g/day are not likely to improve control)

Conversion from insulin to tolazamide:

<20 units day = 100 mg/day

21-<40 units/day = 250 mg/day

≥40 units/day = 250 mg/day and 50% of insulin dose

TOLAZAMIDE

Renal Impairment Conservative initial and maintenance doses are recommended because tolazamide is metabolized to active metabolites, which are eliminated in the urine.

Hepatic Impairment Conservative initial and maintenance doses and careful monitoring of blood glucose are recommended.

Monitoring Parameters Signs and symptoms of hypoglycemia (fatigue, sweating, numbness of extremities); blood glucose; hemoglobin A_{1c}

Reference Range

Recommendations for glycemic control in adults with diabetes:

Hb A_{1c}: <7%

Preprandial capillary plasma glucose: 70-130 mg/dL

Peak postprandial capillary blood glucose: <180 mg/dL

Blood pressure: <130/80 mm Hg

Recommendations for glycemic control in older adults with diabetes:

Relatively healthy, cognitively intact, and with a ≥5-year life expectancy: See Adults

Frail, life expectancy <5-years or those for whom the risks of intensive glucose control outweigh the benefits:

Hb A_{1c}: <8% to 9%

Blood pressure: <140/80 mm Hg or <130/80 mm Hg if tolerated

Pharmacotherapy Pearls Transferring a patient from one sulfonylurea to another does not require a priming dose; doses >1000 mg/day normally do not improve diabetic control.

Special Geriatric Considerations Has not been studied in elderly patients; however, except for drug interactions, it appears to have a safe profile and decline in renal function does not affect its pharmacokinetics. Intensive glucose control (HbA$_{1c}$ <6.5%) has been linked to increased all-cause and cardiovascular mortality, hypoglycemia requiring assistance, and weight gain in adult type 2 diabetes. How "tightly" to control a geriatric patient's blood glucose needs to be individualized. Such a decision should be based on several factors, including the patient's functional and cognitive status, how well he/she recognizes hypoglycemic or hyperglycemic symptoms, and how to respond to them and other disease states. An HbA$_{1c}$ <7.5% is an acceptable endpoint for a healthy older adult, while <8% is acceptable for frail elderly patients, those with a duration of illness >10 years, or those with comorbid conditions and requiring combination diabetes medications. Patients who are unable to accurately draw up their dose will need assistance, such as prefilled syringes. Initial doses may require considerations for renal function in the elderly with dosing adjusted subsequently based on blood glucose monitoring. For elderly patients with diabetes who are relatively healthy, attaining target goals for aspirin use, blood pressure, lipids, smoking cessation, and diet and exercise may be more important than normalized glycemic control.

Dosage Forms Excipient information presented when available (limited, particularly for generics); consult specific product labeling.

Tablet, oral: 250 mg, 500 mg

Selected References

Action to Control Cardiovascular Risk in Diabetes Study Group, Gerstein HC, Miller ME, et al, "Effects of Intensive Glucose Lowering in Type 2 Diabetes," *N Engl J Med*, 2008, 358(24):2545-59.

ADVANCE Collaborative Group, Patel A, MacMahon S, et al, "Intensive Blood Glucose Control and Vascular Outcomes in Patients With Type 2 Diabetes," *N Engl J Med*, 2008, 358(24):2560-72.

American Diabetes Association, "Standards of Medical Care in Diabetes – 2011," *Diabetes Care*, 2011, 34(Suppl 1):11-61.

Brown AF, Mangione CM, Saliba D, et al, "Guidelines for Improving the Care of the Older Person With Diabetes Mellitus," *J Am Geriatr Soc*, 2003, 51(5 Suppl Guidelines):265-80.

"VA/DoD Clinical Practice Guideline for the Management of Diabetes Mellitus," 2010. Available at http://www.healthquality.va.gov/Diabetes_Mellitus.asp

TOLBUTamide (tole BYOO ta mide)

Related Information

Diabetes Mellitus Management, Adults *on page 2073*

Medication Safety Issues

Sound-alike/look-alike issues:

TOLBUTamide may be confused with terbutaline, TOLAZamide

Orinase® may be confused with Orabase®, Ornex®, Tolinase®

High alert medication:

The Institute for Safe Medication Practices (ISMP) includes this medication among its list of drugs which have a heightened risk of causing significant patient harm when used in error.

Brand Names: Canada Apo-Tolbutamide®

Index Terms Orinase; Tolbutamide Sodium

Generic Availability (U.S.) Yes

Pharmacologic Category Antidiabetic Agent, Sulfonylurea

Use Adjunct to diet for the management of type 2 diabetes mellitus (noninsulin dependent, NIDDM)

Contraindications Hypersensitivity to tolbutamide, sulfonylureas, or any component of the formulation; treatment of type 1 diabetes; diabetic ketoacidosis

Warnings/Precautions All sulfonylurea drugs are capable of producing severe hypoglycemia. Hypoglycemia is more likely to occur when caloric intake is deficient, after severe or prolonged exercise, when ethanol is ingested, or when more than one glucose-lowering drug is used. It is also more likely in elderly patients, malnourished patients and in patients with impaired renal or hepatic function; use with caution.

Loss of efficacy may be observed following prolonged use as a result of the progression of type 2 diabetes mellitus which results in continued beta cell destruction. In patients who were previously responding to sulfonylurea therapy, consider additional factors which may be contributing to decreased efficacy (eg, inappropriate dose, nonadherence to diet and exercise regimen). If no contributing factors can be identified, consider discontinuing use of the sulfonylurea due to secondary failure of treatment. Additional antidiabetic therapy (eg, insulin) will be required. It may be necessary to discontinue therapy and administer insulin if the patient is exposed to stress (fever, trauma, infection, surgery).

Chemical similarities are present among sulfonamides, sulfonylureas, carbonic anhydrase inhibitors, thiazides, and loop diuretics (except ethacrynic acid). Use in patients with sulfonylurea allergy is specifically contraindicated in product labeling, however, a risk of cross-reaction exists in patients with allergy to any of these compounds; avoid use when previous reaction has been severe. Patients with G6PD deficiency may be at an increased risk of sulfonylurea-induced hemolytic anemia; however, cases have also been described in patients without G6PD deficiency during postmarketing surveillance. Use with caution and consider a nonsulfonylurea alternative in patients with G6PD deficiency.

Product labeling states oral hypoglycemic drugs may be associated with an increased cardiovascular mortality as compared to treatment with diet alone or diet plus insulin. Data to support this association are limited, and several studies, including a large prospective trial (UKPDS) have not supported an association.

Adverse Reactions (Reflective of adult population; not specific for elderly) Frequency not defined.

Central nervous system: Headache

Dermatologic: Erythema, maculopapular rash, morbilliform rash, pruritus, urticaria, photosensitivity

Endocrine & metabolic: Disulfiram-like reactions, hypoglycemia, hyponatremia, SIADH

Gastrointestinal: Epigastric fullness, heartburn, nausea, taste alteration

Hematologic: Agranulocytosis, aplastic anemia, hemolytic anemia, leukopenia, pancytopenia, thrombocytopenia

Hepatic: Cholestatic jaundice, hepatic porphyria, porphyria cutanea tarda

Miscellaneous: Hypersensitivity reaction

Drug Interactions

Metabolism/Transport Effects Substrate of CYP2C9 (major), 2C19 (minor); **Inhibits** CYP2C8 (weak), 2C9 (strong)

Avoid Concomitant Use There are no known interactions where it is recommended to avoid concomitant use.

Increased Effect/Toxicity

TOLBUTamide may increase the levels/effects of: Alcohol (Ethyl); CYP2C9 Substrates (High risk); Diclofenac; Hypoglycemic Agents; Leflunomide; Porfimer

The levels/effects of TOLBUTamide may be increased by: Beta-Blockers; Chloramphenicol; Cimetidine; Cyclic Antidepressants; CYP2C9 Inhibitors (Moderate); CYP2C9 Inhibitors (Strong); Fibric Acid Derivatives; Fluconazole; GLP-1 Agonists; Herbs (Hypoglycemic Properties); Leflunomide; Pegvisomant; Quinolone Antibiotics; Ranitidine; Salicylates; Sulfonamide Derivatives; Voriconazole

Decreased Effect

The levels/effects of TOLBUTamide may be decreased by: Aprepitant; Corticosteroids (Orally Inhaled); Corticosteroids (Systemic); CYP2C9 Inducers (Highly Effective); Fosaprepitant; Luteinizing Hormone-Releasing Hormone Analogs; Peginterferon Alfa-2b; Quinolone Antibiotics; Rifampin; Somatropin; Thiazide Diuretics

Ethanol/Nutrition/Herb Interactions

Ethanol: Avoid ethanol (possible disulfiram-like reaction).

Herb/Nutraceutical: Herbs with hypoglycemic properties may enhance the hypoglycemic effect of tolbutamide. This includes alfalfa, aloe, bilberry, bitter melon, burdock, celery, damiana, fenugreek, garcinia, garlic, ginger, ginseng (American), gymnema, marshmallow, stinging nettle.

Mechanism of Action Stimulates insulin release from the pancreatic beta cells; reduces glucose output from the liver; insulin sensitivity is increased at peripheral target sites, suppression of glucagon may also contribute

TOLBUTAMIDE

◀ **Pharmacodynamics/Kinetics**
Onset of action: 1 hour
Duration: Oral: 6-24 hours
Absorption: Oral: Rapid
Distribution: V_d: 0.15 L/kg
Protein binding: ~95% (concentration dependent)
Metabolism: Hepatic via CYP2C9 to hydroxymethyltolbutamide (mildly active) and carboxytolbutamide (inactive); metabolism does not appear to be affected by age
Half-life elimination: 4.5-6.5 hours (range: 4-25 hours)
Time to peak, serum: 3-4 hours
Excretion: Urine (75% to 85% primarily as metabolites); feces

Dosage
Geriatric Initial: 250 mg 1-3 times/day; usual: 500-2000 mg; maximum: 3 g/day
Adult Type 2 diabetes: Oral: Initial: 1-2 g/day as a single dose in the morning or in divided doses throughout the day. Maintenance dose: 0.25-3 g/day; however, a maintenance dose >2 g/day is seldom required. **Note:** Divided doses may improve gastrointestinal tolerance
Renal Impairment Adjustment is not necessary.
Hemodialysis: Not dialyzable (0% to 5%)
Hepatic Impairment Reduced dose may be necessary.
Administration Oral: Entire dose can be administered in AM, divided doses may improve GI tolerance
Monitoring Parameters Blood glucose, hemoglobin A_{1c}; signs and symptoms of hypoglycemia

Reference Range
Recommendations for glycemic control in adults with diabetes:
Hb A_{1c}: <7%
Preprandial capillary plasma glucose: 70-130 mg/dL
Peak postprandial capillary blood glucose: <180 mg/dL
Blood pressure: <130/80 mm Hg
Recommendations for glycemic control in older adults with diabetes:
Relatively healthy, cognitively intact, and with a ≥5-year life expectancy: See Adults
Frail, life expectancy <5-years or those for whom the risks of intensive glucose control outweigh the benefits:
Hb A_{1c}: <8% to 9%
Blood pressure: <140/80 mm Hg or <130/80 mm Hg if tolerated
Special Geriatric Considerations Because of its low potency and short duration, it is a useful agent in the elderly if drug interactions can be avoided. Intensive glucose control (HbA_{1c} <6.5%) has been linked to increased all-cause and cardiovascular mortality, hypoglycemia requiring assistance, and weight gain in adult type 2 diabetes. How "tightly" to control a geriatric patient's blood glucose needs to be individualized. Such a decision should be based on several factors, including the patient's functional and cognitive status, how well he/she recognizes hypoglycemic or hyperglycemic symptoms, and how to respond to them and other disease states. An HbA_{1c} <7.5% is an acceptable endpoint for a healthy older adult, while <8% is acceptable for frail elderly patients, those with a duration of illness >10 years, or those with comorbid conditions and requiring combination diabetes medications. Patients who are unable to accurately draw up their dose will need assistance, such as prefilled syringes. Initial doses may require considerations for renal function in the elderly with dosing adjusted subsequently based on blood glucose monitoring. For elderly patients with diabetes who are relatively healthy, attaining target goals for aspirin use, blood pressure, lipids, smoking cessation, and diet and exercise may be more important than normalized glycemic control.
Dosage Forms Excipient information presented when available (limited, particularly for generics); consult specific product labeling.
Tablet, oral: 500 mg

Selected References
Action to Control Cardiovascular Risk in Diabetes Study Group, Gerstein HC, Miller ME, et al, "Effects of Intensive Glucose Lowering in Type 2 Diabetes," N Engl J Med, 2008, 358(24):2545-59.
ADVANCE Collaborative Group, Patel A, MacMahon S, et al, "Intensive Blood Glucose Control and Vascular Outcomes in Patients With Type 2 Diabetes," N Engl J Med, 2008, 358(24):2560-72.
American Diabetes Association, "Standards of Medical Care in Diabetes – 2011," Diabetes Care, 2011, 34(Suppl 1):11-61.
Brown AF, Mangione CM, Saliba D, et al, "Guidelines for Improving the Care of the Older Person With Diabetes Mellitus," J Am Geriatr Soc, 2003, 51(5 Suppl Guidelines):265-80.
Miller AK, Adir J, and Vestal RE, "Effect of Age on the Pharmacokinetics of Tolbutamide in Man," Pharmacologist, 1977, 19:128.
Miller AK, Adir J, and Vestal RE, "Tolbutamide Binding to Plasma Proteins of Young and Old Human Subjects," J Pharm Sci, 1978, 67(8):1192-3.
"VA/DoD Clinical Practice Guideline for the Management of Diabetes Mellitus," 2010. Available at http://www.healthquality.va.gov/Diabetes_Mellitus.asp

◆ **Tolbutamide Sodium** see TOLBUTamide on page 1820

Tolcapone (TOLE ka pone)

Related Information
Antiparkinsonian Agents *on page 1995*
Brand Names: U.S. Tasmar®
Generic Availability (U.S.) No
Pharmacologic Category Anti-Parkinson's Agent, COMT Inhibitor
Use Adjunct to levodopa and carbidopa for the treatment of signs and symptoms of idiopathic Parkinson's disease in patients with motor fluctuations not responsive to other therapies
Prescribing and Access Restrictions A patient signed consent form acknowledging the risks of hepatic injury should be obtained by the treating physician.
Contraindications Hypersensitivity to tolcapone or any component of the formulation; history of liver disease or tolcapone-induced hepatocellular injury; nontraumatic rhabdomyolysis or hyperpyrexia and confusion
Warnings/Precautions [U.S. Boxed Warning]: Due to reports of fatal liver injury associated with use of this drug, the manufacturer is advising that tolcapone be reserved for patients who are experiencing inadequate symptom control or who are not appropriate candidates for other available treatments. Patients must provide written consent acknowledging the risks of hepatic injury. Liver disease should be excluded prior to initiation; laboratory monitoring is recommended. Discontinue if signs and/or symptoms of hepatic injury are noted (eg, transaminases >2 times upper limit of normal) or if clinical improvement is not evident after 3 weeks of therapy. Use with caution in patients with pre-existing dyskinesias; exacerbation of pre-existing dyskinesia and severe rhabdomyolysis has been reported. Levodopa dosage reduction may be required, particularly in patients with levodopa dosages >600 mg daily or with moderate-to-severe dyskinesia prior to initiation.

May cause orthostatic hypotension and syncope; Parkinson's disease patients appear to have an impaired capacity to respond to a postural challenge; use with caution in patients at risk of hypotension (such as those receiving antihypertensive drugs) or where transient hypotensive episodes would be poorly tolerated (cardiovascular disease or cerebrovascular disease). Parkinson's patients being treated with dopaminergic agonists ordinarily require careful monitoring for signs and symptoms of postural hypotension, especially during dose escalation, and should be informed of this risk. May cause hallucinations, which may improve with reduction in levodopa therapy. Use with caution in patients with lower gastrointestinal disease or an increased risk of dehydration; tolcapone has been associated with delayed development of diarrhea (onset after 2-12 weeks).

Tolcapone, in conjunction with other drug therapy that alters brain biogenic amine concentrations (eg, MAO inhibitors, SSRIs), has been associated with a syndrome resembling neuroleptic malignant syndrome (hyperpyrexia and confusion - some fatal) on abrupt withdrawal or dosage reduction. Concomitant use of tolcapone and nonselective MAO inhibitors should be avoided. Selegiline is a selective MAO type B inhibitor (when given orally at ≤10 mg/day) and can be taken with tolcapone. Dopaminergic agents have been associated with compulsive behaviors and/or loss of impulse control, which has manifested as pathological gambling, libido increases (hypersexuality), and/or binge eating. Causality has not been established, and controversy exists as to whether this phenomenon is related to the underlying disease, prior behaviors/addictions and/or drug therapy. Dose reduction or discontinuation of therapy has been reported to reverse these behaviors in some, but not all cases. Risk for melanoma development is increased in Parkinson's disease patients; drug causation or factors contributing to risk have not been established. Patients should be monitored closely and periodic skin examinations should be performed. Dopaminergic agents from the ergot class have also been associated with fibrotic complications, such as retroperitoneal fibrosis, pulmonary infiltrates or effusion and pleural thickening. It is unknown whether non-ergot, pro-dopaminergic agents like tolcapone confer this risk. Use with caution in patients with hepatic impairment or severe renal impairment.
Adverse Reactions (Reflective of adult population; not specific for elderly)
>10%:
   Cardiovascular: Orthostatic hypotension (17%)
   Central nervous system: Somnolence (14% to 32%), sleep disorder (24% to 25%), hallucinations (8% to 24%), excessive dreaming (16% to 21%), dizziness (6% to 13%), headache (10% to 11%), confusion (10% to 11%)
   Gastrointestinal: Nausea (28% to 50%), diarrhea (16% to 34%; approximately 3% to 4% severe), anorexia (19% to 23%)
   Neuromuscular & skeletal: Dyskinesia (42% to 51%), dystonia (19% to 22%), muscle cramps (17% to 18%)

1% to 10%:

Cardiovascular: Syncope (4% to 5%), chest pain (1% to 3%), hypotension (2%), palpitation

Central nervous system: Fatigue (3% to 7%), loss of balance (2% to 3%), agitation (1%), euphoria (1%), hyperactivity (1%), malaise (1%), panic reaction (1%), irritability (1%), mental deficiency (1%), fever (1%), depression, hypoesthesia, tremor, speech disorder, vertigo, emotional lability, hyperkinesia

Dermatologic: Alopecia (1%), bleeding (1%), tumor (1%), rash

Gastrointestinal: Vomiting (8% to 10%), constipation (6% to 8%), xerostomia (5% to 6%), abdominal pain (5% to 6%), dyspepsia (3% to 4%), flatulence (2% to 4%)

Genitourinary: UTI (5%), hematuria (4% to 5%), urine discoloration (2% to 3%), urination disorder (1% to 2%), uterine tumor (1%), incontinence, impotence

Hepatic: Transaminases increased (1% to 3%; 3 times ULN, usually with first 6 months of therapy)

Neuromuscular & skeletal: Paresthesia (1% to 3%), hyper-/hypokinesia (1% to 3%), arthritis (1% to 2%), neck pain (2%), stiffness (2%), myalgia, rhabdomyolysis

Ocular: Cataract (1%), eye inflammation (1%)

Otic: Tinnitus

Respiratory: Upper respiratory infection (5% to 7%), dyspnea (3%), sinus congestion (1% to 2%), bronchitis, pharyngitis

Miscellaneous: Diaphoresis (4% to 7%), influenza (3% to 4%), burning (1% to 2%), flank pain, injury, infection

Drug Interactions

Metabolism/Transport Effects Inhibits CYP2C9 (weak)

Avoid Concomitant Use There are no known interactions where it is recommended to avoid concomitant use.

Increased Effect/Toxicity

Tolcapone may increase the levels/effects of: Alcohol (Ethyl); CNS Depressants; COMT Substrates; MAO Inhibitors; Methotrimeprazine; Selective Serotonin Reuptake Inhibitors

The levels/effects of Tolcapone may be increased by: Droperidol; HydrOXYzine; MAO Inhibitors; Methotrimeprazine

Decreased Effect There are no known significant interactions involving a decrease in effect.

Ethanol/Nutrition/Herb Interactions

Ethanol: May increase CNS depression; monitor for increased effects with coadministration. Caution patients about effects.

Food: Tolcapone, taken with food within 1 hour before or 2 hours after the dose, decreases bioavailability by 10% to 20%.

Avoid valerian, St John's wort, kava kava, gotu kola (may increase CNS depression).

Stability Store at 20°C to 25°C (68°F to 77°F).

Mechanism of Action Tolcapone is a selective and reversible inhibitor of catechol-o-methyltransferase (COMT). In the presence of a decarboxylase inhibitor (eg, carbidopa), COMT is the major degradation pathway for levodopa. Inhibition of COMT leads to more sustained plasma levels of levodopa and enhanced central dopaminergic activity.

Pharmacodynamics/Kinetics

Absorption: Rapid

Distribution: 9 L

Protein binding: >99.0%

Metabolism: Hepatic, via glucuronidation, to inactive metabolite (>99%)

Bioavailability: 65%

Half-life elimination: 2-3 hours

Time to peak: ~2 hours

Excretion: Urine (60% as metabolites, 0.5% as unchanged drug); feces (40%)

Dosage

Geriatric & Adult Note: If clinical improvement is not observed after 3 weeks of therapy (regardless of dose), tolcapone treatment should be discontinued.

Parkinson's Disease: Oral: Initial: 100 mg 3 times/day; may increase as tolerated to 200 mg 3 times/day. **Note:** Levodopa dose may need to be decreased upon initiation of tolcapone (average reduction in clinical trials was 30%). As many as 70% of patients receiving levodopa doses >600 mg daily required levodopa dosage reduction in clinical trials. Patients with moderate-to-severe dyskinesia prior to initiation are also more likely to require dosage reduction.

Renal Impairment No adjustment necessary for mild-moderate impairment. Use caution with severe impairment; no safety information available in patients with Cl_{cr} <25 mL/minute.

Hepatic Impairment Do not use. Discontinue immediately if signs/symptoms of hepatic impairment develop.

Administration May be administered with or without food. In clinical studies, the first dose of the day was given with levodopa/carbidopa and the subsequent doses were given 6 hours and 12 hours later.

Monitoring Parameters Blood pressure, symptoms of Parkinson's disease, liver enzymes at baseline and then every 2-4 weeks for the first 6 months of therapy; thereafter, periodic monitoring should be conducted as deemed clinically relevant. If the dose is increased to 200 mg 3 times/day, reinitiate LFT monitoring every 2-4 weeks for 6 months, and then resume periodic monitoring. Discontinue therapy if the ALT or AST exceeds 2 times ULN or if the clinical signs and symptoms suggest the onset of liver failure.

Pharmacotherapy Pearls If no significant response in 3 weeks, discontinue tolcapone. Patient informed consent forms can be obtained from the manufacturer.

Special Geriatric Considerations No specific data in elderly patients, but based on the pharmacokinetic profile, no dosage adjustment appears necessary.

Dosage Forms Excipient information presented when available (limited, particularly for generics); consult specific product labeling. [DSC] = Discontinued product

Tablet, oral:

Tasmar®: 100 mg, 200 mg [DSC]

Selected References

Olanow CW, Watts RL, and Koller WC, "An Algorithm (Decision Tree) for the Management of Parkinson's Disease (2001): Treatment Guidelines," *Neurology*, 2001, 56(11 Suppl 5):S1-S88.

Pahwa R, Factor SA, Lyons KE, et al, "Practice Parameter: Treatment of Parkinson Disease With Motor Fluctuations and Dyskinesia (An Evidence-Based Review): Report of the Quality Standards Subcommittee of the American Academy of Neurology," *Neurology*, 2006, 66(7):983-95.

◆ **Tolectin** see Tolmetin on page 1825

Tolmetin (TOLE met in)

Index Terms Tolectin; Tolmetin Sodium

Generic Availability (U.S.) Yes

Pharmacologic Category Nonsteroidal Anti-inflammatory Drug (NSAID), Oral

Use Treatment of rheumatoid arthritis and osteoarthritis, juvenile idiopathic arthritis (JIA)

Medication Guide Available Yes

Contraindications Hypersensitivity to tolmetin, aspirin, other NSAIDs, or any component of the formulation; perioperative pain in the setting of coronary artery bypass graft (CABG) surgery

Warnings/Precautions [U.S. Boxed Warning]: NSAIDs are associated with an increased risk of adverse cardiovascular thrombotic events, including MI and stroke. Risk may be increased with duration of use or pre-existing cardiovascular risk factors or disease. Carefully evaluate individual cardiovascular risk profiles prior to prescribing. May cause new-onset hypertension or worsening of existing hypertension. Use caution with fluid retention. Avoid use in heart failure. Concurrent administration of ibuprofen, and potentially other nonselective NSAIDs, may interfere with aspirin's cardioprotective effect. **[U.S. Boxed Warning]: Use is contraindicated for treatment of perioperative pain in the setting of coronary artery bypass graft (CABG) surgery.** Risk of MI and stroke may be increased with use following CABG surgery.

Platelet adhesion and aggregation may be decreased; may prolong bleeding time; patients with coagulation disorders or who are receiving anticoagulants should be monitored closely. Anemia may occur; patients on long-term NSAID therapy should be monitored for anemia. Rarely, NSAID use may cause severe blood dyscrasias (eg, agranulocytosis, aplastic anemia, thrombocytopenia).

NSAID use may compromise existing renal function; dose-dependent decreases in prosta-glandin synthesis may result from NSAID use, reducing renal blood flow which may cause renal decompensation. NSAID use may increase the risk for hyperkalemia. Patients with impaired renal function, dehydration, heart failure, liver dysfunction, those taking diuretics, and ACE inhibitors, and the elderly are at greater risk of renal toxicity and hyperkalemia. Rehydrate patient before starting therapy; monitor renal function closely. Not recommended for use in patients with advanced renal disease. Long-term NSAID use may result in renal papillary necrosis. Acute interstitial nephritis and nephritic syndrome have been reported with tolmetin.

[U.S. Boxed Warning]: NSAIDs may increase risk of gastrointestinal irritation, inflammation, ulceration, bleeding, and perforation. These events may occur at any time during therapy and without warning. Use caution with a history of GI disease (bleeding or ulcers), concurrent therapy with aspirin, anticoagulants and/or corticosteroids, smoking, use of alcohol, the elderly or debilitated patients. When used concomitantly with ≤325 mg of aspirin,

◀ a substantial increase in the risk of gastrointestinal complications (eg, ulcer) occurs; concomitant gastroprotective therapy (eg, proton pump inhibitors) is recommended (Bhatt, 2008).

Use the lowest effective dose for the shortest duration of time, consistent with individual patient goals, to reduce risk of cardiovascular or GI adverse events. Alternate therapies should be considered for patients at high risk.

NSAIDs may cause serious skin adverse events including exfoliative dermatitis, Stevens-Johnson syndrome (SJS) and toxic epidermal necrolysis (TEN); discontinue use at first sign of skin rash or hypersensitivity. Anaphylactoid reactions may occur, even without prior exposure; patients with "aspirin triad" (bronchial asthma, aspirin intolerance, rhinitis) may be at increased risk. Do not use in patients who experience bronchospasm, asthma, rhinitis, or urticaria with NSAID or aspirin therapy.

Use with caution in patients with decreased hepatic function. Closely monitor patients with any abnormal LFT. Severe hepatic reactions (eg, fulminant hepatitis, liver failure) have occurred with NSAID use, rarely; discontinue if signs or symptoms of liver disease develop, or if systemic manifestations occur.

NSAIDS may cause drowsiness, dizziness, blurred vision and other neurologic effects which may impair physical or mental abilities; patients must be cautioned about performing tasks which require mental alertness (eg, operating machinery or driving). Discontinue use with blurred or diminished vision and perform ophthalmologic exam. Monitor vision with long-term therapy.

The elderly are at increased risk for adverse effects (especially peptic ulceration, CNS effects, renal toxicity) from NSAIDs even at low doses.

Withhold for at least 4-6 half-lives prior to surgical or dental procedures.

Adverse Reactions (Reflective of adult population; not specific for elderly)

>10%: Gastrointestinal: Nausea (11%)

1% to 10%:
Cardiovascular: Edema (3% to 9%), hypertension (3% to 9%), chest pain (1% to 3%)
Central nervous system: Dizziness (3% to 9%), headache (3% to 9%), depression (1% to 3%), drowsiness (1% to 3%)
Dermatologic: Skin irritation (1% to 3%)
Endocrine & metabolic: Weight gain/loss (3% to 9%)
Gastrointestinal: Abdominal pain (3% to 9%), diarrhea (3% to 9%), dyspepsia (3% to 9%), flatulence (3% to 9%), gastrointestinal distress (3% to 9%), vomiting (3% to 9%), constipation (1% to 3%), gastritis (1% to 3%), peptic ulcer (1% to 3%)
Genitourinary: Urinary tract infection (1% to 3%)
Hematologic: Hemoglobin/hematocrit decreased (transient; 1% to 3%)
Neuromuscular & skeletal: Weakness (3% to 9%)
Ocular: Visual disturbances (1% to 3%)
Otic: Tinnitus (1% to 3%)
Renal: BUN increased (1% to 3%)

Drug Interactions

Avoid Concomitant Use
Avoid concomitant use of Tolmetin with any of the following: Floctafenine; Ketorolac; Ketorolac (Nasal); Ketorolac (Systemic)

Increased Effect/Toxicity
Tolmetin may increase the levels/effects of: Aminoglycosides; Anticoagulants; Antiplatelet Agents; Bisphosphonate Derivatives; Collagenase (Systemic); CycloSPORINE; Cyclo-SPORINE (Systemic); Deferasirox; Desmopressin; Digoxin; Drotrecogin Alfa; Eplerenone; Haloperidol; Ibritumomab; Lithium; Methotrexate; Nonsteroidal Anti-Inflammatory Agents; PEMEtrexed; Porfimer; Potassium-Sparing Diuretics; PRALAtrexate; Quinolone Antibiotics; Rivaroxaban; Salicylates; Thrombolytic Agents; Tositumomab and Iodine I 131 Tositumomab; Vancomycin; Vitamin K Antagonists

The levels/effects of Tolmetin may be increased by: ACE Inhibitors; Angiotensin II Receptor Blockers; Antidepressants (Tricyclic, Tertiary Amine); Corticosteroids (Systemic); Dasatinib; Floctafenine; Glucosamine; Herbs (Anticoagulant/Antiplatelet Properties); Ketorolac; Ketorolac (Nasal); Ketorolac (Systemic); Nonsteroidal Anti-Inflammatory Agents; Omega-3-Acid Ethyl Esters; Pentosan Polysulfate Sodium; Pentoxifylline; Probenecid; Prostacyclin Analogues; Selective Serotonin Reuptake Inhibitors; Serotonin/Norepinephrine Reuptake Inhibitors; Sodium Phosphates; Treprostinil; Vitamin E

Decreased Effect
Tolmetin may decrease the levels/effects of: ACE Inhibitors; Angiotensin II Receptor Blockers; Antiplatelet Agents; Beta-Blockers; Eplerenone; HydrALAZINE; Potassium-Sparing Diuretics; Salicylates; Selective Serotonin Reuptake Inhibitors; Thiazide Diuretics

The levels/effects of Tolmetin may be decreased by: Bile Acid Sequestrants; Nonsteroidal Anti-Inflammatory Agents; Salicylates

Ethanol/Nutrition/Herb Interactions

Ethanol: Avoid ethanol (may enhance gastric mucosal irritation).

Food: Tolmetin peak serum concentrations may be decreased if taken with food or milk.

Herb/Nutraceutical: Avoid alfalfa, anise, bilberry, bladderwrack, bromelain, cat's claw, celery, chamomile, coleus, cordyceps, dong quai, evening primrose, fenugreek, feverfew, fenugreek, garlic, ginger, ginkgo biloba, ginseng (American, Panax, Siberian), grapeseed, green tea, guggul, horse chestnut seed, horseradish, licorice, prickly ash, red clover, reishi, SAMe (S-adenosylmethionine), sweet clover, turmeric, white willow (all have additional antiplatelet activity).

Stability Store at 15°C to 30°C (59°F to 86°F). Protect from light.

Mechanism of Action Reversibly inhibits cyclooxygenase-1 and 2 (COX-1 and 2) enzymes, which results in decreased formation of prostaglandin precursors; has antipyretic, analgesic, and anti-inflammatory properties.

Other proposed mechanisms not fully elucidated (and possibly contributing to the anti-inflammatory effect to varying degrees) include inhibiting chemotaxis, altering lymphocyte activity, inhibiting neutrophil aggregation/activation, and decreasing proinflammatory cytokine levels.

Pharmacodynamics/Kinetics

Onset of action: Analgesic: 1-2 hours; Anti-inflammatory: Days to weeks

Absorption: Well absorbed, rapid

Bioavailability: Reduced 16% with food or milk

Half-life elimination: Biphasic: Rapid: 1-2 hours; Slow: 5 hours

Time to peak, serum: 30-60 minutes

Excretion: Urine (as inactive metabolites or conjugates) within 24 hours

Dosage

Geriatric & Adult Inflammation, arthritis: Oral: 400 mg 3 times/day; usual dose: 600 mg to 1.8 g/day; maximum: 1.8 g/day

Monitoring Parameters Monitor response (pain, range of motion, grip strength, mobility, ADL function), inflammation; observe for weight gain, edema; monitor renal function; observe for bleeding, bruising; evaluate gastrointestinal effects (abdominal pain, bleeding, dyspepsia); mental confusion, disorientation, CBC, serum, creatinine, BUN, liver function tests

Test Interactions Increased protein, bleeding time; may interfere with urine detection of cannabinoids (false-positive)

Pharmacotherapy Pearls Only NSAID affected by food/milk, which decreases total bioavailability by 16%. If GI upset occurs with tolmetin, take with antacids other than sodium bicarbonate. Each 200 mg of tolmetin contains 0.8 mEq of sodium. There are no clinical guidelines to predict which NSAID will give response in a particular patient. Trials with each must be initiated until response determined. Consider dose, patient convenience, and cost.

Special Geriatric Considerations Elderly are a high-risk population for adverse effects from NSAIDs. As much as 60% of the elderly can develop peptic ulceration and/or hemorrhage asymptomatically. The concomitant use of H_2 blockers and sucralfate is not effective as prophylaxis with the exception of NSAID-induced duodenal ulcers which may be prevented by the use of ranitidine. Misoprostol and proton pump inhibitors are the only agents proven to help prevent the development of NSAID-induced ulcers. Also, concomitant disease and drug use contribute to the risk for GI adverse effects. Use lowest effective dose for shortest period possible. Consider renal function decline with age. Use of NSAIDs can compromise existing renal function especially when $Cl_{cr} \leq 30$ mL/minute. Tinnitus may be a difficult and unreliable indication of toxicity due to age-related hearing loss or eighth cranial nerve damage. CNS adverse effects such as confusion, agitation, and hallucination are generally seen in overdose or high dose situations, but elderly may demonstrate these adverse effects at lower doses than younger adults.

Dosage Forms Excipient information presented when available (limited, particularly for generics); consult specific product labeling.

Capsule, oral: 400 mg

Tablet, oral: 200 mg, 600 mg

♦ **Tolmetin Sodium** see Tolmetin *on page 1825*

Tolnaftate (tole NAF tate)

Medication Safety Issues

Sound-alike/look-alike issues:

Tolnaftate may be confused with Tornalate®

Tinactin® may be confused with Talacen

Brand Names: U.S. Blis-To-Sol® [OTC]; Mycocide® NS [OTC]; Podactin Powder [OTC]; Tinactin® Antifungal Deodorant [OTC]; Tinactin® Antifungal Jock Itch [OTC]; Tinactin® Antifungal [OTC]; Tinaderm [OTC]; Ting® Cream [OTC]; Ting® Spray Liquid [OTC]

Brand Names: Canada Pitrex

Generic Availability (U.S.) Yes: Cream, powder, solution

Pharmacologic Category Antifungal Agent, Topical

Use Treatment of tinea pedis, tinea cruris, tinea corporis

Contraindications Hypersensitivity to tolnaftate or any component of the formulation; nail and scalp infections

Warnings/Precautions For topical use only; avoid contact with eyes. Apply to clean, dry skin. When used for self-medication (OTC use), contact healthcare provider if condition does not improve within 4 weeks. Discontinue if sensitivity or irritation occurs.

Adverse Reactions (Reflective of adult population; not specific for elderly) Frequency not defined.
Dermatologic: Contact dermatitis, pruritus
Local: Irritation, stinging

Drug Interactions

Avoid Concomitant Use There are no known interactions where it is recommended to avoid concomitant use.

Increased Effect/Toxicity There are no known significant interactions involving an increase in effect.

Decreased Effect There are no known significant interactions involving a decrease in effect.

Mechanism of Action Distorts the hyphae and stunts mycelial growth in susceptible fungi

Pharmacodynamics/Kinetics Onset of action: 24-72 hours

Dosage

Geriatric & Adult Tinea infection: Topical: Wash and dry affected area; spray aerosol or apply 1-3 drops of solution or a small amount of cream, or powder and rub into the affected areas 2 times/day

Note: May use for up to 4 weeks for tinea pedis or tinea corporis, and up to 2 weeks for tinea cruris.

Monitoring Parameters Resolution of skin infection

Pharmacotherapy Pearls Usually not effective alone for the treatment of infections involving hair follicles or nails

Special Geriatric Considerations No specific recommendations for use in the elderly.

Dosage Forms Excipient information presented when available (limited, particularly for generics); consult specific product labeling.
Aerosol, topical [powder/spray]:
Tinactin® Antifungal: 1% (133 g) [contains ethanol 11% v/v, talc]
Tinactin® Antifungal Deodorant: 1% (133 g) [contains ethanol 11% v/v, talc]
Tinactin® Antifungal Jock Itch: 1% (133 g) [contains ethanol 11% v/v, talc]
Aerosol, topical [spray]:
Tinactin® Antifungal: 1% (150 g) [contains ethanol 29% v/v]
Ting® Spray Liquid: 1% (128 g) [contains ethanol 41% w/w]
Cream, topical: 1% (15 g, 30 g, 114 g)
Tinactin® Antifungal: 1% (15 g, 30 g)
Tinactin® Antifungal Jock Itch: 1% (15 g)
Ting® Cream: 1% (15 g)
Liquid, topical:
Blis-To-Sol®: 1% (30 mL, 55 mL)
Liquid, topical [spray]:
Tinactin® Antifungal: 1% (59 mL) [contains ethanol 70% v/v]
Powder, topical: 1% (45 g)
Podactin Powder: 1% (60 g)
Tinactin® Antifungal: 1% (108 g)
Solution, topical:
Mycocide® NS: 1% (30 mL)
Tinaderm: 1% (10 mL)

Tolterodine (tole TER oh deen)

Related Information
Beers Criteria – Potentially Inappropriate Medications for Geriatrics *on page 2089*
Pharmacotherapy of Urinary Incontinence *on page 2032*

Medication Safety Issues
Sound-alike/look-alike issues:
Tolterodine may be confused with fesoterodine

Detrol® may be confused with Ditropan

Brand Names: U.S. Detrol®; Detrol® LA

Brand Names: Canada Detrol®; Detrol® LA; Unidet®

Index Terms Tolterodine Tartrate

Generic Availability (U.S.) No

Pharmacologic Category Anticholinergic Agent

Use Treatment of patients with an overactive bladder with symptoms of urinary frequency, urgency, or urge incontinence

Contraindications Hypersensitivity to tolterodine or any component of the formulation; urinary retention; gastric retention; uncontrolled narrow-angle glaucoma

Warnings/Precautions May cause drowsiness and/or blurred vision, which may impair physical or mental abilities; patients must be cautioned about performing tasks which require mental alertness (eg, operating machinery or driving). Use with caution in patients with bladder flow obstruction, may increase the risk of urinary retention. Use with caution in patients with gastrointestinal obstructive disorders (ie, pyloric stenosis), may increase the risk of gastric retention. Use with caution in patients with myasthenia gravis and controlled (treated) narrow-angle glaucoma; metabolized in the liver and excreted in the urine and feces, dosage adjustment is required for patients with renal or hepatic impairment. Tolterodine has been associated with QT_c prolongation at high (supratherapeutic) doses. The manufacturer recommends caution in patients with congenital prolonged QT or in patients receiving concurrent therapy with QT_c-prolonging drugs (class Ia or III antiarrhythmics). However, the mean change in QT_c even at supratherapeutic dosages was less than 15 msec. Individuals who are CYP2D6 poor metabolizers or in the presence of inhibitors of CYP2D6 and CYP3A4 may be more likely to exhibit prolongation. Dosage adjustment is recommended in patients receiving CYP3A4 inhibitors (a lower dose of tolterodine is recommended).

Adverse Reactions (Reflective of adult population; not specific for elderly) As reported with immediate release tablet, unless otherwise specified

>10%: Gastrointestinal: Dry mouth (35%; extended release capsules 23%)

1% to 10%:

Cardiovascular: Chest pain (2%)

Central nervous system: Headache (7%; extended release capsules 6%), somnolence (3%; extended release capsules 3%), fatigue (4%; extended release capsules 2%), dizziness (5%; extended release capsules 2%), anxiety (extended release capsules 1%)

Dermatologic: Dry skin (1%)

Gastrointestinal: Abdominal pain (5%; extended release capsules 4%), constipation (7%; extended release capsules 6%), dyspepsia (4%; extended release capsules 3%), diarrhea (4%), weight gain (1%)

Genitourinary: Dysuria (2%; extended release capsules 1%)

Neuromuscular & skeletal: Arthralgia (2%)

Ocular: Abnormal vision (2%; extended release capsules 1%), dry eyes (3%; extended release capsules 3%)

Respiratory: Bronchitis (2%), sinusitis (extended release capsules 2%)

Miscellaneous: Flu-like syndrome (3%), infection (1%)

Drug Interactions

Metabolism/Transport Effects Substrate of CYP2C9 (minor), 2C19 (minor), 2D6 (major), 3A4 (major)

Avoid Concomitant Use There are no known interactions where it is recommended to avoid concomitant use.

Increased Effect/Toxicity

Tolterodine may increase the levels/effects of: AbobotulinumtoxinA; Anticholinergics; Cannabinoids; OnabotulinumtoxinA; Potassium Chloride; RimabotulinumtoxinB; Warfarin

The levels/effects of Tolterodine may be increased by: Abiraterone Acetate; Antifungal Agents (Azole Derivatives, Systemic); CYP2D6 Inhibitors (Moderate); CYP2D6 Inhibitors (Strong); CYP3A4 Inhibitors (Moderate); CYP3A4 Inhibitors (Strong); Dasatinib; Fluconazole; Pramlintide; VinBLAStine

Decreased Effect

Tolterodine may decrease the levels/effects of: Acetylcholinesterase Inhibitors (Central); Secretin

The levels/effects of Tolterodine may be decreased by: Acetylcholinesterase Inhibitors (Central); CYP3A4 Inducers (Strong); Deferasirox; Herbs (CYP3A4 Inducers); Peginterferon Alfa-2b; Tocilizumab

Ethanol/Nutrition/Herb Interactions
Food: Increases bioavailability (~53% increase) of tolterodine tablets (dose adjustment not necessary); does not affect the pharmacokinetics of tolterodine extended release capsules. As a CYP3A4 inhibitor, grapefruit juice may increase the serum level and/or toxicity of tolterodine, but unlikely secondary to high oral bioavailability.
Herb/Nutraceutical: St John's wort (*Hypericum*) appears to induce CYP3A enzymes.

Stability Store at 25°C (77°F); excursions permitted to 15°C to 30°C (59°F to 86°F). Protect from light.

Mechanism of Action Tolterodine is a competitive antagonist of muscarinic receptors. In animal models, tolterodine demonstrates selectivity for urinary bladder receptors over salivary receptors. Urinary bladder contraction is mediated by muscarinic receptors. Tolterodine increases residual urine volume and decreases detrusor muscle pressure.

Pharmacodynamics/Kinetics
Absorption: Immediate release tablet: Rapid; ≥77%
Distribution: I.V.: V_d: 113 ± 27 L
Protein binding: >96% (primarily to alpha$_1$-acid glycoprotein)
Metabolism: Extensively hepatic, primarily via CYP2D6 to 5-hydroxymethyltolterodine (active) and 3A4 usually (minor pathway). In patients with a genetic deficiency of CYP2D6, metabolism via 3A4 predominates.
Bioavailability: Immediate release tablet: Increased 53% with food
Half-life elimination:
Immediate release tablet: Extensive metabolizers: ~2 hours; Poor metabolizers: ~10 hours
Extended release capsule: Extensive metabolizers: ~7 hours; Poor metabolizers: ~18 hours
Time to peak: Immediate release tablet: 1-2 hours; Extended release tablet: 2-6 hours
Excretion: Urine (77%); feces (17%); primarily as metabolites (<1% unchanged drug) of which the active 5-hydroxymethyl metabolite accounts for 5% to 14% (<1% in poor metabolizers); as unchanged drug (<1%; <2.5% in poor metabolizers)
Note: Mean serum concentrations of tolterodine and its 5-hydroxy metabolite were 20% and 50% higher respectively in older adult patients as compared to young healthy volunteers

Dosage
Geriatric & Adult Treatment of overactive bladder: Oral:
Immediate release tablet: 2 mg twice daily; the dose may be lowered to 1 mg twice daily based on individual response and tolerability
Dosing adjustment in patients concurrently taking CYP3A4 inhibitors: 1 mg twice daily
Extended release capsule: 4 mg once a day; dose may be lowered to 2 mg daily based on individual response and tolerability
Dosing adjustment in patients concurrently taking CYP3A4 inhibitors: 2 mg daily
Renal Impairment Use with caution (studies conducted in patients with Cl_{cr} 10-30 mL/minute):
Immediate release tablet: 1 mg twice daily
Extended release capsule: 2 mg daily
Hepatic Impairment
Immediate release tablet: 1 mg twice daily
Extended release capsule: 2 mg daily

Administration Extended release capsule: Swallow whole; do not crush, chew, or open
Monitoring Parameters Renal function (BUN, creatinine); hepatic function
Pharmacotherapy Pearls Tolterodine can be included in a bladder retraining program.
Special Geriatric Considerations No difference in safety has been noted between elderly and younger patients, therefore, no dosage adjustment is recommended.

Dosage Forms Excipient information presented when available (limited, particularly for generics); consult specific product labeling.
Capsule, extended release, oral, as tartrate:
Detrol® LA: 2 mg, 4 mg
Tablet, oral, as tartrate:
Detrol®: 1 mg, 2 mg

♦ **Tolterodine Tartrate** see Tolterodine on page *1828*

Tolvaptan (tol VAP tan)

Brand Names: U.S. Samsca™
Index Terms OPC-41061
Generic Availability (U.S.) No
Pharmacologic Category Vasopressin Antagonist
Use Treatment of clinically significant hypervolemic or euvolemic hyponatremia (associated with heart failure, cirrhosis or SIADH) with either a serum sodium <125 mEq/L or less marked hyponatremia that is symptomatic and resistant to fluid restriction

Medication Guide Available Yes

Contraindications Hypovolemic hyponatremia; urgent need to raise serum sodium acutely; use in patients unable to sense or appropriately respond to thirst; anuria; concurrent use with strong CYP3A inhibitors (eg, ketoconazole, itraconazole, ritonavir, indinavir, nelfinavir, saquinavir, nefazodone, telithromycin, clarithromycin)

Warnings/Precautions [U.S. Boxed Warning]: Tolvaptan should be initiated and reinitiated in patients only in a hospital where serum sodium can be closely monitored. Too rapid correction of hyponatremia (ie, >12 mEq/L/24 hours) can cause osmotic demyelination resulting in dysarthria, mutism, dysphagia, lethargy, affective changes, spastic quadriparesis, seizures, coma, and death. In susceptible patients (including those with severe malnutrition, alcoholism, or advanced liver disease), slower rates of correction may be advisable. Patients with SIADH or very low baseline serum sodium concentrations may be at greater risk of overly-rapid correction.

Interrupt or discontinue therapy in patients who develop medically significant signs or symptoms of hypovolemia. Patients should ingest fluids in response to thirst. Gastrointestinal bleeding can occur in patients with cirrhosis; use only if the need to treat outweighs the risk. Reductions in extracellular fluid volumes may cause hyperkalemia. Patients with a pretreatment serum potassium >5 mEq/L should be monitored after initiation of therapy.

Use in patients with creatinine clearance <10 mL/minute has not been studied. Do not use in anuric patients. Use with hypertonic saline is not recommended. Use contraindicated in patients taking strong CYP3A inhibitors; avoid use in patients taking moderate CYP3A4 inhibitors. If possible, avoid use with CYP3A4 inducers; if administered with CYP3A4 inducers, dose increases may be necessary. Dose reductions may be necessary if administered with P-gp inhibitors. Consider alternative agents that avoid or lessen the potential for CYP- or P-gp mediated interactions. Patients receiving medications known to increase potassium should be monitored for hyperkalemia.

Monitor closely for rate of serum sodium increase and neurological status; rapid serum sodium correction (>12 mEq/L/24 hours) can lead to permanent neurological damage. Discontinue use if rate of serum sodium increase is undesirable; fluid restriction during the first 24 hours of sodium correction can increase the risk of overly-rapid correction and should generally be avoided; not intended for urgent correction of serum sodium to prevent or treat serious neurologic symptoms; it has not been demonstrated that raising serum sodium with tolvaptan provides a symptomatic benefit.

Adverse Reactions (Reflective of adult population; not specific for elderly)
>10%:
    Gastrointestinal: Nausea (21%), xerostomia (7% to 13%)
    Renal: Pollakiuria (4% to 11%), polyuria (4% to 11%)
    Miscellaneous: Thirst (12% to 16%)
2% to 10%:
    Central nervous system: Pyrexia (4%)
    Endocrine & metabolic: Hyperglycemia (6%)
    Gastrointestinal: Constipation (7%), anorexia (4%)
    Neuromuscular & skeletal: Weakness (9%)

Drug Interactions

Metabolism/Transport Effects Substrate of P-glycoprotein

Avoid Concomitant Use
    Avoid concomitant use of Tolvaptan with any of the following: CYP3A4 Inducers (Strong); CYP3A4 Inhibitors (Moderate); CYP3A4 Inhibitors (Strong); Sodium Chloride

Increased Effect/Toxicity
    Tolvaptan may increase the levels/effects of: ACE Inhibitors; Angiotensin II Receptor Blockers; Digoxin; Potassium-Sparing Diuretics

    The levels/effects of Tolvaptan may be increased by: CYP3A4 Inhibitors (Moderate); CYP3A4 Inhibitors (Strong); Dasatinib; P-Glycoprotein Inhibitors; Sodium Chloride

Decreased Effect
    The levels/effects of Tolvaptan may be decreased by: CYP3A4 Inducers (Strong); Deferasirox; Herbs (CYP3A4 Inducers); P-Glycoprotein Inducers; Tocilizumab

Ethanol/Nutrition/Herb Interactions
Food: Tolvaptan exposure may be doubled when taken with grapefruit juice.
Herb/Nutraceutical: St John's wort may decrease tolvaptan serum concentrations.

Stability Store at 25°C (77°F); excursions permitted between 15°C and 30°C (59°F and 86°F).

Mechanism of Action An arginine vasopressin (AVP) receptor antagonist with affinity for AVP receptor subtypes V_2 and V_{1a} in a ratio of 29:1. Antagonism of the V_2 receptor by tolvaptan promotes the excretion of free water (without loss of serum electrolytes) resulting in net fluid loss, increased urine output, decreased urine osmolality, and subsequent restoration of normal serum sodium levels.

Pharmacodynamics/Kinetics
Onset of action: 2-4 hours
Peak effect: 4-8 hours
Duration: 60% peak serum sodium elevation is retained at 24 hours; urinary excretion of free water is no longer elevated
Distribution: V_d: 3 L/kg
Protein binding: 99%
Metabolism: Hepatic via CYP3A4
Bioavailability: ~40%
Half-life elimination: 5-12 hours; dominant half-life <12 hours
Time to peak, plasma: 2-4 hours
Excretion: Feces

Dosage
Geriatric & Adult Hyponatremia: Oral: Initial: 15 mg once daily; after at least 24 hours, may increase to 30 mg once daily to a maximum of 60 mg once daily titrating at 24-hour intervals to desired serum sodium concentration.

Administration Treatment should be initiated or reinitiated in a hospital. May be administered without regards to meals.

Monitoring Parameters Serum sodium concentration, rate of serum sodium increase, serum potassium concentration (if >5 mEq/L prior to administration or receiving medications known to elevate serum potassium); volume status

Dosage Forms Excipient information presented when available (limited, particularly for generics); consult specific product labeling.
Tablet, oral:
Samsca™: 15 mg, 30 mg

Selected References
Decaux G, Soupart A, Vassart G, "Non-Peptide Arginine-Vasopressin Antagonists: The Vaptans," *Lancet*, 2008, 371 (9624):1624-32.
Gheorghiade M, Konstam MA, Burnett JC Jr, "Short-term Clinical Effects of Tolvaptan, an Oral Vasopressin Antagonist, in Patients Hospitalized for Heart Failure," *JAMA*, 2007, 297(12):1332-43.
Konstam MA, Gheorghiade M, Burnett JC Jr, et al, "Effects of Oral Tolvaptan in Patients Hospitalized for Worsening Heart Failure: The EVEREST Outcome Trial," *JAMA*, 2007, 297(12):1319-31.
Oghlakian G and Klapholz M, "Vasopressin and Vasopressin Receptor Antagonists in Heart Failure," *Cardiol Rev*, 2009, 17(1):10-15.

◆ **Topamax®** *see* Topiramate *on page 1832*
◆ **Topicaine® [OTC]** *see* Lidocaine (Topical) *on page 1064*

Topiramate (toe PYRE a mate)

Medication Safety Issues
Sound-alike/look-alike issues:
Topamax® may be confused with Sporanox®, Tegretol®, Tegretol®-XR, Toprol-XL®
Brand Names: U.S. Topamax®
Brand Names: Canada Apo-Topiramate®; CO Topiramate; Dom-Topiramate; Mint-Topiramate; Mylan-Topiramate; Novo-Topiramate; PHL-Topiramate; PMS-Topiramate; PRO-Topiramate; ratio-Topiramate; Sandoz-Topiramate; Topamax®; ZYM-Topiramate
Generic Availability (U.S.) Yes
Pharmacologic Category Anticonvulsant, Miscellaneous
Use Monotherapy or adjunctive therapy for partial onset seizures and primary generalized tonic-clonic seizures; adjunctive treatment of seizures associated with Lennox-Gastaut syndrome; prophylaxis of migraine headache
Unlabeled/Investigational Use Diabetic neuropathy, neuropathic pain; prophylaxis of cluster headache
Medication Guide Available Yes
Contraindications There are no contraindications listed in the manufacturers' labeling.

Canadian labeling (not in U.S. labeling): Hypersensitivity to topiramate or any component of the formulation or container

Warnings/Precautions Antiepileptics are associated with an increased risk of suicidal behavior/thoughts with use (regardless of indication); patients should be monitored for signs/symptoms of depression, suicidal tendencies, and other unusual behavior changes during therapy and instructed to inform their healthcare provider immediately if symptoms occur. Use with caution in patients with hepatic, respiratory, or renal impairment. Topiramate may decrease serum bicarbonate concentrations (up to 67% of patients); treatment-emergent metabolic acidosis is less common. Risk may be increased in patients with a predisposing condition (organ dysfunction, ketogenic diet, or concurrent treatment with other drugs which may cause acidosis). Metabolic acidosis may occur at dosages as low as 50 mg/day. Monitor serum bicarbonate as well as potential complications of chronic acidosis (nephrolithiasis and osteomalacia). Kidney stones have been reported; the risk of kidney stones is about 2-4 times that of the untreated population; the risk of this event may be reduced by increasing fluid intake.

Cognitive dysfunction, psychiatric disturbances (mood disorders), and sedation (somnolence or fatigue) may occur with topiramate use; incidence may be related to rapid titration and higher doses. Patients must be cautioned about performing tasks which require mental alertness (eg, operating machinery or driving). Topiramate may also cause paresthesia, dizziness, and ataxia. Topiramate has been associated with acute myopia and secondary angle-closure glaucoma, typically within 1 month of initiation; discontinue in patients with acute onset of decreased visual acuity or ocular pain. Hyperammonemia with or without encephalopathy may occur with or without concomitant valproate administration; use with caution in patients with inborn errors of metabolism or decreased hepatic mitochondrial activity. Topiramate may be associated (rarely) with severe oligohydrosis and hyperthermia, most frequently in children; use caution and monitor closely during strenuous exercise, during exposure to high environmental temperature, or in patients receiving receiving other carbonic anhydrase inhibitors and drugs with anticholinergic activity. Concurrent use of topiramate and hydrochlorothiazide may increase the risk for hypokalemia; monitor potassium closely.

Avoid abrupt withdrawal of topiramate therapy, it should be withdrawn/tapered slowly to minimize the potential of increased seizure frequency. Doses were also gradually withdrawn in migraine prophylaxis studies. Effects with other sedative drugs or ethanol may be potentiated.

Adverse Reactions (Reflective of adult population; not specific for elderly) Adverse events are reported for placebo-controlled trials of adjunctive therapy in adult and pediatric patients. Unless otherwise noted, the percentages refer to incidence in epilepsy trials. **Note:** A wide range of dosages were studied; incidence of adverse events was frequently lower in the pediatric population studied.

>10%:
 Central nervous system: Somnolence (15% to 29%), dizziness (4% to 25%; dose dependent), fatigue (9% to 16%; dose-dependent), nervousness (9% to 18%), ataxia (6% to 16%), psychomotor slowing (3% to 13%; dose dependent), speech problems (2% to 13%), memory difficulties (2% to 12%), behavior problems (children 11%), confusion (4% to 11%)
 Endocrine & metabolic: Serum bicarbonate decreased (dose related: 7% to 67%; marked reductions [to <17 mEq/L] 1% to 11%)
 Gastrointestinal: Anorexia (4% to 24%; dose dependent), nausea (6% to 10%; migraine trial: 9% to 14%)
 Neuromuscular & skeletal: Paresthesia (1% to 11%; migraine trial: 35% to 51%)
 Ocular: Abnormal vision (2% to 13%)
 Respiratory: Upper respiratory infection (migraine trial: 12% to 14%)
 Miscellaneous: Injury (14%)
1% to 10%:
 Cardiovascular: Chest pain (2% to 4%), edema (2%), hypertension (1% to 2%), bradycardia (1%), pallor (1%), syncope (1%)
 Central nervous system: Difficulty concentrating (5% to 10%), aggressive reactions (2% to 9%), depression (5% to 9%; dose dependent, insomnia (4% to 8%), mood problems (≤6%), abnormal coordination (4%), agitation (3%), cognitive problems (3%), emotional lability (3%), anxiety (2% to 3%; dose dependent), hypoesthesia (2%; migraine trial: 6% to 8%), stupor (2%), vertigo (2%), fever (migraine trial: 1% to 2%), apathy (1%), hallucination (1%), neurosis (1%), psychosis (1%), seizure (1%), suicide attempt (1%)
 Dermatologic: Pruritus (migraine trial: 2% to 4%), skin disorder (2% to 3%), alopecia (2%), dermatitis (2%), hypertrichosis (2%), rash erythematous (1% to 2%), eczema (1%), seborrhea (1%), skin discoloration (1%)
 Endocrine & metabolic: Breast pain (4%), hot flashes (1% to 2%), libido decreased (<1% to 2%), menstrual irregularities (1% to 2%), hypoglycemia (1%), metabolic acidosis (hyperchloremia, nonanion gap)
 Gastrointestinal: Weight loss (4% to 9%), dyspepsia (2% to 7%), abdominal pain (5% to 6%), salivation increased (6%), constipation (4% to 5%), gastroenteritis (2% to 3%), vomiting (migraine trial: 1% to 3%), diarrhea (2%; migraine trial: 9% to 11%), dysgeusia (2%; migraine trial: 8% to 15%), xerostomia (2%), loss of taste (migraine trial: ≤2%), appetite increased (1%), dysphagia (1%), fecal incontinence (1%), flatulence (1%), GERD (1%), gingivitis (1%), glossitis (1%), gum hyperplasia (1%), weight gain (1%)
 Genitourinary: Incontinence (2% to 4%), UTI (2%), premature ejaculation (migraine trial: ≤3%), cystitis (2%), leukorrhea (2%), impotence (1%), nocturia (1%)
 Hematologic: Purpura (8%), leukopenia (2%), anemia (1%), hematoma (1%), prothrombin time increased (1%), thrombocytopenia (1%)

◀ Neuromuscular & skeletal: Tremor (3% to 9%), gait abnormal (3% to 8%), arthralgia (migraine trial: 1% to 7%), weakness (6%), hyperkinesia (5%), back pain (1% to 5%), involuntary muscle contractions (2%; migraine trial: 2% to 4%), leg cramps (2%), leg pain (2%), myalgia (2%), hyporeflexia (2%), rigors (1%), skeletal pain (1%)

Ocular: Diplopia (1% to 10%), nystagmus (10%), conjunctivitis (1%), lacrimation abnormal (1%), myopia (1%)

Otic: Hearing decreased (2%), tinnitus (2%), otitis media (migraine trial: 1% to 2%)

Renal: Hematuria (2%), renal calculus (migraine trial ≤2%)

Respiratory: Rhinitis (4% to 7%), pharyngitis (6%), sinusitis (5%; migraine trial: 6% to 10%), pneumonia (5%), epistaxis (2% to 4%), cough (migraine trial: 2% to 4%), bronchitis (migraine trial: 3%), dyspnea (migraine trial: 1% to 3%)

Miscellaneous: Viral infection (2% to 7%: migraine trial: 3% to 4%), flu-like syndrome (3%), allergy (2%), infection (2%), thirst (2%), body odor (1%), diaphoresis (1%), moniliasis (1%)

Drug Interactions

Metabolism/Transport Effects Inhibits CYP2C19 (weak); **Induces** CYP3A4 (weak)

Avoid Concomitant Use

Avoid concomitant use of Topiramate with any of the following: Carbonic Anhydrase Inhibitors

Increased Effect/Toxicity

Topiramate may increase the levels/effects of: Alcohol (Ethyl); Alpha-/Beta-Agonists; Amphetamines; Anticonvulsants (Barbiturate); Anticonvulsants (Hydantoin); CarBAMazepine; Carbonic Anhydrase Inhibitors; CNS Depressants; Flecainide; Fosphenytoin; Lithium; Memantine; Methotrimeprazine; Phenytoin; Primidone; QuiNIDine; Selective Serotonin Reuptake Inhibitors; Valproic Acid

The levels/effects of Topiramate may be increased by: Divalproex; Droperidol; HydrOXYzine; Methotrimeprazine; Salicylates; Thiazide Diuretics

Decreased Effect

Topiramate may decrease the levels/effects of: Contraceptives (Estrogens); Contraceptives (Progestins); Lithium; Methenamine; Primidone; Saxagliptin

The levels/effects of Topiramate may be decreased by: CarBAMazepine; Fosphenytoin; Ketorolac; Ketorolac (Nasal); Ketorolac (Systemic); Mefloquine; Phenytoin

Ethanol/Nutrition/Herb Interactions

Ethanol: May increase CNS depression; monitor for increased effects with coadministration. Caution patients about effects.

Food: Ketogenic diet may increase the possibility of acidosis and/or kidney stones.

Herb/Nutraceutical: Avoid evening primrose (seizure threshold decreased).

Stability Store at room temperature of 15°C to 30°C (59°F to 86°F). Protect from moisture.

Mechanism of Action Anticonvulsant activity may be due to a combination of potential mechanisms: Blocks neuronal voltage-dependent sodium channels, enhances GABA(A) activity, antagonizes AMPA/kainate glutamate receptors, and weakly inhibits carbonic anhydrase.

Pharmacodynamics/Kinetics

Absorption: Good, rapid; unaffected by food

Protein binding: 15% to 41% (inversely related to plasma concentrations)

Metabolism: Hepatic via P450 enzymes

Bioavailability: ~80%

Half-life elimination: Mean: Adults: Normal renal function: 21 hours; Elderly: ~24 hours

Time to peak, serum: ~1-4 hours

Excretion: Urine (~70% to 80% as unchanged drug)

Dialyzable: Significantly hemodialyzed; dialysis clearance: 120 mL/minute (4-6 times higher than in adults with normal renal function); supplemental doses may be required

Dosage

Geriatric Most older adults have creatinine clearances <70 mL/minute/1.73 m^2; obtain a serum creatinine and calculate creatinine clearance prior to initiation of therapy. An initial dose of 25 mg/day may be recommended, followed by incremental increases of 25 mg at weekly intervals until an effective dose is reached; refer to adult dosing for titration schedule.

Adult Note: Do not abruptly discontinue therapy; taper dosage gradually to prevent rebound effects. (In clinical trials, adult doses were withdrawn by decreasing in weekly intervals of 50-100 mg/day gradually over 2-8 weeks for seizure treatment, and by decreasing in weekly intervals by 25-50 mg/day for migraine prophylaxis.)

Epilepsy, monotherapy:

Partial onset seizure and primary generalized tonic-clonic seizure: Oral: Initial: 25 mg twice daily; may increase weekly by 50 mg/day up to 100 mg twice daily (week 4 dose); thereafter, may further increase weekly by 100 mg/day up to the recommended maximum of 200 mg twice daily

Canadian labeling: Oral: Initial: 25 mg once daily (in evening); may increase to 25 mg twice daily in weeks 2 or 3 and up to 50 mg twice daily by weeks 3 or 4; may further increase weekly in increments of 50 mg/day up to recommended maximum of 200 mg twice daily

Epilepsy, adjunctive therapy:

Partial onset seizure: Oral: Initial: 25 mg once or twice daily for 1 week; may increase weekly by 25-50 mg/day until response; usual maintenance dose: 100-200 mg twice daily. Doses >1600 mg/day have not been studied

Primary generalized tonic-clonic seizure: Oral: Use initial dose as listed above for partial onset seizures, but use slower initial titration rate; titrate upwards to recommended dose by the end of 8 weeks; usual maintenance dose: 200 mg twice daily. Doses >1600 mg/day have not been studied.

Canadian labeling: Oral: Initial: 25 mg once or twice daily; may increase weekly by 50 mg/day up to the recommended dose of 100-200 mg twice daily (maximum recommended dose: 800 mg/day; doses >400 mg/day have shown no additional benefit)

*Migraine prophylaxis:*Oral: Initial: 25 mg once daily (in evening); may increase weekly by 25 mg/day up to the recommended dose of 100 mg/day given in 2 divided doses. Doses >100 mg/day have shown no additional benefit.

Cluster headache prophylaxis (unlabeled use): Oral: Initial: 25 mg/day, titrated at weekly intervals in 25 mg increments, up to 200 mg/day (Pascual, 2007)

Diabetic neuropathy (unlabeled use): Oral: Initial: 25 mg/day, titrated at weekly intervals in 25-50 mg increments to target dose of 400 mg daily in 2 divided doses (Raskin, 2004; Thienel, 2004)

Renal Impairment Cl$_{cr}$ <70 mL/minute/1.73 m^2: Administer 50% dose and titrate more slowly.

Hemodialysis: Supplemental dose may be needed during hemodialysis

Hepatic Impairment Clearance may be reduced; however the manufacturer's labeling provides no specific dosing recommendations.

Administration Oral: May be administered without regard to meals

Capsule sprinkles: May be swallowed whole or opened to sprinkle the contents on a small amount (~1 teaspoon) of soft food (drug/food mixture should not be chewed; swallow immediately).

Tablet: Because of bitter taste, tablets should not be broken or chewed.

Monitoring Parameters Seizure frequency, hydration status; electrolytes (recommended monitoring includes serum bicarbonate at baseline and periodically during treatment), serum creatinine; monitor for symptoms of acute acidosis and complications of long-term acidosis (nephrolithiasis, osteomalacia); ammonia level in patients with unexplained lethargy, vomiting, or mental status changes; intraocular pressure, symptoms of secondary angle closure glaucoma; suicidality (eg, suicidal thoughts, depression, behavioral changes)

Pharmacotherapy Pearls May be associated with weight loss in some patients

Special Geriatric Considerations This drug may not be a drug of choice in the elderly until all other therapies for seizures have been exhausted. Follow the recommended titration schedule and adjust time intervals to meet patient's needs. Since most elderly will have a Cl$_{cr}$ <70 mL/minute, it is important to either measure or estimate by calculation the Cl$_{cr}$ prior to initiating therapy.

Dosage Forms Excipient information presented when available (limited, particularly for generics); consult specific product labeling.

Capsule, sprinkle, oral: 15 mg, 25 mg

Topamax®: 15 mg, 25 mg

Tablet, oral: 25 mg, 50 mg, 100 mg, 200 mg

Topamax®: 25 mg, 50 mg, 100 mg, 200 mg

Selected References

Carroll DG, Kline KM, and Malnar KF, "Role of Topiramate for the Treatment of Painful Diabetic Peripheral Neuropathy," *Pharmacotherapy*, 2004, 24(9):1186-93.

Chong MS and Libretto SE, " The Rationale and Use of Topiramate for Treating Neuropathic Pain," *Clin J Pain*, 2003, 19(1):59-68.

Dib JG, "Focus on Topiramate in Neuropathic Pain," *Curr Med Res Opin*, 2004, 20(12):1857-61.

◆ **Toprol-XL®** *see* Metoprolol *on page 1195*

◆ **Toradol** *see* Ketorolac (Systemic) *on page 1005*

Toremifene (tore EM i feen)

Brand Names: U.S. Fareston®
Brand Names: Canada Fareston®
Index Terms FC1157a; Toremifene Citrate
Generic Availability (U.S.) No

Pharmacologic Category Antineoplastic Agent, Estrogen Receptor Antagonist; Selective Estrogen Receptor Modulator (SERM)

Use Treatment of metastatic breast cancer in postmenopausal women with estrogen receptor positive or estrogen receptor status unknown

Unlabeled/Investigational Use Treatment of soft tissue sarcoma (desmoid tumors)

Contraindications Hypersensitivity to toremifene or any component of the formulation; long QT syndrome (congenital or acquired QT prolongation), uncorrected hypokalemia, uncorrected hypomagnesemia

Warnings/Precautions Hazardous agent - use appropriate precautions for handling and disposal.

[U.S. Boxed Warning]: May prolong the QT interval; QT$_c$ prolongation is dose-dependent and concentration dependent. Torsade de pointes, syncope, seizure and/or sudden death may occur. Use is contraindicated in patients with congenital or acquired long QT syndrome, uncorrected hypokalemia, or uncorrected hypomagnesemia. Avoid use with other medications known to prolong the QT interval and with strong CYP3A4 inhibitors. Use with caution in patients with heart failure, hepatic impairment, or electrolyte abnormalities. Monitor electrolytes; correct hypokalemia and hypomagnesemia prior to treatment. Obtain ECG at baseline and as clinically indicated in patients at risk for QT prolongation

Hypercalcemia and tumor flare have been reported during the first weeks of treatment in some breast cancer patients with bone metastases; monitor closely for hypocalcemia. Institute appropriate measures if hypercalcemia occurs, and if severe, discontinue treatment. Tumor flare consists of diffuse musculoskeletal pain and erythema with initial increased size of tumor lesions that later regress; is often accompanied by hypercalcemia. Tumor flare does not imply treatment failure or represent tumor progression. Drugs that decrease renal calcium excretion (eg, thiazide diuretics) may increase the risk of hypercalcemia in patients receiving toremifene. Leukopenia and thrombocytopenia have been reported rarely; monitor leukocyte and platelet counts. Endometrial hyperplasia has been reported; some patients have developed endometrial cancer, although a role of toremifene in endometrial cancer development has not been established. Avoid long-term use in patients with pre-existing endometrial hyperplasia. Use with caution in patients with hepatic failure. Avoid use in patients with a history of thromboembolic disease.

Adverse Reactions (Reflective of adult population; not specific for elderly)

>10%:
  Endocrine & metabolic: Hot flashes (35%)
  Gastrointestinal: Nausea (14%)
  Genitourinary: Vaginal discharge (13%)
  Hepatic: Alkaline phosphatase increased (8% to 19%), AST increased (5% to 19%)
  Miscellaneous: Diaphoresis (20%)

1% to 10%:
  Cardiovascular: Edema (5%), arrhythmia (≤2%), CVA/TIA (≤2%), thrombosis (≤2%), cardiac failure (≤1%), MI (≤1%)
  Central nervous system: Dizziness (9%)
  Endocrine & metabolic: Hypercalcemia (≤3%)
  Gastrointestinal: Vomiting (4%)
  Genitourinary: Vaginal bleeding (2%)
  Hepatic: Bilirubin increased (1% to 2%)
  Local: Thrombophlebitis (≤2%)
  Ocular: Cataracts (≤10%), xerophthalmia (≤9%), visual field abnormal (≤4%), corneal keratopathy (≤2%), glaucoma (≤2%), vision abnormal/diplopia (≤2%)
  Respiratory: Pulmonary embolism (≤2%)

Drug Interactions

Metabolism/Transport Effects Substrate of CYP1A2 (minor), 3A4 (major)

Avoid Concomitant Use

  Avoid concomitant use of Toremifene with any of the following: Artemether; CYP3A4 Inhibitors (Strong); Dronedarone; Lumefantrine; Nilotinib; Pimozide; QTc-Prolonging Agents; QUEtiapine; QuiNINE; Tetrabenazine; Thioridazine; Vandetanib; Vemurafenib; Ziprasidone

Increased Effect/Toxicity

  Toremifene may increase the levels/effects of: Dronedarone; Pimozide; QTc-Prolonging Agents; QuiNINE; Tetrabenazine; Thioridazine; Vandetanib; Vemurafenib; Vitamin K Antagonists; Ziprasidone

  The levels/effects of Toremifene may be increased by: Alfuzosin; Artemether; Chloroquine; Ciprofloxacin; Ciprofloxacin (Systemic); CYP3A4 Inhibitors (Strong); Gadobutrol; Lumefantrine; Nilotinib; QTc-Prolonging Agents; QUEtiapine; QuiNINE; Thiazide Diuretics

Decreased Effect
The levels/effects of Toremifene may be decreased by: CYP3A4 Inducers (Strong); Cyproterone; Deferasirox; Herbs (CYP3A4 Inducers); Tocilizumab

Ethanol/Nutrition/Herb Interactions
Food: Avoid grapefruit juice (may increase toremifene levels).
Herb/Nutraceutical: Avoid St John's wort (may decrease toremifene levels).

Stability Store at 25°C (77°F); excursions permitted to 15°C to 30°C (59°F to 86°F); protect from heat. Protect from light.

Mechanism of Action Nonsteroidal, triphenylethylene derivative with potent antiestrogenic properties (also has estrogenic effects). Competitively binds to estrogen receptors on tumors and other tissue targets, producing a nuclear complex that decreases DNA synthesis and inhibits estrogen effects. Competes with estrogen for binding sites in breast and other tissues; cells accumulate in the G_0 and G_1 phases; therefore, toremifene is cytostatic rather than cytocidal.

Pharmacodynamics/Kinetics
Absorption: Well absorbed
Distribution: V_d: 580 L (range: 457-958 L)
Protein binding, plasma: >99.5%, primarily to albumin
Metabolism: Extensively hepatic, principally by CYP3A4 to N-demethyltoremifene (a weak antiestrogen)
Bioavailability: Not affected by food
Half-life elimination: Toremifene: ~5 days; N-demethyltoremifene: 6 days
Time to peak, serum: ≤3 hours
Excretion: Primarily feces; urine (10%) during a 1-week period

Dosage
Geriatric & Adult Metastatic breast cancer (postmenopausal): Oral: 60 mg once daily, continue until disease progression

Administration Administer orally, as a single daily dose, with or without food.

Monitoring Parameters CBC with differential, electrolytes (calcium, magnesium, and potassium), hepatic function. Obtain ECG in patients at risk for QT prolongation. In patients with bone metastases, monitor closely for hypercalcemia during the first few weeks of treatment.

Special Geriatric Considerations No specific information concerning elderly patients.

Dosage Forms Excipient information presented when available (limited, particularly for generics); consult specific product labeling.
Tablet, oral:
Fareston®: 60 mg

Selected References
NCCN (National Comprehensive Cancer Network), "Clinical Practice Guidelines in Oncology™: Breast Cancer, Version 1.2008." Available at http://www.nccn.org/professionals/physician_gls/PDF/breast.pdf
Pagani O, Gelber S, Price K, et al, "Toremifene and Tamoxifen are Equally Effective for Early-Stage Breast Cancer: First Results of International Breast Cancer Study Group Trials 12-93 and 14-93," *Ann Oncol*, 2004, 15(12):1749-59.

◆ **Toremifene Citrate** *see* Toremifene *on page 1835*

Torsemide (TORE se mide)

Medication Safety Issues
Sound-alike/look-alike issues:
Torsemide may be confused with furosemide
Demadex® may be confused with Denorex®

Brand Names: U.S. Demadex®

Generic Availability (U.S.) Yes

Pharmacologic Category Diuretic, Loop

Use Management of edema associated with heart failure and hepatic or renal disease (including chronic renal failure); treatment of hypertension

Contraindications Hypersensitivity to torsemide, any component of the formulation, or any sulfonylurea; anuria

Warnings/Precautions Loop diuretics are potent diuretics; excess amounts can lead to profound diuresis with fluid and electrolyte loss; close medical supervision and dose evaluation are required. Potassium supplementation and/or use of potassium-sparing diuretics may be necessary to prevent hypokalemia. Use with caution in patients with cirrhosis; avoid sudden changes in fluid and electrolyte balance and acid/base status which may lead to hepatic encephalopathy. Administration with an aldosterone antagonist or potassium-sparing diuretic may provide additional diuretic efficacy and maintain normokalemia. Coadministration of antihypertensives may increase the risk of hypotension.

Monitor fluid status and renal function in an attempt to prevent oliguria, azotemia, and reversible increases in BUN and creatinine; close medical supervision of aggressive diuresis required. Ototoxicity has been demonstrated following oral administration of torsemide and following rapid I.V. administration of other loop diuretics. Other possible risk factors may include use in renal impairment, excessive doses, and concurrent use of other ototoxins (eg, aminoglycosides).

Chemical similarities are present among sulfonamides, sulfonylureas, carbonic anhydrase inhibitors, thiazides, and loop diuretics (except ethacrynic acid). Use in patients with sulfonylurea allergy is specifically contraindicated in product labeling; a risk of cross-reaction exists in patients with allergy to any of these compounds; avoid use when previous reaction has been severe. Discontinue if signs of hypersensitivity are noted.

Adverse Reactions (Reflective of adult population; not specific for elderly)

1% to 10%:

Cardiovascular: ECG abnormality (2%), chest pain (1%)

Central nervous system: Nervousness (1%)

Gastrointestinal: Constipation (2%), diarrhea (2%), dyspepsia (2%), nausea (2%), sore throat (2%)

Genitourinary: Excessive urination (7%)

Neuromuscular & skeletal: Arthralgia (2%), myalgia (2%), weakness (2%)

Respiratory: Rhinitis (3%), cough (2%)

Drug Interactions

Metabolism/Transport Effects Substrate of CYP2C8 (minor), CYP2C9 (major), SLCO1B1; **Inhibits** CYP2C19 (weak)

Avoid Concomitant Use There are no known interactions where it is recommended to avoid concomitant use.

Increased Effect/Toxicity

Torsemide may increase the levels/effects of: ACE Inhibitors; Allopurinol; Amifostine; Aminoglycosides; Antihypertensives; Cardiac Glycosides; CISplatin; Dofetilide; Hypotensive Agents; Lithium; Methotrexate; Neuromuscular-Blocking Agents; RisperiDONE; RiTUXimab; Salicylates; Sodium Phosphates; Warfarin

The levels/effects of Torsemide may be increased by: Alfuzosin; Beta2-Agonists; Corticosteroids (Orally Inhaled); Corticosteroids (Systemic); CycloSPORINE (Systemic); CYP2C9 Inhibitors (Moderate); CYP2C9 Inhibitors (Strong); Diazoxide; Eltrombopag; Herbs (Hypotensive Properties); Licorice; MAO Inhibitors; Methotrexate; Pentoxifylline; Phosphodiesterase 5 Inhibitors; Probenecid; Prostacyclin Analogues

Decreased Effect

Torsemide may decrease the levels/effects of: Lithium; Neuromuscular-Blocking Agents

The levels/effects of Torsemide may be decreased by: Bile Acid Sequestrants; CYP2C9 Inducers (Highly Effective); Fosphenytoin; Herbs (Hypertensive Properties); Methotrexate; Methylphenidate; Peginterferon Alfa-2b; Phenytoin; Probenecid; Salicylates; Yohimbine

Ethanol/Nutrition/Herb Interactions Herb/Nutraceutical: Avoid herbs with *hypertensive* properties (bayberry, blue cohosh, cayenne, ephedra, ginger, ginseng [American], kola, licorice); may diminish the antihypertensive effect of torsemide. Avoid herbs with *hypotensive* properties (black cohosh, California poppy, coleus, golden seal, hawthorn, mistletoe, periwinkle, quinine, shepherd's purse); may enhance the hypotensive effect of torsemide.

Stability

I.V.: Store at 15°C to 30°C (59°F to 86°F). If torsemide is to be administered via continuous infusion, stability has been demonstrated through 24 hours at room temperature in plastic containers for the following fluids and concentrations:

200 mg torsemide (10 mg/mL) added to 250 mL D_5W, 250 mL NS or 500 mL 0.45% sodium chloride

50 mg torsemide (10 mg/mL) added to 500 mL D_5W, 500 mL NS, or 500 mL 0.45% sodium chloride

Tablets: Store at 15°C to 30°C (59°F to 86°F).

Mechanism of Action Inhibits reabsorption of sodium and chloride in the ascending loop of Henle and distal renal tubule, interfering with the chloride-binding cotransport system, thus causing increased excretion of water, sodium, chloride, magnesium, and calcium; does not alter GFR, renal plasma flow, or acid-base balance

Pharmacodynamics/Kinetics

Onset of action: Diuresis: Oral: Within 1 hour

Peak effect: Diuresis: Oral: 1-2 hours; Antihypertensive: Oral: 4-6 weeks (up to 12 weeks)

Duration: Diuresis: Oral: ~6-8 hours

Absorption: Oral: Rapid

Distribution: V_d: 12-15 L; Cirrhosis: Approximately doubled

Protein binding: >99%

Metabolism: Hepatic (~80%) via CYP
Bioavailability: ~80%
Half-life elimination: ~3.5 hours; Cirrhosis: 7-8 hours
Time to peak, plasma: Oral: 1 hour; delayed ~30 minutes when administered with food
Excretion: Urine (~20% as unchanged drug)

Dosage
Geriatric & Adult Note: I.V. and oral dosing are equivalent.
  Edema:
    Chronic renal failure: Oral, I.V.: Initial: 20 mg once daily; may increase gradually by doubling dose until the desired diuretic response is obtained (maximum recommended daily dose: 200 mg)
    Heart failure:
      Oral: Initial: 10-20 mg once daily; may increase gradually by doubling dose until the desired diuretic response is obtained. **Note:** ACC/AHA 2009 guidelines for heart failure maximum daily dose: 200 mg (Hunt, 2009)
      I.V.: Initial: 10-20 mg; may repeat every 2 hours with double the dose as needed. **Note:** ACC/AHA 2009 guidelines for heart failure recommend maximum single dose: 100-200 mg (Hunt, 2009)
      Continuous I.V. infusion (unlabeled dose): Initial: 20 mg I.V. load, then 5-20 mg/hour (Hunt, 2009)
  Hepatic cirrhosis: Oral: Initial: 5-10 mg once daily; may increase gradually by doubling dose until the desired diuretic response is obtained (maximum recommended single dose: 40 mg). **Note:** Administer with an aldosterone antagonist or a potassium-sparing diuretic.
  Hypertension: Oral: Initial: 5 mg once daily; may increase to 10 mg once daily after 4-6 weeks if adequate antihypertensive response is not apparent; if still not effective, an additional antihypertensive agent may be added. Usual dosage range (JNC 7): 2.5-10 mg once daily. **Note:** Thiazide-type diuretics are preferred in the treatment of hypertension (Chobanian, 2003)

Administration Administer the I.V. dose slowly over 2 minutes

Monitoring Parameters Renal function, electrolytes, and fluid status (weight and I & O), blood pressure

Pharmacotherapy Pearls 10-20 mg torsemide is approximately equivalent to:
Furosemide 40 mg
Bumetanide 1 mg

Special Geriatric Considerations Loop diuretics are potent diuretics; excess amounts can lead to profound diuresis with fluid and electrolyte loss. Close medical supervision and dose evaluation is required, particularly in the elderly. Severe loss of sodium and/or increase in BUN can cause confusion; for any change in mental status, monitor electrolytes and renal function.

Dosage Forms Excipient information presented when available (limited, particularly for generics); consult specific product labeling.
Injection, solution: 10 mg/mL (2 mL, 5 mL)
Tablet, oral: 5 mg, 10 mg, 20 mg, 100 mg
  Demadex®: 5 mg, 10 mg, 20 mg, 100 mg [scored]

TraMADol (TRA ma dole)

Medication Safety Issues
  Sound-alike/look-alike issues:
    TraMADol may be confused with tapentadol, Toradol®, Trandate®, traZODone, Voltaren®
    Ultram® may be confused with Ultane®, Ultracet®, Voltaren®
  International issues:
    Theradol [Netherlands] may be confused with Foradil brand name for formoterol [U.S., Canada, and multiple international markets], Terazol brand name for terconazole [U.S. and Canada], and Toradol brand name for ketorolac [Canada and multiple international markets]
    Trexol [Mexico] may be confused with Trexall brand name for methotrexate [U.S.]; Truxal brand name for chlorprothixene [multiple international markets]
Brand Names: U.S. Rybix™ ODT; Ryzolt™; Ultram®; Ultram® ER
Brand Names: Canada Ralivia™ ER; Tridural™; Zytram® XL
Index Terms Tramadol Hydrochloride
Generic Availability (U.S.) Yes: Excludes orally disintegrating tablet

◀ **Pharmacologic Category** Analgesic, Opioid

Use Relief of moderate to moderately-severe pain

Extended release formulations are indicated for patients requiring around-the-clock management of moderate to moderately-severe pain for an extended period of time

Contraindications Hypersensitivity to tramadol, opioids, or any component of the formulation; opioid-dependent patients; acute intoxication with alcohol, hypnotics, centrally-acting analgesics, opioids, or psychotropic drugs

Additional contraindications for Ryzolt™: Severe/acute bronchial asthma, hypercapnia, or significant respiratory depression in the absence of appropriately monitored setting and/or resuscitative equipment

Canadian product labeling:

Tramadol is contraindicated during or within 14 days following MAO inhibitor therapy

Extended release formulations (Ralivia™ ER [CAN], Tridural™[CAN], and Zytram® XL [CAN]): Additional contraindications: Severe (Cl_{cr} <30 mL/minute) renal dysfunction, severe (Child-Pugh class C) hepatic dysfunction

Warnings/Precautions Rare but serious anaphylactoid reactions (including fatalities) often following initial dosing have been reported. Pruritus, hives, bronchospasm, angioedema, toxic epidermal necrolysis (TEN) and Stevens-Johnson syndrome also have been reported with use. Previous anaphylactoid reactions to opioids may increase risks for similar reactions to tramadol. Caution patients to swallow extended release tablets whole. Rapid release and absorption of tramadol from extended release tablets that are broken, crushed, or chewed may lead to a potentially lethal overdose. May cause CNS depression, which may impair physical or mental abilities; patients must be cautioned about performing tasks which require mental alertness (eg, operating machinery or driving). May cause CNS depression and/or respiratory depression, particularly when combined with other CNS depressants. Use with caution and reduce dosage when administered to patients receiving other CNS depressants. An increased risk of seizures may occur in patients receiving serotonin reuptake inhibitors (SSRIs or anorectics), tricyclic antidepressants or other cyclic compounds (including cyclobenzaprine, promethazine), neuroleptics, drugs which may lower seizure threshold, or drugs which impair metabolism of tramadol (ie, CYP2D6 and 3A4 inhibitors). Patients with a history of seizures, or with a risk of seizures (head trauma, metabolic disorders, CNS infection, or malignancy, or during ethanol/drug withdrawal) are also at increased risk. Avoid use, if possible, with serotonergic agents such as TCAs, MAO inhibitors (use with extreme caution; contraindicated in Canadian product labeling), triptans, venlafaxine, trazodone, lithium, sibutramine, meperidine, dextromethorphan, St John's wort, SNRIs, and SSRIs; use caution with drugs which impair metabolism of tramadol (ie, CYP2D6 and 3A4 inhibitors); concomitant may increase the risk of serotonin syndrome.

Elderly (particularly >75 years of age), debilitated patients and patients with chronic respiratory disorders may be at greater risk of adverse events. Use with caution in patients with increased intracranial pressure or head injury. Avoid use in patients who are suicidal or addiction prone; use with caution in patients taking tranquilizers and/or antidepressants, or those with an emotional disturbance including depression. Healthcare provider should be alert to problems of abuse, misuse, and diversion. Use caution in heavy alcohol users. Use caution in treatment of acute abdominal conditions; may mask pain. Use tramadol with caution and reduce dosage in patients with liver disease or renal dysfunction. Avoid using extended release tablets in severe hepatic impairment. Do not use Ryzolt™ in any degree of hepatic impairment. Tolerance or drug dependence may result from extended use (withdrawal symptoms have been reported); abrupt discontinuation should be avoided. Tapering of dose at the time of discontinuation limits the risk of withdrawal symptoms. Some products may contain phenylalanine.

Adverse Reactions (Reflective of adult population; not specific for elderly)

>10%:

Cardiovascular: Flushing (8% to 16%)

Central nervous system: Dizziness (10% to 33%), headache (4% to 32%), somnolence (7% to 25%), insomnia (2% to 11%)

Dermatologic: Pruritus (5% to 12%)

Gastrointestinal: Constipation (10% to 46%), nausea (15% to 40%), vomiting (5% to 17%), dyspepsia (1% to 13%)

Neuromuscular & skeletal: Weakness (4% to 12%)

1% to 10%:

Cardiovascular: Postural hypotension (2% to 5%), chest pain (1% to <5%), vasodilation (1% to <5%)

Central nervous system: Anxiety (1% to <5%), confusion (1% to <5%), coordination impaired (1% to <5%), depression (1% to <5%), euphoria (1% to <5%), hypoesthesia (1% to <5%), lethargy (1% to <5%), nervousness (1% to <5%), pain (1% to <5%), pyrexia (1% to <5%), restlessness (1% to <5%), malaise (<1% to <5%), fatigue (2%), vertigo (2%)

Dermatologic: Dermatitis (1% to <5%), rash (1% to <5%)

Endocrine & metabolic: Hot flashes (2% to 9%), menopausal symptoms (1% to <5%)

Gastrointestinal: Diarrhea (5% to 10%), xerostomia (3% to 10%), anorexia (1% to <6%), abdominal pain (1% to <5%), appetite decreased (1% to <5%), weight loss (1% to <5%), flatulence (<1% to <5%)

Genitourinary: Urinary tract infection (1% to <5%), urinary frequency (<1% to <5%), urinary retention (<1% to <5%)

Neuromuscular & skeletal: Arthralgia (1% to <5%), back pain (1% to <5%), hypertonia (1% to <5%), rigors (1% to <5%), paresthesia (1% to <5%), tremor (1% to <5%), creatine phosphokinase increased (1% to <5%)

Ocular: Blurred vision (1% to <5%), miosis (1% to <5%)

Respiratory: Bronchitis (1% to <5%), congestion (nasal/sinus) (1% to <5%), cough (1% to <5%), dyspnea (1% to <5%), nasopharyngitis (1% to <5%), rhinorrhea (1% to <5%), sinusitis (1% to <5%), sneezing (1% to <5%), sore throat (1% to <5%), upper respiratory infection (1% to <5%)

Miscellaneous: Diaphoresis (2% to 9%), flu-like syndrome (1% to < 5%), shivering (<1% to <5%)

A withdrawal syndrome may occur with abrupt discontinuation; includes anxiety, diarrhea, hallucinations (rare), nausea, pain, piloerection, rigors, sweating, and tremor. Uncommon discontinuation symptoms may include severe anxiety, panic attacks, or paresthesia.

Drug Interactions

Metabolism/Transport Effects Substrate of CYP2D6 (major), 3A4 (major)

Avoid Concomitant Use

Avoid concomitant use of TraMADol with any of the following: Conivaptan; Sibutramine

Increased Effect/Toxicity

TraMADol may increase the levels/effects of: Alcohol (Ethyl); Alvimopan; CNS Depressants; Desmopressin; MAO Inhibitors; Selective Serotonin Reuptake Inhibitors; Serotonin Modulators; Thiazide Diuretics; Vitamin K Antagonists

The levels/effects of TraMADol may be increased by: Amphetamines; Antipsychotic Agents (Phenothiazines); Conivaptan; CYP3A4 Inhibitors (Moderate); CYP3A4 Inhibitors (Strong); Dasatinib; Droperidol; HydrOXYzine; Selective Serotonin Reuptake Inhibitors; Sibutramine; Succinylcholine; Tricyclic Antidepressants

Decreased Effect

TraMADol may decrease the levels/effects of: Pegvisomant

The levels/effects of TraMADol may be decreased by: Ammonium Chloride; CYP2D6 Inhibitors (Moderate); CYP2D6 Inhibitors (Strong); CYP3A4 Inducers (Strong); Deferasirox; Mixed Agonist / Antagonist Opioids; Tocilizumab

Ethanol/Nutrition/Herb Interactions

Ethanol: May increase CNS depression; monitor for increased effects with coadministration. Caution patients about effects.

Food:

Immediate release: Does not affect the rate or extent of absorption.

Extended release: Reduced C_{max} and AUC and T_{max} occurred 3 hours earlier when taken with a high-fat meal.

Ryzolt™: Increased C_{max}; no effect on AUC.

Herb/Nutraceutical: Avoid valerian, St John's wort, kava kava, gotu kola (may increase CNS depression).

Stability Store at 25°C (77°F); excursions permitted to 15°C to 30°C (59°F to 86°F).

Mechanism of Action Tramadol and its active metabolite (M1) binds to μ-opiate receptors in the CNS causing inhibition of ascending pain pathways, altering the perception of and response to pain; also inhibits the reuptake of norepinephrine and serotonin, which also modifies the ascending pain pathway

Pharmacodynamics/Kinetics

Onset of action: Immediate release: ~1 hour

Duration: 9 hours

Absorption: Immediate release formulation: Rapid and complete; Extended release formulation: Delayed

Distribution: V_d: 2.5-3 L/kg

Protein binding, plasma: 20%

Metabolism: Extensively hepatic via demethylation (mediated by CYP3A4 and CYP2B6), glucuronidation, and sulfation; has pharmacologically active metabolite formed by CYP2D6 (M1; O-desmethyl tramadol)

Bioavailability: Immediate release: 75%; Extended release: Ultram® ER: 85% to 90% (as compared to immediate release), Zytram® XL, Tridural™: 70%, Ryzolt™: ~95% (as compared to immediate release)

◀ Half-life elimination: Tramadol: ~6-8 hours; Active metabolite: 7-9 hours; prolonged in elderly, hepatic or renal impairment; Zytram® XL: ~16 hours; Ralivia™ ER, Ryzolt™, Tridural™: ~5-9 hours

Time to peak: Immediate release: ~2 hours; Extended release: Ultram® ER: ~12 hours, Ryzolt™, Tridural™: ~4 hours

Excretion: Urine (30% as unchanged drug; 60% as metabolites)

Dosage

Geriatric Elderly >65 years: Oral: Use caution and initiate at the lower end of the dosing range. Refer to adult dosing.

Immediate release: Elderly >75 years: Do not exceed 300 mg/day; see Dosage: Renal Impairment and Dosage: Hepatic Impairment.

Extended release formulation: Elderly >75 years: Use with great caution; see Dosage: Adult, Dosage: Renal Impairment, and Dosage: Hepatic Impairment.

Adult Moderate-to-severe pain: Oral:

Immediate release formulation: 50-100 mg every 4-6 hours (not to exceed 400 mg/day)

For patients not requiring rapid onset of effect, tolerability may be improved by starting dose at 25 mg/day and titrating dose by 25 mg every 3 days, until reaching 25 mg 4 times/day. The total daily dose may then be increased by 50 mg every 3 days as tolerated, to reach dose of 50 mg 4 times/day. After titration, 50-100 mg may be given every 4-6 hours as needed up to a maximum 400 mg/day.

Extended release formulation:

Ultram® ER:

Patients not currently on immediate-release: 100 mg once daily; titrate every 5 days (maximum: 300 mg/day)

Patients currently on immediate-release: Calculate 24-hour immediate release total dose and initiate total extended release daily dose (round dose to the next lowest 100 mg increment); titrate (maximum: 300 mg/day)

Ralivia™ ER (Canadian labeling, not available in U.S.): 100 mg once daily; titrate every 5 days as needed based on clinical response and severity of pain (maximum: 300 mg/day)

Ryzolt™:

Patients not currently on immediate-release: 100 mg once daily; titrate every 2-3 days by 100 mg/day increments; usual daily dose: 200-300 mg/day (maximum: 300 mg/day)

Patients currently on immediate-release: Calculate 24 hour immediate release total dose and initiate total extended release daily dose (round dose to the next lowest 100 mg increment); titrate (maximum: 300 mg/day)

Tridural™ (Canadian labeling, not available in U.S.): 100 mg once daily; titrate by 100 mg/day every 2 days as needed based on clinical response and severity of pain (maximum: 300 mg/day)

Zytram® XL (Canadian labeling, not available in U.S.): 150 mg once daily; if pain relief is not achieved may titrate by increasing dosage incrementally, with sufficient time to evaluate effect of increased dosage; generally not more often than every 7 days (maximum: 400 mg/day)

Renal Impairment

Immediate release: Cl$_{cr}$ <30 mL/minute: Administer 50-100 mg dose every 12 hours (maximum: 200 mg/day).

Extended release: Should not be used in patients with Cl$_{cr}$ <30 mL/minute.

Hepatic Impairment

Immediate release: Cirrhosis: Recommended dose: 50 mg every 12 hours.

Extended release: Should not be used in patients with severe (Child-Pugh class C) hepatic dysfunction; Ryzolt™ should not be used in any degree of hepatic impairment

Administration

Extended release tablet: Swallow whole; do not crush, chew, or split. Administer without regard to meals, but consistently administering with or without meals.

Orally-disintegrating tablet: Remove from foil blister by peeling back (do not push tablet through the foil). Place tablet on tongue and allow to dissolve (may take ~1 minute); water is not needed, but may be administered with water. Do not chew, break, or split tablet.

Monitoring Parameters Pain relief, respiratory rate, blood pressure, and pulse; signs of tolerance, abuse, or suicidal ideation

Reference Range 100-300 ng/mL; however, serum level monitoring is not required

Test Interactions May interfere with urine detection of PCP (false-positive).

Special Geriatric Considerations One study in the elderly found that tramadol 50 mg was similar in efficacy as acetaminophen 300 mg with codeine 30 mg. In Ultram® ER trials, elderly patients experienced more adverse effects than younger adults, particularly constipation, fatigue, weakness, postural hypotension, and dyspepsia. For this reason, the extended release formulation should probably be avoided in the elderly, or only used with great caution.

Dosage Forms Excipient information presented when available (limited, particularly for generics); consult specific product labeling.
Tablet, oral, as hydrochloride: 50 mg
Ultram®: 50 mg [scored]
Tablet, extended release, oral, as hydrochloride: 100 mg, 200 mg
Ryzolt™: 100 mg, 200 mg, 300 mg
Ultram® ER: 100 mg, 200 mg, 300 mg
Tablet, orally disintegrating, oral, as hydrochloride:
Rybix™ ODT: 50 mg [contains aspartame; mint flavor]
Dosage Forms: Canada Excipient information presented when available (limited, particularly for generics); consult specific product labeling.
Tablet, extended release, as hydrochloride
Ralivia™ ER: 100 mg, 200 mg, 300 mg
Tridural™: 100 mg, 200 mg, 300 mg
Zytram® XL: 75 mg, 150 mg, 200 mg, 300 mg, 400 mg
Selected References

American Geriatrics Society Panel on Pharmacological Management of Persistent Pain in Older Persons, "Pharmacological Management of Persistent Pain in Older Persons," *J Am Geriat Soc*, 2009, 57(8):1331-46.
Rauck RL, Ruoff GE, and McGillen, "Comparison of Tramadol and Acetaminophen With Codeine for Long-Term Pain Management in Elderly Patients," *Curr Ther Res*, 1994, 556:1417-31.

◆ **Tramadol Hydrochloride** *see* TraMADol *on page 1839*
◆ **Trandate®** *see* Labetalol *on page 1015*

Trandolapril (tran DOE la pril)

Related Information
Angiotensin Agents *on page 1985*
Brand Names: U.S. Mavik®
Brand Names: Canada Mavik®
Generic Availability (U.S.) Yes
Pharmacologic Category Angiotensin-Converting Enzyme (ACE) Inhibitor
Use Treatment of hypertension alone or in combination with other antihypertensive agents; treatment of heart failure (HF) or left ventricular (LV) dysfunction after myocardial infarction (MI)
Unlabeled/Investigational Use As a class, ACE inhibitors are recommended in the treatment of heart failure; to delay the progression of nephropathy and reduce risks of cardiovascular events in hypertensive patients with type 1 or 2 diabetes mellitus
Contraindications Hypersensitivity to trandolapril or any component of the formulation; history of angioedema related to previous treatment with an ACE inhibitor
Warnings/Precautions Anaphylactic reactions may occur rarely with ACE inhibitors. At any time during treatment (especially following first dose) angioedema may occur rarely with ACE inhibitors; it may involve the head and neck (potentially compromising the airway) or the intestine (presenting with abdominal pain). African-Americans and patients with idiopathic or hereditary angioedema may be at an increased risk. Prolonged frequent monitoring may be required especially if tongue, glottis, or larynx are involved as they are associated with airway obstruction. Patients with a history of airway surgery may have a higher risk of airway obstruction. Aggressive early and appropriate management is critical. Use in patients with previous angioedema associated with ACE inhibitor therapy is contraindicated. Severe anaphylactoid reactions may be seen during hemodialysis (eg, CVVHD) with high-flux dialysis membranes (eg, AN69). Rare cases of anaphylactoid reactions have been reported in patients undergoing sensitization treatment with hymenoptera (bee, wasp) venom while receiving ACE inhibitors.

Symptomatic hypotension with or without syncope can occur with ACE inhibitors (usually with the first several doses); effects are most often observed in volume-depleted patients; correct volume depletion prior to initiation; close monitoring of patient is required especially with initial dosing and dosing increases; blood pressure must be lowered at a rate appropriate for the patient's clinical condition. Initiation of therapy in patients with ischemic heart disease or cerebrovascular disease warrants close observation due to the potential consequences posed by falling blood pressure (eg, MI, stroke). Use with caution in hypertrophic cardiomyopathy with outflow tract obstruction, severe aortic stenosis, or before, during, or immediately after major surgery.

Hyperkalemia may occur with ACE inhibitors; risk factors include renal dysfunction, diabetes mellitus, concomitant use of potassium-sparing diuretics, potassium supplements, and/or potassium-containing salts. Use cautiously, if at all, with these agents and monitor potassium closely. Cough may occur with ACE inhibitors. Other causes of cough should be considered (eg, pulmonary congestion in patients with heart failure) and excluded prior to discontinuation.

◀ Dosage adjustment needed in severe renal dysfunction (Cl_{cr} <30 mL/minute) or hepatic cirrhosis. May be associated with deterioration of renal function and/or increases in serum creatinine, particularly in patients with low renal blood flow (eg, renal artery stenosis, heart failure) whose glomerular filtration rate (GFR) is dependent on efferent arteriolar vasoconstriction by angiotensin II; deterioration may result in oliguria, acute renal failure, and progressive azotemia. Small increases in serum creatinine may occur following initiation; consider discontinuation only in patients with progressive and/or significant deterioration in renal function. Use with caution in patients with unstented unilateral/bilateral renal artery stenosis. When unstented bilateral renal artery stenosis is present, use is generally avoided due to the elevated risk of deterioration in renal function unless possible benefits outweigh risks. Concurrent use of angiotensin receptor blockers may increase the risk of clinically-significant adverse events (eg, renal dysfunction, hyperkalemia).

Rare toxicities associated with ACE inhibitors include cholestatic jaundice (which may progress to fulminant hepatic necrosis), agranulocytosis, neutropenia, or leukopenia with myeloid hypoplasia. Patients with collagen vascular diseases (especially with concomitant renal impairment) or renal impairment alone may be at increased risk for hematologic toxicity; periodically monitor CBC with differential in these patients.

Adverse Reactions (Reflective of adult population; not specific for elderly) Note: Frequency ranges include data from hypertension and heart failure trials. Higher rates of adverse reactions have generally been noted in patients with CHF. However, the frequency of adverse effects associated with placebo is also increased in this population.

>1%:
   Cardiovascular: Hypotension (<1% to 11%), syncope (6%), bradycardia (<1% to 5%), intermittent claudication (4%)
   Central nervous system: Dizziness (1% to 23%)
   Endocrine & metabolic: Uric acid increased (15%), hyperkalemia (5%), hypocalcemia (5%)
   Gastrointestinal: Diarrhea (1%)
   Neuromuscular & skeletal: Myalgia (5%)
   Renal: BUN increased (9%), serum creatinine increased (1% to 5%)
   Respiratory: Cough (2% to 35%)

Worsening of renal function may occur in patients with bilateral renal artery stenosis or hypovolemia. In addition, a syndrome which may include fever, myalgia, arthralgia, interstitial nephritis, vasculitis, rash, eosinophilia and positive ANA, and elevated ESR has been reported with ACE inhibitors. Eosinophilic pneumonitis has also been reported with other ACE inhibitors.

Drug Interactions
   Avoid Concomitant Use There are no known interactions where it is recommended to avoid concomitant use.
   Increased Effect/Toxicity
   Trandolapril may increase the levels/effects of: Allopurinol; Amifostine; Antihypertensives; AzaTHIOprine; CycloSPORINE; CycloSPORINE (Systemic); Ferric Gluconate; Gold Sodium Thiomalate; Hypotensive Agents; Iron Dextran Complex; Lithium; Nonsteroidal Anti-Inflammatory Agents; RiTUXimab; Sodium Phosphates

   The levels/effects of Trandolapril may be increased by: Alfuzosin; Angiotensin II Receptor Blockers; Diazoxide; DPP-IV Inhibitors; Eplerenone; Everolimus; Herbs (Hypotensive Properties); Loop Diuretics; MAO Inhibitors; Pentoxifylline; Phosphodiesterase 5 Inhibitors; Potassium Salts; Potassium-Sparing Diuretics; Prostacyclin Analogues; Sirolimus; Temsirolimus; Thiazide Diuretics; TiZANidine; Tolvaptan; Trimethoprim
   Decreased Effect
   The levels/effects of Trandolapril may be decreased by: Antacids; Aprotinin; Herbs (Hypertensive Properties); Icatibant; Lanthanum; Methylphenidate; Nonsteroidal Anti-Inflammatory Agents; Salicylates; Yohimbine

Ethanol/Nutrition/Herb Interactions Herb/Nutraceutical: Avoid bayberry, blue cohosh, cayenne, ephedra, ginger, ginseng (American), kola, licorice (may worsen hypertension). Avoid black cohosh, California poppy, coleus, golden seal, hawthorn, mistletoe, periwinkle, quinine, shepherd's purse (may have increased antihypertensive effect).

Stability Store at controlled room temperature of 20°C to 25°C (68°F to 77°F).

Mechanism of Action Trandolapril is an ACE inhibitor which prevents the formation of angiotensin II from angiotensin I. Trandolapril must undergo enzymatic hydrolysis, mainly in liver, to its biologically active metabolite, trandolaprilat. A CNS mechanism may also be involved in the hypotensive effect as angiotensin II increases adrenergic outflow from the CNS. Vasoactive kallikrein's may be decreased in conversion to active hormones by ACE inhibitors, thus reducing blood pressure.

Pharmacodynamics/Kinetics
Onset of action: 1-2 hours
  Peak effect: Reduction in blood pressure: 6 hours
Duration: Prolonged; 72 hours after single dose
Absorption: Rapid
Distribution:
  Trandolapril: ~18L
  Trandolaprilat (active metabolite) is very lipophilic in comparison to other ACE inhibitors
Protein binding:
  Trandolapril: ~80%
  Trandolaprilat: 65% to 94% (concentration dependent)
Metabolism: Hepatically hydrolyzed to active metabolite, trandolaprilat
Bioavailability:
  Trandolapril: 10%
  Trandolaprilat: 70%
Half-life elimination:
  Trandolapril: 6 hours; Trandolaprilat: Effective: 22.5 hours
Time to peak: Parent: 1 hour; Active metabolite trandolaprilat: 4-10 hours
Excretion: Urine (33%); feces (66%)
  Clearance: Reduce dose in renal failure; creatinine clearances ≤30 mL/minute result in accumulation of active metabolite

Dosage
Geriatric & Adult
  Hypertension: Initial dose in patients not receiving a diuretic: Oral: 1 mg once daily (2 mg/day in black patients). Adjust dosage at intervals of ≥1 week according to blood pressure response; most patients require 2-4 mg/day. There is little experience with doses >8 mg/day. Patients inadequately treated with once daily dosing at 4 mg may be treated with twice daily dosing. If blood pressure is not adequately controlled with trandolapril monotherapy, a diuretic may be added.
  Usual dose range (JNC 7): 1-4 mg once daily
  Post-MI heart failure or LV dysfunction: Oral: Initial: 1 mg once daily; titrate (as tolerated) towards target dose of 4 mg/day. If 4 mg dose is not tolerated, patients may continue therapy with the greatest tolerated dose.
Renal Impairment Cl_{cr} <30 mL/minute: Recommended starting dose: 0.5 mg once daily.
Hepatic Impairment Cirrhosis: Recommended starting dose: 0.5 mg once daily.
Monitoring Parameters Blood pressure; serum creatinine and potassium; if patient has collagen vascular disease and/or renal impairment, periodically monitor CBC with differential
Pharmacotherapy Pearls Patients taking diuretics are at risk for developing hypotension on initial dosing; to prevent this, discontinue diuretics 2-3 days prior to initiating trandolapril; may restart diuretics if blood pressure is not controlled by trandolapril alone. Watch for hypotensive effect within 1-3 hours of first dose or new higher dose.
Special Geriatric Considerations Due to frequent decreases in glomerular filtration (also creatinine clearance) with aging, elderly patients may have exaggerated responses to ACE inhibitors; differences in clinical response due to hepatic changes are not observed. ACE inhibitors may be preferred agents in elderly patients with CHF and diabetes mellitus. Diabetic proteinuria is reduced and insulin sensitivity is enhanced. In general, the side effect profile is favorable in the elderly and causes little or no CNS confusion; use lowest dose recommendations initially. Adjust for renal function. Many elderly may be volume depleted due to diuretic use and/or blunted thirst reflex resulting in inadequate fluid intake.
Dosage Forms Excipient information presented when available (limited, particularly for generics); consult specific product labeling.
  Tablet, oral: 1 mg, 2 mg, 4 mg
    Mavik®: 1 mg [scored]
    Mavik®: 2 mg, 4 mg

Selected References
American Diabetes Association, "Standards of Medical Care in Diabetes Mellitus – 2009," *Diabetes Care*, 2009, 32 (Suppl 1):13-61.
Chobanian AV, Bakris GL, Black HR, et al, "The Seventh Report of the Joint National Committee on Prevention, Detection, Evaluation, and Treatment of High Blood Pressure: The JNC 7 Report," *JAMA*, 2003, 289(19):2560-71.

Trandolapril and Verapamil (tran DOE la pril & ver AP a mil)

Related Information
  Trandolapril *on page 1843*
  Verapamil *on page 1909*
  Brand Names: U.S. Tarka®
  Brand Names: Canada Tarka®

◄ **Index Terms** Verapamil and Trandolapril
Generic Availability (U.S.) Yes
Pharmacologic Category Angiotensin-Converting Enzyme (ACE) Inhibitor; Calcium Channel Blocker
Use Treatment of hypertension; however, not indicated for initial treatment of hypertension
Dosage
Geriatric Refer to dosing in individual monographs.
Adult Hypertension: Oral: Individualize dose. Patients receiving trandolapril (up to 8 mg) and verapamil (up to 240 mg) in separate tablets may wish to receive Tarka® at equivalent dosages once daily.
Renal Impairment Usual regimen need not be adjusted unless patient's creatinine clearance is <30 mL/minute. Titration of individual components must be done prior to switching to combination product
Hepatic Impairment Has not been evaluated in hepatic impairment. Verapamil is hepatically metabolized, adjustment of dosage in hepatic impairment is recommended.
Special Geriatric Considerations Combination products are not recommended as first-line treatment. Use only if doses of individual agents correspond to the combination available.
Dosage Forms Excipient information presented when available (limited, particularly for generics); consult specific product labeling.
Tablet, variable release: Trandolapril 2 mg [immediate release] and verapamil hydrochloride 180 mg [sustained release]; Trandolapril 2 mg [immediate release] and verapamil hydrochloride 240 mg [sustained release]; Trandolapril 4 mg [immediate release] and verapamil hydrochloride 240 mg [sustained release]
Tarka®:
1/240: Trandolapril 1 mg [immediate release] and verapamil hydrochloride 240 mg [sustained release]
2/180: Trandolapril 2 mg [immediate release] and verapamil hydrochloride 180 mg [sustained release]
2/240: Trandolapril 2 mg [immediate release] and verapamil hydrochloride 240 mg [sustained release]
4/240: Trandolapril 4 mg [immediate release] and verapamil hydrochloride 240 mg [sustained release]

◆ **Transamine Sulphate** *see* Tranylcypromine *on page 1846*
◆ **Transderm Scōp®** *see* Scopolamine (Systemic) *on page 1661*
◆ **Trans-Ver-Sal® [OTC]** *see* Salicylic Acid *on page 1648*
◆ **Tranxene T-Tab** *see* Clorazepate *on page 396*
◆ **Tranxene® T-Tab®** *see* Clorazepate *on page 396*

Tranylcypromine (tran il SIP roe meen)

Related Information
Antidepressant Agents *on page 1991*
Brand Names: U.S. Parnate®
Brand Names: Canada Parnate®
Index Terms Transamine Sulphate; Tranylcypromine Sulfate
Generic Availability (U.S.) No
Pharmacologic Category Antidepressant, Monoamine Oxidase Inhibitor
Use Treatment of major depressive episode without melancholia
Unlabeled/Investigational Use Treatment of post-traumatic stress disorder
Medication Guide Available Yes
Contraindications
Cardiovascular disease (including hypertension); cerebrovascular defect; history of headache; history of hepatic disease or abnormal liver function tests; pheochromocytoma
Concurrent use of antihistamines, antihypertensives, antiparkinson drugs, bupropion, buspirone, caffeine (excessive use), CNS depressants (including ethanol and narcotics), dextromethorphan, diuretics, elective surgery requiring general anesthesia (discontinue tranylcypromine ≥10 days prior to elective surgery), local vasoconstrictors, meperidine, MAO inhibitors or dibenzazepine derivatives (eg, amitriptyline, clomipramine, desipramine, imipramine, nortriptyline, protriptyline, doxepin, carbamazepine, cyclobenzaprine, amoxapine, maprotiline, trimipramine), SSRIs or SNRIs, spinal anesthesia (hypotension may be exaggerated), sympathomimetics (including amphetamines, cocaine, phenylephrine, pseudoephedrine) or related compounds (methyldopa, reserpine, levodopa, tryptophan), or foods high in tyramine content
Bupropion: At least 14 days should elapse between MAO inhibitor discontinuation and bupropion initiation.

Buspirone: At least 10 days should elapse between tranylcypromine discontinuation and buspirone initiation.

MAO inhibitors or dibenzazepine derivatives: At least 1-2 weeks should elapse between the use of another MAO inhibitor or dibenzazepine derivative and tranylcypromine use.

Meperidine: At least 2-3 weeks should elapse between MAO inhibitor discontinuation and meperidine use.

SSRIs or SNRIs: At least 2 weeks should elapse between the discontinuation of sertraline or paroxetine and the initiation of tranylcypromine. At least 5 weeks should elapse between the discontinuation of fluoxetine and the initiation of tranylcypromine. At least 1 week should elapse between discontinuation of a SNRI and the initiation of tranylcypromine. At least 2 weeks should elapse between the discontinuation of tranylcypromine and the initiation of SNRIs and SSRIs.

Warnings/Precautions Risk of suicide: [U.S. Boxed Warning]: Antidepressants increase the risk of suicidal thinking and behavior in children, adolescents, and young adults (18-24 years of age) with major depressive disorder (MDD) and other psychiatric disorders; consider risk prior to prescribing. Short-term studies did not show an increased risk in patients >24 years of age and showed a decreased risk inpatients >65 years. Closely monitor for clinical worsening, suicidality, or unusual changes in behavior such as anxiety, agitation, panic attacks, insomnia, irritability, hostility, impulsivity, akathisia, hypomania, and mania. The patient's family or caregiver should be instructed to closely observe the patient and communicate condition with healthcare provider. Such observation would generally include at least weekly face-to-face contact with patients or their family members or caregivers during the first 4 weeks of treatment, then every other week visits for the next 4 weeks, then at 12 weeks, and as clinically indicated beyond 12 weeks. Additional contact by telephone may be appropriate between face-to-face visits. A medication guide should be dispensed with each prescription. **Tranylcypromine is not FDA approved for treatment of children and adolescents.**

All patients treated with antidepressants should be observed similarly for clinical worsening and suicidality, especially during the initial few months of a course of drug therapy, or at times of dose changes, either increases or decreases. The possibility of a suicide attempt is inherent in major depression and may persist until remission occurs. Worsening depression and severe abrupt suicidality that are not part of the presenting symptoms may require discontinuation or modification of drug therapy. Use caution in high-risk patients during initiation of therapy. Prescriptions should be written for the smallest quantity consistent with good patient care.

Hypertensive crisis may occur with foods/supplements high in tyramine, tryptophan, phenyl-alanine, or tyrosine content; treatment with phentolamine is recommended for hypertensive crisis. Use with caution in patients who have glaucoma, hyperthyroidism, diabetes or hypotension. May cause orthostatic hypotension (especially at dosages >30 mg/day). Use with caution in patients at risk of seizures, or in patients receiving other drugs which may lower seizure threshold. Use with caution in patients with a history of drug abuse or acute alcoholism; potential for drug dependency exists especially in patients using excessive doses. Discontinue at least 48 hours prior to myelography. May increase the risks associated with electroconvulsive therapy. Consider discontinuing, when possible, prior to elective surgery. Use with caution in patients with renal impairment. Do not use with other MAO inhibitors or antidepressants. Avoid products containing sympathomimetic stimulants or dextromethorphan. Concurrent use with antihypertensive agents may lead to exaggeration of hypotensive effects. Tranylcypromine is not generally considered a first-line agent for the treatment of depression; tranylcypromine is typically used in patients who have failed to respond to other treatments. May worsen psychosis in some patients or precipitate a shift to mania or hypomania in patients with bipolar disorder. **Tranylcypromine is not FDA approved for the treatment of bipolar depression.**

Adverse Reactions (Reflective of adult population; not specific for elderly) Frequency not defined.

Cardiovascular: Edema, orthostatic hypotension, palpitation, tachycardia

Central nervous system: Agitation, anxiety, chills, dizziness, drowsiness, headache, insomnia, mania, restlessness

Dermatologic: Alopecia (rare), rash (rare), urticaria

Endocrine & metabolic: Sexual dysfunction (anorgasmia, ejaculatory disturbances, impotence); SIADH

Gastrointestinal: Abdominal pain, anorexia, constipation, diarrhea, nausea, xerostomia

Genitourinary: Urinary retention

Hematologic: Agranulocytosis, anemia, leukopenia, thrombocytopenia

Hepatic: Hepatitis (rare)

Neuromuscular & skeletal: Muscle spasm, myoclonus, numbness, paresthesia, tremor, weakness

◀ Ocular: Blurred vision
Otic: Tinnitus
Miscellaneous: Diaphoresis

Drug Interactions

Metabolism/Transport Effects Inhibits CYP1A2 (moderate), 2A6 (strong), 2C8 (weak), 2C9 (weak), 2C19 (moderate), 2D6 (moderate), 2E1 (weak), 3A4 (weak)

Avoid Concomitant Use

Avoid concomitant use of Tranylcypromine with any of the following: Alpha-/Beta-Agonists (Indirect-Acting); Alpha1-Agonists; Alpha2-Agonists (Ophthalmic); Amphetamines; Anilidopiperidine Opioids; Atomoxetine; Bezafibrate; Buprenorphine; BuPROPion; BusPIRone; CarBAMazepine; Clopidogrel; Cyclobenzaprine; Dexmethylphenidate; Dextromethorphan; Diethylpropion; HYDROmorphone; Linezolid; Maprotiline; Meperidine; Methyldopa; Methylene Blue; Methylphenidate; Mirtazapine; Oxymorphone; Pizotifen; Propoxyphene; Selective Serotonin Reuptake Inhibitors; Serotonin 5-HT1D Receptor Agonists; Serotonin/Norepinephrine Reuptake Inhibitors; Sibutramine; Tapentadol; Tetrabenazine; Tetrahydrozoline; Tetrahydrozoline (Nasal); Thioridazine; Tricyclic Antidepressants; Tryptophan

Increased Effect/Toxicity

Tranylcypromine may increase the levels/effects of: Alpha-/Beta-Agonists (Direct-Acting); Alpha-/Beta-Agonists (Indirect-Acting); Alpha1-Agonists; Alpha2-Agonists (Ophthalmic); Amphetamines; Anticholinergics; Antihypertensives; Atomoxetine; Beta2-Agonists; Bezafibrate; BuPROPion; CYP1A2 Substrates; CYP2A6 Substrates; CYP2C19 Substrates; CYP2D6 Substrates; Dexmethylphenidate; Dextromethorphan; Diethylpropion; Doxapram; Fesoterodine; HYDROmorphone; Linezolid; Lithium; Meperidine; Methadone; Methyldopa; Methylene Blue; Methylphenidate; Mirtazapine; Orthostatic Hypotension Producing Agents; Pizotifen; Reserpine; Selective Serotonin Reuptake Inhibitors; Serotonin 5-HT1D Receptor Agonists; Serotonin Modulators; Serotonin/Norepinephrine Reuptake Inhibitors; Tamoxifen; Tetrahydrozoline; Tetrahydrozoline (Nasal); Thioridazine; Tricyclic Antidepressants

The levels/effects of Tranylcypromine may be increased by: Altretamine; Anilidopiperidine Opioids; Buprenorphine; BusPIRone; CarBAMazepine; COMT Inhibitors; Cyclobenzaprine; Levodopa; MAO Inhibitors; Maprotiline; Oxymorphone; Pramlintide; Propoxyphene; Sibutramine; Tapentadol; Tetrabenazine; TraMADol; Tryptophan

Decreased Effect

Tranylcypromine may decrease the levels/effects of: Acetylcholinesterase Inhibitors (Central); Clopidogrel; Codeine

The levels/effects of Tranylcypromine may be decreased by: Acetylcholinesterase Inhibitors (Central)

Ethanol/Nutrition/Herb Interactions

Ethanol: May increase CNS depression; monitor for increased effects with coadministration. Caution patients about effects. Avoid beverages containing tyramine (hearty red wine and beer).

Food: Concurrent ingestion of foods rich in tyramine may cause sudden and severe high blood pressure (hypertensive crisis). Avoid tyramine-containing foods with MAO-Is.

Herb/Nutraceutical: Avoid valerian, St John's wort, SAMe, kava kava (may increase risk of serotonin syndrome and/or excessive sedation); Avoid supplements containing caffeine, tyrosine, tryptophan, or phenylalanine. Ingestion of large quantities may increase the risk of severe side effects (eg, hypertensive reactions, serotonin syndrome).

Stability Store at room temperature of 15°C to 30°C (59°F to 86°F).

Mechanism of Action Tranylcypromine is a nonhydrazine monoamine oxidase inhibitor. It increases endogenous concentrations of epinephrine, norepinephrine, dopamine, and serotonin through inhibition of the enzyme (monoamine oxidase) responsible for the breakdown of these neurotransmitters.

Pharmacodynamics/Kinetics

Onset of action: Therapeutic: 2 days to 3 weeks continued dosing

Duration: MAO inhibition may persist for up to 10 days following discontinuation

Half-life elimination: 90-190 minutes

Time to peak, serum: ~2 hours

Excretion: Urine

Dosage

Geriatric & Adult Depression: Oral: Usual effective dose: 30 mg/day in divided doses; if symptoms don't improve after 2 weeks, increase by 10 mg increments at 1- to 3-week intervals; maximum: 60 mg/day

Transitioning from another MAO inhibitor or dibenzazepine derivative (eg, TCAs, carbamazepine, cyclobenzaprine) to tranylcypromine therapy: Allow at least 1 medication-free week, then initiate tranylcypromine at 50% of usual starting dose for at least 1 week.

Administration Administer second dose before 4 PM to avoid insomnia

Monitoring Parameters Blood pressure, mental status, suicide ideation (especially at the beginning of therapy or when doses are increased or decreased)

Pharmacotherapy Pearls Has a more rapid onset of therapeutic effect than other MAO inhibitors, but causes more severe hypertensive reactions

Special Geriatric Considerations MAO inhibitors are effective and generally well tolerated by older patients. Potential interactions with tyramine- or tryptophan-containing foods, other drugs, and adverse effects on blood pressure have limited use of MAO inhibitors. They are usually reserved for patients who do not tolerate or respond to traditional "cyclic" or "second generation" antidepressants. Tranylcypromine is the preferred MAO inhibitor because its enzymatic-blocking effects are more rapidly reversed.

Dosage Forms Excipient information presented when available (limited, particularly for generics); consult specific product labeling.

Tablet, oral: 10 mg
  Parnate®: 10 mg

Selected References

Georgotas A, Friedman E, McCarthy M, et al, "Resistant Geriatric Depression and Therapeutic Response to Monoamine-Oxidase Inhibitors," *Biol Psychiatry*, 1983, 18:195-205.

Goff DC and Jenike MA, "Treatment-Resistant Depression in the Elderly," *J Am Geriatr Soc*, 1986, 34(1):63-70.

Jenike MA, "MAO Inhibitors as Treatment for Depressed Patients With Primary Degenerative Dementia (Alzheimer's Disease)," *Am J Psychiatry* 1985, 142:763.

◆ **Tranylcypromine Sulfate** *see* Tranylcypromine *on page 1846*
◆ **Trav-L-Tabs® [OTC]** *see* Meclizine *on page 1118*
◆ **Travatan® [DSC]** *see* Travoprost *on page 1849*
◆ **Travatan Z®** *see* Travoprost *on page 1849*

Travoprost (TRA voe prost)

Related Information
  Glaucoma Drug Therapy *on page 2008*

Medication Safety Issues
  Sound-alike/look-alike issues:
    Travatan® may be confused with Xalatan®

Brand Names: U.S. Travatan Z®; Travatan® [DSC]

Brand Names: Canada Travatan Z®; Travatan®

Generic Availability (U.S.) No

Pharmacologic Category Ophthalmic Agent, Antiglaucoma; Prostaglandin, Ophthalmic

Use Reduction of elevated intraocular pressure in patients with open-angle glaucoma or ocular hypertension who are intolerant of the other IOP-lowering medications or insufficiently responsive (failed to achieve target IOP determined after multiple measurements over time) to another IOP-lowering medication

Contraindications Hypersensitivity to travoprost or any component of the formulation

Warnings/Precautions May permanently change/increase brown pigmentation of the iris, the eyelid skin, and eyelashes. In addition, may increase the length and/or number of eyelashes (may vary between eyes); changes occur slowly and may not be noticeable for months or years. Bacterial keratitis, caused by inadvertent contamination of multiple-dose ophthalmic solutions, has been reported. Use caution in patients with intraocular inflammation, aphakic patients, pseudophakic patients with a torn posterior lens capsule, or patients with risk factors for macular edema. Contact with contents of vial should be avoided in women who are pregnant or attempting to become pregnant; in case of accidental exposure to the skin, wash the exposed area with soap and water immediately. Safety and efficacy have not been determined for use in patients with renal or hepatic impairment, angle-closure-, inflammatory-, or neovascular glaucoma.

Travatan®: Contains benzalkonium chloride which may be absorbed by contact lenses; remove contacts prior to administration and wait 15 minutes before reinserting.

Adverse Reactions (Reflective of adult population; not specific for elderly)
  >10%: Ocular: Hyperemia (35% to 50%)
  5% to 10%: Ocular: Decreased visual acuity, eye discomfort, foreign body sensation, pain, pruritus
  1% to 5%:
    Cardiovascular: Angina pectoris, bradycardia, hyper-/hypotension
    Central nervous system: Depression, pain, anxiety, headache
    Endocrine & metabolic: Hypercholesterolemia
    Gastrointestinal: Dyspepsia
    Genitourinary: Prostate disorder, urinary incontinence
    Neuromuscular & skeletal: Arthritis, back pain, chest pain

◀ Ocular (1% to 4%): Abnormal vision, blepharitis, blurred vision, conjunctivitis, dry eye, iris discoloration, keratitis, lid margin crusting, photophobia, subconjunctival hemorrhage, cataract, tearing, periorbital skin discoloration (darkening), eyelash darkening, eyelash growth increased

Respiratory: Bronchitis, sinusitis

Drug Interactions

Avoid Concomitant Use There are no known interactions where it is recommended to avoid concomitant use.

Increased Effect/Toxicity There are no known significant interactions involving an increase in effect.

Decreased Effect There are no known significant interactions involving a decrease in effect.

Stability Store between 2°C to 25°C (36°F to 77°F).

Mechanism of Action A selective FP prostanoid receptor agonist which lowers intraocular pressure by increasing trabecular meshwork and outflow

Pharmacodynamics/Kinetics

Onset of action: ~2 hours

Peak effect: 12 hours

Duration: Plasma levels decrease to <10 pg/mL within 1 hour

Absorption: Absorbed via cornea

Metabolism: Hydrolyzed by esterases in the cornea to active free acid; systemically; the free acid is metabolized to inactive metabolites

Dosage

Geriatric & Adult Glaucoma (open angle) or ocular hypertension: Ophthalmic: Instill 1 drop into affected eye(s) once daily in the evening; do not exceed once-daily dosing (may decrease IOP-lowering effect). If used with other topical ophthalmic agents, separate administration by at least 5 minutes.

Administration May be used with other eye drops to lower intraocular pressure. If using more than one ophthalmic product, wait at least 5 minutes in between application of each medication. Travatan®: Remove contact lenses prior to administration and wait 15 minutes before reinserting.

Pharmacotherapy Pearls The IOP-lowering effect was shown to be 7-8 mm Hg in clinical studies. The mean IOP reduction in African-American patients was up to 1.8 mm Hg greater than in non-African-American patients. The reason for this effect is unknown.

Healthcare professionals who are pregnant (or attempting to become pregnant) and accidentally come into contact with the solution, should wash skin with soap and water immediately.

Available in Canada in combination with timolol as DuoTrav™.

Special Geriatric Considerations Evaluate the patient's or caregiver's ability to safely administer the correct dose of ophthalmic medication.

Dosage Forms Excipient information presented when available (limited, particularly for generics); consult specific product labeling. [DSC] = Discontinued product

Solution, ophthalmic [drops]:

Travatan Z®: 0.004% (2.5 mL, 5 mL)

Travatan®: 0.004% (2.5 mL [DSC], 5 mL [DSC]) [contains benzalkonium chloride]

TraZODone (TRAZ oh done)

Related Information

Antidepressant Agents on page 1991

Medication Safety Issues

Sound-alike/look-alike issues:

Desyrel may be confused with Demerol®, Delsym®, Zestril®

TraZODone may be confused with traMADol, ziprasidone

International issues:

Desyrel [Canada, Turkey] may be confused with Deseril brand name for methysergide [Australia, Belgium, Great Britain, Netherlands]

Brand Names: U.S. Oleptro™

Brand Names: Canada Apo-Trazodone D®; Apo-Trazodone®; Dom-Trazodone; Mylan-Trazodone; Novo-Trazodone; Nu-Trazodone; Nu-Trazodone D; Oleptro™; PHL-Trazodone; PMS-Trazodone; ratio-Trazodone; Teva-Trazodone; Trazorel®; ZYM-Trazodone

Index Terms Desyrel; Trazodone Hydrochloride

Generic Availability (U.S.) Yes: Excludes extended release tablet

Pharmacologic Category Antidepressant, Serotonin Reuptake Inhibitor/Antagonist

Use Treatment of major depressive disorder

Unlabeled/Investigational Use Potential augmenting agent for antidepressants, hypnotic

Medication Guide Available Yes

Contraindications Hypersensitivity to trazodone or any component of the formulation

Warnings/Precautions [U.S. Boxed Warning]: Antidepressants increase the risk of suicidal thinking and behavior in children, adolescents, and young adults (18-24 years of age) with major depressive disorder (MDD) and other psychiatric disorders; consider risk prior to prescribing. Short-term studies did not show an increased risk in patients >24 years of age and showed a decreased risk in patients ≥65 years of age. Closely monitor for clinical worsening, suicidality, or unusual changes in behavior; the patient's family or caregiver should be instructed to closely observe the patient and communicate condition with healthcare provider. A medication guide should be dispensed with each prescription. **Trazodone is not FDA approved for use in children.**

The possibility of a suicide attempt is inherent in major depression and may persist until remission occurs. Monitor for worsening of depression or suicidality, especially during initiation of therapy (generally first 1-2 months) or with dose increases or decreases. Use caution in high-risk patients. Worsening depression and severe abrupt suicidality that are not part of the presenting symptoms may require discontinuation or modification of drug therapy. The patient's family or caregiver should be alerted to monitor patients for the emergence of suicidality and associated behaviors (such as agitation, irritability, hostility, impulsivity, and hypomania) and call healthcare provider.

May worsen psychosis in some patients or precipitate a shift to mania or hypomania in patients with bipolar disorder. Patients presenting with depressive symptoms should be screened for bipolar disorder. Monotherapy in patients with bipolar disorder should be avoided. **Trazodone is not FDA approved for the treatment of bipolar depression.**

Priapism, including cases resulting in permanent dysfunction, has occurred with the use of trazodone. Instruct patient to seek medical assistance for erection lasting >4 hours; use with caution in patients who have conditions which may predispose them to priapism (eg, sickle cell anemia, multiple myeloma, leukemia). Not recommended for use in a patient during the acute recovery phase of MI. The risks of sedation, postural hypotension, and/or syncope are high relative to other antidepressants. Trazodone frequently causes sedation, which may result in impaired performance of tasks requiring alertness (eg, operating machinery or driving). Sedative effects may be additive with other CNS depressants and ethanol.

Use with caution in patients with a history of cardiovascular disease (including previous MI, stroke, tachycardia, or conduction abnormalities). Although the risk of conduction abnormalities with this agent is low relative to other antidepressants, QT prolongation (with or without torsade de pointes), ventricular tachycardia, and other arrhythmias have been observed with the use of trazodone (reports limited to immediate-release formulation); use with caution in patients with pre-existing cardiac disease. Concurrent use of CYP3A4 inhibitors may increase the risk of QT prolongation and/or proarrhythmia. Concurrent use with other drugs known to prolong QT_c interval is not recommended. May impair platelet aggregation resulting in increased risk of bleeding events (eg, epistaxis, life threatening bleeding), particularly if used concomitantly with aspirin, NSAIDs, warfarin or other anticoagulants. Trazodone should be initiated with caution in patients who are receiving concurrent or recent therapy with a MAO inhibitor. Oleptro™: Avoid use in combination with or within 14 days of an MAO inhibitor.

Serotonin syndrome (SS)/neuroleptic malignant syndrome (NMS)-like reactions may occur with trazodone when used alone, particularly if used with other serotonergic agents (eg, serotonin/norepinephrine reuptake inhibitors [SNRIs], selective serotonin reuptake inhibitors [SSRIs], or triptans), drugs that impair serotonin metabolism (eg, MAO inhibitors), or antidopaminergic agents (eg, antipsychotics). If concurrent use is clinically warranted, carefully observe patient during treatment initiation and dose increases. Do not use concurrently with serotonin precursors (eg, tryptophan).

May cause SIADH and hyponatremia, predominantly in the elderly; volume depletion and/or concurrent use of diuretics likely increases risk. Use with caution in patients taking antihypertensives; may increase the risk of hypotension or syncope. Use with caution in patients taking strong CYP3A4 inhibitors and moderate or strong CYP3A4 inducers; monitor or consider alternative agents that avoid or lessen the potential for CYP-mediated interactions.

Therapy should not be abruptly discontinued in patients receiving high doses for prolonged periods; gradually reduce dosage prior to complete discontinuation to avoid withdrawal symptoms (eg, anxiety, agitation, sleep disturbance). Use caution in patients with a previous seizure disorder or condition predisposing to seizures such as brain damage, alcoholism, or concurrent therapy with other drugs which lower the seizure threshold. Use with caution in patients with hepatic or renal dysfunction and in elderly patients.

◀ **Adverse Reactions (Reflective of adult population; not specific for elderly)**
>10%:
Central nervous system: Sedation (≤46%), headache (10% to 33%), dizziness (20% to 28%), fatigue (6% to 15%)
Gastrointestinal: Xerostomia (15% to 34%), nausea (10% to 21%)
Ocular: Blurred vision (5% to 15%)
1% to 10%:
Cardiovascular: Edema (3% to 7%), hypotension (≤7%), syncope (≤5%), hypertension (1% to 2%)
Central nervous system: Confusion (5% to 6%), incoordination (2% to 5%), concentration decreased (1% to 3%), disorientation (≤2%), memory impairment (≤1%), agitation, migraine
Endocrine & metabolic: Libido decreased (1% to 2%)
Gastrointestinal: Diarrhea (5% to 9%), constipation (7% to 8%), abdominal pain, abnormal taste, flatulence, vomiting, weight gain/loss
Genitourinary: Ejaculation disorder (2%), urinary urgency
Neuromuscular & skeletal: Back pain (≤5%), tremor (1% to 5%), paresthesia (≤1%), myalgia
Ocular: Visual disturbance
Respiratory: Nasal congestion (3% to 6%), dyspnea
Miscellaneous: Night sweats

Drug Interactions
Metabolism/Transport Effects Substrate of CYP2D6 (minor), 3A4 (major); **Inhibits** CYP3A4 (weak); **Induces** P-glycoprotein
Avoid Concomitant Use
Avoid concomitant use of TraZODone with any of the following: Conivaptan; Dabigatran Etexilate; Methylene Blue; Saquinavir; Sibutramine
Increased Effect/Toxicity
TraZODone may increase the levels/effects of: Methylene Blue; Serotonin Modulators

The levels/effects of TraZODone may be increased by: BusPIRone; Conivaptan; CYP3A4 Inhibitors (Moderate); CYP3A4 Inhibitors (Strong); Dasatinib; MAO Inhibitors; Protease Inhibitors; Saquinavir; Selective Serotonin Reuptake Inhibitors; Sibutramine; Telaprevir; Venlafaxine
Decreased Effect
TraZODone may decrease the levels/effects of: Dabigatran Etexilate; Linagliptin; P-Glycoprotein Substrates

The levels/effects of TraZODone may be decreased by: CYP3A4 Inducers (Strong); Deferasirox; Peginterferon Alfa-2b; Tocilizumab
Ethanol/Nutrition/Herb Interactions
Ethanol: May increase CNS depression; monitor for increased effects with coadministration. Caution patients about effects.
Food: Time to peak serum levels may be increased if immediate release trazodone is taken with food.
Herb/Nutraceutical: Avoid valerian, St John's wort, SAMe, kava kava (may increase risk of serotonin syndrome and/or excessive sedation).
Stability
Immediate release tablet: Store at room temperature; avoid temperatures >40°C (>104°F). Protect from light.
Extended release tablet: Store at room temperature of 15°C to 30°C (59°F to 86°F). Protect from light.
Mechanism of Action Inhibits reuptake of serotonin, causes adrenoreceptor subsensivity, and induces significant changes in 5-HT presynaptic receptor adrenoreceptors. Trazodone also significantly blocks histamine (H_1) and alpha$_1$-adrenergic receptors.
Pharmacodynamics/Kinetics
Onset of action: Therapeutic (antidepressant): Up to 6 weeks; sleep aid: 1-3 hours
Absorption: Well absorbed; Extended release: C_{max} increases ~86% when taken shortly after ingestion of a high-fat meal compared to fasting conditions
Protein binding: 85% to 95%
Metabolism: Hepatic via CYP3A4 (extensive) to an active metabolite (mCPP)
Half-life elimination: 7-10 hours
Time to peak, serum:
Immediate release: 30-100 minutes; delayed with food (up to 2.5 hours)
Extended release: 9 hours; not significantly affected by food
Excretion: Primarily urine (<1% excreted unchanged); secondarily feces

Dosage
Geriatric
Immediate release: Oral: 25-50 mg at bedtime with 25-50 mg/day dose increase every 3 days for inpatients and weekly for outpatients, if tolerated; usual dose: 75-150 mg/day
Extended release: Refer to adult dosing. Use with caution in the elderly; clinical experience is limited.

Adult
Depression: Oral: Initial: 150 mg/day in 3 divided doses (may increase by 50 mg/day every 3-7 days); maximum dose: 600 mg/day

Extended release formulation: Initial: 150 mg once daily at bedtime (may increase by 75 mg/day every 3 days); maximum dose: 375 mg/day; once adequate response obtained, gradually reduce with adjustment based on therapeutic response

Note: Therapeutic effects may take up to 6 weeks. Therapy is normally maintained for 6-12 months after optimum response is reached to prevent recurrence of depression.

Sedation/hypnotic (unlabeled use): Oral: 25-50 mg at bedtime (often in combination with daytime SSRIs). May increase up to 200 mg at bedtime.

Administration
Immediate release tablet: Dosing after meals may decrease lightheadedness and postural hypotension

Extended release tablet: Take on an empty stomach; swallow whole or as a half tablet without food. Tablet may be broken along the score line, but do not crush or chew.

Monitoring Parameters Suicide ideation (especially at the beginning of therapy or when doses are increased or decreased)

Reference Range
Plasma levels do not always correlate with clinical effectiveness
Therapeutic: 0.5-2.5 mcg/mL
Potentially toxic: >2.5 mcg/mL
Toxic: >4 mcg/mL

Test Interactions May interfere with urine detection of amphetamine/methamphetamine (false-positive).

Special Geriatric Considerations Very sedating, but little anticholinergic effects.

Dosage Forms Excipient information presented when available (limited, particularly for generics); consult specific product labeling.
Tablet, oral, as hydrochloride: 50 mg, 100 mg, 150 mg, 300 mg
Tablet, extended release, oral, as hydrochloride:
Oleptro™: 150 mg, 300 mg [scored]

Selected References
Bayer AJ, Pathy MS, and Ankier SI, "Pharmacokinetic and Pharmacodynamic Characteristics of Trazodone in the Elderly," *Br J Clin Pharmacol*, 1983, 16(4):371-6.

Triamcinolone (Systemic) (trye am SIN oh lone)

Related Information
Asthma on page 2016
Corticosteroids on page 2005
Inhalant Agents on page 2010
Medication Safety Issues
Sound-alike/look-alike issues:
Kenalog® may be confused with Ketalar®
Other safety concerns:
TAC (occasional abbreviation for triamcinolone) is an error-prone abbreviation (mistaken as tetracaine-adrenaline-cocaine)

Brand Names: U.S. Aristospan®; Kenalog®-10; Kenalog®-40
Brand Names: Canada Aristospan®
Index Terms Triamcinolone Acetonide, Parenteral; Triamcinolone Hexacetonide
Generic Availability (U.S.) No
Pharmacologic Category Corticosteroid, Systemic

◀ **Use**

Intra-articular (soft tissue): Acute gouty arthritis, acute/subacute bursitis, acute tenosynovitis, epicondylitis, rheumatoid arthritis, synovitis of osteoarthritis

Intralesional: Alopecia areata, discoid lupus erythematosus, keloids, granuloma annulare lesions (localized hypertrophic, infiltrated, or inflammatory), lichen planus plaques, lichen simplex chronicus plaques, psoriatic plaques, necrobiosis lipoidica diabeticorum, cystic tumors of aponeurosis or tendon (ganglia)

Systemic: Adrenocortical insufficiency, dermatologic diseases, endocrine disorders, gastrointestinal diseases, hematologic and neoplastic disorders, nervous system disorders, nephrotic syndrome, rheumatic disorders, allergic states, respiratory diseases, systemic lupus erythematosus (SLE), and other diseases requiring anti-inflammatory or immunosuppressive effects

Contraindications Hypersensitivity to triamcinolone or any component of the formulation; systemic fungal infections; cerebral malaria; idiopathic thrombocytopenic purpura (I.M. injection)

Warnings/Precautions May cause hypercorticism or suppression of hypothalamic-pituitary-adrenal (HPA) axis, particularly in patients receiving high doses for prolonged periods. HPA axis suppression may lead to adrenal crisis. Withdrawal and discontinuation of a corticosteroid should be done slowly and carefully. Particular care is required when patients are transferred from systemic corticosteroids to inhaled products due to possible adrenal insufficiency or withdrawal from steroids, including an increase in allergic symptoms. Patients receiving >20 mg per day of prednisone (or equivalent) may be most susceptible. Fatalities have occurred due to adrenal insufficiency in asthmatic patients during and after transfer from systemic corticosteroids to aerosol steroids; aerosol steroids do not provide the systemic steroid needed to treat patients having trauma, surgery, or infections.

Bronchospasm may occur with wheezing after inhalation; if this occurs, stop steroid and treat with a fast-acting bronchodilator (eg, albuterol). Supplemental steroids (oral or parenteral) may be needed during stress or severe asthma attacks. Not to be used in status asthmaticus or for the relief of acute bronchospasm. Acute myopathy has been reported with high-dose corticosteroids, usually in patients with neuromuscular transmission disorders; may involve ocular and/or respiratory muscles; monitor creatine kinase; recovery may be delayed. Corticosteroid use may cause psychiatric disturbances, including depression, euphoria, insomnia, mood swings, and personality changes. Pre-existing psychiatric conditions may be exacerbated by corticosteroid use. Prolonged use of corticosteroids may also increase the incidence of secondary infection, mask acute infection (including fungal infections), prolong or exacerbate viral infections, or limit response to vaccines. Exposure to chickenpox should be avoided; corticosteroids should not be used to treat ocular herpes simplex. Corticosteroids should not be used for cerebral malaria or viral hepatitis. Close observation is required in patients with latent tuberculosis and/or TB reactivity; restrict use in active TB (only in conjunction with antituberculosis treatment). Use with caution in patients with threadworm infection; may cause serious hyperinfection. Prolonged treatment with corticosteroids has been associated with the development of Kaposi's sarcoma (case reports); if noted, discontinuation of therapy should be considered. Avoid use in head injury patients.

Use with caution in patients with thyroid disease, hepatic impairment, renal impairment, cardiovascular disease, diabetes, myasthenia gravis, patients at risk for osteoporosis, patients at risk for seizures, or GI diseases (diverticulitis, peptic ulcer, ulcerative colitis) due to perforation risk. Avoid use in head injury patients. Use caution following acute MI (corticosteroids have been associated with myocardial rupture). Because of the risk of adverse effects, systemic corticosteroids should be used cautiously in the elderly in the smallest possible effective dose for the shortest duration. Azmacort® (metered dose inhaler) comes with its own spacer device attached and may be easier to use in older patients. Patients should not be immunized with live, viral vaccines while receiving immunosuppressive doses of corticosteroids. The ability to respond to dead viral vaccines is unknown.

Adverse Reactions (Reflective of adult population; not specific for elderly) Frequency not defined; reactions reported with corticosteroid therapy in general:

Cardiovascular: Arrhythmia, bradycardia, cardiac arrest, cardiac enlargement, CHF, circulatory collapse, edema, hypertension, hypertrophic cardiomyopathy (premature infants), myocardial rupture (following recent MI), syncope, tachycardia, thromboembolism, vasculitis

Central nervous system: Arachnoiditis (I.T.), depression, emotional instability, euphoria, headache, insomnia, intracranial pressure increased, malaise, meningitis (I.T.), mood changes, neuritis, neuropathy, personality change, pseudotumor cerebri (with discontinuation), seizure, vertigo

Dermatologic: Abscess (sterile), acne, allergic dermatitis, angioedema, atrophy (cutaneous/subcutaneous), bruising, dry skin, erythema, hair thinning, hirsutism, hyper-/hypopigmentation, hypertrichosis, impaired wound healing, lupus erythematosus-like lesions, petechiae, purpura, rash, skin test suppression, striae, thin skin

Endocrine & metabolic: Carbohydrate intolerance, Cushingoid state, diabetes mellitus, fluid retention, glucose intolerance, growth suppression (children), hypokalemia, hypokalemic alkalosis, menstrual irregularities, negative nitrogen balance, sodium retention, sperm motility altered

Gastrointestinal: Abdominal distention, appetite increased, GI hemorrhage, GI perforation, nausea, pancreatitis, peptic ulcer, ulcerative esophagitis, weight gain

Hepatic: Hepatomegaly, liver function tests increased

Local: Thrombophlebitis

Neuromuscular & skeletal: Aseptic necrosis of femoral and humeral heads, calcinosis, Charcot-like arthropathy, fractures, joint tissue damage, muscle mass loss, myopathy, osteoporosis, parasthesia, tendon rupture, vertebral compression fractures, weakness

Ocular: Cataracts, exophthalmos, glaucoma, ocular pressure increased, papilledema

Renal: Glycosuria

Respiratory: Pulmonary edema

Miscellaneous: Abnormal fat deposits, anaphylactoid reaction, anaphylaxis, diaphoresis, hiccups, infection, moon face

Drug Interactions

Avoid Concomitant Use

Avoid concomitant use of Triamcinolone (Systemic) with any of the following: Aldesleukin; BCG; Natalizumab; Pimecrolimus; Tacrolimus (Topical)

Increased Effect/Toxicity

Triamcinolone (Systemic) may increase the levels/effects of: Acetylcholinesterase Inhibitors; Amphotericin B; Deferasirox; Leflunomide; Loop Diuretics; Natalizumab; NSAID (COX-2 Inhibitor); NSAID (Nonselective); Thiazide Diuretics; Vaccines (Live); Warfarin

The levels/effects of Triamcinolone (Systemic) may be increased by: Antifungal Agents (Azole Derivatives, Systemic); Aprepitant; Calcium Channel Blockers (Nondihydropyridine); Denosumab; Estrogen Derivatives; Fluconazole; Fosaprepitant; Macrolide Antibiotics; Neuromuscular-Blocking Agents (Nondepolarizing); Pimecrolimus; Quinolone Antibiotics; Roflumilast; Salicylates; Tacrolimus (Topical); Telaprevir; Trastuzumab

Decreased Effect

Triamcinolone (Systemic) may decrease the levels/effects of: Aldesleukin; Antidiabetic Agents; BCG; Calcitriol; Corticorelin; Isoniazid; Salicylates; Sipuleucel-T; Telaprevir; Vaccines (Inactivated)

The levels/effects of Triamcinolone (Systemic) may be decreased by: Aminoglutethimide; Barbiturates; Echinacea; Mitotane; Primidone; Rifamycin Derivatives

Stability Injection, suspension:

Acetonide injectable suspension: Kenalog®: Store at 20°C to 25°C (68°F to 77°F); avoid freezing. Protect from light.

Hexacetonide injectable suspension: Store at 20°C to 25°C (68°F to 77°F); avoid freezing. Protect from light. Avoid diluents containing parabens, phenol, or other preservatives (may cause flocculation). Diluted suspension stable up to 1 week. Suspension for intralesional use may be diluted with D_5NS, $D_{10}NS$, NS, or SWFI to a 1:1, 1:2, or 1:4 concentration. Solutions for intra-articular use, may be diluted with lidocaine 1% or 2%.

Mechanism of Action Decreases inflammation by suppression of migration of polymorphonuclear leukocytes and reversal of increased capillary permeability; suppresses the immune system by reducing activity and volume of the lymphatic system; suppresses adrenal function at high doses

Pharmacodynamics/Kinetics

Distribution: V_d: 99.5 L

Protein binding: ~68%

Half-life elimination: Biologic: 18-36 hours

Time to peak: I.M.: 8-10 hours

Excretion: Urine (~40%); feces (~60%)

Dosage

Geriatric & Adult The lowest possible dose should be used to control the condition; when dose reduction is possible, the dose should be reduced gradually.

Dermatoses (steroid-responsive, including contact/atopic dermatitis): Injection:

Acetonide: Intradermal: Initial: 1 mg

Hexacetonide: Intralesional, sublesional: Up to 0.5 mg/square inch of affected skin; range: 2-48 mg/day

Hay fever/pollen asthma: I.M.: 40-100 mg as a single injection/season

Multiple sclerosis (acute exacerbation): I.M.: 160 mg daily for 1 week, followed by 64 mg every other day for 1 month

Rheumatic or arthritic disorders:
Intra-articular (or similar injection as designated):
Acetonide: Intra-articular, intrabursal, tendon sheaths: Initial: Smaller joints: 2.5-5 mg, larger joints: 5-15 mg; may require up to 10 mg for small joints and up to 40 mg for large joints; maximum dose/treatment (several joints at one time): 20-80 mg
Hexacetonide: Intra-articular: Average dose: 2-20 mg; smaller joints: 2-6 mg; larger joints: 10-20 mg. Frequency of injection into a single joint is every 3-4 weeks as necessary; to avoid possible joint destruction use as infrequently as possible.
I.M.: Acetonide: Range: 2.5-100 mg/day; Initial: 60 mg
See table.

Triamcinolone Dosing

	Acetonide	Hexacetonide
Intrasynovial	5-40 mg	
Intralesional	1-30 mg (usually 1 mg per injection site); 10 mg/mL suspension usually used	Up to 0.5 mg/sq inch affected area
Sublesional	1-30 mg	
Systemic I.M.	2.5-60 mg/dose (usual adult dose: 60 mg; may repeat with 20-100 mg dose when symptoms recur)	
Intra-articular	2.5-40 mg	2-20 mg average
large joints	5-15 mg	10-20 mg
small joints	2.5-5 mg	2-6 mg
Tendon sheaths	2.5-10 mg	
Intradermal	1 mg/site	

Administration Injection: Shake well prior to use. Avoid injecting into a previously infected joint; do not inject into unstable joints
I.M.: Inject deep in large muscle mass, avoid deltoid.
SubQ: Avoid subcutaneous administration.
Pharmacotherapy Pearls No geriatric-specific information.
Special Geriatric Considerations Because of the risk of adverse effects, corticosteroids should be used cautiously in the elderly, in the smallest possible dose, and for the shortest possible time.
Dosage Forms Excipient information presented when available (limited, particularly for generics); consult specific product labeling.
Injection, suspension, as acetonide:
Kenalog®-10: 10 mg/mL (5 mL) [contains benzyl alcohol, polysorbate 80; not for I.V. or I.M. use]
Kenalog®-40: 40 mg/mL (1 mL, 5 mL, 10 mL) [contains benzyl alcohol, polysorbate 80; not for I.V. or intradermal use]
Injection, suspension, as hexacetonide:
Aristospan®: 5 mg/mL (5 mL); 20 mg/mL (1 mL, 5 mL) [contains benzyl alcohol, polysorbate 80; not for I.V. use]
Selected References
McGee S and Hirschmann J, "Use of Corticosteroids in Treating Infectious Diseases," *Arch Intern Med*, 2008, 168 (10):1034-46.

Triamcinolone (Nasal) (trye am SIN oh lone)

Medication Safety Issues
Sound-alike/look-alike issues:
Nasacort® may be confused with NasalCrom®
Other safety concerns:
TAC (occasional abbreviation for triamcinolone) is an error-prone abbreviation (mistaken as tetracaine-adrenaline-cocaine)
Brand Names: U.S. Nasacort® AQ
Brand Names: Canada Nasacort® AQ; Trinasal®
Index Terms Triamcinolone acetonide

Generic Availability (U.S.) Yes
Pharmacologic Category Corticosteroid, Nasal
Use Management of seasonal and perennial allergic rhinitis
Dosage
Geriatric & Adult Allergic rhinitis (perennial or seasonal):
Nasal spray: 220 mcg/day as 2 sprays in each nostril once daily; once symptoms controlled reduce to 110 mcg/day
Nasal inhaler: Initial: 220 mcg/day as 2 sprays in each nostril once daily; may increase dose to 440 mcg/day (given once daily or divided and given 2 or 4 times/day)
Dosage Forms Excipient information presented when available (limited, particularly for generics); consult specific product labeling.
Suspension, intranasal, as acetonide [spray]: 55 mcg/inhalation (16.5 g)
Nasacort® AQ: 55 mcg/inhalation (16.5 g) [chlorofluorocarbon free; contains benzalkonium chloride; 120 actuations]

Triamcinolone (Ophthalmic) (trye am SIN oh lone)

Related Information
Corticosteroids *on page 2005*
Medication Safety Issues
Other safety concerns:
TAC (occasional abbreviation for triamcinolone) is an error-prone abbreviation (mistaken as tetracaine-adrenaline-cocaine)
Brand Names: U.S. Triesence™
Index Terms Triamcinolone acetonide
Generic Availability (U.S.) No
Pharmacologic Category Corticosteroid, Ophthalmic
Use
Intravitreal: Treatment of sympathetic ophthalmia, temporal arteritis, uveitis, ocular inflammatory conditions unresponsive to topical corticosteroids
Triesence™: Visualization during vitrectomy
Dosage
Geriatric & Adult
Ocular disease: Intravitreal: Initial: 4 mg as a single dose; additional doses may be given as needed
Visualization during vitrectomy: Intravitreal (Triesence™): 1-4 mg
Dosage Forms Excipient information presented when available (limited, particularly for generics); consult specific product labeling.
Injection, suspension, ophthalmic, as acetonide:
Triesence™: 40 mg/mL (1 mL) [contains polysorbate 80; not for I.V. use]

Triamcinolone (Topical) (trye am SIN oh lone)

Related Information
Corticosteroids *on page 2005*
Medication Safety Issues
Sound-alike/look-alike issues:
Kenalog® may be confused with Ketalar®
Other safety concerns:
TAC (occasional abbreviation for triamcinolone) is an error-prone abbreviation (mistaken as tetracaine-adrenaline-cocaine)
Brand Names: U.S. Kenalog®; Oralone®; Pediaderm™ TA; Trianex™; Triderm®; Zytopic™
Brand Names: Canada Kenalog®; Oracort; Triaderm
Generic Availability (U.S.) Yes: Excludes aerosol
Pharmacologic Category Corticosteroid, Topical
Use
Oral topical: Adjunctive treatment and temporary relief of symptoms associated with oral inflammatory lesions and ulcerative lesions resulting from trauma
Topical: Inflammatory dermatoses responsive to steroids
Dosage
Geriatric & Adult
Dermatoses (steroid-responsive, including contact/atopic dermatitis): Topical:
Cream, Ointment:
0.025%: Apply thin film to affected areas 2-4 times/day
0.1% or 0.5%: Apply thin film to affected areas 2-3 times/day

Spray: Apply to affected area 3-4 times/day

Oral inflammatory lesions/ulcers: Oral topical: Press a small dab (about $^1/_4$ inch) to the lesion until a thin film develops; a larger quantity may be required for coverage of some lesions. For optimal results, use only enough to coat the lesion with a thin film; do not rub in.

Dosage Forms Excipient information presented when available (limited, particularly for generics); consult specific product labeling.

Aerosol, topical, as acetonide:
Kenalog®: 0.2 mg/2-second spray (63 g) [contains dehydrated ethanol 10.3%]

Cream, topical, as acetonide: 0.025% (15 g, 80 g, 454 g); 0.1% (15 g, 30 g, 80 g, 454 g); 0.5% (15 g)
Triderm®: 0.1% (30 g, 85 g)

Cream, topical, as acetonide [kit]:
Pediaderm™ TA: 0.1% (30 g) [packaged with protective emollient]
Zytopic™: 0.1% (85 g) [packaged with cleanser and moisturizer]

Lotion, topical, as acetonide: 0.025% (60 mL); 0.1% (60 mL)

Ointment, topical, as acetonide: 0.025% (15 g, 80 g, 454 g); 0.05% (430 g); 0.1% (15 g, 80 g, 454 g); 0.5% (15 g)
Trianex™: 0.05% (17 g, 85 g)

Paste, oral topical, as acetonide: 0.1% (5 g)
Oralone®: 0.1% (5 g)

◆ **Triamcinolone acetonide** *see* Triamcinolone (Nasal) *on page 1856*
◆ **Triamcinolone acetonide** *see* Triamcinolone (Ophthalmic) *on page 1857*
◆ **Triamcinolone Acetonide, Parenteral** *see* Triamcinolone (Systemic) *on page 1853*
◆ **Triamcinolone and Nystatin** *see* Nystatin and Triamcinolone *on page 1324*
◆ **Triamcinolone Hexacetonide** *see* Triamcinolone (Systemic) *on page 1853*
◆ **Triaminic® Children's Cough Long Acting [OTC]** *see* Dextromethorphan *on page 490*
◆ **Triaminic™ Children's Fever Reducer Pain Reliever [OTC]** *see* Acetaminophen *on page 33*
◆ **Triaminic Thin Strips® Children's Cold with Stuffy Nose [OTC]** *see* Phenylephrine (Systemic) *on page 1440*
◆ **Triaminic Thin Strips® Children's Cough & Runny Nose [OTC]** *see* DiphenhydrAMINE (Systemic) *on page 520*
◆ **Triaminic Thin Strips® Children's Long Acting Cough [OTC]** *see* Dextromethorphan *on page 490*

Triamterene (trye AM ter een)

Medication Safety Issues
Sound-alike/look-alike issues:
Triamterene may be confused with trimipramine
Dyrenium® may be confused with Pyridium®
Brand Names: U.S. Dyrenium®
Generic Availability (U.S.) No
Pharmacologic Category Diuretic, Potassium-Sparing
Use Alone or in combination with other diuretics in treatment of edema and hypertension; decreases potassium excretion caused by kaliuretic diuretics
Contraindications Hypersensitivity to triamterene or any component of the formulation; patients receiving other potassium-sparing diuretics; anuria; severe hepatic disease; hyperkalemia or history of hyperkalemia; severe or progressive renal disease
Warnings/Precautions [U.S. Boxed Warning]: Hyperkalemia can occur; patients at risk include those with renal impairment, diabetes, the elderly, and the severely ill. Serum potassium levels must be monitored at frequent intervals especially when dosages are changed or with any illness that may cause renal dysfunction. Avoid potassium supplements, potassium-containing salt substitutes, a diet rich in potassium, or other drugs that can cause hyperkalemia. Monitor for fluid and electrolyte imbalances. Diuretic therapy should be carefully used in severe hepatic dysfunction; electrolyte and fluid shifts can cause or exacerbate encephalopathy. Use cautiously in patients with history of kidney stones and diabetes. Can cause photosensitivity.
Adverse Reactions (Reflective of adult population; not specific for elderly)
1% to 10%:
Cardiovascular: Hypotension, edema, CHF, bradycardia
Central nervous system: Dizziness, headache, fatigue
Gastrointestinal: Constipation, nausea
Respiratory: Dyspnea

Drug Interactions

Avoid Concomitant Use

Avoid concomitant use of Triamterene with any of the following: Tacrolimus

Increased Effect/Toxicity

Triamterene may increase the levels/effects of: ACE Inhibitors; Amifostine; Ammonium Chloride; Antihypertensives; Cardiac Glycosides; Dofetilide; Hypotensive Agents; RiTUXimab; Sodium Phosphates; Tacrolimus

The levels/effects of Triamterene may be increased by: Alfuzosin; Angiotensin II Receptor Blockers; Diazoxide; Drospirenone; Eplerenone; Herbs (Hypotensive Properties); Indomethacin; MAO Inhibitors; Nonsteroidal Anti-Inflammatory Agents; Pentoxifylline; Phosphodiesterase 5 Inhibitors; Potassium Salts; Prostacyclin Analogues; Tolvaptan

Decreased Effect

Triamterene may decrease the levels/effects of: Cardiac Glycosides; QuiNIDine

The levels/effects of Triamterene may be decreased by: Herbs (Hypertensive Properties); Methylphenidate; Nonsteroidal Anti-Inflammatory Agents; Yohimbine

Mechanism of Action Blocks epithelial sodium channels in the late distal convoluted tubule (DCT) and collecting duct which inhibits sodium reabsorption from the lumen. This effectively reduces intracellular sodium, decreasing the function of Na+/K+ ATPase, leading to potassium retention and decreased calcium, magnesium, and hydrogen excretion. As sodium uptake capacity in the DCT/collecting duct is limited, the natriuretic, diuretic, and antihypertensive effects are generally considered weak.

Pharmacodynamics/Kinetics

Onset of action: Diuresis: 2-4 hours

Duration: 7-9 hours

Absorption: Unreliable

Dosage

Geriatric Refer to adult dosing. In the management of hypertension, consider lower initial doses and titrate to response (Aronow, 2011).

Adult Edema, hypertension: Oral: 100-300 mg/day in 1-2 divided doses; maximum dose: 300 mg/day; usual dosage range (JNC 7): 50-100 mg/day

Renal Impairment Cl_{cr} <10 mL/minute: Avoid use.

Hepatic Impairment Dose reduction is recommended in patients with cirrhosis.

Administration May be administered with food.

Monitoring Parameters Blood pressure, serum electrolytes (especially potassium), renal function, weight, I & O

Test Interactions Interferes with fluorometric assay of quinidine

Special Geriatric Considerations Monitor serum potassium.

Dosage Forms Excipient information presented when available (limited, particularly for generics); consult specific product labeling.

Capsule, oral:

Dyrenium®: 50 mg, 100 mg

◆ **Triamterene and Hydrochlorothiazide** *see* Hydrochlorothiazide and Triamterene *on page 879*

◆ **Trianex™** *see* Triamcinolone (Topical) *on page 1857*

Triazolam (trye AY zoe lam)

Related Information

Anxiolytic, Sedative / Hypnotic, and Miscellaneous Benzodiazepines *on page 2000*

Beers Criteria − Potentially Inappropriate Medications for Geriatrics *on page 2089*

Medication Safety Issues

Sound-alike/look-alike issues:

Triazolam may be confused with alPRAZolam

Halcion® may be confused with halcinonide, Haldol®

BEERS Criteria medication:

This drug may be inappropriate for use in geriatric patients (high severity risk).

Brand Names: U.S. Halcion®

Brand Names: Canada Apo-Triazo®; Gen-Triazolam; Halcion®; Mylan-Triazolam

Generic Availability (U.S.) Yes

Pharmacologic Category Hypnotic, Benzodiazepine

Use Short-term treatment of insomnia

Unlabeled/Investigational Use Treatment of anxiety before dental procedures

Medication Guide Available Yes

Contraindications Hypersensitivity to triazolam or any component of the formulation (cross-sensitivity with other benzodiazepines may exist); concurrent therapy with itraconazole, ketoconazole, nefazodone, and other moderate/strong CYP3A4 inhibitors

Warnings/Precautions As a hypnotic, should be used only after evaluation of potential causes of sleep disturbance. Failure of sleep disturbance to resolve after 7-10 days may indicate psychiatric or medical illness. A worsening of insomnia or the emergence of new abnormalities of thought or behavior may represent unrecognized psychiatric or medical illness and requires immediate and careful evaluation. Prescription should be written for a maximum of 7-10 days and should not be prescribed in quantities exceeding a 1-month supply. Abrupt discontinuation after sustained use (generally >10 days) may cause withdrawal symptoms.

An increase in daytime anxiety may occur after as few as 10 days of continuous use, which may be related to withdrawal reaction in some patients. Anterograde amnesia may occur at a higher rate with triazolam than with other benzodiazepines. Use with caution in elderly or debilitated patients, patients with hepatic disease (including alcoholics), or renal impairment. Due to increased sensitivity in the elderly, smaller doses of benzodiazepines may be safer and as effective. Avoid using doses >0.25 mg daily of triazolam (Beers Criteria). Use with caution in patients with respiratory disease or impaired gag reflex. Avoid use in patients with sleep apnea.

Causes CNS depression (dose-related) resulting in sedation, dizziness, confusion, or ataxia which may impair physical and mental capabilities. Patients must be cautioned about performing tasks which require mental alertness (eg, operating machinery or driving). Use with caution in patients receiving other CNS depressants or psychoactive agents. Postmarketing studies have indicated that the use of hypnotic/sedative agents for sleep has been associated with hypersensitivity reactions including anaphylaxis as well as angioedema. An increased risk for hazardous sleep-related activities such as sleep-driving; cooking and eating food, and making phone calls while asleep have also been noted. Effects with other sedative drugs or ethanol may be potentiated. Benzodiazepines have been associated with falls and traumatic injury and should be used with extreme caution in patients who are at risk of these events (especially the elderly).

Use caution with potent CYP3A4 inhibitors, as they may significantly decreased the clearance of triazolam. Use caution in patients with suicidal risk. Use with caution in patients with a history of drug dependence. Benzodiazepines have been associated with dependence and acute withdrawal symptoms on discontinuation or reduction in dose. Acute withdrawal, including seizures, may be precipitated after administration of flumazenil to patients receiving long-term benzodiazepine therapy.

Paradoxical reactions, including hyperactive or aggressive behavior have been reported with benzodiazepines, particularly in psychiatric patients. Does not have analgesic, antidepressant, or antipsychotic properties.

Adverse Reactions (Reflective of adult population; not specific for elderly)
>10%: Central nervous system: Drowsiness (14%)
1% to 10%:
Central nervous system: Headache (10%), dizziness (8%), nervousness (5%), lightheadedness (5%), ataxia (5%)
Gastrointestinal: Nausea (5%), vomiting (5%)

Drug Interactions

Metabolism/Transport Effects Substrate of CYP3A4 (major); **Inhibits** CYP2C8 (weak), 2C9 (weak)

Avoid Concomitant Use
Avoid concomitant use of Triazolam with any of the following: Boceprevir; Conivaptan; Efavirenz; OLANZapine; Protease Inhibitors; Telaprevir

Increased Effect/Toxicity
Triazolam may increase the levels/effects of: Alcohol (Ethyl); CloZAPine; CNS Depressants; Fosphenytoin; Methotrimeprazine; Phenytoin; Selective Serotonin Reuptake Inhibitors

The levels/effects of Triazolam may be increased by: Antifungal Agents (Azole Derivatives, Systemic); Aprepitant; Boceprevir; Calcium Channel Blockers (Nondihydropyridine); Cimetidine; Conivaptan; Contraceptives (Estrogens); Contraceptives (Progestins); CYP3A4 Inhibitors (Moderate); CYP3A4 Inhibitors (Strong); Dasatinib; Droperidol; Efavirenz; Fluconazole; Fosaprepitant; Grapefruit Juice; HydrOXYzine; Isoniazid; Macrolide Antibiotics; Methotrimeprazine; Nefazodone; OLANZapine; Protease Inhibitors; Proton Pump Inhibitors; Selective Serotonin Reuptake Inhibitors; Telaprevir

Decreased Effect

The levels/effects of Triazolam may be decreased by: CarBAMazepine; CYP3A4 Inducers (Strong); Deferasirox; Rifamycin Derivatives; St Johns Wort; Theophylline Derivatives; Tocilizumab; Yohimbine

Ethanol/Nutrition/Herb Interactions

Ethanol: May increase CNS depression; monitor for increased effects with coadministration. Caution patients about effects.

Food: Food may decrease the rate of absorption. Benzodiazepine serum concentrations may be increased by grapefruit juice; monitor.

Herb/Nutraceutical: St John's wort may decrease levels/effects of benzodiazepines. Avoid valerian, St John's wort, kava kava, gotu kola (may increase CNS depression).

Stability Store at controlled room temperature of 20°C to 25°C (68°F to 77°F).

Mechanism of Action Binds to stereospecific benzodiazepine receptors on the postsynaptic GABA neuron at several sites within the central nervous system, including the limbic system, reticular formation. Enhancement of the inhibitory effect of GABA on neuronal excitability results by increased neuronal membrane permeability to chloride ions. This shift in chloride ions results in hyperpolarization (a less excitable state) and stabilization.

Pharmacodynamics/Kinetics

Onset of action: Hypnotic: 15-30 minutes

Duration: 6-7 hours

Distribution: V_d: 0.8-1.8 L/kg

Protein binding: 89%

Metabolism: Extensively hepatic

Half-life elimination: 1.5-5.5 hours

Excretion: Urine as unchanged drug and metabolites

Dosage

Geriatric Oral: Insomnia (short-term use): Initial: 0.125 mg at bedtime; maximum dose: 0.25 mg/day

Adult Note: Onset of action is rapid, patient should be in bed when taking medication.

Insomnia (short-term): Oral: 0.125-0.25 mg at bedtime (maximum dose: 0.5 mg/day)

Dental (preprocedure) (unlabeled use): Oral: 0.25 mg taken the evening before oral surgery; or 0.25 mg 1 hour before procedure

Hepatic Impairment Reduce dose or avoid use in cirrhosis.

Administration May take with food. Tablet may be crushed or swallowed whole. Onset of action is rapid, patient should be in bed when taking medication.

Monitoring Parameters Respiratory, cardiovascular and mental status

Pharmacotherapy Pearls Onset of action is rapid, patient should take triazolam right before going to bed

Special Geriatric Considerations Due to the higher incidence of CNS adverse reactions and its short half-life, this benzodiazepine is not a drug of first choice. For short-term only.

This medication is considered to be potentially inappropriate in this patient population (Beers Criteria severity: High).

Controlled Substance C-IV

Dosage Forms Excipient information presented when available (limited, particularly for generics); consult specific product labeling.

Tablet, oral: 0.125 mg, 0.25 mg

Halcion®: 0.25 mg [scored]

Selected References

Greenblatt DJ, Harmatz JS, Shapiro L, et al, "Sensitivity to Triazolam in the Elderly," *N Engl J Med*, 1991, 324 (24):1691-8.

Trifluoperazine (trye floo oh PER a zeen)

Related Information
Antipsychotic Agents *on page 1997*
Liquid Compatibility of Antidepressants, Antipsychotics, and Mood Stabilizers *on page 2111*

Medication Safety Issues
Sound-alike/look-alike issues:
Trifluoperazine may be confused with trifluopromazine, trihexyphenidyl
Stelazine® may be confused with selegiline
International issues:
Eskazine [Spain] may be confused with Ecazide, a brand name for captopril/hydrochlorothiazide [France, Spain]

Brand Names: Canada Apo-Trifluoperazine®; Novo-Trifluzine; PMS-Trifluoperazine; Terfluzine

Index Terms Trifluoperazine Hydrochloride

Generic Availability (U.S.) Yes

Pharmacologic Category Antipsychotic Agent, Typical, Phenothiazine

Use Treatment of schizophrenia; short-term treatment of generalized nonpsychotic anxiety

Unlabeled/Investigational Use Management of psychotic disorders; behavioral symptoms associated with dementia behavior (elderly); psychosis/agitation related to Alzheimer's dementia

Contraindications Hypersensitivity to trifluoperazine or any component of the formulation (cross-reactivity between phenothiazines may occur); severe CNS depression; bone marrow suppression; blood dyscrasias; severe hepatic disease; coma

Warnings/Precautions [U.S. Boxed Warning]: Elderly patients with dementia-related psychosis treated with antipsychotics are at an increased risk of death compared to placebo. Most deaths appeared to be either cardiovascular (eg, heart failure, sudden death) or infectious (eg, pneumonia) in nature. Trifluoperazine is not approved for the treatment of dementia-related psychosis.

Leukopenia, neutropenia, and agranulocytosis (sometimes fatal) have been reported in clinical trials and postmarketing reports with antipsychotic use; presence of risk factors (eg, pre-existing low WBC or history of drug-induced leuko-/neutropenia) should prompt periodic blood count assessment. Discontinue therapy at first signs of blood dyscrasias or if absolute neutrophil count <1000/mm^3.

May be sedating, use with caution in disorders where CNS depression is a feature. Use with caution in Parkinson's disease. Caution in patients with hemodynamic instability; predisposition to seizures; subcortical brain damage; severe cardiac or renal disease. Liver damage and jaundice of the cholestatic type of hepatitis have been reported with use; use is contraindicated in patients with pre-existing hepatic disease. Esophageal dysmotility and aspiration have been associated with antipsychotic use - use with caution in patients at risk of pneumonia (ie, Alzheimer's disease). Use associated with increased prolactin levels; clinical significance of hyperprolactinemia in patients with breast cancer or other prolactin-dependent tumors is unknown. May alter temperature regulation or mask toxicity of other drugs due to antiemetic effects. May alter cardiac conduction - life-threatening arrhythmias have occurred with therapeutic doses of phenothiazines. May cause orthostatic hypotension - use with caution in patients at risk of this effect or those who would tolerate transient hypotensive episodes (cerebrovascular disease, cardiovascular disease or other medications which may predispose).

Due to anticholinergic effects, should be used with caution in patients with decreased gastrointestinal motility, urinary retention, BPH, xerostomia, visual problems, narrow-angle glaucoma, and myasthenia gravis. Relative to other antipsychotics, trifluoperazine has a low potency of cholinergic blockade.

May cause extrapyramidal symptoms (EPS), including pseudoparkinsonism, acute dystonic reactions, akathisia, and tardive dyskinesia. Risk of dystonia (and possibly other EPS) may be greater with increased doses, use of conventional antipsychotics, males, and younger patients. Use caution in the elderly. May be associated with neuroleptic malignant syndrome (NMS) or pigmentary retinopathy.

Adverse Reactions (Reflective of adult population; not specific for elderly) Frequency not defined.
Cardiovascular: Cardiac arrest, hypotension, orthostatic hypotension
Central nervous system: Dizziness; extrapyramidal symptoms (akathisia, dystonias, pseudoparkinsonism, tardive dyskinesia); headache, impairment of temperature regulation, lowering of seizure threshold, neuroleptic malignant syndrome (NMS)

Dermatologic: Discoloration of skin (blue-gray), increased sensitivity to sun, photosensitivity, rash

Endocrine & metabolic: Breast pain, galactorrhea, gynecomastia, hyperglycemia, hypoglycemia, lactation, libido (changes in), menstrual cycle (changes in)

Gastrointestinal: Constipation, nausea, stomach pain, vomiting, weight gain, xerostomia

Genitourinary: Difficulty in urination, ejaculatory disturbances, priapism, urinary retention

Hematologic: Agranulocytosis, aplastic anemia, eosinophilia, hemolytic anemia, leukopenia, pancytopenia, thrombocytopenic purpura

Hepatic: Cholestatic jaundice, hepatotoxicity

Neuromuscular & skeletal: Tremor

Ocular: Cornea and lens changes, pigmentary retinopathy

Respiratory: Nasal congestion

Drug Interactions

Metabolism/Transport Effects Substrate of CYP1A2 (major)

Avoid Concomitant Use

Avoid concomitant use of Trifluoperazine with any of the following: Metoclopramide

Increased Effect/Toxicity

Trifluoperazine may increase the levels/effects of: Alcohol (Ethyl); Analgesics (Opioid); Anticholinergics; Anti-Parkinson's Agents (Dopamine Agonist); Beta-Blockers; CNS Depressants; Methotrimeprazine; Methylphenidate; Porfimer; Selective Serotonin Reuptake Inhibitors

The levels/effects of Trifluoperazine may be increased by: Abiraterone Acetate; Acetylcholinesterase Inhibitors (Central); Antimalarial Agents; Beta-Blockers; CYP1A2 Inhibitors (Moderate); CYP1A2 Inhibitors (Strong); Deferasirox; Droperidol; Lithium formulations; Methotrimeprazine; Methylphenidate; Metoclopramide; Pramlintide; Tetrabenazine

Decreased Effect

Trifluoperazine may decrease the levels/effects of: Amphetamines; Quinagolide

The levels/effects of Trifluoperazine may be decreased by: Antacids; Anti-Parkinson's Agents (Dopamine Agonist); CYP1A2 Inducers (Strong); Cyproterone; Lithium formulations

Ethanol/Nutrition/Herb Interactions

Ethanol: May increase CNS depression; monitor for increased effects with coadministration. Caution patients about effects.

Herb/Nutraceutical: Avoid kava kava, gotu kola, valerian, St John's wort (may increase CNS depression). Avoid dong quai, St John's wort (may also cause photosensitization).

Mechanism of Action Trifluoperazine is a piperazine phenothiazine antipsychotic which blocks postsynaptic mesolimbic dopaminergic receptors in the brain; exhibits alpha-adrenergic blocking effect and depresses the release of hypothalamic and hypophyseal hormones

Pharmacodynamics/Kinetics

Absorption: May be affected by the inherent anticholinergic action on the gastrointestinal tissue causing variable absorption. Absorption from tablets is erratic with less variation seen with solutions. These agents are widely distributed in tissues with CNS concentrations exceeding that of plasma due to their lipophilic characteristics.

Protein binding: Antipsychotic agents are bound 90% to 99% to plasma proteins; highly bound to brain and lung tissue and other tissues with a high blood perfusion.

Half-life: >24 hours with chronic use

Time to peak concentration: Oral: 2-4 hours

Elimination: Occurs through hepatic metabolism (oxidation) where numerous active metabolites are produced; active metabolites excreted in urine; elimination half-lives of antipsychotics ranges from 20-40 hours which may be extended in older adults due to decline in oxidative hepatic reactions (phase I) with age.

Biologic effect of a single dose persists for 24 hours. When the patient has accommodated to initial side effects (sedation), once daily dosing is possible due to the long half-life of antipsychotics.

Steady-state plasma concentrations are achieved in 4-7 days; therefore, if possible, do not make dose adjustments more than once in a 7-day period. Due to the long half-lives of antipsychotics, as needed (prn) use is ineffective since repeated doses are necessary to achieve therapeutic tissue concentrations in the CNS.

Dosage

Geriatric

Schizophrenia/psychoses: Oral: Refer to adult dosing. Dose selection should start at the low end of the dosage range and titration must be gradual.

Behavioral symptoms associated with dementia behavior (unlabeled use): Oral: Initial: 0.5-1 mg 1-2 times/day; increase dose at 4- to 7-day intervals by 0.5-1 mg/day; increase dosing intervals (bid, tid, etc) as necessary to control response or side effects. Maximum daily dose: 40 mg. Gradual increases (titration) may prevent some side effects or decrease their severity.

Adult

Schizophrenia/psychoses: Oral:

Outpatients: 1-2 mg twice daily

Hospitalized or well supervised patient: Initial: 2-5 mg twice daily with optimum response in the 15-20 mg/day range; do not exceed 40 mg/day.

Nonpsychotic anxiety: Oral: 1-2 mg twice daily; maximum: 6 mg/day; therapy for anxiety should not exceed 12 weeks; do not exceed 6 mg/day for longer than 12 weeks when treating anxiety; agitation, jitteriness, or insomnia may be confused with original neurotic or psychotic symptoms.

Renal Impairment Not dialyzable (0% to 5%)

Administration Administer I.M. injection deep in upper outer quadrant of buttock

Monitoring Parameters Orthostatic blood pressures; tremors, gait changes, abnormal movement in trunk, neck, buccal area, or extremities; monitor target behaviors for which the agent is given. Monitor orthostatic blood pressures 3-5 days after initiation of therapy or a dose increase.

Reference Range Therapeutic response and blood levels have not been established

Test Interactions False-positive for phenylketonuria

Pharmacotherapy Pearls Do not exceed 6 mg/day for longer than 12 weeks when treating anxiety; drug-induced agitation, jitteriness, or insomnia may be confused with original anxious or psychotic symptoms

Special Geriatric Considerations Elderly are more susceptible to hypotension and neuro-muscular reactions.

Many elderly patients receive antipsychotic medications for inappropriate nonpsychotic behavior. Before initiating antipsychotic medication, the clinician should investigate any possible reversible cause; any stress or stress from any disease can cause acute "confusion" or worsening of baseline nonpsychotic behavior. Most commonly acute changes in behavior are due to increases in drug dose or addition of new drug to regimen; fluid electrolyte loss; infections; and changes in environment.

Any changes in disease status in any organ system can result in behavior changes.

In the treatment of agitated, demented, elderly patients, authors of meta-analysis of controlled trials of the response to the traditional antipsychotics (phenothiazines, butyrophenones) in controlling agitation have concluded that the use of neuroleptics results in a response rate of 18%. Clearly neuroleptic therapy for behavior control should be limited with frequent attempts to withdraw the agent given for behavior control.

Dosage Forms Excipient information presented when available (limited, particularly for generics); consult specific product labeling.

Tablet, oral: 1 mg, 2 mg, 5 mg, 10 mg

Selected References

Rabins PV, Blacker D, Rovner BW, et al, "Practice Guidelines for the Treatment of Patients With Alzheimer's Disease and Other Dementias," *Am J Psychiatry*, 2007, 164(12 Suppl):5-56. Available at http://www.psych.org/psych_pract/treatg/pg/prac_guide.cfm.

Schneider LS, Tariot PN, Dagerman KS, et al, "Effectiveness of Atypical Antipsychotic Drugs in Patients With Alzheimer's Disease," *N Engl J Med*, 2006, 355(15):1525-38.

♦ **Trifluoperazine Hydrochloride** *see* Trifluoperazine *on page 1862*
♦ **Trifluorothymidine** *see* Trifluridine *on page 1864*

Trifluridine (trye FLURE i deen)

Medication Safety Issues

Sound-alike/look-alike issues:

Viroptic® may be confused with Timoptic®

Brand Names: U.S. Viroptic®

Brand Names: Canada Sandoz-Trifluridine; Viroptic®

Index Terms F_3T; Trifluorothymidine

Generic Availability (U.S.) Yes

Pharmacologic Category Antiviral Agent, Ophthalmic

Use Treatment of primary keratoconjunctivitis and recurrent epithelial keratitis caused by herpes simplex virus types I and II

Dosage

Geriatric & Adult Herpes keratoconjunctivitis, keratitis: Ophthalmic: Instill 1 drop into affected eye every 2 hours while awake, to a maximum of 9 drops/day, until re-epithelialization of corneal ulcer occurs. Then use 1 drop every 4 hours for another 7 days. Do **not** exceed 21 days of treatment. If improvement has not taken place in 7-14 days, consider another form of therapy.

Special Geriatric Considerations Evaluate the patient's or caregiver's ability to safely administer the correct dose of ophthalmic medication.

Dosage Forms Excipient information presented when available (limited, particularly for generics); consult specific product labeling.

Solution, ophthalmic [drops]: 1% (7.5 mL)

Viroptic®: 1% (7.5 mL)

♦ **Triglide®** see Fenofibrate on page 701

Trihexyphenidyl (trye heks ee FEN i dil)

Related Information

Antiparkinsonian Agents on page 1995

Medication Safety Issues

Sound-alike/look-alike issues:

Trihexyphenidyl may be confused with trifluoperazine

Brand Names: Canada PMS-Trihexyphenidyl; Trihexyphen; Trihexyphenidyl

Index Terms Artane; Benzhexol Hydrochloride; Trihexyphenidyl Hydrochloride

Generic Availability (U.S.) Yes

Pharmacologic Category Anti-Parkinson's Agent, Anticholinergic; Anticholinergic Agent

Use Adjunctive treatment of Parkinson's disease; treatment of drug-induced extrapyramidal symptoms

Contraindications There are no contraindications listed within the manufacturer's labeling.

Warnings/Precautions Use with caution in hot weather or during exercise, especially when administered concomitantly with other atropine-like drugs to chronically-ill patients, alcoholics, patients with CNS disease, or persons doing manual labor in a hot environment. Use with caution in patients with cardiovascular disease (including hypertension), glaucoma, prostatic hyperplasia or any tendency toward urinary retention, liver or kidney disorders, and obstructive disease of the GI tract. May exacerbate mental symptoms when used to treat extrapyramidal symptoms. When given in large doses or to susceptible patients, may cause weakness. May impair physical or mental abilities; patients must be cautioned about performing tasks which require mental alertness (eg, operating machinery or driving). Does not improve symptoms of tardive dyskinesias. Elderly patients require strict dosage regulation.

Adverse Reactions (Reflective of adult population; not specific for elderly) Frequency not defined.

Cardiovascular: Tachycardia

Central nervous system: Agitation, confusion, delusions, dizziness, drowsiness, euphoria, hallucinations, headache, nervousness, paranoia, psychiatric disturbances

Dermatologic: Rash

Gastrointestinal: Constipation, dilatation of colon, ileus, nausea, parotitis, vomiting, xerostomia

Genitourinary: Urinary retention

Neuromuscular & skeletal: Weakness

Ocular: Blurred vision, glaucoma, intraocular pressure increased, mydriasis

Drug Interactions

Avoid Concomitant Use There are no known interactions where it is recommended to avoid concomitant use.

Increased Effect/Toxicity

Trihexyphenidyl may increase the levels/effects of: AbobotulinumtoxinA; Anticholinergics; Cannabinoids; OnabotulinumtoxinA; Potassium Chloride; RimabotulinumtoxinB

The levels/effects of Trihexyphenidyl may be increased by: Pramlintide

Decreased Effect

Trihexyphenidyl may decrease the levels/effects of: Acetylcholinesterase Inhibitors (Central); Secretin

The levels/effects of Trihexyphenidyl may be decreased by: Acetylcholinesterase Inhibitors (Central)

Ethanol/Nutrition/Herb Interactions Ethanol: Avoid ethanol (may increase CNS depression).

Stability Store at 20°C to 25°C (68°F to 77°F).

Mechanism of Action Exerts a direct inhibitory effect on the parasympathetic nervous system. It also has a relaxing effect on smooth musculature; exerted both directly on the muscle itself and indirectly through parasympathetic nervous system (inhibitory effect)

◀ **Pharmacodynamics/Kinetics**
Half-life: 5.6-10.2 hours
Time to peak serum concentrations: Oral: Within 60-90 minutes
Elimination: Primarily in urine

Dosage
Geriatric Parkinson's disease: Refer to adult dosing. **Note:** Conservative initial doses and gradual titration is especially important in patients >60 years of age.

Adult
Parkinson's disease: Oral: Initial: 1 mg/day, increase by 2 mg increments at intervals of 3-5 days; usual dose: 6-10 mg/day in 3-4 divided doses; doses of 12-15 mg/day may be required

Drug-induced EPS: Oral: Initial: 1 mg/day; increase as necessary to usual range: 5-15 mg/day in 3-4 divided doses
Use in combination with levodopa: Usual range: 3-6 mg/day in divided doses

Administration Tolerated best if given in 3 daily doses and with food; high doses may be divided into 4 doses, at meal times and at bedtime

Monitoring Parameters IOP monitoring and gonioscopic evaluations should be performed periodically

Pharmacotherapy Pearls Incidence and severity of side effects are dose related; patients may be switched to sustained-action capsules when stabilized on conventional dosage forms

Special Geriatric Considerations Anticholinergic agents are generally not well tolerated in the elderly (eg, confusion, constipation, urinary retention) and their use should be avoided when possible. In elderly, anticholinergic agents should not be used as prophylaxis against extrapyramidal symptoms.

Dosage Forms Excipient information presented when available (limited, particularly for generics); consult specific product labeling.
Elixir, oral, as hydrochloride: 2 mg/5 mL (473 mL)
Tablet, oral, as hydrochloride: 2 mg, 5 mg

Selected References
Feinberg M, "The Problems of Anticholinergic Adverse Effects in Older Patients," *Drugs Aging*, 1993, 3(4):335-48.
Olanow CW, Watts RL, and Koller WC, "An Algorithm (Decision Tree) for the Management of Parkinson's Disease (2001): Treatment Guidelines," *Neurology*, 2001, 56(11 Suppl 5):S1-S88.

◆ **Trihexyphenidyl Hydrochloride** see Trihexyphenidyl on page 1865
◆ **Trileptal®** see OXcarbazepine on page 1362
◆ **TriLipix®** see Fenofibric Acid on page 704
◆ **Trilisate** see Choline Magnesium Trisalicylate on page 349

Trimethobenzamide (trye meth oh BEN za mide)

Related Information
Beers Criteria – Potentially Inappropriate Medications for Geriatrics on page 2089

Medication Safety Issues
Sound-alike/look-alike issues:
Tigan® may be confused with Tiazac®, Ticar®, Ticlid®
Trimethobenzamide may be confused with metoclopramide, trimethoprim
BEERS Criteria medication:
This drug may be inappropriate for use in geriatric patients (high severity risk).

Brand Names: U.S. Tigan®
Brand Names: Canada Tigan®
Index Terms Trimethobenzamide Hydrochloride
Generic Availability (U.S.) Yes
Pharmacologic Category Antiemetic
Use Treatment of postoperative nausea and vomiting; treatment of nausea associated with gastroenteritis
Contraindications Hypersensitivity to trimethobenzamide or any component of the formulation

Warnings/Precautions May mask emesis due to Reye's syndrome or mimic CNS effects of Reye's syndrome in patients with emesis of other etiologies. Antiemetic effects may mask toxicity of other drugs or conditions (eg, intestinal obstruction). May cause drowsiness; patient should avoid tasks requiring alertness (eg, driving, operating machinery). May cause extrapyramidal symptoms (EPS) which may be confused with CNS symptoms of primary disease responsible for emesis. May be inappropriate for use in the elderly due to the risk of EPS adverse effects combined with lower efficacy, as compared to other antiemetics (Beers Criteria). Risk of CNS adverse effects (eg, coma, EPS, seizure) may be increased in patients with acute febrile illness, dehydration, electrolyte imbalance, encephalitis, or gastroenteritis; use caution. Allergic-type skin reactions have been reported with use; discontinue with signs of sensitization. Trimethobenzamide clearance is predominantly renal; dosage reductions may be recommended in patient with renal impairment.

Adverse Reactions (Reflective of adult population; not specific for elderly) Frequency not defined.

Cardiovascular: Hypotension (I.V. administration)

Central nervous system: Coma, depression, disorientation, dizziness, drowsiness, EPS, headache, Parkinson-like symptoms, seizure

Dermatologic: Allergic-type skin reactions

Gastrointestinal: Diarrhea

Hematologic: Blood dyscrasias

Hepatic: Jaundice

Local: Injection site burning, pain, redness, stinging, or swelling

Neuromuscular & skeletal: Muscle cramps, opisthotonos

Ocular: Blurred vision

Miscellaneous: Hypersensitivity reactions

Drug Interactions

Avoid Concomitant Use There are no known interactions where it is recommended to avoid concomitant use.

Increased Effect/Toxicity

Trimethobenzamide may increase the levels/effects of: AbobotulinumtoxinA; Anticholinergics; Cannabinoids; OnabotulinumtoxinA; Potassium Chloride; RimabotulinumtoxinB

The levels/effects of Trimethobenzamide may be increased by: Pramlintide

Decreased Effect

Trimethobenzamide may decrease the levels/effects of: Acetylcholinesterase Inhibitors (Central); Secretin

The levels/effects of Trimethobenzamide may be decreased by: Acetylcholinesterase Inhibitors (Central)

Ethanol/Nutrition/Herb Interactions Ethanol: Concomitant use should be avoided (sedative effects may be additive).

Stability Store capsules and injection solution at room temperature of 25°C (77°F); excursions permitted to 15°C to 30°C (59°F to 86°F).

Mechanism of Action Acts centrally to inhibit the medullary chemoreceptor trigger zone by blocking emetic impulses to the vomiting center

Pharmacodynamics/Kinetics

Onset of action: Antiemetic: Oral: 10-40 minutes; I.M.: 15-35 minutes

Duration: 3-4 hours

Metabolism: Via oxidation, forms metabolite trimethobenzamide N-oxide

Bioavailability: Oral: 60% to 100%

Half-life elimination: 7-9 hours

Time to peak: Oral: ~45 minutes; I.M.: ~30 minutes

Excretion: Urine (30% to 50%, as unchanged drug)

Dosage

Geriatric Refer to adult dosing. Consider dosage reduction or increasing dosing interval in elderly patients with renal impairment (specific adjustment guidelines are not provided in the manufacturer's labeling).

Adult

Nausea, vomiting:

Oral: 300 mg 3-4 times/day

I.M.: 200 mg 3-4 times/day

Postoperative nausea and vomiting (PONV): I.M.: 200 mg, followed 1 hour later by a second 200 mg dose

Renal Impairment Cl_{cr} ≤70 mL/minute: Consider dosage reduction or increasing dosing interval (specific adjustment guidelines are not provided in the manufacturer's labeling)

Administration Administer I.M. only; not for I.V. administration. Inject deep into upper outer quadrant of gluteal muscle.

Monitoring Parameters Renal function (at baseline)

Pharmacotherapy Pearls Note: Less effective than phenothiazines but may be associated with fewer side effects; rectal is ~60% absorbed

Special Geriatric Considerations No specific data for use in the elderly have been established; as with any drug which has EPS adverse effects and possibility of confusion, caution should be used when administering to elderly.

This medication is considered to be potentially inappropriate in this patient population (Beers Criteria severity: High).

TRIMETHOBENZAMIDE

Dosage Forms Excipient information presented when available (limited, particularly for generics); consult specific product labeling. [DSC] = Discontinued product
Capsule, oral, as hydrochloride: 300 mg
  Tigan®: 300 mg
Injection, solution, as hydrochloride: 100 mg/mL (2 mL [DSC])
  Tigan®: 100 mg/mL (20 mL)
Injection, solution, as hydrochloride [preservative free]:
  Tigan®: 100 mg/mL (2 mL)

◆ **Trimethobenzamide Hydrochloride** see Trimethobenzamide on page 1866

Trimethoprim (trye METH oh prim)

Medication Safety Issues
  Sound-alike/look-alike issues:
    Trimethoprim may be confused with trimethaphan
Brand Names: U.S. Primsol®
Brand Names: Canada Apo-Trimethoprim®
Index Terms TMP
Generic Availability (U.S.) Yes: Tablet
Pharmacologic Category Antibiotic, Miscellaneous
Use Treatment of urinary tract infections due to susceptible strains of *E. coli*, *P. mirabilis*, *K. pneumoniae*, *Enterobacter* spp and coagulase-negative *Staphylococcus* including *S. saprophyticus*
Unlabeled/Investigational Use Alternative agent for *Pneumocystis jirovecii* pneumonia (in combination with dapsone)
Contraindications Hypersensitivity to trimethoprim or any component of the formulation; megaloblastic anemia due to folate deficiency
Warnings/Precautions Use with caution in patients with impaired renal or hepatic function or with possible folate deficiency. Prolonged use may result in fungal or bacterial superinfection, including *C. difficile*-associated diarrhea (CDAD) and pseudomembranous colitis; CDAD has been observed >2 months postantibiotic treatment.
Adverse Reactions (Reflective of adult population; not specific for elderly) Frequency not defined.
Central nervous system: Aseptic meningitis (rare), fever
Dermatologic: Maculopapular rash (3% to 7% at 200 mg/day; incidence higher with larger daily doses), erythema multiforme (rare), exfoliative dermatitis (rare), pruritus (common), phototoxic skin eruptions, Stevens-Johnson syndrome (rare), toxic epidermal necrolysis (rare)
Endocrine & metabolic: Hyperkalemia, hyponatremia
Gastrointestinal: Epigastric distress, glossitis, nausea, vomiting
Hematologic: Leukopenia, megaloblastic anemia, methemoglobinemia, neutropenia, thrombocytopenia
Hepatic: Cholestatic jaundice (rare), liver enzymes increased
Renal: BUN and creatinine increased
Miscellaneous: Anaphylaxis, hypersensitivity reactions
Drug Interactions
  Metabolism/Transport Effects Substrate (major) of CYP2C9, 3A4; **Inhibits** CYP2C8 (moderate), 2C9 (moderate)
  Avoid Concomitant Use
    Avoid concomitant use of Trimethoprim with any of the following: BCG; Dofetilide
  Increased Effect/Toxicity
    Trimethoprim may increase the levels/effects of: ACE Inhibitors; Amantadine; Angiotensin II Receptor Blockers; Antidiabetic Agents (Thiazolidinedione); AzaTHIOprine; Carvedilol; CYP2C8 Substrates (High risk); CYP2C9 Substrates (High risk); Dapsone; Dapsone (Systemic); Dapsone (Topical); Dofetilide; Fosphenytoin; LamiVUDine; Memantine; Methotrexate; Phenytoin; PRALAtrexate; Procainamide; Repaglinide; Varenicline

    The levels/effects of Trimethoprim may be increased by: Amantadine; Conivaptan; CYP2C9 Inhibitors (Moderate); CYP2C9 Inhibitors (Strong); Dapsone; Dapsone (Systemic); Memantine
  Decreased Effect
    Trimethoprim may decrease the levels/effects of: BCG; Typhoid Vaccine

    The levels/effects of Trimethoprim may be decreased by: CYP2C9 Inducers (Highly Effective); CYP3A4 Inducers (Strong); Deferasirox; Herbs (CYP3A4 Inducers); Leucovorin Calcium-Levoleucovorin; Peginterferon Alfa-2b; Tocilizumab

Stability
  Solution: Store between 15°C to 25°C (59°F to 77°F). Protect from light.
  Tablets: Store at 20°C to 25°C (68°F to 77°F). Protect from light.
Mechanism of Action Inhibits folic acid reduction to tetrahydrofolate, and thereby inhibits microbial growth
Pharmacodynamics/Kinetics
  Absorption: Oral: Readily and extensively
  Protein binding: 42% to 46%
  Metabolism: Partially in the liver
  Half-life: 8-14 hours, prolonged with renal impairment
  Time to peak serum concentration: Within 1-4 hours
  Elimination: Significantly in urine (60% to 80% as unchanged drug); in older adults, the area under the curve and peak concentration have been reported to be greater compared to younger subjects
Dosage
  Geriatric & Adult
    ***Pneumocystis jirovecii* pneumonia, mild-to-moderate (unlabeled use) (CDC, 2009):** Oral: 15 mg/kg/day in 3 divided doses in combination with dapsone
    Susceptible infections: Oral: 100 mg every 12 hours or 200 mg every 24 hours for 10 days
  Renal Impairment
    Cl_{cr} 15-30 mL/minute: Administer 50 mg every 12 hours.
    Cl_{cr} <15 mL/minute: Not recommended.
    Moderately dialyzable (20% to 50%)
Administration Administer with milk or food.
Monitoring Parameters Obtain culture and sensitivity results; repeat after treatment has concluded
Reference Range Therapeutic: Peak: 5-15 mg/L; Trough: 2-8 mg/L
Test Interactions May falsely increase creatinine determination measured by the Jaffé alkaline picrate assay; may interfere with determination of serum methotrexate when measured by methods that use a bacterial dihydrofolate reductase as the binding protein (eg, the competitive binding protein technique); does **not** interfere with RIA for methotrexate
Special Geriatric Considerations Trimethoprim is often used in combination with sulfamethoxazole; it can be used alone in patients who are allergic to sulfonamides; adjust dose for renal function (see Pharmacodynamics/Kinetics and Dosage).
Dosage Forms Excipient information presented when available (limited, particularly for generics); consult specific product labeling.
  Solution, oral:
    Primsol®: 50 mg (base)/5 mL (473 mL) [dye free, ethanol free; contains propylene glycol, sodium benzoate; bubblegum flavor]
  Tablet, oral: 100 mg
Selected References
Varoquaux O, Lajoie D, Gobert C, et al, "Pharmacokinetics of the Trimethoprim-Sulfamethoxazole Combination in the Elderly," *Br J Clin Pharmacol*, 1985, 20(6):575-81.

◆ **Trimethoprim and Sulfamethoxazole** *see* Sulfamethoxazole and Trimethoprim *on page 1714*

Trimipramine (trye MI pra meen)

Related Information
  Antidepressant Agents *on page 1991*
Medication Safety Issues
  Sound-alike/look-alike issues:
    Trimipramine may be confused with triamterene, trimeprazine
Brand Names: U.S. Surmontil®
Brand Names: Canada Apo-Trimip®; Nu-Trimipramine; Rhotrimine®; Surmontil®
Index Terms Trimipramine Maleate
Generic Availability (U.S.) No
Pharmacologic Category Antidepressant, Tricyclic (Tertiary Amine)
Use Treatment of depression
Medication Guide Available Yes
Contraindications Hypersensitivity to trimipramine, any component of the formulation, or other dibenzodiazepines; use of MAO inhibitors within 14 days; use in a patient during the acute recovery phase of MI

◄ **Warnings/Precautions [U.S. Boxed Warning]: Antidepressants increase the risk of suicidal thinking and behavior in children, adolescents, and young adults (18-24 years of age) with major depressive disorder (MDD) and other psychiatric disorders;** consider risk prior to prescribing. Short-term studies did not show an increased risk in patients >24 years of age and showed a decreased risk in patients ≥65 years. Closely monitor for clinical worsening, suicidality, or unusual changes in behavior; the patient's family or caregiver should be instructed to closely observe the patient and communicate condition with healthcare provider. A medication guide should be dispensed with each prescription. **Trimipramine is not FDA approved for use in children.**

The possibility of a suicide attempt is inherent in major depression and may persist until remission occurs. Monitor for worsening of depression or suicidality, especially during initiation of therapy (generally first 1-2 months) or with dose increases or decreases. Use caution in high-risk patients. Worsening depression and severe abrupt suicidality that are not part of the presenting symptoms may require discontinuation or modification of drug therapy. The patient's family or caregiver should be alerted to monitor patients for the emergence of suicidality and associated behaviors (such as agitation, irritability, hostility, impulsivity, and hypomania) and call healthcare provider.

May worsen psychosis in some patients or precipitate a shift to mania or hypomania in patients with bipolar disorder. Patients presenting with depressive symptoms should be screened for bipolar disorder. Monotherapy in patients with bipolar disorder should be avoided. **Trimipramine is not FDA approved for the treatment of bipolar depression.**

The degree of sedation, anticholinergic effects, orthostasis, and conduction abnormalities are high relative to other antidepressants. Trimipramine often causes drowsiness/sedation, resulting in impaired performance of tasks requiring alertness (eg, operating machinery or driving). Sedative effects may be additive with other CNS depressants and/or ethanol. Use with caution in patients with a history of cardiovascular disease (including previous MI, stroke, tachycardia, or conduction abnormalities). Use with caution in patients with urinary retention, benign prostatic hyperplasia, narrow-angle glaucoma, xerostomia, visual problems, constipation, or a history of bowel obstruction.

May alter glucose control - use with caution in patients with diabetes. Consider discontinuing, when possible, prior to elective surgery. Therapy should not be abruptly discontinued in patients receiving high doses for prolonged periods. May lower seizure threshold - use caution in patients with a previous seizure disorder or condition predisposing to seizures such as brain damage, alcoholism, or concurrent therapy with other drugs which lower the seizure threshold. May increase the risks associated with electroconvulsive therapy. Use with caution in hyperthyroid patients or those receiving thyroid supplementation. Use with caution in patients with hepatic or renal dysfunction and in elderly patients.

Adverse Reactions (Reflective of adult population; not specific for elderly) Frequency not defined.

Cardiovascular: Arrhythmias, facial edema, flushing, heart block, hyper-/hypotension, MI, palpitation, stroke, tachycardia

Central nervous system: Agitation, anxiety, confusion, delusions, disorientation, dizziness, drowsiness, EEG abnormalities, exacerbation of psychosis, fatigue, hallucinations, headache, hypomania, insomnia, nightmares, restlessness, seizure

Dermatologic: Alopecia, itching, petechiae, photosensitivity, rash, urticaria

Endocrine & metabolic: Breast enlargement, galactorrhea, gynecomastia, hyper-/hypoglycemia, libido (changes in), parotid swelling, syndrome of inappropriate ADH secretion (SIADH)

Gastrointestinal: Abdominal cramps, anorexia, black tongue, constipation, diarrhea, epigastric distress, nausea, paralytic ileus, stomatitis, tongue edema, unpleasant taste, tongue edema, vomiting, weight gain/loss, xerostomia

Genitourinary: Delayed/difficult urination, impotence, polyuria, testicular edema, urinary retention

Hematologic: Agranulocytosis, eosinophilia, purpura, thrombocytopenia

Hepatic: Cholestatic jaundice, liver enzymes increased

Neuromuscular & skeletal: Ataxia, extrapyramidal symptoms, incoordination, numbness, paresthesia, peripheral neuropathy, tingling, tremor, weakness

Ocular: Blurred vision, disturbances in accommodation, mydriasis

Otic: Tinnitus

Miscellaneous: Diaphoresis, withdrawal syndrome

Drug Interactions

Metabolism/Transport Effects Substrate (major) of CYP2C19, 2D6, 3A4

Avoid Concomitant Use

Avoid concomitant use of Trimipramine with any of the following: Artemether; Conivaptan; Dronedarone; Iobenguane I 123; Lumefantrine; MAO Inhibitors; Methylene Blue; Nilotinib; Pimozide; QUEtiapine; QuiNINE; Sibutramine; Tetrabenazine; Thioridazine; Toremifene; Vandetanib; Vemurafenib; Ziprasidone

Increased Effect/Toxicity

Trimipramine may increase the levels/effects of: Alpha-/Beta-Agonists (Direct-Acting); Alpha1-Agonists; Amphetamines; Anticholinergics; Aspirin; Beta2-Agonists; Desmopressin; Dronedarone; Methylene Blue; NSAID (COX-2 Inhibitor); NSAID (Nonselective); Pimozide; QTc-Prolonging Agents; QuiNIDine; QuiNINE; Serotonin Modulators; Sodium Phosphates; Sulfonylureas; Tetrabenazine; Thioridazine; Toremifene; TraMADol; Vandetanib; Vemurafenib; Vitamin K Antagonists; Yohimbine; Ziprasidone

The levels/effects of Trimipramine may be increased by: Abiraterone Acetate; Alfuzosin; Altretamine; Artemether; BuPROPion; Chloroquine; Cimetidine; Cinacalcet; Ciprofloxacin; Ciprofloxacin (Systemic); Conivaptan; CYP2C19 Inhibitors (Moderate); CYP2C19 Inhibitors (Strong); CYP2D6 Inhibitors (Moderate); CYP2D6 Inhibitors (Strong); CYP3A4 Inhibitors (Moderate); CYP3A4 Inhibitors (Strong); Dexmethylphenidate; Divalproex; DULoxetine; Gadobutrol; Lithium; Lumefantrine; MAO Inhibitors; Methylphenidate; Metoclopramide; Nilotinib; Pramlintide; Propoxyphene; Protease Inhibitors; QUEtiapine; QuiNIDine; QuiNINE; Selective Serotonin Reuptake Inhibitors; Sibutramine; Terbinafine; Terbinafine (Systemic); Valproic Acid

Decreased Effect

Trimipramine may decrease the levels/effects of: Acetylcholinesterase Inhibitors (Central); Alpha2-Agonists; Iobenguane I 123

The levels/effects of Trimipramine may be decreased by: Acetylcholinesterase Inhibitors (Central); Barbiturates; CarBAMazepine; CYP2C19 Inducers (Strong); CYP3A4 Inducers (Strong); Deferasirox; Peginterferon Alfa-2b; St Johns Wort; Tocilizumab

Ethanol/Nutrition/Herb Interactions

Ethanol: May increase CNS depression; monitor for increased effects with coadministration. Caution patients about effects.

Food: Grapefruit juice may inhibit the metabolism of some TCAs and clinical toxicity may result.

Herb/Nutraceutical: Avoid valerian, St John's wort, SAMe, kava kava (may increase risk of serotonin syndrome and/or excessive sedation).

Stability Solutions stable at a pH of 4-5. Turns yellowish or reddish on exposure to light. Slight discoloration does not affect potency; marked discoloration is associated with loss of potency. Capsules stable for 3 years following date of manufacture.

Mechanism of Action Increases the synaptic concentration of serotonin and/or norepinephrine in the central nervous system by inhibition of their reuptake by the presynaptic neuronal membrane

Pharmacodynamics/Kinetics

Distribution: V_d: 17-48 L/kg

Protein binding: 95%; free drug: 3% to 7%

Metabolism: Hepatic; significant first-pass effect

Bioavailability: 18% to 63%

Half-life elimination: 16-40 hours

Excretion: Urine

Dosage

Geriatric Oral: 50 mg/day; gradually increase dose to 100 mg/day

Adult Depression: Oral:

Outpatients: Initial: 75 mg/day in divided doses; may increase to 150 mg/day; Maintenance: 50-150 mg/day as a single bedtime dose; maximum: 200 mg/day

Inpatients: Initial: 100 mg /day in divided doses; may increase to 200 mg/day; if no improvement after 2-3 weeks, dose may be increased to 250-300 mg/day

Monitoring Parameters Blood pressure and pulse rate prior to and during initial therapy; evaluate mental status, suicide ideation (especially at the beginning of therapy or when doses are increased or decreased); monitor weight; ECG in older adults

Pharmacotherapy Pearls May cause alterations in bleeding time

Special Geriatric Considerations Similar to doxepin in its side effect profile; has not been well studied in the elderly; very anticholinergic and, therefore, not considered a drug of first choice in the elderly when selecting an antidepressant.

Dosage Forms Excipient information presented when available (limited, particularly for generics); consult specific product labeling. [DSC] = Discontinued product

Capsule, oral: 25 mg [DSC], 50 mg [DSC]

Surmontil®: 25 mg, 50 mg, 100 mg

Triprolidine and Pseudoephedrine (trye PROE li deen & soo doe e FED rin)

Related Information
Pseudoephedrine *on page 1545*
Medication Safety Issues
Sound-alike/look-alike issues:
Aprodine® may be confused with Aphrodyne®
Brand Names: U.S. Allerfrim [OTC]; Aprodine [OTC]; Genac™ [OTC] [DSC]; Pediatex® TD; Silafed [OTC]; Tripohist™ D
Brand Names: Canada Actifed®
Index Terms Pseudoephedrine and Triprolidine
Generic Availability (U.S.) Yes
Pharmacologic Category Alkylamine Derivative; Alpha/Beta Agonist; Decongestant; Histamine H_1 Antagonist; Histamine H_1 Antagonist, First Generation
Use Temporary relief of nasal congestion, decongest sinus openings, running nose, sneezing, itching of nose or throat and itchy, watery eyes due to common cold, hay fever, or other upper respiratory allergies
Dosage
Geriatric & Adult Cold, allergy symptoms: Oral:
Liquid:
Pediatex® TD: 2.67 mL every 6 hours (maximum: 4 doses/24 hours)
Tripohist™ D: 5-10 mL every 4-6 hours (maximum pseudoephedrine: 240 mg/24 hours)
Syrup (Allerfrim, Aprodine®): 10 mL every 4-6 hours; do not exceed 4 doses in 24 hours
Tablet (Aprodine®): One tablet every 4-6 hours; do not exceed 4 doses in 24 hours
Special Geriatric Considerations Use with caution in patients with cardiovascular disease; the anticholinergic action of triprolidine may cause confusion, constipation, or urinary retention in the elderly. Also refer to Pseudoephedrine on page 1545.
Dosage Forms Excipient information presented when available (limited, particularly for generics); consult specific product labeling. [DSC] = Discontinued product
Liquid, oral:
Pediatex® TD: Triprolidine hydrochloride 0.938 mg and pseudoephedrine hydrochloride 10 mg per 1 mL (30 mL) [cotton candy flavor]
Tripohist™ D: Triprolidine hydrochloride 1.25 mg and pseudoephedrine hydrochloride 45 mg per 5 mL (473 mL) [ethanol free, sugar free; contains sodium benzoate; blueberry flavor]
Syrup, oral: Triprolidine hydrochloride 1.25 mg and pseudoephedrine hydrochloride 30 mg per 5 mL (120 mL) [DSC]
Allerfrim: Triprolidine hydrochloride 1.25 mg and pseudoephedrine hydrochloride 30 mg per 5 mL (118 mL [DSC], 473 mL [DSC]) [contains sodium benzoate]
Aprodine: Triprolidine hydrochloride 1.25 mg and pseudoephedrine hydrochloride 30 mg per 5 mL (120 mL)
Silafed: Triprolidine hydrochloride 1.25 mg and pseudoephedrine hydrochloride 30 mg per 5 mL (120 mL, 240 mL)
Tablet, oral:
Allerfrim, Aprodine, Genac™ [DSC]: Triprolidine hydrochloride 2.5 mg and pseudoephedrine hydrochloride 60 mg

- **TripTone® [OTC]** *see* DimenhyDRINATE *on page 518*

Triptorelin (trip toe REL in)

Brand Names: U.S. Trelstar®
Brand Names: Canada Trelstar®
Index Terms AY-25650; CL-118,532; D-Trp(6)-LHRH; Detryptoreline; Triptorelin Pamoate; Tryptoreline
Generic Availability (U.S.) No
Pharmacologic Category Gonadotropin Releasing Hormone Agonist
Use Palliative treatment of advanced prostate cancer
Unlabeled/Investigational Use Treatment of endometriosis, hyperandrogenism, uterine sarcoma

Contraindications Hypersensitivity to triptorelin or any component of the formulation, other GnRH agonists or GnRH

Warnings/Precautions Hazardous agent - use appropriate precautions for handling and disposal. Transient increases in testosterone can lead to worsening symptoms (bone pain, hematuria, bladder outlet obstruction, neuropathy, spinal cord compression) of prostate cancer during the first few weeks of therapy. Androgen-deprivation therapy may increase the risk for cardiovascular disease (Levine, 2010). Hyperglycemia has been reported with androgen deprivation therapy (in prostate cancer) and may manifest as diabetes or worsening of pre-existing diabetes; monitor blood glucose and/or Hb A_{1c}. Cases of spinal cord compression have been reported with GnRH agonists. Closely observe (during the first 2 weeks of treatment) patients with metastatic vertebral lesions or urinary tract obstruction. Hypersensitivity reactions including angioedema, anaphylaxis and anaphylactic shock have rarely occurred; discontinue if severe reaction occurs. Rare cases of pituitary apoplexy (frequently secondary to pituitary adenoma) have been observed with leuprolide administration (onset from 1 hour to usually <2 weeks); may present as sudden headache, vomiting, visual or mental status changes, and infrequently cardiovascular collapse; immediate medical attention required.

Adverse Reactions (Reflective of adult population; not specific for elderly) As reported with all strengths; frequency of effect may vary by strength:

>10%:

Endocrine & metabolic: Hot flashes (59% to 73%), glucose increased, testosterone levels increased (peak: days 2-4; decline to low levels by weeks 3-4)

Hematologic: Hemoglobin decreased, RBC count decreased

Hepatic: Alkaline phosphatase increased (2% to >10%), ALT increased, AST increased

Neuromuscular & skeletal: Skeletal pain (12% to 13%)

Renal: BUN increased

1% to 10%:

Cardiovascular: Leg edema (6%), hypertension (1% to 4%), chest pain (2%), edema (2%), peripheral edema (≤1%)

Central nervous system: Headache (2% to 7%), pain (2% to 3%), dizziness (1% to 3%), fatigue (2%), insomnia (1% to 2%), emotional lability (1%)

Dermatologic: Rash (2%), pruritus (1%)

Endocrine & metabolic: Breast pain (2%), gynecomastia (2%), libido decreased (2%)

Gastrointestinal: Nausea (3%), anorexia (2%), constipation (2%), dyspepsia (2%), vomiting (2%), abdominal pain (1%), diarrhea (1%)

Genitourinary: Erectile dysfunction (10%), testicular atrophy (8%), impotence (2% to 7%), dysuria (5%), urinary retention (≤1%), urinary tract infection (≤1%)

Hematologic: Anemia (1%)

Local: Injection site pain (4%)

Neuromuscular & skeletal: Leg pain (2% to 5%), back pain (1% to 3%), leg cramps (2%), arthralgia (1% to 2%), extremity pain (1%), myalgia (1%), weakness (1%)

Ocular: Conjunctivitis (1%), eye pain (1%)

Respiratory: Cough (2%), dyspnea (1%), pharyngitis (1%)

Drug Interactions

Avoid Concomitant Use There are no known interactions where it is recommended to avoid concomitant use.

Increased Effect/Toxicity There are no known significant interactions involving an increase in effect.

Decreased Effect

Triptorelin may decrease the levels/effects of: Antidiabetic Agents

Stability Store at 20°C to 25°C (68°F to 77°F). Do not freeze MIXJECT® system. Reconstitute with 2 mL sterile water for injection. Shake well to obtain a uniform suspension. Solution will appear milky. Administer immediately after reconstitution.

MIXJECT® System: Follow manufacturer's instructions for mixing prior to use.

Mechanism of Action Causes suppression of ovarian and testicular steroidogenesis due to decreased levels of LH and FSH with subsequent decrease in testosterone (male) and estrogen (female) levels. After chronic and continuous administration, usually 2-4 weeks after initiation, a sustained decrease in LH and FSH secretion occurs.

Pharmacodynamics/Kinetics

Distribution: V_d: 30-33 L

Protein binding: None

Metabolism: Unknown; unlikely to involve CYP; no known metabolites

Half-life elimination: 2.8 ± 1.2 hours

Moderate-to-severe renal impairment: 6.5-7.7 hours

Hepatic impairment: 7.6 hours

Time to peak: 1-3 hours

Excretion: Urine (42% as intact peptide); hepatic

◀ **Dosage**

Geriatric & Adult Advanced prostate carcinoma: I.M.:

3.75 mg once every 4 weeks **or**

11.25 mg once every 12 weeks **or**

22.5 mg once every 24 weeks

Administration Administer by I.M. injection into the buttock; alternate injection sites. Administer immediately after reconstitution.

Monitoring Parameters Serum testosterone levels, prostate-specific antigen; blood pressure; monitor for bone pain and spinal symptoms of compression; urinary retention

Test Interactions Pituitary-gonadal function may be suppressed with chronic administration and for up to 8 weeks after triptorelin therapy has been discontinued.

Special Geriatric Considerations No dosage adjustments are needed in the elderly. Monitoring for bone density changes, serum lipid, hemoglobin A_{1c}, blood pressure, and serum calcium changes is recommended.

Dosage Forms Excipient information presented when available (limited, particularly for generics); consult specific product labeling.

Injection, powder for reconstitution:

Trelstar®: 3.75 mg, 11.25 mg, 22.5 mg [contains polylactide-co-glycolide, polysorbate 80]

◆ **Triptorelin Pamoate** *see* Triptorelin *on page 1872*

◆ **Trivalent Inactivated Influenza Vaccine** *see* Influenza Virus Vaccine (Inactivated) *on page 936*

◆ **Trocal® [OTC]** *see* Dextromethorphan *on page 490*

◆ **Tronolane® Suppository [OTC]** *see* Phenylephrine (Topical) *on page 1443*

Trospium (TROSE pee um)

Related Information

Pharmacotherapy of Urinary Incontinence *on page 2032*

Brand Names: U.S. Sanctura®; Sanctura® XR

Brand Names: Canada Sanctura® XR; Trosec

Index Terms Trospium Chloride

Generic Availability (U.S.) Yes: Tablet

Pharmacologic Category Anticholinergic Agent

Use Treatment of overactive bladder with symptoms of urgency, incontinence, and urinary frequency

Contraindications Hypersensitivity to trospium or any component of the formulation; urinary retention; gastric retention; uncontrolled narrow-angle glaucoma

Warnings/Precautions Cases of angioedema involving the face, lips, tongue, and/or larynx have been reported. Immediately discontinue if tongue, hypopharynx, or larynx are involved. May cause drowsiness and/or blurred vision, which may impair physical or mental abilities; patients must be cautioned about performing tasks which require mental alertness (eg, operating machinery or driving). May occur in the presence of increased environmental temperature; use caution in hot weather and/or exercise. Use with caution in patients with bladder flow obstruction, may increase the risk of urinary retention. Use with caution in patients with gastrointestinal obstructive disorders (eg, pyloric stenosis); may increase the risk of gastric retention. Use caution in patients with decreased GI motility (eg, myasthenia gravis, ulcerative colitis). Avoid use of extended release formulation in severe renal impairment (Cl_{cr} <30 mL/minute). Use immediate release formulation with caution in renal dysfunction; dosage adjustment is required. Ethanol should not be ingested within 2 hours of the administration of the extended release formulation. Concurrent ethanol use may increase the incidence of drowsiness. Active tubular secretion (ATS) is a route of elimination; use caution with other medications that are eliminated by ATS (eg, procainamide, pancuronium, vancomycin, morphine, metformin, and tenofovir). Use with extreme caution in patients with controlled (treated) narrow-angle glaucoma. Use caution in patients with moderate or severe hepatic dysfunction. Use caution in Alzheimer's patients. Use caution in the elderly (≥65 years of age); increased anticholinergic side effects are seen.

Adverse Reactions (Reflective of adult population; not specific for elderly)

>10%: Gastrointestinal: Xerostomia (9% to 22%)

1% to 10%:

Cardiovascular: Tachycardia

Central nervous system: Headache (4% to 7%), fatigue (2%)

Dermatologic: Dry skin

Gastrointestinal: Constipation (9% to 10%), abdominal pain (1% to 3%), dyspepsia (1% to 2%), flatulence (1% to 2%), nausea (1%), abdominal distention (<2%), taste abnormal, vomiting

Genitourinary: Urinary tract infection (1% to 7%), urinary retention (≤1%)

Ocular: Dry eyes (1% to 2%), blurred vision (1%)
Respiratory: Nasopharyngitis (3%), nasal dryness (1%)
Miscellaneous: Influenza (2%)

Drug Interactions

Avoid Concomitant Use There are no known interactions where it is recommended to avoid concomitant use.

Increased Effect/Toxicity

Trospium may increase the levels/effects of: AbobotulinumtoxinA; Anticholinergics; Cannabinoids; OnabotulinumtoxinA; Potassium Chloride; RimabotulinumtoxinB

The levels/effects of Trospium may be increased by: Pramlintide

Decreased Effect

Trospium may decrease the levels/effects of: Acetylcholinesterase Inhibitors (Central); Secretin

The levels/effects of Trospium may be decreased by: Acetylcholinesterase Inhibitors (Central)

Ethanol/Nutrition/Herb Interactions

Ethanol: Avoid use since ethanol may enhance the sedative effects of trospium. Ethanol should not be ingested within 2 hours of the administration of the trospium extended release formulation.

Food: Administration with a fatty meal reduces the absorption and bioavailability of trospium.

Stability Store at 20°C to 25°C (68°F to 77°F).

Mechanism of Action Trospium antagonizes the effects of acetylcholine on muscarinic receptors in cholinergically innervated organs. It reduces the smooth muscle tone of the bladder.

Pharmacodynamics/Kinetics

Absorption: <10%; decreased with food

Distribution: V_d: 395 - >600 L, primarily in plasma

Protein binding: 48% to 85% *in vitro*

Metabolism: Hypothesized to be via esterase hydrolysis and conjugation; forms metabolites

Bioavailability: Immediate release formulation: ~10% (range: 4% to 16%)

Half-life elimination: Immediate release formulation: 20 hours

Severe renal insufficiency (Cl_{cr} <30 mL/minute): ~33 hours; extended release formulation: ~35 hours

Time to peak, plasma: 5-6 hours

Excretion: Feces (85%); urine (~6%; mostly as unchanged drug) primarily via active tubular secretion

Dosage

Geriatric ≥75 years: Immediate release formulation: Consider initial dose of 20 mg once daily (based on tolerability) at bedtime

Adult Overactive bladder: Oral: Immediate release formulation: 20 mg twice daily; extended release formulation: 60 mg once daily

Renal Impairment Cl_{cr} ≤30 mL/minute: Immediate release formulation: 20 mg once daily at bedtime; Extended release formulation: Use not recommended

Administration Administer 1 hour prior to meals or an empty stomach. Administer extended release capsules in the morning with a full glass of water.

Monitoring Parameters Monitor incontinence episodes, postvoid residual (PVR)

Special Geriatric Considerations In studies, the incidence of anticholinergic side effects was higher in patients ≥65 years of age as compared to younger adults. The extended release formulation should be avoided in patients with Cl_{cr} <30 mL/minute.

Dosage Forms Excipient information presented when available (limited, particularly for generics); consult specific product labeling.

Capsule, extended release, oral, as chloride:

Sanctura® XR: 60 mg

Tablet, oral, as chloride: 20 mg

Sanctura®: 20 mg

Selected References

Chancellor M and de Miguel F, "Treatment of Overactive Bladder Selective Use of Anticholinergic Agents With Low Drug-Drug Interaction Potential," *Geriatrics*, 2007, 62(5):15-24.

◆ **Trospium Chloride** *see* Trospium *on page 1874*

◆ **Trusopt®** *see* Dorzolamide *on page 560*

Trypsin, Balsam Peru, and Castor Oil
(TRIP sin, BAL sam pe RUE, & KAS tor oyl)

Related Information
Castor Oil *on page 287*

Medication Safety Issues
Sound-alike/look-alike issues:
Granulex® may be confused with Regranex®

Brand Names: U.S. Granulex®; Optase™; TBC; Vasolex™; Xenaderm®

Index Terms Balsam Peru, Castor Oil, and Trypsin; Castor Oil, Trypsin, and Balsam Peru

Generic Availability (U.S.) No

Pharmacologic Category Protectant, Topical

Use Treatment of decubitus ulcers, varicose ulcers, debridement of eschar, dehiscent wounds and sunburn; promote wound healing; reduce odor from necrotic wounds

Contraindications Hypersensitivity to trypsin, balsam peru, castor oil, or any component of the formulation

Warnings/Precautions For external use only. Do not apply to fresh arterial clots. Wound healing may be retarded in the presence of hemoglobin or zinc deficiency.

Adverse Reactions (Reflective of adult population; not specific for elderly) Frequency not defined: Local: Temporary stinging at application site

Drug Interactions
Avoid Concomitant Use There are no known interactions where it is recommended to avoid concomitant use.

Increased Effect/Toxicity There are no known significant interactions involving an increase in effect.

Decreased Effect There are no known significant interactions involving a decrease in effect.

Stability Store at controlled room temperature; do not freeze. Do not expose spray to fire, open flame, or temperatures >120°F.

Mechanism of Action Trypsin is used to debride necrotic tissue; balsam peru stimulates circulation at the wound site and may be mildly bactericidal; castor oil improves epithelialization, acts as a protectant covering and helps reduce pain

Dosage
Geriatric & Adult Dermatologic conditions: Topical: Apply a minimum of twice daily or as often as necessary

Administration Clean wound prior to application and at each redressing; shake well before spraying; hold can upright ~12" from area to be treated.

Monitoring Parameters Size of the ulcer, skin integrity

Special Geriatric Considerations Preventive skin care should be instituted in all elderly patients at high risk for decubitus ulcers. Practical experience with Granulex® has found that it is not as effective in debriding wounds as compared to other enzymatic products. Therefore, Granulex® may be more appropriately used on stage 1 and 2 decubiti.

Dosage Forms Excipient information presented when available (limited, particularly for generics); consult specific product labeling.
Aerosol, topical:
Granulex®: Trypsin 0.12 mg, balsam Peru 87 mg, and castor oil 788 mg per gram (60 g, 120 g)
TBC: Trypsin 0.1 mg, balsam Peru 72.5 mg, and castor oil 650 mg per 0.82 mL (60 g, 120 g)
Gel, topical:
Optase™: Trypsin 0.12 mg, balsam Peru 87 mg, and castor oil 788 mg per gram (95 g)
Ointment, topical:
Vasolex™: Trypsin 90 USP units, balsam Peru 87 mg, and castor oil 788 mg per gram (5 g, 30 g, 60 g)
Xenaderm®: Trypsin 90 USP units, balsam Peru 87 mg, and castor oil 788 mg per gram (30 g, 60 g)

◆ **Tryptoreline** *see* Triptorelin *on page 1872*
◆ **TST** *see* Tuberculin Tests *on page 1877*
◆ **TT** *see* Tetanus Toxoid (Adsorbed) *on page 1769*
◆ **Tuberculin Purified Protein Derivative** *see* Tuberculin Tests *on page 1877*
◆ **Tuberculin Skin Test** *see* Tuberculin Tests *on page 1877*

Tuberculin Tests (too BER kyoo lin tests)

Medication Safety Issues
  Sound-alike/look-alike issues:
  Aplisol® may be confused with Anusol®, A.P.L.®, Aplitest®, Atropisol®
  Administration issues:
  Tuberculin products may be confused with tetanus toxoid products, poliovirus vaccine (inactivated), and influenza virus vaccine. Medication errors have occurred when tuberculin skin tests (PPD) have been inadvertently administered instead of tetanus toxoid products and influenza virus vaccine. These products are refrigerated and often stored in close proximity to each other.

Brand Names: U.S. Aplisol®; Tubersol®

Index Terms Mantoux; PPD; TB Skin Test; TST; Tuberculin Purified Protein Derivative; Tuberculin Skin Test

Generic Availability (U.S.) No

Pharmacologic Category Diagnostic Agent

Use Skin test in diagnosis of tuberculosis

Contraindications Hypersensitivity to tuberculin purified protein derivative (PPD) or any component of the formulation; previous severe reaction to tuberculin PPD skin test (TST)

Warnings/Precautions Patients with a previous severe reaction to TST (vesiculation, ulceration, necrosis) at the injection site should not receive tuberculin PPD again. Do not administer to persons with documented tuberculosis or a clear history of treatment for tuberculosis; persons with extensive burns or eczema. Skin testing may be deferred with major viral infections or live-virus vaccination within 1 month. Tuberculous or other bacterial infections, viral infection, live virus vaccination, malignancy, immunosuppressive agents, and conditions which impair immune response may cause a decreased response to test. For intradermal administration only; do not administer I.V., I.M., or SubQ. Epinephrine (1:1000) should be available to treat possible allergic reactions.

Adverse Reactions (Reflective of adult population; not specific for elderly) Suspected adverse reactions should be reported to the Food and Drug Administration (FDA) MedWatch Program at 1-800-332-1088

Frequency not defined:
  Dermatologic: Rash
  Local: Injection site reactions: Bleeding, bruising, discomfort, erythematous reaction, hematoma, necrosis, pain, pruritus, redness, scarring, ulceration, vesiculation
  Miscellaneous: Anaphylaxis

Drug Interactions

  Avoid Concomitant Use There are no known interactions where it is recommended to avoid concomitant use.

  Increased Effect/Toxicity There are no known significant interactions involving an increase in effect.

  Decreased Effect
    The levels/effects of Tuberculin Tests may be decreased by: Vaccines (Live)

Stability Aplisol®, Tubersol®: Store under refrigeration at 2°C to 8°C (36°F to 46°F); do not freeze. Protect from light. Opened vials should be discarded after 30 days.

Mechanism of Action Tuberculosis results in individuals becoming sensitized to certain antigenic components of the *M. tuberculosis* organism. Culture extracts called tuberculins are contained in tuberculin skin test preparations. Upon intracutaneous injection of these culture extracts, a classic delayed (cellular) hypersensitivity reaction occurs. This reaction is characteristic of a delayed course (peak occurs >24 hours after injection, induration of the skin secondary to cell infiltration, and occasional vesiculation and necrosis). Delayed hypersensitivity reactions to tuberculin may indicate infection with a variety of nontuberculosis mycobacteria, or vaccination with the live attenuated mycobacterial strain of *M. bovis* vaccine, BCG, in addition to previous natural infection with *M. tuberculosis*.

Pharmacodynamics/Kinetics
  Onset of action: Delayed hypersensitivity reactions: 5-6 hours
  Peak effect: 48-72 hours
  Duration: Reactions subside over a few days

◀ **Dosage**
Geriatric & Adult
Diagnosis of tuberculosis, cell-mediated immunodeficiencies: Intradermal: 0.1 mL

TST interpretation: Criteria for positive TST read at 48-72 hours (see Note below for healthcare workers):
Induration ≥5 mm: Persons with HIV infection (or risk factors for HIV infection, but unknown status), recent close contact to person with known active TB, persons with chest x-ray consistent with healed TB, persons who are immunosuppressed
Induration ≥10 mm: Persons with clinical conditions which increase risk of TB infection, recent immigrants, I.V. drug users, residents and employees of high-risk settings
Induration ≥15 mm: Persons who do not meet any of the above criteria (no risk factors for TB)
Note: A two-step test is recommended when testing will be performed at regular intervals (eg, for healthcare workers). If the first test is negative, a second TST should be administered 1-3 weeks after the first test was read.

TST interpretation (CDC guidelines) in a healthcare setting:
Baseline test: ≥10 mm is positive (either first or second step)
Serial testing without known exposure: Increase of ≥10 mm is positive
Known exposure:
≥5 mm is positive in patients with baseline of 0 mm
≥10 mm is positive in patients with negative baseline or previous screening result of ≥0mm
Read test at 48-72 hours following placement. Test results with 0 mm induration or measured induration less than the defined cutoff point are considered to signify absence of infection with *M. tuberculosis*. Test results should be documented in millimeters even if classified as negative. Erythema and redness of skin are not indicative of a positive test result.

Administration For intradermal administration only. Administer to upper third of forearm (palm up) ≥2 inches from elbow, wrist, or other injection site. If neither arm can be used, may administer to back of shoulder. Administer using inch ¼ to ½ inch 27-gauge needle or finer tuberculin syringe. Should form wheal (6-10 mm in diameter) as liquid is injected which will remain ~10 minutes. Avoid pressure or bandage at injection site. Document date and time of injection, person placing TST, location of injection site and lot number of solution.

Monitoring Parameters Monitor for immediate hypersensitivity reactions for ~15 minutes following injection.

Test Interactions False-positive reactions may occur with BCG vaccination or previous mycobacteria (nonTB) infection (previous BCG vaccination is not a contraindication to testing). False-negative reactions may occur with impaired cell mediated immunity.

Pharmacotherapy Pearls Situations where risk of tuberculosis infection may be increased are with contacts of recently-diagnosed persons with active disease, contact with immigrants from countries where tuberculosis is still common, or reactivation with impaired immunity (HIV infection, diabetes, renal failure, immunosuppressant use, pulmonary silicosis). Healthcare workers, staff of correctional facilities, and travelers at high risk of exposure should have routine testing. Patients with HIV infection should be tested as soon as possible following diagnosis.

The date of administration, the product manufacturer, and lot number of product must be entered into the patient's permanent medical record. Results should be recorded in millimeters (even if 0), not "negative" or "positive".

Special Geriatric Considerations Due to changes in the immune system with age, skin test response may be delayed or reduced in magnitude; therefore when testing, use a two-step test procedure; repeat test 2-4 weeks after reading first test dose; this elicits a "booster effect".

Dosage Forms Excipient information presented when available (limited, particularly for generics); consult specific product labeling.
Injection, solution:
Aplisol®: 5 TU/0.1 mL (1 mL, 5 mL) [contains polysorbate 80]
Tubersol®: 5 TU/0.1 mL (1 mL, 5 mL) [contains polysorbate 80]

◆ **Tubersol®** *see* Tuberculin Tests *on page 1877*
◆ **Tums® [OTC]** *see* Calcium Salts (Oral) *on page 256*
◆ **Tums® Dual Action [OTC]** *see* Famotidine, Calcium Carbonate, and Magnesium Hydroxide *on page 696*
◆ **Tums® E-X Extra Strength Tablet [OTC]** *see* Calcium Salts (Oral) *on page 256*
◆ **Tums® Extra Strength Liquid [OTC]** *see* Calcium Salts (Oral) *on page 256*
◆ **Tums® Ultra [OTC]** *see* Calcium Salts (Oral) *on page 256*
◆ **Tusal®** *see* Salicylates (Various Salts) *on page 1647*
◆ **Tussi-Bid®** *see* Guaifenesin and Dextromethorphan *on page 848*

Typhoid Vaccine (TYE foid vak SEEN)

Related Information
Immunization Administration Recommendations on page 2037
Immunization Recommendations on page 2043
Brand Names: U.S. Typhim Vi®; Vivotif®
Brand Names: Canada Typherix®; Typhim Vi®; Vivotif®
Index Terms Ty21a Vaccine; Typhoid Vaccine Live Oral Ty21a; Vi Vaccine
Generic Availability (U.S.) No
Pharmacologic Category Vaccine, Inactivated (Bacterial); Vaccine, Live (Bacterial)
Use Active immunization against typhoid fever caused by *Salmonella typhi*
Not for routine vaccination. In the United States and Canada, use should be limited to:
 – Travelers to areas with a prolonged risk of exposure to *S. typhi*
 – Persons with intimate exposure to a *S. typhi* carrier
 – Laboratory technicians with exposure to *S. typhi*
 – Travelers with achlorhydria or hypochlorhydria (Canadian recommendation)
Contraindications Hypersensitivity to any component of the vaccine. In addition, the oral vaccine is contraindicated with congenital or acquired immunodeficient state, acute febrile illness
Warnings/Precautions Not all recipients of typhoid vaccine will be fully protected against typhoid fever. Travelers should take all necessary precautions to avoid contact or ingestion of potentially contaminated food or water sources. Should not be used to treat typhoid fever.

Injection: Administer at least 2 weeks prior to expected exposure. Vaccination may be deferred during acute infection or febrile illness. Immune response may be decreased in those receiving immunosuppressive therapy or are otherwise immunocompromised. In general, household and close contacts of persons with altered immunocompetence may receive all age appropriate vaccines. Use caution with coagulation disorders (including thrombocytopenia) where intramuscular injections should not be used. Epinephrine 1:1000 should be readily available.

Oral: Full immunization schedule should be completed at least 1 week prior to expected exposure. The complete immunization schedule must be followed to achieve optimum immune response. Do not administer during acute GI illness; vaccination may be deferred with persistent diarrhea or vomiting.

In order to maximize vaccination rates, the ACIP recommends simultaneous administration of all age-appropriate vaccines (live or inactivated) for which a person is eligible at a single clinic visit, unless contraindications exist.

◀ **Adverse Reactions (Reflective of adult population; not specific for elderly)** In the U.S., all serious adverse reactions must be reported to the Department of Health and Human Services (DHHS) Vaccine Adverse Event Reporting System (VAERS) 1-800-822-7967 or online at https://vaers.hhs.gov/esub/index. In Canada, adverse reactions may be reported to local provincial/territorial health agencies or to the Vaccine Safety Section at Public Health Agency of Canada (1-866-844-0018).

Oral:
1% to 10%:
Central nervous system: Headache (5%), fever (3%)
Dermatologic: Rash (1%)
Gastrointestinal: Abdominal pain (6%), nausea (6%), diarrhea (3%), vomiting (2%)
Postmarketing and/or case reports: Anaphylactic reaction, demyelinating disease, myalgia, pain, RA, urticaria, sepsis, weakness
Injection (incidence may vary based on age and/or product used):
>10%:
Central nervous system: Fever (undefined; 2% to 32%), malaise (4% to 24%), headache (16% to 20%)
Local: Injection site: Tenderness (97% to 98%), pain (27% to 41%), soreness (up to 16%), induration (5% to 15%)
Neuromuscular & skeletal: General aches (1% to 13%)
1% to 10%:
Central nervous system: Fever ≥100°F (2%), >102°F (2%)
Dermatologic: Pruritus (up to 8%)
Gastrointestinal: Nausea (up to 8%), vomiting (2%)
Local: Injection site: Erythema (up to 5%), swelling (up to 4%)
Neuromuscular & skeletal: Myalgia (3% to 7%)

Drug Interactions

Avoid Concomitant Use
Avoid concomitant use of Typhoid Vaccine with any of the following: Belimumab; Fingolimod; Immunosuppressants

Increased Effect/Toxicity
The levels/effects of Typhoid Vaccine may be increased by: AzaTHIOprine; Belimumab; Corticosteroids (Systemic); Fingolimod; Hydroxychloroquine; Immunosuppressants; Leflunomide; Mercaptopurine; Methotrexate

Decreased Effect
Typhoid Vaccine may decrease the levels/effects of: Tuberculin Tests

The levels/effects of Typhoid Vaccine may be decreased by: Antibiotics; Fingolimod; Immune Globulins; Immunosuppressants

Ethanol/Nutrition/Herb Interactions Ethanol: Avoid alcohol within 2 hours of taking the capsule; may disrupt the enteric coating

Stability
Typherix®: Store between 2°C to 8°C (35°F to 46°F); do not freeze. Discard if vaccine has been frozen. Protect from light.
Typhim Vi®: Store between 2°C to 8°C (35°F to 46°F); do not freeze.
Vivotif®: Store between 2°C to 8°C (35°F to 46°F).

Mechanism of Action Virulent strains of *Salmonella typhi* cause disease by penetrating the intestinal mucosa and entering the systemic circulation via the lymphatic vasculature. One possible mechanism of conferring immunity may be the provocation of a local immune response in the intestinal tract induced by oral ingesting of a live strain with subsequent aborted infection. The ability of *Salmonella typhi* to produce clinical disease (and to elicit an immune response) is dependent on the bacteria having a complete lipopolysaccharide. The live attenuate Ty21a strain lacks the enzyme UDP-4-galactose epimerase so that lipopolysaccharide is only synthesized under conditions that induce bacterial autolysis. Thus, the strain remains avirulent despite the production of sufficient lipopolysaccharide to evoke a protective immune response. Despite low levels of lipopolysaccharide synthesis, cells lyse before gaining a virulent phenotype due to the intracellular accumulation of metabolic intermediates.

Pharmacodynamics/Kinetics
Onset of action: Immunity to *Salmonella typhi*: Oral: ~1 week
Duration: Immunity: Oral: ~4-7 years; Parenteral: Typhim Vi®: >17-21 months, Typherix®: ~3 years

Dosage

Geriatric & Adult Immunization:

Oral:

Primary immunization: One capsule on alternate days (day 1, 3, 5, and 7) for a total of 4 doses; all doses should be complete at least 1 week prior to potential exposure

Booster immunization (with repeated or continued exposure to typhoid fever):

U.S. labeling: Repeat full course of primary immunization every 5 years

Canadian labeling: Repeat full course of primary immunization every 7 years

I.M.:

Initial: 0.5 mL given at least 2 weeks prior to expected exposure

Reimmunization:

Typhim Vi®: 0.5 mL; optimal schedule has not been established; a single dose every 2 years is currently recommended for repeated or continued exposure

Typherix® (Canadian labeling; not available in U.S.): 0.5 mL every 3 years

Administration

Injection: Typhim Vi® and Typherix® may be given I.M. and are indicated for children ≥2 years of age; administer as a single 0.5 mL (25 mcg) injection in deltoid muscle. **Do not administer Typhim Vi® or Typherix® intravascularly. Note:** For patients at risk of hemorrhage following intramuscular injection, the ACIP recommends "it should be administered intramuscularly if, in the opinion of the physician familiar with the patients bleeding risk, the vaccine can be administered by this route with reasonable safety. If the patient receives antihemophilia or other similar therapy, intramuscular vaccination can be scheduled shortly after such therapy is administered. A fine needle (23 gauge or smaller) can be used for the vaccination and firm pressure applied to the site (without rubbing) for at least 2 minutes. The patient should be instructed concerning the risk of hematoma from the injection." Patients on anticoagulant therapy should be considered to have the same bleeding risks and treated as those with clotting factor disorders (CDC, 2011).

Oral: Swallow capsule whole soon after placing into mouth; do not chew or open capsule. Capsule should be taken with a cold or lukewarm beverage (≤37°C/98.6°F). Take 1 hour prior to a meal. Avoid alcohol 1 hour before or 2 hours after administration.

Simultaneous administration of vaccines helps ensure patients will be fully vaccinated by the appropriate age. Simultaneous administration of vaccines is defined as administering >1 vaccine on the same day at different anatomic sites. The ACIP prefers each dose of a specific vaccine in a series come from the same manufacturer when possible. Adolescents and adults should be vaccinated while seated or lying down. In general, preterm infants should be vaccinated at the same chronological age as full-term infants (CDC, 2011).

Antipyretics have not been shown to prevent febrile seizures. Antipyretics may be used to treat fever or discomfort following vaccination (CDC, 2011). One study reported that routine prophylactic administration of acetaminophen to prevent fever prior to vaccination decreased the immune response of some vaccines; the clinical significance of this reduction in immune response has not been established (Prymula, 2009).

Monitoring Parameters Monitor for syncope for ≥15 minutes following vaccination

Pharmacotherapy Pearls Federal law requires that the name of medication, date of administration, the vaccine manufacturer, lot number of vaccine, and the administering person's name, title, and address be entered into the patient's permanent medical record.

Special Geriatric Considerations Vaccinating elderly is often overlooked; if no record of immunization can be recalled, repeat primary series.

Dosage Forms Excipient information presented when available (limited, particularly for generics); consult specific product labeling.

Capsule, enteric coated [live]:

Vivotif®: Viable *S. typhi* Ty21a 2-6.8 x 10^9 colony-forming units and nonviable *S. typhi* Ty21a 5-50 x 10^9 bacterial cells [contains lactose 100-180 mg/capsule and sucrose 26-130 mg/capsule]

Injection, solution [inactivated]:

Typhim Vi®: Purified Vi capsular polysaccharide 25 mcg/0.5 mL (0.5 mL, 10 mL) [derived from *S. typhi* Ty2 strain]

Dosage Forms: Canada Excipient information presented when available (limited, particularly for generics); consult specific product labeling.

Injection, solution:

Typherix®: Vi capsular polysaccharide 25 mcg/0.5 mL (0.5 mL) [derived from *S. typhi* Ty2 strain]

Selected References

Begier EM, Burewn DR, Haber P, et al, "Postmarketing Safety Surveillance for Typhoid Fever Vaccines From the Vaccine Adverse Event Reporting System, July 1990 Through June 2002," *Clin Infect Dis*, 2004, 38(6):771-9.

"Canadian Immunization Guide, Seventh Edition, 2006," Ottawa, ONT: Minister of Public Works and Government Services Canada, Public Health Agency of Canada, National Advisory Committee on Immunization, 2006. Available at http://www.phac-aspc.gc.ca/publicat/cig-gci/index.html

Centers for Disease Control, "Recommendations of the Advisory Committee on Immunization Practices (ACIP): General Recommendations on Immunization," *MMWR Recomm Rep*, 2006, 55(RR-15):1-48.

Guzman CA, Borsutzky S, Griot-Wenk M, et al, "Vaccines Against Typhoid Fever," *Vaccine*, 2006, 24(18):3804-11.

Parry CM, Hien TT, Dougan G, et al, "Typhoid Fever," *N Engl J Med*, 2002, 347(22):1770-82.

Ursodiol (ur soe DYE ol)

Medication Safety Issues
Sound-alike/look-alike issues:
Ursodiol may be confused with ulipristal
Brand Names: U.S. Actigall®; Urso 250®; Urso Forte®
Brand Names: Canada Dom-Ursodiol C; PHL-Ursodiol C; PMS-Ursodiol C; Urso®; Urso® DS
Index Terms Ursodeoxycholic Acid
Generic Availability (U.S.) Yes
Pharmacologic Category Gallstone Dissolution Agent
Use
Actigall®: Gallbladder stone dissolution; prevention of gallstones in obese patients experiencing rapid weight loss
Urso®, Urso Forte®: Primary biliary cirrhosis
Unlabeled/Investigational Use Liver transplantation
Contraindications Hypersensitivity to ursodiol or any component of the formulation; not to be used with cholesterol, radiopaque, bile pigment stones; patients with unremitting acute cholecystitis, cholangitis, biliary obstruction, gallstone pancreatitis, or biliary-gastrointestinal fistula; allergy to bile acids
Warnings/Precautions Gallbladder stone dissolution may take several months of therapy. Complete dissolution may not occur and recurrence of stones within 5 years has been observed in 50% of patients. Use with caution in patients with a nonvisualizing gallbladder and those with chronic liver disease.

Adverse Reactions (Reflective of adult population; not specific for elderly)
>10%:
  Central nervous system: Headache (up to 25%), dizziness (17%)
  Gastrointestinal: Diarrhea (up to 27%), constipation (up to 26%), dyspepsia (17%), nausea
    (up to 17%), vomiting (up to 14%)
  Neuromuscular & skeletal: Back pain (up to 12%)
  Respiratory: Upper respiratory tract infection (up to 16%)
1% to 10%:
  Dermatologic: Alopecia (5%), rash (3%)
  Endocrine & metabolic: Hyperglycemia (1%)
  Gastrointestinal: Flatulence (up to 8%), peptic ulcer (1%)
  Genitourinary: Urinary tract infection (7%)
  Hematologic: Leukopenia (3%), thrombocytopenia (1%)
  Hepatic: Cholecystitis (5%)
  Neuromuscular & skeletal: Arthritis (6%), myalgia (6%)
  Renal: Serum creatinine increased (1%)
  Respiratory: Pharyngitis (up to 8%), bronchitis (7%), cough (7%)
  Miscellaneous: Viral infection (9%), flu-like syndrome (7%), allergy (5%)
Drug Interactions
  Avoid Concomitant Use There are no known interactions where it is recommended to
    avoid concomitant use.
  Increased Effect/Toxicity There are no known significant interactions involving an increase
    in effect.
  Decreased Effect
    Ursodiol may decrease the levels/effects of: Nitrendipine

    The levels/effects of Ursodiol may be decreased by: Aluminum Hydroxide; Bile Acid
    Sequestrants; Estrogen Derivatives; Fibric Acid Derivatives
Stability
  Actigall®: Store at 25°C (77°F); excursions permitted to 15°C to 30°C (59°F to 86°F).
  Urso®: Store at 20°C to 25°C (68°F to 77°F).
  Urso Forte®: Store at 20°C to 25°C (68°F to 77°F). When broken in half, scored Urso Forte®
    500 mg tablets maintain quality for up to 28 days when kept in current packaging and stored
    at 20°C to 25°C (68°F to 77°F). Split tablets should be stored separately from whole tablets
    due to bitter taste.
Mechanism of Action Decreases the cholesterol content of bile and bile stones by reducing
  the secretion of cholesterol from the liver and the fractional reabsorption of cholesterol by the
  intestines. Mechanism of action in primary biliary cirrhosis is not clearly defined.
Pharmacodynamics/Kinetics
  Protein binding: ~70%
  Metabolism: Undergoes extensive enterohepatic recycling; following hepatic conjugation and
    biliary secretion, the drug is hydrolyzed to active ursodiol, where it is recycled or transformed
    to lithocholic acid by colonic microbial flora
  Excretion: Feces; urine (<1%)
Dosage
  Geriatric & Adult
    Gallstone dissolution (Actigall®): Oral: 8-10 mg/kg/day in 2-3 divided doses; use beyond
      24 months is not established
    Gallstone prevention (Actigall®): Oral: 300 mg twice daily
    Primary biliary cirrhosis (Urso®, Urso Forte®): Oral: 13-15 mg/kg/day in 2-4 divided
      doses (with food)
Administration Oral: Do not administer with aluminum-based antacids. If aluminum-based
  antacids are needed, administer 2 hours after ursodiol.
Monitoring Parameters
  Gallstone disease: ALT, ALP, AST at initiation, 1 and 3 months and every 6 months thereafter,
    sonogram
  Hepatic disease: Monitor hepatic function tests frequently
Special Geriatric Considerations No specific clinical studies in the elderly. Would recom-
  mend starting at lowest recommended dose with scheduled monitoring.
Dosage Forms Excipient information presented when available (limited, particularly for
  generics); consult specific product labeling.
  Capsule, oral: 300 mg
    Actigall®: 300 mg
  Tablet, oral: 250 mg, 500 mg
    Urso 250®: 250 mg
    Urso Forte®: 500 mg [scored]

◆ **Urso Forte®** *see* Ursodiol *on page 1882*

Ustekinumab (yoo stek in YOO mab)

Medication Safety Issues
Sound-alike/look-alike issues:
Stelara™ may be confused with Aldara®
Ustekinumab may be confused with infliximab, rituximab
Brand Names: U.S. Stelara™
Brand Names: Canada Stelara™
Index Terms CNTO 1275
Generic Availability (U.S.) No
Pharmacologic Category Antipsoriatic Agent; Interleukin-12 Inhibitor; Interleukin-23 Inhibitor; Monoclonal Antibody
Use Treatment of moderate-to-severe plaque psoriasis
Medication Guide Available Yes
Contraindications There are no contraindications listed within the manufacturer's labeling.

Canadian labeling (not in U.S. labeling): Hypersensitivity to ustekinumab or any component of the formulation; severe infections such as sepsis, tuberculosis and opportunistic infections
Warnings/Precautions May increase the risk for malignancy although the impact on the development and course of malignancies is not fully defined. In clinical trials, the incidence of malignancy associated with therapy was comparable to that of the general population. Use with caution in patients with prior malignancy (use not studied in this population).

Infrequent, but serious bacterial, fungal, and viral infections have been observed with use. Avoid use in patients with clinically important active infection. Caution should be exercised when considering use in patients with a history of new/recurrent infections, with conditions that predispose them to infections (eg, diabetes or residence/travel from areas of endemic mycoses), or with chronic, latent, or localized infections. Patients who develop a new infection while undergoing treatment should be monitored closely. If a patient develops a serious infection, therapy should be discontinued or withheld until successful resolution of infection.

Avoid use in patients with active tuberculosis (TB). Patients should be evaluated for latent tuberculosis infection with a tuberculin skin test prior to starting therapy. Treatment of latent TB should be initiated before ustekinumab therapy is used.

Antibody formation to ustekinumab has been observed with therapy and has been associated with decreased serum levels and therapeutic response in some patients. Discontinue immediately with signs/symptoms of hypersensitivity reaction and treat appropriately as indicated. Use in combination with other immunosuppressive drugs or phototherapy has not been studied. Patients should be brought up to date with all immunizations before initiating therapy. **Live vaccines should not be given concurrently;** inactivated or nonlive vaccines may be given concurrently. BCG vaccines should not be given 1 year prior to, during, or 1 year following treatment. Patients >100 kg may require higher dose to achieve adequate serum levels. Use in hepatic or renal impairment has not been studied.

The packaging may contain latex. Product may contain polysorbate 80.
Adverse Reactions (Reflective of adult population; not specific for elderly)
>10%: Miscellaneous: Infection (27% to 61%)
1% to 10%:
Central nervous system: Headache (5%), fatigue (3%), dizziness (1% to 2%), depression (1%)
Dermatologic: Pruritus (1% to 2%), rash (<2%), urticaria (<2%)
Local: Injection site erythema (1% to 2%)
Neuromuscular & skeletal: Back pain (1% to 2%)
Respiratory: Pharyngolaryngeal pain (1% to 2%)
Miscellaneous: Antibody formation (3% to 5%)
Drug Interactions
Avoid Concomitant Use
Avoid concomitant use of Ustekinumab with any of the following: BCG; Belimumab; Natalizumab; Pimecrolimus; Tacrolimus (Topical); Vaccines (Live)
Increased Effect/Toxicity
Ustekinumab may increase the levels/effects of: Belimumab; Leflunomide; Natalizumab; Vaccines (Live)

The levels/effects of Ustekinumab may be increased by: Abciximab; Denosumab; Pimecrolimus; Roflumilast; Tacrolimus (Topical); Trastuzumab

Decreased Effect

Ustekinumab may decrease the levels/effects of: BCG; Sipuleucel-T; Vaccines (Inactivated); Vaccines (Live)

The levels/effects of Ustekinumab may be decreased by: Echinacea

Stability Store vials refrigerated at 2°C to 8°C (36°F to 46°F); do not freeze. Do not shake. Protect from light; store in original container. Discard any unused portion.

Mechanism of Action Ustekinumab is a human monoclonal antibody that binds to and interferes with the proinflammatory cytokines, interleukin (IL)-12 and IL-23. Biological effects of IL-12 and IL-23 include natural killer (NK) cell activation, CD4+ T-cell differentiation and activation. Ustekinumab also interferes with the expression of monocyte chemotactic protein-1 (MCP-1), tumor necrosis factor-alpha (TNF-α), interferon-inducible protein-10 (IP-10), and interleukin-8 (IL-8). Significant clinical improvement in psoriasis patients is seen in association with reduction of these proinflammatory signalers.

Pharmacodynamics/Kinetics

Distribution: V_d (terminal elimination phase): 0.096-0.264 L/kg

Bioavailability: Absolute bioavailability: SubQ: ~57%

Half-life elimination: 10-126 days

Time to peak, plasma: 7-13.5 days

Dosage

Geriatric & Adult Plaque psoriasis: SubQ:

Initial and maintenance: **Note:** Following an interruption in therapy, retreatment may be initiated at the initial dosing interval. Consider therapy discontinuation in any patient failing to demonstrate a response after 12 weeks of therapy.

≤100 kg: 45 mg at 0- and 4 weeks, and then every 12 weeks thereafter

>100 kg: 45 mg or 90 mg at 0- and 4 weeks, and then every 12 weeks thereafter

Per Canadian labeling, if response inadequate on every 12 week therapy, may increase to every 8 weeks.

Renal Impairment Use has not been studied in renal dysfunction.

Hepatic Impairment Use has not been studied in hepatic dysfunction.

Administration Do not use if cloudy or discolored. Administer by subcutaneous injection into the top of the thigh, abdomen, upper arms, or buttocks. Rotate sites. Avoid areas of skin where psoriasis is present.

Monitoring Parameters Place and read PPD prior to initiating therapy; monitor for signs/symptoms of infection; CBC; Ustekinumab-antibody formation

Special Geriatric Considerations Studies to date have not had sufficient numbers of elderly to demonstrate differences in safety and efficacy between elderly and younger adults.

Dosage Forms Excipient information presented when available (limited, particularly for generics); consult specific product labeling.

Injection, solution [preservative free]:

Stelara™: 45 mg/0.5 mL (0.5 mL) [contains natural rubber/natural latex in packaging, polysorbate 80, sucrose 38 mg/syringe]

Stelara™: 90 mg/mL (1 mL) [contains natural rubber/natural latex in packaging, polysorbate 80, sucrose 76 mg/syringe]

Dosage Forms: Canada Excipient information presented when available (limited, particularly for generics); consult specific product labeling.

Injection, solution [preservative free]:

Stelara™: 45 mg/0.5 mL (0.5 mL)

Selected References

Leonardi CL, Kimball AB, Papp KA, et al, "Efficacy and Safety of Ustekinumab, a Human Interleukin-12/23 Monoclonal Antibody, in Patients With Psoriasis: 76-Week Results from a Randomised, Double-Blind, Placebo-Controlled Trial (PHOENIX 1)," Lancet, 2008, 371(9625): 1665-74.

Papp KA, Langley RG, Lebwohl M, et al, "Efficacy and Safety of Ustekinumab, a Human Interleukin-12/23 Monoclonal Antibody, in Patients With Psoriasis: 52-Week Results from a Randomised, Double-Blind, Placebo-Controlled Trial (PHOENIX 2)," Lancet, 2008, 371(9625): 1675-84.

Reddy M, Davis C, Wong J, et al, "Modulation of CLA, IL-12R, CD40L, and II-2Rα Expression and Inhibition of IL-12- and IL-23-Induced Cytokine Secretion by CNTO 1275," Cell Immunol, 2007, 247(1): 1-11.

◆ **UTI Relief® [OTC]** *see* Phenazopyridine *on page 1433*

◆ **Vagifem®** *see* Estradiol (Topical) *on page 648*

◆ **Vagistat®-1 [OTC]** *see* Tioconazole *on page 1803*

ValACYclovir (val ay SYE kloe veer)

Medication Safety Issues

Sound-alike/look-alike issues:

Valtrex® may be confused with Keflex®, Valcyte®, Zovirax®

ValACYclovir may be confused with acyclovir, valGANciclovir, vancomycin

Brand Names: U.S. Valtrex®

◀ **Brand Names: Canada** Apo-Valacyclovir®; Mylan-Valacyclovir; PHL-Valacyclovir; PMS-Valacyclovir; PRO-Valacyclovir; Riva-Valacyclovir; Valtrex®

Index Terms Valacyclovir Hydrochloride

Generic Availability (U.S.) Yes

Pharmacologic Category Antiviral Agent; Antiviral Agent, Oral

Use Treatment of herpes zoster (shingles) in immunocompetent patients; treatment of first-episode and recurrent genital herpes; suppression of recurrent genital herpes and reduction of heterosexual transmission of genital herpes in immunocompetent patients; suppression of genital herpes in HIV-infected individuals; treatment of herpes labialis (cold sores)

Unlabeled/Investigational Use Prophylaxis of cancer-related HSV, VZV, and CMV infections; treatment of cancer-related HSV, VZV infection

Contraindications Hypersensitivity to valacyclovir, acyclovir, or any component of the formulation

Warnings/Precautions Thrombotic thrombocytopenic purpura/hemolytic uremic syndrome has occurred in immunocompromised patients (at doses of 8 g/day). Safety and efficacy have not been established for treatment/suppression of recurrent genital herpes or disseminated herpes in patients with profound immunosuppression (eg, advanced HIV with CD4 <100 cells/mm^3). CNS adverse effects (including agitation, hallucinations, confusion, delirium, seizures, and encephalopathy) have been reported. Use caution in patients with renal impairment, the elderly, and/or those receiving nephrotoxic agents. Acute renal failure has been observed in patients with renal dysfunction; dose adjustment may be required. Decreased precipitation in renal tubules may occur leading to urinary precipitation; adequately hydrate patient. For cold sores, treatment should begin at with earliest symptom (tingling, itching, burning). For genital herpes, treatment should begin as soon as possible after the first signs and symptoms (within 72 hours of onset of first diagnosis or within 24 hours of onset of recurrent episodes). For herpes zoster, treatment should begin within 72 hours of onset of rash. For chickenpox, treatment should begin with earliest sign or symptom. Use with caution in the elderly; CNS effects have been reported. Safety and efficacy have not been established in patients <2 years of age.

Adverse Reactions (Reflective of adult population; not specific for elderly)

>10%:
  Central nervous system: Headache (13% to 38%)
  Gastrointestinal: Nausea (5% to 15%), abdominal pain (1% to 11%)
  Hematologic: Neutropenia (≤18%)
  Hepatic: ALT increased (≤14%), AST increased (2% to 16%)
  Respiratory: Nasopharyngitis (≤16%)

1% to 10%:
  Central nervous system: Fatigue (≤8%), depression (≤7%), fever (children 4%), dizziness (2% to 4%)
  Dermatologic: Rash (≤8%)
  Endocrine: Dysmenorrhea (≤1% to 8%), dehydration (children 2%)
  Gastrointestinal: Vomiting (<1% to 6%), diarrhea (children 5%; adults <1%)
  Hematologic: Thrombocytopenia (≤3%)
  Hepatic: Alkaline phosphatase increased (≤4%)
  Neuromuscular & skeletal: Arthralgia (<1 to 6%)
  Respiratory: Rhinorrhea (children 2%)
  Miscellaneous: Herpes simplex (children 2%)

Drug Interactions

  Avoid Concomitant Use
  Avoid concomitant use of ValACYclovir with any of the following: Zoster Vaccine

  Increased Effect/Toxicity
  ValACYclovir may increase the levels/effects of: Mycophenolate; Tenofovir; Zidovudine

  The levels/effects of ValACYclovir may be increased by: Mycophenolate

  Decreased Effect
  ValACYclovir may decrease the levels/effects of: Zoster Vaccine

Stability Store at 15°C to 25°C (59°F to 77°F).

Mechanism of Action Valacyclovir is rapidly and nearly completely converted to acyclovir by intestinal and hepatic metabolism. Acyclovir is converted to acyclovir monophosphate by virus-specific thymidine kinase then further converted to acyclovir triphosphate by other cellular enzymes. Acyclovir triphosphate inhibits DNA synthesis and viral replication by competing with deoxyguanosine triphosphate for viral DNA polymerase and being incorporated into viral DNA.

Pharmacodynamics/Kinetics

  Absorption: Rapid
  Distribution: Acyclovir is widely distributed throughout the body including brain, kidney, lungs, liver, spleen, muscle, uterus, vagina, and CSF

Protein binding: ~14% to 18%

Metabolism: Hepatic; valacyclovir is rapidly and nearly completely converted to acyclovir and L-valine by first-pass effect; acyclovir is hepatically metabolized to a very small extent by aldehyde oxidase and by alcohol and aldehyde dehydrogenase (inactive metabolites)

Bioavailability: ~55% once converted to acyclovir

Half-life elimination: Normal renal function: Adults: Acyclovir: 2.5-3.3 hours, Valacyclovir: ~30 minutes; End-stage renal disease: Acyclovir: 14-20 hours; During hemodialysis: 4 hours

Excretion: Urine, primarily as acyclovir (89%). Note: Following oral administration of radio-labeled valacyclovir, 46% of the label is eliminated in the feces (corresponding to non-absorbed drug), while 47% of the radiolabel is eliminated in the urine.

Dosage

Geriatric & Adult

CMV prophylaxis in allogeneic HSCT recipients (unlabeled use): 2 g 4 times/day

Herpes labialis (cold sores): Oral: 2 g twice daily for 1 day (separate doses by ~12 hours)

Herpes zoster (shingles): Oral: 1 g 3 times/day for 7 days

HSV, VZV in cancer patients (unlabeled use):
  Prophylaxis: 500 mg 2-3 times/day
  Treatment: 1 g 3 times/day

Genital herpes: Oral:
  Initial episode: 1 g twice daily for 10 days
  Recurrent episode: 500 mg twice daily for 3 days
  Reduction of transmission: 500 mg once daily (source partner)
  Suppressive therapy:
    Immunocompetent patients: 1000 mg once daily (500 mg once daily in patients with <9 recurrences per year)
    HIV-infected patients (CD4 ≥100 cells/mm^3): 500 mg twice daily

Renal Impairment

Herpes zoster: Adults:
  Cl_{cr} 30-49 mL/minute: 1 g every 12 hours
  Cl_{cr} 10-29 mL/minute: 1 g every 24 hours
  Cl_{cr} <10 mL/minute: 500 mg every 24 hours

Genital herpes: Adults:
  Initial episode:
    Cl_{cr} 10-29 mL/minute: 1 g every 24 hours
    Cl_{cr} <10 mL/minute: 500 mg every 24 hours
  Recurrent episode: Cl_{cr} <29 mL/minute: 500 mg every 24 hours
  Suppressive therapy: Cl_{cr} <29 mL/minute:
    For usual dose of 1 g every 24 hours, decrease dose to 500 mg every 24 hours
    For usual dose of 500 mg every 24 hours, decrease dose to 500 mg every 48 hours
    HIV-infected patients: 500 mg every 24 hours

Herpes labialis:
  Cl_{cr} 30-49 mL/minute: 1 g every 12 hours for 2 doses
  Cl_{cr} 10-29 mL/minute: 500 mg every 12 hours for 2 doses
  Cl_{cr} <10 mL/minute: 500 mg as a single dose

Hemodialysis: Dialyzable (~33% removed during 4-hour session); administer dose post-dialysis

Chronic ambulatory peritoneal dialysis/continuous arteriovenous hemofiltration dialysis: Pharmacokinetic parameters are similar to those in patients with ESRD; supplemental dose not needed following dialysis

Hepatic Impairment No adjustment required.

Administration If GI upset occurs, administer with meals.

Monitoring Parameters Urinalysis, BUN, serum creatinine, liver enzymes, and CBC

Special Geriatric Considerations More convenient dosing and increased bioavailability, without increasing side effects, make valacyclovir a favorable choice compared to acyclovir. Has been shown to accelerate resolution of postherpetic pain. Adjust dose for renal impairment.

Dosage Forms Excipient information presented when available (limited, particularly for generics); consult specific product labeling.
Caplet, oral: 500 mg, 1 g
  Valtrex®: 500 mg
  Valtrex®: 1 g [scored]
Tablet, oral: 500 mg, 1 g

Extemporaneously Prepared To prepare a valacyclovir 25 mg/mL oral suspension, crush five valacyclovir 500 mg caplets (10 caplets for 50 mg/mL suspension) into a fine powder in a mortar. Gradually add 5 mL aliquots of Suspension Structured Vehicle USP-NF (SSV) to powder and triturate until a paste is formed. Continue adding 5 mL aliquots of SSV to the mortar until a suspension is formed (minimum 20 mL SSV and maximum 40 mL SSV).

◄ Transfer to 100 mL bottle. Add the cherry flavor (amount recommended on package) to the mortar and dissolve in ~5 mL of SSV. Add to bottle once dissolved. Rinse the mortar at least 3 times with ~5 mL of SSV, transferring contents between additions of SSV. Continue to add the SSV to bring final volume to 100 mL. The preparation is stable for 28 days under refrigeration; shake well before using. (Refer to manufacturer's current labeling.)

Selected References

Beutner KR, Friedman DJ, Forszpaniak C, et al, "Valacyclovir Compared With Acyclovir for Improved Therapy for Herpes Zoster in Immunocompetent Adults," *Antimicrob Agents Chemother*, 1995, 39(7):1546-53.

National Comprehensive Cancer Network (NCCN), "Clinical Practice Guidelines in Oncology™: Prevention and Treatment of Cancer-Related Infections," Version 1, 2008. Available at http://www.nccn.org/professionals/physician_gls/PDF/infections.pdf.

◆ **Valacyclovir Hydrochloride** see ValACYclovir on page 1885

◆ **23-Valent Pneumococcal Polysaccharide Vaccine** see Pneumococcal Polysaccharide Vaccine (Polyvalent) on page 1474

◆ **Valium®** see Diazepam on page 493

◆ **Valorin [OTC]** see Acetaminophen on page 33

◆ **Valorin Extra [OTC]** see Acetaminophen on page 33

◆ **Valproate Semisodium** see Divalproex on page 541

◆ **Valproate Semisodium** see Valproic Acid on page 1888

◆ **Valproate Sodium** see Valproic Acid on page 1888

Valproic Acid (val PROE ik AS id)

Related Information

Liquid Compatibility of Antidepressants, Antipsychotics, and Mood Stabilizers on page 2111

Medication Safety Issues

Sound-alike/look-alike issues:

Depakene® may be confused with Depakote®

Valproate sodium may be confused with vecuronium

Brand Names: U.S. Depacon®; Depakene®; Stavzor™

Brand Names: Canada Apo-Valproic®; Depakene®; Epival® I.V.; Mylan-Valproic; PHL-Valproic Acid; PHL-Valproic Acid E.C.; PMS-Valproic Acid; PMS-Valproic Acid E.C.; ratio-Valproic; ratio-Valproic ECC; Rhoxal-valproic; Sandoz-Valproic

Index Terms 2-Propylpentanoic Acid; 2-Propylvaleric Acid; Dipropylacetic Acid; DPA; Valproate Semisodium; Valproate Sodium

Generic Availability (U.S.) Yes: Excludes delayed release capsule

Pharmacologic Category Anticonvulsant, Miscellaneous; Antimanic Agent; Histone Deacetylase Inhibitor

Use Monotherapy and adjunctive therapy in the treatment of patients with complex partial seizures; monotherapy and adjunctive therapy of simple and complex absence seizures; adjunctive therapy in patients with multiple seizure types that include absence seizures

Stavzor™: Mania associated with bipolar disorder; migraine prophylaxis

Unlabeled/Investigational Use Status epilepticus, diabetic neuropathy

Contraindications Hypersensitivity to valproic acid, derivatives, or any component of the formulation; hepatic disease or significant impairment; urea cycle disorders

Warnings/Precautions

[U.S. Boxed Warning]: Hepatic failure resulting in fatalities has occurred in patients. Other risk factors include organic brain disease, mental retardation with severe seizure disorders, congenital metabolic disorders, and patients on multiple anticonvulsants. Hepatotoxicity has usually been reported within 6 months of therapy initiation. Monitor patients closely for appearance of malaise, weakness, facial edema, anorexia, jaundice, and vomiting; discontinue immediately with signs/symptom of significant or suspected impairment. Liver function tests should be performed at baseline and at regular intervals after initiation of therapy, especially within the first 6 months. Hepatic dysfunction may progress despite discontinuing treatment. Should only be used as monotherapy in patients at high risk for hepatotoxicity. Contraindicated with severe impairment.

[U.S. Boxed Warning]: Cases of life-threatening pancreatitis, occurring at the start of therapy or following years of use, have been reported in adults and children. Some cases have been hemorrhagic with rapid progression of initial symptoms to death. Promptly evaluate symptoms of abdominal pain, nausea, vomiting, and/or anorexia; should generally be discontinued if pancreatitis is diagnosed.

May cause severe thrombocytopenia, inhibition of platelet aggregation, and bleeding. Tremors may indicate overdosage; use with caution in patients receiving other anticonvulsants. Hypersensitivity reactions affecting multiple organs have been reported in association with valproic acid use; may include dermatologic and/or hematologic changes (eosinophilia, neutropenia, thrombocytopenia) or symptoms of organ dysfunction.

Hyperammonemia and/or encephalopathy, sometimes fatal, have been reported following the initiation of valproic acid therapy and may be present with normal transaminase levels. Ammonia levels should be measured in patients who develop unexplained lethargy and vomiting, changes in mental status, or in patients who present with hypothermia (unintentional drop in core body temperature to <35°C/95°F). Discontinue therapy if ammonia levels are increased and evaluate for possible urea cycle disorder (UCD); contraindicated in patients with UCD. Evaluation of UCD should be considered for the following patients prior to the start of therapy: History of unexplained encephalopathy or coma; encephalopathy associated with protein load; unexplained mental retardation; history of elevated plasma ammonia or gluta-mine; history of cyclical vomiting and lethargy; episodic extreme irritability, ataxia; low BUN or protein avoidance; family history of UCD or unexplained infant deaths (particularly male); or signs or symptoms of UCD (hyperammonemia, encephalopathy, respiratory alkalosis). Hypo-thermia has been reported with valproic acid therapy; may or may not be associated with hyperammonemia; may also occur with concomitant topiramate therapy.

In vitro studies have suggested valproic acid stimulates the replication of HIV and CMV viruses under experimental conditions. The clinical consequence of this is unknown, but should be considered when monitoring affected patients.

Antiepileptics are associated with an increased risk of suicidal behavior/thoughts with use (regardless of indication); patients should be monitored for signs/symptoms of depression, suicidal tendencies, and other unusual behavior changes during therapy and instructed to inform their healthcare provider immediately if symptoms occur.

Use of Depacon® injection is not recommended for post-traumatic seizure prophylaxis following acute head trauma. Anticonvulsants should not be discontinued abruptly because of the possibility of increasing seizure frequency; valproic acid should be withdrawn gradually to minimize the potential of increased seizure frequency, unless safety concerns require a more rapid withdrawal. Concomitant use with carbapenem antibiotics may reduce valproic acid levels to subtherapeutic levels; monitor levels frequently and consider alternate therapy if levels drop significantly or lack of seizure control occurs. Concomitant use with clonazepam may induce absence status. Patients treated for bipolar disorder should be monitored closely for clinical worsening or suicidality; prescriptions should be written for the smallest quantity consistent with good patient care.

CNS depression may occur with valproic acid use. Patients must be cautioned about performing tasks which require mental alertness (operating machinery or driving). Effects with other sedative drugs or ethanol may be potentiated. Use with caution in the elderly.

Adverse Reactions (Reflective of adult population; not specific for elderly)
>10%:
  Central nervous system: Headache (≤31%), somnolence (≤30%), dizziness (12% to 25%), insomnia (>1% to 15%), nervousness (>1% to 11%), pain (1% to 11%)
  Dermatologic: Alopecia (>1% to 24%)
  Gastrointestinal: Nausea (15% to 48%), vomiting (7% to 27%), diarrhea (7% to 23%), abdominal pain (7% to 23%), dyspepsia (7% to 23%), anorexia (>1% to 12%)
  Hematologic: Thrombocytopenia (1% to 24%; dose related)
  Neuromuscular & skeletal: Tremor (≤57%), weakness (6% to 27%)
  Ocular: Diplopia (>1% to 16%), amblyopia/blurred vision (≤12%)
  Miscellaneous: Infection (≤20%), flu-like syndrome (12%)
1% to 10%:
  Cardiovascular: Peripheral edema (>1% to 8%), chest pain (>1% to <5%), edema (>1% to <5%), facial edema (>1% to <5%), hypertension (>1% to <5%), hypotension (>1% to <5%), palpitation (>1% to <5%), postural hypotension (>1% to <5%), tachycardia (>1% to <5%), vasodilation (>1% to <5%), arrhythmia
  Central nervous system: Ataxia (>1% to 8%), amnesia (>1% to 7%), emotional lability (>1% to 6%), fever (>1% to 6%), abnormal thinking (≤6%), depression (>1% to 5%), abnormal dreams (>1% to <5%), agitation (>1% to <5%), anxiety (>1% to <5%), catatonia (>1% to <5%), chills (>1% to <5%), confusion (>1% to <5%), coordination abnormal (>1% to <5%), hallucination (>1% to <5%), malaise (>1% to <5%), personality disorder (>1% to <5%), speech disorder (>1% to <5%), tardive dyskinesia (>1% to <5%), vertigo (>1% to <5%), euphoria (1%), hypoesthesia (1%)
  Dermatologic: Rash (>1% to 6%), bruising (>1% to 5%), discoid lupus erythematosus (>1% to <5%), dry skin (>1% to <5%), furunculosis (>1% to <5%), petechia (>1% to <5%), pruritus (>1% to <5), seborrhea (>1% to <5%)
  Endocrine & metabolic: Amenorrhea (>1% to <5%), dysmenorrhea (>1% to <5%), metror-rhagia (>1% to <5%), hypoproteinemia

Gastrointestinal: Weight gain (4% to 9%), weight loss (6%), appetite increased (≤6%), constipation (>1% to 5%), xerostomia (>1% to 5%), eructation (>1% to <5%), fecal incontinence (>1% to <5%), flatulence (>1% to <5%), gastroenteritis (>1% to <5%), glossitis (>1% to <5%), hematemesis (>1% to <5%), pancreatitis (>1% to <5%), periodontal abscess (>1% to <5%), stomatitis (>1% to <5%), taste perversion (>1% to <5%), dysphagia, gum hemorrhage, mouth ulceration

Genitourinary: Cystitis (>1% to 5%), dysuria (>1% to 5%), urinary frequency (>1% to <5%), urinary incontinence (>1% to <5%), vaginal hemorrhage (>1% to 5%), vaginitis (>1% to <5%)

Hepatic: ALT increased (>1% to <5%), AST increased (>1% to <5%)

Local: Injection site pain (3%), injection site reaction (2%), injection site inflammation (1%)

Neuromuscular & skeletal: Back pain (≤8%), abnormal gait (>1% to <5%), arthralgia (>1% to <5%), arthrosis (>1% to <5%), dysarthria (>1% to <5%), hypertonia (>1% to <5%), hypokinesia (>1% to <5%), leg cramps (>1% to <5%), myalgia (>1% to <5%), myasthenia (>1% to <5%), neck pain (>1% to <5%), neck rigidity (>1% to <5%), paresthesia (>1% to <5%), reflex increased (>1% to <5%), twitching (>1% to <5%)

Ocular: Nystagmus (1% to 8%), dry eyes (>1% to 5%), eye pain (>1% to 5%), abnormal vision (>1% to <5%), conjunctivitis (>1% to <5%)

Otic: Tinnitus (1% to 7%), ear pain (>1% to 5%), deafness (>1% to <5%), otitis media (>1% to <5%)

Respiratory: Pharyngitis (2% to 8%), bronchitis (5%), rhinitis (>1% to 5%), dyspnea (1% to 5%), cough (>1% to <5%), epistaxis (>1% to <5%), pneumonia (>1% to <5%), sinusitis (>1% to <5%)

Miscellaneous: Diaphoresis (1%), hiccups

Drug Interactions

Metabolism/Transport Effects For valproic acid: **Substrate** (minor) of CYP2A6, 2B6, 2C9, 2C19, 2E1; **Inhibits** CYP2C9 (weak), 2C19 (weak), 2D6 (weak), 3A4 (weak); **Induces** CYP2A6 (weak)

Avoid Concomitant Use There are no known interactions where it is recommended to avoid concomitant use.

Increased Effect/Toxicity

Valproic Acid may increase the levels/effects of: Barbiturates; Ethosuximide; LamoTRIgine; LORazepam; Paliperidone; Primidone; RisperiDONE; Rufinamide; Temozolomide; Tricyclic Antidepressants; Vorinostat; Zidovudine

The levels/effects of Valproic Acid may be increased by: ChlorproMAZINE; Felbamate; GuanFACINE; Salicylates; Topiramate

Decreased Effect

Valproic Acid may decrease the levels/effects of: CarBAMazepine; Fosphenytoin; OXcarbazepine; Phenytoin

The levels/effects of Valproic Acid may be decreased by: Barbiturates; CarBAMazepine; Carbapenems; Cyproterone; Ethosuximide; Fosphenytoin; Methylfolate; Phenytoin; Primidone; Protease Inhibitors; Rifampin

Ethanol/Nutrition/Herb Interactions

Ethanol: Avoid ethanol (may increase CNS depression).

Food: Food may delay but does not affect the extent of absorption. Valproic acid serum concentrations may be decreased if taken with food. Milk has no effect on absorption.

Herb/Nutraceutical: Avoid evening primrose (seizure threshold decreased).

Stability

Depakene® solution: Store below 30°C (86°F).

Stavzor™: Store at controlled room temperature of 25°C (77°F).

Depakene® capsule: Store at controlled room temperature of 15°C to 25°C (59°F to 77°F).

Depacon®: Store vial at room temperature of 15°C to 30°C (59°F to 86°F). Injection should be diluted in 50 mL of a compatible diluent. Stable in D_5W, NS, and LR for at least 24 hours when stored in glass or PVC.

Mechanism of Action Causes increased availability of gamma-aminobutyric acid (GABA), an inhibitory neurotransmitter, to brain neurons or may enhance the action of GABA or mimic its action at postsynaptic receptor sites

Pharmacodynamics/Kinetics

Distribution: Total valproate: 11 L/1.73 m²; free valproate 92 L/1.73 m²

Protein binding (dose dependent): 80% to 90%; decreased in the elderly and with hepatic or renal dysfunction

Metabolism: Extensively hepatic via glucuronide conjugation and mitochondrial beta-oxidation. The relationship between dose and total valproate concentration is nonlinear; concentration does not increase proportionally with the dose, but increases to a lesser extent due to saturable plasma protein binding. The kinetics of unbound drug are linear.

Half-life elimination (increased with liver disease): Adults: 9-16 hours

Time to peak, serum: Stavzor™: 2 hours

Excretion: Urine (30% to 50% as glucuronide conjugate, 3% as unchanged drug)

Dosage

Geriatric Initiate at lower doses; dose escalation should be managed more slowly (in persons of advanced age). Refer to adult dosing.

Adult

Seizures: Administer doses >250 mg/day in divided doses.

Oral:

Simple and complex absence seizure: Initial: 15 mg/kg/day; increase by 5-10 mg/kg/day at weekly intervals until therapeutic levels are achieved; maximum: 60 mg/kg/day.

Complex partial seizure: Initial: 10-15 mg/kg/day; increase by 5-10 mg/kg/day at weekly intervals until therapeutic levels are achieved; maximum: 60 mg/kg/day.

Note: Regular release and delayed release formulations are usually given in 2-4 divided doses/day

I.V.: Administer as a 60-minute infusion (≤20 mg/minute) with the same frequency as oral products; switch patient to oral products as soon as possible. Rapid infusions ≤45 mg/kg over 5-10 minutes (1.5-6 mg/kg/minute) were generally well tolerated in clinical trials.

Rectal (unlabeled): Dilute syrup 1:1 with water for use as a retention enema; loading dose: 17-20 mg/kg one time; maintenance: 10-15 mg/kg/dose every 8 hours

Status epilepticus (unlabeled use):

Loading dose: I.V.: 15-45 mg/kg administered at ≤6 mg/kg/minute

Maintenance dose: I.V. infusion: 1-4 mg/kg/hour; titrate dose as needed based upon patient response and evaluation of drug-drug interactions

Mania (Stavzor™): *Oral:* Initial: 750 mg/day in divided doses; dose should be adjusted as rapidly as possible to desired clinical effect; maximum recommended dosage: 60 mg/kg/day

Migraine prophylaxis (Stavzor™): *Oral:* 250 mg twice daily; adjust dose based on patient response, up to 1000 mg/day

Diabetic neuropathy (unlabeled use): *Oral:* 500-1200 mg/day (Bril, 2011)

Renal Impairment A 27% reduction in clearance of unbound valproate is seen in patients with Cl_{cr} <10 mL/minute. Hemodialysis reduces valproate concentrations by 20%, therefore, no dose adjustment is needed in patients with renal failure. Protein binding is reduced, monitoring only total valproate concentrations may be misleading.

Hepatic Impairment Dosage reduction is required. Clearance is decreased with liver impairment. Hepatic disease is also associated with decreased albumin concentrations and 2- to 2.6-fold increase in the unbound fraction. Free concentrations of valproate may be elevated while total concentrations appear normal. Use is contraindicated in severe impairment.

Administration

Depacon®: Following dilution to final concentration, administer over 60 minutes at a rate ≤20 mg/minute. Alternatively, single doses up to 45 mg/kg have been administered as a rapid infusion over 5-10 minutes (1.5-6 mg/kg/minute).

Depakene® capsule, Stavzor™: Swallow whole; do not chew.

Monitoring Parameters Liver enzymes (at baseline and during therapy), CBC with platelets (baseline and periodic intervals), PT/PTT (especially prior to surgery), serum ammonia (with symptoms of lethargy, mental status change), serum valproate levels; suicidality (eg, suicidal thoughts, depression, behavioral changes)

Reference Range

Therapeutic:

Epilepsy: 50-100 mcg/mL (SI: 350-690 µmol/L)

Mania: 85-125 mcg/mL (SI: 350-860 µmol/L)

Toxic: Some laboratories may report >200 mcg/mL (SI: >1390 µmol/L) as a toxic threshold, although clinical toxicity can occur at lower concentrations. Probability of thrombocytopenia increases with total valproate levels ≥110 mcg/mL in females or ≥135 mcg/mL in males.

Seizure control: May improve at levels >100 mcg/mL (SI: 690 µmol/L), but toxicity may occur at levels of 100-150 mcg/mL (SI: 690-1040 µmol/L)

Mania: Clinical response seen with trough levels between 85-125 mcg/mL; risk of toxicity increases at levels >125 mcg/mL

Test Interactions False-positive result for urine ketones; altered thyroid function tests

Special Geriatric Considerations Although there is little data in elderly for the use of valproic acid in the treatment of seizures, there are a number of studies which demonstrate its benefit in the treatment of agitation and dementia and other psychiatric disorders. It is important that the clinician understand that serum concentrations do not correlate with behavior response; likewise, it is imperative to monitor LFTs and CBC during the first 6 months of therapy. See Warnings/Precautions and Monitoring Parameters.

Elimination is decreased in elderly. Studies of older adults with dementia show a high incidence of somnolence (which is usually transient); cognitive side effects generally minimal. In some patients, this was associated with weight loss. Starting doses should be lower and increased slowly, with careful monitoring of nutritional intake and dehydration. Safety and efficacy for use in patients >65 years of age have not been studied for migraine prophylaxis.

Dosage Forms Excipient information presented when available (limited, particularly for generics); consult specific product labeling. [DSC] = Discontinued product

Capsule, softgel, oral: 250 mg [strength expressed as valproic acid]

Depakene®: 250 mg [strength expressed as valproic acid]

Capsule, softgel, delayed release, oral:

Stavzor™: 125 mg, 250 mg, 500 mg [strength expressed as valproic acid]

Injection, solution, as valproate sodium [preservative free]: 100 mg/mL (5 mL) [strength expressed as valproic acid]

Depacon®: 100 mg/mL (5 mL) [contains edetate disodium; strength expressed as valproic acid]

Solution, oral, as valproate sodium: 250 mg/5 mL (473 mL, 480 mL [DSC]) [strength expressed as valproic acid]

Syrup, oral, as valproate sodium: 250 mg/5 mL (5 mL, 10 mL, 473 mL) [strength expressed as valproic acid]

Depakene®: 250 mg/5 mL (473 mL) [strength expressed as valproic acid]

Selected References

Limdi NA, Shimpi AV, Faught E, et al, "Efficacy of Rapid I.V. Administration of Valproic Acid for Status Epilepticus," *Neurology*, 2005, 64(2):353-5.

Limdi NA, Knowlton RK, Cofield SS, et al, "Safety of Rapid Intravenous Loading of Valproate," *Epilepsia*, 2007, 48 (3):478-83.

Loy R and Tariot PN, "Neuroprotective Properties of Valproate: Potential Benefit for AD and Tauopathies," *J Mol Neurosci*, 2002, 19(3):303-7.

Meierkord H, Boon P, Engelsen B, et al, "EFNS Guideline on the Management of Status Epilepticus," *Eur J Neurol*, 2006,13(5):445-50.

Pratt CE and Davis SM, "Divalproex Sodium Therapy in Elderly With Dementia-Related Agitation," *Ann Pharmacother*, 2002, 36(10):1625-28.

Sink KM, Holden KF, and Yaffe K, "Pharmacological Treatment of Neuropsychiatric Symptoms of Dementia. A Review of Evidence," *JAMA*, 2005, 293(5):596-608.

◆ **Valproic Acid Derivative** *see* Divalproex *on page 541*

Valsartan (val SAR tan)

Related Information

Angiotensin Agents *on page 1985*

Medication Safety Issues

Sound-alike/look-alike issues:

Valsartan may be confused with losartan, Valstar™, Valturna®

Diovan® may be confused with Darvon®, Dioval®, Zyban®

International issues:

Diovan [U.S., Canada, and multiple international markets] may be confused with Dianben, a brand name for metformin [Spain]

Brand Names: U.S. Diovan®

Brand Names: Canada CO Valsartan; Diovan®; Ran-Valsartan; Sandoz-Valsartan; Teva-Valsartan

Generic Availability (U.S.) No

Pharmacologic Category Angiotensin II Receptor Blocker

Use Alone or in combination with other antihypertensive agents in the treatment of essential hypertension; reduction of cardiovascular mortality in patients with left ventricular dysfunction postmyocardial infarction; treatment of heart failure (NYHA Class II-IV)

Contraindications

There are no contraindications listed in manufacturer's labeling.

Canadian labeling: Hypersensitivity to valsartan or any component of the formulation

Warnings/Precautions May cause hyperkalemia; avoid potassium supplementation unless specifically required by healthcare provider. During the initiation of therapy, hypotension may occur, particularly in patients with heart failure or post-MI patients. Use extreme caution with concurrent administration of potassium-sparing diuretics or potassium supplements, in patients with mild-to-moderate hepatic dysfunction (adjust dose), in those who may be sodium/water depleted (eg, on high-dose diuretics), and in the elderly; correct depletion first.

Use caution with unstented unilateral/bilateral renal artery stenosis. When unstented bilateral renal artery stenosis is present, use is generally avoided due to the elevated risk of deterioration in renal function unless possible benefits outweigh risks. Use with caution with preexisting renal insufficiency; significant aortic/mitral stenosis. May be associated with deterioration of renal function and/or increases in serum creatinine, particularly in patients with low renal blood flow (eg, renal artery stenosis, heart failure) whose glomerular filtration rate (GFR) is dependent on efferent arteriolar vasoconstriction by angiotensin II. Use caution in patients with severe renal impairment or significant hepatic dysfunction. Monitor renal function closely in patients with severe heart failure; changes in renal function should be anticipated and dosage adjustments of valsartan or concomitant medications may be needed. Concurrent use of ACE inhibitors may increase the risk of clinically-significant adverse events (eg, renal dysfunction, hyperkalemia).

Adverse Reactions (Reflective of adult population; not specific for elderly)
>10%:
  Central nervous system: Dizziness (heart failure trials 17%)
  Renal: BUN increased >50% (heart failure trials 17%)
1% to 10%:
  Cardiovascular: Hypotension (heart failure trials 7%; MI trial 1%), postural hypotension (heart failure trials 2%), syncope (up to >1%)
  Central nervous system: Dizziness (hypertension trial 2% to 8%), fatigue (heart failure trials 3%; hypertension trial 2%), postural dizziness (heart failure trials 2%), headache (heart failure trials >1%), vertigo (up to >1%)
  Endocrine & metabolic: Serum potassium increased by >20% (4% to 10%), hyperkalemia (heart failure trials 2%)
  Gastrointestinal: Diarrhea (heart failure trials 5%), abdominal pain (2%), nausea (heart failure trials >1%), upper abdominal pain (heart failure trials >1%)
  Hematologic: Neutropenia (2%)
  Neuromuscular & skeletal: Arthralgia (heart failure trials 3%), back pain (up to 3%)
  Ocular: Blurred vision (heart failure trials >1%)
  Renal: Creatinine doubled (MI trial 4%), creatinine increased >50% (heart failure trials 4%), renal dysfunction (up to >1%)
  Respiratory: Cough (1% to 3%)
  Miscellaneous: Viral infection (3%)

Drug Interactions
  Metabolism/Transport Effects Substrate of SLCO1B1; **Inhibits** CYP2C9 (weak)
  Avoid Concomitant Use There are no known interactions where it is recommended to avoid concomitant use.
  Increased Effect/Toxicity
    Valsartan may increase the levels/effects of: ACE Inhibitors; Amifostine; Antihypertensives; Hypotensive Agents; Lithium; Nonsteroidal Anti-Inflammatory Agents; Potassium-Sparing Diuretics; RiTUXimab; Sodium Phosphates

    The levels/effects of Valsartan may be increased by: Alfuzosin; Diazoxide; Eltrombopag; Eplerenone; Herbs (Hypotensive Properties); MAO Inhibitors; Pentoxifylline; Phosphodiesterase 5 Inhibitors; Potassium Salts; Prostacyclin Analogues; Tolvaptan; Trimethoprim
  Decreased Effect
    The levels/effects of Valsartan may be decreased by: Herbs (Hypertensive Properties); Methylphenidate; Nonsteroidal Anti-Inflammatory Agents; Yohimbine

Ethanol/Nutrition/Herb Interactions
  Food: Decreases the peak plasma concentration and extent of absorption by 50% and 40%, respectively.
  Herb/Nutraceutical: Avoid bayberry, blue cohosh, cayenne, ephedra, ginger, ginseng (American), kola, licorice (may worsen hypertension). Avoid black cohosh, California poppy, coleus, golden seal, hawthorn, mistletoe, periwinkle, quinine, shepherd's purse (may have increased antihypertensive effect).

Stability Store at 25°C (77°F); excursions permitted to 15°C to 30°C (59°F to 86°F). Protect from moisture.

Mechanism of Action Valsartan produces direct antagonism of the angiotensin II (AT2) receptors, unlike the ACE inhibitors. It displaces angiotensin II from the AT1 receptor and produces its blood pressure-lowering effects by antagonizing AT1-induced vasoconstriction, aldosterone release, catecholamine release, arginine vasopressin release, water intake, and hypertrophic responses. This action results in more efficient blockade of the cardiovascular effects of angiotensin II and fewer side effects than the ACE inhibitors.

Pharmacodynamics/Kinetics
  Onset of action: ~2 hours
  Duration: 24 hours
  Distribution: V_d: 17 L (adults)
  Protein binding: 95%, primarily albumin
  Metabolism: To inactive metabolite
  Bioavailability: Tablet: 25% (range: 10% to 35%); suspension: ~40% (~1.6 times more than tablet)

◀ Half-life elimination: ~6 hours
Time to peak, serum: 2-4 hours
Excretion: Feces (83%) and urine (13%) as unchanged drug

Dosage

Geriatric & Adult

Hypertension: Initial: 80 mg or 160 mg once daily (in patients who are not volume depleted); dose may be increased to achieve desired effect; maximum recommended dose: 320 mg/day

Heart failure: Initial: 40 mg twice daily; titrate dose to 80-160 mg twice daily, as tolerated; maximum daily dose: 320 mg

Left ventricular dysfunction after MI: Initial: 20 mg twice daily; titrate dose to target of 160 mg twice daily as tolerated; may initiate ≥12 hours following MI

Renal Impairment

No dosage adjustment necessary if Cl_{cr} >10 mL/minute.

Dialysis: Not significantly removed.

Hepatic Impairment In mild-to-moderate liver disease no adjustment is needed. Use caution in patients with liver disease. Patients with mild-to-moderate chronic disease have twice the exposure as healthy volunteers.

Administration Administer with or without food.

Monitoring Parameters Baseline and periodic electrolyte panels, renal function, BP; in CHF, serum potassium during dose escalation and periodically thereafter

Pharmacotherapy Pearls Valsartan may have an advantage over losartan due to minimal metabolism requirements and consequent use in mild-to-moderate hepatic impairment.

Special Geriatric Considerations No dosage adjustment is necessary when initiating angiotensin II receptor antagonists in the elderly. In clinical studies, no differences between younger adults and elderly were demonstrated. Many elderly may be volume depleted due to diuretic use and/or blunted thirst reflex resulting in inadequate fluid intake.

Dosage Forms Excipient information presented when available (limited, particularly for generics); consult specific product labeling.

Tablet, oral:

Diovan®: 40 mg [scored]

Diovan®: 80 mg, 160 mg, 320 mg

Extemporaneously Prepared To prepare valsartan suspension, add 80 mL of Ora-Plus® to an 8-ounce amber glass bottle containing eight (8) valsartan 80 mg tablets. Shake well ≥2 minutes. Allow the suspension to stand for a minimum of 1 hour then shake for 1 minute. Then add 80 mL of Ora-Sweet SF® to the bottle and shake for at least 10 seconds. Resulting 160 mL suspension will contain valsartan 4 mg/mL. Store for either up to 30 days at room temperature (below 30°C/86°F) or up to 75 days under refrigeration (2-8°C/35-46°F) in the glass bottle. Shake well before use.

Product information, December, 2007; Novartis Pharmaceuticals Corp.

Selected References

Cohn JN and Tognoni G, "A Randomized Trial of the Angiotensin-Receptor Blocker Valsartan in Chronic Heart Failure," *N Engl J Med*, 2001, 345(23):1667-75.

Pfeffer MA, McMurray JJ, Velazquez EJ, et al, "Valsartan, Captopril, or Both in Myocardial Infarction Complicated by Heart Failure, Left Ventricular Dysfunction, or Both," *N Engl J Med*, 2003, 349(20):1893-1906.

◆ **Valsartan and Aliskiren** *see* Aliskiren and Valsartan *on page 64*
◆ **Valsartan and Amlodipine** *see* Amlodipine and Valsartan *on page 109*

Valsartan and Hydrochlorothiazide (val SAR tan & hye droe klor oh THYE a zide)

Related Information

Hydrochlorothiazide *on page 876*
Valsartan *on page 1892*

Medication Safety Issues

Sound-alike/look-alike issues:

Diovan® may be confused with Darvon®, Dioval®, Zyban®

Brand Names: U.S. Diovan HCT®

Brand Names: Canada Diovan HCT®; Sandoz Valsartan HCT; Teva-Valsartan HCTZ; Valsartan-HCTZ

Index Terms Hydrochlorothiazide and Valsartan

Generic Availability (U.S.) No

Pharmacologic Category Angiotensin II Receptor Blocker; Diuretic, Thiazide

Use Treatment of hypertension

Dosage

Geriatric & Adult Note: Dose is individualized; combination product may be used as initial therapy or substituted for individual components in patients currently maintained on both agents separately or in patients not adequately controlled with monotherapy (using one of the agents or an agent within same antihypertensive class).

Hypertension: Oral:

Initial therapy: Valsartan 160 mg and hydrochlorothiazide 12.5 mg once daily; dose may be titrated after 1-2 weeks of therapy. Maximum recommended daily doses: Valsartan 320 mg; hydrochlorothiazide 25 mg.

Add-on/replacement therapy: Valsartan 80-160 mg and hydrochlorothiazide 12.5-25 mg once daily; dose may be titrated after 3-4 weeks of therapy. Maximum recommended daily dose: Valsartan 320 mg; hydrochlorothiazide 25 mg.

Renal Impairment

Cl_{cr} >30 mL/minute: No adjustment needed

Cl_{cr} ≤30 mL/minute: Use of combination not recommended. Contraindicated in patients with anuria.

Hepatic Impairment Use with caution; initiate at lower dose and titrate slowly.

Special Geriatric Considerations Combination products are not recommended as first-line treatment. Use only if doses of individual agents correspond to the combination available.

Dosage Forms Excipient information presented when available (limited, particularly for generics); consult specific product labeling.

Tablet:

Diovan HCT® 80 mg/12.5 mg: Valsartan 80 mg and hydrochlorothiazide 12.5 mg

Diovan HCT® 160 mg/12.5 mg: Valsartan 160 mg and hydrochlorothiazide 12.5 mg

Diovan HCT® 160 mg/25 mg: Valsartan 160 mg and hydrochlorothiazide 25 mg

Diovan HCT® 320 mg/12.5 mg: Valsartan 320 mg and hydrochlorothiazide 12.5 mg

Diovan HCT® 320 mg/25 mg: Valsartan 320 mg and hydrochlorothiazide 25 mg

◆ **Valsartan, Hydrochlorothiazide, and Amlodipine** see Amlodipine, Valsartan, and Hydrochlorothiazide on page 110

◆ **Valtrex®** see ValACYclovir on page 1885

◆ **Valturna®** see Aliskiren and Valsartan on page 64

◆ **Vancenase** see Beclomethasone (Oral Inhalation) on page 184

◆ **Vancocin®** see Vancomycin on page 1895

Vancomycin (van koe MYE sin)

Related Information

Antibiotic Treatment of Adults With Infective Endocarditis on page 2053

Community-Acquired Pneumonia in Adults on page 2059

Prevention of Infective Endocarditis on page 2064

Medication Safety Issues

Sound-alike/look-alike issues:

I.V. vancomycin may be confused with Invanz®

Vancomycin may be confused with clindamycin, gentamicin, tobramycin, valACYclovir, vecuronium, Vibramycin®

High alert medication:

The Institute for Safe Medication Practices (ISMP) includes this medication (intrathecal administration) among its list of drug classes which have a heightened risk of causing significant patient harm when used in error.

Brand Names: U.S. Vancocin®

Brand Names: Canada PMS-Vancomycin; Sterile Vancomycin Hydrochloride, USP; Val-Vanco; Vancocin®; Vancomycin Hydrochloride for Injection, USP

Index Terms Vancomycin Hydrochloride

Generic Availability (U.S.) Yes: Excludes capsule

Pharmacologic Category Glycopeptide

Use Treatment of patients with infections caused by staphylococcal species and streptococcal species; used orally for staphylococcal enterocolitis or for antibiotic-associated pseudomembranous colitis produced by *C. difficile*

Unlabeled/Investigational Use Bacterial endophthalmitis; treatment of infections caused by gram-positive organisms in patients who have serious allergies to beta-lactam agents; treatment of beta-lactam resistant gram-positive infections

Contraindications Hypersensitivity to vancomycin or any component of the formulation; avoid in patients with previous severe hearing loss

Warnings/Precautions May cause nephrotoxicity although limited data suggest direct causal relationship; usual risk factors include pre-existing renal impairment, concomitant nephrotoxic medications, advanced age, and dehydration. If multiple sequential (≥2) serum creatinine

◄ concentrations demonstrate an increase of 0.5 mg/dL or ≥50% increase from baseline (whichever is greater) in the absence of an alternative explanation, the patient should be identified as having vancomycin-induced nephrotoxicity (Rybak, 2009). Discontinue treatment if signs of nephrotoxicity occur; renal damage is usually reversible. May cause neurotoxicity; usual risk factors include pre-existing renal impairment, concomitant neuro-/nephrotoxic medications, advanced age, and dehydration. Ototoxicity, although rarely associated with monotherapy, is proportional to the amount of drug given and the duration of treatment. Tinnitus or vertigo may be indications of vestibular injury and impending bilateral irreversible damage. Discontinue treatment if signs of ototoxicity occur. Prolonged therapy (>1 week) or total doses exceeding 25 g may increase the risk of neutropenia; prompt reversal of neutropenia is expected after discontinuation of therapy. Prolonged use may result in fungal or bacterial superinfection, including *C. difficile*-associated diarrhea (CDAD) and pseudomembranous colitis; CDAD has been observed >2 months postantibiotic treatment. Use with caution in patients with renal impairment or those receiving other nephrotoxic or ototoxic drugs; dosage modification required in patients with impaired renal function (especially elderly). Rapid I.V. administration may result in hypotension, flushing, erythema, urticaria, and/or pruritus. Oral vancomycin is only indicated for the treatment of pseudomembranous colitis due to *C. difficile* and enterocolitis due to *S. aureus* and is not effective for systemic infections; parenteral vancomycin is not effective for the treatment of colitis due to *C. difficile* and enterocolitis due to *S. aureus*. **Note:** The Infectious Disease Society of America (IDSA) recommends the use of oral metronidazole for initial treatment of mild-to-moderate *C. difficile* infection and the use of oral vancomycin for initial treatment of severe *C. difficile* infection (Cohen, 2010).

Adverse Reactions (Reflective of adult population; not specific for elderly)
Oral:
>10%: Gastrointestinal: Bitter taste, nausea, vomiting
1% to 10%:
Central nervous system: Chills, drug fever
Hematologic: Eosinophilia
Parenteral:
>10%:
Cardiovascular: Hypotension accompanied by flushing
Dermatologic: Erythematous rash on face and upper body (red neck or red man syndrome - infusion rate related)
1% to 10%:
Central nervous system: Chills, drug fever
Dermatologic: Rash
Hematologic: Eosinophilia, reversible neutropenia
Local: Phlebitis

Drug Interactions
Avoid Concomitant Use
Avoid concomitant use of Vancomycin with any of the following: BCG; Gallium Nitrate
Increased Effect/Toxicity
Vancomycin may increase the levels/effects of: Aminoglycosides; Colistimethate; Gallium Nitrate; Neuromuscular-Blocking Agents

The levels/effects of Vancomycin may be increased by: Nonsteroidal Anti-Inflammatory Agents
Decreased Effect
Vancomycin may decrease the levels/effects of: BCG; Typhoid Vaccine

Stability
Reconstituted 500 mg and 1 g vials are stable at either room temperature or under refrigeration for 14 days. **Note:** Vials contain no bacteriostatic agent. Solutions diluted for administration in either D_5W or NS are stable under refrigeration for 14 days or at room temperature for 7 days. Reconstitute vials with 20 mL of SWFI for each 1 g of vancomycin (10 mL/500 mg vial; 20 mL/1 g vial; 100 mL/5 g vial; 200 mL/10 g vial). The reconstituted solution must be further diluted with at least 100 mL of a compatible diluent per 500 mg of vancomycin prior to parenteral administration.

Intrathecal (unlabeled route): Vancomycin is available as a powder for injection and may be diluted to 1-5 mg/mL concentration in preservative free 0.9% sodium chloride for administration into the CSF.

Mechanism of Action
Inhibits bacterial cell wall synthesis by blocking glycopeptide polymerization through binding tightly to D-alanyl-D-alanine portion of cell wall precursor

Pharmacodynamics/Kinetics
Absorption: Oral: Poor; I.M.: Erratic; Intraperitoneal: ~38%
Distribution: V_d: 0.4-1 L/kg; Distributes widely in body tissue and fluids, except for CSF
Relative diffusion from blood into CSF: Good only with inflammation (exceeds usual MICs)
Uninflamed meninges: 0-4 mcg/mL; serum concentration dependent

Inflamed meninges: 6-11 mcg/mL; serum concentration dependent
CSF:blood level ratio: Normal meninges: Nil; Inflamed meninges: 20% to 30%
Protein binding: ~50%
Half-life elimination: Biphasic: Terminal:
  Adults: 5-11 hours; significantly prolonged with renal impairment
  End-stage renal disease: 200-250 hours
Time to peak, serum: I.V.: Immediately after completion of infusion
Excretion: I.V.: Urine (80% to 90% as unchanged drug); Oral: Primarily feces

Dosage
Geriatric & Adult
Usual dosage range: Initial intravenous dosing should be based on actual body weight; subsequent dosing adjusted based on serum trough vancomycin concentrations.
  I.V.: 2-3 g/day (or 30-60 mg/kg/day) in divided doses every 8-12 hours (Rybak, 2009);
    Note: Dose requires adjustment in renal impairment
  Oral: 500-2000 mg/day in divided doses every 6 hours

Indication-specific dosing:

Catheter-related infections: Antibiotic lock technique (Mermel, 2009): 2 mg/mL ± 10 units heparin/mL **or** 2.5 mg/mL ± 2500 **or** 5000 units heparin/mL **or** 5 mg/mL ± 5000 units heparin/mL (preferred regimen); instill into catheter port with a volume sufficient to fill the catheter (2-5 mL). **Note:** May use SWFI/NS or D_5W as diluents. Do not mix with any other solutions. Dwell times generally should not exceed 48 hours before renewal of lock solution. Remove lock solution prior to catheter use, then replace.

***C. difficile*-associated diarrhea (CDAD):**
  Oral:
    Manufacturer recommendations: 500-2000 mg/day in 3-4 divided doses for 7-10 days (usual dose: 125-500 mg every 6 hours)
    IDSA guideline recommendations: Severe infection: 125 mg every 6 hours for 10-14 days; Severe, complicated infection: 500 mg every 6 hours with or without concurrent I.V. metronidazole. May consider vancomycin retention enema (in patients with complete ileus) (Cohen, 2010).
  Rectal (unlabeled route): Retention enema (in patients with complete ileus): SHEA/IDSA guideline recommendations: Severe, complicated infection in patients with ileus: 500 mg every 6 hours (in 100 mL 0.9% sodium chloride) with oral vancomycin with or without concurrent I.V. metronidazole (Cohen, 2010)

Complicated infections in seriously-ill patients: I.V.: Loading dose: 25-30 mg/kg (based on actual body weight) may be used to rapidly achieve target concentration; then 15-20 mg/kg/dose every 8-12 hours (Rybak, 2009)

Enterocolitis *(S. aureus)*: Oral: 500-2000 mg/day in 3-4 divided doses for 7-10 days (usual dose: 125-500 mg every 6 hours)

Endophthalmitis (unlabeled use): Intravitreal: Usual dose: 1 mg/0.1 mL NS instilled into vitreum; may repeat administration if necessary in 3-4 days, usually in combination with ceftazidime or an aminoglycoside. **Note:** Some clinicians have recommended using a lower dose of 0.2 mg/0.1 mL, based on concerns for retinotoxicity.

Hospital-acquired pneumonia (HAP): I.V.: 15-20 mg/kg/dose every 8-12 hours (American Thoracic Society [ATS], 2005 guidelines; Rybak, 2009)

Meningitis:
  I.V.: 30-60 mg/kg/day in divided doses every 8-12 hours (Rybak, 2009) **or** 500-750 mg every 6 hours (with third-generation cephalosporin for PCN-resistant *Streptococcus pneumoniae*)
  Intrathecal, intraventricular (unlabeled route): 5-20 mg/day

MRSA infections: I.V.:
  Bacteremia (Liu, 2011): 15-20 mg/kg/dose every 8-12 hours for 2-6 weeks depending on severity
  Brain abscess, subdural empyema, spinal epidural abscess (Liu, 2011): 15-20 mg/kg/dose every 8-12 hours for 4-6 weeks (some experts combine with rifampin)
  Complicated skin and skin structure infections (Liu, 2011): 15-20 mg/kg/dose every 8-12 hours for 7-14 days
  Endocarditis, native valve (Liu, 2011): 15-20 mg/kg/dose every 8-12 hours for 6 weeks
  Endocarditis, prosthetic valve (Liu, 2011): 15-20 mg/kg/dose every 8-12 hours for at least 6 weeks (combine with rifampin for the entire duration of therapy and gentamicin for the first 2 weeks)
  Meningitis (Liu, 2011): 15-20 mg/kg/dose every 8-12 hours for 2 weeks (some experts combine with rifampin)
  Osteomyelitis (Liu, 2011): 15-20 mg/kg/dose every 8-12 hours for a minimum of 8 weeks (some experts combine with rifampin)
  Pneumonia (Liu, 2011): 15-20 mg/kg/dose every 8-12 hours for 7-21 days depending on severity

Septic arthritis (Liu, 2011): 15-20 mg/kg/dose every 8-12 hours for 3-4 weeks

Septic thrombosis of cavernous or dural venous sinus (Liu, 2011): 15-20 mg/kg/dose every 8-12 hours for 4-6 weeks (some experts combine with rifampin)

Prophylaxis against infective endocarditis:

Dental, oral, or upper respiratory tract surgery: 1 g 1 hour before surgery. **Note:** AHA guidelines now recommend prophylaxis only in patients undergoing invasive procedures and in whom underlying cardiac conditions may predispose to a higher risk of adverse outcomes should infection occur

GI/GU procedure: 1 g plus 1.5 mg/kg gentamicin 1 hour prior to surgery. **Note:** As of April 2007, routine prophylaxis no longer recommended by the AHA.

Susceptible (MIC ≤1 mcg/mL; Rybak, 2009) gram-positive infections: 15-20 mg/kg/dose (usual: 750-1500 mg) every 8-12 hours. **Note:** If MIC ≥2 mcg/mL, alternative therapies are recommended.

Renal Impairment Vancomycin levels should be monitored in patients with any renal impairment:

Cl_{cr} >50 mL/minute: Start with 15-20 mg/kg/dose (usual: 750-1500 mg) every 8-12 hours

Cl_{cr} 20-49 mL/minute: Start with 15-20 mg/kg/dose (usual: 750-1500 mg) every 24 hours

Cl_{cr} <20 mL/minute: Will need longer intervals; determine by serum concentration monitoring

Note: In the critically-ill patient with renal insufficiency, the initial loading dose (25-30 mg/kg) should not be reduced. However, subsequent dosage adjustments should be made based on renal function and trough serum concentrations.

Poorly dialyzable by intermittent hemodialysis (0% to 5%); however, use of high-flux membranes and continuous renal replacement therapy (CRRT) increases vancomycin clearance, and generally requires replacement dosing.

Intermittent hemodialysis (IHD) (administer after hemodialysis on dialysis days): Following loading dose of 15-25 mg/kg, give either 500 mg to 1 g **or** 5-10 mg/kg after each dialysis session. (Heintz, 2009). **Note:** Dosing dependent on the assumption of 3 times/week, complete IHD sessions.

Redosing based on pre-HD concentrations:

<10 mg/L: Administer 1g after HD

10-25 mg/L: Administer 500-750 mg after HD

>25 mg/L: Hold vancomycin

Redosing based on post-HD concentrations: <10-15 mg/L: Administer 0.5-1 g

Peritoneal dialysis (PD):

Administration via PD fluid: 15-30 mg/L (15-30 mcg/mL) of PD fluid

Systemic: Loading dose of 1 g, followed by 500 mg to 1 g every 48-72 hours with close monitoring of levels

Continuous renal replacement therapy (CRRT) (Heintz, 2009; Trotman, 2005): Drug clearance is highly dependent on the method of renal replacement, filter type, and flow rate. Appropriate dosing requires close monitoring of pharmacologic response, signs of adverse reactions due to drug accumulation, as well as drug concentrations in relation to target trough (if appropriate). The following are general recommendations only (based on dialysate flow/ultrafiltration rates of 1-2 L/hour and minimal residual renal function) and should not supersede clinical judgment:

CVVH: Loading dose of 15-25 mg/kg, followed by either 1 g every 48 hours **or** 10-15 mg/kg every 24-48 hours

CVVHD: Loading dose of 15-25 mg/kg, followed by either 1 g every 24 hours **or** 10-15 mg/kg every 24 hours

CVVHDF: Loading dose of 15-25 mg/kg, followed by either 1 g every 24 hours **or** 7.5-10 mg/kg every 12 hours

Note: Consider redosing patients receiving CRRT for vancomycin concentrations <10-15 mg/L.

Administration

Intravenous: Administer vancomycin with a final concentration not to exceed 5 mg/mL by I.V. intermittent infusion over at least 60 minutes (recommended infusion period of ≥30 minutes for every 500 mg administered).

If a maculopapular rash appears on the face, neck, trunk, and/or lower extremities (red man syndrome), slow the infusion rate to over 1½ to 2 hours and increase the dilution volume. Hypotension, shock, and cardiac arrest (rare) have also been reported with too rapid of infusion. Reactions are often treated with antihistamines and steroids.

Intrathecal (unlabeled route): Vancomycin is available as a powder for injection and may be diluted to 1-5 mg/mL concentration in preservative free 0.9% sodium chloride for intrathecal administration.

Intravitreal: May be administered by intravitreal injection (unlabeled use).

Oral: May be administered with food. If patient cannot swallow capsules, the powder for injection (not premixed solution) may be diluted in 30 mL of water for oral administration; flavoring may be added to improve taste. The unflavored, diluted solution may also be administered via nasogastric tube.

Rectal (unlabeled route): May be administered as a retention enema per rectum (Cohen, 2010)

Not for I.M. administration.

Extravasation treatment: Monitor I.V. site closely; extravasation will cause serious injury with possible necrosis and tissue sloughing. Rotate infusion site frequently.

Monitoring Parameters Periodic renal function tests, urinalysis, WBC; serum trough vancomycin concentrations in select patients (eg, aggressive dosing, unstable renal function, concurrent nephrotoxins, prolonged courses)

Suggested frequency of trough vancomycin concentration monitoring (Rybak, 2009):

Hemodynamically stable patients: Draw trough concentrations at least once-weekly.

Hemodynamically unstable patients: Draw trough concentrations more frequently or in some instances daily.

Prolonged courses (>3-5 days): Draw at least one steady-state trough concentration; repeat as clinically appropriate.

Note: Drawing >1 trough concentration prior to the fourth dose for short course (<3 days) or lower intensity dosing (target trough concentrations <15 mcg/mL) is not recommended.

Reference Range

Timing of serum samples: Draw trough just before next dose at steady-state conditions (approximately after the fourth dose). Drawing peak concentrations is no longer recommended.

Therapeutic levels: Trough: ≥10 mcg/mL. For pathogens with an MIC ≤1 mcg/mL, the minimum trough concentration should be 15 mcg/mL to meet target AUC/MIC of ≥400 (see 'Note' below). For complicated infections (eg, bacteremia, endocarditis, osteomyelitis, meningitis, and hospital-acquired pneumonia caused by *S. aureus*), trough concentrations of 15-20 mcg/mL are recommended to improve penetration and improve clinical outcomes (Liu, 2011; Rybak, 2009). The American Thoracic Society (ATS) guidelines for hospital-acquired pneumonia and the Infectious Disease Society of America (IDSA) meningitis guidelines also recommend trough concentrations of 15-20 mcg/mL.

Note: Although AUC/MIC is the preferred pharmacokinetic-pharmacodynamic parameter used to determine clinical effectiveness, trough serum concentrations may be used as a surrogate marker for AUC and are recommended as the most accurate and practical method of vancomycin monitoring (Liu, 2011; Rybak, 2009).

Toxic: >80 mcg/mL (SI: >54 µmol/L)

Pharmacotherapy Pearls Because of its long half-life, vancomycin should be dosed on an every 8- to 12-hour basis. Monitoring of trough serum concentrations is advisable in certain situations. "Red man syndrome", characterized by skin rash and hypotension, is not an allergic reaction but rather is associated with too rapid infusion of the drug. To alleviate or prevent the reaction, infuse vancomycin at a rate of ≥30 minutes for each 500 mg of drug being administered (eg, 1 g over ≥60 minutes); 1.5 g over ≥90 minutes.

Special Geriatric Considerations As a result of age-related changes in renal function and volume of distribution, accumulation and toxicity are a risk in the elderly. Careful monitoring and dosing adjustment is necessary.

Dosage Forms Excipient information presented when available (limited, particularly for generics); consult specific product labeling.

Capsule, oral:

Vancocin®: 125 mg, 250 mg

Infusion, premixed iso-osmotic dextrose solution: 500 mg (100 mL); 750 mg (150 mL); 1 g (200 mL)

Injection, powder for reconstitution: 500 mg, 750 mg, 1 g, 5 g, 10 g

Selected References

Cutler NR, Narang PK, Lesko LJ, et al, "Vancomycin Disposition: The Importance of Age," *Clin Pharmacol Ther*, 1984, 36(6):803-10.

Rybak M, Lomaestro B, Rotschafer JC, et al, "Therapeutic Monitoring of Vancomycin in Adult Patients: A Consensus Review of the American Society of Health-System Pharmacists, the Infectious Diseases Society of America, and the Society of Infectious Diseases Pharmacists," *Am J Health-Syst Pharm*, 2009, 66(1):82-98

Vardenafil (var DEN a fil)

Medication Safety Issues

Sound-alike/look-alike issues:

Vardenafil may be confused with sildenafil, tadalafil

Levitra® may be confused with Kaletra®, Lexiva®

Brand Names: U.S. Levitra®; Staxyn™

Brand Names: Canada Levitra®

Index Terms Vardenafil Hydrochloride

Generic Availability (U.S.) No

Pharmacologic Category Phosphodiesterase-5 Enzyme Inhibitor

Use Treatment of erectile dysfunction (ED)

Contraindications Hypersensitivity to vardenafil or any component of the formulation; concurrent (regular or intermittent) use of organic nitrates in any form (eg, nitroglycerin, isosorbide dinitrate)

Warnings/Precautions There is a degree of cardiac risk associated with sexual activity; therefore, physicians may wish to consider the patient's cardiovascular status prior to initiating any treatment for erectile dysfunction. Use caution in patients with anatomical deformation of the penis (angulation, cavernosal fibrosis, or Peyronie's disease) and in patients who have conditions which may predispose them to priapism (sickle cell anemia, multiple myeloma, leukemia). Instruct patients to seek immediate medical attention if erection persists >4 hours.

Use is not recommended in patients with hypotension (<90/50 mm Hg); uncontrolled hypertension (>170/100 mm Hg); unstable angina or angina during intercourse; life-threatening arrhythmias, stroke, or MI within the last 6 months; cardiac failure or coronary artery disease causing unstable angina. Safety and efficacy have not been studied in these patients. Use caution in patients with left ventricular outflow obstruction (eg, aortic stenosis). Use caution with alpha-blockers, effective CYP3A4 inhibitors, the elderly, or those with hepatic impairment (Child-Pugh class B); dosage adjustment is needed.

Rare cases of nonarteritic ischemic optic neuropathy (NAION) have been reported; risk may be increased with history of vision loss. Other risk factors for NAION include heart disease, diabetes, hypertension, smoking, age >50 years, or history of certain eye problems. Sudden decrease or loss of hearing has been reported rarely; hearing changes may be accompanied by tinnitus and dizziness.

Safety and efficacy have not been studied in patients with the following conditions, therefore, use in these patients is not recommended at this time: Congenital QT prolongation, patients taking medications known to prolong the QT interval (avoid use in patients taking Class Ia or III antiarrhythmics); severe hepatic impairment (Child-Pugh class C); end-stage renal disease requiring dialysis; retinitis pigmentosa or other degenerative retinal disorders. The safety and efficacy of vardenafil with other treatments for erectile dysfunction have not been studied and are not recommended as combination therapy. Concomitant use with all forms of nitrates is contraindicated. If nitrate administration is medically necessary, it is not known when nitrates can be safely administered following the use of vardenafil; the ACC/AHA 2007 guidelines support administration of nitrates only if 24 hours have elapsed. Potential underlying causes of erectile dysfunction should be evaluated prior to treatment. Some products may contain phylalanine. Some products may contain sorbitol; do not use in patients with fructose intolerance.

Adverse Reactions (Reflective of adult population; not specific for elderly)

>10%:
  Cardiovascular: Flushing (8% to 11%)
  Central nervous system: Headache (14% to 15%)
2% to 10%:
  Central nervous system: Dizziness (2%)
  Gastrointestinal: Dyspepsia (3% to 4%), nausea (2%)
  Neuromuscular & skeletal: Back pain (2%), CPK increased (2%)
  Respiratory: Rhinitis (9%), nasal congestion (3%), sinusitis (3%)
  Miscellaneous: Flu-like syndrome (3%)

Drug Interactions

Metabolism/Transport Effects Substrate of CYP2C (minor), 3A4 (major)

Avoid Concomitant Use

Avoid concomitant use of Vardenafil with any of the following: Amyl Nitrite; Phosphodiesterase 5 Inhibitors; Vasodilators (Organic Nitrates)

Increased Effect/Toxicity

Vardenafil may increase the levels/effects of: Alpha1-Blockers; Amyl Nitrite; Antihypertensives; Bosentan; Phosphodiesterase 5 Inhibitors; Vasodilators (Organic Nitrates)

The levels/effects of Vardenafil may be increased by: Antifungal Agents (Azole Derivatives, Systemic); Boceprevir; CYP3A4 Inhibitors (Moderate); CYP3A4 Inhibitors (Strong); Dasatinib; Erythromycin; Protease Inhibitors; Sapropterin; Telaprevir

Decreased Effect

The levels/effects of Vardenafil may be decreased by: Bosentan; Etravirine; Tocilizumab

Ethanol/Nutrition/Herb Interactions Food: High-fat meals decrease maximum serum concentration 18% to 50%. Serum concentrations/toxicity may be increased with grapefruit juice; avoid concurrent use.

Stability Store at controlled room temperature of 25°C (77°F); excursions permitted to 15°C to 25°C (59°F to 86°F). Keep oral disintegrating tablets sealed in blisterpack until ready to use.

Mechanism of Action Does not directly cause penile erections, but affects the response to sexual stimulation. The physiologic mechanism of erection of the penis involves release of nitric oxide (NO) in the corpus cavernosum during sexual stimulation. NO then activates the enzyme guanylate cyclase, which results in increased levels of cyclic guanosine monophosphate (cGMP), producing smooth muscle relaxation and inflow of blood to the corpus cavernosum. Vardenafil enhances the effect of NO by inhibiting phosphodiesterase type 5 (PDE-5), which is responsible for degradation of cGMP in the corpus cavernosum; when sexual stimulation causes local release of NO, inhibition of PDE-5 by vardenafil causes increased levels of cGMP in the corpus cavernosum, resulting in smooth muscle relaxation and inflow of blood to the corpus cavernosum; at recommended doses, it has no effect in the absence of sexual stimulation.

Pharmacodynamics/Kinetics
Onset of action: ~60 minutes
Absorption: Rapid
Distribution: V_d: 208 L
Protein binding: ~95% (parent drug and metabolite)
Metabolism: Hepatic via CYP3A4 (major), CYP2C and 3A5 (minor); forms metabolite (active)
Bioavailability: ~15%
Film-coated tablet: Elderly (≥65 years): AUC increased by 52%; Hepatic impairment (moderate, Child-Pugh class B): AUC increased by 160%
Oral disintegrating tablet: Elderly (≥65 years): AUC increased by 21% more compared to film-coated tablet. When administered with water, AUC decreases by 29%.
Half-life elimination: Terminal: Vardenafil and metabolite: 3-6 hours
Time to peak, plasma: 0.5-2 hours
Excretion: Feces (~91% to 95% as metabolites); urine (~2% to 6%)

Dosage
Geriatric Erectile dysfunction: Elderly ≥65 years: Oral: Initial: 5 mg 60 minutes prior to sexual activity; to be given as one single dose and not given more than once daily.

Adult Note: Oral disintegrating tablets should not be used interchangeably with film-coated tablets; patients requiring a dose other than 10 mg should use the film-coated tablets.
Erectile dysfunction: Oral:
Film-coated tablet (Levitra®): 10 mg 60 minutes prior to sexual activity; dosing range: 5-20 mg; to be given as one single dose and not given more than once daily
Oral disintegrating tablet (Staxyn™): 10 mg 60 minutes prior to sexual activity; maximum: 10 mg/day

Dosing adjustment with concomitant medications:
Alpha-blocker (dose should be stable at time of vardenafil initiation):
Film-coated tablet (Levitra®): Initial vardenafil dose: 5 mg/24 hours; if an alpha-blocker is added to vardenafil therapy, it should be initiated at the smallest possible dose and titrated carefully.
Oral disintegrating tablet (Staxyn™): Do not use to initiate therapy. Initial therapy should be with film-coated tablets at lower doses. Patients who have previously used film-coated tablets may be switched to oral disintegrating tablets as recommended by healthcare provider.
Film-coated tablet (Levitra®):
Atazanavir: Maximum vardenafil dose: 2.5 mg/24 hours
Clarithromycin: Maximum vardenafil dose: 2.5 mg/24 hours
Darunavir: Maximum vardenafil dose: 2.5 mg/72 hours
Erythromycin: Maximum vardenafil dose: 5 mg/24 hours
Fosamprenavir: Maximum vardenafil dose: 2.5 mg/24 hours
Fosamprenavir/ritonavir: Maximum vardenafil dose: 2.5 mg/72 hours
Indinavir: Maximum vardenafil dose: 2.5 mg/24 hours
Itraconazole:
200 mg/day: Maximum vardenafil dose: 5 mg/24 hours
400 mg/day: Maximum vardenafil dose: 2.5 mg/24 hours
Ketoconazole:
200 mg/day: Maximum vardenafil dose: 5 mg/24 hours
400 mg/day: Maximum vardenafil dose: 2.5 mg/24 hours
Lopinavir/ritonavir: Maximum vardenafil dose: 2.5 mg/72 hours
Nelfinavir: Maximum vardenafil dose: 2.5 mg/24 hours
Ritonavir: Maximum vardenafil dose: 2.5 mg/72 hours
Saquinavir: Maximum vardenafil dose: 2.5 mg/24 hours

Tipranavir: Maximum vardenafil dose: 2.5 mg/72 hours

Oral disintegrating tablet (Staxyn™): Concurrent use not recommended with potent or moderate CYP3A4 inhibitors (atazanavir, clarithromycin, erythromycin, indinavir, itraconazole, ketoconazole, ritonavir, saquinavir)

Renal Impairment Dose adjustment not needed for mild, moderate, or severe impairment; use not recommended in patients on hemodialysis.

Hepatic Impairment

Child-Pugh class A: No adjustment required

Child-Pugh class B:

Film-coated tablet (Levitra®): Initial: 5 mg 60 minutes prior to sexual activity (maximum dose: 10 mg); to be given as one single dose and not given more than once daily

Oral disintegrating tablet (Staxyn™): Use not recommended

Child-Pugh class C: Has not been studied; use is not recommended by the manufacturer

Administration Administer 60 minutes prior to sexual activity.

Monitoring Parameters Monitor for response, adverse reactions, blood pressure, and heart rate.

Special Geriatric Considerations In adults ≥65 years of age, vardenafil plasma concentrations were higher than younger males (mean C_{max} was 34% higher), therefore, initial dose should be lower than the usual adult dose. Since the elderly often have concomitant diseases, many of which may be contraindicated with the use of vardenafil, a thorough knowledge of disease and medications must be accessed.

Dosage Forms Excipient information presented when available (limited, particularly for generics); consult specific product labeling.

Tablet, oral:

Levitra®: 2.5 mg, 5 mg, 10 mg, 20 mg

Tablet, orally disintegrating, oral:

Staxyn™: 10 mg [contains phenylalanine 1.01 mg/tablet; peppermint flavor]

♦ **Vardenafil Hydrochloride** *see* Vardenafil *on page 1899*

Varenicline (var e NI kleen)

Brand Names: U.S. Chantix®
Brand Names: Canada Champix®
Index Terms Varenicline Tartrate
Generic Availability (U.S.) No
Pharmacologic Category Partial Nicotine Agonist; Smoking Cessation Aid
Use Treatment to aid in smoking cessation
Medication Guide Available Yes
Contraindications Known history of serious hypersensitivity or skin reactions to varenicline
Warnings/Precautions [U.S. Boxed Warning]: Serious neuropsychiatric events (including depression, suicidal thoughts, and suicide) have been reported with use; some cases may have been complicated by symptoms of nicotine withdrawal following smoking cessation. Smoking cessation (with or without treatment) is associated with nicotine withdrawal symptoms and the exacerbation of underlying psychiatric illness; however, some of the behavioral disturbances were reported in treated patients who continued to smoke. Neuropsychiatric symptoms (eg, mood disturbances, psychosis, hostility) have occurred in patients with and without pre-existing psychiatric disease; many cases resolved following therapy discontinuation although in some cases, symptoms persisted. Ethanol consumption may increase the risk of psychiatric adverse events. Monitor all patients for behavioral changes and psychiatric symptoms (eg, agitation, depression, suicidal behavior, suicidal ideation); inform patients to discontinue treatment and contact their healthcare provider immediately if they experience any behavioral and/or mood changes. **[U.S. Boxed Warning]: Before prescribing, the risks of serious neuropsychiatric events must be weighed against the immediate and long term benefits of smoking abstinence for each patient.**

Hypersensitivity reactions (including angioedema) and rare cases of serious skin reactions (including Stevens-Johnson syndrome and erythema multiforme) have been reported. Patients should be instructed to discontinue use and contact healthcare provider if signs/symptoms occur. Treatment may increase risk of cardiovascular events (eg, angina pectoris, nonfatal MI, nonfatal stroke, need for coronary revascularization, new diagnosis of or treatment for PVD). Varenicline was not studied in patients with unstable cardiovascular disease or in patients experiencing recent events (<2 months) prior to treatment. Dose-dependent nausea may occur; both transient and persistent nausea has been reported. Dosage reduction may be considered for intolerable nausea. May cause sedation, which may impair physical or mental abilities; patients must be cautioned about performing tasks which require mental alertness (eg, operating machinery or driving).

Use caution in renal dysfunction; dosage adjustment required. Safety and efficacy of varenicline with other smoking cessation therapies have not been established; increased adverse events when used concurrently with nicotine replacement therapy.

Adverse Reactions (Reflective of adult population; not specific for elderly)

>10%:

Central nervous system: Insomnia (18% to 19%), headache (15% to 19%), abnormal dreams (9% to 13%)

Gastrointestinal: Nausea (16% to 40%; dose related)

1% to 10%:

Central nervous system: Malaise (≤7%), sleep disorder (≤5%), somnolence (3%), night-mares (1% to 2%), lethargy (1% to 2%)

Dermatologic: Rash (≤3%)

Gastrointestinal: Flatulence (6% to 9%), constipation (5% to 8%), abnormal taste (5% to 8%), abdominal pain (≤7%), xerostomia (≤6%), dyspepsia (5%), vomiting (≤5%), appetite increased (3% to 4%), anorexia (≤2%), gastroesophageal reflux (1%)

Respiratory: Upper respiratory tract disorder (5% to 7%), dyspnea (≤2%), rhinorrhea (≤1%)

Drug Interactions

Avoid Concomitant Use There are no known interactions where it is recommended to avoid concomitant use.

Increased Effect/Toxicity

The levels/effects of Varenicline may be increased by: Alcohol (Ethyl); H2-Antagonists; Trimethoprim

Decreased Effect There are no known significant interactions involving a decrease in effect.

Ethanol/Nutrition/Herb Interactions Ethanol: May increase the risk of psychiatric adverse events. Caution patients about the potential effects of ethanol consumption during therapy.

Stability Store at 25°C (77°F); excursions permitted to 15°C to 30°C (59°F to 86°F).

Mechanism of Action Partial neuronal α_4 β_2 nicotinic receptor agonist; prevents nicotine stimulation of mesolimbic dopamine system associated with nicotine addiction. Also binds to 5 HT_3 receptor (significance not determined) with moderate affinity. Varenicline stimulates dopamine activity but to a much smaller degree than nicotine does, resulting in decreased craving and withdrawal symptoms.

Pharmacodynamics/Kinetics

Absorption: Well absorbed; unaffected by food

Protein binding: ≤20%

Metabolism: Minimal (<10% of clearance is through metabolism)

Half-life elimination: ~24 hours

Time to peak, plasma: ~3-4 hours

Excretion: Urine (92% as unchanged drug)

Dosage

Geriatric & Adult Smoking cessation: Oral:

Initial:

Days 1-3: 0.5 mg once daily

Days 4-7: 0.5 mg twice daily

Maintenance (≥ Day 8):

U.S. labeling: 1 mg twice daily for 11 weeks

Canadian labeling: 0.5-1 mg twice daily for 11 weeks

Note: Start 1 week before target quit date. Alternatively, patients may consider setting a quit date up to 35 days after initiation of varenicline (some data suggest that an extended pretreatment regimen may result in higher abstinence rates [Hajek, 2011]). If patient successfully quits smoking at the end of the 12 weeks, may continue for another 12 weeks to help maintain success. If not successful in first 12 weeks, then stop medication and reassess factors contributing to failure.

Renal Impairment

Cl_{cr} ≥30 mL/minute: No adjustment required

Cl_{cr} <30 mL/minute: Initiate: 0.5 mg once daily; maximum dose: 0.5 mg twice daily

Hemodialysis: Maximum dose: 0.5 mg once daily

Hepatic Impairment Dosage adjustment not required

Administration Administer with food and a full glass of water.

Monitoring Parameters Monitor for behavioral changes and psychiatric symptoms (eg, agitation, depression, suicidal behavior, suicidal ideation)

Pharmacotherapy Pearls In all studies, patients received an educational booklet on smoking cessation and received up to 10 minutes of counseling at each weekly visit. Dosing started 1 week before target quit date. Successful cessation of smoking may alter pharmacokinetic properties of other medications (eg, theophylline, warfarin, insulin).

Special Geriatric Considerations Dosage adjustment for renal function may be necessary. Although studies to date do not demonstrate any significant pharmacokinetic differences between elderly (65-75 years of age) and younger adults.

VARENICLINE

Dosage Forms Excipient information presented when available (limited, particularly for generics); consult specific product labeling.

Combination package, oral [dose-pack]:
Chantix®: Tablet: 0.5 mg (11s) [white tablets] and Tablet: 1 mg (42s) [light blue tablets]
Tablet, oral:
Chantix®: 0.5 mg, 1 mg

Selected References

Fiore M, Jaen CR, Baker TB, et al, "A Clinical Practice Guideline for Treating Tobacco Use and Dependence: 2008 Update. A U.S. Public Health Service Report," *Am J Prev Med*, 2008, 35(2):158-76.

Gonzales D, Rennard SI, Nides M, et al, "Varenicline, an Alpha4beta2 Nicotinic Acetylcholine Receptor Partial Agonist, vs Sustained-Release Bupropion and Placebo for Smoking Cessation: A Randomized Controlled Trial," *JAMA*, 2006, 296(1):47-55.

Henningfield JE, Fant RV, Buchhalter JR, et al, "Pharmacotherapy for Nicotine Dependence," *CA Cancer J Clin*, 2005, 55(5):281-99.

Jorenby DE, Hays JT, Rigotti NA, et al, "Efficacy of Varenicline, an Alpha4beta2 Nicotinic Acetylcholine Receptor Partial Agonist, vs Placebo or Sustained-Release Bupropion for Smoking Cessation: A Randomized Controlled Trial," *JAMA*, 2006, 296(1):56-63.

Tonstad S, Tønneson P, Hajek P, et al, "Effect of Maintenance Therapy With Varenicline on Smoking Cessation: A Randomized Controlled Trial," *JAMA*, 2006, 296(1):64-71.

♦ **Varenicline Tartrate** see Varenicline on page 1902
♦ **Varicella-Zoster (VZV) Vaccine (Zoster)** see Zoster Vaccine on page 1965
♦ **Vaseretic®** see Enalapril and Hydrochlorothiazide on page 597
♦ **Vasodilan** see Isoxsuprine on page 992
♦ **Vasolex™** see Trypsin, Balsam Peru, and Castor Oil on page 1876

Vasopressin (vay soe PRES in)

Medication Safety Issues
Administration issues:
Use care when prescribing and/or administering vasopressin solutions. Close attention should be given to concentration of solution, route of administration, dose, and rate of administration (units/minute, units/kg/minute, units/kg/hour).

Brand Names: U.S. Pitressin®
Brand Names: Canada Pressyn®; Pressyn® AR
Index Terms 8-Arginine Vasopressin; ADH; Antidiuretic Hormone; AVP
Generic Availability (U.S.) Yes
Pharmacologic Category Antidiuretic Hormone Analog; Hormone, Posterior Pituitary
Use Treatment of central diabetes insipidus; differential diagnosis of diabetes insipidus
Unlabeled/Investigational Use Adjunct in the treatment of GI hemorrhage and esophageal varices; pulseless arrest (ventricular tachycardia [VT]/ventricular fibrillation [VF], asystole/pulseless electrical activity [PEA]); vasodilatory shock (septic shock); donor management in brain-dead patients (hormone replacement therapy)
Contraindications Hypersensitivity to vasopressin or any component of the formulation
Warnings/Precautions Use with caution in patients with seizure disorders, migraine, asthma, vascular disease, renal disease, cardiac disease; chronic nephritis with nitrogen retention, goiter with cardiac complications, or arteriosclerosis. I.V. infiltration may lead to severe vasoconstriction and localized tissue necrosis, gangrene of extremities, tongue, and ischemic colitis. May cause water intoxication; early signs include drowsiness, listlessness, and headache, these should be recognized to prevent coma and seizures. Elderly patients should be cautioned not to increase their fluid intake beyond that sufficient to satisfy their thirst in order to avoid water intoxication and hyponatremia; under experimental conditions, the elderly have shown to have a decreased responsiveness to vasopressin with respect to its effects on water homeostasis.

Adverse Reactions (Reflective of adult population; not specific for elderly) Frequency not defined.
Cardiovascular: Arrhythmia, asystole (>0.04 units/minute), blood pressure increased, cardiac output decreased (>0.04 units/minute), chest pain, MI, vasoconstriction (with higher doses), venous thrombosis
Central nervous system: Pounding in the head, fever, vertigo
Dermatologic: Ischemic skin lesions, circumoral pallor, urticaria
Gastrointestinal: Abdominal cramps, flatulence, mesenteric ischemia, nausea, vomiting
Genitourinary: Uterine contraction
Neuromuscular & skeletal: Tremor
Respiratory: Bronchial constriction
Miscellaneous: Diaphoresis
Drug Interactions
Avoid Concomitant Use There are no known interactions where it is recommended to avoid concomitant use.

Increased Effect/Toxicity There are no known significant interactions involving an increase in effect.

Decreased Effect There are no known significant interactions involving a decrease in effect.

Ethanol/Nutrition/Herb Interactions Ethanol: Avoid ethanol (due to effects on ADH).

Stability Store injection at room temperature; do not freeze. Protect from heat. Use only clear solutions.

Mechanism of Action Increases cyclic adenosine monophosphate (cAMP) which increases water permeability at the renal tubule resulting in decreased urine volume and increased osmolality; causes peristalsis by directly stimulating the smooth muscle in the GI tract; direct vasoconstrictor without inotropic or chronotropic effects

Pharmacodynamics/Kinetics

Onset of action: Nasal: 1 hour

Duration: Nasal: 3-8 hours; I.M., SubQ: 2-8 hours

Metabolism: Nasal/Parenteral: Hepatic, renal

Half-life elimination: Nasal: 15 minutes; Parenteral: 10-20 minutes

Excretion: Nasal: Urine; SubQ: Urine (5% as unchanged drug) after 4 hours

Dosage

Geriatric & Adult

Central diabetes insipidus: Note: Dosage is highly variable; titrated based on serum and urine sodium and osmolality in addition to fluid balance and urine output. Use of vasopressin is impractical for chronic therapy.

I.M., SubQ: 5-10 units 2-4 times/day as needed

Continuous I.V. infusion (unlabeled route): Continuous infusion has not been formally evaluated in the post-neurosurgical adult. However, some convert I.M./SubQ requirement to an hourly continuous I.V. infusion rate.

Central diabetes insipidus, post-traumatic (unlabeled use): *I.V.:* Initial: 2.5 units/hour; titrate to adequately reduce urine output (Levitt, 1984)

Donor management in brain-dead patients (hormone replacement therapy) (unlabeled use): *I.V.:* Initial: 1 unit bolus followed by 0.5-4 units/hour (Rosendale, 2003; UNOS Critical Pathway, 2002)

Variceal hemorrhage (unlabeled use): *Continuous I.V. infusion:* Dilute in NS or D_5W to 0.1-1 unit/mL. **Note:** Other therapies may be preferred.

[AASLD guidelines, 2007]: *Continuous I.V. infusion:* Initial: 0.2-0.4 units/minute, may titrate dose as needed to a maximum dose of 0.8 units/minute; maximum duration: 24 hours at highest effective dose continuously (to reduce incidence of adverse effects). Patient should also receive I.V. nitroglycerin concurrently to prevent myocardial ischemic complications. Monitor closely for signs/symptoms of ischemia (myocardial, peripheral, bowel).

Pulseless arrest (unlabeled use) [ACLS, 2010]: I.V., I.O.: 40 units; may give 1 dose to replace first or second dose of epinephrine. I.V./I.O. drug administration is preferred, but if no access, may give endotracheally. ACLS guidelines do not recommend a specific endotracheal dose; however, may be given endotracheally using the same I.V. dose (ACLS, 2010; Wenzel, 1997).

Vasodilatory shock/septic shock (unlabeled use): *I.V.:* 0.01-0.04 units/minute for the treatment of septic shock. **Note:** Recommended as a second-line vasopressor in addition to norepinephrine (Dellinger, 2008). Doses >0.04 units/minute may have more cardiovascular side effects. Most case reports have used 0.04 units/minute continuous infusion as a fixed dose.

Hepatic Impairment Some patients respond to much lower doses with cirrhosis.

Administration

I.V.: Use extreme caution to avoid extravasation because of risk of necrosis and gangrene. In treatment of varices, infusions are often supplemented with nitroglycerin infusions to minimize cardiac effects.

Usual concentration: 100 units in 500 mL D_5W. **Note:** In one clinical trial with lower dosing (eg, 0.0005 units/kg/hour) in pediatric patients, a more dilute solution (eg, 20 units in 500 mL D_5W) was employed (Wise-Faberowski, 2004).

Vasodilatory shock: Administration through a central catheter is recommended.

Intranasal (topical administration on nasal mucosa): Administer injectable vasopressin on cotton plugs, as nasal spray, or by dropper. Should not be inhaled.

Endotracheal: If no I.V./I.O. access may give endotracheally. ACLS guidelines do not recommend a specific endotracheal dose; however, may be given endotracheally using the same I.V. dose (Wenzel, 1997). Mix with 5-10 mL of water or normal saline, and administer down the endotracheal tube.

Monitoring Parameters Serum and urine sodium, urine specific gravity, urine and serum osmolality; urine output, fluid input and output, blood pressure, heart rate

Reference Range Plasma: 0-2 pg/mL (SI: 0-2 ng/L) if osmolality <285 mOsm/L; 2-12 pg/mL (SI: 2-12 ng/L) if osmolality >290 mOsm/L

◀ **Pharmacotherapy Pearls** Vasopressin increases factor VIII levels and may be useful in hemophiliacs.

Special Geriatric Considerations Elderly patients should be cautioned not to increase their fluid intake beyond that sufficient to satisfy their thirst in order to avoid water intoxication and hyponatremia. Under experimental conditions, the elderly have shown to have a decreased responsiveness to vasopressin with respect to its effects on water homeostasis.

Dosage Forms Excipient information presented when available (limited, particularly for generics); consult specific product labeling.
Injection, solution: 20 units/mL (0.5 mL, 1 mL, 10 mL)
    Pitressin®: 20 units/mL (1 mL)

Selected References
Miller JH and Shock NW, "Age Differences in the Renal Tubular Response to Antidiuretic Hormone," *J Gerontol*, 1953, 8:446-50.

◆ **Vasotec®** *see* Enalapril *on page* 594
◆ **Vectical™** *see* Calcitriol *on page* 243
◆ **Veltin™** *see* Clindamycin and Tretinoin *on page* 380
◆ **Veltin™** *see* Clindamycin and Tretinoin *on page* 380

Venlafaxine (ven la FAX een)

Related Information
Antidepressant Agents *on page* 1991

Medication Safety Issues
Sound-alike/look-alike issues:
Effexor® may be confused with Effexor XR®

Brand Names: U.S. Effexor XR®; Effexor®

Brand Names: Canada CO Venlafaxine XR; Effexor XR®; Mylan-Venlafaxine XR; PMS-Venlafaxine XR; ratio-Venlafaxine XR; Riva-Venlafaxine XR; Sandoz-Venlafaxine XR; Teva-Venlafaxine XR; Venlafaxine XR

Generic Availability (U.S.) Yes

Pharmacologic Category Antidepressant, Serotonin/Norepinephrine Reuptake Inhibitor

Use Treatment of major depressive disorder, generalized anxiety disorder (GAD), social anxiety disorder (social phobia), panic disorder

Unlabeled/Investigational Use Obsessive-compulsive disorder (OCD); hot flashes; neuropathic pain (including diabetic neuropathy); attention attention-deficit/hyperactivity disorder (ADHD); post-traumatic stress disorder (PTSD)

Medication Guide Available Yes

Contraindications Hypersensitivity to venlafaxine or any component of the formulation; use of MAO inhibitors within 14 days; should not initiate MAO inhibitor within 7 days of discontinuing venlafaxine

Warnings/Precautions [U.S. Boxed Warning]: Antidepressants increase the risk of suicidal thinking and behavior in children, adolescents, and young adults (18-24 years of age) with major depressive disorder (MDD) and other psychiatric disorders; consider risk prior to prescribing. Short-term studies did not show an increased risk in patients >24 years of age and showed a decreased risk in patients ≥65 years. Closely monitor for clinical worsening, suicidality, or unusual changes in behavior; the patient's family or caregiver should be instructed to closely observe the patient and communicate condition with healthcare provider. Reduced growth rate has been observed with venlafaxine therapy in children. A medication guide should be dispensed with each prescription. **Venlafaxine is not FDA approved for use in children.**

The possibility of a suicide attempt is inherent in major depression and may persist until remission occurs. Monitor for worsening of depression or suicidality, especially during initiation of therapy (generally first 1-2 months) or with dose increases or decreases. Use caution in high-risk patients. Worsening depression and severe abrupt suicidality that are not part of the presenting symptoms may require discontinuation or modification of drug therapy. The patient's family or caregiver should be alerted to monitor patients for the emergence of suicidality and associated behaviors (such as agitation, irritability, hostility, impulsivity, and hypomania) and call healthcare provider.

May worsen psychosis in some patients or precipitate a shift to mania or hypomania in patients with bipolar disorder. Patients presenting with depressive symptoms should be screened for bipolar disorder. Monotherapy in patients with bipolar disorder should be avoided. **Venlafaxine is not FDA approved for the treatment of bipolar depression.**

Serotonin syndrome and neuroleptic malignant syndrome (NMS)-like reactions have occurred with serotonin/norepinephrine reuptake inhibitors (SNRIs) and selective serotonin reuptake inhibitors (SSRIs) when used alone, and particularly when used in combination with serotonergic agents (eg, triptans) or antidopaminergic agents (eg, antipsychotics). Concurrent use with MAO inhibitors is contraindicated. May cause sustained increase in blood pressure or tachycardia; dose related and increases are generally modest (12-15 mm Hg diastolic). Control pre-existing hypertension prior to initiation of venlafaxine. Use caution in patients with recent history of MI, unstable heart disease, or hyperthyroidism; may cause increase in anxiety, nervousness, insomnia; may cause weight loss (use with caution in patients where weight loss is undesirable); may cause increases in serum cholesterol. Use caution with hepatic or renal impairment; dosage adjustments recommended. May cause hyponatremia/SIADH (elderly at increased risk); volume depletion (diuretics may increase risk).

May impair platelet aggregation resulting in increased risk of bleeding events, particularly if used concomitantly with aspirin or NSAIDs. Bleeding related to SSRI or SNRI use has been reported to range from relatively minor bruising and epistaxis to life-threatening hemorrhage. Interstitial lung disease and eosinophilic pneumonia have been rarely reported; may present as progressive dyspnea, cough, and/or chest pain. Prompt evaluation and possible discontinuation of therapy may be necessary. Venlafaxine may increase the risks associated with electroconvulsive therapy. Use cautiously in patients with a history of seizures. The risks of cognitive or motor impairment, as well as the potential for anticholinergic effects are very low. May cause or exacerbate sexual dysfunction.

Abrupt discontinuation or dosage reduction after extended (≥6 weeks) therapy may lead to agitation, dysphoria, nervousness, anxiety, and other symptoms. When discontinuing therapy, dosage should be tapered gradually over at least a 2-week period. If intolerable symptoms occur following a decrease in dosage or upon discontinuation of therapy, then resuming the previous dose with a more gradual taper should be considered. Use caution in patients with increased intraocular pressure or at risk of acute narrow-angle glaucoma.

Adverse Reactions (Reflective of adult population; not specific for elderly) Note: Actual frequency may be dependent upon formulation and/or indication

>10%:

Central nervous system: Headache (25% to 38%), somnolence (12% to 26%), dizziness (11% to 24%), insomnia (15% to 24%), nervousness (6% to 21%), anxiety (2% to 11%),

Gastrointestinal: Nausea (21% to 58%), xerostomia (12% to 22%), anorexia (8% to 17%), constipation (8% to 15%)

Genitourinary: Abnormal ejaculation/orgasm (2% to 19%)

Neuromuscular & skeletal: Weakness (8% to 19%)

Miscellaneous: Diaphoresis (7% to 19%)

1% to 10%:

Cardiovascular: Vasodilation (2% to 6%), hypertension (dose related; 3% in patients receiving <100 mg/day, up to 13% in patients receiving >300 mg/day), palpitation (3%), tachycardia (2%), chest pain (2%), postural hypotension (1%), edema

Central nervous system: Yawning (3% to 8%), abnormal dreams (3% to 7%), chills (2% to 7%), agitation (2% to 5%), confusion (2%), abnormal thinking (2%), depersonalization (1%), depression (1% to 3%), fever, migraine, amnesia, hypoesthesia, vertigo

Dermatologic: Rash (3%), pruritus (1%), bruising

Endocrine & metabolic: Libido decreased (2% to 8%), hypercholesterolemia (5%), triglycerides increased

Gastrointestinal: Abdominal pain (8%), diarrhea (8%), vomiting (3% to 8%), dyspepsia (5% to 7%), weight loss (1% to 6%), flatulence (3% to 4%), taste perversion (2%), appetite increased, belching, weight gain

Genitourinary: Impotence (4% to 6%), urinary frequency (3%), urination impaired (2%), urinary retention (1%), metrorrhagia, prostatic disorder, vaginitis

Neuromuscular & skeletal: Tremor (1% to 10%), hypertonia (3%), paresthesia (2% to 3%), twitching (1% to 3%), arthralgia, neck pain, trismus

Ocular: Accommodation abnormal (6% to 9%), abnormal or blurred vision (4% to 6%), mydriasis (2%)

Otic: Tinnitus (2%)

Renal: Albuminuria

Respiratory: Pharyngitis (7%), sinusitis (2%), bronchitis, cough increased, dyspnea

Miscellaneous: Infection (6%), flu-like syndrome (2%), trauma (2%)

Drug Interactions

Metabolism/Transport Effects Substrate of CYP2C9 (minor), 2C19 (minor), 2D6 (major), 3A4 (major); **Inhibits** CYP2B6 (weak), 2D6 (weak), 3A4 (weak)

Avoid Concomitant Use

Avoid concomitant use of Venlafaxine with any of the following: Conivaptan; Iobenguane I 123; MAO Inhibitors; Methylene Blue; Sibutramine

Increased Effect/Toxicity

Venlafaxine may increase the levels/effects of: Alpha-/Beta-Agonists; Aspirin; Methylene Blue; NSAID (Nonselective); Serotonin Modulators; TraZODone; Vitamin K Antagonists

◀ *The levels/effects of Venlafaxine may be increased by:* Abiraterone Acetate; Alcohol (Ethyl); Conivaptan; CYP2D6 Inhibitors (Moderate); CYP2D6 Inhibitors (Strong); CYP3A4 Inhibitors (Moderate); CYP3A4 Inhibitors (Strong); Darunavir; Dasatinib; MAO Inhibitors; Metoclopramide; Propafenone; Sibutramine; Voriconazole

Decreased Effect

Venlafaxine may decrease the levels/effects of: Alpha2-Agonists; Indinavir; Iobenguane I 123

The levels/effects of Venlafaxine may be decreased by: CYP3A4 Inducers (Strong); Deferasirox; Peginterferon Alfa-2b; Tocilizumab

Ethanol/Nutrition/Herb Interactions

Ethanol: May increase CNS depression; monitor for increased effects with coadministration. Caution patients about effects.

Herb/Nutraceutical: Avoid valerian, St John's wort, SAMe, kava kava, tryptophan (may increase risk of serotonin syndrome and/or excessive sedation).

Stability Store at controlled room temperature of 20°C to 25°C (68°F to 77°F).

Mechanism of Action Venlafaxine and its active metabolite, O-desmethylvenlafaxine (ODV), are potent inhibitors of neuronal serotonin and norepinephrine reuptake and weak inhibitors of dopamine reuptake. Venlafaxine and ODV have no significant activity for muscarinic cholinergic, H_1-histaminergic, or alpha$_2$-adrenergic receptors. Venlafaxine and ODV do not possess MAO-inhibitory activity.

Pharmacodynamics/Kinetics

Absorption: Oral: ≥92%; food has no significant effect on absorption or formation of active metabolite

Distribution: V_{dss}: Venlafaxine 7.5 ± 3.7 L/kg, ODV 5.7 ± 1.8 L/Kg

Protein binding: Venlafaxine 27% ± 2%, ODV 30% ± 12%

Metabolism: Hepatic via CYP2D6 to active metabolite, O-desmethylvenlafaxine (ODV); other metabolites include N-desmethylvenlafaxine and N,O-didesmethylvenlafaxine

Bioavailability: Oral: ~45%

Half-life elimination: Venlafaxine: 5 ± 2 hours; ODV: 11 ± 2 hours; prolonged with cirrhosis (venlafaxine: ~30%, ODV: ~60%), renal impairment (venlafaxine: ~50%, ODV: ~40%), and during dialysis (venlafaxine: ~180%, ODV: ~142%)

Time to peak:

Immediate release: Venlafaxine: 2 hours, ODV: 3 hours

Extended release: Venlafaxine: 5.5 hours, ODV: 9 hours

Excretion: Urine (~87%; 5% of total dose as unchanged drug; 29% of total dose as unconjugated ODV; 26% of total dose as conjugated ODV; 27% of total dose as minor inactive metabolites)

Dosage

Geriatric Refer to adult dosing. No specific recommendations for elderly, but may be best to start lower at 25-50 mg twice daily and increase as tolerated by 25 mg/dose. Extended-release formulation: 37.5 mg once daily, increase by 37.5 mg every 4-7 days as tolerated

Alzheimer's dementia-related depression (unlabeled use; Rabins, 2007):

Immediate-release tablets: Initial: 25 mg/day; may increase at weekly intervals to maximum of 375 mg/day in divided doses

Extended-release capsules: Initial: 37.5 mg/day; may increase at weekly intervals to maximum of 225 mg/day

Adult

Depression: Oral:

Immediate-release tablets: Initial: 75 mg/day, administered in 2 or 3 divided doses; may increase in ≤75 mg/day increments at intervals of ≥4 days as tolerated (maximum daily dose: 225-375 mg)

Extended-release capsules or tablets: Initial: 37.5-75 mg once daily; in patients who are initiated at 37.5 mg once daily, may increase to 75 mg once daily after 4-7 days; dose may then be increased by ≤75 mg/day increments at intervals of ≥4 days as tolerated (maximum daily dose: 225 mg)

Generalized anxiety disorder: Oral: *Extended-release capsules:* Initial: 37.5-75 mg once daily; in patients who are initiated at 37.5 mg once daily, may increase to 75 mg once daily after 4-7 days; may then be increased by ≤75 mg/day increments at intervals of ≥4 days as tolerated (maximum daily dose: 225 mg)

Panic disorder: Oral: *Extended-release capsules:* Initial: 37.5 mg once daily for 1 week; may increase to 75 mg once daily after 7 days, may then be increased by ≤75 mg/day increments at intervals of ≥7 days (maximum daily dose: 225 mg)

Social anxiety disorder: Oral: *Extended-release capsules or tablets:* 75 mg once daily (maximum daily dose: 75 mg); no evidence that doses >75 mg/day offer any additional benefit

Obsessive-compulsive disorder (unlabeled use): Oral: Titrate to usual dosage range of 150-300 mg/day; however, doses up to 375 mg/day have been used; response may be seen in 4 weeks (Phelps, 2005)

Neuropathic pain (unlabeled use): Oral: Dosages evaluated varied considerably based on etiology of chronic pain, but efficacy has been shown for many conditions in the range of 75-225 mg/day; onset of relief may occur in 1-2 weeks, or take up to 6 weeks for full benefit (Grothe, 2004).

Diabetic neuropathy (unlabeled use): Oral: 75-225 mg/day (Bril, 2011)

Hot flashes (unlabeled use): Oral: Doses of 37.5-75 mg/day have demonstrated significant improvement of vasomotor symptoms after 4-8 weeks of treatment; in one study, doses >75 mg/day offered no additional benefit (Evans, 2005; Loprinzi, 2000); however, higher doses (225 mg/day) may be beneficial in patients with perimenopausal depression.

Attention-deficit disorder (unlabeled use): Oral: Initial: Doses vary between 18.75 to 75 mg/day; may increase after 4 weeks to 150 mg/day; if tolerated, doses up to 225 mg/day have been used (Maidment, 2003)

Post-traumatic stress disorder (PTSD) (unlabeled use): Oral: *Extended release formulation:* 37.5-300 mg/day (Bandelow, 2008; Benedek, 2009)

Note: When discontinuing this medication after more than 1 week of treatment, it is generally recommended that the dose be tapered. If venlafaxine is used for 6 weeks or longer, the dose should be tapered over 2 weeks when discontinuing its use.

Renal Impairment
GFR: 10-70 mL/minute: Reduce total daily dose by 25% to 50%
Hemodialysis: Reduce total daily dose by 50%

Hepatic Impairment Mild-to-moderate hepatic impairment: Reduce total daily dose by 50%; further reductions may be necessary in some patients

Administration May be administered with food. Swallow extended release capsule whole; do not crush or chew. Alternatively, contents may be sprinkled on a spoonful of applesauce and swallowed immediately without chewing; followed with a glass of water to ensure complete swallowing of the pellets. If switching from a MAO inhibitor to venlafaxine, allow 2 weeks "washout" period before starting venlafaxine; allow 7 days "washout" if switching venlafaxine therapy to a MAO inhibitor.

Monitoring Parameters Blood pressure should be regularly monitored, especially in patients with a high baseline blood pressure; may cause mean increase in heart rate of 4-9 beats/minute; cholesterol; mental status for depression, suicide ideation (especially at the beginning of therapy or when doses are increased or decreased), anxiety, social functioning, mania, panic attacks

Test Interactions May interfere with urine detection of PCP (false-positive).

Special Geriatric Considerations Venlafaxine's low anticholinergic activity, minimal sedation, and hypotension properties makes this a valuable antidepressant in treating elderly with depression or anxiety disorders. No dose adjustment is necessary for age alone; adjust dose for renal function in the elderly. The elderly are more prone to SSRI/SNRI-induced hyponatremia.

Dosage Forms Excipient information presented when available (limited, particularly for generics); consult specific product labeling.
Capsule, extended release, oral: 37.5 mg, 75 mg, 150 mg
Effexor XR®: 37.5 mg, 75 mg, 150 mg
Tablet, oral: 25 mg, 37.5 mg, 50 mg, 75 mg, 100 mg
Effexor®: 50 mg [scored]
Tablet, extended release, oral: 37.5 mg, 75 mg, 150 mg, 225 mg

◆ **Venofer®** see Iron Sucrose *on page 980*
◆ **Ventolin® HFA** see Albuterol *on page 50*
◆ **Veracolate® [OTC]** see Bisacodyl *on page 205*
◆ **Veramyst®** see Fluticasone (Nasal) *on page 771*

Verapamil (ver AP a mil)

Related Information
Calcium Channel Blockers *on page 2003*
Medication Safety Issues
Sound-alike/look-alike issues:
Calan® may be confused with Colace®, diltiazem
Covera-HS® may be confused with Provera®
Isoptin® may be confused with Isopto® Tears

◀ Verelan® may be confused with Virilon®, Voltaren®

High alert medication:
The Institute for Safe Medication Practices (ISMP) includes this medication (I.V. formulation) among its list of drug classes which have a heightened risk of causing significant patient harm when used in error.

Administration issues:
Significant differences exist between oral and I.V. dosing. Use caution when converting from one route of administration to another.

International issues:
Dilacor [Brazil] may be confused with Dilacor XR brand name for diltiazem [U.S.]

Brand Names: U.S. Calan®; Calan® SR; Covera-HS®; Isoptin® SR; Verelan®; Verelan® PM

Brand Names: Canada Apo-Verap®; Apo-Verap® SR; Covera-HS®; Covera®; Dom-Verapamil SR; Isoptin® SR; Mylan-Verapamil; Mylan-Verapamil SR; Novo-Veramil; Novo-Veramil SR; Nu-Verap; Nu-Verap SR; PHL-Verapamil SR; PMS-Verapamil SR; PRO-Verapamil SR; Riva-Verapamil SR; Verapamil Hydrochloride Injection, USP; Verapamil SR; Verelan SRC

Index Terms Iproveratril Hydrochloride; Verapamil Hydrochloride

Generic Availability (U.S.) Yes: Excludes caplet (sustained release) and tablet (extended release, controlled onset)

Pharmacologic Category Antiarrhythmic Agent, Class IV; Calcium Channel Blocker; Calcium Channel Blocker, Nondihydropyridine

Use
Oral: Treatment of hypertension; angina pectoris (vasospastic, chronic stable, unstable) (Calan®, Covera-HS®); supraventricular tachyarrhythmia (PSVT, atrial fibrillation/flutter [rate control])

I.V.: Supraventricular tachyarrhythmia (PSVT, atrial fibrillation/flutter [rate control])

Unlabeled/Investigational Use Migraine; hypertrophic cardiomyopathy; bipolar disorder (manic manifestations)

Contraindications Hypersensitivity to verapamil or any component of the formulation; severe left ventricular dysfunction; hypotension (systolic pressure <90 mm Hg) or cardiogenic shock; sick sinus syndrome (except in patients with a functioning artificial ventricular pacemaker); second- or third-degree AV block (except in patients with a functioning artificial ventricular pacemaker); atrial flutter or fibrillation and an accessory bypass tract (Wolff-Parkinson-White [WPW] syndrome, Lown-Ganong-Levine syndrome)

I.V.: Additional contraindications include concurrent use of I.V. beta-blocking agents; ventricular tachycardia

Warnings/Precautions Avoid use in heart failure; can exacerbate condition; use is contraindicated in severe left ventricular dysfunction. Symptomatic hypotension with or without syncope can rarely occur; blood pressure must be lowered at a rate appropriate for the patient's clinical condition. Rare increases in hepatic enzymes can be observed. Can cause first-degree AV block or sinus bradycardia; use is contraindicated in patients with sick sinus syndrome, second- or third-degree AV block (except in patients with a functioning artificial pacemaker), or an accessory bypass tract (eg, WPW syndrome). Other conduction abnormalities are rare. Use caution when using verapamil together with a beta-blocker. Administration of I.V. verapamil and an I.V. beta-blocker within a few hours of each other may result in asystole and should be avoided; simultaneous administration is contraindicated. Use with caution in patients with hypertrophic cardiomyopathy with outflow tract obstruction (especially those with resting outflow obstruction and severe limiting symptoms); may be used in patients who cannot tolerate beta-blockade.

Decreased neuromuscular transmission has been reported with verapamil; use with caution in patients with attenuated neuromuscular transmission (Duchenne's muscular dystrophy, myasthenia gravis); dosage reduction may be required. Use with caution in renal impairment; monitor hemodynamics and possibly ECG if severe impairment, particularly if concomitant hepatic impairment. Use with caution in patients with hepatic impairment; dosage reduction may be required; monitor hemodynamics and possibly ECG if severe impairment. May prolong recovery from nondepolarizing neuromuscular-blocking agents. Use Covera-HS® (extended-release delivery system) with caution in patients with severe GI narrowing. In patients with extremely short GI transit times (eg, <7 hours), dosage adjustment may be required.

Adverse Reactions (Reflective of adult population; not specific for elderly)
>10%:
Central nervous system: Headache (1% to 12%)
Gastrointestinal: Gingival hyperplasia (≤19%), constipation (7% to 12%)
1% to 10%:
Cardiovascular: Peripheral edema (1% to 4%), hypotension (3%), CHF/pulmonary edema (2%), AV block (1% to 2%), bradycardia (HR <50 bpm: 1%), flushing (1%)
Central nervous system: Fatigue (2% to 5%), dizziness (1% to 5%), lethargy (3%), pain (2%), sleep disturbance (1%)

Dermatologic: Rash (1% to 2%)

Gastrointestinal: Dyspepsia (3%), nausea (1% to 3%), diarrhea (2%)

Hepatic: Liver enzymes increased (1%)

Neuromuscular & skeletal: Myalgia (1%), paresthesia (1%)

Respiratory: Dyspnea (1%)

Miscellaneous: Flu-like syndrome (4%)

Drug Interactions

Metabolism/Transport Effects Substrate of CYP1A2 (minor), CYP2B6 (minor), CYP2C9 (minor), CYP2C18 (minor), CYP2E1 (minor), CYP3A4 (major), P-glycoprotein; **Inhibits** CYP1A2 (weak), CYP2C9 (weak), CYP2D6 (weak), CYP3A4 (moderate), P-glycoprotein

Avoid Concomitant Use

Avoid concomitant use of Verapamil with any of the following: Conivaptan; Disopyramide; Dofetilide; Tolvaptan; Topotecan

Increased Effect/Toxicity

Verapamil may increase the levels/effects of: Alcohol (Ethyl); Aliskiren; Amifostine; Amiodarone; Antihypertensives; Atorvastatin; Benzodiazepines (metabolized by oxidation); Beta-Blockers; Budesonide (Systemic, Oral Inhalation); BusPIRone; Calcium Channel Blockers (Dihydropyridine); CarBAMazepine; Cardiac Glycosides; Colchicine; Corticosteroids (Systemic); CycloSPORINE; CycloSPORINE (Systemic); CYP3A4 Substrates; Dabigatran Etexilate; Disopyramide; Dofetilide; Dronedarone; Eletriptan; Eplerenone; Everolimus; Fexofenadine; Fingolimod; Flecainide; Fosphenytoin; Halofantrine; Hypotensive Agents; Lithium; Lovastatin; Lurasidone; Magnesium Salts; Midodrine; Neuromuscular-Blocking Agents (Nondepolarizing); Nitroprusside; P-Glycoprotein Substrates; Phenytoin; Pimecrolimus; QuiNIDine; Ranolazine; Red Yeast Rice; RisperiDONE; RiTUXimab; Rivaroxaban; Salicylates; Salmeterol; Saxagliptin; Simvastatin; Tacrolimus; Tacrolimus (Systemic); Tacrolimus (Topical); Tolvaptan; Topotecan; Vilazodone

The levels/effects of Verapamil may be increased by: Alpha1-Blockers; Anilidopiperidine Opioids; Antifungal Agents (Azole Derivatives, Systemic); Atorvastatin; Calcium Channel Blockers (Dihydropyridine); Cimetidine; Conivaptan; CycloSPORINE; CycloSPORINE (Systemic); CYP3A4 Inhibitors (Moderate); CYP3A4 Inhibitors (Strong); Dasatinib; Diazoxide; Dronedarone; Fluconazole; Grapefruit Juice; Herbs (Hypotensive Properties); Macrolide Antibiotics; Magnesium Salts; MAO Inhibitors; Pentoxifylline; P-Glycoprotein Inhibitors; Phosphodiesterase 5 Inhibitors; Prostacyclin Analogues; Protease Inhibitors; QuiNIDine; Telithromycin

Decreased Effect

Verapamil may decrease the levels/effects of: Clopidogrel

The levels/effects of Verapamil may be decreased by: Barbiturates; Calcium Salts; CarBAMazepine; CYP3A4 Inducers (Strong); Cyproterone; Deferasirox; Herbs (CYP3A4 Inducers); Herbs (Hypertensive Properties); Methylphenidate; Nafcillin; P-Glycoprotein Inducers; Rifamycin Derivatives; Tocilizumab; Yohimbine

Ethanol/Nutrition/Herb Interactions

Ethanol: Avoid or limit ethanol (may increase ethanol levels).

Food: Grapefruit juice may increase the serum concentration of verapamil; use with caution and monitor for increased verapamil effects.

Herb/Nutraceutical: St John's wort may decrease levels. Avoid herbs with hypertensive properties (bayberry, blue cohosh, cayenne, ephedra, ginger, ginseng [American], kola, licorice); may diminish the antihypertensive effect of verapamil. Avoid herbs with hypotensive properties (black cohosh, California poppy, coleus, golden seal, hawthorn, mistletoe, periwinkle, quinine, shepherd's purse); may enhance the hypotensive effect of verapamil.

Stability Store at controlled room temperature of 15°C to 30°C (59°F to 86°F). Protect from light.

Mechanism of Action Inhibits calcium ion from entering the "slow channels" or select voltage-sensitive areas of vascular smooth muscle and myocardium during depolarization; produces relaxation of coronary vascular smooth muscle and coronary vasodilation; increases myocardial oxygen delivery in patients with vasospastic angina; slows automaticity and conduction of AV node.

Pharmacodynamics/Kinetics

Onset of action: Peak effect: Oral: Immediate release: 1-2 hours; I.V.: 1-5 minutes

Duration: Oral: Immediate release tablets: 6-8 hours; I.V.: 10-20 minutes

Absorption: Well absorbed

Distribution: V_d: 3.89 L/kg (Storstein, 1984)

Protein binding: ~90%

Metabolism: Hepatic (extensive first-pass effect) via multiple CYP isoenzymes; primary metabolite is norverapamil (20% pharmacologic activity of verapamil)

Bioavailability: Oral: 20% to 35%

◀ Half-life elimination: Adults: Single dose: 3-7 hours, Multiple doses: 4.5-12 hours; severe hepatic impairment: 14-16 hours

Time to peak, serum: Oral:

Immediate release: 1-2 hours

Extended release (Covera-HS®, Verelan PM®): ~11 hours, drug release delayed ~4-5 hours

Sustained release: 5.21 hours (Calan® SR, Isoptin® SR); 7-9 hours (Verelan®)

Excretion: Urine (70% as metabolites, 3% to 4% as unchanged drug); feces (16%)

Dosage

Geriatric

Refer to adult dosing.

Hypertension: Oral: **Note:** When switching from immediate release to extended or sustained release formulations, the total daily dose remains the same unless formulation strength does not allow for equal conversion.

Manufacturer's recommendations:

Immediate release: Initial: 40 mg 3 times daily

Sustained release: Calan® SR, Isoptin® SR, Verelan®: Initial: 120 mg once daily in the morning

Extended release:

Covera-HS®: Initial: 180 mg once daily at bedtime

Verelan® PM: Initial: 100 mg once daily at bedtime

ACCF/AHA Expert Consensus recommendations: Consider lower initial doses and titrating to response (Aronow, 2011)

Adult

Angina: Oral: **Note:** When switching from immediate-release to extended/sustained release formulations, the total daily dose remains the same unless formulation strength does not allow for equal conversion.

Immediate release: Initial: 80-120 mg 3 times/day (elderly or small stature: 40 mg 3 times/day); Usual dose range (Gibbons, 2002): 80-160 mg 3 times/day

Extended release (Covera-HS®): Initial: 180 mg once daily at bedtime; if inadequate response, may increase dose at weekly intervals to 240 mg once daily, then 360 mg once daily, then 480 mg once daily; maximum dose: 480 mg/day

Chronic atrial fibrillation (rate-control), PSVT prophylaxis: Oral: Immediate release: 240-480 mg/day in 3-4 divided doses; Usual dose range (Fuster, 2006): 120-360 mg/day in divided doses

Hypertension: Oral: **Note:** When switching from immediate-release to extended/sustained release formulations, the total daily dose remains the same unless formulation strength does not allow for equal conversion.

Immediate release: 80 mg 3 times/day; usual dose range (JNC 7): 80-320 mg/day in 2 divided doses

Sustained release: Usual dose range (JNC 7): 120-480 mg/day in 1-2 divided doses; **Note:** There is no evidence of additional benefit with doses >360 mg/day.

Calan® SR, Isoptin® SR: Initial: 180 mg once daily in the morning (elderly or small stature: 120 mg/day); if inadequate response, may increase dose at weekly intervals to 240 mg once daily, then 180 mg twice daily (or 240 mg in the morning followed by 120 mg in the evening); maximum dose: 240 mg twice daily.

Verelan®: Initial: 180 mg once daily in the morning (elderly or small stature: 120 mg/day); if inadequate response, may increase dose at weekly intervals to 240 mg once daily, then 360 mg once daily, then 480 mg once daily; maximum dose: 480 mg/day

Extended release: Usual dose range (JNC 7): 120-360 mg once daily (once-daily dosing is recommended at bedtime)

Covera-HS®: Initial: 180 mg once daily at bedtime; if inadequate response, may increase dose at weekly intervals to 240 mg once daily, then 360 mg once daily, then 480 mg once daily; maximum dose: 480 mg/day

Verelan® PM: Initial: 200 mg once daily at bedtime (elderly or small stature: 100 mg/day); if inadequate response, may increase dose at weekly intervals to 300 mg once daily, then 400 mg once daily; maximum dose: 400 mg/day

SVT (ACLS, 2010): I.V.: 2.5-5 mg over 2 minutes; second dose of 5-10 mg (~0.15 mg/kg) may be given 15-30 minutes after the initial dose if patient tolerates, but does not respond to initial dose; maximum total dose: 20-30 mg

Renal Impairment Manufacturer recommends caution and additional ECG monitoring in patients with renal insufficiency. The manufacturer of Verelan PM® recommends an initial dose of 100 mg/day at bedtime. **Note:** A multiple dose study in adults suggests reduced renal clearance of verapamil and its metabolite (norverapamil) with advanced renal failure (Storstein, 1984). Additionally, several clinical papers report adverse effects of verapamil in patients with chronic renal failure receiving recommended doses of verapamil (Pritza, 1991; Váquez, 1996). In contrast, a number of single dose studies show no difference in verapamil (or norverapamil metabolite) disposition between chronic renal failure and control patients (Beyerlein, 1990; Hanyok, 1988; Mooy, 1985; Zachariah, 1991).

Dialysis: Not removed by hemodialysis (Mooy, 1985); supplemental dose is not necessary.

Hepatic Impairment In cirrhosis, reduce dose to 20% and 50% of normal for oral and intravenous administration, respectively, and monitor ECG (Somogyi, 1981). The manufacturer of Verelan PM® recommends an initial daily dose of 100 mg/day at bedtime. The manufacturers of Calan®, Calan® SR, Covera-HS®, Isoptin® SR, and Verelan® recommend giving 30% of the normal dose to patients with severe hepatic impairment.

Administration

Oral: Do not crush or chew sustained or extended release products.

Calan® SR, Isoptin® SR: Administer with food.

Verelan®, Verelan® PM: Capsules may be opened and the contents sprinkled on 1 tablespoonful of applesauce, then swallowed immediately without chewing. Do not subdivide contents of capsules.

I.V.: Rate of infusion: Over 2 minutes; over 3 minutes in older patients (ACLS, 2010)

Monitoring Parameters Monitor blood pressure and heart rate; periodic liver function tests; ECG, especially with renal and/or hepatic impairment

Test Interactions May interfere with urine detection of methadone (false-positive).

Pharmacotherapy Pearls Incidence of adverse reactions is most common with I.V. administration; discontinue disopyramide 48 hours before starting therapy, do not restart therapy until 24 hours after verapamil has been discontinued

Special Geriatric Considerations Elderly may experience a greater hypotensive response. Constipation may be more of a problem in the elderly. Calcium channel blockers are no more effective in the elderly than other therapies; however, they do not cause significant CNS effects which is an advantage over some antihypertensive agents. Generic verapamil products which are bioequivalent in young adults may not be bioequivalent in the elderly; use generics cautiously.

Dosage Forms Excipient information presented when available (limited, particularly for generics); consult specific product labeling. [DSC] = Discontinued product

Caplet, sustained release, oral, as hydrochloride:

Calan® SR: 120 mg

Calan® SR: 180 mg, 240 mg [scored]

Capsule, extended release, oral, as hydrochloride: 120 mg, 180 mg, 240 mg

Capsule, extended release, controlled onset, oral, as hydrochloride: 100 mg, 200 mg, 300 mg

Verelan® PM: 100 mg, 200 mg, 300 mg

Capsule, sustained release, oral, as hydrochloride: 120 mg, 180 mg, 240 mg, 360 mg

Verelan®: 120 mg, 180 mg, 240 mg, 360 mg

Injection, solution, as hydrochloride: 2.5 mg/mL (2 mL, 4 mL)

Tablet, oral, as hydrochloride: 40 mg, 80 mg, 120 mg

Calan®: 80 mg, 120 mg [scored]

Tablet, extended release, oral, as hydrochloride: 120 mg, 180 mg, 240 mg

Tablet, extended release, controlled onset, oral, as hydrochloride:

Covera-HS®: 180 mg, 240 mg

Tablet, sustained release, oral, as hydrochloride: 120 mg [DSC], 180 mg [DSC], 240 mg

Isoptin® SR: 120 mg

Isoptin® SR: 180 mg, 240 mg [scored]

Extemporaneously Prepared To prepare a verapamil 50 mg/mL liquid, crush 75 verapamil hydrochloride 80 mg tablets into a fine powder. Add ~40 mL of either Ora-Sweet® and Ora-Plus® (1:1 preparation), or Ora-Sweet® SF and Ora-Plus® (1:1 preparation), or cherry syrup. Mix to a uniform paste. Continue to add the vehicle to bring the final volume to 120 mL. The preparation is stable for 60 days; shake well before using and protect from light.

Allen LV and Erickson III MA, "Stability of Labetalol Hydrochloride, Metoprolol Tartrate, Verapamil Hydrochloride, and Spironolactone With Hydrochlorothiazide in Extemporaneously Compounded Oral Liquids," *Am J Health Syst Pharm*, 1996, 53:304-9.

Selected References

Black HR, Elliott WJ, Grandits G, et al, "Principal Results of the Controlled Onset Verapamil Investigation of Cardiovascular End Points (CONVINCE) Trial," *JAMA*, 2003, 289(16):2073-82.

Chobanian AV, Bakris GL, Black HR, et al, "The Seventh Report of the Joint National Committee on Prevention, Detection, Evaluation, and Treatment of High Blood Pressure: The JNC 7 Report," *JAMA*, 2003, 289(19):2560-71.

Fuster V, Ryden LE, Cannom DS, et al, "ACC/AHA/ESC 2006 Guidelines for the Management of Patients With Atrial Fibrillation-Executive Summary. A Report of the American College of Cardiology/American Heart Association Task Force on Practice Guidelines and the European Society of Cardiology Committee for Practice Guidelines (Writing Committee to Revise the 2001 Guidelines for the Management of Patients With Atrial Fibrillation). Developed in Collaboration With the European Heart Rhythm Association and the Heart Rhythm Society," *J Am Coll Cardiol*, 2006, 48(4):854-906.

Maron BJ, McKenna WJ, Danielson GK, et al, "American College of Cardiology/European Society of Cardiology Clinical Expert Consensus Document on Hypertrophic Cardiomyopathy. A Report of the American College of Cardiology Foundation Task Force on Clinical Expert Consensus Documents and the European Society of Cardiology Committee for Practice Guidelines," *J Am Coll Cardiol*, 2003, 42(9):1687-713.

Nishimura RA and Holmes DR Jr, "Clinical Practice. Hypertrophic Obstructive Cardiomyopathy," *N Engl J Med*, 2004, 350(13):1320-7.

◆ **Verapamil and Trandolapril** *see* Trandolapril and Verapamil *on page 1845*
◆ **Verapamil Hydrochloride** *see* Verapamil *on page 1909*
◆ **Verelan®** *see* Verapamil *on page 1909*
◆ **Verelan® PM** *see* Verapamil *on page 1909*
◆ **Veripred™ 20** *see* PrednisoLONE (Systemic) *on page 1507*
◆ **Versed** *see* Midazolam *on page 1209*

Verteporfin (ver te POR fin)

Brand Names: U.S. Visudyne®
Brand Names: Canada Visudyne®
Generic Availability (U.S.) No
Pharmacologic Category Ophthalmic Agent
Use Treatment of predominantly classic subfoveal choroidal neovascularization due to macular degeneration, presumed ocular histoplasmosis, or pathologic myopia
Unlabeled/Investigational Use Predominantly **occult** subfoveal choroidal neovascularization
Contraindications Hypersensitivity to verteporfin or any component of the formulation; porphyria
Warnings/Precautions Avoid exposing skin or eyes to direct sunlight or bright indoor light for 5 days following treatment. In case of emergency surgery within 48 hours of treatment, protect as much of the internal tissue as possible from intense light. Do not retreat patients who experience a decrease of vision ≥4 lines within 1 week of treatment unless vision recovers and the potential benefits and risks are carefully considered. Use of incompatible lasers (which do not provide the required light for photoactivation) can result in incomplete treatment, overtreatment, or damage to normal tissue.

Use in more than one eye has not been studied; however, it is recommended that if required, initial treatment should be applied to the more aggressive lesion first, followed by the second eye a week later (subsequent treatment may be concurrent). Standard precautions should be taken to avoid extravasation (eg free-flowing I.V. line, use of largest arm vein). Chest pain, vasovagal and hypersensitivity reactions have occurred rarely; observation of patient during infusion is suggested.

Use in patients with moderate-to-severe hepatic impairment, biliary obstruction, or under anesthesia has not been studied. Patients with dark irides, occult lesions, <50% classic choroidal neovascularization, or patients ≥75 years of age are less likely to benefit from therapy. Safety and efficacy of use for longer than 2 years have not been established.

Adverse Reactions (Reflective of adult population; not specific for elderly)
>10%:
  Central nervous system: Headache
  Local: Injection site reactions (including injection site extravasation, injection site rash)
  Ocular: Blurred vision, visual acuity decreased, visual field defects, visual disturbances
1% to 10%:
  Cardiovascular: Atrial fibrillation, hypertension, peripheral vascular disorder, varicose veins
  Central nervous system: Fever, hypoesthesia, sleep disturbance, vertigo
  Dermatologic: Eczema, photosensitivity
  Gastrointestinal: Constipation, gastrointestinal cancers, nausea
  Genitourinary: Prostatic disorder
  Hematologic: Anemia, leukocytosis, leukopenia
  Hepatic: Liver function tests increased
  Neuromuscular & skeletal: Arthralgia, arthrosis, back pain (primarily during infusion), myasthenia, weakness
  Ocular: Diplopia, lacrimation disorder
    Treatment site: Blepharitis, cataracts, conjunctivitis/conjunctival injection, dry eyes, ocular itching, severe vision loss (1% to 4%, decrease in 4 lines or more within 7 days of treatment, partial recovery seen in many patients), subconjunctival, subretinal or vitreous hemorrhage.
  Otic: Hearing loss
  Renal: Albuminuria, creatinine increased
  Respiratory: Cough, pharyngitis, pneumonia
  Miscellaneous: Flu-like syndrome
Drug Interactions
  Avoid Concomitant Use There are no known interactions where it is recommended to avoid concomitant use.
  Increased Effect/Toxicity There are no known significant interactions involving an increase in effect.

Decreased Effect There are no known significant interactions involving a decrease in effect.

Ethanol/Nutrition/Herb Interactions Ethanol: Ethanol may decrease efficacy of verteporfin.

Stability Store vial at 20°C to 25°C (68°F to 77°F). Each vial should be reconstituted with 7 mL of sterile water for injection, providing a total volume of 7.5 mL. Resulting solution will be 2 mg/mL. Solution should be protected from light and used within 4 hours. Once reconstituted, verteporfin will be an opaque dark green solution. The total volume of solution needed to administer the dose should be withdrawn from the vial and further diluted with D_5W to a total volume of 30 mL. Infuse at 3 mL/minute over 10 minutes, using syringe pump and in-line filter.

Mechanism of Action Following intravenous administration, verteporfin is transported by lipoproteins to the neovascular endothelium in the affected eye(s), including choroidal neovasculature and the retina. Verteporfin then needs to be activated by nonthermal red light, which results in local damage to the endothelium, leading to temporary choroidal vessel occlusion.

Pharmacodynamics/Kinetics
Metabolism: Hepatic and by plasma esterases to diacid metabolite
Half-life elimination: Terminal: 5-6 hours, biexponential
Excretion: Feces

Dosage
Geriatric Refer to adult dosing. Patients ≥75 years were less likely to benefit from therapy in clinical trials.

Adult Therapy is a two-step process; first the infusion of verteporfin, then the activation of verteporfin with a nonthermal diode laser (for light administration details, see Administration).

Subfoveal choroidal neovascularization: I.V.: 6 mg/m² body surface area

Note: Treatment in more than one eye: Patients who have lesions in both eyes should be evaluated and treatment should first be done to the more aggressive lesion. Following safe and acceptable treatment, the second eye can be treated one week later. Patients who have had previous verteporfin therapy, with an acceptable safety profile, may then have both eyes treated concurrently. Treat the more aggressive lesion followed immediately with the second eye. The light treatment to the second eye should begin no later than 20 minutes from the start of the infusion.

Hepatic Impairment Half-life is increased by 20% with mild hepatic impairment. There are no clinical studies in patients with moderate-to-severe hepatic impairment.

Administration A free-flowing I.V. line should be established prior to starting infusion. Use of the largest arm vein, especially in the elderly, is suggested; avoid small veins in the back of the hand. Reconstituted solution should be given at 3 mL/minute over 10 minutes using a syringe pump and an in-line filter. If extravasation occurs, protect the site from light. Use of rubber gloves and eye protection is recommended. Skin and eye contact should be avoided and all materials should be disposed of properly.

Light administration: Following intravenous infusion, verteporfin must be light activated using a nonthermal diode laser. The system must provide a stable power output at a wavelength of 689±3 nm. Approved laser systems are listed in manufacturer's package insert. Light delivery should begin 15 minutes following the start of the 10-minute infusion. The light dose is J/cm² of neovascular lesion administered over 83 seconds at an intensity of 600 mW/cm². Instructions for determining lesion size and treatment spot size can also be found in the package insert.

Monitoring Parameters Intravenous site during infusion, to avoid extravasation; fluorescein angiography every 3 months to monitor choroidal neovascular leakage

Pharmacotherapy Pearls Verteporfin also contains lactose, egg phosphatidylglycerol.

Dosage Forms Excipient information presented when available (limited, particularly for generics); consult specific product labeling.
Injection, powder for reconstitution:
Visudyne®: 15 mg [contains egg phosphatidylglycerol]

♦ **Vicks® DayQuil® Sinus [OTC]** *see* Acetaminophen and Phenylephrine *on page 38*
♦ **Vicks® Pediatric Formula 44E [OTC]** *see* Guaifenesin and Dextromethorphan *on page 848*
♦ **Vicks® Sinex® VapoSpray™ 4 Hour Decongestant [OTC]** *see* Phenylephrine (Nasal) *on page 1442*
♦ **Vicks® Sinex® VapoSpray 12-Hour** *see* Oxymetazoline (Nasal) *on page 1374*
♦ **Vicks® Sinex® VapoSpray 12-Hour UltraFine Mist [OTC]** *see* Oxymetazoline (Nasal) *on page 1374*
♦ **Vicks® Sinex® VapoSpray Moisturizing 12-Hour UltraFine Mist [OTC]** *see* Oxymetazoline (Nasal) *on page 1374*
♦ **Vicks® Vitamin C [OTC]** *see* Ascorbic Acid *on page 149*
♦ **Vicodin®** *see* Hydrocodone and Acetaminophen *on page 880*
♦ **Vicodin® ES** *see* Hydrocodone and Acetaminophen *on page 880*
♦ **Vicodin® HP** *see* Hydrocodone and Acetaminophen *on page 880*
♦ **Victoza®** *see* Liraglutide *on page 1077*

Vigabatrin (vye GA ba trin)

Medication Safety Issues
  Sound-alike/look-alike issues:
  Vigabatrin may be confused with Vibativ™
Brand Names: U.S. Sabril®
Brand Names: Canada Sabril®
Generic Availability (U.S.) No
Pharmacologic Category Anticonvulsant, Miscellaneous
Use Treatment of refractory complex partial seizures not controlled by usual treatments

Additional uses in Canadian labeling (not in U.S. labeling): Active management of partial or secondary generalized seizures not controlled by usual treatments
Unlabeled/Investigational Use Spasticity, tardive dyskinesias
Prescribing and Access Restrictions As a requirement of the REMS program, access to this medication is restricted. Vigabatrin is only available in the U.S. under a special restricted distribution program (SHARE). Under the SHARE program, only prescribers and pharmacies registered with the program are able to prescribe and distribute vigabatrin. Vigabatrin may only be dispensed to patients who are enrolled in and meet all conditions of SHARE. Contact the SHARE program at 1-888-45-SHARE.
Medication Guide Available Yes
Contraindications There are no contraindications listed within the FDA-approved manufacturer's labeling.

Canadian labeling (not in U.S. labeling): Hypersensitivity to vigabatrin or any component of the formulation
Warnings/Precautions Use has been associated with decreased hemoglobin and hematocrit; cases of significantly reduced hemoglobin (<8 g/dL) and/or hematocrit (<24%) have been reported. Somnolence and fatigue can occur with use; patients must be cautioned about performing tasks which require mental alertness (eg, operating machinery or driving). Peripheral edema independent of hypertension, heart failure, weight gain, renal or hepatic dysfunction has been reported. Neurotoxicity: Patients must be closely monitored for potential neurotoxicity (observed in animal models but not established in humans). Peripheral neuropathy and manifesting as numbness or tingling in the toes or feet, reduced distal lower limb vibration or position sensation, or progressive loss of reflexes, starting at the ankles has been reported in adult patients. Pooled analysis of trials involving various antiepileptics (regardless of indication) showed an increased risk of suicidal thoughts/behavior (incidence rate: 0.43% treated patients compared to 0.24% of patients receiving placebo); risk observed as early as 1 week after initiation and continued through duration of trials (most trials ≤24 weeks). Monitor all patients for notable changes in behavior that might indicate suicidal thoughts or depression; notify healthcare provider immediately if symptoms occur. Use has been associated with an average weight gain of 3.5 kg in adults.

[U.S. Boxed Warning]: Vigabatrin causes permanent vision loss in infants, children and adults. Due to the risk of vision loss and because vigabatrin, provides an observable symptomatic benefit when it is effective, the patient who fails to show substantial clinical benefit within a short period of time after initiation of treatment -4 weeks for infantile spasms; <3 months in adults), should be withdrawn from therapy. If in the clinical judgment of the prescriber evidence of treatment failure becomes obvious earlier in treatment, vigabatrin should be discontinued at that time. Patient response to and continued need for treatment should be periodically assessed. The onset of vision loss is unpredictable, and can occur within weeks of starting treatment or sooner, or at any time during treatment, even after months or years. The risk of vision loss increases with increasing dose and cumulative exposure, but there is no dose or exposure known to be free of risk of vision loss. It is possible that vision loss can worsen despite discontinuation. Most data are available in adult patients. Vigabatrin causes permanent bilateral concentric visual field constriction in >30% of patients ranging in severity from mild to severe, including tunnel vision to within 10 degrees of visual fixation, and can result in disability. In some cases, vigabatrin can damage the central retina and may decrease visual acuity. Patient response to and continued need for vigabatrin should be periodically reassessed. Vision loss of milder severity, although potentially unrecognized by the parent or caregiver, may still adversely affect function. Vision should be assessed to the extent possible at baseline (no later than 4 weeks after initiation), at least every 3 months during therapy and at 3-6 months after discontinuation. Once detected, vision loss is not reversible. Vigabatrin should not be used in patients with, or at high risk of, other types of irreversible vision loss unless the benefits of treatment clearly outweigh the risks. The interaction of other types of irreversible vision damage with vision damage from vigabatrin has not been well-characterized, but is likely adverse. Vigabatrin should not be used with other drugs associated with serious adverse ophthalmic effects such as retinopathy or glaucoma unless the benefits clearly outweigh the risks. The lowest dose and shortest exposure should be used that is consistent with clinical objectives.

Use with caution in patients with a history of psychosis (psychotic/agitated reactions may occur more frequently), depression, or behavioral problems. Use with caution in patients with renal impairment; modify dose in renal impairment (Cl$_{cr}$ <80 mL/minute). May cause an increase in seizure frequency in some patients; use with particular caution in patients with myoclonic seizures, which may be more prone to this effect. Effects with other sedative drugs or ethanol may be potentiated. Use with caution in the elderly as severe sedation and confusion have been reported; consider dose and/or frequency adjustments as renal clearance may be decreased.

Abnormal MRI changes have been reported in some infants. Resolution of MRI changes usually occurs with discontinuation of therapy. MRI changes were not seen in older children and adult patients. In the U.S., vigabatrin is only available under a special restricted distribution program (SHARE). Under the SHARE program, only prescribers and pharmacies registered with the program are able to prescribe and distribute vigabatrin. Vigabatrin may only be dispensed to patients who are enrolled in and meet all conditions of SHARE. Anticonvulsants should not be discontinued abruptly because of the possibility of increasing seizure frequency; therapy should be withdrawn gradually to minimize the potential of increased seizure frequency, unless safety concerns require a more rapid withdrawal.

Adverse Reactions (Reflective of adult population; not specific for elderly) Note: Adult and pediatric information presented combined unless significantly different.

>10%:
  Central nervous system: Somnolence (adults 17% to 24%; infants 17% to 45%), headache (18% to 33%), fatigue (16% to 28%), fever (adults 4% to 6%; infants 19% to 29%), dizziness (15% to 24%), irritability (adults 7%; infants 16% to 23%), sedation (adults 4%; infants 17% to 19%), nystagmus (7% to 15%), tremor (7% to 15%), insomnia (10% to 12%), seizure (4% to 11%)
  Dermatologic: Rash (4% to 11%)
  Gastrointestinal: Vomiting (adults 6% to 7%; infants 14% to 20%), weight gain (6% to 17%), constipation (6% to 14%), diarrhea (7% to 13%)
  Neuromuscular & skeletal: Tremor (7% to 15%)
  Ocular: Blurred vision (6% to 13%)
  Otic: Otitis media (infants 7% to 44%)
  Respiratory: Upper respiratory tract infection (adults 7% to 10%; infants 46% to 51%), bronchitis (infants 30%), pharyngitis (10% to 14%), pneumonia (infants 11% to 13%), nasal congestion (infants 4% to 13%)
  Miscellaneous: Viral infection (infants 19% to 20%)
1% to 10%:
  Cardiovascular: Peripheral edema (2% to 5%), chest pain (1%)
  Central nervous system: Irritability (adults 7% to 10%; infants 16% to 23%), memory impairment (7% to 10%), coordination impaired (7% to 9%), disturbance in attention (5% to 9%), depression (4% to 8%), lethargy (4% to 7%), confusional state (4% to 6%), hypotonia (4% to 6%), status epilepticus (2% to 6%), weakness (5%), hyporeflexia (4% to 5%), sensory disturbance (4% to 5%), anxiety (4%), hypoesthesia (3% to 4%), abnormal behavior (3%), abnormal thinking (3%), aggression (2%), nervousness (2%), postictal state (2%), vertigo (2%), abnormal dreams (1%), dystonia (1%), expressive language disorder (1%), hypertonia (1%)
  Dermatologic: Contusion (3% to 4%)
  Endocrine & metabolic: Dysmenorrhea (7% to 9%), fluid retention (2%)

◀

Gastrointestinal: Nausea (7% to 10%), decreased appetite (7% to 9%), viral gastroenteritis (infants 5% to 6%), abdominal pain (3% to 5%), dyspepsia (4%), abdominal distention (2%), hemorrhoidal symptoms (2%), toothache (2%), increased appetite (1% to 2%)

Genitourinary: Urinary tract infection (4% to 6%)

Neuromuscular & skeletal: Arthralgia (8% to 10%), gait disturbance (6%), paresthesia (5% to 7%), pain in extremity (5% to 6%), back pain (4% to 6%), hyper-reflexia (4%), myalgia (3%), muscle spasms (2% to 3%), dysarthria (2%), joint swelling (2%), shoulder pain (2%), joint sprain (1%), muscle strain (1%), muscle twitching (1%)

Ocular: Visual field defect (9%), diplopia (3% to 7%), strabismus (5%), conjunctivitis (2% to 5%), eye strain (2%)

Otic: Tinnitus (2%)

Respiratory: Pharyngolaryngeal pain (7% to 9%), sinusitis (5% to 9%), cough (2% to 8%), sinus headache (4% to 6%), dyspnea (2%)

Miscellaneous: Candidiasis (3% to 8%), influenza (3% to 6%), croup (1% to 5%), thirst (2%)

Drug Interactions

Avoid Concomitant Use There are no known interactions where it is recommended to avoid concomitant use.

Increased Effect/Toxicity

Vigabatrin may increase the levels/effects of: Alcohol (Ethyl); CNS Depressants; Methotrimeprazine; Selective Serotonin Reuptake Inhibitors

The levels/effects of Vigabatrin may be increased by: Droperidol; HydrOXYzine; Methotrimeprazine

Decreased Effect

Vigabatrin may decrease the levels/effects of: Fosphenytoin; Phenytoin

The levels/effects of Vigabatrin may be decreased by: Ketorolac; Ketorolac (Nasal); Ketorolac (Systemic); Mefloquine

Ethanol/Nutrition/Herb Interactions

Ethanol: May increase CNS depression; monitor for increased effects with coadministration. Caution patients about effects.

Herb/Nutraceutical: Avoid evening primrose (seizure threshold decreased). Avoid valerian, St John's wort, kava kava, gotu kola (may increase CNS depression).

Stability Store tablet and powder for oral solution at 20°C to 25°C (68°F to 77°F).

Mechanism of Action Irreversibly inhibits gamma-aminobutyric acid transaminase (GABA-T), increasing the levels of the inhibitory compound gamma amino butyric acid (GABA) within the brain. Duration of effect is dependent upon rate of GABA-T resynthesis.

Pharmacodynamics/Kinetics

Duration (rate of GABA-T resynthesis dependent): Variable (not strictly correlated to serum concentrations)

Absorption: Rapid

Distribution: V_d: 1.1 L/kg

Metabolism: Insignificant

Half-life elimination: Adults: 7.5 hours; Elderly: 12-13 hours

Time to peak: Adults: 1 hour

Excretion: Urine (80%, as unchanged drug)

Dosage

Geriatric Refractory complex partial seizures: Refer to adult dosing. Initiate at low end of dosage range; monitor closely for sedation and confusion.

Adult Refractory complex partial seizures: Oral: Initial: 500 mg twice daily; increase daily dose by 500 mg at weekly intervals based on response and tolerability. Recommended dose: 3 g/day

Note: To taper, decrease dose by 1 g/day on a weekly basis

Renal Impairment

Cl_{cr} >50-80 mL/minute: Decrease dose by 25%

Cl_{cr} >30-50 mL/minute: Decrease dose by 50%

Cl_{cr} >10-30 mL/minute: Decrease dose by 75%

Administration May be administered without regard to meals.

Packet: Dissolve each 500 mg powder packet in 10 mL of cold or room temperature water to make a 50 mg/mL solution. Use immediately. The appropriate aliquot may be administered using an oral syringe.

Monitoring Parameters Ophthalmologic examination by an ophthalmic professional with expertise in visual field interpretation and the ability to perform dilated indirect ophthalmoscopy of the retina at baseline (no later than 4 weeks after therapy initiation), periodically during therapy (every 3 months), and 3-6 months after discontinuation of therapy; assessment should include visual acuity and visual field whenever possible including mydriatic peripheral fundus examination and visual field perimetry. Observe patient for excessive sedation, especially when instituting or increasing therapy; hemoglobin and hematocrit

Test Interactions Vigabatrin has been reported to decrease AST and ALT activity in the plasma in up to 90% of patients, causing the enzymes to become undetectable in some patients; this may preclude use of AST and ALT as markers for hepatic injury. Vigabatrin may increase amino acids in the urine leading to false-positive tests for rare genetic metabolic disorders

Special Geriatric Considerations Vigabatrin has not been studied exclusively in the elderly. Clinical trials included an insufficient number of elderly to determine if their response differed from younger adults. Moderate-to-severe sedation and confusion, lasting up to 5 days, was seen in elderly patients with Cl_{cr} <50 mL/minute after a single 1.5 g dose.

Dosage Forms Excipient information presented when available (limited, particularly for generics); consult specific product labeling.

Powder for solution, oral:
Sabril®: 500 mg/packet (50s)
Tablet, oral:
Sabril®: 500 mg [scored]

Dosage Forms: Canada Excipient information presented when available (limited, particularly for generics); consult specific product labeling.

Powder for suspension, oral [sachets]:
Sabril®: 0.5 g

Selected References
Sabers A and Gram L, "Newer Anticonvulsants: Comparative Review of Drug Interactions and Adverse Effects," *Drugs*, 2000, 60(1):23-33.

◆ **Vigamox®** *see* Moxifloxacin (Ophthalmic) *on page 1249*
◆ **Viibryd™** *see* Vilazodone *on page 1919*

Vilazodone (vil AZ oh done)

Related Information
Antidepressant Agents *on page 1991*
Brand Names: U.S. Viibryd™
Index Terms EMD 68843; SB659746-A; Vilazodone Hydrochloride
Generic Availability (U.S.) No
Pharmacologic Category Antidepressant, Selective Serotonin Reuptake Inhibitor/5-HT$_{1A}$ Receptor Partial Agonist
Use Treatment of major depressive disorder
Medication Guide Available Yes
Contraindications Concomitant use with MAO inhibitors or within 2 weeks of discontinuing MAO inhibitors
Warnings/Precautions [U.S. Boxed Warning]: Antidepressants increase the risk of suicidal thinking and behavior in children, adolescents, and young adults (18-24 years of age) with major depressive disorder (MDD) and other psychiatric disorders; consider risk prior to prescribing. Short-term studies did not show an increased risk in patients >24 years of age and showed a decreased risk in patients ≥65 years. Closely monitor patients for clinical worsening, suicidality, or unusual changes in behavior, particularly during the initial 1-2 months of therapy or during periods of dosage adjustments (increases or decreases); the patient's family or caregiver should be instructed to closely observe the patient and communicate condition with healthcare provider. A medication guide concerning the use of antidepressants should be dispensed with each prescription. **Vilazodone is not FDA approved for use in children.**

The possibility of a suicide attempt is inherent in major depression and may persist until remission occurs. Use caution in high-risk patients. Worsening depression and severe abrupt suicidality that are not part of the presenting symptoms may require discontinuation or modification of drug therapy. The patient's family or caregiver should be alerted to monitor patients for the emergence of suicidality and associated behaviors (such as agitation, irritability, hostility, impulsivity, and hypomania) and call healthcare provider.

May worsen psychosis in some patients or precipitate a shift to mania or hypomania in patients with bipolar disorder. Patients presenting with depressive symptoms should be screened for bipolar disorder. Monotherapy in patients with bipolar disorder should be avoided. **Vilazodone is not FDA approved for the treatment of bipolar depression.**

Serotonin syndrome and neuroleptic malignant syndrome (NMS)-like reactions have occurred with serotonin/norepinephrine reuptake inhibitors (SNRIs) and selective serotonin reuptake inhibitors (SSRIs) when used alone, and particularly when used in combination with serotonergic agents (eg, triptans) or antidopaminergic agents (eg, antipsychotics). Concurrent use or use within 2 weeks of discontinuing MAO inhibitors is contraindicated. In addition, allow at least 14 days after stopping vilazodone before starting an MAO inhibitor. High potential for interaction with concomitant medications (see Drug Interactions); monitor closely for toxicity or adverse effects. Dose reductions are recommended with concomitant use of strong or moderate CYP3A4 inhibitors. May increase the risks associated with electroconvulsive therapy. Has a low potential to impair cognitive or motor performance; caution operating hazardous machinery or driving.

Use with caution in patients with hepatic impairment, seizure disorder, in elderly patients, or on concomitant CNS depressants. Use caution with concomitant use of aspirin, NSAIDs, warfarin, or other drugs that affect coagulation; the risk of bleeding may be potentiated. May cause hyponatremia/SIADH (elderly at increased risk); volume depletion and diuretics may increase risk. May cause or exacerbate sexual dysfunction. Upon discontinuation of vilazodone therapy, gradually taper dose. If intolerable symptoms occur following a decrease in dosage or upon discontinuation of therapy, consider resuming the previous dose with a more gradual taper.

Adverse Reactions (Reflective of adult population; not specific for elderly)
>10%:
  Gastrointestinal: Diarrhea (28%), nausea (23%)
1% to 10%:
  Cardiovascular: Palpitation (2%)
  Central nervous system: Dizziness (9%), insomnia (6%), dreams abnormal (4%), fatigue (4%), restlessness (3%), somnolence (3%), migraine (≥1%), sedation (≥1%)
  Dermatologic: Hyperhidrosis (≥1%)
  Endocrine & metabolic: Libido decreased (3% to 5%), orgasm abnormal (2% to 4%), sexual dysfunction (≤2%)
  Gastrointestinal: Xerostomia (8%), vomiting (5%), dyspepsia (3%), flatulence (3%), gastroenteritis (3%), appetite increased (2%), appetite decreased (≥1%)
  Genitourinary: Ejaculation delayed (2%), erectile dysfunction (2%)
  Neuromuscular & skeletal: Arthralgia (3%), paresthesia (3%), jittery (2%), tremor (2%)
  Ocular: Blurred vision (≥1%), dry eyes (≥1%)
  Miscellaneous: Night sweats (≥1%)

Drug Interactions
  Metabolism/Transport Effects Substrate (major) of CYP3A4; (minor) of CYP2C19, 2D6; **Inhibits** CYP2C8, 2C19 (moderate), 2D6 (moderate); **Induces** CYP2C19 (weak)
  Avoid Concomitant Use
  Avoid concomitant use of Vilazodone with any of the following: Iobenguane I 123; MAO Inhibitors; Methylene Blue; Pimozide; Sibutramine; Thioridazine; Tryptophan
  Increased Effect/Toxicity
  Vilazodone may increase the levels/effects of: Alpha-/Beta-Blockers; Anticoagulants; Antidepressants (Serotonin Reuptake Inhibitor/Antagonist); Antiplatelet Agents; Aspirin; Benzodiazepines (metabolized by oxidation); Beta-Blockers; BusPIRone; CarBAMazepine; CloZAPine; Collagenase (Systemic); CYP2D6 Substrates; Desmopressin; Dextromethorphan; Drotrecogin Alfa; Fesoterodine; Galantamine; Haloperidol; Ibritumomab; Lithium; Methadone; Methylene Blue; Mexiletine; NSAID (COX-2 Inhibitor); NSAID (Nonselective); Pimozide; RisperiDONE; Rivaroxaban; Salicylates; Serotonin Modulators; Tamoxifen; Thioridazine; Thrombolytic Agents; Tositumomab and Iodine I 131 Tositumomab; TraMADol; Tricyclic Antidepressants; Vitamin K Antagonists

  The levels/effects of Vilazodone may be increased by: Alcohol (Ethyl); Analgesics (Opioid); BusPIRone; Cimetidine; CNS Depressants; CYP3A4 Inhibitors (Moderate); CYP3A4 Inhibitors (Strong); Dasatinib; Glucosamine; Herbs (Anticoagulant/Antiplatelet Properties); Macrolide Antibiotics; MAO Inhibitors; Metoclopramide; Omega-3-Acid Ethyl Esters; Pentosan Polysulfate Sodium; Pentoxifylline; Prostacyclin Analogues; Sibutramine; TraMADol; Tryptophan; Vitamin E
  Decreased Effect
  Vilazodone may decrease the levels/effects of: Iobenguane I 123

  The levels/effects of Vilazodone may be decreased by: CarBAMazepine; CYP3A4 Inducers (Strong); Cyproheptadine; Deferasirox; NSAID (Nonselective); Peginterferon Alfa-2b; Tocilizumab
  Ethanol/Nutrition/Herb Interactions Ethanol: May increase CNS depression; monitor for increased effects with coadministration. Caution patients about effects.
  Stability Store at 25°C (77°F); excursions permitted to 15°C to 30°C (50°F to 86°F).
  Mechanism of Action Vilazodone inhibits CNS neuron serotonin uptake; minimal or no effect on reuptake of norepinephrine or dopamine. It also binds selectively with high affinity to 5-HT$_{1A}$ receptors and is a 5-HT$_{1A}$ receptor partial agonist. 5-HT$_{1A}$ receptor activity may be altered in depression and anxiety.

Pharmacodynamics/Kinetics
Protein binding: ~96% to 99%
Metabolism: Extensively hepatic, via CYP3A4 (major pathway) and 2C19 and 2D6 (minor pathways)
Bioavailability: 72% (with food); blood concentrations (AUC) may be decreased ~50% in the fasted state
Half-life elimination: Terminal: ~25 hours
Time to peak, serum: 4-5 hours
Excretion: Urine (1% as unchanged drug); feces (2% as unchanged drug)

Dosage
Geriatric & Adult Depression: Oral: Initial: 10 mg once daily for 7 days, then increase to 20 mg once daily for 7 days, then to recommended dose of 40 mg once daily
Dosing adjustment for concomitant medications:
Strong CYP3A4 inhibitors: Reduce vilazodone dose to 20 mg once daily
Moderate CYP3A4 inhibitors (eg, erythromycin): Reduce vilazodone dose to 20 mg once daily in patients with intolerable side effects
Hepatic Impairment
Mild-to-moderate impairment (Child-Pugh class A or B): No adjustment needed
Severe impairment (Child-Pugh class C): Not studied

Administration Administer with food.

Monitoring Parameters Monitor patient periodically for symptom resolution, mental status for depression, suicidal ideation (especially at the beginning of therapy or when doses are increased or decreased), anxiety, social functioning, mania, panic attacks, akathisia

Special Geriatric Considerations Results of a single dose pharmacokinetic study suggest that a dose adjustment is not necessary for persons ≥65 years of age; however, there is limited experience with vilazodone in this age group as <2% of subjects in the clinical trials were ≥65 years. The elderly are more prone to SSRI/SNRI-induced hyponatremia.

Dosage Forms Excipient information presented when available (limited, particularly for generics); consult specific product labeling.
Tablet, oral, as hydrochloride:
Viibryd™: 10 mg, 20 mg, 40 mg

Vitamin E (VYE ta min ee)

Medication Safety Issues
Sound-alike/look-alike issues:
Aquasol E® may be confused with Anusol®

Brand Names: U.S. Alph-E [OTC]; Alph-E-Mixed [OTC]; Aqua Gem-E™ [OTC]; Aquasol E® [OTC]; d-Alpha Gems™ [OTC]; E-Gems® Elite [OTC]; E-Gems® Plus [OTC]; E-Gems® [OTC]; E-Gem® Lip Care [OTC]; E-Gem® [OTC]; Ester-E™ [OTC]; Gamma E-Gems®

[OTC]; Gamma-E PLUS [OTC]; High Gamma Vitamin E Complete™ [OTC]; Key-E® Kaps [OTC]; Key-E® Powder [OTC]; Key-E® [OTC]

Index Terms *d*-Alpha Tocopherol; *dl*-Alpha Tocopherol

Generic Availability (U.S.) Yes

Pharmacologic Category Vitamin, Fat Soluble

Use Dietary supplement

Unlabeled/Investigational Use Prevention and treatment of tardive dyskinesia

Contraindications Hypersensitivity to vitamin E or any component of the formulation

Warnings/Precautions May induce vitamin K deficiency. Necrotizing enterocolitis has been associated with oral administration of large dosages (eg, >200 units/day) of a hyperosmolar vitamin E preparation in low birth weight infants.

Adverse Reactions (Reflective of adult population; not specific for elderly) Frequency not defined.

Central nervous system: Fatigue, headache

Dermatologic: Contact dermatitis with topical preparation

Endocrine & metabolic: Gonadal dysfunction

Gastrointestinal: Diarrhea, intestinal cramps, nausea

Neuromuscular & skeletal: Weakness

Ocular: Blurred vision

Drug Interactions

Avoid Concomitant Use There are no known interactions where it is recommended to avoid concomitant use.

Increased Effect/Toxicity

Vitamin E may increase the levels/effects of: Antiplatelet Agents; Vitamin K Antagonists

The levels/effects of Vitamin E may be increased by: Tipranavir

Decreased Effect

Vitamin E may decrease the levels/effects of: CycloSPORINE; CycloSPORINE (Systemic)

The levels/effects of Vitamin E may be decreased by: Orlistat

Stability Protect from light.

Mechanism of Action Prevents oxidation of vitamin A and C; protects polyunsaturated fatty acids in membranes from attack by free radicals and protects red blood cells against hemolysis

Pharmacodynamics/Kinetics

Absorption: Oral: Depends upon the presence of bile; absorption is reduced in conditions of malabsorption, and as dosage increases; water miscible preparations are better absorbed than oil preparations

Distribution: Distributes to all body tissues, especially adipose tissue, where it is stored

Metabolism: In the liver to glucuronides

Elimination: In feces and bile

Dosage

Geriatric & Adult Vitamin E may be expressed as alpha-tocopherol equivalents (ATE), which refer to the biologically-active (R) stereoisomer content. Oral:

Recommended daily allowance (RDA): 15 mg; upper limit of intake should not exceed 1000 mg/day

Vitamin E deficiency: 60-75 units/day

Prevention of vitamin E deficiency: Oral: 30 units/day

Cystic fibrosis: Oral: 100-400 units/day

Beta-thalassemia: Oral: 750 units/day

Sickle cell disease: Oral: 450 units/day

Tardive dyskinesia (unlabeled use): Oral: 1600 units/day

Superficial dermatologic irritation: Topical: Apply a thin layer over affected area.

Administration Swallow capsules whole; do not crush or chew.

Monitoring Parameters Plasma tocopherol concentrations (normal range: 6-14 mcg/mL)

Reference Range Therapeutic: 0.8-1.5 mg/dL (SI: 19-35 µmol/L), some method variation

Pharmacotherapy Pearls The 2R-stereoisomeric forms of α-tocopherol are used to define vitamin E intake and RDA. While international units are no longer recognized, many fortified foods and supplements continue to use this term although USP units are now used by the pharmaceutical industry when labeling vitamin E supplements. Both IUs and USP units are based on the same equivalency. The following can be used to convert international units (IU) of vitamin E (and esters) to milligrams α-tocopherol in order to meet recommended daily intake:

Synthetic (eg, all-racemic α-tocopherol):

dl-α-tocopherol:

USP: 1.10 IU / mg; 0.91 mg / IU

Molar: 2.12 µmol / IU

α-tocopherol: 0.45 mg / IU
dl-α-tocopherol acetate:
  USP: 1 IU / mg; 1 mg / IU
  Molar: 2.12 μmol / IU
  α-tocopherol: 0.45 mg / IU
dl-α-tocopherol succinate:
  USP: 0.89 IU / mg; 1.12 mg / IU
  Molar: 2.12 μmol / IU
  α-tocopherol: 0.45 mg / IU

Natural (eg, RRR-α-tocopherol):
d-α-tocopherol:
  USP: 1.49 IU / mg; 0.67 mg / IU
  Molar: 1.56 μmol / IU
  α-tocopherol: 0.67 mg / IU
d-α-tocopherol acetate:
  USP: 1.36 IU / mg; 0.74mg / IU
  Molar: 1.56 μmol / IU
  α-tocopherol: 0.67 mg / IU
d-α-tocopherol succinate:
  USP: 1.21 IU / mg; 0.83 mg / IU
  Molar: 1.56 μmol / IU
  α-tocopherol: 0.67 mg / IU

Historically, vitamin E supplements have been labeled (incorrectly) as *d*- or *dl*-α-tocopherol. Synthetic vitamin E compounds are racemic mixtures, and may be designated as all-racemic (all rac-α-tocopherol). The natural form contains the only RRR-α-tocopherol. All of these compounds may be present in fortified foods and multivitamins. Not all stereoisomers are capable of performing physiological functions in humans; therefore, cannot be considered to meet vitamin E requirements.

Special Geriatric Considerations Elderly may have vitamin E prescribed for those with cardiovascular disease. Elderly should be advised not to take more than prescribed.

Dosage Forms Excipient information presented when available (limited, particularly for generics); consult specific product labeling. [DSC] = Discontinued product
Capsule, oral: 400 int. units [DSC], 1000 int. units
  Key-E® Kaps: 200 int. units, 400 int. units [derived from or manufactured using soybean oil]
Capsule, liquid, oral: 400 int. units
Capsule, softgel, oral: 100 int. units, 200 int. units, 400 int. units, 600 int. units, 1000 int. units, 200 units, 1000 units
  Alph-E: 200 int. units, 400 int. units
  Alph-E: 400 int. units [contains soybean oil]
  Alph-E: 1000 int. units
  Alph-E-Mixed: 200 int. units, 400 int. units
  Alph-E-Mixed: 1000 int. units [sugar free]
  Aqua Gem-E™: 200 int. units, 400 int. units
  d-Alpha Gems™: 400 int. units [derived from or manufactured using soybean oil]
  E-Gems®: 30 int. units, 100 int. units, 200 int. units, 400 int. units, 600 int. units, 800 int. units, 1000 int. units, 1200 int. units [derived from or manufactured using soybean oil]
  E-Gems® Elite: 400 int. units
  E-Gems® Plus: 200 int. units, 400 int. units, 800 int. units [derived from or manufactured using soybean oil]
  Ester-E™: 400 int. units
  Gamma E-Gems®: 90 int. units
  Gamma-E PLUS: 200 int. units [contains soybean oil]
  High Gamma Vitamin E Complete™: 200 int. units [contains soybean oil]
Cream, topical: 1000 int. units/120 g (120 g); 100 int. units/g (57 g, 60 g); 30,000 int. units/57 g (57 g)
  Key-E®: 30 int. units/g (57 g, 120 g, 600 g)
Lip balm, topical:
  E-Gem® Lip Care: 1000 int. units/tube [contains aloe, vitamin A]
Liquid, oral/topical: 1150 int. units/1.25 mL (30 mL, 60 mL, 120 mL)
Oil, oral/topical: 100 int. units/0.25 mL (74 mL)
Oil, oral/topical [drops]:
  E-Gem®: 10 int. units/drop (15 mL, 60 mL)

Oil, topical: 100 int. units/5 drops (60 mL [DSC])
  Alph-E: 28,000 int. units/30 mL (30 mL)
Ointment, topical:
  Key-E®: 30 int. units/g (57 g, 113 g, 500 g)
Powder, oral:
  Key-E® Powder: (15 g, 75 g, 1000 g) [derived from or manufactured using soybean oil]
Solution, oral [drops]: 15 int. units/0.3 mL (30 mL)
  Aquasol E®: 15 int. units/0.3 mL (12 mL, 30 mL)
Suppository, rectal/vaginal:
  Key-E®: 30 int. units (12s, 24s) [contains coconut oil]
Tablet, oral: 100 int. units, 200 int. units, 400 int. units, 500 int. units
  Key-E®: 200 int. units, 400 int. units [derived from or manufactured using soybean oil]

- ◆ **Vitamin K₁** *see* Phytonadione *on page 1450*
- ◆ **Vitrase®** *see* Hyaluronidase *on page 873*
- ◆ **Vitrasert®** *see* Ganciclovir (Ophthalmic) *on page 811*
- ◆ **Vi Vaccine** *see* Typhoid Vaccine *on page 1879*
- ◆ **Vivactil®** *see* Protriptyline *on page 1542*
- ◆ **Viva-Drops® [OTC]** *see* Artificial Tears *on page 148*
- ◆ **Vivaglobin® [DSC]** *see* Immune Globulin *on page 922*
- ◆ **Vivelle-Dot®** *see* Estradiol (Systemic) *on page 641*
- ◆ **Vivotif®** *see* Typhoid Vaccine *on page 1879*
- ◆ **Voltaren** *see* Diclofenac (Systemic) *on page 496*
- ◆ **Voltaren® Gel** *see* Diclofenac (Topical) *on page 500*
- ◆ **Voltaren Ophthalmic®** *see* Diclofenac (Ophthalmic) *on page 500*
- ◆ **Voltaren®-XR** *see* Diclofenac (Systemic) *on page 496*

Voriconazole (vor i KOE na zole)

Brand Names: U.S. VFEND®
Brand Names: Canada VFEND®
Index Terms UK109496
Generic Availability (U.S.) Yes: Tablet
Pharmacologic Category Antifungal Agent, Oral; Antifungal Agent, Parenteral
Use Treatment of invasive aspergillosis; treatment of esophageal candidiasis; treatment of candidemia (in non-neutropenic patients); treatment of disseminated *Candida* infections of the skin and viscera; treatment of serious fungal infections caused by *Scedosporium apiospermum* and *Fusarium* spp (including *Fusarium solani*) in patients intolerant of, or refractory to, other therapy
Unlabeled/Investigational Use Fungal infection prophylaxis in intermediate or high risk neutropenic cancer patients with myelodysplastic syndrome (MDS) or acute myelogenous leukemia (AML), neutropenic allogeneic hematopoietic stem cell recipients, and patients with significant graft-versus-host disease; empiric antifungal therapy (second-line) for persistent neutropenic fever
Contraindications Hypersensitivity to voriconazole or any component of the formulation (cross-reaction with other azole antifungal agents may occur but has not been established, use caution); coadministration of CYP3A4 substrates which may lead to QT$_c$ prolongation (cisapride, pimozide, or quinidine); coadministration with barbiturates (long acting), carbamazepine, efavirenz (with standard [eg, not adjusted] voriconazole and efavirenz doses), ergot derivatives, rifampin, rifabutin, ritonavir (≥800 mg/day), sirolimus, St John's wort
Warnings/Precautions Visual changes, including blurred vision, changes in visual acuity, color perception, and photophobia, are commonly associated with treatment. Patients should be warned to avoid tasks which depend on vision, including operating machinery or driving. Changes are reversible on discontinuation following brief exposure/treatment regimens (≤28 days).

Serious hepatic reactions (including hepatitis, cholestasis, and fulminant hepatic failure) have occurred during treatment, primarily in patients with serious concomitant medical conditions. However, hepatotoxicity has occurred in patients with no identifiable risk factors. Use caution in patients with pre-existing hepatic impairment (dose adjustment or discontinuation may be required).

Voriconazole tablets contain lactose; avoid administration in hereditary galactose intolerance, Lapp lactase deficiency, or glucose-galactose malabsorption. Suspension contains sucrose; use caution with fructose intolerance, sucrose-isomaltase deficiency, or glucose-galactose malabsorption. Avoid/limit use of intravenous formulation in patients with renal impairment; intravenous formulation contains excipient cyclodextrin (sulfobutyl ether beta-cyclodextrin), which may accumulate in renal insufficiency. Acute renal failure has been observed in severely ill patients; use with caution in patients receiving concomitant nephrotoxic medications. Anaphylactoid-type infusion-related reactions may occur with intravenous dosing. Consider discontinuation of infusion if reaction is severe.

Use caution in patients taking strong cytochrome P450 inducers, CYP2C9 inhibitors, and major 3A4 substrates (see Drug Interactions); consider alternative agents that avoid or lessen the potential for CYP-mediated interactions. QT interval prolongation has been associated with voriconazole use; rare cases of arrhythmia (including torsade de pointes), cardiac arrest, and sudden death have been reported, usually in seriously ill patients with comorbidities and/or risk factors (eg, prior cardiotoxic chemotherapy, cardiomyopathy, electrolyte imbalance, or concomitant QT_c-prolonging drugs). Use with caution in these patient populations; correct electrolyte abnormalities (eg, hypokalemia, hypomagnesemia, hypocalcemia) prior to initiating therapy. Do not infuse concomitantly with blood products or short-term concentrated electrolyte solutions, even if the two infusions are running in separate intravenous lines (or cannulas).

Rare cases of malignancy (melanoma, squamous cell carcinoma) have been reported in patients (mostly immunocompromised) with prior onset of severe photosensitivity reactions and exposure to long-term voriconazole therapy. Other serious cutaneous reactions, including Stevens-Johnson syndrome, have also been reported. Patient should avoid strong, direct exposure to sunlight; may cause photosensitivity, especially with long-term use. Consider discontinuing in patients developing a rash. Periodic total body skin examinations should be performed, particularly with prolonged use.

Monitor pancreatic function in patients at risk for acute pancreatitis (eg, recent chemotherapy or hematopoietic stem cell transplantation); there have been postmarketing reports of pancreatitis in children.

Adverse Reactions (Reflective of adult population; not specific for elderly)
>10%:
  Central nervous system: Hallucinations (4% to 12%; auditory and/or visual and likely serum concentration-dependent)
  Ocular: Visual changes (dose related; photophobia, color changes, increased or decreased visual acuity, or blurred vision occur in ~21%)
  Renal: Creatinine increased (1% to 21%)
2% to 10%:
  Cardiovascular: Tachycardia (≤2%)
  Central nervous system: Fever (≤6%), chills (≤4%), headache (≤3%)
  Dermatologic: Rash (≤7%)
  Endocrine & metabolic: Hypokalemia (≤2%)
  Gastrointestinal: Nausea (1% to 5%), vomiting (1% to 4%)
  Hepatic: Alkaline phosphatase increased (4% to 5%), AST increased (2% to 4%), ALT increased (2% to 3%), cholestatic jaundice (1% to 2%)
  Ocular: Photophobia (2% to 3%)

Drug Interactions
Metabolism/Transport Effects Substrate of CYP2C9 (major), 2C19 (major), 3A4 (minor); **Inhibits** CYP2C9 (moderate), 2C19 (weak), 3A4 (moderate)

Avoid Concomitant Use
Avoid concomitant use of Voriconazole with any of the following: Alfuzosin; Artemether; Barbiturates; CarBAMazepine; Cisapride; Conivaptan; Crizotinib; Darunavir; Dofetilide; Dronedarone; Eplerenone; Ergot Derivatives; Everolimus; Fluconazole; Fluticasone (Oral Inhalation); Halofantrine; Lapatinib; Lopinavir; Lovastatin; Lumefantrine; Lurasidone; Nilotinib; Nisoldipine; Pimozide; QUEtiapine; QuiNIDine; QuiNINE; Ranolazine; Rifamycin Derivatives; Ritonavir; Rivaroxaban; RomiDEPsin; Salmeterol; Silodosin; Simvastatin; Sirolimus; St Johns Wort; Tamsulosin; Tetrabenazine; Thioridazine; Ticagrelor; Tolvaptan; Toremifene; Vandetanib; Vemurafenib; Ziprasidone

Increased Effect/Toxicity
Voriconazole may increase the levels/effects of: Alfentanil; Alfuzosin; Almotriptan; Alosetron; Antineoplastic Agents (Vinca Alkaloids); Aprepitant; Benzodiazepines (metabolized by oxidation); Boceprevir; Bortezomib; Bosentan; Brentuximab Vedotin; Brinzolamide; Budesonide (Nasal); Budesonide (Systemic, Oral Inhalation); BusPIRone; Busulfan; Calcium Channel Blockers; CarBAMazepine; Carvedilol; Ciclesonide; Cilostazol; Cinacalcet; Cisapride; Colchicine; Conivaptan; Contraceptives (Estrogens); Contraceptives (Progestins); Corticosteroids (Orally Inhaled); Corticosteroids (Systemic); Crizotinib; CycloSPORINE; CycloSPORINE (Systemic); CYP2C9 Substrates (High risk); CYP3A4 Substrates; Diclofenac; Diclofenac (Systemic); Diclofenac (Topical); Dienogest; DOCEtaxel; Dofetilide; Dronedarone; Dutasteride; Eletriptan; Eplerenone; Ergot Derivatives; Erlotinib; Eszopiclone; Etravirine; Everolimus; FentaNYL; Fesoterodine; Fluticasone (Nasal); Fluticasone (Oral Inhalation); Fosaprepitant; Fosphenytoin; Gefitinib; GuanFACINE; Halofantrine; HMG-CoA Reductase Inhibitors; Ibuprofen; Iloperidone; Imatinib; Irinotecan; Ixabepilone; Lapatinib; Losartan; Lovastatin; Lumefantrine; Lurasidone; Macrolide Antibiotics; Maraviroc;

Meloxicam; Methadone; MethylPREDNISolone; Nilotinib; Nisoldipine; OxyCODONE; Paricalcitol; Pazopanib; Phenytoin; Phosphodiesterase 5 Inhibitors; Pimecrolimus; Pimozide; Protease Inhibitors; QTc-Prolonging Agents; QuiNIDine; QuiNINE; Ramelteon; Ranolazine; Repaglinide; Reverse Transcriptase Inhibitors (Non-Nucleoside); Rifamycin Derivatives; Rivaroxaban; RomiDEPsin; Salmeterol; Saxagliptin; Sildenafil; Silodosin; Simvastatin; Sirolimus; Solifenacin; SORAfenib; SUNItinib; Sulfonylureas; SUNItinib; Tacrolimus; Tacrolimus (Systemic); Tacrolimus (Topical); Tadalafil; Tamsulosin; Telaprevir; Tetrabenazine; Thioridazine; Ticagrelor; Tolterodine; Tolvaptan; Toremifene; Vandetanib; Vardenafil; Vemurafenib; Venlafaxine; Vilazodone; Vitamin K Antagonists; Ziprasidone; Zolpidem

The levels/effects of Voriconazole may be increased by: Alfuzosin; Artemether; Boceprevir; Chloramphenicol; Chloroquine; Ciprofloxacin; Ciprofloxacin (Systemic); Contraceptives (Estrogens); Contraceptives (Progestins); CYP2C19 Inhibitors (Moderate); CYP2C19 Inhibitors (Strong); CYP2C9 Inhibitors (Moderate); CYP2C9 Inhibitors (Strong); Etravirine; Fluconazole; Gadobutrol; Grapefruit Juice; Lumefantrine; Macrolide Antibiotics; Nilotinib; Protease Inhibitors; Proton Pump Inhibitors; QUEtiapine; QuiNINE; Telaprevir

Decreased Effect

Voriconazole may decrease the levels/effects of: Amphotericin B; Prasugrel; Saccharomyces boulardii; Ticagrelor

The levels/effects of Voriconazole may be decreased by: Barbiturates; CarBAMazepine; CYP2C19 Inducers (Strong); CYP2C9 Inducers (Highly Effective); Darunavir; Didanosine; Etravirine; Fosphenytoin; Lopinavir; Peginterferon Alfa-2b; Phenytoin; Reverse Transcriptase Inhibitors (Non-Nucleoside); Rifamycin Derivatives; Ritonavir; St Johns Wort; Sucralfate; Telaprevir; Tocilizumab

Ethanol/Nutrition/Herb Interactions

Food: May decrease voriconazole absorption. Oral voriconazole should be taken 1 hour before or 1 hour after a meal. Avoid grapefruit juice (may decrease voriconazole levels).

Herb/Nutraceutical: St John's wort may decrease voriconazole levels; concurrent use with voriconazole is contraindicated.

Stability

Powder for injection: Store at 15°C to 30°C (59°F to 86°F). Reconstitute 200 mg vial with 19 mL of sterile water for injection (use of automated syringe is not recommended). Resultant solution (20 mL) has a concentration of 10 mg/mL. Prior to infusion, must dilute to 0.5-5 mg/mL with NS, LR, D_5WLR, $D_5W^1/_2$NS, D_5W, D_5W with KCl 20 mEq, $^1/_2$NS, or D_5WNS. Do not dilute with 4.2% sodium bicarbonate infusion. Reconstituted solutions are stable for up to 24 hours under refrigeration at 2°C to 8°C (36°F to 46°F).

Powder for oral suspension: Store at 2°C to 8°C (36°F to 46°F). Add 46 mL of water to the bottle to make 40 mg/mL suspension. Reconstituted oral suspension may be stored at 15°C to 30°C (59°F to 86°F). Discard after 14 days.

Tablets: Store at 15°C to 30°C (59°F to 86°F).

Mechanism of Action
Interferes with fungal cytochrome P450 activity (selectively inhibits 14-alpha-lanosterol demethylation), decreasing ergosterol synthesis (principal sterol in fungal cell membrane) and inhibiting fungal cell membrane formation.

Pharmacodynamics/Kinetics

Absorption: Well absorbed after oral administration; administration of crushed tablets is considered bioequivalent to whole tablets

Distribution: V_d: 4.6 L/kg

Protein binding: 58%

Metabolism: Hepatic, via CYP2C19 (major pathway) and CYP2C9 and CYP3A4 (less significant); saturable (may demonstrate nonlinearity)

Bioavailability: 96%

Half-life elimination: Variable, dose-dependent

Time to peak: Oral: 1-2 hours; 0.5 hours (crushed tablet)

Excretion: Urine (as inactive metabolites; <2% as unchanged drug)

Dosage

Geriatric & Adult

Aspergillosis, invasive, including disseminated and extrapulmonary infection: Duration of therapy should be a minimum of 6-12 weeks or throughout period of immunosuppression (Walsh, 2008):

I.V.: Initial: Loading dose: 6 mg/kg every 12 hours for 2 doses; followed by maintenance dose of 4 mg/kg every 12 hours

Oral: Maintenance dose:

Manufacturer's recommendations:

Patients <40 kg: 100 mg every 12 hours; maximum: 300 mg/day

Patients ≥40 kg: 200 mg every 12 hours; maximum: 600 mg/day

IDSA recommendations (Walsh, 2008): May consider oral therapy in place of I.V. with dosing of 4 mg/kg (rounded up to convenient tablet dosage form) every 12 hours; however, I.V. administration is preferred in serious infections since comparative efficacy with the oral formulation has not been established.

Scedosporiosis, fusariosis:

I.V.: Initial: Loading dose: 6 mg/kg every 12 hours for 2 doses; followed by maintenance dose of 4 mg/kg every 12 hours

Oral: Maintenance dose:

Patients <40 kg: 100 mg every 12 hours; maximum 300 mg/day

Patients ≥40 kg: 200 mg every 12 hours; maximum: 600 mg/day

Candidemia and other deep tissue *Candida* infections: Treatment should continue for a minimum of 14 days following resolution of symptoms or following last positive culture, whichever is longer.

I.V.: Initial: Loading dose 6 mg/kg every 12 hours for 2 doses; followed by maintenance dose of 3-4 mg/kg every 12 hours

Oral:

Manufacturer's recommendations: Maintenance dose:

Patients <40 kg: 100 mg every 12 hours; maximum: 300 mg/day

Patients ≥40 kg: 200 mg every 12 hours; maximum: 600 mg/day

IDSA recommendations (Pappas, 2009): Initial: Loading dose: 400 mg every 12 hours for 2 doses; followed by 200 mg every 12 hours

Endophthalmitis, fungal (unlabeled use; Pappas, 2009): I.V.: 6 mg/kg every 12 hours for 2 doses, then 3-4 mg/kg every 12 hours

Esophageal candidiasis: Oral: Treatment should continue for a minimum of 14 days, and for at least 7 days following resolution of symptoms:

Patients <40 kg: 100 mg every 12 hours; maximum: 300 mg/day

Patients ≥40 kg: 200 mg every 12 hours; maximum: 600 mg/day

Dosage adjustment in patients unable to tolerate treatment:

I.V.: Dose may be reduced to 3 mg/kg every 12 hours

Oral: Dose may be reduced in 50 mg decrements to a minimum dosage of 200 mg every 12 hours in patients weighing ≥40 kg (100 mg every 12 hours in patients <40 kg)

Dosage adjustment in patients receiving concomitant CYP450 enzyme inducers or substrates:

Cyclosporine: Reduce cyclosporine dose by one-half and monitor closely; upon discontinuation of voriconazole, monitor cyclosporine concentrations and escalate the cyclosporine dose as needed

Efavirenz: Oral: Increase maintenance dose of voriconazole to 400 mg every 12 hours and reduce efavirenz dose to 300 mg once daily; upon discontinuation of voriconazole, return to the initial dose of efavirenz

Omeprazole: Reduce omeprazole dose by one-half in patients maintained on ≥40 mg/day of omeprazole

Phenytoin:

I.V.: Increase voriconazole maintenance dosage to 5 mg/kg every 12 hours

Oral: Increase voriconazole dose to 400 mg every 12 hours in patients ≥40 kg (200 mg every 12 hours in patients <40 kg)

Tacrolimus: Reduce tacrolimus dose by one-third and monitor closely; upon discontinuation of voriconazole, monitor tacrolimus concentrations and escalate the tacrolimus dose as needed.

Renal Impairment In patients with Cl_{cr} <50 mL/minute, accumulation of the intravenous vehicle (cyclodextrin) occurs. After initial I.V. loading dose, oral voriconazole should be administered to these patients, unless an assessment of the benefit:risk to the patient justifies the use of I.V. voriconazole. Monitor serum creatinine and change to oral voriconazole therapy when possible.

Oral: Poorly dialyzed; no supplemental dose or dosage adjustment necessary, including patients on intermittent hemodialysis, peritoneal dialysis, or continuous renal replacement therapy (eg, CVVHD).

Note: I.V. dosing **NOT** recommended since cyclodextrin vehicle is cleared at half the rate of voriconazole and may accumulate.

Hepatic Impairment

Mild-to-moderate hepatic dysfunction (Child-Pugh class A and B): Following standard loading dose, reduce maintenance dosage by 50%

Severe hepatic impairment: Should only be used if benefit outweighs risk; monitor closely for toxicity

◀ **Administration**
Oral: Administer 1 hour before or 1 hour after a meal.
I.V.: Infuse over 1-2 hours (rate not to exceed 3 mg/kg/hour). Do not infuse concomitantly into same line or cannula with other drug infusions, including TPN.

Monitoring Parameters Hepatic function at initiation and during course of treatment; renal function; serum electrolytes (particularly calcium, magnesium and potassium) prior to therapy initiation; visual function (visual acuity, visual field and color perception) if treatment course continues >28 days; may consider obtaining voriconazole trough level in patients failing therapy or exhibiting signs of toxicity; pancreatic function (in patients at risk for acute pancreatitis); total body skin examination yearly (more frequently if lesions noted)

Special Geriatric Considerations The manufacturer reports that median voriconazole plasma concentrations were increased in patients 65 years and older compared to those 65 years and younger. The recommendation that a dose adjustment is not needed for the elderly was based on a similar safety profile between young and older patients.

Dosage Forms Excipient information presented when available (limited, particularly for generics); consult specific product labeling.
Injection, powder for reconstitution:
VFEND®: 200 mg [contains cyclodextrin]
Powder for suspension, oral:
VFEND®: 40 mg/mL (70 mL) [contains sodium benzoate, sucrose; orange flavor]
Tablet, oral: 50 mg, 200 mg
VFEND®: 50 mg, 200 mg [contains lactose]

◆ **VoSpire ER®** see Albuterol on page 50
◆ **VSL #3® [OTC]** see Lactobacillus on page 1020
◆ **VSL #3®-DS** see Lactobacillus on page 1020
◆ **Vytorin®** see Ezetimibe and Simvastatin on page 691
◆ **VZV Vaccine (Zoster)** see Zoster Vaccine on page 1965

Warfarin (WAR far in)

Related Information
Anticoagulants, Injectable on page 1989
Medication Safety Issues
Sound-alike/look-alike issues:
Coumadin® may be confused with Avandia®, Cardura®, Compazine®, Kemadrin®
Jantoven® may be confused with Janumet®, Januvia®
High alert medication:
The Institute for Safe Medication Practices (ISMP) includes this medication among its list of drugs which have a heightened risk of causing significant patient harm when used in error.
2009 National Patient Safety Goals:
The Joint Commission on Accreditation of Healthcare Organizations requires healthcare organizations that provide anticoagulant therapy to have a process in place to reduce the risk of anticoagulant-associated patient harm. Patients receiving anticoagulants should receive individualized care through a defined process that includes standardized ordering, dispensing, administration, monitoring and education. This does not apply to routine short-term use of anticoagulants for prevention of venous thromboembolism when the expectation is that the patient's laboratory values will remain within or close to normal values (NPSG.03.05.01).

Brand Names: U.S. Coumadin®; Jantoven®
Brand Names: Canada Apo-Warfarin®; Coumadin®; Mylan-Warfarin; Novo-Warfarin; Taro-Warfarin
Index Terms Warfarin Sodium
Generic Availability (U.S.) Yes: Tablet
Pharmacologic Category Anticoagulant, Coumarin Derivative; Vitamin K Antagonist
Use Prophylaxis and treatment of thromboembolic disorders (eg, venous, pulmonary) and embolic complications arising from atrial fibrillation or cardiac valve replacement; adjunct to reduce risk of systemic embolism (eg, recurrent MI, stroke) after myocardial infarction
Unlabeled/Investigational Use Prevention of recurrent transient ischemic attacks
Medication Guide Available Yes

Contraindications Hypersensitivity to warfarin or any component of the formulation; hemorrhagic tendencies (eg, patients bleeding from the GI, respiratory, or GU tract; aneurysm; cerebrovascular hemorrhage; following spinal puncture and other diagnostic or therapeutic procedures with potential for significant bleeding; history of bleeding diathesis); recent or potential surgery of the eye or CNS; major regional lumbar block anesthesia or surgery resulting in large, open surfaces; blood dyscrasias; severe uncontrolled or malignant hypertension; pericarditis or pericardial effusion; subacute bacterial endocarditis; history of warfarin-induced necrosis; an unreliable, noncompliant patient; alcoholism; patient who has a history of falls or is a significant fall risk; unsupervised senile or psychotic patient

Warnings/Precautions Use care in the selection of patients appropriate for this treatment. Ensure patient cooperation especially from the alcoholic, illicit drug user, demented, or psychotic patient; ability to comply with routine laboratory monitoring is essential. Use with caution in trauma, acute infection, moderate-severe renal insufficiency, prolonged dietary insufficiencies, moderate-severe hypertension, polycythemia vera, vasculitis, open wound, active TB, any disruption in normal GI flora, history of PUD, anaphylactic disorders, indwelling catheters, severe diabetes, thyroid disease, and menstruating and postpartum women. Use with caution in protein C deficiency. Use with caution in patients with heparin-induced thrombocytopenia and DVT. Warfarin monotherapy is contraindicated in the initial treatment of active HIT. Reduced liver function, regardless of etiology, may impair synthesis of coagulation factors leading to increased warfarin sensitivity.

[U.S. Boxed Warning]: May cause major or fatal bleeding. Risk factors for bleeding include high intensity anticoagulation (INR >4), age (>65 years), variable INRs, history of GI bleeding, hypertension, cerebrovascular disease, serious heart disease, anemia, malignancy, trauma, renal insufficiency, drug-drug interactions, long duration of therapy, or known genetic deficiency in CYP2C9 activity. Patient must be instructed to report bleeding, accidents, or falls. Unrecognized bleeding sites (eg, colon cancer) may be uncovered by anticoagulation. Patient must also report any new or discontinued medications, herbal or alternative products used, or significant changes in smoking or dietary habits. Necrosis or gangrene of the skin and other tissue can occur, usually in conjunction with protein C or S deficiency. "Purple toes syndrome," due to cholesterol microembolization, may rarely occur. Women may be at risk of developing ovarian hemorrhage at the time of ovulation. The elderly may be more sensitive to anticoagulant therapy.

Presence of the CYP2C9*2 or *3 allele and/or polymorphism of the vitamin K oxidoreductase (VKORC1) gene may increase the risk of bleeding. Lower doses may be required in these patients; genetic testing may help determine appropriate dosing.

Adverse Reactions (Reflective of adult population; not specific for elderly) Bleeding is the major adverse effect of warfarin. Hemorrhage may occur at virtually any site. Risk is dependent on multiple variables, including the intensity of anticoagulation and patient susceptibility.

Cardiovascular: Angina, chest pain, edema, hemorrhagic shock, hypotension, pallor, syncope, vasculitis

Central nervous system: Coma, dizziness, fatigue, fever, headache, lethargy, malaise, pain, stroke

Dermatologic: Alopecia, bullous eruptions, dermatitis, rash, pruritus, urticaria

Gastrointestinal: Abdominal cramps, abdominal pain, anorexia, diarrhea, flatulence, gastrointestinal bleeding, mouth ulcers, nausea, taste disturbance, vomiting

Genitourinary: Hematuria, priapism

Hematologic: Agranulocytosis, anemia, leukopenia, retroperitoneal hematoma, unrecognized bleeding sites (eg, colon cancer) may be uncovered by anticoagulation

Hepatic: Cholestatic jaundice, hepatic injury, hepatitis, transaminases increased

Neuromuscular & skeletal: Joint pain, muscle pain, osteoporosis (potential association with long-term use), paralysis, paresthesia, weakness

Respiratory: Dyspnea, tracheobronchial calcification

Miscellaneous: Anaphylactic reaction, cold intolerance, hypersensitivity/allergic reactions, skin necrosis, gangrene, "purple toes" syndrome

Drug Interactions

Metabolism/Transport Effects Substrate of CYP1A2 (minor), 2C9 (major), 2C19 (minor), 3A4 (minor); **Inhibits** CYP2C9 (moderate), 2C19 (weak)

Avoid Concomitant Use

Avoid concomitant use of Warfarin with any of the following: Rivaroxaban; Tamoxifen

◄ **Increased Effect/Toxicity**

Warfarin may increase the levels/effects of: Anticoagulants; Collagenase (Systemic); Deferasirox; Drotrecogin Alfa; Ethotoin; Fosphenytoin; Phenytoin; Rivaroxaban

The levels/effects of Warfarin may be increased by: Acetaminophen; Allopurinol; Amiodarone; Androgens; Antineoplastic Agents; Antiplatelet Agents; Atazanavir; Bicalutamide; Boceprevir; Capecitabine; Cephalosporins; Chloral Hydrate; Chloramphenicol; Cimetidine; Clopidogrel; Corticosteroids (Systemic); Cranberry; CYP2C9 Inhibitors (Moderate); CYP2C9 Inhibitors (Strong); Desvenlafaxine; Dexmethylphenidate; Disulfiram; Dronedarone; Efavirenz; Erythromycin (Ophthalmic); Esomeprazole; Ethacrynic Acid; Ethotoin; Etoposide; Exenatide; Fenofibrate; Fenofibric Acid; Fenugreek; Fibric Acid Derivatives; Fluconazole; Fluorouracil; Fluorouracil (Systemic); Fluorouracil (Topical); Fosamprenavir; Fosphenytoin; Gefitinib; Ginkgo Biloba; Glucagon; Green Tea; Herbs (Anticoagulant/Antiplatelet Properties); HMG-CoA Reductase Inhibitors; Ifosfamide; Imatinib; Itraconazole; Ivermectin; Ketoconazole; Ketoconazole (Systemic); Lansoprazole; Leflunomide; Macrolide Antibiotics; Methylphenidate; MetroNIDAZOLE; MetroNIDAZOLE (Systemic); Miconazole (Oral); Miconazole (Topical); Milnacipran; Mirtazapine; Nelfinavir; Neomycin; NSAID (COX-2 Inhibitor); NSAID (Nonselective); Omega-3-Acid Ethyl Esters; Omeprazole; Orlistat; Pentosan Polysulfate Sodium; Pentoxifylline; Phenytoin; Posaconazole; Propafenone; Propoxyphene; Prostacyclin Analogues; QuiNIDine; QuiNINE; Quinolone Antibiotics; Ranitidine; RomiDEPsin; Salicylates; Saquinavir; Selective Serotonin Reuptake Inhibitors; Sitaxentan; SORAfenib; Sulfinpyrazone [Off Market]; Sulfonamide Derivatives; Tamoxifen; Telaprevir; Tetracycline Derivatives; Thrombolytic Agents; Thyroid Products; Tigecycline; Tolterodine; Toremifene; Torsemide; TraMADol; Tricyclic Antidepressants; Venlafaxine; Vitamin E; Voriconazole; Vorinostat; Zafirlukast; Zileuton

Decreased Effect

The levels/effects of Warfarin may be decreased by: Aminoglutethimide; Antineoplastic Agents; Antithyroid Agents; Aprepitant; AzaTHIOprine; Barbiturates; Bile Acid Sequestrants; Boceprevir; Bosentan; CarBAMazepine; Coenzyme Q-10; Contraceptives (Estrogens); Contraceptives (Progestins); CYP2C9 Inducers (Highly Effective); Cyproterone; Darunavir; Dicloxacillin; Efavirenz; Fosaprepitant; Ginseng (American); Glutethimide; Green Tea; Griseofulvin; Lopinavir; Mercaptopurine; Nafcillin; Nelfinavir; Peginterferon Alfa-2b; Phytonadione; Rifamycin Derivatives; Ritonavir; St Johns Wort; Sucralfate; Telaprevir; Tocilizumab

Ethanol/Nutrition/Herb Interactions

Ethanol: Avoid ethanol. Acute ethanol ingestion (binge drinking) decreases the metabolism of warfarin and increases PT/INR. Chronic daily ethanol use increases the metabolism of warfarin and decreases PT/INR.

Food: The anticoagulant effects of warfarin may be decreased if taken with foods rich in vitamin K. Vitamin E may increase warfarin effect. Cranberry juice may increase warfarin effect.

Herb/Nutraceutical: Cranberry, fenugreek, ginkgo biloba, glucosamine, may enhance bleeding or increase warfarin's effect. Ginseng (American), coenzyme Q$_{10}$, and St John's wort may decrease warfarin levels and effects. Avoid alfalfa, anise, bilberry, bladderwrack, bromelain, cat's claw, celery, chamomile, coleus, cordyceps, dong quai, evening primrose oil, fenugreek, feverfew, garlic, ginger, ginkgo biloba, ginseng (American), ginseng (Panax), ginseng (Siberian), grapeseed, green tea, guggul, horse chestnut seed, horseradish, licorice, omega-3-acids, prickly ash, red clover, reishi, SAMe (s-adenosylmethionine), sweet clover, turmeric, and white willow (all have additional antiplatelet activity).

Stability

Injection: Prior to reconstitution, store at 15°C to 30°C (59°F to 86°F). Following reconstitution with 2.7 mL of sterile water (yields 2 mg/mL solution), stable for 4 hours at 15°C to 30°C (59°F to 86°F). Protect from light.

Tablet: Store at 15°C to 30°C (59°F to 86°F). Protect from light.

Mechanism of Action Hepatic synthesis of coagulation factors II, VII, IX, and X, as well as proteins C and S, requires the presence of vitamin K. These clotting factors are biologically activated by the addition of carboxyl groups to key glutamic acid residues within the proteins' structure. In the process, "active" vitamin K is oxidatively converted to an "inactive" form, which is then subsequently reactivated by vitamin K epoxide reductase complex 1 (VKORC1). Warfarin competitively inhibits the subunit 1 of the multi-unit VKOR complex, thus depleting functional vitamin K reserves and hence reduces synthesis of active clotting factors.

Pharmacodynamics/Kinetics

Onset of action: Anticoagulation: Oral: 24-72 hours

Peak effect: Full therapeutic effect: 5-7 days; INR may increase in 36-72 hours

Duration: 2-5 days

Absorption: Oral: Rapid, complete

Distribution: 0.14 L/kg

Protein binding: 99%

Metabolism: Hepatic, primarily via CYP2C9; minor pathways include CYP2C8, 2C18, 2C19, 1A2, and 3A4

Genomic variants: Approximately 37% reduced clearance of S-warfarin in patients heterozygous for 2C9 (*1/*2 or *1/*3), and ~70% reduced in patients homozygous for reduced function alleles (*2/*2, *2/*3, or *3/*3)

Half-life elimination: 20-60 hours; Mean: 40 hours; highly variable among individuals

Time to peak, plasma: Oral: ~4 hours

Excretion: Urine (92%, primarily as metabolites)

Dosage

Geriatric Oral: Initial dose ≤5 mg. Usual maintenance dose: 2-5 mg/day. The elderly tend to require lower dosages to produce a therapeutic level of anticoagulation (due to changes in the pattern of warfarin metabolism).

Adult Note: Labeling identifies genetic factors which may increase patient sensitivity to warfarin. Specifically, genetic variations in the proteins CYP2C9 and VKORC1, responsible for warfarin's primary metabolism and pharmacodynamic activity, respectively, have been identified as predisposing factors associated with decreased dose requirement and increased bleeding risk. Genotyping tests are available, and may provide important guidance on initiation of anticoagulant therapy.

Prevention/treatment of thrombosis/embolism:

I.V. (administer as a slow bolus injection): 2-5 mg/day

Oral: Initial dosing must be individualized. Consider the patient (hepatic function, cardiac function, age, nutritional status, concurrent therapy, risk of bleeding) in addition to prior dose response (if available) and the clinical situation. Start 2-5 mg daily for 2 days **or** 5-10 mg daily for 1-2 days (Ansell, 2008). Adjust dose according to INR results; usual maintenance dose ranges from 2-10 mg daily (individual patients may require loading and maintenance doses outside these general guidelines).

Note: Lower starting doses may be required for patients with hepatic impairment, poor nutrition, CHF, elderly, high risk of bleeding, or patients who are debilitated, or those with reduced function genomic variants of the catabolic enzymes CYP2C9 (*2 or *3 alleles) or VKORC1 (-1639 polymorphism); see table. Higher initial doses may be reasonable in selected patients (ie, receiving enzyme-inducing agents and with low risk of bleeding).

Range[1] of Expected Therapeutic Maintenance Dose Based on CYP2C9[2] and VKORC1[3] Genotypes

VKORC1	CYP2C9					
	*1/*1	*1/*2	*1/*3	*2/*2	*2/*3	*3/*3
GG	5-7 mg	5-7 mg	3-4 mg	3-4 mg	3-4 mg	0.5-2 mg
AG	5-7 mg	3-4 mg	3-4 mg	3-4 mg	0.5-2 mg	0.5-2 mg
AA	3-4 mg	3-4 mg	0.5-2 mg	0.5-2 mg	0.5-2 mg	0.5-2 mg

Note: Must also take into account other patient related factors when determining initial dose (eg, age, body weight, concomitant medications, comorbidities).

[1]Ranges derived from multiple published clinical studies.

[2]Patients with CYP2C9 *1/*3, *2/*2, *2/*3, and *3/*3 alleles may take up to 4 weeks to achieve maximum INR with a given dose regimen.

[3]VKORC1 -1639G>A (rs 9923231) variant is used in this table; other VKORC1 variants may also be important determinants of dose.

Renal Impairment No adjustment required, however, patients with renal failure have an increased risk of bleeding complications. Monitor closely.

Hepatic Impairment Monitor effect at usual doses. The response to oral anticoagulants may be markedly enhanced in obstructive jaundice, hepatitis, and cirrhosis. INR should be closely monitored.

Administration

Oral: Administer with or without food. Take at the same time each day.

I.V.: Administer as a slow bolus injection over 1-2 minutes; avoid all I.M. injections

Monitoring Parameters Prothrombin time, hematocrit, INR; consider genotyping of CYP2C9 and VKORC1 prior to initiation of therapy, if available

Reference Range

INR = patient prothrombin time/mean normal prothrombin time

ISI = international sensitivity index

INR should be increased by 2-3.5 times depending upon indication. An INR >4 does not generally add additional therapeutic benefit and is associated with increased risk of bleeding. **Note:** To prevent gastrointestinal bleeding events in patients receiving the combination of warfarin, aspirin, and clopidogrel, an INR of 2-2.5 is recommended unless condition requires a higher INR target (eg, certain mechanical heart valves) (Bhatt, 2008).

◀ **Adult INR ranges based upon indication:** See table.

Adult Target INR Ranges Based Upon Indication

Indication	Targeted INR	Targeted INR Range
Cardiac		
Acute myocardial infarction (high risk)[1]	2.5	2-3[2,3]
Atrial fibrillation or atrial flutter	2.5	2-3
Valvular		
Bileaflet or Medtronic Hall tilting disk mechanical aortic valve in normal sinus rhythm and normal LA size	2.5	2-3
Bileaflet or tilting disk mechanical mitral valve	3	2.5-3.5
Caged ball or caged disk mechanical valve	3	2.5-3.5
Mechanical prosthetic valve with systemic embolism despite adequate anticoagulation	3 or 3.5[4]	2.5-3.5[4] or 3-4[4]
Mechanical valve and risk factors for thromboembolism (eg, AF, MI[5], LA enlargement, hypercoagulable state, low EF) or history of atherosclerotic vascular disease	3	2.5-3.5[6]
Bioprosthetic mitral valve	2.5	2-3[7]
Bioprosthetic mitral or aortic valve with prior history of systemic embolism	2.5	2-3[7]
Bioprosthetic mitral or aortic valve with evidence of LA thrombus at surgery	2.5	2-3[8]
Bioprosthetic mitral or aortic valve with risk factors for thromboembolism (eg, AF, hypercoagulable state or low EF)	2.5	2-3[9]
Prosthetic mitral valve thrombosis (resolved)	4	3.5-4.5[3]
Prosthetic aortic valve thrombosis (resolved)	3.5	3-4[3]
Rheumatic mitral valve disease and normal sinus rhythm (LA diameter >5.5 cm), AF, previous systemic embolism, or LA thrombus	2.5	2-3
Thromboembolism Treatment		
Venous thromboembolism	2.5	2-3[10,11]
Thromboprophylaxis		
Chronic thromboembolic pulmonary hypertension (CTPH)	2.5	2-3
Idiopathic pulmonary artery hypertension (IPAH)[12]	2	1.5-2.5
Lupus inhibitor (no other risk factors)	2.5	2-3
Lupus inhibitor and recurrent thromboembolism	3	2.5-3.5
Major trauma patients with impaired mobility undergoing rehabilitation	2.5	2-3
Spinal cord injury (acute) undergoing rehabilitation	2.5	2-3
Total hip or knee replacement (elective) or hip fracture surgery	2.5	2-3[13]
Other Indications		
Cerebral venous sinus thrombosis	2.5	2-3[14]
Ischemic stroke due to AF	2.5	2-3

[1]High-risk includes large anterior MI, significant heart failure, intracardiac thrombus, atrial fibrillation, history of thromboembolism.

[2]Maintain anticoagulation for 3 months.

[3]Combine with aspirin 81 mg/day.

[4]Combine with aspirin 81 mg/day, if not previously receiving, **and/or** if previous target INR was 2.5, then new target INR should be 3 (2.5-3.5). If previous target INR was 3, then new target INR should be 3.5 (3-4).

[5]MI refers to anterior-apical ST-segment elevation myocardial infarction.

[6]Combine with aspirin 81 mg/day unless patient is at high risk of bleeding (eg, history of GI bleed, age >80 years).

[7]Maintain anticoagulation for 3 months after valve insertion then switch to aspirin 81 mg/day if no other indications for warfarin exist or clinically reassess need for warfarin in patients with prior history of systemic embolism.

[8]Maintain anticoagulation with warfarin until thrombus resolution.

[9]If patient has history of atherosclerotic vascular disease, combine with aspirin 81 mg/day unless patient is at high risk of bleeding (eg, history of GI bleed, age >80 years).

[10]Treat for 3 months in patients with VTE due to transient reversible risk factor. Treat for a minimum of 3 months in patients with unprovoked VTE and evaluate for long term therapy. Other risk groups (eg, cancer) may require >3 months of therapy.

[11]In patients with unprovoked VTE who prefer less frequent INR monitoring, low-intensity therapy (INR range: 1.5-1.9) with less frequent monitoring is recommended over stopping treatment.

[12]Recommendation from the ACCF/AHA 2009 Expert Consensus Document on Pulmonary Hypertension (McLaughlin, 2009)

[13]Continue for at least 10 days and up to 35 days after surgery.

[14]Continue for up to 12 months.

Warfarin levels are not used for monitoring degree of anticoagulation. They may be useful if a patient with unexplained coagulopathy is using the drug surreptitiously or if it is unclear whether clinical resistance is due to true drug resistance or lack of drug intake.

Normal prothrombin time (PT): 10.9-12.9 seconds.

Pharmacotherapy Pearls Prospective genotyping is available, and may provide important guidance on initiation of anticoagulant therapy. Commercial testing with PGxPredict™: WARFARIN is available from PGxHealth™ (Division of Clinical Data, Inc, New Haven, CT). The test genotypes patients for presence of the CYP2C9*2 or *3 alleles and the VKORC1 - 1639G>A polymorphism. The results of the test allow patients to be phenotyped as extensive, intermediate, or poor metabolizers (CYP2C9) and as low, intermediate, or high warfarin sensitivity (VKORC1). Ordering information is available at 888-592-7327 or warfarininfo@pgxhealth.com.

Special Geriatric Considerations Before committing an elderly patient to long-term anti-coagulation therapy, the risk for bleeding complications secondary to falls, drug interactions, living situation, and cognitive status should be considered. A risk of bleeding complications has been associated with increased age.

Dosage Forms Excipient information presented when available (limited, particularly for generics); consult specific product labeling.
Injection, powder for reconstitution, as sodium:
Coumadin®: 5 mg
Tablet, oral, as sodium: 1 mg, 2 mg, 2.5 mg, 3 mg, 4 mg, 5 mg, 6 mg, 7.5 mg, 10 mg
Coumadin®: 1 mg, 2 mg, 2.5 mg, 3 mg, 4 mg, 5 mg, 6 mg, 7.5 mg [scored]
Coumadin®: 10 mg [scored; dye free]
Jantoven®: 1 mg, 2 mg, 2.5 mg, 3 mg, 4 mg, 5 mg, 6 mg, 7.5 mg [scored]
Jantoven®: 10 mg [scored; dye free]

Selected References

Ansell J, Hirsh J, Hylek E, et al, "Pharmacology and Management of the Vitamin K Antagonists: American College of Chest Physicians Evidence-Based Clinical Practice Guidelines (8th Edition)," Chest, 2008, 133:160-98.

Gurwitz JH, Avorn J, Ross-Degnan D, et al, "Aging and the Anticoagulant Response to Warfarin Therapy," Ann Intern Med, 1992, 116(11):901-4.

Harrington RA, Becker RC, Ezekowitz M, et al, "Antithrombotic Therapy for Coronary Artery Disease: The Seventh ACCP Conference on Antithrombotic and Thrombolytic Therapy," Chest, 2004, 126(3 Suppl):514-38

McLaughlin VV, Archer SL, Badesch DB, et al, "ACCF/AHA 2009 Expert Consensus Document on Pulmonary Hypertension. A Report of the American College of Cardiology Foundation Task Force on Expert Consensus Documents and the American Heart Association," Circulation, 2009, 119(16):2250-94.

Redwood M, Taylor C, Bain BJ, et al, "The Association of Age With Dosage Requirement for Warfarin," Age Ageing, 1991, 20(3):217-20.

Salem DN, Stein PD, Al-Ahmad A, et al, "Antithrombotic Therapy in Valvular Heart Disease – Native and Prosthetic: The Seventh ACCP Conference on Antithrombotic and Thrombolytic Therapy," Chest, 2004, 126(3 Suppl):457-82.

Shepherd AM, Hewick DS, Moreland TA, et al, "Age as a Determinant of Sensitivity to Warfarin," Br J Clin Pharmacol, 1977, 4(3):315-20.

◆ **Warfarin Sodium** see Warfarin on page 1928
◆ **Wart-Off® Maximum Strength [OTC]** see Salicylic Acid on page 1648
◆ **4-Way® 12 Hour [OTC]** see Oxymetazoline (Nasal) on page 1374
◆ **4 Way® Fast Acting [OTC]** see Phenylephrine (Nasal) on page 1442
◆ **4 Way® Menthol [OTC]** see Phenylephrine (Nasal) on page 1442
◆ **4-Way® Saline Moisturizing Mist [OTC]** see Sodium Chloride on page 1690
◆ **Welchol®** see Colesevelam on page 412
◆ **Wellbutrin®** see BuPROPion on page 229
◆ **Wellbutrin XL®** see BuPROPion on page 229
◆ **Wellbutrin SR®** see BuPROPion on page 229
◆ **Westcort®** see Hydrocortisone (Topical) on page 886
◆ **Westhroid™** see Thyroid, Desiccated on page 1786

Wheat Dextrin (weet DEKS trin)

Related Information
Laxatives, Classification and Properties on page 2012
Brand Names: U.S. Benefiber® Plus Calcium [OTC]; Benefiber® [OTC]
Index Terms Dextrin; Resistant Dextrin; Resistant Maltodextrin
Generic Availability (U.S.) No
Pharmacologic Category Fiber Supplement; Laxative, Bulk-Producing
Use OTC labeling: Dietary fiber supplement
Unlabeled/Investigational Use Treatment of constipation; aid to enhance LDL lowering to reduce the risk of coronary heart disease
Warnings/Precautions Use with caution in patients with esophageal strictures, ulcers, stenosis, intestinal adhesions, GI obstruction, fecal impaction, or difficulty swallowing. Use with caution in the elderly; may have insufficient fluid intake which may predispose them to fecal impaction and bowel obstruction. To aid in reducing the risk of CHD, the soluble fiber from wheat dextrin should be used in conjunction with a diet low in saturated fat and cholesterol. Some products may contain calcium, potassium, sodium, aspartame, or phenyl-alanine.

◄ **Adverse Reactions (Reflective of adult population; not specific for elderly)** Frequency not defined: Gastrointestinal: Bloating, flatulence, GI discomfort

Drug Interactions

Avoid Concomitant Use There are no known interactions where it is recommended to avoid concomitant use.

Increased Effect/Toxicity There are no known significant interactions involving an increase in effect.

Decreased Effect There are no known significant interactions involving a decrease in effect.

Stability Store at 20°C to 25°C (68°F to 77°F). Protect from moisture.

Mechanism of Action Wheat dextrin is a soluble fiber. It absorbs water in the intestine to form a viscous liquid which promotes peristalsis and reduces transit time.

Dosage

Geriatric & Adult General dosing guidelines; consult specific product labeling.

Adequate intake for total fiber: Oral: **Note:** The definition of "fiber" varies; however, the soluble fiber in wheat dextrin is only one type of fiber which makes up the daily recommended intake of total fiber.

Adults 19-50 years: Male: 38 g/day; Female: 25 g/day

Adults ≥51 years: Male: 30 g/day; Female: 21 g/day

Administration Powder can be mixed into hot or cold beverages (eg, water, coffee, juice), soft foods (eg, applesauce, pudding, yogurt), or cooked into recipes for foods; not recommended for use in carbonated beverages. Caplets should be swallowed with liquid.

Special Geriatric Considerations Elderly may have insufficient fluid intake which may predispose them to fecal impaction and bowel obstruction. Patients should have a 1-month trial, with at least 14 g/day, before effects in bowel function are determined. Bloating and flatulence are mostly a problem in first 4 weeks of therapy.

Dosage Forms Excipient information presented when available (limited, particularly for generics); consult specific product labeling.

Caplet, oral:

Benefiber®: 1.3 g [gluten free, sugar free; provides dietary fiber 3 g and soluble fiber 3 g per 3 caplets]

Powder, oral:

Benefiber®: (80 g, 155 g, 245 g, 350 g, 477 g) [gluten free, sugar free; original flavor]

Benefiber®: (161 g, 267 g, 529 g) [gluten free, sugar free; contains aspartame; orange flavor]

Benefiber®: 3.5 g/packet (28s) [gluten free, sugar free; original flavor; provides dietary fiber 3 g and soluble fiber 3 g per packet]

Benefiber®: 3.5 g/packet (16s) [sugar free; contains phenylalanine; kiwi-strawberry flavor; provides dietary fiber 3 g and soluble fiber 3 g per packet]

Benefiber®: 3.5 g/packet (8s) [sugar free; contains phenylalanine; raspberry tea flavor; provides dietary fiber 3 g and soluble fiber 3 g per packet]

Benefiber®: 3.5 g/packet (8s) [sugar free; contains phenylalanine, sodium 20 mg/packet; cherry-pomegranate flavor; provides dietary fiber 3 g and soluble fiber 3 g per packet]

Benefiber®: 3.5 g/packet (16s) [sugar free; contains phenylalanine, soy; citrus punch flavor; provides dietary fiber 3 g and soluble fiber 3 g per packet]

Benefiber® Plus Calcium: (424 g) [gluten free, sugar free]

Tablet, chewable, oral:

Benefiber®: 2.7 g [gluten free, sugar free; contains phenylalanine, soy; assorted fruit flavor; provides dietary fiber 3 g and soluble fiber 3 g per 3 tablets]

Benefiber®: 2.7 g [gluten free, sugar free; contains phenylalanine, soy; orange créme flavor; provides dietary fiber 3 g and soluble fiber 3 g per 3 tablets]

Benefiber® Plus Calcium: 2.7 g [gluten free, sugar free; contains calcium 100 mg/tablet, phenylalanine, soy; wildberry flavor; provides dietary fiber 3 g and soluble fiber 3 g per 3 tablets]

Selected References

Slavin JL, Savarino V, Paredes-Diaz A, et al, "A Review of the Role of Soluble Fiber in Health With Specific Reference to Wheat Dextrin," *J Int Med Res*, 2009, 37(1):1-17.

"Dietary Reference Intakes for Energy, Carbohydrate, Fiber, Fat, Fatty Acids, Cholesterol, Protein and Amino Acids," Standing Committee on the Scientific Evaluation of Dietary Reference Intakes, Food and Nutrition Board, Institute of Medicine, National Academy of Sciences, Washington, DC: National Academy Press, 2005. Available at http://www.nap.edu.

James SL, Muir JG, Curtis SL, et al, "Dietary Fibre: A Roughage Guide," *Intern Med J*, 2003, 33(7):291-6.

Yellow Fever Vaccine (YEL oh FEE ver vak SEEN)

Related Information
Immunization Administration Recommendations *on page 2037*
Immunization Recommendations *on page 2043*
Brand Names: U.S. YF-VAX®
Brand Names: Canada YF-VAX®
Generic Availability (U.S.) No
Pharmacologic Category Vaccine, Live (Viral)
Use Induction of active immunity against yellow fever virus, primarily among persons traveling or living in areas where yellow fever infection exists and laboratory workers who may be exposed to the virus; vaccination may also be required for some international travelers

The Advisory Committee on Immunization Practices (ACIP) recommends vaccination for:
• Persons traveling to or living in areas at risk for yellow fever transmission
• Persons traveling to countries which require vaccination for international travel
• Laboratory personnel who may be exposed to the yellow fever virus or concentrated preparations of the vaccine
Contraindications Hypersensitivity to egg or chick embryo protein, or any component of the formulation; acute or febrile disease; immunosuppressed patients

Per ACIP provisional guidelines, use is contraindicated in patients with symptomatic HIV infection or CD4+ counts <15% total; thymus disorders associated with abnormal immune cell function (eg, thymomas); primary immunodeficiencies; malignant neoplasms; transplant patients; concurrent immunosuppressive and immunomodulatory therapies (eg, radiation therapy or drugs)
Warnings/Precautions Patients who are immunosuppressed have a theoretical risk of encephalitis with yellow fever vaccine administration; consider delaying travel or obtaining a waiver letter. Patients on low-dose or short-term corticosteroids are not considered immunosuppressed and may be offered the vaccine. If vaccination is only to satisfy an international requirement (as opposed to decreasing risk of infection), efforts should be made to obtain a waiver letter. Per ACIP provisional guidelines, caution should be used if administering the vaccine to asymptomatic patients with HIV infection and CD4+ T-lymphocytes of 15% to 24%.

Immediate treatment (including epinephrine 1:1000) for anaphylactoid and/or hypersensitivity reactions should be available during vaccine use.

Chicken embryos are used in the manufacture of this vaccine. Use is contraindicated in patients with immediate-type hypersensitivity reactions to eggs; in general, persons who are able to eat eggs or egg products may receive the vaccine. The vial stopper contains latex; product may contain gelatin. Immunization should be delayed during the course of an acute or febrile illness. The presence of a low-grade fever is generally not a reason to postpone vaccination. Use with caution in the elderly; the risk of adverse events is increased in patients ≥65 years of age (per manufacturer). The ACIP provisional guidelines note that caution be used if administering to patients ≥60 years, especially those who have not previously received the yellow fever vaccine. In order to maximize vaccination rates, the ACIP recommends simultaneous administration of all age-appropriate vaccines (live or inactivated) for which a person is eligible at a single clinic visit, unless contraindications exist.

Adverse Reactions (Reflective of adult population; not specific for elderly) All serious adverse reactions must be reported to the U.S. Department of Health and Human Services (DHHS) Vaccine Adverse Event Reporting System (VAERS) 1-800-822-7967 or online at https://vaers.hhs.gov/esub/index. In Canada, adverse reactions may be reported to local provincial/territorial health agencies or to the Vaccine Safety Section at Public Health Agency of Canada (1-866-844-0018).

Frequency not defined (adverse reactions may be increased in patients <9 months or ≥60 years of age)

Central nervous system: Chills, fever (incidence of these reactions have been reported to be as low as <5% and as high as 10% to 30% depending on the study), focal neurological defects, headache, malaise, seizure

Dermatologic: Rash, urticaria

Local: Injection site reactions (edema, erythema, hypersensitivity, mass, pain, pruritus, rash, warmth)

Neuromuscular & skeletal: Myalgia, weakness

Miscellaneous: Guillain-Barré syndrome (GBS), hypersensitivity (immediate), vaccine-associated neurotropic disease (rare), viscerotropic disease (rare; may be associated with multiorgan failure)

Vaccine-associated neurologic disease (YEL-AND) may manifest as meningoencephalitis (neurotropic disease), GBS, acute disseminated encephalomyelitis, and bulbar palsy. Vaccine-associated viscerotropic disease (YEL-AVD) mimics naturally-acquired yellow fever disease; risk may be increased in older patients and those with a history of thymus disease or thymectomy.

Drug Interactions

Avoid Concomitant Use

Avoid concomitant use of Yellow Fever Vaccine with any of the following: Belimumab; Fingolimod; Immunosuppressants

Increased Effect/Toxicity

The levels/effects of Yellow Fever Vaccine may be increased by: AzaTHIOprine; Belimumab; Corticosteroids (Systemic); Fingolimod; Hydroxychloroquine; Immunosuppressants; Leflunomide; Mercaptopurine; Methotrexate

Decreased Effect

Yellow Fever Vaccine may decrease the levels/effects of: Tuberculin Tests

The levels/effects of Yellow Fever Vaccine may be decreased by: Fingolimod; Immunosuppressants

Stability Store at 2°C to 8°C (35°F to 46°F); do not freeze. Reconstitute only with diluent provided. Inject diluent slowly into vial and allow to stand for 1-2 minutes. Gently swirl until a uniform suspension forms; swirl well before withdrawing dose. Avoid vigorous shaking to prevent foaming of suspension. Vaccine must be used within 60 minutes of reconstitution. Keep suspension refrigerated until used.

Pharmacodynamics/Kinetics

Onset of action: Seroconversion: 10-14 days

Duration: ≥30 years

Dosage

Geriatric Refer to adult dosing. Monitor closely due to an increased incidence of serious adverse events in patients ≥60 years of age, particularly in patients receiving their first dose. The ACIP guidelines note that if travel is unavoidable, the decision to vaccinate travelers ≥60 years should be made after weighing the risks vs benefits.

Adult Immunization: SubQ: One dose (0.5 mL) ≥10 days before travel; Booster: Every 10 years for those at continued risk of exposure

Administration For SubQ injection only. Do not administer I.M. or I.V.; if inadvertently administered I.M., the dose does not need repeated. Use of expired vaccine is not considered a valid dose and should be repeated after 28 days. For booster doses, if the date of previous vaccination cannot be determined and the patient requires vaccination, the booster dose can be given.

Blood donation following vaccine administration: Transfusion-related transmission of yellow fever vaccine virus has been reported; wait 2 weeks after immunization with yellow fever vaccine to donate blood.

Simultaneous administration of vaccines helps ensure the patients will be fully vaccinated by the appropriate age. Simultaneous administration of vaccines is defined as administering >1 vaccine on the same day at different anatomic sites. Separate vaccines should not be combined in the same syringe unless indicated by product specific labeling. Separate needles and syringes should be used for each injection. The ACIP prefers each dose of a specific vaccine in a series come from the same manufacturer when possible. Adolescents and adults should be vaccinated while seated or lying down. In general, preterm infants should be vaccinated at the same chronological age as full-term infants (CDC, 2011).

Antipyretics have not been shown to prevent febrile seizures. Antipyretics may be used to treat fever or discomfort following vaccination (CDC, 2011). One study reported that routine prophylactic administration of acetaminophen to prevent fever prior to vaccination decreased the immune response of some vaccines; the clinical significance of this reduction in immune response has not been established (Prymula, 2009).

Monitoring Parameters Monitor for syncope for ≥15 minutes following vaccination. Monitor for adverse effects 10 days after vaccination (specifically in the elderly).

Pharmacotherapy Pearls Federal law requires that the name of medication, date of administration, the vaccine manufacturer, lot number of vaccine, and the administering person's name, title, and address be entered into the patient's permanent medical record. Some countries require a valid International Certification of Vaccination or Prophylaxis (ICVP) showing receipt of vaccine. Certificate is valid beginning 10 days after and for 10 years following vaccination (booster doses received within 10 years are valid from the date of vaccination). The WHO requires revaccination every 10 years to maintain traveler's vaccination certificate. All travelers to endemic areas should be advised of the risks of yellow fever disease and all available methods to prevent it. All travelers should take protective measures to avoid mosquito bites.

The following CDC agencies may be contacted if serologic testing is needed or for advice when administering yellow fever vaccine to pregnant women, children <9 months, or patients with altered immune status:

Division of Vector-Borne Infectious Diseases: 970-221-6400

Division of Global Migration and Quarantine: 404-498-1600

Special Geriatric Considerations The rate of serious adverse events is greater in persons aged ≥60 years than in persons aged 19-29 years. The risk for YEL-AND and YEL-AVD also are increased. Use with caution in older travelers who might be receiving vaccine for the first time.

Dosage Forms Excipient information presented when available (limited, particularly for generics); consult specific product labeling.

Injection, powder for reconstitution [17D-204 strain]:

YF-VAX®: ≥4.74 Log_{10} plaque-forming units (PFU) per 0.5 mL dose [single-dose or 5-dose vial; produced in chicken embryos; contains gelatin; packaged with diluent; vial stopper contains latex]

Selected References

"ACIP Provisional Recommendations for the Use of Yellow Fever Vaccine," December 2009. Available at http://www.cdc.gov/vaccines/recs/provisional/default.htm#acip.

American Red Cross Eligibility Criteria by Alphabetical Listing. Available at http://www.redcrossblood.org/donating-blood/eligibility-requirements/eligibility-criteria-alphabetical-listing.

Centers for Disease Control and Prevention, "General Recommendations on immunization. Recommendations of the Advisory Committee on Immunization Practices (ACIP) and the American Academy of Family Physicians (AAFP)," MMWR, 2002, 51(R-2):1-35.

Centers for Disease Control and Prevention, "Transfusion-Related Transmission of Yellow Fever Vaccine Virus - California, 2009," MMMR Recomm Rep, 2010, 59(2): 34-7. Available at http://www.cdc.gov/mmwr/PDF/wk/mm5902.pdf.

Centers for Disease Control and Prevention, "Yellow Fever Vaccine. Recommendations of the Advisory Committee on Immunization Practices (ACIP)," MMWR, 2002, 51(R-2):1-11.

Centers for Disease Control and Prevention, "Guidelines for Preventing Opportunistic Infections Among Hematopoietic Stem Cell Transplant Recipients. Recommendations of CDC, the Infectious Disease Society of America, and the American Society of Blood and Marrow Transplantation," MMWR, 2004, 49(RR-10):89-90.

◆ **YF-VAX®** see Yellow Fever Vaccine on page 1935

◆ **YM087** see Conivaptan on page 416

◆ **YM905** see Solifenacin on page 1699

◆ **Yodoxin®** see Iodoquinol on page 972

◆ **Zaditor® [OTC]** see Ketotifen on page 1013

Zafirlukast (za FIR loo kast)

Related Information

Asthma on page 2016

Medication Safety Issues

Sound-alike/look-alike issues:

Accolate® may be confused with Accupril®, Accutane®, Aclovate®

Brand Names: U.S. Accolate®

Brand Names: Canada Accolate®

Index Terms ICI-204,219

ZAFIRLUKAST

Generic Availability (U.S.) Yes

Pharmacologic Category Leukotriene-Receptor Antagonist

Use Prophylaxis and chronic treatment of asthma

Contraindications Hypersensitivity to zafirlukast or any component of the formulation; hepatic impairment

Warnings/Precautions Zafirlukast is not FDA approved for use in the reversal of bronchospasm in acute asthma attacks, including status asthmaticus. Therapy with zafirlukast can be continued during acute exacerbations of asthma.

Hepatic adverse events (including hepatitis, hyperbilirubinemia, and hepatic failure) have been reported; female patients may be at greater risk. Discontinue immediately if liver dysfunction is suspected. Periodic testing of liver function may be considered (early detection is generally believed to improve the likelihood of recovery). If hepatic dysfunction is suspected (due to clinical signs/symptoms), liver function tests should be measured immediately. Do not resume or restart if hepatic function studies are consistent with dysfunction. Use caution in patients with alcoholic cirrhosis; clearance is reduced. Postmarketing reports of behavioral changes (ie, depression, insomnia) have been noted. Monitor INR closely with concomitant warfarin use. Rare cases of eosinophilic vasculitis (Churg-Strauss) have been reported in patients receiving zafirlukast (usually, but not always, associated with reduction in concurrent steroid dosage). No causal relationship established. Monitor for eosinophilic vasculitis, rash, pulmonary symptoms, cardiac symptoms, or neuropathy.

An increased proportion of zafirlukast patients >55 years of age reported infections as compared to placebo-treated patients. These infections were mostly mild or moderate in intensity and predominantly affected the respiratory tract. Infections occurred equally in both sexes, were dose-proportional to total milligrams of zafirlukast exposure, and were associated with coadministration of inhaled corticosteroids.

Adverse Reactions (Reflective of adult population; not specific for elderly)

>10%: Central nervous system: Headache (13%)

1% to 10%:

Central nervous system: Dizziness (2%), pain (2%), fever (2%)

Gastrointestinal: Nausea (3%), diarrhea (3%), abdominal pain (2%), vomiting (2%), dyspepsia (1%)

Hepatic: ALT increased (2%)

Neuromuscular & skeletal: Back pain (2%), myalgia (2%), weakness (2%)

Miscellaneous: Infection (4%)

Drug Interactions

Metabolism/Transport Effects Substrate of CYP2C9 (major); **Inhibits** CYP1A2 (weak), 2C8 (weak), 2C9 (moderate), 2C19 (weak), 2D6 (weak), 3A4 (weak)

Avoid Concomitant Use There are no known interactions where it is recommended to avoid concomitant use.

Increased Effect/Toxicity

Zafirlukast may increase the levels/effects of: Carvedilol; CYP2C9 Substrates (High risk); Theophylline Derivatives; Vitamin K Antagonists

The levels/effects of Zafirlukast may be increased by: CYP2C9 Inhibitors (Moderate); CYP2C9 Inhibitors (Strong)

Decreased Effect

The levels/effects of Zafirlukast may be decreased by: CYP2C9 Inducers (Highly Effective); Erythromycin; Erythromycin (Systemic); Peginterferon Alfa-2b; Theophylline Derivatives

Ethanol/Nutrition/Herb Interactions Food: Decreases bioavailability of zafirlukast by 40%.

Stability Store tablets at controlled room temperature of 20°C to 25°C (68°F to 77°F). Protect from light and moisture; dispense in original airtight container.

Mechanism of Action Zafirlukast is a selectively and competitive leukotriene-receptor antagonist (LTRA) of leukotriene D4 and E4 (LTD4 and LTE4), components of slow-reacting substance of anaphylaxis (SRSA). Cysteinyl leukotriene production and receptor occupation have been correlated with the pathophysiology of asthma, including airway edema, smooth muscle constriction, and altered cellular activity associated with the inflammatory process, which contribute to the signs and symptoms of asthma.

Pharmacodynamics/Kinetics

Distribution: V_{dss}: 70 L

Protein binding: >99%, primarily to albumin

Metabolism: Extensively hepatic via CYP2C9

Bioavailability: Reduced 40% with food

Half-life elimination: 10 hours

Time to peak, serum: 3 hours

Excretion: Urine (10%); feces

Dosage

Geriatric & Adult Asthma: Oral: 20 mg twice daily

Renal Impairment Dosage adjustment not required.

Hepatic Impairment Use is contraindicated.

Administration Administer at least 1 hour before or 2 hours after a meal

Monitoring Parameters Monitor for improvements in air flow; monitor closely for sign/symptoms of hepatic injury; periodic monitoring of LFTs may be considered (not proved to prevent serious injury, but early detection may enhance recovery)

Special Geriatric Considerations The mean dose (mg/kg) normalized AUC and C_{max} increase and plasma clearance decreases with increasing age. In patients >65 years of age, there is a two- to threefold greater C_{max} and AUC compared to younger adults. Some studies have demonstrated slightly higher adverse effect reports in elderly compared to younger adults: Headache (4.7%), diarrhea and nausea (1.8%), and pharyngitis (1.3%). No changes in dose recommended for elderly.

Dosage Forms Excipient information presented when available (limited, particularly for generics); consult specific product labeling.

Tablet, oral: 10 mg, 20 mg
    Accolate®: 10 mg, 20 mg

Zaleplon (ZAL e plon)

Medication Safety Issues

Sound-alike/look-alike issues:

Sonata® may be confused with Soriatane®

Zaleplon may be confused with Zelapar®, Zemplar®, zolpidem, ZyPREXA® Zydis®

Brand Names: U.S. Sonata®

Generic Availability (U.S.) Yes

Pharmacologic Category Hypnotic, Nonbenzodiazepine

Use Short-term (7-10 days) treatment of insomnia (has been demonstrated to be effective for up to 5 weeks in controlled trial)

Medication Guide Available Yes

Contraindications Hypersensitivity to zaleplon or any component of the formulation

Warnings/Precautions Symptomatic treatment of insomnia should be initiated only after careful evaluation of potential causes of sleep disturbance. Failure of sleep disturbance to resolve after 7-10 days may indicate psychiatric and/or medical illness.

Use with caution in patients with depression, particularly if suicidal risk may be present. Use with caution in patients with a history of drug dependence. Abrupt discontinuance may lead to withdrawal symptoms. Hypnotics/sedatives have been associated with abnormal thinking and behavior changes including decreased inhibition, aggression, bizarre behavior, agitation, hallucinations, and depersonalization. These changes may occur unpredictably and may indicate previously unrecognized psychiatric disorders; evaluate appropriately. May impair physical and mental capabilities. Patients must be cautioned about performing tasks which require mental alertness (operating machinery or driving). Amnesia can occur. Use with caution in patients receiving other CNS depressants or psychoactive medications. Effects with other sedative drugs or ethanol may be potentiated. Postmarketing studies have indicated that the use of hypnotic/sedative agents for sleep has been associated with hypersensitivity reactions including anaphylaxis as well as angioedema. An increased risk for hazardous sleep-related activities such as sleep-driving, cooking and eating food, and making phone calls while asleep have been noted.

Use with caution in the elderly, those with compromised respiratory function, or hepatic impairment (dosage adjustment recommended in mild-to-moderate hepatic impairment; avoid use in severe impairment). Because of the rapid onset of action, zaleplon should be administered immediately prior to bedtime or after the patient has gone to bed and is having difficulty falling asleep. Capsules contain tartrazine (FDC yellow #5); avoid in patients with sensitivity (caution in patients with asthma).

Adverse Reactions (Reflective of adult population; not specific for elderly)

>10%: Central nervous system: Headache (30% to 42%)

1% to 10%:

Cardiovascular: Chest pain (≥1%), peripheral edema (≤1%)

Central nervous system: Dizziness (7% to 9%), somnolence (5% to 6%), amnesia (2% to 4%), depersonalization (<1% to 2%), hypoesthesia (<1% to 2%), malaise (<1% to 2%), abnormal thinking (≥1%), anxiety (≥1%), depression (≥1%), fever (≥1%), migraine (≥1%), nervousness (≥1%), confusion (≤1%), hallucination (≤1%), vertigo (≤1%)

Dermatologic: Pruritus (≥1%), rash (≥1%), photosensitivity reaction (≤1%)

Endocrine & metabolic: Dysmenorrhea (3% to 4%)

Gastrointestinal: Nausea (6% to 8%), abdominal pain (6%), anorexia (<1% to 2%), constipation (≥1%), dyspepsia (≥1%), taste perversion (≥1%), xerostomia (≥1%), colitis (up to 1%)

Neuromuscular & skeletal: Weakness (5% to 7%), paresthesia (3%), tremor (2%), arthralgia (≥1%), arthritis (≥1%), back pain (≥1%), myalgia (≥1%), hypertonia (1%)

Ocular: Eye pain (3% to 4%), abnormal vision (<1% to 2%), conjunctivitis (≥1%)

Otic: Hyperacusis (1% to 2%), ear pain (≤1%)

Respiratory: Bronchitis (≥1%), epistaxis (≤1%)

Miscellaneous: Parosmia (<1% to 2%)

Drug Interactions

Metabolism/Transport Effects Substrate of CYP3A4 (minor)

Avoid Concomitant Use There are no known interactions where it is recommended to avoid concomitant use.

Increased Effect/Toxicity

Zaleplon may increase the levels/effects of: Alcohol (Ethyl); CNS Depressants; Methotrimeprazine; Selective Serotonin Reuptake Inhibitors

The levels/effects of Zaleplon may be increased by: Cimetidine; Conivaptan; Droperidol; HydrOXYzine; Methotrimeprazine

Decreased Effect

The levels/effects of Zaleplon may be decreased by: Flumazenil; Rifamycin Derivatives; Tocilizumab

Ethanol/Nutrition/Herb Interactions

Ethanol: May increase CNS depression; monitor for increased effects with coadministration. Caution patients about effects.

Food: High fat meal prolonged absorption; delayed T_{max} by 2 hours, and reduced C_{max} by 35%.

Herb/Nutraceutical: St John's wort may decrease zaleplon levels. Avoid valerian, St John's wort, kava kava, gotu kola (may increase CNS depression).

Stability Store at controlled room temperature of 20°C to 25°C (68°F to 77°F). Protect from light.

Mechanism of Action Zaleplon is unrelated to benzodiazepines, barbiturates, or other hypnotics. However, it interacts with the benzodiazepine GABA receptor complex. Nonclinical studies have shown that it binds selectively to the brain omega-1 receptor situated on the alpha subunit of the GABA-A receptor complex.

Pharmacodynamics/Kinetics

Onset of action: Rapid

Duration: 6-8 hours

Absorption: Rapid and almost complete; high-fat meal delays absorption

Distribution: V_d: ~1.4 L/kg

Protein binding: ~45% to 75%

Metabolism: Extensive, primarily via aldehyde oxidase to form 5-oxo-zaleplon and, to a lesser extent, by CYP3A4 to desethylzaleplon; all metabolites are pharmacologically inactive

Bioavailability: ~30%

Half-life elimination: 1 hour

Time to peak, serum: 1 hour

Excretion: Urine (~70% primarily metabolites, <1% as unchanged drug); feces (~17%)

Clearance: Plasma: Oral: 3 L/hour/kg

Dosage

Geriatric Reduce dose to 5 mg at bedtime; recommended maximum: 10 mg/day

Adult Insomnia (short-term use): Oral: 10 mg at bedtime (range: 5-20 mg)

Renal Impairment No adjustment for mild-to-moderate renal impairment; use in severe renal impairment has not been adequately studied.

Hepatic Impairment Mild-to-moderate impairment: 5 mg; not recommended for use in patients with severe hepatic impairment.

Administration Immediately before bedtime or when the patient is in bed and cannot fall asleep

Monitoring Parameters Mental status

Pharmacotherapy Pearls Prescription quantities should not exceed a 1-month supply. Zaleplon is primarily used to decrease sleep latency.

Special Geriatric Considerations In clinical trials, elderly responded to the 5 mg dose with decreased sleep latency. As with all hypnotics, assess underlying cause of insomnia.

Controlled Substance C-IV

Dosage Forms Excipient information presented when available (limited, particularly for generics); consult specific product labeling.
Capsule, oral: 5 mg, 10 mg
   Sonata®: 5 mg
   Sonata®: 10 mg [contains tartrazine]

◆ **Zamicet™** *see* Hydrocodone and Acetaminophen *on page 880*
◆ **Zanaflex®** *see* TiZANidine *on page 1808*
◆ **Zanaflex Capsules®** *see* TiZANidine *on page 1808*

Zanamivir (za NA mi veer)

Related Information
  Community-Acquired Pneumonia in Adults *on page 2059*
Medication Safety Issues
  Sound-alike/look-alike issues:
   Relenza® may be confused with Albenza®, Aplenzin™
Brand Names: U.S. Relenza®
Brand Names: Canada Relenza®
Generic Availability (U.S.) No
Pharmacologic Category Antiviral Agent; Neuraminidase Inhibitor
Use Treatment of uncomplicated acute illness due to influenza virus A and B in patients who have been symptomatic for no more than 2 days; prophylaxis against influenza virus A and B

The Advisory Committee on Immunization Practices (ACIP) recommends that **treatment** be considered for the following:
• Persons with severe, complicated or progressive illness
• Hospitalized persons
• Persons at higher risk for influenza complications:
  - Adults ≥65 years of age
  - Persons with chronic disorders of the pulmonary (including asthma) or cardiovascular systems (except hypertension)
  - Persons with chronic metabolic diseases (including diabetes mellitus), hepatic disease, renal dysfunction, hematologic disorders (including sickle cell disease), or immunosuppression (including immunosuppression caused by medications or HIV)
  - Persons with neurologic/neuromuscular conditions (including conditions such as spinal cord injuries, seizure disorders, cerebral palsy, stroke, mental retardation, moderate to severe developmental delay, or muscular dystrophy) which may compromise respiratory function, the handling of respiratory secretions, or that can increase the risk of aspiration
  - American Indians and Alaskan Natives
  - Persons who are morbidly obese (BMI ≥40)
  - Residents of nursing homes or other chronic care facilities
• Use may also be considered for previously healthy, nonhigh-risk outpatients with confirmed or suspected influenza based on clinical judgment when treatment can be started within 48 hours of illness onset.

The ACIP recommends that **prophylaxis** be considered for the following:
• Postexposure prophylaxis may be considered for family or close contacts of suspected or confirmed cases, who are at higher risk of influenza complications, and who have not been vaccinated against the circulating strain at the time of the exposure.
• Postexposure prophylaxis may be considered for unvaccinated healthcare workers who had occupational exposure without protective equipment.
• Pre-exposure prophylaxis should only be used for persons at very high risk of influenza complications who cannot be otherwise protected at times of high risk for exposure.
• Prophylaxis should also be administered to all eligible residents of institutions that house patients at high risk when needed to control outbreaks.
Prescribing and Access Restrictions Zanamivir *aqueous solution* intended for nebulization or intravenous (I.V.) administration is **not** currently approved for use. Data on safety and efficacy via these routes of administration are limited. However, limited supplies of zanamivir aqueous solution may be made available through the Zanamivir Compassionate Use Program for qualifying patients for the treatment of serious influenza illness. For information, contact the GlaxoSmithKline Clinical Support Help Desk at 1-866-341-9160 or gskclinicalsupportHD@gsk.com.
Contraindications Hypersensitivity to zanamivir or any component of the formulation
Warnings/Precautions Allergic-like reactions, including anaphylaxis, oropharyngeal edema, and serious skin rashes have been reported. Rare occurrences of neuropsychiatric events (including confusion, delirium, hallucinations, and/or self-injury) have been reported from postmarketing surveillance; direct causation is difficult to establish (influenza infection may

also be associated with behavioral and neurologic changes). Patients must be instructed in the use of the delivery system. Antiviral treatment should begin within 48 hours of symptom onset. However, the CDC recommends that treatment may still be beneficial and should be started in hospitalized patients with severe, complicated or progressive illness if >48 hours. Nonhospitalized persons who are not at high risk for developing severe or complicated illness and who have a mild disease are not likely to benefit if treatment is started >48 hours after symptom onset. Nonhospitalized persons who are already beginning to recover do not need treatment. Effectiveness has not been established in patients with significant underlying medical conditions or for prophylaxis of influenza in nursing home patients (per manufacturer). The CDC recommends zanamivir to be used to control institutional outbreaks of influenza when circulating strains are suspected of being resistant to oseltamivir (refer to current guidelines). Not recommended for use in patients with underlying respiratory disease, such as asthma or COPD, due to lack of efficacy and risk of serious adverse effects. Bronchospasm, decreased lung function, and other serious adverse reactions, including those with fatal outcomes, have been reported in patients with and without airway disease; discontinue with bronchospasm or signs of decreased lung function. For a patient with an underlying airway disease where a medical decision has been made to use zanamivir, a fast-acting bronchodilator should be made available, and used prior to each dose. Not a substitute for annual flu vaccination; has not been shown to reduce risk of transmission of influenza to others. Consider primary or concomitant bacterial infections. Powder for oral inhalation contains lactose. The inhalation powder should only be administered via inhalation using the provided Diskhaler® delivery device. The commercially available formulation is **not** intended to be solubilized or administered via any nebulizer/mechanical ventilator; inappropriate administration has resulted in death. Safety and efficacy of repeated courses or use with hepatic impairment or severe renal impairment have not been established.

Adverse Reactions (Reflective of adult population; not specific for elderly) Most adverse reactions occurred at a frequency which was less than or equal to the control (lactose vehicle).

>10%:
  Central nervous system: Headache (prophylaxis 13% to 24%; treatment 2%)
  Gastrointestinal: Throat/tonsil discomfort/pain (prophylaxis 8% to 19%)
  Respiratory: Nasal signs and symptoms (prophylaxis 12% to 20%; treatment 2%), cough (prophylaxis 7% to 17%; treatment ≤2%)
  Miscellaneous: Viral infection (prophylaxis 3% to 13%)

1% to 10%:
  Central nervous system: Fever/chills (prophylaxis 5% to 9%; treatment <1.5%), fatigue (prophylaxis 5% to 8%; treatment <1.5%), malaise (prophylaxis 5% to 8%; treatment <1.5%), dizziness (treatment 1% to 2%)
  Dermatologic: Urticaria (treatment <1.5%)
  Gastrointestinal: Anorexia/appetite decreased (prophylaxis 2% to 4%), appetite increased (prophylaxis 2% to 4%), nausea (prophylaxis 1% to 2%; treatment ≤3%), diarrhea (prophylaxis 2%; treatment 2% to 3%), vomiting (prophylaxis 1% to 2%; treatment 1% to 2%), abdominal pain (treatment <1.5%)
  Neuromuscular & skeletal: Muscle pain (prophylaxis 3% to 8%), musculoskeletal pain (prophylaxis 6%), arthralgia/articular rheumatism (prophylaxis 2%), arthralgia (treatment <1.5%), myalgia (treatment <1.5%)
  Respiratory: Infection (ear/nose/throat; prophylaxis 2%; treatment 1% to 5%), sinusitis (treatment 3%), bronchitis (treatment 2%), nasal inflammation (prophylaxis 1%)

Drug Interactions

  Avoid Concomitant Use There are no known interactions where it is recommended to avoid concomitant use.

  Increased Effect/Toxicity There are no known significant interactions involving an increase in effect.

  Decreased Effect
    Zanamivir may decrease the levels/effects of: Influenza Virus Vaccine (Live/Attenuated)

Stability Store at 25°C (77°F); excursions permitted to 15°C to 30°C (59°F to 86°F). Do not puncture blister until taking a dose using the Diskhaler®.

Mechanism of Action Zanamivir inhibits influenza virus neuraminidase enzymes, potentially altering virus particle aggregation and release.

Pharmacodynamics/Kinetics
  Absorption: Inhalation: Systemic: ~4% to 17%
  Protein binding, plasma: <10%
  Metabolism: None
  Half-life elimination, serum: 2.5-5.1 hours; Mild-to-moderate renal impairment: 4.7 hours; Severe renal impairment: 18.5 hours
  Time to peak, plasma: 1-2 hours
  Excretion: Urine (as unchanged drug); feces (unabsorbed drug)

Dosage

Geriatric & Adult Influenza virus A and B:

Prophylaxis: Oral inhalation:

Household setting: Two inhalations (10 mg) once daily for 10 days. Begin within 36 hours following onset of signs or symptoms of index case.

Institutional outbreak, CDC 2011 recommendations: Continue for ≥2 weeks and until ~10 days after identification of illness onset in the last patient. Zanamivir is to be used to control institutional outbreaks of influenza when circulating strains are suspected of being resistant to oseltamivir.

Community outbreak: Two inhalations (10 mg) once daily for 28 days. Begin within 5 days of outbreak.

Treatment: Oral inhalation: Two inhalations (10 mg total) twice daily for 5 days. Doses on first day should be separated by at least 2 hours; on subsequent days, doses should be spaced by ~12 hours. Begin within 2 days of signs or symptoms. Longer treatment may be considered for patients who remain severely ill after 5 days.

Renal Impairment Adjustment not necessary following a 5-day course of treatment due to low systemic absorption; however the potential for drug accumulation should be considered.

Administration Inhalation: Must be used with Diskhaler® delivery device. The foil blister disk containing zanamivir inhalation powder should not be manipulated, solubilized, or administered via a nebulizer. Patients who are scheduled to use an inhaled bronchodilator should use their bronchodilator prior to zanamivir. With the exception of the initial dose when used for treatment, administer at the same time each day.

Pharmacotherapy Pearls Majority of patients included in clinical trials were infected with influenza A, however, a number of patients with influenza B infections were also enrolled. Patients with lower temperature or less severe symptoms appeared to derive less benefit from therapy. No consistent treatment benefit was demonstrated in patients with chronic underlying medical conditions.

The absence of symptoms does not rule out viral influenza infection and clinical judgment should guide the decision for therapy. Treatment should not be delayed while waiting for the results of diagnostic tests. Treatment should be considered for high-risk patients with symptoms despite a negative rapid influenza test when the illness cannot be contributed to another cause. Use of zanamivir is not a substitute for vaccination (when available); susceptibility to influenza infection returns once therapy is discontinued.

Special Geriatric Considerations A study demonstrated that most elderly were unable to use an inhaler device effectively. Evaluate the patient's or caregiver's ability to safely administer the correct dose of medication.

Dosage Forms Excipient information presented when available (limited, particularly for generics); consult specific product labeling.

Powder, for oral inhalation:

Relenza®: 5 mg/blister (20s) [contains lactose 20 mg/blister; 4 blisters per Rotadisk® foil pack, 5 Rotadisk® per package; packaged with Diskhaler® inhalation device]

Selected References

Centers for Disease Control, "Interim Guidance on Antiviral Recommendations for Patients With Novel Influenza A (H1N1) Virus Infection and Close Contacts," May 6, 2009. Available at http://www.cdc.gov/h1n1flu/recommendations.htm

Diggory P, Fernandez C, Humphrey A, et al, "Comparison of Elderly People's Technique in Using Two Dry Powder Inhalers to Deliver Zanamivir: Randomised Controlled Trial," *BMJ*, 2001, 322(7286):577-9.

- **Zenpep™** *see Pancrelipase on page 1387*
- **Zestoretic®** *see Lisinopril and Hydrochlorothiazide on page 1082*
- **Zestril®** *see Lisinopril on page 1079*
- **Zetia®** *see Ezetimibe on page 689*
- **Ziana™** *see Clindamycin and Tretinoin on page 380*

Ziconotide (zi KOE no tide)

Medication Safety Issues
High alert medication:
The Institute for Safe Medication Practices (ISMP) includes this medication among its list of drugs which have a heightened risk of causing significant patient harm when used in error.

Brand Names: U.S. Prialt®

Generic Availability (U.S.) No

Pharmacologic Category Analgesic, Nonopioid; Calcium Channel Blocker, N-Type

Use Management of severe chronic pain in patients requiring intrathecal (I.T.) therapy and who are intolerant or refractory to other therapies

Contraindications Hypersensitivity to ziconotide or any component of the formulation; history of psychosis; I.V. administration

I.T. administration is contraindicated in patients with infection at the injection site, uncontrolled bleeding, or spinal canal obstruction that impairs CSF circulation

Warnings/Precautions [U.S Boxed Warning]: Severe psychiatric symptoms and neurological impairment have been reported; interrupt or discontinue therapy if cognitive impairment, hallucinations, mood changes, or changes in consciousness occur. May cause or worsen depression and/or risk of suicide. Cognitive impairment may appear gradually during treatment and is generally reversible after discontinuation (may take up to 2 weeks for cognitive effects to reverse). Use caution in the elderly; may experience a higher incidence of confusion. Patients should be instructed to use caution in performing tasks which require alertness (eg, operating machinery or driving). May have additive effects with opiates or other CNS-depressant medications; may potentiate opioid-induced decreased GI motility; does not interact with opioid receptors or potentiate opiate-induced respiratory depression. Will not prevent or relieve symptoms associated with opiate withdrawal and opiates should not be abruptly discontinued. Unlike opioids, ziconotide therapy can be interrupted abruptly or discontinued without evidence of withdrawal.

Meningitis may occur with use of I.T. pumps; monitor for signs and symptoms of meningitis; treatment of meningitis may require removal of system and discontinuation of intrathecal therapy. Elevated serum creatine kinase can occur, particularly during the first 2 months of therapy; consider dose reduction or discontinuing if combined with new neuromuscular symptoms (myalgias, myasthenia, muscle cramps, weakness) or reduction in physical activity. Safety and efficacy have not been established with renal or hepatic dysfunction. Should not be used in combination with intrathecal opiates.

Adverse Reactions (Reflective of adult population; not specific for elderly)

>10%:
Central nervous system: Dizziness (46%), confusion (15% to 33%), memory impairment (7% to 22%), somnolence (17%), ataxia (14%), speech disorder (14%), headache (13%), aphasia (12%), hallucination (12%; including auditory and visual)
Gastrointestinal: Nausea (40%), diarrhea (18%), vomiting (16%)
Neuromuscular & skeletal: Creatine kinase increased (40%; ≥3 times ULN: 11%), weakness (18%), gait disturbances (14%)
Ocular: Blurred vision (12%)

2% to 10%:
Cardiovascular: Hypotension, peripheral edema, postural hypotension
Central nervous system: Abnormal thinking (8%), amnesia (8%), anxiety (8%), vertigo (7%), insomnia (6%), fever (5%), paranoid reaction (3%), delirium (2%), hostility (2%), stupor (2%), agitation, attention disturbance, balance impaired, burning sensation, coordination abnormal, depression, disorientation, fatigue, fever, hypoesthesia, irritability, lethargy, mental impairment, mood disorder, nervousness, pain, sedation
Dermatologic: Pruritus (7%)
Gastrointestinal: Anorexia (6%), taste perversion (5%), abdominal pain, appetite decreased, constipation, xerostomia
Genitourinary: Urinary retention (9%), dysuria, urinary hesitance
Neuromuscular & skeletal: Dysarthria (7%), paresthesia (7%), rigors (7%), tremor (7%), muscle spasm (6%), limb pain (5%), areflexia, muscle cramp, muscle weakness, myalgia
Ocular: Nystagmus (8%), diplopia, visual disturbance
Respiratory: Sinusitis (5%)
Miscellaneous: Diaphoresis (5%)

Drug Interactions

Avoid Concomitant Use There are no known interactions where it is recommended to avoid concomitant use.

Increased Effect/Toxicity

Ziconotide may increase the levels/effects of: Alcohol (Ethyl); CNS Depressants; Methotrimeprazine; Selective Serotonin Reuptake Inhibitors

The levels/effects of Ziconotide may be increased by: Droperidol; HydrOXYzine; Methotrimeprazine

Decreased Effect There are no known significant interactions involving a decrease in effect.

Ethanol/Nutrition/Herb Interactions Ethanol: May increase CNS depression; monitor for increased effects with coadministration. Caution patients about effects.

Stability Prior to use, store vials at 2°C to 8°C (36°F to 46°F). Once diluted, may be stored at 2°C to 8°C (36°F to 46°F) for 24 hours; refrigerate during transit. Do not freeze. Protect from light.

Preservative free NS should be used when dilution is needed.

CADD-Micro® ambulatory infusion pump: Initial fill: Dilute to final concentration of 5 mcg/mL. Medtronic SynchroMed® EL or SynchroMed® II infusion system: Prior to initial fill, rinse internal pump surfaces with 2 mL ziconotide (25 mcg/mL), repeat twice. Only the 25 mcg/mL concentration (undiluted) should be used for initial pump fill. When using the Medtronic SynchroMed® EL or SynchroMed® II Infusion System, solutions expire as follows:

25 mcg/mL: Undiluted:
    Initial fill: Use within 14 days.
    Refill: Use within 84 days.
100 mcg/mL:
    Undiluted: Refill: Use within 84 days.
    Diluted: Refill: Use within 40 days.

Mechanism of Action Ziconotide selectively binds to N-type voltage-sensitive calcium channels located on the nociceptive afferent nerves of the dorsal horn in the spinal cord. This binding is thought to block N-type calcium channels, leading to a blockade of excitatory neurotransmitter release and reducing sensitivity to painful stimuli.

Pharmacodynamics/Kinetics

Distribution: I.T.: V_d: ~140 mL

Protein binding: ~50%

Metabolism: Metabolized via endopeptidases and exopeptidases present on multiple organs including kidney, liver, lung; degraded to peptide fragments and free amino acids

Half-life elimination: I.V.: 1-1.6 hours (plasma); I.T.: 2.9-6.5 hours (CSF)

Excretion: I.V.: Urine (<1%)

Dosage

Geriatric Refer to adult dosing. Use with caution.

Adult Chronic pain: I.T.: Initial dose: ≤2.4 mcg/day (0.1 mcg/hour)

Dose may be titrated by ≤2.4 mcg/day (0.1 mcg/hour) at intervals ≤2-3 times/week to a maximum dose of 19.2 mcg/day (0.8 mcg/hour) by day 21; average dose at day 21: 6.9 mcg/day (0.29 mcg/hour). A faster titration should be used only if the urgent need for analgesia outweighs the possible risk to patient safety.

Administration Not for I.V. administration. For I.T. administration only using Medtronic SynchroMed® EL, SynchroMed® II Infusion System, or CADD-Micro® ambulatory infusion pump.

Medtronic SynchroMed® EL or SynchroMed® II Infusion Systems:

Naive pump priming (first time use with ziconotide): Use 2 mL of undiluted ziconotide 25 mcg/mL solution to rinse the internal surfaces of the pump; repeat twice for a total of 3 rinses

Initial pump fill: Use only undiluted 25 mcg/mL solution and fill pump after priming. Following the initial fill only, adsorption on internal device surfaces will occur, requiring the use of the undiluted solution and refill within 14 days.

Pump refills: Contents should be emptied prior to refill. Subsequent pump refills should occur at least every 40 days if using diluted solution or at least every 84 days if using undiluted solution.

CADD-Micro® ambulatory infusion pump: Refer to manufacturers' manual for initial fill and refill instructions

Monitoring Parameters Monitor for psychiatric or neurological impairment; signs and symptoms of meningitis or other infection; serum CPK (every other week for first month then monthly); pain relief

Special Geriatric Considerations Manufacturer reports that in all trials there was a higher incidence of confusion in the elderly compared to younger adults.

Dosage Forms Excipient information presented when available (limited, particularly for generics); consult specific product labeling.
Injection, solution, as acetate [preservative free]:
Prialt®: 25 mcg/mL (20 mL); 100 mcg/mL (1 mL, 5 mL)

Selected References
Wermeling D, Drass M, Ellis D, et al, "Pharmacokinetics and Pharmacodynamics of Intrathecal Ziconotide in Chronic Pain Patients," *J Clin Pharmacol*, 2003, 43(6):624-36.

Zileuton (zye LOO ton)

Related Information
Asthma *on page 2016*
Brand Names: U.S. Zyflo CR®; Zyflo®
Generic Availability (U.S.) No
Pharmacologic Category 5-Lipoxygenase Inhibitor
Use Prophylaxis and chronic treatment of asthma
Contraindications Hypersensitivity to zileuton or any component of the formulation; active liver disease or transaminase elevations ≥3 times ULN
Warnings/Precautions Not appropriate or indicated for the reversal of bronchospasm in acute asthma attacks, including status asthmaticus; therapy may be continued during acute asthma exacerbations. Hepatic adverse effects have been reported (elevated transaminase levels); females >65 years and patients with pre-existing elevated transaminases may be at greater risk. Serum ALT should be monitored. Discontinue zileuton and follow transaminases until normal if patients develop clinical signs/symptoms of liver dysfunction or with transaminase levels >5 times ULN (use caution with history of liver disease and/or in those patients who consume substantial quantities of ethanol). Postmarketing reports of behavioral changes and sleep disorders have been noted.

Adverse Reactions (Reflective of adult population; not specific for elderly)
>10%: Central nervous system: Headache (23% to 25%)
1% to 10%:
  Cardiovascular: Chest pain
  Central nervous system: Pain (8%), dizziness, fever, insomnia, malaise, nervousness, somnolence
  Dermatologic: Pruritus, rash
  Gastrointestinal: Dyspepsia (8%), diarrhea (5%), nausea (5% to 6%), abdominal pain (5%), constipation, flatulence, vomiting
  Genitourinary: Urinary tract infection, vaginitis
  Hematologic: Leukopenia (1% to 3%)
  Hepatic: ALT increased (≥3 x ULN: 2% to 5%), hepatotoxicity
  Neuromuscular & skeletal: Myalgia (7%), weakness (4%), arthralgia, hypertonia, neck pain/rigidity
  Ocular: Conjunctivitis
  Respiratory: Upper respiratory tract infection (9%), sinusitis (7%), pharyngolaryngeal pain (5%)
  Miscellaneous: Hypersensitivity reactions, lymphadenopathy

Drug Interactions
  Metabolism/Transport Effects Substrate (minor) of CYP1A2, 2C9, 3A4; **Inhibits** CYP1A2 (moderate)
  Avoid Concomitant Use There are no known interactions where it is recommended to avoid concomitant use.
  Increased Effect/Toxicity
    Zileuton may increase the levels/effects of: Propranolol; Theophylline; Warfarin

    The levels/effects of Zileuton may be increased by: Conivaptan
  Decreased Effect
    The levels/effects of Zileuton may be decreased by: Cyproterone; Tocilizumab

Ethanol/Nutrition/Herb Interactions
  Ethanol: Avoid ethanol (may increase CNS depression; may increase risk of hepatic toxicity).
  Food: Zyflo CR®: Improved absorption when administered with food.
  Herb/Nutraceutical: St John's wort may decrease zileuton levels.

Stability Store tablets at 20°C to 25°C (68°F to 77°F). Protect from light.

Mechanism of Action Specific 5-lipoxygenase inhibitor which inhibits leukotriene formation. Leukotrienes augment neutrophil and eosinophil migration, neutrophil and monocyte aggregation, leukocyte adhesion, increased capillary permeability, and smooth muscle contraction (which contribute to inflammation, edema, mucous secretion, and bronchoconstriction in the airway of the asthmatic.)

Pharmacodynamics/Kinetics
Distribution: 1.2 L/kg
Protein binding: 93%, primarily albumin
Metabolism: Hepatic and gastrointestinal; zileuton and N-dehydroxylated metabolite can be
metabolized by CYP1A2, 2C9, and 3A4
Half-life elimination: ~3 hours
Time to peak: Immediate release: 1.7 hours
Excretion: Urine (~95% primarily as metabolites); feces (~2%)
Dosage
Geriatric & Adult Asthma: Oral:
Immediate release: 600 mg 4 times/day
Extended release: 1200 mg twice daily
Renal Impairment Adjustment not necessary in renal dysfunction or with hemodialysis.
Hepatic Impairment Contraindicated with hepatic dysfunction.
Administration
Immediate release: Administer without regard to meals.
Extended release: Do not crush, cut, or chew tablet; administer within 1 hour after morning
and evening meals.
Monitoring Parameters Hepatic transaminases (prior to initiation and during therapy),
specifically monitor serum ALT (prior to initiation, once-a-month for the first 3 months, every
2-3 months for the remainder of the first year, and periodically thereafter for patients receiving
long-term therapy)
Special Geriatric Considerations No differences in the pharmacokinetics found between
younger adults and elderly; no dosage adjustments necessary. However, monitor liver effects
closely as with any patient regardless of age.
Dosage Forms Excipient information presented when available (limited, particularly for
generics); consult specific product labeling.
Tablet, oral:
Zyflo® 600 mg [scored]
Tablet, extended release, oral:
Zyflo CR® 600 mg

◆ **Zinacef®** see Cefuroxime on page 316
◆ **Zinc 15 [OTC]** see Zinc Sulfate on page 1947
◆ **Zincate®** see Zinc Sulfate on page 1947

Zinc Sulfate (zink SUL fate)

Medication Safety Issues
Sound-alike/look-alike issues:
$ZnSO_4$ is an error-prone abbreviation (mistaken as morphine sulfate)
Brand Names: U.S. Orazinc® 110 [OTC]; Orazinc® 220 [OTC]; Zinc 15 [OTC]; Zincate®
Brand Names: Canada Anuzinc; Rivasol
Index Terms $ZnSO_4$ (error-prone abbreviation)
Generic Availability (U.S.) Yes
Pharmacologic Category Trace Element
Use Zinc supplement (oral and parenteral); may improve wound healing in those who are
deficient
Adverse Reactions (Reflective of adult population; not specific for elderly) Fre-
quency not defined.
Central nervous system: Dizziness, restlessness
Gastrointestinal: Diarrhea, gastric ulcers, nausea, vomiting
Drug Interactions
Avoid Concomitant Use There are no known interactions where it is recommended to
avoid concomitant use.
Increased Effect/Toxicity There are no known significant interactions involving an increase
in effect.
Decreased Effect
Zinc Sulfate may decrease the levels/effects of: Eltrombopag; Quinolone Antibiotics;
Tetracycline Derivatives; Trientine
The levels/effects of Zinc Sulfate may be decreased by: Trientine
Ethanol/Nutrition/Herb Interactions Food: Avoid foods high in calcium or phosphorus.
Stability Store oral liquid (injectable used orally) in refrigerator.
Pharmacodynamics/Kinetics
Absorption: Zinc and its salts are poorly absorbed from the gastrointestinal tract (20% to 30%)
Elimination: In feces with only traces appearing in urine

◄ **Dosage**
Geriatric & Adult
Recommended Daily Allowance (RDA): Oral: 15 mg elemental zinc/day
Zinc deficiency: Oral: 110-220 mg zinc sulfate (25-50 mg elemental zinc)/dose 3 times/day
Parenteral TPN: I.V.:
Acute metabolic states: 4.5-6 mg/day
Metabolically stable: 2.5-4 mg/day
Replacement for small bowel fluid loss (metabolically stable): An additional 12.2 mg zinc/L of fluid lost, or an additional 17.1 mg zinc per kg of stool or ileostomy output
Monitoring Parameters Skin integrity
Pharmacotherapy Pearls Zinc acetate can be used as an alternative to zinc sulfate in patients who cannot tolerate the gastrointestinal irritant effects of the sulfate salt
Special Geriatric Considerations May be useful to promote wound healing in patients with pressure sores.
Dosage Forms Excipient information presented when available (limited, particularly for generics); consult specific product labeling.
Capsule, oral: 220 mg [elemental zinc 50 mg]
  Orazinc® 220: 220 mg [elemental zinc 50 mg]
  Zincate®: 220 mg [elemental zinc 50 mg]
Injection, solution [preservative free]: Elemental zinc 1 mg/mL (10 mL)
Injection, solution [concentrate, preservative free]: Elemental zinc 5 mg/mL (5 mL)
Tablet, oral: 220 mg [elemental zinc 50 mg]
  Orazinc® 110: 110 mg [elemental zinc 25 mg]
  Zinc 15: 66 mg [elemental zinc 15 mg]

Ziprasidone (zi PRAS i done)

Related Information
  Antipsychotic Agents *on page 1997*
  Atypical Antipsychotics *on page 1999*
Medication Safety Issues
  Sound-alike/look-alike issues:
  Ziprasidone may be confused with TraZODone
Brand Names: U.S. Geodon®
Brand Names: Canada Zeldox®
Index Terms Zeldox; Ziprasidone Hydrochloride; Ziprasidone Mesylate
Generic Availability (U.S.) No
Pharmacologic Category Antipsychotic Agent, Atypical
Use Treatment of schizophrenia; treatment of acute manic or mixed episodes associated with bipolar disorder with or without psychosis; maintenance treatment of bipolar disorder as an adjunct to lithium or valproate; acute agitation in patients with schizophrenia
Unlabeled/Investigational Use Tourette's syndrome; psychosis/agitation related to Alzheimer's dementia
Contraindications Hypersensitivity to ziprasidone or any component of the formulation; history of (or current) prolonged QT; congenital long QT syndrome; recent myocardial infarction; uncompensated heart failure; concurrent use of other QT$_c$-prolonging agents including arsenic trioxide, chlorpromazine, class Ia antiarrhythmics (eg, disopyramide, quinidine, procainamide), class III antiarrhythmics (eg, amiodarone, dofetilide, ibutilide, sotalol), dolasetron, droperidol, gatifloxacin, levomethadyl, mefloquine, mesoridazine, moxifloxacin, pentamidine, pimozide, probucol, tacrolimus, and thioridazine
Warnings/Precautions [U.S. Boxed Warning]: Elderly patients with dementia-related behavioral disorders treated with antipsychotics are at an increased risk of death compared to placebo. Most deaths appeared to be either cardiovascular (eg, heart failure, sudden death) or infectious (eg, pneumonia) in nature. Ziprasidone is not approved for the treatment of dementia-related psychosis.

May result in QT$_c$ prolongation (dose related), which has been associated with the development of malignant ventricular arrhythmias (torsade de pointes) and sudden death. Note contraindications related to this effect. Observed prolongation was greater than with other atypical antipsychotic agents (risperidone, olanzapine, quetiapine), but less than with thioridazine. Correct electrolyte disturbances, especially hypokalemia or hypomagnesemia, prior to use and throughout therapy. Use caution in patients with bradycardia. Discontinue in patients found to have persistent QT$_c$ intervals >500 msec. Patients with symptoms of dizziness, palpitations, or syncope should receive further cardiac evaluation. May cause orthostatic hypotension. Use is contraindicated in patients with recent acute myocardial infarction (MI), QT prolongation, or uncompensated heart failure. Avoid use in patients with a history of cardiac arrhythmias; use with caution in patients with history of MI or unstable heart disease.

Leukopenia, neutropenia, and agranulocytosis (sometimes fatal) have been reported in clinical trials and postmarketing reports with antipsychotic use; presence of risk factors (eg, pre-existing low WBC or history of drug-induced leuko-/neutropenia) should prompt periodic blood count assessment. Discontinue therapy at first signs of blood dyscrasias or if absolute neutrophil count <1000/mm³.

May cause extrapyramidal symptoms (EPS). Risk of dystonia (and probably other EPS) may be greater with increased doses, use of conventional antipsychotics, males, and younger patients. Impaired core body temperature regulation may occur; caution with strenuous exercise, heat exposure, dehydration, and concomitant medication possessing anticholinergic effects; not reported in premarketing trials of ziprasidone. Antipsychotic use may also be associated with neuroleptic malignant syndrome (NMS). Use with caution in patients at risk of seizures.

Atypical antipsychotics have been associated with development of hyperglycemia. There is limited documentation with ziprasidone and specific risk associated with this agent is not known. Use caution in patients with diabetes or other disorders of glucose regulation; monitor for worsening of glucose control. May increase prolactin levels; clinical significance of hyperprolactinemia in patients with breast cancer or other prolactin-dependent tumors is unknown.

Cognitive and/or motor impairment (sedation) is common with ziprasidone. Use with caution in disorders where CNS depression is a feature. Use with caution in Parkinson's disease. Antipsychotic use has been associated with esophageal dysmotility and aspiration; use with caution in patients at risk of pneumonia (ie, Alzheimer's disease). Use caution in hepatic impairment. Ziprasidone has been associated with a fairly high incidence of rash (5%). Significant weight gain has been observed with antipsychotic therapy; incidence varies with product. Monitor waist circumference and BMI. Rare cases of priapism have been reported. Use the intramuscular formulation with caution in patients with renal impairment; formulation contains cyclodextrin, an excipient which may accumulate in renal insufficiency.

The possibility of a suicide attempt is inherent in psychotic illness or bipolar disorder; use caution in high-risk patients during initiation of therapy. Prescriptions should be written for the smallest quantity consistent with good patient care.

Adverse Reactions (Reflective of adult population; not specific for elderly) Note: Although minor QT_c prolongation (mean: 10 msec at 160 mg/day) may occur more frequently (incidence not specified), clinically-relevant prolongation (>500 msec) was rare (0.06%) and less than placebo (0.23%).

>10%:
  Central nervous system: Extrapyramidal symptoms (2% to 31%), somnolence (8% to 31%), headache (3% to 18%), dizziness (3% to 16%)
  Gastrointestinal: Nausea (4% to 12%)
1% to 10%:
  Cardiovascular: Postural hypotension (5%), chest pain (3%), hypertension (2% to 3%), tachycardia (2%), bradycardia (≤2%), facial edema (1%), vasodilation (≤1%), orthostatic hypotension
  Central nervous system: Akathisia (2% to 10%), anxiety (2% to 5%), insomnia (3%), agitation (2%), speech disorder (2%), personality disorder (2%), akinesia (≥1%), amnesia (≥1%), ataxia (≥1%), confusion (≥1%), coordination abnormal (≥1%), delirium (≥1%), dystonia (≥1%), hostility (≥1%), oculogyric crisis (≥1%), vertigo (≥1%), chills (1%), fever (1%), hypothermia (1%), psychosis (1%)
  Dermatologic: Rash (4% to 5%), fungal dermatitis (2%)
  Endocrine & metabolic: Dysmenorrhea (2%)
  Gastrointestinal: Weight gain (6% to 10%), constipation (2% to 9%), dyspepsia (1% to 8%), diarrhea (3% to 5%), vomiting (3% to 5%), xerostomia (1% to 5%), salivation increased (4%), tongue edema (≤3%), anorexia (2%), abdominal pain (≤2%), dysphagia (≤2%), rectal hemorrhage (≤2%), buccoglossal syndrome (≥1%)
  Genitourinary: Priapism (1%)
  Local: Injection site pain (7% to 9%)
  Neuromuscular & skeletal: Weakness (2% to 6%), hypoesthesia (2%), myalgia (2%), paresthesia (2%), abnormal gait (≥1%), choreoathetosis (≥1%), dysarthria (≥1%), dyskinesia (≥1%), hyper-/hypokinesia (≥1%), hypotonia (≥1%), neuropathy (≥1%), tremor (≥1%), twitching (≥1%), back pain (1%), cogwheel rigidity (1%), hypertonia (1%)
  Ocular: Vision abnormal (3% to 6%), diplopia (≥1%)

◀

Respiratory: Infection (8%), rhinitis (1% to 4%), cough (3%), pharyngitis (3%), dyspnea (2%)

Miscellaneous: Diaphoresis (2%), furunculosis (2%), withdrawal syndrome (≥1%), flank pain (1%), flu-like syndrome (1%), photosensitivity reaction (1%),

Drug Interactions

Metabolism/Transport Effects Substrate (minor) of CYP1A2, 3A4; **Inhibits** CYP2D6 (weak), 3A4 (weak)

Avoid Concomitant Use

Avoid concomitant use of Ziprasidone with any of the following: Artemether; Dronedarone; Lumefantrine; Metoclopramide; Nilotinib; Pimozide; QTc-Prolonging Agents; QUEtiapine; QuiNINE; Tetrabenazine; Thioridazine; Toremifene; Vandetanib; Vemurafenib

Increased Effect/Toxicity

Ziprasidone may increase the levels/effects of: Alcohol (Ethyl); CNS Depressants; Dronedarone; Methylphenidate; Pimozide; QTc-Prolonging Agents; QuiNINE; Selective Serotonin Reuptake Inhibitors; Tetrabenazine; Thioridazine; Toremifene; Vandetanib; Vemurafenib

The levels/effects of Ziprasidone may be increased by: Acetylcholinesterase Inhibitors (Central); Alfuzosin; Antifungal Agents (Azole Derivatives, Systemic); Artemether; Chloroquine; Ciprofloxacin; Ciprofloxacin (Systemic); Conivaptan; Gadobutrol; HydrOXYzine; Lithium formulations; Lumefantrine; Methylphenidate; Metoclopramide; Nilotinib; QTc-Prolonging Agents; QUEtiapine; QuiNINE; Tetrabenazine

Decreased Effect

Ziprasidone may decrease the levels/effects of: Amphetamines; Anti-Parkinson's Agents (Dopamine Agonist); Quinagolide

The levels/effects of Ziprasidone may be decreased by: CarBAMazepine; Cyproterone; Lithium formulations; Tocilizumab

Ethanol/Nutrition/Herb Interactions

Ethanol: May increase CNS depression; monitor for increased effects with coadministration. Caution patients about effects.

Food: Administration with food increases serum levels twofold. Grapefruit juice may increase serum concentration of ziprasidone.

Herb/Nutraceutical: St John's wort may decrease serum levels of ziprasidone, due to a potential effect on CYP3A4. This has not been specifically studied. Avoid kava kava, chamomile (may increase CNS depression).

Stability

Capsule: Store at 25°C (77°F); excursion permitted to 15°C to 30°C (59°F to 86°F).

Vials for injection: Store at 25°C (77°F); excursion permitted to 15°C to 30°C (59°F to 86°F). Protect from light. Each vial should be reconstituted with 1.2 mL SWFI. Shake vigorously; will form a pale, pink solution containing 20 mg/mL ziprasidone. Following reconstitution, injection may be stored at room temperature up to 24 hours or under refrigeration for up to 7 days. Protect from light.

Mechanism of Action

Ziprasidone is a benzylisothiazolylpiperazine antipsychotic. The exact mechanism of action is unknown. However, *in vitro* radioligand studies show that ziprasidone has high affinity for D_2, D_3, 5-HT_{2A}, 5-HT_{1A}, 5-HT_{2C}, 5-HT_{1D}, and alpha$_1$-adrenergic; moderate affinity for histamine H_1 receptors; and no appreciable affinity for alpha$_2$-adrenergic receptors, beta-adrenergic, 5-HT_3, 5-HT_4, cholinergic, mu, sigma, or benzodiazepine receptors. Ziprasidone functions as an antagonist at the D_2, 5-HT_{2A}, and 5-HT_{1D} receptors and as an agonist at the 5-HT_{1A} receptor. Ziprasidone moderately inhibits the reuptake of serotonin and norepinephrine.

Pharmacodynamics/Kinetics

Absorption: Well absorbed

Distribution: V_d: 1.5 L/kg

Protein binding: >99%, primarily to albumin and alpha$_1$-acid glycoprotein

Metabolism: Extensively hepatic, primarily via aldehyde oxidase; less than 1/3 of total metabolism via CYP3A4 and CYP1A2 (minor)

Bioavailability: Oral (with food): 60% (up to twofold increase with food); I.M.: 100%

Half-life elimination: 2-7 hours

Time to peak: Oral: 6-8 hours; I.M.: ≤60 minutes

Excretion: Feces (~66%; <4% of total dose as unchanged drug); urine (~20%; <1% of total dose as unchanged drug)

Dosage

Geriatric No dosage adjustment is recommended; consider initiating at a low end of the dosage range, with slower titration.

Adult

Bipolar mania (acute): Oral: Initial: 40 mg twice daily

Adjustment: May increase to 60 mg or 80 mg twice daily on second day of treatment; average dose 40-80 mg twice daily.

Bipolar disorder (maintenance; as adjunct to lithium or valproate): Oral: Continue ziprasidone dose at which the patient was initially stabilized; usual dosage range: 40-80 mg twice daily

Schizophrenia: Oral: Initial: 20 mg twice daily

Adjustment: Increases (if indicated) should be made no more frequently than every 2 days; ordinarily patients should be observed for improvement over several weeks before adjusting the dose.

Maintenance: Range: 20-100 mg twice daily; however, dosages >80 mg twice daily are generally not recommended.

Acute agitation (schizophrenia): I.M.: 10 mg every 2 hours **or** 20 mg every 4 hours (maximum: 40 mg/day). Oral therapy should replace I.M. administration as soon as possible.

Renal Impairment

Oral: No dosage adjustment is recommended

I.M.: Cyclodextrin, an excipient in the I.M. formulation, is cleared by renal filtration; use with caution.

Ziprasidone is not removed by hemodialysis.

Hepatic Impairment No adjustment necessary.

Administration

Oral: Administer with food.

Injection: For I.M. administration only.

Monitoring Parameters Blood pressure, heart rate; temperature; serum potassium and magnesium; fasting lipid profile and fasting blood glucose/Hgb A_{1c} (prior to treatment, at 3 months, then annually); BMI; waist circumference; mental status, abnormal involuntary movement scale (AIMS), extrapyramidal symptoms. Weight should be assessed prior to treatment, at 4 weeks, 8 weeks, 12 weeks, and then at quarterly intervals. Consider titrating to a different antipsychotic agent for a weight gain ≥5% of the initial weight. The value of routine ECG screening or monitoring has not been established.

Test Interactions Increased cholesterol, triglycerides, eosinophils

Pharmacotherapy Pearls Blocks a number of CNS receptors, including dopamine, serotonin, alpha$_1$ adrenergic, and histamine receptors. Also inhibits reuptake of serotonin and epinephrine. Results in improvement in positive and negative symptoms of schizophrenia. The increased potential to prolong QT_c, as compared to other available antipsychotic agents, should be considered in the evaluation of available alternatives.

Special Geriatric Considerations Extrapyramidal syndrome symptoms occur less with this agent than phenothiazine and butyrophenone classes of antipsychotics.

Many elderly patients receive antipsychotic medications for inappropriate nonpsychotic behavior. Before initiating antipsychotic medication, the clinician should investigate any possible reversible cause; any stress or stress from any disease can cause acute "confusion" or worsening of baseline nonpsychotic behavior. Most commonly, acute changes in behavior are due to increases in drug dose or addition of a new drug to regimen, fluid electrolyte loss, infection, and changes in environment. Any changes in disease status and any organ system can result in behavior changes.

In the treatment of agitated, demented, elderly patients, authors of meta-analysis of controlled trials of the response to the traditional antipsychotics (phenothiazines, butyrophenones) in controlling agitation have concluded that the use of neuroleptics results in a response rate of 18%. Clearly, neuroleptic therapy for behavior control should be limited with frequent attempts to withdraw the agent given for behavior control. In light of significant risks and adverse effects in elderly population compared with limited data demonstrating efficacy in the treatment of dementia related psychosis, aggression, and agitation, an extensive risk:benefit analysis should be performed prior to use.

Since diabetes is prevalent in elderly, monitor closely when using this agent in this population.

Dosage Forms Excipient information presented when available (limited, particularly for generics); consult specific product labeling.

Capsule, oral, as hydrochloride:

Geodon®: 20 mg, 40 mg, 60 mg, 80 mg

Injection, powder for reconstitution, as mesylate [strength expressed as base]:

Geodon®: 20 mg [contains cyclodextrin]

Selected References

American Diabetes Association; American Psychiatric Association; American Association of Clinical Endocrinologists; North American Association for the Study of Obesity, "Consensus Development Conference on Antipsychotic Drugs and Obesity and Diabetes," *Diabetes Care*, 2004, 27(2):596-601.

Rabins PV, Blacker D, Rovner BW, et al, "Practice Guidelines for the Treatment of Patients With Alzheimer's Disease and Other Dementias," *Am J Psychiatry*, 2007, 164(12 Suppl):5-56. Available at http://www.psych.org/psych_pract/treatg/pg/prac_guide.cfm.

Schneider LS, Tariot PN, Dagerman KS, et al, "Effectiveness of Atypical Antipsychotic Drugs in Patients With Alzheimer's Disease," *N Engl J Med*, 2006, 355(15):1525-38.

- **Ziprasidone Hydrochloride** *see* Ziprasidone *on page 1948*
- **Ziprasidone Mesylate** *see* Ziprasidone *on page 1948*
- **Zipsor™** *see* Diclofenac (Systemic) *on page 496*
- **Zirgan®** *see* Ganciclovir (Ophthalmic) *on page 811*
- **Zithromax®** *see* Azithromycin (Systemic) *on page 175*
- **Zithromax TRI-PAK™** *see* Azithromycin (Systemic) *on page 175*
- **Zithromax® TRI-PAK™** *see* Azithromycin (Systemic) *on page 175*
- **Zithromax Z-PAK®** *see* Azithromycin (Systemic) *on page 175*
- **Zithromax® Z-PAK®** *see* Azithromycin (Systemic) *on page 175*
- **Zmax®** *see* Azithromycin (Systemic) *on page 175*
- **ZnSO₄ (error-prone abbreviation)** *see* Zinc Sulfate *on page 1947*
- **Zocor®** *see* Simvastatin *on page 1681*
- **Zofran®** *see* Ondansetron *on page 1347*
- **Zofran® ODT** *see* Ondansetron *on page 1347*
- **Zol 446** *see* Zoledronic Acid *on page 1952*
- **Zoladex®** *see* Goserelin *on page 840*
- **Zoledronate** *see* Zoledronic Acid *on page 1952*

Zoledronic Acid (zoe le DRON ik AS id)

Related Information
Osteoporosis Management *on page 2027*
Medication Safety Issues
Sound-alike/look-alike issues:
Zometa® may be confused with Zofran®, Zoladex®
Other safety concerns:
Duplicate therapy issues: Reclast® and Aclasta® contain zoledronic acid, which is the same ingredient contained in Zometa®; patients receiving Zometa® should not be treated with Reclast® or Aclasta®
Brand Names: U.S. Reclast®; Zometa®
Brand Names: Canada Aclasta®; Zometa®
Index Terms CGP-42446; Zol 446; Zoledronate
Generic Availability (U.S.) No
Pharmacologic Category Antidote; Bisphosphonate Derivative
Use
Oncology-related uses: Treatment of hypercalcemia of malignancy (albumin-corrected serum calcium >12 mg/dL); treatment of multiple myeloma; treatment of bone metastases of solid tumors
Nononcology uses: Treatment of Paget's disease of bone; treatment of osteoporosis in postmenopausal women (to reduce the incidence of fractures or to reduce the incidence of new clinical fractures in patients with low-trauma hip fracture); prevention of osteoporosis in postmenopausal women, treatment of osteoporosis in men (to increase bone mass); treatment and prevention of glucocorticoid-induced osteoporosis (in patients initiating or continuing prednisone ≥7.5 mg/day [or equivalent] and expected to remain on glucocorticoids for at least 12 months)
Unlabeled/Investigational Use Prevention of bone loss associated with aromatase inhibitor therapy in postmenopausal women with breast cancer; prevention of bone loss associated with androgen deprivation therapy in prostate cancer
Medication Guide Available Yes
Contraindications Hypersensitivity to zoledronic acid or any component of the formulation; hypocalcemia (Reclast®)

Canadian labeling: Hypersensitivity to other bisphosphonates. Aclasta® is also contraindicated with uncorrected hypocalcemia at the time of infusion.
Warnings/Precautions Osteonecrosis of the jaw (ONJ) has been reported in patients receiving bisphosphonates. Risk factors include invasive dental procedures (eg, tooth extraction, dental implants, boney surgery); a diagnosis of cancer, with concomitant chemotherapy, radiotherapy, or corticosteroids; poor oral hygiene, ill-fitting dentures; and comorbid disorders (anemia, coagulopathy, infection, pre-existing dental disease). Most reported cases occurred after I.V. bisphosphonate therapy; however, cases have been reported following oral therapy. A dental exam and preventative dentistry should be performed prior to placing patients with risk factors on chronic bisphosphonate therapy. The manufacturer's labeling states that there are no data to suggest whether discontinuing bisphosphonates in patients requiring invasive dental procedures reduces the risk of ONJ. However, other experts suggest that there is no evidence that discontinuing therapy reduces the risk of developing ONJ

(Assael, 2009). The benefit/risk must be assessed by the treating physician and/or dentist/ surgeon prior to any invasive dental procedure. Patients developing ONJ while on bisphosph- onates should receive care by an oral surgeon.

Atypical, low energy, or low trauma femur fractures have been reported in patients receiving bisphosphonates for treatment/prevention of osteoporosis. The fractures include subtrochan- teric femur (bone just below the hip joint) and diaphyseal femur (long segment of the thigh bone). Some patients experience prodromal pain weeks or months before the fracture occurs. It is unclear if bisphosphonate therapy is the cause for these fractures; atypical femur fractures have also been reported in patients not taking bisphosphonates, and in patients receiving glucocorticoids. Patients receiving long-term (>3-5 years) bisphosphonate therapy may be at an increased risk. Patients presenting with thigh or groin pain with a history of receiving bisphosphonates should be evaluated for femur fracture. Consider interrupting bisphospho- nate therapy in patients who develop a femoral shaft fracture; assess for fracture in the contralateral limb.

Infrequently, severe (and occasionally debilitating) musculoskeletal (bone, joint, and/or muscle) pain have been reported during bisphosphonate treatment. The onset of pain ranged from a single day to several months. Consider discontinuing therapy in patients who experience severe symptoms; symptoms usually resolve upon discontinuation. Some patients experienced recurrence when rechallenged with same drug or another bisphosphonate; avoid use in patients with a history of these symptoms in association with bisphosphonate therapy.

May cause a significant risk of hypocalcemia in patients with Paget's disease, in whom the pretreatment rate of bone turnover may be greatly elevated. Hypocalcemia must be corrected before initiation of therapy in patients with Paget's disease and osteoporosis. Ensure adequate calcium and vitamin D intake during therapy. Use caution in patients with dis- turbances of calcium and mineral metabolism (eg, hypoparathyroidism, thyroid/parathyroid, surgery, malabsorption syndromes, excision of small intestine).

Reclast®: Use is not recommended in patients with Cl_{cr} <35 mL/minute. Re-evaluate the need for continued therapy for the treatment of osteoporosis periodically; the optimal duration of treatment has not yet been determined.

Zometa®: Use caution in mild-to-moderate renal dysfunction; dosage adjustment required. In cancer patients, renal toxicity has been reported with doses >4 mg or infusions administered over 15 minutes. Risk factors for renal deterioration include pre-existing renal insufficiency and repeated doses of zoledronic acid and other bisphosphonates. Dehydration and the use of other nephrotoxic drugs which may contribute to renal deterioration should be identified and managed. Use is not recommended in patients with severe renal impairment (serum creatinine >3 mg/dL or Cl_{cr} <30 mL/minute) and bone metastases (limited data); use in patients with hypercalcemia of malignancy and severe renal impairment (serum creatinine >4.5 mg/dL for hypercalcemia of malignancy) should only be done if the benefits outweigh the risks. Renal function should be assessed prior to treatment; if decreased after treatment, additional treatments should be withheld until renal function returns to within 10% of baseline. Diuretics should not be used before correcting hypovolemia. Renal deterioration, resulting in renal failure and dialysis has occurred in patients treated with zoledronic acid after single and multiple infusions at recommended doses of 4 mg over 15 minutes.

Aclasta® [CAN; not available in U.S.]: Use is not recommended in patients with Cl_{cr} <30 mL/ minute.

According to the American Society of Clinical Oncology (ASCO) guidelines for bisphospho- nates in multiple myeloma, treatment with zoledronic acid is not recommended for asympto- matic (smoldering) or indolent myeloma or with solitary plasmacytoma (Kyle, 2007). The National Comprehensive Cancer Network® (NCCN) multiple myeloma guidelines (v.1.2011) also do not recommend the use of bisphosphonates in stage 1 or smoldering disease, unless part of a clinical trial.

Adequate hydration is required during treatment (urine output ~2 L/day); avoid overhydration, especially in patients with heart failure. Pre-existing renal compromise, severe dehydration, and concurrent use with diuretics or other nephrotoxic drugs may increase the risk for renal impairment. Single and multiple infusions in patients with both normal and impaired renal function have been associated with renal deterioration, resulting in renal failure and dialysis (rare). Use caution in patients with aspirin-sensitive asthma (may cause bronchoconstriction) and the elderly. Rare cases of urticaria and angioedema and very rare cases of anaphylactic reactions/shock have been reported. Do not administer Zometa® and Reclast® to the same patient for different indications.

◄ **Adverse Reactions (Reflective of adult population; not specific for elderly)** Note: An acute reaction (eg, arthralgia, fever, flu-like symptoms, myalgia) may occur within the first 3 days following infusion in up to 44% of patients; usually resolves within 3-4 days of onset, although may take up to 14 days to resolve. The incidence may be decreased with acetaminophen (prior to infusion and for 72 hours postinfusion).

Zometa®:
>10%:
Cardiovascular: Leg edema (5% to 21%), hypotension (11%)
Central nervous system: Fatigue (39%), fever (32% to 44%), headache (5% to 19%), dizziness (18%), insomnia (15% to 16%), anxiety (11% to 14%), depression (14%), agitation (13%), confusion (7% to 13%), hypoesthesia (12%)
Dermatologic: Alopecia (12%), dermatitis (11%)
Endocrine & metabolic: Dehydration (5% to 14%), hypophosphatemia (13%), hypokalemia (12%), hypomagnesemia (11%)
Gastrointestinal: Nausea (29% to 46%), vomiting (14% to 32%), constipation (27% to 31%), diarrhea (17% to 24%), anorexia (9% to 22%), abdominal pain (14% to 16%), weight loss (16%), appetite decreased (13%)
Genitourinary: Urinary tract infection (12% to 14%)
Hematologic: Anemia (22% to 33%), neutropenia (12%)
Neuromuscular & skeletal: Bone pain (55%), weakness (5% to 24%), myalgia (23%), arthralgia (5% to 21%), back pain (15%), paresthesia (15%), limb pain (14%), skeletal pain (12%), rigors (11%)
Renal: Renal deterioration (8% to 17%; up to 40% in patients with abnormal baseline creatinine)
Respiratory: Dyspnea (22% to 27%), cough (12% to 22%)
Miscellaneous: Cancer progression (16% to 20%), moniliasis (12%)
1% to 10%:
Cardiovascular: Chest pain (5% to 10%)
Central nervous system: Somnolence (5% to 10%)
Endocrine & metabolic: Hypocalcemia (5% to 10%; grades 3/4: ≤1%), hypermagnesemia (grade 3: 2%)
Gastrointestinal: Dysphagia (5% to 10%), dyspepsia (10%), mucositis (5% to 10%), stomatitis (8%), sore throat (8%)
Hematologic: Granulocytopenia (5% to 10%), pancytopenia (5% to 10%), thrombocytopenia (5% to 10%)
Renal: Serum creatinine increased (grades 3/4: ≤2%)
Respiratory: Upper respiratory tract infection (10%)
Miscellaneous: Infection (nonspecific; 5% to 10%)

Reclast®:
>10%:
Cardiovascular: Hypertension (5% to 13%)
Central nervous system: Pain (2% to 24%), fever (9% to 22%), headache (4% to 20%), chills (2% to 18%), fatigue (2% to 18%)
Endocrine & metabolic: Hypocalcemia (≤3%; Paget's disease 21%)
Gastrointestinal: Nausea (5% to 18%)
Neuromuscular & skeletal: Arthralgia (9% to 27%), myalgia (5% to 23%), back pain (4% to 18%), limb pain (3% to 16%), musculoskeletal pain (≤12%)
Miscellaneous: Acute phase reaction (4% to 25%), flu-like syndrome (1% to 11%)
1% to 10%:
Cardiovascular: Chest pain (1% to 8%), peripheral edema (3% to 6%), atrial fibrillation (1% to 3%), palpitation (≤3%)
Central nervous system: Dizziness (2% to 9%), malaise (1% to 7%), hypoesthesia (≤6%), lethargy (3% to 5%), vertigo (1% to 4%), hyperthermia (≤2%)
Dermatologic: Rash (2% to 3%), hyperhidrosis (≤3%)
Gastrointestinal: Abdominal pain (1% to 9%), diarrhea (5% to 8%), vomiting (2% to 8%), constipation (6% to 7%), dyspepsia (2% to 7%), abdominal discomfort/distension (1% to 2%), anorexia (1% to 2%)
Neuromuscular & skeletal: Bone pain (3% to 9%), arthritis (2% to 9%), rigors (8%), shoulder pain (≤7%), neck pain (1% to 7%), weakness (2% to 6%), muscle spasm (2% to 6%), stiffness (1% to 5%), jaw pain (2% to 4%), joint swelling (≤3%), paresthesia (2%)
Ocular: Eye pain (≤2%)
Renal: Serum creatinine increased (2%)
Respiratory: Dyspnea (5% to 7%)
Miscellaneous: C-reactive protein increased (≤5%)

Drug Interactions

Avoid Concomitant Use There are no known interactions where it is recommended to avoid concomitant use.

Increased Effect/Toxicity

Zoledronic Acid may increase the levels/effects of: Deferasirox; Phosphate Supplements

The levels/effects of Zoledronic Acid may be increased by: Aminoglycosides; Nonsteroidal Anti-Inflammatory Agents; Thalidomide

Decreased Effect

The levels/effects of Zoledronic Acid may be decreased by: Proton Pump Inhibitors

Stability

Aclasta® [CAN]: Store at room temperature of 15°C to 30°C (59°F to 86°F).

Reclast®: Store at room temperature of 25°C (77°F); excursions permitted to 15°C to 30°C (59°F to 86°F). After opening, stable for 24 hours at 2°C to 8°C (36°F to 46°F).

Zometa®: Store vials at 25°C (77°F); excursions permitted to 15°C to 30°C (59°F to 86°F). Dilute solution for injection in 100 mL NS or D_5W prior to administration. Solutions for infusion which are not used immediately after preparation should be refrigerated at 2°C to 8°C (36°F to 46°F). Infusion of solution must be completed within 24 hours of preparation.

Mechanism of Action A bisphosphonate which inhibits bone resorption via actions on osteoclasts or on osteoclast precursors; inhibits osteoclastic activity and skeletal calcium release induced by tumors. Decreases serum calcium and phosphorus, and increases their elimination. In osteoporosis, zoledronic acid inhibits osteoclast-mediated resorption, therefore reducing bone turnover.

Pharmacodynamics/Kinetics

Distribution: Binds to bone

Protein binding: 28% to 53%

Half-life elimination: Triphasic; Terminal: 146 hours

Excretion: Urine (39% ± 16% as unchanged drug) within 24 hours; feces (<3%)

Dosage

Geriatric Refer to adult dosing. **Note:** Acetaminophen administration after infusion may reduce symptoms of acute-phase reactions. Patients treated for multiple myeloma, osteoporosis, and Paget's disease should receive a daily calcium supplement with vitamin D.

Adult Note: Acetaminophen administration after the infusion may reduce symptoms of acute-phase reactions. Patients treated for multiple myeloma, osteoporosis, and Paget's disease should receive a daily calcium supplement and multivitamin containing vitamin D (if dietary intake is inadequate).

Hypercalcemia of malignancy (albumin-corrected serum calcium ≥12 mg/dL) (Zometa®): I.V.: 4 mg (maximum) given as a single dose. Wait at least 7 days before considering retreatment. Dosage adjustment may be needed in patients with decreased renal function following treatment.

Multiple myeloma or metastatic bone lesions from solid tumors (Zometa®): I.V.: 4 mg every 3-4 weeks

Osteoporosis, glucocorticoid-induced, treatment and prevention (Reclast®, Aclasta® [CAN]): 5 mg infused over at least 15 minutes once a year

Osteoporosis, prevention (Reclast®): 5 mg infused over at least 15 minutes every 2 years

Osteoporosis, treatment (Reclast®, Aclasta® [CAN]): 5 mg infused over at least 15 minutes once a year

Paget's disease: I.V.: 5 mg infused over at least 15 minutes. **Note:** Data concerning retreatment is not available; retreatment may be considered for relapse (increase in alkaline phosphatase) if appropriate, for inadequate response, or in patients who are symptomatic.

Prevention of aromatase inhibitor-induced bone loss in breast cancer (unlabeled use): 4 mg every 6 months (Brufsky, 2007)

Prevention of androgen deprivation-induced bone loss in nonmetastatic prostate cancer (unlabeled use): 4 mg every 3 months for 1 year (Smith, 2003) or 4 mg every 12 months (Michaelson, 2007)

Renal Impairment

Reclast®:

Cl_{cr} ≥35 mL/minute: No adjustment required.

Cl_{cr} <35 mL/minute: Use is contraindicated.

Zometa®: Multiple myeloma and bone metastases (at treatment initiation):

Cl_{cr} >60 mL/minute: 4 mg

Cl_{cr} 50-60 mL/minute: 3.5 mg

Cl_{cr} 40-49 mL/minute: 3.3 mg

Cl_{cr} 30-39 mL/minute: 3 mg

Cl_{cr} <30 mL/minute: Use is not recommended.

◄ Zometa®: Hypercalcemia of malignancy (at treatment initiation):
Mild-to-moderate impairment: No adjustment necessary.
Severe impairment (serum creatinine >4.5 mg/dL): Evaluate risk versus benefit.
Aclasta® [CAN]:
Cl_{cr} ≥30 mL/minute: No adjustment required.
Cl_{cr} <30 mL/minute: Use is not recommended.

Renal toxicity (during treatment):
Hypercalcemia of malignancy: Evidence of renal deterioration: Evaluate risk versus benefit.
Multiple myeloma and bone metastases: Evidence of renal deterioration: Withhold dose until renal function returns to within 10% of baseline: renal deterioration defined as follows:
Normal baseline creatinine: Increase of 0.5 mg/dL
Abnormal baseline creatinine: Increase of 1 mg/dL
Reinitiate dose at the same dose administered prior to treatment interruption.
Multiple myeloma: Albuminuria >500 mg/24 hours (unexplained): Withhold dose until return to baseline, then re-evaluate every 3-4 weeks; consider reinitiating with a longer infusion time of at least 30 minutes (Kyle, 2007).

Hepatic Impairment Specific guidelines are not available.

Administration Infuse over at least 15 minutes. Flush I.V. line with 10 mL NS flush following infusion. Infuse in a line separate from other medications. Patients should be appropriately hydrated prior to treatment.
Reclast®, Zometa®: If refrigerated, allow to reach room temperature prior to administration. Acetaminophen after administration may reduce the incidence of acute reaction (eg, arthralgia, fever, flu-like symptoms, myalgia).

Monitoring Parameters Prior to initiation of therapy, dental exam and preventative dentistry for patients at risk for osteonecrosis, including all cancer patients
Aclasta® [CAN], Reclast®: Serum creatinine prior to each dose, especially in patients with risk factors, calculate creatinine clearance before each treatment (consider interim monitoring in patients at risk for acute renal failure), evaluate fluid status and adequately hydrate patients prior to and following administration.
Osteoporosis: Bone mineral density as measured by central dual-energy x-ray absorptiometry (DXA) of the hip or spine (prior to initiation of therapy and at least every 2 years; after 6-12 months of combined glucocorticoid and zoledronic acid treatment); annual measurements of height and weight, assessment of chronic back pain; serum calcium and 25(OH)D; phosphorus and magnesium; may consider monitoring biochemical markers of bone turnover
Paget's disease: Alkaline phosphatase; pain; serum calcium and 25(OH)D; phosphorus and magnesium
Zometa®: Serum creatinine prior to each dose; serum electrolytes, phosphate, magnesium, and hemoglobin/hematocrit should be evaluated regularly. Monitor serum calcium to assess response and avoid overtreatment. In patients with multiple myeloma, monitor urine every 3-6 months for albuminuria.

Test Interactions Bisphosphonates may interfere with diagnostic imaging agents such as technetium-99m-diphosphonate in bone scans.

Pharmacotherapy Pearls Oncology Comment:
Metastatic breast cancer: The American Society of Clinical Oncology (ASCO) guidelines on the role of bone-modifying agents (BMAs) in the prevention and treatment of skeletal-related events for metastatic breast cancer patients were updated (Van Poznak, 2011). The guidelines recommend initiating a BMA (denosumab, pamidronate, zoledronic acid) in patients with a diagnosis of metastatic breast cancer to the bone. There is currently no literature indicating the superiority of one particular BMA over another. The optimal duration has yet to be defined; however, the guidelines recommend continuing therapy until substantial decline in patient's performance status. In patients with normal creatinine clearance (>60 mL/minute), no dosage/interval/infusion rate changes for pamidronate or zoledronic acid are necessary. For patients with Cl_{cr} <30 mL/minute, pamidronate and zoledronic acid are not recommended. While no renal dose adjustments are recommended for denosumab, close monitoring is advised for risk of hypocalcemia in patients with Cl_{cr} <30 mL/minute or on dialysis. The ASCO guidelines are in alignment with package insert guidelines for dosing, renal dose adjustments, infusion times, prevention and management of osteonecrosis of the jaw, and monitoring of laboratory parameter recommendations. BMAs are not the first-line therapy for pain. BMAs are to be used as adjunctive therapy for cancer-related bone pain associated with bone metastasis, demonstrating a modest pain control benefit. BMAs should be used in conjunction with agents such as NSAIDS, opioid and nonopioid analgesics, corticosteroids, radiation/surgery, interventional procedures.

Multiple myeloma: The American Society of Clinical Oncology (ASCO) also has guidelines published on the use of bisphosphonates for prevention and treatment of bone disease in multiple myeloma (Kyle, 2007). Pamidronate or zoledronic acid use is recommended in multiple myeloma patients with lytic bone destruction or compression spine fracture from osteopenia. Clodronate (not available in the U.S.; available in Canada), administered orally or I.V., is an alternative treatment. The use of the bisphosphonates pamidronate and zoledronic acid may be considered in patients with pain secondary to osteolytic disease, adjunct therapy to stabilize fractures or impending fractures, and I.V. bisphosphonates for multiple myeloma patients with osteopenia but no radiographic evidence of lytic bone disease. Bisphosphonates are not recommended in patients with solitary plasmacytoma, smoldering (asymptomatic) or indolent myeloma, or monoclonal gammopathy of undetermined significance. The guidelines recommend monthly treatment for a period of 2 years. At that time, physicians need to consider discontinuing in responsive and stable patients, and reinitiate if new-onset skeletal-related event occurs. The ASCO guidelines are in alignment with package insert guidelines for dosing, renal dose adjustments, infusion times, prevention and management of osteonecrosis of the jaw, and monitoring of laboratory parameter recommendations. The guidelines also state in patients with a serum creatinine >3 mg/dL or Cl_{cr} <30 mL/minute or extensive bone disease, pamidronate at a dose of 90 mg over 4-6 hours is recommended (unless pre-existing renal disease at which a reduced dose should be considered). The ASCO committee also recommends monitoring for the presence of albuminuria every 3-6 months. In patients with albuminuria >500 mg/24 hours, withhold the dose until level returns to baseline, then recheck every 3-4 weeks. Pamidronate may be reinitiated at a dose not to exceed 90 mg every 4 weeks with a longer infusion time of at least 4 hours. The committee also recommends considering increasing the infusion time of zoledronic acid to at least 30 minutes. However, one study has demonstrated that extending the infusion to 30 minutes did not change the safety profile (Berenson, 2011).

Special Geriatric Considerations The elderly are frequently treated long-term for osteoporosis. Elderly patients should be advised to report any lower extremity, jaw (osteonecrosis), or muscle pain that cannot be explained or lasts longer than 2 weeks. Additionally, elderly often receive concomitant diuretic therapy and therefore their electrolyte status (eg, calcium, phosphate) should be periodically evaluated.

Dosage Forms Excipient information presented when available (limited, particularly for generics); consult specific product labeling.

Infusion, solution, premixed:
 Reclast® 5 mg (100 mL)
Injection, solution:
 Zometa® 4 mg/5 mL (5 mL)

Dosage Forms: Canada Excipient information presented when available (limited, particularly for generics); consult specific product labeling.

Infusion, solution [premixed]:
 Aclasta® 5 mg (100 mL)

Selected References

Body JJ, "Clinical Research Update: Zoledronate," *Cancer*, 1997, 80(Suppl):1699-701.

Boonen S, Sellmeyer DE, Lippuner K, et al, "Renal Safety of Annual Zoledronic Acid Infusions in Osteoporotic Postmenopausal Women," *Kidney Int*, 2008, 74(5):641-8.

Brufsky A, Harker WG, Beck JT, et al, "Zoledronic Acid Inhibits Adjuvant Letrozole-Induced Bone Loss in Postmenopausal Women With Early Breast Cancer," *J Clin Oncol* 2007, 25(7):829-36.

Cheer SM and Noble S, "Zoledronic Acid," *Drugs*, 2001, 61(6):799-805.

Coleman RE and Seaman JJ, "The Role of Zoledronic Acid in Cancer: Clinical Studies in the Treatment and Prevention of Bone Metastases," *Semin Oncol*, 2001, 28(2 Suppl 6):11-6.

Gatti D and Adami S, "New Bisphosphonates in the Treatment of Bone Diseases," *Drugs Aging*, 1999, 15(4):285-96.

Hillner BE, Ingle JN, Chlebowski RT, et al, "American Society of Clinical Oncology 2003 Update on the Role of Bisphosphonates and Bone Health Issues in Women With Breast Cancer," *J Clin Oncol*, 2003, 21(21):4042-57.

Lipton A, Small E, Saad F, et al, " The New Bisphosphonate, Zometa (Zoledronic Acid), Decreases Skeletal Complications in Both Osteolytic and Osteoblastic Lesions: A Comparison to Pamidronate," *Cancer Invest*, 2002, 20 Suppl 2:45-54.

Major PP and Coleman RE, "Zoledronic Acid in the Treatment of Hypercalcemia of Malignancy: Results of the International Clinical Development Program," *Semin Oncol*, 2001, 28(2 Suppl 6):17-24.

National Comprehensive Cancer Network® (NCCN), "Clinical Practice Guidelines in Oncology™: Breast Cancer," Version 1.2010. Available at http://www.nccn.org/professionals/physician_gls/PDF/breast.pdf.

National Comprehensive Cancer Network® (NCCN), "Clinical Practice Guidelines in Oncology™: Prostate Cancer," Version 1.2010. Available at http://www.nccn.org/professionals/physician_gls/PDF/prostate.pdf

Reid DM, Devogelaer JP, Saag K, et al, "Zoledronic Acid and Risedronate in the Prevention and Treatment of Glucocorticoid-Induced Osteoporosis (HORIZON): A Multicentre, Double-Blind, Double-Dummy, Randomised Controlled Trial," *Lancet*, 2009, 373(9671):1253-63.

Reid IR, Miller P, Lyles K, et al, "Comparison of a Single Infusion of Zoledronic Acid With Risedronate for Paget's Disease," *N Engl J Med*, 2005, 353(9):898-908.

ZOLMitriptan (zohl mi TRIP tan)

Medication Safety Issues

Sound-alike/look-alike issues:

ZOLMitriptan may be confused with SUMAtriptan

Brand Names: U.S. Zomig-ZMT®; Zomig®

Brand Names: Canada Mylan-Zolmitriptan; PMS-Zolmitriptan; PMS-Zolmitriptan ODT; Sandoz-Zolmitriptan; Sandoz-Zolmitriptan ODT; Teva-Zolmitriptan; Teva-Zolmitriptan OD; Zomig®; Zomig® Nasal Spray; Zomig® Rapimelt

Index Terms 311C90

Generic Availability (U.S.) No

Pharmacologic Category Antimigraine Agent; Serotonin 5-HT$_{1B, 1D}$ Receptor Agonist

Use Acute treatment of migraine with or without aura

Contraindications Hypersensitivity to zolmitriptan or any component of the formulation; ischemic heart disease or vasospastic coronary artery disease, including Prinzmetal's angina; signs or symptoms of ischemic heart disease; uncontrolled hypertension; symptomatic Wolff-Parkinson-White syndrome or arrhythmias associated with other cardiac accessory conduction pathway disorders; use with ergotamine derivatives (within 24 hours of); use within 24 hours of another 5-HT$_1$ agonist; concurrent administration or within 2 weeks of discontinuing an MAO inhibitor; management of hemiplegic or basilar migraine

Nasal spray: Additional contraindications with nasal spray: Cerebrovascular syndromes (eg, stroke, TIA); peripheral vascular disease (including ischemic bowel disease)

Warnings/Precautions Zolmitriptan is indicated only in patient populations with a clear diagnosis of migraine. Not for prophylactic treatment of migraine headaches. Cardiac events (coronary artery vasospasm, transient ischemia, myocardial infarction, ventricular tachycardia/fibrillation, cardiac arrest, and death) have been reported with 5-HT$_1$ agonist administration. Patients who experience sensations of chest pain/pressure/tightness or symptoms suggestive of angina following dosing should be evaluated for coronary artery disease or Prinzmetal's angina before receiving additional doses; if dosing is resumed and similar symptoms recur, monitor with ECG. Should not be given to patients who have risk factors for CAD (eg, hypertension, hypercholesterolemia, smoker, obesity, diabetes, strong family history of CAD, menopause, male >40 years of age) without adequate cardiac evaluation. Patients with suspected CAD should have cardiovascular evaluation to rule out CAD before considering zolmitriptan's use; if cardiovascular evaluation negative, first dose would be safest if given in the healthcare provider's office (consider ECG monitoring). Periodic evaluation of those without cardiovascular disease, but with continued risk factors, should be done. Significant elevation in blood pressure, including hypertensive crisis, has also been reported on rare occasions in patients with and without a history of hypertension. Vasospasm-related reactions have been reported other than coronary artery vasospasm. Peripheral vascular ischemia and colonic ischemia with abdominal pain and bloody diarrhea have occurred. Cerebral/subarachnoid hemorrhage and stroke have been reported with 5-HT$_1$ agonist administration; nasal spray contraindicated in patients with cerebrovascular syndromes. Rarely, partial vision loss and blindness (transient and permanent) have been reported with 5-HT$_1$ agonists. Use with caution in patients with hepatic impairment. Zomig-ZMT™ tablets contain phenylalanine. Symptoms of agitation, confusion, hallucinations, hyper-reflexia, myoclonus, shivering, and tachycardia (serotonin syndrome) may occur with concomitant proserotonergic drugs (eg, SSRIs/SNRIs or triptans) or agents which reduce zolmitriptan's metabolism. Concurrent use of serotonin precursors (eg, tryptophan) is not recommended.

Adverse Reactions (Reflective of adult population; not specific for elderly) Percentages noted from oral preparations.

1% to 10%:

Cardiovascular: Chest pain (2% to 4%), palpitation (up to 2%)

Central nervous system: Dizziness (6% to 10%), somnolence (5% to 8%), pain (2% to 3%), vertigo (≤2%)

Gastrointestinal: Nausea (4% to 9%), xerostomia (3% to 5%), dyspepsia (1% to 3%), dysphagia (≤2%)

Neuromuscular & skeletal: Paresthesia (5% to 9%), weakness (3% to 9%), warm/cold sensation (5% to 7%), hypoesthesia (1% to 2%), myalgia (1% to 2%), myasthenia (up to 2%)

Miscellaneous: Neck/throat/jaw pain (4% to 10%), diaphoresis (up to 3%), allergic reaction (up to 1%)

Drug Interactions

Metabolism/Transport Effects Substrate of CYP1A2 (minor)

Avoid Concomitant Use

Avoid concomitant use of ZOLMitriptan with any of the following: Ergot Derivatives; MAO Inhibitors; Sibutramine

Increased Effect/Toxicity

ZOLMitriptan may increase the levels/effects of: Ergot Derivatives; Serotonin Modulators

The levels/effects of ZOLMitriptan may be increased by: Cimetidine; Ergot Derivatives; MAO Inhibitors; Propranolol; Sibutramine

Decreased Effect

The levels/effects of ZOLMitriptan may be decreased by: Cyproterone

Ethanol/Nutrition/Herb Interactions Ethanol: Limit use (may have additive CNS toxicity).

Stability Store at 20°C to 25°C (68°F to 77°F). Protect from light and moisture.

Mechanism of Action Selective agonist for serotonin (5-HT$_{1B}$ and 5-HT$_{1D}$ receptors) in cranial arteries; causes vasoconstriction and reduces sterile inflammation associated with antidromic neuronal transmission correlating with relief of migraine

Pharmacodynamics/Kinetics

Onset of action: 0.5-1 hour

Absorption: Well absorbed

Distribution: V_d: 7 L/kg

Protein binding: 25%

Metabolism: Converted to an active N-desmethyl metabolite (2-6 times more potent than zolmitriptan)

Bioavailability: 40%

Half-life elimination: 2.8-3.7 hours

Time to peak, serum: Tablet: 1.5 hours; Orally-disintegrating tablet and nasal spray: 3 hours

Excretion: Urine (~60% to 65% total dose); feces (30% to 40%)

Dosage

Geriatric Refer to adult dosing. No dosage adjustment needed, but elderly patients are more likely to have underlying cardiovascular disease and should have careful evaluation of cardiovascular system before prescribing.

Adult

Migraine headache:

Oral:

Tablet: Initial: ≤2.5 mg at the onset of migraine headache; may break 2.5 mg tablet in half

Orally-disintegrating tablet: Initial: 2.5 mg at the onset of migraine headache

Nasal spray: Initial: 1 spray (5 mg) at the onset of migraine headache

Note: Use the lowest possible dose to minimize adverse events. If the headache returns, the dose may be repeated after 2 hours; do not exceed 10 mg within a 24-hour period. Controlled trials have not established the effectiveness of a second dose if the initial one was ineffective.

Renal Impairment No dosage adjustment recommended. There is a 25% reduction in zolmitriptan's clearance in patients with severe renal impairment (Cl$_{cr}$ 5-25 mL/minute).

Hepatic Impairment Administer with caution in patients with liver disease, generally using doses <2.5 mg (doses <5 mg can only be achieved using oral tablets). Patients with moderate-to-severe hepatic impairment may have decreased clearance of zolmitriptan, and significant elevation in blood pressure was observed in some patients.

Administration Administer as soon as migraine headache starts.

Tablets: May be broken

Orally-disintegrating tablets: Must be taken whole; do not break, crush or chew; place on tongue and allow to dissolve; administration with liquid is not required

Nasal spray: Blow nose gently prior to use. After removing protective cap, instill device into nostril. Block opposite nostril; breathe in gently through nose while pressing plunger of spray device. One dose (5 mg) is equal to 1 spray in 1 nostril.

Pharmacotherapy Pearls Not recommended if the patient has risk factors for heart disease (high blood pressure, high cholesterol, obesity, diabetes, smoking, strong family history of heart disease, postmenopausal woman, or a male >40 years of age).

This agent is intended to relieve migraine, but not to prevent or reduce the number of attacks. Use only to treat an actual migraine attack.

Special Geriatric Considerations No dosage adjustment needed, but elderly patients are more likely to have underlying cardiovascular disease and should have careful evaluation of the cardiovascular system before prescribing.

Dosage Forms Excipient information presented when available (limited, particularly for generics); consult specific product labeling.

Solution, intranasal [spray]:

Zomig®: 5 mg/0.1 mL (0.1 mL)

Tablet, oral:

Zomig®: 2.5 mg [scored]

Zomig®: 5 mg

◀ Tablet, orally disintegrating, oral:
Zomig-ZMT®: 2.5 mg [contains phenylalanine 2.81 mg/tablet; orange flavor]
Zomig-ZMT®: 5 mg [contains phenylalanine 5.62 mg/tablet; orange flavor]

◆ **Zoloft®** see Sertraline *on page 1669*

Zolpidem (zole Pl dem)

Medication Safety Issues
Sound-alike/look-alike issues:
Ambien® may be confused with Abilify®, Ativan®, Ambi 10®
Zolpidem may be confused with lorazepam, zaleplon
International issues:
Ambien® may be confused with Ambyen which is a brand name for amiodarone in Great Britain

Brand Names: U.S. Ambien CR®; Ambien®; Edluar™; Zolpimist®
Index Terms Zolpidem Tartrate
Generic Availability (U.S.) Yes: Excludes oral spray, sublingual tablet
Pharmacologic Category Hypnotic, Nonbenzodiazepine
Use
Ambien®, Edluar™, Zolpimist®: Short-term treatment of insomnia (with difficulty of sleep onset)
Ambien CR®: Treatment of insomnia (with difficulty of sleep onset and/or sleep maintenance)
Medication Guide Available Yes
Contraindications Hypersensitivity to zolpidem or any component of the formulation
Warnings/Precautions Should be used only after evaluation of potential causes of sleep disturbance. Failure of sleep disturbance to resolve after 7-10 days may indicate psychiatric or medical illness. Hypnotics/sedatives have been associated with abnormal thinking and behavior changes including decreased inhibition, aggression, bizarre behavior, agitation, hallucinations, and depersonalization. These changes may occur unpredictably and may indicate previously unrecognized psychiatric disorders; evaluate appropriately. Sedative/hypnotics may produce withdrawal symptoms following abrupt discontinuation. Use with caution in patients with depression; worsening of depression, including suicide or suicidal ideation has been reported with the use of hypnotics. Intentional overdose may be an issue in this population. The minimum dose that will effectively treat the individual patient should be used. Prescriptions should be written for the smallest quantity consistent with good patient care. Causes CNS depression, which may impair physical and mental capabilities. Zolpidem should only be administered when the patient is able to stay in bed a full night (7-8 hours) before being active again. Effects with other sedative drugs or ethanol may be potentiated.

Use caution in patients with myasthenia gravis. Avoid use in patients with sleep apnea or a history of sedative-hypnotic abuse. Postmarketing studies have indicated that the use of hypnotic/sedative agents for sleep has been associated with hypersensitivity reactions including anaphylaxis as well as angioedema. An increased risk for hazardous sleep-related activities such as sleep-driving; cooking and eating food, and making phone calls while asleep have also been noted; amnesia may also occur. Discontinue treatment in patients who report any sleep-related episodes.

Use caution with respiratory disease. Use caution with hepatic impairment; dose adjustment required. Because of the rapid onset of action, administer immediately prior to bedtime or after the patient has gone to bed and is having difficulty falling asleep.

Use caution in the elderly; dose adjustment recommended. Closely monitor elderly or debilitated patients for impaired cognitive or motor performance.
Adverse Reactions (Reflective of adult population; not specific for elderly) Actual frequency may be dosage form, dose, and/or age dependent
>10%: Central nervous system: Headache (7% to 19%), somnolence (6% to 15%), dizziness (1% to 12%)
1% to 10%:
Cardiovascular: Blood pressure increased, chest discomfort/pain, palpitation
Central nervous system: Abnormal dreams, anxiety, apathy, amnesia, ataxia, attention disturbance, body temperature increased, burning sensation, confusion, depersonalization, depression, disinhibition, disorientation, drowsiness, drugged feeling, euphoria, fatigue, fever, hallucinations, hypoesthesia, insomnia, lethargy, lightheadedness, memory disorder, mood swings, sleep disorder, stress
Dermatologic: Rash, urticaria, wrinkling
Endocrine & metabolic: Menorrhagia

Gastrointestinal: Abdominal discomfort, abdominal pain, abdominal tenderness, appetite disorder, constipation, diarrhea, dyspepsia, flatulence, gastroenteritis, gastroesophageal reflux, hiccup, nausea, vomiting, xerostomia

Genitourinary: Urinary tract infection, vulvovaginal dryness

Neuromuscular & skeletal: Arthralgia, back pain, balance disorder, involuntary muscle contractions, myalgia, neck pain, paresthesia, psychomotor retardation, tremor, weakness

Ocular: Asthenopia, blurred vision, depth perception altered, diplopia, red eye, visual disturbance

Otic: Labyrinthitis, tinnitus, vertigo

Renal: Dysuria

Respiratory: Pharyngitis, sinusitis, throat irritation, upper respiratory tract infection

Miscellaneous: Allergy, binge eating, flu-like syndrome

Drug Interactions

Metabolism/Transport Effects Substrate of CYP1A2 (minor), 2C9 (minor), 2C19 (minor), 2D6 (minor), 3A4 (major)

Avoid Concomitant Use

Avoid concomitant use of Zolpidem with any of the following: Conivaptan

Increased Effect/Toxicity

Zolpidem may increase the levels/effects of: Alcohol (Ethyl); CarBAMazepine; CNS Depressants; Methotrimeprazine; Selective Serotonin Reuptake Inhibitors

The levels/effects of Zolpidem may be increased by: Antifungal Agents (Azole Derivatives, Systemic); Conivaptan; CYP3A4 Inhibitors (Moderate); CYP3A4 Inhibitors (Strong); Dasatinib; Droperidol; HydrOXYzine; Methotrimeprazine

Decreased Effect

The levels/effects of Zolpidem may be decreased by: CarBAMazepine; CYP3A4 Inducers (Strong); Cyproterone; Deferasirox; Flumazenil; Herbs (CYP3A4 Inducers); Peginterferon Alfa-2b; Rifamycin Derivatives; Telaprevir; Tocilizumab

Ethanol/Nutrition/Herb Interactions

Ethanol: May enhance the adverse/toxic effects of zolpidem; avoid use.

Food: Maximum plasma concentration and bioavailability are decreased with food; time to peak plasma concentration is increased; half-life remains unchanged. Grapefruit juice may decrease the metabolism of zolpidem.

Herb/Nutraceutical: St John's wort may decrease the levels/effects of zolpidem; avoid concomitant use. In addition, concomitant use of valerian, kava kava, and gotu kola should be avoided due to the risk of increased CNS depression.

Stability

Ambien®, Edluar™: Store at 20°C to 25°C (68°F to 77°F). Protect sublingual tablets from light and moisture.

Ambien CR®: Store at 15°C to 25°C (59°F to 77°F); limited excursions permitted up to 30°C (86°F).

Zolpimist®: Store at 25°C (77°F); do not freeze. Avoid prolonged exposure to temperatures >30°C (86°F).

Mechanism of Action Zolpidem, an imidazopyridine hypnotic that is structurally dissimilar to benzodiazepines, enhances the activity of the inhibitory neurotransmitter, γ-aminobutyric acid (GABA), via selective agonism at the benzodiazepine-1 (BZ_1) receptor; the result is increased chloride conductance, neuronal hyperpolarization, inhibition of the action potential, and a decrease in neuronal excitability leading to sedative and hypnotic effects. Because of its selectivity for the BZ_1 receptor site over the BZ_2 receptor site, zolpidem exhibits minimal anxiolytic, myorelaxant, and anticonvulsant properties (effects largely attributed to agonism at the BZ_2 receptor site).

Pharmacodynamics/Kinetics

Onset of action: Immediate release: 30 minutes

Duration: Immediate release: 6-8 hours

Absorption: Rapid

Distribution: V_d: 0.54 L/kg

Protein binding: ~93%

Metabolism: Hepatic methylation and hydroxylation via CYP3A4 (~60%), CYP2C9 (~22%), CYP1A2 (~14%), CYP2D6 (~3%), and CYP2C19 (~3%) to three inactive metabolites

Bioavailability: 70%

Half-life elimination:

Immediate release, Extended release: ~2.5 hours (range 1.4-4.5 hours); Cirrhosis: Up to 9.9 hours; Elderly: Prolonged up to 32%

Spray: ~3 hours (range: 1.7-8.4)

Sublingual: ~3 hours (range: 1.6-6.7 hours)

Time to peak, plasma:

Immediate release: 1.6 hours; 2.2 hours with food

Extended release: 1.5 hours; 4 hours with food

Spray: ~0.9 hours
Sublingual: ~1.4 hours; ~1.8 hours with food
Excretion: Urine (48% to 67%, primarily as metabolites); feces (29% to 42%, primarily as metabolites)

Dosage

Geriatric

Immediate release tablet, spray, sublingual tablet: 5 mg immediately before bedtime
Extended release tablet: 6.25 mg immediately before bedtime

Adult Insomnia: Oral:

Immediate release tablet, spray, sublingual tablet: 10 mg immediately before bedtime; maximum dose: 10 mg
Extended release tablet: 12.5 mg immediately before bedtime

Renal Impairment Dose adjustment not required; monitor closely.
Not dialyzable

Hepatic Impairment

Immediate release tablet, spray, sublingual tablet: 5 mg
Extended release tablet: 6.25 mg

Administration Ingest immediately before bedtime due to rapid onset of action.
Ambien CR® tablets should be swallowed whole; do not divide, crush, or chew.
Edluar™ sublingual tablets should be placed under the tongue and allowed to disintegrate; do not swallow or administer with water.
Zolpimist® oral spray should be sprayed directly into the mouth over the tongue. Prior to initial use, pump should be primed by spraying 5 times. If pump is not used for at least 14 days, re-prime pump with 1 spray.

Monitoring Parameters Daytime alertness; respiratory rate; behavior profile

Test Interactions Increased aminotransferase [ALT/AST], bilirubin (S); decreased RAI uptake

Pharmacotherapy Pearls Causes fewer disturbances in sleep stages as compared to benzodiazepines. Time spent in sleep stages 3 and 4 are maintained; zolpidem decreases sleep latency; should not be prescribed in quantities exceeding a 1-month supply.

Special Geriatric Considerations In doses >5 mg, there was subjective evidence of impaired sleep on the first post-treatment night. There have been few reports of increased hypotension and/or falls in the elderly with this drug. Can be considered a drug of choice in the elderly when a hypnotic is indicated. With Ambien CR®, the adverse event profile of 6.25 mg in elderly patients was similar to the 12.5 mg dose in younger adults. Until there is more experience with this dosage form, use with caution in the elderly.

Controlled Substance C-IV

Dosage Forms Excipient information presented when available (limited, particularly for generics); consult specific product labeling.

Solution, oral, as tartrate [spray]:
Zolpimist®: 5 mg/actuation (8.2 g) [contains benzoic acid, propylene glycol; cherry flavor; 60 metered actuations]
Tablet, oral, as tartrate: 5 mg, 10 mg
Ambien®: 5 mg, 10 mg
Tablet, sublingual, as tartrate:
Edluar™: 5 mg, 10 mg
Tablet, extended release, oral, as tartrate: 6.25 mg, 12.5 mg
Ambien CR®: 6.25 mg, 12.5 mg

Selected References

Holm KJ and Goa KL, "Zolpidem: An Update of Its Pharmacology, Therapeutic Efficacy and Tolerability in the Treatment of Insomnia," *Drugs*, 2000, 59(4):865-89.
Simcox DA, "Zolpidem-Associated Falls," *Consult Pharm*, 1995, 10:1378-80.

- ♦ **Zolpidem Tartrate** *see* Zolpidem *on page 1960*
- ♦ **Zolpimist®** *see* Zolpidem *on page 1960*
- ♦ **Zolvit™** *see* Hydrocodone and Acetaminophen *on page 880*
- ♦ **Zometa®** *see* Zoledronic Acid *on page 1952*
- ♦ **Zomig®** *see* ZOLMitriptan *on page 1958*
- ♦ **Zomig-ZMT®** *see* ZOLMitriptan *on page 1958*
- ♦ **Zonalon®** *see* Doxepin (Topical) *on page 567*
- ♦ **Zonatuss™** *see* Benzonatate *on page 191*
- ♦ **Zonegran®** *see* Zonisamide *on page 1962*

Zonisamide (zoe NIS a mide)

Medication Safety Issues

Sound-alike/look-alike issues:

Zonegran® may be confused with SINEquan®
Zonisamide may be confused with lacosamide

Brand Names: U.S. Zonegran®
Generic Availability (U.S.) Yes
Pharmacologic Category Anticonvulsant, Miscellaneous
Use Adjunct treatment of partial seizures in adults with epilepsy
Unlabeled/Investigational Use Treatment of bipolar disorder
Medication Guide Available Yes
Contraindications Hypersensitivity to zonisamide, sulfonamides, or any component of the formulation
Warnings/Precautions Rare, but potentially fatal sulfonamide reactions have occurred following the use of zonisamide. These reactions include Stevens-Johnson syndrome, fulminant hepatic necrosis, agranulocytosis, aplastic anemia, and toxic epidermal necrolysis, usually appearing within 2-16 weeks of drug initiation. Discontinue zonisamide if rash develops. Chemical similarities are present among sulfonamides, sulfonylureas, carbonic anhydrase inhibitors, thiazides, and loop diuretics (except ethacrynic acid). Use in patients with sulfonamide allergy is specifically contraindicated in product labeling, however, a risk of cross-reaction exists in patients with allergy to any of these compounds; avoid use when previous reaction has been severe. Use may be associated with the development of metabolic acidosis (generally dose-dependent) in certain patients; predisposing conditions/therapies include renal disease, severe respiratory disease, diarrhea, surgery, ketogenic diet, and other medications. Serum bicarbonate should be monitored in all patients prior to and during use; if metabolic acidosis occurs, consider decreasing the dose or tapering the dose to discontinue. If use continued despite acidosis, alkali treatment should be considered. Untreated metabolic acidosis may increase the risk of developing nephrolithiasis, nephrocalcinosis, osteomalacia, or osteoporosis.

Pooled analysis of trials involving various antiepileptics (regardless of indication) showed an increased risk of suicidal thoughts/behavior (incidence rate: 0.43% treated patients compared to 0.24% of patients receiving placebo); risk observed as early as 1 week after initiation and continued through duration of trials (most trials ≤24 weeks). Monitor all patients for notable changes in behavior that might indicate suicidal thoughts or depression; notify healthcare provider immediately if symptoms occur.

Discontinue zonisamide in patients who develop acute renal failure or a significant sustained increase in creatinine/BUN concentration. Kidney stones have been reported. Do not use in patients with renal impairment (GFR <50 mL/minute); use with caution in patients with hepatic impairment.

Significant CNS effects include psychiatric symptoms, psychomotor slowing, and fatigue or somnolence. Fatigue and somnolence occur within the first month of treatment, most commonly at doses of 300-500 mg/day. Effects with other sedative drugs or ethanol may be potentiated. May cause sedation, which may impair physical or mental abilities; patients must be cautioned about performing tasks which require mental alertness (eg, operating machinery or driving). Abrupt withdrawal may precipitate seizures; discontinue or reduce doses gradually.

Adverse Reactions (Reflective of adult population; not specific for elderly) Adjunctive therapy: Frequencies noted in patients receiving other anticonvulsants:

>10%:
Central nervous system: Somnolence (17%), dizziness (13%)
Gastrointestinal: Anorexia (13%)
1% to 10%:
Central nervous system: Headache (10%), agitation/irritability (9%), fatigue (8%), tiredness (7%), ataxia (6%), confusion (6%), concentration decreased (6%), memory impairment (6%), depression (6%), insomnia (6%), speech disorders (5%), mental slowing (4%), anxiety (3%), nervousness (2%), schizophrenic/schizophreniform behavior (2%), difficulty in verbal expression (2%), status epilepticus (1%), convulsion (1%), hyperesthesia (1%), incoordination (1%)
Dermatologic: Rash (3%), bruising (2%), pruritus (1%)
Gastrointestinal: Nausea (9%), abdominal pain (6%), diarrhea (5%), dyspepsia (3%), weight loss (3%), constipation (2%), taste perversion (2%), xerostomia (2%), vomiting (1%)
Neuromuscular & skeletal: Paresthesia (4%), abnormal gait (1%), tremor (1%), weakness (1%)
Ocular: Diplopia (6%), nystagmus (4%), amblyopia (1%)
Otic: Tinnitus (1%)
Respiratory: Rhinitis (2%), pharyngitis (1%), increased cough (1%)
Miscellaneous: Flu-like syndrome (4%) accidental injury (1%)
Drug Interactions
Metabolism/Transport Effects Substrate of CYP2C19 (minor), 3A4 (major)

ZONISAMIDE

Avoid Concomitant Use

Avoid concomitant use of Zonisamide with any of the following: Carbonic Anhydrase Inhibitors; Conivaptan

Increased Effect/Toxicity

Zonisamide may increase the levels/effects of: Alcohol (Ethyl); Alpha-/Beta-Agonists; Amphetamines; Anticonvulsants (Barbiturate); Anticonvulsants (Hydantoin); CarBAMazepine; Carbonic Anhydrase Inhibitors; CNS Depressants; Flecainide; Memantine; Methotrimeprazine; Primidone; QuiNIDine; Selective Serotonin Reuptake Inhibitors

The levels/effects of Zonisamide may be increased by: Conivaptan; CYP3A4 Inhibitors (Moderate); CYP3A4 Inhibitors (Strong); Dasatinib; Droperidol; HydrOXYzine; Methotrimeprazine; Salicylates

Decreased Effect

Zonisamide may decrease the levels/effects of: Lithium; Methenamine; Primidone

The levels/effects of Zonisamide may be decreased by: CYP3A4 Inducers (Strong); Deferasirox; Fosphenytoin; Herbs (CYP3A4 Inducers); Ketorolac; Ketorolac (Nasal); Ketorolac (Systemic); Mefloquine; PHENobarbital; Phenytoin; Tocilizumab

Ethanol/Nutrition/Herb Interactions

Ethanol: May increase CNS depression; monitor for increased effects with coadministration. Caution patients about effects.

Food: Food delays time to maximum concentration, but does not affect bioavailability.

Stability Store at controlled room temperature 25°C (77°F). Protect from moisture and light.

Mechanism of Action The exact mechanism of action is not known. May stabilize neuronal membranes and suppress neuronal hypersynchronization through action at sodium and calcium channels. Does not affect GABA activity.

Pharmacodynamics/Kinetics

Distribution: V_d: 1.45 L/kg

Protein binding: 40%

Metabolism: Hepatic via CYP3A4; forms N-acetyl zonisamide and 2-sulfamoylacetyl phenol (SMAP)

Half-life elimination: Plasma: ~63 hours

Time to peak: 2-6 hours

Excretion: Urine (62%, 35% as unchanged drug, 65% as metabolites); feces (3%)

Dosage

Geriatric Data from clinical trials is insufficient for patients older than 65. Begin dosing at the low end of the dosing range.

Adult

Adjunctive treatment of partial seizures: Oral: Initial: 100 mg/day. Dose may be increased to 200 mg/day after 2 weeks. Further dosage increases to 300 mg and 400 mg/day can then be made with a minimum of 2 weeks between adjustments, in order to reach steady state at each dosage level. Doses of up to 600 mg/day have been studied, however, there is no evidence of increased response with doses >400 mg/day.

Mania (unlabeled use): Oral: Initial: 100-200 mg/day; maximum: 600 mg/day (Kanba, 1994)

Renal Impairment Slower titration and frequent monitoring are indicated in patients with renal disease. Use is not recommended in patients with GFR <50 mL/minute. Marked renal impairment (Cl_{cr} <20 mL/minute) was associated with a 35% increase in AUC.

Hepatic Impairment Slower titration and frequent monitoring are indicated.

Administration Capsules should be swallowed whole. Dose may be administered once or twice daily. Doses of 300 mg/day and higher are associated with increased side effects. Steady-state levels are reached in 14 days.

Monitoring Parameters Metabolic profile, specifically BUN, serum creatinine; serum bicarbonate (prior to initiation and periodically during therapy); suicidality (eg, suicidal thoughts, depression, behavioral changes)

Special Geriatric Considerations Consider the CNS effects commonly experienced in the first month of therapy.

Dosage Forms Excipient information presented when available (limited, particularly for generics); consult specific product labeling.

Capsule, oral: 25 mg, 50 mg, 100 mg

Zonegran®: 25 mg, 100 mg

◆ **ZOS** see Zoster Vaccine on page 1965

◆ **Zostavax®** see Zoster Vaccine on page 1965

Zoster Vaccine (ZOS ter vak SEEN)

Medication Safety Issues

Administration issues:

Both varicella vaccine and zoster vaccine are live, attenuated strains of varicella-zoster virus. Their indications, dosing, and composition are distinct. Varicella vaccine is indicated for the prevention of chickenpox, while zoster vaccine is indicated in older individuals to prevent reactivation of the virus which causes shingles. Zoster vaccine is **not** a substitute for varicella vaccine and should not be used in children.

Brand Names: U.S. Zostavax®

Brand Names: Canada Zostavax®

Index Terms Shingles Vaccine; Varicella-Zoster (VZV) Vaccine (Zoster); VZV Vaccine (Zoster); ZOS

Generic Availability (U.S.) No

Pharmacologic Category Vaccine, Live (Viral)

Use Prevention of herpes zoster (shingles) in patients ≥50 years of age

The Advisory Committee on Immunization Practices (ACIP) recommends routine vaccination of all patients ≥60 years of age, including:

- Patients who report a previous episode of zoster.
- Patients with chronic medical conditions (eg, chronic renal failure, diabetes mellitus, rheumatoid arthritis, chronic pulmonary disease) unless those conditions are contraindications.
- Residents of nursing homes and other long-term care facilities ≥60 years of age, without contraindications.

Contraindications Hypersensitivity to any component of the vaccine; individuals with leukemia, lymphomas, or other malignant neoplasms affecting the bone marrow or lymphatic systems; primary and acquired immunodeficiency states including AIDS or clinical manifestations of HIV; those receiving immunosuppressive therapy (including high-dose corticosteroids); pregnancy

In addition, ACIP recommends that the following immunocompromised patients should not receive zoster vaccine:

Patients undergoing hematopoietic stem cell transplant (limited data; assess risk:benefit, if needed, administer ≥24 months after transplantation);

Patients receiving recombinant human immune modulators, particularly antitumor necrosis factor agents (eg, adalimumab, infliximab, etanercept). Safety and efficacy of concurrent administration is unknown and not recommended. Defer vaccination for ≥1 month after discontinuation.

Patients with unspecified cellular immunodeficiency (exception, patients with impaired humoral immunity may receive vaccine).

Warnings/Precautions Zoster vaccine is not a substitute for varicella vaccine. Not for use in the treatment of active zoster outbreak, the treatment of postherpetic neuropathy (PHN), or prevention of primary varicella infection (chickenpox). Avoid administration in patients with acute febrile illness; consider deferral of vaccination; may administer to patients with mild acute illness (with or without fever). Defer treatment in patients with active untreated tuberculosis. May be used in patients with a history of zoster infection.

Medications active against the herpesvirus family (eg, acyclovir, famciclovir, valacyclovir) may interfere with the zoster vaccine. In patients where immunosuppressant therapy is anticipated, zoster vaccine should be given at least 14 days to 1 month prior to beginning therapy when possible Use is contraindicated in severely immunocompromised patients (eg, patients receiving chemo-/radiation therapy or other immunosuppressive therapy [including high-dose corticosteroids]); may have a reduced response to vaccination. Patients receiving corticosteroids in low-to-moderate doses, topical (inhaled, nasal, skin), local injection (intra-articular, bursal, tendon) may receive vaccine. Vaccinated individuals do not need to take precautions against spreading varicella following vaccination; transmission of virus is rare unless rash develops. In case of rash, standard contact precautions should be followed. In general, household and close contacts of persons with altered immunocompetence may receive all age-appropriate vaccines.

Immediate treatment for anaphylactoid reaction should be available during vaccine use. Contains gelatin and neomycin; do not use in patients with a history of anaphylactic/anaphylactoid reaction. Contact dermatitis to neomycin is not a contraindication to the vaccine. Not for use in patients <50 years of age. The ACIP does not recommend zoster vaccination in patients of any age who have received the varicella vaccine.

◄ **Adverse Reactions (Reflective of adult population; not specific for elderly)** All serious adverse reactions must be reported to the U.S. Department of Health and Human Services (DHHS) Vaccine Adverse Event Reporting System (VAERS) 1-800-822-7967 or online at https://vaers.hhs.gov/esub/index.

>10%: Local: Injection site reaction (48% to 64%; includes erythema, tenderness, pain, swelling, hematoma, pruritus, and/or warmth)

1% to 10% (**Note:** Rates similar to placebo):

Central nervous system: Fever (2%), headache (1% to 9%)

Dermatologic: Skin disorder (1%)

Gastrointestinal: Diarrhea (2%)

Neuromuscular & skeletal: Weakness (1%)

Respiratory: Respiratory tract infection (2%), rhinitis (1%)

Miscellaneous: Flu-like syndrome (2%)

Drug Interactions

Avoid Concomitant Use

Avoid concomitant use of Zoster Vaccine with any of the following: Acyclovir-Valacyclovir; Belimumab; Famciclovir; Fingolimod; Immunosuppressants

Increased Effect/Toxicity

The levels/effects of Zoster Vaccine may be increased by: AzaTHIOprine; Belimumab; Corticosteroids (Systemic); Fingolimod; Hydroxychloroquine; Immunosuppressants; Leflunomide; Mercaptopurine; Methotrexate

Decreased Effect

Zoster Vaccine may decrease the levels/effects of: Tuberculin Tests

The levels/effects of Zoster Vaccine may be decreased by: Acyclovir-Valacyclovir; Famciclovir; Fingolimod; Immune Globulins; Immunosuppressants; Pneumococcal Polysaccharide Vaccine (Polyvalent)

Stability To maintain potency, the lypholyzed vaccine must be stored frozen between -50°C to -15°C (-58°F to 5°F). Temperatures below -50°C (-58°F) may occur if stored in dry ice. During shipment, should be maintained at -15°C (5°F) or colder. Store powder in freezer at -15°C (5°F). Protect from light. Store diluent separately at room temperature of 20°C to 25°C (68°F to 77°F) or in refrigerator at 2°C to 8°C (36°F to 46°F). Products with 15-month expiry dating may also be transported/stored under refrigeration at 2°C to 8°C (36°F to 46°F) for up to 72 hours prior to reconstitution; discard if stored under refrigeration and not used within 72 hours.

Withdraw entire contents of the vial containing the provided diluent to reconstitute vaccine. Gently agitate to mix thoroughly. Withdraw entire contents of reconstituted vaccine vial for administration. Discard if reconstituted vaccine is not used within 30 minutes. Do not freeze reconstituted vaccine.

Mechanism of Action As a live, attenuated vaccine (Oka/Merck strain of varicella-zoster virus), zoster virus vaccine stimulates active immunity to disease caused by the varicella-zoster virus. Administration has been demonstrated to protect against the development of herpes zoster, with the highest efficacy in patients 60-69 years of age. It may also reduce the severity of complications, including postherpetic neuralgia, in patients who develop zoster following vaccination.

Pharmacodynamics/Kinetics

Onset of action: Seroconversion: ~6 weeks

Duration: Not established; protection has been demonstrated for at least 4 years

Dosage

Geriatric & Adult Shingles: Adults ≥50 years: SubQ: 0.65 mL administered as a single dose; there are no data to support readministration of the vaccine

Renal Impairment No adjustment required.

Administration Do not administer I.V. or I.M.; inject immediately after reconstitution. Inject SubQ into the deltoid region of the upper arm, if possible. In persons anticipating immunosuppression, give at least 14 days to 1 month prior to starting immunosuppressant.

Administration with chronic use of acyclovir, famciclovir, or valacyclovir: Discontinue ≥24 hours before administration of zoster vaccine. Do not use for ≥14 days after vaccination.

Simultaneous administration of vaccines helps ensure the patients will be fully vaccinated by the appropriate age. Simultaneous administration of vaccines is defined as administering >1 vaccine on the same day at different anatomic sites. Separate vaccines should not be combined in the same syringe unless indicated by product specific labeling. Separate needles and syringes should be used for each injection. The ACIP prefers each dose of a specific vaccine in a series come from the same manufacturer when possible. Adolescents and adults should be vaccinated while seated or lying down (CDC, 2011).

Antipyretics have not been shown to prevent febrile seizures. Antipyretics may be used to treat fever or discomfort following vaccination (CDC, 2011). One study reported that routine prophylactic administration of acetaminophen to prevent fever prior to vaccination decreased the immune response of some vaccines; the clinical significance of this reduction in immune response has not been established (Prymula, 2009).

Monitoring Parameters Fever, rash; monitor for syncope for ≥15 minutes following vaccination

Pharmacotherapy Pearls Federal law requires that the name of medication, date of administration, the vaccine manufacturer, lot number of vaccine, and the administering person's name, title, and address be entered into the patient's permanent medical record.

The varicella-zoster virus (VZV) is capable of causing two distinct manifestations of infection. Primary infection results in chickenpox (varicella). These infections tend to occur in young children or younger adults. Reactivation of latent infection (painful vesicular cutaneous eruption usually in a dermatomal pattern) occurs in older patients or in immunosuppressed populations. This is commonly referred to as shingles (herpes zoster). Although the vaccines are directed against the same causative organism, healthcare workers should be aware of differences in indications, dosing, populations, and composition of the vaccine. Neither vaccine is intended for administration during active outbreaks.

Special Geriatric Considerations This vaccine is intended for those ≥50 years of age. This live attenuated vaccine should be used with caution in patients with neoplastic disease or those who are immunosuppressed.

Dosage Forms Excipient information presented when available (limited, particularly for generics); consult specific product labeling.

Injection, powder for reconstitution [preservative free]:

Zostavax®: 19,400 PFU [contains bovine serum, gelatin, neomycin (may have trace amounts), sucrose (31.16 mg/vial)]

Selected References

Oxman MN, Levin MJ, Johnson GR, et al, "A Vaccine to Prevent Herpes Zoster and Postherpetic Neuralgia in Older Adults," N Engl J Med, 2005, 352(22):2271-84.

APPENDIX TABLE OF CONTENTS

ABBREVIATIONS, ACRONYMS, AND SYMBOLS

Abbreviations Which May Be Used in This Reference

Abbreviation	Meaning
5-HT	5-hydroxytryptamine
AAP	American Academy of Pediatrics
ABG	arterial blood gases
ABW	adjusted body weight
AACT	American Academy of Clinical Toxicology
ACC	American College of Cardiology
ACE	angiotensin converting enzyme
ACLS	advanced cardiac life support
ACOG	American College of Obstetricians and Gynecologists
ACTH	adrenocorticotrophic hormone
ADH	alcohol dehydrogenase
ADHD	attention-deficit/hyperactivity disorder
ADLs	activities of daily living
AED	antiepileptic drug
AHA	American Heart Association
AIDS	acquired immune deficiency syndrome
AIMS	Abnormal Involuntary Movement Scale
ALS	amyotrophic lateral sclerosis
ALT	alanine aminotransferase
AMA	American Medical Association
ANC	absolute neutrophil count
aPTT	activated partial thromboplastin
ARB	angiotensin receptor blocker
ARDS	acute respiratory distress syndrome
AST	aspartate aminotransferase
AUC	area under the curve
BDI	Beck Depression Inventory
BEC	blood ethanol concentration
BLS	basic life support
BMI	body mass index
BMT	bone marrow transplant
BP	blood pressure
BPH	benign prostatic hyperplasia
BPRS	Brief Psychiatric Rating Scale
BSA	body surface area
BUN	blood urea nitrogen
CABG	coronary artery bypass graft
CAD	coronary artery disease
CAN	Canadian
CAPD	continuous ambulatory peritoneal dialysis
CAS	chemical abstract service
CBC	complete blood count
CBT	cognitive behavioral therapy
Cl_{cr}	creatinine clearance

Abbreviations Which May Be Used in This Reference *(continued)*

Abbreviation	Meaning
CDC	Centers for Disease Control and Prevention
CF	cystic fibrosis
CGI	Clinical Global Impression
CHD	coronary heart disease
CHF	congestive heart failure; chronic heart failure
CIE	chemotherapy-induced emesis
C-II	schedule two controlled substance
C-III	schedule three controlled substance
C-IV	schedule four controlled substance
C-V	schedule five controlled substance
CIV	continuous I.V. infusion
C_{max}	maximum plasma concentration
C_{min}	minimum plasma concentration
CMV	cytomegalovirus
CNS	central nervous system or coagulase negative staphylococcus
COLD	chronic obstructive lung disease
COPD	chronic obstructive pulmonary disease
COX	cyclooxygenase
CPK	creatine phosphokinase
CRF	chronic renal failure
CRP	C-reactive protein
CRRT	continuous renal replacement therapy
CSF	cerebrospinal fluid
CSII	continuous subcutaneous insulin infusion
CT	computed tomography
CVA	cerebrovascular accident
CVVH	continuous venovenous hemofiltration
CVVHD	continuous venovenous hemodialysis
CVVHDF	continuous venovenous hemodiafiltration
CYP	cytochrome
D_5W	dextrose 5% in water
DBP	diastolic blood pressure
DEHP	di(3-ethylhexyl)phthalate
DIC	disseminated intravascular coagulation
DM	diabetes mellitus
DMARD	disease modifying antirheumatic drug
DSC	discontinued
DSM-IV	Diagnostic and Statistical Manual
DVT	deep vein thrombosis
EBV	Epstein-Barr virus
ECG	electrocardiogram
ECMO	extracorporeal membrane oxygenation
ECT	electroconvulsive therapy
ED	emergency department
EEG	electroencephalogram
EF	ejection fraction
EG	ethylene glycol
EGA	estimated gestational age
EIA	enzyme immunoassay
ELISA	enzyme-linked immunosorbent assay

Abbreviations Which May Be Used in This Reference *(continued)*

Abbreviation	Meaning
EPS	extrapyramidal side effects
ESR	erythrocyte sedimentation rate
ESRD	end stage renal disease
EtOH	alcohol
FDA	Food and Drug Administration
FTT	failure to thrive
GABA	gamma-aminobutyric acid
GAD	generalized anxiety disorder
GERD	gastroesophageal reflux disease
GFR	glomerular filtration rate
GGT	gamma-glutamyltransferase
GI	gastrointestinal
GU	genitourinary
GVHD	graft versus host disease
HAM-A	Hamilton Anxiety Scale
HAM-D	Hamilton Depression Scale
HDL	high density lipoprotein
HF	heart failure
HFSA	Heart Failure Society of America
HIV	human immunodeficiency virus
HMG-CoA	3-hydroxy-3-methylglutaryl-coenzyme A
HOCM	hypertrophic obstructive cardiomyopathy
HPA	hypothalamic-pituitary-adrenal
HSV	herpes simplex virus
HTN	hypertension
HUS	hemolytic uremic syndrome
IBD	inflammatory bowel disease
IBS	irritable bowel syndrome
IBW	ideal body weight
ICD	implantable cardioverter defibrillator
ICH	intracranial hemorrhage
ICP	intracranial pressure
IDDM	insulin dependent diabetes mellitus
IDSA	Infectious Diseases Society of America
IHSS	idiopathic hypertrophic subaortic stenosis
I.M.	intramuscular
INR	international normalized ration
Int. unit	international unit
IOP	intraocular pressure
IUGR	intrauterine growth retardation
I.V.	intravenous
IVP	intravenous push
IVPB	intravenous piggyback
JIA	juvenile idiopathic arthritis
JNC	Joint National Committee
KIU	kallikrein inhibitor unit
LAMM	L-α-acetyl methadol
LDH	lactate dehydrogenase
LDL	low density lipoprotein
LFT	liver function test

Abbreviations Which May Be Used in This Reference *(continued)*

Abbreviation	Meaning
LGA	large for gestational age
LR	lactated ringers
LVEF	left ventricular ejection fraction
LVH	left ventricular hypertrophy
MADRS	Montgomery Asbery Depression Rating Scale
MAOIs	monamine oxidase inhibitors
MDD	major depressive disorder
MDRD	modification of diet in renal disease
MDRSP	multidrug resistant *streptococcus pneumoniae*
mEq	milliequivalent
mg	milligram
MI	myocardial infarction
mL	milliliter
mm	millimeter
mM	millimolar
mm Hg	millimeters of mercury
MMSE	mini mental status examination
M/P	milk to plasma ratio
MPS I	mucopolysaccharidosis I
MRHD	maximum recommended human dose
MRI	magnetic resonance imaging
MUGA	multiple gated acquisition scan
NAS	neonatal abstinence syndrome
NF	National Formulary
NFD	Nephrogenic fibrosing dermopathy
ng	nanogram
NIDDM	Noninsulin dependent diabetes mellitus
NKA	no known allergies
NKDA	No known drug allergies
NMDA	n-methyl-d-aspartic acid
NMS	neuroleptic malignant syndrome
NNRTI	non-nucleoside reverse transcriptase inhibitor
NRTI	nucleoside reverse transcriptase inhibitor
NS	normal saline
NSAID	nonsteroidal anti-inflammatory drug
NSF	nephrogenic systemic fibrosis
NSTEMI	Non-ST-elevation myocardial infarction
OA	osteoarthritis
OCD	obsessive-compulsive disorder
OHSS	ovarian hyperstimulation syndrome
OTC	over-the-counter
PAT	paroxysmal atrial tachycardia
PD	Parkinson's disease; peritoneal dialysis
PDA	patent ductus arteriosus
PDE-5	phosphodiesterase-5
PE	pulmonary embolus
PEG tube	percutaneous endoscopic gastrostomy tube
PHN	post-herpetic neuralgia
PID	pelvic inflammatory disease
PMDD	premenstrual dysphoric disorder

ABBREVIATIONS, ACRONYMS, AND SYMBOLS

Abbreviations Which May Be Used in This Reference *(continued)*

Abbreviation	Meaning
PONV	postoperative nausea and vomiting
PPN	peripheral parenteral nutrition
PROM	premature rupture of membranes
PSVT	paroxysmal supraventricular tachycardia
PT	prothrombin time
PTSD	post-traumatic stress disorder
PTT	partial thromboplastin time
PUD	peptic ulcer disease
PVD	peripheral vascular disease
QT_c	corrected QT interval
QT_c-F	corrected QT interval by Fredricia's formula
RA	rheumatoid arthritis
REM	rapid eye movement
REMS	risk evaluation and mitigation strategies
RPLS	reversible posterior leukoencephalopathy syndrome
SA	sinoatrial
SAD	seasonal affective disorder
SAH	subarachnoid hemorrhage
SBE	subacute bacterial endocarditis
SBP	systolic blood pressure
S_{Cr}	serum creatinine
SERM	selective estrogen receptor modulator
SGA	small for gestational age
SGOT	serum glutamic oxaloacetic aminotransferase
SGPT	serum glutamic pyruvate transaminase
SI	International System of Units or Systeme international d'Unites
SIADH	syndrome of inappropriate antidiuretic hormone secretion
SLE	systemic lupus erythematosus
SNRI	serotonin norepinephrine reuptake inhibitor
SSKI	saturated solution of potassium iodide
SSRIs	selective serotonin reuptake inhibitors
STD	sexually transmitted disease
STEM I	ST-elevation myocardial infarction
SubQ	subcutaneous
supp	suppository
SVT	supraventricular tachycardia
SWFI	sterile water for injection
syr	syrup
$T_{1/2}$	half-life
tab	tablet
TB	tuberculosis
TC	total cholesterol
TCA	tricyclic antidepressant
TD	tardive dyskinesia
TG	triglyceride
TIA	transient ischemic attack
TMA	thrombotic microangiopathy
T_{max}	time to maximum observed concentration, plasma
TNF	Tumor necrosis factor
TPN	total parenteral nutrition

Abbreviations Which May Be Used in This Reference (continued)

Abbreviation	Meaning
tr, tinct	tincture
tsp	teaspoonful
UC	ulcerative colitis
ULN	upper limits of normal
URI	upper respiratory infection
USAN	United States Adopted Names
USP	United States Pharmacopeia
UTI	urinary tract infection
UV	ultraviolet
V_d	volume of distribution
VEGF	vascular endothelial growth factor
VF	ventricular fibrillation
VT	ventricular tachycardia
VTE	venous thromboembolism
vWD	von Willebrand disease
VZV	varicella zoster virus
YBOC	Yale Brown Obsessive-Compulsive Scale
YMRS	Young Mania Rating Scale

Common Weights, Measures, or Apothecary Abbreviations

Abbreviation	Meaning
<[1]	less than
>[1]	greater than
≤	less than or equal to
≥	greater than or equal to
ac	before meals or food
ad	to, up to
ad lib	at pleasure
AM	morning
AMA	against medical advice
amp	ampul
amt	amount
aq	water
aq. dest.	distilled water
ASAP	as soon as possible
a.u.[1]	each ear
bid	twice daily
bm	bowel movement
C	Celsius, centigrade
cal	calorie
cap	capsule
cc[1]	cubic centimeter
cm	centimeter
comp	compound
cont	continue
d	day
d/c[1]	discharge
dil	dilute

Common Weights, Measures, or Apothecary Abbreviations *(continued)*

Abbreviation	Meaning
disp	dispense
div	divide
dtd	give of such a dose
Dx	diagnosis
elix, el	elixir
emp	as directed
et	and
ex aq	in water
F	Fahrenheit
f, ft	make, let be made
g	gram
gr	grain
gtt	a drop
h	hour
hs[1]	at bedtime
kcal	kilocalorie
kg	kilogram
L	liter
liq	a liquor, solution
M	molar
mcg	microgram
m. dict	as directed
mEq	milliequivalent
mg	milligram
microL	microliter
mL	milliliter
mm	millimeter
mM	millimolar
mm Hg	millimeters of mercury
ng	nanogram
no.	number
noc	in the night
non rep	do not repeat, no refills
NPO	nothing by mouth
NV	nausea and vomiting
O, Oct	a pint
o.d.[1]	right eye
o.l.	left eye
o.s.[1]	left eye
o.u.[1]	each eye
pc, post cib	after meals
PM	afternoon or evening
P.O.	by mouth
P.R.	rectally
prn	as needed
pulv	a powder
q	every
qad	every other day
qd[1,2]	every day, daily
qh	every hour

Common Weights, Measures, or Apothecary Abbreviations *(continued)*

Abbreviation	Meaning
qid	four times a day
qod[1,2]	every other day
qs	a sufficient quantity
qs ad	a sufficient quantity to make
Rx	take, a recipe
SL	sublingual
stat	at once, immediately
SubQ	subcutaneous
supp	suppository
syr	syrup
tab	tablet
tal	such
tid	three times a day
tr, tinct	tincture
trit	triturate
tsp	teaspoon
u.d.	as directed
ung	ointment
v.o.	verbal order
w.a.	while awake
x3	3 times
x4	4 times

[1]ISMP error-prone abbreviation.

[2]JCAHO Do Not Use list.

Additional abbreviations used and defined within a specific monograph or text piece may only apply to that text.

REFERENCES

The Institute for Safe Medication Practices (ISMP) list of Error-Prone Abbreviations, Symbols, and Dose Designations. Available at http://www.ismp.org/Tools/errorproneabbreviations.pdf

The Joint Commission Official "Do Not Use" list. Available at http://www.jointcommission.org/Do_Not_Use_List_o-f_Abbreviations/

BODY SURFACE AREA (BSA)

$$BSA\ (m^2) = (kg^{0.425} \times cm^{0.725} \times 71.84) / 10,000$$

or

$$\log BSA\ (m^2) = [(\log kg \times 0.425) + (\log cm \times 0.725) + 1.8564] / 10,000$$

DuBois D and DuBois EF, "A Formula to Estimate the Approximate Surface Area if Height and Weight Be Known," *Arch Intern Med*, 1916, 17:863-71.

$$BSA\ (m^2) = \sqrt{\frac{ht\ (in)\ x\ wt\ (lb)}{3131}} \quad \textit{or} \quad BSA\ (m^2) = \sqrt{\frac{ht\ (cm)\ x\ wt\ (kg)}{3600}}$$

Lam TK and Leung DT, "More on Simplified Calculation of Body-Surface Area," *N Engl J Med*, 1988, 318(17):1130.
Mosteller RD, "Simplified Calculation of Body Surface Area," *N Engl J Med*, 1987, 317(17):1098.

BODY MASS INDEX (BMI)

$$BMI = \frac{weight\ (kg)}{[height\ (m)]^2}$$

CALCULATIONS

Ideal Body Weight

Adults (18 years and older) (IBW is in kg)
  IBW (male) = 50 + (2.3 x height in inches over 5 feet)
  IBW (female) = 45.5 + (2.3 x height in inches over 5 feet)

Lean Body Weight

Adults: Determination of lean body weight (LBW) in kg.
  LBW = IBW + 0.4(actual body weight - IBW)

Millimoles and Milliequivalent

Definitions

mole	=	gram molecular weight of a substance (aka molar weight)
millimole (mM)	=	milligram molecular weight of a substance (a millimole is 1/1000 of a mole)
equivalent weight	=	gram weight of a substance which will combine with or replace 1 gram (1 mole) of hydrogen; an equivalent weight can be determined by dividing the molar weight of a substance by its ionic valence
milliequivalent (mEq)	=	milligram weight of a substance which will combine with or replace 1 milligram (1 millimole) of hydrogen (a milliequivalent is 1/1000 of an equivalent)

Calculations

moles	=	$\dfrac{\text{weight of a substance (grams)}}{\text{molecular weight of that substance (grams)}}$
millimoles	=	$\dfrac{\text{weight of a substance (milligrams)}}{\text{molecular weight of that substance (milligrams)}}$
equivalents	=	moles x valence of ion
milliequivalents	=	millimoles x valence of ion
moles	=	$\dfrac{\text{equivalents}}{\text{valence of ion}}$
millimoles	=	$\dfrac{\text{milliequivalents}}{\text{valence of ion}}$
millimoles	=	moles x 1000
milliequivalents	=	equivalents x 1000

Note: Use of equivalents and milliequivalents is valid only for those substances which have fixed ionic valences (eg, sodium, potassium, calcium, chlorine, magnesium bromine, etc). For substances with variable ionic valences (eg, phosphorous), a reliable equivalent value cannot be determined. In these instances, one should calculate millimoles (which are fixed and reliable) rather than milliequivalents.

Approximate Milliequivalents — Weights of Selected Ions

Salt	mEq/g Salt	mg Salt/mEq
Calcium carbonate [$CaCO_3$]	20	50
Calcium chloride [$CaCl_2 \cdot 2H_2O$]	14	74
Calcium gluceptate [$Ca(C_7H_{13}O_8)_2$]	4	245
Calcium gluconate [$Ca(C_6H_{11}O_7)_2 \cdot H_2O$]	5	224
Calcium lactate [$Ca(C_3H_5O_3)_2 \cdot 5H_2O$]	7	154
Magnesium gluconate [$Mg(C_6H_{11}O_7)_2 \cdot H_2O$]	5	216
Magnesium oxide [MgO]	50	20
Magnesium sulfate [$MgSO_4$]	17	60
Magnesium sulfate [$MgSO_4 \cdot 7H_2O$]	8	123
Potassium acetate [$K(C_2H_3O_2)$]	10	98
Potassium chloride [KCl]	13	75
Potassium citrate [$K_3(C_6H_5O_7) \cdot H_2O$]	9	108
Potassium iodide [KI]	6	166
Sodium acetate [$Na(C_2H_3O_2)$]	12	82
Sodium acetate [$Na(C_2H_3O_2) \cdot 3H_2O$]	7	136
Sodium bicarbonate [$NaHCO_3$]	12	84
Sodium chloride [$NaCl$]	17	58
Sodium citrate [$Na_3(C_6H_5O_7) \cdot 2H_2O$]	10	98
Sodium iodine [NaI]	7	150
Sodium lactate [$Na(C_3H_5O_3)$]	9	112
Zinc sulfate [$ZnSO_4 \cdot 7H_2O$]	7	144

Valences and Atomic Weights of Selected Ions

Substance	Electrolyte	Valence	Molecular Wt
Calcium	Ca^{++}	2	40
Chloride	Cl^-	1	35.5
Magnesium	Mg^{++}	2	24
Phosphate	HPO_4^{--} (80%)	1.8	96[1]
pH = 7.4	$H_2PO_4^-$ (20%)	1.8	96[1]
Potassium	K^+	1	39
Sodium	Na^+	1	23
Sulfate	SO_4^{--}	2	96[1]

[1]The molecular weight of phosphorus only is 31, and sulfur only is 32.

CONVERSIONS

Apothecary-Metric Exact Equivalents

1 gram (g)	=	15.43 grains	0.1 mg	=	1/600 gr
1 milliliter (mL)	=	16.23 minims	0.12 mg	=	1/500 gr
1 grain (gr)	=	64.8 milligrams	0.15 mg	=	1/400 gr
1 fluid ounce (fl. oz)	=	29.57 mL	0.2 mg	=	1/300 gr
1 pint (pt)	=	473.2 mL	0.3 mg	=	1/200 gr
1 ounce (oz)	=	28.35 grams	0.4 mg	=	1/150 gr
1 pound (lb)	=	453.6 grams	0.5 mg	=	1/120 gr
1 kilogram (kg)	=	2.2 pounds	0.6 mg	=	1/100 gr
1 quart (qt)	=	946.4 mL	0.8 mg	=	1/80 gr
			1 mg	=	1/65 gr

Apothecary-Metric Approximate Equivalents[1]

Liquids			Solids		
1 teaspoonful	=	5 mL	¼ grain	=	15 mg
1 tablespoonful	=	15 mL	½ grain	=	30 mg
			1 grain	=	60 mg
			1½ grain	=	100 mg
			5 grains	=	300 mg
			10 grains	=	600 mg

[1]Use exact equivalents for compounding and calculations requiring a high degree of accuracy.

Pounds-Kilograms

1 pound = 0.45359 kilograms
1 kilogram = 2.2 pounds

Temperature

Celsius to Fahrenheit = (°C x 9/5) + 32 = °F
Fahrenheit to Celsius = (°F - 32) x 5/9 = °C

RENAL FUNCTION ESTIMATION IN ADULT PATIENTS

Evaluation of a patient's renal function often includes the use of equations to estimate glomerular filtration rate (GFR) (eg, estimated GFR [eGFR] creatinine clearance [Cl_{Cr}]) using an endogenous filtration marker (eg, serum creatinine) and other patient variables. For example, the Cockcroft-Gault equation estimates renal function by calculating Cl_{Cr} and is typically used to steer medication dosing. Equations which calculate eGFR are primarily used to categorize chronic kidney disease (CKD) staging. The rate of creatinine clearance does not always accurately represent GFR; creatinine may be cleared by other renal mechanisms in addition to glomerular filtration and serum creatinine concentrations may be affected by non-renal factors (eg, age, gender, race, body habitus, illness, diet). In addition, these equations were developed based on studies in limited populations and may either over- or underestimate the renal function of a specific patient.

Nevertheless, most clinicians estimate renal function using Cl_{Cr} as an indicator of actual renal function for the purpose of adjusting medication doses. For medications that require dose adjustment for renal impairment, utilization of eGFR (ie, Modification of Diet in Renal Disease [MDRD]) may overestimate renal function by up to 40% which may result in supratherapeutic medication doses (Hermsen, 2009). These equations should only be used in the clinical context of patient-specific factors noted during the physical exam/work-up. Decisions regarding drug therapy and doses must be based on clinical judgment.

RENAL FUNCTION ESTIMATION EQUATIONS

Commonly used equations include the Cockcroft-Gault, Jelliffe, four-variable Modification of Diet in Renal Disease (MDRD), and six-variable MDRD (aka, MDRD extended). All of these equations were originally developed using a serum creatinine assay measured by the alkaline picrate-based (Jaffe) method. Many substances, including proteins, can interfere with the accuracy of this assay and overestimate serum creatinine concentration. The National Kidney Foundation and The National Kidney Disease Education Program (NDKEP) advocate for a universal creatinine assay, in order to ensure an accurate estimate of renal function in patients. As a result, a more specific enzymatic assay with an isotope dilution mass spectrometry (IDMS)-traceable international standard has been developed. Compared to the older methods, IDMS-traceable assays may report lower serum creatinine values and may, therefore, overestimate renal function when used in the original equations (eg, Cockcroft-Gault, Jelliffe, original MDRD). Updated four-variable MDRD and six-variable MDRD equations based on serum creatinine measured by the IDMS-traceable method has been proposed for adults (Levey, 2006); the Cockcroft-Gault and Jelliffe equations have not been re-expressed and may overestimate renal function when used with a serum creatinine measured by the IDMS-traceable method. Clinicians should be aware of the serum creatinine assay used by their institution and the ramifications the assay may have on the equations used for renal function estimation.

Regardless of the serum creatinine assay used, the following factors may contribute to an inaccurate estimation of renal function (Stevens, 2006):

- Increased creatinine generation (may underestimate renal function):
    - Black or African American patients
    - Muscular body habitus
    - Ingestion of cooked meats
- Decreased creatinine generation (may overestimate renal function):
    - Increased age
    - Female patients
    - Hispanic patients
    - Asian patients
    - Amputees
    - Malnutrition, inflammation, or deconditioning (eg, cancer, severe cardiovascular disease, hospitalized patients)
    - Neuromuscular disease
    - Vegetarian diet

- Rapidly changing serum creatinine (either up or down): In patients with rapidly rising serum creatinines (ie, increasing by >0.5-0.7 mg/dL/day), it is best to assume that the patient's renal function is severely impaired

Use extreme caution when estimating renal function in the following patient populations:

- Low body weight (actual body weight < ideal body weight)
- Liver transplant
- Elderly (>90 years old)
- Dehydration
- Recent kidney transplantation (serum creatinine values may decrease rapidly and can lead to renal function underestimation; conversely, delayed graft function may be present)

Note: In most situations, the use of the patient's ideal body weight (IBW) is recommended for estimating renal function, except when the patient's actual body weight (ABW) is less than ideal. Use of actual body weight (ABW) in obese patients (and possibly patients with ascites) may significantly overestimate renal function. Some clinicians prefer to use an adjusted body weight in such cases [eg, IBW + 0.4 (ABW - IBW)]; the adjustment factor may vary based on practitioner and/or institutional preference.

Alkaline picrate-based (Jaffe) methods

Note: These equations have not been updated for use with serum creatinine methods traceable to IDMS. Use with IDMS-traceable serum creatinine methods may overestimate renal function; use with caution.

Method 1: MDRD equation:

$eGFR = 186 \times (Creatinine)^{-1.154} \times (Age)^{-0.203} \times (Gender) \times (Race)$

where:
  eGFR = estimated GFR; calculated in mL/minute/1.73 m^2
  Creatinine is input in mg/dL
  Age is input in years
  Gender: Females: Gender = 0.742; Males: Gender = 1
  Race: Black: Race = 1.212; White or other: Race = 1

Method 2: MDRD Extended equation:

$eGFR = 170 \times (Creatinine)^{-0.999} \times (Age)^{-0.176} \times (SUN)^{-0.170} \times (Albumin)^{0.318} \times (Gender) \times (Race)$

where:
  eGFR = estimated GFR; calculated in mL/minute/1.73 m^2
  Creatinine is input in mg/dL
  Age is input in years
  SUN = Serum Urea Nitrogen; input in mg/dL
  Albumin = Serum Albumin; input in g/dL
  Gender: Females: Gender = 0.762; Males: Gender = 1
  Race: Black: Race = 1.18; White or other: Race = 1

Method 3: Cockroft-Gault equation[1]

Males: $Cl_{Cr} = [(140 - Age) \times Weight] / (72 \times Creatinine)$
Females: $Cl_{Cr} = \{[(140 - Age) \times Weight] / (72 \times Creatinine)\} \times 0.85$
where:
  Cl_{Cr} = creatinine clearance; calculated in mL/minute
  Age is input in years
  Weight is input in kg
  Creatinine is input in mg/dL

Method 4: Jelliffe equation

Males: $Cl_{Cr} = \{98 - [0.8 \times (Age - 20)]\} / (Creatinine)$
Females: Cl_{Cr} = Use above equation, then multiply result by 0.9
where:
  Cl_{Cr} = creatinine clearance; calculated in mL/minute/1.73m^2
  Age is input in years
  Creatinine is input in mg/dL

◀ IDMS-traceable methods

Method 1: MDRD equation[2]:

$$eGFR = 175 \times (Creatinine)^{-1.154} \times (Age)^{-0.203} \times (Gender) \times (Race)$$

where:
eGFR = estimated GFR; calculated in mL/minute/1.73 m^2
Creatinine is input in mg/dL
Age is input in years
Gender: Females: Gender = 0.742; Males: Gender = 1
Race: Black: Race = 1.212; White or other: Race = 1

Method 2: MDRD Extended equation:

$$eGFR = 161.5 \times (Creatinine)^{-0.999} \times (Age)^{-0.176} \times (SUN)^{-0.170} \times (Albumin)^{0.318} \times (Gender) \times (Race)$$

where:
eGFR = estimated GFR; calculated in mL/minute/1.73 m^2
Creatinine is input in mg/dL
Age is input in years
SUN = Serum Urea Nitrogen; input in mg/dL
Albumin = Serum Albumin; input in g/dL
Gender: Females: Gender = 0.762; Males: Gender = 1
Race: Black: Race = 1.18; White or other: Race = 1

FOOTNOTES

[1]Equation typically used for adjusting medication doses
[2]Preferred equation for CKD staging National Kidney Disease Education Program

REFERENCES

Cockcroft DW and Gault MH, "Prediction of Creatinine Clearance From Serum Creatinine," *Nephron*, 1976, 16 (1):31-41.

Dowling TC, Matzke GR, Murphy JE, et al, "Evaluation of Renal Drug Dosing: Prescribing Information and Clinical Pharmacist Approaches," *Pharmacotherapy*, 2010, 30(8):776-86.

Hermsen ED, Maiefski M, Florescu MC, et al, "Comparison of the Modification of Diet in Renal Disease and Cockcroft-Gault Equations for Dosing Antimicrobials," *Pharmacotherapy*, 2009, 29(6):649-55.

Jelliffe RW, "Letter: Creatinine Clearance: Bedside Estimate," *Ann Intern Med*, 1973, 79(4):604-5.

Levey AS, Bosch JP, Lewis JB, et al, "A More Accurate Method to Estimate Glomerular Filtration Rate From Serum Creatinine: A New Prediction Equation. Modification of Diet in Renal Disease Study Group," *Ann Intern Med*, 1999, 16;130(6):461–70.

Levey AS, Coresh J, Greene T, et al, "Using Standardized Serum Creatinine Values in the Modification of Diet in Renal Disease Study Equation for Estimating Glomerular Filtration Rate," *Ann Intern Med*, 2006, 145(4):247-54.

National Kidney Disease Education Program, "GFR Calculators." Available at: http://www.nkdep.nih.gov/professionals/gfr_calculators. Last accessed: January 20, 2011.

Stevens LA, Coresh J, Greene T, et al, "Assessing Kidney Function - Measured and Estimated Glomerular Filtration Rate," *N Engl J Med*, 2006, 354(23):2473-83.

ANGIOTENSIN AGENTS

Comparison of Indications and Adult Dosages

Drug	Hypertension	HF	Renal Dysfunction	Dialyzable	Strengths (mg)
ACE Inhibitors					
Benazepril (Lotensin®)	10-40 mg/day	Not FDA-approved	Cl_{cr} <30 mL/min: 5 mg/day initially Maximum: 40 mg/day	Yes	Tablets 5, 10, 20, 40
Captopril (Capoten® [DSC])	25-100 mg/day bid-tid	6.25-100 mg tid Maximum: 450 mg/day	Cl_{cr} 10-50 mL/min: 75% of usual dose Cl_{cr} <10 mL/min: 50% of usual dose	Yes	Tablets 12.5, 25, 50, 100
Cilazapril (Inhibace®) **Note:** Not available in U.S.	2.5-10 mg/day	0.5-2.5 mg/day	Cl_{cr} 10-40 mL/min: Initial: 0.5 mg/day (0.25-0.5 mg/day for HF) (maximum: 2.5 mg/day) Cl_{cr} <10 mL/minute: 0.25-0.5 mg once or twice weekly	Yes	Tablets 1, 2.5, 5
Enalapril (Vasotec®)	2.5-4 mg/day qd-bid	2.5-20 mg bid Maximum: 20 mg bid	Cl_{cr} 30-80 mL/min: 5 mg/day initially Cl_{cr} <30 mL/min: 2.5 mg/day initially	Yes	Tablets 2.5, 5, 10, 20
Enalaprilat[1]	0.625 mg, 1.25 mg, 2.5 mg q6h Maximum: 5 mg q6h	Not FDA-approved	Cl_{cr} <30 mL/min: 0.625 mg q6h	Yes	1.25 mg/mL (1 mL, 2 mL vials)
Fosinopril (Monopril®)	10-40 mg/day	10-40 mg/day	No dosage reduction necessary	Not well dialyzed	Tablets 10, 20, 40
Lisinopril (Prinivil®, Zestril®)	10-40 mg/day Maximum: 40 mg/day	5-40 mg/day	Cl_{cr} 10-30 mL/min: 5 mg/day initially Cl_{cr} <10 mL/min: 2.5 mg/day initially	Yes	Tablets 2.5, 5, 10, 20, 30, 40
Moexipril (Univasc®)	7.5-30 mg/day qd-bid Maximum: 30 mg/day	LV dysfunction (post-MI): 7.5-30 mg/day	Cl_{cr} <40 mL/min: 3.75 mg/day initially Maximum: 15 mg/day	Unknown	Tablets 7.5, 15
Perindopril (Aceon®)	4-8 mg/day	4-8 mg/day Maximum: 16 mg/day	Cl_{cr} 30-60 mL/min: 2 mg/day Cl_{cr} 15-29 mL/min: 2 mg qod Cl_{cr} <15 mL/min: 2 mg on dialysis days	Yes	Tablets 2, 4, 8
Quinapril (Accupril®)	10-40 mg/day qd-bid	5-20 mg bid	Cl_{cr} 30-60 mL/min: 5 mg/day initially Cl_{cr} <10-30 mL/min: 2.5 mg/day initially	Not well dialyzed	Tablets 5, 10, 20, 40
Ramipril (Altace®)	2.5-20 mg/day qd-bid	2.5-10 mg/day	Cl_{cr} <40 mL/min: 25% of normal dose	Unknown	Capsules 1.25, 2.5, 5, 10

Comparison of Indications and Adult Dosages *continued*

Drug	Hypertension	HF	Renal Dysfunction	Dialyzable	Strengths (mg)
Trandolapril (Mavik®)	1-4 mg/day Maximum: 8 mg/day qd-bid	LV dysfunction (post-MI): 1-4 mg/day	Cl$_{cr}$ <30 mL/min: 0.5 mg/day initially	No	Tablets 1, 2, 4
Angiotensin II Receptor Blockers					
Azilsartan (Edarbi™)	40-80 mg/day	Not FDA-approved	No dosage adjustment necessary	Unknown	Tablets 40, 80
Candesartan (Atacand®)	8-32 mg/day	Target: 32 mg once daily	No dosage adjustment necessary	No	Tablets 4, 8, 16, 32
Eprosartan (Teveten®)	400-800 mg/day qd-bid	Not FDA-approved	No dosage adjustment necessary	Unknown	Tablets 400, 600
Irbesartan (Avapro®)	150-300 mg/day	Not FDA-approved	No dosage reduction necessary	No	Tablets 75, 150, 300
Losartan (Cozaar®)	25-100 mg qd or bid	Not FDA-approved	No dosage adjustment necessary	No	Tablets 25, 50, 100
Olmesartan (Benicar®)	20-40 mg/day	Not FDA-approved	No dosage adjustment necessary	Unknown	Tablets 5, 20, 40
Telmisartan (Micardis®)	20-80 mg/day	Not FDA-approved	No dosage reduction necessary	No	Tablets 20, 40, 80
Valsartan (Diovan®)	80-320 mg/day	Target: 160 mg bid	Decrease dose only if Cl$_{cr}$ <10 mL/minute	No	Tablets 40, 80, 160, 320
Renin Inhibitors					
Aliskiren (Tekturna®)	150-300 mg once daily	Not FDA-approved	No dosage adjustment necessary in mild-to-moderate impairment; not adequately studied in severe impairment	Unknown	Tablets 150, 300

Dosage is based on 70 kg adult with normal hepatic and renal function.

[1] Enalaprilat is the only available ACE inhibitor in a parenteral formulation.

ACE Inhibitors: Comparative Pharmacokinetics

Drug	Prodrug	Absorption (%)	Serum $t_{1/2}$ (h) Normal Renal Function	Serum Protein Binding (%)	Elimination	Onset of BP Lowering Action (h)	Peak BP Lowering Effects (h)	Duration of BP Lowering Effects (h)
Benazepril	Yes	37		~97	Renal (32%), biliary (~12%)	1	2-4	24
Benazeprilat			10-11 (effective)	~95%				
Captopril	No	60-75 (fasting)	1.9 (elimination)	25-30	Renal	0.25-0.5	1-1.5	~6
Enalapril	Yes	55-75	2	50-60	Renal (60%-80%), fecal	1	4-6	12-24
Enalaprilat			11 (effective)			0.25	1-4	~6
Fosinopril		36			Renal (~50%), biliary (~50%)	1		24
Fosinoprilat	No		12 (effective)	>99			6	
Lisinopril	No	25	11-12	25	Renal	1	6	24
Moexipril	Yes		1	90	Fecal (53%), renal (8%)		1-2	>24
Moexiprilat			2-10	50				
Perindopril	Yes		1.5-3	60	Renal		3-7	
Perindoprilat			3-10 (effective)	10-20				
Quinapril	Yes	>60	0.8	97	Renal (~60%) as metabolite, fecal	1	2-4	24
Quinaprilat			2					
Ramipril	Yes	50-60	1-2	73	Renal (60%), fecal (40%)	1-2	3-6	24
Ramiprilat			13-17 (effective)	56				
Trandolapril	Yes		6	80	Renal (33%), fecal (66%)	1-2	6	≥24
Trandolaprilat			10	65-94				

Angiotensin II Receptor Blockers and Renin Inhibitors: Comparative Pharmacokinetics

Drug	Prodrug	Time to Peak	Bio-availability	Food "Area-under-the-Curve"	Elimination Half-Life	Elimination Altered in Renal Dysfunction	Precautions in Severe Renal Dysfunction	Elimination Altered in Hepatic Dysfunction	Precautions in Hepatic Dysfunction	Protein Binding
Angiotensin II Receptor Blockers										
Azilsartan (Edarbi™)	Yes	1.5-3 h	60%	No effect	11 h	No	Yes	No	No	>99%
Candesartan (Atacand®)	Yes[1]	3-4 h	15%	No effect	9 h	Yes[2]	Yes	No	Yes	>99%
Eprosartan (Teveten®)	No	1-2 h	13%	No effect	5-9 h	No	Yes	No	Yes	98%
Irbesartan (Avapro®)	No	1.5-2 h	60%-80%	No effect	11-15 h	No	Yes	No	No	90%
Losartan (Cozaar®)	Yes[3]	1 h / 3-4 h[3]	33%	9%-10%	1.5-2 h / 6-9 h[3]	No	Yes	Yes	Yes	~99%
Olmesartan (Benicar®)	Yes	1-2 h	26%	No effect	13 h	Yes	Yes	Yes	No	99%
Telmisartan (Micardis®)	No	0.5-1 h	42%-58%	9.6%-20%	24 h	No	Yes	Yes	Yes	>99.5%
Valsartan (Diovan®)	No	2-4 h	25%	9%-40%	6 h	No	Yes	Yes	Yes	95%
Renin Inhibitors										
Aliskiren (Tekturna®)	No	1-3 h	~3%	85% (high-fat meal)	16-32 h	Yes[4]	Yes	No	No	?

[1] Candesartan cilexetil: Active metabolite candesartan.

[2] Dosage adjustments are not necessary.

[3] Losartan: Active metabolite E-3174.

[4] No initial dosage adjustment in mild-to-moderate impairment.

ANTICOAGULANTS, INJECTABLE

Name	Use	Limitation	Dose (SubQ unless otherwise noted)	Average MW Range (in Daltons)
Low Molecular Weight Heparins				
Dalteparin (Fragmin®) **Note:** Dose may require adjustment according to renal function	Prophylaxis	Abdominal surgery[1] Abdominal surgery[2]	2500 int. units/day 5000 int. units/day	2000-9000
		Hip surgery[1]	5000 int. units/day postoperatively	
	Treatment	DVT or PE (in patients with cancer)	Month 1: 200 int. units/kg once daily (max: 18,000 units) Months 2-6: 150 int. units/kg once daily (max: 18,000 units)	
		Unstable angina NSTEMI	120 int. units/kg (max: 10,000 int units) q12h	
Enoxaparin (Lovenox®) **Note:** Dose may require adjustment according to renal function	Prophylaxis	Hip replacement	30 mg q12h or 40 mg once daily	2000-8000
		Knee replacement	30 mg q12h	
		Abdominal surgery	40 mg once daily	
	Treatment	DVT or PE	1 mg/kg q12h or 1.5 mg/kg once daily	
		Unstable angina/ NSTEMI	1 mg/kg q12h	
		STEMI	<75 years: 1 mg/kg q12h ≥75 years: 0.75 mg/kg q12h	
Tinzaparin (Innohep®) **Note:** Dose may require adjustment according to renal function	Treatment	DVT or PE	175 anti-Xa int. units/kg/day	5500-7500
Heparin				
Heparin	Prophylaxis	Risk of thromboembolic disease	5000 units q8-12h	3000-30,000
	Treatment	DVT or PE[3]	80 units/kg (**or** 5000 units) IVP then 18 units/kg/hour (**or** 1300 units/hour)	
		STEMI/Unstable angina/NSTEMI[4,5]	60 units/kg IVP (max: 4000 units) then 12 units/kg/hour (max: 1000 units/hour)	
Selective Anti-Xa Inhibitor				
Fondaparinux[6] (Arixtra®) **Note:** Dose may require adjustment according to renal function	Prophylaxis	Abdominal surgery Hip fracture Hip or knee replacement	≥50 kg: 2.5 mg once daily	1728
	Treatment	DVT or PE	<50 kg: 5 mg once daily	
			50-100 kg: 7.5 mg once daily	
			>100 kg: 10 mg once daily	

ANTICOAGULANTS, INJECTABLE

(continued)

Name	Use	Limitation	Dose (SubQ unless otherwise noted)	Average MW Range (in Daltons)
Coumarin Derivatives				
Warfarin (Coumadin®)	Prophylaxis	NS	Variable	NS
	Treatment		2-5 mg/day	

NS = not stated in labeling, DVT = Deep venous thrombosis, NSTEMI = Non-ST-elevation MI, STEMI = ST-elevation MI, PE = Pulmonary embolism

[1]Patients with low risk of DVT.

[2]Patients with high risk of DVT.

[3]Dosing according to current clinical practice guidelines (Kearon, 2008).

[4]Not an FDA-approved indication; dosing according to current clinical practice guidelines (Anderson, 2007; Antman, 2004).

[5]Elderly patients may require a lower bolus dose of heparin.

[6]Synthetic pentasaccharide.

Anderson JL, Adams CD, Antman EM, et al, "ACC/AHA 2007 Guidelines for the Management of Patients With Unstable Angina/Non-ST-Elevation Myocardial Infarction: A Report of the American College of Cardiology/American Heart Association Task Force on Practice Guidelines (Writing Committee to Revise the 2002 Guidelines for the Management of Patients With Unstable Angina/Non-ST-Elevation Myocardial Infarction) Developed in Collaboration With the American College of Emergency Physicians, the Society for Cardiovascular Angiography and Interventions, and the Society of Thoracic Surgeons Endorsed by the American Association of Cardiovascular and Pulmonary Rehabilitation and the Society for Academic Emergency Medicine," *J Am Coll Cardiol*, 2007, 50(7):e1-e157.

Antman EM, Anbe DT, Armstrong PW, et al, "ACC/AHA Guidelines for the Management of Patients With ST-Elevation Myocardial Infarction: A Report of the American College of Cardiology/American Heart Association Task Force on Practice Guidelines (Committee to Revise the 1999 Guidelines for the Management of Patients With Acute Myocardial Infarction)," *Circulation*, 2004, 110(9):e82-292.

Kearon C, Kahn SR, Agnelli G, et al, "Antithrombotic Therapy for Venous Thromboembolic Disease: American College of Chest Physicians Evidence-Based Clinical Practice Guidelines (8th Edition)," *Chest*, 2008, 133(6 Suppl):454S-545S.

ANTIDEPRESSANT AGENTS

Comparison of Usual Adult Dosage, Mechanism of Action, and Adverse Effects

Drug	Initial Adult Dose	Usual Adult Dosage (mg/d)	Dosage Forms	ACH	Drowsiness	Orthostatic Hypotension	Conduction Abnormalities[1]	GI Distress	Weight Gain	Comments
Tricyclic Antidepressants and Related Compounds[1]										
Amitriptyline	25-75 mg qhs	100-300	T	4+	4+	3+	3+	1+	4+	Also used in chronic pain, migraine, and as a hypnotic; contraindicated with cisapride
Amoxapine	50 mg bid	100-400	T	2+	2+	2+	2+	0	2+	May cause extrapyramidal symptom (EPS)
ClomiPRAMINE[2] (Anafranil®)	25-75 mg qhs	100-250	C	4+	4+	2+	3+	1+	4+	Only approved for OCD
Desipramine (Norpramin®)	25-75 mg qhs	100-300	T	1+	2+	2+	2+	0	1+	Blood levels useful for therapeutic monitoring
Doxepin	25-75 mg qhs	100-300	C, L	3+	4+	2+	2+	0	4+	
Imipramine (Tofranil®, Tofranil-PM®)	25-75 mg qhs	100-300	T, C	3+	3+	4+	3+	1+	4+	Blood levels useful for therapeutic monitoring
Maprotiline	25-75 mg qhs	100-225	T	2+	3+	2+	2+	0	2+	
Nortriptyline (Pamelor®)	25-50 mg qhs	50-150	C, L	2+	2+	1+	2+	0	1+	Blood levels useful for therapeutic monitoring
Protriptyline (Vivactil®)	15 mg qAM	15-60	T	2+	1+	2+	3+	1+	1+	
Trimipramine (Surmontil®)	25-75 mg qhs	100-300	C	4+	4+	3+	3+	0	4+	
Selective Serotonin Reuptake Inhibitors[3]										
Citalopram (Celexa®)	20 mg qAM	20-60	T, L	0	0	0	0	3+[4]	1+	
Escitalopram (Lexapro®)	10 mg qAM	10-20	T, L	0	0	0	0	3+	1+	S-enantiomer of citalopram

Comparison of Usual Adult Dosage, Mechanism of Action, and Adverse Effects *continued*

Drug	Initial Adult Dose	Usual Adult Dosage (mg/d)	Dosage Forms	ACH	Drowsiness	Orthostatic Hypotension	Conduction Abnormalities	GI Distress	Weight Gain	Comments
							Adverse Effects			
FLUoxetine (PROzac®, PROzac® Weekly™, Sarafem®, Selfemra®)	10-20 mg qAM	20-80	C, CDR, L, T	0	0	0	0	$3+^4$	1+	CYP2B6 and 2D6 inhibitor
FluvoxaMINE[2] (Luvox® CR)	50 mg qhs	100-300	T, CXR	0	0	0	0	$3+^4$	1+	Contraindicated with pimozide, thioridazine, mesoridazine; CYP1A2, 2B6, 2C19, and 3A4 inhibitors
PARoxetine (Paxil®, Paxil CR®, Pexeva®)	10-20 mg qAM	20-50	T, CXR, L	1+	1+	0	0	$3+^4$	2+	CYP2B6 and 2D6 inhibitor
Sertraline (Zoloft®)	25-50 mg qAM	50-200	T, L	0	0	0	0	$3+^4$	1+	CYP2B6 and 2C19 inhibitor
Vilazodone (Viibryd™)	10 mg qAM	10-40	T	0	0	0	0	3+	0	CYP2C8, 2C19, and 2D6 inhibitor; also is a 5-HT$_{1A}$ partial agonist
Dopamine-Reuptake Blocking Compounds										
BuPROPion (Aplenzin™, Buproban®, Budeprion SR®, Budeprion XL®, Wellbutrin®, Wellbutrin SR®, Wellbutrin XL®, Zyban®)	100 mg bid-tid IR[5] 150 mg qAM-bid SR[5]	300-450	T, TSR, TXR	0	0	0	1+/0	1+	0	Contraindicated with seizures, bulimia, and anorexia; low incidence of sexual dysfunction IR: A 6-h interval between doses preferred SR: An 8-h interval between doses preferred XL: Administer once daily

Comparison of Usual Adult Dosage, Mechanism of Action, and Adverse Effects *continued*

Drug	Initial Adult Dose	Usual Adult Dosage (mg/d)	Dosage Forms	Adverse Effects						Comments
				ACH	Drowsiness	Orthostatic Hypotension	Conduction Abnormalities[7]	GI Distress	Weight Gain	
Serotonin / Norepinephrine Reuptake Inhibitors[7]										
Desvenlafaxine (Pristiq®)	50 mg/d	50–100	TXR	0	1+	1+	0	3+,[4]	0	Active metabolite of venlafaxine
DULoxetine (Cymbalta®)	40–60 mg/d	40–60	CDR	1+	1+	0	1+	3+	0	Also indicated for GAD, management of pain associated with diabetic neuropathy, and management of fibromyalgia
Milnacipran[8] (Savella™)	12.5 mg/d	100–200	T	2+	1+	0	1+	3+	0	Only indicated for fibromyalgia
Venlafaxine (Effexor®, Effexor XR®)	25 mg bid-tid IR 37.5 mg qd XR	75–375 IR 75–225 XR	T, TXR, CXR	1+	1+	0	1+	3+,[4]	0	High-dose may be useful to treat refractory depression; frequency of hypertension increases with dosage >225 mg/d
5-HT₂ Receptor Antagonist Properties										
Nefazodone	100 mg bid	300–600	T	1+	1+	2+	1+	1+	0	Contraindicated with carbamazepine, pimozide, astemizole, cisapride, and terfenadine; caution with triazolam and alprazolam; low incidence of sexual dysfunction
TraZODone	50 mg tid	150–600	T	0	4+	3+	1+	1+	2+	
Noradrenergic Antagonist										
Mirtazapine (Remeron®, Remeron SolTab®)	15 mg qhs	15–45	T, TOD	1+	3+	1+	1+	0	3+	Dose >15 mg/d less sedating, low incidence of sexual dysfunction

Comparison of Usual Adult Dosage, Mechanism of Action, and Adverse Effects *continued*

Drug	Initial Adult Dose	Usual Adult Dosage (mg/d)	Dosage Forms	Adverse Effects							Comments
				ACH	Drowsiness	Orthostatic Hypotension	Conduction Abnormalities	GI Distress	Weight Gain		
Monoamine Oxidase Inhibitors											
Isocarboxazid (Marplan®)	10 mg tid	10-30	T	2+	2+	2+	1+	1+	2+		Diet must be low in tyramine; contraindicated with sympathomimetics and other antidepressants
Phenelzine (Nardil®)	15 mg tid	15-90	T	2+	2+	2+	0	1+	3+	
Tranylcypromine (Parnate®)	10 mg bid	10-60	T	2+	1+	2+	1+	1+	2+	
Selegiline (EmSam®)	6 mg/d	6-12	Trans-dermal	2+	1+	2+	0	1+	0	Low tyramine diet not required for 6 mg/d dosage

ACH = anticholinergic effects (dry mouth, blurred vision, urinary retention, constipation); 0 - 4+ = absent or rare - relatively common. T = tablet, TSR - tablet, sustained release. TXR - tablet, extended release. TOD = tablet, orally disintegrating. L = liquid, C = capsule, CDR = capsule, delayed release, CXR = capsule, extended release; IR = immediate release, SR = sustained release, XR = extended release.

[1] **Important note:** A 1-week supply taken all at once in a patient receiving the maximum dose can be fatal.

[2] Not approved by FDA for depression. Approved for OCD.

[3] Flat dose response curve, headache, nausea, and sexual dysfunction are common side effects for SSRIs.

[4] Nausea is usually mild and transient.

[5] R: 100 mg bid, may be increased to 100 mg tid no sooner than 3 days after beginning therapy.

[6] SR: 150 mg qAM, may be increased to 150 mg bid as early as day 4 of dosing. To minimize seizure risk, do not exceed SR 200 mg/dose.

[7] Do not use with sibutramine; relatively safe in overdose.

[8] Milnacipran is only approved for fibromyalgia.

ANTIPARKINSONIAN AGENTS

Drugs Used for the Treatment of Parkinsonian Symptoms[1]

Drug	Mechanism	Initial Dose	Titration Schedule	Usual Daily Dosage	Recommended Dosing Schedule
Dopaminergic Agents					
Amantadine (Symmetrel®)	NMDA receptor antagonist and inhibits neuronal reuptake of dopamine	100 mg every other day	100 mg/dose every week, up to 300 mg 3 times/d	100–200 mg	Twice daily
Apomorphine (Apokyn®)	D_2 receptors (caudate-putamen)	1–2 mg	Complex; based on tolerance and response to test dose(s)	Variable; <20 mg	Individualized; 3–5 times/d prn
Bromocriptine (Parlodel®)	Moderate affinity for D_2 and D_3 dopamine receptors	1.25 mg twice daily	2.5 mg/d every 2–4 wk	2.5–100 mg	3 times/d
Carbidopa/levodopa (Sinemet®)	Converts to dopamine; binds to all CNS dopamine receptors	10-25/100 mg 2-4 times/d CR: 50/200 mg 2 times/d	0.5–1 tablet (10 or 25/100 mg) every 1–2 d	50/200 to 200/2000 mg (3–8 tablets)	3 times/d or twice daily (for controlled release)
Entacapone (Comtan®)	COMT enzyme inhibitor	200 mg 3 times/d	Titrate down the doses of carbidopa/levodopa as required	600–1600 mg	3 times/d; up to 8 times/d
Levodopa/carbidopa/ entacapone (Stalevo®)	Converts to dopamine; binds to all CNS dopamine receptors; COMT enzyme inhibitor	1 tablet 3-4 times/d (to replace previous dosing with individual agents)	As tolerated based on response and presence of dyskinesias	3–8 tablets per day	3–4 times/d
Pramipexole (Mirapex®)	High affinity for D_2 and D_3 dopamine receptors	0.125 mg 3 times/d	0.125 mg/dose every 5–7 d	1.5–4.5 mg	3 times/d
Rasagiline (Azilect®)	Inhibits MAO-B	0.5–1 mg once daily	≤1 mg daily	0.5–1 mg	Once daily
Ropinirole (Requip®)	High affinity for D_2 and D_3 dopamine receptors	0.25 mg 3 times/d	0.25 mg/dose weekly for 4 wk, then 1.5 mg/d every week up to 9 mg/d; 3 mg/d up to a max of 24 mg/d	0.75–24 mg	3 times/d
Selegiline (Eldepryl®)	Inhibits MAO-B	5–10 mg twice daily	Titrate down the doses of carbidopa/levodopa as required	5–10 mg	Twice daily
Tolcapone (Tasmar®)	COMT enzyme inhibitor	100 mg 3 times/d	Titrate down the doses of carbidopa/levodopa as required	300–600 mg	3 times/d

Drugs Used for the Treatment of Parkinsonian Symptoms[1] *continued*

Anticholinergic Agents

Drug	Mechanism	Initial Dose	Titration Schedule	Usual Daily Dosage	Recommended Dosing Schedule
Benztropine (Cogentin®)	Blocks cholinergic receptors, also has antihistamine effects	0.5-2 mg/d in 1-4 divided doses	0.5 mg/dose every 5-6 d	2-6 mg	1-2 times/d
Procyclidine (Kemadrin®)	Blocks cholinergic receptors	2.5 mg 3 times/d	Gradually as tolerated	7.5-20 mg	3 times/d
Trihexyphenidyl (Artane)	Blocks cholinergic receptors; also some direct effects	1-2 mg/d	2 mg/d at intervals of 3-5 d	5-15 mg	3-4 times/d

[1]The medications listed in the table represent treatment options for both idiopathic Parkinson's disease, as well as Parkinsonian symptoms resulting from other drug therapy.

[2]Cabergoline is not FDA approved for the treatment of Parkinson's disease.

ANTIPSYCHOTIC AGENTS

Antipsychotic Agent	Dosage Forms	I.M./P.O. Potency	Equiv. Dosages (approx) (mg/d)	Usual Adult Daily Maint. Dose (mg)	Sedation (Incidence)	Extrapyramidal Side Effects	Anticholinergic Side Effects	Orthostatic Hypotension	Comments
ARIPiprazole (Abilify®)	Solution; tablet; tablet, orally disintegrating; injection		7.5	10-30	Low	Low	Very low	Very low	Low weight gain; activating
Asenapine (Saphris®)	Tablet, sublingual			10-20	Moderate	Low	Very low	Low / moderate	Low weight gain; activating
ChlorproMAZINE	Injection; tablet	4:1	100	200-1000	High	Moderate	Moderate	Moderate / high	
CloZAPine (Clozaril®, FazaClo®)	Tablet; tablet, orally disintegrating		100	75-900	High	Very low	High	High	~1% incidence of agranulocytosis; weekly-biweekly CBC required; potential for weight gain, lipid abnormalities, and diabetes
FluPHENAZine	Solution, concentrate; injection; tablet	2:1	2	0.5-20	Low	High	Low	Low	
	Injection, long-acting			12.5-25*					
Haloperidol (Haldol®)	Solution, concentrate; injection; tablet	2:1	2	0.5-20	Low	High	Low	Low	
(Haldol® Decanoate)	Injection, long-acting			50-200*					
Iloperidone (Fanapt™)	Tablet			12-24	Low	Low	Very low	Low / moderate	
Loxapine (Loxitane®)	Capsule		10	25-250	Moderate	Moderate	Low	Low	
Lurasidone (Latuda®)	Tablet			40-80	Moderate	Low/Moderate	Low	Low	Contraindicated with strong CYP3A4 inducers and inhibitors. Take with food.
OLANZapine (Zyprexa®)	Injection; tablet; tablet, orally disintegrating		5	5-20	Moderate / high	Low	Moderate	Moderate	Potential for weight gain, lipid abnormalities, diabetes
(Zyprexa® Relprevv™)	Injection, long-acting			210-405*					

1997

Antipsychotic Agent	Dosage Forms	I.M./P.O. Potency	Equiv. Dosages (approx) (mg/d)	Usual Adult Daily Maint. Dose (mg)	Sedation (Incidence)	Extrapyramidal Side Effects	Anticholinergic Side Effects	Orthostatic Hypotension	Comments
Paliperidone (Invega®)	Tablet, extended release			3-12	Low / moderate	Low	Very low	Moderate	Active metabolite of risperidone
(Invega® Sustenna®)	Injection, long-acting			39-234*					
Perphenazine	Tablet		10	16-64	Low	Moderate	Low	Low	
Pimozide (Orap®)	Tablet		2	1-10	Moderate	High	Moderate	Low	Contraindicated with CYP3A inhibitors
QUEtiapine (Seroquel®, Seroquel XR®)	Tablet; tablet, extended release		75	50-800	Moderate / high	Very low	Moderate	Moderate	Moderate weight gain; potential for lipid abnormalities; diabetes
RisperiDONE (Risperdal®)	Solution; tablet, tablet, orally disintegrating		2	0.5-6	Low / moderate	Low	Very low	Moderate	Low to moderate weight gain; potential for diabetes
(Risperdal® Consta®)	Injection, long-acting			25-50*					
Thioridazine	Tablet		100	200-800	High	Low	High	Moderate / high	May cause irreversible retinitis pigmentosa at doses >800 mg/d; prolongs QTc; use only in treatment of refractory illness
Thiothixene (Navane®)	Capsule	4:1	4	5-40	Low	High	Low	Low / moderate	
Trifluoperazine	Tablet		5	2-40	Low	High	Low	Low	
Ziprasidone (Geodon®)	Capsule; injection; powder	2:1	60	40-160	Low / moderate	Low	Very low	Low / moderate	Low weight gain; contraindicated with QTc-prolonging agents. Take with food.

* Administered every 2 or 4 weeks; consult drug monograph for specific dosage detailsWoods SW, "Chlorpromazine Equivalent Doses for the Newer Atypical Antipsychotics," *J Clin Psychiatry*, 2003, 64(6):663-7.

ATYPICAL ANTIPSYCHOTICS

Drug[1]	DR EPS	PROL	TD[2]	ACH	SZ	OH	LFTs	SED	WT GAIN	NMS	AGRAN	TX REFR	Lipid	DM	QTc
ARIPiprazole (Abilify®)	No	No	Uncommon	Very low	Low	Low	Low	Low	Very low	Yes	?	Maybe	Very low	Very low	Low
Asenapine (Saphris®)	Yes	No	Uncommon	Very low	Low	Low / moderate	Low	Moderate	Low	Yes	?	No	Very low	Very low	Low
CloZAPine (Clozaril®)	No	No	Uncommon	High	DD	High	Low	High	High	Yes	Yes	Yes	High	High	Low
Iloperidone (Fanapt™)	No	No	Uncommon	Very low	Low	Low / moderate	Low	Low	Low / moderate	Yes	?	No	Very low	Very low	Moderate
Lurasidone (Latuda®)	Yes	Yes	Uncommon	Very low	Low	Low	Low	Moderate	Very low	Yes	?	No	Very low	Very low	Low
OLANZapine ZyPREXA®, ZyPREXA®, Zydis®)	Yes	Yes	Uncommon	Moderate	Low	Low / moderate	Low / moderate	Moderate	High	Yes	Yes[3]	Maybe	High	High	Low
Paliperidone (Invega™)	Yes	Yes	Uncommon	Very low	Low	Moderate	Low	Low	Low	Yes	?	Maybe	Low	Low	Low
QUEtiapine (SEROquel®)	No	No	Uncommon	Moderate	Low	Moderate	Low / moderate	Moderate	Moderate	Yes	Yes[3]	Maybe	Moderate	Low / moderate	Moderate
RisperiDONE (RisperDAL®)	Yes	Yes	Uncommon	Very low	Low	Moderate	Low	Low	Low / moderate	Yes	Yes[3]	Maybe	Low	Low / moderate	Low
Ziprasidone (Geodon®)	Yes	Yes	Uncommon	Very low	Low	Low	Low	Low	Very low	Yes	Yes[3]	Maybe	Very low	Very low	Moderate[4]

DR EPS = dose related extrapyramidal symptoms; **PROL** = prolactin elevation (may cause amenorrhea, galactorrhea, gynecomastia, impotence); **TD** = tardive dyskinesia; **ACH** = anticholinergic side effects (dry mouth, blurred vision, constipation, urinary hesitancy); **SZ** = seizures; **OH** = orthostatic hypotension (blood pressure drops upon standing); **LFTs** = increased liver function test results; **SED** = sedation; **WT GAIN** = weight gain; **NMS** = neuroleptic malignant syndrome; **AGRAN** = agranulocytosis (without white blood cells to fight infection); **TX REFR** = efficacy in treatment refractory schizophrenia; **Lipid** = lipid abnormalities, cholesterol and/or triglyceride elevations; **DM** = diabetes (based on case reports); **QTc** = QTc prolongation; **DD** = dose dependent

[1] Defined as 1) decrease or no EPS at doses producing antipsychotic effect; 2) minimum or no increase in prolactin; 3) decrease in both positive and negative symptoms of schizophrenia.

[2] Rate of TD ~½ that seen with conventional antipsychotics.

[3] Case reports.

[4] Dose related within 40-160 mg dosage range.

ANXIOLYTIC, SEDATIVE / HYPNOTIC, AND MISCELLANEOUS BENZODIAZEPINES

	Peak Blood Concentration (oral) (h)	Protein Binding %	Major Active Metabolite	Half-Life (parent) Adults (h)	Half-Life[1] (metabolite) Adults (h)	Adult Oral Dosage Range	Geriatric Oral Dosage Range
Anxiolytic							
ALPRAZolam (Alprazolam Intensol®, Xanax®)	1-2	80	No	12-15	—	0.75-4 mg/d	0.25-0.75 mg/d
ChlordiazePOXIDE (Librium®)	2-4	90-98	Yes	5-30	24-96	15-100 mg/d	10-20 mg/d[2]
Diazepam (Diastat® Rectal Delivery System, Diazepam Intensol®, Valium®)	0.5-2	98	Yes	20-80	50-100	4-40 mg/d	1-20 mg/d[2]
LORazepam (Ativan®)[3]	1-6	88-92	No	10-20	—	2-4 mg/d	0.5-4 mg/d
Oxazepam (Serax®)	2-4	86-99	No	5-20	—	30-120 mg/d	20-45 mg/d
Sedative / Hypnotic							
Estazolam (ProSom®)	2	93	No	10-24	—	1-2 mg	0.5-1 mg
Flurazepam (Dalmane®)	0.5-2	97	Yes	Not significant	40-114	15-60 mg	15 mg[2]
Quazepam (Doral®)	2	95	Yes	25-41	28-114	7.5-15 mg	7.5 mg[2]
Temazepam (Restoril®)	2-3	96	No	10-40	—	15-30 mg; Transient insomnia: 7.5 mg	7.5-15 mg
Triazolam (Halcion®)	1	89-94	No	2.3	—	0.125-0.5 mg	0.0625-0.25 mg
Miscellaneous							
ClonazePAM (Klonopin®)	1-2	86	No	18-50	—	1.5-20 mg/d	0.5-20 mg/d
Clorazepate (Tranxene®)	1-2	80-95	Yes	Not significant	50-100	15-60 mg/d	7.5-15 mg/d[2]
Midazolam	0.4-0.7[4]	95	No	2-5	—	NA	NA

[1] Significant metabolite.

[2] Not recommended for use in geriatric patients.

[3] Reliable bioavailability when given I.M.

[4] I.V. only.

NA = not available.

BETA-BLOCKERS

Agent	Adrenergic Receptor Blocking Activity	Intrinsic Sympathomimetic Activity (ISA)	Lipid Solubility	Protein Bound (%)	Half-Life (h)	Bioavailability (%)	Primary Site of Metabolism	Primary (Secondary) Route of Elimination	Indications	Usual Dosage
Acebutolol (Sectral®)	beta1	Yes	Low	15-25	3-4	40 7-fold[1]	Hepatic	Feces (renal)	Hypertension, arrhythmias	P.O.: 400-1200 mg/d
Atenolol (Tenormin®)	beta1	No	Low	<5-10	6-9	50-60 4-fold[1]	Hepatic (limited)	Feces (renal)	Hypertension, angina pectoris, acute MI	P.O.: 50-200 mg/d I.V. Acute MI: 5 mg x 2 doses
Betaxolol (Kerlone®)	beta1	No	Low	50-55	14-22	84-94	Hepatic	Renal	Hypertension	P.O.: 5-20 mg/d
Bisoprolol (Zebeta®)	beta1	No	Low	26-33	9-12	80	Hepatic	Renal	Hypertension, heart failure	P.O.: HF: 2.5-10 mg/d HTN: 2.5-20 mg/d
Carvedilol (Coreg®, Coreg CR®)	alpha1 beta1 beta2	No	ND	98	7-10	25-35	Hepatic	Feces	Hypertension, heart failure (mild to severe)	P.O.: 3.125-25 mg twice daily
Esmolol (Brevibloc)	beta1	No	Low	55	0.15	NA 5-fold[1]	Red blood cell esterase	Renal	Supraventricular tachycardia, sinus tachycardia, atrial fibrillation/flutter, hypertension	I.V. infusion: 25-300 mcg/kg/min
Labetalol (Trandate®)	alpha1 beta1 beta2	No	Moderate	50	5.5-8	18-30 10-fold[1]	Hepatic	Renal	Hypertension	P.O.: 200-2400 mg/d I.V.: 20-80 mg at 10-min intervals up to a maximum of 300 mg or continuous infusion of 2-6 mg/min
Metoprolol (Lopressor®, Toprol-XL®)	beta1	No	Moderate	10-12	3-7	50 7- to 10-fold[1] (Toprol XL®: 77)	Hepatic	Renal	Hypertension, angina pectoris, acute MI, heart failure (mild to moderate; XL formulation only), atrial tachyarrhythmias (rate control)	P.O.: 100-450 mg/d HF: (Toprol-XL®): 12.5-200 mg/d I.V. Acute MI: 5 mg q2 min x 3 doses AF (rate control): 2.5-5 mg q2-5 min (max total dose: 15 mg over 0-15 min)

BETA-BLOCKERS

Agent	Adrenergic Receptor Blocking Activity	Intrinsic Sympathomimetic Activity (ISA)	Lipid Solubility	Protein Bound (%)	Half-Life (h)	Bioavailability (%)	Primary Site of Metabolism	Primary (Secondary) Route of Elimination	Indications	Usual Dosage
Nadolol (Corgard®)	beta$_1$ beta$_2$	No	Low	25-30	20-24	30 5- to 8-fold[1]	None	Renal	Hypertension, angina pectoris	P.O.: 40-320 mg/d
Nebivolol (Bystolic®)	beta$_1$	No	High	98	10-32	12-96	Hepatic	Renal (feces)	Hypertension	P.O.: 5-40 mg/d
Penbutolol (Levatol®)	beta$_1$ beta$_2$	Yes	High	80-98	5	~100	Hepatic	Renal	Hypertension	P.O.: 20-80 mg/d
Pindolol	beta$_1$ beta$_2$	Yes	Moderate	57	3-4	90 2- to 2.5-fold[1]	Hepatic	Renal (feces)	Hypertension	P.O.: 20-60 mg/d
Propranolol (Inderal®, various)	beta$_1$ beta$_2$	No	High	90	3-5	25 2- to 3-fold[1]	Hepatic	Renal	Hypertension, angina pectoris, arrhythmias, prophylaxis (post-MI)	P.O.: 40-480 mg/d I.V.: Tachyarrhythmias: 1-3 mg q2-5 min (max: 5 mg)
Propranolol long-acting (Inderal-LA®, InnoPran XL™)	beta$_1$ beta$_2$	No	High	90	9-18	25 2- to 3-fold[1]	Hepatic	Renal	Hypertrophic cardiomyopathy with outflow tract obstruction, prophylaxis (post-MI)	P.O.: 180-240 mg/d
Sotalol (Betapace®, Betapace AF®, Sorine®)	beta$_1$ beta$_2$	No	Low	0	12	90-100	None	Renal	Atrial and ventricular tachyarrhythmias	P.O.: 160-320 mg/d
Timolol (Biocadren®)	beta$_1$ beta$_2$	No	Low to moderate	<10	4	75 7-fold[1]	Hepatic	Renal	Hypertension, prophylaxis (post-MI)	P.O.: 20-60 mg/d

Dosage is based on 70 kg adult with normal hepatic and renal function.

Note: All beta$_1$-selective agents will inhibit beta$_2$ receptors at higher doses.

[1] Interpatient variations in plasma levels.

CALCIUM CHANNEL BLOCKERS

Comparative Pharmacokinetics

Agent	Bioavailability (%)	Protein Binding (%)	Onset of BP Effect (min)	Duration of BP Effect (h)	Half-Life (h)	Volume of Distribution	Route of Metabolism	Route of Excretion
Dihydropyridines								
AmLODIPine (Norvasc®)	64-90	93-98	30-50	24	30-50	21 L/kg	Hepatic; inactive metabolites	Urine: 10% as parent
Clevidipine (Cleviprex™)	>99.5	2-4	5-15 min	1-15 min	0.17 L/kg	Blood and extravascular tissue esterases	Urine (63% to 74%; as metabolites); feces (7% to 22%)
Felodipine (Plendil)	20	>99	2-5 h	24	11-16	10 L/kg	Hepatic; CYP3A4 substrate (major); inactive metabolites; extensive first pass	Urine (70%; as metabolites); feces 10%
Isradipine (DynaCirc CR®)	15-24	95	20	>12	8	3 L/kg	Hepatic; CYP3A4 substrate (major); inactive metabolites; extensive first pass	Urine as metabolites
NiCARdipine (Cardene®)	35	>95	30	≤8	2-4		Hepatic; CYP3A4 substrate (major); saturable first pass	Urine (60%; as metabolites); feces 35%
NIFEdipine (Procardia®)	40-77	92-98	Within 20		2-5		Hepatic; CYP3A4 substrate (major); inactive metabolites	Urine as metabolites
NiMODipine (Nimotop®)	13	>95	ND	4-6	1-2		Hepatic; CYP3A4 substrate (major); metabolites inactive or less active than parent; extensive first pass	Urine (50%; as metabolites); feces 32%
Nisoldipine (Sular®)	5	>99	ND	6-12	7-12		Hepatic; CYP3A4 substrate (major); 1 active metabolite (10% of parent); extensive first pass	Urine as metabolites

2003

Comparative Pharmacokinetics *continued*

Agent	Bioavailability (%)	Protein Binding (%)	Onset of BP Effect (min)	Duration of BP Effect (h)	Half-Life (h)	Volume of Distribution	Route of Metabolism	Route of Excretion
Phenylalkylamines								
Verapamil (Calan®, Verelan®)	20-35	90	30	6-8	4.5-12		Hepatic; CYP3A4 substrate (major); 1 active metabolite (20% of parent); extensive first pass	Urine (70%; 3%-4% as unchanged drug); feces 16%
Benzothiazepines								
Diltiazem (Cardizem®)	~40	70-80	30-60	6-8	3-4.5	3-13 L/kg	Hepatic; CYP3A4 substrate (major); 1 major metabolite (20%-50% of parent); extensive first pass	Urine as metabolites

CORTICOSTEROIDS

Corticosteroids, Systemic Equivalencies

Glucocorticoid	Approximate Equivalent Dose (mg)	Routes of Administration	Relative Anti-inflammatory Potency	Relative Mineralocorticoid Potency	Protein Binding (%)	Half-life Plasma (min)
Short-Acting						
Cortisone	25	P.O., I.M.	0.8	0.8	90	30
Hydrocortisone	20	I.M., I.V.	1	1	90	90
Intermediate-Acting						
MethylPREDNISolone[1]	4	P.O., I.M., I.V.	5	0	—	180
PrednisoLONE	5	P.O., I.M., I.V., intra-articular, intradermal, soft tissue injection	4	0.8	90-95	200
PredniSONE	5	P.O.	4	0.8	70	60
Triamcinolone[1]	4	I.M., intra-articular, intradermal, intrasynovial, soft tissue injection	5	0	—	300
Long-Acting						
Betamethasone	0.75	P.O., I.M., intra-articular, intradermal, intrasynovial, soft tissue injection	25	0	64	100-300
Dexamethasone	0.75	P.O., I.M., I.V., intra-articular, intradermal, soft tissue injection	25-30	0	—	100-300
Mineralocorticoids						
Fludrocortisone	—	P.O.	10	125	42	200

[1]May contain propylene glycol as an excipient in injectable forms.

Asare K, "Diagnosis and Treatment of Adrenal Insufficiency in the Critically Ill Patient," *Pharmacotherapy*, 2007, 27(11):1512-28.

GUIDELINES FOR SELECTION AND USE OF TOPICAL CORTICOSTEROIDS

The quantity prescribed and the frequency of refills should be monitored to reduce the risk of adrenal suppression. In general, short courses of high-potency agents are preferable to prolonged use of low potency. After control is achieved, control should be maintained with a low potency preparation.

1. Low-to-medium potency agents are usually effective for treating thin, acute, inflammatory skin lesions; whereas, high or super-potent agents are often required for treating chronic, hyperkeratotic, or lichenified lesions.

2. Since the stratum corneum is thin on the face and intertriginous areas, low-potency agents are preferred but a higher potency agent may be used for 2 weeks.

3. Because the palms and soles have a thick stratum corneum, high or super-potent agents are frequently required.

4. Low potency agents are preferred for infants and the elderly. Infants have a high body surface area to weight ratio; elderly patients have thin, fragile skin.

5. The vehicle in which the topical corticosteroid is formulated influences the absorption and potency of the drug. Ointment bases are preferred for thick, lichenified lesions; they enhance penetration of the drug. Creams are preferred for acute and subacute dermatoses; they may be used on moist skin areas or intertriginous areas. Solutions, gels, and sprays are preferred for the scalp or for areas where a nonoil-based vehicle is needed.

6. In general, super-potent agents should not be used for longer than 2-3 weeks unless the lesion is limited to a small body area. Medium-to-high potency agents usually cause only rare adverse effects when treatment is limited to 3 months or less, and use on the face and intertriginous areas are avoided. If long-term treatment is needed, intermittent vs continued treatment is recommended.

7. Most preparations are applied once or twice daily. More frequent application may be necessary for the palms or soles because the preparation is easily removed by normal activity and penetration is poor due to a thick stratum corneum. Every-other-day or weekend-only application may be effective for treating some chronic conditions.

Corticosteroids, Topical

	Steroid	Dosage Form
Very High Potency		
0.05%	Betamethasone dipropionate, augmented	Cream, gel, lotion, ointment
0.05%	Clobetasol propionate	Cream, foam, gel, lotion, ointment, shampoo, spray
0.05%	Diflorasone diacetate	Ointment
0.05%	Halobetasol propionate	Cream, ointment
High Potency		
0.1%	Amcinonide	Cream, ointment, lotion
0.05%	Betamethasone dipropionate, augmented	Cream
0.05%	Betamethasone dipropionate	Cream, ointment
0.1%	Betamethasone valerate	Ointment
0.05%	Desoximetasone	Gel
0.25%	Desoximetasone	Cream, ointment
0.05%	Diflorasone diacetate	Cream, ointment
0.05%	Fluocinonide	Cream, ointment, gel
0.1%	Halcinonide	Cream, ointment
0.5%	Triamcinolone acetonide	Cream, spray

Corticosteroids, Topical *(continued)*

	Steroid	Dosage Form
	Intermediate Potency	
0.05%	Betamethasone dipropionate	Lotion
0.1%	Betamethasone valerate	Cream
0.1%	Clocortolone pivalate	Cream
0.05%	Desoximetasone	Cream
0.025%	Fluocinolone acetonide	Cream, ointment
0.05%	Flurandrenolide	Cream, ointment, lotion, tape
0.005%	Fluticasone propionate	Ointment
0.05%	Fluticasone propionate	Cream, lotion
0.1%	Hydrocortisone butyrate[1]	Ointment, solution
0.2%	Hydrocortisone valerate[1]	Cream, ointment
0.1%	Mometasone furoate[1]	Cream, ointment, lotion
0.1%	Prednicarbate	Cream, ointment
0.025%	Triamcinolone acetonide	Cream, ointment, lotion
0.1%	Triamcinolone acetonide	Cream, ointment, lotion
	Low Potency	
0.05%	Alclometasone dipropionate[1]	Cream, ointment
0.05%	Desonide	Cream, ointment
0.01%	Fluocinolone acetonide	Cream, solution
0.5%	Hydrocortisone[1]	Cream, ointment, lotion
0.5%	Hydrocortisone acetate[1]	Cream, ointment
1%	Hydrocortisone acetate[1]	Cream, ointment
1%	Hydrocortisone[1]	Cream, ointment, lotion, solution
2.5%	Hydrocortisone[1]	Cream, ointment, lotion

[1]Not fluorinated.

GLAUCOMA DRUG THERAPY

Ophthalmic Agent (Brand)	Reduces Aqueous Humor Production	Increases Aqueous Humor Outflow[1]	Average Duration of Action	Strengths Available
Cholinesterase Inhibitors[1]				
Echothiophate iodide (Phospholine Iodide®)	No data	Significant	2 wk	0.125%
Direct-Acting Cholinergic Miotics				
Carbachol (Isopto® Carbachol)	Some activity	Significant	8 h	1.5%, 3%
Pilocarpine (Isopto® Carpine, Pilopine HS®)	Some activity	Significant	5 h	0.5%, 1%, 2%, 3%, 4%, 6%
Sympathomimetics				
Apraclonidine (Iopidine®)	Moderate	Moderate	4 h	0.5%, 1%
Brimonidine (Alphagan® P)	Moderate	Moderate	8 h	0.1%, 0.15%
Dipivefrin (Propine®)	Some activity	Moderate	12 h	0.1%
Beta-Blockers				
Betaxolol (Betoptic® S, Kerlone®)	Significant	Some activity	≥12 h	0.25%, 0.5%
Carteolol	Yes	No	12 h	1%
Levobunolol (Betagan®)	Significant	Some activity	24 h	0.25%, 0.5%
Metipranolol (OptiPranolol®)	Significant	Some activity	18 h	0.3%
Timolol (Betimol®, Timoptic®)	Significant	Some activity	24 h	0.25%, 0.5%
Carbonic Anhydrase Inhibitors				
Acetazolamide (Diamox® Sequels®)	Significant	No data	10 h	125 mg tab, 250 mg tab; 500 mg cap
Brinzolamide (Azopt®)	Yes	No data	8 h	1%
Dorzolamide (Trusopt®)	Yes	No	8 h	2%
Methazolamide	Significant	No data	14 h	25 mg, 50 mg
Prostaglandin Agonists				
Bimatoprost (Lumigan®)		Yes	≥24 h	0.03%
Latanoprost (Xalatan®)		Yes	≥24 h	0.005%
Travoprost (Travatan®)		Yes	24 h	0.004%

[1]All miotic drugs significantly affect accommodation.

HELICOBACTER PYLORI TREATMENT IN ADULT PATIENTS

Medication Regimen	Dosages	Duration of Therapy
First-Line Therapy (Option 1)		
H$_2$-Receptor antagonist (H$_2$RA) **or** proton pump inhibitor (PPI)	Standard dose of H$_2$RA or PPI[1]	10-14 days
plus		
Bismuth subsalicylate	525 mg 4 times/day	10-14 days
plus		
MetroNIDAZOLE	250 mg 4 times/day	10-14 days
plus		
Tetracycline	500 mg 4 times/day	10-14 days
First-Line Therapy (Option 2)		
PPI	Standard dose[1]	10-14 days
plus		
Clarithromycin	500 mg 2 times/day	10-14 days
plus		
Amoxicillin	1000 mg 2 times/day	10-14 days
First-Line Therapy (Option 3)		
PPI	Standard dose[1]	10-14 days
plus		
Clarithromycin	500 mg 2 times/day	10-14 days
plus		
MetroNIDAZOLE	500 mg 2 times/day	10-14 days
Salvage Therapy for Persistent Infection (Option 1)		
PPI (once daily), bismuth, metroNIDAZOLE, and tetracycline (4 times/day) for 7-14 days		
Salvage Therapy for Persistent Infection (Option 2)		
PPI (standard dose[1]), levofloxacin 500 mg (once daily), and amoxicillin 1000 mg (2 times/day) for 10 days		

[1]Standard proton pump inhibitor dose: Esomeprazole = 40 mg once daily; Lansoprazole = 30 mg 2 times/day; Omeprazole = 20 mg 2 times/day; RABEprazole = 20 mg 2 times/day

REFERENCES

Chey WD, Wong BC, and Practice Parameters Committee of the American College of Gastroenterology, "American College of Gastroenterology Guideline on the Management of *Helicobacter pylori* Infection," *Am J Gastroenterol*, 2007, 102(8):1808-25.

Saad RJ, Schoenfeld P, Kim HM, et al, "Levofloxacin-Based Triple Therapy Versus Bismuth-Based Quadruple Therapy for Persistent *Helicobacter pylori* Infection: A Meta-Analysis," *Am J Gastroenterol*, 2006, 101(3):488-96.

INHALANT AGENTS

Medications Commonly Used for Asthma, Bronchospasm, and COPD

Agent	Indications	Onset	Duration	Frequency	Comments
Anticholinergics					
Ipratropium bromide (Atrovent®)	Bronchospasm associated with COPD; severe asthma exacerbation (Asthma Guidelines, 2007)	1-3 min	≤4 h	4 times/day	Asthma: Should be used as adjunct therapy to SABA in severe exacerbations. May not provide further benefit if patient hospitalized.
Tiotropium (Spiriva®)	Bronchospasm associated with COPD			Daily	For COPD only.
Short-Acting Beta$_2$-Agonists (SABA)[1]					
Albuterol (Proventil®, Proventil® HFA, Ventolin® HFA)	Prevention of EIB; relief and prevention of bronchospasm	5 min	6-8 h	q4-6h	
Levalbuterol (Xopenex®)	Relief and prevention of bronchospasm	6-17 min	3-6 h	6-8 h intervals (nebulization); 4-6 h (inhaler)	May be used as SABA in asthma exacerbations
Pirbuterol acetate (Maxair™ Autohaler™)	Treatment and prevention of bronchospasm	Within 5 min	4-6 h	q4-6h	Not studied in severe exacerbations
Long-Acting Beta$_2$-Agonists (LABA)[2]					
Arformoterol (Brovana™)	Long-term maintenance treatment in COPD	7-20 min	12 h	q12h	Not to be used for treatment of episodes of acute bronchospasm as rescue therapy
Formoterol (Foradil® Aerolizer™)	Long-term maintenance treatment of asthma; prevention of EIB; maintenance treatment of COPD	Within 3 min	12 h	q12h	Not meant to relieve acute asthmatic symptoms
Salmeterol (Serevent® Diskus®)	Long-term maintenance treatment of asthma; prevention of EIB; maintenance treatment of COPD	20 min	12 h	q12h	Not meant to relieve acute asthmatic symptoms

Medications Commonly Used for Asthma, Bronchospasm, and COPD *(continued)*

Agent	Indications	Onset	Duration	Frequency	Comments
Inhalation Corticosteroids[3]					
Beclomethasone dipropionate (various)	Maintenance and prevention of asthma		6-8 h	Twice daily	Adjustable dose approach may enable reduction in cumulative dose over time without decreasing asthma control
Budesonide (Pulmicort®)	Maintenance and prevention of asthma		12 h	Twice daily	
Flunisolide (various)	Maintenance and prevention of asthma		12 h	Twice daily	
Fluticasone (Flovent®)	Maintenance and prevention of asthma		—	Twice daily	
Mometasone	Maintenance and prevention of asthma		—	Once or twice daily	
Mast Cell Stabilizers[3]					
Nedocromil sodium (Alocril®)	Maintenance treatment of mild-to-moderate asthma		2 h	4 times/day	

EIB = exercise-induced bronchospasm.

[1]Asthma: Only selective beta$_2$-agonists are recommended.

[2]Asthma: Should not be used for symptom relief or exacerbations. Use only with ICS.

[3]Asthma: Should not be used for symptom relief or exacerbations.

Reference:

Expert Panel Report 3, "Guidelines for the Diagnosis and Management of Asthma," *Clinical Practice Guidelines*, National Institutes of Health, National Heart, Lung, and Blood Institute, NIH Publication No. 08-4051, prepublication 2007. Available at http://www.nhlbi.nih.gov/guidelines/asthma/asthgdln.htm.

LAXATIVES, CLASSIFICATION AND PROPERTIES

Laxative	Onset of Action	Site of Action	Mechanism of Action
Saline			
Magnesium citrate Magnesium hydroxide (Phillips'® Milk of Magnesia)	30 min to 3 h	Small and large intestine	Attract/retain water in intestinal lumen increasing intraluminal pressure; cholecystokinin release
Sodium phosphates (Fleet® Enema)	2-15 min	Colon	
Irritant / Stimulant			
Senna (Senokot®)	6-10 h	Colon	Direct action on intestinal mucosa; stimulate myenteric plexus; alter water and electrolyte secretion
Bisacodyl (Dulcolax®) tablets, suppositories	15 min to 1 h	Colon	
Castor oil	2-6 h	Small intestine	
Bulk-Producing			
Methylcellulose (Citrucel®) Psyllium (Metamucil®) Wheat dextrin (Benefiber®)	12-24 h (up to 72 h) 24-48 h	Small and large intestine	Holds water in stool; mechanical distention
Lubricant			
Mineral oil	6-8 h	Colon	Lubricates intestine; retards colonic absorption of fecal water; softens stool
Surfactants / Stool Softener			
Docusate/senna (Peri-Colace®)	8-12 h	Small and large intestine	Senna – mild irritant; docusate – stool softener
Docusate sodium (Colace®) Docusate calcium (Surfak®)	24-72 h	Small and large intestine	Detergent activity; facilitates admixture of fat and water to soften stool
Osmotic Laxatives			
Glycerin suppository	15-30 min	Colon	Local irritation; hyperosmotic action
Lactulose	24-48 h	Colon	Delivers osmotically active molecules to colon
Polyethylene glycol 3350 (GlycoLax™, MiraLax™)	48 h	Small and large intestine	Nonabsorbable solution which acts as an osmotic agent
Sodium sulfate, potassium sulfate, and magnesium sulfate (Suprep®)	24 h	Small and large intestine	Hyperosmotic action
Sorbitol 70%	24-48 h	Colon	Delivers osmotically active molecules to colon
Miscellaneous Laxatives			
Lubiprostone (Amitiza®)	24-48 h	Apical membrane of the GI epithelium	Activates intestinal chloride channels increasing intestinal fluid

OPIOID ANALGESICS

This table serves as a general guide to opioid conversion. Utilization of a direct conversion without a detailed patients and medication assessment is not recommended and may result in over- or underdosing. Chronic administration may alter pharmacokinetics and change parenteral: oral ratio.

Opioid Analgesics – Initial Oral Dosing Commonly Used for Severe Pain

Drug	Equianalgesic Dose (mg)		Initial Oral Dose	
	Oral[1]	Parenteral[2]	Children[3] (mg/kg)	Adults (mg)
Buprenorphine	—	0.4	—	—
Butorphanol	—	2	—	—
FentaNYL	—	0.1	—	—
HYDROmorphone	7.5	1.5	0.06	4-8
Levorphanol	Acute: 4 Chronic: 1	Acute: 2 Chronic: 1	0.04	2-4
Meperidine[4]	300	75	Not recommended	
Methadone[5]	See Guidelines for Conversion to Oral Methadone in Adults	Variable	0.2	5-10
Morphine	30	10	0.3	15-30
Nalbuphine	—	10	—	—
OxyCODONE	20	—	0.2	10-20
Oxymorphone	10	1	—	5-10
Pentazocine	50	30	—	—

Guidelines for Conversion to Oral Methadone in Adults[5]

Oral Morphine Dose or Equivalent (mg/day)	Oral Morphine:Oral Methadone (Conversion Ratio)
<90	4:1
90-300	8:1
>300	12:1

[1]Elderly: Starting dose should be lower for this population group.

[2]Standard parenteral doses (I.M.) for acute pain in adults; can be used to convert doses for I.V. infusions and repeated small I.V. boluses. For single I.V. boluses, use half the I.M. dose.

[3]The pharmacokinetics of opioids in children and infants >6 months old are similar to adults but infants <6 months old, especially premature or physically compromised ones, are at risk of apnea.

[4]Not recommended for routine use.

[5]Conversion of higher doses may be guided by the following (consult a pain or palliative care specialist if unfamiliar with methadone prescribing): As the total daily chronic dose of morphine increases, the equianalgesic dose ratio (morphine:methadone) changes (American Pain Society, 2008). Total daily dose should be divided by 3; delivered every 8 hours. Methadone is significantly more potent with repetitive dosing (due to its active metabolite). Begin methadone at lower doses and gradually titrate. Applicability to pediatric patients is unknown.

REFERENCES

National Cancer Institute, "Pain (PDQ®)," Last Modified 5/7/09. Available at http://www.cancer.gov/cancertopics/pdq/supportivecare/pain/HealthProfessional/page1

National Comprehensive Cancer Network® (NCCN), "Clinical Practice Guidelines in Oncology™: Adult Cancer Pain," Version 1, 2009. Available at http://www.nccn.org/professionals/physician_gls/PDF/pain.pdf

Patanwala AE, Duby J, Waters D, et al, "Opioid Conversions in Acute Care," *Ann Pharmacother*, 2007, 41(2):255-66.

Principles of Analgesic Use in the Treatment of Acute Pain and Cancer Pain, 6th ed, Glenview, IL: American Pain Society, 2008.

SOME POTENTIAL PHOTOSENSITIZING AGENTS

Analgesics
Almotriptan
Nonsteroidal anti-inflammatory drugs[1]
  Celecoxib
  Diclofenac
  Flurbiprofen
  Ibuprofen
  Ketoprofen
  Meloxicam
  Nabumetone
  Naproxen
  Oxaprozin
  Piroxicam
  Tiaprofenic acid
Pentosan polysulfate sodium
SulfaSALAzine
SUMAtriptan
ZOLMitriptan

Antineoplastics
Capecitabine
Dacarbazine
Dasatinib
Epirubicin
Floxuridine
Flucytosine
Fluorouracil
Flutamide
Imatinib
Leuprolide
Methotrexate
Porfimer
Thioguanine
UFT
VinBLAStine

Antimicrobials
Amantadine
Atazanavir
Atovaquone and proguanil
Chloroquine
Dapsone
Demeclocycline[1]
Doxycycline[1]
Gentamicin
Griseofulvin
Interferon alpha-n3
Interferon beta-1b
Itraconazole
Kanamycin
Minocycline
Oxytetracycline
Pyrazinamide
Quinolones[1]
  Ciprofloxacin
  Gemifloxacin
  Levofloxacin
  Lomefloxacin
  Nalidixic acid
  Norfloxacin
  Ofloxacin
  Sparfloxacin
SulfADIAZINE

Sulfadoxine and pyrimethamine
Sulfamethoxazole and trimethoprim
Sulfisoxazole
Tetracycline
Valacyclovir
Voriconazole

Cardiovascular Agents
Antilipemic agents
  Atorvastatin
  Fenofibrate
  Fluvastatin
  Gemfibrozil
  Lovastatin
  Pravastatin
  Simvastatin
ACE inhibitors
  Benazepril
  Enalapril
  Fosinopril
  Lisinopril
  Quinapril
  Ramipril
Beta-Blockers
  Carvedilol
  Metoprolol
  Sotalol
Calcium channel blockers
  Diltiazem
  NIFEdipine
Diuretics
  AcetaZOLAMIDE
  Furosemide
  Methazolamide
  Metolazone
  Thiazides[1]
    Chlorothiazide
    Chlorthalidone
    Hydrochlorothiazide
    Methyclothiazide
    Polythiazide
Miscellaneous cardiovascular agents
  Amiodarone[1]
  Losartan
  QuiNIDine[1]

CNS Agents
Antidepressants, tricyclic[1]
  Amitriptyline
  Amoxapine
  ClomiPRAMINE
  Desipramine
  Doxepin
  Imipramine
  Loxapine
  Maprotiline
  Nortriptyline
  Protriptyline
  Trimipramine
Antidepressants, SSRI
  FLUoxetine
  Sertraline

Antidepressants, miscellaneous
 BuPROPion
 DULoxetine
 Mirtazapine
 Nefazodone
Antihistamines
 Cetirizine
 Clemastine
 Cyproheptadine
 DiphenhydrAMINE
 Loratadine
 Meclizine
Antipsychotic, miscellaneous
 Flupenthixol
 Haloperidol
 Molindone
 QUEtiapine
 RisperiDONE
 Thiothixene
 Ziprasidone
 Zuclopenthixol
Antipsychotic, phenothiazine
 ChlorproMAZINE
 FluPHENAZine
 Methotrimeprazine
 Perphenazine
 Pipotiazine
 Prochlorperazine
 Promethazine
 Trifluoperazine
Antiseizure agents
 CarBAMazepine
 Felbamate
 LamoTRIgine
 OXcarbazepine
 Topiramate
 Valproic acid

Miscellaneous CNS agents
 ChlordiazePOXIDE
 Ropinirole
 Zaleplon

Hypoglycemic Agents
 ChlorproPAMIDE
 Gliclazide
 Glimepiride
 GlipiZIDE
 GlyBURIDE
 TOLAZamide
 TOLBUTamide

Skin Agents
 Acitretin
 Coal tar
 Hexachlorophene
 Silver sulfADIAZINE
 Tretinoin
 Triamcinolone

Miscellaneous Agents
 Acamprosate
 Alendronate
 Anagrelide
 Cevimeline
 Cromolyn
 Danazol
 Droperidol
 Glatiramer
 Pilocarpine
 Rabeprazole
 Sildenafil
 Tacrolimus
 Thalidomide
 Vardenafil
 Verteporfin

[1]A 2004 NEJM paper identifies the marked drugs as being established as photosensitizing (Morison WL, "Clinical Practice. Photosensitivity," *N Engl J Med*, 2004, 350(11):1111-7). In light of sporadic and limited case reports, most other drugs labeled as photosensitizing are apparently only weakly and rarely so.

ASTHMA

MANAGEMENT OF ASTHMA IN ADULTS

Goals of Asthma Treatment

- Prevent chronic and troublesome symptoms: Minimal or no chronic symptoms day or night
- No limitations on activities; no work missed
- Minimal use of inhaled short-acting beta$_2$-agonist (≤2 days/week, <1 canister/month) (not including prevention of exercise induced asthma)
- Minimal or no adverse effects from medications
- Maintain (near) normal pulmonary function
- Prevent recurrent exacerbations (ie, trips to emergency department or hospitalizations)

All Patients

- Short-acting bronchodilator: **Inhaled beta$_2$-agonists** as needed for symptoms.
- Intensity of treatment will depend on severity of exacerbation; see "Management of Asthma Exacerbations".
- Use of short-acting inhaled beta$_2$-agonists on a daily basis, or increasing use, indicates the need to initiate or titrate long-term control therapy.

Education

- Teach self-management.
- Teach about controlling environmental factors (avoidance of allergens or other factors that contribute to asthma severity).
- Review administration technique and compliance with patient.
- Use a written action plan to help educate.

Stepwise Approach for Managing Asthma in Adults

Symptoms	Lung Function	Daily Medications
STEP 6: Severe Asthma		
Day: Throughout the day Night: Often 7 times/week SABA use: Several times/day	FEV$_1$ <60% predicted FEV$_1$/FVC reduced 5%	**Preferred:** High dose ICS plus LABA plus oral corticosteroid AND Consider: Omalizumab (in those with allergies)[1]
STEP 5: Severe Asthma		
Day: Throughout the day Night: Often 7 times/week SABA use: Several times/day	FEV$_1$ <60% predicted FEV$_1$/FVC reduced 5%	**Preferred:** High dose ICS plus LABA AND Consider: Omalizumab (in those with allergies)[1]
STEP 4: Severe Asthma		
Day: Throughout the day Night: Often 7 times/week SABA use: Several times/day	FEV$_1$ <60% predicted FEV$_1$/FVC reduced 5%	**Preferred:** Medium dose ICS plus LABA **Alternatives[2]:** Medium dose ICS plus either LTRA, theophylline, or zileuton[3]
STEP 3: Moderate Asthma		
Day: Daily Night: >1 night/week (not nightly) SABA use: Daily	FEV$_1$ >60%, <80% predicted FEV$_1$/FVC reduced 5%	**Preferred:** Low dose ICS plus LABA OR Medium dose ICS **Alternatives[2]:** Low dose ICS plus either LTRA, theophylline, or zileuton[3]

Stepwise Approach for Managing Asthma in Adults *(continued)*

Symptoms	Lung Function	Daily Medications
STEP 2: Mild Asthma		
Day: >2 days/week (not daily) Night: 3-4 times/month SABA use: >2 days/week, no more than once per day (not daily)	FEV$_1$ <80% FEV$_1$/FVC normal	**Preferred:** Low dose ICS **Alternatives[2]:** LTRA, nedocromil, or theophylline
STEP 1: Intermittent Asthma		
Day: ≤2 days/week Night: ≤2 nights/month SABA use: ≤2 days/week	FEV$_1$ normal between exacerbations FEV$_1$ >80% predicted FEV$_1$/FVC normal	Preferred: SABA as needed

Note: Treatment options within each step are listed in alphabetical order.

Steps 2-4: Consider subcutaneous allergen immunotherapy for patients with allergic asthma.[1]

Consult with asthma specialist if Step 4 or higher care is needed.

FEV$_1$ = forced expiratory volume in 1 second; FVC = forced vital capacity; ICS = inhaled corticosteroid; LABA = long-acting inhaled beta$_2$-agonist; SABA = short-acting inhaled beta$_2$-agonist; LTRA = leukotriene receptor antagonist.

[1]When using immunotherapy or omalizumab, clinicians should be prepared to identify and treat anaphylaxis in the event it occurs.

[2]If alternative treatment is used and response is inadequate, discontinue it and use preferred treatment before stepping up.

[3]Zileuton is less desirable alternative due to limited studies and need to monitor liver function.

Notes:

- **The stepwise approach presents general guidelines to assist clinical decision making; it is not intended to be a specific prescription. Asthma is highly variable; clinicians should tailor specific medication plans to the needs and circumstances of individual patients.**

- Gain control as quickly as possible; then decrease treatment to the least medication necessary to maintain control.

- A rescue course of systemic corticosteroids may be needed at any time and at any step.

- Some patients with intermittent asthma experience severe and life-threatening exacerbations separated by long periods of normal lung function and no symptoms. This may be especially common with exacerbations provoked by respiratory infections.

- At each step, patient education, environmental control, management of comorbidities emphasized.

- Antibiotics are not recommended for treatment of acute asthma exacerbations except where there is evidence or suspicion of bacterial infection.

- Consultation with an asthma specialist is recommended for moderate or severe persistent asthma.

- Peak flow monitoring for patients with moderate-severe persistent asthma and patients who have a history of severe exacerbations should be considered.

Management of Asthma Exacerbations: Home Treatment

Assess Severity

- **Patients at high risk for a fatal attack require immediate medical attention after initial treatment.**

- Symptoms and signs suggestive of a more serious exacerbation such as marked breathlessness, inability to speak more than short phrases, use of accessory muscles, or drowsiness should result in initial treatment while immediately consulting with a clinician.

- If available, measure PEF—values of 50% to 79% predicted or personal best indicate the need for quick-relief mediation. Depending on the response to treatment, contact with a clinician may also be indicated. Values below 50% indicate the need for immediate medical care.

↓

Initial Treatment

- Inhaled SABA: Up to two treatments 20 minutes apart of 2–6 puffs by metered-dose inhaler (MDI) or nebulizer treatments.

- Note: Medication delivery is highly variable. Children and individuals who have exacerbations of lesser severity may need fewer puffs than suggested above.

Good Response	Incomplete Response	Poor Response
No wheezing or dyspnea (assess tachypnea in young children).	Persistent wheezing and dyspnea (tachypnea).	Marked wheezing and dyspnea.
PEF ≥80% predicted or personal best.	PEF 50% to 79% predicted or personal best.	PEF <50% predicted or personal best.
• Contact clinician for followup instructions and further management.	• Add oral systemic corticosteroid.	• Add oral systemic corticosteroid
• May continue inhaled SABA every 3–4 hours for 24–48 hours.	• Continue inhaled SABA.	• Repeat inhaled SABA immediately.

• Consider short course of oral systemic corticosteroids.	• Contact clinician urgently (this day) for further instruction.	• If distress is severe and nonresponsive to initial treatment:
		  – Call your doctor AND
		  – **PROCEED TO EMERGENCY DEPARTMENT;**
		  – Consider calling 911 (ambulance transport

↓

- To emergency department.

MDI: Metered-dose inhaler; PEF: Peak expiratory flow; SABA: Short-acting beta₂-agonist (quick relief inhaler)

2018

Management of Asthma Exacerbations: Emergency Department and Hospital-Based Care

Initial Assessment
Brief history, physical examination (auscultation, use of accessory muscles, heart rate, respiratory rate), PEF or FEV_1, oxygen saturation, and other tests as indicated

FEV_1 or PEF ≥40% (Mild-to-Moderate)
- Oxygen to achieve SaO_2 ≥90%
- Inhaled SABA by nebulizer or MDI with valved holding chamber, up to 3 doses in first hour
- Oral systemic corticosteroids if no immediate response or if patient recently took oral systemic corticosteroids

FEV_1 or PEF <40% (Severe)
- Oxygen to achieve SaO_2 ≥90%
- High-dose inhaled SABA plus ipratropium by nebulizer or MDI plus valved holding chamber, every 20 minutes or continuously for 1 hour
- Oral systemic corticosteroids

Impending or Actual Respiratory Arrest
- Intubation and mechanical ventilation with 100% oxygen
- Nebulized SABA and ipratropium
- I.V. corticosteroids
- Consider adjunct therapies

Repeat Assessment
Symptoms, physical examination, PEF, O_2 saturation, other tests as needed

Admit to Hospital Intensive Care
(see box)

Moderate Exacerbation
FEV_1 or PEF 40% to 69% predicted/personal best
Physical exam: Moderate symptoms
- Inhaled SABA every 60 minutes
- Oral systemic corticosteroid
- Continue treatment 1-3 hours, provided there is improvement; make admit decision in <4 hours

Severe Exacerbation
FEV_1 or PEF <40% predicted/personal best
Physical exam: Severe symptoms at rest, accessory muscle use, chest retraction
History: High-risk patient
No improvement after initial treatment
- Oxygen
- Nebulized SABA plus ipraropium, hourly or continuous
- Oral systemic corticosteroids
- Concider adjunct therapies

Good Response
- FEV_1 or PEF ≥70%
- Response sustained 60 minutes after last treatment
- No distress
- Physical exam: Normal

Incomplete Response
- FEV_1 or PEF 40% to 69%
- Mild-to-moderate symtoms

Individualized decision re: Hospitalization (see text)

Poor Response
- FEV_1 or PEF <40%
- PCO_2 ≥42 mm Hg
- Physical exam: Symptoms severe, drowsiness, confusion

Discharge Home
- Continue treatment with inhaled SABA.
- Continue course of oral systemic corticosteroid.
- Consider initiation of an ICS.
- Patient Education
  - Review medications, including inhaler technique.
  - Review/initiate action plan.
  - Recommend close medical follow-up.

Admit to Hospital Ward
- Oxygen
- Inhaled SABA
- Systemic (oral or intravenous) corticosteroid
- Consider adjunct therapies
- Monitor vital signs, FEV_1 or PEF, SaO_2

Improve

Admit to Hospital Intensive Care
- Oxygen
- Inhaled SABA hourly or continuously
- Intravenous corticosteroid
- Consider adjunct therapies
- Possible intubation and mechanical ventilation

Improve

Discharge Home
- Continue treatment with inhaled SABAs.
- Continue course of oral systemic corticosteroid.
- Continue on ICS. For those not on long-term control therapy, consider initiation of an ICS.
- Patient education (eg, review medications, including inhaler technique and, whenever possible, environmental control measures; review/initiate action plan; recommend close medical follow-up).
- Before discharge, schedule follow-up appointment with primary care provider and/or asthma specialist in 1-4 weeks.

FEV_1 = forced expiratory volume in 1 second; ICS = inhaled corticosteroid; MDI = metered dose inhaler; PCO_2 = partial pressure carbon dioxide; PEF = peak expiratory flow; SABA = short-acting beta$_2$-agonist; SaO_2 = oxygen saturation

ESTIMATED COMPARATIVE <u>DAILY</u> DOSAGES FOR INHALED CORTICOSTEROIDS

Adults

Drug	Low Daily Dose	Medium Daily Dose	High Daily Dose
Beclomethasone HFA 40 mcg/puff 80 mcg/puff	80-240 mcg	>240-480 mcg	>480 mcg
Budesonide DPI 90 mcg/puff 180 mcg/puff 200 mcg/puff	180-600 mcg	>600-1200 mcg	>1200 mcg
Flunisolide 250 mcg/puff	500-1000 mcg	>1000-2000 mcg	>2000 mcg
Flunisolide HFA 80 mcg/puff	320 mcg	>320-640 mcg	>640 mcg
Fluticasone HFA 44 mcg/puff 110 mcg/puff 220 mcg/puff	88-264 mcg	>264-440 mcg	>440 mcg
Mometasone DPI 220 mcg/puff	220 mcg	440 mcg	>440 mcg

DPI = dry powder inhaler; HFA = hydrofluoroalkane.

Reference

Expert Panel Report 3, "Guidelines for the Diagnosis and Management of Asthma," *Clinical Practice Guidelines*, National Institutes of Health, National Heart, Lung, and Blood Institute, NIH Publication No. 08-4051, prepublication 2007. Available at http://www.nhlbi.nih.gov/guidelines/asthma/asthgdln.htm.

HYPERLIPIDEMIA MANAGEMENT

MORTALITY

There is a strong link between serum cholesterol and cardiovascular mortality. This association becomes stronger in patients with established coronary artery disease. Lipid-lowering trials show that reductions in LDL cholesterol are followed by reductions in mortality. In general, each 1% fall in LDL cholesterol confers a 2% reduction in cardiovascular events. The aim of therapy for hyperlipidemia is to decrease cardiovascular morbidity and mortality by lowering cholesterol to a target level using safe and cost-effective treatment modalities. The target LDL cholesterol is determined by the number of patient risk factors (see the following Risk Factors and Goal LDL Cholesterol tables). The goal is achieved through diet, lifestyle modification, and drug therapy. The basis for these recommendations is provided by longitudinal interventional studies, demonstrating that lipid-lowering in patients with prior cardiovascular events (secondary prevention) and in patients with hyperlipidemia but no prior cardiac event (primary prevention) lowers the occurrence of future cardiovascular events, including stroke.

Major Risk Factors That Modify LDL Goals

Positive risk factors	Male ≥45 years
	Female ≥55 years
	Family history of premature coronary heart disease, defined as CHD in male first-degree relative <55 years; CHD in female first-degree relative <65 years
	Cigarette smoking
	Hypertension (blood pressure ≥140/90 mm Hg) or taking antihypertensive medication
	Low HDL (<40 mg/dL [1.03 mmol/L])
Negative risk factors	High HDL (≥60 mg/dL [1.6 mmol/L])[1]

[1]If HDL is ≥60 mg/dL, may subtract one positive risk factor.

Adult Treatment Panel (ATP) III LDL-C Goals and Cutpoints for Therapeutic Lifestyle Changes (TLC) and Drug Therapy in Different Risk Categories

Risk Category	LDL-C Goal	Initiate TLC	Consider Drug Therapy[1]
High risk: CHD[2] or CHD risk equivalents[3] (10-year risk >20%)	<100 mg/dL (optional goal: <70 mg/dL)[4]	≥100 mg/dL[5]	≥100 mg/dL[6] (<100 mg/dL: Consider drug options)[1]
Moderately high risk: ≥2 risk factors[7] (10-year risk 10% to 20%)[8]	<130 mg/dL[9]	≥130 mg/dL[5]	≥130 mg/dL (100-120 mg/dL: Consider drug options)[10]
Moderate risk: ≥2 risk factors[7] (10-year risk <10%)[8]	<130 mg/dL	≥130 mg/dL	≥160 mg/dL
Lower risk: 0-1 risk factor[11]	<160 mg/dL	≥160 mg/dL	≥190 mg/dL (160-189 mg/dL: LDL-lowering drug optional)

[1]When LDL-lowering drug therapy is employed, it is advised that intensity of therapy be sufficient to achieve at least a 30% to 40% reduction in LDL-C levels.

[2]CHD includes history of myocardial infarction, unstable angina, stable angina, coronary artery procedures (angioplasty or bypass surgery), or evidence of clinically significant myocardial ischemia.

[3]CHD risk equivalents include clinical manifestations of noncoronary forms of atherosclerotic disease (peripheral arterial disease, abdominal aortic aneurysm, and carotid artery disease [transient ischemic attacks or stroke of carotid origin or >50% obstruction of a carotid artery]), diabetes, and 2+ risk factors with 10-year risk for hard CHD >20%.

[4]Very high risk favors the optional LDL-C goal of <70 mg/dL, and in patients with high triglycerides, non-HDL-C <100 mg/dL.

[5]Any person at high risk or moderately high risk who has lifestyle-related risk factors (eg, obesity, physical inactivity, elevated triglyceride, low HDL-C, or metabolic syndrome) is a candidate for therapeutic lifestyle changes to modify these risk factors regardless of LDL-C level.

(See additional footnotes on next page.)

(Footnotes continued from previous page.)

[6]If baseline LDL-C is <100 mg/dL, institution of an LDL-lowering drug is a therapeutic option on the basis of available clinical trial results. If a high-risk person has high triglycerides or low HDL-C, combining a fibrate or nicotinic acid with an LDL-lowering drug can be considered.

[7]Risk factors include cigarette smoking, hypertension (BP ≥140/90 mm Hg or on antihypertensive medication), low HDL cholesterol (<40 mg/dL), family history of premature CHD (CHD in male first-degree relative <55 years of age; CHD in female first-degree relative <65 years of age), and age (men ≥45 years; women ≥55 years).

[8]Electronic 10-year risk calculators are available at www.nhlbi.nih.gov/guidelines/cholesterol.

[9]Optional LDL-C goal <100 mg/dL.

[10]For moderately high-risk persons, when LDL-C level is 100-129 mg/dL, at baseline or on lifestyle therapy, initiation of an LDL-lowering drug to achieve an LDL-C level <100 mg/dL is a therapeutic option on the basis of available clinical trial results.

[11]Almost all people with zero or 1 risk factor have a 10-year risk <10%, and 10-year risk assessment in people with zero or 1 risk factor thus not necessary.

Any person with elevated LDL cholesterol or other form of hyperlipidemia should undergo evaluation to rule out secondary dyslipidemia. Causes of secondary dyslipidemia include diabetes, hypothyroidism, obstructive liver disease, chronic renal failure, and drugs that increase LDL and decrease HDL (progestins, anabolic steroids, corticosteroids).

Elevated Serum Triglyceride Levels

Elevated serum triglyceride levels may be an independent risk factor for coronary heart disease. Factors that contribute to hypertriglyceridemia include obesity, inactivity, cigarette smoking, excess alcohol intake, high carbohydrate diets (>60% of energy intake), type 2 diabetes, chronic renal failure, nephrotic syndrome, certain medications (corticosteroids, estrogens, retinoids, higher doses of beta-blockers), and genetic disorders. Non-HDL cholesterol (total cholesterol minus HDL cholesterol) is a secondary focus for clinicians treating patients with high serum triglyceride levels (≥200 mg/dL). The goal for non-HDL cholesterol in patients with high serum triglyceride levels can be set 30 mg/dL higher than usual LDL cholesterol goals. Patients with serum triglyceride levels <200 mg/dL should aim for the target LDL cholesterol goal.

ATP classification of serum triglyceride levels:
- Normal triglycerides: <150 mg/dL
- Borderline-high: 150-199 mg/dL
- High: 200-499 mg/dL
- Very high: ≥500 mg/dL

NONDRUG THERAPY

Dietary therapy and lifestyle modifications should be individualized for each patient. A total lifestyle change is recommended for all patients. Dietary and lifestyle modifications should be tried for 3 months, if deemed appropriate. Nondrug and drug therapy should be initiated simultaneously in patients with highly elevated cholesterol (see LDL Cholesterol Goals and Cutpoints for Therapeutic Lifestyle Changes and Drug Therapy in Different Risk Categories table). Increasing physical activity and smoking cessation will aid in the treatment of hyperlipidemia and improve cardiovascular health.

Note: Refer to the National Cholesterol Education Program reference for details concerning the calculation of 10-year risk of CHD using Framingham risk scoring. Risk assessment tool is available on-line at http://hin.nhlbi.nih.gov/atpiii/calculator.asp?usertype=prof, last accessed March 14, 2002.

Total Lifestyle Change (TLC) Diet

	Recommended Intake
Total fat	25%-35% of total calories
Saturated fat[1]	<7% of total calories
Polyunsaturated fat	≤10% of total calories
Monounsaturated fat	≤20% of total calories
Carbohydrates[2]	50%-60% of total calories
Fiber	20-30 g/day
Protein	~15% of total calories
Cholesterol	<200 mg/day
Total calories[3]	Balance energy intake and expenditure to maintain desirable body weight/prevent weight gain

[1] *Trans* fatty acids (partially hydrogenated oils) intake should be kept low. These are found in potato chips, other snack foods, margarines and shortenings, and fast-foods.

[2] Complex carbohydrates including grains (especially whole grains, fruits, and vegetables).

[3] Daily energy expenditure should include at least moderate physical activity.

DRUG THERAPY

Drug therapy should be selected based on the patient's lipid profile, concomitant disease states, and the cost of therapy. The following table lists specific advantages and disadvantages for various classes of lipid-lowering medications. The expected reduction in lipids with therapy is listed in the Lipid-Lowering Agents table. Refer to individual drug monographs for detailed information.

Advantages and Disadvantages of Specific Lipid-Lowering Therapies

	Advantages	Disadvantages
Bile acid sequestrants	Good choice for ↑ LDL, especially when combined with a statin (↓ LDL ≤50%); low potential for systemic side effects; good choice for younger patients	May increase triglycerides; higher incidence of adverse effects; moderately expensive; drug interactions; inconvenient dosing
Niacin	Good choice for almost any lipid abnormality; inexpensive; greatest increase in HDL	High incidence of adverse effects; may adversely affect type 2 DM (with high dose >1.5 g/day) and gout; sustained release niacin may decrease the incidence of flushing and circumvent the need for multiple daily dosing; sustained release niacin may not increase HDL cholesterol or decrease triglycerides as well as immediate release niacin
HMG-CoA reductase inhibitors	Produces greatest ↓ in LDL; generally well-tolerated; convenient once-daily dosing; proven decrease in mortality	Expensive
Fibric acid derivatives	Good choice in patients with ↑ triglycerides where niacin is contraindicated or not well-tolerated	Variable effects on LDL
Ezetimibe	Additional cholesterol-lowering effects when combined with HMG-CoA reductase inhibitors	Effects similar to bile acid sequestrants

Lipid-Lowering Agents

Drug	Dose / Day	Effect on LDL (%)	Effect on HDL (%)	Effect on TG (%)
HMG-CoA Reductase Inhibitors				
Atorvastatin	10 mg	-39	+6	-19
	20 mg	-43	+9	-26
	40 mg	-50	+6	-29
	80 mg	-60	+5	-37
Fluvastatin	20 mg	-22	+3	-12
	40 mg	-25	+4	-14
	80 mg	-36	+6	-18
Lovastatin	10 mg	-21	+5	-10
	20 mg	-24	+7	-10
	40 mg	-30	+7	-14
	80 mg	-40	+9.5	-19
Pitavastatin	1 mg	-32	+8	-15
	2 mg	-36	+7	-19
	4 mg	-43	+5	-18
Pravastatin	10 mg	-22	+7	-15
	20 mg	-32	+2	-11
	40 mg	-34	+12	-24
	80 mg	-37	+3	-19
Rosuvastatin	5 mg	-45	+13	-35
	10 mg	-52	+14	-10
	20 mg	-55	+8	-23
	40 mg	-63	+10	-28
Simvastatin	5 mg	-26	+10	-12
	10 mg	-30	+12	-15
	20 mg	-38	+8	-19
	40 mg	-41	+13	-28
	80 mg	-47	+16	-33
Bile Acid Sequestrants				
Cholestyramine	4-24 g	-15 to -30	+3 to +5	+0 to +20
Colesevelam	6 tablets	-15	+3	+10
	7 tablets	-18	+3	+9
Colestipol	7-30 g	-15 to -30	+3 to +5	+0 to +20
Fibric Acid Derivatives				
Fenofibrate	67-200 mg	-20 to -31	+9 to +14	-30 to -50
Gemfibrozil	600 mg twice daily	-5 to -10[1]	+10 to +20	-40 to -60
Niacin	1.5-6 g	-5 to -25	+15 to +35	-20 to -50
2-Azetidinone				
Ezetimibe	10 mg	-15 to -20	+1 to +4	-5 to -8
Omega-3-Acid Ethyl Esters	4 g	+44.5	+9.1	-44.9
Combination Products				
Ezetimibe and simvastatin	10/10 mg	-45	+8	-23
	10/20 mg	-52	+10	-24
	10/40 mg	-55	+6	-23
	10/80 mg	-60	+6	-31
Niacin and lovastatin	1000/20 mg	-30	+20	-32
	1000/40 mg	-36	+20	-39
	1500/40 mg	-37	+27	-44
	2000/40 mg	-42	+30	-44
Niacin and simvastatin	1000/20 mg	-12	+21	-27
	1000/40 mg	-7	+15	-23
	2000/20 mg	-14	+29	-38
	2000/40 mg	-5	+24	-32

[1]May increase LDL in some patients.

Progression of Drug Therapy in Primary Prevention

Initiate LDL-lowering drug therapy	• Start statin or bile acid sequestrant or nicotinic acid
↓ 6 wk	
If LDL goal not achieved, intensify LDL-lowering therapy	• Consider higher dose of statin or add a bile acid sequestrant or nicotinic acid
↓ 6 wk	
If LDL goal not achieved, intensify drug therapy or refer to a lipid specialist	• If LDL goal achieved, treat other lipid risk factors
↓ q4-6mo	
Monitor response and adherence to therapy	

DRUG SELECTION

Lipid Profile	Monotherapy	Combination Therapies
Increased LDL with normal HDL and triglycerides (TG)	Resin Niacin[1] Statin	Resin plus niacin[1] or statin Statin plus niacin[1,2]
Increased LDL and increased TG (200-499 mg/dL)[2]	Intensify LDL-lowering therapy	Statin plus niacin[1,3] Statin plus fibrate[3]
Increased LDL and increased TG (≥500 mg/dL)[2]	Consider combination therapy (niacin,[1] fibrates, statin)	
Increased TG	Niacin[1] Fibrates	Niacin[1] plus fibrates
Increased LDL and low HDL	Niacin[1] Statin	Statin plus niacin[1,2]

[1]Avoid in diabetics.

[2]Emphasize weight reduction and increased physical activity.

[3]Risk of myopathy with combination.

Resins = bile acid sequestrants; statins = HMG-CoA reductase inhibitors; fibrates = fibric acid derivatives (eg, gemfibrozil, fenofibrate).

COMBINATION DRUG THERAPY

If after at least 6 weeks of therapy at the maximum recommended or tolerated dose, the patient's LDL cholesterol is not at target, consider optimizing nondrug measures, prescribing a higher dose of current lipid-lowering drug, or adding another lipid-lowering medication to the current therapy. Successful drug combinations include statin and niacin, statin and bile acid sequestrant, or niacin and bile acid sequestrant. At maximum recommended doses, LDL cholesterol may be decreased by 50% to 60% with combination therapy. This is the same reduction achieved by atorvastatin 40 mg twice daily. If a bile acid sequestrant is used with other lipid-lowering agents, space doses 1 hour before or 4 hours after the bile acid sequestrant administration. Statins combined with either fenofibrate, gemfibrozil, or niacin increase the risk of rhabdomyolysis. In this situation, patient education (muscle pain/weakness) and careful follow-up are warranted.

HYPERLIPIDEMIA MANAGEMENT

References

Guidelines

American Diabetes Association, "Standards of Medical Care in Diabetes - 2010," *Diabetes Care*, 2010, 33(Suppl 1): S11-61.

Brunzell JD, Davidson M, Furberg CD, et al, "Lipoprotein Management in Patients With Cardiometabolic Risk: Consensus Statement From the American Diabetes Association and the American College of Cardiology Foundation," *Diabetes Care*, 2008, 31(4):811-22.

Grundy SM, Cleeman JI, Merz CN, et al, "Implications of Recent Clinical Trials for the National Cholesterol Education Program Adult Treatment Panel III Guidelines," *J Am Coll Cardiol*, 2004, 44(3):720-32.

National Cholesterol Education Program, "Third Report of the Expert Panel on Detection, Evaluation, and Treatment of High Blood Cholesterol in Adults (Adult Treatment Panel III)," *JAMA*, 2001, 285(19):2486-97.

Others

Berthold HK, Sudhop T, and von Bergmann K, "Effect of a Garlic Oil Preparation on Serum Lipoproteins and Cholesterol Metabolism: A Randomized Controlled Trial," *JAMA*, 1998, 279(23):1900-2.

Bertolini S, Bon GB, Campbell LM, et al, "Efficacy and Safety of Atorvastatin Compared to Pravastatin in Patients With Hypercholesterolemia," *Atherosclerosis*, 1997, 130(1-2):191-7.

Blankenhorn DH, Nessim SA, Johnson RL, et al, "Beneficial Effects of Combined Colestipol-Niacin Therapy on Coronary Atherosclerosis and Venous Bypass Grafts," *JAMA*, 1987, 257(23):3233-40.

Bradford RH, Shear CL, Chremos AN, et al, "Expanded Clinical Evaluation of Lovastatin (EXCEL) Study Results. I. Efficacy in Modifying Plasma Lipoproteins and Adverse Event Profile in 8245 Patients With Moderate Hypercholesterolemia," *Arch Intern Med*, 1991, 151(1):43-9.

Brown G, Albers JJ, Fisher LD, et al, "Regression of Coronary Artery Disease as a Result of Intensive Lipid-Lowering Therapy in Men With High Levels of Apolipoprotein B," *N Engl J Med*, 1990, 323(19):1289-98.

Capuzzi DM, Guyton JR, Morgan JM, et al, "Efficacy and Safety of an Extended-Release Niacin (Niaspan®): A Long-Term Study," *Am J Cardiol*, 1998, 82(12A):74U-81U.

Coronary Drug Project Research Program, "Clofibrate and Niacin in Coronary Heart Disease," *JAMA*, 1975, 231(4):360-81.

Dart A, Jerums G, Nicholson G, et al, "A Multicenter, Double-Blind, One-Year Study Comparing Safety and Efficacy of Atorvastatin Versus Simvastatin in Patients With Hypercholesterolemia," *Am J Cardiol*, 1997, 80(1):39-44.

Davidson MH, Dillon MA, Gordon B, et al, "Colesevelam Hydrochloride (Cholestagel): A New Potent Bile Acid Sequestrant Associated With a Low Incidence of Gastrointestinal Side Effects," *Arch Intern Med*, 1999, 159(16):1893-900.

Davidson M, McKenney J, Stein E, et al, "Comparison of One-Year Efficacy and Safety of Atorvastatin Versus Lovastatin in Primary Hypercholesterolemia," *Am J Cardiol*, 1997, 79(11):1475-81.

Frick MH, Heinonen OP, Huttunen JK, et al, "Helsinki Heart Study: Primary-Prevention Trial With Gemfibrozil in Middle-Aged Men With Dyslipidemia," *N Engl J Med*, 1987, 317(20):1237-45.

Garber AM, Browner WS, and Hulley SB, "Clinical Guideline, Part 2: Cholesterol Screening in Asymptomatic Adults, Revisited," *Ann Intern Med*, 1995, 124(5):518-31.

Johannesson M, Jonsson B, Kjekshus J, et al, "Cost-Effectiveness of Simvastatin Treatment to Lower Cholesterol Levels in Patients With Coronary Heart Disease. Scandinavian Simvastatin Survival Study Group," *N Engl N Med*, 1997, 336(5):332-6.

Jones P, Kafonek S, Laurora I, et al, "Comparative Dose Efficacy Study of Atorvastatin Versus Simvastatin, Pravastatin, Lovastatin, and Fluvastatin in Patients With Hypercholesterolemia," *Am J Cardiol*, 1998, 81(5):582-7.

Kasiske BL, Ma JZ, Kalil RS, et al, "Effects of Antihypertensive Therapy on Serum Lipids," *Ann Intern Med*, 1995, 122(2):133-41.

Lipid Research Clinics Program, "The Lipid Research Clinics Coronary Primary Prevention Trial Results: I. Reduction in Incidence of Coronary Heart Disease," *JAMA*, 1984, 251(3):351-64.

Mauro VF and Tuckerman CE, "Ezetimibe for Management of Hypercholesterolemia," *Ann Pharmacother*, 2003, 37(6):839-48.

Multiple Risk Factor Intervention Trial Research Group, "Multiple Risk Factor Intervention Trial: Risk Factor Changes and Mortality Results," *JAMA*, 1982, 248(12):1465-77.

Pitt B, Waters D, Brown WV, et al, "Aggressive Lipid-Lowering Therapy Compared With Angioplasty in Stable Coronary Artery Disease. Atorvastatin Versus Revascularization Treatment Investigators," *N Engl J Med*, 1999, 341(2):70-6.

Ross SD, Allen IE, Connelly JE, et al, "Clinical Outcomes in Statin Treatment Trials: A Meta-Analysis," *Arch Intern Med*, 1999, 159(15):1793-802.

Sacks FM, Pfeffer MA, Moye LA, et al, "The Effect of Pravastatin on Coronary Events After Myocardial Infarction in Patients With Average Cholesterol Levels," *N Engl J Med*, 1996, 335(14):1001-9.

Scandinavian Simvastatin Survival Study, "Randomized Trial of Cholesterol Lowering in 4444 Patients With Coronary Heart Disease: The Scandinavian Simvastatin Survival Study (4S)," *Lancet*, 1994, 344(8934):1383-9.

Schrott HG, Bittner V, Vittinghoff E, et al, "Adherence to National Cholesterol Education Program Treatment Goals in Postmenopausal Women With Heart Disease. The Heart and Estrogen/Progestin Replacement Study (HERS)," *JAMA*, 1997, 277(16):1281-6.

Shepherd J, Cobbe SM, Ford I, et al, "Prevention of Coronary Heart Disease With Pravastatin in Men With Hypercholesterolemia, The West of Scotland Coronary Prevention Study Group," *N Engl J Med*, 1995, 333(20):1301-7.

Stein EA, Davidson MH, Dobs AS, et al, "Efficacy and Safety of Simvastatin 80 mg/day in Hypercholesterolemic Patients. The Expanded Dose Simvastatin U.S. Study Group," *Am J Cardiol*, 1998, 82(3):311-6.

OSTEOPOROSIS MANAGEMENT

PREVALENCE

Osteoporosis affects more than 10 million Americans. An additional 34 million Americans have low bone density of the hip. An osteoporosis-related fracture will occur in approximately one out of every two Caucasian females at some point in her lifetime, and will occur in approximately one in five men.

CONSEQUENCES

Fractures and the complications resulting from fractures are the clinically significant sequelae of osteoporosis. Fractures may result in pain, physical limitations, lifestyle changes, and decreased quality of life. In particular, hip fractures result in a 10% to 20% excess mortality in one year. In the U.S., osteoporosis-related fractures result in heavy economic burden caused by the >432,000 hospitalizations, almost 2.5 million medical office visits, and ~180,000 nursing home admissions that occur annually as a result.

RISK FACTORS

Conditions, Diseases, and Medications

- Postmenopausal women and men ≥50 years of age
- Endocrine disorders, such as adrenal insufficiency, Cushing's disease, diabetes mellitus, hyperparathyroidism, thyrotoxicosis
- Excessive alcohol intake (≥3 drinks/day)
- Excessive vitamin A intake
- Falls
- Parental history of hip fracture
- Genetic factors, due to conditions such as cystic fibrosis, Ehlers-Danlos, Gaucher's disease, glycogen storage diseases, hemochromatosis, homocystinuria, hypophosphatasia, idiopathic hypercalciuria, Marfan syndrome, Menkes steely hair syndrome, osteogenesis imperfecta, porphyria, Riley-Day syndrome
- Gastrointestinal disorders, such as celiac disease, gastric bypass, GI surgery, inflammatory bowel disease, malabsorption, pancreatic disease, primary biliary cirrhosis
- Hematologic disorders, such as hemophilia, leukemia/lymphoma, multiple myeloma, sickle cell disease, systemic mastocytosis, thalassemia
- High caffeine and/or sodium intake
- Hypogonadal states, due to conditions such as androgen insensitivity, anorexia, athletic amenorrhea, hyperprolactinemia, panhypopituitarism, premature ovarian failure, Turner's and Klinefelter's syndrome
- Low calcium and/or vitamin D intake
- Medications: Aluminum-containing antacids (excessive use), anticoagulants (heparin), anticonvulsants, aromatase inhibitors, barbiturates, chemotherapy, cyclosporine A, depo-medroxyprogesterone, glucocorticoids (≥5 mg/day of prednisone or equivalent for ≥3 months), gonadotropin-releasing hormone agonists, heparin, lithium, parenteral nutrition, tacrolimus
- Miscellaneous conditions/diseases, including amyloidosis, chronic metabolic acidosis, depression, emphysema, end-stage renal disease, epilepsy, heart failure, idiopathic scoliosis, multiple sclerosis, muscular dystrophy, post-transplant bone disease, sarcoidosis
- Previous fracture as an adult
- Rheumatic/autoimmune diseases, such as ankylosing spondylitis, lupus, rheumatoid arthritis
- Sedentary lifestyle or immobilization
- Smoking (active or passive)
- Thinness (low body mass index)

◀ DIAGNOSIS / MONITORING

- Bone mineral density (BMD) measurement using Dual-energy x-ray absorptiometry (DXA) bone density scan[1]

- U.S.-adapted WHO Fracture Risk Algorithm (FRAX®; www.nof.org and www.shef.ac.uk/FRAX)[2]

[1]BMD measurement by DXA at the hip or spine is used to establish or confirm an osteoporosis diagnosis.

[2]US-FRAX® is designed to calculate the 10 year probability of a hip fracture and the 10 year probability of a major osteoporotic fracture (vertebral, hip, forearm, or humerus fracture). Application of Frax™ is intended for postmenopausal women and men ≥50 years of age (not for younger adults or pediatrics) and results apply only to previously untreated patients.

Definition of Osteoporosis[1]

Normal: T score at -1.0 and above
Low bone mass or "osteopenia": T score between -1.0 and -2.5
Osteoporosis: T score at -2.5 or below

[1]Based on World Health Organization (WHO) established definition of osteoporosis using BMD measurements by DXA devices at the spine, hip or forearm. T-score values are based on standard deviations (SD) below that of a "young normal" adult. The WHO diagnostic classification only applies to postmenopausal women and men ≥50 years of age; not applicable for premenopausal women, men <50 years of age or pediatrics.

Bone mineral density (BMD) testing

Recommend for the following patients:

- All women ≥65 years and men ≥70 years

- High risk postmenopausal women and men aged 50-69 years

- Women in menopausal transition if increased fracture risk present (eg, low body weight, prior low-trauma fracture, receiving high risk medication)

- Patients with a history of a fracture (occurring after age 50)

- Adults with a predisposing condition associated with low bone mass or loss (see Risk Factors)

- Any patient being considered for pharmacologic therapy for osteoporosis or receiving treatment for osteoporosis (monitoring typically performed every 2 years unless more frequent testing warranted)

- Any patient not receiving therapy but evidence of bone loss would lead to treatment

Consider for the following patients:

- Postmenopausal women discontinuing estrogen

PREVENTION / TREATMENT

- Fall prevention (eg, visual/hearing checks, minimizing pharmacologic agents that contribute to fall risk, checking environment for safety hazards)

- Weight-bearing exercise (eg, walking) and muscle strengthening, as tolerated

- Avoidance of tobacco use and excessive alcohol intake

- Adequate intake of at least 1200 mg **elemental** calcium daily in the form of dietary calcium or calcium supplementation, particularly women ≥50 years of age. Intakes exceeding 1200-1500 mg offer limited additional benefit and may increase the risk for cardiovascular disease or kidney stones. Also refer to table located at the end of appendix piece for selected calcium supplement information.

- Adequate intake of at least 800-1000 int. units of vitamin D for adults ≥50 years of age. Measuring serum vitamin D concentrations may be warranted, particularly in those at greatest risk for deficiency, to allow for the administration of vitamin D replacement. **Note:** Certain patients at risk for vitamin D deficiency (eg, elderly, diseases associated with malabsorption, chronic renal insufficiency) may require higher intakes.

Pharmacologic Therapy

- Consider using FDA approved pharmacologic therapy in postmenopausal women and men ≥50 years with a hip or vertebral fracture **or** those with a T score ≤ -2.5 at the femoral neck or spine (after excluding secondary causes) **or** those with low bone mass (T score between -1.0 and -2.5 at the femoral neck or spine) in combination with a 10-year hip fracture probability of ≥3% or a 10-year osteoporosis-related major fracture probability of ≥20% (based on the U.S.-adapted WHO algorithm)

1. Bisphosphonates: Oral bisphosphonates should be administered ≥30 minutes before first food or drink (except water) with 6-8 ounces tap water (**not** mineral water) and patients should remain upright (or raise head of bed to at least a 30° angle) to avoid ulcerative esophagitis. Consult individual monographs for details regarding use, precautions, and dosing and administration of any of the specific drugs mentioned below.

   Osteoporosis prevention: Postmenopausal females:

   - Alendronate: Oral: 5 mg once daily or 35 mg once weekly
   - Ibandronate: Oral: 2.5 mg once daily or 150 mg once per month
   - Risedronate: Oral: 5 mg once daily or 35 mg once weekly or one 75 mg tablet once daily on two consecutive days per month (total of 2 tablets/month) or 150 mg once per month
   - Zoledronic acid (Reclast®): I.V.: 5 mg infused over at least 15 minutes every 2 years

   Osteoporosis treatment:

   - Alendronate: Males and Postmenopausal females: Oral: 10 mg once daily or 70 mg once weekly
   - Ibandronate: Postmenopausal females:
     - Oral: 2.5 mg once daily or 150 mg once per month
     - I.V.: 3 mg every 3 months
   - Risedronate:
     - Postmenopausal females: Oral: 5 mg once daily or 35 mg once weekly or one 75 mg tablet once daily on two consecutive days per month (total of 2 tablets/month) or 150 mg once monthly
     - Males: Oral: 35 mg once weekly
   - Zoledronic acid (Reclast®): Males and Postmenopausal females: I.V.: 5 mg infused over at least 15 minutes every 12 months

   Glucocorticoid-induced osteoporosis prevention:

   - Risedronate: Oral: 5 mg once daily
   - Zoledronic acid (Reclast®): I.V.: 5 mg infused over at least 15 minutes every 12 months (in patients initiating or continuing prednisone ≥7.5 mg/day [or equivalent] and expected to remain on glucocorticoids for at least 12 months)

   Glucocorticoid-induced osteoporosis treatment:

   - Alendronate: Oral: 5 mg once daily; Postmenopausal women not receiving estrogen: 10 mg once daily
   - Risedronate: Oral: 5 mg once daily
   - Zoledronic acid (Reclast®): I.V.: 5 mg infused over at least 15 minutes every 12 months (in patients initiating or continuing prednisone ≥7.5 mg/day [or equivalent] and expected to remain on glucocorticoids for at least 12 months)

2. Estrogen agonist/antagonist (previously known as selective estrogen receptor modulators)

   Osteoporosis prevention and treatment: Postmenopausal females:

   - Raloxifene: Oral: 60 mg once daily; may be taken any time of the day without regard to meals but should be stopped 72 hours prior to or during immobilization due to risk of thromboembolic events.

3. Estrogens/hormone therapy: Should not be considered first agents for preventing osteoporosis due to increased risk of breast cancer, heart disease, stroke, and deep-vein thrombosis (DVT) found in the Women's Health Initiative study. Estrogens, as well as various combination therapies, including ethinyl estradiol and norethindrone (femhrt®) and estradiol and norgestimate (Prefest™), have been approved for the prevention of

◄

osteoporosis. The FDA recommends that approved nonestrogen treatments should be considered before the use of estrogen/hormone therapy for the sole purpose of prevention of osteoporosis.

Note: In women with an intact uterus, administer estrogen with oral progesterone; unopposed estrogen can cause endometrial cancer.

4. Calcitonin: Adequate dietary or supplemental calcium and vitamin D are essential.
    Osteoporosis treatment: Postmenopausal females (>5 years postmenopause):

    *   Calcitonin (Miacalcin®): I.M., SubQ: 100 units every other day (I.M. route is preferred if volume exceeds 2 mL)

    *   Calcitonin (Fortical®, Miacalcin®): Intranasal: 200 units (1 spray) in one nostril daily, alternate right and left nostril daily

5. Parathyroid hormone: Initial administration of teriparatide should occur under circumstances in which the patient may sit or lie down, in the event of orthostasis
    Osteoporosis treatment: Postmenopausal women at high risk of fracture or treatment of primary or hypogonadal osteoporosis in men at high risk of fracture:

    *   Teriparatide: SubQ: 20 mcg once daily

    Glucocorticoid induced osteoporosis treatment: Men and women:

    *   Teriparatide: SubQ: 20 mcg once daily

Calcium Type	Elemental Calcium	Equivalent Elemental Calcium	Example Brands
Acetate	25%	667 mg = 169 mg	Phos-Lo®
Carbonate	40%	364 mg = 145.6 mg	Florical®
		500 mg = 200 mg	Tums® chewable tablets
		1000 mg = 400 mg	Tums® Ultra chewable tablets
		1500 mg = 600 mg	Calcarb 600, Caltrate® 600, Nephro-Calci®
Citrate	21%	950 mg = 200 mg	Citracal®
Glubionate	6.5%	1.8 g/5 mL = 115 mg/5 mL	Various OTC and generic brands available
Gluconate	9%	500 mg = 45 mg	
Lactate	13%	650 mg = 84.5 mg	
Phosphate (tribasic)	39%	1565.2 mg = 600 mg	Posture®

References

Ashworth A, "Focus on Alendronate. A Nonhormonal Option for the Treatment of Osteoporosis in Postmenopausal Women," *Formulary*, 1996, 31:23-30.

Barrett-Connor E, Grady D, Sashegyi A, et al, "Raloxifene and Cardiovascular Events in Osteoporotic Postmenopausal Women: Four-Year Results From the MORE (Multiple Outcomes of Raloxifene Evaluation) Randomized Trial," *JAMA*, 2002, 287(7):847-57.

Hully S, Grady D, Bush T, et al, "Randomized Trial of Estrogen Plus Progestin for Secondary Prevention of Coronary Heart Disease in Postmenopausal Women. Heart and Estrogen/Progestin Replacement Study (HERS) Research Group," *JAMA*, 1998, 280(7):605-13.

Johnson SR, "Should Older Women Use Estrogen Replacement," *J Am Geriatr Soc*, 1996, 44(1):89-90.

NIH Consensus Development Panel on Optimal Calcium Intake, *JAMA*, 1994, 272(24):1942-8.

National Osteoporosis Foundation, "Clinician's Guide to Prevention and Treatment of Osteoporosis," Washington, DC: National Osteoporosis Foundation, 2010, 1-44. Available at http://www.nof.org/sites/default/files/pdfs/NOF_ClinicianGuide2009_v7.pdf.

Rossouw JE, Anderson GL, Prentice RL, et al, "Risks and Benefits of Estrogen Plus Progestin in Healthy Postmenopausal Women: Principle Results From the Women's Health Initiative Randomized Controlled Trial,"- *JAMA*, 2002, 288(3):321-33.

PARKINSON'S DISEASE MANAGEMENT

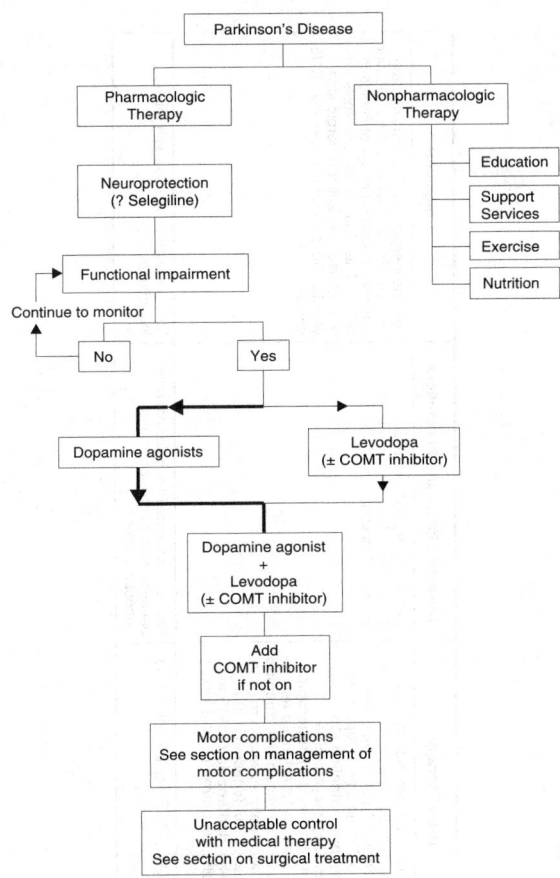

Recommendations for PD management are as follows:
- Ensure that correct diagnosis is made.
- Consider neuroprotective therapy as soon as diagnosis is made.
- Initiate symptomatic therapy with a dopamine agonist as appropriate.
- Supplement with levodopa when dopamine agonist monotherapy no longer provides satisfactory clinical control.
- Consider introducing supplemental levodopa therapy in combination with a COMT inhibitor to extend its elimination half-life.
- Consider surgical intervention when parkonsonism cannot be satisfactorily controlled with medical therapies.

Adapted from Olanow CW, Watts RL, and Koller WC, "An Algorithm (Decision Tree) for the Management of Parkinson's Disease (2001): Treatment Guidelines," *Neurology*, 2001, 56(11; Suppl 5):54.

PHARMACOTHERAPY OF URINARY INCONTINENCE

Incontinence Type	Drug Class	Drug Therapy	Adverse Effects and Precautions	Comments
Urge incontinence	Anticholinergic agents (antimuscarinic effects)	**Oxybutynin** (2.5 mg 2-3 times/day, extended release 5-30 mg once daily, or transdermal 1 patch twice weekly delivering 3.9 mg/day, or topical gel 1 g daily), **propantheline** (15-30 mg 3-5 times/day), **dicyclomine** (10-20 mg 3 times/day), **tolterodine** (1-2 mg twice daily; extended release capsule: 2-4 mg once daily), **trospium** (20 mg twice daily, extended release 60 mg daily), **solifenacin** (5-10 mg once daily), **darifenacin** (7.5-15 mg once daily), **fesoterodine** (4-8 mg once daily)	Dry mouth, blurred vision, constipation, dry skin, decreased cognitive function	Anticholinergics are the first-line drug therapy. Propantheline and dicyclomine are not considered drugs of choice in older adults. Darifenacin and solifenacin may cause less anticholinergic side effects. Trospium may cause less CNS effects.
	Tricyclic antidepressants (TCAs)	Imipramine (10-25 mg 1-4 times/day)	Not recommended for older patients because of anticholinergic and orthostatic effects.	May be used in women with mixed incontinence.

Incontinence Type	Drug Class	Drug Therapy	Adverse Effects and Precautions	Comments
Stress or combined urge/stress incontinence	Estrogen	Topical, intravaginal, dissolving tablets in postmenopausal women; administered with varying dosing intervals (twice weekly to once daily)	Should not be used if suspected or confirmed breast or endometrial cancer, active or past thromboembolism with past oral contraceptive, estrogen, or pregnancy	Medications may not play a strong role in treatment of stress incontinence. Oral estrogen should not be prescribed for this indication; may worsen incontinence.
	Tricyclic antidepressants (TCAs)	Imipramine (10-25 mg 1-4 times/day)	May worsen cardiac conduction abnormalities, postural hypotension, anticholinergic effects	TCAs are generally reserved for patients with an additional indication (eg, depression, neuralgia) at an initial dose of 10-25 mg 1-4 times/day.
Overflow	Alpha-adrenergic antagonists	**Terazosin** (1 mg at bedtime with first dose in supine position and increase by 1 mg every 4 days to maximum 10 mg/day); **doxazosin** (1 mg at bedtime with first dose in supine position and increase by 1 mg every 7-14 days to maximum 8 mg/day); **tamsulosin** (0.4 mg-0.8 mg daily); **alfuzosin** (10 mg daily); **silodosin** (8 mg daily)	Postural hypotension, headache, dizziness	Effective in men with overactive bladder symptoms associated with benign prostatic hypertrophy.

PHARMACOTHERAPY OF URINARY INCONTINENCE

References

Chapple C, Khullar V, Gabriel Z, et al, "The Effects of Antimuscarinic Treatments in Overactive Bladder: A Systematic Review and Meta-Analysis," *Eur Urol*, 2005, 48(1):5-26.

Herbison P, Hay-Smith J, Ellis G, et al, "Effectiveness of Anticholinergic Drugs Compared With Placebo in the Treatment of Overactive Bladder: Systematic Review," *BMJ*, 2003, 326(7394):841-4.

Resnick NM, "Urinary Incontinence," *Lancet*, 1995, 346(8967):94-9.

Rossouw JE, Anderson GL, Prentice RL, et al, "Risks and Benefits of Estrogen Plus Progestin in Healthy Postmenopausal Women: Principal Results From the Women's Health Initiative Randomized Controlled Trial," *JAMA*, 2002, 288(3):321-33.

TREATMENT OPTIONS FOR CONSTIPATION

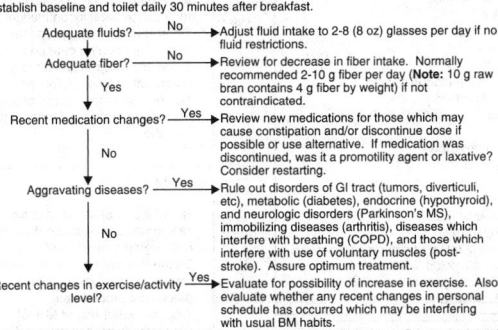

- Define constipation as no more than two bowel movements per week, or straining upon defecation 25% of the time or more. If possible, educate resident about this definition to develop cooperation.
- Verify constipation with digital exam and/or x-ray (radiography) if impaction is suspected.

Establish baseline and toilet daily 30 minutes after breakfast.

Adequate fluids? — No → Adjust fluid intake to 2-8 (8 oz) glasses per day if no fluid restrictions.

Adequate fiber? — No → Review for decrease in fiber intake. Normally recommended 2-10 g fiber per day (**Note:** 10 g raw bran contains 4 g fiber by weight) if not contraindicated.

Yes

Recent medication changes? — Yes → Review new medications for those which may cause constipation and/or discontinue dose if possible or use alternative. If medication was discontinued, was it a promotility agent or laxative? Consider restarting.

No

Aggravating diseases? — Yes → Rule out disorders of GI tract (tumors, diverticuli, etc), metabolic (diabetes), endocrine (hypothyroid), and neurologic disorders (Parkinson's MS), immobilizing diseases (arthritis), diseases which interfere with breathing (COPD), and those which interfere with use of voluntary muscles (post-stroke). Assure optimum treatment.

No

Recent changes in exercise/activity level? — Yes → Evaluate for possibility of increase in exercise. Also evaluate whether any recent changes in personal schedule has occurred which may be interfering with usual BM habits.

Once constipation is identified and contributing factors are ruled out, determine if any signs or symptoms of fecal impaction are exhibited (distended abdomen, fever, vomiting, confusion).

Not impacted ↓ Impacted

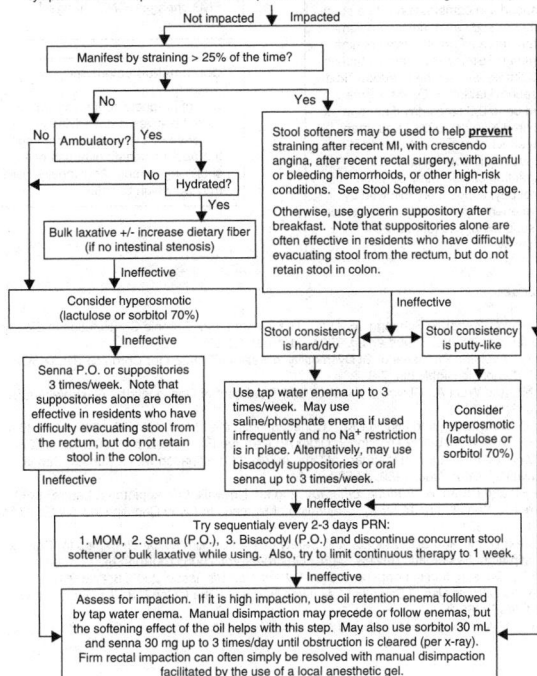

Manifest by straining > 25% of the time?

No ↓ Yes ↓

No — Ambulatory? — Yes

No — Hydrated? — Yes

Bulk laxative +/- increase dietary fiber (if no intestinal stenosis)
↓ Ineffective

Stool softeners may be used to help **prevent** straining after recent MI, with crescendo angina, after recent rectal surgery, with painful or bleeding hemorrhoids, or other high-risk conditions. See Stool Softeners on next page.

Otherwise, use glycerin suppository after breakfast. Note that suppositories alone are often effective in residents who have difficulty evacuating stool from the rectum, but do not retain stool in colon.

Consider hyperosmotic (lactulose or sorbitol 70%)
↓ Ineffective

Senna P.O. or suppositories 3 times/week. Note that suppositories alone are often effective in residents who have difficulty evacuating stool from the rectum, but do not retain stool in the colon.

Ineffective

↓ Ineffective

Stool consistency is hard/dry ←→ Stool consistency is putty-like

Use tap water enema up to 3 times/week. May use saline/phosphate enema if used infrequently and no Na+ restriction is in place. Alternatively, may use bisacodyl suppositories or oral senna up to 3 times/week.

Consider hyperosmotic (lactulose or sorbitol 70%)

↓ Ineffective ←

Try sequentially every 2-3 days PRN:
1. MOM, 2. Senna (P.O.), 3. Bisacodyl (P.O.) and discontinue concurrent stool softener or bulk laxative while using. Also, try to limit continuous therapy to 1 week.

↓ Ineffective

Assess for impaction. If it is high impaction, use oil retention enema followed by tap water enema. Manual disimpaction may precede or follow enemas, but the softening effect of the oil helps with this step. May also use sorbitol 30 mL and senna 30 mg up to 3 times/day until obstruction is cleared (per x-ray). Firm rectal impaction can often simply be resolved with manual disimpaction facilitated by the use of a local anesthetic gel.

TREATMENT OPTIONS FOR CONSTIPATION

One should expect gradual rather than immediate results from a newly instituted laxative regimen. Additionally, nondrug interventions should be maintained during pharmacologic treatment of constipation as this is one of the cornerstones of long-term management.

Constipating Drugs

Aluminum (antacids, sucralfate)
Anticholinergics (antiparkinsons)
Antihistamines
CCBs
Levodopa
Opiates
MAOIs
Tricyclic antidepressants
Aluminum
Calcium (supplements & antacids)
Iron
Phenothiazines
Diuretics
Clonidine
Guanabenz
Guanfacine
Disopyramide
Irritant laxatives (with cathartic colon)
Vinca alkaloids
5-HT$_3$ antagonists
Anticonvulsants

Stool Softeners

Stool softeners have no laxative action and are not helpful in alleviating chronic constipation and may cause fecal incontinence. Short-term use is appropriate to minimize straining caused by hard stools following rectal surgery or recent MI or when defecation causes hemorrhoidal pain, rectal bleeding, crescendo angina, or other high risk condition.

Saline Laxatives

Regular use of saline laxatives is not recommended because their risks outweigh the benefits of the laxative. Saline laxatives are only indicated for acute bowel evacuation for diagnostic procedures.
Also, note that use of Milk of Magnesia in renally impaired residents can result in Mg^{++} toxicity (hypotension, muscle weakness, EKG changes, CNS changes).

Opioid-Induced Constipation

Stimulant laxatives such as senna or bisacodyl in combination with a stool softener such as docusate sodium often serve as an effective first-line regimen. Senna P.O. up to 4 tablets 2-3 times/day may be needed. Next, bisacodyl tablets P.O. at bedtime and up to 2-3 times/day if needed. If desired, use docusate to augment the effect of one or both medications, especially if stool is hard. If impaction can be ruled out, use bisocodyl suppository followed by fleet enema (if needed). If impaction is suspected, see last step of pathway.

Combination Laxatives

Use of products containing two or more laxatives is not advised because of a lack of documented therapeutic benefit over use of a single ingredient. Additionally, risks may outweigh benefits.

References

Bosshard W, Dreher R, Schnegg JF, et al, "The Treatment of Chronic Constipation in Elderly People: An Update," *Drugs Aging,* 2004, 21(14):911-30.

Burke C, "Avoiding Problems of GI Dysmotility in Patients Treated for Chronic Pain," *ASCP* 1995 Symposia Highlights, 7-8.

Floch MH and Wald A, "Clinical Evaluation and Treatment of Constipation," *Gastrolenterologist,* 1994, 2(1):50-60.

Harari D, Gurwitz JH, and Minaker KL, "Constipation in the Elderly," *JAGS,* 1993; 41:1130-40.

Hsieh C, "Treatment of Constipation in Older Adults," *Am Fam Physician,* 2005, 72(11):2277-84.

Izard MW and Ellison FS, "Treatment of Drug Induced Constipation with a Purified Senna Derivative," *Conn Med,* 1962; 26:589.

Lange RL and DiPiro JT, *Pharmacotherapy,* 2nd ed, Norwalk, CT: Appleton & Lange, 1993.

Maguire LC, Yon JL, and Miller E, "Prevention of Narcotic-Induced Constipation," *N Eng J Med,* 1981; 305:1651.

Ramkumar D and Rao SS, "Efficacy and Safety of Traditional Medical Therapies for Chronic Constipation: Systematic Review," *Am J Gastroenterol,* 2005, 100(4):936-71.

Tariq SH, "Constipation in Long-Term Care," *J Am Med Dir Assoc,* 2007, 8(4):209-18.

Wald A, "Is Chronic Use of Stimulant Laxatives Harmful to the Colon?" *J Clin Gastroenterol,* 2003, 36(5):386-9.

Wrenn K, "Fecal Impaction," *N Engl J Med,* 1989; 321:658-61.

IMMUNIZATION ADMINISTRATION RECOMMENDATIONS

The following tables are taken from the General Recommendations on Immunization, 2011:

- Guidelines for Spacing of Live and Inactivated Antigens
- Guidelines for Administering Antibody-Containing Products and Vaccines
- Recommended Intervals Between Administration of Antibody-Containing Products and Measles- or Varicella-Containing Vaccine, by Product and Indication for Vaccination
- Vaccination of persons with Primary and Secondary Immunodeficiencies
- Needle length and Injection Site of I.M. injections

Guidelines for Spacing of Live and Inactivated Antigens

Antigen Combination	Recommended Minimum Interval Between Doses
Two or more inactivated[1]	May be administered simultaneously or at any interval between doses
Inactivated and live	May be administered simultaneously or at any interval between doses
Two or more live injectable[2]	28 days minimum interval, if not administered simultaneously

[1]Certain experts suggest a 28-day interval between tetanus toxoid, reduced diphtheria toxoid, and reduced acellular pertussis (Tdap) vaccine and tetravalent meningococcal conjugate vaccine if they are not administered simultaneously.

[2]Live oral vaccines (eg, Ty21a typhoid vaccine and rotavirus vaccine) may be administered simultaneously or at any interval before or after inactivated or live injectable vaccines.

Adapted from American Academy of Pediatrics, Pertussis. In: Pickering LK, Baker CJ, Kimberlin DW, Long SS, eds, Red Book: 2009 Report of the Committee on Infectious Diseases, 28th ed, Elk Grove Village, IL: American Academy of Pediatrics, 2009, 22.

Guidelines for Administering Antibody-Containing Products[1] and Vaccines

Simultaneous Administration (during the same office visit)	
Products Administered	Recommended Minimum Interval Between Doses
Antibody-containing products and inactivated antigen	Can be administered simultaneously at different anatomic sites or at any time interval between doses.
Antibody-containing products and live antigen	Should **not** be administered simultaneously.[2] If simultaneous administration of measles-containing vaccine or varicella vaccine is unavoidable, administer at different sites and revaccinate or test for seroconversion after the recommended interval.

Nonsimultaneous Administration		
Products Administered		Recommended Minimum Interval Between Doses
Administered first	Administered second	
Antibody-containing products	Inactivated antigen	No interval necessary
Inactivated antigen	Antibody-containing products	No interval necessary
Antibody-containing products	Live antigen	Dose-related[2,3]
Live antigen	Antibody-containing products	2 weeks[2]

[1]Blood products containing substantial amounts of immune globulin include intramuscular and intravenous immune globulin, specific hyperimmune globulin (eg, hepatitis B immune globulin, tetanus immune globulin, varicella zoster immune globulin, and rabies immune globulin), whole blood, packed red blood cells, plasma, and platelet products.

[2]Yellow fever vaccine; rotavirus vaccine; oral Ty21a typhoid vaccine; live-attenuated influenza vaccine; and zoster vaccine are exceptions to these recommendations. These live-attenuated vaccines can be administered at any time before, after, or simultaneously with an antibody-containing product.

[3]The duration of interference of antibody-containing products with the immune response to the measles component of measles-containing vaccine, and possibly varicella vaccine, is dose-related.

Recommended Intervals Between Administration of Antibody-Containing Products and Measles- or Varicella-Containing Vaccine, by Product and Indication for Vaccination

Product / Indication	Dose (mg IgG/kg) and Route[1]	Recommended Interval Before Measles- or Varicella-Containing Vaccine[2] Administration (mo)
Tetanus IG	I.M.: 250 units (10 mg IgG/kg)	3
Hepatitis A IG		
Contact prophylaxis	I.M.: 0.02 mL/kg (3.3 mg IgG/kg)	3
International travel	I.M.: 0.06 mL/kg (10 mg IgG/kg)	3
Hepatitis B IG	I.M.: 0.06 mL/kg (10 mg IgG/kg)	3
Rabies IG	I.M.: 20 int. units/kg (22 mg IgG/kg)	4
Varicella IG	I.M.: 125 units/10 kg (60-200 mg IgG/kg) (maximum: 625 units)	5
Measles prophylaxis IG		
Standard (ie, nonimmunocompromised) contact	I.M.: 0.25 mL/kg (40 mg IgG/kg)	5
Immunocompromised contact	I.M.: 0.50 mL/kg (80 mg IgG/kg)	6
Blood transfusion		
Red blood cells (RBCs), washed	I.V.: 10 mL/kg (negligible IgG/kg)	None
RBCs, adenine-saline added	I.V.: 10 mL/kg (10 mg IgG/kg)	3
Packed RBCs (hematocrit 65%)[3]	I.V.: 10 mL/kg (60 mg IgG/kg)	6
Whole blood cells (hematocrit 35% to 50%)[3]	I.V.: 10 mL/kg (80-100 mg IgG/kg)	6
Plasma/platelet products	I.V.: 10 mL/kg (160 mg IgG/kg)	7
Cytomegalovirus intravenous immune globulin (IGIV)	150 mg/kg maximum	6
IGIV		
Replacement therapy for immune deficiencies[4]	I.V.: 300-400 mg/kg[4]	8
Immune thrombocytopenic purpura treatment	I.V.: 400 mg/kg	8
Postexposure varicella prophylaxis[5]	I.V.: 400 mg/kg	8
Immune thrombocytopenic purpura treatment	I.V.: 1000 mg/kg	10
Kawasaki disease	I.V.: 2 g/kg	11
Monoclonal antibody to respiratory syncytial virus F protein (Synagis® [Medimmune])[6]	I.M.: 15 mg/kg	None

HIV = human immunodeficiency virus; IG = immune globulin; IgG = immune globulin G; IGIV = intravenous immune globulin; mg IgG/kg = milligrams of immune globulin G per kilogram of body weight; I.M. = intramuscular; I.V. = intravenous; RBCs = red blood cells

[1] This table is not intended for determining the correct indications and dosages for using antibody-containing products. Unvaccinated persons might not be fully protected against measles during the entire recommended interval, and additional doses of IG or measles vaccine might be indicated after measles exposure. Concentrations of measles antibody in an IG preparation can vary by manufacturer's lot. Rates of antibody clearance after receipt of an IG preparation also might vary. Recommended intervals are extrapolated from an estimated half-life of 30 days for passively acquired antibody and an observed interference with the immune response to measles vaccine for 5 months after a dose of 80 mg IgG/kg.

[2] Does not include zoster vaccine. Zoster vaccine may be given with antibody-containing blood products.

[3] Assumes a serum IgG concentration of 16 mg/mL.

[4] Measles and varicella vaccinations are recommended for children with asymptomatic or mildly symptomatic HIV infection but are contraindicated for persons with severe immunosuppression from HIV or any other immunosuppressive disorder.

[5] The investigational product VariZIG™, similar to licensed varicella-zoster IG (VZIG), is a purified human IG preparation made from plasma containing high levels of anti-varicella antibodies (IgG). The interval between VariZIG™ and varicella vaccine (Var or MMRV) is 5 months.

[6] Contains antibody only to respiratory syncytial virus.

Vaccination of Persons With Primary and Secondary Immunodeficiencies

Category	Specific Immunodeficiency	Contraindicated Vaccines[1]	Risk-Specific Recommended Vaccines[1]	Effectiveness and Comments
Primary				
B-lymphocyte (humoral)	Severe antibody deficiencies (eg, X-linked agammaglobulinemia and common variable immunodeficiency)	Oral poliovirus (OPV)[2] Smallpox Live-attenuated influenza vaccine (LAIV) BCG Ty21a (live oral typhoid) Yellow fever	Pneumococcal Consider measles and varicella vaccination	The effectiveness of any vaccine is uncertain if it depends only on the humoral response (eg, PPSV or MPSV4) IGIV interferes with the immune response to measles vaccine and possibly varicella vaccine.
	Less severe antibody deficiencies (eg, selective IgA deficiency and IgG subclass deficiency)	OPV[2] BCG Yellow Fever Other live-vaccines appear to be safe	Pneumococcal	All vaccines likely effective; immune response may be attenuated.
T-lymphocyte (cell-mediated and humoral)	Complete defects (eg, severe combined immunodeficiency [SCID] disease, complete DiGeorge syndrome)	All live vaccines[3,4,5]	Pneumococcal	Vaccines might be ineffective.
	Partial defects (eg, most patients with DiGeorge syndrome, Wiskott-Aldrich syndrome, ataxia-telangiectasia)	All live vaccines[3,4,5]	Pneumococcal Meningococcal Hib (if not administered in infancy)	Effectiveness of any vaccine depends on degree of immune suppression.
Complement	Persistent complement, properdin, or factor B deficiency	None	Pneumococcal Meningococcal	All routine vaccines likely effective.
Phagocytic function	Chronic granulomatous disease, leukocyte adhesion defect, and myeloperoxidase deficiency	Live bacterial vaccines[3]	Pneumococcal[6]	All inactivated vaccines safe and likely effective. Live viral vaccines likely safe and effective.

Vaccination of Persons With Primary and Secondary Immunodeficiencies *continued*

Category	Specific Immunodeficiency	Contraindicated Vaccines[1]	Risk-Specific Recommended Vaccines[1]	Effectiveness and Comments
Secondary				
	HIV/AIDS	OPV[2] Smallpox BCG LAIV Withhold MMR and varicella in severely immunocompromised persons Yellow fever vaccine might have a contraindication or a precaution depending on clinical parameters of immune function[9]	Pneumococcal Consider Hib (if not administered in infancy) and meningococcal vaccination.	MMR, varicella, rotavirus, and all inactivated vaccines, including inactivated influenza, might be effective.[7]
	Malignant neoplasm, transplantation, immunosuppressive or radiation therapy	Live viral and bacterial, depending on immune status[3,4]	Pneumococcal	Effectiveness of any vaccine depends on degree of immune suppression.

Vaccination of Persons With Primary and Secondary Immunodeficiencies *continued*

Category	Specific Immunodeficiency	Contraindicated Vaccines[1]	Risk-Specific Recommended Vaccines[1]	Effectiveness and Comments
	Asplenia	None	Pneumococcal Meningococcal Hib (if not administered in infancy)	All routine vaccines likely effective.
	Chronic renal disease	LAIV	Pneumococcal Hepatitis B[8]	All routine vaccines likely effective.

AIDS = acquired immunodeficiency syndrome; BCG = bacille Calmette-Guérin; Hib = *Haemophilus influenzae* type b; HIV = human immunodeficiency virus; IG = immunoglobulin; IGIV = immune globulin intravenous; LAIV = live, attenuated influenza vaccine; MMR = measles, mumps, and rubella; MPSV4 = quadrivalent meningococcal polysaccharide vaccine; OPV = oral poliovirus vaccine (live); PPSV = pneumococcal polysaccharide vaccine; TIV = trivalent inactivated influenza vaccine

[1] Other vaccines that are universally or routinely recommended should be administered if not contraindicated.

[2] OPV is no longer available in the United States.

[3] Live bacterial vaccines: BCG and oral Ty21a *Salmonella typhi* vaccine.

[4] Live viral vaccines: MMR, MMRV, OPV, LAIV, yellow fever, zoster, rotavirus, varicella, and vaccinia (smallpox). Smallpox vaccine is not recommended for children or the general public.

[5] Regarding T-lymphocyte immunodeficiency as a contraindication for rotavirus vaccine, data exist only for severe combined immunodeficiency.

[6] Pneumococcal vaccine is not indicated for children with chronic granulomatous disease beyond age-based universal recommendations for PCV. Children with chronic granulomatous disease are not at increased risk for pneumococcal disease.

[7] HIV-infected children should receive IG after exposure to measles, and may receive varicella and measles vaccine if CD4[+] lymphocyte count is ≥15%.

[8] Indicated based on the risk from dialysis-based bloodborne transmission.

[9] Symptomatic HIV infection or CD4[+] T-lymphocyte count of <200/mm[3] or <15% of total lymphocytes for children aged <6 years is a contraindication to yellow fever vaccine administration. Asymptomatic HIV infection with CD4[+] T-lymphocyte count of 200-499/mm[3] for persons aged ≥6 years or 15% to 24% of total lymphocytes for children aged <6 years is a precaution for yellow fever vaccine administration. Details of yellow fever vaccine recommendations are available from CDC. (CDC. Yellow fever vaccine: recommendations of the Advisory Committee on Immunization Practices [ACIP]. MMWR 2010, 59[No. RR-7])

Adapted from American Academy of Pediatrics. Passive Immunization. In: Pickering LK, Baker CJ, Kimberline DW, Long SS, eds. Red Book: 2009 Report of the Committee on Infectious Diseases, 28th ed, Elk Grove Village, IL: American Academy of Pediatrics, 2009, 74-5.

Needle Length and Injection Site of I.M. for Children Aged ≤18 years (by age) and Adults Aged ≥19 years (by sex and weight)

Age Group	Needle Length	Injection Site
Children (birth to 18 y)		
Neonates[1]	5/8" (16 mm)[2]	Anterolateral thigh
Infant 1-12 mo	1" (25 mm)	Anterolateral thigh
Toddler 1-2 y	1-1¼" (25-32 mm)	Anterolateral thigh[3]
	5/8²-1" (16-25 mm)	Deltoid muscle of the arm
Children 3-18 y	5/8²-1" (16-25 mm)	Deltoid muscle of the arm[3]
	1-1¼" (25-32 mm)	Anterolateral thigh
Adults ≥19 y		
Men and women <60 kg (130 lb)	1" (25 mm)[4]	Deltoid muscle of the arm
Men and women 60-70 kg (130-152 lb)	1" (25 mm)	
Men 70-118 kg (152-260 lb)	1-1½" (25-38 mm)	
Women 70-90 kg (152-200 lb)		
Men >118 kg (260 lb)	1½" (38 mm)	
Women >90 kg (200 lb)		

I.M. = intramuscular

[1] First 28 days of life.

[2] If skin is stretched tightly and subcutaneous tissues are not bunched.

[3] Preferred site.

[4] Some experts recommend a 5/8" needle for men and women who weigh <60 kg.

Adapted from Poland GA, Borrud A, Jacobsen RM, et al, "Determination of Deltoid Fat Pad Thickness: Implications for Needle Length in Adult Immunization," *JAMA*, 1997, 277:1709-11.

RECOMMENDATIONS FOR TRAVELERS

The Centers for Disease Control and Prevention (CDC) also provides guidance to assist travelers and their healthcare providers in deciding the vaccines, medications, and other measures necessary to prevent illness and injury during international travel. Information can be found on the following website: http://wwwnc.cdc.gov/travel/

Reference:
Centers for Disease Control, "Recommendations of the Advisory Committee on Immunization Practices (ACIP): General Recommendations on Immunization," *MMWR Recomm Rep*, 2011, 60 (2):1-61.

IMMUNIZATION RECOMMENDATIONS

This schedule includes recommendations in effect as of December 21, 2010. Any dose not administered at the recommended age should be administered at a subsequent visit, when indicated and feasible. The use of a combination vaccine generally is preferred over separate injections of its equivalent component vaccines. Considerations should include provider assessment, patient preference, and the potential for adverse events. Providers should consult the relevant Advisory Committee on Immunization Practices statement for detailed recommendations: **http://www.cdc.gov/vaccines/pubs/acip-list.htm**. Clinically significant adverse events that follow immunization should be reported to the Vaccine Adverse Event Reporting System (VAERS) at http://www.vaers.hhs.gov or by telephone, **800-822-7967**.

Recommended adult immunization schedule, by vaccine and age group—United States, 2011

VACCINE ▼ AGE GROUP▶	19–26 years	27–49 years	50–59 years	60–64 years	≥65 years
Influenza[1],*			1 dose annually		
Tetanus, diphtheria, pertussis (Td/Tdap)[2],*		Substitute 1-time dose of Tdap for Td booster; then boost with Td every 10 years			Td booster every 10 years
Varicella[3],*			2 doses		
Human papillomavirus (HPV)[4],*	3 doses (females)				
Zoster[5]				1 dose	
Measles, mumps, rubella (MMR)[6],*	1 or 2 doses		1 dose		
Pneumococcal (polysaccharide)[7,8]		1 or 2 doses			1 dose
Meningococcal[9],*		1 or more doses			
Hepatitis A[10],*		2 doses			
Hepatitis B[11],*		3 doses			

* Covered by the Vaccine Injury Compensation Program | For all persons in this category who meet the age requirements and who lack evidence of immunity (e.g., lack documentation of vaccination or have no evidence of previous infection) | Recommended if some other risk factor is present (e.g., based on medical, occupational, lifestyle, or other indications) | No recommendation

Vaccines that might be indicated for adults, based on medical and other indications—United States, 2011

INDICATION▶ VACCINE ▼	Pregnancy	Immunocompromising conditions (excluding human immunodeficiency virus [HIV])[3,5,6,13]	HIV infection[3,6,12,13] CD4+T lymphocyte count <200 cells/μL	HIV infection[3,6,12,13] CD4+T lymphocyte count ≥200 cells/μL	Diabetes, heart disease, chronic lung disease, chronic alcoholism	Asplenia[12] (including elective splenectomy) and persistent complement component deficiencies	Chronic liver disease	Kidney failure, end-stage renal disease, receipt of hemodialysis	Health-care personnel
Influenza[1],*				1 dose TIV annually					1 dose TIV or LAIV annually
Tetanus, diphtheria, pertussis (Td/Tdap)[2],*	Td		Substitute 1-time dose of Tdap for Td booster; then boost with Td every 10 years						
Varicella[3],*	Contraindicated				2 doses				
Human papillomavirus (HPV)[4],*				3 doses through age 26 years					
Zoster[5]	Contraindicated					1 dose			
Measles, mumps, rubella[6],*	Contraindicated				1 or 2 doses				
Pneumococcal (polysaccharide)[7,8]				1 or 2 doses					
Meningococcal[9],*		1 or more doses							
Hepatitis A[10],*			2 doses						
Hepatitis B[11],*			3 doses						

* Covered by the Vaccine Injury Compensation Program | For all persons in this category who meet the age requirements and who lack evidence of immunity (e.g., lack documentation of vaccination or have no evidence of previous infection) | Recommended if some other risk factor is present (e.g., on the basis of medical, occupational, lifestyle, or other indications) | No recommendation

Footnotes to Recommended Adult Immunization Schedule

[1]Influenza vaccination.

- Annual vaccination against influenza is recommended for all persons aged 6 months and older, including all adults. Healthy, nonpregnant adults aged less than 50 years without high-risk medical conditions can receive either intranasally administered live, attenuated influenza vaccine (FluMist®), or inactivated vaccine. Other persons should receive the inactivated vaccine. Adults aged 65 years and older can receive the standard influenza vaccine or the high-dose (Fluzone®) influenza vaccine. Additional information about influenza vaccination is available at http://www.cdc.gov/vaccines/vpd-vac/flu/default.htm.

[2]Tetanus, diphtheria, and acellular pertussis (Td/Tdap) vaccination.

- Administer a one-time dose of Tdap to adults aged less than 65 years who have not received Tdap previously or for whom vaccine status is unknown to replace one of the 10-year Td boosters, and as soon as feasible to all 1) postpartum women, 2) close contacts of infants younger than age 12 months (eg, grandparents and child-care providers), and 3) health-care personnel with direct patient contact. Adults aged 65 years and older who have not previously received Tdap and who have close contact with an infant aged less than 12 months also should be vaccinated. Other adults aged 65 years and older may receive Tdap. Tdap can be administered regardless of interval since the most recent tetanus or diphtheria-containing vaccine.

- Adults with uncertain or incomplete history of completing a 3-dose primary vaccination series with Td-containing vaccines should begin or complete a primary vaccination series. For unvaccinated adults, administer the first 2 doses at least 4 weeks apart and the third dose 6–12 months after the second. If incompletely vaccinated (ie, less than 3 doses), administer remaining doses. Substitute a one-time dose of Tdap for one of the doses of Td, either in the primary series or for the routine booster, whichever comes first.

- If a woman is pregnant and received the most recent Td vaccination 10 or more years previously, administer Td during the second or third trimester. If the woman received the most recent Td vaccination less than 10 years previously, administer Tdap during the immediate postpartum period. At the clinician's discretion, Td may be deferred during pregnancy and Tdap substituted in the immediate postpartum period, or Tdap may be administered instead of Td to a pregnant woman after an informed discussion with the woman.

- The ACIP statement for recommendations for administering Td as prophylaxis in wound management is available at http://www.cdc.gov/vaccines/pubs/acip-list.htm.

[3]Varicella vaccination.

- All adults without evidence of immunity to varicella should receive 2 doses of single-antigen varicella vaccine if not previously vaccinated or a second dose if they have received only 1 dose, unless they have a medical contraindication. Special consideration should be given to those who 1) have close contact with persons at high risk for severe disease (eg, health-care personnel and family contacts of persons with immunocompromising conditions) or 2) are at high risk for exposure or transmission (eg, teachers; child-care employees; residents and staff members of institutional settings, including correctional institutions; college students; military personnel; adolescents and adults living in households with children; nonpregnant women of childbearing age; and international travelers).

- Evidence of immunity to varicella in adults includes any of the following: 1) documentation of 2 doses of varicella vaccine at least 4 weeks apart; 2) U.S.-born before 1980 (although for health-care personnel and pregnant women, birth before 1980 should not be considered evidence of immunity); 3) history of varicella based on diagnosis or verification of varicella by a health-care provider (for a patient reporting a history of or having an atypical case, a mild case, or both, health-care providers should seek either an epidemiologic link with a typical varicella case or to a laboratory-confirmed case or evidence of laboratory confirmation, if it was performed at the time of acute disease); 4) history of herpes zoster based on diagnosis or verification of herpes zoster by a health-care provider; or 5) laboratory evidence of immunity or laboratory confirmation of disease.

- Pregnant women should be assessed for evidence of varicella immunity. Women who do not have evidence of immunity should receive the first dose of varicella vaccine upon completion or termination of pregnancy and before discharge from the health-care facility. The second dose should be administered 4–8 weeks after the first dose.

[4]Human papillomavirus (HPV) vaccination.

- HPV vaccination with either quadrivalent (HPV4) vaccine or bivalent vaccine (HPV2) is recommended for females at age 11 or 12 years and catch-up vaccination for females aged 13-26 years.

- Ideally, vaccine should be administered before potential exposure to HPV through sexual activity; however, females who are sexually active should still be vaccinated consistent with age-based recommendations. Sexually active females who have not been infected with any of the four HPV vaccine types (types 6, 11, 16, and 18, all of which HPV4 prevents) or any of the two HPV vaccine types (types 16 and 18, both of which HPV2 prevents) receive the full benefit of the vaccination. Vaccination is less beneficial for females who have already been infected with one or more of the HPV vaccine types. HPV4 or HPV2 can be administered to persons with a history of genital warts, abnormal Papanicolaou test, or positive HPV DNA test, because these conditions are not evidence of previous infection with all vaccine HPV types.

- HPV4 may be administered to males aged 9-26 years to reduce their likelihood of genital warts. HPV4 would be most effective when administered before exposure to HPV through sexual contact.
- A complete series for either HPV4 or HPV2 consists of 3 doses. The second dose should be administered 1–2 months after the first dose; the third dose should be administered 6 months after the first dose.
- Although HPV vaccination is not specifically recommended for persons with the medical indications described in Figure 2, "Vaccines that might be indicated for adults based on medical and other indications," it may be administered to these persons because the HPV vaccine is not a live-virus vaccine. However, the immune response and vaccine efficacy might be less for persons with the medical indications described in Figure 2 than in persons who do not have the medical indications described or who are immunocompetent.

[5]Herpes zoster vaccination.

- A single dose of zoster vaccine is recommended for adults aged 60 years and older regardless of whether they report a previous episode of herpes zoster. Persons with chronic medical conditions may be vaccinated unless their condition constitutes a contraindication.

[6]Measles, mumps, rubella (MMR) vaccination.

- Adults born before 1957 generally are considered immune to measles and mumps. All adults born in 1957 or later should have documentation of 1 or more doses of MMR vaccine unless they have a medical contraindication to the vaccine, laboratory evidence of immunity to each of the three diseases, or documentation of provider-diagnosed measles or mumps disease. For rubella, documentation of provider-diagnosed disease is not considered acceptable evidence of immunity.
- *Measles component:* A second dose of MMR vaccine, administered a minimum of 28 days after the first dose, is recommended for adults who 1) have been recently exposed to measles or are in an outbreak setting; 2) are students in postsecondary educational institutions; 3) work in a health-care facility; or 4) plan to travel internationally. Persons who received inactivated (killed) measles vaccine or measles vaccine of unknown type during 1963–1967 should be revaccinated with 2 doses of MMR vaccine.
- *Mumps component:* A second dose of MMR vaccine, administered a minimum of 28 days after the first dose, is recommended for adults who 1) live in a community experiencing a mumps outbreak and are in an affected age group; 2) are students in postsecondary educational institutions; 3) work in a health-care facility; or 4) plan to travel internationally. Persons vaccinated before 1979 with either killed mumps vaccine or mumps vaccine of unknown type who are at high risk for mumps infection (eg, persons who are working in a health-care facility) should be revaccinated with 2 doses of MMR vaccine.
- *Rubella component:* For women of childbearing age, regardless of birth year, rubella immunity should be determined. If there is no evidence of immunity, women who are not pregnant should be vaccinated. Pregnant women who do not have evidence of immunity should receive MMR vaccine upon completion or termination of pregnancy and before discharge from the health-care facility.
- *Healthcare personnel born before 1957:* For unvaccinated healthcare personnel born before 1957 who lack laboratory evidence of measles, mumps, and/or rubella immunity or laboratory confirmation of disease, healthcare facilities should 1) consider routinely vaccinating personnel with 2 doses of MMR vaccine at the appropriate interval (for measles and mumps) and 1 dose of MMR vaccine (for rubella), and 2) recommend 2 doses of MMR vaccine at the appropriate interval during an outbreak of measles or mumps, and 1 dose during an outbreak of rubella. Complete information about evidence of immunity is available at http://www.cdc.gov/vaccines/recs/provisional/default.htm.

[7]Pneumococcal polysaccharide (PPSV) vaccination.

- Vaccinate all persons with the following indications:
    - *Medical:* Chronic lung disease (including asthma); chronic cardiovascular diseases; diabetes mellitus; chronic liver diseases; cirrhosis; chronic alcoholism; functional or anatomic asplenia (eg, sickle cell disease or splenectomy [if elective splenectomy is planned, vaccinate at least 2 weeks before surgery]); immunocompromising conditions (including chronic renal failure or nephrotic syndrome); and cochlear implants and cerebrospinal fluid leaks. Vaccinate as close to HIV diagnosis as possible.

- *Other:* Residents of nursing homes or long-term care facilities and persons who smoke cigarettes. Routine use of PPSV is not recommended for American Indians/ Alaska Natives or persons aged less than 65 years unless they have underlying medical conditions that are PPSV indications. However, public health authorities may consider recommending PPSV for American Indians/Alaska Natives and persons aged 50-64 years who are living in areas where the risk for invasive pneumococcal disease is increased.

[8]**Revaccination with PPSV.**

- One-time revaccination after 5 years is recommended for persons aged 19-64 years with chronic renal failure or nephrotic syndrome; functional or anatomic asplenia (eg, sickle cell disease or splenectomy); and for persons with immunocompromising conditions. For persons aged 65 years and older, one-time revaccination is recommended if they were vaccinated 5 or more years previously and were aged less than 65 years at the time of primary vaccination.

[9]**Meningococcal vaccination.**

- Meningococcal vaccine should be administered to persons with the following indications:
  - *Medical:* A 2-dose series of meningococcal conjugate vaccine is recommended for adults with anatomic or functional asplenia, or persistent complement component deficiencies. Adults with HIV infection who are vaccinated should also receive a routine 2-dose series. The 2 doses should be administered at 0 and 2 months.
  - *Other:* A single dose of meningococcal vaccine is recommended for unvaccinated first-year college students living in dormitories; microbiologists routinely exposed to isolates of *Neisseria meningitidis*; military recruits; and persons who travel to or live in countries in which meningococcal disease is hyperendemic or epidemic (eg, the "meningitis belt" of sub-Saharan Africa during the dry season [December through June]), particularly if their contact with local populations will be prolonged. Vaccination is required by the government of Saudi Arabia for all travelers to Mecca during the annual Hajj.
- Meningococcal conjugate vaccine, quadrivalent (MCV4) is preferred for adults with any of the preceding indications who are aged 55 years and younger; meningococcal polysaccharide vaccine (MPSV4) is preferred for adults aged 56 years and older. Revaccination with MCV4 every 5 years is recommended for adults previously vaccinated with MCV4 or MPSV4 who remain at increased risk for infection (eg, adults with anatomic or functional asplenia, or persistent complement component deficiencies).

[10]**Hepatitis A vaccination.**

- Vaccinate persons with any of the following indications and any person seeking protection from hepatitis A virus (HAV) infection:
  - *Behavioral:* Men who have sex with men and persons who use injection drugs.
  - *Occupational:* Persons working with HAV-infected primates or with HAV in a research laboratory setting.
  - *Medical:* Persons with chronic liver disease and persons who receive clotting factor concentrates.
  - *Other:* Persons traveling to or working in countries that have high or intermediate endemicity of hepatitis A (a list of countries is available at http://wwwn.cdc.gov/travel/contentdiseases.aspx).
- Unvaccinated persons who anticipate close personal contact (eg, household or regular babysitting) with an international adoptee during the first 60 days after arrival in the United States from a country with high or intermediate endemicity should be vaccinated. The first dose of the 2-dose hepatitis A vaccine series should be administered as soon as adoption is planned, ideally 2 or more weeks before the arrival of the adoptee.
- Single-antigen vaccine formulations should be administered in a 2-dose schedule at either 0 and 6–12 months (Havrix®), or 0 and 6–18 months (VAQTA®). If the combined hepatitis A and hepatitis B vaccine (Twinrix®) is used, administer 3 doses at 0, 1, and 6 months; alternatively, a 4-dose schedule may be used, administered on days 0, 7, and 21–30, followed by a booster dose at month 12.

[11]**Hepatitis B vaccination.**

- Vaccinate persons with any of the following indications and any person seeking protection from hepatitis B virus (HBV) infection:
  - *Behavioral:* Sexually active persons who are not in a long-term, mutually monogamous relationship (eg, persons with more than one sex partner during the previous 6 months); persons seeking evaluation or treatment for a sexually transmitted disease (STD); current or recent injection-drug users; and men who have sex with men.
  - *Occupational:* Health-care personnel and public-safety workers who are exposed to blood or other potentially infectious body fluids.
  - *Medical:* Persons with end-stage renal disease, including patients receiving hemodialysis; persons with HIV infection; and persons with chronic liver disease.

- *Other:* Household contacts and sex partners of persons with chronic HBV infection; clients and staff members of institutions for persons with developmental disabilities; and international travelers to countries with high or intermediate prevalence of chronic HBV infection (a list of countries is available at http://wwwn.cdc.gov/travel/contentdiseases.aspx).

- Hepatitis B vaccination is recommended for all adults in the following settings: STD treatment facilities; HIV testing and treatment facilities; facilities providing drug-abuse treatment and prevention services; health-care settings targeting services to injection-drug users or men who have sex with men; correctional facilities; end-stage renal disease programs and facilities for chronic hemodialysis patients; and institutions and nonresidential day-care facilities for persons with developmental disabilities.

- Administer missing doses to complete a 3-dose series of hepatitis B vaccine to those persons not vaccinated or not completely vaccinated. The second dose should be administered 1 month after the first dose; the third dose should be given at least 2 months after the second dose (and at least 4 months after the first dose). If the combined hepatitis A and hepatitis B vaccine (Twinrix®) is used, administer 3 doses at 0, 1, and 6 months; alternatively, a 4-dose Twinrix® schedule, administered on days 0, 7, and 21-30, followed by a booster dose at month 12 may be used.

- Adult patients receiving hemodialysis or with other immunocompromising conditions should receive 1 dose of 40 µg/mL (Recombivax HB®) administered on a 3-dose schedule or 2 doses of 20 µg/mL (Engerix-B®) administered simultaneously on a 4-dose schedule at 0, 1, 2, and 6 months.

[12]**Selected conditions for which *Haemophilus influenzae* type b (Hib) vaccine may be used.**
- 1 dose of Hib vaccine should be considered for persons who have sickle cell disease, leukemia, or HIV infection, or who have had a splenectomy, if they have not previously received Hib vaccine.

[13]**Immunocompromising conditions.**
- Inactivated vaccines generally are acceptable (eg, pneumococcal, meningococcal, influenza [inactivated influenza vaccine]) and live vaccines generally are avoided in persons with immune deficiencies or immunocompromising conditions. Information on specific conditions is available at http://www.cdc.gov/vaccines/pubs/acip-list.htm.

Reference

"Recommended Adult Immunization Schedule - United States, 2011," *MMWR*, 2011, 60(4):Q1-4.

These schedules indicate the recommended age groups and medical indications for which administration of currently licensed vaccines is commonly indicated for adults ages 19 years and older, as of January 1, 2011. For all vaccines being recommended on the adult immunization schedule: a vaccine series does not need to be restarted, regardless of the time that has elapsed between doses. Licensed combination vaccines may be used whenever any components of the combination are indicated and when the vaccine's other components are not contraindicated. For detailed recommendations on all vaccines, including those used primarily for travelers or that are issued during the year, consult the manufacturers' package inserts and the complete statements from the Advisory Committee on Immunization Practices (http:// www.cdc.gov/vaccines/pubs/acip-list.htm).

Report all clinically significant postvaccination reactions to the Vaccine Adverse Event Reporting System (VAERS). Reporting forms and instructions on filing a VAERS report are available at http://www.vaers.hhs.gov or by telephone, 800-822-7967.

Information on how to file a Vaccine Injury Compensation Program claim is available at http://www.hrsa.gov/vaccinecompensation or by telephone, 800-338-2382. Information about filing a claim for vaccine injury is available through the U.S. Court of Federal Claims, 717 Madison Place, N.W., Washington, D.C. 20005; telephone, 202-357-6400.

Additional information about the vaccines in this schedule, extent of available data, and contraindications for vaccination also is available at http://www.cdc.gov/vaccines or from the CDC-INFO Contact Center at 800-CDC-INFO (800-232-4636) in English and Spanish, 24 hours a day, 7 days a week.

Use of trade names and commercial sources is for identification only and does not imply endorsement by the U.S. Department of Health and Human Services.

The recommendations in this schedule were approved by ACIP, the American Academy of Family Physicians, the American College of Obstetricians and Gynecologists, and the American College of Physicians.

VACCINE INJURY TABLE

The Vaccine Injury Table makes it easier for some people to get compensation. The table lists and explains injuries/conditions that are presumed to be caused by vaccines. It also lists time periods in which the first symptom of these injuries/conditions must occur after receiving the vaccine. If the first symptom of these injuries/conditions occurs within the listed time periods, it is presumed that the vaccine was the cause of the injury or condition unless another cause is found. For example, if the patient received the tetanus vaccines and had a severe allergic reaction (anaphylaxis) within 4 hours after receiving the vaccine, then it is presumed that the tetanus vaccine caused the injury if no other cause is found.

If the injury/condition is not on the table or if the injury/condition did not occur within the time period on the table, it must be proven that the vaccine caused the injury/condition. Such proof must be based on medical records or opinion, which may include expert witness testimony.

Vaccine Injury Table[1]

Vaccine		Adverse Event	Time Interval
Tetanus toxoid-containing vaccines (eg, DTaP, Tdap, DTP-Hib, DT, Td, TT)	A.	Anaphylaxis or anaphylactic shock	0-4 hours
	B.	Brachial neuritis	2-28 days
	C.	Any acute complication or sequela (including death) of above events	Not applicable
Pertussis antigen-containing vaccines (eg, DTaP, Tdap, DTP, P, DTP-Hib)	A.	Anaphylaxis or anaphylactic shock	0-4 hours
	B.	Encephalopathy (or encephalitis)	0-72 hours
	C.	Any acute complication or sequela (including death) of above events	Not applicable
Measles, mumps, and rubella virus-containing vaccines in any combination (eg, MMR, MR, M, R)	A.	Anaphylaxis or anaphylactic shock	0-4 hours
	B.	Encephalopathy (or encephalitis)	5-15 days
	C.	Any acute complication or sequela (including death) of above events	Not applicable
Rubella virus-containing vaccines (eg, MMR, MR, R)	A.	Chronic arthritis	7-42 days
	B.	Any acute complication or sequela (including death) of above events	Not applicable
Measles virus-containing vaccines (eg, MMR, MR, M)	A.	Thrombocytopenic purpura	7-30 days
	B.	Vaccine-strain measles viral infection in an immunodeficient recipient	0-6 months
	C.	Any acute complication or sequela (including death) of above events	Not applicable
Polio live virus-containing vaccines (OPV)	A.	Paralytic polio	
	•	In a nonimmunodeficient recipient	0-30 days
	•	In an immunodeficient recipient	0-6 months
	•	In a vaccine associated community case	Not applicable
	B.	Vaccine-strain polio viral infection	
	•	In a nonimmunodeficient recipient	0-30 days
	•	In an immunodeficient recipient	0-6 months
	•	In a vaccine associated community case	Not applicable
	C.	Any acute complication or sequela (including death) of above events	Not applicable
Polio inactivated-virus containing vaccines (eg, IPV)	A.	Anaphylaxis or anaphylactic shock	0-4 hours
	B.	Any acute complication or sequela (including death) of above events	Not applicable
Hepatitis B antigen-containing vaccines	A.	Anaphylaxis or anaphylactic shock	0-4 hours
	B.	Any acute complication or sequela (including death) of above events	Not applicable

Vaccine Injury Table[1] *(continued)*

Vaccine		Adverse Event	Time Interval
Hemophilus influenzae (type b polysaccharide conjugate vaccines)	A.	No condition specified for compensation	Not applicable
Varicella vaccine	A.	No condition specified for compensation	Not applicable
Rotavirus vaccine	A.	No condition specified for compensation	Not applicable
Pneumococcal conjugate vaccines	A.	No condition specified for compensation	Not applicable
Any new vaccine recommended by the Centers for Disease Control and Prevention for routine administration to children, after publication by Secretary, HHS of a notice of coverage[2,3]	A.	No condition specified for compensation	Not applicable

[1]Effective date: November 10, 2008.

[2]As of **December 1, 2004**, hepatitis A vaccines have been added to the Vaccine Injury Table under this category. As of **July 1, 2005**, trivalent influenza vaccines have been added to the table under this category. Trivalent influenza vaccines are given annually during the flu season either by needle and syringe or in a nasal spray. All influenza vaccines routinely administered in the U.S. are trivalent vaccines covered under this category. See Federal Register Notice: April 12, 2005.

[3]As of February 1, 2007, meningococcal (conjugate and polysaccharide) and human papillomavirus (HPV) vaccines have been added to the table under this category.

See *News* on the VICP website for more information. Available at: http://www.hrsa.gov/vaccinecompensation.

AMINOGLYCOSIDE DOSING AND MONITORING

All aminoglycoside therapy should be individualized for specific patients in specific clinical situation. The following are guidelines for initiating therapy.

1. Loading dose based on estimated ideal body weight (IBW). **All patients require a loading dose independent of renal function**.

Agent	Dose
Gentamicin	2 mg/kg
Tobramycin	2 mg/kg
Amikacin	7.5 mg/kg

    Significantly higher loading doses may be required in severely ill intensive care unit patients.

2. Initial maintenance doses as a percent of loading dose according to desired dosing interval and creatinine clearance (Cl_{cr}):
    Male Cl_{cr} (mL/min) = (140 − age) x IBW / 72 x serum creatinine
    Female = 0.85 x Cl_{cr} males

Cl_{cr} (mL/min)	Dosing Interval (h)		
	8	12	24
90	84%	—	—
80	80%	—	—
70	76%	88%	—
60	—	84%	—
50	—	79%	—
40	—	72%	92%
30	—	—	86%
25	—	—	81%
20	—	—	75%

    Patients >65 years of age should not receive initial aminoglycoside maintenance dosing more often than every 12 hours.

3. Serum concentration monitoring

    *   Serum concentration monitoring is necessary for **safe** and **effective** therapy, particularly in patients with serious infections and those with risk factors for toxicity.

    *   Peak serum concentrations should be drawn 30 minutes after the completion of a 30-minute infusion. Trough serum concentrations should be drawn within 30 minutes prior to the administered dose.

    *   Serum concentrations should be drawn after 5 half-lives, usually around the third dose or thereafter.

4. Desired measured serum concentrations

	Peak (mcg/mL)	Trough (mcg/mL)
Gentamicin	6-10	0.5-2
Tobramycin	6-10	0.5-2
Amikacin	20-30	<5

5. For patients receiving hemodialysis:

    - administer the **same** loading dose

    - administer ⅔ of the loading dose after each dialysis

    - **serum concentrations must be monitored**

    - watch for ototoxicity from accumulation of drug

6. For individual clinical situations the prescribing physician should feel free to consult Infectious Disease, the Pharmacology Service, or the Pharmacy.

"Once Daily" Aminoglycosides

High dose, "once daily" aminoglycoside therapy for treatment of gram-negative bacterial infections has been studied and remains controversial. The pharmacodynamics of aminoglycosides reveal dose-dependent killing which suggests an efficacy advantage of "high" peak serum concentrations. It is also suggested that allowing troughs to fall to unmeasurable levels decreases the risk of nephrotoxicity without detriment to efficacy. Because of a theoretical saturation of tubular cell uptake of aminoglycosides, decreasing the number of times the drug is administered in a particular time period may play a role in minimizing the risk of nephrotoxicity. Ototoxicity has not been sufficiently formally evaluated through audiometry or vestibular testing comparing "once daily" to standard therapy. Over 100 letters, commentaries, studies and reviews have been published on the topic of "once daily" aminoglycosides with varying dosing regimens, monitoring parameters, inclusion and exclusion criteria, and results (most of which have been favorable for the "once daily" regimens). The caveats of this simplified method of dosing are several, including assurance that creatinine clearances be calculated, that all patients are not candidates and should not be considered for this regimen, and that "once daily" is a semantic misnomer.

Because of the controversial nature of this method, it is beyond the scope of this book to present significant detail and dosing regimen recommendations. Considerable experience with two methods warrants mention. The Hartford Hospital has experience with over 2000 patients utilizing a 7 mg/kg dose, a dosing scheme for various creatinine clearance estimates, and a serum concentration monitoring nomogram.[1] Providence Medical Center utilizes a 5 mg/kg dosing regimen but only in patients with excellent renal function; serum concentrations are monitored 4-6 hours prior to the dose administered.[2] Two excellent reviews discuss the majority of studies and controversies regarding these dosing techniques.[3,4] An editorial accompanies one of the reviews and is worth examination.[5]

"Once daily" dosing may be a safe and effective method of providing aminoglycoside therapy to a large number of patients who require these efficacious yet toxic agents. As with any method of aminoglycoside administration, dosing must be individualized and the caveats of the method considered.

Footnotes

1. Nicolau DP, Freeman CD, Belliveau PP, et al, "Experience With a Once-Daily Aminoglycoside Program Administered to 2,184 Patients," *Antimicrob Agents Chemother*, 1995, 39(3):650-5.
2. Gilbert DN, "Once-Daily Aminoglycoside Therapy," *Antimicrob Agents Chemother*, 1991, 35(3):399-405.
3. Preston SL and Briceland LL, "Single Daily Dosing of Aminoglycosides," *Pharmacotherapy*, 1995, 15(3):297-316.
4. Bates RD and Nahata MC, "Once-Daily Administration of Aminoglycosides," *Ann Pharmacother*, 1994, 28 (6):757-66.
5. Rotschafer JC and Rybak MJ, "Single Daily Dosing of Aminoglycosides: A Commentary," *Ann Pharmacother*, 1994, 28(6):797-801.

Aminoglycoside Penetration Into Various Tissues

Site	Extent of Distribution
Eye	Poor
CNS	Poor (<25%)
Pleural	Excellent
Bronchial secretions	Poor
Sputum	Fair (10%-50%)
Pulmonary tissue	Excellent
Ascitic fluid	Variable (43%-132%)
Peritoneal fluid	Poor
Bile	Variable (25%-90%)
Bile with obstruction	Poor
Synovial fluid	Excellent
Bone	Poor
Prostate	Poor
Urine	Excellent
Renal tissue	Excellent

Adapted from Neu HC, "Pharmacology of Aminoglycosides," *The Aminoglycosides*, Whelton E and Neu HC, eds, New York, NY: Marcel Dekker, Inc, 1981.

ANTIBIOTIC TREATMENT OF ADULTS WITH INFECTIVE ENDOCARDITIS

Table 1. Suggested Regimens for Therapy of Native Valve Endocarditis Due to Penicillin-Susceptible Viridans Streptococci and *Streptococcus bovis*

(Minimum Inhibitory Concentration ≤0.12 mcg/mL)[1]

Antibiotic	Dosage and Route	Duration (wk)	Comments
Aqueous crystalline penicillin G sodium **or**	12-18 million units/24 h I.V. either continuously or in 4-6 equally divided doses	4	Preferred in most patients older than 65 y and in those with impairment of the 8th cranial nerve or renal function
CefTRIAXone sodium	2 g once daily I.V. or I.M.[2]	4	
Either penicillin or cefTRIAXone regimen above with gentamicin sulfate[3]	3 mg/kg/24 h I.M./I.V. as single daily dose	2	When using combination therapy, both β-lactam and aminoglycoside regimen duration is 2 weeks; 2-week regimen not intended if known cardiac or extracardiac abscess, Cl_{cr} <20 mL/min, 8th cranial nerve impairment or *Abiotrophia*, *Granulicatella*, or *Gemella* spp
Vancomycin hydrochloride[4]	30 mg/kg/24 h I.V. in 2 equally divided doses, not to exceed 2 g/24 h unless serum levels are monitored	4	Vancomycin therapy is recommended for patients allergic to β-lactams; peak serum concentrations of vancomycin should be obtained 1 h after completion of the infusion and should be in the range of 30-45 mcg/mL and trough of 10-15 mcg/mL for twice-daily dosing

[1]Dosages recommended are for patients with normal renal function. For nutritionally variant streptococci, see Table 3. I.V. indicates intravenous; I.M., intramuscular.

[2]Patients should be informed that I.M. injection of cefTRIAXone is painful.

[3]Dosing of gentamicin on a mg/kg basis will produce higher serum concentrations in obese patients than in lean patients. Therefore, in obese patients, dosing should be based on ideal body weight. (Ideal body weight for men is 50 kg + 2.3 kg per inch over 5 feet, and ideal body weight for women is 45.5 kg + 2.3 kg per inch over 5 feet.) Relative contraindications to the use of gentamicin are age >65 years, renal impairment, or impairment of the eighth nerve. Other potentially nephrotoxic agents (eg, nonsteroidal anti-inflammatory drugs) should be used cautiously in patients receiving gentamicin.

[4]Vancomycin dosage should be reduced in patients with impaired renal function. Vancomycin given on a mg/kg basis will produce higher serum concentrations in obese patients than in lean patients. Therefore, in obese patients, dosing should be based on ideal body weight. Each dose of vancomycin should be infused over at least 1 hour to reduce the risk of the histamine-release "red man" syndrome.

Table 2. Therapy for Native Valve Endocarditis Due to Strains of Viridans Streptococci and *Streptococcus bovis* Relatively Resistant to Penicillin G (Minimum Inhibitory Concentration >0.12 mcg/mL and ≤0.5 mcg/mL)[1]

Antibiotic	Dosage and Route	Duration (wk)	Comments
Aqueous crystalline penicillin G sodium	24 million units/24 h I.V. either continuously or in 4-6 equally divided doses	4	CeFAZolin or other first-generation cephalosporins may be substituted for penicillin in patients whose penicillin hypersensitivity is not of the immediate type.
With gentamicin sulfate[2]	3 mg/kg/24 h I.M./I.V. as single daily dose	2	
CefTRIAXone sodium	2 g once daily I.V. or I.M.[2]	4	
With gentamicin sulfate[2]	3 mg/kg/24 h I.M./I.V. as single daily dose	2	
Vancomycin hydrochloride[3]	30 mg/kg/24 h I.V. in 2 equally divided doses, not to exceed 2 g/24 h unless serum levels are monitored	4	Vancomycin therapy is recommended for patients allergic to β-lactams

[1]Dosages recommended are for patients with normal renal function. I.V. indicates intravenous; I.M., intramuscular.

[2]For specific dosing adjustment and issues concerning gentamicin (obese patients, relative contraindications), see Table 1 footnotes.

[3]For specific dosing adjustment and issues concerning vancomycin (obese patients, length of infusion), see Table 1 footnotes.

Table 3. Standard Therapy for Endocarditis Due to Enterococci[1]

Antibiotic	Dosage and Route	Duration (wk)	Comments
Aqueous crystalline penicillin G sodium	18-30 million units/24 h I.V. either continuously or in 6 equally divided doses	4-6	Native valve: 4-week therapy recommended for patients with symptoms ≤3 months in duration; 6-week therapy recommended for patients with symptoms >3 months in duration
With gentamicin sulfate[2]	1 mg/kg I.M. or I.V. every 8 h	4-6	
Ampicillin sodium	12 g/24 h I.V. in 6 equally divided doses	4-6	Prosthetic valve or other prosthetic material: 6-week minimum therapy recommended
With gentamicin sulfate[2]	1 mg/kg I.M. or I.V. every 8 hours	4-6	
			Target gentamicin peak concentration of 3-4 mcg/mL and trough of <1 mcg/mL
Vancomycin hydrochloride[2,3]	30 mg/kg/24 h I.V. in 2 equally divided doses, not to exceed 2 g/24 h unless serum levels are monitored	6	Vancomycin therapy is recommended for patients allergic to β-lactams; cephalosporins are not acceptable alternatives for patients allergic to penicillin
With gentamicin sulfate[2]	1 mg/kg I.M. or I.V. every 8 h	6	

[1]All enterococci causing endocarditis must be tested for antimicrobial susceptibility in order to select optimal therapy. This table is for endocarditis due to penicillin-, gentamicin-, and vancomycin-susceptible enterococci, viridans streptococci with a minimum inhibitory concentration of >0.5 mcg/mL, nutritionally variant viridans streptococci, or prosthetic valve endocarditis caused by viridans streptococci or *Streptococcus bovis*. If penicillin-resistant organisms, use vancomycin/gentamicin regimen above, or may use ampicillin/sulbactam (12 g/24 h in 4 divided doses) with gentamicin for 6 weeks. Antibiotic dosages are for patients with normal renal function. I.V. indicates intravenous; I.M., intramuscular.

[2]For specific dosing adjustment and issues concerning gentamicin (obese patients, relative contraindications), see Table 1 footnotes.

[3]For specific dosing adjustment and issues concerning vancomycin (obese patients, length of infusion), see Table 1 footnotes.

Table 4. Therapy for Native or Prosthetic Valve Endocarditis Due to Enterococci[1] Resistant to Vancomycin, Aminoglycosides, and Penicillin[2]

Antibiotic	Dosage and Route	Duration (wk)	Comments
E. faecium			
Linezolid	1200 mg/24 h P.O./I.V. in 2 divided doses	≥8	May cause severe, but reversible thrombocytopenia, particularly with extended therapy >2 weeks.
Quinupristin-dalfopristin	22.5 mg/kg/24 h I.V. in 3 divided doses	≥8	May cause severe myalgia; not effective against *E. faecalis*.
E. faecalis			
Imipenem/cilastatin	2 g/24 h I.V. in 4 divided doses	≥8	Limited patient experience with these regimens.
With ampicillin sodium	12 g/24 h in 6 divided doses	≥8	
or			
CefTRIAXone sodium	2 g/24 h I.V./I.M.[3] once daily	≥8	Limited patient experience with these regimens.
With ampicillin sodium	12 g/24 h in 6 divided doses	≥8	

[1]Endocarditis caused by the organisms should be treated in consultation with an infectious disease specialist; bacteriologic cure with antimicrobial therapy alone may be <50% and valve replacement may be required.

[2]Dosages recommended are for patients with normal renal function. I.V. = intravenous; I.M. = intramuscular.

[3]Patients should be informed that I.M. injection of cefTRIAXone is painful.

Table 5. Therapy for Endocarditis Due to *Staphylococcus* in the Absence of Prosthetic Material[1]

Antibiotic	Dosage and Route	Duration	Comments
Methicillin-Susceptible Staphylococci			
Regimens for non-β-lactam-allergic patients			
Nafcillin sodium or oxacillin sodium	12 g/24 h I.V. in 4-6 divided doses	6 wk	Uncomplicated right side endocarditis may be treated for 2 weeks.
With optional addition of gentamicin sulfate[2]	3 mg/kg/24 h I.M./I.V. in 2-3 divided doses	3-5 d	Benefit of additional aminoglycosides has not been established.
Regimens for β-lactam-allergic patients (nonanaphylactic)			
CeFAZolin (or other first-generation cephalosporins in equivalent dosages)	2 g I.V. every 8 h	6 wk	Cephalosporins should be avoided in patients with immediate-type hypersensitivity to penicillin; if penicillin-sensitive, vancomycin should be used.
With optional addition of gentamicin[2]	3 mg/kg/24 h I.M./I.V. in 2-3 divided doses	3-5 d	Benefit of additional aminoglycosides has not been established.
Methicillin-Resistant Staphylococci			
Vancomycin hydrochloride[3]	30 mg/kg/24 h I.V. in 2 equally divided doses; not to exceed 2 g/24 h unless serum levels are monitored	4-6 wk	Vancomycin therapy is recommended for patients allergic to β-lactams; peak serum concentrations of vancomycin should be obtained 1 h after completion of the infusion and should be in the range of 30-45 mcg/mL and trough of 10-15 mcg/mL for twice-daily dosing.

[1]For treatment of endocarditis due to penicillin-susceptible staphylococci (minimum inhibitory concentration ≤0.1 mcg/mL and non-beta-lactamase producing), aqueous crystalline penicillin G sodium 24 million units/24 h can be used instead of nafcillin or oxacillin. Shorter antibiotic courses have been effective in some drug addicts with right-sided endocarditis due to *Staphylococcus aureus*. I.V. indicates intravenous; I.M., intramuscular.

[2]For specific dosing adjustment and issues concerning gentamicin (obese patients, relative contraindications), see Table 1 footnotes.

[3]For specific dosing adjustment and issues concerning vancomycin (obese patients, length of infusion), see Table 1 footnotes.

Table 6. Treatment of Staphylococcal Endocarditis in the Presence of a Prosthetic Valve or Other Prosthetic Material[1]

Antibiotic	Dosage and Route	Duration (wk)	Comments
Methicillin-Susceptible Staphylococci			
Nafcillin sodium or oxacillin sodium[2]	12 g/24 h I.V. in 6 divided doses	≥6	First-generation cephalosporins or vancomycin should be used in patients allergic to β-lactam. Cephalosporins should be avoided in patients with immediate-type hypersensitivity to penicillin or with methicillin-resistant staphylococci.
With rifampin[3]	300 mg P.O./I.V. every 8 h	≥6	–
And with gentamicin sulfate[4,5]	3 mg/kg I.M./I.V. in 2-3 divided doses	2	Aminoglycoside should be administered in close proximity to vancomycin, nafcillin, or oxacillin.
Methicillin-Resistant Staphylococci			
Vancomycin hydrochloride[6]	30 mg/kg/24 h I.V. in 2 equally divided doses, not to exceed 2 g/24 h unless serum levels are monitored	≥6	–
With rifampin[3]	300 mg P.O./I.V. every 8 h	≥6	Rifampin increases the amount of warfarin sodium required for antithrombotic therapy.
And with gentamicin sulfate[4,5]	3 mg/kg I.M./I.V. in 2-3 divided doses	2	Aminoglycoside should be administered in close proximity to vancomycin, nafcillin, or oxacillin.

[1]Dosages recommended are for patients with normal renal function. I.V. = intravenous; I.M. = intramuscular.

[2]May use aqueous penicillin G 24 million units/24 h in 4-6 divided doses if strain is penicillin susceptible (MIC ≤0.1 mcg/mL and non-beta-lactamase producing).

[3]Rifampin plays a unique role in the eradication of staphylococcal infection involving prosthetic material; combination therapy is essential to prevent emergence of rifampin resistance.

[4]For a specific dosing adjustment and issues concerning gentamicin (obese patients, relative contraindications), see Table 1 footnotes.

[5]Use during initial 2 weeks.

[6]For specific dosing adjustment and issues concerning vancomycin (obese patients, relative contraindications), see Table 1 footnotes.

Table 7. Therapy for Native or Prosthetic Valve Endocarditis Due to HACEK Microorganisms (*Haemophilus parainfluenzae, Haemophilus aphrophilus, Actinobacillus actinomycetemcomitans, Cardiobacterium hominus, Eikenella corrodens*, and *Kingella kingae*)[1]

Antibiotic	Dosage and Route	Duration (wk)	Comments
CefTRIAXone sodium[2]	2 g once daily I.V. or I.M.[2]	4	Cefotaxime sodium or other third- or fourth-generation cephalosporins may be substituted.
Ampicillin/ sulbactam[3]	12 g/24 h I.V. in 6 equally divided doses	4	
Ciprofloxacin	1000 mg/24 h orally or 800 mg/24 h I.V. in 2 divided doses	4	Use of fluoroquinolone recommended only if patient intolerant to ampicillin or cephalosporins; may substitute fluoroquinolone with equivalent coverage (eg, levofloxacin, moxifloxacin); if prosthetic material involved, treatment duration should be 6 weeks.

[1]Antibiotic dosages are for patients with normal renal function. I.V. indicates intravenous; I.M. intramuscular.

[2]Patients should be informed that I.M. injection of cefTRIAXone is painful.

[3]Ampicillin should not be used if laboratory tests show β-lactamase production.

REFERENCE

Baddour LM, Wilson WR, Bayer AS, et al, "Infective Endocarditis. Diagnosis, Antimicrobial Therapy, and Management of Complications. A Statement for Healthcare Professionals from the Committee on Rheumatic Fever, Endocarditis, and Kawasaki Disease, Council on Cardiovascular Disease in the Young, and the Councils on Clinical Cardiology, Stroke, and Cardiovascular Surgery and Anesthesia, American Heart Association," *Circulation*, 2005, 111(23): e394-434.

COMMUNITY-ACQUIRED PNEUMONIA IN ADULTS

Alternative methods exist to facilitate the objective rating of disease severity in community-acquired pneumonia patients in order to guide appropriate site of care and aggressiveness of treatment. The first option, the Pneumonia Severity Index (PSI) was derived from the Pneumonia Patient Outcomes Research Team (PORT). This is a well-validated instrument which stratifies patients based on risk of mortality; however, calculation of the patient's score requires assessment of 19 variables. The second method is referred to as the "Confusion, Uremia, Respiratory rate, Blood pressure, and age >65 years (CURB-65)" score. This system has fewer variables to evaluate and focuses more on assessment of disease severity, but is less well validated. In either case, these measures should not be used in exclusion to appropriate clinical judgement.

PNEUMONIA SEVERITY INDEX (PSI)

The initial site of treatment should be based on a 3-step process:
1. Assessment of pre-existing conditions that compromise safety of home care
2. Calculation of the Pneumonia Severity Index with recommendation for home care for risk classes I, II, and III, and
3. Clinical judgment

Algorithm

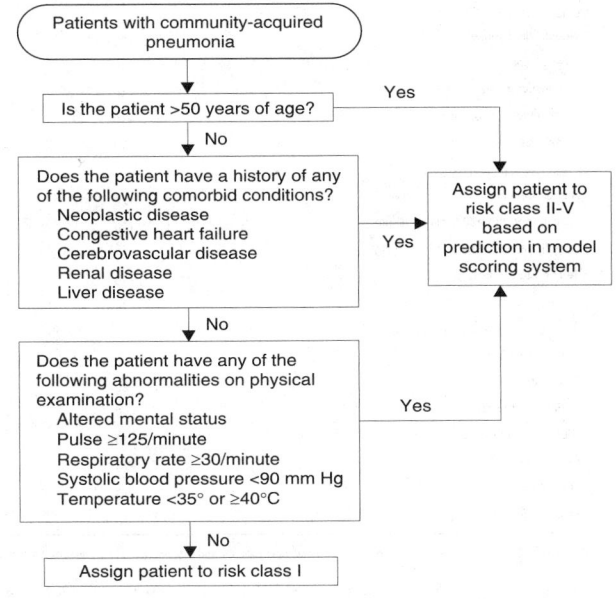

Stratification of Risk Score

Risk	Risk Class	Based on
	I	Algorithm
Low	II	≤70 total points
	III	71-90 total points
Moderate	IV	91-130 total points
High	V	>130 total points

Risk-Class Mortality Rates for Patients With Pneumonia

Risk Class	No. of Points	Validation Cohort		Recommended Site of Care
		No. of Patients	Mortality (%)	
I	No predictors	3034	0.1	Outpatient
II	≤70	5778	0.6	Outpatient
III	71-90	6790	2.8	Outpatient or brief inpatient
IV	91-130	13,104	8.2	Inpatient
V	>130	9333	29.2	Inpatient

Scoring System: Assignment to Risk Classes II-V

Patient Characteristic	Points Assigned[1]
Demographic factors	
Age	
Male	No. of years
Female	No. of years -10
Nursing home resident	+10
Comorbid illnesses	
Neoplastic disease[2]	+30
Liver disease[3]	+20
Congestive heart failure[4]	+10
Cerebrovascular disease[5]	+10
Renal disease[6]	+10
Physical examination findings	
Altered mental status[7]	+20
Respiratory rate >30 breaths/minute	+20
Systolic blood pressure <90 mm Hg	+20
Temperature <35°C or >40°C	+15
Pulse >125 beats/minute	+10
Laboratory or radiographic findings	
Arterial pH <7.35	+30
BUN >30 mg/dL	+20
Sodium <130 mEq/L	+20
Glucose >250 mg/dL	+10
Hematocrit <30%	+10
pO_2 <60 mm Hg[8]	+10
Pleural effusion	+10

[1]A total point score for a given patient is obtained by adding the patient's age in years (age -10, for females) and the points for each applicable patient characteristic.

[2]Any cancer, except basal or squamous cell cancer of the skin, that was active at the time of presentation or diagnosed within 1 year of presentation.

[3]A clinical or histologic diagnosis of cirrhosis or other form of chronic liver disease such as chronic active hepatitis.

[4]Systolic or diastolic ventricular dysfunction documented by history and physical examination, as well as chest radiography, echocardiography, Muga scanning, or left ventriculography.

[5]A clinical diagnosis of stroke, transient ischemic attack, or stroke documented by MRI or computed axial tomography.

[6]A history of chronic renal disease or abnormal blood urea nitrogen (BUN) and creatinine values documented in the medical record.

[7]Disorientation (to person, place, or time; not known to be chronic), stupor, or coma.

[8]In the Pneumonia Patient Outcome Research Team cohort study, an oxygen saturation value <90% on pulse oximetry or intubation before admission was also considered abnormal.

CONFUSION, UREMIA, RESPIRATORY RATE, BLOOD PRESSURE, AND AGE >65 YEARS (CURB-65)

Risk factors:

1. Presence of confusion (based on specific tests or noted disorientation to people, place, or time)
2. Blood urea nitrogen (BUN) of >7mmol/L (20 mg/dL)
3. Respiratory rate >30 breaths/minute
4. Systolic blood pressure <90 mmHg or diastolic <60 mmHg
5. Age >65 years

Number of Risk Factors	30-Day Mortality Risk (%)
0	0.7
1	2.1
2	9.2
3	14.5
4	40
5	57

Scoring:

0-1 risk factors: Treat as outpatient.

2 risk factors: Treat as inpatient.

3-5 risk factors: Treat as inpatient; likely requires more aggressive management, possibly ICU.

Epidemiological Conditions Related to Specific Pathogens in Patients With Selected Community-Acquired Pneumonia

Condition	Commonly Encountered Pathogens
Alcoholism	Streptococcus pneumoniae, anaerobes
COPD and/or smoker	S. pneumoniae, Haemophilus influenzae, Moraxella catarrhalis, Legionella species
Nursing home residency	S. pneumoniae, gram-negative bacilli, H. influenzae, Staphylococcus aureus, anaerobes, Chlamydia pneumoniae
Poor dental hygiene	Anaerobes
Epidemic Legionnaires' disease	Legionella species
Exposure to bats or soil enriched with bird droppings	Histoplasma capsulatum
Exposure to birds	Chlamydia psittaci
Exposure to rabbits	Francisella tularensis
HIV infection (early stage)	S. pneumoniae, H. influenzae, Mycobacterium tuberculosis
HIV infection (late stage)	Above plus P. carinii, Cryptococcus, Histoplasma species
Travel to southwestern United States	Coccidioides species
Exposure to farm animals or parturient cats	Coxiella burnetii (Q fever)
Influenza active in community	Influenza, S. pneumoniae, S. aureus, Streptococcus pyogenes, H. influenzae
Suspected large-volume aspiration	Anaerobes (chemical pneumonitis, obstruction)
Structural disease of the lung (bronchiectasis, cystic fibrosis, etc)	Pseudomonas aeruginosa, Burkholderia (Pseudomonas) cepacia, S. aureus
Injection drug use	S. aureus, anaerobes, M. tuberculosis, S. pneumoniae
Airway obstruction	Anaerobes, S. pneumoniae, H. influenzae, S. aureus

COPD = chronic obstructive pulmonary disease.

Initial Empiric Therapy for Suspected Bacterial Community-Acquired Pneumonia (CAP) in Immunocompetent Adults

Patient Variable	Preferred Treatment Options
Outpatient	
Previously healthy	
No recent antibiotic therapy or risk for DRSP	A macrolide[1] or doxycycline
Comorbidities[2]; recent antibiotic therapy[3]; risk factors for DRSP[4]	A respiratory fluoroquinolone[5] alone, or an advanced macrolide[6] plus high-dose amoxicillin,[7] high-dose amoxicillin-clavulanate,[8] cefpodoxime, cefTRIAXone, or cefuroxime.
Suspected aspiration with infection	Amoxicillin-clavulanate or clindamycin
Influenza with bacterial superinfection	Antiviral agent oseltamivir or zanamivir, plus a cefotaxime or cefTRIAXone or a respiratory fluoroquinolone[5]
Inpatient	
Non-ICU	A respiratory fluoroquinolone alone or macrolide plus a β-lactam[9]
ICU	
Pseudomonas infection is not an issue	Cefotaxime, cefTRIAXone, or ampicillin-sulbactam plus either azithromycin or a respiratory fluoroquinolone[5]
Pseudomonas infection is not an issue but patient has a β-lactam allergy	A respiratory fluoroquinolone,[5] with aztreonam
Pseudomonas infection is an issue[10]	Either (1) an antipseudomonal agent[11] plus ciprofloxacin or levofloxacin, or (2) an antipseudomonal agent plus an aminoglycoside[12] plus a respiratory fluoroquinolone[5] or azithromycin
Pseudomonas infection is an issue but the patient has a β-lactam allergy	Substitute aztreonam for any β-lactam antipseudomonal agent[11]
Nursing home	
Receiving treatment in nursing home	A respiratory fluoroquinolone[5] alone or amoxicillin-clavulanate plus an advanced macrolide
Suspicion or MRSA	Add vancomycin or linezolid to any suggested regimens

DRSP = drug-resistant *Streptococcus pneumoniae*; ICU = intensive care unit.

[1]Erythromycin, azithromycin, or clarithromycin.

[2]Chronic heart, lung, liver, and/or renal disease, diabetes, malignancy, or immunosuppressive medication and/or conditions.

[3]That is, the patient was given a course of antibiotic(s) for treatment of any infection within the past 3 months, excluding the current episode of infection. Such treatment is a risk factor for drug-resistant *Streptococcus pneumoniae* and possibly for infection with gram-negative bacilli. Depending on the class of antibiotics recently given, one or other of the suggested options may be selected. Recent use of a fluoroquinolone should dictate selection of a nonfluoroquinolone regimen, and vice versa.

[4]Risk factors for β-lactam-resistant *S. pneumoniae* include age <2 or >65 years, recent antimicrobial therapy (within previous 3 months, and especially to repeated courses of same antibiotic class), alcoholism, comorbidities, immunosuppressive illness or therapy, and exposure to child care centers.

[5]Moxifloxacin, levofloxacin, or gemifloxacin.

[6]Azithromycin or clarithromycin.

[7]Dosage, 1 g P.O. 3 times/day.

[8]Dosage, 2 g P.O. twice daily.

[9]Cefotaxime, cefTRIAXone, ampicillin (or ampicillin-sulbactam), or ertapenem; ertapenem was recently approved for such use (in once-daily parenteral treatment), but there is little experience thus far. **Note:** The 2007 CAP guidelines excluded ampicillin-sulbactam in favor of the single agent without the lactamase inhibitor. While this may be useful in specific situations, the prevalence of beta-lactamase-producing *H. influenzae* should be a concern, and thus the use of ampicillin-sulbactam may be more appropriate for empiric use.

[10]The antipseudomonal agents chosen reflect this concern. Risk factors for *Pseudomonas* infection include severe structural lung disease (eg, bronchiectasis), and recent antibiotic therapy or stay in hospital (especially in the ICU). For patients with CAP in the ICU, coverage for *S. pneumoniae* and *Legionella* species must always be assured. Piperacillin-tazobactam, imipenem, meropenem, and cefepime are excellent β-lactams and are adequate for most *S. pneumoniae* and *Haemophilus influenzae* infections. They may be preferred when there is concern for relatively unusual CAP pathogens, such as *Pseudomonas aeruginosa*, *Klebsiella* species, and other gram-negative bacteria.

[11]Piperacillin-tazobactam, imipenem, meropenem, or cefepime.

[12]Data suggest that elderly patients receiving aminoglycosides have worse outcomes.

REFERENCES

Bartlett JG, Breiman RF, Mandell LA, et al, "Community-Acquired Pneumonia in Adults: Guidelines for Management. The Infectious Diseases Society of America," *Clin Infect Dis*, 1998, 26(4):811-38.

Mandell LA, Bartlett JG, Dowell SF, et al, "Update of Practice Guidelines for the Management of Community-Acquired Pneumonia in Immunocompetent Adults," *Clin Infect Dis*, 2003, 37(11):1405-33.

Mandell LA, Wunderink RG, Anzueto A, et al, "Infectious Diseases Society of America/American Thoracic Society Consensus Guidelines on the Management of Community-Acquired Pneumonia in Adults," *Clin Infect Dis*, 2007, 44 (Suppl 2):S27-72.

PREVENTION OF INFECTIVE ENDOCARDITIS

Recommendations by the American Heart Association
(*Circulation* , 2007, 116(15):1736-54.)

Consensus Process – The recommendations were formulated by a writing group under the auspices of the American Heart Association (AHA), and included representation from the Infectious Diseases Society of America (IDSA), the American Academy of Pediatrics (AAP), and the American Dental Association (ADA). Additionally, input was received from both national and international experts on infective endocarditis (IE). These guidelines are based on expert interpretation and review of scientific literature from 1950 through 2006. The consensus statement was subsequently reviewed by outside experts not affiliated with the writing group and by the Science Advisory and Coordinating Committee of the American Heart Association. These guidelines are meant to aid practitioners but are not intended as the standard of care or as a substitute for clinical judgment.

Significant change from the previous 1997 guidelines – The previously published guidelines identified a broad range of cardiac conditions thought to predispose patients to a higher risk of IE. The document stratified these conditions into high-, moderate-, and low-risk categories, based on the likelihood of developing IE. The subsequent recommendations for prophylaxis were based on this classification, in conjunction with specification of numerous invasive procedures which were assumed to confer a higher risk of bacteremia, and therefore a higher risk of endocarditis. However, it is the consensus of the current writing group that existing data fail to show a clear link between many of these procedures, preexisting cardiovascular condition and IE. In the case of dental procedures, it was determined that the cumulative lifetime risk of developing bacteremia as a result of normal hygiene measures (eg, teeth brushing, flossing) vastly exceeded the risk associated with many of the procedures for which prophylaxis was previously recommended. Similarly, the writing group estimated that the absolute risk of developing IE as a result of dental procedures in patients with preexisting cardiac conditions was quite low, and there was little evidence to support the value of prophylactic antimicrobial efficacy in these cases.

In a major departure from the former recommendations, the current guidelines have been greatly simplified to place a much greater emphasis on a very limited number of underlying cardiac conditions (see below). These specific conditions have been associated with the highest risk of adverse outcomes due to IE. Patients should receive IE prophylaxis only if they are undergoing certain invasive procedures (see Table 1) and have one of the underlying cardiovascular conditions specified below.

Common situations for which routine prophylaxis was previously, but no longer recommended, include mitral valve prolapse, general dental cleanings and local anesthetic administration (noninfected tissue), and bronchoscopy (see Table 1).

Specific cardiac conditions for which IE antibiotic prophylaxis is recommended:

- Previous infective endocarditis

- Prosthetic cardiac valve or prosthetic material used for cardiac valve repair

- Cardiac transplantation patients who develop valvulopathy

- Congenital heart disease (CHD), only under the following conditions:

  – Unrepaired cyanotic CHD, including palliative shunts and conduits

  – Completely repaired defects (with prosthetic materials/devices), regardless of method of repair, within the first 6 months after the procedure

  – Repaired CHD with residual defects at or adjacent to the site of repair

Table 1. Guidance for Use of Prophylactic Antibiotic Therapy Based on Procedure or Condition[1]

Location of Procedure	Prophylaxis Recommended	Prophylaxis NOT Recommended
Dental	All invasive manipulations of the gingival or periapical region or perforation of oral mucosa	Anesthetic injections (through noninfected tissue), radiographs, placement/adjustment/removal prosthodontic/orthodontic appliances or brackets, shedding of deciduous teeth, trauma-induced bleeding from lips, gums, or oral mucosa
Respiratory tract	Biopsy/incision of respiratory mucosa (eg, tonsillectomy/adenoidectomy); drainage of abscess or empyema[2]	Bronchoscopy (unless incision of mucosa required)
Gastrointestinal (GI) or genitourinary (GU) tract	Established GI/GU infection or prevention of infectious sequelae[3]; elective cystoscopy or other urinary tract procedure with established enterococci infection/colonization[3,4]	Routine diagnostic procedures, including esophagogastroduodenoscopy or colonoscopy in the absence of active infection; vaginal delivery and hysterectomy
Skin, skin structure, or musculoskeletal	Any surgical procedure involving infected tissue	Procedures conducted in noninfected tissue; tattoos and ear/body piercing

[1]Patients should receive prophylactic antibiotic therapy if they meet the criteria for a specified procedure/condition in this table and they have a high-risk cardiovascular condition listed in the preceding text.

[2]If treating an infection of known staphylococcal origin, consider antistaphylococcal penicillin or cephalosporin, or vancomycin in beta-lactam-sensitive patients.

[3]Alternative agents with activity against enterococci to consider: Vancomycin (for beta-lactam-sensitive patients) or piperacillin.

[4]Eradication of enterococci from the urinary tract should be considered.

Table 2. Prophylactic Regimens for Oral / Dental, Respiratory Tract, Genitoruinary Tract, or Esophageal Procedures

Situation	Agent	Regimen to Be Given 30-60 Minutes Before Procedure	
		Adults	Children[1]
Standard general prophylaxis	Amoxicillin	2 g P.O.	50 mg/kg P.O.
Unable to take oral medications	Ampicillin **or**	2 g I.M./I.V.	50 mg/kg I.M./I.V.
	CeFAZolin or cefTRIAXone	1 g I.M./I.V.	50 mg/kg I.M./I.V.
Allergic to penicillin	Clindamycin **or**	600 mg P.O.	20 mg/kg P.O.
	Cephalexin[2] or other dose-equivalent first/ second generation cephalosporin **or**	2 g P.O	50 mg/kg P.O.
	Azithromycin or clarithromycin	500 mg P.O.	15 mg/kg P.O.
Allergic to penicillin and unable to take oral medications	Clindamycin **or**	600 mg I.V.	20 mg/kg I.V.
	CeFAZolin or cefTRIAXone[2]	1 g I.M./I.V.	50 mg/kg I.M./I.V.

[1]Total children's dose should not exceed adult dose.

[2]Cephalosporins should not be used in individuals with immediate-type hypersensitivity reaction (urticaria, angioedema, or anaphylaxis) to penicillins.

REFERENCE

Wilson W, Taubert KA, Gewitz M, et al, "Prevention of Infective Endocarditis. Guidelines From the American Heart Association. A Guideline From the American Heart Association Rheumatic Fever, Endocarditis, and Kawasaki Disease Committee, Council on Cardiovascular Disease in the Young, and the Council on Clinical Cardiology, Council on Cardiovascular Surgery and Anesthesia, and the Quality of Care and Outcomes Research Interdiscipli-nary Working Group," *Circulation*, 2007, 116(15):1736-54.

REFERENCE VALUES FOR ADULTS

CHEMISTRY

Test	Values	Remarks
Serum / Plasma		
Acetone	Negative	
Albumin	3.2-5 g/dL	
Alcohol, ethyl	Negative	
Aldolase	1.2-7.6 IU/L	
Ammonia	20-70 mcg/dL	Specimen to be placed on ice as soon as collected.
Amylase	30-110 units/L	
Bilirubin, direct	0-0.3 mg/dL	
Bilirubin, total	0.1-1.2 mg/dL	
Calcium	8.6-10.3 mg/dL	
Calcium, ionized	2.24-2.46 mEq/L	
Chloride	95-108 mEq/L	
Cholesterol, total	≤200 mg/dL	Fasted blood required – normal value affected by dietary habits. This reference range is for a general adult population.
HDL cholesterol	40-60 mg/dL	Fasted blood required – normal value affected by dietary habits.
LDL cholesterol	<160 mg/dL	If triglyceride is >400 mg/dL, LDL cannot be calculated accurately (Friedewald equation). Target LDL-C depends on patient's risk factors.
CO_2	23-30 mEq/L	
Creatine kinase (CK) isoenzymes		
CK-BB	0%	
CK-MB (cardiac)	0%-3.9%	
CK-MM (muscle)	96%-100%	
CK-MB levels must be both ≥4% and 10 IU/L to meet diagnostic criteria for CK-MB positive result consistent with myocardial injury.		
Creatine phosphokinase (CPK)	8-150 IU/L	
Creatinine	0.5-1.4 mg/dL	
Ferritin	13-300 ng/mL	
Folate	3.6-20 ng/dL	
GGT (gamma-glutamyltranspeptidase)		
male	11-63 IU/L	
female	8-35 IU/L	
GLDH	To be determined	
Glucose (preprandial)	<115 mg/dL	Goals different for diabetics.
Glucose, fasting	60-110 mg/dL	Goals different for diabetics.
Glucose, nonfasting (2-h postprandial)	<120 mg/dL	Goals different for diabetics.
Hemoglobin A_{1c}	<8	

CHEMISTRY *(continued)*

Test	Values	Remarks
Hemoglobin, plasma free	<2.5 mg/100 mL	
Hemoglobin, total glycosolated (Hb A_1)	4%-8%	
Iron	65-150 mcg/dL	
Iron binding capacity, total (TIBC)	250-420 mcg/dL	
Lactic acid	0.7-2.1 mEq/L	Specimen to be kept on ice and sent to lab as soon as possible.
Lactate dehydrogenase (LDH)	56-194 IU/L	
Lactate dehydrogenase (LDH) isoenzymes		
LD_1	20%-34%	
LD_2	29%-41%	
LD_3	15%-25%	
LD_4	1%-12%	
LD_5	1%-15%	

Flipped LD_1/LD_2 ratios (>1 may be consistent with myocardial injury) particularly when considered in combination with a recent CK-MB positive result.

Lipase	23-208 units/L	
Magnesium	1.6-2.5 mg/dL	Increased by slight hemolysis.
Osmolality	289-308 mOsm/kg	
Phosphatase, alkaline		
adults 25-60 y	33-131 IU/L	
adults ≥61 y	51-153 IU/L	
infancy-adolescence	Values range up to 3-5 times higher than adults	
Phosphate, inorganic	2.8-4.2 mg/dL	
Potassium	3.5-5.2 mEq/L	Increased by slight hemolysis.
Prealbumin	>15 mg/dL	
Protein, total	6.5-7.9 g/dL	
AST	<35 IU/L (20-48)	
ALT (10-35)	<35 IU/L	
Sodium	134-149 mEq/L	
Thyroid stimulating hormone (TSH)		
adults ≤20 y	0.7-6.4 mIU/L	
21-54 y	0.4-4.2 mIU/L	
55-87 y	0.5-8.9 mIU/L	
Transferrin	>200 mg/dL	
Triglycerides	45-155 mg/dL	Fasted blood required.
Troponin I	<1.5 ng/mL	
Urea nitrogen (BUN)	7-20 mg/dL	
Uric acid		
male	2-8 mg/dL	
female	2-7.5 mg/dL	

CHEMISTRY *(continued)*

Test	Values	Remarks
Cerebrospinal Fluid		
Glucose	50-70 mg/dL	
Protein	15-45 mg/dL	CSF obtained by lumbar puncture.

Note: Bloody specimen gives erroneously high value due to contamination with blood proteins

Urine
(24-hour specimen is required for all these tests unless specified)

Test	Values	Remarks
Amylase	32-641 units/L	The value is in units/L and **not** calculated for total volume.
Amylase, fluid (random samples)		Interpretation of value left for physician, depends on the nature of fluid.
Calcium	Depends upon dietary intake	
Creatine		
male	150 mg/24 h	Higher value on children and during pregnancy.
female	250 mg/24 h	
Creatinine	1000-2000 mg/24 h	
Creatinine clearance (endogenous)		
male	85-125 mL/min	A blood sample must accompany urine specimen.
female	75-115 mL/min	
Glucose	1 g/24 h	
5-hydroxyindoleacetic acid	2-8 mg/24 h	
Iron	0.15 mg/24 h	Acid washed container required.
Magnesium	146-209 mg/24 h	
Osmolality	500-800 mOsm/kg	With normal fluid intake.
Oxalate	10-40 mg/24 h	
Phosphate	400-1300 mg/24 h	
Potassium	25-120 mEq/24 h	Varies with diet; the interpretation of urine electrolytes and osmolality should be left for the physician.
Sodium	40-220 mEq/24 h	
Porphobilinogen, qualitative	Negative	
Porphyrins, qualitative	Negative	
Proteins	0.05-0.1 g/24 h	
Salicylate	Negative	
Urea clearance	60-95 mL/min	A blood sample must accompany specimen.
Urea N	10-40 g/24 h	Dependent on protein intake.
Uric acid	250-750 mg/24 h	Dependent on diet and therapy.
Urobilinogen	0.5-3.5 mg/24 h	For qualitative determination on random urine, send sample to urinalysis section in Hematology Lab.
Xylose absorption test		
children	16%-33% of ingested xylose	

CHEMISTRY *(continued)*

Test	Values	Remarks
Feces		
Fat, 3-day collection	<5 g/d	Value depends on fat intake of 100 g/d for 3 days preceding and during collection.
Gastric Acidity		
Acidity, total, 12 h	10-60 mEq/L	Titrated at pH 7.

Blood Gases

	Arterial	Capillary	Venous
pH	7.35-7.45	7.35-7.45	7.32-7.42
pCO_2 (mm Hg)	35-45	35-45	38-52
pO_2 (mm Hg)	70-100	60-80	24-48
HCO_3 (mEq/L)	19-25	19-25	19-25
TCO_2 (mEq/L)	19-29	19-29	23-33
O_2 saturation (%)	90-95	90-95	40-70
Base excess (mEq/L)	-5 to +5	-5 to +5	-5 to +5

HEMATOLOGY

Complete Blood Count

Age	Hgb (g/dL)	Hct (%)	RBC (mill/mm^3)	RDW
0-3 d	15.0-20.0	45-61	4.0-5.9	<18
1-2 wk	12.5-18.5	39-57	3.6-5.5	<17
1-6 mo	10.0-13.0	29-42	3.1-4.3	<16.5
7 mo to 2 y	10.5-13.0	33-38	3.7-4.9	<16
2-5 y	11.5-13.0	34-39	3.9-5.0	<15
5-8 y	11.5-14.5	35-42	4.0-4.9	<15
13-18 y	12.0-15.2	36-47	4.5-5.1	<14.5
Adult male	13.5-16.5	41-50	4.5-5.5	<14.5
Adult female	12.0-15.0	36-44	4.0-4.9	<14.5

Age	MCV (fL)	MCH (pg)	MCHC (%)	Plts (x 10^3/mm^3)
0-3 d	95-115	31-37	29-37	250-450
1-2 wk	86-110	28-36	28-38	250-450
1-6 mo	74-96	25-35	30-36	300-700
7 mo to 2 y	70-84	23-30	31-37	250-600
2-5 y	75-87	24-30	31-37	250-550
5-8 y	77-95	25-33	31-37	250-550
13-18 y	78-96	25-35	31-37	150-450
Adult male	80-100	26-34	31-37	150-450
Adult female	80-100	26-34	31-37	150-450

WBC and Differential

Age	WBC (x 10³/mm³)	Segs	Bands	Lymphs	Monos
0-3 d	9.0-35.0	32-62	<18	19-29	5-7
1-2 wk	5.0-20.0	14-34	<14	36-45	6-10
1-6 mo	6.0-17.5	13-33	<12	41-71	4-7
7 mo to 2 y	6.0-17.0	15-35	<11	45-76	3-6
2-5 y	5.5-15.5	23-45	<11	35-65	3-6
5-8 y	5.0-14.5	32-54	<11	28-48	3-6
13-18 y	4.5-13.0	34-64	<11	25-45	3-6
Adults	4.5-11.0	35-66	<11	24-44	3-6

Age	Eosinophils	Basophils	Atypical Lymphs	No. of NRBCs
0-3 d	0-2	0-1	0-8	0-2
1-2 wk	0-2	0-1	0-8	0
1-6 mo	0-3	0-1	0-8	0
7 mo to 2 y	0-3	0-1	0-8	0
2-5 y	0-3	0-1	0-8	0
5-8 y	0-3	0-1	0-8	0
13-18 y	0-3	0-1	0-8	0
Adults	0-3	0-1	0-8	0

Segs = segmented neutrophils.

Bands = band neutrophils.

Lymphs = lymphocytes.

Monos = monocytes.

Erythrocyte Sedimentation Rates and Reticulocyte Counts

Sedimentation rate, Westergren

Children 0-20 mm/h

Adult male 0-15 mm/h

Adult female 0-20 mm/h

Sedimentation rate, Wintrobe

Children 0-13 mm/h

Adult male 0-10 mm/h

Adult female 0-15 mm/h

Reticulocyte count

Newborns 2%-6%

1-6 mo 0%-2.8%

Adults 0.5%-1.5%

CMS GUIDELINES FOR GRADUAL DOSE REDUCTION OF PSYCHOPHARMACOLOGICAL AGENTS IN NURSING FACILITY RESIDENTS

http://www.cms.hhs.gov/transmittals/downloads/R22SOMA.pdf
Section 483.25(l)

The following is an excerpt from Appendix PP of the Centers for Medicare and Medicaid Services (CMS) State Operations Manual concerning gradual dose reduction in relation to specific classes of psychopharmacologic agents. The reader is referred to Table 1 (Medication Issues of Particular Relevance) in the above document, for further information regarding the use of psychopharmacological agents in nursing facilities.

CONSIDERATIONS SPECIFIC TO ANTIPSYCHOTICS

The regulation addressing the use of antipsychotic medications identifies the process of tapering as a "gradual dose reduction (GDR)" and requires a GDR, unless clinically contraindicated.

Within the first year in which a resident is admitted on an antipsychotic medication or after the facility has initiated an antipsychotic medication, the facility must attempt a GDR in two separate quarters (with at least one month between the attempts), unless clinically contraindicated. After the first year, a GDR must be attempted annually, unless clinically contraindicated.

For any individual who is receiving an antipsychotic medication to treat behavioral symptoms related to dementia, the GDR may be considered clinically contraindicated if:

- The resident's target symptoms returned or worsened after the most recent attempt at a GDR within the facility; and

- The physician has documented the clinical rationale for why any additional attempted dose reduction at that time would be likely to impair the resident's function or increase distressed behavior.

For any individual who is receiving an antipsychotic medication to treat a psychiatric disorder other than behavioral symptoms related to dementia (for example, schizophrenia, bipolar mania, or depression with psychotic features), the GDR may be considered contraindicated, if:

- The continued use is in accordance with relevant current standards of practice and the physician has documented the clinical rationale for why any attempted dose reduction would be likely to impair the resident's function or cause psychiatric instability by exacerbating an underlying psychiatric disorder; or

- The resident's target symptoms returned or worsened after the most recent attempt at a GDR within the facility and the physician has documented the clinical rationale for why any additional attempted dose reduction at that time would be likely to impair the resident's function or cause psychiatric instability by exacerbating an underlying medical or psychiatric disorder.

ATTEMPTED TAPERING RELATIVE TO CONTINUED INDICATION OR OPTIMAL DOSE

As noted, attempted tapering is one way to determine whether a specific medication is still indicated, and whether target symptoms and risks can be managed with a lesser dose of a medication. As noted, many medications in various categories can be tapered safely. The following examples of tapering relate to two common categories of concern: sedatives/hypnotics and psychopharmacologic medications (other than antipsychotic and sedatives/hypnotics medications).

TAPERING CONSIDERATIONS SPECIFIC TO SEDATIVES / HYPNOTICS

For as long as a resident remains on a sedative/hypnotic that is used routinely and beyond the manufacturer's recommendations for duration of use, the facility should attempt to taper the medication quarterly unless clinically contraindicated. Clinically contraindicated means:

- The continued use is in accordance with relevant current standards of practice and the physician has documented the clinical rationale for why any attempted dose reduction would be likely to impair the resident's function or cause psychiatric instability by exacerbating an underlying medical or psychiatric disorder; or

- The resident's target symptoms returned or worsened after the most recent attempt at tapering the dose within the facility and the physician has documented the clinical rationale for why any additional attempted dose reduction at that time would be likely to impair the resident's function or cause psychiatric instability by exacerbating an underlying medical or psychiatric disorder.

CONSIDERATIONS SPECIFIC TO PSYCHOPHARMACOLOGICAL MEDICATIONS (OTHER THAN ANTIPSYCHOTICS AND SEDATIVES / HYPNOTICS)

During the first year in which a resident is admitted on a psychopharmacological medication (other than an antipsychotic or a sedative/hypnotic), or after the facility has initiated such medication, the facility should attempt to taper the medication during at least two separate quarters (with at least one month between the attempts), unless clinically contraindicated. After the first year, a tapering should be attempted annually, unless clinically contraindicated. The tapering may be considered clinically contraindicated, if:

- The continued use is in accordance with relevant current standards of practice and the physician has documented the clinical rationale for why any attempted dose reduction would be likely to impair the resident's function or cause psychiatric instability by exacerbating an underlying medical or psychiatric disorder; or

- The resident's target symptoms returned or worsened after the most recent attempt at tapering the dose within the facility and the physician has documented the clinical rationale for why any additional attempted dose reduction at that time would be likely to impair the resident's function or cause psychiatric instability by exacerbating an underlying medical or psychiatric disorder.

DIABETES MELLITUS MANAGEMENT, ADULTS

OVERVIEW

Diabetes represents a significant health care problem in the United States and worldwide. Of the nearly 23.6 million Americans (7.8% of the population) with diabetes, the majority (90% to 95%) have type 2 diabetes. Of this number, nearly one-quarter are undiagnosed. The incidence of type 2 diabetes is increasing around the world. There is strong evidence to support an interaction between a genetic predisposition and behavioral or environmental factors, such as obesity and physical inactivity, in the development of this disease. In individuals at high risk of developing type 2 diabetes, it has been shown that the development of diabetes may be prevented or delayed by changes in lifestyle or pharmacologic intervention.

Within the United States, type 1 diabetes is estimated to comprise 5% to 10% of those with diabetes, and therefore represents the minority of individuals with diabetes. In addition to type 1 and type 2 diabetes, approximately 7% of pregnancies are complicated by the development of gestational diabetes. Gestational diabetes mellitus is defined as the first onset or recognition of glucose intolerance during pregnancy. Women who have had gestational diabetes are at an increased risk for later development of type 2 diabetes. In addition to the causes noted above, diabetes may result from genetic syndromes, surgery (pancreatectomy), chemicals and/or drugs, recurrent pancreatitis, malnutrition, and viral infections.

Additional information available at: http://care.diabetesjournals.org/content/34/Supplement_1

COMPLICATIONS OF DIABETES

Diabetes was listed as the seventh leading cause of death in the United States in 2007. Complications of diabetes are often contributing factors in the death of these patients; the most frequently reported diabetes complications on the death certificates of patients with diabetes in 2004 were heart disease and stroke, which were listed as contributing factors in 68% and 16% of diabetes-related deaths, respectively.

In addition to cardiovascular effects, diabetes is the leading cause of new blindness in people 20-74 years old, and diabetic nephropathy is the most common cause of end-stage renal disease. Mild to severe forms of diabetic neuropathy are common. Neuropathy and circulatory insufficiency combine to make diabetes the most frequent cause of nontraumatic lower-limb amputations (60% of cases). The rate of impotence in diabetic males over 50 years old has been estimated to be as high as 35% to 50%. Control of hyperglycemia may significantly decrease the rate at which diabetic complications develop; this provides compelling justification for early diagnosis and management of this disorder.

DIAGNOSIS

Diabetes

Diagnosis of diabetes in nonpregnant adults is made by any of the four criteria described below. In the absence of unequivocal hyperglycemia with acute metabolic decompensation, these criteria should be confirmed by repeat testing on a different day. New in the 2010 American Diabetes Association (ADA) Standards of Medical Care is the recommendation for the use of Hb A_{1c} for the diagnosis of diabetes; the method used should be certified by the National Glycohemoglobin Standardization Program (NGSP) and standardized to the Diabetes Control and Complications Trial (DCCT) assay. Screening should be considered in overweight adult patients (BMI ≥25 kg/m^2) who have at least one risk factor for diabetes (eg, physical inactivity, first-degree relative with diabetes, history of cardiovascular disease, etc). In patients without risk factors, testing should begin at age 45. Repeat testing should occur at least every 3 years in patients with normal test results.

Criteria for Diagnosis

1. Hb A$_{1c}$ ≥6.5%

   OR

2. Fasting plasma glucose (no caloric intake for at least 8 hours) ≥126 mg/dL (7 mmol/L)
   OR

3. Casual plasma glucose concentration≥200 mg/dL (11.1 mmol/L) in patients with symptoms of hyperglycemia (polydipsia, polyuria, unexplained weight loss) or hyperglycemic crisis. **Note:** Casual plasma glucose is defined as any time of day without regard to time of last meal.
   OR

4. A 2-hour plasma glucose ≥200 mg/dL (11.1 mmol/L) during an oral glucose tolerance test (OGTT) in accordance with the standards set forth by the World Health Organization (WHO) using a 75 g anhydrous glucose load (or equivalent) dissolved in water. **Note:** OGTT is not recommended for routine clinical use.

Note: In the absence of unequivocal hyperglycemia, criteria 1, 2, and 4 should be confirmed by repeat testing.

Categories of Increased Risk for Diabetes

Patients with impaired fasting glucose (IFG), impaired glucose tolerance (IGT), or an intermediately high Hb A$_{1c}$ are considered to be in a group whose glucose levels do not meet the criteria for diabetes, yet are higher than normal. Patients who meet any of the following criteria are considered to be at high risk for developing diabetes and cardiovascular disease, and are referred to as having "prediabetes":

1. IFG: Fasting plasma glucose (no caloric intake for at least 8 hours) 100-125 mg/dL (5.6-6.9 mmol/L)

   OR

2. IGT: A 2-hour plasma glucose 140-199 mg/dL (7.8-11 mmol/L) during an oral glucose tolerance test (OGTT) in accordance with the standards set forth by the World Health Organization (WHO) using a 75 g anhydrous glucose load (or equivalent) dissolved in water.
   OR

3. Hb A$_{1c}$: 5.7% to 6.4%; **Note:** Patients with an Hb A$_{1c}$ >6% should be considered at very high risk for diabetes and receive intensive interventions and monitoring.

The International Expert Committee consisting of members of the ADA, the European Association for the Study of Diabetes (EASD), and the International Diabetes Federation (IDF) recently recommended that the clinical states "prediabetes," IFG, and IGT be phased out as the Hb A1c becomes the preferred diagnostic test (International Expert Committee, 2009).

GOALS

The goals of diabetes treatment include normalization of hyperglycemia, avoidance of hypo-glycemia, and slowing the development of diabetic complications. The following is a summary of recommendations for nonpregnant adults with diabetes.

2011 ADA Summary of Recommendations for Adults With Diabetes

Glycemic control

Hb A$_{1c}$	<7%[1]
Preprandial capillary plasma glucose	70-130 mg/dL
Peak postprandial capillary plasma glucose[2]	<180 mg/dL

Blood pressure[7]

	<130/80 mm Hg

Lipids[3]

LDL[4]	<100 mg/dL
Triglycerides	<150 mg/dL
HDL	Male: >40 mg/dL Female: >50 mg/dL
Non-HDL chloesterol[5]	<130 mg/dL
Apolipoprotein B[6]	<90 mg/dL

[1]Referenced to a nondiabetic range of 4% to 6% using a DCCT-based assay. **Note:** The Hb A$_{1c}$ goal for patients in general is <7%; an even lower goal may be appropriate for selected individuals (eg, short duration of diabetes, long life expectancy, and no significant cardiovascular disease) so long as a lower goal can be achieved without significant hypoglycemia or other adverse effects. Conversely, a less stringent goal may be appropriate in certain patients (eg, history of severe hypoglycemia, limited life expectancy, advanced micro- or macrovascular complications, extensive comorbid conditions, longstanding diabetes in whom the general goal is difficult to attain despite appropriate diabetes management).

[2]Postprandial glucose measurements should be made 1-2 hours after the beginning of the meal, generally peak levels in patients with diabetes.

[3]Current NCEP/ATP III guidelines suggest that in patients with triglycerides ≥200 mg/dL, the non-HDL cholesterol (total cholesterol minus HDL) be used. The goal is <130 mg/dL.

[4]In patients with overt CVD or cardiometabolic risk factors (eg, central obesity, insulin resistance, hypertension), a lower LDL goal of <70 mg/dL is an option.

[5]In patients with overt CVD or cardiometabolic risk factors (eg, central obesity, insulin resistance, hypertension) with an LDL goal of <70 mg/dL, the non-HDL cholesterol goal is <100 mg/dL

[6]In patients on a statin with an LDL goal of <70 mg/dL or patients with cardiometabolic risk factors (eg, central obesity, insulin resistance, hypertension), the apolipoprotein B goal is <80 mg/dL

[7]Higher or lower systolic blood pressure targets may be appropriate based on individual patient characteristics and response to therapy.

Key concepts in setting glycemic goals:

- Hb A$_{1c}$ is the primary target for glycemic control.

- Goals should be individualized.

- Certain populations (children, pregnant women, and elderly) require special consider-ations.

- Less intensive glycemic goals may be indicated in patients with severe or frequent hypoglycemia.

- A lower glycemic goal (eg, Hb A$_{1c}$ <6%) may further reduce the risk of microvascular complications at the cost of an increased risk of hypoglycemia (particularly in those with type 1 diabetes). However, recent studies (eg, ACCORD and VADT) have highlighted certain patient populations in which the risks of intensive glycemic control may outweigh the benefits, including patients with a very long duration of diabetes, history of severe hypoglycemia, advanced atherosclerosis, and advanced age or frailty.

- Postprandial glucose may be targeted if Hb A$_{1c}$ goals are not met despite reaching preprandial glucose goals.

MANAGEMENT

Multidisciplinary approach necessary. Patient education:

- Wearing appropriate identification of disease
- Foot care
- Eye care
- Acute illness management
- Hypoglycemia recognition and management
- Weight monitoring and management, including diet and exercise and bariatric surgery options (BMI >35 kg/m^2)

TYPE 1 DIABETES DRUG TREATMENT

Intensive insulin therapy: ≥3 injections/day of basal and prandial insulin or continuous subcutaneous infusion. If hypoglycemia is problematic, the use of insulin analogs may be helpful.

Monitoring

Self-monitoring of blood glucose (SMBG) should be carried out three or more times daily for patients using multiple insulin injections or insulin pump therapy. For patients using less frequent insulin injections, noninsulin therapies, or medical nutrition therapy (MNT) alone, SMBG may be useful as a guide to the success of therapy. To achieve postprandial glucose targets, postprandial SMBG may be appropriate.

Continuous glucose monitoring (CGM) in conjunction with intensive insulin regimens can be a useful tool to lower A1C in selected adults (age ≥25 years) with type 1 diabetes. CGM may be a supplemental tool in those with hypoglycemia episodes.

Insulin

Insulin therapy is required in type 1 diabetes, and may be necessary in some individuals with type 2 diabetes. The general objective of insulin replacement therapy is to approximate the physiologic pattern of insulin secretion which is characterized by two distinct phases. Phase 1 insulin secretion suppresses hepatic glucose production and phase 2 insulin secretion occurs in response to carbohydrate ingestion. This requires a basal level of insulin throughout the day (such as intermediate- or long-acting insulin or continuous insulin infusion administered via an external SubQ insulin infusion pump), supplemented by additional insulin at mealtimes (eg, short- or rapid-acting insulin).

Multiple daily doses guided by blood glucose monitoring are the standard of diabetes care. Combinations of insulin are commonly used. The number and size of daily doses, time of administration, and diet and exercise require continuous medical supervision. In addition, specific formulations may require distinct administration procedures/timing (refer to individual monographs).

There is solid scientific documentation of the benefit of tight glucose control, either by insulin pump or multiple daily injections (4-6 times daily). However, the benefits must be balanced against the risk of hypoglycemia, the patient's ability to adhere to the regimen, and other issues regarding the complexity of management. Diabetes self-management education (DSME) and medical nutrition therapy (MNT) are essential to maximize the effectiveness of therapy. In addition to the educational issues outlined above, patients should be instructed in insulin administration techniques, timing of administration, and sick-day management.

The initial dose of insulin in type 1 diabetes is typically 0.5-1 units/kg/day in divided doses. Conservative initial doses of 0.2-0.4 units/kg/day are often recommended to avoid the potential for hypoglycemia. Generally, one-half to three-fourths of the daily insulin dose is given as an intermediate- or long-acting form of insulin (in 1-2 daily injections). The remaining portion of the 24-hour insulin requirement is divided and administered as a rapid-acting or short-acting form of insulin. These may be given with meals (before or at the time of meals depending on the form of insulin) or at the same time as injections of intermediate forms (some premixed combinations are intended for this purpose). Some patients may benefit from the use of continuous subcutaneous insulin infusion (CSII) which delivers rapid-acting insulin as a continuous infusion throughout the day and as boluses at mealtimes via an external pump device.

Since combinations of agents are frequently used, dosage adjustment must address the individual component of the insulin regimen which most directly influences the blood glucose value in question, based on the known onset and duration of the insulin component (see table). The frequency of doses and monitoring must also be individualized in consideration of the patient's ability to manage therapy.

Types of Insulin	Onset (h)	Peak Glycemic Effect (h)	Duration (h)
Rapid-Acting			
Insulin lispro (HumaLOG®)	0.25-0.5	0.5-2.5	≤5
Insulin aspart (NovoLOG®)	0.2-0.3	1-3	3-5
Insulin glulisine (Apidra®)	0.2-0.5	1.6-2.8	3-4
Short-Acting			
Insulin regular (HumuLIN® R, NovoLIN® R)	0.5	2.5-5	4-12 – U-100 Up to 24 – U-500
Intermediate-Acting			
Insulin NPH (isophane suspension) (HumuLIN® N, NovoLIN® N)	1-2	4-12	14-24
Intermediate- to Long-Acting			
Insulin detemir (Levemir®)	3-4	3-9	6-23 (duration is dose-dependent)
Long-Acting			
Insulin glargine (Lantus®)	3-4	*	10.8-≥24
Combinations			
Insulin aspart protamine suspension and insulin aspart (NovoLOG® Mix 70/30)	0.17-0.33	1-4	18-24
Insulin lispro protamine and insulin lispro (HumaLOG® Mix 75/25™)	0.25-0.5	1-6.5	14-24
Insulin NPH suspension and insulin regular solution (NovoLIN® 70/30)	0.5	2-12	18-24

*Insulin glargine has no pronounced peak.

Maintenance Dosing

Typical maintenance insulin doses are between 0.5 and 1.2 units/kg/day in divided doses. Adolescents may require as much as 1.5 units/kg/day during puberty; whereas prepubescent individuals may only require 0.7-1 unit/kg/day.

As stated above, the general objective of insulin replacement therapy is to approximate the physiologic pattern of insulin secretion. This requires a basal level of insulin throughout the day, supplemented by additional insulin at mealtimes. Combination regimens which exploit differences in the onset and duration of different insulin products are commonly used to approximate physiologic secretion. Frequently, split-mixed or basal-bolus regimens are used to approximate physiologic secretion.

Split-mixed regimens: In split-mixed regimens, an intermediate-acting insulin (eg, NPH insulin) is administered once or twice daily and supplemented by short-acting (regular) or rapid-acting (lispro, aspart, or glulisine) insulin. Blood glucose measurements are completed several times daily. Dosages are adjusted emphasizing the individual component of the regimen which most directly influences the blood sugar in question (either the intermediate-acting component or the shorter-acting component). Fixed-ratio formulations (eg, 70/30 mix) may be used as twice daily injections in this scenario; however, the ability to titrate the dosage of an individual component is limited. An example of a "split-mixed" regimen would be 21 units of NPH plus 9 units of regular in the morning and an evening meal dose consisting of 14 units of NPH plus 6 units of regular insulin.

Basal-bolus regimens: Basal-bolus regimens are designed to more closely mimic physiologic secretion. These regimens employ intermediate- to long-acting insulins (eg, glargine, detemir) or a continuous insulin infusion administered via an external SubQ insulin infusion pump to simulate basal insulin secretion. The basal component is frequently administered at bedtime or in the early morning or as a continuous insulin infusion and then supplemented by multiple daily injections of rapid-acting products (lispro, glulisine, or aspart) immediately prior to a meal; thereby, providing insulin at the time when nutrients are absorbed. An example of a basal-bolus regimen would be 30 units of glargine at bedtime and 12 units of lispro insulin prior to each meal.

Adjustment of Insulin Dose

Dosage must be titrated to achieve glucose control and avoid hypoglycemia. In general, dosage is adjusted to maintain recommendations for glycemic control. Since treatment regimens often consist of multiple formulations, dosage adjustments must address the specific phase of insulin release that is primarily contributing to the patient's impaired glycemic control. Treatment and monitoring regimens must be individualized.

Estimation of the effect per unit: A "Rule of 1500" has been frequently used as a means to estimate the change in blood sugar relative to each unit of insulin administered. In fact, the recommended values used in these calculations may vary from 1500-2200 (a value of at least 1800 is recommended for lispro). The higher values lead to more conservative estimates of the effect per unit of insulin, and therefore lead to more cautious adjustments. The effect per unit of insulin (aka, correction factor) is approximated by dividing the selected numerical value (eg, 1500-2200) by the number of units/day received by the patient. The correction factor may be used as a crude approximation of the patient's insulin sensitivity to determine the correction doses of insulin or adjust the current insulin regimen. Each additional unit of insulin added to the corresponding insulin dose may be expected to lower the blood glucose by the value of the correction factor.

To illustrate, in the "basal-bolus" regimen which includes 30 units of glargine at bedtime and 12 units of lispro insulin prior to each meal, the rule of 1800 would indicate an expected change of 27 mg/dL per unit of insulin (the total daily insulin dose is 66 units; using the formula: correction factor = 1800/66 = 27). A patient may be instructed to add additional insulin if the preprandial glucose is >125 mg/dL. For a prelunch glucose of 195 mg/dL (70 mg/dL higher than goal), this would mean the patient would administer the scheduled 12 units of lispro along with an additional "correction dose" of 3 units (70 divided by the correction factor of 27 derived from the formula) for a total of 15 units prior to the meal. If correction doses are required on a consistent basis, an adjustment of the patient's diet and/or scheduled insulin dose may be necessary.

Hypoglycemia

Hypoglycemia is the leading limiting factor in the treatment of diabetes. A patient experiencing an episode of acutely low blood sugar can perceive the event as an inconvenience in milder cases to a real threat of falls, motor vehicle accidents, etc. in severe cases.

Management of hypoglycemia:

- Conscious individual: Oral glucose: 15-20 g (any form of carbohydrate that contains glucose may be used). If a self-measurement of blood glucose (SMBG) 15 minutes after treatment shows continued hypoglycemia, the treatment should be repeated. Once SMBG glucose returns to normal, the individual should consume a meal or snack to prevent recurrence of hypoglycemia.

- Glucagon should be prescribed for all individuals at significant risk of severe hypoglycemia, and caregivers or family members should be instructed in administration.

- Patients with hypoglycemia unawareness or one or more episodes of severe hypoglycemia should be advised to raise their glycemic targets to avoid further hypoglycemia at least for a short period of time.

- Re-enforce education about prevention of hypoglycemia.

TYPE 2 DIABETES DRUG TREATMENT

Insulin therapy

Several suggested algorithms for management of adult nonpregnant patients may be found (Nathan, 2009; Rodbard, 2009). Insulin may be used in type 2 diabetes as a means to augment response to oral antidiabetic agents or as monotherapy in selected patients. According to a consensus statement developed by the ADA and the European Association for the Study of Diabetes, basal insulin (eg, glargine, detemir) should be considered in patients who have failed to achieve their glycemic goals following lifestyle interventions and the administration of the maximal tolerated dose of metformin (ADA, 2009; Rodbard, 2009). Furthermore, intensive insulin therapy (eg, basal-bolus regimens) should be considered in patients who have failed to achieve their glycemic goals with an optimized two- or three-drug regimen (ADA, 2009; Rodbard, 2009). Augmentation to control postprandial glucose may be accomplished with regular, glulisine, aspart, or lispro insulin. Dosage must be carefully adjusted.

When used as monotherapy, the requirements for insulin are highly variable. An empirically defined scheme for dosage estimation based on fasting plasma glucose and degree of obesity has been published with recommended doses ranging from 6-77 units/day (Holman, 1995). In the setting of glucose toxicity (loss of beta-cell sensitivity to glucose concentrations), insulin therapy may be used for short-term management to restore sensitivity of beta-cells; in these cases, the dose may need to be rapidly reduced/withdrawn when sensitivity is re-established.

Oral Agents

A large number of drugs for oral administration have become available for the management of type 2 diabetes. Oral antidiabetic agents include sulfonylureas, meglitinides, alpha-glucosidase inhibitors, biguanides, thiazolidinediones (TZDs), and dipeptidyl peptidase IV (DPP-IV) inhibitors. The drug classes vary in terms of their magnitude of effect on glycemic control, mechanism of action, and adverse effect profiles. In many cases, the adverse effect profile may influence the selection of a particular drug. The risk of hypoglycemia is higher for drugs which promote insulin secretion (particularly sulfonylureas or insulin secretagogues). Drug selection is based on patient-specific factors and anticipated tolerance of adverse effects.

Metformin is currently the drug of choice if the patient has no contraindications. If lifestyle intervention and the maximal tolerated dose of metformin fail to achieve or sustain the glycemic goals, another medication should be added in several months. Another medication may also be necessary if metformin is contraindicated or not tolerated. Insulin or a sulfonylurea may be considered the next step if metformin and lifestyle changes are not adequate.

Combination therapy may be necessary to achieve glycemic goals. The risk of additive or additional adverse effects must be balanced with the desire to achieve goals of glycemic control as well as normalization of other metabolic parameters. In particular, weight gain and lipid disturbances may complicate drug treatment.

Oral Antidiabetic Agents for Type 2 Diabetes

Generic Name (Brand Name)	Expected Decrease (%) in Hb A_{1c} With Monotherapy	Key Adverse Effects
Alpha-Glucosidase Inhibitors		
Acarbose (Precose®)	0.5-0.8	GI distress, bloating, flatulence
Miglitol (Glyset®)		
Antilipemic Agent (Adjunct Therapy)		
Colesevelam (WelChol®)	0.5-1 (not for use as monotherapy)	Constipation, dyspepsia
Biguanide		
Metformin (Fortamet™; Glucophage® XR; Glucophage®; Glumetza®; Riomet®)	1-2	**Lactic acidosis [BOXED WARNING]**, GI distress, weakness
Dipeptidyl Peptidase IV (DPP-IV) Inhibitors		
Linagliptin (Tradjenta™)	0.4	Headache, nasopharyngitis, arthralgia, back pain
Saxagliptin (Onglyza™)	0.4-0.5	Headache, UTI, sinusitis
Sitagliptin (Januvia™)	0.5-0.8	Nasopharyngitis, GI distress, nausea, peripheral edema, hypoglycemia
Dopamine agonists		
Bromocriptine (Cycloset®)	0.1	Nausea, dizziness, somnolence, postural hypotension, headache
Meglitinide Derivatives		
Nateglinide (Starlix®)	0.5-1.5 (repaglinide may be more effective)	Upper respiratory infection, flu-like syndrome, headache, hypoglycemia
Repaglinide (Prandin®)		
Sulfonylurea, 1st Generation		
ChlorproPAMIDE (Diabinese®)	1-2	Hypoglycemia, dizziness, headache, GI distress, SIADH
Tolazamide		
TOLBUTamide		
Sulfonylurea, 2nd Generation		
Glimepiride (Amaryl®)	1-2	Hypoglycemia, dizziness, headache, GI distress, SIADH
GlipiZIDE (Glucotrol® XL; Glucotrol®)		
GlyBURIDE (DiaBeta®; Glynase® PresTab®; Micronase®)		
Thiazolidinediones		
Pioglitazone (Actos®)	0.5-1.4	**May cause or exacerbate heart failure [BOXED WARNING]**, hepatic dysfunction, weight gain, edema, lipid changes
Rosiglitazone (Avandia®)		

Injectable Agents (Noninsulin)

In addition to insulin and oral agents, three injectable products are available for the management of diabetes. Exenatide (Byetta®) and liraglutide (Victoza®) are GLP-1 receptor agonists FDA-approved for the treatment of type 2 diabetes. Exenatide is used as an adjunct to diet and exercise to improve glycemic control in patients with type 2 diabetes mellitus. The manufacturer of liraglutide states that it is an injectable prescription medicine that may improve blood sugar in adults with type 2 diabetes when used along with diet and exercise. GLP-1 agonists increase insulin secretion, increase B-cell growth/replication, slow gastric emptying, and may decrease food intake.

Pramlintide (Symlin®) is FDA approved for the treatment of type 1 and type 2 diabetes. In type 1 diabetes, it is approved for use in patients who have failed to achieve glucose control despite optimal insulin therapy. When used for type 2 diabetes, pramlintide is approved for use in patients who have failed to achieve desired glucose control despite optimal insulin therapy, with or without concurrent sulfonylurea and/or metformin. Pramlintide is a synthetic analog of human amylin cosecreted with insulin by pancreatic beta cells. It reduces postprandial glucose increases by prolonging gastric emptying time, reducing postprandial glucagon secretion, and reducing caloric intake through centrally-mediated appetite suppression. It should be noted that the concentration of this product is in mcg/mL; patients and healthcare providers should exercise caution when administering this product to avoid inadvertent calculation of the dose based on "units," which could result in a sixfold overdose.

Injectable Agents (Non-Insulin) for Type 2 Diabetes

Generic Name (Brand Name)	Expected Decrease (%) in Hb A_{1c} With Monotherapy	Key Adverse Effects
Glucagon-Like Peptide 1 (GLP-1) Agonist		
Exenatide (Byetta®)	0.5-1	Hypoglycemia, nausea, vomiting, pancreatitis, headache, jittery feeling
Liraglutide (Victoza®)	1	Thyroid C-cell Tumors [BOXED WARNING], nausea, vomiting, diarrhea, constipation, headache, pancreatitis
Amylin Agonists		
Pramlintide (Symlin®)	0.4-0.6	Coadministration with insulin may induce severe hypoglycemia [BOXED WARNING], nausea, vomiting, hypoglycemia, headache, anorexia

Additional Management Issues

Recommendation by the ADA include glycemic control, as well as the following:

*   Monitoring: In all patients with diabetes, cardiovascular risk factors should be assessed at least annually.

*   Cardiovascular risk management

    –   Use an ACEI or ARB in patients with diabetes who have hypertension and micro- or macroalbuminuria to slow the progression of nephropathy, unless contraindicated (eg, pregnancy); additional agents (eg, thiazide or loop diuretics) may be added as needed to achieve blood pressure goals.

    –   Consider statin use in all patients with diabetes and cardiovascular disease or in patients with diabetes >40 years old without cardiovascular disease but have at least one other cardiovascular disease risk factor, irrespective of lipoprotein levels (exception: Statin use is contraindicated in pregnancy). For patients without overt CVD and <40 years old, statin therapy may be considered if LDL remains >100 mg/dL with lifestyles changes or in those with multiple cardiovascular risk factors. In individuals with overt CVD, lower LDL goals (<70 mg/dL) are suggested.

    –   Use of low-dose aspirin (75-162 mg daily) is reasonable for primary prevention in all patients with diabetes at increased cardiovascular disease (CVD) risk (10-year risk >10%), including most men >50 years old and most women >60 years old who have at least one additional risk factor (eg, hypertension, smoking, family history of CVD, dyslipidemia, albuminuria), unless contraindicated. Low-dose aspirin may be considered for those at intermediate CVD risk (younger patients with ≥1 risk factor, older patients without risk factors, or patients with 10-year CVD risk of 5% to 10%).

Aspirin is not recommended for primary prevention in patients with lower risk for CVD (eg, men <50 years old and women <60 years old without additional risk factor; 10-year CVD risk <5%). In secondary prevention, all patients with a history of CVD should receive aspirin (75-162 mg daily). Given the risk of Reye syndrome with the use of aspirin in patients <21 years old, aspirin is not recommended in this population for primary or secondary prevention. In patients unable to take aspirin (eg, documented allergy), the use of clopidogrel is considered a reasonable alternative.

- Coronary heart disease (CHD): In patients with known cardiovascular disease (CVD), ACE inhibitor therapy and aspirin and statin therapy (if not contraindicated) should be used to reduce the risk of cardiovascular events. In patients with a prior myocardial infarction, beta-blockers should be continued for at least 2 years after the event. Avoid thiazolidinedione (TZD) treatment in patients with symptomatic heart failure. Metformin may be used in patients with stable congestive heart failure (CHF) if renal function is normal; however, it should be avoided in unstable or hospitalized patients with CHF.

- Other preventative actions

  - Immunize against pneumococcal disease ≥2 years old. One time revaccination is recommended for individuals >64 years old if they were <65 years old when previously immunized >5 years ago.

  - Influenza immunization annually for all diabetic patients ≥6 months old.

  - Patients should be advised not to smoke.

  - Patients should be advised to perform at least 150 minutes/week of moderate-intensity aerobic physical activity (50% to 70% of maximal heart rate). In the absence of contradictions, patients with type 2 diabetes should be encouraged to perform resistance training 3 times/week.

  - Eye care: To reduce the risk or slow the progression of retinopathy, optimize glycemic and blood pressure control. Adults and children ≥10 years old with type 1 diabetes should have an initial dilated and comprehensive eye examination within 5 years after the onset of diabetes (if type 2, exam should occur shortly after the diagnosis of diabetes). Subsequent examinations should be repeated annually. Promptly refer patients with any level of macular edema, severe non-proliferative diabetic retinopathy (NPDR), or any proliferative diabetic retinopathy (PDR) to an ophthalmologist who is knowledgeable and experienced in the management and treatment of diabetic retinopathy.

  - Nephropathy: To reduce the risk or slow the progression of nephropathy, optimize glucose and blood pressure control. In the treatment of the nonpregnant patient with micro- or macroalbuminuria, either ACE inhibitors or ARBs should be used (if one class is not tolerated, the other should be substituted). When estimated GFR (eGFR) is <60 mL/minute/1.73 m^2, evaluate and manage potential complications of CKD. Consider referral to a physician experienced in the care of kidney disease when there is uncertainty about the etiology of the disease (heavy proteinuria, active urine sediment, absence of retinopathy, rapid decline in GFR), difficult management issues, or advanced kidney disease.

  - Neuropathy: All patients should be screened for distal symmetric polyneuropathy (DPN) at diagnosis and at least annually thereafter, using simple clinical tests. Screening for signs and symptoms of cardiovascular autonomic neuropathy should be instituted at diagnosis of type 2 and 5 years after the diagnosis of type 1 diabetes.

  - Foot care: Perform general foot self-care education to all patients with diabetes. For all patients with diabetes, perform an annual comprehensive foot examination. The foot examination should include inspection, assessment of foot pulses, and testing for loss of protective sensation (10 g monofilament, plus testing any one of: Vibration using a 128-Hz tuning fork, pinprick sensation, ankle reflexes, or vibration perception threshold).

  - Thyroid: TSH concentrations should be measured after metabolic control has been established. If normal, they should be rechecked every 1-2 years or if the patient develops symptoms of thyroid dysfunction, thyromegaly, or an abnormal growth rate.

◀ REFERENCES

Action to Control Cardiovascular Risk in Diabetes Study Group, "Effects of Intensive Glucose Lowering in Type 2 Diabetes," *N Engl J Med*, 2008, 358(24):2545-59.

ADVANCE Collaborative Group, "Intensive Blood Glucose Control and Vascular Outcomes in Patients With Type 2 Diabetes," *N Engl J Med*, 2008, 358(24):2560-72.

American Diabetes Association, "Diagnosis and Classification of Diabetes Mellitus," *Diabetes Care*, 2011, 34(Suppl 1): S62-9.

American Diabetes Association, "Standards of Medical Care in Diabetes - 2011," *Diabetes Care*, 2011, 34(Suppl 1): S11-61.

Brunzell JD, Davidson M, Furberg CD, et al, "Lipoprotein Management in Patients With Cardiometabolic Risk: Consensus Statement From the American Diabetes Association and the American College of Cardiology Foundation," *Diabetes Care*, 2008, 31(4):811-22.

Centers for Disease Control (CDC), "National Diabetes Fact Sheet: 2007 General Information," Available at: http://www.cdc.gov/diabetes/pubs/pdf/ndfs_2007.pdf. Accessed January 9, 2009.

Colhoun HM, Betteridge DJ, Durrington PN, et al, "Primary Prevention of Cardiovascular Disease With Atorvastatin in Type 2 Diabetes in the Collaborative Atorvastatin Diabetes Study (CARDS): Multicentre Randomised Placebo-Controlled Trial," *Lancet*, 2004, 364(9435):685-96.

Dailey G, "New Strategies for Basal Insulin Treatment in Type 2 Diabetes Mellitus," *Clin Ther*, 2004, 26(6):889-901.

DeFronzo RA, "Pharmacologic Therapy for Type 2 Diabetes Mellitus," *Ann Intern Med*, 1999, 131(4):281-303.

DeFronzo RA, "Pharmacologic Therapy for Type 2 Diabetes Mellitus," *Ann Intern Med*, 2000, 133(1):73-4.

Duckworth W, Abraira C, Moritz T, et al, "Glucose Control and Vascular Complications in Veterans With Type 2 Diabetes," *N Engl J Med*, 2009, 360(2):129-39.

Holman RR and Turner RC, "Insulin Therapy in Type II Diabetes," *Diabetes Res Clin Pract*, 1995, (28 Suppl):S179-84.

International Expert Committee, "International Expert Committee Report on the Role of the A1C Assay in the Diagnosis of Diabetes," *Diabetes Care*, 2009, 32(7):1327-34.

Kitabchi AE, Umpierrez GE, Murphy MB, et al, "Hyperglycemic Crises in Diabetes," *Diabetes Care*, 2004, 27(Suppl 1): S94-102.

Nathan DM, Buse JB, Davidson MB, et al, "Medical Management of Hyperglycemia in Type 2 Diabetes: A Consensus Algorithm for the Initiation and Adjustment of Therapy: A Consensus Statement of the American Diabetes Association and the European Association for the Study of Diabetes," *Diabetes Care*, 2009, 32(1):193-203.

National Institute of Diabetes and Kigestive and Kidney Diseases, "Erectile Dysfunction," available at http://kidney.niddk.nih.gov/kudiseases/pubs/pdf/ErectileDysfunction.pdf. Accessed January 9, 2009.

Oiknine R, Bernbaum M, and Mooradian AD, "A Critical Appraisal of the Role of Insulin Analogues in the Management of Diabetes Mellitus," *Drugs*, 2005, 65(3):325-40.

Pignone M, Alberts MJ, Colwell JA, et al, "Aspirin for Primary Prevention of Cardiovascular Events in People With Diabetes: A Position Statement of the American Diabetes Association, a Scientific Statement of the American Heart Association, and an Expert Consensus Document of the American College of Cardiology Foundation," *Circulation*, 2010, 121(24):2694-701.

Rodbard HW, Jellinger PS, Davidson JA, et al, "Statement by an American Association of Clinical Endocrinologists/American College of Endocrinology Consensus Panel on Type 2 Diabetes Mellitus: An Algorithm for Glycemic Control," *Endocr Pract*, 2009, 15(6):540-59.

Scheife RT (editor), "Liraglutide: A New Option for the Treatment of Type 2 Diabetes Mellitus," *Pharmacotherapy*, 2009, 29(12 part 2): 23s-67s.

Sherifali D, Nerenberg K, Pullenayegum E, et al, "The Effect of Oral Antidiabetic Agents on A1C Levels: A Systematic Review and Meta-Analysis," *Diabetes Care*, 2010, 33(8):1859-64.

Silverstein J, Klingensmith G, Copeland K, et al, "Care of Children and Adolescents With Type 1 Diabetes: A Statement of the American Diabetes Association," *Diabetes Care*, 2005, 28(1):186-212.

The Diabetes Control and Complications Trial Research Group, "The Effect of Intensive Treatment of Diabetes on the Development and Progression of Long-Term Complications in Insulin-dependent Diabetes Mellitus," *N Engl J Med*, 1993, 329(14):977-86.

Tuomilehto J, Lindstrom J, Eriksson JG, et al, "Prevention of Type 2 Diabetes Mellitus by Changes in Lifestyle Among Subjects With Impaired Glucose Tolerance," *N Engl J Med*, 2001, 344(18):1343-50.

UK Prospective Diabetes Study Group, "Intensive Blood Glucose Control With Sulphonylureas or Insulin Compared With Conventional Treatment and Risk of Complications in Patients With Type 2 Diabetes (UKPDS 33)," *Lancet*, 1998, 352(9131):837-53.

HEART FAILURE (SYSTOLIC)

INTRODUCTORY COMMENTS

This summarizes the pharmacotherapy of patients with systolic heart failure with respect to treating mild-to-moderate exacerbations and chronic therapy. A more detailed discussion is available at http://content.onlinejacc.org/cgi/content/full/j.jacc.2008.11.013.

It should be recognized that the most common cause for exacerbations of patients' heart failure is poor adherence to therapy (medications and diet restriction). Healthcare providers need to educate patients about the importance of adherence to medical regimens.

For many years, therapy of heart failure focused on correcting the hemodynamic imbalances that occurred in heart failure. It is now recognized that heart failure triggers the release of several neurohormones that, in the short-run, help the patient; but, in the long-run, are detrimental. Newer pharmacotherapeutic approaches address counteracting the actions of these harmful neuro-hormones as well as address hemodynamic issues.

DIURETICS

Although data have yet to demonstrate that diuretics reduce the mortality associated with heart failure, they relieve symptoms seen in heart failure. Diuretics should only be used in patients experiencing congestion with their heart failure. Although not usually the case, some patients do have heart failure without congestion. In such rare instances, diuretic therapy is not indicated since they further stimulate the deleterious neurohormonal responses seen.

Although some heart failure patients with congestion can be controlled with thiazide diuretics, most will require the more potent loop diuretics, either because a strong diuretic effect is needed or renal function is compromised (thus limiting the effectiveness of the thiazide diuretic). When patients with heart failure are discovered to have mild-to-moderate worsening congestion, they often can be controlled by adjusting their oral loop diuretic dose or, if applicable, initiating a loop diuretic regimen. If a more aggressive diuresis is indicated, especially if the patient is suffering from pulmonary congestion, intravenous loop diuretics would be indicated. When loop diuretics are given intravenously, before any diuretic effect occurs, they benefit the patient by dilating veins and reducing preload, thus relieving pulmonary congestion. Intravenous loop diuretics may also be considered in a patient where concerns exist about the ability to absorb orally administered medication.

If already on an oral loop diuretic, the dosage should be increased (generally, 1.5-2 times their current regimen) in an effort for the patient to lose about 1-1.5 liters of fluid per day (about equivalent to 1-1.5 kg of weight per day). If the patient had yet to be started on a diuretic or was previously receiving a thiazide diuretic, initiating furosemide at 20-40 mg once or twice daily is a reasonable consideration. If the initial increase (or initiation) in dosage fails to induce a diuretic response, the dosage may be increased. If the initial increase (or initiation) does induce a diuretic response but the patient fails to lose weight or is not losing more fluids than taking in, the frequency of giving the loop diuretic may be increased. When an effective regimen is achieved, this regimen should be continued until the patient achieves a goal "dry" weight. Once this weight is attained, a decision needs to be made on how to continue the patient on diuretic therapy. If the patient had not been on a diuretic at home, continuation of the loop diuretic at a reduced dose is a worthy consideration. If the exacerbation was related to nonadherence with the diuretic or diet, the previous home dose might be continued with education on adherence to the prescribed diet and medication use. If the exacerbation was caused by an inadequate pharmacotherapeutic regimen (such as vasodilator was not being use), the previous home dose might be continued in conjunction with a more complete pharmacotherapeutic regimen. If the patient was compliant and on an acceptable pharmacotherapeutic regimen, the patient's original diuretic dose would be increased to some dosage greater than their home regimen, yet generally less than what was just used to achieve their dry weight.

The use of loop diuretics can lead to hypokalemia and/or hypomagnesemia. Electrolyte disturbances can predispose a patient to serious cardiac arrhythmias particularly if the patient is concurrently receiving digoxin. Fluid depletion, hypotension, and azotemia can also result from excessive use of diuretics. In contrast to thiazide diuretics, a loop diuretic can also lower serum calcium concentrations. For some patients, despite higher doses of loop diuretic treatment, an adequate diuretic response cannot be attained. Diuretic resistance can usually be overcome by intravenous administration (including continuous infusion), the use of 2 diuretics together (eg, furosemide and metolazone), or the use of a diuretic with a positive inotropic agent. When such combinations are used, serum electrolytes need to be monitored even more closely.

When loop diuretics are used in patients with renal dysfunction, to achieve the desired diuretic response, dosages typically will need to be greater than what is used in patients with normal renal function.

Due to its long existence and inexpensive price, furosemide tends to be the loop diuretic most commonly used. Bumetanide and torsemide are now available as generics and their use, especially bumetanide, has increased. The oral bioavailability of bumetanide and torsemide are nearly 100%; whereas, furosemide's oral bioavailability averages about 50%. A useful rule of thumb for conversion of intravenous loop diuretics is 40 mg of furosemide is equal to 1 mg bumetanide is equal to 20 mg torsemide. A few patients have allergies to diuretics because many contain a sulfur element. The only loop diuretic that lacks a sulfur element is ethacrynic acid.

VASODILATORS

Combination Hydralazine and Isosorbide Dinitrate

Vasodilator therapy, specifically the combination of hydralazine and isosorbide dinitrate, was the first pharmacotherapeutic treatment demonstrated to enhance survival of heart failure patients. The use of hydralazine 75 mg (which reduces afterload) and isosorbide dinitrate 40 mg 4 times a day (which reduces preload) demonstrated enhanced survival compared to placebo and prazosin. Unfortunately, many patients were unable to tolerate this regimen (primarily due to headaches and gastrointestinal disturbances) and the magnitude of benefit in survival dissipated with time.

The African-American Heart Failure Trial (A-HeFT) demonstrated mortality benefit with the use of a fixed combination of hydralazine and isosorbide dinitrate in combination with standard heart failure therapies, including ACE inhibitors, in self-identified African-American heart failure patients. The use of the commercially available combination of hydralazine and isosorbide dinitrate may be cost prohibitive in some patients; therefore, the use of the individually separate products is justifiable.

ACE Inhibitors

A series of investigations demonstrated that enalapril (which reduces both afterload and preload) enhances the survival of heart failure patients. Dosages used in these trials averaged about 10 mg twice daily. Since these trials, other ACE inhibitors were proven to benefit heart failure patients.

This led to the question – which is superior, ACE inhibitor or the combination of hydralazine and isosorbide dinitrate? In a comparative trial, using doses described above, enalapril was superior to the combination of hydralazine and isosorbide dinitrate, making an ACE inhibitor the vaso-dilator of choice in heart failure patients. An ACE inhibitor can alleviate symptoms, improve clinical status, and enhance a patient's quality of life. In addition an ACE inhibitor can reduce the risk of death and the combined risk of death or hospitalization.

Adverse effects associated with ACE inhibitors include hyperkalemia, rash, dysgeusia, dry cough, and (rarely) angioedema. Patients sometime develop renal dysfunction with the initiation of ACE inhibitors. This is not due to direct nephrotoxicity but is related to the ACE inhibitor dilating the efferent renal artery of the kidney, thus shunting blood away from being filtered in the glomerulus. The risk for renal dysfunction is increased when the ACE inhibitor is introduced to a patient who is hypovolemic, is being aggressively diuresed, is on an NSAID (which should be avoided in heart failure patients), or has bilateral renal artery stenosis (unilateral if only one kidney is present). ACE inhibitors should be avoided in patients with known renal artery stenosis. Monitor renal function and serum potassium within 1-2 weeks of initiation of therapy and routinely thereafter especially in patients with pre-existing hypotension, hyponatremia, diabetes, azotemia, or those taking potassium supplements. Some patients will have an exaggerated hypotensive response following the initial doses (especially the first dose) of an ACE inhibitor.

Angiotensin Receptor Blockers

A major limitation to using ACE inhibitors treatment in heart failure can be the dry cough that some patients develop. Lowering the ACE inhibitor dose sometimes can control it, but this may limit the effectiveness of the ACE inhibitor treatment. The development of angiotensin receptor blockers (ARBs) has helped address this issue. ARBs were demonstrated to enhance survival of heart failure patients. Although they are not the vasodilator of first choice in heart failure, they are a reasonable alternative in patients who cannot tolerate an ACE inhibitor due to the cough or some other adverse effect (with the exception of hyperkalemia and renal dysfunction; ARBs can induce as well). ARBs do not cause an accumulation of kinins as ACE inhibitors do.

Can ARBs be used in patients who suffer angioedema with ACE inhibitors? Reports are available in the literature describing patients who experienced angioedema with both ACE inhibitors and ARBs. These cases do not indicate the safety of an ARB when used in a patient who has experienced ACE inhibitor-induced angioedema. The CHARM-Alternative trial confirmed that only one of 39 patients (~2.6%) who experienced angioedema with an ACE inhibitors also experienced it with an ARB.

Concurrent Use of an ACE Inhibitor and an ARB

In Val-HeFT, valsartan added to conventional treatment (included ACE inhibitor treatment) did not impact survival but did reduce morbidity. Of note, a subgroup analysis of this trial suggested the combination of valsartan and an ACE inhibitor may be detrimental to patients also receiving a beta-blocker. In CHARM-Added, candesartan added to ACE inhibitor therapy was of benefit to heart failure patients (modest reduction in hospitalization; increased risk of hyperkalemia and renal dysfunction), even for those receiving a beta-blocker. As a result, the ACCF/AHA Practice Guidelines do not speak against using the combination of ACE inhibitors and ARBs. However, few patients in these trials were receiving an aldosterone blocker (such as spironolactone), which is now known to be of benefit to heart failure patients. Since there is enhanced risk for hyperkalemia and outcome data are currently unknown, the ACCF/AHA Practice Guidelines for heart failure do not advocate the combined use of ACE inhibitors, ARBs, and an aldosterone inhibitor.

In summary, vasodilator therapy should initially consist of an ACE inhibitor. If such therapy cannot be tolerated due to renal failure or hyperkalemia, the combination of hydralazine and isosorbide dinitrate may be considered as ARBs can also cause renal failure and hyperkalemia. If the ACE inhibitor cannot be tolerated due to adverse effects such as dry cough, an ARB may be considered. If an ACE inhibitor and beta-blocker have been maximized yet heart failure symptoms persist, consider adding hydralazine and isosorbide dinitrate. This approach, in fact, has been demonstrated to enhance the survival of African-American patients with heart failure. Another approach may be to add an ARB to the ACE inhibitor; but caution should occur, due to the risk of hyperkalemia.

BETA-BLOCKERS

Despite being negative inotropes, beta-blockers have been demonstrated to enhance the survival of systolic heart failure patients. Their benefit is attributed to their ability to protect the myocardium from the "bombardment" of catecholamines present in heart failure that can lead to ventricular remodeling. Bisoprolol, metoprolol succinate (extended release), and carvedilol have been demonstrated in trials to improve survival. Carvedilol is also available as a once-a-day extended-release preparation; but, its daily cost is considerably greater than generically-available immediate-release carvedilol that is given twice a day. At present, superiority of a particular beta-blocker over another has not been definitively demonstrated. For patients to be able to tolerate this therapy, beta-blocker treatment needs to be initiated at low doses and titrated slowly (generally, the dose is double every two weeks). Following the initiation of treatment and increase in dosage, patients may feel that their disease is worsening but this should dissipate after a few days. If this ill feeling continues beyond a few days, consideration should be given to regimen adjustments. If the patient is congested, increase the diuretic dosage. If the patient's discomfort is related to hypotension, staggering the beta-blocker dose with the vasodilator dose and/or lowering the vasodilator dosage may be helpful. If these approaches are ineffective or cannot explain the patient's ill feeling, consideration should be given to lowering the beta-blocker dosage and attempt a dose titration increase later on. Sometimes, a patient may not be able to tolerate "goal" doses of both beta-blockers and concurrent vasodilator treatment due to hypotension. It is the consensus opinion that a reduced dose of each agent is better than a goal dose of just one agent. Beta-blockers are not necessarily contraindicated but need to be used cautiously in patients with bronchospastic disease, peripheral arterial disease, or diabetes mellitus.

ALDOSTERONE BLOCKERS

It has been demonstrated, especially in the more severe forms of heart failure, that spirono-lactone, at an average dose of 25 mg daily, enhances the survival of heart failure patients. In patients who suffer hyperkalemia at this relatively low dosage, lowering the dose to 25 mg every other day may be attempted. In patients who remain symptomatic with their heart failure and have maximized the other proven treatments of heart failure and whose potassium concentrations can tolerate increases, the spironolactone dose may be increased to 50 mg daily.

Obviously, hyperkalemia is a concern with this treatment, especially since patients generally will also be receiving an ACE inhibitor or ARB. It has been demonstrated that the number of emergency visits related to hyperkalemia in heart failure has increased with the introduction of aldosterone blocking therapy in treating heart failure. About 10% of patients will experience endocrinological effects with spironolactone. In men, breast tenderness and gynecomastia may occur. In women, menstrual irregularities may be seen. In such instances, the use of eplerenone may be considered. Eplerenone is less apt to induce endocrinological effects but it is more expensive. A typical dose is 25-50 mg daily. Eplerenone has been demonstrated to enhance survival of post-MI patients with reduced ejection fractions. Spironolactone has not been studied in this patient group.

These medications should not be started in patients with renal insufficiency. These medications should be avoided if the serum creatinine exceeds 2.5 mg/dL in men (2 mg/dL in women) or if baseline potassium ≥5 mEq/L.

DIGOXIN

The value of digoxin in heart failure has crossed the spectrum. In the late 1980s, further investigation with digoxin suggested that indeed it may have a role in heart failure treatment, but the methods of these trials were not ideal (digoxin was taken away from stabilized patients to see if the condition of patients worsened – it did). Finally, digoxin was studied in a prospective manner where patients were on known optimal heart failure treatment at the time and randomized to placebo or digoxin. The digoxin dosage used resulted in digoxin steady-state concentrations of 1 mcg/L. This trial revealed that digoxin did not impact survival but reduced the number of patient hospitalizations, suggesting digoxin has a morbidity benefit. Many are of the opinion that digoxin's benefit is unrelated to its positive inotropic activity but related to inhibiting neuro-hormonal activity. Healthcare providers may consider adding digoxin in patients with persistent heart failure symptoms as a fourth line agent.

Digoxin is primarily renally eliminated; therefore, renal function of patients should be closely monitored and the dose adjusted. Digoxin does become difficult to use in patients whose renal function is unstable. In the DIG trial, effective digoxin steady-state concentrations ranged between 0.7-1 mcg/L. Concentrations much beyond 1 mcg/L were associated with worsened outcomes, especially in women. Since digoxin's benefit is long-term, a loading dose is not necessary. When checking a digoxin serum concentration, the sample should not be obtained until 12 hours after a dose, especially if it was oral, since digoxin has a relatively long distribution phase. It should also be assured that the patient is at steady-state (recall that the half-life of digoxin in a patient with normal renal function is approximately 36 hours and that patients with heart failure generally have worsened renal function).

Hypokalemia, hypomagnesia, hypercalcemia, and hypothyroidism can precipitate digoxin toxicity in the presence of a therapeutic digoxin concentration. This toxicity can be alleviated by correcting the electrolyte abnormality. In acute digoxin overdoses, hyperkalemia can occur since digoxin inhibits the sodium-potassium ATPase pump. For this reason, one should not assume potassium is given to just **any** patient with digoxin toxicity. Digoxin toxicity can present as bradyarrhythmias, heart blocks, ventricular tachyarrhythmias, and atrial tachyarrhythmias (PAT with block is pathognomonic). Other toxic manifestations include visual disturbances (including greenish-yellowish vision and halos around lights), gastrointestinal disturbances, anorexia, and altered mental status. Many medications elevate digoxin concentrations and a patient's regimen should be assessed for potential interactions.

OTHER HEART FAILURE THERAPEUTIC CONSIDERATIONS

- If a calcium channel blocker is desired, amlodipine or felodipine are preferred choices.

- To treat arrhythmias, amiodarone and dofetilide are best documented to lack significant proarrhythmic propensity in heart failure patients. Dronedarone, a newer antiarrhythmic agent structurally similar to amiodarone, is contraindicated in patients with NYHA Class IV heart failure or Class II-III heart failure with recent decompensation requiring hospitalization or referral to a specialized heart failure clinic.

- In heart failure patients with diabetes mellitus, metformin should not be used and "glitazones" should not be used in severe heart failure (NYHA III and IV) and used cautiously, if at all, in mild-to-moderate heart failure.

- The use of cilostazol, because it has type III phosphodiesterase-inhibiting properties, is contraindicated in heart failure. This is because the chronic use of *oral* milrinone and inamrinone, also type III phosphodiesterase inhibitors, resulted in enhanced mortality in heart failure patients (and therefore, these two agents were never FDA-approved for oral use).

- NSAID use should be avoided or used minimally as these agents antagonize the effects of diuretics and ACE inhibitors.

- Retrospective data suggests that daily aspirin may also negate the effects of ACE inhibitors but this has yet to be definitively proven in prospective trials. Using the lowest possible aspirin dose with the highest possible ACE inhibitor dose has been suggested as a way to best circumvent this issue.

- Routine intermittent intravenous infusions of positive inotropes are not recommended; but their use may be considered as palliative therapy in end-stage disease when ordinary therapy is insufficient.

CLASS I RECOMMENDATIONS FOR THE HOSPITALIZED PATIENT WITH ACUTE DECOMPENSATED HEART FAILURE

- Patients presenting to the hospital with fluid overload should be treated immediately with intravenous loop diuretics (eg, furosemide) since earlier treatment may be associated with better outcomes. If chronically receiving oral loop diuretic therapy, the initial intravenous dose should equal or exceed their chronic oral daily dose and titrated to relieve symptoms and reduce fluid excess. If this is inadequate, use of higher doses of loop diuretics, adding a second diuretic (eg, intravenous chlorothiazide), or a continuous infusion of the loop diuretic may improve diuresis.

- If evidence of hypotension with associated hypoperfusion and elevated cardiac filling pressures (eg, increase JVP) exists, intravenous inotropic support (eg, dobutamine) or vasopressor drugs (eg, dopamine) should be administered. Use of intravenous inotropes in patients without evidence of hypoperfusion is not recommended.

- In the absence of hemodynamic instability or contraindications, the use of therapies known to improve outcomes (eg, ACE inhibitors or ARBs, and beta-blockers) should be continued during the hospital stay. When appropriate, these agents should be initiated or reinitiated to stabilized patients prior to hospital discharge. Beta-blockers should only be initiated upon successful discontinuation of intravenous diuretics, vasodilators, and inotropic agents in the stabilized patient; initiate at a low dose and use caution in those patients who required inotropic support during their hospital course.

Dosing of ACE Inhibitors in Heart Failure[1]

ACEI	Initial Dose	Maximum Dose[2]
Captopril	6.25 mg tid	50 mg tid
Enalapril	2.5 mg bid	10-20 mg bid
Fosinopril	5-10 mg daily	40 mg daily
Lisinopril	2.5-5 mg daily	20-40 mg daily
Perindopril	2 mg daily	8-16 mg daily
Quinapril	5 mg bid	20 mg bid
Ramipril	1.25-2.5 mg daily	10 mg daily
Trandolapril	1 mg daily	4 mg daily

[1]From ACCF/AHA Guidelines.

[2]Maximum/target dose recommendation may vary between guidelines (also see Heart Failure Society of America, 2010)

Dosing of ARBs in Heart Failure[1]

ARB	Initial Dose	Maximum Dose[2]
Candesartan	4-8 mg daily	32 mg daily
Losartan	25-50 mg daily	50-100 mg daily
Valsartan	20-40 mg bid	160 mg bid

[1]From ACCF/AHA Guidelines.

[2]Maximum/target dose recommendation may vary between guidelines (also see Heart Failure Society of America, 2010)

Initial and Target Doses for Beta-Blocker Therapy in Heart Failure[1]

Beta-Blocker	Starting Dose	Target Dose	Comment
Bisoprolol	1.25 mg daily	10 mg daily	β_1-Selective blocker Inconvenient dosage forms for initial dose titration
Carvedilol	3.125 mg bid	25 mg bid (≤85 kg) 50 mg bid (>85 kg)	β-Nonselective blocker α_1-Blocking properties
Carvedilol phosphate, extended release	10 mg daily	80 mg daily[2]	
Metoprolol succinate, extended release	12.5-25 mg daily	200 mg daily	β_1-Selective blocker

[1]From ACCF/AHA Guidelines.

[2]Equivalent to carvedilol immediate release 25 mg twice daily

Conversion From Immediate Release to Extended Release Carvedilol (Coreg CR®)

Carvedilol Immediate Release Dose	Carvedilol Phosphate Extended Release Dose
3.125 mg twice daily	10 mg once daily
6.25 mg twice daily	20 mg once daily
12.5 mg twice daily	40 mg once daily
25 mg twice daily	80 mg once daily

REFERENCES

Brater DC, "Diuretic Therapy," *N Engl J Med*, 1998, 339(6):387-95.
Granger CB, McMurray JJ, Yusuf S, et al, "Effects of Candesartan in Patients With Chronic Heart Failure and Reduced Left-Ventricular Systolic Function Intolerant to Angiotensin-Converting-Enzyme Inhibitors: The CHARM-Alternative Trial," *Lancet*, 2003, 362(9386):772-6.
Heart Failure Society of America, Lindenfeld J, Albert NM, et al, "HFSA 2010 Comprehensive Heart Failure Practice Guideline," *J Card Fail*, 2010, 16(6):e1-194.
Hunt SA, Abraham WT, Chin MH, et al, "2009 Focused Update Incorporated Into the ACC/AHA 2005 Guidelines for the Diagnosis and Management of Heart Failure in Adults A Report of the American College of Cardiology Foundation/ American Heart Association Task Force on Practice Guidelines Developed in Collaboration With the International Society for Heart and Lung Transplantation," *J Am Coll Cardiol*, 2009, 53(15):e1-e90.
McMurray JJ, Ostergren J, Swedberg K, et al, "Effects of Candesartan in Patients With Chronic Heart Failure and Reduced Left-Ventricular Systolic Function Taking Angiotensin-Converting-Enzyme Inhibitors: The CHARM-Added Trial," *Lancet*, 2003, 362(9386):767-71.
Taylor AL, Ziesche S, Yancy C, et al, "Combination of Isosorbide Dinitrate and Hydralazine in Blacks With Heart Failure," *N Engl J Med*, 2004, 351(20):2049-57.

BEERS CRITERIA – POTENTIALLY INAPPROPRIATE MEDICATIONS FOR GERIATRICS

Table 1. Criteria Independent of Diagnoses or Conditions

Applicable Medication	Summary of Prescribing Concern	Severity
Amiodarone (Cordarone®)	Associated with QT interval problems and risk of provoking torsade de pointes. Lack of efficacy in older adults.	High
Amitriptyline (Elavil®), amitriptyline and chlordiazepoxide (Limbitrol®), and amitriptyline and perphenazine (Triavil®)	Because of its strong anticholinergic and sedation properties, amitriptyline is rarely the antidepressant of choice for elderly patients.	High
Amphetamines (excluding methylphenidate hydrochloride and anorexics)	CNS stimulant adverse effects.	High
Amphetamines and anorexic agents	These drugs have potential for causing dependence, hypertension, angina, and myocardial infarction.	High
Anticholinergics and antihistamines: Chlorpheniramine (Chlor-Trimeton®), diphenhydrAMINE (Benadryl®), hydrOXYzine (Vistaril®, Atarax®), cyproheptadine (Periactin®), promethazine (Phenergan®), tripelennamine, dexchlorpheniramine (Polaramine®)	All nonprescription and many prescription antihistamines may have potent anticholinergic properties. Nonanticholinergic antihistamines are preferred in elderly patients when treating allergic reactions.	High
Barbiturates (all, except PHENobarbital) except when used to control seizures	Are highly addictive and cause more adverse effects than most sedative or hypnotic drugs in elderly patients.	High
Benzodiazepines, long-acting: ChlordiazePOXIDE (Librium®), amitriptyline and chlordiazepoxide (Limbitrol®), clidinium and chlordiazepoxide (Librax®), diazepam (Valium®), quazepam (Doral®), halazepam (Paxipam®), and chlorazepate (Tranxene®)	These drugs have a long half-life in elderly patients (often several days), producing prolonged sedation and increasing the risk of falls and fractures. Short- and intermediate-acting benzodiazepines are preferred if a benzodiazepine is required.	High
Benzodiazepines, short-acting (doses greater than): Alprazolam (Xanax®) 2 mg; oxazepam (Serax®) 60 mg; LORazepam (Ativan®) 3 mg; temazepam (Restoril®) 15 mg; and triazolam (Halcion®) 0.25 mg	Because of increased sensitivity to benzodiazepines in elderly patients, smaller doses may be effective as well as safer. Total daily doses should rarely exceed the suggested maximums.	High
Chlorpropamide (Diabinese®)	It has prolonged half-life in elderly patients and could cause prolonged hypoglycemia. Additionally, it is the only oral hypoglycemic agent that causes SIADH.	High
Cimetidine (Tagamet®)	CNS adverse effects including confusion.	Low
CloNIDine (Catapres®)	Potential for orthostatic hypotension and CNS adverse effects.	Low
Cyclandelate (Cyclospasmol®)	Lack of efficacy.	Low
Desiccated thyroid	Concerns about cardiac effects. Safer alternatives available.	High
Digoxin (Lanoxin®) (should not exceed >0.125 mg/day except when treating atrial arrhythmias)	Decreased renal clearance may lead to increased risk of toxic effects	Low
DiphenhydrAMINE (Benadryl®)	May cause confusion and sedation. Should not be used as a hypnotic, and when used to treat emergency allergic reactions, it should be used in the smallest possible dose.	High

Table 1. Criteria Independent of Diagnoses or Conditions *(continued)*

Applicable Medication	Summary of Prescribing Concern	Severity
Dipyridamole, short-acting (Persantine®). Do not consider the long-acting dipyridamole (which has better properties than the short-acting in older adults) except with patients with artificial heart valves	May cause orthostatic hypotension.	Low
Disopyramide (Norpace®, Norpace® CR)	Of all antiarrhythmic drugs, this is the most potent negative inotrope and therefore may induce heart failure in elderly patients. It is also strongly anticholinergic. Other antiarrhythmic drugs should be used.	High
Doxazosin (Cardura®)	Potential for hypotension, dry mouth, and urinary problems.	Low
Doxepin (SINEquan®)	Because of its strong anticholinergic and sedating properties, doxepin is rarely the antidepressant of choice for elderly patients.	High
Ergot mesyloids (Hydergine®) and cyclandelate (Cyclospasmol®)	Have not been shown to be effective in the doses studied.	Low
Estrogens only (oral)	Evidence of the carcinogenic (breast and endometrial cancer) potential of these agents and lack of cardioprotective effect in older women.	Low
Ethacrynic acid (Edecrin®)	Potential for hypertension and fluid imbalances. Safer alternatives available.	Low
Ferrous sulfate >325 mg/day	Doses >325 mg/day do not dramatically increase the amount absorbed but greatly increase the incidence of constipation.	Low
FLUoxetine, daily (PROzac®)	Long half-life of drug and risk of producing excessive CNS stimulation, sleep disturbances, and increasing agitation. Safer alternatives exist.	High
Flurazepam (Dalmane®)	This benzodiazepine hypnotic has an extremely long half-life in elderly patients (often days), producing prolonged sedation and increasing the incidence of falls and fracture. Medium- or short-acting benzodiazepines are preferable.	High
Gastrointestinal antispasmodic drugs: Dicyclomine (Bentyl®), hyoscyamine (Levsin® and Levsinex®), propantheline (Pro-Banthine®), belladonna alkaloids (Donnatal® and others), and clidinium and chlordiazepoxide (Librax®)	GI antispasmodic drugs are highly anticholinergic and have uncertain effectiveness. These drugs should be avoided (especially for long-term use).	High
Guanadrel (Hylorel®)	May cause orthostatic hypotension.	High
Guanethidine (Ismelin®)	May cause orthostatic hypotension. Safer alternatives exist.	High
Indomethacin (Indocin® and Indocin® SR)	Of all available NSAIDs, this drug produces the most CNS adverse effects.	High
Isoxsuprine (Vasodilan®)	Lack of efficacy.	Low
Ketorolac (Toradol®)	Immediate and long-term use should be avoided in older persons, since a significant number have asymptomatic GI pathologic conditions.	High
Long-term use of full-dosage, longer half-life, non-COX-selective NSAIDs: Naproxen (Naprosyn®, Avaprox, and Aleve®), oxaprozin (Daypro®), and piroxicam (Feldene®)	Have the potential to produce GI bleeding, renal failure, high blood pressure, and heart failure.	High
Long-term use of stimulant laxatives: Bisacodyl (Dulcolax®), cascara sagrada, and Neoloid except in the presence of opiate analgesic use	May exacerbate bowel dysfunction.	High
Meperidine (Demerol®)	Not an effective oral analgesic in doses commonly used. May cause confusion and has many disadvantages to other narcotic drugs.	High

Table 1. Criteria Independent of Diagnoses or Conditions *(continued)*

Applicable Medication	Summary of Prescribing Concern	Severity
Meprobamate (Miltown®)	This is a highly addictive and sedating anxiolytic. Those using meprobamate for prolonged periods may become addicted and may need to be withdrawn slowly.	High
Mesoridazine (Serentil®)	CNS and extrapyramidal adverse effects.	High
Methyldopa (Aldomet) and methyldopa and hydrochlorothiazide (Aldoril®)	May cause bradycardia and exacerbate depression in elderly patients.	High
Methyltestosterone (Android®, Testrad®, Virilon®)	Potential for prostatic hypertrophy and cardiac problems.	High
Mineral oil	Potential for aspiration and adverse effects. Safer alternatives available.	High
Muscle relaxants and antispasmodics: Methocarbamol (Robaxin®), carisoprodol (Soma®), chlorzoxazone (Paraflex®), metaxalone (Skelaxin®), cyclobenzaprine (Flexeril®), and oxybutynin (Ditropan®). Do not consider the extended-release Ditropan® XL.	Most muscle relaxants and antispasmodic drugs are poorly tolerated by elderly patients, since these cause anticholinergic adverse effects, sedation, and weakness. Additionally, their effectiveness at doses tolerated by elderly patients is questionable.	High
NIFEdipine, short-acting (Adalat®, Procardia®)	Potential for hypotension and constipation.	High
Nitrofurantoin (Macrodantin®)	Potential for renal impairment. Safer alternatives available.	High
Orphenadrine (Norflex™)	Causes more sedation and anticholinergic adverse effects than safer alternatives.	High
Pentazocine (Talwin®)	Narcotic analgesic that causes more CNS adverse effects, including confusion and hallucinations, more commonly than other narcotic drugs. Additionally, it is a mixed agonist and antagonist.	High
Propoxyphene (Darvon®) and combination products (Darvon® with ASA, Darvon-N®, and Darvocet-N®)	Offers few analgesic advantages over acetaminophen, yet has the adverse effects of other narcotic drugs.	Low
Reserpine at doses >0.25 mg	May induce depression, impotence, sedation, and orthostatic hypotension.	Low
Thioridazine (Mellaril®)	Greater potential for CNS and extrapyramidal adverse effects.	High
Ticlopidine (Ticlid®)	Has been shown to be no better than aspirin in preventing clotting and may be considerably more toxic. Safer, more effective alternatives exist.	High
Trimethobenzamide (Tigan®)	One of the least effective antiemetic drugs, yet it can cause extrapyramidal adverse effects.	High

Table 2. Final Criteria Considering Diagnoses or Conditions

Disease or Condition	Drug	Concern	Severity
Anorexia and malnutrition	CNS stimulants: Dextroamphetamine and amphetamine (Adderall®), methylphenidate (Ritalin®), methamphetamine (Desoxyn®), pemolin, and FLUoxetine (PROzac®)	Concern due to appetite suppressing effects	High
Arrhythmias	Tricyclic antidepressants (imipramine hydrochloride, doxepin hydrochloride, and amitriptyline hydrochloride)	Concern due to proarrhythmic effects and ability to produce QT interval changes.	High
Bladder outflow obstruction	Anticholinergics and antihistamines, gastrointestinal antispasmodics, muscle relaxants, oxybutynin (Ditropan®), flavoxATE (Urispas®), anticholinergics, antidepressants, decongestants, and tolterodine (Detrol®)	May decrease urinary flow, leading to urinary retention.	High
Blood clotting disorders or receiving anticoagulant therapy	Aspirin, NSAIDs, dipyridamole (Persantine®), ticlopidine (Ticlid®), and clopidogrel (Plavix®)	May prolong clotting time and elevate INR values or inhibit platelet aggregation, resulting in an increased potential for bleeding.	High
Chronic constipation	Calcium channel blockers, anticholinergics, and tricyclic antidepressant (imipramine hydrochloride, doxepin hydrochloride, and amitriptyline hydrochloride)	May exacerbate constipation	Low
Cognitive impairment	Barbiturates, anticholinergics, antispasmodics, and muscle relaxants, CNS stimulants: Dextroamphetamine and amphetamine (Adderall®), methylphenidate (Ritalin®), methamphetamine (Desoxyn®), and pemolin	Concern due to CNS-altering effects	High
COPD	Benzodiazepines, long-acting: ChlordiazePOXIDE (Librium®), amitriptyline and chlordiazepoxide (Limbitrol®), clidinium and chlordiazepoxide (Librax®), diazepam (Valium®), quazepam (Doral®), and chlorazepate (Tranxene®). Beta-blockers: Propranolol	CNS adverse effects. May induce respiratory depression. May exacerbate or cause respiratory depression.	High
Depression	Long-term benzodiazepine use. Sympatholytic agents: Methyldopa (Aldomet®), reserpine, and guanethidine (Ismelin)	May produce or exacerbate depression.	High
Gastric or duodenal ulcers	NSAIDs and aspirin (>325 mg) (coxibs excluded)	May exacerbate existing ulcers or produce new/additional ulcers.	High

Table 2. Final Criteria Considering Diagnoses or Conditions *(continued)*

Disease or Condition	Drug	Concern	Severity
Heart failure	Disopyramide (Norpace®), and high sodium content drugs (sodium and sodium salts [alginate bicarbonate, biphosphate, citrate, phosphate, salicylate, and sulfate])	Negative inotropic effect. Potential to promote fluid retention and exacerbation of heart failure.	High
Hypertension	Phenylpropanolamine hydrochloride (removed from the market in 2001), pseudoephedrine; diet pills, and amphetamines	May produce elevation of blood pressure secondary to sympathomimetic activity.	High
Insomnia	Decongestants, theophylline (Theodur), methylphenidate (Ritalin®), MAOIs, and amphetamines	Concern due to CNS stimulant effects	High
Obesity	OLANZapine (ZyPREXA®)	May stimulate appetite and increase weight gain.	Low
Parkinson disease	Metoclopramide (Reglan®), conventional antipsychotics, and tacrine (Cognex®)	Concern due to their antidopaminergic/ cholinergic effects	High
Seizures or epilepsy	CloZAPine (Clozaril®), chlorproMAZINE (Thorazine®), thioridazine (Mellaril®), thiothixene (Navane®)	May lower seizure thresholds.	High
Seizure disorder	BuPROPion (Wellbutrin®)	May lower seizure threshold.	High
SIADH/ hyponatremia	SSRIs: FLUoxetine (PROzac®), citalopram (CeleXA™), fluvoxaMINE (Luvox®), paroxetine (Paxil®), and sertraline (Zoloft®)	May exacerbate or cause SIADH.	Low
Stress incontinence	α-Blockers (doxazosin, prazosin, and terazosin), anticholinergic, tricyclic antidepressants (imipramine hydrochloride, doxepin hydrochloride, and amitriptyline hydrochloride), and long-acting benzodiazepines	May produce polyuria and worsening of incontinence	High
Syncope or falls	Short- to intermediate-acting benzodiazepine and tricyclic antidepressants (imipramine hydrochloride, doxepin hydrochloride, and amitriptyline hydrochloride)	May produce ataxia, impaired psychomotor function, syncope, and additional falls.	High

Reference

Fick DM, Cooper JW, Wade WE, et al, "Updating the Beers Criteria for Potentially Inappropriate Medication Use in Older Adults: Results of a U.S. Consensus Panel of Experts," *Arch Intern Med*, 2003, 163(22):2716-24.

TARGET INR RANGES FOR ADULT PATIENTS WITH PROSTHETIC HEART VALVES

PROSTHETIC HEART VALVES

Patients with mechanical prosthetic valves require life-long anticoagulation therapy. The optimal intensity of anticoagulation is not established. The risk of thromboembolism is greater in valve patients who have atrial fibrillation (AF); have an enlarged left atrium (>5.5 cm); have a history of systemic embolism, left ventricular systolic dysfunction, coronary artery disease, left atrial thrombus; have ball valve; or have more than one mechanical valve. The risk for thromboembolism is also higher for mechanical valves in the mitral position compared to aortic. These factors should be weighed in each patient before deciding the desired level of anticoagulation to prevent thromboembolism and to avoid bleeding complications. Ranges for anticoagulation intensity in patients with prosthetic valves are described in the following table.

Anticoagulation Management of Mechanical and Bioprosthetic Valves With Warfarin

Valve Type	Location and Specific Valve Type / Clinical Situation	Recommended INR Range / Therapy
Mechanical	Mitral − bileaflet or tilting disk	2.5-3.5
	Aortic − bileaflet or Medtronic Hall® tilting disk in normal sinus rhythm and normal LA size	2-3
	Mitral or aortic − caged ball or disk	2.5-3.5
	Mitral or aortic − with systemic embolism despite adequate warfarin therapy	2.5-3.5[2] or 3-4[2]
	Mitral or aortic (or both) − with risk factors for thromboembolism (eg, AF, MI[3], LA enlargement, hypercoagulable state, low EF) or a history of atherosclerotic vascular disease	2.5-3.5[4]
Bioprosthetic	Mitral valve	2-3; Maintain for 3 months after valve insertion then aspirin 81 mg/day if no other indications for warfarin
	Aortic valve in normal sinus rhythm	Aspirin 81 mg/day
	Mitral or aortic valve with evidence of LA thrombus at surgery	2-3; Maintain until thrombus resolution
	Mitral or aortic valve with risk factors for thromboembolism (eg, AF, hypercoagulable state, or low EF)	2-3[5]
	Mitral or aortic valve with history of systemic embolism	2-3; Maintain for 3 months after valve insertion then clinically reassess

AF=atrial fibrillation; EF=ejection fraction; LA=left atrial; MI=myocardial infarction

[1]Combine with aspirin 81 mg/day, if not previously receiving

[2]Combine with aspirin 81 mg/day, if not previously receiving, **and/or** if previous target INR was 2.5, then new target INR should be 3 (2.5-3.5). If previous target INR was 3, then new target INR should be 3.5 (3-4).

[3]MI refers to anterior-apical ST-segment elevation myocardial infarction

[4]Combine with aspirin 81 mg/day unless patient is at high risk of bleeding (eg, history of GI bleed, age >80 years)

[5]If patient has a history of atherosclerotic vascular disease, combine with aspirin 81 mg/day unless patient is at high risk of bleeding (eg, history of GI bleed, age >80 years)

As a general rule, concomitant warfarin and aspirin therapy should be avoided, except in special situations. The combination of warfarin and low-dose aspirin in all mechanical valve patients is uncertain; patients at the highest risk (eg, AF, hypercoagulable state, or low EF) for thromboembolism should be considered. For patients with mechanical prosthetic valves who suffer a systemic thromboembolism despite adequate anticoagulation therapy, low-dose aspirin should be added if not on previously and/or the INR should be maintained between 2.5 and 3.5 or between 3 and 4, depending on previous target INR.

In some situations aspirin alone with or without initial treatment with warfarin is appropriate. Patients with bioprosthetic mitral valves should be initially treated with warfarin for 3 months after insertion due to the higher rate of thromboembolism during this time and then switched to low-dose aspirin. For patients with bioprosthetic aortic valves, treatment with warfarin is not recommended at any time since treatment with warfarin in the postoperative period has not shown a reduction in thromboembolism compared to aspirin alone and may increase the risk of bleeding. Therefore, patients with a bioprosthetic aortic valve should be treated with low dose aspirin only unless other indications exist.

REFERENCE

Salem DN, O'Gara PT, Madias C, et al, "Valvular and Structural Heart Disease: American College of Chest Physicians Evidence-Based Clinical Practice Guidelines (8th Edition)," *Chest*, 2008, 133(6 Suppl):593S-629S.

TREATMENT OF ELEVATED INR DUE TO WARFARIN

Eighth ACCP Consensus Conference on Antithrombotic Therapy: Recommendations on Managing Elevated INR In Patients Taking Warfarin

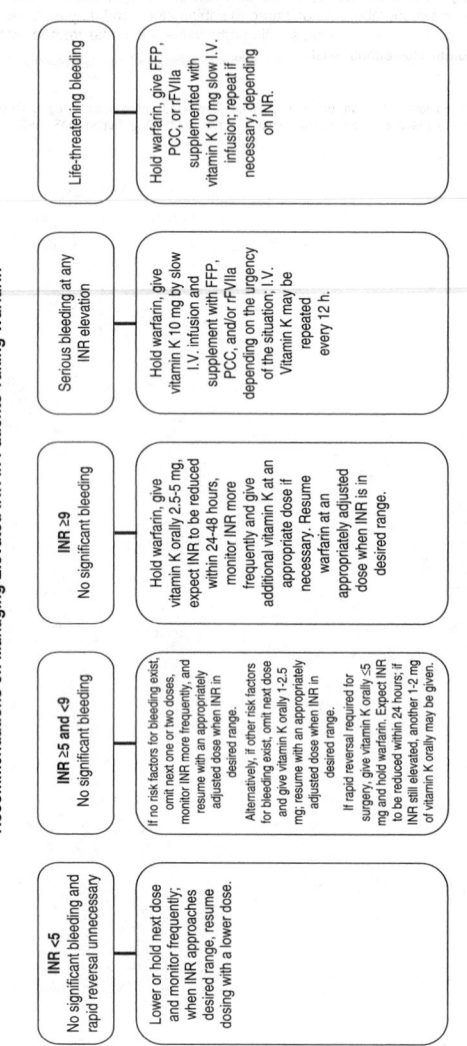

INR <5 No significant bleeding and rapid reversal unnecessary	INR ≥5 and <9 No significant bleeding	INR ≥9 No significant bleeding	Serious bleeding at any INR elevation	Life-threatening bleeding
Lower or hold next dose and monitor frequently; when INR approaches desired range, resume dosing with a lower dose.	If no risk factors for bleeding exist, omit next one or two doses, monitor INR more frequently, and resume with an appropriately adjusted dose when INR in desired range. Alternatively, if other risk factors for bleeding exist, omit next dose and give vitamin K orally 1-2.5 mg; resume with an appropriately adjusted dose when INR in desired range. If rapid reversal required for surgery, give vitamin K orally ≤5 mg and hold warfarin. Expect INR to be reduced within 24 hours; if INR still elevated, another 1-2 mg of vitamin K orally may be given.	Hold warfarin, give vitamin K orally 2.5-5 mg, expect INR to be reduced within 24-48 hours; monitor INR more frequently and give additional vitamin K at an appropriate dose if necessary. Resume warfarin at an appropriately adjusted dose when INR is in desired range.	Hold warfarin, give vitamin K 10 mg by slow I.V. infusion and supplement with FFP, PCC, and/or rFVIIa depending on the urgency of the situation; I.V. Vitamin K may be repeated every 12 h.	Hold warfarin, give FFP, PCC, or rFVIIa supplemented with vitamin K 10 mg slow I.V. infusion; repeat if necessary, depending on INR.

FFP = fresh frozen plasma; INR = international normalized ratio; PCC = prothrombin complex concentrate; rFVIIa = recombinant factor VIIa

Note 1: If mild-moderate INR elevation without major bleeding occurs, give vitamin K orally instead of subcutaneously.

Note 2: Use of high doses of vitamin K (eg, 10-15 mg) may cause warfarin resistance for ≥1 week. During this period of resistance, heparin or low molecular weight heparin may be given until INR responds.

Note 3: PCC may contain II, IX, X; Factor VII is not currently contained in U.S. products.

WARFARIN THERAPY

Patients should **not** receive loading doses of warfarin (ie, doses >10 mg) as the steady-state INR is not achieved more quickly. In general, most patients should receive doses between 5 mg and 10 mg for the first 1-2 days with the addition of heparin or low molecular weight heparin when a more rapid anticoagulant effect is required. Initial warfarin doses of 5 mg usually results in an INR>2 in 4-5 days. Initial doses of 10 mg usually results in a therapeutic INR in 3-4 days; however, 10 mg doses may be associated with more excessive anticoagulation. Patients who are debilitated, malnourished, have heart failure, have had recent surgery, or are taking medications known to increase the effects of warfarin should begin treatment with a dose ≤5 mg. The intensity of anticoagulation therapy should be monitored closely until the patient has reached a stable PT/INR. Once the patient is stabilized on a fixed dose of warfarin, the PT/INR can be monitored on a monthly basis if the patient demonstrates a stable PT/INR on chronic therapy. If dosage adjustments are made, PT/INR should be evaluated in approximately 2 weeks.

Supratherapeutic INR values are managed based on the presence and severity of bleeding (see chart). Determinants of bleeding due to warfarin therapy include intensity of treatment, patient characteristics, concomitant use of drugs that interfere with hemostasis, and the length therapy. The target INR should be established with consideration of these factors. Patients on warfarin should be warned to seek medical evaluation if they develop a very severe headache, abdominal pain, unusual bleeding, backache, or if they experience significant trauma, particularly head injuries. Please refer to the Warfarin monograph on page 1928 for complete drug information.

REFERENCE

Ansell J, Hirsh J, Hylek E, et al, "Pharmacology and Management of the Vitamin K Antagonists: American College of Chest Physicians Evidence-Based Clinical Practice Guidelines (8th Edition)," Chest, 2008, 133:160-98.

CYTOCHROME P450 ENZYMES: SUBSTRATES, INHIBITORS, AND INDUCERS

INTRODUCTION

Most drugs are eliminated from the body, at least in part, by being chemically altered to less lipid-soluble products (ie, metabolized), and thus are more likely to be excreted via the kidneys or the bile. Phase I metabolism includes drug hydrolysis, oxidation, and reduction, and results in drugs that are more polar in their chemical structure, while Phase II metabolism involves the attachment of an additional molecule onto the drug (or partially metabolized drug) in order to create an inactive and/or more water soluble compound. Phase II processes include (primarily) glucuronidation, sulfation, glutathione conjugation, acetylation, and methylation.

Virtually any of the Phase I and II enzymes can be inhibited by some xenobiotic or drug. Some of the Phase I and II enzymes can be induced. Inhibition of the activity of metabolic enzymes will result in increased concentrations of the substrate (drug), whereas induction of the activity of metabolic enzymes will result in decreased concentrations of the substrate. For example, the well-documented enzyme-inducing effects of phenobarbital may include a combination of Phase I and II enzymes. Phase II glucuronidation may be increased via induced UDP-glucuronosyl-transferase (UGT) activity, whereas Phase I oxidation may be increased via induced cytochrome P450 (CYP) activity. However, for most drugs, the primary route of metabolism (and the primary focus of drug-drug interaction) is Phase I oxidation.

CYP enzymes may be responsible for the metabolism (at least partial metabolism) of approximately 75% of all drugs, with the CYP3A subfamily responsible for nearly half of this activity. Found throughout plant, animal, and bacterial species, CYP enzymes represent a superfamily of xenobiotic metabolizing proteins. There have been several hundred CYP enzymes identified in nature, each of which has been assigned to a family (1, 2, 3, etc), subfamily (A, B, C, etc), and given a specific enzyme number (1, 2, 3, etc) according to the similarity in amino acid sequence that it shares with other enzymes. Of these many enzymes, only a few are found in humans, and even fewer appear to be involved in the metabolism of xenobiotics (eg, drugs). The key human enzyme subfamilies include CYP1A, CYP2A, CYP2B, CYP2C, CYP2D, CYP2E, and CYP3A. However, the number of distinct isozymes (eg, CYP2C9) found to be functionally active in humans, as well as, the number of genetically variant forms of these isozymes (eg, CYP2C9*2) in individuals continues to expand.

CYP enzymes are found in the endoplasmic reticulum of cells in a variety of human tissues (eg, skin, kidneys, brain, lungs), but their predominant sites of concentration and activity are the liver and intestine. Though the abundance of CYP enzymes throughout the body is relatively equally distributed among the various subfamilies, the relative contribution to drug metabolism is (in decreasing order of magnitude) CYP3A4 (nearly 50%), CYP2D6 (nearly 25%), CYP2C8/9 (nearly 15%), then CYP1A2, CYP2C19, CYP2A6, and CYP2E1. Owing to their potential for numerous drug-drug interactions, those drugs that are identified in preclinical studies as substrates of CYP3A enzymes are often given a lower priority for continued research and development in favor of drugs that appear to be less affected by (or less likely to affect) this enzyme subfamily.

Each enzyme subfamily possesses unique selectivity toward potential substrates. For example, CYP1A2 preferentially binds medium-sized, planar, lipophilic molecules, while CYP2D6 preferentially binds molecules that possess a basic nitrogen atom. Some CYP subfamilies exhibit polymorphism (ie, genetic variation that results in a modified enzyme with small changes in amino acid sequences that may manifest differing catalytic properties). The best described polymorphisms involve CYP2C9, CYP2C19, and CYP2D6. Individuals possessing "wild type" genes exhibit normal functioning CYP capacity. Others, however, possess genetic variants that leave the person with a subnormal level of catalytic potential (so called "poor metabolizers"). Poor metabolizers would be more likely to experience toxicity from drugs metabolized by the affected enzymes (or less effects if the enzyme is responsible for converting a prodrug to it's active form as in the case of codeine). The percentage of people classified as poor metabolizers varies by enzyme and population group. As an example, approximately 7% of Caucasians and only about 1% of Asians appear to be CYP2D6 poor metabolizers.

CYP enzymes can be both inhibited and induced by other drugs, leading to increased or decreased serum concentrations (along with the associated effects), respectively. Induction occurs when a drug causes an increase in the amount of smooth endoplasmic reticulum, secondary to increasing the amount of the affected CYP enzymes in the tissues. This "revving up" of the CYP enzyme system may take several days to reach peak activity, and likewise, may take several days, even months, to return to normal following discontinuation of the inducing agent.

CYP inhibition occurs via several potential mechanisms. Most commonly, a CYP inhibitor competitively (and reversibly) binds to the active site on the enzyme, thus preventing the substrate from binding to the same site, and preventing the substrate from being metabolized. The affinity of an inhibitor for an enzyme may be expressed by an inhibition constant (Ki) or IC50 (defined as the concentration of the inhibitor required to cause 50% inhibition under a given set of conditions). In addition to reversible competition for an enzyme site, drugs may inhibit enzyme activity by binding to sites on the enzyme other than that to which the substrate would bind, and thereby cause a change in the functionality or physical structure of the enzyme. A drug may also bind to the enzyme in an irreversible (ie, "suicide") fashion. In such a case, it is not the concentration of drug at the enzyme site that is important (constantly binding and releasing), but the number of molecules available for binding (once bound, always bound).

Although an inhibitor or inducer may be known to affect a variety of CYP subfamilies, it may only inhibit one or two in a clinically important fashion. Likewise, although a substrate is known to be at least partially metabolized by a variety of CYP enzymes, only one or two enzymes may contribute significantly enough to its overall metabolism to warrant concern when used with potential inducers or inhibitors. Therefore, when attempting to predict the level of risk of using two drugs that may affect each other via altered CYP function, it is important to identify the relative effectiveness of the inhibiting/inducing drug on the CYP subfamilies that significantly contribute to the metabolism of the substrate. The contribution of a specific CYP pathway to substrate metabolism should be considered not only in light of other known CYP pathways, but also other nonoxidative pathways for substrate metabolism (eg, glucuronidation) and transporter proteins (eg, P-glycoprotein) that may affect the presentation of a substrate to a metabolic pathway.

HOW TO USE THIS TABLE

The following table provides a clinically relevant perspective on drugs that are affected by, or affect, cytochrome P450 (CYP) enzymes. Not all human, drug-metabolizing CYP enzymes are specifically (or separately) included in the table. Some enzymes have been excluded because they do not appear to significantly contribute to the metabolism of marketed drugs (eg, CYP2C18). In the case of CYP3A4, the industry routinely uses this single enzyme designation to represent all enzymes in the CYP3A subfamily. CYP3A7 is present in fetal livers. It is effectively absent from adult livers. CYP3A4 (adult) and CYP3A7 (fetal) appear to share similar properties in their respective hosts. The impact of CYP3A7 in fetal and neonatal drug interactions has not been investigated.

An enzyme that appears to play a clinically significant (major) role in a drug's metabolism is indicated by "S". A clinically significant designation is the result of a two-phase review. The first phase considered the contribution of each CYP enzyme to the overall metabolism of the drug. The enzyme pathway was considered potentially clinically relevant if it was responsible for at least 30% of the metabolism of the drug. If so, the drug was subjected to a second phase. The second phase considered the clinical relevance of a substrate's concentration being increased twofold, or decreased by one-half (such as might be observed if combined with an effective CYP inhibitor or inducer, respectively). If either of these changes was considered to present a clinically significant concern, the CYP pathway for the drug was designated "major." If neither change would appear to present a clinically significant concern, or if the CYP enzyme was responsible for a smaller portion of the overall metabolism (ie, <30%), then no association between the enzyme and the drug will appear in the table.

Enzymes that are strongly or moderately inhibited by a drug are indicated by "↓". Enzymes that are weakly inhibited are not identified in the table. The designations are the result of a review of published clinical reports, available Ki data, and assessments published by other experts in the field. As it pertains to Ki values set in a ratio with achievable serum drug concentrations ([I]) under normal dosing conditions, the following parameters were employed: [I]/Ki ≥1 = strong; [I]/Ki 0.1-1 = moderate; [I]/Ki <0.1 = weak.

Enzymes that appear to be effectively induced by a drug are indicated by "↑". This designation is the result of a review of published clinical reports and assessments published by experts in the field.

CYTOCHROME P450 ENZYMES: SUBSTRATES, INHIBITORS, AND INDUCERS

In general, clinically significant interactions are more likely to occur between substrates ("S") and either inhibitors or inducers of the same enzyme(s), which have been indicated by "↓" and "↑", respectively. However, these assessments possess a degree of subjectivity, at times based on limited indications regarding the significance of CYP effects of particular agents. An attempt has been made to balance a conservative, clinically-sensitive presentation of the data with a desire to avoid the numbing effect of a "beware of everything" approach. It is important to note that information related to CYP metabolism of drugs is expanding at a rapid pace, and thus, the contents of this table should only be considered to represent a "snapshot" of the information available at the time of publication.

SELECTED READINGS

Bjornsson TD, Callaghan JT, Einolf HJ, et al, "The Conduct of *in vitro* and *in vivo* Drug-Drug Interaction Studies: A PhRMA Perspective," *J Clin Pharmacol*, 2003, 43(5):443-69.

Drug-Drug Interactions, Rodrigues AD, ed, New York, NY: Marcel Dekker, Inc, 2002.

Levy RH, Thummel KE, Trager WF, et al, eds, *Metabolic Drug Interactions*, Philadelphia, PA: Lippincott Williams & Wilkins, 2000.

Michalets EL, "Update: Clinically Significant Cytochrome P-450 Drug Interactions," *Pharmacotherapy*, 1998, 18 (1):84-112.

Thummel KE and Wilkinson GR, "*In vitro* and *in vivo* Drug Interactions Involving Human CYP3A," *Annu Rev Pharmacol Toxicol*, 1998, 38:389-430.

Zhang Y and Benet LZ, "The Gut as a Barrier to Drug Absorption: Combined Role of Cytochrome P450 3A and P-Glycoprotein," *Clin Pharmacokinet*, 2001, 40(3):159-68.

SELECTED WEBSITES

http://www.imm.ki.se/CYPalleles
http://medicine.iupui.edu/flockhart
http://www.fda.gov/Drugs/DevelopmentApprovalProcess/DevelopmentResources/DrugInteractionsLabeling/ucm080499.htm

CYP: Substrates, Inhibitors, Inducers

S = substrate; ↓ = inhibitor; ↑ = inducer

Drug	1A2	2A6	2B6	2C8	2C9	2C19	2D6	2E1	3A4
Acenocoumarol	S				S				
Alfentanil									S
Alfuzosin									S
Alosetron	S								
ALPRAZolam									S
Ambrisentan						S			S
Aminophylline	S								
Amiodarone		↓		S	↓		↓		S, ↓
Amitriptyline							S		
AmLODIPine	↓								S
Amobarbital		↑							
Amoxapine							S		
Aprepitant									S, ↓
ARIPiprazole							S		S
Armodafinil						↓			S, ↑
Atazanavir									S, ↓
Atomoxetine							S		
Atorvastatin									S
Benzphetamine									S
Betaxolol	S						S		
Bisoprolol									S
Bortezomib						S, ↓			S
Bosentan					S, ↑				S, ↑
Bromazepam									S

CYP: Substrates, Inhibitors, Inducers (continued)

Drug	1A2	2A6	2B6	2C8	2C9	2C19	2D6	2E1	3A4
Bromocriptine									S
Budesonide									S
Buprenorphine									S
BuPROPion			S						
BusPIRone									S
Busulfan									S
Caffeine	S								↓
Captopril							S		
CarBAMazepine	↑		↑	↑	↑	↑			S, ↑
Carisoprodol						S			
Carvedilol					S		S		
Celecoxib				↓	S				
ChlordiazePOXIDE									S
Chloroquine							S, ↓		S
Chlorpheniramine									S
ChlorproMAZINE							S, ↓		
Chlorzoxazone								S	
Ciclesonide									S
Cilostazol									S
Cimetidine	↓					↓	↓		↓
Cinacalcet							↓		
Ciprofloxacin	↓								
Cisapride									S
Citalopram						S			S
Clarithromycin									S, ↓
Clobazam						S			S
ClomiPRAMINE	S					S	S, ↓		
ClonazePAM									S
Clorazepate									S
Clotrimazole									↓
CloZAPine	S						↓		
Cocaine							↓		S
Codeine[1]							S		
Colchicine									S
Conivaptan									S, ↓
Cyclobenzaprine	S								
Cyclophosphamide[2]			S						S
CycloSPORINE									S, ↓
Dacarbazine	S							S	
Dantrolene									S
Dapsone					S				S
Darifenacin							↓		S
Darunavir									S
Dasatinib									S
Delavirdine					↓	↓	↓		S, ↓

CYP: Substrates, Inhibitors, Inducers *(continued)*

Drug	1A2	2A6	2B6	2C8	2C9	2C19	2D6	2E1	3A4
Desipramine		↓	↓				S, ↓		↓
Desogestrel						S			
Dexamethasone									S, ↑
Dexlansoprazole						S, ↓			S
Dexmedetomidine		S					↓		
Dextromethorphan							S		
Diazepam						S			S
Diclofenac	↓								
Dihydroergotamine									S
Diltiazem									S, ↓
DiphenhydrAMINE							↓		
Disopyramide									S
Disulfiram								↓	
DOCEtaxel									S
Doxepin							S		
DOXOrubicin			↓				S		S
Doxycycline									↓
DULoxetine	S						S, ↓		
Efavirenz[3]			S		↓	↓			S, ↓, ↑
Eletriptan									S
Enflurane								S	
Eplerenone									S
Ergoloid mesylates									S
Ergonovine									S
Ergotamine									S
Erlotinib									S
Erythromycin									S, ↓
Escitalopram						S			S
Esomeprazole						S, ↓			S
Estradiol	S								S
Estrogens, conjugated A/synthetic	S								S
Estrogens, conjugated equine	S								S
Estrogens, esterified	S								S
Estropipate	S								S
Eszopiclone									S
Ethinyl estradiol									S
Ethosuximide									S
Etoposide									S
Exemestane									S
Felbamate									S
Felodipine				↓					S
FentaNYL									S
Flecainide							S		
Fluconazole					↓	↓			↓
Flunisolide									S

CYP: Substrates, Inhibitors, Inducers *(continued)*

Drug	1A2	2A6	2B6	2C8	2C9	2C19	2D6	2E1	3A4
FLUoxetine	↓				S	↓	S, ↓		
FluPHENAZine							S		
Flurazepam									S
Flurbiprofen					↓				
Flutamide	S								S
Fluticasone									S
Fluvastatin					S, ↓				
FluvoxaMINE	S, ↓					↓	S		
Fosamprenavir (as amprenavir)									S, ↓
Fosaprepitant									S, ↓
Fosphenytoin (as phenytoin)			↑	↑	S, ↑	S, ↑			↑
Fospropofol	↓		S		S	↓			↓
Gefitinib									S
Gemfibrozil	↓			↓	↓	↓			
Glimepiride					S				
GlipiZIDE					S				
Guanabenz	S								
Haloperidol							S, ↓		S, ↓
Halothane								S	
Ibuprofen					↓				
Ifosfamide[4]		S				S			S
Imatinib							↓		S, ↓
Imipramine						S	S, ↓		
Indinavir									S, ↓
Indomethacin					↓				
Irbesartan				↓	↓				
Irinotecan			S						S
Isoflurane								S	
Isoniazid		↓				↓	↓	S, ↓	
Isosorbide dinitrate									S
Isosorbide mononitrate									S
Isradipine									S
Itraconazole									S, ↓
Ixabepilone									S
Ketamine			S		S				S
Ketoconazole	↓	↓			↓	↓	↓		S, ↓
Lansoprazole						S, ↓			S
Lapatinib									S
Letrozole		↓							
Levonorgestrel									S
Lidocaine	↓						S, ↓		S, ↓
Lomustine							S		
Lopinavir									S
Loratadine						↓			
Losartan				↓	S, ↓				S

CYP: Substrates, Inhibitors, Inducers *(continued)*

Drug	1A2	2A6	2B6	2C8	2C9	2C19	2D6	2E1	3A4
Lovastatin									S
Maprotiline							S		
Maraviroc									S
MedroxyPROGESTERone									S
Mefenamic acid					↓				
Mefloquine									S
Mephobarbital						S			
Mestranol[5]					S				S
Methadone							↓		S
Methamphetamine							S		
Methimazole							↓		
Methoxsalen	↓	↓							
Methsuximide						S			
Methylergonovine									S
MethylPREDNISolone									S
Metoprolol							S		
MetroNIDAZOLE									↓
Mexiletine	S, ↓						S		
Miconazole	↓	↓			↓	↓	↓	↓	S, ↓
Midazolam									S
Mirtazapine	S						S		S
Moclobemide						S	S		
Modafinil						↓			S
Montelukast					S				S
Nafcillin									↑
Nateglinide					S				S
Nebivolol							S		
Nefazodone							S		S, ↓
Nelfinavir						S			S, ↓
Nevirapine			↑						S, ↑
NiCARdipine					↓	↓	↓		S, ↓
NIFEdipine	↓								S
Nilotinib									S
Nilutamide					S				
NiMODipine									S
Nisoldipine									S
Norethindrone									S
Norfloxacin	↓								↓
Norgestrel									S
Nortriptyline							S		
Ofloxacin	↓								
OLANZapine	S								
Omeprazole					↓	S, ↓			S
Ondansetron									S
OXcarbazepine									↑

CYP: Substrates, Inhibitors, Inducers *(continued)*

Drug	1A2	2A6	2B6	2C8	2C9	2C19	2D6	2E1	3A4
PACLitaxel				S	S				S
Pantoprazole						S			
Paricalcitol									S
PARoxetine			↓				S, ↓		
Pazopanib									S
Pentamidine						S			
PENTobarbital		↑							↑
Perphenazine							S		
PHENobarbital	↑	↑	↑	↑	↑	S			↑
Phenytoin			↑	↑	S, ↑	S, ↑			↑
Pimozide	S								S
Pindolol							S		
Pioglitazone				S, ↓					
Piroxicam					↓				
Posaconazole									↓
Primaquine	↓								S
Primidone	↑		↑	↑	↑				↑
Procainamide							S		
Progesterone						S			S
Promethazine			S				S		
Propafenone							S		
Propofol	↓		S		S	↓			↓
Propranolol	S						S		
Protriptyline							S		
Pyrimethamine					↓		↓		
Quazepam						S			S
QUEtiapine									S
QuiNIDine							↓		S, ↓
QuiNINE				↓	↓		↓		S
RABEprazole				↓		S, ↓			S
Ramelteon	S								
Ranolazine							↓		S
Rasagiline	S								
Repaglinide				S					S
Rifabutin									S, ↑
Rifampin	↑	↑	↑	↑	↑	↑			↑
Rifapentine				↑	↑				↑
Riluzole	S								
RisperiDONE							S		
Ritonavir				↓			S, ↓		S, ↓
ROPINIRole	S								
Ropivacaine	S								
Rosiglitazone				S, ↓					
Salmeterol									S
Saquinavir									S, ↓

CYP: Substrates, Inhibitors, Inducers *(continued)*

Drug	1A2	2A6	2B6	2C8	2C9	2C19	2D6	2E1	3A4
Secobarbital		↑		↑	↑				
Selegiline			S						
Sertraline			↓			S, ↓	S, ↓		↓
Sevoflurane								S	
Sibutramine									S
Sildenafil									S
Simvastatin									S
Sirolimus									S
Sitaxsentan					↓	↓			↓
Solifenacin									S
SORAfenib			↓	↓	↓				
Spiramycin									S
SUFentanil									S
SulfADIAZINE					S, ↓				
Sulfamethoxazole					S, ↓				
SUNItinib									S
Tacrine	S								
Tacrolimus									S
Tadalafil									S
Tamoxifen				↓	S		S		S
Tamsulosin							S		S
Telithromycin									S, ↓
Temsirolimus									S
Teniposide									S
Terbinafine							↓		
Tetracycline									S, ↓
Theophylline	S							S	S
Thiabendazole	↓								
Thioridazine							S, ↓		
Thiotepa			↓						
Thiothixene	S								
TiaGABine									S
Ticlopidine						↓	↓		S
Timolol							S		
Tinidazole									S
Tipranavir									S
TiZANidine	S								
TOLBUTamide					S, ↓				
Tolterodine							S		S
Toremifene									S
Torsemide					S				
TraMADol[1]							S		S
Tranylcypromine	↓	↓				↓	↓		
TraZODone									S
Tretinoin				S					

CYP: Substrates, Inhibitors, Inducers *(continued)*

Drug	1A2	2A6	2B6	2C8	2C9	2C19	2D6	2E1	3A4
Triazolam									S
Trifluoperazine	S								
Trimethoprim				↓	S, ↓				S
Trimipramine						S	S		S
Vardenafil									S
Venlafaxine							S		S
Verapamil									S, ↓
VinBLAStine									S
VinCRIStine									S
Vinorelbine									S
Voriconazole					S	S			↓
Warfarin					S, ↓				
Zafirlukast					S, ↓				
Zileuton	↓								
Zolpidem									S
Zonisamide									S
Zopiclone					S				S
Zuclopenthixol							S		

[1]This opioid analgesic is bioactivated *in vivo* via CYP2D6. Inhibiting this enzyme would decrease the effects of the analgesic. The active metabolite might also affect, or be affected by, CYP enzymes.

[2]Cyclophosphamide is bioactivated *in vivo* to acrolein via CYP2B6 and 3A4. Inhibiting these enzymes would decrease the effects of cyclophosphamide.

[3]Data have shown both induction (*in vivo*) and inhibition (*in vitro*) of CYP3A4.

[4]Ifosfamide is bioactivated *in vivo* to acrolein via CYP3A4. Inhibiting this enzyme would decrease the effects of ifosfamide.

[5]Mestranol is bioactivated *in vivo* to ethinyl estradiol via CYP2C8/9.

DEPRESSION SCALES

Short Form Geriatric Depression Scale*

NAME _____ AGE _____ SEX _____ DATE _____

WING _____ ROOM _____ PHYSICIAN _____

SCORING SYSTEM

Answers indicating depression are highlighted. Each BOLD-FACED answer counts one (1) point.   Score greater than 5 indicates probable depression

1.	Are you basically satisfied with your life?	YES / **NO**
2.	Have you dropped any of your activities and interests?	**YES** / NO
3.	Do you feel that your life is empty?	**YES** / NO
4.	Do you often get bored?	**YES** / NO
5.	Are you in good spirits most of the time?	YES / **NO**
6.	Are you afraid that something bad is going to happen to you?	**YES** / NO
7.	Do you feel happy most of the time?	YES / **NO**
8.	Do you often feel helpless?	**YES** / NO
9.	Do you prefer to stay in your room/facility, rather than going out and doing new things?	**YES** / NO
10.	Do you feel you have more problems with memory than most?	**YES** / NO
11.	Do you think it is wonderful to be alive?	YES / **NO**
12.	Do you feel worthless the way you are now?	**YES** / NO
13.	Do you feel full of energy?	YES / **NO**
14.	Do you feel that your situation is hopeless?	**YES** / NO
15.	Do you think that most people are better off than you?	**YES** / NO

SCORE

NOTES / CURRENT MEDICATIONS:
ASSESSOR:

*This scale may be used when evaluating residents who do not have limited cognition.

The following Patient Health Questionnaire - 9 (PHQ-9) is intended to assist clinicians with diagnosing depressive behavior, as well as determining depressive symptom severity for monitoring treatment. The nine items are based directly on the nine signs and symptoms of major depression. Patients should not be diagnosed solely on the basis of a PHQ-9 score. The clinician should corroborate the score with clinical determination that a significant depressive syndrome is present. Scores of 5, 10, 15, and 20 represent cutpoints for mild, moderate, moderately severe, and severe depression, respectively. Table 2 directs the clinician in determining the patient's depression severity and a treatment plan, if necessary, based on the total score of the PHQ-9.

Table 1: Patient Health Questionnaire - 9 (PHQ-9)

Over the last 2 weeks, how often have you been bothered by any of the following problems? (Check to indicate your answer.)	Not at all	Several days	More than half the days	Nearly every day
	(0)	(1)	(2)	(3)
1. Little interest or pleasure in doing things	0	0	0	0
2. Feeling down, depressed, or hopeless	0	0	0	0
3. Trouble falling or staying asleep, or sleeping too much	0	0	0	0
4. Feeling tired or having little energy	0	0	0	0
5. Poor appetite or overeating	0	0	0	0
6. Feeling bad about yourself – or that you are a failure or have let yourself or your family down	0	0	0	0
7. Trouble concentrating on things, such as reading the newspaper or watching television	0	0	0	0
8. Moving or speaking so slowly that other people could have noticed, or the opposite – being so fidgety or restless that you have been moving around a lot more than usual	0	0	0	0
9. Thoughts that you would be better off dead or of hurting yourself in some way	0	0	0	0
For office coding:	0	+ ___	+ ___	+ ___
				= Total score: ___

If you checked off any problems, how difficult have these problems made it for you to do your work, take care of things at home, or get along with other people?			
0 Not difficult at all	0 Somewhat difficult	0 Very difficult	0 Extremely difficult

Developed by Spitzer RL, Williams JBW, Kroenke K, et al, with an educational grant from Pfizer, Inc. Available at http://www.phqscreeners.com/pdfs/02_PHQ-9/English.pdf

Table 2: PHQ-9 Scores and Proposed Treatment Actions

PHQ-9 Score	Depression Severity	Proposed Treatment Actions
0 - 4	None - minimal	None
5 - 9	Mild	Watchful waiting; repeat PHQ-9 at follow-up
10 - 14	Moderate	Treatment plan; considering counseling, follow-up, and/or pharmacotherapy
15 - 19	Moderately Severe	Active treatment with pharmacotherapy and/or psychotherapy
20 - 27	Severe	Immediate initiation of pharmacotherapy and, if severe impairment or poor response to therapy, expedited referral to a mental health specialist for psychotherapy and/or collaborative management

Developed by Spitzer RL, Williams JBW, Kroenke K, et al, with an educational grant from Pfizer, Inc. Available at http://www.phqscreeners.com/instructions/instructions.pdf

LIQUID COMPATIBILITY OF ANTIDEPRESSANTS, ANTIPSYCHOTICS, AND MOOD STABILIZERS

Fruit and Vegetable Juices

Drug	Apple Juice	Grape Juice	Grapefruit Juice	Lemonade	Orange Juice	Pineapple Juice	Prune Juice	Tomato Juice
ARIPiprazole								
CarBAMazepine[1]								
ChlorproMAZINE[1]	X	X	C		C		U	
Citalopram	C				C			
Doxepin			C		C	C	C	C
Escitalopram	C				C			
FLUoxetine								
FluPHENAZine	X		C		C		C	
Haloperidol	C		X		C			
Lithium	X	C	C		C		C	
Loxapine			C		C			
PARoxetine								
RisperiDONE					C			
Sertraline				C	C			
Thioridazine	X	X	C		C		X	
Thiothixene	X		C		C		C	
Trifluoperazine	X	X	C		C		C	
Valproic acid[2]								

C = compatible; X = incompatible; U = conflicting data; Blank = no data.

[1] CarBAMazepine is not compatible with chlorproMAZINE.

[2] Only where syrup is available.

LIQUID COMPATIBILITY OF ANTIDEPRESSANTS, ANTIPSYCHOTICS, AND MOOD STABILIZERS

Other Beverages

Drug	Water	Saline	Milk	Coffee	Tea	Cola	Gingerale	7-Up / Sprite
ARIPiprazole								
CarBAMazepine[1]	C	C						
ChlorproMAZINE[1]	C	C	C	U	U	U	C	
Citalopram	C							
Doxepin	C		C			X		
Escitalopram	C							
FLUoxetine								
FluPHENAZine	C	C	C	X	X	X	X	
Haloperidol	C	X	X	X	X	C		
Lithium	C	C	C	C	C	C	C	
Loxapine				C		C	C	
PARoxetine								
RisperiDONE	C	C	C	C	X	X		
Sertraline	C						C	C
Thioridazine	C	C	X	X	X	X	C	
Thiothixene	C		C	X	X	X		
Trifluoperazine	C	C	C	U	C	C	C	
Valproic acid[2]	C	C				X	X	

C = compatible; X = incompatible; U = conflicting data; Blank = no data.

[1]CarBAMazepine is not compatible with chlorproMAZINE.

[2]Only where syrup is available.

ORAL MEDICATIONS THAT SHOULD NOT BE CRUSHED OR ALTERED

There are a variety of reasons for crushing tablets or capsule contents prior to administering to the patient. Patients may have nasogastric tubes which do not permit the administration of tablets or capsules; an oral solution for a particular medication may not be available from the manufacturer or readily prepared by pharmacy; patients may have difficulty swallowing capsules or tablets; or mixing of powdered medication with food or drink may make the drug more palatable.

Generally, medications which should not be crushed fall into one of the following categories.

- **Extended-Release Products**. The formulation of some tablets is specialized as to allow the medication within it to be slowly released into the body. This may be accomplished by centering the drug within the core of the tablet, with a subsequent shedding of multiple layers around the core. Wax melts in the GI tract releasing drug contained within the wax matrix (eg, OxyCONTIN®). Capsules may contain beads which have multiple layers which are slowly dissolved with time.

Common Abbreviations for Extended-Release Products

CD	Controlled dose
CR	Controlled release
CRT	Controlled-release tablet
LA	Long-acting
SR	Sustained release
TR	Timed release
TD	Time delay
SA	Sustained action
XL	Extended release
XR	Extended release

- **Medications Which Are Irritating to the Stomach**. Tablets which are irritating to the stomach may be enteric-coated which delays release of the drug until the time when it reaches the small intestine. Enteric-coated aspirin is an example of this.

- **Foul-Tasting Medication**. Some drugs are quite unpleasant to taste so the manufacturer coats the tablet in a sugar coating to increase its palatability. By crushing the tablet, this sugar coating is lost and the patient tastes the unpleasant tasting medication.

- **Sublingual Medication**. Medication intended for use under the tongue should not be crushed. While it appears to be obvious, it is not always easy to determine if a medication is to be used sublingually. Sublingual medications should indicate on the package that they are intended for sublingual use.

- **Effervescent Tablets**. These are tablets which, when dropped into a liquid, quickly dissolve to yield a solution. Many effervescent tablets, when crushed, lose their ability to quickly dissolve.

- **Potentially hazardous substances**. Certain drugs including antineoplastic agents, hormonal agents, some antivirals, some bioengineered agents, and other miscellaneous drugs are considered potentially hazardous when used in humans based on their characteristics. Examples of these characteristics include carcinogenicity, teratogenicity, reproductive toxicity, organ toxicity at low doses, or genotoxicity. Exposure to these substances can result in adverse effects and should be avoided. Crushing or breaking a tablet or opening a capsule of a potentially hazardous substance may increase the risk of exposure to the substance through skin contact, inhalation, or accidental ingestion. The extent of exposure, potency, and toxicity of the hazardous substance determines the health risk. Institutions have policies and procedures to follow when handling any potentially hazardous substance. **Note:** All potentially hazardous substances may not be represented in this table. Refer to institution-specific guidelines for precautions to observe when handling hazardous substances.

RECOMMENDATIONS

1. It is not advisable to crush certain medications.

2. Consult individual monographs prior to crushing capsule or tablet.

3. If crushing a tablet or capsule is contraindicated, consult with your pharmacist to determine whether an oral solution exists or can be compounded.

Drug Product	Dosage Form	Dosage Reasons / Comments
Accutane®	Capsule	Mucous membrane irritant; teratogenic potential
Aciphex®	Tablet	Slow release
Actiq®	Lozenge	Slow release. This lollipop delivery system requires the patient to dissolve it slowly.
Actoplus Met® XR	Tablet	Slow release
Actonel®	Tablet	Irritant. Chewed, crushed, or sucked tablets may cause oropharyngeal irritation.
Adalat® CC	Tablet	Slow release
Adderall XR®	Capsule	Slow release[1]
Adenovirus (Types 4, 7) Vaccine	Tablet	Teratogenic potential; enteric-coated; do not disrupt tablet to avoid releasing live adenovirus in upper respiratory tract
Advicor®	Tablet	Slow release
AeroHist Plus™	Tablet	Slow release[8]
Afeditab® CR	Tablet	Slow release
Afinitor®	Tablet	Mucous membrane irritant; teratogenic potential; potentially hazardous substance[10]
Aggrenox®	Capsule	Slow release. Capsule may be opened; contents include an aspirin tablet that may be chewed and dipyridamole pellets that may be sprinkled on applesauce.
Alavert™ Allergy Sinus 12 Hour	Tablet	Slow release
Allegra-D®	Tablet	Slow release
Allfen Jr	Tablet	Slow release
Alophen®	Tablet	Enteric-coated
ALPRAZolam ER	Tablet	Slow release
Altoprev®	Tablet	Slow release
Ambien CR®	Tablet	Slow release
Amitiza®	Capsule	Slow release
Amrix®	Capsule	Slow release
Aplenzin™	Tablet	Slow release
Apriso™	Capsule	Slow release[1]
Aptivus®	Capsule	Taste. Oil emulsion within spheres
Aricept® 23 mg	Tablet	Film-coated; chewing or crushing may increase rate of absorption
Arava®	Tablet	Teratogenic potential; hazardous substance[10]
Arthrotec®	Tablet	Enteric-coated

Drug Product	Dosage Form	Dosage Reasons / Comments
Asacol®	Tablet	Slow release
Ascriptin® A/D	Tablet	Enteric-coated
Atelvia™	Tablet	Slow release; tablet coating is an important part of the delayed release
Augmentin XR®	Tablet	Slow release[2, 8]
AVINza™	Capsule	Slow release[1] (applesauce)
Avodart®	Capsule	Capsule should not be handled by pregnant women due to teratogenic potential[9]; hazardous substance[10]
Azulfidine® EN-tabs®	Tablet	Enteric-coated
Bayer® Aspirin EC	Caplet	Enteric-coated
Bayer® Aspirin, Low Adult 81 mg	Tablet	Enteric-coated
Bayer® Aspirin, Regular Strength 325 mg	Caplet	Enteric-coated
Biaxin® XL	Tablet	Slow release
Biltricide®	Tablet	Taste[8]
Biohist LA	Tablet	Slow release[8]
Bisa-Lax	Tablet	Enteric-coacted[3]
Bisac-Evac™	Tablet	Enteric-coated[3]
Bisacodyl	Tablet	Enteric-coated[3]
Boniva®	Tablet	Irritant. Chewed, crushed, or sucked tablets may cause oropharyngeal irritation.
Bontril® Slow-Release	Capsule	Slow release
Bromfed®	Capsule	Slow release
Bromfed®-PD	Capsule	Slow release
Budeprion™ SR, XL	Tablet	Slow release
Buproban®	Tablet	Slow release
BuPROPion SR	Tablet	Slow release
Campral®	Tablet	Enteric-coated; slow release
Calan® SR	Tablet	Slow release[8]
Caprelsa®	Tablet	Teratogenic potential; hazardous substance[10]
Carbatrol®	Capsule	Slow release[1]
Cardene® SR	Capsule	Slow release
Cardizem®	Tablet	Not described as slow release but releases drug over 3 hours.
Cardizem® CD	Capsule	Slow release
Cardizem® LA	Tablet	Slow release
Cardura® XL	Tablet	Slow release
Cartia® XT	Capsule	Slow release
Casodex®	Tablet	Teratogenic potential; hazardous substance[10]
CeeNU®	Capsule	Teratogenic potential; hazardous substance[10]
Cefaclor extended release	Tablet	Slow release
Ceftin®	Tablet	Taste[2]. Use suspension for children.
Cefuroxime	Tablet	Taste[2]. Use suspension for children.
CellCept®	Capsule, tablet	Teratogenic potential; hazardous substance[10]
Charcoal Plus®	Tablet	Enteric-coated

ORAL MEDICATIONS THAT SHOULD NOT BE CRUSHED OR ALTERED

Drug Product	Dosage Form	Dosage Reasons / Comments
Chlor-Trimeton® 12-Hour	Tablet	Slow release[2]
Cipro® XR	Tablet	Slow release
Claritin-D® 12-Hour	Tablet	Slow release
Claritin-D® 24-Hour	Tablet	Slow release
Colace®	Capsule	Taste[5]
Colestid®	Tablet	Slow release
Commit®	Lozenge	Integrity compromised by chewing or crushing.
Concerta®	Tablet	Slow release
Coreg CR®	Capsule	Slow release[1]
Cotazym-S®	Capsule	Enteric-coated[1]
Covera-HS®	Tablet	Slow release
Creon®	Capsule	Slow release[1]
Crixivan®	Capsule	Taste. Capsule may be opened and mixed with fruit puree (eg, banana).
Cymbalta®	Capsule	Enteric-coated
Cytoxan®	Tablet	Drug may be crushed, but manufacturer recommends using injection; hazardous substance[10]
Dallergy®	Caplet	Slow release[2,8]
Depakene®	Capsule	Slow release; mucous membrane irritant[2]
Depakote®	Tablet	Slow release
Depakote® ER	Tablet	Slow release
Detrol® LA	Capsule	Slow release
Dexedrine® Spansule®	Capsule	Slow release
Dexilant™	Capsule	Slow release[1]
Diamox® Sequels®	Capsule	Slow release
Dilacor® XR	Capsule	Slow release
Dilatrate-SR®	Capsule	Slow release
Dilt-CD	Capsule	Slow release
Dilt-XR	Capsule	Slow release
Diltia XT®	Capsule	Slow release
Ditropan® XL	Tablet	Slow release
Divalproex ER	Tablet	Slow release
Donnatal® Extentab®	Tablet	Slow release[2]
Doxidan®	Tablet	Enteric-coated[3]
Drisdol®	Capsule	Liquid filled[4]
Drixoral® Allergy Nondrowsy	Tablet	Slow release
Drixoral® Cold and Allergy	Tablet	Slow release
Drixoral® Nondrowsy	Tablet	Slow release
Droxia®	Capsule	May be opened; wear gloves to handle; hazardous substance[10]
Drysec	Tablet	Slow release[8]
Dulcolax®	Capsule	Liquid-filled
Dulcolax®	Tablet	Enteric-coated[3]
DuraHist™ PE	Tablet	Slow release[8]
Duraphen™ II DM	Tablet	Slow release[8]

Drug Product	Dosage Form	Dosage Reasons / Comments
Duraphen™ Forte	Tablet	Slow release[8]
Duratuss®	Tablet	Slow release[8]
Duratuss® A	Tablet	Slow release[8]
DynaCirc® CR	Tablet	Slow release
Easprin®	Tablet	Enteric-coated
EC-Naprosyn®	Tablet	Enteric-coated
Ecotrin® Adult Low Strength	Tablet	Enteric-coated
Ecotrin® Maximum Strength	Tablet	Enteric-coated
Ecotrin® Regular Strength	Tablet	Enteric-coated
Ed A-Hist™	Caplet	Slow release[2]
E.E.S.® 400	Tablet	Enteric-coated[2]
Effer-K™	Tablet	Effervescent tablet[6]
Effervescent Potassium	Tablet	Effervescent tablet[6]
Effexor® XR	Capsule	Slow release
Embeda™	Capsule	Slow release; can open capsule and sprinkle on applesauce; do not give via NG tube
E-Mycin®	Tablet	Enteric-coated
Enablex®	Tablet	Slow release
Entex® LA	Capsule	Slow release[2]
Entocort® EC	Capsule	Enteric-coated[1]
Equetro®	Capsule	Slow release[1]
Ergomar®	Tablet	Sublingual form[7]
Ery-Tab®	Tablet	Enteric-coated
Erythrocin Stearate	Tablet	Enteric-coated
Erythromycin Base	Tablet	Enteric-coated
Erythromycin Delayed-Release	Capsule	Enteric-coated pellets[1]
Etoposide	Capsule	Hazardous substance[10]
Evista®	Tablet	Taste; teratogenic potential; hazardous substance[10]
ExeFen-PD	Tablet	Slow release[8]
Extendryl JR	Capsule	Slow release
Extendryl SR	Capsule	Slow release[2]
Fareston®	Tablet	Teratogenic potential; hazardous substance[10]
Feen-A-Mint®	Tablet	Enteric-coated[3]
Feldene®	Capsule	Mucous membrane irritant
Fentora®	Tablet	Buccal tablet
Feosol®	Tablet	Enteric-coated[2]
Feratab®	Tablet	Enteric-coated[2]
Fergon®	Tablet	Enteric-coated
Fero-Grad 500®	Tablet	Slow release
Ferro-Sequels®	Tablet	Slow release
Flagyl ER®	Tablet	Slow release
Flomax®	Capsule	Slow release
Focalin® XR	Capsule	Slow release[1]
Fosamax®	Tablet	Mucous membrane irritant

ORAL MEDICATIONS THAT SHOULD NOT BE CRUSHED OR ALTERED

Drug Product	Dosage Form	Dosage Reasons / Comments
Fosamax Plus D™	Tablet	Mucous membrane irritant
Gengraf®	Capsule	Teratogenic potential; hazardous substance[10]
Gleevec®	Tablet	Taste[8]. May be dissolved in water or apple juice; hazardous substance[10]
GlipiZIDE	Tablet	Slow release
Glucophage® XR	Tablet	Slow release
Glucotrol® XL	Tablet	Slow release
Glumetza™	Tablet	Slow release
Guaifed®	Capsule	Slow release
Guaifed®-PD	Capsule	Slow release
Guaifenex® DM	Tablet	Slow release[8]
Guaifenex® PSE	Tablet	Slow release[8]
Guaimax-D®	Tablet	Slow release[8]
Halfprin®	Tablet	Enteric coated
Hexalen®	Capsule	Teratogenic potential; hazardous substance[10]
Hista-Vent® DA	Tablet	Slow release[8]
Horizant™	Tablet	Slow release
Hycamtin®	Capsule	Teratogenic potential; hazardous substance[10]
Hydrea®	Capsule	Can be opened and mixed with water; wear gloves to handle; hazardous substance[10]
Imdur®	Tablet	Slow release[8]
Inderal® LA	Capsule	Slow release
Indocin® SR	Capsule	Slow release[1,2]
InnoPran XL®	Capsule	Slow release
Intelence™	Tablet	Tablet should be swallowed whole and not crushed; tablet may be dispersed in water
Intuniv™	Tablet	Slow release
Invega®	Tablet	Slow release
Ionamin®	Capsule	Slow release
Isochron™	Tablet	Slow release
Isoptin® SR	Tablet	Slow release[8]
Isordil® Sublingual	Tablet	Sublingual form[7]
Isosorbide Dinitrate Sublingual	Tablet	Sublingual form[7]
Isosorbide SR	Tablet	Slow release
Jalyn®	Capsule	Capsule should not be handled by pregnant women due to teratogenic potential[9]; hazardous substance[10]
Kadian®	Capsule	Slow release[1]. Do not give via NG tubes.
Kaletra®	Tablet	Film coated
Kaon-Cl®	Tablet	Slow release[2]
Kapidex™	Capsule	Slow release[1]
Kapvay™	Tablet	Slow release
K-Dur®	Tablet	Slow release
Keppra®	Tablet	Taste[2]
Keppra® XR	Tablet	Slow release

Drug Product	Dosage Form	Dosage Reasons / Comments
Ketek®	Tablet	Slow release
Klor-Con®	Tablet	Slow release[2]
Klor-Con® M	Tablet	Slow release[2]; some strengths are scored
Klotrix®	Tablet	Slow release[2]
K-Lyte®	Tablet	Effervescent tablet[6]
K-Lyte/Cl®	Tablet	Effervescent tablet[6]
K-Lyte DS®	Tablet	Effervescent tablet[6]
Kombiglyze™ XR	Tablet	Slow release; tablet matrix may remain in stool
K-Tab®	Tablet	Slow release[2]
LaMICtal® XR™	Tablet	Slow release
Lescol® XL	Tablet	Slow release
Letairis®	Tablet	Film coated
Leukeran®	Tablet	Teratogenic potential; hazardous substance[10]
Levbid®	Tablet	Slow release[8]
Levsinex® Timecaps®	Capsule	Slow release
Lexxel®	Tablet	Slow release
Lialda™	Tablet	Delayed release, enteric coated
Lipram 4500	Capsule	Enteric-coated[1]
Lipram-PN	Capsule	Slow release[1]
Lipram-UL	Capsule	Slow release[1]
Liquibid-D®	Tablet	Slow release
Lithobid®	Tablet	Slow release
Lodrane® 24	Capsule	Slow release
Lodrane® 24D	Capsule	Slow release
LoHist 12D	Tablet	Slow release
Lovaza®	Capsule	Contents of capsule may erode walls of styrofoam or plastic materials
Luvox® CR	Capsule	Slow release
Lysodren®	Tablet	Hazardous substance[10]
Mag-Tab® SR	Tablet	Slow release
Matulane®	Capsule	Teratogenic potential; hazardous substance[10]
Maxifed DM	Tablet	Slow release[8]
Maxifed DMX	Tablet	Slow release[8]
Maxifed-G®	Tablet	Slow release
Maxiphen DM	Tablet	Slow release[8]
Medent-DM	Tablet	Slow release
Mestinon® Timespan®	Tablet	Slow release[2]
Metadate® CD	Capsule	Slow release[1]
Metadate® ER	Tablet	Slow release
Methylin® ER	Tablet	Slow release
Metoprolol ER	Tablet	Slow release
MicroK® Extencaps	Capsule	Slow release[1,2]
Minocin	Capsule	Slow release
Miraphen PSE	Tablet	Slow release

Drug Product	Dosage Form	Dosage Reasons / Comments
Morphine sulfate extended-release	Tablet	Slow release
Motrin®	Tablet	Taste[5]
Moxatag™	Tablet	Slow release
MS Contin®	Tablet	Slow release[2]
Mucinex®	Tablet	Slow release
Mucinex® DM	Tablet	Slow release[2]
Myfortic®	Tablet	Slow release; teratogenic potential; hazardous substance[10]
Namenda® XR	Capsule	Slow release[1]
Naprelan®	Tablet	Slow release
Nasatab® LA	Tablet	Slow release[8]
Neoral®	Capsule	Teratogenic potential; hazardous substance[10]
NexAVAR®	Tablet	Teratogenic potential; hazardous substance[10]
NexIUM®	Capsule	Slow release[1]
Niaspan®	Tablet	Slow release
Nicotinic Acid	Capsule, Tablet	Slow release[8]
Nifediac® CC	Tablet	Slow release
Nifedical® XL	Tablet	Slow release
NIFEdipine ER	Tablet	Slow release
Nitrostat®	Tablet	Sublingual route[7]
Norflex™	Tablet	Slow release
Norpace® CR	Capsule	Slow release
Nucynta® ER	Tablet	Slow release; tablet disruption may cause a potentially fatal overdose
Oforta™	Tablet	Teratogenic potential; hazardous substance[10]
Oleptro™	Tablet	Slow release[8]
Opana® ER	Tablet	Slow release; tablet disruption may cause a potentially fatal overdose
Oracea™	Capsule	Slow release
Oramorph SR®	Tablet	Slow release[2]
Orphenadrine citrate ER	Tablet	Slow release
OxyCONTIN®	Tablet	Slow release; surrounded by wax matrix; tablet disruption may cause a potentially fatal overdose
Pancrease MT®	Capsule	Enteric-coated[1]
Pancreaze™	Capsule	Enteric-coated[1]
Pancrelipase™	Capsule	Enteric-coated[1]
Paxil CR®	Tablet	Slow release
Pentasa®	Capsule	Slow release
Plendil®	Tablet	Slow release
Pradaxa®	Capsule	Bioavailability increases by 75% when the pellets are taken without the capsule shell
Prevacid®	Capsule	Slow release[1]
Prevacid®	Suspension	Slow release. Contains enteric-coated granules. Not for use in NG tubes.

Drug Product	Dosage Form	Dosage Reasons / Comments
Prevacid® SoluTab™	Tablet	Orally disintegrating. Do not swallow; dissolve in water only and dispense via dosing syringe or NG tube.
PriLOSEC®	Capsule	Slow release
PriLOSEC OTC™	Tablet	Slow release
Pristiq®	Tablet	Slow release
Procardia XL®	Tablet	Slow release
Profen II®	Tablet	Slow release[8]
Profen II DM®	Tablet	Slow release[8]
Profen Forte™ DM	Tablet	Slow release
Propecia®	Tablet	Women who are, or may become, pregnant should not handle crushed or broken tablets due to teratogenic potential[9]; hazardous substance[10]
Proquin® XR	Tablet	Slow release
Proscar®	Tablet	Women who are, or may become, pregnant should not handle crushed or broken tablets due to teratogenic potential[9]; hazardous substance[10]
Protonix®	Tablet	Slow release
PROzac® Weekly™	Capsule	Enteric coated
Pseudovent™	Capsule	Slow release
Pseudovent™-Ped	Capsule	Slow release
Purinethol®	Tablet	Teratogenic potential[9]; hazardous substance[10]
QDALL® AR	Capsule	Slow release
QuiNIDine ER	Tablet	Slow release[8]; enteric-coated
Ralix	Tablet	Slow release
Ranexa®	Tablet	Slow release
Rapamune®	Tablet	Taste; hazardous substance[10]
Razadyne™ ER	Capsule	Slow release
Renagel®	Tablet	Expands in liquid if broken/crushed.
Renvela	Tablet	Enteric-coated
Requip® XL™	Tablet	Slow release
Rescon®	Tablet	Slow release
Rescon-Jr	Tablet	Slow release
Rescon® MX	Tablet	Slow release[8]
Rescriptor®	Tablet	If unable to swallow, may dissolve 100 mg tablets in water and drink; 200 mg tablets must be swallowed whole
Respa®-1st	Tablet	Slow release[2,8]
Respa-DM®	Tablet	Slow release[2,8]
Respahist®	Capsule	Slow release[2,8]
Respaire®-60 SR/-120 SR	Capsule	Slow release[2]
Revlimid®	Capsule	Teratogenic potential; hazardous substance[10]; healthcare workers should avoid contact with capsule contents/body fluids
RisperDAL® M-Tab	Tablet	Orally disintegrating. Do not chew or break tablet; after dissolving under tongue, tablet may be swallowed
Ritalin® LA	Capsule	Slow release[1]

Drug Product	Dosage Form	Dosage Reasons / Comments
Ritalin-SR®	Tablet	Slow release
R-Tanna	Tablet	Slow release
Rythmol® SR	Capsule	Slow release
Ryzolt™	Tablet	Slow release; tablet disruption may cause overdose
SandIMMUNE®	Capsule	Teratogenic potential; hazardous substance[10]
Saphris®	Tablet	Sublingual form[7]
SEROquel® XR	Tablet	Slow release
Sinemet® CR	Tablet	Slow release
SINUvent® PE	Tablet	Slow release[8]
Slo-Niacin®	Tablet	Slow release[8]
Slow-Mag®	Tablet	Slow release
Solodyn®	Tablet	Slow release
Somnote®	Capsule	Liquid filled
Sprycel®	Tablet	Film coated. Active ingredients are surrounded by a wax matrix to prevent healthcare exposure. Women who are, or may become pregnant, should not handle crushed or broken tablets; teratogenic potential; hazardous substance[10]
Stavzor™	Capsule	Slow release
Strattera®	Capsule	Capsule contents can cause ocular irritation.
Sudafed® 12-Hour	Capsule	Slow release[2]
Sudafed® 24-Hour	Capsule	Slow release[2]
Sulfazine EC	Tablet	Delayed release, enteric coated
Sular®	Tablet	Slow release
Sustiva®	Tablet	Tablets should not be broken (capsules should be used if dosage adjustment needed)
Symax® Duotab	Tablet	Slow release
Symax® SR	Tablet	Slow release
Syprine®	Capsule	Potential risk of contact dermatitis
Tabloid®	Tablet	Teratogenic potential; hazardous substance[10]
Tamoxifen®	Tablet	Teratogenic potential; hazardous substance[10]
Tasigna®	Capsule	Potentially hazardous substance[10]; altering capsule may lead to high blood levels, increasing the risk of toxicity
Taztia XT®	Capsule	Slow release[1]
TEGretol®-XR	Tablet	Slow release
Temodar®	Capsule	Teratogenic potential; hazardous substance[10]. **Note:** If capsules are accidentally opened or damaged, rigorous precautions should be taken to avoid inhalation or contact of contents with the skin or mucous membranes.
Tessalon®	Capsule	Swallow whole; pharmacologic action may cause choking if chewed or opened and swallowed.
Thalomid®	Capsule	Teratogenic potential; hazardous substance[10]
Theo-24®	Tablet	Slow release[2]

Drug Product	Dosage Form	Dosage Reasons / Comments
Theochron™	Tablet	Slow release[2]
Tiazac®	Capsule	Slow release[1]
Topamax®	Capsule	Taste[1]
Topamax®	Tablet	Taste
Toprol XL®	Tablet	Slow release[8]
Touro® CC/CC-LD	Caplet	Slow release[2,8]
Touro LA®	Caplet	Slow release
Toviaz™	Tablet	Slow release
Tracleer®	Tablet	Teratogenic potential; hazardous substance[10].
TRENtal®	Tablet	Slow release
Treximet™	Tablet	Unique formulation enhances rapid drug absorption
Tylenol® Arthritis Pain	Caplet	Slow release
Tylenol® 8 Hour	Caplet	Slow release
Ultram® ER	Tablet	Slow release. Tablet disruption my cause a potentially fatal overdose.
Ultrase®	Capsule	Enteric-coated[1]
Ultrase® MT	Capsule	Enteric-coated[1]
Uniphyl®	Tablet	Slow release
Urocit®-K	Tablet	Wax-coated
Uroxatral®	Tablet	Slow release
Valcyte®	Tablet	Irritant potential; teratogenic potential; hazardous substance[10]
Verapamil SR	Tablet	Slow release[8]
Verelan®	Capsule	Slow release[1]
Verelan® PM	Capsule	Slow release[1]
Vesanoid®	Capsule	Teratogenic potential; hazardous substance[10]
VESIcare®	Tablet	Enteric-coated
Videx® EC	Capsule	Slow release
Vimovo™	Tablet	Slow release
Voltaren®-XR	Tablet	Slow release
VoSpire ER®	Tablet	Slow release
Votrient™	Tablet	Crushing significantly increases AUC and T_{max}
Wellbutrin SR®	Tablet	Slow release
Wellbutrin XL™	Tablet	Slow release
Xalkori®	Capsule	Teratogenic potential; hazardous substance[10]
Xanax XR®	Tablet	Slow release
Xeloda®	Tablet	Teratogenic potential; hazardous substance[10].
Zelboraf™	Tablet	Teratogenic potential; hazardous substance[10]
ZENPEP®	Capsule	Slow release[1]
Zolinza®	Capsule	Irritant; avoid contact with skin or mucous membranes; use gloves to handle; teratogenic potential; hazardous substance[10]
Zomig-ZMT®	Tablet	Sublingual form[7]

ORAL MEDICATIONS THAT SHOULD NOT BE CRUSHED OR ALTERED

Drug Product	Dosage Form	Dosage Reasons / Comments
ZORprin®	Tablet	Slow release
Zortress®	Tablet	Mucous membrane irritant; teratogenic potential; potentially hazardous substance[10]
Zyban®	Tablet	Slow release
Zyflo CR®	Tablet	Slow release
ZyrTEC-D® Allergy & Congestion	Tablet	Slow release
Zytiga™	Tablet	Teratogenic potential; hazardous substance[10]

[1]Capsule may be opened and the contents taken without crushing or chewing; soft food such as applesauce or pudding may facilitate administration; contents may generally be administered via nasogastric tube using an appropriate fluid, provided entire contents are washed down the tube.

[2]Liquid dosage forms of the product are available; however, dose, frequency of administration, and manufacturers may differ from that of the solid dosage form.

[3]Antacids and/or milk may prematurely dissolve the coating of the tablet.

[4]Capsule may be opened and the liquid contents removed for administration.

[5]The taste of this product in a liquid form would likely be unacceptable to the patient; administration via nasogastric tube should be acceptable.

[6]Effervescent tablets must be dissolved in the amount of diluent recommended by the manufacturer.

[7]Tablets are made to disintegrate under (or on) the tongue.

[8]Tablet is scored and may be broken in half without affecting release characteristics.

[9]Prescribing information recommends that women who are, or may become, pregnant should not handle medication especially if crushed or broken; avoid direct contact.

[10]Potentially hazardous or hazardous substance; refer to institution-specific guidelines for precautions to observe when handling this substance.

REFERENCES

Mitchell JF, "Oral Dosage Forms That Should Not Be Crushed." Available at: http://www.ismp.org/tools/DoNotCrush.-pdf. Last accessed July 29, 2010.

National Institute for Occupational Safety and Health, "NIOSH List of Antineoplastic and Other Hazardous Drugs in Healthcare Settings 2010." Available at: http://www.cdc.gov/niosh/docs/2010-167/. Last accessed September 20, 2010.

PATIENT INFORMATION FOR DISPOSAL OF UNUSED MEDICATIONS

Federal guidelines and the Food and Drug Administration (FDA) recommend that disposal of most unused medications should NOT be accomplished by flushing them down the toilet or drain unless specifically stated in the drug label prescribing information. (See "Disposal of Unused Medications Not Specified to be Flushed" below.)

However, certain drugs can potentially harm an individual for whom it is not intended, even in a single dose, depending on the size of the individual and strength of the medication. Accidental (or intentional) ingestion of one of these drugs by an unintended individual (eg, child or pet) can cause hypotension, somnolence, respiratory depression, or other severe adverse events that could lead to coma or death. For this reason, certain unused medications **should** be disposed of by flushing them down a toilet or sink.

Disposal by flushing of these medications is not believed to pose a risk to human health or the environment. Trace amounts of medicine in the water system have been noted, mainly from the body's normal elimination through urine or feces, but there has been no evidence of these small amounts being harmful. Disposal by flushing of these select, few medications contributes a small fraction to the amount of medicine in the water system. The FDA believes that the benefit of avoiding a potentially life-threatening overdose by accidental ingestion outweighs the potential risk to the environment by flushing these medications.

Medications Recommended for Disposal by Flushing

Medication	Active Ingredient
Actiq®, oral transmucosal lozenge	FentaNYL citrate
AVINza®, capsule (extended release)	Morphine sulfate
Daytrana™, transdermal patch	Methylphenidate
Demerol®, tablet[1]	Meperidine hydrochloride
Demerol®, oral solution[1]	Meperidine hydrochloride
Diastat® / Diastat® AcuDial™, rectal gel	Diazepam
Dilaudid®, tablet[1]	HYDROmorphone hydrochloride
Dilaudid®, oral liquid[1]	HYDROmorphone hydrochloride
Dolophine®, tablet (as hydrochloride)[1]	Methadone hydrochloride
Duragesic®, patch (extended release)[1]	FentaNYL
Embeda™, capsule (extended release)	Morphine sulfate and naltrexone hydrochloride
Fentora®, tablet (buccal)	FentaNYL citrate
Kadian®, capsule (extended release)	Morphine sulfate
Methadone hydrochloride (oral solution)[1]	Methadone hydrochloride
Methadose®, tablet[1]	Methadone hydrochloride
Morphine sulfate, tablet (immediate release)[1]	Morphine sulfate
Morphine sulfate, oral solution[1]	Morphine sulfate
MS Contin®, tablet (extended release)[1]	Morphine sulfate
Onsolis™, soluble film (buccal)	FentaNYL citrate
Opana®, tablet (immediate release)	Oxymorphone hydrochloride
Opana® ER, tablet (extended release)	Oxymorphone hydrochloride
Oramorph® SR, tablet (sustained release)	Morphine sulfate
OxyCONTIN®, tablet (extended release)[1]	OxyCODONE hydrochloride
Percocet®, tablet[1]	Oxycodone hydrochloride and acetaminophen
Percodan®, tablet[1]	Oxycodone hydrochloride and aspirin
Xyrem®, oral solution	Sodium oxybate

[1]Medications available in generic formulations.

◀ DISPOSAL OF UNUSED MEDICATIONS NOT SPECIFIED TO BE FLUSHED

The majority of medications should be disposed of without flushing them down a toilet or drain. These medications should be removed from the original container, mixed with an unappealing substance (eg, coffee grounds, cat litter), sealed in a plastic bag or other closable container, and disposed of in the household trash.

Another option for disposal of unused medications is through drug take-back programs. For information on availability of drug take-back programs in your area, contact city or county trash and recycling service.

For more information on unused medication disposal, see specific drug product labeling information or call the FDA at 1-888-INFO-FDA (1-888-463-6332).

REFERENCE

U.S. Food and Drug Administration (FDA), "Disposal by Flushing of Certain Unused Medicines: What You Should Know." Available at: http://www.fda.gov/Drugs/ResourcesForYou/Consumers/BuyingUsingMedicineSafely/Ensuring-SafeUseofMedicine/SafeDisposalofMedicines/ucm186187.htm Lasted accessed October 20, 2009.

PRESSURE ULCER TREATMENT

Specific Treatment Options by Category	Description by Category	Advantages by Category	Disadvantages by Category
Surgical Debridement Indicated when there is evidence of cellulitis or sepsis	Surgical excision of eschar by physician; may require concomitant treatment with systemic antimicrobials.	Repaid removal of necrotic tissue. Large wounds may be partially debrided reducing risk to resident.	May require hospitalization for procedure. Caution must be used with those who are immunosuppressed, debilitated, or have bleeding disorders. May leave some necrotic debris in place.
Autolytic Debriders Absorption, hydrocolloid, and transparent dressings Indicated in wounds with minimal exudate. Do not use in presence of infection.	Use of occlusive dressings or dressings which impart moisture to soften and liquefy necrotic tissue.	Selective form of debridement (does not harm healing tissue). Effective alternative for debridement of small wounds. Readily available.	May lead to infection in large necrotic wounds. Not indicated for clinically infected wounds due to increased bacterial growth beneath dressing.
Enzymatic Debriders Uses topical agents such as collagenase, papain, fibrinolysin, and deoxyribonuclease; promotes growth of granulation tissue. Indicated in patients in long-term care or who cannot tolerate surgery. Granulex® Santyl® Xenaderm™	Enzyme topically applied to necrotic surface; usually covered with wet gauze and/or transparent dressing; applying a protectant (ie, moisture barrier cream) to surrounding tissue may be indicated; often requires concomitant treatment with topical or systemic antimicrobials; discontinue when wound is red and granulating or if it bleeds easily when cleansed.	Less traumatic than surgical debriding. Ease of application. Cost-effective debridement therapy.	Cross-hatching recommended if thick eschar is present. Some detergents and antiseptics may inactivate certain products. Effect on viable tissue varies by product. Takes longer than surgical debridement. May need barrier cream around wound to protect healthy skin. Requires secondary dressing.
Mechanical Debriders Wet-to-dry gauze dressings, hydrotherapy, wound irrigation and scrubbing the wound with gauze. Best for wounds with thick exudate, slough on loose necrotic tissue.	Removal of eschar using mechanical forces that pull off necrotic tissue; discontinue when wound is red and granulating or if it bleeds easily when cleansed.	Promotes softening and loosening of eschar. Potentially less traumatic than surgical debridement. Economical. Readily available.	Generally not as effective in severely necrotic wounds. Must monitor for signs of injury to healthy tissue.
Cleansing Solutions Acetic acid Hydrogen peroxide Lactated Ringer's Normal saline	Cleansing solution that also hydrates; some products are bactericidal.	Cleanses wound. Maintains moist environment.	Can disturb granulation tissue. Can be cytotoxic if not diluted or used too vigorously.

Specific Treatment Options by Category	Description by Category	Advantages by Category	Disadvantages by Category
Topical Antibiotics Betadine® Gentamicin Mupirocin Neosporin® Silvadene®	Antimicrobial solutions, ointments and creams; indicated for prophylaxis or for treatment of an infected wound.	Easy to apply. Water miscible creams easy to remove. Helps control bacterial growth until necrotic tissue can be debrided.	May have cytotoxic effects which may delay wound healing. Ointments are difficult to remove. Allergic reactions may occur. Bacteria may become resistant with prolonged use.
Absorption Dressings DuoDERM® FlexiGel Strands® Intrasite® Kaltostat® Sorbsan®	Includes granules, flakes, paste, and pads; placed directly into wound bed to absorb exudate; provides minor debriding action by retaining wound debris.	Absorbs wound exudate while maintaining wound moisture. Cleanses wound bed. Reduces wound odor.	Some dressings require irrigation to remove from wound. May increase time for dressing changes. May impair granulation and epithelialization by drying wound bed, if exudate is minimal. Permeable to fluids and bacteria. Contraindicated with tunneling. May sting upon application. Requires secondary dressing.
Gauze Dressings	Fine mesh gauze dressing used as vehicle for soaks, lubricants, or antimicrobials.	Economical. Readily available. Effective delivery of solution if kept moist. Cost-effective filler for large wounds.	May cause bleeding, pain, and remove healthy granulation tissue if allowed to dry. Requires increased nursing time to keep dressing moist.
Hydrocolloid Dressings DuoDERM®	Dressing that reacts with exudate to form a gel; creates a physical barrier and maintains a moist/acidic environment.	Totally occlusive; protects wound from physical injury and contamination.- Maintains moist environment. Easy removal without adhesion to wound surface. May remain on wound for up to 5 days. Waterproof dressing allows resident to shower.	Difficult to observe wound. May promote development of infection in deep wounds. May accumulate excess fluid and macerate tissue. Dressing may soften, and wrinkles may increase pressure on wound base.
Nonadherent Dressings ABD Pads Telfa® Vaseline® Gauze	Nonocclusive, absorbent dressing; may be used with topical medications.	Easy to use. Inexpensive. Nontraumatic.	Nonocclusive. Does not physically protect wound site from injury. Less absorptive than plain gauze. Need secondary dressing.
Transparent Dressings Bioclusive® Op-Site® Tegaderm® Uniflex®	Adhesive, transparent, thin film-type semipermeable dressing; semipermeable membrane allows moisture and oxygen exchange.	A barrier to contamination that also keeps wound moist. Allows for easy visual inspection. Good adhesive properties. Waterproof dressing allows resident to shower. Reduces pain. Time saving.	May lead to tissue maceration in extremely moist wounds. Some products are difficult to apply, and wrinkling may occur. May promote infection if necrotic tissue is present. Potential for adhesive injury. Expensive.

Specific Treatment Options by Category	Description by Category	Advantages by Category	Disadvantages by Category
Hydrogels Curasol® Gel Intrasite® Gel	Topicals with absorptive and moisturizing properties.	Nonadherent. May cool and/or soothe wound. Easy to apply. Conforms to wound bed.	Usually requires protective outer dressing. May require multiple daily dressing changes. May macerate surrounding tissue.
Pain Pain may be present in pressure ulcers and does not respond well to oral drugs at doses low enough to avoid side effects	Extemporaneous preparation may be helpful topically. 1 mL injectable morphine sulfate in 8 g of Intrasite® gel applied topically once daily; cover with Tegaderm® dressing.		

REFERENCES

Flock P, "Pilot Study to Determine the Effectiveness of Diamorphine Gel to Control Pressure Ulcer Pain," *J Pain Symptom Manage*, 2003, 25(6):547-54.

Lyder CH, "Pressure Ulcer Prevention and Management," *JAMA*, 2003, 289(2):223-6.

Pullen R, Popp R, Volkers P, et al, "Prospective Randomized Double-Blind Study of the Wound-Debriding Effects of Collagenase and Fibrinolysin/Deoxyribonuclease in Pressure Ulcers," *Age Ageing*, 2002, 31(2):126-30.

Zeppetella G, Paul J, and Ribeiro MD, "Analgesic Efficacy of Morphine Applied Topically to Painful Ulcers," *J Pain Symptom Manage*, 2003, 25(6):555-8.

PHARMACOLOGIC CATEGORY INDEX

NOTES

Other Products Offered by Lexicomp

Anesthesiology & Critical Care Drug Handbook

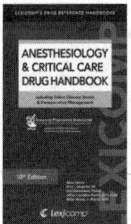

Designed for anesthesiologists, critical care practitioners, and all healthcare professionals involved in the treatment of surgical or ICU patients.

Includes: Comprehensive drug information to ensure appropriate clinical management of patients; Intensivist and Anesthesiologist perspective; Over 2000 medications most commonly used in the preoperative and critical care setting; Special Topics/Issues addressing frequently encountered patient conditions.

Drug Information Handbook

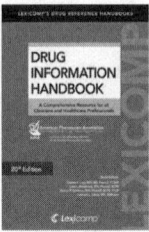

An easy-to-use reference for pharmacists, physicians and other healthcare professionals requiring fast access to comprehensive drug information. This handbook presents over 1400 drug monographs, each with up to 37 fields of information. A valuable appendix includes hundreds of charts and reviews of special topics such as guidelines for treatment and therapy recommendations. A pharmacologic category index is also provided.

Drug Information Handbook with International Trade Names Index

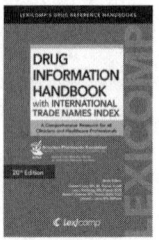

The *Drug Information Handbook with International Trade Names Index* includes the content of our *Drug Information Handbook*, plus international drug monographs for use worldwide! This easy-to-use reference is complied especially for the pharmacist, physician or other healthcare professional seeking quick access to comprehensive drug information.

Drug Information Handbook for Advanced Practice Nursing

Designed to assist the advanced practice nurse with prescribing for, monitoring and educating patients.

Includes: Over 4800 generic and brand names cross-referenced by page number; generic drug names and cross-references highlighted in RED; Labeled and Investigational indications; Adult, Geriatric and Pediatric dosing; up to 60 fields of information per monograph, including Patient Education and Physical Assessment.

Other Products Offered by Lexicomp

Drug Information Handbook for Nursing

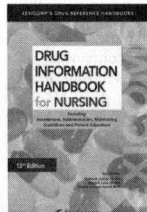

Designed for registered professional nurses and upper-division nursing students requiring dosing, administration, monitoring and patient education information.

Includes: Over 4800 generic and brand name drugs, cross-referenced by page number; drug names and specific nursing fields highlighted in RED for easy reference; Nursing Actions field includes Physical Assessment and Patient Education guidelines.

Drug Information Handbook for Oncology

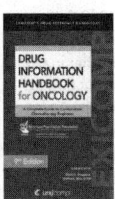

Designed for oncology professionals requiring information on combination chemotherapy regimens and dosing protocols.

Includes: Monographs containing warnings, adverse reaction profiles, drug interactions, dosing for specific indications, vesicant, emetic potential, combination regimens and more; where applicable, a special Combination Chemotherapy field links to specific oncology monographs; Special Topics such as Cancer Treatment Related Complications, Bone Marrow Transplantation and Drug Development.

Drug Information Handbook for Psychiatry

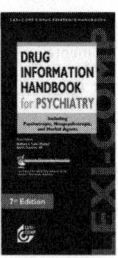

Designed for any healthcare professional requiring quick access to comprehensive drug information as it relates to mental health issues.

Includes: Drug monographs for psychotropic, nonpsychotropic and herbal medications; Special fields such as Mental Health Comment (useful clinical pearls), Medication Safety Issues, Effects on Mental Status and Effects on Psychiatric Treatment.

Pediatric Dosage Handbook

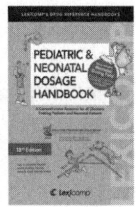

This book is designed for healthcare professionals requiring quick access to comprehensive pediatric drug information. Each monograph contains multiple fields of content, including usual dosage by age group, indication and route of administration. Drug interactions, adverse reactions, extemporaneous preparations, pharmacodynamics/pharmacokinetics data and medication safety issues are covered.

Also available:
Manual de Prescripción Pediátrica (Spanish version)

Other Products Offered by Lexicomp

Pediatric Dosage Handbook with International Trade Names Index

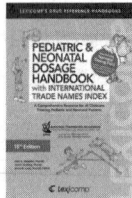

The *Pediatric Dosage Handbook with International Trade Names Index* is the trusted pediatric drug resource of medical professionals worldwide. The International Edition contains all the content of Lexicomp's *Pediatric Dosage Handbook,* plus an International Trade Names Index including trade names from over 100 countries.

Pharmacogenomics Handbook

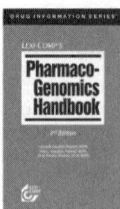

Ideal for any healthcare professional or student wishing to gain insight into the emerging field of pharmacogenomics.

Includes: Information concerning key genetic variations that may influence drug disposition and/or sensitivity; brief introduction to fundamental concepts in genetics and genomics. A foundation for all clinicians who will be called on to integrate rapidly-expanding genomics knowledge into the management of drug therapy.

Rating Scales in Mental Health

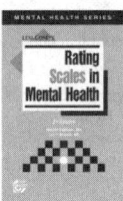

Ideal for clinicians as well as administrators, this book provides an overview of over 100 recommended rating scales for mental assessment.

Includes: Rating scales for conditions such as General Anxiety, Social/Family Functioning, Eating Disorders and Sleep Disorders; Monograph format covering such topics as Overview of Scale, General Applications, Psychometric Properties and References.

Other Products Offered by Lexicomp

Lexicomp On-Hand™

Available for tablets, smartphones and other mobile devices

At Lexicomp, we take pride in creating quality drug information for use at the point-of-care. Our content is not subject to third party recommendations, but based on the contributions of our respected authors and editors, internal clinical team and thousands of professionals within the healthcare industry who continually review and validate our data.

With Lexicomp On-Hand, you can be confident you are accessing the most timely drug information available for mobile devices. All updates are included with your annual subscription.

Lexicomp On-Hand databases include:

- Lexi-Drugs®
- Pediatric & Neonatal Lexi-Drugs™
- Lexi-Drugs® para Pediatría (Spanish Version)
- Lexi-Interact™
- Lexi-Natural Products™
- Lexi-Tox™
- Household Products
- Lexi-Infectious Diseases™
- Lexi-Lab & Diagnostic Procedures™
- Nursing Lexi-Drugs®
- Dental Lexi-Drugs®
- Oral Soft Tissue Diseases
- Lexi-Pharmacogenomics™
- Lexi-Patient Education™
- Lexi-Drug ID™

- Lexi-CALC™
- Lexi-I.V. Compatibility™*
- Lexi-Companion Guides™
- Drug Allergy & Idiosyncratic Reactions
- Lexi-Pregnancy & Lactation™
- The 5-Minute Pediatric Consult
- AHFS Essentials
- Harrison's Practice
- Stedman's Medical Dictionary for the Health Professions and Nursing
- Stedman's Medical Abbreviations

* I.V. compatibility information © copyright King Guide Publications, Inc.

Visit www.lexi.com for more information and device compatibility!

To order, call Customer Service at 1-866-397-3433 or visit www.lexi.com.
Outside of the U.S., call 330-650-6506 or visit www.lexi.com.